ROCKWOOD AND WILKINS'

FRACTURES IN CHILDREN

SEVENTH EDITION

ROCKWOOD AND WILKINS'

FRACTURES IN CHILDREN

SEVENTH EDITION

EDITORS

James H. Beaty, MD
Professor of Orthopaedics
Department of Orthopaedic Surgery,
University of Tennessee-Campbell Clinic;
Chief of Staff, Campbell Clinic,
Memphis, Tennessee

James R. Kasser, MD
John E. Hall Professor of Orthopaedic Surgery
Harvard Medical School; Orthopaedic Surgeon-in-Chief,
Children's Hospital Boston, Boston, Massachusetts

ASSOCIATE EDITORS

David L. Skaggs, MD
Chief of Orthopaedic Surgery
Childrens Hospital Los Angeles
Professor of Orthopaedic Surgery
University of Southern California School of Medicine
Los Angeles, California

John M. (Jack) Flynn, MD
Associate Professor of Orthopaedic Surgery
University of Pennsylvania School of Medicine
Associate Chief of Orthopaedic Surgery
The Children's Hospital of Philadelphia
Philadelphia, Pennsylvania

Peter M. Waters, MD
Clinical Chief of Orthopaedic Surgery
Children's Hospital Boston
Professor of Orthopaedic Surgery
Harvard Medical School
Boston, Massachusetts

Wolters Kluwer Health | Lippincott Williams & Wilkins
Philadelphia • Baltimore • New York • London
Buenos Aires • Hong Kong • Sydney • Tokyo

Acquisitions Editor: Robert Hurley
Product Manager: Dave Murphy
Senior Manufacturing Manager: Benjamin Rivera
Marketing Manager: Lisa Lawrence
Design Coordinator: Doug Smock
Production Service: Absolute Service/Maryland Composition

530 Walnut Street
Philadelphia, PA 19106 USA
LWW.com

Printed in China

Library of Congress Cataloging-in-Publication Data

Rockwood and Wilkins' fractures in children. — 7th ed. / editors, James H. Beaty, James R. Kasser ; associate editors, David L. Skaggs, John M. Flynn, Peter M. Waters.
p. ; cm.
Includes bibliographical references and index.
ISBN 978-1-58255-784-7
1. Fractures in children. 2. Children—Wounds and injuries. I. Rockwood, Charles A., 1936- II. Beaty, James H. III. Kasser, James R. IV. Title: Fractures in children.
[DNLM: 1. Fractures, Bone. 2. Adolescent. 3. Child. 4. Dislocations. 5. Infant. WE 175 R6842 2010]
RD101.F74 2010
617.1'5083—dc22

2009039361

Care has been taken to confirm the accuracy of the information presented and to describe generally accepted practices. However, the authors, editors, and publisher are not responsible for errors or omissions or for any consequences from application of the information in this book and make no warranty, expressed or implied, with respect to the currency, completeness, or accuracy of the contents of the publication. Application of the information in a particular situation remains the professional responsibility of the practitioner.

The authors, editors, and publisher have exerted every effort to ensure that drug selection and dosage set forth in this text are in accordance with current recommendations and practice at the time of publication. However, in view of ongoing research, changes in government regulations, and the constant flow of information relating to drug therapy and drug reactions, the reader is urged to check the package insert for each drug for any change in indications and dosage and for added warnings and precautions. This is particularly important when the recommended agent is a new or infrequently employed drug.

Some drugs and medical devices presented in the publication have Food and Drug Administration (FDA) clearance for limited use in restricted research settings. It is the responsibility of the health care provider to ascertain the FDA status of each drug or device planned for use in their clinical practice.

To purchase additional copies of this book, call our customer service department at (800) 638-3030 or fax orders to (301) 223-2320. International customers should call (301) 223-2300.

Visit Lippincott Williams & Wilkins on the Internet: at LWW.com. Lippincott Williams & Wilkins customer service representatives are available from 8:30 am to 6 pm, EST.

10 9 8 7 6 5 4 3 2 1

As we have worked on several editions of this text, we have come to appreciate more fully the extraordinary support and encouragement given to us by our institutions and by our colleagues. Their willingness to allow us time to complete these massive projects, their understanding when we are frantically working to make a deadline, their cooperation with endless requests for just one more x-ray "for the book," and their continued assurances that the result is worth all the effort have made our editorial duties possible. In appreciation for years of unwavering support and belief in our abilities to produce yet another edition, we dedicate this text to our colleagues and our respective institutions:

The Campbell Clinic and Foundation, Memphis, Tennessee
Children's Hospital, Boston, Massachusetts

We also dedicate this text to all of the orthopaedic fellows and residents we have had the privilege of teaching. Their enthusiasm, knowledge, and vision have been impressive and humbling and have reassured us that our specialty of pediatric orthopaedics is in good hands for the future.

CONTENTS

Dedication v
Contributing Authors ix
Preface xi
Acknowledgments xiii

SECTION ONE: BASIC PRINCIPLES

1 **Epidemiology of Fractures in Children** 3
Michael Vitale

2 **The Biologic Aspects of Children's Fractures** 18
Cory J. Xian and Bruce K. Foster

3 **Pain Relief and Related Concerns in Children's Fractures** 45
Gregory A. Mencio

4 **Management of the Multiply Injured Child** 71
Frances A. Farley and Robert M. Kay

5 **Physeal Injuries and Growth Disturbances** 91
Karl E. Rathjen and John G. Birch

6 **Pathologic Fractures Associated with Tumors and Unique Conditions of the Musculoskeletal System** 120
Alexandre Arkader and John P. Dormans

7 **The Orthopaedic Recognition of Child Maltreatment** 192
Richard M. Schwend, Laurel C. Blakemore, and Lisa Lowe

SECTION TWO: UPPER EXTREMITY

8 **Fractures and Dislocations of the Hand and Carpus in Children** 225
Scott H. Kozin and Peter M. Waters

9 **Fractures of the Distal Radius and Ulna** 292
Peter M. Waters and Donald S. Bae

10 **Injuries to the Shafts of the Radius and Ulna** 347
Charles T. Mehlman and Eric J. Wall

11 **Fractures of the Proximal Radius and Ulna** 405
Mark Erickson and Steven Frick

12 **Monteggia Fracture-Dislocation in Children** 446
Peter M. Waters

13 **The Elbow Region: General Concepts in the Pediatric Patient** 475
James H. Beaty and James R. Kasser

14 **Supracondylar Fractures of the Distal Humerus** 487
David L. Skaggs and John M. Flynn

15 **The Elbow: Physeal Fractures, Apophyseal Injuries of the Distal Humerus, Osteonecrosis of the Trochlea, and T-condylar Fractures** 533
James H. Beaty and James R. Kasser

16 **Dislocations of the Elbow** 594
Anthony A. Stans

17 **Proximal Humerus, Scapula, and Clavicle** 620
John F. Sarwark, Erik C. King, and Joseph A. Janicki

SECTION THREE: SPINE

18 **Cervical Spine Injuries in Children** 685
William C. Warner Jr. and Daniel J. Hedequist

19 **Thoracolumbar Spine Fractures** 723
Peter O. Newton and Scott J. Luhmann

SECTION FOUR: LOWER EXTREMITY

20 **Fractures of the Pelvis** 743
Ernest L. Sink and Dale Blaiser

21 **Fractures and Traumatic Dislocations of the Hip in Children** 769
James McCarthy and Kenneth Noonan

22 **Femoral Shaft Fractures** 797
John M. Flynn and David L. Skaggs

23 **Extra-Articular Injuries of the Knee** 842
Charles T. Price and Jose Herrera-Soto

24 **Intra-Articular Injuries of the Knee** 886
Mininder S. Kocher

25 **Fractures of the Shaft of the Tibia and Fibula** 930
Stephen D. Heinrich and James F. Mooney

26 **Distal Tibial and Fibular Fractures** 967
R. Jay Cummings and Kevin G. Shea

27 **Fractures and Dislocations of the Foot** 1017
Haemish Crawford

Index *1059*

CONTRIBUTING AUTHORS

Alexandre Arkader, MD Assistant Professor of Clinical Orthopaedic Surgery, Keck School of Medicine at the University of Southern California, Director of Orthopaedic Oncology Program, Department of Orthopaedic Surgery, Childrens Hospital Los Angeles, Los Angeles, California

James H. Beaty, MD Professor of Orthopaedics, Department of Orthopaedic Surgery, University of Tennessee-Campbell Clinic, Chief of Staff, Campbell Clinic, Memphis, Tennessee

Donald S. Bae, MD Department of Orthopaedic Surgery, Children's Hospital Boston, Boston, Massachusetts

John G. Birch, MD, FRCS(C) Professor of Orthopaedic Surgery, University of Texas Southwestern Medical School, Assistant Chief of Staff, Orthopaedics Department, Texas Scottish Rite Hospital for Children, Dallas, Texas

Laurel C. Blakemore, MD Associate Professor of Orthopaedic Surgery, George Washington University, Chief of Orthopaedic Surgery and Sports Medicine, Children's National Medical Center, Washington, DC

R. Dale Blasier, MD, FRCS(C), MBA Professor of Orthopaedic Surgery, The University of Arkansas for Medical Sciences, Chief of Orthopaedic Trauma, Arkansas Children's Hospital, Little Rock, Arkansas

Haemish A. Crawford, MB, ChB, FRACS Pediatric Orthopaedic Surgeon, Department of Pediatric Orthopaedic Surgery, Starship Children's Hospital, Auckland, New Zealand

R. Jay Cummings, MD Associate Professor of Orthopaedics, Mayo Clinic Medical School, Vice President of Florida Physician Practices, Nemours Foundation, Jacksonville, Florida

John P. Dormans, MD Professor of Orthopaedic Surgery, University of Pennsylvania School of Medicine, Chief of Orthopaedic Surgery, Children's Hospital of Philadelphia, Philadelphia, Pennsylvania

Mark Erickson, MD Associate Professor of Orthopaedic Surgery, University of Colorado Denver School of Medicine, Rose Brown Chairman of Orthopaedic Surgery, The Children's Hospital, Aurora, Colorado

Frances A. Farley, MD Associate Professor of Orthopaedic Surgery, University of Michigan, Chief of Section of Pediatric Orthopaedic Surgery, Department of Orthopaedic Surgery, University of Michigan, Ann Arbor, Michigan

Bruce K. Foster, MD, FRACS Clinical Associate Professor of Pediatrics and Orthopaedics, University of Adelaide, Deputy Director and Senior Specialist, Department of Orthopaedic Surgery, Women's and Children's Hospital, North Adelaide, Australia

John M. (Jack) Flynn, MD Associate Professor of Orthopaedic Surgery, University of Pennsylvania School of Medicine, Associate Chief of Orthopaedic Surgery, The Children's Hospital of Philadelphia, Philadelphia, Pennsylvania

Steven Frick, MD Residency Program Director, Carolinas Medical Center Department of Orthopaedic Surgery, Charlotte, North Carolina

Daniel J. Hedequist, MD Assistant Professor of Orthopaedic Surgery, Harvard Medical School, Attending Orthopaedic Surgeon, Division of Spinal Surgery, Children's Hospital, Boston, Massachusetts

Stephen D. Heinrich, MS, MD Chairman, Department of Orthopaedic Surgery, Children's Hospital, Clinical Professor, Louisiana State University Health Sciences Center, New Orleans, Louisiana

Jose Herrera-Soto, MD Director of Orthopaedic Research, Assistant Program Director, Pediatric Orthopaedic Fellowship, Orlando Health, Orlando Florida

Joseph A. Janicki, MD Attending Physician, Orthopaedic Surgery, Assistant Professor of Orthopaedic Surgery, Northwestern University's Feinberg School of Medicine Chicago, Illinois

James R. Kasser, MD John E. Hall Professor of Orthopaedic Surgery, Harvard Medical School; Orthopaedic Surgeon-in-Chief, Children's Hospital Boston, Boston, Massachusetts

Robert M. Kay, MD Associate Professor of Orthopaedic Surgery, University of Southern California Keck School of Medicine, Vice Chief of Pediatric Orthopaedics, Childrens Hospital Los Angeles, Los Angeles, California

Erik C. King, MD, MS Pediatric Orthopaedic Surgeon, Department of Orthopaedic Surgery, Children's Memorial Hospital, Chicago, Illinois

Mininder S. Kocher, MD, MPH Associate Professor of Orthopaedic Surgery, Harvard Medical School, Associate Director, Division of Sports Medicine, Children's Hospital Boston, Boston, Massachusetts

Scott H. Kozin, MD Associate Professor of Orthopaedic Surgery, Temple University, Director of Upper Extremity Center for Excellence, Shriners Hospitals for Children, Philadelphia, Pennsylvania

Lisa Lowe, MD, FAAP Professor and Academic Chair, Department of Radiology, University of Missouri-Kansas City, Pediatric Radiologist, Department of Radiology, Children's Mercy Hospitals and Clinics, Kansas City, Missouri

Scott J. Luhmann, MD Associate Professor of Orthopaedic Surgery, Washington University, Associate Professor, Department of Orthopaedic Surgery, St. Louis Children's Hospital, St. Louis, Missouri

James McCarthy, MD Associate Professor, Department of Orthopaedics and Rehabilitation, University of Wisconsin School of Medicine and Public Health, Department of Orthopaedics and Rehabilitation, Madison, Wisconsin

Charles T. Mehlman, DO, MPH Professor of Pediatric Orthopaedic Surgery, Cincinnati Children's Hospital Medical Center, University of Cincinnati College of Medicine, Director of Musculoskeletal Outcomes Research and Director of Pediatric Orthopaedic Resident Education, Division of Pediatric Orthopaedic Surgery, Cincinnati Children's Hospital Medical Center, University of Cincinnati College of Medicine, Cincinnati, Ohio

Gregory A. Mencio, MD Professor of Orthopaedics, Vanderbilt University, Chief of Pediatric Orthopaedics, Monroe Carell Jr. Children's Hospital at Vanderbilt, Nashville, Tennessee

James F. Mooney, MD Professor of Orthopaedic Surgery, Medical University of South Carolina, Chief of Pediatric Orthopaedics, Medical University of South Carolina, Charleston, South Carolina

Peter O. Newton, MD Associate Clinical Professor of Orthopaedic Surgery, University of California San Diego, Rady Children's Hospital, San Diego, California

Kenneth Noonan, MD Associate Professor of Orthopaedics, University of Wisconsin

Charles T. Price, MD Professor of Orthopaedic Surgery, University of Central Florida College of Medicine, Director of Pediatric Orthopaedic Education, Associate Director of Orthopaedic Residency Program, Orlando Health/Arnold Palmer Hospital for Children, Orlando, Florida

Karl E. Rathjen, MD Assistant Professor of Orthopaedic Surgery, University of Texas Southwestern Medical School, Staff Pediatric Orthopaedist, Texas Scottish Rite Hospital for Children, Dallas, Texas

John F. Sarwark, MD Professor of Orthopaedic Surgery, Northwestern University Feinberg School of Medicine, Head of Pediatric Orthopaedic Surgery, Children's Memorial Hospital, Chicago, Illinois

Kevin G. Shea, MD Associate Clinical Faculty, Department of Orthopaedics, University of Utah School of Medicine, Medical Staff, St. Luke's Children's Hospital, Boise, Idaho

Richard M. Schwend, MD Professor of Orthopaedic Surgery, University of Missouri-Kansas City, Pediatric Orthopaedic Surgeon, Orthopaedic Surgery Department, Children's Mercy Hospital, Kansas City, Missouri

Ernest L. Sink, MD Associate Professor of Orthopaedic Surgery, University of Colorado Denver, Associate Professor of Orthopaedic Surgery, The Children's Hospital, Aurora, Colorado

David L. Skaggs, MD Chief of Orthopaedic Surgery, Childrens Hospital Los Angeles, Professor of Orthopaedic Surgery, University of Southern California School of Medicine, Los Angeles, California

Anthony A. Stans, MD Chair, Division of Pediatric Orthopaedics, Department of Orthopaedic Surgery, Mayo Clinic, Rochester, Minnesota

Michael Vitale, MD, MPH Ana Lucia Associate Professor of Pediatric Orthopaedic Surgery, Columbia University Medical Center, Associate Chief of Pediatric Orthopaedics and Chief of Pediatric Spine and Scoliosis Service, Morgan Stanley Children's Hospital of New York – Presbyterian, New York, New York

Eric J. Wall, MD Assistant Professor of Orthopaedic Surgery, University of Cincinnati College of Medicine, Director of Orthopaedic Surgery, Cincinnati Children's Hospital Medical Center, Cincinnati, Ohio

William C. Warner, Jr., MD Professor, University of Tennessee-Campbell Clinic, Department of Orthopaedic Surgery Staff, Campbell Clinic, Memphis, Tennessee

Peter M. Waters, MD Clinical Chief of Orthopaedic Surgery, Children's Hospital Boston, Professor of Orthopaedic Surgery, Harvard Medical School, Boston, Massachusetts

Cory J. Xian, PhD Affiliate Senior Lecturer of Pediatrics, University of Adelaide, Principal Scientist, Department of Orthopaedic Surgery, Women's and Children's Hospital, North Adelaide, Australia

PREFACE

With this seventh edition of *Rockwood & Wilkins' Fractures in Children*, we are grateful to have had the assistance of three new section editors: Jack Flynn, David Skaggs, and Peter Waters. In addition to contributing excellent chapters, each has taken on a portion of the editing duties, helping us integrate the vast amounts of new information about children's fractures into the text. All of our contributors, both old and new, have made substantial updates to their chapters to ensure that the most current findings are available about new techniques, clinical outcomes, and basic science research.

As with every edition, we have tried to improve not only the information presented but also the way it is presented, to make access and understanding easier. More color illustrations, new graphics, and new formatting have been used in an effort to make this edition more "user-friendly" for our readers.

We hope that this edition continues the tradition of excellence begun by Drs. Rockwood, Wilkins, and King, and that all those who treat children's fractures will find valuable information to improve their decision-making and treatment skills.

ACKNOWLEDGMENTS

As always, the most important contributors to this text are our chapter authors who so willingly share their knowledge and expertise. Without their conscientious efforts to review the literature, gather illustrations, and compile their chapters in a timely fashion this publication would not have been possible. We are most grateful to all of them for their hard work and dedication. We also thank our associate editors, Drs. Flynn, Skaggs, and Waters, for their skillful assistance in editing and for their commitment to the lengthy process.

The staff at Lippincott Williams & Wilkins again provided their excellent guidance and support, as well as organization and encouragement. Our thanks to Bob Hurley for having confidence in our ability to see this project through, to Dave Murphy for putting all the pieces together to make a coherent whole, and to Eileen Wolfberg for keeping all of us informed and "on task." Personnel at our respective institutions provided invaluable assistance in editing, illustrating, verifying references, and keeping us organized and on track: from the Campbell Foundation in Memphis, Kay Daugherty (Editorial), Barry Burns (Graphics), and Joan Crowson (Library); and from Boston, Kathryn Macdonald (Editorial) and Alison Clapp (Library).

Throughout the four years spent in preparation of this text, our families have provided encouragement and empathy as we struggled to meet deadlines. They were understanding about missed dinners, lengthy phone calls, late nights with manuscripts, and working weekends. We are especially grateful to our wives, Terry Beaty and Candace Kasser, for allowing us to "go do our little thing" with their blessing and support.

James H. Beaty
James R. Kasser

I would like to thank my wife Val for supporting me and enabling me to work on such enjoyable and meaningful projects, while being such a good friend and so fun to be around. To my children Kira, Jamie, and Clay – when you hear Dad upstairs typing before the sun rises on weekends, this is what I am doing. I love you.

David L. Skaggs

I would like to thank my wife, Mary, and children, Erin, Colleen, John, and Kelly, for appreciating the importance of Dad's writing and editing "homework," and for tolerating the early morning noise that results from his reliance on voice-recognition software. That is why Dad required them to master typing in elementary school.

John M. (Jack) Flynn

I do not have enough words to express gratitude to my wife Janet for her support of all my adventures, including academic work; to my children Rebecca and James for always being willing to join me and keep me honest along the way; and to my colleagues for the joy of our lively professional exchanges.

Peter M. Waters, M.D.

SECTION

ONE

BASIC PRINCIPLES

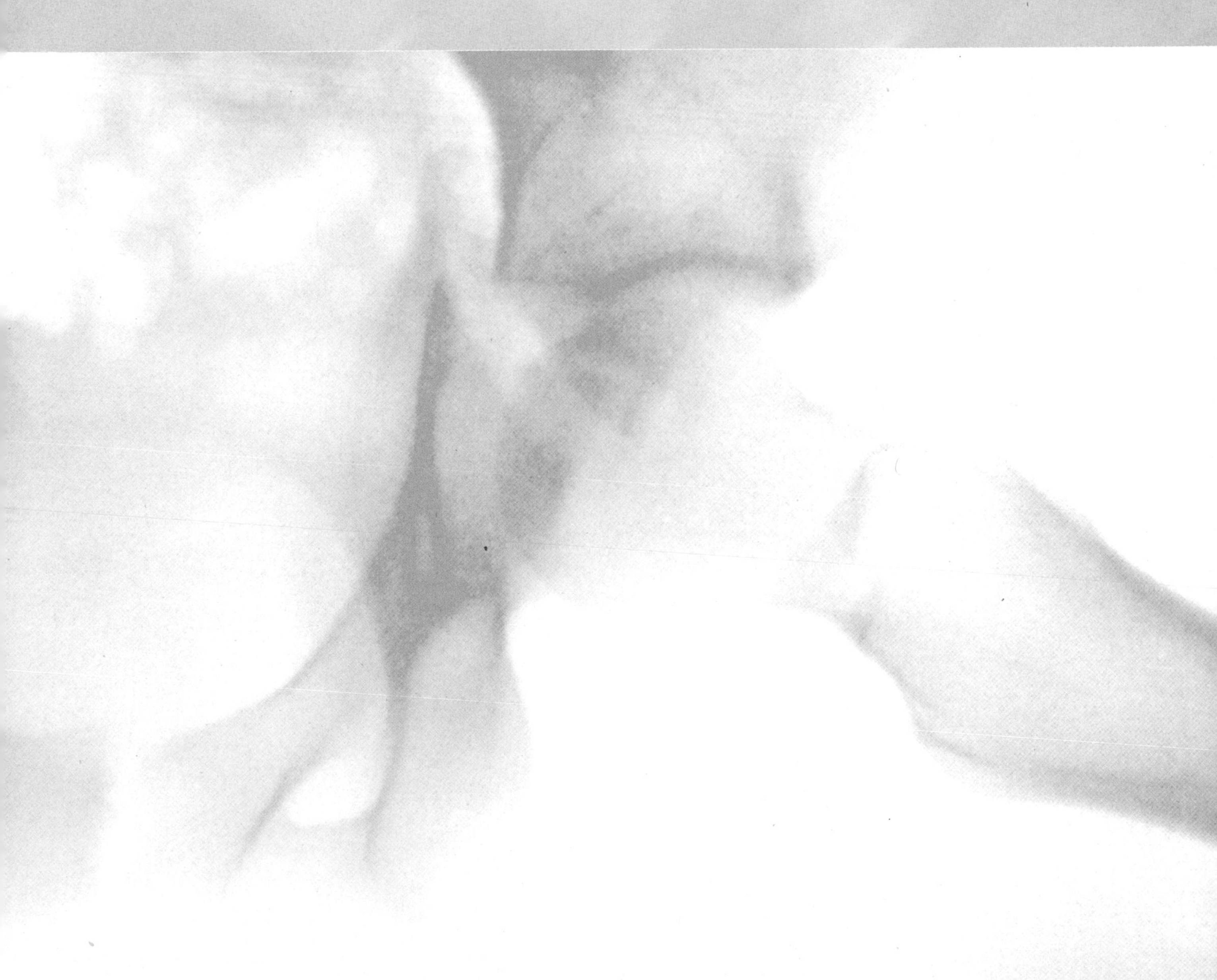

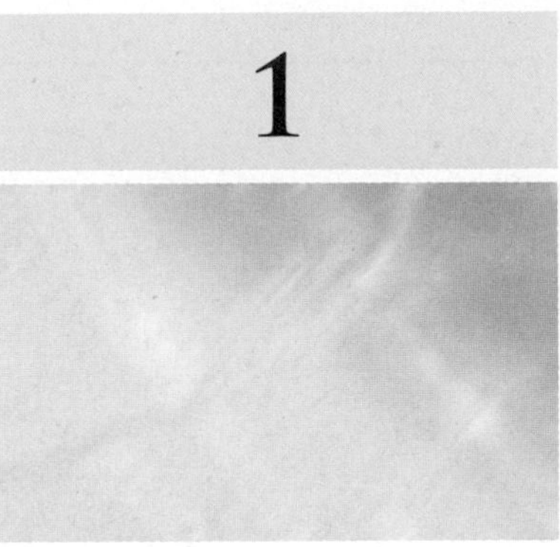

EPIDEMIOLOGY OF FRACTURES IN CHILDREN

Michael Vitale

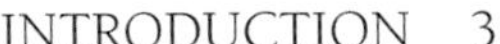

INTRODUCTION 3

CHANGES IN THE PHILOSOPHY OF MANAGEMENT OF FRACTURES IN CHILDREN 4
- Changes from Previous Editions 4
- Improvements in Technology 4
- Rapid Healing 4
- Minimal Hospitalization 4
- The Perfect Result 4
- Phases in the Development of New Operative Techniques 4

EPIDEMIOLOGY OF FRACTURES IN CHILDREN 5
- Fracture Incidence and Fracture Patterns Are Driven by Many Socioclinical Factors 5
- "Classification Bias": Difficulties Defining Disease 5
- Incidence of Fractures 6
- Frequency of Childhood Fractures 6
- Incidences by Specific Fracture Categories 9

ETIOLOGY OF FRACTURES 11
- Studies Essential for Prevention 11
- Three Broad Causes 11
- Fractures Resulting from Accidental Trauma 11

PREVENTIVE PROGRAMS 15
- National Campaigns 16
- Local Community Participation 16

INTRODUCTION

Epidemiology is the field of science that examines factors affecting health and disease in populations. As such, epidemiology is the cornerstone of an evidence-based approach to preventing disease and to optimizing treatment strategies. The term "epidemiology" is derived from the Greek roots *epi* = upon, *demos* = people, *logos* = study, meaning "the study of what is upon the people." An understanding of the epidemiology of pediatric trauma is a prerequisite for the timely evolution of optimal care strategies and for the development of effective prevention strategies.

As the leading cause of death and disability in children, pediatric trauma presents one of the largest challenges to the health of children, as well as a great opportunity for positive impact. It is estimated that more than 11 million hospitalizations and 15,000 deaths result from childhood injury every year. While children more often survive significant injury than adults, survivors of significant trauma may be left with long-term functional problems.[1]

It has been estimated that up to 25% of children sustain an injury every year, with 10% to 25% of these injuries consisting of a fracture. In fact, on both the outpatient and inpatient sides, musculoskeletal trauma makes up the largest share of pediatric injuries.[106]

The incidence of pediatric trauma in the United States is among the highest in the developing world, reflecting the realities of urban violence, firearms, and the dangers of a highly mechanized society. Given the wide-reaching impact that pediatric musculoskeletal injury has on public health, an understanding of the epidemiology of pediatric fractures provides an opportunity to maximize efforts aimed at prevention and optimal treatment. In the years since the production of the first edition of *Fractures in Children*, there have been many changes in the incidence, etiology, and philosophy of management of children's fractures.

CHANGES IN THE PHILOSOPHY OF MANAGEMENT OF FRACTURES IN CHILDREN

Recent years have witnessed a shift toward a greater role for operative management for many children's fractures. In most instances, operative management produces better results than nonoperative treatment, but this shift in treatment has not been without some controversy.

Changes from Previous Editions

The trend toward surgical intervention can be seen in the changes in the previous editions of this textbook. In the first edition,[100] very little mention was made regarding intramedullary (IM) fixation of either femoral or radial and ulnar shaft fractures. There was an extensive discussion of methods of traction for femoral shaft fractures and supracondylar fractures. In the fifth edition,[10] the reverse was true. There was considerable discussion of IM fixation and very little mention of traction techniques.

This trend toward more operative intervention has been the result of four factors: (i) improvements in technology, (ii) rapid healing that allows minimal and temporary fixation, (iii) financial and social pressures to limit the hospitalization of children, and (iv) an expectation by the public for a "perfect outcome" in every case.

Improvements in Technology

The use of the image intensifier has greatly improved the ease of reducing and internally stabilizing fractures with percutaneous methods. Other technical advances, such as widespread access to computed tomography (CT) and magnetic resonance imaging (MRI), have expanded the ability to better define the fracture patterns. The use of powered instruments and cannulated implants, coupled with the use of radiographic real time images, has greatly facilitated the accuracy of applying fixation devices with percutaneous techniques.

Rapid Healing

Because children's bones heal and remodel rapidly, fixation devices often need to be used for only a short time. Children tolerate all types of casts well for short periods of time, which allows a minimally stabilized fracture to be immobilized with a cast until there is sufficient internal callous to supplement the limited internal fixation.

Minimal Hospitalization

The rising costs of hospitalization have created a trend to mobilize children to an outpatient setting as soon as possible. This is reinforced by the fact that in two thirds of the families in the United States, both parents are wage earners. There are both social and financial pressures to mobilize the child early. The trend now is to surgically stabilize these fractures so that the patient can be discharged early. The shift away from traction and toward IM fixation for femoral fractures in intermediate aged children is but one example of this dynamic at work.

The Perfect Result

Modern parents have become very sophisticated and now often expect a perfect outcome for their child. They inspect the radiographs, question the alignment, and expect the alignment to be perfect. These pressures often direct the treating physician toward operative intervention to obtain a perfect alignment.

Are the Results Better with Operative Intervention?

Yes, Results are Definitely Better for Many Injuries, such as Supracondylar Humeral Fractures. The superiority of operative treatment of supracondylar fractures of the distal humerus was clearly demonstrated in a report published in 1988 from Toronto, Canada, in which treatment in traction, treatment with a cast alone, and treatment with percutaneous pin fixation were compared.[92] The worst results were in patients treated with only a cast. The best results were achieved in those stabilized with percutaneous pin fixation. The universal acceptance of percutaneous pin fixation of these fractures is evidence of the superiority of operative management.

Cox and Clarke, in evaluating the fracture management in their hospital in Southampton, England, found a high incidence of secondary hospital treatment for fractures initially managed nonoperatively.[28] There was a 12% readmission rate to correct late displacement of fractures of the radius and distal humerus. In addition, 24% of their internal fixation procedures were to salvage unacceptable results of nonoperative management. They concluded that more selective initial operative intervention in radial and distal humeral fractures could decrease the incidence of costly readmissions to the hospital.

Maybe, Depending on What You Call Results. A 7-year-old with a midshaft fracture of the femur may have had the same excellent bony alignment and healing when treated with 6 weeks of skeletal traction as when treated with IM fixation. However, quality of life during treatment, burden of care on the family, and costs are markedly different in these two scenarios.

In some cases, operative fixation has created a new set of iatrogenic problems that result in less favorable outcomes for some children. Some of the specific problems that have occurred over the years are: (i) ulnar nerve injury with medial pin fixation of supracondylar fractures,[67] (ii) high refracture rate with external fixation of femoral shaft fractures,[94] and (iii) osteonecrosis of the femoral head following the use of interlocking IM nails inserted through the piriformis fossa.[9,77]

Phases in the Development of New Operative Techniques

Often, when a new procedure becomes widely used, there is an initial wave of enthusiasm. However, with more widespread use, problems become more apparent and modifications are made to the original technique. Thus, it takes time before the technique becomes relatively complication free.

Nonoperative Techniques Need to Be Maintained

With emphasis on operative management, the fact that most children's fractures can be managed by nonoperative techniques has become obscured. As a result, many recent orthopaedic trainees are less exposed to and less comfortable with nonoperative technical skills.

In fact, several articles have demonstrated excellent results of treating children's fractures by focusing on improvements in nonoperative methods, "pleading for conservatism."[47] Chess et al.[23] showed that when properly applied, a well-molded short-arm cast provides just as good a result as a long-arm cast in treating displaced fractures of the distal radial metaphysis. These authors believed the key to success in using a short-arm cast is in a careful molding of the cast at the fracture site so there is the proper cast index of 0.7 or less. Walker and Rang challenged traditional thinking by demonstrating that unstable fractures of the radius and ulna could be treated with a lower frequency of remanipulation if immobilized in elbow extension rather than flexion.[127]

It is important to remember that most children's fractures are still treated by nonoperative methods.

EPIDEMIOLOGY OF FRACTURES IN CHILDREN

Despite the importance of understanding the epidemiology of pediatric fractures, there are still significant gaps in our knowledge base, and there is much work to be done. There are several challenges to gathering appropriate data in this area: risk factors for pediatric injury are diverse and heterogenous, practice patterns vary across countries and even within countries, and the available infrastructure to support data collection for pediatric trauma is far from ideal.

Fracture Incidence and Fracture Patterns Are Driven by Many Socioclinical Factors

Cultural Differences

The incidence of pediatric fracture varies in different cultural settings. For instance, Cheng and Shen studied children in Hong Kong who lived in confined high-rise apartments.[22] Their risk of exposure to injury differed from the study by Reed of children living in the rural environment of Winnipeg, Canada.[97] Two separate reviews by Laffoy[55] and Westfelt[86] found that children in a poor social environment (as defined by a lower social class or by dependence on public assistance) had more frequent accidents than more affluent children. In England, children from single-parent families were found to have higher accident and infection rates than children from two parent families.[36]

Two additional studies in the United Kingdom looked at the relationship of affluence to the incidence of fractures in children. Lyons et al.[68] found no difference in the fracture rates of children in affluent population groups compared to those of children in nonaffluent families. On the other hand, Stark et al.[119] in Scotland found that the fracture rates in children from nonaffluent social groups was significantly higher than those in affluent families.

Climatic Differences

The climate may be a strong factor as well. Children in colder climates, with ice and snow, are exposed to risks different from those of children living in warmer climates. The exposure time to outdoor activities may be greater for children who live in warmer climates. For example, the incidence of chronic overuse elbow injuries in young baseball players (Little League elbow) is far greater in the southern United States than in the northern part of the country.

Pediatric trauma should be viewed as a disease where there are direct and predictable relationships between exposure and incidence.

"Classification Bias": Difficulties Defining Disease

Rigorous epidemiological studies demand consistent information about how we define and classify a given disease state. This is a challenge in pediatric trauma, making it difficult to compare studies. Some studies extend the pediatric age group to only 16 years, for example, while others include patients up to 21 years of age. Moreover, it is particularly difficult to examine injuries that only sometimes result in admission. Many studies[17,66,110] are limited to injuries that require hospital admission, despite the fact that most injuries in children do not. Reports vary in the precision of their defined types of fracture patterns. In the older series, reports were only of the long bone involved, such as the radius. Series that are more recent have emphasized a more specific location, separating the radius, for example, into physeal, distal, shaft, and proximal fracture types.

Thus, in trying to define the exact incidence of pediatric fractures, it is difficult to compare series because of cultural, environmental, and age differences. In the following synopsis, these differences were considered in grouping the results and producing average figures. These data are presented in an attempt to provide a reasonable and accurate reflection of the overall incidence of injuries and fractures in all children.

Modern Day Data Systems May Provide Expanded Opportunities to Examine the Epidemiology of Pediatric Trauma

Several sources of administrative, national, and regional data have recently become available providing significantly improved investigation into various areas within pediatric trauma. The Healthcare Cost and Utilization Project (HCUP) is a family of databases including the State Inpatient Databases (SID), the Nationwide Inpatient Sample (NIS), and the Kids' Inpatient Database (KID). While administrative data may lack clinical detail for certain purposes, these datasets provide a comprehensive overview of healthcare utilization in the United States and are available without purchase (http://www.ahrq.gov/data/hcup/hcupnet.htm).[120] The KID database has been increasingly used to examine the incidence of pediatric trauma as well as practice patterns in pediatric trauma. Data for KIDS are collected and published every 3 years, with data currently available for 1997, 2000, 2003, and 2006. KIDS is "nationally representatative," meaning that the database contains a large but incomplete sample of the hospital discharge records (3.1 million in 2006), which are then statisticaly weighted upward to reflect the complete population of pediatric discharges (7.6 million in 2006). Several other databases including the National Electronic Injury Surveillance System (http://www.cpsc.gov/library/neiss.html) have also been useful in providing information about the epidemiology of pediatric trauma.

Currently available data sources provide scant clinical detail, limiting broader utility as a source of health outcomes data in the field. Constructed in an attempt to fill such a role, the National Pediatric Trauma Registry (NPTR) is a multi-institutional database designed to provide a snapshot of physiological and clinical information. The NPTR was functional for about 15 years and provided a source of important data in the realm of pediatric trauma.[122] The NPTR is currently being redesigned into an even more powerful database that will be called the National Trauma Registry for Children, which should serve as a powerful reference for contributors to future editions of this book.

Incidence of Fractures

Earlier Studies Defined the Remodeling Processes

Early reviews primarily developed a knowledge base of fracture healing in children. In 1941, Beekman and Sullivan published an extensive review of the incidence of children's fractures.[11] Their pioneering work—still quoted today—included a study of 2094 long bone fractures seen over a 10-year period at Bellevue Hospital in New York City. The major purpose of their study was to develop basic principles for treating children's fractures.

In 1954, two reports, one by Hanlon and Estes[41] and the other by Lichtenberg,[62] confirmed the findings of the previous studies with regard to the general incidence of children's long bone fractures and their ability to heal and readily remodel. These initial reviews were mainly statistical analyses and did not delve deeply into the true epidemiology of children's fractures. In 1965, Wong explored the effect of cultural factors on the incidence of fractures by comparing Indian, Malay, and Swedish children.[133] In the 1970s, two other studies, one by Iqbal[44] and another by Reed,[97] added more statistics regarding the incidence of the various long bone fractures.

More Recent Studies

Landin's 1983 report on 8682 fractures remains a landmark on this subject.[58] He reviewed the data on all fractures in children that occurred in Malmo, Sweden, over 30 years and examined the factors affecting the incidence of children's fractures. By studying two populations, 30 years apart, he determined that fracture patterns were changing and suggested reasons for such changes. His initial goal was to establish data for preventive programs, so he focused on fractures that produced clean, concise, concrete data.

In 1997, Landin updated his work, re-emphasizing the statistics from his previous publication.[57] He suggested that the twofold increase in fracture rate during the 30 years from 1950 to 1979 in Malmo was due mainly to an increased participation in sports. In 1999, in cooperation with Tiderius and Duppe, Landin[123] studied the incidence in the same age group again in Malmo and found that the rate had actually declined by 9% in 1993 and 1994. The only exception was an increase of distal forearm fractures in girls, which he attributed to their increased participation in sporting events.

Cheng and Shen,[66] in their 1993 study from Hong Kong, also set out to define children's fractures by separating the incidences into age groups. They tried to gather epidemiologic data on which to build preventive programs. In 1999, this study was expanded to include almost 6500 fractures in children 16 and younger over a 10-year period.[21] The fracture patterns changed little over those 10 years. What did change was the increased frequency of closed reduction and percutaneous pin fixation of fractures, with a corresponding decrease in open reductions. There also was a marked decrease in the hospital stay of their patients.

More recently, using the HCUP's KIDS dataset, Galano et al.[40] examined the face of pediatric inpatient trauma in 1997. They estimated that roughly 84,000 children were admitted for fracture care which resulted in about 1 billion dollars in hospital charges. Of some interest, more than 70% of children were treated at non-children's hospitals.

Frequency of Childhood Fractures

Overall Incidence

In Landin's series from Malmo, Sweden, the chance of a child sustaining a fracture during childhood (birth to age 16) was 42% for boys and 27% for girls.[58] When considered on an annual basis, 2.1% of all the children (2.6% for boys; 1.7% for girls) sustained at least one fracture each year. These figures were for all fracture types and included those treated on an inpatient basis and an outpatient basis. The overall chance of fracture per year was 1.6% for both girls and boys in a study from England of both outpatients and inpatients by Worlock and Stower.[134] The chance of a child sustaining a fracture severe enough to require inpatient treatment during the first 16 years of life is 6.8%.[22] Thus, on an annual basis, 0.43% of the children in an average community will be admitted for a fracture-related problem during the year.

In a series of 23,915 patients seen at four major hospitals for injury-related complaints, 4265 (17.8%) had fractures.[17,41,75,86] Thus, close to 20% of the patients who present to hospitals with injuries have a fracture.

It is interesting to note that, in a follow-up study by Tiderius, Landin, and Duppe[123] in the years 1993 and 1994, 13 years after the termination of the original 30-year study by Landin,[58] there was an almost 10% decrease in the incidence of fractures in the 0- to 16-year age group. They attributed this to less physical activity on the part of modern-day children coupled with better protective sports equipment and increased traffic safety (e.g., stronger cars and use of auto restraint systems). The overall incidence of children's fractures is summarized in Table 1-1.

Age Groups

Fractures Show a Linear Increase with Age. Starting with birth and extending to age 12, all the major series that segregated patients by age have demonstrated a linear increase in the annual incidence of fractures with age (Fig. 1-1).[16,21,22,44,58,134]

Although there is a high incidence of injuries in children ages 1 to 2, the incidence of fractures is low.[55] Most injuries in children of this age are nonorthopaedic entities such as head injuries, lacerations, and abrasions. In fact, the incidence of lacerations in both sexes peaks at this age.[99]

Nonaccidental Trauma

In 1962, Kempe et al.[49] called attention to the frequency of fractures and other injuries in young children that were due to nonaccidental trauma. They termed these injuries part of the

TABLE 1-1 Overall Frequency of Fractures*

Percentage of children sustaining at least one fracture from 0 to 16 years of age: boys, 42%; girls, 27%

Percentage of children sustaining a fracture in 1 year: 1.6% to 2.1%

Percentage of patients with injuries (all types) who have fractures: 17.8%

*8,44,55,57,59,75,86,97,119

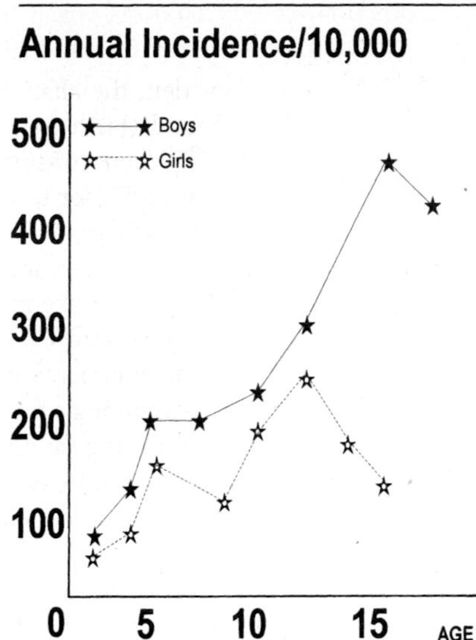

FIGURE 1-1 Incidence of fractures by age. Boys peak at 15 years while girls peak earlier, at 12 years, and then decline. (Reprinted from Landin LA. Fracture patterns in children. Acta Orthop Scand 1983;202:13; with permission.)

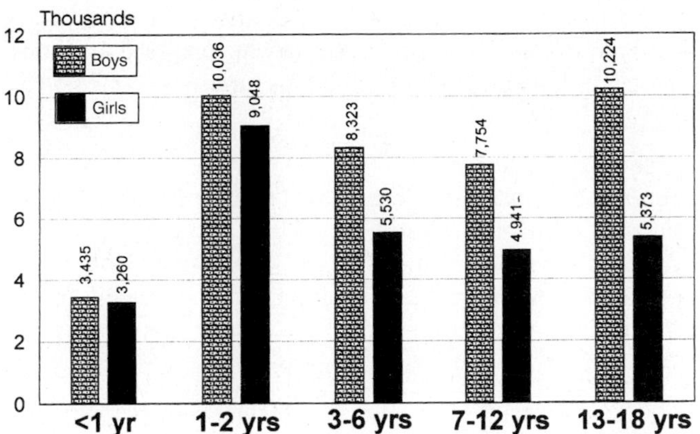

FIGURE 1-2 Injuries per 100,000 children per year. Estimated US injury rates in children by age and sex, 1978. (Reprinted from Rivara FP, Bergman AB, LoGerfo JP, et al. Epidemiology of childhood injuries. Am J Dis Child 1982;136:503; with permission.)

battered child syndrome. Arkbania et al.[2] later defined the specific fracture patterns seen in victims of child abuse. The high rate of fractures from nonaccidental trauma has been shown to extend to age 3.[52]

Not all fractures in the first year of life can be attributed to abuse. In a review of fractures occurring in the first year of life, McClelland and Heiple found that fully 44% were from documented accidental and nonabusive etiologies.[74] They also noted that 23% of these patients had generalized conditions that predisposed them to fractures. Thus, although nonaccidental trauma remains the leading cause of fractures during the first year of life, other general and metabolic conditions may predispose children to fractures from accidental causes.

Information from the 2000 KIDS database indicates that about half of abused hospitalized children older than 3 years of age have concomitant psychiatric or neurological conditions, reminding caretakers to maintain vigilance in this at risk population.[65] For example, a nonambulatory child with cerebral palsy is expected to have osteopenia and be at increasd risk for fracture. The orthopaedic surgeon should not fall into the trap, however, of assuming that all fractures in children with cerebral palsy are accidents, because children with cerebral palsy also are at an increased risk of child abuse.

Gender

Males Predominate in Late Age Groups. The male predominance of injury and fracture victims has been discussed (see Table 1-1; Figs. 1-1 and 1-2). For all age groups, the overall ratio of boys to girls who sustain a single fracture is 2.7:1.[22] In girls, fracture incidence peaks just before adolescence and then decreases during adolescence.[22,58,97] In the 10-year study from Hong Kong by Chang et al.,[21] the male incidence in the 12- to 16-year age group was 83%. The incidence of fractures in girls steadily declined from their peak in the birth to 3-year age group.

In some areas, there is little difference in the incidence of fractures between boys and girls. For example, during the first 2 years of life, the overall incidence of injuries and fractures in both genders is nearly equal. During these first 2 years, the injury rates for foreign body ingestion, poisons, and burns have no significant gender differences. With activities in which there is a male difference in participation, such as with sports equipment and bicycles, there is a marked increase in the incidence of injuries in boys.[21,99]

Role of Behavior. The injury incidence may not be due to the rate of exposure alone; behavior may be a major factor. For example, one study found that the incidence of auto/pedestrian childhood injuries peaks in both sexes at ages 5 to 8.[104] When the total number of street crossings per day was studied, both sexes did so equally. Despite this equal exposure, boys had a higher number of injuries. Thus, the difference in the rate between the sexes begins to develop a male predominance when behaviors change. The difference in the injury rate between the genders may change in the future as more girls participate in activities with increased physical risk.[21,99]

Right versus Left Frequency

In most series, the left upper extremity demonstrates a slight but significant predominance.[14,27,30,31,34,39] The ratio of left to right overall averages 1.3:1. In some fractures, however, especially those of supracondylar bones, lateral condyles, and the distal radius, the incidence is far greater, increasing to as much as 2.3:1 for the lateral condyle. In the lower extremity, the incidence of injury on the right side is slightly increased.[41,58]

The reasons for the predominance of the left upper extremity have been studied, but no definite answers have been found. Rohl[102] speculated that the right upper extremity is often being used actively during the injury, so the left assumes the role of protection. In a study examining the left-sided predominance in the upper extremity, Mortensson and Thonell[80] questioned patients and their parents on arrival to the emergency department about which arm was used for protection and the position of the fractured extremity at the time of the accident. They found two trends: regardless of handedness, the left arm was used more often to break the fall, and when exposed to trauma, the left arm was more likely to be fractured.

Frequency by Season

Summertime Increase. Fractures are more common during the summer, when children are out of school and exposed to more vigorous physical activities (Fig. 1-3). Five studies from the northern hemisphere have confirmed this summertime increase.[21,22,102,129,134]

Hours of Sunshine. The most consistent climatic factor appears to be the number of hours of sunshine. Masterson et al,[73] in a study from Ireland, found a strong positive correlation between monthly sunshine hours and monthly fracture admissions. There was also a weak negative correlation with monthly rainfall. Overall, the average number of fractures in the summer was 2.5 times that in the winter. In days with more sunshine hours than average, the average fracture admission rate was 2.31 per day; on days with fewer sunshine hours than average, the admission rate was 1.07 per day.

In Sweden, the incidence of fractures in the summer had a bimodal pattern that seemed to be influenced by cultural traditions. In two large series of both accidents and fractures in Sweden by Westfelt[86] and Landin,[58] the researchers noticed increases in May and September and significant decreases in June, July, and August. Both writers attributed this to the fact that children in their region left the cities to spend the summer in the countryside. Thus, the decrease in the overall fracture rate was probably due to a decrease in the number of children at risk remaining in the city.

Masterson et al.[73] speculated that because the rate of growth increases during the summer, the number of physeal fractures should also increase, as the physes would be weaker during this time. For example, the incidence of slipped capital femoral epiphysis, which is related to physeal weakness, increases during the summer.[7] However, Landin, in his study of more than 8000 fractures of all types, found the overall seasonal incidence of physeal injuries to be exactly the same as nonphyseal injuries.[58]

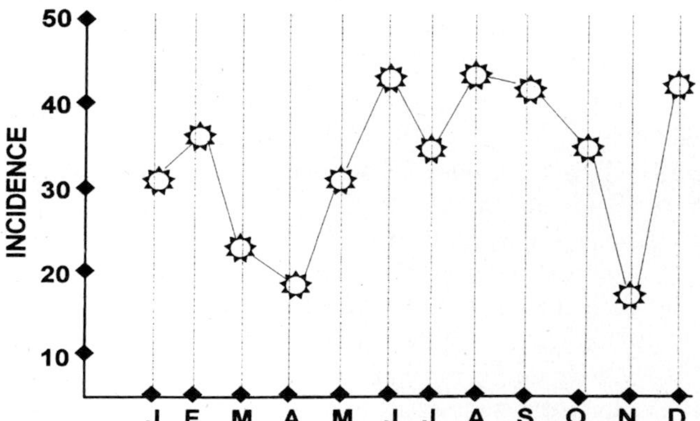

FIGURE 1-3 Distribution of children's fractures on a monthly basis. Note the general increase from May to October. (Reprinted from Reed MH. Fractures and dislocations of the extremities in children. J Trauma 1977; 17:353; with permission.)

Younger Age Groups Unaffected. Thus, it appears that climate, especially in areas where there are definite seasonal variations, influences the incidence of fractures in all children, especially in older children. However, in small children and infants, whose activities are not seasonally dependent, there appears to be no significant seasonal influence.

Time of Day

The time of day in which children are most active seems to correlate with the peak time for fracture occurrence. In Sweden, the incidence peaked between 2 and 3 PM.[86] In a well-documented study from Texas by Shank et al.,[110] the hourly incidence of fractures formed a well-defined bell curve peaking at about 6 PM (Fig. 1-4).

Long-Term Trends

Increase in Minor Trauma. Landin's study is the only one that has compared the changes over a significant time span: his data were collected over 30 years.[58] He classified the degree of trauma as slight, moderate, or severe. The incidence of all trauma in both boys and girls increased significantly over the 30-year study period, but the incidence of severe trauma increased only slightly. The greatest increase was in the "slight" category. Landin attributed the increase in this category to the introduction of subsidized medical care. Because expense was not a factor, parents were more inclined in the later years of the study to seek medical attention for relatively minor complaints. Physicians, likewise, were more inclined to order radiographs. Thus, many of the minor injuries, such as torus fractures, which were often ignored in the earlier years, were seen more often at medical facilities during the later years.

Likewise, the overall incidence of fractures in Malmo, Sweden (the same city as Landin's original study),[58] had decreased significantly (10%) in the more recent years.[123]

The one fracture type that exhibited a true increase over this period was that of the femoral shaft. This increase was thought to be influenced by new types of play activities and increased participation in sports.

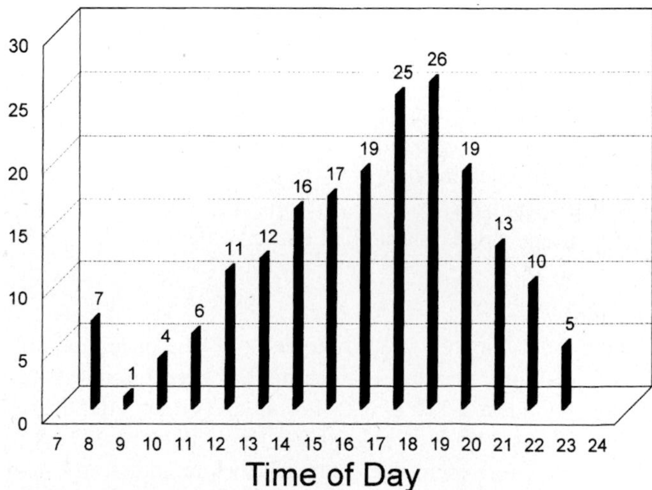

FIGURE 1-4 Incidence of children's fractures per time of day. There is an almost bell-shaped curve with a peak at around 6 PM. (Reprinted from Shank LP, Bagg RJ, Wagnon J. Etiology of pediatric fractures: the fatigue factors in children's fractures. Presented at the National Conference on Pediatric Trauma, Indianapolis, 1992; with permission.)

Increase in Child Abuse. The number of fractures due to nonaccidental causes (child abuse) has risen consistently in the past decades. In the study of fractures in children ages birth to 3 years old by Kowal-Vern et al.,[52] the number of fractures due to abuse increased almost 150 times from 1984 to 1989. This increase was attributed to a combination of improved recognition, better social resources, and a true increase in the number of cases of child abuse.

Incidences by Specific Fracture Categories

Age Variations in Fracture Location

The anatomic areas most often fractured seem to be the same in the major series, but these rates change with age. For example, supracondylar fractures of the humerus are most common in the first decade, with a peak at age 7. Fractures of the femur are most common in children ages 0 to 3. Fractures of the physis are more common just before skeletal maturity. This variation is best illustrated in Cheng and Shen's data (Fig. 1-5).[22]

Landin's Age Patterns. Landin found a similar age variability and divided it into six distinct patterns (Fig. 1-6).[58] When he compared these variability patterns with the common etiologies, he found some correlation. For example, late-peak fractures (distal forearm, phalanges, proximal humerus) were closely correlated with sports and equipment etiologies. Bimodal pattern fractures (clavicle, femur, radius and ulna, diaphyses) showed an early increase from lower energy trauma, then a late peak in incidence due to injury from high- or moderate-energy trauma. Early peak fractures (supracondylar humeral fractures are a classic example) were due mainly to falls from high levels.

The overall incidence of fractures occurring because of play activity in the home environment increases with age. Only 15% occur in toddlers, but 56% occur during older years.[134]

Locations

Early reports of children's fractures lumped the areas fractured together, and fractures were reported only as to the long bone involved (e.g., radius, humerus, femur).[11,41,44,62,66] More recent reports have split fractures into the more specific areas of the long bone involved (e.g., the distal radius, the radial neck, the supracondylar area of the humerus).[22,44,58,97,134]

Single Bones

In children, fractures in the upper extremity are much more common than those in the lower extremity.[41,44] Overall, the radius is the most commonly fractured long bone, followed by the humerus. In the lower extremity, the tibia is more commonly fractured than the femur (Table 1-2).

Specific Areas Fractured

Given the fact that different reports classify fractures somewhat differently, it is somewhat of a challenge to distill detailed and accurate prevalence data for specific fractures In trying do so, we have identified areas common to a number of recent reports,[22,44,58,97,134] but have taken some liberties in doing so. For example, distal radial metaphyseal and physeal fractures were combined as the distal radial fractures. Likewise, the carpals, metacarpals, and phalanges were combined to form the region of the hand and wrist. All the fractures around the elbow, from those of the radial neck to supracondylar fractures, were grouped as elbow fractures. This grouping allows comparison of the regional incidence of specific fracture types in children (Table 1-3).

The individual reports agreed that the most common area fractured was the distal radius. The next most common area, however, varied from the hand in Landin's series[58] to the elbow (mainly supracondylar fractures) in Cheng and Shen's series.[21,22]

Physeal Injuries

The incidence of physeal injuries overall varied from 14.5%[24] to a high of 27.6%.[72] To obtain an overall incidence of physeal fractures, six reports totaling 6479 fractures in children were combined.[13,24,72,79,97,134] In this group, 1404 involved the phy-

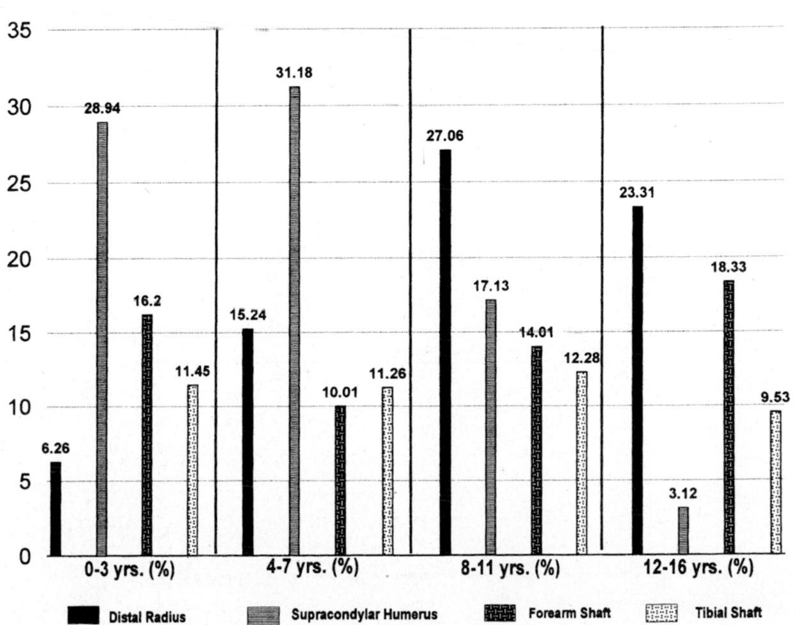

FIGURE 1-5 The frequency of occurrence of the most common fracture areas in children. The frequency of each fracture pattern differs with the various age groups. The figures express the percentage of total fractures for that age group and represent boys and girls combined. (Reprinted from Cheng JC, Shen WY. Limb fracture pattern in different pediatric age groups: a study of 3350 children. J Orthop Trauma 1993;7:17; with permission.)

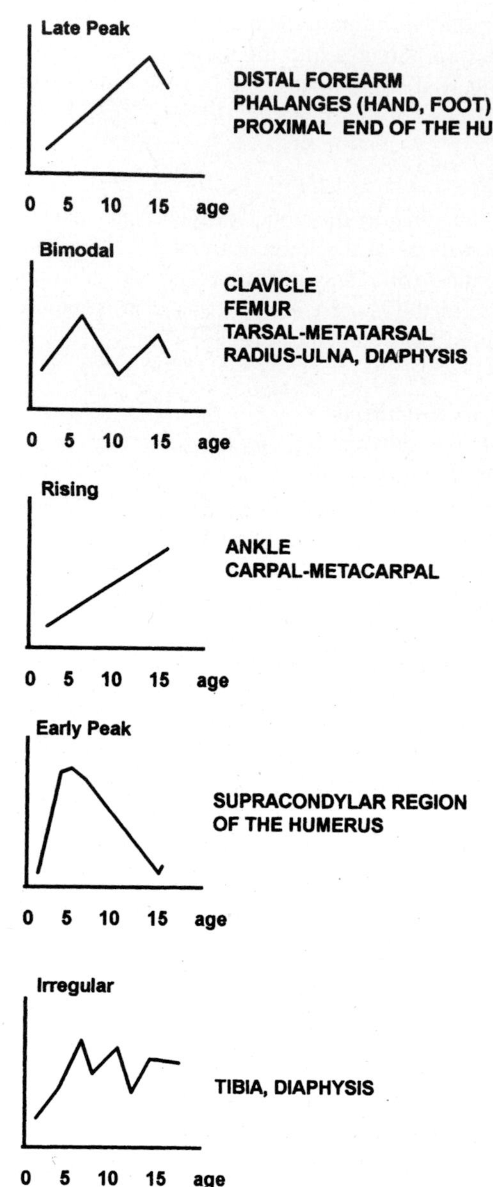

FIGURE 1-6 Patterns of fracture: variations with age. The peak ages for the various fracture types occur in one of five patterns. (Reprinted from Landin LA. Fracture patterns in children. Acta Orthop Scand 1983;202:73; with permission.)

TABLE 1-2 Incidence of Fractures in Long Bones*

Bone	%
Radius	45.1
Humerus	18.4
Tibia	15.1
Clavicle	13.8
Femur	7.6

*36,49,55,62,99,102

TABLE 1-3 Incidence of Specific Fracture Types*

Fracture	%
Distal radius and physis	23.3
Hand (carpals, metacarpals, and phalanges)	20.1
Elbow area (distal humerus, proximal radius, and ulna)	12.0
Clavicle	6.4
Radial shaft	6.4
Tibial shaft	6.2
Foot (metatarsals and phalanges)	5.9
Ankle (distal tibia)	4.4
Femur (neck and shaft)	2.3
Humerus (proximal and shaft)	1.4
Other	11.6

*8,36,57,75,129

sis, producing an average overall incidence of 21.7% for physeal fractures (Table 1-4).

Open Fractures

The overall incidence of open fractures in children is consistent. The data were combined from the four reports in which the incidence of open fractures was reported.[22,41,72,134] The incidence in these reports varied from 1.5% to 2.6%. Combined, these reports represented a total of 8367 fractures with 246 open fractures, resulting in an average incidence of 2.9% (Table 1-5).

Regional trauma centers often see patients exposed to more severe trauma, so there may be a higher incidence of open fractures in these patients. The incidence of open fractures was 9% in a report of patients admitted to the trauma center of the Children's National Medical Center, Washington, DC.[17]

Multiple Fractures

Multiple fractures in children are uncommon: the incidence ranges in the various series from 1.7% to as much as 9.7%. In four major reports totaling 5262 patients, 192 patients had more than one fracture (Table 1-6).[22,41,44,134] The incidence in these multiple series was 3.6%.

Fractures in Weak Bones. Children with generalized bone dysplasias and metabolic diseases that produce osteopenia (such as osteogenesis imperfecta) are expected to have recurrent frac-

TABLE 1-4 Incidence of Physeal Fractures*

Total fractures = 6477
Number of physeal injuries = 1404
Percentage of physeal injuries = 21.7%

*8,52,102,123,129,133

TABLE 1-5 Incidence of Open Fractures*

Total number of fractures = 8367
Total open fractures = 246
Percentage = 2.9%

*8,17,52,55

tures. In these patients, the etiology is understandable and predictable. However, some children with normal osseous structures are prone to recurrent fractures for reasons that remain unclear. The incidence of recurrent fractures in children is about 1%.[32]

Landin and Nilsson[59] found that children who sustained fractures with relatively little trauma had a lower mineral content in their forearms, but they could not correlate this finding with subsequent fractures. Thus, in children who seem to be structurally normal, there does not appear to be a physical reason for their recurrent fractures.

Repeat Fractures

Failure to find a physical cause for repeat fractures shifts the focus to a psychological or social cause. The one common factor in accident repeaters has been a high incidence of dysfunctional families.[46] In Sweden, Westfelt found that children who were accident repeaters came from "socially handicapped" families (i.e., those on public assistance or those with a caregiver who was an alcoholic).[86] Thus, repeat fractures are probably due more to behavioral or social causes than physical causes. Landin, in his follow-up article,[57] followed children with repeat fractures (four or more) into adolescence and adulthood. He found these children had a significantly increased incidence of convictions for serious criminal offenses when compared with children with only one lifetime fracture.

ETIOLOGY OF FRACTURES

Studies Essential for Prevention

While studying the epidemiology of fractures, it is important to focus on the etiology of fractures and the settings in which they occur. Fractures do not occur in a vacuum, and well-researched studies that analyze the physical and social environment in which they occur are extremely valuable. Efforts can be made toward creating a safer environment for play and recreation. Studies that identify risky patterns of use or unsafe playground behavior can significantly influence preventive health measures. Recommendations can be made to manufacturers regarding modification of a product, and education can be imparted to parents, school authorities, healthcare professionals, physical trainers, and children.

TABLE 1-6 Incidence of Multiple Fractures*

Total fractures = 5262
Total number of multiple fractures = 192
Percentage = 3.6%

*8,36,55,57

Three Broad Causes

Broadly, fractures have three main causes: (i) accidental trauma, (ii) nonaccidental trauma (child abuse), and (iii) pathologic conditions. Accidental trauma forms the largest etiologic group. Nonaccidental trauma and fractures resulting from pathologic conditions are discussed in later chapters of this book.

Fractures Resulting from Accidental Trauma

Accidental trauma can occur in a variety of settings, some often overlapping others. However, for purposes of simplicity, fractures can be considered to occur in the following five environments: (i) home environment, (ii) school environment, (iii) play and recreational activities, (iv) motor vehicle and road accidents, and (v) uncommon situations involving such causes as ice cream trucks, water tubing, and gunshot and missile injuries.

Home Environment

Fractures sustained in the home environment are defined as those that occur in the house and surrounding vicinity. These generally occur in a fairly supervised environment and are mainly due to falls from furniture, stairs, fences, and trees.

Falls from Heights. Falls can vary in severity from a simple fall while running to a fall of great magnitude, such as from a third story window. In falling from heights, adults often land on their lower extremities, accounting for the high number of lower extremity fractures, especially the calcaneus. Children tend to fall head first, using the upper extremities to break the fall. This accounts for the larger number of skull and radial fractures in children. Femoral fractures also are common in children falling from great heights. In contrast to adults, spinal fractures are rare in children who fall from great heights.[8,76,114,117] In one study, children falling three stories or less all survived. Falls from the fifth or sixth floor resulted in a 50% mortality rate.[8]

Social Factors. Interestingly, a Swedish study[86] showed that an increased incidence of fractures in a home environment did not necessarily correlate with the physical attributes or poor safety precautions of the house. Rather, it appears that a disruption of the family structure and presence of social handicaps (alcoholism, welfare recipients, etc.) is an important risk factor for pediatric fracture.

School Environment

The supervised environments at school are generally safe, and the overall annual rate of injury (total percentage of children injured in a single year) in the school environment ranges from 2.8% to 9.2%.[15,60,86,112] True rates may be higher because of inaccurate reporting, especially of mild injuries. In one series, the official rate was 5.6%, but when the parents were closely questioned, the incidence of unreported, trivial injuries was as much as 15%.[34] The annual fracture rate of school injuries is low. Of all injuries sustained by children at school in a year, only 5% to 10% involved fractures.[34,60,112] In Worlock and

Stower's series of children's fractures from England,[134] only 20% occurred at school. Most injuries (53%) occurring in school are related to athletics and sporting events,[60] and injuries are highest in the middle-school children. The peak time of day for injuries at school is in the morning, which differs from the injury patterns of children in general.[60]

Play and Recreational Activities

Playground Equipment. Play is an essential element of a child's life. It enhances physical development and fosters social interaction. Unfortunately, unsupervised or careless use of some play equipment can endanger life and limb. When Mott et al.[81] studied the incidence and pattern of injuries to children using public playgrounds, they found that approximately 1% of children using playgrounds sustained injuries. Swings, climbers, and slides are the pieces of playground equipment associated with 88% of the playground injuries.[69]

In a study of injuries resulting from playground equipment, Waltzman et al.[128] found that most injuries occurred in boys (56%) with a peak incidence in the summer months. Fractures accounted for 61% of these injuries, 90% of which involved the upper extremity and were sustained in falls from playground equipment such as monkey bars and climbing frames. Younger children (1 to 4 years old) were more likely to sustain fractures than older children.

Similar observations were made in a study by Lillis and Jaffe[63] in which upper extremity injuries, especially fractures, accounted for most of hospitalizations resulting from injuries on playground equipment. Older children sustained more injuries on climbing apparatus, whereas younger children sustained more injuries on slides.

Loder et al.[64] utilized the National Electronic Injury Surveillance System (NEISS) dataset to explore the demographics of playground equipment injuries in children. Monkey bars were the most common cause of fractures. In another study looking specifically at injuries from monkey bars, the peak age group was the 5- to 12-year-old group, with supracondylar humeral fractures being the most common fracture sustained.[70]

The correlation of the hardness of the playground surface with the risk of injury has been confirmed in numerous studies.[56,64,82,83] Changing playground surfaces from concrete to more impact-absorbing surfaces such as bark reduced the incidence and severity of head injury but increased the tendency for long bone fractures (40%), bruises, and sprains. Chalmers et al.[19] determined that the height of the equipment was just as great a risk factor as the surface composition.

Public playgrounds appear to have a higher risk for injuries than private playgrounds because they usually have harder surfaces and higher pieces of equipment,[90] although playground injury was most likely to occur at school compared to home, public, and other locations.[91]

Bicycle Injuries. Bicycle injuries are a significant cause of mortality and morbidity for children.[96] Bicycle mishaps are the most common causes of serious head injury in children.[131] Boys in the 5- to 14-year age group are at greatest risk for bicycle injury (80%). Puranik et al.[96] studied the profile of pediatric bicycle injuries in a sample of 211 children who were treated for bicycle-related injury at their trauma center over a 4-year period. They found that bicycle injuries accounted for 18% of all pediatric trauma patients. Bicycle/motor vehicle collisions caused 86% of injuries. Sixty-seven percent had head injuries and 29% sustained fractures. More than half of the incidents occurred on the weekend. Sixteen percent were injured by ejection from a bicycle after losing control, hitting a pothole, or colliding with a fixed object or another bicycle. Fractures mainly involved the lower extremity, upper extremity, skull, ribs, and pelvis in decreasing order of incidence.

Low Helmet Use. More importantly, the study detected that the use of safety helmets was disturbingly low (<2%). Other studies confirm the observation that fewer than 13% to 15% of children wear helmets while riding bicycles.[35,101] The Year 2000 Health Objectives called for helmet use by 50% of bicyclists.[95] Even as recently as 2003, the use of bicycle helmets was still below 20%.[42] Research has shown that legislation, combined with education and helmet subsidies, is the most effective strategy to increase use of safety helmets in child bicyclists.[18] As public awareness of both the severity and preventability of bicycle-related injuries grows, the goal of safer bicycling practices and lower injury rates can be achieved.[96]

Injuries from Bicycle Parts. Bicycle spokes and handle bars also are responsible for many fractures and soft tissue injuries in children. D'Souza et al.[29] and Segers et al.[109] found that bicycle spoke injuries are typically sustained when the child's foot is caught in the spokes of the rotating wheel. Of 130 children with bicycle spoke injuries, 29 children sustained fractures of the tibia, fibula, or foot bone. Several had lacerations and soft tissue defects. D'Souza et al.[29] suggested that a mesh cover to prevent the toes from entering between the spokes and a plastic shield to bridge the gap between the fork and horizontal upright could substantially decrease the incidence of these injuries.

Skateboarding. Skateboarding and in-line skating have experienced a renewed surge in popularity over the past three decades. With the increasing number of participants, high-tech equipment development, and vigorous advertising, skateboard and skating injuries are expected to increase. There was an initial increase in the early 1980s, with a decrease after 1993. Since 1998, there has been an increase in the number of skateboard injuries.[75] Because the nature of skateboarding encompasses both high speed and extreme maneuvers, high-energy fractures and other injuries can occur, as highlighted by several studies.[37,88,93] Studies have shown that skateboarding-related injuries are more severe and have more serious consequences than roller-skating or in-line skating injuries.[88] In a study of skateboarding injuries, Fountain et al.[37] found that fractures of the upper or lower extremity accounted for 50% of all skateboarding injuries. Interestingly, more than one third of those injured sustained injuries within the first week of skateboarding. Most injuries occurred in preadolescent boys (75%) 10 to 16 years of age; 65% sustained injuries on public roads, footpaths, and parking lots. Several reports[37,108] have recommended safety guidelines and precautions such as use of helmets, knee and elbow pads, and wrist guards, but such regulations seldom are enforced.

Roller Skates and Inline Skates. In a study of in-line skate and roller skate injuries in childhood, Jerosch et al.[45] found that in a group of 1036 skaters, 60% had sustained injuries. Eight percent of these were fractures, mostly involving the elbow, forearm, wrist, and fingers (78%). Fewer than 20% used protective devices, and most lacked knowledge of the basic techniques of skating, braking, and falling. In a larger study of 60,730 skating injuries in children, Powell and Tanz[93] found that 68% of the children were preadolescent boys with a mean age of 11.8 years. Fractures were the most common injury (65%) and two thirds of these involved the distal forearm. Two and a half percent required hospital admissions; 90% of these admissions were for a fracture. Similarly, Mitts and Hennrikus[78] found that 75% of in-line skating fractures in children occurred in the distal forearm as a result of falls on the out-stretched hand. One in eight children sustained a fracture during the first attempt at the sport. The orthopaedic community has an obligation to educate the public on the need for wearing wrist guards when using in-line skates or roller skates.

Skate Parks Actually Increase the Injury Rate. It was thought that formal skate parks could decrease the injury rate. However, a study by Sheehan et al.[111] demonstrated that dedicated skate parks led to an increase in pediatric fractures referred to the hospital. The authors suggested that there should be closer supervision and training of children and more emphasis on limb protective gear.

Inline Scooters. Since 2000, a substantial increase in injuries related to nonmotorized scooters (kickboards) has been observed among children. Most of the scooter-related accidents were caused by the wheels of the scooter getting caught by uneven ground, whereas most skateboard accidents occurred during attempted trick maneuvers. Protective gear was seldom used.[20,71,105] Scooters seem to have a high incidence of collisions with motor vehicles.[71] The recent motorizing of the scooters will only increase the severity of the injuries sustained.

Trampoline-Related Injuries. Trampolines enjoyed increasing popularity in the 1990s and are a significant cause of morbidity in children. Several studies have noted a dramatic increase in the number of pediatric trampoline injuries during the past 10 years, rightfully deeming it as a "national epidemic."[39,115]

Using the NEISS data, Smith et al.[115] estimated that there are roughly 40,000 pediatric trampoline injuries per year. Furnival et al.,[39] in a retrospective study over a 7-year period, found that the annual number of pediatric tramopoline injuries tripled between 1990 and 1997. In contrast to other recreational activities in which boys constitute the population at risk, patients with pediatric tramopoline injuries were predominantly girls, with a median age of 7 years. Nearly a third of the injuries resulted from falling off the trampoline. Fractures of the upper and lower extremities occurred in 45% and were more frequently associated with falls off the trampoline. In another excellent study on pediatric tramopoline injuries, Smith[115] found that there was virtually a 100% increase in injuries from 1990 to 1995, with an average of more than 60,000 injuries per year. Younger children had a higher incidence of upper extremity fractures and other injuries. In a later study, Smith and Shields[116] reported that fractures, especially involving the upper extremity, accounted for 35% of all injuries. Interestingly, more than 50% of the injuries occurred under direct adult supervision. More disturbingly, 73% of the parents were aware of the potential dangers of trampolines, and 96% of the injuries occurred in the home backyard. These researchers, along with others,[39] rightly concluded that use of warning labels, public education, and even direct adult supervision were inadequate in preventing these injuries and have called for a total ban on the recreational, school, and competitive use of trampolines by children.[115,116]

Skiing Injuries. In a study of major skiing injuries in children and adolescents, Shorter et al.[113] found more than 90% of injured children were boys 5 to 18 years of age. Sixty percent of the accidents occurred in collisions with stationary objects such as trees, poles, and stakes. Most injuries occurred in the afternoon, among beginners, and in the first week of skiing season. Fractures accounted for one third of the total injuries sustained. The two main factors implicated in skiing injuries are excessive speed and loss of control; effective prevention efforts should target both of these factors.

Snowboarding Injuries. Snowboarding runs a risk similar to skiing. Bladin et al.[14] found that approximately 60% of snowboarding injuries involved the lower limbs and occurred in novices. The most common injuries were sprains (53%) and fractures (26%). Compared with skiers, snowboarders had 2½ times as many fractures, particularly to the upper limb, as well as more ankle injuries and higher rates of head injury. The absence of ski poles and the fixed position of the feet on the snowboard mean that the upper limbs absorb the full impact of any fall. Wrist braces can decrease the incidence of wrist injuries in snowboarding.[103] Of some concern, a recent study has shown that rates of snowboard injuries seem to be rising, while rates of ski injuries have been flat.[43]

Motor Vehicle Accidents

This category includes injuries sustained by occupants of a motor vehicle and victims of vehicle-pedestrian accidents.

The injury patterns of children involved in motor vehicle accidents differ from those of adults. In all types of motor vehicle accidents for all ages, children constitute a little over 10% of the total number of patients injured.[58,105] Of all the persons injured as motor vehicle occupants, only about 17% to 18% are children. Of the victims of vehicle-versus-pedestrian accidents, about 29% are children. Of the total number of children involved in motor vehicle accidents, 56.4% were vehicle-pedestrian accidents, and 19.6% were vehicle-bicycle accidents.[31]

The fracture rate of children in motor vehicle accidents is less than that of adults. Of the total number of vehicle-pedestrian accidents, about 22% of the children sustained fractures; 40% of the adults sustained fractures in the same type of accident. This has been attributed to the fact that children are more likely to "bounce" when hit.[31]

Children are twice as likely as adults to sustain a femoral fracture when struck by an automobile; in adults, tibial and knee injuries are more common in the same type of accident. This seems to be related to where the car's bumper strikes the victim.[17,124] Motor vehicle accidents do produce a high proportion of spinal and pelvic injuries.[17]

Recreational all-terrain vehicles (ATVs) have emerged as a new cause of serious pediatric injury. Using the KID dataset, Killingsworth et al.[50] showed that 5292 children were admitted to a hospital in 1997 and 2000 (the two years for which KID data was available) resulting in 74 million dollars in hospital charges, with rates of hospitalization increasing 80% between these 2 years. In fact, using the Oregon state database, Mullins et al.[85] showed that the number of patients who sought tertiary care for severe injuries caused by off-road vehicles doubled over a period of 4 years. In contrast to other etiologies of injury, children who sustained ATV-related fractures had more severe injuries and a higher percentage of significant head trauma, with 1% of these injuries resulting in in-hospital death. These statisitics point to the failure of voluntary safety efforts to date and argue for much stronger regulatory control.

According to the 2007 report of the CPSC, serious ATV injuries in children younger than 16 years requiring emergency room treatment rose from 146,000 in 2006 to 150,900 in 2007. In their 11-year review of ATV injuries treated at al level 1 pediatric trauma center, Kute et al.[53] determined that ATV accident-related admissions increased almost five times and overall fracture number increased four times over the study period; 63% of the 238 patients sustatined at least one fracture.

In a review of 96 children who sustained injuries in ATV-related accidents during a 30-month period, Kellum et al.[48] noted age-related patterns of injury. Younger children (≤12 years) were more likely to sustain an isolated fracture and were more likely to sustain a lower extremity fracture, specifically a femoral fracture, than older children. Older children were more likely to sustain a pelvic fracture. Kirkpatrick et al.[51] expressed concern about the frequency and severity of fractures about the elbow in their 73 patients injured in ATV accidents between 2001 and 2007: all six open fractures involving the upper extremity involved the elbow.

The etiologic aspects of children's fractures are summarized in Figure 1-7 and Table 1-7.

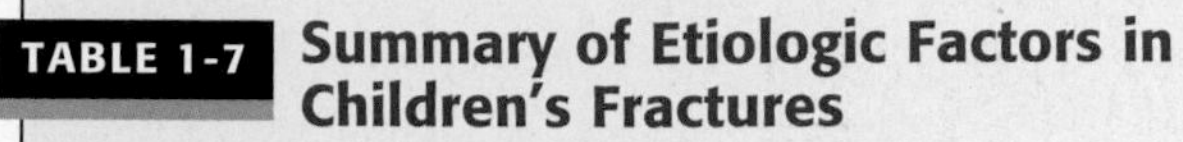

TABLE 1-7 Summary of Etiologic Factors in Children's Fractures

Home environment
Injuries
83% of all children's injuries
Fractures
37% of all children's fractures
School environment
Injuries
Overall rate, 2.8% to 9.2% annually
53% related to athletic events
Peak age: middle-school group
Fractures
Occur in only 5% to 10% of all school-related injuries
About 20% of all children's fractures
Motor vehicle accidents (MVA)
Injuries
Children only 10% of all MVAs
Of children's MVAs, only 17% to 18% were occupants; remainder were vehicle/pedestrian or vehicle/bicycle
Fractures
High incidence of femoral fractures in vehicle-pedestrian accidents in children
Children have a more spinal and pelvic fractures with MVAs than with other mechanisms

Gunshot and Firearm Injuries

Gunshot or missile wounds arise from objects projected into space by an explosive device. Gunshot wounds have become

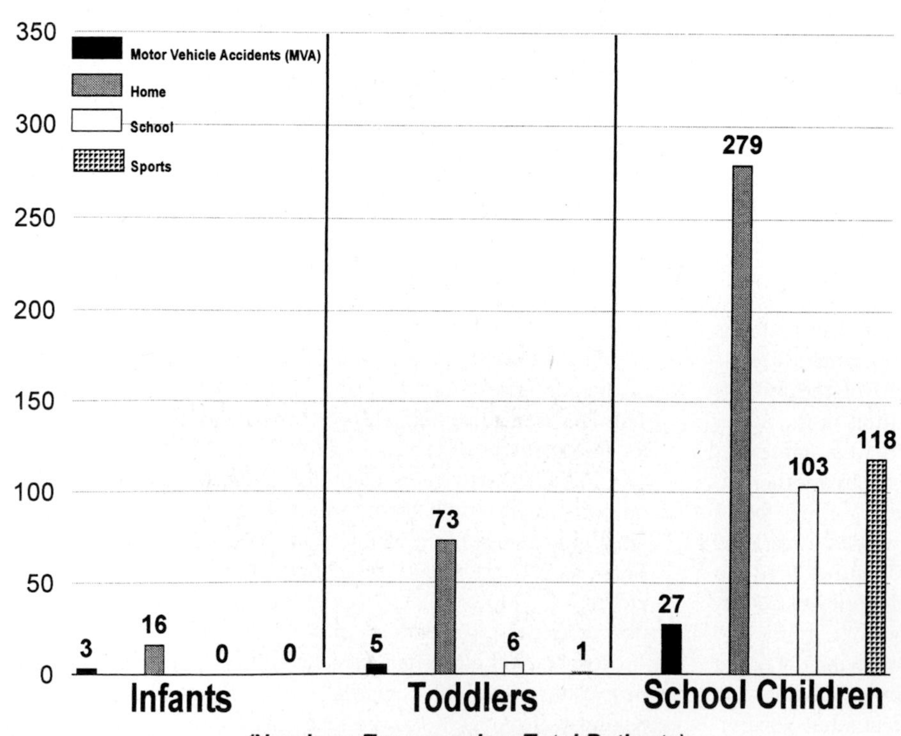

FIGURE 1-7 The incidence of fractures in children expressed as the four common etiologic categories. Most fractures occur at home. The numbers are expressed as total patients per each age category. (Reprinted from Worlock P, Stower M. Fracture patterns in Nottingham children. J Pediatr Orthop 1986;6:656; with permission.)

increasingly common in children in the United States.[130] In a sad reflection of the changing times and the newly pervasive gun culture, firearms are determined to be second only to motor vehicles as the leading cause of death in youths. In considering the prevalence of firearms in the United States, it has been estimated that there are about 200 million privately owned guns in the United States and that approximately 40% of US households contain firearms of some type.[26]

Etiology. In two reports from inner-city hospitals in the United States in the 1990s, most injuries resulted from random violence to innocent bystanders; the prime example was "drive-by shootings."[121,130] Few were self-inflicted, either voluntarily or accidentally. In a 1976 report on patients in a relatively rural setting in Canada, almost all the missile injuries were accidental, having been caused by the patient or a close friend or relative.[61]

In the urban setting, handguns and rifles are the most common weapons.[121,125,130] In the rural setting, the most common weapon is a shotgun.[61] The firepower of these weapons has changed over the years. In one urban hospital reporting gunshot wounds from 1973 to 1983, most of the injuries were from .32- or .38-caliber weapons; only 5% were high-caliber or high-velocity weapons.[87] In a later study of gunshot wounds from the same institution from 1991 to 1994, the incidence of injuries from high-caliber and high-velocity weapons (e.g., .357 magnum, AK-47, and other assault rifles) had increased to 35%.[113]

In the urban setting, the victims' ages ranged from 1 to 17 years, and most of the injuries were in children aged 12 to 14.[87,121,125,130] In the rural setting, the patients were younger; the average age was 9 years.[61]

Of 839 children sustaining gunshot wounds, 274 (32.6%) involved the extremities.[87,121,125,130] Of the gunshot wounds that involved the extremities, 51.3% produced significant fractures.[61,121,130] No single bone seemed to predominate, although most of the fractures were distal to the elbow.[87,121,125,130]

Complications of Gunshot Wounds. The two most common complications were growth arrest and infection. Other complications included delayed union and malunion. Considering the magnitude of many of these injuries, the infection rate for extremity wounds was low (about 7.3%). The type of missile did not seem to have any relation to the development of an infection.[130]

In Letts and Miller's 1976 series, one sixth of the patients had some type of growth disturbance.[61] In a third of their patients, the missile was only in close proximity to the physis, but still appeared to cause a growth disturbance. In a 1995 report by Washington et al.,[130] the incidence of missiles' growth arrest was exactly the same; however, all were a result of a direct injury to the physis by the missile. None of their patients with growth arrest had proximity missile wounds. The higher incidence of growth abnormalities in the 1976 series was due to the larger number of shotgun and hunting rifle injuries, which dissipate more of their energy peripheral to the missile track.

In two of the studies in which patients were followed closely, all of the fractures ultimately healed.[61,130] On the other hand, DiScala and Sege[33] found in their review of children and adolescents who required hospitalization for gunshot wounds that almost half of them were discharged with disabilities.

Prevention. In a 1999 report, Freed et al.[38] analyzed the magnitude and implications of the increasing incidence of firearm-related injuries in children. They suggested a product-oriented approach, focusing on the gun, in an attempt to provide an efficient strategy of gun control and hence reduce the disturbing trend of firearm-related injuries and death among youths. Rather than modifying behavioral or environmental issues, which are more complex, they suggested focusing primarily on strategies that offset the accessibility and design of firearms. In brief, these strategies included reducing the number of guns in the environment through restrictive legislation, gun buy-back programs, gun taxes, physician counseling, and modifying the design of guns to make them more child-proof and prevent unauthorized and unintended use.

Intrinsic Causes

Nutrition. In a study in Spain, a significant difference in fracture rates was found when cities with a high calcium content in their water were compared with those with a lower calcium content. With all other factors being equal (e.g., fluoride content, socioeconomic background), children who lived in the cities with a lower calcium content had a higher fracture rate.[126]

An increase in the consumption of carbonated beverages has been shown to produce an increased incidence of fractures in adolescents.[135]

Bone Density. Bone density may be a factor, but the data are unclear. Landin and Nilsson[59] found that the mineral content of the forearms was lower in children who sustained fractures from mild trauma than in children who had never sustained fractures. It was not significantly different, however, in those sustaining fractures from severe trauma. This study used measurements of bone density of the cortical bone in the forearms. Cook et al.,[27] using measurements of bone density obtained from trabecular bone in the spine and femoral neck, found no difference between children who had sustained fractures and those who had not.

Premature Infants

Fractures not related to birth trauma reportedly occur in 1% to 2% of low-birth-weight or premature infants during their stay in a neonatal intensive care unit.[6] A combination of clinical history, radiographic appearance, and laboratory data has shown evidence of bone loss from inadequate calcium and phosphorus intake in these infants. Correcting the metabolic status of these low–birth-weight infants, with special emphasis on calcium and phosphorus intake, appears to decrease the incidence of repeat fractures and to improve the radiographic appearance of their bony tissues. Once the metabolic abnormalities are corrected, this temporary deficiency seems to have no long-term effects. When premature infants were followed into later years, there was no difference in their fracture rate compared with that of children of normal birth weight.[30]

PREVENTIVE PROGRAMS

One of the major goals of studying the incidence of fractures is to identify problem areas. It is hoped that by targeting these areas, programs can be designed to decrease the risk factors.

National Campaigns

Several national organizations have developed safety programs. The foremost is the American Academy of Pediatrics, which has committees on accident and poisoning prevention, and has produced guidelines for athletics,[5] playgrounds,[98,132] trampolines,[3,4] ATVs, and skateboards.[25] The American Academy of Orthopaedic Surgeons has produced a program designed to decrease the incidence of playground injuries. These programs offer background data and guidelines for various activities, but their effectiveness has not been fully studied.

Local Community Participation

To be effective, accident prevention programs require local participation and cooperation. They must be broad-based, and they require considerable effort by members of the local community. In the United States, one effective program is the New York Health Department's "Kids Can't Fly" campaign, developed in response to the large number of injuries and deaths from children falling out of apartment house windows in the 1970s.[118] This extensive program consisted of a good reporting system from hospital emergency rooms, with follow-up by public health personnel; a strong media campaign to educate the public; a door-to-door hazard identification program; and the distribution of low- or no-cost, easily installed window guards to families in high-rise apartments. The city required property owners to provide window guards in apartments where children 10 years or younger lived. The success of this program was demonstrated by a 50% decrease in reported falls after 3 years and a 96% decrease after 7 years.[8,118]

Over the past 30 years, Sweden has developed broader-based, community-oriented programs to decrease the incidence of all types of childhood injuries.[12] The development of these pilot programs has been relatively easy in a country like Sweden because the population is homogeneous, the incidence of poverty is low, and the government is stable. The Swedish program had a three-pronged approach: injury surveillance and prevention research; establishment of a safer environment for children through legislative regulation; and a broad-based safety education campaign. These programs have produced positive results. Schelp demonstrated a 27% reduction in home accidents in the municipality of Falkoping only 3 years after the establishment of a community-wide campaign.[107]

Effective prevention programs require local community participation and education. All the articles, lectures, and pamphlets in the world cannot help unless local communities make the necessary changes to decrease accident risks.

ACKNOWLEDGMENTS

With appreciation to Kaye Wilkins for previous work on this chapter.

REFERENCES

1. Aitken ME, Jaffe KM, DiScala C, et al. Functional outcome in children with multiple trauma without significant head injury. Arch Phys Med Rehabil 1999;80(8):889–895.
2. Akbarnia B, Torg JS, Kirkpatrick J, et al. Manifestations of the battered-child syndrome. 1974;56(6):1159–1166.
3. American Academy of Pediatrics. Committee on Pediatric Aspects of Physical Fitness, Recreation, and Sports. Competitive athletics for children of elementary school age. Pediatrics 1981:67(6):927–928.
4. American Academy of Pediatrics, Committee on Accident and Poison Prevention. Trampolines. News and Comment. September 1977.
5. American Academy of Pediatrics, Committee on Accident and Poison Prevention and Committee on Pediatric Aspects of Physical Fitness, Recreation, and Sports. Trampolines II. Pediatrics 1981; 67:438–439.
6. Amir J, Katz K, Grunebaum M, et al. Fractures in premature infants. J Pediatr Orthop 1988;8(1):41–44
7. Andren L, Borgstrom KE. Seasonal variation of epiphysiolysis of the hip and possibility of causal factor. Acta Orthop Scand 1958;28(1):22–26.
8. Barlow B, Niemirska M, Gandhi RP, et al. Ten years of experience with falls from a height in children. J Pediatr Surg 1983;18(4):509–511.
9. Beaty JH, Austin SM, Warner WC, et al. Interlocking intramedullary nailing of femoral shaft fractures in adolescents: preliminary results and complications. J Pediatr Orthop 1994;14(2):178–183.
10. Beaty JH, Kasser JR, eds. Rockwood & Wilkins fractures in children. 5th ed. Philadelphia: Lippincott Williams & Wilkins, 2001.
11. Beekman F, Sullivan JE. Some observations on fractures of long bones in children. Am J Surg 1941;51:722–738.
12. Bergman AB, Rivara FP. Sweden's experience in reducing childhood injuries. Pediatrics 1991;88(1):69–74.
13. Bisgard JD, Martenson L. Fractures in children. Surg Gynec Obstet 1937;65:464–474.
14. Bladin C, Giddings P, Robinson M. Australian snowboard injury data base study. A 4-year prospective study. Am J Sports Med 1993;21(5):701–704.
15. Boyce WT, Sprunger LW, Sobolewski S, et al. Epidemiology of injuries in a large, urban school district. Pediatrics 1984;74(3):342–349.
16. Brinker MR, O'Connor DP. The incidence of fractures and dislocations referred for orthopaedic services in a capitated population. J Bone Joint Surg Am 2004;86-A(2): 290–297.
17. Buckley SL, Gotschall C, Robertson W Jr, et al. The relationships of skeletal injuries with trauma score, injury severity score, length of hospital stay, hospital charges, and mortality in children admitted to a regional pediatric trauma center. J Pediatr Orthop 1994;14(4):449–453.
18. Cameron M, Vulcan AP, Finch CF, et al. Mandatory bicycle helmet use following a decade of helmet promotion in Victoria, Australia—an evaluation. Accid Anal Prev 1996;26(3):325–337.
19. Chalmers DJ, Marshall SW, Langley JD, et al. Height and surfacing as risk factors for injury in falls from playground equipment: a case-control study. Inj Prev 1996;2(2): 98–104.
20. Chapman S, Webber S, O'Meara M. Scooter injuries in children. J Pediatr Child Health 2001;37(6):567–570.
21. Cheng JC, Ng BK, Ying SY, et al. A 10-year study of the changes in the pattern and treatment of 6493 fractures. J Pediatr Orthop 1999;19:344–350.
22. Cheng JC, Shen WY. Limb fracture pattern in different pediatric age groups: a study of 3350 children. J Orthop Trauma 1993;7(1):15–22.
23. Chess DG, Hyndman JC, Leahey JL, et al. Short-arm plaster for pediatric distal forearm fractures. J Pediatr Orthop 1994;14(2):211–213.
24. Compere EL. Growth arrest in long bones as result of fractures that include the epiphysis. JAMA 1935;105:2140–2146.
25. Committee on Accident and Poison Prevention: Skateboard Injuries. Pediatrics 1989; 83:1070–1071.
26. Cook PJ, Ludwig J. Guns in America: Results of a Comprehensive National Survey on Firearms Ownership and Use. Washington, DC: Police Foundation, 1996.
27. Cook SD, Harding AF, Morgan EL, et al. Association of bone mineral density and pediatric fractures. J Pediatr Orthop 1987;7(4):424–427.
28. Cox PJ, Clarke NM. Improving the outcome of paediatric orthopaedic trauma: an audit of inpatient management in Southampton. Ann R Coll Surg Engl 1997;79(6):441–446.
29. D'Souza LG, Hynes DE, McManus F, et al. The bicycle spoke injury: an avoidable accident? Foot Ankle Int 1996;17(3):170–173.
30. Dahlenburg SL, Bishop NJ, Lucas A. Are preterm infants at risk for subsequent fractures? Arch Dis Child 1989;64(10 Spec No):1384–1385.
31. Derlet RW, Silva J Jr, Holcroft J. Pedestrian accidents: adult and pediatric injuries. J Emerg Med 1989;7(1):5–8.
32. Dershewitz R. Is it of any practical value to identify "accident-prone" children? Pediatrics 1977;60(5):786.
33. DiScala C, Sege R. Outcomes in children and young adults who are hospitalized for firearms-related injuries. Pediatrics 2004;113(5):1306–1312.
34. Feldman W, Woodward CA, Hodgson C, et al. Prospective study of school injuries: incidence, types, related factors, and initial management. Can Med Assoc J 1983; 129(12):1279–1283.
35. Finvers KA, Strother RT, Mohtadi N. The effect of bicycling helmets in preventing significant bicycle-related injuries in children. Clin J Sport Med 1996;6(2):102–107.
36. Fleming DM, Charlton JR. Morbidity and healthcare utilization of children in households with one adult: comparative observational study. BMJ 1988;316(7144): 1572–1576.
37. Fountain JL, Meyers MC. Skateboarding injuries. Sports Med 1996;22(6):360–366.
38. Freed LH, Vernick JS, Hargarten SW. Prevention of firearm-related injuries and deaths among youth. A product-oriented approach. Pediatr Clin North Am 1998;45(2): 427–438.
39. Furnival RA, Street KA, Schunk JE. Too many pediatric trampoline injuries. Pediatrics 1999;103(5):e57.
40. Galano GJ, Vitale MA, Kessler MW, et al. The most frequent traumatic orthopaedic injuries from a national pediatric inpatient population. J Pediatr Orthop 2005;25(1): 39–44.
41. Hanlon CR, Estes WL Jr. Fractures in childhood—a statistical analysis. Am J Surg 1954;87(3):312–323.
42. Hansen KS, Engesaeter LB, Viste A. Protective effect of different types of bicycle helmets. Traffic Inj Prev 2003;4(4):285–290.
43. Hayes JR, Groner JI. The increasing incidence of snowboard-related trauma. J Pediatr Surg 2008;43(5):928–930.
44. Iqbal QM. Long-bone fractures among children in Malaysia. Int Surg 1975;59(8): 410–415.
45. Jerosch J, Heidjann J, Thorwesten L, et al. Injury patterns in acceptance of passive and

active injury prophylaxis for inline skating. Knee Surg Sports Traumatol Arthrosc 1998; 6(1):44–49.
46. Jones JG. The child accident repeater, a review. Clin Pediatr (Phila) 1980;19(4): 284–288.
47. Jones K, Weiner DS. The management of forearm fractures in children: a plea for conservatism. J Pediatr Orthop 1999;19(6):811–815.
48. Kellem E, Creek A, Dawkins R, et al. Age-related patterns of injury in children involved in all-terrain vehicle accidents. J Peditr Orthop 2008;28:854–858.
49. Kempe CH, Silverman FN, Steele BF, et al. The battered-child syndrome. JAMA 1962; 181:17–24.
50. Killingsworth JB, Tilford JM, Parker JG, et al. National hospitalization impact of pediatric all-terrain vehicle injuries. Pediatrics 2005;115(3):e316–e321.
51. Kirkpatrick R, Puffinbarger W, Sullivan JA. All-terrain vehicle injuries in children. j Pediatr Orthop 2007;27:725–728.
52. Kowal-Vern A, Paxton TP, Ros SP, et al. Fractures in the under-3-year-old age cohort. Clin Pediatr (Phila) 1992;31(11):653–659.
53. Kute B, Nyland JA, Roberts CS, et al. Recreational all-terrain vehicle injuries among children: an 11-year review of a Central Kentucky level 1 pediatric trauma center database. J Pediatr Orthop 2007;27:851–855.
54. Kyle SB, Nance ML, Rutherford GW Jr, et al. Skateboard-associated injuries: participation-based estimates and injury characteristics. J Trauma 2002;53(4):686–690.
55. Laffoy M. Childhood accidents at home. Ir Med J 1997;90(1):26–27.
56. Laforest S, Robitaille Y, Lesage D, et al. Playground injuries: surface characteristics, equipment height, and the occurrence and severity of playground injuries. Inj Prev 2001;7(1):35–40.
57. Landin LA. Epidemiology of children's fractures. J Pediatr Orthop B 1997;6(2):79–83.
58. Landin LA. Fracture patterns in children. Analysis of 8682 fractures with special reference to incidence, etiology, and secular changes in a Swedish urban population 1950–1979. Acta Orthop Scand Suppl 1983;64(suppl 202):1–109.
59. Landin LA, Nilsson BE. Bone mineral content in children with fractures. Clin Orthop Relat Res 1983;178:292–296.
60. Lenaway DD, Ambler AG, Beaudoin DE. The epidemiology of school-related injuries: new perspectives. Am J Prev Med 1992;8(3):193–198.
61. Letts RM, Miller D. Gunshot wounds of the extremities in children. J Trauma 1976; 16(10):807–811.
62. Lichtenberg RP. A study of 2532 fractures in children. Am J Surg 1954;87(3):330–338.
63. Lillis KA, Jaffe DM. Playground injuries in children. Pediatr Emerg Care 1997;13(2): 149–153.
64. Loder RT. The demographics of playground equipment injuries in children. J Pediatr Surg 2008;43(4):691–699.
65. Loder RT, Feinberg JR. Orthopaedic injuries in children with nonaccidental trauma: demographics and incidence from the 2000 kids' inpatient database. J Pediatr Orthop 2007;27(4):421–6.
66. Lopez AA, Rennie TF. A survey of accidents to children aged under 15 years seen at a district hospital in Sydney in 1 year. Med J Aust 1969;1(16):806–809.
67. Lyons JP, Ashley E, Hoffer M. Ulnar nerve palsies after percutaneous cross-pinning of supracondylar fractures in children's elbows. J Pediatr Orthop 1998;18(1):43–45.
68. Lyons RA, Delahunty AM, Heaven M, et al. Incidence of fractures in affluent and deprived areas population based study. BMJ 2000;320(7228):149.
69. Mack MG, Hudson S, Thompson D. A descriptive analysis of children's playground injuries in the United States 1990–1994. Inj Prev 1997;3(2):100–103.
70. Mahadev A, Soon MY, Lam KS. Monkey bars are for monkeys: a study on playground equipment-related extremity fractures in Singapore. Singapore Med J 2004;45(1):9–13.
71. Mankovsky AB, Mendoza-Sagaon M, Cardinaux C, et al. Evaluation of scooter-related injuries in children. J Pediatr Surg 2002;37(5):755–759.
72. Mann DC, Rajmaira S. Distribution of physeal and nonphyseal fractures in 2650 long-bone fractures in children aged 0–16 years. J Pediatr Orthop 1990;10(6):713–716.
73. Masterson E, Borton D, O'Brien T. Victims of our climate. 1993;24(4):247–248.
74. McClelland CQ, Heiple KG. Fractures in the first year of life. A diagnostic dilemma. Am J Dis Child 1982;136(1):26–29.
75. Melin G, Melin KA. Accidents in childhood. J Insur Med 1950;5(3):35–37.
76. Meller JL, Shermeta DW. Falls in urban children. A problem revisited. Am J Dis Child 1987;141(12):1271–1275.
77. Mileski RA, Garvin KL, Huurman WW. Avascular necrosis of the femoral head after closed intramedullary shortening in an adolescent. J Pediatr Orthop 1995;15(1):24–26.
78. Mitts KG, Hennrikus WL. Inline skating fractures in children. J Pediatr Orthop 1996; 16(5):640–643.
79. Mizuta T, Benson WM, Foster BK, et al. Statistical analysis of the incidence of physeal injuries. J Pediatr Orthop 1987;7(5):518–523.
80. Mortensson W, Thönell S. Left-side dominance of upper extremity fracture in children. Acta Orthop Scand 1991;62(2):154–155.
81. Mott A, Evans R, Rolfe K, et al. Patterns of injuries to children on public playgrounds. Arch Dis Child 1994;71(4):328–330.
82. Mott A, Rolfe K, James R, et al. Safety of surfaces and equipment for children in playgrounds. Lancet 1997;349(9069):1874–1876.
83. Mowat DL, Wang F, Pickett W, et al. A case-control study of risk factors for playground injuries among children in Kingston and area. Inj Prev 1998;4(1):39–43.
84. Mubarak SJ, Lavernia C, Silva PD. Ice cream truck–related injuries to children. J Pediatr Orthop 1998;18(1):46–48.
85. Mullins, RJ, Brand D, Lenfesty B, et al. Statewide assessment of injury and death rates among riders of off-road vehicles treated at trauma centers. J Am Coll Surg 2007; 204(2):216–224.
86. Nathorst Westfelt JA. Environmental factors in childhood accidents: a prospective study in Göteborg, Sweden. 1982;291:1–75.
87. Ordog GJ, Prakash A, Wasserberger J, et al. Pediatric gunshot wounds. J Trauma 1987; 27(11):1272–1278.
88. Osberg JS, Schneps SC, Di Scala C, et al. Skateboarding: more dangerous than roller skating or inline skating. Arch Pediatr Adolesc Med 1998;152(10):985–991.
89. Parmar P, Letts M, Jarvis J. Injuries caused by water tubing. J Pediatr Orthop 1998; 18(1):49–53.
90. Petridou E, Sibert J, Dedoukou X, et al. Injuries in public and private playgrounds: the relative contribution of structural, equipment, and human factors. Acta Paediatr 2002;91(6):691–697.
91. Phelan KJ, Khoury J, Kalkwarf HJ, et al. Trends and patterns of playground injuries in United States children and adolescents. Ambul Pediatr 2001;1(4):227–233.
92. Pirone AM, Graham HK, Krajbich JI. Management of displaced extension-type supracondylar fractures of the humerus in children. J Bone Joint Surg Am 1988;70(5): 641–650.
93. Powell EC, Tanz RR. Inline skate and rollerskate injuries in childhood. Pediatr Emerg Care 1996;12(4):259–262.
94. Probe R, Lindsey RW, Hadley NA, et al. Refracture of adolescent femoral shaft fractures: a complication of external fixation: a report of two cases. J Pediatr Orthop 1993;13(1): 102–105.
95. Public Health Service. Healthy people 2000: national health promotion and disease prevention objectives. Washington, DC: US Department of Health and Human Services, Public Health Service, 1990; DHHS publication no. (PHS)90-50212.
96. Puranik S, Long J, Coffman S. Profile of pediatric bicycle injuries. South Med J 1998; 91(11):1033–1037.
97. Reed MH. Fractures and dislocations of the extremities in children. J Trauma 1977; 17(5):351–354.
98. Reichelderfer TE, Overbach A, Greensher J. Unsafe playgrounds. Pediatrics 1979;64(6): 962–963.
99. Rivara FP, Bergman AB, LoGerfo JP, et al. Epidemiology of childhood injuries. II. Sex differences in injury rates. Am J Dis Child 1982;136(6):502–506.
100. Rockwood CA, Wilkins KE, King RE, eds. Fractures in children. Philadelphia: JB Lippincott,1984.
101. Rogers GB. Bicycle helmet use patterns among children. Pediatrics 1996;97(2): 166–173.
102. Rohl L. On fractures through the radial condyle of the humerus in children. Acta Chir Scand 1952;104(1):74–80.
103. Rønning R, Rønning I, Gerner T, et al. The efficacy of wrist protectors in preventing snowboarding injuries. Am J Sports Med 2001;29(5):581–585.
104. Routledge DA, Repett-Wright R, Howarth CI. The exposure of young children to accident risk as pedestrians. Ergonomics 1974;17(4):457–480.
105. Schalamon J, Sarkola T, Nietosvaara Y. Injuries in children associated with the use of nonmotorized scooters. J Pediatr Surg 2003;38(11):1612–1615.
106. Scheidt PC, Harel Y, Trumble AC, et al. The epidemiology of nonfatal injuries among US children and youth. Am J Public Health 1995;85(7):932–938.
107. Schelp L. The role of organizations in community participation–prevention of accidental injuries in a rural Swedish municipality. Soc Sci Med 1988;26(11):1087–1093.
108. Schieber RA, Olson SJ. Developing a culture of safety in a reluctant audience. West J Med 2002;176(3):E1–2.
109. Segers MJM, Wink D, Clevers GJ. Bicycle-spoke injuries: a prospective study. Injury 1997;28(4):267–269.
110. Shank LP, Bagg RJ, Wagnon J. Etiology of pediatric fractures: the fatigue factors in children's fractures. Presented at National Conference on Pediatric Trauma, Indianapolis, 1992.
111. Sheehan E, Mulhall KJ, Kearns S, et al. Impact of dedicated skate parks on the severity and incidence of skateboard- and rollerblade-related pediatric fractures. J Pediatr Orthop 2003;23(4):440–442.
112. Sheps SB, Evans GD. Epidemiology of school injuries: a 2-year experience in a municipal health department. Pediatrics 1987;79(1):69–75.
113. Shorter NA, Jensen PE, Harmon BJ, et al. Skiing injuries in children and adolescents. J Trauma 1996;40(6):997–1001.
114. Sieben RL, Leavitt JD, French JH. Falls as childhood accidents: an increasing urban risk. Pediatrics 1971;47(5):886–892.
115. Smith GA. Injuries to children in the United States related to trampolines, 1990–1995: a national epidemic. Pediatrics 1998;101(3 Pt 1):406–412.
116. Smith GA, Shields BJ. Trampoline-related injuries to children. Arch Pediatr Adolesc Med 1998;152(7):694–699.
117. Smith MD, Burrington JD, Woolf AD. Injuries in children sustained in free falls: an analysis of 66 cases. J Trauma 1975;15(11):987–991.
118. Spiegel CN, Lindaman FC. Children can't fly: a program to prevent childhood morbidity and mortality from window falls. Am J Public Health 1977;67(12):1143–1147.
119. Stark AD, Bennet GC, Stone DH, et al. Association between childhood fractures and poverty: population-based study. BMJ 2002;324(7335):457.
120. Steiner C, Elixhauser A, Schnaier J. The healthcare cost and utilization project: an overview. Eff Clin Pract 2002;5(3):143–151.
121. Stucky W, Loder RT. Extremity gunshot wounds in children. J Pediatr Orthop 1991; 11(1):64–71.
122. Tepas JJ 3rd. The national pediatric trauma registry: a legacy of commitment to control of childhood injury. Semin Pediatr Surg 2004;13(2):126–132.
123. Tiderius CJ, Landin L, Duppe H. Decreasing incidence of fractures in children—an epidemiological analysis of 1673 fractures in Malmö, Sweden, 1993–1994. Acta Orthop Scand 1999;70(6):622–626.
124. Topoleski T, et al. Motor vehicle injuries in pediatric trauma patients. Presented at the American Academy of Orthopaedic Surgeons Annual Meeting, Orlando, 1995.
125. Valentine J, Blocker S, Chang JH. Gunshot injuries in children. J Trauma 1984;24(11): 952–956.
126. Verd Vallespir S, Domínguez Sánchez J, González Quintial M, et al. Association between calcium content of drinking water and fractures in children. (Article in Spanish) An Esp Pediatr 1992;37(6):461–465.
127. Walker JL, Rang M. Forearm fractures in children. Cast treatment with elbow extension. J Bone Joint Surg Br 1991;73(2):299–301
128. Waltzman ML, Shannon M, Bowen AP, et al. Monkeybar injuries: complications of play. Pediatrics 1999;103(5):e58.
129. Wareham K, Johansen A, Stone MD, et al. Seasonal variation in the incidence of wrist and forearm fractures, and its consequences. Injury 2003;34(3):219–222.
130. Washington ER, Lee WA, Ross WA Jr. Gunshot wounds to the extremities in children and adolescents. Orthop Clin North Am 1995;26(1):19–28.
131. Weiss BD. Bicycle-related head injuries. Clin Sports Med 1994;13(1):99–112.
132. Werner P. Playground injuries and voluntary product standards for home and public playgrounds. Pediatrics 1982;69(1):18–20.
133. Wong PCN. A comparative epidemiologic study of fractures among Indian, Malay, and Swedish children. Med J Malaya 1965;20(2):132–143.
134. Worlock P, Stower M. Fracture patterns in Nottingham children. J Peditr Orthop 1986; 6(6):656–660.
135. Wyshak G, Frisch RE. Carbonated beverages, dietary calcium, the dietary calcium/phosphorus ratio, and bone fractures in girls and boys. J Adolesc Health 1994;15(3): 210–215.

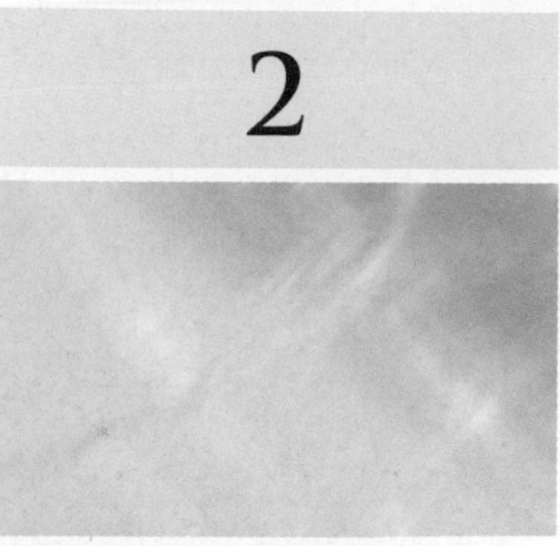

THE BIOLOGIC ASPECTS OF CHILDREN'S FRACTURES

Cory J. Xian and Bruce K. Foster

THE IMMATURE SKELETON 18

ANATOMIC REGIONS OF THE CHILD'S BONE 19
- Epiphysis 19
- Physis 20
- Metaphysis 21
- Diaphysis 24
- Periosteum 24
- Apophysis 26

THE MOLECULAR BONE 26
- Molecules of the Cartilage and Bone Matrices 26

MECHANISMS OF BONE GROWTH 31
- Endochondral Ossification 31
- Regulatory Mechanisms in the Physis 32
- Membranous Ossification 34
- Remodeling of Bones 34

FRACTURE REPAIR 35
- Osseous Healing 35
- Cellular Response to Trauma 35
- Physeal Healing Patterns 38
- Remodeling of Bones in Children After Injury 40

THE FUTURE OF FRACTURE REPAIR 40
- Growth Factor Therapy 40
- Tissue Engineering, Stem Cell and Gene Therapies 41
- Regeneration of Injured Physeal Cartilage 41

THE IMMATURE SKELETON

Compared with the relatively static, mature bone of adults, the changing structure and function, both physiologic and biomechanical, of immature bones make them susceptible to different patterns of failure. Even the types of fracture patterns within a given bone demonstrate temporal (chronobiologic) variations that may be correlated with progressive anatomic changes affecting the epiphysis, physis, metaphysis, and diaphysis at macroscopic and microscopic levels.

Skeletal trauma accounts for 10% to 15% of all childhood injuries.[66,141,142,144] Fractures of the immature skeleton differ from those of the mature skeleton.[9,141,142] Fractures in children are more common and are more likely to occur after seemingly insignificant trauma. Physeal disruptions make up about 15% of all skeletal injuries in children.[126,141,142,144,150,182] Damage involving specific growth regions, such as the physis or epiphyseal ossification center, may lead to acute or chronic growth disturbances.[140,141,194,221] The physis is constantly changing, both with active longitudinal and latitudinal (diametric) growth and in mechanical relation to other components. Physeal fracture patterns vary with the extent of chondro-osseous maturation. Salter-Harris type I injuries are common in infants, and types II, III, and IV become more common as the secondary ossification center enlarges and physeal undulations develop. Although joint injuries, dislocations, and ligamentous disruptions are much less common in children, it is more likely that one of the contiguous physes will be damaged. Changing trabecular and cortical structures affect metaphyseal and diaphyseal fracture patterns, and the variable size of the secondary ossification center affects susceptibility to physeal and epiphyseal injuries.

Due to increased research into the injury/healing responses in fractures and strategies for enhancing bone and physis repair in children, the treatment options available for skeletal injuries in children are expanding. Most notable is the introduction of growth factors, such as the bone morphogenic proteins (BMPs), for the induction of bone formation in nonunions and large segmental bone defects, and for the repair of cartilage defects,[78] and the research and development of stem-cell–based therapy for bone and cartilage regeneration[157] and physeal repair.[31,81,101] Due to these new developments, it has become necessary for the orthopaedic surgeon to understand the biological aspects of the skeletal injury responses and new treatment options for fracture repair. This chapter covers the basic biology and regulation of bone growth, bone fracture repair responses, physeal injury and physeal bar formation, roles of growth factors and cytokines in regulating injury/repair responses, and future therapeutic strategies for bone/articular cartilage/physis regeneration using growth factors, tissue engineering, stem cells, and gene therapy.

ANATOMIC REGIONS OF THE CHILD'S BONE

The major long bones of children can be divided into four distinct, anatomic areas: the epiphysis, physis, metaphysis, and diaphysis.[95] Each region is prone to certain patterns of injury, and the intrinsic injury susceptibility varies with physiologic and biomechanical changes during postnatal development. The four regions originate and become modified as a result of the basic endochondral ossification process. Subsequently, they are supplemented by membranous bone formation along the metaphyseal and diaphyseal shafts. Finally, the regions are remodeled to create mature cortical and trabecular bone.

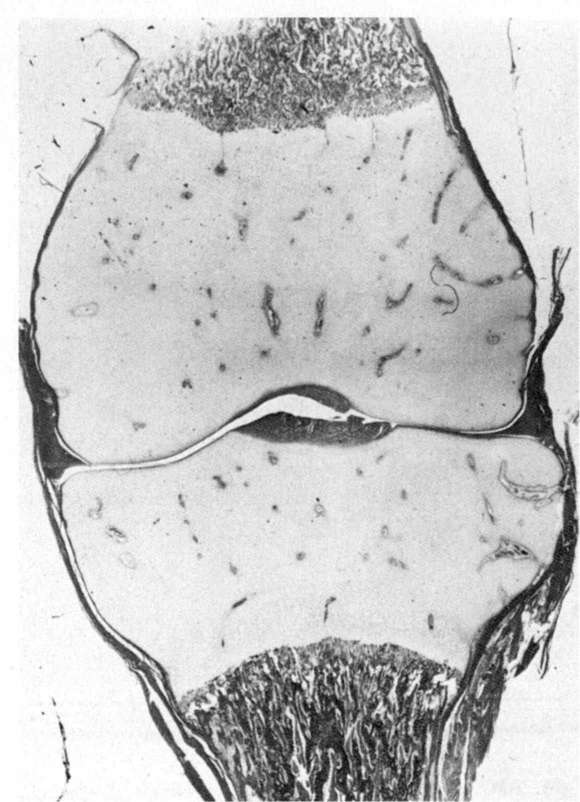

FIGURE 2-1 Chondroepiphyses of the distal femur and proximal tibia. These structures have an extensively developed vascular system (cartilage canals) before secondary ossification.

Epiphysis

At birth, each epiphysis (except the distal femur) consists of a completely cartilaginous structure at the end of each long bone (Fig. 2-1), the chondroepiphysis. At a time characteristic for each of these chondroepiphyses, a secondary center of ossification forms and gradually enlarges until the cartilaginous area has been almost completely replaced by bone at skeletal maturity. This chondro-osseous transformation is vascular-dependent (Fig. 2-2). Only articular cartilage remains at maturity.

As the ossification center expands, it undergoes structural modifications. The region adjacent to the physis forms a distinct subchondral plate parallel to the metaphysis, creating the radiographically characteristic lucent physeal line. The appearance of the ossification centers differ in certain chondroepiphyses, a factor that must be considered when diagnosing fractures of these regions. The ossification center imparts increasing rigidity to the more resilient epiphyseal cartilage as the secondary osseous tissue expands.[203]

The external surface of an epiphysis is composed of either articular cartilage or perichondrium (Fig. 2-3). Muscle fibers, tendons, and ligaments may attach directly to the perichondrium, which is densely contiguous with the underlying hyaline cartilage. The perichondrium contributes to the continued centrifugal enlargement of the epiphysis. It also blends imperceptibly into the periosteum. This perichondrial/periosteal tissue continuity contributes to the biomechanical strength of the epiphyseal/metaphyseal junction at the zone of Ranvier.

When the hyaline cartilage of the chondroepiphysis first forms, there are no easily demonstrable histologic differences between the cells of the joint surface and the rest of the epiphyseal cartilage. However, at some point, a finite cell population becomes stabilized and physiologically different from the remaining epiphyseal cartilage. McKibbin[120] established that these two cartilage types are different physiologically and biochemically. If a contiguous core of articular and hyaline cartilage is removed, turned 180°, and reinserted, the transposed hyaline cartilage eventually will form bone at the joint surface, whereas the transposed articular cartilage remains cartilaginous and becomes surrounded by the enlarging secondary ossification center. Normally, articular cartilage does not appear capable of

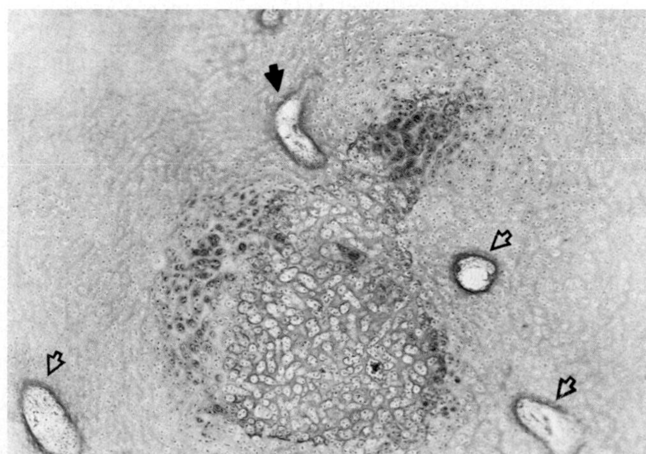

FIGURE 2-2 Early formation of the secondary ossification center within the epiphyseal cartilage. This usually occurs in a region well vascularized by cartilage canals (*open arrows*). One of the canals sends a branch into the hypertrophic cells (*solid arrow*), triggering the ossification process.

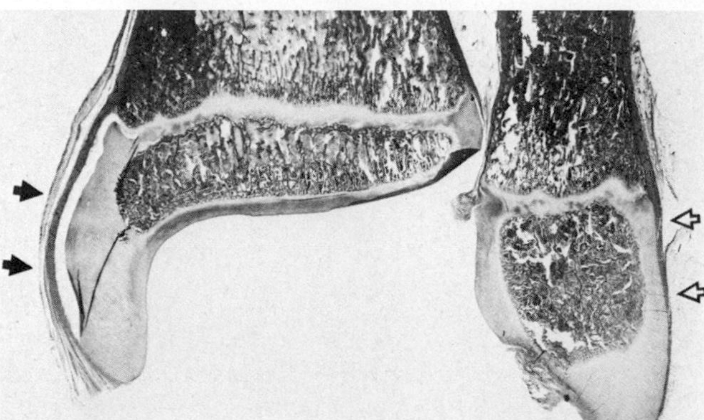

FIGURE 2-3 As the epiphysis matures, the ossification center expands and progressively follows the contours of the chondroepiphysis. The epiphyseal surface is either articular cartilage or perichondrium along the outer surfaces, as in the medial (*solid arrows*) and lateral (*open arrows*) malleoli.

calcification and ossification. As skeletal maturity is reached, a tide mark progressively develops as a demarcation between the articular and calcified epiphyseal hyaline cartilage.

An important aspect of McKibbin's experiment was an explanation of nonunion of certain fractures in which the fragment may be rotated, causing the articular surface to lie against metaphyseal and epiphyseal bone. Union is unlikely in such a situation because the articular surface is incapable of a reparative osteogenic response, an essential component of bone healing.

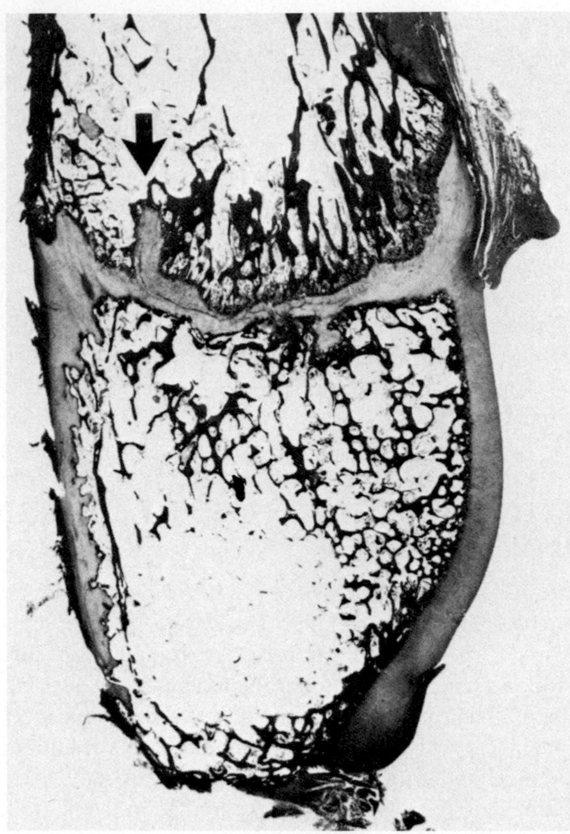

FIGURE 2-4 Distal fibula, showing the variably undulated physis, including a mammillary process (*arrow*). The physeal and epiphyseal cartilage turns proximally at the medial region (lappet formation) to participate in the formation of the distal tibiofibular articulation. Note the difference in the subarticular subchondral bone, which has formed a thick plate, compared with the thin, outer subchondral bone.

Physis

The growth plate, or physis, is the essential structure adding bone through endochondral ossification.[139,143,148,194] The primary function of the physis is rapid, integrated longitudinal and latitudinal growth. Injuries to this component are unique to skeletally immature patients.

Because the physeal cartilage remains radiolucent, except for the final stages of physiologic epiphysiodesis, its exact location must be inferred from the metaphyseal contour, which follows the physeal contour. The changing size of the secondary ossification center more effectively demarcates the physeal contour on the epiphyseal (germinal layer) side. As this center of ossification enlarges centrifugally to approach the physis, the original spherical shape of the ossification center flattens and gradually develops a contour paralleling the metaphyseal contour. Similar contouring also occurs as the ossification center approaches the lateral and subarticular regions of the epiphysis (Fig. 2-4). The region of the ossification center juxtaposed to the physis forms a discrete subchondral bone plate that the essential epiphyseal blood vessels must penetrate to reach the physeal germinal zone (Fig. 2-5). Damage to this osseous plate in a fracture may cause localized physeal ischemia.

If a segment of the epiphyseal vasculature is compromised, whether temporarily or permanently, the zones of cellular growth associated with these particular vessels cannot undergo appropriate cell division. In contrast, unaffected regions of the physis continue longitudinal and latitudinal growth, leaving the affected region behind (Figs. 2-6 and 2-7). The growth rates of the cells directly adjacent to the affected area are more mechanically compromised than cellular areas farther away. The differential rather than uniform growth results in an angular or longitudinal growth deformity, or both.[24,150]

Interruption of the metaphyseal circulation has no effect on chondrogenesis within the germinal zone or the sequential cartilage maturation within the hypertrophic zone of the physis (see

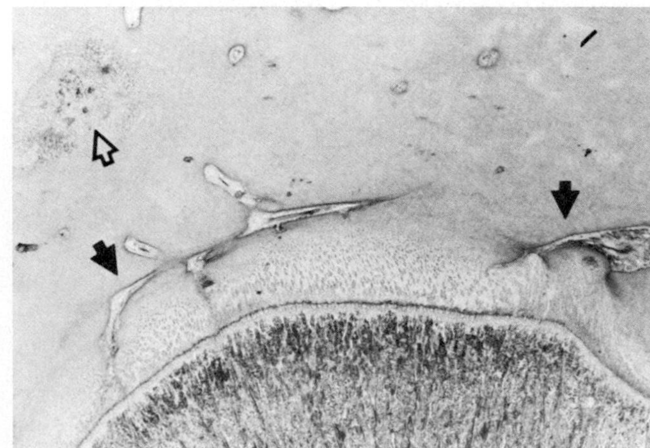

FIGURE 2-5 Epiphyseal circulation (*solid arrows*) in a toddler. These supply the germinal/dividing zones of the physis. The open arrow indicates the early ossification center. As this area enlarges, it will incorporate the epiphyseal vessels.

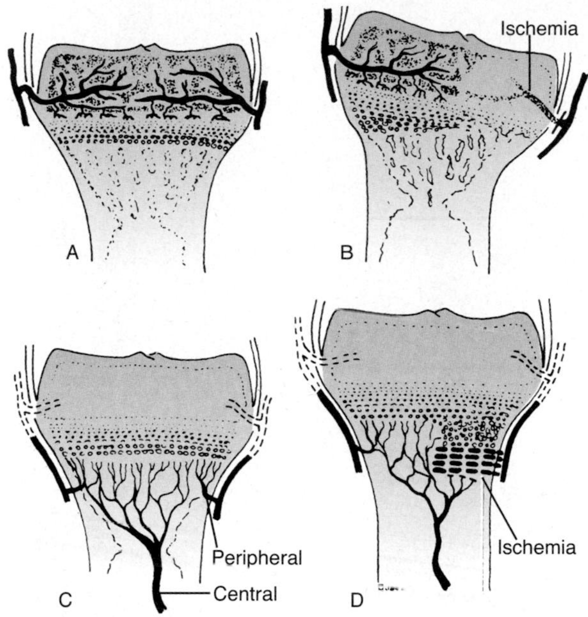

FIGURE 2-6 Patterns of response to ischemia of the epiphyseal **(A,B)** versus metaphyseal **(C,D)** circulatory systems. Metaphyseal ischemia is usually transient; epiphyseal ischemia is usually severe and permanent.

Fig. 2-6). However, the subsequent transformation of cartilage to bone (primary spongiosa) is blocked. This causes widening of the affected area, because more cartilage is added to the cell columns but none is replaced by invasive metaphyseal vessels and bone. Once the disrupted metaphyseal circulation is reestablished, this widened, calcified region of the physis is rapidly penetrated and ossified, returning the physis to its normal width. This is the mechanism seen in physeal and metaphyseal fractures. The metaphyseal blood supply is temporarily blocked by separation or impaction and requires 3 to 4 weeks for restoration. If the circulatory compromise has been caused by a metaphyseal fracture, there also may be a temporary halt to bone formation in the transiently ischemic portion of the metaphysis. This leads to an apparent sclerosis when the bone is compared with the adjacent vascularized metaphysis, which undergoes a relative disuse osteoporosis. Compromise of the metaphyseal circulation has minimal, if any, effect on physeal development, particularly when compared with the major detrimental effects of epiphyseal circulatory compromise.

The effects of physeal ischemia have been studied extensively by Trueta and coworkers.[209–212] Disrupting the epiphyseal circulation leads to either partial or complete cessation of growth. The central region seems more sensitive to ischemia than the periphery, which may have a variable capacity to recover through continued latitudinal growth.[128,138] Ischemic compromise leads to different rates of growth across the affected physis and significant changes in physeal contour.[19] Some changes may be caused by venous stasis rather than arterial damage.[86]

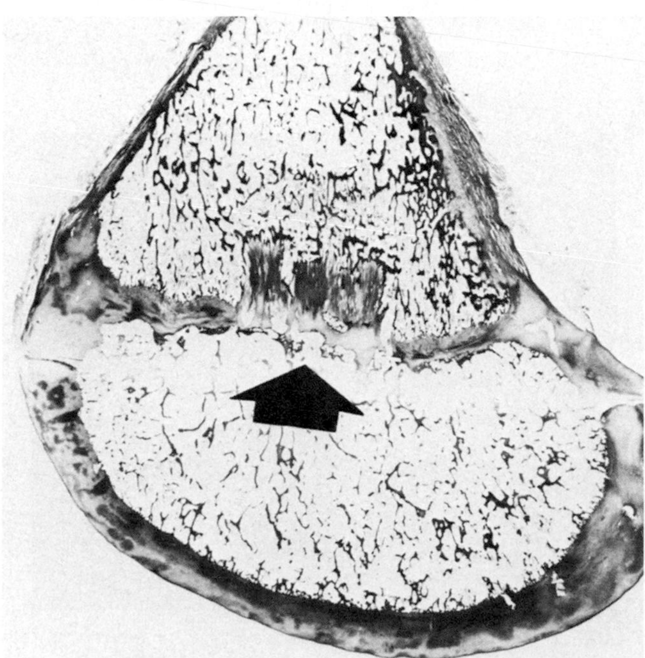

FIGURE 2-7 Histologic section showing an area of central ischemic growth arrest (*arrow*). The infarcted area of cartilage is left behind as the rest of the physis continues longitudinal growth.

Metaphysis

The metaphysis is a variably contoured flare at each end of the diaphysis. Its major characteristics are decreased thickness of the cortical bone and increased trabecular bone in the secondary spongiosa. Extensive endochondral modeling centrally and peripherally initially forms the primary spongiosa, which then is remodeled into the more mature secondary spongiosa, a process that involves osteoclastic and osteoblastic activity. Therefore, the metaphyses exhibit considerable bone turnover compared with other regions of the bone, and this factor is responsible for the increased uptake of radionuclides in technetium 99m bone scans.[80]

The metaphyseal cortex also changes with time. Compared with the confluent diaphysis, the metaphyseal cortex is thinner and is more porous (trabecular fenestration; Fig. 2-8). These cortical fenestrations contain fibrovascular soft-tissue elements that connect the metaphyseal marrow spaces with the subperiosteal region. The metaphyseal cortex exhibits greater fenestration near the physis than in the diaphysis, with which it gradually blends as an increasingly thicker, dense bone (Fig. 2-9). As longitudinal growth continues, cortical fenestration becomes a less dominant feature, and the overall width of the cortex increases, creating a greater morphologic transition between the juxtaphyseal and juxtadiaphyseal cortices. The metaphyseal region does not develop extensive secondary and tertiary Haversian systems until the late stages of skeletal maturation. These microscopic anatomic changes appear to be directly correlated with changing fracture patterns and are the reason why torus (buckle) fractures are more likely to occur than complete metaphyseal or epiphyseal/physeal fractures.

Another microscopic anatomic variation in the metaphysis occurs at the junction of the primary spongiosa and the hypertrophic region of the physis. In most rapidly growing bones, the trabeculae tend to be longitudinally oriented. However, in shorter growing bones, such as the metacarpals and phalanges,

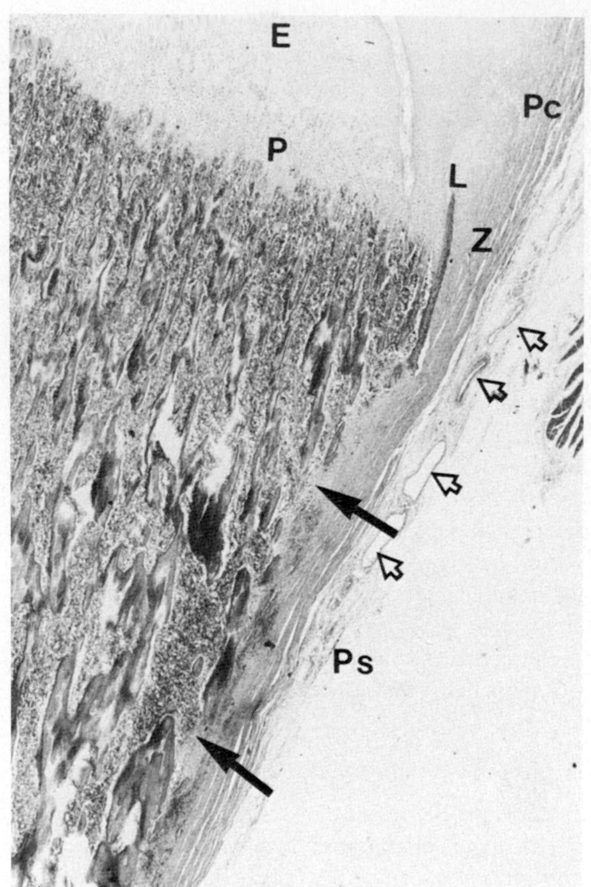

FIGURE 2-8 Cortical fenestration (*solid arrows*) of a metaphysis. Note the interdigitation of periosteal (Ps) tissue with the fenestrations. The periosteum blends into the perichondrium (Pc). Extensive vascularity is often present in this region (*open arrows*). (E, epiphysis; P, physis; Z, zone of Ranvier; L, ring of Lacroix.)

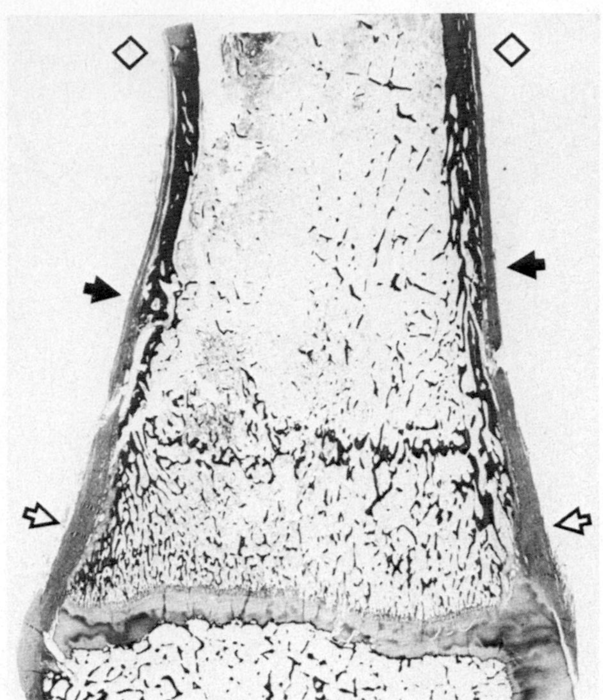

FIGURE 2-9 Section of distal tibia showing the transition (*solid arrows*) of cortical bone from the dense, remodeled diaphysis (diamonds) to the fenestrated metaphysis (*open arrows*). Note the progressive change from a relatively thin periosteum over the diaphysis to a much thicker one at the metaphysis.

trabecular formation is predominantly horizontal. As growth decelerates in adolescence, a similar horizontal orientation may be seen in the major long bones. These variations in trabecular orientation affect the responsiveness of metaphyseal and physeal regions to abnormal stress and predispose to certain fracture modes.

Although the periosteum is attached relatively loosely to the diaphysis, it is firmly fixed to the metaphysis because of the increasingly complex continuity of fibrous tissue through the metaphyseal fenestrations. Such intermingling of endosteal and interosseous fibrous tissues with the periosteal tissue imparts additional biomechanical strength to the region.[198] The periosteum subsequently attaches densely into the peripheral physis, blending into the zone of Ranvier as well as the epiphyseal perichondrium. The fenestrated metaphyseal cortex extends to the physis as the thin osseous ring of Lacroix.

The metaphysis is the site of extensive osseous modeling and remodeling, both peripherally and centrally (Fig. 2-10). The metaphyseal cortex is fenestrated, modified trabecular bone on which the periosteum deposits membranous bone to thicken the cortex progressively. Similar endosteal bone formation occurs. As this metaphyseal region thickens, the trabecular bone is progressively invaded by diaphyseal osteon systems, not unlike osteons traversing the fracture site in primary bone healing. This converts peripheral trabecular (woven or fiber) bone to lamellar (osteonal) bone, which has different biomechanical capacities, and thus progressively transforms metaphyseal cortex into diaphyseal cortex as longitudinal growth continues. A torus (buckle) fracture is most likely to occur in a metaphyseal region with a trabecular, fenestrated, compressible cortex.

As in the diaphysis, there are no significant direct muscle attachments to the metaphyseal bone. Instead, muscle fibers

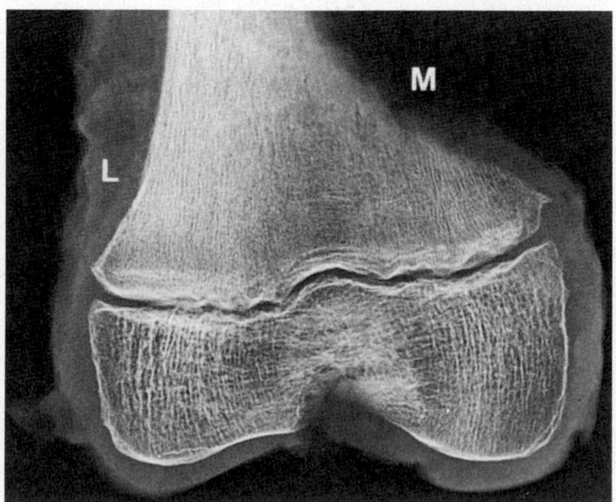

FIGURE 2-10 Extensive modeling and remodeling of the medial (M) versus the lateral (L) cortex of the distal femur may create irregularities that have been misinterpreted as fracture, stress fracture, infection, and tumor. Note the well-formed subchondral bone at the periphery of the epiphyseal ossification center.

primarily blend into the periosteum. The medial distal femoral attachment of the adductor muscles is a significant exception. Because of extensive remodeling and insertion of muscle and tendon in this area, the bone often appears irregular and may be misinterpreted as showing chronic trauma (i.e., a stress fracture), infection, or a tumor.

Transverse Lines of Park and Harris

Many bones exhibit transversely oriented, dense trabecular linear bone patterns within the metaphysis. These lines usually duplicate the contiguous physeal contour. They may appear after trauma, particularly when the child has been immobilized in bed (e.g., traction for femoral fracture), and they also may appear after generalized illnesses or even localized processes within the bone (e.g., osteomyelitis).[1,67,160,161] The lines result from a temporary slowdown of normal longitudinal growth after injury or illness, and they often are called Harris or Park growth slowdown or arrest lines (Fig. 2-11). Because of the slowdown, the trabeculae of the primary spongiosa become more transversely than longitudinally oriented, creating a temporary thickening in the primary spongiosa adjacent to the physis. Once the normal longitudinal growth rate resumes, longitudinal trabecular orientation is restored. The thickened, transversely oriented osseous plate is left behind, and will be gradually remodeled as primary spongiosa becomes secondary spongiosa.

Usually, transverse lines are distributed relatively symmetrically throughout the skeleton and occupy identical sites in the corresponding bones on the two sides of the body. They are thickest in metaphyses that grow most rapidly, such as the distal femur and proximal tibia, as more primary spongiosa bone is formed in a transverse orientation in these growing regions.[140] In the metaphyses with slowest growth, they may not form at all, or they are exceedingly thin and lie at the very end of the shaft, directly under the provisional zone of calcification. These transverse lines parallel the contours of the physeal provisional zone of calcification. When several transverse lines are present, they tend to be parallel. The lines nearest the end of the shaft ordinarily are the thickest and widest, whereas lines away from the physes tend to be thinner and less distinct and are usually broken and irregular. As remodeling occurs, with migration of the epiphysis away from this region, and with conversion of primary spongiosa to secondary spongiosa, there is a gradual breakup of this transverse trabecular orientation. As they eventually become part of the elongating diaphysis, they disappear completely with endosteal remodeling.

Although the more rapidly growing bones are associated with longitudinally oriented trabeculae in the juxtaphyseal region, slower growing bones, particularly the proximal radius, metacarpals, metatarsals, and phalanges, normally have a greater amount of transversely oriented primary spongiosa,[145] making transverse septa a normal finding. These particular bones do not have a sufficient difference in the orientation of trabeculae to manifest transverse lines on radiographs.

In response to administration of bisphosphonate treatment in children with osteogenesis imperfecta, there are some distinct metaphyseal bands in the growing skeleton, which may vary in spacing according to the regimens of treatment, age of the patient, rate of growth, and the location of the metaphysis. The bands may reflect decreased osteoclastic activity occurring in response to drug administration, and the spacing between the bands indicates resumption of osteoclastic activity and linear growth of the bone between treatments. As with growth arrest lines, the migration of these treatment bands varies with the rate of the bone growth of the patient and the particular physis.[62]

Useful to Assess Growth After Injury. These biologic marker lines are important in analyzing the effects of a fracture on growth. They can be measured and the sides compared to corroborate femoral overgrowth after diaphyseal fracture and eccentric overgrowth medially after proximal tibial metaphyseal frac-

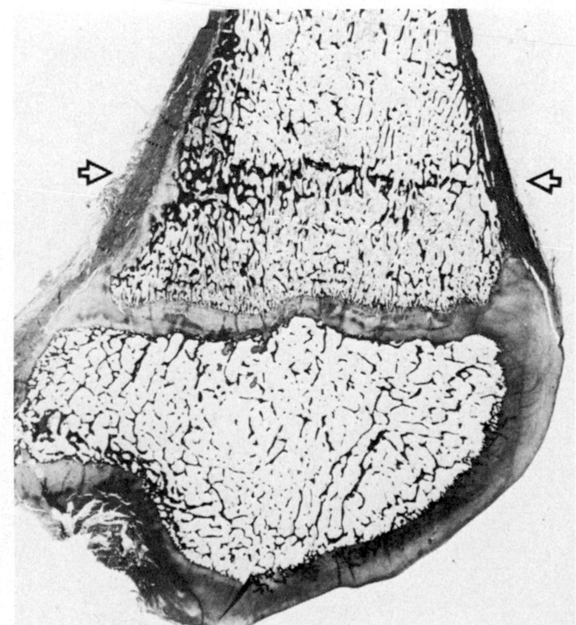
A

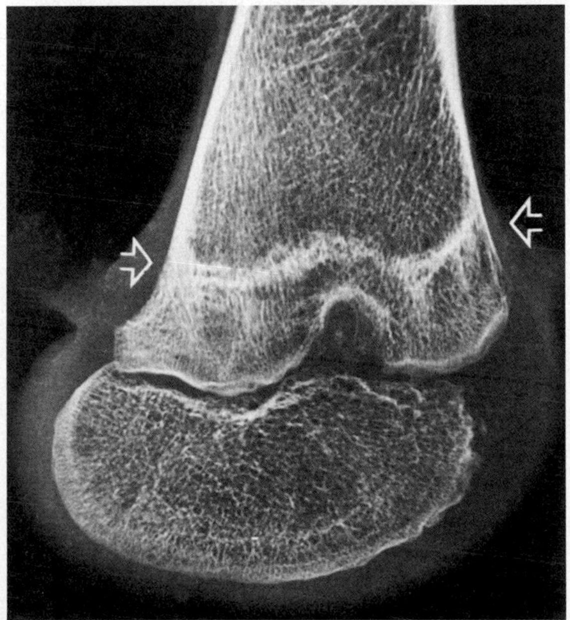
B

FIGURE 2-11 Histologic section **(A)** and x-ray study **(B)** of a distal femur showing a typical Harris line (*arrows*). This formed during an acute illness and chemotherapy for leukemia. The child then resumed a more normal pattern of growth until her death from leukemia about 14 months later.

ture. A line that converges toward a physis suggests localized growth damage that may result in an osseous bridge and the risk of angular deformity.

Diaphysis

The diaphysis constitutes the major portion of each long bone. It is principally a product of periosteal, membranous osseous tissue apposition on the original endochondral model. This leads to the gradual replacement of the endochondrally derived primary ossification center and primary spongiosa; the latter is replaced by secondary spongiosa in the metaphyseal region. At birth, the diaphysis is composed of laminar (fetal, woven) bone that characteristically lacks Haversian systems. The neonatal femoral diaphysis appears to be the only area exhibiting any significant change from this fetal osseous state to a more mature bone with osteon systems (lamellar bone) before birth (Fig. 2-12).

Periosteum-mediated, membranous, appositional bone formation with concomitant endosteal remodeling leads to enlargement of the overall diameter of the shaft, variably increased width of the diaphyseal cortices, and formation of the marrow cavity. Mature, lamellar bone with intrinsic but constantly remodeling osteonal patterns progressively becomes the dominant feature (Fig. 2-13).

The developing diaphyseal bone in a neonate or young child is extremely vascular. When analyzed in cross section, it appears much less dense than the maturing bone of older children, adolescents, and adults. Subsequent growth leads to increased complexity of the Haversian (osteonal) systems and the formation of increasing amounts of extracellular matrix, causing a relative decrease in cross-sectional porosity and an increase in hardness, factors that constantly change the child's susceptibility to different fracture patterns. Certain bones, especially the tibia, exhibit a significant decrease in vascularity as the bone matures; this factor affects the rate of healing and risk of nonunion.

The vascularity of the developing skeleton constantly changes. In experimental studies, significant chronobiologic changes in flow patterns were found in the developing canine tibia and femur.[102–104,121,187,188,222] In particular, there was a dramatic decrease in tibial circulation with increasing skeletal maturation.[188] This also occurs in humans, which helps to explain the increasing delay in fracture healing and the increased incidence of nonunion of the tibia in adolescents and adults. A poor vascular response could impair the early, crucial stages of callus formation.

Other researchers have suggested that adequate vascularity was a major factor in fracture healing,[107,177,178,213,221,227] but they did not consider chronobiologic changes in blood flow patterns.

Periosteum

A child's periosteum is thicker, is more readily elevated from the diaphyseal and metaphyseal bone, and exhibits greater os-

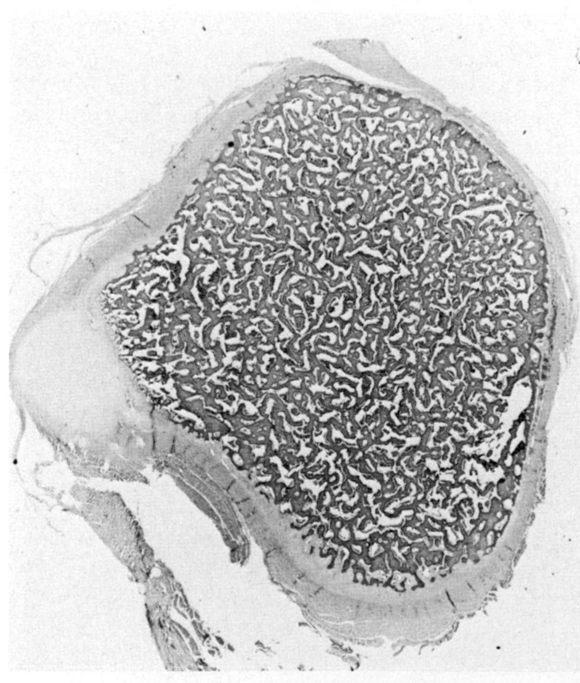

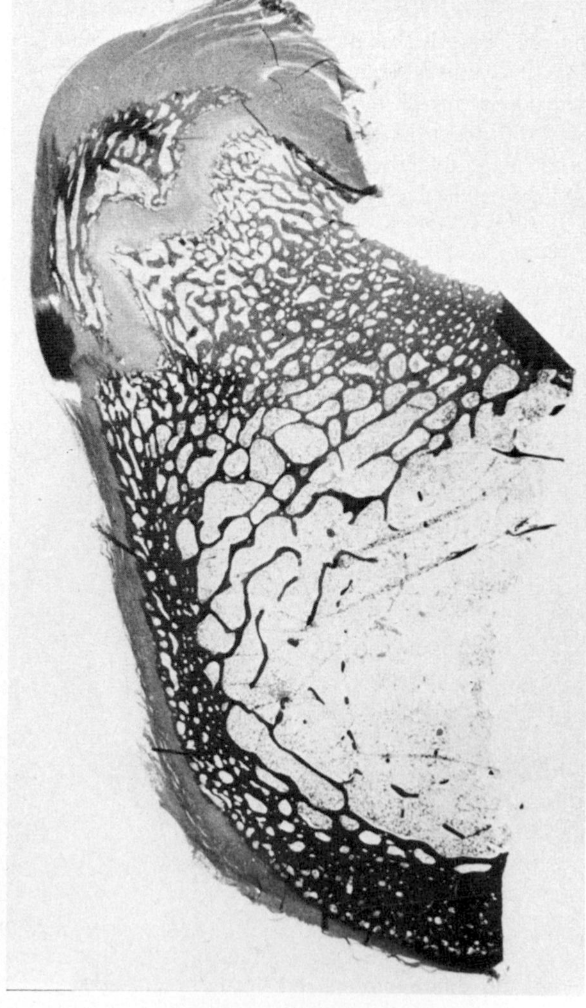

FIGURE 2-12 Sections of the femur at the level of the lesser trochanter at birth **(A)** and age 7 years **(B)**. At birth, some cortical thickening and osteon remodeling is evident laterally; the rest of the cortex is irregular. By age 7 years, extensive thickening and remodeling of the cortex has taken place.

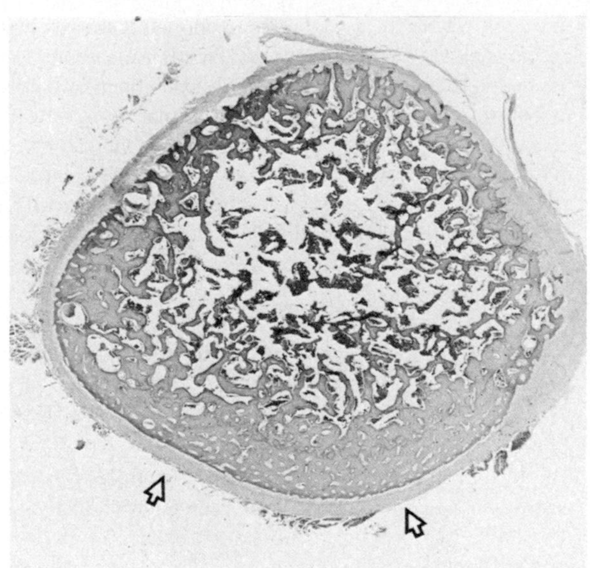

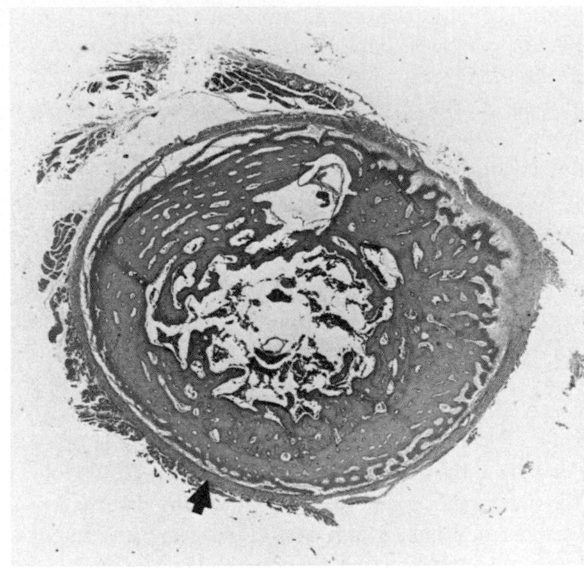

FIGURE 2-13 Transverse sections of the tibial diaphysis in a neonate **(A)** and at age 2 years **(B)**. A thick periosteum is evident in **(A)** (*open arrows*), in association with a rapidly forming anterior cortex. At age 2 years, new subperiosteal (membranous) bone is being added to the cortex (*solid arrow*).

teogenic potential than that of an adult.[139] The periosteum is loosely attached to much of the shaft of the bone, but it attaches densely into the physeal periphery (the zone of Ranvier; Fig. 2-14) through intricate collagen meshwork, thereby playing a role in fracture mechanics and treatment of growth mechanism injuries.[198] The thicker, stronger, more biologically active periosteum affects fracture displacement, reduction, and the rate of subperiosteal callus formation. It also may serve as an effective internal restraint in closed reductions.

Because of its contiguity with the underlying bone, the periosteum is usually injured to some extent in all fractures in children. However, because the periosteum more easily separates from the bone in children, there is much less likelihood of complete circumferential rupture. A significant portion of the periosteum usually remains intact on the concave (compression) side of an injury. This intact periosteal hinge or sleeve may lessen the extent of displacement of the fracture fragments, and it also can be used to assist in the reduction, because the intact portion contributes to the intrinsic stability. Because the periosteum allows some tissue continuity across the fracture, the subperiosteal new bone that forms quickly bridges the fracture gap and leads to more rapid long-term stability. The periosteum may be specifically damaged, with or without concomitant injury to the contiguous bone. Such avulsion injuries may lead to the formation of ectopic bone.[147] In contrast, severe disruption of the periosteum, as in an open injury, may impair the fracture healing response. Complete loss of a bone segment, with the periosteal sleeve reasonably intact, may be followed by complete reformation of the missing bone.[15]

Histologically, periosteum comprises two tissue layers. While the outer fibroblast layer provides fibrous attachment to subcutaneous connective tissue, muscles, tendons, and ligaments, the inner cambium layer contains a pool of undifferentiated mesenchymal cells that support bone formation and repair.[193] During embryonic and postnatal bone growth, mesenchymal osteoprogenitor cells at the inner layer differentiate directly into bone-forming cells (osteoblasts) and form

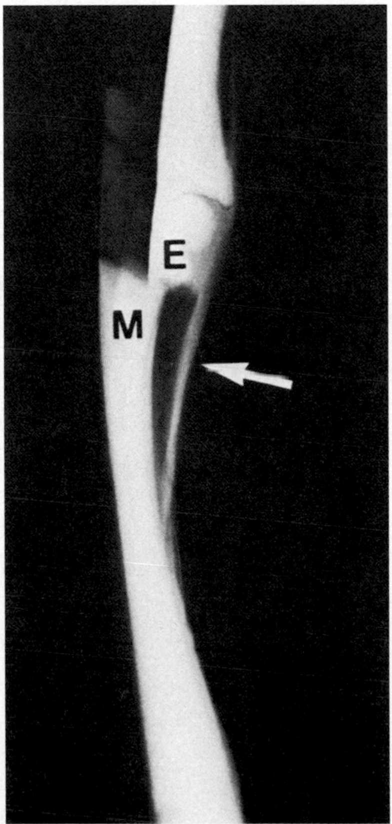

FIGURE 2-14 Simulated type 1 epiphyseal (E) displacement from the metaphysis (M). Note the thick periosteum (*arrow*) and its contiguity with the cartilage of the epiphysis (radiopaque here because of the cartilage and air contrast). In the body, however, the similar soft-tissue radiodensities of cartilage, ligament, muscle, and so forth blend together, making them radiolucent.

periosteal bone collar by the intramembranous method.[164] Formation of new periosteal bone keeps pace with formation of new endochondral bone. During fracture healing, the mesenchymal cells at the cambium layer undergo both intramembranous ossification and chondrogenic differentiation with subsequent endochondral ossification.[170] Due to the osteochondrogenic potential of these cells from the inner periosteal layer, there has been a lot of interest surrounding the use periosteum as graft tissues or as sources of osteochondroprogenitor cells for repairing cartilage/bone defects or for tissue engineering.[130,134,136,199,226]

The periosteum, rather than the bone itself, serves as the origin for most muscle fibers along the metaphysis and diaphysis. This mechanism allows coordinated growth of bone and muscle units; this would be impossible if all the muscle tissue attached directly to the developing bone or cartilage. Exceptions include the attachment of muscle fibers near the linea aspera and into the medial distal femoral metaphysis. The latter pattern of direct metaphyseal osseous attachment may be associated with significant irregularity of cortical and trabecular bone. Radiographs of this area often are misinterpreted as showing a neoplastic, osteomyelitic, or traumatic response, even though they exhibit only a variation of skeletal development.

Apophysis

Because of the differing histologic composition of the tibial tuberosity (fibrocartilage instead of columnar cartilage; Fig. 2-15), failure patterns differ from those in other physes. This area develops primarily as a tensile-responsive structure (i.e., an apophysis). However, the introduction of an osseous secondary ossification center, initially in the distal tuberosity, interposes osseous tissue, which tends to fail in tension and thus may lead to avulsion of part of this ossification center (Fig. 2-16). Healing of the displaced fragment to the underlying undisplaced secondary center creates the symptomatic reactive overgrowth known as an Osgood-Schlatter lesion.[146,151] Similarly, in adolescents, excessive tensile stress may avulse the entire tuberosity during the late stages of closure.[152]

THE MOLECULAR BONE

Molecules of the Cartilage and Bone Matrices

The Cartilage Matrix

The cartilage matrix is synthesized by chondrocytes. The main constituents of the cartilaginous matrix are collagens (mainly type II) and proteoglycans. Although collagen type II provides structural strength, the proteoglycans have structural and regulatory effects. The structural effects of proteoglycans arise through binding to the collagen components and the water-binding properties that provide resilience to compression. Regulatory effects include growth factor interactions, cell-matrix interactions, and regulation of collagen fibril size. Specific molecules expressed and their functions are listed in Table 2-1.

The Bone Matrix

Except for a small percentage of molecules from the circulation and preexistent matrices that may become entrapped, the bone

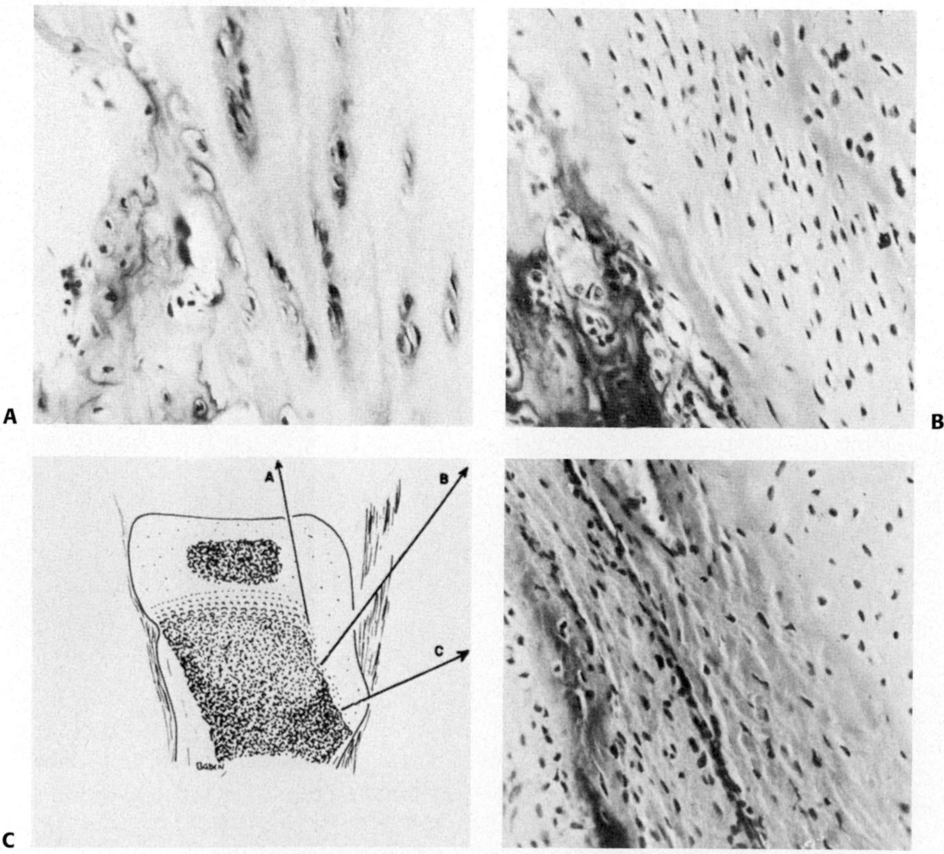

FIGURE 2-15 Histology of a typical apophysis, the tibial tuberosity (tubercle). **A.** Attenuated columnar cartilage adjacent to the main proximal tibial physis. **B.** Fibrocartilage and minimal hypertrophic matrix in the mid-tuberosity region. **C.** Fibrocartilage and membranous ossification in the distal end of the tuberosity.

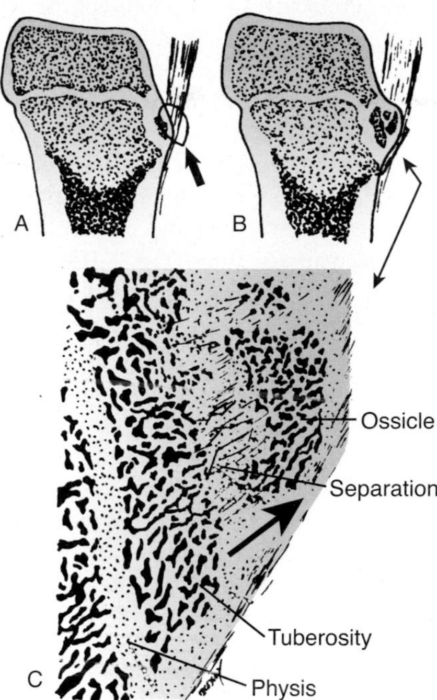

FIGURE 2-16 Avulsion (tension) failure of the developing ossification center of an apophysis. The degree of displacement determines the likelihood of healing and the symptoms and size of the final lump, typical of an Osgood-Schlatter injury.

matrix is almost entirely synthesized by osteoblasts. The composition of the bone matrix was outlined by Buckwalter and associates.[20] Briefly, bone matrix is a composite material composed of an inorganic (mineral) portion and an organic portion. The composite structure provides physical strength and resilience to fracture. Bone with deficient inorganic mineral content is pliable, and bone with deficient organic content is brittle.

The composition of living bone is 60% to 70% inorganic components, 5% to 8% water, and the remainder 22% to 35% is organic.[83] The inorganic portion is mainly hydroxyapatite, with some carbonate and acid phosphate groups. It has also been suggested that bone crystals do not contain hydroxyl groups and should be termed apatite rather than hydroxyapatite.[20] The organic portion is composed of collagen type I (90%) and noncollagenous proteins. The noncollagenous protein portion includes a number of proteins and proteoglycans that perform structural and regulatory functions. Actual molecules and functions are outlined in Table 2-2 and in the following section.

Matrix Constituents

Although it is not a complete list, the following provides an example of the major proteins found within bone and cartilage matrices.

Collagens. Collagens are a family of proteins coded by at least 19 distinct genes. Members are expressed in most tissues. Collagens have a triple helical region that arises from the repeated winding of three collagen molecules around a common axis. Collagens are synthesized as propeptides that are often glycosylated. Collagen is secreted from cells and is processed in the extracellular space. The processed collagen forms into subunits that then undergo fibrillogenesis (Fig. 2-17). The fact that the final fiber is composed of many individual molecules accounts for the dominant negative mutations that can be observed within the collagen family.[79] The incorporation of individual molecules containing mutations that affect the packing of the peptides into the triple helix can disturb the structure of the whole fiber. The molecular structures that arise are in the form of fibrils or netlike structures. In reality, the multimeric fibers observed in vivo are often composed of a number of different collagens.[8]

Collagen type I is the main collagen found in bone and other tissues. It is composed of two $\alpha 1$(I) and one $\alpha 2$(I) polypeptides.

TABLE 2-1 Matrix Molecules of Cartilage

Component	Site of Expression Within Physis and Proposed Functions	
Collagens		
Collagen II (fibril)	Predominate collagen of all cartilage; physeal proliferative zone	Imparts strength, site of initial mineralization[129,167,184]
Collagen IX	Proliferative zone of the physis	Associates with the surface of the collagen II fibril[87]
Collagen X (short chain collagen)	Hypertrophic cartilage	Mineralization[59,88,184]
Collagen XI (fibril)	Proliferative and hypertrophic zone of the physis	Collagen fibril size[184]
Proteoglycans		
Aggrecan	Throughout cartilage	Imparts resistance to compression. Forms aggregates with hyaluronic acid and link proteins[23,129,184]
Decorin (DS-PG2)	Within chondrocytes and the interterritorial capsules of the upper proliferative chondrocytes	Influences collagen fibril size and TGF-β activity.[10,72]
Biglycan (DS-PG1)	Territorial capsules of the upper proliferative chondrocytes	TGT-β activity[72]
Fibromodulin	Physeal cartilage	Influences collagen fibril diameter and binding of cells to the matrix[24]
Matrix Gla protein	Cartilage	Inhibits mineralization[68,109,172]

TABLE 2-2 Composition of Bone

Component	Proposed Functions
Collagens	
Collagen I	Imparts strength, site of initial mineralization
Collagen V	Provides the inner core of the collagen fibril[11,50]
Collagen VI	Cell attachment
Collagen XII	Collagen fibril size
Proteoglycans	
Decorin (DS-PG2)	Influences collagen fibril size and TGF-β activity[71,189,190]
Biglycan (DS-PG1)	Influences collagen fibril assembly and TGF-β activity[191,229]
Fibromodulin	Influences collagen fibril diameter and binding of cells to matrix molecules[71]
Osteocalcin (bone Gla protein)	Binds hydroxyapatite[12,171]
Matrix Gla protein	Controls mineralization[171]
Osteonectin	Binds calcium[12]
Osteopontin	Cell attachment[74,176]

The collagen type I fibers act as sites for initial mineralization and provide tensile strength to the bone. Mutations in the propeptides can cause a variety of phenotypes affecting mineralization and bone fragility, the most severe being osteogenesis imperfecta. In contrast, collagen type II is a triple helical molecule that is composed of three $\alpha 1$(II) polypeptides and is expressed in cartilage, particularly within the proliferative zone of the physis. It is the main fibril-forming collagen in cartilage. Mutations cause Langer-Saldino achondrogenesis and spondyloepiphyseal dysplasia congenita.[28,49]

Other collagen types, such as V, IX, and XI, associate with the collagen fibers.[87,165] They may influence collagen diameters and interact with other matrix molecules.[11] Mutations in types IX and XI can result in a number of clinical manifestations.[154] Collagen type X is associated with the matrix of hypertrophic chondrocytes and is involved with the mineralization process of cartilage matrix.[88,89,162,167] Mutation of collagen X causes spondylometaphyseal dysplasia,[80] but the deletion of the encoding gene results in mild changes.[80,181]

Proteoglycans. Proteoglycans are present in large amounts within all connective tissues. Proteoglycans are proteins that have either one or a number of polysaccharide chains linked to a protein core. The polysaccharide's glycosaminoglycan side chains are heparin, heparin sulfate, chondroitin sulfate, dermatan sulfate, or keratan sulfate. The glycosaminoglycans differ in the composition of their constituent disaccharide structures. They can combine with other molecules within the matrix to form macromolecular structures (Fig. 2-18).[52]

Proteoglycans are critical components of cartilage and bone.[23,129,168,229] The proteoglycans present in the physis include large proteoglycans like aggrecan as well as smaller proteoglycans, such as decorin, biglycan, and possibly, fibromodulin. Decorin and biglycan have side chains of dermatan sulfate, and betaglycan has chondroitin and heparin sulfate chains. Fibromodulin has side chains of keratan sulfate. The territorial capsules of the chondrocytes in the upper proliferative region of the physis stain for biglycan, and the interterritorial matrix stains for decorin.[10] These proteoglycans have a structural role but are also known to interact with growth factors.[10,72,168,189]

Other Noncollagenous Proteins. Osteocalcin is also known as bone Gla protein. It has three residues of gamma-carboxyglutamic acid that enable it to bind to hydroxyapatite. It is thought to play a role in mineralization of the bone matrix,[171,172] but the exact mechanism and function are undetermined.[40,68] Osteonectin has the ability to bind calcium and collagen type I, and may enable the process of mineralization that is initiated on the collagen type I fibers.[12] Osteopontin is thought to be critically involved with the binding of osteoclasts,[74,176] the cells that degrade the bone and physeal matrix.[119] Matrix Gla protein is an inhibitor of calcification. The cartilage of mice lacking this protein undergoes spontaneous calcification.[109]

Growth Factors

Within an individual, cell-to-cell communication occurs between neighboring cells and between cells that are separated by up to an almost complete body length. Communication signals take the form of diffusible molecules, which pass between the cells, or by cell surface–bound receptor-ligand interactions.[100,225] In addition, neighboring cells can pass information between one another via their gap junctions.[51] These channels enable the passage of small molecules, including calcium ions,

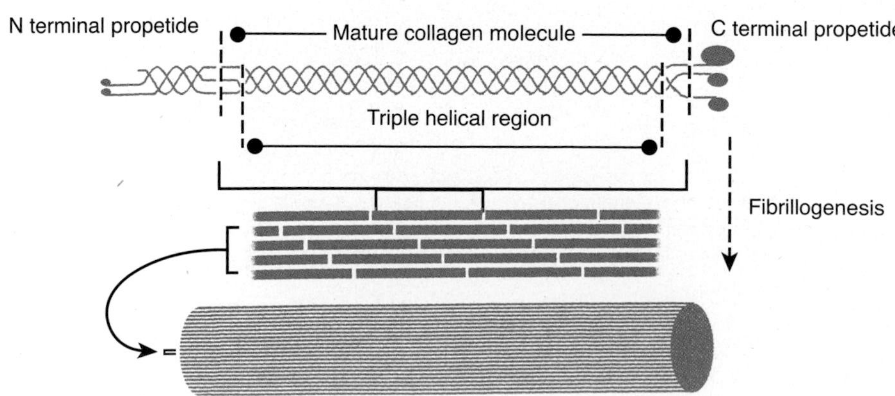

FIGURE 2-17 Collagens are synthesized as a propeptide that is often glycosylated (not shown). The collagen molecule has a triple helical region that arises from the repeated winding of three collagen molecules around a common axis. The processed collagen forms into subunits that then undergo fibrillogenesis.

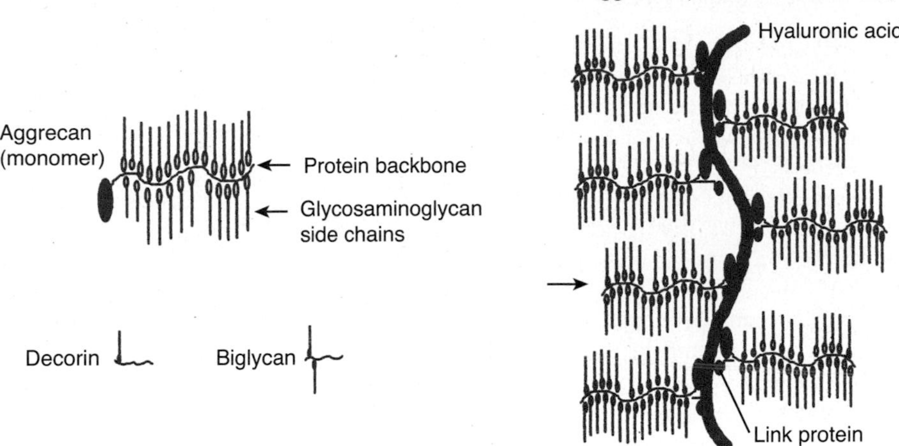

FIGURE 2-18 Proteoglycans are proteins that have either one or a number of polysaccharide (glycosaminoglycan) chains linked to a protein core. Aggrecan is present in cartilage and has the ability to form macromolecular structures with hyaluronic acid and link protein. Decorin and biglycan are present in bone and cartilage matrix.

between neighboring cells. Calcium is a key second messenger that provokes a number of cellular events.[127]

Hormones are a group of diverse molecules that are secreted by endocrine glands and are transported by body fluids. They coordinate body functions in complex organisms. Hormones can be in the form of amino acid derivatives (e.g., epinephrine), polypeptides (e.g., somatotropin or growth hormone), glycoproteins (e.g., follicle-stimulating hormone), steroids (e.g., testosterone), or fatty acids (e.g., prostaglandins).

Growth factors and hormones may circulate in a free form or be bound to carrier molecules or to the extracellular matrix.[159] The binding of growth factors and hormones to other molecules may facilitate their transportation to their target tissues, increase their survival by inhibiting their proteolytic degradation, and control their activities. Many growth factors, including the fibroblast growth factors (FGFs), transforming growth factor-β (TGF-β), and insulin-like growth factors (IGFs), can be bound to the matrix molecules. Cell activation usually requires the factors to bind to their receptors on the cell surface, although a number of hydrophobic hormones pass directly through the outer cell membrane and bind to intracellular receptors[34,48,117,133] (Fig. 2-19).

A degree of redundancy often exists in that a gene knockout for one particular growth factor may result in only slight changes

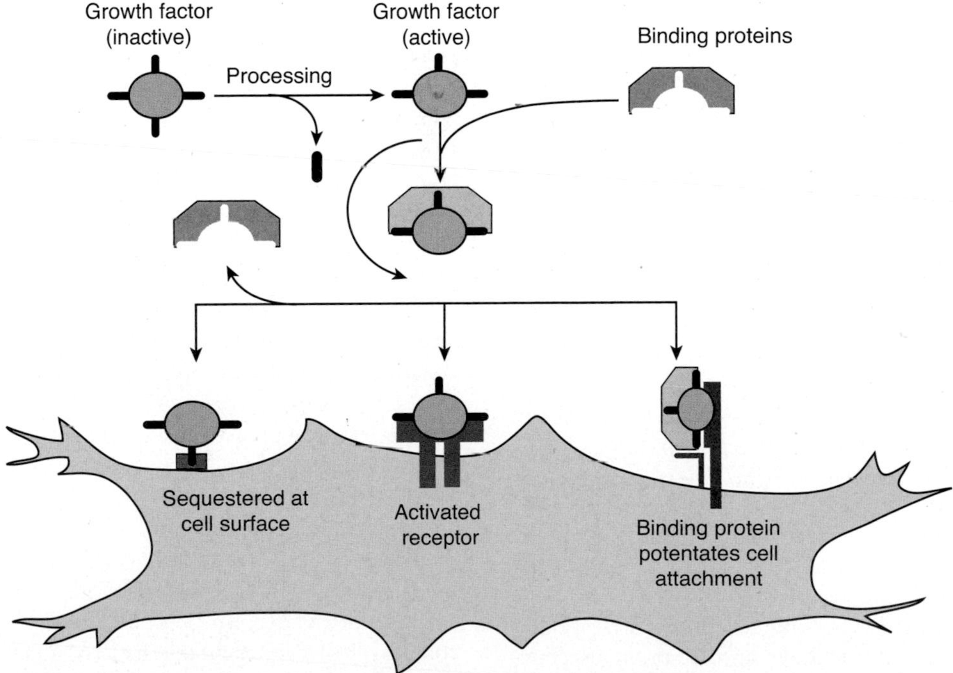

FIGURE 2-19 The figure shows aspects of growth factor interactions. Any particular growth factor will possess only a subset of such interactions. Growth factors may require activation (e.g., TGF-β). Binding proteins may sequester or protect the growth factor. The binding protein may also potentate the binding of the growth factor to the surface receptor (e.g., FGF and heparin). Cells may also sequester the growth factor at the cell surface.

in the phenotype observed. A good example is the double mutant of BMP-5 and BMP-7, which is lethal during embryonic development, but a null mutation in either one has little effect.[197]

Fibroblast Growth Factors. The biologic effects of the fibroblast growth factors (FGFs) are widespread. FGFs are angiogenic and can influence mitosis, differentiation, migration, and survival in many cell types. FGFs can activate one of four high-affinity FGF receptors (FGFRs). Point mutations of these receptors have been implicated in a number of skeletal deformities including Pfeiffer syndrome (FGFR1), Crouzon and Jackson-Weiss syndromes (FGFR2), and achondroplasia (FGFR3),[156] suggesting that FGFR signaling is an essential regulatory component for skeletal growth and development.[132]

The ligands activating the FGFRs in the developing skeleton remain largely unknown. To date, the FGF family comprises 22 members including acidic FGF (FGF-1), basic FGF (FGF-2).[155] FGF-1 and FGF-2 are present in the extracellular matrix of bone.[69] More recent data reveal that FGF-18 may be a physiological ligand for FGFR-3 in regulating bone lengthening, but it may also signal through another FGFR to regulate osteoblast growth.[106]

The FGFs are also complicated by the presence of alternative forms of the specific forms of FGF-1 and FGF-2. FGF-1 is typically 140 amino acids in length, but larger forms of 160 and 154 amino acids have been identified. FGF-2 is normally translated as a 155 amino acid molecule, but through the use of alternative start codons, three higher molecular weight forms have been identified.

The acidic (FGF-1) and basic (FGF-2) forms of FGFs are well conserved across species. Comparing the amino acid composition of FGF-1 and FGF-2 from different species, Hearn found a 92% sequence identity between human and bovine FGF-1. Only 2/155 and 3/155 amino acids differ in human and bovine, and human and ovine, forms of FGF-2, respectively.[70]

Insulin-Like Growth Factor. Insulin-like growth factor-1 (IGF-1) is critical for normal bone growth as has been confirmed by the severe growth retardation in the IGF-1 and its receptor gene knockout mice.[4,105] Genetic studies with various mutant, knock out, and congenic mice have revealed that there is a clear relationship between circulating IGF-1 concentrations and bone volume.[230] Consistently, delivery of exogenous IGF-1 stimulated growth of physeal height in normal rats, enhanced chondrocyte maturation and thus longitudinal growth in hypophysectomized rats,[75] and stimulated longitudinal and circumferential growth and increased bone mineral density.[230]

Cell-surface receptor for IGF-1 has been found present on chondrocytes at all stages of differentiation in growth plate cartilage.[207] Expression of IGF-1 mRNA and protein has also been localized in all chondrocyte layers of the physis,[175] suggesting that locally produced IGF-1 acts at the chondrocyte level in a paracrine/autocrine manner to stimulate longitudinal growth. In primary cultures, IGF-1 stimulates proliferation and matrix synthesis in physeal chondrocytes.[208] Consistently, in rodent in vivo studies, infused IGF-1 not only stimulates physeal chondrocytes at all stages of differentiation, but also promotes chondrogenic differentiation via its effects on resting stem-like cells of the physis.[75]

In bone, there is a high level of IGF-1 protein deposited in bone matrix, and it has been demonstrated that the vast majority of IGF-1 in bone is derived locally from osteoblastic synthesis.[230] Osteoblasts appear to be the major target of IGF-1 as IGF-1 type 1 receptor is present on osteoblasts and IGF-1 stimulates osteoblast proliferation and its recruitment.[233] Since IGF-1 is stored within the skeletal matrix and is released during bone resorption, IGF-1 may be a critical coupling factor that keeps bone formation closely linked to bone remodeling[230] (see Bone Remodeling section later).

Transforming Growth Factor-Beta. The transforming growth factor-beta (TGF-β) superfamily is composed of more than 24 members.[73] They are subdivided into families including TGF-β, inhibin, decapentaplegic protein/vegetal hemisphere 1 (DPP/Vg1), and müllerian-inhibiting substance. Members of the TGF-β and the DPP/Vg1 families have critical functions in the development of the skeleton, its growth and maintenance, and fracture repair. The bone morphogenic proteins (except for BMP-1) are members of the DPP/Vg1 family and are discussed in the next section.

Previous studies indicated that TGF-β stimulates bone formation when injected into rodent bones and induces endochondral bone formation in adult non-human primates. Most fracture healing studies have also demonstrated positive effects of TGF-β in stimulating bone repair and its potential usefulness in implant fixation.[25]

There are at least nine receptors for TGF-β. However, most of the TGF-β functions are mediated through two receptors termed receptor 1 and 2, which are members of the serine/threonine kinase family.[115] TGF-β receptor type 3 is a membrane-bound proteoglycan termed betaglycan. Betaglycan is thought to act as a TGF-β cell surface reservoir and is not involved with signal transduction itself.

Of the five TGF-β family members, four members including three identified in mammals (TGF-β1, -β2 and -β3) and one in amphibians (TGF-β5) are synthesized as large precursor forms that are processed to active forms. Members of the TGF-β family (TGF-β1, TBG-β2) are highly expressed in bone, and like IGF-1, the proteins are sequestered in the matrix. Important in fracture repair, TGF-β1 and TGF-β2 are also released in large quantities during platelet activation. The active form is either a heterodimer or homodimer. It is thought that the pro-region may either help in the folding of the proteins during synthesis or control TGF-β activity. In the case of TGF-β1, the proregion and a second glycoprotein can also bind to the active factor to form a latent complex. Apart from the presence of the growth factor itself, the presence or absence of the latent complex controls the activity of TGF-β1. The active TGF-β1 complex can be released from the latent complex by extreme pH or by catalytic methods. This is particularly important in fracture repair and bone remodeling. The activation of latent TGF-β is likely to be critical in the induction of fracture repair and osteoblast function.

The active TGF-β molecules may also be bound and their activity controlled by a number of matrix molecules, including betaglycan and decorin.[115,231] Betaglycan has the possibility of binding FGFs through the heparin sulfate chains and may present TGF-β in conjunction with FGFs to the cell.[115] TGF-β also binds to the small proteoglycans: biglycan, decorin, and fibromodulin.[72,189] The small proteoglycans bind TGF-β through the leucine-rich repeats in their protein cores and are thought to sequester TGF-β in the matrix. They also compete with betaglycan in binding TGF-β. Decorin has the ability to negatively regulate the activity of TGF-β.[14,186]

Bone Morphogenic Proteins. The bone morphogenic proteins (BMPs) and their orthopaedic relevance and applications have been reviewed previously.[25,78,186] The BMPS (except BMP-1) represent a group of related growth factors that have critical roles in the cell proliferation and differentiation of a number of cell types including mesenchymal cells, chondrocytes, and osteoblasts.[25,30,78,90,91,182,186,216,232] They have roles in embryo and fetal development, bone growth, and fracture repair. Several BMPs produce ectopic cartilage or bone when implanted subcutaneously.[2,219,224]

BMPs exist as glycosylated dimers. Like the other growth factors discussed so far, the BMPs have a number of binding proteins both in the extracellular matrix and on the cell surface. A secreted glycoprotein termed noggin can bind and inactivate BMPs.[55] Chordin is a similar protein that most likely has a similar function.[166] It has been proposed that these proteins control BMP activity and may also serve as a mechanism for establishing gradients of BMPs across the embryo during development. Active BMPs bind to heterotetrameric serine/threonine kinase receptors. The nonactivated receptors exist as type 1 and 2 receptor proteins, with the type 2 receptor being able to autophosphorylate. Once the ligand binds, the two receptors are brought together and the receptor type 1 receptor is phosphorylated. Only after the receptor type 1 is phosphorylated is a cellular response achieved. Intracellular activation is via the intracellular proteins termed SMADs, but other inhibitors can still come into play. Exposure of the cell to a number of other growth factors (including cer-1) can inhibit the activation of the cell by BMPs.[163,186]

Angiogenic Growth Factors. The invasion of the metaphyseal vascular supply is crucial to endochondral ossification, and fracture repair does not occur without an adequate vascular supply. Bone fracture disrupts the marrow architecture and blood vessels within and around the fracture site. During fracture healing, regeneration of three normal blood supplies (the medullary, periosteal, and osseous) to the callus and cortical bone need to be coordinated.[177]

Angiogenic factors are growth factors that promote neovascularization. They are essential for neovascularization during the normal bone lengthening and fracture repair. Previous studies have shown that the key angiogenic growth factor, vascular endothelial growth factor (VEGF), is essential for blood vessel invasion of the growth plate mineralized hypertrophic cartilage, cartilage remodeling, and bone formation during normal endochondral bone lengthening.[56] Endogenous VEGF also plays a key role in bone repair, as blocking VEGF activity inhibited repair of femoral fractures and cortical defects in rodents.[200] At the bone fracture site, VEGF activity is essential for appropriate angiogenesis, callus architecture, and mineralization.[25] Several studies have demonstrated that local delivery of exogenous VEGF promotes angiogenesis and bone formation at the bone fracture site.[25]

Apart from VEGF, several other growth factors are also important angiogenic factors, including FGF-2, TGF-β, platelet-derived growth factor (PDGF). It is probably not by accident that a number of angiogenic factors such as TGF-β and FGF-2 are sequestered in the bone matrix. Angiogenic factors act directly (such as VEGF and FGF-2) or indirectly (such as TGF-β and tumor necrosis factor-α) on endothelial cells, promoting proliferation and migration of the cells into areas in which they are released at the injury site.[174] Angiogenic factors acting indirectly by recruiting macrophages and monocytes, in turn, release their own direct-acting angiogenic factors.[192] During angiogenesis, while VEGF and FGF-2 induce angioblast differentiation and TGF-β1 enhances smooth muscle cell differentiation from mesenchymal cells, PDGF-B stimulates recruitments of smooth muscle cells and pericytes around nascent vessels.[35]

MECHANISMS OF BONE GROWTH

Because bone is rigid, it cannot grow by internal expansion and bone growth is achieved by adding newly synthesized bone to existing bone by two mechanisms: *endochondral ossification* and *intramembranous ossification*. These mechanisms are named by the intermediate structures that must be passed to form the bone. The production of any particular bone after initial differentiation may involve discrete, juxtaposed, or interspersed areas of each basic pattern. Endochondral-derived bones generally have membranous ossification by appositional bone growth from the periosteum. Similarly, membrane-derived bones may grow and elongate by an endochondral process.[139,147]

Endochondral Ossification

Endochondral ossification is the process by which bone forms via a cartilaginous intermediate. The physis (or the growth plate) best reflects this process. Physes are temporary cartilaginous tissue situated between the primary and secondary ossification centers of all long bones. From 9 to 10 weeks' gestational age to skeletal maturity at 15 to 17 years, they are responsible for the longitudinal growth of bone. The physis can be divided into at least three zones. The reserve or resting zone is situated on the epiphyseal side and contains small, spherical cells in groups of two or three cells randomly distributed throughout the zone. These cells are stem cell–like, responsible for generating new chondrocytes of the physis. In the adjacent proliferative zone, chondrocytes undergo mitosis and are organized into columns running parallel to the axis of bone growth. Cells in the proliferative zone mature and eventually increase to five to ten times their volume in the hypertrophic region. Matrix vesicles are also deposited within the longitudinal septa of the physis. Matrix vesicles are membrane-encapsulated structures that are thought to concentrate calcium and phosphate. Enzymes such as alkaline phosphatase convert organic phosphates to inorganic phosphates. The longitudinal septum around the terminal hypertrophic chondrocytes mineralizes, and this mineralized matrix forms the template for new bone deposition in the metaphysis (Fig. 2-20).

Associated with these changes in cellular arrangement and volume, the matrix in the physis also undergoes a continual modification in content. The two major macromolecules of cartilage matrix produced by the chondrocytes are the proteoglycans (predominantly aggrecan and with lesser amounts of decorin, biglycan, and fibromodulin) and the collagens (types II, IX, X, and XI). The major change in physeal proteoglycan structure occurs as chondrocytes organize into columns in the proliferative zone. Additional variation occurs in the hypertrophic region, where the glycosaminoglycan sulfation pattern demon-

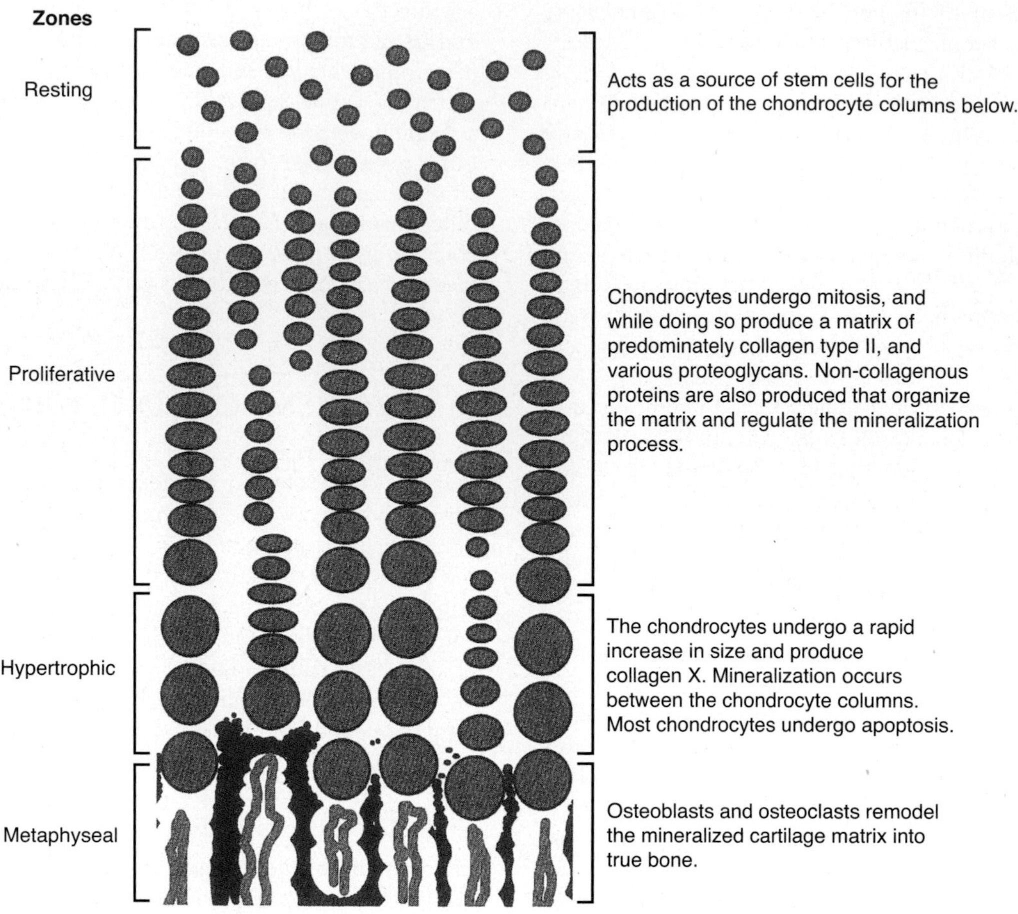

Zones
Resting
Acts as a source of stem cells for the production of the chondrocyte columns below.
Proliferative
Chondrocytes undergo mitosis, and while doing so produce a matrix of predominately collagen type II, and various proteoglycans. Non-collagenous proteins are also produced that organize the matrix and regulate the mineralization process.
Hypertrophic
The chondrocytes undergo a rapid increase in size and produce collagen X. Mineralization occurs between the chondrocyte columns. Most chondrocytes undergo apoptosis.
Metaphyseal
Osteoblasts and osteoclasts remodel the mineralized cartilage matrix into true bone.

FIGURE 2-20 The figure shows the process of endochondral ossification within the physis. Although not as organized, endochondral ossification follows a similar pattern during fracture repair.

strates differences between the pericellular and extracellular spaces and the appearance of a unique collagen (type X) is observed. The small proteoglycans—decorin, biglycan, and fibromodulin—are also differentially expressed across the physis, although detailed studies of these proteoglycans have not been done (see Table 2-1).

Regulatory Mechanisms in the Physis

The normal process of endochondral bone formation is tightly regulated by endocrine/paracrine/autocrine factors, such as hormones, vitamins, transcriptional factors, and growth factors, and involves coordinated and sequential expression of growth-regulatory factors. Although growth hormone (GH) in the circulation has a global effect on physeal function throughout the body, many locally produced growth factors act locally. Many hormones (such as GH, thyroid hormone, estrogen, glucocorticoids, calcitonin), vitamins (vitamin D3, ascorbate, retinoic acid), morphorgens (Indian hedgehog [IHH], BMPs), growth factors (IGFs, BMPs, FGFs, parathyroid hormone-related peptide [PTHrP], PDGF, TGF-β, VEGF) and their binding proteins (such as IGFBPs, chordin, noggin), and cytokines (tumor necrosis factor-α, interleukin IL-1, and others) have now been shown to have important roles in regulating various processes of the endochondral ossification (Fig. 2-21).[5] Cellular response is determined by parallel processing of the intracellular signals that are induced by a number of active growth factors binding

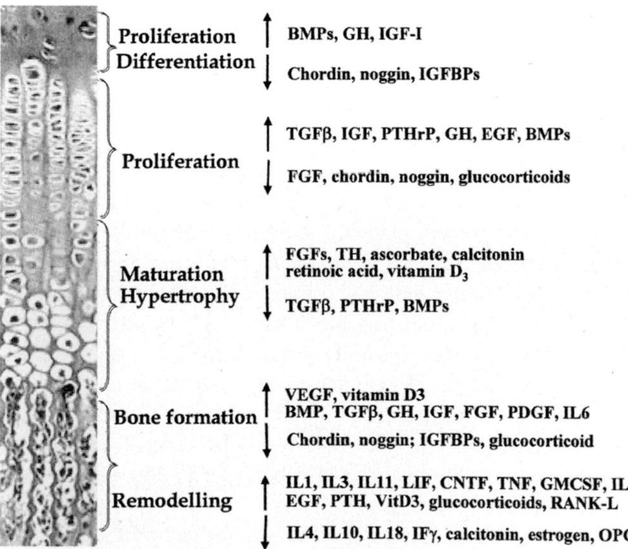

FIGURE 2-21 Systemic and local factors including hormones, vitamins, cytokines, and growth factors that control or influence chondrocyte differentiation, proliferation, and maturation, as well as bone formation and remodeling.

to their specific receptors. Presented below is an outline of the likely actions of a number of key growth factors on endochondral ossification.

It is well known that growth hormone (GH) and IGF-1 are two major factors regulating postnatal growth. In skeletal tissues, both chondrocytes and osteoblasts synthesize IGF-1, and GH modulates its synthesis in both cell populations. According to the original somatomedin hypothesis, GH stimulates skeletal growth through IGF-1 that is produced in the liver under the influence of GH and secreted into the circulation.[39] Upon reaching target tissues, IGF-1 interacts with its receptors and induces a cellular growth signal. However, normal postnatal growth achieved in liver-IGF-1 null mice (in which hepatic IGF-1 expression was abolished specifically) suggests the importance of extrahepatic IGF-1 expression and an autocrine-paracrine role for IGF-1 in normal skeletal growth.[196] Therefore, both circulating and locally expressed IGF-1 play important roles in longitudinal bone growth and the maintenance of bone mass, and IGF-1 plays an essential role in longitudinal bone growth in response to GH exposure.[195]

GH controls stem cell maturation and this action is at least partially mediated via local production and action of IGF-1 at the stem cell zone.[175] GH receptor has been localized in the physeal chondrocytes particularly in the proliferative zone,[6,41,223] and it is generally accepted that GH acts at both the stem and proliferative phases of chondrocyte differentiation.[75] At present, apart from the IGF-1-mediated effects on the stem cells of the physis, GH also stimulates proliferation of the prechondrocytes in the resting zone[153] and has some priming effect on these stem cells to promote their differentiation independently of IGF-1, as proposed by the dual effector theory. In addition, there is genetic evidence that supports this dual, IGF-1-independent and IGF-1-dependent roles for GH in promoting longitudinal bone growth.[220]

Apart from IGF-1 and GH, BMP-2 and BMP-7 also promote proliferation, differentiation, and matrix synthesis in undifferentiated chondrocytes in the resting zone.[45,90] It is believed that once the chondrocytes start differentiating, the expression of noggin inhibits the continual outgrowth of the undifferentiated chondrocytes.[18] Once the chondrocyte has lost its resting phenotype, IGF-1 may act as a stimulator of proliferation and differentiation.[135,203] Epidermal growth factor (EGF) can augment IGF stimulation by increasing the expression of the IGF-1 receptor.[13] Although the chondrocytes synthesize large quantities of matrix molecules, they also synthesize FGF-1, FGF-2, TGF-*β*, VEGF, and a number of the BMPs.[15,26,32] These molecules can act in an autocrine or paracrine manner, but many are sequestered into the newly formed cartilage matrix. While FGF-2 in low doses is mitogenic for the chondrocytes,[110] as occurs in achondroplasia, constant activation of FGF receptor (FGFR3) inhibits chondrocyte proliferation and accelerates terminal differentiation of chondrocytes.[93,99,111] FGF/heparin sulfate interaction is probable in the differentiation of the physeal chondrocytes because the continuous exposure of FGF-2 inhibits chondrocyte differentiation in vitro and inhibitors of glycosaminoglycan sulfation (including heparin sulfate) restore the differentiation process. Additional sulfate permits glycosaminoglycan sulfation and returns the effect of FGF-2.[33]

Parathyroid hormone (PTH) and parathyroid hormone–related protein (PTHrP) act to maintain the proliferative state of and inhibit the maturation of chondrocytes. It is postulated that two negative feedback loops involving actions of PTHrP regulate the pace of chondrocyte differentiation in the postnatal growth plate.[215] The first loop is confined to the proliferative-hypertrophic transition zone and early hypertrophic chondrocytes, which express morphogen Indian hedgehog (IHH), its receptor Patched, and PTH/PTHrP receptor. IHH, which stimulates chondrocyte proliferation and inhibits hypertrophic differentiation, binds Patched in the hypertrophic zone resulting in a stimulated production of PTHrP. PTHrP then acts on its receptor at the proliferating chondrocytes to keep them proliferating and, thereby to delay the production of IHH, thus closing the IHH-PTHrP feedback loop (Fig. 2-22). In the second feedback loop, IHH can bind Patched in the resting stem cell zone, and this may stimulate PTHrP production, which then diffuses to its receptor leading to IHH down-regulation. These two IHH-PTHrP signaling cascade feedback loops limit maturation of proliferative chondrocytes to hypertrophic form.[94,215,217]

Studies have shown that several signaling pathways regulating chondrocyte proliferation and hypertrophic differentiation interact with the IHH-PTHrP feedback loops (Fig. 2-22). Apart from inhibiting chondrocyte proliferation, part of the effects of FGF signaling in positively affecting chondrocyte maturation is mediated by the suppression of IHH expression.[125] However, FGF effects on chondrocytes can occur independently of PTHrP/IHH action.[185] In the physis, expression of the mRNA for BMP-2 and BMP-6 peaks in hypertrophic chondrocytes before mineralization.[26] Studies have demonstrated that BMPs act on chondrocytes to induce proliferation through the induction of IHH expression by prehypertrophic chondrocytes, suggesting that BMP signaling modulates the IHH/PTHrP signaling pathway that regulates the rate of chondrocyte differentiation.[93,234] In addition, in vitro studies have suggested that during embryonic development, signaling of TGF-*β*2 may act as a critical

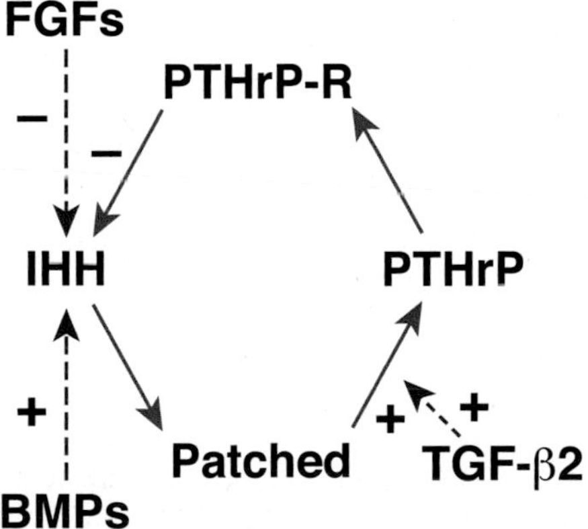

FIGURE 2-22 Schematic representation of an IHH-PTHrP feedback loop controlling the rate of chondrocyte hypertrophic maturation and its modulation by BMPs, TGF-*β*2, and FGFs in a postnatal growth plate. PTHrP is secreted from hypertrophic chondrocytes and acts on PTHrP receptor on proliferating chondrocytes to keep the chondrocytes proliferating. When PTHrP expression is low, IHH is produced by the maturing cells. IHH binds to its receptor Patched on the hypertrophic cells, resulting in a stimulation of PTHrP expression. Activation of PTHrP receptor by PTHrP in turn represses IHH expression, thus closing a negative feedback loop. FGFs and BMPs interact with this negative feedback loop through their activities in inhibiting and stimulating the production of IHH, respectively. Evidence has suggested that TGF-*β*2 mediates the function of IHH in stimulating the production of PTHrP.

signal relay between IHH and PTHrP. It mediates the effects of IHH inhibiting hypertrophic differentiation and induces PTHrP expression, maintaining the chondrocytes in proliferative state and slowing down the pace of their maturation.[2]

Although the chondrocytes of the physis will proliferate and form a cartilaginous matrix with only the epiphyseal vascular supply, the metaphyseal vessels are critical for the mineralization process.[212] Metaphyseal vascular invasion occurs at the hypertrophic-metaphyseal interface. The endothelial cells invade most likely as a consequence of angiogenic factors present in the matrix or secreted by the chondrocytes themselves. VEGF, TGF-β, and FGFs are known to be present in the physeal cartilage matrix and are angiogenic. It is interesting that an oversupply of FGF-2 infused into the physis induces vascular invasion from the metaphysis only; even if the FGF-2 is present at the epiphyseal side of the physis, the epiphyseal vessel will not invade.[7] Apart from providing the necessary nutrients for the mineralization process, the metaphyseal vessels also bring in osteoblasts, osteoclasts, and other cell types. The osteoclasts degrade the mineralized cartilage matrix while osteoblasts lay down new bone that is also rich in growth factors such as TGF-β, FGF-2, IGF-1, and BMPs.

Membranous Ossification

All axial and appendicular skeletal elements are involved in secondary membranous ossification. The diaphyseal cortex of developing tubular bone is progressively formed (modeled) by the periosteum and modified (remodeled) by the re-formation of osteons. This peripheral periosteal process of membrane-derived ossification is extensive and rapid in fracture healing in infants and young children. The replacement process also may be seen when portions of the developing metaphysis or diaphysis are removed for use as bone grafts.

Intramembranous ossification occurs when osteoprogenitor cells are formed from the overlying tissue, the inner cambium layer of the periosteum[193] (see Periosteum section earlier). The osteoprogenitor cells continue to differentiate into osteoblasts, which produce and add new bone matrix peripherally that later undergoes mineralization.

Remodeling of Bones

The first bone to be laid down either from the physis at the metaphysis or in the fracture callus is woven bone, which is remodeled to lamellar bone. At the metaphysis, the trabeculae of bone-covered calcified cartilage (primary spongiosa) are resorbed by osteoclasts and the calcified cartilage template is replaced by lamellar bone and remodeled into more mature bone trabeculae (secondary spongiosa). The deposited secondary bone trabeculae at the metaphyseal-diaphyseal junction is further remodeled and incorporated into the diaphysis, in a process in which osteoclasts remove bone from the periphery of the metaphysis and new bone is formed at the endosteal surfaces. Although cancellous bone can be remodeled and obtain its nutrients from the surface, cortical bone is remodeled into a complex structure of osteons that together form the cortical bone. Osteons are tubular structures that interconnect. They consist of layers of ordered lamellar bone around a central canal. The central canal contains blood vessels, lymphatics, and in some cases, nerves.[20]

Bone is constantly remodeled by osteoclasts and osteoblasts. The bone is encapsulated by bone-lining cells that have the potential to become activated osteoblasts. The bone-lining cells have slender cellular processes that make contact with the osteocytes within the mineralized bone. Osteocytes are thought to arise from osteoblasts that have become entrapped during bone formation. It has been proposed that the bone-lining cells need to erode the osteoid that covers the underling bone for osteoclasts to bind.[122,123] Osteoclasts are bone-degrading cells that are produced from the hematopoietic pathway. Upon activation, they bind to the surface of the bone and secrete enzymes into the space beneath. The space is acidic and contains many proteolytic and bone degrading enzymes.[114] The acidic pH and proteases are thought to release and activate the sequestered growth factors IGF-1 and TGF-β, resulting in the recruitment, proliferation, differentiation, and activation of the stromal osteoprogenitor cells and bone-lining cells to become active osteoblasts, synthesizing bone matrix and increasing their survival (Fig. 2-23).[46,47,116,118] The newly laid osteoid by osteoblasts is subsequently mineralized to become bone.

It is now generally accepted that the osteoblast activity and osteoclast activity are linked during the bone remodeling. On the one hand, osteoclastic activity releases growth factors IGF-1 and TGF-β stimulating osteoblastic differentiation and activity as described above (Fig. 2-23), and on the other, cells of the osteoblast lineage provide factors essential for the differentiation of osteoclasts. The discovery of the interaction between the receptor activator of NF-kappaB (RANK) ligand (RANKL) expressed by osteoblasts and its receptor RANK expressed on osteoclast precursors confirms the well-known hypothesis that osteoblasts play an essential role in osteoclast differentiation (Fig. 2-23).[201] It is now known that two hematopoietic factors, namely RANKL and macrophage colony-stimulating factor (M-CSF), together are necessary and sufficient for osteoclast formation.[16] Several factors have now been identified that can modulate RANK-induced osteoclastogenesis. Although vitamin D3 metabolite, PTH, PTHrP, PGE2, cytokines IL-1, IL-6, TNF, LIF, and IL-11, and corticosteroids have been shown to induce the expression of RANKL in stromal/osteoblastic cells and thus stimulate osteoclast formation, osteoprotegerin (OPG), a decoy receptor for RANKL, blocks the RANKL-RANK interaction and inhibits osteoclastogenesis.[16,112] Recent studies have also shown that lipopolysaccharide and inflammatory cytokines such as TNF-α and IL-1 can also directly regulate osteoclast differentiation and function through a mechanism independent of the RANKL-RANK interaction.[92] TGF-β superfamily members and interferon-gamma (INF-γ) are also shown to be important regulators in osteoclastogenesis.[84] Estrogens, calcitonin, BMP2/4, TGF-β, IL-17, PDGF, and calcium have been shown to be anabolic or inhibit osteoclastogenesis[16] (Fig. 2-21). In addition, EGF receptor signaling has been shown to be important for the secretion of matrix metalloproteases (MMPs)[124] and maintenance of osteoclast activity,[29] both of which are important for the bone remodeling.

The osteocytes may serve as the mechanosensory system that may be associated with bone remodeling. Osteocytes also possess cellular processes that connect osteocytes to one another and to the bone-lining cells above.[36] It is possible that the osteocytes are responsible for sensing bone stress; if undue stress is detected, they favor bone deposition, whereas if a lack of stress is detected, they favor bone resorption.

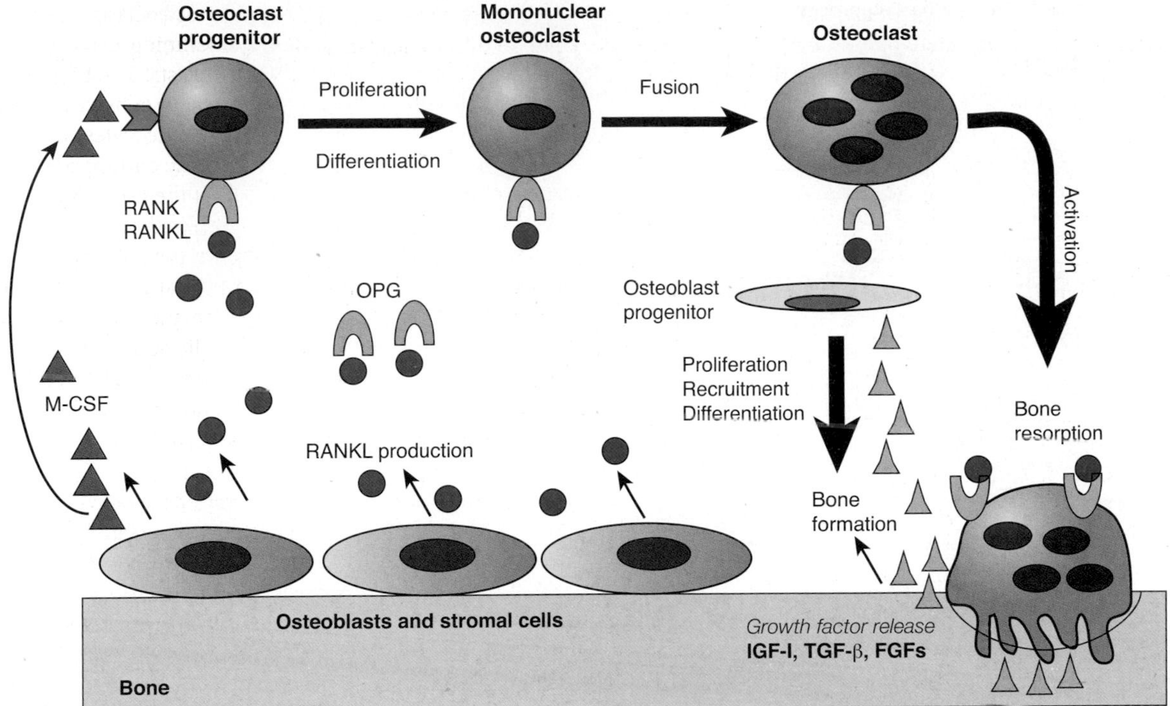

FIGURE 2-23 The linked activities of osteoclast bone resorption and osteoblast bone formation during bone remodeling. Bone-lining cells, osteoblasts or some marrow stromal cells express RANKL, which activates receptor RANK on osteoclast progenitors of the monocyte-macrophage lineage and stimulates the osteoclast differentiation and activation. M-CSF is another essential factor for osteoclast differentiation. However, decoy receptor OPG binds RANKL and antagonizes RANK function and thus inhibits osteoclast formation. Activated osteoclasts secret acid and proteases and erode bone on the surface. During the resorption process, sequestered growth factors, such as IGF-I, TGF-β and FGFs, are released from the bone matrix and activated, which results in the recruitment, differentiation, and activation of the osteoprogenitors to become osteoblasts to initiate bone matrix synthesis and bone formation.

FRACTURE REPAIR

Injuries to the developing skeleton may involve osseous, fibrous, and cartilaginous tissues. Healing of these tissues differs, depending on both the type of tissue and the temporal maturation.

Osseous Healing

The progressive changes of the normal process of osseous fracture healing, whether in the diaphysis, metaphysis, or epiphyseal ossification center, can be grouped conveniently into a series of phases that occur in a reasonably chronologic sequence.[120,180] Several factors that influence bone healing have been identified from clinical observation as well as experimental work[160,214] and must be taken into account when treating childhood fractures on a rational basis. However, certain areas of the developing skeleton, particularly the physis and epiphyseal hyaline cartilage, probably do not heal by classic callus formation. In fact, when this type of osseous (callus) repair occurs in these cartilaginous regions, significant growth deformities may result due to formation of an osseous bridge between the secondary ossification center and the metaphysis (see "Physeal Healing Patterns").

As in adults, there are three basic mechanisms of fracture repair: primary osteonal, secondary osteonal, and nonosteonal. Primary osteonal fracture healing occurs when cortical bone is laid down without any intermediate, and therefore hardly any callus forms; it is only possible if cortical bone is repositioned and fixed in close proximity. Secondary osteonal union occurs if cortical bone is laid down between two segments of fractured cortical bone before callus formation. Nonosteonal union occurs through endosteal and periosteal callus formation.[183]

Fracture repair by callus production in the immature skeleton can be divided into three closely integrated, but sequential, phases: the inflammatory phase, the reparative phase, and the remodeling phase (Fig. 2-24). In children, the remodeling phase is temporally much more extensive and physiologically more active (depending on the child's age) than the comparable phase in adults. The remodeling phase is further modified by the effects of the physis responding to changing joint reaction forces and biologic stresses to alter angular growth dynamics. This occurs even when the fracture is mid-diaphyseal.

Cellular Response to Trauma

Inflammatory Phase

Immediately after a fracture through any of the osseous portions of the developing skeleton (diaphysis, metaphysis, or epiphyseal ossification center), disruption of blood vessels leads to activation of the coagulation cascade and formation of a hematoma enclosing the fracture area.

Hematoma Formation. Bleeding of the damaged periosteum, contiguous bone, and soft tissues starts the process of repair

Non-osteoneal healing process
Monocytes
Mesenchymal cells
Macrophages
Recruitment
PDGF → Neovascularization
TGF-β etc...
Platelets
Removal of necrosed tissue and synthesis of a matrix permissive for chondrogenesis and osteoblast mediated bone formation.
Coagulation ← Hemorrhage
Cell necrosis
A

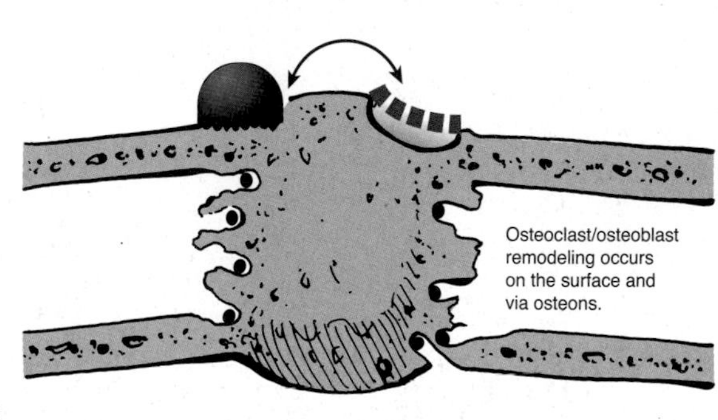

Osteoclast/osteoblast remodeling occurs on the surface and via osteons.
C

FIGURE 2-24 The figure demonstrates the three phases of fracture repair **(A)** inflammatory phase, **(B)** reparative phase, and **(C)** remodeling phase. The inflammatory cells remove the debris from the fracture site and, together with the fibroblastic cells, develop the site into a matrix that will support the cells that enable new bone to be formed. The mesenchymal cells are recruited by the release of growth factors in the fracture site. The mesenchymal cells may differentiate into osteoblasts that produce bone in a membranous fashion. Alternately the mesenchymal cell may become chondrogenic and produce bone by the endochondral pathway. Remodeling begins with resorption of mechanically unnecessary, inefficient portions of the callus and the subsequent orientation of trabecular bone along the lines of stress.

through the release of growth factors, cytokines, and prostaglandins. If the fracture is localized to the maturing diaphysis, there is bleeding from the Haversian systems, as well as from the multiple small blood vessels of the microcirculatory systems of the endosteal and periosteal surfaces and contiguous soft-tissue anastomoses.[61] In the region of the metaphysis, this bleeding may be extensive because of the anastomotic ramifications of the peripheral and central metaphyseal vascular systems. A hematoma accumulates within the medullary canal at the fracture site, beneath the elevated periosteum, and extraperiosteally whenever the periosteum is disrupted during the fracture. In contrast to adults, the periosteum strips away easily from the underlying bone in children, allowing the fracture hematoma to dissect along the diaphysis and metaphysis; and this is evident in the subsequent amount of new bone formation along the shaft.

However, the dense attachments of the periosteum into the zone of Ranvier limit subperiosteal hematoma formation to the metaphysis and diaphysis. Because the perichondrium is densely attached, this type of hemorrhagic response is uncharacteristic of the epiphyseal ossification center, thus limiting its contributions to callus formation and any intrinsic stabilization effect. Further, because of the partially or completely intracapsular nature of some epiphyses, propagation of a fracture into the joint allows decompression of some of the bleeding into the joint, again limiting the potential volume for eventual callus formation.

Coagulation and platelet activation stop the blood loss but also produce both inflammatory mediators and angiogenic factors. Endothelial cells respond and increase the vascular permeability, and allow the passage of inflammatory cells (leukocytes, monocytes, and macrophages), fibroblasts, and stem cells into the fracture site. Neovascularization is also initiated. Angiogenic factors like platelet-derived growth factor (PDGF), VEGF, and TGF-*β* also promote osteoblast recruitment and activation.

Local Necrosis. The blood supply is temporarily disrupted for a few millimeters on either side of the fracture, creating juxtaposed, avascular trabecular and cortical bone[60] and producing local necrosis. It is likely that the necrosis also results in the release of sequestered growth factors (e.g., IGF-1, TGF-*β*, FGF-1, and FGF-2) from the bone. These growth factors may help in promoting differentiation of the surrounding mesenchymal cells into bone-forming cells.

The inflammatory response results in the release of several growth factors and cytokines that have important roles in repair. The inflammatory cells remove the debris from the fracture site and, with the fibroblastic cells, develop the site into a matrix that will support the cells that enable new bone to be formed. This initial matrix often contains collagens type I, III, and V.

Organization of Hematoma. The initial cellular repair process involves organization of the fracture hematoma.[169] Fibrovascular tissue replaces the clot with a matrix rich in collagens I, III, and V. This matrix allows chondrogenesis or intramembranous bone formation. Such mechanisms eventually lead to mineralization and the formation of the woven bone of the provisional (primary) callus. Initial invasion and cell division are around the damaged bone ends but proceed centrifugally away from the fracture site, thus placing the most mature repair process closest to the fracture site. However, bone formation occurs only in the presence of an intact, functional microvascular supply. If the vascular supply is deficient, then this modulation of cartilaginous to osseous tissue cannot readily occur.

Reparative Phase

The fracture hematoma is the area in which the early stages of healing occur.[169] Osteogenic cells proliferate from the periosteum to form an external callus and, to a lesser extent, from the endosteum to form an internal callus. However, when the periosteum is severely disrupted, healing cells must differentiate from the ingrowth of undifferentiated mesenchymal cells throughout the hematoma. By 10 to 14 days in a child, the fracture callus consists of a thick, enveloping mass of peripheral osteogenic tissue that is beginning to be evident radiographically. This new bone is primarily woven (fiber) bone.[177,178]

The next step in osseous fracture healing is cellular organization.[37] During this stage, the circumferential tissues serve primarily as a fibrous scaffold over which cells migrate and orient to induce a stable repair. This pluripotential mesenchyme is theoretically capable of modulation into cartilage, bone, or fibrous tissue.[158] The mesenchymal cells are recruited by the released growth factors within the fracture site. Members of the BMP family, and possibly their inhibitors, are likely to be involved in the recruitment and differentiation of the mesenchymal cells. The mesenchymal cells may differentiate into osteoblasts that produce bone in a membranous fashion or may become chondrogenic and produce bone by the endochondral pathway. Both mechanisms usually are present in a fracture callus, and the degree to which each is present depends on the type of bone, age, degree of fixation, level of bone loss, and trauma. In children, because of the osteoblastic activity, the periosteum contributes significantly to new bone formation by accentuating the normal process of membranous ossification to supplement the cellular organization within the hematoma, which is going through a cartilaginous phase.[64,65] The region around the fracture site thus repeats the process of endochondral ossification, in close juxtaposition to membranous ossification from the elevated periosteum. Similar processes occur within the medullary cavity. An integral part of the reparative process at this stage is microvascular invasion, which occurs very readily in children because of the state of vascularity within the bone and surrounding soft tissues.[27] Vessels come from the periosteal region as well as from the nutrient artery and endosteal vessels.

Until this healing bone goes through the final stages of maturation, it is still biologically plastic and, if not protected, may gradually deform, especially in an active young child after early release from an immobilization device. Even in a cast, this plasticity may allow deformation from isometric muscle activity.

Clinical union is attained when the fracture site no longer moves and is not painful to attempts at manipulation, although it is by no means restored to its original strength at this time. With time, the primary callus is gradually replaced. This is enhanced in the child because as appositional growth and increasing diameter envelop the original fracture region, the cartilage and woven bone are replaced by mature, lamellar bone, and the fracture is consolidated and essentially returns to most of its normal biologic standards and response to stress.

Remodeling Phase

The last phase (remodeling) begins with resorption of mechanically unnecessary, inefficient portions of the callus and the subsequent orientation of trabecular bone along the lines of stress. The remodeling phase is the longest of the three phases and in children may continue until (and beyond) skeletal maturation in response to constantly changing stress patterns imposed by continued skeletal growth and development. Initially, new bone is laid down by both the fracture callus and subperiosteal tissue. This bone is randomly oriented and cannot withstand all stresses imposed on it. However, as the bone grows diametrically in the diaphyseal or metaphyseal regions, this new bone is gradually and increasingly incorporated into the preexisting cortical bone, aligned in accord with predominant stress patterns, and replaced by physiologic remodeling processes. The degree of remodeling and progressive replacement of fracture callus is greater in younger children, who have an immense capacity for growth and change.

The critical step between the reparative and remodeling phases is the establishment of an intact bony bridge between the fragments. Because this involves the joining of separated segments of hard tissue, the whole system must become immobile. Once the bridge has been established—provided that adequate, continued mechanical protection is given—subsequent biologic failure is unlikely. If the two or more fracture fragments remain connected by the periosteum or related material, as is likely in a child, it is easy to see how reparative activity could be conducted from one side to the other relatively easily and rapidly.

The intact bone must then readapt to functional demands. This is much easier in children, whose skeletons are actively and continually remodeling in response to stress, than in adults, who have more static skeletons. The processes of replacement and repair are continuous and concomitant in the normally developing skeleton. The mechanisms involved in fracture healing essentially are no different than most of the active maturational processes. These processes are much more active in children and are more active in the metaphysis than in the diaphysis.

The fracture remodeling process differs in cortical or cancellous bone. Both involve a process of simultaneous bone removal and replacement by the osteoclasts and osteoblasts through the accompanying blood vessels. In cancellous bone of the metaphysis or the endosteal surface of the diaphysis, the cells are never very far away from blood vessels, and the whole process of apposition and replacement may occur on the surface of the trabeculae. However, in compact bone, the more deeply placed cells require the presence of an adequately functioning perfusion system that must be replaced. This is a much longer sequence of events and is not a major method of bone repair in children, except when the fracture involves densely cortical regions, such as the femoral or tibial shafts. McKibbin[120] presented an extensive discussion of this process, which is sometimes referred to as *primary bone union* because no intermediate cells are involved.

Gerstenfeld et al[57] reviewed the molecular, spatial, and temporal aspects of the regulation of bone facture healing in animal models. It is now clear that fracture healing is a specialized postnatal repair process that recapitulates aspects of embryological skeletal development. It is also becoming increasingly evident that the sequential cellular responses in the different phases of bone fracture healing are intricately regulated by many molecules, including (a) M-CSF, IL-1, IL-6, IL-11, RANKL, OPG, INF-γ, TNF, TGF-β1, BMP-2, and growth and differentiation factor GDF-8 after the initial injury and during the inflammatory response; (b) M-CSF, RANKL, OPG, TGF-β2, TGF-β3, BMP-3, BMP-4, BMP-5, BMP-6, BMP-7, BMP-8, GDF-1, GDF-10, VEGF, and matrix metalloproteases MMP-2, MMP-8, MMP-9, MMP-13, MMP-14 during the repair phase; and (c) all the cytokines listed above (except IL-11 and INF-γ), GDF-10, TGF-β1, MMP-9, MMP-13, and all BMP members previously listed in the remodeling phase.

Physeal Healing Patterns

The physis has a limited ability to repair; it primarily heals by increased endochondral bone and cartilage formation, and gradual reinvasion by the disrupted metaphyseal vessels to replace the temporarily widened physis eventually. Very little experimental work, mostly in rats, has been directed at assessing the post-traumatic cellular response patterns of the physis.[17,97,228]

Depending on the level of cellular injury within the physis, *three types of chondro-osseous healing* may occur. First, when the fracture occurs through the cell columns, healing occurs primarily by continued, relatively rapid increases in the number of cells within the columns, causing moderate widening of the physis. Because there are some small epiphyseal vessels in this region, some damaged tissue may be resorbed early in the healing process. These vessels also exhibit a hyperemic response, increasing cellular proliferation rates, especially in the peripheral zone of Ranvier. The metaphyseal response parallels this, in that an increased rate of bone replacement of the hypertrophic cartilage also occurs. Once the level of fracture fibrosis and debris within the physis is encountered, the vessels rapidly invade to reach the rest of the maturing cell columns. These cellular response patterns lead to restoration of normal anatomy within 3 to 4 weeks.[179]

Second, when the fracture occurs through the transition of hypertrophic cells to primary spongiosa (the most commonly involved cellular level), there may be marked separation, with the gap filled by hemorrhagic and fibroblastic tissue. This region may progressively form disorganized cartilaginous tissue, which is similar to the initial, disorganized cartilaginous callus around a diaphyseal fracture. Meanwhile, cellular proliferation, cell column formation, hypertrophy, and calcification continue on the epiphyseal side of the disorganized callus, leading to widening of the physis. Vascular invasion of the remnants of hypertrophic, calcified cartilage also rapidly occurs on the metaphyseal side of the fracture. However, once metaphyseal vessel invasion reaches the disorganized cartilaginous callus, vascular-mediated bone replacement is temporarily slowed, because there is no pattern of cell columns to invade in an organized fashion. As the callus cartilage matures and calcifies, the metaphyseal vessels begin to invade and replace the cartilage with bone irregularly.[21] This callus may be variably thick, depending on the degree of longitudinal and lateral displacement and periosteal continuity with the physeal periphery. The callus is replaced at different rates, and the invading metaphyseal vessels reach the normal cell columns, which have been maturing in a normal sequence but without osseous replacement. This widened physis is rapidly invaded by the vessels and replaced by primary spongiosa, and normal physeal width is progressively restored.

The callus in the subperiosteal region of the metaphysis contributes to early stability. This region heals by vascular invasion of the callus to form trabecular bone between the original metaphyseal cortex and the subperiosteal membranous bone forming continuously external to the metaphyseal cartilaginous callus. These three microscopic bone regions progressively merge and remodel, strengthening the bone. These initial cellular replacement processes in both metaphyseal and physeal regions probably take 3 to 6 weeks. However, remodeling may continue for months to years, and it enhances the capacity for spontaneous correction of many residual deformities.

Third, when the injury extends across all cell layers of the physis, the repair processes differ slightly. Fibrous tissue initially fills the gap between separated physeal components, whereas typical callus formation occurs in the contiguous metaphyseal spongiosa or epiphyseal ossification center. If large surfaces of nonossified epiphyseal cartilage also are involved, fibrous tissue initially forms in the intervening region. The reparative response shows irregular healing of the epiphyseal and physeal cartilage, with loss of normal cellular architecture. Within the central physeal regions, diametric expansion of cell columns is minimal, so closure of a large defect by physeal cartilage is unlikely. The gap will remain fibrous, but with the potential to ossify. Toward the physeal periphery, diametric expansion is more likely, but still may not lead to closure of large cartilage gaps by progressive replacement of fibrous tissue. This replacement process essentially requires the germinal and hypertrophic cell regions to diametrically expand by cell division, maturation, and matrix expansion. The intervening fibrous tissue may disappear through growth, but only if the gap is narrow. Because blood supply is minimal in this region, the fibrous tissue similarly is not well vascularized, and significant cell modulation, especially to osteoblastic tissue, is less likely in the short term. However, the larger the gap filled with fibrous tissue and the longer the time from fracture to skeletal maturity, the greater the likelihood of developing sufficient vascularity to commence an osteoblastic response and to form an osseous bridge. Further, in young children with minimal epiphyseal ossification, the blood supply to the physeal germinal region is not as well defined, whereas once the ossification center expands and forms a subchondral plate over the germinal region, microvascularity probably increases and the chances for vascularization and ossification of the fibrous region increase. This explains the delayed appearance of the osseous bridge.

If accurate anatomic reduction is performed, a thin gap should be present that should fill in with minimal fibrous tissue, allowing progressive replacement of the tissue by diametric expansion of the physis and contiguous epiphysis. However, if the fragment has been partially or completely devascularized by either the initial trauma or subsequent dissection to effect an open reduction, cellular growth and diametric and longitudinal expansion may not occur. This increases the chances of cellular disorganization, fibrosis, and eventual osteoblastic response. Failure to correct anatomic displacement, especially in Salter-Harris type IV growth mechanism injuries, increases the possibility of apposition of the epiphyseal ossification center and metaphyseal bone, and thereby enhances the risk of forming an osseous bridge between the two regions. When the defect was large enough and the fracture involved the whole width of the physis extending from the metaphysis to the epiphysis, the injured physis will have structural disorganization, formation of vertical septa, and finally formation of a bone bridge. When the bone bridge is large enough, particularly in Salter-Harris types III and IV injuries, the defect will result in a growth arrest. While growth arrest at the peripheral portions of the physis results in angular deformities, centrally located lesions may cause longitudinal shortening.[141]

The cellular and molecular mechanisms for the bone bridge formation at the site of physeal injury site remain largely unknown. Using a proximal tibial drill-hole transphyseal injury model in rats, a study from the authors' laboratory characterized the injury-induced responses and cellular mechanisms for the

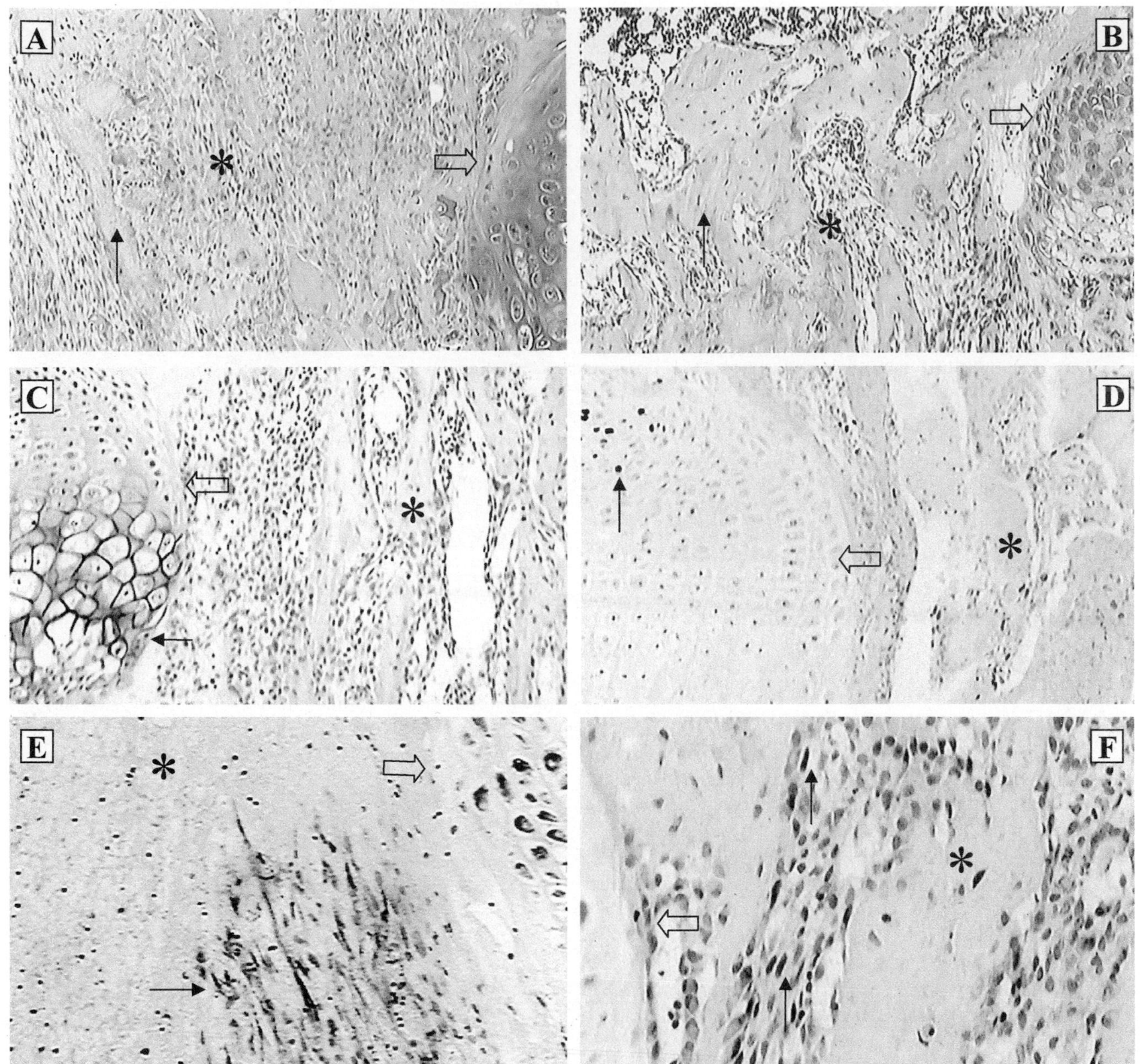

FIGURE 2-25 Intramembranous ossification mechanism for bone bridge formation at the growth plate injury site. Histologically (Barbara's histology stain), bony bridge trabeculae start to appear on day 7 postinjury **(A)**, and become well-constructed on day 14 with marrow **(B)**. Prior to and during physeal bar formation, there is no new cartilage formation, no collagen-X synthesis (as examined by immunostaining) at the injury site **(C)**, and no expansion of chondrocyte proliferation (as examined by BrdU labeling) from adjacent physeal cartilage **(D)**. Starting from day 3 **(E)** until day 14, there is infiltration of marrow-derived fibroblast-like mesenchymal cells (as examined by vimentin immunostaining), some of which are osteoblast precursor cells displaying positive immunostaining for bone cell differentiation transcription factor cbf-a1 **(F)** and *(continues)*

bone bridge formation (Fig. 2-25).[228] At the physeal injury site, this study demonstrated an early acute inflammatory response (up to day 3 postinjury). Straight after this inflammatory response, the injury site was filled by mesenchymal infiltrate (days 3 to 14) and subsequently was repaired by bone bridge formation (starting from day 7). Histologically, bony bridge trabeculae appeared on day 7 (Fig. 2-25A) and became well-constructed on day 14 with marrow (Fig. 2-25B). Before and during physeal bar formation, there were no new cartilage formation, no collagen-X synthesis at the injury site (Fig. 2-25C), and no expansion of chondrocyte proliferation from adjacent physeal cartilage (Fig. 2-25D), suggesting that the bone bridge formation did not involve endochondral ossification in this rat model. These results are consistent with an earlier study that reported a lack of increased expression of IHH and collagen-2, two molecules typically involved in endochondral ossification.[98] Furthermore, Xian et al's[228] study also demonstrated infiltration of marrow-derived fibroblast-like mesenchymal cells starting from day 3 (Fig. 2-25E), presence of osteoblast precursor cells among the mesenchymal infiltrates and their close proximity to bone bridge trabeculae (Fig. 2-25F, Fig. 2-25G), and production of bone matrix protein osteocalcin during for-

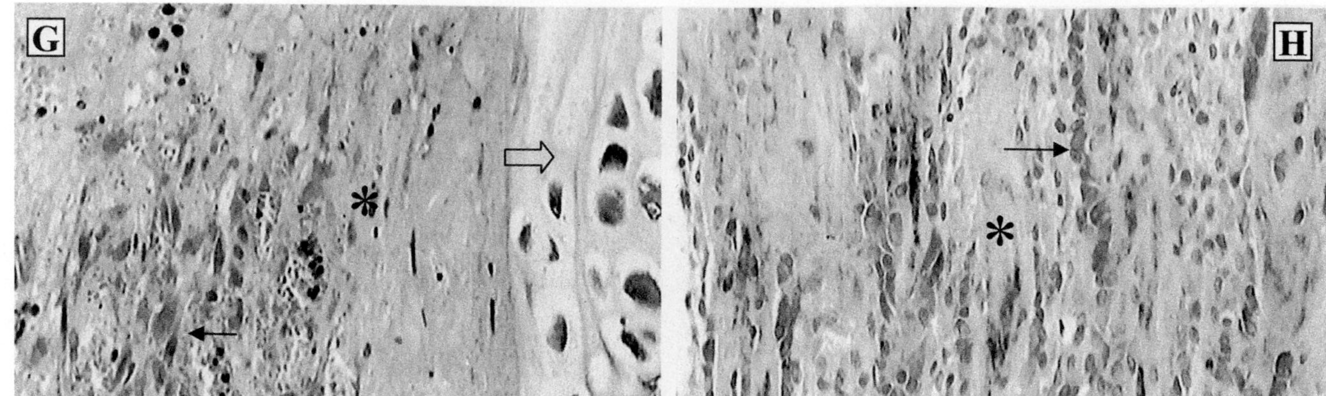

FIGURE 2-25 (*continued*) osteoblast/osteoprogenitor maturation marker alkaline phosphatase **(G)**. During bone bridge formation, bone matrix protein osteocalcin is produced by osteoblasts on bone bridge trabeculae (immunostaining) **(H)**. *, injury site; *block arrow*, pointing to adjacent growth plate cartilage; *small arrow*, pointing to bone bridge trabeculae or immunostained positive cells. This photo-composite is derived from the authors' previous study. (From Xian CJ, Zhou FH, McCarty RC, et al. Intramembranous ossification mechanism for bone bridge formation at the growth plate cartilage injury site. *J Orthop Res* 2004;22:417–426; with permission from copyright 2004 Orthopaedic Research Society.)

mation of bone bridge trabeculae (Fig. 2-25H). These results suggested that bone bridge formation after physeal injury in this rat model occurs directly via intramembranous ossification through recruitment of marrow-derived osteoprogenitor cells.[228]

Remodeling of Bones in Children after Injury

In a growing child, the normal process of bone remodeling in the diaphysis and metaphysis (particularly the latter) may realign initially malunited fragments, making anatomic reduction less important than in a comparable injury in an adult. However, although some residual angular deformities undergo spontaneous correction, accurate anatomic reduction should be the goal whenever possible.[58,142,149] Bone and cartilage generally remodel in response to normal stresses of body weight, muscle action, and joint reaction forces, as well as intrinsic control mechanisms such as the periosteum. The potential for spontaneous, complete correction is greater if the child is younger, the fracture site is closer to the physis, and there is relative alignment of the angulation in the normal plane of motion of the joint. This is particularly evident in fractures involving hinge joints such as the knee, ankle, elbow, or wrist, in which corrections are relatively rapid if the angulation is in the normal plane of motion. However, spontaneous correction of angular deformities is unlikely in other directions, such as a cubitus varus deformity following a supracondylar fracture of the humerus. Similarly, rotational deformities usually do not correct spontaneously.

Growth Stimulation

Fractures may stimulate longitudinal growth by increasing the blood supply to the metaphysis, physis, and epiphysis, and at least on an experimental basis, by disrupting the periosteum and its physiologic restraint on the rates of longitudinal growth of the physes.[38] Such increased growth may make the bone longer than it would have been without an injury.[42,213] Eccentric overgrowth may also occur; this is particularly evident in tibia valgum following an incomplete fracture of the proximal tibial metaphysis.

THE FUTURE OF FRACTURE REPAIR

Bone grafts contain bone growth factors that normally induce bone formation and have the appropriate osteoconductive matrix. Autogenic grafts also contain osteogenic cells. Bone grafts are effective, but there are difficulties in obtaining safe and reliable source tissue. Although the mechanisms of fracture repair are not fully understood, the level of understanding has enabled key molecules or cells to be targeted as therapeutic in controlling and promoting fracture repair. Filler compounds have been developed that stimulate proliferation of mesenchymal cells, and/or enhance their osteoblast or chondrocyte differentiation, leading to formation of new bone or cartilage (osteoinductive or chondrogenic) or enabling the cells to infiltrate and incorporate into bone (osteoconductive) or cartilage. Further studies on repair of bone, articular cartilage, or physis are required to understand the contribution of different cell types (inflammatory, endothelial, chondrocytic, osteoblastic and osteoclastic cells) to the repair process and their associated regulatory molecular pathways. In order to develop the most optimal strategies to treat fracture-associated complications that allow for lower effective doses and fewer side effects, more studies should also be carried out to identify and to test the optimal growth factors, novel factors, inhibitors or their small-molecule mimetics, cell-based therapy including stem cells, and/or gene therapy and their delivery systems.

Growth Factor Therapy

Specific growth factors have been targeted for their ability to promote bone formation. Due to their ability to stimulate proliferation and differentiation of mesenchymal and osteoprogenitor cells, two bone morphogenic proteins (BMP-2 and BMP-7) have shown great promise and acceptance for their ability to promote fracture repair.[90,91,103,104,113,202,224] BMP-2 promotes bone formation and repair in critical size defects, fractures and spinal fusions in human, and has been recently approved for clinical use in fracture repair (Wyeth Pharmaceutical) and spinal fusion (Medtronic Sofamor Danek, Memphis, TN). Like BMP-2, BMP-7 (also called osteogenic protein-1, OP-1) induces ectopic bone formation in vivo and enhances bone repair in preclinical models and clinical studies.[25] Clinically, OP-1, delivered with a type-1 collagen carrier, induced bone repair, which was found to be equivalent to autogenous bone graft in a clinical trial of patients with tibial nonunions.[54] OP-1 has now been approved for use in the treatment of established nonunions (Stryker Biotech).

A number of other growth factors, such as TGF-β, IGF-1, PDGFs, and FGF-2, also may prove to be useful. TGF-β plays a major role in fracture repair by promoting proliferation and differentiation of the mesenchymal cells. Exogenous TGF-β administration can initiate the repair process and callus formation in uninjured bone.[82] The addition of TGF-β to fractures results in a larger, stronger callus.[82] It also may be of use in promoting repair in nonhealing bone defects. PDGF also increases callus size but does not improve the fracture mechanically.[131] Growth hormone and IGF-1 have also been tested to determine their effects on fracture repair. Although growth hormone produces inconsistent results,[3] the administration of IGF-1 increases intramembranous bone formation.[205] The FGFs stimulate mitogenesis of mesenchymal cells and osteoblasts, increase the callus size and mineral content, and improve mechanical stability at early stages of fracture repair.[77,85,218] FGF-2 also increases osteoclastic bone remodeling.[131] In addition, it is possible that the effects of FGFs[22] and of a number of the other growth factors are a result of the angiogenic properties of such growth factors, as most osteogenic factors also stimulate angiogenesis, if not directly, then indirectly, through production of angiogenic molecules, such as VEGF. The potential synergism between potent pro-angiogenic factors (such as VEGF) and strong osteoinductive factors (such as BMPs) suggest that combination therapies might produce optimal results, particularly for individuals at risk of delayed repair or nonunions.[25]

Although there have been many studies and reviews on the use of growth factors for fracture repair[25,43,44,103,104,173,204] and some successful clinical applications of BMP-2 and OP-1 in inducing bone formation and repair, more research is required to establish the most effective delivery devices for these growth factors.[76] Apart from the requirements of biocompatibility and effectiveness, the growth factor carriers or delivery matrix systems or devices need to make the growth factor delivery cost-effective and practical in their clinical applications to induce bone formation in vivo, which should allow the application of relatively low doses of growth factors for optimal bone or cartilage regeneration in clinical contexts.

Tissue Engineering, Stem Cell and Gene Therapies

In the past decade, there has been an increasing interest in tissue engineering and mesenchymal stem cells for bone reconstruction of nonunion defects and for articular cartilage regeneration. Using tissue-engineering technologies, it is now possible to enhance bone repair and/or replace bone defect; and using the patient's own articular chondrocytes retrieved during arthroscopy and expanded in vitro, it is now possible to repair full-thickness articular cartilage defects with satisfactory clinical results.[137] Researchers worldwide are working to prepare the three fundamental components for the successful orthopaedic tissue engineering: (a) appropriate biological or artificial carriers or delivery systems or extracellular matrix scaffolds, and (b) the right set of viable responding cells (such as mesenchymal stem cells) in combination with (c) appropriate soluble inductive signal molecules or growth factors that, once transplanted, will ensure bone repair and/or cartilage regeneration.[173]

In particular, due to the capacity of self expansion in vitro, the less stringent ethical and regulatory issues and the lack of immunologic implications, mesenchymal stem cells derived from autologous bone marrow stroma have been the research focus for their potential applications, which have offered a new perspective for bone and cartilage tissue engineering. There have been some excellent advances in understanding the stem cells, their interactions with their matrix, particularly stimuli or signal molecules controlling their proliferation (such as LIF, FGF-2, HGF, Wnt and Dickkopt-1), osteogenic differentiation (such as IHH, Notch-1 and PPARgamma), and chondrogenic differentiation (such as BMP-4 and TGF-β3).[157] However, preclinical and clinical evaluations of the stromal stem cells or their derived osteoblasts or chondrocytes or the engineered bone or cartilage tissues will yet have to prove their efficacy, biocompatibility, safety, practicality, and reproducibility in bone and cartilage regeneration.[108]

Genetic engineering or gene transfer technology has also opened novel treatment avenues for the regeneration or repair of damaged articular cartilage, as gene transfer provides the capability to deliver bioactive proteins or gene products to sites of tissue damage locally and in a sustained manner. Previous research has already convincingly demonstrated the principle of gene delivery to synovium, chondrocytes and mesenchymal progenitor cells, and efficacy studies provide optimism that this gene transfer approach can be used to enhance articular cartilage repair.[206]

Regeneration of Injured Physeal Cartilage

Biological regeneration of physeal cartilage remains a great challenge. Foster and colleagues[53] have used a sheep tibial physeal injury model to investigate therapeutic potential of transplanted chondrocytes or periosteum,[226] and more recently growth factor OP-1.[81] They unfortunately found that these treatments under the experimental conditions were not preventative of bony bridge formation. Similarly, in a rat tibial physeal fracture model, Gruber et al[63] found that interposed periosteum at the fracture site could not enhance healing of the fractured physis, and in a rabbit tibial physeal injury model, Lee et al[97] observed that BMP-2 gene therapy delivered via adenoviral vectors within muscle implant caused increased osteogenic activity in the injured physis. Previous work has demonstrated that implantation of cultured chondrocytes embedded in agarose into physeal defects resulted in a partial correction of angular deformity and a significant reduction in growth arrest in a rabbit model,[96] and muscle-based gene therapy with adenoviral vectors encoding for IGF-1 restored the injured physeal cartilage.[97] More recently, direct transfer of periosteum-derived mesenchymal stem cells embedded in agarose into the tibial physeal defect resulted in regeneration of the physis, preventing growth arrest or angular deformity of the tibia.[31,101] The search for the optimal treatment options to achieve correction of angular deformity and to prevent limb length discrepancy using tissue engineering will continue and is not clinically applicable at this time.

ACKNOWLEDGMENTS

Supported in part by the Bone Growth Foundation (Australia), Channel-7 Children's Research Foundation of South Australia, National Health and Medical Research Council of Australia, Skeletal Educational Association, and the Foundation for Musculoskeletal Research and Education. The authors would like to acknowledge the contribution of Drs. Edward W. Johnstone, John A. Ogden, Timothy M. Ganey, and Dali A. Ogden, writers of the previous two editions, of which parts have been updated and carried forward.

REFERENCES

1. Acheson RM. Effects of starvation, septicaemia, and chronic illness on the growth cartilage plate and metaphysis of the immature rat. J Anat 1959;93:123–130.
2. Alvarez J, Sohn P, Zeng X, et al. TGFbeta2 mediates the effects of hedgehog on hypertrophic differentiation and PTHrP expression. Development 2002;129:1913–1924.
3. Bak B. Fracture healing and growth hormone. A biochemical study in the rat. Dan Med Bull 1993;40:519–536.
4. Baker J, Liu JP, Robertson EJ, et al. Role of insulin-like growth factors in embryonic and postnatal growth. Cell 1993;75:73–82.
5. Ballock RT, O'Keefe RJ. The biology of the growth plate. J Bone Joint Surg Am 2003; 85A:715–726.
6. Barnard R, Haynes KM, Werther GA, et al. The ontogeny of growth hormone receptors in the rabbit tibia. Endocrinology 1988;122:2562–2569.
7. Baron J, Klein KO, Yanovski JA, et al. Induction of growth plate cartilage ossification by basic fibroblast growth factor. Endocrinology 1994;135:2790–2793.
8. Bateman JF, Lamande SR, Ramshaw JAM. Collagen superfamily. In: Comper WD, ed. Extracellular matrix. Amsterdam: Harwood Academic Publishers, 1996:22–67.
9. Beckman F, Sullivan J. Some observations of fractures of long bones in the child. Am J Surg 1941;51:722–738.
10. Bianco P, Fisher LW, Young MF, et al. Expression and localization of the two small proteoglycans biglycan and decorin in developing human skeletal and nonskeletal tissues. J Histochem Cytochem 1990;38:1549–1563.
11. Birk DE, Fitch JM, Babiarz JP, et al. Collagen fibrillogenesis in vitro: interaction of types I and V collagen regulates fibril diameter. J Cell Sci 1990;95:649–657.
12. Bolander ME, Young MF, Fisher LW, et al. Osteonectin cDNA sequence reveals potential binding regions for calcium and hydroxyapatite and shows homologies with both a basement membrane protein (SPARC) and a serine proteinase inhibitor (ovomucoid). Proc Natl Acad Sci USA 1998;85:2919–2923.
13. Bonassar LJ, Trippel SB. Interaction of epidermal growth factor and insulin-like growth factor-I in the regulation of growth plate chondrocytes. Exp Cell Res 1997;234:1–6.
14. Border WA, Noble NA, Yamamoto T, et al. Natural inhibitor of transforming growth factor-beta protects against scarring in experimental kidney disease. Nature 1992;360: 361–364.
15. Boyan BD, Schwartz Z, Park-Snyder S, et al. Latent transforming growth factor-beta is produced by chondrocytes and activated by extracellular matrix vesicles upon exposure to 1,25-(OH)2D3. J Biol Chem 1994;269:28374–28381.
16. Boyle WJ, Simonet WS, Lacey DL. Osteoclast differentiation and activation. Nature 2003;423:337–342.
17. Brashear HR Jr. Epiphyseal fractures—a microscopic study of the healing process in rats. J Bone Joint Surg Am 1959;41A:1055–1064.
18. Brunet LJ, McMahon JA, McMahon AP, et al. Noggin, cartilage morphogenesis, and joint formation in the mammalian skeleton. Science 1998,280:1455–1457.
19. Bucholz RW, Ogden JA. Patterns of ischemic necrosis of the proximal femur in nonoperatively treated congenital hip disease. In: Nelson CL, ed. The hip: Proceedings of the Hip Society, vol 6. St. Louis: CV Mosby, 1978:43–63.
20. Buckwalter JA, Glimcher MJ, Cooper RR, et al. Bone biology. I: structure, blood supply, cells, matrix, and mineralization. Instr Course Lect 1996;45:371–386.
21. Burger M, Sherman BS, Sobel AE. Observations on the influence of chondroitin sulphate on the rate of bone repair. J Bone Joint Surg 1962;44B:675–687.
22. Burgess WH, Mehlman T, Marshak DR, et al. Structural evidence that endothelial cell growth factor is the precursor of both endothelial cell growth factor and acidic fibroblast growth factor. Proc Natl Acad Sci USA 1986;83:7216–7220.
23. Byers S, van Rooden JC, Foster BK. Structural changes in the large proteoglycan, aggrecan, in different zones of the ovine growth plate. Calcif Tissue Int 1997;60:71–78.
24. Calandruccio RA, Gilmer WS. Proliferation, regeneration, and repair of articular cartilage of immature animals. J Bone Joint Surg 1962;44A:431–455.
25. Carano RA, Filvaroff EH. Angiogenesis and bone repair. Drug Discov Today 2003;8: 980–989.
26. Carey DE, Liu X. Expression of bone morphogenetic protein-6 messenger RNA in bovine growth plate chondrocytes of different size. J Bone Miner Res 1995;10:401–405.
27. Chalmers J, Gray DH, Rush J. Observations on the induction of bone in soft tissues. J Bone Joint Surg Br 1975;57:36–45.
28. Chan D, Taylor TK, Cole WG. Characterization of an arginine 789 to cysteine substitution in alpha-1(II) collagen chains of a patient with spondyloepiphyseal dysplasia. J Biol Chem 1993;268:15238–15245.
29. Chan SY, Wong RW. Expression of epidermal growth factor in transgenic mice causes growth retardation. J Biol Chem 2000;275:38693–38698.
30. Cheifetz S, Li IW, McCulloch CA, et al. Influence of osteogenic protein-1 (OP-1,P-7) and transforming growth factor-beta 1 on bone formation in vitro. Connect Tissue Res 1996;35:71–78.
31. Chen F, Hui JH, Chan WK, et al. Cultured mesenchymal stem cell transfers in the treatment of partial growth arrest. J Pediatr Orthop 2003;23:425–429.
32. Chintala SK, Miller RR, McDevitt CA. Basic fibroblast growth factor binds to heparan sulfate in the extracellular matrix of rat growth plate chondrocytes. Arch Biochem Biophys 1994;310:180–186.
33. Chintala SK, Miller RR, McDevitt CA. Role of heparan sulfate in the terminal differentiation of growth plate chondrocytes. Arch Biochem Biophys 1995;316:227–234.
34. Cohen S, Ushiro H, Stoscheck C, et al. A native 170,000 epidermal growth factor receptor-kinase complex from shed plasma membrane vesicles. J Biol Chem 1982;257: 1523–1531.
35. Conway EM, Collen D, Carmeliet P. Molecular mechanisms of blood vessel growth. Cardiovasc Res 2001;49:507–521.
36. Cowin SC, Moss-Salentijn L, Moss ML. Candidates for the mechanosensory system in bone. J Biomech Eng 1991;113:191–197.
37. Crelin ES, White AA, Panjabi MM, et al. Microscopic changes in fractured rabbit tibias. Conn Med 1978;42:561–569.
38. Crilly RG. Longitudinal overgrowth of chicken radius. J Anat 1972;112:11–18.
39. Daughaday WH, Hall K, Raben MS, et al. Somatomedin: proposed designation for sulphation factor. Nature 1972;235:107.
40. Ducy P, Desbois C, Boyce B, et al. Increased bone formation in osteocalcin-deficient mice. Nature 1996;382(6590):448–452.
41. Edmondson SR, Baker NL, Oh J, et al. Growth hormone receptor abundance in tibial growth plates of uremic rats: GH/IGF-I treatment. Kidney Int 2000;58:62–70.
42. Edvardson P, Syversen SM. Overgrowth of the femur after fractures of the shaft in childhood. J Bone Joint Surg Br 1976;58:339–346.
43. Einhorn TA. Enhancement of fracture healing. Instr Course Lect 1996;45:401–416.
44. Einhorn TA, Trippel SB. Growth factor treatment of fractures. Instr Course Lect 1997; 46:483–486.
45. Erickson DM, Harris SE, Dean DD, et al. Recombinant bone morphogenetic protein (BMP)-2 regulates costochondral growth plate chondrocytes and induces expression of BMP-2 and BMP-4 in a cell maturation–dependent manner. J Orthop Res 1997;15: 371–380.
46. Erlebacher A, Derynck R. Increased expression of TGF-beta 2 in osteoblasts results in an osteoporosis-like phenotype. J Cell Biol 1996;132:195–210.
47. Erlebacher A, Filvaroff EH, Ye JQ, et al. Osteoblastic responses to TGF-beta during bone remodeling. Mol Biol Cell 1998;9:1903–1918.
48. Evans RM. The steroid and thyroid hormone receptor superfamily. Science 1988;240: 889–895.
49. Eyre DR, Upton MP, Shapiro FD, et al. Nonexpression of cartilage type II collagen in a case of Langer-Saldino achondrogenesis. Am J Hum Genet 1986;39:52–67.
50. Fichard A, Kleman JP, Ruggiero F. Another look at collagen V and XI molecules. Matrix Biol 1994;14:515–531.
51. Finkbeiner S. Calcium waves in astrocytes-filling in the gaps. Neuron 1992;8: 1101–1108.
52. Fosang A, Hardingham T. Matrix proteoglycans. In: Comper WD, ed. Extracellular matrix. Amsterdam: Harwood Academic Publishers, 1996:200–229.
53. Foster BK, Hansen AL, Gibson GJ, et al. Reimplantation of growth plate chondrocytes into growth plate defects in sheep. J Orthop Res 1990;8:555–564.
54. Friedlaender GE, Perry CR, Cole JD, et al. Osteogenic protein-1 (bone morphogenetic protein-7) in the treatment of tibial nonunions. J Bone Joint Surg Am 2001;83A(Suppl 1):S151–S158.
55. Gazzerro E, Gangji V, Canalis E. Bone morphogenetic proteins induce the expression of noggin, which limits their activity in cultured rat osteoblasts. J Clin Invest 1998; 102:2106–2114.
56. Gerber HP, Vu TH, Ryan AM, et al. VEGF couples hypertrophic cartilage remodeling, ossification and angiogenesis during endochondral bone formation. Nat Med 1999;5: 623–628.
57. Gerstenfeld LC, Cullinane DM, Barnes GL, et al. Fracture healing as a postnatal developmental process: molecular, spatial, and temporal aspects of its regulation. J Cell Biochem 2003;88:873–884.
58. Giberson RG, Ivins JC. Fractures of the distal part of the forearm in children: correction of deformity by growth. Minn Med 1952;35:744.
59. Gibson G, Lin DL, Francki K, et al. Type X collagen is colocalized with a proteoglycan epitope to form distinct morphological structures in bovine growth cartilage. Bone 1996;19:307–315.
60. Goldhaber P. Osteogenic induction across millipore filters in vivo. Science 1961;133: 2065–2067.
61. Gotham L. Vascular reactions in experimental fractures: microangiographic and radioisotope studies. Acta Chir Scand Suppl 1961;284(Suppl):1–34.
62. Grissom LE, Harcke HT. Radiographic features of bisphosphonate therapy in pediatric patients. Pediatr Radiol 2003;33:226–229.
63. Gruber HE, Phieffer LS, Wattenbarger JM. Physeal fractures, part II: fate of interposed periosteum in a physeal fracture. J Pediatr Orthop 2002;22:710–716.
64. Ham AW. A histological study of the early phase of bone repair. J Bone Joint Surg 1930;12:827–844.
65. Ham AW. Histology. 6th ed. Philadelphia: JB Lippincott, 1969.
66. Hanlon CR, Estes WL Jr. Fractures in childhood—A statistical analysis. Am J Surg 1954;87:312–323.
67. Harris HA. The growth of long bones in childhood with special reference to certain bony striations of the metaphysis and to the role of vitamins. Arch Intern Med 1926; 38:785–806.
68. Hauschka PV, Lian JB, Cole DE, et al. Osteocalcin and matrix Gla protein: vitamin K-dependent proteins in bone. Physiol Rev 1989;69:990–1047.
69. Hauschka PV, Mavrakos AE, Iafrati MD, et al. Growth factors in bone matrix. Isolation of multiple types by affinity chromatography on heparin-Sepharose. J Biol Chem 1986; 261:12665–12674.
70. Hearn MT. Structure and function of the heparin-binding (fibroblast) growth factor family. Baillieres Clin Endocrinol Metab 1991;5:571–593.

71. Hedbom E, Heinegård D. Binding of fibromodulin and decorin to separate sites on fibrillar collagens. J Biol Chem 1993;268:27307–27312.
72. Hildebrand A, Romarís M, Rasmussen LM, et al. Interaction of the small interstitial proteoglycans biglycan, decorin, and fibromodulin with transforming growth factor beta. Biochem J 1994;302:527–534.
73. Hogan BL, Blessing M, Winnier GE, et al. Growth factors in development: the role of TGF-beta related polypeptide signalling molecules in embryogenesis. Dev Suppl 1994; 53–60.
74. Hultenby K, Reinholt FP, Heinegård D, et al. Osteopontin: a ligand for the alpha v beta 3 integrin of the osteoclast clear zone in osteopetrotic (ia/ia) rats. Ann N Y Acad Sci 1995;760:315–318.
75. Hunziker EB, Wagner J, Zapf J. Differential effects of insulin-like growth factor I and growth hormone on developmental stages of rat growth plate chondrocytes in vivo. J Clin Invest 1994;93:1078–1086.
76. Illi OE, Feldmann CP. Stimulation of fracture healing by local application of humoral factors integrated in biodegradable implants. Eur J Pediatr Surg 1998;8:251–255.
77. Inui K, Maeda M, Sano A, et al. Local application of basic fibroblast growth factor minipellet induces the healing of segmental bony defects in rabbits. Calcif Tissue Int 1998;63:490–495.
78. Issack PS, DiCesare PE. Recent advances toward the clinical application of bone morphogenetic proteins in bone and cartilage repair. Am J Orthop 2003;32:429–436.
79. Jacenko O, Ito S, Olsen BR. Skeletal and hematopoietic defects in mice transgenic for collagen X. Ann N Y Acad Sci 1996;785:278–280.
80. Jacenko O, LuValle PA, Olsen BR. Spondylometaphyseal dysplasia in mice carrying a dominant negative mutation in a matrix protein specific for cartilage-to-bone transition. Nature 1993;365:56–61.
81. Johnstone EW, McArthur M, Solly PB, et al. The effect of osteogenic protein 1 in an in vivo physeal injury model. Clin Orthop Relat Res 2002;395:234–240.
82. Joyce ME, Jingushi S, Scully SP, et al. Role of growth factors in fracture healing. Prog Clin Biol Res 1991;365:391–416.
83. Kaplan FS, Hayes WC, Keaveny TM, et al. Form and function of bone. In: Simon SR, ed. Orthopaedic basic science: American Academy of Orthopaedic Surgeons. Rosemont, IL: Port City Press, 1994:127–184.
84. Katagiri T, Takahashi N. Regulatory mechanisms of osteoblast and osteoclast differentiation. Oral Dis 2002;8:147–159.
85. Kato T, Kawaguchi H, Hanada K, et al. Single local injection of recombinant fibroblast growth factor-2 stimulates healing of segmental bone defects in rabbits. J Orthop Res 1998;16:654–659.
86. Keck SW, Kelly PJ. The effect of venous stasis on intraosseous pressure and longitudinal bone growth in the dog. J Bone Joint Surg Am 1965;47A:539–544.
87. Keene DR, Oxford JT, Morris NP. Ultrastructural localization of collagen types II, IX, and XI in the growth plate of human rib and fetal bovine epiphyseal cartilage: type XI collagen is restricted to thin fibrils. J Histochem Cytochem 1995;43:967–979.
88. Kielty CM, Kwan AP, Holmes DF, et al. Type X collagen, a product of hypertrophic chondrocytes. Biochem J 1985;227:545–554.
89. Kirsch T, von der Mark K. Isolation of bovine type X collagen and immunolocalization in growth-plate cartilage. Biochem J 1990;265:453–459.
90. Klein-Nulend J, Louwerse RT, Heyligers IC, et al. Osteogenic protein (OP-1, BMP-7) stimulates cartilage differentiation of human and goat perichondrium tissue in vitro. J Biomed Mater Res 1998;40:614–620.
91. Klein-Nulend J, Semeins CM, Mulder JW, et al. Stimulation of cartilage differentiation by osteogenic protein-1 in cultures of human perichondrium. Tissue Eng 1998;4: 305–313.
92. Kobayashi K, Takahashi N, Jimi E, et al. Tumor necrosis factor alpha stimulates osteoclast differentiation by a mechanism independent of the ODF/RANKL-RANK interaction. J Exp Med 2000;191:275–286.
93. Kronenberg HM. Developmental regulation of the growth plate. Nature 2003;423: 332–336.
94. Kronenberg HM, Lanske B, Kovacs CS, et al. Functional analysis of the PTH/PTHrP network of ligands and receptors. Recent Prog Horm Res 1998;53:283–301; discussion 301–303.
95. Lacroix P. The organization of Bone. Philadelphia: Blakiston, 1951.
96. Lee EH, Chen F, Chan J, et al. Treatment of growth arrest by transfer of cultured chondrocytes into physeal defects. J Pediatr Orthop 1998;18:155–160.
97. Lee CW, Martinek V, Usas A, et al. Muscle-based gene therapy and tissue engineering for treatment of growth plate injuries. J Pediatr Orthop 2002;22:565–572.
98. Lee MA, Nissen TP, Otsuka NY. Utilization of a murine model to investigate the molecular process of transphyseal bone formation. J Pediatr Orthop 2000;20:802–806.
99. Legeai-Mallet L, Benoist-Lasselin C, Delezoide AL, et al. Fibroblast growth factor receptor 3 mutations promote apoptosis but do not alter chondrocyte proliferation in thanatophoric dysplasia. J Biol Chem 1998;273:13007–13014.
100. Levi-Montalcini R, Hamburger V. Selective growth stimulating effects of mouse sarcoma on the sensory and sympathetic nervous system of the chick embryo. J Exp Zool 1951; 116:321–362.
101. Li L, Hui JH, Goh JC, et al. Chitin as a scaffold for mesenchymal stem cells transfers in the treatment of partial growth arrest. J Pediatr Orthop 2004;24:205–210.
102. Light TR, McKinstry MP, Schnitzer J, et al. Bone blood flow: regional variation with skeletal maturation. In: Arlet J, Ficat RP, Hungerford DS, eds. Bone circulation. Baltimore: Williams & Wilkins, 1984.
103. Lind M. Growth factor stimulation of bone healing. Effects on osteoblasts, osteomies, and implants fixation. Acta Orthop Scand Suppl 1998;283:2–37.
104. Lind M. Growth factors: possible new clinical tools. A review. Acta Orthop Scand 1996; 67:407–417.
105. Liu JP, Baker J, Perkins AS, et al. Mice carrying null mutations of the genes encoding insulin-like growth factor I (Igf-1) and type 1 IGF receptor (Igf1r). Cell 1993;75:59–72.
106. Liu Z, Xu J, Colvin JS, et al. Coordination of chondrogenesis and osteogenesis by fibroblast growth factor 18. Genes Dev 2002;16:859–869.
107. Lockwood R, Latta LL. Bone blood flow changes with diaphyseal fracture. Trans Orthop Res Soc 1980;5:158.
108. Lucarelli E, Donati D, Cenacchi A, et al. Bone reconstruction of large defects using bone marrow derived autologous stem cells. Transfus Apheresis Sci 2004;30:169–174.
109. Luo G, Ducy P, McKee MD, et al. Spontaneous calcification of arteries and cartilage in mice lacking matrix GLA protein. Nature 1997;385:78–81.
110. Makower AM, Wroblewski J, Pawlowski A. Effects of IGF-I, rGH, FGF, EGF and NCS on DNA-synthesis, cell proliferation and morphology of chondrocytes isolated from rat rib growth cartilage. Cell Biol Int Rep 1989;13:259–270.
111. Mancilla EE, De Luca F, Uyeda JA, et al. Effects of fibroblast growth factor-2 on longitudinal bone growth. Endocrinology 1998;139:2900–2904.
112. Manolagas SC. Birth and death of bone cells: basic regulatory mechanisms and implications for the pathogenesis and treatment of osteoporosis. Endocr Rev 2000;21: 115–137.
113. Margolin MD, Cogan AG, Taylor M, et al. Maxillary sinus augmentation in the non-human primate: a comparative radiographic and histologic study between recombinant human osteogenic protein-1 and natural bone mineral. J Periodontol 1998;69:911–919.
114. Marks SC Jr. Osteoclast biology: lessons from mammalian mutations. Am J Med Genet 1998;34:43–54.
115. Massagué J. Receptors for the TGF-beta family. Cell 1992;69:1067–1070.
116. Massagué J. The transforming growth factor-β family. J Biol Chem 1990;6:597–641.
117. Massagué J, Weis-Garcia F. Serine/threonine kinase receptors: mediators of transforming growth factor beta family signals. Cancer Surv 1996;27:41–64.
118. McCarthy TL, Centrella M. Local IGF-I expression and bone formation. Growth Horm IGF Res 2001;11:213–219.
119. McKee MD, Nanci A. Osteopontin at mineralized tissue interfaces in bone, teeth, and osseointegrated implants: ultrastructural distribution and implications for mineralized tissue formation, turnover, and repair. Microsc Res Tech 1996;33:141–164.
120. McKibbin B. The biology of fracture healing in long bones. J Bone Joint Surg Br 1978; 60B:150–162.
121. McKinstry P, Schnitzer JE, Light TR, et al. Relationship of 99mTC-MDP uptake to regional osseous circulation in skeletally immature and mature dogs. Skeletal Radiol 1982;8:115–121.
122. Meikle MC, Bord S, Hembry RM, et al. Human osteoblasts in culture synthesize collagenase and other matrix metalloproteinases in response to osteotropic hormones and cytokines. J Cell Sci 1992;103:1093–1099.
123. Meikle MC, McGarrity AM, Thomson BM, et al. Bone-derived growth factors modulate collagenase and TIMP (tissue inhibitor of metalloproteinases) activity and type I collagen degradation by mouse calvarial osteoblasts. Bone Miner 1991;12:41–55.
124. Miettinen PJ, Chin JR, Shum L, et al. Epidermal growth factor receptor function is necessary for normal craniofacial development and palate closure. Nat Genet 1999;22: 69–73.
125. Minina E, Kreschel C, Naski MC, et al. Interaction of FGF, Ihh/Pthlh, and BMP signaling integrates chondrocyte proliferation and hypertrophic differentiation. Dev Cell 2002; 3:439–449.
126. Mizuta T, Benson WM, Foster BK, et al. Statistical analysis of the incidence of physeal injuries. J Pediatr Orthop 1987;7:518–523.
127. Moolenaar WH, Defize LH, de Laat SW. Calcium in the action of growth factors. Ciba Found Symp 1986;122:212–231.
128. Morscher E. Posttraumatic zapfenepiphyse. Arch Orthop Unfallchir 1967;61:128–136.
129. Muir H. The chondrocyte, architect of cartilage. Biomechanics, structure, function, and molecular biology of cartilage matrix macromolecules. Bioessays 1995;17:1039–1048.
130. Nakahara H, Goldberg VM, Caplan AI. Culture-expanded human periosteal-derived cells exhibit osteochondral potential in vivo. J Orthop Res 1991;9:465–476.
131. Nash TJ, Howlett CR, Martin C, et al. Effect of platelet-derived growth factor on tibial osteotomies in rabbits. Bone 1994;15:203–208.
132. Naski MC, Ornitz DM. FGF signaling in skeletal development. Front Biosci 1998;3: D781–D794.
133. Neufeld G, Gospodarowicz D. The identification and partial characterization of the fibroblast growth factor receptor of baby hamster kidney cells. J Biol Chem 1985;260: 13860–13868.
134. Niedermann B, Boe S, Lauritzen J, et al. Glued periosteal grafts in the knee. Acta Orthop Scand 1985;56:457–460.
135. Nilsson A, Ohlsson C, Isaksson OG, et al. Hormonal regulation of longitudinal bone growth. Eur J Clin Nutr 1994;48(Supp l)1:S150–S158; discussion S158–S160.
136. O'Driscoll SW, Fitzsimmons JS. The role of periosteum in cartilage repair. Clin Orthop Relat Res 2001;391:S190–S207.
137. Oakes BW. Orthopaedic tissue engineering: from laboratory to the clinic. Med J Aust 2004;180:S35–S38.
138. Ogden JA. An anatomical and histological study of the factors affecting development and evolution of avascular necrosis in congenital dislocation of the hip. In: Harris WH, ed. The hip: proceedings of the Hip Society, vol 2. St. Louis: CV Mosby, 1974:125–153.
139. Ogden JA. Chondro-osseous development and growth. In: Urist MR, ed. Fundamental and clinical bone physiology. Philadelphia: JB Lippincott, 1980.
140. Ogden JA. Growth slowdown and arrest lines. J Pediatr Orthop 1984;4:409–415.
141. Ogden JA. Injury to the immature skeleton. In: Touloukian R, ed. Pediatric Trauma, 2nd ed. New York: John Wiley & Sons, 1990.
142. Ogden JA. Skeletal Injury in the Child, 2nd ed. Philadelphia: WB Saunders, 1990.
143. Ogden JA. The development and growth of the musculoskeletal system. In: Albright JA, Brand RA, eds. The Scientific Basis of Orthopaedics. New York: Appleton-Century-Crofts, 1979.
144. Ogden JA. The role of orthopaedic surgery in sports medicine. Yale J Biol Med 1980; 53:281–288.
145. Ogden JA, Grogan DP, Light TR. Postnatal skeletal development and growth of musculoskeletal system. In: Albright JA, Brand RD, eds. The scientific Basis of Orthopaedics. New York: Appleton & Lange, 1987.
146. Ogden JA, Hempton RJ, Southwick WO. Development of the tibial tuberosity. Anat Rec 1975;182:431–445.
147. Ogden JA, Pais MJ, Murphy MJ, et al. Ectopic bone secondary to avulsion of periosteum. Skeletal Radiol 1979;4:124–128.
148. Ogden JA, Rosenberg LC. Defining the growth plate. In: Uhthoff HK, Wiley JJ, eds. Behavior of the Growth Plate. New York: Raven Press, 1988.
149. Ogden JA, Southwick WO. Adequate reduction of fractures and dislocations. Radiol Clin North Am 1973;11:667–681.
150. Ogden JA, Southwick WO. Electrical injury involving the immature skeleton. Skeletal Radiol 1981;6:187–192.
151. Ogden JA, Southwick WO. Osgood-Schlatter disease and tibial tuberosity development. Clin Orthop Relat Res 1976;116:180–189.

152. Ogden JA, Tross RB, Murphy MJ. Fractures of the tibial tuberosity in adolescents. J Bone Joint Surg Am 1980;62A:205–215.
153. Ohlsson C, Nilsson A, Isaksson O, et al. Growth hormone induces multiplication of the slowly cycling germinal cells of the rat tibial growth plate. Proc Natl Acad Sci USA 1992;89:9826–9830.
154. Olsen BR. Mutations in collagen genes resulting in metaphyseal and epiphyseal dysplasias. Bone 1995;17:S45–S49.
155. Ornitz DM, Itoh N. Fibroblast growth factors. Genome Biol 2001;2:REVIEWS3005.
156. Ornitz DM, Marie PJ. FGF signaling pathways in endochondral and intramembranous bone development and human genetic disease. Genes Dev 2002;16:1446–1465.
157. Otto WR, Rao J. Tomorrow's skeleton staff: mesenchymal stem cells and the repair of bone and cartilage. Cell Prolif 2004;37:97–110.
158. Owen M. The origin of bone cells. Int Rev Cytol 1970;28:213–238.
159. Pardridge WM. Transport of protein-bound hormones into tissues in vivo. Endocr Rev 1981;2:103–123.
160. Park EA. Bone growth in health and disease. Arch Dis Child 1954;29:269–281.
161. Park EA. The imprinting of nutritional disturbances on growing bone. Pediatrics 1964; 33:815–862.
162. Paschalis EP, Jacenko O, Olsen B, et al. The role of type X collagen in endochondral ossification as deduced by Fourier transform infrared microscopy analysis. Connect Tissue Res 1996;35:371–377.
163. Pearce JJ, Penny G, Rossant J. A mouse cerberus/Dan-related gene family. Dev Biol 1999;209:98–110.
164. Pechak DG, Kujawa MJ, Caplan AI. Morphology of bone development and bone remodeling in embryonic chick limbs. Bone 1986;7:459–472.
165. Petit B, Ronzière MC, Hartmann DJ, et al. Ultrastructural organization of type XI collagen in fetal bovine epiphyseal cartilage. Histochemistry 1993;100:231–239.
166. Piccolo S, Sasai Y, Lu B, et al. Dorsoventral patterning in Xenopus: inhibition of ventral signals by direct binding of chordin to BMP-4. Cell 1996;86:589–598.
167. Poole AR, Matsui Y, Hinek A, et al. Cartilage macromolecules and the calcification of cartilage matrix. Anat Rec 1989;224:167–179.
168. Poole AR, Webber C, Pidoux I, et al. Localization of a dermatan sulfate proteoglycan (DS-PGII) in cartilage and the presence of an immunologically related species in other tissues. J Histochem Cytochem 1986;34:619–625.
169. Potts WJ. The role of the hematoma in fracture healing. Surg Gynecol Obstet 1933; 57:318–324.
170. Poussa M, Ritsilä V. The osteogenic capacity of free periosteal and osteoperiosteal grafts. A comparative study in growing rabbits. Acta Orthop Scand 1979;50:491–499.
171. Price PA. Gla-containing proteins of bone. Connect Tissue Res 1989;21:51–57.
172. Price PA, Williamson MK. Primary structure of bovine matrix Gla protein, a new vitamin K–dependent bone protein. J Biol Chem 1985;260:14971–14975.
173. Ramoshebi LN, Matsaba TN, Teare J, et al. Tissue engineering: TGF-beta superfamily members and delivery systems in bone regeneration. Expert Rev Mol Med 2002;4: 1–11.
174. Rappolee DA, Mark D, Banda MJ, et al. Wound macrophages express TGF-alpha and other growth factors in vivo: analysis by mRNA typing. Science 1988;241:708–712.
175. Reinecke M, Schmid AC, Heyberger-Meyer B, et al. Effect of growth hormone and insulin-like growth factor I (IGF-I) on the expression of IGF-I messenger ribonucleic acid and peptide in rat tibial growth plate and articular chondrocytes in vivo. Endocrinology 2000;141:2847–2853.
176. Reinholt FP, Hultenby K, Oldberg A, et al. Osteopontin—a possible anchor of osteoclasts to bone. Proc Natl Acad Sci USA 1990;87:4473–4475.
177. Rhinelander FW. Tibial blood supply in relation to fracture healing. Clin Orthop Relat Res 1974;105:34–81.
178. Rhinelander FW, Phillips RS, Steel WM, et al. Microangiography and bone healing. II. Displaced closed fractures. J Bone Joint Surg Am 1968;50(4):643–662 passim.
179. Röhlig H. Perlost und langenwachstum. Beitr Orthop Traumatol 1966;13:603–606.
180. Rokkanen P, Slaetis P. The repair of experimental fractures during long-term anticoagulant treatment. An experimental study on rats. Acta Orthop Scand 1964;35:21–38.
181. Rosati R, Horan GS, Pinero GJ, et al. Normal long bone growth and development in type X collagen-null mice. Nat Genet 1994;8:129–135.
182. Ryöppy S. Injuries of the growing skeleton. Ann Chir Gynaecol Fenn 1972;61:3–10.
183. Sandberg MM, Aro HT, Vuorio EI. Gene expression during bone repair. Clin Orthop Relat Res 1993;289:292–312.
184. Sandell LJ, Sugai JV, Trippel SB. Expression of collagens I, II, X, and XI and aggrecan mRNAs by bovine growth plate chondrocytes in situ. J Orthop Res 1994;12:1–14.
185. Schipani E, Provot S. PTHrP, PTH, and the PTH/PTHrP receptor in endochondral bone development. Birth Defects Res Part C Embryo Today 2003;69:352–362.
186. Schmitt JM, Hwang K, Winn SR, et al. Bone morphogenetic proteins: an update on basic biology and clinical relevance. J Orthop Res 1999;17:269–278.
187. Schnitzer JE, McKinstry P, Light TR, et al. Quantitation of regional chondro-osseous circulation in canine tibia and femur. Am J Physiol 1982;242:H365–H375.
188. Schnitzer JE, McKinstry P, Light TR, et al. Quantitation of regional osseous circulation in the maturing canine tibia and femur. Surg Forum 1980;31:509–511.
189. Schönherr E, Broszat M, Brandan E, et al. Decorin core protein fragment Leu155-Val260 interacts with TGF-beta but does not compete for decorin binding to type I collagen. Arch Biochem Biophys 1998;355:241–248.
190. Schönherr E, Hausser H, Beavan L, et al. Decorin-type I collagen interaction. Presence of separate core protein-binding domains. J Biol Chem 1995;270:8877–8883.
191. Schönherr E, Witsch-Prehm P, Harrach B, et al. Interaction of biglycan with type I collagen. J Biol Chem 1995;270:2776–2783.
192. Schultz GS, Grant MB. Neovascular growth factors. Eye 1991;5:170–180.
193. Scott-Savage P, Hall BK. Differentiative ability of the tibial periosteum for the embryonic chick. Acta Anat (Basel) 1980;106:129–140.
194. Siffert RS. The effect of trauma to the epiphysis and growth plate. Skeletal Radiol 1977; 2:21–30.
195. Sims NA, Clement-Lacroix P, Da Ponte F, et al. Bone homeostasis in growth hormone receptor-null mice is restored by IGF-I but independent of Stat5. J Clin Invest 2000; 106:1095–1103.
196. Sjögren K, Liu JL, Blad K, et al. Liver-derived insulin-like growth factor I (IGF-I) is the principal source of IGF-I in blood but is not required for postnatal body growth in mice. Proc Natl Acad Sci USA 1999;96:7088–7092.
197. Solloway MJ, Robertson EJ. Early embryonic lethality in Bmp5;Bmp7 double mutant mice suggests functional redundancy within the 60A subgroup. Development 1999; 126:1753–1768.
198. Speer DP. Collagenous architecture of the growth plate and perichondral ossification groove. J Bone Joint Surg Am 1982;64A:399–407.
199. Stevens MM, Qanadilo HF, Langer R, et al. A rapid-curing alginate gel system: utility in periosteum-derived cartilage tissue engineering. Biomaterials 2004;25:887–894.
200. Street J, Bao M, deGuzman L, et al. Vascular endothelial growth factor stimulates bone repair by promoting angiogenesis and bone turnover. Proc Natl Acad Sci USA 2002; 99:9656–9661.
201. Suda T, Takahashi N, Udagawa N, et al. Modulation of osteoclast differentiation and function by the new members of the tumor necrosis factor receptor and ligand families. Endocr Rev 1999;20:345–357.
202. Takiguchi T, Kobayashi M, Suzuki R, et al. Recombinant human bone morphogenetic protein-2 stimulates osteoblast differentiation and suppresses matrix metalloproteinase-1 production in human bone cells isolated from mandibulae. J Periodontal Res 1998; 33:476–485.
203. Treharne RW. Review of Wolff's law and its proposed means of operation. Orthop Rev 1981;10:35–44.
204. Trippel SB. Growth factors as therapeutic agents. Instr Course Lect 1997;46:473–476.
205. Trippel SB. Potential role of insulin-like growth factors in fracture healing. Clin Orthop Relat Res 1998;355:S301–S313.
206. Trippel SB, Ghivizzani SC, Nixon AJ. Gene-based approaches for the repair of articular cartilage. Gene Ther 2004;11:351–359.
207. Trippel SB, Van Wyk JJ, Foster MB, et al. Characterization of a specific somatomedin-c receptor on isolated bovine growth plate chondrocytes. Endocrinology 1983;112: 2128–2136.
208. Trippel SB, Wroblewski J, Makower AM, et al. Regulation of growth-plate chondrocytes by insulin-like growth-factor I and basic fibroblast growth factor. J Bone Joint Surg Am 1993;75:177–189.
209. Trueta J. Studies of the development and decay of the human frame. Philadelphia: WB Saunders, 1968.
210. Trueta J, Amato MP. The vascular contribution to osteogenis. III. Changes in the growth cartilage caused by experimentally induced ischaemia. J Bone Joint Surg Br 1960;42B: 571–587.
211. Trueta J, Cavadias AX. A study of the blood supply of the long bones. Surg Gynecol Obstet 1964;118:485–498.
212. Trueta J, Morgan JD. The vascular contribution to osteogenesis. I. Studies by the injection method. J Bone Joint Surg Br 1960;42B:97–109.
213. Tscherne H, Suren EG. Fehlstellungen, wachstumsstorungen, and pseudoarthrosen nach kindlichen frakturen. Langenbecks Arch Chir 1976;342:299–304.
214. Uhthoff HK, Rahn B. Healing patterns of metaphyseal fractures. Clin Orthop Relat Res 1981;(160)295–303.
215. van der Eerden BC, Karperien M, Gevers EF, et al. Expression of Indian hedgehog, parathyroid hormone-related protein, and their receptors in the postnatal growth plate of the rat: evidence for a locally acting growth restraining feedback loop after birth. J Bone Miner Res 2000;15:1045–1055.
216. Volk SW, Luvalle P, Leask T, et al. A BMP responsive transcriptional region in the chicken type X collagen gene. J Bone Miner Res 1998;13:1521–1529.
217. Vortkamp A, Lee K, Lanske B, et al. Regulation of rate of cartilage differentiation by Indian hedgehog and PTH-related protein. Science 1996;273:613–622.
218. Wang JS. Basic fibroblast growth factor for stimulation of bone formation in osteoinductive or conductive implants. Acta Orthop Scand Suppl 1996;269:1–33.
219. Wang EA, Rosen V, D'Alessandro JS, et al. Recombinant human bone morphogenetic protein induces bone formation. Proc Natl Acad Sci USA 1990;87:2220–2224.
220. Wang J, Zhou J, Cheng CM, et al. Evidence supporting dual, IGF-I-independent and IGF-I-dependent, roles for GH in promoting longitudinal bone growth. J Endocrinol 2004;180:247–255.
221. Warrell E, Taylor JF. The effect of trauma on tibial growth. J Bone Joint Surg 1976; 58B:375.
222. Weinman DT, Kelly PJ, Owen CA Jr. Blood flow in bone distal to a femoral arteriovenous fistula in dogs. J Bone Joint Surg Am 1964;46A:1676–1682.
223. Werther GA, Haynes KM, Barnard R, et al. Visual demonstration of growth hormone receptors on human growth plate chondrocytes. J Clin Endocrinol Metab 1990;70: 1725–1731.
224. Whang K, Tsai DC, Nam EK, et al. Ectopic bone formation via rhBMP-2 delivery from porous bioabsorbable polymer scaffolds. J Biomed Mater Res 1998;42:491–499.
225. Wieser RJ, Janik-Schmitt B, Renauer D, et al. Contact-dependent inhibition of growth of normal diploid human fibroblasts by plasma membrane glycoproteins. Biochimie 1988;70:1661–1671.
226. Wirth T, Byers S, Byard RW, et al. The implantation of cartilaginous and periosteal tissue into growth plate defects. Int Orthop 1994;18:220–228.
227. Wray JB. Acute changes in femoral arterial blood flow after closed tibial fracture in dogs. J Bone Joint Surg Am 1964;46A:1262–1268.
228. Xian CJ, Zhou FH, McCarty RC, et al. Intramembranous ossification mechanism for bone bridge formation at the growth plate cartilage injury site. J Orthop Res 2004;22: 417–426.
229. Xu T, Bianco P, Fisher LW, et al. Targeted disruption of the biglycan gene leads to an osteoporosis-like phenotype in mice. Nat Genet 1998;20:78–82.
230. Yakar S, Rosen CJ. From mouse to man: redefining the role of insulin-like growth factor-I in the acquisition of bone mass. Exp Biol Med (Maywood) 2003;228:245–252.
231. Yamaguchi Y, Mann DM, Ruoslahti E. Negative regulation of transforming growth factor-beta by the proteoglycan decorin. Nature 1990;346:281–284.
232. Yamamoto N, Akiyama S, Katagiri T, et al. Smad1 and smad5 act downstream of intracellular signalings of BMP-2 that inhibits myogenic differentiation and induces osteoblast differentiation in C2C12 myoblasts. Biochem Biophys Res Commun 1997; 238:574–580.
233. Zapf J, Froesch ER. Insulin-like growth factor I actions on somatic growth. In: Kostyo JL, ed. Handbook of Physiology. New York and Oxford: Oxford University Press, 1999.
234. Zhang D, Schwarz EM, Rosier RN, et al. ALK2 functions as a BMP type I receptor and induces Indian hedgehog in chondrocytes during skeletal development. J Bone Miner Res 2003;18:1593–1604.

3

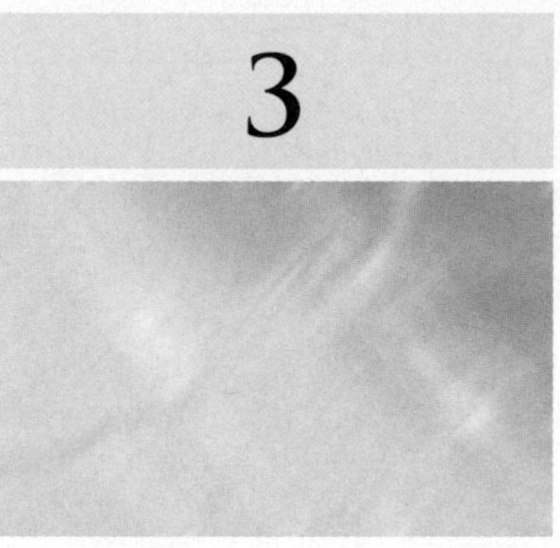

PAIN RELIEF AND RELATED CONCERNS IN CHILDREN'S FRACTURES

Gregory A. Mencio

INTRODUCTION 45

PRINCIPLES OF SEDATION AND PAIN MANAGEMENT IN CHILDREN 46

GUIDELINES OF SEDATION IN CHILDREN 46
Definitions 46
Monitoring 47
Patient Assessment 49
Oral Intake Precautions 49
Hemodynamic Status 49
Coexisting Nonmusculoskeletal Injuries 49
Status of the Airway 49
Treatment Facility 50

SEDATIVE MEDICATIONS 50
Pediatric Cocktail 50
Chloral Hydrate 50
Barbiturates 51
Nitrous Oxide 51
Benzodiazepines and Opioids 52
Ketamine 56
Propofol 57
Comparative Studies of Sedative Medications 58

REGIONAL ANESTHESIA IN THE CHILD WITH A MUSCULOSKELETAL INJURY 58
Local/Regional Anesthetic Agents 58
Intravenous Regional Anesthesia 59
Local Infiltration Anesthesia: Hematoma Block 62
Axillary Block 62
Wrist and Digital Blocks 63
Femoral Nerve Block 64

POSTOPERATIVE ANALGESIA IN THE CHILD WITH A MUSCULOSKELETAL INJURY 65
Postoperative Analgesia with Opioids 65
Postoperative Analgesia with Nonsteroidal Anti-inflammatory Drugs 67
Postoperative Analgesia with Local Anesthetic Agents 67

TREATMENT OF POSTOPERATIVE NAUSEA 68

INTRODUCTION

Providing pain relief is one of the many important parts of the management of children's fractures. In order to be able to perform satisfactory closed treatment of musculoskeletal injuries, effective and safe levels of sedation and analgesia are essential in order to minimize pain and allay apprehensions of the child.[127,184] Optimal pain management in the emergency room or other setting is delivered by the combined efforts of the orthopaedic surgeon and anesthesiologist or emergency medicine specialist. Numerous techniques, short of general anesthesia, are available to control pain associated with fractures in children including local, regional, and intravenous blocks and moderate or deep sedation. Important factors in choosing a particular technique include efficacy, safety, ease of administration, cost, and patient/parent acceptance. The correct use of any of the available medications for obtaining these goals necessitates an appropriate understanding of proper dose, desired effects, and untoward side effects. The purpose of this chapter is to provide a source of information regarding safe and effective analgesia and sedation for children with fractures. The definitions of the various levels of sedation and the medications used to achieve the desired sedation state are discussed. Local and regional anesthetic techniques including intravenous (IV) regional anesthesia (Bier blocks), hematoma blocks, and femoral nerve blocks (for femoral fractures) are discussed in depth. The management of postoperative pain and the treatment of the troublesome side effect of postoperative nausea are discussed. The hope is that the concepts discussed in this chapter will aid the orthopaedic surgeon in managing fractures in the emergency room, office, and hospital setting.

PRINCIPLES OF SEDATION AND PAIN MANAGEMENT IN CHILDREN

Children with fractures typically have a great deal of pain and apprehension. Psychologically, their perceptions of the emergency department, office, or hospital and the impending treatment of their injury often exacerbate their level of discomfort and anxiety.[148] Children with painful injuries about to undergo additionally painful treatment are entitled to adequate analgesia and sedation. Despite the rationale of this concept, the problem of undertreatment of pain in children in the emergency department and postoperative setting has been documented and is still an all-too-common occurrence.[14,80,90,130,151,152,157,158,204] Ignorance of the problem of pain in children, lack of familiarity with the methods of anesthesia and sedation for children, and apprehension of complications such as respiratory depression and hypotension are reasons for the often inadequate management of pain in the pediatric population.[80,90,130,137,147,148,151,153,157,165,204]

In recognition of the increase in the number of painful procedures performed on children in a variety of ambulatory settings, the American Academy of Pediatrics (AAP) has developed goals for sedation and analgesia in children. Their purpose is to ensure the child's safety and welfare while minimizing the physical discomfort and negative psychologic impact frequently associated with treatment of painful injuries, to control the child's behavior, and to return the child to a state in which safe discharge is possible.[5] From a practical perspective, the method of analgesia/sedation must also allow for the satisfactory treatment of the primary problem. Thus, efficacy, safety, ease of administration, patient/parent acceptance, and cost are important factors to be considered in selecting a technique.[184]

From an orthopaedic perspective, the ultimate goal of anesthesia for the child with a closed fracture requiring manipulation is to facilitate satisfactory closed treatment of the injury and obviate the need for a trip to the operating room. The ideal method of analgesia/sedation would be efficacious and safe in eliminating pain, promoting patient compliance, and producing amnesia of the procedure. It would be easy to administer, predictable in its action, and reliable for a wide range of ages. It would have a rapid onset and short duration of action, result in no complications or side effects, and be rapidly reversible. Finally, it would be relatively inexpensive to administer and completely satisfactory to the child and his or her parents.[13,22,35,37,39,46,50,73–75,83,84,93,136,137,147,148,162,184]

A variety of techniques short of general anesthesia have been used to achieve analgesia and sedation in children with closed fractures requiring treatment in the ambulatory setting. The techniques can be grouped into two broad categories: *blocks* (local, regional, and intravenous) and *sedation*, either moderate (formerly referred to as conscious) or deep (anxiolytics, narcotic analgesics, or dissociative agents alone or in combination). Each technique incorporates various aspects of the ideal method described above. It is incumbent upon the person treating children's fractures to be aware of the various techniques, their relative merits, and the potential side effects and complications of each in order to be able to make an educated decision about which to use in a particular situation.[96,114,115]

GUIDELINES OF SEDATION IN CHILDREN

Definitions

Sedation describes a continuum ranging from near wakefulness to complete loss of consciousness (Fig. 3-1). Terms used to describe various stages along this continuum have included *conscious sedation, deep sedation,* and *general anesthesia*.[5] Strictly speaking, the term *conscious sedation* means a pharmacologically controlled, altered state of consciousness in which patients maintain their ability to respond purposefully to verbal commands. For nonverbal patients or young infants, conscious sedation implies the ability to respond purposefully to physical stimulation, not simply by reflex withdrawal to pain. Unfortunately, most physicians and nurses tend to use conscious sedation to mean anything short of a general anesthetic. For such reasons, the consensus of the 1996 report by the American Society of Anesthesiologists Task Force on Sedation and Analgesia by Non-Anesthesiologists is that the term conscious sedation, although in common use, is imprecise. This report recommends replacing the term with the more descriptive term *sedation analgesia* (see Fig. 3-1).[7]

Current classification and terminology recognizes two levels of sedation: *moderate* (previously termed *conscious*) and *deep*. All levels of sedation short of deep are characterized by a state of depressed consciousness in which a patent airway and protective reflexes are maintained and from which the individual can be aroused by physical stimulation or verbal command. *Deep sedation* is a more profound state of unconsciousness with loss of protective airway reflexes. Sedation can be achieved using inhalational agents such as nitrous oxide or parenteral tech-

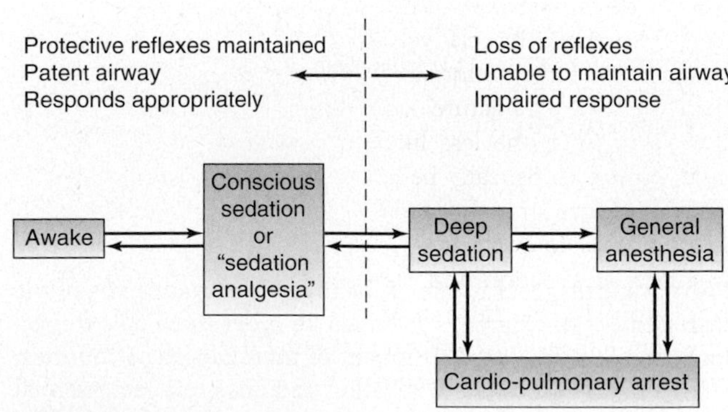

FIGURE 3-1 Sedation and analgesia for procedures is a continuum. (Reproduced with permission from American Society of Anesthesiologists, from Kaplan RK, Yang CI. Sedation and analgesia in pediatric patients for procedures outside the operating room. Anesthesiol Clin North America. 2002;20(1):181–194, vii.)

TABLE 3-1 Recommended Discharge Criteria after Sedation

1. Cardiovascular function and airway patency are satisfactory and stable.
2. The patient is easily arousable, and protective reflexes are intact.
3. The patient can talk (if age-appropriate).
4. The patient can sit up unaided (if age-appropriate).
5. For a very young or handicapped child incapable of the usually expected responses, the presedation level of responsiveness or a level as close as possible to the normal level for that child should be achieved.
6. The state of hydration is adequate.*

*Adequate hydration may be achieved with IV fluids. There is no specific requirement that children be able to tolerate oral fluids before discharge from a treatment facility. Children who are nauseated or actively vomiting should be treated and observed until this problem resolves (see "Treatment of Postoperative Nausea").
American Academy of Pediatrics Committee on Drugs. Guidelines for monitoring and management of pediatric patients during and after sedation for diagnostic and therapeutic procedures. Pediatrics 1992;89:110–115, with permission.

niques including opioids, benzodiazepines, propofol, or neuroleptic drugs (Ketamine), alone or in combination. The AAP has established guidelines for equipment and monitoring for all levels and methods of sedation in an attempt to guard patients' welfare during sedation and emergence and allow safe discharge home afterward (Table 3-1).[5,115] The safe and efficacious use of procedural sedation and analgesia (PSA), specifically by non-anesthesiologists, in a pediatric emergency department has been demonstrated. In a study performed at Children's Hospital of Pittsburgh, PSA was successfully provided in 1177 (98.6%) of 1194 sedation events, a little more than half of which were for fracture reduction (643 patients or 52.9%), using parenteral (intramuscular [IM] or IV) ketamine hydrochloride, fentanyl citrate, and/or midazolam in various combinations. Complications occurred in about 18% of patients, but most commonly consisted of hypoxia that was easily treated.[134]

Whatever the preferred term, the important point to recognize is that the safest level of sedation is that which permits purposeful response to verbal or physical stimulation. It is at this level of sedation that the risk of hypoventilation, apnea, or cardiovascular instability is minimal. Unfortunately, and realistically speaking, such relatively light levels of sedation are totally inadequate for the performance of a painful procedure such as the reduction of a fracture. Also, the younger and less cooperative the patient, the less likely it is that so-called conscious sedation can realistically be achieved at all.[113] Therefore, it is very likely that for orthopaedic procedures, children may have to be sedated to levels at which they are not easily responsive to verbal stimulation and, as such, are at increased risk for respiratory and cardiovascular compromise. Even in children in whom light levels of sedation (true conscious sedation) are possible, unintended oversedation may occur without warning. Over-sedation may lead to (a) loss of the airway, (b) impaired protective reflexes, leading to the possibility of aspiration of gastric contents, and (c) cardiopulmonary arrest (see Fig. 3-1). It is for these reasons that careful monitoring of sedated patients, as prescribed in the standard guidelines, is imperative.[5,7]

Monitoring

The purpose for monitoring sedated patients is to provide timely detection and correction of abnormalities in respiratory and cardiovascular function. The monitoring process begins before the administration of any sedative medications. Monitoring continues unabated until the patient returns to his or her baseline presedation level of consciousness and is ready for discharge. Acceptable discharge criteria are noted later (see Table 3-1). Vital to the monitoring process is the presence of qualified personnel who are competent in the use of monitoring devices and capable of recognizing the clinical signs of airway or hemodynamic instability. Although skill in at least pediatric basic life support is necessary, training in pediatric advanced life support is certainly desirable.[5,147,148] It is imperative that these skilled health professionals, either physicians or nurses, are completely dedicated to administering drugs and observing the patient and monitors during procedures requiring medications that are known to depress respiratory or cardiovascular function. Having one person performing both the surgical procedure and monitoring the patient is a practice that should be strongly discouraged, as both tasks may be compromised.

Oxygenation, ventilation, and circulation are the three parameters that require careful assessment. Monitoring temperature is usually of minimal importance; the major exceptions are children who arrive in the hospital either severely hypothermic or febrile.

Monitoring oxygenation requires continuous pulse oximetry and continual visual inspection of the patient. The term *continuous monitoring* refers to a constant measurement undertaken for a period of time without interruption. *Continual monitoring* refers to an assessment taken at frequent, regular intervals. The value of pulse oximetry as an early detector of impeding hypoxemia has been well demonstrated.[43] The problem with relying on visual inspection alone to determine the adequacy of oxygenation is that cyanosis is both a late and variable sign of hypoxemia. Demonstrable cyanosis requires the presence of at least 5 g of desaturated hemoglobin per deciliter. Therefore, as an example, a patient with a hemoglobin level of 10 g/dL would theoretically not even appear cyanotic until the oxygen saturation level plummets to 50%. For this same reason, a severely anemic patient may never develop visible cyanosis even at profound levels of hypoxemia. To add to a potentially confusing situation, the ambient light (especially fluorescent light) in many clinical environments may make any patient appear cyanotic.[42,43] Therefore, pulse oximetry is essential in all patients with the potential of becoming heavily sedated to detect abnormalities of oxygenation rapidly. The pulse oximeter is not perfect, however, and factors such as patient movement, direct bright light on the probe, and malposition of the probe can affect the accuracy of pulse oximetry readings.[12,26,42] Simple measures like correct probe placement, shielding the probe site from bright light, and gentle restraint of the monitoring site can improve the dependability of this all-important monitor.

Monitoring ventilation goes hand in hand with monitoring oxygenation and requires close observation of the patient and either intermittent or continuous auscultation of breath sounds. A sedated child's head may flex forward easily, producing airway obstruction as the child begins to fall asleep.[42] Maintaining patients in the so-called "sniffing" position helps prevent airway

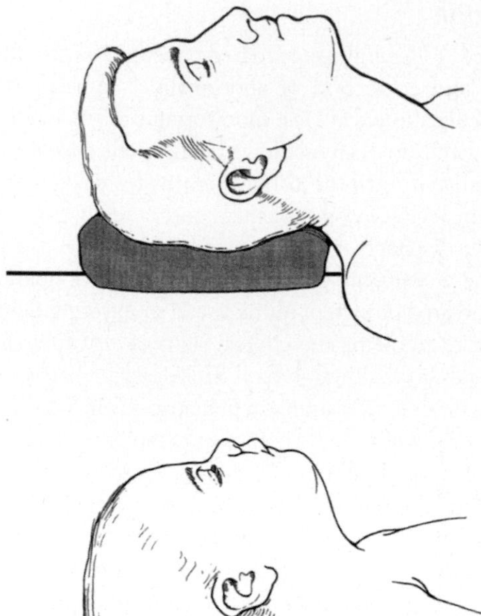

FIGURE 3-2 The sniffing position. In an adult or in an older child, a folded sheet or towel under the occiput, plus moderate head extension at the atlanto-occipital joint, helps to maintain an open airway. In a child younger than 3 years of age, the relatively large head size in proportion to the trunk makes occipital padding unnecessary.[44]

obstruction (Fig. 3-2). The sniffing position consists of elevating the patient's head with pads under the occiput, keeping the shoulders flat on the table, and extending the head at the atlanto-occipital junction.[169] Children younger than 3 years of age have a relatively large head in proportion to the size of their trunk and do not require padding under the occiput.[44] Along with continual assessment of the child's head position, any restraining devices should be checked to ensure that they are not contributing to either airway obstruction or restriction of chest movement.[5] Auscultation with the precordial stethoscope is valuable in the monitoring of both ventilation (breath sounds) and circulation (heart sounds). Its use is encouraged in the monitoring of deeply sedated patients.[5]

Monitoring circulation for most sedated children consists of intermittent determination of heart rate and blood pressure. In children, normal values for heart rate (Table 3-2) and blood pressure (Table 3-3) vary with age. A simple formula for calculating the normal systolic blood pressure and lower limit of normal for systolic blood pressure in children by age is worth memorizing (Table 3-4). Electrocardiographic (ECG) monitoring is especially important for the child with an underlying history of a significant cardiac dysrhythmia or known ECG abnormality such as long QT syndrome or a history of Wolff-Parkinson-White syndrome. In the absence of monitor artifact, the pulse oximeter provides a continuous assessment of heart rate. Deeply sedated children should have blood pressure and heart rate and respiratory rate measurements determined and recorded at least at 5-minute intervals.[5] For children undergoing more moderate procedural sedation/analgesia, the frequency of vital sign determination is at the discretion of the physician or practitioner in responsible for monitoring.[5]

TABLE 3-2 Normal Values for Heart Rate by Age

Age	Range (beats/min)
Newborn	110–150
1–11 months	80–150
2 years	85–125
4 years	75–115
6 years	65–110
8 years	60–110

Rasch DK, Webster DE. Clinical Manual of Pediatric Anesthesia. New York: McGraw-Hill, 1994:16, with permission.

TABLE 3-3 Normal Values for Blood Pressure by Age

	Blood Pressure (mm Hg)	
Age	Systolic	Diastolic
Full-term infant	60[121]	35
3–10 days	70–75[180]	40
6 months	95[143]	45
4 years	98	57
6 years	110	60
8 years	112	60
12 years	115	65
16 years	120	65

The numbers in parentheses refer to mean arterial blood pressure. Steward DJ. Manual of pediatric anesthesia. New York: Churchill-Livingstone, 1990:24 and Rasch DK, Webster DE. Clinical Manual of Pediatric Anesthesia. New York: McGraw-Hill, 1994:17, with permission.

TABLE 3-4 Calculation of Normal Blood Pressure by Age

80 + (2 × age in years) = normal systolic blood pressure for age

70 + (2 × age in years) = lower limit of normal systolic blood pressure for age

Rasch DK, Webster DE. Clinical Manual of Pediatric Anesthesia. New York: McGraw-Hill, 1994:197, with permission.

Monitoring must continue until the patient meets preset discharge criteria (see Table 3-1).[5] It is important to be cognizant of the possibility that, when the surgical procedure is over and patients are no longer being actively stimulated, unintentional deep sedation with resulting airway obstruction and apnea may occur. Therefore, it is essential to remain vigilant until the patient emerges completely from the sedative medications. The time to recovery varies depending on the amount and type of sedative medication given, and this point should be taken into account when planning a sedation regimen. The durations of action of particular sedatives and sedative combinations are discussed separately.

Patient Assessment

Careful patient assessment is critical in order to determine whether administering sedative medications to a child in an ambulatory setting, where the airway is uncontrolled and unprotected, is feasible and safe. It is important first to be aware of the child's medical history, previous allergic or adverse drug reactions, current medications, and presence of coexisting diseases.[5] In addition to these basic details, other important factors including time of last oral (PO) intake, hemodynamic status, presence of other injuries, and status of the airway must be assessed before considering sedation for children with musculoskeletal injuries.

Oral Intake Precautions

Significant pulmonary aspiration is rare in children following anesthesia or sedation for elective procedures.[176] Multiple studies support and encourage the liberal intake of clear liquids up until 2 to 3 hours before the start of a scheduled procedure in otherwise healthy children.[41,120,154,164] Acceptable clear liquids are apple juice, water, sugar water, sport/electrolyte drinks, and gelatin. Milk (including breast milk), milk products, and juices with pulp are not considered clear liquids. For elective procedures in children, most anesthesia and nursing protocols now adhere to the so-called "2-4-6-8 rule" regarding PO intake. This rule restricts clear liquids to 2 hours before the start of an elective procedure requiring anesthesia, breast milk to 4 hours, baby formula (cow's milk) to 6 hours, and solid food to 8 hours prior.[61]

In contrast to children receiving sedation for scheduled, elective procedures, those requiring sedation for emergency procedures are at higher risk for aspiration, so caution is necessary when considering administration of drugs that may depress protective airway reflexes.[5,176] In trauma patients, the time interval between last PO intake and time of injury is a critical factor in the retention of gastric contents.[123] Children injured within 1 to 2 hours after eating have been shown to have large gastric volumes.[24] Gastric emptying may be further slowed in a child with a fracture by the presence of pain and anxiety and the administration of opioid pain relievers.[69] At present, there is no reliable method of assessing the volume of gastric contents, although different methods have been suggested.[67] Patient hunger on presentation for surgical treatment has been shown not to be a good indicator of an empty stomach.[120]

Although fasting can reduce an injured child's gastric volume, the ideal duration is not clear.[120] If circumstances of the injury permit and the procedure can wait, a minimal fasting period of 4 hours is generally recommended before administering sedative medications. IV fluids should be given to prevent dehydration, medications to reduce gastric volume (metoclopramide) or to decrease gastric acidity (histamine-2–receptor blockers) should be administered intravenously 1 hour before sedative medications, and sedation should be titrated tightly, utilizing the minimal levels possible to allow completion of the procedure. The appropriate dose of metoclopramide is 0.15 mg/kg. Famotidine, a histamine-2–receptor blocker, may be given in a dose of 0.3 to 0.4 mg/kg IV, with a maximal dose of 20 mg. Pregnancy, morbid obesity, gastroesophageal reflux, bowel obstruction, and increased intracranial pressure all magnify the risk of regurgitation and aspiration of gastric contents. Therefore, additional caution is necessary in managing patients with any of these conditions. Patients with coexisting bowel obstruction should not be sedated, and patients with increased intracranial pressure should not be sedated without neurosurgical evaluation and input. If treatment cannot wait and the procedure or the patient is not appropriate for regional anesthesia, the safest approach is to utilize general anesthesia with a rapid sequence induction and a protected airway (endotracheal tube).

Hemodynamic Status

The magnitude of blood loss from a child's injuries is not always readily apparent. In children, long bone fractures and head injuries may easily have associated large, concealed hemorrhages.[174,191] It is important to assess the patient's volume status accurately before administering sedative medications. In a child who is hypovolemic, sedatives may interfere with catecholamine-mediated compensatory mechanisms and produce profound hemodynamic instability, leading to cardiovascular collapse.

In an injured child, blood pressure monitoring alone does not provide a good indication of the patient's underlying volume status.[131,194] Children maintain a normal blood pressure for their age in the face of large intravascular volume deficits.[194] More reliable signs of ongoing hypovolemia in children include tachycardia, mottling, cool extremities, poor urine output (less than 1 to 2 mL/kg/hour), and altered level of consciousness. Each of these signs can imply poor perfusion of different organ systems (skin, musculoskeletal system, kidneys, and central nervous system, respectively). Volume replacement, not sedation, should be the initial goal in the management of hypovolemic children.

Coexisting Nonmusculoskeletal Injuries

Serious head injury accounts for 70% of pediatric trauma deaths.[38,131] Respiratory depression from sedation, with resultant hypercapnia and hypoxia, may aggravate an underlying closed head injury and worsen its prognosis.[191] In addition, any pharmacologic change in the patient's state of consciousness may confuse the neurologic evaluation. Other injuries to major body cavities or injuries associated with major blood loss should be assessed carefully before any sedative medications are administered.

Status of the Airway

A tenuous airway can easily become a completely obstructed airway in a sedated child. Several common conditions in children may predispose to breathing difficulty and airway obstruc-

TABLE 3-5 Airway Management Equipment

Airway Management Equipment
Ventilation face masks* (infant, child, small adult, medium adult, large adult)
Breathing bag and valve set
Oral airways (infant, child, small adult, medium adult, large adult)
Nasal airways (small, medium, large)
Laryngoscope handles
Laryngoscope blades: straight (Miller) number 1, 2, 3; curved (Macintosh) number 1, 2, 3
Endotracheal tubes: 2.5–6.0 uncuffed; 6.0–8.0 cuffed
Appropriate-sized stylets for endotracheal tubes (*must be lubricated before insertion*)
Appropriate-sized suction catheters for endotracheal tubes
Yankauer-type suction
Nasogastric tubes (10–18 French)
Nebulizer set-up for treatment of bronchospasm

*The correct-sized ventilation facemask will fit over the child's face from the bridge of the nose to the cleft of the chin. This guideline is also correct when using patient-administered nitrous oxide analgesia.
American Academy of Pediatrics Committee on Drugs. Guidelines for monitoring and management of pediatric patients during and after sedation for diagnostic and therapeutic procedures. Pediatrics 1992;89:1110–1115, with permission.

TABLE 3-6 Vascular Access Equipment

Vascular Access Equipment
IV catheters (24–16 gauge)*
Intraosseous bone-marrow needle
IV tubing: pediatric drip (60 drops/mL); pediatric burette-type; adult drip (10 drips/mL)
IV fluids: lactated Ringer's; normal saline
Miscellaneous equipment: tourniquets, alcohol wipes, arm boards

*In resuscitation situations, no more than 90 seconds should be spent attempting to gain peripheral venous access. If attempts have been unsuccessful, then central venous cannulation, intraosseous cannulation, or peripheral venous cutdown should be done according to the expertise of available personnel.
American Academy of Pediatrics Committee on Drugs. Guidelines for monitoring and management of pediatric patients during and after sedation for diagnostic and therapeutic procedures. Pediatrics 1992;89:1110–1115, with permission.

tion following sedation. For example, children with large tonsils and adenoids may have obstructive sleep apnea.[110] Obstructive sleep apnea, which is associated with a history of loud snoring and daytime sleepiness, may be acutely exacerbated with the administration of sedative medications.[45] Other conditions that may predispose to airway patency following sedation include micrognathia (short jaw), limited ability to open the mouth (arthrogryposis), and limited movement of the neck, either congenital or acquired.[17]

Treatment Facility

The facility where the child is receiving treatment should be appropriately equipped to ensure optimal patient care and safety. Equipment for resuscitation, airway management (Table 3-5), and vascular access (Table 3-6) must be immediately available for children of all ages and sizes.[5] In addition, a positive-pressure oxygen delivery system capable of delivering at least 90% oxygen for at least 60 minutes must also be readily available A working suction apparatus must be easily accessible to handle patient secretions, as well as for unexpected regurgitation and vomiting.[5]

SEDATIVE MEDICATIONS

Having considered the preliminary step of patient assessment, the practitioner must now decide which sedative or sedatives to use. The ideal sedative should be easy to administer, quick in onset, devoid of side effects, and rapid in termination of effects. The abundance of references in the literature extolling the virtues of different sedative drugs and drug combinations is the best indicator that there is no one ideal choice. Since each drug has only some of the properties of an ideal sedative medication and individual patients may demonstrate considerable variability in response to the same drugs, it is unwise and perhaps unsafe to try to fit every child with a fracture into a particular sedation regimen. It is equally important to remember that for those patients who cannot be adequately sedated safely, fracture reduction should be performed under general anesthesia.

Pediatric Cocktail

The so-called pediatric cocktail (DPT) or "lytic" cocktail is a mixture of meperidine (Demerol) and two phenothiazines: promethazine (Phenergan) and chlorpromazine (Thorazine). For multiple reasons, this sedative regimen should be avoided.[6] Prolonged and profound sedation occurs, often far outlasting the procedure for which the sedation was intended. One study reported a mean total recovery time of 19 hours, plus or minus 15 hours, in children receiving DPT in the emergency department.[175] Orthostatic hypotension is possible because promethazine and chlorpromazine are alpha-adrenergic blockers.[42] Severe respiratory depression and death, both during and after the procedure, have occurred in patients sedated with DPT. All three medications in this mixture lower the seizure threshold, and phenothiazines can produce dystonic reactions.[42] There is no reversal agent for phenothiazine overdose.

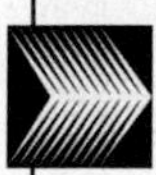

AUTHORS' PREFERRED TREATMENT

Use of the pediatric cocktail should be abandoned.[162]

Chloral Hydrate

Chloral hydrate was introduced in 1832 and continues to be a commonly used sedative for children undergoing painless diagnostic procedures, such as radiographic studies.[21,109] Chloral hydrate may be administered orally or rectally in a dose of 20 to 75 mg/kg. The maximal single dose is 1 g. If more than one dose has to be given, the upper limit for the total dose is either 100 mg/kg or 2 g, whichever is lower. Children receiving chloral hydrate must be observed for at least several hours. Respiratory depression is unusual, but children with sleep apnea and adenoid and tonsillar hypertrophy may be particularly vulnerable to airway obstruction after sedation with chloral hydrate.[20] At least one death has been reported following its use.[89] These problems emphasize that even sedatives thought to have little risk of producing respiratory depression must be administered under properly supervised conditions and with strict adherence to dosage guidelines.[5]

Although chloral hydrate may be effective for the sedation of young children (< 6 years old) undergoing therapeutic procedures, it has several disadvantages for the management of fractures in children.[147] First, the onset of sedation is slow (40 to 60 minutes). Second, chloral hydrate has no analgesic properties, and children can become disinhibited and agitated in response to painful stimuli while under the influence of the drug. Finally, recovery can be prolonged, taking up to several hours with residual effects lasting as long as 24 hours. For these reasons, chloral hydrate is not a preferred technique for sedation in the management of fractures in children.[21,109,136,137,147,148,157,158]

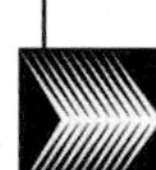

AUTHORS' PREFERRED TREATMENT

Chloral hydrate is of minimal use in the sedation and treatment of patients with fractures. It provides no analgesia, and it lacks the rapidity of onset and titratability of IV opioids and benzodiazepines. The practitioner should be familiar with this medication, however, because it remains in common use for nonpainful pediatric procedures. Salient features regarding its administration are summarized in Table 3-7.

Barbiturates

In general, barbiturates have a lower margin of safety than benzodiazepines (discussed below).[168,170] In addition, barbiturates seem to lower the pain threshold and are therefore a poor choice for producing sedation in the presence of a painful condition such as a fracture. With these points in mind, barbiturates should not be used for sedating children with fractures.

TABLE 3-7 Chloral Hydrate in Pediatric Sedation

I. Method of Administration
   20 to 75 mg/kg orally or rectally (maximum single dose, 1.0 g; if a second dose is given, the maximum total dose is either 100 mg/kg or 2.0 g, whichever is lower)

II. Contraindications
   A. Compromised hepatic function
   B. History of obstructive sleep apnea*
   C. Previous unfavorable experience with chloral hydrate

III. Advantages
   No specific advantages for sedation and treatment of children with fractures

IV. Disadvantages
   A. Prolonged time to peak effect (as long as 60 min)
   B. Difficult to titrate
   C. Prolonged observation period required

*Caution is required when using any sedative medication in patients with obstructive sleep apnea.

Nitrous Oxide

Dentists have used nitrous oxide extensively since the 1950s to provide anesthesia for patients undergoing office dental procedures. Its use in the ambulatory setting for fracture management is more recent.[83,84,190] Nitrous oxide is a relatively weak inhalational anesthetic with low solubility. It has weak sedative and analgesic properties. It acts quickly on the central nervous system (CNS) and has a fairly short duration of action, making it a good anesthetic option for fracture treatment. Other desirable effects of nitrous oxide include a variable degree of analgesia, sedation, anxiolysis, and amnesia.[56,83,84,109,147,148] It does have the advantages of rapid onset, relative ease of use, and rapid termination of effects. Because it diffuses rapidly into enclosed air-filled spaces, its use is contraindicated in patients with bowel obstruction or pneumothorax. Nitrous oxide is also contraindicated in patients with altered intracranial compliance.[109]

Nitrous oxide has been shown to be most effective when it is administered as a 50% mixture of nitrous oxide and oxygen.[147,148,190] This mixture of gases is most commonly delivered through a machine which controls the rate of flow of the gases, regulates the mix, and scavenges stray nitrous oxide from the surrounding environment. The gas is self-administered through inspiratory effort with the child holding the facemask. Once adequate sedation occurs, the child relaxes and drops the mask. When the mask seal is broken, the flow of nitrous is stopped. As a safeguard against overdosing, it is important that the mask not be held by anyone but the patient. Fracture reduction can begin within a few minutes of administration of the nitrous oxide.[147,148] After the fracture has been immobilized, 100% oxygen is administered to the child for approximately 5 minutes to wash out the nitrous oxide and prevent diffusion hypoxia.[56,84,148,190]

This technique of sedation is relatively easy to administer, works quickly, and does appear to be safe. Nitrous oxide is quickly eliminated and does not appear to suppress laryngeal reflexes. The child does not have to have an empty stomach, and intravenous access is not required.[84,190] This method is not region specific and can be used for fractures in all extremities. On the negative side, administration of nitrous can be a problem in the child who is uncooperative or anxious with the face mask and in the child who has difficulty obtaining a tight seal with the mask.[83,84,190] Other potential problems are nausea, vomiting, diffusion hypoxia, and respiratory depression. Contraindications to the use of nitrous oxide include the presence of significant cardiac or pulmonary disease, prior administration of narcotics or sedatives, presence of a pneumothorax or abdominal distension, middle ear infection, or altered mental status.

Studies suggest that nitrous oxide does provide effective sedation for the management of fractures but that its analgesic effects are variable.[56,76,84,190] Evans et al.[56] found nitrous oxide to provide similar analgesia but also to have a faster onset of action, a shorter recovery time, and better patient satisfaction compared to IM meperidine. Gregory and Sullivan[76] compared nitrous oxide to IV regional anesthesia (Bier block) in a prospective study of 28 children with upper extremity fractures and found that fracture reduction was completed in less time with nitrous oxide although the pain response, as measured by a visual analog scale, was worse. In two separate studies by Hennrikus et al.[84] and Wattenmaker et al.[190] with a combined total of 76 children, in whom nitrous oxide was used as the sole anesthetic agent, fracture reduction was successful in 95% and no complications were encountered. However, "moderate" or "significant" pain was observed in 41% of the patients during fracture reduction, and in the Wattenmaker study, analgesia was completely ineffective in 9%.

Nitrous Oxide and Hematoma Block Combination

Because of the unpredictable nature of analgesia with nitrous oxide alone, some have suggested that it be combined with regional anesthesia. Hennrikus et al.[83] reported on the use of nitrous oxide and hematoma block in 100 children from 4 to 17 years old with various closed fractures treated in the emergency department. When the techniques are combined, preliminary administration of nitrous oxide provides sedation and anxiolysis that facilitates placement of the regional block as well as an amnestic response to fracture reduction. The hematoma block provides additional analgesia both during and after the reduction. The study found a significant decrease in behavior suggestive of pain with this technique compared to an earlier study using nitrous oxide alone.[83,190] This study illustrates the important point that where possible, the use of regional anesthesia, in combination with almost any sedation regimen, is an excellent way to enhance pain relief and minimize the need for systemic sedative and analgesics.

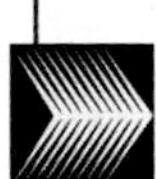

AUTHORS' PREFERRED TREATMENT

Since analgesia is somewhat unpredictable with nitrous oxide, it is probably best used in conjunction with regional anesthesia.

Benzodiazepines and Opioids

Narcotics and benzodiazepines have been safely administered to children with painful injuries to provide analgesia or to supplement other methods of anesthesia in the emergency department setting for many years.[66,97–99,115,119,136,147,184] Narcotics produce analgesia by reversibly binding to opioid receptors. In higher doses, they also have some sedative properties. Benzodiazepines are primarily sedatives. They produce hypnosis, anxiolysis, muscle relaxation, and some amnesia but have no analgesic properties. When these two different classes of drugs are given in combination, they act synergistically to induce a deep level of sedation and analgesia.[136]

The IV route of administration is preferred over others (IM, nasal, PO, and rectal) because it is the most reliable and manageable.[147] The effect following IV administration is rapid in onset, can be readily titrated, and is reversible if necessary. IV access should be obtained in a noninjured extremity and the guidelines for conscious sedation should be adhered to. The benzodiazepine is ideally administered prior to the narcotic in order to provide a sedative effect. Low doses of medications should be given initially and titrated for effect within recommended dosage levels.[115] Supplemental oxygen should be administered if oxygen saturation falls below 90%. Reversal agents such as naloxone for the narcotic and flumazenil for the benzodiazepine should be readily available. Fracture reduction typically can begin when the patient becomes drowsy.[183] As a cautionary note, IV sedation should never be used in children with history of apnea or airway disease, altered mental status, or hemodynamic instability or in infants less than 2 months old.

Benzodiazepines

Initial interest in the use of benzodiazepines developed when these drugs were noted to exert taming effects in animals.[170] Benzodiazepines provide anxiolysis, hypnosis, centrally mediated relaxation of muscle tone, antegrade and retrograde amnesia, and anticonvulsant activity.[52,140,170] Benzodiazepines have no analgesic activity and require supplementation for painful procedures.[170]

Pharmacology. Midazolam is the primary benzodiazepine used for pediatric sedation. It offers several advantages over other benzodiazepines.[199] It is water soluble and therefore usually relatively painless on injection,[140,199] in contradistinction to diazepam, which can be quite painful on parenteral administration. At physiologic pH, midazolam becomes highly lipid soluble, facilitating transport into the CNS and onset of sedative effects.[199] Initial recovery, which is due to redistribution of the drug away from the CNS, occurs in about 30 minutes. On a milligram-per-milligram basis, midazolam is at least two to three times as potent as diazepam, and the elimination half-life of midazolam is significantly shorter than that of diazepam, which is approximately 24 hours.[68] Because of these characteristics, midazolam has supplanted diazepam as the benzodiazepine of choice for noxious procedural sedation in most emergency departments.[103] However, despite its relative pharmacokinetic deficiencies, diazepam is an excellent muscle relaxant and continues to be a good choice for fracture and/or joint reduction.[147,148] Electroencephalographic studies indicate that the blood-brain equilibration time is 4.8 minutes for midazolam versus 1.6 minutes for diazepam.[29] Therefore, when titrating midazolam for sedation, it is important to wait 5 minutes between doses.

Central Nervous System Effects. Anxiolysis and centrally mediated relaxation of skeletal muscle tone are presumed to occur from a benzodiazepine-induced increase in the availability of glycine inhibitory neurotransmitters.[170] The sedative effects of benzodiazepines are caused by facilitation of the action of the inhibitory neurotransmitter gamma-aminobutyric acid. However, the exact mechanism responsible for causing amnesia is not known.[170]

Midazolam and diazepam produce direct depression of the central respiratory drive.[65] Oxygen desaturation and apnea may occur, especially after parenteral administration of these drugs.[23,88,140] Although generally considered very safe, orally administered midazolam has been reported to produce airway obstruction in a child with congenital airway anomalies.[105] In general, the incidence of respiratory complications increases with the presence of major vital organ disease.[88] However, even in healthy adult volunteers, IV sedation with midazolam (0.1 mg/kg) can depress the ventilatory response to hypoxia.[3] Concomitant administration of opioids greatly increases the risk of respiratory complications.[88,170,202] Therefore, extra vigilance and careful titration of medications to effect are even more important when using more than one sedative or analgesic medication. As a general rule, all patients who receive parenteral benzodiazepines (either IV or IM) must be monitored with pulse oximetry.[159]

Other Systemic Effects. With careful titration, significant hemodynamic changes are unusual with midazolam.[140] Loss of protective airway reflexes is also unlikely under these circumstances as long as the physician pays careful attention to the effects of each incremental dose on the patient's state of consciousness.[140] Caution is always urged if the patient's stomach is full. Slurring of speech is a typical sign of sedation with benzodiazepines. Children may also exhibit loss of anxiety, unsolicited smiling, and even laughter.[140] In reporting their experience with 2617 children sedated for endoscopic procedures, Massanari et al.[112] noted that 36 patients exhibited paradoxical reactions to midazolam, including inconsolable crying, combativeness, and agitation. These adverse responses were effectively reversed with flumazenil, a benzodiazepine antagonist, which is discussed below.

Review of Relevant Literature. In children, midazolam can be administered by PO, nasal, sublingual, IV, IM, and rectal routes.[109] A liquid PO formulation, whose concentration is 2 mg/mL, is available as Midazolam Hydrochloride Syrup 2 mg/mL. If this formulation is not available at a particular location, then the practitioner can order the parenteral form (usually the 5 mg/mL concentration) to be mixed in 5 to 10 mL of a sweet-tasting syrup.[132] Acetaminophen and ibuprofen syrup are useful vehicles for the purpose of concocting an elixir containing parenteral midazolam, keeping in mind the appropriate pediatric doses of acetaminophen and ibuprofen. The midazolam can be mixed in 3 to 5 mL of either syrup, and the mixture is very palatable. Nasal administration of the parenteral preparation (with no additives) is another option, though one that is not often used as most children find its administration via this route to be very unpleasant. In one study, 84% of children given intranasal midazolam cried in response to administration of the medication.[96] Although sublingual administration is a good idea from a pharmacologic point of view (see discussion under morphine), it requires a degree of patient cooperation that may be difficult to obtain in children, who may be unwilling or unable to hold the medication under his or her tongue.

PO midazolam has been shown to be effective in allaying the anxiety of children undergoing laceration repair in the emergency department.[58,82] The recommended dose of PO midazolam is 0.5 to 0.75 mg/kg, with a waiting period of 10 to 30 minutes to allow adequate onset of effect.[59] The maximal amount of midazolam that should be administered orally has not been determined, but in practice the total dose is usually limited to 20 to 25 mg. However, analgesic supplementation in the form of local anesthetics, opioids, or both is required for painful procedures.

Drug Reversal. Flumazenil reverses the sedative effects of benzodiazepines.[92,100,133] The initial flumazenil dose for children is 10 μg/kg IV, and it may then be continued at 5 μg/kg/minute until the child awakens, or until a total dose of 1 mg has been given.[92] The elimination half-life of flumazenil is 30 minutes, compared with 1 to 2 hours for midazolam. Therefore, patients who receive flumazenil should be observed for at least 2 hours before discharge to ensure that resedation from the original benzodiazepine does not occur. Generally, the use of flumazenil should be limited to situations of relative or absolute benzodiazepine overdose leading to respiratory or hemodynamic compromise. Routinely reversing benzodiazepines is both unnecessary and, in the absence of persistent monitoring, potentially dangerous.

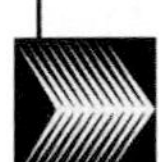

AUTHORS' PREFERRED TREATMENT

Salient points regarding the use of midazolam and other benzodiazepines are summarized in Table 3-8. The anxiolysis and amnesia that midazolam produces make it an excellent medication for procedural sedation, but supplemental analgesia is required for painful procedures, such as the reduction of fractures. For emergency procedures, IV titration is the best and most efficient way to achieve desirable levels of patient sedation and cooperation. IV midazolam may be titrated in increments of 0.05 mg/kg in combination with the administration of opioids (discussed in the next section), ketamine or a regional anesthetic block (e.g., Bier block, hematoma block) for pain relief. Oral midazolam, with its mandatory 10- to 30-minute waiting period and limited ability to be titrated effectively, is probably best reserved for use as a preoperative medication before elective surgical procedures.

TABLE 3-8 Benzodiazepines in Pediatric Sedation

I. Method of Administration
   A. Diazepam: 0.1 to 0.3 mg/kg IV or PO. IM administration should be avoided because it is painful.
   B. Midazolam
      1. PO: 0.5–0.75 mg/kg
      2. Nasal: 0.3–0.4 mg/kg*
      3. IM: 0.03–0.1 mg/kg
      4. IV: 0.05–0.1 mg/kg

II. Contraindications
   A. Previous unfavorable experience with benzodiazepines
   B. (?) Early pregnancy (possible teratogenicity)
   C. Altered state of consciousness

III. Advantages
   A. Generally provide excellent sedation and amnesia
   B. Reversible if necessary (flumazenil, 10 μg/kg, up to a total dose of 1.0 mg)

IV. Disadvantages
   A. No analgesic effect
   B. Respiratory depression, especially with parenteral administration
   C. Combination with narcotics may lead to oversedation or respiratory arrest.

*Many children find the intranasal administration of midazolam to be very unpleasant. This method of administering midazolam is not recommended.

Opioids

Opioids include all exogenous substances, natural or synthetic, that bind to specific receptors and produce morphine-like effects. There are several types and subtypes of opioid receptors.[11,172] Opioids vary in their respective affinity for receptor types, accounting for differences in side effects. Opioids are classified as pure receptor agonists (e.g., morphine, meperidine, fentanyl), agonist-antagonists (e.g., nalbuphine), or pure antagonists (e.g., naloxone).[172]

Opioid Agonists. All opioid agonists produce dose-dependent respiratory depression and apnea.[172] Nausea and vomiting occur because of direct stimulation of the chemoreceptor trigger zone in the floor of the fourth ventricle of the medulla oblongata.[172] Morphine sulphate, meperidine, and fentanyl citrate are the most common narcotics used for intravenous management of acute pain and painful procedures in the emergency department.[147]

Morphine. Morphine is the standard by which other narcotics are compared. It tends to be more effective for continuous dull pain than the sharp pain typically associated with fractures.[136,137] It is the least lipid soluble of the narcotics listed and, as a consequence, has a slower onset and longer duration of action (3 to 4 hours). As a result, it is difficult to titrate.[136] Although morphine is usually administered parenterally (IV or IM), sublingual and rectal routes have been described.[42] Oral morphine is usually used for long-term pain control in patients with severe, chronic pain. Rectal morphine is unpredictably absorbed, as is the case with most medications given via this route, and has been associated with delayed onset of respiratory depression and death, making it both impractical and unsafe.[42,71]

The usual starting dose for IV or IM morphine is 0.05 to 0.1 mg/kg. In infants younger than 3 months, the dose should be reduced by at least one half because of increased susceptibility to respiratory depression. Morphine should be reserved for painful procedures lasting at least 30 minutes.[42] Morphine is not very lipid soluble so CNS clearance is slow, which accounts for a potential duration of action of 3 to 4 hours.[11,42] Hypotension secondary to vasodilation, histamine release, or vagally mediated bradycardia can occur even with the administration of small doses of morphine.[11] Allergic reactions are triggered by release of histamines and can cause symptoms ranging from erythema along the course of the vein in which the morphine is injected to pruritis to anaphylactic reactions, although the latter are very rare.[172]

Meperidine. Meperidine has historically been a commonly used narcotic in the emergency department, although it has some characteristics that make it less desirable than other narcotics. It is one tenth as potent as morphine but has better euphoric properties. It has a slightly faster onset and shorter duration of action (2 to 3 hours) than morphine. Like morphine, meperidine is also difficult to titrate. When used for initial pain management, both drugs, but meperidine in particular, have been shown to cause a significant increase in sedation recovery times.[108]

The initial IV or IM dose of meperidine is 0.5 to 1.0 mg/kg. As with morphine, the dose should be reduced by at least one half in infants younger than 3 months.[143] Normeperidine, a metabolic breakdown product of meperidine, has been associated with seizures, agitation, tremors, and myoclonus.[85,94] Meperidine is not recommended for patients with an underlying seizure disorder. Accumulation of normeperidine is more likely in situations of prolonged meperidine administration. Therefore, meperidine should be used cautiously, if at all, in the treatment of chronic pain.[42] As with morphine, meperidine may produce hypotension due to various mechanisms including vasodilation, histamine release, or vagally mediated bradycardia.[11] Like morphine, allergic reactions mediated by histamine release can also occur with meperidine.[11]

Fentanyl. Fentanyl is a narcotic analgesic that is 100 times more potent than morphine and 1000 times more potent than meperidine on a milligram-to-milligram basis. It is highly lipid soluble and rapidly penetrates the CNS. It has a rapid onset of action with peak analgesia in 2 to 3 minutes. When administered in low doses, its duration of action (approximately 30 minutes) is shorter than the either meperidine or morphine, and it can be titrated more easily. For sedation, fentanyl is given IV in increments of 0.5 to 1 μg/kg. The maximal total dose is 4 to 5 μg/kg.[42,136,137,147,148] Infants less than 6 months old metabolize fentanyl more slowly than older children and should be dosed more conservatively (one-third normal).[147,148] Fentanyl is also available in an oral raspberry-flavored lollipop known as the Fentanyl Oralet, available in 200 μg, 300 μg, and 400 μg amounts.[109] The recommended dose ranges from 10 to 20 μg/kg. Troublesome side effects of this preparation include nausea and vomiting, pruritus, and oxygen desaturation.[153]

Repeat onset of respiratory depression up to 4 hours after fentanyl administration has been reported.[167] Glottic closure[8] and muscular rigidity[9,150,163] can occur, especially, although not exclusively, at higher doses. Respiratory arrest may occur, especially with the coadministration of other sedatives.[202] For these reasons, fentanyl should be titrated slowly to effect.

Opioid Agonists-Antagonists.

Nalbuphine and Butorphanol. Nalbuphine and butorphanol are the most commonly used opioid agonists-antagonists. Nalbuphine and morphine have the same analgesic potency on a milligram-per-milligram basis.[143] Nalbuphine has a shorter elimination half-life. Despite the fact that this group of drugs has a so-called ceiling effect or limit on the degree of respiratory depression, opioid agonist-antagonists have no particular advantage over properly dosed opioids.[49] The major problem with opioid agonist-antagonists is that their ceiling effect on respiratory depression is often accompanied by a ceiling effect for analgesia.[172] A further disadvantage of agonist-antagonists is that they can reduce the analgesic effectiveness of pure agonists (e.g., morphine, meperidine, fentanyl, codeine) if additional analgesia is required.[49] Yet another potential problem is that administration of opioid agonist-antagonists can precipitate acute withdrawal symptoms in patients receiving opioids on a long-term basis.[49]

Drug Reversal—Opioid Antagonists.

Naloxone. Naloxone is an opioid antagonist. It has no agonist activity of its own and works by displacing opioids from their receptors.[172] It is indicated as a reversal agent in the event of respiratory depression associated with narcotic overdose. Rapid reversal of narcotic effects may precipitate severe hypertension, pulmonary edema, ventricular or supraventricular irritability, seizures, and cardiac arrest.[10,55] Dysphoria, nausea, and vomiting may also occur. These side effects of acute narcotic withdrawal are caused by sympathetic nervous system stimulation from abrupt reversal of analgesia and the sudden perception of pain.[11] In attempting to reverse narcotic overdose, one must therefore be cautious to not precipitate acute narcotic withdrawal. Accordingly, administration of naloxone should be titrated to effect (relief of respiratory depression) in increments of 1 to 5 μg/kg IV. It is equally important to remember that naloxone has duration of action of 30 to 45 minutes, which may be shorter than the drug it is being used to reverse. To prevent resedation, close patient observation is required, and supplemental dosing of naloxone may be necessary.

If respiratory depression occurs when administering IV sedation with *both* a narcotic and a benzodiazepine and reversal is necessary, the narcotic should be reversed first with naloxone. If respiratory depression persists after 1 to 2 minutes, the benzodiazepine should be reversed with flumazenil.[134,136,137,184] Both reversal agents have a shorter half-life than the drugs they are reversing. Therefore, monitoring must continue until all respiratory effects have dissipated.

As was previously discussed with flumazenil for reversal of benzodiazepines, the routine use of naloxone to reverse narcotic sedative medications is unwarranted and, for reasons noted earlier, potentially dangerous. Naloxone use should be reserved for situations of airway compromise brought on by relative opioid overdose, and it should never be used as a way of expediting patient discharge after procedural sedation.

Review of Relevant Literature. In the absence of specific contraindications, including tenuous airway status, unstable hemodynamic status, history of specific allergic reactions, or age of less than 2 months old, and with careful monitoring and judicious administration of drugs, IV sedation (opioids for analgesia and benzodiazepines for amnesia and anxiolysis) has proven to be safe and effective for the management of fractures in children of various ages.[39,42,95,97,119,134,136,137,147,184,202] In a study by Varela et al.,[184] 104 children (ages 2 months to 15 years) received IV meperidine (average dose 1.47 mg/kg) and midazolam (average dose 0.11mg/kg) prior to fracture manipulation in an ambulatory setting. Physician satisfaction with the sedation was good or excellent for 94% of the reductions. Most of the children did display some signs of pain as the fracture was manipulated; however, 93% had amnesia for the event. Minor side effects including oversedation, hallucinations, and pruritus, and emesis occurred in 14% of the patients. There were no episodes of apnea or cardiorespiratory complications. Eighty-two of 86 parents (98%) contacted were satisfied with the sedation as well. The authors stressed the importance of careful patient monitoring, both during and after the procedure.

IV sedation with morphine (0.1 mg/kg) plus midazolam (0.1 mg/kg) combined with a hematoma block is another effective technique for fracture reduction in an ambulatory setting. With this particular method of sedation, the midazolam is administered first, followed by the morphine about 5 minutes later. The hematoma block is performed, and the fracture is then reduced. As previously outlined, careful patient monitoring is essential.

AUTHORS' PREFERRED TREATMENT

Salient points regarding the use of opioids as well as opioid and benzodiazepine combinations for pediatric sedation are summarized in Tables 3-9 and 3-10. Opioid and benzodiaze-

TABLE 3-9 Opioids in Pediatric Sedation

I. Method of Administration
 A. Morphine: 0.05–0.1 mg/kg IM or IV
 B. Meperidine: 0.5–1.0 mg/kg IM or IV
 C. Fentanyl: In increments of 0.001 mg/kg IV (maximum *total* dose, 0.004–0.005 mg/kg)
 D. Nalbuphine: 0.1 mg/kg IM or IV

Patients younger than 3 months old should be given no more than half of these doses initially. IV titration to desired effect is the ideal way to administer *all* sedative medications.

II. Contraindications
 A. Altered state of consciousness
 B. Previous unfavorable experience (excludes that medication only)
 C. Sedation for nonpainful procedure

III. Advantages
 A. Provide excellent analgesia
 B. Reversible if necessary (naloxone 0.001–0.005 mg/kg IV *titrated to effect*)

IV. Disadvantages
 A. Risk of respiratory depression and apnea
 B. Increased risk of respiratory depression and apnea when combined with other sedatives
 C. No amnestic effects

V. Additional side effects (more likely when used in recurrent doses for treatment of pain)

Nausea, vomiting, pruritus, constipation, decreased gastric motility

TABLE 3-10 Fentanyl and Midazolam in Pediatric Sedation*

I. Method of Administration IV titration to effect
 A. Midazolam: In increments of 0.05 mg/kg to a maximum of 0.1 mg/kg. Wait 5 min between doses.
 B. Fentanyl: Begin 5 min after last midazolam dose. Give in increments of 0.001 mg/kg to a maximum of 0.003 mg/kg. Wait 2 to 3 min between doses.

II. Contraindications
 A. Altered state of consciousness
 B. Previous unfavorable experience with either medication
 C. Specific contraindications to benzodiazepines or opioids (see Tables 3-8 and 3-9)

III. Advantages
 A. Provides sedation, amnesia (midazolam), and analgesia (fentanyl)
 B. Reversible if necessary (see Tables 3-8 and 3-9)

IV. Disadvantages
 A. Additive respiratory depressant effects
 B. Additive depressant effects on protective airway reflexes with increased risk for regurgitation and aspiration of gastric contents

*An excellent review of the advantages and problems associated with this drug regimen is provided in Yaster M, Nichols DG, Deshpande JK, Wetzel RC. Midazolam–fentanyl intravenous sedation in children: case report of respiratory arrest. Pediatrics 1990;86:463–467.

pine combinations provide amnesia, analgesia, and sedation; the tradeoff is additive respiratory depression and additive depression of protective airway reflexes. In both elective and emergent situations, the practitioner must:

1. Thoroughly evaluate the patient, as discussed earlier in the chapter.
2. Follow standard practice guidelines for deep sedation.[5]
3. Pay careful attention to dosing limits (see Table 3-10).
4. Be certain that both flumazenil and naloxone are available. These medications are to be used strictly for the treatment of absolute or relative overdose of benzodiazepines and opioids, respectively. They should never be used routinely to expedite discharge from the emergency room.

Ketamine

Ketamine, which is structurally related to phencyclidine, was first synthesized in 1963. It was developed to produce the "anesthetic state (analgesia, amnesia, loss of consciousness, and immobility)" without total CNS depression and was approved for general clinical use in 1970.[40,196] The commercial preparation of ketamine is a racemic mixture of two optical isomers with differing activity.[196] Ketamine is typically administered via IV or IM routes,[72–74] although rectal,[149] oral,[79,178] and intranasal[193] routes of administration have been described in the literature (Table 3-11).

The IV route is attractive because dosing can be titrated and a smaller cumulative dose given to achieve the desired effect. The onset of action is also quicker and recovery is more rapid.[73,116] The IV dose of ketamine is 1 to 2 mg/kg and should be administered slowly to avoid respiratory depression. The IM route can be used when IV access is unobtainable. The IM dose is 4 mg/kg. Pain reduction has actually been shown to be better following IM administration, but recovery times are significantly longer and nausea and vomiting are more common, making the IV route more preferable.[144] Typically, fracture manipulation may begin within 1 to 2 minutes following IV administration and 5 minutes after IM administration. A repeat IM dose can be given after 10 to 15 minutes if the initial effect is inadequate.[73,74,115,116]

TABLE 3-11 Ketamine in Pediatric Sedation

I. Methods of Administration and Dosage
   A. IM: 4 mg/kg
   B. IV: 1–2 mg/kg
   C. PO: 6–10 mg/kg
   D. Rectal: 5–10 mg/kg

II. Contraindications
   A. Altered state of consciousness
   B. Increased intracranial pressure
   C. Active upper respiratory infections (increased quantity of secretions and possible increased risk of laryngospasm)
   D. Full stomach
   E. Prior unfavorable experience with ketamine
   F. Patients older than 16 yrs old (increased incidence of emergence phenomena)

III. Advantages
   A. Provides sedation, amnesia, intense analgesia
   B. Sympathetic-mediated activity may be beneficial for children with asthma.

IV. Disadvantages
   A. Increases production of saliva and tracheobronchial secretions; coadministration of glycopyrrolate 0.01 mg/kg recommended
   B. Potential for loss of the airway from:
      1. Laryngospasm secondary to increased secretions
      2. Aspiration from laryngeal incompetence
      3. Apnea
   C. Emergence phenomena: Rare in young children. No advantage to quiet environment. Midazolam may help, but may contribute to oversedation.

Pharmacology

Ketamine is metabolized in the liver, primarily by *N*-methylation to nor-ketamine. Nor-ketamine has about one third the sedative and analgesic potency of ketamine. As such, ketamine should be administered cautiously or in reduced doses to patients with impaired hepatic function. IV ketamine, given in a dose of 1 to 2 mg/kg, produces unconsciousness within 30 to 60 seconds. Peak plasma concentrations occur within 1 minute. Return of consciousness occurs within 10 to 15 minutes, although complete recovery may be delayed.[170] Dose requirements and recovery times from ketamine are age related.[107]

Ketamine has been found to have interactions at multiple binding sites, including *N*-methyl-D-aspartate (NMDA) and non-NMDA receptors, nicotinic and muscarinic cholinergic receptors, and opioid receptors. Agonist actions of ketamine on opioid receptors play only a minor role in its analgesic effects. The main site of analgesic action is the NMDA receptor, which explains why naloxone, a narcotic antagonist, does not reverse the analgesic effect of ketamine. The psychotomimetic effects of ketamine, however, may involve interaction with a specific subclass of opioid receptors known as kappa receptors.[101]

Central Nervous System Effects of Ketamine

Ketamine produces a state known as dissociative anesthesia. Dissociative anesthesia refers to a cataleptic state characterized by functional and electrophysiologic dissociation between the thalamo-neocortical and limbic systems.[196] Patients keep their eyes open and exhibit a slow nystagmic gaze. Corneal and pupillary reflexes remain intact. Generalized hypertonicity associated with ketamine are thought to be due primarily to effects on the CNS and to a lesser extent on nicotinic acetylcholine receptors in skeletal muscle.[101] Patients receiving ketamine may exhibit purposeful movements but not necessarily in response to surgical stimulation.[196]

The analgesic effect of ketamine is intense and may outlast its sedative effect.[72] In one study of minor surgical procedures with ketamine anesthesia, no additional analgesics were required for 24 hours postoperatively.[86] Amnesia persists for about 1 hour after apparent recovery from ketamine.[170]

Emergence phenomena are relatively rare in children, although young adults are especially susceptible to this problem.[86] Changes in mood and body image, out-of-body experiences, floating sensations, and frank delirium are all possible. Emergence phenomena result from misinterpretation of auditory and visual stimuli at the neurologic level.[196] Although they usually terminate within 24 hours, prolonged emergence phenomena lasting as long as 10 to 12 months have been reported in children.[126,170] The incidence of emergence reactions is higher in patients older than 16 years, females, patients who have received ketamine doses above 2 mg/kg IV, and patients with a history of abnormal personalities.[75,196] There is no evidence that emergence in a quiet environment decreases the incidence of this problem.[196] Benzodiazepines (e.g., diazepam and midazolam) are the most effective treatment for ketamine-induced delirium and hallucinations,[115,116,196] and administration of a benzodiazepine 3 to 5 minutes before ketamine is effective in almost entirely eliminating the possibility of emergence delirium.[188]

Transient diplopia,[40] ataxia, and disequilibrium[73,74] may occur after ketamine use, and early attempts at ambulation should be discouraged. Ketamine does not induce seizures and is not necessarily contraindicated in patients with an underlying seizure disorder.[196] Ketamine is, however, contraindicated in patients with increased intracranial pressure or with abnormal intracerebral compliance. Thus, patients with head injuries should not receive this drug, despite some reports that have suggested a neuroprotective effect for ketamine.[101,177]

Respiratory Effects of Ketamine

Ketamine can have some potentially troublesome effects on the airway. It causes the production of increased salivary and tracheobronchial secretions, which can lead to coughing, laryngospasm, and airway obstruction. This problem may be especially treacherous in patients with an ongoing respiratory infection. Glycopyrrolate, an antisialogogue, should be administered 3 to 5 minutes before ketamine (at the same time that the benzodiazepine is given) to ameliorate this problem.[109,115,116] The dose for glycopyrrolate is 5 to 10 μg/kg IV. For large children, a dose of 0.2 mg (200 μg) of glycopyrrolate given IV is sufficient. Unless there is some other strong indication for its use, ketamine should be avoided in patients with ongoing infections of the respiratory tract.

Although ketamine does not usually produce significant depression of ventilation,[170] apnea has been reported with its administration.[47] Apnea is more likely to occur when the drug is given IV in rapid boluses[47] or in combination with other respiratory depressants,[170] but has also been reported following IM administration with appropriate dosing in the emergency department.[121,160] In addition, ketamine may not protect against aspiration of gastric contents. In this regard, ketamine is no different from any other sedative and analgesic except maybe for self-administered 50% nitrous oxide in oxygen. Ketamine should never be given in an unmonitored setting, such as a patient's room on a regular hospital ward, or in a clinic area that does not have appropriate monitoring and resuscitation equipment.

Cardiovascular Effects of Ketamine

Ketamine stimulates the sympathetic nervous system and leads to the release of endogenous catecholamines. Through such an effect, ketamine produces a dose-dependent increase in heart rate and blood pressure; therefore, it is useful in patients with mild hypovolemia. However, ketamine is also a direct myocardial depressant and can lead to cardiovascular collapse in patients who are profoundly hypovolemic, and whose sympathetic nervous system is already maximally stimulated. Ketamine also causes bronchodilation by the same mechanism of sympathetic stimulation and, as such, may be used in children with asthma.[109]

Review of Relevant Literature

Ketamine has been in clinical use for more than 30 years. During that time, the safety and efficacy of ketamine sedation for children undergoing painful procedures in an emergency department setting has been established.[73,74,136,137,141,147,148] In 1990, Green et al.[73] performed a meta-analysis of 97 studies of ketamine sedation that included administration to 11,589 children. Only two children (0.017%) required intubation for laryngospasm. The incidence of emesis was 8.5%, but there were no cases of aspiration. Because of its unique properties and safe track record, ketamine is in many ways an ideal drug for procedural sedation and analgesia in children in the emergency department.[147]

Until the past decade, there had been limited experience with ketamine for sedation of children during fracture treatment or management of other musculoskeletal problems. Of the studies reviewed by Green et al. in their extensive analysis of the literature on ketamine use in the emergency department, only one mentioned fracture treatment as one of the indications for sedation by this method.[30] A subsequent investigation by Green et al.[73,74] on the use of IM ketamine sedation in the emergency department reported successful utilization in seven children (out of 108 children) with fractures. Physician satisfaction with the sedation was excellent. Most of the patients (82.9%) were able to undergo fracture reduction within 5 minutes of ketamine injection. Several minor complications, including hypersalivation, hypertonicity, rash, and vomiting, did occur but no major problems were reported. Overall parental satisfaction was high in this study.

In the early 1970s, there were several reports in the European literature regarding use of ketamine in children with fractures.[31,125,129] More recently, Vas[185] and McCarty et al.[116] have reported the efficacy and safety of ketamine sedation for fracture reduction in the emergency department. In the McCarty et al. study, which included 114 children with a variety of fractures, the time from administration of the ketamine to manipulation of the fracture averaged less than 2 minutes following IV dosing and less than 5 minutes following IM administration.[116] Pain scale scores reflected minimal or no pain during fracture reduction. Parental satisfaction was high, and 99% of parents responded that they would allow it to be used again in a similar situation. Airway patency and independent respiration were maintained. Minor adverse effects including nausea (13 patients) and vomiting (eight patients) occurred but only well into the emergence phase of the sedation. No major problems were encountered.

Propofol

Propofol is a nonopioid, nonbarbiturate, short-acting anesthetic agent. Chemically, propofol is a substituted isopropylphenol that is virtually insoluble in aqueous solutions and has to be dissolved in lecithin-containing formulations, gaining it the popular name of "milk of anesthesia."[170] Although originally used almost exclusively in operating rooms and intensive care units, it has become increasingly popular in the ambulatory-care setting for procedural sedation because it has advantage of rapid induction, owing to its lipid solubility, and short duration of action. Propofol has comparable amnestic properties to midazolam with the advantages of more rapid onset (about 40 seconds) of sedation, faster recovery, smoother emergence, and antiemetic properties.[81,109,161,183] There are several potential disadvantages of propofol, causing some to suggest that only an anesthesiologist use it.[95] First, airway patency can be rapidly lost. Second, propofol has vasodilatory and negative inotropic effects, which can lead to hypotension.[109] Third, as propofol does not have analgesic properties, the concurrent use of an opioid analgesic such as fentanyl or morphine is required, further increasing the risk of respiratory depression and hypotension. Fourth, propofol may be associated with opisthotonic posturing and myoclonus, neither of which is desirable in a child with a fracture, and it also may cause seizures.[109] Finally, there is no reversal agent for propofol, so adverse events must be treated supportively until the drug is completely metabolized. It is the author's opinion that in children with fractures, propofol should be reserved for administration in the operating room as part of a regimen of general anesthesia by an anesthesiologist.

Comparative Studies of Sedative Medications

Kennedy et al.[99] compared the safety and efficacy of ketamine- versus fentanyl-based protocols in the emergency management of pediatric fractures. In this study, patients 5 to 15 years of age needing emergency fracture or joint reduction were randomized to receive intravenous midazolam plus either fentanyl or ketamine. During fracture reduction, ketamine subjects (n = 130) had lower distress scores and parental ratings of pain and anxiety than did fentanyl subjects (n = 130). Although both regimens equally facilitated fracture treatment, deep sedation, and procedural amnesia, orthopaedists favored the ketamine-based technique. Recovery was 14 minutes longer for ketamine but fewer ketamine subjects had hypoxia (6% vs. 25%), needed breathing cues (1% vs. 12%), or required oxygen (10% vs. 20%) than did fentanyl subjects. Two ketamine subjects did require assisted ventilation briefly and more ketamine subjects vomited. Adverse emergence reactions were rare but equivalent between regimens. The authors concluded that ketamine was more effective for pediatric fracture reduction than fentanyl for pain and anxiety relief and was associated with fewer respiratory complications, although vomiting was slightly more frequent and recovery more prolonged (mean 15 minutes) with ketamine.

Roback et al.[144] compared the frequency and severity of adverse events associated with four major parenteral drug combinations used for procedural sedation in the emergency department in 2500 children (mean age 6.7 years old): ketamine alone (n = 1492; 59.7%), ketamine/midazolam (n = 299; 12.0%), midazolam/fentanyl (n = 336; 13.4%), and midazolam alone (n = 260; 10.4%). They identified a total of 458 adverse events (respiratory or nausea/vomiting) in 426 patients (17%), and that patients receiving ketamine with or without midazolam experienced fewer respiratory adverse events than those sedated with the combination of midazolam and fentanyl. Patients who received ketamine did experience more vomiting, although none aspirated.

In a systematic review of the literature to assess safety and efficacy of various forms of analgesia and sedation for fracture reduction in the emergency department, Migita et al.[119] identified eight randomized, controlled trials with a total of 1086 patients that showed, among parenteral drug combinations, ketamine-midazolam to be associated with less distress during fracture manipulation than fentanyl citrate-midazolam or propofol-fentanyl and that patients receiving ketamine-midazolam required significantly fewer airway interventions than those in whom either fentanyl-midazolam or propofol-fentanyl were used. In another comparative study of ketamine-midazolam versus propofol-fentanyl, Godambe et al. found that propofol-fentanyl was comparable to ketamine in reducing procedural distress associated with painful orthopaedic procedures in children in an emergency department setting and that propofol-fentanyl was associated with a shorter recovery time than ketamine. However, propofol had a greater potential for respiratory depression and airway obstruction than ketamine.

Administering ketamine and propofol simultaneously, a combination referred to as "ketofol," has been shown to be very effective for procedural sedation.[197] This combination of drugs takes advantage of the rapid onset and short duration of both ketamine and propofol, eliminates the need for adjunctive benzodiazepine or opioid sedatives, and reduces the potential adverse synergistic interactions associated with administration of those drugs.

REGIONAL ANESTHESIA IN THE CHILD WITH A MUSCULOSKELETAL INJURY

Local/Regional Anesthetic Agents

A number of local and regional techniques including hematoma, intravenous regional, and regional nerve blocks have been shown to be variably effective in providing anesthesia for fracture treatment in children. These methods require the surgeon to be familiar with regional anatomy, have working knowledge of the pharmocokinetics and dosing of local anesthetic drugs, and be proficient in the techniques of administering them. Compared to adults, these techniques are often technically easier to perform in children because anatomic landmarks are more readily identifiable,[77] and physiologically, the relatively smaller calibers of the peripheral nerves in children are more susceptible to the pharmacologic actions of anesthetic agents.[192] Local and regional anesthetic drugs work by blocking the conduction of nerve impulses. At the cellular level, they depress sodium ion flux across the nerve cell membrane and, in this way, inhibit the initiation and propagation of action potentials.[173,198] After injection, local anesthetics diffuse toward their intended site of action and also towards nearby vasculature where uptake is determined by the number of capillaries, the local blood flow, and the affinity of the drug for the tissues. Elimination occurs following vascular uptake by metabolism in the plasma or liver. Vasoconstrictors such as epinephrine are mixed with local anesthetics to decrease the vascular uptake and prolong the anesthetic effect.

Local anesthetics are classified chemically as either amides or esthers based on their molecular structure.[179] Amino amide local anesthetics include lidocaine, bupivacaine, mepivacaine, prilocaine, etidocaine, and the relatively new agent ropivacaine. Amino ester local anesthetics include procaine, chloroprocaine, tetracaine, benzocaine, and cocaine. Following absorption in the blood, esters are broken down by plasma cholinesterase while amides are bound by plasma proteins and then metabolized in the liver. Medications within each group have important intrinsic differences in potency, duration of action, and potential for toxicity.[45,179] For example, lidocaine is significantly less toxic a drug than bupivacaine, but it also has a shorter duration of action. An important feature of ropivacaine is that even though its duration of action is similar to bupivacaine, it produces less CNS toxicity and less cardiac toxicity.[155]

Duration of action for the various local anesthetic medications is also determined in part by the type of regional block performed. For example, single-dose brachial plexus blocks tend to have a far longer duration than do single-dose epidural or subarachnoid blocks.[45] Local adverse effects include erythema, swelling, and, rarely, ischemia when injected into tissues supplied by terminal arteries. Adverse systemic effects are caused by high blood levels of local anesthetics and include tinnitus, drowsiness, visual disturbances, muscle twitching, seizures, respiratory depression, and cardiac arrest. Bupivicaine is particularly dangerous because it binds with high affinity to myocardial contractile proteins and can cause cardiac arrest.

Local Anesthesia Toxicity

At least three types of adverse reactions can occur from local anesthetic agents. Clinically, the most important is systemic toxicity of the CNS and cardiovascular system from relative overdose into the circulation (Table 3-12). This type of reaction is not a medication allergy but simply a function of placing too much medication into the bloodstream. In the presence of a major artery, even a few drops of local anesthetic can lead to seizure activity. In most cases, however, the severity of systemic toxicity is directly related to the concentration of local anesthetic in the bloodstream.[45] Seizures and cardiac arrest may be the initial manifestations of systemic toxicity in patients who rapidly attain a high serum level of medication.[54,122,135] Agents with greater intrinsic potency, such as bupivacaine and etidocaine, require lower levels for production of symptoms.[45] Dysrhythmias and cardiovascular toxicity may be especially severe with bupivacaine, and resuscitation of these patients may be prolonged and difficult.[2,45] The prevention and treatment of acute local anesthetic systemic toxicity are outlined in Table 3-13. Although the potential for CNS toxicity may be diminished with barbiturates or benzodiazepines, given either as premedications or during treatment of convulsions, these measures do not alter the cardiotoxic threshold of local anesthetic agents. With rapid and appropriate treatment, the fatality rate from local anesthetic convulsions can be greatly decreased.[45] It is essential to stay within accepted dose limits when using any local anesthetic (Table 3-14). To aid in dose calculations, a simple formula for converting percent concentration to milligrams per milliliter is provided in Table 3-15. Although rare, true immune-mediated allergic reactions to local anesthetics are possible and more likely to occur with amino esters than with amino amides.[27,63] Local nerve damage and reversible skeletal muscle changes have been reported from the use of local anesthetics.[45]

TABLE 3-13 Prevention and Treatment of Acute Local Anesthetic Systemic Toxicity

Preventive Measures

1. Ensure availability of oxygen administration equipment, airway equipment, suction equipment, and medications for treatment of seizures (diazepam or midazolam, thiopental, succinylcholine).
2. Ensure constant verbal contact with patient (for symptoms of toxicity) and monitor cardiovascular signs and oxygen saturation.
3. Personally prepare the dose of local anesthetic and ensure it is within the accepted dosage range.
4. Give the anesthetic slowly, and fractionate the dose.

Treatment

1. Establish a clear airway; suction if required.
2. Give oxygen by facemask. Begin artificial ventilation if necessary.
3. Give diazepam 0.1–0.3 mg/kg IV in incremental doses until convulsions cease. Midazolam (0.05–0.1 mg/kg) may be used instead, also in increments until convulsions cease.
4. Thiopental in increments of 1–2 mg/kg IV may be used to control the seizures.
5. Succinylcholine (1 mg/kg IV) may be used if there is inadequate control of ventilation with the other medications. Artificial ventilation and possibly endotracheal intubation are required after using succinylcholine.
6. Use advanced cardiac life-support measures as necessary to support the cardiovascular system (more likely with local anesthetics of increased potency, such as bupivacaine).

TABLE 3-12 Manifestations of Local Anesthetic Toxicity*

1. Numbness of the lips and tongue, metallic taste in the mouth
2. Lightheadedness
3. Visual and auditory disturbances (double vision and tinnitus)
4. Shivering, muscle twitching, tremors (initial tremors may involve the muscles of the face and distal parts of the extremities)
5. Unconsciousness
6. Convulsions
7. Coma
8. Respiratory arrest
9. Cardiovascular depression and collapse

*With gradual increases in plasma concentration, these signs and symptoms may occur in order as listed. With the sudden development of high plasma concentrations of a local anesthetic agent, the first manifestation of toxicity may be a convulsion, respiratory arrest, or cardiovascular collapse. In young children, or in children who are heavily sedated, subjective evidence of impending local anesthetic toxicity (manifestations 1, 2, 3) may be difficult to elicit.

Intravenous Regional Anesthesia

IV regional anesthesia was originally described in 1908 by August Bier who used IV cocaine to obtain analgesia.[19,22,93] Although it declined in popularity as brachial plexus blocks were developed, it was revived in 1963, when its safe and successful use for the reduction of forearm fractures in adults was reported.[87] Subsequently, a number of studies have described the effective use of this technique of anesthesia for the treatment of upper extremity fractures in children in an ambulatory setting.[13,15,22,32,36,37,57,64,70,93,87,104,128,180] The block has also been described for use in lower extremity fractures but is less commonly utilized.[104]

The technique for administering the Bier block in the upper extremity involves placement of a deflated pneumatic cuff above the elbow of the injured extremity. Holmes[87] introduced the

TABLE 3-14 Maximal Recommended Doses of Commonly Used Local Anesthetics in Children

Agent	Injection Dose (mg/kg) Plain	With Epinephrine*
Lidocaine† (Xylocaine)	5	7
Bupivacaine‡ (Marcaine, Sensorcaine)	2.5	3
Mepivacaine (Carbocaine)	4	7
Prilocaine‡‡	5.5	8.5

*The addition of epinephrine (vasoconstrictor) reduces the rate of local anesthetic absorption into the bloodstream, permitting use of a higher dose.
†For IV regional anesthesia (Bier blocks), the maximal lidocaine dose is 3 mg/kg. Preservative-free lidocaine without epinephrine should be used for either Bier blocks or hematoma blocks.
‡Owing to its cardiotoxicity, bupivacaine should never be used for IV regional anesthesia or for hematoma blocks.
‡‡Of the amide local anesthetics, prilocaine is the least likely to produce CNS and cardiovascular toxicity. However, a byproduct of prilocaine metabolism may lead to severe methemoglobinemia in young children. Prilocaine is, therefore, contraindicated in children younger than 6 months old.

concept of two cuffs in an effort to minimize tourniquet discomfort with prolonged inflation, but the practice has not proven to be necessary for the limited amount of time it takes for fracture reduction in a child.[13,22,37] The tourniquet should be secured with tape to prevent Velcro failure.[128] IV access is established in a vein on the dorsum of the hand of the injured extremity with a 22- or 23-gauge butterfly needle. The arm is exsanguinated by elevating it for 1 to 2 minutes. Although exsanguination with a circumferential elastic bandage is described classically, this method can be more painful and difficult to perform in an injured extremity and is no more efficacious than the gravity method.[22,37,76,93] The blood pressure cuff is then rapidly inflated to either 100 mm Hg above systolic blood pressure or between 200 and 250 mm Hg.[13,22,37,76,93,128] The arm is lowered after cuff inflation. Lidocaine is administered, the IV catheter removed, and reduction of the fracture performed. In the traditional technique, the lidocaine dose is 3 to 5 mg/kg[13,37,128] and, in the "mini-dose" technique, 1 to 1.5 mg/kg.[22,57,76,93]

The tourniquet is kept inflated until the fracture is immobilized and radiographs are obtained, in case repeat manipulation is necessary. In any event, the tourniquet should remain inflated for at least 20 minutes to permit the lidocaine to diffuse and become adequately fixed to the tissues, thus minimizing the risk of systemic toxicity.[128,182] The blood pressure cuff may be deflated in either a single stage or graduated fashion, although single stage release has proven to be clinically safe and technically easier.[57,93,128] During the entire procedure, basic monitoring is required, and cardiac monitoring is suggested in case toxicity occurs. Routine IV access in the noninjured extremity may be beneficial but is not required.[13,76] Patients should be observed for at least 30 minutes following cuff deflation for any adverse systemic reactions. Motor and sensory function typically returns during this period, allowing assessment of neurovascular status of the injured extremity prior to discharge.[182]

The literature within the past decade certainly speaks to the effectiveness of the traditional Bier block, utilizing a lidocaine dose of 3 to 5 mg/kg, in managing forearm fractures in children. Four large series with a total of 895 patients undergoing this technique demonstrated satisfactory anesthesia and successful fracture reduction in over 90% of cases.[13,37,128,180] The most common adverse effect of the procedure in these studies was tourniquet pain in about 6% of patients.[37,180] One patient experienced transient dizziness and circumoral parenthesis.[180] One patient developed persistent myoclonic twitching following tourniquet deflation and was admitted for observation.[128]

Despite the efficacy and relatively low number of complications with the "traditional" Bier block (lidocaine, 3 to 5 mg/kg), concerns and anecdotal reports of systemic lidocaine toxicity (i.e., seizures, hypotension, tachycardia, arrhythmias) have prompted development of a "mini-dose" (lidocaine, 1 to 1.5 mg/kg) technique of IV regional anesthesia.[22,57,93] Reports by Farrell et al.[57] and Bolte et al.[22] utilizing a lidocaine dose of 1.5 mg/kg and by Juliano et al.[93] using a dose of 1.0 mg/kg in a total of 218 patients have shown the mini-dose Bier block to be effective in achieving adequate anesthesia in 94% of children studied. Although the exact mechanism of action is uncertain, the primary site of action of the IV regional block is thought to be the small peripheral nerve branches. At this anatomic level, blockade is better achieved with a larger volume of anesthetic that can be distributed more completely to the peripheral nerve receptors. It appears to be the quantity (i.e., volume) and not the dose of anesthetic that predicates success of the block. For any given dose of lidocaine, diluting the concentration permits the administration of a larger volume of fluid (see Table 3-4). This mechanism explains the success of the mini-dose technique. In the series by Juliano et al.,[93] forearm fracture reduction was pain free in 43 of 44 patients (98%) following IV regional block achieved with a very dilute lidocaine solution (0.125%) and a relatively small total dose (1 mg/kg).

IV regional anesthesia, using either the traditional or mini-dose technique, has several advantages. The technique is fairly easy to administer. The onset of action of the block is relatively fast (<10 minutes) but also of relatively short duration, allowing for assessment of neurovascular function in the extremity after fracture reduction and immobilization. However, rapid recovery may also be considered a disadvantage as the analgesic effect of the local anesthetic is lost once the tourniquet is deflated. A recent report in adults examined the addition of the nonsteroidal anti-inflammatory drug (NSAID) ketorolac to the local anesthetic solution and found that patients did obtain prolonged analgesia after the tourniquet was released.[156] However, no pediatric studies have been performed on this technique. An empty stomach is not required. Tourniquet discomfort is the

TABLE 3-15 Conversion Formula From % Concentration to Milligrams/Milliliter

Percentage concentration × 10 = Number of mg/mL

Examples: 0.25% bupivacaine has 2.5 mg bupivacaine/mL; 2% lidocaine has 20 mg lidocaine/mL

Decreasing the % concentration of anesthetic (as is done in the mini-dose Bier block technique) permits the infusion of a larger volume (mL) of drug with lower risk of systemic toxicity because the total amount (mg) of lidocaine is lower.

most common adverse side effect. Inadvertent cuff deflation with loss of analgesia or systemic toxicity is a potentially significant problem. Compartment syndrome has also been reported. Technically, placing the tourniquet and obtaining IV access in the injured extremity can be a challenge in the uncooperative child, and application of the splint or cast can be cumbersome with the tourniquet in place. IV regional anesthesia is unsuitable for lesions above the elbow.[87] The technique is contraindicated in patients with underlying heart block, known hypersensitivity to local anesthetic agents, and seizure disorders. Although not totally contraindicated, caution is urged when using this technique in patients with underlying hemoglobinopathies such as sickle cell disease.

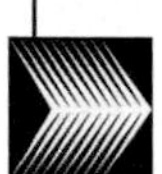

AUTHORS' PREFERRED TREATMENT

The basic steps involved in performing an IV regional block are as follows:

1. Confirm the immediate availability of a functioning positive-pressure oxygen delivery system, as well as appropriate airway management equipment (see Table 3-5).[5] Also, confirm the immediate availability of medications for the treatment of anesthetic-induced convulsions (see Table 3-13).
2. Start an IV infusion in the contralateral arm. A patent IV line is of paramount importance in treating the complications of this block. Obtain a baseline set of vital signs, including systolic and diastolic blood pressure. Monitor pulse oximetry as well as the ECG continuously.
3. Select an appropriate tourniquet. An orthopaedic tourniquet that can be fastened securely should be used. Because Velcro may become less adhesive with time, check the tenacity of the tourniquet before use. As an added safety measure, the tourniquet may be covered with strong adhesive tape or an elastic bandage after application. The tourniquet should fully encircle the arm and overlap back on itself by at least 6 cm. The arm may be minimally padded with cast padding underneath the tourniquet.[22] If a pneumatic tourniquet is used, the physician must be familiar with the location of the tourniquet pressure gauge[37] and valves, because these features vary in location from model to model. Narrow-cuffed double tourniquets may not effectively occlude arterial flow, and their use has been discouraged.[87] Tourniquet discomfort should not be a problem during short procedures, but if this develops, a second tourniquet can be applied distally over the anesthetized area of the arm.
4. Palpate the radial pulse of the injured limb.
5. Place and secure a short 22-gauge cannula or 23-gauge butterfly needle in a vein on the dorsum of the hand of the fractured limb. IV catheters can be secured more readily. If a distal vein is unavailable, a proximal vein or even an antecubital vein can be used, but may result in a less effective block.[87]
6. With the tourniquet deflated, exsanguinate the limb by vertically elevating it above the level of the heart for 60 seconds.
7. Rapidly inflate the tourniquet to a pressure of 225 to 250 mm Hg or 150 mm Hg above the patient's systolic blood pressure.[62] Check for disappearance of the radial pulse. Cross-clamping the tubing of the cuff after inflation is discouraged because it might prevent detection of a small leak.[87] Constant observation of the cuff pressure gauge is recommended.
8. Lower the extremity and slowly inject the local anesthetic. This injection should be done over a period of 60 seconds. A concentration of 0.125 to 0.5% plain lidocaine (1.25 to 5 mg/mL) is used. (Bupivacaine is contraindicated for this block because of its cardiotoxicity.) To prevent thrombophlebitis, the local anesthetic solution must be free of any additives or preservatives.[87] In different studies, the recommended dose of lidocaine has varied from 1.5 to 3.0 mg/kg.[13,22,37,57,64,93,128,180] A dose of 1.5 mg/kg appears to be safe and effective and may produce a decreased incidence of complications.[22] One study has recommended a maximal lidocaine dose of 100 mg for this block.[57] The skin of the extremity becomes mottled as the drug is injected. The patient, unless he or she is very sedated, and the parents, if they are watching, should be warned that the extremity will look and feel strange. Analgesia and muscle relaxation develop within 5 minutes of injection.[87] For fractures at the wrist, placement of a regular Penrose drain tourniquet around the distal forearm may improve distribution of the local anesthetic solution at the fracture site (Fig. 3-3).
9. To improve analgesia for fracture reduction, the last 2 mL of local anesthetic solution may be injected directly into the fracture hematoma (Fig. 3-4). The technique of local infiltration anesthesia, or hematoma block, is discussed later in this chapter.
10. Reduce the fracture and apply the cast or splint.
11. Leave the cuff inflated for at least 15 minutes, even if the surgical procedure takes less time to prevent significant entry of local anesthetic into the general circulation.[87]
13. Monitor the patient closely for at least 15 minutes for any complications related to the block. The treatment of local anesthetic-induced systemic toxicity has been discussed (see Table 3-12).
14. Depending on whatever sedation has been administered, the patient should be monitored until discharge criteria are met (see Table 3-1). An assistant must be present to watch the patient, the tourniquet, and the monitors at all times.

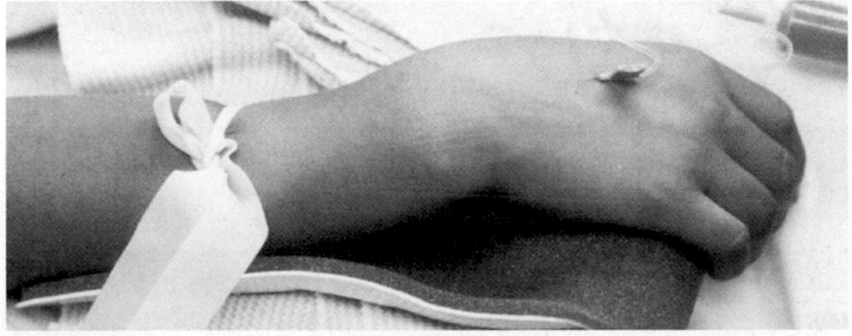

FIGURE 3-3 Penrose drain tourniquet on the forearm to improve distribution of local anesthetic at the fracture site.

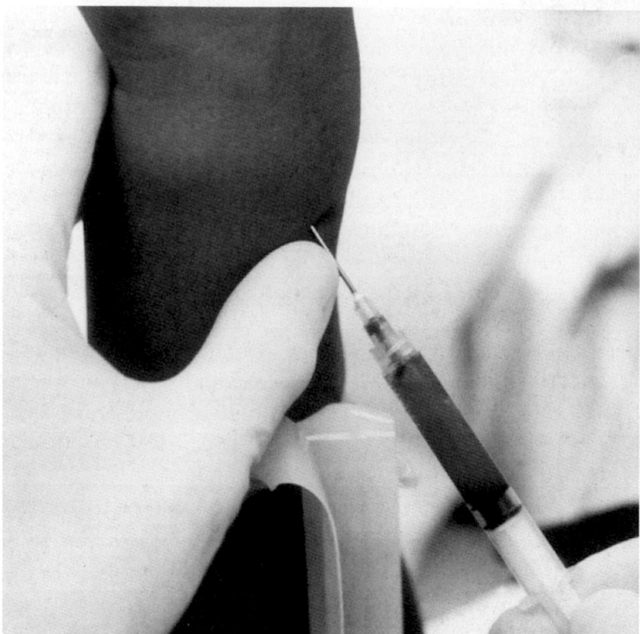

FIGURE 3-4 Hematoma block performed by barbotage. Half the anesthetic is injected into the hematoma and then withdrawn from the fracture site until original volume is regained. The mixed material is then repeatedly aspirated and injected until the anesthetic is dispersed in the hematoma about the fracture site.

Local Infiltration Anesthesia: Hematoma Block

The hematoma block has been a popular method of anesthesia for the reduction of fractures, particularly in the distal radius but also about the ankle.[1,4,33,50,91] In this technique, a local anesthetic agent is injected directly into the hematoma surrounding the fracture, the location of which is confirmed by aspirating blood into the syringe (see Fig. 3-4). This block is quick and relatively simple to administer. The skin is prepped with a bactericidal agent and draped at the site of infiltration. The fracture hematoma is aspirated with a 20- or 22-gauge needle and then injected with plain lidocaine. The typical dose of lidocaine is 1 to 3 mg/kg, which should be concentrated so as to limit the total amount of fluid injected to less than 10 mL in order to avoid elevating soft-tissue compartment pressures and minimize the risk of creating a compartment syndrome or other neurovascular problem.[203] Although the medication is rapidly absorbed into the circulation, the resulting systemic blood levels of local anesthetic have been shown to be well below those required for CNS toxicity.[118] The anesthetic inhibits the generation and conduction of painful impulses primarily in small nonmyelinated nerve fibers in the periosteum and local tissues.[136] Although direct injection of the hematoma theoretically converts a closed fracture into an open one, there have been no reports of infection with this technique.[33] Reported complications with hematoma blocks in the upper extremity include compartment syndrome,[203] temporary paralysis of the anterior interosseous nerve,[203] and acute carpal tunnel syndrome.[102]

Although children as young as 2 years old have been included in reports of this method, there are no studies of hematoma block anesthesia administered exclusively to a pediatric population. In three separate studies authored by Dinley and Michelinakis,[50] Case,[33] and Johnson and Noffsinger[91] with a combined total of 491 adult *and* pediatric patients, hematoma block was shown to be effective for the reduction of a variety of fractures of the distal upper extremity in patients of all ages. Despite the generally favorable experience with hematoma block anesthesia, other methods of regional anesthesia have been shown to be more effective for the management of upper extremity fractures. A study by Abbaszadegan and Johnson[1] found that analgesia during fracture reduction was superior with IV regional (Bier block) anesthesia compared to hematoma block and that fracture alignment following reduction was better as well. The authors concluded that the more favorable outcomes achieved with Bier block were related to better analgesia and muscle relaxation.[1] Alioto et al.[4] described the use of an intra-articular hematoma block in the lower extremity for the manipulative reduction of ankle fractures in a population that included both children and adults. The youngest patient in their study group was 12 years old. The authors recommended that the block be administered via a slow direct injection with careful ECG monitoring for any evidence of dysrhythmias, and with this method, found the technique to be safe, effective, and well tolerated by patients.[4]

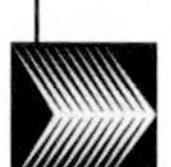

AUTHORS' PREFERRED TREATMENT

Full aseptic technique, including adequate skin preparation and the use of sterile gloves, is recommended.[91] The hematoma is localized by aspirating blood into the syringe. The local anesthetic solution is given gradually by barbotage—the alternate injection of a small amount of medication and withdrawal of a small amount of hematoma—until all of the medication has been given.

Axillary Block

Axillary block provides excellent anesthesia for the forearm and hand. Initial use of the technique is attributed to Halsted and Hall, who first utilized axillary block for outpatient procedures in 1884. The technique has since proven to be a safe and reliable method of anesthesia for a variety of outpatient surgical procedures in the upper extremity in both adults and children.[192] It is an excellent choice of anesthesia for treatment of fractures below the elbow because it provides muscle relaxation in addition to analgesia. Cramer et al.[46] reported on the successful use of axillary anesthesia by orthopaedic surgeons in the emergency department for the reduction of forearm fractures in children. In this study, effective anesthesia was achieved in 105 of 111 (95%) children with no complications.

Axillary block anesthesia is administered by placing the child in a supine position with the injured arm abducted and externally rotated 90 degrees. IV access is usually established in the uninjured extremity. Mild sedation may be helpful prior to the procedure. The axilla is prepped with a bactericidal solution and draped with sterile towels. The block is performed using a 1.0 % lidocaine solution at a dose of 3 to 5 mg/kg. As with the Bier block, a larger volume of local anesthetic is preferable and can be achieved by using a more dilute concentration of drug. The target for delivery of the anesthetic agent is the axillary sheath, which contains the axillary artery and vein surrounded by the radial nerve (behind), median nerve (above), and ulnar nerve (below). The musculocutaneous nerve courses outside of this sheath through the coracobrachialis muscle and, for this reason, may escape blockade, explaining the unreliability of this technique for anesthesia above the elbow.

Several techniques have been described to ensure accurate delivery of the anesthetic into the axillary sheath including blind injection into the neurovascular sheath, patient-reported paresthesia, use of a nerve stimulator, and transarterial puncture. Elicitation of paresthesias provides reliable evidence of position within the neurovascular sheath but may be uncomfortable and requires a conscious and cooperative patient. For these reasons, it cannot be used in most children. The use of a nerve stimulator and insulated needle to elicit a motor response is another effective method to determine accurate location within the sheath. However, this technique requires special equipment (nerve stimulator and insulated needles), which may not be readily available in an ambulatory setting, and threshold stimulation of the nerves may be distressful to the conscious patient.

The transarterial method is the most popular technique of axillary block and, as described in the study by Cramer et al.,[46] has been shown to be an effective way to administer this block in children (Fig. 3-5). With this method, the axillary artery is palpated, and a 23-gauge butterfly needle, connected via extension tubing to a syringe containing lidocaine, is inserted perpendicular to the artery. The needle is advanced while being continuously aspirated until a flash of arterial blood is seen and then advanced through the artery. Approximately two thirds of the lidocaine is injected into the sheath deep to the artery, checking by aspiration after every 5 cc to ensure extravascular positioning. The needle is withdrawn to the superficial side of the artery and the remaining lidocaine is injected. Pressure is held over the puncture site for 5 minutes, and fracture manipulation can usually begin shortly thereafter.

In most children, the axillary sheath is superficial because of the dearth of subcutaneous fat making for a technically easier procedure in a child than an adult. Of course, this advantage can be offset if the child is obese or uncooperative. From a pharmacokinetic standpoint, the local anesthetic diffuses more rapidly and with enhanced blockade of the nerves, which are smaller in diameter in children compared to adults.[192] The duration of the block is usually prolonged enough to allow repeat manipulation of the fracture in the event of an unsatisfactory reduction.

Potential complications of axillary block anesthesia include systemic lidocaine toxicity, hematoma formation, and persistent neurologic symptoms. Horner's syndrome has also been reported. In actuality, complications of axillary block anesthesia are rare.[192] None were encountered in the series reported by Cramer et al.[46] of 111 children with displaced forearm fractures treated in an emergency department setting. Contraindications to axillary block anesthesia are the presence of a coagulopathy of any type, a pre-existing neurologic or vascular abnormality of the extremity, axillary lymphadenitis, or an uncooperative or combative patient.

Wrist and Digital Blocks

While brachial plexus anesthesia may be efficacious for any fracture of the upper extremity below the elbow, more-distal upper extremity blocks at the wrist or of the digital nerves in the hand may be useful for treatment of fractures or minor surgical procedures of the hand. Anesthesia to the digits can be achieved by block of the common digital nerves near the point of bifurcation at the level of the metacarpal heads or by block of the radial and ulnar digital nerves at the base of each finger. This technique is most useful for treatment of phalangeal fracture(s) of a single digit. For injuries involving multiple digits or the metacarpals, anesthesia of the hand can be achieved by blocking the three major nerves of the upper extremity at the wrist (wrist block). The median nerve is located on the radial side of the palmaris longus tendon approximately 2 cm proximal to the wrist crease and can be blocked with 3 to 5 mL of local anesthetic (Fig. 3-6A). The ulnar nerve is blocked on the radial side of the flexor carpi ulnaris about 2 cm proximal to the volar wrist crease with 3 to 5 mL of local anesthetic, and the dorsal and volar cutaneous branches of the nerve are blocked by subcu-

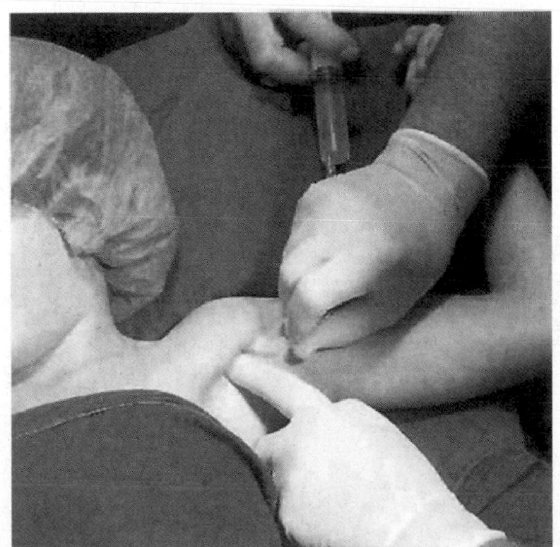

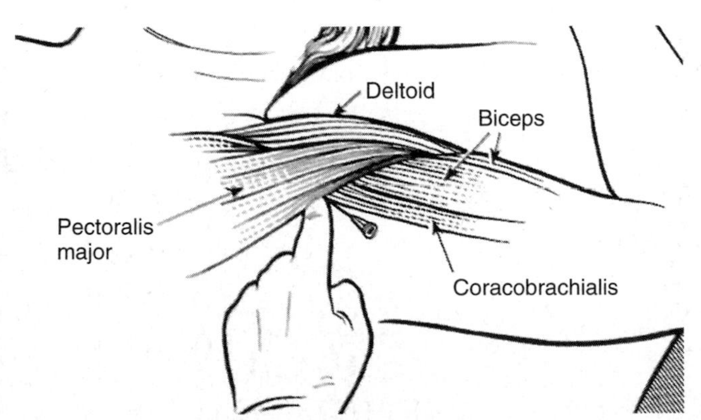

FIGURE 3-5 Technique of needle insertion for axillary block. The axillary artery is palpated and the needle inserted at the lateral edge of the pectoralis major and parallel to the coracobrachialis. (Adapted from McCarty EC, Mencio GA. Anesthesia and analgesia for the ambulatory management of children's fractures. In: Green NE, Swiontkowski MF, eds. Skeletal Trauma in Children. 3rd ed. Philadelphia: Saunders, 2003.)

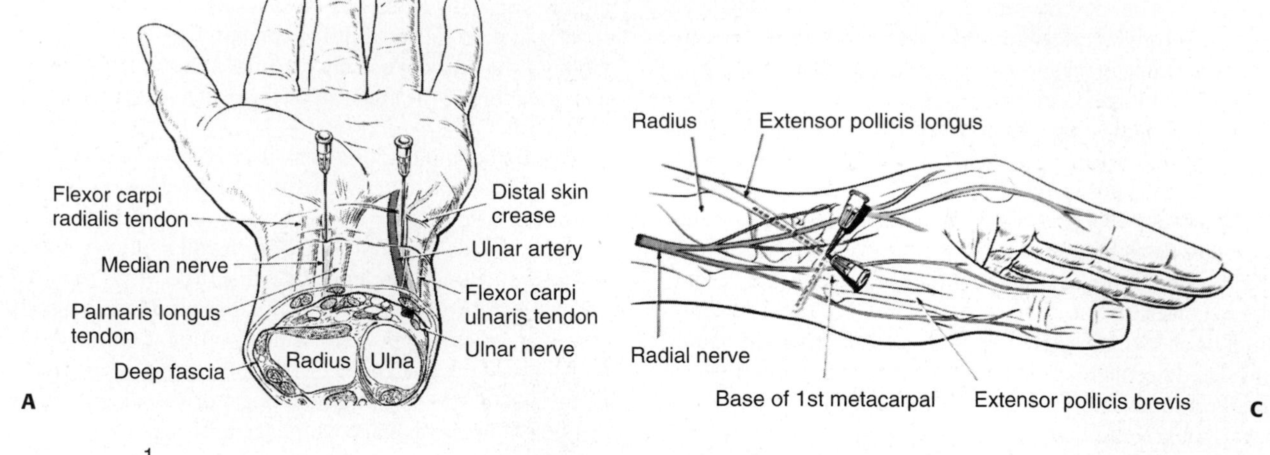

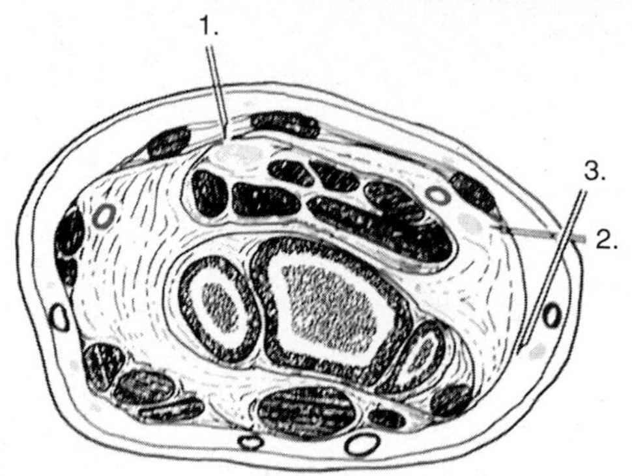

FIGURE 3-6 A. Technique for median and ulnar nerve blockade at the wrist. The median nerve is approached from the palmar side of the wrist between the palmaris longus and flexor carpi radialis. The ulnar nerve can be approached between the flexor carpi ulnaris tendon and the ulnar artery. **B.** Alternative method for ulnar nerve blockade. The ulnar can also be approached from the ulnar side of the wrist just dorsal to the flexor carpi ulnaris tendon. **C.** Technique for radial nerve block at the wrist. Needle is inserted where the extensor pollicis longus tendon crosses the base of the first metacarpal and approximately 2 to 3 mm of local anesthetic injected as the needle is advanced along the tendon to the radial tubercle. The needle is then redirected at a right angle across the anatomical "snuff box" and an additional 1 to 2 mm injected to the radial border of the extensor pollicis longus tendon. (From McCarty EC, Mencio GA. Anesthesia and analgesia for the ambulatory management of children's fractures. In: Green NE, Swiontkowski MF, eds. Skeletal Trauma in Children, 3rd ed. Philadelphia: Saunders, Philadelphia, 2003.)

taneous injection of an additional 2 to 3 mL of anesthetic (Fig. 3-6A). Alternatively, the ulnar nerve may be approached from the ulnar side of the wrist, just dorsal to the flexor carpi ulnaris tendon (Fig. 3-6B). The terminal branches of the radial nerve are blocked by injection of 1 to 2 mL of anesthetic along the extensor pollicis longus tendon as it crosses the base of the first metacarpal and across the "snuff box" to the radial side of the extensor pollicis brevis tendon (Fig. 3-6C).

Femoral Nerve Block

Femoral nerve blockade is another type of regional anesthesia that has been used in the treatment of femoral fractures.[18,34,48,78,142,143,188] Although the majority of children with femoral fractures are not managed on an outpatient basis, femoral nerve blockade can provide excellent anesthesia and analgesia for the initial management of this injury including manipulation of the fracture, application of an immediate spica cast, or placement of a traction pin. It is a good option for children unable to undergo general anesthesia or for those who cannot be sedated for any reason. This technique is most effective for fractures of the middle third of the femur but less so for fractures of the proximal and distal thirds of the bone, as these areas also receive sensory innervation from branches of the obturator and sciatic nerves, respectively.

Blockade of the femoral nerve is performed by preparing and draping the inguinal area and palpating the femoral artery. A 22- or 23-gauge needle on a syringe containing an appropriately dosed local anesthetic agent (typically either 1% to 1.5% lidocaine with 1:200,000 epinephrine, dosed up to 7 mg/kg[18] or 0.5% bupivicaine, dosed at 1 to 1.5 mg/kg[145]) is inserted one fingerbreadth lateral to the artery and 1 to 2 centimeters below the inguinal ligament (Fig. 3-7). The needle is advanced at a 30 to 45-degree angle to the skin and the syringe aspirated as the needle passes through the deep fascia into the femoral triangle. If no blood is aspirated, the anesthetic agent is injected

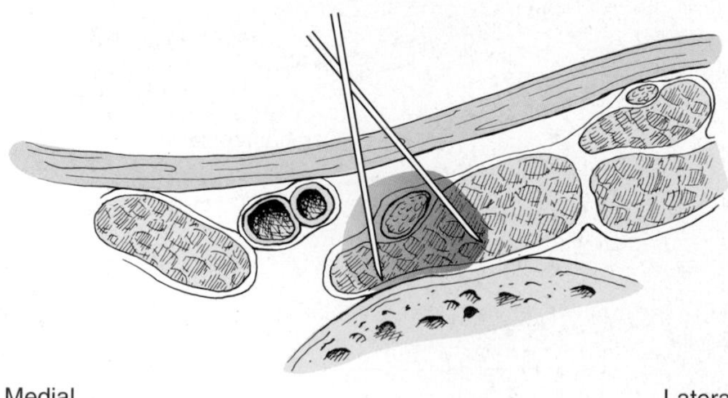

FIGURE 3-7 Section of right thigh immediately below the inguinal ligament, showing femoral nerve under cover of fascia iliaca and its block by a barrage technique. (Reproduced with permission from Berry FR. Analgesia in patients with fractured shaft of femur. Anesthesia 1977;32:577.)

around the femoral nerve. Alternatively, the nerve can be blocked more proximally within the fascia iliaca compartment by entering just above the inguinal ligament with the advantage of accessing all branches of the nerve before it starts to arborize. As with axillary block, the volume of the anesthetic is the key to achieving anesthesia with this technique. The onset of analgesia occurs within 10 minutes and, with the use of long-acting agents such as bupivicaine, may last up to 8 hours.[48] In one randomized control study, regional blockade of the femoral nerve was shown to provide clinically superior pain relief compared with IV morphine sulfate throughout the initial 6 hours of management in children aged 16 months to 15 years with isolated femoral shaft fractures.[188]

In the reports of this technique, there have been few inadvertent arterial punctures with no long-term sequelae and no neurologic complications.[48,78,145] Other potential complications include systemic toxicity from intravascular injection, infection, and injury to the nerve. As with the axillary block, this method may be difficult in obese children as well as the young and/or uncooperative child. Contraindications include any preexisting neurologic abnormality of the injured lower extremity and the inability to manage complications of systemic toxicity.

POSTOPERATIVE ANALGESIA IN THE CHILD WITH A MUSCULOSKELETAL INJURY

Safe and effective postoperative analgesia in children with musculoskeletal injuries can be accomplished with opioids, NSAIDs, or local anesthetic agents. Simultaneous use of more than one modality may be beneficial to minimize the side effects from any one particular approach (e.g., the use of NSAIDs to decrease the incidence of nausea, vomiting, or even respiratory depression from opioids). The end point is to make patients comfortable while minimizing adverse reactions.

Postoperative Analgesia with Opioids

Opioids have long been the mainstay of postoperative analgesia. It is important for the practitioner to understand the rationale behind different dosage regimens to maximize pain relief for the patient.

Intermittent Dosing

Although commonly used, traditional intermittent as-needed dosing of IM and IV opioids (Table 3-16) makes little pharmacologic sense for control of severe pain.[60,181] Wide variations in plasma opioid levels occur, leading to periods of sedation alternating with prolonged periods of no pain relief at all.[60] In addition, for pediatric care, IM dosing is a particularly poor choice because children often choose to hide their pain rather than risk having to undergo an injection. The end result with intermittent dosing, especially with IM narcotics, is undertreatment of pain.

Patient-Controlled Analgesia

Patient-controlled analgesia (PCA) is a sensible approach to the problems inherent with intermittent dosing of opioids.[60] With PCA, intravenous self-titration of small doses of opioids at frequent intervals eliminates the wide variations in plasma drug levels seen with intermittent dosing. It also allows patients to gain control over their pain management, which may be of psychologic importance to the patient's well-being. PCA was first evaluated in adolescents in 1987, after several years of successful use in adults.[28] Since then, this modality has been used for children as young as 6 years of age.[16] Depending on the intelligence and cooperative ability of the child, it is conceivable that PCA could be used for younger individuals, although careful assessment of each individual situation is required.

TABLE 3-16 Parenteral Opioid Dosing Schedule for Analgesia in Children*

IM†: Morphine, 0.1–0.15 mg/kg q3–4h; Meperidine, 1.0–1.5 mg/kg q3–4h

IV: Morphine, 0.05–0.1 mg/kg q2h; Meperidine, 0.5–1.0 mg/kg q2h

*Infants less than 3 mos old should be dosed in increments of one third to one half because of increased risk of respiratory depression.
†IM dosing should rarely be used.
Adapted from Roger L, Moro M. Acute postoperative and chronic pain in children. In: Rasch DK, Webster DE, eds. Clinical Manual of Pediatric Anesthesia. New York: McGraw-Hill, 1994:297, with permission.

When compared with traditional intermittent dosing, improved pain control and greater patient satisfaction have been demonstrated.[16] Further improvement in pain relief may be achieved with the addition of a continuous background infusion of opioids to maintain the plasma concentrations of the analgesic during sleep. However, adding a background infusion may increase the risk of opioid-associated nausea, sedation, and hypoxemia.[51,200] Conceivably, for younger children or for children incapable of reliably pushing the button on the PCA cord, "parent-controlled analgesia" may be useful. This approach has led to many instances of oversedation. In general, PCA is safest when only the patient is operating the device.

Parameters that must be considered are the loading dose, the maintenance dose, the lockout interval (the period during which no further administration of medication will occur despite attempts to do so by the patient), and the 4-hour maximum dose (Table 3-17). For PCA, morphine is more effective than meperidine.[186] Opioids other than morphine should be used only for patients allergic to morphine, or in whom morphine produces intolerable side effects. Whenever possible, the persistent use of one medication helps avoid dosing errors.[25] The use of the PCA pump should be explained to patients preoperatively. Effective use of a loading dose will avoid the problem of having to "catch up" with soaring levels of pain. Mishaps have occurred with PCA pumps due to programming errors, so staff must be well-trained in safe use of the equipment.[195] Treatment of opioid-related side effects is outlined in Table 3-17.

Oral Administration of Opioids

Oral dosing of opioids is extremely useful for the continued management of diminishing postoperative pain, as soon as oral intake is tolerated. Several oral analgesics are available, and their appropriate use is summarized in Table 3-18. All of these drugs have side effects including mood changes, nausea, vomiting, constipation, dizziness, and pruritus. The occurrence and degree of side effects vary from patient to patient, so the physician should be prepared to change dosing regimens based on patient

TABLE 3-17 Patient-Controlled Analgesia in Children

Loading dose: Morphine, 0.025–0.05 mg/kg

Maintenance dose: Morphine, 0.01–0.02 mg/kg

Lockout interval: 6–10 min

4-hr maximum: Morphine, 0.4 mg/kg/4 h

Treatment of Side Effects

Pruritus: Diphenhydramine (0.5 mg/kg IV) OR low-dose naloxone (0.5–1.0 μg/hr)

Nausea/vomiting: Metoclopramide (0.1 mg/kg IV) OR droperidol (10–30 μg/kg IV or IM) OR ondansetron (0.15 mg/kg IV over 15 min) OR low-dose naloxone as for pruritus

Urinary retention (<1 mL/kg/h in the face of adequate fluid intake): Low-dose naloxone infusion as above

Respiratory depression: Specify vital sign parameters that require treatment and method for contracting responsible physician. Stop PCA pump. Give 100% oxygen and maintain the airway. Give naloxone (1–5 μg/kg IV bolus); repeat as needed. Consider naloxone infusion (3–5 μg/kg/h).

From Rogers J, Moro M. Acute postoperative and chronic pain in children. In: Rasch DR, Webster DE, eds. Clinical Manual of Pediatric Anesthesia. New York: McGraw-Hill, 1994:298, with permission.

TABLE 3-18 Dosing Schedules and Formulations for Oral Opioids in Children

Agent	Dose	Pediatric Formulations*
Codeine†	0.5–1.0 mg/kg q4 to 6h (max. single dose, 60 mg)	15 mg/5 mL oral solution
Codeine with acetaminophen (Tylenol with Codeine, Phenaphen with Codeine, Capital with Codeine)	0.5–1.0 mg/kg codeine q4 to 6h + 10–15 mg/kg acetaminophen q4 to 6h	12 mg codeine + 120 mg acetaminophen/5 mL solution Tylenol (300 mg) + Codeine tablets #1: 7.5 mg, #2: 15 mg, #3: 30 mg, #4: 60 mg
Hydrocodone with acetaminophen (Lortab, Anexsia, Co-Gesic, DuoCet, Hy-Phen, Vicodin)	Adult dose: hydrocodone 5–10 mg q4 to 6h Children (only antitussive dose is published): 0.6 mg/kg day divided in three to four doses/day. <2 yr: Do not exceed 1.25 mg/dose. 2–12 yr: Do not exceed 5 mg/single dose. >12 yr: Do not exceed 10 mg/single dose.	2.5 mg hydrocodone/5 mL + acetaminophen 120 mg/5 mL (Lortab Liquid)
Meperidine (Meperidine HCl, Demerol HCl)†	1.1–1.8 mg/kg q3 to 4h Max. single dose 100 mg	50 mg meperidine/5 mL solution
Morphine (morphine sulfate, Raxanol)†	0.2–0.4 mg/kg q4h (adult dose is 10–30 mg q4h) Absorption from the gastrointestinal tract is variable.	10 mg/5 mL and 20 mg/5 mL solution
Hydromorphone (Dilaudid, Hydromorphone HCl)†	Optimal pediatric dosage for analgesia not established. Antitussive dose is: 6–12 yr: 0.5 mg q3–4h >12 yr: 1 mg q3–4h	5 mg hydromorphone/5 mL solution
Oxycodone and Aspirin‡ (Percodan-Demi)† ‡‡	6–12 yr: 1/4 tablet q6h >12 yr: 1/2 tablet q6h	Oxycodone‡‡ + 325 mg aspirin

*This table does not provide an exhaustive list of all available oral opioids and oral opioid/nonsteroidal anti-inflammatory drug combinations. A complete discussion and complete lists of all respective formulations may be found in AHFS Drug Information 1994.
†Denotes a schedule 1 drug, for which a triplicate prescription is required.
‡Owing to an association with Reyes syndrome, medications containing aspirin should be expressly avoided in children with flulike symptoms or children with chickenpox.
‡‡Percodan-Demi contains 2.25 mg oxycodone hydrochloride and 0.19 mg oxycodone terephthalate + 325 mg aspirin.
Adapted from Opiate Agonists. In McEvoy CK, Litvak K, Weish OH, Jr, eds. AHFS Drug Information 1994. Bethesda, MD American Society of Hospital Pharmacists, 1994; Taketomo CK, Hodding JHJ, Kraus DM. Pediatric Dosage Handbook. 2nd ed. Hudson, OH. Lexi-Comp, 1993; Ragers J, Moro M. Acute postoperative and chronic pain in children. In Rasch DK, Webster DE (eds.). Clinical Manual of Pediatric Anesthesia. New York: McGraw-Hill, 1994, with permission.

response. The use of NSAIDs (see the following section) as part of the analgesic regimen may be helpful in reducing or eliminating troublesome opioid-related side effects.

Other Modes of Opioid Administration

Epidural opioids are being used in children after major surgery with excellent results. Communication and cooperation between surgeons and anesthesiologists is critical to identify appropriate candidates for this modality of analgesia whenever feasible.[139]

Postoperative Analgesia with Nonsteroidal Anti-inflammatory Drugs

NSAIDs have good analgesic properties.[181] Unlike opioids, which produce analgesia by effects on CNS receptors, NSAIDs act peripherally by inhibiting prostaglandin synthesis and decreasing inflammation. Inflammatory mechanisms play an important part in the pathogenesis of postoperative pain[18]; therefore, the use of NSAIDs makes good sense in the postoperative setting. Also, although NSAIDs have some troubling side effects of their own, they do not produce respiratory depression, nausea, and vomiting, which are some of the bothersome features of opioids. Thus, using NSAIDs either as an adjunct or as a substitute for opioids when feasible should help lessen opioid-induced nausea, vomiting, and respiratory depression in the surgical patient.[18]

Potential side effects of this class of drugs include platelet dysfunction, gastritis, and acute renal dysfunction.[117,187] A history of sensitivity to aspirin or a history of nasal polyps may be associated with potentially fatal cross-sensitivity to other NSAIDs.[171] In children with asthma, the prevalence of aspirin sensitivity may be as high as 28%.[138] Therefore, asthmatic children should probably receive only those NSAIDs that do not cross-react with aspirin. These medications include acetaminophen, salsalate, and choline magnesium trisalicylate (see Table 3-18).[166] In a child with a chronic underlying bleeding disorder, NSAIDs are not necessarily contraindicated. Consultation with the child's hematologist is advised regarding the use of specific medications in this class.

Ketorolac, unlike other NSAIDs, can be administered not only orally but also IV and IM. A loading dose of 1.0 mg/kg may provide similar analgesia as 0.1 mg/kg of morphine.[111] The pharmacology of ketorolac has been extensively reviewed and both its mode of action and adverse reactions are generally typical of NSAIDs.[106] The major controversy with this drug remains its effect on hemostasis and bleeding. Rusy et al.[146] found that ketorolac contributed to increased blood loss and more difficulty in achieving surgical hemostasis in pediatric tonsillectomy patients. Caution is advised in administering ketorolac or any other NSAID in a perioperative situation in which bleeding has been or can be significant. Ketorolac has been associated with an increased incidence of nonunion in patients undergoing spine fusion. Suggested dosing schedules for some of the more common NSAIDs are listed in Table 3-19. Acetaminophen is considered a member of this class of medications, although its mechanism of action is central and its effects on prostaglandin synthesis and the inflammatory response are comparatively very weak.[187]

Postoperative Analgesia with Local Anesthetic Agents

Regional anesthesia is an excellent means of providing postoperative analgesia without respiratory depression and with minimal

TABLE 3-19 Dosing Schedules and Formulations for Nonsteroidal Anti-inflammatory Drugs in Children

Agent	Dose	Formulations*
Ibuprofen (oral)	5–10 mg/kg q6h (published dose is for treatment of fever, not specifically for analgesia)	100 mg/5 mL suspension Tablets: 200, 300, 400, 600, 800 mg
Naproxen (oral)	5–7.5 mg/kg q12h	125 mg/5 mL suspension Tablets: 250, 375, 500 mg
Ketorolac (IM, IV)	0.5 mg/kg q6h	Injectable 30 mg/mL
Choline Magnesium	50 mg/kg/day	500 mg salicylate/5 mL solution
Trisalicylate (Trilisate) (oral)†	Divided into 2 or 3 doses (maximum daily dose, 2.25 g)	Tablets: 500, 750, 1000 mg
Salsalatel† (oral) (Disalcid)	Pediatric dose not published; adult maintenance dose is 2–4 g/day.	Tablets: 500, 750 mg
Acetaminophen‡ (oral, rectal)	10–15 mg/kg q4–6h	80mg/0.8mL drops 80mg chewable tablets 160mg/5mL solution 325-, 500-mg tablets 120-, 325-, 650-mg suppositories

*An exhaustive listing of available formulations for NSAIDs may be found in AHFS Drug Information 1994.
†Although they are salicylates, choline magnesium trisalicylate, and salsalate do not cross-react with aspirin and may be used in patients allergic to aspirin. As many as 28% of children with asthma may be in this group of patients. Owing to an association with Reye syndrome, salicylates should be avoided in children with flu-like symptoms or chickenpox.
‡Acetaminophen is considered a member of this class of medications, even though it mainly acts centrally and it only very weakly inhibits prostaglandin synthesis. Acetaminophen also does not cross-react with aspirin and may be used in patients allergic to aspirin.
Adapted from Nonsteroidal Anti-Inflammatory Agents. In McEvoy GK, Litvak K, Welsh OH Jr, eds. AHFS Drug Information 1994. Bethesda, MD: American Society of Hospital Pharmacists, 1994; Walson PD, Mortensen ME. Pharmacokinetics of common analgesics, anti-inflammatories, and antipyretics in children. Clin Pharmacokinet 1989;17:116–137, with permission.

physiologic alterations.[201] Both central (epidural) and peripheral (e.g., brachial plexus) nerve blocks may be used for this purpose. The physician must ensure that the pain relief achieved does not mask the signs and symptoms of developing vascular or neurologic compromise.[53,124]

TREATMENT OF POSTOPERATIVE NAUSEA

Postoperative nausea is common in children, although not particularly after peripheral orthopaedic procedures.[111] The pharmacologic treatment is outlined in Table 3-19. Additional helpful measures include not forcing intake of oral fluids until the child is hungry and minimizing early postoperative ambulation, especially when opioids have been given.[17]

REFERENCES

1. Abbaszadegan H, Jonsson U. Regional anesthesia preferable for Colles' fracture: controlled comparison with local anesthesia. Acta Orthop Scand 1990;61:348–349.
2. Albright G. Cardiac arrest following regional anesthesia with etidocaine or bupivacaine [editorial]. Anesthesiology 1979;51:285–287.
3. Alexander C, Gross J. Sedative doses of midazolam depress hypoxic ventilatory responses in humans. Anesth Analg 1988;67:377–382.
4. Alioto R, Furia J, Marquardt J. Hematoma block for ankle fractures: a safe and efficacious technique for manipulations. J Orthop Trauma 1995;9:113–116.
5. American Academy of Pediatrics Committee of Drugs. Guidelines for monitoring and management of pediatric patients during and after sedation for diagnostic and therapeutic procedures. Pediatrics 1992;6:1110–1115.
6. American Academy of Pediatrics Committee of Drugs. Reappraisal of lytic cocktail/demerol, phenergen, and thorazine (DPT) for the sedation of children. Pediatrics 1995; 95:598–602.
7. American Society of Anesthesiologists Task Force on Sedation and Analgesia by Non-Anesthesiologists. Practice guidelines for sedation and analgesia by non-anesthesiologists. Anesthesiology 1996;84:459–471.
8. Arandia H, Patil V. Glottic closure following large doses of fentanyl [letter]. Anesthesiology 1987;66:574–575.
9. Askgaard B, Nilsson T, Ibler M, et al. Muscle tone under fentanyl-nitrous oxide anaesthesia measured with a transducer apparatus in cholecystectomy incisions. Acta Anaesthesiol Scand 1977;21(1):1–4.
10. Azar I, Turndorf H. Severe hypertension and multiple atrial premature contractions following naloxone administration. Anesth Anal 1979;58:524–525.
11. Bailey P, Stanley T. Pharmacology of intravenous narcotic anesthetics. In: Miller R, ed. Anesthesia. 2nd ed. New York: Churchill-Livingstone, 1986.
12. Barker S, Hyatt J, Shah N, et al. The effect of sensor malpositioning of pulse oximeter accuracy during hypoxemia. Anesthesiology 1993;79:248–254.
13. Barnes C, Blasier R, Dodge B. Intravenous regional anesthesia: a safe and cost-effective outpatient anaesthetic for upper extremity fracture treatment in children. J Pediatr Orthop 1991;11:717–720.
14. Beales J, Kean J, Lennox-Holt P. The child's perception of the diseases and experience of pain in juvenile chronic arthritis. J Rheumatol 1983;10(1):61–65.
15. Bell H, Slater E, Harris W. Regional anesthesia with intravenous lidocaine. JAMA 1963; 186:544–549.
16. Berde C, Lehn B, Yee J, et al. Patient-controlled analgesia in children and adolescents: a prospective comparison with intramuscular administration of morphine for postoperative analgesia. J Pediatr 1991;118:461–466.
17. Berry F. Anesthesia for the child with a difficult airway. In: Berry F, ed. Anesthetic management of difficult and routine pediatric patients. New York: Churchill-Livingstone, 1990.
18. Berry F. Analgesia in patients with fractured shaft of femur. Anesthesia 1977;32: 576–577.
19. Bier A. Ueber einen neuen weg local anasthesie an den gliedmassen zu enzeugen. Arch Klin Chir 1908;86:1007–1016.
20. Bilban P, Baraldi E, Pattenazzo A, et al. Adverse effect of chloral hydrate in two young children with obstructive sleep apnea. Pediatrics 1993;92:461–463.
21. Binder L, Leake L. Chloral hydrate for emergent pediatric procedural sedation: a new look at an old drug. Am J Emerg Med 1991;9:530–534.
22. Bolte R, Stevens P, Scott S, et al. Mini-dose Bier block intravenous regional anesthesia in the emergency department treatment of pediatric upper-extremity injuries. J Pediatr Orthop 1994;14:534–537.
23. Braunstein M. Apnea with maintenance of consciousness following intravenous diazepam. Anesth Analg 1979;58:52–53.
24. Bricker S, McLuckie A, Nightingale D. Gastric aspirates after trauma in children. Anesthesia 1989;44:721–724.
25. Broadman L. Patient-controlled analgesia in children and adolescents. In: Ferrante FM, Ostheimer GW, Covino BG, eds. Patient-Controlled Analgesia. Boston: Blackwell Scientific Publishing, 1990:129–138.
26. Brooks T, Paulus D, Winkle W. Infrared heat lamps interfere with pulse oximeters (letter). Anesthesiology 1984;61:630.
27. Brown D, Beamish D, Wildsmith J. Allergic reaction to an amide local anaesthetic. Br J Anaesth 1981;53:435–437.
28. Brown R Jr, Broadman L. Patient-controlled analgesia for postoperative pain control in adolescents [abstract]. Anesth Anal 1987;66:S22.
29. Buhrer M, Maitre P, Crevoisier C, et al. EEG effects of benzodiazepines. II. Pharmacodynamic modeling of the EEG effects of midazolam and diazepam. Clin Pharmacol Ther 1990;48:555–567.
30. Caro D. Trial of ketamine in an accident and emergency department. Anaesthesia 1974; 29:227–229.
31. Caroli G, Lari S, Serra G. La ketamina in ortopedia e traumatologia: indicazioni e limiti. Chir Degli Organi Movimento 1972;61:99–104.
32. Carrel E, Eyring E. Intravenous regional anesthesia for childhood fractures. J Trauma 1971;11:301–305.
33. Case R. Haematoma block—a safe method of reducing Colles' fractures. Injury 1985; 16:469–470.
34. Chu RS, Browner GJ, Cheng NG, et al. Femoral nerve block for femoral shaft fractures in a paediatric Emergency department: can it be done better? Eur J Emerg Med 2003; 10:258–263.
35. Chudnofsky C, Wright S, Pronen S. The safety of fentanyl use in the emergency department. Ann Emerg Med 1989;18:635.
36. Colbern E. The Bier block for intravenous regional anesthesia: technic and literature review. Anesth Analg 1970;49(6):935–940.
37. Colizza W, Said E. Intravenous regional anesthesia in the treatment of forearm and wrist fractures and dislocations in children. Can J Surg 1993;36:225–228.
38. Coln D. Trauma in children. In: Levin D, Morris F, eds. Essentials of Pediatric Intensive Care. St. Louis: Quality Medical Publishing, 1990:671–676.
39. Cook B, Bass J, Nomizu S, et al. Sedation of children for technical procedures. Clin Pediatr 1992;31:137–142.
40. Corssen G. Dissociative anesthesia. In: Corssen G, Reves J, Stanley T, eds. Intravenous anesthesia and analgesia. Philadelphia: Lea & Febiger, 1988.
41. Cote CJ. NPO after midnight for children—a reappraisal. Anesthesiology 1990;72: 589–592.
42. Cote CJ. Sedation for the pediatric patient: a review. Pediatr Clin North Am 1994;41: 31–51.
43. Cote CJ, Goldstein E, Cote M, et al. A single-blind study of pulse oximetry in children. Aneshesiology 1988;68:184–188.
44. Cote CJ, Todres ID. The pediatric airway. In: Cote CJ, Todres ID, Ryan JF, et al., eds. Practice of Anesthesia for Infants and Children. New York: Elsevier Health Services, 1986:31–51.
45. Covino B. Clinical pharmacology of local anesthetic agents. In: Cousins M, Bridenbaugh P, eds. Neural Blockade in Clinical Anesthesia and Management of Pain. 2nd ed. Philadelphia: J.B. Lippincott, 1988:111–144.
46. Cramer K, Glasson S, Mencio GA, et al. Reduction of forearm fractures in children using axillary block anesthesia. J Orthop Trauma 1995;9(5):407–410.
47. Dachs RJ, Innes GM. Intravenous ketamine sedation of pediatric patients in the emergency department. Ann Emerg Med 1997;29:146–150.
48. Denton J, Manning M. Femoral nerve block for femoral shaft fractures in children: brief report. J Bone Joint Surg 1988;70-B:84.
49. Deshpande J, Anand K. Basic aspects of acute pediatric pain and sedation. In: Deshpande J, Tobias, JD, eds. The Pediatric Pain Handbook. St. Louis: Mosby, 1996:48.
50. Dinley R, Michelinakis E. Local anesthesia in the reduction of Colles' fractures. Injury 1973;4:345–346.
51. Doyle E, Robinson D, Morton N. Comparison of patient-controlled analgesia with and without a background infusion after lower abdominal surgery in children. Br J Anaesth 1993;71:670–673.
52. Dretchen K, Ghoneim M, Long J. The interaction of diazepam with myoneural blocking agents. Anesthesiology 1971;34:463–468.
53. Dunwoody J, Reichert C, Brown K. Compartment syndrome associated with bupivacaine and fentanyl analgesia in pediatric orthopaedics. 1997;17:285–288.
54. Eddie R, Deutsch S. Cardiac arrest after interscalene brachial-plexus block. Anesth Anal 1977;56:446–447.
55. Estilo A, Cottrell J. Hemodynamic and catecholamine changes after administration of naloxone. Anesth Anal 1965;61:349–353.
56. Evans J, Buckley S, Alexander A, et al. Analgesia for the reduction of fractures in children: a comparison of nitrous oxide with intramuscular sedation. J Pediatr Orthop 1995;15:73–77.
57. Farrell R, Swanson S, Walter J. Safe and effective iv regional anesthesia for use in the emergency department. Ann Emerg Med 1984;14:239–241.
58. Fatovich D, Jacobs I. A randomized, controlled trial of oral midazolam and buffered lidocaine for suturing lacerations in children (the SLIC trial). Ann Emerg Med 1995; 25:209–214.
59. Feld L, Negus J, White P. Oral midazolam preanesthetic medication in pediatric outpatients. Anesthesiology 1990;73:831–834.
60. Ferrante F. Patient Characteristics Influencing Effective Use of Patient-Controlled Analgesia. Boston: Blackwell Scientific Publications, 1990.
61. Ferrari LR, Rooney FM, Rockoff MA. Preoperative fasting practices in pediatrics. Anesthesiology 1999;90:978–980.
62. Finegan B, Bukht M. Venous pressure in the isolated upper limb during saline injection. Can Anaesth Soc J 1984;31:364–367.
63. Fisher M, Graham R. Adverse responses to local anesthetics. Anesthesia Intensive Care 1984;12:325–327.
64. Fitzgerald B. Intravenous regional anaesthesia in children. Br J Anaesth 1976;48: 485–486.
65. Forster A, Gardaz J, Sutter P, et al. Respiratory depression by midazolam and diazepam. Anesthesiology 1980;53:494–497.
66. Friedland L, Kulick R. Emergency department analgesic use in pediatric trauma victims with fractures. Ann Emerg Med 1994;23:203–207.
67. Fujigaki T, Fukusaki M, Nakamura H, et al. Quantitative evaluation of gastric contents using ultrasound. J Clin Anesth 1993;5:451–455.
68. Galletly D, Forrest P, Purdie G. Comparison of the recovery characteristics of diazepam and midazolam. Br J Anesthe 1988;60:520–524.
69. Gibbs PC, Modell JH. Aspiration pneumonitis In: Miller R, New Y, eds. Anesthesia. New York: Churchill-Livingstone, 1986.
70. Gingrich T. Intravenous regional anaesthesia of the upper extremity in children. JAMA 1967;200:235.

71. Gourlay G, Boas R. Fatal outcome with use of rectal morphine for postoperative pain control in an infant. Br Med J 1992;304:766–767.
72. Grant I, Nimmo W, McNicol L, et al. Ketamine disposition in children and adults. Br J Anesthe 1983;55:1107–1111.
73. Green SM, Johnson N. Ketamine sedation for pediatric procedures: part 2, review and implications. Ann Emerg Med 1990;19:1033–1046.
74. Green SM, Nakamura R, Johnson NE. Ketamine sedation for pediatric procedures: part 1, a prospective series. Ann Emerg Med 1990;19:1024–1032.
75. Green SM, Sherwin TS. Incidence and severity of recovery agitation after ketamine sedation in young adults. Am J Emerg Med 2005;23:142–144.
76. Gregory P, Sullivan J. Nitrous oxide compared with intravenous regional anesthesia in pediatric forearm fracture management. J Pediar Orthop 1996;16:187–191.
77. Grey W. Regional blocks and their difficulties. Aust Fam Physician 1977;6:900–906.
78. Grossbard G, Love B. Femoral nerve block: a simple and safe method of instant analgesia for femoral shaft fractures in children. Aust NZ J Surg 1979;49:592–594.
79. Gutstein H, Johnson K, Heard M, et al. Oral ketamine preanesthetic medication in children. Anesthesiology 1992;76:28–33.
80. Haslam D. Age and the perception of pain. Psychonomic Sci 1969;15:86–87.
81. Havel CJ, Strait RT, Hennes H. A clinical trial of propofol vs midazolam for procedural sedation in a pediatric emergency department. Acad Emerg Med 1999;6:989–997.
82. Hennes H, Wagner V, Bonadio W, et al. The effect of oral midazolam on anxiety of preschool children during laceration repair. Ann Emerg Med 1990;19:1006–1009.
83. Hennrikus W, Shin A, Klingelberger C. Self-administered nitrous oxide and a hematoma block for analgesia in the outpatient reduction of fractures in children. J Bone Joint Surg 1995;77-A:335–339.
84. Hennrikus W, Simpson R, Klingelberger C, et al. Self-administered nitrous oxide analgesia for pediatric reductions. J Pediatr Orthop 1994;14:538–542g.
85. Hershey L. Meperidine and central nervous system toxicity [editorial]. Ann Intern Med 1983;98:548–549.
86. Hollister G, Burn J. Side effects of ketamine in pediatric anesthesia. Anesth Analg 1974; 53:264–267.
87. Holmes C. Intravenous regional analgesia: a useful method of producing analgesia of the limbs. Lancet 1963;1:245–247.
88. Iber F, Livak A, Kruss D. Apnea and cardiopulmonary arrest during and after endoscopy. J Clin Gastroenterol 1992;14:109–113.
89. Jastak J, Pallasch J. Death after chloral hydrate sedation: report of a case. J Am Dent Assoc 1988;116:345–347.
90. Jay S, Ozolins M, Elliott C, et al. Assessment of children's distress during painful medical procedures. Health Psych 1983;2:133–147.
91. Johnson P, Noffsinger M. Hematoma block of distal forearm fractures: is it safe? Orthop Rev 1991;20:977–979.
92. Jones R, Chan K, Roulson C, et al. Pharmacokinetics of flumazenil and midazolam. Br J Anesthe 1993;70:286–292.
93. Juliano P, Mazur J, Cummings R, et al. Low-dose lidocaine intravenous regional anesthesia for forearm fractures in children. J Pediatr Orthop 1992;12:633–635.
94. Kaiko R, Foley K, Gabrinsky P, et al. Central nervous system excitatory effects of meperidine in cancer patients. Ann Neurol 1983;13:180–185.
95. Kaplan R, Yang CI. Sedation and analgesia in pediatric patients for procedures outside the operating room. Anesthesiol Clin North America. 2002;20(1):181–194, vii.
96. Karl H, Keifer A, Rosenberger J, et al. Comparison of the safety and efficacy of intranasal midazolam or sufentanil for preinduction of anesthesia in pediatric patients. Anesthesiology 1989;76:209–215.
97. Kennedy RM, Luhmann JD, Luhmann SJ. Emergency department management of pain-and anxiety-related to orthopedic fracture care: a guide to analgesic techniques and procedural sedation in children. Paediatr Drugs 2004;6:11–31.
98. Kennedy RM, Porter FL, Miller JP, et al. Comparison of fentanyl/midazolam with ketamine/midazolam for pediatric orthopedic emergencies. Pediatrics 1998;102: 956–963.
99. Kennedy RM, Porter FL, Miller JP, et al. Comparison of fentanyl/midazolam with ketamine/midazolam for pediatric orthopedic emergencies (comment). Pediatrics 1999; 104:1167–1168.
100. Klotz U, Kanto J. Pharmacokinetics and clinical use of flumazenil (Ro 15-1788). Clin Pharmacokinet 1988;14:1–12.
101. Kohrs R, Durieux M. Ketamine: teaching and old dog new tricks. Anesth Analg 1998; 87:264–267.
102. Kongsholm J, Olerud C. Neurological complications of dynamic reduction of Colles' fractures without anesthesia compared with traditional manipulation after local infiltration anesthesia. J Orthop Trauma 1987;1:43–47.
103. Krauss B, Zurakowski D. Sedation patterns in pediatric and general community hospital emergency departments. Pediatr Emerg Care 1998;14:99–103.
104. Lehman W, Jones W. Intravenous lidocaine for anesthesia in the lower extremity. A prospective study. J Bone J Surg 1984;66:1056–1060.
105. Litman RS. Airway obstruction after oral midazolam [letter]. Anesthesiology 1996;85: 1217–1218.
106. Litvak K, McEvoy G. Ketorolac, an injectable nonnarcotic analgesic. Clin Pharm 1987; 9:921–935.
107. Lockhart C, Nelson W. The relationship of ketamine requirement to age in pediatric patients. Anesthesiology 1974;40:507–508.
108. Losek JD, Reid S. Effects of initial pain treatment on sedation recovery time in pediatric emergency care. Pediatr Emerg Care 2006;22:100–103.
109. Lowe S, Hershey S. Sedation for imaging and invasive procedures. In: Deshpande J, Tobias J, eds. The pediatric pain handbook. St. Louis: Mosby, 1996:263–317.
110. Magnat D, Orr W, Smith R. Sleep apnea, hypersomnolence, and upper airway obstruction secondary to adenotonsillar enlargement. Arch Otolaryngol Head Neck Surg 1977; 103:383–386.
111. Mason L. Challenges in pediatric anesthesia. International Anesthesia Research Society Review Course Lectures 1999;:64–70.
112. Massanari M, Novitsky J, Reinstein L. Paradoxical reaction in children associated with midazolam use during endoscopy. Clin Pediatr 1997;36:681–684.
113. Maxwell LG, Yaster Y. The myth of conscious sedation. Arch Pediatr Adolesc Med 1996;150:665–667.
114. McCarty EC, Mencio GA. Anesthesia and analgesia for the ambulatory management of children's fractures. Philadelphia: Saunders, 2003:606–617.
115. McCarty EC, Mencio GA, Green NE. Anesthesia and analgesia for the ambulatory management of fractures in children. J Am Acad Orthop Surg 1999;7:81–91.
116. McCarty EC, Mencio GA, Walker LA, et al. Ketamine sedation for the reduction of children's fractures in the emergency department. J Bone Joint Surg 2000;82:912–918.
117. McIntire S, Rubenstein R, Gartner J, et al. Acute flank pain and reversible renal dysfunction associated with nonsteroidal anti-inflammatory drug use. Pediatrics 1993;92: 459–460.
118. Meinig R, Quick A, Lobmeyer L. Plasma lidocaine levels following hematoma block for distal radius fractures. J Orthop Trauma 1989;3:187–189.
119. Migita RT, Klein EJ, Garrison MM. Sedation and analgesia for pediatric fracture reduction in the emergency department: a systematic review. Arch Pediatr Adolesc Med 2006;160:46–51.
120. Miller M, Wishar HY, Nummo WS. Gastric contents at induction of anesthesia—is a 4-hour fast necessary. Br J Anesthe 1983;55:1185–1187.
121. Mitchell R, Koury S. Respiratory arrest after intramuscular ketamine injection in a 2-year-old child. Am J Emerg Med 1996;14:580–581.
122. Moore D, Crawford R, Scurlock J. Severe hypoxia and acidosis following local anesthetic-induced convulsions. Anesthesiology 1983;53:1185–1187.
123. Morris R, Miller G. Preoperative management of the patient with a full stomach. Clin Anesth 1976;11:25–29.
124. Mubarak S, Wilton NC. Compartment syndromes and epidural anesthesia [editorial]. J Pediatr Orthop 1997;17:282–284.
125. Muncibi S, Santoni R. Utilizzazione della Ketamina in ortopedia e traumatologia. Minerva Anes 1973;39:370–376.
126. Myers E, Charles P. Prolonged adverse reactions to ketamine in children. Anesthesiology 1978;49:39–40.
127. Ogden J. Skeletal Injury in the Child. Philadelphia: W.B. Saunders Company, 1990.
128. Olney B, Lugg P, Turner P, et al. Outpatient treatment of upper extremity injuries in childhood using intravenous regional anaesthesia. J Pediatr Orthop 1988;8:576–579.
129. Pagnani I, Ramaioli F, Mapelli A. Prospettive sull'impiego clinico della Ketamina cloridrato in ortopedia e traumatologia pediatrica. Minerva Anes 1974;40:159–162.
130. Paris P. Pain management in children. Emerg Med Clin North Am 1987;5:699–707.
131. Perkin R, Levin D. Shock. In: Levin D, Morris F, eds. Essentials of Pediatric Intensive Care. St. Louis: Quality Medical Publishing, 1990.
132. Peterson M. Making oral midazolam palatable for children [letter]. Anesthesiology 1990;73:1053.
133. Philip B, Simpson T, Hauch MA, et al. Flumazenil reverses sedation after midazolam-induced general anesthesia in ambulatory surgery patients. Anesth Analg 1990;71(4): 371–376.
134. Pitetti RD, Singh S, Pierce MC. Safe and efficacious use of procedural sedation and analgesia by nonanesthesiologists in a pediatric emergency department. Arch Pediatr Adolesc Med 2003;157:1090–1096.
135. Prentiss J. Cardiac arrest following caudal anesthesia. Anesthesiology 1979;50:51–53.
136. Proudfoot J. Analgesia, anesthesia, and conscious sedation. Emerg Med Clin North Am 1995;13:357–378.
137. Proudfoot J, Roberts M. Providing safe and effective sedation and analgesia for pediatric patients. Emerg Med Reports 1993;14:207–217.
138. Rachelefsky G, Coulson A, Siegel SC, et al. Aspirin intolerance in chronic childhood asthma: detected by oral challenge. Pediatrics 1975;56:443–448.
139. Rasmussen G. Epidural and spinal anesthesia and analgesia. St. Louis: Mosby, 1996.
140. Reeves J, Fragen R, Vinik H, et al. Midazolam: pharmacology and uses. Anesthesiology 1999;62:310–324.
141. Reich D, Silvay G. Ketamine: an update on the first 25 years of clinical experience. Can J Anaesth 1989;36:186–197.
142. Riou B, Barriot P, Viars P. Femoral nerve block in fractured shaft of femur. Anesthesiology 1988;69:A375.
143. Rita L, Seleny F, Goodarzi M. Comparison of the calming and sedative effects of nalbuphine and pentazocine for paediatric premedication. Can Anaesth Soc J 1980;27: 546–549.
144. Roback M, Wathen J, Bajaj L, et al. Adverse events associated with procedural sedation and analgesia in a pediatric emergency department: a comparison of common parenteral drugs. Acad Emerg Med 2005;12:508–513.
145. Ronchi L, Rosenbaum D, Athouel A, et al. Femoral nerve blockade in children using bupivacaine. Anesthesiology 1989;70:622–624.
146. Rusy L, Houck C, Sullivan L, et al. A double-blind evaluation of ketorolac tromethamine versus acetaminophen in pediatric tonsillectomy patients, effects on analgesia, and bleeding. 1995;80:226–229.
147. Sacchetti A. Pediatric sedation and analgesia. Acad Emerg Med 1995;2(3):240–241.
148. Sacchetti A, Schafermeyer R, Gerardi M, et al. Pediatric analgesia and sedation. Ann Emerg Med 1994;23(2):237–250.
149. Saint-Maurice C, Laguenie G, Couturier C, et al. Rectal ketamine in pediatric anesthesia (letter). Br J Anesthe 1979;51:573–574.
150. Scamman F. Fentanyl-oxygen-nitrous oxide rigidity and pulmonary compliance. Anesth Analg 1983;62:332–334.
151. Schecter N. Pain and pain control in children. Curr Probl Pediatr 1985;15:1–67.
152. Schecter N. The undertreatment of pain in children: an overview. Pediatr Clin North Am 1989;36:781–794.
153. Schechter N, Weisman S, Rosenblum M, et al. The use of oral transmucosal fentanyl citrate for painful procedures in children. Pediatrics 1995;95:335–339.
154. Schreiner M, Triebwasser A, Keon T. Ingestion of liquids compared to preoperative fasting in paediatric outpatients. Anesthesiology 1990;72:593–597.
155. Scott D. Acute toxicity of ropivacaine compared with that of bupivacaine. Anesth Anal 1989;69:563–569.
156. Scott R, Steinberg R, Kreitzer J, et al. Intravenous regional anesthesia using lidocaine and ketorolac. Anesth Anal 1995;81:110–113.
157. Selbst S. Managing pain in the pediatric emergency department. Pediatr Emerg Care 1989;5:56–63.
158. Selbst S, Henretig F. The treatment of pain in the emergency department. Pediatr Clin North Am 1989;36:965–977.
159. Sievers T, Yee J, Foley M, et al. Midazolam for conscious sedation during pediatric oncology procedures: safety and recovery parameters. 1990;88:1172–1179.
160. Smith J, Santer L. Respiratory arrest following intramuscular ketamine injection in a 4-year-old child. Ann Emerg Med 1993;22:613–615.

161. Skokan EG, Pribble C, Bassett F, et al. Use of propofol sedation in a pediatric emergency department: A prospective study. Clin Pediatr 2001;40:663–671.
162. Snodgrass W, Dodge W. Lytic/"DPT" cocktail: time for rational and safe alternatives. Pediatr Clin North Am 1989;36:1285–1291.
163. Sokoll M, Hoyt J, Gergis S. Studies in muscle rigidity, nitrous oxide, and narcotic analgesic agents. Anesth Analg 1972;51:16–20.
164. Splinter W, Stewart J, Muir J. The effect of preoperative apple juice on gastric contents, thirst, and hunger in children. Can J Anaesth 1989;36:55–58.
165. Stehling L. Anesthesia update #11—unique considerations in pediatric orthopaedics. Orthop Rev 1981;10:95–99.
166. Stevenson D, Simon R. Aspirin sensitivity: respiratory and cutaneous manifestations. In: Middleton E Jr, ed. Allergy: Principles and Practice. 3rd ed. St. Louis: Elsevier, 1988:1537–1554.
167. Stoeckel H, Hengstmann J, Shuttler J. Pharmacokinetics of fentanyl as a possible explanation for recurrent respiratory depression. Br J Anaesth 1979;51:741–745.
168. Stoelting RK. Barbiturates. In: Pharmacology and Psychology in Anesthetic Practice: J.B. Lippincott, 1987:107–116.
169. Stoelting RK. Endotracheal intubation. In: Miller R, New Y, eds. Anesthesia. New York: Churchill-Livingstone, 1986.
170. Stoelting RK. Nonbarbiturate Induction Drugs. Philadelphia: J.B. Lippincott, 1987: 134–147.
171. Stoelting RK. Nonopioid and Nonsteroidal Analgesic, Antipyretic, and Anti-inflammatory Drugs. Philadelphia: J.B. Lippincott, 1987:240–250.
172 Stoelting RK. Opioid Agonists and Antagonists. Philadelphia: J.B. Lippincott, 1987.
173. Strichartz G. Neural physiology and local anesthetic action. In: Cousins MB, Bridenbaugh PO, eds. Neural Blockade in Clinical Anesthesia and Management of Pain. Philadelphia: J.B. Lippincott, 1987.
174. Striker T. Anesthesia for trauma in the pediatric patient. In: Gregory G, ed. Pediatric Anesthesia. New York: Churchill-Livingstone, 1989.
175. Tendrup T. Pain control, analgesia, and sedation. In: Barkin R, Asch S, Caputo G, et al., eds. Pediatric Emergency Medicine: Concepts and Clinical Practice. St. Louis: Mosby Year-Book, 1992.
176. Tiret L. Complications related to anaesthesia in infants and children. A prospective survey of 40,240 anaesthetics. Br J Anesth 1988;61:263–269.
177. Tobias J. Sedation in the pediatric intensive care unit. In: Deshpande J, Tobias J, eds. The Pediatric Pain Handbook. St. Louis: Mosby, 1996:255–261.
178. Tobias J, Phipps S, Smith B, et al. Oral ketamine premedication to alleviate the distress of invasive procedures in pediatric oncology patients. Pediatrics 1992;90:537–541.
179. Tucker G, Mather L. Properties, absorption, and disposition of local anesthetic agents. In: Cousins MB, Bridenbaugh PO, eds. Neural Blockade in Clinical Anesthesia and Management of Pain. Philadelphia: J.B. Lippincott, 1987.
180. Turner P, Batten J, Hjorth D, et al. Intravenous regional anaesthesia for the treatment of upper limb injuries in childhood. Aust NZ J Surg 1986;56:153–155.
181. Tyler D. Pharmacology of pain management. Pediatr Clin North Am 1994;41:59–69.
182. Urban B, McKain C. Onset and progression of intravenous regional anesthesia with dilute lidocaine. Anesth Analg 1982;61:834–838.
183. Vardi A, Salem Y, Padeh S, et al. Is propofol safe for procedural sedation in children. A prospective evaluation of propofol vs ketaminein pediatric critical care. Crit Care Med 2002;30:1231–1236.
184. Varela C, Lorfing K, Schmidt T. Intravenous sedation for the closed reduction of fractures in children. J Bone J Surg 1995;77(3):340–345.
185. Vas L. The safety of ketamine sedation in the treatment of traumatic fractures in children. J Bone Joint Surg Am 2001;83-A:1593–1594.
186. Vetter T. Pediatric patient-controlled analgesia with morphine versus meperidine. J Pain Symptom Manage 1992;7:204–208.
187. Walson P, Mortensen M. Pharmacokinetics of common analgesics, anti-inflammatories and antipyretics in children. Clin Pharmacokniet 1989;17(Suppl 1):116–137.
188. Wathen JE, Gao D, Merritt G, et al. A randomized controlled trial comparing a fascia iliaca compartment nerve block to a traditional systemic analgesic for femur fractures in a pediatric emergency department. Ann Emerg Med 2007;50:162–171.
189. Wathen JE, Roback MG, Mackenzie T, et al. Does midazolam alter the clinical effects of intravenous ketamine sedation in children? A double-blind, randomized, controlled, emergency department trial. Ann Emerg Med 2000;36:579–588.
190. Wattenmaker I, Kasser J, McGravey A. Self-administered nitrous oxide for fracture reduction in children in an emergency room setting. J Orthop Trauma 1990;4:35–38.
191. Webster D. The pediatric trauma patient. In: Rasch D, Webster D, eds. Clinical Manual of Pediatric Anesthesia. New York: McGraw-Hill, 1994.
192. Wedel D, Krohn J, Hall J. Brachial plexus anesthesia in pediatric patients. Mayo Clin Proc 1991;66:583–588.
193. Weksler N, Ovadia L, Mutai G, et al. Nasal ketamine for pediatric premedication. Can J Anaesth 1993;40:119–121.
194. Wertzel R. Anesthesia for pediatric trauma. In: Stene JK, Grande CM, eds. Trauma Anesthesia. Baltimore: Williams & Wilkins, 1991.
195. White P. Mishaps with patient-controlled analgesia. Anesthesiology 1987;66:81–83.
196. White P, Way W, Trevor A. Ketamine—its pharmacology and therapeutic uses. Anesthesiology 1982;56:119–136.
197. Willman EV, Andolfatto G. A prospective evaluation of "ketofol" (ketamine/propofol combination) for procedural sedation and analgesia in the emergency department. Ann Emerg Med 2007;49:23–30.
198. Winnie A. Regional anesthesia. Surg Clin North Am 1975;54:861–892.
199. Wright S, Chudnofsky C, Dronen S. Comparison of midazolam and diazepam for conscious sedation in the emergency department. Ann Emerg Med 1993;22:201–205.
200. Wu M, Purcell G. Patient-controlled analgesia—the value of a background infusion [letter]. Anaesthesia Intensive Care 1990;18:575–576.
201. Yaster M, Maxwell L. Pediatric regional anesthesia. Anesthesiology 1989;70:324–338.
202. Yaster M, Nichols D, Deshpande J, et al. Midazolam-fentanyl intravenous sedation in children: case report of respiratory arrest. Pediatrics 1990;86:463–467.
203. Younge D. Haematoma block for fractures of the wrist: a cause of compartment syndrome. J Hand Surg 1989;14B:194–195.
204. Zeltzer L, Jay S, Fisher D. The management of pain associated with pediatric procedures. Pediatr Clin North Am 1989;36:941–963.

SUGGESTED READINGS

Bassett KE, Anderson JL, Pribble CG, et al. Propofol for procedural sedation in children in the emergency department. Ann Emerg Med 2003;42:773–782.

Carre P, Joly A, Cluzel Field B, et al. Axillary block in children: single or multiple injection? Paediatr Anaesth 2000;10:35–39.

Davidson AJ, Eyres RL, Cole WG. A comparison of prilocaine and lidocaine for intravenous regional anaesthesia for forearm fracture reduction in children. Paediatr Anaesth 2002; 12:146–150.

Dial S, Silver P, Bock K, et al. Pediatric sedation for procedures titrated to a desired degree of immobility results in unpredictable depth of sedation. Pediatr Emerg Care 2001;17: 414–420.

Ecoffey C. Local anesthetics in pediatric anesthesia: an update. Minerva Anesthesiol 2005; 71:357–360.

Fleischmann E, Marhofer P, Greher M, et al. Brachial plexus anaesthesia in children: lateral infraclavicular vs. axillary approach. Paediatr Anaesth 2003;13:103–108.

Herrera JA, Wall EJ, Foad SL. Hematoma block reduces narcotic pain medication after femoral elastic nailing in children. J Pediatr Orthop 2004;24:254–256.

Hoffman GM, Nowakowski R, Troshynski TJ, et al. Risk reduction in pediatric procedural sedation by application of an American Academy of Pediatrics/American Society of Anesthesiologists process model. Pediatrics 2002;109:236–243.

Kennedy RM, Luhmann JD, Luhmann SJ. Emergency department management of pain and anxiety related to orthopedic fracture care: a guide to analgesic techniques and procedural sedation in children. Paediatr Drugs 2004;6:11–31.

Marcus RJ, Thompson JP. Anaesthesia for manipulation of forearm fractures in children: a survey of current practice. Paediatr Anaesth 2000;10:273–277.

McCarty EC, Mencio GA, Green NE. Anesthesia and analgesia for the ambulatory management of fractures in children. J Am Acad Orthop Surg 1999;7:81–91.

4

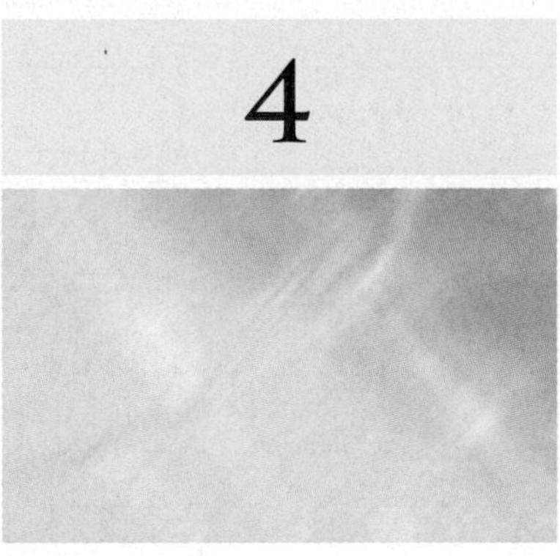

MANAGEMENT OF THE MULTIPLY INJURED CHILD

Frances A. Farley and Robert M. Kay

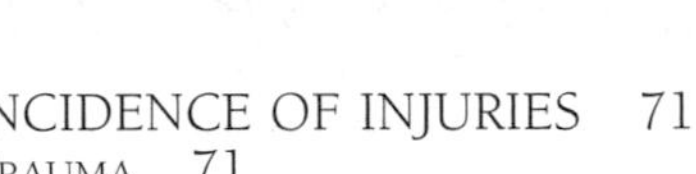

INCIDENCE OF INJURIES 71
Trauma 71
Fractures 72
Child Abuse 72

COMMON MECHANISMS OF INJURY 72
Falls 72
Motor Vehicles 72

ROLE OF THE PEDIATRIC TRAUMA CENTER 73

INITIAL RESUSCITATION AND EVALUATION 73
The Child Is Different 73
Fluid Replacement 73

EVALUATION AND ASSESSMENT 74
Trauma Rating Systems 74
Physical Assessment 74
Imaging Studies 75

NONORTHOPAEDIC CONDITIONS IN THE MULTIPLY INJURED CHILD 77
Head Injury 77
Peripheral Nerve Injuries 79
Abdominal Injuries 79
Genitourinary Injuries 79
Fat Embolism and Pulmonary Embolism 79
Nutritional Requirements 80

ORTHOPAEDIC MANAGEMENT OF THE MULTIPLY INJURED CHILD 80
Timing 80
Pelvic Fractures 80
Open Fractures 80

STABILIZATION OF FRACTURES 84
Beneficial Effects 84
Outcomes of Treatment of the Multiply Injured Child 87

INCIDENCE OF INJURIES

Trauma

The most common cause of death in children over the age of 1 year is trauma, not only in the United States, but worldwide. Estimates of cost to the American public for the care of pediatric trauma range from over $1 billion[112] to $13.8 billion[114] annually. A 1997 national pediatric inpatient database reported 84,000 orthopaedic trauma admissions, with a cost of $932.8 million in hospital charges.[54] Hospital charges for treatment of children with femoral fractures in the United States in 2000 was over $222 million.[109] In 2003, the mean hospitalization expenditure was $28,137 for injury discharges, with a median of $10,808.[136] Although isolated long-bone fractures still comprise the bulk of orthopaedic injuries in children, a surprising number of these young patients have multiple system injuries.

More than 1.5 million pediatric injuries have been reported to occur annually in the United States, resulting in more than 500,000 hospitalizations and 15,000 to 20,000 pediatric deaths.[135,140,150] In an urban practice at a level 1 trauma center, 1903 new fractures accounted for 5698 work relative value units.[195] Boys are injured twice as often as girls and may account for an even greater proportion of hospital admissions related to pediatric trauma.[151,169] Blunt trauma is the mechanism of injury in most children and preadolescents, whereas penetrating trauma more often is the source of multiple injuries in adults. Although blunt trauma in the youngest children is often due to child abuse, vehicular accidents and falls from a height account for the more severe multiple injuries in the rest of childhood.[23] The cause of death from trauma in children is generally severe head injury or severe combined head, chest, and abdominal trauma.[83,156]

The causes of multiple injuries in teenagers more closely mirror those in adults. In the adolescent age group, alcohol abuse is now considered a major factor in more than one third of injuries resulting from accidents.[113] Orthopaedists treating teenagers involved in vehicular accidents need to be aware of the potential alcohol use in this age group and be prepared to refer adolescents for appropriate counseling to avoid future accidents and injuries.[159]

Fractures

Although rarely the cause of mortality in a child with multiple injuries, fractures and other musculoskeletal injuries are common in multitrauma and contribute significantly to the associated morbidity.[23,37,39,128] In one series from a pediatric trauma center treating children with polytrauma, femoral shaft fractures accounted for 22% of the fractures; 9% of these fractures were open.[23] Although less common, fractures of the spine, pelvis, and scapula and clavicle were associated with longer stays in the hospital and in the intensive care unit, in addition to having the highest associated mortality rates.

Knowledge of fracture associations leads to improved diagnostic skill and fracture care. For example, calcaneal fractures often result from axial loading and most commonly occur after a fall from a height (40%) or from a motor vehicle accident (MVA) (15%).[152,153] Associated fractures have been reported in approximately one third of children with calcaneal fractures, including spine fractures in 5%.[152,153]

Femoral and adjacent pelvic fractures often occur together. If a pedestrian child has been struck by an automobile, there are often fractures in the ipsilateral upper and lower extremity.[21] In one study, 58% (87/149) of children with femoral fractures due to MVAs were noted to have associated injuries, including 14% with head injuries, 6% with chest injuries, 5% with abdominal injuries, and 4% with genitourinary injuries.[77] The coexistence of a femoral fracture and a head injury indicates substantial high-energy trauma and has a more guarded prognosis than does either of these injuries alone.

Child Abuse

Child abuse continues to be a societal problem that crosses all socioeconomic and ethnic groups and is the most common cause of traumatic death in infants and toddlers. Currently, child abuse is estimated to occur in 15 to 42 of every 1000 children in the United States annually, resulting in more than 1200 deaths.[88] Nonaccidental trauma has higher mortality and morbidity than accidental trauma.[141] This diagnosis must be suspected in all cases of multiple injuries in children younger than 2 years old if there is no obvious and witnessed plausible explanation of the injuries. Abuse should be considered a possible cause of injury in all young children with multiple long-bone fractures in association with head injury. Pediatrician confidence in identifying these injuries remains low.[182] Even a single long-bone fracture associated with a head injury or abdominal injury should raise suspicion of child abuse. Although the corner fracture usually is thought of as being most characteristic of child abuse, the most common extremity fracture caused by abuse is a single transverse fracture of the femur or humerus, not multiple fractures.[84] There is no fracture that is absolutely diagnostic of abuse; the entire clinical and social picture needs to be taken into consideration. Orthopaedic surgeons have difficulty distinguishing accidental from nonaccidental trauma when faced with a long-bone fracture.[93] Although rib fractures occur in only about 5% of children with multiple injuries from trauma of other causes, they are more common in child abuse.[55,128] Whereas blunt compressive trauma to the thorax from other causes may result in lateral rib fractures, the rib fractures seen in child abuse are often posterolateral and adjacent to the transverse processes of the thoracic spine.[10,88,200]

A skeletal survey is routinely performed in suspected cases of abuse. Some authors have recommended a bone scan in conjunction with the skeletal survey,[115] although this recommendation is controversial since the addition of a bone scan requires sedation, elevates radiation exposure, and increases cost.[2,84]

COMMON MECHANISMS OF INJURY

Falls

A fall is one of the two primary mechanisms of multiple injuries in children.[23,59,92,146,194] Falls occur more often in younger children. One unfortunate example is children who fall out of a second story window that is adjacent to a bed. Injuries from falls result from direct impact or from deceleration forces present at the time of landing. Direct impact usually causes fractures, whereas internal injury more often results from the impact forces. Although a variety of injuries can result from these falls, the position of the body at impact and the surface on which the child lands are important factors that affect the injury severity.[59] Injuries associated with falls from heights include head injuries in 39% of children,[92] orthopaedic injuries in 34% to 65%,[92,132] and mortality in 5%.[44]

Motor Vehicles

Accidents involving motor vehicles account for most multiple-system injuries in school-age children and preadolescents. These injuries occur when a vehicle strikes a child on foot or riding a bicycle, or when the child is a passenger in a car involved in an accident. In 2002, more than 300,000 children aged 15 years and younger were injured and more than 2500 were killed in such MVAs in the United States.[185]

More than 250,000 injuries and 1700 deaths in this age group in 2002 occurred in passengers in cars and light trucks.[185] More than half of the children killed in these accidents were unrestrained at the time of the accident.[185] For childhood passengers injured or killed in car accidents, the risk of death is six times greater for those unrestrained than for those restrained at the time of injury.[185]

Noncompliance with car seat use is a major contributor to morbidity and mortality following MVAs. Thompson et al.[175] reported that 80% of children treated at a trauma center following MVAs were unrestrained at the time of injury. Vaca et al.[187] noted that many parents in California with children aged 6 years and younger were unaware of basic safety information regarding child car seats and airbags, and that they were also unaware of state laws regarding child seat restraints. Severe injuries are higher for children in the front seat.[22] In Arizona, a comparison of injuries sustained in children in MVAs who were restrained or unrestrained showed higher mortality, longer mean hospital stays, higher mean hospital charges, more hospital admissions, and more fractures, intraabdominal injuries, and head injuries in unrestrained passengers.[31]

Even with appropriate use of car seats, properly restrained

children may be severely injured. Zuckerbraun et al.[208] noted a higher incidence of cervical spine injuries in younger children. Others have noted the importance of padding in child seats in potentially decreasing the risk of head injury in children restrained in child safety seats.[91]

Although most states require that infants and toddlers be restrained in car seats when riding in a car, standard adult shoulder and lap belts do not adequately restrain children who are too big for car seats and too small for the standard restraints. Age and size appropriate car seats and restraints are essential for child occupant safety. Adjustable restraints to better accommodate the size of the car occupant have been proposed to solve this problem. In addition, there is increasing public sentiment to require seat belt use on school buses, a policy that has been in place for physically disabled student transport for some time.

Although teaching children better safety while on foot and on bicycles is a laudable and important goal, the safety of automobile travel can be dramatically improved with appropriate parent education regarding child safety seats and airbags and by enforcement of current laws.

ROLE OF THE PEDIATRIC TRAUMA CENTER

After the rapid transport of wounded soldiers to a specialized treatment center proved effective in improving survival in the military setting, trauma centers, using the same principles of rapid transport and immediate care, have been established throughout the United States. These trauma centers are supported by the states on the premise that the first hour after injury is the most critical in influencing the rates of survival from the injuries. Rapid helicopter or ambulance transport to an onsite team of trauma surgeons in the trauma center has led to an improvement in the rates of acute survival after multiple injuries have occurred.

The first trauma centers focused on adult patients because more adults than children are severely injured. However, pediatric trauma centers have been established at numerous medical centers across the United States with the idea that the care of pediatric polytrauma patients differs from the care given to adults and that special treatment centers are important for optimal results.[65,67,80] The American College of Surgeons has established specific criteria for pediatric trauma centers, which include the same principles of rapid transport and rapid treatment by an in-house surgical team as in adult trauma centers. A pediatric general surgeon is in the hospital at all times and heads the pediatric trauma team. This surgeon evaluates the child first, and the other surgical specialists are immediately available. General radiographic services and computed tomography (CT) capability must be available at all times for patient evaluation, and an operating room must be immediately available.

Although there is some evidence that survival rates for severely injured children are improved if the children are brought to a pediatric trauma center rather than a community hospital,[164] the costs associated with such a center (particularly the on-call costs of personnel) have limited the number of pediatric trauma centers. Younger and more seriously injured children have improved outcomes at children's hospitals.[45] Given the limited number of pediatric trauma centers, patients frequently are often either stabilized at other hospitals before transfer to a pediatric trauma center or treated at an adult trauma center.

Larson et al.[94] reported that there did not appear to be better outcomes for pediatric trauma patients flown directly to a pediatric trauma center than for those stabilized at nontrauma centers before transfer to the same pediatric trauma center. Other centers have documented the need for improved transfer coordination.[147,167]

Knudson et al.[87] studied the results of pediatric multiple injury care in an adult level 1 trauma center and concluded that the results were comparable to national standards for pediatric trauma care. Sanchez et al.[149] reported that adolescent trauma patients admitted to an adult surgical intensive care unit (SICU) had similar outcomes to comparable patients admitted to a pediatric intensive care unit (PICU) in a single institution. However, those admitted to the SICU were more likely to be intubated and to have a Swan-Ganz catheter placed and had longer ICU stays and longer hospital stays.[149] The use of a general trauma center for pediatric trauma care may be an acceptable alternative if it is not feasible to fund a separate pediatric trauma center.

INITIAL RESUSCITATION AND EVALUATION

Regardless of the mechanism causing the multiple injuries, the initial medical management focuses on the life-threatening, nonorthopaedic injuries to stabilize the child's condition.[114] The responsibility for initial lifesaving resuscitation is rarely the responsibility of the orthopaedist; however, such resuscitative efforts by the orthopaedist may be more commonly required in nontrauma centers and those in rural settings.

The Child Is Different

The initial steps in resuscitation of a child are essentially the same as those used for an adult.[4,39,114] In severe injuries, the establishment of an adequate airway immediately at the accident site often means the difference between life and death. The cervical spine needs to be stabilized for transport if the child is unconscious or if neck pain is present. A special transport board with a cutout for the occipital area is recommended for children younger than 6 years of age because the size of the head at this age is larger in relation to the rest of the body. Because of this larger head size, if a young child is placed on a normal transport board, the cervical spine is flexed, a position that is best avoided if a neck injury is suspected.[71]

Fluid Replacement

Once an adequate airway is established, the amount of hemorrhage from the injury, either internally or externally, is assessed. This blood loss is replaced initially with intravenous crystalloid solution. In younger children, rapid intravenous access may be difficult. In this situation, the use of intraosseous fluid infusion should be considered for administration of both fluid and medications. Guy et al.[64] reported successful intraosseous infusion into the tibias of 15 children between the ages of 3 months and 10 years. In this series, intraosseous needles were placed by prehospital and hospital personnel and colloid, crystalloid solution, and blood were all given by this route; no complications occurred in the surviving children. Bielski et al.,[15] in a rabbit tibia model, likewise demonstrated no adverse effects on the histology of bone or the adjacent physis with intraosseous injection of various resuscitation drugs and fluids.

Because death is common if hypovolemic shock is not rapidly reversed, the child's blood pressure must be maintained at an adequate level for organ perfusion. Most multiply injured children have sustained blunt trauma rather than penetrating injuries, and most of the blood loss from visceral injury or from pelvic and femoral fractures is internal and may be easily underestimated at first. The "triad of death," consisting of acidosis, hypothermia, and coagulopathy, has been described in trauma patients as a result of hypovolemia and the systemic response to trauma.[198] Peterson et al.[129] reported that an initial base deficit of 8 portends an increased mortality risk.

Despite the need to stabilize the child's blood pressure, caution needs to be exercised in children with head injuries so that overhydration is avoided because cerebral edema is better treated with relative fluid restriction. Excessive fluid replacement also may lead to further internal fluid shifts, which often produce a drop in the arterial oxygenation from interstitial pulmonary edema, especially when there has been direct trauma to the thorax and lungs. In some instances, in order to accurately assess the appropriate amount of fluid replacement, a central venous catheter is inserted during initial resuscitation. A urinary catheter is essential during the resuscitation to monitor urine output as a means of gauging adequate organ perfusion.

EVALUATION AND ASSESSMENT

Trauma Rating Systems

After initial resuscitation has stabilized the injured child's condition, it is essential to perform a quick but thorough check for other injuries. A number of injury rating systems have been proposed, but the Injury Severity Score (ISS) is a valid, reproducible rating system that can be widely applied in the pediatric polytrauma setting (Table 4-1).[197] Another injury rating system for children that has been shown to be valid and reproducible is the Pediatric Trauma Score (PTS) (Table 4-2).[197] The injury rating system chosen varies among trauma centers, but whether the ISS or PTS is used, each allows an objective means to assess mortality risk at the time of initial treatment, as well as allowing some degree of prediction of future disability.[126,169,204]

Head injury is most often evaluated and rated by the Glasgow Coma Scale (GCS), which evaluates eye opening (1 to 4 points), motor function (1 to 6 points), and verbal function (1 to 5 points) on a total scale of 3 to 15 points (Table 4-3).[174] There are some limitations in the use of the GCS in children who are preverbal or who are in the early verbal stages of development, but in other children this rating system has been a useful guide for predicting early mortality and later disability. A relative head injury severity scale (RHISS) is currently being validated[40] and is available in trauma registries. As a rough guide in verbal children, a GCS score of less than 8 points indicates a significantly worse chance of survival for these children than for those with a GCS of more than 8. The GCS should be noted on arrival in the trauma center and again 1 hour after the child arrives at the hospital (Fig. 4-1). Serial changes in the GCS correlate with improvement or worsening of the neurologic injury. Repeated GCS assessments over the initial 72 hours after injury may be of prognostic significance. In addition to the level of oxygenation present at the initial presentation to the hospital, the 72-hour GCS motor response score has been noted to be very predictive of later permanent disability as a sequel to the head injury.[117]

Physical Assessment

In a child with multiple injuries, a careful abdominal examination is essential to allow early detection of injuries to the liver, spleen, pancreas, or kidneys.

Ecchymosis on the abdominal wall must be noted, because this is often a sign of significant visceral or spinal injury.[26,161] In one series, 48% (22/46) of children with such ecchymosis required abdominal exploration,[26] while in another series 23% (14/61) of children were noted to have spine fractures.[161]

Swelling, deformity, or crepitus in any extremity is noted, and appropriate imaging studies are arranged to evaluate potential extremity injuries more fully. If extremity deformity is present, it is important to determine whether the fracture is open or closed. Sites of external bleeding are examined, and pressure dressings are applied if necessary to prevent further blood loss. A pelvic fracture combined with one or more other skeletal injuries has been suggested to be a marker for the presence of head and abdominal injuries.[190] Major arterial injuries associated with fractures of the extremity are usually diagnosed early by the lack of a peripheral pulse. However, abdominal venous injuries caused by blunt trauma are less common and are less commonly diagnosed before exploratory laparotomy. About half of abdominal venous injuries have been reported to be fatal, so the trauma surgeon needs to consider this diagnosis in children who continue to require substantial blood volume support after the initial resuscitation has been completed.[51]

Initial splinting of suspected extremity fractures is routinely done in the field. However, once the injured child is in the hospital, the orthopaedist should personally inspect the extremities to determine the urgency with which definitive treatment is needed. Most important are whether a vascular injury has occurred and whether the fracture is open or closed. The back and spine should be carefully examined. If there is not an open fracture and if the peripheral vascular function is normal, there is less urgency in treating the fracture and splinting will suffice until the other organ system injuries are stabilized.

Splinting decreases the child's pain while the child is resuscitated and stabilized and minimizes additional trauma to the soft tissue envelope surrounding the fracture. Splinting also facilitates transport of the child within the hospital while the trauma work-up, including appropriate imaging studies, is completed. If the child is to be transferred to a trauma center, splints are invaluable for patient comfort and safety during transfer.

Any evident neurologic deficit is noted in order to document the extremity function before any treatment. It is important to remember that a detailed neurologic examination may not be possible since these are often young and scared children who are in pain and may have a central nervous system injury. The inability to obtain a reliable examination should also be documented.

Head injuries and extreme pain in certain locations can result in some injuries being missed initially. In a series of 149 pediatric polytrauma patients, 13 injuries were diagnosed an average of 15 days following injury, including five fractures (one involving the spine), four abdominal injuries, two aneurysms, one head injury, and one facial fracture.[101] Given this 9% incidence of delayed diagnosis, it is imperative that polytrauma patients be reexamined once they are more comfortable to reassess for

TABLE 4-1 Injury Severity Score

Abbreviated Injury Scale (AIS)

The AIS classifies injuries as moderate, severe, serious, critical, and fatal for each of the five major body systems. The criteria for each system into the various categories is listed in a series of charts for each level of severity. Each level of severity is given a numerical code (1–5). The criteria for severe level (Code 4) is listed below.

Severity Code	(AIS) Severity Category/Injury Description	Policy Code
4	Severe (Life-Threatening, Survival Probable)	B

General

Severe lacerations and/or avulsions with dangerous hemorrhage; 30%–50% surface second- or third-degree burns.

Head and Neck

Cerebral injury with or without skull fracture, with unconsciousness >15 min, with definite abnormal neurologic signs; posttraumatic amnesia 3–12 hr; compound skull fracture.

Chest

Open chest wounds; flail chest; pneumomediastinum; myocardial contusion without circulatory embarrassment; pericardial injuries.

Abdomen

Minor laceration of intra-abdominal contents (ruptured spleen, kidney, and injuries to tail of pancreas); intraperitoneal bladder rupture; avulsion of the genitals.
Thoracic and/or lumbar spine fractures with paraplegia.

Extremities

Multiple closed long-bone fractures; amputation of limbs.

Injury Severity Score (ISS)

The injury severity score (ISS) is a combination of values obtained from the AIS. The ISS is the sum of the squares of the highest AIS grade in each of the three most severely injured areas. For example, a person with a laceration of the aorta (AIS = 5), multiple closed long-bone fractures (AIS = 4), and retroperitoneal hemorrhage (AIS = 3) would have an injury severity score of 50 (25 + 16 + 9). The highest possible score for a person with trauma to a single area is 25. The use of the ISS has dramatically increased the correlation between the severity and mortality. The range of severity is from 0 to 75.

Committee on Medical Aspects of Automotive Safety. Rating the severity of tissue damage I. The abbreviated scale. JAMA 1971;215:277–280; Baker SP, O'Neill B, Haddon W Jr, et al. The Injury Severity Score: a method for describing patients with multiple injuries and evaluating emergency care. J Trauma 1974;14:187–196.

potential sites of injury. In some cases, despite careful inpatient re-evaluations, some pediatric injuries escape detection until later follow-up visits. In addition, children with head injuries need to be reassessed once they awaken enough to cooperate with re-examination. Families and patients need to be informed of the frequency of delayed diagnosis of some injuries in polytrauma patients so that they can partner with the medical team in recognizing such injuries (often evident as previously undetected sites of pain or dysfunction).

Imaging Studies

Radiographs

Imaging studies should be obtained as quickly as possible after the initial resuscitation and physical examination. Any extremity suspected of having a significant injury should be examined on radiograph. If the child has a head injury or if neck pain is noted on the examination, a lateral cervical spine radiograph is obtained. Some centers evaluate the cervical spine with a CT scan in children with polytrauma who have neck pain, a traumatic brain injury (TBI), or who have been drinking alcohol.[148] Further work-up with cervical spine magnetic resonance imaging (MRI) is necessary before cervical spine clearance in those who have persistent neck pain or tenderness and should be considered in patients who remain obtunded (see "Magnetic Resonance Imaging").

If a cervical spine injury is present, the lateral radiograph of this area almost always will detect it. If there is suspicion of a cervical spine injury on the neutral lateral view, a lateral flexion

TABLE 4-2 Pediatric Trauma Score

Component	Category		
	+2	+1	−1
Size	≥20 kg	10–20 kg	<10 kg
Airway	Normal	Maintainable	Unmaintainable
Systolic Blood Pressure	≥90 mm Hg	90–50 mm Hg	<50 mm Hg
Central Nervous System	Awake	Obtunded/LOC	Coma/decerebrate
Open Wound	None	Minor	Major/penetrating
Skeletal	None	Closed fracture	Open/multiple fractures

This scoring system includes six common determinants of the clinical condition in the injured child. Each of the six determinants is assigned a grade: +2, minimal or no injury; +1, minor or potentially major injury; −1, major, or immediate life-threatening injury. The scoring system is arranged in a manner standard with advanced trauma life-support protocol, and thereby provides a quick assessment scheme. The ranges are from −6 for a severely traumatized child to +12 for a least traumatized child. This system has been confirmed in its reliability as a predictor of injury severity.
From Tepas JJ, Mollitt DL, Talbers JL, et al. The Pediatric Trauma Score as a predictor of injury severity in the injured child. J Pediatr Surg 1987;22:14–18, with permission.

radiograph of the cervical spine taken in an awake patient will help detect any cervical instability. The cervical spine of a young child is much more flexible than the cervical spine in an adult. Under the age of 12 years, the movement of C1 on C2 during flexion of the neck can normally be up to 5 mm, whereas in adults, this distance should be less than 3 mm. Likewise in this young age group, the distance between C2 and C3 is up to 3 mm in flexion. No forward movement of C2 on C3 should be present in a skeletally mature individual when the neck is flexed. This so-called pseudosubluxation of C2 on C3 in a child should not be diagnosed as instability that requires treatment because this is a normal finding in most young children.[30] Because it is difficult to detect a fracture of the thoracic or lumbar spine clinically, radiographs of this area, primarily a lateral view, should be carefully evaluated, particularly in a comatose child.

TABLE 4-3 Glasgow Coma Scale

Response	Action	Score
Best motor response	Obeys	M6
	Localizes	5
	Withdraws	4
	Abnormal flexion	3
	Extensor response	2
	Nil	1
Verbal response	Oriented	V5
	Confused conversation	4
	Inappropriate words	3
	Incomprehensible sounds	2
	Nil	1
Eye opening	Spontaneous	E4
	To speech	3
	To pain	2
	Nil	1

This scale is used to measure the level of consciousness using the eye opening, best verbal, and best motor responses. The range of scores is from 3 for the most severe to 15 for the least severe. This is a measure of level and progression of changes in consciousness.
From Jennett B, Teasdale G, Galbraith S, et al. Severe head injuries in three countries. J Neurol Neurosurg Psychiatry 1977;40:291–298, with permission.

Computed Tomography

CT is essential in evaluating a child with multiple injuries. If a head injury is present, CT of the head will detect skull fractures and intracranial bleeding. With abdominal swelling, pain, or bruising, CT of the abdomen provides excellent visualization of the liver and spleen and allows quantification of the amount of hemorrhage present. Because most hepatic and splenic lacerations are treated nonoperatively,[26,73,143] the CT scan and serial hematocrit levels are used to determine whether surgical treatment of these visceral lacerations is needed.

CT of the pelvis is more sensitive for pelvic fractures than is a screening pelvic radiograph (Fig. 4-2). In one study, a screening pelvic radiograph only demonstrated 54% of pelvic fractures identified on CT scan.[61] CT also is useful for thoroughly evaluating fracture configuration and determining appropriate treatment options, both surgical and nonsurgical. If

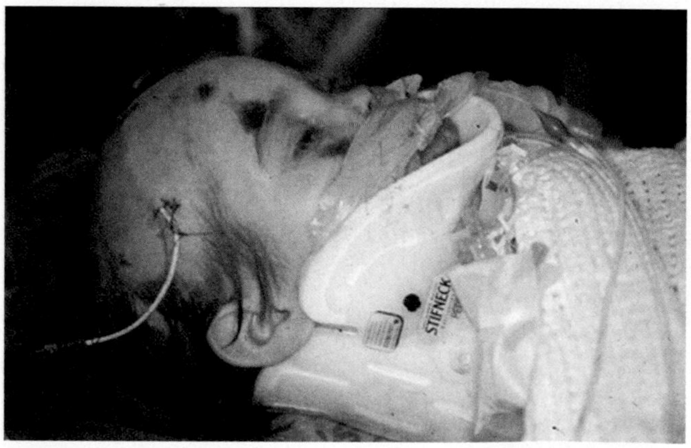

FIGURE 4-1 Temporary cervical spine stabilization is imperative in any child with multitrauma, especially those who are unconscious or complain of neck pain.

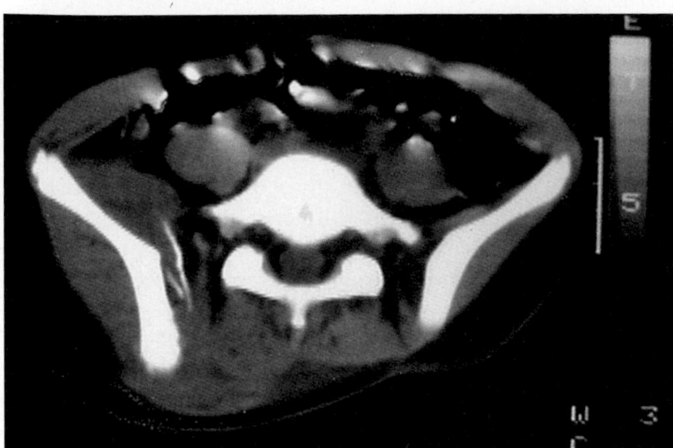

FIGURE 4-2 CT is an excellent addition to radiographs for evaluation of pelvic fractures.

abdominal CT is being done to evaluate visceral injury, it is simple to request that the abdominal CT be extended distally to include the pelvis. CT of a fractured vertebra will provide the information needed to classify the fracture as stable or unstable and determine whether operative treatment is needed.

Intravenous Pyelography

There is a strong correlation of urologic injury with anterior pelvic fractures, as well as with liver and spleen injury. Although CT and ultrasonography are used to evaluate renal injuries, the intravenous pyelogram still has a role in helping to diagnose bladder and urethral injuries.[125] Regardless of the methods of imaging, the anatomy of the urethral disruption often cannot be accurately demonstrated preoperatively.[3]

Radionuclide Scans

Bone scans have a limited role in the acute evaluation of a child with multiple injuries. In conjunction with a skeletal survey, a technetium-99m bone scan is sometimes used in children with suspected child abuse to detect previously undetected new or old fractures.[2,84,115]

Heinrich et al.[69] reported that bone scans in 48 children with multiple injuries often demonstrated an unsuspected injury. Nineteen previously unrecognized fractures were identified by obtaining radiographs of the areas with increased isotope uptake. In addition, there were 66 false-positive areas of increased uptake in the 48 patients. Of their 48 patients, six had a change in their orthopaedic care as a result of this bone scan, although this treatment was usually simple cast immobilization of a nondisplaced fracture. Nonetheless, the bone scan can be a valuable screening tool in a child with multiple injuries from any cause. In some instances, the bone scan can be useful to differentiate a normal variation in skeletal ossification (normal uptake) from a fracture (increased uptake), particularly in an extremity or a spinal area where pain is present. Areas of increased uptake require further imaging studies to determine if orthopaedic treatment is required.

Magnetic Resonance Imaging

MRI is used primarily for the detection of injury to the brain or the spine and spinal cord. In young children, the bony spine is more elastic than the spinal cord. As a result, a spinal cord injury can occur without an obvious spinal fracture in children with multiple injuries, particularly in automobile accidents.[7,20,49] In the spinal cord injury without radiographic abnormality (SCIWORA) syndrome, MRI is valuable in demonstrating the site and extent of spinal cord injury and in defining the level of injury to the disks or vertebral apophysis. A fracture through the vertebral apophysis is similar to a fracture through the physis of a long bone and may not be obvious on planar radiographs. MRI in obtunded and intubated pediatric trauma patients has been reported to lead to a quicker cervical spine clearance with a resulting decrease in hospital stay and cost.[53]

MRI is also useful in evaluating knee injuries,[110] particularly when a hemarthrosis is present. If blood is present on knee arthrocentesis, MRI can assist in diagnosing an injury to the cruciate ligaments or menisci. In addition, a chondral fracture that cannot be seen on routine radiographss may be demonstrated by MRI.

Ultrasonography

Ultrasound evaluation has been shown to be an accurate means of detecting hemoperitoneum following injury. Some trauma centers have replaced peritoneal lavage and laparoscopy with serial ultrasound evaluations to monitor liver, spleen, pancreas, and kidney injury in children with multiple injuries.[24,73,143] One problem with ultrasonography is the operator-dependent nature of this imaging study. Another is the fact that, unlike CT, ultrasonography cannot be used to rule out the frequently concomitant pelvic fractures. As a result, CT is more often used for assessment and monitoring of visceral injury in children sustaining multiple injuries. Comparisons of CT and ultrasonography have demonstrated the superiority of CT for diagnosing visceral injury in children with polytrauma.[36,122,138,170]

NONORTHOPAEDIC CONDITIONS IN THE MULTIPLY INJURED CHILD

Head Injury

Prognosis for Recovery

Head injuries occur in children with multiple injuries even more often than orthopaedic injuries. In a review of 494 pediatric polytrauma patients, Letts et al.[101] reported closed head injuries in 17% and skull fractures in 12%, while Schalamon et al.[151] reported injuries to the head and neck region in 87% of pediatric polytrauma patients. It has been clearly demonstrated that a child recovers more quickly and more fully from a significant head injury than does an adult.[37,104,201] Even children who are in a coma for several hours to several days often recover full motor function. Mild cognitive or learning deficits may persist, however, so educational testing needs to be considered for children who have had head injury and coma. Two factors that have been linked to poorer functional recovery and more severe permanent neurologic deficits are a low oxygen saturation level at the time of presentation to the hospital and a low GCS score 72 hours after the head injury. Because children with head injuries are often transported long distances, it is difficult for them to have evacuation of a cerebral hematoma within 4 hours.[172]

Despite the fact that excellent motor recovery is expected in most children after a head injury, children are often left with some residual deficits. Many children who sustain TBIs are unaware of their residual cognitive limitations and tend to overestimate their mental capacities.[66] Children who have had a TBI also often have behavioral problems, the presence of which may be predictive of behavioral problems in uninjured siblings as well.[171] Greenspan and MacKenzie[60] reported that 55% of children in their series had one or more health problems at 1-year follow-up, many of which were relatively minor. Headaches were present in 32% and extremity complaints in 13% of patients. The presence of a lower extremity injury with a head injury led to a higher risk of residual problems.

Because of the more optimistic outlook for children with head injuries than for adults with similar injuries, orthopaedic care should be provided in the most timely way possible, and the orthopaedist should base the orthopaedic care on the assumption of full neurologic recovery. Waiting for a child to recover from a coma is not appropriate, and comatose children tolerate general anesthesia well. The treatment undertaken for the orthopaedic injury is designed to optimize the orthopaedic outcome from the injury, with the assumption that the child will make a full neurologic recovery. Unless the musculoskeletal injuries are treated with the assumption that full neurologic recovery will take place, long-bone fractures may heal in angled or shortened positions. Once neurologic recovery occurs, the primary functional deficit will be from ill-managed orthopaedic injuries rather than from the neurologic injury.

Intracranial Pressure

After a head injury, intracranial pressure is commonly monitored to prevent excessive pressure, which may lead to further permanent disability or death. Normally, intracranial pressure does not exceed 15 mm Hg, and all attempts should be made to keep the pressure under 30 mm Hg after a head injury. This is accomplished by elevating the head of the bed to 30 degrees, lowering the PCO2, and restricting intravenous fluid administration. Ventilator assistance is used to lower the PCO2, which helps lessen cerebral edema. Fluid restriction also is recommended if peripheral perfusion can be maintained despite the polytrauma. Elevation of serum norepinephrine has been shown to correlate well with the severity of head injury in patients with injury of multiple organ systems.[202]

Motion at the site of a long-bone fracture will cause an elevation of the intracranial pressure in children with multiple injuries. Because of this problem, long-bone fractures must be immobilized to limit fracture motion until definitive fracture care can be provided. Initial immobilization is usually accomplished by splinting or casting of the fractures, or by use of traction for femoral shaft fractures. The use of external or internal fixation of fractures should be strongly considered to help control elevation of intracranial pressure. Fracture stabilization also facilitates dressing changes for the treatment of adjacent soft tissue injury as well as allowing in-hospital transport for imaging studies and other necessary treatments.[178,179]

Secondary Orthopaedic Effects of Head Injuries

A head injury can have later impact on the management of musculoskeletal injuries, even after the acute phase has passed. Persistent spasticity, the development of contractures, heterotopic bone formation in soft tissue, and changes in fracture healing rates are all sequelae of a head injury in children.

Spasticity. Spasticity may develop within a few days of head injury. The early effect of this spasticity is to cause shortening at the sites of long-bone fractures if traction or splint or cast immobilization is being used. If fracture displacement or shortening occurs in a circumferential cast, the bone ends may cause pressure points between the bone and the cast, leading to skin breakdown at the fracture site, with a higher risk for deep infection. Even with skeletal traction for femoral fractures, fracture shortening and displacement will occur as the spasticity overcomes the traction forces. Once spasticity develops and long-bone fractures displace, internal or external fixation is needed to maintain satisfactory reduction. This operative stabilization should be done as soon as the spasticity becomes a problem for fracture reduction because fracture healing is accelerated by a head injury.[177–179]

Contractures. The persistence of spasticity in the extremities often leads to subsequent contractures of the joints spanned by the spastic muscles. Contractures can develop quickly, and early preventative stretching or splinting should begin while the child is in the intensive care unit. Nonselective mass action muscle activity associated with brain injury can be used to help prevent these early contractures. If the child lies in bed with the hips and knees extended, there will usually be a strong plantarflexion of the feet at the ankles. If the hip and knee are flexed, it will be much easier to dorsiflex the foot at the ankle, so part-time positioning in this way will prevent early equinus contractures from developing. Stretching and splinting can often be effective in preventing contractures, and casting may be needed if contractures develop. If these measures are not successful and are interfering with rehabilitation, there should be no hesitation to treat these contractures surgically.

Heterotopic Bone Formation. Heterotopic bone may form in the soft tissues of the extremity as early as a few weeks after a head injury with persistent coma.[86] Although any joint can be affected, the most common sites are the hip and elbow. There is some evidence that heterotopic bone formation can be stimulated by surgical incisions. In head-injured teenagers who undergo antegrade reamed femoral intramedullary nailing of femoral fractures, heterotopic bone that later restricts hip motion can form at the nail insertion site.[81] A sudden increase of alkaline phosphatase a few weeks after the onset of coma, even with fractures coexisting, may mean that heterotopic bone is starting to form and a more careful examination of the extremities is indicated.[119] Technetium-99 bone scans show increased isotope uptake in the soft tissue where heterotopic bone forms, and this imaging study should be considered if new swelling is noted in the extremity of a comatose child. Other diagnoses that must be considered in a comatose child with new swelling of the extremity are a new long-bone fracture and deep venous thrombosis.[166]

Observation and excision are the two primary approaches taken in managing heterotopic bone formation in an injured child. If the child remains comatose, usually little treatment is administered. There are no conclusive data to support medical treatment if an early diagnosis of heterotopic bone formation is made. However, it may be useful to try to block some of the heterotopic bone formation by use of salicylates or nonsteroidal antiinflammatory medication once an early diagnosis is established. If the child has recovered from the head injury and has heterotopic bone that does not interfere with rehabilitation, no intervention is required. If there is significant restriction of joint motion from the heterotopic bone, this bone should be excised to facilitate rehabilitation. The timing of the heterotopic bone excision is somewhat controversial, but resection should be considered whenever heterotopic bone significantly interferes with rehabilitation, rather than waiting for 12 to 18 months until the bone is more mature. After surgical excision, early postoperative prophylaxis with local low-dose radiation therapy or medications (salicylates or nonsteroidal antiinflammatory drugs) is needed to minimize the risk of recurrence. Mital et al.[119] reported success in preventing recurrence of heterotopic bone after excision by use of salicylates at a dosage of 40 mg/kg/day in divided doses for 6 weeks postoperatively.

Fracture Healing Rates. Long-bone fractures heal more quickly in children and adults who have associated head injuries.[207] It has been demonstrated that polytrauma patients in a coma have a much higher serum calcitonin level than do conscious patients with similar long-bone fractures, but how or whether this finding influences fracture healing is still unclear.[43]

Peripheral Nerve Injuries

Although TBI most often accounts for persistent neurologic deficits in a child with multiple injuries, peripheral nerve injury should be considered as well during the rehabilitation process. In one clinical review of brain-injured children, 7% had evidence of an associated peripheral nerve injury documented by electrodiagnostic testing.[130] For closed injuries, the peripheral nerve injury is typically associated with an adjacent fracture or with a stretching injury of the extremity. In most cases, observation is indicated since these injuries often recover spontaneously. However, if the nerve injury is at the level of an open fracture, then exploration of the nerve is indicated. In children being observed following a nerve injury, if function does not return within 2 to 3 months, then electrodiagnostic testing should be undertaken. It is important to recognize these injuries because surgical peripheral nerve repair with nerve grafts offers an excellent chance of nerve function recovery in young patients.

Abdominal Injuries

Studies have reported abdominal injuries in 8%[101] to 27%[46] of pediatric polytrauma patients. Abdominal swelling, tenderness, or bruising are all signs of injury. CT evaluation has largely replaced peritoneal lavage or laparoscopy as the initial method of evaluation of abdominal injury.[173] Abdominal injury is not unusual if a child in an accident has been wearing a lap seat belt, regardless of whether a contusion is evident.[26,184] Bond et al.[19] noted that the presence of multiple pelvic fractures strongly correlated (80%) with the presence of abdominal or genitourinary injury, whereas the child's age or mechanism of injury had no correlation with abdominal injury rates. Although hepatic and splenic injuries are much more common, 22% of pediatric cases of pancreatitis have been reported to result from trauma.[14]

The usual practice is to treat hepatic and splenic lacerations nonoperatively, by monitoring the hematocrit, by repeating the abdominal examination frequently, and by serial CT scans or ultrasound examinations.[28,33–35,100,173,186] Once the child's overall condition has stabilized, and the child is stable to undergo general anesthesia, the presence of nonoperative abdominal injuries should not delay fracture care.

Genitourinary Injuries

Genitourinary system injuries are rare in the pediatric polytrauma population, with Letts[101] reporting an incidence of 1% in these patients. However, genitourinary injuries have been reported in 9%[158] to 24%[180] of children with pelvic fractures. Most injuries to the bladder and urethra are associated with fractures of the anterior pelvic ring (Fig. 4-3).[11] Such injuries are more common in males and usually occur at the bulbourethra, but the bladder, prostate, and other portions of the urethra can also be injured.[11,125] Although less common following pelvic fracture in girls, such injuries are often associated with severe injuries, including those to the vagina and rectum, with long-term concerns regarding continence, stricture formation, and childbearing.[133,145] If the iliac wings are displaced or the pelvic ring shape is changed, it may be necessary to reduce these fractures in order to reconstitute the birth canal in female patients. There are increased rates of caesarean section in young women who have had a pelvic fracture.[38] Adolescent females with displaced pelvic fractures should be informed of this potential problem with vaginal delivery. If the injury is severe, kidney injury may also occur, but most urologic injuries that occur with pelvic fractures are distal to the ureters.[1]

Fat Embolism and Pulmonary Embolism

Although fat embolism and acute respiratory distress syndrome are relatively common in adults with multiple long-bone fractures, they are rare in young children.[106,142] When fat embolism occurs, the signs and symptoms are the same as in adults: axillary petechiae, hypoxemia, and radiograph changes of pulmonary infiltrates appearing within several hours of the fractures. It is likely that some degree of hypoxemia develops in some children after multiple fractures, but the full clinical picture of fat embolism seldom develops. If a child with multiple fractures without a head injury develops a change in sensorium and orientation, hypoxemia is most likely the cause, and arterial blood gases are essential to determine the next step in management.

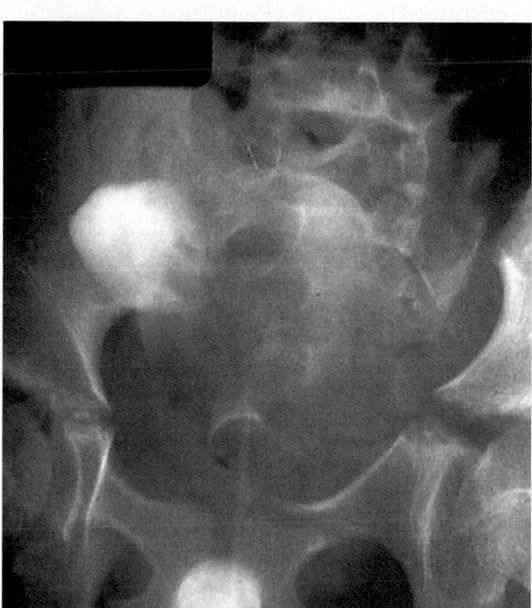

FIGURE 4-3 Most injuries to the bladder and urethra are associated with anterior pelvic ring fractures and should be suspected with these injuries.

The other primary cause of mental status change after fractures is overmedication with narcotics.

If fat embolism is diagnosed by low levels of arterial oxygenation, the treatment is the same as in adults, generally with endotracheal intubation, positive pressure ventilation, and hydration with intravenous fluid. The effect of early fracture stabilization, intravenous alcohol, or high-dose corticosteroids on fat embolism syndrome has not been studied well in children with multiple injuries.

Deep venous thrombosis and pulmonary thromboembolism also are rare, but are reported in children.[8,9,42,105,183] Previously, pulmonary embolism was rarely reported in association with pediatric trauma, but literature reports have increased. The risk of deep venous thrombosis and pulmonary embolism is increased with older children, a higher ISS, and central venous catheter placement.[42]

Nutritional Requirements

Pediatric polytrauma patients have high caloric demands. If an injured child requires ventilator support for several days, caloric intake through a feeding tube or a central intravenous catheter is necessary to avoid catabolism, improve healing, and help prevent complications. The baseline caloric needs of a child can be determined based on the weight and age of the child. Children on mechanical ventilation in a PICU have been shown to require 150% of the basal energy or caloric requirements for age and weight.[176] The daily nitrogen requirement for a child in the acute injury phase is 250 mg/kg.

ORTHOPAEDIC MANAGEMENT OF THE MULTIPLY INJURED CHILD

Timing

Because fractures are rarely life-threatening, splinting generally suffices as the initial orthopaedic care while the child's overall condition is stabilized. Loder[107] reported that, in 78 children with multiple injuries, early operative stabilization of fractures within the first 2 or 3 days after injury led to a shorter hospital stay, a shorter stay in the intensive care unit, and a shorter time on ventilator assistance. In addition, there were fewer complications in those who had surgical treatment of the fractures less than 72 hours after injury. In a more recent study, Loder et al.[108] reported a trend toward a higher rate of complications of immobilization (including pulmonary complications) in fractures treated late (after 72 hours), but the difference did not reach statistical significance. In this more recent study, age greater than 7 years and Modified Injury Severity Score (MISS) ≥140 were predictive of an increased rate of complications of immobilization. A mixed series of adults and children demonstrated comparable results for early (within 24 hours) and late (after 24 hours) fixation of fractures in the setting of blunt trauma and severe head injuries.[191]

Pelvic Fractures

Pelvic fractures are common in children and adolescents with multiple injuries and have been reported in up to 7% of children referred to level 1 regional trauma centers.[165,193] Survival is related to ISS and type of hospital.[193] In two series, 60%–87% of pelvic fractures involved a pedestrian struck by a motor vehicle.[158,168] Other common mechanisms include being a passenger in a MVA or falling from a height.[158,168] Although many of these pelvic injuries are stable, unstable patterns have been reported in up to 30% of cases.[17]

Injuries to the axial skeleton have been reported to be associated with the most intense hospital care and higher mortality rates than other injury combinations.[23] In their series of 166 consecutive pelvic fractures, Silber et al.[158] reported associated substantial head trauma in 39%, chest trauma in 20%, visceral/abdominal injuries in 19%, and a mortality rate of 3.6% (Fig. 4-4). In this same series,[158] 12% (20/166) had acetabular fractures, while in another series, 62% of children (8/13) with pelvic fractures had other orthopaedic injuries.[168]

Control of bleeding, either from the retroperitoneum near the fracture or from the peritoneum from injured viscera, may present an immediate threat.[76] However, death of children with pelvic fractures appears to be caused more often by an associated head injury rather than an injury to the adjacent viscera or vessels.[121]

Anterior pelvic ring fractures are the primary cause of urethral injury,[1,11,133,145] although urethral injuries are reported to occur less frequently in children than in adults.[158] Bilateral anterior and posterior pelvic fractures are most likely to cause severe bleeding,[116] but death from blood loss in children is uncommon.[44,121] Injury to the sciatic nerve or the lumbosacral nerve roots may result from hemipelvis displacement through a vertical shear fracture. Nonorthopaedic injuries associated with pelvic fractures led to long-term morbidity or mortality in 31% (11/36) of patients in one review of pediatric pelvic fractures.[56] Most pelvic fractures in children are treated nonoperatively. However, in a child or preadolescent, an external fixator can be used to close a marked pubic diastasis or to control bleeding by stabilizing the pelvis for transport and other injury care. The external fixator will not reduce a displaced vertical shear fracture, but the stability provided is helpful to control the hemorrhage while the child's condition is stabilized.[137,180] Operative treatment can result in healing by 10 weeks with a low complication rate.[79]

Open Fractures

Background

Most serious open fractures in children result from high-velocity blunt injury involving vehicles. Penetrating injuries are much less common in children than in adults; however, many low-

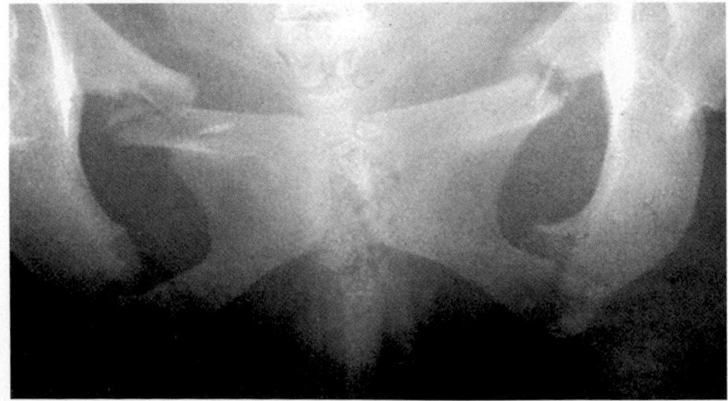

FIGURE 4-4 Bilateral superior and inferior pubic rami fractures. Genitourinary and abdominal injuries must be ruled out with severe pelvic fractures.

energy blunt injuries can cause puncture wounds in the skin adjacent to fractures, especially displaced radial, ulnar, and tibial fractures. In children with multiple injuries, approximately 10% of the fractures are open.[23,151] When open fractures are present, 25% to 50% of patients have additional injuries involving the head, chest, abdomen, and other extremities.[151]

Wound Classification

The classification used to describe the soft tissues adjacent to an open fracture is based on the system described by Gustilo and Anderson[62] and Gustilo and colleagues.[63] Primary factors that are considered and ranked in this classification system are the size of the wound, the degree of wound contamination, and the presence or absence of an associated vascular injury (Table 4-4).

Type I. Type I fractures usually result from a spike of bone puncturing the skin (from the inside to the outside). The wound is less than 1 cm in size, and there is minimal local soft tissue damage or contamination.

Type II. A type II wound is generally larger than 1 cm and is typically associated with a transverse or oblique fracture with minimal comminution. There is adjacent soft-tissue injury, including skin flaps or skin avulsion, and a moderate crushing component of adjacent soft tissue usually is present. Skin grafts or flaps should not be needed for coverage.

Type III and Subgroups. The most severe open fractures are classified as type III, with associated subgroups A, B, or C; the letters indicate increasing severity of injury. These fractures typically result from high-velocity trauma and are associated with extensive soft tissue injury, a large open wound, and significant wound contamination. In a type IIIA fracture, there is soft-tissue coverage over the bone, which is often a segmental fracture. In a type IIIB fracture, bone is exposed at the fracture site, with treatment typically requiring skin or muscle flap coverage of the bone. Type IIIC fractures are defined as those with an injury to a major artery in that segment of the extremity, regardless of wound size or the other soft-tissue disruption. Although these injuries are commonly associated with extensive soft-tissue loss and contamination, a type IIIC injury may, in fact, be associated with even a small wound in some cases.

This classification is widely used and has been shown to correlate in adults with sequelae of the injury, including the potential for infection, delayed union, nonunion, amputation, and residual impairment. The final functional results of type III fractures in children appear to be superior to results after similar fractures in adults, likely due to their better peripheral vascular supply.

TABLE 4-4 Classification of Open Fractures

Type I	An open fracture with a wound <1 cm long and clean
Type II	An open fracture with a laceration >1 cm long without extensive soft-tissue damage, flaps, or avulsions
Type III	Massive soft tissue damage, compromised vascularity, severe wound contamination marked fracture instability
Type IIIA	Adequate soft tissue coverage of a fractured bone despite extensive soft tissue laceration or flaps, or high-energy trauma irrespective of the size of the wound
Type IIIB	Extensive soft-tissue injury loss with periosteal stripping and bone exposure; usually associated with massive contamination
Type IIIC	Open fracture associated with arterial injury requiring repair

Adapted from Gustilo RB, Mendoza RM, Williams DN. Problems in the management of type III (severe) open fractures: a new classification of type III open fractures. J Trauma 1984;24:742–746; and Gustilo RB, Anderson JT. Prevention of infection in the treatment of 1025 open fractures of long bones, retrospective and prospective analyses. J Bone Joint Surg Am 1976;58:453–458.

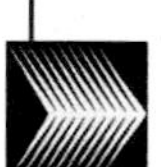

AUTHORS' PREFERRED METHOD

Three Stages

The treatment of open fractures in children is similar to that for open fractures in adults. The primary goals are to prevent infection of the wound and fracture site, while allowing soft tissue healing, fracture union, and eventual return of optimal function. Initial emergency care includes the ABCs of resuscitation, application of a sterile povidone-iodine dressing, and preliminary alignment and splinting of the fracture. If profuse bleeding is present, a compression dressing is applied to limit blood loss. In the emergency department, masks and gloves should be worn as each wound is thoroughly inspected. Tetanus prophylaxis is provided, and the initial dose of intravenous antibiotics is given. The dose of tetanus toxoid is 0.5 mL intramuscularly to be given if the patient's immunization status is unknown, or if it is more than 5 years since the last dose. The second stage of management is the primary surgical treatment, including initial and (if necessary) repeat débridement of the tissues in the area of the open fracture until the entire wound appears viable. The fracture is reduced and stabilized at this time. If the bone ends are not covered with viable soft tissue, muscle or skin flap coverage is considered. Vacuum-assisted closure (VAC) Therapy (Kinetic Concepts, Inc., San Antonio, TX) may be a useful adjunct to facilitate coverage and obviate the need for flaps in some patients.[70,120,196] VAC has been shown to shorten time of healing of wounds associated with open fractures.[99] The third and final stage of this management is bony reconstruction as needed if bone loss has occurred and, ultimately, rehabilitation of the child.

Cultures

Previous studies have demonstrated poor correlation of growth on routine cultures with wound infections.[97,188] Lee[97] reported that neither pre- nor postdébridement cultures accurately predicted the risk of infection in open fractures. He noted that only 20% of wounds (24/119) with positive predébridement cultures and only 28% (9/32) with positive postdébridement cultures became infected.[97] Although postdébridement cultures were more predictive of infection, these cultures identified the causative organism in only 42% (8/19) of infected wounds. Valenziano et al.[188] found that cultures at the time of presentation to the trauma center also were of no value, with only two of 28 patients (7%) with positive cultures becoming infected, in comparison to five of 89 patients (6%) with negative initial cultures. Initial cultures were positive in only two of seven of cases that became infected. Open fractures do not need to be routinely cultured. Cultures should only be obtained only at the time of reoperation in patients with clinical evidence of infection.

Antibiotic Therapy

Antibiotic therapy decreases the risk of infection in children with open fractures. Wilkins and Patzakis[199] reported a 13.9% infection rate in 79 patients who received no antibiotics after open fractures, and a 5.5% rate in 815 patients with similar injuries who had antibiotic prophylaxis. Bacterial contamination has been noted in 70% of open fractures in children, with both Gram-positive and Gram-negative organisms noted, depending on the degree of wound contamination and adjacent soft tissue injury. We limit antibiotic administration generally to 48 hours after surgical treatment of the open fracture.[96]

For all type I and some type II fractures, we use a first-generation cephalosporin (cefazolin 100 mg/kg/day divided q 8 hr, maximal daily dose 6 g).[96] For more severe type II fractures and for type III fractures, we use a combination of a cephalosporin and aminoglycoside (gentamicin 5–7.5 mg/kg/day divided q 8 hr).[96]

For farm injuries or grossly contaminated fractures, penicillin (150,000 units/kg/day divided q 6 hr, maximal daily dose 24 million units) is added to the cephalosporin and aminoglycoside. All antibiotics are given intravenously for 48 hours. Oral antibiotics are occasionally used if significant soft tissue erythema at the open fracture site remains after the intravenous antibiotics have been completed. Gentamicin levels should be checked after 4 or 5 doses (and doses adjusted as necessary) during therapy to minimize the risk of ototoxicity.

An additional 48-hour course is given around subsequent surgeries, such as those for repeat irrigation and débridement, delayed wound closure, open reduction and internal fixation of fractures, and secondary bone reconstruction procedures.

Débridement and Irrigation

We consider débridement and irrigation of the open fracture in the operating room to be the most important step in the primary management of open fractures in children. Some authors have reported that significantly higher infection rates occurred if débridement and irrigation were done more than 6 hours after open fractures in children.[89] A multicenter report, however, demonstrated an overall infection rate of 1% to 2% after open long-bone fractures, with no difference in infection rates between groups of patients treated with irrigation and débridement within 6 hours of injury and those treated between 6 and 24 hours following injury.[162] Another study of pediatric type I open fractures reported a 2.5% infection rate with nonoperative treatment.[75] One likely reason for the low rates of infection in these two series is the early administration of intravenous antibiotics in both groups. Although up to a 24-hour delay does not appear to have adverse consequences regarding infection rates, it may be necessary to perform an earlier irrigation and débridement to minimize compromise of the soft tissue envelope. The débridement needs to be performed carefully and systematically to remove all foreign and nonviable material from the wound. The order of débridement typically is (a) excision of the necrotic tissue from the wound edges; (b) extension of the wound to adequately explore the fracture ends; (c) débridement of the wound edges to bleeding tissue; (d) resection of necrotic skin, fat, muscle, and contaminated fascia; (e) fasciotomies as needed; and (f) thorough irrigation of the fracture ends and wound.

Because secondary infection in ischemic muscle can be a major problem in wound management and healing, all ischemic muscle is widely débrided back to muscle that bleeds at the cut edge and contracts when pinched with the forceps.

When débriding and irrigating an open diaphyseal fracture, we bring the proximal and distal bone ends into the wound to allow visual inspection and thorough irrigation and débridement. This often necessitates extension of the open wound, but is preferable to leaving the fracture site contaminated. We carefully remove devitalized bone fragments and contaminated cortical bone with curettes or a small rongeur. If there is a possible nonviable bone fragment, judgment is needed as to whether this bone fragment should be removed or left in place. Small fracture fragments without soft tissue attachments are removed, whereas very large ones may be retained if they are not significantly contaminated. Reconstruction of a large segmental bone loss has a better outcome in children than in adults because children have a better potential for bone regeneration and a better vascular supply to their extremities. Nearby major neurovascular structures in the area of the fracture are identified and protected. Débridement is complete when all contaminated, dead, and ischemic tissues have been excised; the bones ends are clean with bleeding edges; and only viable tissue lines the wound bed.

We usually use a lavage system to irrigate the open fracture with sterile normal saline, although lavage using wide-bore cystoscopy tubing is a reasonable alternative. We routinely use 9 L of solution for the lower extremities and 6 L in the upper extremities because of the smaller compartment size.

After the débridement and irrigation are complete, local soft tissue is used to cover the neurovascular structures, tendons, and bone ends. If local soft tissue coverage is inadequate, consideration should be given to local muscle flaps or other coverage methods, including VAC. The area of the wound that has been incised to extend the wound for fracture inspection can be primarily closed. The traumatic wound should either be left open to drain or may be closed over one or more drains. Wounds that are left open can be dressed with a moistened povidone-iodine or saline dressing. Types II and III fractures are routinely reoperated on every 48 to 72 hours for repeat irrigation and débridement until the wounds appear clean and the tissue viable. This cycle is repeated until the wound can be sutured closed or a split-thickness skin graft or local flap is used to cover it. If flap coverage is necessary, this is optimally accomplished within 1 week of injury.

Fracture Stabilization

Fracture stabilization in children with open fractures decreases pain, protects the soft tissue envelope from further injury, decreases the spread of bacteria, allows stability important for early soft tissue coverage, and improves the fracture union rate.

Principles for stabilization of open fractures in children include allowing access to the soft tissue wound and the extremity for débridement and dressing changes, allowing weight-bearing when appropriate, and preserving full motion of the adjacent joints to allow full functional recovery.

Although casts or splints can be used to stabilize type I fractures and occasionally type II fractures with relatively small wounds and minimal soft-tissue involvement, difficulties with soft-tissue management and loss of alignment as swelling subsides are common with such closed treatment. Most of these injuries involve the radius or ulna in the upper extremity or the tibia in the lower extremity. Splint or cast immobilization is generally not satisfactory for the more unstable type II and most type III injuries.

For diaphyseal forearm fractures, a flexible intramedullary implant in the radius and/or ulna commonly provides enough stability of the fracture to allow dressing changes through the cast or splint. For intramedullary fixation, we prefer 2- to 4-mm-diameter flexible titanium implants for stabilizing open fractures in the forearm when reduction of either the radial or ulnar fracture is unstable. Since the ulnar canal is straight, the implant chosen is often at least 80% of the narrowest canal diameter, while the implant for the radius is generally 50% to 60% of the narrowest canal diameter. The ulnar implant is inserted antegrade, and the radial implant is inserted retrograde just proximal to the distal radial physis. One or both bones can be stabilized, and the implants can be removed easily after fracture healing.

For distal forearm fractures, percutaneous pinning of the radius (and, occasionally, the ulna) generally is appropriate and provides sufficient stability. A short-arm cast usually is sufficient to maintain appropriate alignment following such fixation. The pins are removed in the office at 3 to 4 weeks, but the cast is used for a total of 6 weeks.

We also use flexible intramedullary nails for most open fractures of the femoral shaft. For type III fractures, especially if there is a large or contaminated soft tissue wound present, external fixation may be indicated. Trochanteric antegrade nails are gaining popularity and may be considered in children 10 years old or older or those who weigh 50 kilograms (110 lbs) or more.

Flexible intramedullary rod fixation has replaced external fixation as our treatment of choice for most open tibial and femoral fractures in children. Both intramedullary rodding and external fixation allow access to the wound for débridement and dressing changes as well as any soft tissue reconstruction needed.[123] Wound access, however, may be limited with external fixators, especially when there are extensive soft tissue wounds. Intramedullary rods generally are better tolerated by patients and families, do not require daily care, leave more cosmetic scars, and are load-sharing devices. With intramedullary rodding, the child is allowed to weight bear as tolerated following transverse or short oblique fractures, but weight-bearing is protected for 4 to 6 weeks following comminuted or spiral fractures.

External fixation is preferable for fractures with segmental bone loss, and ring fixators may even be used in such instances for bone transport. External fixation allows weight bearing relatively soon after the injury. We find that a uniplanar frame is best for most fractures and is relatively easy to apply. For some segmental fractures in the metaphysis and diaphysis, as well as soft tissue injuries, a ring fixator may be a better choice.

We use open reduction and internal fixation for open intra-articular fractures. When feasible, fixation should be parallel to (and avoid) the physis. Cannulated screws often are used in such instances. Screws or threaded pins should never be placed across the physis. If fixation across the physis is necessary, smooth pins are used; they should be removed 3 to 4 weeks after injury to minimize the risk of growth disturbance.

For fractures that involve both the metaphysis and diaphysis, open reduction and internal fixation can be combined with external fixation. For diaphyseal fractures in skeletally immature children, we prefer flexible intramedullary nails to compression plates for internal fixation of type I, type II, and some type III fractures. The superiority of intramedullary or external fixation for type IIIB fractures has not been firmly established. For treatment of a floating joint, usually the knee or elbow, we almost always stabilize both fractures operatively.[18,103]

Wound Management

Serial irrigation and débridement are done every 2 to 3 days until the wounds are clean and all remaining tissue appears viable. Fracture fixation at the time of initial surgery (as described previously) facilitates wound management. We prefer to provide soft tissue coverage of the open fracture and adjacent soft-tissue defect by 5 to 7 days after the injury to limit the risk of later infection. Most type I wounds heal with local dressing changes. For some type II and type IIIA fractures, we use delayed wound closure or a split-thickness skin graft over underlying muscle cover.

Large soft-tissue loss is most often a problem with types IIIB and IIIC fractures. In the proximal tibia, plastic surgeons may be needed to provide a gastrocnemius rotational flap, followed by secondary coverage of the muscle with a skin graft. In the middle third of the leg, a soleus flap is used with skin graft coverage, and a vascularized free muscle transfer is necessary if local coverage is inadequate. Free flaps may be required for coverage of the distal third of the tibia, especially in adolescents,[139] although there is a 60% postoperative complication rate. VAC sometimes can reduce the need for free tissue transfers. The VAC can convert wounds that need free tissue to ones that need split-thickness skin graft or can heal completely.[29,120]

The flaps and grafts used for reconstructing severe injuries are either muscle flaps or composite grafts. For a massive loss of soft tissue and bone, composite grafts of muscle and bone often are necessary. The younger the child, the better the likelihood that autogenous graft will fill in a bone defect if there is a well-vascularized bed from the muscle flap. Free flaps, especially from the latissimus dorsi, are useful in the midtibial and distal tibial regions to decrease infection rates and improve union rates. Vascularized fibular grafts rarely are used acutely to reconstruct bone defects, but may be useful after soft tissue healing.

For the rare case of significant bone defect in a child, we rely on the healing capacity of young periosteum and bone and the vascular supply of a child's extremity. An external fixator is used to hold the bone shortened about 1 to 2 cm to decrease the size of the bone loss. In a growing child, 1 to 2 cm of overgrowth can be expected in the subsequent 2 years after these severe injuries, so the final leg length will be satisfactory. Autogenous bone graft can be used early, but if there is surviving periosteum at this site, spontaneous bone formation often is surprisingly robust and may preclude the need for bone grafting. In teenagers with bone loss, once the soft tissue has healed, bone transport using either a uniplanar lengthening device or an Ilizarov device is our preferred method of reconstruction, although use of an allograft or vascularized fibular graft may be considered.

Amputation

In children, attempts should generally be made to preserve all extremities, even with type IIIC open fractures that are usually treated with primary amputation in adults. Wounds and fractures that do not heal in adults often heal satisfactorily in children and preservation of limb length and physes are important in young children. Although the Mangled Extremity Severity Score (MESS) correlates well with the need for amputation in adults, the correlation is less in children.[50] In one series,[50] the MESS predicted limb amputation or salvage correctly in 86% (31/36) of children, with 93% accuracy in salvaged limbs but only 63% in amputated limbs.

If amputation is absolutely necessary, as much length as possible should be preserved. For example, if the proximal tibial physis is preserved in a child with a below knee amputation at age 7 years, 3 to 4 inches more growth of the tibial stump can be expected by skeletal maturity. Thus, even a very short tibial stump in a skeletally immature child may grow to an appropriate length by skeletal maturity. As a result, even a short below-knee amputation at the time of injury would likely be superior to a knee disarticulation in final function.

Although amputations to treat congenital limb deficits usually are done through the joint to limit bone spike formation (overgrowth) at the end of the stump, we prefer to maintain maximal possible length if amputation becomes necessary as a result of a severe injury.

Management of Other Fractures

When a child with an open fracture is brought to the operating room for irrigation and débridement of the open fracture, the orthopaedist may use this opportunity to treat the other fractures as well, whether operative treatment or closed reduction and casting are needed. To facilitate patient care and rehabilitation, most long-bone fractures in these children are treated surgically.

STABILIZATION OF FRACTURES

Beneficial Effects

Fracture stabilization also provides a number of nonorthopaedic benefits to a child with multiple injuries. Among the potential benefits are ease of patient mobilization, ease of nursing care, decreased risks of pressure sores, and better access to the wounds. Pulmonary contusions at the time of injury often lead to increasing respiratory problems in the first few days after injury.[131] If the lungs have been severely contused, protein leaks into the alveolar spaces, making ventilation more difficult. This may be exacerbated by the systemic inflammatory response syndrome, which is commonly seen following severe trauma.[142,198] Surfactant dysfunction follows and is most abnormal in patients with the most severe respiratory failure.[131] As the time from the injury increases, pulmonary function deteriorates and general anesthesia becomes more risky. Orthopaedic surgical treatment before such pulmonary deterioration limits the anesthetic risks in these patients. In patients with severe pulmonary contusions and multiple fractures, the use of extracorporeal life support may be the only treatment available to allow patient survival.[155]

In adults with multiple injuries, early operative stabilization of fractures decreases pulmonary and other medical complications associated with prolonged bed rest that is a part of nonoperative fracture treatment.[13] Most adult trauma centers follow the treatment protocol of early fracture stabilization, even though Poole et al.[134] reported that, despite early fracture stabilization simplifying patient care, pulmonary complications in patients with marked chest trauma were not prevented and the course of the head injury was not affected. In children, medical complications are less common, so the recommendations that mandate early fracture stabilization are somewhat more difficult to support in young patients. Nonetheless, bruises on the chest or rib fractures should alert the orthopaedist to potential pulmonary contusions as a part of the injury complex.[127] Initial chest radiographs may not clearly demonstrate the degree of pulmonary parenchymal injury, and arterial blood gas determinations are more useful in estimating the anesthetic risk of these patients during operative care of the fractures.

Timing

As noted, splinting is needed at the time of the initial resuscitation. In a child with multiple closed fractures, definitive treatment should proceed expeditiously once the child's condition has been stabilized. Loder[107] reported that operative stabilization of fractures within the first 2 or 3 days after injury led to fewer complications, shorter hospital and intensive care unit stays, and a shorter time on ventilator assistance in children with multiple injuries. A more recent study by Loder et al.[108] reported a trend toward a higher rate of complications in fractures treated after 72 hours. Although there appear to be other factors besides the timing of surgery that affect the eventual outcomes of polytrauma patients, the timing of surgery is a variable that can be controlled by the surgeon, and it seems prudent to complete fracture stabilization within 2 to 3 days of injury when possible.

Operative Fixation

The type of operative stabilization used in multiply injured children commonly depends on the training, experience, and personal preference of the orthopaedist. The most common methods used are intramedullary rod fixation, external fixation, compression plating, and locking plating; Kirschner-wires or Steinmann pins may be used in conjunction with casts.

Intramedullary Rod Fixation

There has been an increase in the use of 2- to 4-mm-diameter flexible titanium intramedullary rods for stabilization of long-bone fractures of the upper and lower extremities. Intramedullary rodding is most commonly used for unstable closed fractures of the radius and ulna in patients through adolescence and for femoral shaft fractures in patients between the ages of 5 and skeletal maturity.[179,192] A trochanteric antegrade nails often is a viable option in children 10 years old or older or in those with comminuted femoral fractures. The tibia also can be fixed with intramedullary rods in children with an open fracture, polytrauma, a "floating knee" injury (concurrent femur fracture), or a high-energy, unstable injury (especially during adolescence). A diaphyseal fracture of the humerus can be treated with intramedullary fixation in the presence of a "floating" shoulder or elbow.[144]

Common indications for intramedullary fixation of forearm fractures include unstable diaphyseal fractures (especially in adolescents) and open fractures.[58,95,98,111] Forearm fractures can generally be reduced closed, with the intramedullary implant passed across the fracture site under fluoroscopy to stabilize the fracture.[95] In one study,[98] 23% (10/43) of closed forearm fractures treated with intramedullary rod fixation required open reduction. The ulnar implant is placed in antegrade fashion and can be inserted through the lateral proximal metaphyseal area or the tip of the olecranon. The radial implant is inserted retrograde and is contoured to conform to the normal radial bow before insertion. The insertion point is proximal to the distal radial physis and the rod can be inserted from the radial aspect of the distal radius or dorsally (slightly ulnar to Lister's tubercle). Stability of both fractures may be achieved by instrumenting only the radius or the ulna in younger children, but both bones are more commonly fixed in adolescents. Intramedullary fixation of open forearm fractures appears to decrease the rate of loss of reduction.[58,111] In one series,[98] reduction was maintained in all 27 patients treated with rodding of both bones or of only the radius, compared with loss of reduction in 32% (7/22) of patients in whom only the ulna was rodded. The high rate of failure may be due to the small diameter pins (1.6 or 2.0 mm) used to fix the ulna in this series.[98] A cast is used for further immobilization.

The implants are easily removed from the wrist area and the elbow region 6 to 12 months after insertion. Despite the utility of flexible intramedullary implants for stabilizing forearm fractures in children, the radius and ulna in young patients have significant remodeling capacity and not all fractures require anatomic reduction. A closed reduction and cast immobilization may suffice. Displaced distal forearm fractures in polytrauma patients are often well treated with closed reduction and percutaneous pinning, thus affording sufficient stability for use of a short-arm cast in these polytrauma patients.

In a series of 20 pediatric patients treated with intramedullary rodding of forearm fractures, 50% of patients had complications including loss of reduction, infection, hardware migration, nerve injury, and delayed union, although 95% (19/20) of patients had excellent or good results at follow-up.[41] In another series,[205] compartment syndromes occurred in six of 80 (7.5%) patients with forearm fractures treated with intramedullary fixation; risk factors in this study were reported to be increased operative time and increased intraoperative use of fluoroscopy.

If flexible intramedullary nails are used in the femur, the most common technique is retrograde insertion from the medial and lateral metaphyseal region of the distal femur, 2 to 3 cm proximal to the physis. Two rods are used to cross the fracture site and obtain purchase in the proximal femur, usually with one at the base of the femoral neck and the other at the base of the greater trochanter. Rod diameter is generally 40% of the intramedullary diameter of the femoral isthmus, up to a maximum rod size of 4 to 4.5 mm (depending on manufacturer). A cast is not necessary postoperatively, although a fracture brace can be used to help control rotation at the fracture site and provide some patient comfort during early walking, especially for proximal third fractures or those with significant comminution. The implants usually are removed within 1 year of the fracture.[68,74] One study showed that intramedullary nailing of the femur had more complications in comminuted fractures and children weighing over 100 pounds,[52] while another noted higher complication rates in children 10 years old or older at the time of surgery.[72]

The use of reamed antegrade intramedullary rods to treat femoral shaft fractures in the pediatric population should be reserved for those with a closed proximal femoral physis. In younger children, rod insertion at the piriformis fossa may interfere with the vascular supply to the femoral epiphysis, may cause growth arrest of the greater trochanter (i.e., apophysis with resultant coxa valga), or may interfere with the appositional bone growth at the base of the femoral neck, thereby thinning this region and potentially predisposing the child to a femoral neck fracture.[12,27,102,118,124] Some authors have advocated rigid intramedullary rodding using an entrance point at the tip of the greater trochanter.[57,181] Although the use of trochanteric antegrade nails is increasingly common, there are not yet sufficient data to confirm the safety and efficacy of such an approach. The specific indications for intramedullary fixation of the femur are discussed in more detail in Chapter 22.

Flexible intramedullary rod fixation is becoming increasingly common for diaphyseal tibial fractures. The most common indications currently are open fractures, "floating knee" injuries, and unstable diaphyseal fractures in adolescents. The rods are inserted in antegrade fashion, with medial and lateral entrance points distal to the physis and avoiding the tibial tubercle. As with femoral fractures, rod diameter is 40% of the narrowest intramedullary diameter, with a maximum rod size of 4 to 4.5 mm (depending on implant manufacturer). A short-leg walking cast or fracture boot often is used for comfort for the first 4 to 6 weeks postoperatively, although a splint may be used initially to allow access to wounds associated with an open fracture or degloving injury.

Compression Plates

Some authors have advocated the use of compression plates to stabilize long-bone fractures, especially in the femoral shaft, in children with multiple injuries.[25,90] Kregor et al.[90] reported an average overgrowth of the femur of 9 mm, and all fractures healed in a near anatomic position. Caird et al.[25] noted that 3% of patients (2/60) had a limb length discrepancy of greater than 2.5 cm following femoral plating, including a 5-cm discrepancy in one child. The disadvantages of compression plating include the need for more extensive operative exposure at the site of

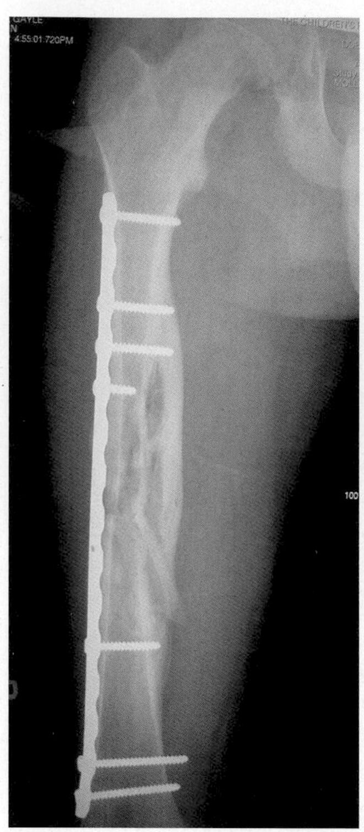

FIGURE 4-5 Stabilization of femoral shaft fractures in children with multi-trauma can be obtained with several methods. Minimally invasive percutaneous submuscular plating techniques can occasionally be used. (Courtesy of Steven T. Morgan, MD, Denver, CO.)

the fracture, the fact that they are not load-sharing devices, and the usual need to remove the plate through a relatively long incision once healing is complete. Newer minimally invasive percutaneous submuscular plating techniques have eliminated some of the problems associated with traditional plating (Fig. 4-5).[78,160] Refracture may occur through the screw holes left after plate removal if physical activity is resumed too quickly.[78] Stiffness of adjacent joints is rarely a problem in children unless there has been an associated severe soft tissue injury. The number of cortices the screws cross on each side of the fracture may be fewer in children than in adults, because a cast or splint is routinely used in young patients. Kanlic et al.[78] reported an 8% incidence of leg length discrepancy after submuscular bridge plating.

Although some authors have recommended open reduction and compression plate fixation of displaced radial and ulnar fractures,[203] we prefer flexible intramedullary nails, as noted earlier. The use of compression plates in the forearm requires a larger operative incision with a resultant scar, a second extensive procedure for plate removal, and a significant risk of refracture following hardware removal. We do not believe that the healing capability of the young child requires the rigid fixation of compression plating to obtain fracture union.

External Fixation

Traditional indications for external fixation in a child with multiple injuries are open fractures with significant soft tissue injury, fractures in children with a head injury and coma, and "floating knee" fractures of the femur and tibia (Fig. 4-6).[5,6,16,18,85,103,144,154,178,206] With advances in intramedullary rod techniques, external fixation is now uncommon. A uni-

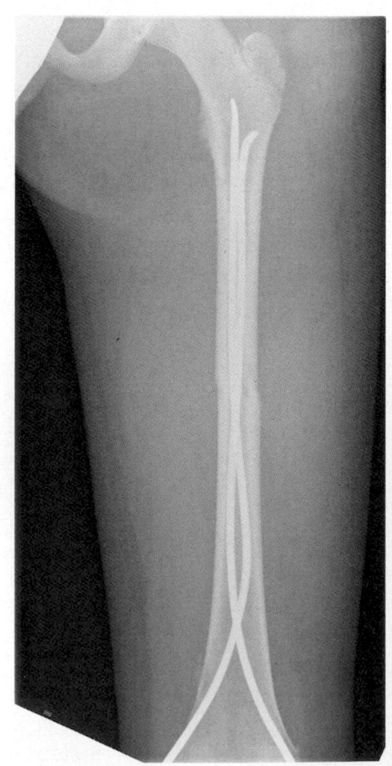

A

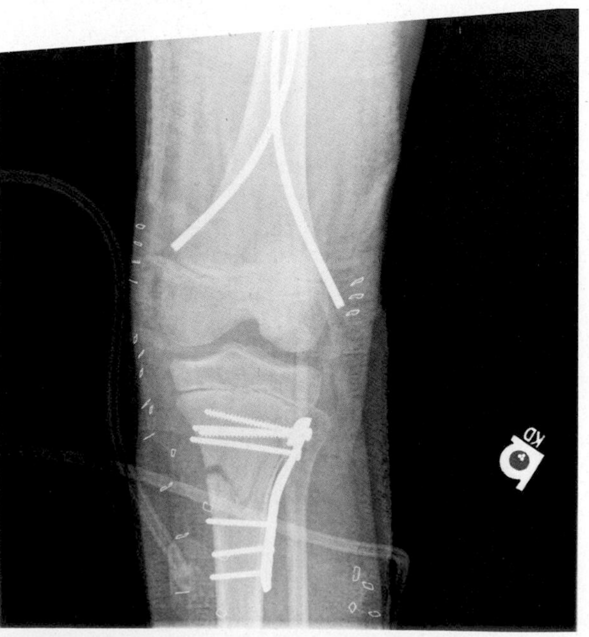

B

FIGURE 4-6 "Floating knee" injury in a 12-year-old child included **(A)** a femoral shaft fracture, the femoral physeal fracture was reduced with flexible IM nails. **B.** Open fractures of the tibia were treated with débridement and irrigation and stabilization with internal fixation. (Courtesy of Michelle Caird, MD, Ann Arbor, MI.)

lateral fixator generally is sufficient to hold the fracture reduced in this age group.

If external fixation is used, the pin sites should be predrilled and the pins placed in the operating room under fluoroscopic control. The caliber of the pin should be less than 30% of the diameter of the bone into which it is to be inserted to minimize the risk of fracture through a pin site. The distal and proximal pins must be inserted at a level to avoid the physis, and we recommend leaving at least 1 to 2 cm between the pin and physis, partly to avoid any adverse effect on the physis should a pin track infection occur. The proximal tibial physis is more distal anteriorly below the tibial tubercle, and this area must be avoided or a recurvatum deformity of the proximal tibia and knee will result. The external fixator is usually left in place until fracture healing is complete, but it can be removed once the reason for placement has resolved (such as waking from coma or healing of a skin wound).[48,201] If the fixator is removed early, a walking cast is applied. Transverse open fractures reduced out to length take longer to heal than do oblique fractures reduced with slight overlap. Refracture is a well-described risk following fixator removal. However, refracture rates have been variable, with a 21% rate noted in a series in which a rigid transfixion type of fixator was used[177] and a 1.4% rate in a series with more flexible unilateral frames.[16] One report indicated that if 3 of the 4 cortices at the fracture site appear to be healing on anteroposterior and lateral radiographs of the fracture, the refracture rate after frame removal should be low.[163]

Laboratory studies have suggested that dynamization of external fixators may stimulate early fracture healing.[32,94] We prefer to dynamize the fixator early to stimulate callus formation, although the effect of dynamization on refracture rates is unclear.[47,82]

Outcomes of Treatment of the Multiply Injured Child

In one review of 74 children with multiple injuries, 59 (80%) survived, but after 1 year, 22% were disabled, mainly from a brain injury.[189] At 9 years after the injuries, 12% had significant physical disability, whereas 42% had cognitive impairment. In this group, however, the SF-36 or functional outcome survey did not differ from the control population. The best predictor of long-term disability was the Glasgow Outcome Scale from 6 weeks after injury and later.[189] Letts et al.[101] reported that 71.6% of multiply injured children made a full recovery, with a mean of 28 weeks until full recovery. Of the 53 residual deficits in 48 patients, the common deficits were neurologic (38%), psychosocial (34%), and musculoskeletal (24%).[101] Outcomes of children with pelvic fractures were near normal status at 6 months.[157]

Whether operative or nonoperative fracture treatment is chosen for a child with multiple injuries, it is important that an orthopaedist be involved in the care of the child from the start. While recognizing the need to care for the other organ system injuries the child has sustained, it is important to advocate for the expeditious and appropriate treatment of the fractures that are present. Failure to do so will leave the multiply injured child with musculoskeletal disability once healing of the other injuries occurs.

After multiple injuries, the most common long-term problems relate to either sequelae of the head injury or of the orthopaedic injuries.

ACKNOWLEDGMENTS

The authors gratefully acknowledge Vernon T. Tolo, MD, for his past contributions to this chapter. We thank Donna M. Zink and Kristi A. Overgaard for their assistance during preparation of this chapter.

REFERENCES

1. Abou-Jaoude WA, Sugarman JM, Fallat ME, et al. Indicators of genitourinary tract injury or anomaly in cases of pediatric blunt trauma. J Pediatr Surg 1996;31(1): 86–89,discussion 90.
2. American Academy of Pediatrics. Diagnostic imaging of child abuse. Pediatrics 2000; 105(6):1345–1348.
3. Andrich DE, O'Malley KJ, Summerton DJ, et al. The type of urethroplasty for a pelvic fracture urethral distraction defect cannot be predicted preoperatively. J Urol 2003; 170(2 Pt 1):464–467.
4. Armstrong PF. Initial management of the multiply injured child: the ABCs. Instr Course Lect 1992;41:347–350.
5. Aronson J, Tursky EA. External fixation of femur fractures in children. J Pediatr Orthop 1992;12(2):157–163.
6. Arslan H, Kapukaya A, Kesemenli C, et al. Floating knee in children. J Pediatr Orthop 2003;23(4):458–463.
7. Aufdermaur M. Spinal injuries in juveniles. Necropsy findings in 12 cases. J Bone Joint Surg Br 1974;56B(3):513–519.
8. Azu MC, McCormack JE, Scriven RJ, et al. Venous thromboembolic events in pediatric trauma patients: is prophylaxis necessary? J Trauma 2005;59(6):1345–1349.
9. Babyn PS, Gahunia HK, Massicotte P. Pulmonary thromboembolism in children. Pediatr Radiol 2005;35(3):258–274.
10. Barsness KA, Cha ES, Bensard DD, et al. The positive predictive value of rib fractures as an indicator of nonaccidental trauma in children. J Trauma 2003;54(6):1107–1110.
11. Batislam E, Ates Y, Germiyanoglu C, et al. Role of Tile classification in predicting urethral injuries in pediatric pelvic fractures. J Trauma 1997;42(2):285–287.
12. Beaty JH, Austin SM, Warner WC, et al. Interlocking intramedullary nailing of femoral-shaft fractures in adolescents: preliminary results and complications. J Pediatr Orthop 1994;14(2):178–183.
13. Beckman SB, Scholten DJ, Bonnell BW, et al. Long-bone fractures in the polytrauma patient. The role of early operative fixation. Am Surg 1989;55(6):356–358.
14. Benifla M, Weizman Z. Acute pancreatitis in childhood: analysis of literature data. J Clin Gastroenterol 2003;37(2):169–172.
15. Bielski RJ, Bassett GS, Fideler B, et al. Intraosseous infusions: effects on the immature physis—an experimental model in rabbits. J Pediatr Orthop 1993;13(4):511–515.
16. Blasier RD, Aronson J, Tursky EA. External fixation of pediatric femur fractures. J Pediatr Orthop 1997;17(3):342–346.
17. Blasier RD, McAtee J, White R, et al. Disruption of the pelvic ring in pediatric patients. Clin Orthop Relat Res 2000;376:87–95.
18. Bohn WW, Durbin RA. Ipsilateral fractures of the femur and tibia in children and adolescents. J Bone Joint Surg Am 1991;73(3):429–439.
19. Bond SJ, Gotschall CS, Eichelberger MR. Predictors of abdominal injury in children with pelvic fracture. J Trauma 1991;31(8):1169–1173.
20. Bosch PP, Vogt MT, Ward WT. Pediatric spinal cord injury without radiographic abnormality (SCIWORA): the absence of occult instability and lack of indication for bracing. Spine 2002;27(24):2788–2800.
21. Brainard BJ, Slauterbeck J, Benjamin JB. Fracture patterns and mechanisms in pedestrian motor-vehicle trauma: the ipsilateral dyad. J Orthop Trauma 1992;6(3):279–282.
22. Brown JK, Jing Y, Wang S, et al. Patterns of severe injury in pediatric car crash victims: Crash Injury Research Engineering Network database. J Pediatr Surg 2006;41(2): 362–367.
23. Buckley SL, Gotschall C, Robertson W Jr, et al. The relationships of skeletal injuries with trauma score, injury severity score, length of hospital stay, hospital charges, and mortality in children admitted to a regional pediatric trauma center. J Pediatr Orthop 1994;14(4):449–453.
24. Buess E, Illi OE, Soder C, et al. Ruptured spleen in children—15-year evolution in therapeutic concepts. Eur J Pediatr Surg 1992;2(3):157–161.
25. Caird MS, Mueller KA, Puryear A, et al. Compression plating of pediatric femoral shaft fractures. J Pediatr Orthop 2003;23(4):448–452.
26. Campbell DJ, Sprouse LR 2nd, Smith LA, et al. Injuries in pediatric patients with seatbelt contusions. Am Surg 2003;69(12):1095–1099.
27. Canale ST, Tolo VT. Fractures of the femur in children. Instr Course Lect 1995;44: 255–273.
28. Canarelli JP, Boboyono JM, Ricard J, et al. Management of abdominal contusion in polytraumatized children. Int Surg 1991;76(2):119–121.
29. Caniano DA, Ruth B, Teich S. Wound management with vacuum-assisted closure: experience in 51 pediatric patients. J Pediatr Surg 2005;40(1):128–132.
30. Cattell HS, Filtzer DL. Pseudosubluxation and other normal variations in the cervical spine in children. A study of 160 children. J Bone Joint Surg Am 1965;47(7): 1295–1309.
31. Chan L, Reilly KM, Telfer J. Odds of critical injuries in unrestrained pediatric victims of motor vehicle collision. Pediatr Emerg Care 2006;22(9):626–629.
32. Claes LE, Wilke HJ, Augat P, et al. Effect of dynamization on gap healing of diaphyseal fractures under external fixation. Clin Biomech (Bristol, Avon) 1995;10(5):227–234.

33. Cloutier DR, Baird TB, Gormley P, et al. Pediatric splenic injuries with a contrast blush: successful nonoperative management without angiography and embolization. J Pediatr Surg 2004;39(6):969–971.
34. Coburn MC, Pfeifer J, DeLuca FG. Nonoperative management of splenic and hepatic trauma in the multiply injured pediatric and adolescent patient. Arch Surg 1995;130(3): 332–338.
35. Cochran A, Mann NC, Dean JM, et al. Resource utilization and its management in splenic trauma. Am J Surg 2004;187(6):713–719.
36. Coley BD, Mutabagani KH, Martin LC, et al. Focused abdominal sonography for trauma (FAST) in children with blunt abdominal trauma. J Trauma 2000;48(5):902–906.
37. Colombani PM, Buck JR, Dudgeon DL, et al. One-year experience in a regional pediatric trauma center. J Pediatr Surg 1985;20(1):8–13.
38. Copeland CE, Bosse MJ, McCarthy ML, et al. Effect of trauma and pelvic fracture on female genitourinary, sexual, and reproductive function. J Orthop Trauma 1997;11(2): 73–81.
39. Cramer KE. The pediatric polytrauma patient. Clin Orthop Relat Res 1995;318: 125–135.
40. Cuff S, DiRusso S, Sullivan T, et al. Validation of a relative head injury severity scale for pediatric trauma. J Trauma 2007;63(1):172–177,discussion 177–178.
41. Cullen MC, Roy DR, Giza E, et al. Complications of intramedullary fixation of pediatric forearm fractures. J Pediatr Orthop 1998;18(1):14–21.
42. Cyr C, Michon B, Pettersen G, et al. Venous thromboembolism after severe injury in children. Acta Haematol 2006;115(3–4):198–200.
43. De Bastiani G, Mosconi F, Spagnol G, et al. High calcitonin levels in unconscious polytrauma patients. J Bone Joint Surg Br 1992;74(1):101–104.
44. Demetriades D, Karaiskakis M, Velmahos GC, et al. Pelvic fractures in pediatric and adult trauma patients: are they different injuries? J Trauma 2003;54(6):1146–1151,discussion 1151.
45. Densmore JC, Lim HJ, Oldham KT, et al. Outcomes and delivery of care in pediatric injury. J Pediatr Surg 2006;41(1):92–98.
46. Dereeper E, Ciardelli R, Vincent JL. Fatal outcome after polytrauma: multiple-organ failure or cerebral damage? Resuscitation 1998;36(1):15–18.
47. Domb BG, Sponseller PD, Ain M, et al. Comparison of dynamic versus static external fixation for pediatric femur fractures. J Pediatr Orthop 2002;22(4):428–430.
48. Evanoff M, Strong ML, MacIntosh R. External fixation maintained until fracture consolidation in the skeletally immature. J Pediatr Orthop 1993;13(1):98–101.
49. Evans DL, Bethem D. Cervical spine injuries in children. J Pediatr Orthop 1989;9(5): 563–568.
50. Fagelman MF, Epps HR, Rang M. Mangled extremity severity score in children. J Pediatr Orthop 2002;22(2):182–184.
51. Fayiga YJ, Valentine RJ, Myers SI, et al. Blunt pediatric vascular trauma: analysis of 41 consecutive patients undergoing operative intervention. J Vasc Surg 1994;20(3): 419–424,discussion 424–425.
52. Flynn JM, Luedtke L, Ganley TJ, et al. Titanium elastic nails for pediatric femur fractures: lessons from the learning curve. Am J Orthop 2002;31(2):71–74.
53. Frank JB, Lim CK, Flynn JM, et al. The efficacy of magnetic resonance imaging in pediatric cervical spine clearance. Spine 2002;27(11):1176–1179.
54. Galano GJ, Vitale MA, Kessler MW, et al. The most frequent traumatic orthopaedic injuries from a national pediatric inpatient population. J Pediatr Orthop 2005;25(1): 39–44.
55. Garcia VF, Gotschall CS, Eichelberger MR, et al. Rib fractures in children: a marker of severe trauma. J Trauma 1990;30(6):695–700.
56. Garvin KL, McCarthy RE, Barnes CL, et al. Pediatric pelvic ring fractures. J Pediatr Orthop 1990;10(5):577–582.
57. Gordon JE, Swenning TA, Burd TA, et al. Proximal femoral radiographic changes after lateral transtrochanteric intramedullary nail placement in children. J Bone Joint Surg Am 2003;85-A(7):1295–1301.
58. Greenbaum B, Zionts LE, Ebramzadeh E. Open fractures of the forearm in children. J Orthop Trauma 2001;15(2):111–118.
59. Greenberg MI. Falls from heights. JACEP 1978;7(8):300–301.
60. Greenspan AI, MacKenzie EJ. Functional outcome after pediatric head injury. Pediatrics 1994;94(4 Pt 1):425–432.
61. Guillamondegui OD, Mahboubi S, Stafford PW, et al. The utility of the pelvic radiograph in the assessment of pediatric pelvic fractures. J Trauma 2003;55(2):236–239, discussion 239–240.
62. Gustilo RB, Anderson JT. Prevention of infection in the treatment of 1025 open fractures of long bones: retrospective and prospective analyses. J Bone Joint Surg Am 1976; 58(4):453–458.
63. Gustilo RB, Mendoza RM, Williams DN. Problems in the management of type III (severe) open fractures: a new classification of type III open fractures. J Trauma 1984; 24(8):742–746.
64. Guy J, Haley K, Zuspan SJ. Use of intraosseous infusion in the pediatric trauma patient. J Pediatr Surg 1993;28(2):158–161.
65. Haller JA Jr, Shorter N, Miller D, et al. Organization and function of a regional pediatric trauma center: does a system of management improve outcome? J Trauma 1983;23(8): 691–696.
66. Hanten G, Dennis M, Zhang L, et al. Childhood head injury and metacognitive processes in language and memory. Dev Neuropsychol 2004;25(1–2):85–106.
67. Harris BH. Creating pediatric trauma systems. J Pediatr Surg 1989;24(2):149–152.
68. Heinrich SD, Drvaric DM, Darr K, et al. The operative stabilization of pediatric diaphyseal femur fractures with flexible intramedullary nails: a prospective analysis. J Pediatr Orthop 1994;14(4):501–507.
69. Heinrich SD, Gallagher D, Harris M, et al. Undiagnosed fractures in severely injured children and young adults. Identification with technetium imaging. J Bone Joint Surg Am 1994;76(4):561–572.
70. Herscovici D Jr, Sanders RW, Scaduto JM, et al. Vacuum-assisted wound closure (VAC therapy) for the management of patients with high-energy soft tissue injuries. J Orthop Trauma 2003;17(10):683–688.
71. Herzenberg JE, Hensinger RN, Dedrick DK, et al. Emergency transport and positioning of young children who have an injury of the cervical spine. The standard backboard may be hazardous. J Bone Joint Surg Am 1989;71(1):15–22.
72. Ho CA, Skaggs DL, Tang CW, et al. Use of flexible intramedullary nails in pediatric femur fractures. J Pediatr Orthop 2006;26(4):497–504.
73. Hoffmann R, Nerlich M, Muggia-Sullam M, et al. Blunt abdominal trauma in cases of multiple trauma evaluated by ultrasonography: a prospective analysis of 291 patients. J Trauma 1992;32(4):452–458.
74. Huber RI, Keller HW, Huber PM, et al. Flexible intramedullary nailing as fracture treatment in children. J Pediatr Orthop 1996;16(5):602–605.
75. Iobst CA, Tidwell MA, King WF. Nonoperative management of pediatric type I open fractures. J Pediatr Orthop 2005;25(4):513–517.
76. Ismail N, Bellemare JF, Mollitt DL, et al. Death from pelvic fracture: children are different. J Pediatr Surg 1996;31(1):82–85.
77. Jawadi AH, Letts M. Injuries associated with fracture of the femur secondary to motor vehicle accidents in children. Am J Orthop 2003;32(9):459–462,discussion 462.
78. Kanlic EM, Anglen JO, Smith DG, et al. Advantages of submuscular bridge plating for complex pediatric femur fractures. Clin Orthop Relat Res 2004;426:244–251.
79. Karunakar MA, Goulet JA, Mueller KL, et al. Operative treatment of unstable pediatric pelvis and acetabular fractures. J Pediatr Orthop 2005;25(1):34–38.
80. Kay RM, Skaggs DL. Pediatric polytrauma management. J Pediatr Orthop 2006;26(2): 268–277.
81. Keret D, Harcke HT, Mendez AA, et al. Heterotopic ossification in central nervous system–injured patients following closed nailing of femoral fractures. Clin Orthop Relat Res 1990;256:254–259.
82. Kesemenli CC, Subasi M, Arslan H, et al. Is external fixation in pediatric femoral fractures a risk factor for refracture? J Pediatr Orthop 2004;24(1):17–20.
83. Kim KA, Wang MY, Griffith PM, et al. Analysis of pediatric head injury from falls. Neurosurg Focus 2000;8(1):e3.
84. King J, Diefendorf D, Apthorp J, et al. Analysis of 429 fractures in 189 battered children. J Pediatr Orthop 1988;8(5):585–589.
85. Kirschenbaum D, Albert MC, Robertson WW Jr, et al. Complex femur fractures in children: treatment with external fixation. J Pediatr Orthop 1990;10(5):588–591.
86. Kluger G, Kochs A, Holthausen H. Heterotopic ossification in childhood and adolescence. J Child Neurol 2000;15(6):406–413.
87. Knudson MM, Shagoury C, Lewis FR. Can adult trauma surgeons care for injured children? J Trauma 1992;32(6):729–737,discussion 737–739.
88. Kocher MS, Kasser JR. Orthopaedic aspects of child abuse. J Am Acad Orthop Surg 2000;8(1):10–20.
89. Kreder HJ, Armstrong P. A review of open tibia fractures in children. J Pediatr Orthop 1995;15(4):482–488.
90. Kregor PJ, Song KM, Routt ML, Jr., et al. Plate fixation of femoral shaft fractures in multiply injured children. J Bone Joint Surg Am 1993;75(12):1774–1780.
91. Kumaresan S, Sances A Jr, Carlin F. Biomechanical analysis of padding in child seats and head injury. Biomed Sci Instrum 2002;38:453–458.
92. Lallier M, Bouchard S, St-Vil D, et al. Falls from heights among children: a retrospective review. J Pediatr Surg 1999;34(7):1060–1063.
93. Lane WG, Dubowitz H. What factors affect the identification and reporting of child abuse–related fractures? Clin Orthop Relat Res 2007;461:219–225.
94. Larson JT, Dietrich AM, Abdessalam SF, et al. Effective use of the air ambulance for pediatric trauma. J Trauma 2004;56(1):89–93.
95. Lascombes P, Prevot J, Ligier JN, et al. Elastic stable intramedullary nailing in forearm shaft fractures in children: 85 cases. J Pediatr Orthop 1990;10(2):167–171.
96. Lavelle WF, Uhl R, Krieves M, et al. Management of open fractures in pediatric patients: current teaching in Accreditation Council for Graduate Medical Education (ACGME) accredited residency programs. J Pediatr Orthop B 2008;17(1):1–6.
97. Lee J. Efficacy of cultures in the management of open fractures. Clin Orthop Relat Res 1997;339:71–75.
98. Lee S, Nicol RO, Stott NS. Intramedullary fixation for pediatric unstable forearm fractures. Clin Orthop Relat Res 2002;402:245–250.
99. Leininger BE, Rasmussen TE, Smith DL, et al. Experience with wound VAC and delayed primary closure of contaminated soft tissue injuries in Iraq. J Trauma 2006;61(5): 1207–1211.
100. Leinwand MJ, Atkinson CC, Mooney DP. Application of the APSA evidence-based guidelines for isolated liver or spleen injuries: a single institution experience. J Pediatr Surg 2004;39(3):487–490.
101. Letts M, Davidson D, Lapner P. Multiple trauma in children: predicting outcome and long-term results. Can J Surg 2002;45(2):126–131.
102. Letts M, Jarvis J, Lawton L, et al. Complications of rigid intramedullary rodding of femoral shaft fractures in children. J Trauma 2002;52(3):504–516.
103. Letts M, Vincent N, Gouw G. The "floating knee" in children. J Bone Joint Surg Br 1986;68(3):442–446.
104. Levin HS, High WM Jr, Ewing-Cobbs L, et al. Memory functioning during the first year after closed head injury in children and adolescents. Neurosurgery 1988;22(6 Pt 1):1043–1052.
105. Levy ML, Granville RC, Hart D, et al. Deep venous thrombosis in children and adolescents. J Neurosurg 2004;101(1 Suppl):32–37.
106. Limbird TJ, Ruderman RJ. Fat embolism in children. Clin Orthop Relat Res 1978;136: 267–269.
107. Loder RT. Pediatric polytrauma: orthopaedic care and hospital course. J Orthop Trauma 1987;1(1):48–54.
108. Loder RT, Gullahorn LJ, Yian EH, et al. Factors predictive of immobilization complications in pediatric polytrauma. J Orthop Trauma 2001;15(5):338–341.
109. Loder RT, O'Donnell PW, Feinberg JR. Epidemiology and mechanisms of femur fractures in children. J Pediatr Orthop 2006;26(5):561–566.
110. Luhmann SJ, Schootman M, Gordon JE, et al. Magnetic resonance imaging of the knee in children and adolescents. Its role in clinical decision-making. J Bone Joint Surg Am 2005;87(3):497–502.
111. Luhmann SJ, Schootman M, Schoenecker PL, et al. Complications and outcomes of open pediatric forearm fractures. J Pediatr Orthop 2004;24(1):1–6.
112. MacKenzie EJ, Morris JA Jr, de Lissovoy GV, et al. Acute hospital costs of pediatric trauma in the United States: how much and who pays? J Pediatr Surg 1990;25(9): 970–976.
113. Maio RF, Portnoy J, Blow FC, et al. Injury type, injury severity, and repeat occurrence of alcohol-related trauma in adolescents. Alcohol Clin Exp Res 1994;18(2):261–264.
114. Maksoud JG Jr, Moront ML, Eichelberger MR. Resuscitation of the injured child. Semin Pediatr Surg 1995;4(2):93–99.
115. Mandelstam SA, Cook D, Fitzgerald M, et al. Complementary use of radiological skeletal

survey and bone scintigraphy in detection of bony injuries in suspected child abuse. Arch Dis Child 2003;88(5):387–390.
116. McIntyre RC Jr, Bensard DD, Moore EE, et al. Pelvic fracture geometry predicts risk of life-threatening hemorrhage in children. J Trauma 1993;35(3):423–429.
117. Michaud LJ, Rivara FP, Grady MS, et al. Predictors of survival and severity of disability after severe brain injury in children. Neurosurgery 1992;31(2):254–264.
118. Mileski RA, Garvin KL, Crosby LA. Avascular necrosis of the femoral head in an adolescent following intramedullary nailing of the femur. A case report. J Bone Joint Surg Am 1994;76(11):1706–1708.
119. Mital MA, Garber JE, Stinson JT. Ectopic bone formation in children and adolescents with head injuries: its management. J Pediatr Orthop 1987;7(1):83–90.
120. Mooney JF 3rd, Argenta LC, Marks MW, et al. Treatment of soft tissue defects in pediatric patients using the V.A.C. system. Clin Orthop Relat Res 2000;376:26–31.
121. Musemeche CA, Fischer RP, Cotler HB, et al. Selective management of pediatric pelvic fractures: a conservative approach. J Pediatr Surg 1987;22(6):538–540.
122. Mutabagani KH, Coley BD, Zumberge N, et al. Preliminary experience with focused abdominal sonography for trauma (FAST) in children: is it useful? J Pediatr Surg 1999; 34(1):48–52,discussion 52–54.
123. Myers SH, Spiegel D, Flynn JM. External fixation of high-energy tibia fractures. J Pediatr Orthop 2007;27(5):537–539.
124. O'Malley DE, Mazur JM, Cummings RJ. Femoral head avascular necrosis associated with intramedullary nailing in an adolescent. J Pediatr Orthop 1995;15(1):21–23.
125. Onuora VC, Patil MG, al-Jasser AN. Missed urological injuries in children with polytrauma. Injury 1993;24(9):619–621.
126. Ott R, Kramer R, Martus P, et al. Prognostic value of trauma scores in pediatric patients with multiple injuries. J Trauma 2000;49(4):729–736.
127. Peclet MH, Newman KD, Eichelberger MR, et al. Patterns of injury in children. J Pediatr Surg 1990;25(1):85–90,discussion 90–91.
128. Peclet MH, Newman KD, Eichelberger MR, et al. Thoracic trauma in children: an indicator of increased mortality. J Pediatr Surg 1990;25(9):961–965,discussion 965–966.
129. Peterson DL, Schinco MA, Kerwin AJ, et al. Evaluation of initial base deficit as a prognosticator of outcome in the pediatric trauma population. Am Surg 2004;70(4): 326–328.
130. Philip PA, Philip M. Peripheral nerve injuries in children with traumatic brain injury. Brain Inj 1992;6(1):53–58.
131. Pison U, Seeger W, Buchhorn R, et al. Surfactant abnormalities in patients with respiratory failure after multiple trauma. Am Rev Respir Dis 1989;140(4):1033–1039.
132. Pitone ML, Attia MW. Patterns of injury associated with routine childhood falls. Pediatr Emerg Care 2006;22(7):470–474.
133. Podesta ML, Jordan GH. Pelvic fracture urethral injuries in girls. J Urol 2001;165(5): 1660–1665.
134. Poole GV, Miller JD, Agnew SG, et al. Lower-extremity fracture fixation in head-injured patients. J Trauma 1992;32(5):654–659.
135. Potoka DA, Schall LC, Gardner MJ, et al. Impact of pediatric trauma centers on mortality in a statewide system. J Trauma 2000;49(2):237–245.
136. Pressley JC, Trieu L, Kendig T, et al. National injury-related hospitalizations in children: public versus private expenditures across preventable injury mechanisms. J Trauma 2007;63(3 Suppl):S10–S19.
137. Reff RB. The use of external fixation devices in the management of severe lower-extremity trauma and pelvic injuries in children. Clin Orthop Relat Res 1984;188:21–33.
138. Richardson MC, Hollman AS, Davis CF. Comparison of computed tomography and ultrasonographic imaging in the assessment of blunt abdominal trauma in children. Br J Surg 1997;84(8):1144–1146.
139. Rinker B, Valerio IL, Stewart DH, et al. Microvascular free flap reconstruction in pediatric lower extremity trauma: a 10-year review. Plast Reconstr Surg 2005;115(6): 1618–1624.
140. Rivara FP. Pediatric injury control in 1999: where do we go from here? Pediatrics 1999;103(4 Pt 2):883–888.
141. Roaten JB, Partrick DA, Nydam TL, et al. Nonaccidental trauma is a major cause of morbidity and mortality among patients at a regional level 1 pediatric trauma center. J Pediatr Surg 2006;41(12):2013–2015.
142. Robinson CM. Current concepts of respiratory insufficiency syndromes after fracture. J Bone Joint Surg Br 2001;83(6):781–791.
143. Roche BG, Bugmann P, Le Coultre C. Blunt injuries to liver, spleen, kidney, and pancreas in pediatric patients. Eur J Pediatr Surg 1992;2(3):154–156.
144. Roposch A, Reis M, Molina M, et al. Supracondylar fractures of the humerus associated with ipsilateral forearm fractures in children: a report of 47 cases. J Pediatr Orthop 2001;21(3):307–312.
145. Rourke KF, McCammon KA, Sumfest JM, et al. Open reconstruction of pediatric and adolescent urethral strictures: long-term follow-up. J Urol 2003;169(5):1818–1821, discussion 1821.
146. Rozycki GS, Maull KI. Injuries sustained by falls. Arch Emerg Med 1991;8(4):245–252.
147. Sabharwal S, Zhao C, McClemens E, et al. Pediatric orthopaedic patients presenting to a university emergency department after visiting another emergency department: demographics and health insurance status. J Pediatr Orthop 2007;27(6):690–694.
148. Sanchez B, Waxman K, Jones T, et al. Cervical spine clearance in blunt trauma: evaluation of a computed tomography-based protocol. J Trauma 2005;59(1):179–183.
149. Sanchez JL, Lucas J, Feustel PJ. Outcome of adolescent trauma admitted to an adult surgical intensive care unit versus a pediatric intensive care unit. J Trauma 2001;51(3): 478–480.
150. Schafermeyer R. Pediatric trauma. Emerg Med Clin North Am 1993;11(1):187–205.
151. Schalamon J, v Bismarck S, Schober PH, et al. Multiple trauma in pediatric patients. Pediatr Surg Int 2003;19(6):417–423.
152. Schantz K, Rasmussen F. Calcaneus fracture in the child. Acta Orthop Scand 1987; 58(5):507–509.
153. Schmidt TL, Weiner DS. Calcaneal fractures in children. An evaluation of the nature of the injury in 56 children. Clin Orthop Relat Res 1982;171:150–155.
154. Schranz PJ, Gultekin C, Colton CL. External fixation of fractures in children. Injury 1992;23(2):80–82.
155. Senunas LE, Goulet JA, Greenfield ML, et al. Extracorporeal life support for patients with significant orthopaedic trauma. Clin Orthop Relat Res 1997;339:32–40.
156. Sharma OP, Oswanski MF, Stringfellow KC, et al. Pediatric blunt trauma: a retrospective analysis in a Level I trauma center. Am Surg 2006;72(6):538–543.
157. Signorino PR, Densmore J, Werner M, et al. Pediatric pelvic injury: functional outcome at 6-month follow-up. J Pediatr Surg 2005;40(1):107–112,discussion 112–113.
158. Silber JS, Flynn JM, Koffler KM, et al. Analysis of the cause, classification, and associated injuries of 166 consecutive pediatric pelvic fractures. J Pediatr Orthop 2001;21(4): 446–450.
159. Sindelar HA, Barnett NP, Spirito A. Adolescent alcohol use and injury. A summary and critical review of the literature. Minerva Pediatr 2004;56(3):291–309.
160. Sink EL, Hedequist D, Morgan SJ, et al. Results and technique of unstable pediatric femoral fractures treated with submuscular bridge plating. J Pediatr Orthop 2006; 26(2):177–181.
161. Sivit CJ, Taylor GA, Newman KD, et al. Safety-belt injuries in children with lap-belt ecchymosis: CT findings in 61 patients. AJR Am J Roentgenol 1991;157(1):111–114.
162. Skaggs DL, Kautz SM, Kay RM, et al. Effect of delay of surgical treatment on rate of infection in open fractures in children. J Pediatr Orthop 2000;20(1):19–22.
163. Skaggs DL, Leet AI, Money MD, et al. Secondary fractures associated with external fixation in pediatric femur fractures. J Pediatr Orthop 1999;19(5):582–586.
164. Smith JS Jr, Martin LF, Young WW, et al. Do trauma centers improve outcome over non-trauma centers: the evaluation of regional trauma care using discharge abstract data and patient management categories. J Trauma 1990;30(12):1533–1538.
165. Smith WR, Oakley M, Morgan SJ. Pediatric pelvic fractures. J Pediatr Orthop 2004; 24(1):130–135.
166. Sobus KM, Sherman N, Alexander MA. Coexistence of deep venous thrombosis and heterotopic ossification in the pediatric patient. Arch Phys Med Rehabil 1993;74(5): 547–551.
167. Soundappan SV, Holland AJ, Fahy F, et al. Transfer of pediatric trauma patients to a tertiary pediatric trauma centre: appropriateness and timeliness. J Trauma 2007;62(5): 1229–1233.
168. Spiguel L, Glynn L, Liu D, et al. Pediatric pelvic fractures: a marker for injury severity. Am Surg 2006;72(6):481–484.
169. Sullivan T, Haider A, DiRusso SM, et al. Prediction of mortality in pediatric trauma patients: new injury severity score outperforms injury severity score in the severely injured. J Trauma 2003;55(6):1083–1087,discussion 1087–1088.
170. Suthers SE, Albrecht R, Foley D, et al. Surgeon-directed ultrasound for trauma is a predictor of intra-abdominal injury in children. Am Surg 2004;70(2):164–167,discussion 167–168.
171. Swift EE, Taylor HG, Kaugars AS, et al. Sibling relationships and behavior after pediatric traumatic brain injury. J Dev Behav Pediatr 2003;24(1):24–31.
172. Tasker RC, Gupta S, White DK. Severe head injury in children: geographical range of an emergency neurosurgical practice. Emerg Med J 2004;21(4):433–437.
173. Tataria M, Nance ML, Holmes JHT, et al. Pediatric blunt abdominal injury: age is irrelevant and delayed operation is not detrimental. J Trauma 2007;63(3):608–614.
174. Teasdale G, Jennett B. Assessment of coma and impaired consciousness. A practical scale. Lancet 1974;2(7872):81–84.
175. Thompson EC, Perkowski P, Villarreal D, et al. Morbidity and mortality of children following motor vehicle crashes. Arch Surg 2003;138(2):142–145.
176. Tilden SJ, Watkins S, Tong TK, et al. Measured energy expenditure in pediatric intensive care patients. Am J Dis Child 1989;143(4):490–492.
177. Tolo VT. External skeletal fixation in children's fractures. J Pediatr Orthop 1983;3(4): 435–442.
178. Tolo VT. External fixation in multiply injured children. Orthop Clin North Am 1990; 21(2):393–400.
179. Tolo VT. Orthopaedic treatment of fractures of the long bones and pelvis in children who have multiple injuries. Instr Course Lect 2000;49:415–423.
180. Torode I, Zieg D. Pelvic fractures in children. J Pediatr Orthop 1985;5(1):76–84.
181. Townsend DR, Hoffinger S. Intramedullary nailing of femoral shaft fractures in children via the trochanter tip. Clin Orthop Relat Res 2000;376:113–118.
182. Trowbridge MJ, Sege RD, Olson L, et al. Intentional injury management and prevention in pediatric practice: results from 1998 and 2003 American Academy of Pediatrics Periodic Surveys. Pediatrics 2005;116(4):996–1000.
183. Truitt AK, Sorrells DL, Halvorson E, et al. Pulmonary embolism: which pediatric trauma patients are at risk? J Pediatr Surg 2005;40(1):124–127.
184. Tso EL, Beaver BL, Haller JA Jr. Abdominal injuries in restrained pediatric passengers. J Pediatr Surg 1993;28(7):915–919.
185. U.S. Department of Transportation NHTSA. Traffic safety facts 2002. DOT HS 809 620. 2004;1–202. Available at: http://www.nrd.nhtsa.dot.gov/Pubs/TSF2004.PDF. Accessed June 29,2009.
186. Uranus S, Pfeifer J. Nonoperative treatment of blunt splenic injury. World J Surg 2001; 25(11):1405–1407.
187. Vaca F, Anderson CL, Agran P, et al. Child safety seat knowledge among parents utilizing emergency services in a level I trauma center in Southern California. Pediatrics 2002;110(5):e61.
188. Valenziano CP, Chattar-Cora D, O'Neill A, et al. Efficacy of primary wound cultures in long bone open extremity fractures: are they of any value? Arch Orthop Trauma Surg 2002;122(5):259–261.
189. van der Sluis CK, Kingma J, Eisma WH, et al. Pediatric polytrauma: short-term and long-term outcomes. J Trauma 1997;43(3):501–506.
190. Vazquez WD, Garcia VF. Pediatric pelvic fractures combined with an additional skeletal injury is an indicator of significant injury. Surg Gynecol Obstet 1993;177(5):468–472.
191. Velmahos GC, Arroyo H, Ramicone E, et al. Timing of fracture fixation in blunt trauma patients with severe head injuries. Am J Surg 1998;176(4):324–329, discussion 329–330.
192. Verstreken L, Delronge G, Lamoureux J. Orthopaedic treatment of paediatric multiple trauma patients. A new technique. Int Surg 1988;73(3):177–179.
193. Vitale MG, Kessler MW, Choe JC, et al. Pelvic fractures in children: an exploration of practice patterns and patient outcomes. J Pediatr Orthop 2005;25(5):581–587.
194. Wang MY, Kim KA, Griffith PM, et al. Injuries from falls in the pediatric population: an analysis of 729 cases. J Pediatr Surg 2001;36(10):1528–1534.
195. Ward WT, Rihn JA. The impact of trauma in an urban pediatric orthopaedic practice. J Bone Joint Surg Am 2006;88(12):2759–2764.
196. Webb LX. New techniques in wound management: vacuum-assisted wound closure. J Am Acad Orthop Surg 2002;10(5):303–311.

197. Wesson DE, Spence LJ, Williams JI, et al. Injury scoring systems in children. Can J Surg 1987;30(6):398–400.
198. Wetzel RC, Burns RC. Multiple trauma in children: critical care overview. Crit Care Med 2002;30(11 Suppl):S468–S477.
199. Wilkins J, Patzakis M. Choice and duration of antibiotics in open fractures. Orthop Clin North Am 1991;22(3):433–437.
200. Williams RL, Connolly PT. In children undergoing chest radiography what is the specificity of rib fractures for nonaccidental injury? Arch Dis Child 2004;89(5):490–492.
201. Winogron HW, Knights RM, Bawden HN. Neuropsychological deficits following head injury in children. J Clin Neuropsychol 1984;6(3):267–286.
202. Woolf PD, McDonald JV, Feliciano DV, et al. The catecholamine response to multisystem trauma. Arch Surg 1992;127(8):899–903.
203. Wyrsch B, Mencio GA, Green NE. Open reduction and internal fixation of pediatric forearm fractures. J Pediatr Orthop 1996;16(5):644–650.
204. Yian EH, Gullahorn LJ, Loder RT. Scoring of pediatric orthopaedic polytrauma: correlations of different injury scoring systems and prognosis for hospital course. J Pediatr Orthop 2000;20(2):203–209.
205. Yuan PS, Pring ME, Gaynor TP, et al. Compartment syndrome following intramedullary fixation of pediatric forearm fractures. J Pediatr Orthop 2004;24(4):370–375.
206. Yue JJ, Churchill RS, Cooperman DR, et al. The floating knee in the pediatric patient. Nonoperative versus operative stabilization. Clin Orthop 2000;376:124–136.
207. Zhao XG, Zhao GF, Ma YF, et al. Research progress in mechanism of traumatic brain injury affecting speed of fracture healing. Chin J Traumatol 2007;10(6):376–380.
208. Zuckerbraun BS, Morrison K, Gaines B, et al. Effect of age on cervical spine injuries in children after motor vehicle collisions: effectiveness of restraint devices. J Pediatr Surg 2004;39(3):483–486.

5

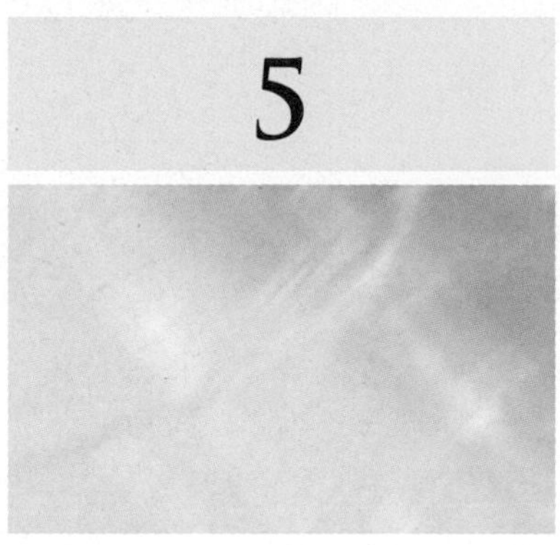

PHYSEAL INJURIES AND GROWTH DISTURBANCES

Karl E. Rathjen and John G. Birch

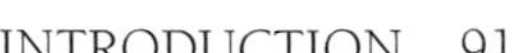

INTRODUCTION 91

PHYSEAL ANATOMY 91
Normal Physeal Anatomy 91
Mechanical Features of the Physis and Patterns of Injury 92
Contributions to Longitudinal Growth and Maturation Characteristics of Selected Physes 94

PHYSEAL INJURIES 94
Etiology of Physeal Injuries 94
Historical Review of Physeal Fractures 97
Classification of Physeal Fractures 97
Epidemiology of Physeal Fractures 105
Evaluation of Physeal Fractures 105
Treatment 106
Complications of Physeal Fractures 107

PHYSEAL GROWTH DISTURBANCE 108
Etiology 108
Evaluation 108
Physeal Arrests 110
Physeal Arrest Resection 111
Preoperative Planning and Surgical Principles 112
Growth Disturbance without Arrest 115

SUMMARY 117

INTRODUCTION

One of the unique aspects of pediatric orthopaedics is the presence of the physis (or growth plate), which provides longitudinal growth of children's long bones. Physeal injuries are a common and unique feature of children's bony injuries, in part because the physis is structurally more susceptible to loads that would produce metaphyseal or juxta-articular fractures in adults.[13,26,59,76,102,106,122,124,129] Physeal injury may occur in a variety of ways in addition to trauma.[12,13,17,21,24,30,36,49,61,73,81,83,111,115,123,135,138,140] Although physes, similar to the children with them, are resilient to permanent injury, uneventful outcomes are by no means assured.[1,8,15,18,23,28,57,71,86,94,96,100,103,110,121,130] In this discussion of management of physeal injuries and associated growth disturbances the term *epiphysis* is used to refer to the bulbous end of a long bone incorporating the "growth plate" or "physis" and the secondary ossification center, and the term *physis* is used rather than "growth plate."

PHYSEAL ANATOMY

Normal Physeal Anatomy

Gross

Five regions characterize long bones: the bulbous, articular cartilage-covered ends (epiphyses) tapering to the funnel-shaped metaphyses, with the central diaphysis interposed between the metaphyses. During growth, the epiphyseal and metaphyseal regions are separated by the organized cartilaginous physis, which is the major contributor to longitudinal growth of the bone. The larger long bones (clavicle, humerus, radius, ulna, femur, tibia, and fibula) have physes at both ends, whereas the smaller tubular bones (metacarpals, metatarsals, and phalanges) usually have a physis at one end only.

At birth, with the exception of the distal femur and occasionally the proximal tibia, all of the above-mentioned epiphyses are purely cartilaginous. At various stages of postnatal growth and development, a secondary ossification center forms within

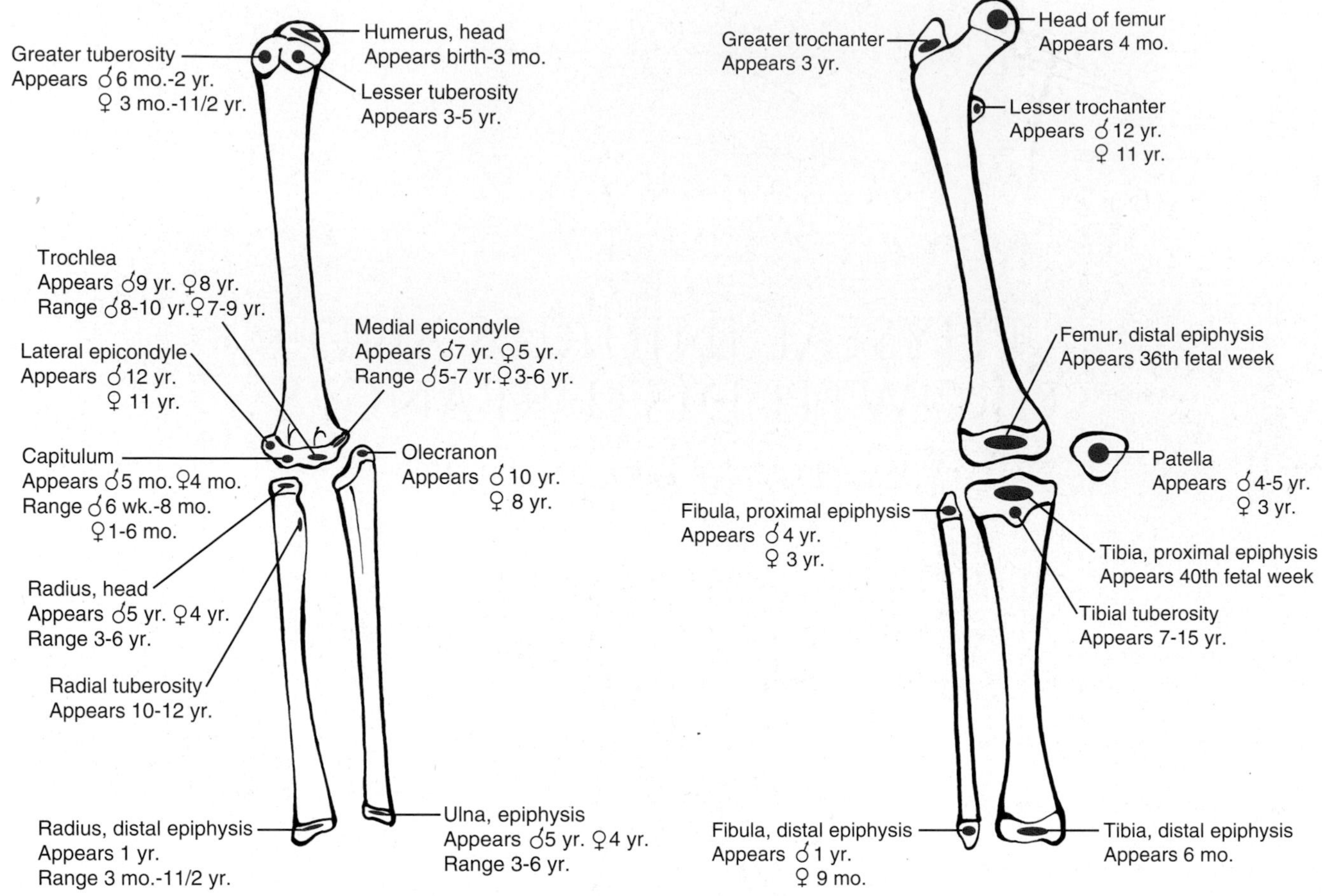

Figure 5-1 Typical age (and range) of development of the secondary ossification centers of the epiphyses in the **(A)** upper extremity and **(B)** lower extremity.

the epiphysis. This development helps define the radiolucent zone of the physis, which persists until the physis closes at skeletal maturation. Typical ages for appearance of the major secondary ossification centers and physeal closure are summarized in Figures 5-1 and 5-2.

Microscopic

The microscopic architecture of the physis is highly organized and germane to an understanding of physeal injuries.[122] Traditionally, the physis is divided into four zones from the center of the epiphysis to the metaphysis: germinal, proliferative, hypertrophic, and provisional calcification (or enchondral ossification) (Fig. 5-3). The germinal and proliferative zones are the location of cellular proliferation, whereas the hypertrophic and provisional calcification zones are characterized by matrix production, cellular hypertrophy, apoptosis, and matrix calcification. Normal longitudinal growth is dependent on the interaction of many factors, both hormonal and mechanical.

The peripheral margin of the physis comprises two specialized areas important to the mechanical integrity and peripheral growth of the physis (see Fig. 5-3). The zone (or groove) of Ranvier is a triangular microscopic structure at the periphery of the physis, containing fibroblasts, chondroblasts, and osteoblasts. It is responsible for peripheral growth of the physis. The perichondral ring of LaCroix is a fibrous structure overlying the zone of Ranvier, connecting the metaphyseal periosteum and cartilaginous epiphysis, and has the important mechanical function of stabilizing the epiphysis to the metaphysis.

The epiphysis and secondary ossific nucleus must receive blood supply for viability.[139] Dale and Harris[43] identified two types of blood supply to the epiphysis (Fig. 5-4). Type A epiphyses (such as the proximal humeral and proximal femoral epiphyses) are nearly completely covered with articular cartilage; therefore, most of the blood supply must enter from the perichondrium. The blood supply to these epiphyses may be easily compromised by epiphyseal separation. Type B epiphyses (such as the proximal and distal tibia and the distal radius) have only a portion of their surface covered with articular cartilage and are theoretically less susceptible to devascularization from epiphyseal separation.

Mechanical Features of the Physis and Patterns of Injury

An understanding of the microscopic characteristics of the physeal zones permits an understanding of the theoretical line of least resistance (and hence fracture) within the physis. The germinal and proliferative zones are characterized by an abundance of extracellular matrix, whereas the hypertrophic and enchondral ossification zones are primarily apoptotic cells and vascular channels. As a consequence, fracture lines can be predicted to pass through the hypertrophic and enchondral ossification zones, a finding that Salter and Harris reported in their experimental investigation in rats.[125] Theoretically, Salter-Harris types I and II fractures should involve these zones only, not affecting

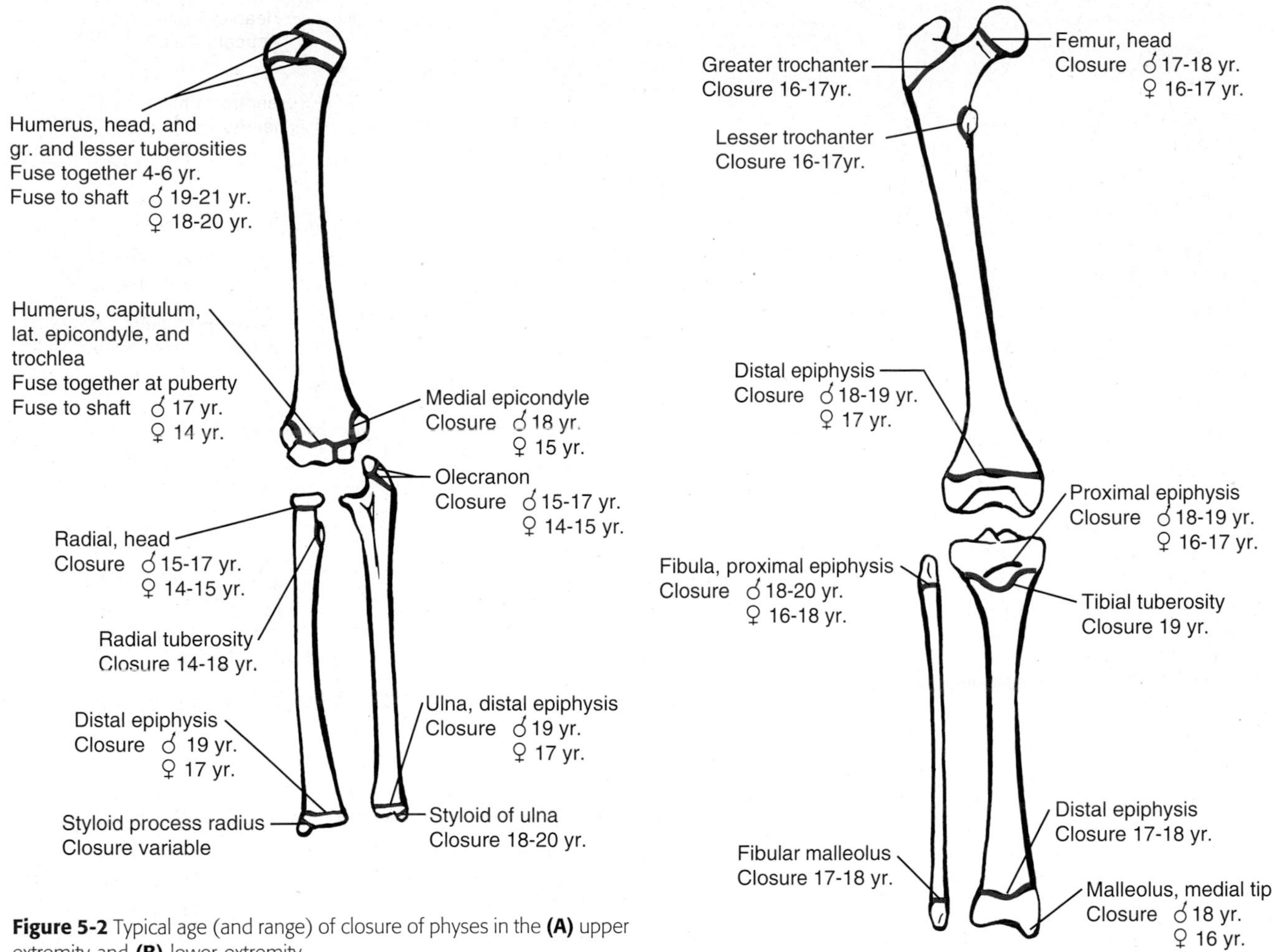

Figure 5-2 Typical age (and range) of closure of physes in the **(A)** upper extremity and **(B)** lower extremity.

Figure 5-3 Schematic diagram of the organization of the physis. Four zones are illustrated: the germinal, proliferative, hypertrophic, and provisional calcification (or enchondral ossification) layers. Note also the groove of Ranvier and the perichondral ring of LaCroix.

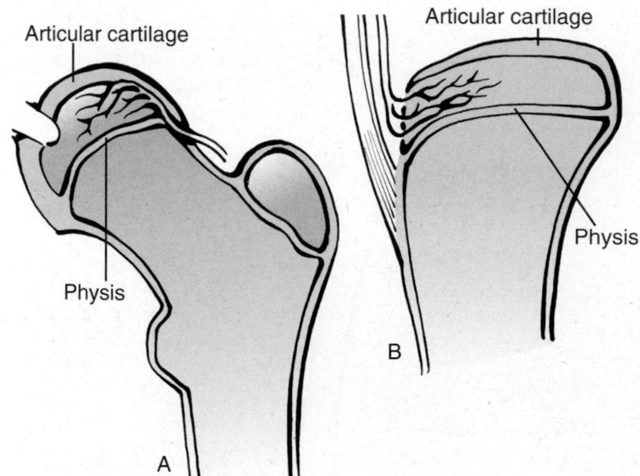

Figure 5-4 Classification of epiphyseal blood supply according to Dale and Harris. **A.** Type A epiphyses are nearly completely covered by articular cartilage. Blood supply must enter via the perichondrium. This blood supply is susceptible to disruption by epiphyseal separation. The proximal femur and proximal humerus are examples of type A epiphyses. **B.** Type B epiphyses are only partially covered by articular cartilage. Such epiphyses are more resistant to blood supply impairment by epiphyseal separation. The distal femur, proximal and distal tibia, and distal radius are clinical examples of type B epiphyses.

the germinal and proliferative zones, and thus should be at lower risk for subsequent growth disturbance. However, types III and IV physeal fractures traverse the entire physis, including the germinal and proliferative zones. In addition, displacement between bone fragments containing portions of the physis may occur. Consequently, growth disturbance is more likely from type III or IV injuries.

Not surprisingly, mechanical and clinical studies of microscopic fracture patterns have demonstrated that fracture lines through the physeal layers are more complex than this simplistic view, and often undulate through the various zones.[26,59,75,102,134,142] Smith et al.[134] reported a Salter-Harris type I fracture of the distal tibia examined microscopically after associated traumatic lower leg amputation. In this high-energy injury, they found that the fracture line involved all four layers of the physis, in part because of the relatively straight plane of fracture and the undulations of the physis. Bright et al.,[26] in a study of experimentally induced physeal fractures in immature rats, found that not only was the fracture line usually complex, involving all four layers of the physis, but also that the physis contained a number of horizontal "cracks" separate from the fracture itself. They also observed a statistically significant lower force required to produce a physeal fracture in male and prepubescent animals, which might have clinical relevance to the epidemiologic aspects of physeal fractures (see "Epidemiology"). The rate, direction, and magnitude of force are also factors that contribute to the histologic pattern of physeal fractures. Moen and Pelker,[102] in an experimental study in calves, found that compression forces produced fractures in the zone of provisional calcification and metaphysis, shear caused fractures in the proliferative and hypertrophic zones, and torque produced fracture lines involving all four layers of the physis. Finally, the energy of injury is a factor in the extent of physeal injury. Distal femoral physeal fractures are a good example of the overriding significance of the energy of injury in potential for subsequent growth disturbance. High-energy mechanisms of injury are frequent in this region, and the risk of subsequent growth disturbance is high.[121,91]

Contributions to Longitudinal Growth and Maturation Characteristics of Selected Physes

Growth of long bones is more complex than simple elongation occurring at their ends. However, as a generality, the physes at the end of long bones contribute known average lengths in percentage of total bone growth and percentage contributions to the total length between two physes at either end of a long bone. This information has come from observations of longitudinal growth by a number of authors.[9–11,60,67,93] Knowledge of this information is paramount for the surgeon managing physeal injuries to long bones. Figure 5-5 outlines the generally accepted percentage of longitudinal growth contribution of pairs of physes for each long bone in the upper and lower extremities. Table 5-1 outlines the average amount of growth in millimeters per year of skeletal growth contributed by these same physes. These are estimations only, and growth tables should be consulted when more specific information is required.[10,11,60,67,93]

PHYSEAL INJURIES

Etiology of Physeal Injuries

Physes can be injured in many ways, both obvious and subtle. Obviously, the most frequent mechanism of injury is fracture. Most commonly, fracture injury is direct, with the fracture pattern involving the physis itself. Occasionally, physeal injury from trauma is indirect and associated with a fracture elsewhere in the limb segment, either as a result of ischemia[115] or perhaps compression[1,8,23,71,97,103,141] (see discussion of Salter-Harris type V physeal fractures below). Other mechanisms of injuries to the physes include infection,[17,21,83,111] disruption by tumor, cysts,[135] and tumor-like disorders, vascular insult,[115] repetitive stress,[7,24,37,38,90,146] irradiation,[32,123] and other rare etiologies.[16,30,36,126]

Infection

Long bone osteomyelitis or septic arthritis (particularly of the shoulder, hip, and knee) can cause physeal damage resulting in either physeal growth disturbance or frank growth arrest.[12,17,21,49,61,73,81,83,111] These septic injuries may be further complicated by joint disruption resulting from associated epiphyseal destruction, articular cartilage damage, and capsular adhesions, particularly in the hip and shoulder.

Multifocal septic arrests can produce significant deformity requiring multiple surgical procedures. The most common causes are fulminant neonatal sepsis, particularly in premature infants or those with neonatal sepsis associated with maternal diabetes, and multiple septic arrests associated with meningococcemia (Fig. 5-6). In the latter case, physeal damage may also result from the cardiovascular collapse and disseminated intravascular coagulation known as purpura fulminans.[12,61,73,81]

Tumor

Both malignant and benign tumors and tumor-like disorders can disrupt normal physeal architecture, resulting in direct physeal destruction. In the case of malignant tumors, the extent of growth lost as the result of local irradiation or limb salvage

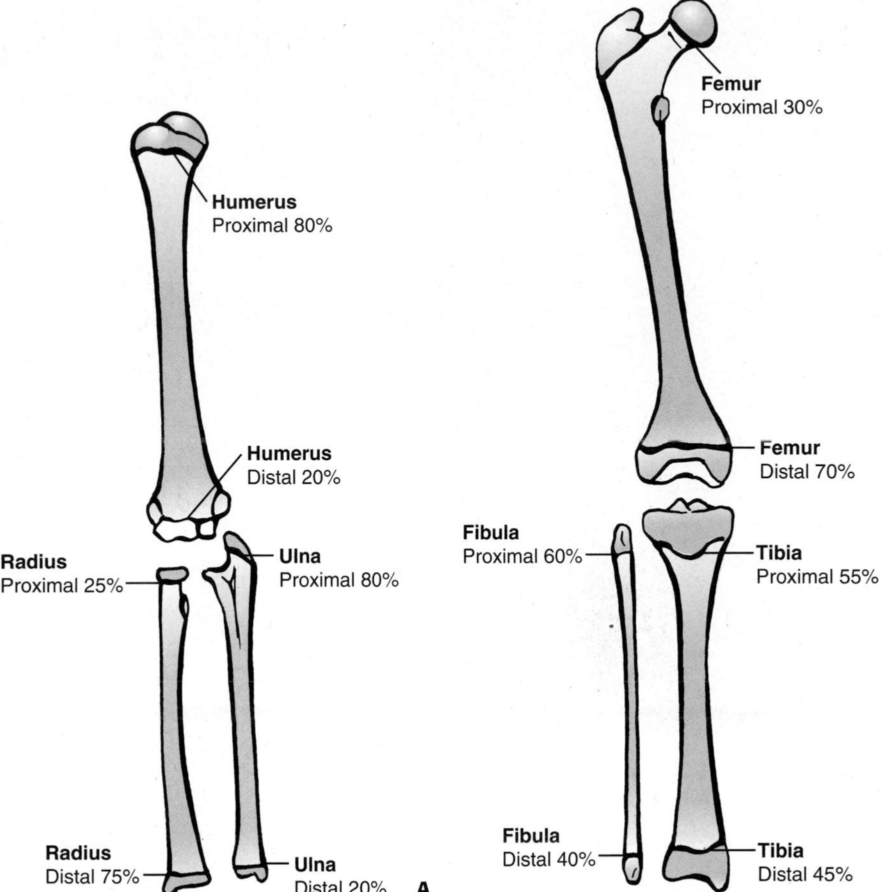

Figure 5-5 Approximate percentage of longitudinal growth provided by the proximal and distal physes for each long bone in the upper **(A)** and lower **(B)** extremities.

TABLE 5-1 Average Growth Per Year (in millimeters) of Specific Physes of the Upper and Lower Extremities*

Location	Average Growth (mm/yr)
Proximal humerus	7
Distal humerus	2
Proximal radius	1.75
Distal radius	5.25
Proximal ulna	5.5
Distal ulna	1.5
Proximal femur	3.5
Distal femur	9
Proximal tibia	6
Distal tibia	5
Proximal fibula	6.5
Distal fibula	4.5

*Estimations only. Gender, skeletal age, percentile height, and epiphyseal growth all influence magnitude of individual bone growth. Growth tables should be consulted when specific calculations are required.
Adapted from growth studies.[1–9]

surgery must be taken into consideration in planning and recommending the therapeutic reconstruction to be undertaken.

Benign tumors and tumor-like conditions can result in destruction of all or part of a physis. Examples include enchondromata, either isolated or multiple (Ollier disease) (Fig. 5-7), and unicameral bone cysts.[135] Growth disturbance as a consequence of physeal damage from these disorders generally cannot be corrected by surgical physeal arrest resection (see "Physeal Arrests"), and other treatment strategies must be adopted as clinically indicated.

Vascular Insult

Known vascular insult is a rare cause of physeal injury.[115] Partial or complete growth arrests can occur from a pure vascular injury to an extremity (Fig. 5-8). Unrecognized vascular insult may represent the mechanism of subsequent growth disturbance after an injury in an adjacent part of a limb and may represent Salter-Harris type V injuries; the most common location for this is the tibial tubercle after femoral shaft or distal femoral physeal fractures. In addition, ischemia may be the cause of physeal damage associated with purpura fulminans.[12,61,73,81]

Repetitive Stress

Repetitious physical activities in skeletally immature individuals can result in physeal stress-fracture equivalents.[7,37,38] The most common location for such injuries are in the distal radius or ulna, as seen in competitive gymnasts (Fig. 5-9); the proximal tibia, as in running and kicking sports such as soccer (Fig.

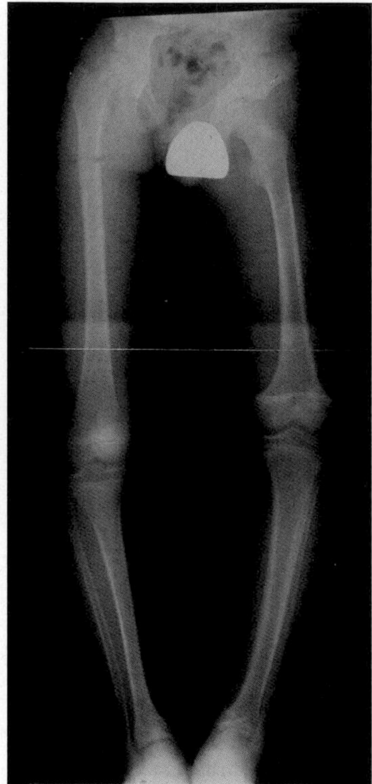

Figure 5-6 Standing anteroposterior lower extremity radiograph of a 12-year-old boy with multifocal physeal disturbance from purpura fulminans associated with meningococcemia. Radiograph abnormalities are present in the left proximal femur; both distal femoral epiphyses, including partial arrest of the left distal femoral physis; and both distal tibial epiphyses. The patient also has digital amputations and extensive soft-tissue scarring resulting from this septic event.

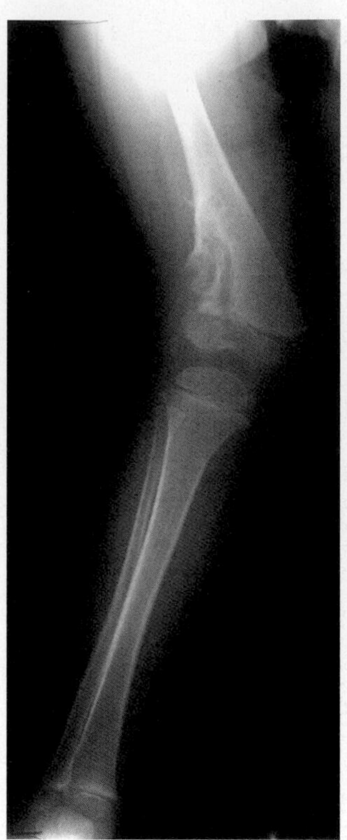

Figure 5-7 Valgus deformity of the distal femur associated with the presence of an enchondroma of the distal lateral femur involving the lateral physis.

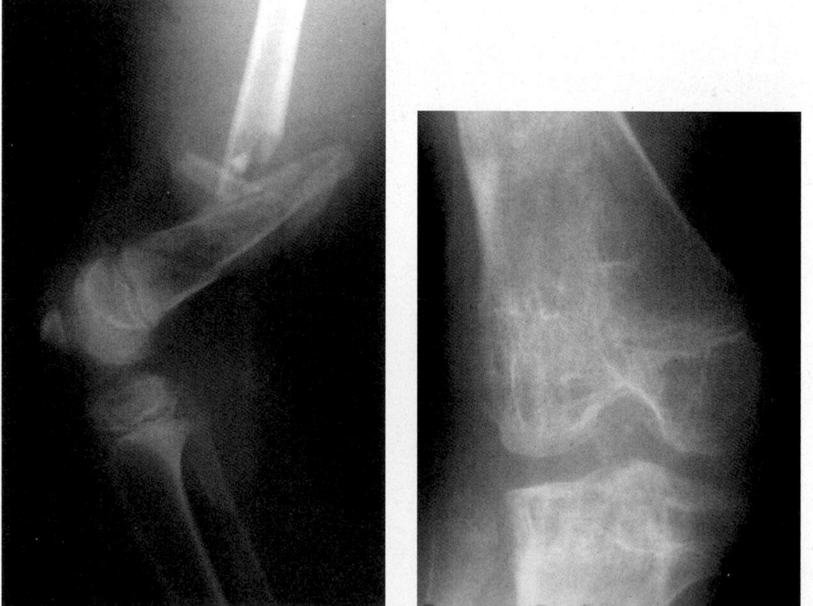

Figure 5-8 Physeal injury from presumed vascular insult. **A.** The patient's leg was caught under heavy pipes rolling off a rack, resulting in stripping of the soft tissues from the distal thigh, open comminuted fracture of the distal femur, and popliteal artery injury. **B.** In follow-up, after arterial and soft tissue reconstruction, the patient has physeal growth arrests of the distal femur and proximal tibia. The mechanism of injury to the proximal tibial physis was presumed to be vascular because of the associated femoral artery injury.

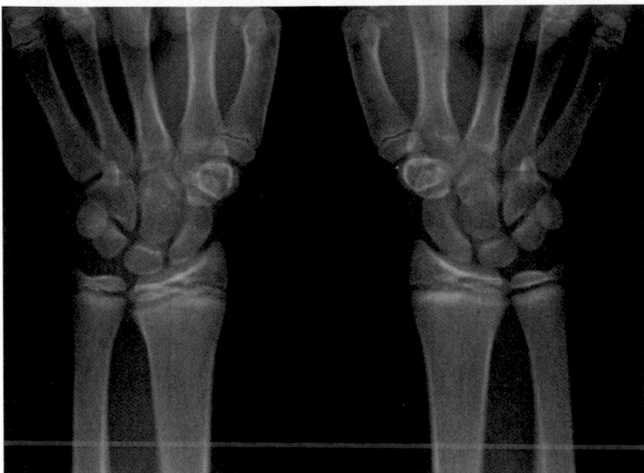

Figure 5-9 Stress injury of the distal radius and ulna in both wrists of a competitive gymnast. There was no history of specific injury. The wrists were tender to touch. Note distal radial and ulnar physeal widening and irregularity.

5-10); and the proximal humerus, as in baseball pitchers.[37] These injuries should be managed by rest, judicious resumption of activities, and longitudinal observation to monitor for potential physeal growth disturbance.

Miscellaneous (Irradiation, Thermal Injury, Electrical, Unrecognized)

Rare causes of physeal injury, usually recognized from consequent growth disturbance, include irradiation (Fig. 5-11)[32,123]; thermal injury, especially phalangeal physeal injury from frostbite (Fig. 5-12)[30,36]; burns; and electrical injuries. On rare occasions, physeal growth disturbance noted on clinical findings and radiographs has no identifiable cause. Presumably, such events represent unrecognized trauma or infection involving the physis.

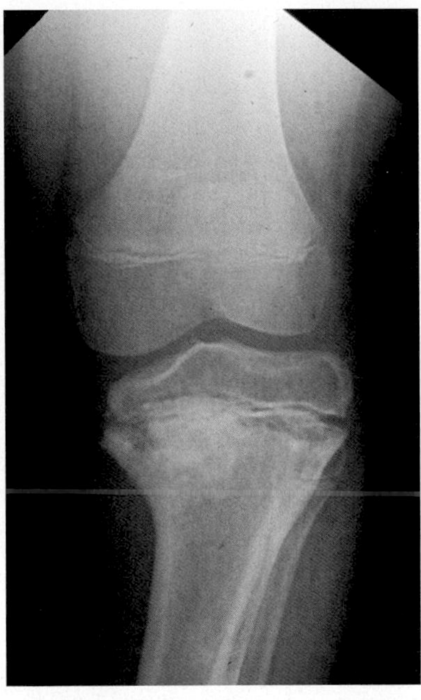

Figure 5-11 Proximal tibial physeal growth disturbance with angular deformity after irradiation for Ewing sarcoma.

Historical Review of Physeal Fractures

Physeal fractures have been recognized as unique since ancient times. Hippocrates is credited with the first written account of this injury. Poland (see "Classification of Physeal Fractures") reviewed accounts of physeal injuries in his 1898 book, *Traumatic Separation of the Epiphysis*.[119] Poland is also credited with the first classification of the patterns of physeal fracture, and the publication of his text closely followed Roentgen's discovery of radiographs in 1895.

Classification of Physeal Fractures

Poland[119] proposed the first classification of physeal fractures in 1898. Modifications to Poland's original scheme have been pro-

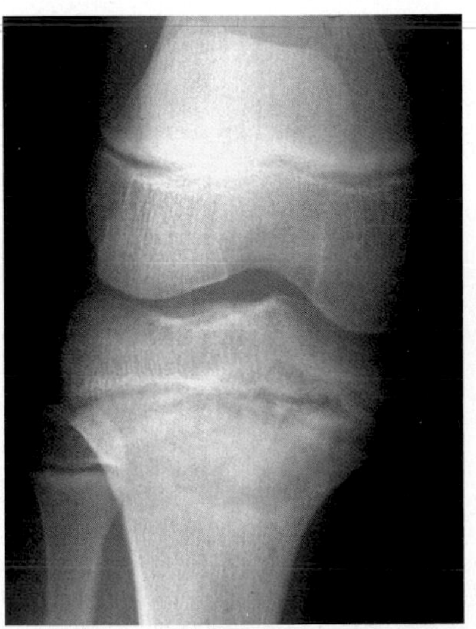

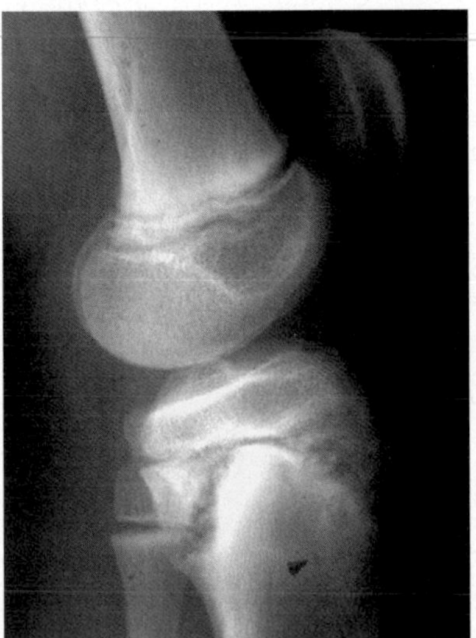

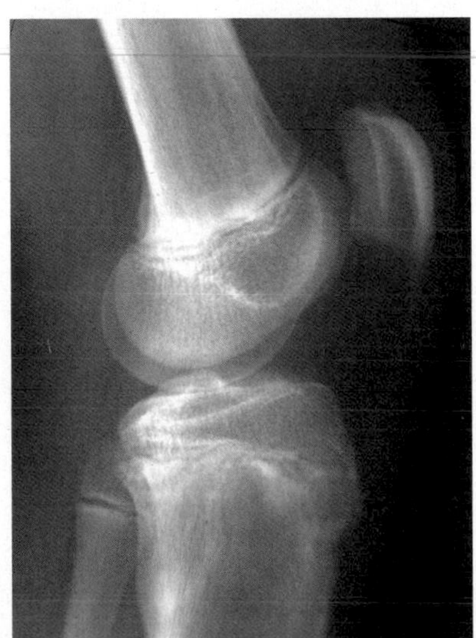

Figure 5-10 Stress injury of the proximal tibia in an elite soccer player. **A.** Anteroposterior radiograph film demonstrates subtle proximal tibial physeal widening. **B.** Lateral radiograph shows widening, a metaphyseal Thurston-Holland fragment, and some posterior displacement of the proximal epiphysis. **C.** Significant radiograph improvement noted after discontinuing athletic activities for 3 months.

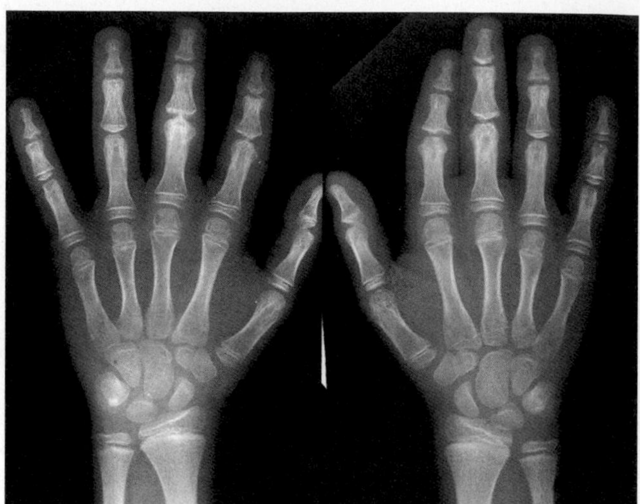

Figure 5-12 Premature closure of the distal phalangeal physes after a frostbite injury to the digits.

posed by a number of authors,[2–5,43,46,92,106,107,113,114,118,125] including Aitken,[4] Salter and Harris,[125] Ogden et al.,[107] and Peterson.[113,114] Classifications of physeal fractures are important because they alert the practitioner to potentially subtle radiographic fracture patterns, can be of prognostic significance with respect to growth disturbance potential, and guide general treatment principles based on that risk and associated joint disruption. To some extent, fracture pattern provides some insight into mechanism of injury and the extent of potential physeal microscopic injury ("Normal Physeal Anatomy" and "Mechanical Features of the Physis and Patterns of Injury").

Currently, the Salter-Harris classification, first published in 1963,[125] is firmly entrenched in the literature and most orthopaedists' minds. Therefore, evolution and specifics of the nature of physeal fractures of the various classification schemes are discussed relative to the Salter-Harris classification. The reader also should be aware of some deficiencies in that classification, as pointed out by Peterson.[113,114,116]

Poland Classification of Physeal Fractures

Poland's classification, published in 1898,[119] consisted of four types of physeal fractures (Fig. 5-13). Types I, II, and III were the foundation of the Salter-Harris classification, as described below. Poland's type IV fracture was effectively a T-condylar fracture of the epiphysis and physis.

Aitken Classification of Physeal Fractures

Aitken in 1936[4] included three patterns of physeal fracture in his classification (Fig. 5-14). His type I corresponded to Poland and Salter-Harris type II fractures, his type II to Poland and Salter-Harris type III fractures, and his type III was an intra-articular transphyseal metaphyseal-epiphyseal fracture equivalent to a Salter-Harris type IV fracture.

Salter-Harris Classification of Physeal Fractures

Salter and Harris published their commonly used five-part classification of physeal injuries in 1963.[125] The first four types were adopted from Poland (types I, II, and III) and Aitken (Aitken type III became Salter-Harris type IV) (Fig. 5-15). Salter and Harris added a fifth type, which they postulated was an unrecognized compression injury characterized by normal radiographs and late physeal closure. Peterson challenged the existence of true type V injuries,[116] but other authors have subsequently documented its existence in some form.[1,8,15,23,70,71,80,141,116] Because we believe that delayed physeal closure can occur after some occult injuries, we have chosen to retain this type of injury in our preferred classification scheme.

Type I. Salter-Harris type I injuries are characterized by a transphyseal plane of injury, with no bony fracture line through either the metaphysis or the epiphysis. Radiographs of undisplaced type I physeal fractures, therefore, are normal except for associated soft tissue swelling, making careful patient examination particularly important in this injury. In the Olmstead County Survey of physeal fractures,[117] type I fractures occurred most frequently in the phalanges, metacarpals, distal tibia, and distal ulna. Epiphyseal separations in infants occur most commonly in the proximal humerus, distal humerus, and proximal femur. If an urgency to make the diagnosis is deemed necessary for patients suspected of having a type I injury, further imaging by ultrasound, magnetic resonance imaging (MRI),[34,41,74,118,133] or arthrography may be helpful.[6,63,95,145] Stress radiographs to document displacement are generally unnecessary and probably unwise. Ultrasound is particularly helpful for assessing epiphyseal separations in infants (especially in the proximal femur and elbow regions) without the need for sedation, anesthetic, or invasive procedure.[29,45,47,69,128]

The fracture line of type I injuries is usually in the zone of hypertrophy of the physis, as the path of least resistance during the propagation of the injury (see "Normal Physeal Anatomy") (Fig. 5-16). As a consequence, in theory, the essential resting and proliferative zones are relatively spared, and, assuming that there is no vascular insult to these zones as a consequence of the injury, subsequent growth disturbance is relatively uncommon. As discussed above, however, studies have shown this to be a simplistic view of the fracture line through a physis, and that, due to uneven loading and macroscopic undulations in

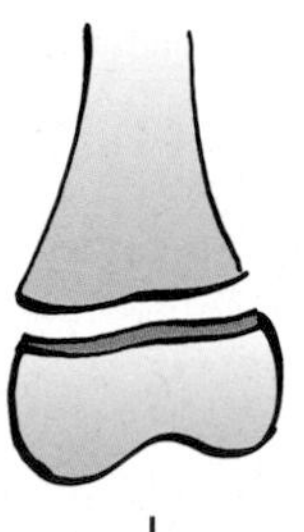

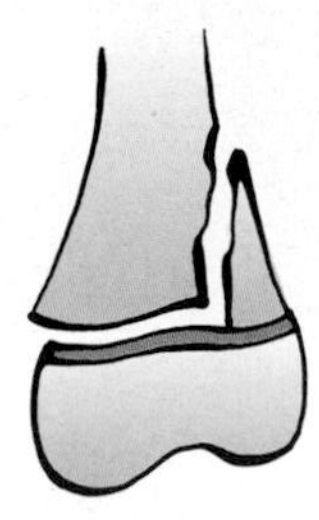

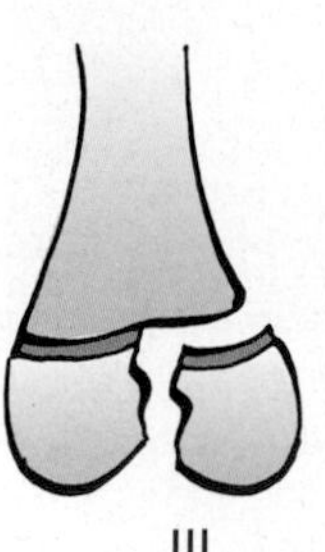

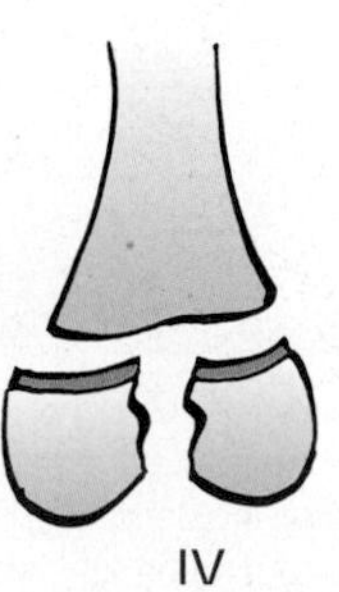

Figure 5-13 Poland classification of physeal fractures. Compare to the Salter-Harris classification. Poland type I: epiphyseal separation without metaphyseal fragment, or extension into the epiphysis. Poland type II: physeal fracture line extends into the metaphysis. Poland type III: fracture extends from the articular surface to the physis and continues peripherally through the physis. Poland type IV: T-condylar fracture of the epiphysis and physis.

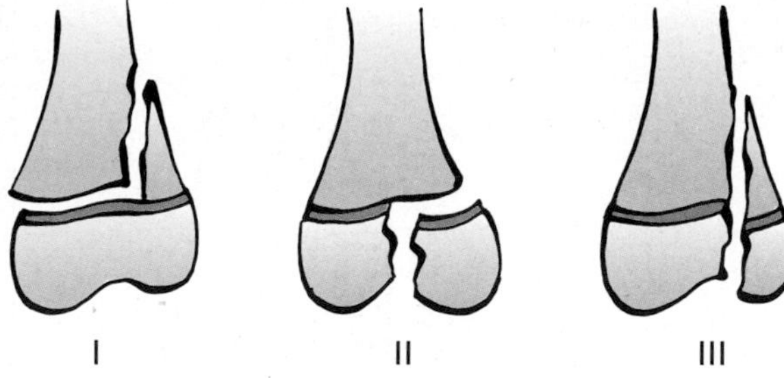

Figure 5-14 Aitken classification of physeal fractures: types I, II, and III. Type III is equivalent of Salter-Harris type IV.

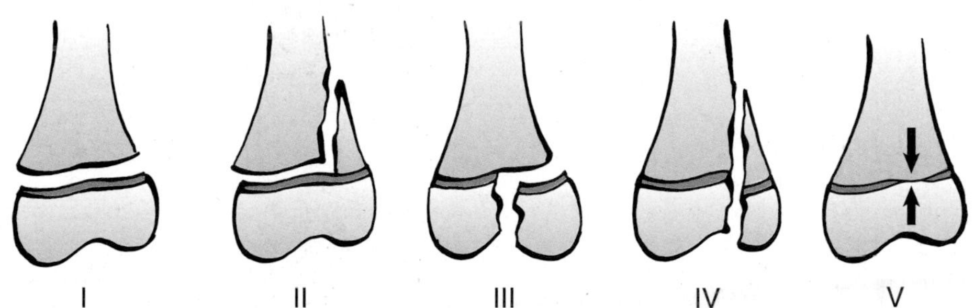

Figure 5-15 Salter-Harris classification of physeal fractures. In Salter-Harris type I fractures, the fracture line is entirely within the physis, referred to by Poland as type I. In Salter-Harris type II fractures, the fracture line extends from the physis into the metaphysis; described by Poland as type II and Aitken as type I. In Salter-Harris type III fractures, the fracture enters the epiphysis from the physis and almost always exits the articular surface. Poland described this injury as type III and Aitken as type II. In Salter-Harris type IV, the fracture extends across the physis from the articular surface and epiphysis, to exit in the margin of the metaphysis. Aitken described this as a type III injury in his classification. Salter-Harris type V fractures were described by Salter and Harris as a crush injury to the physis with initially normal radiographs with late identification of premature physeal closure.

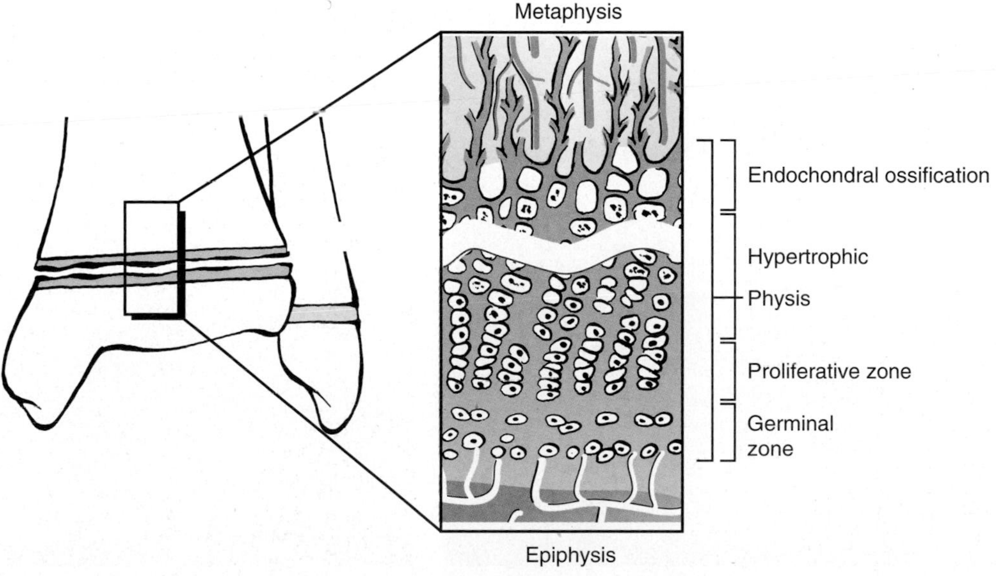

Figure 5-16 Scheme of theoretic fracture plane of Salter-Harris type I fractures. Because the hypertrophic zone is the weakest zone structurally, separation should occur at this level. Experimental and clinical studies have confirmed that the fracture plane is more complex than this concept and frequently involves other physeal zones as well.

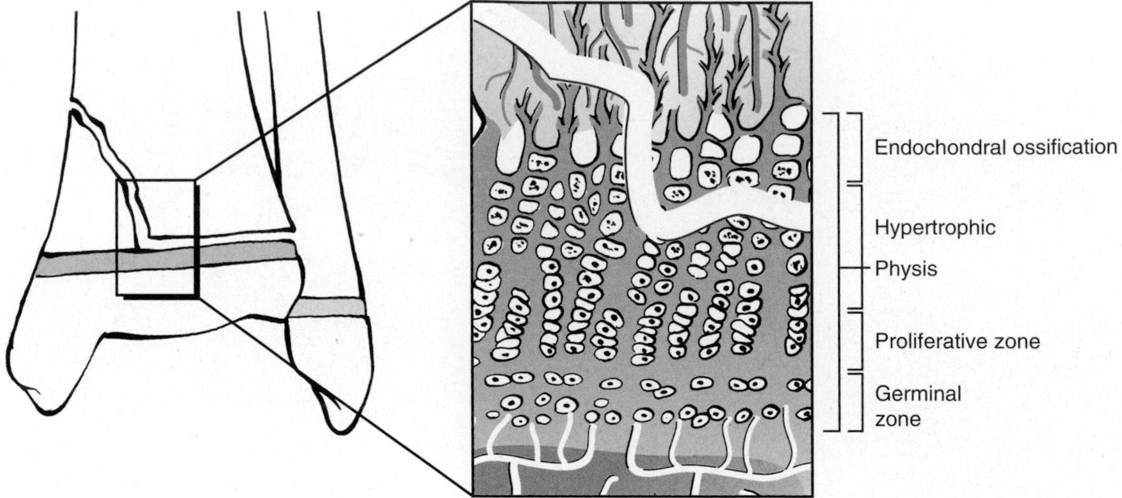

Figure 5-17 Fracture plane of Salter-Harris type II fractures. The fracture extends from the physis into the periphery of the metaphysis.

the physis, any zone of the physis can be affected by the fracture line.[26,75,102,124,129,134]

Because the articular surface and, at least in theory, the germinal and proliferative layers of the physis are not displaced, the general principles of fracture management are to secure a gentle and adequate reduction of the epiphysis on the metaphysis and stabilize the fragments as needed.

Type II. Type II injuries have physeal and metaphyseal components; the fracture line extends from the physeal margin peripherally across a variable portion of the physis and exits into the metaphysis at the opposite end of the fracture (Fig. 5-17). The epiphyseal fragment thus comprises all of the epiphysis and some portion of the peripheral metaphysis (the Thurston-Holland fragment or sign). The physeal portion of this fracture has microscopic characteristics similar to those of type I injuries, but the fracture line exits the physis to enter the metaphysis (i.e., away from the germinal and proliferative layers) at one margin. Similar to type I injuries, these fractures should have a limited propensity to subsequent growth disturbance as a consequence of direct physeal injury. However, the metaphyseal "spike" of the diaphyseal/metaphyseal fragment may be driven into the physis of the epiphyseal fragment, which can damage the physis (Fig. 5-18). Similar to type I injuries, the articular surface is not affected and the general principles of fracture management are effectively the same.

Type III. Salter-Harris type III fractures begin in the epiphysis (with only rare exception) as a fracture through the articular surface and extend vertically toward the physis. The fracture

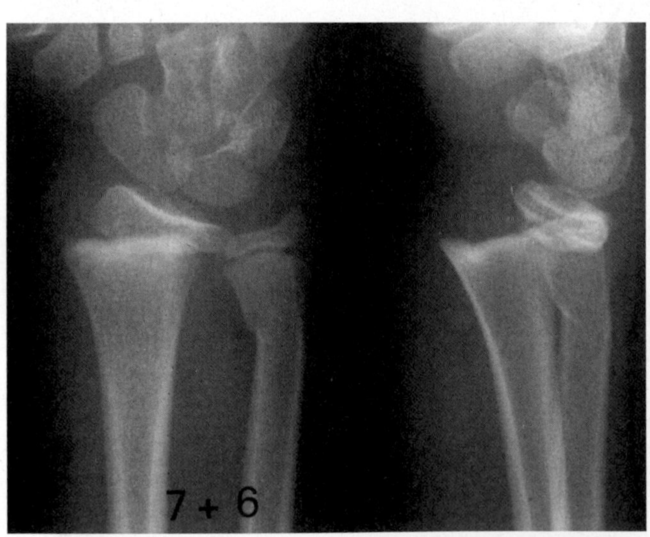

A

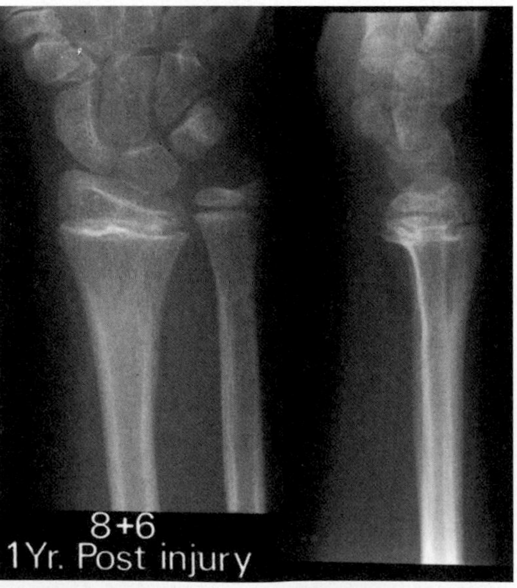

B

Figure 5-18 Potential mechanism of physeal arrest development after Salter-Harris type II fracture of the distal radius. **A.** Dorsally displaced type II fracture of the distal radius. Note the evidence of impaction of the epiphyseal fragment (with the physis) by the dorsal margin of the proximal fragment metaphysis. **B.** One year later, there is radiographic evidence of physeal arrest formation in the distal radial physis.

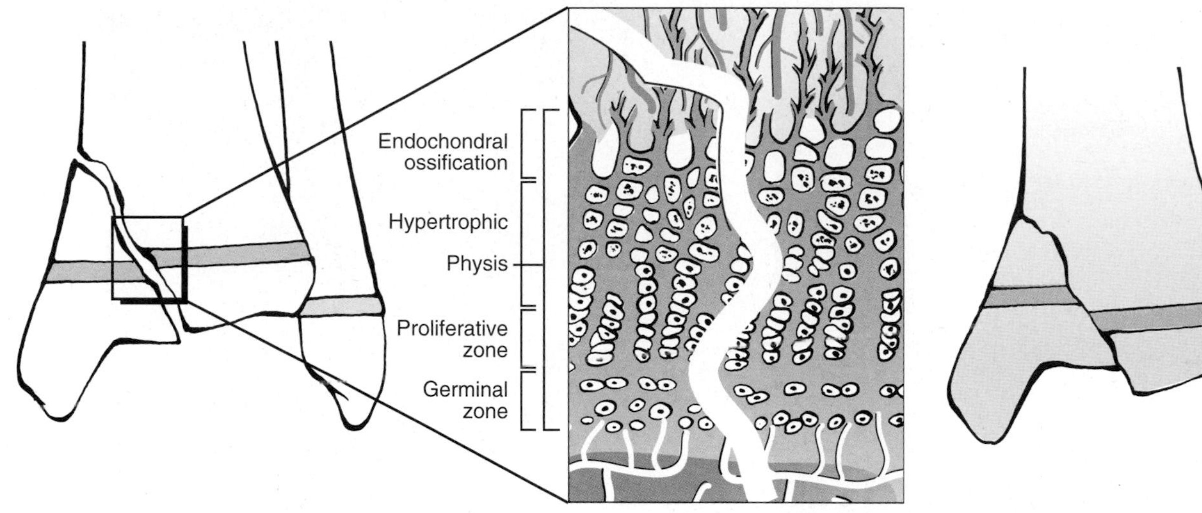

Figure 5-22 Scheme of the Salter-Harris type IV fracture. **A.** The fracture line extends across the physis from the epiphysis and articular surface into the peripheral metaphysis. **B.** Displacement of the fragments can lead to horizontal apposition (and cross union) of the epiphyseal and metaphyseal bone.

of recurvatum deformity of the proximal tibia, after fractures of the femur or distal femoral epiphysis (Fig. 5-23).[23,70,80] While the mechanism of such injuries may be unclear (perhaps vascular rather than compression trauma), the traditionally held view that such injuries occurred as a result of inadvertent direct injury during the insertion of proximal tibial skeletal traction pins has been unequivocally discounted in some cases.[23,70,80] Other locations and case reports of late physeal closure after extremity injury and apparently normal initial radiographs exist in the literature.[1,8,15,71,101,141] By definition, this pattern of injury is unrecognized on initial radiographs. Undoubtedly, more sophisticated imaging of injured extremities (such as with MRI) will identify physeal injuries in the presence of normal plain radiographs (Fig. 5-24). Although the mechanism of injury in type V injuries may be in dispute, in our opinion, the existence of such injuries is not.

Peterson Classification of Physeal Fractures

In an epidemiologic study of physeal injuries, Peterson et al[117] identified several deficiencies of the Salter-Harris classification and subsequently developed a new classification of physeal fractures (Fig. 5-25). They were not able to identify any Salter-Harris type V injuries caused by compression in this epidemiologic study, challenged their existence, and excluded that type from the classification. This classification retained Salter-Harris types I through IV as Peterson types II, III, IV, and V and added two new types.[113,114] It is important to be cognizant of the two new patterns that Peterson et al described, because they are clinically relevant.

Peterson's type I is a transverse metaphyseal fracture with a longitudinal extension to the physis (Fig. 5-26). This pattern of injury is subclassified into four types, based on the extent of metaphyseal comminution and fracture pattern.[114]

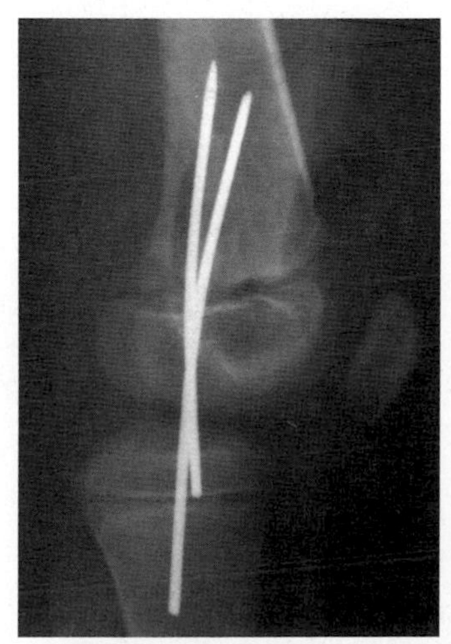

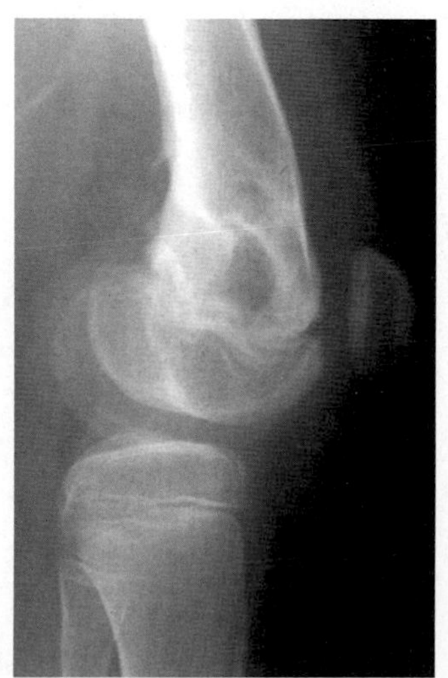

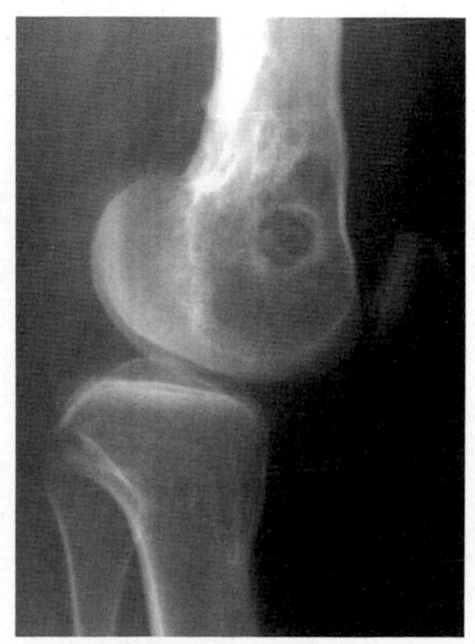

Figure 5-23 Posttraumatic closure of the anterior proximal tibial physis after displaced Salter-Harris type II fracture of the distal femoral physis. **A.** Lateral radiographs after reduction. No injury to the proximal tibia was noted at the time of treatment of the distal femoral injury. **B.** At follow-up, distal femoral physeal growth disturbance with flexion deformity is apparent. **C.** At skeletal maturity, proximal tibial extension deformity with sclerosis of the tibial tubercle area is evident, suggestive of arrest in this area. The patient has undergone a distal femoral extension osteotomy.

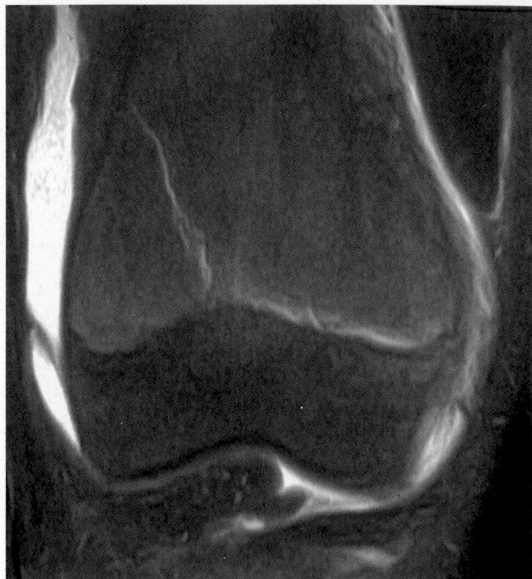

Figure 5-24 MRI of patient after injury with normal radiographs. MRI clearly documents the presence of a Salter-Harris type II fracture of the distal femur.

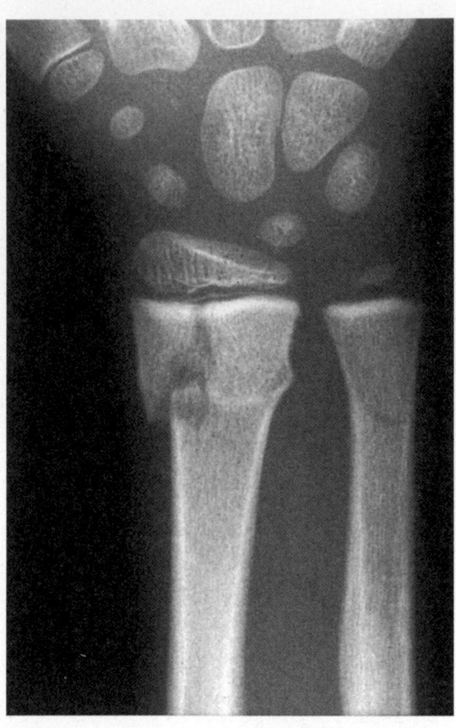

Figure 5-26 Peterson type I injury of the distal radius. These injuries typically have a benign course with respect to subsequent growth disturbance.

Peterson's type VI is a partial physeal loss (Fig. 5-27). Unfortunately, this pattern of injury currently is common, largely as a consequence of lawnmower injuries. Soft tissue loss, neurovascular injury, and partial physeal loss (usually including the epiphysis so that articular impairment also results) further complicate this often-devastating injury.

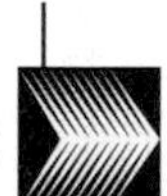

AUTHORS' PREFERRED TREATMENT

We believe that the Salter-Harris classification remains an easily recognized and recalled classification scheme embracing most physeal injuries and continue to use it to describe most physeal fracture patterns. It provides generally useful prognostic and treatment guidelines. We encourage the continued recognition of the Salter-Harris type V physeal injury as a delayed, indirect, or occult injury–induced physeal closure, whose mechanism may be compression, other unrecognized direct injury, or vascular insult. We also believe that Peterson types I and VI physeal fractures are not classifiable by the Salter-Harris scheme and refer to them as Peterson type I and VI fractures, respectively.

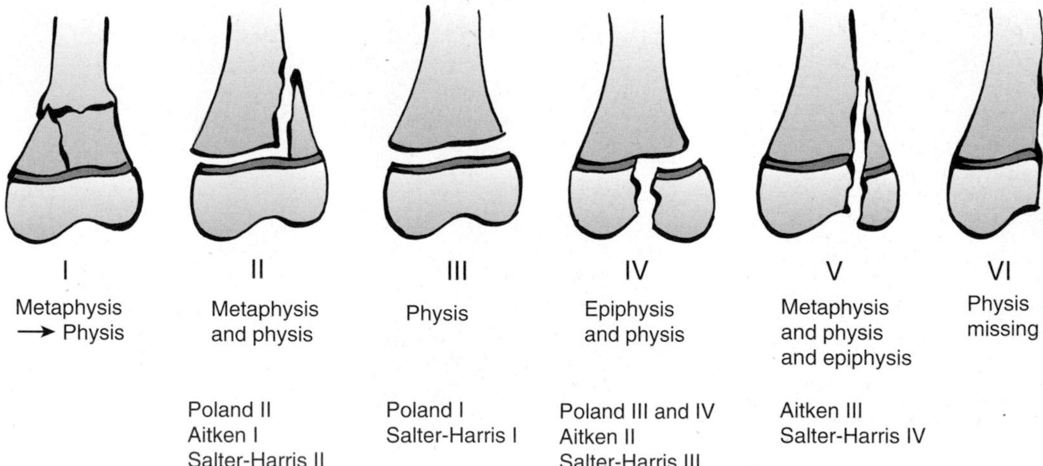

Figure 5-25 Peterson classification of physeal fractures. Type I is a fracture of the metaphysis extending to the physis. Types II to V are the equivalents of Salter-Harris types I, II, III, and IV, respectively. Peterson type VI is epiphyseal (and usually articular surface) loss. Lawnmower injuries are a frequent mechanism for type VI injuries (see text for further discussion).

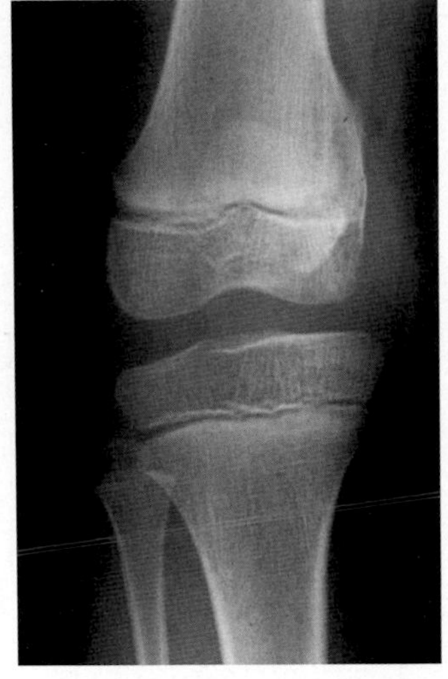

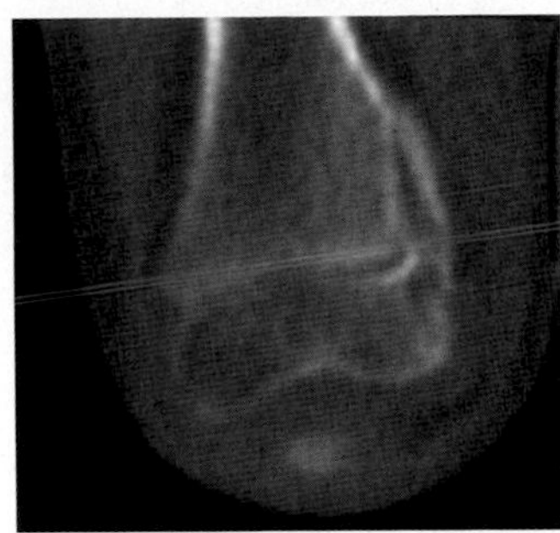

Figure 5-27 Sequelae of a Peterson type VI physeal injury. **A.** Anteroposterior radiograph of distal femur of a young girl who suffered a Peterson type VI injury. This particular injury was the result of direct abrasion of the distal femur when the unrestrained child was ejected from a car. **B.** CT scan 1 year after injury demonstrates the development of a peripheral physeal arrest with valgus deformity.

Epidemiology of Physeal Fractures

In several population surveys reporting the frequency and distribution of childhood fractures, including physeal injuries,[92,101,117,144] 20% to 30% of all childhood fractures were physeal injuries. The phalanges represent the most common location of physeal injuries.

In our opinion, the most useful epidemiologic study of physeal fractures is the Olmstead County Survey.[117] This study of the frequency of physeal fractures in a stable population base was performed between 1979 and 1988, in Olmstead County, Minnesota. The most relevant components are summarized in Tables 5-2 and 5-3. During the study period, 951 physeal fractures were identified: 37% of fractures occurred in the finger phalanges, with the next most common site the distal radius; 71% fractures occurred in the upper extremity, 28% in the lower, and 1% in the axial skeleton. Other salient findings of the Olmstead County survey included a 2:1 male to female ratio and age-related incidence by gender (peak incidence at age 14 in boys and 11 to 12 in girls) (Fig. 5-28). The Adelaide, Australia, survey by Mizuta et al.[101] had similar findings: 30% of physeal fractures were phalangeal, males outnumbered females approximately 2:1, and the prepubertal age groups had the highest relative frequency of physeal fracture.

TABLE 5-2 Frequency of Physeal Fracture by Location

Skeletal Site	Number	Percent
Phalanges (fingers and toes)	411	43.4
Distal radius	170	17.9
Distal tibia	104	11.0
Distal fibula	68	7.2
Metacarpal	61	6.4
Distal humerus	37	3.9
Distal ulna	27	2.8
Proximal humerus	18	1.9
Distal femur	13	1.4
Metatarsal	13	1.4
Proximal tibia	8	0.8
Proximal radius	6	0.6
Clavicle (medial and lateral)	6	0.6
Proximal ulna	4	0.4
Proximal femur	1	0.1
Proximal fibula	1	0.1

Modified from Peterson HA, Madhok R, Benson JT, et al. Physeal fractures. I. Epidemiology in Olmsted County, Minnesota, 1979–1988. J Pediatr Orthopedics 1994;14:423–430.

Evaluation of Physeal Fractures

Modalities available for the evaluation of physeal injuries include plain radiographs, computed tomography scans (CT), and MRI scans,[34,41,56,74,75,118,133] arthrography,[6,44,63,95,145] and ultrasound.[29,45,47,69,128] Plain radiographs remain the preferred initial modality for the assessment of most physeal injuries. Radiographs should be taken in true orthogonal views and include the joint both above and below the fracture. If a physeal injury is suspected, dedicated views centered over the suspected physis

TABLE 5-3 Distribution of Physeal Fracture Patterns by Salter-Harris and Peterson Types I and VI Classification*

Fracture Type	Number	Percent
Salter-Harris I	126	13.2
Salter-Harris II	510	53.6
Salter-Harris III	104	10.9
Salter-Harris IV	62	6.5
Peterson I	147	15.5
Peterson VI	2	0.2

*See text for description of physeal fracture classification.
Modified from Peterson HA, Madhok R, Benson JT, et al. Physeal fractures. I. Epidemiology in Olmsted County, Minnesota, 1979–1988. J Pediatr Orthopedics 1994;14:423–430.

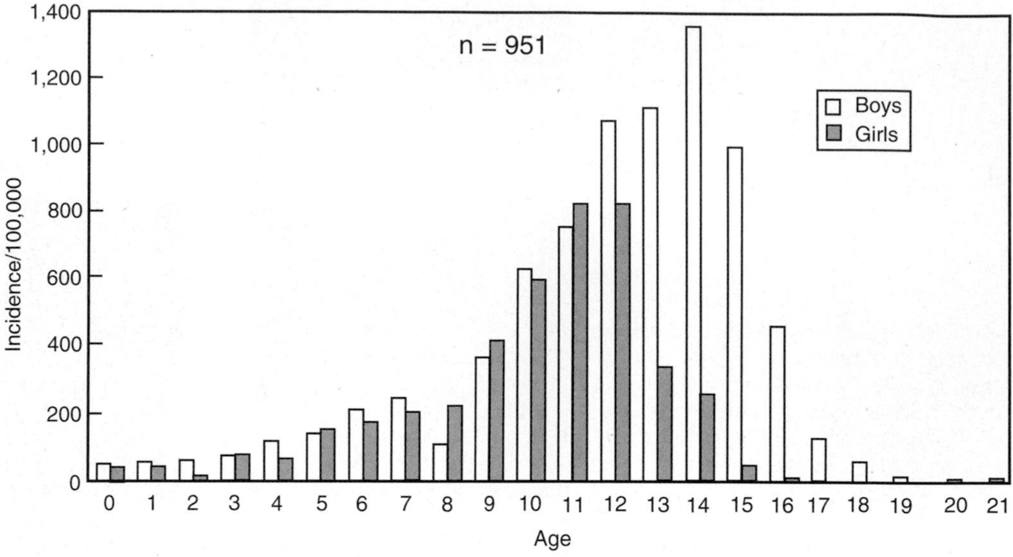

Figure 5-28 Relative frequency of physeal fractures by age and sex according to the Olmstead County survey by Peterson et al.[81] Peak incidence age 14 in boys, and 11 to 12 in girls.

should be obtained to decrease parallax and increase detail. Oblique views may be of value in assessing minimally displaced injuries.

Although plain radiographs provide adequate detail for the assessment and treatment of most physeal injuries, occasionally greater anatomic detail is necessary. CT scans provide excellent definition of bony anatomy, particularly using reconstructed images. They may be helpful in assessing complex or highly comminuted fractures, as well as the articular congruency of minimally displaced fractures (Fig. 5-29). MRI scans are excellent for demonstrating soft tissue lesions and "minor osseous injuries," which may not be seen using standard radiation techniques.

Both arthrography and ultrasound have been used to assess the congruency of articular surfaces. Arthrography may help define the anatomy in young patients with small or no secondary ossification centers in the epiphyses.[6,44,63,95,145] Ultrasonography is occasionally useful for diagnostic purposes to identify epiphyseal separation in infants (Fig. 5-30).[29,44,45,47,69]

Treatment

The general tenets of physeal fracture management are essentially the same as those for injuries not involving the physis, including radiographs of all areas with abnormal physical findings. Once the patient has been stabilized and the initial assessment completed, further studies may be obtained as indicated. Open physeal injuries and those involving neurovascular compromise or impending compartment syndrome should be managed emergently. In most cases, stabilization of the physeal fractures will help facilitate management of the soft tissue injury. All trauma patients should be reassessed as their condition stabilizes to identify occult injuries not identified in the initial assessment.

General Principles of Treatment

In general, fractures in children, including physeal injuries, heal more rapidly than in adults, and they are less likely to experience morbidity or mortality from prolonged immobilization. Additionally, children are also often less compliant with postoperative activity restrictions, making cast immobilization a frequently necessary adjunct to therapy.

Physeal fractures, like all fractures, should be managed in a consistent methodical manner that includes a general assessment and stabilization of the polytraumatized patient, evaluation of the neurovascular and soft tissue status of the traumatized limb, and reduction and stabilization of the fracture. What

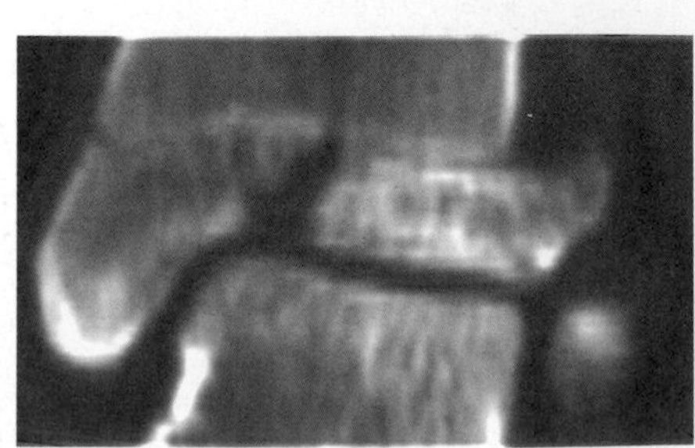

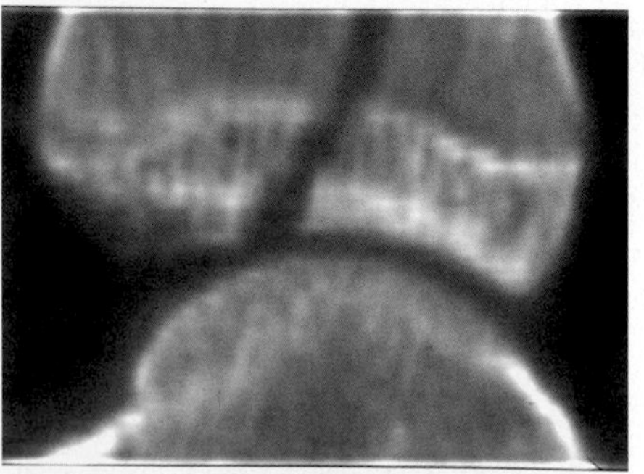

Figure 5-29 CT scans with or without reconstructed images can be helpful in the assessment of physeal fractures. Coronal **(A)** and sagittal **(B)** plane reconstructions of a triplane fracture of the distal tibia.

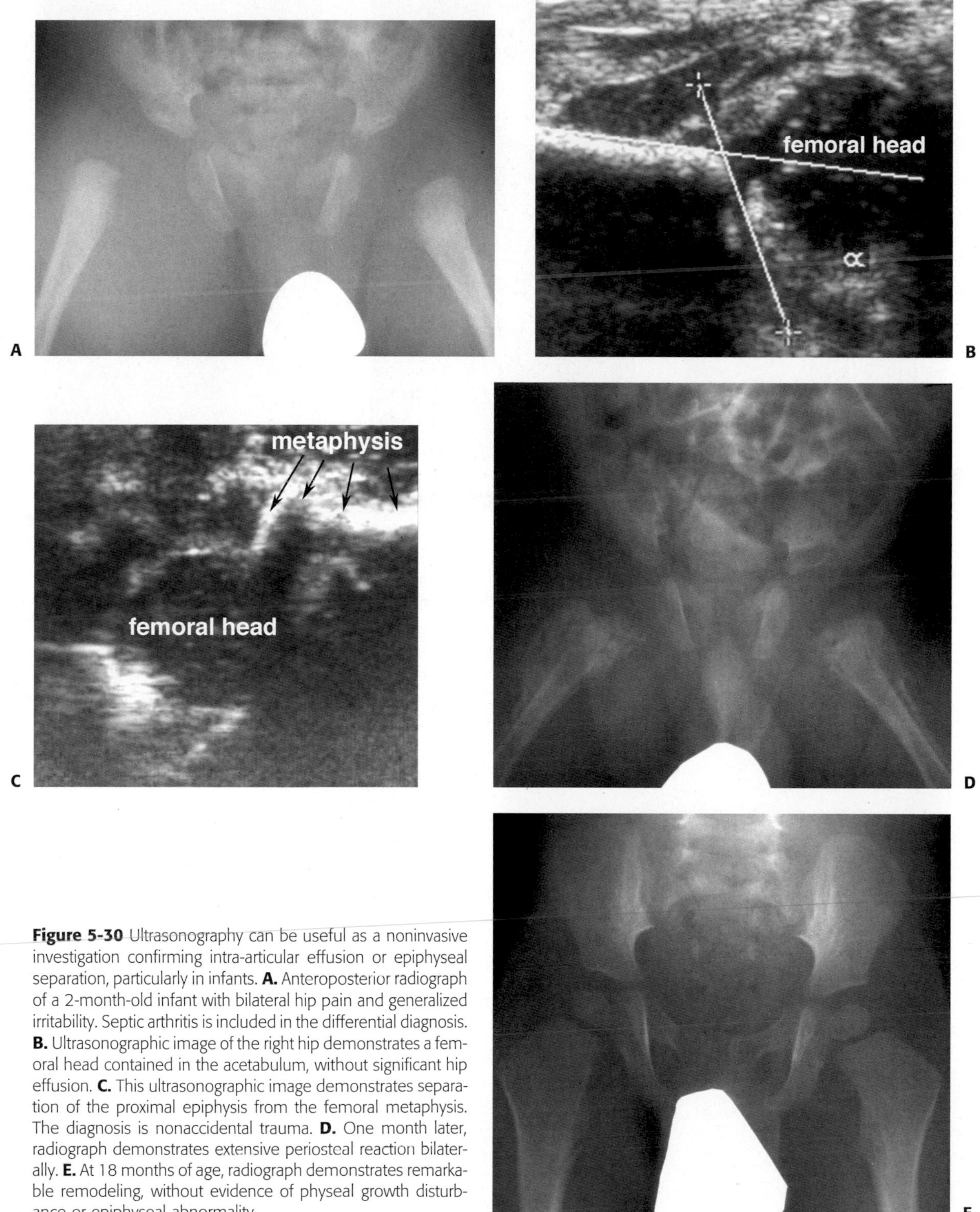

Figure 5-30 Ultrasonography can be useful as a noninvasive investigation confirming intra-articular effusion or epiphyseal separation, particularly in infants. **A.** Anteroposterior radiograph of a 2-month-old infant with bilateral hip pain and generalized irritability. Septic arthritis is included in the differential diagnosis. **B.** Ultrasonographic image of the right hip demonstrates a femoral head contained in the acetabulum, without significant hip effusion. **C.** This ultrasonographic image demonstrates separation of the proximal epiphysis from the femoral metaphysis. The diagnosis is nonaccidental trauma. **D.** One month later, radiograph demonstrates extensive periosteal reaction bilaterally. **E.** At 18 months of age, radiograph demonstrates remarkable remodeling, without evidence of physeal growth disturbance or epiphyseal abnormality.

constitutes an "acceptable" reduction is dictated in part by the fracture pattern and remodeling potential of the fracture. Intra-articular fractures (such as Salter-Harris types III and IV) require anatomic reduction to restore the articular surface and prevent epiphyseal–metaphyseal cross union. Salter-Harris types I and II fractures, particularly those that are the result of low-energy injuries, have minimal risk of growth disturbance (excepting injuries of the distal femur and proximal tibia) and excellent remodeling potential in most patients; in such patients, the surgeon must be cautious not to *create* physeal injury by excessively forceful or invasive reductions.

Complications of Physeal Fractures

Except for the possibility of subsequent growth disturbance, the potential complications of physeal injuries are no different than other traumatic musculoskeletal injuries. Neurovascular

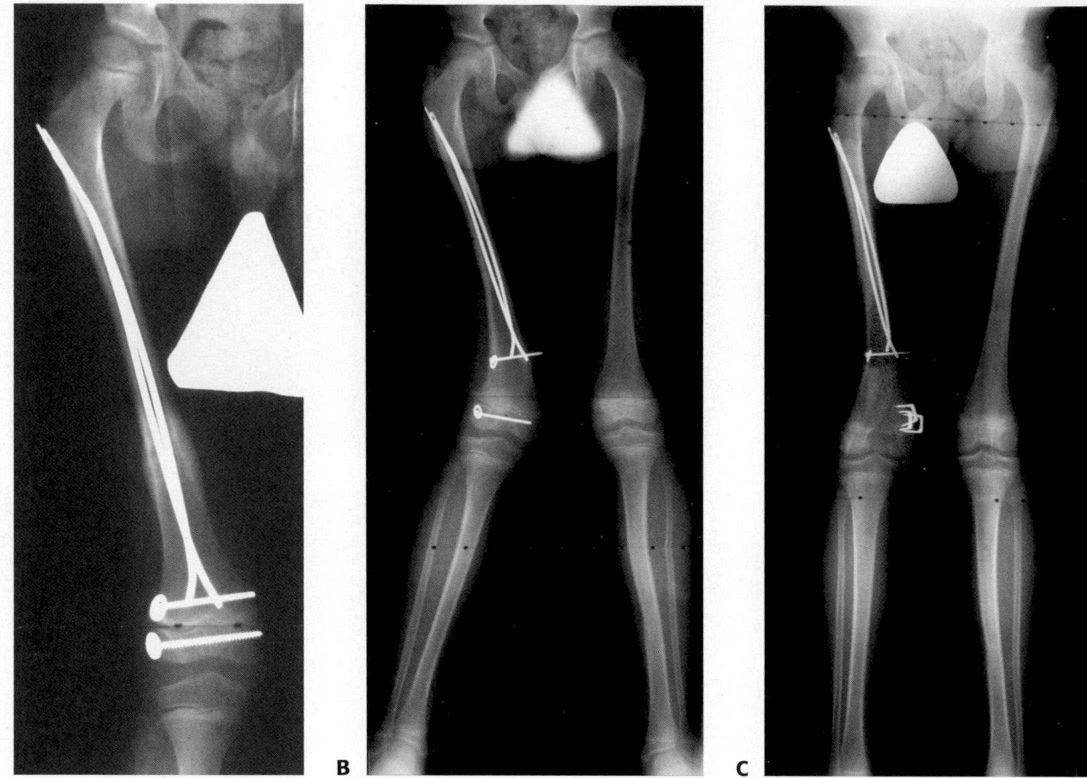

Figure 5-31 Growth deceleration in the absence of a true physeal arrest. This patient sustained concurrent ipsilateral femoral shaft and Salter-Harris type IV distal femoral epiphyseal fractures. **A.** Anteroposterior radiograph of the healed femur. Both fractures were treated with internal fixation. **B.** The patient developed valgus deformity of the distal femur due to asymmetric growth of the distal femoral physis. Note that the distance between the screws on either side of the physis has increased asymmetrically, confirming asymmetric growth rather than cessation of growth laterally. **C.** The angular deformity was treated with medial distal femoral epiphyseal stapling.

compromise and compartment syndrome represent the most serious potential complications.[28,110] It is important to remember that, although a high degree of suspicion and diligence may avoid some of these potentially devastating complications, they can occur even with "ideal" management. Infection and soft tissue loss can complicate physeal fracture management, just as they can in other fractures. The one complication unique to physeal injuries is growth disturbance. Most commonly, this "disturbance" is the result of a tethering (physeal bar or arrest) that may produce angular deformity or shortening. However, growth disturbance may occur without an obvious tether or bar and growth acceleration also occurs (Fig. 5-31). Finally, growth disturbance may occur without injury to the physis.

PHYSEAL GROWTH DISTURBANCE

An uncommon but important complication of physeal fracture is physeal growth disturbance.[96,103,121] The potential consequences of physeal growth disturbance include the development of angular deformity, limb length inequality, epiphyseal distortion, or various combinations of these. Development of these abnormalities, if any, depends on the physis affected, location within the affected physis, the duration of time present, and the skeletal maturity of the patient. Frequently, further surgery, often repeated and extensive, is required to correct or prevent deformity caused by an established growth disturbance.[25,27,64,78,82,84,127,143]

Etiology

Disturbance of normal physeal growth may result from physical loss of the physis (such as after Peterson type VI injuries), from disruption of normal physeal architecture and function without actual radiograph loss of the physis, or by the formation of a physeal arrest, also called bony bridges or physeal bars.[142] Careful identification of the nature of physeal growth disruption is important, because treatment strategies may differ based on the etiology of growth disturbance and the presence or absence of a true growth arrest.

Growth disturbance as a result of physeal injury may result from direct trauma (physeal fracture)[96,103,121] or associated vascular disruption.[115] Infection,[17,21] destruction by a space-occupying lesion such as unicameral bone cyst or enchondroma,[135] infantile Blount disease,[16] other vascular disturbances (such as purpura fulminans),[12,61,73,81] irradiation,[15,123] and other rare causes[19,30,36,] also may result in physeal growth disturbance or physeal arrest.

Evaluation

Physeal growth disturbance may present as a radiographic abnormality noted on serial radiographs in a patient known to be at risk after fracture or infection, clinically with established limb deformity (angular deformity, shortening, or both), or occasionally incidentally on radiographs obtained for other reasons. The hallmark of plain radiographic features of physeal growth dis-

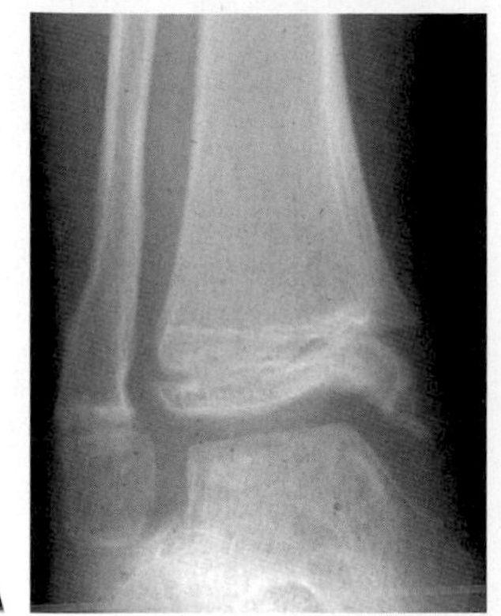
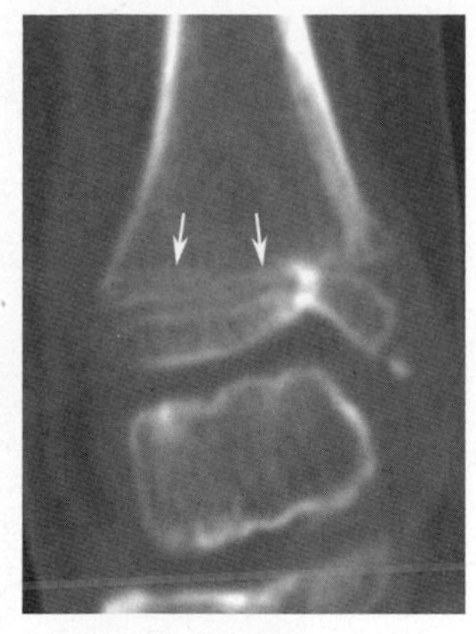
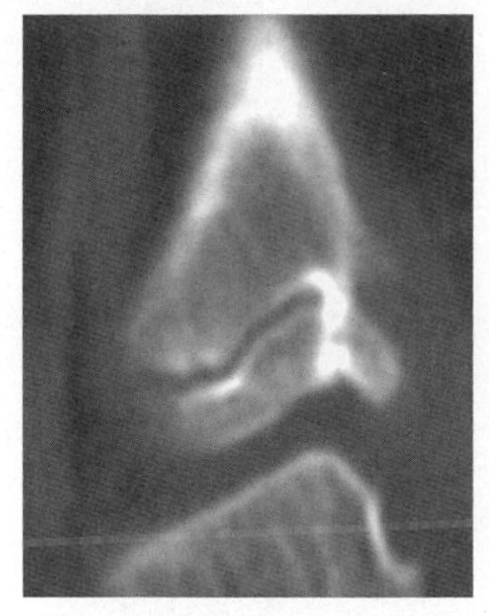
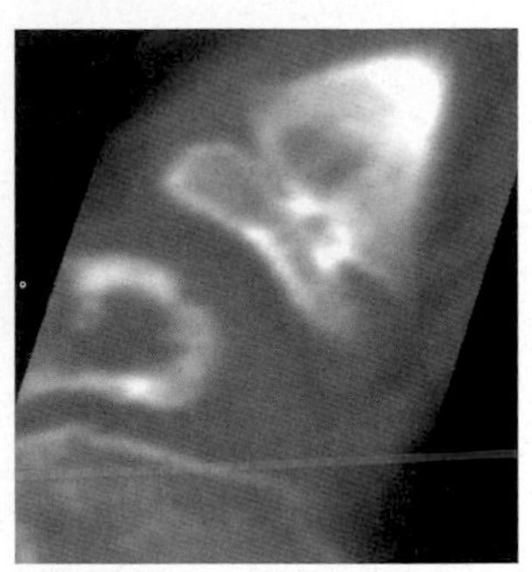

Figure 5-32 Harris growth arrest line tapering to the physis at the level of the growth arrest can serve as an excellent radiograph confirmation of the presence of the true growth arrest. Although most commonly noted on plain radiographs, these arrest lines can be seen on CT scans and MRIs as well. **A.** Anteroposterior radiograph of the distal tibia after Salter-Harris type IV fracture demonstrates a Harris growth arrest line tapering to the medial distal tibial physis, where a partial physeal arrest has formed. **B.** Harris growth arrest line as noted on CT. CT scans with coronal **(C)** and sagittal **(D)** reconstructions corrected for bone distortion provide excellent images of the location and size of arrest.

turbance is the loss of normal physeal contour and the sharply defined radiolucency between epiphyseal and metaphyseal bone. Frank physeal arrests typically are characterized by sclerosis in the region of the arrest. If asymmetric growth has occurred, there may be tapering of a growth arrest line to the area of arrest,[65,105] angular deformity, epiphyseal distortion, or shortening (Fig. 5-32). Physeal growth disturbance without frank arrest typically appears on plain radiographs as a thinner or thicker physeal area with an indistinct metaphyseal border because of alteration in normal enchondral ossification. There may be an asymmetric growth arrest line indicating angular deformity, but the arrest line will not taper to the physis itself (Fig. 5-33).[105] This indicates altered physeal growth (either asymmetric acceleration or deceleration) but not a complete cessation of growth. This distinction is important, because the consequences and treatment are different from those caused by complete growth arrest.

If a growth arrest is suspected on plain radiographs in a skeletally immature child, further evaluation often is warranted. CT scanning with sagittal and coronal reconstructions (orthogonal to the area of interest) may demonstrate clearly an area of bone bridging the physis between the epiphysis and metaphysis (see Fig. 5-32C,D). MRI is also a sensitive method of assessing normal physeal architecture (Fig. 5-34).[34,48,56] Revealing images of the physis and the region of physeal growth disturbance can be obtained using three-dimensional spoiled recalled gradient echo images with fat saturation or fast spin echo proton density images with fat saturation (Fig. 5-35). MRI has the additional advantage of the opportunity to assess the organization of the residual physis that may indicate its relative "health." This assessment may be helpful in cases of infection, irradiation, or tumor to determine if arrest resection is feasible based on the integrity of the remaining physis. With either CT or MRI, physeal arrests are characterized by an identifiable bridge of bone between the epiphysis and metaphysis, whereas growth disruption without arrest demonstrates some degree of loss of normal physeal contour and architecture without the bony bridge or physeal bar.

Although definitive assessment of physeal growth disturbance or arrest usually requires advanced imaging, further evalu-

Figure 5-33 Asymmetric growth arrest line that does not taper to the physis is a strong indication of the presence of physeal growth disturbance without frank physeal arrest. In this case, the asymmetric growth arrest line is noted in the proximal tibial metaphysis on CT scan.

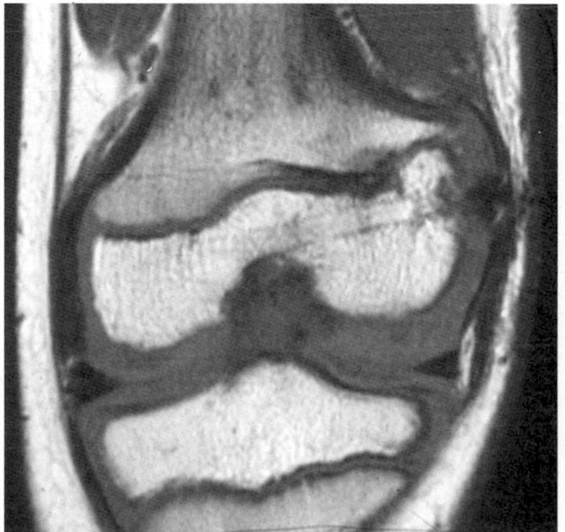

Figure 5-34 MRI scan of a patient with traumatic lateral distal femoral partial growth arrest. Note Harris arrest line tapering to the site of the arrest.

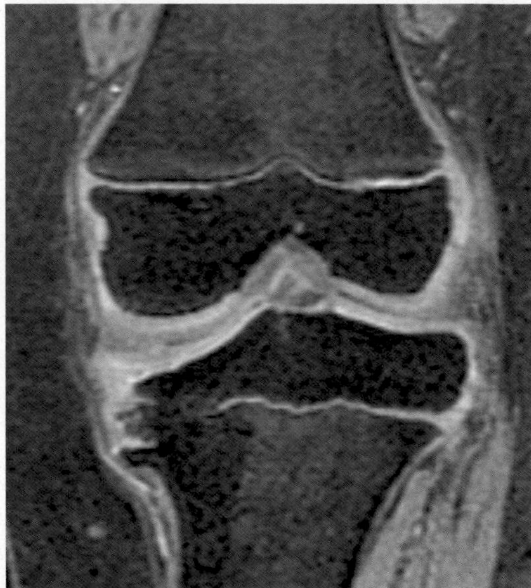

Figure 5-35 MRI scan (three-dimensional spoiled recalled gradient echo images with fat saturation) provides excellent visualization of the affected area and some sense of the integrity of the residual physis. This patient has infantile Blount disease.

ation by plain radiographs is also beneficial. Radiographs of the entire affected limb should be obtained to document the magnitude of angular deformity. Existing limb length inequality should be assessed by scanogram. An estimation of predicted growth remaining in the contralateral unaffected physis should be made based on a determination of the child's skeletal age and reference to an appropriate growth table.[9–11,60,67,68,93]

Physeal Arrests

Whenever a bridge of bone develops across a portion of physis, tethering of the metaphyseal and epiphyseal bone together may result (Table 5-4). These partial physeal arrests can result in angular deformity, joint distortion, limb length inequality, or combinations of these, depending on the location of the arrest, the rate and extent of growth remaining in the physis involved, and the health of the residual affected physis. Although these partial arrests are not common, their presence usually requires preventive or corrective treatment to minimize the long-term sequelae of the disturbance of normal growth they can create (Fig. 5-36).

TABLE 5-4 Potential Causes of Physeal Arrest Formation

Potential Causes of Physeal Arrest
Physeal fracture
Traumatic vascular disruption
Transphyseal infection
Vascular collapse associated with infection (purpura fulminans)
Infantile Blount disease
Irradiation
Unicameral bone cyst
Enchondroma

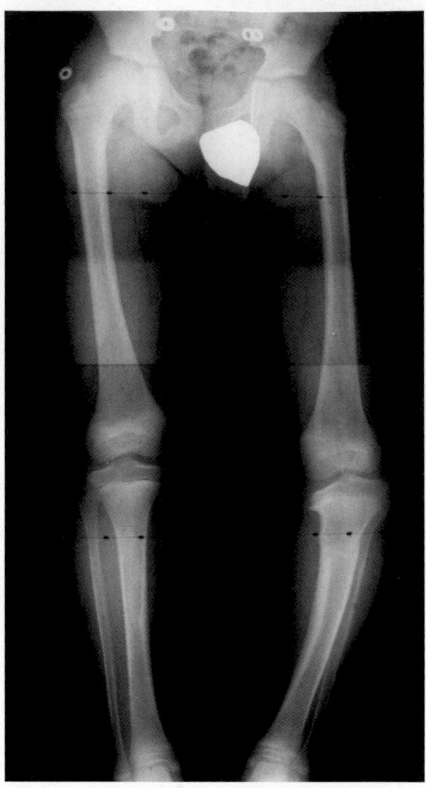

Figure 5-36 Physeal arrests create variable amounts of limb shortening, angular deformity, and epiphyseal distortion, depending on the duration of the arrest, the physis affected, and the size of the arrest. A long, standing film of the lower extremities with the hip, knee, and ankle joints included provides an overall assessment of angular deformity and shortening.

Classification

Partial physeal arrests can be classified by etiology and by anatomic pattern. Potential etiologies of physeal arrest are summarized in Table 5-4 and include physeal fracture, Langenskiöld stage VI infantile Blount disease, infection, tumor, and irradiation. Physeal arrests also can be classified based on the anatomic relationship of the arrest to the residual "healthy" physis. Three basic patterns are recognized (Fig. 5-37): central, peripheral, and linear. A *central* arrest is surrounded by a perimeter of normal physis, like an island within the remaining physis. Central arrests are most likely to cause tenting of the articular surface, but also may result in angular deformity if eccentrically located and limb length inequality (Fig. 5-38). A *peripheral* arrest is located at the perimeter of the affected physis. This type of arrest primarily causes progressive angular deformity and variable shortening. A *linear* arrest is a "through-and-through" lesion with anatomic characteristics of both a central and peripheral arrest; specifically, the affected area includes the perimeter of the physis, but there is normal physis on either side of the affected area. Linear arrests most commonly develop after Salter-Harris type III or IV physeal fractures of the medial malleolus.

Management

Several management alternatives are available. It is important to be aware of these and to weigh carefully the appropriateness of each for the individual situation.

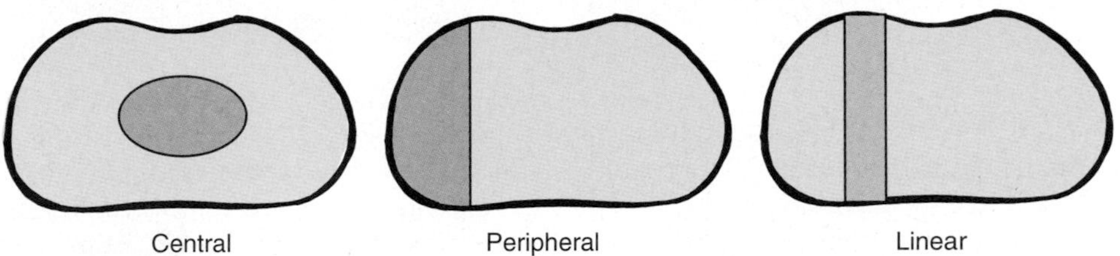

Figure 5-37 Anatomic classification of physeal arrests. Central arrests are surrounded by a perimeter of normal physis. Peripheral arrests are located at the perimeter of the physis. Linear arrests are "through-and-through" lesions with normal physis on either side of the arrest area.

Prevention of Arrest Formation. Ideally, the surgeon should be proactive in the prevention of physeal arrest formation. Most commonly, this can be accomplished by adhering to the general treatment principles of physeal fractures: gentle, anatomic, and secure reduction of the fracture, especially Salter-Harris types III and IV injuries. Damaged, exposed physes can be protected by immediate fat grafting,[53] similar to the principle of interposition material insertion for the resection of established arrests (see following discussion). The most common situation in which this can be considered appropriately is during open reduction of medial malleolar fractures, where comminution or partial physeal damage is identified during reduction.

Some experimental work[137] indicates that nonsteroidal anti-inflammatory medications (specifically indomethacin) given for a period of time after physeal injury may prevent formation of physeal arrest. There is, however, no clinical study supporting this experimental study, so the use of nonsteroidal antiinflammatory medications is empiric and not common clinical practice.

Partial Physeal Arrest Resection. Conceptually, surgical resection of a physeal arrest (sometimes referred to as *physiolysis* or *epiphysiolysis*) restoring normal growth of the affected physis is the ideal treatment for this condition.[25,27,39,55,78,82,84,85,96,109,143] The principle is to remove the bony tether between the metaphysis and physis and fill the physeal defect with a bone reformation retardant, anticipating that the residual healthy physis will resume normal longitudinal growth.[25,55,82,84,85,109]

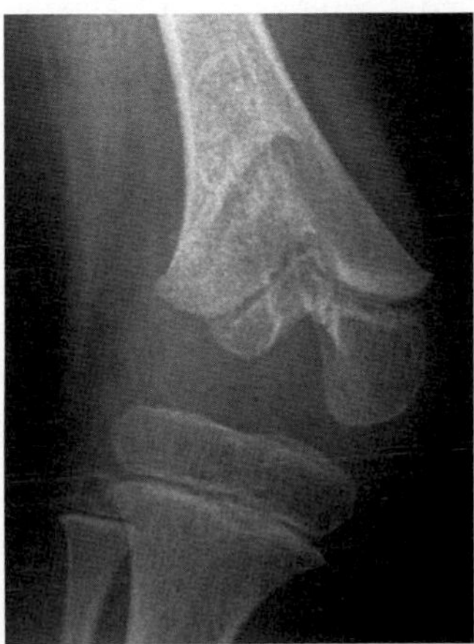

Figure 5-38 Central arrests are characterized by tenting of the articular surface. Variable shortening and angular deformity will develop, depending on the size and location of the arrest.

However, this procedure can be technically demanding, and results in our practice are modest. To determine if this procedure is indicated, careful consideration must be given to the location and extent of the arrest and the amount of longitudinal growth to be potentially salvaged.

Physeal Distraction. Physeal arrests have been treated with the application of an external fixator spanning the arrest and gradual distraction until the arrest "separates."[33,42] Angular deformity correction and lengthening can be accomplished after separation as well. However, distraction injury usually results in complete cessation of subsequent normal physeal growth at the distracted level.[51] Furthermore, the fixation wires or halfpins may have tenuous fixation in the epiphysis or violate the articular space, risking septic arthritis. Thus, this modality is rarely used in patients near the end of growth.

Repeated Osteotomies during Growth. The simplest method to correct angular deformity associated with physeal arrests is corrective osteotomy in the adjacent metaphysis. Of course, neither significant limb length inequality nor epiphyseal distortion that may result from the arrest is corrected by this strategy. However, in young patients with a great deal of growth remaining in whom previous physeal arrest resection has been unsuccessful or is technically not possible, this treatment may be a reasonable interim alternative until more definitive completion of arrest and management of limb length inequality is feasible.

Completion of Epiphysiodesis and Management of Resulting Limb Length Discrepancy. An alternative strategy for the management of physeal arrests is to complete the epiphysiodesis to prevent recurrent angular deformity or epiphyseal distortion and manage the existing or potential limb length discrepancy appropriately. Management of the latter may be by simultaneous or subsequent lengthening of the affected limb segment or contralateral epiphysiodesis if the existing discrepancy is tolerable and lengthening is not desired. We believe that this course of management is specifically indicated if arrest resection has failed to result in restoration of longitudinal growth and in patients in whom the amount of growth remaining does not warrant an attempt at arrest resection. In our opinion, this treatment should be considered carefully in all patients with a physeal arrest.

Physeal Arrest Resection

Based on our experience with the results of physeal arrest resection, the factors discussed in the following sections should be considered before determining if physeal arrest resection is indicated.

Etiology of the Arrest

Arrests caused by trauma or infantile Blount disease have a relatively good prognosis for resumption of normal growth, whereas those secondary to infection, tumor or tumorlike conditions, or irradiation are less likely to demonstrate growth after resection.

Anatomic Type of the Arrest

Central and linear arrests have been reported to be more likely to demonstrate resumption of growth after resection,[27] but our experience has not supported this observation.

Physis Affected

Because proximal humeral and proximal femoral lesions are difficult to expose, a technically adequate resection is less likely in these areas. Distal femoral bars have a poorer prognosis for growth after resection, whereas those of the distal tibia have a more favorable prognosis for the resumption of growth.

Extent of the Arrest

The potential for resumption of longitudinal growth after arrest resection is influenced by the amount of physeal surface area affected.[25,27,78] Arrests affecting more than 25% of the total surface area are unlikely to grow, and, except in patients in whom significant growth potential remains, alternative treatment strategies should be used.

Amount of Growth Remaining in the Physis Affected

Some authors[27,78,82,84,85,112] have stated that 2 years of growth remaining based on skeletal age determination is a prerequisite for arrest resection to be considered. Based on our results with this procedure, we find that 2 years of growth remaining is an inadequate indication for physeal arrest resection. We believe that the decision to perform arrest resection should be made on a combination of the calculated amount of growth remaining in the affected physis and the likelihood of resumption of growth. Scanogram and determination of skeletal age (Fig. 5-39) will document the existing discrepancy, and consultation with the growth remaining tables for the affected physis[9–11,57,70,93] will allow calculation of growth remaining in the affected physis.

Preoperative Planning and Surgical Principles

If physeal arrest resection is considered appropriate, some planning is required to maximize the opportunity for resumption of longitudinal growth.

First, the extent and location of the arrest relative to the rest of the physis must be carefully documented. The most cost-effective method to accurately evaluate an arrest is with reconstructed sagittal and coronal CT images to provide views orthogonal to the affected physis. MRI may also be used and, with

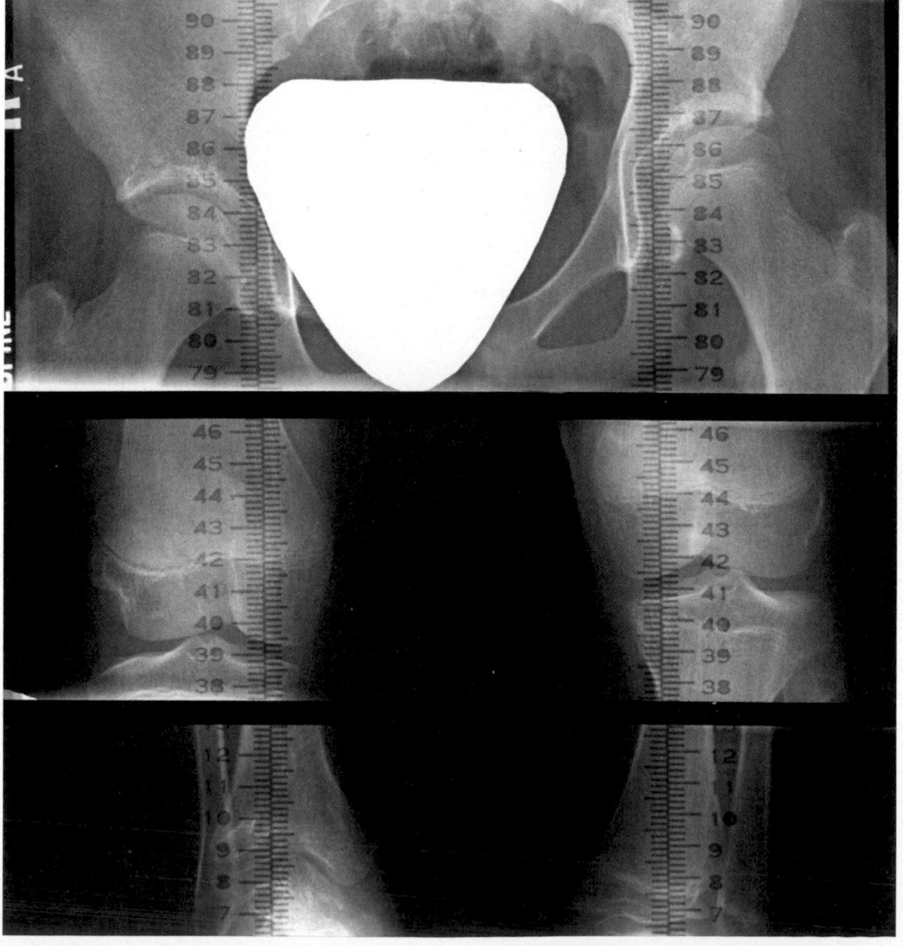

Figure 5-39 Scanogram indicates the existing limb length inequality. Bone age determination and growth contribution per year of the affected physis will allow calculation of the extent of limb segment shortening to be expected.

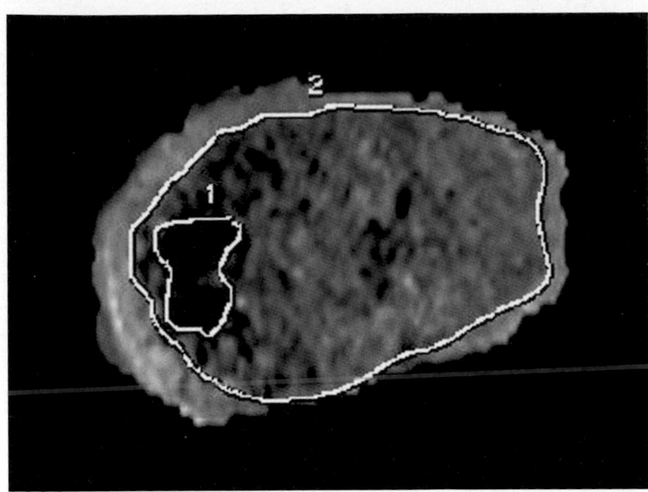

Figure 5-40 Reconstructed MRIs allow estimation of the percentage of surface area of the physis affected by a growth arrest. This workstation reconstruction delineates the perimeter of normal physis (*border 2*) and that of the physeal arrest (*border 1*). Surface area affected can be calculated from these reconstructions.

recent advancements in the capability to identify and quantify physeal arrests, may soon become the imaging study of choice. We currently prefer three-dimensional spoiled recalled gradient echo images with fat saturation or fast spin echo proton density images with fat saturation to visualize the physis. CT images allow precise delineation of bony margins and, at the current time, is cheaper than MRI. An estimation of the affected surface area can be computed with the assistance of the radiologist using a modification of the method of Carlson and Wenger (Fig. 5-40).[35] The procedure should be planned with consideration of the principles discussed in the following section.

Minimize Trauma. The arrest must be resected in a manner that minimizes trauma to the residual physis. Central lesions should be approached through either a metaphyseal window (Fig. 5-41) or through the intramedullary canal after a metaphyseal osteotomy. Peripheral lesions are approached directly, resecting the overlying periosteum to help prevent reformation of the arrest. Intraoperative imaging (fluoroscopy) is needed to keep the surgeon oriented properly to the arrest and the residual healthy physis. Care to provide adequate visualization of the surgical cavity is essential, because visualization is usually difficult even under "ideal" circumstances. A brilliant light source, magnification, and a dry surgical field are very helpful. An arthroscope can be inserted into a metaphyseal cavity to permit a circumferential view of the resection area. A high-speed burr worked in a gentle to-and-fro movement perpendicular to the physis is usually the most effective way to gradually remove the bone composing the arrest and expose the residual healthy physis (Fig. 5-42). By the end of the resection, all of the bridging bone between the metaphysis and epiphysis should be removed, leaving a void in the physis where the arrest had been, and the perimeter of the healthy residual physis should be visible circumferentially at the margins of the surgically created cavity (Fig. 5-43).

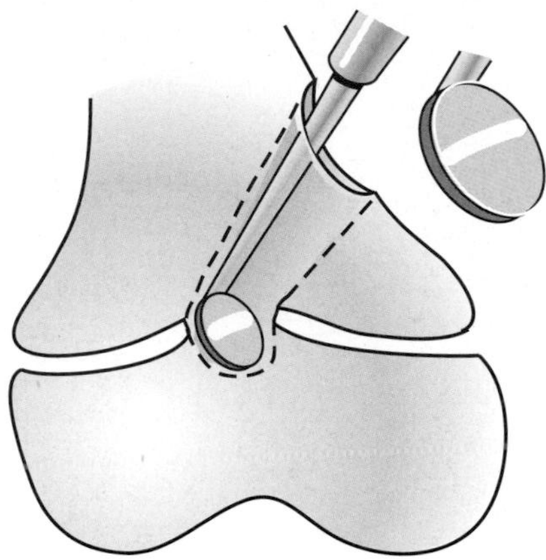

Figure 5-42 The arrest is removed, leaving in its place a metaphyseal-epiphyseal cavity with intact physis surrounding the area of resection.

Prevent Re-forming of Bridge between Metaphysis and Epiphysis. A bone-growth retardant or "spacer" material should be placed in the cavity created by the arrest resection to prevent re-forming of the bony bridge between the metaphysis and epiphysis. Four compounds have been used for this purpose either clinically or experimentally: autogenous fat,[27,78,82,84,85,87,88,143]

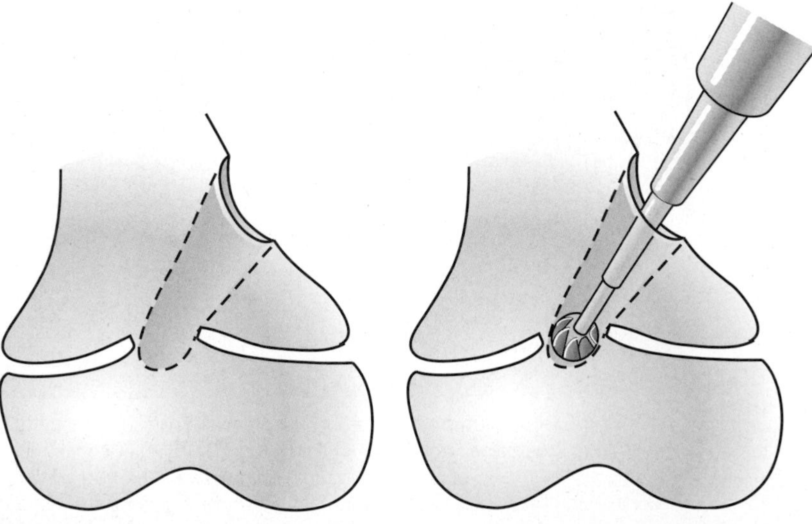

Figure 5-41 Central arrests are approached through a metaphyseal "window" or the medullary canal after metaphyseal osteotomy.

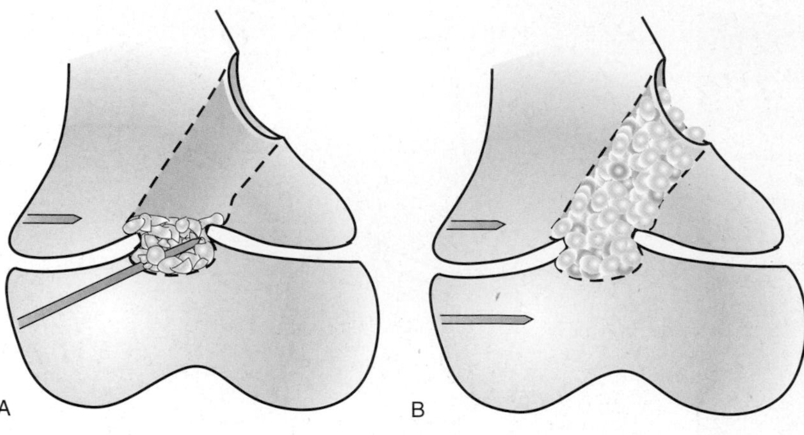

Figure 5-43 After complete resection, the healthy physis should be evident circumferentially within the cavity produced by the arrest resection.

methylmethacrylate,[20,78,112] silicone rubber,[25] and autogenous cartilage.[14,16,52,62,79,89] Silicone rubber is no longer available and, to our knowledge, autogenous cartilage has been used only experimentally as a press-fit plug or cultured chondroblasts. Currently, only autogenous fat graft, harvested either locally or from the buttock, and methylmethacrylate are used clinically. Autogenous fat has at least a theoretic advantage of the ability to hypertrophy and migrate with longitudinal and interstitial growth (Fig. 5-44).[87,88] Methylmethacrylate is inert, but provides some immediate structural stability.[31] This feature may be important with large arrest resections in weight-bearing areas, as in the proximal tibia in association with infantile Blount disease (Fig. 5-45). However, embedded methylmethacrylate, especially products without barium to clearly delineate its location on radiograph, can be extremely difficult to remove and can jeopardize bone fixation if subsequent surgery is required.

Marker Implantation. Metallic markers should implanted in the epiphysis and metaphysis at the time of arrest resection to allow reasonably accurate estimation of the amount of longitudinal growth that occurs across the operated physis, as well as to identify the deceleration or cessation of that growth (Fig. 5-46). We believe that precise monitoring of subsequent longitudinal growth is an important aspect of the management of patients after arrest resection. First, resumption of longitudinal growth may not occur despite technically adequate arrest resection in patients with good clinical indications. Perhaps more importantly, resumption of normal or even accelerated longitudinal growth may be followed by late deceleration or cessation of that growth.[64] It is imperative that the treating surgeon be alert to those developments, so that proper intervention can be instituted promptly. Embedded metallic markers serve those purposes admirably.

Authors' Observation. It has been our clinical observation that even patients who have significant resumption of growth following arrest resection will experience premature cessation of longitudinal growth of the affected physis relative to the contralateral uninvolved physis. We believe that even if growth resumes after bar resection, the previously injured physis will cease growing before the contralateral physis. Thus, the percent of predicted growth might be expected to decrease over the length of follow-up.

Our experience with physeal arrest resection prompted several conclusions and treatment recommendations:

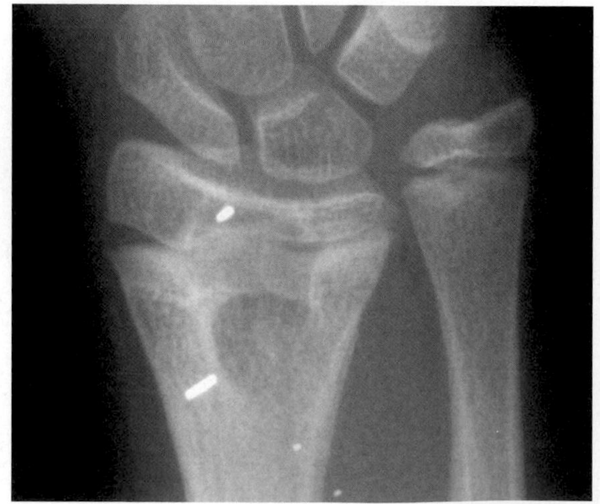

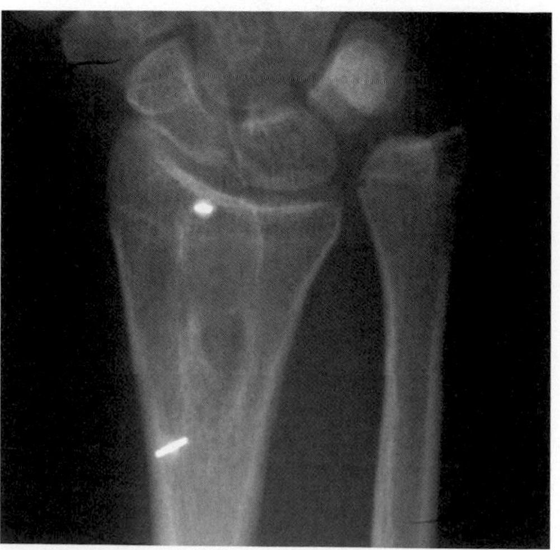

Figure 5-44 Fat used as an interposition material in partial physeal arrest resection can persist and hypertrophy during longitudinal growth. **A.** Radiograph appearance after traumatic distal radial physeal arrest resection. **B.** Appearance 5 years later. Longitudinal growth between the metallic markers is obvious. The fat-filled cavity created at physeal arrest resection has persisted and elongated with distal radial growth.

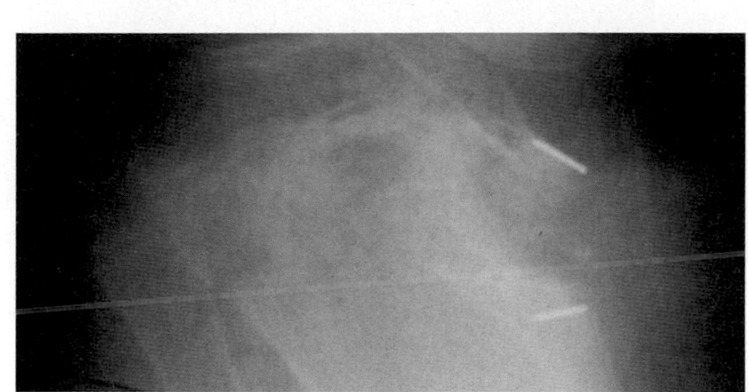
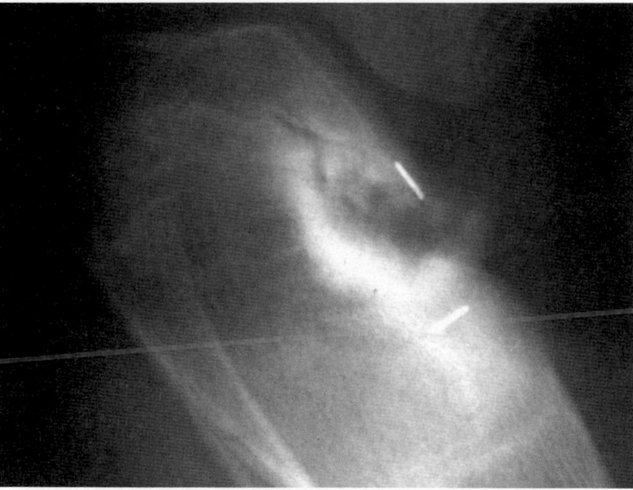

Figure 5-45 Resection of substantial physeal arrests in weight-bearing areas may allow subsidence of the articular surface. This is of particular concern in the proximal tibia of patients with infantile Blount disease. **A.** Early postoperative radiograph after partial physeal arrest resection in an obese patient with infantile Blount disease. **B.** One year later, the metallic markers are actually closer together, in addition to demonstrating increased varus. Subsidence of the medial proximal tibial articular surface is the likely explanation of this radiograph finding. Protected weight-bearing or methylmethacrylate as the interposition material may be indicated in such cases.

- On average, approximately 60% of physeal arrests demonstrate clear radiograph evidence of resumption of longitudinal growth of the affected physis after physeal arrest resection.
- There is a correlation between the amount of surface area of the physis affected and the prognosis for subsequent longitudinal growth after arrest resection. Physeal arrests affecting less than 10% of the surface area of the physis have a better prognosis than larger arrests.
- Langenskiöld stage VI infantile Blount disease has results comparable to posttraumatic physeal arrests.
- Etiologies other than posttraumatic and infantile Blount disease have poor prognoses for subsequent growth.
- Central and peripheral arrests have equivalent prognoses with respect to resumption of growth.
- Early growth resumption may be followed by cessation of longitudinal growth before skeletal maturity. As a consequence, patients must be evaluated regularly until skeletal maturity with some reliable method (such as metaphyseal and epiphyseal radiograph markers) to detect such development as promptly as possible.

We believe that physeal bar resection has a role to play in patients with significant longitudinal growth remaining. However, the benefits of such surgery must be weighed against the actual amount of growth remaining, and the etiology, location, and extent of the physeal arrest must be considered. The appropriate time to add a corrective osteotomy to bony bar resection is controversial. Generally, when the angular deformity is more than 10 to 15 degrees from normal, corrective osteotomy should be considered.

Growth Disturbance without Arrest

Recognition

Growth disturbance may also occur without physeal arrest. Both growth deceleration and, less frequently, acceleration have been reported. Growth deceleration without arrest is characterized radiographically by the appearance of an injured physis (usually relative widening of the physis with indistinct metaphyseal boundaries). There may be associated clinical or radiographic deformity if the disturbance is severe and long standing. It is important to make a distinction between growth deceleration without complete cessation and true physeal arrest, because management and outcome are typically different in these two disorders. The concept of growth deceleration without arrest is most readily appreciated in patients with adolescent Blount disease and the milder stages of infantile Blount disease. Recently, growth deceleration without physeal arrest has also been reported to produce distal femoral valgus deformity in obese adolescents.[146] Growth deceleration may also occur after infection and physeal fracture. In contrast to physeal arrests, there is no sclerotic area of arrest on plain radiographs (see Fig. 5-33). A growth arrest line, if present, may be asymmetric but will not taper to the physis, thereby suggesting growth asymmetry but not complete arrest. Furthermore, in some cases, deformity will not be relentlessly progressive and can actually improve over time.

Growth acceleration most classically occurs following proximal tibial fracture in young patients resulting in valgus deformity which usually spontaneously resolves.[72,77,108,131,132,147] Interestingly, it has also recently been reported to occur in patients younger than 10 years who have had curettage of benign lesions of the proximal tibial metaphysis.[66]

Management

The diagnosis of physeal growth disturbance is usually made incidentally by noting physeal abnormality on radiographs during physeal fracture follow-up or after a diagnosis of frank physeal arrest has been excluded during the evaluation of a patient with angular deformity and physeal abnormality on plain radiographs. Once a growth disturbance has been identified in a patient, its full impact should be assessed by determining the

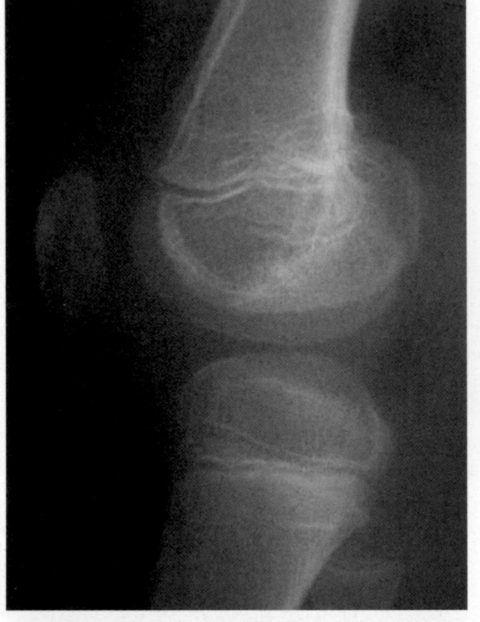

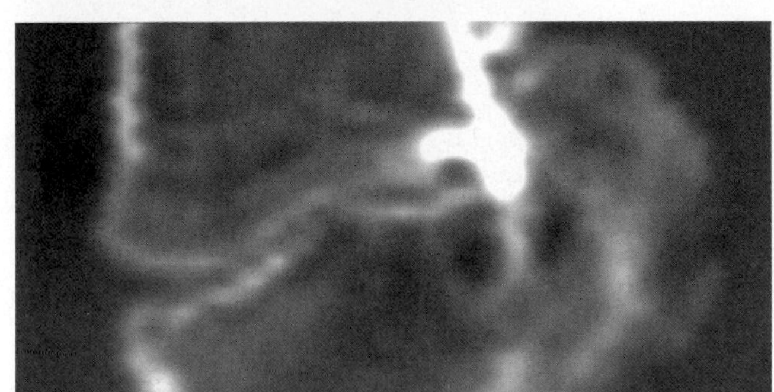

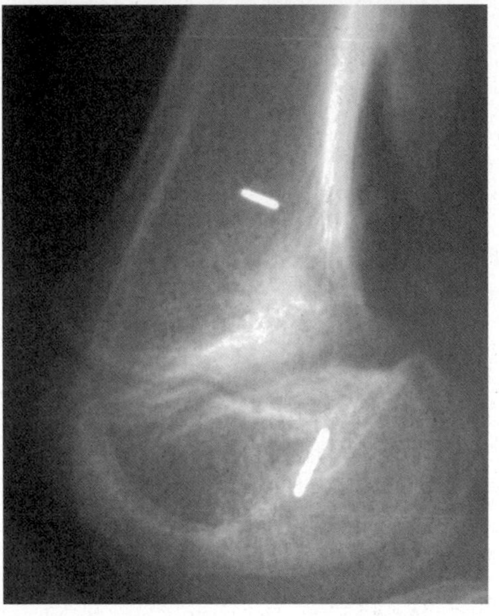

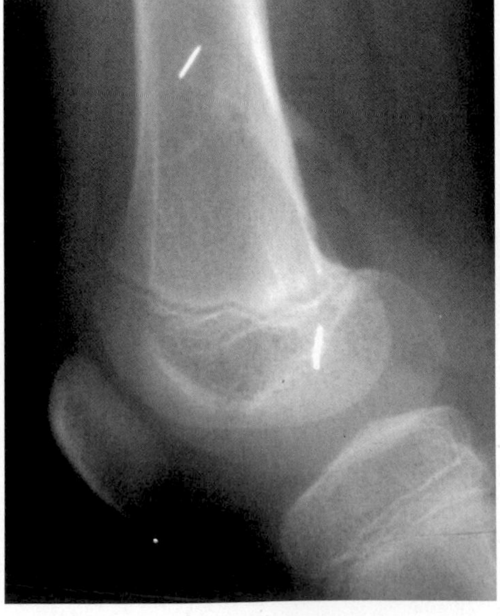

Figure 5-46 Intraosseous metallic markers in the epiphysis and metaphysis spanning the area of arrest resection allow sensitive radiographic documentation of the presence and extent of growth after arrest resection and permit early detection of the cessation of restored longitudinal growth. This patient had a small central arrest of the lateral portion of the distal femoral physis after a Salter-Harris type IV fracture. **A.** Injury films show a mildly displaced Salter-Harris type IV fracture of the lateral distal femur. **B.** Several years later, a small central arrest has developed involving a portion of the lateral distal femoral physis. A tapering growth arrest line is faintly visible. **C.** The posterior location of the partial arrest can be seen on the sagittal CT reconstructions. **D.** After arrest resection through a metaphyseal window, a cavity is evident in the region of the original bar. Metallic markers have been placed in the metaphysis and epiphysis. **E.** Three years after arrest resection, substantial growth has occurred, as documented by the increased distance between the markers. However, on radiographs taken at 4 years postoperatively, no further growth was documented. This event was treated by completion of the epiphysiodesis and contralateral distal femoral epiphysiodesis to prevent the development of limb length discrepancy from developing.

presence and extent of limb length inequality and the calculated amount of potential growth remaining for the affected physis.

In some cases, the radiographic abnormality is stable and only longitudinal observation is required. This observation must be regular and careful, because progressive deformity will require treatment. If angular deformity is present or progressive, treatment options include hemiepiphysiodesis or physeal "tethering" with staples, screws, or tension plates[22,40,50,54,98,99,104,136] and corrective osteotomy, with or without completion of the epiphysiodesis.

In the absence of frank arrest formation, hemiepiphysiodesis or "tethering" the affected physis with staples, screws, or tension plates on the convex side may result in gradual correction of the deformity. If correction occurs, options include completion of the epiphysiodesis (with contralateral epiphysiodesis if necessary to prevent the development of significant leg length deformity) and removal of the tethering device with careful longitudinal observation for recurrence or overcorrection of deformity.

Corrective osteotomy is the other option for the management of growth disturbance with established angular deformity. Angular deformity correction in the early stages of infantile and adolescent Blount disease is known to result in resolution of the physeal growth disturbance in some patients, both on radiographs and clinically. We are unaware of confirmation of similar outcome when the etiology of growth disturbance is infection or trauma, although it may occur. Thus, the treating surgeon must decide whether to perform epiphysiodesis of the affected physis (with contralateral epiphysiodesis, if appropriate) to prevent recurrence or to ensure careful longitudinal observation of the growth performance of the affected physis until skeletal maturity.

SUMMARY

Physeal fractures are one of the unique aspects of pediatric orthopaedics. These injuries are common and usually have a favorable outcome without long-term sequelae. Physeal fractures must be treated gently and expertly to maximize restoration of normal limb function and longitudinal growth. Depending on the severity and nature of physeal injury, longitudinal follow-up to identify the development of physeal growth disturbance is important.

REFERENCES

1. Abram LJ, Thompson GH. Deformity after premature closure of the distal radial physis following a torus fracture with a physeal compression injury. Report of a case. J Bone Joint Surg Am 1987;69(9):1450–1453.
2. Aitken AP. The end result of the fractured distal tibial epiphysis. J Bone Joint Surg Am 1936;18:685–691.
3. Aitken AP. Fractures of the epiphyses. Clin Orthop Relat Res 1965;41:19–23.
4. Aitken AP. Fractures of the proximal tibial epiphysial cartilage. Cline Orthop Relat Res 1965;41:92–97.
5. Aitken AP, Magill HK. Fractures involving the distal femoral epiphyseal cartilage. J Bone Joint Surg Am 1952;34-A(1):96–108.
6. Akbarnia BA, Silvrestein MJ, Rende RJ, et al. Arthrography in the diagnosis of fractures of the distal end of the humerus in infants. J Bone Joint Surg Am 1986;68(4):599–602.
7. Albanese SA, Palmer AK, Kerr DR, et al. Wrist pain and distal growth plate closure of the radius in gymnasts. J Pediatr Orthop 1989;9(1):23–28.
8. Aminian A, Schoenecker PL. Premature closure of the distal radial physis after fracture of the distal radial metaphysis. J Pediatr Orthop 1995;15(4):495–498.
9. Anderson M, Green WT. Length of femur and tibia; norms derived from orthoroentgenogram of children from 5 years of age until epiphyseal closure. Am J Dis Child 1948;75(3):279–290.
10. Anderson M, Green WT, Messner M Growth and predictions of growth in the lower extremities. J Bone Joint Surg Am 1963;45-A:1–14.
11. Anderson M, Messner MB, Green WT. Distribution of lengths of the normal femur and tibia in children from 1 to 18 years of age. J Bone Joint Surg Am 1964;46:1197–1202.
12. Appel M, Pauleto AC, Cunha LAM. Osteochondral sequelae of meningococcemia: radiographic aspects. J Pediatr Orthop 2002;22(4):511–516.
13. Arriola F, Forriol F, Cañadell J. Histomorphometric study of growth plate subjected to different mechanical conditions (compression, tension, and neutralization): an experimental study in lambs. Mechanical growth plate behavior. J Pediatr Orthop B 2001; 10(4):334–338.
14. Barr SJ, Zaleske DJ. Physeal reconstruction with blocks of cartilage of varying developmental time. J Pediatr Orthop 1992;12(6):766–773.
15. Beals RK. Premature closure of the physis following diaphyseal fractures. J Pediatr Orthop 1990;10(6):717–720.
16. Beck CL, Burke SW, Roberts JM, et al. Physeal bridge resection in infantile Blount disease. J Pedaitr Orthop 1987;7(2):161–163.
17. Bergdahl S, Ekengren K, Eriksson M. Neonatal hematogenous osteomyelitis: risk factors for long-term sequelae. J Pediatr Orthop 1985;5(5):564–568.
18. Bertin KC, Goble EM. Ligament injuries associated with physeal fractures about the knee. Clin Orthop Relat Res 1983;177:188–195.
19. Bigelow DR, Ritchie GW. The effects of frostbite in childhood. J Bone Joint Surg Br 1963;45-B(1):122–131.
20. Bollini G, Tallet JM, Jacquemier M, et al. New procedure to remove a centrally located bone bar. J Pediatr Orthop 1990;10(5):662–666.
21. Bos CF, Mol LJ, Obermann WR, et al. Late sequelae of neonatal septic arthritis of the shoulder. J Bone Joint Surg Br 1998;80(4):645–650.
22. Bowen JR, Torres RR, Forlin E. Partial epiphysiodesis to address genu varum or genu valgum. J Pediatr Orthop 1992;12(3):359–364.
23. Bowler JR, Mubarak SJ, Wenger DR. Tibial physeal closure and genu recurvatum after femoral fracture: occurrence without a tibial traction pin. J Pediatr Orthop 1990;10(5): 653–657.
24. Boyd KT, Batt ME. Stress fracture of the proximal humeral epiphysis in an elite junior badminton player. Br J Sports Med 1997;31(3):252–253.
25. Bright RW. Operative correction of partial epiphyseal plate closure by osseous-bridge resection and silicone-rubber implant. An experimental study in dogs. J Bone Joint Surg Am 1974;56(4):655–664.
26. Bright, RW, Burstein AH, Elmore SM. Epiphyseal-plate cartilage. A biomechanical and histological analysis of failure modes. J Bone Joint Surg Am 1974;56(4):688–703.
27. Broughton NS, Dickens DR, Cole WG, et al. Epiphysiolysis for partial growth plate arrest. Results after 4 years or at maturity. J Bone Joint Surg Br 1989;71(1):13–16.
28. Brogle PJ, Gaffney JT, Denton JR. Acute compartment syndrome complicating a distal tibial physeal fracture in a neonate. Am J Orthop 1999;28(10):587–589.
29. Broker FH, Burbach T. Ultrasonic diagnosis of separation of the proximal humeral epiphysis in the newborn. J Bone Joint Surg Am 1990;72(2):187–191.
30. Brown FE, Spiegel PK, Boyle WE Jr. Digital deformity: an effect of frostbite in children. Pediatrics 1983;71(6):955–959.
31. Bueche MJ, Phillips WA, Gordon J, et al. Effect of interposition material on mechanical behavior in partial physeal resection: a canine model. J Pediatr Orthop 1990;10(4): 459–462.
32. Butler MS, Robertson WW Jr, Rate W, et al. Skeletal sequelae of radiation therapy for malignant childhood tumors. Clin Orthop Relat Res 1990;251:235–240.
33. Canadell J, de Pablos J. Breaking bony bridges by physeal distraction: a new approach. Int Orthop 1985;9(4):223–229.
34. Carey J, Spence L, Blickman H, et al. MRI of pediatric growth plate injury: correlation with plain film radiographs and clinical outcome. Skeletal Radiol 1998;27(5):250–255.
35. Carlson WO, Wenger DR. A mapping method to prepare for surgical excision of a partial physeal arrest. J Pediatr Orthop 1984;4(2):232–238.
36. Carrera GF, Kozin F, Flaherty L et al. Radiographic changes in the hands following childhood frostbite injury. Skeletal Radiol 1981;6(1):33–37.
37. Carson WG Jr, Gasser SI. Little Leaguer's shoulder. A report of 23 cases. Am J Sports Med 1998;26(4):575–580.
38. Carter SR, Aldridge MJ. Stress injury of the distal radial growth plate. I Bone Joint Surg Br 1988;70(5):834–836.
39. Cass JR, Peterson HA. Salter-Harris type-IV injuries of the distal tibial epiphyseal growth plate, with emphasis on those involving the medial malleolus. J Bone Joint Surg Am 1983;65(8):1059–1070.
40. Castañeda P, Urquhart B, Sullivan E, et al. Hemiepiphysiodesis for the correction of angular deformity about the knee. J Pediatr Orthop 2008;28(2):188–191.
41. Close BJ, Strouse PJ. MR of physeal fractures of the adolescent knee. Pediatr Radiol 2000;30(11):756–762.
42. Connolly JF, Huurman WW, Ray S. Physeal distraction treatment of fracture deformities. Orthopaedic Transactions 1991;3(2):231–232.
43. Dale G, Harris W. Prognosis of epiphyseal separations. An experimental study. J Bone Joint Surg 1958;40B:116–122.
44. Davidson RS, Markowitz RI, Dormans J, et al. Ultrasonographic evaluation of the elbow in infants and young children after suspected trauma. J Bone Joint Surg Am 1994; 76(12):1804–1813.
45. Dias JJ, Lamont AC, Jones JM. Ultrasonic diagnosis of neonatal separation of the distal humeral epiphysis. J Bone Joint Surg Br 1988;70(5):825–828.
46. Dias LS, Tachdjian MO. Physeal injuries of the ankle in children: classification. Clin Orthop Relat Res 1978;136:230–233.
47. Diaz MJ, Hedlund GL. Sonographic diagnosis of traumatic separation of the proximal femoral epiphysis in the neonate. Pediatr Radiol 1991;21(3):238–240.
48. Ecklund K, Jaramillo D. Patterns of premature physeal arrest: MR imaging of 111 children. AJR Am J Roentgenol 2002;178(4):967–72.
49. Ellefsen BK, Frierson MA, Raney EM, et al. Humerus varus: a complication of neonatal, infantile, and childhood injury and infection. J Pediatr Orthop 1994;14(4):479–486.
50. Ferrick MR, Birch JG, Albright M. Correction of non-Blount's angular knee deformity by permanent hemiepiphysiodesis. J Pediatr Orthop 2004;24(4):397–402.
51. Fjeld TO, Steen H. Growth retardation after experimental limb lengthening by epiphyseal distraction. J Pediatr Orthop 1990;10(4):463–466.
52. Foster BK, Hansen AL, Gibson GJ, et al. Reimplantation of growth plate chondrocytes into growth plate defects in sheep. J Orthop Res 1990;8(4):555–564.

53. Foster BK, John B, Hasler C. Free fat interpositional graft in acute physeal injuries: the anticipatory Langenskiöld procedure. J Pediatr Orthop 2000;20(3):282–285.
54. Fraser RK, Dickens DR, Cole WG. Medial physeal stapling for primary and secondary genu valgum in late childhood. J Bone Joint Surg Br 1995;77(5):733–735.
55. Freidenberg ZB. Reaction of the epiphysis to partial surgical resection. J Bone Joint Surg Am 1957;39-A(2):332–340.
56. Gabel GT, Peterson HA, Berquist TH. Premature partial physeal arrest. Diagnosis by magnetic resonance imaging in two cases. Clin Orthop Relat Res 1991;272:242–247.
57. Goldfarb CA, Bassett GS, Sullivan S, et al. Retrosternal displacement after physeal fracture of the medial clavicle in children treatment by open reduction and internal fixation. J Bone Joint Surg Br2001;83(8):1168–1172.
58. Gomes LS, Volpon JB. Experimental physeal fracture-separations treated with rigid internal fixation. J Bone Joint Surg Am 1993;75(12):1756–1764.
59. Gomes LS, Volpon JB, Goncalves RP. Traumatic separation of epiphyses. An experimental study in rats. Clin Orthop Relat Res 1988;236:286–295.
60. Green WT, Anderson M. Skeletal age and the control of bone growth. Instr Course Lect 1960;17:199–217.
61. Grogan DP, Love SM, Ogden JA, et al. Chondro-osseous growth abnormalities after meningococcemia. A clinical and histopathological study. J Bone Joint Surg Am 1989; 71(6):920–928.
62. Hansen AL, Foster BK, Gibson GJ, et al. Growth-plate chondrocyte cultures for reimplantation into growth-plate defects in sheep: characterization of cultures. Clin Orthop Relat Res 1990;256:286–298.
63. Hansen PE, Barnes DA, Tullos HS. Arthrographic diagnosis of an injury pattern in the distal humerus of an infant. J Pediatr Orthop 1982;2(5):569–572.
64. Hasler CC, Foster BK. Secondary tethers after physeal bar resection: a common source of failure. Clin Orthop Relat Res 2002;405:242–249.
65. Harris H. Lines of arrested growth in the long bones in childhood: the correlation of histological and radiographic appearance in clinical and experimental conditions. Br J Radiol 1931;4:561–588.
66. Heck RK Jr, Sawyer JR, Warner WC, et al. Progressive valgus deformity after curettage of benign lesions of the proximal. J Pediatr Orthop 2008;28(7):757–760.
67. Hensinger R. Linear growth of long bones of the lower extremity form infancy to adolescence. In: Hensinger R, Raven P, eds. Standards in Pediatric Orthopaedics: Tables, Charts, and Graphs Illustrating Growth. New York: Raven Press Books, 1986, 232–233.
68. Hensinger R. Standards in Pediatric Orthopaedics: Tables, Charts, and Graphs Illustrating Growth. New York: Raven Press Books, 1986.
69. Howard CB, Shinwell E, Nyska M, et al. Ultrasound diagnosis of neonatal fracture separation of the upper humeral epiphysis. J Bone Joint Surg Br 1992;74(3):471–472.
70. Hresko MT, Kasser JR. Physeal arrest about the knee associated with nonphyseal fractures in the lower extremity. J Bone Joint Surg Am 1989;71(5):698–703.
71. Hunter LY, Hensinger RN. Premature monomelic growth arrest following fracture of the femoral shaft: a case report. J Bone Joint Surg Am 1978;60(6):850–852.
72. Ippolito E, Pentimalli G. Posttraumatic valgus deformity of the knee in proximal tibial metaphyseal fractures in children. Ital J Orthop Traumatol 1984;10(1):103–108.
73. Jacobsen ST, Crawford AH. Amputation following meningococcemia. A sequela to purpura fulminans. Clin Orthop Relat Res 1984;185:214–219.
74. Jain R, Bielski RJ. Fracture of lower femoral epiphysis in an infant at birth: a rare obstetrical injury. J Perinatol 2001;21(8):550–552.
75. Jaramillo D, Kammen BF, Shapiro F. Cartilaginous path of physeal fracture-separations: evaluation with MR imaging—an experimental study with histologic correlation in rabbits. Radiology 2000;215(2):504–511.
76. Johnston RM, James WW. Fractures through human growth plates. Orthop Trans 1980; 4:295.
77. Jordan SE, Alonso JE, Cook FF. The etiology of valgus angulation after metaphyseal fractures of the tibia in children. J Pediatr Orthop 1987;7(4):450–457.
78. Kasser JR. Physeal bar resections after growth arrest about the knee. Clin Orthop Relat Res 1990;255:68–74.
79. Kawabe N, Ehrlich MG, Mankin HJ. Growth plate reconstruction using chondrocyte allograft transplants. J Pediatr Orthop 1987;7(4):381–388.
80. Keret D, Mendez AA, Harcke HT, et al. Type V physeal injury: a case report. J Pediatr Orthop 1990;10(4):545–548.
81. Kruse RW, Tassanawipas A, Bowen JR. Orthopedic sequelae of meningococcemia. Orthopedics 1991;14(2):174–178.
82. Langenskiöld A. Growth disturbance after osteomyelitis of femoral condyles in infants. Acta Orthop Scand 1984;55(1):1–13.
83. Langenskiöld A. An operation for partial closure of an epiphysial plate in children, and its experimental basis. J Bone Joint Surg Br 1975;57(3):325–330.
84. Langenskiöld A. The possibilities of eliminating premature partial closure of an epiphyseal plate caused by trauma or disease. Acta Orthop Scand 1967;38:267–279.
85. Langenskiöld A. Surgical treatment of partial closure of the growth plate. J Pediatr Orthop 1981;1(1):3–11.
86. Langenskiöld A. Traumatic premature closure of the distal tibial epiphyseal plate. Acta Orthop Scand 1967;38(4):520–531.
87. Langenskiöld A, Osterman K, Valle M. Growth of fat grafts after operation for partial bone growth arrest: demonstration by computed tomography scanning. J Pedaitr Orthop 1987;7(4):389–394.
88. Langenskiöld A, Videman T, Nevalainen T. The fate of fat transplants in operations for partial closure of the growth plate. Clinical examples and an experimental study. J Bone Joint Surg Br 1986;68(2):234–238.
89. Lennox DW, Goldner RD, Sussman MD. Cartilage as an interposition material to prevent transphyseal bone bridge formation: an experimental model. J Pediatr Orthop 1983;3(2):207–210.
90. Liebling MS, Berdon WE, Ruzal-Shapiro C, et al. Gymnast's wrist (pseudorickets growth plate abnormality) in adolescent athletes: findings on plain films and MR imaging. AJR Am J Roentgenol 1995;164(1):157–159.
91. Lombardo S, Harvey J. Fractures of the distal femoral epiphysis. Factors influencing prognosis: a review of 34 cases. J Bone Joint Surg Am 1977;59(6):742–751.
92. Mann DC, Rajmaira S. Distribution of physeal and nonphyseal fractures in 2650 long-bone fractures in children aged 0 to 16 years. J Pediatr Orthop 1990;10(6):713–716.
93. Maresh MM. Linear growth of long bones of the extremities from infancy through adolescence. AMA Am J Dis Child 1955;89(6):725–742.
94. Martin RP, Parsons DL. Avascular necrosis of the proximal humeral epiphysis after physeal fracture. A case report. J Bone Joint Surg Am 1997;79(5):760–762.
95. Marzo JM, d'Amato C, Strong M, et al. Usefulness and accuracy of arthrography in management of lateral humeral condyle fractures in children. J Pediatr Orthop 1990; 10(3):317–321.
96. Mayer V, Marchisello PJ. Traumatic partial arrest of tibial physis. Clin Orthop Relat Res 1984;183:99–104.
97. Mendez AA, Bartal E, Grillot MB, et al. Compression (Salter-Harris type V) physeal fracture: an experimental model in the rat. J Pediatr Orthop 1992;12(1):29–37.
98. Métaizeau JP, Wong-Chung J, Bertrand H, et al. Percutaneous epiphysiodesis using transphyseal screws (PETS). J Pediatr Orthop 1998;18(3):363–369.
99. Mielke CH, Stevens PM. Hemiepiphyseal stapling for knee deformities in children younger than 10 years: a preliminary report. J Pediatr Orthop 1996;16(4):423–429.
100. Minami A, Sugawara M. Humeral trochlear hypoplasia secondary to epiphyseal injury as a cause of ulnar nerve palsy. Clin Orthop Relat Res 1988;228:227–232.
101. Mizuta T, Benson WM, Foster BK, et al. Statistical analysis of the incidence of physeal injuries. J Pedaitr Orthop 1987;7(5):518–523.
102. Moen, CT, Pelker RR. Biomechanical and histological correlations in growth plate failure. J Pediatr Orthop 1984;4(2):180–184.
103. Navascués JA, González-López JL, López-Valverde S, et al. Premature physeal closure after tibial diaphyseal fractures in adolescents. J Pediatr Orthop 2000;20(2):193–196.
104. Nouth F, Kuo LA. Percutaneous epiphysiodesis using transphyseal screws (PETS): prospective case study and review. J Pediatr Orthop 2004;24(6):721–725.
105. Ogden JA. Growth slowdown and arrest lines. J Pediatr Orthop 1984;4(4):409–415.
106. Ogden, JA. Skeletal growth mechanism injury patterns. J Pediatr Orthop 1982;2(4): 371–377.
107. Ogden JA, Ganey T, Light TR, et al. The pathology of acute chondro-osseous injury in the child. Yale J Biol Med 1993;66(3):219–233.
108. Ogden JA, Ogden DA, Pugh L, et al. Tibia valga after proximal metaphyseal fractures in childhood: a normal biologic response. J Pediatr Orthop 1995;15(4):489–494.
109. Osterman K. Operative elimination of partial premature epiphyseal closure: an experimental study. Acta Orthop Scand Suppl 1972;3–79.
110. Pape JM, Goulet JA, Hensinger RN. Compartment syndrome complicating tibial tubercle avulsion. Clin Orthop Relat Res 1993;295:201–204.
111. Peters W, Irving J, Letts M. Long-term effects of neonatal bone and joint infection on adjacent growth plates. J Pediatr Orthop 1992;12(6):806–810.
112. Peterson HA. Partial growth plate arrest and its treatment. J Pedaitr Orthop 1984;4(2): 246–258.
113. Peterson HA. Physeal fractures: part 2. Two previously unclassified types. J Pediatr Orthop 1994;14(4):431–438.
114. Peterson HA. Physeal fractures: part 3. Classification. J Pediatr Orthop 1994;14(4): 439–448.
115. Peterson HA. Premature physeal arrest of the distal tibia associated with temporary arterial insufficiency. J Pediatr Orthop 1993;13(5):672–675.
116. Peterson HA, Burkhart SS. Compression injury of the epiphyseal growth plate: fact or fiction? J Pediatr Orthop 1981;1(4):377–384.
117. Peterson HA, Madhok R, Benson JT, et al. Physeal fractures: part 1. Epidemiology in Olmsted County, Minnesota, 1979–1988. J Pediatr Orthop 1994;14(4):423–430.
118. Petit P, Panuel M, Faure F, et al. Acute fracture of the distal tibial physis: role of gradient-echo MR imaging versus plain film examination. AJR Am J Roentgenol 1996; 166(5):1203–1206.
119. Poland J, ed. Traumatic Separation of the Epiphysis. London; E. Smith and Company, 1898.
120. Rang M, ed. Injuries of the epiphyses, the growth plate, and the perichondral ring. Children's Fractures. Philadelphia: JB Lippincott, 1983, 10–25.
121. Riseborough EJ, Barrett IR, Shapiro F. Growth disturbances following distal femoral physeal fracture-separations. J Bone Joint Surg Am 1983;65(7):885–893.
122. Rivas R, Shapiro F. Structural stages in the development of the long bones and epiphyses: a study in the New Zealand white rabbit. J Bone Joint Surg Am 2002;84A-1: 85–100.
123. Robertson WW Jr, Butler MS, D'Angio GJ, et al. Leg length discrepancy following irradiation for childhood tumors. J Pediatr Orthop 1991;11(3):284–287.
124. Rudicel S, Pelker RR, Lee KE, et al. Shear fractures through the capital femoral physis of the skeletally immature rabbit. J Pediatr Orthop 1985;5(1):27–31.
125. Salter R, Harris W. Injuries involving the epiphyseal plate. J Bone Joint Surg 1963;45: 587–622.
126. Saltzman MD, King EC. Central physeal arrests as a manifestation of hypervitaminosis A. J Pediatr Orthop 2007;27(3):351–353.
127. Scheffer MM, Peterson HA. Opening-wedge osteotomy for angular deformities of long bones in children. J Bone Joint Surg Am 1994;76(3):325–334.
128. Sferopoulos NK. Fracture separation of the medial clavicular epiphysis: ultrasonography findings. Arch Orthop Trauma Surg 2003;123(7):367–369.
129. Shapiro F. Epiphyseal growth plate fracture-separation: a pathophysiologic approach. Orthopaedics 1982;5:720–736.
130. Shelton WR, Canale ST. Fractures of the tibia through the proximal tibial epiphyseal cartilage. J Bone Joint Surg Am 1979;61(2):167–173.
131. Skak SV. Valgus deformity following proximal tibial metaphyseal fracture in children. Acta Orthop Scand 1982;53(1):141–147.
132. Skak SV, Jensen TT, Poulsen TD. Fracture of the proximal metaphysis of the tibia in children. Injury 1987;18(3):149–156.
133. Smith BG, Rand F, Jaramillo D, et al. Early MR imaging of lower-extremity physeal fracture-separations: a preliminary report. J Pediatr Orthop 1994;14(4):526–533.
134. Smith DG, Geist RW, Cooperman DR. Microscopic examination of a naturally occurring epiphyseal plate fracture. J Pediatr Orthop 1985;5(3):306–308.
135. Stanton RP, Abdel-Mota'al MM. Growth arrest resulting from unicameral bone cyst. J Pediatr Orthop 1998;18(2):198–201.
136. Stevens PM, Pease F. Hemiepiphysiodesis for posttraumatic tibial valgus. J Pediatr Orthop 2006;26(3):385–392.
137. Sudmann E, Husby OS, Bang G. Inhibition of partial closure of epiphyseal plate in rabbits by indomethacin. Acta Orthop Scand 1982;53(4):507–511.

138. Trueta J, Amato VP. The vascular contribution to osteogenesis. III. Changes in the growth cartilage caused by experimentally induced ischaemia. J Bone Joint Surg Br 1960;42-B:571–587.
139. Trueta J, Morgan J. The vascular contribution to osteogenesis. I. Studies by the injection method. J Bone Joint Surg Br 1960;42-B:97–109.
140. Trueta J, Trias A. The vascular contribution to osteogenesis. IV. The effect of pressure upon the epiphyseal cartilage of the rabbit. J Bone Joint Surg Br 1961;43-B:800–813.
141. Valverde JA, Albiñana J, Certucha JA. Early posttraumatic physeal arrest in distal radius after a compression injury. J Pediatr Orthop B 1996;5(1):57–60.
142. Wattenbarger JM, Gruber HE, Phieffer LS. Physeal fractures, part I: histologic features of bone, cartilage, and bar formation in a small animal model. J Pediatr Orthop 2002; 22(6):703–709.
143. Williamson RV, Staheli LT. Partial physeal growth arrest: treatment by bridge resection and fat interposition. J Pediatr Orthop 1990;10(6):769–776.
144. Worlock P, Stower M. Fracture patterns in Nottingham children. J Pediatr Orthop 1986;6(6):656–660.
145. Yates C, Sullivan JA. Arthrographic diagnosis of elbow injuries in children. J Pediatr Orthop 1987;7(1):54–60.
146. Zhang AL, Exner GU, Wenger DR. Progressive genu valgum resulting from idiopathic lateral distal femoral physeal. J Pediatr Orthop 2008;28(7):752–756.
147. Zionts LE, Harcke HT, Brooks KM, et al. Posttraumatic tibia valga: a case demonstrating asymmetric activity at the proximal growth plate on technetium bone scan. J Pediatr Orthop 1987;7(4):458–462.

6

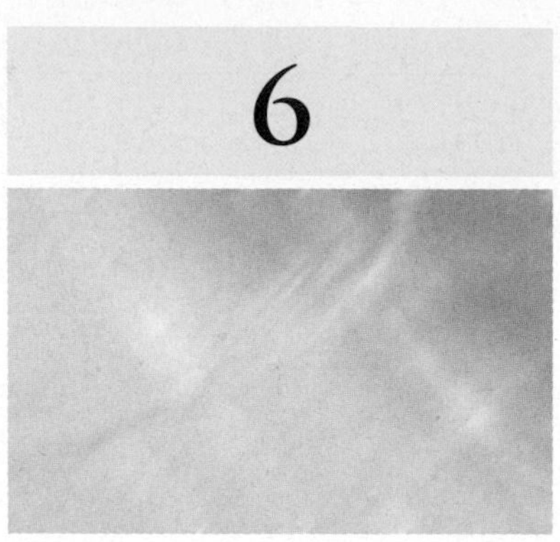

PATHOLOGIC FRACTURES ASSOCIATED WITH TUMORS AND UNIQUE CONDITIONS OF THE MUSCULOSKELETAL SYSTEM

Alexandre Arkader and John P. Dormans

INTRODUCTION 121

TUMORS OR TUMOR-LIKE PROCESSES 122
Unicameral Bone Cyst 122
Aneurysmal Bone Cyst 125
Fibrous Cortical Defects and Nonossifying Fibromas 129
Giant Cell Tumors of Bone 131
Enchondroma 132
Osteochondroma 135
Eosinophilic Granuloma (Langerhans Cell Histiocytosis) 135
Malignant Bone Tumors and Metastasis 138
Fibrous Dysplasia 141
Osteofibrous Dysplasia 143
Neurofibromatosis 143
Congenital Insensitivity to Pain 148

DISEASES OF THE BONE MARROW 148
Gaucher Disease 148
Sickle Cell Disease 150
Leukemia 151
Hemophilia 151
Osteomyelitis 153

PATHOLOGIC FRACTURES AFTER LIMB LENGTHENING 156

FRACTURES IN CONDITIONS THAT WEAKEN BONE 158
Osteogenesis Imperfecta 158
Osteopetrosis 163
Pyknodysostosis 164
Rickets 165
Idiopathic Osteoporosis 170
Iatrogenic Osteoporosis 170
Primary Hyperparathyroidism 171
Cushing Syndrome 173
Scurvy 173
Copper Deficiency and Scurvy-Like Syndrome 174

FRACTURES IN NEUROMUSCULAR DISEASE 175
Cerebral Palsy 175
Myelomeningocele 177
Muscular Dystrophy 181
Arthrogryposis and Poliomyelitis 181
Spinal Cord Injury 184

INTRODUCTION

Children and adolescents are often prone to musculoskeletal injuries and fractures due to their high activity level during recreational and sports activities. Whenever the structural characteristics and the inherited strength of the bone are compromised by a localized or generalized underlying disorder, the risk of fractures is increased. The combination of a previous bone abnormality and a fracture poses special challenges in the decision-making and management of these injuries. The definition of a pathologic fracture is one that occurs through abnormal bone. These abnormalities cause the bone to lack its normal biomechanical and viscoelastic properties. Pathologic fractures may result from localized or generalized bone weakness that originates from intrinsic or extrinsic processes. Examples of localized causes of bone weakness caused by an intrinsic process are tumors or tumor-like lesions; generalized causes due to an extrinsic process include osteopenia or osteoporosis of different etiologies.

This chapter describes the clinical and radiographic features of the most common causes of pediatric pathologic fractures, including specific patterns of injury and special concerns of treatment. The goals are to warn and prepare the orthopaedic surgeon for the correct diagnostic approach and management of these lesions.

The evaluation of a child with a pathologic fracture should start with a thorough history and physical examination. A well-taken history may especially help in the development of an accurate differential diagnosis. Key points that should be investigated include:

- Patient's age: Some lesions are more common in specific age groups, including benign and malignant tumors, as well as other generalized causes of bone weakness (Table 6-1).
- Characterization of the pain, if any:
  - Length: Although most bone tumors present with increasing pain of several days or weeks of duration, some present with recent pain. Chronic diseases or processes may also present with a chronic, intermittent pain.
  - Factors that make the pain better or worse, such as resting, pain medications (e.g., osteoid osteoma is a classic example of pain that improves rapidly with aspirin or nonsteroidal anti-inflammatory drugs).
  - Inflammatory signs: The presence of a bony lesion in view of increased temperature, redness, and swelling may indicate an infection.
  - Neurologic signs: Large lesions may present with compressive neurologic changes.
- Radiographic evaluation:
  - Where is the lesion? Different bone lesions are seen more frequently in specific areas of the body and the bone (Figs. 6-1 and 6-2).
  - What is the lesion's size and extent? Aggressive lesions tend to be larger and grow faster. Exceptions include fibrous dysplasia that may involve not only the entire bone but also several bones at the same time and nonetheless is a benign condition. Multiple lesions or generalized bone weakness may pose another challenge in the prevention and management of pathologic fractures.
  - What is the lesion doing to the bone? The pattern of bone involvement and/or destruction plays an important role in the bone strength. For example, lytic lesions (e.g., uni-

TABLE 6-1 Common Predisposing Factors for Pathologic Fractures by Peak Age Incidence

Age (Years)	Benign Lesions	Malignant Tumors	Generalized Causes
0–5	Eosinophilic granuloma Osteomyelitis	Metastatic tumors (neuroblastoma, Wilm) Leukemia Ewing sarcoma	Neuromuscular diseases (medications, disuse osteopenia) Osteogenesis imperfecta
5–10	Unicameral bone cyst Aneurysmal bone cyst Nonossifying fibroma Osteochondroma Fibrous dysplasia Enchondromatosis/Ollier Neurofibromatosis/Congenital pseudarthrosis of the tibia	Leukemia Osteogenic sarcoma Ewing sarcoma	Neuromuscular diseases (medications, disuse osteopenia) Osteogenesis imperfecta Other medications (e.g., steroids) Rickets Dietary deficiencies Osteopetrosis Bone marrow diseases
10–20	Unicameral bone cyst Aneurysmal bone cyst Nonossifying fibroma Osteochondroma Fibrous dysplasia Chondroblastoma Giant cell tumor	Leukemia Lymphoma Osteogenic sarcoma Ewing sarcoma	Neuromuscular diseases (medications, disuse osteopenia) Other medications (e.g., steroids) Stress fractures Dietary deficiencies Bone marrow diseases

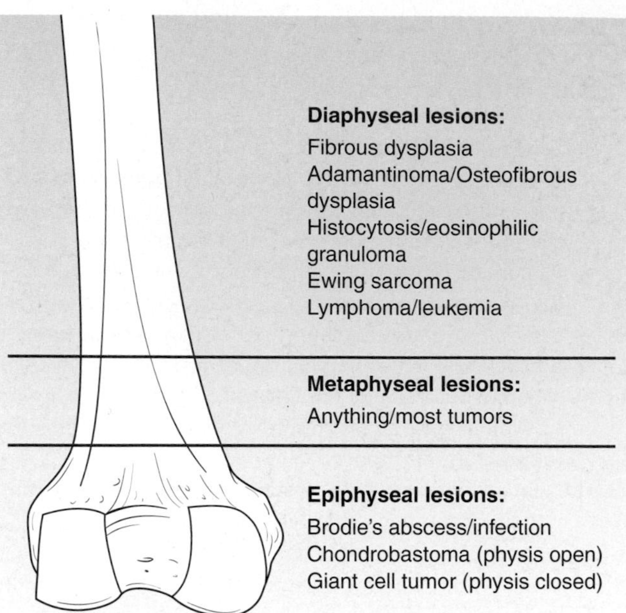

FIGURE 6-1 Schematic distribution of the most common benign and malignant bone lesions seen in the long bones in children.

cameral bone cyst) put the bone at a much higher risk of pathologic fracture than blastic lesions (e.g., osteoblastoma).

- What is the bone's response? If the bone has time to "compensate" for its destruction caused by a lesional process, new bone formation and cortical thickening may be observed and will to some point prevent or delay a pathologic fracture.
- Soft tissue mass? The presence of an associated soft tissue mass may be an indication of a more aggressive, perhaps malignant process; furthermore, the cortical adjacent to the associated soft tissue mass will often be severely weakened or destructed.

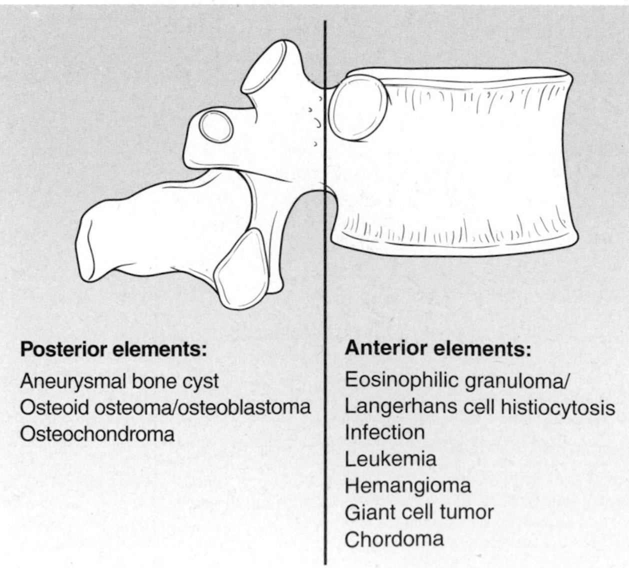

FIGURE 6-2 Schematic distribution of the most common benign and malignant bone tumors seen in the spine in children.

Several authors have attempted to predict the likelihood of a "weakened" to fracture due to a minor trauma. Most studies, however, are based in the study of metastatic disease in adults.[220] More recently, quantitative computerized tomography (CT) has been used with success to predict the risk of pathologic fractures in children with cystic lesions of the bone. The combination of bending and torsional a rigidity measured noninvasively with quantitative CT was found to be more accurate (97%) for predicting pathologic fracture through benign bone lesions in children than the standard radiographic criteria (42% to 61% accuracy).[223,479]

Another important consideration in the management of pathologic fracture is that usually the underlying cause has to be addressed in order to achieve a successful healing of the fracture. For that reason, is not uncommon that some of the classic principles of fracture treatment in children are often altered in order to adapt to this new situation. In another words, the treatment plan must consider both the treatment of the fracture and the its underlying cause.

TUMORS OR TUMOR-LIKE PROCESSES

Benign tumors can be classified according to their aggressiveness (Table 6-2). Stage 1, or latent benign lesions, are usually asymptomatic, discovered incidentally, and seldom associated with pathologic fracture. Stage 2 lesions are intermediate in behavior, and stage 3, or aggressive benign lesions, are usually symptomatic, grow rapidly, and may be associated with pathologic fracture.

Unicameral Bone Cyst

Unicameral bone cyst (UBC), also known as simple bone cyst, is a benign, active or latent, solitary cystic lesion that usually involves the metaphysis or metadiaphysis of long bones. Approximately 40% to 80% of these lesions are seen in the proximal humerus and proximal femur.[374,375] In order of decreasing frequency, UBCs are most commonly seen in the proximal humerus, proximal femur, proximal tibia, distal tibia, distal femur, calcaneous, distal humerus, radius, fibula, ilium, ulna, and rib.[374,375] Although its etilogy is still unknown, theories range

TABLE 6-2 Classification of Benign Lesions According to Their Aggressiveness

Stage 1, Latent Benign
Asymptomatic
Often discovered incidentally
Seldom associated with pathologic fracture
Stage 2, Active Benign
Majority
Tend to grow steadily
May be symptomatic
Stage 3, Aggressive Benign
Generally symptomatic
Discomfort, usually tender
May be associated with pathologic fracture
Growth rapid

from UBC being a reactive or developmental process caused by obstruction to the drainage of intersticial fluid, to a true neoplasm.[91,96] Isolated cytogenetic analysis have reported on the presence of a translocation t(16;20)(p11.2;q13) and TP53 mutations in recurrent cases of UBC.[506] It is unclear whether genetic alterations truly play a role in its pathogenesis.

UBCs may be classified as to their relationship to the growth plate: inactive or latent cysts tend to "migrate" away from the growth plate as longitudinal growth occurs and therefore are far from the epiphysis; active cysts are in close relationship with the physeal line and growth arrest may occur prior to treatment.[374,375]

Approximately 90% of the patients diagnosed with UBC are younger than 20 years old; furthermore, UBCs may regress spontaneously after skeletal maturity.[91,521] The male to female ratio is about 2:1.[78,375] UBCs are often asymptomatic and, in more than 70% of cases, the initial presentation is with a pathologic fracture following minor trauma.[82,130,131,521] The fractures are usually incomplete or minimally displaced. The fractures tend to heal in approximately 6 weeks, and in less than 10% of the cases the cyst will heal following fracture healing.[8,126,129] Lower extremity fractures, particularly around the hip, often need surgical intervention.

Plain radiographs are usually sufficient for the diagnosis. UBC is a well defined, centrally located, radiolucent/lytic cystic lesion, usually surrounded by a sclerotic margin and narrow zone of transition. Cortical thinning and mild expansion are common. When a pathologic fracture occurs, there is periosteal reaction and occasionally the typical "fallen fragment" sign is visualized (fragment of bone "floating" inside the fluid-filled cystic cavity). CT is useful for lesions located in areas that are of difficult visualization on plain films (e.g., spine, pelvis) and to rule out minimally displaced fractures. Magnetic resonance imaging (MRI) is sometimes used for differential diagnosis of atypical UBCs. Although the characteristics are nonspecific, UBCs usually present as low to intermediate signals on T1-weighted images and a bright and homogeneous signals on T2-weighted images (Fig. 6-3).[330]

Although the radiographic appearance of UBCs is very typical, the differential diagnoses include aneurysmal bone cyst,[484] nonossifying fibroma, fibrous dysplasia, brown tumor of hyperparathyroidism, bone abscess, and, for calcaneous lesions, chondroblastoma and giant cell tumor. Diaphyseal tumors may look very similar to fibrous dysplasia.

Natural History

With time, UBCs tend to stabilize in size and "migrate" away from the growth plate. Although some lesions heal or disappear spontaneously at puberty,[374,375] the majority will persist into adulthood (Table 6-3).

Lesions that have the typical radiographic appearance and therefore do not warrant biopsy for diagnostic confirmation, particularly those lesions in non–weight-bearing bones, can be followed with serial radiographs.

Large lesions that involve more than 50% to 80% of the bone diameter and lesions that are associated with marked cortical thinning are at high risk of fractures and warrant prophylactic treatment.[215,481] Lesions of weight-bearing bones, especially around the hip, need to be addressed (Fig. 6-4). Although several attempts have been made to predict the true risk of pathologic fracture associated with bone cysts, most of the data are related to other lesions, particularly among adults. More recently, CT has been shown to be useful predicting the likelihood of fracture. This method uses a computerized regression system and may help deciding which cysts warrant intervention.[481]

Although spontaneous resolution of UBCs following fracture may occur in up to 15% of the cases (Fig. 6-5), pathologic fractures associated with UBCs do not always heal uneventfully. Malunion, growth arrest, and osteonecrosis (ON) (proximal femoral fractures) are some of the commonly reported complications.[244,321]

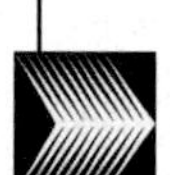

AUTHORS' PREFERRED METHOD

Our preferred treatment involves percutaneous intramedullary decompression, curettage, and grafting with medical-grade calcium-sulfate pellets.[126,130]

Some authors believe that relieving the pressure of the intersticial fluid in the lesions can heal the cyst. Chigira et al.[91] used multiple Kirschner-wires to decompress the cyst; Santori et al.[452] used Enders or Rush nails to decompress the cyst. Other methods have been used including cannulated screws. New grafting materials have also been used including demineralized bone matrix,[445] medical-grade calcium sulfate, and others. Dormans et al.[130] described a new minimally invasive technique that combines the different steps of several techniques and is done percutaneously under image guidance.

Surgical Technique

- Under fluoroscopic guidance, a Jamshidi trocared needle (CardinalHalth, Dublin, OH) is percutaneously inserted into the cyst cavity, preferably in the middle of the cyst.
- The cyst is aspirated to confirm the presence of straw-colored fluid.
- Three to 10 mL of Renografin dye (E.R. Squibb, Princeton, NJ) are injected to perform a cystogram and confirm the single fluid-filled cavity.
- A 0.5-cm longitudinal incision is then made over the site of the aspiration and a 6-mm arthroscopy trocar is advanced into the cyst cavity through the same cortical hole. The cortical entry is then enlarged manually.
- Under fluroscopic guidance, percutaneous removal of the cyst lining is done with curved curettes and a pituitary rongeur.
- An angled curette and/or flexible intramedullary nail is used to perform the intramedullary decompression in one direction (toward diaphysis) or in both directions (if the growth plate is far enough to avoid injury).
- Bone grafting is done with medical-grade calcium sulfate pellets (Osteoset, Wright Medical Technology, Arlington, TN) inserted through the same cortical hole and deployed to completely fill the cavity. The pellets do not offer structural support but act as a scaffolding for new bone formation and cyst healing. Angled curettes can be used to

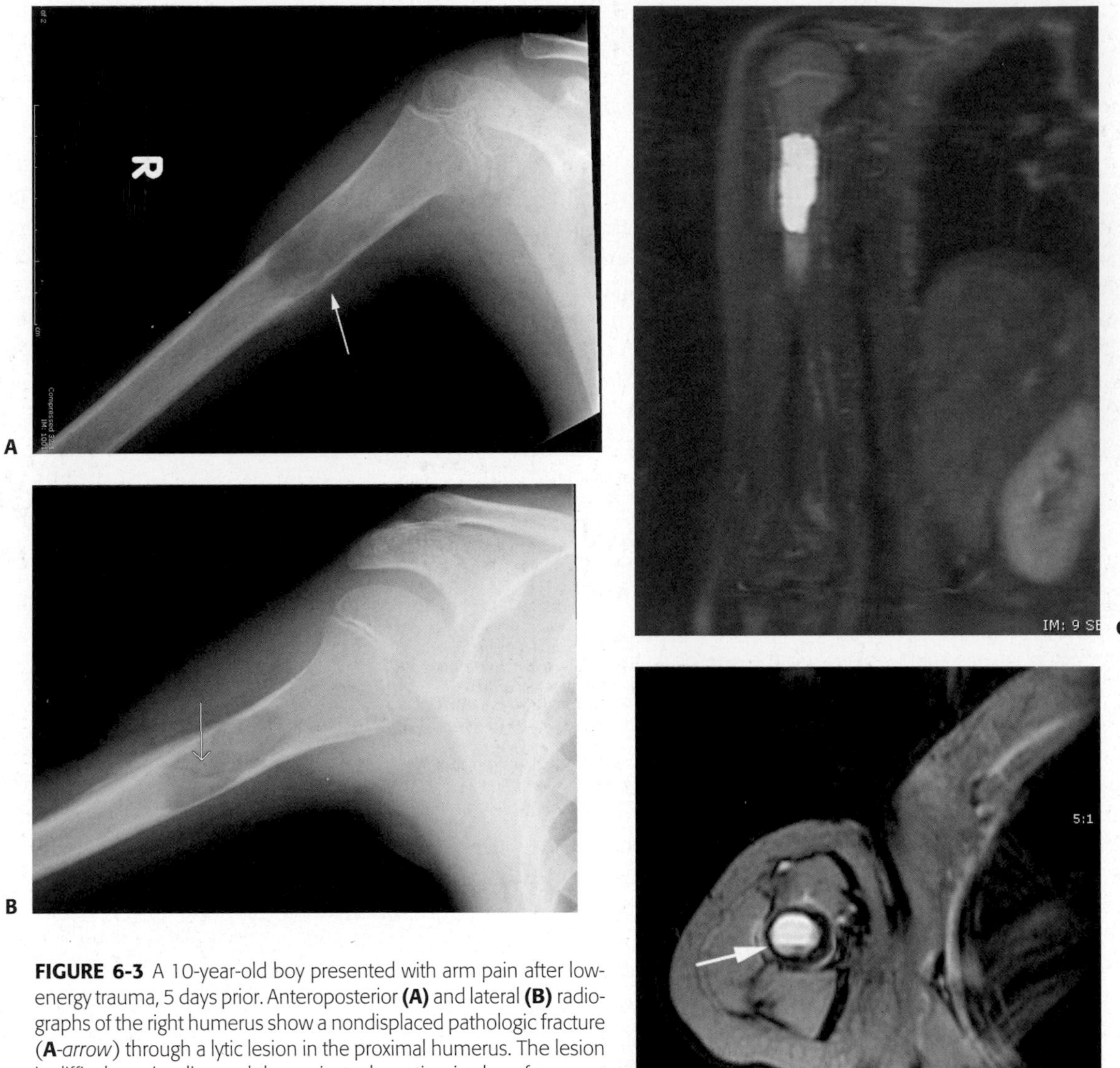

FIGURE 6-3 A 10-year-old boy presented with arm pain after low-energy trauma, 5 days prior. Anteroposterior **(A)** and lateral **(B)** radiographs of the right humerus show a nondisplaced pathologic fracture (**A**-*arrow*) through a lytic lesion in the proximal humerus. The lesion is difficult to visualize and the periosteal reaction is also of concern (**B**-*arrow*). T2-weighted MRI images show a well-defined, fluid-filled cystic lesion, with fluid–fluid levels (**D**-*arrow*) and no soft tissue mass or other worrisome signs in the coronal **(C)** and axial **(D)** cuts. The diagnosis was consistent with unicameral bone cyst and conservative treatment was recommended. (Figures reproduced with permission from The Childrens Orthopaedic Center, Los Angeles, CA.)

TABLE 6-3 Staging of Unicameral Bone Cysts

	Active	Inactive or "Latent"
Age of the patient	<10–12 years	>12 years
Location	Abutting the physis	Separated from physis by a zone of normal cancellous bone
Radiographic appearance	Single cavity	Multiloculated cavity
Intralesional pressure	>30 cm H_2O	6–10 cm H_2O
Pathology	Thin shiny membrane, few osteocytes, little or no hemosiderin, osteoclasts	Thick membrane, frequent giant cells, cholesterol slits, hemosiderin, osteoblasts

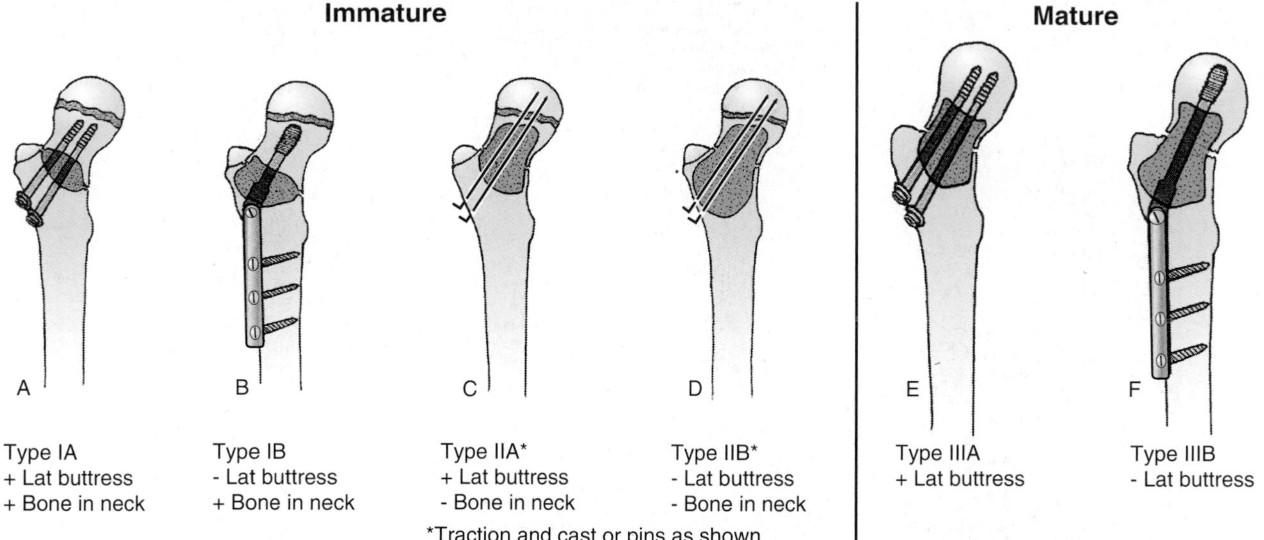

FIGURE 6-4 Classification system for the treatment of pathologic fractures of the proximal femur associated with bone cysts in children. **A.** In type IA, a moderately sized cyst is present in the middle of the femoral neck. There is enough bone in the femoral neck and lateral proximal femur (lateral buttress) to allow fixation with cannulated screws, avoiding the physis, after curettage and bone grafting. **B.** In type IB, a large cyst is present at the base of the femoral neck. There is enough bone proximally in the femoral neck but there is loss of lateral buttress, so a pediatric hip screw and a side plate should be considered rather than cannulated screws after curettage and bone grafting. **C,D.** In type II A-B, a large lesion is present in the femoral neck, so there is not enough bone beneath the physis to accept screws. There are two options for treatment of these bone cysts: (i) after curettage and bone grafting, parallel smooth pins across the physis can be used in combination with spica cast; (ii) the patient can be treated in traction until the fracture heals (with subsequent spica cast) followed by curettage and bone grafting. **E,F.** In type IIIA-B, the physis is closing or closed. The lateral buttress is present in type IIIA hips, so cannulated screws can be used to stabilize the fracture after curettage and bone grafting. In type IIIB hips, the loss of lateral buttress makes it necessary to use a pediatric hip screw and a side plate following curettage and bone grafting. In all types, we recommend spica cast immobilization after surgery.

advance pellets into the medullary canal, which also confirms adequate decompression. Tight packing of the cyst is preferred.

- The wound is closed in a layered fashion.

Aneurysmal Bone Cyst

Aneurysmal bone cysts (ABCs)[484] are benign, locally aggressive bone tumors. They are well-defined, eccentric or central, expansile, osteolytic, blood-filled lesions usually seen in the metaphyseal region of long bones or in the posterior elements of the spine. ABCs have a tendency to expand beyond the width of the epiphyseal plate. Approximately 75% of ABCs are seen in patients younger than 20 years old, and 50% are seen in individuals between 10 and 20 years of age.[78,103,297] The estimated incidence ABCs is of approximately 1.4 cases per 100,000, representing around 1.5% of all primary bone tumors.[103,297]

The long bones are involved in approximately 65% of patients.[103,455] In order of decreasing frequency, the most commonly involved bones are the femur (~20%), tibia (~17%), spine (~15%), humerus (~13%), pelvis (~8%), and fibula (~7%).[103,455] The vertebrae are involved in 12% to 27% of patients.[78,103,455] The lumbar vertebrae are most commonly affected.[63] The primary site of involvement is the posterior elements of the spine with frequent extension into the vertebral body.[63,169,394,397]

The lesions are not true cysts but rather sponge-like collections of interconnected fibrous tissue and blood-filled spaces.[109] They tend to be destructive lesions, which replace bone and thin the cortices of the host bone. The elevated viable periosteum usually maintains a thin osseous shell.

The etiology of ABCs is still unknown. The neoplastic basis of primary ABCs has been in part demonstrated by the chromossomal translocation t(16;17)(q22;p13) that places the ubiquitin protease USP6 gene under the regulatory influence of the highly active osteoblast cadherin 11 gene, which is strongly expressed in bones.[388] There is a fairly high incidence of ABCs associated with other benign and malignant tumors such as UBCs, nonossifying fibromas, fibrous dysplasia, and osteogenic sarcoma.[109,303,335] The most common presenting symptom is localized pain and/or swelling of less than 6 months duration. Spinal lesions may present with radicular pain.[78,115,169,178,275,394]

On plain radiographs, ABCs present as an eccentric lytic lesion. Although usually the overlying cortex is intact, sometimes a cortical disruption is identified. When that occurs, a reactive periosteal reaction is seen.[60,275,493] Cystic septation is common, giving rise to the so-called soap bubble or honeycomb appearance. Lesions in the short tubular bones, such as the metacarpals and metatarsals, are commonly more central. Spine involvement is characteristically of the posterior elements; how-

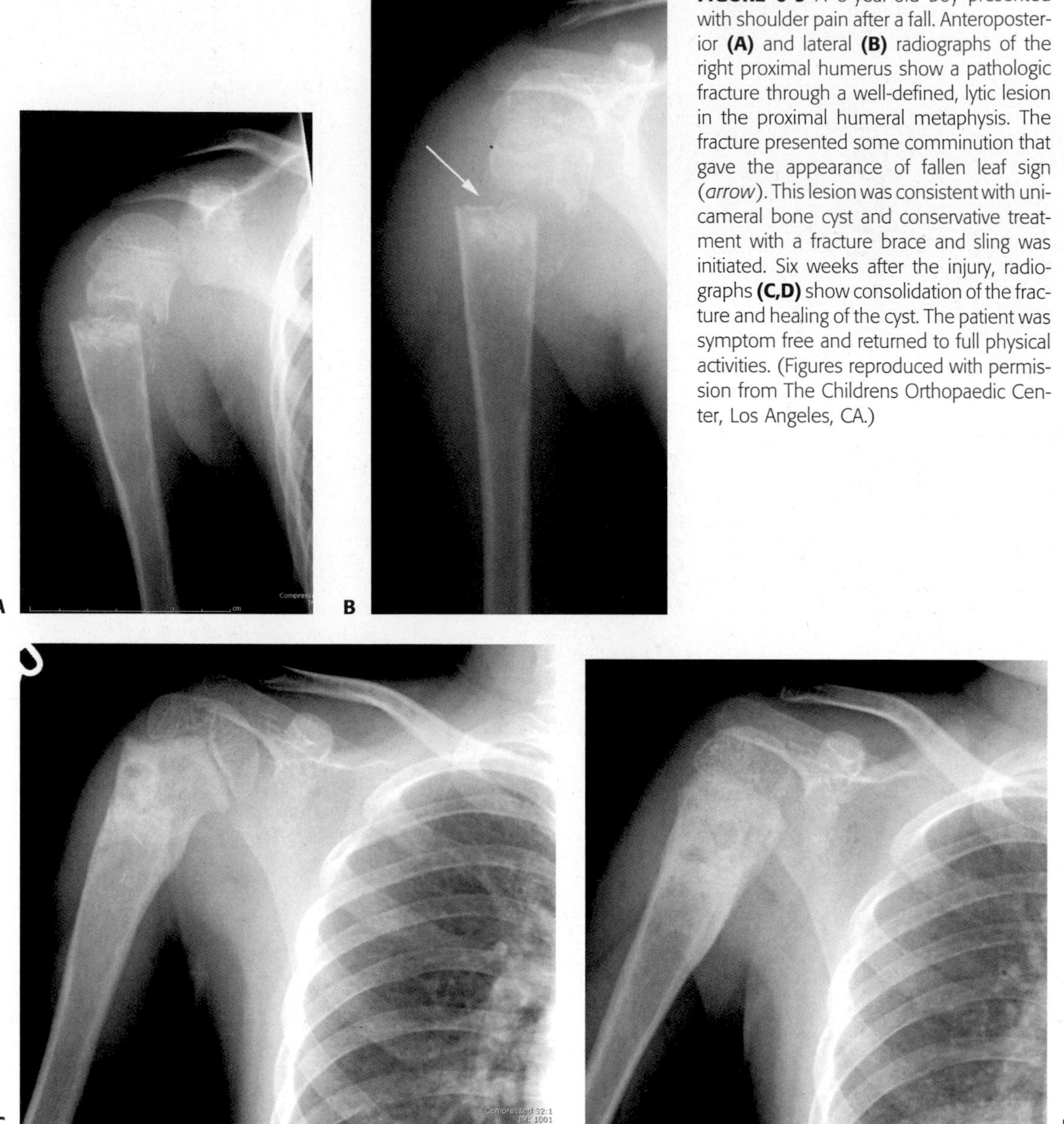

FIGURE 6-5 A 6-year-old boy presented with shoulder pain after a fall. Anteroposterior **(A)** and lateral **(B)** radiographs of the right proximal humerus show a pathologic fracture through a well-defined, lytic lesion in the proximal humeral metaphysis. The fracture presented some comminution that gave the appearance of fallen leaf sign (*arrow*). This lesion was consistent with unicameral bone cyst and conservative treatment with a fracture brace and sling was initiated. Six weeks after the injury, radiographs **(C,D)** show consolidation of the fracture and healing of the cyst. The patient was symptom free and returned to full physical activities. (Figures reproduced with permission from The Childrens Orthopaedic Center, Los Angeles, CA.)

ever, extension to the anterior body may occur. Pathologic fracture and vertebral collapse may occur and vertebra plana has been described.[60,63,95,178,398]

The radiographic picture evolves with time. Initially, the lesion is mostly lytic; with growth there is progressive destruction of bone with poorly demarcated margins. This is followed by a stabilization phase, with formation of a bone shell with septa. Later, with further ossification, a bony mass begins to form.[109] Characteristically, lesions near the growth plate tend to expand beyond the width of the adjacent epiphysis (Fig. 6-6). MRI is often helpful in obtaining better definition of axial lesions and in demonstrating the characteristic double density fluid level, septation, low signal on T1 images, and high intensity on T2 images; however, these findings are not pathognomonic for ABC.[493]

Campanacci et al.[78] have classified the ABCs into three groups. An aggressive cyst has signs of reparative osteogenesis with ill-defined margins and no periosteal shell. An active cyst has an incomplete periosteal shell and a defined margin between the lesion and the host bone. An inactive cyst has a complete periosteal shell and a sclerotic margin between the cyst and the long bone (Fig. 6-7).

Natural History

ABCs are benign but locally aggressive tumors. Pathologic fractures occur in 11% to 35% of patients with ABCs of the long bones.[129,169,275,394] The humerus and femur are the most commonly fractured long bones.[169,274,394] The incidence of pathologic fracture associated with spinal lesions is approximately 20%.[63,115,178] Epiphyseal involvement due to extension of metaphyseal/juxtaepiphyseal lesions may occur, and although it is rare, it may cause growth disturbance.[83] Conservative treatment with immobilization is inappropriate as a definitive treatment for pathologic fractures of ABCs. Although the pathologic fracture will heal, the ABC will persist, if not enlarge, and a recurrent pathologic fracture will most likely occur.

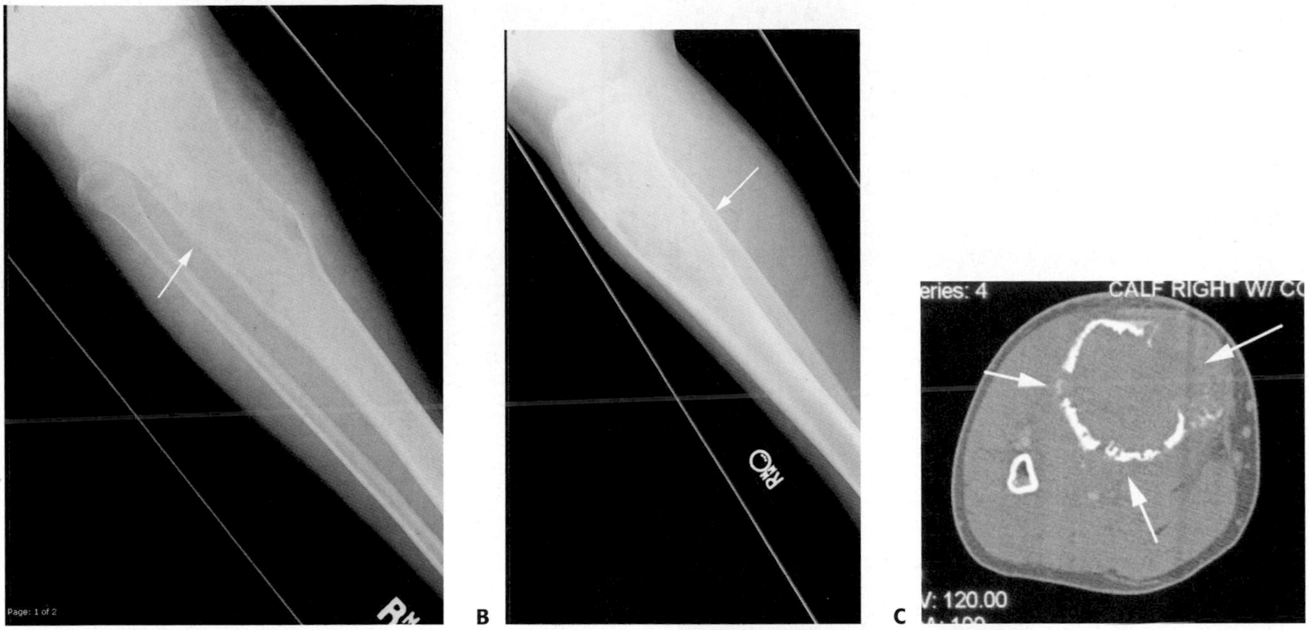

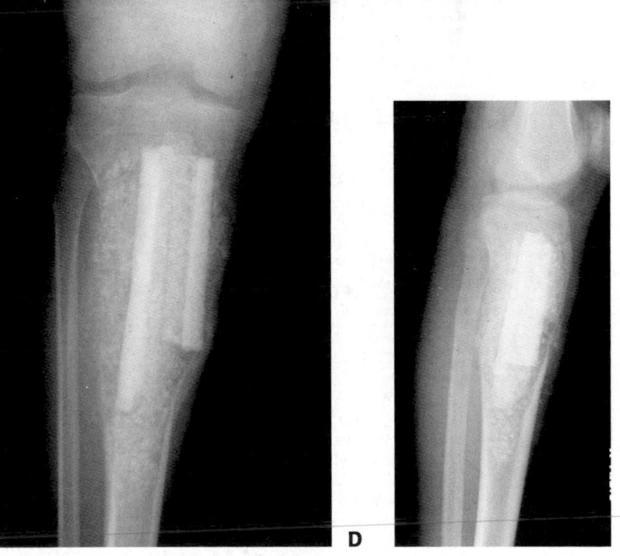

FIGURE 6-6 A 14-year-old boy presented with acute right leg pain following a fall from his bicycle. He reported previous intermittent pain over that same area. On initial plain radiographs **(A,B)** there is a large, expansile, and destructive lesion in the proximal tibial metaphysis. The bone is mildly expanded and there is a minimally displaced pathologic fracture (*arrow*). Axial CT image **(C)** better defines the extensive cortical disruption and soft tissue involvement postfracture anterior–medially. The patient underwent biopsy confirming the diagnosis of aneurysmal bone cyst. After the final pathology report was available, he underwent intralesional excision of the mass with curettage, high-speed burr, electro-cauterization, cryosurgery, and bone grafting with a combination of a strut allograft and crushed cancellous allograft **(D,E).** (Figures reproduced with permission from the Childrens Orthopaedic Center, Los Angeles, CA.)

Although simple intralesional curettage and bone grafting has been advised by many authors, recurrence rates are as high as 30%.[127,183,507] Several authors have shown that the recurrence is higher among younger children.[39,99,127,169,394] Freiberg et al.[169] treated ABCs with curettage and bone grafting in seven patients younger than 10 years of age and noted recurrence in five of the seven patients at an average of 8 months after the first procedure.

Due to the high recurrence rate, several authors attempted the use of surgical adjuvant. Cryotherapy in conjunction with

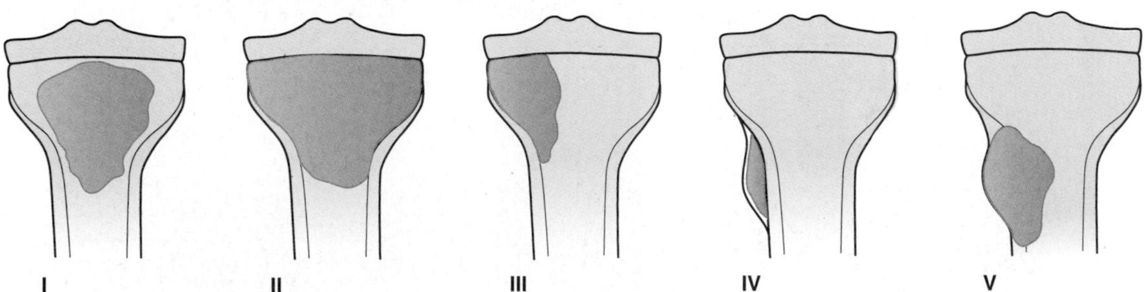

FIGURE 6-7 Classification of morphologic types of aneurysmal bone cyst. (From Campanna R, Bettelli G, Biagini R, et al. Aneurysmal cysts of long bones. Ital J Orthop Traumatol 1985;XI:421–429, with permission.)

curettage has a recurrence rate of between 8% and 14%.[329,455] Polymethylmethacrylate cementation has also been described as an adjuvant to curettage.

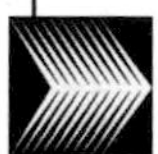

AUTHORS' PREFERRED METHOD

Four-Step Approach Resection[127,178]

This technique has been previously described and it is based on the notion that there is high recurrence rate associated with simple intralesional curettage. In the reported series, the recurrence rate for appendicular lesions was as low as 8%.[127] It also takes into account the advent of modern imaging techniques that help with preoperative planning as well as intraoperative guidance.[127,178] We recommend the use of headlamps for enhanced illumination and loupes for magnification. An image intensifier is available for intraoperative confirmation of complete tumor excision and appropriate bone grafting. Diagnostic tissue confirmation is essential part of this technique. For large spinal tumors, preoperative embolization is recommended (Fig. 6-8). If instrumentation is needed after spine tumors resection, we recommend titanium instrumentation that gives a much better visualization of the spine (less artifact) than stainless steel (Fig. 6-9).

Surgical Technique

- Under fluoroscopic guidance, a small longitudinal incision is made over the cyst. No flaps are created, and the dissection is carried down to the lesion level. The cyst wall is usually easily penetrated with curettes. Care should be taken to control eventual significant bleeding at the time of cyst penetration.
- Lesional tissue is than retrieved and sent for frozen section for diagnostic confirmation.
- Upon diagnostic confirmation, the cortical window is enlarged using roungers or a high-speed burr to allow appropriate visualization and excision. Using angled and straight curettes of different sizes, the intralesional resection/curettage is performed (Step 1).
- After the first step, the high speed burr is used to extend the intralesional margins as well to excise any residual tumoral cells (Step 2).
- Step 3 entails the use of electrocautery. This has two goals: first, it helps identify residual tumor pockets and second, has the theoretical capability of killing residual tumor cells.
- Adjuvant in the form of phenol solution 5% is used for appendicular lesions (Step 4).
- The lesion is now completely excised and bone grafting is performed, usually using a combination of allograft cancellous cubes and demineralized bone matrix paste. Tight packing of the cyst is preferred.
- Internal fixation is done on case-by-case basis. Lesions of weight-bearing bones, particularly of the proximal femur, and some large vertebral lesions may warrant internal fixation/instrumentation following the 4-step approach.
- The wound is closed in a layered fashion.

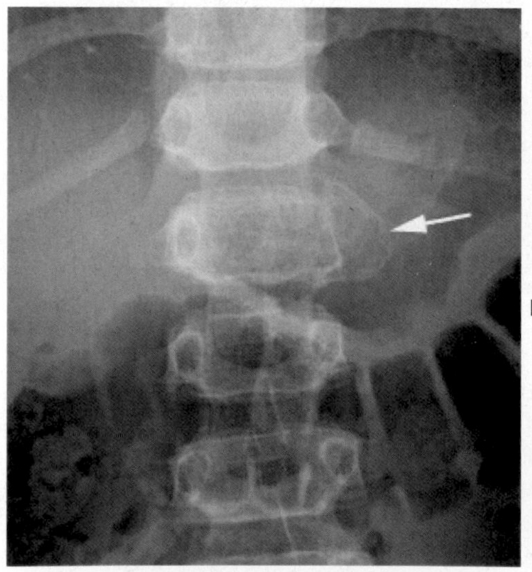

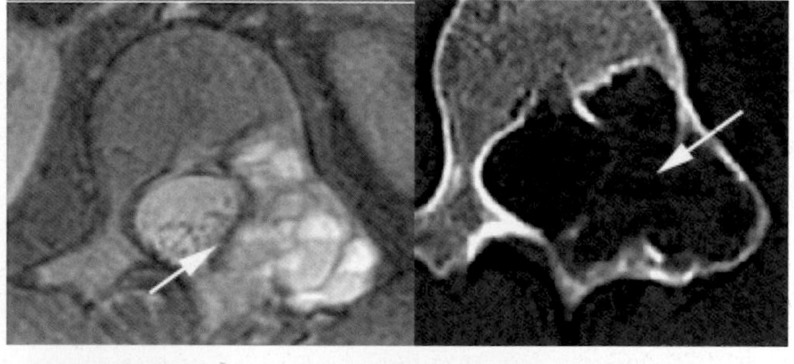

FIGURE 6-8 A 9-year-old boy presented with low back pain and abdominal discomfort. On plain radiographs of the abdomen **(A)**, an expansile lesion involving the left posterior elements of L1 was visualized. Axial T2-weighted MRI **(B)** and an axial CT scan image **(C)** show the microfractures at the pedicle and lamina level (*arrow*) and the fluid–fluid levels. The patient underwent open biopsy that confirmed the diagnosis of aneurysmal bone cyst, followed by a 4-step approach excision and bone grafting. Limited instrumentation of the spine was performed due to stability compromise **(D)**. (Permission)

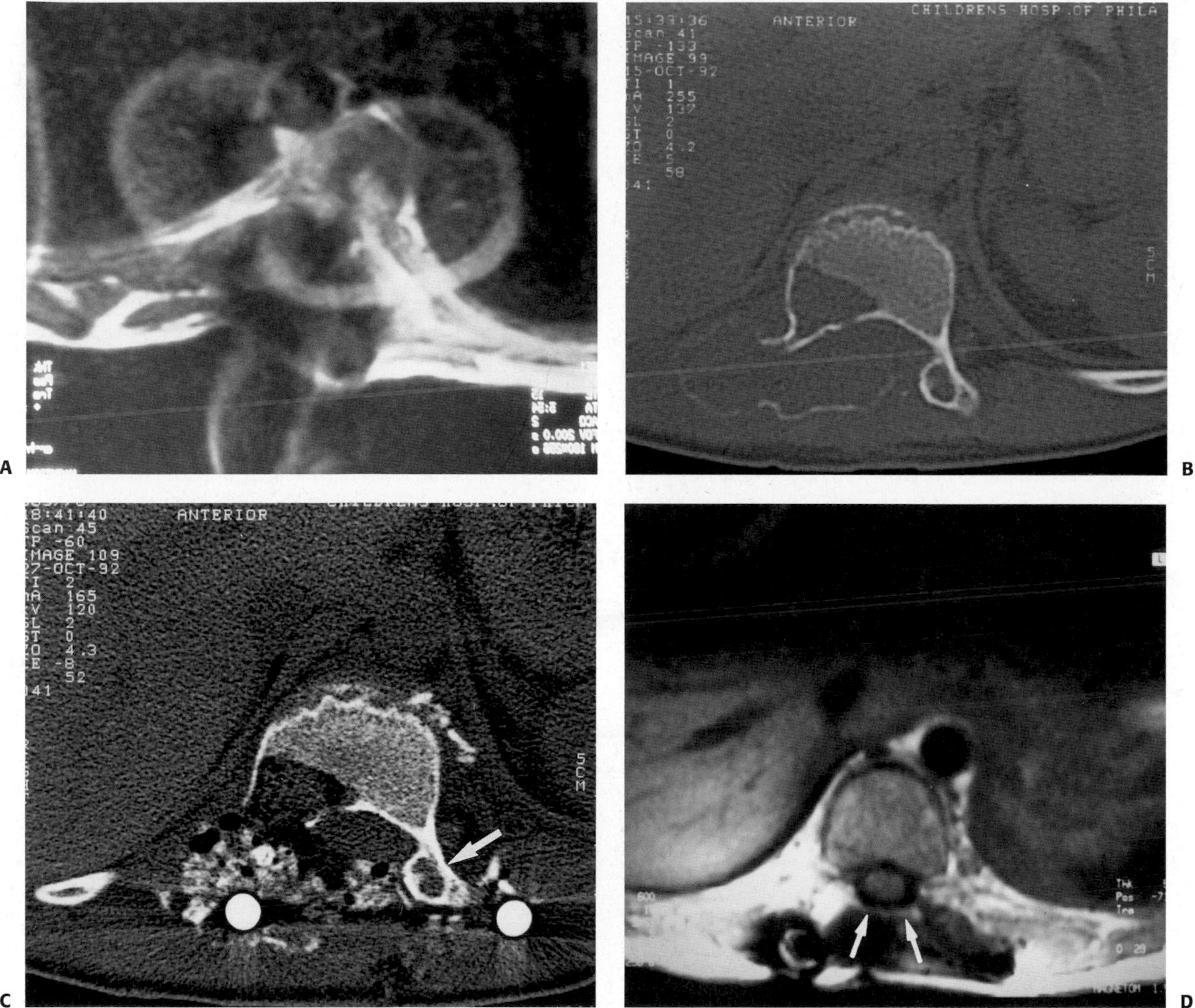

FIGURE 6-9 When dealing with pathologic fractures secondary to tumors or tumor-like processes of the spine, if instrumentation is needed, titanium instrumentation allows much better postoperative visualization with both CT and MRI for the detection of tumor recurrence as compared with standard stainless-steel instrumentation. **A.** Postoperative MRI of the spine with standard stainless-steel instrumentation showing a large degree of artifact that makes interpretation difficult. **B.** Preoperative CT scan of a patient with an ABC of the spine. **C.** Postoperative CT scan of the same patient showing an adequate view of the surgical area. **D.** Postoperative MRI of a patient with a previous spinal tumor again adequately showing the surgical site to monitor for recurrence or persistent tumor.

Fibrous Cortical Defects and Nonossifying Fibromas

Fibrous cortical defects (FCDs) are the most common bone tumor or tumor-like condition seen in the growing child. Both FCDs and the larger variant known as nonossifying fibroma (NOF) may be associated with pathologic fractures in children. These lesions are characterized by the presence of fibrous tissue, foam cells, and multinucleated giant cells.[107] Pathologic fractures through these lesions occur more commonly in boys between 6 and 14 years old.[80]

FCDs are small, well-defined, intracortical, metaphyseal lesions surrounded by a sclerotic rim with localized cortical thinning, ranging from 1 to 2 cm in diameter and most commonly found in the distal femur, proximal tibia, and fibula. FCDs can be seen on radiographic studies of the lower extremity in approximately 25% of pediatric patients.[80,107,432] In view of their usually asymptomatic nature, it is difficult to estimate the true incidence. They usually require no treatment other than observation.

NOFs present at a similar age as FCDs and follow a similar distribution of bone involvement; however, multiple lesions are present in approximately one third of patients.[80,133] Radiographically, they present as a well-defined, eccentric radiolucent cystlike lesion of the metaphysis that may be mostly intracortical or intramedullary and are usually larger than 4 cm,[21] sometimes extending across a substantial portion of the width of the long bone.[107] NOFs are usually asymptomatic unless a pathologic fracture is present.[21,107]

Natural History

Several authors have suggested that FCDs and NOFs regress spontaneously[80,133,139,432] with time, the defects become sclerotic and resolve.[432] Typically, this tumor remains asymptomatic and is commonly an incidental radiographic finding. However, lesions with extensive cortical involvement can cause pathologic fractures.

Previous reports suggest that the absolute size of the lesion correlates directly with the risk of pathologic fracture.[21] Based on this factor, prophylactic curettage and bone grafting of larger NOFs have been recommended. Arata et al.[21] noted that all pathologic fractures associated with NOFs in the lower extremity occurred through lesions involving more than 50% of the transverse cortical diameter. These large lesions were defined as exhibiting more than 50% cortical involvement on anteroposterior (AP) and lateral radiographic studies and a height measurement of more than 33 mm.[21] In their series, 43% of the pathologic fractures through NOFs were in the distal tibia. Although the authors recommended careful observation of these large NOFs, they suggested that "prophylactic curettage and bone grafting be considered if there is a reasonable chance of fracture."[21] Their series does not include any large lesions meeting their size criteria that did not fracture, and their hypothesis has never been tested in any published series. Drennan et al.[133] suggested that large NOFs causing pain might predispose to fracture and recommended prophylactic curettage and bone grafting for selected larger lesions.

Operative Treatment

Fractures through NOFs exhibit excellent healing potential,[21,107,133] but the lesion usually persists after healing of the fracture (Fig. 6-10). Recurrent fractures have been reported, but the incidence of refracture is low.[21,133] In theory, since fracture healing does not usually obliterate the lesions (lesion healing), recurrent fracture can occur.[21,139]

Large lesions, defined as having a diameter more than 50% of the width of a long bone on both AP and lateral radiographs, are believed to be prone to pathologic fracture, and most authors have recommended curettage and bone grafting for these large lesions.[21,107,133,139]

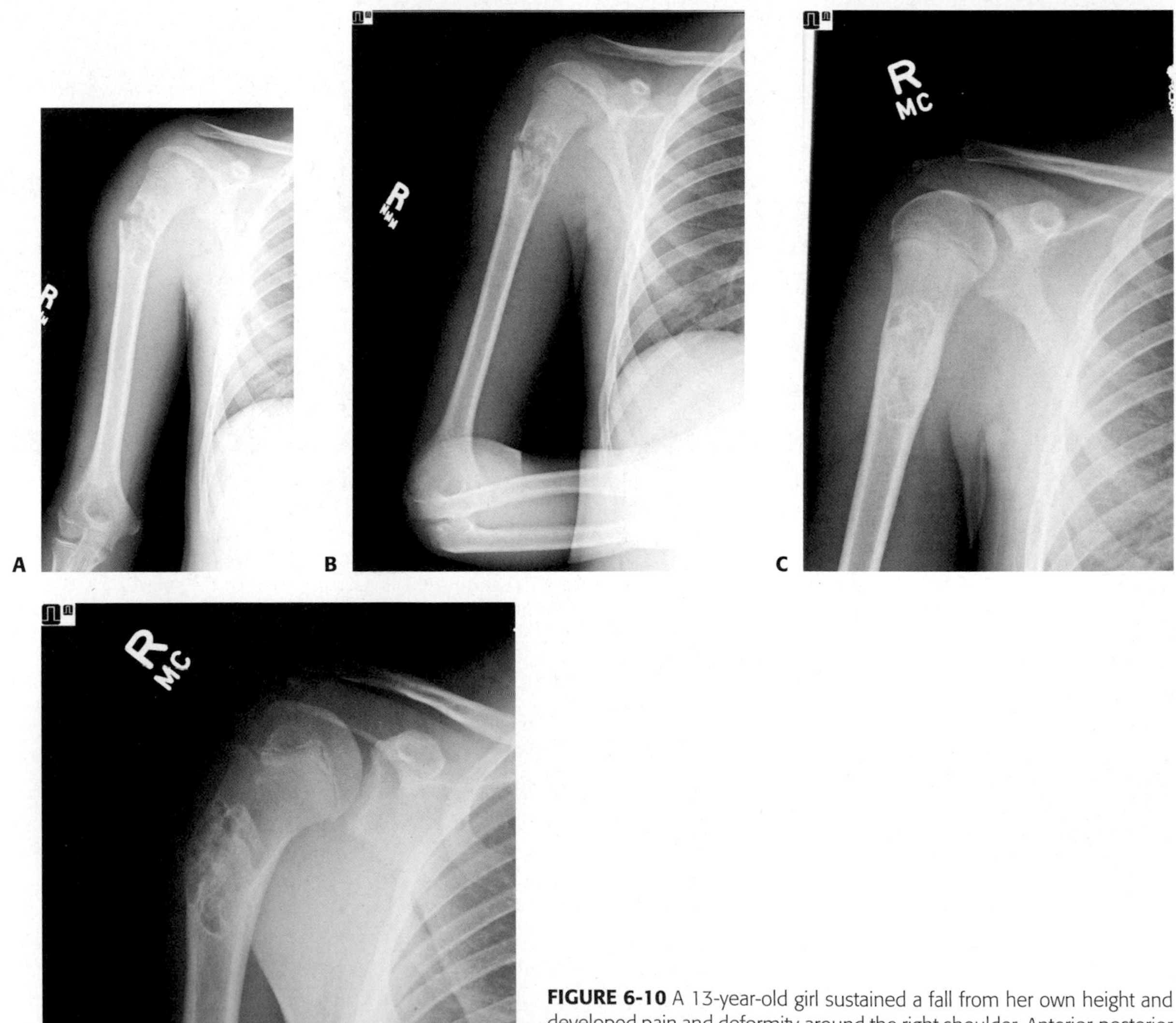

FIGURE 6-10 A 13-year-old girl sustained a fall from her own height and developed pain and deformity around the right shoulder. Anterior-posterior **(A)** and lateral **(B)** plain films show a pathologic fracture through a well-defined, eccentric, cortical based lesion in the proximal humerus metaphysis. There is sharp sclerotic rim and the lesion was clinically diagnosed as nonossifying fibroma. After 4 weeks of conservative treatment, the fractured healed **(C,D)** in a few degrees of varus and the lesion persisted.

Easley and Kneisel[139] reported that although absolute size parameters were helpful in predicting pathologic fracture, they did not imply a requirement for prophylactic curettage and bone grafting. In their series, 13 (59%) large NOFs had not had pathologic fracture despite exceeding the previously established size threshold. In the nine (41%) patients in whom pathologic fracture occurred, healing was uneventful after closed reduction and cast immobilization, and no refractures occurred. They suggested that most patients with large NOFs can be monitored without intervention, because previous studies support spontaneous resolution of most of these lesions.[21,107,133] All fractured NOFs in their series healed with closed reduction and immobilization. It may be reasonable to restrict the activity of patients with large NOFs based on the nine patients in their study with pathologic fractures caused by trauma.

Fractures are usually treated with immobilization until healing is obtained.[80] Surgery is necessary only if the residual lesion of significant size to predispose the patient to further pathologic fractures or there is doubt about the nature of the lesion.[21,139] Displaced pathologic supracondylar fractures of the distal femur may require open reduction, bone grafting, and intramedullary fixation.[133]

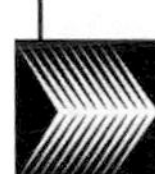

AUTHORS' PREFERRED METHOD

Treatment is based on the size and location of the lesion and the type of pathologic fracture. Small lesions without fracture can be observed and may require 1 to 3 years to spontaneously resolve.[80] Substantial lesions of the lower extremity in active children, even if they are assymptomatic, should either be followed carefully with serial radiographic studies or should undergo curettage and bone grafting to avoid pathologic fracture. Although absolute size parameters may be useful in predicting pathologic fracture, they do not imply a requirement for prophylactic curettage and bone grafting. Most patients with large NOFs can be monitored without surgical intervention, and fractures can be successfully managed with nonoperative treatment. Our experience is that a considerable number of incidentally discovered large NOFs do not fracture. Although we cannot readily identify an accurate denominator, we infer that many large NOFs remain unindentified and nonproblematic. Patient and family wishes and the individual's activity demands also influence the decision. Given the historic evidence for spontaneous resolution and favorable healing characteristics of NOFs, patients with lesions larger than 50% of the width of the bone should be approached individually, especially in the presence of clinical symptoms (Fig. 6-11).

Giant Cell Tumors of Bone

Giant cell tumors of bone are benign-aggressive tumors that usually involve the epiphysis of long bones following closure of the growth plate. Therefore, they are rarely seen in the pediatric population. In a series of 221 patients with giant cell tumors of bone,[344] only 20% of patients were younger than 20 years of age. In decreasing order of frequency, these tumors most commonly occur in the distal femur, proximal tibia, proximal humerus, and distal radius. The incidence of pathologic fractures with giant cell tumors is up to 30%.[77,116,373,494,503]

Radiographically, they are well-defined, osteolytic, epiphyseal lesions that extend into the metaphysis, usually after physeal closure. Although they start as an eccentric lesion, with growth, larger lesions can involve the full width of the bone. Little or no sclerosis is present around the margins and heavy trabeculation may be present. Periosteal reaction with new bone formation is seen with pathologic fractures.

Pathologic fractures are associated with giant cell tumors in 6% to 30% of patients. The complexity of treatment is markedly increased if a pathologic fracture is present. Management

FIGURE 6-11 An 11-year-old boy fell while playing baseball and developed acute pain over the right distal leg/ankle area. Anteroposterior **(A)** and lateral **(B)** radiographs of the right ankle show a spiral fracture through a well-defined, eccentric lesion in the lateral distal aspect of the tibia metaphysis. There is narrow zone of transition and a sclerotic border. The lesion was thought to be consistent with a nonossifying fibroma, and the fracture was allowed to heal for 5 weeks **(C,D)**. *(continues)*

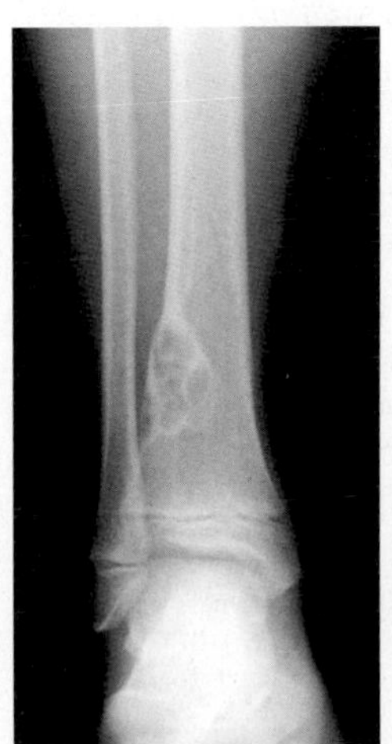

A

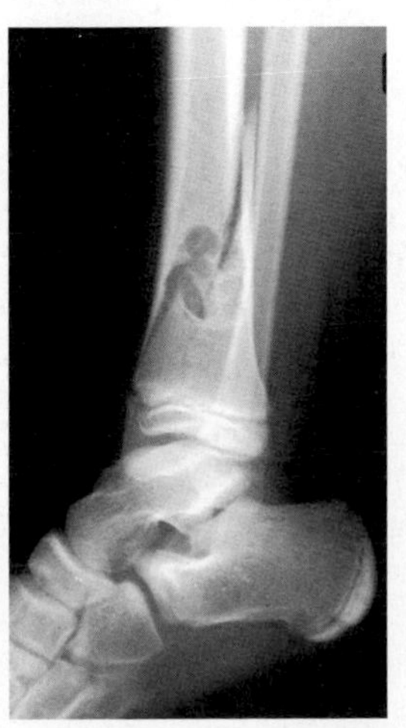

B

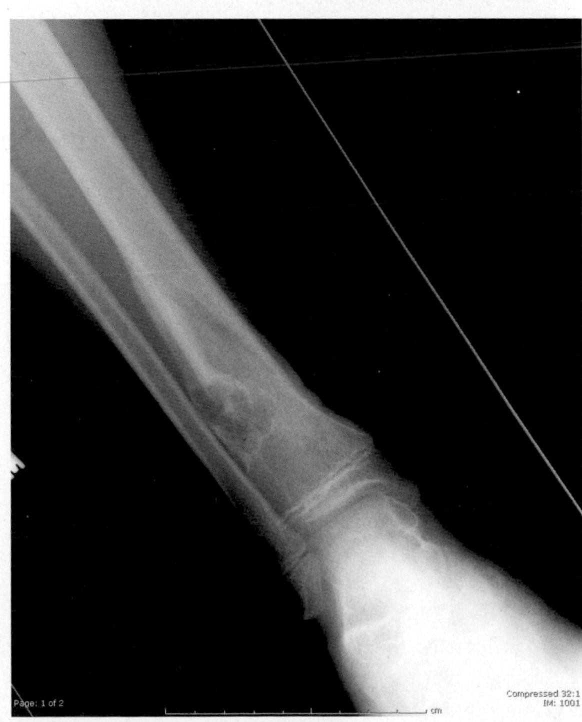

C

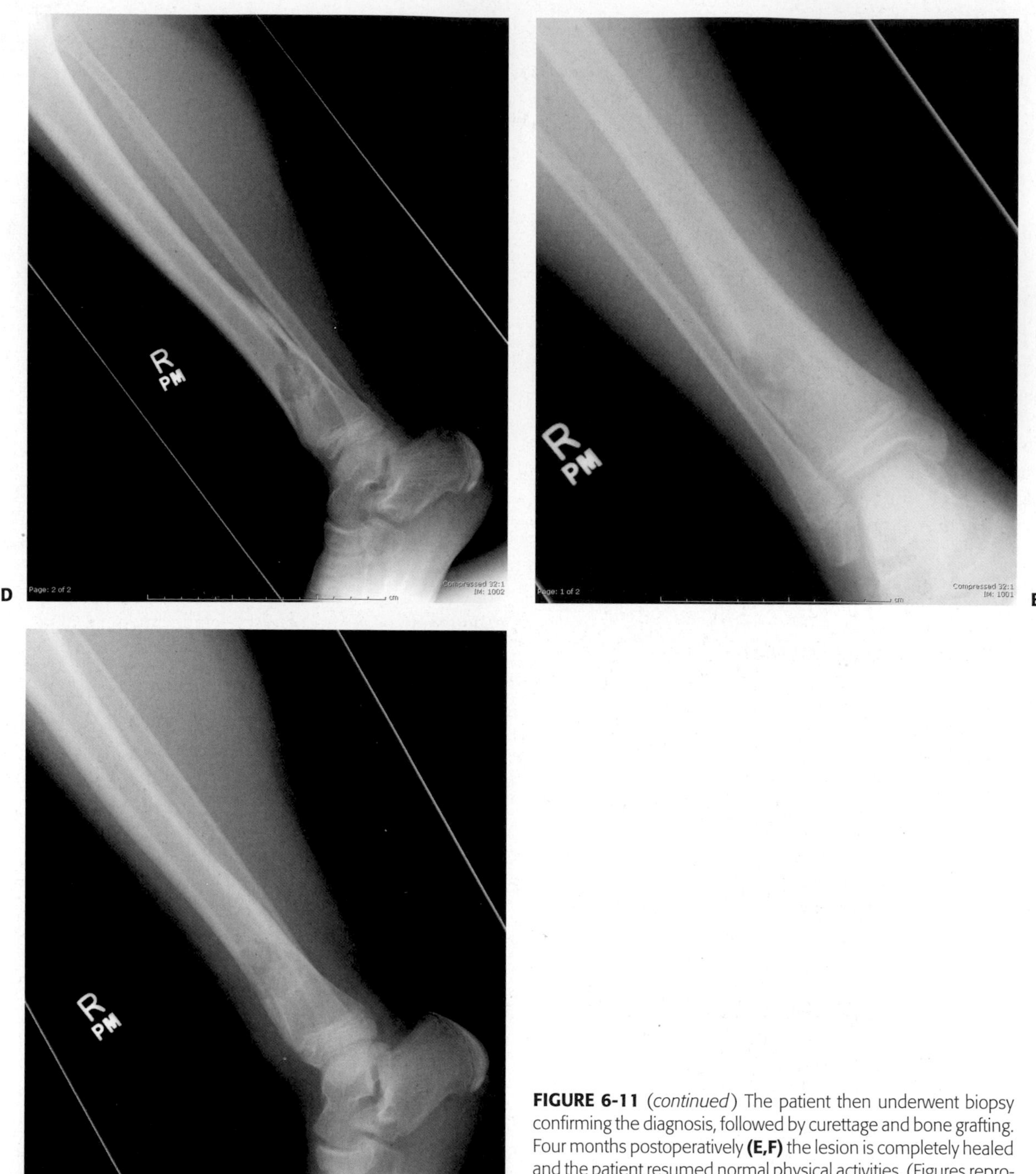

FIGURE 6-11 (*continued*) The patient then underwent biopsy confirming the diagnosis, followed by curettage and bone grafting. Four months postoperatively **(E,F)** the lesion is completely healed and the patient resumed normal physical activities. (Figures reproduced with permission from The Childrens Orthopaedic Center, Los Angeles, CA.)

depends on the type of fracture and fracture displacement (Table 6-4).

A biopsy is usually recommended before fracture treatment, especially if the diagnosis is not certain. Most pathologic fractures are minimally displaced or nonarticular and require no change in the treatment plan. For more significant fractures, an attempt at preserving the joint should be made (Fig. 6-12). It is still debatable whether the presence of a pathologic fracture itself directly influences the recurrence rate of giant cell tumors[116,503]; however, it does influence the reconstruction options and perhaps the overall functional result.

Enchondroma

Enchondromas are benign cartilaginous tumors. Solitary enchondroma is a rare lesion in children. The common presenting symptom is pain, usually associated with a pathologic fracture. The most common sites of involvement in decreasing order of frequency are the phalanges, metacarpals, metatarsals, humerus, and femur. Pathologic fracture is commonly the presenting symptom for enchondromas located in the phalanges of the hands or feet, but is rare for enchondromas in other locations.[42,179]

On plain radiographs, enchondromas are usually central in-

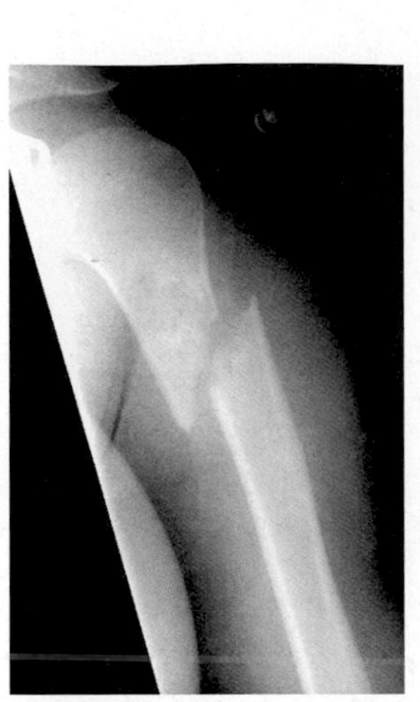

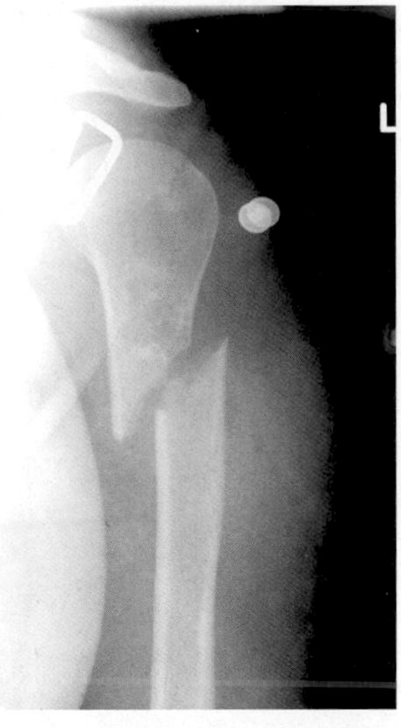

FIGURE 6-13 A 17-year-old girl with developmental delays sustained a fall and developed pain and deformity around the right proximal humerus. Radiographs of the proximal humerus **(A,B)** demonstrated a pathologic fracture through a right proximal humerus metaphyseal lesion. There is some matrix formation with speckled calcification, some cortical thinning/scalloping, but no soft tissue mass, gross cortical disruption, or other worrisome signs. The lesion was clinically consistent with enchondroma. (Figures reproduced with permission from The Childrens Orthopaedic Center, Los Angeles, CA.)

tage and bone grafting are necessary for those lesions with acute or impending pathologic fracture, or in cases of continued pain. Fixation is not necessary for those lesions of the short tubular bones but may be necessary for lesions of the proximal femur or long bone of the lower extremity. Standard fracture care is adequate to treat most injuries.

Osteochondroma

Osteochondromas are one of the most common tumors of bone in children, and clinical symptoms are usually related to irritation of the surrounding soft tissue structures. Peroneal nerve palsy may occur in association with osteochondroma of the proximal fibula.[85] Radiation induced osteochondromas also can occur.[318]

Although fractures associated with osteochondromas are rare, they may occur through the base or stalk of a pedunculated tumor (Fig. 6-16).[86] Fractures through osteochondromas should be observed, and excision should be reserved for those patients with persistent symptoms after healing or worsening of symptoms prior to healing (functional compromise).

Eosinophilic Granuloma (Langerhans Cell Histiocytosis)

Langerhans cell histiocytosis (LCH) is a rare group of disorders with a wide spectrum of clinical presentation, where the constant

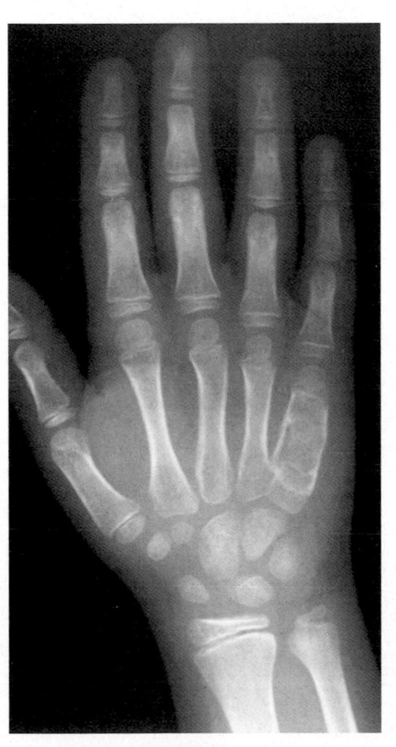

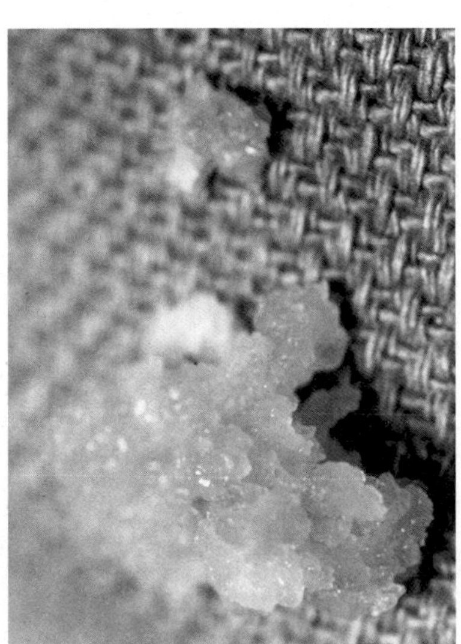

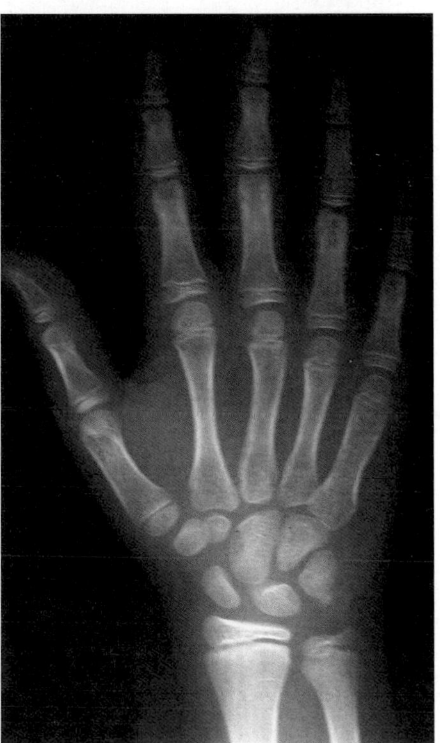

FIGURE 6-14 An 8-year-old boy presented with pain and swelling of the ulnar border of his right hand. **A.** Radiographic studies showed an expansile, lucent lesion of the diaphysis of the patient's right fifth metacarpal with microfractures. The patient had an open incisional biopsy with frozen section, which was consistent with enchondroma with subsequent curettage and bone grafting. **B.** Gross appearance of material removed at the time of surgery, which is consistent with enchondroma. **C.** At 6-month follow-up, the fracture is well healed, and there is no sign of recurrent tumor.

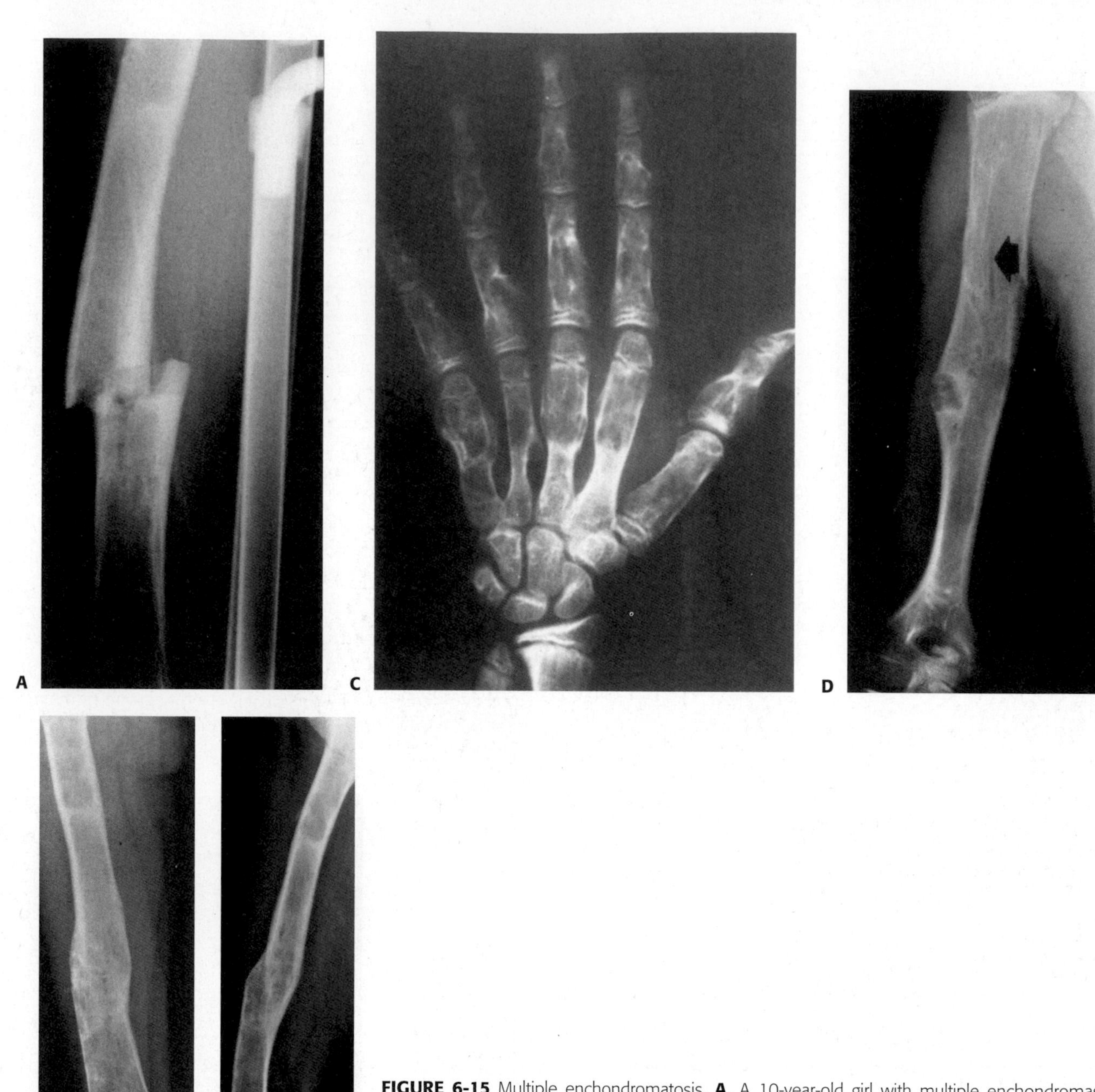

FIGURE 6-15 Multiple enchondromatosis. **A.** A 10-year-old girl with multiple enchondromas sustained a spontaneous pathologic fracture of the femur while running. The lateral radiograph shows overriding of the fracture. **B.** At 3-year follow-up, the fracture is well healed. **C.** The anteroposterior radiograph of the hand in this patient demonstrated multiple expansile enchondromas of the small bones. **D.** A radiograph of the humerus shows the streaked-mud appearance of the lateral humerus (*arrow*).

pathologic finding is the "Langerhans cell." The present nomenclature defines solitary osseous lesion as eosinophilic granuloma (EG). EG is a benign condition with either solitary or multiple lytic bone lesions. The annual incidence of LCH is at 6 per million children per year.[50] Males are affected to a slightly higher degree than females.[69,228] It is predominantly a disease of childhood, with more than 50% of cases diagnosed between the ages of 1 and 15. There is a peak in incidence between the ages of 1 and 4.[50,69] The clinical course of the disease is quite variable, with some forms undergoing seemingly spontaneous remission. The disease can be localized to a bone or single system, or multifocal involving multiple bones and/or systems. Bone pain is the initial symptom in 50% to 90% of the patients with osseous lesion.[101,124] Other reported symptoms in osseous LCH include night pain, soft tissue swelling, tenderness, pathologic fractures, headaches (skull lesions), diminished hearing, and otitis media (mastoid lesions) or loose teeth (mandible lesions). Dull, aching neck or back pain is usually the presenting symptom of children with spinal LCH.[177] Although neurologic symptoms are rarely seen at presentation, several levels of spinal involvement may occur. Later in the course of the disease, vertebral collapse may produce pain and spasm, torticollis may be seen with cervical spine lesions, and kyphosis might be present with thoracic lesions.[165,303,419] Multisystemic LCH has a wide range of manifestations. It includes the two classic syndromes (Letterer-Siwe disease and Hand-Schuller-Christian) and also several other symptoms, such as diabetes insipidus, ante-

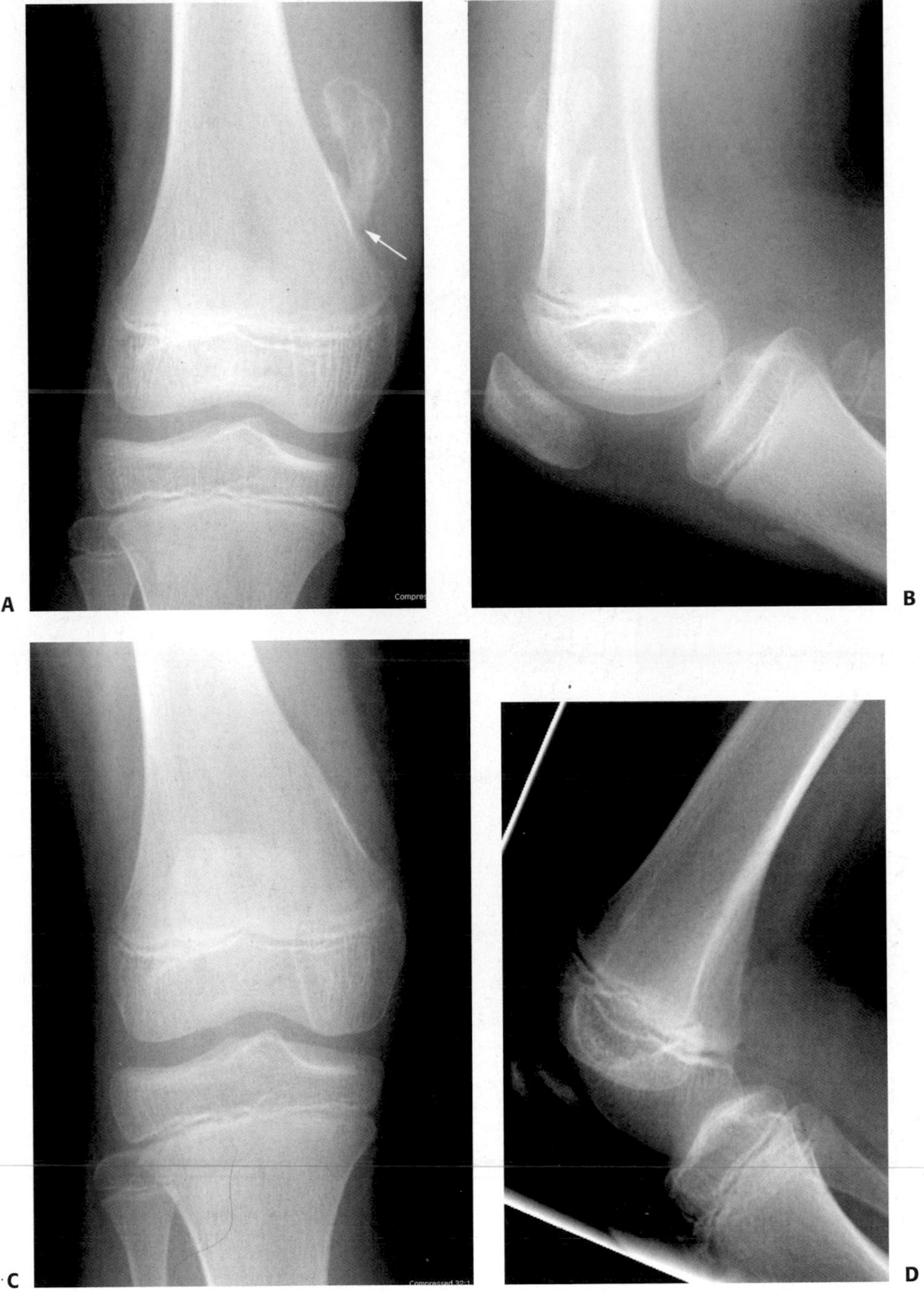

FIGURE 6-16 A 13-year-old girl presented with right knee pain following direct trauma to that area 10 days prior. On anteroposterior **(A)** and lateral **(B)** radiographs, there was a pathologic fracture through the base of a pedunculated osteochondroma (*arrow*). The patient was very tender around that area and elected surgical excision. Immediately after excision **(C,D)**, there was improvement of the symptoms. Four weeks later, she returned to full activities. (Figures reproduced with permission from The Childrens Orthopaedic Center, Los Angeles, CA.)

rior pituitary deficiency (manifested by amenorrhea, hypothyroidism, growth retardation), skin manifestations (eczema, macular rash, ulcers), pulmonary compromise (dyspnea, cough, pleural effusion), lymphadenopathy, hepatosplenomegaly, thrombocytopenia, and anemia.[145,186,228,260,261,355]

Radiographic Findings

The radiographic appearance is highly variable depending on how long the lesion has been present. For this reason, LCH has been traditionally referred to as the "great imitator." On plain radiographs, lesions typically present as radiolucent with well-defined margins, with or without surrounding sclerosis. Skeletal lesions may be solitary or multiple. In children, long bone lesions may occur in both the diaphysis and metaphysis, with destructive osteolysis that erodes the cortex and overlying expansion by periosteal layering.[69,355] Epiphyseal involvement is rare but may occur. The size of the lytic area may vary from 1 to 4 cm. Vertebral destruction with complete collapse of the vertebral body is classically referred to as "vertebra plana." Adjacent intervertebral disc height is usually maintained (Fig. 6-17).

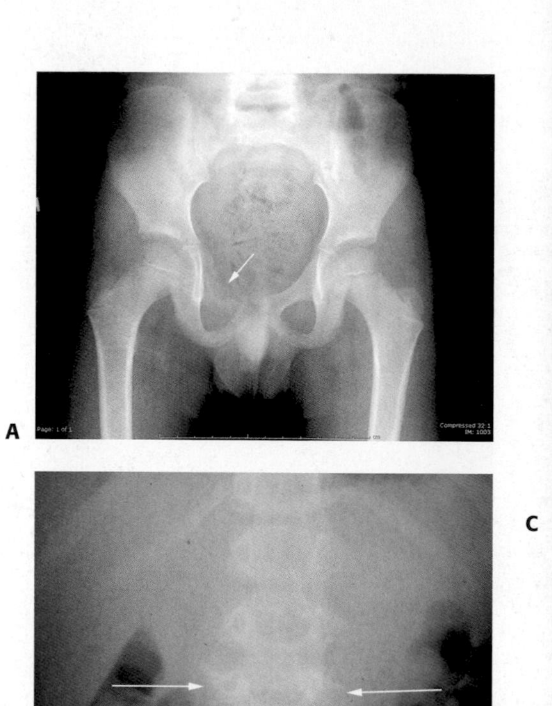

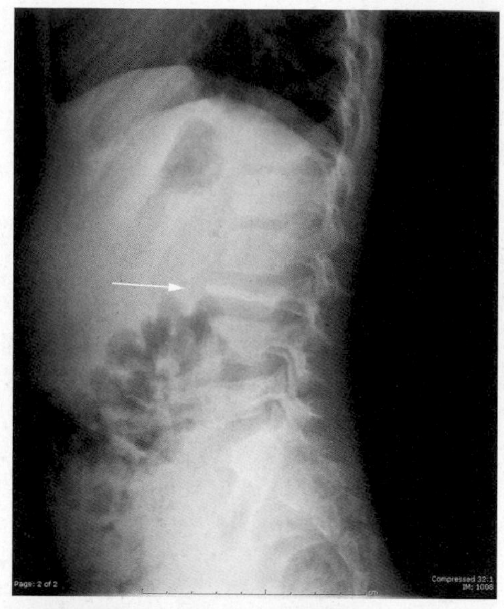

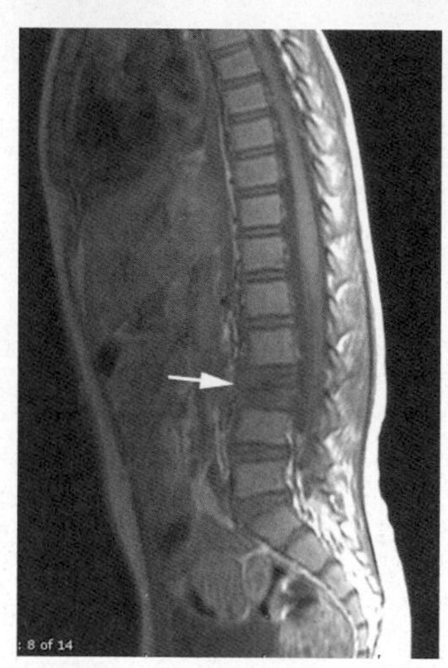

FIGURE 6-17 A 5-year-old boy presented with a history of several months of intermittent back pain and recent development of right inguinal pain. On pelvic radiographs **(A)** a lytic lesion of the right superior pubic rami is visualized (*arrow*). There is no soft-tissue mass, periosteal reaction, or other worrisome signs. The lumbar spine radiographs **(B and C)** show a classic "vertebra plana" of L3 (*arrow*). **(D)** Sagittal T1-weighted MRI shows no soft-tissue mass or other associated lesions, no compromise of the spinal canal and no extension to the posterior elements. The pelvic lesion was biopsied and a diagnosis of polyostotis Langerhans cell histiocytosis was made. (Figures reproduced with permission from The Childrens Orthopaedic Center, Los Angeles, CA.)

Spinal lesions can be classified based on the amount and pattern of maximal vertebral collapse[177]: grade I (0% to 50% of collapse), grade II (51% to 100%), or grade III (limited to the posterior elements); and A (symmetric collapse) or B (asymmetric collapse).

Treatment

Biopsy is usually necessary to confirm the diagnosis and also to differentiate LCH from malignancies that may present with similar radiographic appearance.[355] Once the diagnosis is established, treatment options include curettage, curettage and bone grafting, irradiation, chemotherapy, and steroid injection. All of these forms of treatment have been reported to promote lesion healing.[69,124,182,228] For small lesions with established diagnosis, observation may be the best option; marginal sclerosis about the lytic area suggests healing.[355] Chemotherapy is sometimes indicated, especially in cases of multiple bone involvement or visceral disease. Various agents have been used including carboplatin, cyclophosphamide, etoposide, methotrexate, vinblastine, vincristine, and steroids.[22,145]

Pathologic fracture is uncommon in patients with LCH. The correct diagnosis should be established with biopsy for most lesions, and the use of newer diagnostic methods such as immunohistochemistries (such as CD1A) can be helpful in confirming the diagnosis of these lesions. The natural history is one of gradual regression and healing. Standard fracture care is usually sufficient for pathologic fractures.

Malignant Bone Tumors and Metastasis

The two most common primary sarcomas of the long bones in children are osteogenic sarcoma and Ewing sarcoma. Destructive bone lesions can also be caused by metastatic cancer to bone, being more common than primary tumors in certain age groups. Careful staging[150,337] and subsequent biopsy[28,326,405,475] are critical in the evaluation of children with malignant bone tumors. However, biopsy is not done without risks. One of the main complications following biopsies is pathologic fracture. To avoid a pathologic fracture, an oval hole with smooth edges should be used, preferably in areas of less stress for weight-bearing bones. Sometimes, the biopsy hole can be filled with bone cement.[337] Furthermore, most malignant tumors have a large soft tissue mass that can be sampled, avoiding the need to make a hole in the bone. Pathologic fractures can sometimes be the presenting symptom of a malignant tumor (Fig. 6-18).

There has been a great deal of progress in the understanding of the molecular biology and genetics of cancer.[202,218,277,458] These advances have already led to better diagnostic analysis

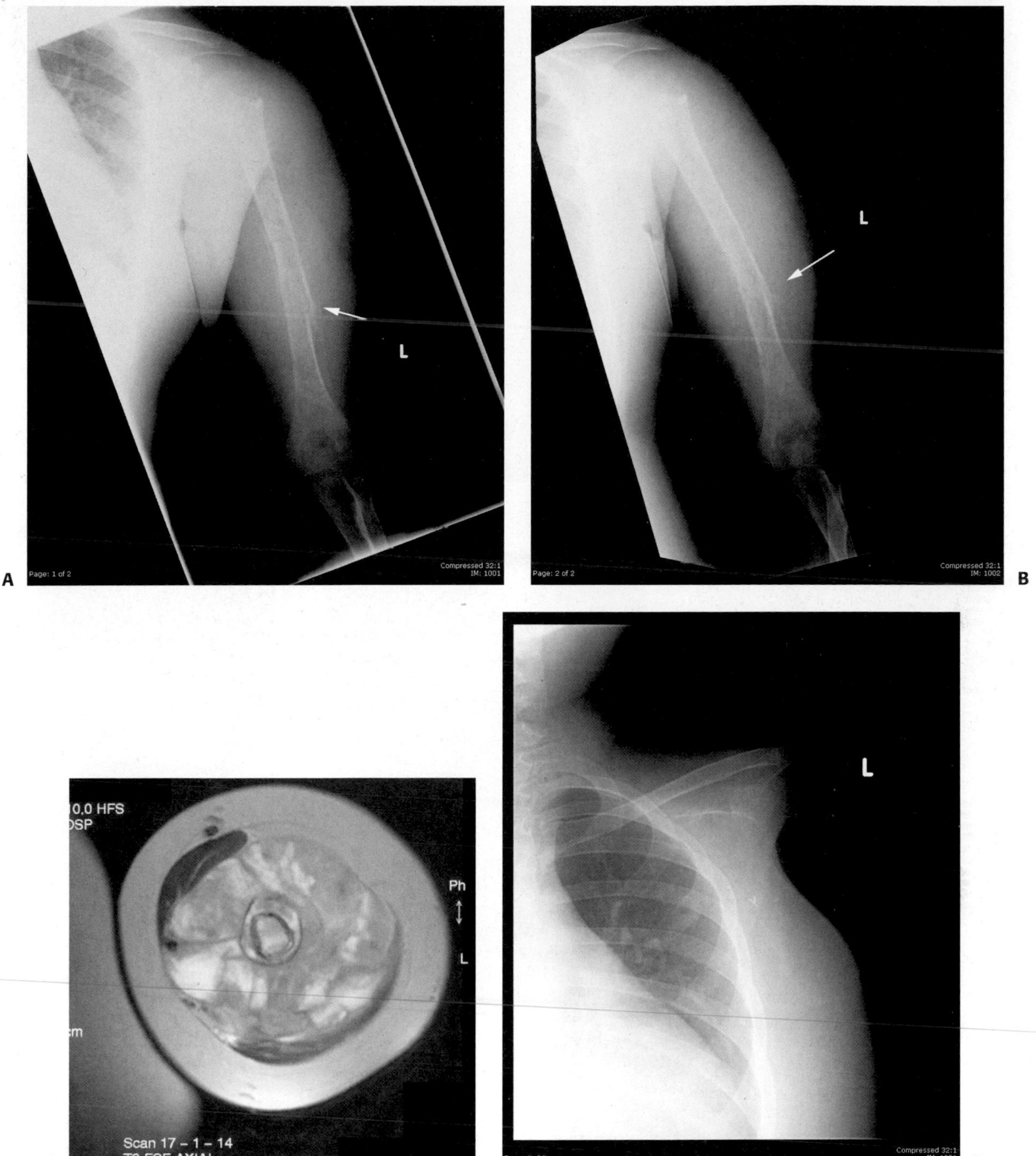

FIGURE 6-18 A 13-year-old boy presented with several months history of right arm pain and recent increase in pain following minor trauma. Anteroposterior **(A)** and lateral **(B)** radiographs show a minimally displaced midshaft humeral pathologic fracture through a poorly defined, permeative, aggressive-looking diaphyseal lesion. **(C)** T2-weighted axial MRI shows a huge soft tissue mass associated with the bone lesion and involvement of the neurovascular bundle. The patient was diagnosed with Ewing sarcoma, received neoadjuvant chemotherapy, and had a shoulder disarticulation **(D)**, followed by postoperative chemotherapy. (Figures reproduced with permission from The Childrens Orthopaedic Center, Los Angeles, CA.)

of these tumors. Immunohistochemical, molecular genetic, and cytogenetic tests are often critical in establishing the correct diagnosis, especially for small round blue cell tumors. The evaluation and biopsy of these children should preferably be done at a tertiary center where these techniques are known and available.[28,300,326,405]

One of the major advances in the care of children with extremity sarcoma has been the development of limb sparing surgical techniques for local control of the tumors. Pathologic fracture has been cited as a contraindication to this procedure because of concerns about tumor dissemination by fracture hematoma. Several studies have shown that pathologic fractures eventually heal with neoadjuvant chemotherapy and may not affect survival rates (Fig. 6-19).[146,409,526] Abudu et al.[2] reviewed

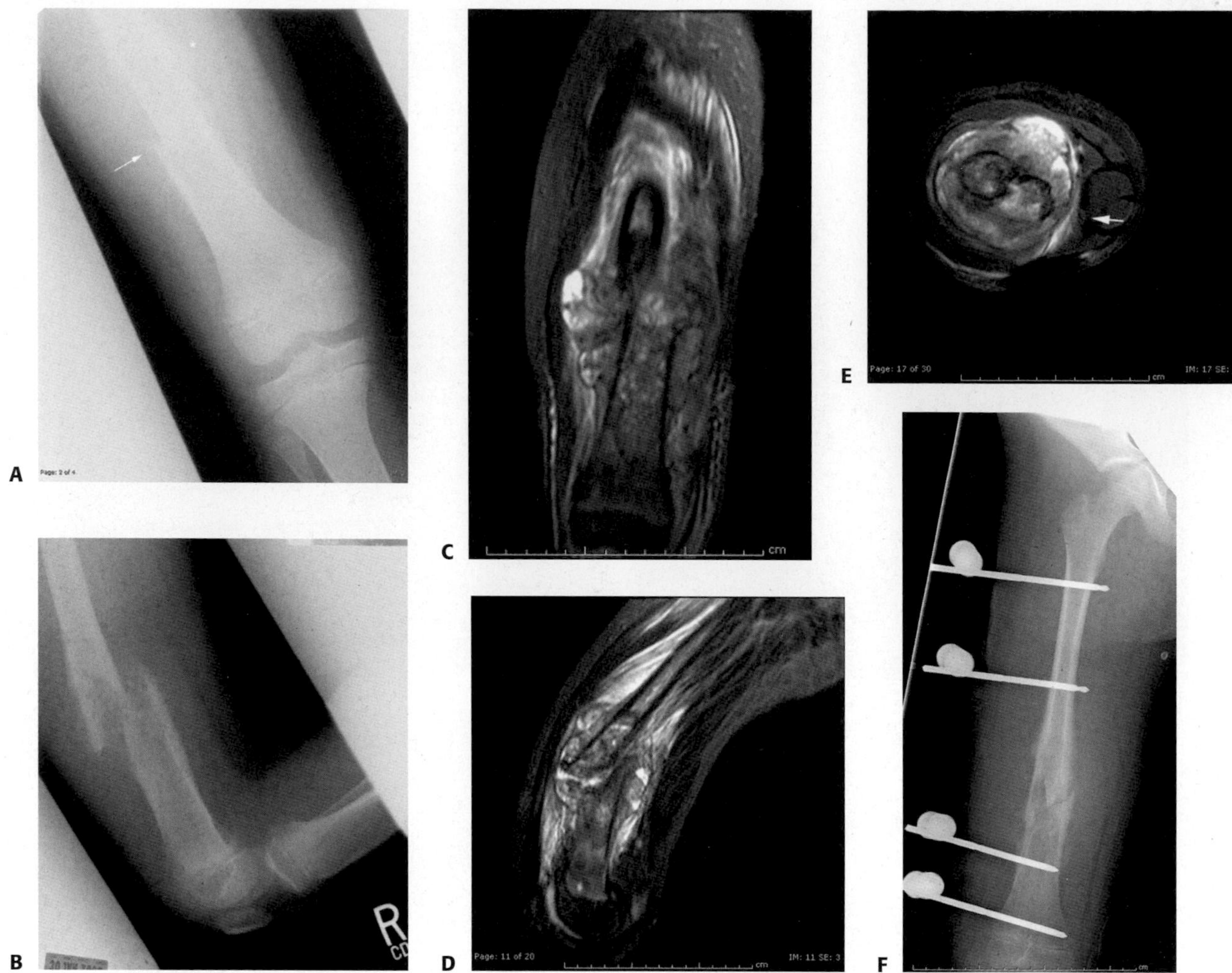

FIGURE 6-19 An 8-year-old girl sustained a pathologic fracture of the femur after falling off her bicycle. She denied symptoms previous to this injury. The radiographs **(A,B)** showed a grossly displaced fracture through a poorly defined, mixed lesion in the midshaft of the femur (*arrow*); there is disorganized periosteal reaction with sunburst sign. T2-weighted coronal **(C)**, sagittal **(D)**, and axial **(E)** MRI showed extensive soft tissue mass; the neurovascular bundle does not seem do be involved by the tumor mass. The patient underwent biopsy that confirmed osteogenic sarcoma and fracture stabilization with an external fixator at a referring institute. Note that the external fixator pins were inappropriately placed too far from the tumor and fracture site **(F)**, increasing the contaminated area. The surgical treatment options were limited to rotationplasty and amputation. (Figures reproduced with permission from The Childrens Orthopaedic Center, Los Angeles, CA.)

the surgical treatment and outcome of pathologic fractures in 40 patients with localized osteosarcoma and found that limb-sparing surgery with adequate margins of excision could be achieved in many patients without compromising survival, but that 19% of those treated with limb-sparing surgery had local recurrences. Scully et al.[458] reviewed the surgical treatment of 18 patients with osteosarcoma pathologic fractures. Of the 10 patients who had limb sparing surgery, three had local recurrences and six had distant recurrences. Although the distant recurrence rate for patients undergoing amputation was no different from the rate for those undergoing limb salvage, the difference in local tumor control approached statistical significance. All patients who developed local recurrence died. The authors stated that surgical treatment should be individualized.[458] Bacci et al.[29] compared the disease free-survival and overall survival of 46 patients with nonmetastatic osteogenic sarcoma of the extremity and pathologic fracture to a cohort of 689 patients without pathologic fracture and found no significant difference. Limb-sparing surgery is possible and appropriate in carefully selected patients as long as wide margins can be safely achieved and the function of the child will be better than that achieved with an amputation and a well-fitting prosthesis.

Pathologic fracture after limb-sparing surgery is another major complication, occurring most commonly after allograft reconstruction but also associated with endoprosthetic reconstruction.[48,451,513] Berrey et al.[48] reviewed 43 patients in whom allograft used in reconstruction after resection of tumors had subsequently fractured. Four fractures healed with immobilization alone, and the remainder of patients attained satisfactory results with open reduction and grafting, replacement of the internal fixation device, or total joint replacement.[48] San-Julian and Canadell[451] reported on 12 patients with 14 fractures (10.2% of 137 patients with allograft for limb sparing surgery in their series). They recommended intramedullary fixation whenever possible to reduce the incidence of allograft fracture.

Pathologic fractures also can occur in children with metastatic disease but are less common in children than in adults. Most are microfractures and can be managed with conservative fracture management techniques.

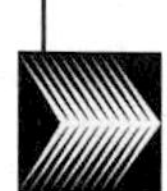

AUTHORS' PREFERRED METHOD

For all suspicious lesions, careful staging and biopsy are the appropriate initial approaches by individuals who have experience in the management of children with musculoskeletal sarcomas. Furthermore, access to special diagnostic modalities, such as immunohistochemistry and cytogenetics, will decrease the chances of misdiagnosis. The decision for or against limb-sparing surgery in patients with pathologic fracture associated with a bone sarcoma should be individualized based on factors such as the fracture displacement, fracture stability, histologic and radiographic response to chemotherapy, and, most important, the ability to achieve wide margins for local tumor control. Pathologic fractures that occur after reconstruction through allograft or endoprosthetic reconstruction often can be successfully treated with bone grafting or exchange of allograft or endoprosthesis.

Fibrous Dysplasia

Fibrous dysplasia (FD) is a developmental abnormality of bone characterized by replacement of normal bone and marrow by fibrous-osseous tissue resulting in decrease of bone strength, pathologic fracture, and deformity. The disease process may be limited to a single bone (monostotic FD) or disseminated (poliostotic FD). When the bone disease is associated with café-au-lait skin hyperpigmentation and endocrine dysfunction, it is known as McCune-Albright syndrome. Hyperthyroidism, growth hormone excess, hyperparathyroidism, hyperprolactinemia, and/or hypercortisolism may be present in any combination.[386,430] The common factor is expansile fibrous tissue lesions of the bone, which contain woven bone formed by metaplasia with poorly oriented bone trabeculae.

Clinical Presentation

The diagnosis of FD is usually made between 5 and 15 years of age, although neonatal fibrous dysplasia has been reported.[219] Often, the lesions are asymptomatic and a pathologic fracture may be the presenting symptom. Fractures of the long bones are generally not displaced or incomplete, many being microfractures and presenting with pain and swelling, usually between ages 6 and 10 with a decline thereafter.[296] The sites of fracture in decreasing order of frequency are the proximal femur, tibia, ribs, and bones of the face. The age of first fracture, number of fractures, and fracture rate are related to the severity of the metabolic derangement. The endocrinopathies are often associated with phosphaturia that has a deleterious effect on the normal skeleton and seems to be related to the incidence of fractures.[296] Although the fractures heal rapidly, endosteal callus is poorly formed and periosteal callus is normal.[206] With mild deformity, the cortex thickens on the concave side of the long bone. Nonunion is rare in monostotic FD. Most patients with polyostotic FD are diagnosed before age 10 years with pain, limp, deformity, or pathologic fracture.[219,306] The bones most commonly affected are the femur, tibia, humerus, radius, facial bones, pelvis, ribs, and phalanges. Involvement is often unilateral, usually affecting a single extremity. Spine involvement occurs with polyostotic FD, and limb-length discrepancy is common.[206,219] Some authors believe that polyostotic FD usually does not progress significantly after adulthood,[219,514] but others believe that puberty does not affect the bone lesions. In one series of 37 patients with polyostotic FD, nearly 85% had at least one fracture and 40% had an average of three fractures.[206] Fractures are most common in the femur, humerus, radius, and wrist.[305,306] Similar to monostotic FD, the fractures in the polyostotic form are generally nondisplaced and healing is not delayed; however, nonunion can occur.[206]

Cutaneous lesions are usually absent in monostotic FD. Although pregnancy may stimulate these lesions,[104] overall progression is rare after initial presentation.

FD lesions have an incidence of sarcomatous degeneration of approximately 0.5% and that generally occurs approximately 15 years after the initial diagnosis. Osteogenic sarcoma, fibrosarcoma, and malignant fibrous histiocytoma are the most common.[225] The warning signs for sarcoma in existing lesions of fibrous dysplasia are pain and rapid enlargement of the lesion.[225]

On plain radiographs, FD is seen as well-defined, central lesions often located in the diaphysis. The borders are commonly sclerotic, and the lesion is mainly lytic with trabeculation. The metaplastic woven bone comprising the lesion creates the ground-glass appearance on radiograph (Fig. 6-20). Bowing and/or angular deformity of tibia and femur are often seen. Distinguishing polyostotic from monostotic FD may be difficult. Plain radiograph skeletal surveys usually are done; technetium bone scans are helpful in identifying multiple lesions that may not be present on plain radiographic studies.[119,216]

Treatment

Conservative treatment with immobilization is indicated for most fractures that occur in conjunction with monostotic fibrous dysplasia. Traction with subsequent casting can be used for femoral shaft fractures in young children; casts or cast-bracing for upper and other lower extremity fractures is often appropriate.[190] Operative intervention is indicated for fractures of severely deformed long bones and those through large cystic areas, especially in the lower extremities.

The fractures of polyostotic FD usually occur through very diseased bone and are associated with marked deformity. They often require more aggressive treatment than fractures seen in the monostotic form. Conservative immobilization techniques are usually appropriate for most shaft fractures in children before puberty. Fractures of the femur can be treated with traction and subsequent casting in young patients. After adolescence, however, the recurrence of deformity after surgery is less, and curettage and grafting should be considered for fractures, especially for large lesions with associated deformity.[206,307] Stephenson et al.[485] found that in patients younger than 18 years of age, closed treatment or curettage and bone grafting of lower extremity fractures gave unsatisfactory results, but internal fixation produced more satisfactory outcomes.

The greatest challenge is treatment of fractures of the proximal femur. With recurrent fracture and deformity, a severe coxa vara resembling a shepherd's crook develops. Curettage of the lesion with bone grafting has been recommended for mild de-

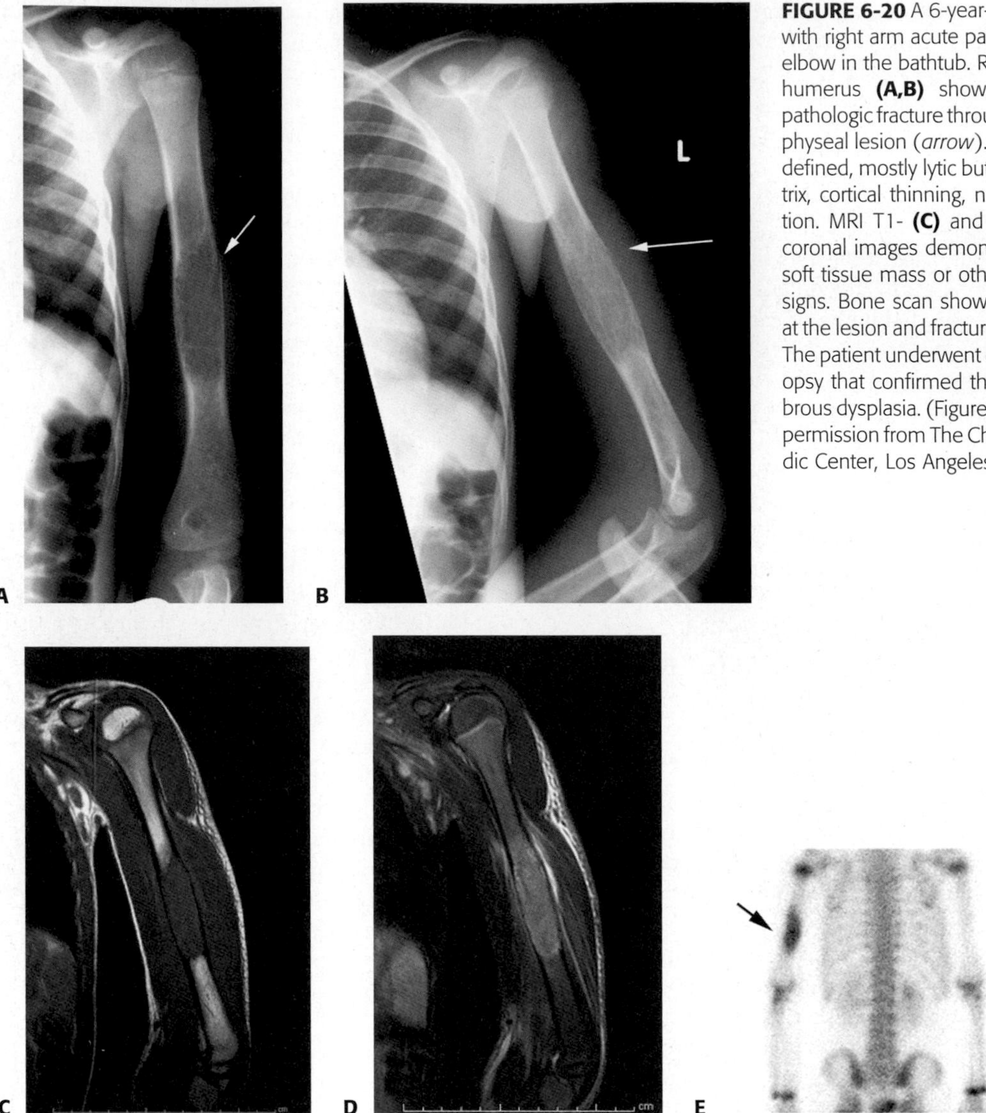

FIGURE 6-20 A 6-year-old girl presented with right arm acute pain after hitting the elbow in the bathtub. Radiographs of the humerus **(A,B)** show a nondisplaced pathologic fracture through a humeral diaphyseal lesion (*arrow*). The lesion is well defined, mostly lytic but with definite matrix, cortical thinning, no periosteal reaction. MRI T1- **(C)** and T2-weighted **(D)** coronal images demonstrate absence of soft tissue mass or other aggressiveness signs. Bone scan shows increase activity at the lesion and fracture site (*arrow*) **(E)**. The patient underwent open incisional biopsy that confirmed the diagnostic of fibrous dysplasia. (Figures reproduced with permission from The Childrens Orthopaedic Center, Los Angeles, CA.)

formities,[216,307] and fixation is usually needed for large lesions. Femoral neck fracture or osteotomy for deformity can be stabilized with internal fixation. For severe shepherd's crook deformity, medial displacement valgus osteotomies with plate fixations are needed to restore the biomechanical stability of the hip.[258] For severe lesions, Funk and Wells[172] recommended complete excision of the intertrochanteric area and advancement of the psoas and gluteus medius tendons. Breck[70] recommended securing the side plate of the femoral nail with bolts and washers rather than with screws to obtain better stability.

Deformity can occur, and internal fixation may be required for stabilization. Complete en bloc extraperiosteal excision with grafting has been shown to be successful for severe lesions but is seldom needed. Both painful lesions without fracture and impending pathologic fractures can be treated with bone grafting. Proximal femoral lesions with pathologic fracture are especially troublesome because of the propensity for malunion with coxa vara. For fractures through small lesions, either cast immobilization or curettage with grafting can be used; osteotomy can be done for residual deformity.[172] For larger lesions, internal fixation is necessary. Proximal femoral pathologic fractures have been stabilized with lag screws, blade plates,[190] intramedullary nails, and Enders nails. Cast immobilization and protected weight bearing are necessary after these procedures to protect the reduction. Spine fractures are rare but can be treated with bed rest followed by immobilization with an orthosis.[190] The main limitation of bone grafting is the potential resorbtion and transformation into FD. Autogenous cancellous graft has the higher likelihood to become FD, and cortical allograft is the least likely to be transformed.[121,151,199]

The use of bisphosphonates, primarily pamidronate, may offer hope for a medical treatment for patients with severe FD. Pamidronate is a second-generation bisphosphonate that has had documented success in selected patients with the disease. It is a potent inhibitor of bone resorption and has a lasting effect on bone turnover. The major effect is decreased bone pain. A few studies have demonstrated improved bone density with pamidronate therapy in patients with FD.[385]

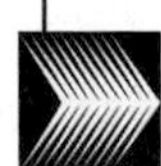

AUTHORS' PREFERRED METHOD OF TREATMENT

Conservative treatment with immobilization is indicated for most fractures in children with monostotic FD. In younger children, immediate casting or traction and subsequent casting are used for most femoral shaft fractures. Because fractures in patients with polyostotic FD usually occur through very abnormal bone and can result in marked deformity, they often require more aggressive treatment (e.g., internal fixation).

After adolescence, the occurrence of deformity after surgery is less frequent. Nonoperative treatment of fractures and curettage and cancellous bone grafting do not generally produce satisfactory results in children with FD of the lower extremity. Curettage and grafting are indicated for fractures of severely deformed long bones and those through large cystic areas, with internal fixation appropriate for the location and age. Bone graft can be reabsorbed after placement in extensive lesions, and proximal deformity can occur after corrective osteotomy. Allograft has a lower likelihood to be reabsorbed than autograft. Recently, the use of coral as bone substitute has been shown to be effective.[121]

One of the most common sites of fracture and deformity is the proximal femur. Proximal femoral lesions with pathologic fracture are especially difficult to treat because of the tendency for varus deformity and refracture. Stable fractures through small lesions can be treated with cast immobilization, but one must be vigilant and ready to intervene at any sign of varus displacement. Femoral neck fractures can be stabilized in situ with a cannulated screw or compression screw and side plate, depending on the extent of involvement and the nature and location of the fracture. Fixation can be combined with valgus osteotomy if there is pre-existing deformity or with curettage and grafting if there is a large area of bone loss. Postoperative cast immobilization and protected weight bearing usually are necessary. Varus deformity is best treated with valgus osteotomy of the subtrochanteric region and internal fixation early in the course of the disease to restore the normal neck shaft angle and mechanical axis. Intramedullary load-sharing fixation (such as flexible intramedullary nails) can be used for juvenile patients with femoral shaft fractures. For larger lesions with more severe deformity, and in older patients, rigid fixation often is necessary. Depending on the situation, intramedullary load-sharing fixation devices that support not only the femoral neck but also the shaft of the femur (such as second-generation intramedullary nails) are better and should be used when possible. For severe shepherd's crook deformity, medial displacement osteotomies are needed to restore the biomechanical stability of the hip.

Osteofibrous Dysplasia

Osteofibrous dysplasia (OD) is an unusual developmental tumor-like fibro-osseous condition. Most patients present before the age of 5 years, ranging from 5 weeks to 15 years of age.[79,401] Clinically, there is usually a painless enlargement of the tibia with slight to moderate anterior or anterolateral bowing. The disease process is almost always confined to one tibia, but the ipsilateral fibula can also be involved. Solitary involvement of the fibula is infrequent, and bilateral involvement of both tibias is rare. Both distal and proximal lesions can occur, and with fibular involvement, the lesion is located distally. Pathologic fractures may be present in nearly one third of patients[79]; however, these fractures are usually incomplete (e.g., stress fractures, microfractures) or minimally displaced and heal well with conservative treatment.[79] Pseudarthrosis is rare but sometimes delayed union may be a problem.

OD presents as a well-defined, eccentric, intracortical, lytic lesion usually located in the middle third of the tibia, extending proximally or distally.[401] The cortex overlying the lesion is expanded and thinned, and in the medullary canal, a dense band of sclerosis borders the lesion with narrowing of the medullary canal. Single areas of radiolucency may be present and have a ground-glass appearance, but often there are several areas of involvement with a bubble-like appearance (Fig. 6-21).

Intralesional curettage and grafting are associated with a local recurrence rate of up to 64%.[79] Wide extraperiosteal resection can be performed for aggressive lesions and seem to have lower rate of recurrence.[292] Some authors[9,270] believe that bracing until skeletal maturity is preferable to surgery.

Pathologic fractures in this disorder should heal with cast immobilization in plaster casts. If fractures recur, or if the lesion is rapidly progressive, wide extraperiosteal resection with grafting is necessary.[79] Open reduction with bone grafting and internal fixation is recommended for fractures with angular deformity. Early osteotomy is recommended for severe bowing deformity, followed by internal fixation (intramedullary device). Bracing is recommended to prevent fractures and angular deformity.

Neurofibromatosis

Neurofibromatosis (NF), also known as von Recklinghausen disease (NF type-1), is an autosomal dominant condition with variable penetrance that occurs in 1 in 2500 to 3000 live births.[105] It affects neural tissue, vascular structures, skin, and the skeleton. The diagnosis of NF can be based on the presence of two of the four following criteria, according to Crawford and Bagamery[105]:

1. Multiple café-au-lait spots
2. Positive family history for NF
3. Diagnostic biopsy of a neurofibroma
4. Presence of pseudarthrosis of the tibia, hemihypertrophy, or a short, angular scoliosis

Crowe and Schull[106] pointed out that adult patients with NF usually had more than five café-au-lait spots with a diameter of more than 1.5 cm. The presence of café-au-lait spots, however, is not pathognomonic for NF. Whitehouse[519] noted that 23% of normal children have one or two café-au-lait spots with a diameter of more than 0.5 cm, and the presence of five or more café-au-lait spots is needed to suggest the diagnosis of NF. Although café-au-lait spots may be present at birth, usually they are not seen until the patient is 5 or 6 years old.[105] Generalized soft tissue hypertrophy of the limbs is present in 37% of adults with NF,[342] whereas children have an 11% incidence of limb-length discrepancy and only a 3% incidence of soft tissue enlargement of the extremities.[105]

A diagnostic biopsy of a dermal neurofibroma is considered a valuable criterion for the diagnosis of NF. These tumors, however, tend not to be clinically apparent until the child is older than 12 years of age.[105] Plain radiographic studies are not helpful in identifying these soft tissue tumors. MRI can be helpful in identifying the soft tissue masses. Technetium 99m–labeled diethylenetriaminepentaacetic acid accumulates in the soft tissue tumors of NF.[323,324] Routine isotopic imaging with this technique can identify lesions as small as 1.5 cm. Lesions as

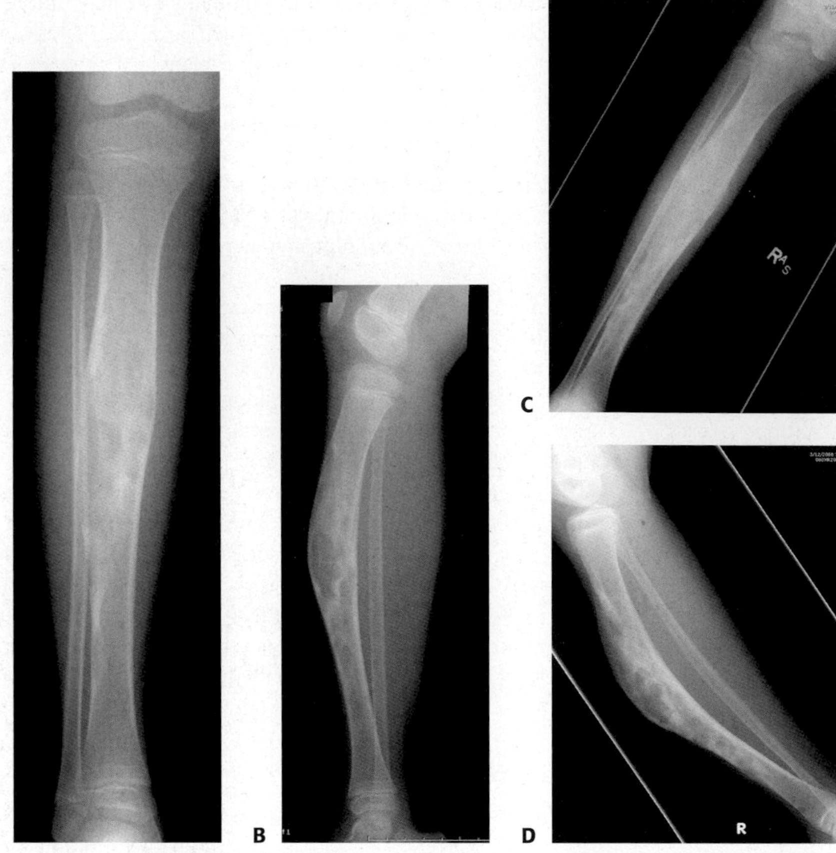

FIGURE 6-21 Anteroposterior **(A)** and lateral **(B)** radiographs of a 4-year-old boy presenting with intermittent leg pain associated with progressive bowing. The images show circumscribed sclerotic and lytic lesion involving the anterior tibial diaphyseal cortex. The patient was thought to have osteofibrous dysplasia and conservative treatment with bracing was elected. Seven years later, the radiographs **(C,D)** show increased bowing of the tibia measuring approximately 40 degrees. The patient was, however, essentially asymptomatic and was not interested in any surgical treatment. (Figures reproduced with permission from The Childrens Orthopaedic Center, Los Angeles, CA.)

small as 0.8 cm were seen through a more advanced technique known as single proton emission computed tomography. Such techniques may be useful in identifying occult NF and pseudarthrosis of the long bones.

Pseudarthrosis of the long bones in patients with NF can be a therapeutic dilemma. The appearance of pseudarthroses and their resistance to treatment has been postulated to be due to a deficiency of bone formation secondary to mesodermal dysplasia. The abnormal soft tissue associated with these pseudarthroses has been postulated to be the major associated factor in causing pseudarthrosis.[525] Approximately 5% of patients with NF eventually develop pseudarthrosis of the long bones. The tibia is the bone most often affected, but only 55% of the cases of congenital pseudarthroses of the tibia are thought to be associated with NF.[104]

The term congenital pseudarthrosis is misleading because the majority of patients do not have a pseudarthrosis at birth but rather develop it later after a pathologic fracture.[369] Brown et al.[72] found that in six children with NF, anterior bowing of the leg developed at an average age of 8 months and then went on to fracture and pseudarthrosis an average of 4.5 months after the initial clinical observation of deformity.

Although most authors focus on the treatment of congenital pseudarthrosis of the tibia,[369] pseudarthroses in other locations in children with NF occur and can be a challenge. Pseudarthroses have been reported in the radius,* ulna,[10,11,43,44,309,372,393] both the radius and the ulna,[11,43,327,338,429,460] femur, clavicle, and humerus.

Children with NF-type 1 have a general tendency toward osteopenia and osteoporosis, suggesting an abnormal underlying bone phenotype. This may be another reason as why there is a high incidence of pseudarthrosis, nonunion, and poor bone healing associated with NF.[137]

Radiographic Findings

Anterolateral bowing of the tibia with loss of the medullary canal is usually present before fracture.[72] Another radiographic characteristic is a prefracture cystic lesion of the tibia with anterolateral bowing.[105] Biopsy specimens of these pseudarthroses invariably reveal fibrous tissue, but there are reports of found evidence of neural tissue in biopsy specimens.[11,336] None of these findings, however, has been confirmed by electron microscopy to document the presence of Schwann cells. Radiographic findings in patients with established pseudarthroses of the tibia include narrowing or obliteration of the medullary canal at the pseudarthrosis site, with sclerosis and anterolateral angulation. Pseudarthrosis of the fibula is associated with valgus deformity of the ankle.

In the upper extremity pseudarthroses of NF, the radiographic signs of the bone at risk are narrowing of the diaphysis,[393] sclerosis and hypoplasia with associated absent medullary canal,[327] and the presence of a cystic lesion in the bone. Once a fracture has occurred, a pseudarthrosis is likely when the fracture line persists for more than 7 weeks after injury.[336] The ends of the fracture gradually become tapered, there is little callus, and the cortex of the healing bone thickens with a decreased diameter of the medullary canal. The cause of these radio-

*References 44,72,194,245,246,249,302,309,319,323,324,327,336, 338

graphic changes is unclear. Pseudarthroses have also developed in children with NF after fracture through normal-appearing forearm bones.[245,246]

Treatment

A tibia with an anterolateral bow in an infant or child will eventually fracture; corrective osteotomy to correct angular deformity will only accelerate the progression to pseudarthrosis and should not be done. Once the fracture occurs, there is little indication for closed treatment. In conjunction with excision of the hypotrophic bone ends, methods of treatment of this congenital pseudarthrosis include intramedullary fixation with iliac bone graft, fixation with vascularized fibular graft, and Ilizarov compression of the pseudarthrosis with callotastic lengthening of the proximal tibia. All of these methods may be complicated by further pathologic fracture and nonunion.

In contrast to pseudarthrosis of the upper extremity, there is substantial experience with treatment of pseudarthrosis of the tibia, but results are still disappointing. Bracing has proved ineffectual in the treatment of an established pseudarthrosis, but may be useful to prevent fracture and deformity. Surgical procedures have included bypass grafts,[345] onlay grafts,[67] grafting with small bone chips, periosteal grafting, intramedullary nailing procedures,[14,34] and intramedullary rod fixation after segmental osteotomies.[483] The rate of union with these procedures ranges from 7% to 90%, and eventual amputation has been common. Electrical stimulation has been used with some success, but most series reporting its use have short patient follow-up and the electrical stimulation was used in combination with other surgical techniques. In one series, a 20% success rate was achieved using direct-current stimulation.[71] In another series, union was achieved in 10 of 12 patients with pseudarthrosis of the tibia through rigid intramedullary rod fixation and electrical stimulation through implanted electrodes.[404] The Farmer procedure, a skin and bone pedicle from the contralateral leg, has a reported union rate approaching 53%.[368] Free vascularized fibular grafts also have been used for reconstruction after excision of the involved tibia.[368] In one series, 11 of 12 patients with NF and pseudarthrosis of the tibia were successfully treated with free vascularized fibular grafts. Union of the pseudarthrosis occurred between 3 to 8 months after surgery.[114,128,516] A free vascularized iliac graft has been used in one patient with NF, resulting in union within 10 weeks.[302] Fabry et al.[156] obtained union of pseudarthrosis of the tibia in two patients with compression through an Ilizarov fixator. In another series,[424] the fractures in three of five patients healed in 4.5 months. The other two patients needed supplementary iliac grafts, and eventually, the bone united. It is important to stress that treatment cannot be considered successful until skeletal maturity has been reached; many of these series included patients with short follow-up, and few included follow-up to skeletal maturity.

A prophylactic bypass grafting of the prepseudarthrotic tibia in NF has been performed with some success (Fig. 6-22). This modification of the original McFarland bypass procedure, which was originally done for established pseudarthrosis, was successful in a series of patients from several centers reviewed by Strong and Wong-Chung.[491] A modified sequential McFarland bypass procedure for prepseudarthrosis of the tibia also has been described.[125] More recently, some authors have been reporting on the use recombinant human bone morphogenetic protein with promising results.[155,290]

Amputation should be considered and discussed with the family early when previous operative interventions have been unsuccessful. Amputation usually is at the Syme level, with prosthetic fitting around the pseudarthrosis. In a gait analysis study, Karol et al.[248] compared 12 patients with previously operated and healed congenital pseudarthroses of the tibia with four children with amputations for final treatment of congenital pseudarthroses of the tibia. They found marked disturbance of gait and muscle strength in patients with healed congenital pseudarthroses of the tibia. They concluded that patients with early onset of disease, early surgery, and transankle fixation had more inefficient gaits than amputees. Patients with forearm pseudarthroses can be pain free and function may be satisfactory with observation or splinting. However, persistence of an ulnar pseudarthrosis in a growing child often leads to bowing of the radius and posterior lateral subluxation or dislocation of the radial head.[11,12,302,393] Healing after 6 months of casting has been reported in a 2-month-old infant with a congenital pseudarthrosis of the radius. There was no clinical evidence of NF at the time of treatment of this patient.[191] Union after conventional bone grafting and fixation has been reported in only a small number of patients with congenital pseudarthrosis of the forearm.[43,44,245,246,327,465] Many of these patients require multiple conventional bone grafting procedures and often years of immobilization. There are more reports of patients (and probably many more patients) with pseudarthroses of the forearm bones who did not respond to multiple grafting procedures.[10,44,72,336,393] The results of treatment of congenital pseudarthrosis of the forearm in NF by free vascularized fibular grafts are encouraging. Allieu et al.[12] treated one patient with radial and ulnar pseudarthroses and another with ulnar pseudarthrosis with free vascularized fibular grafts. They obtained union in the patient with radial and ulnar pseudarthroses in 6 weeks and in the patient with ulnar pseudarthroses in 3 months. Earlier conventional grafting techniques had failed in both. Two additional patients with pseudarthroses of the radius without evidence of NF were treated with free vascularized fibular grafts, resulting union within 6 weeks.[460,525] Mathlin et al.[338] reported six pseudarthroses of the forearm bones treated with vascularized fibular grafting with union in five ranging from 6 to 18 months after surgery. Other surgical options include excision of the ulnar pseudarthrosis to avoid a later tethering effect on the growing radius[10] and fusion of the distal radius and ulnar joint.[393] Creation of a one-bone forearm is often technically successful, but both length and rotation of the forearm are sacrificed with this procedure.[309,393]

Spinal deformity is the most common musculoskeletal abnormality seen in individuals with NF. Although scoliosis was present in 64% of patients with NF in one series,[105] kyphoscoliosis may be the primary contributor to the development of paraplegia.[524] Patients younger than 19 years of age may have paraplegia secondary to vertebral deformity, whereas those patients older than 19 are more likely to have neurologic deficits secondary to a neurofibroma. Complete dislocation of the spine with neurologic defect has been reported in two patients with NF.[438] Rib penetration of the enlarged neural foramen with spinal cord

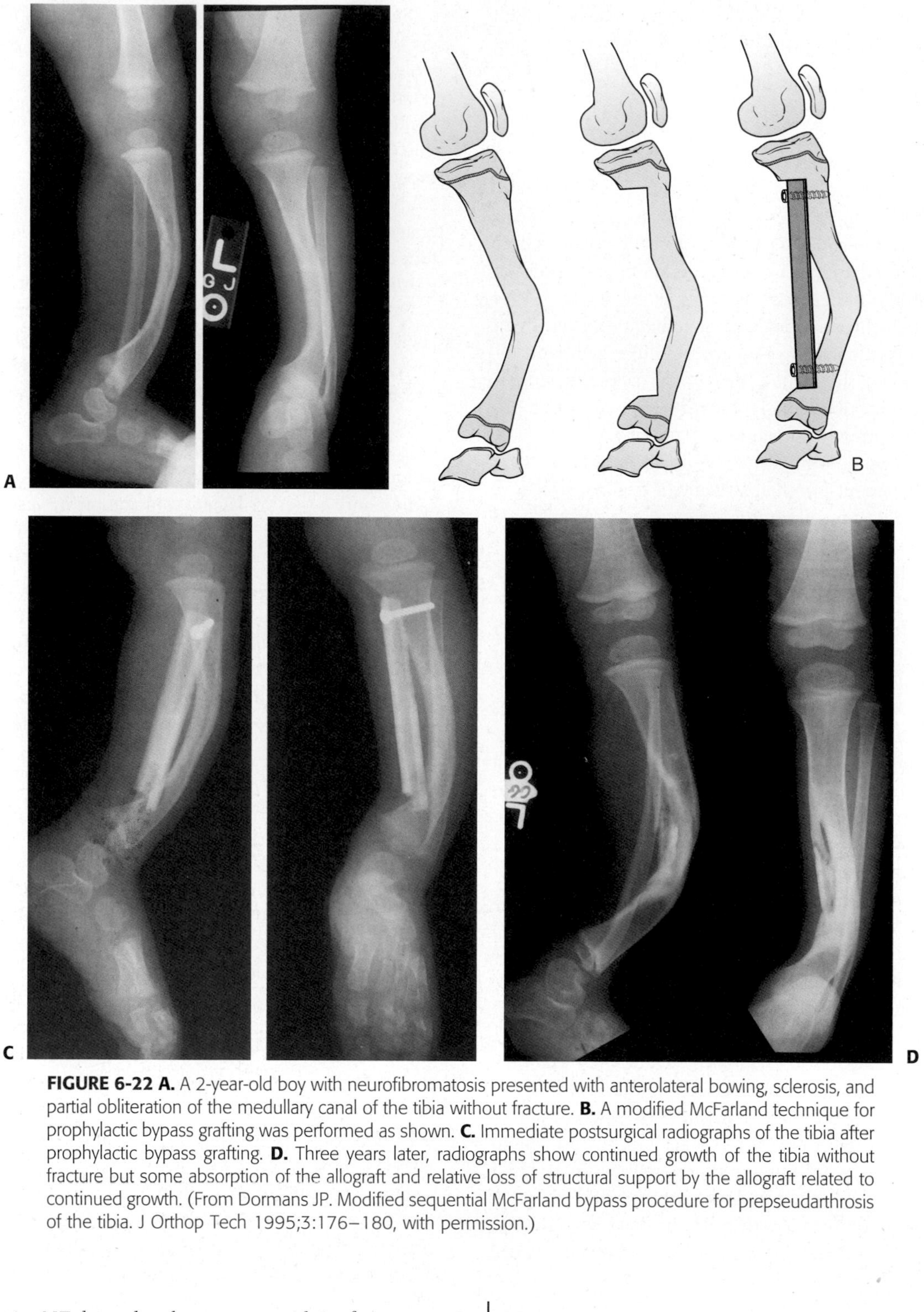

FIGURE 6-22 A. A 2-year-old boy with neurofibromatosis presented with anterolateral bowing, sclerosis, and partial obliteration of the medullary canal of the tibia without fracture. **B.** A modified McFarland technique for prophylactic bypass grafting was performed as shown. **C.** Immediate postsurgical radiographs of the tibia after prophylactic bypass grafting. **D.** Three years later, radiographs show continued growth of the tibia without fracture but some absorption of the allograft and relative loss of structural support by the allograft related to continued growth. (From Dormans JP. Modified sequential McFarland bypass procedure for prepseudarthrosis of the tibia. J Orthop Tech 1995;3:176–180, with permission.)

compression in NF has also been reported in four patients.[167,319] CT and MRI are useful for evaluating these patients. Resection through either an anterior or a posterior approach seems satisfactory.[319]

Extreme care should be taken in surgical treatment of children with NF. Complications are common. The periosteum of the long bones is less adherent to the bone than normal periosteum, and extensive subperiosteal hemorrhage may occur resulting from a trauma or after an osteotomy or other surgical procedure.[528] It is important preoperatively to rule out hypertension in children with NF because 16% of children with NF had hypertension in one series.[509]

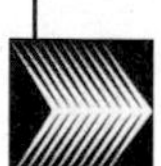

AUTHORS' PREFERRED METHOD OF TREATMENT

The treatment of congenital pseudarthrosis of the tibia remains controversial. When a child presents with prepseudarthrosis (angulation without fracture), either bypass grafting with fibular allograft or bracing are reasonable options. Once pseudarthrosis has developed, our preference is inserting an intramedullary rod and bone grafting of both the tibia and fibula when possible (Fig. 6-23). If these procedures fail, free vascularized fibula transfer or resection and bone trans-

FIGURE 6-23 A 19-month-old girl presented with right leg bowing and recent inability to bear weight on that extremity. The patient has neurofibromatosis type 1 with associated café-au-lait spots **(A)**. Anteroposterior **(B)** and lateral **(C)** radiographs of the tibia and fibula show pseudarthrosis of the tibia diaphysis associated with intramedullary obliteration and bone thinning at the pseudarthrosis level. The fibula presents anterior-lateral deformity and partial obliteration of the medullary canal without fracture. Postoperative images **(D,E)** following excision of the pseudarthrosis, fibular osteotomy, iliac bonegraft and periosteum grafting, and fixation with a William rod. (Figures reproduced with permission from The Childrens Orthopaedic Center, Los Angeles, CA.)

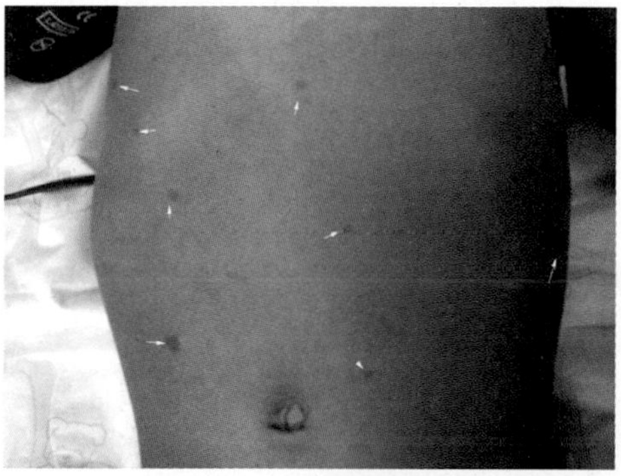

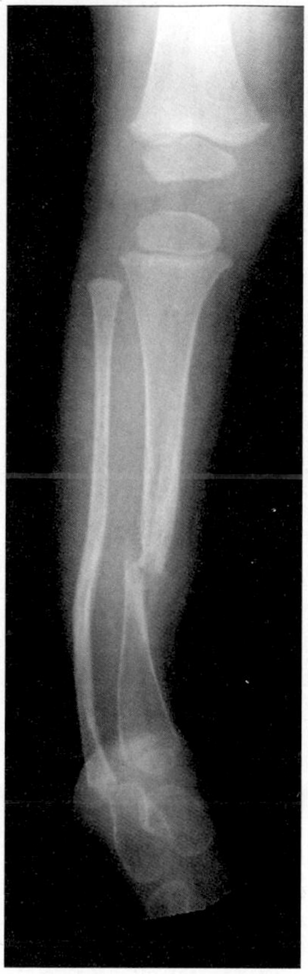

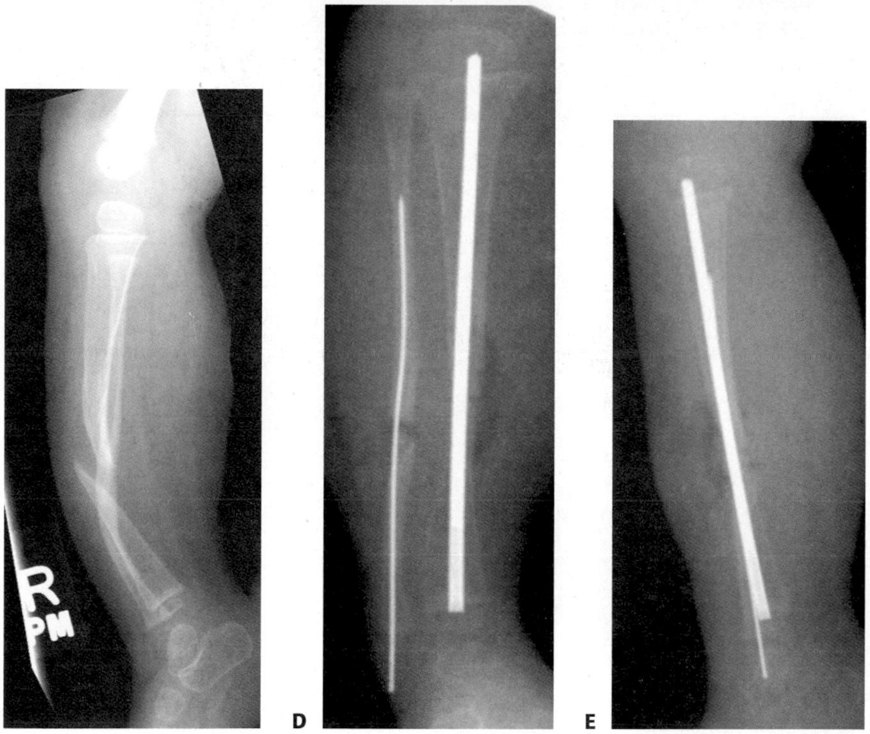

port with circular frame techniques can be considered. Amputation and prosthetic fitting should be considered early in patients with failure of the above-mentioned techniques and severe shortening and a stiff ankle and foot. Conservative options, such as bracing or observation, for upper extremity pseudarthroses may be justified in a patient with a nonprogressive deformity and a satisfactory functional use of the extremity. Conventional bone grafting and fixation procedures for treatment of pseudarthrosis of the upper extremity have very limited success, and other approaches should be considered. Free vascularized fibular grafts seem the treatment of choice for upper extremity pseudarthrosis associated with NF.

Congenital Insensitivity to Pain

Congenital insensitivity to pain is a rare hereditary sensory neuropathy disorder characterized by the absence of normal subjective and objective responses to noxious stimuli in patients with intact central and peripheral nervous systems. The cause is unknown, but sporadic reports have appeared in the orthopaedic literature.[197,198,279,387]

The orthopaedic manifestations of congenital insensitivity to pain include recurrent fractures, osteomyelitis, and neuropathic joints. Although the lower extremities are most commonly affected, the spine could also be involved with gross and unstable spondylolisthesis. Limb-length discrepancy may occur from physeal damage. Lack of pain perception is associated with the development of Charcot joints, which may lead to later neuropathic arthropathy. The weight-bearing joints are usually affected, especially the knees and ankles. Although fracture healing usually occurs, the arthropathy is progressive, eventually resulting in gross deformity and instability. In addition to absence of deep pain, the patients had impaired temperature sensation.[365]

The differential diagnosis includes a spectrum of closely related sensory disorders including congenital sensory neuropathy, hereditary sensory radicular neuropathy, familial sensory neuropathy with anhidrosis, and familial dysautonomia (Riley-Day syndrome). Acquired conditions with pain insensitivity include syringomyelia, diabetes mellitus, tabes dorsalis, alcoholism, and leprosy. Loss of protective sensation promotes self-mutilation, burns, bruises, and fractures. The disease comes to light when the child develops teeth and then bites his or her tongue, lips, and fingers.

Management should aim at education and prevention of injury. Prevention of joint disease is the best early option.[197,387] Joint injury should be recognized and treated early to prevent progression to gross arthropathy. Early diagnosis and treatment of fractures is important, usually by conservative manners.[197,279] In a severely unstable, degenerated joint, arthrodesis may eventually be appropriate; however, poor healing, nonunion, and pseudarthrosis are common in neuropathic joints (Fig. 6-24). Infection rate is also increased, and it is important to make the differentiation between fracture and infection.[36] The condition appears to improve with time with the gradual recovery of pain sensation.

DISEASES OF THE BONE MARROW

Gaucher Disease

Gaucher disease is a hereditary disorder of lipid metabolism. It is the most common lysosomal storage disease and is caused by deficient production and activity of the lysosomal enzyme beta-glucosidase (glucocerebrosidase), resulting in progressive accumulation of glucosylceramide (glucocerebroside) in macrophages of the reticuloendothelial system in the spleen, liver, and bone marrow. The most common sphingolipidosis, it is inherited as an autosomal recessive trait,[251] with most cases noted in Ashkenazic Jews of eastern European origin.[280] There are three types of Gaucher disease: type I represents more than 90% of all cases and is the most common type seen by orthopaedic surgeons. It presents as a chronic nonneuropathic disease with visceral (spleen and liver) and osseous involvement, also known as the adult form, although patients present during childhood[251]; Type II is an acute, neuropathic disease with central nervous system involvement and early infantile death; and type III is a subacute nonneuropathic type with chronic central nervous system involvement. Types II and III are both characterized as either infantile or juvenile, and are notable for severe progressive neurologic disease, usually being fatal.

Osseous lesions are a result of marrow accumulation and present with Erlenmeyer flask appearance, osteonecrosis (particularly of the femoral head), and pathologic fractures, especially of the spine and femoral neck. Bone lesions are most common in the femur, but they also occur in the pelvis, vertebra, humerus, and other locations.[280] Infiltration of bone by Gaucher cells leads to vessel thrombosis, compromising the medullary vascular supply and leading to localized osteonecrosis of the long bones.[442] ON of the femoral head occurs in most patients in whom the disease is diagnosed in childhood.

Pathologic fractures, especially of the femoral neck or shaft after biopsy, and of the spine, are usually best managed conservatively. Katz et al.[251] reported 23 pathologic fractures in nine children with Gaucher disease; seven had multiple fractures. In decreasing order of frequency, the site of involvement included the distal femur, basilar neck of the femur, spine, and proximal tibia. Fractures also occurred infrequently in the distal tibia, proximal humerus, rib, and acetabulum. Fractures of the long bones were transverse and usually in the metaphysis. Fractures of the spine were either wedge-shaped or centrally depressed at the end plate. The factors predisposing these children to fracture included significant medullary space infiltration, cortical bone erosion, osteonecrosis, and associated disuse osteoporosis.[251]

In another report of 53 patients with Gaucher disease aged 9 to 18 years,[253] 11 children had vertebral fractures, usually at two or three sites in each patient, with either anterior wedging, central vertebral collapse, or total rectangular collapse. Most patients had relief of their pain after 1 to 4 months of conservative treatment; two required decompression laminectomies, and one had a posterior lateral fusion to stabilize the spine.

Katz et al.[252] found that fractures of the upper extremities in Gaucher disease were prone to occur in areas of prior crisis. Although external callus formed in 6 to 8 weeks in most patients, complete healing with internal callus took almost 2 years in some. Other authors have found fracture union to be rapid.[187] Both delayed union and nonunion[442] have been reported in older patients with Gaucher's disease.

Pathologic femoral neck fractures with minimal associated trauma in children with Gaucher disease often heal with a varus malunion and minimal subsequent remodeling; osteonecrosis of the femoral head also can be associated with femoral neck fractures.[187,280] Goldman and Jacobs[187] stated that the presence of a mixed density of bone of the femoral neck on radiograph with narrowing of the medial cortex was a risk factor for fracture.

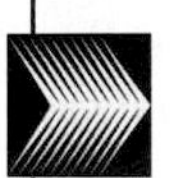

AUTHORS' PREFERRED METHOD OF TREATMENT

Conservative immobilization with nonweight bearing is suggested for long bone fractures when appropriate. Stable fractures of the femoral neck should be treated by immobiliza-

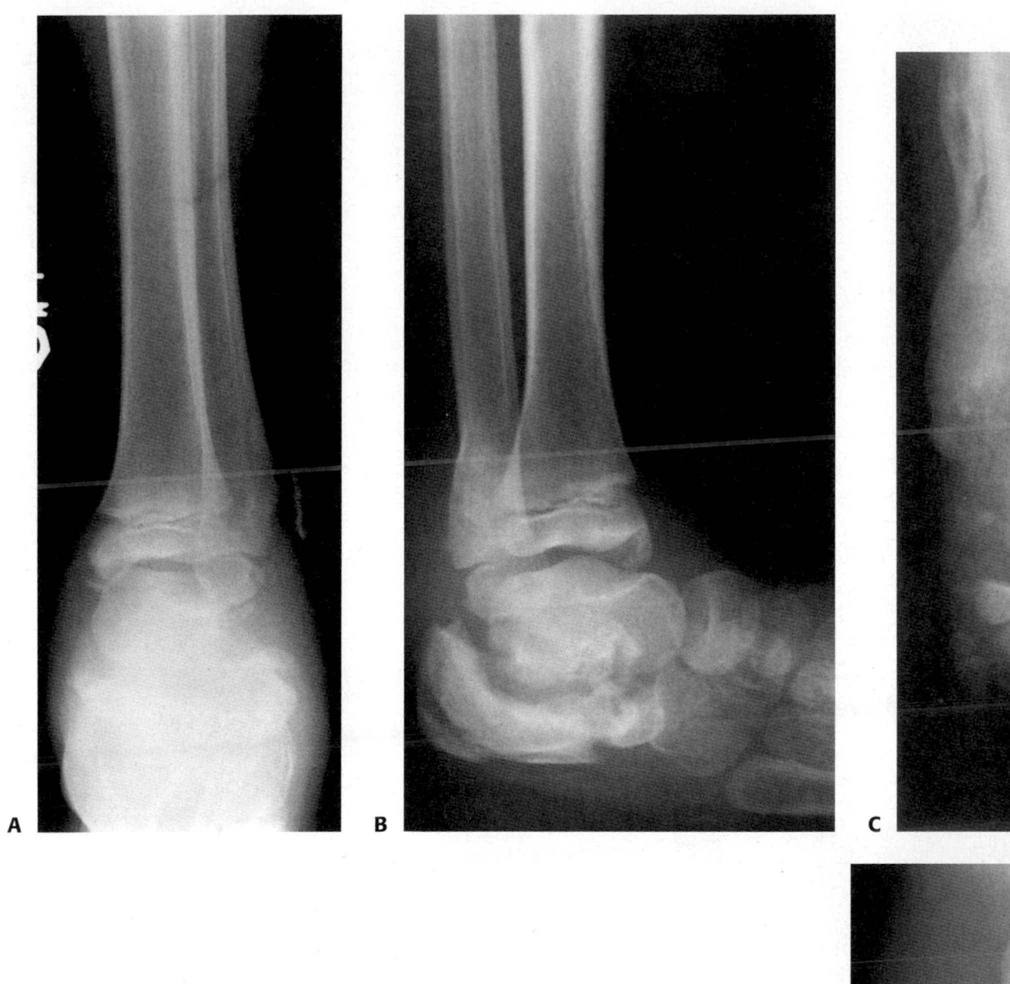

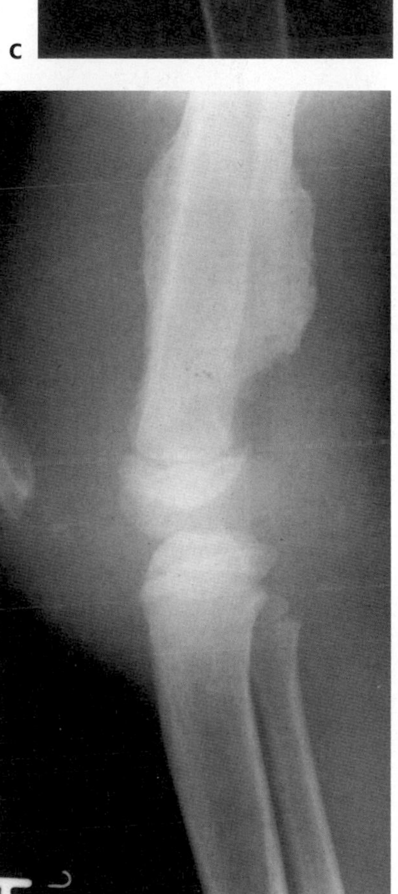

FIGURE 6-24 This 6-year-old child with anhidrosis, congenital insensitivity to pain, and attention deficit disorder presented with a history of swollen ankles and knees. Anteroposterior **(A)** and lateral **(B)** radiographs show Charcot changes in the subtalar joint with calcaneal and distal fibular fractures. Anteroposterior **(C)** and lateral **(D)** radiographs of the right knee show large, loose osteochondral fragments, medial subluxation of the femur on the tibia, and extensive periosteal new bone formation in the distal femur. Soft tissue shadows are consistent with her huge knee hemarthrosis. More than 100 mL of sterile serosan guineous fluid was aspirated from the knee at her initial visit. The effusion quickly returned in the days following the aspiration. Because management with casts at another hospital resulted in significant skin breakdown, we stabilized the knees with removable hinged braces. The effusions improved but did not resolve.

tion with frequent follow-up radiographs. Internal fixation should be used in unstable femoral neck fractures. Preoperative planning is important, and the anesthesiologist must recognize that patients with Gaucher disease may be prone to upper airway obstruction because of infiltration of the upper airway with glycolipids[499] and abnormal clotting function, even when clotting tests are normal.[217]

Sickle Cell Disease

The term sickle cell disease (SCD) characterizes conditions caused by the presence of sickle cell hemoglobin (HbS). The most common type of SCD, HbS-S, is a homozygous recessive condition in which individuals inherit the HbS globin gene from each parent. SCD has systemic effects particularly on splenic function and on the central nervous, renal, hepatic, and musculoskeletal systems. SCD affects approximately one in 400 African Americans. Sickle cell trait affects 8% to 10% of the African American population and other groups less frequently. With sickle cell trait, each individual has inherited a beta-S globin gene and a beta-A globin gene. Clinical manifestations of sickle cell trait usually are not apparent. The presence of this abnormal hemoglobin in red blood cells causes them to be mechanically fragile, and when they are deoxygenated, the cells assume a sickle shape, which makes them prone to clumping with blockage of the small vessels of the spleen, kidneys, and bones.[406] Chronic hemolytic anemia is present in most severely affected patients, and marrow hyperplasia is found in both the long bones and the short tubular bones. The prevalence of osteopenia and osteoporosis in young adults with SCD is extremely high and that can be related or predispose to pathologic fractures.[361] These disorders are diagnosed by hemoglobin electrophoresis.[92]

Pathologic fractures of the long bones in SCD occur frequently[45,61,141,356,477] and may be the first symptom of the disorder.[406] Children with SCD often have undiagnosed osteopenia or osteoporosis (Fig. 6-25).[361] Pathologic fractures are often seen in association with osteomyelitis. In a series of 81 patients with 198 long bone infarcts with occasional concurrent osteo-

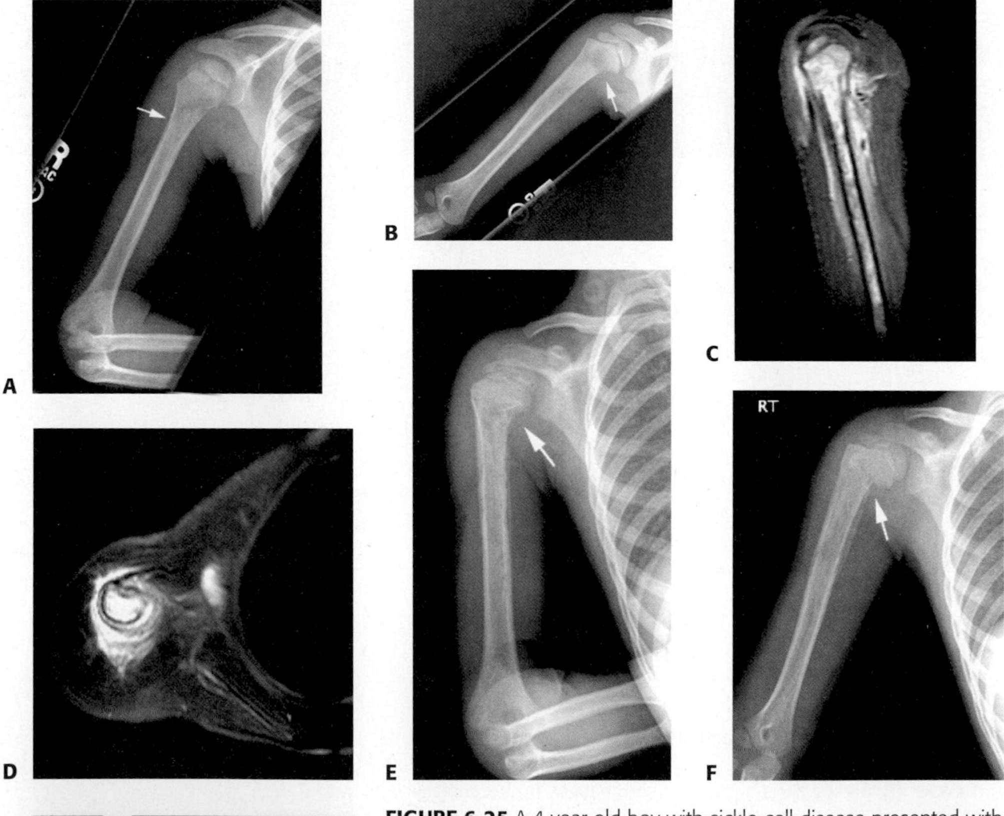

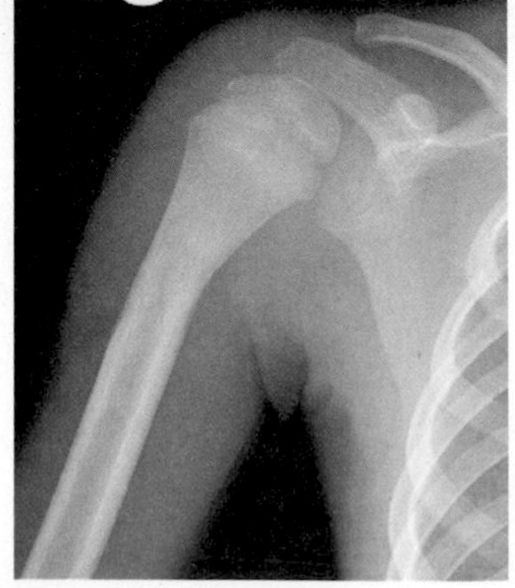

FIGURE 6-25 A 4-year-old boy with sickle cell disease presented with acute onset of right arm pain, swelling, increased warmth, and low-grade fever. The initial radiographs **(A,B)** show a poorly defined area of lucency in the proximal humeral metaphysis (*arrow*). T2-weighted sagittal **(C)** and axial **(D)** MRI show intramedullary changes (enhancement) and periosteal reaction/abscess with no soft tissue mass. The clinical diagnosis of osteomyelitis was initially made and the patient was started on intravenous antibiotics. Three weeks later, there was little clinical improvement and new radiographs showed pathologic fracture/insufficiency fracture through the proximal humeral metaphysis **(E,F)** (*arrow*). The patient underwent a biopsy that showed that this was an infarct with no superimposed infection. After clinical treatment, the patient's symptoms improved. At 6-months follow-up, he was completely asymptomatic and the radiographs showed remodeling and continued growth **(G)**.

myelitis, Bohrer[57] found evidence of fracture in 25% of femoral lesions, 20% of humeral lesions, and a significant percentage also in tibial bone infarcts. Ebong[141] reported pathologic fractures in 20% of patients with SCD and osteomyelitis. The most common site of fracture was the femur. The fractures are transverse and commonly located in the shaft of the long bone,[123] and although minimal trauma is needed to cause them,[356] they often have significant displacement.[57,58] The exact mechanism for pathologic fracture in these patients is unclear; although it is often associated with bone infarct, the fracture itself is seldom through the area of infarction. Marrow hyperplasia may be a major contributing factor; not only does the hypercellular bone marrow expand the medullary canal with thinning of both trabecular and cortical bone, but it also extends into widened Haversian and Volkmann canals.[123] This process probably weakens the bone sufficiently so that fractures occur. Also, children with SCD have significant deficits in the whole body bone mineral content that persist despite adjustment for poor growth and decreased lean mass; therefore, these children may be at increased risk for fragility fractures and suboptimal peak bone mass.[73] The healing process seems unaffected, and union usually occurs normally.[406]

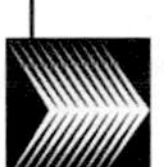

AUTHORS' PREFERRED METHOD OF TREATMENT

Pathologic fractures in patients with SCD usually heal well with conservative treatment. Operative management of fractures in patients with SCD is potentially hazardous. Extreme care must be taken to oxygenate the patient's tissues adequately during the procedure, and ideally, elective procedures should be preceded by multiple transfusions to reduce HbS to less than 30% of total hemoglobin levels. A randomized multicenter study found that a simple conservative transfusion regimen to raise hemoglobin levels to 10 g/dL was as effective as an aggressive exchange transfusion regimen (to reduce HbS to less than 30%) in preventing perioperative complications.

Intravenous hydration is also important, with one and a half to two times the daily fluid requirements needed in addition to routine replacement of fluid losses. The use of a tourniquet in surgery for patients with SCD is somewhat controversial. Osteonecrosis of the femoral head is an especially difficult problem in patients with SCD. Treatment options include conservative measures such as physical therapy and sometimes core decompression, although some have shown no difference in the final outcome.[378] Patients with total head involvement may require femoral or pelvic osteotomies. Athanassiou-Metaxa et al.[27] showed that out of nine children treated with subtrochanteric varus femoral osteotomy for femoral head osteonecrosis, eight children experienced improvements in pain, joint motion, and walking. Total joint replacement is occasionally indicated in young adults. Before general anesthesia, the patient's hematocrit should be raised to more than 30 and hemoglobin to more than 10 g/dL.

Leukemia

Leukemia accounts for over 30% of cases of childhood cancer. Acute lymphocytic leukemia is one of the most common malignant diseases in childhood and accounts for 80% of pediatric leukemias. There is an increased occurrence of lymphoid leukemias in patients with Down syndrome, immunodeficiencies, and ataxic telangiectasia. The peak incidence occurs at 4 years of age.

Leukemic involvement of bones and joints is common. Skeletal lesions occur more frequently in leukemic children than in adults because leukemic cells can quickly replace the smaller marrow reserves in children. Approximately 50% to 75% of children with acute leukemia develop radiographic skeletal manifestations during the course of their disease.[213,351] Pathologic fractures can be seen in up to a third of the patients.[268,439,476]

Skeletal involvement occurs in approximately 50% of patients; however, there are no pathognomonic osseous manifestations.[476] Diffuse osteopenia is the most frequent radiographic finding (Fig. 6-26).[476] Nonspecific juxtaepiphyseal lucent lines are often seen and are a result of generalized metabolic dysfunction. Sclerotic bands of bone trabeculae are more typical in older children. Lucencies and periostitis may mimic osteomyelitis. A characteristic lesion seen within a month of onset of symptoms is a radiolucent metaphyseal band adjacent to the physis[476]; these are usually bilateral and vary from 2 to 15 mm in width. Osteolytic lesions with punctate areas of radiolucency are found in the metaphysis and can either appear moth-eaten or as a confluent radiolucency. Periosteal reaction often is present with osteolytic lesions and is most common in the posterior cortex of the distal femoral metaphysis, the medial neck of the femur, and the diaphysis of the tibia and fibula.[476] Most bone lesions in leukemia improve during remission after treatment and tend to progress with worsening of the disease.

The risk of pathologic fractures usually decreases with treatment. Fracture is most commonly associated with osteoporosis of the spine, resulting in vertebral collapse (compression fracture). The thoracic vertebrae are the most commonly involved. Fractures occasionally occur at other locations and usually after minor trauma.[233,378] A bone scan may aid in identifying clinically silent areas but may not correlate with areas of obvious destruction on radiographs. Spastic paraparesis has been reported in one patient with vertebral fracture due to leukemia.[233]

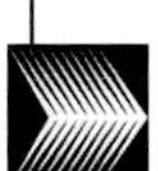

AUTHORS' PREFERRED METHOD OF TREATMENT

Prompt diagnosis and initiation of chemotherapy is the first step in the treatment of pathologic fractures associated with leukemia. Most fractures are stable microfractures and can be treated with conservative immobilization techniques with emphasis on early ambulation to avoid further problems with disuse osteoporosis. Most vertebral fractures can be treated nonoperatively with close observation; however, often a back brace or thoracolumbosacral orthosis is used to alleviate symptoms.

Hemophilia

Hemophilia is a sex-linked recessive disorder of the clotting mechanism that presents most commonly as a functional deficiency of either factor VIII (hemophilia A) or factor IX (hemophilia B). Classic hemophilia, or hemophilia A (factor VIII defi-

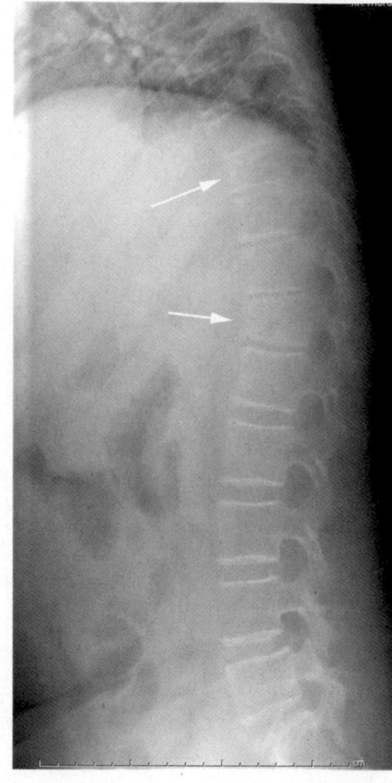

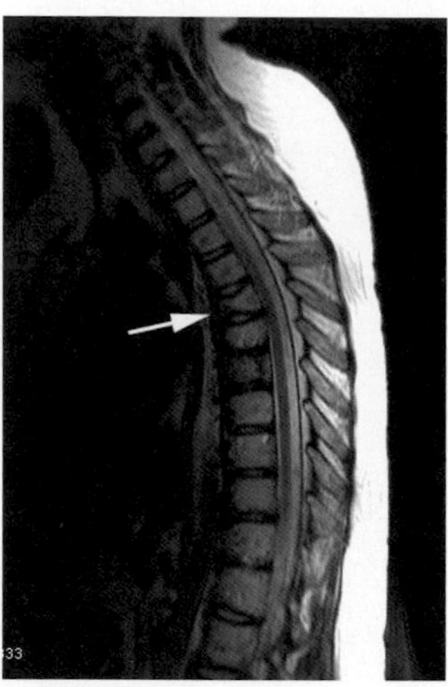

FIGURE 6-26 This 8-year-old girl presented with back pain, fever, malaise, and weight loss. Lateral radiographs **(A)** of the spine showed diffuse osteopenia and compression/insufficiency fractures of the vertebral body (*arrows*). T1-weighted sagittal MRI **(B)** confirms disease process within the vertebral body (*arrow*) and no soft tissue mass or intraspinal involvement. She was diagnosed with acute lymphoblastic leukemia. (Figures reproduced with permission from The Childrens Orthopaedic Center, Los Angeles, CA.)

ciency), is an inherited sex-linked recessive disorder. The incidence is one per 10,000 live male births in the United States.[7] Christmas disease, or hemophilia B, is a sex-linked recessive factor IX deficiency and occurs in one per 40,000 live births.

When hemophilia is suspected, screening tests should be performed, including platelet count, bleeding time, prothrombin time, and partial thromboplastin time. Deficiency of factor VIII, the most common form of hemophilia, causes a marked prolongation in the partial thromboplastin time.[467] Once the disease is suspected, specific factor assays can document the type of hemophilia.

Musculoskeletal complications in a child with hemophilia include acute hemarthroses (knee, elbow, and ankle, in decreasing order of frequency), soft tissue and muscle bleeds, acute compartment syndrome, carpal tunnel syndrome, and femoral nerve neuropraxia (Table 6-5). The severity of the deficiency often is correlated with circulating levels of factors VIII or IX. The disease is classified as severe when clotting activity is less than 1%, moderate when clotting activity is 1% to 5%, and mild when clotting activity is more than 5%. By definition, each milliliter of normal human plasma contains one unit of factor activity, and the clinical severity of hemophilia correlates with the patient's percentage of normal levels of plasma factor activity (Table 6-6). Early diagnosis and aggressive management are the keys to lessening complications.

TABLE 6-5 Grades of Articular Involvement

Grade 1	Transitory synovitis; no bleeding sequelae and with no more than three episodes in 3 months
Grade 2	Permanent synovitis with increased joint size, synovial thickening, and limitation of movement
Grade 3	Chronic arthropathy with axial deformity and muscular atrophy
Grade 4	Ankylosis

Surgery in Hemophilia

Should a child with hemophilia require operative management of a fracture, the orthopaedist and the hematologist should work closely together. Preoperatively, the patient should be tested for the presence of inhibitor and a test dose of factor replacement should be given to determine the biologic half-life of that factor for that particular patient.[7] Elective surgery is usually contraindicated in the presence of inhibitor. Most authors recommend a level of factor activity during surgery ranging from 70% to 100%,[7,283,412] although others believe that approximately 50% is adequate.[402,407] Tourniquets are recommended for extremity surgery. The use of routine drains is not advised, but 24 hours of suction drainage is favored by some.[7,283,412] Factor levels are checked immediately after surgery and then at least daily. Factor VIII is given every 6 hours, and factor IX is given every 8 hours. It is useful to check a trough level factor activity immediately before the next dose of factor supplementation. In the immediate postoperative period, factor levels are maintained at 30% to 40%,[7,283] and these levels should be maintained until sutures are removed. During the rehabilitative period, maintenance levels of factor ranging from 20% to 50% immediately before sessions of physical therapy should be maintained.[7,282,402,412] Intramuscular injections of analgesics should be avoided, as should aspirin compounds and nonsteroidal anti-inflammatory medications that affect platelet function. Both acetaminophen and codeine medications are safe oral analgesics.[249] In the past, hemophiliac patients had an increased risk of operative infections and delayed wound healing, but aggressive replacement therapy has minimized those problems.[412]

Fractures in patients with hemophilia do not appear to happen more or less frequently than in nonhemophilic patients.[56,62,440] Nonetheless, decreased bone mineral density

TABLE 6-6 Severity of Hemophilia Correlated with Plasma Factor Activity Levels

Degree of Hemophilia	Percentage of Factor	Clinical Characteristics
Mild	20%–60%	Usually clinically occult, excessive bleeding after major trauma or surgery
Moderate	5%–20%	Excessive bleeding during surgery and after minor trauma
Moderately severe	1%–5%	Excessive bleeding with mild injury and infrequent spontaneous hemarthrosis
Severe	Less than 1%	Frequent excessive bleeding with trauma and spontaneous bleeding into the soft tissue and joints

(osteopenia and osteoporosis) is frequently diagnosed in hemophiliac patients, especially when there is hepatitis C associated.[37,511] Most authors have noted that healing of fractures proceeds primarily with endosteal callus and very little periosteal callus,[160,163,257] but Lancourt et al.[282] observed significant periosteal calcification in these fractures with a normal rate of healing. Fractures occur in both the upper and lower extremities.[6,56,160,257,437] Joint dislocations are rare in hemophiliac patients. Floman and Niska[166] reported on a 6-year-old boy who sustained a posterior dislocation of the hip with mild trauma that required a closed reduction under general anesthesia and immobilization in a hip spica cast. The joint was found to be enclosed at a 6-year follow-up. Ackroyd and Dinley[3] reported on two patients with the patella locked into the intercondylar notch of the distal femur after sustaining hyperflexion injuries of the knees, which had limited range of motion owing to arthropathy. These injuries were treated by flexion of the knee under general anesthesia, depression of the inferior pole of the patella to unlock it, and then extension of the knee followed by splinting.

Most fractures in hemophiliac patients are treated conservatively with immobilization.[294] Factor replacement is important for about the first week after the fracture, and levels of factor activity recommended vary from 20% to 50%.[6,7,56,160,227,282] Circumferential plaster casts are extremely hazardous in the treatment of these fractures because of the risk of swelling from bleeding as well as subsequent compartment syndrome and skin necrosis.[485] A Robert Jones dressing may be preferable for fracture immobilization immediately after injury, and a cast should be applied once active swelling has stopped.[227] All casts applied should be well padded and split, and the patient should be monitored carefully for swelling. Fractures of the femur can be treated with traction and subsequent spica casting.[56,294] Some authors consider skeletal traction to be hazardous because of the risk of infection or bleeding,[7,227] but Boardman and English[56] suggested that with proper replacement therapy, skeletal pins can be used in the hemophiliac. Replacement therapy is advisable while fractures are manipulated and casts are changed. Most authors think that open reduction and internal fixation should be performed in hemophiliac patients for fractures that would customarily be treated with such methods.[7,56,282] External fixators are not commonly used for patients with hemophilia; however, Lee et al.[295] described the use of external fixators (Ilizarov, AO, uni- and biplanar fixators, and Charnley clamp) in nine patients with hemophilia for arthrodesis of infected joints, treatment of open fractures, and osteoclasis. One major complication related to external fixators occurred in a patient who developed inhibitors. They concluded that external fixators can be used safely in hemophilic patients without inhibitors and does not require prolonged factor replacement.[295]

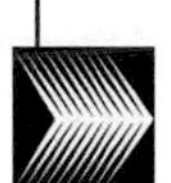

AUTHORS' PREFERRED METHOD OF TREATMENT

Collaboration between the orthopaedist and the hematologist is important in providing care for children with hemophilia. Most fractures in children with hemophilia can be treated with either traction or cast techniques. Care must be taken to avoid complications related to compression in these patients, and a monovalved, well-padded plaster cast provides a safe means of treatment. A fiberglass cast may not be desirable because a simple monovalved will fail to expand the cast completely. Operative treatment should be reserved for fractures that normally require surgery, and the usual precautions for hemophiliac patients for surgery are observed.

Osteomyelitis

The pattern of pediatric acute hematogenous osteomyelitis in North America has changed during the past several decades. Although the typical clinical picture of acute osteomyelitis in children is still seen, subtle presentations and more aggressive pathogens have become more frequent. There are several reasons for this change, including modification of the clinical course by antibiotics given before admission[162] and, possibly, increased awareness and an earlier presentation to a medical facility resulting in earlier diagnosis. Children often present with acute osteomyelitis. Less common variants include Brodie abscess, subacute epiphyseal osteomyelitis, viral osteomyelitis,[474] and chronic recurrent multifocal osteomyelitis.[243] Some patients present with a bone lesion that may be confused with other disease entities, including neoplasm.[75] Biopsy is often needed to clarify the diagnosis. Even with appropriate antibiotic therapy, some patients have recurrent infection, growth disturbance, and pathologic fractures.

Acute hematogenous osteomyelitis can be classified by age (neonatal, childhood, and adult osteomyelitis), organism (pyo-

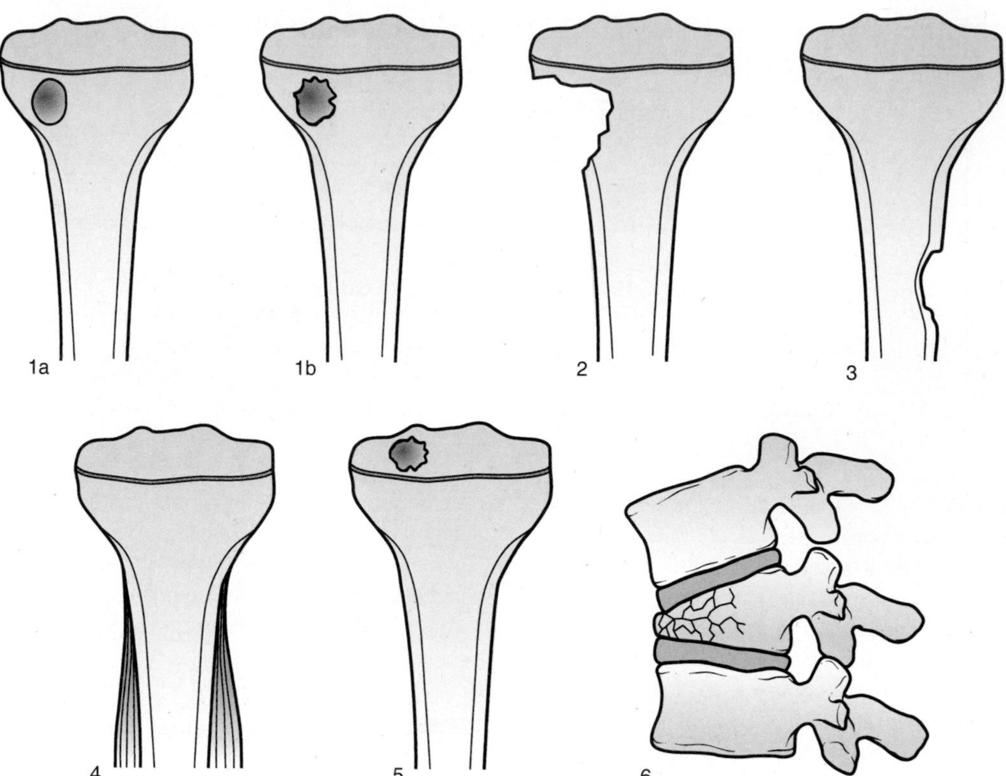

FIGURE 6-27 Classification of subacute osteomyelitis. Type 1A, punched-out radiolucency suggestive of eosinophilic granuloma. Type 1B, similar but with sclerotic margin; classic Brodie abscess. Type II, metaphyseal lesion with loss of cortical bone. Type III, diaphyseal lesion with excessive cortical reaction. Type IV, lesion with onionskin layering of subperiosteal bone. Type V, concentric epiphyseal radiolucency. Type VI, osteomyelitic lesion of vertebral body. (From Dormans JP, Drummond DS. Pediatric hematogenous osteomyelitis: new trends in presentation, diagnosis, and treatment. J Am Acad Orthop Surg 1994;2:333–341, with permission.)

genic and granulomatous infections), onset (acute, subacute, and chronic), and routes of infection (hematogenous and direct inoculation). Chronic osteomyelitis is defined by most authors as osteomyelitis with symptoms that have been present for longer than 1 month (Fig. 6-27 and Table 6-7).

Radiographic Evaluation

Only 20% of patients have plain radiographic findings of osteomyelitis within 10 to 14 days after onset of symptoms; the earliest finding is loss of defined deep soft tissue planes.[236] Because of this early insensitivity of plain radiographic studies, isotope-scanning techniques have been used to aid in diagnosis with varying rates of success. In proven osteomyelitis, abnormal technetium scans are seen in 63% to 90% of patients.[229] MRI detects increased intramedullary water and decreased fat content, which occurs when there is inflammatory exudate, edema, hyperemia, and ischemia, all of which are markers of infection.[274] MRI has up to 98% sensitivity and 100% specificity for the detection of osteomyelitis.[274]

In 1932, Capener and Pierce[84] reviewed 1068 patients with osteomyelitis and found only 18 pathologic fractures, 13 of which occurred in the femur. They thought these fractures were due to delayed recognition of the infection or inadequate treatment. Other factors were disuse osteopenia, presence of a weak involucrum, and excessive surgical removal of involved bone. In that preantibiotic era, most of the fractures were sustained after surgical treatment of the osteomyelitis, and the authors believed that conservation of the involucrum and proper immo-

TABLE 6-7 Comparison of Acute and Subacute Hematogenous Osteomyelitis

Presentation	Subacute	Acute
Pain	Mild	Severe
Fever	Few patients	Majority
Loss of function	Minimal	Marked
Prior antibiotics	Often (30%–40%)	Occasional
Elevated white blood cell count	Few	Majority
Elevated erythrocyte sedimentation rate	Majority	Majority
Blood cultures	Few positive	50% positive
Bone cultures	60% positive	85% positive
Initial x-ray study	Frequently abnormal	Often normal
Site	Any location (may cross physis)	Usually metaphysis

From Dormans JP, Drummond DS. Pediatric hematogenous osteomyelitis: new trends in presentation, diagnosis, and treatment. J Am Acad Ortho Surg 1994;2: 333–341.

bilization could have prevented these injuries. White and Dennison[518] noted that before antibiotics, pathologic fractures of osteomyelitis were common, but union occurred with certainty in the presence of dense involucrum. Daoud and Saighi-Bouaouina[111] reported on 34 patients with hematogenous osteomyelitis complicated by pathologic fracture, pseudarthrosis, or significant segmental bone loss. The tibia was affected in 24 cases, the femur was affected in 8 cases, and the humerus was affected in two cases. A pathologic proximal femoral fracture has been reported in neonatal osteomyelitis.[28] Although extremely rare, hematogenous osteomyelitis has also been reported at the site of a closed fracture.[81,254,459] Canale et al.[81] reported three children with osteomyelitis after closed fracture. They pointed out that progressive pain and swelling at a fracture site during healing are suggestive of possible osteomyelitis. Daoud et al.[110] reported 35 children with upper femoral osteomyelitis with associated septic arthritis. The incidence of osteonecrosis (ON) of the femoral head was approximately 50% both in the group that was treated with arthroscopy and in the group in which no surgery had been done. They postulated that ON of the femoral head may be due to compression by abscess of the vessels lying on the posterior superior femoral neck. The complications of fracture, dislocation, and displacement of the capital femoral epiphysis occurred in two thirds of their patients, and these usually were patients who presented long after an acute phase of the disease. They recommended surgical drainage of septic hips, and reduction and stabilization of hips with ON using skin traction and plaster immobilization for 40 to 60 days. Lewallen and Peterson[459] documented osteomyelitis in 40% of 20 nonunions of diaphyseal open fractures in children. They believed that the presence of infection was a significant factor in their failure to heal. Long bone lesions also may be present in congenital rubella,[446] and pathologic fractures have been reported in congenital cytomegalic inclusion disease.[480]

Treatment

Fractures associated with osteomyelitis may be difficult to treat and may be associated with complications such as malunion and growth disturbance (Fig. 6-28).[367] Pathologic fractures associated with osteomyelitis are rare in North America and usually are associated with neglected or chronic osteomyelitis, neonatal osteomyelitis, or septic arthritis. In children with chronic osteomyelitis, the purulent material elevates the periosteum and a supportive involucrum develops. Sequestrectomy of a portion of the necrotic diaphysis while leaving the supportive involucrum is often needed to bring the infection under control, but the timing of this procedure is controversial. Langenskiold[286] delayed sequestrectomy of a necrotic femoral shaft for 10 months in a 6-year-old patient to allow the involucrum to develop, but Daoud and Saighi-Bouaouina[111] recommended much earlier débridement. In patients with active infection, they performed sequestrectomy with débridement followed by antibiotic therapy for up to 6 months. Prolonged cast immobilization was necessary. They obtained healing in 33 of 34 patients with pathologic fractures or pseudarthroses due to osteomyelitis. The mean healing time of fractures was 5 months in patients with involucrum. Patients with active infection without involucrum required débridement, antibiotics, and subsequent treatment with corticocancellous iliac graft. The mean healing time was 8.7 months. The patients without active infection and no involucrum were treated with prolonged immobilization and cancellous bone graft, supplemented by fixation. Angular deformities were treated with cast manipulation. Tudisco et al.[502] reported on 26 patients with chronic osteomyelitis with average follow-up of 23 years. Approximately 15% had shortening and angular

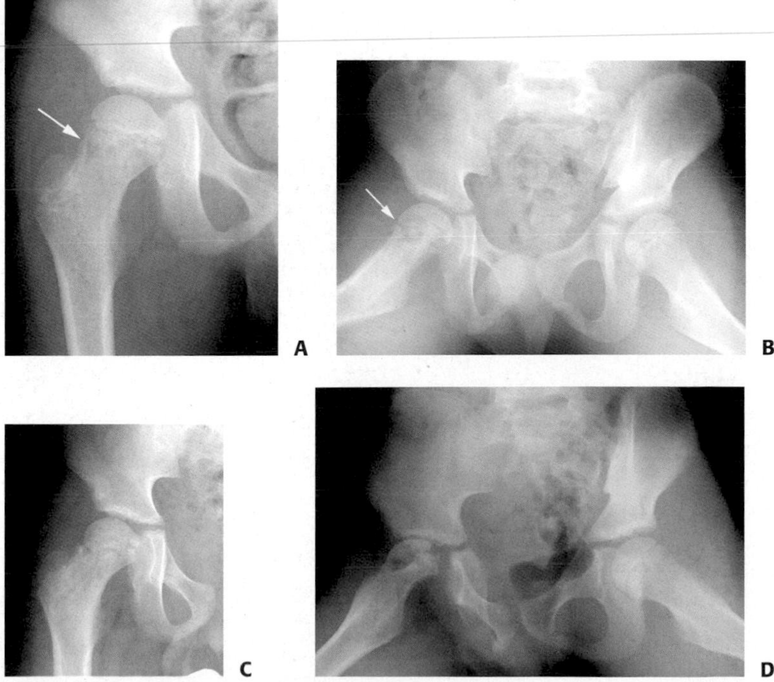

FIGURE 6-28 A 7-year-old boy presented with classic picture of septic arthritis of the right hip. He underwent promptly irrigation and débridement of the hip. On follow-up just a few weeks later, plain radiographs demonstrated a lytic area in the femoral neck **(A,B)** (*arrow*) and blood work showed increased c-reative protein and sedimentation rate. The patient underwent repeated irrigation of the hip and drilling of the lytic area (osteomyelitis) in the femoral neck. Two months later, he developed collapse (pathologic fracture) of the femoral head with gross deformity of the proximal femur **(C,D)**, especially in the lateral views **(D)** with decreased range of motion. (Figures reproduced with permission from The Childrens Orthopaedic Center, Los Angeles, CA.)

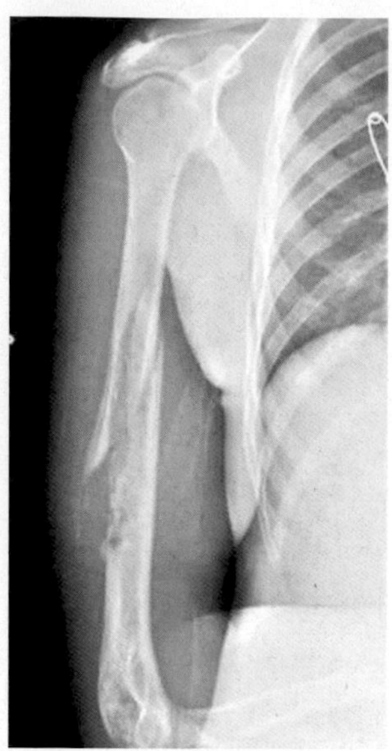

FIGURE 6-29 This lateral radiograph of the humeral shaft of a 17-year-old boy shows a pathologic fracture through chronic osteomyelitis of the humerus. (Case courtesy of B. David Horn, MD.)

deformity of the affected limb. Newer techniques for difficult cases have also been developed.

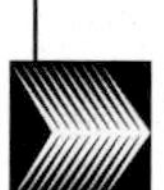

AUTHORS' PREFERRED METHOD OF TREATMENT

With early recognition and appropriate treatment, osteomyelitis leading to pathologic fracture is uncommon. When osteomyelitis is associated with pathologic fracture (Fig. 6-29), it usually is neglected chronic osteomyelitis or, rarely, neonatal osteomyelitis or septic arthritis. The most important step in the treatment of fracture associated with osteomyelitis is to control the underlying infection. At a minimum, this requires biopsy for culture and sensitivities, drainage and débridement of the infection with immobilization in association with antibiotic therapy (Table 6-8). In advanced infections, sequestrectomy may be necessary. MRI is useful in identifying the sequestrum; an attempt should be made to leave as much supporting involucrum as possible at the time of sequestrectomy. Bone transport and lengthening may be valuable in certain cases. Prolonged immobilization with either plaster casts or external fixation devices may be needed, and segmental bone loss can be treated with bone transport or grafting.

PATHOLOGIC FRACTURES AFTER LIMB LENGTHENING

Limb lengthening has evolved dramatically over the past several decades. Surgeons experienced with lengthening techniques can now correct problems that previously had no satisfactory solution. The very high complication rate that has come with these advances has decreased with newer techniques and more extensive surgical experience. Complications with the Wagner method, popular 20 to 30 years ago, were as high as 92%.[224,320] Newer techniques, using gradual lengthening with either monolateral fixators or fine wire fixators, such as the Ilizarov fixator, have decreased the complication rate. Fractures that occur in association with limb lengthening fall into three general categories: (i) fractures through pin tracks, (ii) fractures through regenerate bone, or (iii) fractures through bone weakened by disuse osteoporosis. Fractures that occur through holes left after removal of screws or fine wires generally occur a few weeks after device removal. The incidence of these fractures can be minimized by protective weight bearing after removal of the device and using the smallest possible screw diameter that is appropriate for the fixation device needed.

Fractures through regenerate bone are true pathologic fractures. The bone that is formed by distraction callotasis must be subjected to normal weight-bearing forces over a period of time before normal bony architecture is established. Fractures that occur through the lengthening gap can occur either soon after removal of the fixator or years later (Fig. 6-30). Various reports describe fractures through regenerative bone occurring as late as 2 to 8 years after lengthening.[318,320,370] The incidence of fractures has been reported to be as high as 50% for Wagner lengthening but only 3% for newer

TABLE 6-8 Initial Antibiotic Therapy for Osteomyelitis

Patient Type	Probable Organism	Initial Antibiotic
Neonate	Group B Streptococcus, *S. aureus*, Gram-negative rods (*H. influenza*)	Cefotaxime (100–120 mg/kg/ 24 h) or oxacillin and gentamicin (5–7.5 mg/kg/24 h)
Infants and children	*S. aureus* (90%) if allergic to penicillin* if allergic to penicillin and cephalosporins*	Oxacillin (150 mg/kg/24 h) Cefazolin (100 mg/kg/24 h) Clindamycin (25–40 mg/kg/24 h) or Vancomycin (40 mg/kg/24 h)
Sickle cell disease	*S. aureus* or Salmonella	Oxacillin and ampicillin or chloramphenicol or cefotaxime (100–120 mg/kg/24 h)

*Overall 80% due to *S. aureus*.

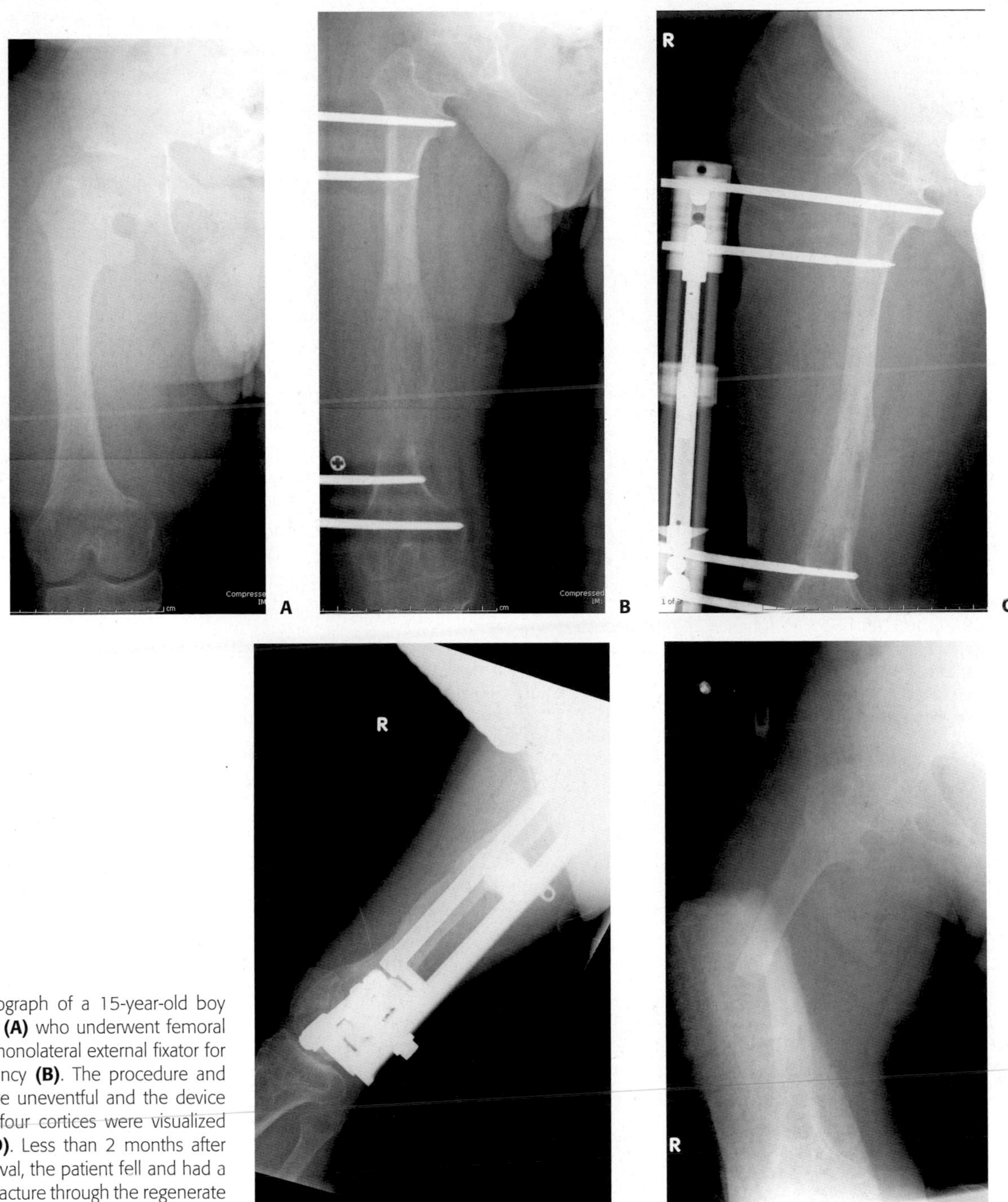

FIGURE 6-30 Radiograph of a 15-year-old boy with achondroplasia **(A)** who underwent femoral lengthening with a monolateral external fixator for limb-length discrepancy **(B)**. The procedure and the lengthening were uneventful and the device was removed after four cortices were visualized on radiographs **(C,D)**. Less than 2 months after external fixator removal, the patient fell and had a pathologic femoral fracture through the regenerate bone **(E)**. *(continues)*

techniques.[148,152,224,315,370,392,416] At present, most lengthenings are performed through the metaphysis, which has a larger bone diameter and better blood supply than the diaphysis (where Wagner lengthening was done).[315,395] When fractures occur in regenerate bone, they can be treated with simple cast immobilization. However, because this method further promotes osteopenia, many surgeons reapply a fixator, correct any malalignment caused by the fracture, and compress at the fracture site until healing. To ensure that the regenerate bone can bear the forces of normal activity, a variety of imaging methods have been used.[53,317] When the regenerate bone attains the density and ultrastructural appearance (development of the cortex and the medullary canal) of the adjacent bone, fixator removal is generally safe. Some authors have reported on decreased incidence of fractures combining lengthening with internal fixation (intramedullary nail or submuscular plating).[235,396]

Pathologic fracture can also be caused by the osteopenia and joint contractures that can occur after months in an external fixation device. Some children, because of pain or anxiety, are reluctant to bear sufficient weight on their fixator devices, putting them at risk for disuse osteoporosis. Joint contractures can be related to either the lengthening itself or insufficient rehabilitation during and after lengthening. Many of the fractures due to these causes are avoidable; when they do occur, appropriate immobilization or internal fixation is used.

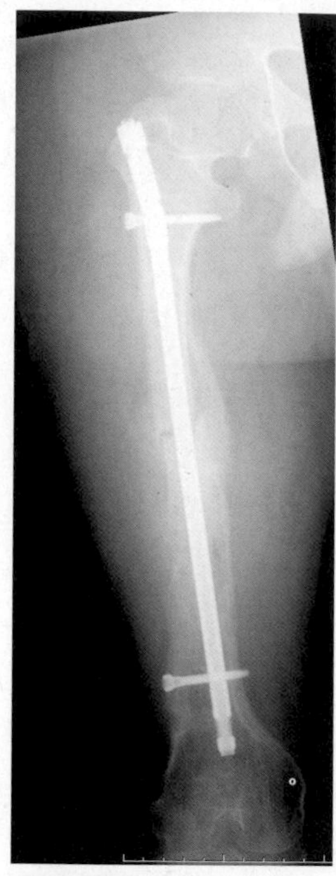

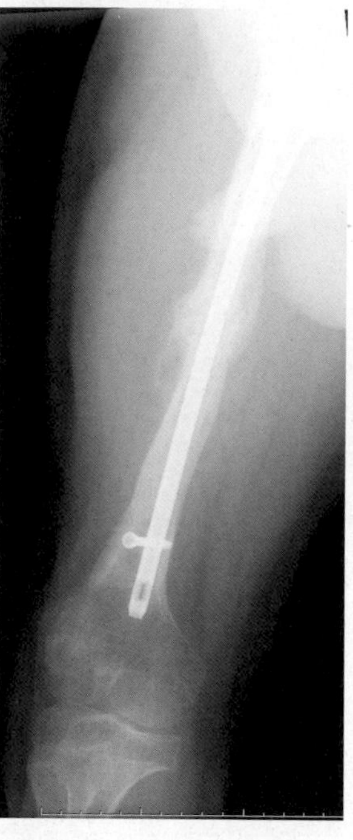

FIGURE 6-30 *(continued)* He underwent open reduction and internal fixation with an intramedullary device and the fracture healed in approximately 3 months **(F,G)**. (Figures reproduced with permission from The Childrens Orthopaedic Center, Los Angeles, CA.)

FRACTURES IN CONDITIONS THAT WEAKEN BONE

Osteogenesis Imperfecta

Osteogenesis imperfecta (OI) are heterogeneous group of inherited disorders in which the structure and function of type I collagen is altered. The fragile bone is susceptible to frequent fractures and progressive deformity.[98,269] OI is identifiable in 1 in 20,000 total births, with an overall prevalence of approximately 16 cases per million index patients.[269,527] The wide spectrum of clinical severity—from perinatal lethal forms to clinically silent forms—reflects the tremendous genotypic heterogeneity (more than 150 different mutations of the type 1 procollagen genes COL1A1 and COL1A2 have been described). Most forms of OI are the result of mutations in the genes that encode the pro alpha1 and pro alpha2 polypeptide chains of type I collagen.[384] As the molecular basis of this continuum of severity is further elucidated, the phenotypic groupings of the various classifications and subclassifications may seem arbitrary. However, these classifications facilitate communication, predict natural history, and help the clinician plan management strategies.[269] From a practical viewpoint of orthopaedic care, patients with OI can be divided into two groups. One group of patients with severe disease develops long-bone deformity through repetitive fractures, eventually requiring open treatment with intramedullary fixation. Another group of patients has mild disease with frequent fractures, but most of their injuries respond well to closed methods of treatment and there is less residual deformity.

Clinical Presentation

Children with severe OI may present with a short trunk, marked deformity of the weight-bearing lower extremities, prominence of the sternum, triangular faces, thin skin, muscle atrophy, and ligamentous laxity; some develop kyphoscoliosis,[46,204,365] basilar impression,[349,466] and deafness (due to otosclerosis).[205] Despite this multitude of physical problems, children with OI usually have normal intelligence. Blue sclera, a classic finding in certain forms of OI, can also be present in normal infants, as well as in children with hypophosphatasia, osteopetrosis, Marfan syndrome, and Ehlers-Danlos syndrome.[262] Osseous histologic findings in severe cases reveal a predominance of woven bone, an absence of lamellar bone, and thinning of the cortical bone with osteopenia. Children with OI also have a greater incidence of airway anomalies, thoracic anatomy abnormalities, coagulation dysfunction, hyperthyroidism, and an increased tendency to develop perioperative hyperthermia.[490]

Patients with OI may present with swelling of the extremity, pain, low-grade fever, and a radiograph showing exuberant, hyperplastic, callus formation. The callus may occur without fracture and can have a distinct butterfly shape,[262] as opposed to the usual fusiform callus of most healing fractures. The femur is most commonly involved, but involvement of the tibia and humerus has been reported.[431] The sedimentation rate and serum alkaline phosphatase may be elevated. Because osteosarcoma has been associated with OI,[240,265] aggressive-appearing lesions may occasionally require biopsy to confirm their benign nature.

Radiographic Findings

Radiographic findings vary (Fig. 6-31). In severe involvement, there is marked osteoporosis, thin cortical bone, and evidence of past fracture with angular malunion. Both anterior and lateral bowing of the femur and anterior bowing of the tibia are common. The long bones may be gracile with multiple cystic areas. Spinal radiographs may show compression of the vertebrae between the cartilaginous disc spaces (so-called codfish vertebra). The presence of wormian bones on a skull radiograph is relatively specific for OI. Subsequent development of multiple pathologic fractures with callus and deformity firmly establishes the diagnosis.

The diagnosis of OI is based on clinical and radiographic findings. There is no specific laboratory diagnostic test, although fibroblast cell culture can detect the collagen abnormality in 85% of OI patients.[97] In the absence of multiple fractures, the initial radiographic diagnosis can be difficult. It is crucial, but often difficult, to distinguish OI from nonaccidental injury.[266,362] Unexplained fractures in mild, undiagnosed OI can drag a family through unnecessary legal proceedings; conversely, a child with OI may be abused but not exhibit classic fracture patterns (e.g., corner fractures) owing to the fragility of their bones. Although no test or finding is specific, skin biopsy plays an important role.[403,486]

Treatment

Multiple fractures in OI usually are transverse, diaphyseal, and seldom displaced, and they usually heal at a relatively normal rate in most patients.[262,466] Most fractures in patients with OI occur before skeletal maturity. In a series of 31 patients, Moorefield and Miller[365] noted 951 fractures, 91% of which occurred before skeletal maturity. Fractures of the femur and tibia predominate. The humerus is the most commonly fractured bone in the upper extremity. Multiple long bone fractures may result in coxa vara, genu valgum, and leg-length discrepancy. Lateral

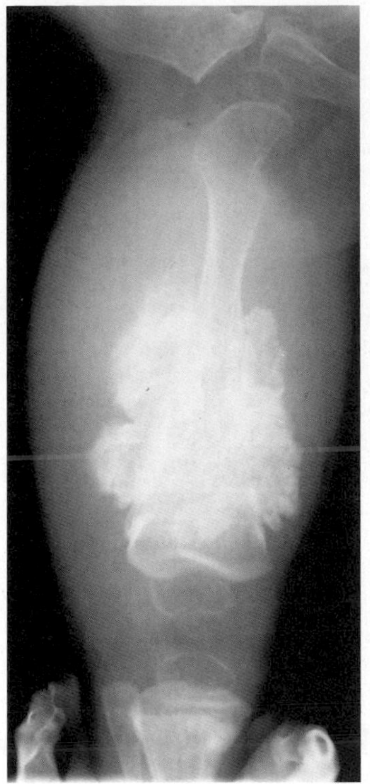
A

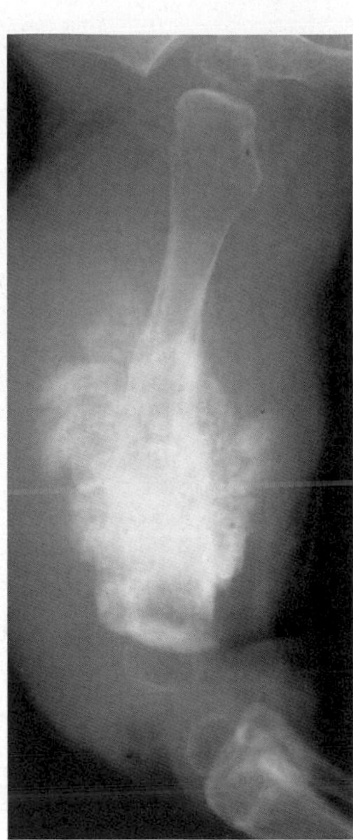
B

FIGURE 6-31 This 10-month-old boy with a history of osteogenesis imperfecta presented with a right thigh pain and swelling and refusal to bear weight. Anteroposterior **(A)** and lateral **(B)** radiographs of the right femur show the extraordinarily abundant, hyperplastic callus—with the characteristic butterfly shape—that can occur in osteogenesis imperfecta. This appearance may be mistaken for an infection or a neoplastic process.

dislocation of the radial head has been noted in some patients.[262] Olecranon sleeve (apophysis) fractures, which are rare in unaffected children, are more common in patients with OI, especially the tarda form (Fig. 6-32).[262,490] Zionts and Moon[531] reviewed 17 fractures of the olecranon apophysis in 10 children with mild OI; 15 of these fractures were treated operatively. The same injury presented in the opposite extremity 1 to 70 months after the initial fracture in seven of the 10 patients. All fractures had healed by the time of cast removal; however, two refractured. The authors concluded that with careful follow-up, cast immobilization can be used for minimally displaced fractures, but operative management is suggested for displaced fractures. The high rate of bilateral injury (70%) suggests that children with OI who sustain this fracture be counselled about the possible risks of injury to the opposite extremity.[531] Also, olecranon fractures in OI children tend to occur at a younger age.[200]

Nonunion may occur in patients with OI; however, callus

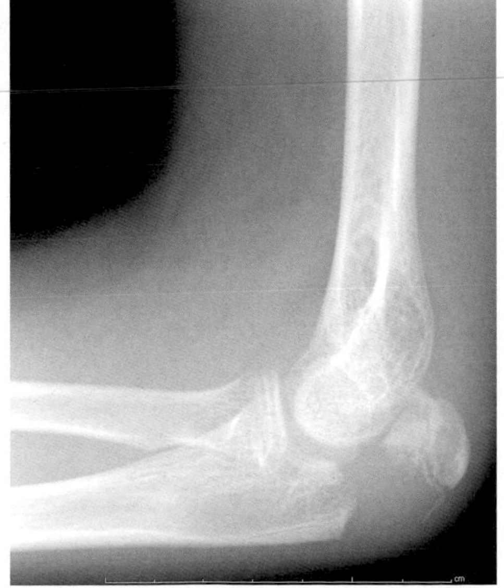
A

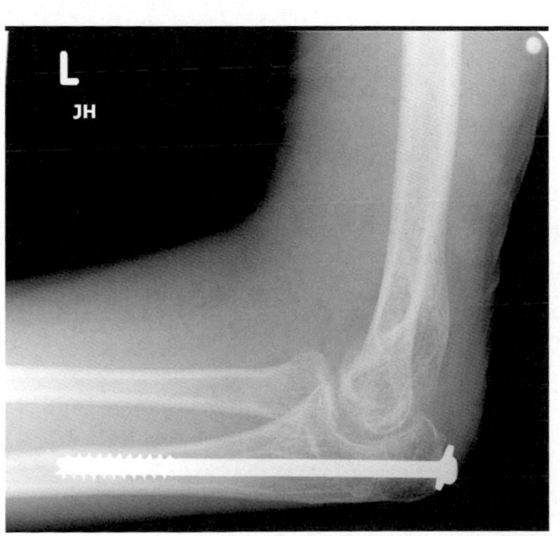

B

FIGURE 6-32 A 13-year-old boy with mild osteogenesis imperfecta presented after a fall on an outstretched arm, with inability to move his elbow, pain, and swelling. Radiographs showed a displaced olecranon fracture **(A)**. This fracture pattern is commonly seen in children with osteogenesis imperfecta and is quite uncommon in healthy children. The patient underwent open reduction and internal fixation. The fracture healed after 6 weeks **(B)**. (Figures reproduced with permission from The Childrens Orthopaedic Center, Los Angeles, CA.)

formation is usually adequate and most nonunions seem to be associated with inadequate fixation and distraction after osteotomies and fractures.[5] Gamble et al.[175] emphasized the problem with a report of 12 nonunions in 10 patients. Almost all had type III OI[470] and presented with nonpainful clinical deformity and decreased functional ability. A history of inadequate treatment of the initial fracture was seen in 50% of these nonunions. One patient eventually required an amputation for a painful nonunion of a distal femoral supracondylar fracture.

The role of medical therapy in the prevention of fractures associated to OI has been well established in the past few years. Bisphosphonates are a potent inhibitor of bone resorption and have been used with good results. Among the advantages of using bisphosphonates are good short-term safety (particularly with regard to renal function), significant reduction in chronic bone pain, decrease in the rate of fractures, gain in muscle force, increase in density and size of vertebral bodies, thickening of bone cortex, and gain in growth rate.[19,184] Some have reported on the negative effects that include decrease in bone remodeling rate, reduction in growth plate cartilage resorption, and delay in the healing of osteotomy sites.[184]

In a trial of 30 children with severe OI, Glorieux et al.[185] showed that cyclic intravenous administration of pamidronate every 4 to 6 months resulted in a 41.9% increase per year in bone mineral density, an increase in metacarpal cortical width, and a decrease in fracture incidence of 1.7 fractures per year. Mobility improved in 16 of the 30 children, and all reported substantial relief of chronic pain. The results of a study performed by Falk et al.[158] supports the findings of Glorieux et al.[185] However, they concluded that long-term follow-up is required to determine whether bisphosphonate therapy will decrease fracture rates and increase mobility in children with moderate to severe OI.[158] Sakkers et al.[447] reported a reduction of fracture risk of long bones in children with OI using oral treatment with olpadronate at a daily dose of 10 mg. However, the issue of whether bisphosphonates will alter the natural course of OI remains unresolved.[447] Zeitlin et al.[530] have also shown that administering cyclical intravenous pamidronate to children with OI reduces bone pain and fracture incidence and increases bone density and level of ambulation, with minimal side effects. Effects on bone include an increase in the size of vertebral bodies as well as thickening of cortical bone, therefore allowing for more effective corrective surgery using intramedullary rodding of the long bones and spinal instrumentation. Specific occupational and physiotherapy programs are important parts of the treatment procedure. This multidisciplinary approach will prevail until strategies aiming at the correction of the basic defect(s) are found.[530]

Gene therapy for OI has been attempted; however, since most of the mutations in OI are dominant negative, supplying the normal gene without silencing the abnormal gene may not be beneficial.[384] Nonetheless, potential new therapies for OI have been tested in cell culture systems, animal models, and patients and may offer hope for the future development of successful therapies.[363]

The orthopaedist caring for children with OI must balance good, standard fracture care (satisfactory reduction and casting) with the goal of minimizing immobilization to avoid a vicious circle: immobilization, weakness, and osteopenia, then refracture.[12,269,366] Plaster splints and casts, braces, and air splints have all been used.[54,74,173,180,365,466] Protected weight bearing is thought to reduce the incidence of lower extremity fractures.[180] Customized splints and braces can add support to limbs weakened by fragile and deformed bone. Letts et al.[301] encouraged weight bearing in patients by protecting them with vacuum pants. The splinting system is a two-layer set of pants with styrofoam beads between the layers. By evacuating the interval between the layers, a form-fitting orthosis results, much like the beanbag seating systems. Both decreased frequency of fracture and increased bone density were reported after use of this support system.

Load-sharing devices (such as intramedullary rods) are used for internal fixation of long bone fractures or osteotomies in children with OI. Plates and screws should be avoided. In patients with OI, most internal fixation is used for stabilization after corrective osteotomies. The goals of these osteotomies are to improve function and reduce fractures in weight-bearing bones by correcting angulation (Fig. 6-33). Porat et al.[411] found that the percentage of ambulatory patients in their series went from 45% to 75% after intramedullary rodding. The amount of bowing that requires osteotomy has not been defined. In one series,[380] the average preoperative bowing was 71 degrees for the femur and 40 degrees for the tibia, but many patients had much less angulation. Traditionally, multiple osteotomy and rodding procedures (Sofield technique) involved extensive incisions with significant soft tissue stripping and blood loss. Sijbrandij[469] reported a percutaneous technique in which the deformity is straightened by closed osteoclasis and Rush pins are inserted along the proximal axis of the long bones, partially transfixing them to stabilize them in a new alignment. Most centers now use limited incisions, thus minimizing blood loss and periosteal stripping, while ensuring optimally placed osteotomies and efficient, controlled instrumentation. The choice of fixation device should be based on the age of the patient and the width of the medullary canal of the bone. Both fixed-length rods[262,410,482] and extensible Bailey-Dubow rods[32,33,174,175,380,381,411] are used. Skeletally mature patients and patients with very small medullary canals are best treated with nonelongating rods, whereas skeletally immature patients with adequate width of the medullary canal are best treated with extensible rods.[175] Luhmann et al.[314] reported a 20-year experience with extensible nails: both overlapping Rush rods and Bailey-Dubow rods. They first implanted the rods at an average age of 7 years and averaged more than 5 years before the first revision. They recommended a posterior position in the canal and using the stronger overlapping Rush rods technique in the femur whenever the canal diameter permitted; they advised against using overlapping Rush rods in the tibia. Malpuri and Joseph[370] reported the results of intramedullary rodding of long bones in 16 children with OI over a 10-year period. Sheffield elongating rods or nonelongating rods were used. The rate of fractures was reduced drastically after insertion of either type of rod, and the ambulatory status improved in all patients. With regard to the frequency of complications requiring reoperations and the longevity of the rods, Mulpuri and Joseph[370] determined results were notably superior after Sheffield rodding.

Displaced fractures of the apophysis of the olecranon in patients with OI can be treated with open reduction and internal fixation using two Kirschner wires and tension band technique by figure-of-eight suture.[490] Tibial tubercle avulsion injuries should be treated by surgical stabilization if displaced.

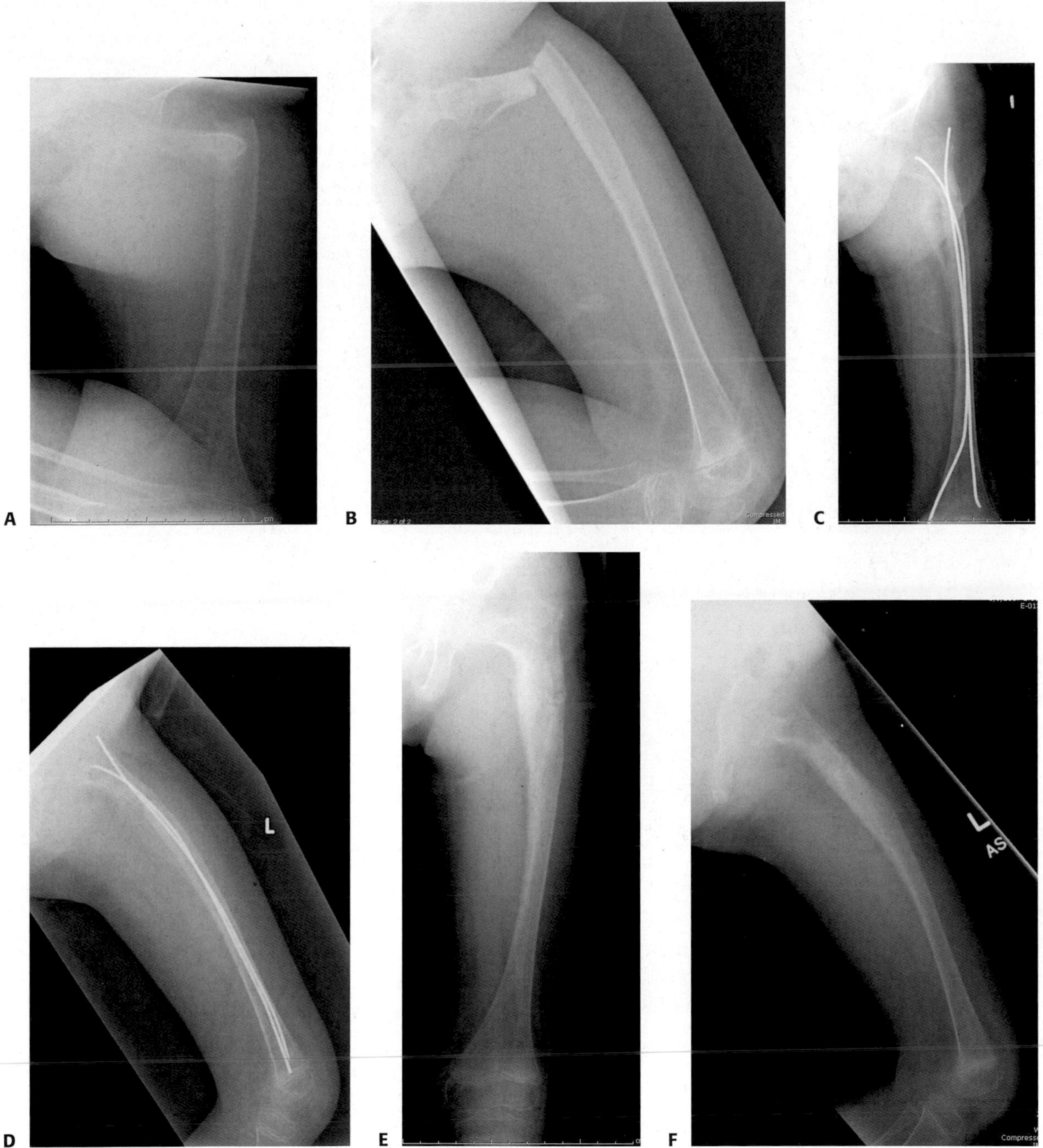

FIGURE 6-33 This 8-year-old girl presented with pain and deformity around the right hip after minor trauma. The patient had a known history of osteogenesis perfecta. Initial radiographs **(A,B)** showed grossly displaced fracture of the proximal femur in the subtrochanteric area. The patient underwent closed reduction and internal fixation with titanium elastic nails, and the fracture healed after 5 weeks, with good alignment in both anteroposterior **(C)** and lateral **(D)** views. The nails were slightly prominent and the family elected removal of the hardware **(E,F)**. *(continues)*

Complication rates are high after osteotomies and intramedullary fixation in OI. Problems include fracture at the rod tip, migration of the fixation device, joint penetration, loosening of components of extensible rods, and fractures through the area of uncoupled rods. Harrison and Rankin[208] compared the complications of 23 extensible rods with those of 27 fixed-length rods. They found that the refracture rate was higher in the fixed-length rods and fewer surgical interventions were necessary when extensible rods were used. Gamble et al.[174] reported that, although the complication rate approached 69% for Bailey-Dubow rods (mostly due to loosening of the T-piece), the fixed-length rods had a complication rate of 55%; however, the replacement rate for nonelongating rods was 24% but only 12% for the Bailey-Dubow rods. They recommended crimping the T-piece to the sleeve and burying it slightly under the bone of the greater trochanter to prevent displacement. Jerosch[239] found a similar 63.5% complication rate for Bailey-Dubow rods but also thought that they were the best device available. Porat et

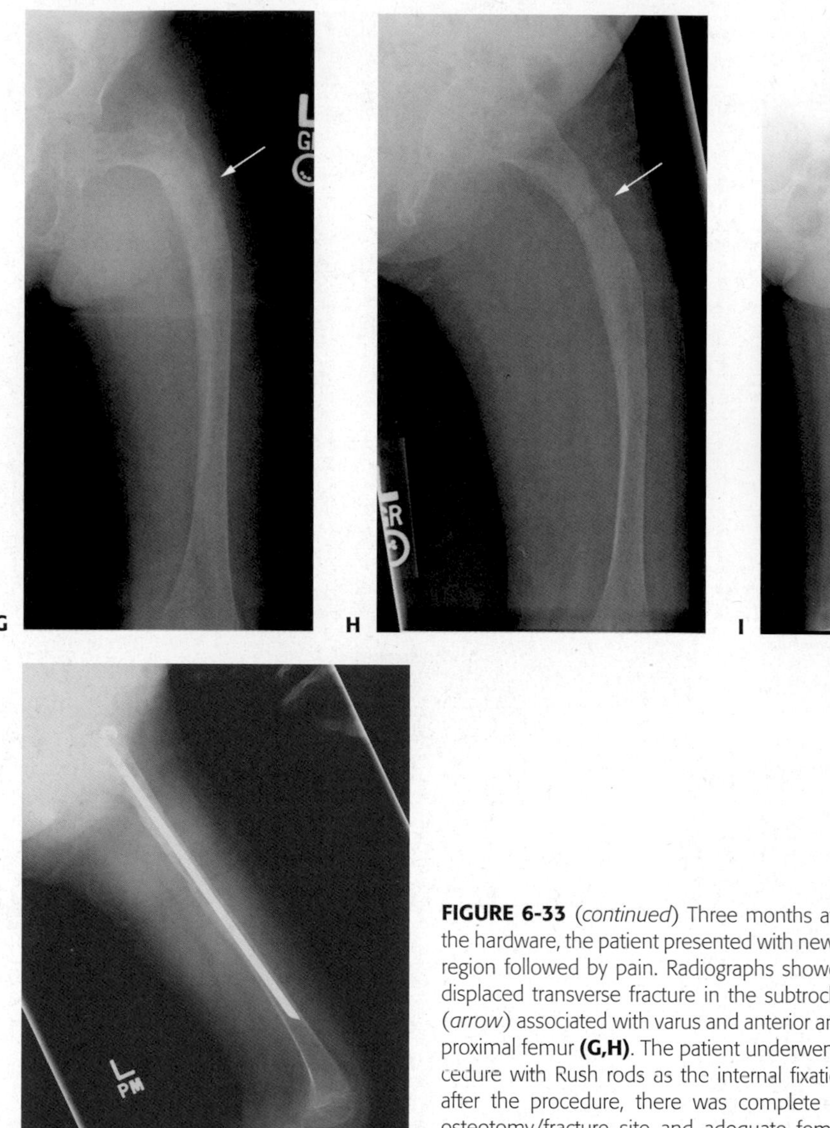

FIGURE 6-33 (*continued*) Three months after removal of the hardware, the patient presented with new trauma to that region followed by pain. Radiographs showed a minimally displaced transverse fracture in the subtrochanteric region (*arrow*) associated with varus and anterior angulation of the proximal femur **(G,H)**. The patient underwent a Sofield procedure with Rush rods as the internal fixation. Ten weeks after the procedure, there was complete healing at the osteotomy/fracture site and adequate femoral alignment **(I,J)**. (Figures reproduced with permission from The Childrens Orthopaedic Center, Los Angeles, CA.)

al.[411] found that the complication rate was 75% for Bailey-Dubow rods and 50% for nonelongating rods, with a similar percentage requiring reoperation for both types of nails. Zionts et al.[529] reported 40 complications in 40 extensible nailings of 15 children, finding a much higher complication rate when insertion of the rods was initiated before 5 years of age. Complications were also higher for tibial nailing.

Postoperative bracing is suggested for lower extremity fractures.[380] Upper extremity fractures should also undergo prolonged splinting after removal of fracture fixation. Immobilization also may be adequate to treat stable, minimally displaced fractures just distal or proximal to the intramedullary rods.[175]

Nonunions, after fracture or surgical intervention, may cause difficulty in both ambulation and transfer. In one series of nonunions,[175] the average age at diagnosis was close to 10 years and most patients responded to treatment with intramedullary rods and bone grafting, with healing in approximately 9 weeks. Nonunion can occur after insertion of rods for upper extremity fractures. Growth arrest also can follow the use of intramedullary rods in the lower extremities.

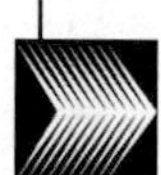

AUTHORS' PREFERRED METHOD OF TREATMENT

Protected weight bearing is the goal for patients with severe OI. Close follow-up is necessary in the first few years of life, with protective posterior plaster splinting for fractures. Orthoses are constructed for bracing of the lower extremities to aid in both standing and ambulation. Standing frames also are used. Once ambulatory, the child is advanced to the use of a walker or independent ambulation. Bisphosphonates should be considered at an early age, prior to fractures and deformity. The length of treatment is still debatable. Severe bowing of the extremities after recurrent fractures is an indication for osteotomy and intramedullary rodding. Whenever possible, surgery is delayed until 6 or 7 years of age. We recommend extensible rods in skeletally immature patients and nonelongating rods both in older patients and in younger patients whose canal is not wide enough for insertion of Bailey-Dubow rods. When possible, we use limited incisions for insertion of Bailey-Dubow rods to minimize blood loss and to avoid devascularization of the long bones, which occurs commonly in the so-called open shish-kabob technique.

Operative Technique–Bailey-Dubow Rod

Multiple small skin incisions are made at the point of maximal deformity of the long bones, and a small periosteal incision is made to permit introduction of a drill bit. After the cortex is drilled repeatedly, manual osteoclasis completes the osteotomy and the long bone is straightened. A guide pin is drilled in to the medial edge of the tip of the greater trochanter, down into the intertrochanteric femur, and then is tapped distally through the intramedullary canal through the knee. If callus from an old fracture halts progress, the guide pin can be drilled through the obstruction and then tapped farther distally into the middle of the distal flexed knee joint. Next, the reamer is advanced over the guide pin and the female portion of the Bailey-Dubow rod is threaded over the guide pin and driven down the canal. The guide pin is pulled out of the knee joint through a small arthrotomy incision, and the T-piece is attached to the Bailey-Dubow sleeve. The T-piece is tapped down into the greater trochanter. The male portion is then slid into the sleeve to complete assembly of the expandable rod.

The patient is immobilized for approximately 4 weeks in a hip spica cast and then in a brace for 3 to 6 months. When there are fractures associated with intramedullary rods, these are treated with either rod revision or immobilization. Every effort should be made to keep patients ambulatory early after fractures occur to minimize disuse osteoporosis.

Osteopetrosis

Osteopetrosis is a condition in which excessive density of bone occurs as a result of abnormal function of osteoclasts.[23,410] The resultant bone of these children is dense, brittle, and highly susceptible to pathologic fracture. The incidence of osteopetrosis is approximately 1 per 200,000 births. The inherent problem is a failure of bone resorption with continuing bone formation and persistent primary spongiosa. The disorder classically has been divided into a severe infantile type and a milder form that presents later in life. Intermediate forms have been identified in which osteopetrosis presents as renal tubular acidosis.[520] Although the number of osteoclasts present in the affected bone is variable,[237,349] in the severe form of this disease, the osteoclasts may be increased but function poorly.[462] Osteopetrosis is a heterogeneous group of disorders classified into three main forms: malignant autosomal recessive, intermediate autosomal recessive, and benign autosomal dominant.

Radiographically, the bones have a dense, chalklike appearance (Fig. 6-34). The spinal column may have a sandwich or "rugger jersey" appearance because of dense, sclerotic bone at each end plate of the vertebrae and less involvement of the central portion. The long bones tend to have a dense, marblelike appearance and may have an Erlenmeyer flask shape at their ends owing to deficient cutback remodeling. Radiolucent transverse bands may be present in the metaphysis of the long bones, and these may represent a variable improvement in the resorption defect during growth of the child.[537] There may be bowing of the bones due to multiple fractures,[210] spondylolysis,[334] or coxa vara.[410] The small bones of the hands and feet may show a bone-within-bone appearance with increased density around the periphery. The unusual radiographic appearance may initially obscure occult non-displaced fractures.

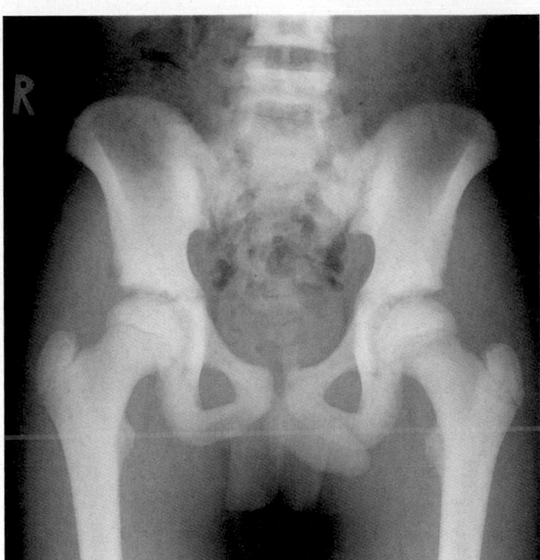

FIGURE 6-34 Anteroposterior radiograph of the pelvis of an 8-year-old boy with osteopetrosis. Note the typical increased bone density and obliteration of the medullary canal. (Figures reproduced with permission from The Childrens Orthopaedic Center, Los Angeles, CA.)

Treatment

Pathologic fractures are quite common in patients with osteopetrosis (Fig. 6-35).[59,210,247,238,349,410,461] Patients with a severe form of the disease have more fractures than those with presentation later in childhood. Concurrent blindness can make patients more susceptible to accidental trauma. Patients with autosomal dominant osteopetrosis with rugger jersey spine and endobones of the pelvis (type II) are six times more likely to have fractures than patients with only sclerosis of the cranial vault (type I).[59]

Patients with the severe, congenital disease have transverse or short oblique fractures of the diaphysis, particularly the femur. Distal physeal fractures with exuberant callus may be confused with osteomyelitis.[357] Common locations for fractures include the inferior neck of the femur, the proximal third of the femoral shaft, and the proximal tibia.[23,357] Although most fractures involve the long bones of the lower extremities, upper extremity fractures also occur frequently.[23,210] The onset of callus formation after fracture in osteopetrosis is variable.[23,218,237] Although many studies state that fractures in osteopetrosis heal at a normal rate,[237,410] others report delayed union and nonunion.[23] In a rat model of osteopetrosis, Marks and Schmidt[332] found delayed fracture healing and remodeling. Hasenhuttl[210] observed that in one patient with recurrent fractures of the forearm, each succeeding fracture took longer to heal, with the last fracture taking nearly 5 months to unite.

The orthopaedist treating fractures in children with osteopetrosis should follow the principles of standard pediatric fracture care, with additional vigilance for possible delayed union and associated rickets (Fig. 6-36).[210,461524] Immobilization is prolonged when delayed union is recognized. Armstrong et al.[23] surveyed the membership of the Pediatric Orthopaedic

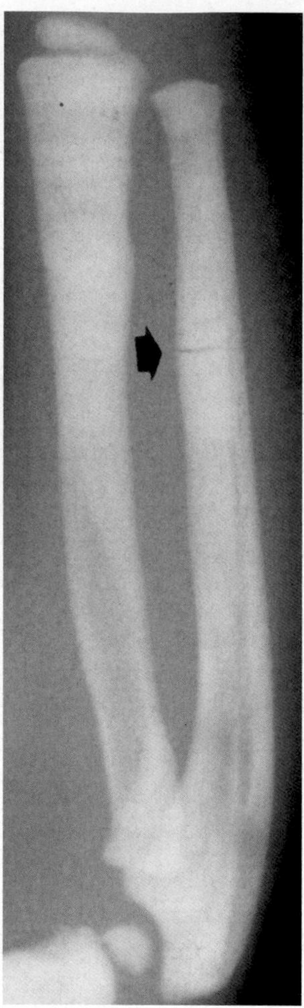

FIGURE 6-35 This 2-year-old with osteopetrosis presented with forearm pain. An anteroposterior radiograph shows the characteristic increased bone density and absence of a medullary canal, especially in the distal radius and ulna. There is a typical transverse, nondisplaced fracture (*arrow*) in the distal ulnar diaphysis.

Society of North America and compiled the combined experience of 58 pediatric orthopaedic surgeons with experience treating pathologic fractures in osteopetrosis. In this comprehensive review, they concluded that nonoperative treatment should be strongly considered for most diaphyseal fractures of the upper and lower limbs in children, but surgical management is recommended for femoral neck fractures and coxa vara.

Open treatment of these fractures with fixation is technically difficult. One author[192] described insertion of fixation into this bone like "drilling into a rock." In intramedullary fixation of femoral fractures, extensive reaming may be required because the intramedullary canal can be completely obliterated by sclerotic bone.[76] Other authors have found fixation of hip fractures with fixation to be a formidable task,[23,357] with damage occurring to the fixation devices on insertion. The bone is hard enough to break the edges off both chisels and drill bits. Armstrong et al.[23] cautioned, "the surgeon should expect to use several drill bits and possibly more than one power driver."

In addition to these technical difficulties, patients with osteopetrosis are at risk for excessive bleeding and infection, probably related to the hematopoietic dysfunction caused by obliteration of the marrow cavity.[461] Procedures should not be performed unless the platelet count is greater than 50,000 mm^3; preoperative platelet transfusions may be necessary.[461] Prophylactic antibiotic coverage is advised. Minor procedures should be performed percutaneously whenever possible.[461]

In the past, primary medical treatment for osteopetrosis included transfusions, splenectomy, calcitriol, and adrenal corticosteroids, but these techniques have proved ineffectual.[428,505] Stimulation of host osteoclasts has been attempted with calcium restriction, calcitriol, steroids, parathyroid hormone, and interferon. Bone marrow transplantation for severe infantile osteopetrosis has proved to be an effective means of treatment for some patients; however, it does not guarantee survival, and it may be complicated by hypercalcaemia.[23,90,94,181,425]

Pyknodysostosis

Pyknodysostosis, also known as Maroteaux-Lamy syndrome, is a rare syndrome of short stature and generalized sclerosis of the entire skeleton. The dense brittle bones of affected children are highly susceptible to pathologic fractures. Pyknodysostosis is inherited as an autosomal recessive trait, with an incidence estimated as 1.7 per 1 million births. Mutations in the gene encoding cathepsin K, a lysosomal cysteine protease localized exclusively in osteoclasts is responsible for this disease.[171] The long bones are sclerotic with poorly formed medullary canals; histologic sections show attenuated Haversian canal systems. Patients with pyknodysostosis have short stature, a hypoplastic face, a nose with a parrot-like appearance, and both frontal and occipital bossing. Bulbous distal phalanges of the fingers and toes with spooning of the nails are common. Coxa vara, coxa valgum, genu valgum, kyphosis, and scoliosis may be present. Failure of segmentation of the lower lumbar spine has been reported.[431] Results of laboratory studies usually are normal.

Radiographs show a sclerotic pattern very similar to that of osteopetrosis. In pyknodysostosis, however, the medullary canals, although poorly formed, are present and a faint trabecular pattern is seen. Such sclerotic bone is also seen in Engelmann's disease, but clinically those patients are tall and eventually develop muscle weakness. The distal femur in a patient with pyknodysostosis usually has an Erlenmeyer flask deformity similar to that found in patients with Gaucher disease.[47]

Treatment

Although pathologic fractures are thought to be less common in pyknodysostosis than in OI, almost all patients with pyknodysostosis reported in the literature have had pathologic fractures.[40] By age 22 years, one patient had sustained more than 100 fractures.[138] The fractures are usually transverse and diaphyseal, and heal with scanty callus.[354] The fracture line can persist for nearly 3 years after clinical union, with an appearance similar to a Looser line. Lower extremity fractures are the most common,[138] and clinical deformity of both the femur and tibia is frequent.

Fracture healing has been described as both normal[496] and delayed.[138] Nonunion is reported in the ulna, clavicle, and tibia.[354] One series[354] with long-term follow-up suggests that fractures tend to heal readily in childhood, but nonunion can be a problem in adulthood. Edelson et al.[142] reported 14 new cases of pyknodysostosis from a small Arab village. They described a hangman fracture of C2 in a 2-year-old child that went on to asymptomatic nonunion. There was 100% incidence of spondylolysis in their patients aged 9 years or older, with

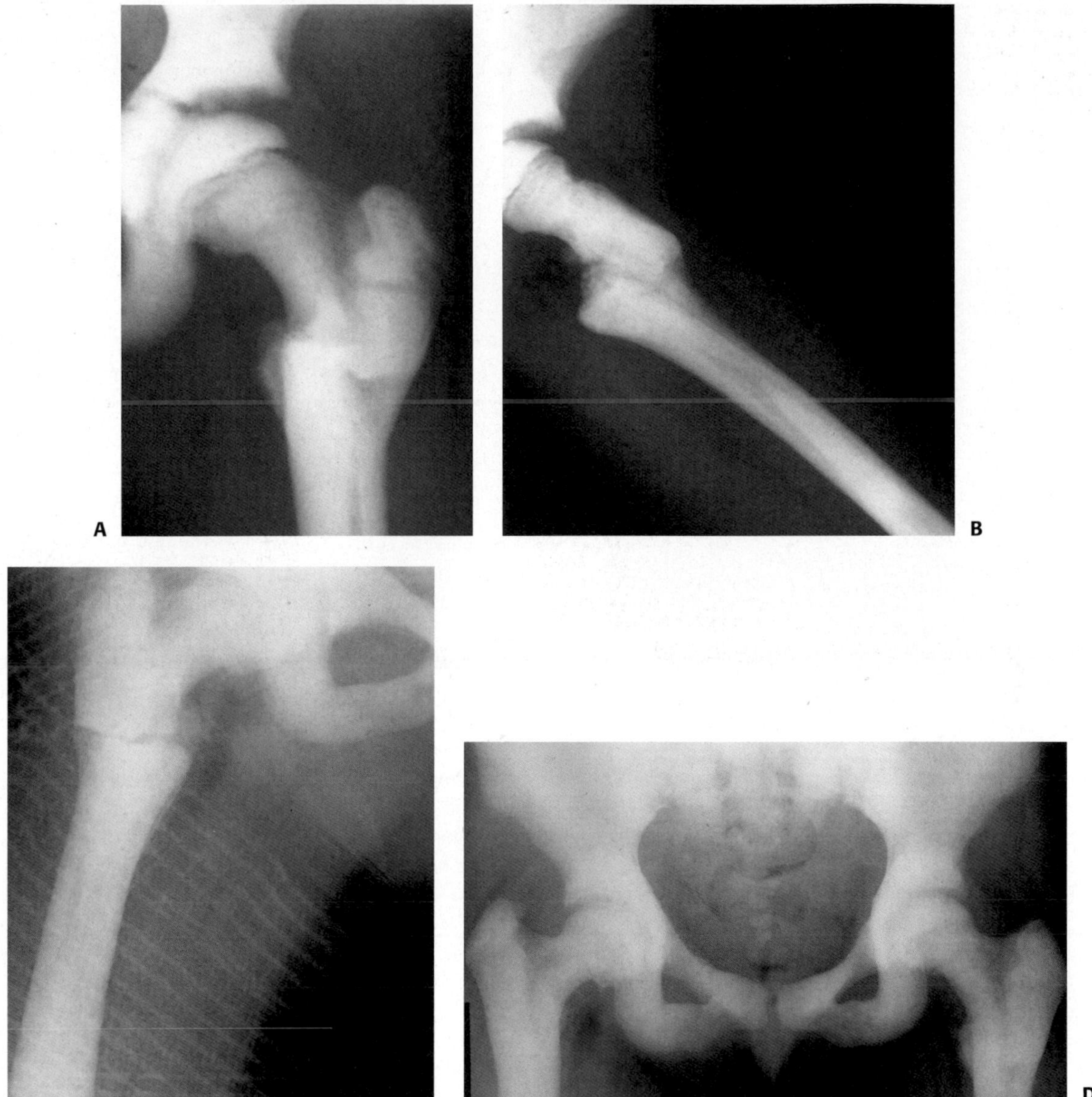

FIGURE 6-36 A. This 9-year-old with osteopetrosis sustained similar bilateral subtrochanteric fractures of the femur over a 2-year period. Anteroposterior **(A)** and lateral **(B)** femoral radiographs show a healing transverse subtrochanteric fracture of the left femoral. **C.** One year later, at age 10, she sustained a similar right transverse minimally displaced subtrochanteric femur fracture, which was treated with reduction and a spica cast. **D.** This anteroposterior radiograph taken at age 14 years shows that both proximal femoral fractures have healed and there is mild residual coxa vara, especially on the right side.

most located at L4–L5. None of the spondylolytic lesions showed uptake on technetium 99m bone scan. Treatment was conservative, with one patient with symptomatic spondylolysis responding to bed rest.

Cast immobilization is successful in the treatment of most of these fractures. Taylor et al.[497] treated a femoral fracture in an 11-year-old boy with skin traction and a one-and-a-half hip spica cast. At 6-month follow-up, clinical union with persistent fracture line was seen. In adults, both plates and screws and hip screws have been used for proximal femoral fractures.[444] Delayed union of tibial fractures has been treated with both compression plating and bone grafting[354] and intramedullary nailing with cast immobilization. Roth[444] noted that treatment of a hip fracture with fixation was technically difficult. Cervical immobilization through a Minerva cast and soft cervical collar has been used for a C2 fracture in a child; the patient did well, although immobilization was prematurely discontinued.[138] Total hip arthroplasty has been performed uneventfully in adults.[510]

Rickets

Rickets is a disease of growing children caused by either a deficiency of vitamin D or an abnormality of its metabolism. The osteoid of the bone is not mineralized, and broad unossified osteoid seams form on the trabeculae. With failure of physeal mineralization, the zone of provisional calcification widens and the ingrowth of blood vessels into the zone is disrupted. In the rickets of renal failure, the effects of secondary hyperparathyroidism (bone erosion and cyst formation) are also present. Be-

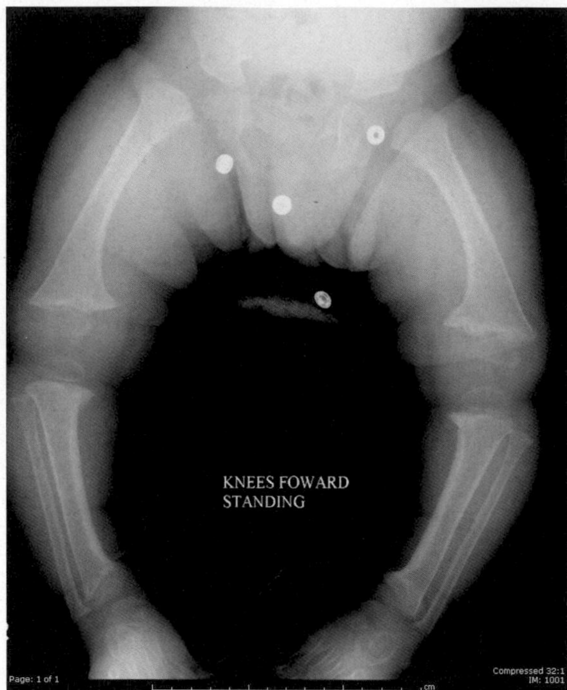

FIGURE 6-37 Lower extremity radiograph of an 18-month-old boy with rickets. Note the severe bowing, physeal irregularities and widening with flaring of distal tibial metaphysis. (Figures reproduced with permission from The Childrens Orthopaedic Center, Los Angeles, CA.)

fore widespread fortification of common foods, vitamin D deficiency was a common cause of rickets, but other diseases affecting the metabolism of vitamin D have become a more common cause. Regardless of the underlying cause, the various types of rickets share similar clinical and radiographic features (Fig. 6-37). Although many of the metabolic findings are the same, there are some differences.

Both pathologic fractures[31,237,337,399,479] and epiphyseal displacement[187,353] can occur in rickets. The treatment of rickets depends on identification of the underlying cause. In addition to nutritional rickets, many diseases of the various organ systems can affect vitamin D metabolism, and their treatment is necessary before the clinical rickets can be resolved (Table 6-9).

Nutritional Rickets

Inadequate dietary vitamin D and lack of exposure to sunlight can lead to a vitamin D deficiency. Pathologic fractures from vitamin D deficiency rickets also occur in children on certain diets: unsupplemented breast milk,[289] diets restricted by religious beliefs,[31] and fat diets.[143] Fractures are treated with both cast immobilization and correction of the vitamin deficiency by oral vitamin D supplementation. Oral calcium supplements also may be necessary, and patients should consume a vitamin D–fortified milk source.[31]

Rickets in Malabsorption

Celiac disease caused by gluten-sensitive enteropathy affects intestinal absorption of fat-soluble vitamins (such as vitamin D), resulting in rickets. Biopsy of the small intestine shows characteristic atrophy of the villi. Treatment is oral vitamin D and a gluten-free diet. Infants with short gut syndrome may have vitamin D-deficiency rickets. This syndrome may develop after intestinal resection in infancy for volvulus or necrotizing enterocolitis, in intestinal atresia, or after resection of the terminal ileum and the ileocecal valve.[500] Pathologic fractures have been reported, and treatment is immobilization and administration of vitamin D_2 with supplemental calcium gluconate.

Hepatobiliary disease is also associated with rickets.[222,273] With congenital biliary atresia, the bile acids, essential for the intestinal absorption of vitamin D, are inadequate. By age 3 months, nearly 60% of patients with biliary atresia may have rickets.[267] Intravenous vitamin D is often needed for effective treatment of these patients. After appropriate surgical correction of the hepatic syndrome, the bone disease gradually improves (Fig. 6-38). The pathologic fractures that develop in these disorders[222] can be treated with immobilization.

Epilepsy may affect bone in a number of ways such as restriction of physical activity, cerebral palsy, or other coexisting morbidities. Also, the use of anticonvulsant therapy can interfere with the hepatic metabolism of vitamin D and result in rickets and pathologic fractures.[450] Fewer fractures occur in institutionalized patients receiving vitamin D prophylaxis.[464]

Ifosfamide, a chemotherapeutic agent used for treatment of different sarcomas, can cause hypophosphatemic rickets in children. The onset of rickets may occur anywhere from 2 to 14

TABLE 6-9 Rickets: Metabolic Abnormalities

Disorder	Cause	1,25 $(OH)_2$ Vitamin D	Parathyroid Hormone	Calcium	P	Alkaline Phosphate
Vitamin D deficiency rickets	Lack of vitamin D in the diet	↓	↑	↓ or →	↓	↑
Gastrointestinal rickets	Decreased gastrointestinal absorption of vitamin D or calcium	↓ or →	↑	↓	↓	↑
Vitamin D–dependent rickets	Reduced 1,25$(OH)_2$ vitamin D production	↓↓	↑	↓	↓	↑
Vitamin D–resistant rickets—end-organ insensitivity	Intestinal cell insensitivity to vitamin D causing decreased calcium absorption	↑ or →	↑	↓	↓	↑
Renal osteodystrophy	Renal failure causing decreased vitamin D synthesis, phosphate retention, hypocalcemia, and secondary hyperparathyroidism	↓↓	↑↑	↓	↑	↑

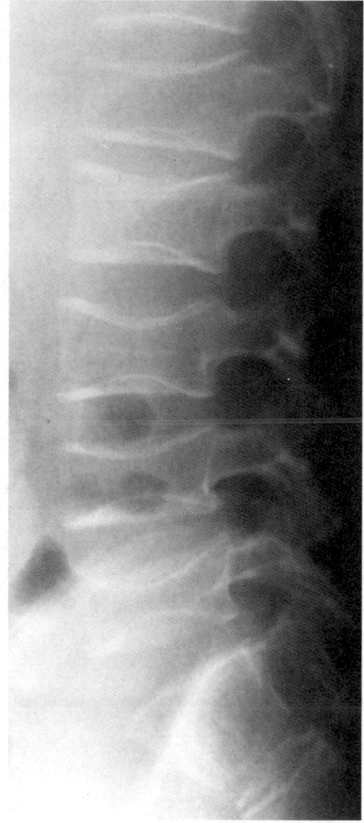
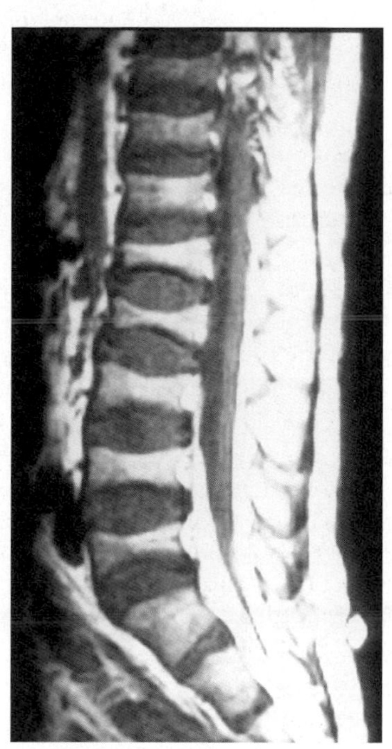

FIGURE 6-38 This 18-year-old boy with sclerosing cholangitis and a history of steroid use presented with several months of worsening low back pain. **A.** Lateral radiograph of his lumbar spine shows marked osteopenia, collapsed codfish vertebrae with sclerotic end plates and widened disc spaces and Schmorl nodes. **B.** This MRI shows flattened concave vertebrae that are smaller in most locations than the adjacent intervertebral discs. He was successfully treated with 3 months in a thoraco-lumbar-sacral-orthosis brace, followed by weaning from the brace and conditioning exercises.

months after chemotherapy and can be corrected with the administration of oral phosphates.[495] Other mineral deficiencies such as magnesium (a cofactor for parathyroid hormone) can cause rare forms of rickets.

Rickets and Very-Low-Birth-Weight Infants

Very-low-birth-weight infants (1500 g or less) can have pathologic fractures. In one study of 12 very-low-birth-weight infants, the incidence of pathologic fracture was 2.1%, nearly twice the rate of other premature infants with a birth weight of more than 1500 g.[13] The fractures are likely caused by a nutritional osteomalacia that may evolve into frank rickets in nearly 30% of very-low-birth-weight infants.[13,211,271,272] During the last trimester of pregnancy, the intrauterine growth rate is exponential—almost two thirds of the birth weight is gained at that time.[434] Eighty percent of both calcium and phosphorus is acquired then.[256] Bone loss can be graded by either loss of cortical bone of the humerus[413] or loss of bone of the distal radius.[271] Other than craniotabes (thinning and softening of the skull bone with widening of the sutures and fontanelles), the clinical signs of rickets are generally lacking in these patients.[211] The risk factors predisposing these patients to both rickets and fractures include hepatobiliary disease,[267,273,495] prolonged total parenteral nutrition,[495] chronic lung disease,[13] necrotizing enterocolitis,[498] patent ductus arteriosus,[64] and physical therapy with passive range-of-motion exercises.[211,272] In a prospective study of 78 low-birth-weight infants, Koo et al.[272] observed a 73% incidence of rickets with associated pathologic fractures in patients with a birth weight of 800 g or less and only a 15% incidence of rickets with fractures in patients with a birth weight ranging from 1000 to 1500 g. In most cases, pathologic fractures in very-low-birth-weight infants are found incidentally on chest radiograph or gastrointestinal studies. The fractures may be suspected when physical examination reveals swelling and decreased movement of an extremity. The differential diagnosis of these fractures is limited but important: OI, copper deficiency syndrome, child abuse, and pathologic fracture from overzealous physical therapy.[211] Recurrent fractures, physical findings, and a positive family history are the hallmarks of OI; serum copper levels are useful in establishing copper deficiency syndrome. Neonatal osteomyelitis may also present a similar radiographic appearance. If risk factors for infection are present, the bone lesion should be aspirated and cultured.[13]

In the series reported by Amir et al.,[13] 12 (1.2%) of 973 preterm infants had fractures; 11 of 12 had more than one fracture. Radiographically, osteopenia is first seen at the 4th week of life. Typically, rib fractures are next seen at 6 to 8 weeks of life, then fractures of the long bones at 11 to 12 weeks.[434] In one study, 54% of fractures were in the upper extremities, 18% in the lower extremities, 22% in the ribs, and approximately 6% in either the scapula or the clavicle.[272] Most long bone fractures are metaphyseal and may be transverse or greenstick with either angulation or complete displacement.[13] Callus is seen at the fracture site in less than a week, and complete remodeling occurs in 6 to 12 months.[13,272] Passive range-of-motion exercises for these infants, by both physical therapists and parents, should be avoided unless it is absolutely necessary.[211] Rib fractures have been associated with vigorous chest physiotherapy.[272] Care also should be taken even with routine manipulation of the extremities during nursing care, and special care should be taken in restraining the extremities during surgical procedures.[272] Splinting is the treatment of choice for pathologic fractures of the long bones in very-low-birth-weight infants.

Hip spica casts are contraindicated because they may compromise cardiopulmonary support and hamper nursing care.[272] Regardless of the means of immobilization, the prognosis is excellent for most of these fractures because they go on to complete remodeling within 12 months; prolonged follow-up is advised. Preventive measures are important to minimize the risk of fracture in low-birth-weight infants. Their nutritional need for high levels of calcium, phosphorus, and vitamin D should be recognized. Alternating high levels of calcium with low levels of phosphorus in hyperalimentation solutions can help meet these needs. Because growth arrest is possible after fractures, follow-up over the first 2 to 3 years of life is advised.

Rickets and Renal Osteodystrophy

Renal osteodystrophy is common in patients with end-stage renal failure.[230] Typically developing about 1.4 years after diagnosis of the kidney disease,[230] the clinical syndrome is a combination of rickets and secondary hyperparathyroidism with marked osteoporosis. Affected children present with short stature, bone pain, muscle weakness, delayed sexual development, and bowing of the long bones.[87] The underlying renal disease may be chronic nephritis, pyelonephritis, congenitally small kidneys, or cystinosis.[479] Identification of the renal disorder is important because patients presenting with rickets due to obstructive uropathy may respond to surgical treatment of the renal disease.

Specific clinical deformities include genu valgum (most common), genu varum, coxa vara, and varus deformities of the ankle.[20,87,113] These deformities are most common in patients diagnosed before 3 years of age. Davids et al.[113] showed that periods of metabolic instability, characterized as an alkaline phosphatase of 500 U for at least 10 months, were associated with progression of deformity. With the adolescent growth spurt, osseous deformities can accelerate rapidly over a matter of weeks.[113]

Radiographs show rickets and osteopenia with osteitis fibrosa cystica.[20] Osteoclastic cysts (brown tumors) may form. Metaphyseal cortical erosions occur in the lateral clavicle, distal ulna and radius, neck of the humerus, medial femoral neck, medial proximal tibia, and middle phalanges of the second and third fingers.[230] The proximal femur may become so eroded with tapering and thinning that it has been likened to a rotting fence post.[498] In renal osteodystrophy, the Looser zone may represent a true stress fracture and, with minor trauma, may extend across the full thickness of the bone with development of a true fracture (Fig. 6-39). Callus may be scanty in patients with fractures who have untreated renal disease, but in patients on hemodialysis, abundant callus may form at the fracture site.[399] Phalangeal quantitative ultrasound may be a useful method to assess bone quality and fracture risk in children and adolescents with bone and mineral disorders.[38]

In renal osteodystrophy, pathologic fractures of the long bones, rib fractures, vertebral compression fractures, and epiphyseal displacement of the epiphyses occur frequently. Fractures occur in areas of metaphyseal erosion or through cysts. Immobilization is used to treat pathologic fractures through both generalized weakened bone and brown tumors. Once the underlying bone disease is under control, open procedures such as curettage of cysts with bone grafting and open reduction of fractures may be considered when appropriate.[399] Internal fixation is preferable to external fixation.[89] Preoperative tests needed for these patients before surgery include electrolytes, calcium, phosphorus, and alkaline phosphatase. Before surgery, these patients may need dialysis, phosphate adjustment, either medical or surgical correction of hyperparathyroidism, or chelation therapy for aluminium toxicity. Supplemental vitamin D should be discontinued or the dose halved 2 to 4 weeks before any procedure that may require immobilization.[87] It is important to rule out dental abscess, which may be present in as many as 25% of patients with vitamin D–resistant rickets.[350] Postoperative infection may be more common in patients who are on corticosteroid therapy after renal transplantation.[376] Prophylactic antibiotics are highly recommended for surgery of all patients with renal osteodystrophy.[154]

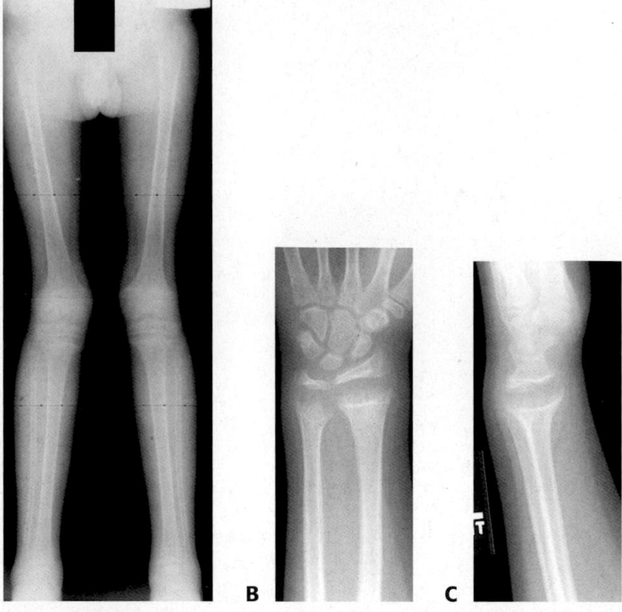

FIGURE 6-39 This 12-year-old girl with rickets associated with chronic kidney disease presented with complaints of knocked knees and wrist pain. Hip to ankle radiographs **(A)** showed typical rickets changes with valgus deformity at the knee level. Looser lines around the distal femur, and physeal widening. Wrist images **(B,C)** demonstrated marked physeal widening and metaphyseal flare of the distal radius and ulna. (Figures reproduced with permission from The Childrens Orthopaedic Center, Los Angeles, CA.)

The incidence of epiphyseal displacement in children with renal osteodystrophy ranges from 20% to 30%.[264,348] Sites of involvement include the distal femur, proximal femur, and proximal humerus, the heads of both the metatarsals and metacarpals, and the distal radial and ulnar epiphyses, which tend to displace in an ulnar direction.[264] In the proximal femur, both femoral neck fractures[188] and slipped capital femoral epiphysis occur. Possible explanations for displacement of the proximal femoral epiphysis include metaphyseal erosion with subsequent fracture,[188,264] and a layer of fibrous tissue that forms between the physis and the metaphysis because of the destructive effects of the renal osteodystrophy.[276] The warning signs and risk factors for slipped capital femoral epiphysis in renal osteodystrophy include subperiosteal erosion of the medial femoral neck, increasing width of the physis, bilateral coxa vara, male gender, and an age between 10 and 20 years (Fig. 6-40).[188] With erosion of the cortex of the inferior medial femoral neck, the femoral head collapses, decreasing the neck shaft angle, and subjecting the physis to shear forces as it assumes a vertical

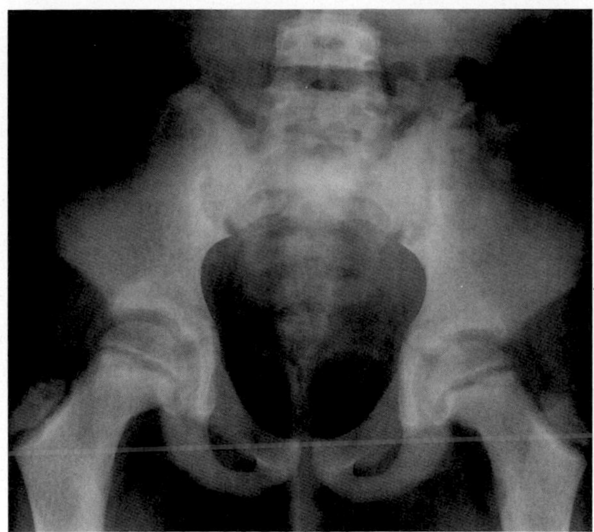

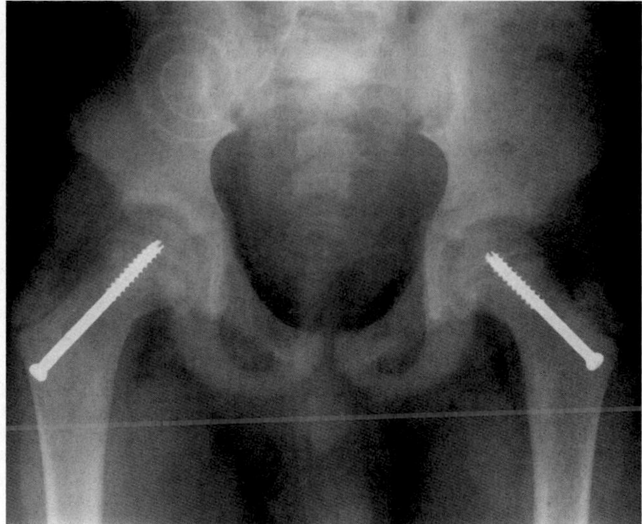

FIGURE 6-40 This 13-year-old boy with renal osteodystrophy presented with bilateral hip and thigh pain. **A.** Anteroposterior pelvic radiograph shows widening of the proximal femoral physes with sclerosis. Slipped capital femoral epiphyses were diagnosed. **B.** This anteroposterior pelvic radiograph taken 9 months after surgery shows narrowing of the physis and no evidence of further displacement of the capital femoral epiphyses.

orientation. The slip is bilateral in up to 95% of the patients and is usually stable.[313,389]

The aggressive medical treatment of renal osteodystrophy, including administration of vitamin D,[308] calcitriol, hemodialysis, renal transplantation, and parathyroidectomy, has improved the long-term survival and quality of life for these patients. Temporary limitation of weight bearing is recommended if there is little metaphyseal erosion, minimal coxa vara, and fusion of the physis is expected within 1 to 2 years.[399] If the primary disease is not readily treated, progression of the displacement will occur.[313,389] With continuing slippage after medical treatment, most authors recommend in situ fixation.[87,188,313,383,388] However, continuing displacement of the proximal femoral epiphysis may occur even after pinning, because the fixation holds poorly, possibly because the wide radiolucent zone of the femoral neck in this disorder is not true physis, but rather poorly mineralized woven bone and fibrous tissue.[350] In a very young child, threaded pin fixation of the proximal femoral epiphysis may result in growth abnormality with trochanteric overgrowth.

Smooth pins can be used to stabilize the epiphysis temporarily until medical treatment resolves the underlying bone disease and avoids definitive physeal closure.[313] For patients younger than 5 years, Hartjen and Koman[209] recommended treatment of slipped capital femoral epiphysis with reduction through Buck traction and fixation with a single specially fabricated 4.5-mm cortical screw. The distal threads of the screw were machined off so that only the smooth shank of the screw extended across the physis. Subtrochanteric osteotomy with fixation or total hip arthroplasty may be necessary in older patients with severe coxa vara after slipped capital femoral epiphysis.[87,188]

Renal Osteodystrophy Complicated by Aluminium Toxicity

Oppenheim et al.[389] noted the contribution of aluminium toxicity to the development of fractures in renal osteodystrophy. Because phosphorus restriction is important in children with renal disease, aluminium hydroxide has been commonly used as a phosphate binder.[16] Aluminium intoxication causes defective mineralization. Multiple pathologic fractures may occur with poor healing. Serum aluminium levels are not diagnostic, but the use of deferoxamine, a chelation agent, in an infusion test may provide the diagnosis.[362] A bone biopsy is often necessary. After treatment of the renal disease with correction of the aluminium toxicity by chelation agents, acute fractures will heal. Severe bowing of the long bones due to fractures can be treated with multiple osteotomies with intramedullary Rush rod or plate fixation.[389] Recurrence of the syndrome is prevented by use of aluminium-free phosphate-binding agents such as calcium carbonate.[449]

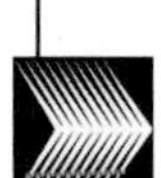

AUTHORS' PREFERRED METHOD OF TREATMENT

Recognition of the underlying metabolic abnormalities is the most important aspect in the care of all of these injuries. Slipped capital femoral epiphysis may be the first presenting sign of renal failure.[188] A slipped capital femoral epiphysis should be stabilized with in situ screw fixation in older children if progression is noted despite medical treatment. Multiple screws should be considered because the underlying metaphyseal bone is quite soft. For treatment of progressive slipped capital femoral epiphysis in very young children, some form of unthreaded fixation seems most logical. Most fractures of the long bones respond readily to cast or splint immobilization, with concurrent aggressive medical treatment of the underlying metabolic disease. Femoral neck fractures are treated with anatomic reduction and internal fixation. The underlying bone disease should be medically treated to ensure success of open procedures. Significant cysts should be treated with curettage and bone grafting. Angular deformities of the long bones should be corrected when the patient is close to maturity.

Idiopathic Osteoporosis

Osteoporosis in a child generally is associated with either congenital disease such as osteogenesis imperfecta or metabolic disorders such as Cushing syndrome. Rarely, children develop idiopathic osteoporosis with pathologic fractures. Idiopathic osteoporosis is characteristically seen 2 years before puberty, but age at presentation may range from 4 to 16 years.[478] Unique metaphyseal impaction fractures are a hallmark of this disorder.[226] It usually presents with bone pain, deformities, and fractures. Biopsy specimens show a quantitative decrease in the amount of bone that has been linked to both increased resorption[241] and primary failure bone formation.[478] Osteoblasts in this disorder seem to function normally when stimulated by oral 1,25-hydroxyvitamin D_3.[49] The etiology in healthy children is likely multifactorial and incompletely understood. Poor calcium intake during the adolescent growth spurt may play some role. Symptoms can persist for 1 to 4 years after diagnosis, with spontaneous resolution in most patients after the onset of puberty. The only consistent metabolic abnormality is a negative calcium balance with high rates of fecal excretion of calcium.[226] This finding supports the hypothesis that idiopathic juvenile osteoporosis results from intestinal malabsorption of calcium.[118]

Rauch et al.[425] suggested a pathogenetic model for idiopathic osteoporosis in which impaired osteoblast team performance decreases the ability of cancellous bone to adapt to the increasing mechanical needs during growth. The result of this impairment is load failure and fractures.[425]

Although many children present with back pain as the only complaint, the most severely affected present with generalized skeletal pain.[117,241,478] Patients have difficulty walking, and their symptoms may be initiated by mild trauma. In a review of 40 patients with idiopathic osteoporosis, Smith[478] observed that 87% had vertebral fractures and 42% had metaphyseal fractures. Symptoms of back or extremity pain can predate fractures by 6 months. Generally, 30% of bone mass must be absent before osteoporosis is detected on radiographs.[284] Serum calcium, phosphorus, and alkaline phosphatase levels are usually normal.[226] Low plasma calcitriol, a vitamin D metabolite that aids calcium absorption in the gut, has been observed in juvenile osteoporosis.[333] Some authors have noticed that it is mostly a disorder of cancellous bone, reflecting a decreased modelling activity on the endocortical surface of the internal cortex.[426]

Some of the issues when dealing with idiopathic osteoporosis in children include the usually difficult interpretation of bone densitometry and turnover markers and poorly established guidelines regarding prevention and treatment of bone fragility. Prospective studies are needed to establish the safety, efficacy, and optimal drug, duration, and dosage for improving bone quality in otherwise healthy children. Most authors believe that the bone health during the first two decades contributes to the lifetime risk of osteoporosis.[30]

Radiographs of the spine show decreased density in the central areas of the vertebral bodies, and clarity of the dense vertebral end plates is increased. The long bones lose trabecular anatomy and show thinning of the cortex.[226,473] Once symptoms begin, a mildly lucent area of newly formed bone, a so-called neo-osseous porosis, is observable in the metaphysis (Fig. 6-41). This is considered weaker than the surrounding bone, which formed before onset of the disease.[478]

Treatment

Lower extremity and vertebral fractures[331] are common, but fractures of the proximal humerus, radius, ulna, and ribs may also occur.[226] Nonunions of the tibia, radius, and ulna have been reported.[118,226] Spinal cord compression has also been reported with vertebral fractures of osteoporosis in a child. Metaphyseal fractures can start as hairline cracks that gradually extend across the width of the shaft, and with further collapse in the femoral shaft, the cracks may telescope into the distal femur, with later distortion of the femoral condyle.[226] Tibial and femoral shaft fractures may heal with bowing. Long bone shaft fractures are either transverse or oblique,[226] and the callus formed seems to be normal.[226,332] A technetium bone scan may be useful in showing healing fractures that are not obvious on plain radiograph studies.[332] No clear-cut effective medical treatment has been found for idiopathic juvenile osteoporosis.[189,226,241] Many patients have been treated by both vitamin D and calcium supplements with equivocal benefit, and usually mineralization of the skeleton does not improve until puberty, when the disease spontaneously resolves. Low-dose pamidronate appears promising in the treatment of childhood osteoporosis.[176]

Dent and Friedman[118] summarized the treatment of fractures in juvenile osteoporosis when they stated that these fractures should undergo anatomic reduction with immobilization "as little as practical." They noted both severe deformity of the long bones and pseudarthrosis when the fractures could not be immobilized. The bones usually are so soft that they are thought to be unsuitable for the usual forms of fixation, but femoral neck fractures in this disorder have been treated with internal fixation.[226]

Iatrogenic Osteoporosis

Osteoporosis Associated With Cancer Treatment

Osteoporosis is commonly seen in children who are undergoing cancer therapy. The cause of reduced bone mineral density is multifactorial. The disease itself may play a role (e.g., acute lymphoblastic leukemia, malignant lymphomas, brain tumors, malignant bone tumors, rhabdomyosarcoma), but specifically the treatment including corticosteroids, chemotherapy (such as methotrexate, ifosfomide) and radiation (such as brain radiation that can reduce growth hormone secretion and cause hypogonadotropic hypogonadism), all contribute to the development of osteoporosis.[448,504] Methotrexate, for example, is believed to inhibit osteogenesis, causing both delayed union and nonunion of fractures.[420] The incidence of pathologic fractures after methotrexate use ranges from 19% to 57%.[285,420,484]

Generalized demineralization of the skeleton is seen with marked radiolucency of the metaphyseal regions of the long bones. Radiographic changes in the metaphysis and epiphysis resemble those seen in scurvy.[420] Minimally displaced transverse fractures occur in the long bones of both the upper and lower extremities and the small bones of the feet.[420,484] Schwartz and Leonidas[456] cautioned that stress fractures of the long bones that can occur after methotrexate therapy can be mistaken for recurrence of leukemia. If feasible from an oncologic viewpoint, methotrexate should be discontinued to allow these fractures to heal in a cast. The cast immobilization itself may result in additional osteopenia and fractures even though methotrexate is discontinued.[456] Persistent nonunion requires open reduction and internal fixation with bone graft.[484] Patients

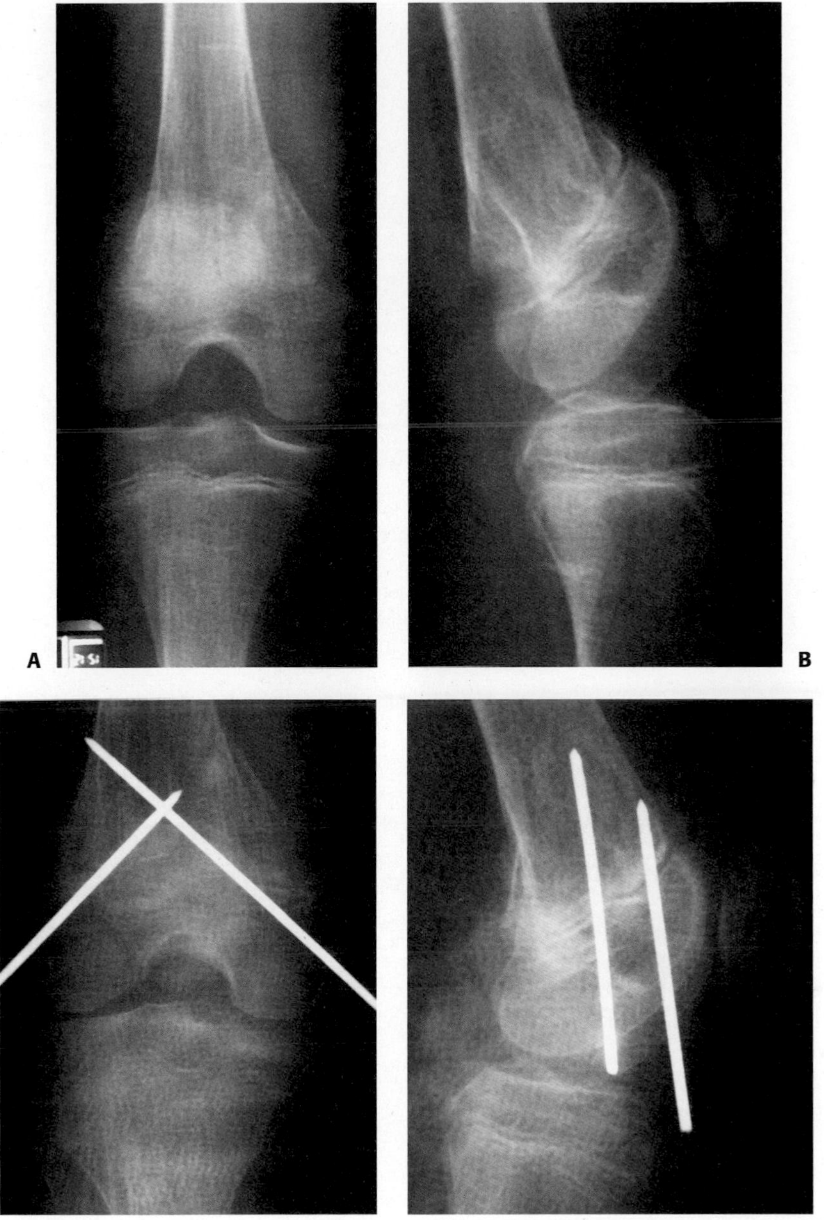

FIGURE 6-41 A. Multiple pathologic fractures in a previously healthy teenage boy who developed idiopathic osteoporosis. This anteroposterior radiograph of the right knee and this lateral radiograph **(B)** demonstrate a displaced distal femoral metaphyseal fracture with apex posterior angulation. **C.** This was treated with closed reduction and percutaneous pinning and application of a cast. **D.** This lateral radiograph shows satisfactory alignment with the pins in place. *(continues)*

with severe osteoporosis and bone pain without fracture also respond to a halt in methotrexate therapy.[420] Prevention is the key and physical activity, adequate vitamin D intake, and sometimes bisphosphonates are some of the options.[448,504]

Immobilization Osteoporosis

Immobilization of an extremity for fracture treatment can result in loss of as much as a 44% of mineralization of trabecular bone. In some patients, osteoporosis may persist for 6 months after injury.[149] Immobilization leads to bone resorption, especially in unstressed areas.[285] In one study,[149] bone density of the distal radius returned to normal in all patients at l-year follow-up. Nilsson and Westlin[382] found a residual decrease in bone mineralization of the distal femur of 7% at nearly 11 years of follow-up in a study of 30 patients. Persistent osteoporosis after cast immobilization for fracture can contribute to refracture.

Primary Hyperparathyroidism

Primary hyperparathyroidism in childhood is extremely rare. Although the exact incidence remains unknown, it results from hyperplasia of the parathyroid gland. Symptoms are associated with high serum calcium and inappropriate parathyroid hormone level, causing increased osteoclastic activity, leading to general demineralization of the skeleton and hypercalcemia. In severely affected patients, osteitis fibrosa cystica may develop with fibrous tissue replacement of bone and formation of cysts. In a large retrospective study, among the 44 children and adolescents, ranging in age from 6 to 18 (mean 13) years, 83% were

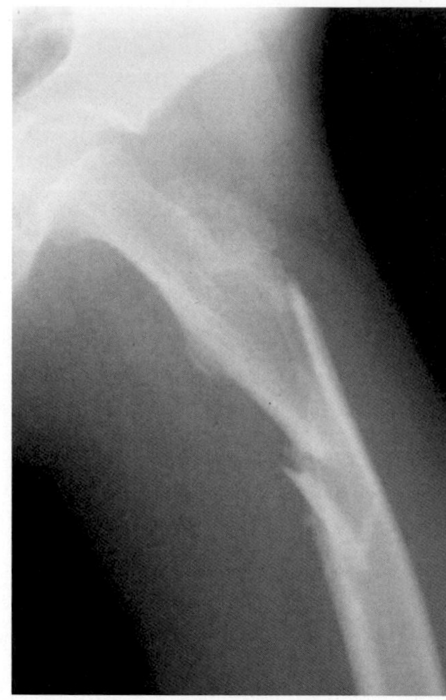

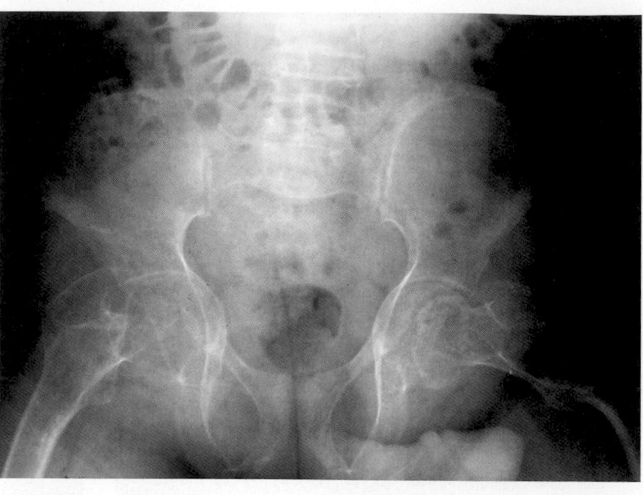

FIGURE 6-41 *(continued)* **E.** A few months later, he sustained a left proximal femoral fracture, which was treated with a spica cast. **F.** This anteroposterior pelvic radiograph taken 3 years later shows healed proximal femoral fractures with varus angulation and severe osteopenia of the pelvis and femora with profusion of both acetabuli.

symptomatic and 43% had nephrolithiasis. Two had multiple endocrine neoplasias.[322]

A particularly severe form of primary hyperparathyroidism seen in infants is congenital primary hyperparathyroidism, which results from an autosomal recessive trait[140] and is lethal without parathyroidectomy. These patients present with respiratory difficulty, hypotonia, poor feeding with constipation, and failure to thrive.[423] Serum calcium is markedly increased in most patients, but a gradual rise above normal serum levels may occur in some infants with serial measurements.[421] Radiographs reveal demineralization of the skeleton. Marked resorption is present in the femoral necks and distal tibiae, with decreased trabeculae and poorly defined cortices.[140] Periosteal elevation is common, and when it is severe, the long bones may actually look cloaked with new bone (Fig. 6-42). Periosteal resorption of the bone of the middle phalanges is believed to be characteristic of this disease. Brown tumors are rare in infancy.

In older children and adolescents, the clinical presentation is subtler. Weakness, anorexia, and irritability are present in 50% of patients, and constipation is present in 28%.[52] Renal calculi also are present in 25% of patients, and polyuria, excessive thirst, bone pain, abdominal distension, pancreatitis, and swelling of the knees are occasionally present.[18,52,112] Approximately 50% of older patients have osteopenia and other osseous

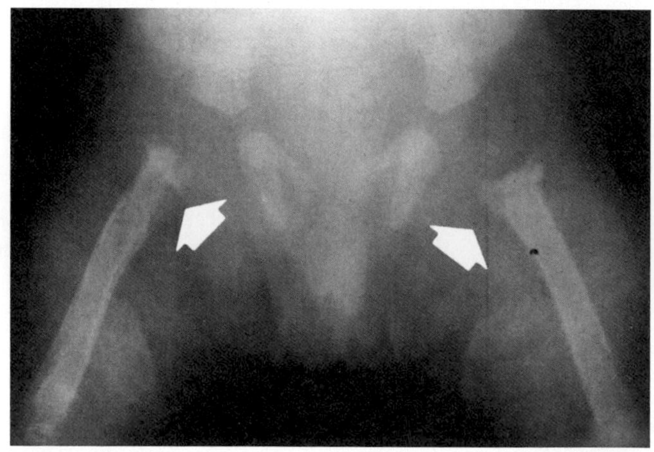

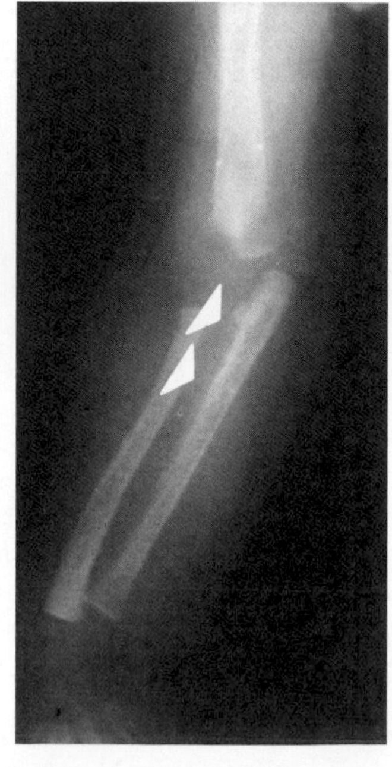

FIGURE 6-42 A. Newborn with hyperparathyroidism. There is marked demineralization of bone, and marked resorption is present in the proximal femurs (*arrows*). **B.** Periosteal elevation is present along the ulna (*arrows*). (Courtesy of Bruce Mewborne, MD.)

signs of hyperparathyroidism.[52] The serum calcium is only moderately elevated in many patients, but 24-hour urine calcium excretion is abnormally high.[52,400] If the diagnosis is uncertain, selective venous catheterization for parathyroid hormone can be done, localizing the gland by either ultrasound, CT, or MRI.[55]

Treatment

Pathologic fractures of the long bones are common in patients with hyperparathyroidism,[4,400] especially in infancy. Vertebral fractures, which occur in 4.4% of adult patients,[93] are rare in infancy. Increased levels of parathyroid hormone results in decreased function and numbers of osteoblasts, and hence delayed union of pathologic fractures,[283] but this problem has only been reported in adults; healing occurred after parathyroidectomy.[237] Most fractures are successfully treated with simple immobilization. Occasionally, a fracture through a cyst or brown tumor requires curettage and bone grafting after a period of initial healing.[522]

Cushing Syndrome

Endogenous Cushing syndrome in children is a rare disorder that is most frequently caused by pituitary or adrenocortical tumors, resulting in excessive production of cortisol and its related compounds. If the hyperactivity of the adrenal cortex is due to pituitary gland stimulation, the syndrome is most precisely known as Cushing disease.[108] In children, hypercortisolism is most often caused by carcinoma, adenoma, hyperplasia of the adrenal cortex,[340] Ewing sarcoma,[414] or exogenous corticosteroid therapy. The elevated adrenal corticosteroids inhibit the formation of osteoblasts,[207] resulting in increased resorption of the bone matrix and decreased bone formation.[242]

Presenting symptoms include failure to thrive, short stature with excessive weight gain, moon facies, presence of a buffalo hump, hirsutism, weakness, and hypertension.[340] Cutaneous striae are rare, and the genitalia are of normal size. Mortality is well over 50%.[340] In older children, the clinical picture is somewhat different: truncal obesity, short stature, a lowered hairline, acne, weakness, emotional lability, hirsutism, cutaneous striae, hypertension, and ecchymosis. Radiographic findings may include severe osteopenia and a retarded bone age. Fractures of the ribs, vertebrae, and long bones have been reported in children with Cushing syndrome.[341] In terms of diagnostic studies, it has been shown that a single cortisol value at midnight followed by overnight high-dosage dexamethasone test led to rapid and accurate confirmation and diagnostic differentiation, respectively, of hypercortisolemia caused by pituitary and adrenal tumors.[41]

Treatment

The primary treatment of Cushing syndrome of childhood is total adrenalectomy.[341] The associated fractures usually can be treated with standard immobilization techniques, but care should be taken not to increase the extent of osteopenia through excessive immobilization. In patients on corticosteroid therapy, the dose should be reduced, converted to an alternate-day schedule, or discontinued, if possible.[414] Also, children and adolescents who have Cushing syndrome may have significant alterations in body composition that result in a small but significant decrease in bone mass and increase in visceral adiposity. Long-term monitoring of body fat and bone mass should be mandatory after treatment.[299]

Scurvy

Scurvy is rare; it occurs in children who eat inadequate amounts of fresh fruit or vegetables leading to depletion in vitamin C. It takes up to 6 to 12 months before symptoms arise, including asthenia, vascular purpura, bleeding, and gum abnormalities. In 80% of cases, the manifestations of scurvy include musculoskeletal symptoms consisting of arthralgia, myalgia, hemarthrosis, and muscular hematomas.[157] Because vitamin C is essential for normal collagen formation, deficiency of the vitamin results in defective osteogenesis, vascular breakdown, delayed healing, and wound dehiscence.[197] Children experience severe lower limb pain related to subperiosteal bleeding. Although scurvy is often due to a dietary deficiency of vitamin C,[197,377,391] both aspirin and phenytoin are associated with decreased plasma levels of ascorbic acid. Vitamin C deficiency also is present in patients with myelomeningocele,[346] although its contribution to fracture in that population is unclear. Infants with scurvy may present with irritability, lower extremities tenderness, weakness, pseudoparalysis, and possibly bleeding gums (if teeth have erupted). Subperiosteal hemorrhages may exist as well as hemorrhage into the subcutaneous tissues, muscles, urinary system, and gastrointestinal tract.[293] Anemia is also a common finding. In developing countries, older children with scurvy presenting with inability to walk may be misdiagnosed as having poliomyelitis.[422]

Radiographs may show osteolysis, joint space loss, osteonecrosis, osteopenia, and/or periosteal proliferation. Trabecular and cortical osteoporosis is common.[157] Profound demineralization is evident. In advanced disease, the long bones become almost transparent with a ground-glass appearance and extreme thinning of the cortex. Calcium accumulates in the zone of provisional calcification adjacent to the physis and becomes densely white (Fränkel line). Fractures generally occur in the scurvy line (Trummerfeld zone)—the radiolucent juxtaepiphyseal area above Fränkel line where the matrix is not converted to bone. Dense lateral spurs, known as the Pelken sign, may be seen.[195] A characteristic finding of scurvy is the corner sign in which a peripheral metaphyseal defect exists where fibrous tissue replaces absorbed cortex and cartilage.[35] Cupping of the metaphysis is common in both scurvy and rickets; in rickets, the metaphysis is ragged, whereas in scurvy, the metaphysis is sharply outlined.[195] The epiphysis becomes ringed with a thin, dense line (Wimberger sign). The periosteal elevation caused by hemorrhage calcifies within 10 days of treatment with vitamin C (Fig. 6-43).

Treatment

Fractures and epiphyseal displacement occur in both infants and older children with scurvy.[35,316,347,457,471] The most common sites of fracture, in order of frequency, are the distal femur, proximal humerus, costochondral junction of the ribs, and distal tibia.[195] Fractures of the long bones generally are nondisplaced metaphyseal buckle fractures with mild angulation. In contrast, marked epiphyseal displacement occurs with a moderate amount of callus present even in untreated patients. Exuberant callus forms once vitamin C is administered. Standard immobilization, with administration of vitamin C, is adequate for most fractures. Remodeling potential is high in these patients.[457] Even healed fractures that appear to have undergone growth arrest should be observed, because the potential for continued growth with medical treatment of the vitamin C deficiency can be nearly normal.[471] For infants who are older than 12 months

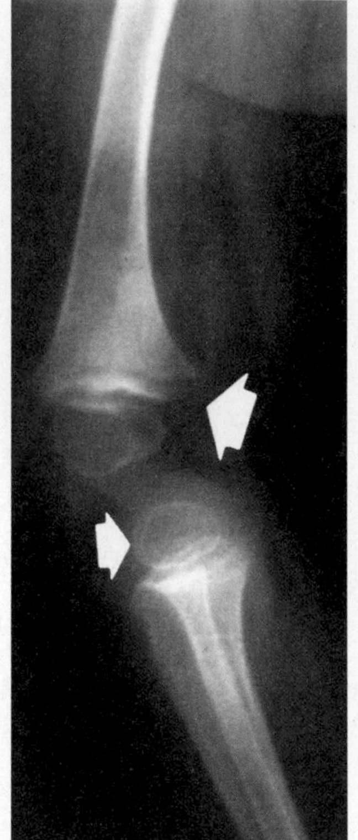
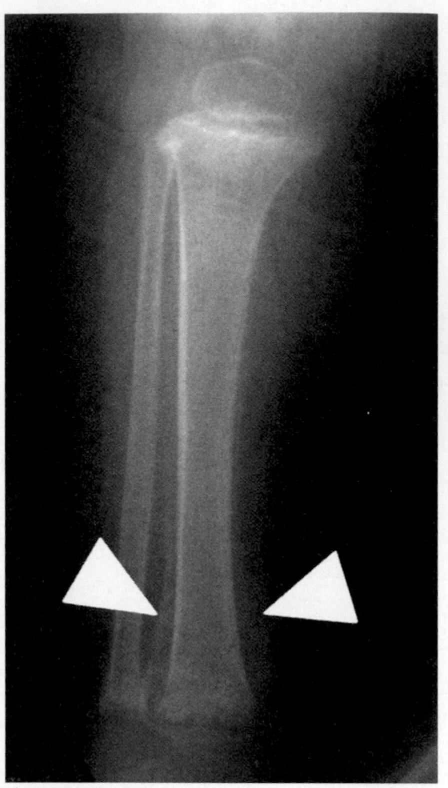
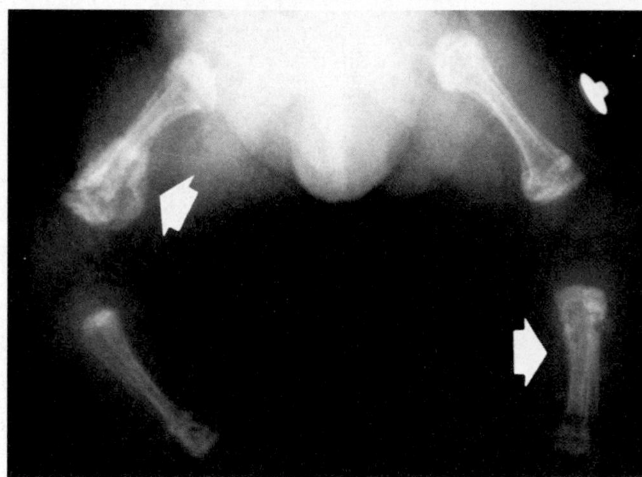

FIGURE 6-43 Scurvy. **A.** A 10-month-old boy presented with a 2-week history of refusal to walk with tenderness of the lower extremities. He had a history of milk and cereal intake only. There are signs of scurvy in the metaphysis (*large arrow*). The dense white line in the zone of the provisional calcification of the distal femur is known as the Fränkel line. The radiolucent juxtaepiphyseal line above the white line is known as the scurvy line. The peripheral metaphyseal defect, where fibrous tissue replaces absorbed cortex in cartilage, is known as the corner sign. Wimberger sign is a thin, dense line surrounding the epiphysis (*small arrow*). **B.** This is a child with healing scurvy. There is marked periosteal calcification around the distal tibia (*arrows*). **C.** A newborn with scurvy. Periosteal hemorrhage has become calcified in the bones of the lower extremity (*arrows*). (Courtesy of Bruce Mewborne, MD.)

of age and have begun weight bearing, spine films are recommended to rule out vertebral fractures.[316]

The literature of fracture treatment in scurvy consists primarily of case reports. Hoeffel et al.[221] reported on a 14-month-old girl with scurvy with bilateral distal femoral epiphysis displacement. This condition resolved after treatment with vitamin C, but limb-length discrepancy developed on one side.[415] In two patients with distal femoral fractures, healing went on to cupping of the metaphysis with an appearance similar to that in central growth arrest.[347,472]

Copper Deficiency and Scurvy-Like Syndrome

Copper is a vital trace element needed in the production of collagen. Copper deficiency results in a decreased number of collagen crosslinks, with adverse effects on both bone and blood vessels.[196] Copper deficiency can occur by 3 months in low-birth-weight infants[214] and after prolonged total parenteral nutrition. Copper deficiency can also develop as a result of excessive supplemental zinc ingestion.[65] Another cause of copper deficiency is disruption of one gene on the X chromosome causing a defect in the process of copper absorption, with consequent deficiency of available copper at the cellular level, resulting in abnormalities of collagen formation and brain maturation, leading to early death.[512]

Infants at risk for nutritional copper deficiency are those who are primarily milk fed and are on semistarvation diets with concurrent vomiting and diarrhea.[102] Both rib and wrist enlargement are frequent,[196] and neutropenia is common.[214] The diagnosis is commonly based on clinical presentation and decreased levels of serum copper.

Rarely, disruption of the copper controlling gene on chromosome 13 is associated with accumulation of excess copper in the body, initially in the liver and brain. With time, copper accumulates in the kidneys, causing renal damage and osteoarticular changes (e.g., osteoporosis, osteomalacia, and pathologic fractures).[512]

Radiographic findings in copper deficiency syndrome are very similar to those in rickets, including metaphyseal cupping, flaring, demineralization of the skeleton, and subperiosteal elevation with calcification.[488] There are some radiographic differences between scurvy and copper deficiency syndrome.[196] The corner sign is frequently absent in copper deficiency, the metaphyseal spurs are not strictly lateral but sickle shaped, and radiolucent bands of the metaphysis are absent. Bone age also is frequently retarded. Pathologic fractures have been reported in copper deficiency syndrome. Cordano et al.[123] noted prompt healing of a distal femoral fracture in an infant, but the fracture recurred before treatment of the copper deficiency. Such injuries can be treated like those in scurvy, with simple immobilization and concurrent correction of the copper deficiency.

FRACTURES IN NEUROMUSCULAR DISEASE

Cerebral Palsy

Children affected with neuromuscular diseases such as cerebral palsy (CP) may develop osteoporosis. The main causes of low bone density and osteoporosis in children and adolescents with CP are lack of activity, nutritional issues, and pharmacologic treatments (e.g., anticonvulsivants drugs).[408]

In a review of 1232 institutionalized patients with cerebral palsy, McIvor and Samilson[348] documented 134 extremity fractures, primarily in quadriplegics. When the mechanism of injury was known, most of these fractures were the consequence of a fall, often associated with seizure activity. Approximately 46% of these fractures involved the femoral shaft, 6% were fractures of the head or neck of the femur, 15% involved the tibia and fibula, and 13% were humeral fractures. These authors believed that contracture or paralytic dislocation of the hip joint predisposed these patients to femoral fractures.

Presedo et al.[415] reported on 156 children with CP who were treated for fractures. The mean age at the time of the first fracture was 10 years; 66% of patients had spastic quadriplegia, of those 83% were nonambulatory. Most fractures (82%) occurred in the lower limbs. The risk factors for fracture were nonambulatory CP child on anticonvulsant therapy, resulting in a high incidence of low-energy fractures.[415]

In another large multicenter study including 364 children with moderate-to-severe motor impairment, the rate of fracture was 4% per year. Children with greater body fat, feeding gastrostomy, and history of fracture were at highest risk of fractures.[489] Leet et al.[297] reported on 418 children with CP: 243 (58%) had quadriplegia, 120 (29%) had diplegia, and 55 (13%) hemiplegia. Of these, 366 were spastic, 23 mixed tone, 13 athetoid, and 16 classified as others. Pathologic fractures were seen in 50 children (12%). Older age at first fracture and use of valproic acid were predictive of fractures and defined a group of children who may benefit from treatment interventions to increase bone density.[297]

Miller and Glazer[360] emphasized that spontaneous fractures can occur in patients with CP without episodes of trauma, and factors such as disuse atrophy, nutritional deficiencies, and preexisting joint contractures contributed to these injuries. Nearly 50% of the full-time bedridden patients they studied developed spontaneous fractures. The diagnosis usually was delayed because the patients were noncommunicative. Anticonvulsant therapy may contribute to osteoporosis in patients with multiple fractures—low levels of serum vitamin D were seen in 42% of patients in one series.[291] One study concluded that unless sunlight exposure can be guaranteed, vitamin D supplementation should be considered for children and adults in residential care, especially if they are on anticonvulsant therapy, even in areas with year-round sunshine.[51] Fractures through osteoporotic bone can occur both above and below fixation devices.

Although long-bone fractures in patients with cerebral palsy heal quickly with abundant callus,[360] their treatment through either closed or open methods can be quite difficult. In a large series of patients, McIvor and Samilson[348] recommended closed treatment through skeletal traction, hip spica cast, or long-leg cast. Approximately 65% of the femoral shaft fractures and 86% of distal femoral fractures went on to malunion. Despite malunion, most patients regained their prefracture function. Nearly 21% of their patients had refractures, and the authors believed that this was due to disuse osteopenia, inadequate reduction, or joint contractures. Closed treatment of these fractures can be complicated by the development of decubitus ulcers. Closed fractures, especially those of the femur, can become open injuries during treatment, owing to spasticity or inadequate immobilization.[348,360] Hip spica casts are difficult to use in patients with severe flexion contractures or dislocation of the hip. The healing time of femoral fractures treated through immobilization varies from 1 to 3.5 months.[348,359] Fractures of the humerus have been treated with light hanging-arm casts or sling-and-swath bandages.[360] Hip nails with side plates, compression plates, and intramedullary fixations also have been used for femoral shaft fractures in patients with CP. The mean healing time has been 5.3 months.[348]

Numerous reports note success in treating fractures of neurologically impaired children with internal or external fixation.[170,212] Heinrich et al.[212] treated four femoral fractures in young patients with CP with flexible intramedullary nails with good outcomes. Femoral neck fractures may require in situ pinning, but observation may be adequate in asymptomatic bedridden patients. Although he advocated open fixation of some lower extremity fractures in patients with mental retardation, Sherk[463] cautioned that some patients may have inadequate motivation to resume ambulation even with successful healing of their injuries. Medical management of these patients must also be emphasized. In patients with cerebral palsy and multiple fractures, Lee and Lyne[291] recommended metabolic supplementation, along with traditional fracture care.

In a randomized controlled trial of standing program impact on bone mineral density in nonambulant children with CP, participation in 50% longer periods of standing (in either upright or semiprone standing frames) improved vertebral but not proximal tibial volumetric trabecular bone mineral density. The authors concluded that such intervention might reduce the risk of vertebral fractures but is unlikely to reduce the risk of lower limb fractures in children with CP.[88]

Fractures of the distal pole of the patella have been reported in children with CP due to spasticity of the extensor mechanism of the knee in the presence of established knee flexion contracture.[255,310,443] Lloyd-Roberts et al.[310] reported on eight patients with this injury who presented with deterioration in walking and decreased endurance. All had knee flexion contractures. Seven of the eight patients complained of pain and local tenderness at the distal pole of the patella. In a series of 88 patients, fragmentation was seen in only 8%.[443] Patella alta and elongation of the patella are frequent in affected patients.[255,443] Children predisposed to distal pole patellar fractures are spastic ambulators with flexion contractures of the knees, patella alta, and a history of falls.[255] Extension casting may be helpful in symptomatic patients.[443] If conservative treatment is unsatisfactory, then hamstring lengthening with correction of the knee flexion contracture can result in both healing of the fracture and relief of symptoms.[310,443] Some authors[255,310] also have excised the avulsed distal pole of the patella to relieve chronic symptoms.

Although less common than metaphyseal and diaphyseal fractures, epiphyseal separations may occur. In a report of nine epiphyseal separations involving the distal femur and proximal humerus in four severely affected children with spastic quadriplegic CP, the clinical-radiologic features confirmed the cause to be scurvy. The fractures healed nicely with treatment with vitamin C and splintage.[24]

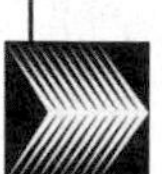

AUTHORS' PREFERRED METHOD OF TREATMENT

The goal of fracture treatment in CP is to restore the child to his or her prefracture level of function. If the patient is ambulatory, conventional forms of fracture treatment should be used (Fig. 6-44). In nonambulatory children with CP, a goal

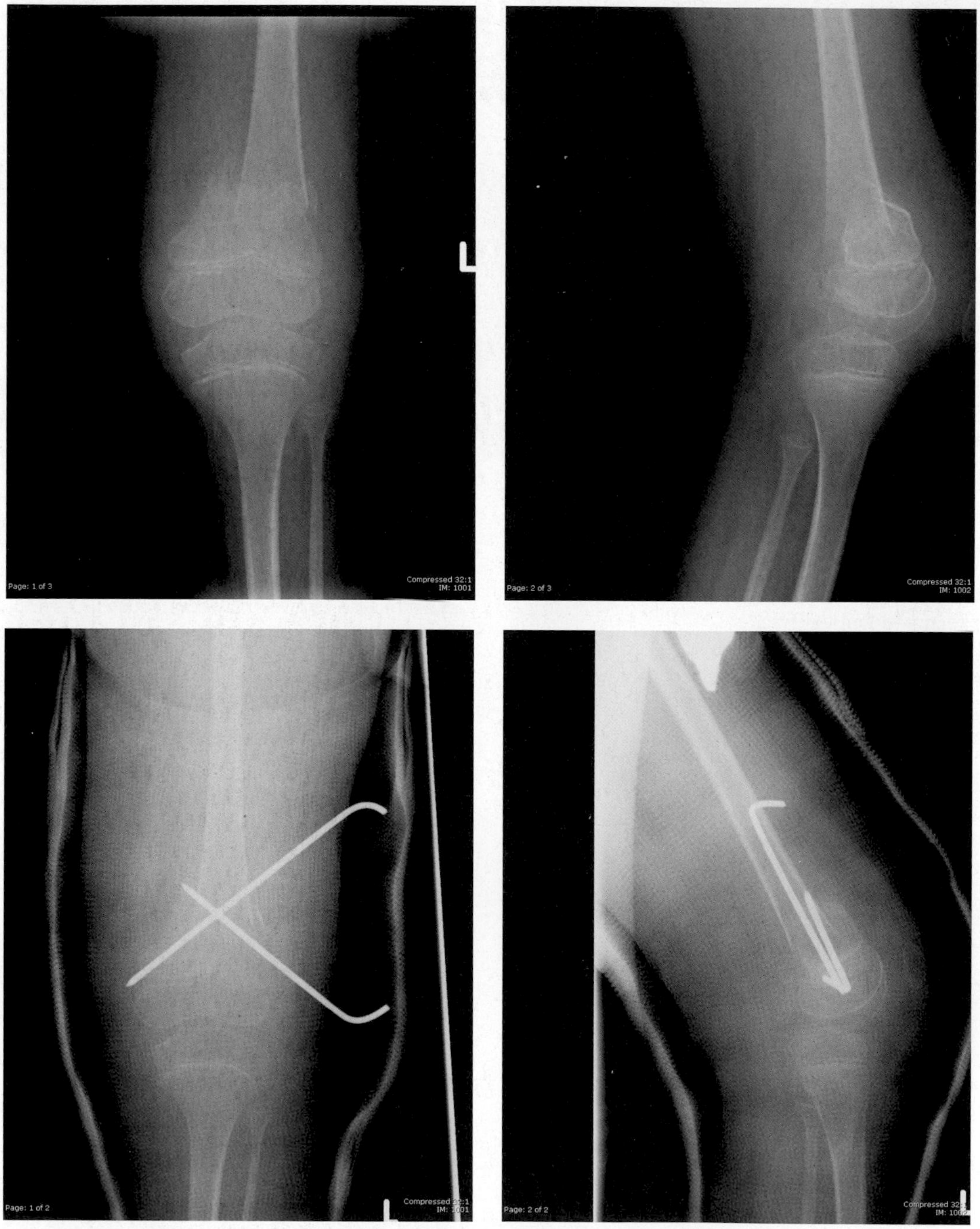

FIGURE 6-44 An 11-year-old boy with total body involvement cerebral palsy was receiving physical therapy when he developed pain and swelling around the left knee. Radiographs showed displaced femoral supracondylar fracture **(A,B)**. In order to be able to fit to the brace adequately, closed reduction and percutaneous pinning was performed **(C,D)**. *(continues)*

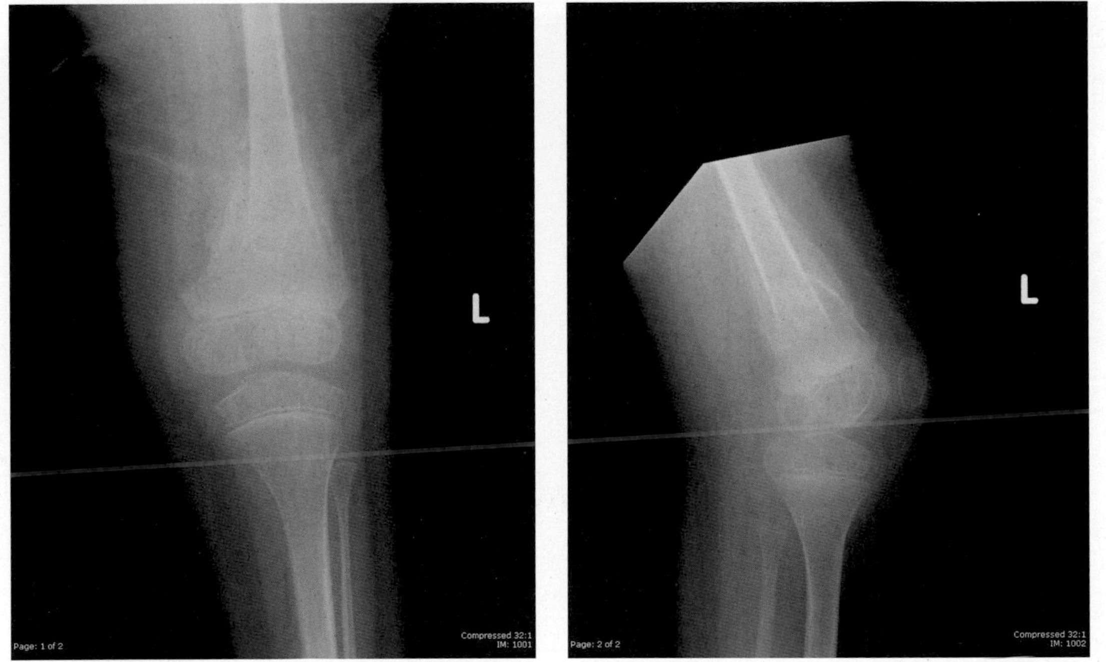

FIGURE 6-44 (*continued*) The fracture healed in good alignment and the pins were removed after 6 weeks **(E,F)**. (Figures reproduced with permission from The Childrens Orthopaedic Center, Los Angeles, CA.)

of fracture care should be to preserve the ability to transfer. Special precautions should be used in closed treatment of fractures in these patients. The patients' spasticity and inability to communicate make them prone to skin problems, so casts should be properly applied and well padded, usually with felt and polyurethane foam. Extra padding should be placed over the patella, anterior ankle, and heel, and a snug cast mould should be placed above the calcaneus to prevent proximal migration of the heel. When indicated, operative fracture fixation should be used in ambulatory patients. Elastic intramedullary nails can be a very effective way to treat femoral fractures in children with spasticity (Fig. 6-45).

Prevention is an important part of managing fractures in children with CP. Traditionally, long-leg casts or spica casts were used after multiple muscle lengthening or hip osteotomies, then after several weeks, the cast was removed and therapy begun. After cast treatment, however, the osteopenia was worse, the joints were stiff, and fractures—especially in the distal femoral metaphysis—occurred during therapy or transfers. We and others[358,359] use foam abduction pillows and knee immobilizers and an intensive therapy program in the immediate postoperative period to avoid the deconditioning, osteopenia, and joint stiffness that develop after prolonged cast immobilization. In ambulatory children who need hip osteotomies, use of rigid internal fixation allows standing and gait training within 2 weeks, preventing not only osteopenia but also the risk that the child may never regain the full level of preoperative function after a prolonged period of cast immobilization.

In nonambulatory children with severe CP, some degree of both malunion and shortening may be accepted. Well-padded splints or casts are adequate treatment for many displaced fractures. Acute femoral shaft fractures can be treated with a heavily padded hip spica cast and distal fractures of the femur by a long-leg cast. Distal femoral buckle fractures in nonambulatory children are safely treated with a knee immobilizer. If a long-leg cast is used for a fracture of the lower extremity and the joint of the involved side is dislocated, the rigid cast may function as a lever arm, with the posterior fracture of the proximal femur beyond the cast (Fig. 6-46).

Myelomeningocele

Children with myelomeningocele are at a high risk of pathologic fractures of the lower extremities. The etiology is multifactorial but results from decreased bone mineral density due to disuse (nonambulators), immobilization after reconstructive surgical procedures, and increased urinary calcium loss.[311] The incidence of fractures in children with myelomeningocele ranges from 12% to 31%.[134,135,161,238,358,359,443,517] The locations of these fractures, in order of decreasing frequency, are midshaft of the femur, distal femur, midshaft of the tibia, proximal femur, femoral neck, distal femoral physis, and proximal tibia.[134] Fractures of the distal tibia also have been reported in numerous series.[144,238,278,501,517] Both metaphyseal and diaphyseal fractures, usually resulting from minor trauma, are often either incomplete or impacted with intact periosteum.[312] They tend to heal rapidly—nonunion is rare.[134] Physeal fractures, however, may take 3 to 33 months to heal.[517]

Numerous factors predispose these patients to fracture. Children with flail limbs tend to pick up one leg and drop it out of the way when they roll over in bed or twist around while in a sitting position, and this may be enough force to cause a fracture.[238] Because protective sensation is absent, the child can neither anticipate impending injury nor be aware of injury once it has occurred. The level of neurologic involvement also affects the incidence of fractures. In a series of 76 fractures, Lock and Aronson[312] found that 41% occurred with neurologic deficit at

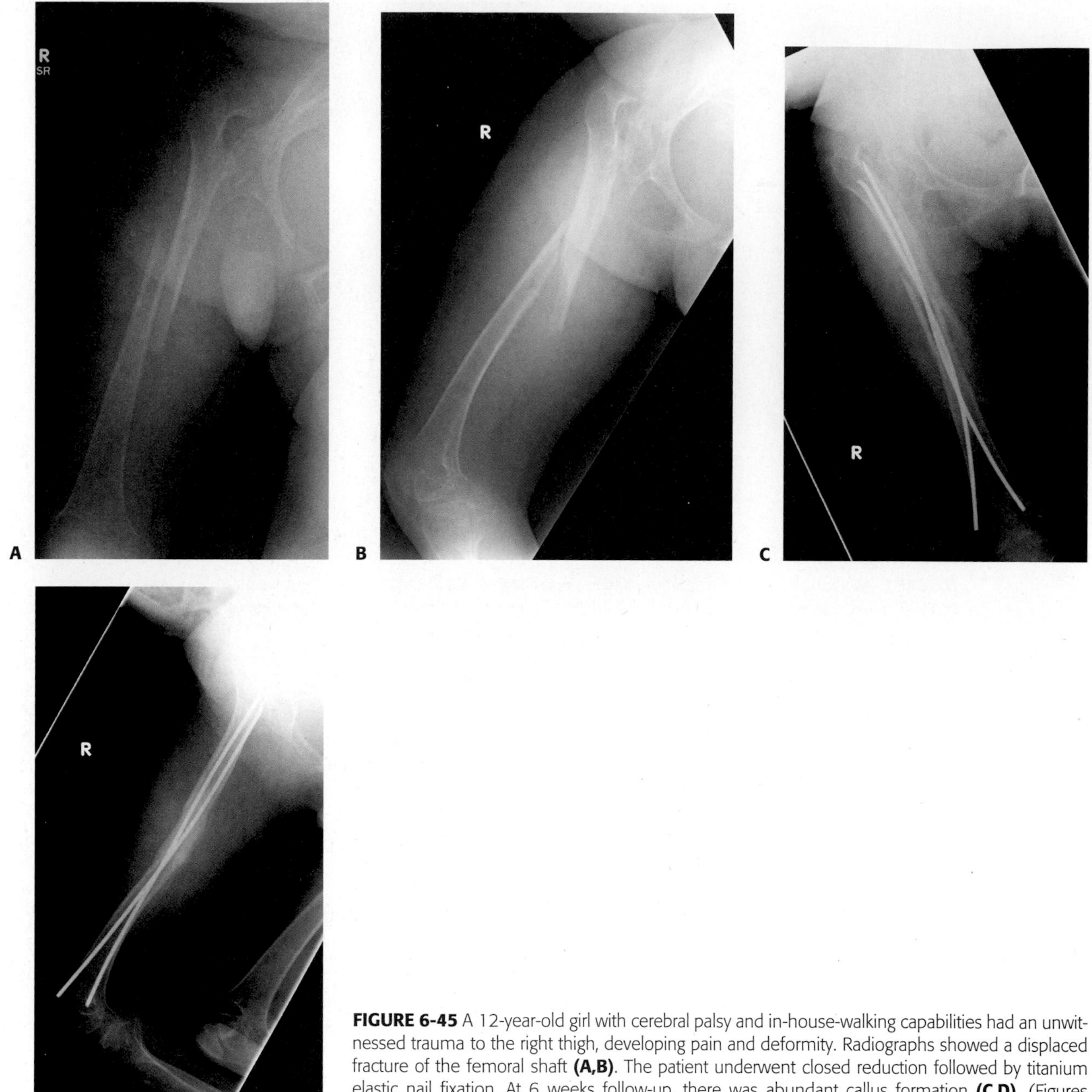

FIGURE 6-45 A 12-year-old girl with cerebral palsy and in-house-walking capabilities had an unwitnessed trauma to the right thigh, developing pain and deformity. Radiographs showed a displaced fracture of the femoral shaft **(A,B)**. The patient underwent closed reduction followed by titanium elastic nail fixation. At 6 weeks follow-up, there was abundant callus formation **(C,D)**. (Figures reproduced with permission from The Childrens Orthopaedic Center, Los Angeles, CA.)

the thoracic level, 36% occurred with deficit at the upper lumbar level, and only 13% occurred in patients with lower lumbar or sacral deficits. Nearly 86% of these fractures occurred before 9 years of age, and 76% were associated with cast immobilization. Most fractures after immobilization occur within 4 weeks of cast removal,[135] and in one series,[312] 30% of patients with casts had multiple cluster fractures of either the casted extremity or the partially casted contralateral extremity. In addition to the inherent disuse osteoporosis from immobilization, casting causes stiffness of joints with concentration of force on the osteoporotic bone adjacent to the joints.[312] Boytim et al.[68] reported neonatal fractures in six infants with myelomeningocele and concluded that the risk of fracture was 17% for patients with thoracic or high lumbar level deficits with significant contracture of the lower extremities. The authors cautioned that particular care must be used to avoid fractures in these patients during physical therapy, positioning for radiographs, or surgical procedures. Fractures associated with spina bifida are, however, most commonly seen in early adolescence.[26]

Stable fractures of the long bones may not require complete immobilization.[135] Femoral shaft fractures have been treated with padding and sandbags.[147] Skin traction of anesthetic limbs may cause massive skin necrosis.[134,147] Skeletal traction usually is inadvisable because of problems with decubitus ulcers and poor fixation in atrophic bone.[134,147] However, Drummond et al.[136] treated nine of 18 patients with skeletal traction without mention of failure or fixation.

Preventive measures include limiting cast immobilization after reconstructive surgery.[10,136] Solid side cushions may prevent fractures that occur when patients catch their lower extremities in bed rails.[417] The most important consideration was noted by Norton and Foley[385] in 1959, when they stated "the

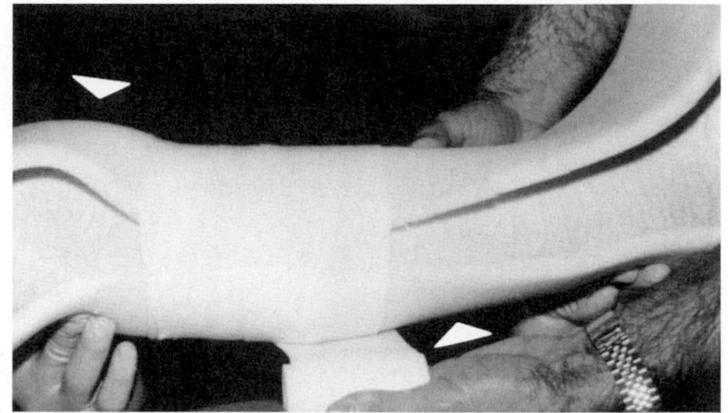

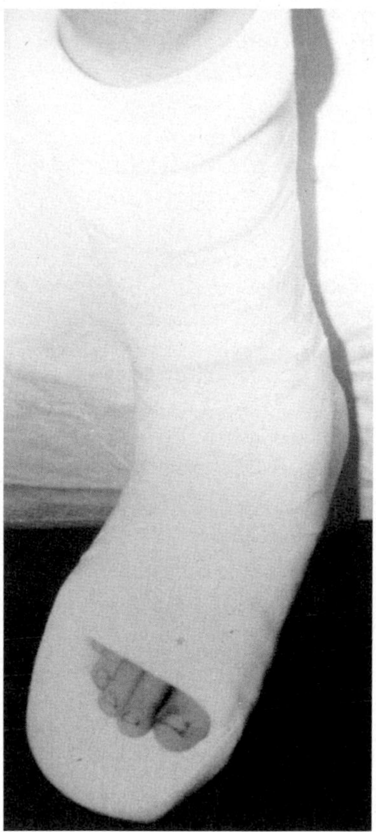

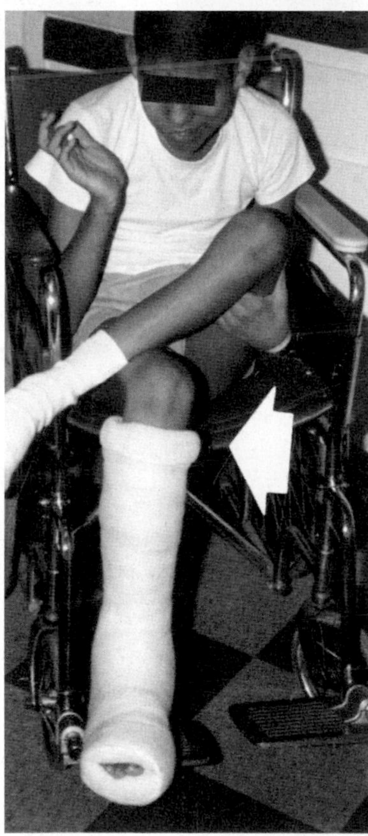

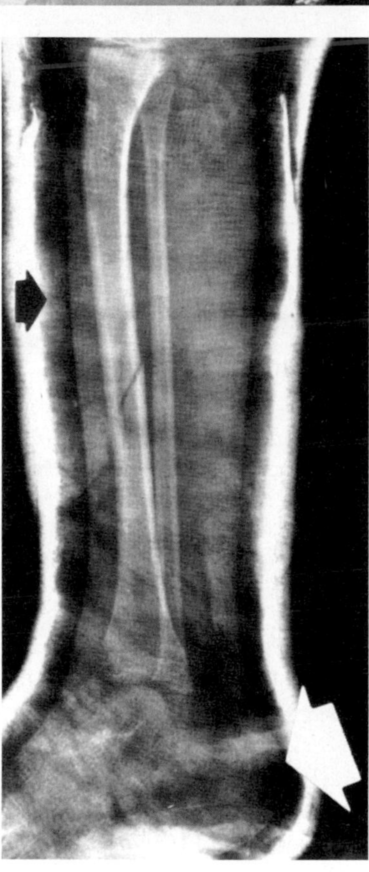

FIGURE 6-46 Casting in neuromuscular fractures. **A.** A polyurethane foam short-leg cast is being placed on a patient. Two long rectangular sheets of foam (*arrows*) are placed anteriorly and posteriorly over the stockinette, and Webril padding is wrapped around the foam. **B.** A long toe plate is needed to prevent injury to the foot of the patient. **C.** A thick, protective cuff of foam is formed by folding the polyurethane toward the center of the cast with the stockinette (*arrow*). **D.** The Webril must be wrapped quite snugly to compress the foam against the underlying extremity evenly (*black arrow*). Extra foam is placed over the anterior ankle and over the Achilles tendon to prevent proximal migration of the foot in the cast. A plaster cast is usually applied and covered with a layer of fiberglass for strength. A lateral radiograph verifies the position of the heel in the cast (*white arrow*).

quality of bone developed by activity appears to be the best protection against pathologic fractures," and the orthopaedist should assist these patients in maintaining the highest activity level possible.

Fractures of the physes in patients with myelomeningocele are relatively uncommon and difficult to diagnose.[259] The clinical presentation may mimic infection, with elevated temperature and swelling, redness, and local warmth at the fracture site.[439,501] Fractures of the proximal tibia may be confused with septic arthritis of the knee, with swelling up to the midthigh and limited knee flexion. Both the white blood cell count and erythrocyte sedimentation rate are often elevated. Immobilization of these injuries usually results in a dramatic decrease in swelling and redness of the extremity within 2 to 3 days of casting. With healing, the radiographic picture can be alarming, with epiphyseal plate widening, metaphyseal fracture, and periosteal elevation.[201] The radiographic differential diagnoses should include osteomyelitis, sarcoma, leukemia, and Charcot joint.[144]

Recurrent trauma to the physis, from either continued walking or passive joint motion after injury, results in an exuberant healing reaction (Fig. 6-47).[144] Repetitive trauma delays resumption of normal endochondral ossification, resulting in abnormal thickening of the cartilage in the zone of hypertrophy and the physeal widening seen on radiographs.[517] In a study of 19 chronic physeal fractures, Rodgers et al.[144] compared MRI with histology and found that adjacent to this thickened, disorganized zone of hypertrophy is juxtametaphyseal fibrovascular tissue that enhances gadolinium on MRI. Delayed union is common, and premature growth arrest occurs in 29% to 55% of patients.[312,516] Anschuetz et al.[17] reported a unique syndrome in three patients with myelomeningocele and fracture. These children sustained fractures of the lower extremities during long-term immobilization and with cast removal went on to dramatic cardiopulmonary distress with increased pulse rate, hypotension, and increased respiratory rate. Fever also developed with decreased hematocrit levels. They suggested that the

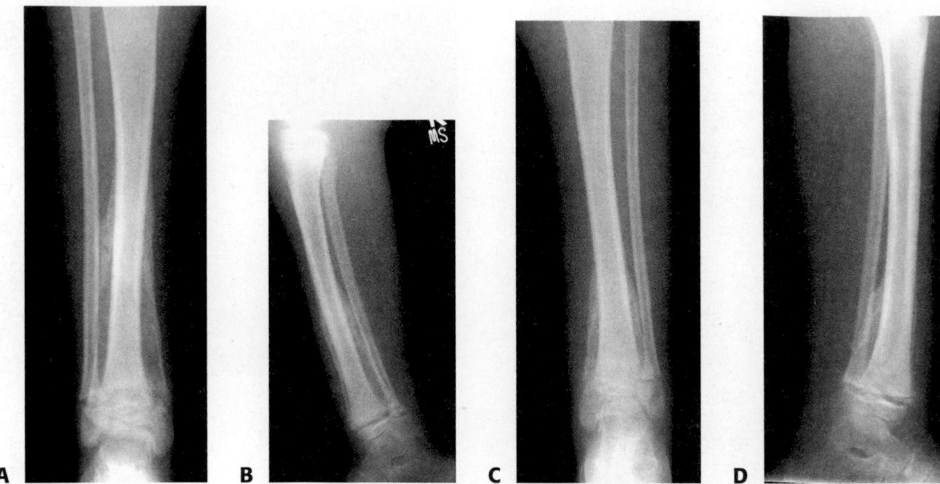

FIGURE 6-47 A 10-year-old boy with low-lumbar spina bifida and community ambulation (with braces) presented with chronic bilateral leg/ankle pain. Anteroposterior **(A,C)** and lateral **(B,D)** radiographs of both tibia and fibula show stress/insufficiency fracture of the distal tibial physis associated with extensive periosteal bone formation, characteristic of myelomeningocele.

etiology of this problem was loss of intravascular volume into the fracture sites and recommended intravenous replacement of fluid losses, along with careful splinting of associated fractures.

Physeal injuries in patients with myelomeningocele are more difficult to treat than metaphyseal or diaphyseal long bone fractures and require lengthy immobilization with strict avoidance of weight bearing to avoid destructive repetitive trauma to the physis.[144] Either a plaster cast or a snug-fitting total-contact orthosis is suggested for immobilization, and union can be determined by return of the physis to normal width on radiographs.[517] Kumar et al.[278] emphasized that application of a long-leg cast for 8 to 12 weeks is necessary to obtain satisfactory healing of physeal fractures of the tibia, and weight bearing is to be avoided until union occurs.

Treatment

Immediate casting[238] and bivalved casting[147] have been used for long-bone fractures in children with myelomeningocele. A bilateral hip spica cast is suggested for supracondylar fractures of the femur, because use of a one-and-a-half hip spica cast may predispose the uninjured side to fracture.[134] A bulky Webril dressing approximately 1.5 cm thick wrapped with an elastic bandage can be used instead of a plaster or fiberglass cast. Lock and Aronson[312] used Webril immobilization for an average of 1 to 3 weeks in their patients with fractures and discontinued immobilization when callus was visible. They found similar outcomes in patients treated with Webril dressings and those treated with casts; however, there was much less difficulty with pressure sores in the group treated with Webril dressings. Kumar et al.[278] used a polyurethane padded long-leg posterior plaster splint for metaphyseal and diaphyseal fractures for 3 weeks, followed by bracing. Drennan and Freehafer[134] recommend a well-padded cast for 2 to 3 weeks for infants with fracture and braces or Webril immobilization for incomplete fractures that followed surgery. Injuries with deformity were placed in a cast. Mobilization was begun as soon as practical to prevent further osteopenia—patients with shaft fractures began ambulation 2 weeks after injury. Shortening was not a problem in their series. Lock and Aronson[312] cautioned that brace treatment of acute fractures may cause pressure sores. Drummond et al.[135] reported on 18 fractures treated by closed techniques that resulted in three malunions, two shortenings, and two episodes of pressure sores; one patient had four refractures. Drabu and Walker[132] noted a mean loss of knee movement of 58 degrees in 67% of fractures about the knee. The stiffness began 2 months after fracture and was well established by 6 months but resolved almost completely in all patients 3 years after injury. They suggested that aggressive physical therapy to restore knee motion is probably not necessary in these injuries.

Operative fixation of fractures in children with myelomeningocele is associated with a high rate of infection.[147] Wenger et al.[517] reported that most patients with proximal femoral epiphyseal displacement can be treated with hip spica casts. Reduction and pinning with subtrochanteric osteotomy may be necessary in certain patients. Bailey-Dubow rods may be valuable in multiple recurrent pathologic fractures of the femoral or tibial shaft.[281] If operative treatment is necessary, it should be noted that the incidence of malignant hyperthermia is higher in patients with myelomeningocele than in other children.[15]

Life-threatening anaphylactic reactions due to latex allergy in children with myelomeningocele have been reported with increasing frequency.[131,312] Minor allergic reactions, such as rash, edema, hives, and respiratory symptoms, are common when children with myelodysplasia are exposed to latex products such as gloves, catheters, and balloons. Between 18% and 40% of children with myelodysplasia are allergic to latex.[159] Meeropol et al.[352] emphasized that every child with myelomeningocele should be screened for latex allergy, and those with a positive history should be evaluated individually by the anesthesiologist for preoperative prophylaxis. Current preoperative prophylaxis begins 24 hours before surgery and is continued for 24 hours after surgery. Medications used include diphenhydramine 1 mg/kg every 6 hours (maximum 50 mg), methylprednisolone 1 mg/kg every 6 hours (maximum 125 mg), and cimetidine 5 mg/kg every 6 hours (maximum 300 mg). A latex-free environment must also be provided throughout the hospitalization.

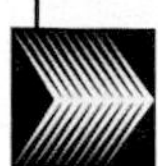

AUTHORS' PREFERRED METHOD OF TREATMENT

In nonambulatory patients, mild malunion and shortening can be tolerated, and stable or minimally angulated fractures can be treated with either polyurethane splints or Webril dressings. Fractures with significant deformity may require reduction and immobilization in a cast heavily padded with polyurethane foam. In children who walk, fractures should be carefully aligned with heavily padded casts that allow continued protective weight bearing, if possible. Hip spica casts may be necessary for femoral shaft fractures. Fractures of the proximal femur should be treated by immobilization and any later deformity corrected by osteotomy. Any patient considered for operative intervention should be treated prophylactly with latex-free gloves and equipment. Physeal fractures are treated with padded long leg casts and nonweight bearing. Long-term follow-up is encouraged for physeal injuries because of the risk of growth arrest. Significant discrepancies can be addressed through contralateral epiphysiodesis or bridge resection.

Muscular Dystrophy

Fractures of the lower extremity in children with Duchenne muscular dystrophy must be managed so as not to cause premature loss of the ability to walk[343,508] or transfer.[232] In patients 9 to 10 years old, increasing muscle weakness and joint contractures contribute to falls, and a loss of normal muscle bulk and fat limit the cushioning on impact.[468] Patients in lower extremity braces seem to sustain few fractures in falls,[508] probably because the overlying orthoses provide some protection.[468] Patients confined to a wheelchair can fall because they have poor sitting balance, and fractures are frequent because these patients are more osteoporotic than ambulatory individuals.[468] In a chart review of 143 boys with genetically confirmed dystrophinopathies, boys treated with steroids ambulated independently 3.3 years longer than the untreated group and had a lower prevalence of scoliosis. However, vertebral compression fractures occurred in 32% of the treated group, whereas no vertebral fractures were seen in the nontreatment group; long-bone fractures were 2.6 times greater in steroid-treated patients.[263]

Concentric "osseous atrophy" occurs in the long bones of patients with Duchenne muscular dystrophy; osteoporosis is also common.[153,339] Osteoporosis is most profound in the lower extremities and begins to develop early while still ambulating. Consequently, frequent fractures may result in loss of ambulation.[287] Larson and Henderson[287] reported that bone density in the proximal femur was profoundly diminished even when gait was minimally affected, and then progressively decreased to nearly four standard deviations below age-matched normal.[287] Fractures are seldom displaced and are frequently minimally painful because there is minimal muscle spasm.[468] Fractures tend to heal rapidly. The most commonly fractured bone is the femur[231,232,467] followed by the proximal humerus.[467]

Corticosteroid therapy given to children with Duchenne muscular dystrophy to prolong mobility has been shown to increase the rate of osteoporosis and consequently, increase the risk of fracture. A study of 33 boys with Duchenne muscular dystrophy demonstrated the incidence of vertebral fractures in these patients after the initiation of corticosteroid treatment; 40 months after commencement of steroids the first vertebral fracture emerged. By 100 months of treatment, approximately 75% of patients had sustained a vertebral fracture.[66]

There are two goals of fracture care in children with muscular dystrophy: limb stability and maintenance of maximal function during fracture healing. In ambulatory patients, treatment methods should allow children to maintain the ability to walk as the fracture heals. When ambulatory ability is tenuous, even minor bruises or ankle sprains[508] may end walking ability. As little as 1 week in a wheelchair can prematurely end ambulation[508]; patients at bed rest for more than 2 weeks will likely lose the ability to ambulate.[343] Hsu[231] reported that 25% of ambulatory patients with muscular dystrophy lost the ability to walk after sustaining fractures. In one of these patients, the ankle was casted in 20 degrees of plantarflexion, and the resulting contracture prevented ambulation at the end of treatment.

Treatment of specific fractures should be individualized. Upper extremity fractures can be treated with lightweight slings.[468] Lower extremity fractures can be treated with either light walking casts or long-leg double upright braces.[468,507] Splints also can be used until the patients are pain free. Routine activities are begun as soon as possible.[231] Protected standing and ambulation with physical therapy are crucial in maintaining independent ambulation (Fig. 6-48).[507]

Hsu and Garcia-Ariz[232] reported on 20 femoral fractures in 16 patients with muscular dystrophy. Six of the seven ambulatory patients were able to walk after treatment. In the nonambulatory patients in this series, most had supracondylar femoral fractures which were splinted for 2 to 3 weeks, with emphasis on physical therapy to maintain functional abilities. Although union was achieved rapidly, hip and knee flexion contractures often increased in these patients and up to 20 degrees of angulation of the fracture was routinely accepted. One patient with slipped capital femoral epiphysis was treated successfully with pinning in situ.

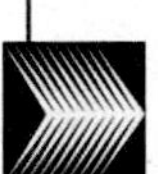

AUTHORS' PREFERRED METHOD OF TREATMENT

The first goal of fracture treatment in children with muscular dystrophy is to avoid making matters worse. The patient should be mobilized as soon as possible in a lightweight cast or orthosis. Aggressive physical therapy should be used to maintain functional status. In a very young child, midshaft femoral fractures can be treated by traction and hip spica techniques, but in an older patient, ambulatory cast bracing might be a better choice.

Arthrogryposis and Poliomyelitis

Arthrogryposis is a group of rare and heterogeneous disorders affecting children in whom there are at least two or more joint contractures in multiple body areas. There are at least a few hundred arthrogrypotic syndromes. Arthrogryposis has an incidence of 3 in 10,000 live births.[523] Although the etiology is unknown and likely multifactorial, there is a lack of fetal joint movement after initially normal development, leading to collagen proliferation, fibrotic replacement of muscle, a marked thickening of joint capsules, taut ligaments, and capsular tightness resulting in joint stiffness.[203] Dislocations can occur with severe shortening of the involved muscles.

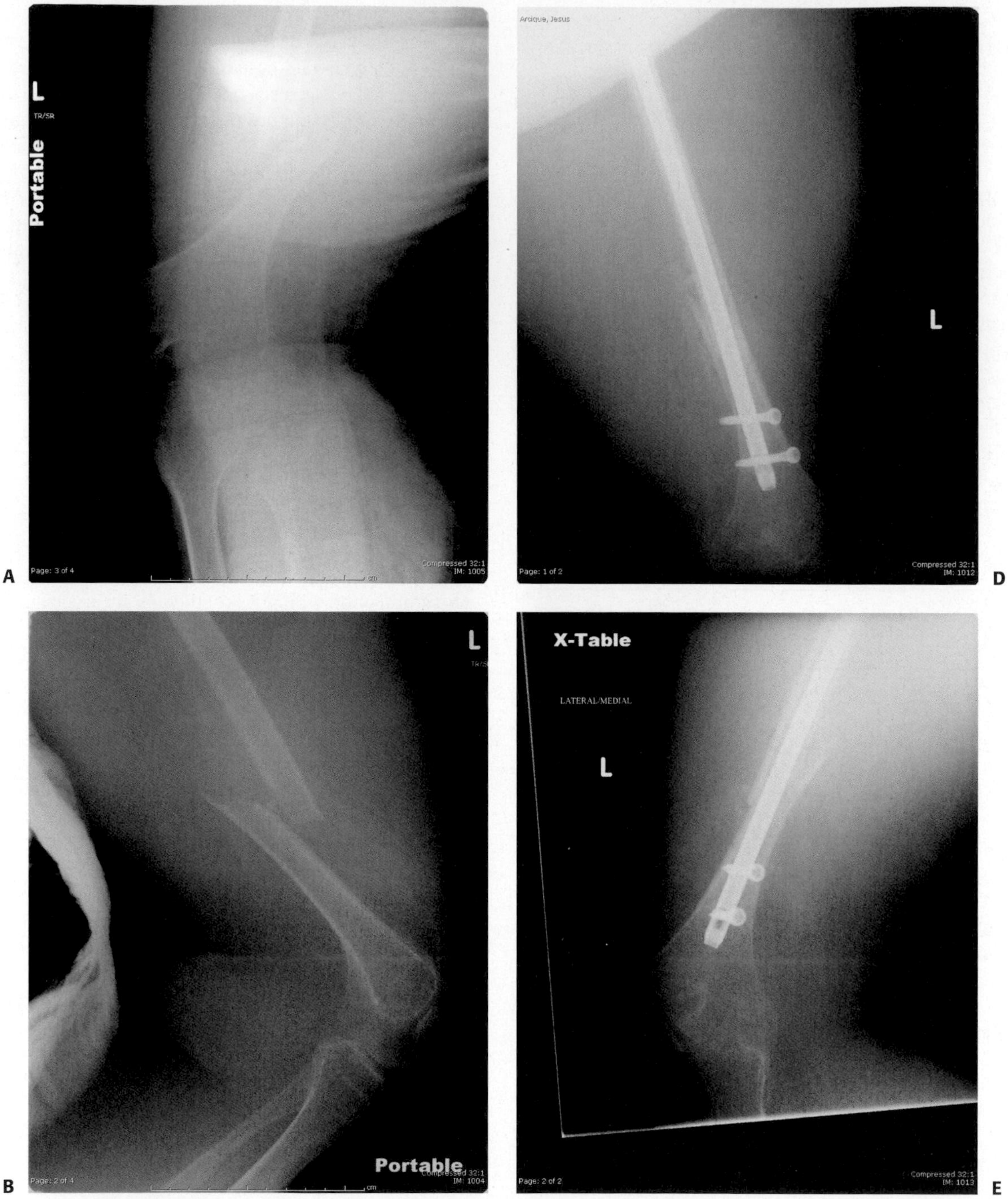

A D

B E

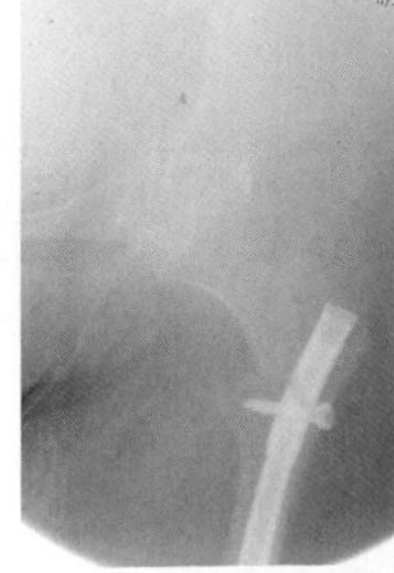

C

FIGURE 6-48 This 15-year-old domiciliary-ambulatory boy with Duchenne muscular dystrophy who sustained a fall at home had this displaced femoral shaft fracture **(A,B)**. Due to his prefracture ambulatory status, he underwent closed reduction and intramedullary fixation of his fracture **(C,D,E)**.

Fractures may occur in 25% of infants with arthrogryposis.[120] A difficult delivery or forceful manipulation of the extremities can lead to fracture.[120] Diamond and Alegado[120] reported 16 fractures in nine infants with arthrogryposis; an ipsilateral dislocated hip was present in 35% of patients. Most fractures involved the femur, with the remainder mostly tibial fractures, one humeral fracture, and one clavicle fracture. Epiphyseal separations occurred in the proximal tibia, distal femur, and proximal humerus. Clinical symptoms included poor feeding, irritability, and fussiness when handled. The involved extremity was thickened, and there was often an increased white blood cell count. Plain radiographs after acute injury, especially with epiphyseal separations, were not helpful, and arthrogram was used in one patient to evaluate a distal femoral epiphyseal separation. With healing, these fractures develop exuberant callus with rapid union and ready remodeling of angulated midshaft fractures.

Short-term immobilization is adequate to treat nondisplaced fractures in these patients (Fig. 6-49). Postnatal fractures are most common in patients with either knee contracture or dislocation of the hip, and postnatal injury could possibly be reduced by avoidance of forceful manipulation of these extremities. Older patients with lower extremity contractures do not seem to have difficulty with pathologic fractures.[482]

Acute poliomyelitis has become a relatively rare disease in most Western countries but occasionally occurs in children who live in less developed countries. There are few reports in the literature concerning fractures in patients with poliomyelitis. Robin[436] reported 62 fractures in patients with poliomyelitis. More than half were fractures of the femur, and 90% of those injuries were supracondylar fractures. More than half of the fractures occurred after cast immobilization, and joint stiffness also was associated with a significant number of fractures. There were no epiphyseal injuries in this series.

Treatment of these fractures is simple immobilization. Because most fractures have very little displacement, reduction is seldom necessary; if there is pre-existing deformity, manual osteoclasis through the fracture site can be used to correct deformities. Robin[436] stressed that joint mobility must be obtained before general mobilization of the patient to reduce the incidence of fracture after plaster immobilization. He also emphasized that fractures in these patients heal rapidly, and immobili-

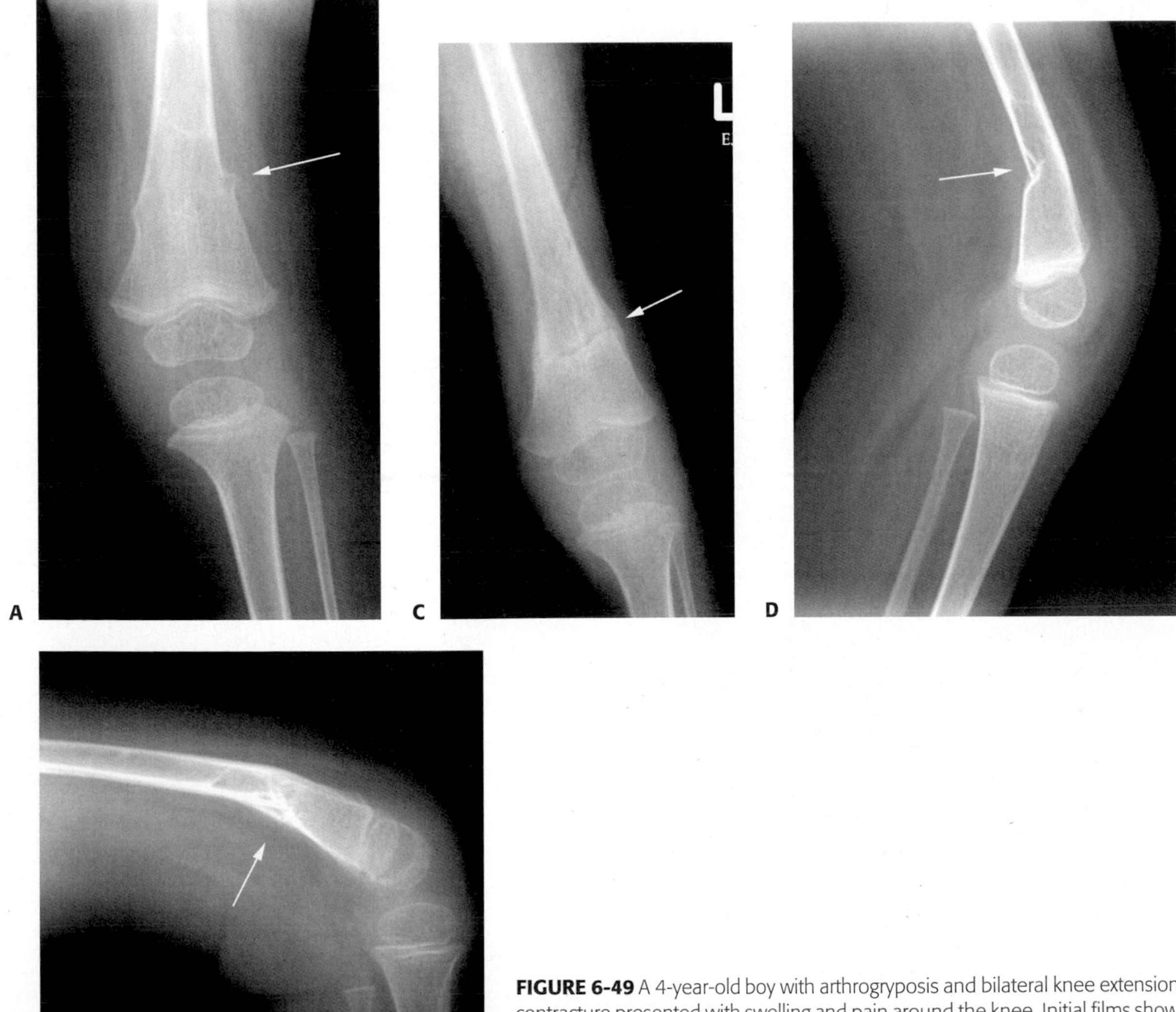

FIGURE 6-49 A 4-year-old boy with arthrogryposis and bilateral knee extension contracture presented with swelling and pain around the knee. Initial films show minimally displaced transverse fracture through the distal femoral metaphysis (*arrow*). After 4 weeks in a long-leg cast, radiographs show new bone formation (*arrow*) and good alignment of the fracture in both views.

zation times should be reduced accordingly, with walking or standing in casts to decrease osteoporosis.

Spinal Cord Injury

Fortunately, childhood spinal cord injury is rare, and reports of pathologic fractures usually are included in larger series of patients with fractures and myelomeningocele because of the clinical similarities in presentation.[250,435] Fractures of the femur, especially supracondylar fractures, are most common,[168] but tibial fractures also are common.[168] In most patients, these are pathologic fractures through osteoporotic bone. Children with a spinal cord injury have a substantially lower bone mineral density at the hip and knee in comparison with children without disability, placing them at least at the same risk for lower extremity fractures as adults with spinal cord injury. Children may actually be much more susceptible to fractures than adults since they lack of activity in a period of their life where exercise is essential for optimal bone health.[288] Although fractures in paraplegics appear to heal rapidly with abundant callus,[168] animal experiments suggest that in denervated limbs, the quality of the callus in fractures is compromised.[234] Children with traumatic peripheral nerve lesions may have distal tibial physeal lesions similar to those in patients with myelomeningocele, neuropathic arthropathy of the small joints of the foot, and soft tissue ulcers.[454]

Conservative treatment of fractures in patients with spinal cord injury is most commonly recommended. Skin traction is contraindicated because of the possibility of skin necrosis.[147] Comarr et al.[100] also used pillow sandbag splints and, for certain fractures, treated patients with a turning frame. Open reduction and internal fixation of these fractures is controversial. The conservative techniques used for the treatment of similar fractures in children with myelomeningocele might best be applied to fractures in children with traumatic paraplegia.[134,250,435]

Although crutch and brace ambulation in paraplegics reportedly restores bone integrity,[1] fractures continue to occur through osteoporotic bone in children actively ambulating with brace support.[250] Some authors advocate light protective braces,[100] but Katz[250] suggested that continuous splinting will worsen the disuse osteoporosis. He recommended careful manipulation of the lower extremities when they are out of ambulatory braces to reduce the incidence of fracture. Robin[435] emphasized that immobilization should be discontinued as soon as possible after fracture healing. Patient activity should be limited until knee motion is restored.

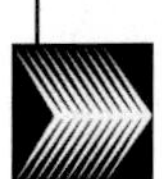

AUTHORS' PREFERRED METHOD OF TREATMENT

Heavily padded casts or splints are recommended for most lower extremity fractures in children with traumatic paraplegia. Returning to ambulation with protection by walking braces is permitted once callus and joint motion are adequate. Every effort should be made to restore the child's prefracture function. Moderate malunion and shortening are acceptable in patients who are nonambulatory. Operative treatment of such fractures should be reserved for selected patients whose function would be significantly compromised by less than anatomic reduction.

REFERENCES

1. Abramson A. Bone disturbances in injuries to the spinal cord and cauda equina (paraplegia): their prevention by ambulation. J Bone Joint Surg Am 1948;30:982–987.
2. Abudu A, Sferopoulos NK, Tillman RM, et al. The surgical treatment and outcome of pathological fractures in localised osteosarcoma. J Bone Joint Surg Br 1996;78(5):694–698.
3. Ackroyd CE, Dinley RJ. The locked patella. An unusual complication of haemophilia. J Bone Joint Surg Br 1976;58-B(4):511–512.
4. Adam A, Ritchie D. Hyperparathyroidism with increased bone density in the areas of growth. J Bone Joint Surg Br 1954;36-B(2):257–260.
5. Agarwal V, Joseph B. Nonunion in osteogenesis imperfecta. J Pediatr Orthop B 2005;14(6):451–455.
6. Ahlberg AK. On the natural history of hemophilic pseudotumor. J Bone Joint Surg Am 1975;57(8):1133–1136.
7. Ahlberg AK, Nilsson IM. Fractures in haemophiliacs with special reference to complications and treatment. Acta Chir Scand 1967;133(4):293–302.
8. Ahn JI, Park JS. Pathological fractures secondary to unicameral bone cysts. Int Orthop 1994;18(1):20–22.
9. Akamatsu N, Hamada Y, Kohno H, et al. Osteofibrous dysplasia of the tibia treated by bracing. Int Orthop 1992;16(2):180–184.
10. Ali MS, Hooper G. Congenital pseudarthrosis of the ulna due to neurofibromatosis. J Bone Joint Surg Br 1982;64(5):600–602.
11. Allieu Y, Gomis R, Yoshimura M, et al. Congenital pseudarthrosis of the forearm—two cases treated by free vascularized fibular graft. J Hand Surg Am 1981;6(5):475–481.
12. Alman B, Frasca P. Fracture failure mechanisms in patients with osteogenesis imperfecta. J Orthop Res 1987;5(1):139–143.
13. Amir J, Katz K, Grunebaum M, et al. Fractures in premature infants. J Pediatr Orthop 1988;8(1):41–44.
14. Anderson DJ, Schoenecker PL, Sheridan JJ, et al. Use of an intramedullary rod for the treatment of congenital pseudarthrosis of the tibia. J Bone Joint Surg Am 1992;74(2):161–168.
15. Anderson TE, Drummond DS, Breed AL, et al. Malignant hyperthermia in myelomeningocele: a previously unreported association. J Pediatr Orthop 1981;1(4):401–403.
16. Andreoli SP, Bergstein JM, Sherrard DJ. Aluminum intoxication from aluminum containing phosphate binders in children with azotemia not undergoing dialysis. N Engl J Med 1984;310(17):1079–1084.
17. Anschuetz RH, Freehafer AA, Shaffer JW, et al. Severe fracture complications in myelodysplasia. J Pediatr Orthop 1984;4(1):22–24.
18. Anspach WC. Hyperparathyrodism in children: a report of two cases. Am J Dis Child 1939;58:540–557.
19. Antoniazzi F, Zamboni G, Lauriola S, et al. Early bisphosphonate treatment in infants with severe osteogenesis imperfecta. J Pediatr 2006;149(2):174–179.
20. Apel DM, Millar EA, Moel DI. Skeletal disorders in a pediatric renal transplant population. J Pediatr Orthop 1989;9(5):505–511.
21. Arata MA, Peterson HA, Dahlin DC. Pathological fractures through nonossifying fibromas. Review of the Mayo Clinic experience. J Bone Joint Surg Am 1981;63(6):980–988.
22. Arceci RJ, Brenner MK, Pritchard J. Controversies and new approaches to treatment of Langerhans cell histiocytosis. Hematol Oncol Clin North Am 1998;12(2):339–357.
23. Armstrong DG, Newfield JT, Gillespie R. Orthopedic management of osteopetrosis: results of a survey and review of the literature. J Pediatr Orthop 1999;19(1):122–132.
24. Aroojis AJ, Gajjar SM, Johari AN. Epiphyseal separations in spastic cerebral palsy. J Pediatr Orthop B 2007;16(3):170–174.
25. Ash JM, Gilday DL. The futility of bone scanning in neonatal osteomyelitis: concise communication. J Nucl Med 1980;21(5):417–420.
26. Asirdizer M, Zeyfeoglu Y. Femoral and tibial fractures in a child with myelomeningocele. J Clin Forensic Med 2005;12(2):93–97.
27. Athanassiou-Metaxa M, Kirkos J, Koussi A, et al. Avascular necrosis of the femoral head among children and adolescents with sickle cell disease in Greece. Haematologica 2002;87(7):771–772.
28. Ayala AG, Ro JY, Fanning CV, et al. Core needle biopsy and fine-needle aspiration in the diagnosis of bone and soft-tissue lesions. Hematol Oncol Clin North Am 1995;9(3):633–651.
29. Bacci G, Ferrari S, Longhi A, et al. Nonmetastatic osteosarcoma of the extremity with pathologic fracture at presentation: local and systemic control by amputation or limb salvage after preoperative chemotherapy. Acta Orthop Scand 2003;74(4):449–454.
30. Bachrach LK. Consensus and controversy regarding osteoporosis in the pediatric population. Endocr Pract 2007;13(5):513–520.
31. Bachrach S, Fisher J, Parks JS. An outbreak of vitamin D deficiency rickets in a susceptible population. Pediatrics 1979;64(6):871–877.
32. Bailey RW. Further clinical experience with the extensible nail. Clin Orthop 1981;(59):171–176.
33. Bailey RW, Dubow HI. Studies of longitudinal bone growth resulting in an extensible nail. Surg Forum 1963;14:455–458.
34. Baker JK, Cain TE, Tullos HS. Intramedullary fixation for congenital pseudarthrosis of the tibia. J Bone Joint Surg Am 1992;74(2):169–178.
35. Banks S. Bone changes in acute and chronic scurvy: an experimental study. J Bone Joint Surg Am 1943;15:553–565.
36. Bar-on E, Weigl D, Parvari R, et al. Congenital insensitivity to pain. Orthopaedic manifestations. J Bone Joint Surg Br 2002;84(2):252–257.
37. Barnes C, Wong P, Egan B, et al. Reduced bone density among children with severe hemophilia. Pediatrics 2004;114(2):e177–e181.
38. Baroncelli GI, Federico G, Bertelloni S, et al. Assessment of bone quality by quantitative ultrasound of proximal phalanges of the hand and fracture rate in children and adolescents with bone and mineral disorders. Pediatr Res 2003;54(1):125–136.
39. Basarir K, Piskin A, Guclu B, et al. Aneurysmal bone cyst recurrence in children: a review of 56 patients. J Pediatr Orthop 2007;27(8):938–943.
40. Bathi RJ, Masur VN. Pyknodysostosis—a report of two cases with a brief review of the literature. Int J Oral Maxillofac Surg 2000;29(6):439–442.
41. Batista DL, Riar J, Keil M, et al. Diagnostic tests for children who are referred for the investigation of Cushing syndrome. Pediatrics 2007;120(3):e575–e586.

42. Bauer RD, Lewis MM, Posner MA. Treatment of enchondromas of the hand with allograft bone. J Hand Surg Am 1988;13(6):908–916.
43. Bayne LG. Congenital pseudarthrosis of the forearm. Hand Clin 1985;1(3):457–465.
44. Bell DF. Congenital forearm pseudarthrosis: report of six cases and review of the literature. J Pediatr Orthop 1989;9(4):438–443.
45. Bennett OM, Namnyak SS. Bone and joint manifestations of sickle cell anaemia. J Bone Joint Surg Br 1990;72(3):494–499.
46. Benson DR, Newman DC. The spine and surgical treatment in osteogenesis imperfecta. Clin Orthop 1981;159:147–153.
47. Benz G, Schmid-Ruter E. Pycnodysostosis with heterozygous beta-thalassemia. Pediatr Radiol 1977;5(3):164–171.
48. Berrey BH Jr, Lord CF, Gebhardt MC, et al. Fractures of allografts. Frequency, treatment, and end-results. J Bone Joint Surg Am 1990;72(6):825–833.
49. Bertelloni S, Baroncelli GI, Di Nero G, et al. Idiopathic juvenile osteoporosis: evidence of normal osteoblast function by 1,25-dihydroxyvitamin D3 stimulation test. Calcif Tissue Int 1992;51(1):20–23.
50. Bhatia S, Nesbit ME Jr, Egeler RM, et al. Epidemiologic study of Langerhans cell histiocytosis in children. J Pediatr 1997;130(5):774–784.
51. Bischof F, Basu D, Pettifor JM. Pathological long-bone fractures in residents with cerebral palsy in a long-term care facility in South Africa. Dev Med Child Neurol 2002; 44(2):119–122.
52. Bjernulf A, Hall K, Sjogren L, et al. Primary hyperparathyroidism in children. Brief review of the literature and a case report. Acta Paediatr Scand 1970;59(3):249–258.
53. Blane CE, Herzenberg JE, Dipietro MA. Radiographic imaging for Ilizarov limb lengthening in children. Pediatr Radiol 1991;21(2):117–120.
54. Bleck EE. Nonoperative treatment of osteogenesis imperfecta: orthotic and mobility management. Clin Orthop 1981;(59):111–122.
55. Bleck EK. Special injuries of the musculoskeletal system. Philadelphia: JB Lippincott, 1984.
56. Boardman KP, English P. Fractures and dislocations in hemophilia. Clin Orthop Relat Res 1980;148:221–232.
57. Bohrer SP. Acute long bone diaphyseal infarcts in sickle cell disease. Br J Radiol 1970; 43(514):685–697.
58. Bohrer SP. Fracture complicating bone infarcts and-or osteomyelitis in sickle-cell disease. Clin Radiol 1971;22(1):83–88.
59. Bollerslev J, Andersen PE Jr. Fracture patterns in two types of autosomal-dominant osteopetrosis. Acta Orthop Scand 1989;60(1):110–112.
60. Bohrer SP. Growth disturbances of the distal femur following sickle cell bone infarcts and-or osteomyelitis. Clin Radiol 1974;25(2):221–235.
61. Bonakdarpour A, Levy WM, Aegerter E. Primary and secondary aneurysmal bone cyst: a radiological study of 75 cases. Radiology 1978;126(1):75–83.
62. Boni M, Ceciliani L. Fractures in haemophilia. Ital J Orthop Traumatol 1976;2(3): 301–310.
63. Boriani S, De Iure F, Campanacci L, et al. Aneurysmal bone cyst of the mobile spine: report on 41 cases. Spine 2001;26(1):27–35.
64. Bosley AR, Verrier-Jones ER, Campbell MJ. Aetiological factors in rickets of prematurity. Arch Dis Child 1980;55(9):683–686.
65. Botash As, Nasca J, Dubowy R, et al. Zinc-induced copper deficiency in an infant. Am J Dis Child 1992;146(6):709–711.
66. Bothwell JE, Gordon KE, Doley JM, et al. Vertebral fractures in boys with Duchenne muscular dystrophy. Clin Pediatr (Phila) 2003;42(4):353–356.
67. Boyd HB, Sage FP. Congenital pseudarthrosis of the tibia. J Bone Joint Surg Am 1958; 40-A(6):1245–1270.
68. Boytim MJ, Davidson RS, Charney E, et al. Neonatal fractures in myelomeningocele patients. J Pediatr Orthop 1991;11(1):28–30.
69. Braier J, Chantada G, Rosso D, et al. Langerhans cell histiocytosis: retrospective evaluation of 123 patients at a single institution. Pediatr Hematol Oncol 1999;16(5):377–385.
70. Breck LW. Treatment of fibrous dysplasia of bone by total femoral plating and hip nailing. A case report. Clin Orthop 1972;82:82–83.
71. Brighton CT, Friedenberg ZB, Zemsky LM, et al. Direct-current stimulation of nonunion and congenital pseudarthrosis. Exploration of its clinical application. J Bone Joint Surg Am 1975;57(3):368–377.
72. Brown GA, Osebold WR, Ponseti IV. Congenital pseudarthrosis of long bones: a clinical, radiographic, histologic and ultrastructural study. Clin Orthop 1977;(128):228–242.
73. Buison AM, Kawchak DA, Schall JI, et al. Bone area and bone mineral content deficits in children with sickle cell disease. Pediatrics 2005;116(4):943–949.
74. Byers PH, Bonadio JF, Steinmann B. Osteogenesis imperfecta: update and perspective. Am J Med Genet 1984;17(2):429–435.
75. Cabanela ME, Sim FH, Beabout JW, et al. Osteomyelitis appearing as neoplasms. A diagnostic problem. Arch Surg 1974;109(1):68–72.
76. Cameron HU, Dewar FP. Degenerative osteoarthritis associated with osteopetrosis. Clin Orthop 1977;27:148–149.
77. Campanacci M, Baldini N, Boriani S, et al. Giant-cell tumor of bone. J Bone Joint Surg Am 1987;69(1):106–114.
78. Campanacci M, Capanna R, Picci P. Unicameral and aneurysmal bone cysts. Clin Orthop Relat Res 1986;204:25–36.
79. Campanacci M, Laus M. Osteofibrous dysplasia of the tibia and fibula. J Bone Joint Surg Am 1981;63(3):367–375.
80. Campbell CJ, Harkess J. Fibrous metaphyseal defect of bone. Surg Gynecol Obstet 1957;104(3):329–336.
81. Canale ST, Puhl J, Watson FM, et al. Acute osteomyelitis following closed fractures. Report of three cases. J Bone Joint Surg Am 1975;57(3):415–418.
82. Capanna R, Dal Monte A, Gitelis S, et al. The natural history of unicameral bone cyst after steroid injection. Clin Orthop Relat Res 1982;166:204–211.
83. Capanna R, Springfield DS, Biagini R, et al. Juxtaepiphyseal aneurysmal bone cyst. Skeletal Radiol 1985;13(1):21–25.
84. Capener MP. Pathological fractures in osteomyelitis. J Bone Joint Surg Am 1932;14: 501–510.
85. Cardelia JM, Dormans JP, Drummond DS, et al. Proximal fibular osteochondroma with associated peroneal nerve palsy: a review of six cases. J Pediatr Orthop 1995;15(5): 574–577.
86. Carpintero P, Leon F, Zafra M, et al. Fractures of osteochondroma during physical exercise. Am J Sports Med 2003;31(6):1003–1006.
87. Cattell HS, Levin S, Kopits S, et al. Reconstructive surgery in children with azotemic osteodystrophy. J Bone Joint Surg Am 1971;53(2):216–228.
88. Caulton JM, Ward KA, Alsop CW, et al. A randomized controlled trial of standing programme on bone mineral density in nonambulant children with cerebral palsy. Arch Dis Child 2004;89(2):131–135.
89. Chalmers J. Subtrochanteric fractures in osteomalacia. J Bone Joint Surg Br 1970;52(3): 509–513.
90. Chen CJ, Chao TY, Chu DM, et al. Osteoblast and osteoclast activity in a malignant infantile osteopetrosis patient following bone marrow transplantation. J Pediatr Hematol Oncol 2004;26(1):5–8.
91. Chigira M, Maehara S, Arita S, et al. The aetiology and treatment of simple bone cysts. J Bone Joint Surg Br 1983;65(5):633–637.
92. Chung SM, Alavi A, Russell MO. Management of osteonecrosis in sickle-cell anemia and its genetic variants. Clin Orthop 1978;130:158–174.
93. Clark OH, Duh QY. Primary hyperparathyroidism. A surgical perspective. Endocrinol Metab Clin North Am 1989;18(3):701–714.
94. Coccia PF, Krivit W, Cervenka J, et al. Successful bone-marrow transplantation for infantile malignant osteopetrosis. N Engl J Med 1980;302(13):701–708.
95. Codd PJ, Riesenburger RI, Klimo P Jr, et al. Vertebra plana due to an aneurysmal bone cyst of the lumbar spine. Case report and review of the literature. J Neurosurgc 2006; 105(6 Suppl):490–495.
96. Cohen J. Simple bone cysts. Studies of cyst fluid in six cases with a theory of pathogenesis. J Bone Joint Surg Am 1960;42-A:609–616.
97. Cohn DH, Byers PH. Clinical screening for collagen defects in connective tissue diseases. Clin Perinatol 1990;17(4):793–809.
98. Cole WG. The Nicholas Andry Award–1996. The molecular pathology of osteogenesis imperfecta. Clin Orthop 1997;343:235–248.
99. Cole WG. Treatment of aneurysmal bone cysts in childhood. J Pediatr Orthop 1986; 6(3):326–329.
100. Comarr AE, Hutchinson RH, Bors E. Extremity fractures of patients with spinal cord injuries. Am J Surg 1962;103:732–739.
101. Copley L, Dormans JP. Benign pediatric bone tumors. Evaluation and treatment. Pediatr Clin North Am 1996;43(4):949–966.
102. Cordano A, Baertl JM, Graham GG. Copper deficiency in infancy. Pediatrics 1964;34: 324–336.
103. Cottalorda J, Kohler R, Sales De Gauzy J, et al. Epidemiology of aneurysmal bone cyst in children: a multicenter study and literature review. J Pediatr Orthop B 2004;13(6): 389–394.
104. Crawford AH Jr. Neurofibromatosis in the pediatric patient. Orthop Clin North Am 1978;9(1):11–23.
105. Crawford AH Jr, Bagamery N. Osseous manifestations of neurofibromatosis in childhood. J Pediatr Orthop 1986;6(1):72–88.
106. Crowe FW, Schull WJ. Diagnostic importance of cafe-au-lait spot in neurofibromatosis. AMA Arch Intern Med 1953;91(6):758–766.
107. Cunningham JB, Ackerman LV. Metaphyseal fibrous defects. J Bone Joint Surg Am 1956;38-A(4):797–808.
108. Cushing H. The basophil adenomas of the pituitary body and their clinical manifestations. Bull Johns Hopkins Hosp 1932;50:137–195.
109. Dabska M, Buraczewski J. Aneurysmal bone cyst. Pathology, clinical course, and radiologic appearances. Cancer 1969;23(2):371–389.
110. Daoud A, Descamps L, Maestro M. Hematogenous osteomyelitis of the femoral neck in children. J Pediatr Orthop B 1993;2:83–95.
111. Daoud A, Saighi-Bouaouina A. Treatment of sequestra, pseudarthroses, and defects in the long bones of children who have chronic hematogenous osteomyelitis. J Bone Joint Surg Am 1989;71(10):1448–1468.
112. Dauphine RT, Riggs BL, Scholz DA. Back pain and vertebral crush fractures: an unemphasized mode of presentation for primary hyperparathyroidism. Ann Intern Med 1975;83(3):365–367.
113. Davids JR, Fisher R, Lum G, et al. Angular deformity of the lower extremity in children with renal osteodystrophy. J Pediatr Orthop 1992;12(3):291–299.
114. De Boer HH, Verbout AJ Nielsen HK, et all. Free vascularized fibular graft for tibial pseudarthrosis in neurofibromatosis. Acta Orthop Scand 1988;59(4):425–429.
115. De Kleuver M, Van Der Heul RO, Veraart BE. Aneurysmal bone cyst of the spine: 31 cases and the importance of the surgical approach. J Pediatr Orthop B 1998;7(4): 286–292.
116. Deheshi BM, Jaffer SN, Griffin AM, et al. Joint salvage for pathologic fracture of giant cell tumor of the lower extremity. Clin Orthop Relat Res 2007;459:96–104.
117. Dent CE. Osteoporosis in childhood. Postgrad Med J 1977;53(622):450–457.
118. Dent CE, Friedman M. Idiopathic juvenile osteoporosis. Q J Med 1965;34:177–210.
119. Depalma AF, Ahmad I. Fibrous dysplasia associated with Shepherd's Crook deformity of the humerus. Clin Ortho. 1973;97:38–39.
120. Diamond LS, Alegado R. Perinatal fractures in arthrogryposis multiplex congenita. J Pediatr Orthop 1981;1(2):189–192.
121. Dicaprio MR, Enneking WF. Fibrous dysplasia. Pathophysiology, evaluation, and treatment. J Bone Joint Surg Am 2005;87(8):1848–1864.
122. Dicesare PE, Sew-Hoy A, Krom W. Bilateral isolated olecranon fractures in an infant as presentation of osteogenesis imperfecta. Orthopedics 1992;15(6):741–743.
123. Diggs LW. Bone and joint lesions in sickle-cell disease. Clin Orthop 1967;52:119–143.
124. Donadieu J, Piguet C, Bernard F, et al. A new clinical score for disease activity in Langerhans cell histiocytosis. Pediatr Blood Cancer 2004;43(7):770–776.
125. Dormans JP. Modified sequential McFarland bypass procedure for prepseudarthrosis of the tibia. J Orthop Tech 1995;3:176–180.
126. Dormans JP, Dormans NJ. Use of percutaneous intramedullary decompression and medical-grade calcium sulfate pellets for treatment of unicameral bone cysts of the calcaneus in children. Orthopedics 2004;27(1 Suppl):s137-s139.
127. Dormans JP, Hanna BG, Johnston DR, et al. Surgical treatment and recurrence rate of aneurysmal bone cysts in children. Clin Orthop Relat Res 2004(421):205–211.
128. Dormans JP, Krajbich JI, Zuker R, et al. Congenital pseudarthrosis of the tibia: treatment with free vascularized fibular grafts. J Pediatr Orthop 1990;10(5):623–628.
129. Dormans JP, Pill SG. Fractures through bone cysts: unicameral bone cysts, aneurysmal bone cysts, fibrous cortical defects, and nonossifying fibromas. Instr Course Lect 2002; 51:457–467.
130. Dormans JP, Sankar WN, Moroz L, et al. Percutaneous intramedullary decompression,

curettage, and grafting with medical-grade calcium sulfate pellets for unicameral bone cysts in children: a new minimally invasive technique. J Pediatr Orthop 2005;25(6): 804–811.
131. Dormans JP, Templeton J, Schreiner MS, et al. Intraoperative latex anaphylaxis in children: classification and prophylaxis of patients at risk. J Pediatr Orthop 1997;17(5): 622–625.
132. Drabu KJ, Walker G. Stiffness after fractures around the knee in spina bifida. J Bone Joint Surg Br 1985;67(2):266–267.
133. Drennan DB, Maylahn DJ, Fahey JJ. Fractures through large nonossifying fibromas. Clin Orthop Relat Res 1974(103):82–88.
134. Drennan JC, Freehafer AA. Fractures of the lower extremities in paraplegic children. Clin Orthop 1971;77:211–217.
135. Drummond DS, Moreau M, Cruess RL. Postoperative neuropathic fractures in patients with myelomeningocele. Dev Med Child Neurol 1981;23(2):147–150.
136. Drummond DS, Moreau M, Cruess RL. The results and complications of surgery for the paralytic hip and spine in myelomeningocele. J Bone Joint Surg Br 1980;62-B(1): 49–53.
137. Dulai S, Briody J, Schindeler A, et al. Decreased bone mineral density in neurofibromatosis type 1: results from a pediatric cohort. J Pediatr Orthop 2007;27(4):472–475.
138. Dusenberry JF Jr, Kane JJ. Pycnodysostosis. Report of three new cases. Am J Roentgenol Radium Ther Nucl Med 1967;99(3):717–723.
139. Easley ME, Kneisl JS. Pathologic fractures through nonossifying fibromas: is prophylactic treatment warranted? J Pediatr Orthop 1997;17(6):808–813.
140. Eaton DG, Hewitt CA. Renal function in hyperparathyroidism with complicating nephrocalcinosis. Acta Paediatr 1993;82(1):111–112.
141. Ebong WW. Pathological fracture complicating long bone osteomyelitis in patients with sickle cell disease. J Pediatr Orthop 1986;6(2):177–181.
142. Edelson JG, Obad S, Geiger R, et al. Pycnodysostosis. Orthopedic aspects with a description of 14 new cases. Clin Orthop 1992;80:263–276.
143. Edidin DV, Levitsky LL Schey W, et al. Resurgence of nutritional rickets associated with breast-feeding and special dietary practices. Pediatrics 1980;65(2):232–235.
144. Edvardsen P. Physeo-epiphyseal injuries of lower extremities in myelomeningocele. Acta Orthop Scand 1972;43(6):550–557.
145. Egeler RM, D'Angio GJ. Langerhans cell histiocytosis. J Pediatr 1995;127(1):1–11.
146. Ehara S, Kattapuram SV, Egglin TK. Ewing sarcoma. Radiographic pattern of healing and bony complications in patients with long-term survival. Cancer 1991;68(7): 1531–1535.
147. Eichenholtz S. Management of long-bone fractures in paraplegic patients. J Bone Joint Surg Am 1963;45:299–310.
148. Eldridge JC, Bell DF. Problems with substantial limb lengthening. Orthop Clin North Am 1991;22(4):625–631.
149. Elsasser U, Ruegsegger P, Anliker M, et al. Loss and recovery of trabecular bone in the distal radius following fracture-immobilization of the upper limb in children. Klin Wochenschr 1979;57(15):763–767.
150. Enneking WF. A system of staging musculoskeletal neoplasms. Instr Course Lect 1988; 37:3–10.
151. Enneking WF, Gearen PF. Fibrous dysplasia of the femoral neck. Treatment by cortical bone-grafting. J Bone Joint Surg Am 1986;68(9):1415–1422.
152. Epps CH Jr, Bowen JR, eds. Complications in pediatric orthopaedic surgery. Philadelphia: J.B. Lippincott, 1995.
153. Epstein BA. Roentgenological changes in the bones in cases of pseudohypertrophic muscular dystrophy. Arch Neurol Psychiatry 1941;46:868–876.
154. Eyres KS, Brown J, Douglas DL. Osteotomy and intramedullary nailing for the correction of progressive deformity in vitamin D-resistant hypophosphatasemic rickets. JR Coll Surg Edinb 1993;38(1):50–54.
155. Fabeck L, Ghafil D, Gerroudj M, et al. Bone morphogenetic protein 7 in the treatment of congenital pseudarthrosis of the tibia. J Bone Joint Surg Br 2006;88(1):116–118.
156. Fabry G, Lammens J, Van M, et al. Treatment of congenital pseudarthrosis with the Ilizarov technique. J Pediatr Orthop 1988;8(1):67–70.
157. Fain O. Musculoskeletal manifestations of scurvy. Joint Bone Spine 2005;72(2): 124–128.
158. Falk MJ, Heeger S, Lynch KA, et al. Intravenous bisphosphonate therapy in children with osteogenesis imperfecta. Pediatrics 2003;111(3):573–578.
159. FDA Allergic Reactions to Latex Containing Medical Devices: FDA Medical Alert. DHHS (NIOSH) 1997:97–135.
160. Feil E, Bentley G, Rizza CR. Fracture management in patients with haemophilia. J Bone Joint Surg Br 1974;56-B(4):643–649.
161. Feiwell E, Sakai D, Blatt T. The effect of hip reduction on function in patients with myelomeningocele. Potential gains and hazards of surgical treatment. J Bone Joint Surg Am 1978;60(2):169–173.
162. Ferguson AB Jr. Osteomyelitis in children. Clin Orthop 1973;96:51–56.
163. Fernandez V, Spain M, Matthews JM. The haemophilic pseudotumour or haemophilic subperiosteal haematoma. J Bone Joint Surg Br 1965;47:256–265.
164. Ferris B, Walker C, Jackson A, et al. The orthopaedic management of hypophosphataemic rickets. J Pediatr Orthop 1991;11(3):367–373.
165. Floman Y, Bar-on E, Mosheiff R, et al. Eosinophilic granuloma of the spine. J Pediatr Orthop B 1997;6(4):260–265.
166. Floman Y, Niska M. Dislocation of the hip joint complicating repeated hemarthrosis in hemophilia. J Pediatr Orthop 1983;3(1):99–100.
167. Flood BM, Butt WP, Dickson RA. Rib penetration of the intervertebral foraminae in neurofibromatosis. Spine 1986;11(2):172–174.
168. Freehafer AA, Mast WA. Lower extremity fractures in patients with spinal-cord injury. J Bone Joint Surg Am 1965;47:683–694.
169. Freiberg AA, Loder RT, Heidelberger KP, et al. Aneurysmal bone cysts in young children. J Pediatr Orthop 1994;14(1):86–91.
170. Fry K, Hoffer MM, Brink J. Femoral shaft fractures in brain-injured children. J Trauma 1976;16(5):371–373.
171. Fujita Y, Nakata K, Yasui N, et al. Novel mutations of the cathepsin K gene in patients with pycnodysostosis and their characterization. J Clin Endocrinol Metab 2000;85(1): 425–431.
172. Funk FJ Jr, Wells RE. Hip problems in fibrous dysplasia. Clin Orthop 1973;90:77–82.
173. Furey JG, McNamee DC. Air splints for long-term management of osteogenesis imperfecta. J Bone Joint Surg Am 1973;55(3):645–649.
174. Gamble JG, Rinsky LA, Strudwick J, et al. Non-union of fractures in children who have osteogenesis imperfecta. J Bone Joint Surg Am 1988;70(3):439–443.
175. Gamble JG, Strudwick WJ, Rinsky LA, et al. Complications of intramedullary rods in osteogenesis imperfecta: Bailey-Dubow rods versus nonelongating rods. J Pediatr Orthop 1988;8(6):645–649.
176. Gandrud LM, Cheung JC, Daniels MW, et al. Low-dose intravenous pamidronate reduces fractures in childhood osteoporosis. J Pediatr Endocrinol Metab 2003;16(6): 887–892.
177. Garg S, Mehta S, Dormans JP. Langerhans cell histiocytosis of the spine in children. Long-term follow-up. J Bone Joint Surg Am 2004;86-A(8):1740–1750.
178. Garg S, Mehta S, Dormans JP. Modern surgical treatment of primary aneurysmal bone cyst of the spine in children and adolescents. J Pediatr Orthop 2005;25(3):387–392.
179. Gaulke R, Suppelna G. Solitary enchondroma at the hand. Long-term follow-up study after operative treatment. J Hand Surg Br 2004;29(1):64–66.
180. Gerber LH, Binder H, Weintrob J, et al. Rehabilitation of children and infants with osteogenesis imperfecta. A program for ambulation. Clin Orthop 1990;(51):254–262.
181. Gerritsen EJ, Vossen JM, Van Loo IH, et al. Autosomal recessive osteopetrosis: variability of findings at diagnosis and during the natural course. Pediatrics 1994;93(2):247–253.
182. Ghanem I, Tolo VT, D'Ambra P, et al. Langerhans cell histiocytosis of bone in children and adolescents. J Pediatr Orthop 2003;23(1):124–130.
183. Gibbs CP Jr, Hefele MC, Peabody TD, et al. Aneurysmal bone cyst of the extremities. Factors related to local recurrence after curettage with a high-speed burr. J Bone Joint Surg Am 1999;81(12):1671–1678.
184. Glorieux FH. Experience with bisphosphonates in osteogenesis imperfecta. Pediatrics 2007;119(Suppl 2):S163–S165.
185. Glorieux FH, Bishop NJ, Plotkin H, et al. Cyclic administration of pamidronate in children with severe osteogenesis imperfecta. N Engl J Med 1998;339(14):947–952.
186. Glotzbecker MP, Carpentieri DF, Dormans JP. Langerhans cell histiocytosis: clinical presentation, pathogenesis, and treatment from the LCH etiology research group at The Children's Hospital of Philadelphia. UPOJ 2002;15:67–73.
187. Goldman AB, Jacobs B. Femoral neck fractures complicating Gaucher disease in children. Skeletal Radiol 1984;12(3):162–168.
188. Goldman AB, Lane JM, Salvati E. Slipped capital femoral epiphyses complicating renal osteodystrophy: a report of three cases. Radiology 1978;126(2):333–339.
189. Gooding CA, Ball JH. Idiopathic juvenile osteoporosis. Radiology 1969;93(6): 1349–1350.
190. Grabias SL, Campbell CJ. Fibrous dysplasia. Orthop Clin North Am 1977;8(4): 771–783.
191. Greenberg LA, Schwartz A. Congenital pseudarthrosis of the distal radius. South Med J 1975;68(8):1053–1054.
192. Greene WB, Torre BA. Femoral neck fracture in a child with autosomal dominant osteopetrosis. J Pediatr Orthop 1985;5(4):483–485.
193. Greene WB, Yankaskas BC, Guilford WB. Roentgenographic classifications of hemophilic arthropathy. Comparison of three systems and correlation with clinical parameters. J Bone Joint Surg Am 1989;71(2):237–244.
194. Gregg PJ, Price BA, Ellis HA, et al. Pseudarthrosis of the radius associated with neurofibromatosis. A case report. Clin Orthop 1982;(171):175–179.
195. Grewar D. Infantile scurvy. Clin Pediatr (Phila) 1965;35:82–89.
196. Grunebaum M, Horodniceanu C, Steinherz R. The radiographic manifestations of bone changes in copper deficiency. Pediatr Radiol 1980;9(2):101–104.
197. Guidera KJ, Multhopp H, Ganey T, et al. Orthopaedic manifestations in congenitally insensate patients. J Pediatr Orthop 1990;10(4):514–521.
198. Guille JT, Forlin E, Bowen JR. Charcot joint disease of the shoulders in a patient who had familial sensory neuropathy with anhidrosis. A case report. J Bone Joint Surg Am 1992;74(9):1415–1417.
199. Guille JT, Kumar SJ, Macewen GD. Fibrous dysplasia of the proximal part of the femur. Long-term results of curettage and bone-grafting and mechanical realignment. J Bone Joint Surg Am 1998;80(5):648–658.
200. Gwynne-Jones DP. Displaced olecranon apophyseal fractures in children with osteogenesis imperfecta. J Pediatr Orthop 2005;25(2):154–157.
201. Gyepes MT, Newbern DH, Neuhauser EB. Metaphyseal and physeal injuries in children with spina bifida and meningomyeloceles. Am J Roentgenol Radium Ther Nucl Med 1965;95:168–177.
202. Hahn M, Dormans JP. Primary bone malignancies in children. Curr Opin Pediatr 1996; 8(1):71–74.
203. Hall JG. Arthrogryposis (multiple congenital contractures). In: Rimoin DL, Connor JM, Pyeritz RE, et al., eds. Emery and Rimion's Principles and Practice of Medical Genetics. Vol. 168. 5th ed. Philadelphia: Churchill Livingstone, 2007:3785–3856.
204. Hanscom DA, Winter RB, Lutter L, et al. Osteogenesis imperfecta. Radiographic classification, natural history, and treatment of spinal deformities. J Bone Joint Surg Am 1992; 74(4):598–616.
205. Harkey HL, Crockard HA, Stevens JM, et al. The operative management of basilar impression in osteogenesis imperfecta. Neurosurgery 1990;27(5):782–786.
206. Harris WH, Dudley HR Jr, Barry RJ. The natural history of fibrous dysplasia. An orthopaedic, pathological, and roentgenographic study. Am J Orthop 1962;44-A:207–233.
207. Harris WH, Heaney RP. Skeletal renewal and metabolic bone disease. N Engl J Med 1969;280(6):303–311.
208. Harrison WJ, Rankin KC. Osteogenesis imperfecta in Zimbabwe: a comparison between treatment with intramedullary rods of fixed-length and self-expanding rods. J R Coll Surg Edinb 1998;43(5):328–332.
209. Hartjen CA, Koman LA. Treatment of slipped capital femoral epiphysis resulting from juvenile renal osteodystrophy. J Pediatr Orthop 1990;10(4):551–554.
210. Hasenhuttl K. Osteopetrosis. Review of the literature and comparative studies on a case with a 24-year follow-up. Am J Orthop 1962;44-A:359–370.
211. Helfer RE, Scheurer SL, Alexander R, et al. Trauma to the bones of small infants from passive exercise: a factor in the etiology of child abuse. J Pediatr 1984;104(1):47–50.
212. Heinrich SD, Drvaric DM, Darr K, et al. The operative stabilization of pediatric diaphyseal femur fractures with flexible intramedullary nails: a prospective analysis. J Pediatr Orthop 1994;14(4):501–507.
213. Heinrich SD, Gallagher D, Warrior R, et al. The prognostic significance of the skeletal manifestations of acute lymphoblastic leukemia of childhood. J Pediatr Orthop 1994; 14(1):105–111.

214. Heller RM, Kirchner SG, O'Neill JA Jr, et al. Skeletal changes of copper deficiency in infants receiving prolonged total parenteral nutrition. J Pediatr 1978;92(6):947–949.
215. Herring JA, Peterson HA. Simple bone cyst with growth arrest. J Pediatr Orthop 1987; 7(2):231–235.
216. Higashi T, Iguchi M, Shimura A, et al. Computed tomography and bone scintigraphy is polyostotic fibrous dysplasia. Report of a case. Oral Surg Oral Med Oral Pathol 1980; 50(6):580–583.
217. Hill SC, Parker CC, Brady RO, et al. MRI of multiple platyspondyly in Gaucher disease: response to enzyme replacement therapy. J Comput Assist Tomogr 1993;17(5): 806–809.
218. Himelstein BP, Dormans JP. Malignant bone tumors of childhood. Pediatr Clin North Am 1996;43(4):967–984.
219. Hindman BW, Bell S, Russo T, et al. Neonatal osteofibrons dysplasia; a case report. Pediatr Radiol 1996;26:303–306.
220. Hipp JA, Springfield DS, Hayes WC. Predicting pathologic fracture risk in the management of metastatic bone defects. Clin Orthop Relat Res 1995(312):120–135.
221. Hoeffel JC, Lascombes P, Mainard L, et al. Cone epiphysis of the knee and scurvy. Eur J Pediatr Surg 1993;3(3):186–189.
222. Holda ME, Ryan JR. Hepatobiliary rickets. J Pediatr Orthop 1982;2(3):285–287.
223. Hong J, Cabe GD, Tedrow JR, et al. Failure of trabecular bone with simulated lytic defects can be predicted non-invasively by structural analysis. J Orthop Res 2004; 22(3):479–486.
224. Hood RW, Riseborough EJ. Lengthening of the lower extremity by the Wagner method. A review of the Boston Children's Hospital Experience. J Bone Joint Surg Am 1981; 63(7):1122–1131.
225. Hoshi M, Matsumoto S, Manabe J, et al. Malignant change secondary to fibrous dysplasia. Int J Clin Oncol 2006;11(3):229–235.
226. Houang MTW, Brenton DP, Renton P, et al. Idiopathic juvenile osteoporosis. Skeletal Radiol 1978;3:17–23.
227. Houghton GR, Duthie RB. Orthopedic problems in hemophilia. Clin Orthop 1979; 138:197–216.
228. Howarth DM, Gilchrist GS, Mullan BP, et al. Langerhans cell histiocytosis: diagnosis, natural history, management, and outcome. Cancer 1999;85(10):2278–2290.
229. Howie DW, Savage JP, Wilson TG, et al. The technetium phosphate bone scan in the diagnosis of osteomyelitis in childhood. J Bone Joint Surg Am 1983;65(4):431–437.
230. Hsu AC, Kooh SW, Fraser D, et al. Renal osteodystrophy in children with chronic renal failure: an unexpectedly common and incapacitating complication. Pediatrics 1982;70(5):742–750.
231. Hsu JD. Extremity fractures in children with neuromuscular disease. Johns Hopkins Med J 1979;145(3):89–93.
232. Hsu JD, Garcia-Ariz M. Fracture of the femur in the Duchenne muscular dystrophy patient. J Pediatr Orthop 1981;1(2):203–207.
233. Hughes RG, Kay HE. Major bone lesions in acute lymphoblastic leukaemia. Med Pediatr Oncol 1982;10(1):67–70.
234. Hulth A, Olerud S. The healing of fractures in denervated limbs. An experimental study using sensory and motor rhizotomy and peripheral denervation. J Trauma 1965;5(5): 571–579.
235. Iobst CA, Dahl MT. Limb lengthening with submuscular plate stabilization: a case series and description of the technique. J Pediatr Orthop 2007;27(5):504–509.
236. Jackson MA, Nelson JD. Etiology and medical management of acute suppurative bone and joint infections in pediatric patients. J Pediatr Orthop 1982;2(3):313–323.
237. Jaffe H. Metabolic, degenerative, and inflammatory diseases of bone and joints. Philadelphia: Lea & Febiger, 1972.
238. James CC. Fractures of the lower limbs in spina bifida cystica: a survey of 44 fractures in 122 children. Dev Med Child Neurol 1970;Suppl 22:88.
239. Jerosch J, Mazzotti I, Tomasevic M. Complications after treatment of patients with osteogenesis imperfecta with a Bailey-Dubow rod. Arch Orthop Trauma Surg 1998; 117(4–5):240–245.
240. Jewell FL. Osteogenetic sarcoma occurring in fragilitas ossium: a case report. Radiology 1940;34:741–743.
241. Jowsey J, Johnson KA. Juvenile osteoporosis: bone findings in seven patients. J Pediatr 1972;81(3):511–517.
242. Jowsey J, Riggs BL. Bone formation in hypercortisonism. Acta Endocrinol (Copenh) 1970;63(1):21–28.
243. Jurik AG, Helmig O, Ternowitz T, et al. Chronic recurrent multifocal osteomyelitis: a follow-up study. J Pediatr Orthop 1988;8(1):49–58.
244. Kaelin AJ, Macewen GD. Unicameral bone cysts. Natural history and the risk of fracture. Int Orthop 1989;13(4):275–282.
245. Kaempffe FA, Gillespie R. Pseudarthrosis of the radius after fracture through normal bone in a child who had neurofibromatosis. A case report. J Bone Joint Surg Am 1989; 71(9):1419–1421.
246. Kameyama O, Ogawa R. Pseudarthrosis of the radius associated with neurofibromatosis: report of a case and review of the literature. J Pediatr Orthop 1990;10(1):128–131.
247. Kaplan FS, August CS, Fallon MD, et al. Osteopetrorickets. The paradox of plenty. Pathophysiology and treatment. Clin Orthop 1993;94:64–78.
248. Karol LA, Haideri NF, Halliday SE, et al. Gait analysis and muscle strength in children with congenital pseudarthrosis of the tibia: the effect of treatment. J Pediatr Orthop 1998;18(3):381–386.
249. Kasper CK, Rapaport SI. Bleeding times and platelet aggregation after analgesics in hemophilia. Ann Intern Med 1972;77(2):189–193.
250. Katz JF. Spontaneous fractures in paraplegic children. J Bone Joint Surg Am 1953;35-A(1):220–226.
251. Katz K, Cohen IJ, Ziv N, et al. Fractures in children who have Gaucher disease. J Bone Joint Surg Am 1987;69(9):1361–1370.
252. Katz K, Horev G, Rivlin E, et al. Upper limb involvement in patients with Gaucher disease. J Hand Surg Am 1993;18(5):871–875.
253. Katz K, Sabato S, Horev G, et al. Spinal involvement in children and adolescents with Gaucher disease. Spine 1993;18(3):332–335.
254. Kavanaugh JH. Occult infected fracture of the femur: report of two cases with longterm followup. J Trauma 1978;18(12):813–815.
255. Kaye JJ, Freiberger RH. Fragmentation of the lower pole of the patella in spastic lower extremities. Radiology 1971;101(1):97–100.
256. Kelly HJ, Sloan RE, Hoffman W, et al. Accumulation of nitrogen and six minerals in the human fetus during gestation. Hum Biol 1951;23(1):61–74.
257. Kemp HS, Matthews JM. The management of fractures in haemophilia and Christmas disease. J Bone Joint Surg Br 1968;50(2):351–358.
258. Kensinger DR, Guille JT, Horn BD, et al. The stubbed great toe: importance of early recognition and treatment of open fractures of the distal phalanx. J Pediatr Orthop 2001;21(1):31–34.
259. Khoury JG, Morcuende JA. Dramatic subperiosteal bone formation following physeal injury in patients with myelomeningocele. Iowa Orthop J 2002;22:94–98.
260. Kilborn TN, Teh J, Goodman TR. Paediatric manifestations of Langerhans cell histiocytosis: a review of the clinical and radiological findings. Clin Radiol 2003;58(4): 269–278.
261. Kilpatrick SE, Wenger DE, Gilchrist GS, et al. Langerhans cell histiocytosis (histiocytosis X) of bone. A clinicopathologic analysis of 263 pediatric and adult cases. Cancer 1995; 76(12):2471–2484.
262. King JB, Bobenchko WP. Osteogenesis imperfecta: an orthopaedic discussion and surgical review. J Bone Joint Surg Br 1971;53:72–89.
263. King WM, Ruttencutter R, Nagaraja HN, et al. Orthopedic outcomes of long-term daily corticosteroid treatment in Duchenne muscular dystrophy. Neurology 2007;68(19): 1607–1613.
264. Kirkwood JR, Ozonoff MB, Steinbach HL. Epiphyseal displacement after metaphyseal fracture in renal osteodystrophy. Am J Roentgenol Radium Ther Nucl Med 1972; 115(3):547–554.
265. Klenerman L, Ockenden BG, Townsend AC. Osteosarcoma occurring in osteogenesis imperfecta. Report of two cases. J Bone Joint Surg Br 1967;49(2):314–323.
266. Knight DJ, Bennet GC. Nonaccidental injury in osteogenesis imperfecta: a case report. J Pediatr Orthop 1990;10(4):542–544.
267. Kobayashi A, Kawai S, Utsunomiya T, et al. Bone disease in infants and children with hepatobiliary disease. Arch Dis Child 1974;49(8):641–646.
268. Kobayashi D, Satsuma S, Kamegaya M, et al. Musculoskeletal conditions of acute leukemia and malignant lymphoma in children. J Pediatr Orthop B 2005;14(3):156–161.
269. Kocher MS, Shapiro F. Osteogenesis imperfecta. J Am Acad Orthop Surg 1998;6(4): 225–236.
270. Komiya S, Inoue A. Aggressive bone tumorous lesion in infancy: osteofibrous dysplasia of the tibia and fibula. J Pediatr Orthop 1993;13(5):577–581.
271. Koo WW, Gupta JM, Nayanar VV, et al. Skeletal changes in preterm infants. Arch Dis Child 1982;57(6):447–452.
272. Koo WW, Oestreich AE, Sherman R, et al. Radiological case of the month. Osteopenia, rickets, and fractures in preterm infants. Am J Dis Child 1985;139(10):1045–1046.
273. Kooh SW, Jones G, Reilly BJ, et al. Pathogenesis of rickets in chronic hepatobiliary disease in children. J Pediatr 1979;94(6):870–874.
274. Kothari NA, Pelchovitz DJ, Meyer JS. Imaging of musculoskeletal infections. Radiol Clin North Am 2001;39(4):653–671.
275. Kransdorf MJ, Sweet DE. Aneurysmal bone cyst: concept, controversy, clinical presentation, and imaging. AJR Am J Roentgenol 1995;164(3):573–580.
276. Krempien B, Mehls O, Ritz E. Morphological studies on pathogenesis of epiphyseal slipping in uremic children. Virchows Arch A Pathol Anat Histol 1974;362(2): 129–143.
277. Kruzelock RP, Hansen MF. Molecular genetics and cytogenetics of sarcomas. Hematol Oncol Clin North Am 1995;9(3):513–540.
278. Kumar SJ, Cowell HR, Townsend P. Physeal, metaphyseal, and diaphyseal injuries of the lower extremities in children with myelomeningocele. J Pediatr Orthop 1984;4(1): 25–27.
279. Kuo RS, Macnicol MF. Congenital insensitivity to pain: orthopaedic implications. J Pediatr Orthop 1996;B-5(4):292–295.
280. Lachiewicz PF. Gaucher disease. Orthop Clin North Am 1984;15(4):765–774.
281. Laidlaw AT, Loder RT, Hensinger R. Telescoping intramedullary rodding with Bailey-Dubow nails for recurrent pathologic fractures in children without osteogenesis imperfecta. J Pediatr Orthop 1998;18(1):4–8.
282. Lancourt JE, Gilbert MS, Posner MA. Management of bleeding and associated complications of hemophilia in the hand and forearm. J Bone Joint Surg Am 1977;59(4): 451–460.
283. Lancourt JE, Hochberg F. Delayed fracture healing in primary hyperparathyroidism. Clin Orthop 1977;124:214–218.
284. Lane JM, Vigorita VJ. Osteoporosis. J Bone Joint Surg Am 1983;65(2):274–278.
285. Lane MN, Hall TC. Chemotherapy: discussion. Cancer 1976;37(Suppl):1055–1057.
286. Langenskiöld A. Femur remodelled during growth after osteomyelitis causing coxa vara and shaft necrosis. J Pediatr Orthop 1982;2(3):289–294.
287. Larson CM, Henderson RC. Bone mineral density and fractures in boys with Duchenne muscular dystrophy. J Pediatr Orthop 2000;20(1):71–74.
288. Lauer R, Johnston TE, Smith BT, et al. Bone mineral density of the hip and knee in children with spinal cord injury. J Spinal Cord Med 2007;30(Suppl 1):S10–S14.
289. Lebrun JB, Moffatt ME, Mundy RJ, et al. Vitamin D deficiency in a Manitoba community. Can J Public Health 1993;84(6):394–396.
290. Lee FY, Sinicropi SM, Lee FS, et al. Treatment of congenital pseudarthrosis of the tibia with recombinant human bone morphogenetic protein-7 (rhBMP-7). A report of five cases. J Bone Joint Surg Am 2006;88(3):627–633.
291. Lee JJ, Lyne ED. Pathologic fractures in severely handicapped children and young adults. J Pediatr Orthop 1990;10(4):497–500.
292. Lee RS, Weitzel S, Eastwood DM, et al. Osteofibrous dysplasia of the tibia. Is there a need for a radical surgical approach? J Bone Joint Surg Br 2006;88(5):658–664.
293. Lee RV. Scurvy: a contemporary historical perspective (3). Conn Med 1984;48(1): 33–35.
294. Lee VN, Srivastava A, Nithyananth M, et al. Fracture neck of femur in haemophilia A—experience from a cohort of 11 patients from a tertiary centre in India. Haemophilia 2007;13(4):391–394.
295. Lee VN, Srivastava A, Palanikumar C, et al. External fixators in haemophilia. Haemophilia 2004;10(1):52–57.
296. Leet AI, Chebli C, Kushner H, et al. Fracture incidence in polyostotic fibrous dysplasia and the McCune-Albright syndrome. J Bone Miner Res 2004;19(4):571–577.
297. Leet AI, Mesfin A, Pichard C, et al. Fractures in children with cerebral palsy. J Pediatr Orthop 2006;26(5):624–627.

298. Leithner A, Windhager R, Lang S, et al. Aneurysmal bone cyst. A population-based epidemiologic study and literature review. Clin Orthop Relat Res 1999;363:176–179.
299. Leong GM, Abad V, Charmandari E, et al. Effects of child- and adolescent-onset endogenous Cushing syndrome on bone mass, body composition, and growth: a 7-year prospective study into young adulthood. J Bone Miner Res 2007;22(1):110–118.
300. Letson GD, Greenfield GB, Heinrich SD. Evaluation of the child with a bone or soft tissue neoplasm. Orthop Clin North Am 1996;27(3):431–451.
301. Letts M, Monson R, Weber K. The prevention of recurrent fractures of the lower extremities in severe osteogenesis imperfecta using vacuum pants: a preliminary report in four patients. J Pediatr Orthop 1988;8(4):454–457.
302. Leung PC. Congenital pseudarthrosis of the tibia. Three cases treated by free vascularized iliac crest graft. Clin Orthop 1983;(175):45–50.
303. Levine SE, Dormans JP, Meyer JS, et al. Langerhans cell histiocytosis of the spine in children. Clin Orthop 1996;323:288–293.
304. Levy WM, Miller AA, Bonakdarpour A, et al. Aneurysmal bone cyst secondary to other osseous lesions. Report of 57 cases. Am J Clin Pathol 1975;63(1):1–8.
305. Lewis RJ, Ketcham AS. Maffucci syndrome: functional and neoplastic significance. Case report and review of the literature. J Bone Joint Surg Am 1973;55(7):1465–1479.
306. Lichtenstein L. Polystotic fibrous dysplasia. Arch Surg 1938;36:874–898.
307. Lichtenstein L, Jaffee HL. Fibrous dysplasia of bone: a condition affecting one, several or many bones, the graver cases of which may present abnormal pigmentation of skin, premature sexual development, hyperthyroidism or still other extra skeletal abnormalities. Arch Pathol 1942;33:777–815.
308. Llach F, Nikakhtar B. Current advances in the therapy of secondary hyperparathyroidism and osteitis fibrosa. Miner Electrolyte Metab 1991;17(4):250–255.
309. Lloyd-Roberts GC. Treatment of defects of the ulna in children by establishing cross-union with the radius. J Bone Joint Surg Br 1973;55(2):327–330.
310. Lloyd-Roberts GC, Jackson AM, Albert JS. Avulsion of the distal pole of the patella in cerebral palsy. A cause of deteriorating gait. J Bone Joint Surg Br 1985;67(2):252–254.
311. Lock TR, Aronson DD. Fractures in patients who have myelomeningocele. J Bone Joint Surg Am 1989;71(8):1153–1157.
312. Loder RT, Hensinger RN. Slipped capital femoral epiphysis associated with renal failure osteodystrophy. J Pediatr Orthop 1997;17(2):205–211.
313. Luhmann SJ, Sheridan JJ, Capelli AM, et al. Management of lower-extremity deformities in osteogenesis imperfecta with extensible intramedullary rod technique: a 20-year experience. J Pediatr Orthop 1998;18(1):88–94.
314. Luke DL, Schoenecker PL, Blair VP 3rd, et al. Fractures after Wagner limb lengthening. J Pediatr Orthop 1992;12(1):20–24.
315. MacLean AD. Spinal changes in a case of infantile scurvy. Br J Radiol 1968;41(485): 385–387.
316. Maffulli N, Hughes T, Fixsen JA. Ultrasonographic monitoring of limb lengthening. J Bone Joint Surg Br 1992;74(1):130–132.
317. Mahboubi S, Dormans JP, D'Angio G. Malignant degeneration of radiation-induced osteochondroma. Skeletal Radiol 1997;26(3):195–198.
318. Major MR, Huizenga BA. Spinal cord compression by displaced ribs in neurofibromatosis. A report of three cases. J Bone Joint Surg Am 1988;70(7):1100–1102.
319. Malhis TM, Bowen JR. Tibial and femoral lengthening: a report of 54 cases. J Pediatr Orthop 1982;2(5):487–491.
320. Malkawi H, Shannak A, Amr S. Surgical treatment of pathological subtrochanteric fractures due to benign lesions in children and adolescents. J Pediatr Orthop 1984; 4(1):63–69.
321. Mallet E. Primary hyperparathyroidism in neonates and childhood. The French experience (1984–2004). Horm Res 2008,69(3):180–188.
322. Mandell GA, Harcke HT, Harkey C, et al. SPECT imaging of para-axial neurofibromatosis with technetium-99m DTPA. J Nucl Med 1987;28(11):1688–1694.
323. Mandell GA, Herrick WC, Harcke HT, et al. Neurofibromas: location by scanning with Tc-99m DTPA. Work in progress. Radiology 1985;157(3):803–806.
324. Mankin HJ. Rickets, osteomalacia, and renal osteodystrophy. Part II. J Bone Joint Surg Am 1974;56(2):352–386.
325. Mankin HJ, Lange TA, Spanier SS. The hazards of biopsy in patients with malignant primary bone and soft-tissue tumors. J Bone Joint Surg Am 1982;64(8):1121–1127.
326. Manske PR. Forearm pseudarthrosis-neurofibromatosis: case report. Clin Orthop 1979; 139:125–127.
327. Manusov EG, Douville DR, Page LV, et al. Osteopetrosis ("marble bone" disease). Am Fam Physician 1993;47(1):175–180.
328. Marcove RC, Sheth DS, Takemoto S, et al. The treatment of aneurysmal bone cyst. Clin Orthop Relat Res 1995(311):157–163.
329. Margau R, Babyn P, Cole W, et al. MR imaging of simple bone cysts in children: not so simple. Pediatr Radiol 2000;30(8):551–557.
330. Marhaug G. Idiopathic juvenile osteoporosis. Scand J Rheumatol 1993;22(1):45–47.
331. Marks SC Jr, Schmidt CJ. Bone remodeling as an expression of altered phenotype: studies of fracture healing in untreated and cured osteopetrotic rats. Clin Orthop 1978; 37:259–264.
332. Marder HK, Tsang RC, Hug G, Et Al. Calcitriol deficiency in idiopathic juvenile osteoporosis. Am J Dis Child 1982;136(10):914–917.
333. Martin RP, Deane RH, Collett V. Spondylolysis in children who have osteopetrosis. J Bone Joint Surg Am 1997;79(11):1685–1689.
334. Martinez V, Sissons HA. Aneurysmal bone cyst. A review of 123 cases including primary lesions and those secondary to other bone pathology. Cancer 1988;61(11):2291–2304.
335. Masihuz Z. Pseudarthrosis of the radius associated with neurofibromatosis. A case report. J Bone Joint Surg Am 1977;59(7):977–978.
336. Massengill AD, Seeger LL, Eckardt JJ. The role of plain radiography, computed tomography, and magnetic resonance imaging in sarcoma evaluation. Hematol Oncol Clin North Am 1995;9(3):571–604.
337. Mathoulin C, Gilbert A, Azze RG. Congenital pseudarthrosis of the forearm: treatment of six cases with vascularized fibular graft and a review of the literature. Microsurgery 1993;14(4):252–259.
338. Maybarduk PL. Osseous atrophy associated with progressive muscular dystrophy. Am J Dis Child 1941;61:565–576.
339. McArthur RG, Bahn RC, Hayles AB. Primary adrenocortical nodular dysplasia as a cause of Cushing syndrome in infants and children. Mayo Clin Proc 1982;57(1):58–63.
340. McArthur RG, Cloutier MD, Hayes AB, et al. Cushing disease in children. Findings in 13 cases. Mayo Clin Proc 1972;47(5):318–326.
341. McCarroll H. Clinical manifestations of congenital neurofibromatosis. J Bone Joint Surg Am 1950;32(A):601–617.
342. McDonald DG, Kinali M, Gallagher AC, et al. Fracture prevalence in Duchenne muscular dystrophy. Dev Med Child Neurol 2002;44(10):695–698.
343. McDonald DJ, Sim FH, Mcleod RA, et al. Giant-cell tumor of bone. J Bone Joint Surg Am 1986;68(2):235–242.
344. McFarland B. Pseudarthrosis of the tibia in childhood. J Bone Joint Surg Br 1951;33-B(1):36–46.
345. McKibbin B, Porter RW. The incidence of vitamin C deficiency in meningomyelocele. Dev Med Child Neurol 1967;9(3):338–344.
346. McLean SM. Healing in infantile scurvy as shown by x-ray. Am J Dis Child 1928;36: 875–930.
347. McIvor WC, Samilson RL. Fractures in patients with cerebral palsy. J Bone Joint Surg Am 1966;48(5):858–866.
348. McKusick V. Heritable Disorders of Connective Tissue. 3rd ed. St. Louis: CV Mosby, 1972.
349. McWhorter AG, Seale NS. Prevalence of dental abscess in a population of children with vitamin D-resistant rickets. Pediatr Dent 1991;13(2):91–96.
350. Meehan PL, Viroslav S, Schmitt EW Jr. Vertebral collapse in childhood leukemia. J Pediatr Orthop 1995;15(5):592–595.
351. Meeropol E, Frost J, Pugh L, et al. Latex allergy in children with myelodysplasia: a survey of Shriners hospitals. J Pediatr Orthop 1993;13(1):1–4.
352. Mehls O, Ritz E, Krempien B, et al. Slipped epiphyses in renal osteodystrophy. Arch Dis Child 1975;50:545–554.
353. Meredith SC, Simon MA, Laros GS, et al. Pycnodysostosis. A clinical, pathological, and ultramicroscopic study of a case. J Bone Joint Surg Am 1978;60(8):1122–1127.
354. Meyer JS, Harty MP, Mahboubi S, et al. Langerhans cell histiocytosis: presentation and evolution of radiologic findings with clinical correlation. Radiographics 1995;15(5): 1135–1146.
355. Middlemiss JH, Raper AB. Skeletal changes in the haemoglobinopathies. J Bone Joint Surg Br 1966;48(4):693–702.
356. Milgram JW, Jasty M. Osteopetrosis. A morphological study of twenty-one cases. J Bone Joint Surg Am 1982;64(6):912–929.
357. Miller F, Cardoso Dias R, Dabney KW, et al. Soft-tissue release for spastic hip subluxation in cerebral palsy. J Pediatr Orthop 1997;17(5):571–584.
358. Miller F, Girardi H, Lipton G, et al. Reconstruction of the dysplastic spastic hip with peri-ilial pelvic and femoral osteotomy followed by immediate mobilization. J Pediatr Orthop 1997;17(5):592–602.
359. Miller PR, Glazer DA. Spontaneous fractures in the brain-crippled, bedridden patient. Clin Orthop 1976;(120):134–137.
360. Miller RG, Segal JB, Ashar BH, et al. High prevalence and correlates of low bone mineral density in young adults with sickle cell disease. Am J Hematol 2006;81(4):236–241.
361. Milliner DS, Nebeker HG, Ott SM, et all. Use of the deferoxamine infusion test in the diagnosis of aluminum-related osteodystrophy. Ann Intern Med 1984;101(6): 775–779.
362. Millington-Ward S, Mcmahon HP, Farrar GJ. Emerging therapeutic approaches for osteogenesis imperfecta. Trends Mol Med 2005;11(6):299–305.
363. Minch CM, Kruse RW. Osteogenesis imperfecta: a review of basic science and diagnosis. Orthopedics 1998;21(5):558–567.
364. Minde J, Svensson O, Holmberg M, et al. Orthopedic aspects of familial insensitivity to pain due to a novel nerve growth factor beta mutation. Acta Orthop 2006;77(2): 198–202.
365. Moorefield WG Jr, Miller GR. Aftermath of osteogenesis imperfecta: the disease in adulthood. J Bone Joint Surg Am 1980;62(1):113–119.
366. Morrey BF, Peterson HA. Hematogenous pyogenic osteomyelitis in children. Orthop Clin North Am 1975;6(4):935–951.
367. Morrissy RT. Congenital pseudarthrosis of the tibia. Factors that affect results. Clin Orthop 1982;(166):21–27.
368. Morrissy RT, Riseborough EJ, Hall JE. Congenital pseudarthrosis of the tibia. J Bone Joint Surg Br 1981;63-B(3):367–375.
369. Mosca VM, Moseley C. Complications of Wagner leg lengthening and their avoidance. Orthop Trans 1986;10:462.
370. Mulpuri K, Joseph B. Intramedullary rodding in osteogenesis imperfecta. J Pediatr Orthop 2000;20(2):267–273.
371. Murray HH, Lovell WW. Congenital pseudarthrosis of the tibia. A long-term follow-up study. Clin Orthop 1982;(166):14–20.
372. Muscolo DL, Ayerza MA, Calabrese ME, et al. The use of a bone allograft for reconstruction after resection of giant-cell tumor close to the knee. J Bone Joint Surg Am 1993; 75(11):1656–1662.
373. Neer CS 2nd, Francis KC, Johnston AS, et al. Current concepts on the treatment of solitary unicameral bone cyst. Clin Orthop Relat Res 1973;97:40–51.
374. Neer CS 2nd, Francis KC, Marcove RC, et al. Treatment of unicameral bone cyst. A follow-up study of one hundred seventy-five cases. J Bone Joint Surg Am 1966;48(4): 731–745.
375. Nelson CL, Evarts CM, Popowniak K. Musculoskeletal complications of renal transplantation. Surg Clin North Am 1971;51(5):1205–1209.
376. Nerubay J, Pilderwasser D. Spontaneous bilateral distal femoral physiolysis due to scurvy. Acta Orthop Scand 1984;55(1):18–20.
377. Neumayr LD, Aguilar C, Earles AN, et al. Physical therapy alone compared with core decompression and physical therapy for femoral head osteonecrosis in sickle cell disease. Results of a multicenter study at a mean of three years after treatment. J Bone Joint Surg Am 2006;88(12):2573–2582.
378. Newman AJ, Melhorn DK. Vertebral compression in childhood leukemia. Am J Dis Child 1973;125(6):863–865.
379. Nicholas RW, James P. Telescoping intramedullary stabilization of the lower extremities for severe osteogenesis imperfecta. J Pediatr Orthop 1990;10(2):219–223.
380. Niemann KM. Surgical treatment of the tibia in osteogenesis imperfecta. Clin Orthop 1981;59:134–140.
381. Nilsson BE, Westlin NE. Restoration of bone mass after fracture of the lower limb in children. Acta Orthop Scand 1971;42(1):78–81.

382. Nixon JR, Douglas JF. Bilateral slipping of the upper femoral epiphysis in end-stage renal failure. A report of two cases. J Bone Joint Surg Br 1980;62-B(1):18–21.
383. Niyibizi C, Smith P, Mi Z, et al. Potential of gene therapy for treating osteogenesis imperfecta. Clin Orthop Relat Res 2000(379 Suppl):S126–S133.
384. Norton PL, Foley JJ. Paraplegia in children. Am J Orthop 1959;41-A:1291–1309.
385. O'Sullivan M, Zacharin M. Intramedullary rodding and bisphosphonate treatment of polyostotic fibrous dysplasia associated with the McCune-Albright syndrome. J Pediatr Orthop 2002;22(2):255–260.
386. Okuno T, Inoue A, Izumo S. Congenital insensitivity to pain with anhidrosis. A case report. J Bone Joint Surg Am 1990;72(2):279–282.
387. Oliveira AM, Perez-Atayde AR, Inwards CY, et al. USP6 and CDH11 oncogenes identify the neoplastic cell in primary aneurysmal bone cysts and are absent in so-called secondary aneurysmal bone cysts. Am J Pathol 2004;165(5):1773–1780.
388. Oppenheim WL, Bowen RE, McDonough PW, et al. Outcome of slipped capital femoral epiphysis in renal osteodystrophy. J Pediatr Orthop 2003;23(2):169–174.
389. Oppenheim WL, Namba R, Goodman WG, et al. Aluminum toxicity complicating renal osteodystrophy. A case report. J Bone Joint Surg Am 1989;71(3):446–452.
390. Ossofsky Hj. Infantile scurvy. Am J Dis Child 1965;109:173–176.
391. Osterman K, Merikanto J. Diaphyseal bone lengthening in children using Wagner device: long-term results. J Pediatr Orthop 1991;11(4):449–451.
392. Ostrowski DM, Eilert RE, Waldstein G. Congenital pseudarthrosis of the ulna: a report of two cases and a review of the literature. J Pediatr Orthop 1985;5(4):463–467.
393. Ozaki T, Hillmann A, Lindner N, et al. Aneurysmal bone cysts in children. J Cancer Res Clin Oncol 1996;122(12):767–769.
394. Paley D. Problems, obstacles, and complications of limb lengthening by the Ilizarov technique. Clin Orthop 1990;250:81–104.
395. Paley D, Herzenberg JE, Paremain G, et al. Femoral lengthening over an intramedullary nail. A matched-case comparison with Ilizarov femoral lengthening. J Bone Joint Surg Am 1997;79(10):1464–1480.
396. Papagelopoulos PJ, Choudhury SN, Frassica FJ, et al. Treatment of aneurysmal bone cysts of the pelvis and sacrum. J Bone Joint Surg Am 2001;83-A(11):1674–1681.
397. Papagelopoulos PJ, Currier BL, Galanis EC, et al. Vertebra plana of the lumbar spine caused by an aneurysmal bone cyst: a case report. Am J Orthop 1999;28(2):119–124.
398. Parfitt AM. The actions of parathyroid hormone on bone: relation to bone remodeling and turnover. Calcium homeostasis and metabolic bone disease. Part III of IV parts; PTH and osteoblasts, the relationship between bone turnover and bone loss, and the state of the bones in primary hyperparathyroidism. Metabolism 1976;25(9):1033–1069.
399. Parfitt AM. Renal osteodystrophy. Orthop Clin North Am 1972;3(3):681–698.
400. Park YK, Unni KK, Mcleod RA, et al. Osteofibrous dysplasia: clinicopathologic study of 80 cases. Hum Pathol 1993;24(12):1339–1347.
401. Patel MR, Pearlman HS, Lavine LS. Arthrodesis in hemophilia. Clin Orthop 1972;86:168–174.
402. Paterson CR, Burns J, McAllion SJ. Osteogenesis imperfecta: the distinction from child abuse and the recognition of a variant form. Am J Med Genet 1993;45(2):187–192.
403. Paterson DC, Simonis RV. Electrical stimulation in the treatment of congenital pseudarthrosis of the tibia. J Bone Joint Surg Br 1985;67(3):454–462.
404. Peabody TD, Simon MA. Making the diagnosis: keys to a successful biopsy in children with bone and soft-tissue tumors. Orthop Clin North Am 1996;27(3):453–459.
405. Piehl FC, Davis RJ, Prugh SI. Osteomyelitis in sickle cell disease. J Pediatr Orthop 1993;13(2):225–227.
406. Pietrogrande V, Dioguardi N, Mannucci PM. Short-term evaluation of synovectomy in haemophilia. Br Med J 1972;2(810):378–381.
407. Plotkin H, Sueiro R. Osteoporosis in children with neuromuscular diseases and inborn errors of metabolism. Minerva Pediatr 2007;59(2):129–135.
408. Pochanugool L, Subhadharaphandou T, Dhanachaim, et al. Prognostic factors among 130 patients with osteosarcoma. Clin Orthop 1997;(345):206–214.
409. Popoff SN, Marks SC Jr. The heterogeneity of the osteopetroses reflects the diversity of cellular influences during skeletal development. Bone 1995;17(5):437–445.
410. Porat S, Heller E, Seidman DS, et al. Functional results of operation in osteogenesis imperfecta: elongating and nonelongating rods. J Pediatr Orthop 1991;11(2):200–203.
411. Post M, Telfer MC. Surgery in hemophilic patients. J Bone Joint Surg Am 1975;57(8):1136–1145.
412. Poznanski AK, Kuhns LR, Guire KE. New standards of cortical mass in the humerus of neonates: a means of evaluating bone loss in the premature infant. Radiology 1980;134(3):639–644.
413. Preeyasombat C, Sirikulchayanonta V, Mahachokelertwattana P, et al. Cushing syndrome caused by Ewing's sarcoma secreting corticotropin releasing factor-like peptide. Am J Dis Child 1992;146(9):1103–1105.
414. Presedo A, Dabney KW, Miller F. Fractures in patients with cerebral palsy. J Pediatr Orthop 2007;27(2):147–153.
415. Price CT, Cole JD. Limb lengthening by callotasis for children and adolescents. Early experience. Clin Orthop 1990; 250:105–111.
416. Quiles M, Sanz TA. Epiphyseal separation in scurvy. J Pediatr Orthop 1988;8(2):223–225.
417. Quilis AN. Fractures in children with myelomeningocele. Acta Orthop Scand 1974;45(6):883–897.
418. Raab P, Hohmann F, Kuhl J, et al. Vertebral remodeling in eosinophilic granuloma of the spine. A long-term follow-up. Spine 1998;23(12):1351–1354.
419. Ragab AH, Frech RS, Vietti TJ. Osteoporotic fractures secondary to methotrexate therapy of acute leukemia in remission. Cancer 1970;25(3):580–585.
420. Rajasuriya K, Peiris OA, Ratnaike VT, et al. Parathyroid adenomas in childhood. Am J Dis Child 1964;107:442–449.
421. Ramar S, Sivaramakrishnan V, Manoharan K. Scurvy—a forgotten disease. Arch Phys Med Rehabil 1993;74(1):92–95.
422. Randall C, Lauchlan SC. Parathyroid hyperplasia in an infant. Am J Dis Child 1963;105:364–367.
423. Rathgeb JM, Ramsey PL, Cowell HR. Congenital kyphoscoliosis of the tibia. Clin Orthop 1974;103:178–190.
424. Rauch F, Travers R, Norman ME, et al. Deficient bone formation in idiopathic juvenile osteoporosis: a histomorphometric study of cancellous iliac bone. J Bone Miner Res 2000;15(5):957–963.
425. Rauch F, Travers R, Norman ME, et al. The bone formation defect in idiopathic juvenile osteoporosis is surface-specific. Bone 2002;31(1):85–89.
426. Rawlinson PG, Green RH, Coggins AM, et al. Malignant osteoporosis: hypercalcaemia after bone marrow transplantation. Arch Dis Child 1995;66:638–639.
427. Reeves JD, Huffer WE, August CS, et al. The hematopoietic effects of prednisone therapy in four infants with osteopetrosis. J Pediatr 1979;94(2):210–214.
428. Richin PF, Kranik A, Van Herpe L, et al. Congenital pseudarthrosis of both bones of the forearm. A case report. J Bone Joint Surg Am 1976;58(7):1032–1023.
429. Riminucci M, Fisher LW, Shenker A, et al. Fibrous dysplasia of bone in the McCune-Albright syndrome: abnormalities in bone formation. Am J Pathol 1997;151(6):1587–1600.
430. Riseborough EJ, Herndon JH. Scoliosis of Other Deformities of the Axial Skeleton. Boston: Little, Brown, and Company, 1975.
431. Ritschl P, Karnel F, Hajek P. Fibrous metaphyseal defects—determination of their origin and natural history using a radiomorphological study. Skeletal Radiol 1988;17(1):8–15.
432. Roberts JB. Bilateral hyperplastic callus formation in osteogenesis imperfecta. J Bone Joint Surg Am 1976;58(8):1164–1166.
433. Roberts WA, Badger VM. Osteomalacia of very-low-birth-weight infants. J Pediatr Orthop 1984;4(5):593–598.
434. Robin GC. Fracture in childhood paraplegia. Paraplegia 1965;3(3):165–170.
435. Robin GC. Fractures in poliomyelitis in children. J Bone Joint Surg Am 1966;48(6):1048–1054.
436. Robins RH, Murrell JS. Traumatic ischaemia in a haemophiliac. Report of a case of prolonged haemostasis with cryoprecipitate during decompression and skin grafting. J Bone Joint Surg Br 1971;53(1):113–117.
437. Rockower S, Mckay D, Nason S. Dislocation of the spine in neurofibromatosis. A report of two cases. J Bone Joint Surg Am 1982;64(8):1240–1242.
438. Rodgers WB, Schwend RM, Jaramillo D, et al. Chronic physeal fractures in myelodysplasia: magnetic resonance analysis, histologic description, treatment, and outcome. J Pediatr Orthop 1997;17(5):615–621.
439. Rodriguez-Merchan EC. Bone fracture in the haemophilic patient. Haemophilia 2002;8:104.
440. Rogalsky RJ, Black GB, Reed MH. Orthopaedic manifestations of leukemia in children. J Bone Joint Surg Am 1986;68(4):494–501.
441. Rosenthal DI, Scott JA, Barranger J, et al. Evaluation of Gaucher disease using magnetic resonance imaging. J Bone Joint Surg Am 1986;68(6):802–808.
442. Rosenthal RK, Levine DB. Fragmentation of the distal pole of the patella in spastic cerebral palsy. J Bone Joint Surg Am 1977;59(7):934–939.
443. Roth VG. Pycnodysostosis presenting with bilateral subtrochanteric fractures: case report. Clin Orthop 1976;17:247–253.
444. Rougraff BT, Kling TJ. Treatment of active unicameral bone cysts with percutaneous injection of demineralized bone matrix and autogenous bone marrow. J Bone Joint Surg Am 2002;84-A(6):921–929.
445. Sacks R, Habermann ET. Pathological fracture in congenital rubella. A case report. J Bone Joint Surg Am 1977;59(4):557–559.
446. Sakkers R, Kok D, Engelbert R, et al. Skeletal effects and functional outcome with olpadronate in children with osteogenesis imperfecta: a 2-year randomized placebo controlled study. Lancet 2004;363(9419):1427–1431.
447. Sala A, Barr RD. Osteopenia and cancer in children and adolescents: the fragility of success. Cancer 2007;109(7):1420–1431.
448. Salusky IB, Coburn JW, Foley J, et al. Effects of oral calcium carbonate on control of serum phosphorus and changes in plasma aluminum levels after discontinuation of aluminum-containing gels in children receiving dialysis. J Pediatr 1986;108(5 Pt 1):767–770.
449. Samaniego EA, Sheth RD. Bone consequences of epilepsy and antiepileptic medications. Semin Pediatr Neurol 2007;14(4):196–200.
450. San-Julian M, Canadell J. Fractures of allografts used in limb preserving operations. Int Orthop 1998;22(1):32–36.
451. Santori F, Ghera S, Castelli V. Treatment of solitary bone cysts with intramedullary nailing. Orthopedics 1988;11(6):873–878.
452. Schein AJ, Arkin AM. The classic: hip-joint involvement in Gaucher disease. Clin Orthop 1973;90:4–10.
453. Schneider R, Goldman AB, Bohne WH. Neuropathic injuries to the lower extremities in children. Radiology 1978;128(3):713–718.
454. Schreuder HW, Veth RP, Pruszczynski M, et al. Aneurysmal bone cysts treated by curettage, cryotherapy and bone grafting. J Bone Joint Surg Br 1997;79(1):20–25.
455. Schwartz AM, Leonidas JC. Methotrexate osteopathy. Skeletal Radiol 1984;11(1):13–16.
456. Scott W. Epiphyseal dislocations in scurvy. J Bone Joint Surg Am 1941;23:314–322.
457. Scully SP, Temple HT, O'Keefe RJ, et al. The surgical treatment of patients with osteosarcoma who sustain a pathologic fracture. Clin Orthop 1996;(324):227–232.
458. Seftion G. Osteomyelitis after closed femoral fracture in a child. J R Coll Surg Edinb 1982;27:113.
459. Sellers DS, Sowa DT, Moore JR, et al. Congenital pseudarthrosis of the forearm. J Hand Surg Am 1988;13(1):89–93.
460. Shapiro F. Osteopetrosis. Current clinical considerations. Clin Orthop 1993;94:34–44.
461. Shapiro F, Glimcher MJ, Holtrop ME, et al. Human osteopetrosis: a histological, ultrastructural, and biochemical study. J Bone Joint Surg Am 1980;62(3):384–399.
462. Sherk HH. Indications for orthopedic surgery in the mentally retarded patient. Clin Orthop 1973;90:174–177.
463. Sherk HH, Cruz M, Stambaugh J. Vitamin D prophylaxis and the lowered incidence of fractures in anticonvulsant rickets and osteomalacia. Clin Orthop 1977;29:251–257.
464. Shertzer JH, Bickel WH, Stubbins SG. Congenital pseudarthrosis of the ulna. Report of two cases. Minn Med 1969;52(7):1061–1066.
465. Shoenfeld Y. Osteogenesis imperfecta. Review of the literature with presentation of 29 cases. Am J Dis Child 1975;129(6):679–687.
466. Shopnick RI, Brettler DB. Hemostasis: a practical review of conservative and operative care. Clin Orthop 1996(328):34–38.
467. Siegel IM. Fractures of long bones in Duchenne muscular dystrophy. J Trauma 1977;17(3):219–222.
468. Sijbrandij S. Percutaneous nailing in the management of osteogenesis imperfecta. Int Orthop 1990;14(2):195–197.

469. Sillence D. Osteogenesis imperfecta: an expanding panorama of variants. Clin Orthop 1981;159:11–25.
470. Silverman FN. Recovery from epiphyseal invagination: sequel to an unusual complication of scurvy. J Bone Joint Surg Am 1970;52(2):384–390.
471. Silverman FN. An unusual osseous sequel to infantile scurvy. J Bone Joint Surg Am 1953;35-A(1):215–220.
472. Singh M, Nagrath AR, Maini PS. Changes in trabecular pattern of the upper end of the femur as an index of osteoporosis. J Bone Joint Surg Am 1970;52(3):457–467.
473. Silverman FN. Virus diseases of bone. Do they exist? The Neuhauser Lecture. Am J Roentgenol 1976;126(4):677–703.
474. Simon MA. Biopsy of musculoskeletal tumors. J Bone Joint Surg Am 1982;64(8): 1253–1257.
475. Sinigaglia R, Gigante C, Bisinella G, et al. Musculoskeletal manifestations in pediatric acute leukemia. J Pediatr Orthop 2008;28(1):20–28.
476. Smith JA. Bone disorders in sickle cell disease. Hematol Oncol Clin North Am 1996; 10(6):1345–1356.
477. Smith R. Idiopathic osteoporosis in the young. J Bone Joint Surg Br 1980;62-B(4): 417–427.
478. Smith R. The pathophysiology and management of rickets. Orthop Clin North Am 1972;3(3):601–621.
479. Smith R, Specht EE. Osseous lesions and pathologic fractures in congenital cytomegalic inclusion disease: report of a case. Clin Orthop 1979;(144):280–283.
480. Snyder BD, Hauser-Kara DA, Hipp JA, et al. Predicting fracture through benign skeletal lesions with quantitative computed tomography. J Bone Joint Surg Am 2006;88(1): 55–70.
481. Sodergard J, Ryoppy S. The knee in arthrogryposis multiplex congenita. J Pediatr Orthop 1990;10(2):177–182.
482. Sofield H, Millar EA. Fragmentation, realignment, and intramedullary rod fixation of deformities of the long bones in children. J Bone Joint Surg Am 1959;41:1371–1391.
483. Stanisavljevic S, Babcock AL. Fractures in children treated with methotrexate for leukemia. Clin Orthop 1977;(25):139–144.
484. Stein H, Dickson RA. Reversed dynamic slings for knee-flexion contractures in the hemophiliac. J Bone Joint Surg Am 1975;57(2):282–283.
485. Stein RE, Urbaniak J. Use of the tourniquet during surgery in patients with sickle cell hemoglobinopathies. Clin Orthop 1980;(151):231–233.
486. Steiner RD, Pepin M, Byers PH. Studies of collagen synthesis and structure in the differentiation of child abuse from osteogenesis imperfecta. J Pediatr 1996;128(4): 542–547.
487. Stephenson RB, London MD, Hankin FM, et al. Fibrous dysplasia. An analysis of options for treatment. J Bone Joint Surg Am 1987;69(3):400–409.
488. Stern PJ, Watts HG. Osteonecrosis after renal transplantation in children. J Bone Joint Surg Am 1979;61(6A):851–856.
489. Stevenson RD, Conaway M, Barrington JW, et al. Fracture rate in children with cerebral palsy. Pediatr Rehabil 2006;9(4):396–403.
490. Stott NS, Zionts LE. Displaced fractures of the apophysis of the olecranon in children who have osteogenesis imperfecta. J Bone Joint Surg Am 1993;75(7):1026–1033.
491. Strong ML, Wong-Chung J. Prophylactic bypass grafting of the prepseudarthrotic tibia in neurofibromatosis. J Pediatr Orthop 1991;11(6):757–764.
492. Stynowick GA, Tobias JD. Perioperative care of the patient with osteogenesis imperfecta. Orthopedics 2007;30(12):1043–1049.
493. Sullivan RJ, Meyer JS, Dormans JP, et al. Diagnosing aneurysmal and unicameral bone cysts with magnetic resonance imaging. Clin Orthop Relat Res 1999(366):186–190.
494. Sung HW, Kuo DP, Shu WP, et al. Giant-cell tumor of bone: analysis of 208 cases in Chinese patients. J Bone Joint Surg Am 1982;64(5):755–761.
495. Sweeney LE. Hypophosphataemic rickets after ifosfamide treatment in children. Clin Radiol 1993;47(5):345–347.
496. Tachdjian M. Pediatric Orthopaedics. 2nd ed. Philadelphia: WB Saunders, 1989.
497. Taylor MM, Moore TM, Harvey JP Jr. Pycnodysostosis. A case report. J Bone Joint Surg Am 1978;60(8):1128–1130.
498. Teall C. A radiological study of the bone changes in renal infantilism. Br J Radiol 1928; 1:49–58.
499. Tobias JD, Atwood R, Lowe S, et al. Anesthetic considerations in the child with Gaucher disease. J Clin Anesth 1993;5(2):150–153.
500. Touloukian RJ, Gertner JM. Vitamin D deficiency rickets as a late complication of the short gut syndrome during infancy. J Pediatr Surg 1981;16(3):230–235.
501. Townsend PF, Cowell HR, Steg NL. Lower extremity fractures simulating infection in myelomeningocele. Clin Orthop 1979;44:255–259.
502. Tudisco C, Farsetti P, Gatti S, et al. Influence of chronic osteomyelitis on skeletal growth: analysis at maturity of 26 cases affected during childhood. J Pediatr Orthop 1991;11(3):358–363.
503. Turcotte RE, Wunder JS, Isler MH, et al. Giant cell tumor of long bone: a Canadian Sarcoma Group study. Clin Orthop Relat Res 2002;397:248–258.
504. Van Der Sluis IM, Van Den Heuvel-Eibrink MM. Osteoporosis in children with cancer. Pediatr Blood Cancer 2008;50(2 Suppl):474–478; discussion 486.
505. Van Lie Peters EM, Aronson DC, Everts V, et al. Failure of calcitriol treatment in a patient with malignant osteopetrosis. Eur J Pediatr 1993;152(10):818–821.
506. Vayego-Lourenco SA. TP53 mutations in a recurrent unicameral bone cyst. Cancer Genet Cytogenet 2001;124(2):175–176.
507. Vergel De Dios AM, Bond JR, Shives TC, et al. Aneurysmal bone cyst. A clinicopathologic study of 238 cases. Cancer 1992;69(12):2921–2931.
508. Vignos PJ Jr, Archibald KC. Maintenance of ambulation in childhood muscular dystrophy. J Chronic Dis 1960;12:273–290.
509. Virdis R, Balestrazzi P, Zampolli M, et al. Hypertension in children with neurofibromatosis. J Hum Hypertens 1994;8(5):395–397.
510. Wadia F, Shah N, Porter M. Bilateral charnley low-friction arthroplasty with cement in a patient with pyknodysostosis. A case report. J Bone Joint Surg Am 2006;88(8): 1846–1848.
511. Wallny TA, Scholz DT, Oldenburg J, et al. Osteoporosis in haemophilia—an underestimated comorbidity? Haemophilia 2007;13(1):79–84.
512. Walshe JM. Copper: not too little, not too much, but just right. Based on the triennial Pewterers Lecture delivered at the National Hospital for Neurology, London, on 23 March 1995. J R Coll Physicians Lond 1995;29(4):280–288.
513. Wang J, Temple HT, Pitcher JD, et al. Salvage of failed massive allograft reconstruction with endoprosthesis. Clin Orthop Relat Res 2006;443:296–301.
514. Warric C. Polystotic fibrous dysplasia—Albright syndrome. A review of the literature and report of four male cases, two of which were associated with precocious puberty. J Bone Joint Surg Am 1949;31:175–183.
515. Watanabe K, Tsuchiya H, Sakurakichi K, et al. Treatment of lower limb deformities and limb-length discrepancies with the external fixator in Ollier's disease. J Orthop Sci 2007;12(5):471–475.
516. Weiland AJ, Daniel RK. Congenital pseudarthrosis of the tibia: treatment with vascularized autogenous fibular grafts. A preliminary report. Johns Hopkins Med J 1980; 147(3):89–95.
517. Wenger DR, Jeffcoat BT, Herring JA. The guarded prognosis of physeal injury in paraplegic children. J Bone Joint Surg Am 1980;62(2):241–246.
518. White M, Dennison WM. Acute haematogenous osteitis in childhood. J Bone Joint Surg Br 1952;34-B(4):608–623.
519. Whitehouse D. Diagnostic value of the cafe-au-lait spot in children. Arch Dis Child 1966;41(217):316–319.
520. Whyte MP. Carbonic anhydrase II deficiency. Clin Orthop 1993;94:52–63.
521. Wilkins RM. Unicameral bone cysts. J Am Acad Orthop Surg 2000;8(4):217–224.
522. Wilkinson H, James J. Self-limiting neonatal primary hyperparathyroidism associated with familial hypocalciuric hypercalcaemia. Arch Dis Child 1993;69(3 Spec No): 319–321.
523. Williams P. The management of arthrogryposis. Orthop Clin North Am 1978;9(1): 67–88.
524. Winter RB, Moe JH, Bradford DS, et al. Spine deformity in neurofibromatosis. A review of 102 patients. J Bone Joint Surg Am 1979;61(5):677–694.
525. Wright J, Dormans J, Rang M. Pseudarthrosis of the rabbit tibia: a model for congenital pseudarthrosis? J Pediatr Orthop 1991;11(3):277–283.
526. Wunder JS, Paulian G, Huvos AG, et al. The histological response to chemotherapy as a predictor of the oncological outcome of operative treatment of Ewing sarcoma. J Bone Joint Surg Am 1998;80(7):1020–1033.
527. Wynne-Davies R, Hall CM, Apley AG. Atlas of skeletal dysplasias. New York: Churchill Livingstone, 1985.
528. Yaghmai I, Tafazoli M. Massive subperiosteal hemorrhage in neurofibromatosis. Radiology 1977;122(2):439–441.
529. Zeitlin L, Fassier F, Glorieux FH. Modern approach to children with osteogenesis imperfecta. J Pediatr Orthop B 2003;12(2):77–87.
530. Zionts LE, Ebramzadeh E, Stott NS. Complications in the use of the Bailey-Dubow extensible nail. Clin Orthop 1998;(48):186–195.
531. Zionts LE, Moon CN. Olecranon apophysis fractures in children with osteogenesis imperfecta revisited. J Pediatr Orthop 2002;22(6):745–750.

SUGGESTED READINGS

Al-Salem AH, Ahmed HA, Qaisruddin S, et al. Osteomyelitis and septic arthritis in sickle cell disease in the eastern province of Saudi Arabia. Int Orthop 1992;16(4):398–402.
Arnold WD, Hilgartner MW. Hemophilic arthropathy. Current concepts of pathogenesis and management. J Bone Joint Surg Am 1977;59(3):287–305.
Aronstam A, Browne RS, Wassef M, et al. The clinical features of early bleeding into the muscles of the lower limb in severe haemophiliacs. J Bone Joint Surg Br 1983;65(1):19–23.
Aur RJ, Westbrook HW, Riggs W Jr. Childhood acute lymphocytic leukemia. Initial radiological bone involvement and prognosis. Am J Dis Child 1972;124(5):653–654.
Bell RS, Mankin HJ, Doppelt SH. Osteomyelitis in Gaucher disease. J Bone Joint Surg Am 1986;68(9):1380–1388.
Bembi B, Ciana G, Mengel E, et al. Bone complications in children with Gaucher disease. Br J Radiol 2002;75(Suppl 1):A37–A44.
Beredjiklian PK, Drummond DS, Dormans J, et al. Orthopaedic manifestations of chronic graft-versus-host disease. J Pediatr Orthop 1998;18(5):572–575.
Berquist TH, Brown ML, Fitzgerald RH Jr, et al. Magnetic resonance imaging: application in musculoskeletal infection. Magn Reson Imaging 1985;3(3):219–230.
Bilchik TR, Heyman S. Skeletal scintigraphy of pseudo-osteomyelitis in Gaucher disease. Two case reports and a review of the literature. Clin Nucl Med 1992;17(4):279–282.
Bizot P, Witvoet J, Sedel L. Avascular necrosis of the femoral head after allogenic bone marrow transplantation. A retrospective study of 27 consecutive THAs with a minimal 2-year follow-up. J Bone Joint Surg Br 1996;78(6):878–883.
Bleyer WA. Acute lymphoblastic leukemia in children. Advances and prospectus. Cancer 1990;65(Suppl 3):689–695.
Bos GD, Simon MA, Spiegel PG, et al. Childhood leukemia presenting as a diaphyseal radiolucency. Clin Orthop 1978;(135):66–68.
Brady RO, Schiffmann R. Enzyme-replacement therapy for metabolic storage disorders. Lancet Neurol 2004;3(12):752–756.
Brant EE, Jordan HH. Radiologic aspects of hemophilic pseudotumors in bone. Am J Roentgenol Radium Ther Nucl Med 1972;115(3):525–539.
Brawley OW, Cornelius LJ, Edwards LR, et al. NIH consensus development statement on hydroxyurea treatment for sickle cell disease. NIH Consens State Sci Statements 2008; 25(1):1–30.
Castaneda VL, Parmley RT, Bozzini M, et al. Radiotherapy of pseudotumors of bone in hemophiliacs with circulating inhibitors to factor VIII. Am J Hematol 1991;36(1):55–59.
Chang CH, Stanton RP, Glutting J. Unicameral bone cysts treated by injection of bone marrow or methylprednisolone. J Bone Joint Surg Br 2002;84(3):407–412.
Cho HS, Oh JH, Kim HS, et al. Unicameral bone cysts: a comparison of injection of steroid and grafting with autologous bone marrow. J Bone Joint Surg Br 2007;89(2):222–226.
Clarke JT, Amato D, Deber RB. Managing public payment for high-cost, high-benefit treatment: enzyme replacement therapy for Gaucher disease in Ontario. CMAJ 2001;165(5): 595–596.
Clausen N, Gotze H, Pedersen A, et al. Skeletal scintigraphy and radiography at onset of acute lymphocytic leukemia in children. Med Pediatr Oncol 1983;11(4):291–296.
Connelly S, Kaleko M. Gene therapy for hemophilia A. Thromb Haemost 1997;78(1):31–36.
Dalton GP, Drummond DS, Davidson RS, et al. Bone infarction versus infection in sickle cell disease in children. J Pediatr Orthop 1996;16(4):540–544.

Davidson JK, Tsakiris D, Briggs JD, et al. Osteonecrosis and fractures following renal transplantation. Clin Radiol 1985;36(1):27–35.

Dietrich AM, James CD, King DR, et al. Head trauma in children with congenital coagulation disorders. J Pediatr Surg 1994;29(1):28–32.

Dormans JP, Drummond DS. Pediatric hematogenous osteomyelitis: new trends in presentation, diagnosis, and treatment. J Am Acad Orthop Surg 1994;2(6):333–341.

Epps CH, Bryant DD Jr, Coles MJ 3rd, et al. Osteomyelitis in patients who have sickle cell disease. Diagnosis and management. J Bone Joint Surg Am 1991;73(9):1281–1294.

Erken EH. Radiocolloids in the management of hemophilic arthropathy in children and adolescents. Clin Orthop 1991;264:129–135191 476. Ferris B, Walker C, Jackson A, et al. The orthopaedic management of hypophosphataemic rickets. J Pediatr Orthop 1991; 11(3):367–373.

Figueroa ML, Rosenbloom BE, Kay AC, et al. A less costly regimen of alglucerase to treat Gaucher disease. N Engl J Med 1992;327(23):1632–1636.

Gallagher DJ, Phillips DJ, Heinrich SD. Orthopedic manifestations of acute pediatric leukemia. Orthop Clin North Am 1996;27(3):635–644.

Goldblatt J, Sacks S, Beighton P. The orthopedic aspects of Gaucher disease. Clin Orthop 1978;(137):208–214.

Golding JS, Maciver JE, Went LN. The bone changes in sickle cell anaemia and its genetic variants. J Bone Joint Surg Br 1959;41-B:711–718.

Gregosiewicz A, Wosko I, Kandzierski G. Intra-articular bleeding in children with hemophilia: the prevention of arthropathy. J Pediatr Orthop 1989;9(2):182–185.

Hann IM, Gupta S, Palmer MK, et al. The prognostic significance of radiological and symptomatic bone involvement in childhood acute lymphoblastic leukaemia. Med Pediatr Oncol 1979;6(1):51–55.

Hutcheson J. Peripelvic new bone formation in hemophilia. Report of three cases. Radiology 1973;109(3):529–530.

Idy-Peretti I, Le Balc'h T, Yvart J, et al. MR imaging of hemophilic arthropathy of the knee: classification and evolution of the subchondral cysts. Magn Reson Imaging 1992;10(1): 67–75.

Ingram GI, Mathews JA, Bennett AE. Controlled trial of joint aspiration in acute haemophilic haemarthrosis. Ann Rheum Dis 1972;31(5):423.

Itzchaki M, Lebel E, Dweck A, et al. Orthopedic considerations in Gaucher disease since the advent of enzyme replacement therapy. Acta Orthop Scand 2004;75(6):641–653.

Journeycake JM, Miller KL, Anderson AM, et al. Arthroscopic synovectomy in children and adolescents with hemophilia. J Pediatr Hematol Oncol 2003;25(9):726–731.

Keeley K, Buchanan GR. Acute infarction of long bones in children with sickle cell anemia. J Pediatr 1982;101(2):170–175.

Kisker CT, Burke C. Double-blind studies on the use of steroids in the treatment of acute hemarthrosis in patients with hemophilia. N Engl J Med 1970;282(12):639–642.

Koc A, Gumruk F, Gurgey A. The effect of hydroxyurea on the coagulation system in sickle cell anemia and beta-thalassemia intermedia patients: a preliminary study. Pediatr Hematol Oncol 2003;20(6):429–434.

Koren A, Garty I, Katzuni E. Bone infarction in children with sickle cell disease: early diagnosis and differentiation from osteomyelitis. Eur J Pediatr 1984;142(2):93–97.

Koren A, Segal-Kupershmit D, Zalman L, et al. Effect of hydroxyurea in sickle cell anemia: a clinical trial in children and teenagers with severe sickle cell anemia and sickle cell beta-thalassemia. Pediatr Hematol Oncol 1999;16(3):221–232.

Krill CE Jr, Mauer AM. Pseudotumor of calcaneus in Christmas disease. J Pediatr 1970;77(5): 848–855.

Kumari S, Fulco JD, Karayalcin G, et al. Gray scale ultrasound: evaluation of iliopsoas hematomas in hemophiliacs. AJR Am J Roentgenol 1979;133(1):103–105.

Lokiec F, Ezra E, Khermosh O, et al. Simple bone cysts treated by percutaneous autologous marrow grafting. A preliminary report. J Bone Joint Surg Br 1996;78(6):934–937.

Lurie A, Bailey BP. The management of acute haemophilic haemarthroses and muscle haematomata. S Afr Med J 1972;46(21):656–659.

Manco-Johnson MJ, Abshire TC, Shapiro AD, et al. Prophylaxis versus episodic treatment to prevent joint disease in boys with severe hemophilia. N Engl J Med 2007;357(6): 535–544.

Masera G, Carnelli V, Ferrari M, et al. Prognostic significance of radiological bone involvement in childhood acute lymphoblastic leukaemia. Arch Dis Child 1977;52(7):530–533.

Meikle PJ, Fietz MJ, Hopwood JJ. Diagnosis of lysosomal storage disorders: current techniques and future directions. Expert Rev Mol Diagn 2004;4(5):677–691.

Miller EH, Flessa HC, Glueck HI. The management of deep soft tissue bleeding and hemarthrosis in hemophilia. Clin Orthop 1972;82:92–107.

Miller JH, Ortega JA, Heisel MA. Juvenile Gaucher disease simulating osteomyelitis. AJR Am J Roentgenol 1981;137(4):880–882.

Moneim MS, Gribble TJ. Carpal tunnel syndrome in hemophilia. J Hand Surg Am 1984; 9(4):580–583.

Mota RM, Mankin H. Use of plain radiography to optimize skeletal outcomes in children with type 1 Gaucher disease in Brazil. J Pediatr Orthop 2007;27(3):347–350.

Norris CF, Smith-Whitley K, Mcgowan KL. Positive blood cultures in sickle cell disease: time to positivity and clinical outcome. J Pediatr Hematol Oncol 2003;25(5):390–395.

Nuss R, Kilcoyne RF, Geraghty S, et al. Utility of magnetic resonance imaging for management of hemophilic arthropathy in children. J Pediatr 1993;123(3):388–392.

Oppenheim WL, Galleno H. Operative treatment versus steroid injection in the management of unicameral bone cysts. J Pediatr Orthop 1984;4(1):1–7.

Park JS, Ryu KN. Hemophilic pseudotumor involving the musculoskeletal system: spectrum of radiologic findings. AJR Am J Roentgenol 2004;183(1):55–61.

Pettersson H, Ahlberg A. Computed tomography in hemophilic pseudotumor. Acta Radiol Diagn (Stockh) 1982;23(5):453–457.

Powars DR, Chan LS, Hiti A, et al. Outcome of sickle cell anemia: a 4-decade observational study of 1056 patients. Medicine (Baltimore) 2005;84(6):363–376.

Rodriguez-Merchan EC. Pathogenesis, early diagnosis, and prophylaxis for chronic hemophilic synovitis. Clin Orthop 1997;343:6–11.

Rosenthal RL, Graham JJ, Selirio E. Excision of pseudotumor with repair by bone graft of pathological fracture of femur in hemophilia. J Bone Joint Surg Am 1973;55(4):827–832.

Ruderman RJ, Poehling GG, Gray R, et al. Orthopedic complications of renal transplantation in children. Transplant Proc 1979;11(1):104–106.

Samuda GM, Cheng MY, Yeung CY. Back pain and vertebral compression: an uncommon presentation of childhood acute lymphoblastic leukemia. J Pediatr Orthop 1987;7(2): 175–178.

Scaglietti O. Sull' azione osteogenice dell'acetato di prednisolone. Boll Soc Tosco-Umbra Chir 1974;35:1.

Scaglietti O, Marchetti PG, Bartolozzi P. Final results obtained in the treatment of bone cysts with methylprednisolone acetate (depo-medrol) and a discussion of results achieved in other bone lesions. Clin Orthop Relat Res 1982(165):33–42.

Schulte CM, Beelen DW. Avascular osteonecrosis after allogeneic hematopoietic stem-cell transplantation: diagnosis and gender matter. Transplantation 2004;78(7):1055–1063.

Septimus EJ, Musher DM. Osteomyelitis: recent clinical and laboratory aspects. Orthop Clin North Am 1979;10(2):347–359.

Shindell R, Huurman WW, Lippiello L, et al. Prostaglandin levels in unicameral bone cysts treated by intralesional steroid injection. J Pediatr Orthop 1989;9(5):516–519.

Shirkhoda A, Mauro MA, Staab EV, et al. Soft-tissue hemorrhage in hemophiliac patients. Computed tomography and ultrasound study. Radiology 1983;147(3):811–814.

Sitarz AL, Berdon WE, Wolff JA, et al. Acute lymphocytic leukemia masquerading as acute osteomyelitis. A report of two cases. Pediatr Radiol 1980;9(1):33–35.

Silverstein MN, Kelly PJ. Leukemia with osteoarticular symptoms and signs. Ann Intern Med 1963;59:637–645.

Skaggs DL, Kim SK, Greene NW, et al. Differentiation between bone infarction and acute osteomyelitis in children with sickle-cell disease with use of sequential radionuclide bone-marrow and bone scans. J Bone Joint Surg Am 2001;83-A(12):1810–1813.

Specht EE. Hemoglobinopathic salmonella osteomyelitis. Orthopedic aspects. Clin Orthop 1971;79:110–118.

Stark JE, Glasier CM, Blaisier RD, et al. Osteomyelitis in children with sickle cell disease: early diagnosis with contrast-enhanced CT. Radiology 1991;179(3):731–733.

Tsai P, Lipton JM, Sahdev I, et al. Allogenic bone marrow transplantation in severe Gaucher disease. Pediatr Res 1992;31(5):503–507.

Umans H, Haramati N, Flusser G. The diagnostic role of gadolinium enhanced MRI in distinguishing between acute medullary bone infarct and osteomyelitis. Magn Reson Imaging 2000;18(3):255–262.

Unkila-Kallio L, Kallio MJ, Eskola J, et al. Serum C-reactive protein, erythrocyte sedimentation rate, and white blood cell count in acute hematogenous osteomyelitis of children. Pediatrics 1994;93(1):59–62.

Vichinsky EP, Haberkern CM, Neumayr L, et al. A comparison of conservative and aggressive transfusion regimens in the perioperative management of sickle cell disease. The Preoperative Transfusion in Sickle Cell Disease Study Group. N Engl J Med 1995;333(4):206–213

Wei SY, Esmail AN, Bunin N, et al. Avascular necrosis in children with acute lymphoblastic leukemia. J Pediatr Orthop 2000;20(3):331–335.

Wilson DJ, Green DJ, Maclamon JC. Arthrosonography of the painful hip. Clin Radiol 1984; 35(1):17–19.

Yandow SM, Lundeen GA, Scott SM, et al. Autogenic bone marrow injections as a treatment for simple bone cyst. J Pediatr Orthop 1998;18(5):616–620.

Zimran A, Elstein D, Kannai R, et al. Low-dose enzyme replacement therapy for Gaucher disease: effects of age, sex, genotype, and clinical features on response to treatment. Am J Med 1994;97(1):3–13.

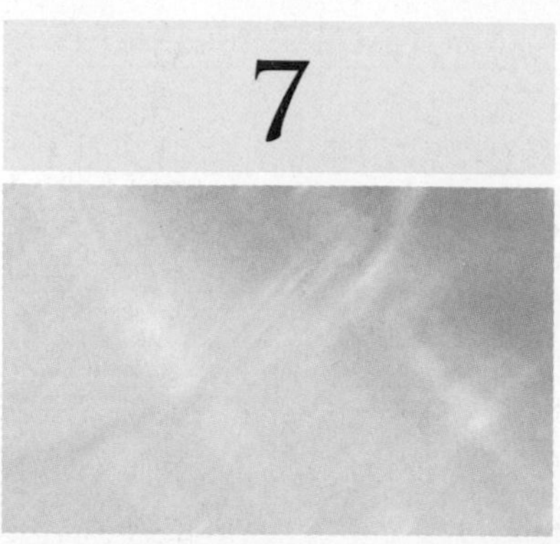

7 THE ORTHOPAEDIC RECOGNITION OF CHILD MALTREATMENT

Richard M. Schwend, Laurel C. Blakemore, and Lisa Lowe

INTRODUCTION 192
Epidemiology 192
Overview 193

THE RISK FACTORS FOR CHILD ABUSE 193
The Home at Risk 193
The Child at Risk 194
The Risk for Child Abuse That Occurs in a Medical Setting 194
The Risk for Sexual Abuse 195

OBTAINING THE HISTORY 195
The Orthopaedic Interview 195
Documentation Requirements 197

PHYSICAL EXAMINATION 197
Soft Tissue Injuries 197
Burns 198
Abusive Head Trauma 199
Abdominal Injuries 202
Genital Injuries 203

FRACTURES IN CHILD ABUSE 204
Overview 204
Dating Fractures 205
The Skeletal Survey 206
Skull Fractures 208
Extremity Fractures 208
Classic Metaphyseal Lesion of Child Abuse 209
Rib Fractures 209
Spinal Fractures 211

LABORATORY STUDIES 212

MULTIDISCIPLINARY APPROACH 212

THE DIFFERENTIAL DIAGNOSIS 212
Osteogenesis Imperfecta 214
Temporary Brittle Bone Disease 216
Sudden Unexpected Death in Infancy 216

POSTEMERGENCY ROOM TREATMENT AND LEGAL REPORTING REQUIREMENTS 217
The Orthopaedic Surgeon's Legal Role in Nonaccidental Injury 217
Disposition Following Custody Hearings 219

PREVENTION OF CHILD ABUSE 219

INTRODUCTION

Epidemiology

Child maltreatment is any act or failure to act on the part of a parent or caretaker which results in death, serious physical or emotional harm, sexual abuse or exploitation; or an act or failure to act which presents an imminent risk of serious harm.[253] Child maltreatment includes all types of abuse and neglect that occur among children under the age of 18 years.[202] The four common types of maltreatment include physical, sexual, and emotional abuse as well as child neglect.[121] Neglect is the most frequently encountered type of child maltreatment.[75] Recent terminology for a battered child, physical abuse, or child abuse include nonaccidental injury (NAI), inflicted injury, or nonaccidental trauma (NAT).[88]

The National Child Abuse and Neglect Data System

(NCANDS) was initiated in response to Public Law 93-247 to collect and analyze child abuse statistics.[254] NCANDS documents that the epidemic of child abuse continues to worsen in the United States, with approximately 3.6 million reports (47.8 per 1000 children) filed in federal fiscal year 2006 compared to 1.2 million in 1982.[253] Approximately one quarter of these children who received an investigation were confirmed to have been abused or neglected. This represents a victim rate of 12.1 per 1000, totaling 905,000 U.S. children in 2006.[253] Approximately 60% of confirmed cases are neglect, 16% physical abuse, 10% sexual abuse, and 7% psychologic abuse.[202] Reports by professionals are more likely to be confirmed. Whereas children under the age of 4 years are at greatest risk for maltreatment, the victim rate is highest for infants, totaling 91,278 (23.2 per 1000 population over the course of less than 1 year). Newborns in the first week of life may be at the highest risk, with a total of 29,881 reported cases, 70% of which were reported for neglect.[202]

One of every 1000 abused children in the United States die.[125] Three children die of abuse or neglect each day,[201] with 50% to 80% having evidence of a prior injury. The World Health Organization estimates that 57,000 children worldwide die from maltreatment, while more than 1500 die in the United States.[149] However, mortality rates are commonly underestimated.[65,108] Nineteen percent of maltreatment fatalities occur in infants; whereas, newborns in the first week of life have greatest risk of death.[202] Abuse is second only to sudden infant death syndrome (SIDS) for mortality in infants 1 to 6 months of age and second only to accidental injury in children older than 1 year. The incidence of abuse is three times that of developmental dysplasia of the hip or clubfoot. Fortunately, there is some evidence that abusive fracture incidence may be decreasing over the past 24 years, possibly due to a general increase in recognition of child maltreatment and more preventive services available to families.[158]

The minimal annual cost of child abuse in the United States is approximately 9 billion dollars,[57] but additional costs, both direct and indirect, exist. The estimated national cost of child abuse for the child welfare system is 14 billion dollars, law enforcement 24 million, and the court system 341 million.[201] The long-term social costs of child abuse are substantial: one third of the victims of child abuse grow up to be seriously dysfunctional, neglectful, or abusive parents; one third are at high risk for eventually becoming abusive parents; and only one third do not repeat the destructive patterns they were exposed to as children.[188,234] Exposure to adverse childhood experiences has a high probability of both recent and lifetime depressive disorders.[56] Direct and indirect total estimated national costs of child abuse, including special education for learning disorders of abused children, maternal mental and health care, legal costs of juvenile delinquency, lost productivity to society of abused and neglected children as unemployed adults, and later adult criminality of abused and neglected children in 2007 is 103.8 billion dollars.

The orthopaedist becomes involved in the care of 30% to 50% of abused children.[6] Early recognition by the orthopaedist is critical because children returned to their homes after an unrecognized episode of child abuse have a 25% risk of serious reinjury and a 5% risk of death.[212] Jenny and Isaac[123] have noted a three fold increased mortality rate of children who have been listed on state abuse registry for all types of abuse. The mortality rate is highest for those who are physically abused, especially infants.[123]

Overview

In 1946, Caffey[43] described 6 infants with long-bone fractures, chronic subdural hematomas, and intraocular bleeding without a history of trauma to explain the injuries; however, he did not speculate about the etiology of the children's injuries. Although his work is cited as the first report in the English literature of child abuse, it was Ambroise Tardieu, the prolific French forensic physician, who during the mid 1800s described in great detail the condition of sexual abuse in children, as well as the battered child syndrome.[151] In 1953, Silverman[222] characterized the unique metaphyseal fractures found in abused children and clearly emphasized that these were due to nonaccidental trauma. Altman and Smith[8] published the first series in the orthopaedic literature of injuries caused by child abuse in 1960. General public awareness of child abuse increased with the 1962 publication of a report by Kempe et al.[130] characterizing the problems as the battered child syndrome. In 1974, Caffey[44] introduced the term "whiplash-shaken infant syndrome" to the literature to emphasize the etiology of subdural hematomas in infants caused by shaking episodes. In 1974, Congress acknowledged the national importance of the prevention of child abuse by the passage of the Child Abuse Prevention and Treatment Act.[254] Since pediatric personnel and hospital-based child protection teams must be aware of reporting requirements for child maltreatment, there are published guidelines for the establishment and management of hospital-based child protection teams.[180]

THE RISK FACTORS FOR CHILD ABUSE

The Home at Risk

In assessing where child abuse may occur, households in turmoil from marital separation, job loss, divorce, family death, housing difficulties, or financial difficulties are more likely to have abusive episodes.[77] One of the most important predictors of abuse is the presence of a nonrelated adult living in the household. Compared to single parent families, death due to child abuse was noted to be 50 times higher in households that had unrelated adults; the perpetrator was the unrelated adult in 83.9% of these cases.[213] Families with two unplanned births are 2.8 times more likely to have an episode of child abuse than families with no unplanned births.[265] Stepparents, babysitters, boyfriends, relatives, and even larger siblings may be abusers.[4,109,185] Young, unmarried mothers are more likely to have an infant death from intentional injury, with a peak incidence of 10.5 intentional deaths per 10,000 live births.[218] In a study of 630 fractures in 194 abused children, the perpetrator was identified in 79% of cases.[230] Sixty-eight percent of the perpetrators were male, and 45% of the time the biologic father was responsible. Abused infants were significantly younger (4.5 months of age) when a male had abused the child, than when a female was the abuser (10 months of age). The parents of battered children may themselves have been abused when they were children.[95] High levels of parental stress and belief in corporal punishment are associated with child abuse.[64] Parental substance abuse, whether alcohol or other drugs, makes child abuse more likely.[105] The risk of physical abuse is fivefold more likely with maternal cocaine use.[255] Violence in the home is not directed solely toward the child. In one study of families with substantiated child abuse, 30% of the mothers had also been abused.[45] Although the youngest, poorest, most socially isolated, and economically frustrated caretakers are the most likely to act violently toward their children,[260] any adult from any social or economic level may abuse a child.[4] Daycare may be an at-risk environment in situations when there is poor supervision of the child caregivers. However, in an analysis of 1362 deaths in daycare, home daycare was a much higher risk than was a formal institutional daycare due to less training and supervision of the adult caregivers and the absence of adult witnesses.[261] Primary parental predictors of child abuse are listed in Table 7-1.

The Child at Risk

Most reported cases of child abuse involve children younger than 3 years of age.[91] In one report of abused children,[29] 78% of all fractures reported were in children younger than 3 years of age and 50% of all fractures occurred in children younger than 1 year of age. Infants younger than 1 year are especially at risk for infant homicide, the most severe form of child abuse.[70,136] The problem may be more widespread than suspected. In one report,[33] covert video recordings of adults attending their children who were hospitalized for suspicious illness documented 14 separate instances of caretaker attempts to cause upper airway obstruction. An infant may present to the emergency room dead or near dead after an apparent "life threatening event." In these cases, it is important to be open to all diagnostic possibilities and use a multidisciplinary team approach to the evaluation.[182] Possible explanations for these events include SIDS, metabolic disease, cardiac disease, infection, as well as accidental or nonaccidental suffocation. Up to 11% of infants treated in the emergency room for apparent life-threatening events are later confirmed to be victims of child abuse.[37] First-born children, premature infants, stepchildren, and disabled children are at a greater risk for child abuse, as are twins and children of multiple births.[29] Benedict et al.,[30] in a longitudinal study of 500 disabled children followed from birth to age 10 years, documented a 4.6% incidence of physical abuse. The most severely disabled children were less likely to be abused, whereas marginally functioning children were at greater risk, with parental frustration considered to be a factor.

TABLE 7-1 Parental Predictors of Child Abuse

General
- Unrelated adult living in the home*
- Parent history of child abuse
- Divorce or separation of mother's parents
- Maternal history of being separated from mother, parental alcohol, or drug abuse
- Maternal history of depression
- Child attends a home daycare

Mother
- Age less than 20 years
- Lower educational achievement
- History of sexual abuse
- Child guidance issues
- Absent father during childhood
- History of psychiatric illness

Father
- Age less than 20 years
- Lower educational achievement
- Child guidance issues
- History of psychiatric illness

*Fifty times the risk of death during infancy due to nonaccidental trauma.
Adapted from: Sidebotham P, Golding J. The ALSPAC Study Team: child maltreatment in the "Children of the Nineties"—a longitudinal study of parental risk factors. Child Abuse Negl 2001;25:1177–1200, with permission.

The Risk for Child Abuse That Occurs in a Medical Setting

Children who are repeatedly presented by parents for medical assessment of vague illness and have a history of multiple diagnostic or therapeutic procedures for unclear reasons are at risk for having a form of child abuse known as "child abuse that occurs in the medical setting."[233] This term has replaced the previously used "Münchhausen Syndrome by Proxy,"[174] which was named after Baron von Münchhausen, an eighteenth-century mercenary whose exaggerated tales of adventure were viewed with great suspicion. In child abuse that occurs in a medical setting, children become the victims of this adult behavior when misguided parents fabricate a wide range of illnesses for their children, often subjecting them to needless diagnostic workups and treatment.[174] Symptoms of the child's "illness" are based on an imaginary medical history given by the parent, with signs of the illness either simulated or induced by the parent. For example, a child may be brought into the emergency room by a parent with a complaint of vomiting. This complaint may either be a total fabrication by the parent or the parent may simulate the complaint by producing "vomitus" from some source as proof of illness. In one report, bloodstained material was presented by a caretaker as proof of a child's "gastrointestinal bleeding," but DNA testing revealed that the source was actually from the caretaker.[256] Conjunctivitis from a caustic agent placed on an infant by a caretaker has been reported.[27] Children have been given clozapine and clonidine by caretakers to simulate illness.[26] A parent has caused vomiting in a child by the administration of salt[173] or ipecac. In other extreme cases, a rodenticide-induced coagulopathy was seen in a 2-year-old child,[17] a deliberate self-induced preterm labor was caused by a parent,[93] and another repeatedly gave insulin to a 1-year-old child.[174] Over half of reported cases of child abuse in the medical setting involve induced symptoms, whereas 25% involve a combination of both simulation and induction of symptoms.[37] In less severe cases, the parent's anxiety can cause them to obtain unnecessary and harmful or potentially harmful medical care, even though the parent believes that he or she is acting in the child's best interest. Physicians need to be vigilant so as not to be an unwary participant of this form of child maltreatment.

The biologic mother is almost always the perpetrator of child abuse in the medical setting,[209] but men can be responsible.[172] Caretakers often have a medical background: 35% to 45% are nurses, 5% are medical office workers, 3% are social workers, and 1% are orderlies.[209] The perpetrator of the child's illness denies the knowledge of its etiology; however, the acute signs and symptoms of the child's illness will resolve if the syndrome is recognized and the child is separated from the parent.[209]

Follow-up of families with this disorder is crucial. Failure to diagnose this condition places a child at risk for either serious long-term sequelae or death in approximately 9% of cases.

The diagnosis of child abuse in the medical setting remains difficult. Healthcare workers must have a high degree of suspicion when children present with repetitive illness with no physiologic explanation. Physicians need to recognize that their perseverance in finding an explanation to a child's illness may contribute to the inflicted harm to the child. When possible, a pediatrician with experience in child abuse should become involved in the evaluation as well as the hospital or community-based multidisciplinary child protection team. A thorough review of all the medical care received by the child and communication among team members is necessary to establish the diagnosis and to recognize patterns of parental behavior that may harm the child. Covert in-hospital video surveillance (CVS) of caretakers with their children may be a valuable means to substantiate or disprove this diagnosis. Hall et al.[97] reported that CVS with audio surveillance allowed diagnosis in 56% of patients monitored and was supportive of the diagnosis in another 22% of children. The approach is expensive, is not covered by third party payers, and so is infrequently used. Effective treatment generally involves assuring the safety of all children in the family and addressing ongoing dysfunctional family behaviors.

The Risk for Sexual Abuse

Although the orthopaedist usually considers child abuse in the context of fractures and other obvious injuries, an increasingly important situation to recognize is sexual abuse. It is estimated that 25% of abused or neglected children have been sexually abused.[130] Physically abused children have a 1 in 6 chance of being sexually abused, whereas sexually abused children have a 1 in 7 risk of being physically abused.[110] Children living with nonbiologic parents or with caretakers who are substance abusers are most at risk. The child usually discloses sexual abuse under three types of circumstances: the child may have just experienced an argument with the abuser and may "accidentally" reveal the existence of the abusive relationship, the child is permanently separated from the abuser, or the abusive adult is shifting attention to a younger sibling.[259] Up to 25% to 83% of children with a disability have been reported to be abused.[239]

OBTAINING THE HISTORY

The history is critical in the diagnosis of child abuse, which is a team effort with the consulting pediatrician, social worker and other personnel from the hospital's child protective team, child protective services worker, law enforcement, and the appropriate consulting service. The orthopaedic surgeon is involved if the child has an injury to the musculoskeletal system. The history is usually taken in the chaotic environment of a busy emergency room, so it is important to find a quiet area for the interview to be conducted calmly and with minimal distractions. The orthopaedic surgeon should focus on the facts of the injury, including the child's ability to get into the injury scenario, details of when, where, and what happened, the child's position and action before the injury, position after the injury, how the child reacted, and how promptly the caregiver responded appropriately. Such detailed interview skills rarely are taught during residency training. In a survey of pediatric residents, 42% of them had 1 hour or less in training for detection of child abuse, and most orthopaedic residents likely have even less.[76] In a study comparing the documentation of physical abuse between 1980 and 1995 in a teaching hospital, very little improvement was noted.[161] Little progress has been made in how frequently physicians inquire about basic historic information such as the timing of the injury and who were the witnesses.[13] The type of hospital that an injured child visits also influences the likelihood that a diagnosis of abuse will be made.[251,252] General hospitals were less likely to diagnose a case of abuse compared to children's hospitals. Use of a structured clinical form can increase the information collected to support the diagnosis of child abuse.[21] Having received recent continuing medical education focused on child abuse was the most important factor for a physician to properly recognize and report child abuse.[84] Precise documentation in child abuse is vital for reasons beyond medical care. Although most subpoenas for testimony by physicians in child abuse cases do not result in courtroom appearances,[193] all documentation in child abuse cases may become evidence in courtroom proceedings. Thus, detailed records are helpful to all in courtroom testimony by physicians.[100] The history needed to document child abuse is termed the investigative interview, is a team effort, and should be led by members of the child protective team and the police when potential child abuse is investigated.

The Orthopaedic Interview

When involved, the orthopaedic surgeon performs a detailed musculoskeletal history and physical examination to characterize the features and mechanism of the obvious injury and to discover evidence of additional undocumented injuries. The interview documents the history (or the lack of history) of the presenting injury and attempts to uncover enough details about the child's life so that plausible scenarios can be evaluated that might explain the injury. The team should determine how the injured child lives, find out which family members, friends, or other caretakers have access to the child, and how likely it is that they might have contributed to the child's injuries. A detailed history of injury is obtained individually from each adult family member in a private setting. If the patient and siblings can communicate, they should be interviewed separately from the parents and other members of the family. The location where the injury occurred and which individuals were actually present are documented. The interviewer should follow a systematic review of symptoms: what happened, who was there, when the injury was recognized, and how long before medical treatment was sought. To avoid provoking emotions, any additional soft tissue or skeletal trauma discovered should be brought up at the end of the interview for explanation once the presentation injury has been thoroughly discussed.

Delay in seeking medical care for an injured child is very suggestive of child abuse.[77] An infant who has sustained abusive head trauma (AHT) typically will develop immediate neurologic change and will invariably show symptoms within a few hours.[35] For a child with head trauma, a caregiver's story that there was a long period after the injury in which the child had no symptoms is suspect. When central nervous injury in child abuse is significant or severe, it is immediately symptomatic; thus, the last caretaker who witnessed the reported injury or found the child immediately after the injury is highly suspected of being the perpetrator.[23] Inconsistencies are not challenged during the interview. Leading questions are avoided in favor of open-end questions. Medical terms should be explained in plain English, with care taken to avoid medical jargon. More plausible explanations for the injury are not volunteered. Open prompts can enhance the interview.[190] If the injury was observed, the caregiver should be able to give a detailed description of the injury mechanism that fits the energy of the fracture and the clinical picture.[198,199] The crucial questions to be answered are not only whether the given history of trauma is sufficient to explain the severity of injury, but what other possible scenarios could explain the injury if the volunteered explanation is not plausible. This requires obtaining a working knowledge of the child's environment, which team members can obtain by asking specific, detailed questions (Table 7-2).

When interviewing injured children, it is essential to be as gentle as possible, asking how they got hurt rather than who hurt them. Questions asked should be appropriate for the child's age. The child's account of what he or she was doing at time of injury should be compared with the accounts of the adult witnesses. If possible, the siblings of the injured child should be interviewed because they also are at risk for child abuse. Nonvisual cues during the interview should be noted (see Table 7-2).

TABLE 7-2 Child Abuse: Investigative Interview

Environmental Issues
Primary Caretakers
- Unsupervised
- Responsible for feeding, discipline, toilet training
- Easy or difficult child

Home Environment
- Place of residence
- Living conditions
- Adults employed or unemployed
- Sleeping arrangements
- Marital status of parents
- Boyfriend or girlfriend of single parent
- Substance abuse

Home Stress Level
- Recent job loss
- Marital problems (separation or divorce)
- Death in the family
- Housing problems
- Inadequate funds for food

Parental or Caregiver Responses and Attitudes
- Evasive, not readily responsive to questions
- Irritated by questioning
- Contradictory in responses
- Hostile and critical toward child
- Fearful of losing child or criminal prosecution, or both
- Unconcerned about child's injuries
- Disinterested in treatment and prognosis
- Intermittently unavailable for interview (without valid reason)
- Unwilling to give medical information
- Unwilling to give consent for tests
- Indifferent to child's suffering (seldom touches or looks at child)

Selected data from Akbarnia BA. The role of the orthopaedic surgeon in child abuse. In: Morrissy RP, ed. Lowell and Winter's Pediatric Orthopaedic. Philadelphia: JB Lippincott; 1990; and Green FC. Child abuse and neglect: a priority problem for the private physician. Pediatr Clin North Am 1975;22: 329–339, with permission.

To make the diagnosis of child abuse, the orthopaedic surgeon or child abuse team must determine if the history of trauma is adequate to explain the severity of injury.[53] This should be based on experience in the care of fractures with knowledge of their mechanisms of injury and special insight into the types of trauma most likely to cause significant injury. In addition, it is extremely important to have knowledge of the developmental abilities of a child when a caretaker states the child's injuries are self-inflicted.[125] For example, if the parents explain that a 4-month-old infant's femoral fracture occurred in a fall while the infant was standing alone, this history is inconsistent with the child's developmental ability.

Details given as the reason for the injury should be carefully considered. Although it is not unusual for a young child to sustain an accidental fall, it is unusual to sustain a serious injury from that fall alone. Infants fall from a bed or a raised surface during a diaper change fairly frequently. In a study of 536 normal infants,[148] nearly 50% of them had fallen accidentally from an elevated surface, usually after the first 5 months of life, when the children were able to roll over and were more active. Significant injury in such falls is, however, extremely rare. Combining two studies of 782 children younger than 5 years of age who accidentally fell off an elevated surface, such as bed or sofa, reveals that injuries were limited to three clavicle fractures, six skull fractures, one humeral fracture, and one subdural hematoma.[106,146] In another report, a much higher rate of fracture was seen in falls from furniture with 98% having fractures, mostly in the upper extremity, due to the child catapulting during play activity rather than sustaining a simple short height fall.[107] More severe injuries occur in falls from greater heights. Stairway falls usually result in low-energy injuries, but there is increased risk of injury if the child is being carried by the caregiver. In a report of 363 stairway injuries,[131] 10 were infants who were dropped by their caretakers and four of those sustained skull fractures. In patients 6 months to 1 year of age, 60% were using walkers at the time of the stairway injury. Only 4% of patients had extremity fractures and 1% had skull fractures. Reported short height falls (<1.5 meters) are rarely documented to cause death.[52] A review of child mortality in infants and young children in California showed the following causes of death/1 million children/year: prematurity 165, congenital malformation 316, neoplasms 33, respiratory 38, accidents 121, homicide 22, and short-height falls 0.48 (a total of six cases, all occurring in the home). Although short-height falls are a rare cause of death, there has been no reported case of short-fall death in an institution-type daycare setting, where witnesses are typically present. A fatally injured child from a reported short-height fall at home must receive expert postmortem investigation for child abuse.

Additional information about the child and the family may be obtained by a review of past medical records or by contacting the patient's primary physician and social workers who may have been involved with the family. The physician or social worker should be asked if there has been any previous pattern of injury, illness, ingestion of objects or medications, or noncompliance with healthcare recommendations; whether the family is receiving counseling or other support from any community groups; and whether the family has any previous involvement with child protective services or law enforcement.[77]

Documentation Requirements

Careful documentation is critical. Chart notes may later be presented as evidence in court for either custodial hearings or criminal trial.[161] Defending inaccurate or partial chart notes in court can be extremely embarrassing as well as placing the child at additional risk. Each account should be recorded in as much detail as possible, using quotation marks for exact quotes and specifying who is giving the history. Particularly with crucial answers, the exact question preceding the response should be documented. In a study of subsequent confessions, the initial history, although not consistently true, did reveal some elements of truth.[83] In addition, the general emotional state of the individual providing the account, as well as the individual's reaction to emotionally charged questions should be documented to assist in later evaluation of the credibility of the account. If the family wishes to change their story after the initial account, no changes should be made to the earlier record, but an addendum should be placed detailing the new account. The completed record should include several specific items such as the timing and mechanism of the injury, who found the child, timing of events, family history of underlying conditions such as osteogenesis imperfecta, radiographs, and documentation of protective services involvement.

PHYSICAL EXAMINATION

After the initial musculoskeletal evaluation for acute fracture assessment, a detailed physical examination should follow, systematically evaluating from head to toes, to detect any signs of additional acute or chronic injury. Acute and subacute fractures may cause local tenderness and swelling, whereas chronic fractures may produce swelling from the presence of callus and clinical deformity from malunion. Radiographs are obtained to confirm clinically suspected fractures. A skeletal survey must be performed in children under 2 years of age when there is reasonable suspicion of abuse[12]: it should be considered an extension of the physical examination for this age group. A thorough examination should focus on the body areas commonly involved in child abuse including the skin, central nervous system, abdomen, and genitalia. Careful evaluation for signs of previous injury is useful since 50% of verified abuse cases show evidence of prior abuse.[95]

Soft Tissue Injuries

In addition to examination of the soft tissue around the acute fracture site for swelling and bruising, the patient's entire body should be systematically evaluated to detect acute and chronic soft tissue trauma. Deliberate soft tissue injuries are present in 81% to 92% of abused patients,[91,171,241] making them the most common abuse-related physical examination finding. The types of skin lesions commonly encountered include bruises, welts, abrasions, lacerations, scars, and burns.

The number and location of bruises relates to the child's development. Seventeen percent of mobile infants, 53% of toddlers, and most school children have bruises.[166] Young infants have a much lower prevalence of accidental bruising (seen in 1%) compared to mobile toddlers.[166] Accidental bruises in babies are also typically noted over bony prominences.[47] The toddler may have multiple accidental bruises over bony prominences such as the chin, brow, knees, and shins.[4,212,237] Bruises on the back of the head, neck,[4] arms, legs, buttocks, abdomen, cheeks, or genitalia may be suspicious for abuse, although accidental bruises can also occur in all these locations.[8] Accidental bruising of the face is much less common and should be carefully evaluated.[166] In the dentistry literature, in a series of 266 children suspected of being abused, Jessee and Rieger[124] reported that bruises were the most common soft tissue injury, with the most common facial. In nonabused children, only 7% had accidental soft tissue injuries of the face and head, with the peak incidence of 17% seen in toddlers; whereas, soft tissue injuries were present on the lower extremities and buttocks in 31% of children and on the upper extremities in 9%.[207] In a study of 1467 patients seen for reasons other than trauma at a medical center over a 1-year period, 76.6% had at least one skin lesion of recent onset, 17% had at least five, 4% had at least 10, and fewer than 1% had more than 15 recent lesions.[152] In children less than 9 months of age, skin lesions were uncommon and were concentrated on the head and face, while in children over 9 months of age, the skin lesions were mostly on the lower extremities.[152] Although any number of bruises may be present in any child, the location and configuration of the bruises and the mobility of the child, taken together with the rest of the medical and social history determines the suspicion for abuse (Fig. 7-1 and Table 7-3).

Although the configuration of abusive bruises may resemble the implement used to inflict the injury, the soft tissue injuries of abuse are weapon specific in fewer than 10% of patients.[171] The weapons used to abuse children often include belt buckles, staplers, ropes, switches, coat hangers, ironing cords, and the open or closed human hand.[126,240] Bruises inflicted by an open hand may appear on the face or a flat area of skin and grasp marks may appear as ovoid lesions when the fingertips are

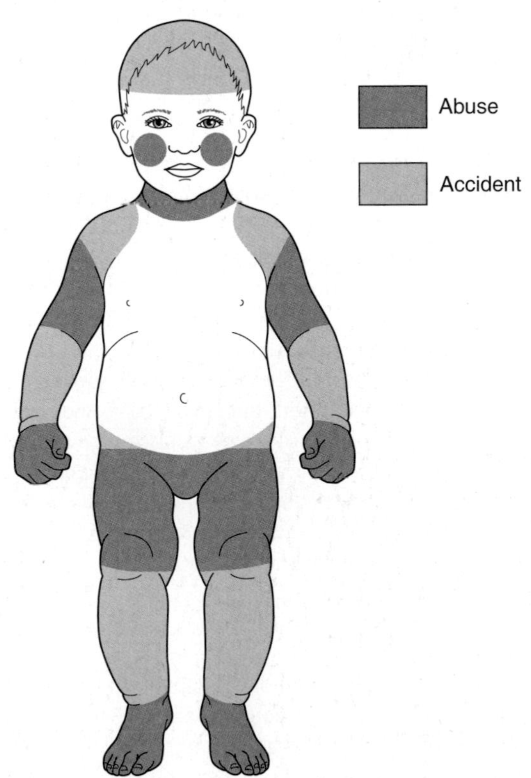

FIGURE 7-1 Schematic illustrates distribution of abusive versus accidental bruising. (Redrawn from original courtesy of Samir Abedin, MD.)

TABLE 7-3 Evaluating Bruising in a Child—Implications for Practice

A bruise must never be interpreted in isolation and must always be assessed in the context of medical and social history, developmental stage, explanation given, full clinical examination, and relevant investigations.

Patterns of bruising that are suggestive of physical child abuse

- Bruising in children who are not independently mobile
- Bruising in babies
- Bruises that are seen away from bony prominences
- Bruises to the face, back, abdomen, arms, buttocks, ears, hands
- Multiple bruises in clusters
- Multiple bruises of uniform shape
- Bruises that carry the imprint of implement used or a ligature

Maguire S, Mann MK, Sibert J, et al. Are there patterns of bruising in childhood which are diagnostic or suggestive of abuse? A systematic review. Arch Dis Child 2005;90:182–186.

deeply embedded in the extremities or the shoulders of the child during extreme shaking.[115] The injury pattern and the severity of the bruising depend on the amount of force used, how directly the instrument made contact, and the specific type of implement used to strike the child.[115]

Other types of skin lesions may be noted. Welts are more complex skin lesions in which swelling accompanies bruising from injury through lashing or whipping. Lacerations, scars, and burns are seen in older abused children, while bruises are seen in all ages.[171] Like bruises, the laceration configuration can resemble the weapon used to inflict the injury on the child. Although minor lacerations around the eye are fairly common, multiple scars from either lacerations or burns are suspicious.[203,247] Displaced fractures may have associated bruising, with or without abuse. Deep bruising after abuse can be so extensive that rhabdomyolysis can occur, detectible by urine dipstick.[196]

The age of a bruise can be roughly estimated by a change in color over the 2 to 4 weeks following injury, with fading of the lesions beginning at the periphery. Acute contusions are blue or reddish purple, gradually changing to green, then to yellow, with final resolution as a brownish stain as hemoglobin is finally broken down.[258] Langlois and Gresham[154] noted that a yellowish bruise must be older than 18 hours; a red, purple, blue, or black coloration of the bruise may be present from 1 hour after injury to resolution; red is always present in bruises regardless of the age; and bruises of identical age and etiology on the same person may be of different appearances and may change at different rates. A deep contusion may take some time to rise to the skin surface because of intervening fascial planes and thus delay its appearance. While the color of a bruise may roughly aid in determining the length of time it has been present, dating bruises based on appearance should be done with caution.[214,232]

Natural skin lesions should not be mistaken for bruises. Mongolian spots, more common in black or Asian infants, are deep-blue pigmented areas that are present on the lower back at birth, usually just proximal to the buttocks.[16] They do not change in color and gradually resolve as the child matures.[115] Cultural differences should be considered when unusual skin lesions are noted. Vietnamese children may be subjected to the folklore medical practice known as cao-gio, which places scratches and bruises on the back of the trunk and may be mistaken for child abuse.[43] Other conditions can mimic inflicted bruising: eczema, coagulation disorders, vasculitis, impetigo, Ehlers-Danlos syndrome, vascular malformations, dye stains, and others.[241] In cases where bruising or bleeding is the only finding of abuse, a family history for bleeding diathesis, using established protocols for hematologic evaluation for an underlying bleeding disorder and involvement of a hematologist, is advised before child maltreatment is diagnosed.[155,244]

Burns

Burns are found in approximately 20% of abused patients[91] and are most likely to occur in patients younger than 3 years of age.[171] Burn evaluation should include configuration, approximate percentage of body surface area, location, distribution, uniformity, length of time the child was in contact with the burning agent, temperature of the burning agent, and presence or absence of splash marks when hot liquids are involved.[115]

Scalds are the most frequent type of abusive burns and are caused either by a spill or an immersion.[147] Accidental spill burns are generally located on the trunk and proximal upper extremities (Fig. 7-2). Most accidental pour or spill burns occur on the front of the child, but accidental burns can also occur on the back as well. In accidental flowing liquid burns, the injury usually has an arrowhead configuration in which the burn becomes shallower and more narrow as it moves downward, and there may be splash marks surrounding the lesion.[115]

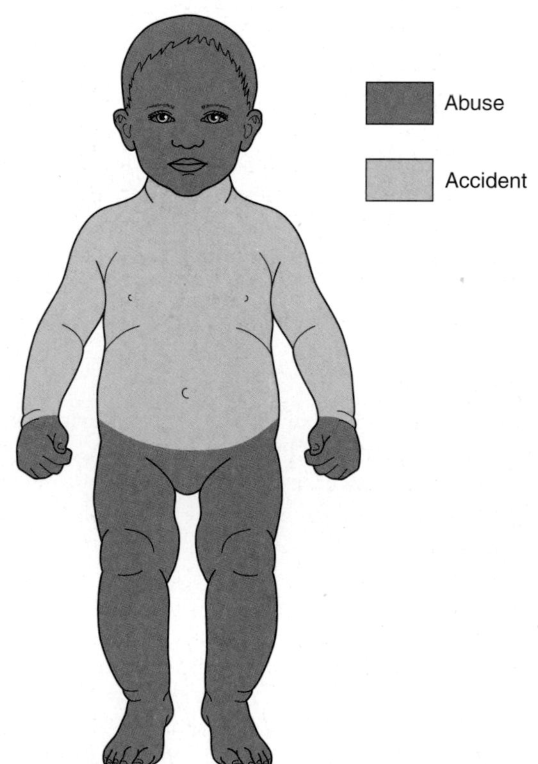

FIGURE 7-2 Schematic illustrates location of accidental versus abusive burns. Note the buttock and lower extremity distribution of nonaccidental immersion burns compared to thoracic distribution accidental burns. (Redrawn from original courtesy of Samir Abedin, MD.)

The pattern in accidental burns may also be indicative of flowing water.[205] Abuse should be suspected when deep second- or third-degree burns are well demarcated with circumferential definition. The typical child abused by scalding burns is an undernourished 2-year-old child with 15% to 20% of the body involved, usually the buttocks, and has a 10% to 15% mortality rate from secondary sepsis.[205]

In accidental hot water immersion, an indistinct stocking or glove configuration may be seen with varying burn depths and indistinct margins. In deliberate immersion burns such as occurs when a child's buttocks are immersed in hot water, the burn demarcation has uniform depth and a well-demarcated water line.[115] The gluteal crease of the buttocks may be spared, giving a doughnut-like appearance to the burn. In accidental hot water immersion, the child is uniformly scalded about the lower extremities as the legs are quickly extended by the child to climb out of the water, but in deliberate, abusive immersion the child is lowered into the water and instinctively flexes the hips and knees, thus sparing the popliteal area.[91]

Burns can be inflicted by many objects commonly found in the household. Intentional burns by cigarettes are circular, deeply excavated, and sometimes repetitive, usually about 8 mm in diameter.[115] Impetigo may resemble scalds or cigarette burns, but is more superficial. Severe eczema may mimic burns suspicious for child abuse.[104] Contact with heated objects may cause burns of unique shape that allow identification of their etiology. Children accidentally grasping curling irons sustain burns of the palms, whereas burns on the dorsum of the hands are more suspicious for abuse.[125] Hair dryers can be used to inflict burns on children, and full-thickness skin burns can result from the heated air or from contact with the grill up to 2 minutes after it has been turned off.[200] Abuse burns have also been inflicted by stun guns.[89] These devices deliver a high-voltage impulse of up to 100,000 volts at 3 to 4 mA, incapacitating the individual and leaving hypopigmented burn scars on the skin 0.5 cm apart. Circular scars about the wrists may be due to rope burns when children are restrained for beatings.[125] Full-thickness skin burns have been reported in small children who were placed in microwave ovens.[7] Certain folklore practices may cause lesions simulating abusive burns. Round burns on the abdomen, buttock, or between the thumb and forefinger of Southeast Asian children may be due to a variant on the Chinese medical practice of moxibustion. Folk medical practitioners' burn balls of the moxa herb on the surface of the skin for therapeutic purposes, and both cigarettes and yarn have been similarly used in refugee camps. The knowledge of these practices may help to avoid inappropriate accusations of child abuse.[81]

The orthopaedic surgeon must examine and carefully document all soft tissue injuries that are present before treating acute fractures. Casts applied in the treatment of fractures, especially a spica cast, may obscure potentially incriminating skin lesions and will preclude other members of the child advocacy team from being able to identify or document them. Photographs taken to document skin lesions must be done before cast placement.

Abusive Head Trauma

Several terms have been used to describe head trauma related to abuse, including the older term shaken baby syndrome (SBS) and the preferred newer terms AHT,[35] inflicted traumatic brain injury (ITBI), inflicted head trauma (IHT), or nonaccidental head trauma.[182] These terms have been used to describe a form of physical nonaccidental trauma in infants with a triad of subdural hemorrhage, retinal hemorrhage, and encephalopathy occurring with an inconsistent or inappropriate history, commonly associated with other inflicted injuries.[101] The American Academy Committee on Child Abuse and Neglect recommends the term "abusive head trauma" to be used in the medical record. Recent excellent review articles discuss fatal AHT[90] and the diagnosis of pediatric head trauma in general.[116,117] A child under the age of 3 years who suffers head trauma from abuse is more likely to have sustained a noncontact injury mechanism (acceleration-deceleration or shaking) resulting in deeper brain injury, cardiorespiratory compromise with diffuse cerebral hypoxia-ischemia, and a worse outcome at 6 months than a child who is accidentally injured.[117] Head injuries can be from indirect noncontact forces such as in shaking or from direct contact from a blow to the head such as occurs when the child is thrown against an object. Indirect trauma is felt to be responsible for the most severe injuries, although the actual injury may be from both mechanisms. Symptoms typically occur early rather than later, although secondary or delayed brain injury may occur with edema and the brain's neurotoxic injury response.

In physical abuse, the most common cause of death is head trauma.[204] In Kleinman's[139] classic postmortem study of 31 infants with an average age of 3 months, head trauma was the cause of death in 18. For children less than 2 years of age dying from a traumatic brain injury, 80% of the deaths are from abuse, with the highest incidence at 6 months.[88] For a child with AHT, the mortality rate is approximately 20%, and survivors have a higher rate of permanent and significant disability than is seen with accidental trauma.[128]

When an infant presents with altered mental status, AHT should be suspected (Table 7-4). Jenny et al.[122] reported that 31% of cases of SBS were misdiagnosed on initial presentation to the emergency room. While early diagnosis of an infant with AHT is essential, primary prevention is the most important new development to occur nationally. There is correlation between peak incidence of infant crying and peak incidence of AHT that occurs 4 to 6 weeks later, suggesting that repeat and prior injuries occur.[24] Dias et al.,[73] utilizing an early postnatal hospital-based program for new parents to learn about shaking impact syndrome and how to appropriately deal with an inconsolable infant, found a 47% decrease in SBS, whereas intervention programs after abuse is recognized have much less success.[163]

As a general principle, a typical short fall in the home is highly unlikely to cause generalized central nervous system (CNS) injury or subdural or retinal hemorrhage, although isolated skull fracture or epidural hemorrhage may be seen. The young infant who is not developmentally mobile enough to cause a fall from a height, having a relatively large head, immature brain, and weak neck muscles, is very vulnerable to the whiplash effects of inflicted violent shaking (Fig. 7-3). In 25% to 54% of confirmed cases of AHT, the abuser described an indirect mechanism by shaking the infant without the head contacting a surface, with resulting immediate onset of symptoms.[34,229] Indirect trauma is responsible for the most severe injuries. There is sudden angular acceleration and deceleration with associated rotation of the head and neck in relation to the thorax, producing inertial shear strain deformation and disrup-

TABLE 7-4 Criteria for Categorizing the Etiology of Head Injuries

Category	Criteria
Noninflicted	Cases in which the child's primary caregiver described an accidental head injury event that was developmentally consistent, historically consistent with repetition over time, could be linked to the child's acute clinical presentation for traumatic cranial injuries, and occurred in the absence of any noncranial injuries considered moderately or highly specific for abuse* Cases in which an accidental head injury event was witnessed independently and could be linked to the child's acute clinical presentation for traumatic cranial injuries (e.g., motor vehicle accident)
Inflicted	Cases in which the child's primary caregiver admitted abusive acts that could be linked to the child's acute clinical presentation for traumatic cranial injuries Cases in which an independent witness verified abusive acts that could be linked to the child's acute clinical presentation for traumatic cranial injuries Cases in which a child not yet cruising or walking became clearly and persistently ill with signs of acute cardiorespiratory compromise† linked to his or her traumatic cranial injuries while in the care of a primary caregiver who denied any knowledge of a head injury event Cases in which the child's primary caregiver provided an explanation for the child's head injury event that was clearly developmentally inconsistent with the parents' description of their child's developmental capabilities Cases in which the child's primary caregiver provided an explanation for the child's head injury event that was highly inconsistent with repetition over time Cases in which the head-injured child also revealed at least two noncranial injuries considered moderately or highly specific for abuse*
Undetermined	Cases meeting criteria for both inflicted and noninflicted etiology Cases not meeting any criteria for either inflicted or noninflicted etiology

*Including classic metaphyseal lesion(s); fractures of the rib(s), scapula, sternum, spinous process(es), or digit(s); vertebral body fracture(s) or dislocation(s); epiphyseal separation(s); noncranial bruising; abrasion(s) or laceration(s) in location(s) other than the knees, shins, or elbows; patterned bruise(s) or dry contact burn(s); scalding burns with uniform depth, clear lines of demarcation, and a paucity of splash marks; intra-abdominal injuries; retinal hemorrhages described by an ophthalmologist as dense, extensive, covering a large surface area of the retina, or extending to the periphery of the retina; and retinoschisis diagnosed by an ophthalmologist.
†Including breathing difficulty, respiratory distress, infrequent respirations, apnea, or cyanosis; clinical manifestations of shock, delayed capillary refill, or cardiac arrest; any requirement for mouth-to-mouth breathing, bag-mask ventilation, intubation, chest compressions, rapid volume expansion, or epinephrine therapy; occurring at the scene of injury, during transport, in the emergency department, or at the time of hospital admission; documented by medical personnel or reported by the child's primary caregiver.
(Source: Hymel KP, Makoroff KL, Laskey AL, et al. Mechanisms, clinical presentations, injuries, and outcomes from inflicted vs noninflicted head trauma during infancy: results of a prospective, multicentered, comparative study. Pediatrics 2007;119(5): 922–929.)

tion leading to diffuse injury.[23] Whereas accidental trauma causes subdural hemorrhage from the translational forces of an impact, inflicted head trauma from rotational and shearing forces may result in more diffuse subdural or intrahemispheric hemorrhage.[112]

The eye of a young infant has a soft sclera: the globe can more easily deform during shaking. This causes vitreo-retinal traction leading to direct hemorrhage in the retina and in the optic nerve sheath.[262] Fundoscopic examination confirms and documents retinal optic nerve as well as orbital hemorrhage.[44] Retinal hemorrhages of abuse classically are multilayered, more anterior, closer to the ora serrata, and are numerous and bilateral. Retinoschisis is a splitting of the layers of the macula forming a cystic cavity caused by shearing and pulling forces of the strong vitreous attachments to the retinal surface and is classic for AHT.[211] Unilateral retinal hemorrhages may occur in 10% to 16% of cases, so unilateral does not rule out SBS.[15] Although retinal hemorrhages resulting from normal vaginal birth are present in 34% of newborns, these resolve by 16 days of age.[113]

Previous clinical studies on SBS do not typically address injury to the cervical spine, so it is not known how frequently the spine also is injured with this mechanism.[20] In very young infants (2 to 3 months of age), forces may be directed to the upper cervical spine leading to spinal cord injury without obvious radiographic abnormality (SCIWORA), cervicomedullary junction cord injury, apnea, and cardiorespiratory arrest.[92,117] Direct head injuries may also occur when the child's head is slammed onto a soft surface such as a mattress.[78] On impact, deceleration forces approaching 400 Gs may occur, tearing the bridging vessels between the skull and the brain and producing intracranial hemorrhage and cerebral edema. Skull fractures are rare unless the child is thrown onto a hard object.

A complete neural examination is required for any child suspected of being abused. This should include assessment of the child's mental status, motor function, sensation, reflexes, and gait, if possible. Any abnormal findings warrant further investigation. Also included should be a dilated fundoscopic examination by an ophthalmologist looking for retinal hemorrhages. For the child with acute neurologic findings suspicious for AHT, a

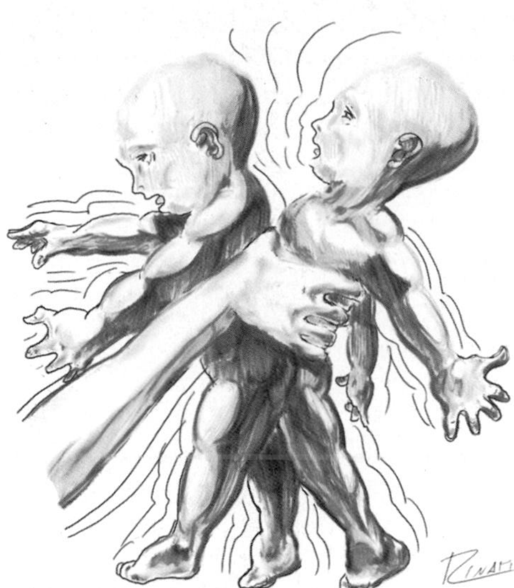

FIGURE 7-3 Illustration of acceleration-deceleration injury sustained by a shaken infant. Shaken infants suffer whiplash injuries due in part to their disproportionately large heads in relation to their bodies. This mechanism is believed responsible for the common association of subdural hematomas, retinal hemorrhages, and posterior rib fractures. (Artwork courtesy of Gholamreza Zinati, MD.)

noncontrast computed tomography (CT) scan is done to evaluate for conditions that may benefit from prompt medical and neurosurgical treatment, such as intracranial hemorrhage-acute parenchymal, subarachnoid, subdural, or epidural (Fig. 7-4). If the head CT scan includes upper cervical spine-associated injuries, pre-existing bony conditions such as Klippel Feil syndrome or occipital cervical assimilation may be detected.[111] Anteroposterior and lateral skull and spinal radiographs are always included as part of the routine skeletal survey for the child less than 2 years of age and should be performed for any aged child with suspected AHT (Table 7-5). CT scans alone may occasionally miss in-plane axial skull fractures. However, these fractures are usually easily seen on the accompanying skeletal survey. Although fine-cut three-dimensional CT skull reconstructions may reveal subtle skull fractures, they may increase delivered radiation by up to 30% over standard head CT. Since the infant is 15 times more sensitive to the effects of radiation than is an adult, fine-cut CT should not be the primary imaging modality for detecting skull fractures. Magnetic resonance imaging (MRI) is best used to fully assess various intracranial pathology and has become the imaging modality of choice for evaluating asymptomatic, nonacute parenchymal brain lesions and for fully documenting the abuse. MRI is also effective for diagnosis of related conditions in the cervical spine, including ligamentous injury and intra-spinal injuries such as SCIWORA.

TABLE 7-5 Standard Skeletal Survey Radiographic Protocol

Minimum required views
- Anteroposterior views of entire skeleton
- Dedicated views of hands and feet
- Lateral views of appendicular skeleton—skull and spine

Imaging also suggested
- Oblique views of the ribs
- Oblique views of the hands and feet

Optional useful images
- Lateral views of the joints-wrists ankles and knees
- Orthogonal views of any fractures found

Adapted from American Academy of Pediatrics. Section on Radiology. Diagnostic imaging of child abuse. Pediatrics 2000;105(6):1345–1348.

Even in abused children without neurologic findings or retinal hemorrhages, occult head injury should always be suspected. At risk children with obvious neurologic findings should be urgently screened with head CT for acute pathology. At risk children without obvious neurologic findings are best imaged initially with MR brain imaging (ACR guidelines).[12] MRI is sensitive for diagnosing small parenchymal hemorrhages[78] and offers the highest sensitivity and specificity for the diagnosis of subacute and chronic head injuries.[12] Diffusion and susceptibility weighted imaging sequences are extremely sensitive for detecting subtle hypoxic-ischemic brain injury and parenchymal hemorrhage[194,238] and are routinely included in imaging protocols when available. MR venography may be used if venous sinus thrombosis is suspected. MR spectroscopy may detect lactate levels, an indicator of prognosis.[82]

Infants with acute head injuries may have fever, bulging fontanelles, and macrocephaly. Paresis may be present, and reflexes may be increased. Older infants and children may have subdural hemorrhages and musculoskeletal injuries.[92] Classic infant AHT with multilayered retinal hemorrhages and acute subdural hematomas has been noted in an autopsy series of four older children between 2.5 and 7 years of age.[211] Cerebral edema may be lethal,[58] so emergency neurosurgical consultation may be needed. Barnes and Krasnokutsky[23] reviewed the radiographic evaluation of a young child with a suspected nonaccidental head injury, including mimicking of conditions, such as accidental injury from short falls, acute CNS infections, coagulopathies, venous thrombosis, metabolic abnormalities, and neoplasms. The diagnosis of these mimics may require

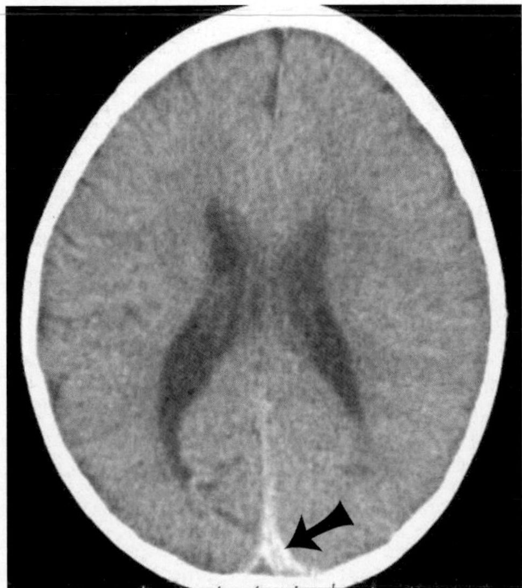

FIGURE 7-4 Interhemispheric subdural hematoma in an 8-month-old female presenting with seizures due to nonaccidental trauma. Axial CT image shows high attenuation blood along the left aspect of the posterior falx (*arrow*).

TABLE 7-6 Differential Diagnosis of Subdural Hemorrhage in Infants and Children

- Accidental or abusive trauma
- Birth trauma (in child <6 weeks of age)
- Congenital malformations (e.g., arteriovenous malformations) in older children
- Coagulopathies (vitamin K deficiency in the newborn, disseminated intravascular coagulation, hemophilia)
- Infection (septicemia, meningitis, necrotizing encephalitis)
- Metabolic disorders (glutaric aciduria type 1, OI, Menke kinky hair syndrome)
- Tumor—very rare. Seen in older child.
- Vasculitis (Kawasaki disease)
- Venous sinus thrombosis with hemorrhagic infarct

From Sirotnak AP, Grigsby T, Krugman RD. Physical abuse of children. Pediatr Rev 2004;25:264–277.

more extensive workup before a diagnosis of AHT is confirmed (Table 7-6).[224] Oehmichen et al.[186] have presented very practical principles for diagnosing AHT (Table 7-7).

Disability after AHT is frequent and ranges from mild to severe. Common late sequelae after AHT include developmental delays, sensory and motor deficits, feeding difficulties, recurrent seizures, attention deficits, and intellectual, educational, and behavioral dysfunctions.[117] In a long-term outcome study, 69% of children had an abnormality and 40% had severe dysfunction.[22] Approximately 50% had visual impairment and another 50% had behavior disorder.[22] Some children seemed normal until 5 years after the inflicted injury, then showed learning disorders, so long-term follow-up is essential. Repeat abuse when AHT is not recognized and the child is returned to the home is too common.[92]

TABLE 7-7 Principles of Diagnosing Inflicted Traumatic Brain Injury in Children

1. Simple injuries are caused by simple mechanism; extreme violence (blows, shaking, impact) is necessary to cause life-threatening injuries.
2. Life-threatening injuries are characterized by the rapid onset of serious clinical symptoms (coma, circulatory and respiratory arrest) without a lucid interval.
3. If a parent or caregiver attributes a severe traumatic brain injury in a child to a household fall, the claim should be regarded as suspect until proven otherwise.
4. If a child is injured by a fall, the parent or caregiver will immediately seek medical care and express extreme anxiety regarding the fate of the child. But if a child is injured by abuse, the perpetrator often waits to see if the child will recover spontaneously.
5. The diagnosis of shaking trauma is rarely based on a confession, more on the implausibility of an explanation. Shaking is hardly ever witnessed
6. The following symptom complex is highly specific to shaking trauma:
   - Intracranial hemorrhage, especially subdural or subarachnoid
   - Retinal hemorrhage
   - Dural bleeding of the cervical cord
   - Bleeding of the throat and neck muscles
   - Gripping marks on the thorax and shoulders
   - Symptoms of recurrent trauma

From Oehmihen M, Meissner C, Saternus KS. Fall or shaken: traumatic brain injury in children caused by falls or abuse at home—a review on biomechanics and diagnosis. Neuropediatrics 2005;36:240–245.

Abdominal Injuries

After AHT, trauma to the abdomen is the second most common reason for death from abuse.[37] In a review of the National Pediatric Trauma Registry, 16% of all blunt abdominal trauma in children 0 to 4 years of age was attributable to child abuse.[250] The pediatric thorax and pelvis are very compliant. The abdominal muscles are pliable with little subcutaneous and omental fat, so there is less protection to the internal abdominal, chest, and pelvic organs. Whereas shaken infants sustain head trauma, toddlers receive abdominal injuries as they are more often punched and beaten. Inflicted abdominal trauma may be due to beatings with the hand, fist, or when the child is thrown into a fixed object. The compliant pediatric abdominal wall does not absorb much of the injury energy, so abdominal bruising is present in only 12% to 15% of major intra-abdominal injury cases.[115] Children with inflicted injuries are more likely to be of a younger age, malnourished, have a pancreatic or hollow viscous injury, have an associated traumatic brain injury, and have higher mortality compared to victims of accidental abdominal injury.[251]

Children with abdominal injury from child abuse may have a wide range of symptoms depending on the organ involved and the severity of the injury. Fever, vomiting, anemia, abdominal distention, localized involuntary spasm, and bowel sounds may be absent.[185] The liver is the most commonly injured solid organ. With a damaged liver, right shoulder pain from hemidiaphragm irritation (Kehr sign) may be associated with abdominal pain and fatal hypovolemic shock.[248] Liver function tests may reveal occult liver injury. In one study,[60] elevated aspartate aminotransferase, alanine aminotransferase, and lactic dehydrogenase enzyme levels were useful markers for occult liver lacerations in abused children who had false-negative abdominal examinations. Blows to the abdomen often injure the pancreas as it is violently compressed against the spine. Blunt pancreatic injury due to nonaccidental injury commonly presents with contusion, transaction, or laceration, all of which are associated with pancreatitis and elevated blood amylase. A pancreatic pseudocyst may form, causing obstructive symptoms several weeks after initial injury.[115] Splenic and renal injuries, rare in child abuse, have a 45% risk of mortality from hemorrhagic or septic shock if care is delayed.[63]

Hollow organ injuries to the upper or lower gastrointestinal tract or bladder are infrequent in accidents but common in child abuse, particularly in the younger child (mean age 2.5 years).[156] Hollow organ abuse injuries, as is true for most abdominal injuries due to nonaccidental injury, present for medical attention late, with an inconsistent or vague history. In a young child with unexplained hollow organ injury, abuse should be suspected and investigated.

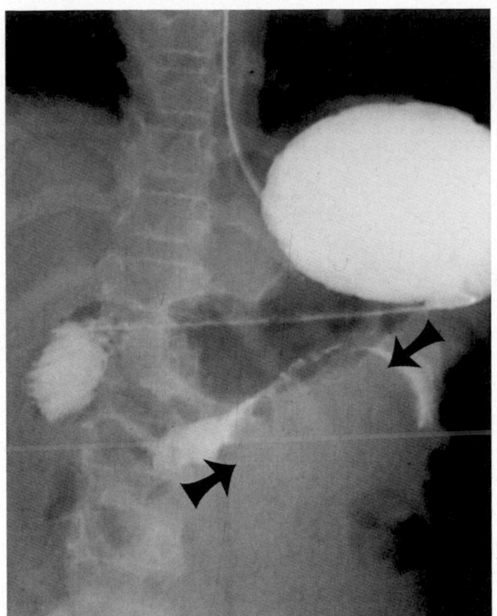
A

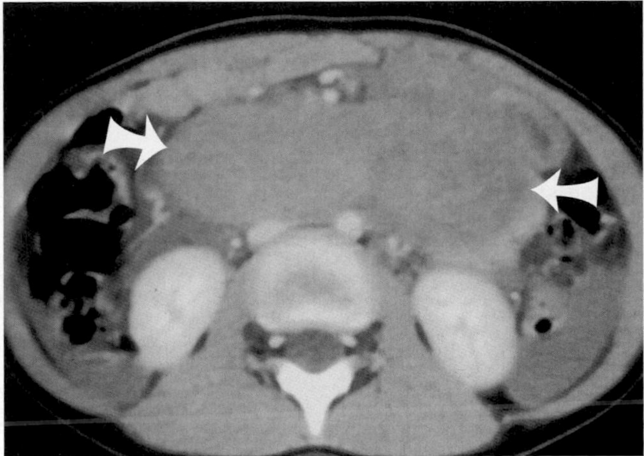
B

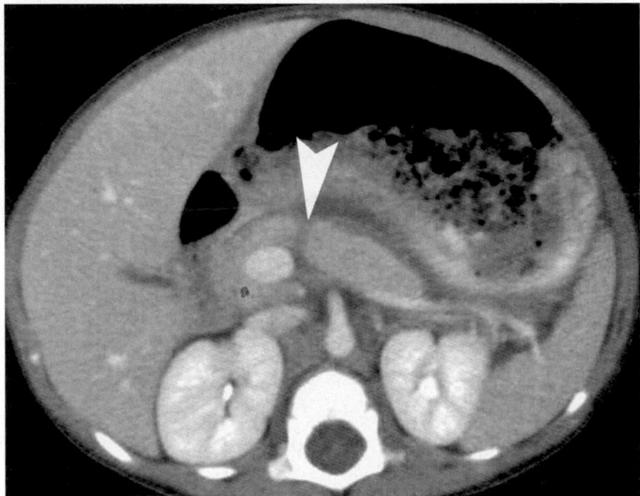
C

FIGURE 7-5 Duodenal hematoma and pancreatic transection in a 4-year-old male presenting with bilious vomiting due to nonaccidental abdominal trauma. **A.** Fluoroscopic upper gastrointestinal image reveals a large, well-defined defect within the third portion of the duodenum (*arrows*). Axial contrast enhanced CT images at the level of the duodenum **(B)** and pancreas **(C)** show a large hyperattenuated retroperitoneal duodenal hematoma (*arrows*) and a linear low attenuation defect (*arrowhead*) in the pancreatic head. Also noted is peripancreatic fluid.

Child abuse is the leading cause of duodenal injury in children less than 4 years of age.[249] Intramural duodenal hematoma may cause obstruction and bilious vomiting.[115] CT, ultrasound imaging, and/or upper gastrointestinal radiography may be diagnostic (Fig. 7-5). More severe trauma may cause duodenal avulsion or transection with nausea, vomiting, and clinical acute abdomen.[162] Frequently, the radiologist first suggests the possibility of nonaccidental trauma by finding a duodenal hematoma with no history by the caregiver of trauma. Blunt trauma to the abdomen may also cause intestinal perforation, usually involving the small intestine, and the physical examination may suggest peritonitis. Previously, plain radiographs were used to search for free air in suspected hollow organ injuries; however, only 19% of radiographs were diagnostic.[39] Today, CT with intravenous contrast enhancement is used for the trauma evaluation. Hollow organ injuries classically manifested with free air on the plain radiographs; however, CT imaging better reveals free fluid, focal bowel wall thickening, inflammation, or ileus. Associated spine injuries, such as Chance flexion-distraction lumbar spine fracture, should be evaluated.

The Academy of Pediatrics Section on Radiology[12] recommends CT scans with nonionic intravenous contrast to define injury to abdominal organs. Contrast should not be used if there is a history of iodine allergy or renal failure. The use of oral contrast is debatable with CT scans and may place the patient at risk of aspiration. Ultrasound and upper gastrointestinal series are most often used to evaluate duodenal hematoma. When abdominal injury is suspected in an abused child, the hematocrit and hemoglobin levels are checked, the child is typed and crossmatched for blood, and two large intravenous lines are placed in anticipation for surgical treatment. General surgery consultation is obtained. The overall mortality rate associated with visceral injury in child abuse is 40% to 50%.[60] In fatal cases with liver injury, hepatic glycogen staining may be helpful in establishing time of death for legal reasons.[243] Occult abdominal trauma is easily missed, so a high index of suspicion with serial abdominal examination and liberal use of abdominal CT should be used in the suspected abused child.[112]

Genital Injuries

Sexual abuse should always be considered when evaluating a physically abused child. Specific guidelines for the evaluation for sexual abuse were revised and published in 2005.[2] Children who have been sexually abused can have symptoms of bed wetting, fecal incontinence, painful defecation, pelvic pain, abdominal pain, vaginal itching and bleeding, sexually transmitted diseases, and pregnancy in postmenarche adolescents. Sexually transmitted diseases found in abused children include gonorrhea, syphilis, chlamydia, trichomoniasis, and lymphogranuloma venereum. Although the percentage of sexually assaulted children with obvious physical trauma to the genitalia is low, failure to document such findings is a serious matter. Sexual abuse is always a criminal offense and must be reported to legal authorities. The physical signs of sexual abuse, including genital trauma, sexually transmitted diseases, or presence of sperm, are present in only 3% to 16% of verified sexual assaults,[28,223] but even this minority of patients will be undiagnosed if sexual abuse is not considered when a child presents with musculoskeletal injury resulting from abuse.

The orthopaedic surgeon should be aware of proper procedure for handling suspected sexual abuse, but is not expected to manage this evaluation. When sexual abuse is suspected, consultation with an experienced medical team will assure competent assessment of the child's physical, emotional, and behavioral needs, manage reporting and legal requirements, and interact with appropriate professionals to provide comprehensive treatment and follow-up.[2] The child's genitalia should always be examined and documented in a chaperoned setting by an appropriate physician consultant such as a pediatrician or a gynecologist in children with physical abuse. If the sexual assault occurred within 72 hours of evaluation, then a rape kit must be used by the evaluating physician or nurse examiner to provide medical evidence of the attack.[150] However, detecting semen on examination for forensic evidence decreases markedly after 24 hours.[192]

Patterns of injury that suggest, but are not specific for, sexually motivated assault include bruises, scratches, and burns around the lower trunk, genitalia, thighs, buttocks, and upper legs, including the knees. Pinch or grip marks may be found where the child was held. Attempted or achieved penetration may involve the mouth, vagina, or anus.[110] Sexually abused boys may have poor rectal sphincter tone, perianal scarring, or urethral discharge. Female genital examination findings that are consistent with sexual abuse include chafing, abrasion, or bruising of the inner thighs or genitalia, distortion of the hymen, decreased or absent hymen, scarring of the external genitalia, and enlargement of the hymenal opening.[9] The size of the transverse hymenal orifice does not correlate as a marker of child abuse.[118] The examination of the female genitalia can be normal even when there has been penetration, because hymen tissue is elastic and there can be rapid healing. In a study of 36 adolescent pregnant girls evaluated for sexual abuse, only 2 of 36 had genital changes diagnostic of penetrating trauma, suggesting that injuries either may not occur or may heal completely.[129] There also is a wide variability of appearance of normal female genitalia,[46,58] but posterior hymen disruption is rare and should raise suspicion for abuse.[31]

FRACTURES IN CHILD ABUSE

Overview

After skin lesions, fractures are the second most common physical presentation of abuse. Fractures, documented on plain radiographs or CT, are present in 11% to 55% of abused children and are most common in children younger than 3 years of age.[4,69,95] The child abuse literature shows varying incidence of abuse-related fractures, depending on the age of the study population, institution, study entry criteria, selection bias, and time period when the study was published.[158] The younger the child with a fracture, especially under 18 months of age, the more likely abuse is the cause.[61] Fractures resulting from abuse should be suspected in young children if a caretaker brings the child for evaluation but reports no history of accidental trauma, especially if the caretaker reports a change in the child such as extremity swelling or decreased movement of the limb. Particularly concerning is a bone that fractures under tension with torsion, rather than the physiologic loading of compression of normal childhood activity or falls. Pierce and Bertocci[199] recommend that the clinician determine if the observed injury of a long bone and the stated mechanism are consistent (Table 7-8).

TABLE 7-8 Considerations When Evaluating a Child with a Long Bone Fracture

1. What are the biodynamics of the injury event, the energies generated by the event, and how could certain factors of the injury environment contribute to the likelihood of injury?
2. What injuries are expected, and what is the likelihood that the event generated the specific load required to cause each and all of the injuries?
3. Did the energy of the event exceed the injury threshold, or was there a biologic abnormality such as decreased bone density that resulted in a lowering of the actual threshold for injury? Is there evidence of bone weakness or disease?
4. Is the fracture morphology consistent with the direction, magnitude, and rate of loading of the described mechanism?
5. Is the facture pattern unusual, and one that requires an extremely unusual loading condition, as is the case with a classic metaphyseal lesion (also termed corner or bucket-handle fracture)?
6. What are the child's developmental capabilities, and could the child have generated the necessary energy independent of "outside" forces to cause the observed injury?
7. Does the fracture reflect a high-energy fracture? Did the event generate enough energy to cause a high-energy fracture? Or is the fracture a small cortical defect, or hairline crack, reflecting a smaller amount of energy required for propagation of the fracture type?
8. What regions of the bone have been injured and what are the structural components that affect the ultimate pattern of fracture that is being observed? Were there structural factors that contributed to the likelihood of fracture?

From Pierce MC, Bertocci GE. Evaluating long bone fractures in children: a biomechanical approach with illustrative cases. Child Abuse & Neglect 2004;28:505–524.

Femoral shaft fractures are common fracture in abuse, and although nonspecific, are always suspicious for child abuse in nonambulatory infants (Fig. 7-6).[215] Accidental femoral frac-

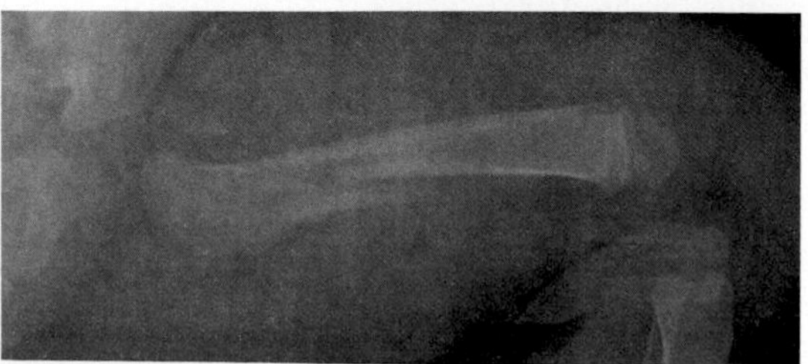

FIGURE 7-6 Femoral fracture in a 3-month-old male victim of nonaccidental trauma. Radiograph of the femur demonstrates an oblique diaphyseal fracture without evidence of periosteal reaction or healing.

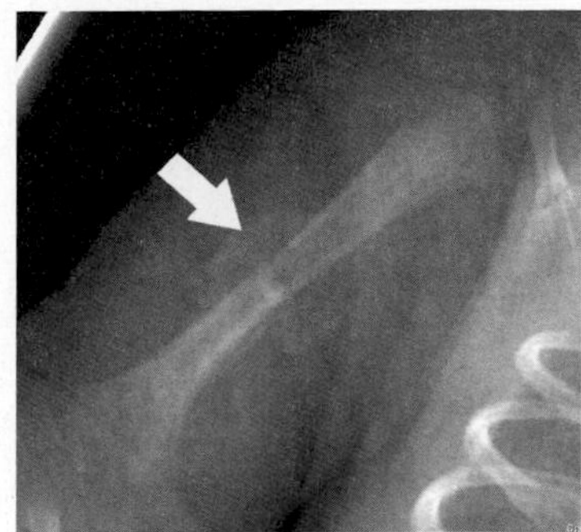

FIGURE 7-7 Humeral fracture in a 3-week-old male after a difficult delivery. Radiograph shows a transverse middiaphyseal fracture with extensive callus (*arrow*).

tures occur in children old enough to stand or run and who may fall with a twisting injury to the lower extremities, but femoral fractures in children younger than 1 year of age are commonly due to abuse.[215,246] However, even among nonambulatory children less than 1 year of age with a femoral fracture, abuse is present in only 42% and other mechanisms need to be considered.[215] Humeral shaft fractures are frequently seen in nonaccidental trauma (Fig. 7-7). Fractures in unusual locations such as the distal clavicle, scapula, acromial tip, proximal humeral metaphysis, or distal humeral physis may result from violent blows or upper extremity traction injury and are suggestive of abuse in young children.[10] Infants may normally have a separate ossification center adjacent to the tip of the acromion, simulating a fracture,[144] but a true fracture has sharp, demarcated edges, may be positive on bone scan, and will show callus or healing. Although fractures of the sternum are believed to be specific for child abuse by Kleinmann,[133] accidental midsternal fractures in children have been reported.[103]

Fractures of the hands and feet are commonly due to accidental trauma in older children,[177] but are suspicious for abuse in infants. Nimkin et al.[184] reviewed 11 hand and foot fractures in abused children younger than 10 months of age and found mostly torus fractures either of the metacarpals or the proximal phalanges of the hand and similar fractures of the first metatarsals of the feet (Fig. 7-8). Clinical signs of fracture were present in only one patient, and bones scans were insensitive to the presence of the fractures in all patients. These injuries are best seen on the oblique views standard in the skeletal survey.

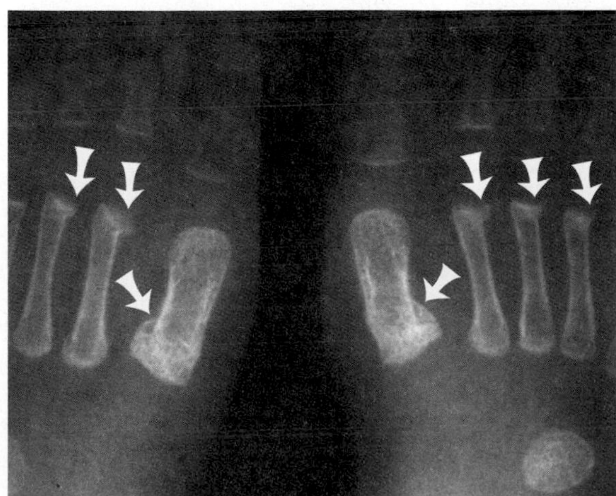

FIGURE 7-8 Metatarsal fractures in a 2-month-old female victim of nonaccidental trauma. Radiographic image from a skeletal survey shows multiple healing, bilateral, and symmetric proximal and distal metatarsal fractures (*arrows*).

All types of fractures have been reported in the child abuse literature, and it is often the presence of multiple fractures that indicates nonaccidental trauma (Fig. 7-9). In one of the largest series, King et al.[132] reported 429 fractures in 189 abused children. Fifty percent of these patients had a single fracture, and 17% had more than three fractures. Approximately 60% of fractures were found in roughly equal numbers in the humerus, femur, and tibia. Fractures also occurred in the radius, skull, spine, ribs, ulna, and fibula, in order of decreasing frequency. Another study[185] found a similar incidence of fractures of the humerus, femur, and tibia in abused children, with skull fractures seen in 14%. In contrast, Akbarnia et al.[3] found that rib fractures in abused patients were twice as prevalent as fractures of any one long bone; the next most frequently fractured bone was the humerus, followed by the femur and the tibia. Nearly a third of these patients had skull fractures. Loder and Bookout[162] reported the tibia to be the bone most commonly fractured in their series of abused children, followed by the humerus, the femur, the radius, and the ulna. In a classic study of 31 postmortem infants, the fracture pattern was very different from clinical studies in living children.[139] Highly detailed skeletal, specimen, and histopathologic analysis revealed 165 total fractures, most commonly ribs, distal femur, the ends of the tibia, and skull (Fig. 7-10). The fact that 29 of the 31 infants had evidence of a healing fracture provides sobering evidence of the need to aggressively diagnose nonaccidental trauma before an infant is killed. Physician education in child abuse is necessary to properly identify and report child abuse,[153] as there are many pitfalls to avoid (Table 7-9). There are several medical conditions that result in weakened bone and predisposition to fracture, such as osteogenesis imperfecta, that should be considered in the evaluation of a young child with multiple fractures.[120]

Dating Fractures

Radiographic proof of unexplained fractures in various stages of healing is believed to be strong evidence of child abuse (Fig. 7-11).[3] The orthopaedist often is asked to determine the age of fractures with some certainty to corroborate a history of injury given by caretakers. Experienced orthopaedists and radiologists can roughly estimate the age range of fractures by their radiographic appearance and their experience reading many radiographs of known dated injuries. Although specific guidelines have been established for estimating the age of fractures in children,[74] there is not good evidence-based data for accurately predicting the age of healing fractures.[202] In general, fractures seen on radiographs are considered acute until callus appears. Classic metaphyseal lesions (CML) are acute until periosteal reaction appears at about 14 days; however, not all CML develop visible callous, so dating in the absence of callous should be done with caution. Skull fractures generally cannot be dated.

In a review of studies that met minimal evidence-based inclusion criteria, the following conclusions were reached: the science of fracture dating is inexact and periosteal reaction is seen as early as 4 days and is present in at least 50% of cases by 2 weeks with remodeling peaking at 8 weeks after the fracture.[202] In dating fractures in infants younger than 6 months, one must be aware of the normal physiologic diaphyseal periosteal reac-

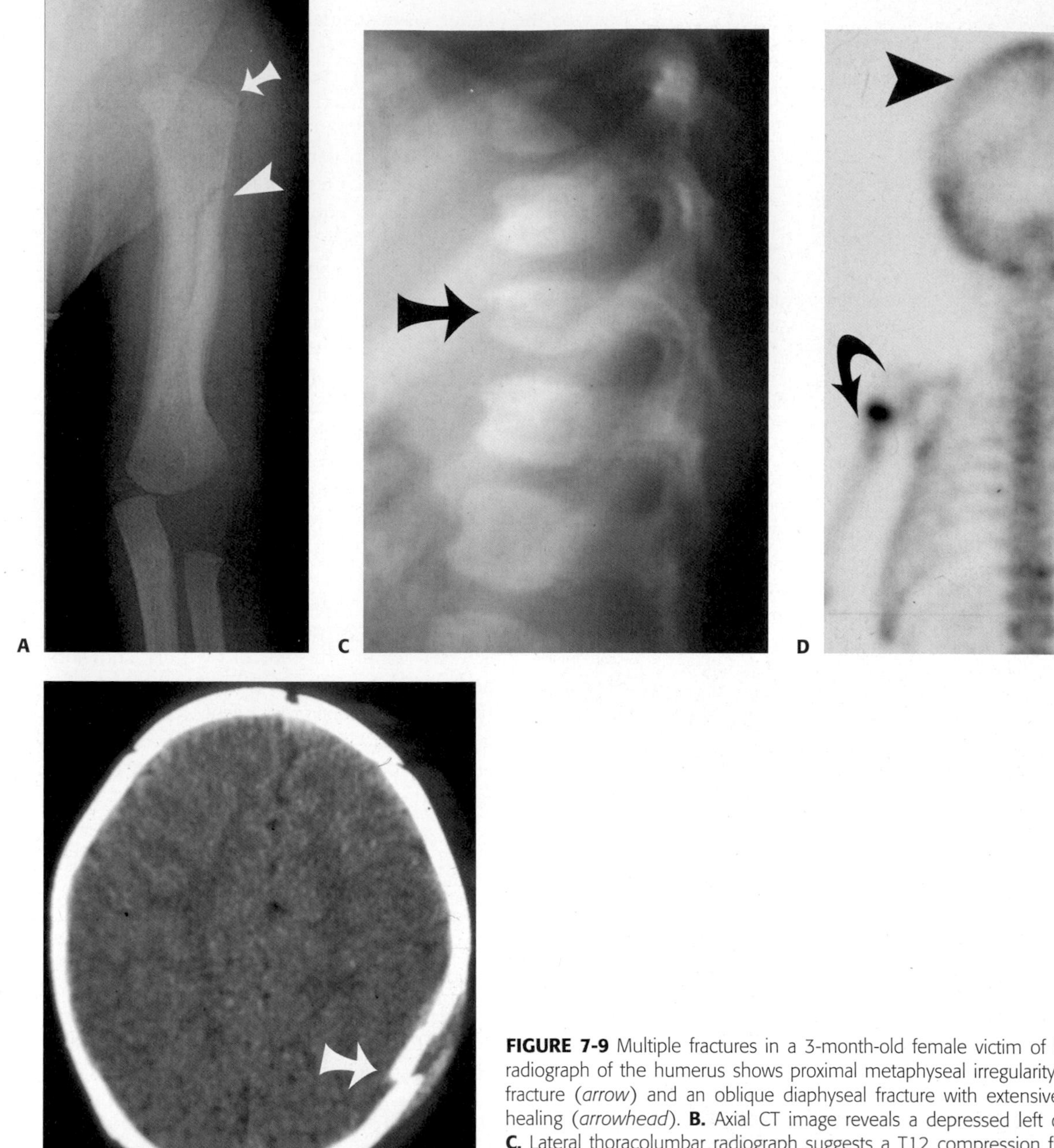

FIGURE 7-9 Multiple fractures in a 3-month-old female victim of inflicted injury. **A.** Frontal radiograph of the humerus shows proximal metaphyseal irregularity consistent with a corner fracture (*arrow*) and an oblique diaphyseal fracture with extensive periosteal reaction and healing (*arrowhead*). **B.** Axial CT image reveals a depressed left calvarial fracture (*arrow*). **C.** Lateral thoracolumbar radiograph suggests a T12 compression fracture (*arrow*), which is confirmed on nuclear bone scintigraphy **(D)** as a region of increased uptake (*arrow*). Bone scan also confirms left parietal (*arrowhead*) and humeral (*curved arrow*) fractures.

tion that is frequently present.[197] This is typically symmetric, diaphyseal only, and seen on the long bones of the extremities. The most difficult fractures to date are those that are completely healed, with substantial remodeling, and often the only sign of a healed fracture is a thickened cortex.

The Skeletal Survey

In addition to standard radiographic studies of the acute injury, a complete skeletal survey should be used to screen for additional fractures in all children younger than age 2 years when abuse is suspected.[12,130] The standard views obtained on a skeletal survey recommended by the American College of Radiology[11] are listed in Table 7-5. Abnormalities of the limbs detected on one view should undergo additional orthogonal views for completeness. Lateral views of the entire spine must always be included in the skeletal survey. Bilateral oblique views of the thorax are helpful, and some authors insist mandatory, in the diagnosis of subtle rib fractures.[130] Oblique thoracic films obtained on 2-week follow-up skeletal survey increased diagnostic yield, with 46% of repeat surveys revealing additional fractures.[141,264] Oblique radiographs of the hands are standard, since they may detect subtle torus fractures of the metacarpals and the phalanges not seen on a plain anteroposterior images.[184] The American Academy of Pediatrics Section on Radiology[12] cautioned that a "baby gram" has no place in diagnosing fractures of child abuse because the obliquity of the angle at which the radiographs transverse the skeleton may obscure many sub-

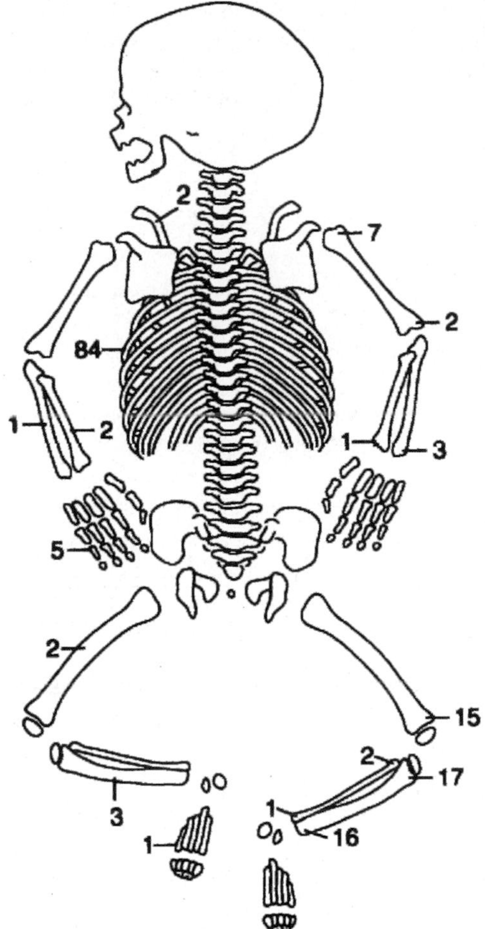

FIGURE 7-10 Schematic representation of the distribution 165 fractures in 31 infant fatalities. Single vertebral fracture and 13 skull fractures in this case series are not shown. (Image reprinted with permission from Kleinmann PK, Marks SC Jr, Richmond JM, et al. Inflicted skeletal injury: a postmortem radiologic-histologic study in 31 infants. AJR September 1995;165(3):647–650).

TABLE 7-9 Pearls and Pitfalls of Nonaccidental Trauma

- Be particularly cautious of a young infant with an injury.
- It is unusual for a young child to sustain a life-threatening injury from a fall alone, and he or she is highly unlikely to die from a short height fall.
- Caregiver should be able to describe in detail the mechanism that is consistent with the observed injury.
- Multiple rib fractures, fractures in various stages of healing, and classic metaphyseal fractures are highly specific.
- Injury mechanism stated by the parents should agree with the type and energy of the fracture.
- Failure to diagnose child abuse may result in 25% risk of repeat abuse and 5% chance of death.
- Concerning bruises and skin lesions are the most common presentation of abuse. However, the child with such bruises should receive a proper evaluation for bleeding disorder.
- Unexplained fractures are much more likely to represent abuse than a rare or diseases such as OI, but always consider OI when multiple fractures are seen.
- Obtain skeletal survey in all children younger than 2 years old, and individualize for 2–5 year olds when child abuse is suspected. Repeat in 2 weeks.
- Involve the hospital child protective team early in the evaluation.
- Prepare records as though everything will be reviewed and read in court.

tle fractures.[62] Imaging systems should have a spatial resolution of at least 10 line pairs per millimeter and should be used without a grid.[11]

The sensitivity of skeletal surveys diminishes in patients older than 2 years of age. They have less value for children older than age 5 years since the older child can describe where the pain is located. For children between the ages of 2 and 5 years, the test should be individualized.[12] The cost-effectiveness of skeletal surveys in the older child appears to be low, but may be helpful for the child with a disability who cannot cooperate with the physical examination. In one study of 331 children, only eight patients without overt physical signs of child abuse had occult fractures revealed by the survey[80]; however, the use of the skeletal survey in these few patients possibly prevented both reinjury and death.

A screening skeletal survey (see Table 7-5) is the standard of care for imaging suspected child abuse in children less than 2 years of age. A radionucleotide bone rarely is used as a complementary and confirmatory test for problem solving some difficult cases.[62] Neither a skeletal survey or a technetium bone scan alone will detect all occult fractures.[130] In Kleinman's postmortem infant study of fractures diagnosed by detailed histopathol-

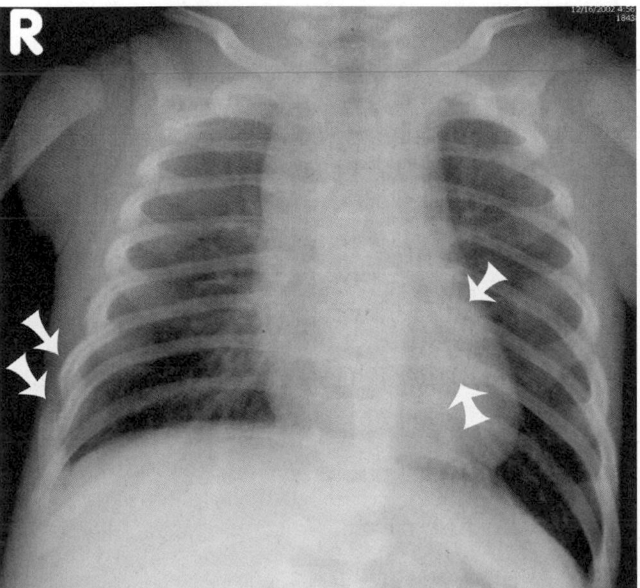

FIGURE 7-11 Rib fractures in multiple stages of healing in a 4-month-old female victim of nonaccidental injury. Frontal chest radiograph reveals acute (no periosteal reaction or healing) and subacute/healing (positive periosteal reaction) rib fractures (*arrows*).

ogy, 58% of these fractures were seen on skeletal survey and 92% were seen by specimen radiographs. Because of a false-negative rate of 12% with skeletal surveys, Sty and Starshak[236] suggested that a technetium bone scan be used as an initial screening test. Technetium bone scintigraphy is very useful in the diagnosis of occult rib fractures[62]; however, there is inconsistent interpretation in children younger than 18 months of age. Bone scintigraphy is not useful for areas that are normally active such as the physis and metaphysis, but is very good when imaging areas away from the physis, such as the shaft of a long bone. Scintigraphy is not reliable to detect skull fractures.[177] Bone scan and skeletal survey may be considered complementary rather than competing imaging modalities; however, the skeletal survey is performed first. Jaudes[119] found that when results of either a bone scan or a skeletal survey were normal in a known abused child, the use of both tests often revealed additional occult fractures. Technetium scans are not useful for dating fractures because increased isotope uptake may occur at a fracture as early as 24 hours after injury and scan abnormalities may persist for years.[87]

Follow-up skeletal survey at 2 weeks increases the diagnosis of occult fractures, since some fractures, especially of the ribs, may not be seen until callus appears at 10 to 14 days. The second look skeletal survey better defines the fracture seen on the original survey and may help determine the age of the fracture.[130] Kleinman et al.[141] reported that a follow-up skeletal survey 2 weeks after the initial series detected 27% more fractures and provided assistance in dating 20% of previously detected fractures.

Digital radiography through the picture archiving and communication system has replaced standard film-screen imaging in most hospitals; however, its role in the detection of the subtle fractures of child abuse needs further study. Child abuse fractures can be missed on digitalized images.[263] Kleinman et al.[142] noted that digital imaging of child abuse fractures had a spatial resolution lower than film-screen imaging, but the difference was not appreciable in detecting rib fractures in a postmortem evaluation. High-quality image screens are necessary for optimal image interpretation.

Skull Fractures

Infants in the first year of life with fractures of the skull or the extremities have an equal risk of the etiology being either accident or abuse.[169] However, 80% of skull fractures from abuse are seen in infants less than 1 year of age. Skull fractures were the most commonly reported fracture in one series.[171] Detailed postmortem analysis of 31 abused infants, with an average age of 3 months, observed confirmed skull fractures in 13.[139] Skeletal surveys missed 26% of skull fractures confirmed on CT scan.[211] Bone scintography is even less sensitive and is notably poor in detection of skull fractures. Skull fractures are nonspecific and the morphology of the fracture does not distinguish accidental from inflicted trauma.[23] Simple linear skull fractures are usually accidental; however, 80% of inflicted skull fractures are also linear.[157] Complex skull fractures without a history of significant trauma, including comminuted, diastatic (separated sutures), displaced fractures, and fractures crossing suture lines, are suspicious, but not diagnostic for abuse.[37] Skull fractures cannot be dated.

Extremity Fractures

There is no predominant pattern of diaphyseal fracture in child abuse. Traditionally, a midshaft spiral fracture was believed to be uniquely caused by a violent abusive twisting injury of the extremity of the child. However, it is now known that this is not true. In a study of 23 long-bone fractures in abused children, spiral fractures were found in 78%.[109] However, others found that 71% of diaphyseal fractures were transverse in abused children.[91] Loder and Bookout[162] reviewed 69 long-bone fractures in abused children and noted that 56% were transverse, 36% oblique, and only 8% spiral. In another study of 429 fractures,[81] 48% of fractures were transverse and 26% were spiral. Most of these long-bone fractures were in either the middle or distal third of the shaft. Transverse fractures are most commonly associated with either a violent bending force or a direct blow to the extremities, whereas spiral or oblique fractures of the long bones are due to axial-loaded, twisting injuries, such as in a fall. Humeral shaft fractures in children under 3 years of age have an 18% risk of being due to probable abuse.[216] In delayed follow-up, long-bone fractures may show exuberant callus because of a lack of immobilization, and multiple fractures may be present in different stages of healing.[6] Juxtacortical calcification may be seen without fracture when there is diaphyseal periosteal separation resulting from tractional or torsional force when the limb is grasped or pulled along the shaft of the bone.[176]

Femoral fractures in infants are especially suspicious for nonaccidental trauma; whereas children old enough to run can fall and accidentally fracture their femurs if there is a significant twisting motion at the time of injury.[246] Despite a high likelihood of nonaccidental trauma in an infant with a femoral fracture, an infant with a femur fracture may have accidental trauma as the cause, if the parent's reported mechanism is consistent with the injury. In a recent case series from Alberta, Canada, only 17% of femoral fractures in infants less than 1 year of age were from abuse, while the author's review of eight previous reports showed that nonaccidental trauma was the cause for 42% to 93% of cases.[114] Scherl et al.[206] reported that there was equal risk of having a spiral or transverse femoral fracture as a result of abuse. As children get older and more active, a femoral fracture is more likely to be from accidental injury than from abuse. Schwend et al.[215] reported that while 42% of femoral fractures in infants not walking were related to nonaccidental injury, only 2.6% of femoral fractures in ambulatory toddlers were. Blakemore et al.[36] noted that only 2% of femoral fractures from age 1 to 5 years were due to abuse. Risk factors for abuse were age younger than 12 months, the child not yet walking, a questionable mechanism, and other associated injuries.

Metaphyseal and epiphyseal fractures of the long bones are classically associated with child abuse.[43,222] In infants and toddlers, these fractures can occur when the child is violently shaken by the extremities with direct violent traction or rotation of the extremity (see Fig. 7-7).[177] Buckle fractures may occur at multiple sites, seldom producing exuberant callus. Repeated injury may cause irregular metaphyseal deformities. Periosteal avulsion typically produces new bone formation within 2 to 3 weeks of injury and may be confused with osteomyelitis.[6] New bone formation may be delayed, particularly in children with malnutrition or rickets. Metaphyseal fractures constituted 40% of fractures in one series,[91] but fewer than 15% in another.[146]

Kleinman[133] ranked the specificity of skeletal trauma for abuse (Table 7-10). Distinguishing between an accident and child abuse is based on the location and the type of fracture. He emphasized that both moderate- and low-specificity radio-

TABLE 7-10 Specificity of Skeletal Trauma for Abuse

High specificity
- Classic metaphyseal lesions
- Posterior rib fracture
- Scapular fracture
- Spinous process fracture
- Sternal fracture

Moderate specificity
- Multiple fractures, especially bilateral
- Fractures in various stages of healing
- Epiphyseal separation
- Vertebral body fracture or subluxation
- Digital fracture
- Complex skull fracture

Low specificity
- Clavicular fracture
- Long-bone shaft fracture
- Linear skull fracture

Data from Kleinman PK, ed. Diagnostic Imaging of Child Abuse. Baltimore: Williams & Wilkins, 1987, with permission.

graphic findings of child abuse become much more specific when there is an inadequate explanation for the injury. The presence of multiple injuries, particularly in the young child, is especially concerning for abuse.

Compared to healthy term infants, premature infants are more susceptible to fractures, both related to their prematurity and to increased risk of child abuse.[49] They may have underlying genetic, metabolic, and nutritional deficiency that predispose to fractures. Underlying osteopenia may lead to insufficiency fractures, both acute and chronic, in various stages of healing. Higher parental stress from caring for a sick or disabled infant may result in higher risk of nonaccidental trauma. In the premature infant with multiple fractures, investigation of the bone health as well as for child abuse is necessary, depending on the clinical context and findings.

Classic Metaphyseal Lesion of Child Abuse

The almost pathognomonic fracture of child abuse is the CML, commonly termed the "corner" or "bucket-handle fracture."[4,6] These fractures are almost exclusively seen in nonaccidental injury, but are not the most common fractures in abused children. The incidence of CML in large series ranges from 15% to 32%.[91,132,146,162] Radiographs show a corner fracture at the edge of the ossified portion of the zone of provisional calcification, *which is the metaphyseal side of the physis as opposed to the epiphyseal side.* If a significant portion of the metaphyseal rim is involved, a bucket-handle fracture pattern is produced. Based on their histopathologic autopsy study of metaphyseal fractures in abused infants, Kleinman et al.[136,138] found that bucket-handle and corner fractures are actually a full-thickness metaphyseal fracture extending through the primary spongiosa of bone just above the zone of provisional calcification (Fig. 7-12). Centrally, the amount of metaphysis remaining attached to the physis was thin, but peripherally the fracture line curved away from the physis so that a substantial metaphyseal rim remained attached to the physis (Fig. 7-13). On radiographic study, this

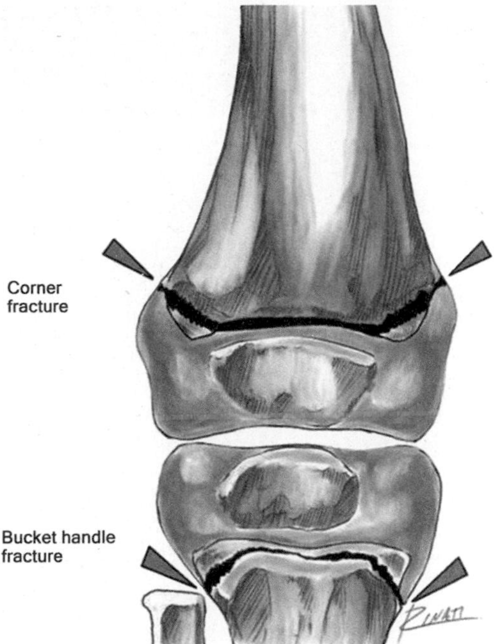

FIGURE 7-12 Schematic representation of classic metaphyseal lesions (CML). Illustration demonstrates the path of the CML. Depending upon the angle at which the CML is viewed from, it may appear to extend across the width of the ossified physis (tibia illustrating a bucket handle fracture) or only the margins of the physis (femur, illustrating a corner fracture). (Artwork courtesy of Gholamreza Zinati, MD.)

metaphyseal rim formed the basis for both corner and bucket-handle fractures. In healing fractures, biopsy specimens showed metaphyseal extension of hypertrophied chondrocytes.[191] Metaphyseal corner fractures are most likely caused by either violent shaking or traction injuries to the extremity.[4] Subepiphyseal-metaphyseal lucency can also be caused by systematic disease such as rickets and leukemia. Corner fractures of the distal radius, ulna, tibia, and proximal humerus also have been reported with developmental coxa vara associated with spondylometaphyseal dysplasia.[68] Since fracture callus does not reliably occur, dating the CML lesion is always unreliable. The presence of callus does indicate that the fracture is greater than 10 to 14 days.

Rib Fractures

Rib fractures are uncommon in childhood accidents, especially when located posterior and associated with other long-bone fractures. Abusive rib fractures may be caused by squeezing of the chest by a caretaker,[44] hitting the child from behind, or stepping on the chest.[141,226] Kleinman et al.[140] postulated that severe shaking of an infant can cause front-to-back chest compression, which levers the posterior rib over the transverse process of the vertebral body, causing fractures of the posterior rib shaft at the transverse process and of the rib head adjacent to the vertebra (Fig. 7-14). One series showed that fractures of the first rib in children were only seen in abuse.[235] Barsness et al.[25] reported that rib fractures had a positive predictive value of nonaccidental injury of 95% in children younger than 3 years of age. In this study, rib fracture(s) were the only skeletal manifestation of nonaccidental injury in 29% of the children. Posterior rib fractures are difficult to diagnose acutely because they lack callus and are rarely displaced. Even with healing, the callus

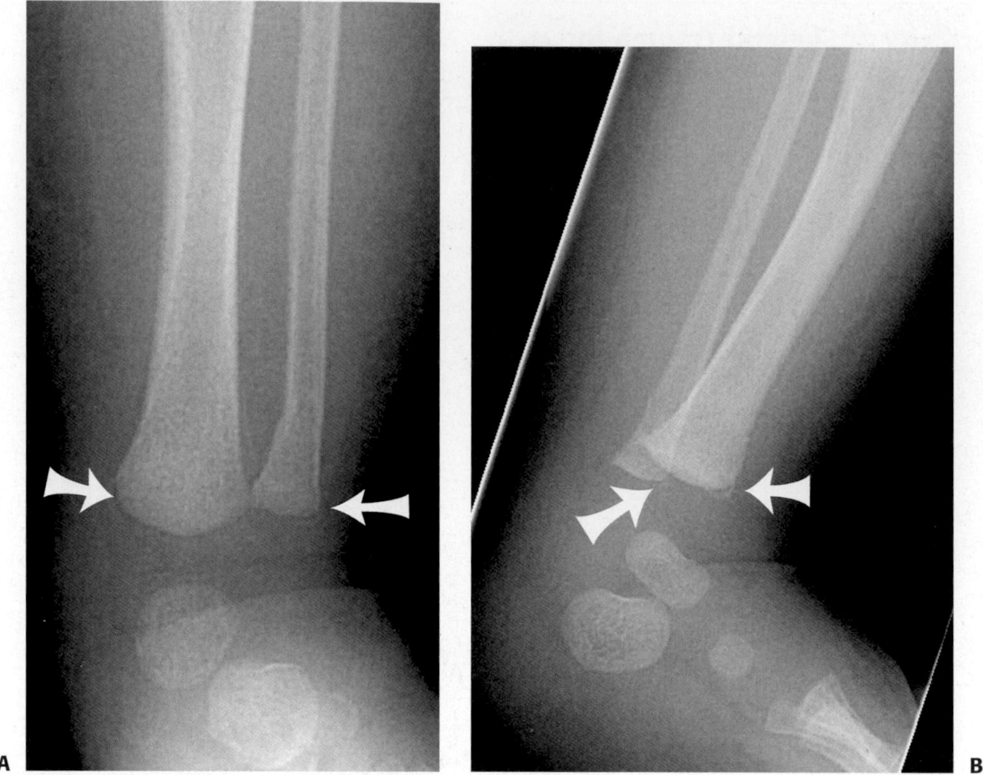

FIGURE 7-13 Classic metaphyseal fracture in a 2.5-month-old male victim of nonaccidental injury. **A.** Frontal radiograph of the tibia and fibula demonstrate transmetaphyseal lucencies, or bucket handle fractures (*arrows*). **B.** A lateral ankle radiograph reveals lucency at the tibial and fibular metaphyseal margins indicating corner fractures (*arrows*).

on radiography may be obscured by the overlying transverse process.[136] Oblique views of the chest are often included in skeletal surveys because they may better show these fractures. Posterior rib fractures are the most common location in child abuse, but fractures may occur anywhere along the arc of the rib, including disruption of the anterior costochondral junction (Fig. 7-15). Posterior rib fractures tend to occur between T4 and T9. Acute anterior costochondral separations of the ribs may be difficult to see on chest radiographs,[225] and with healing, the anterior end of the osseous rib becomes widened and

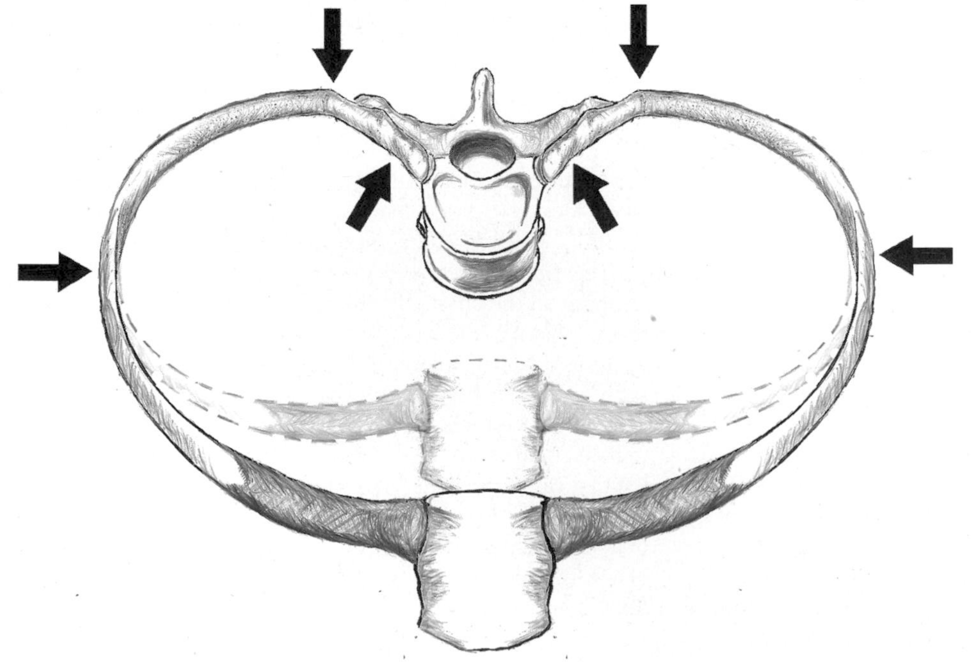

FIGURE 7-14 Schematic representation of rib fracture mechanism. Anterior chest compression causes the posterior ribs to be levered over the transverse processes of the vertebra causing posterior and lateral rib fractures. (Artwork courtesy of Samir Abedin, MD.)

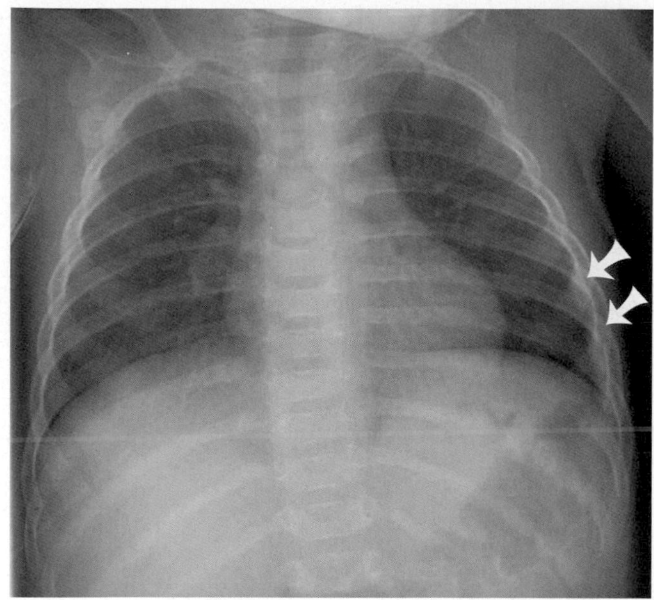

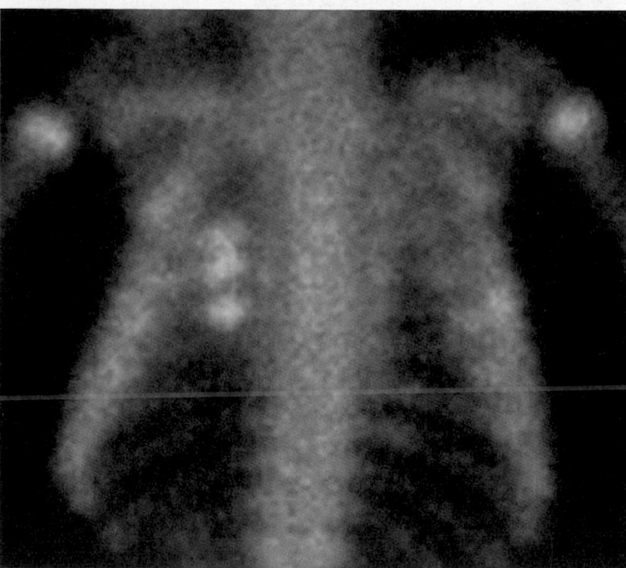

FIGURE 7-15 Rib fractures in a 9-month-old male victim of nonaccidental trauma. **A.** Chest radiograph reveals left lateral sixth and seventh rib fractures (*arrows*). **B.** Nuclear medicine bone scan confirms foci of increased uptake within the left lateral ribs as well as revealing additional hot foci in multiple right posterior lateral ribs.

club shaped.[146,185] Anterior rib fractures are commonly associated with abdominal injury and can be detected on CT scan. Healing fractures show callus, but healed fractures may be subtle, with only a fusiform thickening of the rib. Older fractures of the ribs in nonaccidental trauma may form lytic, expansile lesions.[164]

Rib fractures are rarely discovered in abused infants who have undergone resuscitation for cardiac arrest; in which case, there may be confusion about the etiology of the fractures. However, the elasticity of the infant chest allows a high tolerance to compression, having low reported rates of rib fractures from cardiopulmonary resuscitation between 0.3% and 2%, with none being posterior rib fractures.[165] Cardiopulmonary resuscitation is therefore a very rare cause of rib fractures and seldom causes classic posterior rib fractures. Death from cardiac arrhythmia from a blow to the chest has been reported in a 7-week-old abused infant whose rib fractures at autopsy were initially thought to be due to resuscitation efforts.[18] In addition to rib fractures, abused infants can sustain severe lung contusion and respiratory distress from chest wall trauma,[170] with fatal fat embolus reported.[183]

In infant fatalities of suspicious origin, postmortem high-detailed preautopsy skeletal surveys and specimen radiographs are helpful in fully evaluating and diagnosing child abuse.[134] In a postmortem study of 31 infants who died of inflicted skeletal injury,[139] there were a total of 165 fractures (51% rib fractures, 39% metaphyseal long bone fractures, 5% long-bone shaft fractures, 4% fractures of the hands and feet, 1% clavicular fractures, and less than 1% spinal fractures).

Spinal Fractures

Spinal fractures in abused children are infrequent but important to recognize. Based on autopsy findings,[135] spinal fractures of fatally abused children generally involve 25% or less compression of the vertebrae. In a report of 103 children with cervical spine injury, only three patients had injury due to abuse and all had spinal cord injury without radiographic abnormality (SCIWORA).[40] In another study of fractures of the cervical spine, prevertebral soft tissue edema on radiographs was the only sign of cervical injury, since spontaneous reduction of the cervical vertebrae after dislocation was common.[242] Thomas et al.[245] reported a 9-week-old boy with spinal cord injury resulting from cervical spine fracture who presented as a floppy infant. Although routine cervical radiographs were normal, MRI studies showed retropulsion of a fragment of the primarily cartilaginous C3 vertebrae into the spinal canal. Hangman's type fractures of the posterior elements have been described in infants as a result of child abuse.[143] This must be distinguished from C2 primary spondylolysis which may be associated with pyknodysostosis, both of which are rare disorders associated with wormian bones and pencil pointing of the distal phalanges.[67]

CT is helpful in evaluating pediatric cervical trauma. Rooks et al.[208] reported a compression fracture of C5 with anterior subluxation of C4 on C5 in a 3-month-old abused premature twin requiring decompression and cervical fusion. The other twin had a C5 on C6 fracture-subluxation treated with casting, but later required surgery to reduce and fuse the subluxation. MRI was very helpful in showing spinal cord compression in both cases. Oral[189] reported on an inflicted avulsion fracture of C2 and interspinous ligament injury in a 4-year-old child.

Vertebral compression fractures can occur when a child's buttocks are forcibly slammed onto a flat surface with hyperflexion of the spine.[4,5] Half of these fractures involved the anterosuperior end plate associated with a compression deformity, 30% had pure compression fractures, and 20% had fractures of the superior end plate without significant compression. Positioning premature infants in extreme hyperflexion for lumbar puncture has been reported to cause iatrogenic lumbar spine fracture.[96] Carrion et al.[48] reported circumferential physeal frac-

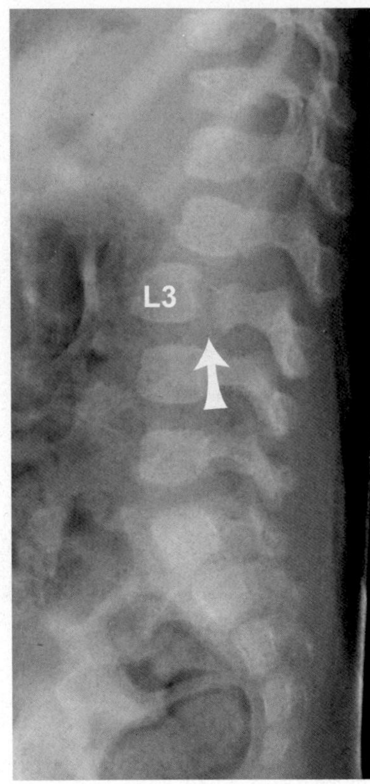

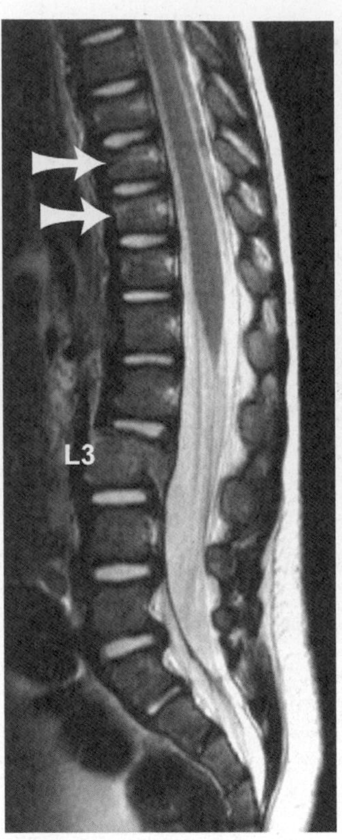

A B

FIGURE 7-16 Lumbar spine fracture in a 16-month-old male victim of nonaccidental trauma. **A.** Lateral lumbar radiograph shows lucency through the L3 synchondrosis (arrow) with anterolisthesis of L3 body on L4. **B.** Sagittal T2-weighted MRI reveals hyperintense signal within the bone marrow of the fractured L3. Slight compression fractures of T10 and T11 are also noted (*arrows*).

tures of the thoracolumbar spine associated with child abuse that required open reduction. Thoracolumbar fracture dislocations may occur in abused children with or without neurologic injury.[159,219] Flexion-distraction Chance fractures and synchondroses injuries (Fig. 7-16) may also be seen in nonaccidental trauma. Although neurologic injury in spinal fractures resulting from child abuse is uncommon,[66] any patient with abusive spinal injury should undergo thorough neurologic examination (see Fig. 7-16).

LABORATORY STUDIES

An abused child should have a complete blood cell count with sedimentation rate, liver function studies, and urinalysis. Clotting studies, including prothrombin time and activated partial thromboplastin time, thrombin time, fibrinogen, factor VIII, factor IX, and von Willebrand factor antigen and activity should be performed in patients with bleeding or ecchymosis to evaluate for bleeding diathesis. If bruising is the only finding of possible abuse, consultation with a hematologist may be necessary to fully evaluate for an unusual bleeding disorder.[244] Infants born prematurely are at risk for rickets and low bone density. Therefore, evaluation of calcium, phosphorous, alkaline phosphatase, and 25-OH vitamin D may be useful in such infants.

Recently, two biomarkers for head injury, neuron-specific enolase S100B and myelin-basic protein, have been found to be released into the peripheral circulation, analogous to cardiac enzyme release after myocardial injury. These two markers when used together are 79% sensitive and 100% specific in diagnosing traumatic brain injury, making them potentially very promising for evaluating suspected mild head trauma.[32] If there is suspicion of substance abuse by any family member, a toxicology screen should also be performed on the patient.[91]

MULTIDISCIPLINARY APPROACH

The most important consultation to request for a child with suspected inflicted injury is the child protective services team. In a study by Banaszkiewicz et al.,[19] three tiers of physicians reviewed the medical records of 74 children under the age of 1 year presenting to the emergency department with fractures: staff clinicians, orthopaedic attendings, and a child protective team pediatrician. In over one fourth of cases of abuse, the possibility was underestimated during the original evaluation. Any suspected abuse should initiate a minimum evaluation that includes an appropriate radiographic evaluation with a skeletal survey in the younger child, dilated fundoscopic examination by an ophthalmologist, and consultation by a child abuse specialist. Any significant nonorthopaedic injury should prompt consultation by the appropriate subspecialty: neurosurgery, general surgery, plastic surgery, ophthalmology, or urology.[6] In cases of suspected sexual abuse, a thorough genital examination will be required, including a gynecologic consultation for girls. This is typically initiated by the child protective services team.

THE DIFFERENTIAL DIAGNOSIS

Although it is extremely important not to miss the diagnosis of child abuse, it is equally important to maintain an objective, critical view and not to make the diagnosis in error.[120] Overdiagnosing child abuse can be harmful to the family, with the parents being placed at risk of losing custody of their children and also facing criminal charges.[127] Even direct allegations of child abuse may turn out to be false. Patients or family friends may make false statements about an abuse situation through misinterpretation, confabulation, fantasy, delusions, and other situations.[33] The American Academy of Child and Adolescent

Psychiatry[43] has published guidelines for the evaluation of abuse, stating that the possibility of false allegations needs to be considered, particularly if the charges are coming from the parent rather than the child, the parents are engaged in a dispute over custody or visitation, or the child is a preschooler.

Normal metaphyseal variations are seen occasionally and should not be confused with corner fractures of child abuse. These variants are seen most commonly in the proximal tibia, distal femur, proximal fibula, distal radius, and distal ulna. A bony beak may be seen medially in the proximal humerus or tibia, and is usually bilateral. Cortical irregularity in the medial proximal tibia may also be seen in 4% of normal infants and young toddlers and is bilateral in 25%. Beaks may extend beyond the metaphyseal margins in both the distal radius and the lateral aspect of the distal femur, with bilateral normal variants in 25% of infants and young toddlers.[187]

The signs of child abuse found on radiographs can overlap with the findings of systemic diseases such as Caffey disease (infantile cortical hyperostosis), osteomyelitis, septic arthritis, insufficiency fracture, hypophosphatasia (Fig. 7-17), leukemia (Fig. 7-18), metastatic neuroblastoma, osteogenesis imperfecta (OI) (Fig. 7-19), scurvy (Fig. 7-20), vitamin D deficient and drug-induced rickets (Fig. 7-21), congenital insensitivity to pain, osteopetrosis, kinky hair syndrome, prostaglandin therapy, osteoid osteoma, and other benign bone tumors.[6] Children with biliary atresia may present with osteopenia and fractures

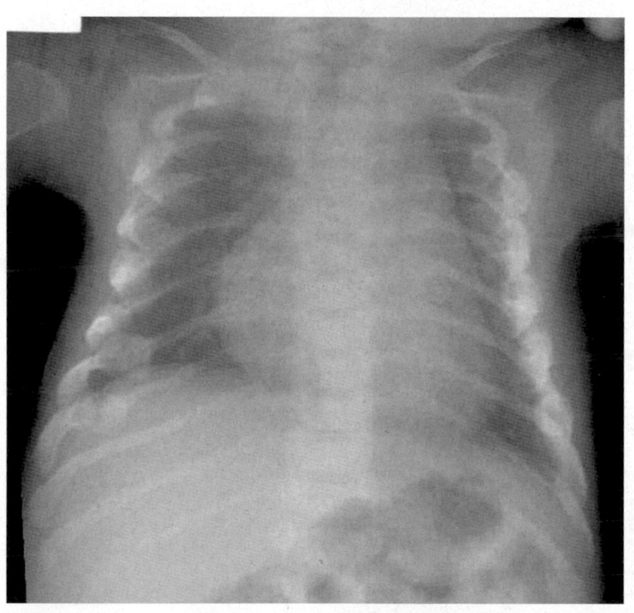
A

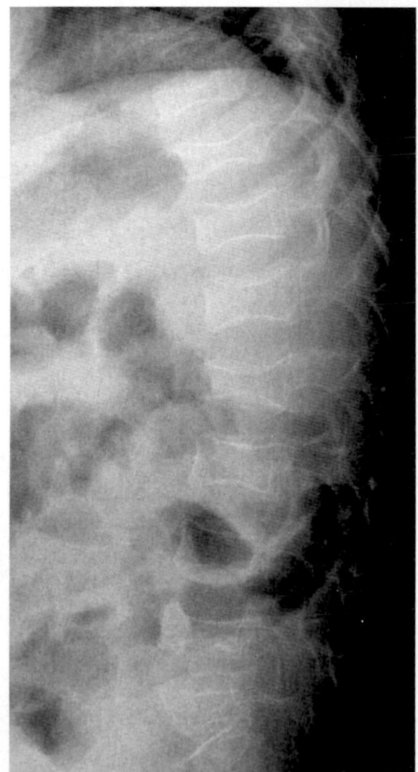
B

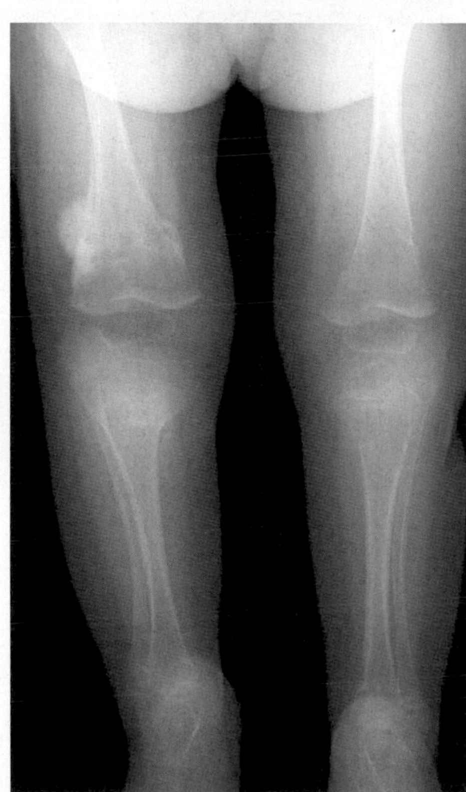
C

FIGURE 7-17 Hypophosphatasia in a 2-month-old female with multiple fractures. **A.** Chest radiograph shows severe osteopenia and multiple bilateral healing rib fractures. **B.** Lateral spine radiograph reveals multiple compressed vertebra. **C.** Lower extremity radiographs demonstrate multiple, bilateral healing femoral and lower leg fractures.

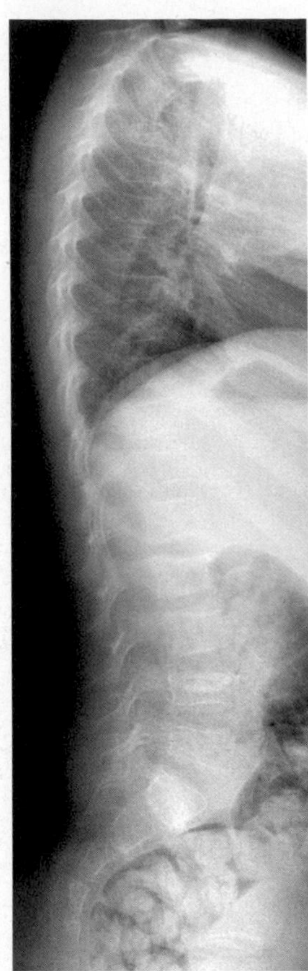

FIGURE 7-18 Leukemia in a 4-year-old boy presenting with back pain. Lateral spine radiograph shows osteopenia and multiple spine compression fractures.

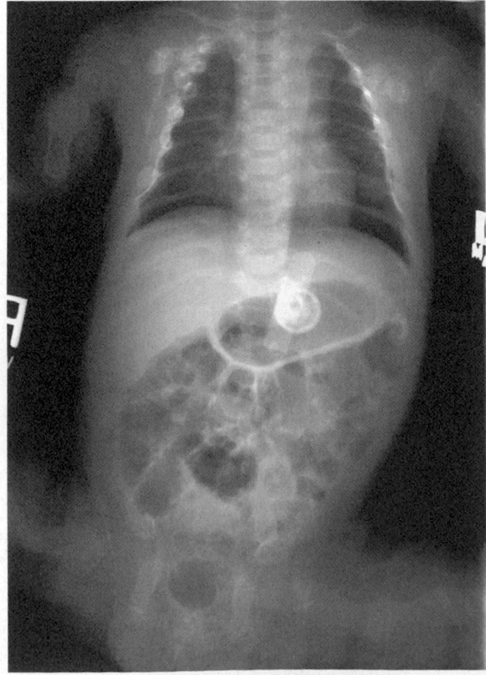

FIGURE 7-19 Osteogenesis imperfecta in a 2-month-old female with multiple rib and extremity fractures. Frontal radiograph of the chest and abdomen reveals diffuse osteopenia as well as multiple bilateral rib and proximal extremity fractures in various stages of healing.

without history of significant injury, which should not be mistaken for child abuse.[72] There has been an increase in the incidence of syphilis in females of childbearing age, and, although extremely rare, congenital syphilis can mimic fractures of child abuse with diaphysitis, metaphysitis, and multiple pathologic fractures in different stages of healing.[160] Physiologic periostitis, in contrast to lesions from child abuse, is seen in young infants of about 6 months of age, is usually bilateral, symmetric, diaphyseal, located on the long bones—humerus, femur, and tibia—and has no periostitis of the metaphysis.[62] Insufficiency rib fractures may be seen in rickets of prematurity as well as rickets of low birth weight and also have been reported after chest physiotherapy.[53] The presence of metabolic disease and pathologic fractures does not exclude the possibility of child abuse. Duncan and Chandry[79] reported a 3-month-old girl with multiple fractures associated with rickets who died suddenly at 5 months of age. Child abuse was suspected but not proven. Three years later, evidence of child abuse was found in a subsequent sibling in the same family.

Several diseases are commonly brought up in custodial hearings as alternative possibilities to nonaccidental traumatic injuries, and these diseases should be objectively considered in the differential diagnosis. Linear lucencies of the proximal tibia noted after intraosseous vascular access needles may mimic fractures, but careful analysis of the imaging studies can determine the actual cause of the lucency.[102] Metaphyseal corner fractures of the distal tibia and fibula were seen in eight children treated with likely forceful serial casting for clubfoot, with only one potentially related to nonaccidental trauma.[94] Leukemia should always be considered in a child with diffuse osteopenia or metaphyseal lucencies. McClain et al.[168] reported a 2-year-old child who died of undiagnosed acute lymphoblastic leukemia, having been earlier reported as a possible victim of child abuse. Ecchymosis on the back and extremities did not initiate an appropriate evaluation for leukemia or bleeding disorder. Clinical signs of leukemia, including fever, pallor, petechia, purpura, adenopathy, hepatosplenomegaly, and bone pain, should be sought in children with bruising of unknown origin. Factor XIII deficiency may cause unexplained bleeding from minor trauma and be mistaken for child abuse because the standard coagulation profile may be negative and factor-specific tests may be negative if performed posttransfusion.[181]

Osteogenesis Imperfecta

Undiagnosed OI should always be considered when a child presents with multiple fractures of unknown etiology, but may be a difficult diagnosis to make. OI caused by spontaneous mutation can occur without a family history.[195] The so-called hallmark of OI is an intensely blue sclerae, but this feature is consistently present only in Sillence type I,[220] may be completely absent in patients with type IV, and is less obvious in type III.[195] Sillence and Butler[221] noted that patients with either type II or III OI may have blue sclerae at birth, but the sclerae can become normal by adolescence. The rare Sillence type II OI, termed Congenta A in the Shapiro classification, has normal sclerae, but bone abnormalities and osteopenia are severe and early death is likely.[195] Blue sclerae may be present in normal young infants and can be misinterpreted as a sign of OI. The presence of abnormal teeth, known as dentinogenesis imperfecta, may be helpful in a diagnosis if the child is old enough

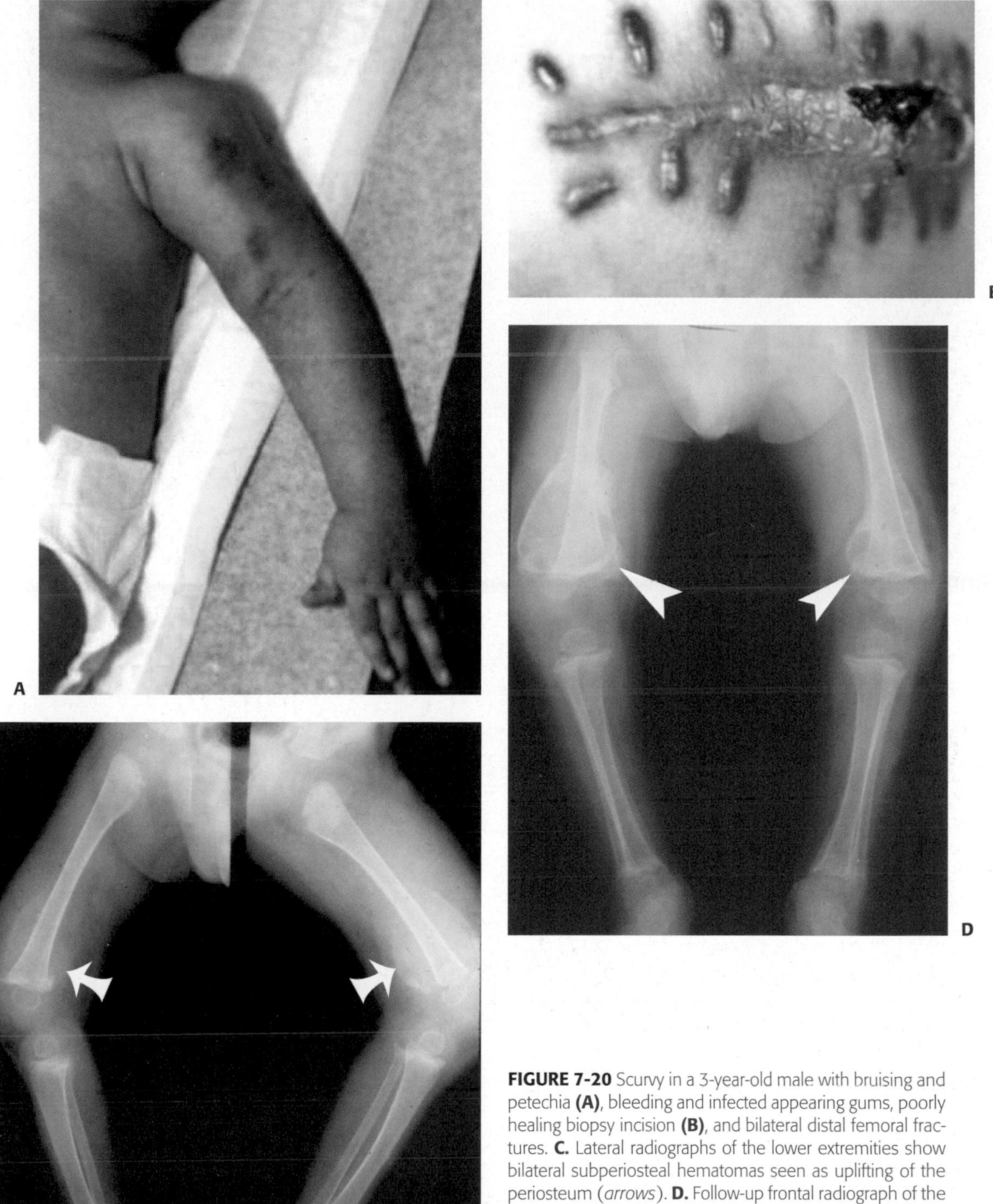

FIGURE 7-20 Scurvy in a 3-year-old male with bruising and petechia **(A)**, bleeding and infected appearing gums, poorly healing biopsy incision **(B)**, and bilateral distal femoral fractures. **C.** Lateral radiographs of the lower extremities show bilateral subperiosteal hematomas seen as uplifting of the periosteum (*arrows*). **D.** Follow-up frontal radiograph of the lower extremities after treatment with vitamin C demonstrates calcification of subperiosteal hematomas, as well as metaphyseal irregularity similar to classic metaphyseal lesions (*arrowheads*).

for teeth to have erupted. Plain radiographs may show long bones of normal density in both types I and IV OI. Another radiographic sign of OI, wormian bones of the skull, is consistently present only in type III and is often absent in types I and IV.[195] Since type IV OI does not have blue sclera or wormian bones and is a milder form of OI than type III, diagnosis may be initially delayed or confused with nonaccidental trauma. Other rare types of OI have been described, which further confounds the medical and legal evaluation. Some authors believe that the presence of metaphyseal fracture is pathognomonic for child abuse and, therefore, helpful to distinguish abuse from OI,[1,14] but others[71,195] believe that there is no particular fracture pattern that renders the diagnosis of OI likely. Children with OI tend to bruise excessively, which overlaps with child abuse.[217] SIDS has also been described in infants with undiagnosed OI.[187]

When the diagnosis of OI cannot be made on clinical grounds, the diagnosis may be made by biochemical assay. Ga-

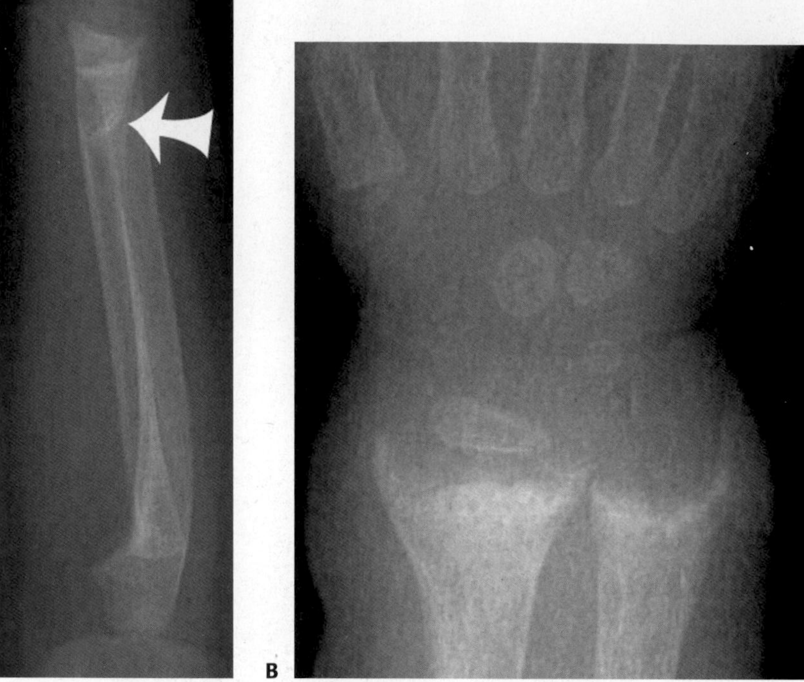

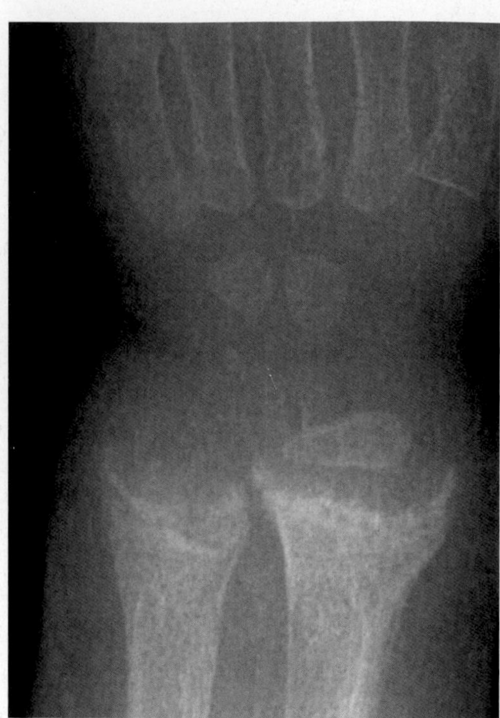

FIGURE 7-21 Rickets in a 16-month-old male who was breast fed. **A.** Lateral forearm radiograph shows osteopenia and a distal radial fracture (*arrow*) with some dorsal angulation **(B,C)**. Metaphyseal cupping and fraying of the distal radius and ulna bilaterally are also noted.

hagan and Rimsza[90] reported that 87% of children with OI have abnormal procollagen that can be detected by a skin biopsy with fibroblast culture. Fibroblasts are assayed for abnormally low levels of procollagen as well as primary abnormal procollagen.[42] Steiner et al.[231] reported that over a 4-year period, 48 patients were referred for collagen analysis to diagnose OI in cases of suspected child abuse. Only 6 of these 48 children had abnormal collagen test results, and in five of the six patients, the diagnosis of OI could have been made on clinical and radiologic findings. More recently, Malowe et al.[166] found 11 of 262 samples submitted to rule out OI had alterations in the amount or structure of type I collagen synthesized, consistent with the diagnosis of OI. In 11 others, OI could not be excluded. Referring physicians correctly diagnosed children with OI in six of the 11 patients clinically. Four children believed to have OI by physical examination had normal biochemical studies, representing a false-positive clinical diagnosis, attributed mostly to the use of sclera hue as a major diagnostic criterion.[167] The authors concluded that laboratory testing for OI remains a valuable adjunct when determining the etiology of fractures in children. Even when a child has OI or other metabolic bone disorders, fractures may be due to comorbid nonaccidental trauma. Knight and Bennett.[145] reported a young child with OI whose abuse could not be proved until linear bruising of the face from being slapped was documented.

Temporary Brittle Bone Disease

In 1993, Patterson et al.[195] described 39 patients with a variant of OI that they described as a temporary brittle bone disease in which fractures were limited to the first year of life followed by spontaneous improvement. However, an extensive review by the Society for Pediatric Radiology[175] concluded that the entity of temporary brittle bone disease has insufficient scientific evidence to warrant this as a plausible diagnosis.

Sudden Unexpected Death in Infancy

The death of an infant is a sentinel event and must be handled appropriately with the medical and the legal systems cooperatively involved.[123] SIDS is a subset of sudden unexpected death in infancy (SUDI) and refers to the death of an infant less than 1 year of age with the onset of the fatal episode apparently occurring during sleep that remains unexplained after a thorough review of the circumstances of death and clinical history.[123,258] Since SIDS is more common than infanticide, death by abuse intentional suffocation is very commonly initially attributed to SIDS before the correct diagnosis is made.[116a] However, other causes of sudden death such as intracranial bleeds must be excluded. Byard et al.[41] reported a 5-month-old girl who died suddenly from spontaneous subarachnoid hemorrhage from undiagnosed Ehlers-Danlos syndrome. They recommended collagen analysis in patients with unexplained multifocal spontaneous hemorrhages to exclude this rare syndrome. Sperry and Pfalzgraf[228] reported a 9-month-old infant whose diagnosis of SIDS became uncertain when postmortem radiographs showed healing symmetric clavicle fractures and a healing left medial humeral condyle fracture. Subsequent investigation showed that the child had undergone "chiropractic" manipulation 4 weeks before death by an unlicensed therapist to correct "shoulder dislocations," with the parents exonerated of abuse charges. When abuse is suspected in an infant fatality, combined radiology, CT scan, detailed forensic autopsy, and osteologic investigation is required to detect all fractures that are present.[50] Detailed examination of organs, such as the orbit, are also becoming the standard in autopsy protocols.[178]

POSTEMERGENCY ROOM TREATMENT AND LEGAL REPORTING REQUIREMENTS

Once nonaccidental trauma is recognized, the first step in treatment is hospital admission. This is therapeutic in that it places the child in a safe, protected environment, provides the opportunity for additional diagnostic workup, and, more importantly, investigation of the family's social situation by appropriate personnel. In tertiary centers, multidisciplinary teams often are available to evaluate and treat such children, but in other circumstances the orthopaedist may be primarily responsible for coordinating both evaluation and treatment. Court custody may be required for children of uncooperative families who refuse admission, and hospitalization should be continued until a full investigation is completed by the appropriate child protective services and a safe disposition is established. In the United States, the physician is required by law to report all suspected abuse to appropriate child protective services or legal authorities. Although physicians have better reporting rates than most other professionals, 27% of injuries considered likely to be caused by abuse and 76% of injuries that were considered possibly related to child abuse were not reported.[85] When the reporting is done in good faith, the physician has immunity against criminal or civil liability for these actions, but in only three states—Ohio, California, and Alabama—does this protection include absolute immunity.[59] The distinction is critical. Absolute immunity means that the physician who reports suspected child abuse cannot ever be held for damages sought by families for allegedly inappropriate reports of child abuse or neglect. The granting of absolute immunity, even for physicians, is not encouraged by the American legal system because in theory it would protect individuals who make false reports of child abuse in order to harass families and would deprive the injured parties their legal right to seek damages for harmful actions. In contrast, physician immunity based on good faith reporting of suspected child abuse is contingent on the physician having a reasonable belief that abuse or neglect has occurred. Although in theory this protection seems to be quite adequate, recently there has been a dramatic rise in the number of lawsuits filed by families seeking damages for alleged, unfounded reports of child abuse and neglect. Although it is true that by the time these lawsuits are eventually resolved, physicians have almost never been held liable for good faith reports of child abuse, in a substantial number of these cases, the physicians first lost at trial level before eventually prevailing at appeal. Considerable expense, frustration, and loss of time can be experienced by the physician in defending against such allegations as the families and their attorneys pursue multiple forms of legal theories in court and attempt to evade the immunity provisions.[59] On the other hand, the stakes for failure to report suspected child abuse are likely much higher, potentially exposing the physician to charges of malpractice.[4]

All states require physicians to report not only cases of definitive child abuse or neglect but also cases when abuse is just suspected or is considered a possibility. Physicians have been held liable for damages for their negligence in failing to diagnose child abuse when the child subsequently was reinjured by further abuse, and, ironically, the parents also may be able to collect additional compensation for losses resulting from medical expenses. For families to be successful in these lawsuits, they must be able to prove that the failure to make the diagnosis of child abuse was negligent and that, had the diagnosis been made, steps would have been taken to protect the child from additional abuse. Although the probability of a physician being held liable under such circumstances is low, the amount of damages can be high if the family does prevail when the child has suffered permanent sequelae.[59]

After admission, the orthopaedist proceeds with care of the child's musculoskeletal injuries and facilitates various medical consultations. Recommendations for disposition of the child after completion of medical treatment may be a group decision through a multidisciplinary team or, more often, the decision of the primary physician, who may be the orthopaedist. Final disposition choices may include return to the family, return to a family member who does not live in the child's home, or placement in a shelter or a foster home setting. The risk of reinjury and death is significant if the abused child is returned to the unsafe home, so the orthopaedist must strongly support child protective services in custodial actions when it is believed that a child's injury truly occurred from abuse at home. Not only must the definitive diagnosis of child abuse be documented in the chart, but a separate notarized affidavit may be necessary. Commonly, custodial actions by child protective services are reviewed in a court hearing in a matter of weeks, and the physician may be called to testify in the hearing. Criminal charges also may be brought against the perpetrator of the child abuse, and the physician likely also serves as a witness in these proceedings.

The Orthopaedic Surgeon's Legal Role in Nonaccidental Injury

The orthopaedist fills a dual role in the courtroom in child abuse proceedings. First, he or she serves as a material witness whose testimony is confined to the physician's personal involvement in the legal matter of the child's evaluation and treatment. The testimony may include clarification to the court of information contained in progress notes in the chart or of other past documentation. As a material witness, the physician cannot render opinions about the facts as stated during his or her testimony. In addition, however, the physician may also be sworn in as an expert witness.[98] This is an individual considered by the court to have special knowledge and experience that qualifies him or her to render opinions about certain facts presented in the courtroom. The limits of the physician's expertise usually are defined by the attorneys in court before the testimony of the expert witness.

Physicians may be reluctant to testify in court for many reasons. The courtroom is an unfamiliar setting for most physicians and the adversarial nature of the American legal system may be perceived as a hostile environment. In the courtroom, opposing attorneys are likely to search for inconsistencies in the testimony or unfamiliarity with the record to discredit the physician witness.

To avoid being a poor witness, the orthopaedist should meticulously prepare to give testimony by conducting a thorough review of the child's medical records and a review of recent medical literature on the subject of child abuse.[98] Often, there is a pretestimony discussion with child protective services counsel in family court cases or the district attorney's office in criminal cases. Such meetings should preferably be in person, and the orthopaedist's professional training and expertise are examined to determine whether he or she may serve as a material witness, an expert witness, or both. The attorney should be provided the orthopaedist's curriculum vitae, and another copy should be made available to the court. If the orthopaedist is to serve as a material witness, the factual information of the case as well as the limitations of the physician's knowledge are discussed, as are questions that may be posed during testimony. Orthopaedists functioning as expert witnesses should indicate relevant information that should be provided through questioning during testimony. In addition, anticipated testimony from any opposing expert witness and cross-examination questions from the opposing attorney should be discussed. The opposing attorney also may request an informal pretestimony meeting. The orthopaedist should request a list of questions that will be asked in this session ahead of time and request that both the prosecution attorney and the opposing attorney be present during the session, which often is recorded.

The next step may be a deposition in which both attorneys question the witness under oath to "discover" the testimony that the witness will provide in court. The primary purpose for a deposition in the discovery process is to keep attorneys from later being surprised in court by testimony of witnesses.[52] Any testimony the physician gives during the deposition will be recorded, and later in court any inconsistencies between testimony and prior depositions will be vigorously attacked by attorneys in cross-examination. Depositions are rarely used in criminal prosecutions[98]; instead, a subpoena is issued requiring a physician witness to appear at the courtroom at a certain time. Often, there may be hours of delay before the testimony actually begins. Through prior arrangements with the attorneys, the orthopaedist may be placed "on call" if he or she works within a reasonable distance of the courtroom and can be available a short time before the actual testimony is needed. The physician has no legal right to such treatment and must be prepared to honor the exact conditions of the subpoena if alternative arrangements cannot be made. If significant delays are encountered to giving testimony and the attorneys are not responsive to physician hardship, then the orthopaedist should contact the judge directly to remedy the situation.[52] In the courtroom, the orthopaedist should be conservatively dressed and appear attentive, competent, poised, and at ease.[52,98]

Once called to the stand, the orthopaedist is sworn in and identified. Next follows qualification, direct examination, and then cross-examination. In the qualification process, the attorney asks the physician fairly detailed questions about the orthopaedist's training and background to establish whether he or she is a credible witness.[98] The attorney wishes to impress the judge or jury with the orthopaedist's qualifications as a witness, whereas the opposing attorney may challenge the witness with questions to cast doubt on his or her expertise.[52] During this phase, the attorneys also may establish the limits of the physician's expertise as an expert medical witness. Next, the attorney will proceed with direct examination. A series of questions are asked that aim at developing a logical and progressive line of thought leading to a conclusion.[52] In child abuse cases, in particular, the testimony will lead to the fact that the abuse has occurred and that it has been appropriately diagnosed. In addition, the physician expert witness may be asked to give an opinion of the risk for subsequent abuse if the child returns to the home where the alleged abuse occurred. The physician witness will almost never be asked about the guilt or innocence of the caretaker accused of abuse, but the orthopaedist in certain circumstances will come close to answering the "ultimate question"[52] by testifying about a child's statement of history if it identifies the abuser. Some states, however, restrict such testimony. In Maryland, a physician may not testify regarding any disclosures made by a child abuse victim unless the disclosure is admissible under a recognized exception to the rule prohibiting hearsay evidence.[237] The orthopaedist should ask about any possible restrictions on his or her testimony with the attorney in pretrial discussion. In testimony, the orthopaedist will want to use the courtroom setting to advocate for the safety and well-being of the child.[98] Questions regarding medical findings often will be prefaced in the courtroom by the words "reasonable medical certainty," a term that is poorly understood by most physicians. Chadwick[52] offered a definition of reasonable medical certainty as "certain as a physician should be in order to recommend and carry out treatment for a given medical condition." He offered an example that the certainty for the diagnosis and treatment of leukemia must be much higher than that for diagnosis and treatment of a viral upper respiratory tract infection.

During testimony, the orthopaedist's words should be carefully chosen and should be understandable by a lay jury. Testimony should be objective, honest, and thorough.[98] Attorneys may frame questions in ways that are difficult to understand, and the orthopaedist should not hesitate to ask the attorney to clarify a question.[52] Answers should be brief, without volunteering extra information, but the perception listeners will have of the answers should be carefully considered by the orthopaedist. In particular, attorneys may phrase yes or no questions that could place misleading words in the mouth of the orthopaedist. In such situations, when neither response is appropriate, the orthopaedist should answer in a sentence that provides an accurate answer.[98] Language should be straightforward, and visual aids may be used in providing clear testimony. The expert should use testimony as an educational process for the court, in which the common experience and knowledge of the jury is used to build understanding with common sense explanations of medical findings.[52]

Cross-examination by the opposing attorney follows direct examination. The opposing attorney's role is to challenge the material presented by the physician witness to protect the defendant.[98] This may involve an attempt to bring into question the physician's credibility, the medical record, the physician's training or expertise, or the physician's objectivity or composure and clarity of thought before the jury.[98] Attorneys may accomplish this by finding inconsistencies with prior statements, asking leading questions as well as questions that allow only certain desired answers, and minimizing physician qualifications.[52] The attorney may frame a question that contains certain elements that the physician agrees with and others that are misleading, and often the question will end with "Isn't that so, doctor?" or "Is that true?" The physician witness should be firm in answering such questions, clearly stating what in the question he or she agrees with and what he or she does not. It is also common to encounter questions from attorneys based on hypotheses that are extremely unlikely, and the physician needs to point out that unlikelihood.[52] Part of the strategy of aggressive cross-examination is to provoke the physician into arguments or unprofessional behavior that could discredit the physician or his or her testimony before the court. In particular, juries will allow aggression on the part of an attorney, but they expect physician witnesses to respond professionally, even under extreme duress.[69] Inexperienced potential physician witnesses can prepare themselves by either watching trials or participating in mock trials.[52] Brent[38] assembled an excellent series of vignettes of expert medical witness case studies in court and provided detailed instructions with regard to the responsibilities of such experts. Both redirect examination and recross-examination may follow cross-examination at the discretion of attorneys, but usually these procedures are very short.[52]

Disposition Following Custody Hearings

After a hearing or trial, the child historically either remains in the protective custody of the state or was returned to the home, but the danger of further abuse exists in both situations. In a study of recurrent maltreatment in 10 states based on the National Child Abuse and Neglect Data System, Fluke et al.[86] found that the recurrence rate was 13% by 6 months after the first episode of reported abuse and return to the home, increasing to 17% by 12 months. In a report of 206 care and protection petitions brought to the Boston juvenile courts,[179] 31 were dismissed with return of the child to the parents. During a 2-year follow-up of these dismissed cases, 29 had reports of further mistreatment, and 16 were returned to court under another care and protection petition. One risk factor identified by the study was a previous appearance in court; half of dismissed cases with this risk factor returned to court again. Children ordered permanently removed from parental custody by the court may still suffer further abuse by a new caretaker. Another alternative pathway of custody is gaining popularity with the court systems in which the abused child is released to the custody of a relative of the family with consideration given to the wishes of the parents or other prior custodians of the child. Although in theory this approach may help preserve the integrity of the family unit, the child may still be in danger in this sort of arrangement. Handy et al.[99] of the Pediatric Forensic Medicine Program of the Kentucky State Medical Examiner's Office noted evidence of recurrent abuse 2 to 9 months after the original injury in six patients out of 316 referrals (1.8%) to the program. They emphasized that in two of these cases, the child was in protective custody of a family relative when the original perpetrator was allowed unsupervised access to the child in violation of court order. It is possible that such reinjuries occur because either the close relatives of the child abuser may not believe that the caretaker committed the original abuse or the relatives are under emotional pressure to allow the caretaker to have access to the child in spite of court order. It is hoped that the court systems can strike a balance between the need to preserve the family unit and the need to protect the child from further abuse.

PREVENTION OF CHILD ABUSE

Prevention of child abuse lies in early intervention. Home visitor programs can contact a mother immediately after the birth of her child and arrange for a visit in which the mother's parenting strengths are assessed. Parents requiring additional support are linked to community agencies and family resources.[10,227] Practicing Safety, a project sponsored by the American Academy of Pediatrics (AAP) and funded by the Doris Duke Charitable Foundation, works to decrease child abuse and neglect by expanding anticipatory guidance and increasing screening by pediatric practices to parents of children aged 0 to 3 years. The AAP website (www.aap.org/practicingsafety) also lists resources for physicians and parents.

Parenting education offers instruction in specific parenting skills such as discipline methods, basic childcare, infant stimulation, child development, education, and familiarity with local support services. Such support seems to enhance parent and child interactions, and mothers report a diminished need to punish or restrict their children. Antivictimization programs teach children certain concepts believed to facilitate self-protection, such as identification of strangers, types of touching, saying "no" to inappropriate advances, and telling someone about inappropriate behavior.

Continuing abuse can be prevented by the orthopaedist's and trauma team's prompt recognition of child abuse in the emergency department or clinic and appropriate intervention.[55] After protecting the welfare of the child, the most important issue in dealing with child abuse is to help both the child and the family through early recognition of the problem and appropriate therapeutic measures by all health personnel.

ACKNOWLEDGMENTS

Special thanks is given to Shelley Sheppard for technical assistance with the manuscript and to Drs. Sami Abedin and Reza Zinati for their medical illustrations.

REFERENCES

1. Ablin DS, Greenspan A, Reinhart M, et al. Differentiation of child abuse from osteogenesis imperfecta. AJR Am J Roentgenol 1990;154(5):1035–1046.
2. Adams JA, Kaplan RA, Starling SP, et al. Guidelines for medical care of children who may have been sexually abused. J Pediatr Adolesc Gynecol 2007;20(3):163–172.
3. Akbarnia B, Torg JS, Kirkpatrick J, et al. Manifestations of the battered-child syndrome. J Bone Joint Surg Am 1974;56(6):1159–1166.
4. Akbarnia BA. The role of the orthopaedic surgeon in child abuse. Philadelphia: Lippincott Williams & Wilkins; 1996.
5. Akbarnia BA. Pediatric spine fractures. Orthop Clin North Am 1999;30(3):521–536.
6. Akbarnia BA, Akbarnia NO. The role of orthopedist in child abuse and neglect. Orthop Clin North Am 1976;7(3):733–742.
7. Alexander RC, Surrell JA, Cohle SD. Microwave oven burns to children: an unusual manifestation of child abuse. Pediatrics 1987;79(2):255–260.
8. Altman DH, Smith RL. Unrecognized trauma in infants and children. J Bone Joint Surg Am 1960;42-A:407–413.
9. American Academy of Pediatrics Committee on Child Abuse and Neglect: Guidelines for the evaluation of sexual abuse of children. Pediatrics 1991;87(2):254–260.
10. American Academy of Pediatrics. A guide to references and resources in child abuse and neglect. In: AAP, ed. American Academy of Pediatrics: Section on Child Abuse and Neglect. Elk Grove Village, IL; Author; 1994:107–190.
11. American College of Radiology. Imaging of the Child with Suspected Child Abuse. Reston, VA: Author; 1997:23.
12. American Academy of Pediatrics Section on Radiology. Diagnostic imaging of child abuse. Pediatrics 2000;105(6):1345–1348.
13. Anderst JD. Assessment of factors resulting in abuse evaluations in young children with minor head trauma. Child Abuse Negl 2008;32(3):405–413.
14. Arkader A, Friedman JE, Warner WC Jr, et al. Complete distal femoral metaphyseal fractures: a harbinger of child abuse before walking age. J Pediatr Orthop 2007;27(7):751–753.
15. Arlotti SA, Forbes BJ, Dias MS, et al. Unilateral retinal hemorrhages in shaken baby syndrome. J AAPOS 2007;11(2):175–178.
16. Asnes RS. Buttock bruises—Mongolian spot. Pediatrics 1984;74(2):321.
17. Babcock J, Hartman K, Pedersen A, et al. Rodenticide-induced coagulopathy in a young child. A case of Munchausen syndrome by proxy. Am J Pediatr Hematol Oncol 1993;15(1):126–130.
18. Baker AM, Craig BR, Lonergan GJ. Homicidal commotio cordis: the final blow in a battered infant. Child Abuse Negl 2003;27(1):125–130.
19. Banaszkiewicz PA, Scotland TR, Myerscough EJ. Fractures in children younger than age 1 year: importance of collaboration with child protection services. J Pediatr Orthop 2002;22(6):740–744.
20. Bandak FA. Shaken baby syndrome: a biomechanics analysis of injury mechanisms. Forensic Sci Int 2005;151(1):71–79.
21. Bar-on ME, Zanga JR. Child abuse: a model for the use of structured clinical forms. Pediatrics 1996;98(3 Pt 1):429–433.
22. Barlow KM, Thomson E, Johnson D, et al. Late neurologic and cognitive sequelae of inflicted traumatic brain injury in infancy. Pediatrics 2005;116(2):e174–185.
23. Barnes PD, Krasnokutsky M. Imaging of the central nervous system in suspected or alleged nonaccidental injury, including the mimics. Top Magn Reson Imaging 2007;18(1):53–74.
24. Barr RG, Trent RB, Cross J. Age-related incidence curve of hospitalized Shaken Baby

Syndrome cases: convergent evidence for crying as a trigger to shaking. Child Abuse Negl 2006;30(1):7–16.
25. Barsness KA, Cha ES, Bensard DD, et al. The positive predictive value of rib fractures as an indicator of nonaccidental trauma in children. J Trauma 2003;54(6):1107–1110.
26. Bartsch C, Risse M, Schutz H, et al. Munchausen syndrome by proxy (MSBP): an extreme form of child abuse with a special forensic challenge. Forensic Sci Int 2003; 137(2–3):147–151.
27. Baskin DE, Stein F, Coats DK, et al. Recurrent conjunctivitis as a presentation of Münchhausen syndrome by proxy. Ophthalmology 2003;110(8):1582–1584.
28. Bays J, Chadwick D. Medical diagnosis of the sexually abused child. Child Abuse Negl 1993;17(1):91–110.
29. Beals RK, Tufts E. Fractured femur in infancy: the role of child abuse. J Pediatr Orthop 1983;3(5):583–586.
30. Benedict MI, White RB, Wulff LM, et al. Reported maltreatment in children with multiple disabilities. Child Abuse Negl 1990;14(2):207–217.
31. Berenson AB, Heger AH, Hayes JM, et al. Appearance of the hymen in prepubertal girls. Pediatrics 1992;89(3):387–394.
32. Berger RP, Dulani T, Adelson PD, et al. Identification of inflicted traumatic brain injury in well-appearing infants using serum and cerebrospinal markers: a possible screening tool. Pediatrics 2006;117(2):325–332.
33. Bernet W. False statements and the differential diagnosis of abuse allegations. J Am Acad Child Adolesc Psychiatry 1993;32(5):903–910.
34. Biron D, Shelton D. Perpetrator accounts in infant abusive head trauma brought about by a shaking event. Child Abuse Negl 2005;29(12):1347–1358.
35. Biron DL, Shelton D. Functional time limit and onset of symptoms in infant abusive head trauma. J Paediatr Child Health 2007;43(1–2):60–65.
36. Blakemore LC, Loder RT, Hensinger RN. Role of intentional abuse in children 1 to 5 years old with isolated femoral shaft fractures. J Pediatr Orthop 1996;16(5):585–588.
37. Bonkowsky JL, Guenther E, Filloux FM, et al. Death, child abuse, and adverse neurological outcome of infants after an apparent life-threatening event. Pediatrics 2008;122(1): 125–131.
38. Brent RL. The irresponsible expert witness: a failure of biomedical graduate education and professional accountability. Pediatrics 1982;70(5):754–762.
39. Brown RA, Bass DH, Rode H, et al. Gastrointestinal tract perforation in children due to blunt abdominal trauma. Br J Surg 1992;79(6):522–524.
40. Brown RL, Brunn MA, Garcia VF. Cervical spine injuries in children: a review of 103 patients treated consecutively at a level 1 pediatric trauma center. J Pediatr Surg 2001; 36(8):1107–1114.
41. Byard RW, Keeley FW, Smith CR. Type IV Ehlers-Danlos syndrome presenting as sudden infant death. Am J Clin Pathol 1990;93(4):579–582.
42. Byers PH. Disorders of Collagen Biosynthesis and Structure. New York: McGraw-Hill; 1989.
43. Caffey J. Mulitple fractures in long bones of infants suffering from chronic subdural hematoma. Am J Roentgenol 1946;56:163–173.
44. Caffey J. The whiplash shaken infant syndrome: manual shaking by the extremities with whiplash-induced intracranial and intraocular bleedings, linked with residual permanent brain damage and mental retardation. Pediatrics 1974;54(4):396–403.
45. Campbell JC. Child abuse and wife abuse: the connections. Md Med J 1994;43(4): 349–350.
46. Cantwell HB. Vaginal inspection as it relates to child sexual abuse in girls under 13. Child Abuse Negl 1983;7(2):171–176.
47. Carpenter RF. The prevalence and distribution of bruising in babies. Arch Dis Child 1999;80(4):363–366.
48. Carrion WV, Dormans JP, Drummond DS, et al. Circumferential growth plate fracture of the thoracolumbar spine from child abuse. J Pediatr Orthop 1996;16(2):210–214.
49. Carroll DM, Doria AS, Paul BS. Clinical-radiological features of fractures in premature infants—a review. J Perinat Med 2007;35(5):366–375.
50. Cattaneo C, Marinelli E, Di Giancamillo A, et al. Sensitivity of autopsy and radiological examination in detecting bone fractures in an animal model: implications for the assessment of fatal child physical abuse. Forensic Sci Int 2006;164(2–3):131–137.
51. Centers for Disease Control and Prevention. Nonfatal maltreatment on infants. United States, October 2005 to September 2006. Morb Mortal Wkly Rep 2008;27:338–339.
52. Chadwick DL. Preparation for court testimony in child abuse cases. Pediatr Clin North Am 1990;37(4):955–970.
53. Chadwick DL, Bertocci G, Castillo E, et al. Annual risk of death resulting from short falls among young children: less than 1 in 1 million. Pediatrics 2008;121(6):1213–1224.
54. Chalumeau M, Foix-L'Helias L, Scheinmann P, et al. Rib fractures after chest physiotherapy for bronchiolitis or pneumonia in infants. Pediatr Radiol 2002;32(9):644–647.
55. Chang DC, Knight V, Ziegfeld S, et al. The tip of the iceberg for child abuse: the critical roles of the pediatric trauma service and its registry. J Trauma 2004;57(6):1189–1198; discussion 1198.
56. Chapman S, Hall CM. Nonaccidental injury or brittle bones. Pediatr Radiol 1997;27(2): 106–110.
57. Children's Health and Safety Initiative: Building Blocks for Healthy Children. In: Health TDO, ed. 1996;24.
58. Cho DY, Wang YC, Chi CS. Decompressive craniotomy for acute shaken/impact baby syndrome. Pediatr Neurosurg 1995;23(4):192–198.
59. Clayton EW. Potential liability in cases of child abuse and neglect. Pediatr Ann 1997; 26(3):173–177.
60. Coant PN, Kornberg AE, Brody AS, et al. Markers for occult liver injury in cases of physical abuse in children. Pediatrics 1992;89(2):274–278.
61. Coffey C, Haley K, Hayes J, et al. The risk of child abuse in infants and toddlers with lower extremity injuries. J Pediatr Surg 2005;40(1):120–123.
62. Conway JJ, Collins M, Tanz RR, et al. The role of bone scintigraphy in detecting child abuse. Semin Nucl Med 1993;23(4):321–333.
63. Cooper A, Floyd T, Barlow B, et al. Major blunt abdominal trauma due to child abuse. J Trauma 1988;28(10):1483–1487.
64. Crouch JL, Behl LE. Relationships among parental beliefs in corporal punishment, reported stress, and physical child abuse potential. Child Abuse Negl 2001;25(3): 413–419.
65. Crume TL, DiGuiseppi C, Byers T, et al. Underascertainment of child maltreatment fatalities by death certificates, 1990 to 1998. Pediatrics 2002;110(2 Pt 1):e18.
66. Cullen JC. Spinal lesions in battered babies. J Bone Joint Surg Br 1975;57(3):364–366.
67. Currarino G. Primary spondylolysis of the axis vertebra (C2) in three children, including one with pyknodysostosis. Pediatr Radiol 1989;19(8):535–538.
68. Currarino G, Birch JG, Herring JA. Developmental coxa vara associated with spondylometaphyseal dysplasia (DCV/SMD): "SMD-corner fracture type" (DCV/SMD-CF) demonstrated in most reported cases. Pediatr Radiol 2000;30(1):14–24.
69. Dalton HJ, Slovis T, Helfer RE, et al. Undiagnosed abuse in children younger than 3 years with femoral fracture. Am J Dis Child 1990;144(8):875–878.
70. de Silva S, Oates RK. Child homicide—the extreme of child abuse. Med J Aust 1993; 158(5):300–301.
71. Dent JA, Paterson CR. Fractures in early childhood: osteogenesis imperfecta or child abuse? J Pediatr Orthop 1991;11(2):184–186.
72. DeRusso PA, Spevak MR, Schwarz KB. Fractures in biliary atresia misinterpreted as child abuse. Pediatrics 2003;112(1 Pt 1):185–188.
73. Dias MS, Smith K, DeGuehery K, et al. Preventing abusive head trauma among infants and young children: a hospital-based, parent education program. Pediatrics 2005; 115(4):e470–477.
74. Dreizen S, Spirakis CN, Stone RE. The influence of age and nutritional status on "bone scar" formation in the distal end of the growing radius. Am J Phys Anthropol 1964; 22:295–305.
75. Dubowitz H, Bennett S. Physical abuse and neglect of children. Lancet 2007;369(9576): 1891–1899.
76. Dubowitz H, Black M. Teaching pediatric residents about child maltreatment. Dev Behav Pediatr 1991;12:305–307.
77. Dubowitz H, Bross DC. The pediatrician's documentation of child maltreatment. Am J Dis Child 1992;146(5):596–599.
78. Duhaime AC, Gennarelli TA, Thibault LE, et al. The shaken baby syndrome. A clinical, pathological, and biomechanical study. J Neurosurg 1987;66(3):409–415.
79. Duncan AA, Chandy J. Case report: multiple neonatal fractures—dietary or deliberate? Clin Radiol 1993;48(2):137–139.
80. Ellerstein NS, Norris KJ. Value of radiologic skeletal survey in assessment of abused children. Pediatrics 1984;74(6):1075–1078.
81. Feldman KW. Pseudoabusive burns in Asian refugees. Am J Dis Child 1984;138(8): 768–769.
82. Fernando S, Obaldo RE, Walsh IR, et al. Neuroimaging of nonaccidental head trauma: pitfalls and controversies. Pediatr Radiol 2008;38(8):827–838.
83. Flaherty EG. Analysis of caretaker histories in abuse: comparing initial histories with subsequent confessions. Child Abuse Negl 2006;30(7):789–798.
84. Flaherty EG, Sege R, Mattson CL, et al. Assessment of suspicion of abuse in the primary care setting. Ambul Pediatr 2002;2(2):120–126.
85. Flaherty EG, Sege RD, Griffith J, et al. From suspicion of physical child abuse to reporting: primary care clinician decision-making. Pediatrics 2008;122(3):611–619.
86. Fluke JD, Yuan YY, Edwards M. Recurrence of maltreatment: an application of the National Child Abuse and Neglect Data System (NCANDS). Child Abuse Negl 1999; 23(7):633–650.
87. Fordham EW, Ramachandran PC. Radionuclide imaging of osseous trauma. Semin Nucl Med 1974;4(4):411–429.
88. Frasier L Rauth-Farley K, Alexander R, et al. Abusive Head Trauma in Infants and Children: A Medical, Legal, and Forensic Reference. St. Louis, MO: GW Medical Publishing; 2006.
89. Frechette A, Rimsza ME. Stun gun injury: a new presentation of the battered child syndrome. Pediatrics 1992;89(5 Pt 1):898–901.
90. Gahagan S, Rimsza ME. Child abuse or osteogenesis imperfecta: how can we tell? Pediatrics 1991;88(5):987–992.
91. Galleno H, Oppenheim WL. The battered child syndrome revisited. Clin Orthop Relat Res 1982(162):11–19.
92. Gerber P, Coffman K. Nonaccidental head trauma in infants. Childs Nerv Syst 2007; 23(5):499–507.
93. Goss PW, McDougall PN. Munchausen syndrome by proxy—a cause of preterm delivery. Med J Aust 1992;157(11–12):814–817.
94. Grayev AM, Boal DK, Wallach DM, et al. Metaphyseal fractures mimicking abuse during treatment for clubfoot. Pediatr Radiol 2001;31(8):559–563.
95. Green FC. Child abuse and neglect. A priority problem for the private physician. Pediatr Clin North Am 1975;22(2):329–339.
96. Habert J, Haller JO. Iatrogenic vertebral body compression fracture in a premature infant caused by extreme flexion during positioning for a lumbar puncture. Pediatr Radiol 2000;30(6):410–411.
97. Hall DE, Eubanks L, Meyyazhagan LS, et al. Evaluation of covert video surveillance in the diagnosis of munchausen syndrome by proxy: lessons from 41 cases. Pediatrics 2000;105(6):1305–1312.
98. Halverson KC, Elliott BA, Rubin MS, et al. Legal considerations in cases of child abuse. Prim Care 1993;20(2):407–416.
99. Handy TC, Nichols GR 2nd, Smock WS. Repeat visitors to a pediatric forensic medicine program. J Forensic Sci 1996;41(5):841–844.
100. Hanes M, McAuliff T. Preparation for child abuse litigation: perspectives of the prosecutor and the pediatrician. Pediatr Ann 1997;26(5):288–295.
101. Harding B, Risdon RA, Krous HF. Shaken baby syndrome. BMJ 2004;328(7442): 720–721.
102. Harty MP, Kao SC. Intraosseous vascular access defect: fracture mimic in the skeletal survey for child abuse. Pediatr Radiol 2002;32(3):188–190.
103. Hechter S, Huyer D, Manson D. Sternal fractures as a manifestation of abusive injury in children. Pediatr Radiol 2002;32(12):902–906.
104. Heider TR, Priolo D, Hultman CS, et al. Eczema mimicking child abuse: a case of mistaken identity. J Burn Care Rehabil 2002;23(5):357–359; discussion 357.
105. Helfer RE. The epidemiology of child abuse and neglect. Pediatr Ann 1984;13(10): 745–751.
106. Helfer RE, Slovis TL, Black M. Injuries resulting when small children fall out of bed. Pediatrics 1977;60(4):533–535.
107. Hennrikus WL, Shaw BA, Gerardi JA. Injuries when children reportedly fall from a bed or couch. Clin Orthop Relat Res 2003(407):148–151.
108. Herman-Giddens ME, Brown G, Verbiest S, et al. Underascertainment of child abuse mortality in the United States. JAMA 1999;282(5):463–467.
109. Herndon WA. Child abuse in a military population. J Pediatr Orthop 1983;3(1):73–76.

110. Hobbs CJ, Wynne JM. The sexually abused battered child. Arch Dis Child 1990;65(4): 423–427.
111. Hosalkar HS, Sankar WN, Wills BP, et al. Congenital osseous anomalies of the upper cervical spine. J Bone Joint Surg Am 2008;90(2):337–348.
112. Hudson M, Kaplan R. Clinical response to child abuse. Pediatr Clin North Am 2006; 53(1):27–39, v.
113. Hughes LA, May K, Talbot JF, et al. Incidence, distribution, and duration of birth-related retinal hemorrhages: a prospective study. J AAPOS 2006;10(2):102–106.
114. Hui C, Joughin E, Goldstein S, et al. Femoral fractures in children younger than three years: the role of nonaccidental injury. J Pediatr Orthop 2008;28(3):297–302.
115. Hyden PW, Gallagher TA. Child abuse intervention in the emergency room. Pediatr Clin North Am 1992;39(5):1053–1081.
116a. Hymel KP, and the Committee on Child abuse and Neglect and National Association of Medical Examiners. Distinguishing sudden infant death syndrome from child abuse fatalities. Pediatrics 2006;118:421–427.
116. Hymel KP, Hall CA. Diagnosing pediatric head trauma. Pediatr Ann 2005;34(5): 358–370.
117. Hymel KP, Makoroff KL, Laskey AL, et al. Mechanisms, clinical presentations, injuries, and outcomes from inflicted versus noninflicted head trauma during infancy: results of a prospective, multicentered, comparative study. Pediatrics 2007;119(5):922–929.
118. Ingram DM, Everett VD, Ingram DL. The relationship between the transverse hymenal orifice diameter by the separation technique and other possible markers of sexual abuse. Child Abuse Negl 2001;25(8):1109–1120.
119. Jaudes PK. Comparison of radiography and radionuclide bone scanning in the detection of child abuse. Pediatrics 1984;73(2):166–168.
120. Jenny C. Evaluating infants and young children with multiple fractures. Pediatrics 2006;118(3):1299–1303.
121. Jenny C. Recognizing and responding to medical neglect. Pediatrics 2007;120(6): 1385–1389.
122. Jenny C, Hymel KP, Ritzen A, et al. Analysis of missed cases of abusive head trauma. JAMA 1999;281(7):621–626.
123. Jenny C, Isaac R. The relation between child death and child maltreatment. Arch Dis Child 2006;91(3):265–269.
124. Jessee SA, Rieger M. A study of age-related variables among physically abused children. ASDC J Dent Child 1996;63(4):275–280.
125. Johnson CF. Inflicted injury versus accidental injury. Pediatr Clin North Am 1990; 37(4):791–814.
126. Johnson CF, Kaufman KL, Callendar C. The hand as a target organ in child abuse. Clin Pediatr (Phila) 1990;29(2):66–72.
127. Kaplan JM. Pseudoabuse—the misdiagnosis of child abuse. J Forensic Sci 1986;31(4): 1420–1428.
128. Keenan HT, Runyan DK, Marshall SW, et al. A population-based study of inflicted traumatic brain injury in young children. JAMA 2003;290(5):621–626.
129. Kellogg ND, Menard SW, Santos A. Genital anatomy in pregnant adolescents: "normal" does not mean "nothing happened." Pediatrics 2004;113(1 Pt 1):e67–69.
130. Kemp AM, Butler A, Morris S, et al. Which radiological investigations should be performed to identify fractures in suspected child abuse? Clin Radiol 2006;61(9):723–736.
131. Kempe CH, Silverman FN, Steele BF, et al. The battered-child syndrome. JAMA 1962; 181:17–24.
132. King J, Diefendorf D, Apthorp J, et al. Analysis of 429 fractures in 189 battered children. J Pediatr Orthop 1988;8(5):585–589.
133. Kleinman P. Dianogstic Imaging of Child Abuse. 2nd ed. St Louis: Mosby; 1998.
134. Kleinman PK, Blackbourne BD, Marks SC, et al. Radiologic contributions to the investigation and prosecution of cases of fatal infant abuse. N Engl J Med 1989;320(8): 507–511.
135. Kleinman PK, Marks SC. Vertebral body fractures in child abuse. Radiologic-histopathologic correlates. Invest Radiol 1992;27(9):715–722.
136. Kleinman PK, Marks SC Jr. Relationship of the subperiosteal bone collar to metaphyseal lesions in abused infants. J Bone Joint Surg Am 1995;77(10):1471–1476.
137. Kleinman PK, Marks SC Jr, Adams VI, et al. Factors affecting visualization of posterior rib fractures in abused infants. AJR Am J Roentgenol 1988;150(3):635–638.
138. Kleinman PK, Marks SC Jr, Blackbourne B. The metaphyseal lesion in abused infants: a radiologic-histopathologic study. AJR Am J Roentgenol 1986;146(5):895–905.
139. Kleinman PK, Marks SC Jr, Richmond JM, et al. Inflicted skeletal injury: a postmortem radiologic-histopathologic study in 31 infants. AJR Am J Roentgenol 1995;165(3): 647–650.
140. Kleinman PK, Marks SC Jr, Spevak MR, et al. Fractures of the rib head in abused infants. Radiology 1992;185(1):119–123.
141. Kleinman PK, Nimkin K, Spevak MR, et al. Follow-up skeletal surveys in suspected child abuse. AJR Am J Roentgenol 1996;167(4):893–896.
142. Kleinman PK, O'Connor B, Nimkin K, et al. Detection of rib fractures in an abused infant using digital radiography: a laboratory study. Pediatr Radiol 2002;32(12): 896–901.
143. Kleinman PK, Shelton YA. Hangman's fracture in an abused infant: imaging features. Pediatr Radiol 1997;27(9):776–777.
144. Kleinman PK, Spevak MR. Variations in acromial ossification simulating infant abuse in victims of sudden infant death syndrome. Radiology 1991;180(1):185–187.
145. Knight DJ, Bennet GC. Nonaccidental injury in osteogenesis imperfecta: a case report. J Pediatr Orthop 1990;10(4):542–544.
146. Kogutt MS, Swischuk LE, Fagan CJ. Patterns of injury and significance of uncommon fractures in the battered child syndrome. Am J Roentgenol Radium Ther Nucl Med 1974;121(1):143–149.
147. Kos L, Shwayder T. Cutaneous manifestations of child abuse. Pediatr Dermatol 2006; 23(4):311–320.
148. Kravitz H, Driessen G, Gomberg R, et al. Accidental falls from elevated surfaces in infants from birth to 1 year of age. Pediatrics 1969;44(5):869–876.
149. Krug EG, Dahlberg LL, Mercy JA, et al. World Report on Violence and Health. Geneva: World Health Organization; 2002.
150. Krugman RD. Recognition of sexual abuse in children. Pediatr Rev 1986;8(1):25–30.
151. Labbe J. Ambroise Tardieu: the man and his work on child maltreatment a century before Kempe. Child Abuse Negl 2005;29(4):311–324.
152. Labbe J, Caouette G. Recent skin injuries in normal children. Pediatrics 2001;108(2): 271–276.
153. Lane WG, Dubowitz H. What factors affect the identification and reporting of child abuse-related fractures? Clin Orthop Relat Res 2007;461:219–225.
154. Langlois NE, Gresham GA. The aging of bruises: a review and study of the color changes with time. Forensic Sci Int 1991;50(2):227–238.
155. Laposata ME, Laposata M. Children with signs of abuse: when is it not child abuse? Am J Clin Pathol 2005;123 Suppl:S119–124.
156. Ledbetter DJ, Hatch EI Jr, Feldman KW, et al. Diagnostic and surgical implications of child abuse. Arch Surg 1988;123(9):1101–1105.
157. Leventhal JM, Thomas SA, Rosenfield SN, et al. Fractures in young children: distinguishing child abuse from unintentional injuries. Am Dis Child 1993;147(1):87–92.
158. Leventhal JM, Larson IA, Abdoo D, et al. Are abusive fractures in young children becoming less common? Changes over 24 years. Child Abuse Negl 2007;31(3): 311–322.
159. Levin TL, Berdon WE, Cassell I, et al. Thoracolumbar fracture with listhesis—an uncommon manifestation of child abuse. Pediatr Radiol 2003;33(5):305–310.
160. Lim HK, Smith WL, Sato Y, et al. Congenital syphilis mimicking child abuse. Pediatr Radiol 1995;25(7):560–561.
161. Limbos MA, Berkowitz CD. Documentation of child physical abuse: how far have we come? Pediatrics 1998;102(1 Pt 1):53–58.
162. Loder RT, Bookout C. Fracture patterns in battered children. J Orthop Trauma 1991; 5(4):428–433.
163. MacMillan HL, Thomas BH, Jamieson E, et al. Effectiveness of home visitation by public-health nurses in prevention of the recurrence of child physical abuse and neglect: a randomised controlled trial. Lancet 2005;365(9473):1786–1793.
164. Magid N, Glass T. A "hole in a rib" as a sign of child abuse. Pediatr Radiol 1990;20(5): 334–336.
165. Maguire S, Mann MK, John N, Ellaway B, et al. Does cardiopulmonary resuscitation cause rib fractures in children? A systematic review. Child Abuse Negl 2006;30(7): 739–751.
166. Maguire S, Mann MK, Sibert J, et al. Are there patterns of bruising in childhood which are diagnostic or suggestive of abuse? A systematic review. Arch Dis Child 2005;90(2): 182–186.
167. Marlowe A, Pepin MG, Byers PH. Testing for osteogenesis imperfecta in cases of suspected nonaccidental injury. J Med Genet 2002;39(6):382–386.
168. McClain JL, Clark MA, Sandusky GE. Undiagnosed, untreated acute lymphoblastic leukemia presenting as suspected child abuse. J Forensic Sci 1990;35(3):735–739.
169. McClelland CQ, Heiple KG. Fractures in the first year of life. A diagnostic dilemma. Am J Dis Child 1982;136(1):26–29.
170. McEniery J, Hanson R, Grigor W, et al. Lung injury resulting from a nonaccidental crush injury to the chest. Pediatr Emerg Care 1991;7(3):166–168.
171. McMahon P, Grossman W, Gaffney M, et al. Soft-tissue injury as an indication of child abuse. J Bone Joint Surg Am 1995;77(8):1179–1183.
172. Meadow R. Munchausen syndrome by proxy abuse perpetrated by men. Arch Dis Child 1998;78(3):210–216.
173. Meadow R. Nonaccidental salt poisoning. Arch Dis Child 1993;68(4):448–452.
174. Mehl AL, Coble L, Johnson S. Munchausen syndrome by proxy: a family affair. Child Abuse Negl 1990;14(4):577–585.
175. Mendelson KL. Critical review of "temporary brittle bone disease." Pediatr Radiol 2005; 35(10):1036–1040.
176. Merten DF, Carpenter BL. Radiologic imaging of inflicted injury in the child abuse syndrome. Pediatr Clin North Am 1990;37(4):815–837.
177. Merten DF, Radkowski MA, Leonidas JC. The abused child: a radiological reappraisal. Radiology 1983;146(2):377–381.
178. Mungan NK. Update on shaken baby syndrome: ophthalmology. Curr Opin Ophthalmol 2007;18(5):392–397.
179. Murphy JM, Bishop SJ, Jellinek MS, et al. What happens after the care and protection petition? Reabuse in a court sample. Child Abuse Negl 1992;16(4):485–493.
180. National Association of Children's Hospital and Related Institutions. Defining the Children's Hospital Role in Child Maltreatment. Alexandria, VA: Author; 2006.
181. Newman RS, Jalili M, Kolls BJ, et al. Factor XIII deficiency mistaken for battered child syndrome: case of "correct" test ordering negated by a commonly accepted qualitative test with limited negative predictive value. Am J Hematol 2002;71(4):328–330.
182. Newton AW, Vandeven AM. Unexplained infant and child death: a review of sudden infant death syndrome, sudden unexplained infant death, and child maltreatment fatalities including shaken baby syndrome. Curr Opin Pediatr 2006;18(2):196–200.
183. Nichols GR II, Corey TS, Davis GJ. Nonfracture-associated fatal fat embolism in a case of child abuse. J Forensic Sci 1990;35(2):493–499.
184. Nimkin K, Spevak MR, Kleinman PK. Fractures of the hands and feet in child abuse: imaging and pathologic features. Radiology 1997;203(1):233–236.
185. O'Neill JA Jr, Meacham WF, Griffin JP, et al. Patterns of injury in the battered child syndrome. J Trauma 1973;13(4):332–339.
186. Oehmichen M, Meissner C, Saternus KS. Fall or shaken: traumatic brain injury in children caused by falls or abuse at home—a review on biomechanics and diagnosis. Neuropediatrics 2005;36(4):240–245.
187. Ojima K, Matsumoto H, Hayase T, et al. An autopsy case of osteogenesis imperfecta initially suspected as child abuse. Forensic Sci Int 1994;65(2):97–104.
188. Oliver JE. Intergenerational transmission of child abuse: rates, research, and clinical implications. Am J Psychiatry 1993;150(9):1315–1324.
189. Oral R, Rahhal R, Elshershari H, et al. Intentional avulsion fracture of the second cervical vertebra in a hypotonic child. Pediatr Emerg Care 2006;22(5):352–354.
190. Orbach Y, Lamb ME. Enhancing children's narratives in investigative interviews. Child Abuse Negl 2000;24(12):1631–1648.
191. Osier LK, Marks SC Jr, Kleinman PK. Metaphyseal extensions of hypertrophied chondrocytes in abused infants indicate healing fractures. J Pediatr Orthop 1993;13(2): 249–254.
192. Palusci VJ, Cox EO, Shatz EM, et al. Urgent medical assessment after child sexual abuse. Child Abuse Negl 2006;30(4):367–380.
193. Palusci VJ, Hicks RA, Vandervort FE. "You are hereby commanded to appear": pediatrician subpoena and court appearance in child maltreatment. Pediatrics 2001;107(6): 1427–1430.
194. Parizel PM, Ceulemans B, Laridon A, et al. Cortical hypoxic-ischemic brain damage in shaken-baby (shaken impact) syndrome: value of diffusion-weighted MRI. Pediatr Radiol 2003;33(12):868–871.

195. Paterson CR, Burns J, McAllion SJ. Osteogenesis imperfecta: the distinction from child abuse and the recognition of a variant form. Am J Med Genet 1993;45(2):187–192.
196. Peebles J, Losek JD. Child physical abuse and rhabdomyolysis: case report and literature review. Pediatr Emerg Care 2007;23(7):474–477.
197. Pergolizzi R Jr, Oestreich AE. Child abuse fracture through physiologic periosteal reaction. Pediatr Radiol 1995;25(7):566–567.
198. Pierce MC, Bertocci GE, Janosky JE, et al. Femur fractures resulting from stair falls among children: an injury plausibility model. Pediatrics 2005;115(6):1712–1722.
199. Pierce MC, Bertocci GE, Vogeley E, et al. Evaluating long bone fractures in children: a biomechanical approach with illustrative cases. Child Abuse Negl 2004;28(5): 505–524.
200. Prescott PR. Hair dryer burns in children. Pediatrics 1990;86(5):692–697.
201. Wang CT, Holton J. The total estimated cost of child abuse and neglect in the United States. Chicago: Prevent Child Abuse America. Available at: http://member.preventchildabuse.org/site/DocServer/cost_analysis.pdf?docID = 144. Accessed August 25, 2009.
202. Prosser I, Maguire S, Harrison SK, et al. How old is this fracture? Radiologic dating of fractures in children: a systematic review. AJR Am J Roentgenol 2005;184(4): 1282–1286.
203. Purdue GF, Hunt JL, Prescott PR. Child abuse by burning—an index of suspicion. J Trauma 1988;28(2):221–224.
204. Reece RM, Sege R. Childhood head injuries: accidental or inflicted? Arch Pediatr Adolesc Med 2000;154(1):11–15.
205. Renz BM, Sherman R. Abusive scald burns in infants and children: a prospective study. Am Surg 1993;59(5):329–334.
206. Rex C, Kay PR. Features of femoral fractures in nonaccidental injury. J Pediatr Orthop 2000;20(3):411–413.
207. Robertson D, Barbor, P. Unusual Injury? Recent injury in normal children and children with suspected nonaccidental trauma. Br Med J (Clin Res Ed) 1982;285:1399–1401.
208. Rooks VJ, Sisler C, Burton B. Cervical spine injury in child abuse: report of two cases. Pediatr Radiol 1998;28(3):193–195.
209. Rosenberg DA. Web of deceit: a literature review of Munchausen syndrome by proxy. Child Abuse Negl 1987;11(4):547–563.
210. Rubin DM, Christian CW, Bilaniuk LT, et al. Occult head injury in high-risk abused children. Pediatrics 2003;111(6 Pt 1):1382–1386.
211. Salehi-Had H, Brandt JD, Rosas AJ, et al. Findings in older children with abusive head injury: does shaken-child syndrome exist? Pediatrics 2006;117(5):e1039–1044.
212. Schmitt B. Child Abuse. Philadelphia: WB Saunders; 1984.
213. Schnitzer P. Child deaths resulting from inflected injuries: household risk factors and perpetrator characteristics. Pediatrics 2005;116:687–693.
214. Schwartz AJ, Ricci LR. How accurately can bruises be aged in abused children? Literature review and synthesis. Pediatrics 1996;97(2):254–257.
215. Schwend RM, Werth C, Johnston A. Femur shaft fractures in toddlers and young children: rarely from child abuse. J Pediatr Orthop 2000;20(4):475–481.
216. Shaw BA, Murphy KM, Shaw A, et al. Humerus shaft fractures in young children: accident or abuse? J Pediatr Orthop 1997;17(3):293–297.
217. Shoenfeld Y. Osteogenesis imperfecta. Review of the literature with presentation of 29 cases. Am J Dis Child 1975;129(6):679–687.
218. Siegel CD, Graves P, Maloney K, et al. Mortality from intentional and unintentional injury among infants of young mothers in Colorado, 1986 to 1992. Arch Pediatr Adolesc Med 1996;150(10):1077–1083.
219. Sieradzki JP, Sarwark JF. Thoracolumbar fracture-dislocation in child abuse: case report, closed reduction technique and review of the literature. Pediatr Neurosurg 2008; 44(3):253–257.
220. Sillence D. Osteogenesis imperfecta: an expanding panorama of variants. Clin Orthop Relat Res 1981(159):11–25.
221. Sillence D, Butler B, Latham M, et al. Natural history of blue sclerae in osteogenesis imperfecta. Am J Med Genet 1993;45(2):183–186.
222. Silverman FN. The roentgen manifestations of unrecognized skeletal trauma in infants. Am J Roentgenol Radium Ther Nucl Med 1953;69(3):413–427.
223. Sinal SH. Sexual abuse of children and adolescents. South Med J 1994;87(12): 1242–1258.
224. Sirotnak A. Medical Disorders that Mimic abusive Head Trauma. St. Louis, MO: GW Medical Publishing; 2006.
225. Smeets AJ, Robben SG, Meradji M. Sonographically detected costo-chondral dislocation in an abused child. A new sonographic sign to the radiological spectrum of child abuse. Pediatr Radiol 1990;20(7):566–567.
226. Smith FW, Gilday DL, Ash JM, et al. Unsuspected costo-vertebral fractures demonstrated by bone scanning in the child abuse syndrome. Pediatr Radiol 1980;10(2): 103–106.
227. Smith PB, Poertner J, Fields JD. Preventing child abuse and neglect in Texas. Tex Med 1990;86(2):44–45.
228. Sperry K, Pfalzgraf R. Inadvertent clavicular fractures caused by "chiropractic" manipulations in an infant: an unusual form of pseudoabuse. J Forensic Sci 1990;35(5): 1211–1216.
229. Starling SP, Patel S, Burke BL, et al. Analysis of perpetrator admissions to inflicted traumatic brain injury in children. Arch Pediatr Adolesc Med 2004;158(5):454–458.
230. Starling SP, Sirotnak AP, Heisler KW, et al. Inflicted skeletal trauma: the relationship of perpetrators to their victims. Child Abuse Negl 2007;31(9):993–999.
231. Steiner RD, Pepin M, Byers PH. Studies of collagen synthesis and structure in the differentiation of child abuse from osteogenesis imperfecta. J Pediatr 1996;128(4): 542–547.
232. Stephenson T, Bialas Y. Estimation of the age of bruising. Arch Dis Child 1996;74(1): 53–55.
233. Stirling J Jr. Beyond Munchausen syndrome by proxy: identification and treatment of child abuse in a medical setting. Pediatrics 2007;119(5):1026–1030.
234. Stirling J Jr, Amaya-Jackson L. Understanding the behavioral and emotional consequences of child abuse. Pediatrics 2008;122(3):667–673.
235. Strouse PJ, Owings CL. Fractures of the first rib in child abuse. Radiology 1995;197(3): 763–765.
236. Sty JR, Starshak RJ. The role of bone scintigraphy in the evaluation of the suspected abused child. Radiology 1983;146(2):369–375.
237. Sugar NF, Taylor JA, Feldman KW. Bruises in infants and toddlers: those who don't cruise rarely bruise. Puget Sound Pediatric Research Network. Arch Pediatr Adolesc Med 1999;153(4):399–403.
238. Suh DY, Davis PC, Hopkins KL, et al. Nonaccidental pediatric head injury: diffusion-weighted imaging findings. Neurosurgery 2001;49(2):309–318; discussion 318–320.
239. Sullivan PM, Brookhouser PE, Scanlan JM, et al. Patterns of physical and sexual abuse of communicatively handicapped children. Ann Otol Rhinol Laryngol 1991;100(3): 188–194.
240. Sussman SJ. Skin manifestations of the battered-child syndrome. J Pediatr 1968;72(1): 99.
241. Swerdlin A, Berkowitz C, Craft N. Cutaneous signs of child abuse. J Am Acad Dermatol 2007;57(3):371–392.
242. Swischuk LE. Spine and spinal cord trauma in the battered child syndrome. Radiology 1969;92(4):733–738.
243. Thogmartin JR, England D, Siebert CF Jr. Hepatic glycogen staining. Applications in injury survival time and child abuse. Am J Forensic Med Pathol 2001;22(3):313–318.
244. Thomas AE. The bleeding child: is it NAI? Arch Dis Child 2004;89(12):1163–1167.
245. Thomas NH, Robinson L, Evans A, et al. The floppy infant: a new manifestation of nonaccidental injury. Pediatr Neurosurg 1995;23(4):188–191.
246. Thomas SA, Rosenfield NS, Leventhal JM, et al. Long-bone fractures in young children: distinguishing accidental injuries from child abuse. Pediatrics 1991;88(3):471–476.
247. Titus MO, Baxter AL, Starling SP. Accidental scald burns in sinks. Pediatrics 2003; 111(2):E191–194.
248. Touloukian RJ. Abdominal visceral injuries in battered children. Pediatrics 1968;42(4): 642–646.
249. Tracy T Jr, O'Connor TP, Weber TR. Battered children with duodenal avulsion and transection. Am Surg 1993;59(6):342–345.
250. Trokel M, DiScala C, Terrin NC, et al. Blunt abdominal injury in the young pediatric patient: child abuse and patient outcomes. Child Maltreat 2004;9(1):111–117.
251. Trokel M, Discala C, Terrin NC, et al. Patient and injury characteristics in abusive abdominal injuries. Pediatr Emerg Care 2006;22(10):700–704.
252. Trokel M, Waddimba A, Griffith J, et al. Variation in the diagnosis of child abuse in severely injured infants. Pediatrics 2006;117(3):722–728.
253. U.S. Department of Health and Human Services. Child Maltreatment. Washington, DC: Author; 2006.
254. U.S. Department of Health and Human Services. The Child Abuse Prevention and Treatment Act (CAPTA). Washington, DC: Author; 2003.
255. Wasserman DR, Leventhal JM. Maltreatment of children born to cocaine-dependent mothers. Am J Dis Child 1993;147(12):1324–1328.
256. Wenk RE. Molecular evidence of Munchausen syndrome by proxy. Arch Pathol Lab Med 2003;127(1):e36–37.
257. Willinger M, James LS, Catz C. Defining the sudden infant death syndrome (SIDS): deliberations of an expert panel convened by the National Institute of Child Health and Human Development. Pediatr Pathol 1991;11(5):677–684.
258. Wilson EF. Estimation of the age of cutaneous contusions in child abuse. Pediatrics 1977;60(5):750–752.
259. Wissow LS. Child abuse and neglect. N Engl J Med 1995;332(21):1425–1431.
260. Wolfner GD, Gelles RJ. A profile of violence toward children: a national study. Child Abuse Negl 1993;17(2):197–212.
261. Wrigley J, Dreby J. Fatalities and the organization of child care in the United States, 1985–2003. Am Sociol Rev 2005;70:729–757.
262. Wygnanski-Jaffe T, Levin AV, Shafiq A, et al. Postmortem orbital findings in shaken baby syndrome. Am J Ophthalmol 2006;142(2):233–240.
263. Youmans DC, Don S, Hildebolt C, et al. Skeletal surveys for child abuse: comparison of interpretation using digitized images and screen-film radiographs. AJR Am J Roentgenol 1998;171(5):1415–1419.
264. Zimmerman S, Makoroff K, Care M, et al. Utility of follow-up skeletal surveys in suspected child physical abuse evaluations. Child Abuse Negl 2005;29(10):1075–1083.
265. Zuravin SJ. Unplanned childbearing and family size: their relationship to child neglect and abuse. Fam Plann Perspect 1991;23(4):155–161.

RECOMMENDED READINGS

Two references invaluable for preparation for testimony in the courtroom about child abuse:

Chadwick DL. Preparation for court testimony in child abuse cases. Pediatr Clin North Am 1990;37:955–970.

Halverson KC, Elliott BA, Rubin MS, et al. Legal considerations in cases of child abuse. Primary Care 1993;20:407–415.

A handy reference for courtroom testimony involving dating fractures:

O'Connor JF, Cohen J. Dating fractures. In: Kleinman PK, ed. Diagnostic Imaging of Child Abuse. Baltimore: Williams & Wilkins; 1987:168–177.

The bible of child abuse radiology:

Kleinman PK. Diagnostic Imaging of Child Abuse. 2nd ed. St. Louis: Mosby; 1998.

A current, concise review of the orthopaedic detection of child abuse:

Kocher MS, Kasser JR. Orthopaedic aspects of child abuse. J Am Acad Orthop Surg 2000; 8:10–20.

Newton AW, Vandeven AM. Update on child maltreatment. Curr Opin Pediatr 2007;19: 223–229.

Illustrates the need to keep open mind regarding other diagnoses and the mimics of child abuse:

Laposata ME, Laposata M. Children with signs of abuse. When is it not child abuse? Am J Clin Path 2005;123(Suppl 1):S1–S6.

OTHER RESOURCES

Visual diagnosis of Child Abuse on CD-ROM. This media from AAP 2008 (www.aap.org) has more than 300 new diagnosis slides.

Child Abuse: Medical Diagnosis and Management. Lecture series of topics in child abuse (www.aap.org).

AAP Section on Child Abuse and Neglect web site: www.aap.org/sections/scan

SECTION

TWO

UPPER EXTREMITY

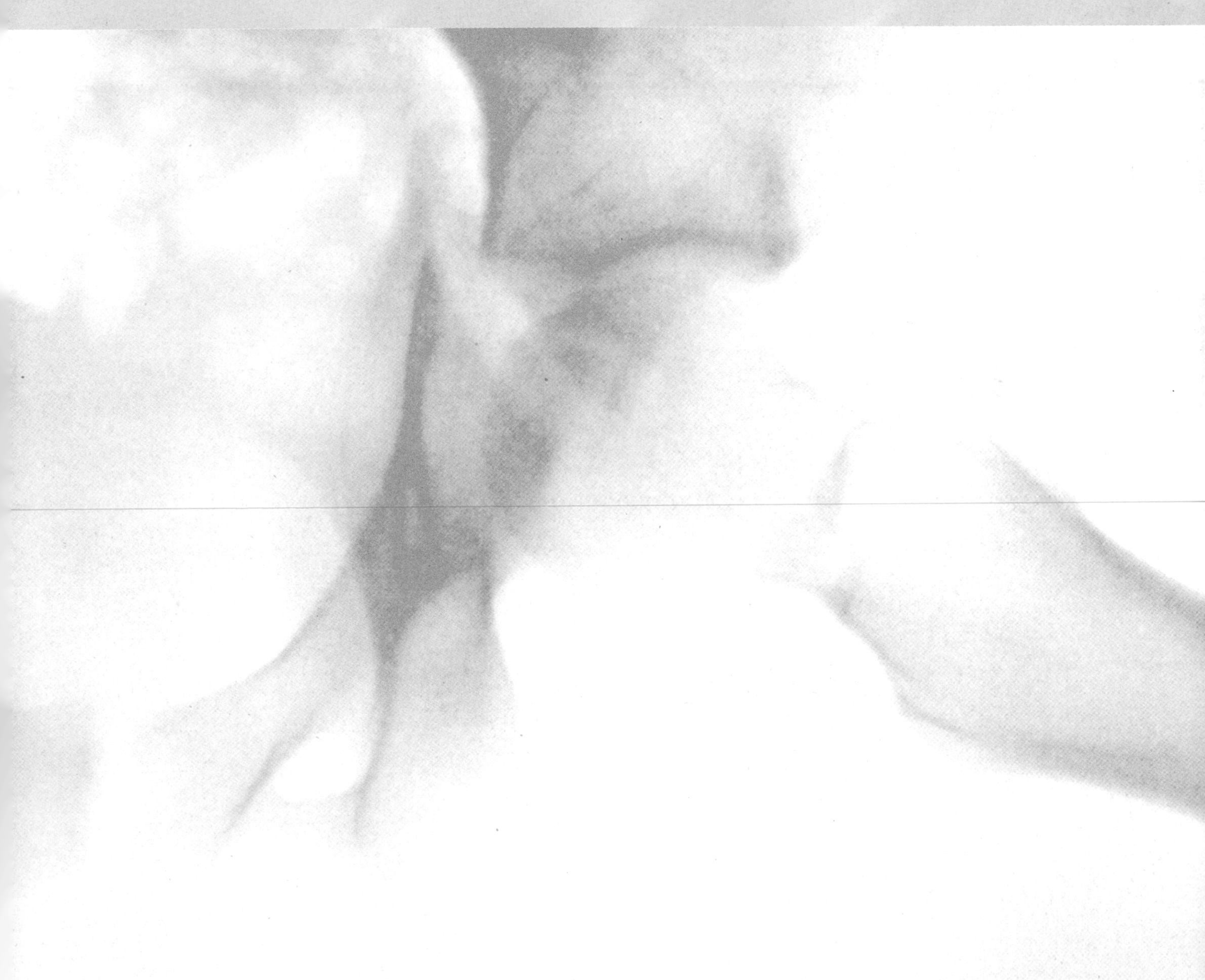

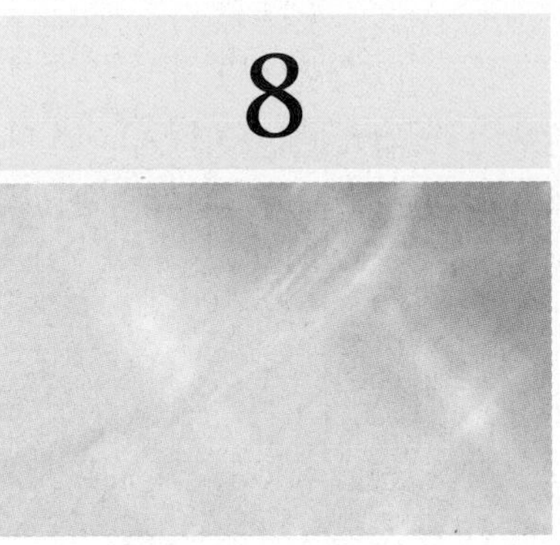

FRACTURES AND DISLOCATIONS OF THE HAND AND CARPUS IN CHILDREN

Scott H. Kozin and Peter M. Waters

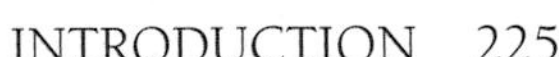

INTRODUCTION 225
Epidemiology 225
Anatomy of the Immature Hand 226
Remodeling 228

EVALUATION OF PEDIATRIC HAND INJURIES 228
Clinical Examination 228
Radiographic Examination 229
Differential Diagnosis 229

GENERAL PRINCIPLES OF TREATMENT 229
Nonoperative Management 229
Surgical Management 232
Rehabilitation 232
Complications 232

SPECIFIC FRACTURES OF THE PEDIATRIC HAND 233
Fractures of the Distal Phalanx 233
Fractures of the Proximal and Middle Phalanges 240
Fractures of the Metacarpals 255
Fractures of the Thumb Metacarpal 262

CARPAL INJURIES IN CHILDREN 267
Epidemiology 267
Anatomy 268

SPECIFIC CARPAL FRACTURES 269
Scaphoid Fractures 269
Capitate Fractures 276
Triquetrum Fractures 278
Hamate, Pisiform, Lunate, and Trapezium Fractures 279
Soft Tissue Injuries about the Carpus 279

TRIANGULAR FIBROCARTILAGE COMPLEX TEARS 280
Epidemiology 280
Anatomic Considerations 280
Classification 280
Diagnosis 281
Treatment 281

DISLOCATIONS OF THE HAND AND CARPUS 281
Dislocations of the Interphalangeal Joints 281
Metacarpophalangeal Joint Dislocations 282

INTRODUCTION

Epidemiology

Incidence

The pediatric hand is vulnerable to injury for several reasons. Usage pattern of the exposed hand and the child's curiosity about the surrounding world are prime factors. Youngsters often are unaware of dangers and place their hands in vulnerable situations.[14,84,196,209,210] Hand and wrist injuries account for up to 25% of pediatric fractures (Table 8-1).[70,84] The annual incidence is approximately 26.4 fractures per 10,000 children.[209]

Biphasic Distribution

Pediatric hand fractures occur primarily in two distinct age groups: the toddler and the adolescent. In the toddler age group, the injury usually is secondary to a crush,[10,56,108,196] often involving a finger caught in a closing door. In the adolescent

TABLE 8-1 Incidence of Pediatric Hand Injuries

Peak age: 13 years

Annual incidence: 26.4 per 10,000 children

Percentage of all pediatric emergency patients: 1.7%

Right side incidence equals left

Male incidence is greater than female incidence

Most common areas
- Nonphyseal: distal phalanx (crush)
- Physeal: proximal phalanx

Index and small fingers most commonly injured

age group, the injury is most commonly from participation in sports.[29,59,66,118,158,204,212] Football and skiing are prime examples of sports prone to athletic hand injuries.[15,27,59]

There are certain high-risk activities for fractures, such as snowboarding, horseback riding, skateboarding, and snowboarding.[119] In addition, overweight adolescents have poorer balance than those of healthy weight, which may explain their propensity for fracture.[69] Hand fractures in children peak around age 13, which coincides with active participation in organized contact sports.

Incidence of Specific Fractures

The most common fractures are distal phalangeal crush injuries and Salter-Harris (S-H) II fractures of the proximal phalangeal base.[70,84,117,152,209,210] The border digits (index and small fingers) are the most commonly injured rays.[14,84,117,152,209,210] Dislocations of the pediatric hand are relatively uncommon injuries. The metacarpophalangeal (MCP) joint is the most commonly dislocated joint in the immature hand.[38,65,110] The proximal interphalangeal (PIP) joint is the most commonly injured joint from volar plate tears or avulsion fractures.

Incidence of Physeal Fractures

Fracture forces often are transmitted through the physis in a child's hand because this course is the path of least resistance.[84,108,118,172,209,210] A S-H II fracture is the predominate type of phalangeal fracture, and the proximal phalanx is the most commonly injured bone.

Anatomy of the Immature Hand

Adults and children have disparate patterns of hand injury because of different usage patterns and differences in underlying skeletal and soft tissue composition. Knowledge of the architecture of the physis, the soft tissue origins and insertions, and the surrounding periosteum is useful for recognition and treatment of children's hand fractures.

Osseous Anatomy

There are potential epiphyses at both the proximal and distal ends of all the tubular hand bones. Secondary ossification centers, however, develop only at the distal ends of the metacarpals of the index, long, ring, and small rays, and at the proximal end of the thumb. Conversely, the secondary centers of ossification are present only at the proximal ends of the phalanges in all digits.[75,118]

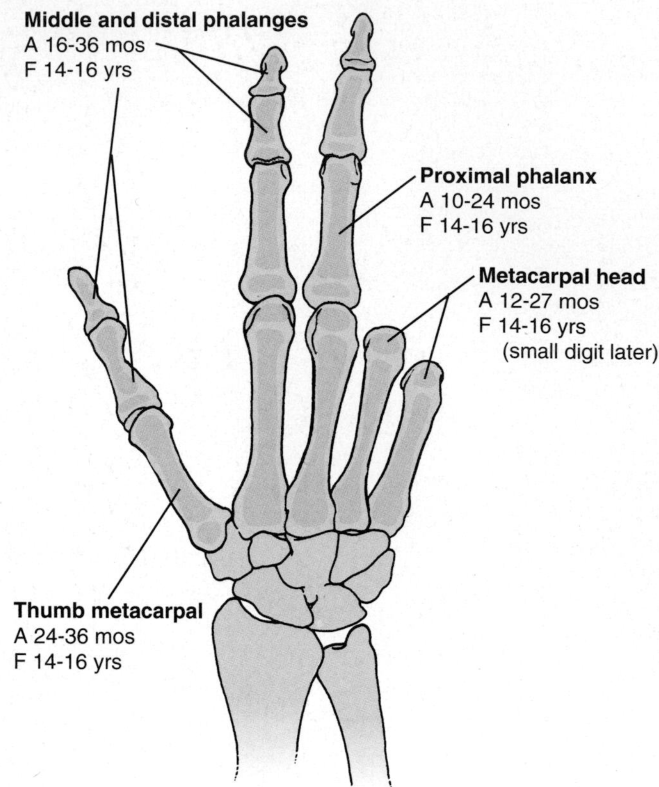

FIGURE 8-1 Appearance of secondary ossification centers (A). Fusion of secondary centers to the primary centers (F).

Secondary Ossification Centers

In boys, the secondary ossification centers within the proximal phalanges appear at 15 to 24 months and fuse at bone age of 16 years (Fig. 8-1).[75,188] In girls, the appearance and fusion occur earlier, at 10 to 15 months and bone age of 14 years, respectively. The appearance of the secondary ossification centers of the middle and distal phalanges is later than the proximal phalanx, usually by 6 to 8 months. Fusion of the secondary ossification centers, however, occurs from distal to proximal.

Within the metacarpal, the secondary ossification centers appear at 18 to 27 months in boys and at 12 to 17 months in girls. The proximal thumb metacarpal secondary ossification center appears 6 to 12 months after the fingers. The secondary centers within the metacarpals fuse between 14 to 16 years of age in girls and boys.

Physeal Anatomy

The physis (or growth plate) provides longitudinal growth. The anatomy of the physis has direct impact on fracture geometry.[133] The physis is divided into four distinct zones: germinal, proliferative, hypertrophic, and provisional calcification. The zone of chondrocyte hypertrophy (zone III) is the least resistant to mechanical stresses. This zone is devoid of the collagen that provides inherent stabilizing properties. The collagen is present in germinal and proliferative (zones I and II), and the calcium present in provisional calcification (zone IV) provides similar structural strength.[70,194] Therefore, the fracture often propagates through the zone of chondrocyte hypertrophy (zone III) as the path of least resistance. However, high-energy injuries may undulate through all four zones of the physis.[133,176]

The irregularity of the physeal zones increases near skeletal maturity.[21] Thus, a fracture line may be transmitted through several zones. This variable path through irregular topography may contribute to partial growth arrest after adolescent fractures that involve the physis.[176] This change in irregularity also explains the differing patterns of physeal injuries dependent on age: S-H I and II fractures tend to occur in younger patients compared to S-H III or IV fractures, which are more prevalent in children close to skeletal maturity.

Pseudoepiphyses and Double Epiphyses

A persistent expression of the distal epiphysis of the thumb metacarpal is called a pseudoepiphysis.[78] The pseudoepiphysis appears earlier than the proximal epiphysis and fuses rapidly. By the sixth or seventh year, the pseudoepiphysis is incorporated within the metacarpal and is inconspicuous. Pseudoepiphyses also have been noted at the proximal ends of the finger metacarpals, usually of the index ray. The only clinical significance is differentiation from an acute fracture (Fig. 8-2).

Double epiphyses can be present in any bone of the hand, but these anomalies are more common in the metacarpals of the index finger and thumb. There are variable expressions of double epiphyses, but the true entity is considered only when a fully developed growth mechanism is present on both ends of a tubular bone. Double epiphyses usually are seen in children with other congenital anomalies, but their presence does not appear to influence overall bone growth. When fractures occur in bones with double epiphyses, growth of the involved bone appears to be accelerated.[208]

Double epiphyses must be delineated from a pseudoepiphysis or metaphyseal "notching."[45,78,198,208] Periphyseal notching can be confused with trauma or double epiphyses. The location of the notches can coincide with the physis or may be slightly more distant from the epiphysis. Notching is a benign condition that does not influence the structural properties of the bone.[208]

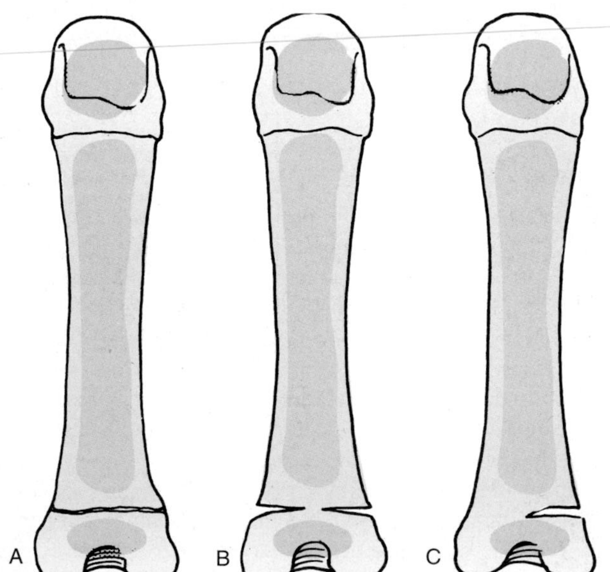

FIGURE 8-2 Abnormal epiphyseal appearance. **A.** Double epiphysis. **B.** Pseudoepiphysis. **C.** Notched epiphysis.

Soft Tissue Anatomy

The tensile strength of a child's soft tissues usually exceeds that of the adjacent physis and epiphysis.[18,133] For this reason, ligament ruptures and tendon avulsions are uncommon compared to physeal or epiphyseal fractures.[18,82]

Tendons

The extensor tendons insert onto the epiphyses. The terminal tendon of the digital extensor mechanism and the extensor pollicis longus insert on the epiphyses of the distal phalanx. The central slip of the extensor mechanism inserts onto the epiphysis of the middle phalanx. The extensor pollicis brevis inserts onto the epiphysis of the proximal phalanx. The abductor pollicis longus has a broad-based insertion onto both the epiphysis and metaphysis of the thumb metacarpal. The extensor digitorum communis connects into the sagittal band at the MCP joint, which in turn lifts the proximal phalanx into extension by its insertion along the volar plate.

The flexor tendons do not insert onto the epiphyses. The long digital flexor tendons (the flexor digitorum profundus and the flexor pollicis longus) insert into the metadiaphyseal region of their respective terminal phalanges.[82] The flexor digitorum superficialis inserts onto the central three fifths of the middle phalanx.

Collateral Ligaments

The collateral ligaments about the interphalangeal joint originate from the collateral recesses of the phalangeal head, span the physis, and insert onto both the metaphysis and epiphysis of the middle and distal phalanges (Fig. 8-3). The collaterals also insert onto the volar plate to create a three-sided box that protects the physes and epiphyses of the interphalangeal joints from laterally directed forces.[38,82] This configuration explains the rarity of S-H III injuries at the interphalangeal joints.

In contrast, the collateral ligaments about the MCP joints originate from the metacarpal epiphysis and insert almost exclusively onto the epiphysis of the proximal phalanx (Fig. 8-4). This anatomic arrangement accounts for the frequency of S-H III injuries at the MCP joint level. The ligamentous anatomy about the thumb MCP joint more closely resembles that of the PIP joints, which mirrors the arrangement of the adjacent physes.

Volar Plate

The volar plate is a stout stabilizer of the interphalangeal joint and MCP joints and resists hyperextension forces. The volar plate originates from the metaphysis of the respective proximal digital segment and inserts onto the epiphysis of the distal segment (Fig. 8-3B). The plate receives insertional fibers from the accessory collateral ligaments to create a three-sided box that protects the joint.

Periosteum

The periosteum is robust in a child's hand and can act as a considerable asset or liability in fracture management. The periosteal sleeve can minimize fracture displacement, aid in fracture reduction, or interpose between displaced fracture fragments and prevent reduction.

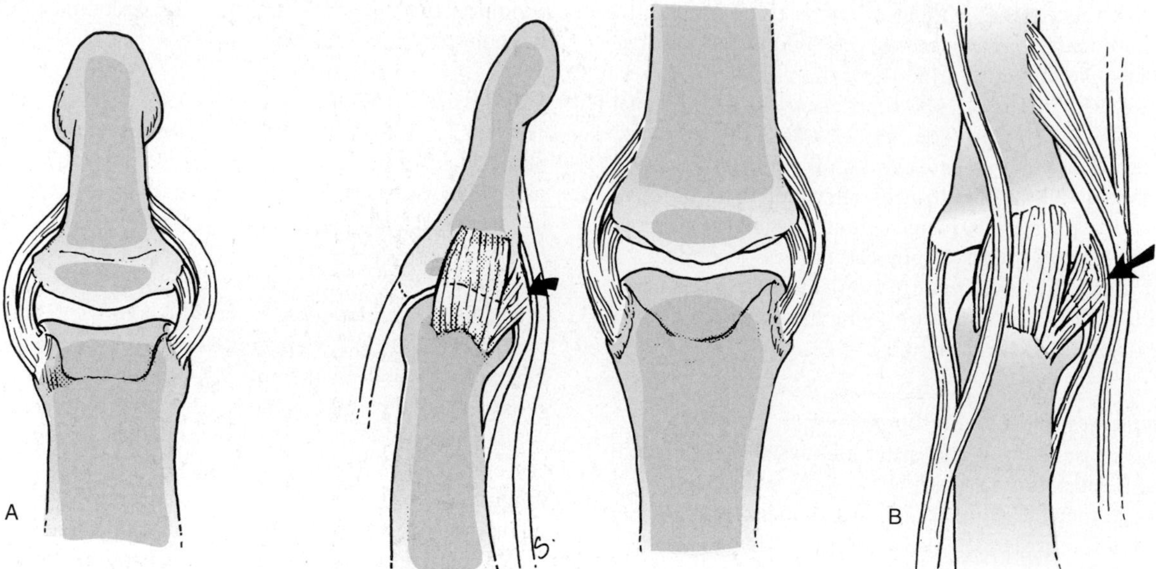

FIGURE 8-3 Anatomy of the collateral ligaments at the distal **(A)** and proximal **(B)** interphalangeal joints. The collateral ligaments at the interphalangeal joints originate in the collateral recesses and insert into both the metaphyses and epiphyses of their respective middle and distal phalanges. Additional insertion into the volar plane (*arrows*) is seen at the interphalangeal joints.

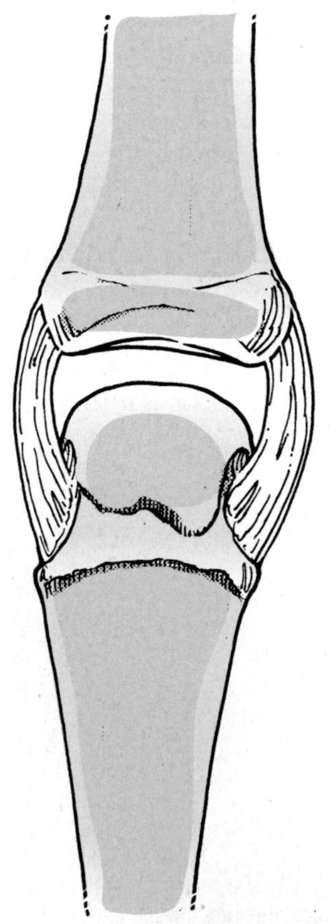

FIGURE 8-4 The collateral ligaments at the MCP joint both originate and insert almost exclusively on the epiphyseal regions of the metacarpal and the proximal phalanx.

Remodeling

Children's ability to remodel must be considered during fracture management. Factors that influence remodeling include the patient's age, the proximity of the fracture to the physis, the plane of motion of the adjacent joint, and the plane of malalignment.[17] The remodeling capacity is greater in younger children, fractures near a physis, and deformity in the plane of motion.[70,71,130,153] Several clinicians have observed remodeling between 20 to 30 degrees in the sagittal plane in children under 10 years of age and about 10 to 20 degrees in older children.[36,130] Remodeling in the coronal or adduction-abduction plane is considerably reduced compared to the sagittal plane. The amount is rarely quantified but is probably 50% or less than remodeling in the sagittal plane. Rotational remodeling does not occur.

EVALUATION OF PEDIATRIC HAND INJURIES

Clinical Examination

The evaluation of a child, especially infants and toddlers, is more difficult than an adult. The child frequently is noncompliant, unable to understand instructions, and fearful of the physician. The physician must be patient and engage the child. Observation and play are the mainstays of the examination. The child's hand posture and movements provide clues about the location and severity of the injury as the child interacts with toys, parents, and the environment in the examining area. Fracture is diagnosed by swelling, ecchymosis, deformity, or limited movement. Fracture malrotation is noted by digital scissoring during active grasp or passive tenodesis. Tendon integrity is observed by digital posture at rest and during active grasp around objects of varying size. Comparison to the uninjured hand is invaluable. A hurried exam or a frightened child can lead an erroneous or missed diagnosis. Passive wrist exam with finger flexion tenodesis is a critical part of the exam to accurately diagnose fracture malrotation.

After the child is relaxed, the physician may palpate areas of tenderness and move injured joints to assess their integrity. Stress testing should be gentle, and joint stability should be recorded in the anteroposterior and lateral directions. Neurologic injuries are especially difficult to detect in a young child. The proper digital artery is dorsal to the proper digital nerve within the finger. Therefore, there is a high concordance between pulsatile bleeding indicative of a digital artery injury and laceration of the digital nerve.

Sensory function is particularly difficult to determine in a young child. Normal discriminatory sensibility does not occur until 5 to 7 years of age. Therefore, meaningful objective data are difficult to obtain. A clinical clue is that children often bypass an anesthetic digit during grasp and pinch. A helpful examination maneuver is the wrinkle test. Immersion of an innervated digit in warm water for 5 minutes usually results in corrugation or wrinkling of the volar skin of the tuft. Wrinkling is often absent in a denervated digit. If there is doubt about the integrity of the nerve, operative exploration is appropriate.

Radiographic Examination

A careful clinical evaluation is a prerequisite for conducting a proper radiographic examination. Localization of areas of tenderness or deformity directs a thorough radiographic assessment. Several pediatric imaging factors complicate interpretation of plain radiographs, including lack of bony detail and normal variations. The normal ossification pattern of the immature hand creates problems with the detection of fractures and also promotes false interpretation of ligamentous injuries. Uncertain interpretation requires comparison to the uninjured hand or consultation with a pediatric atlas of child development and normal radiographic variants.[75,188]

Anteroposterior, lateral, and oblique views are needed for complete evaluation of the injured hand or digit. The phalangeal line test is useful in recognizing displaced fractures and joint malalignment. If a line is drawn from the center of the phalangeal neck through the center of the phalangeal metaphysis at the level of the physis, it should pass through the exact center of the metacarpal or phalangeal head in a normal finger, regardless of joint flexion (Fig. 8-5).[26] Oblique views are particularly useful for assessing displacement and intra-articular extension. A common radiograph pitfall is failure to obtain a true lateral radiograph of the injured digit. Isolation of the affected digit on the film or splaying of the fingers projects a true lateral view. Stress views are rarely used for fracture evaluation. Minifluoroscopy units are invaluable and allow a real-time assessment of articular congruity and joint stability. These units have considerable advantages, including the ability to obtain multiple views and stress views with low-radiation exposure for the patient and physician.

Differential Diagnosis

The differential diagnosis includes nontraumatic entities that may be interpreted as acute injuries. These diagnoses are uncommon but may cause swelling, deformity, or decreased motion.

Congenital

A Kirner deformity is a palmar and radial curving of the terminal phalanx of the small digit distal phalanx. This deformity occurs spontaneously between the ages of 8 and 14 years and may be confused with an acute fracture or epiphyseal separation (Fig. 8-6).[101] A Kirner deformity, however, usually is bilateral and not associated with trauma.[49] A trigger thumb in a young child sometimes is mistaken for an interphalangeal joint dislocation because of the fixed flexion posture and near equivalent clinical feel of "joint reduction" with manipulative digital extension and triggering of the nodule through the A1 pulley. The key diagnostic feature of a trigger thumb is the palpable nodule over the A1 pulley.

Thermal Injury

Thermal injury to the growing hand (e.g., frostbite, burns from flame or radiation) may cause bizarre deformities from altered appositional and interstitial bone growth. An ischemic necrosis of the physes and epiphyses may result (Fig. 8-7). The clinical result may yield altered bone width, length, or angulation secondary to the unpredictable effect on the growing elements that make interpretation of subsequent trauma difficult.[79,138]

Osteochondrosis (Thiemann Disease)

Osteochondrosis of the phalangeal epiphyses may cause epiphyseal narrowing and fragmentation, which are characteristic of Thiemann disease. This hereditary entity usually involves the middle and distal phalanges and typically resolves without treatment, although some permanent joint deformity has been reported.[40,165]

Tumors

A tumor may be discovered after fracture of the weakened bone or confused with fracture secondary to swelling and pain. An enchondroma of the proximal phalanx is the classic benign tumor that may fracture after trivial trauma (Fig. 8-8). The malignant bone, cartilage, or muscle tumors are rare. Radiographs reveal intrinsic destructive bony changes in an osteogenic sarcoma or extrinsic compression with adjacent periosteal reaction secondary to an adjacent rhabdomyosarcoma.

Inflammatory and Infectious Processes

Dactylitis from sickle cell anemia can masquerade as a traumatic injury. The affected digit(s) present(s) with fusiform swelling and decreased motion. The medical history usually is positive for sickle cell disease. The inflammatory arthropathies (e.g., juvenile rheumatoid arthritis, psoriatic arthritis, scleroderma, systemic lupus) may be confused with trauma. A joint effusion and tenosynovitis are common findings that require further diagnostic evaluation. Aside from standard laboratory testing, magnetic resonance imaging (MRI) is important for diagnosis of an inflammatory synovitis or tenosynovitis. An infectious process often can be mistaken for injury, although local and systemic evaluation usually ascertains this diagnosis.

GENERAL PRINCIPLES OF TREATMENT

Nonoperative Management

Most children's hand fractures can be treated without surgery. Children have a remarkable ability to remodel moderate fracture

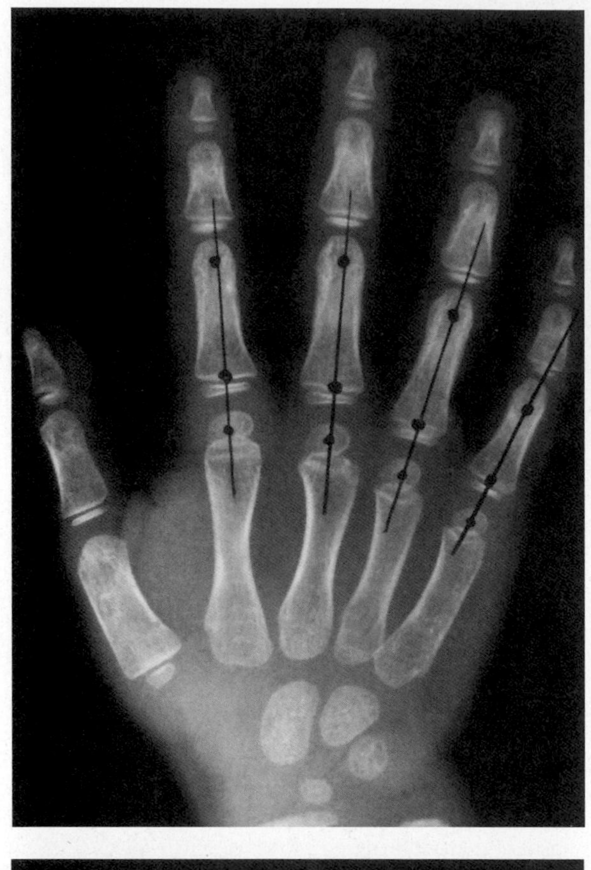
A

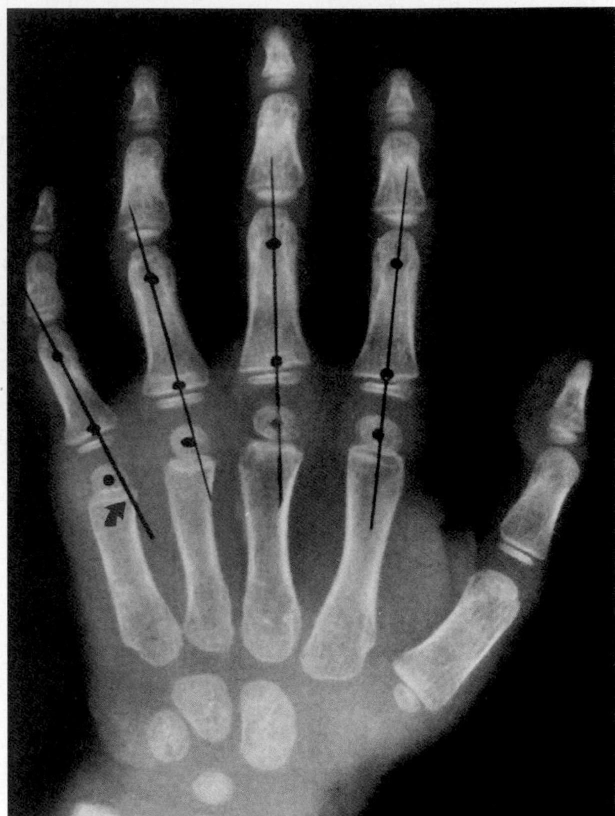
B

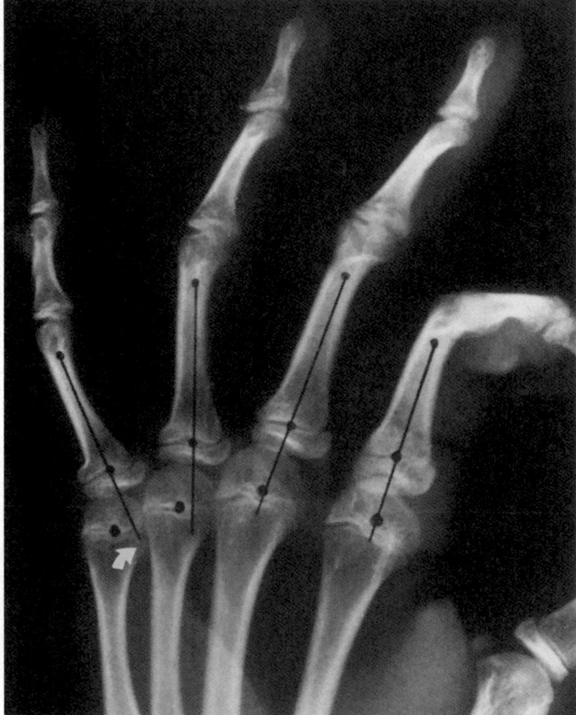
C

FIGURE 8-5 The straight-method of assessing alignment about the MCP joint. The long axes of the metacarpal and proximal phalanx should align, as they do in this normal hand **(A)**. If there is a fracture in the proximal phalanx, as in this patient's opposite or injured hand **(B,C)**, the axes will not be colinear (*arrows*). (Courtesy of Robert M. Campbell, Jr., MD.)

malalignment in the coronal and sagittal planes. In contrast, children cannot remodel malrotation, which requires reduction and stabilization to prevent malunion and digital scissoring. It is essential that the clinician properly diagnose and adequately treat problematic fractures. Anesthesia is required for fracture reduction. A digital block may be used for finger fracture reduction in adolescents. Conscious sedation, regional anesthesia, and general anesthesia are alternatives. Rapid fracture manipulation without anesthesia should be avoided. Immobilization is best applied immediately after reduction. The choice of a splint or cast depends on the degree of swelling, the difficulty of reduction, and the age of the patient. The amount of padding is an important consideration during cast application. Too much padding renders the cast ineffective in maintaining the reduc-

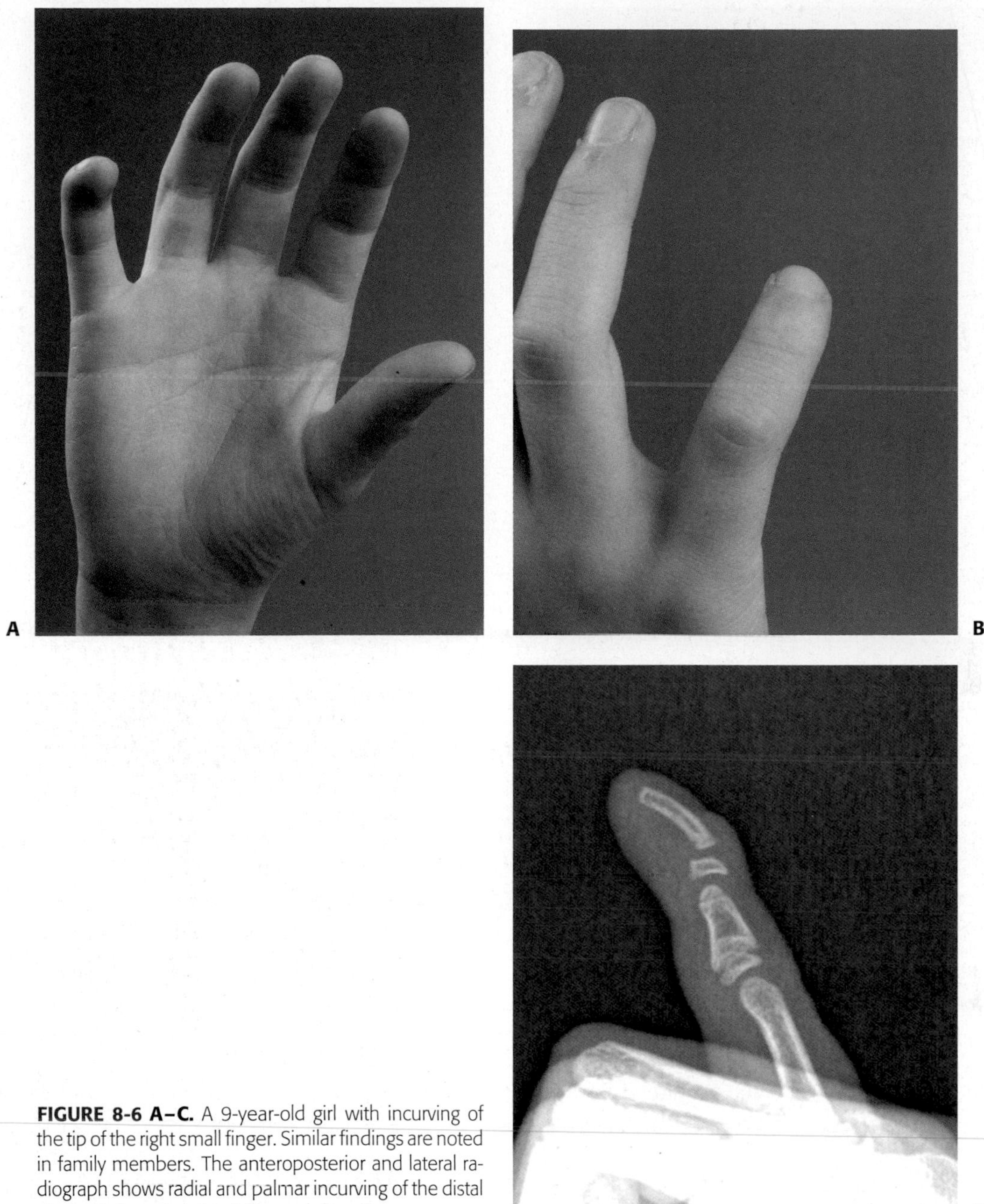

FIGURE 8-6 A–C. A 9-year-old girl with incurving of the tip of the right small finger. Similar findings are noted in family members. The anteroposterior and lateral radiograph shows radial and palmar incurving of the distal phalanx, characteristic of Kirner deformity.

tion. In contrast, too little padding may cause skin compromise from thermal injury or direct pressure. The use of rigid materials other than accepted casting materials (e.g., tongue blades, arm boards, metal rods) should be discouraged. Immobilization of a solitary digit in a child should be avoided because it is ineffective.

Fractures of the phalanges and metacarpals require immobilization of the injured digit with at least one of the adjacent digits. Similar to the adult hand, the child's hand is best immobilized in the "safe position" with the MCP joints in flexion and the interphalangeal joints in extension. Short-arm immobilization usually is adequate for hand fractures, provided cooperation is reasonable. Fractures in infants and toddlers require long-arm immobilization to encircle the elbow and decrease the chances of escaping from the cast.

Fractures that are truly nondisplaced are treated with immobilization and re-evaluation in 3 to 4 weeks for cast or splint removal. Fractures that required reduction necessitate weekly evaluation to ensure maintenance of alignment. The first evaluation should be within a week to allow detection of recurrent displacement and provide ample time to perform repeat reduction before the rapid healing process that occurs in children. To assess for malrotation, it is necessary to remove the immobilization and check alignment by active motion and passive tenodesis because radiographs can be misleading regarding rotational alignment. An unstable malaligned fracture should be treated with pin fixation to avoid malunion.

Children's fractures possess a remarkable propensity to heal. Therefore, delayed union and nonunion are uncommon problems except after open fractures or open surgery that disrupts the inherent blood supply. A frequent concern is growth arrest following a physeal injury. The arrest usually is secondary to

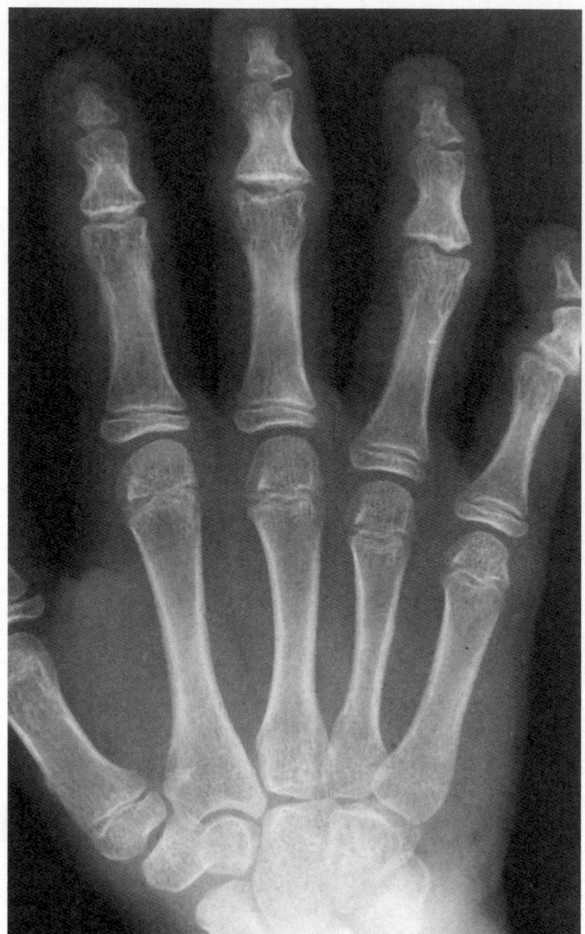

FIGURE 8-7 An 11-year-old girl sustained a frostbite injury to the right hand. Radiograph reveals premature fusion of the physis of the distal and proximal phalanges with irregularity of the bases of the shortened phalanges.

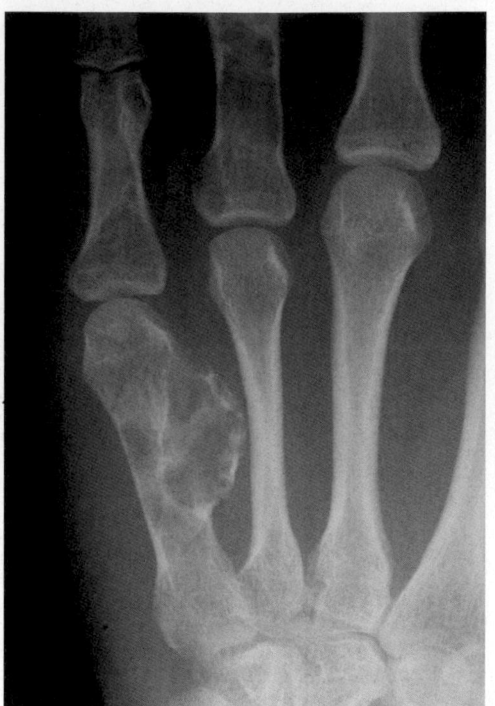

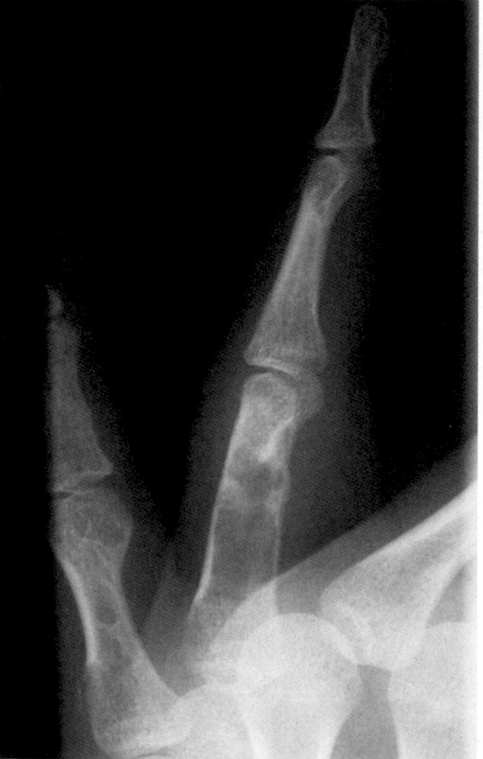

FIGURE 8-8 A,B. A 14-year-old girl with multiple enchondromas (Ollier disease), which weaken the bone and increase the susceptibility to fracture. (Courtesy of Shriners Hospitals for Children, Philadelphia, PA.)

the initial injury, although repeated manipulations impart additional trauma to the damaged physis and should be avoided.

Surgical Management

Surgery in children is different than that in adults. There are inherent differences in anatomy that require special consideration. The periosteum is thick and periosteal flaps can be created and later approximated to enhance healing and remodeling. The periosteal layer also provides excellent coverage for implants and a good sliding surface for tendons.

The physis requires meticulous respect. Surgical dissection around the physis should be minimized to avoid injury. Fixation across a physis requires thoughtful consideration concerning growth arrest. When fixation is necessary, the smallest diameter smooth wire that effectively holds the fracture fragments should be used. Implants, such as plates, should also avoid the physis.

Rehabilitation

Following fracture union, formalized therapy rarely is necessary. Simple liberation from immobilization and instructions to the patient and parents regarding range of motion, strengthening, and activity return usually are sufficient. In uncommon circumstances (e.g., complicated fractures or multiple trauma), formal hand therapy is indicated.

Complications

Complications from pediatric hand fractures are relatively uncommon. However, the physician should avoid being nonchalant in thinking that the pediatric hand is forgiving in its ability to remodel and regain motion. Recognition of the potential pitfalls is important, as is the development of a systematic plan for rectifying complications.

The most common complication of pediatric hand fractures is failure to diagnose the fracture or an underappreciation of the extent of injury. Anteroposterior, lateral, and oblique radiographs are needed for complete evaluation of the injured hand or digit. Imaging of the contralateral hand for comparison and consultation with a pediatric atlas of child development and normal radiographic variants should be done whenever the diagnosis is in question.[75,188]

Once the fracture is recognized, the appropriate treatment is instituted to ensure anatomic healing and return of normal function. Displacement or rotation at the fracture site may be subtle on radiographs. Inspection of the radiographs and a meticulous examination are necessary. Finger fractures must be scrutinized for evidence of malrotation by evaluating the plane of the fingernails with the fingers semiflexed by tenodesis or active motion. A malrotated or markedly displaced fracture requires reduction under anesthesia to regain bony alignment. The degree of reduction required depends on the configuration, location, and extent of the fracture as well as the age of the child. Although sagittal and coronal remodeling can occur in the immature skeleton, rotational malalignment will not remodel.[140] Pin stabilization may be required to maintain reduction. Open reduction and internal fixation may be necessary for displaced intra-articular fractures (i.e., S-H III thumb proximal phalanx fractures).

SPECIFIC FRACTURES OF THE PEDIATRIC HAND

Fractures of the Distal Phalanx

Relevant Anatomy

The skin, nail elements, soft tissues, and bone of the distal digit are closely related (Fig. 8-9). The dorsal periosteum of the distal phalanx is the underlying nutritional and structural support for the sterile matrix and nail bed. The germinal matrix is responsible for generating the nail plate. The volar aspect of the distal phalanx anchors the pulp through tough, fibrous septae that stabilize the skin against shear forces. The terminal extensor tendon inserts onto the epiphysis of the distal phalanx. The flexor digitorum profundus bypasses the physis to insert onto the metadiaphysis of the distal phalanx.

Mechanism of Injury

The primary mechanisms of injury are crush, hyperflexion, and hyperextension. A crush injury creates a spectrum of injury from minor tissue disruption with little need for intervention to severe tissue trauma that requires bony fixation, meticulous nail bed repair, and skin coverage (Fig. 8-10). A flexion force applied to the extended tip of the finger results in a mallet injury to the terminal tendon insertion or physeal separation with nail bed injury (Seymour fracture). The distal interphalangeal (DIP) joint rests in flexion and active extension is impossible in both cases. A hyperextension force can produce a bony avulsion injury of the flexor digitorum profundus tendon (pediatric jersey finger).

Fracture Patterns

Fractures of the distal phalanx can be divided into extraphyseal and physeal injuries (Table 8-2). Extraphyseal fractures are common and range from a simple distal tuft fracture to an unstable diaphyseal fracture underlying a nail bed laceration. The fracture pattern can be divided into three types (Fig. 8-11). A transverse fracture (Fig. 8-11A) may occur either at the distal extent of the terminal phalanx or through the diaphysis. Displaced transverse fractures through the diaphysis are almost always associated with a considerable nail bed injury that requires repair. A longitudinal splitting type fracture is much less common (Fig. 8-11B). This pattern is the result of excessive hoop stress within the tubular distal phalanx at the time of a crush injury. The "cloven-hoof" appearance of the fracture is characteristic (Fig. 8-12). The fracture may be contained within

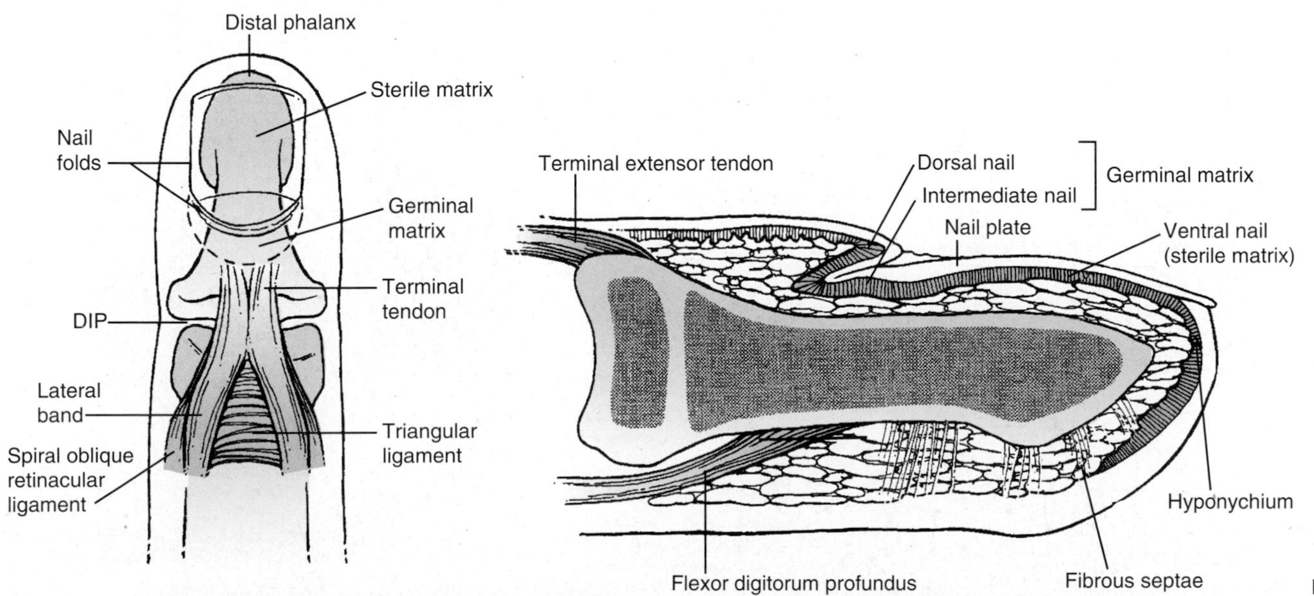

FIGURE 8-9 Anatomy about the distal phalanx. **A.** The skin, nail, and extensor apparatus share a close relationship with the bone of the distal phalanx. Specific anatomic structures at the terminal aspect of the digit are labeled. **B.** This lateral view of the nail demonstrates the tendon insertions and the anatomy of the specialized nail tissues.

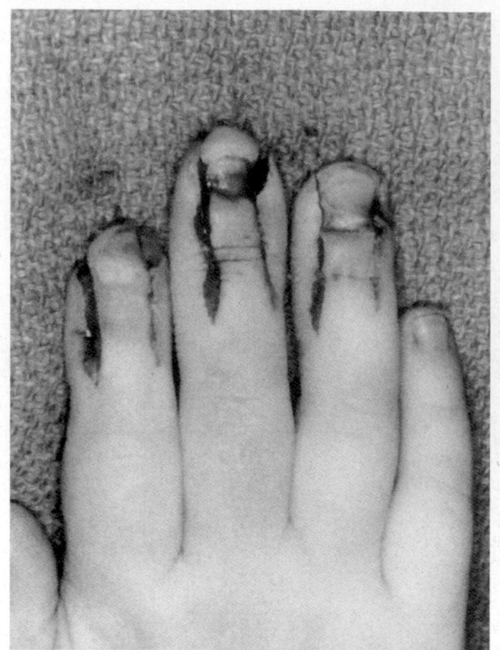

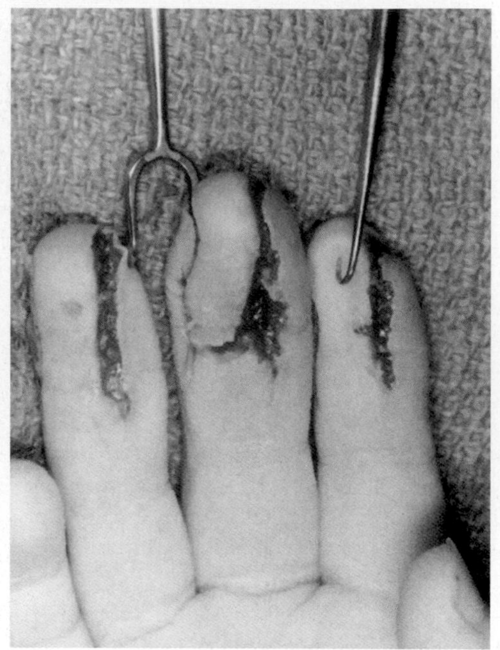

FIGURE 8-10 A,B. Crush injury to the fingers of a 4-year-old with nail bed laceration requiring meticulous repair with absorbable suture.

TABLE 8-2 Classification of Distal Phalangeal Fractures

Extraphyseal (see Fig. 8-10)
- Transverse diaphysis
- Longitudinal splitting
- Comminuted separations
- Avulsion of flexor digitorum profundus tendon with bone (jersey finger) (see Fig. 8-13)

Physeal

Dorsal mallet injuries (see Fig. 8-14)
- Salter-Harris I or II
- Salter-Harris III or IV
- Salter-Harris I or II joint dislocation
- Avulsion of extensor tendon and Salter-Harris fracture

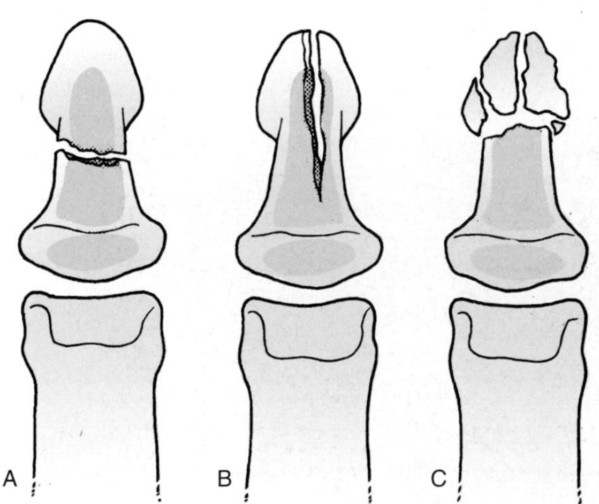

FIGURE 8-11 Three types of extraepiphyseal fractures of the distal phalanx. **A.** Transverse diaphyseal fracture. **B.** Cloven-hoof longitudinal splitting fracture. **C.** Comminuted distal tuft fracture with radial fracture lines.

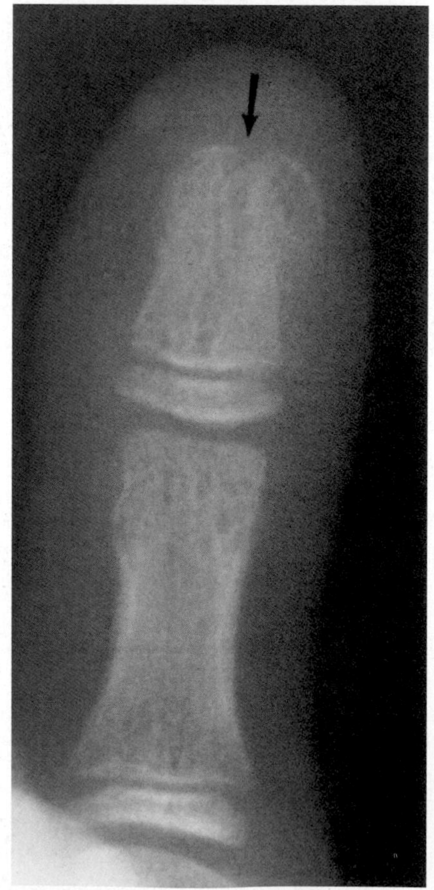

FIGURE 8-12 Extraepiphyseal fracture of the distal phalanx: the cloven-hoof longitudinal splitting fracture. In this patient, the fracture line (*arrow*) does not appear to extend across the physis.

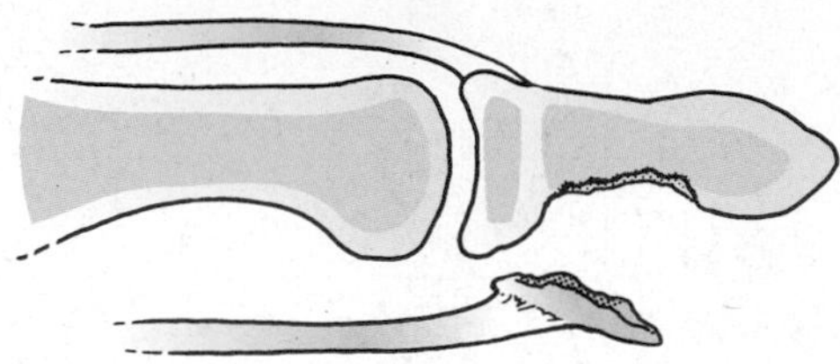

FIGURE 8-13 Flexor digitorum profundus avulsion fracture of the distal phalanx (jersey finger). This bony avulsion is apparent on radiographs, indicating the extent of proximal migration.

the shaft or can propagate through the physis and even into the joint.[10] A comminuted fracture of the distal diaphysis also can occur and usually is accompanied by extensive soft tissue injury (Figs. 8-11C).

A less common etiology of extraphyseal fracture is forced extension of the flexed DIP joint. This mechanism can result in either a bony avulsion injury or a soft tissue disruption of the flexor digitorum profundus (jersey finger) (Fig. 8-13).[106,205] An avulsion fracture often limits flexor digitorum profundus retraction in the pulley system by tethering of the bone fragment on the A5 or A4 pulley. The radiographic location of the bony fragment identifies the level of tendon retraction. In contrast, soft tissue disruption of the flexor digitorum profundus frequently retracts into the palm. Diagnosis of this injury is often missed in the acute setting.

Physeal fractures clinically resemble a mallet finger. There are four basic fracture patterns and all result in a flexed posture of the DIP joint (Fig. 8-14). A S-H I or II fracture with flexion of the distal fragment occurs predominantly in young patients less than 12 years of age. The unopposed flexor digitorum profundus flexes the distal fragment. The injury often is open and associated with a nail bed injury. There is a high risk for incarceration of the germinal or sterile matrix in the fracture site, known as a Seymour fracture.[169] Closed reduction may be blocked by interposition of the nail bed in the dorsal physis deep to the nail plate. Rarely, a S-H I or II fracture causes extrusion of the epiphyseal fragment.[125,199] This "epiphyseal dislocation" is challenging to diagnose with an unossified epiphysis because the remaining distal phalanx remains colinear with the axis of the digit, whereas the displaced unossified epiphysis is dorsally dislocated by traction produced by the extensor tendon. A dorsal S-H III fracture of the distal phalanx occurs in teenagers and results in an extension lag at the DIP joint. Rarely, the epiphysis also may separate from the terminal extensor tendon.[164]

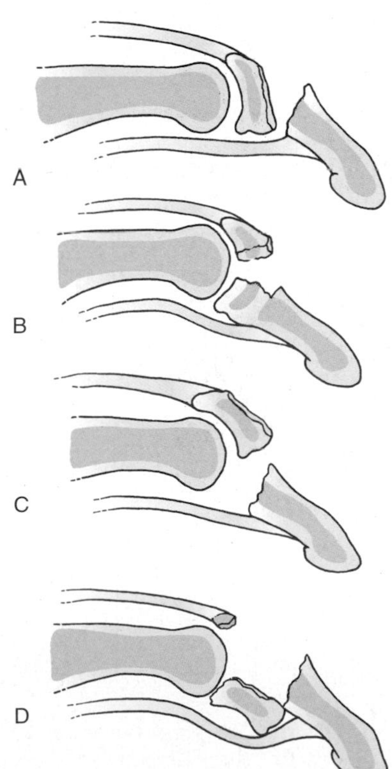

FIGURE 8-14 A–D. Mallet-equivalent fracture types.

Diagnosis

Signs and Symptoms. The diagnosis is usually straightforward. The history and physical examination are consistent with a distal phalanx fracture. A nail bed injury or a subungual hematoma greater than 50% creates a high index of suspicion for bony injury and displaced nail bed laceration (Fig. 8-15).[213] Radiographs are confirmatory and detail the fracture pattern. Antero-

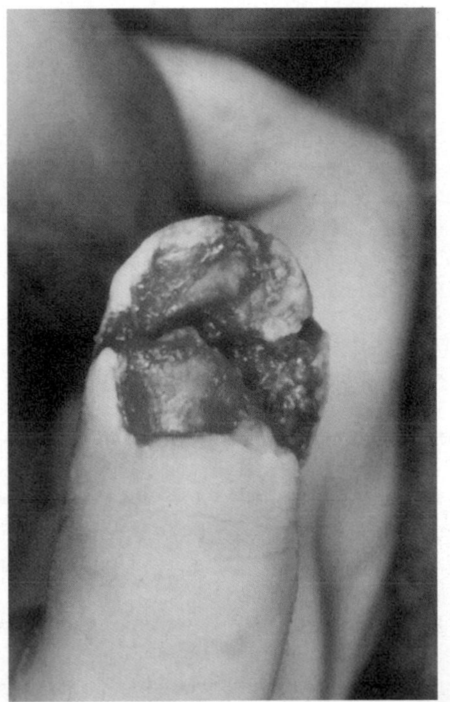

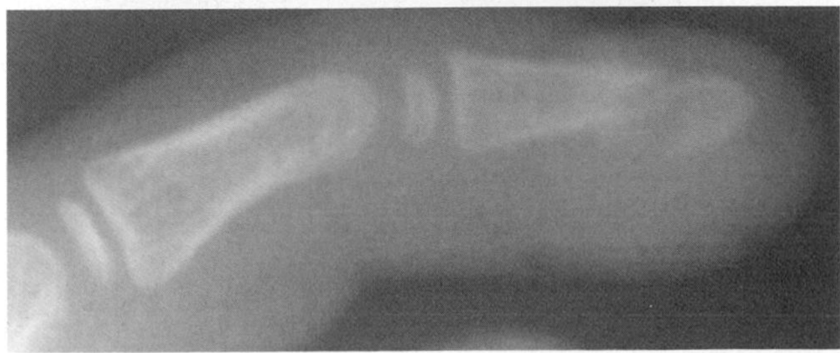

FIGURE 8-15 A. A crush injury to the thumb of a 4-year-old with a stellate nail bed laceration and fracture of the tuft. **B.** Radiograph reveals a comminuted tuft fracture.

posterior and lateral views of the distal phalanx are necessary to ascertain fracture configuration.

Treatment Options

Fractures associated with nail bed lacerations require attention to the soft tissue and bony injuries. The soft tissue repair is as critical to outcome as the bony treatment. Any substantial nail bed laceration requires repair. The distal phalangeal fracture is assessed for alignment and stability. An unstable fracture that cannot support the nail bed necessitates stabilization.

Nonoperative Management. Most distal phalangeal fractures can be treated with nonoperative measures using a splint or cast. Mild and moderate displacement of extraphyseal fractures will heal without difficulty. Even physeal injuries with mild displacement of the dorsal epiphyseal fragment have favorable results with splinting.

Hematoma Evacuation. Indications for a hematoma evacuation include subungual hematoma involving more than 50% of the nail plate or painful pressure under the nail.[42] Decompression can be done with a hypodermic needle that penetrates the nail plate. A heated paper clip or cautery tip may also be used, but the heat can cause further nail bed injury if penetration is too deep.

Nail Bed Repair. Nail bed repair is required for obvious nail bed lacerations and potentially for subungual hematomas that involve more than 50% of the nail plate. A blunt freer elevator is used to remove the nail plate to avoid additional nail bed injury. Partial nail removal is rarely indicated for nail bed repair in children. Proximal exposure of the germinal matrix requires incisions along the eponychial folds and proximal retraction of the eponychial flap. The nail bed is repaired with interrupted 6-0 or 7-0 absorbable sutures under loupe magnification. Following repair, the nail bed is supported using the nail plate or another substitute, such as the foil from the suture pack.[54,163,213]

Operative Management. Extremely unstable extraphyseal fractures with wide displacement may require stabilization. Usually a smooth Kirschner wire can be inserted across the fracture through the tip of the finger. A hypodermic needle can be used as a substitute for the smooth wires.[124] Physeal fractures with a dorsal fragment larger than 50% of the epiphysis or considerable DIP joint subluxation may require operative intervention.[38,80] Closed manipulation and percutaneous Kirschner-wire fixation usually is sufficient.

Open unstable injuries with severe displacement or irreducible fractures require reduction and stabilization (Fig. 8-16).[4,26] The Seymour fracture represents an irreducible fracture that requires open reduction. The sterile matrix must be extricated from the fracture site and repaired beneath the eponychium. Epiphyseal dislocations also require operative intervention to both restore joint congruity and reestablish extensor tendon continuity.

An avulsion of the flexor digitorum profundus is an indication for open repair. Surgery should be done as soon as possible to limit tendon ischemia and shortening. The profundus tendon is identified at the level of retraction and repaired to the distal phalanx (Fig. 8-17). Too often, this diagnosis is made late.

Surgical Approach. A dorsal approach is used for most extraphyseal and physeal fractures that require open reduction (Fig. 8-18). The dorsal fragment is isolated and reduced (Fig. 8-19). A

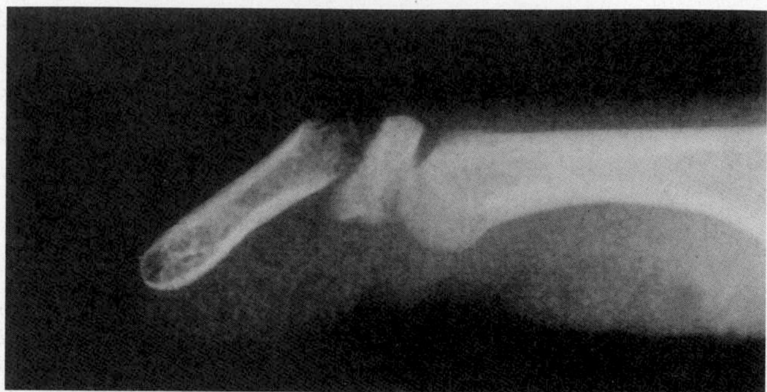

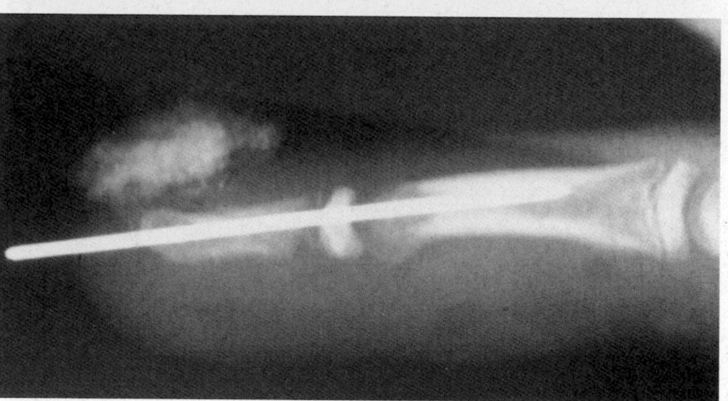

FIGURE 8-16 A. An irreducible distal phalangeal fracture that required extrication of the nail bed from within the fracture site. **B.** Stabilization of the fracture fragments with a longitudinal Kirschner wire across the DIP joint.

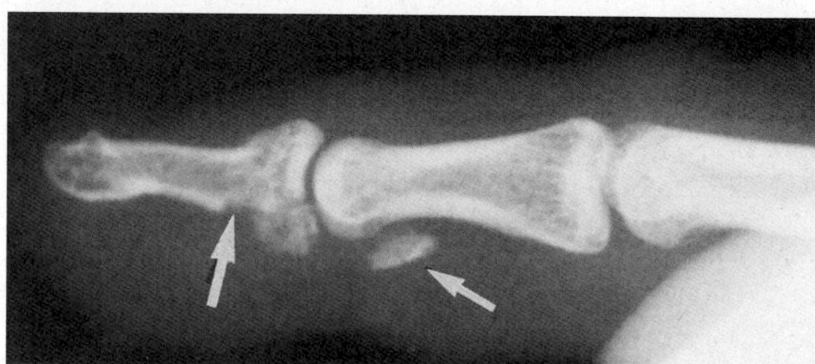

FIGURE 8-17 A 17-year-old athlete with an avulsion fracture from the flexor digitorum profundus tendon. The fracture extends through the epiphysis and into the joint (*large arrow*). The flexor digitorum profundus tendon with its attached bony fragment has retracted to the level of the A4 pulley (*small arrow*).

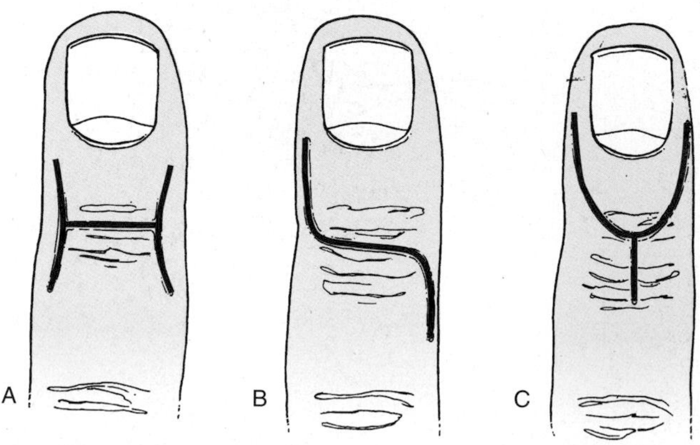

FIGURE 8-18 Exposures to the DIP joint. **A.** H-type flap with the transverse limb over the DIP joint. **B.** S-shaped exposure of the DIP joint. **C.** An extended exposure of the DIP joint. All exposures must avoid injury to the germinal matrix, which is located just proximal to the nail fold.

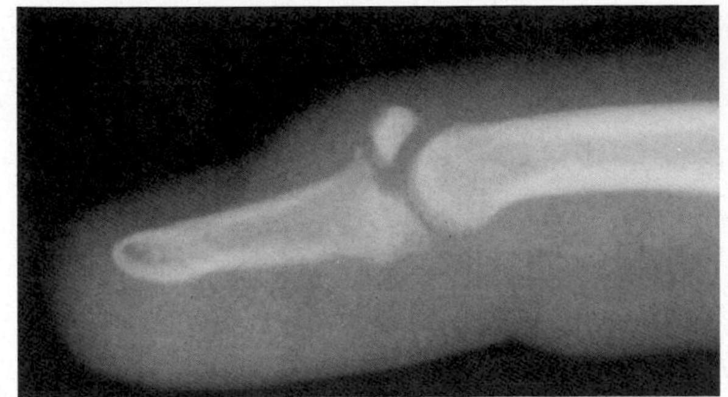

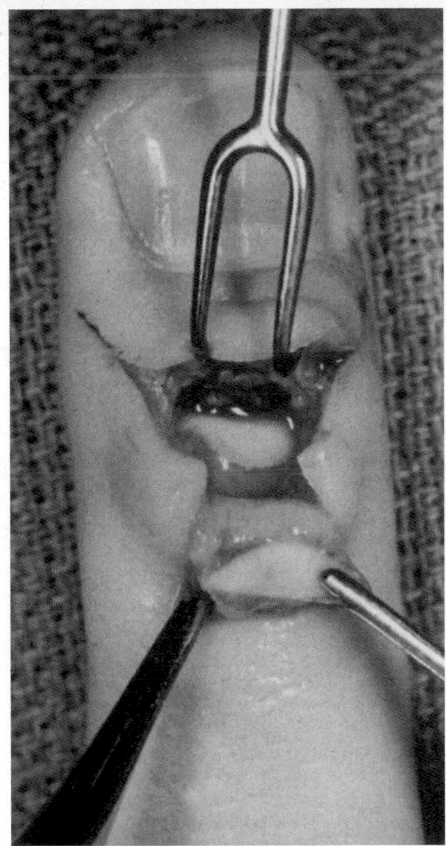

FIGURE 8-19 A. Displaced mallet fracture with considerable articular involvement and dorsal prominence. **B.** Open reduction through a dorsal approach reveals the articular fragment attached to the terminal tendon.

small portion of the collateral ligaments may be recessed to enhance exposure; however, soft tissue dissection should be limited to prevent osteonecrosis of small bony fragments. Fracture fixation can be accomplished with a smooth wire, pullout wire, tension band, or heavy suture.[70,80,84,102,140] Fixation across the DIP joint with a small diameter, smooth wire usually is necessary to maintain joint and physeal congruity. A volar approach is used for avulsion of the flexor digitorum profundus tendon.

Amputations. Amputations of the fingertip often are open distal phalangeal fractures. The injury may involve skin, nail tissue, and bone. Support for nail growth is a primary consideration. Minimal loss of tissue can be treated with local wound care and healing through secondary intention. A small amount of exposed bone does not preclude spontaneous healing in children. The likelihood of nail deformity (hooked or "parrot's beak") is high for amputations that involve more than 50% of the distal phalanx.

Soft Tissue Coverage of Amputations. Soft tissue coverage varies depending on the degree of tissue loss and direction of injury. Simple healing by primary closure is preferred for most volar oblique fingertip amputations. Dorsal oblique amputations are complicated by nail bed injury and are more difficult to cover. Composite grafts of skin and subcutaneous tissue from the amputated part have been used in young children with variable results. Local flaps are another option for coverage of large volar or dorsal oblique amputations. Options include a variety of flaps, such as a V-Y volar advancement, a thenar flap, a cross-finger flap, a pedicled flap, or a neurovascular island flap (Figs. 8-20 and 8-21).[7,98] Fortunately, coverage issues are rare in children. An amputation of the distal thumb also can be covered with a bipedicle (Moberg volar advancement flap) or unipedicle neurovascular flap.[132] The choice of coverage de-

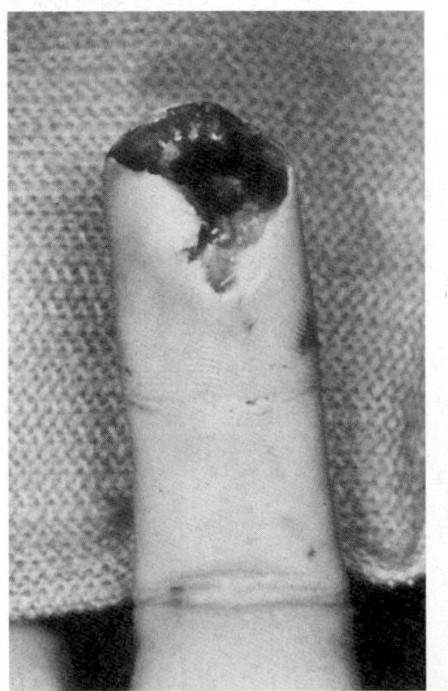

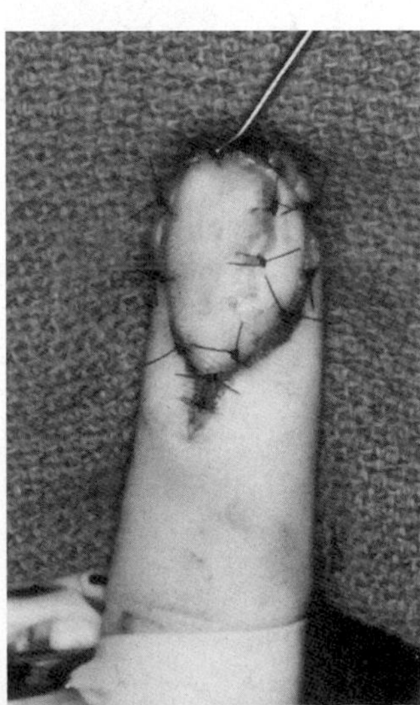

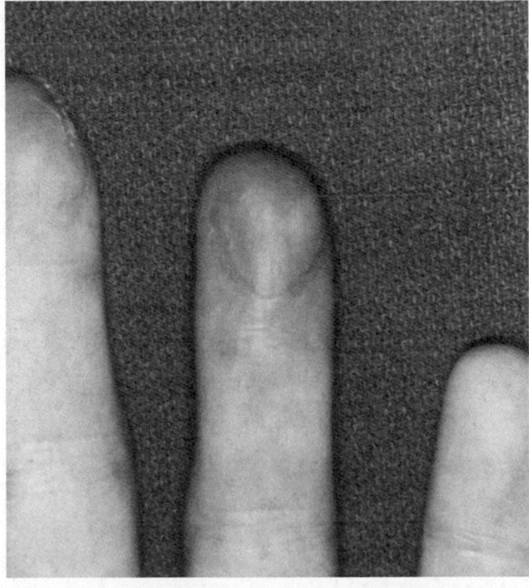

FIGURE 8-20 Volar V-Y advancement flap for coverage. **A.** A volar oblique tissue loss of the ring finger with intact nail bed. **B.** Flap designed with apex at the DIP joint and mobilized to cover the fingertip. The defect is closed proximal to the flap creating the Y. **C.** Satisfactory result with good durability and sensibility.

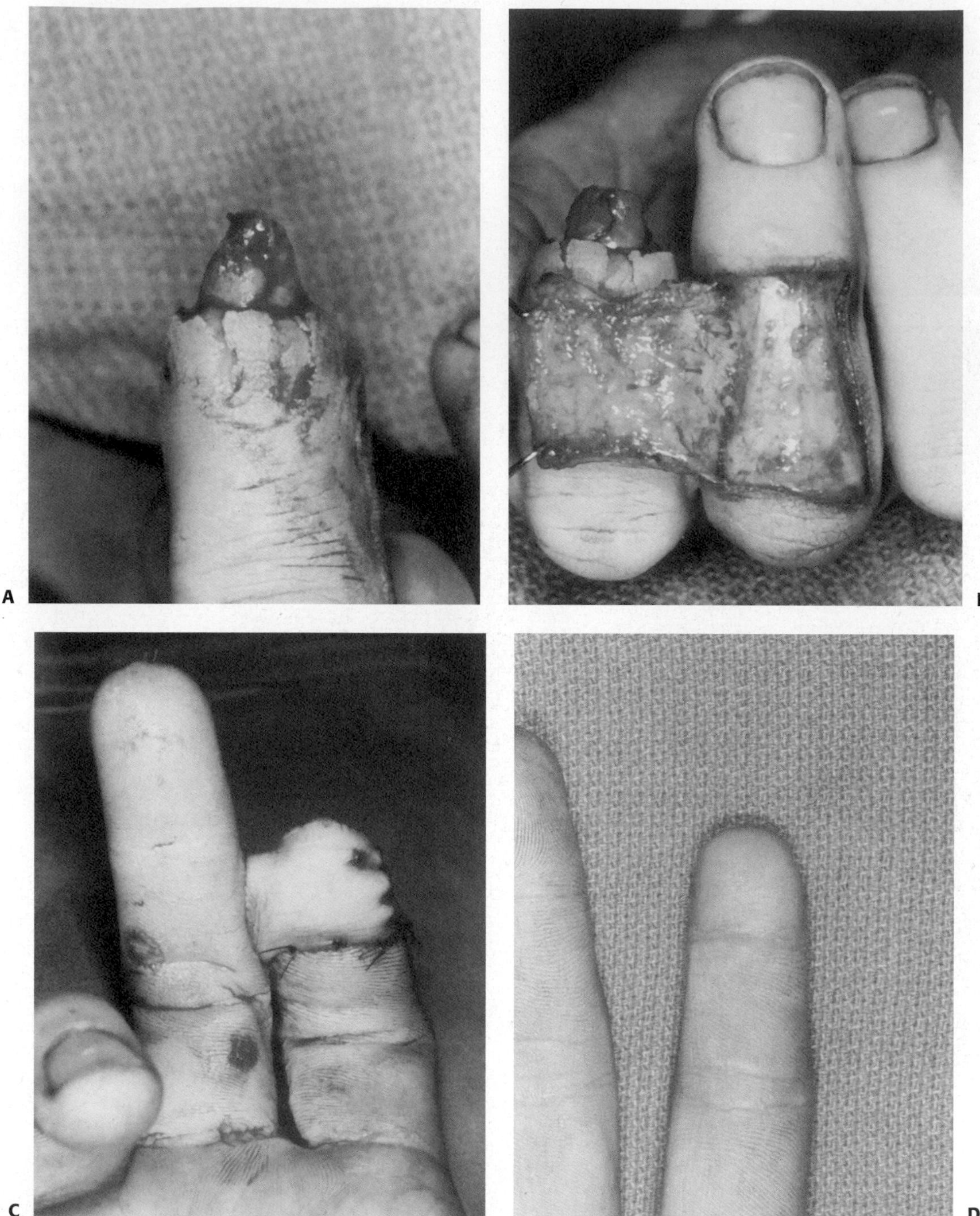

FIGURE 8-21 Cross-finger flap in a 17-year-old male with open distal phalangeal injury and tissue loss. **A.** Extensive volar and distal soft tissue loss with preservation of the bone and nail bed. **B.** A cross-finger flap of skin and subcutaneous tissue is elevated from the dorsal aspect of the adjacent donor digit based on the side of the index finger. **C.** The vascular epitenon is preserved on the donor digit to support a skin graft. The flap is transferred to the volar aspect of the index finger to recreate the tuft. **D.** Satisfactory coverage and functional result.

pends on the degree and direction of soft tissue loss, age of the patient, and preference of the surgeon.

Postoperative Care and Rehabilitation

Children younger than 4 or 5 years are immobilized with long arm mitten casts. As the child ages, the degree of immobilization is decreased. An adolescent with a simple distal phalangeal fracture or nail bed repair usually can be treated similar to an adult with only DIP joint immobilization. Percutaneous fixation is removed in the office 4 to 6 weeks after surgery. Formal hand therapy usually is not required, although an instructed home program with emphasis on DIP joint motion is useful. DIP blocking exercises are particularly helpful to regain full joint movement. Formal therapy is reserved for patients who fail to regain motion and strength after 3 to 4 weeks on a home program.

Prognosis

The overall results following distal phalangeal fractures are favorable. A small loss of motion has little functional impact. A small extensor lag or minor longitudinal nail ridge is well tolerated by most patients. Considerable nail irregularity or deformity is a frequent source of dissatisfaction.

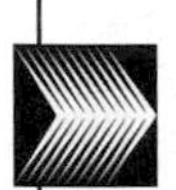

AUTHORS' PREFERRED TREATMENT

Extraphyseal Fractures

Most simple closed fractures are treated with immobilization. Immobilization for 3 to 4 weeks allows clinical union, which proceeds complete radiographic healing by about 1 month. Uncommonly, an unstable distal phalangeal fracture requires percutaneous pinning with a small Kirschner wire. The DIP joint usually is transfixed to provide additional stability. The pin is removed approximately 4 weeks after injury.

Fractures with a nail bed laceration require adequate anesthesia, removal of the nail plate, and nail bed repair. The parents and patient are told that it takes several cycles of nail growth (3 to 6 months) before the final morphology of the nail is known. Fortunately, in properly treated nail bed injuries, chronic deformity is rare.

Physeal Fractures

Most closed pediatric physeal fractures are treated by reduction and splinting. Placement of the DIP joint into extension reduces most fractures. A splint is applied and radiographs are taken to assess the degree of reduction. Adequate alignment requires full-time splinting for 4 to 6 weeks depending on the age of the child, size of the fracture fragment, and amount of bony apposition. The DIP joint is positioned in neutral to 15 degrees of extension. Extreme hyperextension is contraindicated because dorsal skin hypoperfusion and necrosis may result.[155] Careful instructions regarding skin monitoring are given to parents and patients to avoid splint pressure necrosis. Radiographs are taken weekly for the first 2 weeks and then every 2 weeks thereafter to monitor for loss of reduction or volar joint subluxation.

Surgery is indicated for fractures that are open, grossly unstable, irreducible, or have unacceptable alignment. Closed reduction and percutaneous fixation is preferred unless the fracture is irreducible. Additional fixation of the dorsal fragment can be accomplished with a 0.028-inch smooth Kirschner wire placed parallel to the epiphysis. An irreducible fracture requires open reduction. Fixation techniques vary depending on the age of the child and the fracture configuration. Smooth wires, however, are the principle means of fixation.

Physeal fractures with dorsal entrapment of the germinal matrix (Seymour fractures) require nail plate removal, extrication of the nail bed, and repair. Axial alignment after nail bed repair is maintained with a splint or longitudinal fixation for 4 weeks (Fig. 8-22).

Adolescent mallet fingers with soft tissue terminal tendon disruption are treated similarly to adults with 4 to 6 weeks of dorsal DIP joint splint immobilization. Operative repair of soft tissue or bony mallet fingers rarely is indicated, even for chronic injuries. Most chronic mallet injuries will heal with splint immobilization. The loss of digital flexion associated with surgery can be more disabling than a minor extension lag after an untreated injury.

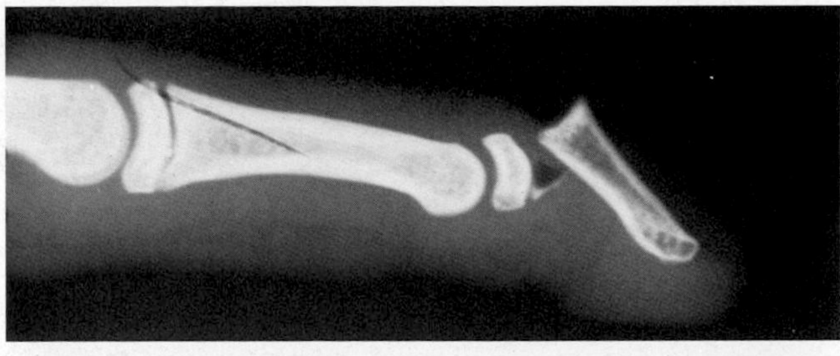

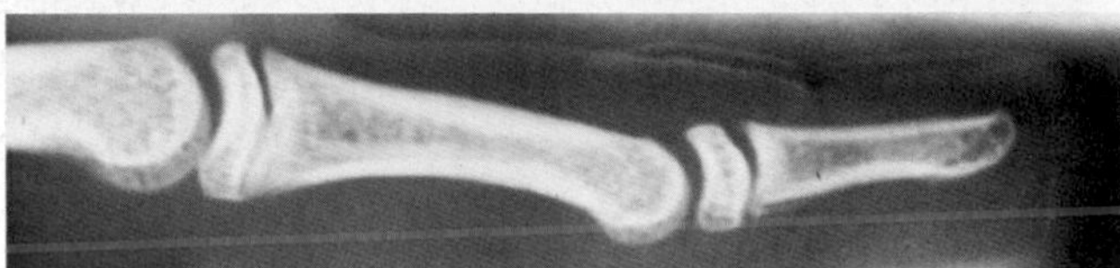

FIGURE 8-22 A. A 13-year-old boy sustained an open S-H type II fracture. **B.** The wound was cleansed, and acceptable alignment was obtained with closed reduction.

Jersey Finger

Flexor digitorum profundus avulsion injuries require open repair (see Fig. 8-17). Too often, this injury is missed in the acute setting. Specific examination for profundus function is necessary for diagnosis. Bone-to-bone fixation is preferred using wires or suture. Fragments that are too small for fixation require bone removal and repair of the tendon directly to the fracture bed. This usually requires transosseous sutures from volar to dorsal, avoiding injury to the germinal nail bed. Repair of long-standing profundus avulsions is controversial and is usually not recommended with an intact and functioning flexor digitorum superficialis tendon.

Amputations

Mild to moderate loss of skin, subcutaneous tissue, and bone is best treated by wound cleansing, dressing changes, and healing by secondary intention. Acceptable functional and cosmetic results are uniform. Skin or composite grafts are rarely necessary for coverage in children and are associated with donor site morbidity, hyperpigmentation, and lack of sensibility. Extensive soft tissue loss with exposed bone requires more innovative coverage. A volar oblique injury usually can be treated with a variety of local flaps, including a V-Y advancement flap, cross finger flap, or thenar flap (see Figs. 8-20 and 8-21).

Dorsal tissue loss is more difficult to reconstruct. The nail bed injury adds additional complexity. Mild loss can be treated by local wound care. Moderate to severe loss may require a reverse cross-finger flap or a more distant flap. Unfortunately, nail bed replacement techniques often result in considerable nail deformity.

Complications

Osseous. Bony complications from distal phalangeal fractures are uncommon. Potential problems include nonunion, malunion, and osteomyelitis. Nonunion and malunion are exceedingly rare, except in open injuries that result in avascular fracture fragments or untreated widely displaced fractures. Osteomyelitis can result from open fractures and requires application of the basic tenets for the treatment of infected bone. Débridement, removal of any sequestrum, and intravenous antibiotics are required to resolve the infection. Additional tissue coverage is necessary in digits with a marginal soft tissue envelope. These infections are rare due to the robust vascularity of a child's hand.

Soft Tissue. Soft tissue complications are more prevalent than bony problems. Difficulties may involve the skin, subcutaneous tissue, nail, and tendons. An inadequate soft tissue envelope can be reconstructed with replacement using a variety of local flaps.

Nail problems depend on the location and degree of nail bed injury. Damage to the germinal matrix produces deficient nail growth and nail ridging. Injury to the sterile matrix causes poor nail adherence or nail ridging. Treatment options are limited and usually involve resection of the damaged segment and replacement with a full-thickness or split-thickness skin graft.[31,170,214] Adjacent digits or toes are potential sources of nail bed transfers. The results in children have been superior to those in adults.[103,170,171,214] The hook-nail or "parrot's beak" nail is a nail plate complication related to the underlying bony deficit and volar, distal soft tissue contracture. The nail plate curves over the abbreviated end of the distal phalanx (Fig. 8-23). Treatment requires restoring length to the shortened distal phalanx and creation of an adequate soft tissue envelope to support the nail plate (Fig. 8-24).[7] Usually, a thenar flap or composite graft is used to provide improved support for the nail bed in these situations.

A mild DIP joint or extensor tendon lag can occur after pediatric mallet fracture treatment. No further treatment is warranted. Severe DIP joint deformities are uncommon but may result in swan-neck positioning of the finger. Reconstruction options are similar to methods used in adults, such as a spiral oblique retinacular ligament reconstruction or central slip tenotomy.[192] In a young child, untreated lacerations proximal to the terminal tendon insertion may result in an extensor lag that can be repaired successfully with a dermodesis repair.[43,99]

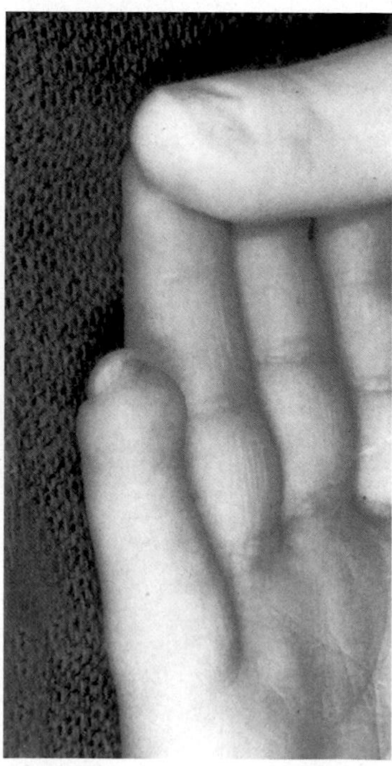

FIGURE 8-23 A hook-nail deformity of the small finger after a distal fingertip amputation.

Fractures of the Proximal and Middle Phalanges

Relevant Anatomy

The physes are located in the proximal aspect of the phalanges. The physis of the thumb metacarpal is also located in the proximal portion, whereas the physes of the finger metacarpals are located in the distal segment (see Fig. 8-1). The collateral ligaments at the PIP and DIP joints originate from the collateral recesses of the proximal bone and insert into both the epiphysis and metaphysis of the distal bone (see Fig. 8-3). The thumb MCP collateral ligaments resemble those of the interphalangeal joints, having epiphyseal and metaphyseal insertions (see Fig. 8-4). The collateral ligaments at the MCP joints of the fingers originate and insert almost exclusively onto the epiphyses of the opposing bones.

The extensor tendons insert onto the dorsal aspect of the epiphysis of the middle and distal phalanges. The flexor digitorum superficialis inserts over about two thirds of the central portion of the middle phalanx. The flexor digitorum profundus has a metaphyseal insertion onto the distal phalanx.

Mechanism of Injury

Most fractures of the proximal and middle phalanges result from some form of axial load combined with a torsional or angular force, such as catching a ball or collision in sports. An isolated lateral force across the PIP or MCP joint can lead to a lateral fracture-dislocation. Crush injuries are less common in the proximal and middle phalanges than in the distal phalanx.

Fracture Patterns

The fracture pattern varies with the direction and amount of force incurred. There are four locations: the physis, the shaft, the neck, and the condylar area (Table 8-3).

Physeal Fractures. Physeal fractures of the proximal phalanx may be the most common pediatric hand fracture.[10,71,84,108,194] Extra-articular S-H II fractures are most prevalent, and intra-articular S-H III and IV fractures are less common. Physeal fractures about the middle phalanx can involve the lateral, dorsal, or volar aspects of the physis. A lateral force across the PIP joint may cause a S-H III or IV fracture. Similarly, a flexion force may produce a dorsal S-H III fracture indicative of a central slip avulsion fracture (pediatric boutonniere injury). A hyperextension injury produces small avulsion fragments from the middle phalangeal epiphysis associated with a volar plate injury.

The thumb proximal phalanx is particularly susceptible to injury. An ulnar collateral ligament avulsion injury at the base of the thumb proximal phalanx is similar to the adult gamekeeper's or skier's thumb. The fracture pattern usually is a S-H III injury. The ligament usually remains attached to the epiphyseal fracture fragment. Fracture displacement with articular incongruity and joint instability is common.[183] Displaced injuries require open reduction and internal fixation to restore articular alignment and joint stability.

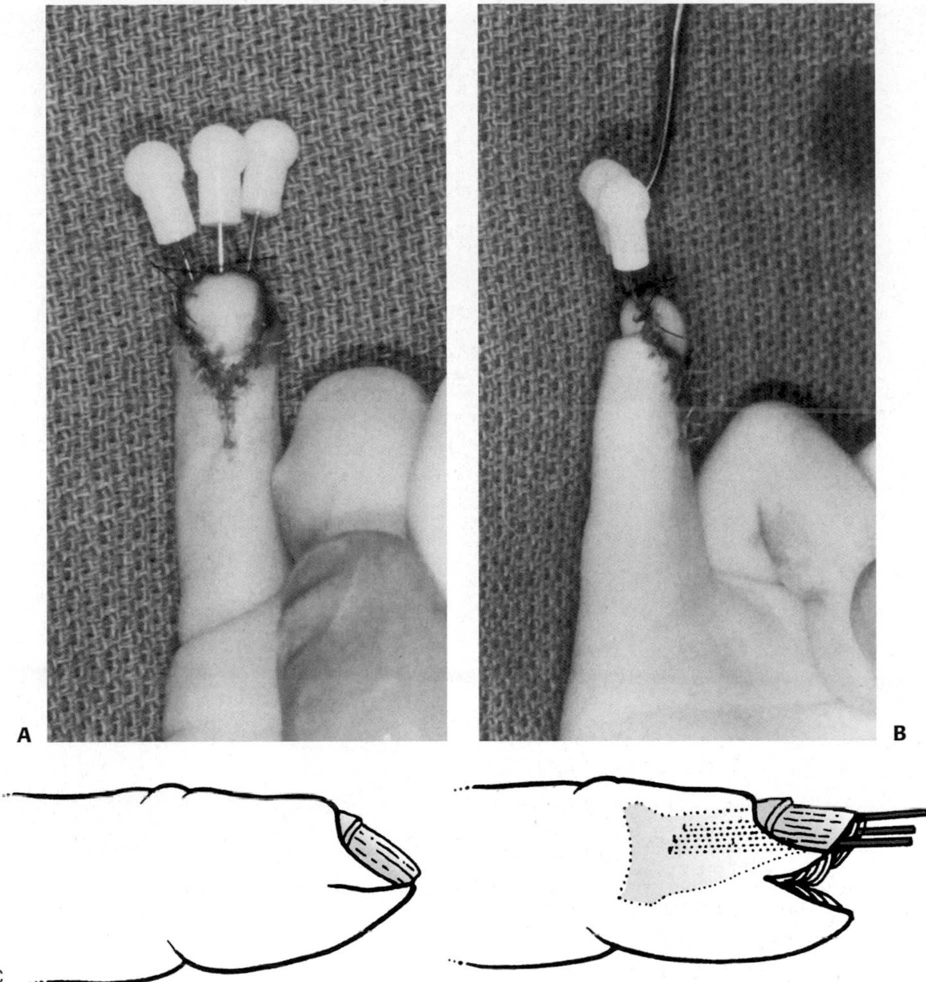

FIGURE 8-24 A,B. Postoperative photographs of the patient shown in Figure 8-25 after the antenna procedure. The procedure involved a volar V-Y advancement flap to cover the distal tip, elevation of the sterile matrix, and the nail supported using three Kirschner-wires. **C.** Line drawings demonstrating technique of elevation and support of the sterile matrix with wires. (A,B. Courtesy of William B. Kleinman, MD. C. Reprinted from Atasoy E, Godfrey A, Kalisman M. The "antenna" procedure for the "hook-nail" deformity. J Hand Surg [Am] 1983;8:55, with permission.)

Children rarely sustain a comminuted intra-articular fracture of the PIP joint, considered "pilon" fractures or fracture-dislocations.[184] These injuries can occur in adolescent athletes and result from an axial load sustained while catching a ball or contacting an opponent. Fracture lines often propagate into the physis. The fracture fragment from the volar side may have the volar plate attached, while the dorsal fragment is likely to have the central slip attached. The central aspect of the joint may be depressed and comminuted. The joint can be unstable and incongruent, requiring careful treatment.

TABLE 8-3 Classification of Proximal and Middle Phalangeal Fractures

- Physeal
- Shaft
- Phalangeal neck
- Intra-articular (condylar)

Shaft Fractures. Shaft fractures in children are less common. The fracture configuration may be transverse, spiral, or spiral oblique. The fracture may be comminuted. Proximal phalangeal fractures usually are angulated in an apex volar pattern because the distal fragment is extended by the central slip and lateral band and the proximal fragment is flexed by the intrinsic musculature (Fig. 8-25). Oblique fractures often rotate and shorten. Careful clinical evaluation of rotational alignment is critical. Comminution is secondary to a high-energy injury or direct trauma to the phalanx (Fig. 8-26).

Neck Fractures. Neck fractures of the phalanx are problematic with regards to treatment and functional outcome. Displaced neck fractures also are referred to as subcondylar fractures and often occur in young children as a result of finger entrapment in a closing door. The head fragment remains attached to the collateral ligaments and tends to rotate into extension.[46] This displacement disrupts the architecture of the subcondylar fossa, which normally accommodates the volar plate and base of the phalanx during interphalangeal joint flexion. Malunited neck fractures, therefore, result in a mechanical block to interphalan-

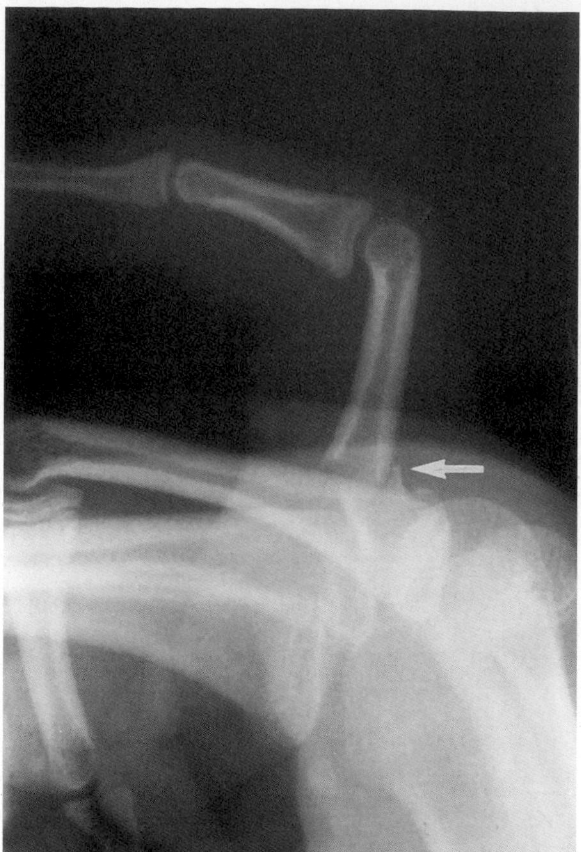

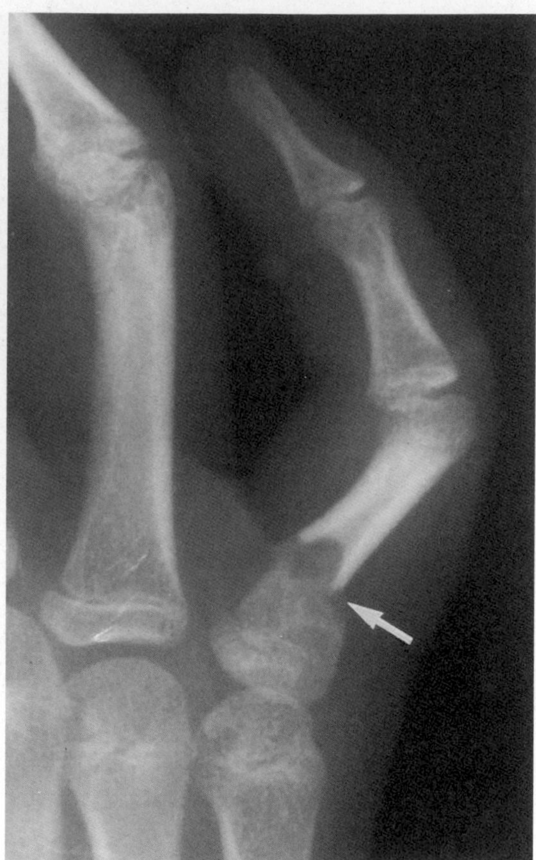

FIGURE 8-25 A,B. Lateral and oblique radiographs of a transverse proximal phalangeal fracture that demonstrates the characteristic apex volar deformity.

geal joint flexion. Frequently, these fractures are inadequately imaged, underappreciated, or misinterpreted as trivial and referred late for care.

Intra-articular (Condylar) Fractures. Condylar fractures involve the joint and represent a constellation of fracture patterns, including small lateral avulsion fractures, unicondylar or intracondylar fractures, bicondylar or transcondylar fractures, and a rare shearing injury of the entire articular surface and its underlying subchondral bone from the distal aspect of the phalanx (Fig. 8-27). Condylar fractures can be associated with subluxations or dislocations of the joint. Many of these fractures are initially misdiagnosed as sprains.[84,108] Restoration of articular alignment and joint stability is critical to a successful outcome.

Diagnosis

Signs and Symptoms. The diagnosis of proximal and middle phalangeal fractures begins with a high index of suspicion based on the history and physical examination. Swelling and ecchymosis are the clinical clues to an underlying fracture. The child usually refuses to move the digit and resists passive motion. Mild fractures may not be clinically apparent, and radiographs should be routinely obtained. Every fracture must be carefully examined for malrotation and rotational deformity regardless of radiographic appearance. Active or passive movement can be used to detect malrotation of the fracture (see Fig. 8-27). Active finger flexion will produce deviation of the plane of the nails or overt digital scissoring. Passive wrist extension will cause long finger flexor tenodesis, and malrotation is evident by an abnormal digital cascade.

Radiographic Findings. Anteroposterior and true lateral views are mandatory. Oblique radiographs are often helpful to determine fracture configuration and alignment. Failure to recognize the extent of injury is an ongoing problem, especially with unicondylar and bicondylar fractures. These fractures may appear fairly normal on the anteroposterior view, but a slight overlap of the subchondral surfaces usually is present on the true lateral projection. This "double density" shadow is made by the offset of the displaced condyle and should not be regarded as a normal finding (Fig. 8-28). Questionable radiographic findings can be further evaluated by additional views, tomograms, or fluoroscopy. Phalangeal neck fractures are too often interpreted as benign injuries.

Treatment Options

The treatment of proximal and middle phalangeal fractures varies greatly with the location of injury. Nonoperative treatment is predictable management for most physeal and shaft fractures. Operative treatment is common for neck and condylar fractures, especially fractures that are displaced or unstable.

Physeal Fractures. Most physeal fractures of the proximal and middle phalanges can be managed by simple immobilization. Displaced fractures often require closed reduction. A common fracture pattern is a S-H II fracture along the ulnar aspect of

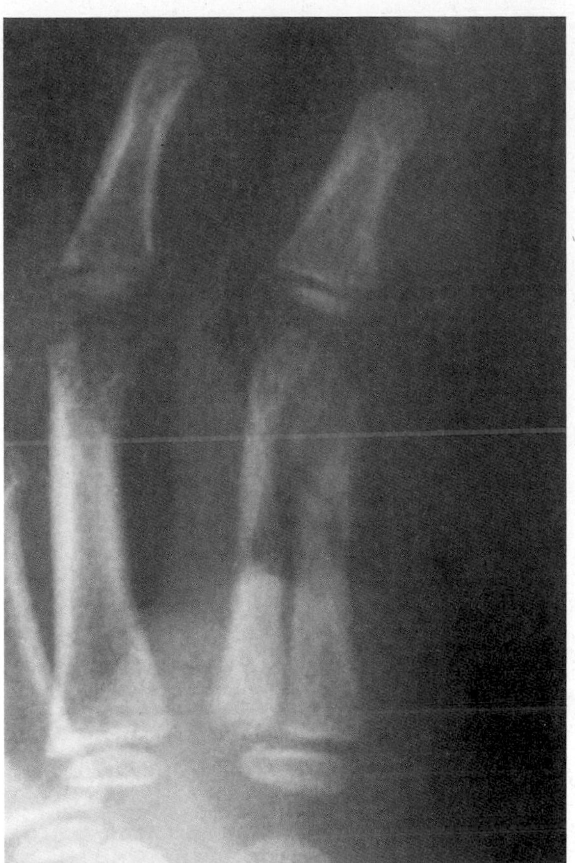

FIGURE 8-26 Comminuted fractures secondary to a crush injury with longitudinal splitting into the physis.

the proximal phalanx of the small digit. The small digit is angulated in an ulnar direction. This fracture has been termed the "extra-octave fracture" to denote its potential benefit to the span of a pianist's hand (Fig. 8-29).[153] Minimal displacement is treated with splinting in the safe position for 3 weeks. Moderate displacement requires closed reduction with local anesthesia or conscious sedation. Placing the MCP joint into flexion to tighten the collateral ligaments and angulating the digit into radial deviation reduces the fracture. Placing a pencil or digit in the web space and using it as a fulcrum to assist reduction has been recommended.[207] Minimal force is necessary to restore alignment.[5,51] Buddy taping and cast immobilization will maintain alignment until healing.

Irreducible fractures of the physis have been reported.[10,37,83,108] A variety of tissues, including periosteum and tendons, may prevent reduction. Open treatment with removal of the impeding tissue and fracture reduction is required for these rare injuries (Fig. 8-30). In addition, some S-H II fractures may be reducible but unstable after reduction. These fractures tend to be higher-energy injuries with more disruption of the supporting soft tissues. Insertion of a smooth Kirschner wire after reduction is required to maintain fracture alignment.[83,167] Another indication for operative management is a displaced S-H III fracture of the proximal phalangeal base with a sizable (more than 25%) epiphyseal fragment. Closed or open reduction may be required to restore articular congruity.[84,167] Small Kirschner wires can be inserted parallel to the joint surface, avoiding the physis. Tension-band wiring[179] techniques can be used for S-H III and IV fractures. Operative exposure and fixation techniques are challenging with nonborder digit proximal phalangeal S-H III fractures.

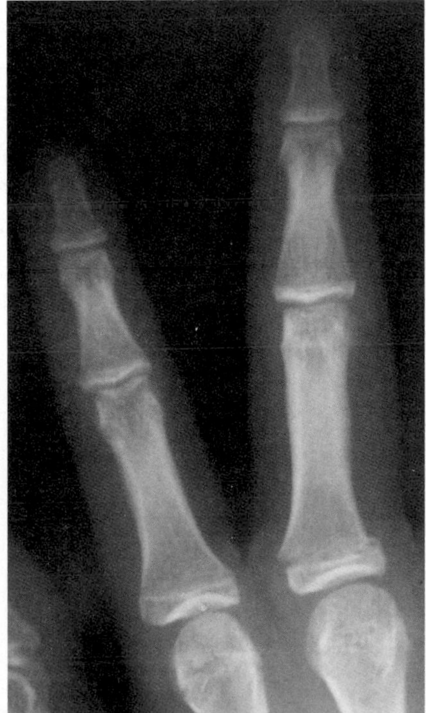

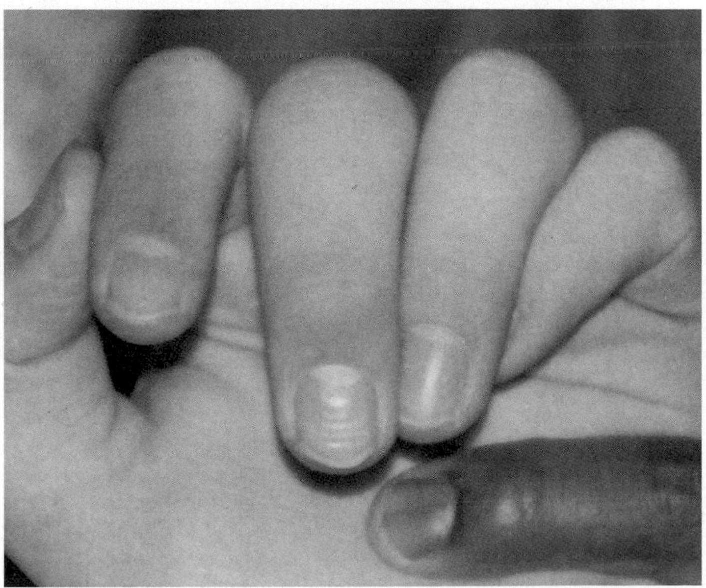

FIGURE 8-27 A. Anteroposterior radiograph of a S-H II fracture at the long finger proximal phalanx. The radiogaph reveals slight angulation and can appear benign. Clinical examination must be done to assess the digital cascade for malrotation. **B.** Tenodesis of the wrist with passive extension reveals unacceptable malrotation as evident by the degree of overlap of the middle finger on the ring finger.

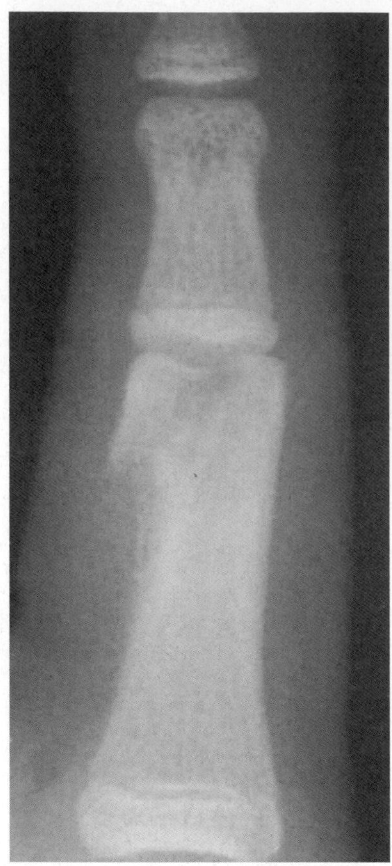

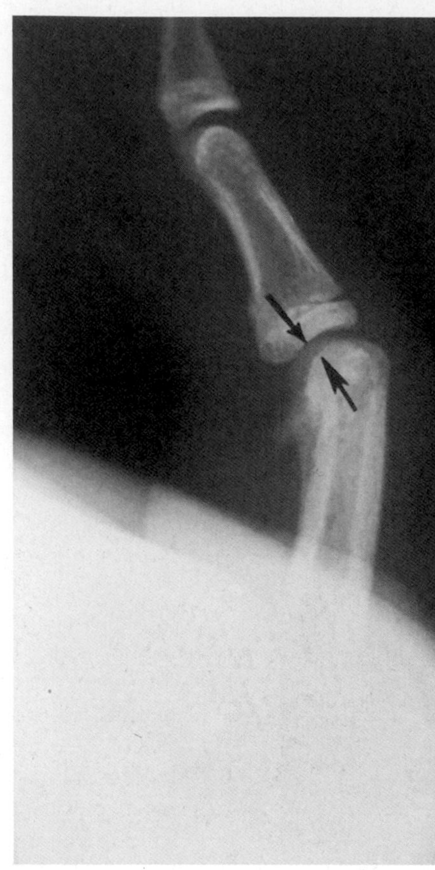

FIGURE 8-28 A. Anteroposterior radiograph reveals intra-articular fracture of the small finger. **B.** Lateral view demonstrates double density sign indicative of displacement (*arrows*).

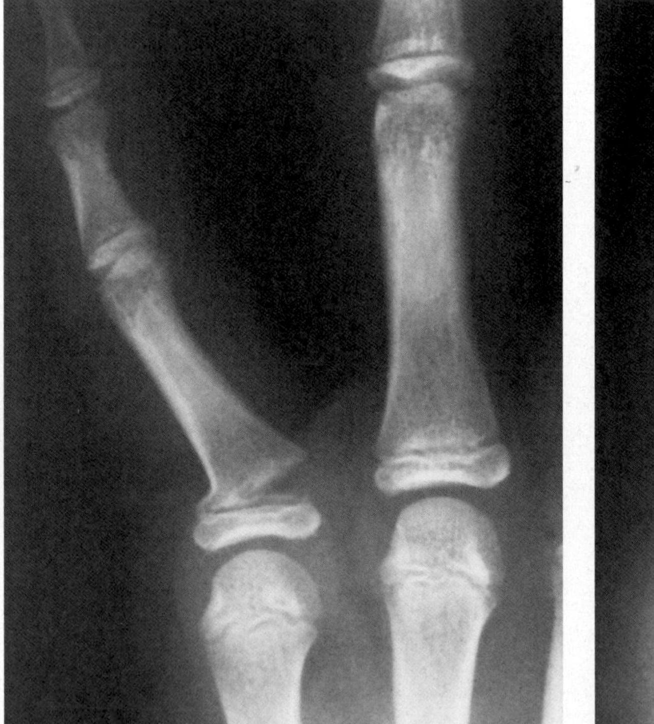

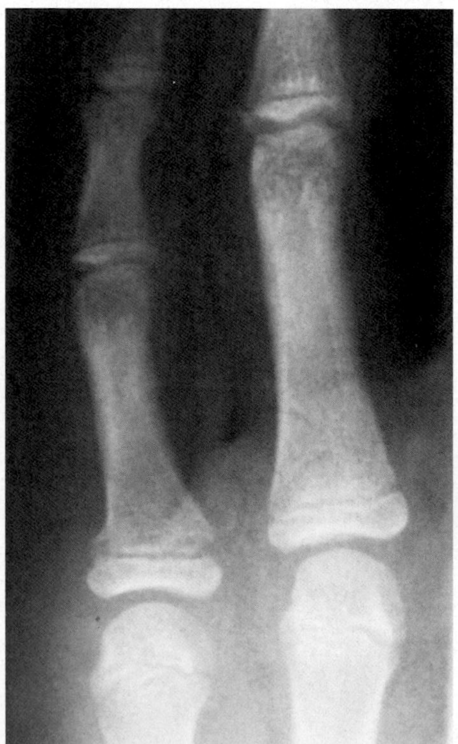

FIGURE 8-29 A. An extra-octave fracture in a 12-year-old girl. **B.** The fracture was reduced with the MCP joint in full flexion.

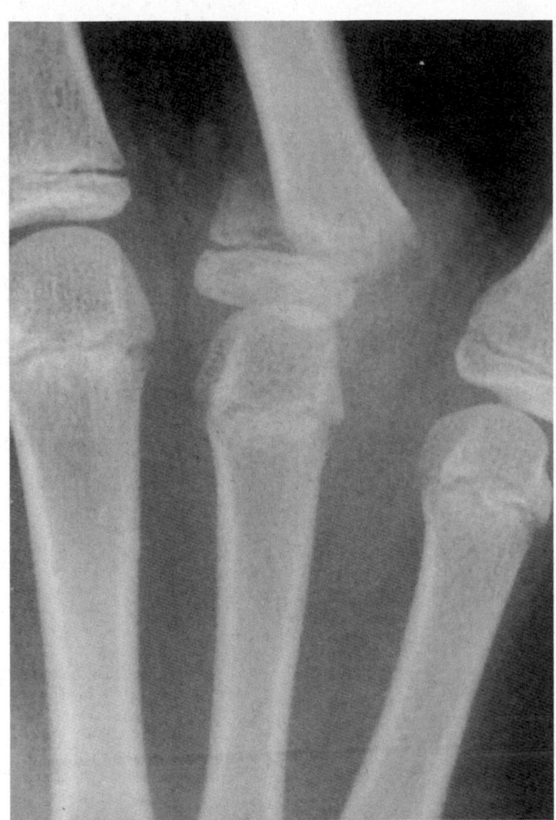

FIGURE 8-30 Displaced S-H II fracture of the proximal phalanx that was irreducible. The distal fragment was herniated through a rent in the periosteum and extensor mechanism that prohibited reduction.

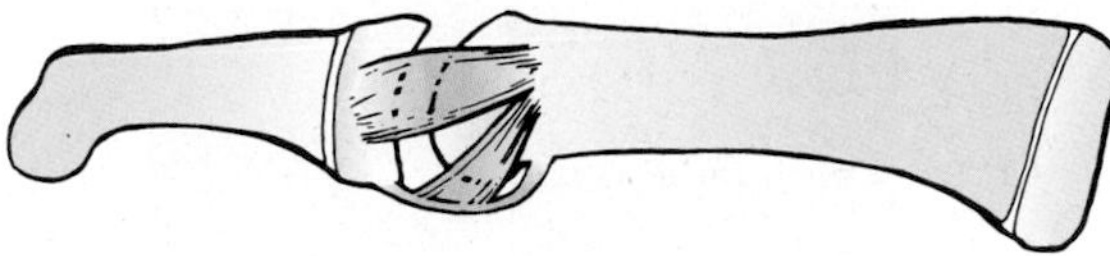

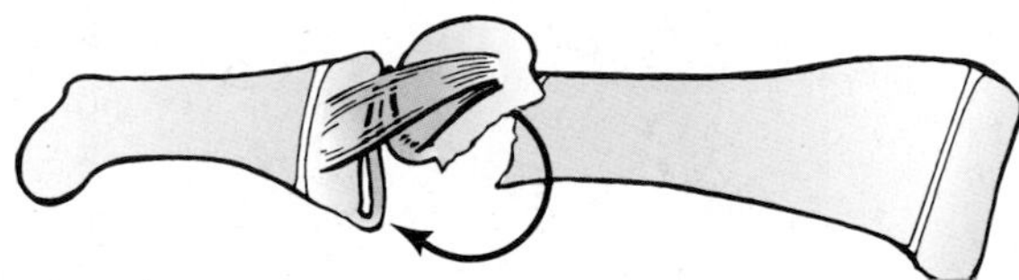

FIGURE 8-31 Phalangeal neck fractures often are unstable and rotated. These fractures are difficult to reduce and control by closed means because of the forces imparted by the volar plate and ligaments. (Reprinted from Wood BE. Fractures of the hand in children. Orthop Clin North Am 1976;7:527–534, with permission.)

Shaft Fractures. Shaft fractures that are nondisplaced and stable can be treated with simple immobilization. Safe position splinting for 3 to 4 weeks should be adequate for clinical union. Displaced or angulated fractures require closed reduction. The amount of acceptable angulation in the plane of motion is controversial.[172] In children less than 10 years of age, 20 to 30 degrees may be acceptable. In children older than 10 years, 10 to 20 degrees angulation is acceptable. Less angulation is acceptable in the coronal plane. Malrotation is unacceptable.

Fractures that are unstable after reduction or irreducible by closed methods require operative intervention. A shaft fracture that is unstable after reduction is managed by Kirschner-wire fixation.[181] Open reduction is indicated for fractures that cannot be reduced. A dorsal approach usually is used for exposure. The extensor tendon is split for proximal phalangeal fractures and elevated for middle phalangeal fractures. The choice of implant depends on the age of the patient and the fracture configuration. Smooth wires or screws are preferable to plates to avoid extensor mechanism adherence.[90] Bone grafting alone has been described to provide rigid fixation to proximal phalangeal base fractures.[186] All malrotated fractures require reduction and fixation.

Phalangeal Neck Fractures. Closed treatment of fractures of the phalangeal neck is difficult because these fractures often are unstable (Fig. 8-31). Closed manipulation is done with digital distraction, a volar-directed pressure on the distal fragment, and hyperflexion of the PIP joint. Percutaneous pinning usually is necessary to maintain the reduced position.[46] Under fluoroscopy, Kirschner wires are inserted through the collateral recesses and across the fracture. These wires should engage the contralateral cortex proximal to the fracture site. An alternative technique with a small distal fragment is to insert the pins through the articular surface of the phalanx in a longitudinal fashion, crossing the fracture to engage the proximal fragment.

Intra-articular Fractures. Nondisplaced fractures can be treated by immobilization. Weekly radiographs are necessary to ensure maintenance of reduction. Displaced intra-articular fractures require closed or open reduction.[167] Closed or percutaneous reduction can be accomplished with traction and use of a percutaneous towel clip or reduction clamp to obtain provisional fracture reduction. Percutaneous fixation is used for definitive fracture fixation. Fractures not appropriate for closed manipulation require open reduction and internal fixation (Fig. 8-32). A dorsal, lateral, or even volar incision is used for direct inspection of the fracture and articular surface. Care is taken to preserve the blood supply of the fracture fragments entering through the collateral ligaments. Fracture stabilization is by either Kirschner wires or miniscrews.

Certain unusual intra-articular fractures are especially difficult to treat. Shear fractures and osteochondral slice fractures are difficult to recognize. Treatment is open reduction and smooth wire fixation. Osteonecrosis, especially of small fragments, is a concern. Some of these fractures require a volar surgical approach. Avoidance of extensive soft tissue dissection lessens the risk of osteonecrosis.

Comminuted pilon fracture-dislocations of the PIP joint are uncommon in children. Operative intervention is usually required to restore articular congruity. Anatomic reduction is preferred whenever possible (Fig. 8-33).[185] Bone grafting may be necessary for stable reduction. Extreme joint comminution may preclude anatomic reduction, and alternative treatment options, such as dynamic traction, may be necessary.[2,166]

Complex Injuries. Combined injuries that affect several tissue systems are common in the digits. Skin, tendon, neurovascular

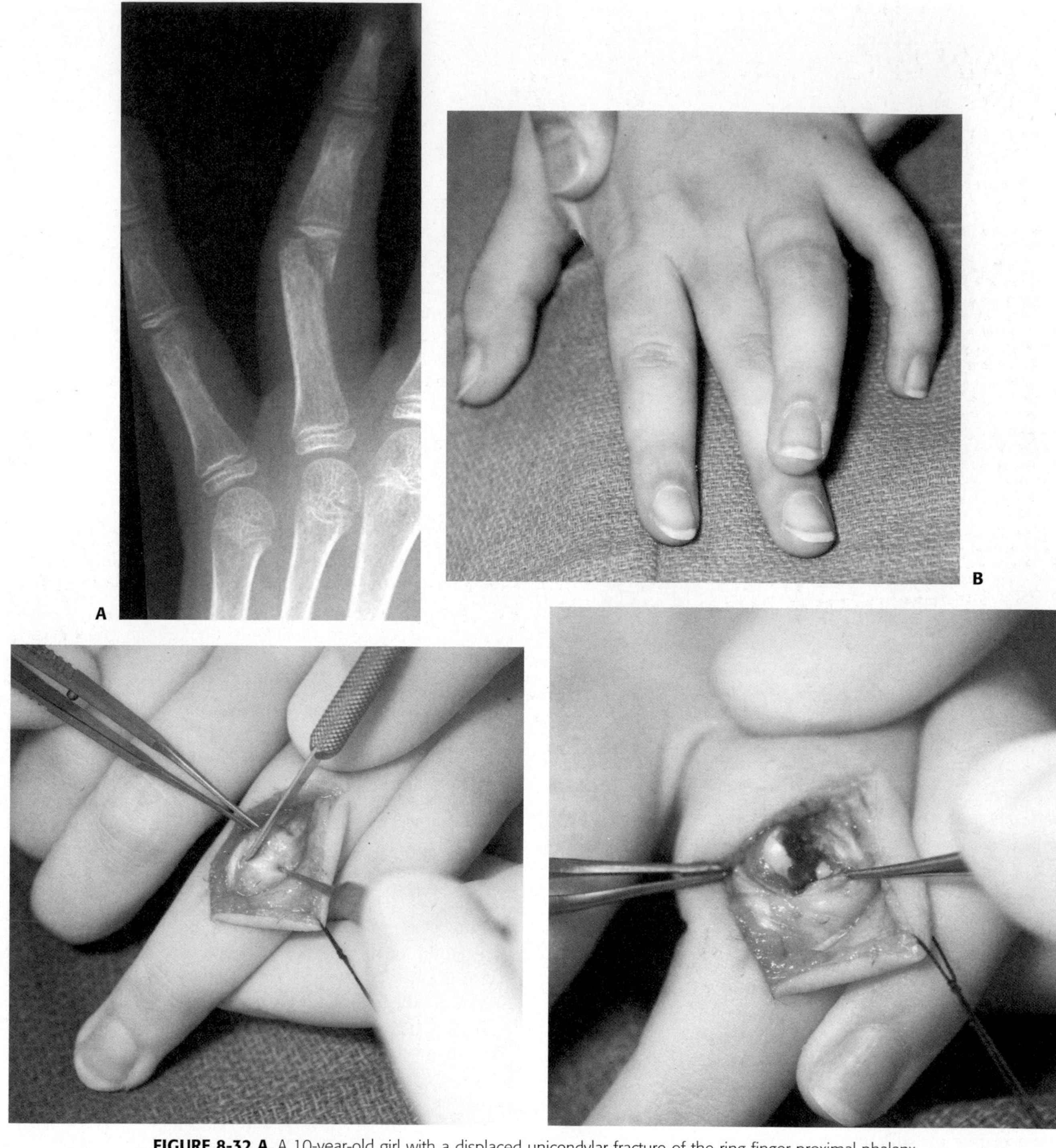

FIGURE 8-32 A. A 10-year-old girl with a displaced unicondylar fracture of the ring finger proximal phalanx. **B.** Clinical examination reveals malrotation of the digit. **C.** Dorsal exposure with incision between lateral band and central slip. **D.** Exposure of displaced fracture fragment. *(continues)*

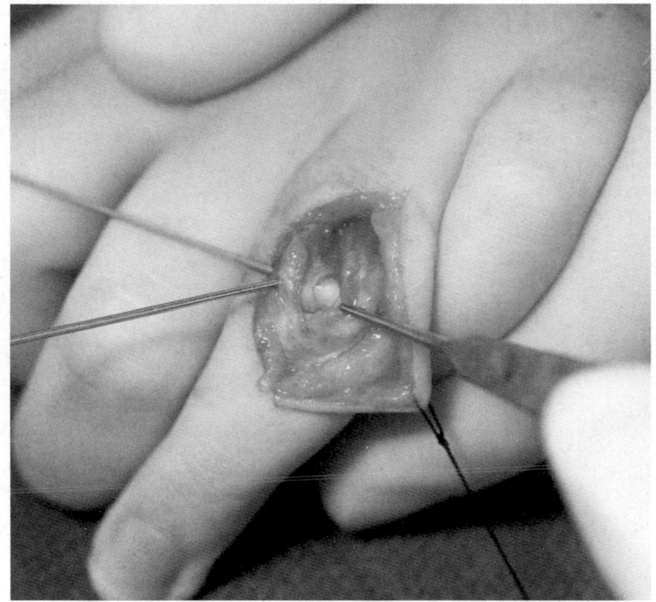

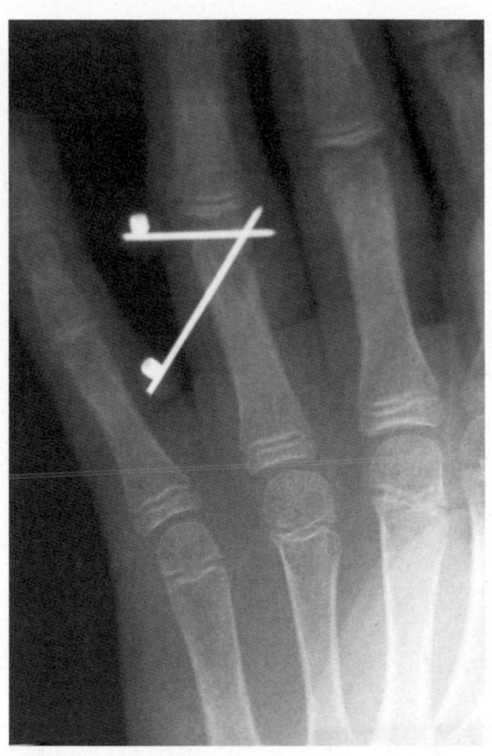

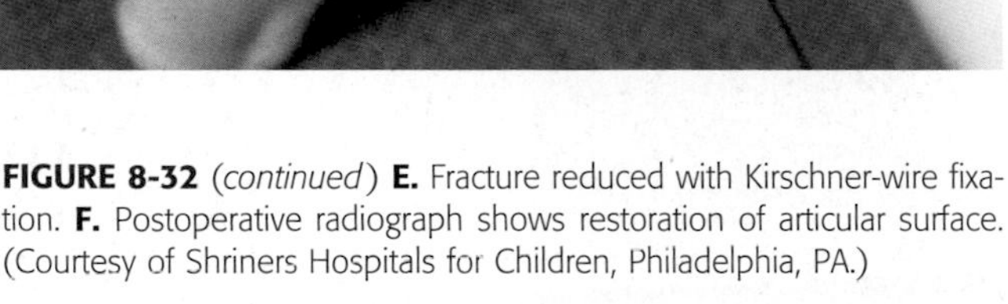

FIGURE 8-32 (*continued*) **E.** Fracture reduced with Kirschner-wire fixation. **F.** Postoperative radiograph shows restoration of articular surface. (Courtesy of Shriners Hospitals for Children, Philadelphia, PA.)

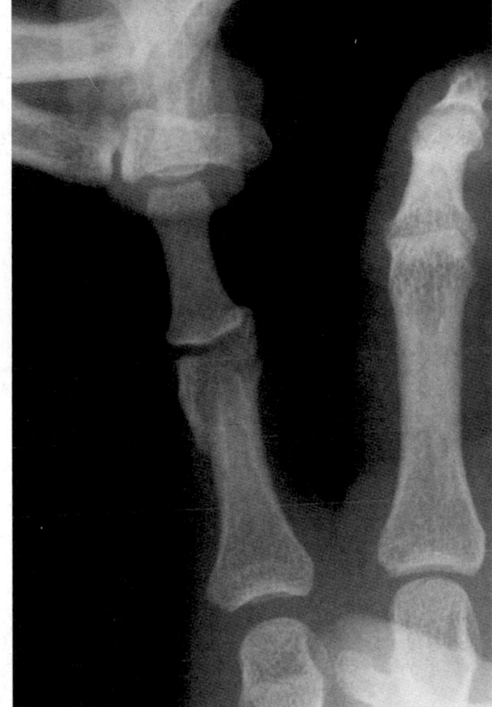

B

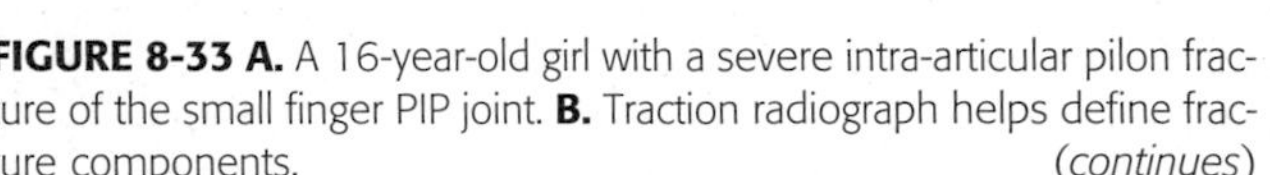

FIGURE 8-33 A. A 16-year-old girl with a severe intra-articular pilon fracture of the small finger PIP joint. **B.** Traction radiograph helps define fracture components. (*continues*)

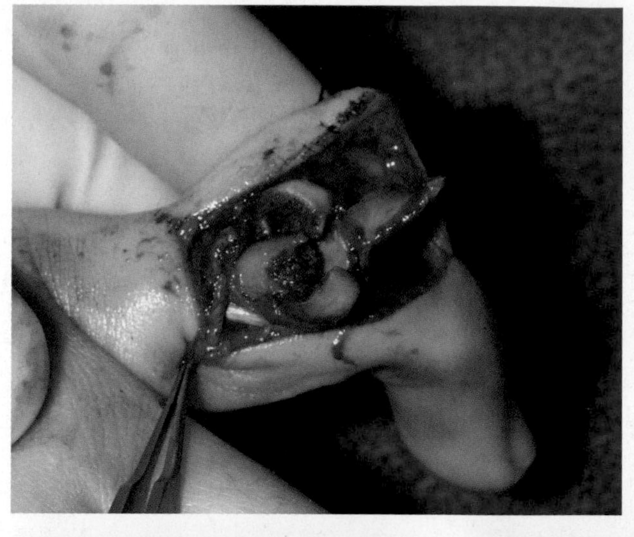
C

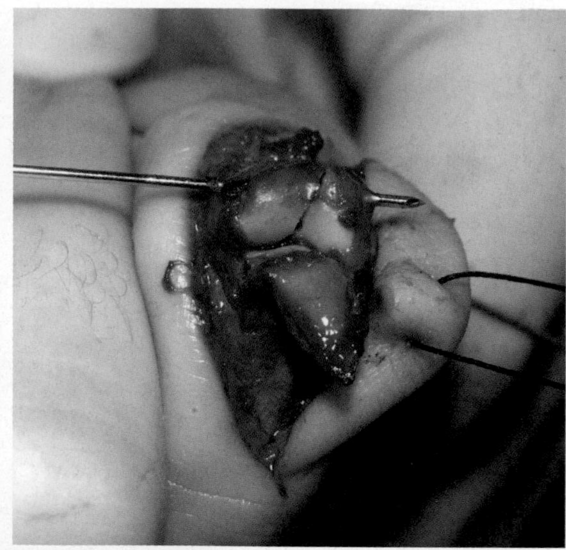
D

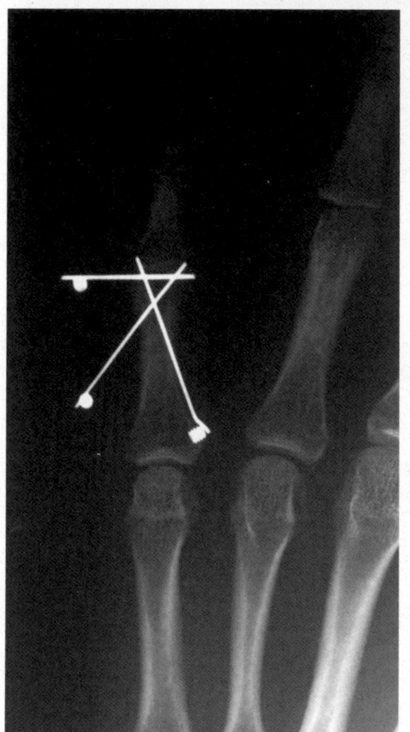
E

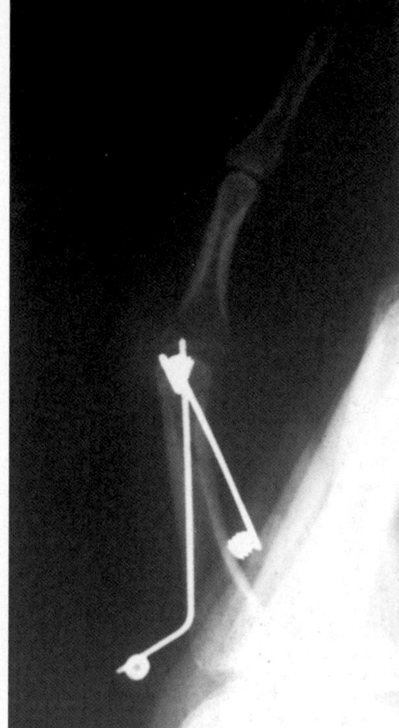
F

FIGURE 8-33 *(continued)* **C.** Dorsal exposure revealed ulnar condyle outside of joint requiring incision of extensor tendon for reduction. **D.** Reduction of joint surface and Kirschner-wire fixation. **E.** Postoperative anteroposterior radiograph shows restoration of articular surface. **F.** Lateral radiograph shows sagittal alignment of condyles. (Courtesy of Shriners Hospitals for Children, Philadelphia, PA.)

structures, and bone may all be injured in the same digit (Fig. 8-34). Open fracture care is mandatory, followed by establishment of a stable bony foundation. Markedly comminuted fractures or injuries with bone loss may require external fixation followed by delayed bony reconstruction. Neurovascular and tendon reconstruction in children follows the same principles as for adults. Rehabilitation of complex injuries in children can be complicated by a lack of cooperation. Vascular injuries can affect subsequent growth.

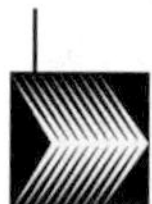

AUTHORS' PREFERRED TREATMENT

Physeal Fractures

Nondisplaced fractures are treated with simple immobilization for 3 weeks. Most displaced S-H I and II fractures can be treated with closed reduction (Fig. 8-35). Alignment and rotation is verified clinically and reduction is assessed with radiographs. The hand is immobilized in a safe-position splint, and a radiograph is obtained 5 to 7 days later to ensure maintenance of reduction. When there is doubt about anatomic alignment, the cast is removed for more thorough clinical and radiographic examinations. Immobilization is continued for 3 to 4 weeks. Physeal fractures that are unstable after closed reduction require percutaneous pin fixation. Small smooth wires are used to secure the reduction. Irreducible fractures require open reduction, removal of any interposed tissue, and fixation.

Displaced S-H III fractures of either the middle or proximal phalanges are difficult to reduce and maintain by closed methods. Dorsal S-H III or IV fractures of the middle phalangeal base often require open reduction and fixation to avoid

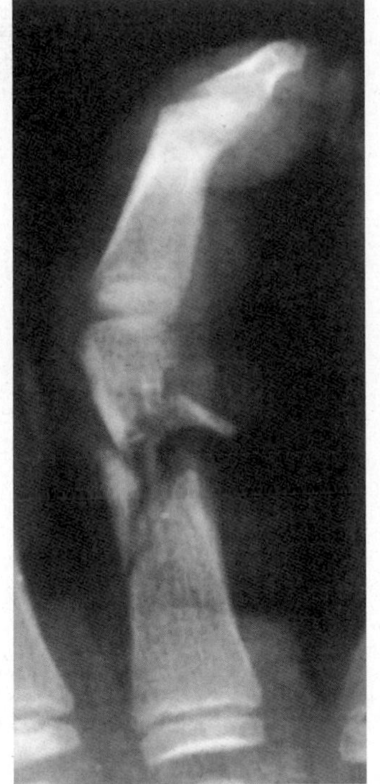

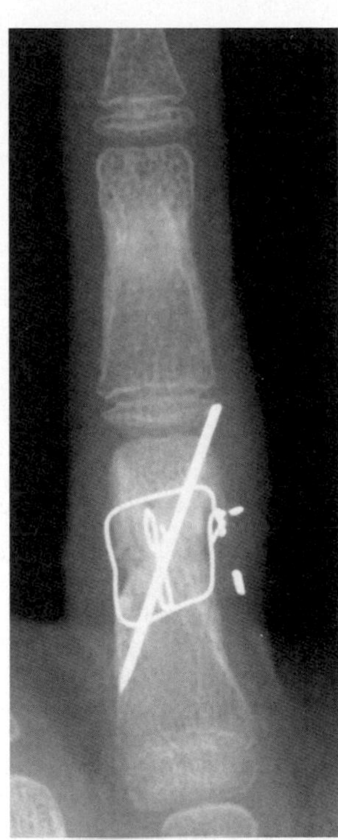

FIGURE 8-34 A. A 14-year-old boy sustained a near-amputation of his ring digit with severe soft tissue injury. **B.** 90-90 intraosseous wiring supplemented with Kirschner-wire fixation to provide a stable base for soft tissue repair.

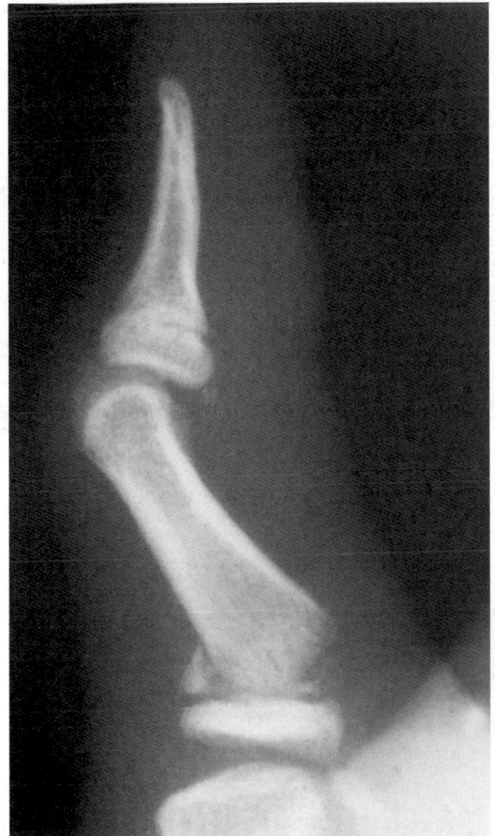

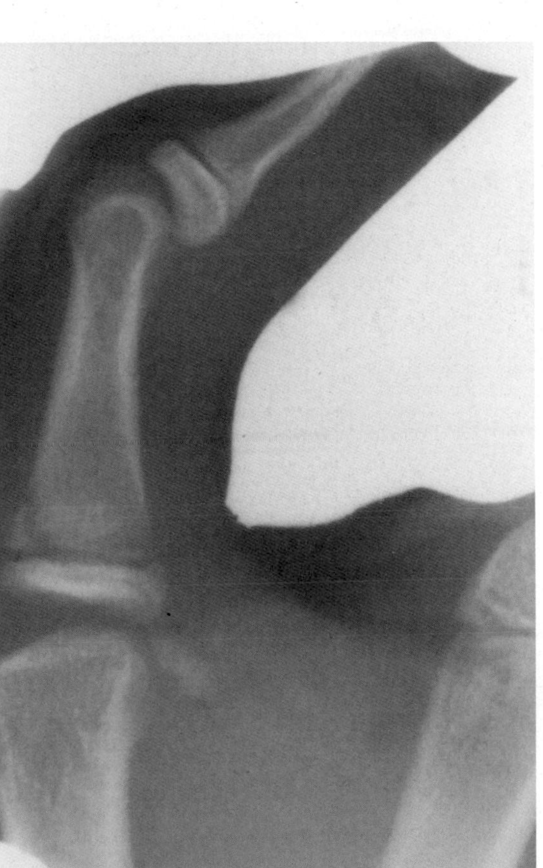

FIGURE 8-35 A. A S-H II fracture of the proximal phalanx of the thumb. **B.** Gentle closed reduction under fluoroscopic control obtained an anatomic reduction.

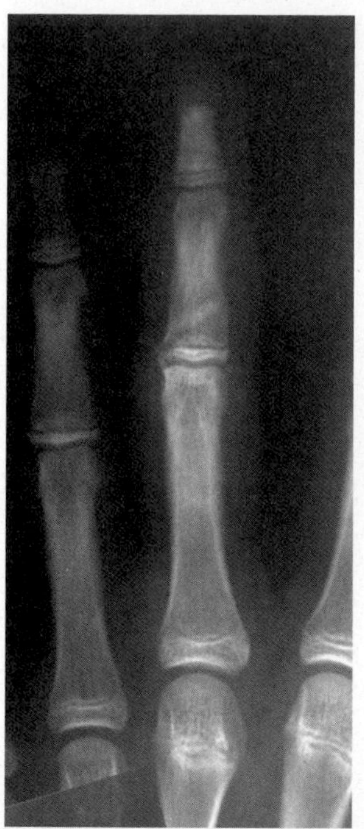

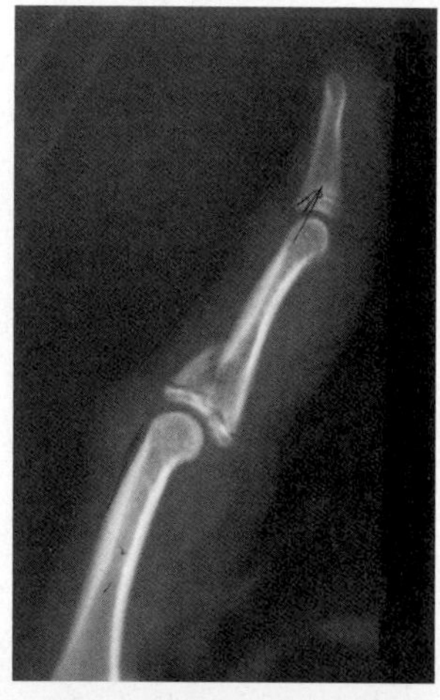

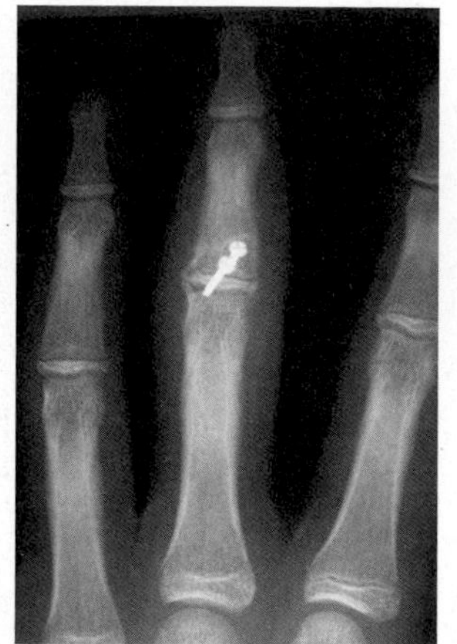

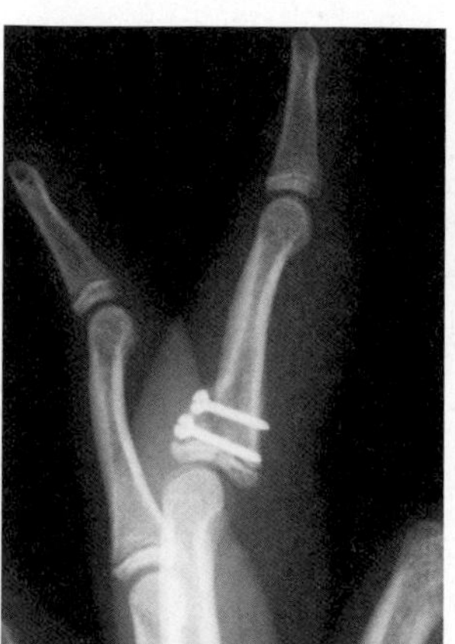

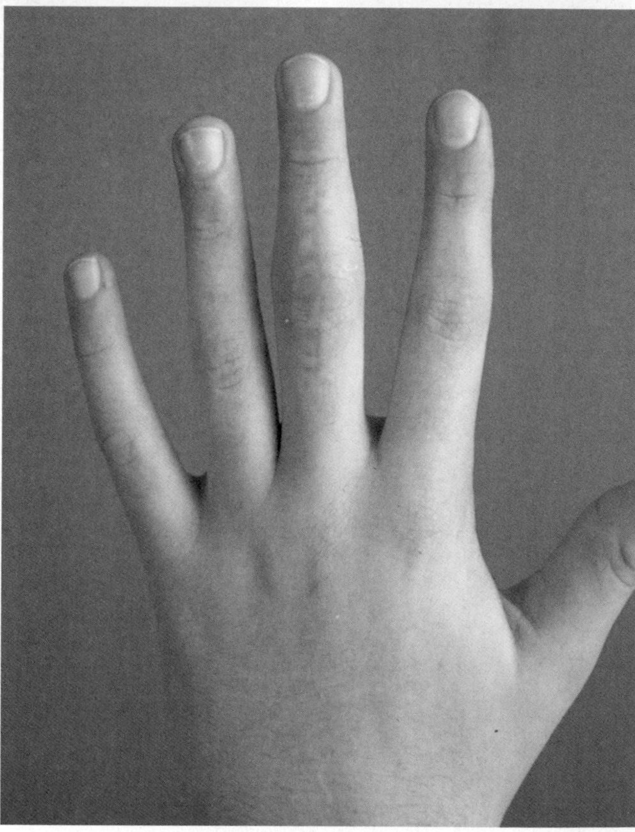

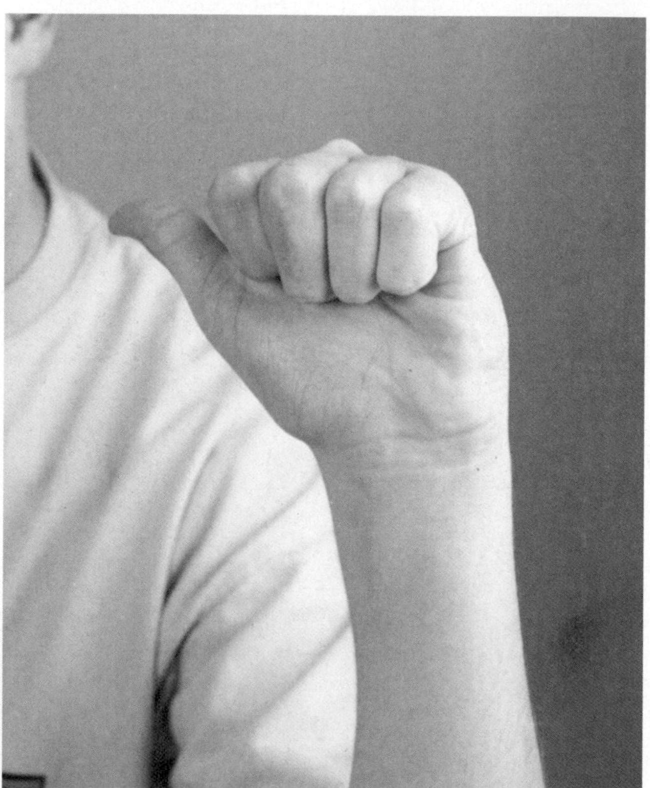

FIGURE 8-36 A,B. A 16-year-old male sustained a dorsal S-H IV fracture of the middle phalanx. **C,D.** Open reduction and internal screw fixation were accomplished through a dorsal approach. Radiographs show reduction of joint subluxation and fixation of fracture fragment. **E,F.** Postoperative extension and flexion with near normal motion. (Courtesy of Shriners Hospitals for Children, Philadelphia, PA.)

the development of a boutonniere deformity (Fig. 8-36). A dorsal approach, with an incision between the central tendon and the lateral band, is preferred. The PIP joint may require supplemental pin fixation for 3 weeks to permit healing. Lateral S-H III fractures that are displaced more than 1.5 mm or involve more than 25% of the articular surface also may require open reduction and internal fixation. This fracture pattern is especially common in the proximal phalanx of the thumb.

Shaft Fractures

Nondisplaced fractures are treated with immobilization for 3 to 4 weeks. Displaced fractures are treated with closed reduction and percutaneous pin fixation.[72] Reduction is accomplished with longitudinal traction and rotation of the distal fragment to approximate the proximal fragment. For a proximal phalangeal fracture, the MCP joint is flexed to relax the intrinsic muscle pull and to stabilize the proximal fragment. The fracture orientation dictates the angle of pin insertion. Optimal pin placement is perpendicular to the fracture line. Placement of the pins in the midaxial line prevents iatrogenic injury of the neurovascular structures or entrapment of the extensor mechanism by the pin. Open reduction is reserved for irreducible fractures.

Neck Fractures

Neck fractures usually require operative intervention. If closed reduction is obtainable, then percutaneous pin fixation is performed. The pins are placed through the collateral recesses to engage the proximal fragment in a crossed fashion. If closed reduction is unsuccessful, open reduction with preservation of the collateral ligaments and similar percutaneous pinning are indicated. However, open reduction should be avoided whenever possible to decrease the chances of osteonecrosis.

Late presentation of a neck fracture requires consideration of the time from injury and fracture displacement. Considerable displacement requires treatment to regain joint flexion (Fig. 8-37). If the fracture line is still visible, a percutaneous pin osteoclasis may be possible. Under fluoroscopy, one or two smooth Kirschner wires are inserted into the fracture site to break up any callus. These Kirschner wires are used to "joystick" the distal fragment into a reduced position.[201] The fracture is then stabilized with additional percutaneous pins. This approach may decrease the risk of osteonecrosis associated with late open reduction. A nascent or established malunion that cannot be reduced by osteoclasis can be treated by late open reduction (Fig. 8-38). The callus is gently removed and the fracture aligned. The risks of osteonecrosis must be weighed against acceptance of the malunion. Mild loss of the condylar recess can be treated with recession of the prominent volar bone rather than risk osteonecrosis associated with extensive fracture mobilization.[173,189] In addition, slow remodeling is feasible in very young children without rotational malalignment and with a family that is willing to wait up to 2 years for remodeling.[36,85]

FIGURE 8-37 Displaced phalangeal neck fracture of the proximal phalanx revealing loss of subchondral fossa at the PIP joint. If this is not corrected to anatomic alignment, there will be a mechanical block to flexion.

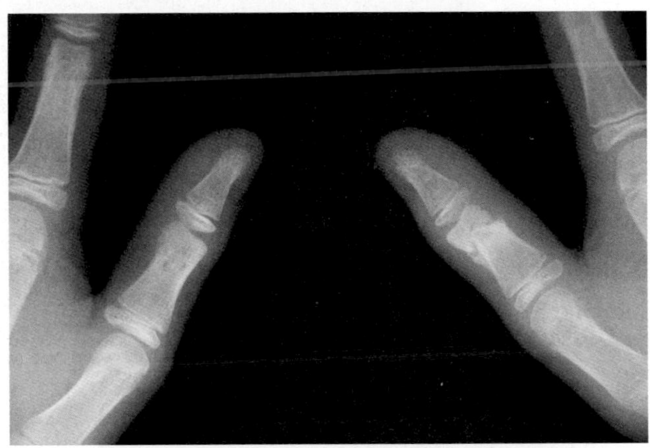

A

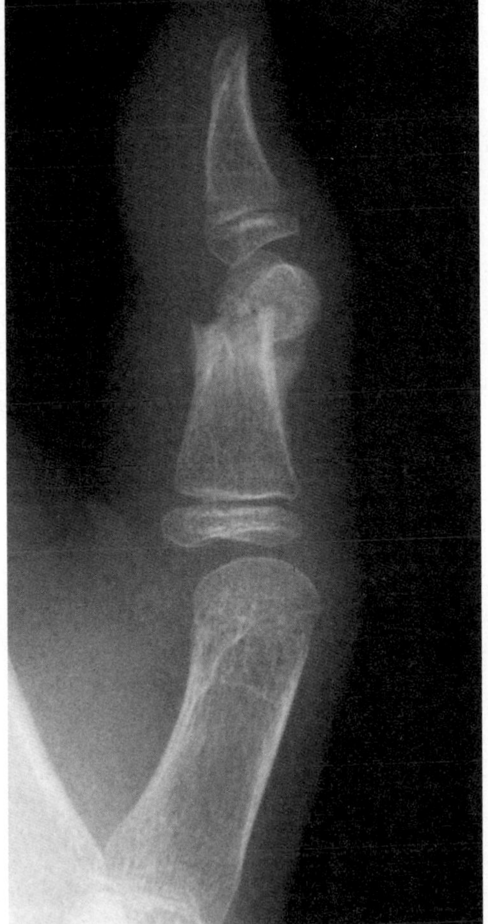

B

FIGURE 8-38 A. A 14-year-old girl with incipient malunion of right thumb proximal phalanx neck fractures that impede flexion. **B.** Lateral radiograph reveals loss of the subchondral fossa. *(continues)*

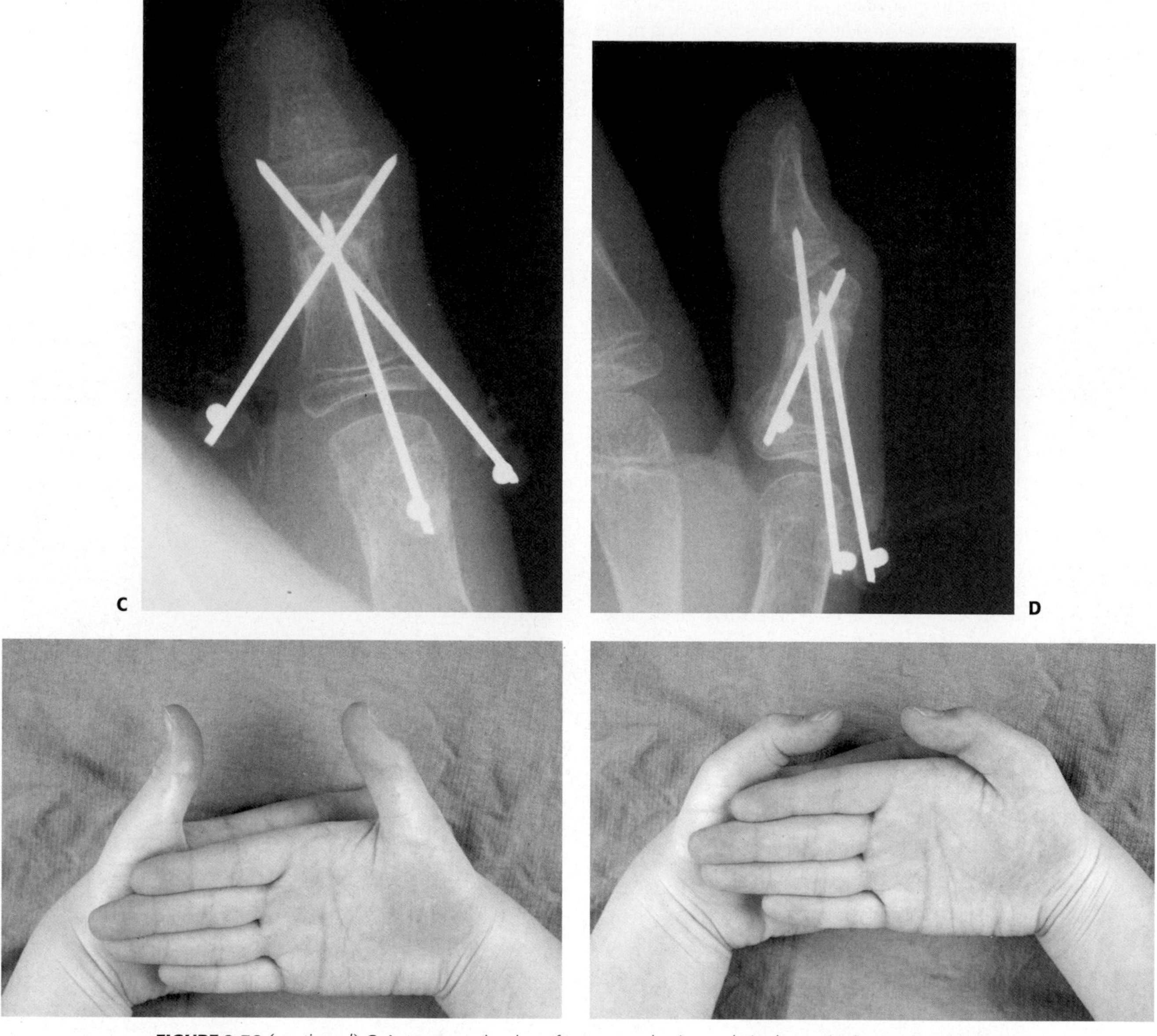

FIGURE 8-38 *(continued)* **C.** Anteroposterior view after open reduction and Kirschner-wire fixation. **D.** Oblique view reveals restoration of subchondral fossa. **E,F.** Postoperative flexion and extension compared to the other side. (Courtesy of Shriners Hospitals for Children, Philadelphia, PA.)

Intra-articular Fractures

Intra-articular fractures of the phalanges usually require percutaneous or open reduction. Unicondylar fractures that are mildly displaced can be treated with closed reduction and percutaneous pinning. Widely displaced unicondylar and bicondylar fractures require open reduction (see Fig. 8-32). A dorsal approach is preferred. Fixation usually is obtained with smooth wires. The placement and direction are dictated by the fracture configuration. Rotational control of the fragment may require multiple wires. The fixation device must avoid tethering of the collateral ligament, which will limit motion. Usually, a pin is placed parallel to the joint to maintain articular alignment, followed by oblique pins to stabilize the articular fragment(s) to the shaft. In adolescents, miniscrew fixation can be used. These screws must avoid impingement of the collateral ligaments, which will impede flexion.

Pilon fractures or intra-articular fracture-dislocations present a management dilemma.[185] Open reduction is worthwhile when the fragments are large and the joint surface can be reconstructed. Bone grafting may be necessary for stable reduction. Severe articular damage and comminution are treated with dynamic traction.

Postoperative Care and Rehabilitation

The duration of immobilization after surgical intervention for phalangeal fractures is usually 3 to 4 weeks. Percutaneous pins are removed at that time and motion instituted. Formal hand therapy usually is not required, although the child must be encouraged to re-establish a normal usage pattern to improve motion and flexibility. Periarticular fractures are monitored closely for persistent loss of motion that would benefit from formal hand therapy. Patients with complex fractures or replantations are more prone to develop stiffness. In these instances, therapy is routinely prescribed to regain motion. Therapy is directed at both flexion and extension of the injured digit. Static or dynamic splinting may be required after fracture healing. Persistent stiffness may require tenolysis and joint release to regain motion (Fig. 8-39).

Prognosis

The overall results following proximal and middle phalangeal fractures are positive. Considering the frequency of these fractures, the occurrence of complications and functional impairment is low. Despite appropriate treatment, however, some children have permanent loss of motion, malunion, or growth disturbance. The major concern is to avoid rotational, articular, or periarticular malunion due to inappropriate diagnosis or treatment.

Complications

Early. Complications associated with proximal and middle phalangeal fractures begin with failure to recognize the injury (Fig. 8-40). Anteroposterior and lateral radiographs must be made

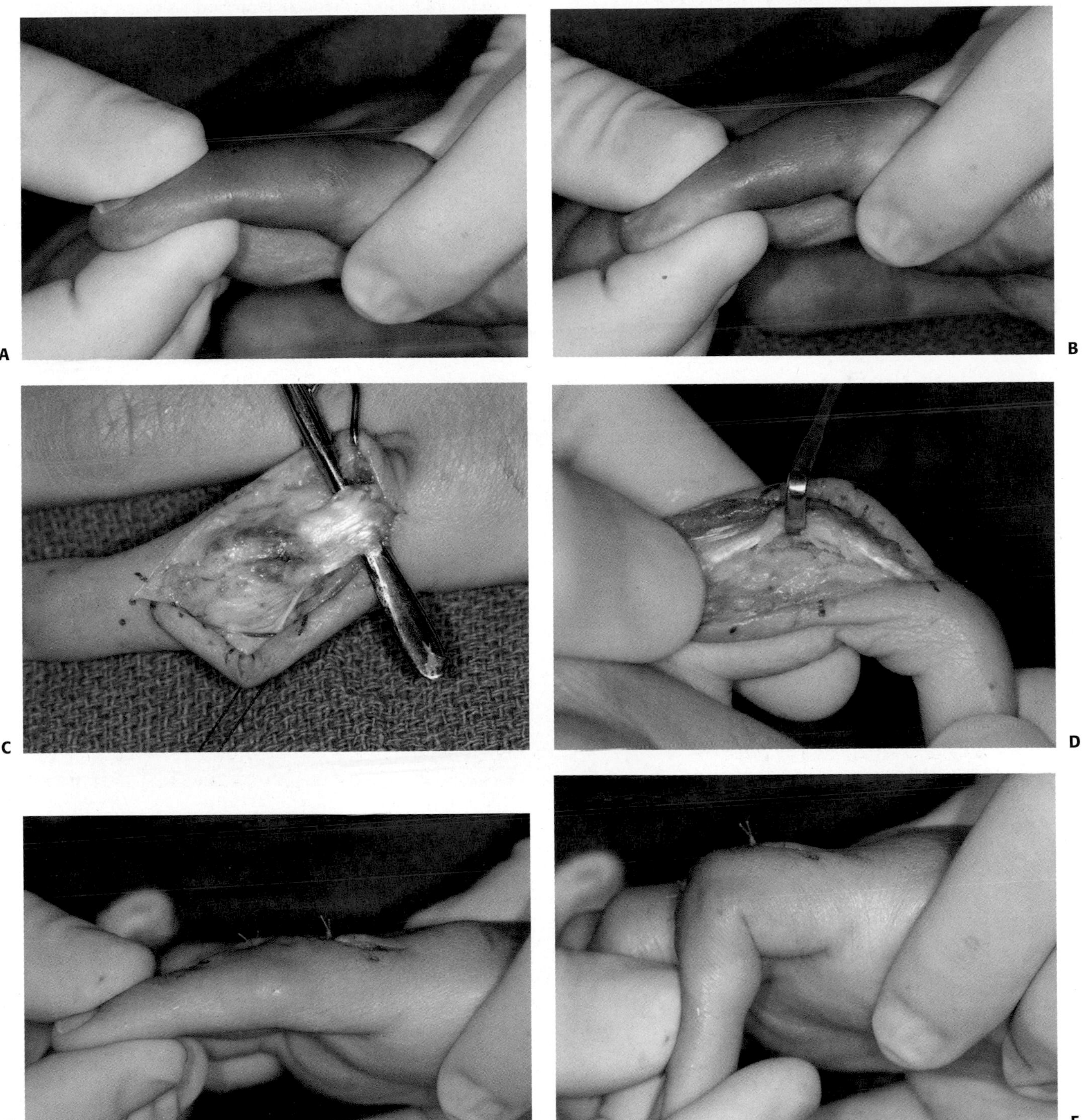

FIGURE 8-39 A 16-year-old girl with a severe intra-articular pilon fracture of the small finger PIP joint depicted in Figure 8-33 with healed fracture, but limited motion after therapy. **A.** Passive extension **B.** Passive flexion. **C.** Dorsal exposure and tenolysis under local anesthesia with sedation. **D.** Joint release. **E.** Passive extension. **F.** Passive flexion. *(continues)*

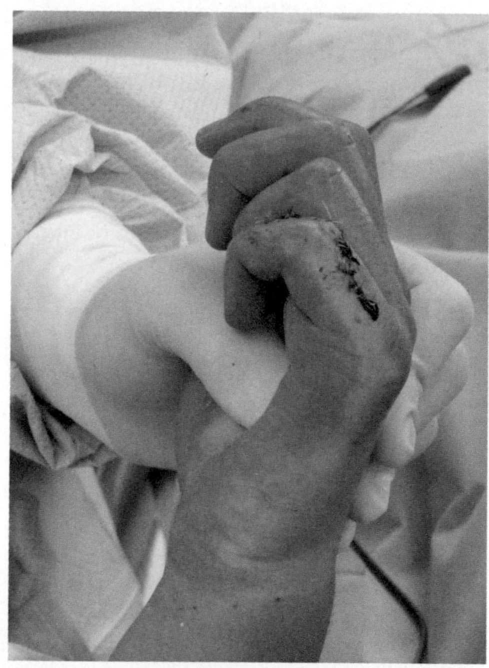

G

FIGURE 8-39 (*continued*) **G.** Active flexion. (Courtesy of Shriners Hospitals for Children, Philadelphia, PA.)

correctly and scrutinized for subtle abnormalities. Questionable findings warrant additional views or advanced imaging studies. A common misdiagnosis is failure to recognize a displaced phalangeal neck fracture because of inadequate lateral radiographs of the fracture.

Another early complication is false interpretation of a "nondisplaced" fracture that is malrotated. All children with phalangeal fractures require careful examination for rotational alignment. The clinical examination is the mainstay for determining fracture rotation. Digital scissoring is indicative of fracture malrotation and requires reduction. Regardless of radiographic appearance, rotational alignment should be evaluated by active finger flexion and passive tenodesis.

Most phalangeal fractures can be maintained in satisfactory alignment after closed reduction. Certain fractures, however, have a propensity for redisplacement (Fig. 8-41). Oblique shaft fractures, unicondylar articular fractures, and neck fractures are prime examples. Early follow-up to ensure maintenance of reduction is paramount if closed treatment is chosen. Displacement requires repeat manipulation and pin fixation. When in doubt, the digit should be examined carefully for malalignment and blocks to motion due to fracture displacement. Most of these fractures do best with pin fixation after acceptable reduction.

Late. Late complications include nonunion, malunion, osteonecrosis, growth disturbance, and arthritis. Nonunion is rare except in combined injuries with devascularization of the frac-

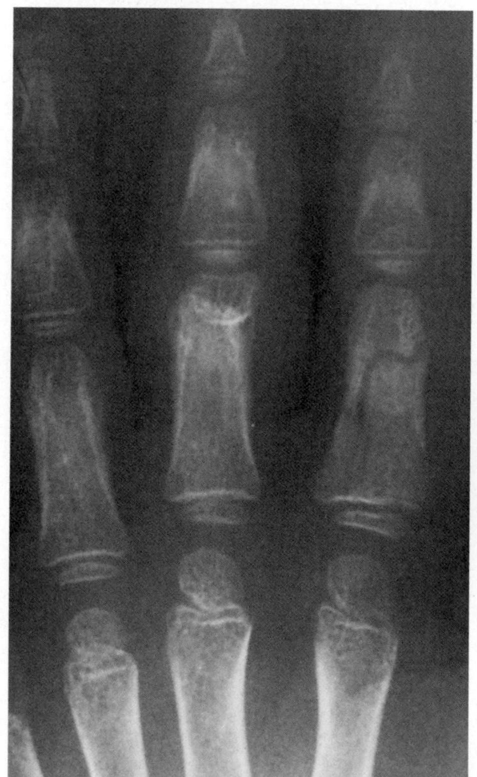

A

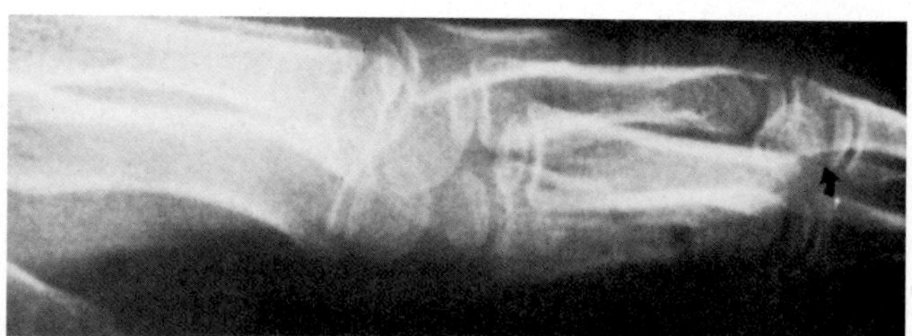

B

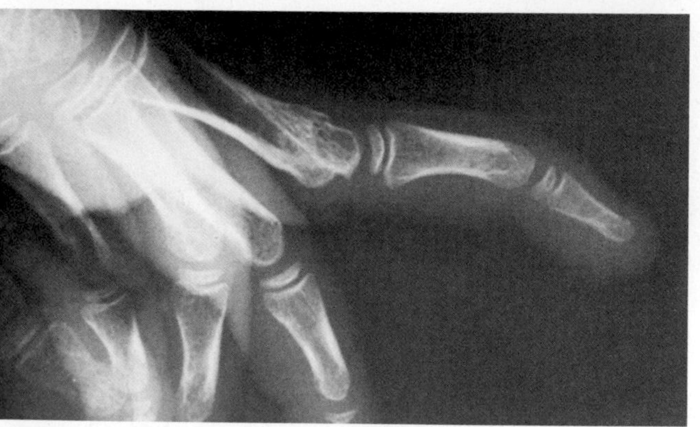

C

FIGURE 8-40 A. A 3-year-old girl sustained a fracture of the neck of the proximal phalanx of the index and middle fingers. The displaced fracture in the middle finger appears similar to an epiphysis at the distal end of the phalanx. **B.** No true lateral radiograph of the injured finger was obtained. Close scrutiny of this lateral view shows a dorsally displaced neck fracture, rotated almost 90 degrees (*arrow*). **C.** Eighteen months later, lateral radiograph reveals malunion with hyperextension of the PIP joint and loss of flexion.

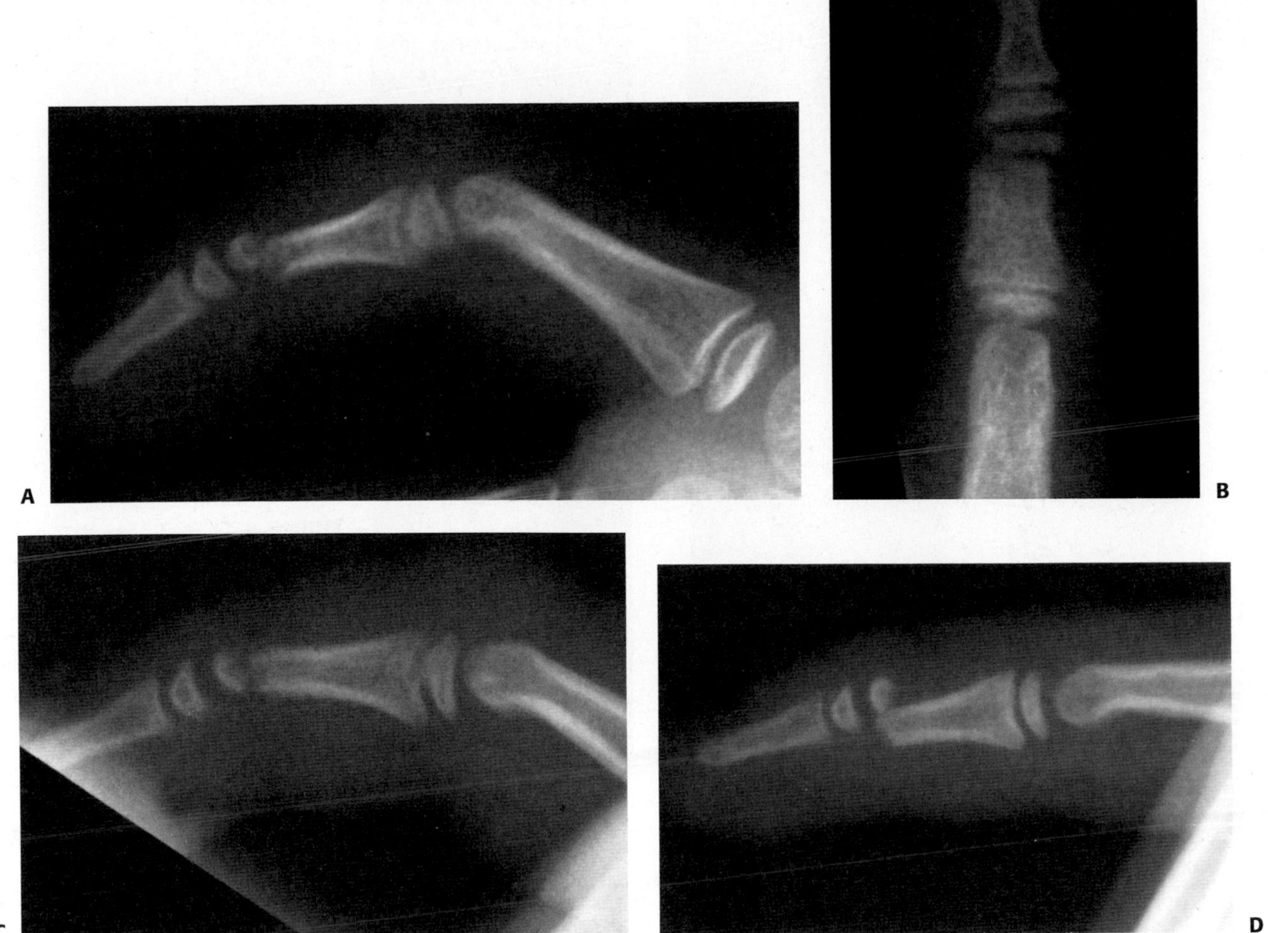

FIGURE 8-41 A,B. An 8-year-old girl with a mildly displaced fracture of the neck of the middle phalanx. **C.** Closed reduction was successful on the day of injury and a plaster splint was applied. **D.** Two weeks later, the fracture had markedly redisplaced.

ture fragments. Bone grafting is usually successful. Malunion can result in angulation or limited motion. Extra-articular malunion can cause angulation or rotational abnormalities. The treatment depends on the child's age and ability to remodel according to fracture location, plane of malunion, and degree of deformity (Fig. 8-42). Considerable deformity may require osteotomy to realign the bone.[67] A subcondylar or intra-articular malunion is particularly difficult to treat. Early diagnosis within the first month offers the possibility of fracture realignment through the site of deformity. Treatment of a late diagnosis must include consideration of the risks and benefits associated with extensive surgery.

Osteonecrosis usually is related to extensive fracture comminution, soft tissue injury, or surgical dissection of an intra-articular fracture. In severe cases, reconstruction is limited to some form of joint transfer. Growth disturbance can result from any injury that involves the physis. A shortened or angulated digit may result. It is fortunate that this complication is rare because reconstruction options for growth are limited. Malangulation is corrected by osteotomy.

Posttraumatic degenerative joint disease is rare in children, but intra-articular injury and sepsis may result in arthrosis. Treatment is directed toward the child's symptoms and not the radiographic findings. Minimal pain and excellent function often accompany considerable arthritic changes on radiographs and warrant no treatment. Pain and functional limitations require treatment; options include a vascularized joint transfer, interposition or distraction arthroplasty, prosthetic joint replacement, and arthrodesis.[174]

Fractures of the Metacarpals

Relevant Anatomy

The metacarpals are surrounded by soft tissue and are relatively protected within the hand. Considerable variation exists in the relative mobility of the metacarpals through the carpometacarpal (CMC) joints. The index and long rays have minimal CMC joint motion (10 to 20 degrees). In contrast, the ring and small rays possess more motion (30 to 40 degrees), and the thumb CMC joint has universal motion.

The neck is the most common site of metacarpal fracture. The metacarpal geometry and composition predispose the metacarpal neck to injury. The distal metacarpal angles as it approaches the MCP joint, and the cortical bone within the subcondylar fossa is relatively thin, which creates a vulnerable area susceptible to injury.

Mechanism of Injury

Direct trauma, rotational forces, and axial loading may all cause fractures of the metacarpal. Contact sports or striking an object are the most common mechanisms.

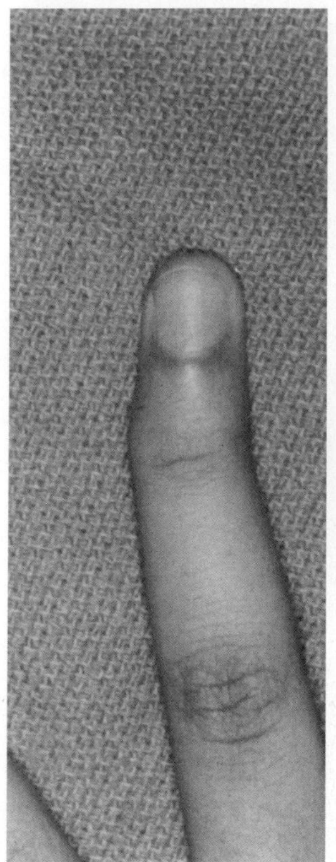

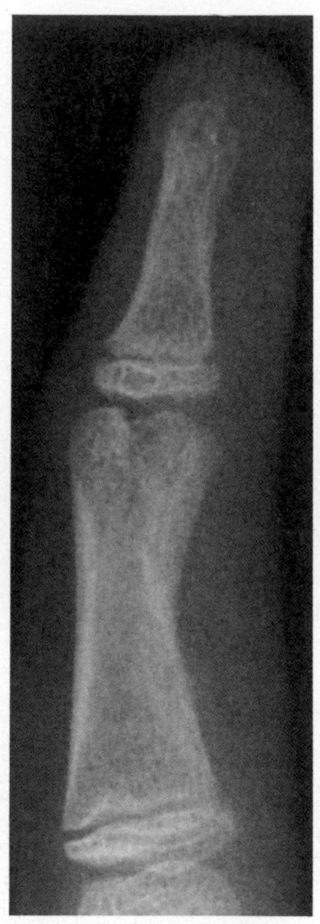

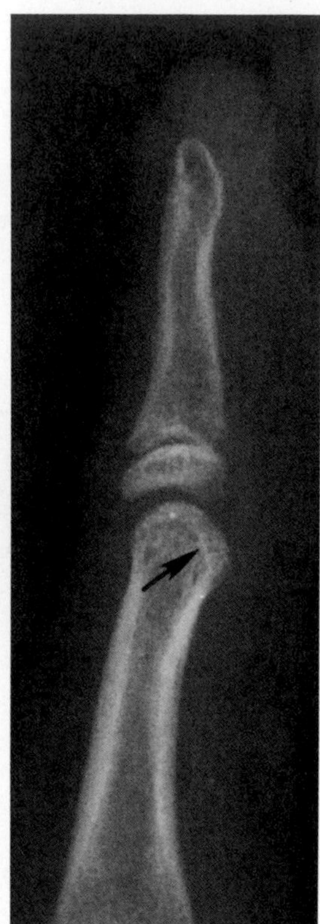

FIGURE 8-42 A. A 13-year-old boy with malunion of the ring finger middle phalanx articular surface. **B,C.** Radiographs reveal slight malunion of the radial condyle with mild intra-articular incongruity. The lateral view suggests a double density shadow (*arrow*). The flexion and extension motion of the digit was normal, and reconstruction was not recommended.

Fracture Patterns

Fractures of the metacarpals can occur at the epiphysis, physis, neck, shaft, or base (Table 8-4).

Epiphyseal and Physeal Fractures. Epiphyseal and physeal fractures of the metacarpal head are rare but occur most often in the small ray.[11,26,84,111] S-H II fractures of the small metacarpal are most common among patients 12 to 16 years of age.[111,122,140] Intra-articular, head-splitting fractures at the metacarpal epiphysis and physis consistent with S-H III and IV patterns seldom occur at the metacarpal level but are problematic when displaced (Fig. 8-43).

Metacarpal Neck Fractures. The metacarpal neck is the most frequent site of metacarpal fractures in children. Neck fractures in children are analogous to boxer's fractures in adults (Fig. 8-44). Neck fractures are more common in the small and ring fingers. Fortunately, these injuries are juxtaphyseal and have considerable remodeling potential.

Metacarpal Shaft Fractures. Metacarpal shaft fractures are relatively common. Torsional forces cause oblique and spiral fractures while direct trauma produces transverse fractures. An isolated shaft fracture of a central ray is suspended by the intermetacarpal ligaments, which limit displacement and shortening. In contrast, the border digits (index and small) displace more readily.

TABLE 8-4 Classification of Finger Metacarpal Fractures

Epiphyseal and physeal fractures
Neck fractures
Shaft fractures
Metacarpal base fractures

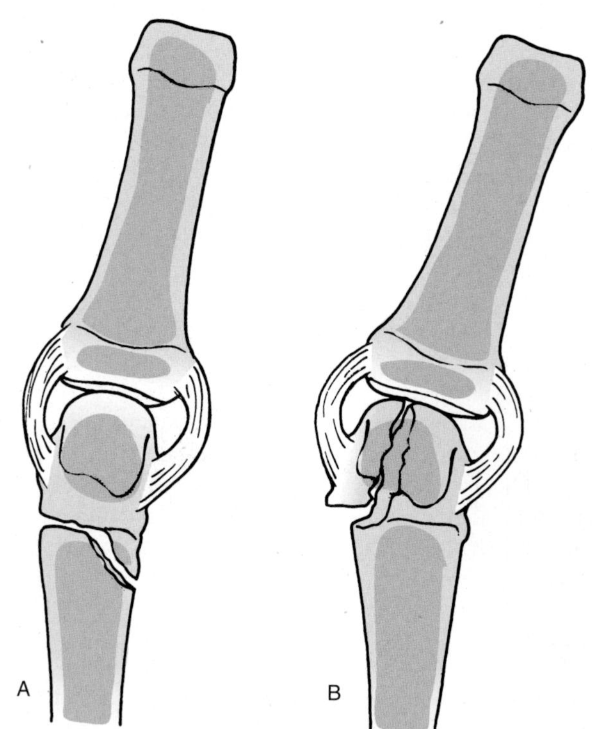

FIGURE 8-43 A. S-H type II fracture of the metacarpal head. **B.** Head-splitting fracture of the metacarpal epiphysis.

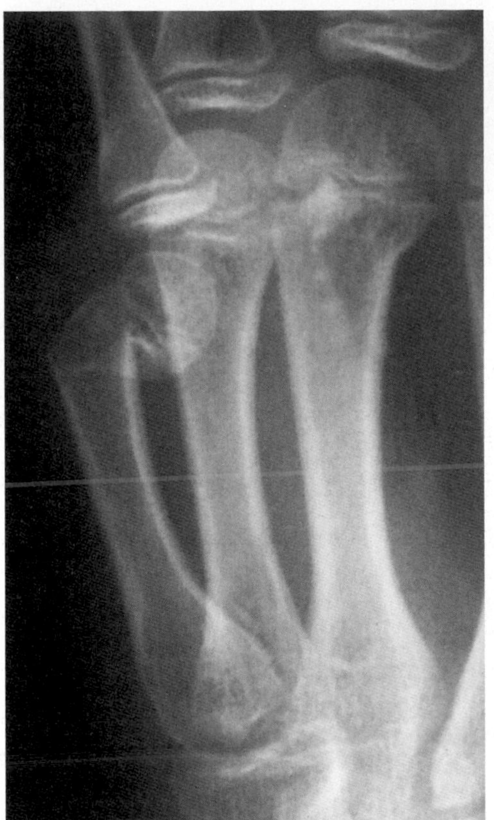
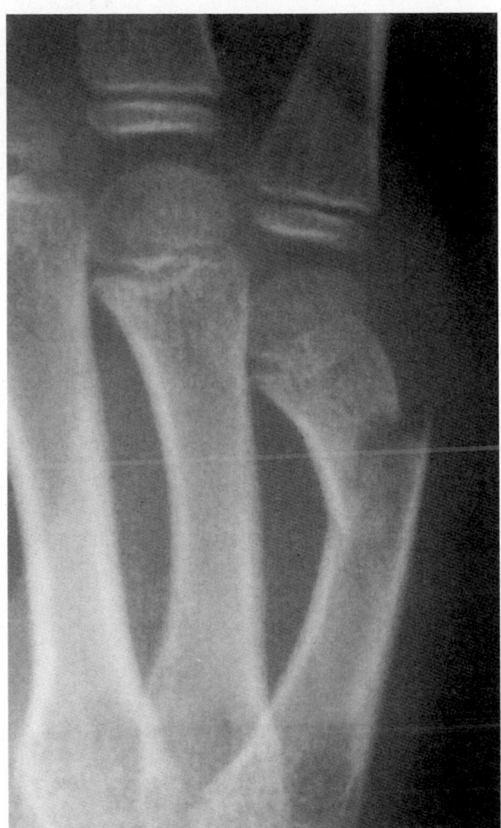

FIGURE 8-44 A. A true boxer's fracture of the metacarpal neck of the fifth ray. **B.** This fracture is more in the diaphysis and should not be considered a boxer's fracture.

Metacarpal Base Fractures. Metacarpal base fractures are uncommon in children. The base is protected from injury by its proximal location in the hand and the stability afforded by the bony congruence and soft tissue restraints. The small finger CMC joint is the most prone to injury. Fracture-dislocations of the small finger CMC joint are often unstable because of the proximal pull of the extensor carpi ulnaris (reverse Bennett fracture).

Diagnosis

Signs and Symptoms. The diagnosis of metacarpal fracture is based on the history and physical examination. Deformity and swelling may be hidden in the dorsal hand. The child usually avoids active movement and resists passive motion. Every metacarpal fracture must be examined for malrotation. Malrotation will result in digital scissoring during active flexion or an abnormal digital cascade with passive tenodesis.

Radiographic Findings. Metacarpal fractures usually are readily visible on radiographs. Anteroposterior and lateral views may be supplemented by an oblique view to assess fracture configuration. A metacarpal head splitting fracture may be difficult to detect and requires special views. The Brewerton view is helpful and is made with the dorsum of the hand against the cassette and the MCP joints flexed about 65 degrees. The central beam is angled 15 degrees to the ulnar side of the hand.[104] This projection focuses on the metacarpal heads and may highlight subtle bony abnormalities. MRI scans to assess articular alignment are diagnostic in complex injuries.

Treatment Options

The treatment of metacarpal fractures varies with the location, extent, and configuration of the fracture. Nonoperative or closed treatment is the primary mode of management for most fractures. Operative intervention is used for multiple metacarpal fractures, extensive soft tissue injury, intra-articular head splitting fractures, malrotated fractures, and irreducible fractures.

Epiphyseal and Physeal Fractures. Management is based on the amount of displacement and fracture stability. Many of these fractures can be treated by closed methods. Gentle reduction under metacarpal or wrist block anesthesia is followed by application of a splint in the safe position. If the fracture is reducible but unstable, percutaneous pin fixation is recommended. If the Thurston-Holland fragment is large enough, the wire can secure the metaphyseal piece and avoid the physis. Otherwise, the wire must cross the physis to obtain stability. A small-diameter smooth wire is advocated, and multiple passes should be avoided.

Displaced intra-articular head-splitting fractures require open reduction and internal fixation to restore articular congruity. Many of these fractures have unrecognized comminution that complicates internal fixation. Wire or screw fixation is used, depending on the age of the patient and size of the fragments. Transosseous suture repair may be necessary. Bone grafting may be necessary for stable reduction. The primary goal of surgical treatment is anatomic reduction of the joint. A secondary goal is stable fixation to allow early motion.

Neck Fracture. Metacarpal neck fractures usually are treated by closed methods. The amount of acceptable apex dorsal angulation is controversial. Greater angulation is allowable in the mobile ring and small rays compared to the index and long. Another consideration is the effect of remodeling over time, which is dependent on the age of the child. In general, 10 to 30 degrees of angulation greater than the corresponding CMC joint motion is acceptable.

Considerable angulation can be treated with closed reduction with local anesthesia or conscious sedation and splint or cast application. The Jahss maneuver is commonly recommended and involves initial flexion of the MCP joint to 90 degrees to relax the deforming force of the intrinsic muscles and tighten the collateral ligaments.[93] Subsequently, upward pressure is applied along the proximal phalanx to push the metacarpal head in a dorsal direction while counterpressure is applied along the dorsal aspect of the proximal metacarpal fracture. Jahss[93] suggested immobilization with the MCP and PIP joints flexed, but this type of immobilization is no longer advocated for fear of stiffness and skin breakdown. Immobilization in the intrinsic plus or safe position is the appropriate position. A well-molded splint or cast is necessary. Three-point modeling over the volar metacarpal head and proximal dorsal shaft is recommended. The PIP joints may or may not be included in the immobilization depending on the status of the reduction and reliability of the patient.

Uncommonly, a neck fracture may be extremely unstable and require percutaneous pinning (Fig. 8-45). Pins can be inserted in a variety of configurations. Extramedullary techniques include crossed pinning or pinning to the adjacent stable metacarpal. Intramedullary techniques also can be used, similar to those used for metacarpal shaft and neck fractures in adults.[57,68] Intramedullary techniques are reserved for patients near physeal closure. Prebent Kirschner wires or commercially available implants are inserted through the metacarpal base in an antegrade fashion. The wires can be used to assist in fracture reduction. Stability is obtained by stacking several wires within the canal and across the fracture site.

Open reduction of metacarpal neck fractures is seldom required in children and is reserved for irreducible fractures, unstable fractures in skeletally mature children, multiple metacarpal fractures, and combination injuries that require a stable bony platform.

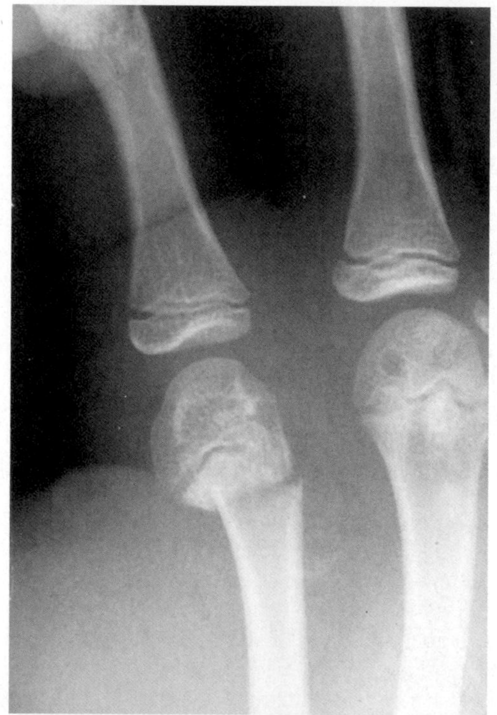
A

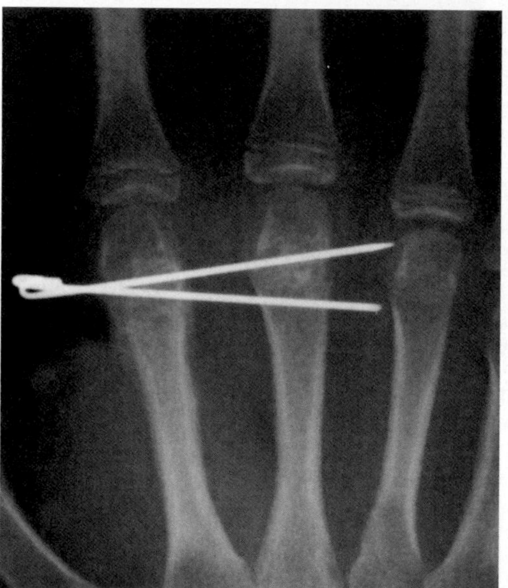
C

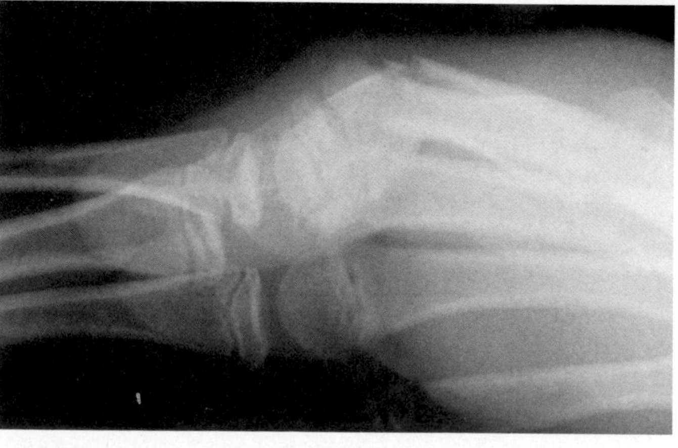
B

FIGURE 8-45 A,B. A 14-year-old boy with a dorsally angulated fracture of the second metacarpal. **C.** Closed reduction was unstable, and percutaneous Kirschner-wire fixation was performed. (Reprinted from O'Brien ET. Fractures of the hand. In: Green DP, ed. Operative Hand Surgery. 2nd ed. New York: Churchill Livingstone, 1988: 715–716, with permission.)

Shaft Fractures. An isolated long or ring metacarpal fracture is often minimally displaced because the metacarpals are suspended by the intermetacarpal ligaments. Immobilization for 4 weeks is usually all that is necessary. In contrast, the index and small digits may require additional treatment, such as closed reduction and immobilization. Percutaneous pinning is reserved for unstable shaft fractures (Fig. 8-46). Pins can be inserted with extramedullary or intramedullary techniques. Diaphyseal fractures are slower to heal and more prone to malunion than neck fractures.

Open reduction and internal fixation of a metacarpal shaft fracture are rarely indicated in children unless there are multiple fractures or extensive soft-tissue damage or the child is skeletally mature. However, a long spiral-oblique fracture with substantial malrotation and shortening may require miniscrew fixation to re-establish alignment.

Metacarpal Base Fractures. Fractures of the metacarpal base or fracture-dislocations at the CMC joint are usually high-energy injuries with substantial tissue disruption. Assessment for signs of compartment syndrome and careful neurovascular assessment are mandatory. Isolated fracture-dislocations of the small ray CMC joint are the most common metacarpal base fractures. CT scans may better define articular congruity and comminution. Closed reduction and percutaneous pinning are usually sufficient to restore alignment and to resist the deforming force of the extensor carpi ulnaris.[162] The pins can be placed transversely between the small and ring metacarpals and/or across the CMC joint.

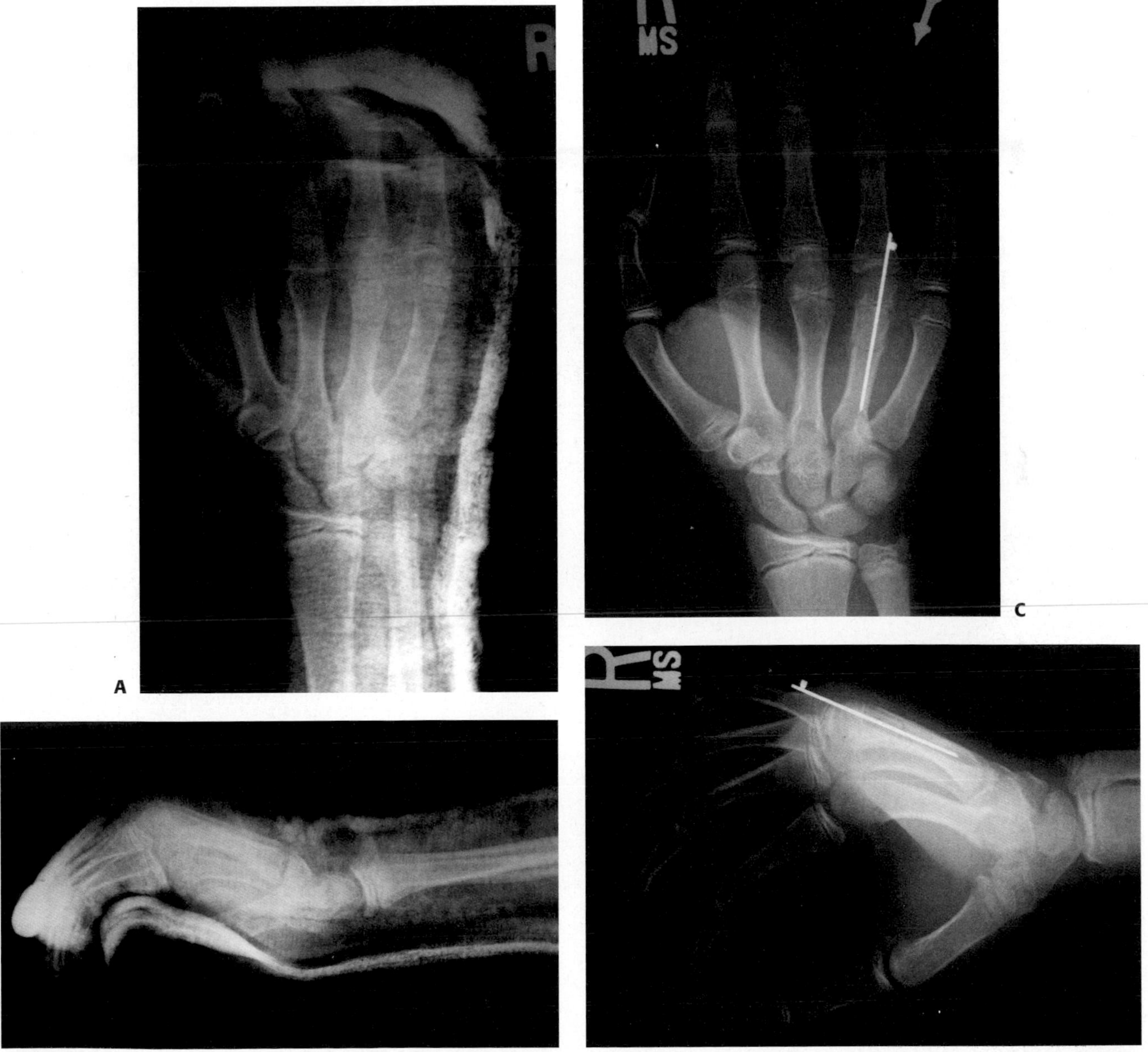

FIGURE 8-46 A 14 year-old boy with a reducible, but unstable, ring finger metacarpal shaft fracture. **A.** Anteroposterior radiograph appears reduced. **B.** Lateral radiograph with persistent apex dorsal angulation. **C.** Anteroposterior radiograph after closed reduction and percutaneous pinning. **D.** Lateral radiograph with anatomic alignment.

(continues)

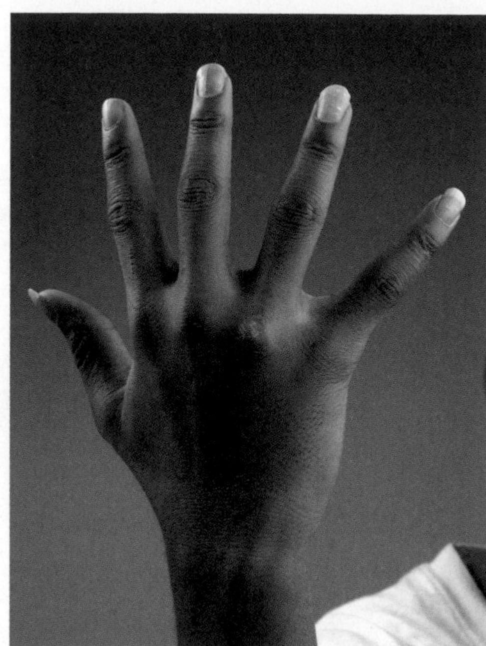

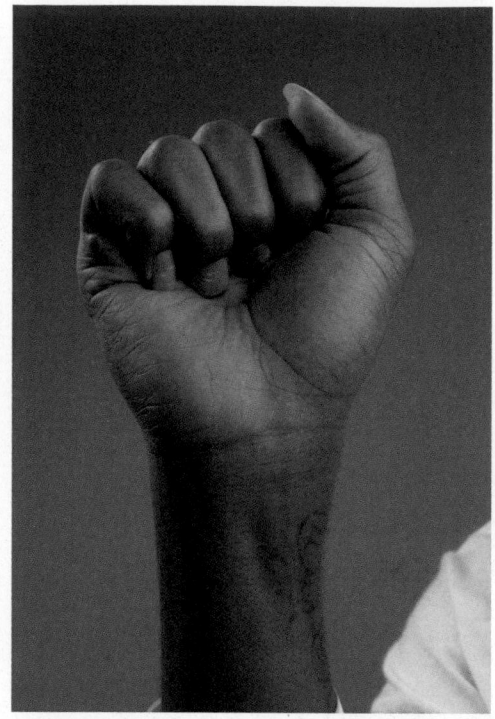

FIGURE 8-46 *(continued)* **E.** Full extension after pin removal and home therapy. **F.** Full flexion with normal digital cascade. (Courtesy of Shriners Hospitals for Children, Philadelphia, PA.)

Open reduction may be necessary to achieve reduction and ensure stable fixation in high-energy injuries. A transverse or longitudinal incision can be used for exposure. Longitudinal incisions are recommended in patients with concomitant compartment syndrome to allow for simultaneous decompression. Fixation options are numerous, depending on the fracture configuration. Supplemental bone graft may be necessary for substantial comminution. Late presentation is especially difficult. Treatment often requires open reduction or CMC arthrodesis (Fig. 8-47).

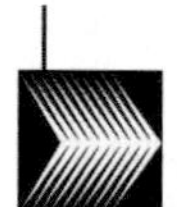

AUTHORS' PREFERRED TREATMENT

Epiphyseal and Physeal Fractures

Most nondisplaced physeal fractures are treated with immobilization. S-H II metacarpal neck fractures seldom require reduction. These fractures typically occur in adolescents who possess enough remodeling to accept 30 to 35 degrees of sagittal angulation as long as rotation is acceptable and there is sufficient growth remaining. A widely displaced fracture that is reducible requires percutaneous pinning to maintain the reduction. Displaced epiphyseal fractures with considerable intra-articular displacement require open reduction and internal fixation through a dorsal approach and splitting of the extensor apparatus over the MCP joint. Anatomic reduction of the articular surface is the objective, and fixation devices vary according to the patient and fracture configuration.

Metacarpal Neck Fractures

Nonoperative and closed methods are the mainstays of treatment. Considerable sagittal angulation is acceptable, especially in the ring and small digits. Small finger angulation up to 30 degrees usually does not necessitate closed reduction as long as there is no malrotation and there is sufficient growth remaining. Greater angulations are treated with closed reduction and cast application. Index and ring finger angulations of more than 20 degrees are treated by closed reduction. Pin fixation is used for unstable fractures that have a tendency to redisplace. Open reduction rarely is necessary.

Metacarpal Shaft Fractures

The number, configuration, and location of the metacarpal shaft fracture(s) dictate treatment. Isolated fractures that are minimally displaced require only immobilization. Isolated fractures that are displaced or malrotated require closed reduction and percutaneous fixation. Rotation is carefully assessed to ensure adequate reduction. An irreducible fracture or multiple fractures usually require open reduction (see Fig. 8-46). The fixation technique varies according to the age of the child and fracture pattern. If open fixation is necessary, stable fixation is the goal. Miniplate and screw fixation is preferred to restore alignment and to allow early mobilization of tendons and soft tissue. The physis should be avoided during plate application to prevent growth disturbance. The operative approach and internal fixation principles are similar in children and adults. Long oblique fractures are managed with interfragmentary screw fixation. Short oblique and transverse fractures require a neutralization plate with purchase of four cortices proximal and distal to the fracture.

Metacarpal Base Fractures

Metacarpal base fractures often are displaced or unstable. Extra-articular fractures can be treated by closed reduction with or without percutaneous pinning. Intra-articular frac-

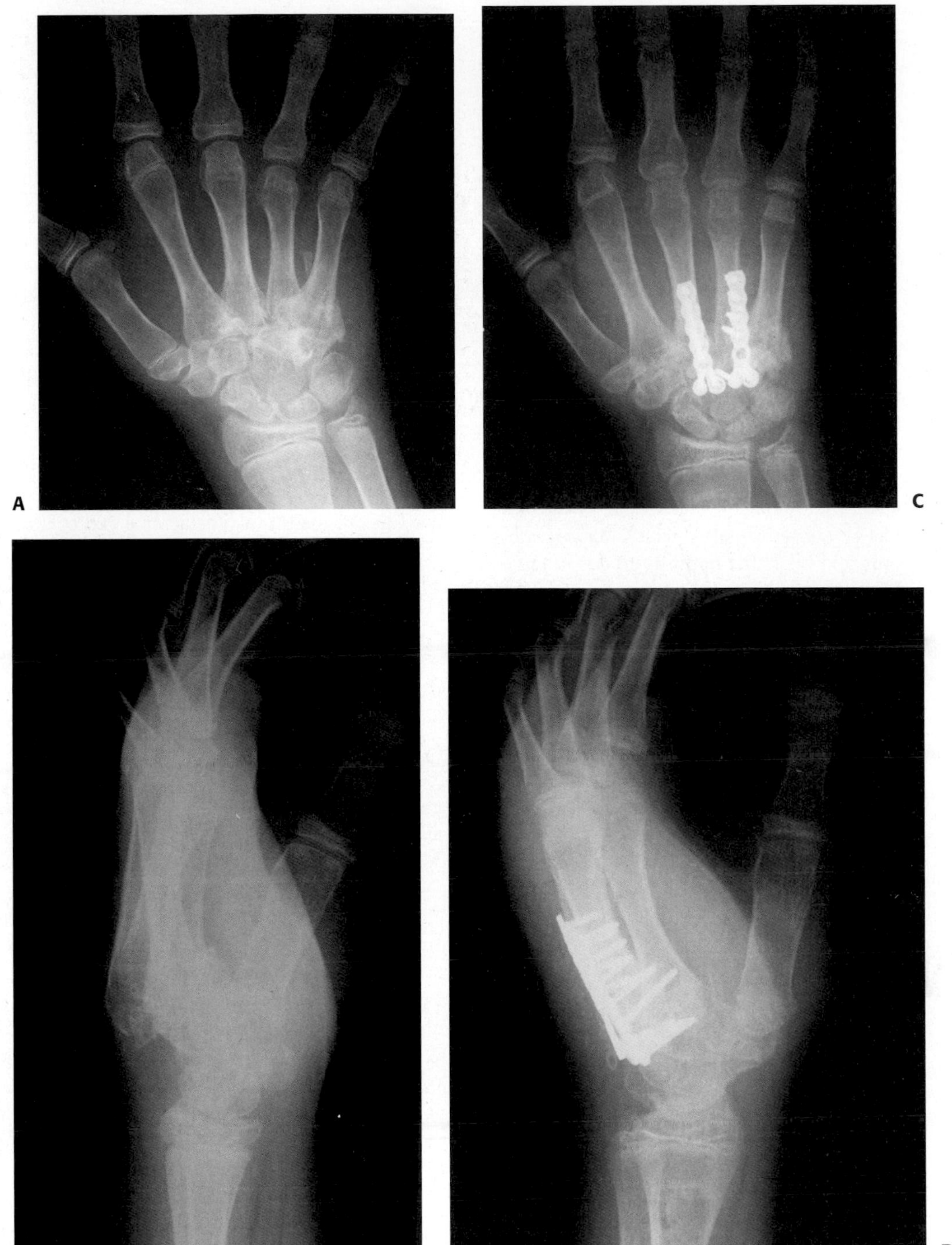

FIGURE 8-47 A 15-year-old boy with crush injury of the right hand requiring compartment release. He presented 6 weeks later with persistent pain and limited motion. **A.** Anteroposterior radiograph with overlapping long, ring, and small CMC joints **B.** Lateral radiographs show fracture-dislocations of long, ring, and small CMC joints. **C.** Postoperative anteroposterior radiograph after reduction and CMC fusion using mini-plates. **D.** Lateral radiograph after reduction and CMC fusion. (Courtesy of Shriners Hospitals for Children, Philadelphia, PA.)

ture-dislocations are more challenging. Percutaneous pinning is often required to stabilize the fracture and to reduce CMC joint subluxation. The wires are placed between the bases of the adjacent metacarpals or across the CMC joint in isolated injuries. Irreducible or multiple fracture-dislocations require open reduction. Late presentation with symptomatic degenerative changes requires CMC arthrodesis (see Fig. 8-47).

Postoperative Care and Rehabilitation

Most metacarpal fractures managed by closed treatment are immobilized for 4 weeks. Subsequently, a home program of range-of-motion exercises is started and formal therapy is not needed. In active children and young athletes, a light splint can be worn for protection and as a peer warning signal for an additional few weeks. If percutaneous pin fixation is used, the wires are removed in the office 4 weeks after surgery.

Rehabilitation of open fracture reduction depends on the stability of the fixation and the dependability of the patient. Older and reliable patients with stable internal fixation are mobilized earlier, usually 5 to 7 days after surgery. A removable splint for protection between exercise sessions is used for 4 to 6 weeks.

Prognosis

Most metacarpal fractures heal without substantial sequelae. Mild deformity in the plane of motion is tolerated and may correct with remodeling. Considerable angulation or rotation creates a functional impairment that requires treatment.

Complications

Bony complications include malunion and osteonecrosis (Table 8-5). Nonunion is rare.[92,140] Even a small amount (less than 10 degrees) of rotational malalignment may create overlap of the digits during flexion and a functional disturbance (Fig. 8-48). Corrective osteotomy to realign the digit is often necessary. The osteotomy for rotational correction can be made at the site of fracture or anywhere along the metacarpal. The proximal shaft or base has certain advantages. This area provides ample bone for healing and offers the opportunity for internal fixation using wires or a plate. Diaphyseal malunions with symptomatic flexion deformity into the palm require a dorsal wedge osteotomy and internal fixation.

Osteonecrosis of the metacarpal head may occur after an intra-articular fracture. Factors include the degree of injury and the intracapsular pressure caused by the hemarthrosis.[39,122,151] Theoretically, early joint aspiration may diminish the intra-articular pressure. Fortunately, partial osteonecrosis in a growing child incites remarkable remodeling of the adjacent articular surface and often results in a functional joint. Part-time splint protection during the remodeling phase is recommended. Considerable joint incongruity is rare, and reconstruction options are limited.[174]

Fractures of the Thumb Metacarpal

Relevant Anatomy

The adductor pollicis, abductor pollicis longus, and thenar muscles play a role in fracture mechanics and can displace metacarpal fractures. Their directions of pull dictate the direction of fracture displacement and deformity. The adductor pollicis inserts onto the proximal phalanx and into the extensor apparatus through the adductor aponeurosis. Epiphyseal fragments of the proximal phalanx base with the attached ulnar collateral ligament (UCL) can displace outside the adductor aponeurosis.[183]

TABLE 8-5 Adverse Factors for Finger Metacarpal Fractures

Epiphyseal and physeal fractures
Osteonecrosis, malreduction/malunion
Neck fractures
Excessive apex dorsal angulation, malrotation
Shaft fractures
Malrotation, soft tissue interposition, nonunion
Metacarpal base fractures
Loss of reduction, malreduction of articular fragments, late instability

This pediatric "Stener lesion" prohibits healing and requires open reduction. The abductor pollicis longus inserts onto the metacarpal base and is the primary deforming force in most fracture-dislocations about the thumb CMC joint (Bennett fractures or pediatric equivalents).

Mechanism of Injury

Direct trauma, rotational forces, and axial loading may all cause thumb metacarpal fractures. Sporting endeavors are the prime events causing fractures. A valgus force to the MCP joint usually produces an epiphyseal fracture. Skiing and extreme biking are specific activities that place the thumb MCP joint and metacarpal shaft in a vulnerable position. Adduction forces, such as direct trauma to a soccer goalie or basketball player during a fall or ball injury, place the thumb CMC joint and base of thumb metacarpal at risk.

Fracture Patterns

Fractures of the thumb metacarpal can occur at the epiphysis, physis, neck, shaft, or base. Fractures of the neck and shaft and their treatment principles are similar to those of the fingers (Table 8-6). Thumb metacarpal base fractures that involve the physis or epiphysis require particular mention (Fig. 8-49).

Thumb Metacarpal Base Fractures. Fractures of the base of the thumb metacarpal are subdivided according to their location. Type A fractures occur between the physis and the junction of the proximal and middle thirds of the bone. They often are transverse or slightly oblique. There often is an element of medial impaction, and the fracture is angulated in an apex lateral direction (Fig. 8-50).

Type B and C fractures are S-H II fractures at the thumb metacarpal base. Most patterns have the metaphyseal fragment on the medial side (type B) (see Fig. 8-49). The shaft fragment is adducted by the pull of the adductor pollicis and shifted in a proximal direction by the pull of the abductor pollicis longus. Although this pattern resembles a Bennett fracture with respect to the deforming forces, there is no intra-articular extension.[13] Type C fractures are the least common and have the reverse pattern, with the metaphyseal fragment on the lateral side and the proximal shaft displacement in a medial direction. This pattern often results from more substantial trauma and does not lend itself to closed treatment.

A type D fracture is a S-H III or IV fracture that most closely resembles the adult Bennett fracture.[17,61,70,167] The deforming forces are similar to a type B injury with resultant adduction and proximal migration of the base-shaft fragment.

Diagnosis

Signs and Symptoms. The diagnosis of thumb metacarpal fracture usually is straightforward. Swelling and ecchymosis are obvious signs of injury. Most of the swelling appears about the thenar eminence and at times can be marked. Active thumb motion is limited, and passive thumb movement is painful. The thumb may appear angulated or rotated. However, thumb motion is oriented differently than finger movement, which makes angulation and malrotation more difficult to judge.

Radiographic Findings. Biplanar images of the thumb are mandatory. Anteroposterior and lateral views of the thumb and not

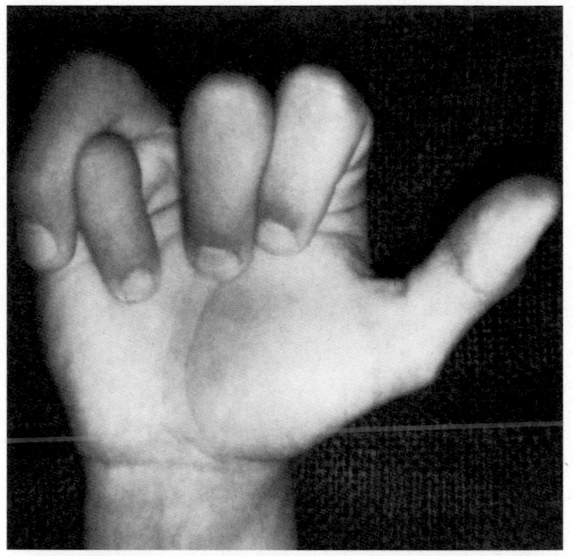

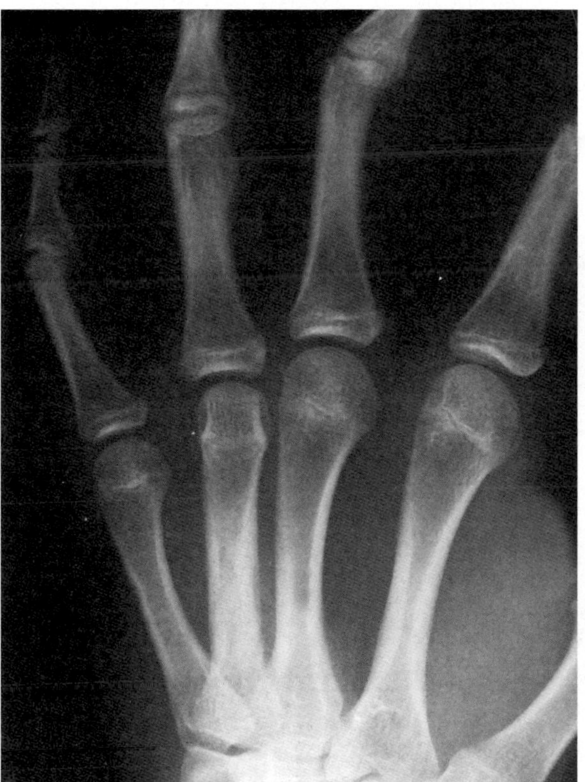

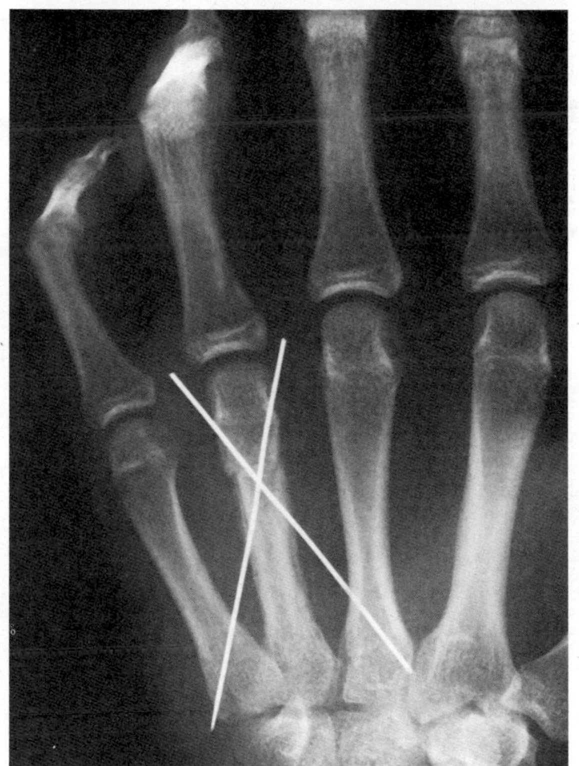

FIGURE 8-48 A,B. A 15-year-old boy with severe overlapping of the ring finger on the little finger secondary to rotatory malunion of a spiral fracture of the ring metacarpal. **C.** Distal osteotomy through the deformity stabilized with pin fixation to correct the malrotation. (Reprinted from O'Brien ET. Fractures of the hand. In: Green DP, ed. Operative Hand Surgery. 2nd ed. New York: Churchill Livingstone, 1988:731, with permission.)

TABLE 8-6 Classification of Thumb Metacarpal Fractures

Fractures of the head

Fractures of the shaft

Fractures of the thumb metacarpal base
- Fractures distal to the physis
- S-H II fractures—metaphyseal medial
- S-H II fractures—metaphyseal lateral

Intra-articular S-H III or IV fractures

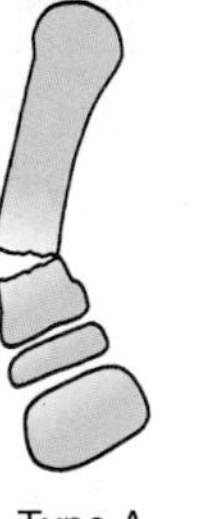

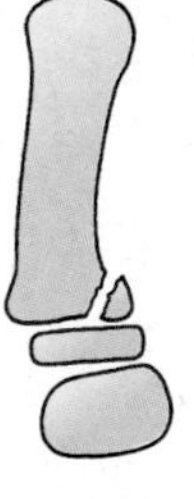

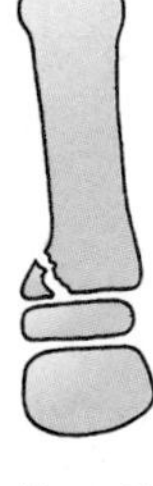

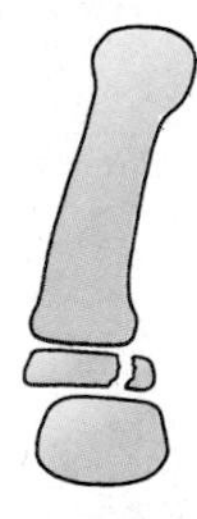

FIGURE 8-49 Classification of thumb metacarpal fractures. Type A: Metaphyseal fracture. Types B and C: S-H type II physeal fractures with lateral or medial angulation. Type D: S-H type III fracture (pediatric Bennett fracture).

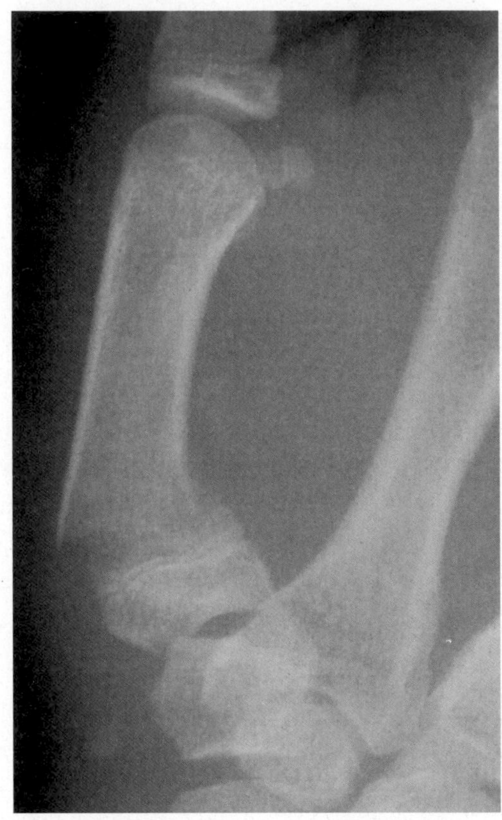

FIGURE 8-50 Metaphyseal thumb metacarpal fracture that does not involve the physis. Treatment consisted of closed reduction and cast immobilization.

the fingers are required. Biplanar radiographs ensure adequate evaluation of fracture position. A hyperpronated view of the thumb accentuates the view of the CMC joint.

Treatment Options

Thumb Metacarpal Base Fractures.

Type A. Type A fractures usually can be treated by closed methods. Although swelling about the thenar eminence limits manipulation of the fracture and diminishes the effectiveness of immobilization, most fractures can still be treated successfully by closed reduction and immobilization. The CMC joint has near universal motion, and the physis is proximal in the metacarpal, so remodeling is extensive in young patients. If reduction is attempted, pressure is applied to the apex of the fracture to affect reduction. Anatomic reduction is not required because remodeling is plentiful.[102,140] Unstable fractures with marked displacement require percutaneous pin fixation to maintain alignment (Fig. 8-51).

Types B and C. Closed reduction is more difficult for type B and C fractures. The mobility of the metacarpal base and the swelling make closed reduction difficult. Comminution, soft tissue interposition, or transperiosteal "buttonholing" in type C fractures may further complicate reduction.[207] If closed reduction is accomplished and stable, then short-arm thumb spica splint or cast immobilization is possible. Repeat radiographic evaluation should be obtained 5 to 7 days later to ensure maintenance of reduction.[11]

If closed reduction is possible but the reduction is unstable, percutaneous pinning is recommended (Fig. 8-52). There are multiple options for pin configuration including direct fixation across the fracture, pinning across the reduced CMC joint, and pinning between the first and second metacarpals. Open reduction is indicated for irreducible fractures. Type C fractures may

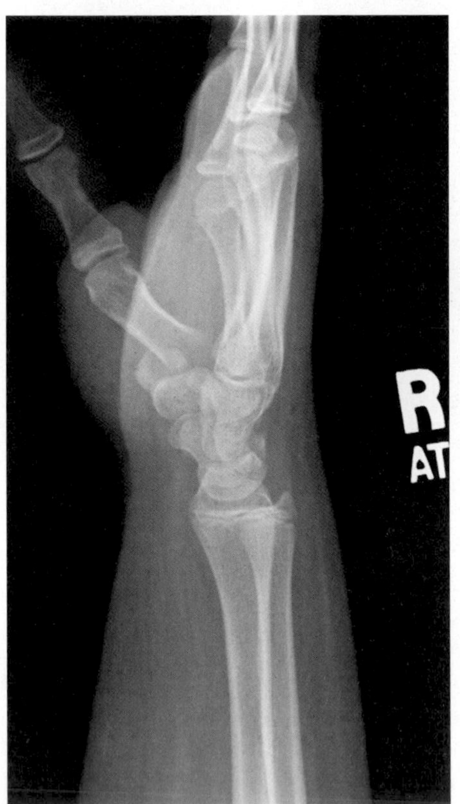

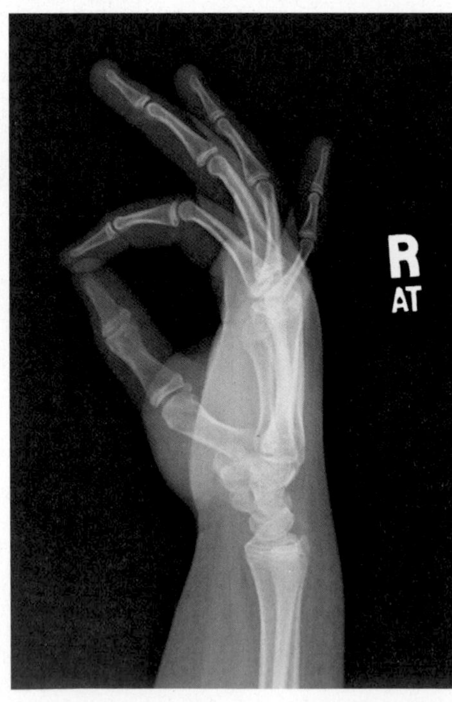

FIGURE 8-51 A 13-year-old boy fell down stairs and injured his right thumb **A.** Anteroposterior radiograph with displaced fracture base of the thumb metacarpal **B.** Lateral radiograph shows considerable angulation. *(continues)*

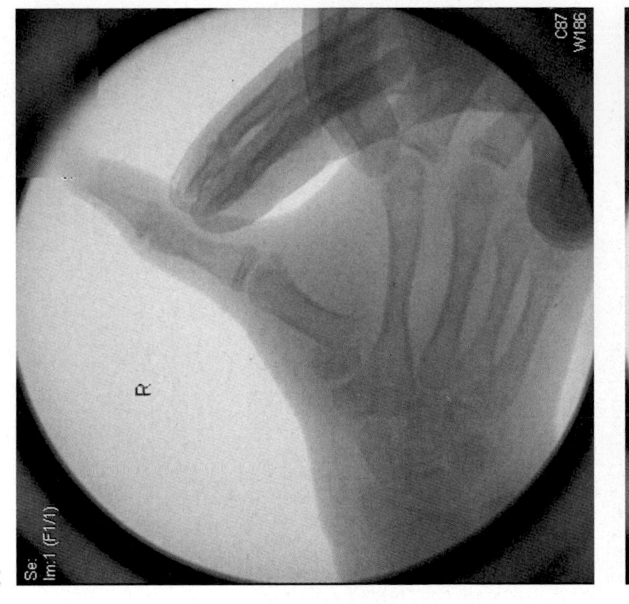

C

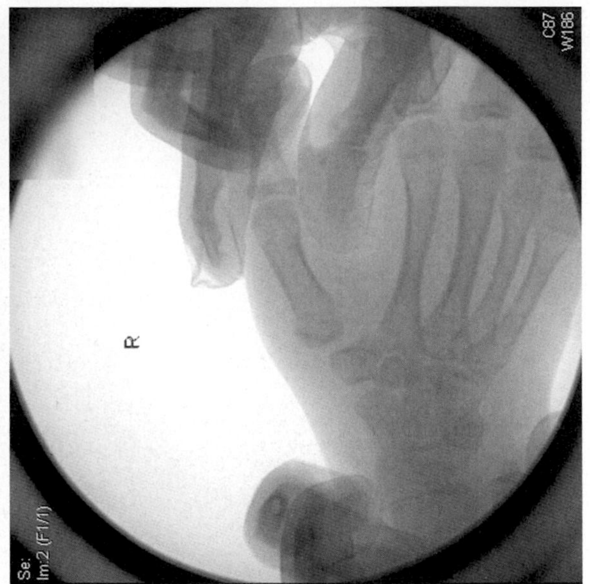

D

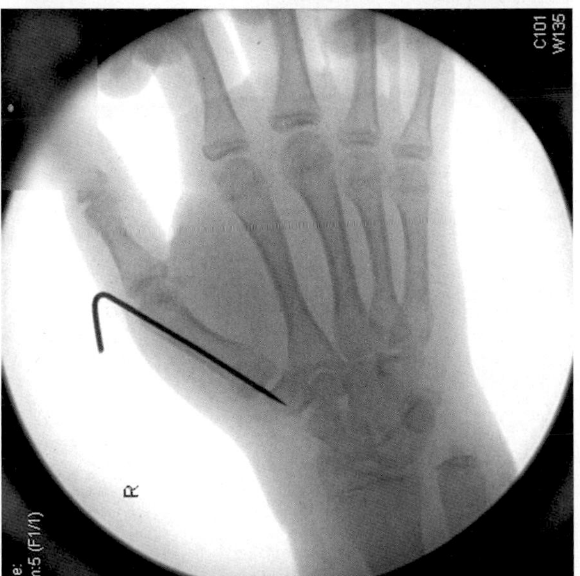

E

FIGURE 8-51 *(continued)* **C.** At time of reduction, fracture was very unstable. **D.** Closed reduction under fluoroscopy **E.** Percutaneous pin fixation to maintain alignment. (Courtesy of Shriners Hospitals for Children, Philadelphia, PA.)

require open reduction to remove any interposed periosteum that blocks reduction (Fig. 8-53).[25,207]

Type D. Type D fractures are unstable and require closed or open reduction to restore physeal and articular alignment.[61,76] An acceptable closed reduction is maintained by percutaneous pin fixation. An unacceptable closed reduction is rare but requires open reduction and fixation.[167] The choice of implant must be individualized, although smooth wires are favored to minimize potential injury to the physis and articular cartilage (Fig. 8-54).[70,167] Skeletal traction is an alternative treatment for complex injuries with severe bony or soft tissue damage.[23,178]

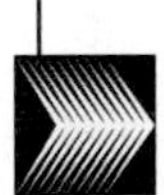

AUTHORS' PREFERRED TREATMENT

Type A

Type A fractures usually can be treated with closed reduction and cast application. Residual angulation between 20 to 30 degrees is acceptable depending on the age of the child and clinical appearance of the thumb. The multiplanar motion of the CMC joint combined with the potential for remodeling makes this degree of angulation inconsequential. Fractures that are reducible, but unstable, require percutaneous pinning (see Fig. 8-51).

Types B and C

Treatment varies with the amount of displacement and degree of periosteal disruption. Mild angulation requires only cast application without reduction. Moderate angulation is treated with closed reduction and immobilization. Severe angulation usually is combined with displacement and requires reduction. A successful closed reduction is often augmented with percutaneous pin fixation due to fracture instability. An unsuccessful closed reduction requires open reduction and fixation.

Type D

Displaced S-H III and IV fractures are rare and require closed or open reduction and internal fixation. The goal is anatomic

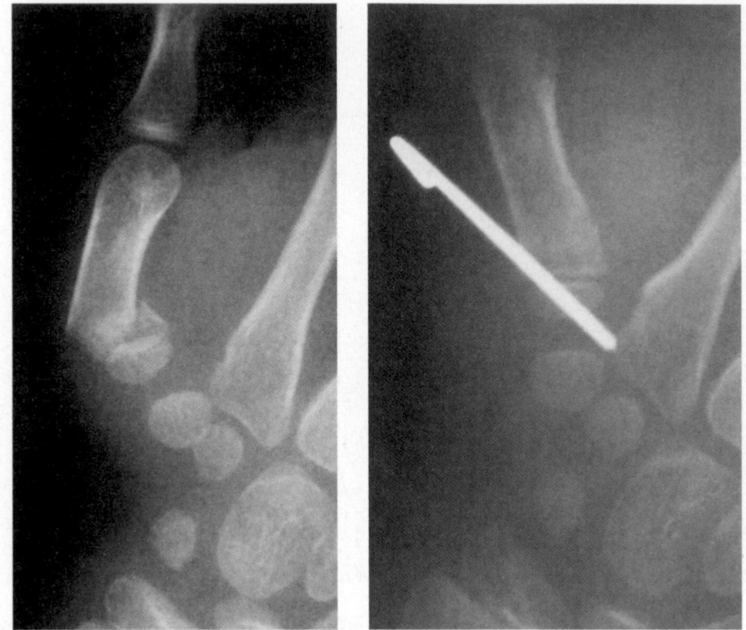

FIGURE 8-52 A. An 8-year-old boy with reducible, but unstable, fracture. **B.** A single percutaneous pin was placed to maintain alignment.

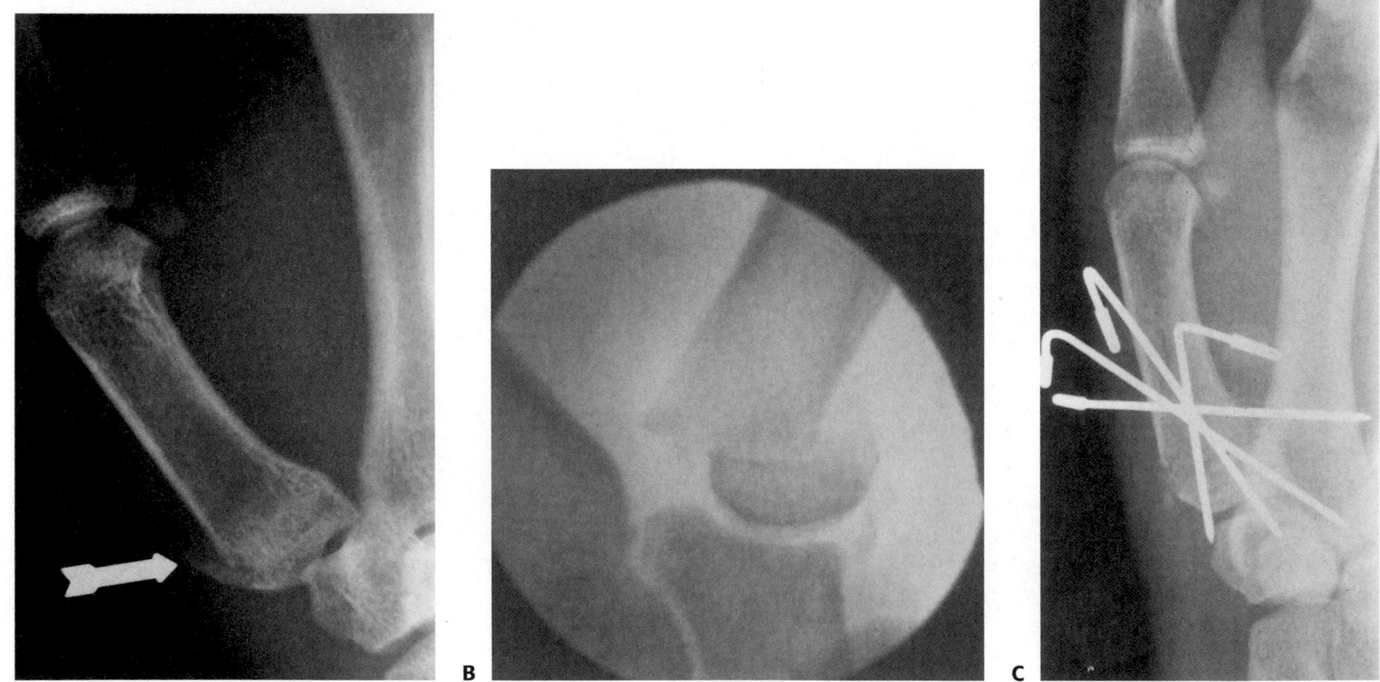

FIGURE 8-53 A. Fracture of the thumb metacarpal base with small lateral metaphyseal flag that appears innocuous on radiograph (*arrow*). **B.** However, additional images revealed marked displacement of the distal fragment. **C.** Closed reduction was unsuccessful, because of interposed tissue. After open reduction, Kirschner wires were used to stabilize the fracture.

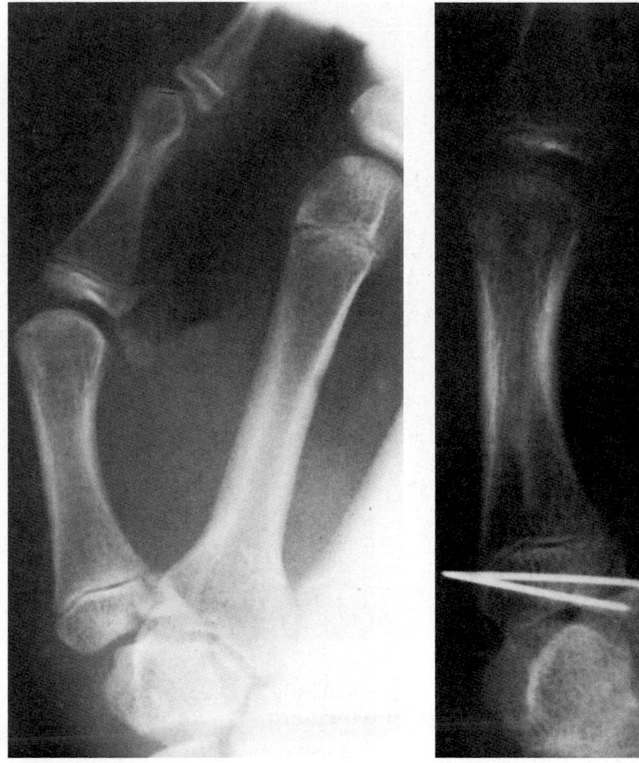

FIGURE 8-54 A. A 14-year-old boy sustained a S-H type III fracture of the proximal thumb metacarpal with lateral subluxation of the carpometacarpal joint. **B.** Open reduction and Kirschner-wire fixation to restore joint alignment and congruity. (Reprinted from O'Brien FT. Fractures of the hand. In: Green DP, ed. Operative Hand Surgery. 2nd ed. New York: Churchill Livingstone, 1988:769, with permission.)

alignment of the joint and physis. If an open reduction is required, the preferred approach is through a gently curved incision overlying the CMC joint along the glabrous border of the skin. The cutaneous nerves are protected. The origins of the thenar eminence muscles are reflected. A CMC joint arthrotomy is made and the articular surface is exposed. The fracture joint surface is reduced and fixed with pins or miniscrews. Additional percutaneous pin fixation of the first to second metacarpal is used to protect the fracture fixation.

Postoperative Care and Rehabilitation

Closed treatment requires immobilization for 4 to 6 weeks, depending on the fracture severity and degree of soft tissue damage. A home program for range of motion is started thereafter. Formal therapy is not instituted unless considerable soft tissue injury occurred. In active children and young athletes, a light splint may be worn for protection for an additional few weeks.

Open fracture management depends on the stability of the fixation and the reliability of the patient. Young children or marginal fixations require 4 to 6 weeks of immobilization. Fracture union with mild stiffness takes precedence over fracture nonunion with excessive motion. Adolescents with stable fixation can be mobilized earlier, usually 5 to 7 days after surgery, provided they are trustworthy in terms of activity restrictions. A removable splint is used for protection between exercise sessions until union.

Prognosis

Thumb metacarpal fractures usually heal without altering hand function. The remodeling capabilities of fractures near or involving the physis are extensive. The basilar thumb joint also allows multiplanar motion and can accommodate moderate fracture malunion. Residual deformity along the thumb metacarpal can be concealed through CMC joint motion, and the thumb tolerates malrotation better than the fingers (Fig.8-55).

Complications

Complications are uncommon. Nonunion, malunion, and articular incongruity are potential problems.[76] Intra-articular incongruity may occur after incomplete reduction of intra-articular fractures or inadequate fixation after satisfactory reduction. Sequelae include pain, diminished motion, and arthrosis. Fortunately, the occurrence of articular malunion and the development of symptoms are uncommon. Available treatment options are limited and include fusion or interposition arthroplasty.

CARPAL INJURIES IN CHILDREN

Epidemiology

Fractures and dislocations about the child's carpus are rare compared to injuries of the adjacent physis of the distal radius.[131,210]

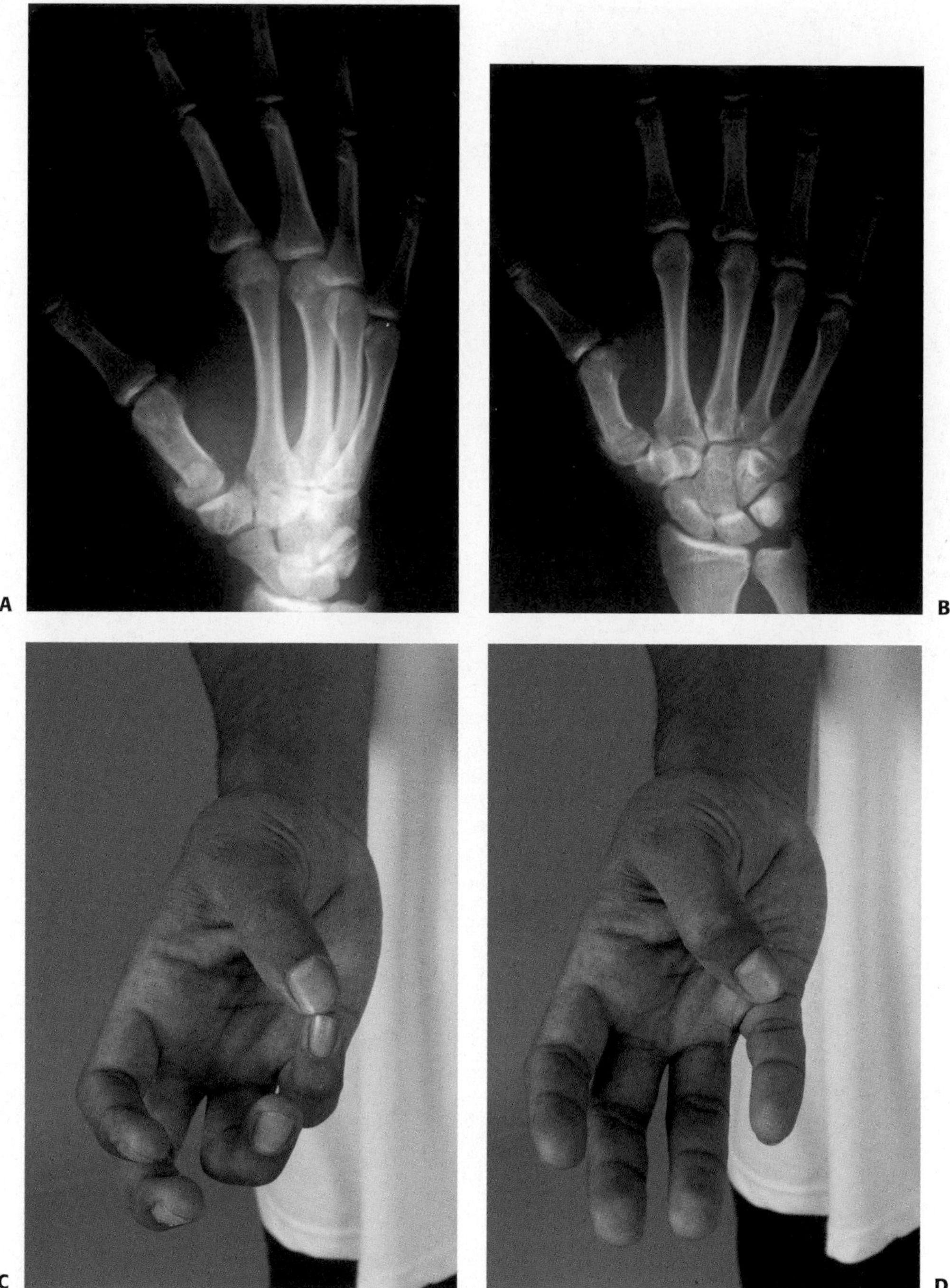

FIGURE 8-55 A 14-year-old boy presents 3 weeks after injury with mild pain and deformity base of right thumb **A.** Anteroposterior radiograph shows moderately displaced fracture base of the thumb metacarpal **B.** Lateral radiograph shows mild angulation. **C.** Follow-up motion after splinting for an additional 2 weeks, and home therapy reveals excellent opposition. **D.** Thumb able to touch base of small finger. (Courtesy of Shriners Hospitals for Children, Philadelphia, PA.)

The detection of injuries to the immature carpus is problematic because of the difficulties in examining an injured child and the limited ability of radiographs to detail the immature skeleton.[11,136,159]

Anatomy

Ossification of the Carpus

The fetal wrist begins as a single cartilaginous mass. By the tenth week of gestation, the carpus transforms into eight distinct entities with definable intercarpal separations. Although there are some minor changes in contour, these precursors greatly resemble the individual carpal bones in their mature form.[109]

The carpal bones ossify in a predictable pattern with only slight variations (Fig. 8-56).[75,188] The capitate is the first bone to ossify, usually within the first few months of life. The pattern of ossification proceeds in a clockwise fashion. The hamate appears next, usually at about 4 months of age. The triquetrum appears during the second year, and the lunate begins ossification around the fourth year. The scaphoid begins to ossify in

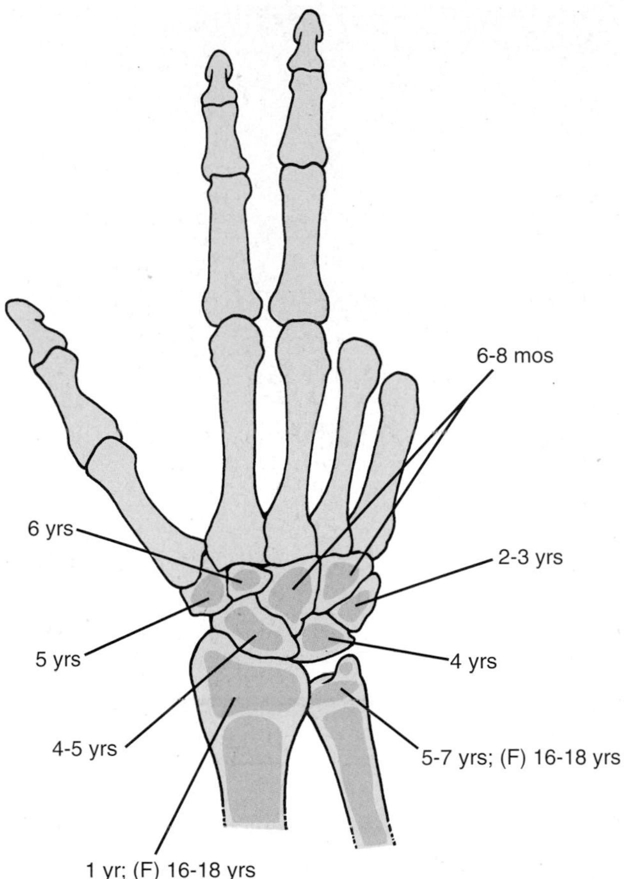

FIGURE 8-56 The age at the time of appearance of the ossific nucleus of the carpal bones and distal radius and ulna. The ossific nucleus of the pisiform (not shown) appears at about 6 to 8 years of age.

the fifth year, usually slightly predating the appearance of the trapezium.[105] Scaphoid ossification begins at the distal aspect and progresses proximally.[140] The trapezium and trapezoid ossify in the fifth year, with the trapezoid lagging slightly behind. The ossification pattern usually concludes with the pisiform in the ninth or tenth year. The scaphoid, trapezoid, lunate, trapezium, and pisiform may demonstrate multiple centers of ossification.[114,140] Although these variations are well recognized, they may be confused with acute trauma by the uninitiated observer.

The ossific nucleus is cloaked in a cartilaginous cover during development. This arrangement is thought to provide a unique shelter from injury.[11,70] This observation is supported by epidemiologic studies of scaphoid fractures that highlight the infrequent incidence in children younger than 7 years of age and the marked increase in teenagers.[74,105]

SPECIFIC CARPAL FRACTURES

Scaphoid Fractures

Epidemiology

The scaphoid is the most frequently injured carpal bone in children.[11,30,74] Pediatric scaphoid fractures have a peak incidence between the ages of 12 and 15 years.[52] Scaphoid fractures are extremely rare during the first decade of life.[16,58,74,105,149,158,172,177,195] Only a few reported cases involve children younger than 8 years of age, and the youngest patient reported is 4 years of age.[52]

Mechanism of Injury: Differences in Children

The low incidence of scaphoid fracture in children is most likely related to the thick peripheral cartilage that covers and protects the ossification center. Therefore, fracture requires a considerable force to disrupt this cartilaginous shell and injure the underlying bone.[41] The pattern of pediatric scaphoid injury differs from that of adults because of the evolving changes in the ossification center.[52] During early stages of ossification, the scaphoid is more susceptible to avulsion fractures about the distal pole fracture.[180,195] As the ossification progresses from distal to proximal, the fracture pattern mirrors the adult forms by early adolescence (Fig. 8-57).

In children, fractures of the distal third of the scaphoid have traditionally been the most common injury pattern and often result from direct trauma.[16,41,195] However, scaphoid waist fractures are increasing in frequency in younger children as participation in contact athletics begins earlier. Proximal pole fractures are rare in children and often represent an avulsion fracture of the scapholunate ligament. These fractures are at higher risk for nonunion and osteonecrosis. The scaphoid also can be fractured as a component of a greater arc perilunate injury.[52]

Mechanism of Injury: Differences in Location

Distal Scaphoid. Distal pole fractures often are secondary to direct trauma or avulsion with a dorsoradial or dorsovolar fragment.[195] The strong scaphotrapezial ligaments and capsular attachments produce mechanical failure through the bone (Figs.

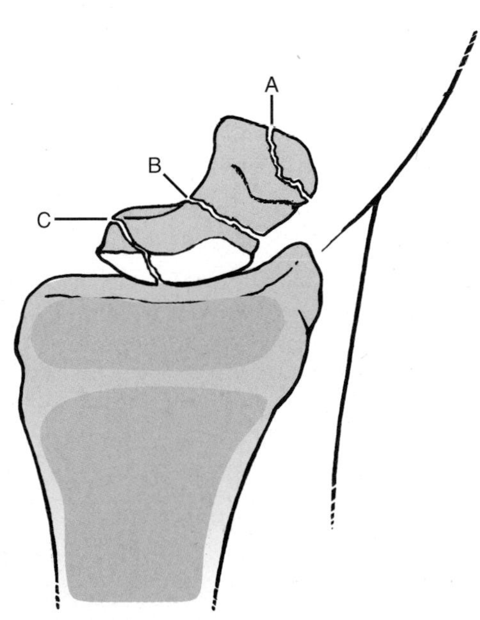

FIGURE 8-57 Three types of scaphoid fractures. **A.** Distal third. **B.** Middle third. **C.** Proximal pole.

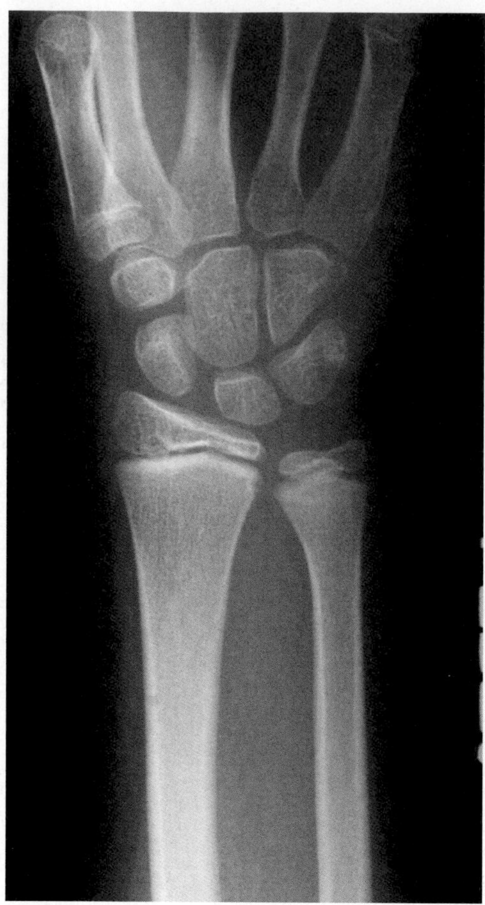

FIGURE 8-58 A 12-year-old boy fell on his right wrist and was tender over scaphoid tubercle. Radiograph reveals small avulsion fracture of distal scaphoid that can easily be overlooked. (Courtesy of Shriners Hospitals for Children, Philadelphia, PA.)

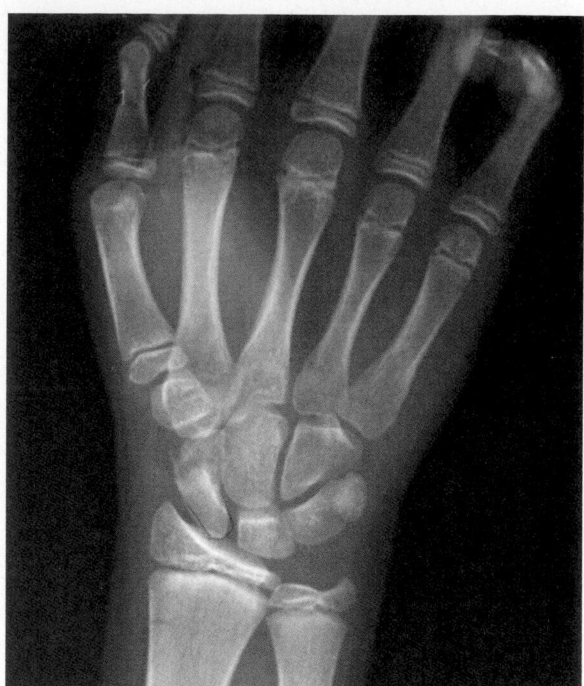

FIGURE 8-59 A 12-year-old boy fell playing ice hockey and complained of right wrist pain. Radiograph reveals a distal pole scaphoid fracture with slight comminution. (Courtesy of Shriners Hospitals for Children, Philadelphia, PA.)

8-58 and 8-59).[33,195] The fracture line and size of the avulsion fragment vary from an isolated chondral injury that is barely visible on radiograph to a large osteochondral fragment.

Middle Third. Middle third fractures do occur in skeletally immature patients. The mechanism of injury usually is a fall onto the outstretched hand and pronated forearm, which exerts tensile forces acting across the volar portion of the scaphoid as the wrist extends.[32,52,203] Bony comminution may be present (Fig. 8-60). A careful scrutiny for other injuries about the carpus is mandatory.[3,30]

Proximal Pole. Proximal pole fractures are rare in children but have been reported in competitive adolescent athletes. The mechanism often is unclear and can be atypical, such as punching game machines or fighting.[193] A proximal pole fracture may propagate through the interface between newly ossified tissue and the cartilaginous anlage, or the injury may be strictly through the cartilage. Proximal fractures may cause destabilization of the scapholunate joint, as the scapholunate interosseous ligament remains attached to the avulsed fragment (Fig. 8-61).

Fracture Patterns (Table 8-7)

Type A: Fractures of the Distal Pole.

Type A1: Extra-articular Distal Pole Fractures. The most important prognostic factor is the presence or absence of joint involvement. Extra-articular fractures may be either volar or dorsal avulsions (see Fig. 8-58). A volar pattern is more common and is attributed to the stout scaphotrapezial ligaments. A dorsal fracture configuration is less common and is attributed to the dorsal intercarpal ligament. The fragments vary in size, and the radiographic appearance is age dependent.

Type A2: Intra-articular Distal Pole Fractures. This type of fracture may be a variation of a type IA fracture with intra-articular extension (Fig. 8-62). Similar types (i.e., volar and dorsal) and mechanisms of injury are possible.

Type B: Middle Third (Waist Fractures). Dividing the bone into thirds or delineating the area bounded by the radioscaphocapitate ligament defines the waist of the scaphoid. Waist fractures occur in many forms. Pediatric fractures are incomplete, minimally displaced, or complete with or without displacement. Comminuted fractures are rare and are associated with higher energy (see Fig. 8-60).

Type C: Proximal Third. Proximal third fractures present diagnostic and therapeutic dilemmas. The proximal pole is the last to ossify, which further complicates diagnosis. The tenuous blood supply of this region presents the same problems in children as adults in terms of nonunion and osteonecrosis risks.

Bipartite Scaphoid Controversy: Traumatic Versus Developmental

A bipartite scaphoid probably exists, but is uncommon (Fig. 8-63).[47,114] Criteria that must be met to diagnose a congenital bipartite scaphoid include: (a) similar bilateral appearance, (b) absence of historical or clinical evidence of antecedent trauma,

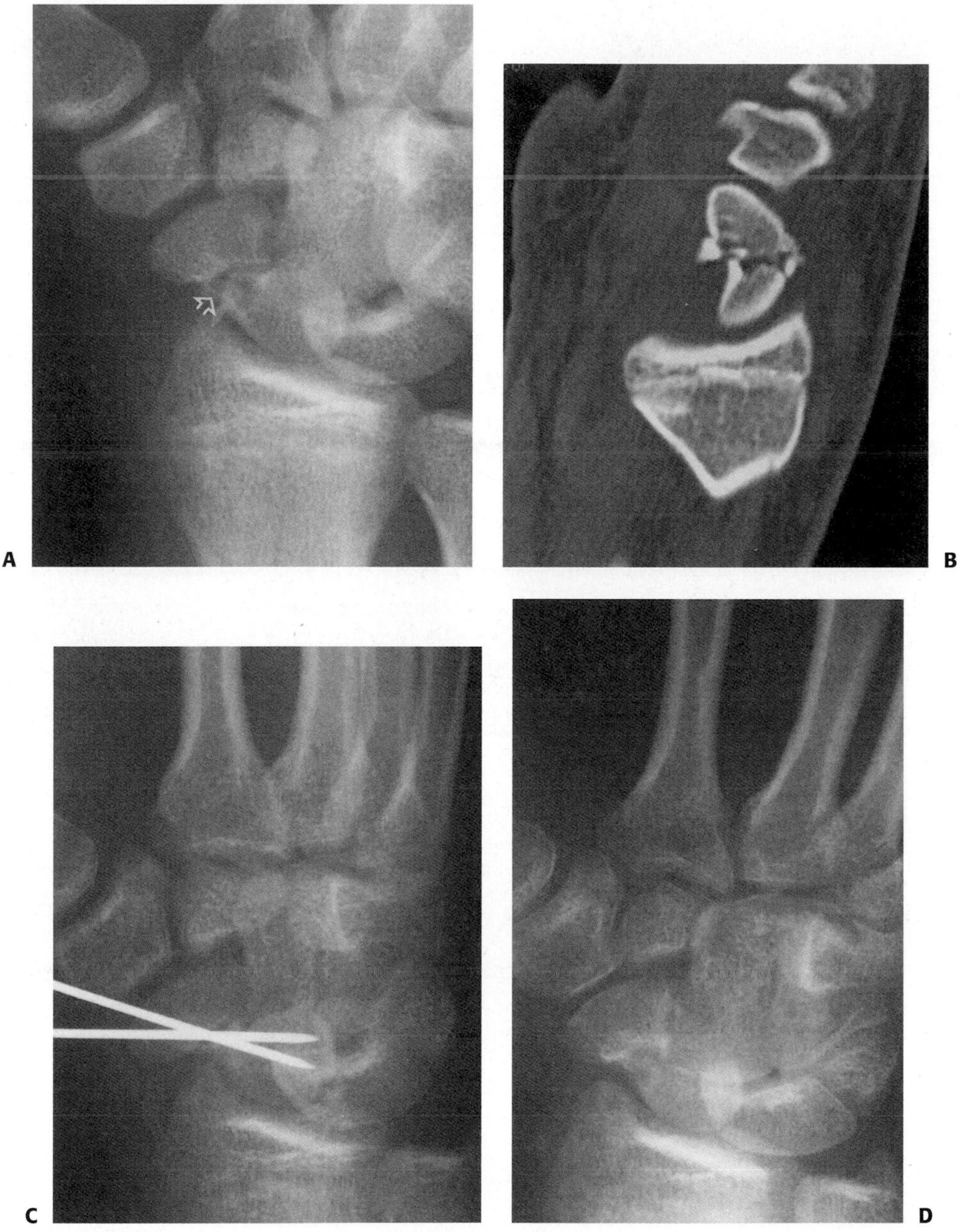

FIGURE 8-60 A. A displaced midwaist scaphoid fracture with comminution, including a butterfly fragment from the volar radial aspect (*arrow*). **B.** CT scan demonstrates the comminution. **C.** Open reduction with internal fixation was performed with two smooth wires and bone graft from the distal radius. **D.** Healing of fracture after pin removal.

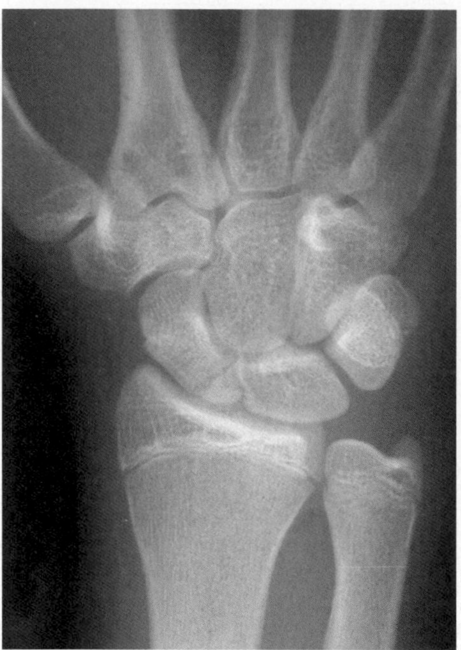

FIGURE 8-61 Anteroposterior radiograph of a 16-year-old male hockey player with a proximal one-third scaphoid fracture. (Courtesy of Shriners Hospitals for Children, Philadelphia, PA.)

TABLE 8-7 Classification of Scaphoid Fractures

Fractures of the Distal Pole
- Extra-articular distal pole fractures
- Intra-articular distal pole fractures

Fractures of the middle third (waist fractures)

Fractures of the proximal third

(c) equal size and uniform density of each component, (d) absence of degenerative change between the scaphoid components or elsewhere in the carpus, and (e) smooth, rounded architecture of each scaphoid component. A unilateral "bipartite scaphoid" should be viewed as a posttraumatic scaphoid nonunion.

Diagnosis

Signs and Symptoms. The history, physical examination, and clinical suspicion are the essential elements to diagnosis of a scaphoid fracture.[148] While the findings are similar in adults and children, they are more difficult to elicit in children. The relative infrequency of this injury and the difficulty in interpreting radiographs of the immature wrist increase the rate of missing a pediatric scaphoid fracture. A distal pole fracture presents with swelling or tenderness over the scaphoid tuberosity. A scaphoid waist fracture presents with pain to palpation within the anatomic snuffbox, scaphoid tubercle, and/or with axial compression of the thumb ray.

Radiographic Findings. Anteroposterior, lateral, and scaphoid views in ulnar deviation of the wrist are routine. Middle third fractures may or may not be evident on initial radiographs. Distal pole fractures are best seen on the lateral view. A pronated oblique view further highlights the CMC joint and distal pole fracture pattern. A scaphoid view places the scaphoid parallel to the film and reveals the scaphoid in its full size. One must be aware of the pseudo-Terry Thomas sign.[107] The scaphoid ossifies from distal to proximal, which changes the distance between the ossified lunate and scaphoid as the child approaches adolescence. This produces an increased distance between the scaphoid and lunate in the immature patient, which

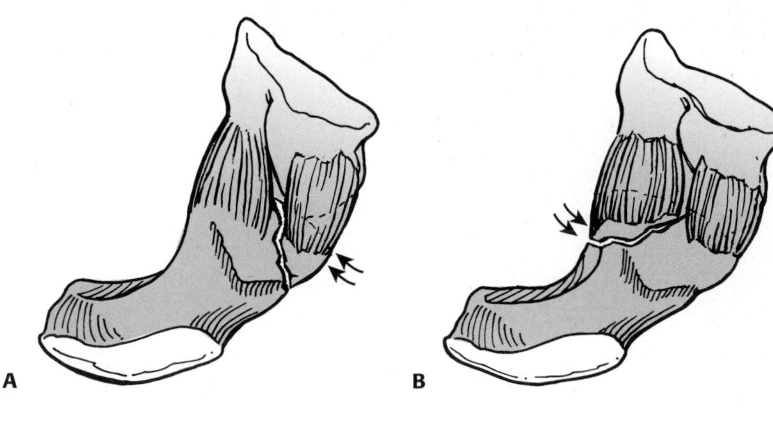

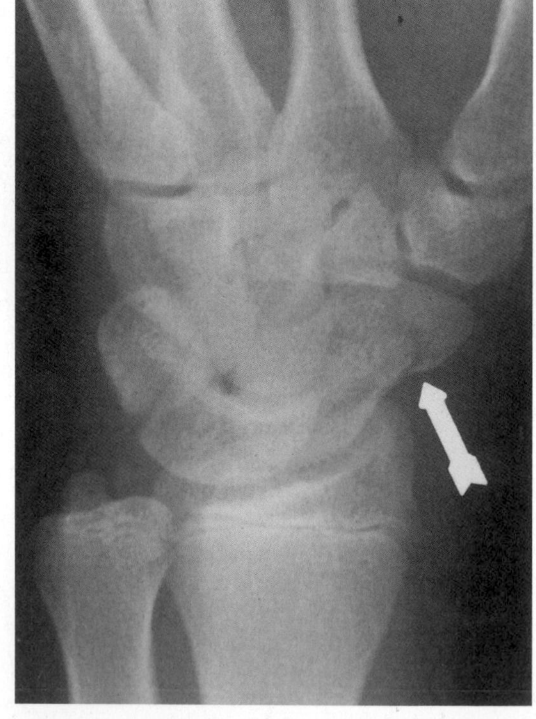

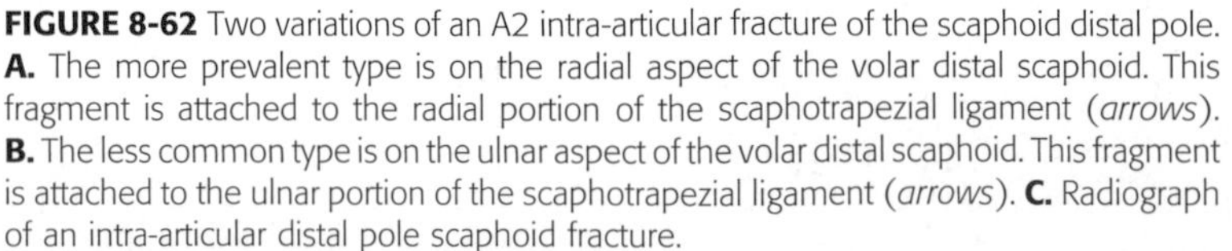

FIGURE 8-62 Two variations of an A2 intra-articular fracture of the scaphoid distal pole. **A.** The more prevalent type is on the radial aspect of the volar distal scaphoid. This fragment is attached to the radial portion of the scaphotrapezial ligament (*arrows*). **B.** The less common type is on the ulnar aspect of the volar distal scaphoid. This fragment is attached to the ulnar portion of the scaphotrapezial ligament (*arrows*). **C.** Radiograph of an intra-articular distal pole scaphoid fracture.

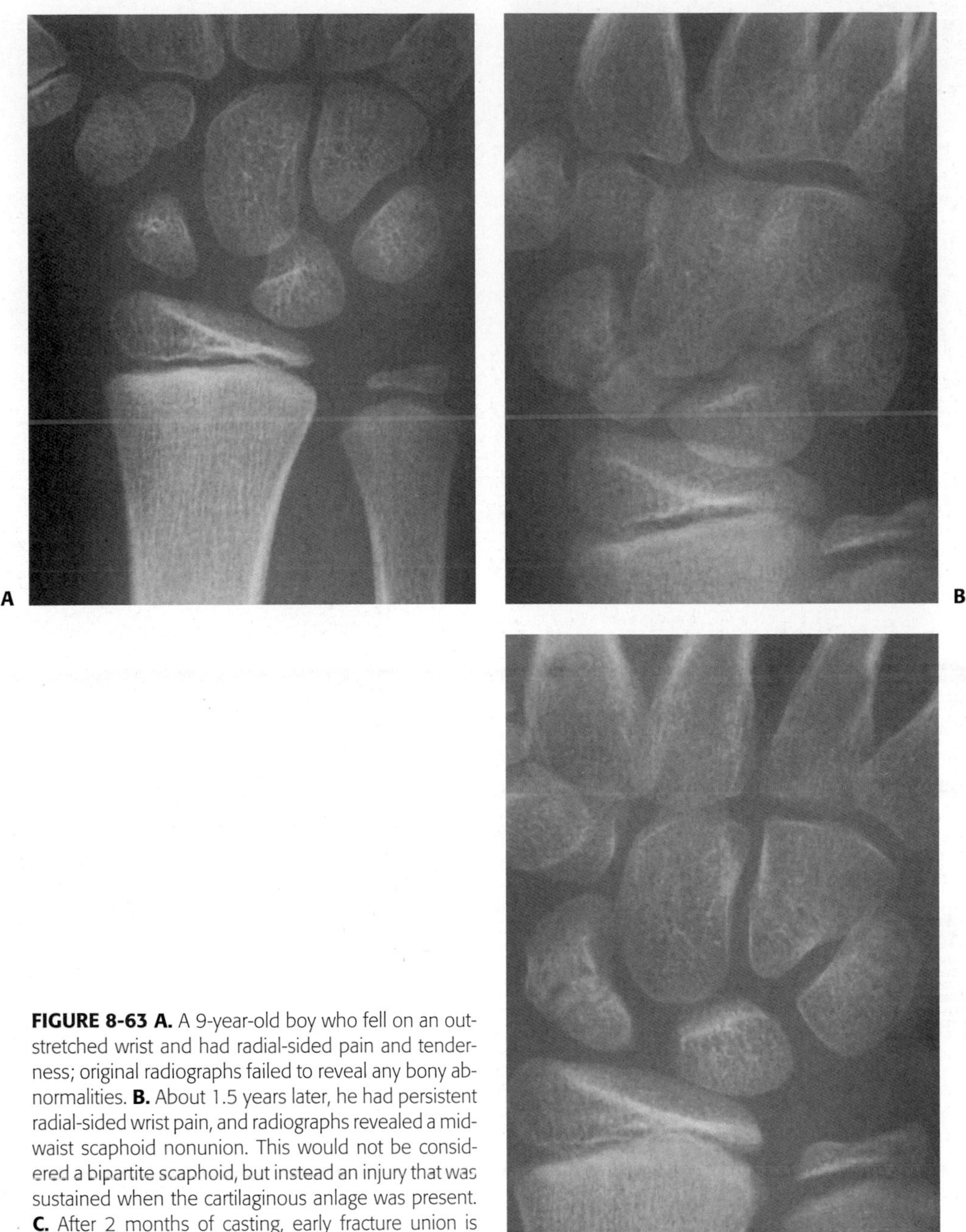

FIGURE 8-63 A. A 9-year-old boy who fell on an outstretched wrist and had radial-sided pain and tenderness; original radiographs failed to reveal any bony abnormalities. **B.** About 1.5 years later, he had persistent radial-sided wrist pain, and radiographs revealed a midwaist scaphoid nonunion. This would not be considered a bipartite scaphoid, but instead an injury that was sustained when the cartilaginous anlage was present. **C.** After 2 months of casting, early fracture union is present.

ranges from 9 mm in a 7-year-old to 3 mm in a 15-year-old.[96,107] Failure to appreciate these normal radiographic variants may lead to an erroneous diagnosis of scapholunate dissociation when the apparent gap is filled with normal cartilage and unossified bone. Comparison to contralateral wrist radiographs is extremely useful in distinguishing abnormal from normal patterns; however, one must keep in mind that carpal ossification is not always symmetric. MRI or CT scans are usually diagnostic.

If the clinical picture is consistent with a scaphoid fracture but the radiographs are negative, the patient should be immobilized. The child should either be instructed to return in 2 weeks for repeat exam and radiographs, or advanced images studies may be ordered. MRI is a useful modality to detect scaphoid fractures that are not visualized on the initial radiographs.[22,35,48,94,116] Johnson et al.[94] evaluated 56 children (57 injuries) with MRI within 10 days of injury. All children had a suspected scaphoid injury but negative radiographs. In 33 (58%) of the 57 injuries, the MRI was normal and the patients were discharged from care. In 16 cases (28%), a fractured scaphoid was diagnosed, and treatment was initiated. MRI does require sedation in the young child and may be overly sensitive in identifying bone edema that never develops into a fracture.

Other advanced imaging studies, such as bone scan, CT, and ultrasound have also been shown to be effective in detecting

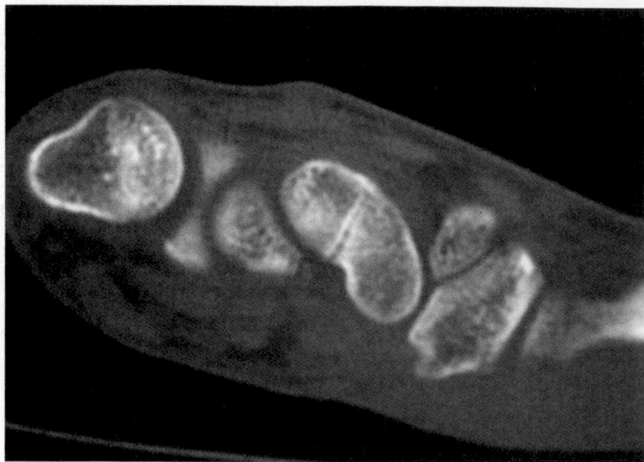

FIGURE 8-64 CT scan of 16-year-old male with negative radiographs but persistent pain. Sagittal image reveals waist fracture without displacement. (Courtesy of Shriners Hospitals for Children, Philadelphia, PA.)

scaphoid fracture (Fig. 8-64).[52] The role of bone scan has been nearly supplanted by MRI. CT scans are most valuable in the assessment of scaphoid fracture displacement for operative indications and in the determination of scaphoid union. The CT images must be made along the longitudinal axis of the scaphoid, which is different than CT imaging of the wrist.[161]

Treatment

Presumed Fracture. Normal radiographs do not preclude the presence of a scaphoid fracture. Clinical suspicion in the presence of normal radiographs warrants immobilization and reevaluation in 2 weeks.[30] The cast is removed, the wrist is examined, and radiographs are obtained. Pain resolution and negative radiographs warrant discontinuation of immobilization and return to normal activities. Persistent pain with normal radiographs requires continued immobilization and advanced imaging studies. MRI scans have been shown to be diagnostically useful in this clinical setting to avoid both misdiagnosis and overtreatment.[22,35,48,94,116] However, MRI may be overly sensitive in identifying bone edema that fails to develop into a fracture.

Confirmed Fracture. If radiographs reveal a fracture, immediate treatment is required. Most pediatric scaphoid fractures can be treated with cast immobilization because children possess a great ability to heal and remodel. In addition, most scaphoid fractures in children are either incomplete (disrupting only a single cortex) or nondisplaced. This principle is especially true for the distal pole, which is a frequent site of scaphoid fracture (Fig. 8-65).[52] Therefore, cast immobilization is the standard of treatment for most nondisplaced or minimally displaced pediatric scaphoid fractures. For avulsion and incomplete fractures, a short thumb spica cast for 4 to 6 weeks is recommended. In the young child, a long arm cast is appropriate to prevent the cast from sliding off the arm. For complete distal third and waist fractures, immobilization is recommended until healing or 6 to 8 weeks of casting.

A longer period of immobilization (8 to 12 weeks) is recommended for proximal pole fractures, delayed diagnosis, or fractures with apparent bony resorption.[52] Immobilization usually begins with 4 to 6 weeks of a long thumb spica cast, followed by up to 6 weeks of a short thumb spica cast. The exact cast position and the joints immobilized are a matter of individual preference.[24,62,81] Most authors favor a long arm thumb spica cast that permits thumb interphalangeal joint motion.[62]

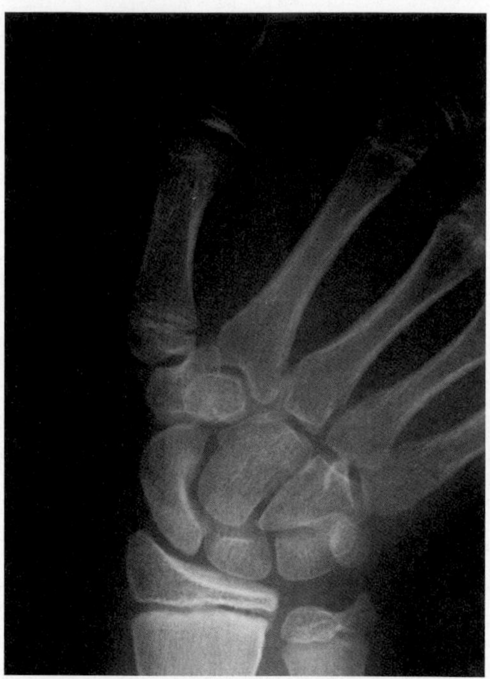

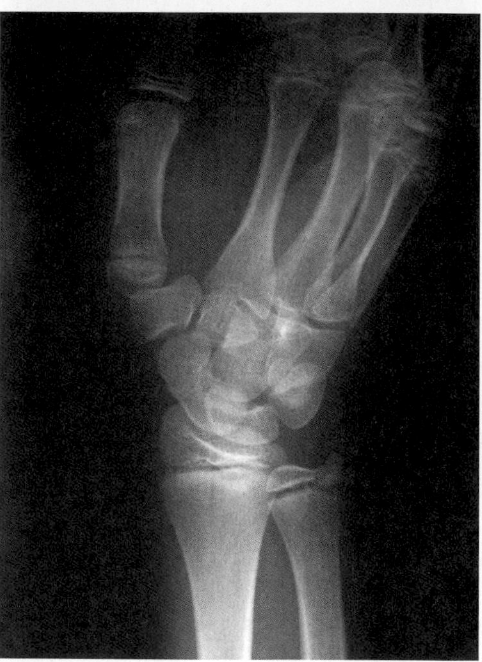

FIGURE 8-65 A 12-year-old boy depicted in Figure 8-59 after 8 weeks of casting. **A.** Scaphoid view demonstrates healing of the fracture. **B.** Pronated oblique radiograph further confirms fracture union. (Courtesy of Shriners Hospitals for Children, Philadelphia, PA.)

Displaced Fractures.

Closed Reduction and Casting. Historically, closed reduction of a displaced scaphoid fracture has been described.[24,81] Currently, open reduction and internal fixation is a more reliable method for restoring alignment and obtaining union.

Percutaneous Screw Fixation. In adults, percutaneous screw fixation for displaced fractures has been advocated.[1,211] However, the fracture must be reduced at the time of screw fixation. Fracture reduction can be accomplished with manipulation, joysticks, or arthroscopic assistance. This technique can be applied to adolescent patients with displaced scaphoid fractures. Screws can be placed under fluoroscopic control either volarly (distal to proximal) or dorsally (proximal to distal) depending on fracture patterns and surgeon preference (Fig. 8-66).[20,175] This procedure is challenging in displaced scaphoid fractures.

Open Reduction and Internal Fixation. Displacement of more than 1 mm or intrascaphoid angulation of more than 10 degrees on any image warrants open reduction and internal fixation. The implant choice is individualized according to the fracture and patient. Scaphoid screws are the primary fixation techniques, although Kirschner wires can be used.[127]

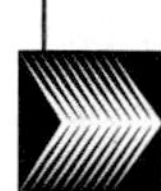

AUTHORS' PREFERRED TREATMENT

Almost all nondisplaced scaphoid fractures are treated with cast immobilization. Indications for open reduction are fractures with more than 1 mm of displacement or an angular deformity of more than 10 degrees. Transscaphoid perilunate injuries also require operative management.

Role of Closed Treatment

The preferred immobilization is a long arm thumb spica cast for the initial 4 to 6 weeks, followed by a short arm cast until clinical and radiographic union. Radiographs are obtained in the first 7 to 10 days to ensure alignment and then monthly until union. If in doubt regarding anatomic alignment or union, a CT scan is obtained.

Percutaneous Screw Fixation

Proximal pole fractures are at high risk for osteonecrosis and nonunion. These injuries are unstable with motion due to the scapholunate ligament insertions. Percutaneous screw fixation stabilizes the fracture fractures without further disruption of the precarious blood supply by operative exposure. Although technically exacting, percutaneous screw fixation of these fractures with protected immobilization until sufficient healing may lessen the risk of osteonecrosis, nonunion, and degenerative changes.

Open Reduction and Internal Fixation

Displaced fractures are treated with open reduction. Fractures of the middle and distal thirds are exposed through a volar approach. Proximal third fractures are exposed through a dorsal approach.[156] The implant depends on the fracture configuration and age of the child. Smooth wires may be necessary in young children. Wires are buried beneath the skin and removed after union. Scaphoid screw fixation is preferred in adolescents.[86,87,129,134] Comminution is treated with bone graft obtained from the metaphysis of the distal radius or iliac crest.

Postoperative Care and Rehabilitation

Nondisplaced fractures are treated with immobilization until union. After the cast is removed, a home therapy program is started. Formal therapy usually is not necessary. Displaced fractures treated with open reduction and internal fixation require variable periods of immobilization. Fixation with

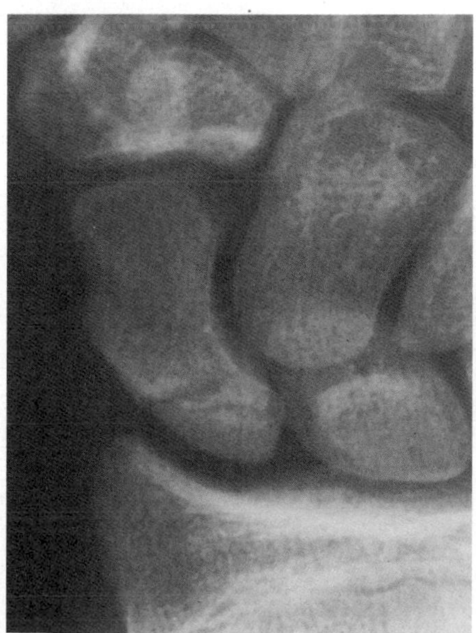

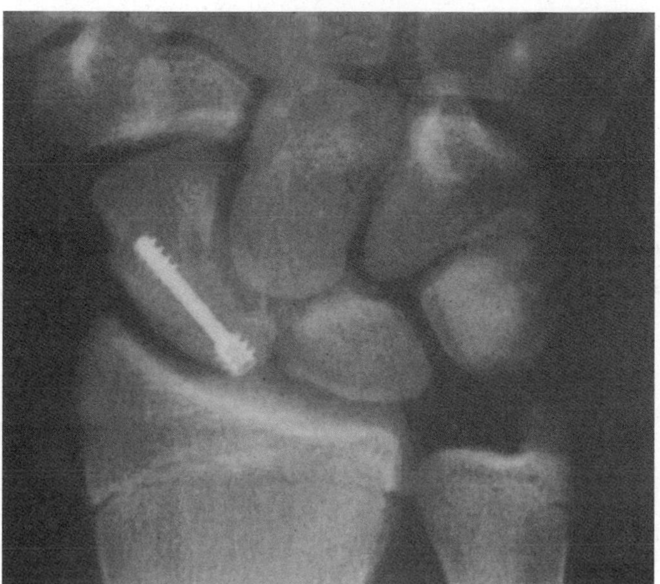

FIGURE 8-66 A. Nondisplaced proximal pole scaphoid fracture in a skeletally mature adolescent athlete. **B.** Treatment by percutaneous screw fixation led to healing.

Kirschner wires requires prolonged immobilization and may require formal therapy to recover motion. Stable screw fixation allows early motion 10 to 14 days after surgery with a short arm thumb spica splint worn for protection during vigorous activity until union. However, many adolescents will not wear the splint dependably and require longer periods of immobilization to prevent loss of screw fixation and nonunion.

Prognosis

Prompt treatment of a nondisplaced scaphoid fracture allows healing in most patients.[30] Nondisplaced pediatric scaphoid fractures have a greater than 95% healing rate. A delay in treatment impedes healing and increases the possibility of displacement.[74,167,195] Displaced fractures require recognition and open reduction because adequate reduction and fixation result in predictable union.

Complications

The most prevalent complications are missed diagnosis and late presentation. Scaphoid nonunions do occur in children, although the incidence is low.[30,44,55,113,120,141,177] There are numerous reasons for late presentation, including a reluctance for children to tell their parents about their mechanism of injury, moderate symptoms that were not severe enough to seek medical attention, and a fear of losing their position on a sporting team.[89] Open reduction, bone grafting, and internal fixation are the standard procedures for treatment of scaphoid nonunions (Fig. 8-67).[55,89,129,193] The approach varies according to the location of fracture and vascularity of the fracture fragments. The principles of operative scaphoid nonunion treatment in children are similar to those in adults. Persistent scaphoid nonunion results in altered kinematics within the wrist and produces degenerative changes over time.[115,202] The goal is to obtain union to prevent long-term arthrosis.

Osteonecrosis may result from a scaphoid fracture. The proximal fragment is more prone to avascular changes. Avascular changes within the proximal fragment do not preclude union after internal fixation. The size of the fragment and the extent of avascularity dictate management. The treatment principles are similar in adults and children. Options to obtain union include conventional or vascularized bone grafting.[200] With nonunion and osteonecrosis of the proximal pole, vascularized bone grafting from the distal radius has been successful.[182,200]

Capitate Fractures

Epidemiology

Isolated fractures of the capitate are rare and usually result from high-energy trauma.[109] Capitate fractures may represent a form of greater arc perilunar injury (Fig. 8-68). The force can propa-

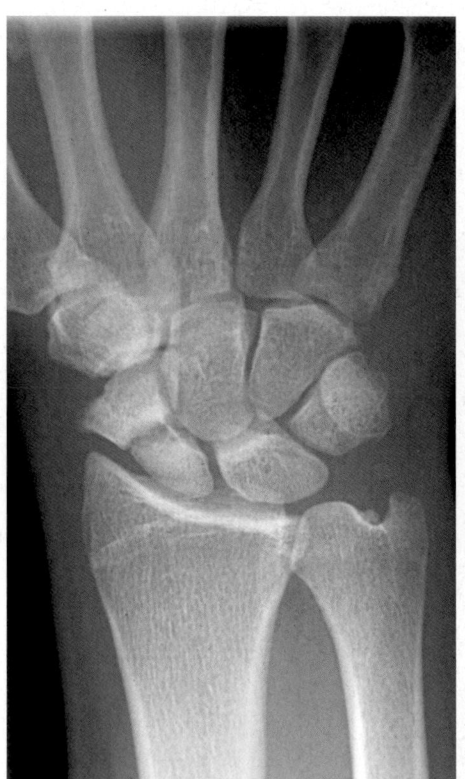

A

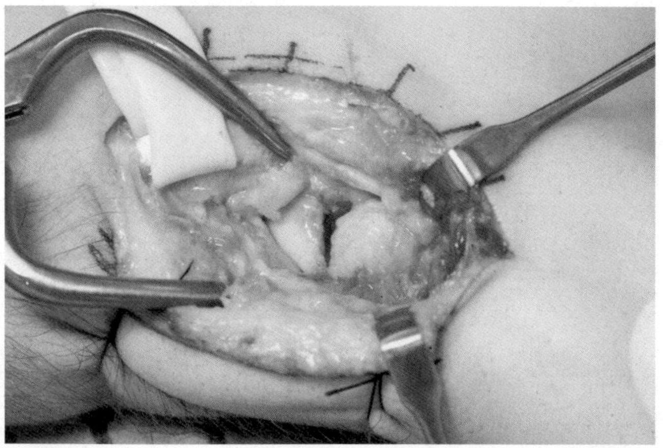

B

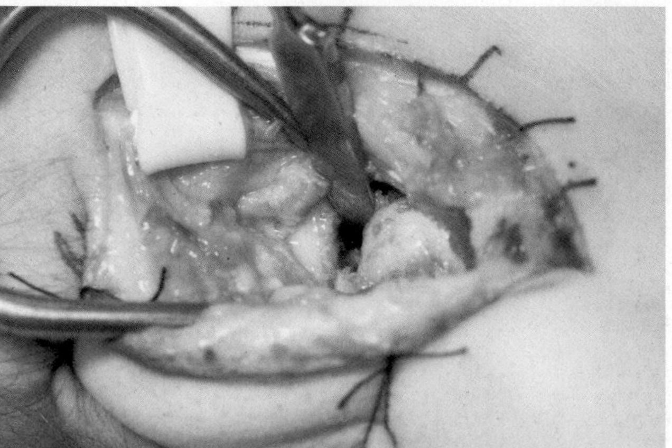

C

FIGURE 8-67 A. A 16-year-old male with a right scaphoid nonunion with resorption at the fracture site. **B.** Volar approach and exposure of the fracture site. **C.** The fracture site was débrided of fibrous material, and the hump back deformity was corrected. *(continues)*

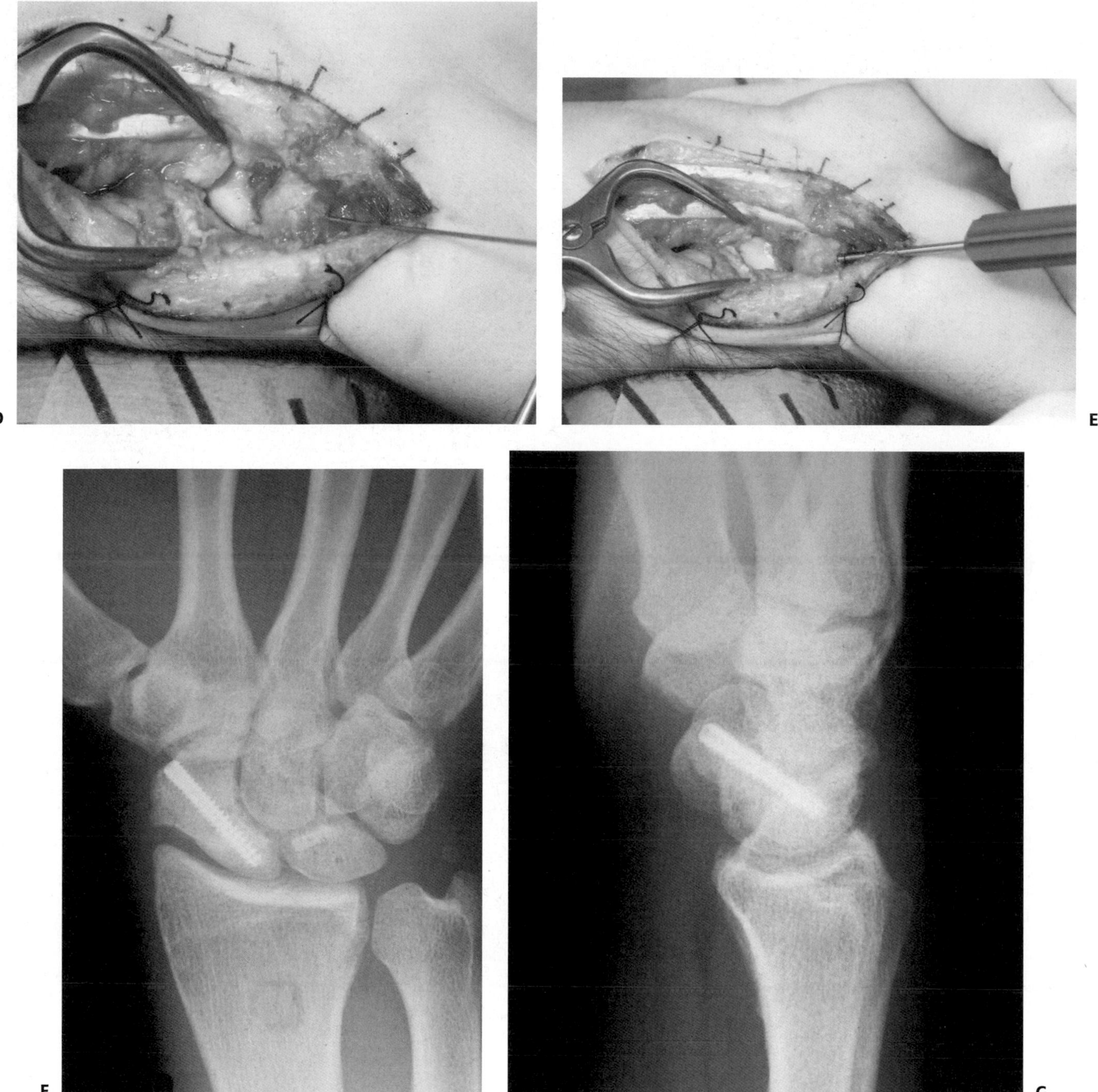

FIGURE 8-67 (*continued*) **D.** The fracture site was packed with bone graft and a guide wire was placed for screw fixation. **E.** The screw was inserted over the guide wire. **F,G.** Anteroposterior and lateral radiographs after fracture reduction, bone grafting, and screw placement. (Courtesy of Shriners Hospitals for Children, Philadelphia, PA.)

gate completely around the lunate and cause a perilunate or lunate dislocation.[30,34,146] The injury also can halt within the capitate and produce a scaphocapitate syndrome.[6,197]

Mechanism of Injury

Excessive dorsiflexion of the wrist is the most common mechanism. The waist of the capitate abuts against the lunate or dorsal aspect of the radius. The fracture occurs through the waist with variable displacement.

Diagnosis

Signs and Symptoms. The wrist usually is markedly swollen and painful to palpation. The clinical presentation varies with the associated carpal injuries. Median nerve paresthesias may be present secondary to swelling within the carpal tunnel.

Radiographic Findings. Standard anteroposterior and lateral views usually are adequate (Fig. 8-69). Careful scrutiny of the radiographs is necessary. The capitate fracture can be subtle,

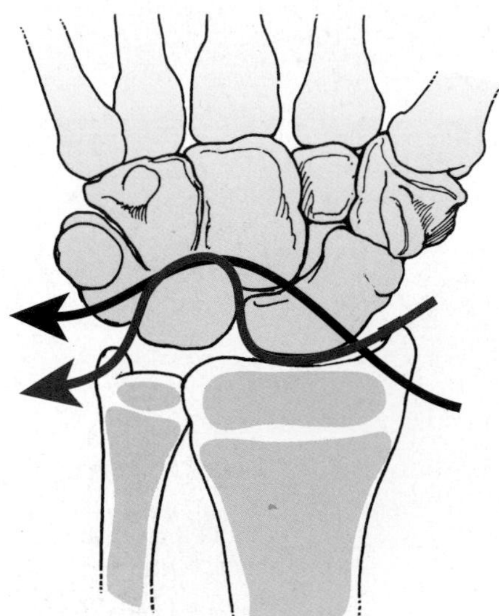

FIGURE 8-68 Progressive perilunar instability. The greater arc (*black arrow*) is associated with fractures of the carpal bones, which may include the scaphoid, lunate, capitate, hamate, and triquetrum. The *red arrow* depicts the lesser arc, in which forces are transmitted only through soft tissue structures. (Reprinted from Mayfield JK, Johnson RP, Kilcoyn RK. Carpal dislocations: pathomechanics and progressive perilunar instability. J Bone Joint Surg Am 1980;5:226–241, with permission.)

or the proximal capitate fragment can rotate 180 degrees. Either scenario can create a confusing image that often results in misinterpretation. Incomplete ossification further complicates radiographic diagnosis and degree of displacement. Small osteochondral fragments in the midcarpal region may indicate a greater arc injury or isolated capitate fracture. In these cases, advanced imaging studies, such as MRI or CT, may be useful (Fig. 8-70).

Treatment

Treatment depends on the fracture pattern, degree of displacement, and associated injuries. Distraction radiographs, MRI, or

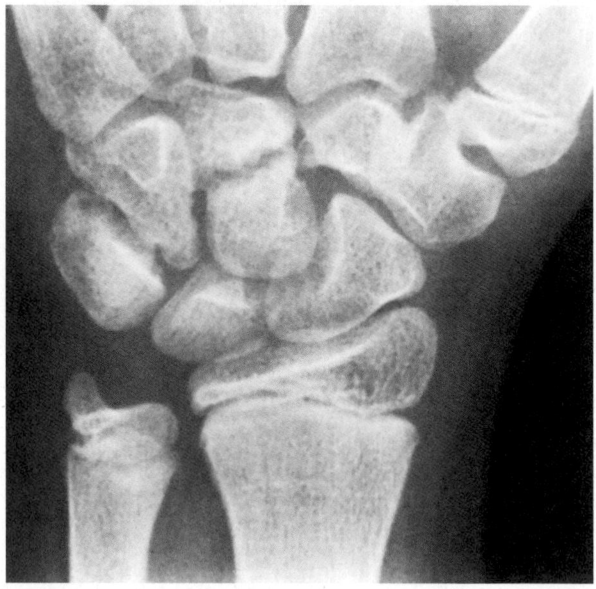

FIGURE 8-69 A 12-year-old boy sustained multiple carpal fractures attributed to a crushing injury. Sixteen months later, an established nonunion of the capitate is present that required bone grafting to obtain union. (Courtesy of James H. Dobyns, MD.)

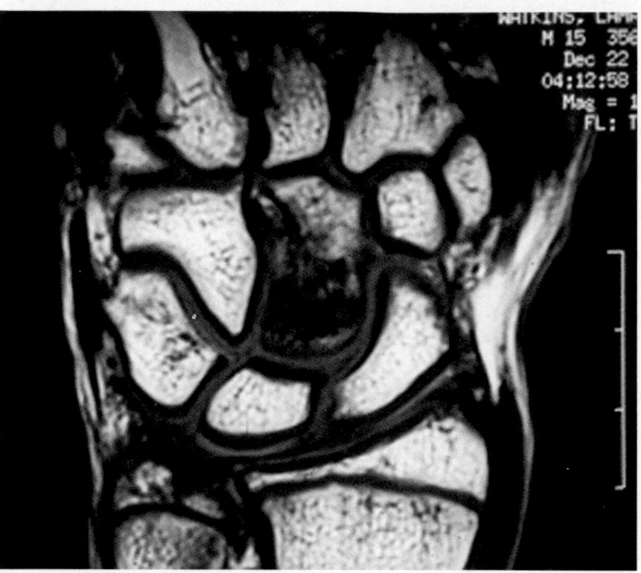

FIGURE 8-70 A 13-year-old boy with persistent midcarpal pain after a fall. MRI shows a capitate fracture. (Courtesy of Shriners Hospitals for Children, Philadelphia, PA.)

CT scans may be necessary to determine the exact pattern of injury.

Nonoperative Treatment. Nondisplaced fractures of the capitate and/or scaphoid can be treated with a long arm cast for 6 to 8 weeks. Closed reduction of displaced fractures is not feasible.[34]

Operative Treatment. Displaced fractures require open reduction, especially the rotated proximal capitate pole. Associated perilunar injuries also require internal fixation and ligamentous repair. The anatomic relationships within the carpus must be restored. Wire or osseous screw fixation is appropriate stabilization after open reduction. Suture repair of ligamentous injuries is performed.

Prognosis and Complications

The rarity of this injury prevents broad generalizations. Early recognition and appropriate treatment lead to an acceptable outcome. Nonunion is rare and requires bone grafting (see Fig. 8-69).[126] Despite the considerable rotation of the proximal pole, osteonecrosis of the capitate is rare.

Triquetrum Fractures

Epidemiology

Avulsion fractures of the triquetrum are more common in adults than in children. The injury may occur in adolescents as carpal ossification nears completion. A fracture through the body of the triquetrum is rare and may occur with a perilunar injury as the path of the greater arc injury passes through the triquetrum.[121]

Mechanism of Injury

A fall on an outstretched wrist is the common event. The probable mechanism for a dorsal triquetrum fracture is a pulling force through the dorsal ligaments or abutment of the ulnar styloid.

Diagnosis

Signs and Symptoms. The wrist is mildly swollen and painful to palpation directly over the dorsal triquetrum. The clinical presentation is more severe with associated carpal injuries.

Radiographic Findings. Anteroposterior and lateral views may not show the avulsion fracture. A pronated oblique view highlights the dorsum of the triquetrum and may reveal the avulsed fragment. At times, CT scans are necessary for accurate diagnosis (Fig. 8-71).

Treatment

An avulsion fracture is treated with a short period of immobilization (3 to 6 weeks) followed by motion and return to activities. A fracture through the body of the triquetrum with a perilunar injury requires open reduction and internal fixation.

Prognosis and Complications

Avulsion fractures are relatively minor injuries. Treatment results in prompt and complete recovery. Body fractures associated with perilunar injures have a guarded prognosis, depending on the extent of concomitant injuries and treatment provided.

Hamate, Pisiform, Lunate, and Trapezium Fractures

Pediatric fractures of the hamate, pisiform, lunate, and trapezium are rare. Hook of the hamate fractures usually occur in adults but may occur in adolescents with traumatic falls. A CT scan may be necessary for diagnosis if the fracture is not visible on the carpal tunnel view. Pisiform fractures are the result of direct trauma. Lunate fractures are associated with Kienböck disease,[154] which is relatively uncommon in children. Trapezium fractures can occur with CMC joint injuries about the thumb.

FIGURE 8-71 A minimally displaced dorsal triquetral avulsion fracture (*arrow*) that was treated with short-term immobilization.

Soft Tissue Injuries about the Carpus

Ligamentous Injuries

Epidemiology. Ligamentous injuries about the pediatric wrist are less common than osseous injuries.[63,64,146] The immature carpus and viscoelastic ligaments are relatively resistant to injury.

Mechanism of Injury. Fracture-dislocations and isolated ligamentous injuries usually are caused by high-energy trauma (Fig. 8-72).[88] Motor vehicle accidents and sports-related injuries are potential causes of the rare fracture-dislocation. However, recurrent or chronic wrist pain is not uncommon in adolescents. Most recurrent ligamentous pain results from hypermobility and overuse during the adolescent growth spurt. This mechanism may result in joint subluxation, chondral impingement, or ligamentous tears similar to patellofemoral injuries in adolescents.

Diagnosis.

Signs and Symptoms. A child with an acute traumatic injury avoids use of the wrist and hand. The wrist is swollen and painful to palpation, making isolation of the injured segment difficult except in extremely cooperative children. Provocative maneuvers for carpal instability usually are not possible because of pain in the injured wrist.

Gross instability without pain on stress testing may indicate a hyperelasticity syndrome that is not related to trauma.[147] However, recurrent pain does occur in children with hypermo-

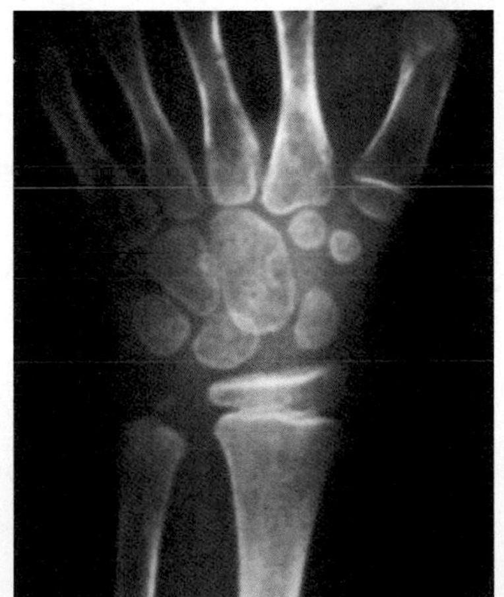

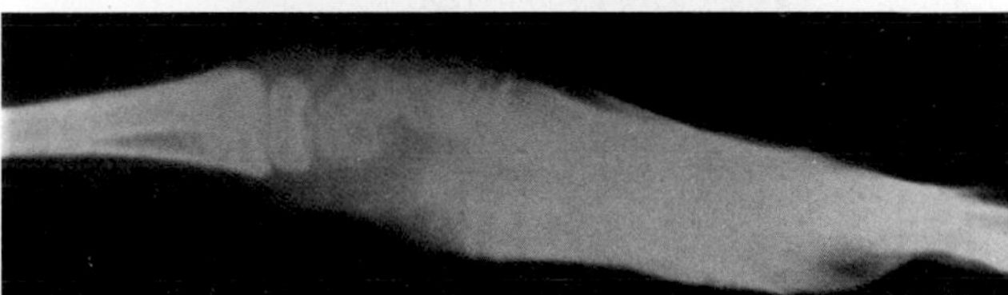

FIGURE 8-72 Anteroposterior **(A)** and lateral **(B)** radiographs of a dorsal perilunar dislocation in a 6-year-old boy. (Courtesy of William F. Benson, MD.)

bility, overuse, and relative muscular weakness. These children complain of diffuse pain, generalized tenderness, and limited strength on examination. Diagnosis is difficult particularly because of concerns regarding emotional overlay.

Radiographic Findings. Anteroposterior and lateral views are routine. The incomplete ossification complicates radiographic interpretation, especially the assessment of carpal widening. Detection of slight widening or malalignment within the carpus often is difficult. Contralateral views are useful to compare ossification and carpal spacing.[96] Suspicion of a fracture warrants advanced imaging studies, such as arthrography, stress radiograph, fluoroscopy, and MRI. MRI scans are used for diagnosis of ligamentous injuries.

Treatment. General treatment recommendations for rare traumatic dislocation injuries are difficult. Decisive factors include the age of child, degree of clinical suspicion, and extent of injury. Minor injuries are treated with immobilization for 3 to 6 weeks and re-examination. Resolution of symptoms and signs allows return to normal activities. Persistent pain warrants further clinical and radiographic evaluation. Overt ligamentous injuries with static instability and malalignment require accurate diagnosis and appropriate treatment. A complete ligament tear (e.g., an adolescent with a scapholunate injury) is treated with principles similar to those for adults. Open reduction, anatomic reduction, and ligament repair are the basic tenets of treatment.

A child or adolescent with ligamentous laxity and persistent activity-related pain is especially difficult to treat. Discerning focal from nonfocal wrist pathology is imperative. Radiographs and MRI scans often are normal. Most of these children respond to therapeutic strengthening. Protective sport-specific wrist protectors or taping may be appropriate (Fig. 8-73). A small subset of children have unresolved pain caused by chondral injuries or ligamentous tears that require arthroscopic treatment.[50]

TRIANGULAR FIBROCARTILAGE COMPLEX TEARS

Epidemiology

Tears of the triangular fibrocartilage complex (TFCC) rarely occur in children.[190] These tears most often are associated with distal radial fractures, radial growth arrest, ulnar overgrowth, and ulnar carpal impaction. Most often these children present late after acute trauma with activity-related pain.

Anatomic Considerations

The TFCC consists of the triangular fibrocartilage (TFC) and the volar ulnocarpal ligaments. The TFC spans the sigmoid notch of the radius to the fovea at the base of the ulnar styloid and provides stability to the distal radioulnar and ulnocarpal joints.

Mechanism of Injury

Rotational forces with axial loading causes tearing of the TFCC. In children with a positive ulnar variance, the TFC is thinner and more susceptible to injury. Similarly, ulnar styloid hypertrophic unions and nonunions increase the risk of TFCC injuries with ulnocarpal impaction.

Classification

TFCC tears are classified according to the location of the tear.[190] Peripheral tears (type B) are most common in adolescents. Tears from the radial insertion (type D) are next in frequency, while central (type A) and volar (type C) tears are rare.[142,144]

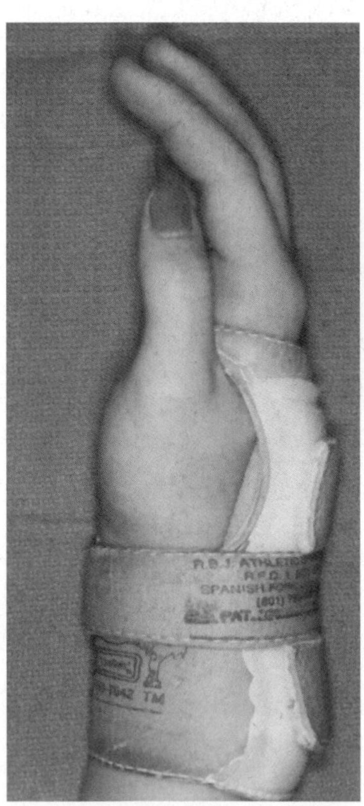

A

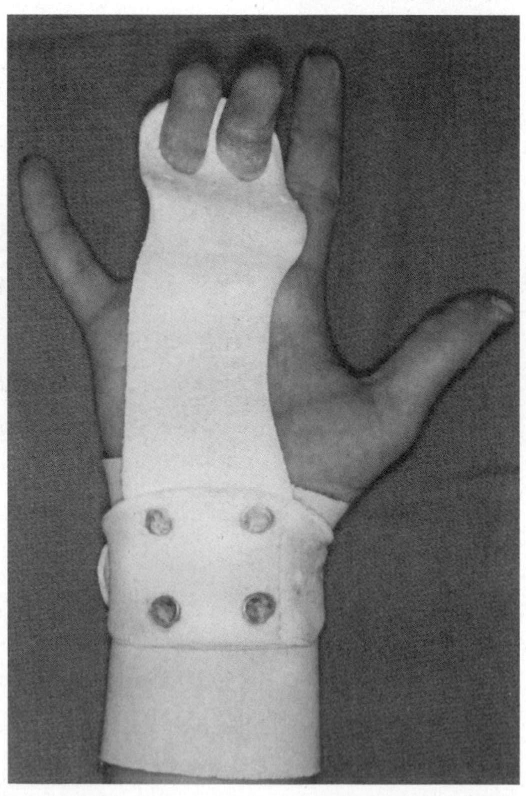

B

FIGURE 8-73 Wrist guards for gymnastics. **A.** The "lion's paw" protector used mainly for vault. **B.** Hand and wrist protectors used primarily for the uneven parallel bars.

Diagnosis

Signs and Symptoms

Pain is localized to the distal ulna and ulnar carpal region. Forearm rotation may be limited and usually reproduces the pain, particularly at the extremes of supination and/or pronation. Compression and ulnar deviation of the carpus against the ulna may reproduce the pain with crepitus. The stability of the distal radioulnar should be compared to the contralateral side.[137,190]

Radiographic Findings

Plain radiographs may reveal an ulnar styloid fracture. An acute displaced fracture at the base of the styloid suggests the likelihood of a TFCC tear. Arthrograms and MRI scans may help in the diagnosis.[28,77]

Treatment

The initial approach to adolescents with chronic wrist pain without instability incorporates rest until symptoms subside followed by a strengthening program. If pain persists after regaining symmetric pinch and grip strength, then further evaluation is appropriate. If clinical examination is consistent with a TFCC tear or ulnar-carpal impaction, MRI and/or arthroscopy is appropriate. Partial TFCC tears or carpal chondromalacia is treated with arthroscopic débridement. Full thickness tears from the fovea (1B) require peripheral repair, usually arthroscopically, to restore stability. Tears from the radial insertion (1D) require a trans-radial repair.

DISLOCATIONS OF THE HAND AND CARPUS

Dislocations of the Interphalangeal Joints

In children, the soft tissue stabilizers about the interphalangeal joints are stronger than the physis, which explains the propensity for fracture rather than dislocation. Occasionally, dislocations and fracture-dislocations occur about the interphalangeal and metacarpophalangeal joints (Fig. 8-74).

Distal Interphalangeal Joint

A hyperextension or lateral force may result in dorsal or lateral DIP joint dislocation. The collateral ligaments and volar plate typically detach from the middle phalanx. Most dislocations can be reduced by longitudinal traction, recreation of the dislocation force, and reduction of the distal phalanx. The DIP joint reduction and congruity are confirmed by clinical motion and radiographs. Two to 3 weeks of DIP joint splinting is sufficient, followed by a home program that focuses on DIP joint motion.

Irreducible or complex dislocations of the DIP occur primarily in adults, but can occur in pediatric patients.[143,150,160,168,187] Open reduction through a dorsal approach is required for removal of the interposed tissue. The volar plate often is the offending agent, although the collateral ligaments and the flexor digitorum profundus can block reduction.[143,150] A stable DIP joint is treated with DIP joint splinting for 3 to 4 weeks. An unstable DIP joint requires pin fixation for 3 to 4 weeks.

Proximal Interphalangeal Joint

Dislocation of the PIP joint may occur in a variety of directions. Dorsal dislocations are the most common, although lateral and volar dislocations also occur. The differential diagnosis includes adjacent bony and tendon injuries.[53] Radiographs are required to assess the physis and to confirm joint alignment. The postreduction lateral radiograph must confirm concentric joint reduction. Subtle joint subluxation is detected by a slight offset between the proximal and middle phalanges along with a dorsal V space instead of smooth articular congruity.

Dorsal PIP Joint Dislocations. The middle phalanx is displaced dorsal to the proximal phalanx. The collateral ligaments and volar plate are disrupted. Many dorsal dislocations probably are joint subluxations that retain some of the collateral ligament or volar plate integrity. Some subluxations are reduced by the patient or trainer and never receive medical evaluation.

Unreduced dorsal dislocations cause pain and obvious deformity. If necessary, anesthesia usually can be accomplished with a digital block. The dislocation is reduced with longitudinal traction, hyperextension, and palmar translation of the middle phalanx onto the proximal phalanx. The quality of the reduction and the stability of the joint must be assessed. Asking the patient to flex and extend the digit evaluates active motion. Most dislocations are stable throughout the normal range of motion, and radiographs confirm a concentric reduction. A stable joint requires a brief period (3 to 5 days) of splinting for comfort, followed by range of motion and buddy taping. Immediate motion may be started, although pain often prohibits movement. Prolonged immobilization leads to PIP joint stiffness.

An unstable reduction tends to subluxate or dislocate during PIP joint extension. The radiographs must be scrutinized for subtle dorsal subluxation and concomitant fracture of the middle phalangeal base. Unstable PIP joint dislocations, with or without small fractures of the middle phalangeal base, have a stable arc of motion that must be defined. This stable arc is typically from full flexion to about 30 degrees of flexion. This arc is used to determine the confines of extension-block splinting.[122] A short arm cast is applied with an aluminum outrigger that positions the MCP joint in flexion and the PIP joint in 10 degrees less than the maximal extension that leads to joint subluxation. Reduction is verified by lateral radiographs. The aluminum splint is modified every 7 to 10 days to increase PIP joint extension 10 degrees. A lateral view or dynamic fluoroscopy is used to confirm concentric reduction. This process

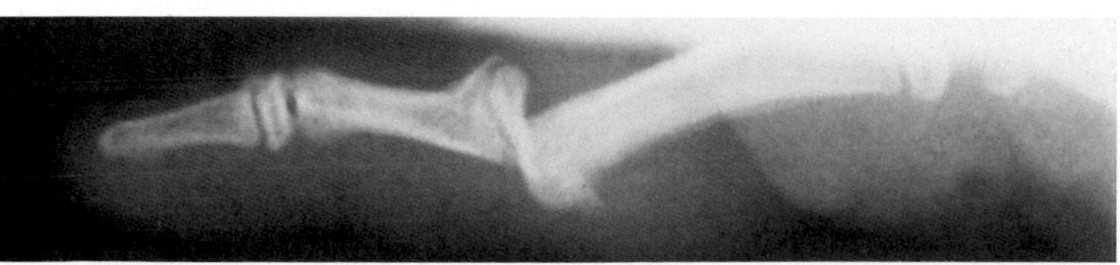

FIGURE 8-74 A dorsal dislocation of the PIP joint with a S-H type II fracture of the middle phalanx in a 15-year-old boy.

is continued over 4 to 5 weeks. The cast and splint are then discontinued and a home therapy program is instituted.

Extremely unstable injuries that dislocate in more than 30 degrees of flexion almost always involve considerable fracture of the middle phalanx. These injuries are regarded as pilon fractures or intra-articular fracture-dislocations. Treatment presents a management dilemma as discussed earlier.[185] Options range from open reduction to dynamic traction. Long-term subluxation, stiffness, and arthrosis are concerns.

Volar PIP Joint Dislocations. Volar PIP joint dislocations are uncommon in children,[95,145] and the diagnosis often is delayed.[145] Interposition of soft tissues or bony fragments can render the dislocation irreducible.[95] The proximal phalangeal head may herniate between the lateral band and the central tendon. In contrast to dorsal dislocations, long-term results often are suboptimal. This outcome may be related to a delay in treatment or the degree of soft tissue involvement, especially the central slip.

Volar dislocations require closed or open reduction. Reducible dislocations are treated with 4 weeks of full-time PIP joint extension splinting to promote healing of the central slip.[191] Radiographs are necessary to confirm concentric reduction. An unstable reduction may require temporary pin fixation across the PIP joint. Irreducible dislocations require open reduction through a dorsal approach to extricate any interposed tissue. The central slip can be repaired to the middle phalanx. Postoperative immobilization consists of 4 weeks of full-time PIP joint extension splinting.

Lateral PIP Joint Dislocations. Pure lateral dislocations are uncommon, although dorsal dislocations may have a lateral component.[60] An isolated lateral dislocation represents severe disruption of the collateral ligament complex. The injury is a spectrum of injury, beginning with damage to the proper and accessory collateral ligaments and culminating in volar plate disruption.[100] Bony avulsion fragments may accompany the ligamentous failure.[37] Closed reduction is uniformly successful. A brief period (5 to 7 days) of immobilization followed by buddy taping to protect the healing collateral ligament complex is the customary treatment.

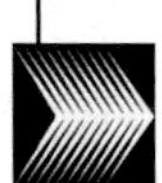

AUTHORS' PREFERRED TREATMENT

Variables that affect treatment of PIP joint dislocations include the extent and anatomic location of soft tissue disruption, presence or absence of fracture, reducibility, and stability after reduction. The initial treatment of almost all PIP dislocations is an attempt at closed reduction followed by a stability assessment. Early mobilization is important to prevent PIP joint stiffness.

Dorsal Dislocation

A stable reduction is treated with brief immobilization followed by early motion. Coban-wrap (3M, St. Paul, Minnesota) buddy taping is used until full stable motion is achieved. Sports are restricted until the patient gains joint stability and full motion. An unstable reduction that can be held reduced in more than 30 to 40 degrees of flexion is treated with extension block splinting. Extremely unstable fracture-dislocations require open treatment, external fixation, or dynamic traction depending on the size of the fracture fragments.

Volar Dislocation

A stable reduction is treated with immobilization for 4 weeks with the PIP joint in extension. Unstable reductions are treated with percutaneous pin fixation to maintain a concentric reduction. Irreducible dislocations require open reduction with repair of the central slip.

Lateral Dislocations

Pure lateral dislocations are rare. Closed reduction usually is obtainable, followed by a brief period of immobilization. Irreducible dislocations require open reduction with or without collateral ligament repair.

Metacarpophalangeal Joint Dislocations

The MCP joint is an uncommon site for dislocation in the child's hand.[65,110] The dislocation may involve a finger or thumb. The gamekeeper's or skier's thumb can be considered a subset of subluxation or dislocation.

Dorsal Metacarpophalangeal Dislocations of the Fingers

The most frequent dislocation of the MCP joint is dorsal dislocation of the index digit (Fig. 8-75), which results from a hyperextension force that ruptures the volar plate. The proximal phalanx is displaced dorsal to the metacarpal head. The diagnosis is readily apparent because the digit is shortened, supinated, and deviated in an ulnar direction. The interphalangeal joints are slightly flexed due to digital flexor tendon tension. The volar skin is tense over the prominent metacarpal head.

MCP joint dislocations are classified as simple or complex. Complex dislocations are irreducible because of volar plate interposition in the joint. The injury can be open with the metacarpal head penetrating the palmar skin (Fig. 8-76). Simple dislocations are in a position of hyperextension on radiographs. Irreducible dislocations have bayonet apposition of the proximal phalanx dorsal to the metacarpal head. The sesamoid bone(s) of the index or thumb may be seen within the joint. The position of the sesamoid bones is indicative of the site of the volar plate.[26,157] The most common irreducible dislocation is at the index MCP joint. Additional structures may impede reduction.[97] The metacarpal head becomes "picture-framed" by the flexor tendon on the ulnar side and the lumbrical on the radial side. The superficial transverse metacarpal ligament and the natatory ligaments also can entrap the metacarpal neck. The collar of retraining tissue is tightened by longitudinal traction, and this reduction maneuver may convert a dislocation from reducible to irreducible.

Most simple dislocations can be reduced with distraction and volar manipulation of the proximal phalanx over the metacarpal head. Avoidance of hyperextension during reduction is important to prevent conversion of a simple to a complex dislocation. These reductions are usually stable. Reduction of a complex dislocation is problematic. The maneuver involves further hy-

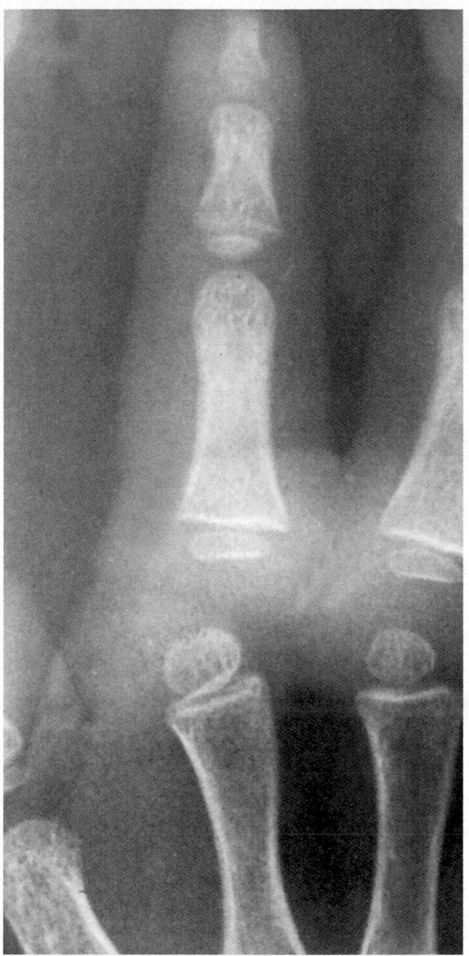

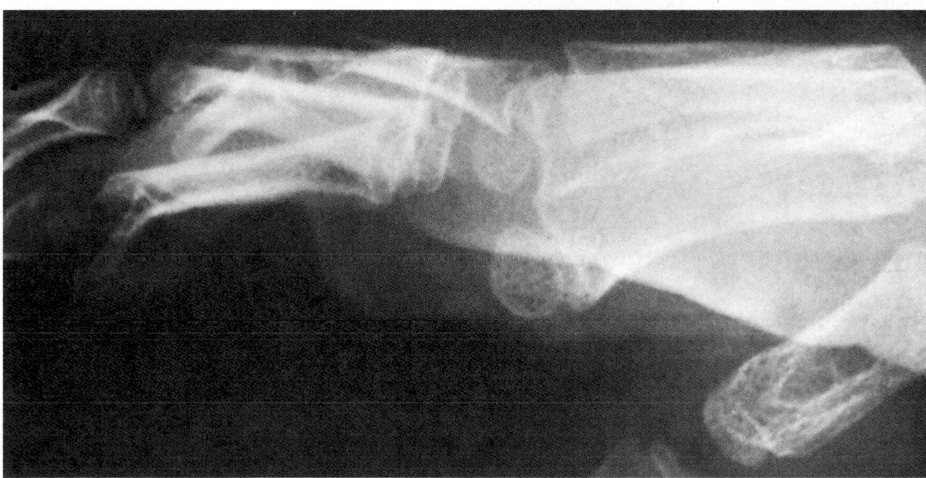

FIGURE 8-75 A. A 3-year-old boy with a complete complex dislocation of the index finger metacarpal joint. **B.** Note the parallelism in this lateral view. Open reduction was done through a volar approach.

perextension of the joint and palmar translation of the proximal phalanx. The goal is to extricate the volar plate with the proximal phalanx during palmar translation. Intra-articular infiltration of anesthetic fluid may assist reduction through joint distention and "floating" of the volar plate from its displaced position. The success rate for conversion of an irreducible dislocation to a reducible dislocation is low; open reduction is necessary in almost all patients.

Open Reduction

Open reduction can be accomplished through a volar or dorsal approach. The volar approach provides excellent exposure of the metacarpal head and the incarcerated structures.[9,12,65,73,97,110,123] However, the digital nerves are draped over the articular surface of the metacarpal head and precariously close to the skin. A deep skin incision can cut these nerves. The skin is gently incised and soft tissue is dissected. The first annular pulley is incised. The metacarpal head is extricated from between the flexor tendon and the lumbrical. The joint is evaluated for interposed structures, such as the volar plate, and then reduced under direct observation.

The dorsal approach offers a less extensive exposure but avoids the risk of digital nerve injury.[12] Through a dorsal incision, the extensor tendon is longitudinally split over the MCP

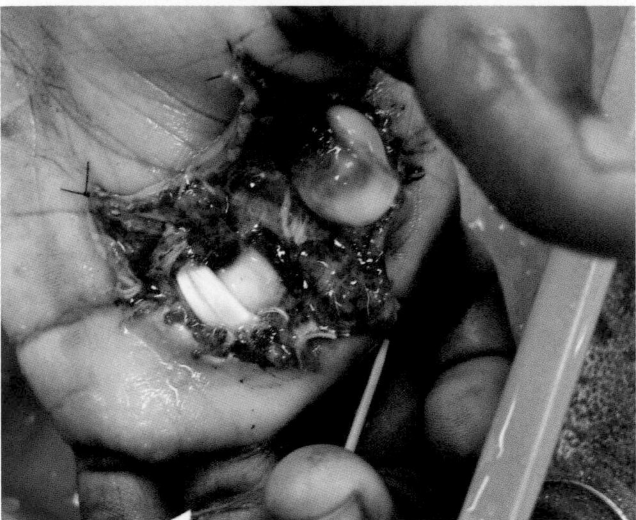

FIGURE 8-76 A 17-year-old male after fall from height with open index and middle finger dorsal dislocations. (Courtesy of Joshua Ratner, MD.)

joint. A transverse or longitudinal capsulotomy is made if the injury has not torn the capsule. A Freer elevator is placed within the joint to clear it of any interposed tissue. Often, the interposed volar plate needs to be split longitudinally to reduce the joint. If the flexor tendon is wrapped around the metacarpal, the Freer is used to extricate the metacarpal head.

Regardless of the approach used, early motion is necessary to optimize outcome.[97,123] The postoperative regimen is a 3 to 5 day immobilization period, followed by active motion. Rarely, a dorsal blocking splint is needed to prevent hyperextension that may foster repeat dislocation.

Dorsal dislocations of the other fingers are uncommon (Fig. 8-77).[8,139] Lateral fracture-dislocations are often S-H III fractures involving the base of the proximal phalanx (Fig. 8-78) and require open reduction and internal fixation of the displaced physeal fracture.

Neglected Metacarpophalangeal Joint Dislocations

Early treatment is preferred for MCP joint dislocations,[91] but delay of a few months may still result in an acceptable outcome. A delay of more than 6 months is associated with joint degeneration and a less predictable result. Late reduction may require a combined dorsal and volar approach for adequate exposure.[9,112,135] Collateral ligament resection and temporary MCP joint pin fixation may be necessary.

Dorsal Dislocation of the Thumb Ray

Thumb MCP joint dislocations are similar to those of the fingers, and hyperextension is the common mechanism. Thumb dislocations are classified according to the integrity and position of the volar plate, the status of the collateral ligaments, and the relative position of the metacarpal and proximal phalanx. The components of the classification are incomplete dislocation, simple complete dislocation, and complex complete dislocation (Fig. 8-79).

Incomplete Thumb Metacarpophalangeal Joint Dislocations. An incomplete dislocation implies rupture of the volar plate with partial preservation of the collateral ligament integrity. The proximal phalanx perches on the dorsum of the metacarpal. Closed reduction is easily accomplished, and a 3-week course of immobilization is adequate. Return to sports requires protection for an additional 3 weeks.

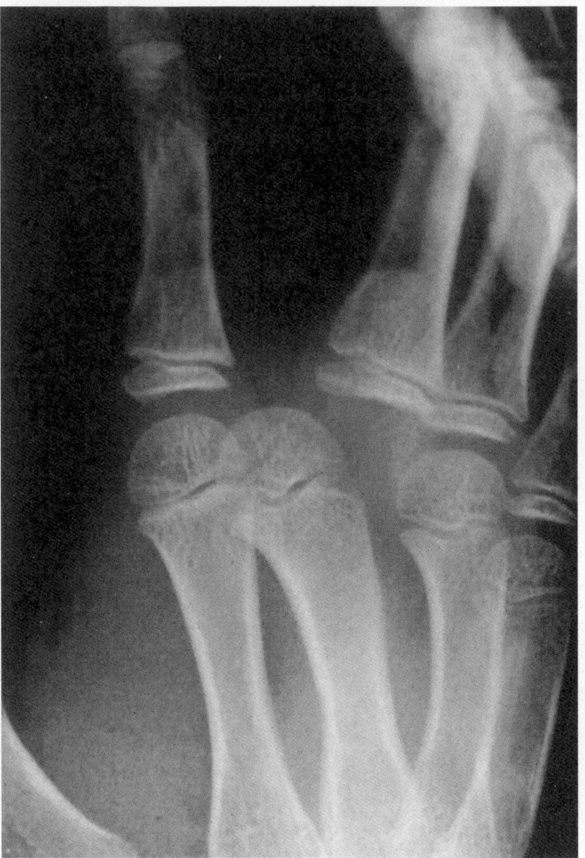

FIGURE 8-77 A rare dorsal dislocation of the long finger that was irreducible by closed means. A dorsal approach permitted inspection of the joint and extrication of the volar plate.

Simple Complete Thumb Metacarpophalangeal Dislocation. A simple, complete dislocation implies volar plate and collateral ligament disruption. The proximal phalanx is displaced in a dorsal direction and is angulated 90 degrees to the long axis of the thumb metacarpal. Many of these dislocations can be reduced by closed means, although unnecessary longitudinal traction may convert a reducible condition into an irreducible situation (Fig. 8-80).[73,123] A successful reduction requires thumb spica immobilization for 3 to 4 weeks to allow healing of the volar plate and collateral ligaments.

Complex Complete Thumb Metacarpophalangeal Joint Dislocation. A complete or irreducible dislocation is the most severe type of injury. The long axes of both the proximal phalanx and metacarpal often are parallel. Open reduction is usually required to extricate the volar plate from within the joint (Fig. 8-81).[19] A dorsal or volar approach is suitable, with concerns similar to those for irreducible index MCP joint dislocations.[184]

Thumb Metacarpophalangeal Ulnar Collateral Ligament Injury (Gamekeeper's Thumb)

UCL injuries are less prevalent in children than adults. Forced abduction stress at a child's thumb MCP joint results in four

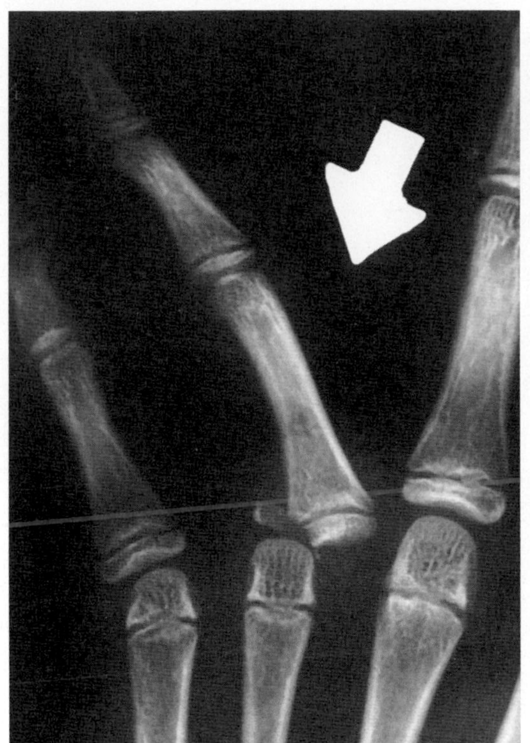
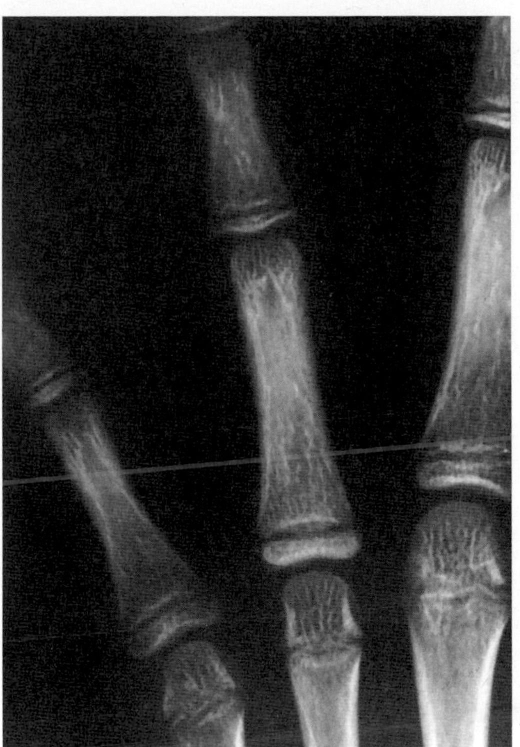

FIGURE 8-78 A. A 9-year-old girl sustained this radial fracture-dislocation of the middle fingers. **B.** Closed reduction restored joint and fracture alignment.

types of injury: (i) a simple sprain of the UCL, (ii) a rupture or avulsion of the insertion or origin of the ligament, (iii) a simple S-H I or II fracture of the proximal physis, or (iv) a S-H III avulsion fracture that involves one fourth to one third of the epiphysis of the proximal phalanx (Figs. 8-82 and 8-83).[128,206]

The injury is most common in preadolescents and adolescents. A history of trauma is customary, especially involving sports. The thumb is swollen about the MCP joint with ecchymosis, and tenderness to palpation is well localized over the UCL. Pain is exacerbated by abduction stress. A complete rupture or displaced fracture lacks a discrete endpoint. Anteroposterior and lateral radiographs are used to diagnosis and delineate fracture configuration. Stress views may be needed if the diagnosis is questionable. MRI can be used to evaluate ligament disruption in complicated injuries.

Cast immobilization for 4 to 6 weeks is adequate for simple sprains, incomplete injuries, and nondisplaced fractures. Complete ruptures or displaced fractures usually require operative intervention. A major concern is displacement of

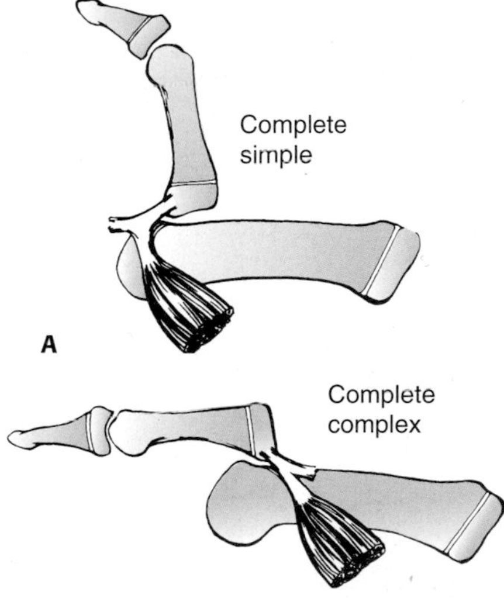

FIGURE 8-79 Simple and complex dorsal dislocations of the thumb MCP joint. Simple dislocations **(A)** are in extension and reducible. Complex dislocations **(B)** are in bayonet apposition and are irreducible because of the interposed volar plate.

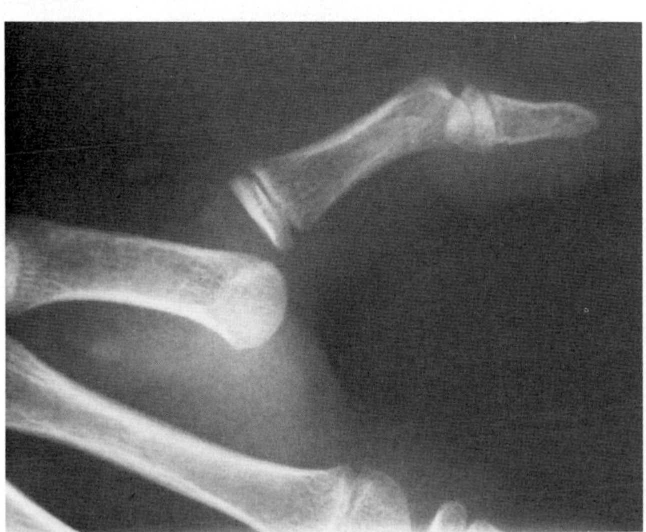

FIGURE 8-80 A 9-year-old boy with a complete simple dorsal dislocation of the thumb MCP joint.

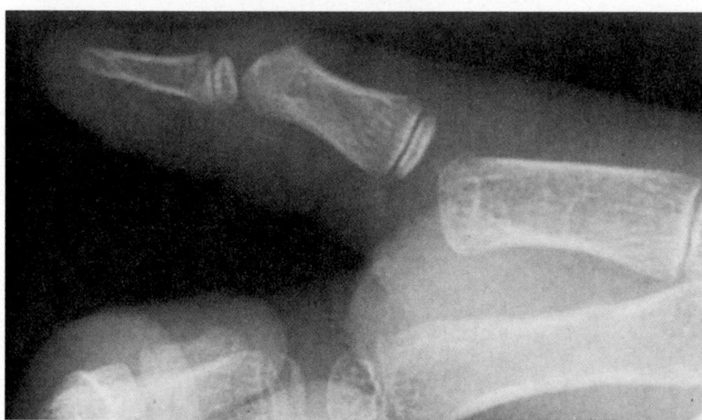

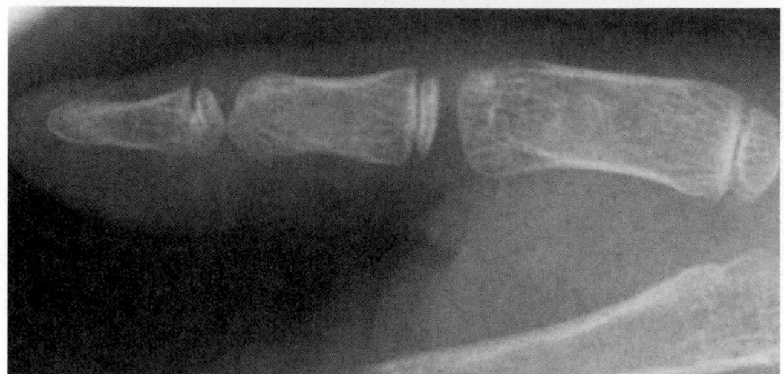

FIGURE 8-81 A. Irreducible dorsal MCP dislocation in a 7-year-old boy. **B.** After open reduction through a volar incision.

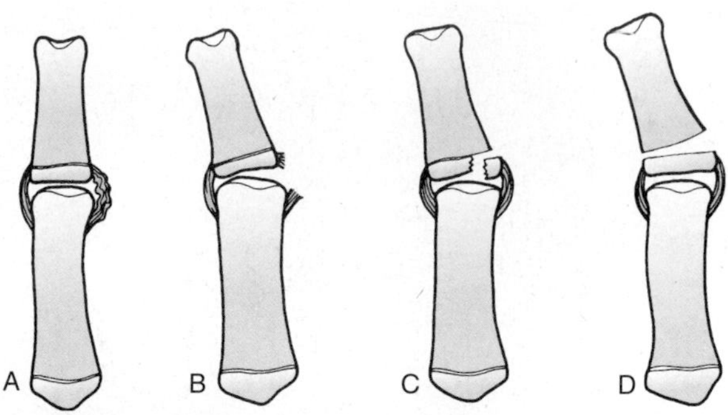

FIGURE 8-82 Ulnar instability of the thumb metacarpal joint. **A.** Simple sprain. **B.** Rupture of the ligament. **C.** Avulsion fracture (S-H type III). **D.** Pseudogamekeeper's injury resulting from a S-H type I or II fracture of the proximal phalanx.

the ligament or fracture fragment behind the adductor aponeurosis, which prohibits healing.[183,184] A S-H III fracture of the ulnar corner of the epiphysis of the proximal phalanx is the most common childhood gamekeeper's injury. A displaced fracture (fragment rotated or displaced more than 1.5 mm) requires open reduction and internal fixation to restore the integrity of the UCL and to obtain a congruous joint surface (Fig. 8-84).

Chronic UCL injuries are more difficult to manage. Treat-

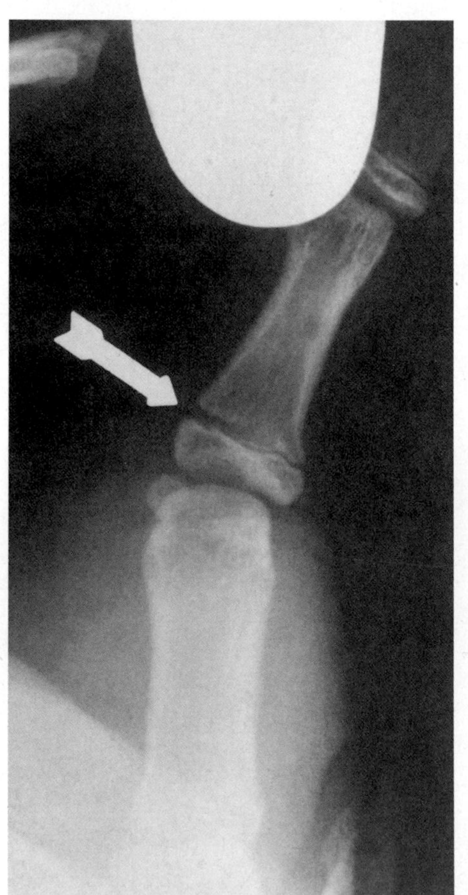

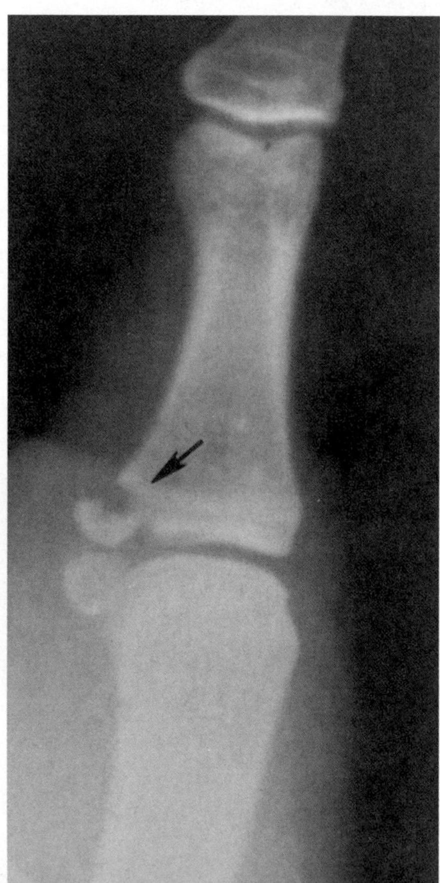

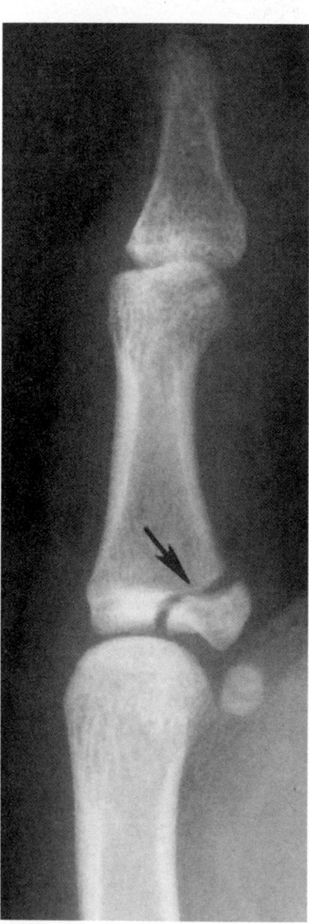

FIGURE 8-83 Spectrum of ulnar collateral ligament injuries of the thumb. **A,B.** On stress examination, a widening of the physis is seen. Varying sizes of fragments **(B,C)** may be associated with ulnar collateral ligament avulsion fractures (*arrows*). The size of the fragment is important with respect to the congruity of the MCP joint.

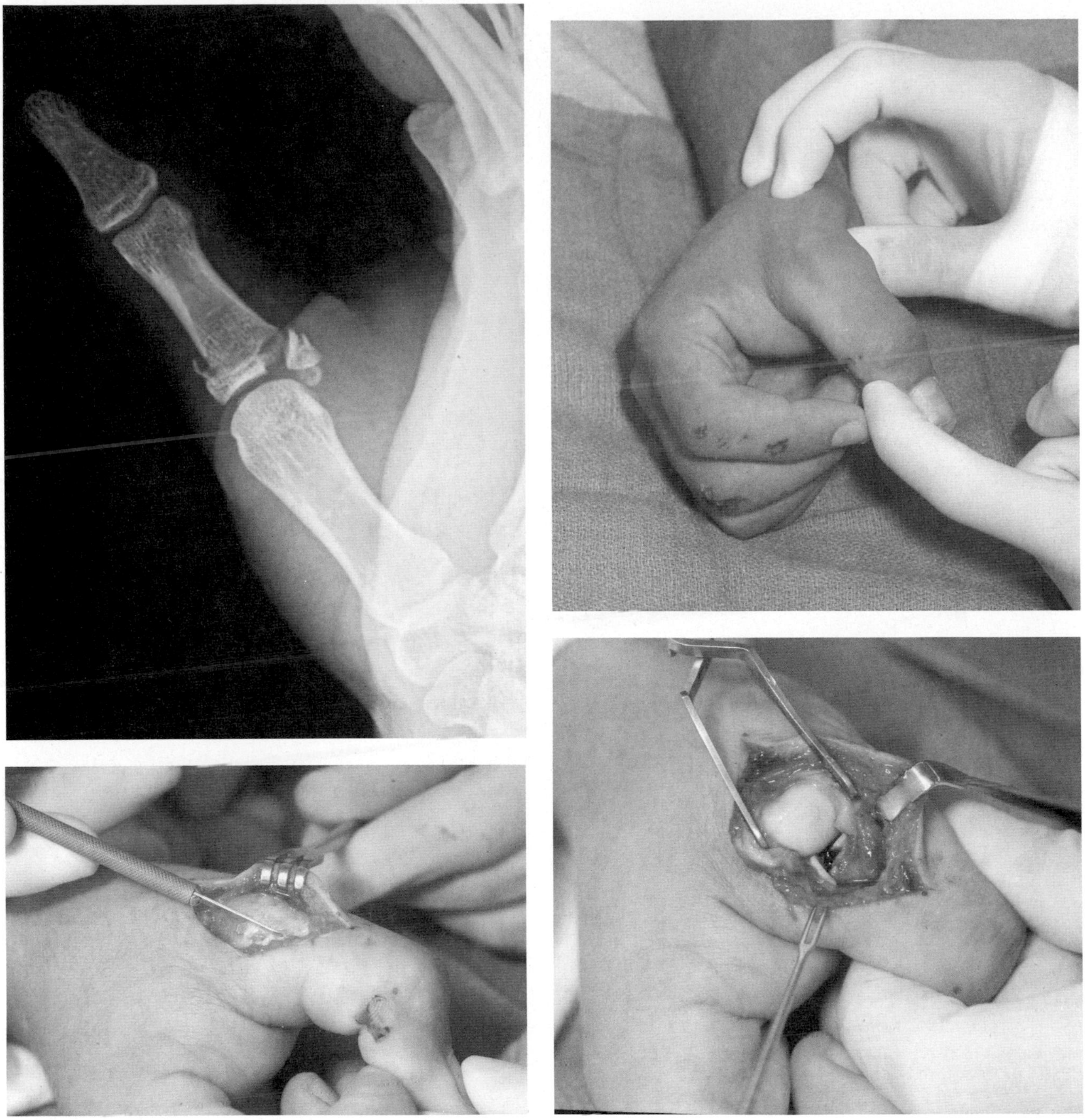

A B C D

FIGURE 8-84 A. A 13-year-old boy with a displaced S-H III fracture of the right thumb proximal phalanx. **B.** Valgus instability on stress testing. **C.** Exposure through an incision of adductor aponeurosis. **D.** Fracture fragment exposed revealing rotation and displacement. *(continues)*

ment depends on the length of time since original injury, age of the patient, and current level of function. Options range from reconstruction to fusion.[174]

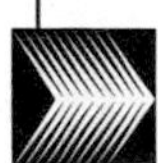

AUTHORS' PREFERRED TREATMENT

The treatment of dorsal MCP joint dislocations of the fingers and thumb should be stepwise and logical. The initial treatment for simple dislocations is usually closed reduction. This requires local anesthesia or conscious sedation to ensure comfort and eliminate resistance. Irreducible dislocations require open reduction. It is important to avoid multiple attempts at closed reduction of an irreducible dislocation. A dorsal or volar approach is used with removal of any interposed structure(s). The volar approach must respect the taut digital nerves overlying the prominent metacarpal head. Postoperative immobilization is used for 7 to 10 days, followed by active motion with splint-protection; athletic activities are restricted until healing is complete.

Ulnar collateral ligament injuries of the thumb are treated according to stability and displacement. Stable ligamentous

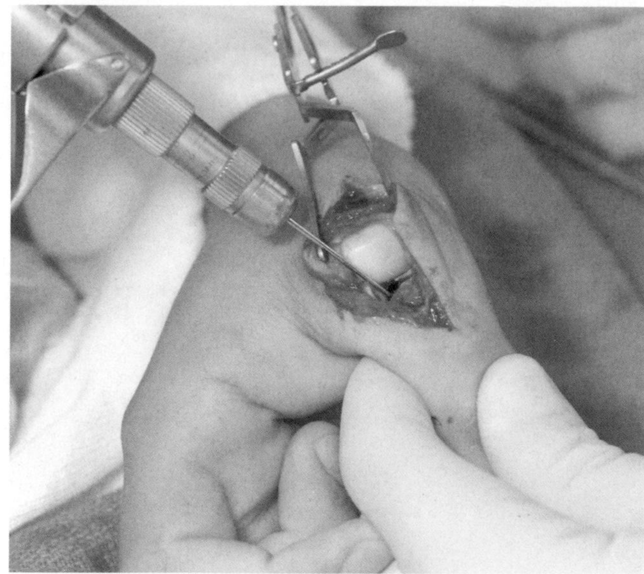

E

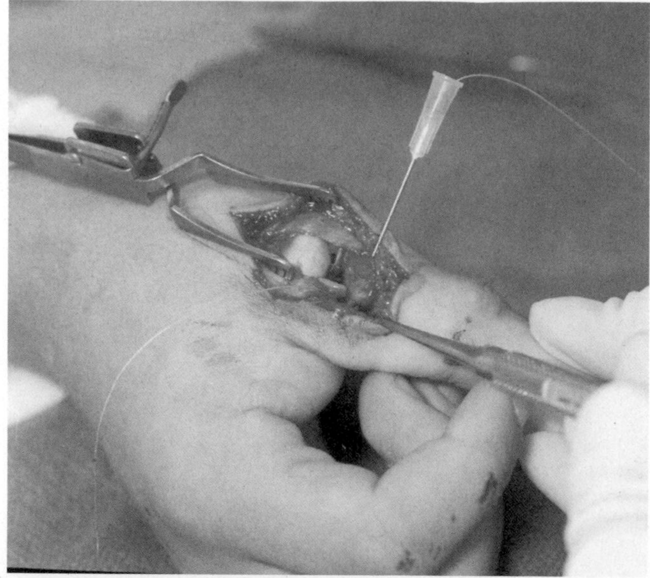

F

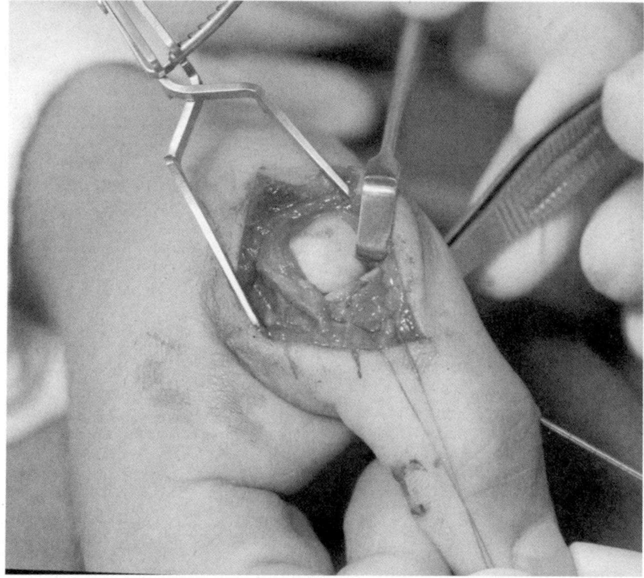

G

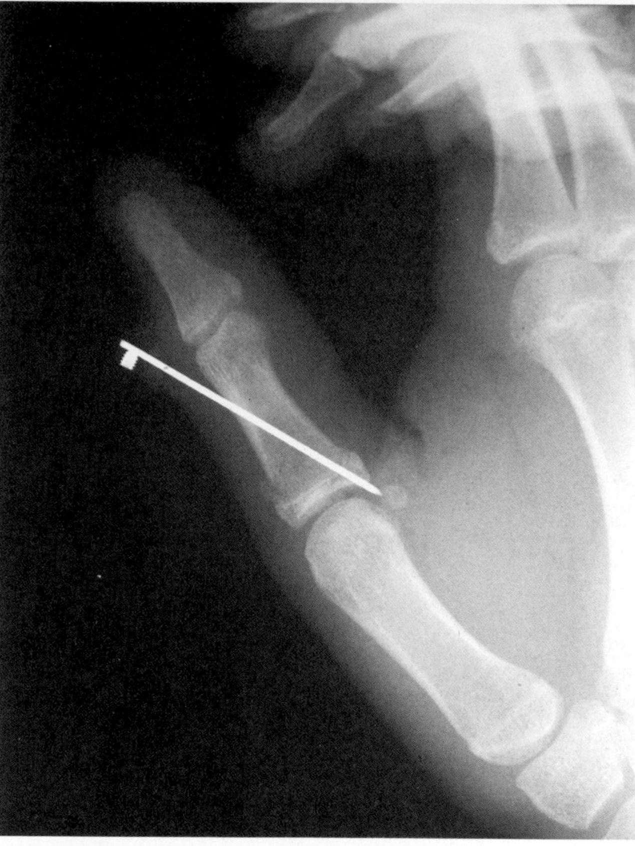

H

FIGURE 8-84 *(continued)* **E.** Antegrade Kirschner wire through fracture site. **F.** Thumb is placed into pronation and suture is passed for tension band fixation. **G.** Fracture reduced, Kirschner wire advanced, and suture tied in a figure-eight fashion. **H.** After tension band fixation with restoration of joint and fracture alignment. (Courtesy of Shriners Hospitals for Children, Philadelphia, PA.)

injuries or minimally displaced fractures are treated with cast immobilization. Unstable ligamentous injuries or displaced fractures are treated with open reduction.

REFERENCES

1. Adolfsson L, Lindau T, Arner M. Acutrak screw fixation versus cast immobilisation for undisplaced scaphoid waist fractures. J Hand Surg Br 2001;26:192–195.
2. Agee JM. Unstable fracture dislocations of the proximal interphalangeal joint of the fingers: a preliminary report of a new treatment technique. J Hand Surg Am 1978;3:386–389.
3. Aggarwal AK, Sangwan SS, Siwach RC. Transscaphoid perilunate dislocation in a child. Contemp Orthop 1993;26:172–174.
4. Al-Qattan MM. Extra-articular transverse fractures of the base of the distal phalanx (Seymour's fracture) in children and adults. J Hand Surg Br 2001;26:201–206.
5. Al-Qattan MM. Juxta-epiphyseal fractures of the base of the proximal phalanx of the fingers in children and adolescents. J Hand Surg Br 2002;27:24–30.
6. Anderson WJ. Simultaneous fracture of the scaphoid and capitate in a child. J Hand Surg Am 1987;12:271–273.
7. Atasoy E, Ioakimidis E, Kasdan ML, et al. Reconstruction of the amputated finger tip with a triangular volar flap. A new surgical procedure. J Bone Joint Surg Am 1970; 52(5):921–926.
8. Baldwin LW, Miller DL, Lockhart LD, et al. Metacarpophalangeal-joint dislocations of the fingers. J Bone Joint Surg Am 1967;49(8):1587–1590.
9. Barenfeld PA, Weseley MS. Dorsal dislocation of the metacarpophalangeal joint of the index finger treated by late open reduction. A case report. J Bone Joint Surg Am 1972; 54-A:1311–1313.
10. Barton NJ. Fractures of the phalanges of the hand in children. Hand 1979;11:134–143.
11. Beatty E, Light TR, Belsole RJ, et al. Wrist and hand skeletal injuries in children. Hand Clin 1990;6(4):723–738.
12. Becton JL, Christian JD Jr, Goodwin HN, et al. A simplified technique for treating the

complex dislocation of the index metacarpophalangeal joint. J Bone Joint Surg Am 1975;57(5):698–700.
13. Bennett EH. Fractures of the metacarpal bones. Dublin J Med Sci 1982;73:72–75.
14. Bhende MS, Dandrea LA, Davis HW. Hand injuries in children presenting to a pediatric emergency department. Ann Emerg Med 1993;22:1519–1523.
15. Blitzer CM, Johnson RJ, Ettlinger CF, et al. Downhill skiing injuries in children. Am J Sports Med 1984;12(2):142–147.
16. Bloem JJ. Fracture of the carpal scaphoid in a child aged 4. Arch Chir Neerl 1971;23: 91–94.
17. Blount WP. Fractures in children. Schweiz Med Wochenschr 1954;84:986–988.
18. Bogumill GP. A morphologic study of the relationship of collateral ligaments to growth plates in the digits. J Hand Surg Am 1983;8:74–79.
19. Bohart PG, Gelberman RH, Vandell RF, et al. Complex dislocations of the metacarpophalangeal joint. Clin Orthop Relat Res 1982(164):208–210.
20. Bond CD, Shin AY, McBride MT, et al. Percutaneous screw fixation or cast immobilization for nondisplaced scaphoid fractures. J Bone Joint Surg Am 2001;83-A(4):483–488.
21. Brighton CT. Clinical problems in epiphyseal plate growth and development. Instr Course Lect 1974;3:105–122.
22. Brydie A, Raby N. Early MRI in the management of clinical scaphoid fracture. Br J Radiol 2003;76:296–300.
23. Buchler U, McCollam SM, Oppikofer C. Comminuted fractures of the basilar joint of the thumb: combined treatment by external fixation, limited internal fixation, and bone grafting. J Hand Surg Am 1991;16(556–560).
24. Burge P. Closed cast treatment of scaphoid fractures. Hand Clin 2001;17:541–552.
25. Butt WD. Rigid wire fixation of fractures of the hand. Henry Ford Hosp Med Bull 1956;4:134–143.
26. Campbell RM Jr. Operative treatment of fractures and dislocations of the hand and wrist region in children. Orthop Clin North Am 1990;21:217–243.
27. Carr D, Johnson RJ, Pope MH. Upper extremity injuries in skiing. Am J Sports Med 1981;12:142–147.
28. Cerezal L, del Pinal F, Abascal F, et al. Imaging findings in ulnar-sided wrist impaction syndromes. Radiographics 2002;22(1):105–121.
29. Chambers RB. Orthopaedic injuries in athletes (ages 6 to 17). Comparison of injuries occurring in six sports. Am J Sports Med 1979;7:195–197.
30. Christodoulou AG, Colton CL. Scaphoid fractures in children. J Pediatr Orthop 1986; 6:37–39.
31. Clayburgh RH, Wood MB, Cooney WP III. Nail bed repair and reconstruction by reverse dermal grafts. J Hand Surg Am 1983;8:594–598.
32. Cobey MC, White RK. An operation for nonunions of the carpal navicular. J Bone Joint Surg 1946;28:757–764.
33. Cockshott WP. Distal avulsion fractures of the scaphoid. Br J Radiol 1980;53: 1037–1040.
34. Compson JP. Transcarpal injuries associated with distal radial fractures in children: a series of three cases. J Hand Surg Br 1992;17:311–314.
35. Cook PA, Yu JS, Wiand W, et al. Suspected scaphoid fractures in skeletally immature patients: application of MRI. J Comput Assist Tomogr 1997;21(4):511–515.
36. Cornwall R, Waters PM. Remodeling of phalangeal neck fracture malunions in children: case report. J Hand Surg Am 2004;29:458–461.
37. Cowen NJ, Kranik AD. An irreducible juxta-epiphyseal fracture of the proximal phalanx. Report of a case. Clin Orthop Relat Res 1975(110):42–44.
38. Crick JC, Franco RS, Conners JJ. Fractures about the interphalangeal joints in children. J Orthop Trauma 1987;1:318–325.
39. Crock HV, Chari PR, Crock MC. The blood supply of the wrist and hand bones in man. In: Tubiana R, ed. The Hand. Philadelphia: W.B. Saunders, 1981, 335–347.
40. Cullen JC. Thiemann disease. Osteochondrosis juvenilis of the basal epiphyses of the phalanges of the hand. Report of two cases. J Bone Joint Surg Br 1970;52:532–534.
41. D'Arienzo M. Scaphoid fractures in children. J Hand Surg Br 2002;27(5):424–426.
42. DaCruz DJ, Slade RJ, Malone W. Fractures of the distal phalanges. J Hand Surg Am 1988;13:350–352.
43. De Boeck H, Jaeken R. Treatment of chronic mallet finger deformity in children by tenodermodesis. J Pediatr Orthop 1992;12:351–354.
44. De Boeck H, Van Wellen P, Haentjens P. Nonunion of a carpal scaphoid fracture in a child. A case report. J Orthop Trauma 1991;5:370–372.
45. de Iturriza JR, Tanner JM. Cone-shaped epiphyses and other minor anomalies in the hands of normal British children. J Pediatr 1969;75:265–272.
46. Dixon GL Jr, Moon NF. Rotational supracondylar fractures of the proximal phalanx in children. Clin Orthop Relat Res 1972;83:151–156.
47. Doman AN, Marcus NW. Congenital bipartite scaphoid. J Hand Surg Am 1990;15: 869–873.
48. Dorsay TA, Major NM, Helms CA. Cost-effectiveness of immediate MR imaging versus traditional follow-up for revealing radiographically occult scaphoid fractures. AJR Am J Roentgenol 2001;177:1257–1263.
49. Dykes RG. Kirner deformity of the little finger. J Bone Joint Surg Br 1978;60:58–60.
50. Earp BE, Waters PM, Wyzykowski RJ. Arthroscopic treatment of partial scapholunate ligament tears in children with chronic wrist pain. J Bone Joint Surg Am 2006;88(11): 2448–2455.
51. Ebinger T, Roesch M, Wachter N, et al. Functional treatment of physeal and periphyseal injuries of the metacarpal and proximal phalangeal bones. J Pediatr Surg 2001;36(4): 611–615.
52. Elhassen BT, Shin AY, Kozin SH. Scaphoid fractures in children. In: Shin AY, ed. Scaphoid Fractures. Rosemont, IL: American Academy of Orthopaedic Surgeons Monograph Series; 2007:85–95.
53. Elson RA. Rupture of the central slip of the extensor hood of the finger. A test for early diagnosis. J Bone Joint Surg Br 1986;68:229–231.
54. Ersek RA, Gadaria U, Denton DR. Nail bed avulsions treated with porcine xenografts. J Hand Surg Am 1985;10:152–153.
55. Fabre O, De Boeck H, Haentjens P. Fractures and nonunions of the carpal scaphoid in children. Acta Orthop Belg 2001;67(2):121–125.
56. Fischer MD, McElfresh EC. Physeal and periphyseal injuries of the hand. Patterns of injury and results of treatment. Hand Clin 1994;10:287–301.
57. Foucher G. "Bouquet" osteosynthesis in metacarpal neck fractures: a series of 66 patients. J Hand Surg Am 1995;20:S86–S90.
58. Gamble JG, Simmons SC III. Bilateral scaphoid fractures in a child. Clin Orthop Relat Res 1982;162:125–128.
59. Garrick JG, Requa RK. Injuries in high school sports. Pediatrics 1978;61:465–469.
60. Garroway RY, Hurst LC, Leppard J, et al. Complex dislocations of the PIP joint. A pathoanatomic classification of the injury. Orthop Rev 1984;13:21–28.
61. Gedda KO. Studies in Bennett fracture: anatomy, roentgenology, and therapy. Acta Chir Scand Suppl 1954;193:1–114.
62. Gellman H, Caputo RJ, Carter V, et al. Comparison of short and long thumb-spica casts for nondisplaced fractures of the carpal scaphoid. J Bone Joint Surg Am 1989; 71(3):354–357.
63. Gerard FM. Posttraumatic carpal instability in a young child. A case report. J Bone Joint Surg Am 1980;62(1):131–133.
64. Giddins GE, Shaw DG. Lunate subluxation associated with a Salter-Harris type 2 fracture of the distal radius. J Hand Surg Br 1994;19:193–194.
65. Gilbert A. Dislocation of the MCP joints in children. In: Tubiana R, ed. The Hand. Philadelphia: W.B. Saunders, 1985, 922–925.
66. Goldberg B, Rosenthal PP, Robertson LS, et al. Injuries in youth football. Pediatrics 1988;81(2):255–261.
67. Gollamudi S, Jones WA. Corrective osteotomy of malunited fractures of phalanges and metacarpals. J Hand Surg Br 2000;25:439–441.
68. Gonzalez MH, Igram CM, Hall RF Jr. Flexible intramedullary nailing for metacarpal fractures. J Hand Surg Am 1995;20(3):382–387.
69. Goulding A, Jones IE, Taylor RW, et al. Dynamic and static tests of balance and postural sway in boys: effects of previous wrist bone fractures and high adiposity. Gait Posture 2003;17(2):136–141.
70. Grad JB. Children's skeletal injuries. Orthop Clin North Am 1986;17:437–449.
71. Green DP. Hand injuries in children. Pediatr Clin North Am 1977;24:903–918.
72. Green DP, Anderson JR. Closed reduction and percutaneous pin fixation of fractured phalanges. J Bone Joint Surg Am 1973;55(8):1651–1654.
73. Green DP, Terry GC. Complex dislocation of the metacarpophalangeal joint. Correlative pathological anatomy. J Bone Joint Surg Am 1973;55:1480–1486.
74. Green MH, Hadied AM, LaMont RL. Scaphoid fractures in children. J Hand Surg Am 1984;9:536–541.
75. Greulich WW, Pyle SI. Radiographic Atlas of Skeletal Development of the Hand and Wrist. Stanford, CA: Stanford University Press; 1959.
76. Griffiths JC. Bennett fracture in childhood. Brit J Clin Pract 1966;20:582–583.
77. Haims AH, Schweitzer ME, Morrison WB, et al. Limitations of MR imaging in the diagnosis of peripheral tears of the triangular fibrocartilage of the wrist. AJR Am J Roentgenol 2002;178(2):419–422.
78. Haines RW. The pseudoepiphysis of the first metacarpal of man. J Anat 1974;117: 145–158.
79. Hakstian RW. Cold-induced digital epiphyseal necrosis in childhood (symmetric focal ischemic necrosis). Can J Surg 1972;15:168–178.
80. Hamas RS, Horrell ED, Pierret GP. Treatment of mallet finger due to intra-articular fracture of the distal phalanx. J Hand Surg Am 1978;3:361–363.
81. Hambidge JE, Desai VV, Schranz PJ, et al. Acute fractures of the scaphoid. Treatment by cast immobilisation with the wrist in flexion or extension? J Bone Joint Surg Br 1999;81(1):91–92.
82. Hankin FM, Janda DH. Tendon and ligament attachments in relationship to growth plate in a child's hand. J Hand Surg Br 1989;14:315–318.
83. Harryman DT II, Jordan TF III. Physeal phalangeal fracture with flexor tendon entrapment. A case report and review of the literature. Clin Orthop Relat Res 1990;250: 194–196.
84. Hastings H II, Simmons BP. Hand fractures in children. A statistical analysis. Clin Orthop Relat Res 1984;188:120–130.
85. Hennrikus WL, Cohen MR. Complete remodeling of displaced fractures of the neck of the phalanx. J Bone Joint Surg Br 2003;85:273–274.
86. Herbert TJ. Use of the Herbert bone screw in surgery of the wrist. Clin Orthop Relat Res 1986;202:79–92.
87. Herbert TJ, Fisher WE. Management of the fractured scaphoid using a new bone screw. J Bone Joint Surg Br 1984;66-B:114–123.
88. Hildebrand KA, Ross DC, Patterson SD, et al. Dorsal perilunate dislocations and fracture-dislocations: questionnaire, clinical, and radiographic evaluation. J Hand Surg Am 2000;25(6):1069–1079.
89. Horii E, Nakamura R, Watanabe K. Scaphoid fracture as a "puncher's fracture." J Orthop Trauma 1994;8:107–110.
90. Horton TC, Hatton M, Davis TR. A prospective, randomized controlled study of fixation of long oblique and spiral shaft fractures of the proximal phalanx: closed reduction and percutaneous Kirschner-wiring versus open reduction and lag screw fixation. J Hand Surg Br 2003;28:5–9.
91. Hunt JC, Watts HB, Glasgow JD. Dorsal dislocation of the metacarpophalangeal joint of the index finger with particular reference to open dislocation. J Bone Joint Surg Am 1967;49(8):1572–1578.
92. Ireland ML, Taleisnik J. Nonunion of metacarpal extraarticular fractures in children: report of two cases and review of the literature. J Pediatr Orthop 1986;6(3):352–355.
93. Jahss SA. Fractures of the metacarpals: a new method of reduction and immobilization. J Bone Joint Surg 1938;20:178–186.
94. Johnson KJ, Haigh SF, Symonds KE. MRI in the management of scaphoid fractures in skeletally immature patients. Pediatr Radiol 2000;30(10):685–688.
95. Jones NF, Jupiter JB. Irreducible palmar dislocation of the proximal interphalangeal joint associated with an epiphyseal fracture of the middle phalanx. J Hand Surg Am 1985;10:261–264.
96. Kaawach W, Ecklund K, Di Canzio J, et al. Normal ranges of scapholunate distance in children 6 to 14 years old. J Pediatr Orthop 2001;21(4):464–467.
97. Kaplan EB. Dorsal dislocation of the metacarpophalangeal joint of the index finger. J Bone Joint Surg Am 1957;39-A(5):1081–1086.
98. Kappel DA, Burech JG. The cross-finger flap. An established reconstructive procedure. Hand Clin 1985;1:677–683.
99. Kardestuncer T, Bae DS, Waters PM. The results of tenodermodesis for severe chronic mallet finger deformity in children. J Pediatr Orthop 2008;28(1):81–85.
100. Kiefhaber TR, Stern PJ. Fracture dislocations of the proximal interphalangeal joint. J Hand Surg Am 1989;23:368–380.

101. Kirner J. Doppelseitige verdrummung des kleinfingr-grundgleides als selbstandiges krankheitsbild. Fortschr Geb Rontgenstr 1927;36:804.
102. Kleinman WB, Bowers WH. Fractures and ligamentous injuries to the hand. In: Bora FW Jr, ed. The Pediatric Upper Extremity: Diagnosis and management. Philadelphia, PA: W.B. Saunders, 1988.
103. Koshima I, Soeda S, Takase T, et al. Free vascularized nail grafts. J Hand Surg Am 1988;13(1):29–32.
104. Lane CS. Detecting occult fractures of the metacarpal head: the Brewerton view. J Hand Surg Am 1977;2:131–133.
105. Larson B, Light TR, Ogden JA. Fracture and ischemic necrosis of the immature scaphoid. J Hand Surg Am 1987;12:122–127.
106. Leddy JP, Packer JW. Avulsion of the profundus tendon insertion in athletes. J Hand Surg Am 1977;2:66–69.
107. Leicht P, Mikkelsen JB, Larsen CF. Scapholunate distance in children. Acta Radiol 1996;37(5):625–626.
108. Leonard MH, Dubravcik P. Management of fractured fingers in the child. Clin Orthop Relat Res 1970;73:160–168.
109. Light TR. Injury to the immature carpus. Hand Clin 1988;4(3):415–424.
110. Light TR, Ogden JA. Complex dislocation of the index metacarpophalangeal joint in children. J Pediatr Orthop 1988;8:300–305.
111. Light TR, Ogden JA. Metacarpal epiphyseal fractures. J Hand Surg Am 1987;12: 460–464.
112. Lipscomb PR, Janes JM. Twenty-year follow-up of an unreduced dislocation of the first metacarpophalangeal joint in a child. Report of a case. J Bone Joint Surg Am 1969; 51(6):1216–1218.
113. Littlefield WG, Friedman RL, Urbaniak JR. Bilateral nonunion of the carpal scaphoid in a child. A case report. J Bone Joint Surg Am 1995;77(1):124–126.
114. Louis DS, Calhoun TP, Garn SM, et al. Congenital bipartite scaphoid—fact or fiction? J Bone Joint Surg Am 1976;58(8):1108–1112.
115. Mack GR, Bosse MJ, Gelberman RH, et al. The natural history of scaphoid nonunion. J Bone Joint Surg Am 1984;66(4):504–509.
116. Mack MG, Keim S, Balzer JO, et al. Clinical impact of MRI in acute wrist fractures. European Radiol 2003;13(3):612–617.
117. Mahabir RC, Kazemi AR, Cannon WG, et al. Pediatric hand fractures: a review. Pediatr Emerg Care 2001;17(3):153–156.
118. Markiewitz AD, Andrish JT. Hand and wrist injuries in the preadolescent and adolescent athlete. Clin Sports Med 1992;11:203–225.
119. Matsumoto K, Sumi H, Sumi Y, et al. Wrist fractures from snowboarding: a prospective study for three seasons from 1998 to 2001. Clin J Sport Med 2004;14(2):64–71.
120. Maxted MJ, Owen R. Two cases of nonunion of carpal scaphoid fractures in children. Injury 1982;13:441–443.
121. Mayfield JK, Johnson RP, Kilcoyne RK. Carpal dislocations: pathomechanics and progressive perilunar instability. J Hand Surg Am 1980;5:226–241.
122. McElfresh EC, Dobyns JH. Intra-articular metacarpal head fractures. J Hand Surg Am 1983;8:383–393.
123. McLaughlin HL. Complex "locked" dislocation of the metacarpophalangeal joints. J Trauma 1965;5:683–688.
124. Melone CP Jr, Grad JB. Primary care of fingernail injuries. Emerg Med Clin North Am 1985;3:255–261.
125. Michelinakis E, Vourexaki H. Displaced epiphyseal plate of the terminal phalanx in a child. Hand 1980;12:51–53.
126. Minami M, Yamazaki J, Chisaka N, et al. Nonunion of the capitate. J Hand Surg Am 1987;12(6):1089–1091.
127. Mintzer CM, Waters PM. Acute open reduction of a displaced scaphoid fracture in a child. J Hand Surg Am 1994;19:760–761.
128. Mintzer CM, Waters PM. Late presentation of a ligamentous ulnar collateral ligament injury in a child. J Hand Surg Am 1994;19:1048–1049.
129. Mintzer CM, Waters PM. Surgical treatment of pediatric scaphoid fracture nonunions. J Pediatr Orthop 1999;19:236–239.
130. Mintzer CM, Waters PM, Brown DJ. Remodelling of a displaced phalangeal neck fracture. J Hand Surg Br 1994;19:594–596.
131. Mizuta T, Benson WM, Foster BK, et al. Statistical analysis of the incidence of physeal injuries. J Pediatr Orthop 1987;7(5):518–523.
132. Moberg E. Aspects of sensation in reconstructive surgery of the upper extremity. J Bone Joint Surg Am 1964;46:817–825.
133. Moen CT, Pelker RR. Biomechanical and histological correlations in growth plate failure. J Pediatr Orthop 1984;4(2):180–184.
134. Muramatsu K, Doi K, Kuwata N, et al. Scaphoid fracture in the young athlete—therapeutic outcome of internal fixation using the Herbert screw. Arch Orthop Trauma Surg 2002;122(9–10):510–513.
135. Murphy AF, Stark HH. Closed dislocation of the metacarpophalangeal joint of the index finger. J Bone Joint Surg Am 1967;49(8):1579–1586.
136. Nafie SA. Fractures of the carpal bones in children. Injury 1987;18:117–119.
137. Nakamura R. Diagnosis of ulnar wrist pain. Nagoya J Med Sci 2001;64:81–91.
138. Nakazato T, Ogino T. Epiphyseal destruction of children's hands after frostbite: a report of two cases. J Hand Surg Am 1986;11:289–292.
139. Nussbaum R, Sadler AH. An isolated, closed, complex dislocation of the metacarpophalangeal joint of the long finger: a unique case. J Hand Surg Am 1986;11:558–561.
140. Ogden JA. Skeletal Injury in the Child. Philadelphia, PA: W.B. Saunders, 1990.
141. Onuba O, Ireland J. Two cases of nonunion of fractures of the scaphoid in children. Injury 1983;15:109–112.
142. Palmer AK. Triangular fibrocartilage complex lesions: a classification. J Hand Surg Am 1989;14:594–606.
143. Palmer AK, Linscheid RL. Irreducible dorsal dislocation of the distal interphalangeal joint of the finger. J Hand Surg Am 1977;2:406–408.
144. Palmer AK, Werner FW. The triangular fibrocartilage complex of the wrist-anatomy and function. J Hand Surg Am 1981;6.
145. Peimer CA, Sullivan DJ, Wild DR. Palmar dislocation of the proximal interphalangeal joint. J Hand Surg Am 1984;9:39–48.
146. Peiro A, Martos F, Mut T, et al. Transscaphoid perilunate dislocation in a child. A case report. Acta Orthop Scand 1981;52(1):31–34.
147. Pennes DR, Braunstein EM, Shirazi KK. Carpal ligamentous laxity with bilateral perilunate dislocation in Marfan syndrome. Skeletal Radiol 1985;13:62–64.
148. Perron AD, Brady WJ, Keats TE, et al. Orthopedic pitfalls in the ED: scaphoid fracture. Am J Emerg Med 2001;19(4):310–316.
149. Pick RY, Segal D. Carpal scaphoid fracture and nonunion in an 8-year-old child. Report of a case. J Bone Joint Surg Am 1983;65(8):1188–1189.
150. Pohl AL. Irreducible dislocation of a distal interphalangeal joint. Br J Plast Surg 1976; 29:227–229.
151. Prosser AJ, Irvine GB. Epiphyseal fracture of the metacarpal head. Injury 1988;19: 34–35.
152. Rajesh A, Basu AK, Vaidhyanath R, et al. Hand fractures: a study of their site and type in childhood. Clin Radiol 2001;56(8):667–669.
153. Rang M. Children's Fractures. Philadelphia, PA: J.B. Lippincott, 1983.
154. Rasmussen F, Schantz K. Lunatomalacia in a child. Acta Orthop Scand 1987;58:82–84.
155. Rayan GM, Mullins PT. Skin necrosis complicating mallet finger splinting and vascularity of the distal interphalangeal joint overlying skin. J Hand Surg Am 1987;12:548–552.
156. Rettig ME, Raskin KB. Retrograde compression screw fixation of acute proximal pole scaphoid fractures. J Hand Surg Am 1999;24:1206–1210.
157. Robins RH. Injuries of the metacarpophalangeal joints. Hand 1971;3:159–163.
158. Roser LA, Clawson DK. Football injuries in the very young athlete. Clin Orthop Relat Res 1970;69:219–223.
159. Roy S, Caine D, Singer KM. Stress changes of the distal radial epiphysis in young gymnasts. A report of 21 cases and a review of the literature. Am J Sports Med 1985; 13:301–308.
160. Salamon PB, Gelberman RH. Irreducible dislocation of the interphalangeal joint of the thumb. J Bone Joint Surg Am 1978;60(3):400–401.
161. Sanders WE. Evaluation of the humpback scaphoid by computed tomography in the longitudinal axial plane of the scaphoid. J Hand Surg Am 1988;13:182–187.
162. Sandzen SC. Fracture of the fifth metacarpal resembling Bennett fracture. Hand 1973; 5:49–51.
163. Sandzen SC, Oakey RS. Crushing injury of the fingertip. Hand 1972;4:253–256.
164. Savage R. Complete detachment of the epiphysis of the distal phalanx. J Hand Surg Br 1990;15:126–128.
165. Schantz K, Rasmussen F. Thiemann finger or toe disease. Follow-up of seven cases. Acta Orthop Scand 1986;57:91–93.
166. Schenck RR. Dynamic traction and early passive movement for fractures of the proximal interphalangeal joint. J Hand Surg Am 1986;11:850–858.
167. Segmuller G, Schonenberger F. Treatment of fractures in children and adolescents. In: Weber BG, Brunner C, Freuler F, eds. Fracture of the Hand. New York: Springer-Verlag, 1980:218–225.
168. Selig S, Schein A. Irreducible buttonhole dislocations of the fingers. J Bone Joint Surg Br 1940;22:436–441.
169. Seymour N. Juxta-epiphysial fracture of the terminal phalanx of the finger. J Bone Joint Surg Br 1966;48:347–349.
170. Shepard GH. Nail grafts for reconstruction. Hand Clin 1990;6:79–102.
171. Shibata M, Seki T, Yoshizu T, et al. Microsurgical toenail transfer to the hand. Plast Reconstr Surg 1991;88(1):102–109; discussion 110.
172. Simmons BP, Lovallo JL. Hand and wrist injuries in children. Clin Sports Med 1988; 7:495–512.
173. Simmons BP, Peters TT. Subcondylar fossa reconstruction for malunion of fractures of the proximal phalanx in children. J Hand Surg Am 1987;12(6):1079–1082.
174. Simmons BP, Stirrat CR. Treatment of traumatic arthritis in children. Hand Clin 1987; 3:611–627.
175. Slade JF III, Geissler WB, Gutow AP, et al. Percutaneous internal fixation of selected scaphoid nonunions with an arthroscopically assisted dorsal approach. J Bone Joint Surg Am 2003;85-A(Suppl 4):20–32.
176. Smith DG, Geist RW, Cooperman DR. Microscopic examination of a naturally occurring epiphyseal plate fracture. J Pediatr Orthop 1985;5(3):306–308.
177. Southcott R, Rosman MA. Nonunion of carpal scaphoid fractures in children. J Bone Joint Surg Br 1977;59:20–23.
178. Spanberg O, Thoren L. Bennett fracture: a new method of treatment with oblique traction. J Bone Joint Surg Br 1963;45:732–736.
179. Stahl S, Jupiter JB. Salter-Harris type II and IV epiphyseal fractures in the hand treated with tension-band wiring. J Pediatr Orthop 1999;19:233–235.
180. Stanciu C, Dumont A. Changing patterns of scaphoid fractures in adolescents. Can J Surg 1994;37(3):214–216.
181. Stein F. Skeletal injuries of the hand in children. Clin Plast Surg 1981;8:65–81.
182. Steinmann SP, Bishop AT, Berger RA. Use of the 1, 2 intercompartmental supraretinacular artery as a vascularized pedicle bone graft for difficult scaphoid nonunion. J Hand Surg Am 2002;27:391–401.
183. Stener B. Displacement of the ruptured ulnar collateral ligament of the MCP joint of the thumb. A clinical and anatomical study. J Bone Joint Surg Br 1962;44:869–879.
184. Stener B. Hyperextension injuries to the metacarpophalangeal joint of the thumb: rupture of ligaments, fracture of sesamoid bones, rupture of flexor pollicis brevis. An anatomical and clinical study. Acta Chir Scand 1963;125:275–293.
185. Stern PJ, Roman RJ, Kiefhaber TR, et al. Pilon fractures of the proximal interphalangeal joint. J Hand Surg Am 1991;16(5):844–850.
186. Strickler M, Nagy L, Buchler U. Rigid internal fixation of basilar fractures of the proximal phalanges by cancellous bone grafting only. J Hand Surg Br 2001;26:455–458.
187. Stripling WD. Displaced intra-articular osteochondral fracture. Cause for irreducible dislocation of the distal interphalangeal joint. J Hand Surg Am 1982;7:77–78.
188. Stuart HC, Pyle SI, Cornoni J, et al. Onsets, completions, and spans of ossification in the 29 bonegrowth centers of the hand and wrist. Pediatrics 1962;29:237–249.
189. Teoh LC, Yong FC, Chong KC. Condylar advancement osteotomy for correcting condylar malunion of the finger. J Hand Surg Br 2002;27:31–35.
190. Terry CL, Waters PM. Triangular fibrocartilage injuries in pediatric and adolescent patients. J Hand Surg Am 1998;23:626–634.
191. Thompson JS, Eaton RG. Volar dislocation of the PIP joint. J Hand Surg Am 1977;2: 232.
192. Thompson JS, Littler JW, Upton J. The spiral oblique retinacular ligament (SORL). J Hand Surg Am 1978;3:482–487.
193. Toh S, Miura H, Arai K, et al. Scaphoid fractures in children: problems and treatment. J Pediatr Orthop 2003;23(2):216–221.
194. Torre BA. Epiphyseal injuries in the small joints of the hand. Hand Clin 1988;4: 113–121.

195. Vahvanen V, Westerlund M. Fracture of the carpal scaphoid in children. A clinical and roentgenological study of 108 cases. Acta Orthop Scand 1980;51(6):909–913.
196. Valencia J, Leyva F, Gomez-Bajo GJ. Pediatric hand trauma. Clin Orthop Relat Res 2005;432:77–86.
197. Vance RM, Gelberman RH, Evans EF. Scaphocapitate fractures. Patterns of dislocation, mechanisms of injury, and preliminary results of treatment. J Bone Joint Surg Am 1980;62(2):271–276.
198. Wakeley CPG. Bilateral epiphysis at the basal end of the second metacarpal. J Anat 1974;58:340–345.
199. Waters PM, Benson LS. Dislocation of the distal phalanx epiphysis in toddlers. J Hand Surg Am 1993;18(4):581–585.
200. Waters PM, Stewart SL. Surgical treatment of nonunion and avascular necrosis of the proximal part of the scaphoid in adolescents. J Bone Joint Surg Am 2002;84-A(6): 915–920.
201. Waters PM, Taylor BA, Kuo AY. Percutaneous reduction of incipient malunion of phalangeal neck fractures in children. J Hand Surg Am 2004;29:707–711.
202. Watson HK, Ballet FL. The SLAC wrist: scapholunate advanced collapse pattern of degenerative arthritis. J Hand Surg Am 1984;9:358–365.
203. Weber ER, Chao EY. An experimental approach to the mechanism of scaphoid waist fractures. J Hand Surg Am 1978;3:142–148.
204. Weiker GG. Hand and wrist problems in the gymnast. Clin Sports Med 1992;11: 189–202.
205. Wenger DR. Avulsion of the profundus tendon insertion in football players. Arch Surg 1973;106:145–149.
206. White GM. Ligamentous avulsion of the ulnar collateral ligament of the thumb of a child. J Hand Surg Am 1986;11:669–672.
207. Wood VE. Fractures of the hand in children. Orthop Clin North Am 1976;7:527–542.
208. Wood VE, Hannah JD, Stilson W. What happens to the double epiphysis in the hand? J Hand Surg Am 1994;19:353–360.
209. Worlock PH, Stower MJ. Fracture patterns in Nottingham children. J Pediatr Orthop 1986;6:656–660.
210. Worlock PH, Stower MJ. The incidence and pattern of hand fractures in children. J Hand Surg Br 1986;11:198–200.
211. Yip HS, Wu WC, Chang RY, et al. Percutaneous cannulated screw fixation of acute scaphoid waist fracture. J Hand Surg Br 2002;27(1):42–46.
212. Zaricznyj B, Shattuck LJ, Mast TA, et al. Sports-related injuries in school-aged children. Am J Sports Med 1980;8(5):318–324.
213. Zook EG, Guy RJ, Russell RC. A study of nail bed injuries: causes, treatment, and prognosis. J Hand Surg Am 1984;9:247–252.
214. Zook EG, Russell RC. Reconstruction of a functional and esthetic nail. Hand Clin 1990; 6:59–68.

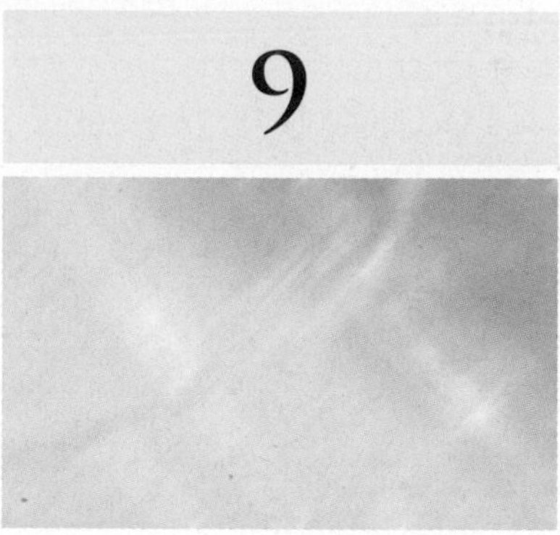

9

FRACTURES OF THE DISTAL RADIUS AND ULNA

Peter M. Waters and Donald S. Bae

INTRODUCTION 292

PRINCIPLES OF MANAGEMENT 292
Mechanism of Injury 292
Signs and Symptoms 293
Associated Injuries 293
Diagnosis and Classification 293

SURGICAL AND APPLIED ANATOMY 294

PHYSEAL INJURIES 294
Diagnosis 294
Current Treatment Options 296

RADIAL PHYSEAL STRESS FRACTURES 312

ULNAR PHYSEAL FRACTURES 313
Current Treatment Options 313

ULNAR STYLOID FRACTURES 313
Complications 314

METAPHYSEAL FRACTURES 316
Mechanism of Injury 317
Signs and Symptoms 318
Associated Injuries 318
Diagnosis and Classification 318
Current Treatment Options 319

COMPLETE FRACTURES 322
Reduction Techniques 323
Complications 331

PEDIATRIC GALEAZZI FRACTURES 338
Mechanism of Injury 338
Signs and Symptoms 339
Classification 339
Anatomy 339
Current Treatment Options 340
Complications 343

INTRODUCTION

Forearm fractures are the most common long bone fractures in children, comprising about 40% of all pediatric fractures.[118,123,222] The distal aspect of the radius and ulna is the most common site of fracture in the forearm.[27,102,118,184,248] These fractures have been reported to be three times more common in boys; however, the increased participation in athletics by girls at a young age may be changing this ratio. Although these fractures occur at any age, they are most frequent during the adolescent growth spurt.[10,103] The fractures are described by location, metaphyseal or physeal, and by severity of displacement. The pediatric Galeazzi injury usually involves a distal radial metaphyseal fracture and a distal ulnar physeal fracture that result in a displaced distal radioulnar joint. These injuries are rare, but need to be identified acutely for proper management. The specifics of fracture patterns for individual fracture types are discussed in separate sections of this chapter. Most of these injuries have traditionally been treated with closed reduction and cast immobilization. Indications for percutaneous pinning and open reduction in pediatric patients are evolving and are discussed in each section.

PRINCIPLES OF MANAGEMENT

Mechanism of Injury

A direct fall is the usual mechanism of injury. With the wrist and hand extended, a fracture occurs if the mechanical force is sufficient. Usually, this is secondary to a sporting event. Snowboarding, skateboarding, soccer goal-keeping, and horseback riding have been shown to be high-risk sports,[19,114,116,138,187,196,197,231] but a severe enough fall in any recreational activity can lead to a fracture. There is seasonal variation, with an increase in both incidence and severity of fractures in summer.[234] Children who are overweight have poor postural balance, ligamentous laxity, or less bone mineralization, and are at increased risk for distal radial fractures.[58,82–84,131,155,176,204] The fractures generally occur with an extension deformity because of the mechanism of a fall on an outstretched hand. Occasionally, a direct blow or a fall onto a flexed wrist and hand causes volar displacement or angulation of the distal fragment. In either case, there may be a rotational component to the fracture pattern.

Repetitive loading of the wrist can lead to physeal stress injuries of the distal radius and, less commonly, the ulna. These injuries are rare and occur most frequently in gymnasts.[5,23,43,51,141,191,223] Any patient with chronic physeal region wrist pain who participates in an activity with repetitive axial loading of the wrist, such as gymnastics or break dancing,[79] should be examined for a stress injury.

Signs and Symptoms

Regardless of the type, these fractures cause pain in the distal forearm, tenderness directly over the fracture site, and limited motion of the forearm, wrist, and hand. Deformity depends on the degree of fracture displacement. Fractures with marked extension displacement can lead to a silver fork deformity similar to an adult Colles fracture. Standard anteroposterior (AP) and lateral radiographs are diagnostic of fracture type and displacement. Metaphyseal fractures are most common, followed by physeal fractures[74,146,222]; the distal fragment in either usually is extended. Neurovascular examination should be performed before treatment to assess for median or ulnar neuropathy or the rare compartment syndrome. Hand and elbow regions need to be examined clinically and, if appropriate, radiographically for associated injuries.

Associated Injuries

Associated fractures of the hand and elbow regions are rare but need to be assessed because their presence implies more severe trauma. The risk of a compartment syndrome is higher with a "floating elbow" combination of radial, ulnar, and elbow fractures.[185] With marked radial or ulnar fracture displacement, neurovascular compromise can occur. Median neuropathy results from contusion at the time of fracture displacement, persistent direct pressure from an unreduced fracture, or an acute compartment syndrome.[239] Ulnar neuropathy has been described with similar mechanisms as well as entrapment. Wrist ligamentous and articular cartilage injuries have been described in association with distal radial and ulnar fractures in adults and less commonly in children.[49,221] Concomitant scaphoid fractures have occurred.[206] Associated wrist injuries need to be treated both in the acute setting and in the patient with persistent pain after fracture healing. Some patients with distal radial and ulnar fractures are multitrauma victims. Their systemic care modifies their distal forearm fracture care.

Diagnosis and Classification

Distal radial and ulnar fractures are defined by their anatomic relationship to the physis. Transphyseal injuries are classified by the widely accepted Salter-Harris system.[194] Metaphyseal injuries may be torus or buckle fractures, greenstick or incomplete fractures, or complete injuries. Pediatric equivalents of adult Galeazzi fracture-dislocations involve a distal radial fracture and either a soft tissue disruption of the distal radioulnar joint (DRUJ) or a transphyseal fracture of the ulna (Table 9-1). In contrast to adults, skeletally immature patients rarely sustain intra-articular fractures of the distal radius. On occasion, a Salter-Harris type III fracture, a triplane fracture,[20] or an adolescent intra-articular Colles fracture occurs.

TABLE 9-1 Distal Forearm Fractures: General Classification

Physeal fractures
Distal radius
Distal ulna
Distal metaphyseal (radius or ulna)
Torus
Greenstick
Complete fractures
Galeazzi fracture-dislocations
Dorsal displaced
Volar displaced

Distal radial fracture stability has been more clearly defined in adults[237] than in children. At present, an unstable fracture in a child is often defined as one in which closed reduction cannot be maintained. Pediatric classification systems have yet to more precisely define fracture stability, but this issue is critical in determining proper treatment management. Distal radial metaphyseal fractures have been shown to have a high degree of recurrent displacement and, therefore, inherent instability.[6,80,136,177,238,248,254]

Fractures also are defined by the degree of displacement and angulation. Static AP and lateral radiographs can be diagnostic of the fracture type and degree of deformity (Fig. 9-1). In adults,

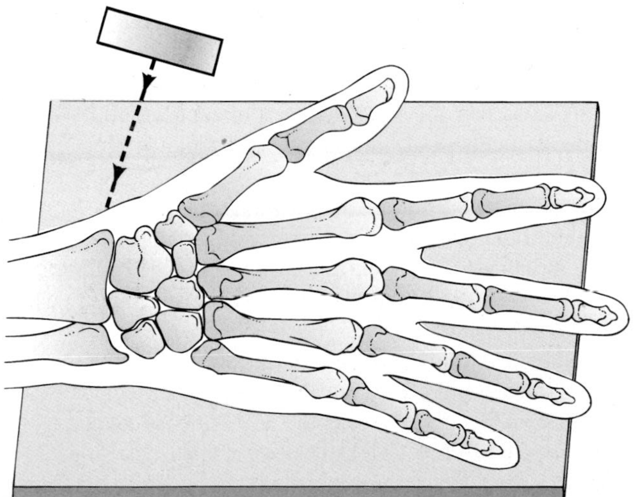

FIGURE 9-1 Angulation of the x-ray beam tangential to the articular surface, providing the optimal lateral view of the distal radius. The wrist is positioned as for the standard lateral radiograph, but the x-ray beam is directed 15 degrees cephalad. (Redrawn from Johnson PG, Szabo RM. Angle measurements of the distal radius: a cadaver study. Skel Radiol 1993;22:243, with permission.)

the distal radial articular alignment averages 22 degrees on the AP view and 11 degrees on the lateral view.[98,145,150,203,228] Radial inclination is a goniometric measurement of the angle between the distal radial articular surface and a line perpendicular to the radial shaft on the AP radiograph. Palmar tilt is measured by a line across the distal articular surface and a line perpendicular to the radial shaft on the lateral view. Pediatric values for radial inclination tend to be less, depending on the degree of skeletal maturity of the patient. Palmar tilt tends to be more consistent regardless of the age of the patient.

Rarely, tomographic views are necessary to assess intra-articular involvement or displacement. This can be by AP and lateral tomograms, computerized tomographic (CT) scans, or magnetic resonance imaging (MRI). Dynamic motion studies with fluoroscopy can provide important information on fracture stability and the success of various treatment options. Dynamic fluoroscopy requires adequate pain relief and has been used more often in adult patients with distal radial fractures. Ultrasound has been used to diagnose fractures in some centers.[52,97]

SURGICAL AND APPLIED ANATOMY

The distal radial epiphysis normally appears between 0.5 and 2.3 years in boys and 0.4 and 1.7 years in girls.[75] Initially transverse in appearance, it rapidly becomes more adultlike with its triangular shape. The contour of the radial styloid progressively elongates with advancing skeletal maturity. The secondary center of ossification for the distal ulna appears at about age 7. Similar to the radius, the ulnar styloid appears with the adolescent growth spurt. It also becomes more elongated and adultlike until physeal closure. On average, the ulnar physis closes at age 16 in girls and age 17 in boys, whereas the radial physis closes on average 6 months later than the ulnar physis.[86,145] The distal radial and ulnar physes contribute approximately 75% to 80% of the growth of the forearm and 40% of the growth of the upper extremity (Fig. 9-2).[158]

The distal radius articulates with the distal ulna at the DRUJ. Both the radius and ulna articulate with the carpus, serving as the support for the hand. The radial joint surface has three concavities for its articulations: the scaphoid and lunate fossa for the carpus and the sigmoid notch for the ulnar head (Fig. 9-3). These joints are stabilized by a complex series of volar and dorsal radiocarpal, ulnocarpal, and radioulnar ligaments. The volar ligaments are the major stabilizers. Starting radially at the radial styloid, the radial collateral, radioscaphocapitate, radiolunotriquetral (long radiolunate), and radioscapholunate (short radiolunate) ligaments volarly stabilize the radiocarpal joint. The dorsal radioscaphoid and radial triquetral ligaments are less important stabilizers.

The triangular fibrocartilage complex (TFCC) is the primary stabilizer of the ulnocarpal and radioulnar articulations. It extends from the sigmoid notch of the radius across the DRUJ and inserts into the base of the ulnar styloid. It also extends distally as the ulnolunate, ulnotriquetral, and ulnar collateral ligaments and inserts into the ulnar carpus and base of the fifth metacarpal.[60] The interosseous ligament of the forearm (Fig. 9-4) helps stabilize the radius and ulna more proximally in the diaphysis of the forearm. The ulna remains relatively immobile as the radius rotates around it. The complex structure of ligaments stabilize the radius, ulna, and carpus through the normal wrist motion of 120 degrees of flexion and extension, 50 degrees of radial and ulnar deviation, and 150 degrees of forearm rotation.[60]

The length relationship between the distal radius and ulna is defined as ulnar variance. In adults, this is measured by the relationship of the radial corner of the distal ulnar articular surface to the ulnar corner of the radial articular surface.[99] However, measurement of ulnar variance in children requires modifications of this technique. Hafner[90] described measuring from the ulnar metaphysis to the radial metaphysis to lessen the measurement inaccuracies related to epiphyseal size and shape (Fig. 9-5). If the ulna and radius are of equal lengths, there is a neutral variance. If the ulna is longer, there is a positive variance. If the ulna is shorter, there is a negative variance. Variance measurement is usually made in millimeters.

Variance is not dependent on the length of the ulnar styloid,[18] but the measurement is dependent on forearm positioning and radiographic technique.[54,70,213] Radiographs of the wrist to determine ulnar variance should be standardized with the hand and wrist pronated on the cassette, the elbow flexed 90 degrees, and the shoulder abducted 90 degrees (Fig. 9-6). The importance of ulnar variance relates to the force transmission across the wrist with axial loading. Normally, the radiocarpal joint bears approximately 80% of the axial load and the ulnocarpal joint bears 20%. Changes in the length relationship of the radius and ulna alter respective load bearing. Biomechanical and clinical studies have shown that this load distribution is important in fractures, TFCC tears (positive ulnar variance), and Kienböck disease (negative ulnar variance).[51,78,162]

PHYSEAL INJURIES

Distal radial physeal injuries were described more than 100 years ago,[33,174] and these early descriptions raised concerns regarding permanent deformity from this injury. In the 1930s, however, Aitken[3,4] concluded from his observations at the Boston City Hospital outpatient clinic that permanent deformity was rare. Instead, he emphasized the remodeling potential of distal radial physeal fractures, even when not reduced. The observations of Aitken have been confirmed throughout the twentieth century (Fig. 9-7). Most researchers agree that as long as there is sufficient growth remaining, a distal radial extension deformity from a fracture malunited in extension has the potential to remodel. Permanent deformity, however, can occur in malunited fractures near the end of growth, with rotational deformity, or fractures that cause distal radial growth arrest.

Diagnosis

Distal radial physeal fractures are far more common than distal ulnar physeal fractures.[118,146,167,172,211] The nondominant arm in boys is most commonly injured. The peak incidence is in the preadolescent growth spurt.[10,103,104,118,248] More than 50% of distal radial physeal fractures have an associated ulnar fracture. This usually is an ulnar styloid fracture but can be a distal ulnar plastic deformation, greenstick, or complete fracture.[8,124,125] The mechanism of injury generally is a fall on an outstretched hand and wrist. Many of the injuries are nondisplaced and present only with pain at the physis.[151,166] With displaced fractures, the distal fragment usually moves dorsally, creating an extension deformity that is usually clinically appar-

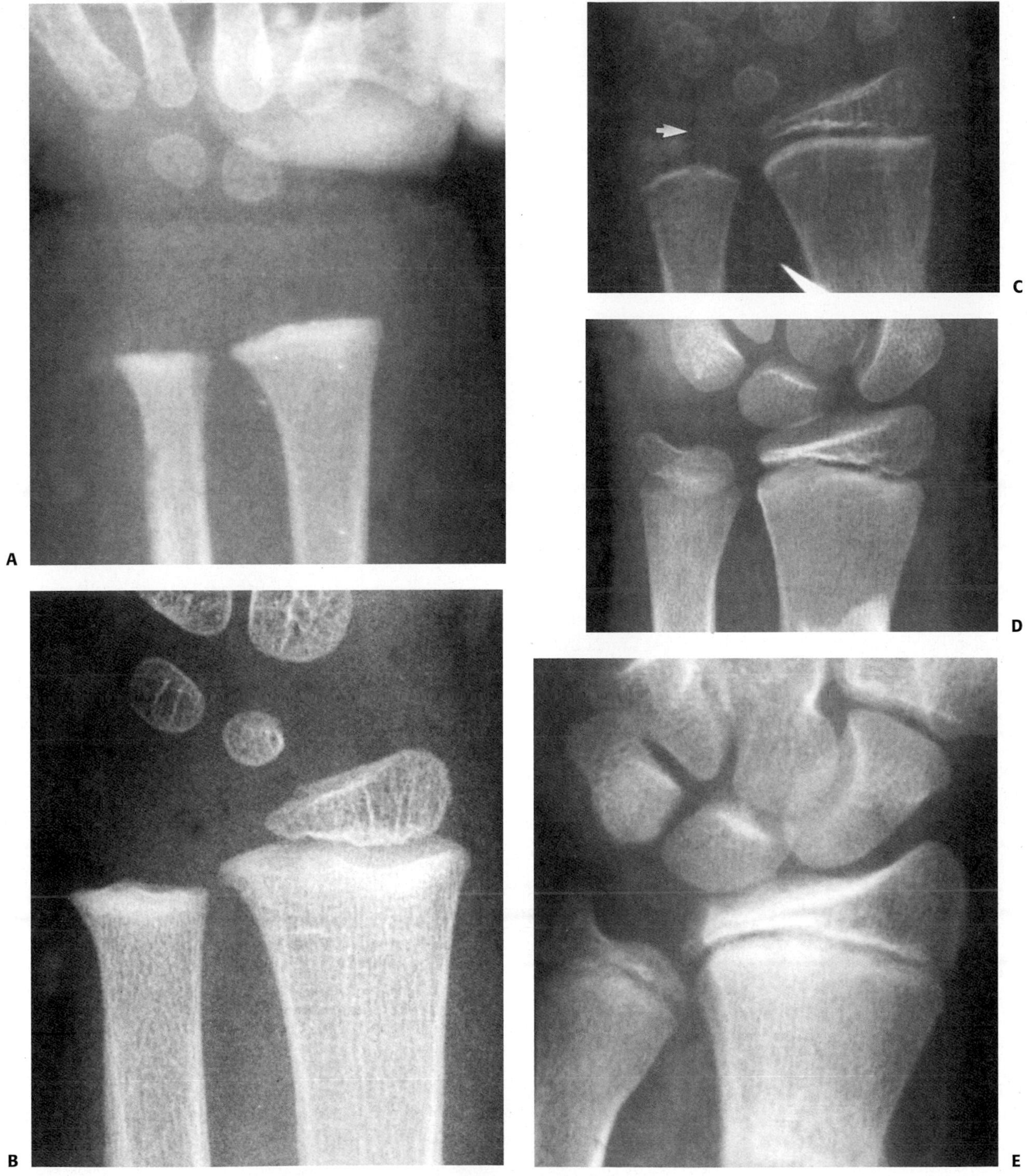

FIGURE 9-2 Ossification of the distal radius. **A.** Preossification distal radius with transverse ossification in a 15-month-old boy. **B.** The triangular secondary ossification center of the distal radius in a 2-year-old girl. **C.** The initial ossification center of the styloid in this 7-year-old girl progresses radially (*arrow*). **D.** Extension of the ulnar ossification center into the styloid process of an 11-year-old. **E.** The styloid is fully ossified and the epiphyses have capped their relative metaphyses in this 13-year-old boy.

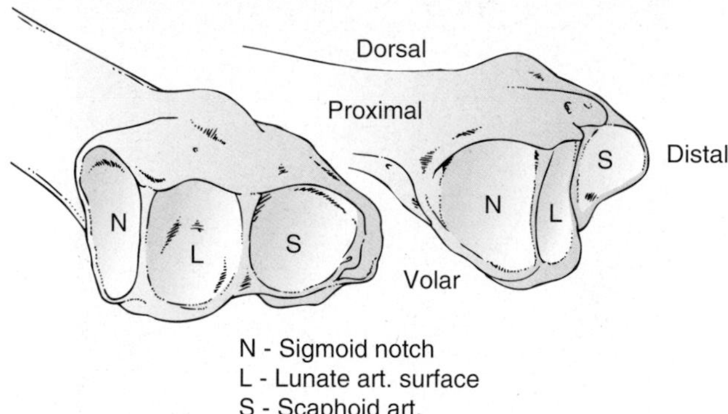

FIGURE 9-3 Articulations of the distal radioulnar joint. (Redrawn from Bowers WH. Green's Operative Hand Surgery. New York: Churchill-Livingstone, 1993:988.)

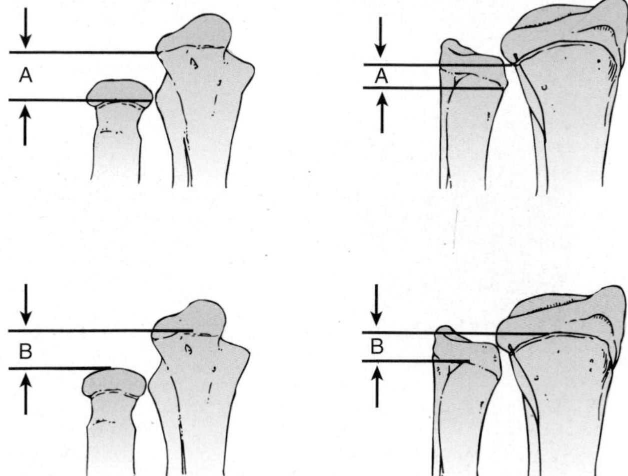

FIGURE 9-5 Hafner's technique to measure ulnar variance. **A.** The distance from the most proximal point of the ulnar metaphysis to the most proximal point of the radial metaphysis. **B.** The distance from the most distal point of the ulnar metaphysis to the most distal point of the radial metaphysis. (From Hafner R, Poznanski AK, Donovan JM. Ulnar variance in children. Standard measurements for evaluation of ulnar shortening in childhood. Skel Radiol 1989;18:514, with permission.)

ent. Patients have pain and tenderness at the fracture site, and the range of motion at the wrist and hand usually is limited by pain. Neurovascular compromise is uncommon but can occur.[239] When present, it usually consists of median nerve irritability or dysfunction caused by direct trauma to the nerve at the time of injury or ongoing ischemic compression from the displaced fracture. Thenar muscle function and discriminatory sensibility (two-point discrimination) should be tested before reduction in the emergency setting. Acute carpal tunnel syndrome or forearm compartment syndrome can occur, but more often is caused by marked volar forearm and wrist swelling that occurs after reduction and application of a well-molded, tight cast.[34,195,239] Open physeal fractures are rare, but the local skin should be examined closely for penetration.

Plain AP and lateral radiographs are diagnostic of the fracture type and deformity. The Salter-Harris system is the basis for classification of physeal fractures.[194] Most are Salter-Harris type II fractures. The dorsal displacement of the distal fragment of the epiphysis and dorsal Thurston-Holland metaphyseal fragment is evident on the lateral view (Fig. 9-8). Salter-Harris type I fractures also usually displace dorsally. Volar displacement of either a Salter-Harris type I or II fracture is less common (Fig. 9-9). Nondisplaced Salter-Harris type I fractures may be indicated only by a displaced pronator fat pad sign (Fig. 9-10)[198,253] or tenderness over the involved physis.[8,181] A scaphoid fat pad sign may indicate a scaphoid fracture (Fig. 9-11). If the acute fracture is unrecognized, a late-appearing periosteal reaction may indicate the fracture.

Salter-Harris type III fractures are rare and may be caused by a compression injury or an avulsion of the radial origin of the volar radiocarpal ligaments (Fig. 9-12).[7,124] Triplane equivalent fractures,[169–171] a combination of Salter-Harris type II and III fractures in different planes, are rare. CT scans may be necessary to define the fracture pattern and degree of intra-articular displacement. Stress injuries to the physis occur most commonly in competitive gymnasts (Fig. 9-13).

Current Treatment Options

Treatment options include no reduction, closed reduction and cast immobilization, closed reduction and pin fixation, and open reduction. Nondisplaced fractures are immobilized until appropriate healing and pain resolution have been achieved.[8,191] If there is a question of fracture stability, these fractures should be treated with a well-molded cast and monitored closely during the first 3 weeks of healing to be certain that there is no loss of alignment. Most acute displaced Salter-Harris type I and II fractures can be treated successfully with gentle closed reduction and cast immobilization. There are advocates for both long-arm and short-arm treatment methods.[28,29,31,89,95,121,212] Closed reduction and percutaneous pin fixation are performed in patients with neurovascular compromise and displaced physeal fractures[239] to lessen the risk of development of a compartment syndrome in the carpal tunnel or forearm. Open reduction is indicated for irreducible frac-

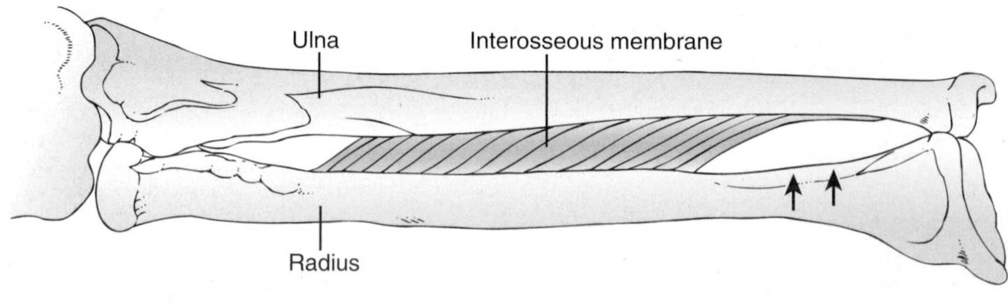

FIGURE 9-4 The attachment and the fibers of the interosseous membrane are such that there is no attachment to the distal radius. (Redrawn from Kraus B, Horne G. Galeazzi fractures. J Trauma 1985;25:1094, with permission.)

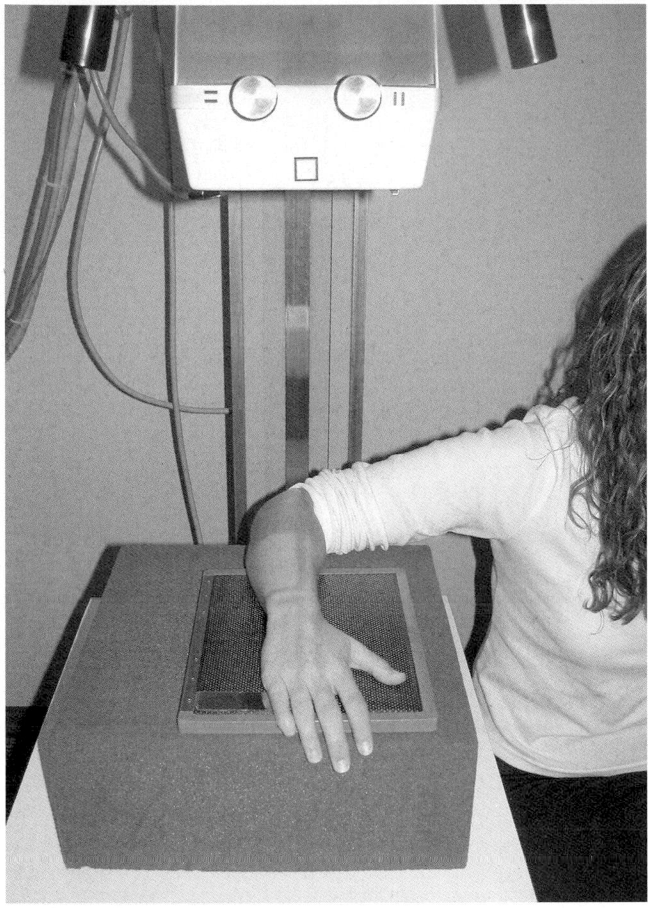

FIGURE 9-6 Technique for neutral rotation radiograph with wrist neutral, forearm pronated, elbow flexed 90 degrees, and shoulder abducted 90 degrees.

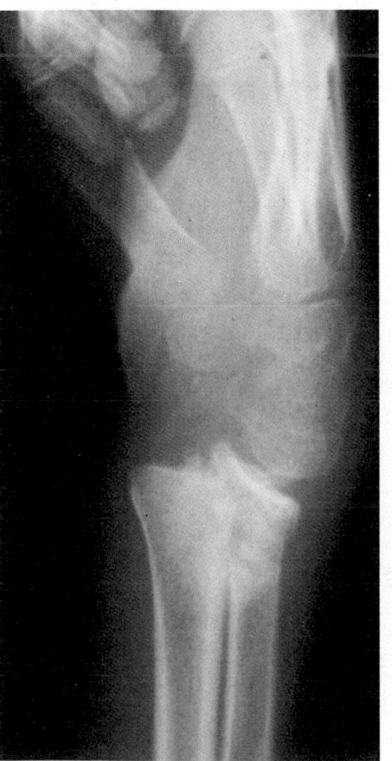

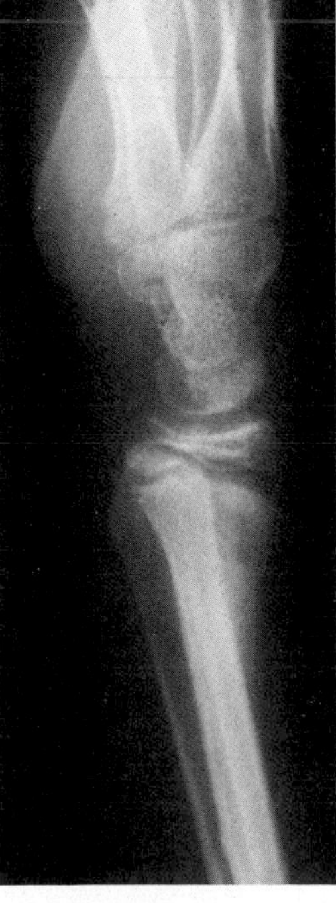

FIGURE 9-7 A. A 13-year-old boy presented 1 month after injury with a displaced and healed Salter-Harris type II distal radial fracture with obvious clinical deformity. **B.** Over the next 6 months, the patient grew 4 inches and the deformity remodeled without intervention.

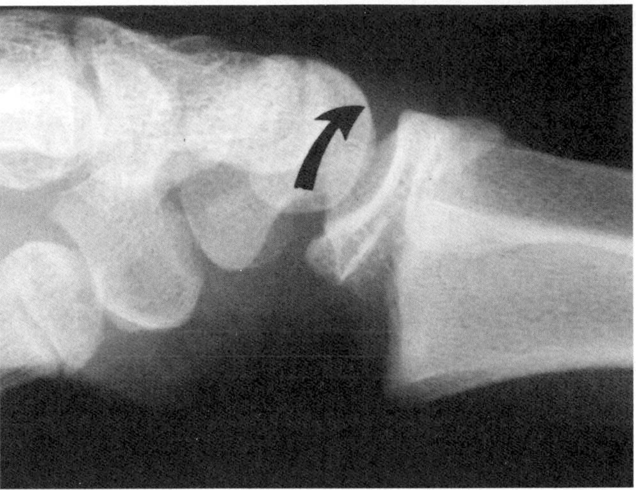

FIGURE 9-8 Dorsally displaced physeal fracture (type A). The distal epiphysis with a small metaphyseal fragment is displaced dorsally (*curved arrow*) in relation to the proximal metaphyseal fragment.

tures, open fractures, displaced Salter-Harris type III and IV fractures, and triplane equivalent fractures. Irreducible fractures usually are due to an entrapped periosteum or pronator quadratus.[137] Internal fixation usually is with smooth, small-diameter pins to lessen the risk of growth arrest. Plates and screws rarely are used unless the patient is near skeletal maturity because of concerns about further physeal injury. In the rare displaced intra-articular Salter-Harris type III or IV fracture, internal fixation can be intraepiphyseal without violating the physis. If it is necessary to cross the physis, then smooth, small diameter pins should be used to lessen the risk of iatrogenic physeal injury. Extra-articular external fixation also can be used to stabilize and align the fracture.

Closed Reduction

Most displaced Salter-Harris I and II fractures are treated with closed reduction and cast stabilization. Closed manipulation of the displaced fracture is performed with appropriate conscious

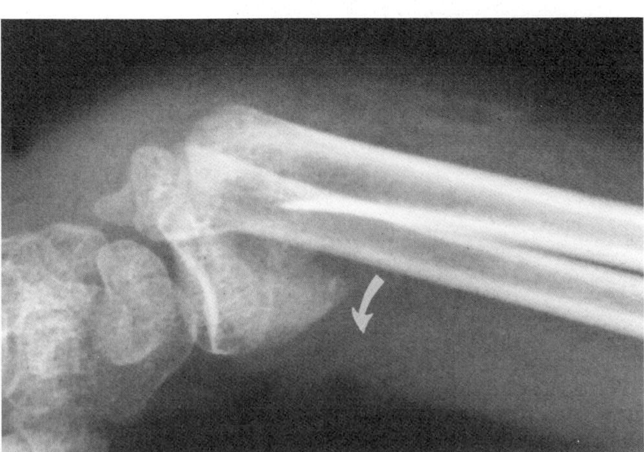

FIGURE 9-9 Volarly displaced physeal fracture (type B). Distal epiphysis with a large volar metaphyseal fragment is displaced in a volar direction (*curved arrow*). (Reprinted from Wilkins KE, ed. Operative Management of Upper Extremity Fractures in Children. Rosemont, IL: American Academy of Orthopaedic Surgeons, 1994:21, with permission.)

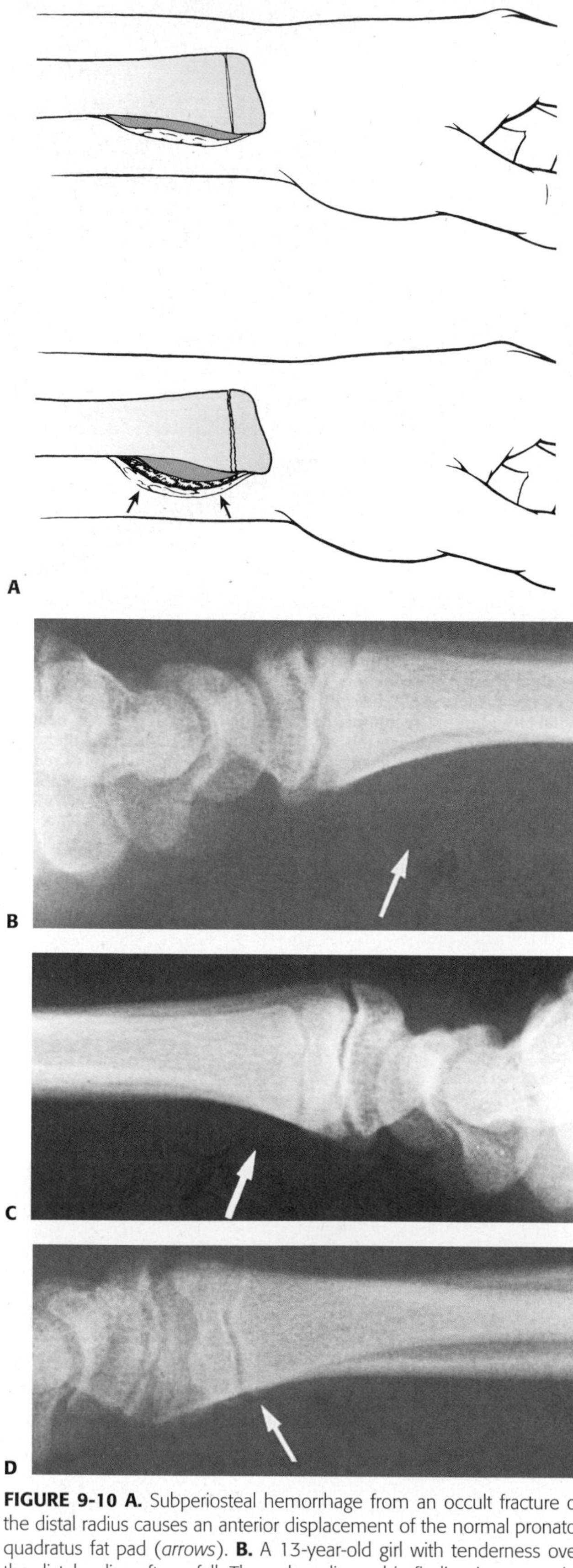

FIGURE 9-10 A. Subperiosteal hemorrhage from an occult fracture of the distal radius causes an anterior displacement of the normal pronator quadratus fat pad (*arrows*). **B.** A 13-year-old girl with tenderness over the distal radius after a fall. The only radiographic finding is an anterior displacement of the normal pronator quadratus fat pad (*arrow*). **C.** The opposite normal side (*arrow* indicates normal fat pad). **D.** Two weeks later, there is a small area of periosteal new bone formation (*arrow*) anteriorly, substantiating that bony injury has occurred.

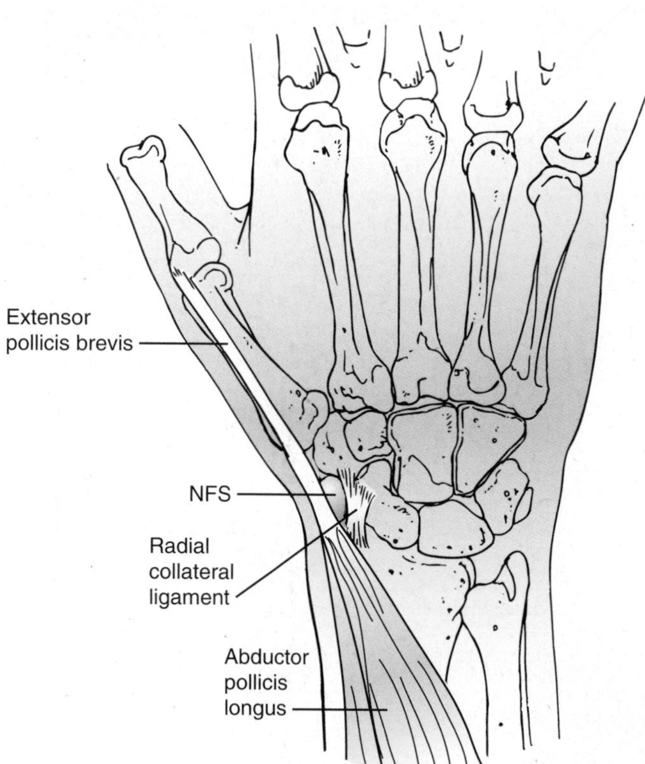

FIGURE 9-11 Anatomic relationships of the navicular fat stripe (NFS). The NFS, shaded black, is located between the combined tendons of the abductor pollicis longus and extensor pollicis brevis, and the lateral surface of the carpal navicular. (Reprinted from Terry DW, Ramen JE. The navicular fat stripe. Ham J Roent Rad Ther Nucl Med 1975;124: 25, with permission.)

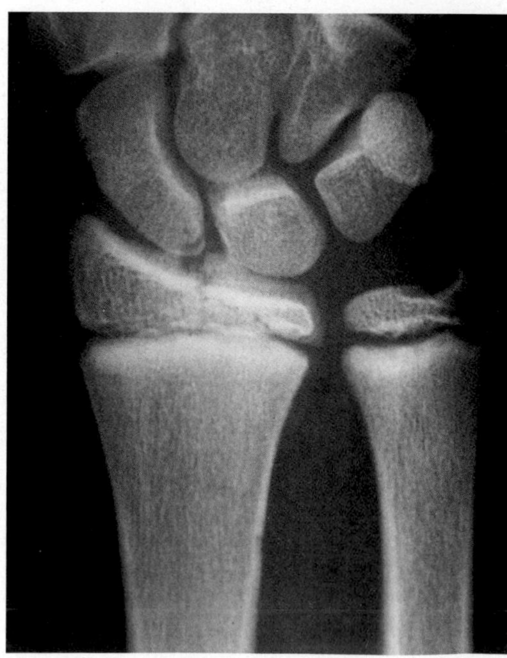

FIGURE 9-12 AP radiograph of Salter-Harris type III fracture of the distal radius.

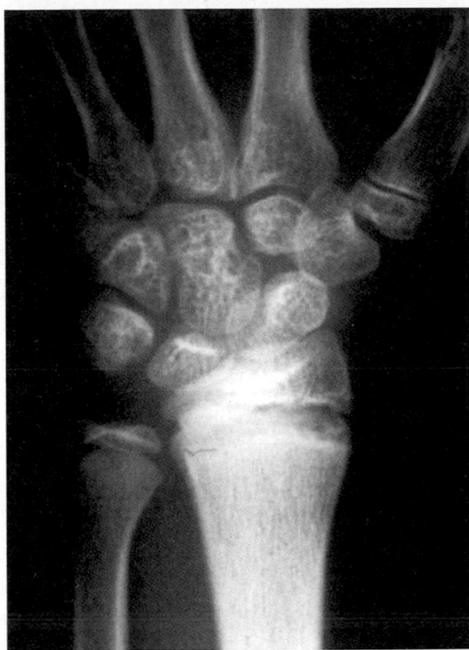

FIGURE 9-13 Stress changes in a female gymnast with widening of the distal radial physis from long-standing high-level performance.

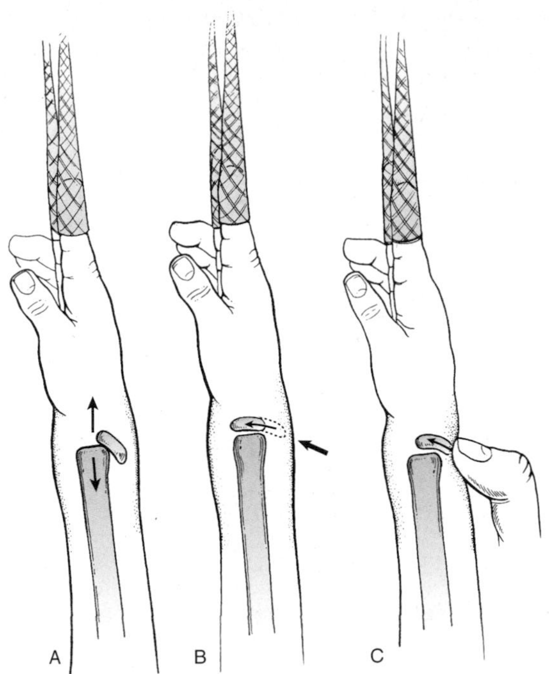

FIGURE 9-14 Acceptable method of closed reduction of distal physeal fractures of the radius. **A.** Position of the fracture fragments as finger trap traction with countertraction is applied (*arrows*). **B.** With traction alone, the fracture will often reduce without external pressure (*arrows*). **C.** If the reduction is incomplete, simply applying direct pressure over the fracture site in a distal and volar direction with the thumb often completes the reduction while maintaining traction. This technique theoretically decreases the shear forces across the physis during the reduction process.

sedation, analgesia, or, rarely, anesthesia to achieve pain relief and an atraumatic reduction.[8,108,191] Most of these fractures involve dorsal and proximal displacement of the epiphysis with an apex–volar extension deformity. Manipulative reduction is by gentle distraction and flexion of the distal epiphysis, carpus, and hand over the proximal metaphysis (Figs. 9-14 and 9-15). The intact dorsal periosteum is used as a tension band to aid in reduction and stabilization of the fracture. Unlike similar fractures in adults, finger trap distraction with pulley weights is often counterproductive. However, finger traps can help stabilize the hand, wrist, and arm for manipulative reduction and casting by applying a few pounds of weight for balance. Otherwise, an assistant is helpful to support the extremity in the proper position for casting.

If portable fluoroscopy is available, immediate radiographic assessment of the reduction is obtained. Otherwise, a well-molded cast is applied and AP and lateral radiographs are obtained to assess the reduction. The cast should provide three-

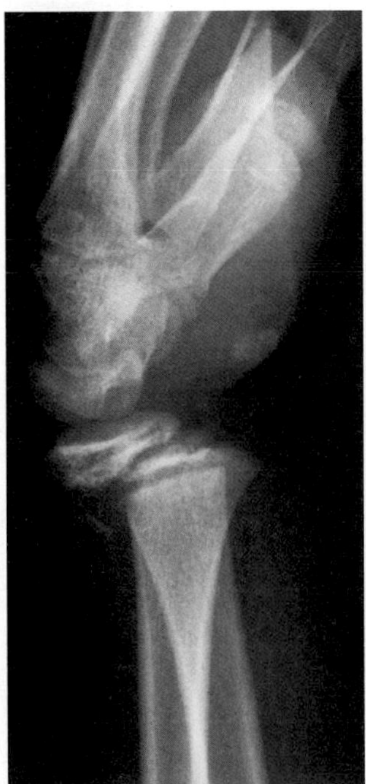
A

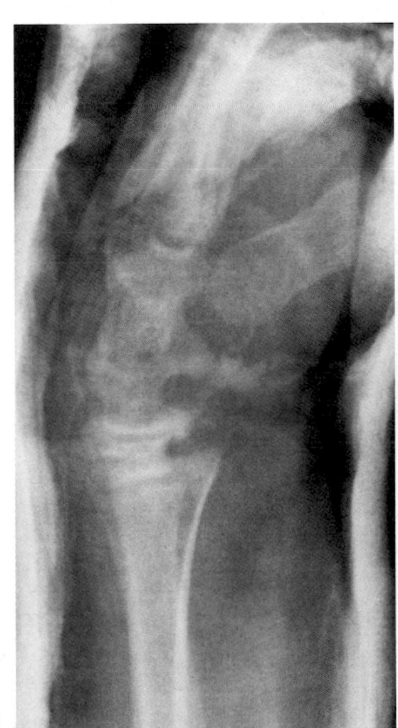
B

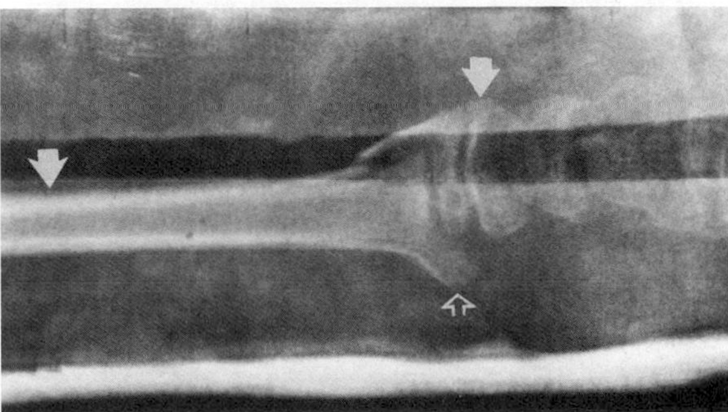
C

FIGURE 9-15 A. Lateral radiograph of dorsally displaced Salter-Harris type II fracture. **B.** Lateral radiograph after closed reduction and cast application. **C.** Reduction of the volar displaced fracture shown in Figure 9-9. The forearm was in supination with three-point molding anterior over the distal epiphysis and proximal shaft (*white arrows*). The third point is placed dorsally over the distal metaphysis (*open arrow*). (The dorsal surface of the cast is oriented toward the bottom of this figure.) (Reprinted from Wilkins KE, ed. Operative Management of Upper Extremity Fractures in Children. Rosemont, IL: American Academy of Orthopaedic Surgeons, 1994:17, with permission.)

point molding over the distal radius to lessen the risk of fracture displacement and should follow the contour of the normal forearm. The distal dorsal mold should not impair venous outflow from the hand, which can occur if the mold is placed too distal and too deep so as to obstruct the dorsal veins. Advocates of short-arm casting[28,29] indicate at least equivalent results with proper casting techniques and more comfort during immobilization due to free elbow mobility. Instructions for elevation and close monitoring of swelling and the neurovascular status of the extremity are critical.

The fracture also should be monitored closely with serial radiographs for the first 3 weeks to be certain that there is no loss of anatomic alignment (Fig. 9-16). Generally, these fractures are stable after closed reduction and cast immobilization. If there is loss of reduction after 7 days, the surgeon should be wary of repeat reduction because of the risk of physeal arrest.[8,194] Fortunately, remodeling of an extension deformity with growth is common if the patient has more than 2 years of growth remaining and the deformity is less than 20 degrees.

Closed Reduction and Percutaneous Pinning

The indications for percutaneous pinning of distal radial physeal fractures are still controversial. The best indication is a displaced radial physeal fracture with median neuropathy and significant volar soft tissue swelling (Fig. 9-17).[239] These patients are at risk for development of an acute carpal tunnel syndrome or forearm compartment syndrome with closed reduction and well-molded cast immobilization.[34,91,195,239] The torn periosteum volarly allows the fracture bleeding to dissect into the volar forearm compartments and carpal tunnel. If a tight cast is applied with a volar mold over that area, compartment pressures can increase dangerously. Percutaneous pin fixation allows the application of a loose dressing, splint, or cast without the risk of loss of fracture reduction.

Pin fixation can be either single or double (Fig. 9-18). Fluoroscopy is used to guide proper fracture reduction and pin placement. Anesthesia is used for adequate pain relief and to lessen the risk of further physeal injury. The fracture is manipulated into anatomic alignment and the initial, and often only, pin

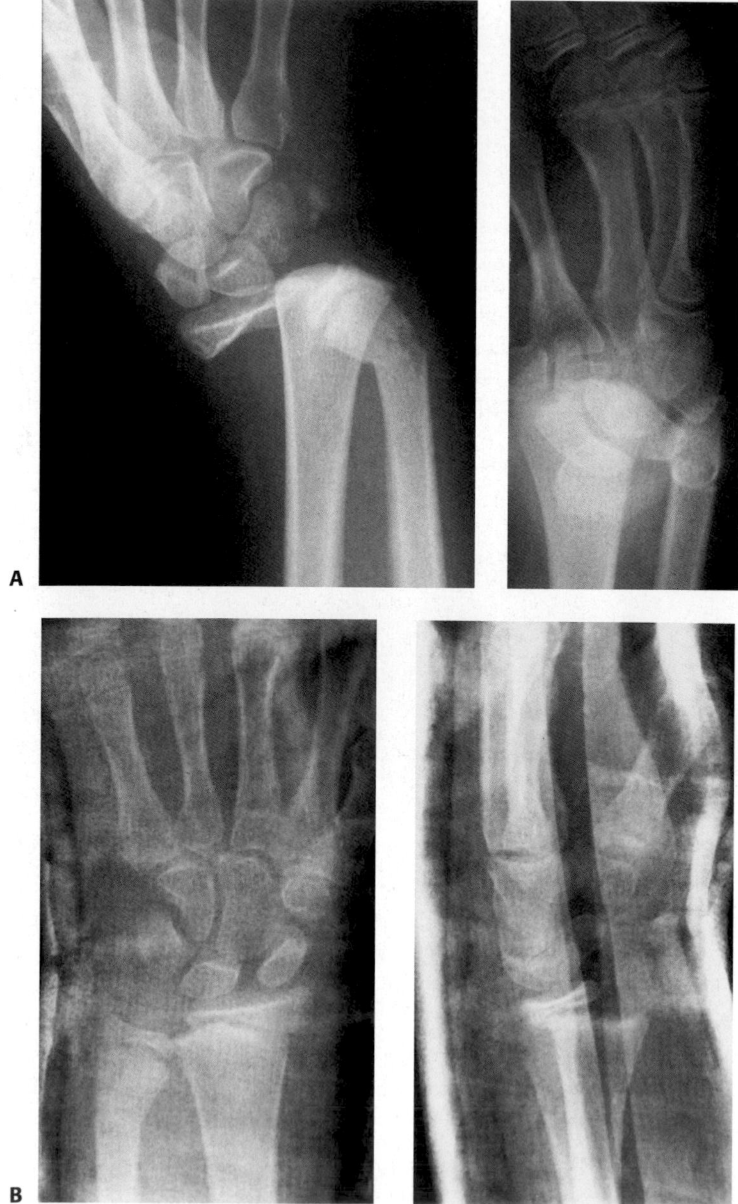

FIGURE 9-16 A. AP and lateral radiographs of severely displaced Salter-Harris type II fracture of the distal radius. **B.** Closed reduction shows marked improvement but not anatomic reduction. The cast had to be bivalved due to excessive swelling. *(continues)*

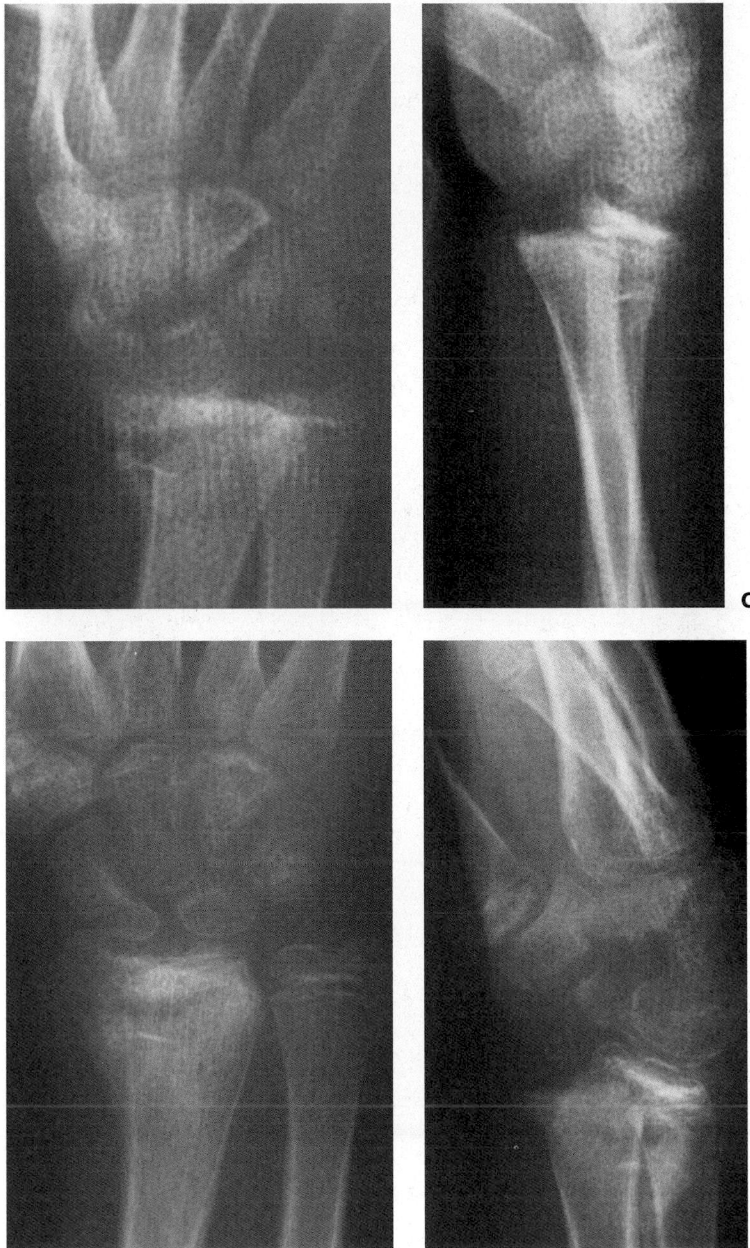

FIGURE 9-16 *(continued)* **C.** Unfortunately, the patient lost reduction after a new fiberglass cast was applied. **D.** Out-of cast-radiographs show a healed malunion in a similar position to the prereduction radiographs.

is placed from the distal epiphysis of the radial styloid obliquely across the physis into the more proximal ulnar aspect of the radial metaphysis (Fig. 9-19). Alternatively, smooth pins may be placed such that they avoid crossing the distal radial physis, theoretically decreasing the risk of physeal disturbance, though this has not been well demonstrated in the published literature.[252] A sufficient skin incision should be made with pin placement to be certain there is no iatrogenic injury to the radial sensory nerve or extensor tendons. Stability of the fracture should be evaluated with flexion and extension and rotatory stress under fluoroscopy. Often in children and adolescents, a single pin and the reduced periosteum provide sufficient stability to prevent redisplacement of the fracture. If fracture stability is questionable with a single pin, a second pin should be placed. The second pin can either parallel the first pin or, to create cross-pin stability, can be placed distally from the ulnar corner of the radial epiphysis between the fourth and fifth dorsal compartments and passed obliquely to the proximal radial portion of the metaphysis. Again, the skin incisions for pin placement should be sufficient to avoid iatrogenic injury to the extensor tendons.

The pins are bent, left out of the skin, and covered with a sterile dressing. Splint or cast immobilization is used but does not need to be tight because fracture stability is provided by the pins. The pins are left in until there is adequate fracture healing (usually 4 weeks). The pins can be removed in the office without sedation or anesthesia.

One of the arguments against pin fixation is the risk of additional injury to the physis by a pin.[20] The risk of physeal arrest is more from the displaced fracture than from a short-term, smooth pin. As a precaution, smooth, small-diameter pins should be used, insertion should be as atraumatic as possible, and removal should be done as soon as there is sufficient fracture healing for fracture stability in a cast or splint alone.

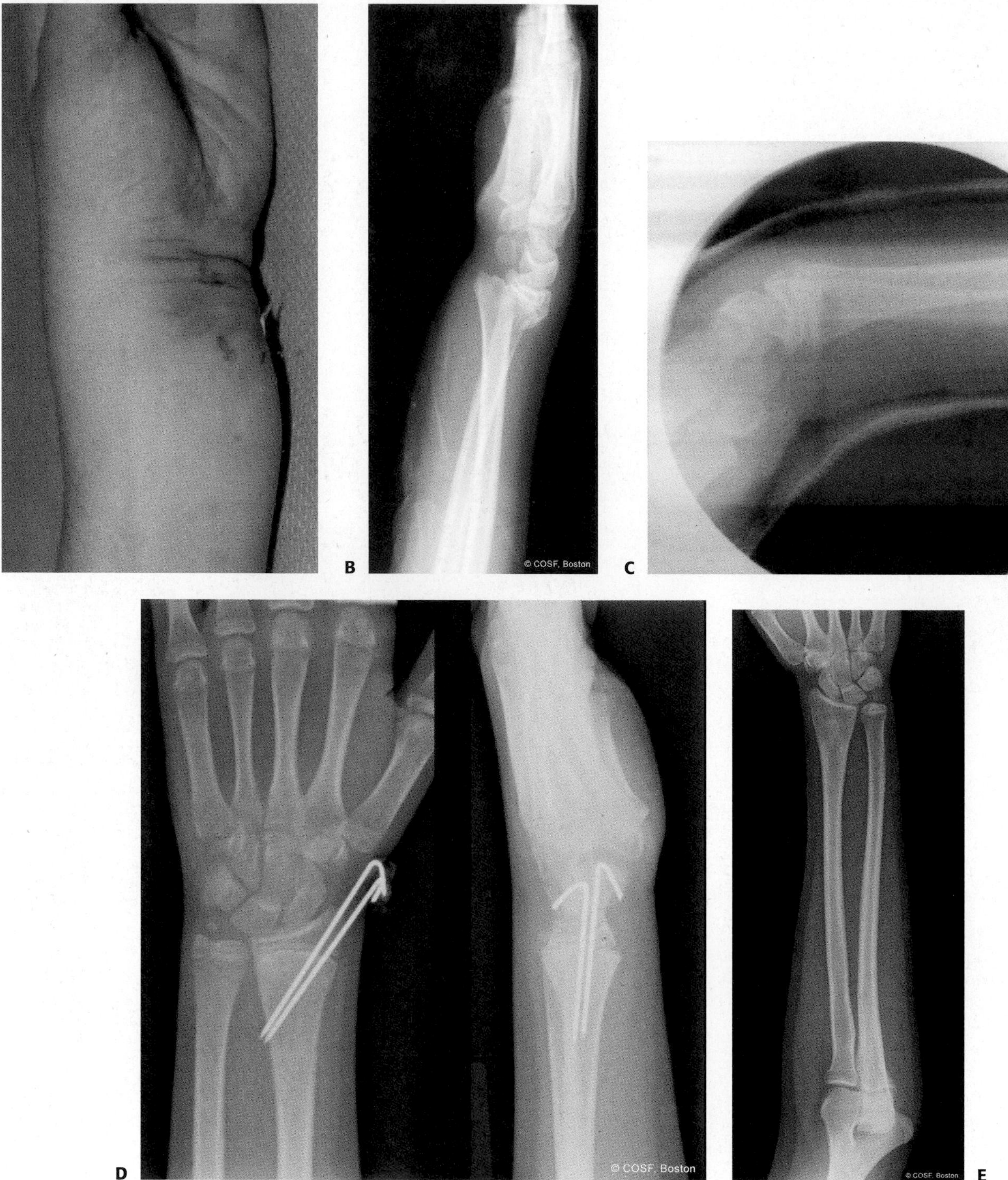

FIGURE 9-17 A. Clinical photograph of patient with a displaced Salter-Harris type II fracture of the distal radius. The patient has marked swelling volarly with hematoma and fracture displacement. The patient had a median neuropathy upon presentation. **B.** Lateral radiograph of the displaced fracture. **C.** Lateral radiograph following closed reduction and cast application. Excessive flexion has been utilized to maintain fracture reduction, resulting in persistent median neuropathy and increasing pain. **D.** Radiographs following urgent closed reduction and percutaneous pinning. **E.** Follow-up radiograph depicting distal radial physeal arrest and increased ulnar variance.

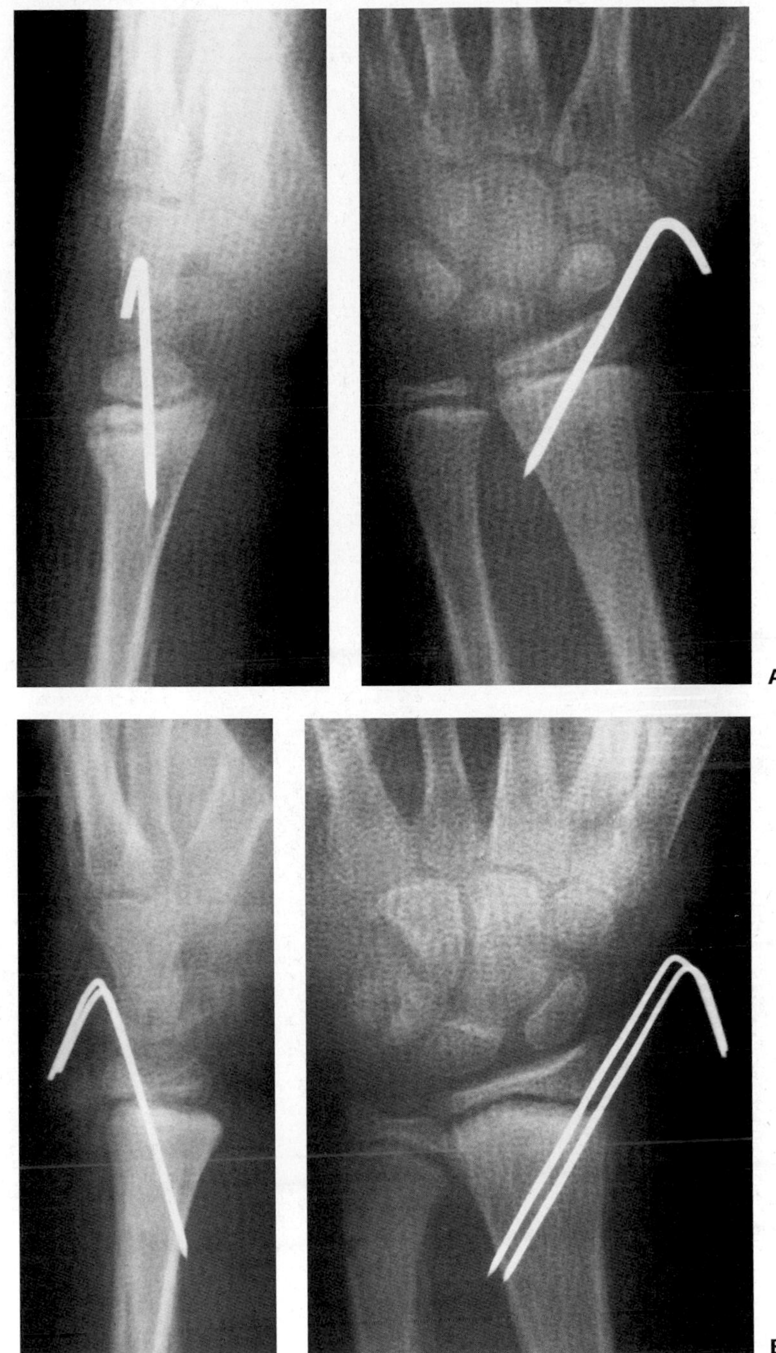

FIGURE 9-18 A. AP and lateral radiographs of displaced Salter-Harris type II fracture pinned with a single pin. **B.** After reduction and pinning with parallel pins.

Open Reduction

The main indication for open reduction of a displaced distal radial Salter-Harris type II physeal fracture is irreducibility. Most often this is caused by interposed periosteum or, less likely, pronator quadratus.[107,137,250] Open reduction is done through a volar approach to the distal radial physis. The interval between the radial artery and the flexor carpi radialis is used. This dissection also can proceed directly through the flexor carpi radialis sheath to protect the artery. The pronator quadratus is isolated and elevated from radial to ulnar. Although this muscle can be interposed in the fracture site, the volar periosteum is more commonly interposed. This is evident only after elevation of the pronator quadratus. The periosteum is extracted from the physis with care to minimize further injury to the physis. The fracture can then be easily reduced. Usually, a percutaneous smooth pin is used for stabilization of the reduction. The method of pin insertion is the same as after closed reduction.

Open physeal fractures are rare but require irrigation and débridement. Care should be taken with mechanical débridement of the physeal cartilage to avoid further risk of growth arrest. Cultures should be taken at the time of operative débridement, and appropriate antibiotics are used to lessen the risk of deep space infection.

The rare Salter-Harris type III or IV fracture or triplane fracture[171] may require open reduction if the joint or physis cannot be anatomically reduced closed. The articular and physeal alignment can be evaluated by radiographic tomograms (trispiral or

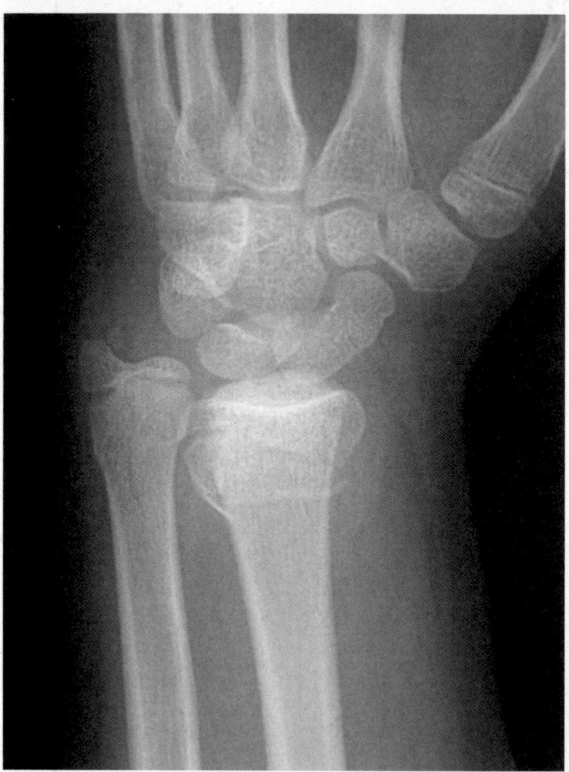

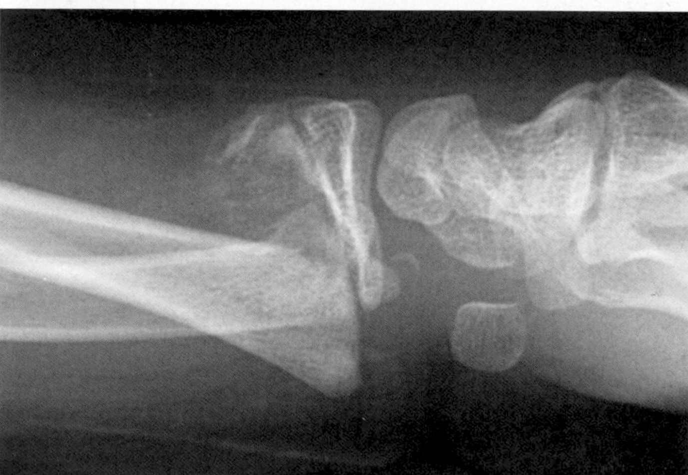

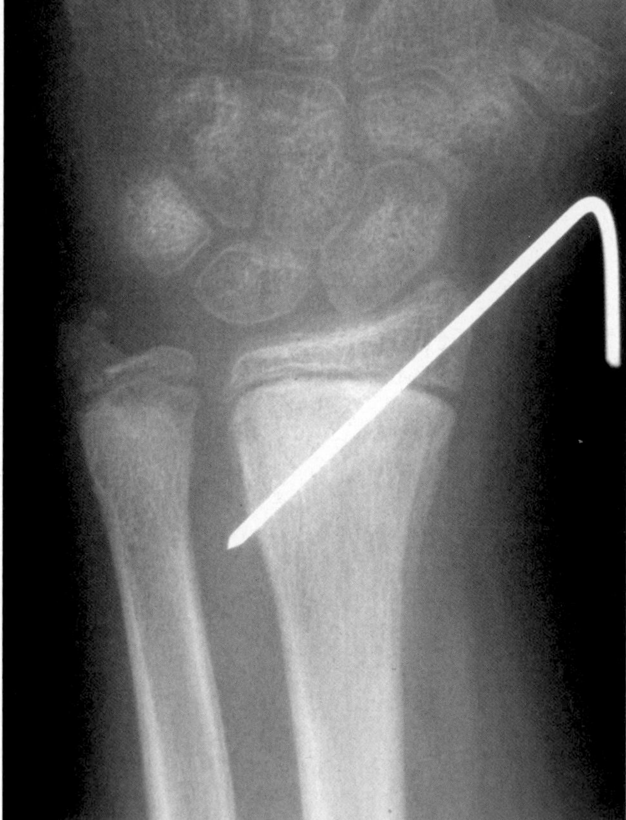

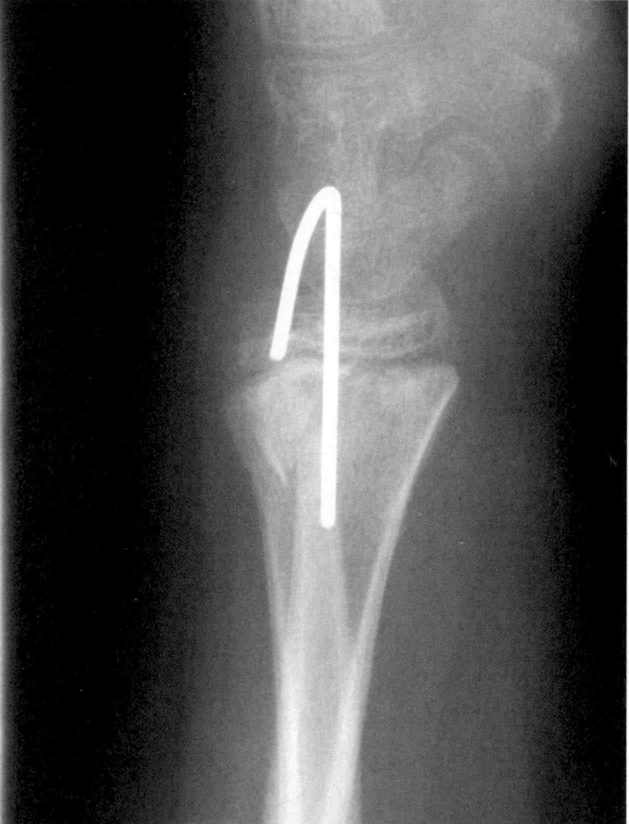

FIGURE 9-19 A. AP and lateral views of a displaced Salter-Harris type II distal radial fracture. **B.** AP and lateral views 1 month after simple pin fixation.

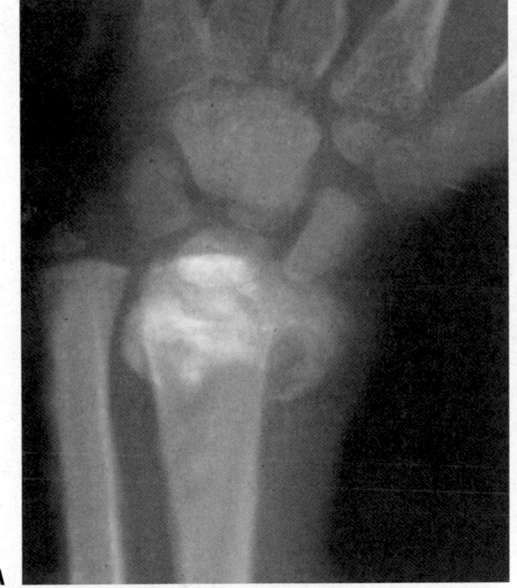

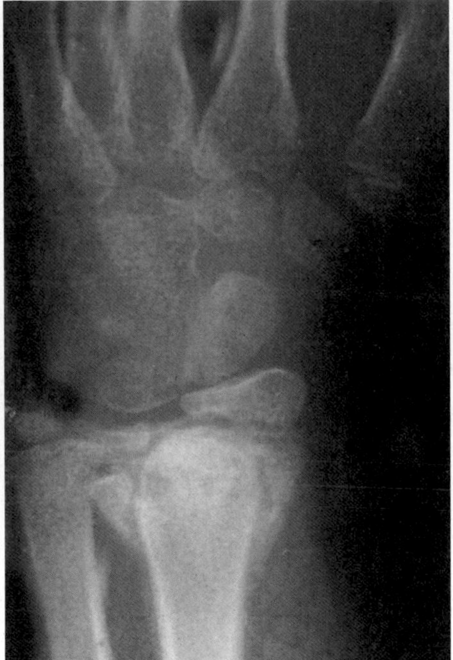

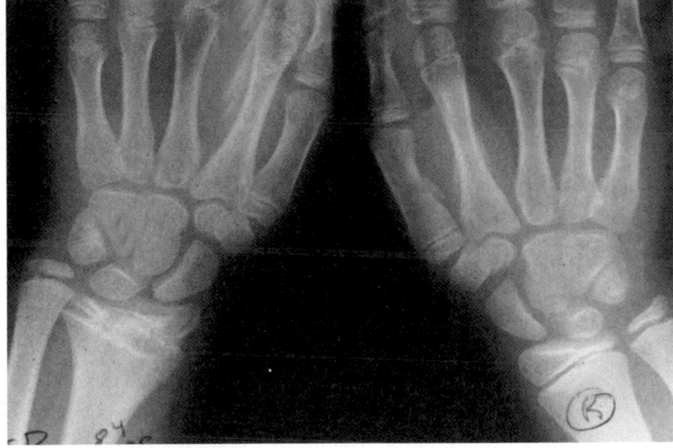

FIGURE 9-20 A. A markedly displaced Salter-Harris type IV fracture of the distal radius in an 11-year-old boy who fell from a horse. **B.** Radiograph taken 3 weeks after closed reduction demonstrates displacement of the comminuted fragments. **C.** Eighteen months after injury, there was 15 mm of radial shortening, and the patient had a pronounced radial deviation deformity of the wrist.

CT), MRI scans, or wrist arthroscopy. If anatomic alignment of the physis and articular surface is not present, the risk of growth arrest, long-term deformity, or limited function is great (Fig. 9-20). Even minimal displacement (more than 1 mm) should not be accepted in this situation. Arthroscopically assisted reduction is helpful to align and stabilize these rare physeal fractures.[48,76] Although it is an equipment intensive operation with arthroscopy, external fixation, transphyseal and transepiphyseal pin or screw fixation, and fluoroscopy, anatomic reduction, and stabilization of the physis and articular surface can be achieved (Fig. 9-21).

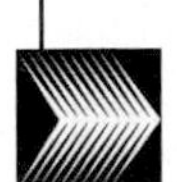

AUTHORS' PREFERRED METHOD OF TREATMENT

Physeal Injuries

Most Salter-Harris type I and II fractures are reduced closed under conscious sedation with the assistance of portable fluoroscopy. A long-arm cast with appropriate three-point molding is applied. This is changed to a short-arm cast when there is sufficient healing for fracture stability, usually after 3 to 4 weeks. Cast immobilization is discontinued when there is clinical and radiographic evidence of fracture healing, generally 4 to 6 weeks after fracture. Range-of-motion and strengthening exercises are begun with a home program. When the child achieves full motion and strength, he or she can return to full activity, including competitive sports. As the risk of posttraumatic physeal disturbance is approximately 4% to 5%, follow-up radiographs are obtained at 6 to 12 months after fracture to be certain there is no growth arrest.[9,24]

A patient with a displaced Salter-Harris type I or II physeal fracture associated with significant volar soft tissue swelling, median neuropathy, or ipsilateral elbow and radial fractures ("floating elbow") is treated with closed reduction and percutaneous pinning (Fig. 9-22). This avoids the increased risk of compartment syndrome in the carpal canal or volar forearm that is present if a well-molded, tight cast is applied. In addition, acute percutaneous pinning of the fracture prevents increased swelling, cast splitting, loss of reduction, and concerns about malunion or growth arrest with repeat reduction. Acute pinning of the fracture with one or two smooth pins through the radial epiphysis provides fracture stability without a compressive cast. The risk of growth arrest from a narrow-diameter, smooth pin left in place for 3 to 4 weeks is exceedingly small.[252]

Open reduction is reserved for irreducible Salter-Harris type I and II fractures, open fractures, fractures with associ-

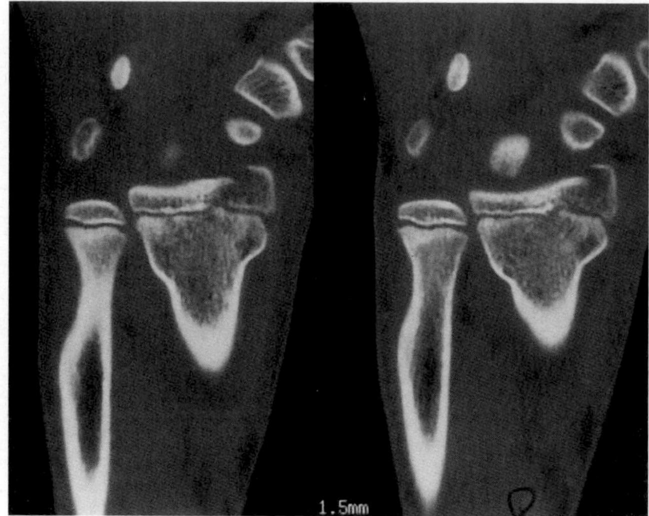

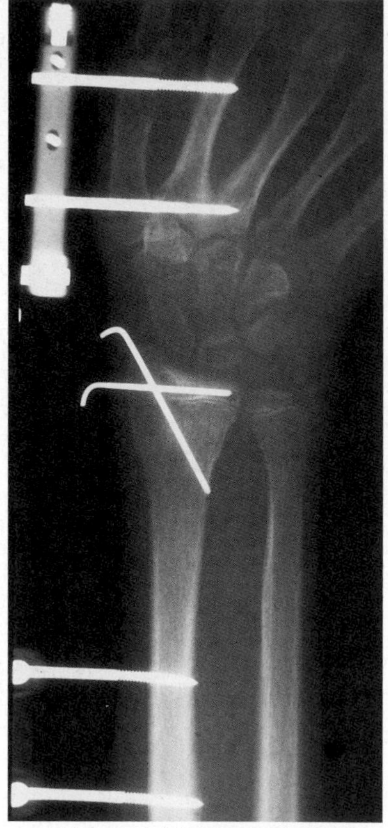

FIGURE 9-21 A. CT scan of displaced Salter-Harris type IV fracture. **B.** Surgical correction included external fixation distraction, arthroscopically assisted reduction, and smooth pin fixation.

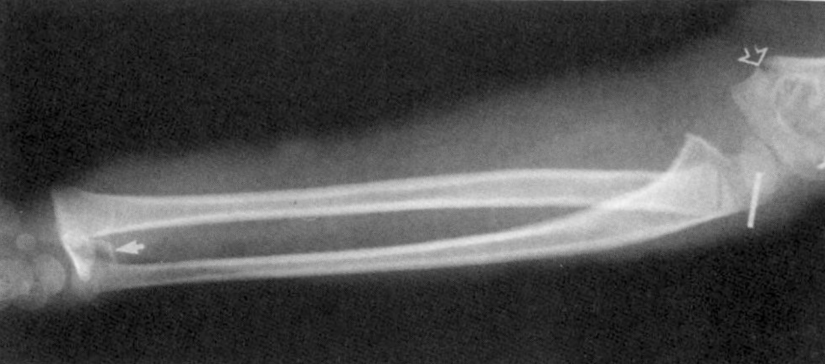

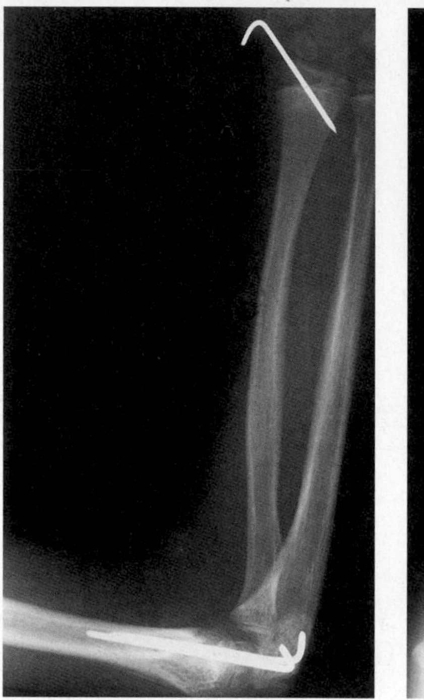

FIGURE 9-22 A. Ipsilateral distal radial physeal and supracondylar fractures. This 6-year-old sustained both a dorsally displaced distal radial physeal fracture (*closed arrow*) and a type II displaced supracondylar fracture of the humerus (*open arrows*). **B.** Similar case treated with percutaneous pinning of radial physeal fracture and supracondylar humeral fracture.

ated acute carpal tunnel or forearm compartment syndrome, displaced (more than 1 mm) Salter-Harris type III or IV fractures, or triplane equivalent fractures. For an irreducible Salter-Harris type I or II fracture, exposure is from the side of the torn periosteum. Because these fractures usually are displaced dorsally, a volar exposure is used. Smooth pins are used for stabilization and are left in for 3 to 4 weeks. Open fractures are exposed through the open wound with proximal and distal extension for adequate débridement. All open débridements are performed in the operating room under general anesthesia. Acute compartment syndromes are treated with immediate release of the transverse carpal ligament or forearm fascia. The transverse carpal ligament is released in a Z-plasty fashion to lengthen the ligament and prevent volar bow-stringing and scarring of the median nerve against the palmar skin. Displaced intra-articular fractures are best treated with arthroscopically assisted reduction and fixation. Distraction across the joint can be achieved with application of an external fixator or wrist arthroscopy traction devices and finger traps. Standard dorsal portals (3/4 and 4/5) are used for viewing the intra-articular aspect of the fracture and alignment of the reduction[66,76] In addition, direct observation through the arthroscope can aid in safe placement of the intraepiphyseal pins.[48,129] Fluoroscopy is used to evaluate the extra-articular aspects of the fracture (triplane equivalent and type IV fractures), the reduction, and placement of fixation pins.

Complications

Malunion. Complications from physeal fractures are relatively rare. The most frequent problem is malunion. Fortunately, these

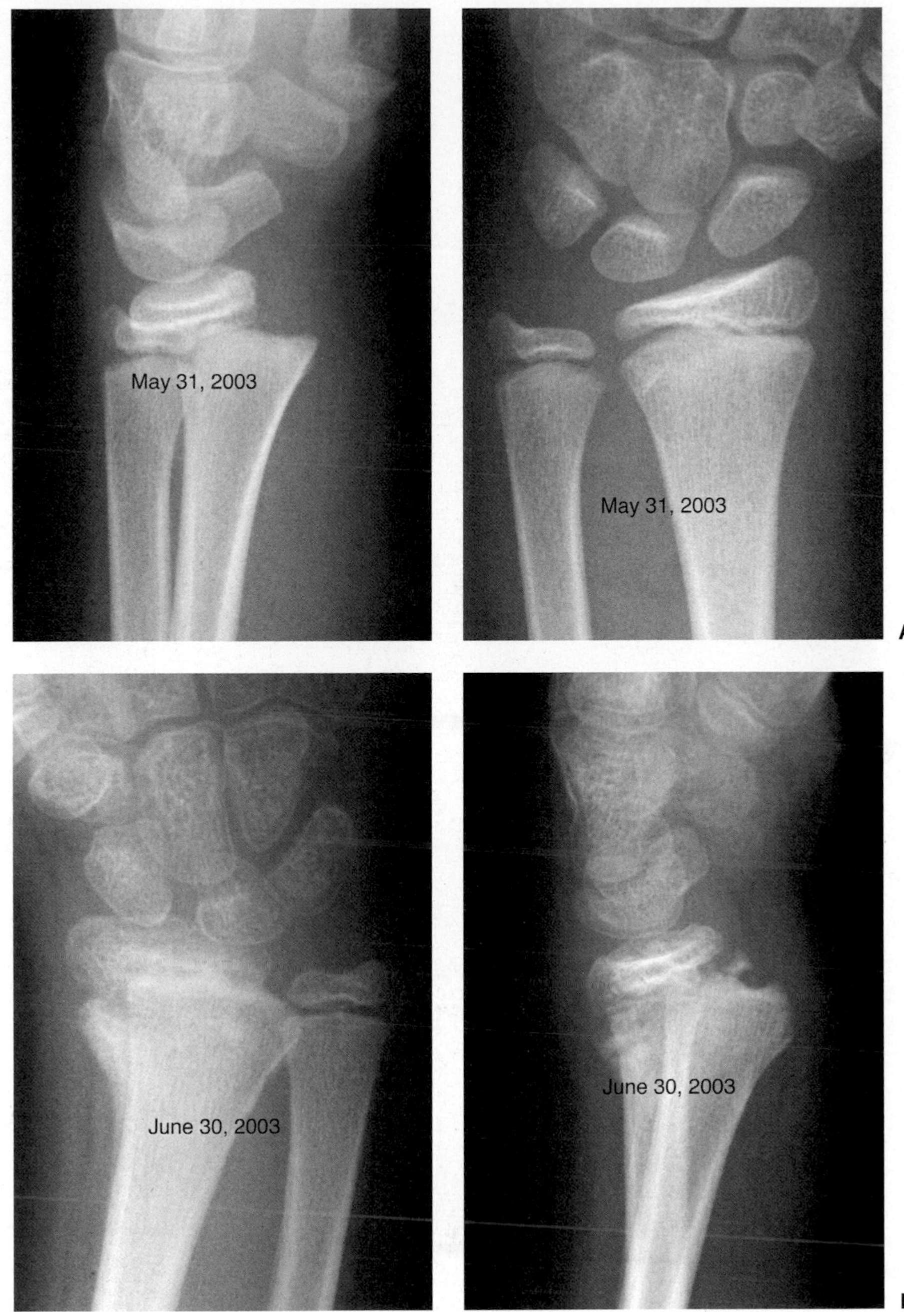

FIGURE 9-23 A. AP and lateral views of displaced radial physeal fracture. **B.** Healed malunion 1 month after radial physeal fracture. *(continues)*

fractures often occur in children with significant growth remaining. The deformity from a Salter-Harris type I or II fracture is in the plane of motion of the wrist joint and, therefore, will remodel with ensuing growth (Fig. 9-23).[8,108,181] Repeat reduction should not be done more than 7 days after fracture because of the risk of growth arrest. The malunited fracture should be monitored over the next 6 to 12 months for remodeling. If the fracture does not remodel, persistent extension deformity of the distal radial articular surface puts the patient at risk for developing midcarpal instability[217] or degenerative arthritis of the wrist, though a recent report has raised the question of whether imperfect final radiographic alignment necessarily leads to symptomatic arthrosis.[64] For malunion correction, an opening-wedge dorsal osteotomy is made, iliac crest bone of appropriate trapezoidal shape to correct the deformity is inserted, and either a plate or external fixator is used to maintain correction until healing.[62]

Intra-articular malunion is more worrisome because of the risk of development of degenerative arthritis if the articular step-off is more than 2 mm.[113] MRI or CT scans can be useful in preoperative evaluations. Arthroscopy allows direct examination of the deformity and areas of impingement or potential degeneration. Intra-articular osteotomy with bone grafting in the metaphysis to support the reconstructed articular surface is controversial and risky; however, it has the potential to restore anatomic alignment to the joint and prevent serious long-term complications. This problem fortunately is uncommon in children because of the rarity of the injury and this type of malunion.

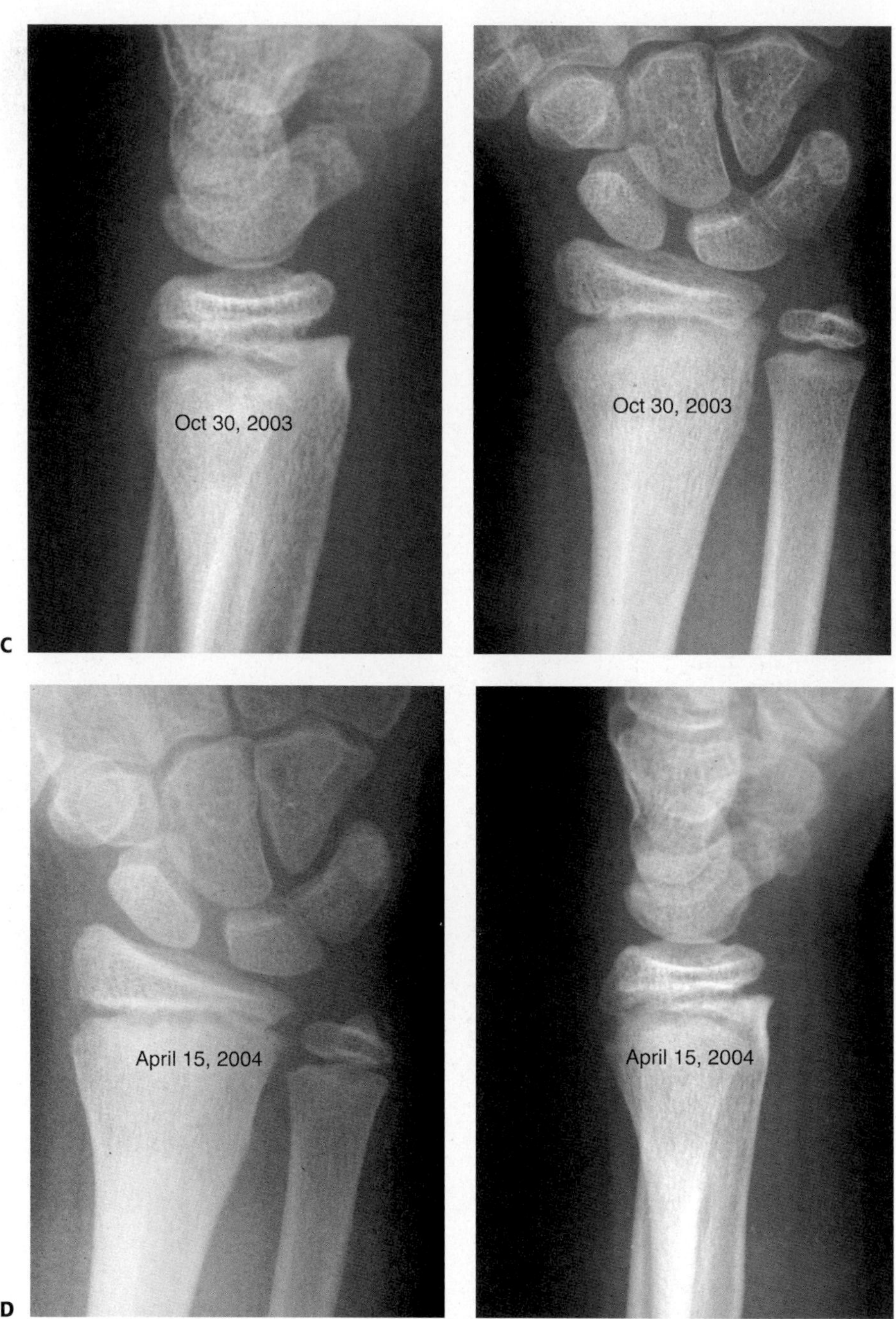

FIGURE 9-23 *(continued)* **C.** Significant remodeling at 5 months after fracture. **D.** Anatomic remodeling with no physeal arrest.

Physeal Arrest. Distal radial physeal arrest can occur from either the trauma of the original injury (Fig. 9-24)[95,124,227] or late (more than 7 days) reduction of a displaced fracture. The incidence of radial growth arrest has been shown to be 4% to 5% of all displaced radial physeal fractures.[9,24,124] The trauma to the physeal cartilage from displacement and compression is a significant risk factor for growth arrest. However, a correlation between the risk of growth arrest and the degree of displacement, type of fracture, or type of reduction has yet to be defined. Similarly, the risk of further compromising the physis with late reduction at various time intervals is still unclear. The current recommendation is for an atraumatic reduction of a displaced physeal fracture less than 7 days after injury.

When a growth arrest develops, the consequences depend on the severity of the arrest and the amount of growth remaining. A complete arrest of the distal radial physis in a skeletally immature patient can be a serious problem. The continued growth of the ulna with cessation of radial growth can lead to incongruity of the DRUJ, ulnocarpal impaction, and development of a TFCC tear (Fig. 9-25).[9,236] The radial deviation deformity at the wrist can be severe enough to cause limitation of wrist and forearm motion. Pain and clicking can develop at the ulnocarpal or radioulnar joints, indicative of ulnocarpal impaction or a TFCC tear. The deformity will progress until the end of growth. Pain and limited motion and function will be present until forearm length is rebalanced, until the radiocarpal, ulnocarpal, and radioulnar joints are restored, and until the TFCC tear and areas of chondromalacia are repaired or débrided.[161,221,236]

Ideally, physeal arrest of the distal radius will be discovered early before the consequences of unbalanced growth develop.

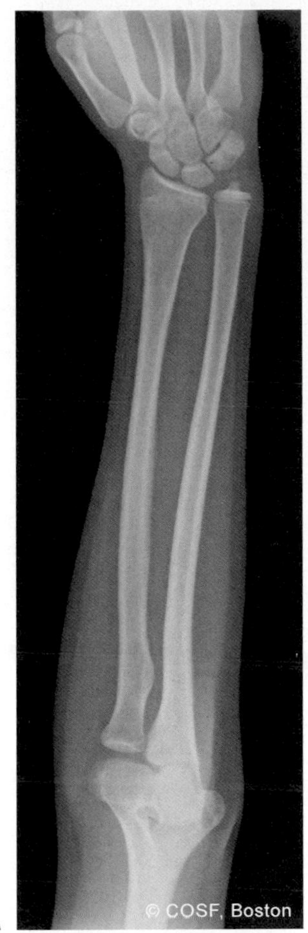

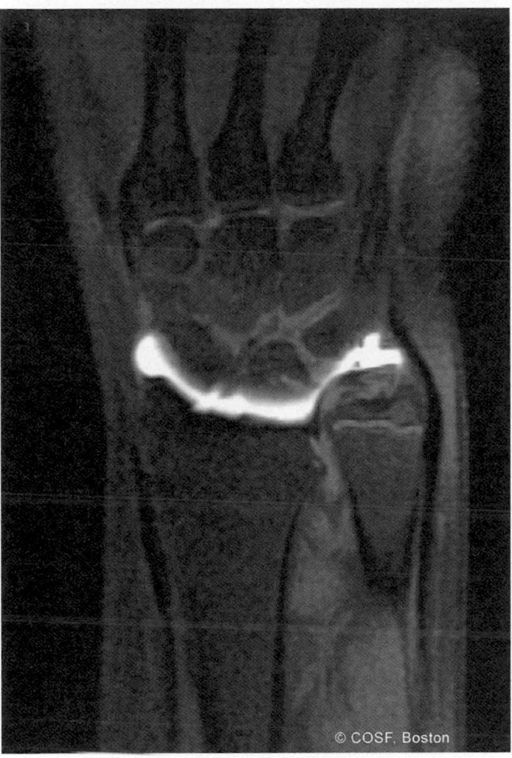

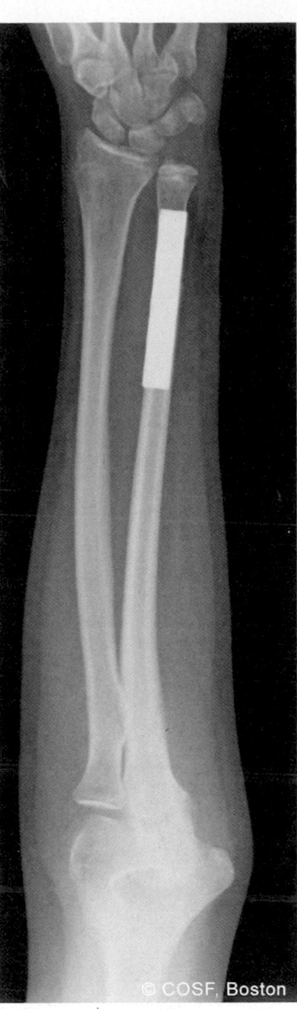

FIGURE 9-24 A. AP radiograph of growth arrest with open ulnar physis. **B.** MRI scan of large area of growth arrest that was not deemed resectable by mapping. Note is made of impaction of the distal ulna against the triquetrum and a secondary peripheral TFCC tear. **C.** Radiograph after ulnar shortening osteotomy, restoring neutral ulnar variance.

Radiographic screening 6 to 12 months after injury can identify the early arrest. A small area of growth arrest in a patient near skeletal maturity may be clinically inconsequential. However, a large area of arrest in a patient with marked growth remaining can lead to ulnocarpal impaction and forearm deformity if intervention is delayed. MRI can map the area of arrest.[168] If it is less than 45% of the physis, a bar resection with fat interposition can be attempted.[120,121] This may restore radial growth and prevent future problems (Fig. 9-26). If the bar is larger than 45% of the physis, bar resection is unlikely to be successful.

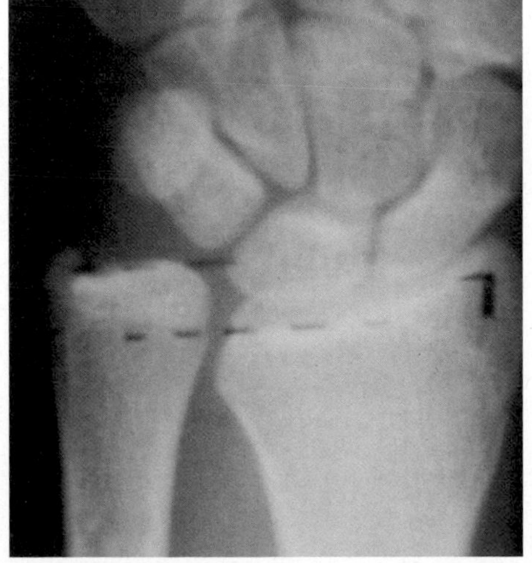

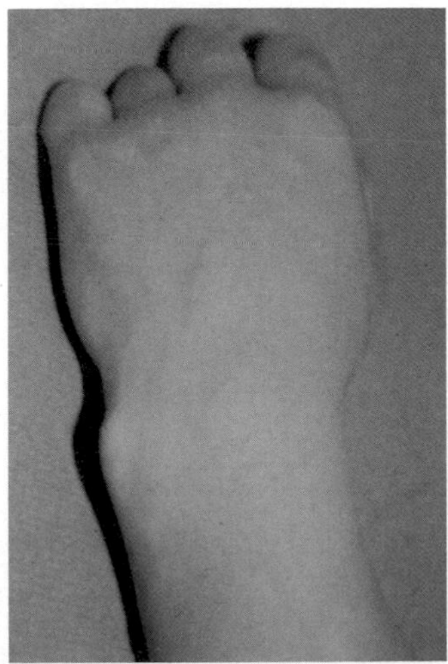

FIGURE 9-25 A. AP radiograph of radial growth arrest and ulnar overgrowth after physeal fracture. Patient complained of ulnar-sided wrist pain and clicking. **B.** Clinical photograph of ulnar overgrowth and radial deviation deformity.

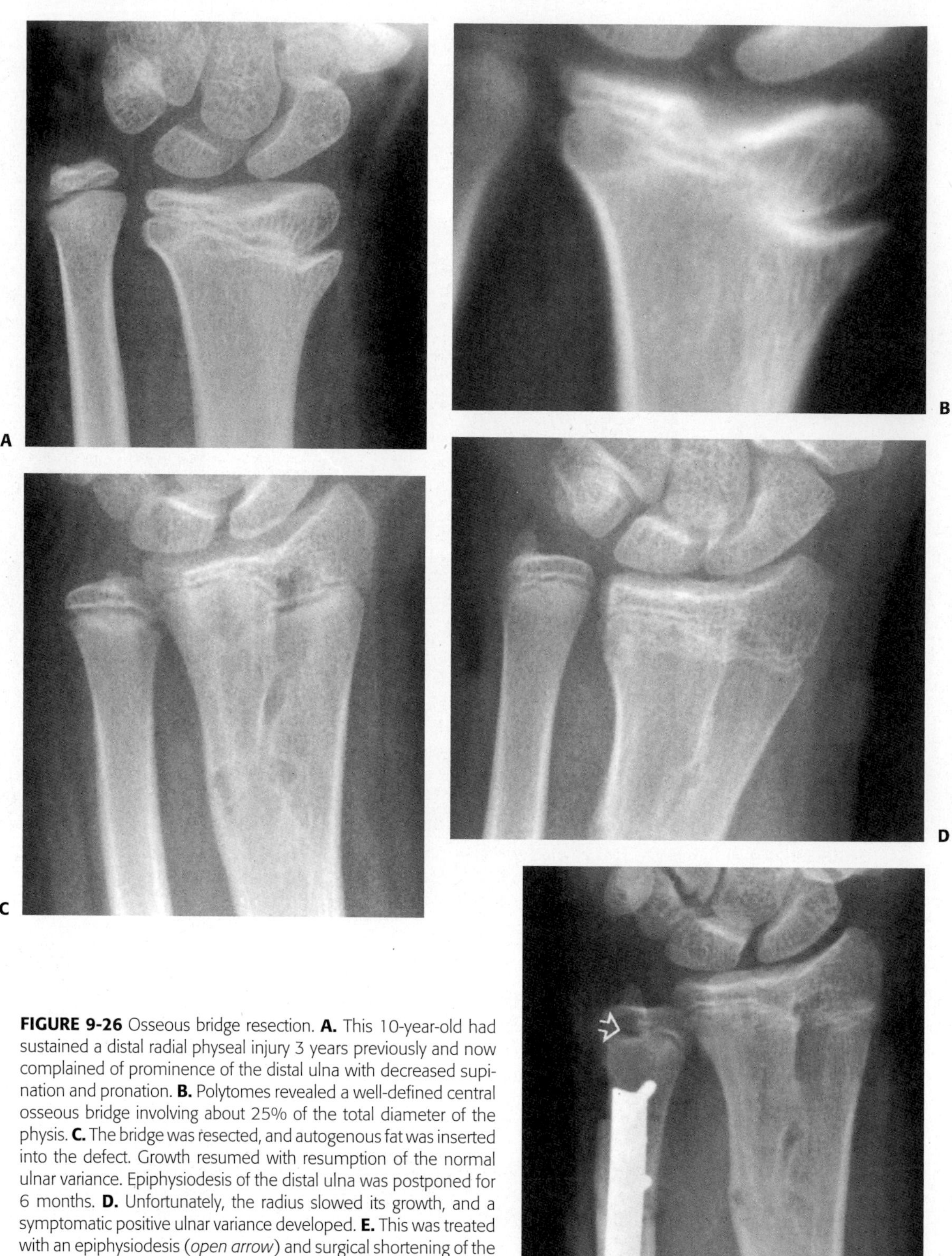

FIGURE 9-26 Osseous bridge resection. **A.** This 10-year-old had sustained a distal radial physeal injury 3 years previously and now complained of prominence of the distal ulna with decreased supination and pronation. **B.** Polytomes revealed a well-defined central osseous bridge involving about 25% of the total diameter of the physis. **C.** The bridge was resected, and autogenous fat was inserted into the defect. Growth resumed with resumption of the normal ulnar variance. Epiphysiodesis of the distal ulna was postponed for 6 months. **D.** Unfortunately, the radius slowed its growth, and a symptomatic positive ulnar variance developed. **E.** This was treated with an epiphysiodesis (*open arrow*) and surgical shortening of the ulna. The clinical appearance and range of motion of the forearm returned to essentially normal.

An early ulnar epiphysiodesis will prevent growth imbalance of the forearm.[236] The growth discrepancy between forearms in most patients is minor and does not require treatment. However, this is not the case for a patient with an arrest at a very young age, for whom complicated decisions regarding forearm lengthening need to occur.

Ulnocarpal Impaction Syndrome. The growth discrepancy between the radius and ulna can lead to relative radial shortening and ulnar overgrowth. The distal ulna can impinge on the lunate and triquetrum and cause pain with ulnar deviation, extension, and compression activities.[12] This is particularly true in repetitive wrist loading sports such as field hockey, lacrosse, and gymnastics.[45] Physical examination loading the ulnocarpal joint in ulnar deviation and compression will recreate the pain. Radiographs show the radial arrest, ulnar overgrowth, and distal ulnocarpal impingement. The ulnocarpal impaction also may be caused by a hypertrophic ulnar styloid fracture union

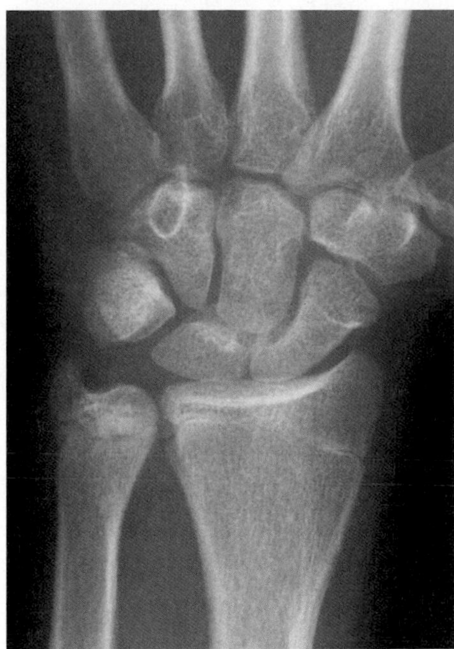

FIGURE 9-27 AP radiograph revealing hypertrophic ulnar styloid healing as the source of the ulnar carpal impaction pain in this patient.

(Fig. 9-27) or an ulnar styloid nonunion.[22,133] MRI may reveal chondromalacia of the lunate or triquetrum, a tear of the TFCC, and the extent of the distal radial physeal arrest.

Treatment should correct all components of the problem. The ulnar overgrowth is corrected by either an ulnar shortening osteotomy or radial lengthening. Most often, a marked degree of positive ulnar variance requires ulnar shortening to neutral or negative variance (Fig. 9-28). If the ulnar physis is still open, a simultaneous arrest should be done to prevent recurrent deformity. If the degree of radial deformity is marked, this should be corrected by a realignment or lengthening osteotomy. Criteria for radial correction is debatable, but we have used radial inclination of less than 11 degrees on the AP radiograph as an indication for correction (Fig. 9-29).[236] In the rare case of complete arrest in a very young patient, radial lengthening is preferable to ulnar shortening to rebalance the forearm.

Triangular Fibrocartilage Complex Tears. Peripheral traumatic TFCC tears should be repaired. The presence of an ulnar styloid nonunion at the base often is indicative of an associated peripheral tear of the TFCC.[1,161,221,236] The symptomatic ulnar styloid nonunion is excised[22,133,159] and any TFCC tear is repaired. If physical examination or preoperative MRI indicates a TFCC tear in the absence of an ulnar styloid nonunion, an initial arthroscopic examination can define the lesion and appropriate treatment. Peripheral tears are the most common TFCC tears in children and adolescents and can be repaired arthroscopically by an outside-in suture technique. Tears off the sigmoid notch are the next most common in adolescents and can be repaired with arthroscopic-assisted, transradial sutures. Central tears are rare in children and, as opposed to adults with degenerative central tears, arthroscopic débridement usually does not result in pain relief in children. Distal volar tears also are rare and are repaired open, at times with ligament reconstruction.[221]

Neuropathy. Median neuropathy can occur from direct trauma from the initial displacement of the fracture, traction ischemia from a persistently displaced fracture, or the development of a compartment syndrome in the carpal canal or volar forear (Fig. 9-30).[239] All patients with displaced distal radial fracturesin

A

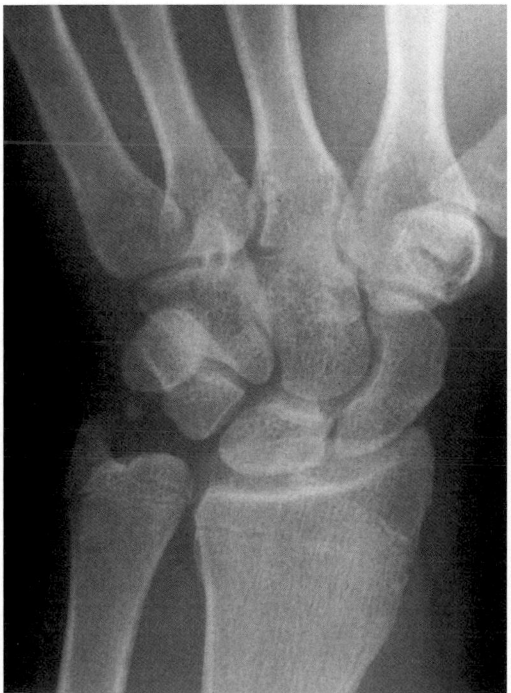

B

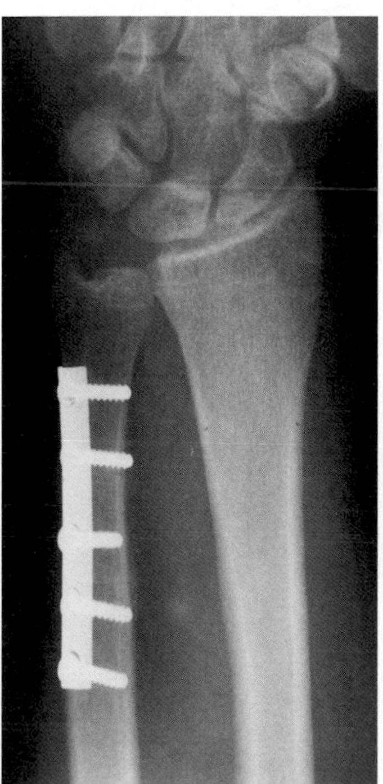

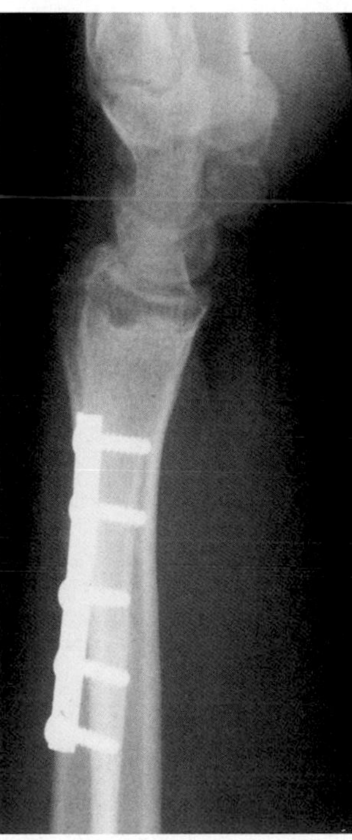

FIGURE 9-28 A. AP radiogaph of distal radial growth arrest, ulnar overgrowth, and an ulnar styloid nonunion. Wrist arthroscopy revealed an intact triangular fibrocartilage complex. **B.** AP and lateral radiographs after ulnar shortening osteotomy.

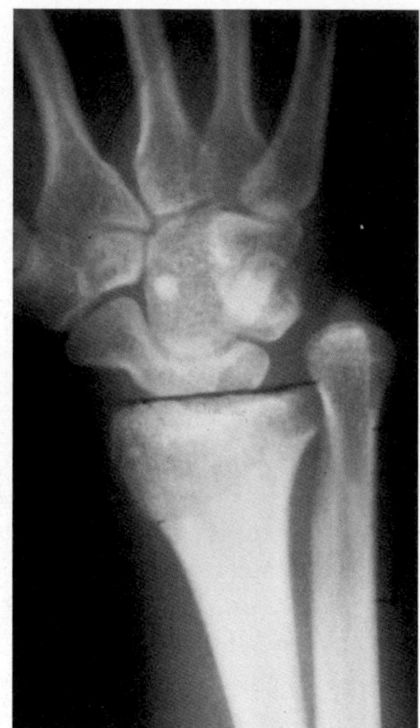

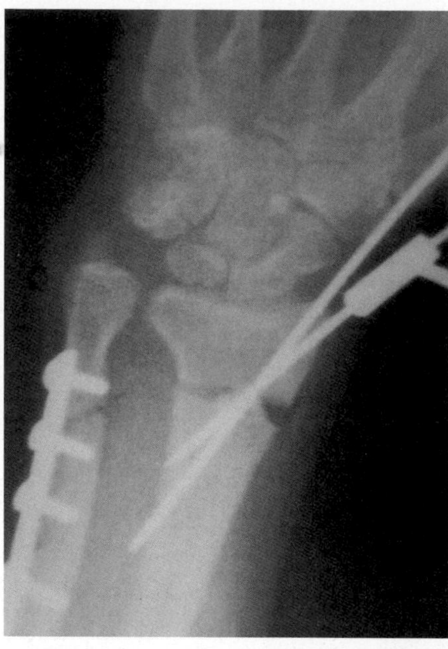

FIGURE 9-29 A. More severe ulnar overgrowth with dislocation of the distal radioulnar joint and flattening of the radial articular surface. **B.** Intraoperative fluoroscopic view of ulnar shortening and radial osteotomy to corrective deformities.

should undergo a careful motor-sensory examination upon presentation to an acute care facility. The flexor pollicis longus, index flexor digitorum profundus, and abductor pollicis brevis muscles should be tested. Light-touch and two-point discrimination sensibility of the thumb and index finger should be tested in any child over 5 years of age with a displaced Salter-Harris type I or II fracture. Median neuropathy and marked volar soft tissue swelling are indications for percutaneous pin stabilization of the fracture to lessen the risk of compartment syndrome in a cast.

Median neuropathy caused by direct trauma or traction ischemia generally resolves after fracture reduction. The degree of neural injury determines the length of time to recovery. Recovery can be monitored with an advancing Tinel sign along the median nerve. Motor-sensory testing can define progressive return of neural function.

Carpal Tunnel Syndrome. Median neuropathy caused by a carpal tunnel syndrome will not recover until the carpal tunnel is decompressed. After anatomic fracture reduction and pin stabilization, volar forearm and carpal tunnel pressures are measured. Gelberman[77] recommended waiting 20 minutes or more to allow for pressure-volume equilibration before measuring pressures. If the pressures are elevated beyond 40 mm Hg or the difference between the diastolic pressure and the compartment pressure is less than 30 mm Hg,[108] an immediate release of the affected compartments should be performed. The carpal tunnel is released through a palmar incision in line with the fourth ray, with care to avoid injuring the palmar vascular arch and the ulnar nerves exiting the Guyon canal. The transverse carpal ligament is released with a Z-plasty closure of the ligament to prevent late bow-stringing of the nerve against the palmar skin. The volar forearm fascia is released in the standard fashion.

RADIAL PHYSEAL STRESS FRACTURES

Repetitive axial loading of the wrist in dorsiflexion can lead to physeal stress injuries, almost always involving the radius.

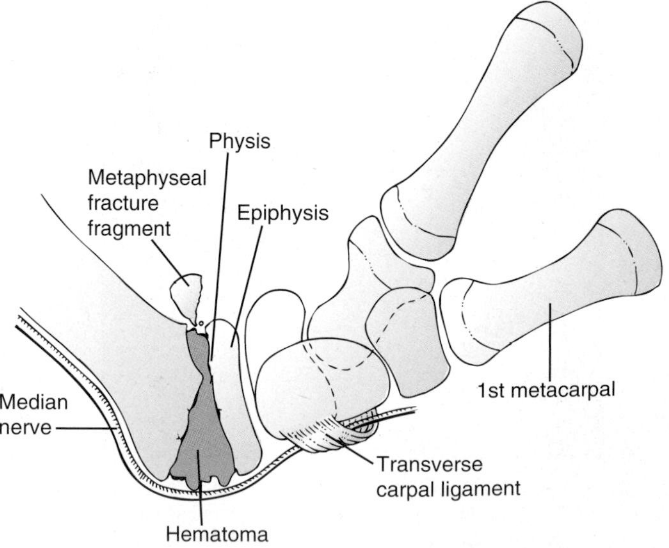

FIGURE 9-30 Volar forearm anatomy outlining the potential compression of the median nerve between the metaphysis of the radius and dorsally displaced physeal fracture. The taut volar transverse carpal ligament and fracture hematoma also are contributing factors. (Redrawn from Waters PM, Kolettis GJ, Schwend R. Acute median neuropathy following physeal fractures of the distal radius. J Pediatr Orthop 1994;14:173–177, with permission.)

Competitive gymnastics is by far the most common cause.[23,43,47,135,192,223] Other activities reported to cause radial physeal stress fractures include break dancing, wrestling, and cheerleading.[79] Factors that predispose to this injury include excessive training, poor techniques, and attempts to advance too quickly in competitive level. Proper coaching is important in preventing these injuries.

A child with a radial physeal stress fracture has recurring, activity-related wrist pain, usually aching and diffuse, in the region of the distal radial metaphysis and physis. Extremes of dorsiflexion and palmar flexion reproduce the pain. There is local tenderness over the dorsal, distal radial physis. Resistive contracture strength testing of the wrist dorsiflexors often reproduces the pain. There may be fusiform swelling about the wrist if there is reactive bone formation. The differential diagnosis includes physeal stress injury, ganglion, ligamentous or TFCC injury, tendonitis or muscle-tendon tear, fracture such as a scaphoid fracture, and osteonecrosis of the scaphoid (Preiser disease) or lunate (Kienböck disease). Radiographs may be diagnostic. Physeal widening and reactive bone formation are indicative of chronic physeal stress fracture. Premature physeal closure indicates long-standing stress.[191,249] In this situation, continued ulnar growth leads to an ulnar positive variance and pain from ulnocarpal impaction or a TFCC tear.[5,45,223] Normal radiographs may not show an early physeal stress fracture. If the diagnosis is suggested clinically, bone scanning or MRI is indicated. Bone scanning is sensitive but nonspecific; MRI usually is diagnostic.

Treatment first and foremost involves rest. This may be difficult depending on the skill level of the athlete and the desires of the child, coach, and parents to maintain constant training. Education regarding the long-term consequences of a growth arrest is important in this emotionally charged situation. Short-arm cast immobilization for several weeks may be the only way to restrict stress to the radial physis in some patients. Splint protection is appropriate in cooperative patients. Protection should continue until there is resolution of pain with examination and activity. The athlete can maintain cardiovascular fitness, strength, and flexibility while protecting the injured wrist. Once the acute physeal injury has healed, return to weight-bearing activities should be gradual. This requires the cooperation of the coach and parents. Adjustment of techniques and training methods often is necessary to prevent recurrence. The major concern is development of a radial growth arrest in a skeletally immature patient. This is an avoidable complication.

If a radial growth arrest has already occurred upon presentation, treatment depends on the degree of deformity and the patient's symptoms. Physeal bar resection often is not possible because the arrest is usually too diffuse in stress injuries. If there is no significant ulnar overgrowth, a distal ulnar epiphysiodesis will prevent the development of an ulnocarpal impaction syndrome. For ulnar overgrowth and ulnocarpal pain, an ulnar shortening osteotomy is indicated. Techniques include transverse, oblique, and Z-shortening osteotomies. Transverse osteotomy has a higher risk of nonunion than either oblique or Z-shortening and should be avoided. Even when oblique or Z-shortenings are used, making the osteotomy more distally in the metaphyseal region will lessen the risk of nonunion, owing to the more robust vascularity of the distal ulna. The status of the TFCC also should be evaluated by MRI or wrist arthroscopy. If there is an associated TFCC tear, it should be repaired as appropriate.

ULNAR PHYSEAL FRACTURES

Isolated ulnar physeal fractures are rare injuries. Most ulnar physeal fractures occur in association with radial metaphyseal or physeal fractures. Physeal separations are classified by the standard Salter-Harris criteria. The rare pediatric Galeazzi injury usually involves an ulnar physeal fracture rather than a soft tissue disruption of the distal radioulnar joint. Another ulnar physeal fracture is an avulsion fracture off the distal aspect of the ulnar styloid.[1,211] Although an ulnar styloid injury is an epiphyseal avulsion, it can be associated with soft tissue injuries of the TFCC and ulnocarpal joint but does not cause growth-related complications.

Physeal growth arrest is frequent with distal ulnar physeal fractures (Fig. 9-31), occurring in 10% to 55% of patients. It is unclear why the distal ulna has a higher incidence of growth arrest after fracture than does the radius. Ulnar growth arrest in a young child leads to relative radial overgrowth and bowing.

Current Treatment Options

Treatment options are similar to those for radial physeal fractures: immobilization alone, closed reduction and cast immobilization, closed reduction and percutaneous pinning, and open reduction. Often, these fractures are minimally displaced or nondisplaced. Immobilization until fracture healing at 3 to 6 weeks is standard treatment. Closed reduction is indicated for displaced fractures with more than 50% translation or 20 degrees of angulation. Most ulnar physeal fractures reduce to a near anatomic alignment with reduction of the radial fracture due to the attachments of the distal radioulnar joint ligaments and TFCC. Failure to obtain a reduction of the ulnar fracture may indicate that there is soft tissue interposed in the fracture site. This is an indication for open reduction. Exposure should be from the side of the torn periosteum, typically opposite the Thurston-Holland fragment or direction of displacement. The interposed soft tissue (periosteum, extensor tendons, abductor digiti quinti, or flexor tendons) must be extracted from the fracture site.[55,117,157] If reduction is not stable, a small-diameter smooth pin can be used to maintain alignment until healing at 3 to 4 weeks. Further injury to the physis should be avoided during operative exposure and reduction because of the high risk of growth arrest.

ULNAR STYLOID FRACTURES

Ulnar styloid avulsion fractures are common in association with radial fractures[211] and represent a soft tissue avulsion of the attachment of the TFCC or ulnocarpal ligaments. Treatment consists of immobilization and monitoring of long-term outcome, and most heal without sequelae.[119] However, an acute displaced fracture of the base of the styloid represents a disruption of the TFCC.[1] Most of these injuries are caused by high-velocity trauma in adolescents at or near skeletal maturity. Treatment should be open reduction with tension band fixation

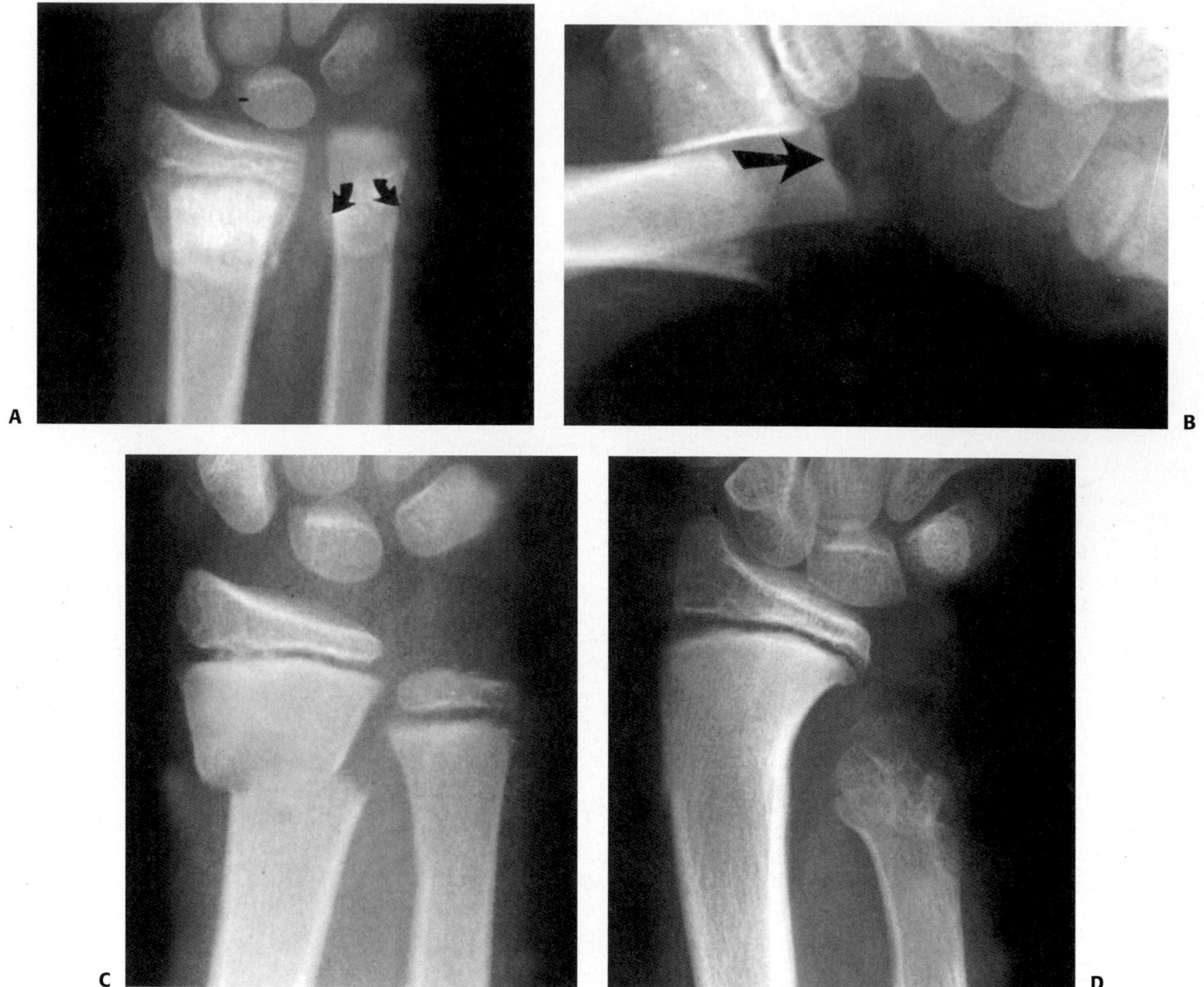

FIGURE 9-31 A,B. A 10-year-old boy sustained a closed Salter-Harris type I separation of the distal ulnar physis (*arrows*) combined with a fracture of the distal radial metaphysis. **C.** An excellent closed reduction was achieved atraumatically. **D.** Long-term growth arrest of the distal ulna occurred.

of the styloid to the metaphysis and repair of the TFCC. The tension band wire is removed at 3 to 6 weeks.

Some ulnar styloid fractures result in nonunion or hypertrophic union.[22,133,159,221] Nonunion may be associated with TFCC tears or ulnocarpal impaction. The hypertrophic healing represents a pseudoulnar positive variance with resultant ulnocarpal impaction. Both cause ulnar-sided wrist pain. Compression of the lunate or triquetrum on the distal ulna reproduces the pain. Clicking with ulnocarpal compression or forearm rotation represents either a TFCC tear or chondromalacia of the lunate or triquetrum. Surgical excision of the nonunion or hypertrophic union with repair of the TFCC to the base of the styloid is the treatment of choice. Postoperative immobilization for 4 weeks in a long-arm cast followed by 2 weeks in a short-arm cast protects the TFCC repair.

Complications

Growth Arrest

The most common complication of distal ulnar physeal fractures is growth arrest. Golz[81] described 18 such fractures, with growth arrest in 10%. If the patient is young enough, continued growth of the radius will lead to deformity and dysfunction. The distal ulnar aspect of the radial physis and epiphysis appears to be tethered by the foreshortened ulna (Fig. 9-32). The radial articular surface develops increased inclination toward the foreshortened ulna. This is similar to the deformity Peinado[164] created experimentally with arrest of the distal ulna in rabbits' forelimbs. The distal ulna loses its normal articulation in the sigmoid notch of the distal radius. The metaphyseal-diaphyseal region of the radius often becomes notched from its articulation with the distal ulna during forearm rotation. Frequently, these patients have pain and limitation of motion with pronation and supination.[12]

Ideally, this problem is identified before the development of marked ulnar foreshortening and subsequent radial deformity. Because it is well known that distal ulnar physeal fractures have a high incidence of growth arrest, these patients should have serial radiographs at 6 to 12 months after fracture for early identification. Unfortunately, in the distal ulnar physis, physeal bar resection generally is unsuccessful. Surgical arrest of the radial physis can prevent radial deformity. Usually, this occurs toward the end of growth so that the forearm length discrepancy is not a problem.

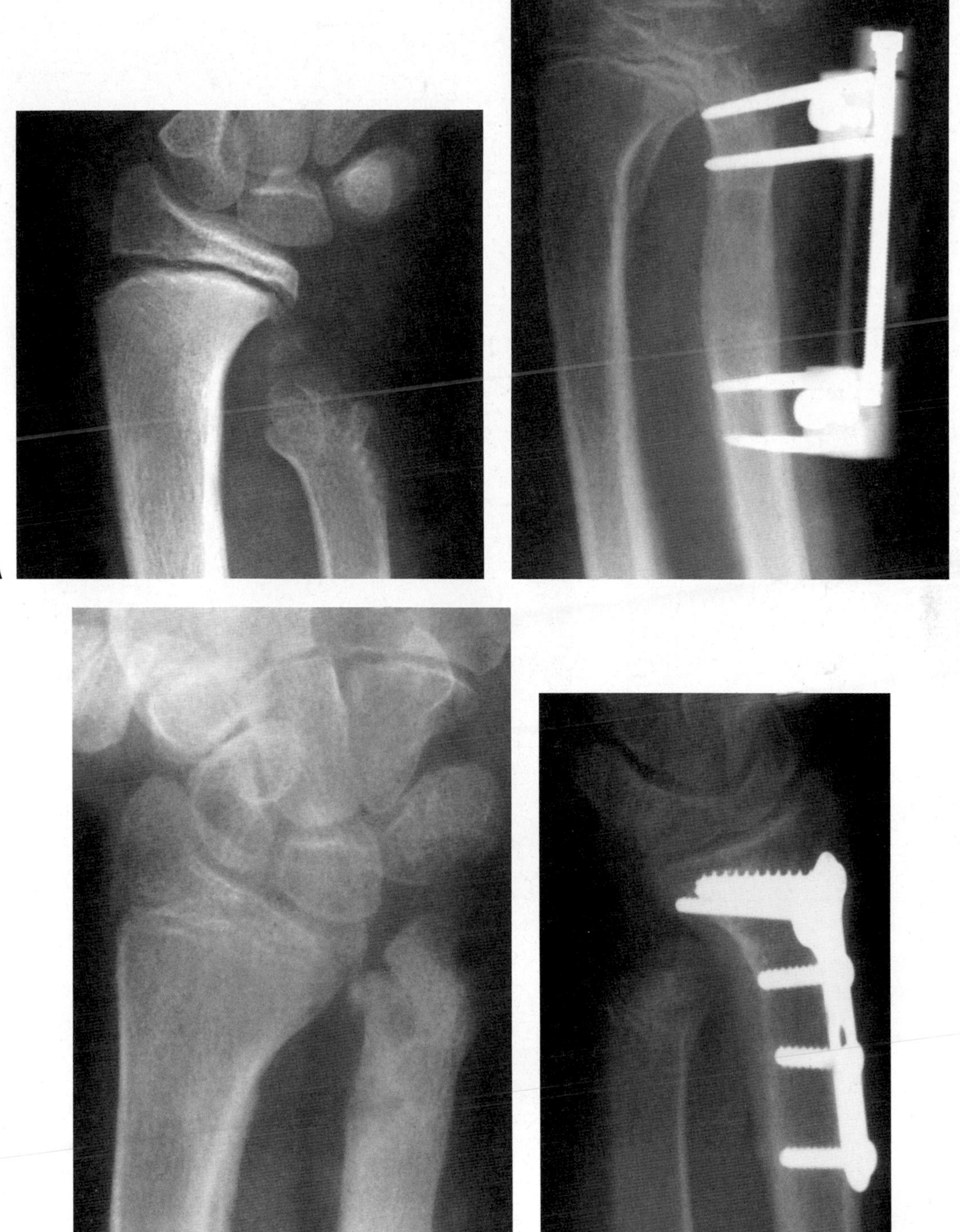

FIGURE 9-32 A. The appearance of the distal ulna in the patient seen in Figure 9-21, 3 years after injury, demonstrating premature fusion of the distal ulnar physis with 3.2 cm of shortening. The distal radius is secondarily deformed, with tilting and translocation toward the ulna. **B.** In the patient in Figure 9-21 with distal ulnar physeal arrest, a lengthening of the distal ulna was performed using a small unipolar distracting device. The ulna was slightly overlengthened to compensate for some subsequent growth of the distal radius. **C.** Six months after the lengthening osteotomy, there is some deformity of the distal ulna, but good restoration of length has been achieved. The distal radial epiphyseal tilt has corrected somewhat, and the patient has asymptomatic supination and pronation to 75 degrees. **D.** Similar case to Figure 9-32A–C, but with more progressive distal radial deformity treated with corrective osteotomy and epiphysiodesis of the distal radius.

Rarely, patients present late with established deformity. Treatment involves rebalancing the length of the radius and ulna. The options include hemiphyseal arrest of the radius, corrective radial closing wedge osteotomy, and ulnar lengthening (Fig. 9-32),[12,81,152] or a combination of these procedures. The painful impingement of the radius and ulna with forearm rotation can be corrected with reconstitution of the distal radioulnar joint. If the radial physis has significant growth remaining, a radial physeal arrest should be done at the same time as the surgical rebalancing of the radius and ulna.[154] Treatment is individualized depending on the age of the patient, degree of deformity, and level of pain and dysfunction.

METAPHYSEAL FRACTURES

The metaphysis of the distal radius is the most common site of forearm fracture in children and adolescents,[111,118,205,222] and recent evidence suggests that the incidence of these fractures is increasing.[110] They occur most commonly in boys in the nondominant arm.[246] These fractures have a peak incidence during the adolescent growth spurt, which in girls is age 11 to 12 years and in boys is 12 to 13 years.[10] During this time of extensive bone remodeling, there is relative osteoporosis of the distal radial metaphysis, which makes this area more susceptible to fracture with a fall.

A

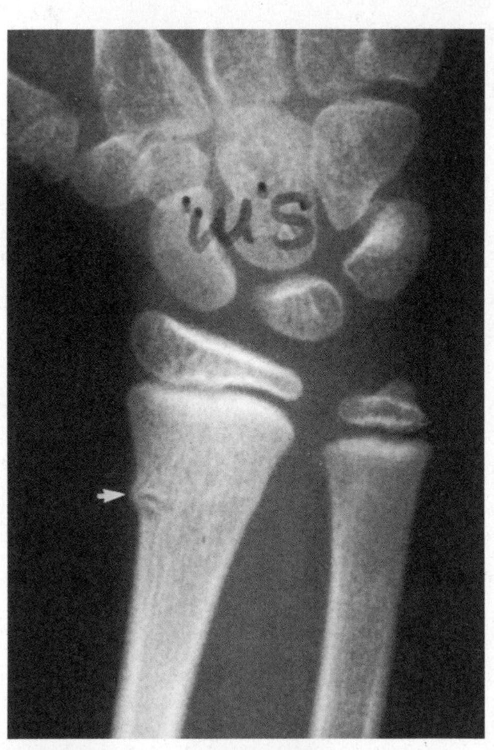

B

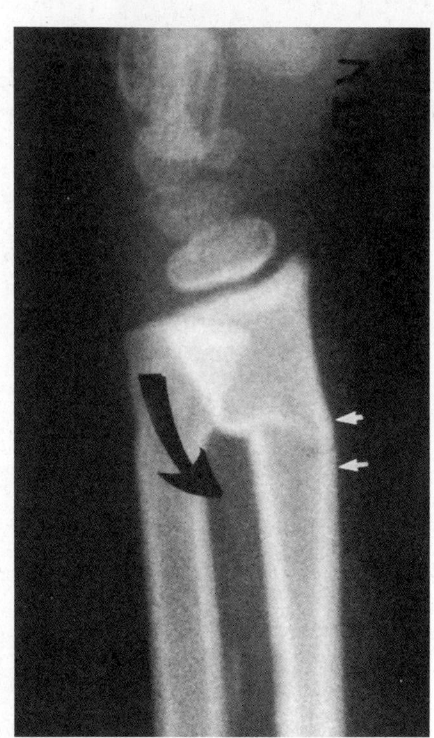

C

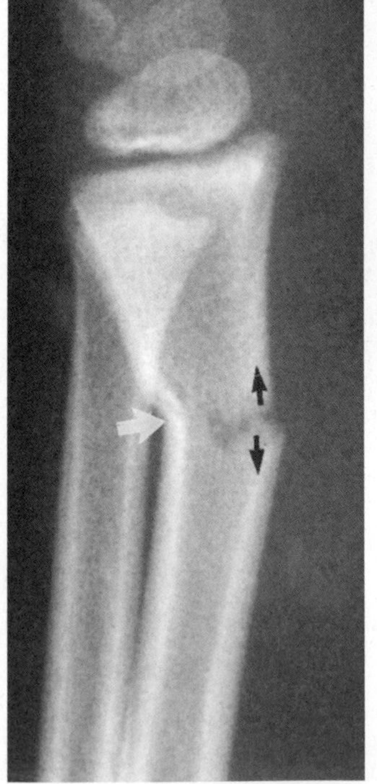

D

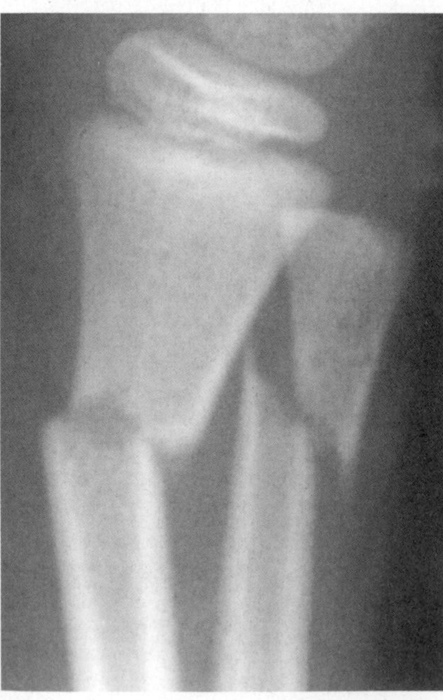

FIGURE 9-33 Metaphyseal biomechanical patterns. **A.** Torus fracture. Simple bulging of the thin cortex (*arrow*). **B.** Compression greenstick fracture. Angulation of the dorsal cortex (*large curved arrow*). The volar cortex is intact but slightly plastically deformed (*small white arrows*). **C.** Tension failure greenstick fracture. The dorsal cortex is plastically deformed (*white arrow*), and the volar cortex is complete and separated (*black arrows*). **D.** Complete length maintained. Both cortices are completely fractured, but the length of the radius has been maintained. (Reprinted from Wilkins KE, ed. Operative Management of Upper Extremity Fractures in Children. Rosemont, IL: American Academy of Orthopaedic Surgeons, 1994:24, with permission.)

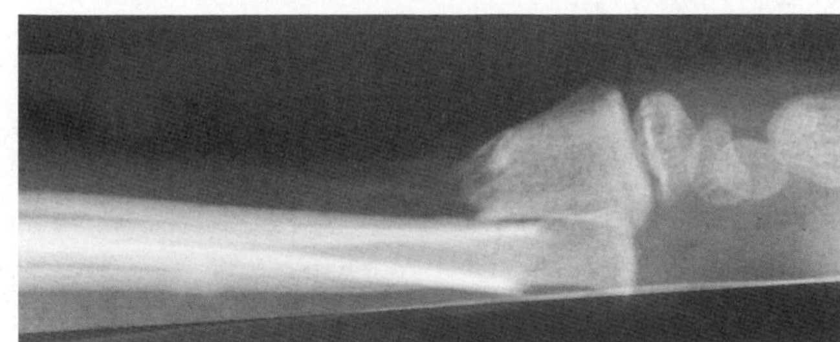

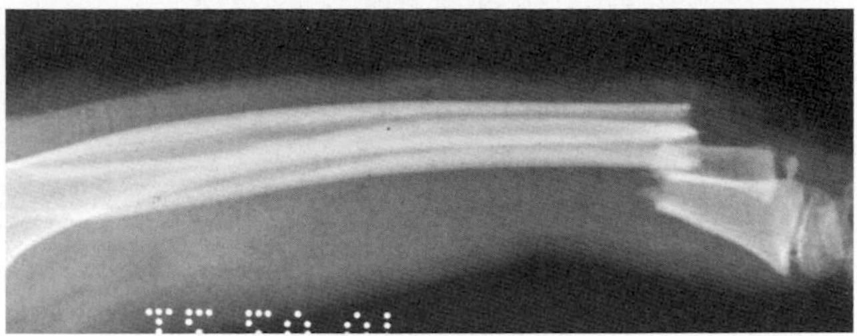

FIGURE 9-34 Complete fractures; bayonet apposition. **A.** Dorsal bayonet. **B.** Volar bayonet.

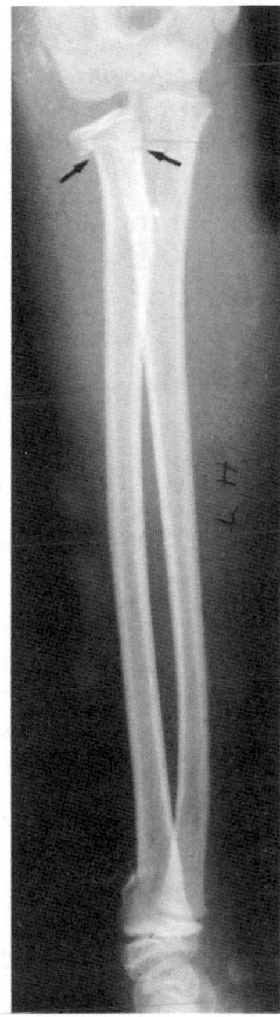

FIGURE 9-35 A 10-year-old girl with an innocuous-appearing distal radial fracture associated with an ipsilateral angulated radial neck fracture (*arrows*).

Mechanism of Injury

The mechanism of injury generally is a fall on an outstretched hand. The usual dorsiflexion position of the wrist leads to tension failure on the volar side. Fracture type and degree of displacement depend on the height and velocity of the fall.[205] These fractures can be nondisplaced torus or buckle injuries (common in younger children with a minimal fall) or dorsally displaced fractures with apex volar angulation (more common in older children with higher velocity injuries) (Fig. 9-33). Displacement may be severe enough to cause foreshortening and bayonet apposition (Fig. 9-34). Rarely, a mechanism such as a fall from a height can cause a distal radial fracture associated with a more proximal fracture of the forearm or elbow (Fig. 9-35).[163,210,241] These "floating elbow" situations are indicative of higher-velocity trauma and risk of compartment syndrome.[185] In addition, a fall with a palmar flexed wrist can produce a volarly displaced fracture with apex dorsal angulation (Fig. 9-36).

Seasonal variation has been noted in these fractures in children younger than 15 years of age.[234] The incidence of wrist and forearm fractures was roughly half (5.7/1000 per year) in the three winter months in Wales compared with the rest of the year (10.7/1000 per year). In addition, the nonwinter month fractures were more severe in terms of requiring reduction and hospitalization in this longitudinal study. Certain sports, such as snowboarding, soccer goal-keeping, and horseback riding, have been shown to have an increased risk of distal radial fracture.[104,116,138,187,197,215] Protective wrist guards have been shown to decrease the injury rate in snowboarders, especially beginners and persons with rental equipment.[187]

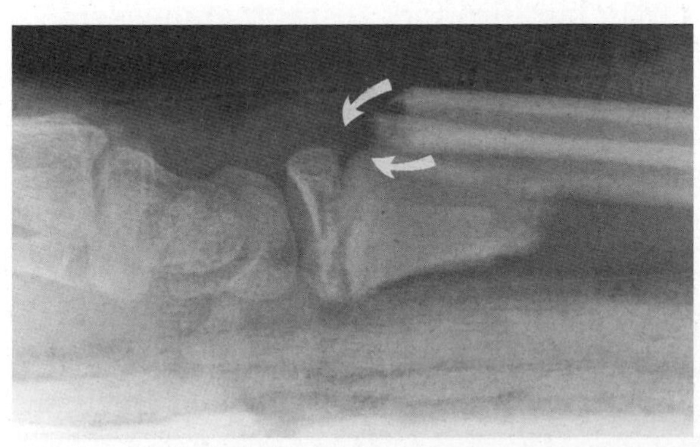

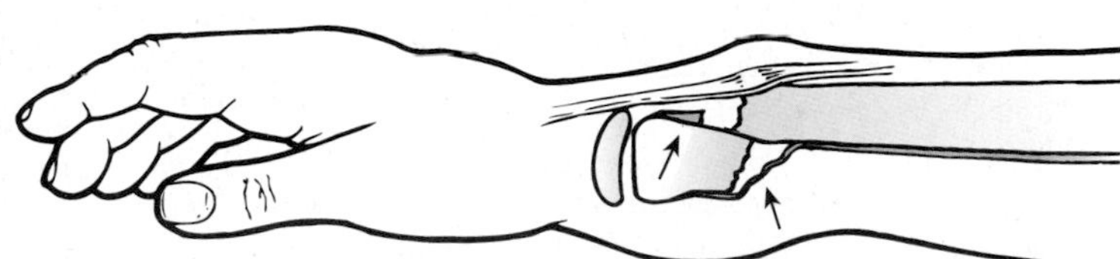

FIGURE 9-36 Reverse bayonet. **A.** Typical volar bayonet fracture. Often the distal end of the proximal fragment is buttonholed through the extensor tendons (*arrows*). (Reprinted from Wilkins KE, ed. Operative Management of Upper Extremity Fractures in Children. Rosemont, IL: American Academy of Orthopaedic Surgeons, 1994:27, with permission.) **B.** Intact volar periosteum and disrupted dorsal periosteum (*arrows*). The extensor tendons are displaced to either side of the proximal fragment.

A

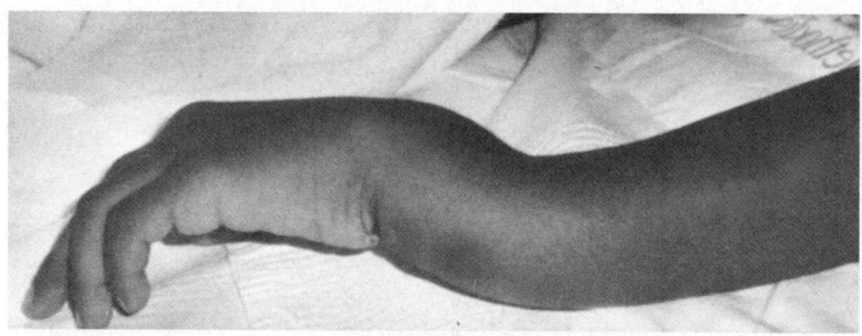

B

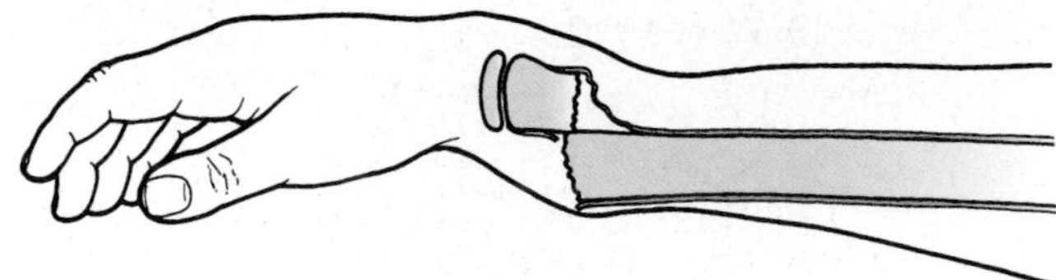

FIGURE 9-37 Dorsal bayonet deformity. **A.** Typical distal metaphyseal fracture with dorsal bayonet showing a dorsal angulation of the distal forearm. **B.** Usually, the periosteum is intact on the dorsal side and disrupted on the volar side.

Signs and Symptoms

Children with distal radial fractures present with pain, swelling, and deformity of the distal forearm (Fig. 9-37). The clinical signs depend on the degree of fracture displacement. With a nondisplaced torus fracture in a young child, medical attention may not be sought until several days after injury, because the intact periosteum is protective in this situation, lessening pain and the child's restriction of activities. Most children with distal radial fractures, however, present acutely after the fall with an obvious deformity. Physical examination is limited by the patient's pain and anxiety, but it is imperative to obtain an accurate examination of the motor and sensory components of the radial, median, and ulnar nerves before treatment. Median nerve motor function is evaluated by testing the abductor pollicis brevis (intrinsic) and flexor pollicis longus (extrinsic) muscles. Ulnar nerve motor evaluation includes testing the first dorsal interosseous (intrinsic), abductor digit quinti (intrinsic), and flexor digitorum profundus to the small finger (extrinsic) muscles. Radial nerve evaluation involves testing the common digital extensors for metacarpophalangeal joint extension. Sensibility to light touch and two-point discrimination should be tested. Normal two-point discrimination is less than 5 mm but is not present until age 5 to 7 years. Pin-prick sensibility testing will only hurt and scare the already anxious child and should be avoided. A prospective study indicated an 8% incidence of nerve injury in children with distal radial fractures.[246]

Associated Injuries

The ipsilateral extremity should be carefully examined for fractures of the carpus,[206] forearm, or elbow[31,85,87,96,188,210,220,225,226] because 3% to 13% of distal radial fractures have associated ipsilateral extremity fractures,[65,210] increasing the risk of neurovascular compromise and compartment syndrome.[158,163,210] In the multitrauma patient, fracture care is appropriately modified to coincide with appropriate systemic care.

Diagnosis and Classification

Radiographs are diagnostic of the fracture type and degree of displacement. Standard AP and lateral radiographs usually are sufficient. Complete wrist, forearm, and elbow views are necessary for high-velocity injuries or when there is clinical tenderness. More extensive radiographic studies (CT scan, tomography) usually are not necessary unless there is intra-articular extension of the metaphyseal fracture in a skeletally mature adolescent.

These fractures are classified by fracture pattern, type of associated ulnar fracture, and direction of displacement. Fracture displacement is broadly classified as dorsal or volar. Most distal radial metaphyseal fractures are displaced dorsally with apex volar angulation.[222] Volar displacement with apex dorsal angulation can occur with palmar flexion injuries.

Metaphyseal fracture patterns are torus, incomplete or greenstick, and complete fractures (see Fig. 9-33). Torus fractures are axial compression injuries. The site of cortical failure is the transition from metaphysis to diaphysis.[128] These injuries are stable because of the intact periosteum. Rarely, they may extend into the physis, putting them at risk for growth impairment.[168,169] Incomplete or greenstick fractures occur with a combination of compressive and rotatory forces, generally a dorsiflexion force and supination deforming force. This leads to a volar tension side failure and a dorsal compression injury. The degree of force determines the amount of plastic deformation, dorsal comminution, and fracture angulation and rotation. If the force is sufficient, a complete fracture occurs with disruption of both the volar and dorsal cortices. Length may be maintained with apposition of the proximal and distal fragments. Frequently, the distal fragment lies proximal and dorsal to the proximal fragment in bayonet apposition (Table 9-2).

The ulnar fracture often associated with radial metaphyseal fracture can be metaphyseal or physeal or an ulnar styloid avulsion. Similar to radial metaphyseal fractures, the ulnar fracture can be complete or incomplete.

Distal radial fractures also can occur in conjunction with more proximal forearm fractures,[11] Monteggia fracture-dislocations,[13] supracondylar distal humeral fractures,[158,163,188] or carpal fractures.[13,85,87,96,206,225,226] The combination of a displaced supracondylar distal humeral fracture and a displaced distal radial metaphyseal fracture has been called the pediatric floating elbow. This injury combination is unstable and has an increased risk for malunion and neurovascular compromise.

Pediatric distal radial metaphyseal fractures are not classified by degree of instability. Unstable fractures have been predominately defined by the failure to maintain a successful closed re-

TABLE 9-2 Classification: Distal Metaphyseal Fractures

Directional displacement	Biomechanical patterns
Dorsal	Torus
Volar	Greenstick
Fracture combinations	One cortex
Isolated radius	Two cortices
Radius with ulna	Complete fracture
Ulnar styloid	Length maintained
Ulnar physis	Bayonet apposition
Ulnar metaphysis, incomplete	
Ulnar metaphysis, complete	

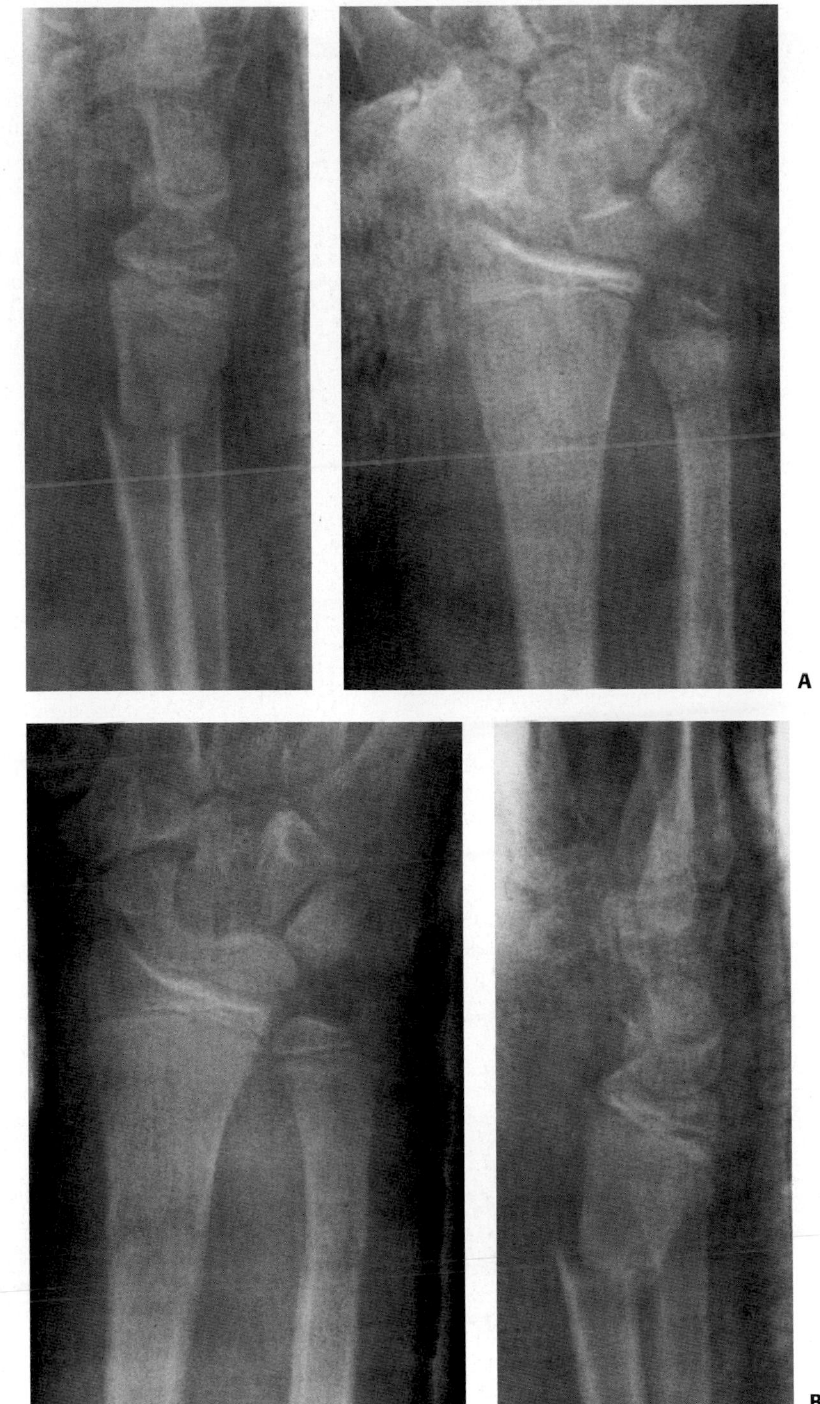

FIGURE 9-38 A. Serial radiographs at 3 days and 10 days **(B)** revealing slow loss of reduction that is common after closed reduction of distal radial metaphyseal fractures.

duction (Fig. 9-38). This occurs in approximately 30% of complete distal radial metaphyseal fractures.[136,177,244] This high percentage of loss of alignment has been tolerated because of the remodeling potential of the distal radius. Anatomic remodeling is possible because the extension deformity is in the plane of motion of the wrist joint, the metaphyseal fracture is juxtaphyseal, and most of these fractures occur while there is still significant growth remaining. However, concern has increased about the high failure rate of closed reduction to maintain anatomic alignment of these fractures. Factors that have been identified as increasing the risk of loss of reduction with closed manipulation and casting include poor casting, bayonet apposition, translation of more than 50% the diameter of the radius, apex volar angulation of more than 30 degrees, isolated radial fractures, and radial and ulnar metaphyseal fractures at the same level.[6,136,177,244,254]

Current Treatment Options

Treatment options are the same as those for radial physeal fractures: immobilization alone, closed reduction and cast immobilization, closed reduction and percutaneous pinning, and open reduction. The fracture type, degree of fracture instability, associated soft tissue or skeletal trauma, and the age of the patient all influence choice of treatment.

TABLE 9-3 Acceptable Angular Corrections in Degrees

Age (yr)	Sagittal Plane Boys	Sagittal Plane Girls	Frontal Plane
4–9	20	15	15
9–11	15	10	5
11–13	10	10	0
>13	5	0	0

Acceptable residual angulation is that which will result in total radiographic and functional correction. (Courtesy of B. deCourtivron, MD. Centre Hospitalie Universitaire de Tours. Tours, France.)

Torus Fractures

Torus fractures are compression injuries with minimal cortical disruption. As failure occurs in compression, by definition these are inherently stable injuries. Treatment should consist of protected immobilization to prevent further injury and relieve pain.[39,109,156,173,208,215,243] Once the patient is comfortable, range-of-motion exercises and nontraumatic activities can begin. Fracture healing usually occurs in 2 to 4 weeks.[8,123,133,157] Simple torus fractures usually heal without long-term sequelae.

Bicortical disruption on both the AP and lateral views indicates a more severe injury than a stable torus fracture. Splint or limited immobilization in this situation puts the child at risk for displacement. More prolonged, long-arm cast protection in a young patient who can wiggle out of a short-arm cast and closer follow-up generally are recommended to lessen the risk of malunion. These fractures generally heal in 3 to 6 weeks.

Incomplete/Greenstick Fractures

Immobilization Alone. Treatment of incomplete distal radial and ulnar fractures depends on the age of the patient, the degree and direction of fracture displacement and angulation, the surgeon's biases regarding remodeling, and the surgeon's and community's biases regarding deformity. In younger patients, the remodeling potential of an acute distal radial malunion is extremely high. Acceptable sagittal plane angulation of an acute distal radial metaphyseal fracture has been reported to be from 10 to 35 degrees in patients under 5 years of age.[16,32,132,157,175,202,246] Similarly, in patients under 10 years of age, the degree of acceptable angulation has ranged from 10 to 25 degrees.[16,32,132,157,175,202,246] In patients over 10 years of age, acceptable alignment has ranged from 5 to 20 degrees depending on the skeletal maturity of the patient (Table 9-3).[16,32,41,132,157,175,202,244,246]

The high potential for remodeling of a distal radial metaphyseal malunion has led some clinicians to recommend immobilization alone.[46] As mentioned, the range of accepted sagittal malalignment has been broad and is age and clinician dependent (Figs. 9-39 and 9-40).

Acceptable frontal plane deformity has been more uniform. The fracture tends to displace radially with an apex ulnar angulation. This does have the potential to remodel,[165] but less so than sagittal plane deformity. Most researchers agree that only 10 degrees or less of acute malalignment in the frontal plane should be accepted. More malalignment than this may not remodel and may result in loss of forearm rotation because of the loss of interosseous space between the radius and ulna (see Table 9-3).[245]

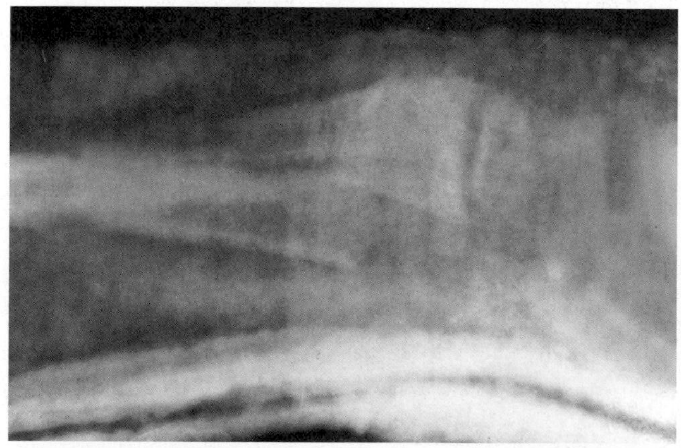

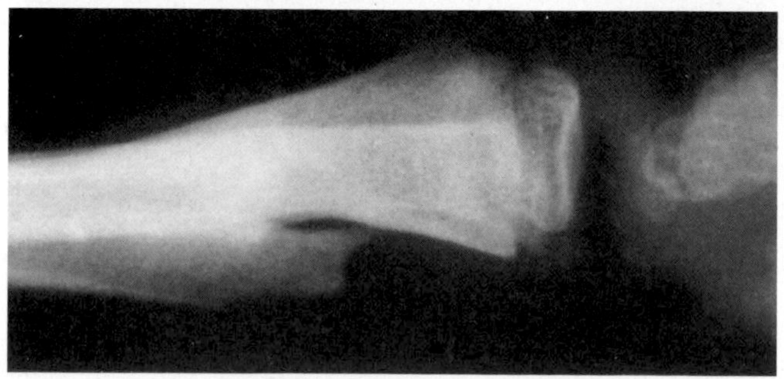

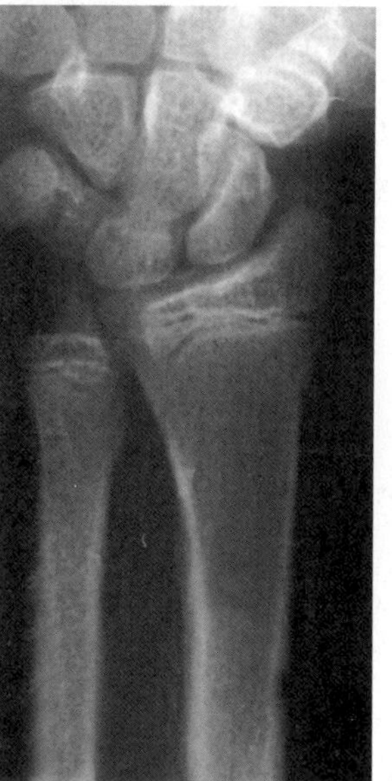

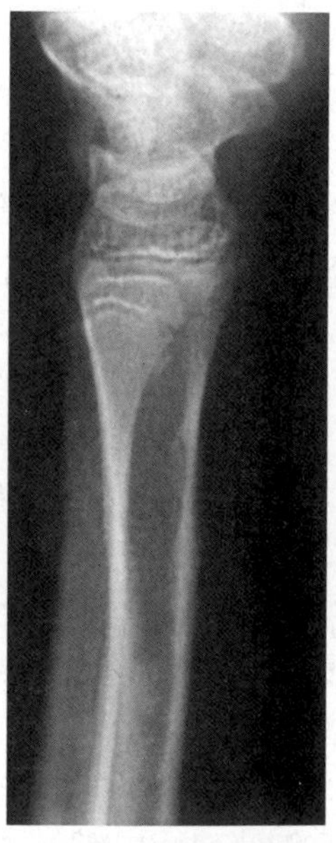

FIGURE 9-39 Bayonet remodeling. **A.** After numerous attempts at closed reduction, the best alignment that could be obtained was dorsal bayonet apposition in this 8-year-old. **B.** Three months after fracture, there is good healing and early remodeling. **C,D.** Five years after the injury (age 13), remodeling was complete and the patient had normal appearance and forearm motion.

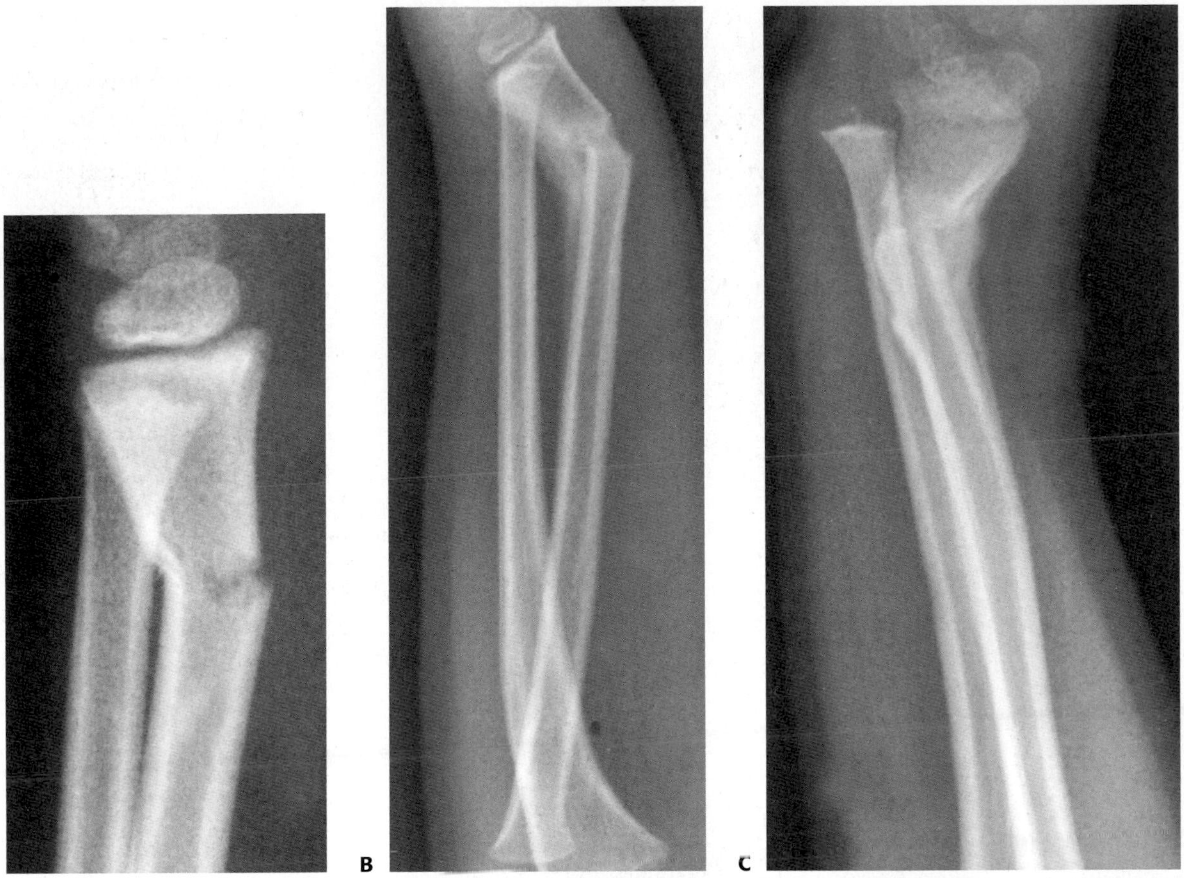

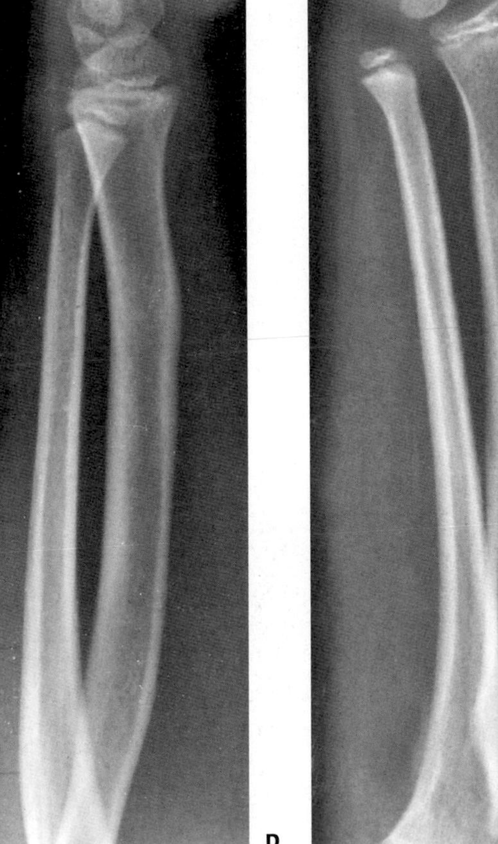

FIGURE 9-40 Extensive remodeling. **A.** Injury film of a 7-year-old with a tension failure greenstick fracture. **B,C.** Lateral and AP views of the same patient taken 1 month later showing development of 45-degree angulation in the sagittal plane and 40 degrees in the coronal plane. **D,E.** True appearance taken 4 years later shows only residual angulation of 10 degrees in the sagittal plane and full correction of radial angulation in the coronal plane. The patient had a range of forearm motion equal to that of the opposite extremity and was asymptomatic.

Closed Reduction. Most displaced and malaligned incomplete fractures should be reduced closed. The areas of controversy are the degree of acceptable deformity, whether the intact cortex should be fractured, and the position and type of immobilization.

Controversies about acceptable angulation of the fracture after closed reduction involve the same differences discussed in the immobilization section. As mentioned, more malalignment can be accepted in younger patients, in those with sagittal plane deformity, and in those without marked cosmetic deformity. Malaligned apex volar incomplete fractures are less obvious than the less common apex dorsal fractures.

As Evans[56] and Rang[181] emphasized, incomplete forearm fractures have a rotatory component to their malalignment. The more common apex volar fractures represent a supination deformity, whereas the less common apex dorsal fractures are malrotated in pronation. Correction of the malrotation is necessary to achieve anatomic alignment. Controversy exists regarding completion of greenstick fractures.[40,61,102,181,199] Although some researchers advocate completion of the fracture to reduce the risk of subsequent loss of reduction from the intact periosteum and concave deformity acting as a tension band[214,246] to redisplace the fracture, completing the fracture increases the risk of instability and malunion.

The position and type of immobilization after reduction also have been controversial. Recommendations for the position of postreduction immobilization include supination, neutral, and pronation. The rationale for immobilization in pronation is that reduction of the more common apex volar fractures requires correction of the supination deformity.[56] Following this rationale, apex dorsal fractures should be reduced and immobilized in supination. Pollen[175] believed that the brachioradialis was a deforming force in pronation and was relaxed in supination (Fig. 9-41) and advocated immobilization in supination for all displaced distal radial fractures. Kasser[108] recommended immobilization in slight supination to allow better molding of the volar distal radius. Some researchers advocate immobilization in a neutral position, believing this is best at maintaining the interosseous space and has the least risk of disabling loss of forearm rotation in the long term.[44,132,216] Davis and Green[40] and Ogden[157] advocated that each fracture seek its own preferred position of stability. Gupta and Danielsson[89] randomized immobilization of distal radial metaphyseal greenstick fractures in neutral, supination, or pronation to try to determine the best position of immobilization. Their study showed a statistical improvement in final healing with immobilization in supination. More recently, Boyer et al.[21] prospectively randomized 109 distal third forearm fractures into long-arm casts with the forearm in neutral rotation, supination, or pronation following closed reduction. No significant differences in final radiographic position were noted among the differing positions of forearm rotation.

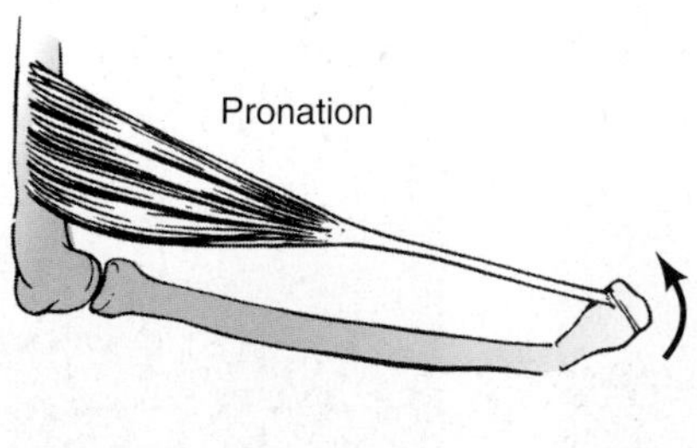

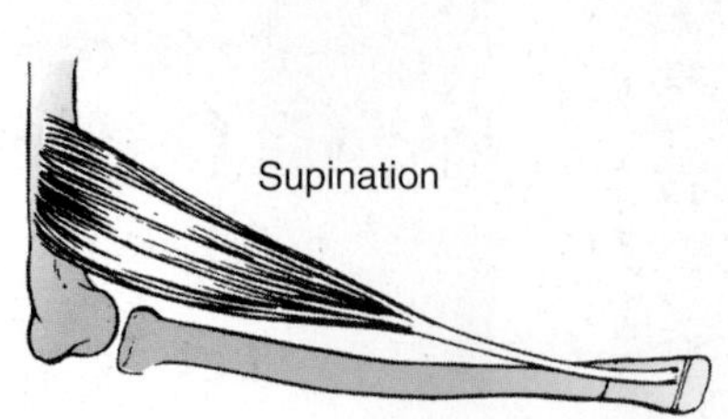

FIGURE 9-41 The brachioradialis is relaxed in supination but may become a deforming force in pronation. (Reprinted from Pollen AG. Fractures and Dislocations in Children. Baltimore: Williams & Wilkins, 1973, with permission.)

Another area of controversy is whether long-arm or short-arm cast immobilization is better. Historically, most publications on pediatric distal radial fracture treatment advocated long-arm cast treatment for the first 3 to 4 weeks of healing.[8,16,108,123,157,216] The rationale is that elbow flexion reduces the muscle forces acting to displace the fracture. In addition, a long-arm cast may further restrict the child's activity and therefore decrease the risk of displacement. However, Chess et al.[28,29] reported redisplacement and reduction rates with well-molded short-arm casts similar to those with long-arm casts. They used a cast index (sagittal diameter divided by coronal diameter at the fracture site) of 0.7 or less to indicate a well-molded cast. Wilkins[246] achieved similar results with short-arm cast treatment. The short-arm cast offers the advantage of elbow mobility and better patient acceptance of casting. Despite these data, historically most centers continue to use long-arm cast immobilization.[8,16,108,123,216]

Two recent randomized prospective clinical trials compared the efficacy of short- and long-arm cast immobilization following closed reduction for pediatric distal radial fractures.[17,240] Bohm et al.[17] randomized 102 patients over the age of 4 years to either short- or long-arm casts following closed reduction of displaced distal radial metaphyseal fractures. No statistically significant difference was seen in loss of reduction rate between the two treatment groups. Webb et al.[240] similarly randomized 103 patients to short- or long-arm casts after reduction of distal radial fractures. No significant difference in rate of lost reduction was seen between the two cohorts. Patients in short-arm casts, however, missed fewer days of school and required less assistance with activities of daily living than those with long-arm casts. In both of these studies, quality of fracture reduction and cast mold were influential factors in loss of reduction rates. These studies have challenged the traditional teaching regarding the need for elbow immobilization to control distal radial fracture alignment.

In addition to the cast index,[28,29,240] a number of other radiographic parameters have been proposed to quantify the quality of reduction and cast molding. These include the gap index, the three-point index, and axis deviation.[6,134,251] Three-point index was the most sensitive, specific, and predictive in a study by Ameldaroglu et al.[6]

COMPLETE FRACTURES

Complete fractures of the distal radius, with or without an associated displaced ulnar fracture, are unstable fractures. Generally, these fractures are displaced dorsally, tearing the volar periosteum and soft tissues. The distal fragment of epiphysis and metaphysis often is in bayonet apposition with the proximal fragment. Concomitant radial and ulnar fractures at the same level may be more unstable than isolated fractures.[244] However, Gibbons et al.[80] reported loss of reduction in 91% of isolated radial fractures after closed reduction. Although a rare fracture with bayonet apposition in a very young patient may remodel,[246] the standard treatment for completely displaced fractures is reduction and stabilization. The current controversy is whether cast immobilization alone is adequate stabilization or whether percutaneous pin fixation is more appropriate for displaced, complete, distal radial metaphyseal fractures.[25,74,140]

Reduction Techniques

Techniques of reduction have included initial distraction with finger traps[40,214] followed by direct manipulation of the fracture by accentuating the deformity. Both Rang[181] and Fernandez[61] expressed concern about the success of finger trap distraction because the intact dorsal periosteum will not stretch adequately to allow reduction. They advocated sequential reduction maneuvers: initial manipulation of the distal fragment dorsally to accentuate the deformity (Fig. 9-42), thumb pressure on the relaxed dorsal edge of the distal fragment to correct the overriding, and reduction of the fracture by application of distal and volar pressure (Fig. 9-43). Anatomic reduction may require repetitive "toggling" of the distal fragment volarly. Reduction is then assessed with fluoroscopic imaging (Fig. 9-44).

There is considerable controversy about what constitutes an acceptable reduction.[38,67,68,92,122,186,190,229] This is clearly age dependent, because the younger the patient, the greater the potential for remodeling. Volar–dorsal malalignment has the greatest potential for remodeling because this is in the plane of predominant motion of the joint. Marked radioulnar malalignment is less likely to remodel. Malrotation will not remodel. The ranges for acceptable reduction according to age are given in the immobilization section on incomplete fractures and apply to complete fractures as well.

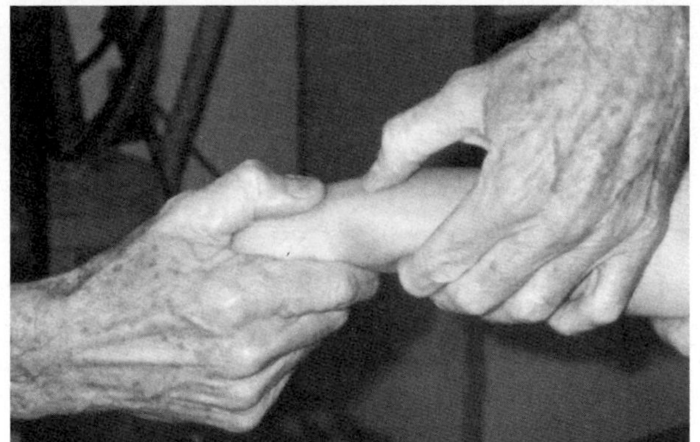

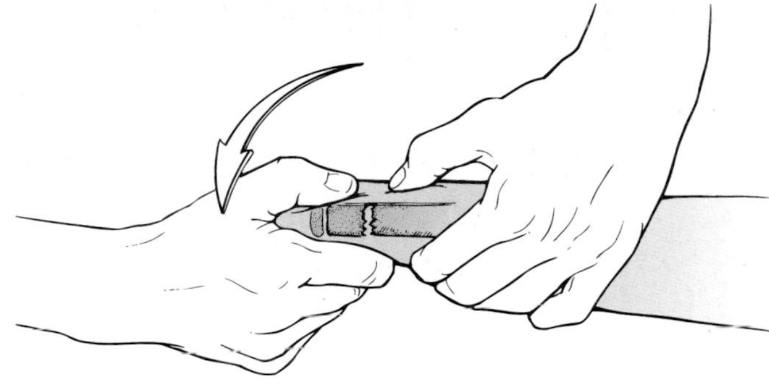

FIGURE 9-43 A,B. Once length has been re-established, the distal fragment is flexed into the correct position. Alignment is checked by determining the position of the fragments with the thumb and forefingers of each hand.

Cast Immobilization

As discussed earlier, there is controversy regarding short-arm or long-arm cast immobilization.[28,29,246] However, regardless of the length of the cast, it is imperative to have a well-molded cast over the fracture site (Fig. 9-45). After reduction of a dorsally displaced fracture, three-point fixation is used with dorsal pressure proximal and distal to the fracture site and volar pressure over the reduced fracture (Fig. 9-46). The cast should be molded to the normal contour of the forearm. An extension

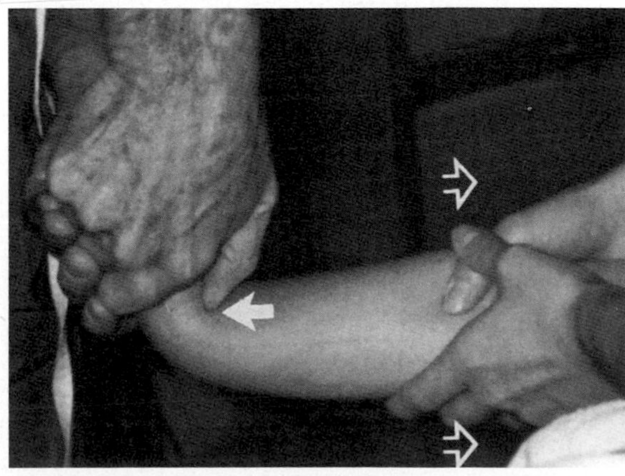

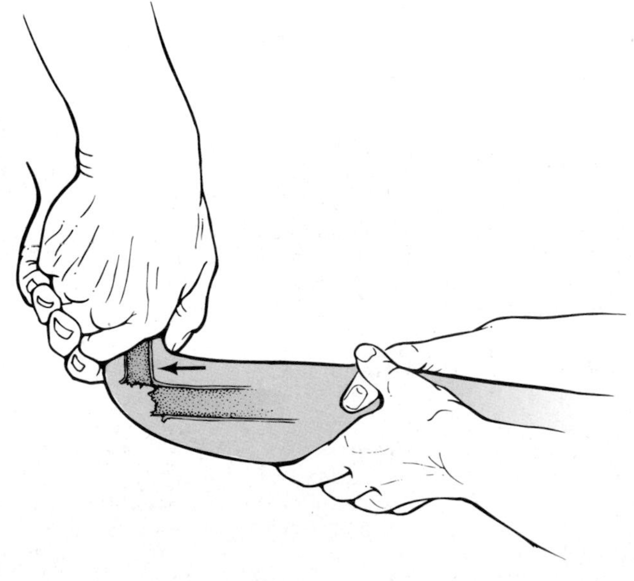

FIGURE 9-42 A,B. Use of the thumb to push the distal fragment hyperdorsiflexed 90 degrees (*solid arrow*) until length is re-established. Countertraction is applied in the opposite direction (*open arrows*).

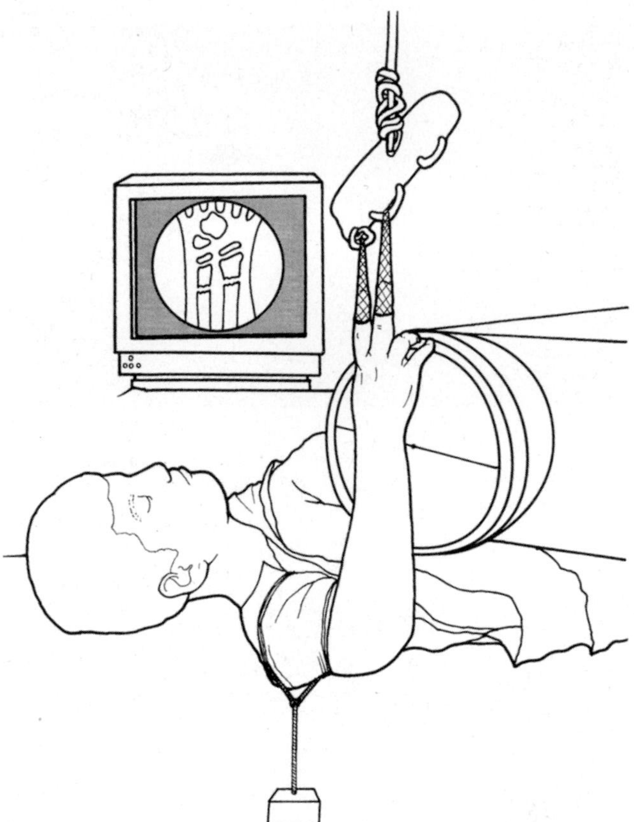

FIGURE 9-44 Once reduced, the fracture is maintained with finger trap traction and countertraction on the arm. The quality of reduction is assessed quickly with the image intensifier.

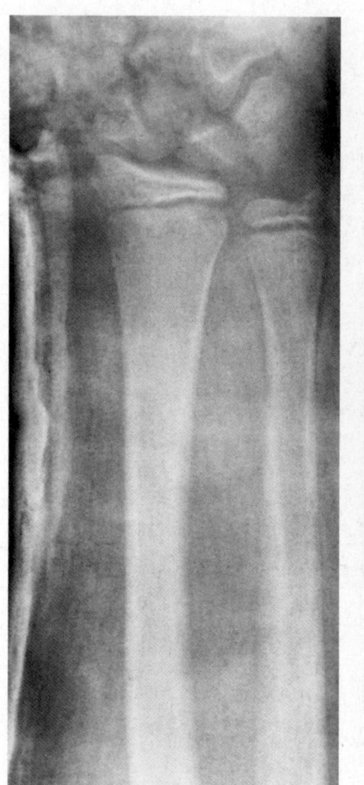

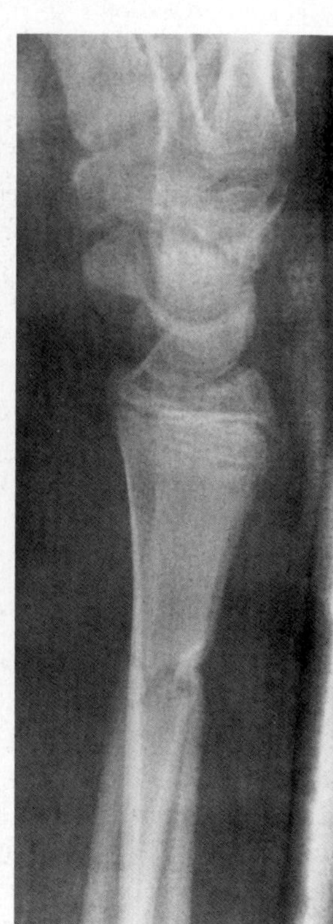

FIGURE 9-46 AP and lateral radiographs of anatomic alignment with closed reduction of a distal radial metaphyseal fracture.

long-arm cast can be used in younger children to better maintain reduction of the ulnar bow. A thumb spica component with felt over the dorsum of the thumb and wrist prevents distal migration of cast and skin irritation. Excessive swelling should be monitored due to dependency of the hand. If there is any concern regarding impending compartment syndrome, the cast and Webril (Kendall, Mansfield, MA) should be immediately bivalved and the patient's clinical status monitored closely. In general, closed reduction and well-molded casting will result in successful healing of the fracture in desired alignment (Fig. 9-47).

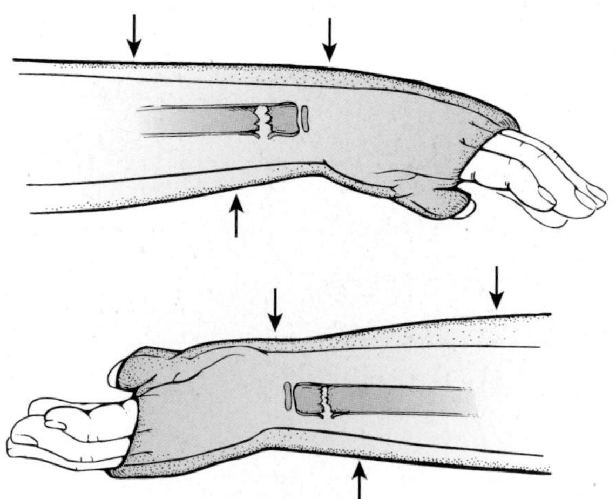

FIGURE 9-45 Three-point molding. **Top:** Three-point molding for dorsally angulated (apex volar) fractures, with the proximal and distal points on the dorsal aspect of the cast and the middle point on the volar aspect just proximal to the fracture site. **Bottom:** For volar angulated fractures, where the periosteum is intact volarly and disrupted on the dorsal surface, three-point molding is performed with the proximal and distal points on the volar surface of the cast and the middle point just proximal to the fracture site on the dorsal aspect of the cast.

The primary problem with closed reduction and cast immobilization is loss of reduction (Fig. 9-48). There are many studies that indicate an incidence of loss of reduction in the 20% to 30% range.[136,177,216] Mani et al.[136] and Proctor et al.[177] described remanipulation rates of 21% and 23%, respectively. Mani et al.[136] concluded that initial displacement of the radial shaft of over 50% was the single most reliable predictor of failure of reduction. Proctor et al.[177] found that complete initial displacement resulted in a 52% incidence of redisplacement of distal radial fractures in children. Gibbons et al.[80] noted that completely displaced distal radial fractures with intact ulnas had a remanipulation rate of 91% after closed reduction and cast immobilization alone compared to a 0% rate of remanipulation when the same fractures were treated with closed reduction, Kirschner wire fixation, and cast immobilization. All three studies strongly advocated percutaneous pinning of distal radial fractures at risk of redisplacement. Two prospective studies confirmed the risk of loss of reduction with cast immobilization. Miller et al.[144] reported a study of distal radial metaphyseal fractures treated by either closed reduction and cast immobilization or closed reduction and percutaneous pinning. Selection criteria were a closed metaphyseal fracture angulated more than 30 degrees in a skeletally immature patient over 10 years of age. To maximize the outcome of the cast immobilization group, these patients were treated by a member of the Pediatric Orthopedic Society of North America with expertise in trauma

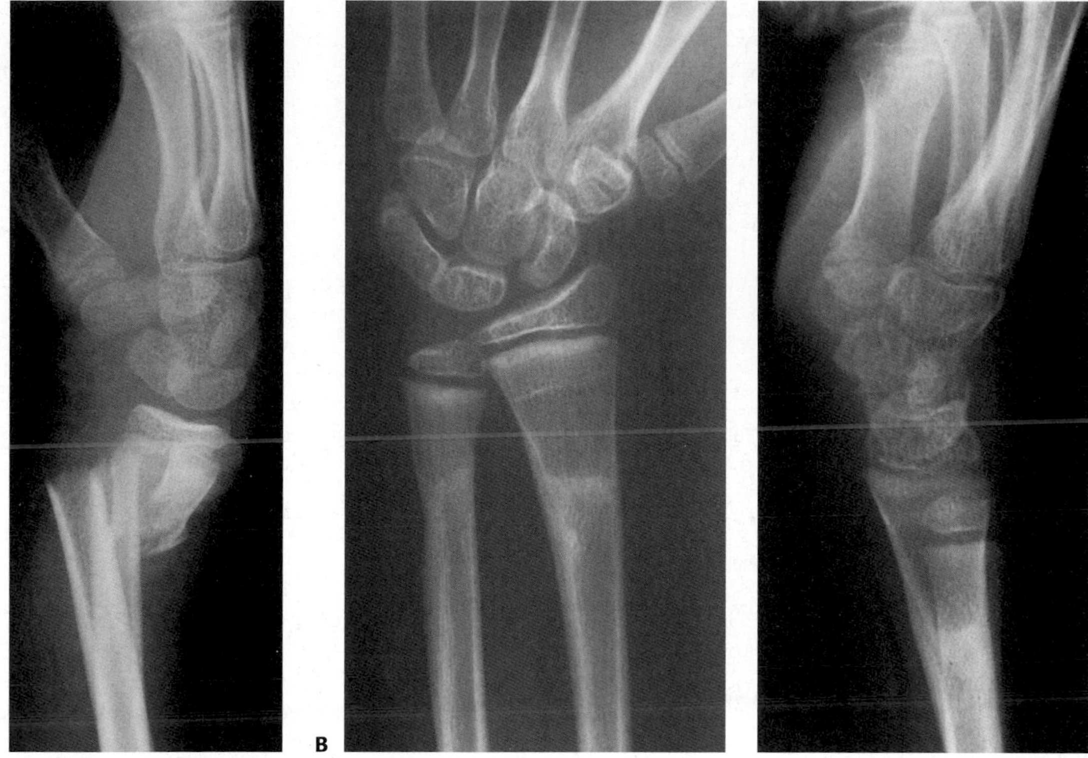

FIGURE 9-47 A. Lateral radiograph of displaced metaphyseal radial and ulnar fractures. **B.** AP and lateral radiographs show anatomic alignment after closed reduction.

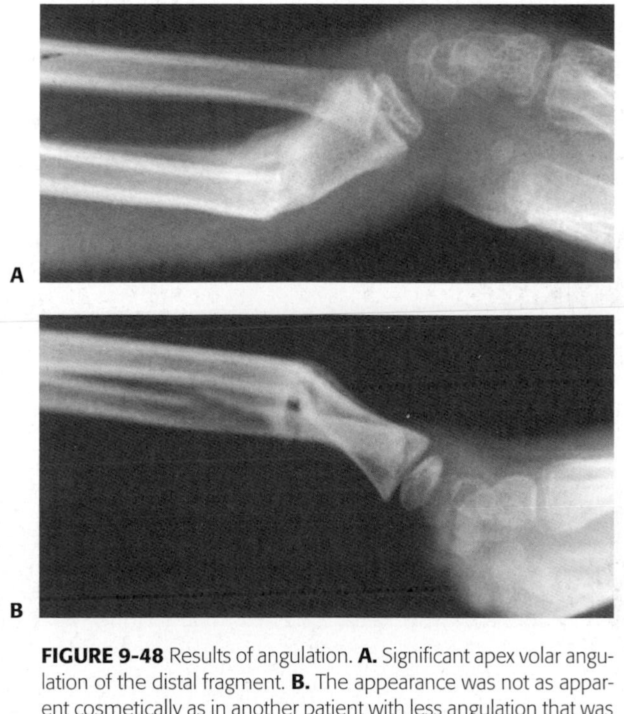

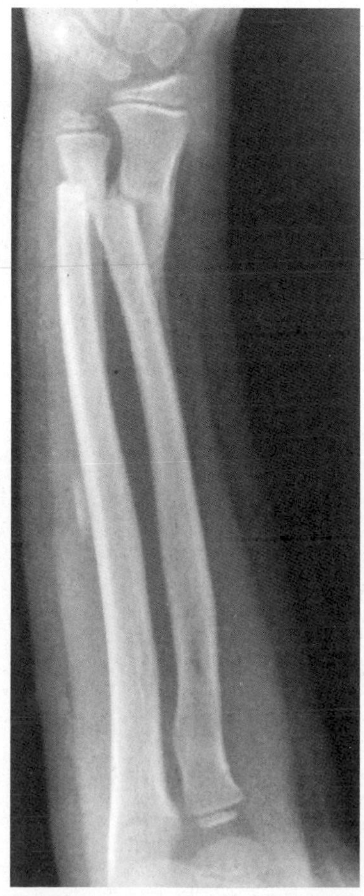

FIGURE 9-48 Results of angulation. **A.** Significant apex volar angulation of the distal fragment. **B.** The appearance was not as apparent cosmetically as in another patient with less angulation that was directed apex dorsally. (Reprinted from Wilkins KE, ed. Operative Management of Upper Extremity Fractures in Children. Rosemont, IL: American Academy of Orthopaedic Surgeons, 1994:27, with permission.) **C.** Radial deviation constricts the interosseous space, which may decrease forearm rotation. (Reprinted from Wilkins KE, ed. Operative Management of Upper Extremity Fractures in Children. Rosemont, IL: American Academy of Orthopaedic Surgeons, 1994:28, with permission.)

care. General anesthesia, fluoroscopic control, and well-molded cast immobilization were used. Despite these optimal conditions, 30% of the patients in the cast immobilization group lost reduction and required remanipulation. These findings were similar to the prospective study of pinning and cast treatment of distal radial metaphyseal fractures.[140] Again, closed reduction and cast immobilization had a loss of reduction rate of 21%, whereas pinning maintained reduction. The authors of these prospective, randomized studies concluded that pinning is a safe, effective means of treating distal radial metaphyseal fractures; however, in both prospective studies, results of casting and pinning were equivalent after 2 years postfracture.[140,144]

The results of all of these studies indicate that distal radial metaphyseal fractures with initial displacement of more than 30 degrees are inherently unstable. Loss of reduction is common, with the risk in the 20%-to-60% range. Incomplete reduction[136,177] and poor casting techniques[28,29,246] increase the risk of loss of reduction. In addition, the risk of loss of reduction increases with the age of the patient and the degree of initial displacement. Bayonet apposition in a child older than 10 years is the highest risk.

Loss of reduction requires repeat manipulation to avoid a malunion. Although the rate of malunion is frequent after these fractures,[8,28,29,34,35,40,91,108,125,195,232] because of the potential for remodeling in skeletally immature patients it has not been considered a serious problem (Fig. 9-49).[3,4,16,67,68,71,98] Distal radial fractures are juxtaphyseal, the malunion often is in the plane of motion of the wrist joint (dorsal displacement with apex volar angulation), and the distal radius accounts for 60% to 80% of the growth of the radius. All these factors favor remodeling of a malunion.

However, De Courtivron et al.[41] reported that of 602 distal radial fractures, 14% had an initial malunion of more than 5 degrees. Of these, 78% corrected the frontal plane deformity, and only 53% remodeled completely in the sagittal plane. In addition, 37% had loss of forearm rotation. Do et al.[46] came to similar conclusions in their analysis of 34 pediatric distal radial metaphyseal fractures that lost reduction and healed with angulation and/or shortening. Alemdaroglu et al.[6] determined that initial complete displacement and initial fracture obliquity of more than 30 degrees were the greatest risk factors for redisplacement after closed reduction.

Closed Reduction and Percutaneous Pinning

In the past decade or two, closed reduction and percutaneous pinning have become more common as the primary treatment of distal radial metaphyseal fractures in children and adolescents.[88,136,177,238,244] The indications cited include fracture instability and high risk of loss of reduction,[88,136,177] excessive local swelling that increases the risk of neurovascular compromise,[238,239,246] ipsilateral fractures of the distal radius and elbow region (floating elbow) that increase the risk of compartment syndrome,[210,245] and the likelihood that remanipulation will be required.[244,246] In addition, surgeon's preference for pinning in a busy office practice has been considered an acceptable indication because of similar complication rates and long-term outcomes with pinning and casting[140,144] and the avoidance of remanipulation because alignment is secure.

Pinning usually is done from distal to proximal under fluoroscopic guidance. When possible, the physis is avoided. Adequate exposure through a small incision over the radial styloid should be obtained to avoid radial sensory nerve or extensor tendon injury. Smooth Kirschner or C-wires are used. In younger patients, a single pin with supplemental cast immobilization may be adequate fixation (Fig 9-50). Crossed pins are more stable provided they do not cross at the fracture site (Fig. 9-51). The first pin, or single pin, enters from the radial side distal to the fracture and passes obliquely to the ulnar aspect of the radius proximal to the fracture. The second pin enters the radius distal to the fracture between the fourth and fifth compartments and passes obliquely across the fracture into the proximal radial side of the radius. The pins are left out through

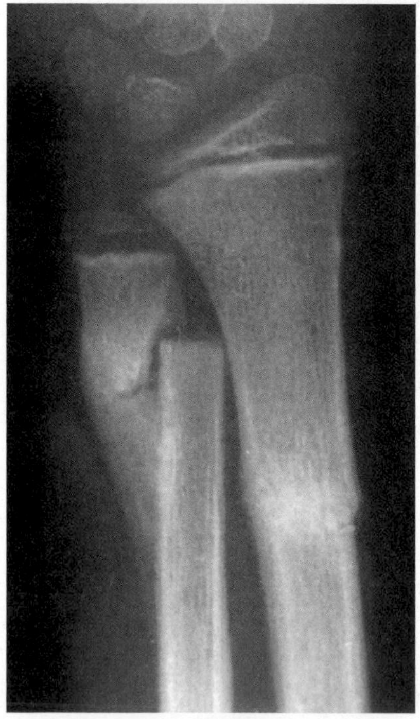

A

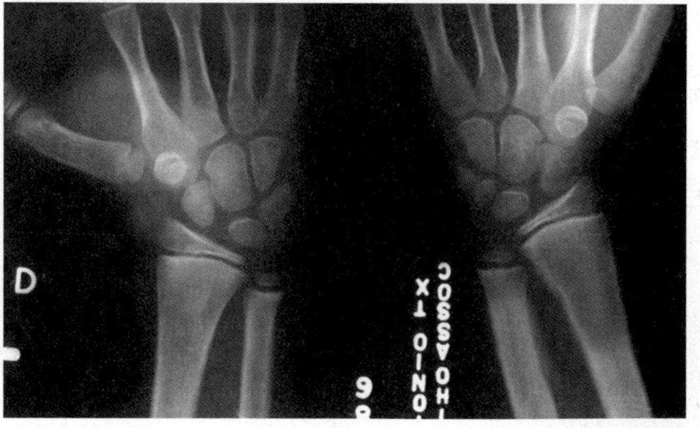

B

FIGURE 9-49 A. Appearance 6 weeks after closed reduction of a distal forearm fracture in an 8½-year-old boy. The radius was reduced, and the ulnar fracture remained overriding. **B.** Eighteen months after injury, the ulnar fracture had remodeled completely with symmetric distal radioulnar joints.

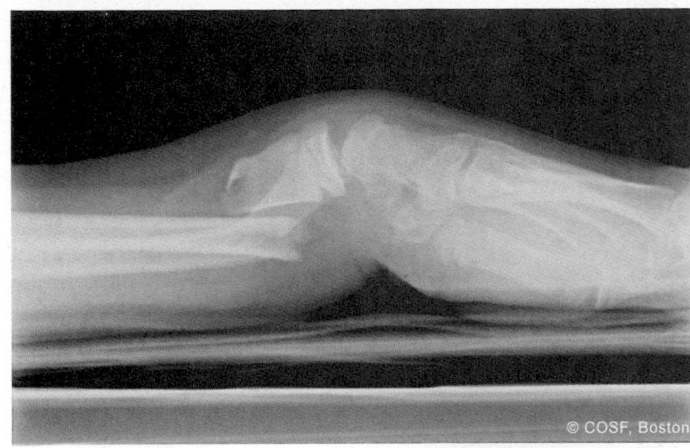

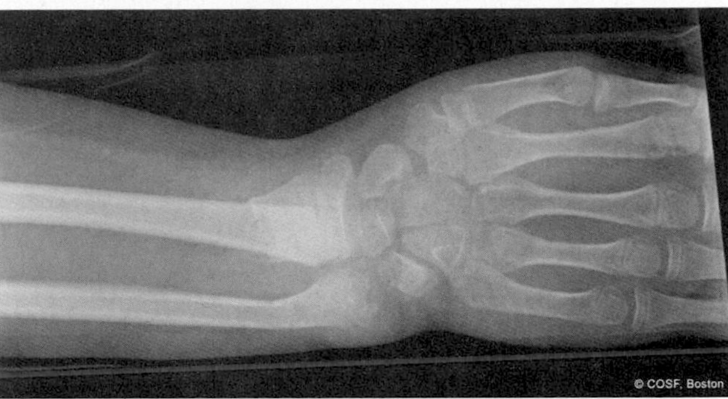

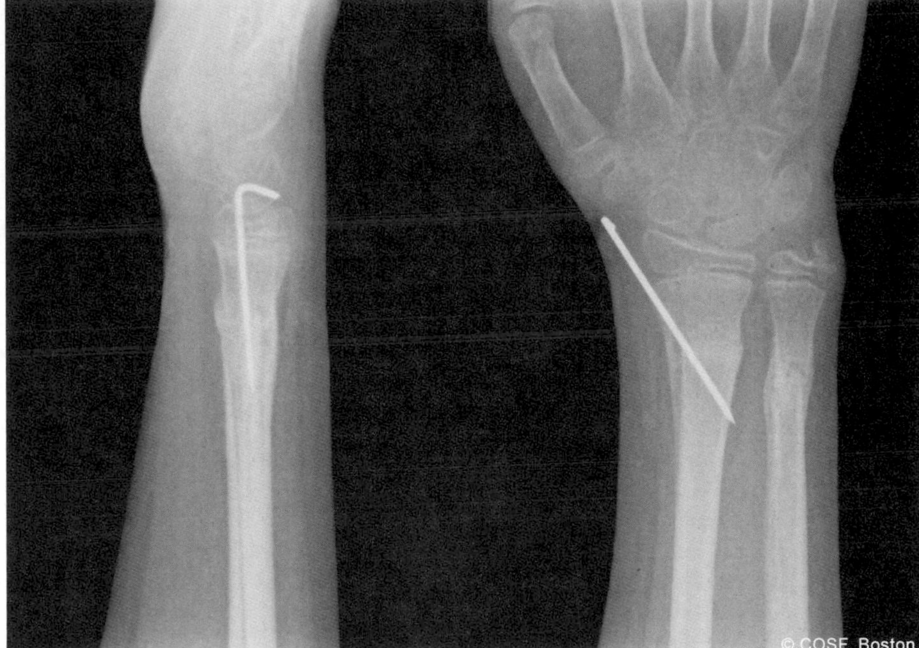

FIGURE 9-50 Severe swelling. **A,B.** Complete displacement and bayonet apposition of a distal radial fracture associated severe swelling from a high-energy injury. **C.** Once reduced, the fragment was secured with an oblique percutaneous pin across the fracture site, sparing the distal radial physis.

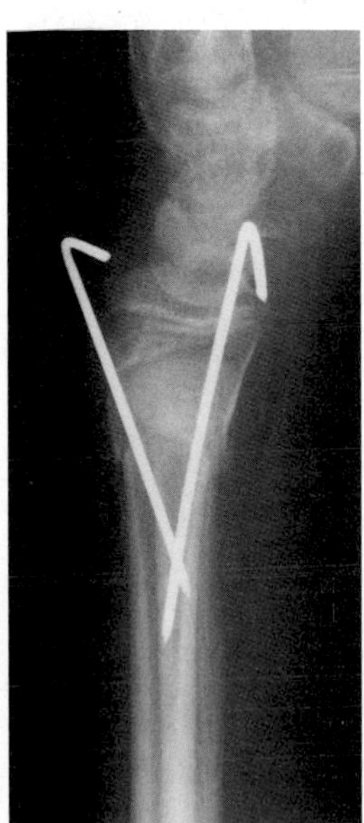

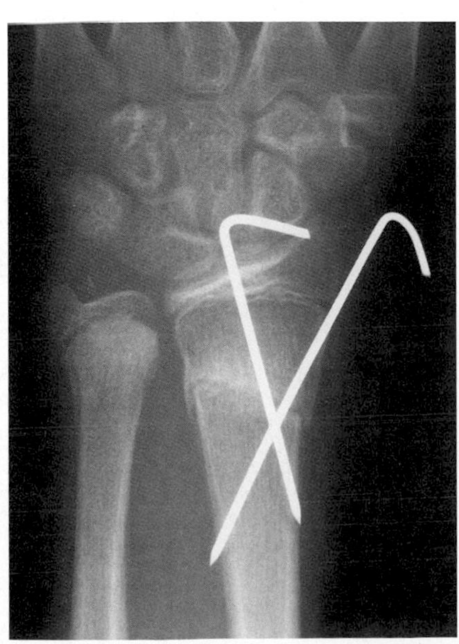

FIGURE 9-51 Crossed-pin technique for stabilization of distal radial metaphyseal fracture in a skeletally immature patient.

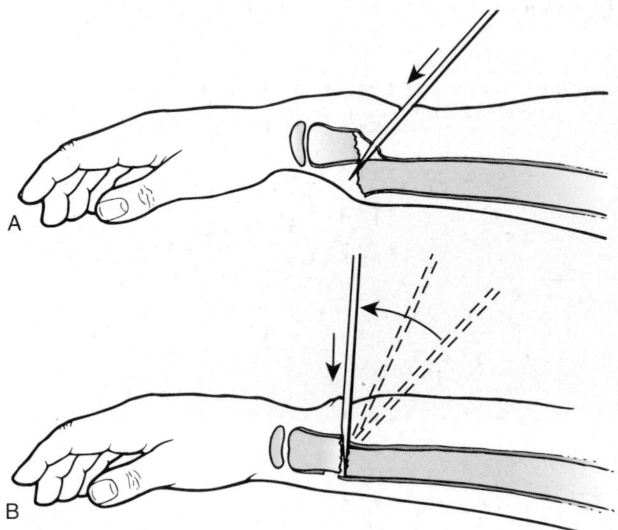

FIGURE 9-52 Pin leverage. **A.** If a bayonet is irreducible, after sterile preparation, a chisel-point Steinmann pin can be inserted between the fracture fragments from a dorsal approach. Care must be taken not to penetrate too deeply past the dorsal cortex of the proximal fragment. **B.** Once the chisel is across the fracture site, it is levered into position and supplementary pressure is placed on the dorsum of the distal fragment (*arrow*) to slide it down the skid into place. This procedure is usually performed with an image intensifier.

the skin to allow easy removal. Another technique of pinning is intrafocal placement of multiple pins into the fracture site to lever the distal fragment into anatomic reduction (Kapandji technique, Fig. 9-52). The pins are then passed through the opposing cortex for stability.[130,224] A supplemental, loose-fitting cast is applied. The advantage of pin fixation is that a tight, well-molded cast is not necessary to maintain reduction. This lessens the risk of neurovascular compromise with associated excessive swelling or ipsilateral fractures. Obviously, pin fixation avoids the risk of loss of reduction in an unstable fracture. Pinning does have the risk of infection and concerns regarding growth injury.

External Fixation

Unlike distal radial fractures in adults, external fixation rarely is indicated for similar fractures in skeletally immature patients. Although it can be used successfully,[201,232] the success rates of both closed reduction and percutaneous pinning techniques make it unnecessary for uncomplicated distal radial fractures in children. The best indication is severe associated soft tissue injuries. A severe crush injury, open fracture, or replantation after amputation that requires extensive soft tissue care and surgery are all indications for the use of external fixation. Supplemental external fixation also may be necessary for severely comminuted fractures to maintain length and provide additional stability to pin fixation. Standard application of the specific fixator chosen is done with care to avoid injury to the adjacent sensory nerves and extensor tendons.

Open Reduction

Open reduction is indicated for open or irreducible fractures. Open fractures constitute approximately 1% of all distal radial metaphyseal fractures. All open fractures, regardless of grade of soft tissue injury, should be irrigated and débrided in the operating room (Fig. 9-53). The open wound should be enlarged adequately to débride the contaminated and nonviable tissues and protect the adjacent neurovascular structures. After thorough irrigation and débridement, the fracture should be anatomically reduced and stabilized, usually with two smooth pins. If the soft tissue injury is severe, supplemental external fixation allows observation and treatment of the wound without jeopardizing the fracture reduction. The original open wound should not be closed primarily. Appropriate prophylactic antibiotics should be used depending on the severity of the open fracture.

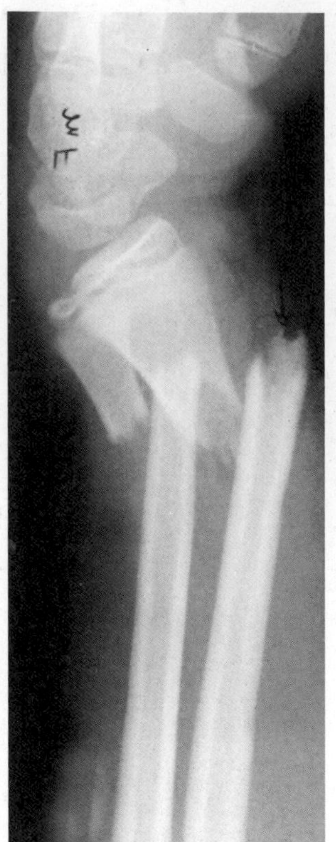
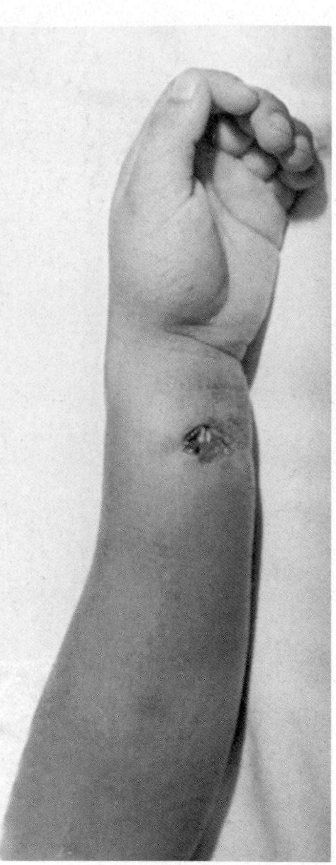

A B

FIGURE 9-53 Open fractures. Radiograph **(A)** and clinical photo **(B)** of an open fracture of the distal radius. This patient needs formal irrigation and débridement in the operating room.

Irreducible fractures are rare (Fig. 9-54) and generally are secondary to interposed soft tissues. With dorsally displaced

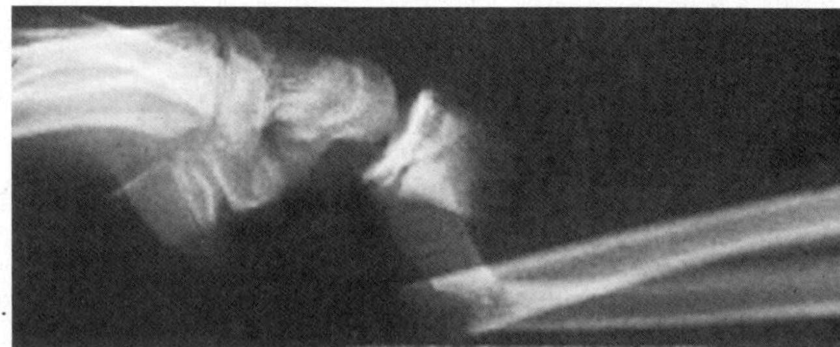

FIGURE 9-54 A 10-year-old girl with a markedly displaced closed fracture of the distal radius with an angulated ulnar fracture. Note the wide separation between the radial fragments. Dimpling of the skin was noted when longitudinal traction was applied, and reduction was impossible. At open reduction, the proximal fragment was buttonholed through the forearm fascia and located between the median nerve and finger flexor tendons. The pronator quadratus muscle was also interposed between the two fragments.

fractures, the interposed structure usually is the volar periosteum or pronator quadratus[93] and rarely the flexor tendons or neurovascular structures. In volarly displaced fractures, the periosteum or extensor tendons may be interposed. The fracture should be approached in a standard fashion opposite the side of displacement (i.e., volar approach for an irreducible dorsal fracture). The adjacent neurovascular and tendinous structures are protected and the offending soft tissue is extracted from the fracture site. Pin stabilization is recommended to prevent problems with postoperative swelling or loss of reduction in cast.

Closed reduction rarely fails if there is no interposed soft tissue. Occasionally, however, multiple attempts at reduction of a bayonet apposition fracture can lead to significant swelling that makes closed reduction impossible. If the patient is too old to remodel bayonet apposition, open reduction is appropriate. Pin fixation without violating the physis is recommended.

Plate fixation can be used in more skeletally mature adolescents. Low profile, fragment specific fixation methods and locking plates also are now commonly used for internal fixation of distal radial fractures in adults. The utility of these anatomically contoured locking plates in children and skeletally immature adolescents is unknown, as is the deleterious effect, if any, on growth potential. Furthermore, the advantage of these more rigid constructs in younger patients in whom adequate stability may be achieved with pins is unclear, particularly given the reports of late tendon rupture and other soft tissue complications associated with fixed-angle volar plates,[36,112,180] Indications for skeletally mature adolescents are the same as for adults. Articular malalignment and comminution are assessed by CT preoperatively, and fracture-specific fixation is used as appropriate.

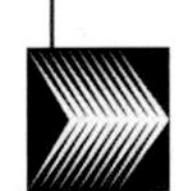

AUTHORS' PREFERRED METHOD OF TREATMENT

Nondisplaced Fractures

Nondisplaced metaphyseal compression fractures, including torus and unicortical compression greenstick fractures, are inherently stable. Immobilization is used until resolution of pain (generally about 3 weeks). Depending on the activity level of the patient, a volar wrist splint or a short-arm cast can be used. Immobilization provides comfort from pain during healing and protects against displacement with secondary injury. It is important that an unstable bicortical fracture be recognized on radiograph. Bicortical fractures need more protection, longer restriction of activity, and closer follow-up to avoid displacement and malunion. A well-molded short- or long-arm cast, depending on the age of the patient, is applied and radiographs obtained every 7 to 10 days until evidence of early healing is seen. A short-arm cast is then worn until clinical and radiographic healing is complete. Any loss of reduction is treated with repeat reduction. Return to contact sports is restricted until the patient regains full motion and strength.

Minimally Displaced Fractures

Displaced greenstick fractures that are reduced are at risk for redisplacement. If left unreduced or poorly immobilized, a mild deformity can become severe during the course of healing. Therefore, closed anatomic reduction is indicated in all bicortical fractures with more than 10 degrees of malalignment. Generally, these fractures have apex volar angulation and dorsal displacement. Conscious sedation is used with portable fluoroscopy in the emergency care setting. The distal fragment and hand are distracted and then reduced volarly. With isolated distal radial fractures, it is imperative to reduce the DRUJ with appropriate forearm rotation. For apex volar fractures, this usually is with pronation. If the fracture is apex dorsal with volar displacement, the reduction forces are the opposite. A long-arm cast with three-point molding is used for 3 to 4 weeks. Radiographs are obtained every 7 to 10 days until there is sufficient callus formation. A short-arm cast or volar wrist splint is used until full healing, generally at 4 to 6 weeks after fracture reduction. The patient is then restricted from contact sports until full motion and strength are regained, which may take up to 3 weeks after cast removal. Formal therapy rarely is required. The patient and parents should be warned at the start of treatment of the risk of redisplacement of the fracture.

Bayonet Apposition

Marked displacement of distal radial metaphyseal fractures usually results in foreshortening and dorsal overlap of the distal fragment on the proximal fragment. This often is associated with a same-level ulnar metaphyseal fracture, similarly in bayonet apposition. Rarely, the distal fragment is in volar bayonet apposition. Both of these situations require more skill of reduction and complete analgesia at the fracture site. At our institution, we reduce this fracture in the emergency room with conscious sedation and supplemental local hematoma block or in the operating room with general anesthesia. In either situation, portable fluoroscopy is used. The fracture usually is reduced in the emergency room in young patients with minimal swelling and no neurovascular compromise and in whom cast treatment will be sufficient. Reduction with general anesthesia is preferred for older patients and for those with marked displacement, swelling, or associated neurovascular compromise in whom percutaneous pin treatment is chosen.

The reduction maneuver is the same regardless of anesthesia type or stabilization method. As opposed to a Colles fracture in an adult, traction alone will not reduce the fracture because the dorsal periosteum acts as a tension band that does not respond to increasing linear traction with weights. Finger traps with minimal weight (less than 10 lb) can be used to balance the hand and help with rotational alignment (the "steel resident") (see Fig. 9-14). However, applying progressive weight will only distract the carpus and will not alter the fracture alignment.

After applying preliminary traction with either light-weight finger traps or hand traction, a hyperdorsiflexion maneuver is performed. The initial deformity is accentuated and the distal fragment is brought into marked dorsiflexion. The dorsum of the hand should be brought more than 90 degrees and at times parallel to the dorsum of the forearm to lessen the tension on the dorsal forearm. Thumb pressure is used on the distal fragment while still in this deformed position to restore length by bringing the distal fragment beyond the proximal fragment. Reduction is then obtained by flexing the distal fragment while maintaining length.

Often, this initial reduction maneuver restores length and alignment, but translational reduction is incomplete. The fracture should be completely reduced by toggling the distal fragment all the way volarly by repetitive slight dorsiflexion positioning of the distal fragment followed by volar pressure with the thumbs. It is important to anatomically reduce the fracture. Loss of reduction with cast immobilization is more likely if the fracture remains translated or malaligned.

If the patient presents late with marked swelling and the reduction is difficult, it is useful to try to lever the proximal fragment distally with percutaneous smooth wire(s). This may prevent an unnecessary open reduction. Percutaneous pin fixation is used after reduction, either by standard pinning or intrafocal techniques.

Cast Treatment

If the patient is under 10 years of age, has no prereduction signs or symptoms of neurovascular impairment, or has minimal swelling, then cast immobilization is used. The cast is applied with the aid either of an assistant or finger traps and balancing counterweights on the upper arm. The advantage of the finger-trap steel resident is that there is no risk of muscle fatigue, mental distraction, or failure to maintain elbow flexion at 90 degrees that can occur with a human assistant. A long-arm cast is applied with the elbow flexed 90 degrees, the wrist in slight palmar flexion, and the forearm in the desired rotation for stability and alignment. Rotational positioning and short- versus long-arm casting varies with each fracture and each surgeon. Our preference is neutral forearm rotation unless the fracture dictates differently. This allows excellent molding against the volar aspect of the distal radius at the fracture site.

One of the most important elements in a successful casting for a forearm fracture is the application of the Webril (Kendall, Mansfield, MA). The Webril should be applied in a continuous roll with overlap of one third to one half its width. Extra padding is applied over the olecranon when a long-arm cast is used, along the volar and dorsal forearm where the cast may have to be split, and at the ends of the cast to prevent irritation from fraying. Plaster of Paris can be used for the cast to obtain the best mold possible. Initially, a single layer is applied, followed by splints five layers thick along the volar and dorsal forearm and the extension region of the elbow. This lessens the bulk of the cast and still allows deep molds. The cast is completed with plaster of Paris rolls over the splints. A three-point mold is applied at the fracture site as the cast hardens. In addition, molds are applied to maintain a straight ulnar border, the interosseous space, and straight posterior humeral line. This creates the classic "box" long-arm cast rather than the all too frequent "banana" cast that allows displacement. Final radiographs are obtained, and if the reduction is anatomic, the cast is overwrapped with fiberglass to lessen the weight, increase patient satisfaction, and prevent cast breakdown that could lead to loss of reduction.

Patients are either discharged or admitted to the hospital depending on the degree of concern regarding risk of excessive swelling, neurovascular compromise, and patient and parental reliability. If there is any doubt, the patient is admitted for observation. The cast is split anytime there are signs of neurovascular compromise or excessive swelling. The patient is instructed to maintain elevation for at least 48 to 72 hours after discharge and return immediately if excessive swelling or neurovascular compromise occurs. The patient and family are warned of the risk of loss of reduction and the need for close follow-up. We inform our patients and parents that the risk of return to the day surgery unit for repeat reduction or pinning is approximately 20% to 30% during the first 3 weeks.

Follow-up examinations and radiographs are obtained every 7 to 10 days for 3 weeks. If there is loss of reduction, we individualize treatment depending on the patient's age, degree of deformity, time since fracture, and remodeling potential. If restoration of alignment with growth occurs, we reassure the family that the child should achieve anatomic alignment over time with growth. If the child is older, there is risk of further displacement, or the deformity is marked, repeat reduction is done in the day surgery unit with fluoroscopy. Most often, a percutaneous pin is used for the second reduction (Fig. 9-55). Occasionally, in pure bending injuries, loss of reduction can be corrected with cast wedging.

Cast immobilization usually is for 4 to 6 weeks. The molded cast is changed at 3 to 4 weeks. With clinical and radiograph healing, a protective volar splint is used and activities are restricted until the patient regains full motion and strength, usually in 1 to 3 weeks after cast removal. As with other distal radial fractures, formal physical therapy rarely is required.

Percutaneous Pin Fixation

Percutaneous pinning of distal radial metaphyseal fractures is most often used in patients with excessive swelling or signs of neurologic injury. In these situations, the patient is at risk for development of a forearm or carpal tunnel compartment syndrome with a well-molded, tight-fitting cast. Similarly, concurrent displaced supracondylar and distal radial fractures are treated with percutaneous fixation of both fractures to lessen the risk of neurovascular compromise (Fig. 9-56). Older patients near the end of growth with bayonet apposition fractures also are treated with percutaneous pin fixation because they have less ability to remodel and their fractures are very unstable with a high risk of displacement. Finally, open fractures usually are treated with pin fixation.

The pinning technique for the radius is either a single radial-sided pin or crossed radial- and ulnar-sided pins. Fixation of the ulna rarely is necessary. Stability with a single pin is checked with fluoroscopy, and if further fixation is needed, a second pin is added. The physis is avoided if possible. Intrafocal pins are used if reduction is not possible without levering the distal fragment into a reduced position. A small incision is made for the insertion of each pin to protect the radial sensory nerve and adjacent extensor tendons. Smooth pins are used and are removed in the office as soon as there is sufficient healing to make the fracture stable in a cast or splint (usually at 4 weeks). Rehabilitation is similar to that for cast-treated fractures.

Open Reduction

The two most common indications for open reduction in the skeletally immature patient are an open fracture and

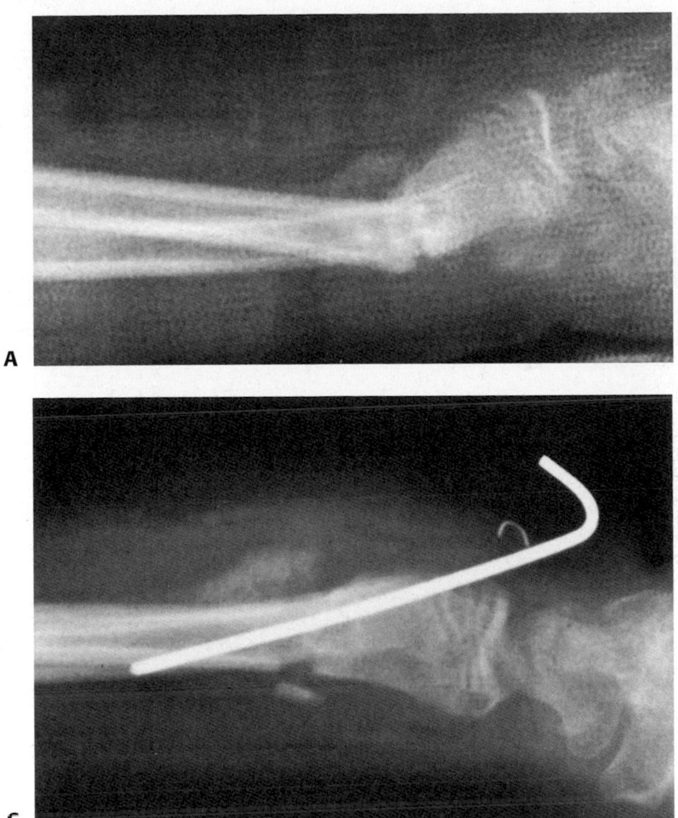

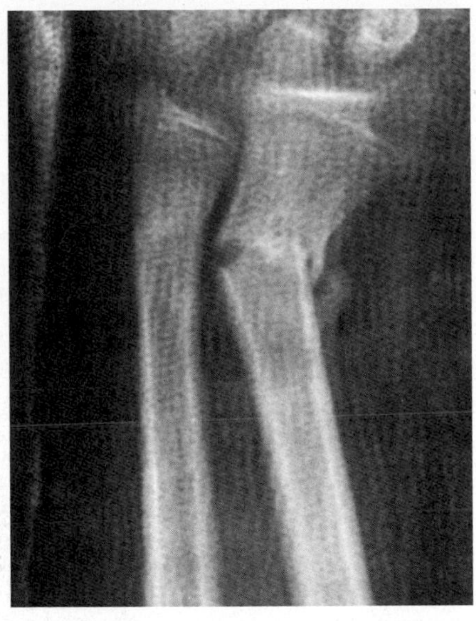

FIGURE 9-55 Remanipulation. **A,B.** Two weeks after what initially appeared to be an undisplaced greenstick fracture, a 14-year-old boy was found to have developed late angulation of 30 degrees in both the coronal and sagittal planes. **C.** Because this was beyond the limits of remodeling, a remanipulation was performed. To prevent reangulation, the fracture was secured with a pin placed percutaneously obliquely through the dorsal cortex.

an irreducible fracture. All open fractures are irrigated and débrided in the operating room. The initial open wound is extended adequately to inspect and cleanse the open fracture site. After thorough irrigation and débridement, the fracture is reduced and stabilized. A cast rarely is applied in this situation because of concern about fracture stability, soft tissue care, and excessive swelling. Crossed-pin fixation often is used with Gustilo grade 1 or 2 open fractures. More severe soft tissue injuries usually require external fixation with a unilateral frame, with care taken to avoid soft tissue impingement during pin placement. If flap coverage is necessary for the soft tissue wounds, the fixator pins should be placed in consultation with the microvascular surgeon planning the soft tissue coverage.

Irreducible fractures usually are secondary to soft tissue entrapment. With dorsal displacement, this is most often either the volar periosteum or pronator quadratus, and open reduction through a volar approach is necessary to extract the interposed soft tissues and reduce the fracture (Fig. 9-57). Percutaneous pin fixation usually is used to stabilize the fracture in patients with open physes. If plate fixation is used, it should avoid violation of the physis (Fig. 9-58). Displaced intra-articular injuries in skeletally immature adolescents are adultlike and require standard treatment, such as open reduction and internal fixation (Fig. 9-59). Lower profile and locking plates have been used more recently (Fig. 9-60).

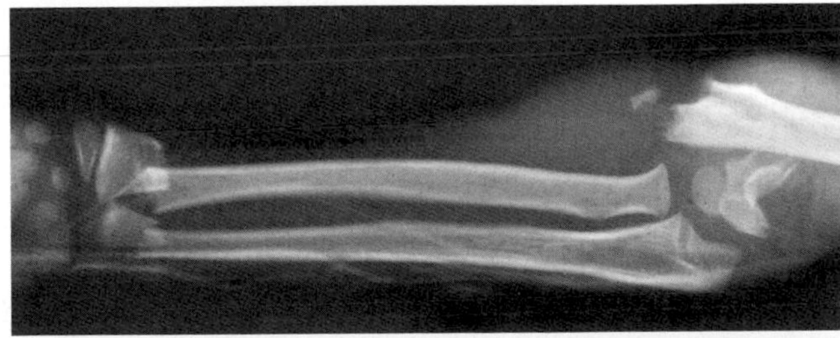

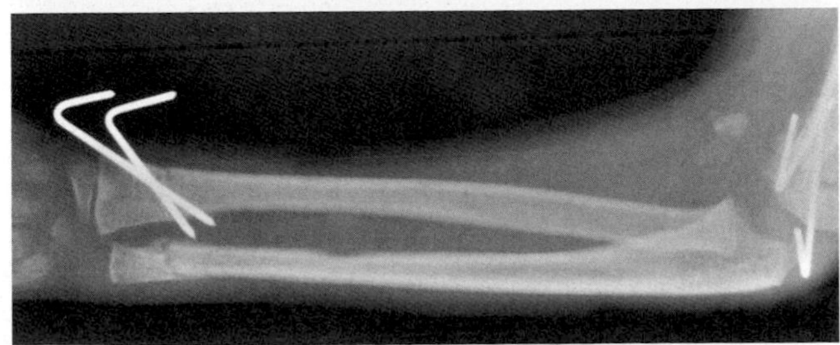

FIGURE 9-56 Ipsilateral fractures. **A.** Markedly displaced ipsilateral distal radial and supracondylar fractures. **B.** Both fractures were reduced and stabilized with pins placed percutaneously. (Wilkins KE, ed. Operative Management of Upper Extremity Fractures in Children. Rosemont, IL: American Academy of Orthopaedic Surgeons, 1994:29, with permission.)

Complications

Distal radial metaphyseal fractures have complications similar to physeal fractures but with different frequencies. Loss of reduction and malunion are the most common problems, and growth-related complications are infrequent. Neurovascular compromise does occur and should be considered in the acute management of this fracture.

Malunion

Loss of reduction is a common complication of distal radial metaphyseal fractures treated with cast immobilization. Because

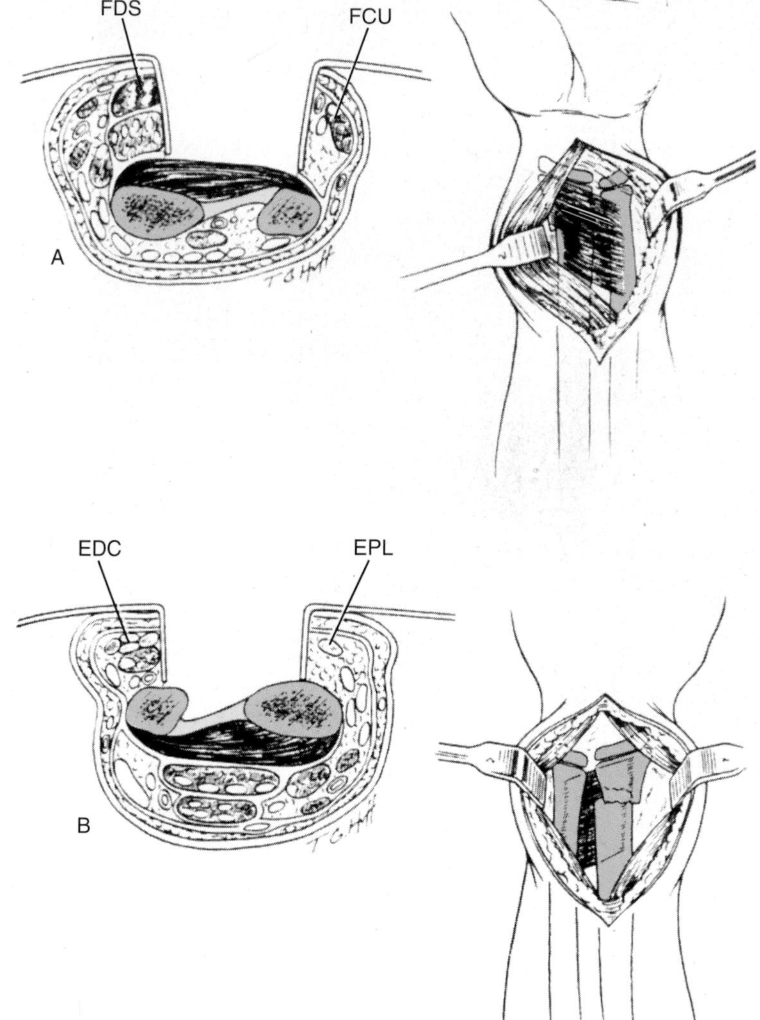

FIGURE 9-57 A. Volar approach through the interval between the digital flexors and ulnar neurovascular bundle. FCU, flexor carpi ulnaris; FDS, flexor digitorum superficialis. **B.** Dorsal approach between the third and fourth dorsal compartments. EDC, extensor digitorum communis; EPL, extensor pollicis longus. (Reprinted from Holmes JR, Luis DS. Entrapment of pronator quadratus in pediatric distal-radius fractures: recognition and treatment. J Pediatr Orthop 1994, 14:498–500, with permission.)

this complication occurs in at least 30% of bayonet apposition fractures,[80,136,177,234,244] many surgeons treat this fracture primarily with pin fixation to avoid the problems that can occur with malunion. Otherwise, it is clear that patients treated with cast immobilization need to be monitored closely.[251]

Fortunately, many angular malunions of the distal radius will remodel,* probably because of asymmetric physeal growth.[106,122] True growth arrest associated with a distal radial metaphyseal fracture is very rare.[218] The younger the patient, the less the deformity, and the closer the fracture is to the physis, the greater the potential for remodeling. It is unclear whether there is any capacity for rotational malunion remodeling.[71,193] Angular and rotational malunion that does not remodel can lead to loss of motion. The degree and plane of loss of motion, as well as the individual affected, determine if this is functionally significant.[251] In cadaver studies, malangulation of more than 20 degrees of the radius or ulna caused loss of forearm rotation,[139,216,219] whereas less than 10 degrees of malangulation did not alter forearm rotation significantly. Distal third malunion affected rotation less than middle or proximal third malunion. Radioulnar malunion affected forearm rotation more than volar–dorsal malunion. Excessive angulation may lead to a loss of rotation at a 1:2 degree ratio, whereas malrotation may lead to rotational loss at only a 1:1 degree loss.[181] The functional loss associated with rotational motion loss is difficult to predict. This has led some clinicians to recommend no treatment,[38,40] arguing that most of these fractures will remodel, and those that do not remodel will not cause a functional problem.[101] However, a significant functional problem is present if shoulder motion cannot compensate for loss of supination.

We prefer to reduce forearm fractures as near to perfect alignment as possible. No element of malrotation is accepted in the reduction. As indicated in the treatment sections, fractures at high risk of loss of reduction and malunion are treated with anatomic reduction and pin or, rarely, plate fixation. Fractures treated in a cast are followed closely and rereduced for any loss of alignment of more than 10 degrees. Although loss of forearm rotation can occur with anatomic healing,[153,222,246] it is less likely than with malunions.

Unfortunately, not all fractures heal anatomically or remodel to anatomic alignment. Long-term malunion is a concern for

*References 16,40,67–69,75,122,157,159,165,179,190,214.

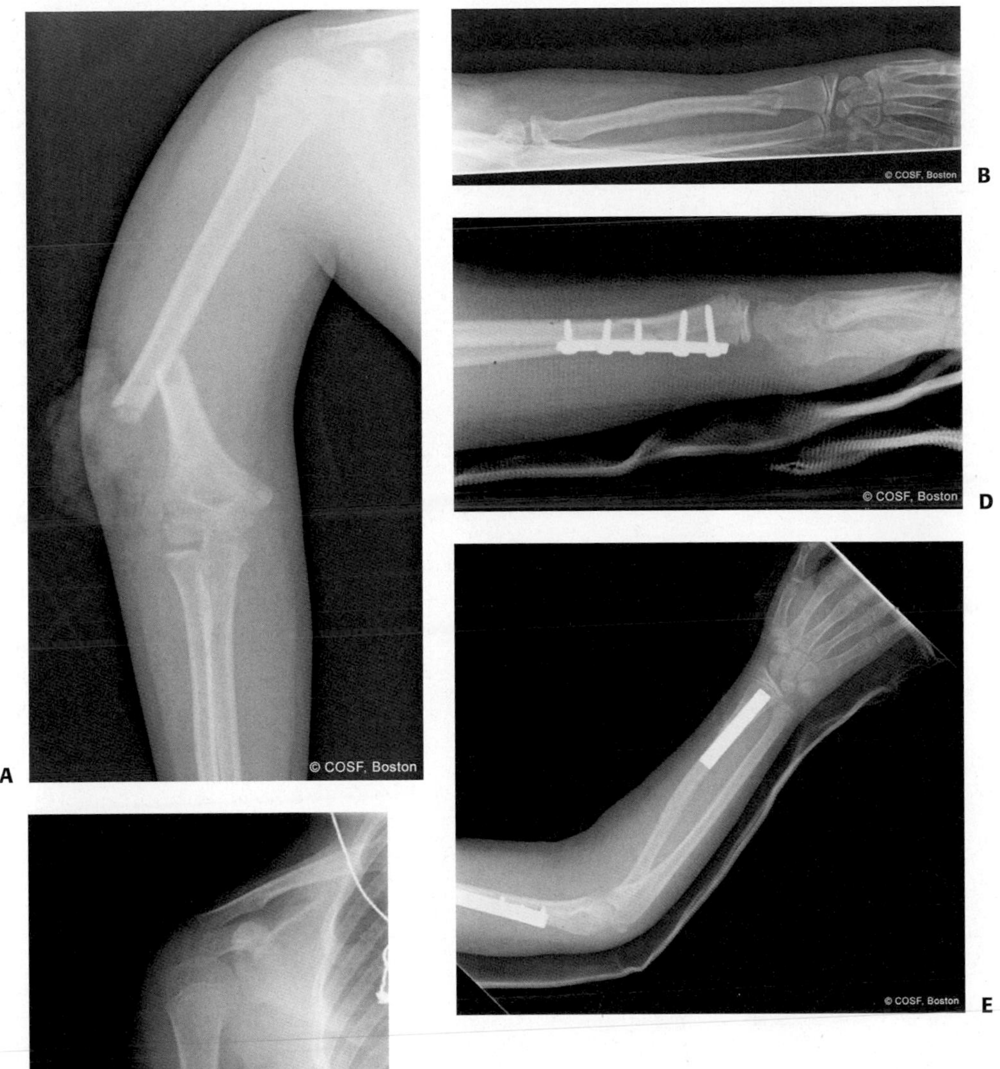

FIGURE 9-58 A. Radiograph of an open humeral diaphyseal fracture in the setting of a "floating elbow injury." **B.** Radiograph depicting a displaced distal radial metaphyseal fracture. **C.** Plate fixation following irrigation and débridement of the humerus fracture. **D,E.** Radiographs following open reduction and plate fixation of the radius fracture, sparing the distal radial physis.

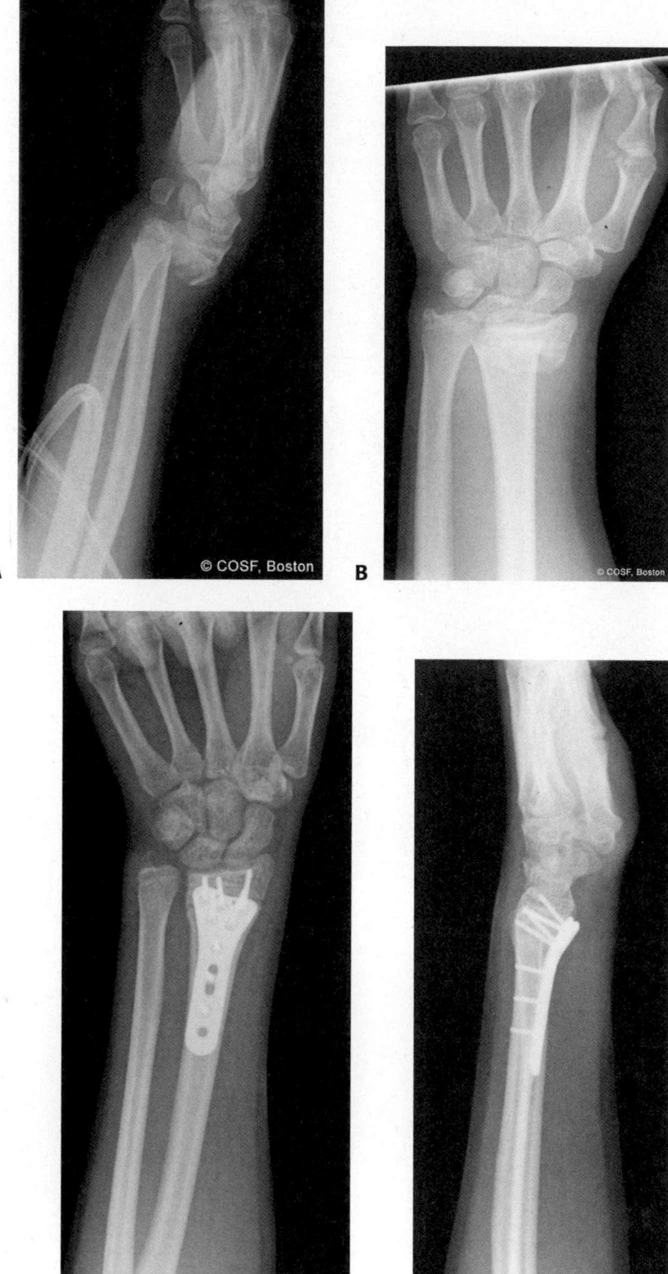

FIGURE 9-59 A,B. AP and lateral radiographs of a 14-year-old skeletally mature female with a displaced extra-articular fracture. **C,D.** This fracture was treated with a fixed-angle volar locking plate, with distal screws crossing the physis. The long-term effects of this type of fixation are unknown.

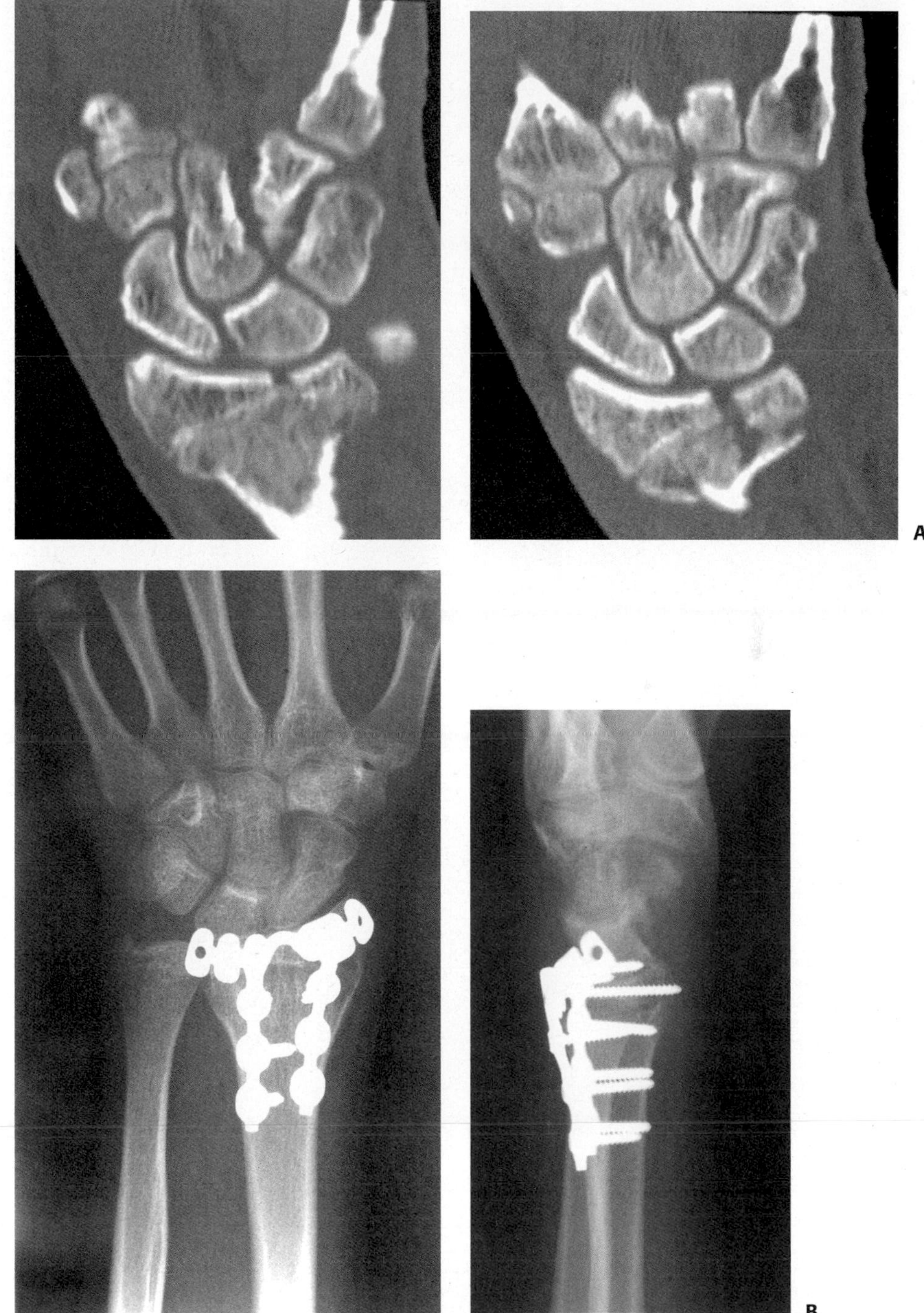

FIGURE 9-60 A. CT scan of a displaced intra-articular fracture of a nearly skeletally mature adolescent. **B.** Dorsal plating with a low profile system to achieve anatomic reduction and stable fixation.

midcarpal instability[217] and long-term arthrosis. A distal radial malunion in a skeletally mature adolescent should be treated with an opening wedge osteotomy, bone graft, and internal fixation (Fig. 9-61).[62,142,178]

Nonunion

Nonunion of a closed radial or ulnar fracture is rare. In children, nonunion has been universally related to a pathologic condition of the bone or vascularity.[246] Congenital pseudarthrosis or neurofibromatosis (Fig. 9-62) should be suspected in a patient with a nonunion after a benign fracture.[105] This occurs most often after an isolated ulnar fracture. The distal bone is often narrowed, sclerotic, and plastically deformed. These fractures rarely heal with immobilization. Vascularized fibular bone grafting usually is necessary for healing of a nonunion associated with neurofibromatosis or congenital pseudarthrosis. If the patient is very young, this may include a vascularized epiphyseal transfer to restore distal growth.

Vascular impairment also can lead to nonunion. Distal radial nonunion has been reported in a child with an ipsilateral supracondylar fracture with brachial artery occlusion. Revascularization of the limb led to eventual union of the fracture. Nonunion also can occur with osteomyelitis and bone loss.[22] Débridement of the necrotic bone and either traditional bone grafting, os-

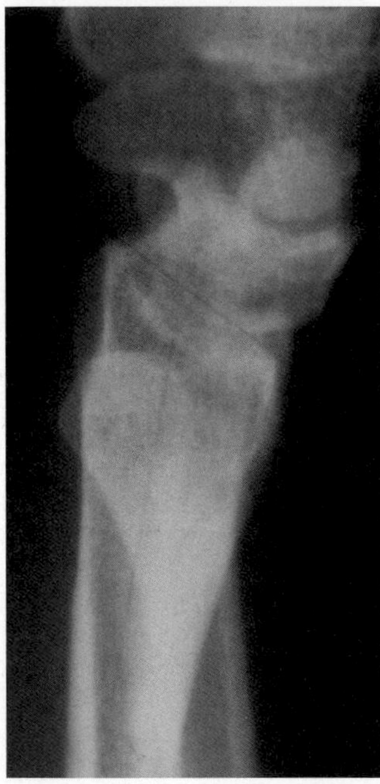

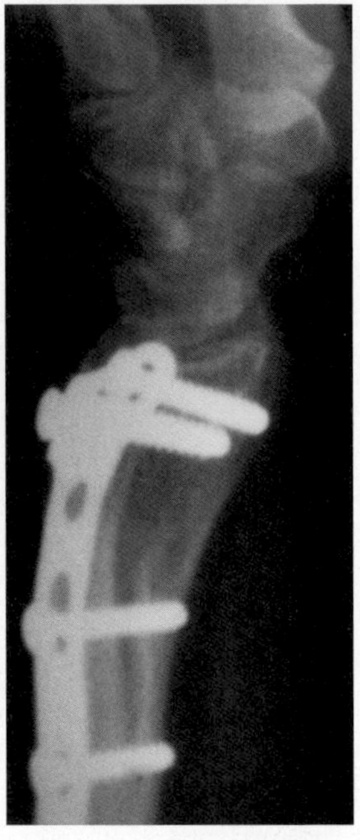

FIGURE 9-61 A. Radial metaphyseal fracture that did not remodel in a now 16-year-old skeletally mature boy. **B.** Corrective osteotomy with iliac crest bone graft and internal fixation was performed.

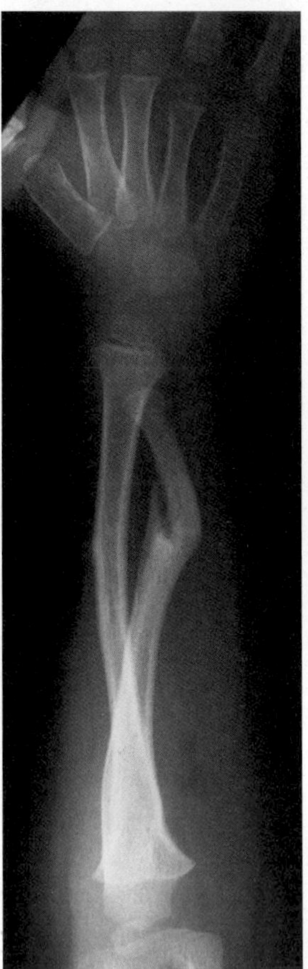

FIGURE 9-62 This 3-year-old presented to the emergency room with pain after an acute fall on his arm. The ulna is clearly pathologic with thinning and deformity before this injury. This represents neurofibromatosis.

teoclasis lengthening, vascularized bone grafting, or creation of a single-bone forearm are surgical options. The choice depends on the individual patient.

Cross-Union

Cross-union is a rare complication of pediatric distal radial and ulnar fractures. It has been described after high-energy trauma and internal fixation.[230] A single-pin crossing both bones increases the risk of cross-union.[230] Synostosis take-down can be performed, but the results usually are less than full restoration of motion. It is important to determine if there is an element of rotational malunion with the cross-union because this will affect the surgical outcome.

Soft tissue contraction across both bones also has been described.[57] Contracture release resulted in restoration of forearm motion.

Refracture

Fortunately, refractures after metaphyseal radial fractures are rare and much less common than after diaphyseal level radial and ulnar fractures. Most commonly, refracture occurs with premature discontinuation of immobilization or early return to potentially traumatic activities. It is advisable to protectively immobilize the wrist until full radiograph and clinical healing (usually 6 weeks) and to restrict activities until full motion and strength are regained (usually an additional 1 to 6 weeks). Individuals involved in high-risk activities, such as downhill ski racing, snowboarding, or skateboarding, should be protected with a splint during those activities for much longer.

Growth Disturbance

Growth arrest of the distal radius after metaphyseal fracture is rare. Abram, Thompson, and Connolly et al.[2,31a] each reported one patient with physeal arrest after nondisplaced torus fractures. Two additional patients were reported in a series of 150 distal radial metaphyseal fractures.[63] Wilkins and O'Brien[246] proposed that these arrests may be in fractures that extend from the metaphysis to the physis. This coincides with a Peterson type I fracture (Fig. 9-63)[169,170] and in essence is a physeal fracture. These fractures should be monitored for growth arrest.

Both undergrowth and overgrowth of the distal radius after fracture were described by DePablos.[42] The average difference in growth was 3 mm, with a range of -5 to +10 mm of growth disturbance compared with the contralateral radius. Maximal overgrowth occurred in the 9- to 12-year-old age group. As long as the patient is asymptomatic, under- or overgrowth is not a problem. If ulnocarpal impaction or DRUJ disruption occurs, then surgical rebalancing of the radius and ulna may be necessary.

Neurovascular Injuries

Both the median and ulnar[30,229] nerves are less commonly injured in metaphyseal fractures than in physeal fractures. The mechanisms of neural injury in a metaphyseal fracture include direct contusion from the displaced fragment, traction ischemia from tenting of the nerve over the proximal fragment,[11,165] entrapment of the nerve in the fracture site,[8,247] rare laceration of the nerve (Fig. 9-64), and the development of an acute compartment syndrome. If signs or symptoms of neuropathy are present, a prompt closed reduction should be performed. Extreme

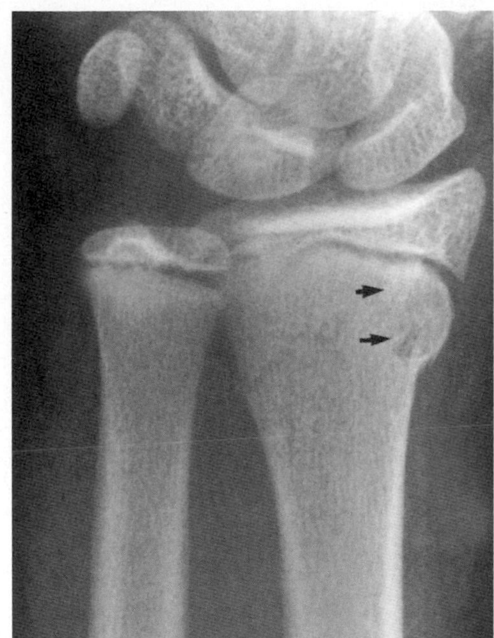
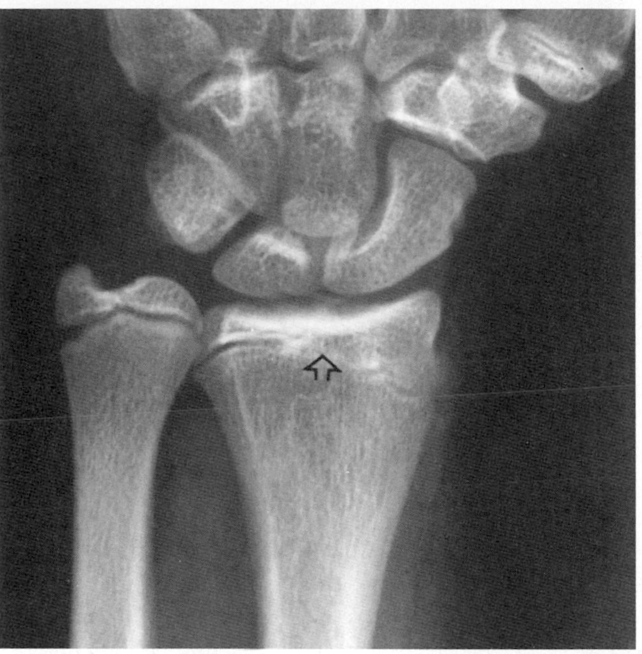

FIGURE 9-63 Physeal arrest in a Peterson type I fracture. **A.** Injury film showing what appears to be a benign metaphyseal fracture. Fracture line extends into the physis (*arrows*). **B.** Two years postinjury, a central arrest (*open arrow*) has developed, with resultant shortening of the radius. (Reprinted from Wilkins KE, ed. Operative Management of Upper Extremity Fractures in Children. Rosemont, IL: American Academy of Orthopaedic Surgeons, 1994:21, with permission.)

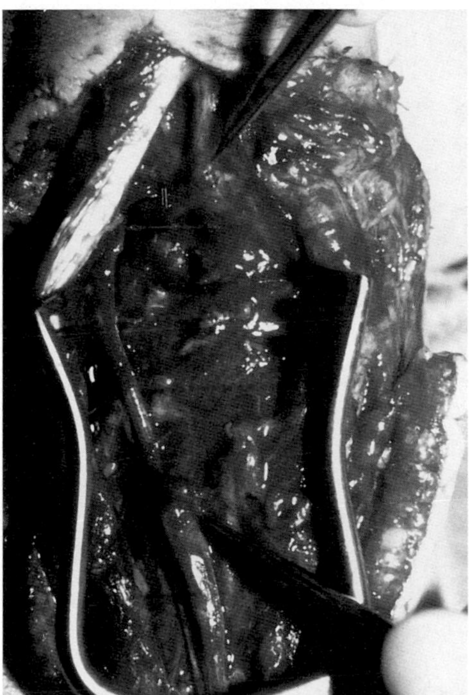
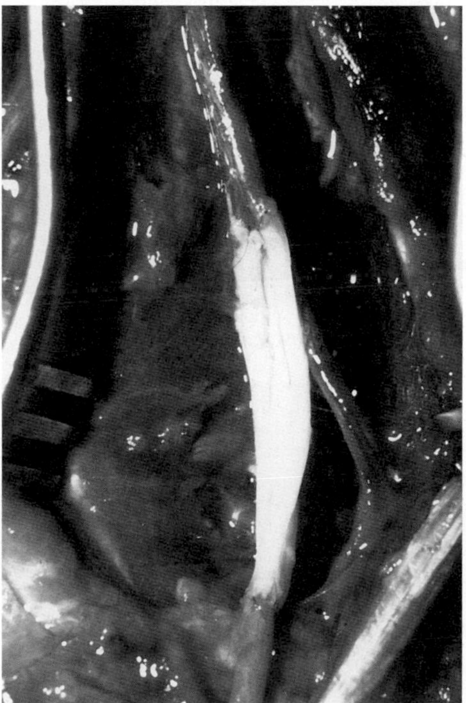

FIGURE 9-64 A grade III open fracture of the radius resulted in complete disruption of the ulnar nerve. Intraoperative photographs of the nerve deficit between the operative jeweler's forceps **(A)** and sural nerve grafting **(B)** after the wound was clean enough to allow for nerve reconstruction.

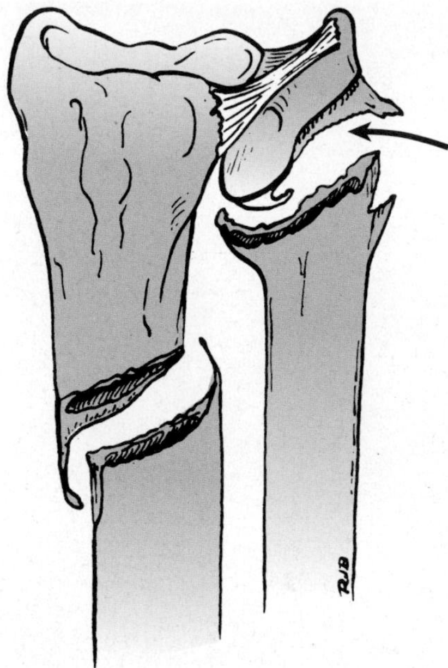

FIGURE 9-65 Galeazzi fracture-dislocation variant. Interposed periosteum can block reduction of the distal ulnar physis (*arrow*). This destabilizes the distal radial metaphyseal fracture. (Reprinted from Lanfried MJ, Stenclik M, Susi JG. Variant of Galeazzi fracture–dislocation in children. J Pediatr Orthop 1991;11:333, with permission.)

positions of immobilization should be avoided because this can lead to persistent traction or compression ischemia and increase the risk of compartment syndrome. If there is marked swelling, it is better to percutaneously pin the fracture than to apply a constrictive cast. If there is concern about compartment syndrome, the forearm and carpal canal pressures should be measured immediately. If pressures are markedly elevated, appropriate fasciotomies and compartment releases should be performed immediately. Finally, if the nerve was intact before reduction and is out after reduction, neural entrapment should be considered, and surgical exploration and decompression may be required. Fortunately, most median and ulnar nerve injuries recover after anatomic reduction of the fracture.

Infection

Infection after distal radial fractures is rare and is associated with open fractures or surgical intervention. Fee et al.[59] described the development of gas gangrene in four children after minor puncture wounds or lacerations associated with distal radial fractures. Treatment involved only local cleansing of the wound in all four and wound closure in one. All four developed life-threatening clostridial infections. Three of the four required upper limb amputations, and the fourth underwent multiple soft tissue and bony procedures for coverage and treatment of osteomyelitis.

Infections related to surgical intervention also are rare. Superficial pin site infections can occur and should be treated with pin removal and antibiotics. Deep-space infection from percutaneous pinning of the radius has not been described.

PEDIATRIC GALEAZZI FRACTURES

Fractures of the distal radius associated with DRUJ disruption have been called Galeazzi fracture-dislocations. Although Sir Ashley Cooper is credited with the first description of this injury in 1824, Riccardo Galeazzi[72,183] gave this fracture-dislocation its name with his 1934 report of 18 such injuries. In children, this injury may involve either disruption of the DRUJ ligaments or, more commonly, a distal ulnar physeal fracture (Fig. 9-65).[1,15,117,127,182,183] Galeazzi fracture-dislocations are relatively rare injuries in children. Walsh and McLaren[233] cited an occurrence of 3% of pediatric distal radial fractures in their study. Eberl et al.[50] reported 26 cases in a series of 198 forearm fractures (13%). Most series of Galeazzi fractures contain a relatively small number of pediatric patients.[127,143,170,233]

Mechanism of Injury

The mechanism of injury is axial loading in combination with extremes of forearm rotation (Fig. 9-66).[37,182,189,207] In adults, the mechanism of injury usually is an axially loading fall with hyperpronation. This results in a distal radial fracture with a

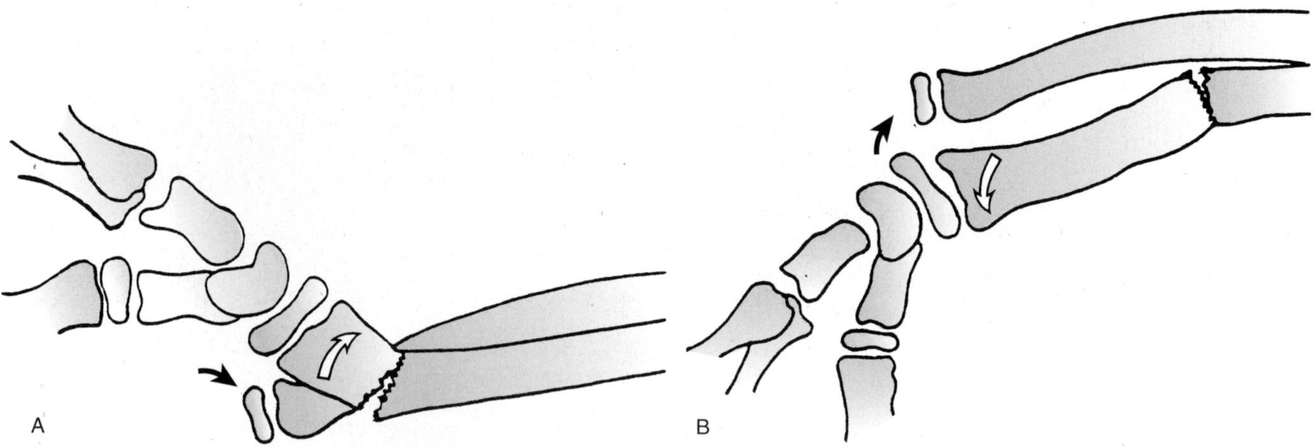

FIGURE 9-66 Walsh classification. **A.** The most common pattern, in which there is dorsal displacement with supination of the distal radius (*open arrow*). The distal ulna (*black arrow*) lies volar to the dorsally displaced distal radius. **B.** The least common pronation pattern. There is volar or anterior displacement of the distal radius (*open arrow*), and the distal ulna lies dorsal (*black arrow*). (Reprinted from Walsh HPJ, McLaren CANP. Galeazzi fractures in children. J Bone Joint Surg Br 1987;69:730–733, with permission.)

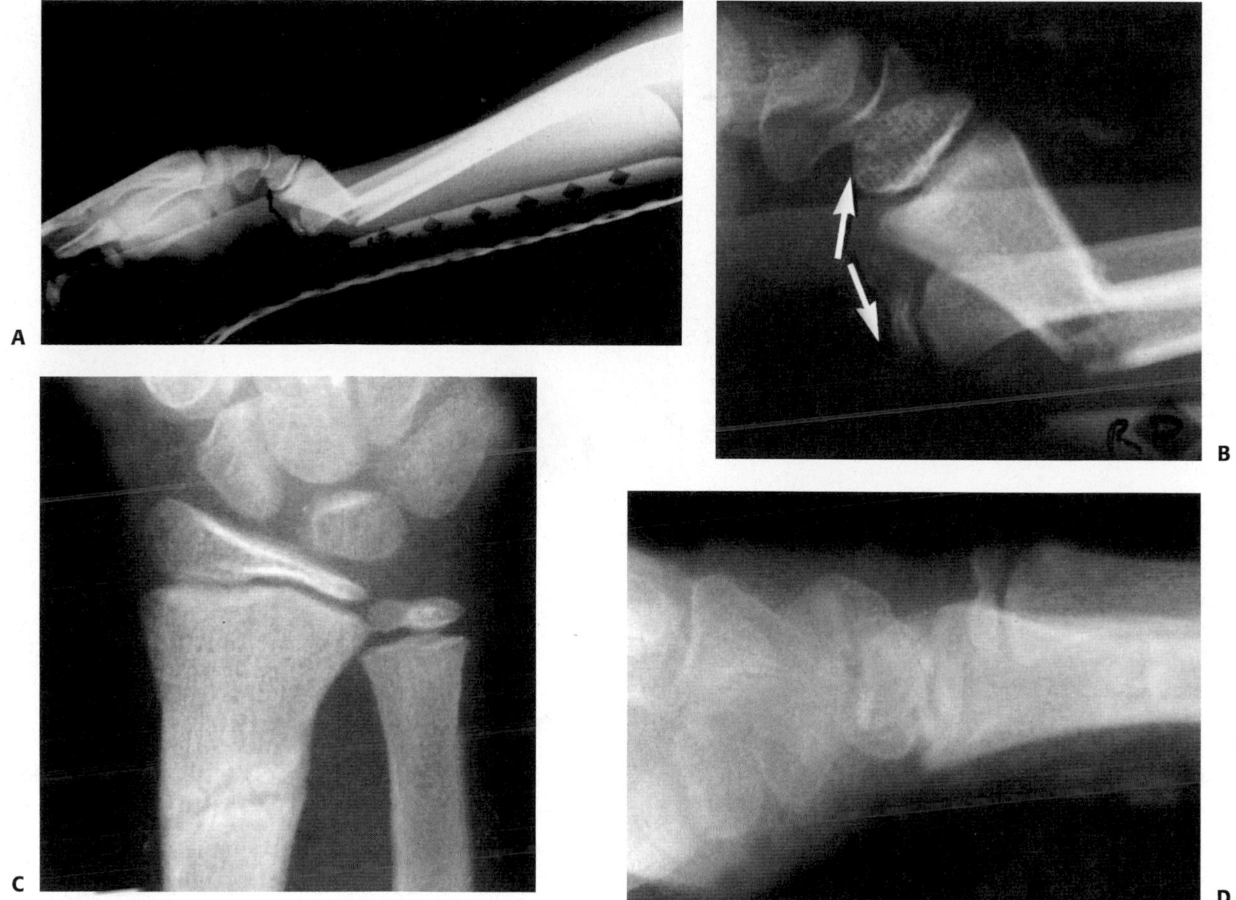

FIGURE 9-67 Supination-type Galeazzi fracture. **A.** View of the entire forearm of an 11-year-old boy with a Galeazzi fracture-dislocation. **B.** Close-up of the distal forearm shows that there has been disruption of the distal radioulnar joint (*arrows*). The distal radial fragment is dorsally displaced (apex volar), making this a supination type of mechanism. Note that the distal ulna is volar to the distal radius. **C,D.** The fracture was reduced by pronating the distal fragment. Because the distal radius was partially intact by its greenstick nature, the length was easily maintained, re-establishing the congruity of the distal radioulnar joint. The patient was immobilized in supination for 6 weeks, after which full forearm rotation and function returned.

dorsal ulnar dislocation. However, in children, both supination (apex volar) and pronation (apex dorsal) deforming forces have been described.[126,182,233] The mechanism of injury is most obvious when the radial fracture is an incomplete fracture. With an apex volar (supination) radial fracture, the distal ulna is displaced volarly, whereas with an apex dorsal (pronation) radial fracture, the distal ulna is displaced dorsally (Fig. 9-67). This is evident both on clinical and radiographic examinations. In addition, the radius is foreshortened in a complete fracture, causing more radial deviation of the hand and wrist (Fig. 9-68).

Signs and Symptoms

A child with a Galeazzi injury has pain and limitation of forearm rotation and wrist flexion and extension. Neurovascular impairment is rare. The radial deformity usually is clinically evident. The DRUJ disruption may be obvious by the prominence of the ulnar head. A subtle ligament disruption may be evident only by local tenderness and instability to testing on the DRUJ.

The radial fracture is evident on radiographs, and concurrent injuries to the ulna or DRUJ should be identified. A true lateral view is necessary to identify the direction of displacement, which is imperative to determine the method of reduction. Rarely are special radiographs, such as a CT scan, necessary.

Classification

Galeazzi fracture-dislocations are most commonly described by direction of displacement of either the distal ulnar dislocation or the radial fracture. Letts[126,127] preferred to describe the direction of the ulna: volar or dorsal. Walsh and McLaren[233] classified pediatric Galeazzi injuries by the direction of displacement of the distal radial fracture. Dorsal displacement (apex volar) fractures were more common than volar displacement (apex dorsal) fractures in their series. Wilkins and O'Brien[246] modified the Walsh and McLaren method by classifying radial fractures as incomplete and complete fractures and ulnar injuries as true dislocations and physeal fractures (Table 9-4). DRUJ dislocations are called true Galeazzi lesions and distal ulnar physeal fractures are called Galeazzi equivalent lesions.[94,117,126,127]

Anatomy

The distal radius normally rotates around the relatively stationary ulna. The two bones of the forearm articulate at the proximal

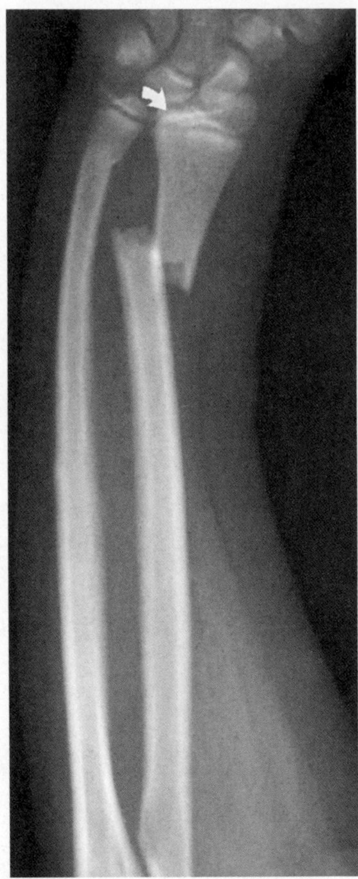

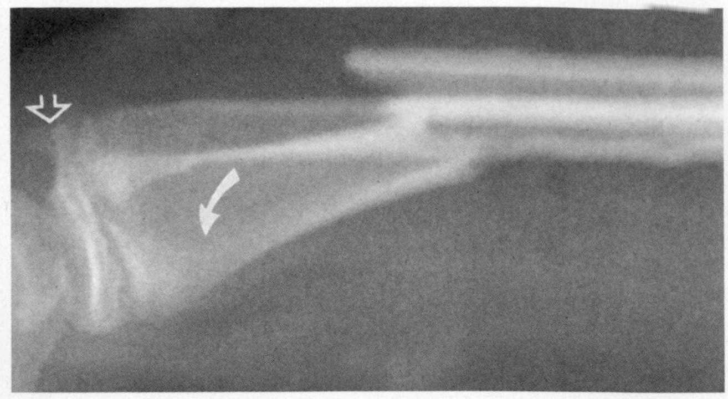

FIGURE 9-68 Pronation Galeazzi. This 8-year-old sustained a pronation Galeazzi fracture. **A.** The AP view shows some shortening of the distal radius (*arrow*) in relation to the distal ulna, which has a small greenstick component. **B.** The pronation component (*arrow*) is better appreciated on this lateral view. The distal ulna lies dorsal to the distal radius (*open arrow*).

and distal radioulnar joints. In addition, proximally the radius and ulna articulate with the distal humerus and distally with the carpus. These articulations are necessary for forearm pronation and supination. At the DRUJ, the concave sigmoid notch of the radius incompletely matches the convex, asymmetric, semicylindrical shape of the distal ulnar head.[18] This allows some translation at the DRUJ with rotatory movements. The

TABLE 9-4 Classification: Galeazzi Fractures in Children

Type I: Dorsal (apex volar) displacement of distal radius
- Radius fracture pattern
  - Greenstick
  - Complete
- Distal ulna physis
  - Intact
  - Disrupted (equivalent)

Type II: Volar (apex dorsal) displacement of distal radius
- Radius fracture pattern
  - Greenstick
  - Complete
- Distal ulna physis
  - Intact
  - Disrupted

Reprinted from Walsh HPJ, McLaren CAN, Owen R. Galeazzi fractures in children. J Bone Joint Surg Br 1987;69B:730–733.

ligamentous structures are critical in stabilizing the radius as it rotates about the ulna (Fig. 9-69).

The DRUJ includes multiple soft tissue attachments, the most important of which is the TFCC. The TFCC includes the volar and dorsal ligamentous attachments of the distal ulna to the radial sigmoid notch, as well as the distal extension to the ulnar styloid, carpus, and base of the fifth metacarpal. The volar ulnocarpal ligaments (V ligament) from the ulna to the lunate and triquetrum are important ulnocarpal stabilizers.[18,200,242] The central portion of the TFCC is the articular disk (Fig. 9-70). The interaction between the bony articulation and the soft tissue attachments accounts for stability of the DRUJ during pronation and supination. At the extremes of rotation, the joint is most stable. The compression loads between the radius and ulna are aided by the tensile loads of the TFCC to maintain stability throughout rotation.

Throughout the midforearm, the interosseous ligament connects the radius to the ulna. It passes obliquely from the proximal radius to the distal ulna. However, the interosseous ligament is not present in the distal radius. Moore et al.[149] found that injuries to the TFCC and interosseous ligament were responsible for progressive shortening of the radius with fracture in a cadaveric study. The soft tissue component to the injury is a major factor in the deformity and instability in a Galeazzi fracture-dislocation.

Current Treatment Options

Pediatric Galeazzi fractures have a higher success rate with nonoperative treatment than similar injuries in adults.[50,143,182] In

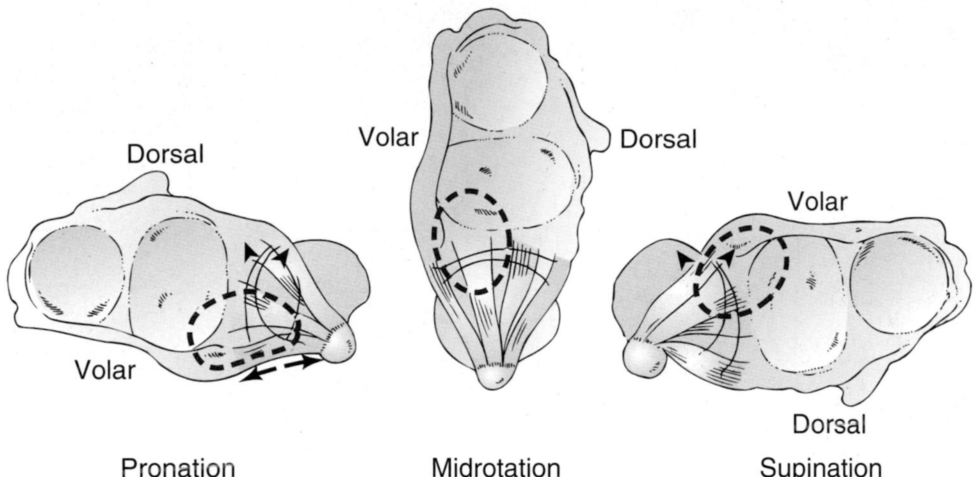

FIGURE 9-69 Distal radioulnar joint stability in pronation (*left*) is dependent on (a) tension developed in the volar margin of the triangular fibrocartilage (TFCC, *small arrows*) and (b) compression between the contact areas of the radius and ulna (volar surface of ulnar articular head and dorsal margin of the sigmoid notch, *large arrows*). Disruption of the volar TFCC would therefore allow dorsal displacement of the ulna in pronation. The reverse is true in supination, where disruption of the dorsal margin of the TFCC would allow volar displacement of the ulna relative to the radius as this rotational extreme is reached. The dark area of the TFCC emphasizes the portion of the TFCC that is not supported by the ulnar dome. The dotted circle is the arc of load transmission (lunate to TFCC) in that position. (Redrawn from Bowers WH. Green's Operative Hand Surgery. New York: Churchill-Livingstone, 1993.)

adults, it is imperative to anatomically reduce and internally fix the distal radial fracture.[115,143,147,148,182] Generally, the DRUJ is reduced with reduction and fixation of the radius. In pediatric patients, the distal radial fracture often is a greenstick type that is stable after reduction; cast immobilization is sufficient.[143,233]

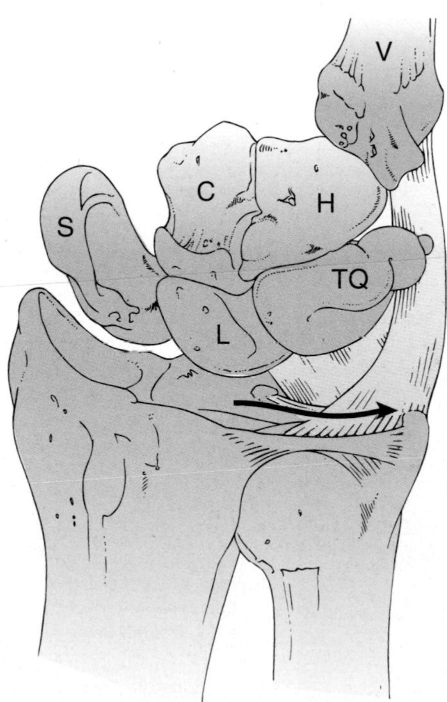

FIGURE 9-70 Diagrammatic drawing of the TFCC and the prestyloid recess. The meniscal reflection runs from the dorsoulnar radius to the ulnovolar carpus. The arrow denotes access under the reflection to the tip of the styloid—the so-called prestyloid recess. (Redrawn from Bowers WH. Green's Operative Hand Surgery. New York: Churchill-Livingstone, 1993.)

Adolescents with complete fractures should be treated with internal fixation similar to adults.

Closed Reduction

The method of reduction for greenstick radial fractures depends on the type of displacement. With apex volar dorsally displaced fractures of the radius, the rotatory deformity is supination. Pronating the radius and applying a dorsal-to-volar reduction force should align the fracture and reduce the DRUJ. Similarly, if the incomplete radial fracture is an apex dorsal volar displaced fracture, the rotatory deformity is pronation. Supinating the forearm and applying a volar-to-dorsal force should reduce the incomplete fracture of the radius and the DRUJ dislocation.[126,127,144,246] In both these situations, portable fluoroscopy can be used to evaluate the fracture-dislocation reduction and to test the stability of the distal ulna. If anatomically reduced and stable, a long-arm cast is applied with appropriate rotation and three-point molds. The cast is left in place for 6 weeks to allow the soft tissue injuries to heal.

In a Galeazzi equivalent injury with a radial fracture and an ulnar physeal fracture, both bones should be reduced. Usually, this can be accomplished with the same methods of reduction as when the radial fracture is incomplete. The distal ulnar physis can remodel a nonanatomic reduction if there is sufficient growth remaining and the ulnar physis continues to grow normally. Unfortunately, the risk of ulnar growth arrest after a Galeazzi equivalent has been reported to be as high as 55%.[81]

Complete fractures of the distal radius have a higher rate of loss of reduction after closed treatment than do incomplete fractures (Fig. 9-71).[246] If not monitored closely and rereduced if necessary, loss of reduction can lead to malunion with loss of motion and function. These injuries may be best treated with open reduction as in adults.

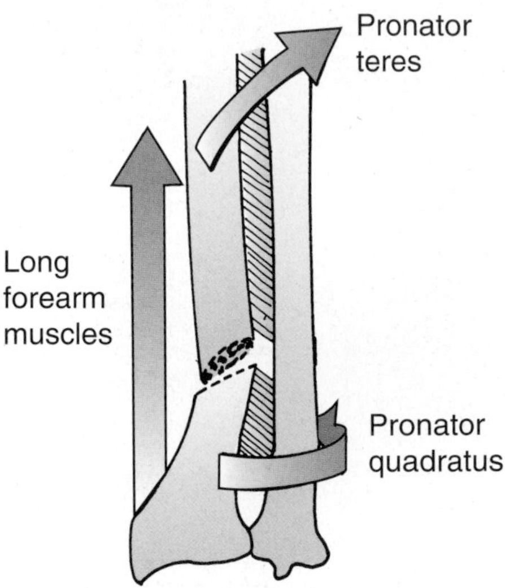

FIGURE 9-71 Fractures of the distal radius are angulated toward the ulna due to the pull of the long forearm muscles and the pronator quadratus. (Redrawn from Cruess RL. The management of forearm injuries. Orthop Clin North Am 1973;4:969–982, with permission.)

Open Reduction

The indication for open reduction of the radial fracture is failure to obtain or maintain fracture reduction. This most often occurs with unstable complete fractures. Open reduction and internal fixation of the radius are done through an anterior approach. Standard compression plating is preferred to intramedullary or cross-pinning techniques (Fig. 9-72). Stable, anatomic reduction of the radius almost always leads to stable reduction of the DRUJ dislocation. A long-arm cast is used for 6 weeks to allow fracture and soft tissue healing.

Occasionally, the DRUJ dislocation cannot be reduced (Fig. 9-73) because of interposed soft tissues, most commonly the periosteum, extensor tendons (extensor carpi ulnaris, extensor digit quinti), TFCC, or other ligamentous structures.[14,26,100,127] The easiest approach for open reduction of the DRUJ is an extended ulnar approach. Care should be taken to avoid injury to the ulnar sensory nerve. This approach allows exposure both volarly and dorsally to extract the interposed soft tissues and repair the torn structures. Alternatively, a Bowers approach to the distal radioulnar joint may be used, providing the advantage of more direct visualization and extraction of interposed soft tissues in irreducible cases. Smooth pin fixation of the DRUJ can be used to maintain reduction and allow application of a loose-fitting cast. The pin is removed in the office at 4 weeks with continuation of the cast for 6 weeks.

Similarly, the ulnar physeal fracture can be irreducible in a Galeazzi equivalent injury. This also has been reported to be secondary to interposed periosteum,[117,182] extensor tendons,[160] or joint capsule.[53] Open reduction must be executed with care to avoid further violating the physis.

Incomplete Fractures

Incomplete fractures of the distal radius with either a true dislocation of the DRUJ or an ulnar physeal fracture are treated with closed reduction and long-arm cast immobilization. This can be done in the emergency room with conscious sedation or in the operating room with general anesthesia. Portable fluoroscopy is used. If the fracture is apex volar with dorsal displacement of the radius and volar dislocation of the DRUJ, then

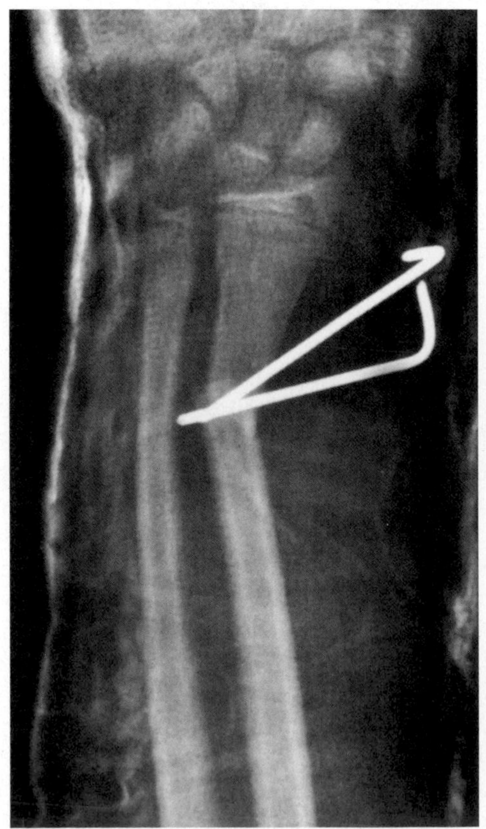

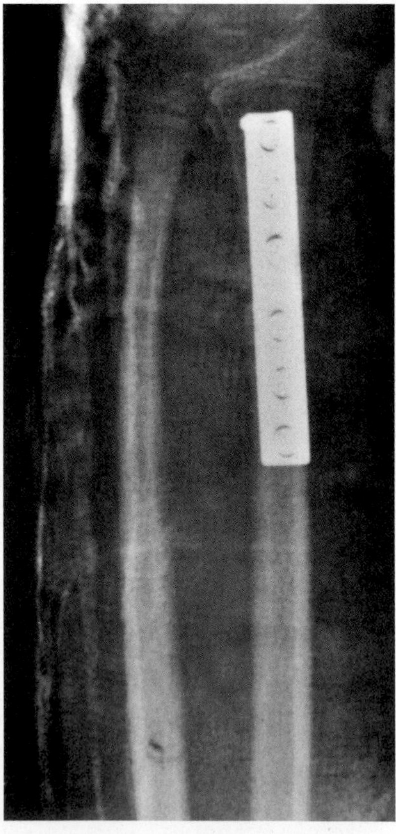

FIGURE 9-72 A. The patient with the pronation injury shown in Figure 9-68 had a closed reduction and attempted fixation with pins placed percutaneously across the fracture site. However, this was inadequate in maintaining the alignment and length of the fracture of the distal radius. **B.** The length of the radius and the distal radioulnar relationship were best re-established after internal fixation of the distal radius with a plate placed on the volar surface. The true amount of shortening present on the original injury film (see Fig. 9-68A) is not really appreciated until the fracture of the distal radius is fully reduced. (Reprinted from Wilkins KE, ed. Operative Management of Upper Extremity Fractures in Children. Rosemont, IL: American Academy of Orthopaedic Surgeons, 1994:34, with permission.)

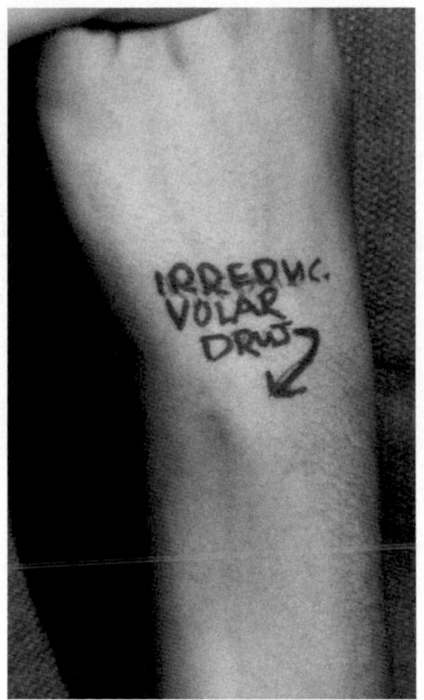

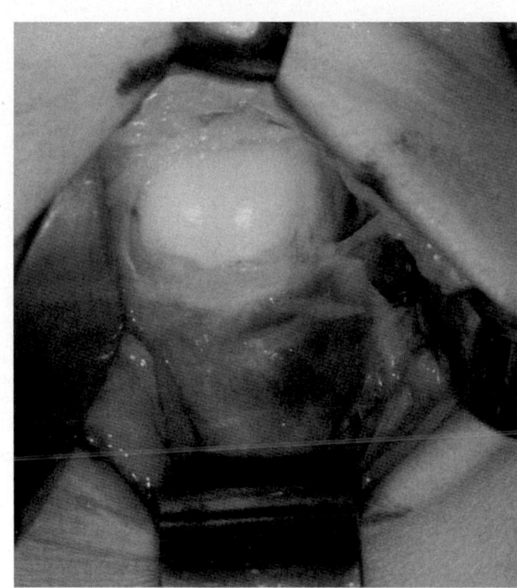

FIGURE 9-73 An adolescent girl presented 4 weeks after injury with a painful, stiff wrist. **A.** By examination, she was noted to have a volar distal radioulnar dislocation that was irreducible even under general anesthesia. **B.** At the time of surgery, the distal ulna was found to have buttonholed out of the capsule, and there was entrapped triangular fibrocartilage and periosteum in the joint.

pronation and volar-to-dorsal force on the radial fracture is used for reduction. If the fracture is apex dorsal with volar displacement of the radius and dorsal dislocation of the DRUJ, then supination and dorsal-to-volar force is applied to the distal radius for reduction. The reduction and stability of the fracture and DRUJ dislocation are checked on dynamic fluoroscopy before long-arm cast immobilization. If both are anatomically reduced and stable, the cast is used for 6 weeks to allow soft tissue and fracture healing. In a Galeazzi equivalent injury, there is potential for remodeling of the physeal fracture if sufficient growth remains. As long as the DRUJ is reduced, malalignment of less than 10 degrees can remodel in a young child. The risk of physeal growth arrest is high with this physeal injury, and operative exposure may increase the risk of growth impairment. If the fracture is severely malaligned, the DRUJ cannot be reduced, or the patient is older and remodeling is unlikely, open reduction and smooth pin fixation are indicated.[246]

Complete Fractures

Open reduction and internal fixation with an anterior plate and screws are used for complete Galeazzi fractures of the radius. The DRUJ usually reduces anatomically and is stable with reduction and fixation of the radius. The patient is immobilized in a long-arm cast for 4 weeks and a short-arm cast for 2 more weeks. Return to unrestricted activities and sports depends on restoration of full motion and strength.

Irreducible Dislocations

Irreducible dislocations are treated with open reduction. Extensile exposure is necessary to define the pathologic anatomy and carefully reduce the DRUJ. The interposed soft tissues are extracted and repaired. Depending on the stability of the reduction and repair, a supplemental smooth pin may be used across the DRUJ for 4 weeks to maintain the joint reduction. This is particularly true if the patient presents late.

Complications

Malunion and Distal Radioulnar Joint Subluxation

Malunion of the radius can lead to subluxation of the DRUJ, limited forearm rotation, and pain, usually secondary to persistent shortening and malrotation of the radial fracture. Most often, this occurs when complete fractures are treated with closed reduction and there is failure to either obtain or maintain reduction of the radial fracture. The ulna remains subluxed and heals with an incongruent joint. Treatment of this requires proper recognition and corrective osteotomy. If physical examination is not definitive for diagnosis, then a CT scan in pronation, neutral rotation, or supination may be helpful. MRI or wrist arthroscopy will aid in the diagnosis and management of associated ligamentous, chondral, or TFCC injuries that will benefit from débridement or repair. It is important to understand that if the DRUJ subluxation is caused by a radial malunion, a soft tissue reconstruction of the DRUJ alone will fail.[18] In the true soft tissue disruption, repair of the TFCC will often stabilize the DRUJ. If there is no TFCC tear, soft tissue reconstruction of the DRUJ ligaments with extensor retinaculum or local tendon is appropriate.

Ulnar Physeal Arrest

Golz et al.[81] cited ulnar physeal arrest in 55% of Galeazzi equivalent fractures. If the patient is young enough, this ulnar growth arrest in the presence of ongoing radial growth will lead to deformity. Initially, there will be ulnar shortening. Over time, the foreshortened ulna can act as a tether, causing asymmetric growth of the radius. There will be increased radial articular inclination on the AP radiograph and subluxation of the DRUJ. Operative choices include ulnar lengthening, radial closing wedge osteotomy, radial epiphysiodesis, and a combination of the above procedures that is appropriate for the individual patient's age, deformity, and disability.

Nerve Injury

Injuries to the ulnar nerve[143] and anterior interosseous nerve[209,235] have been described with Galeazzi fracture-dislocations. These injuries have had spontaneous recovery. Moore et al.[148] described an 8% rate of injury to the radial nerve with operative exposure of the radius for internal fixation in their series. Careful surgical exposure, dissection, and retraction can decrease this risk.

REFERENCES

1. Abid A, Accadbled F, Kany J, et al. Ulnar styloid fracture in children: a retrospective study of 46 cases. J Pediatr Orthop B 2008;17:15–19.
2. Abram LJ, Thompson GH. Deformity after premature closure of the distal radial physis following a torus fracture with a physeal compression injury. Report of a case. J Bone Joint Surg Am 1987;69:1450–1453.
3. Aitken AP. The end results of the fractured distal radial epiphysis. Bone Joint Surg 1935;17:302–308.
4. Aitken AP. Further observations on the fractured distal radial epiphysis. J Bone and Joint Surg 1935;17:922–927.
5. Albanese SA, Palmer AK, Kerr DR, et al. Wrist pain and distal growthplate closure of the radius in gymnasts. J Pediatr Orthop 1989;9:23–28.
6. Alemdaroğlu KB, Iltar S, Cimen O, et al. Risk factors in redisplacement of distal radial fractures in children. J Bone Joint Surg Am 2008;90:1224–1230.
7. Arima J, Uchida Y, Miura H, et al. Osteochondral fracture in the distal end of the radius. J Hand Surg Am 1993;18:489–491.
8. Armstrong P, Joughlin J, Clarke H. Pediatric fractures of the forearm, wrist, and hand in skeletal trauma in children. In: Green N, Swiontkowski M, eds. Skeletal Trauma in Children. Philadelphia: WB Saunders, 1994:161–257.
9. Bae DS, Waters PM. Pediatric distal radius fractures and triangular fibrocartilage complex injuries. Hand Clin 2006;22:43–53.
10. Bailey DA, Wedge JH, McCulloch RG, et al. Epidemiology of fractures of the distal end of the radius in children as associated with growth. J Bone Joint Surg Am 1989; 71:1225–1231.
11. Banas MP, Dalldorf PG, Marquardt JD. Skateboard and in-line skate fractures: a report of one summer's experience. J Orthop Trauma 1992;6:301–305.
12. Bell MJ, Hill RJ, McMurtry RY. Ulnar impingement syndrome. J Bone Joint Surg Br 1985;67:126–129.
13. Biyani A. Ipsilateral Monteggia equivalent injury and distal radial and ulnar fracture in a child. J Orthop Trauma 1994;8:431–433.
14. Biyani A, Bhan S. Dual extensor tendon entrapment in Galeazzi fracture-dislocation: a case report. J Trauma 1989;29:1295–1297.
15. Bley L, Seitz WH Jr. Injuries about the distal ulna in children. Hand Clin 1998;14: 231–237.
16. Blount WP. Fractures in Children. Baltimore: Williams & Wilkins, 1955.
17. Bohm ER, Bubbar V, Yong Hing K, et al. Above and below-the-elbow plaster casts for distal forearm fractures in children. A randomized controlled trial. J Bone Joint Surg Am 2006;88:1–8.
18. Bowers W. The distal radioulnar joint. In: Green D, Hotchkiss R, Pederson W, ed. Green's Operative Hand Surgery. New York: Churchill-Livingstone, 1999:986–1032.
19. Boyd KT, Brownson P, Hunter JB. Distal radial fractures in young goalkeepers: a case for an appropriately sized soccer ball. Br J Sports Med 2001;35:409–411.
20. Boyden EM, Peterson HA. Partial premature closure of the distal radial physis associated with Kirschner wire fixation. Orthopedics 1991;14:585–588.
21. Boyer BA, Overton B, Schrader W, et al. Position of immobilization for pediatric forearm fractures. J Pediatr Orthop 2002;22:185–187.
22. Burgess RC, Watson HK. Hypertrophic ulnar styloid nonunions. Clin Orthop Relat Res 1988;228:215–217.
23. Caine D, Roy S, Singer KM, et al. Stress changes of the distal radial growth plate. A radiographic survey and review of the literature. Am J Sports Med 1992;20:290–298.
24. Cannata G, DeMaio F, Mancini F, et al. Physeal fractures of the distal radius and ulna: long-term prognosis. J Orthop Trauma 2003; 17:172–179.
25. Carpenter C, Williams P. Management of completely displaced metaphyseal fractures of the distal radius in children. J Bone Joint Surg Br 2003;85:933.
26. Cetti NE. An unusual cause of blocked reduction of the Galeazzi injury. Injury 1977; 9:59–61.
27. Cheng JC, Shen WY. Limb fracture pattern in different pediatric age groups: a study of 3350 children. J Orthop Trauma 1993;7(1):15–22.
28. Chess DG, Hyndman JC, Leahey JL, et al. Short-arm plaster cast for distal pediatric forearm fractures. J Pediatr Orthop 1994;14:211–213.
29. Chess DG, Hyndman JC, Leahey JL. Short-arm plaster for paediatric distal forearm fractures. J Bone Joint Surg Br 1987;69:506.
30. Clarke AC, Spencer RF. Ulnar nerve palsy following fractures of the distal radius: clinical and anatomical studies. J Hand Surg Br 1991;16:438–440.
31. Compson JP. Transcarpal injuries associated with distal radial fractures in children: a series of three cases. J Hand Surg Br 1992;17:311–314.

31a. Connolly JF, Eastman T, Haverman WW. Torus fracture of the distal radius producing growth arrest. Nebr Med J 1985;70:204–207.

32. Cooper RR. Management of common forearm fractures in children. J Iowa Med Soc 1964;54:689–698.
33. Cotton FJ. Dislocations and Joint Fractures. Philadelphia: WB Saunders, 1924:370.
34. Crawford AH. Pitfalls and complications of fractures of the distal radius and ulna in childhood. Hand Clin 1988;4:403–413.
35. Creasman C, Zaleske DJ, Ehrlich MG. Analyzing forearm fractures in children. The more subtle signs of impending problems. Clin Orthop Relat Res 1984;188:40–53.
36. Cross AW, Schmidt CC. Flexor tendon injuries following locked volar plating of distal radius fractures. J Hand Surg Am 2008;33:164–167.
37. Dameron TB Jr. Traumatic dislocation of the distal radioulnar joint. Clin Orthop Relat Res 1972;83:55–63.
38. Daruwalla JS. A study of radioulnar movements following fractures of the forearm in children. Clin Orthop Relat Res 1979;139:114–120.
39. Davidson JS, Brown DJ, Barnes SN, et al. Simple treatment for torus fractures of the distal radius. J Bone Joint Surg Br 2001;83:1173–1175.
40. Davis DR, Green DP. Forearm fractures in children: pitfalls and complications. Clin Orthop Relat Res 1976;120:172–183.
41. De Courtivron B. Spontaneous correction of the distal forearm fractures in children. Presented at the European Pediatric Orthopaedic Society Annual Meeting; Brussels, Belgium, 1995.
42. de Pablos J, Franzreb M, Barrios C. Longitudinal growth pattern of the radius after forearm fractures conservatively treated in children. J Pediatr Orthop 1994;14: 492–495.
43. De Smet L, Claessens A, Lefevre J, et al. Gymnast wrist: an epidemiologic survey of ulnar variance and stress changes of the radial physis in elite female gymnasts. Am J Sports Med 1994;22:846–850.
44. Deffer PA, Schonholtz G, Litchman HM. Displaced distal forearm fractures in children. Bull Hosp Joint Dis 1963;24:42–47.
45. DiFiori JP, Puffer JC, Aish B, et al. Wrist pain, distal radial physeal injury, and ulnar variance in young gymnasts: does a relationship exist? Am J Sports Med 2002;30: 879–885.
46. Do TT, Strub WM, Foad SL, et al. Reduction versus remodeling in pediatric distal forearm fractures: a preliminary cost analysis. J Pediatr Orthop Br 2003;12:109–115.
47. Dobyns JH, Gabel GT. Gymnast's wrist. Hand Clin 1990;6:493–505.
48. Doi K, Hattori Y, Otsuka K, et al. Intra-articular fractures of the distal aspect of the radius: arthroscopically assisted reduction compared with open reduction and internal fixation. J Bone Joint Surg Am 1999;81:1093–1110.
49. Earp BE, Waters PW, Wyzokowski RJ. Arthroscopic treatment of partial scapholunate tears in children with chronic wrist pain. J Bone Joint Surg Am 2006;88(11): 2448–2455.
50. Eberl R, Singer G, Schalamon J, et al. Galeazzi lesions in children and adolescents. Clin Orthop Relat Res 2008;466:1705–1709.
51. Ekenstrom F. The anatomy of the distal radioulnar joint. Clin Orthop Relat Res 1992; 275:14–18.
52. Ekşioğlu F, Altinok D, Uslu MM, et al. Ultrasonographic findings in pediatric fractures. Turk J Pediatr 2003;45:136–140.
53. Engber WD, Keene JS. Irreducible fracture-separation of the distal ulnar epiphysis. Report of a case. J Bone Joint Surg Am 1985;67:1130–1132.
54. Epner RA, Bowers WH, Guilford WB. Ulnar variance—the effect of wrist positioning and roentgen filming technique. J Hand Surg Am 1982;7:298–305.
55. Evans DL, Stauber M, Frykman GK. Irreducible epiphyseal plate fracture of the distal ulna due to interposition of the extensor carpi ulnaris tendon. A case report. 1990; 251:162–165.
56. Evans EM. Fractures of the radius and ulna. J Bone Joint Surg Br 1951;33B:548–561.
57. Fatti JF, Mosher JF. An unusual complication of fracture of both bones of the forearm in a child. A case report. J Bone Joint Surg Am 1986;68:451–453.
58. Faulkner RA, Davison KS, Bailey DA, et al. Size-corrected BMD decreases during peak linear growth: implications for fracture incidence during adolescence. J Bone Miner Res 2006;21(12):1864–1870.
59. Fee NF, Dobranski A, Bisla RS. Gas gangrene complicating open forearm fractures. Report of five cases. J Bone Joint Surg Am 1977;59:135–138.
60. Fernandez DL, Palmer AK. Fractures of the distal radius. In: Green D, Hotchkiss R, Pederson W, eds. Green's Operative Hand Surgery. New York: Churchill-Livingstone, 1999:929–985.
61. Fernandez DL. Conservative treatment of forearm fractures in children. In: Chapchal G, ed. Fractures in Children. New York: Thieme-Stratton, 1981.
62. Fernandez DL. Correction of posttraumatic wrist deformity in adults by osteotomy, bone-grafting, and internal fixation. J Bone Joint Surg Am 1982;64;1164–1178.
63. Fodden DI. A study of wrist injuries in children: the incidence of various injuries and of premature closure of the distal radial growth plate. Arch Emerg Med 1992;9:9–13.
64. Forward DP, Davis TRC, Sithole JS. Do young patients with malunited fractures of the distal radius inevitably develop symptomatic posttraumatic osteoarthritis? J Bone Joint Surg Br 2008;90:629–637.
65. Fowles JV, Kassab MT. Displaced supracondylar fractures of the elbow in children. A report on the fixation of extension and flexion fractures by two lateral percutaneous pins. J Bone Joint Surg Br 1974;56B:490–500.
66. Freeland AE, Geissler WB. The arthroscopic management of intra-articular distal radius fractures. Hand Surg 2000;5:93–102.
67. Friberg KS. Remodelling after distal forearm fractures in children. I. The effect of residual angulation on the spatial orientation of the epiphyseal plates. Acta Orthop Scand 1979;50:537–546.
68. Friberg KS. Remodelling after distal forearm fractures in children. II. The final orientation of the distal and proximal epiphyseal plates of the radius. Acta Orthop Scand 1979;50:731–739.
69. Friberg KS. Remodelling after distal forearm fractures in children. III. Correction of residual angulation in fractures of the radius. Acta Orthop Scand 1979;50:741–749.
70. Friedman SL, Palmer AK, Short WH, et al. The change in ulnar variance with grip. J Hand Surg Am 1993;19:713–716.
71. Fuller DJ, McCullough CJ. Malunited fractures of the forearm in children. J Bone Joint Surg Br 1982;64:364–367.
72. Galeazzi R. Di una particulare sindrome, traumatica delle scheletro dell avambraccio. Atti Mem Soc Lomb Chir 1934;2:12.
73. Gambhir AK, Fischer J, Waseem M. Management of completely displaced metaphyseal fractures of the distal radius in children. J Bone Joint Surg Br 2003;85:463.
74. Gandhi RK, Wilson P, Mason Brown JJ, et al. Spontaneous correction of deformity following fractures of the forearm in children. Br J Surg 1962;50:5–10.
75. Garn SM, Rohmann CG, Silverman FN. Radiographic standards for postnatal ossification and tooth calcification. Med Radiogr Photogr 1967;43:45–66.
76. Geissler W, Freeland A, Weiss AP, et al. Techniques of wrist arthroscopy. Instructional course lecture. J Bone Joint Surg Am 1999;81:1184–1197.
77. Gelberman RH. Acute carpal tunnel syndrome. In: Gelbern AN, ed. Operative Nerve Repair and Reconstruction. Philadelphia: JB Lippincott, 1991:937–948.
78. Gelberman RH, Salamon PB, Jurist JM, et al. Ulnar variance in Kienbock's disease. J Bone Joint Surg Am 1975;57:674–676.
79. Gerber SD, Griffin PP, Simmons BP. Break dancer's wrist. J Pediatr Orthop 1986;6: 98–99.
80. Gibbons CL, Woods DA, Pailthorpe C, et al. The management of isolated distal radius fractures in children. J Pediatr Orthop 1994;14:207–210.
81. Golz RJ, Grogan DP, Greene TL, et al. Distal ulnar physeal injury. J Pediatr Orthop 1991;11:318–326.
82. Goulding A, Jones IE, Taylor RW, et al. Bone mineral density and body composition in boys with distal forearm fractures: a dual-energy x-ray absorptiometry study. J Pediatr 2001;139:509–515.
83. Goulding A, Jones IE, Taylor RW, et al. Dynamic and static tests of balance and postural sway in boys: effects of previous wrist bone fractures and high adiposity. Gait Posture 2003;17:136–141.
84. Goudling A, Jones IE, Taylor RW, et al. More broken bones: a 4-year double cohort study of young girls with and without distal forearm fractures. J Bone Miner Res 2000; 15:2011–2018.

85. Greene WB, Anderson WJ. Simultaneous fracture of the scaphoid and radius in a child. J Pediatr Orthop 1982;2:191–194.
86. Greulich W, Pyle SI. Radiographic atlas of skeletal development of the hand and wrist. Stanford: Stanford University Press; 1959.
87. Grundy M. Fractures of the carpal scaphoid in children. A series of eight cases. Br J Surg 1969;56:523–524.
88. Guero S. Fractures and epiphyseal fracture separation of the distal bones of the forearm in children. In: Saffar P, Cooney WP, eds. Fractures of the Distal Radius. Philadelphia: JB Lippincott, 1995.
89. Gupta RP, Danielsson LG. Dorsally angulated solitary metaphyseal greenstick fractures in the distal radius: results after immobilization in pronated, neutral, and supinated position. J Pediatr Orthop 1990;10:90–92.
90. Hafner R, Poznanski AK, Donovan JM. Ulnar variance in children-standard measurements for evaluation of ulnar shortening in juvenile rheumatoid arthritis, hereditary multiple exostosis and other bone or joint disorders in childhood. Skeletal Radiol1989; 18:513–516.
91. Hernandez J Jr, Peterson HA. Fracture of the distal radial physis complicated by compartment syndrome and premature physeal closure. J Pediatr Orthop 1986;6:627–630.
92. Högström H, Nilsson BE, Willner S. Correction with growth following diaphyseal forearm fracture. Acta Orthop Scand 1976;47:229–303.
93. Holmes JR, Louis DS. Entrapment of pronator quadratus in pediatric distal-radius fractures: recognition and treatment. J Pediatr Orthop 1994;14:498–500.
94. Homans J, Smith JA. Fracture of the lower end of the radius associated with fracture or dislocation of the lower end of the ulna. Boston Med Surg J 1922;187:401–407.
95. Horii E, Tamura Y, Nakamura R, et al. Premature closure of the distal radial physis. J Hand Surg Br 1993;18:11–16.
96. Hove LM. Simultaneous scaphoid and distal radial fractures. J Hand Surg Br 1994;19: 384–388.
97. Hubner U, Schlicht W, Outzen S, et al. Ultrasound in the diagnosis of fractures in children. J Bone Joint Surg Br 2000;82:1170–1173.
98. Hughston JC. Fractures of the forearm. J Bone Joint Surg Am 1962;44:1664–1667.
99. Hulten O. Uber anatomische variationen der hand-gelenkknochen. Acta Radiol 1928; 9:155–168.
100. Itoh Y, Horiuchi Y, Takahashi M, et al. Extensor tendon involvement in Smith's and Galeazzi's fractures. J Hand Surg Am 1987;12.535–540.
101. Johari AN, Sinha M. Remodeling of forearm fractures in children. J Pediatr Orthop B 1999;8:84–87.
102. Johnson PG, Szabo RM. Angle measurements of the distal radius: a cadaver study. Skeletal Radiol 1993;22(4):243–246.
103. Jones IE, Cannan R, Goulding A. Distal forearm fractures in New Zealand children: annual rates in a geographically defined area. N Z Med J 2000;113:443–445.
104. Jones IE, Williams SM, Dow N, et al. How many children remain fracture-free during growth? A longitudinal study of children and adolescents participating in the Dunedin Multidisciplinary Health and Development Study. Osteoporos Int 2002;13:990–995.
105. Kameyama O, Ogawa R. Pseudarthrosis of the radius associated with neurofibromatosis: report of a case and review of the literature. J Pediatr Orthop 1990;10:128–131.
106. Karaharju EO, Ryöppy SA, Mäkinen RJ. Remodelling by asymmetrical epiphysial growth. An experimental study in dogs. J Bone Joint Surg Br 1976;58:122–126.
107. Karlsson J, Appelqvist R. Irreducible fracture of the wrist in a child. Entrapment of the extensor tendons. Acta Orthop Scand 1987;58:280–281.
108. Kasser JR. Forearm fractures. In: MacEwen GD, Kasser JR, Heinrich SD, eds. Pediatric Fractures: A Practical Approach to Assessment and Treatment. Baltimore: Williams & Wilkins, 1993:165–190.
109. Khan KS, Grufferty A, Gallagher O, et al. A randomized trial of "soft cast" for distal radius buckle fractures in children. Acta Orthop Belg 2007;73:594–597.
110. Khosla S, Melton LJ 3rd, Dekutoski MB, et al. Incidence of childhood distal forearm fractures over 30 years: a population based study. JAMA 2003;290:1479–1485.
111. Kiely PD, Kiely PJ, Stephens MM, et al. Atypical distal radial fractures in children. J Pediatr Orthop B 2004;13:202–205.
112. Klug RA, Press CM, Gonzalez MH. Rupture of the flexor pollicis longus tendon after volar fixed-angle plating of a distal radius fracture: a case report. J Hand Surg Am 2007;32:984–988.
113. Knirk JL, Jupiter JB. Intra-articular fractures of the distal end of the radius in young adults. J Bone Joint Surg Am 1986;68:647–659.
114. Kocher MS. Waters PM, Micheli LJ. Upper extremity injuries in the paediatric athlete. Sports Med 2000;30:117–135.
115. Kraus B, Horne G. Galeazzi fractures. J Trauma 1985;25:1093–1095.
116. Kyle SB, Nance ML, Rutherford GW Jr, et al. Skateboard-associated injuries: participation-based estimates and injury characteristics. J Trauma 2002;53:686–690.
117. Landfried MJ, Stenclik M, Susi JG. Variant of Galeazzi fracture-dislocation in children. J Pediatr Orthop 1991;11:332–335.
118. Landin LA. Fracture patterns in children. Analysis of 8682 fractures with special reference to incidence, etiology and secular changes in a Swedish urban population 1950–1979. Acta Orthop Scand Suppl 1983;202:1–109.
119. Langenberg R. Fracture of the ulnar styloid process. Effect on wrist function in the presence of distal radius fracture [in German]. Zentralbl Chir 1989;114:1006–1011.
120. Langenskiöld A. Surgical treatment of partial closure of the growth plate. J Pediatr Orthop 1981;1:3–11.
121. Langenskiöld A, Osterman K. Surgical treatment of partial closure of the epiphysial plate. Reconstr Surg Traumatol 1979;17:48–64.
122. Larsen E, Vittas D, Torp-Pedersen S. Remodeling of angulated distal forearm fractures in children. Clin Orthop Relat Res 1988;237:190–195.
123. Lawton L. Fractures of the distal radius and ulna in management of pediatric fractures. In: Letts M, ed. Management of Pediatric Fractures. New York: Churchill-Livingstone, 1994:345–368.
124. Lee BS, Esterhai JL Jr, Das M. Fracture of the distal radial epiphysis. Characteristics and surgical treatment of premature, posttraumatic epiphyseal closure. Clin Orthop Relat Res 1984;(185):90–96.
125. Lesko PD, Georgis T, Slabaugh P. Irreducible Salter-Harris type II fracture of the distal radial epiphysis. J Pediatr Orthop 1987;7:719–721.
126. Letts M, Rowhani N. Galeazzi-equivalent injuries of the wrist in children. J Pediatr Orthop 1993;13:561–566.
127. Letts RM. Monteggia and Galeazzi fractures. In: Letts RM, ed. Management of Pediatric Fractures. New York: Churchill-Livingstone, 1994:313–321.
128. Light TR, Ogden DA, Ogden JA. The anatomy of metaphyseal torus fractures. Clin Orthop Relat Res 1984;188:103–111.
129. Lindau T. Wrist arthroscopy in distal radial fractures using a modified horizontal technique. Arthroscopy 2001;17:E5.
130. Low CK, Liau KH, Chew WY. Results of distal radial fractures treated by intrafocal pin fixation. Ann Acad Med Singapore 2001;30:573–576.
131. Ma D, Jones G. The association between bone mineral density, metacarpal morphometry, and upper limb fractures in children: a population-based case-control study. J Clin Endocrinol Metab 2003;88:1486–1491.
132. MacLaughlin HL. Trauma. Philadelphia: WB Saunders, 1959.
133. Maffulli N, Fixsen JA. Painful hypertrophic nonunion of the ulnar styloid. J Hand Surg Br 1990;15:355–357.
134. Malviya A, Tsintzas D, Mahawar K, et al. Gap index: a good predictor of failure of plaster cast in distal third radius fractures. J Pediatr Orthop Br 2007;16:48–52.
135. Mandelbaum BR, Bartolozzi AR, Davis CA, et al. Wrist pain syndrome in the gymnast. Pathogenetic, diagnostic, and therapeutic considerations. Am J Sports Med 1989;17: 305–317.
136. Mani GV, Hui PW, Cheng JC. Translation of the radius as a predictor of outcome in distal radial fractures of children. J Bone Joint Surg Br 1993;75:808–811.
137. Manoli A. Irreducible fracture-separation of the distal radial epiphysis. J Bone Joint Surg Am 1982;64:1095–1096.
138. Matsumoto K, Sumi H, Sumi Y, et al. Wrist fractures from snowboarding: a prospective study for 3 seasons from 1998 to 2001. Clin J Sport Med 2004;14:64–71.
139. Matthews LS, Kaufer H, Garver DF, et al. The effect on supination-pronation of angular malalignment of fractures of both bones of the forearm. J Bone Joint Surg Am 1982; 64:14–17.
140. McLauchlan GJ, Cowan B, Annan IH, et al. Management of completely displaced metaphyseal fractures of the distal radius in children. A prospective, randomized controlled trial. J Bone Joint Surg Br 2002;84:413–417.
141. Meeusen R, Borms J. Gymnastic injuries. Sports Med 1992;13:337–356.
142. Meier R, Prommersberger KJ, van Griensven M, et al. Surgical correction of deformities of the distal radius due to fractures in pediatric patients. Arch Orthop Trauma Surg 2004;124:1–9.
143. Mikić ZD. Galeazzi fracture-dislocations. J Bone Joint Surg Am 1975;57:1071–1080.
144. Miller BS, Taylor B, Widmann RF, et al. Cast immobilization versus percutaneous pin fixation of displaced distal radius fractures in children: a prospective, randomized study. J Pediatr Orthop 2005;25(4):490–494.
145. Mino DE, Palmer AK, Levinsohn EM. Radiography and computerized tomography in the diagnosis of incongruity of the distal radioulnar joint. A prospective study. J Bone Joint Surg Am 1985;67:247–252.
146. Mizuta T, Benson WM, Foster BK, et al. Statistical analysis of the incidence of physeal injuries. J Pediatr Orthop 1987;7:518–523.
147. Mohan K, Gupta AK, Sharma J, et al. Internal fixation in 50 cases of Galeazzi fracture. Acta Orthop Scand 1988;59:318–320.
148. Moore TM, Lester DK, Sarmiento A. The stabilizing effect of soft-tissue constraints in artificial Galeazzi fractures. Clin Orthop Relat Res 1985;194:189–194.
149. Moore TM, Klein JP, Patzakis MJ, et al. Results of compression-plating of closed Galeazzi fractures. J Bone Joint Surg Am 1985;67:1015–1021
150. Morton R. A radiographic survey of 170 clinically diagnosed as "Colles' fracture." Lancet 1907;1:731–732.
151. Musharafieh RS, Macari G. Salter-Harris I fractures of the distal radius misdiagnosed as wrist sprain. J Emerg Med 2000;19:265–270.
152. Nelson DA, Buchanan JR, Harrison CS. Distal ulnar growth arrest. Hand Surg Am 1984;9:164–171.
153. Nilsson BE, Obrant K. The range of motion following fracture of the shaft of the forearm in children. Acta Orthop Scand 1977;48;600–602.
154. Noonan KJ. Ulnar growth arrest after distal radius and ulna fracture. In Price CT ed. Complications in Orthopaedics. Pediatric upper extremity fractures. Rosemont, IL. American Academy of Orthopaedic Surgeons; 2004:12–20.
155. Nork SE, Hennrikus WL, Loncarich DP, et al. Relationship between ligamentous laxity and the site of upper extremity fractures in children: extension supracondylar fracture versus distal forearm fracture. J Pediatr Orthop B 1999;8:90–92.
156. Oakley EA, Ooi KS, Barnett PL. A randomized controlled trial of two methods of immobilizing torus fractures of the distal forearm. Pediatr Emerg Care 2008;24:65–70.
157. Ogden JA. Skeletal Injury in the Child. Philadelphia: WB Saunders, 1990.
158. Ogden JA, Beall JK, Conlogue GJ, et al. Radiology of postnatal skeletal development. IV. Distal radius and ulna. Skeletal Radiol 1981;6:255–266.
159. Onne L, Sandblom PH. Late results in fractures of the forearm in children. Acta Chir Scand 1949;98:549–567.
160. Ooi LH, Toh CL. Galeazzi-equivalent fracture in children associated with tendon entrapment—report of two cases. Ann Acad Med Singapore 2001;30:51–54.
161. Palmer AK, Glisson RR, Werner FW. Relationship between ulnar variance and triangular fibrocartilage complex thickness. J Hand Surg Am 1984;9:681–682.
162. Palmer AK, Werner FW. The triangular fibrocartilage complex of the wrist-anatomy and function. 1981;6:153–162.
163. Papavasiliou V, Nenopoulos S. Ipsilateral injuries of the elbow and forearm in children. J Pediatr Orthop 1986;6:58–60.
164. Peinado A. Distal radial epiphyseal displacement after impaired distal ulnar growth. J Bone Joint Surg Am 1979;61:88–92.
165. Perona PG, Light TR. Remodeling of the skeletally immature distal radius. J Orthop Trauma 1990;4:356–361.
166. Pershad J, Monroe K, King W, et al. Can clinical parameters predict fractures in acute pediatric wrist injuries? Acad Emerg Med 2000;7:1152–1155.
167. Peterson CA, Peterson HA. Analysis of the incidence of injuries to the epiphyseal growth plate. J Trauma 1972;12:275–281.
168. Peterson HA. Partial growthplate arrest and its treatment. J Pediatr Orthop 1984;4: 246–258.
169. Peterson HA. Physeal fractures: Part 2. Two previously unclassified types. J Pediatr Orthop 1994;14:431–438.
170. Peterson HA. Physeal fractures: Part 3. Classification. J Pediatr Orthop 1994;14: 439–448.

171. Peterson HA. Triplane fracture of the distal radius: case report. J Pediatr Orthop 1996; 16:192–194.
172. Peterson HA, Madhok R, Benson JT, et al. Physeal fractures: Part 1. Epidemiology in Olmsted County, Minnesota, 1979-1988. J Pediatr Orthop 1994;14:423–430.
173. Plint AC, Perry JJ, Correll R, et al. A randomized, controlled trial of removable splinting versus casting for wrist buckle fractures in children. Pediatrics 2006;117:691–697.
174. Poland J. Traumatic Separation of the Epiphysis. London: Smith, Elder & Co, 1898.
175. Pollen AG. Fractures and Dislocations in Children. Baltimore: Williams & Wilkins, 1973.
176. Prais D, Diamond G, Kattan A, et al. The effect of calcium intake and physical activity on bone quantitative ultrasound measurements in children: a pilot study. J Bone Miner Metab 2008;26:248–253.
177. Proctor MT, Moore DJ, Paterson JM. Redisplacement after manipulation of distal radial fractures in children. J Bone Joint Surg Br 1993;75:453–454.
178. Prommersberger KJ, Van Schoonhoven J, Lanz UB. Outcome after corrective osteotomy for malunited fractures of the distal end of the radius. J Hand Surg Br 2002;27:55–60.
179. Qairul IH, et al. Early remodeling in children's forearm fractures. Med J Malaysia 2001; 56(Suppl D):34–37.
180. Rampoldi M, Marsico S. Complications of volar plating of distal radius fractures. Acta Orthop Belg 2007;73:714–719.
181. Rang M. Children's Fractures. 2nd ed. Philadelphia: JB Lippincott, 1983.
182. Reckling FW, Cordell LD. Unstable fracture-dislocations of the forearm. The Monteggia and Galeazzi lesions. Arch Surg 1968;96:999–1007.
183. Reckling FW, Peltier LF. Riccardo Galeazzi and Galeazzi's fracture. Surgery 1965;58: 453–459.
184. Reed MH. Fractures and dislocations of the extremities in children. J Trauma 1977; 17:351–354.
185. Ring D, Waters PM, Hotchkiss RN, et al. Pediatric floating elbow. J Pediatr Orthop 2001;21:456–459.
186. Roberts JA. Angulation of the radius in children's fractures. J Bone Joint Surg Br 1986; 68:751–754.
187. Rønning R, Rønning I, Gerner T, et al. The efficacy of wrist protectors in preventing snowboarding injuries. Am J Sports Med 2001;29:581–585.
188. Roposch A, Reis M, Molina M, et al. Supracondylar fractures of the humerus associated with ipsilateral forearm fractures in children. J Pediatr Orthop 2001;21:307–312.
189. Rose-Innes AP. Anterior dislocation of the ulna at the inferior radioulnar joint. Case report, with a discussion of the anatomy of rotation of the forearm. J Bone Joint Surg Br 1960;42-B:515–521.
190. Roy DR. Completely displaced distal radius fractures with intact ulnas in children. Orthopedics 1989;12:1089–1092.
191. Roy S, Caine D, Singer KM. Stress changes of the distal radial epiphysis in young gymnasts. A report of 21 cases and a review of the literature. Am J Sports Med 1985; 13:301–308.
192. Ruggles DL, Peterson HA, Scott SG. Radial growthplate injury in a female gymnast. Med Sci Sports Exerc 1991;23:393–396.
193. Ryöppy S, Karaharju EO. Alteration of epiphyseal growth by an experimentally produced angular deformity. Acta Orthop Scand 1974;45:490–498.
194. Salter RB, Harris WR. Injuries involving the epiphyseal plate. J Bone Joint Surg Am 1963;45:587–622.
195. Santoro V, Mara J. Compartmental syndrome complicating Salter-Harris type II distal radius fracture. Clin Orthop Relat Res 1988;226–229.
196. Sasaki K, Takagi M, Ida H, et al. Severity of upper limb injuries in snowboarding. Arch Orthop Trauma Surg 1999;119:292–295.
197. Sasaki K, Takagi M, Kiyoshige Y, et al. Snowboarder's wrist: its severity compared with Alpine skiing. J Trauma 1999;46:1059–1061.
198. Sasaki Y, Sugioka Y. The pronator quadratus sign: its classification and diagnostic usefulness for injury and inflammation of the wrist. J Hand Surg Br 1989;14:80–83.
199. Schranz PJ, Fagg PS. Undisplaced fractures of the distal third of the radius in children: an innocent fracture? Injury 1992;23:165–167.
200. Schuind F, An KN, Berglund L, et al. The distal radioulnar ligaments: a biomechanical study. J Hand Surg Am 1991;16:1106–1114.
201. Schuind F, Cooney WP 3rd, Burny F, et al. Small external fixation devices for the hand and wrist. Clin Orthop Relat Res 1993;293;77–82.
202. Sharrard WJW. Paediatric Orthopaedics and Fractures. Oxford: Blackwell Scientific Publications, 1971.
203. Short WH, Palmer AK, Werner FW, et al. A biomechanical study of the distal radius. J Hand Surg Am 1897;12:529–534.
204. Skaggs DL, Loro ML, Pitukcheewanont P, et al. Increased body weight and decreased radial cross-sectional dimensions in girls with forearm fractures. J Bone Miner Res 2001;16:1337–1342.
205. Skillern PG. Complete fracture of the lower third of the radius in childhood, with greenstick fracture of the ulna. Ann Surg 1915;61:209–225.
206. Smida M, et al. Combined fracture of the distal radius and scaphoid in children. Report of two cases. Acta Orthop Belg 2003;69:79–81.
207. Snook GA, Chrisman OD, Wilson TC, et al. Subluxation of the distal radioulnar joint by hyperpronation. J Bone Joint Surg Am 1969;51:1315–1323.
208. Solan MC, Rees R, Daly K. Current management of torus fractures of the distal radius. Injury 2002;33:503–505.
209. Stahl S, Freiman S, Volpin G. Anterior interosseous nerve palsy associated with Galeazzi fracture. J Pediatr Orthop B 2000;9:45–46.
210. Stanitski CL, Micheli LJ. Simultaneous ipsilateral fractures of the arm and forearm in children. Clin Orthop Relat Res 1980;218–222.
211. Stansberry SD, Swischuk LE, Swischuk JL, et al. Significance of ulnar styloid fractures in childhood. Pediatr Emerg Care 1990;6:99–103.
212. Stein AH Jr, Katz SF. Stabilization of comminuted fractures of the distal inch of the radius: percutaneous pinning. Clin Orthop Relat Res 1975;174–181.
213. Steyers CM, Blair WF. Measuring ulnar variance: a comparison of techniques. J Hand Surg Am 1989;14:607–612.
214. Stuhmer KG. Fractures of the distal forearm. In: Weber BG, Burner C, Freuler F, eds. Treatment of Fractures in Children and Adolescents. New York: Springer-Verlag, 1980: 203–217.
215. Symons S, Rowsell M, Bhowal B, et al. Hospital versus home management of children withbuckle fractures of the distal radius. A prospective, randomised trial. J Bone Joint Surg Br 2001;83:556–560.
216. Tachdjian MO. Pediatric Orthopedics. 2nd ed. Philadelphia: WB Saunders; 1990.
217. Talesnik J, Watson HK. Midcarpal instability caused by malunited fracture of the distal radius. J Hand Surg Am 1984;9(3):350–357.
218. Tang CW, Kay RM, Skaggs DL. Growth arrest of the distal radius following a metaphyseal fracture: case report and review of the literature. J Pediatr Orthop B 2002;11: 89–92.
219. Tarr RR, Garfinkel AI, Sarmiento A. The effects of angular and rotational deformities of bothbones of the forearm. An in vitro study. J Bone Joint Surg Am 1984;66:65–70.
220. Templeton PA, Graham HK. The "floating elbow" in children. Simultaneous supracondylar fractures of the humerus and of the forearm in the same upper limb. J Bone Joint Surg Br 1995;77:791–796.
221. Terry CL, Waters PM. Triangular fibrocartilage injuries in pediatric and adolescent patients. J Hand Surg Am 1998;23:626–634.
222. Thomas EM, Tuson TW, Browne PS. Fractures of the radius and ulna in children. Injury 1975;7:120–124.
223. Tolat AR, Sanderson PL, De Smet L, et al. The gymnast's wrist: acquired positive ulnar variance following chronic epiphyseal injury. J Hand Surg Br 1992;17:678–681.
224. Trumble TE, Wagner W, Hanel DP, et al. Intrafocal (Kapandji) pinning of distal radius fractures withand without external fixation. J Hand Surg Am 1998;23:381–394.
225. Trumble TE, Benirschke SK, Vedder NB. Ipsilateral fractures of the scaphoid and radius. J Hand Surg Am 1993;18:8–14.
226. Vahvanen V, Westerlund M. Fracture of the carpal scaphoid in children. A clinical and roentgenological study of 108 cases. Acta Orthop Scand 1980;51:909–913.
227. Valverde JA, Albiñana J, Certucha JA. Early posttraumatic physeal arrest in distal radius after a compression injury. J Pediatr Orthop B 1996;5:57–60.
228. van der Linden W, Ericson R. Colles' fracture. How should its displacement be measured and how should it be immobilized? J Bone Joint Surg Am 1981;63:1285–1288.
229. Vance RM, Gelberman RH. Acute ulnar neuropathy with fractures at the wrist. J Bone Joint Surg Am 1978;60:962–965.
230. Vince KG, Miller JE. Cross-union complicating fracture of the forearm. Part II: children. J Bone Joint Surg Am 1987;69:654–661.
231. Vioreanu M, Sheehan E, Glynn A, et al. Heelys and street gliders injuries: a new type of pediatric injury. Pediatrics 2007;119:e1294–e1298.
232. Voto SJ, Weiner DS, Leighley B. Redisplacement after closed reduction of forearm fractures in children. J Pediatr Orthop 1990;10:79–84.
233. Walsh HP, McLaren CA, Owen R. Galeazzi fractures in children. J Bone Joint Surg Br 1987;69:730–733.
234. Wareham K, Johansen A, Stone MD, et al. Seasonal variation in the incidence of wrist and forearm fractures, and its consequences. Injury 2003;34:219–222.
235. Warren JD. Anterior interosseous nerve palsy as a complication of forearm fractures. J Bone Joint Surg Br 1963;45:511–512.
236. Waters PM, Bae DS, Montgomery KD. Surgical management of posttraumatic distal radial growth arrest in adolescents. J Pediatr Orthop 2002;22:717–724.
237. Waters PM, Mintzer CM, Hipp JA, et al. Noninvasive measurement of distal radius instability. J Hand Surg Am 1997;22:572–579.
238. Waters PM, et al. Prospective study of displaced radius fractures in adolescents treated with casting vs. percutaneous pinning. 2000.
239. Waters PM, Kolettis GJ, Schwend R. Acute median neuropathy following physeal fractures of the distal radius. J Pediatr Orthop 1994;14:173–177.
240. Webb GR, Galpin RD, Armstrong DG. Comparison of short- and long-arm plaster casts for displaced fractures in the distal third of the forearm in children. J Bone Joint Surg Am 2006;88:9–17.
241. Weiker GG. Hand and wrist problems in the gymnast. Clin Sports Med 1992;11: 189–202.
242. Werner FW, Palmer AK, Fortino MD, et al. Force transmission through the distal ulna: effect of ulnar variance, lunate fossa angulation, and radial and palmar tilt of the distal radius. J Hand Surg Am 1992;17:423–428.
243. West S, Andrews J, Bebbington A, et al. Buckle fractures of the distal radius are safely treated in a soft bandage: a randomized prospective trail of bandage versus plaster cast. J Pediatr Orthop 2005;25:322–325.
244. Widmann R, Waters PM, Reeves S. Complications of closed treatment of distal radius fractures in children. Presented at the POSNA annual meeting, Miami, 1995.
245. Wilkins KE. Operative Management of Upper Extremity Fractures in Children. American Academy of Orthopaedic Surgeons. Chicago, IL: Rosemont, 1994.
246. Wilkins KE, O'Brien E. Distal radius and ulnar fractures. In: Bucholz RW, Heckman JD, eds. Rockwood and Green's Fractures in Adults. Philadelphia: Lippincott Williams & Wilkins, 2002.
247. Wolfe JS, Eyring EJ. Median-nerve entrapment within a greenstick fracture; a case report. J Bone Joint Surg Am 1974;56:1270–1272.
248. Worlock P, Stower M. Fracture patterns in Nottingham children. J Pediatr Orthop 1986;6:656–660.
249. Yong-Hing K, Wedge JH, Bowen CV. Chronic injury to the distal ulnar and radial growthplates in an adolescent gymnast. A case report. J Bone Joint Surg Am 1988;70: 1087–1089.
250. Young TB. Irreducible displacement of the distal radial epiphysis complicating a fracture of the lower radius and ulna. Injury 1984;16:166–168.
251. Younger AS, Tredwell SJ, Mackenzie WG, et al. Accurate prediction of the outcome after pediatric forearm fracture. J Pediatr Orthop 1994;14:200–206.
252. Yung PS, Lam CY, Ng BK, et al. Percutaneous transphyseal intramedullary Kirschner wire pinning: a safe and effective procedure for treatment of displaced diaphyseal forearm fracture in children. J Pediatr Orthop 2004;24:7–12.
253. Zammit-Maempel I, Bisset RA, Morris J, et al. The value of soft-tissue signs in wrist trauma. Clin Radiol 1988;39:664–668.
254. Zamzam MM, Khoshhal KI. Displaced fracture of the distal radius in children: factors responsible for redisplacement after closed reduction. J Bone Joint Surg Br 2005;87: 841–843.

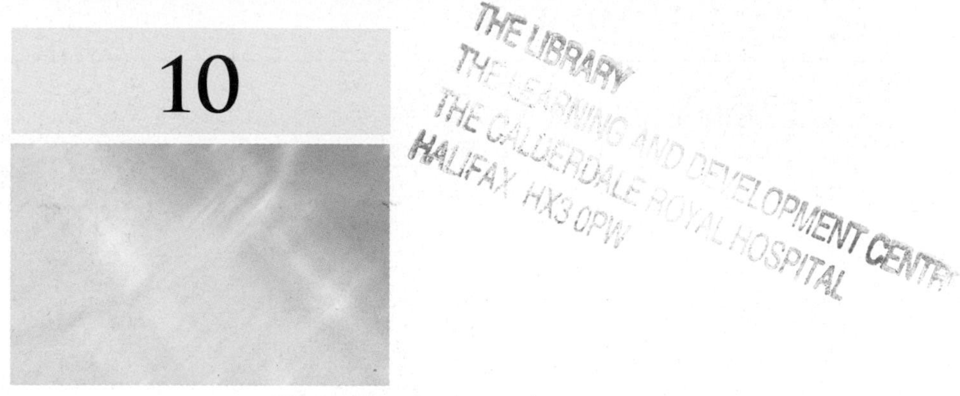

INJURIES TO THE SHAFTS OF THE RADIUS AND ULNA

Charles T. Mehlman and Eric J. Wall

INTRODUCTION 347

HISTORY 348

EPIDEMIOLOGY 350

PRINCIPLES OF MANAGEMENT 350
Mechanism of Injury 350
Signs and Symptoms 352
Associated Injuries 353
Diagnosis and Classification 354
Rationale 355

SURGICAL AND APPLIED ANATOMY 360
Bony Anatomy and Static Restraints 360
Pertinent Anatomy of the Muscles and Nerves 361
Common Surgical Approaches 364

CURRENT CLOSED TREATMENT OPTIONS 365
Overview of Closed Fracture Treatment 365
Traumatic Bowing/Plastic Deformation 366
Greenstick Fractures 366
Complete Fractures 367
Comminuted Fractures 368

CURRENT SURGICAL TREATMENT OPTIONS 368
Overview of Surgical Treatment 368
Plate Fixation 369
Kirschner Wire, Rush Rod, and Steinmann Pin Intramedullary Fixation 369
Elastic Stable Intramedullary Nailing 369
Management of Open Fractures 374

COMPLICATIONS 381
Redisplacement/Malalignment 381
Forearm Stiffness 383
Refracture 383
Malunion 384
Delayed Union/Nonunion 396
Cross-Union/Synostosis 396
Infection 397
Neurapraxia 397
Muscle or Tendon Entrapment/Tendon Rupture 397
Compartment Syndrome 398
Complex Regional Pain Syndromes 398

CONTROVERSIES AND FUTURE DIRECTIONS 399
Fracture Risk/Fracture Prevention 399
Parental Presence during Fracture Reduction 399

INTRODUCTION

Injuries to the shafts of the radius and ulna are the most common reasons for children to receive orthopaedic care[62,64,200] and are among the most challenging to the orthopaedist because of their treatment complexity and risk of complications.[80,230,255] Because of numerous differences in both treatment and prognosis, shaft fractures are considered to be clinically distinct from fractures of the distal (metaphyseal fractures and physeal fractures) and proximal (radial neck fractures and physeal fractures) ends of the same bones.[72,144,281,322,326,329] Most shaft injuries require nothing more than skillful closed fracture care.[161,254,356] The remainder are a subset of malaligned fractures that raise concerns with the orthopaedist and parents about remodeling potential, loss of motion, and long-term outcome. Issues regarding reduction, remanipulation, recasting, open treatment, and refracture must be mastered. Shaft fractures of the forearm also are the most common reason for orthopaedic surgery of the forearm in children.[62,128] Thus, it is very important for orthopaedic surgeons who treat children to skillfully manage the cognitive and technical aspects of both nonoperative and operative treatment for injuries to the shafts of the radius and ulna.

HISTORY

Forearm fractures in children are common both in contemporary and ancient terms. In one of the oldest examples, the remains of a 15-year-old from the Paleolithic period (the Stone Age) demonstrate posttraumatic forearm deformity.[106] Among the skeletons of children from medieval England (circa 950 A.D.) acute trauma and new bone formation were most common in 6- to 10-year-olds.[190] Other archeological reports from the medieval period (circa 1100–1550 A.D.) indicate that forearm fractures were not only common but also presumably well treated, based on absence of substantial deformity.[126] This latter finding may simply be an early testament to pediatric remodeling potential.

The contemporary history of pediatric forearm fracture care bears the marks of many orthopaedic icons. The Austrian surgeon Lorenz Böhler (1885–1973) had a world-wide impact on fracture care.[239,309] In the late 1920s, he published his important book *The Treatment of Fractures*, and it flourished for nearly three decades. It was translated into 8 different languages and published in 13 German and 5 English editions.[309] Böhler recognized that reduction tactics that used exaggeration of the deformity and re-engagement of the bone ends often were effective in distal-third forearm fractures, but longitudinal traction was his main tool for reducing fractures in the middle and proximal thirds (Fig.10-1).[309] His protocol for forearm fracture reduction included belted countertraction of the humerus above the flexed elbow while exerting "steady (not jerky) strong traction by pulling on the thumb with one hand and on the second to fourth fingers with the other hand. Traction on the thumb must be stronger than that on the other fingers" (Fig. 10-2).[309] Böhler believed that forearm fracture reduction would occur within 5 to 10 minutes when using this technique, and he favored skin-tight plasters (i.e., form-fitting casts with little to no padding) for immobilization.[264,309] He stated that "it is unimportant whether lateral displacement of half or even of the entire width of the diaphysis is corrected, because such displacement usually disappears within a year. The same is true of angulation up to 10 or 15 degrees. More marked angulation and rotation must be corrected. Shortening is of no importance. There is never any necessity in adolescents to reduce closed forearm fractures operatively, or to unite the fragments with nails, wires or plates and screws."[309] Böhler's outspoken criticism of pediatric forearm surgery continued, "Operative treatment, as bourne out by x-ray pictures in the literature, is very often practiced in children, and consists of osteosynthesis of different types as well

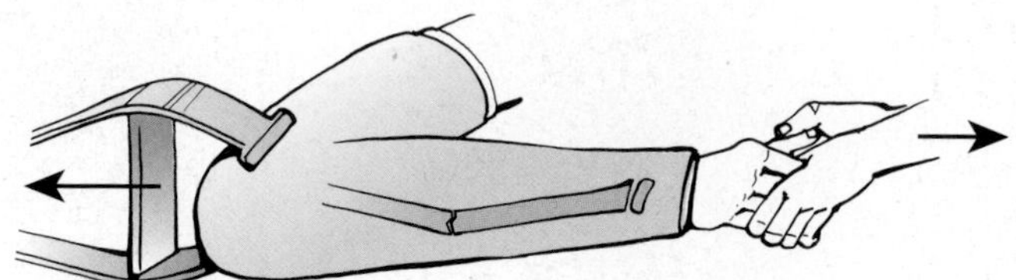

FIGURE 10-2 Böhler's horizontal traction/countertraction method.

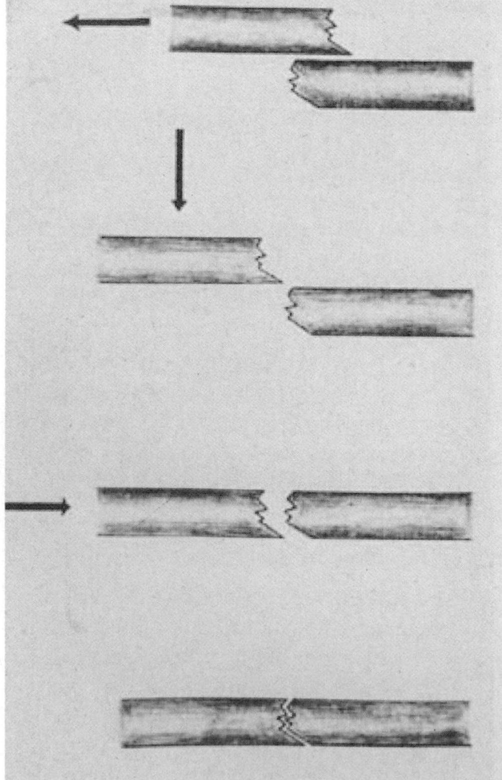

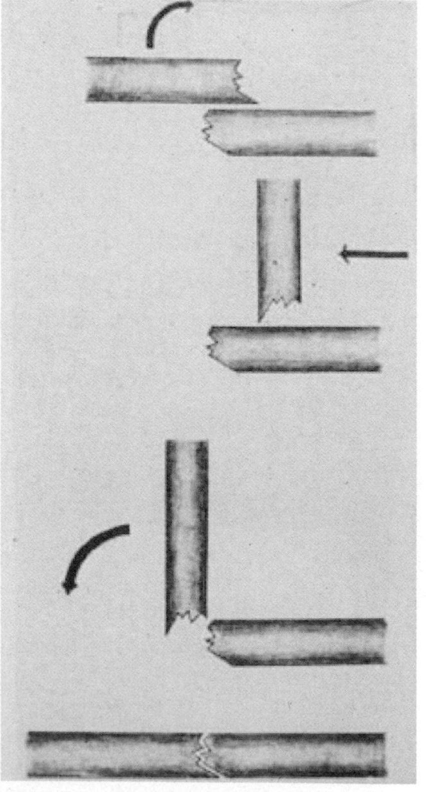

FIGURE 10-1 Fracture reduction techniques for complete fractures from Böhler's original textbook. **A.** Longitudinal traction method. **B.** Exaggeration of deformity method. (Reproduced from Böhler L. The Treatment of Fractures. 5th English ed. New York: Grune & Stratton, 1956.)

as open reduction. It is superfluous, because conservative treatment is always successful. Moreover, operative treatment is dangerous in that infection with all its consequences may ensue. Pseudarthroses have also been reported following operative treatment, which are unknown in children."[23]

Despite high-profile critics such as Böhler, enthusiasm for internal fixation in children grew, reflecting the resurgent interest in osteosynthesis in adults that occurred in the late 1930s.[286] With the publication of his highly regarded textbook *Operative Orthopaedics* in 1939, the American Willis Campbell (1880–1941) tacitly approved operations on children's forearm fractures by illustrating open reduction and internal fixation of a distal-third forearm shaft fracture in a patient who was perhaps as young as 11 or 12 years of age (Fig. 10-3). He stated, "When satisfactory alignment or fixation in fractures of both bones of the forearm is not possible by conservative measures, skeletal traction or open reduction is required. This is particularly true of oblique or spiral fractures. Internal fixation, preferably by a vitallium plate, should be applied to prevent bowing."[50] Later advocates of osteosynthesis such as the Belgian Jean Verbrugge (1896–1964) also reported on internal fixation for fractures in children, listing forearm fractures as one of the most common indications.[336] The rather indiscriminate application of surgical techniques (by some surgeons of the day) to children helps explain the criticism from Böhler and other authors who followed.[23,24,33,36,152]

In the 1950s, two important authors influenced pediatric forearm fracture care. The Englishman Sir John Charnley (1911–1982) in his textbook *The Closed Treatment of Common Fractures* challenged the utility of Böhler's horizontal traction approach to forearm reduction and advocated his preferred method of vertical traction (Fig. 10-4).[61] Charnley did not accept Böhler's concept of skin-tight plasters and favored padded plasters with three-point molding instead (Fig. 10-5). This concept was embodied by Charnley's maxim: "A curved plaster is necessary in order to make a straight limb."[61]

The American Walter Blount (1900–1992), in his book on children's fractures,[34] offered strong recommendations for nonoperative treatment of nearly all children's fractures (especially fractures of the middle third of the forearm). He was an outspoken critic of most surgical treatment of children's fractures and offered impressive illustrations of successful nonoperative care of forearm shaft fractures in children (Fig. 10-6).[34] Blount's frustration regarding the state of affairs of children's fractures is captured in this 1967 quote: "The ever-changing crop of fledgling surgeons of trauma must learn anew that fractures in children are different from those in adults. This is particularly true of fractures of the forearm."[33] The reduction technique he advocated was one of manually exaggerating the fracture deformity while simultaneously applying traction and using the surgeon's thumbs as a fulcrum. Regarding forearm fractures in children Blount also stated, "Bayonet apposition in good alignment is not to be confused with angular deformity. . . . Too many men treat roentgenograms instead of children."[34]

By the mid-1960s, another important personality entered the world of pediatric fractures: the Englishman Mercer Rang (1933–2003). Rang first published a book entitled *The Growth Plate and Its Disorders*, which was aimed at orthopaedists who cared for children, and later his classic text *Children's Fractures*, in which he highlighted many of the practical aspects of caring

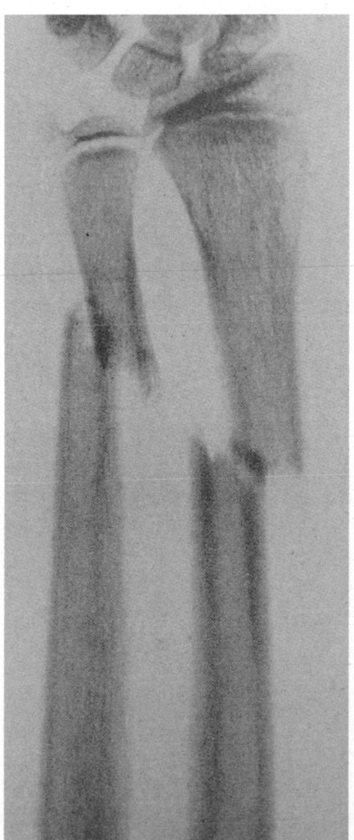

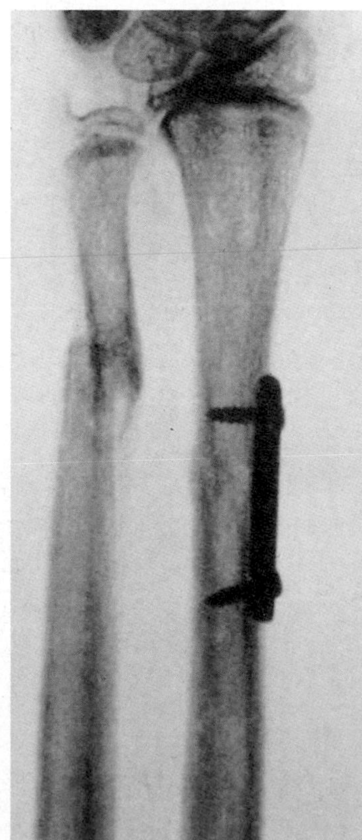

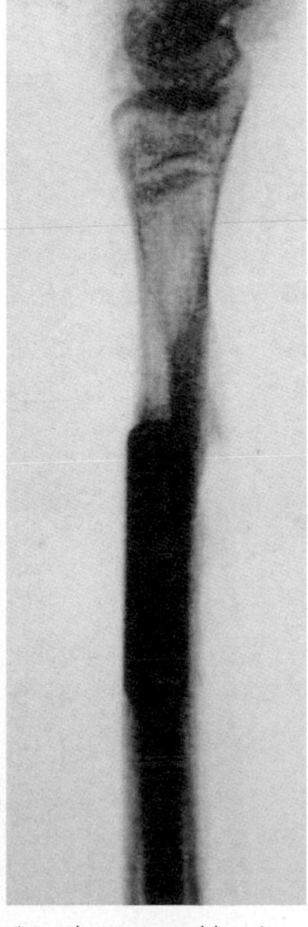

FIGURE 10-3 Original illustration from Campbell's 1939 textbook. **A.** An approximately 12-year-old patient with distal-third radius and ulna shaft fracture. **B.** Postoperative radiographs after plate fixation of radius.

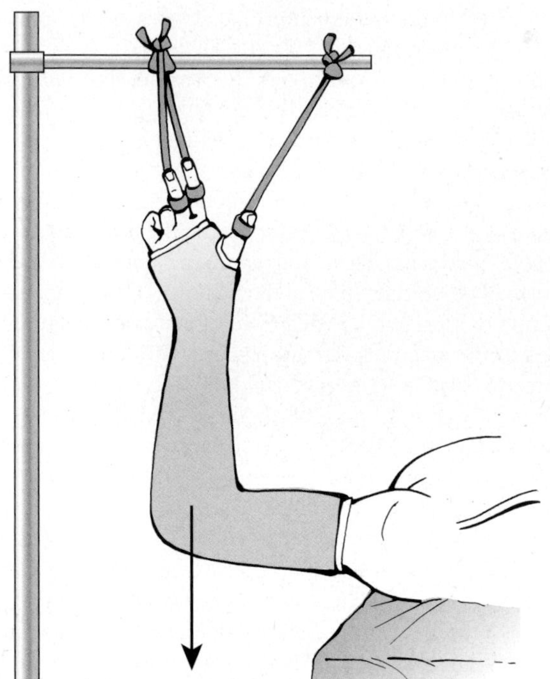

FIGURE 10-4 Charnley's vertical traction.

for children's fractures, including forearm fractures. Contrary to the forearm shaft fracture rotational dogma of others, Rang said, "Immobilize the fracture in the position—any position—in which the alignment is correct and the reduction feels stable."[262] He also discussed the value of single-bone internal fixation with a Kirschner wire in selected patients when open reduction was preferable to malunion.[262] The bulk of his discussion of reduction techniques and casting techniques was not new (it reflected the work of those who had come before him), but it was effectively illustrated (with his own artwork) and communicated to generations of orthopaedic surgeons around the world.[220]

EPIDEMIOLOGY

Risk is a central concept in clinical epidemiology.[210] Landin[181] has shown that the overall risk of fracture in children slowly increases for both males and females until they are 11 or 12 years old and then drops for females and increases further for males (Fig. 10-7). This risk difference is starkly illustrated by the fact that males who are 13 or older have approximately double the fracture rate of their female peers.[181] Forearm fractures have been reported to be the most common pediatric fracture associated with backyard trampoline use[28] and the second most common one (supracondylar humeral fractures were first) associated with monkeybars.[345] Using a national database, Chung and Spilson[64] looked at the frequency of upper extremity fractures in the United States and found that the single largest demographic group was fractures of the radius and ulna in children aged 14 years or less, with a rate approaching 1 in 100.

Large studies that distinguish distal radial fractures from forearm shaft fractures indicate that overall, radial shaft injuries rank as the third most common fracture of childhood (behind distal radial and supracondylar humeral fractures).[62] Open fractures in children are most often fractures of the shaft of the radius and ulna or tibial shaft fractures.[62] Among pediatric fractures, forearm shaft injuries are the most common site of refracture.[181] Forearm shaft fractures have been shown to occur most commonly in the 12- to 16-year-old age group, a challenging age group to treat.[62]

The impact of increasing age on fracture incidence is further illustrated by Worlock and Stower,[355] who showed that the rate of forearm shaft fractures in school-age children (more than 5 years old) is more than double that in toddlers (1.5 to 5 years old). Age also may have an effect on injury severity. Many experienced clinicians have pointed out the increasing level of treatment difficulty as the level of forearm fracture moves proximally,[72,144,241,326,329] and more proximal fractures tend to occur in older patients.[72]

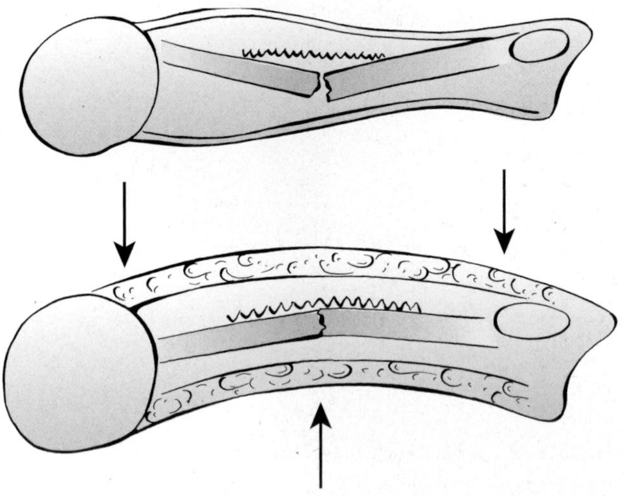

FIGURE 10-5 Charnley's three-point mold illustration.

PRINCIPLES OF MANAGEMENT

Mechanism of Injury

The primary mechanism of injury associated with radial and ulnar shaft fractures is a fall on an outstretched hand that transmits indirect force to the bones of the forearm.[3,70,165] Biomechanic studies have suggested that the junction of the middle and distal thirds of the radius and a substantial portion of the shaft of the ulna have an increased vulnerability to fracture.[150] Often, a significant rotational component is associated with the fall, causing the radius and ulna to fracture at different levels (Fig. 10-8).[93,207] If the radial and ulnar fractures are near the same level, a minimal torsional component can be inferred (Fig. 10-9). If comminution is present, higher-energy trauma should be suspected.[85] Significant hyperpronation forces are associated with isolated shaft fractures of either the radius or the ulna and concomitant dislocation of either the distal or the proximal radioulnar joint. Thus, in any single-bone forearm shaft fracture, these important joints need to be closely scrutinized. Galeazzi and Monteggia fracture–dislocations are discussed in Chapters 9 and 12, respectively.

A direct force to the arm (such as being hit by a baseball bat) can fracture a single bone (usually the ulna) without injury to the adjacent distal or proximal radioulnar joints.[36] Isolated ulnar shaft fractures have been referred to as "nightstick fractures." Alignment of the radial head should be confirmed in

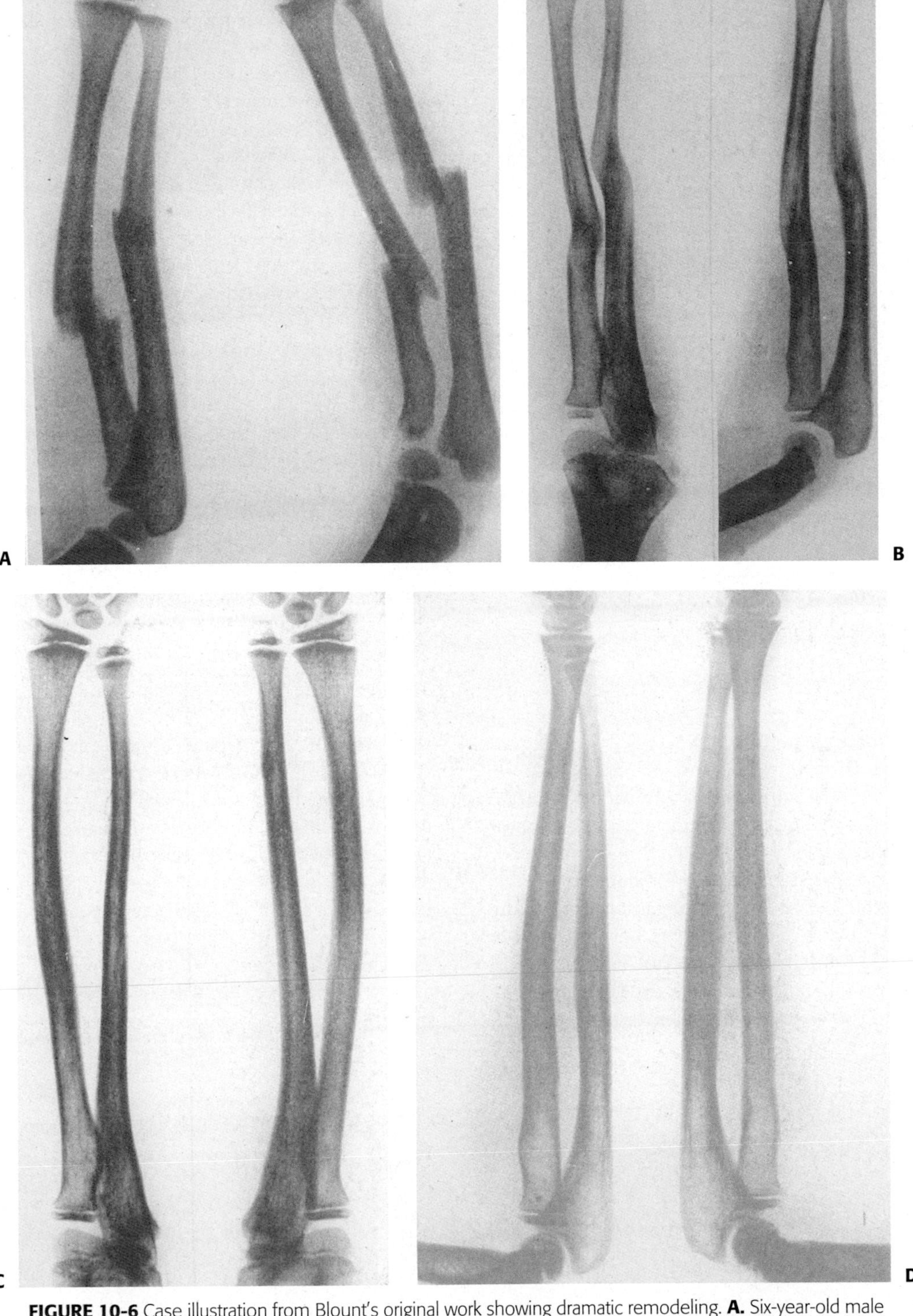

FIGURE 10-6 Case illustration from Blount's original work showing dramatic remodeling. **A.** Six-year-old male with both-bone forearm fracture. **B.** Six months after injury. Comparison of AP **(C)** and lateral **(D)** radiographs of both forearms at 5-years follow-up.

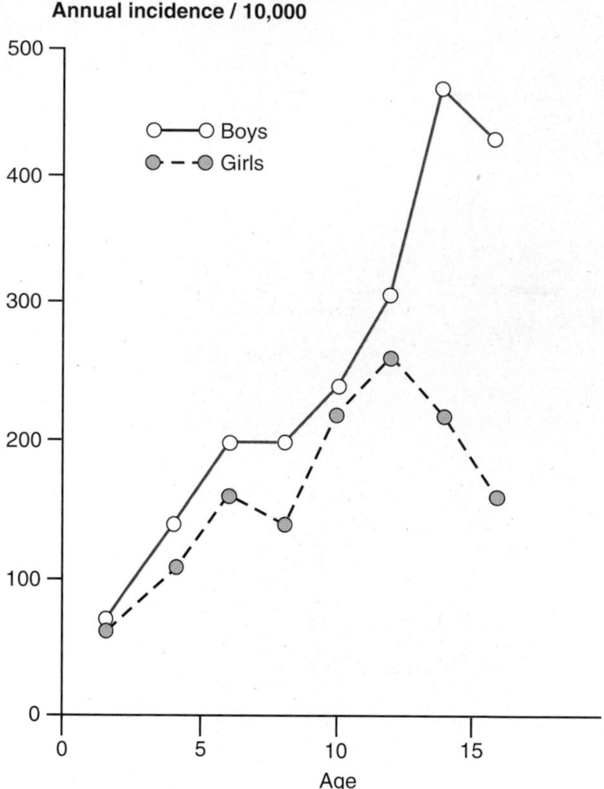

FIGURE 10-7 Annual incidence of all fractures in children. (From Landin LA. Epidemiology of children's fractures. J Pediatr Orthop B 1997;6: 79–83.)

any child with such a fracture to avoid a "missed Monteggia" injury.[148] Isolated radial shaft fractures are rare but notoriously difficult to reduce with closed methods.[68,92] Rang[263] referred to apex volar greenstick fractures of the distal radial shaft near the metaphysis as "the slipper" because of its annoying tendency to lose position after otherwise satisfactory reduction.

The mechanisms of injury of two particular forearm fracture patterns, traumatic bowing (also known as bow fractures or plastic deformation)[263] and greenstick fracture, also bear mentioning. Bone behaves differently based on the direction of the forces applied to it. This is the so-called anisotropic property of bone, and it can be simply explained as follows: bone is more resistant to axial forces than to bending and rotational forces.[54] Pediatric bone also is much more porous than its adult counterpart and behaves somewhat differently from a biomechanic standpoint.[57,232] Because of its porosity, pediatric bone absorbs significantly more energy prior to failure than does adult bone.[75] When relatively slowly applied, longitudinal forces bend immature bone beyond its elastic limits and into its plastic zone, resulting in traumatic bowing.[40,198] Thus, when a bending force is applied relatively slowly, many microfractures occur along the length of the bone, leading to macroscopic deformity without discernible radiographic fracture. This bending can usually be seen radiographically if suspected.

Greenstick fractures represent an intermediate step between plastic deformation and complete fractures.[55] On anteroposterior (AP) and lateral radiographs, greenstick fractures show cortical violation of one, two, or three of their radiographic cortices, and thus some bony continuity is preserved. Rotational deformity is considered to be intimately related to the clinical deformity seen with greenstick fractures of the forearm, and the analogy of a cardboard tube that tends to bend as it is twisted has been offered by Holdsworth.[144] Specifically, hyperpronation injuries usually are associated with apex-dorsal greenstick fractures of the forearm, and hypersupination injuries usually are associated with the opposite, apex-volar injuries.[92,220] The treatment of these greenstick fractures requires a derotation maneuver in addition to correction of any angulation.[55,133]

Signs and Symptoms

The signs and symptoms indicating fracture of the shafts of the radius and ulna usually are not subtle. Deformity and pain are the classic findings. Patients typically experience exquisite pain emanating from the involved area. Decreased pronation and supination motion are also usually noted.[308] Neither practitioners nor parents are always reliable assessors of children's pain, and ideally patients should rate their own pain.[170,301] Significant anxiety and muscle spasm almost always amplify a child's painful experience.[49,116] It has been suggested that muscle spasm is a protective effort by the body to splint or otherwise protect the injured body part.[116] When such muscle spasm occurs in association with certain fracture patterns (e.g., a radial shaft fracture proximal to the pronator teres insertion), it produces

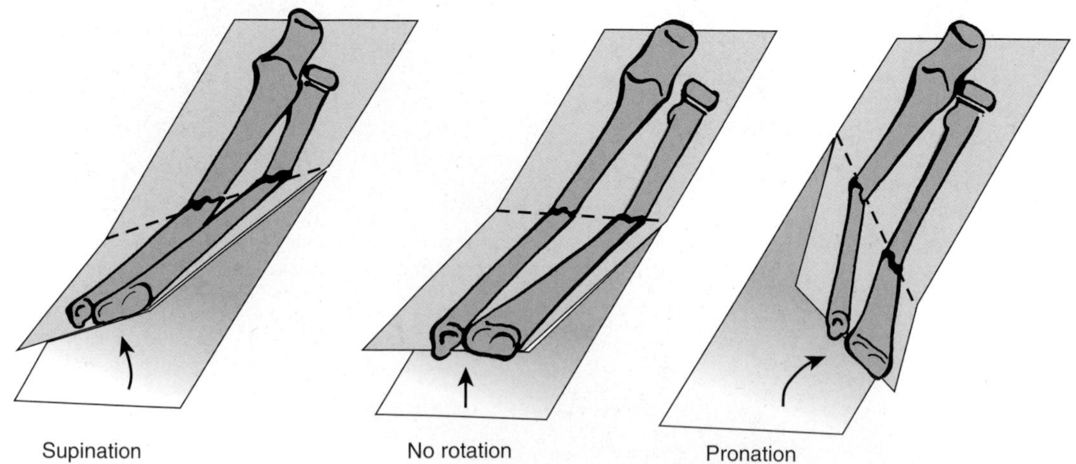

FIGURE 10-8 Radius and ulna shaft fractures occurring at different levels, implying rotational mechanism.

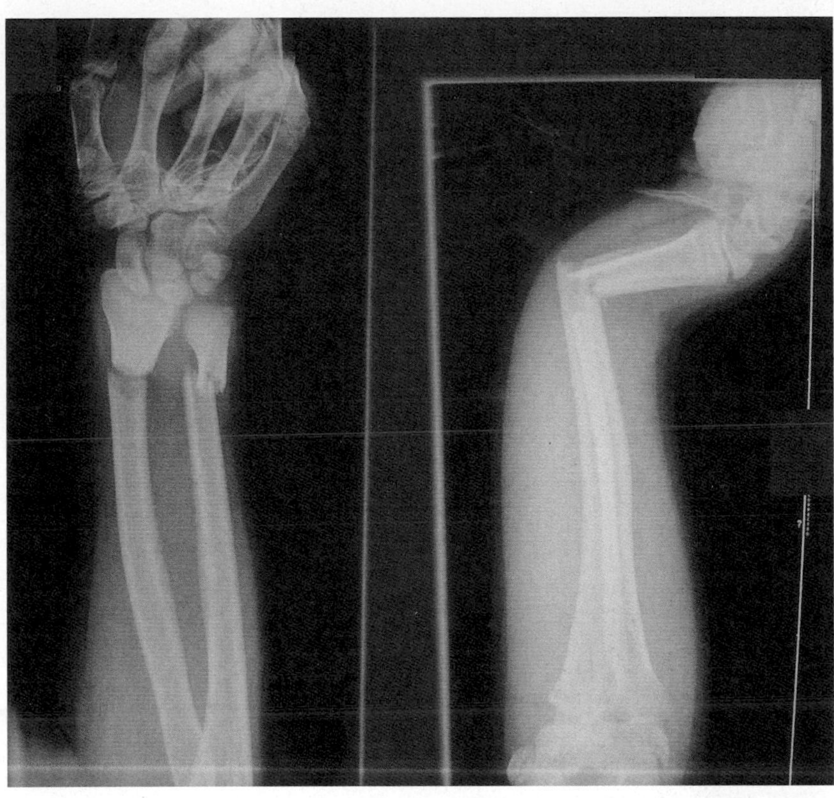

FIGURE 10-9 Radial and ulnar shaft fractures occurring at same level, implying no significant rotation.

predictable fracture displacement (e.g., a pronated distal radial fragment and a supinated proximal fragment).

More subtle fractures present special diagnostic challenges. Certain pathologic fractures of the forearm may occur in the absence of overt trauma.[156,178] Many minimally displaced fractures of the shafts of the radius and ulna can be mistaken for a "sprain" or "just a bruise" for several days to several weeks. This usually occurs in young children who continue to use the fractured arm during low-level play activities. As a general rule, a fracture should be suspected if the child has not resumed all normal arm function within 1 or 2 days of injury.

Associated Injuries

Most fractures of the shafts of the radius and ulna occur as isolated injuries, but wrist and elbow fractures may occur in conjunction with forearm fractures, and the elbow and wrist region needs to be included on standard forearm radiographs.[27,76,165,353,313,359] If clinical suspicion is high, then dedicated wrist and elbow films are necessary. The so-called floating elbow injury (fracture of the bones of the forearm along with ipsilateral supracondylar humeral fracture) is a well-described entity that must not be missed.[27,272,313,353] Surgical stabilization of both the supracondylar fracture and the forearm fractures has been recommended by multiple authors in recent years[31,138,271,272,318,321] to avoid the risk of a compartment syndrome. Galeazzi and Monteggia fracture-dislocations also must be ruled out. Compartment syndrome also can occur in conjunction with any forearm shaft fracture.[74,363] This rare but potentially devastating complication can lead to a Volkmann ischemic contracture, which has been shown to occur after forearm shaft fractures almost as often as it does after supracondylar humeral fractures in children.[221] Patients with severe pain unrelieved by immobilization and mild narcotic medication should be reassessed for excessive swelling and tight forearm compartments. If loosening of the splint, cast, and underlying cast materials fails to relieve pain, then measurement of compartment pressures and subsequent fasciotomy may be necessary.

Abrasions or seemingly small unimportant lacerations that occur in conjunction with forearm fractures must be carefully evaluated because they may be an indication of an open fracture. Clues to the presence of an open fracture include persistent slow bloody ooze from a small laceration near the fracture site and subcutaneous emphysema on injury films. Careful evaluation and, in some situations, sterile probing of suspicious wounds will be necessary. Open forearm fractures are discussed later in this chapter.

Vascular or neurologic injuries rarely are associated with forearm shaft fractures, but the consequences of such injuries are far-reaching. Serial neurovascular examinations should be performed and documented. Radial and ulnar pulses along with distal digital capillary refill should be routinely evaluated. Davis and Green[80] reported nerve injuries in 1% (5/547) of their pediatric forearm fracture patients, with the most commonly injured nerve being the median nerve. Combined data from three large series of pediatric open forearm fractures reveal an overall nerve injury rate at presentation of 10% (17/173), with the median nerve once again being the one most commonly injured.[128,135,195] To screen for these rare but significant injuries, every child with a forearm fracture should routinely have evaluation of the radial, ulnar, and median nerves.[68] Nerve injuries occurring at the time of injury must be differentiated from treatment-related or iatrogenic neurologic deficits.

Davidson[79] suggested using the game of "rock-paper-scissors" for testing the median, radial, and ulnar nerves (Fig. 10-10). The pronated fist is the rock and tests median nerve

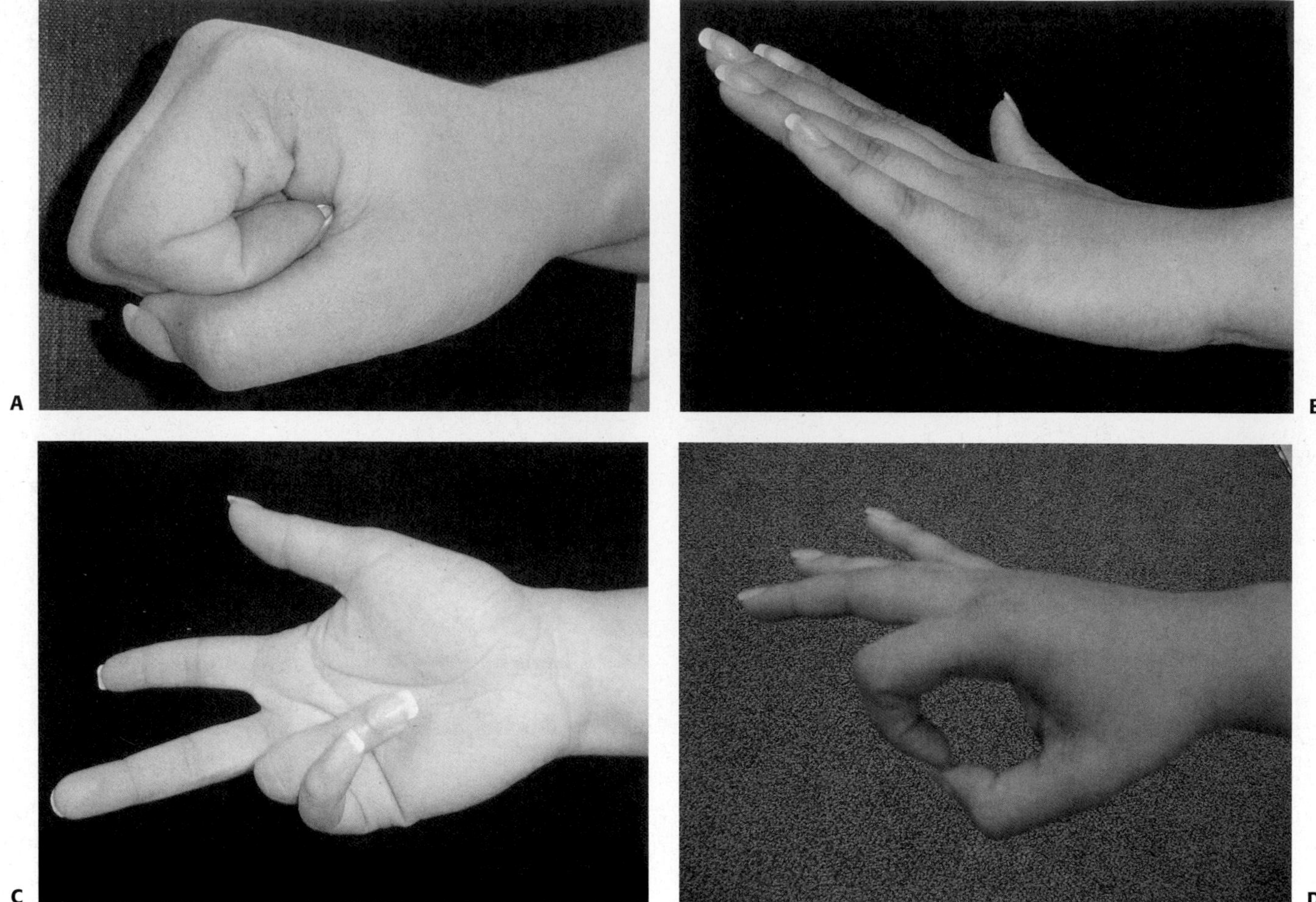

FIGURE 10-10 Upper extremity motor nerve physical examination. **A.** Rock position demonstrates median nerve motor function. **B.** Paper position demonstrates radial nerve motor function. **C.** Scissor position demonstrates ulnar nerve motor function. **D.** "OK" sign demonstrates function of anterior interosseus nerve.

function. The extended fingers and wrist depict paper and test radial nerve function. Fully flexed small and ring fingers, an adducted thumb, and spreading the index and ring fingers mimic scissors and test ulnar nerve function. Further focused testing should also be done on two important nerve branches: the anterior interosseous nerve (branch of median nerve) and the posterior interosseous nerve (branch of radial nerve). The anterior interosseous nerve provides motor function to the index flexor digitorum profundus, the flexor pollicis longus, and pronator quadratus and is best tested by having the patient make an "OK" sign. The posterior interosseous nerve typically innervates the extensor carpi ulnaris, extensor digitorum communis, extensor digiti minimi, extensor indicis, and the three out-cropping muscles of the thumb (abductor pollicis longus, extensor pollicis brevis, and extensor pollicis longus).[45] Its function is best documented by full extension of the phalangeal and metacarpophalangeal joints. This is especially difficult to test in a patient in a cast or splint that partially covers the fingers. Most injuries that occur in association with forearm fractures are true neurapraxias and typically resolve over the course of days to weeks.[74,80]

Diagnosis and Classification

Fractures of the shafts of the radius and ulna often are described in rather imprecise terms such as "both-bone forearm fracture" and "greenstick fracture." Radiographs confirm the diagnosis of forearm shaft fracture and are the basis for most classification systems. The most comprehensive classification of forearm fractures is the one adopted by the Orthopaedic Trauma Association (OTA).[12] Although this system is sound in concept, its 36 discrete subtypes[12] make it impractical for everyday clinical use, and it has not been widely used by clinical researchers.[269] Despite its complexity, the OTA classification does not account for one of the most important prognostic factors in pediatric forearm shaft fracture: location of the fracture in the distal, middle, or proximal third of the shaft.

Clinicians and clinical researchers have favored simpler descriptions of forearm shaft fractures. An orderly and practical approach to forearm shaft fracture classification should provide information about the bone (single bone, both bones), the level (distal, middle, or proximal third), and the pattern (plastic deformation, greenstick, complete, comminuted). Bone involvement is important because it not only indicates the severity of injury but also influences suspicion regarding additional soft tissue injury (e.g., single-bone injury increases the likelihood of a Monteggia or Galeazzi injury)[335] and affects reduction tactics (unique single-bone fracture reduction strategies can be used) (Fig. 10-11). Single-bone shaft fractures occur, but both-bone fractures are more common. Level is important for anatomic reasons relative to muscle and interosseous ligament attach-

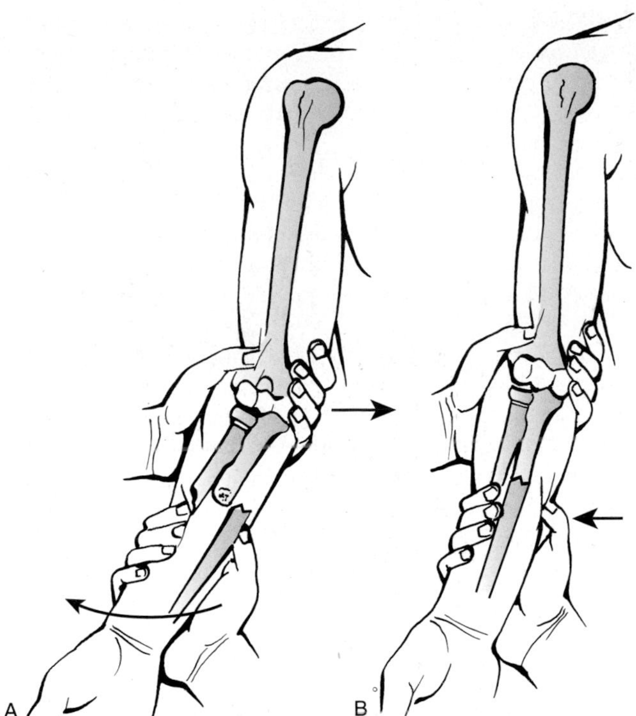

FIGURE 10-11 Isolated ulnar shaft reduction technique (Blount). Valgus force applied to fracture site and direct thumb pressure over distal ligament.

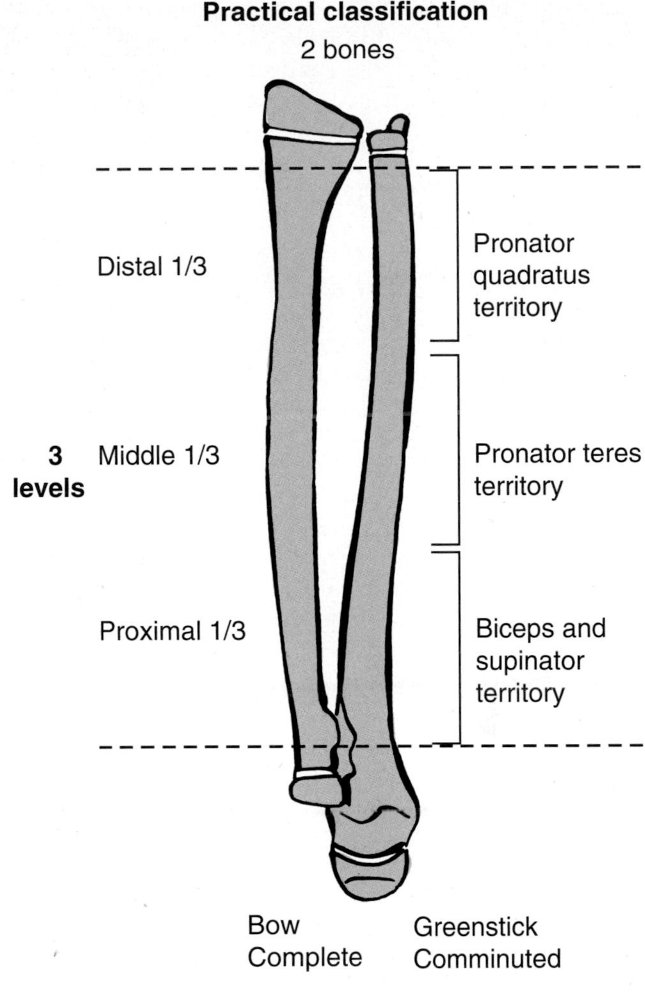

FIGURE 10-12 Practical classification of forearm shaft fractures. (Distal dotted line defined by proximal extent of Lister's tubercle and proximal dotted line defined by proximal extent of bicipital tuberosity.)

ments, as well as differences in prognosis for distal-, middle-, and proximal-third shaft fractures. Pattern is important because it significantly alters the treatment approach. For example, the primary reduction strategy is very different for greenstick fractures (rotation) compared to that for complete fractures (vertical traction). Certain comminuted fractures (e.g., comminution of both bones) may preclude reduction and casting and require plate fixation.[103,104] Fortunately, comminuted fracture patterns are rare in children. For all practical purposes, the buckle fracture pattern that is common in the distal radial metaphysis never occurs in isolation in the shaft region. The typical buckle fracture "speed bump" may accompany either plastic deformation or greenstick fractures. Thus, there are two bones, three levels, and four common fracture patterns (Fig. 10-12). We believe this is a practical and clinically relevant way to describe forearm shaft fractures.[211]

Once the forearm fracture has been described in the terms of this practical classification, fracture displacement must be evaluated. Fracture displacement can occur as angulation, rotation, shortening, or translation. Angulation is important in treatment decision-making and can be measured with reasonable reliability.[185,319] Rotation is a simple concept, but it is difficult to assess clinically.[93,255] The best that usually can be done is to roughly estimate rotation within a 45-degree margin of error.[72,255] Based on available clinical studies, it appears that less than 1 cm of shortening should be accepted in either single-bone or both-bone fracture patterns.[53,81,86,213,273] It also has been suggested that the shortening that accompanies displaced fractures may help preserve future motion through interosseous membrane relaxation.[255] Translation also is a simple concept and can be easily measured. Completely (100%) translated fractures of the middle third[72,255] and distal third[86,213,273] of the forearm have been shown to reliably remodel. Certain situations may raise concern regarding complete translation, such as isolated middle-third radial fractures with medial (ulnar) displacement that significantly narrows the interosseous space and translation in children who have less than 2 full years of growth remaining, because remodeling of the translated fracture site is less predictable than in younger children.[230,232]

Rationale

The fundamental reason for treating fractures of the shafts of the radius and ulna relates to the likelihood of bad results in the absence of adequate care. Data from certain developing countries may be as close as we come to natural history studies of untreated fractures. Archibong and Onuba[14] reported on 102 pediatric fracture patients treated in southeastern Nigeria. Their patients most commonly had upper extremity fractures, and they frequently experienced significant delays in seeking medical treatment, which led to high rates of malunion requiring surgical treatment.[14] Other Nigerian authors have found that young age was not protective against fracture malunion (more than 50%) and nonunion (25%) following traditional bonesetter treatment.[236] It is unclear whether children treated in this fashion are better or worse off than if they had received no treatment at all. The rationale for treating pediatric forearm shaft fractures is thus based on the premise that the results of modern orthopaedic treatment will exceed "pseudonatural histories" such as these.

The consequences of excessively crooked (and malrotated) forearm bones are both cosmetic and functional (Fig. 10-13).[29,35,144,206,229,329] Limited forearm supination following a forearm shaft malunion is illustrated in Figure 10-14. Despite their great concern to parents, cosmetic issues have not been formally studied, and as a result the practitioner must interpret forearm cosmetic issues on a case-by-case basis. Clinical experience has shown that the ulna appears to be less forgiving from a cosmetic standpoint because of its long subcutaneous border. Early and repeated involvement of the parents (or other legal guardians) in an informed and shared decision-making process is essential.

Bony malunion and soft tissue fibrosis have both been implicated as causes of limited forearm motion after forearm shaft fractures.[143,229] Limited forearm pronation and supination can have significant effects on upper extremity function.[27,243,255] Inability to properly pronate often can be compensated for with shoulder abduction, but no easy compensatory mechanism exists for supination deficits.[68,144,243,255] Daruwalla[76] identified a nearly 53% rate of limited forearm rotation (subtle in some, dramatic in others) in his series of 53 children with forearm fractures and attributed it to angular deformity and rotational malalignment. Several patients in Price's[255] classic series of pediatric forearm malunions had severe forearm range-of-motion losses that significantly limited vocational and avocational activities. Trousdale and Linscheid[329] reported range-of-motion losses severe enough to prompt corrective osteotomies in many of their predominantly pediatric (less than 14 years old at time of injury) patients with forearm malunions. Meier[214] also reported significant range-of-motion deficits in association with pediatric forearm malunion.

Range-of-motion losses due to deformity have been studied by numerous authors using adult cadaveric forearm specimens. Matthews et al.[206] studied 10- and 20-degree midshaft angular deformities of the radius and ulna in 10 forearm specimens. They found that 10-degree deformities of either bone individually resulted in little or no measurable motion loss (in the range of 3 degrees or less). When both bones were angulated 10 degrees dorsal, volar, or toward the interosseous membrane, larger motion losses were documented (approximately 10 degrees pronation and 20 degrees supination). Significantly greater losses of motion occurred when one or both bones were angulated 20 degrees (approximately 40 degrees for both pronation and supination). Some of the 10-degree angulated specimens demonstrated "cosmetically unacceptable deformity."[206] These findings indicate that relatively small angular deformities can be clinically significant.

Additional important information about the influence of fracture level on forearm motion was provided by a series of experiments conducted by Sarmiento et al.[280,320] They found that fracture angulation of 15 to 30 degrees led to greater supination losses when the deformity was in the middle third of the forearm (40 to 90 degrees) and greater pronation losses when in the distal third (30 to 80 degrees).[320] Fracture angulation of 10 degrees or less in the proximal or middle forearm rarely resulted in more than 15 degrees of motion loss,[280,320] but the same angulation in the distal third of the forearm was at times

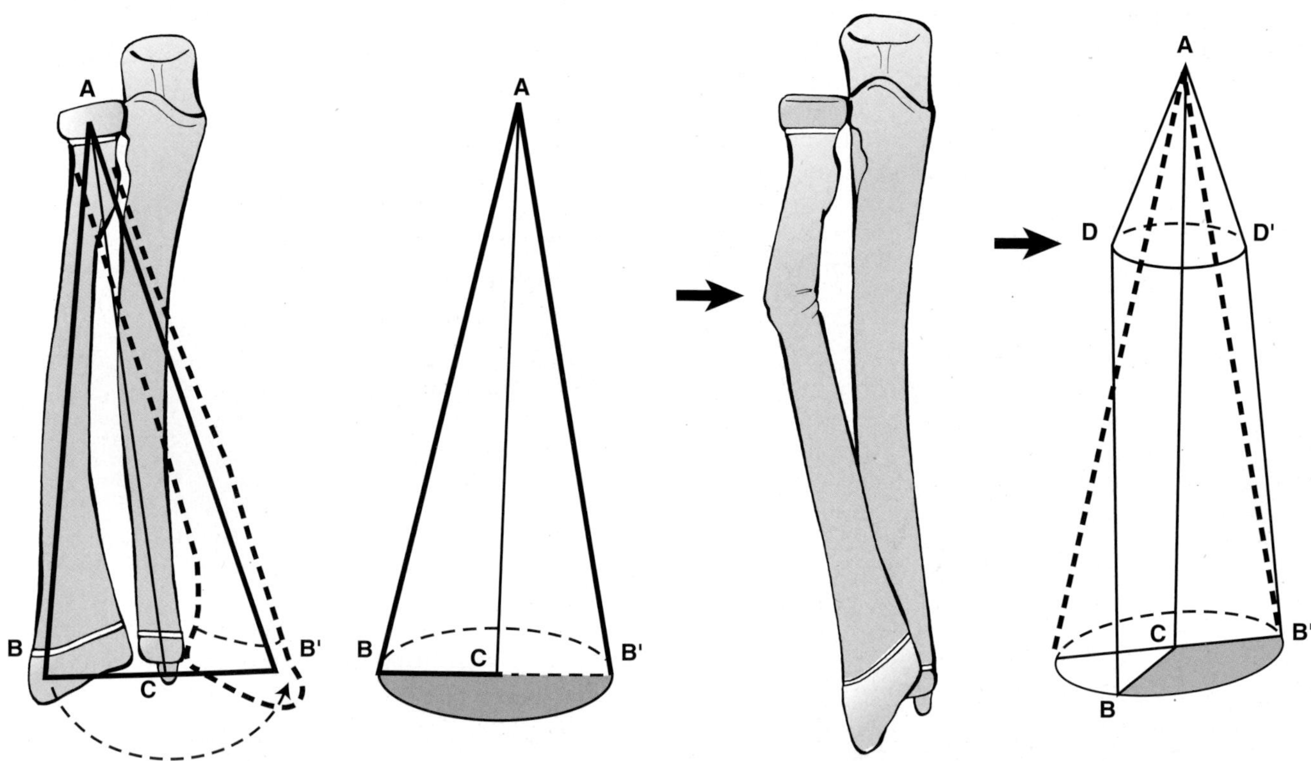

FIGURE 10-13 Effect of forearm malunion on forearm motion. **A.** Normal arc of forearm motion. **B.** Angulated radius leads to diminished arc of forearm motion. (Ogden JA. Skeletal Injury in the Child. Philadelphia: Lea & Febiger, 1982.)

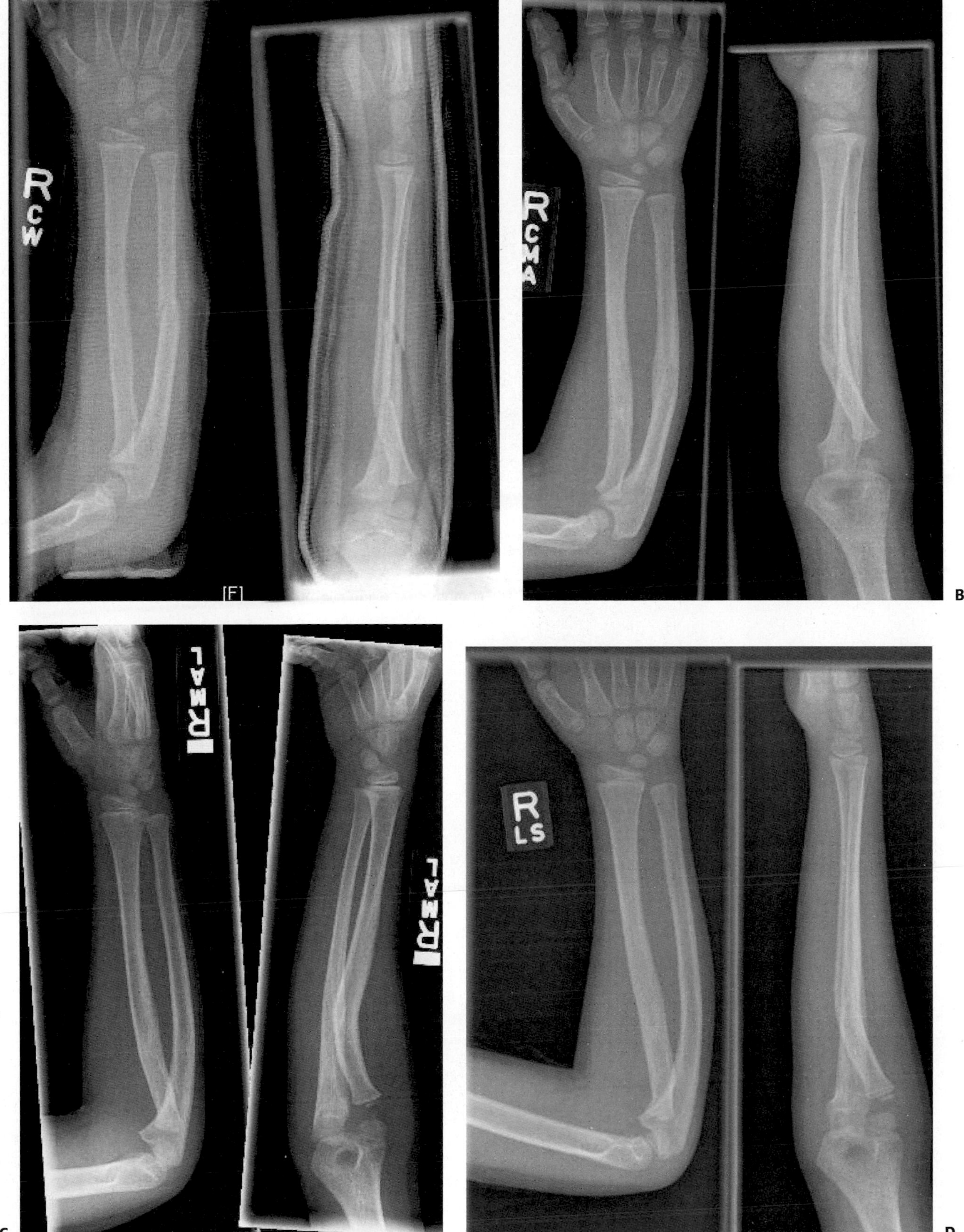

FIGURE 10-14 A 6-year-old male who suffered a right forearm shaft malunion. **A.** Radiograph one week after fracture showing complete midshaft ulnar and proximal third radial fractures. **B.** Healed fractures at 6-month follow-up. **C.** Twenty month follow-up. **D.** Twenty-six month follow-up. *(continues)*

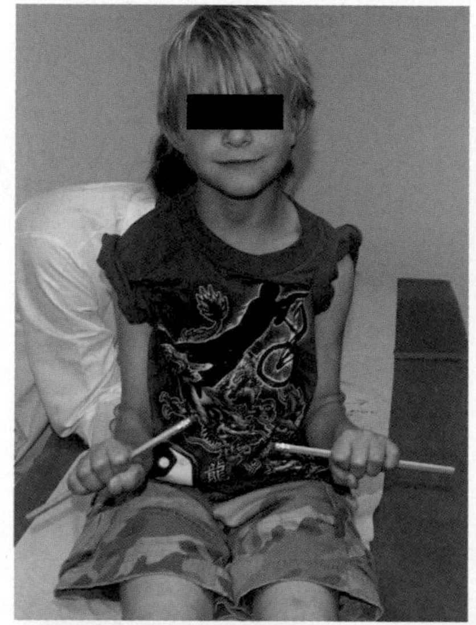
E

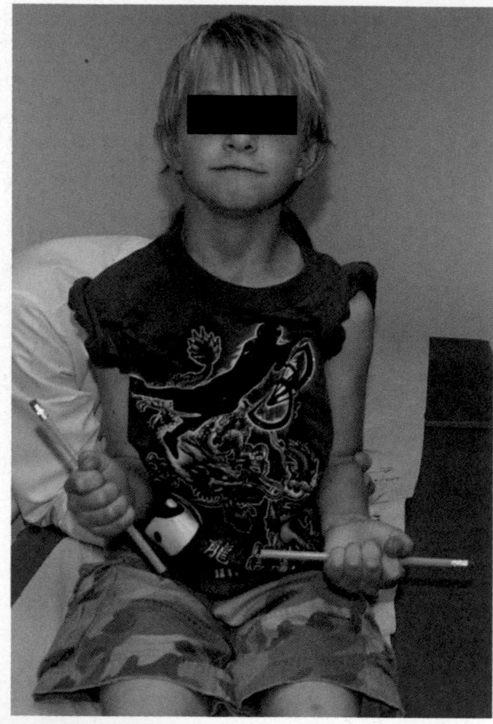
F

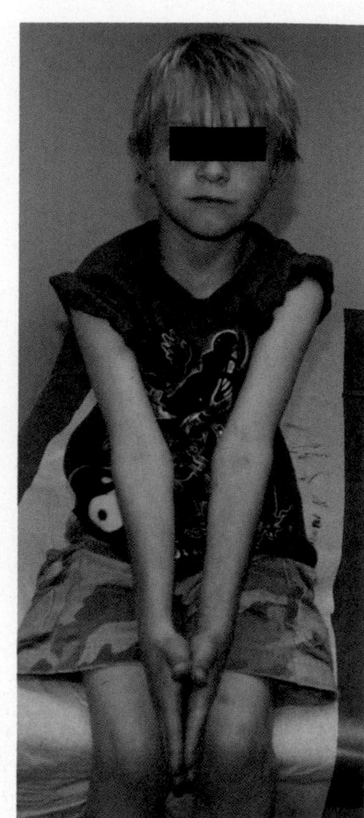
G

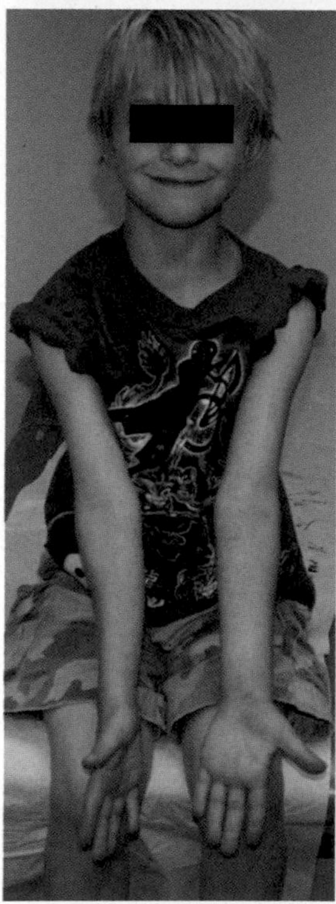
H

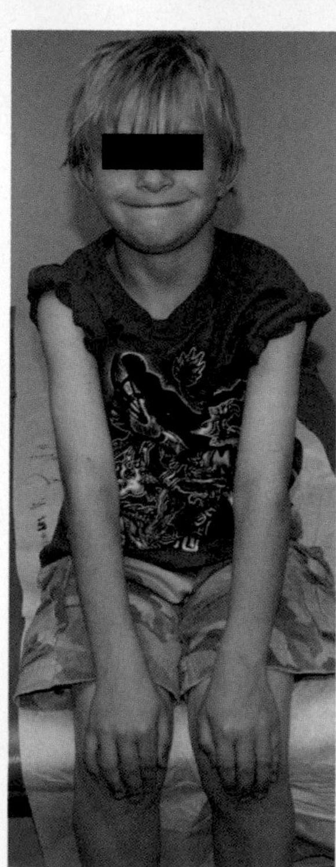
I

FIGURE 10-14 (*continued*) **E.** Symmetrical pronation. **F.** Limited supination on the right **G.** Axial alignment with palms together. **H.** An effort at supination. **I.** Axial alignment in pronation.

(usually with isolated radius fracture) associated with pronation losses of 20 degrees.[280,320] These findings challenge commonly held beliefs that the distal third of the forearm is the most forgiving. These same authors asserted that rotational malalignment led to rotational motion losses that usually were equal in magnitude and opposite in direction to the deformity (e.g., a 10-degree pronation deformity led to a 10-degree loss of supination).[320]

Rotational malalignment of the forearm has been studied in greater detail in recent years.[88,167,331] In isolated midshaft radial fractures, more than 30 degrees of malrotation was a threshold for significant losses in motion (approximately 15 degrees).[167] Isolated midshaft ulnar fracture malrotation did not alter the total arc of forearm motion but did change the set point (e.g., a 30-degree pronation deformity took away 30 degrees of pronation and added 30 degrees of supination).[331] Larger ulnar axial malalignment of 45 degrees decreased overall forearm rotation by no more than 20 degrees.[331] Large residual ulnar shaft translation has similarly been found to have little impact on forearm rotation.[209] Simulated combined radial and ulnar midshaft rota-

TABLE 10-1 Condensed Range-of-Motion Information

Ulna 40 degrees pronated
Radius 40 degrees pronated
102/52
105/57
62/65
Ulna 0 degrees neutral
Radius neutral
97/58
90/90
69/107
Ulna 40 degrees supinated
Radius 40 degrees supinated
53/55
52/95
46/110

Numerator is pronation while denominator is supination.
From Dumont CE, Thalmann R, Macy JC. The effect of rotational malunion of the radius and ulna on supination and pronation. J Bone Joint Surg Br 2002;84: 1070–1074.

tional malunions resulted in the worst motion (more than 50% losses of pronation and supination when 60-degree rotational malunions were in opposite directions).[88] Rotational malunions that approximated recommended limits in the literature (45 degrees)[255] produced less extreme but real limitations of motion (Table 10-1).[88] From these studies and our clinical experience, it appears that the radius is more sensitive to rotational problems and less sensitive regarding cosmetic issues, while the ulna is exactly the opposite.

Several generations of orthopaedic surgeons have been taught that 50 degrees of pronation and 50 degrees of supination represent adequate forearm motion.[219] It must be remembered that this classic study performed by Morrey and his Mayo Clinic colleagues involving 33 normal subjects (18 female, 15 male) from 21 to 75 years of age is not the only study that addresses forearm motion. The average arc of normal forearm motion for the Mayo group (68 degrees pronation to 74 degrees supination)[219] was approximately 20 degrees less than that measured in 53 healthy male subjects who were no older than 19 years old (77 degrees pronation to 83 degrees supination) by Boone and Azen[39] and 35 degrees less than that reported by Rickert et al.[270] (75 degrees pronation to 100 degrees supination) in 141 subjects of both sexes between 20 and 30 years of age. Contemporary three-dimensional motion analysis has revealed that maximal pronation occurs when pouring liquid from a pitcher and maximal supination commonly occurs during personal hygiene activities.[261] Thus, it seems clear that the forearm motion "goals" reported by Morrey et al.[219] are not necessarily ideal or even optimal, but rather they may be considered as the minimal limits of forearm function. Stated another way, losing 20 degrees or 30 degrees of either pronation or supination carries the potential for significant functional impact upon important activities of daily living.

The goal of treatment is to achieve satisfactory healing of the forearm injury within established anatomic and functional guidelines while also taking into account the reasonable degree of remodeling that can be expected in growing children.[154] Most of the time, these goals can be achieved with closed fracture care, and little or no radiographic or clinical abnormality can be detected following healing. A paradox exists in pediatric forearm fractures whereby anatomic radiographic alignment is not always associated with normal motion, and normal motion often is associated with nonanatomic radiographic healing.[143,225,229,320] Herein lies the inherent controversy between operative and nonoperative treatment approaches (Table 10-2). In patients with anatomic radiographs, range-of-motion problems usually have been attributed to scarring of the interosseous membrane.[168,243,255] With nonanatomic radiographs (incomplete remodeling), range-of-motion deficits usually are attributed to the radiographic abnormalities. Thus, treatment of forearm shaft fracture must balance the risk of allowing stiffness to occur secondary to malunion against the risk of creating stiffness secondary to surgical procedures.

The rationalization for remodeling of pediatric forearm fractures has strong historical support,[23,36,51,239] but knowledge of the limits of remodeling must be taken into consideration. Established reduction criteria state that complete (100%) translation is acceptable,[213,255] as well as up to 15 degrees of angulation and up to 45 degrees of malrotation.[255] Because important forearm fracture treatment decisions frequently are based on radiographic measurement of angular deformities, it must be remembered that these angles are projected shadows that are affected by rotation.[102] If angulation is present on both AP and lateral views (commonly called two orthogonal views), the true deformity is out of the plane of the radiographs, and its true magnitude is greater than that measured on each individual view. Certain forearm shaft fracture deformities are clearly "two-plane deformities" whose maximal angular magnitude is in some plane other than the standard AP or lateral plane (Fig. 10-15).[17] Bär and Breitfuss[17] produced a table (based on the Pythagorean Theorem) that predicts the true maximal angulation. Accurate deformity measurement can be made when angulation is seen on only one view and there is no angulation on the other orthogonal view. A cast change with molding, remanipulation under analgesia or anesthesia, or surgical fixation may become necessary, but even with anatomic reduction patients may not regain full pronation and supination.[229,243] Most series of pediatric forearm fractures document excellent subjective results, and

TABLE 10-2 Pros and Cons of Cast versus Surgical Treatment

Pros and Cons
Cast Treatment
Long track record
Anatomic reduction rare
Negligible infection risk
Stiffness may still occur
Fine-tuning possible
Frequent follow-up visits
Surgical Treatment
Anatomic reduction
Risk of infection
Minimize immobilization
Need for implant removal
Fewer follow-up visits
Stiffness from surgery

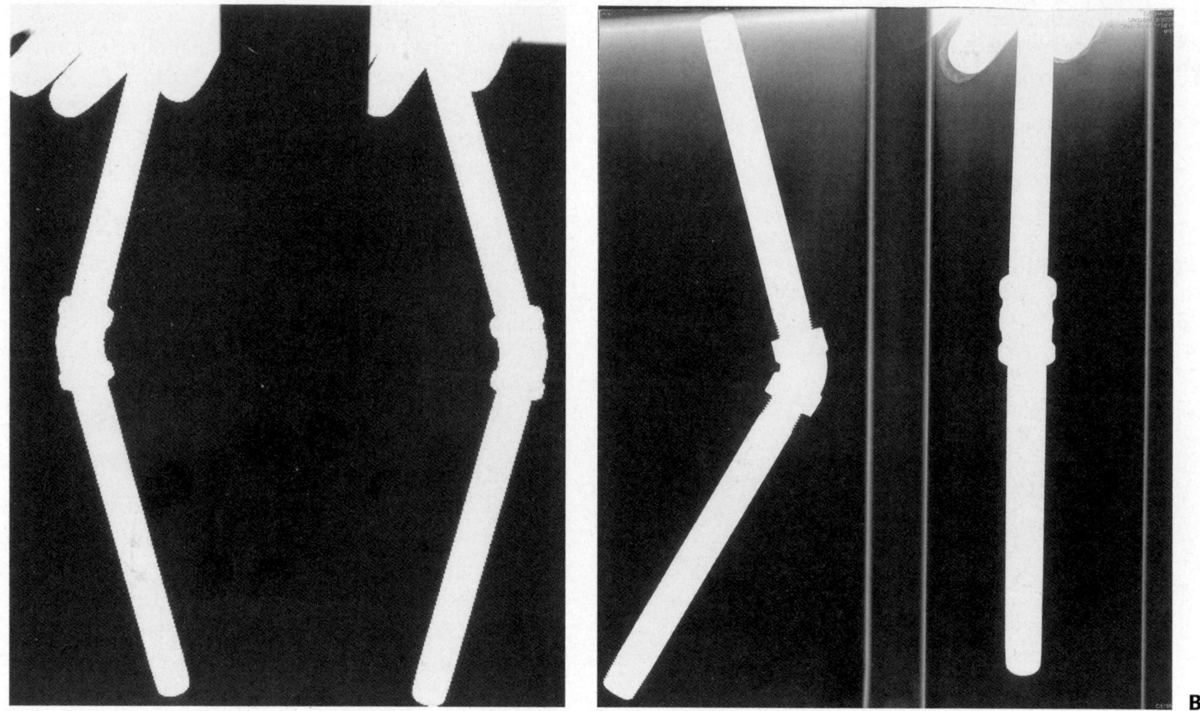

FIGURE 10-15 Underestimation of true angulation. **A.** "Out of the AP and lateral plane" underestimates angulation at 30 degrees. **B.** True AP and lateral demonstrates that true maximal angulation is 40 degrees.

only with special goniometric testing is a decreased range of motion detected objectively.[72]

Published clinical studies have shown that pediatric forearm shaft fractures have great remodeling potential that occurs through several mechanisms.[289] The distal radial epiphysis will redirect itself toward normal at about 10 degrees per year. As long as the physis is open, this rate is independent of age. Although the epiphysis will return to normal direction, it will have much less effect on correcting an angular deformity at the midshaft compared to fractures at the subphyseal level. Remodeling also occurs with lengthening of the bone through growth, which produces an apparent decrease in angulation, especially if measured as the difference between the proximal and distal ends of the bone. Bone also remodels by intramembranous apposition on the concave side and resorption on the convex side.[75,154,289] This occurs throughout life, but more rapidly when driven by the thick periosteum found in children. Larsen[182] found that although the epiphyseal angle realigns quickly, children older than 11 years correct bone angulation less than the younger children. Thomas stated the following regarding pediatric forearm remodeling potential: "We should not fail to recall that the remodeling capabilities of the bones of children have not changed in the last million years and that open reduction and internal fixation must be undertaken only after due deliberation."[322] Others such as Ashok Johari[157] would state that if one critically evaluates the limits of forearm shaft remodeling capacity you will find a much higher rate (approximately 50%) of incomplete remodeling in children over 10 years of age.

SURGICAL AND APPLIED ANATOMY

Bony Anatomy and Static Restraints

The forearm is a large nonsynovial joint with nearly a 180-degree arc of motion. Its bones, the radius and ulna, are not simple straight bony tubes. The shaft of the radius is a three-sided structure with two prominent curvatures. One major gradual convexity (approximately 10 degrees with its apex lateral-radial) is present along its midportion; a second, more acute curve of approximately 15 degrees with its apex medial occurs proximally near the bicipital tuberosity.[100,127,277] The deviation along the midportion is commonly referred to as the radial bow, and maintenance of this normal contour is a goal of forearm shaft fracture care.[259,284,285] The most important bony landmarks of the radius are the radial styloid (lateral prominence) and the bicipital tuberosity (anteromedial prominence), which are oriented somewhat less than 180 degrees away from each other (Fig. 10-16).[217] Anthropologists consider a full 180-degree relationship to be characteristic of Neanderthal osteology.[327] Maintenance of the styloid-tuberosity rotational relationship is another forearm shaft fracture principle. The nutrient artery of the radius enters the bone in its proximal half and courses anterior to ulnar (medial).[119] Such nutrient vessels typically are seen on only one orthogonal view and should not be confused with fracture lines. In cross section, most of the shaft of the ulna also is shaped like a classic three-sided prism, while its more distal and proximal portions are much more circular. The most important bony landmarks of the ulna are its styloid process (distally) and its coronoid process (proximally). These two landmarks are oriented nearly 180 degrees from one another, with the styloid aimed in a posterior (dorsal) direction and the coronoid in an anterior (volar) direction.[217] Tracking styloid-coronoid rotational alignment of the ulna is another part of forearm shaft fracture care. The ulnar shaft has mild curvatures in both its proximal (apex lateral/radial) and distal (apex medial/ulnar) portions but is otherwise relatively straight.[127,277] The nutrient artery to the ulna enters the bone in its proximal half and courses anterior to radial (lateral).[119]

The classic works of Evans helped focus attention on rota-

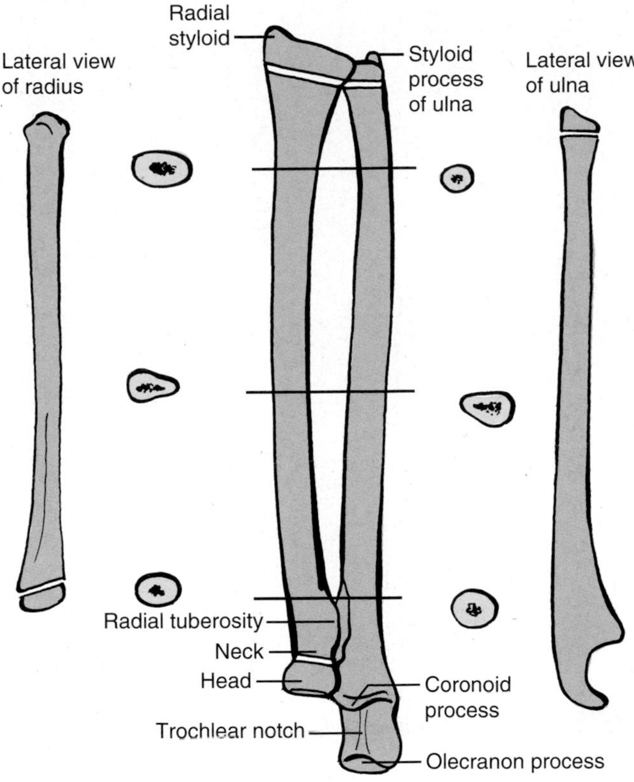

FIGURE 10-16 Radial and ulnar anatomy.

tional deformity associated with fractures of both bones of the forearm.[94,207,263] Evans stated, "The orthodox position in which to immobilize these fractures is that of full supination for the upper third, and the midposition for fractures of the middle and lower thirds, these positions being based on the anatomical arrangement of the pronators and supinators of the forearm. However, it is unreasonable to suppose that all fractures at a given level will present the same degree of rotational deformity."[94] He pointed out the importance of tracking the rotational alignment of the free-moving radial fragment by ascertaining the relative location of the bicipital tuberosity. This was a major step forward in refining the orthopaedic care of these forearm injuries. On a fully supinated AP radiograph of an unfractured forearm, the bicipital tuberosity points predominantly in a medial direction (nearly 180 degrees opposite of the radial tuberosity).[94] The radius and ulna also are nearly parallel to each other on such a view. On a fully pronated AP radiograph of an unfractured forearm, the bicipital tuberosity points in a lateral direction and the radial tuberosity is situated medially.[94] The radius also crosses over the ulna in a pronated AP view. Rang[262] noted that in an unfractured limb, the bicipital tuberosity tended to align with a point near the thenar eminence (Fig. 10-17), more nearly a 165-degree relationship than a true 180-degree one. These relationships are best assessed on standard radiographs that include the entire forearm on one film[76,255,329] rather than the specialized bicipital tuberosity view originally suggested by Evans.[94]

Some generalities regarding the appearance and closure of secondary ossification centers of the radius and ulna should be kept in mind because these growth areas must be respected during both surgical and nonsurgical fracture care.[244,256,364,365] The secondary center (epiphysis) of the distal radius is the first to appear at around 1 year of age.[32,233] Next are the epiphyses of the proximal radius and distal ulna, which appear by about 4 to 6 years of age.[299] The proximal ulna is last and appears at around 9 years of age.[298] Physeal closure occurs in two stages, with the proximal radius and proximal ulna closing by about 15 years of age and the distal radius and ulna by about 18 years of age.[231] It must be remembered that females' physes close 1 to 2 years before their male counterparts.

The radius and ulna are joined by three major passive restraints: the proximal radioulnar joint (PRUJ), the distal radioulnar joint (DRUJ), and the interosseous membrane complex, all of which have important stabilizing and load-transferring functions. These structures allow rotation of the radius about the ulna along an axis that runs approximately from the center of the radial head to the center of the distal ulna.[145,243] The PRUJ and DRUJ are discussed elsewhere in this book (Chapters 9 and 11). The structure and biomechanic function of the interosseous membrane have been studied extensively in recent years. Hotchkiss et al.[149] showed that the central band of the interosseous membrane (the interosseous ligament) courses from a point near the junction of the proximal and middle thirds of the radius to a point near the junction of the middle and distal thirds of the ulna. It is an important longitudinal stabilizer of the forearm in that 71% of forearm longitudinal stiffness is provided by the interosseous ligament after radial head excision.[149] Transverse vectors also have been identified[246] and reflect the stabilizing effect of the interosseous ligament during pronation and supination movements. The interosseous ligament demonstrates tensile properties comparable to the patellar tendon and the anterior cruciate ligament,[247] indicative of the magnitude of the arm forces to which this structure is subjected.

Although some difference of opinion still exists,[82,109,304] multiple studies have shown that the most strain in the central band of the interosseous membrane is generated when the forearm is in the neutral position.[203,204,304] These findings of maximal strain in neutral in cadaver studies also are consistent with radiographic measurement studies[72] and dynamic magnetic resonance imaging studies of the forearm showing that the interosseous space is maximal near a neutral position.[226] This may help explain certain pathologic situations such as the fixed supination deformity of neonatal brachial plexus palsy[208] as well as limitations of pronation and supination due to encroachment on the interosseous space from malangulated fractures (Fig. 10-18).[360] The interosseous membrane also serves as an important anchoring point for several forearm muscles: the flexor digitorum profundus, flexor pollicis longus, extensor indicis, and the outcropping muscles (extensor digitorum brevis, abductor pollicus longus).

Pertinent Anatomy of the Muscles and Nerves

The paired and seemingly balanced radial and ulnar bones have an unbalanced number of muscular connections. The ulna typically has 14 attached muscles and the radius only 10 (Tables 10-3 and 10-4).[87,127] Powerful supinators attach to the proximal third of the forearm, while important pronators attach to its middle and distal thirds (Fig. 10-19). The accompanying vasculature of the forearm is complex: these muscles are supplied by more than 248 vascular pedicles arising from the brachial artery, its branches, or other collateral vessels.[268] The radial, ulnar,

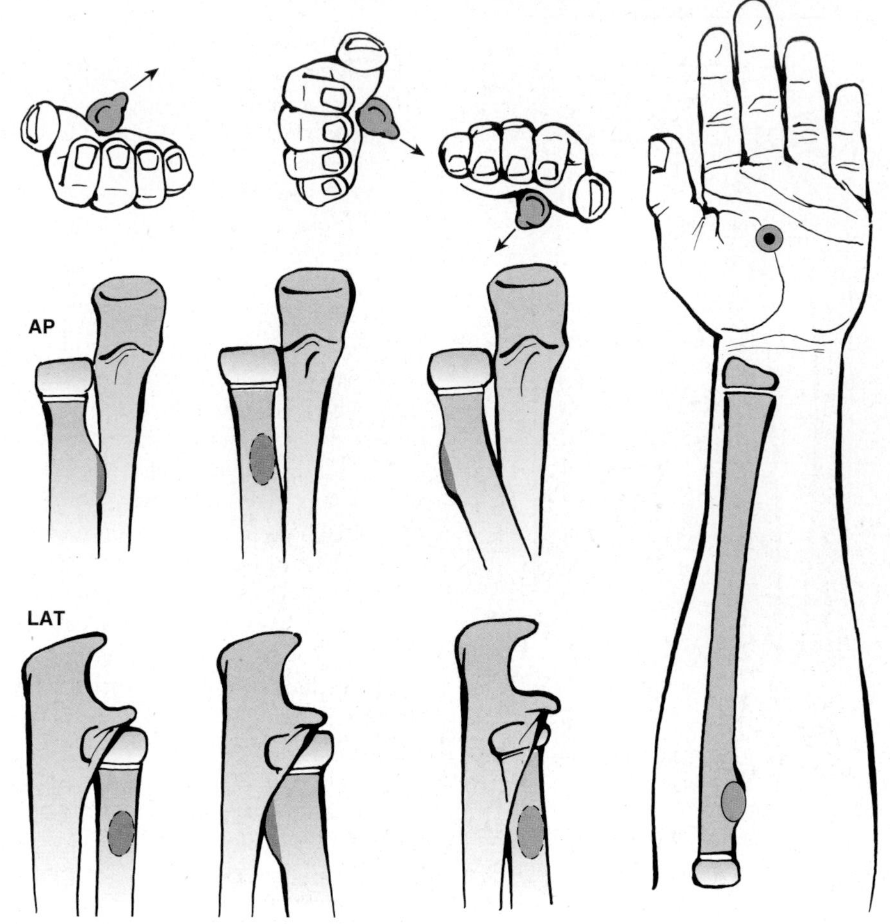

FIGURE 10-17 Rang's illustration depicting the position of the bicipital tuberosity on AP and lateral views with the forearm in pronation, supination, and neutral position. (From Rang M. Children's Fractures. Philadelphia: JB Lippincott, 1974.)

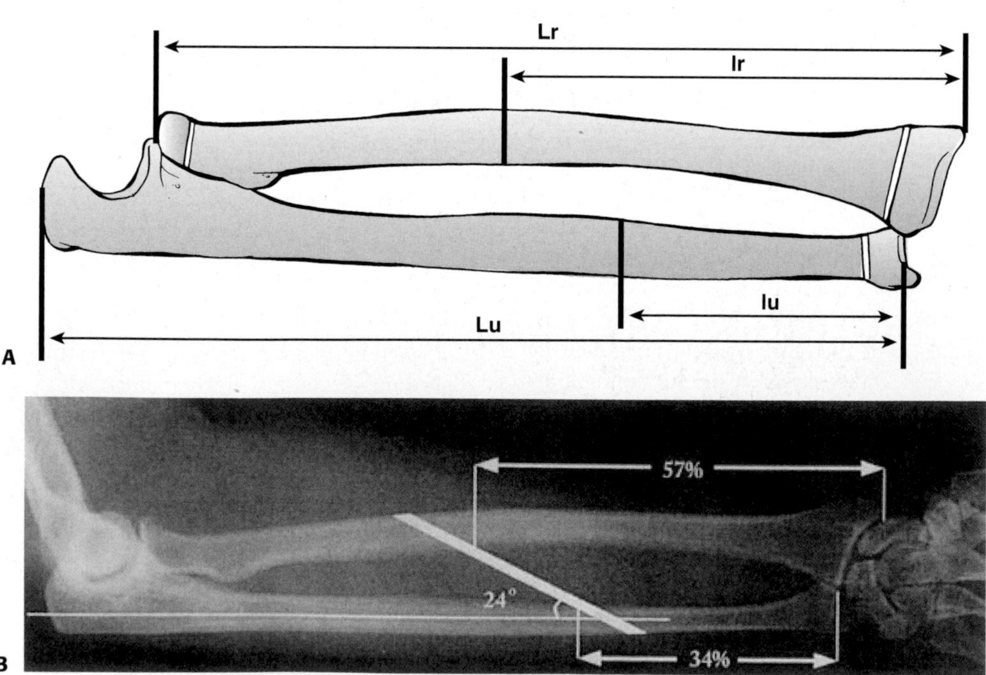

FIGURE 10-18 Anatomy of interosseous ligament. **A.** Central oblique orientation of interosseous ligament. **B.** Interosseous ligament attachment in terms of percentage forearm length. (From Skahen JR 3rd, Palmer AK, Werner FW, et al. Reconstruction of the interosseous membrane of the forearm in cadavers. J Hand Surg Am 1997;22:986–994.)

TABLE 10-3 Ten Muscles That Attach to the Radius (and Their Innervation)

1. Abductor pollicis longus (PIN)
2. Biceps (musculocutaneous nerve)
3. Brachioradialis (radial nerve)
4. Extensor pollicis brevis (PIN)
5. Extensor pollicis longus (PIN)
6. Flexor digitorum superficialis (median nerve)
7. Flexor pollicis longus (AIN)
8. Pronator quadratus (AIN)
9. Pronator teres (median nerve)
10. Supinator (PIN)

AIN, anterior interosseous innervation; PIN, posterior interosseous nerve.

and median nerves (or their branches) along with the musculocutaneous nerve provide all of the key innervations to the motors that attach to the forearm bones. As mentioned earlier, the median nerve is the most commonly injured nerve with forearm fractures.[79,80,128,135]

The radial nerve proceeds from a posterior to anterior direction and enters the forearm after passing the lateral epicondyle between the brachialis and brachioradialis muscles. Near this same level, it divides into superficial and deep terminal branches. The deep motor branch of the radial nerve also is known as the posterior interosseous nerve. In addition to its

TABLE 10-4 Fourteen Muscles That Attach to the Ulna (and Their Innervation)

1. Abductor pollicis longus (PIN)
2. Anconeus (radial nerve)
3. Biceps (musculocutaneous nerve)
4. Brachialis (musculocutaneous and small branches; median and radial nerves)
5. Extensor carpi ulnaris (PIN)
6. Extensor indicis proprius (PIN)
7. Extensor pollicis longus (PIN)
8. Flexor carpi ulnaris (ulnar nerve)
9. Flexor digitorum profundus (AIN, index and long; ulnar nerve, ring and small)
10. Flexor digitorum superficialis (median nerve)
11. Pronator teres (median nerve)
12. Pronator quadratus (AIN)
13. Supinator (PIN)
14. Triceps (radial nerve)

AIN, anterior interosseous innervation; PIN, posterior interosseous nerve. Occasionally, the accessory head flexor pollicis longus (aka Gantzer's muscle; from coronoid region in 15% of specimens) is innervated by AIN.

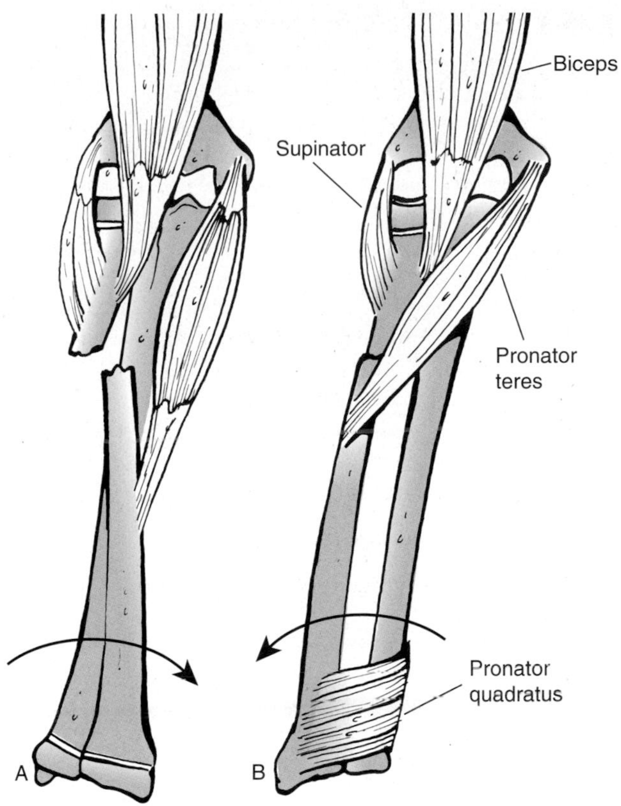

FIGURE 10-19 Muscle forces acting in proximal, middle, and distal thirds.

routine innervation of the brachioradialis and extensor carpi radialis longus, most commonly (55% of the time) a motor branch arises from the radial nerve proper or its superficial terminal branch to innervate the extensor carpi radialis brevis, while the rest of the time (45%) this motor branch comes from the posterior interosseous nerve.[2] The superficial branch travels along with and beneath the brachioradialis. The posterior interosseous nerve enters the supinator muscle, passing the fibrous thickening called the arcade of Frohse shortly after branching from the radial nerve proper. It courses within the supinator past the proximal radius, later exiting this muscle dorsally (posteriorly) near the junction of the proximal and middle thirds of the radius. Following its emergence from the supinator, the posterior interosseous nerve branches repetitively to the superficial extensors and the deeper outcropping muscles. The ulnar nerve enters the forearm between the two heads of the flexor carpi ulnaris.[121] It traverses the forearm between the flexor carpi ulnaris and the flexor digitorum profundus. In the distal forearm, it lays just beneath the flexor carpi ulnaris. The median nerve enters the forearm as it passes between the two heads of the pronator teres.[59] It next passes beneath the archway created by the two heads of the flexor digitorum superficialis. The median nerve then continues down the course of the forearm nestled between the flexor digitorum superficialis and the flexor digitorum profundus. It becomes much more superficial as it nears the level of the carpal tunnel. The anterior interosseous branch arises from the median nerve at the level of the pronator and travels deep with the anterior interosseous vessels. Abundant muscle shields the radial, ulnar, and median nerves from the shafts of the radius and ulna through most of the forearm.

Common Surgical Approaches

The large exposure required for plate fixation of pediatric forearm fractures can be achieved with three surgical approaches: the Henry (anterior) and Thompson (posterior) approaches to the radial shaft and the direct (medial) approach to the ulnar shaft.[73,223] Compartment syndrome release usually requires the serpentine incision of McConnell's combined approach.[141] These approaches and their variations are well described and illustrated in detail elsewhere.[5,19,90,147,296] For open reduction of both the radius and the ulna, most authors favor separate incisions to minimize the possibility of communicating hematoma and the development of a radioulnar synostosis.[180,259,333] The Thompson approach to the radius generally is used for fractures of its proximal third[358] but requires special care to protect the posterior interosseous nerve.[84,215,317] Other authors have emphasized the utility of the Henry approach for plating of the proximal radius.[215] When open reduction is done in conjunction with other internal fixation techniques (e.g., intramedullary fixation), limited versions of the same surgical approaches are used.

Indirect reduction and internal fixation of forearm fractures requires knowledge of appropriate physeal-sparing entry portals about the distal and proximal forearm. Because of the relative inaccessibility of its proximal end, the radius usually is approached only distally through either a dorsal or radial entry point. The dorsal entry point is near the proximal base of Lister's tubercle or just lateral to it in a small bare area between the second and third dorsal compartments. This location is a short distance proximal to the physis of the distal radius. Another dorsal alternative is pin entry just medial to Lister's tubercle, between the third and fourth dorsal compartments,[275] but this may entail greater tendon risk. The most commonly used radial entry point is located in line with the styloid process just proximal to the physis.[356] Entry in this area passes adjacent to the first dorsal compartment, and thus the tendons of abductor pollicis longus and extensor pollicis brevis (as well as branches of the superficial radial nerve) must be protected (Fig. 10-20). Because of its extensive branching pattern, portions of the superficial branch of the radial nerve may be at risk when dorsal or radial intramedullary entry points are used.[1,16]

Both distal and proximal intramedullary entry sites for the ulna have been described.[188,194,254,297,337] In the distal portion of the ulna, an entry site can be made proximal to the physis and in the interval between the extensor carpi ulnaris and flexor carpi ulnaris tendons. Care must be taken to avoid branches of the dorsal cutaneous sensory nerve. Ulnar entry is most easily accomplished in the proximal portion of the bone along its lateral metaphyseal border (just distal to the olecranon apo-

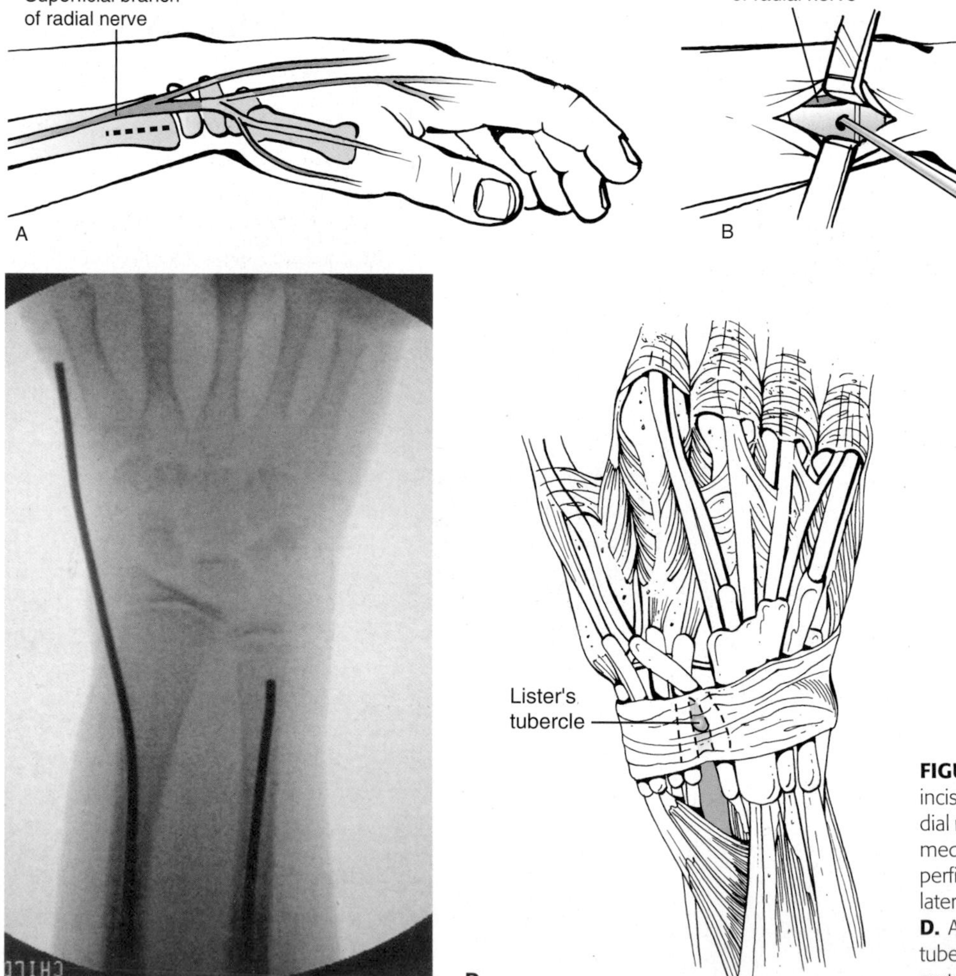

FIGURE 10-20 Distal radial entry. **A.** Distal radial incision in proximity to superficial branch of radial nerve. **B.** Distal radial entry position for intramedullary rod placement in relationship to superficial branch of radial nerve. **C.** Radiograph of lateral starting point for intramedullary nail. **D.** Alternate entry point just proximal to Lister tubercle between second and third dorsal compartment.

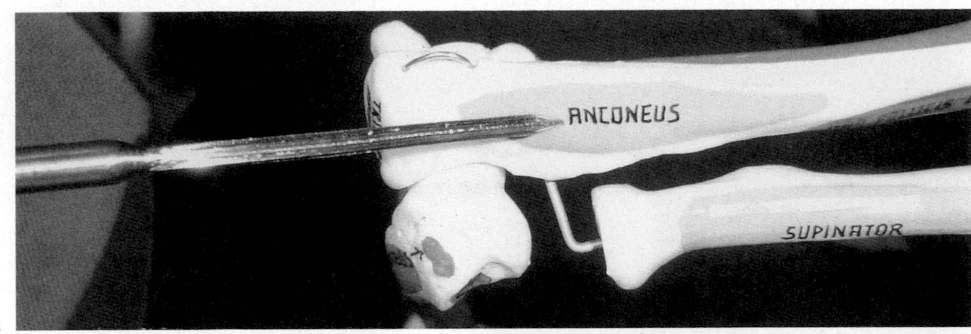

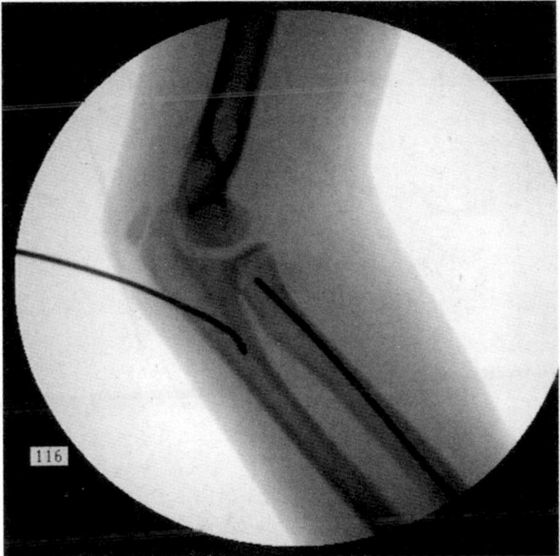

FIGURE 10-21 Proximal ulnar entry. **A.** Anconeus entry point. **B.** Radiograph of proximal ulnar entry point.

physis), piercing peripheral fibers of the anconeus (Fig. 10-21).[48,184,191] This anconeus entry site described by the Nancy group avoids the physis and avoids the painful bursa that tends to form over "tip of the olecranon" pins.

Transphyseal approaches to both the distal radius[364,365,366] and the proximal ulna[10,215,194] have been suggested by some authors. Significant growth potential exists at the distal radius (approximately 10 mm per year), while there is proportionately less from the olecranon apophysis (approximately 2 mm per year). There is an unnecessary risk to the radial physis and few if any technical advantages to transphyseal entry of the radius in diaphyseal level fracture fixation. The ulna apophyseal entry site is used in many centers.

CURRENT CLOSED TREATMENT OPTIONS

Overview of Closed Fracture Treatment

Most pediatric radial and ulnar shaft fractures can be treated by nonoperative methods.[366] Low-energy, undisplaced, and minimally displaced forearm fractures can be immediately immobilized in a properly molded (three-point mold concept of Charnley) above-elbow cast.[10] If posttraumatic tissue swelling is a concern, noncircumferential splint immobilization (e.g., sugar tong splint) can be used initially.[68,324,362] For fractures in the distal third of the forearm, below-elbow casting has been shown to be as effective as above-elbow casting in maintenance of satisfactory fracture alignment.[63,112] Appropriate follow-up is important for these undisplaced fractures (an initial follow-up radiograph usually is taken 7 to 14 days after injury) because displacement may still occur for a variety of reasons: new trauma to the extremity, male gender, and poor casting technique.[68,113,290,362]

Good casting technique is infrequently discussed in contemporary orthopaedic textbooks and sometimes is underemphasized during orthopaedic residency training. The principles of good forearm casting technique include: (a) interosseous molding, (b) supracondylar molding, (c) appropriate padding, (d) evenly distributed cast material, (e) straight ulnar border, and (f) three-point molding (Fig. 10-22). The risk of excessive cast tightness can be minimized through the use of the stretch-relax fiberglass casting technique described by Davids et al.[77] Chess et al.[63] described a cast index for distal radial fractures defined as the sagittal cast width divided by the coronal cast width at the level of the fracture site; a normal ratio is considered to be 0.70. The cast index has not been validated for forearm shaft fractures, but it embodies the sound concept of good interosseous molding. Advanced techniques such as pins and plaster and cast wedging also have a role to play.[18,89] Cast wedging is almost always done with an opening wedge technique because this entails less risk of soft tissue impingement.[169]

Displaced fractures usually require reduction following appropriate analgesia.[86,334] Options include hematoma block,[107,140,159] regional intravenous anesthesia,[46,78,163] and inhalational methods.[95,129,140] After informed consent for the sedation and reduction is obtained, monitored sedation can be used in the emergency department with a combination of narcotics and anxiolytics.[173] This typically requires a dedicated nurse to administer oxygen and perform appropriate monitoring functions

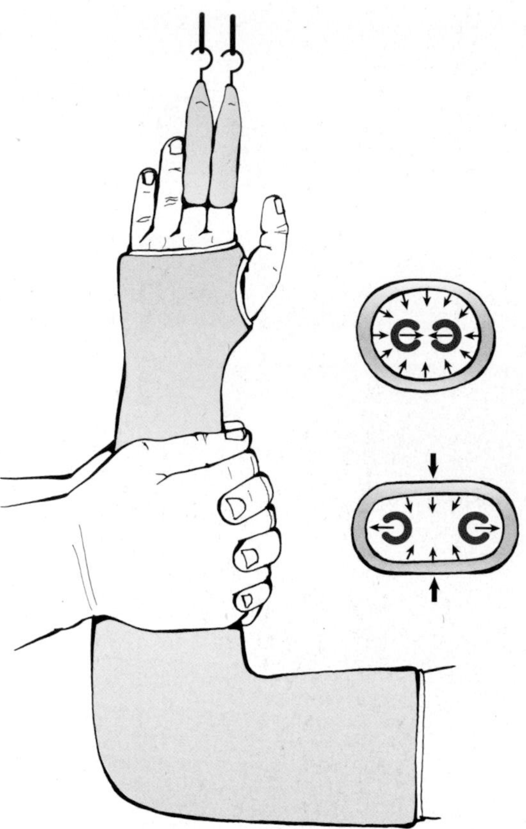

FIGURE 10-22 Interosseous mold technique.

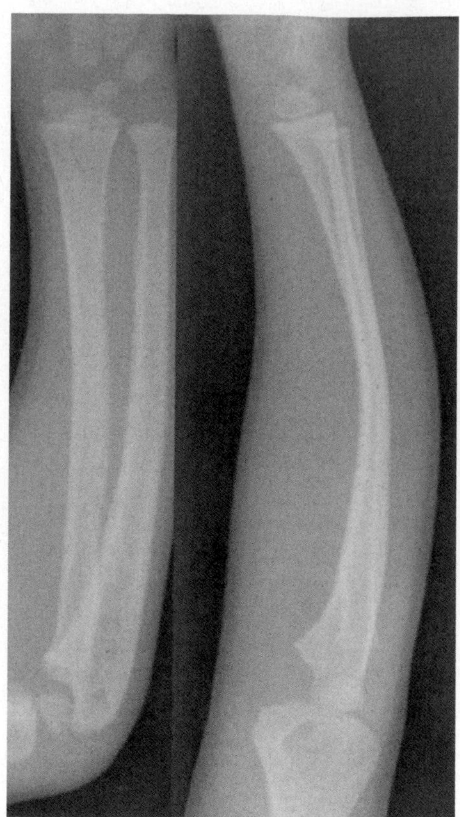

FIGURE 10-23 Bow fracture: approximately 15 degrees of apex dorsal bowing of radius and ulna shaft.

(vital signs, continuous electrocardiogram, and pulse oximetry).[8,9,142] Ketamine protocols also are being used with increased frequency.[120,173] Young children with less than 5 or 10 degrees of angulation in the plane of wrist and elbow motion probably do not require the additional trauma, time, expense, and sedation risk involved in a formal reduction because of the predictable remodeling in this age group.[14] It has been shown that the more displaced the fracture, the more likely that formal monitored sedation techniques will be used for pediatric forearm fracture reduction as opposed to other techniques.[334]

More specific closed treatment options are discussed for pediatric forearm injuries in terms of their common fracture patterns: bow (plastic deformation), greenstick, complete, and comminuted.

Traumatic Bowing/Plastic Deformation

Although traumatic bowing was described by Rauber in 1876,[300] it was not widely recognized until Spencer Borden's classic paper was published in 1974.[40] This injury occurs almost exclusively with children's forearm fractures.[176] Bow fractures (Fig. 10-23) show no obvious macroscopic fracture line or cortical discontinuity, but they do demonstrate multiple microfractures (slip lines) along the length of the bow.[279] At times, a nearly classic buckle fracture (torus fracture) coexists with a bow fracture. The most common clinical scenario is a plastically deformed ulna along with a more typical fracture of the radius.[198]

Borden[40] and subsequent authors stressed the importance of natural remodeling potential in these injuries but voiced concern about this approach in older children (especially those over 10 years of age).[40,198,279] Vorlat and DeBoeck[340] reported incomplete remodeling in 3 of 11 children at long-term follow-up (average 6.7 years) after traumatic bowing of the forearm. Because these three children were between the ages of 7 and 10 at the time of injury, the authors recommended more aggressive efforts at reduction in all patients with clinically significant deformity (more than 10 degrees) older than 6 years of age.[340] Traumatic bowing that causes cosmetically or functionally unacceptable angular deformity[276] must be manipulated under general anesthesia or deep sedation because strong (20 to 30 kg) gradual force applied over 2 to 3 minutes is required to obtain acceptable alignment (Fig. 10-24).[279] Application of this reductive pressure over a rolled towel, block, or surgeon's knee fulcrum followed by a three-point molded cast can substantially (although at times still incompletely) correct the deformity. Care must be taken to avoid direct pressure over adjacent epiphyses for fear of creating a physeal fracture.

Greenstick Fractures

Greenstick fractures present special issues in terms of diagnosis and treatment. Angulated greenstick fractures of the shafts of the radius and ulna at different levels indicate a significant rotational component to the injury (see Fig. 10-8). Evans, Rang, and others have stated that the apex-volar angulation pattern usually is associated with a supination-type injury mechanism, while most apex-dorsal greenstick fractures involve a pronation-type injury mechanism (Fig. 10-25),[92,94,230,262] although exceptions certainly occur.[92,132] Often, the apparent angular deformity can be corrected by simply reversing the forearm rotational forces (e.g., reducing an apex-dorsal pronation-type injury with supi-

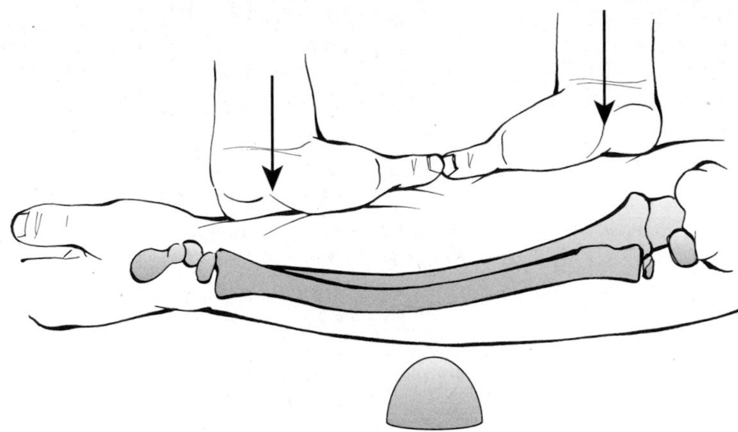

FIGURE 10-24 Reduction technique of bow fracture over fulcrum. (From Sanders WE, Heckman JD. Traumatic plastic deformation of the radius and ulna: a closed method of correction of deformity. Clin Orthop 1984;188:58–67.)

nation). Noonan and Price[230] observed that it is difficult to remember whether to use pronation or supination reductive forces and suggested that most fractures can be reduced by rotating the palm toward the deformity. They also noted that most greenstick fractures are supination injuries with apex-volar angulation and thus can be reduced by a pronation movement.[230]

Greenstick fractures that occur near the same level probably have little to no rotational component and are best corrected by manipulative reduction and three-point molding techniques (see Fig. 10-9). Charnley believed that greenstick fractures of the forearm in children perfectly illustrated his dictum that "A curved plaster is necessary in order to make a straight limb."[61] He also stated that "The unsuspected recurrence of angular deformity in greenstick fractures of the forearm, while concealed in plaster, is an annoying event if it takes the surgeon by surprise and is not discovered until the plaster is removed. Parents, quite understandably, may be more annoyed about this happening to their children than if it had happened to themselves, and do not easily forgive the surgeon."[61] Despite these concerns, it is clear from large published reports that greenstick fractures can almost always be successfully treated with nonoperative methods.[365]

Two philosophies are reflected in the literature regarding greenstick fracture reduction: one in which the greenstick fracture is purposely completed and another in which it is not. Those who favor completing the fracture (dating back at least to the 1859 work of Malgaigne) cite concerns about lost reduction and recurrent deformity that can be prevented only by converting the greenstick into a complete fracture.[24,36,103,152] Others prefer to maintain and perhaps exploit some of the inherent stability of the greenstick fracture.[6,63,80,92,322] In addition to the traditional view that loss of reduction is less likely if a greenstick fracture is completed, there also is the theoretical advantage of a lower refracture rate because of more exuberant callus formation.[63,230] To the best of our knowledge, these theories have not been validated in any controlled clinical studies. Davis and Green[80] advocated a derotational approach to greenstick fracture reduction and reported a 10% (16/151) reangulation rate in their series of patients with greenstick fracture. They compared this to the 25% (12/47) reangulation rate in patients with complete fractures and questioned the wisdom of routinely completing greenstick fractures.[80] In a prospective study, Boyer et al.[44] showed statistically that greenstick fractures maintain their reduction better than complete forearm fractures.

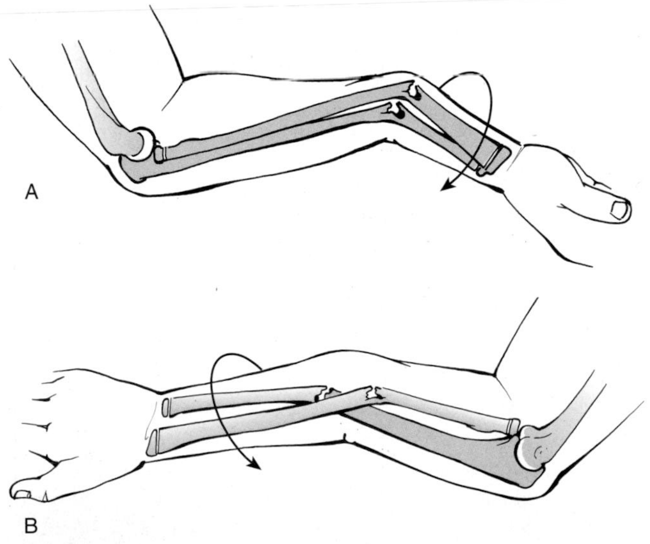

FIGURE 10-25 Shaft fractures at different levels implies rotational mechanism. **A.** Apex-volar angulation with supination deformity of the forearm. **B.** Apex-dorsal angulation with pronation deformity of forearm.

Complete Fractures

Complete fractures in different regions of the shaft of the forearm behave differently from a clinical perspective and have classically been divided into distal-, middle-, and proximal-third fractures. Single-bone complete fractures usually are caused by direct trauma (nightstick fracture) and are difficult to reduce. Blount described a reduction technique that may be effective for reduction of a displaced single-bone shaft fracture.[34] The intact bone is used as a lever to re-establish length of the fractured bone, and then transverse forces are applied to realign the bone ends (see Fig. 10-11). Both-bone complete fractures (often with bayonet shortening) are common and are best treated with finger-trap or arm traction applied over 5 to 10 minutes. This stretches out the soft tissue envelope and aids in both reduction and cast or splint application. Traction allows complete fractures to "seek their own level of rotation" and allows correction of rotational malalignment.[80]

The position of immobilization for forearm fractures has

been an area of debate since the days of Hippocrates.[36] Theoretically, the position of forearm rotation in an above-elbow cast or splint affects rotational alignment of complete fractures at all levels; however, a study of distal-third forearm fractures found no significant effect of forearm rotation position on ultimate alignment.[44] We are aware of no similar studies analyzing the effects of forearm position on middle- or proximal-third shaft fractures, and treatment is influenced by certain anatomic considerations. Because of the strong supination pull of the biceps, aided by the supinator, complete proximal radial fractures may be best immobilized in supination so that the distal forearm rotation matches that of the proximal forearm (see Fig. 10-19). The position of immobilization of fractures in the middle third of the forearm commonly is dictated by whether the radial fracture occurs distal or proximal to the insertion of the pronator teres. Fractures proximal to its insertion are best treated by fully supinating the distal fragment, while those distal to its insertion are probably best treated in a neutral position.

Manipulated fractures should be evaluated weekly for the first 2 to 3 weeks because most position loss can be recognized and corrected during this time.[179,341] Any significant shift in position between visits necessitates cast wedging or a cast change, with remolding and possible fracture remanipulation if unacceptable displacement is present. Voto et al.[341] found that, in general, 7% of forearm fractures redisplace; this can occur up to 24 days after the initial manipulation. Davis[80] reported a 25% reangulation rate in complete fractures. Remanipulation can be done in the office following administration of oral analgesics. Judicious use of benzodiazepines may also be valuable because of their anxiolytic effects.

Although in adults the above-elbow cast generally is changed to a below-elbow cast after 3 to 4 weeks, this is unnecessary in most children because they heal more quickly and permanent elbow stiffness is rare.[171] A cast change at week 3 or 4 also can be traumatic to a young child and carries the additional small risk of cast saw injury. Once the fracture shows good callus formation, the cast can be removed. Because shaft fractures of the radius and ulna in children have a significant rate of refracture,[15,181,326] they should be splinted for an additional period of time.[67] Parents should be warned of the risk of refracture.

Above-elbow casting with the elbow in extension has been suggested for some complete fractures of the middle and proximal thirds.[293,344,348] The supination moment exerted by the biceps has been shown to be diminished when the elbow is extended.[224] Walker and Rang[344] reported successful treatment of 13 middle- or proximal-third forearm shaft fractures with this method (some following failed flexed-elbow casting). They suggested that the "short fat forearms" of some young children prevented successful flexed-elbow casting.[344] Shaer et al.[293] also reported 20 children treated with this method and emphasized full supination of the forearm. Three of their patients required cast wedging, but at final follow-up 19 of the 20 patients had excellent results.[293] One patient who was lost to follow-up for 6 months (presumably removing his own cast) did suffer "mild residual deformity."[293] Walker and Rang[344] recommended that benzoin be applied to the skin, in addition to creation of an adequate supracondylar mold, to further secure the cast. Casting the thumb in abduction with extra padding may prevent the cast from sliding. Turco[330] suggested that reduction should be obtained with horizontal traction applied to the extended upper extremity, followed by additional steps outlined in Table 10-5. Based on published clinical results, concerns related to cast slippage and elbow stiffness appear to have been overstated.[293,344] The main drawback of this technique is its awkwardness as compared to flexed-elbow casting.[344]

TABLE 10-5 Turco Technique for Extended Elbow Cast Treatment

1. Closed reduction under sedation
   a. Supine patient, fully supinated forearm
   b. Abducted shoulder
   c. Elbow extended (approximately 170 degrees)
2. Above-elbow cast applied
   a. Interosseous mold
   b. Supracondylar mold
3. Weekly radiographs first 3 weeks
4. Cast changes based on "Rule of 3s"
   a. 3 weeks at 170 degrees
   b. 3 weeks at 135 degrees
   c. 3 weeks at 90 degrees

Comminuted Fractures

Although comminuted forearm fractures are less common in children than in adults,[322] they do occur.[25,103,104,152,180,358] Comminuted fractures tend to occur in conjunction with high-energy injuries, such as open fractures.[152,205] Comminuted forearm fractures deserve special attention because they often require specially tailored treatment approaches. If satisfactory reduction cannot be achieved or maintained by closed methods, then other treatment alternatives should be considered.

One option is to accept some shortening; according to Price,[255] this may help maintain motion through interosseous membrane slackening. Shortening of more than 1 cm is unacceptable in either single-bone or both-bone comminuted patterns. Standard closed fracture treatment generally is unsuccessful when both bones are comminuted, and surgical stabilization may be necessary.[103] Bellemans and Lamoureux[25] reported intramedullary nailing of all comminuted forearm fractures in their pediatric series. Other reported fixation methods for comminuted forearm fractures in children include plate-and-screw devices,[103,104] flexible intramedullary nailing for single-bone comminution,[269] and pins-and-plaster techniques.[342] Bone grafting is rarely if ever indicated in acute comminuted forearm features in children.

CURRENT SURGICAL TREATMENT OPTIONS

Overview of Surgical Treatment

Duncan and Weiner[89] cited an "aggressive surgical mentality" as the reason for frequent operative treatment of pediatric forearm fractures, and Wilkins[352] expressed concern about "impetuous" surgeons who are too eager to operate. Cheng et al.[62] documented a more than 10-fold increase in the rate of operative treatment of forearm shaft fractures in children, but it is unclear as to whether this increase in operative treatment has led to a commensurate improvement in clinical outcomes.

Operative treatment of radial and ulnar shaft fractures usually is reserved for open fractures, those associated with compartment syndrome, floating elbow injuries, and fractures that develop unacceptable displacement during nonoperative management. Residual angulation after closed treatment is much better tolerated by younger children than older adolescents and adults because of the increased remodeling potential in the younger age group.[168] As a consequence, adolescents are more likely to benefit from surgical treatment of their forearm fractures than are younger children. Although internal fixation is the standard of care for displaced forearm fractures in adults, the success of nonoperative methods and the complications associated with internal fixation have tempered enthusiasm for its application to pediatric forearm fractures. Compared to closed treatment methods, healing is slower after open reduction and internal fixation,[25] no matter what type of implant is used.[103] Crossed Kirschner wire fixation techniques that often are used successfully in the distal radius are technically difficult in the shaft region of the radius and ulna. In rare situations, external fixation has been used for pediatric forearm fixation.[291]

Preoperative planning is essential regardless of which surgical technique is chosen. Assessment of the fracture, including rotation and the presence or absence of comminution, is important. Bone-plate mismatch (due to narrow bones and wide plates) and extensive soft tissue dissection are risks when adult-sized plates are applied to pediatric bones.[356] Before intramedullary nailing of fractures, the forearm intramedullary canal diameter should be measured, especially at the narrowest canal dimension; typically this is the central portion of the radius[305] and the distal portion of the ulna near the junction of its middle and distal thirds. Precise canal measurement can be difficult,[277,306] and the consequences of a nail or pin that is too large are probably worse than those of a nail or pin that is too small.[234,288] Modern digital radiography systems have made these measurements easier.[242]

Plate Fixation

Open reduction and internal fixation of pediatric forearm shaft fractures with plates and screws is a well-documented procedure in both pediatric series[240,310,323,333] and adult series that include patients as young as 13[60] and even 7[60] years of age. In one of the early series of pediatric forearm fractures fixed with plates,[83] dynamic compression plates and one-third tubular plates applied with standard atlas orthogonal technique (six cortices above and below the fracture site) obtained good results.[227] Four-cortex fixation on either side of the fracture site has been shown to be equally effective in pediatric forearm fractures.[358]

Plate fixation uses the standard adult approach and technique except that smaller plates (2.7-mm compression and stacked one-third tubular), fewer screws, and single-bone fixation often are acceptable.[358] Plate fixation may allow more anatomic and stable correction of rotational and angular abnormalities and restoration of the radial bow than with noncontoured intramedullary rods; however, the larger incisions and extensive surgical exposures required for plate fixation have raised concerns regarding unsightly scars[275,333,356] and muscle fibrosis with consequent motion loss.[358] While the cosmetic concerns seem valid, ultimate forearm motion is similar with the two techniques, with only minor losses reported in the literature after both plating and intramedullary nailing.[74,168,297,332] Fernandez et al.[97] recently documented these precise issues very nicely in that they found no significant differences in functional outcome in their plate fixation versus intramedullary nailing patients, but they noted the longer operating room time and inferior cosmesis of the plated patients.

Open reduction and internal fixation with plates and screws may be appropriate in the management of fractures with delayed presentation or fractures that angulate late in the course of cast care,[135,358] when significant fracture callus makes closed reduction and percutaneous passage of intramedullary nails difficult or impossible.[13] Other indications for plate fixation include shaft fractures with significant comminution[103] and impending or established malunion[329] or nonunion.[136,189,234] Several authors have reported good results with plate fixation of the radius only[50,105,240,262] or the ulna only (Fig. 10-26).[26] Bhaskar and Roberts[26] compared 20 children with both-bone plate fixation to 12 with ulna-only fixation and found significantly more complications in the dual plating group, although motion was equal at 1-year follow-up. Single-bone fixation requires satisfactory reduction of both bones. Flynn and Waters[105] stated that they would preferentially plate the radius only when the fracture could not be reduced by closed means. Two patients in Bhaskar and Roberts'[26] study required open reduction and internal fixation of the radius when it was not adequately reduced after plate fixation of the ulna.

Kirschner Wire, Rush Rod, and Steinmann Pin Intramedullary Fixation

Currently, intramedullary fixation is the preferred method for internal fixation of forearm fractures in children.[10,48,180,188,194,259,260,337] Intramedullary fixation of children's forearm fractures dates back at least to Fleischer's 1975 report in the German literature in which he called it "marrow wiring."[101] Closed intramedullary nailing (also known as indirect reduction and internal fixation) of diaphyseal forearm fractures in adolescents was later reported in the English language literature by Ligier et al.,[191] Amit et al.,[10] and others.[30,184,356] A variety of implants have been used for forearm intramedullary nailing, including Kirschner wires, Rush rods, and Steinmann pins. Continued favorable reports from around the world (e.g., England, Germany, New Zealand, Turkey, and the United States) have established intramedullary fixation as the surgical treatment of choice.[56,115,162,188,267]

Intramedullary fixation has several advantages over plate fixation, including improved cosmesis because of smaller incisions and less deep tissue dissection, potentially leading to a lower risk of stiffness.[74,180,297,356] Contoured pins are used in the radius to preserve its natural anatomic bow[10,74,259,267,346]; contoured pins are not necessary for the ulna.[10] Although the rotational stability of pediatric forearm fractures treated with intramedullary fixation has been questioned, Blasier and Salaman[30] suggested that the strong periosteum in children resists torsional stresses. In a cadaver study of the rotational stability of fractures of the ulna and radius treated with Rush rods, Ono et al.[238] found that intramedullary fixation of both bones reduced fracture rotation to one eighth of that in unfixed fractures.

Elastic Stable Intramedullary Nailing

In the early 1980s, Metaizeau et al.[216] described elastic stable intramedullary nailing (ESIN) of pediatric forearm fractures

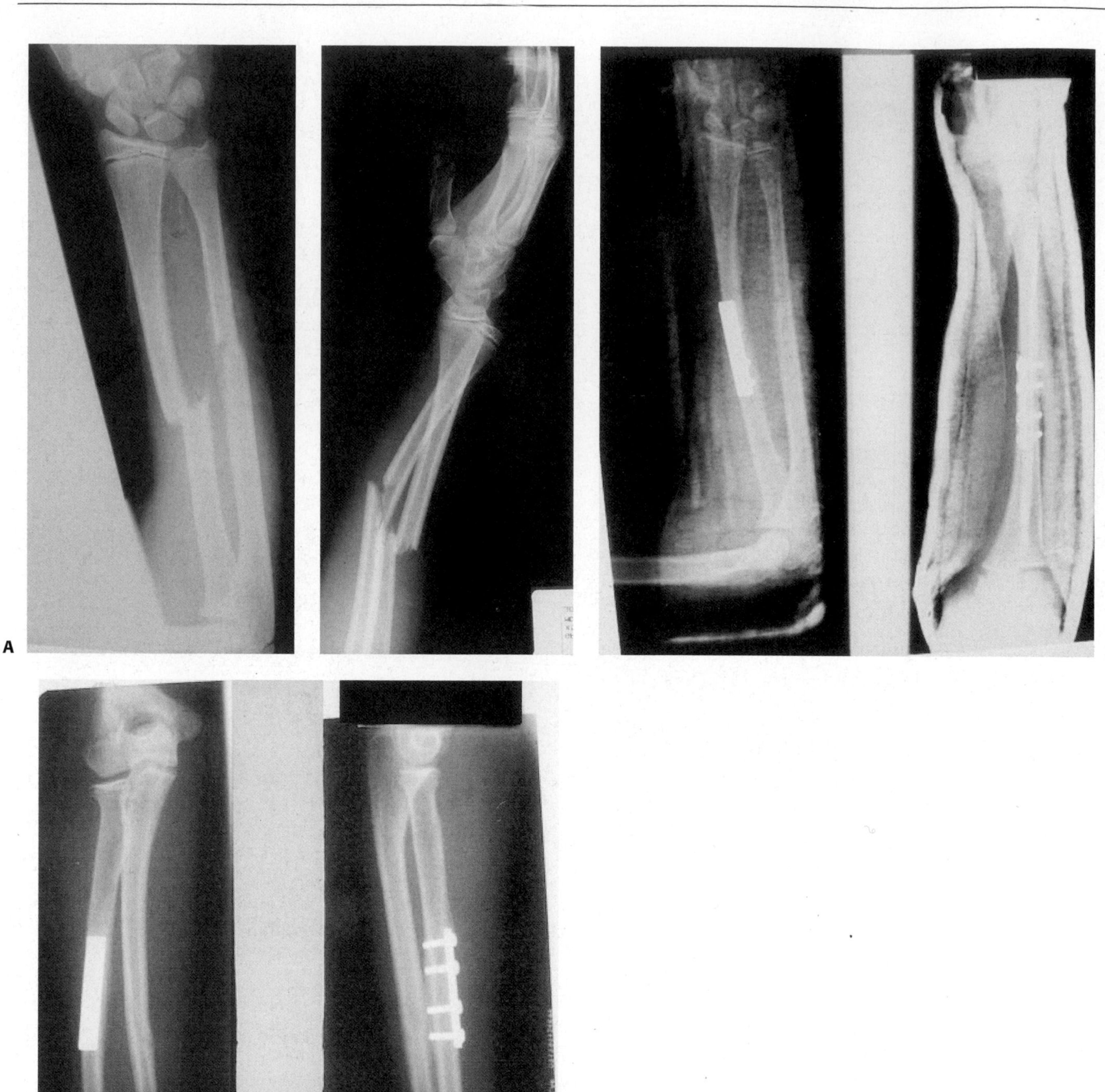

FIGURE 10-26 Single-bone plate fixation (radius only). **A.** A 12-year-old female with both-bone forearm fracture (AP and lateral). **B.** Immediate postoperative images. **C.** Two-year follow-up images. (Courtesy of Tom Welle, DO.)

with small-diameter (1.5- to 2.5-mm) contoured implants.[191] No effort was made to fill the medullary canal as with other intramedullary nailing techniques,[269] and the "summit of the curve must be calculated preoperatively to lie at the level of the fracture."[184] The prebent flexible rods (known as Nancy nails) were reported to maintain satisfactory fracture alignment while encouraging development of normal physiologic fracture callus.[191,216,251] Biomechanically, these implants have been shown to act as internal splints provided the nails extend three or more diameters beyond the fracture site.[158] Good results with this technique have been reported by numerous authors (Figs. 10-27 and 10-28).[131,225,269,287,294,325,328,357]

Because the ESIN technique emphasizes the interdependence of the radius and ulna, if both bones are fractured, both

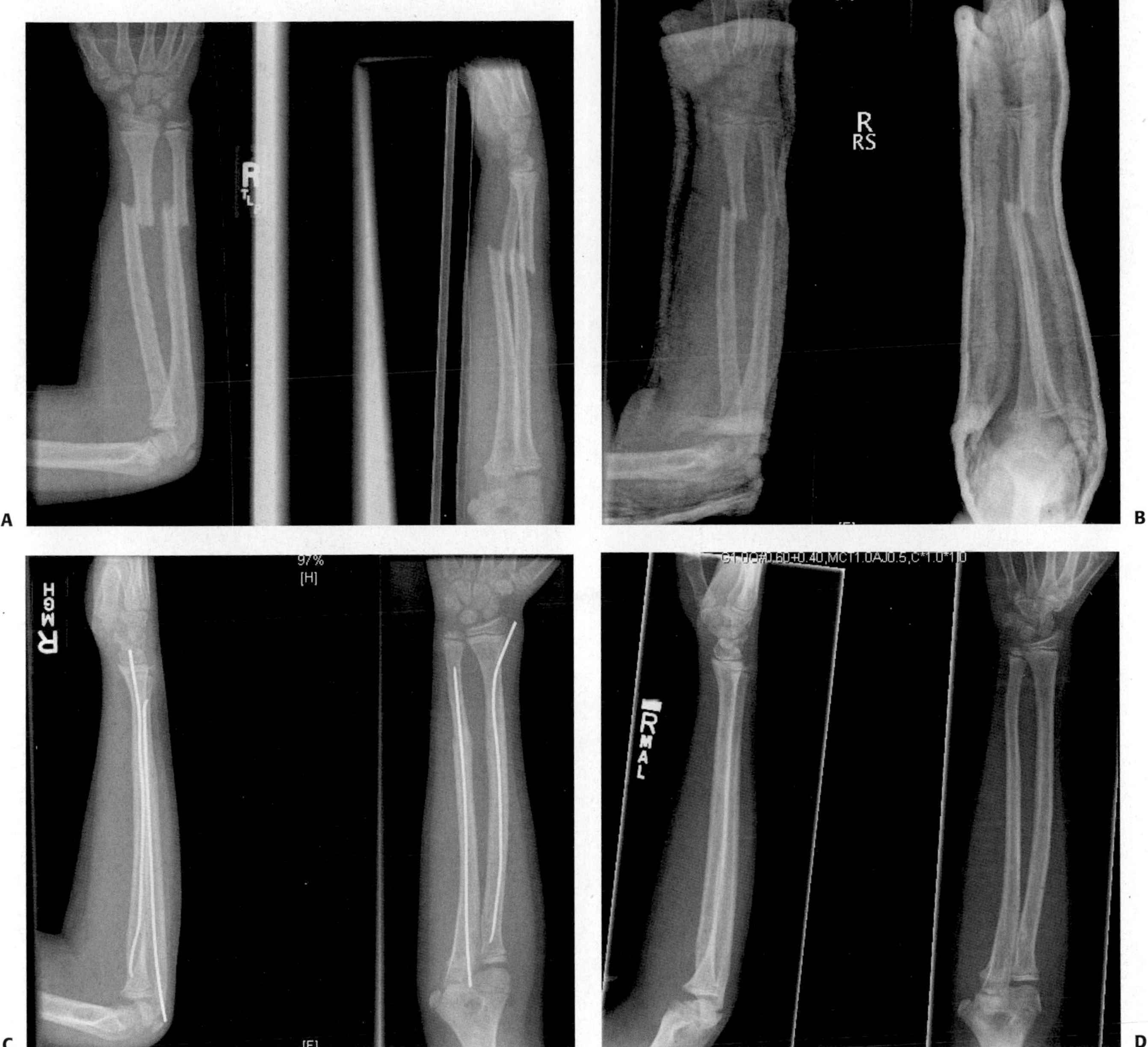

FIGURE 10-27 A 10-year-old male whose both-bone complete forearm fracture near the junction of the middle and distal thirds was treated with elastic stable intramedullary nailing. **A.** Injury radiographs demonstrating completely displaced radial and ulnar shaft fractures. **B.** Postreduction radiographs reveal unsatisfactory angular alignment as well as significant loss of radial bow. **C.** Anatomic appearance following ESIN. **D.** One and a half year follow-up radiographs. Nails were removed 6 months postoperatively. *(continues)*

bones are internally fixed.[184] It also is dependent on anchorage of the nails in the upper and lower metaphyseal portions of the bone to produce an internal three-point fixation construct.[184] Technique principles include fixing first the bone that is easiest to reduce, using physeal-sparing entry points, and using small nails varying in diameter from 1.5 to 2.5 mm.[184] A nail that is too large may lead to nail incarceration and distraction at the fracture site, especially in the ulna.[234] Contouring of both nails is recommended, with particular attention to restoration of the appropriate radial bow (Fig. 10-29). Initially, nails were removed by about the fourth postoperative month, but several refractures led the originators of the technique to delay nail removal until 1 full year after surgery.[184] Pin ends should be cut short and buried to maintain prolonged fixation.

Immediate motion has been recommended by some authors after ESIN of pediatric forearm fractures,[25,131,184,337] while others have recommended immobilization for variable periods of time.[48] Early refracture with nails in place has been reported. Bellemans and Lamoureux[25] considered displaced oblique or comminuted midshaft forearm fractures in children older than 7 years of age to be an indication for ESIN. They considered bayonet apposition (overriding) to be unacceptable at any age because of concerns about rotational malalignment and frequent narrowing of the interosseous space.[25] Their fixation technique

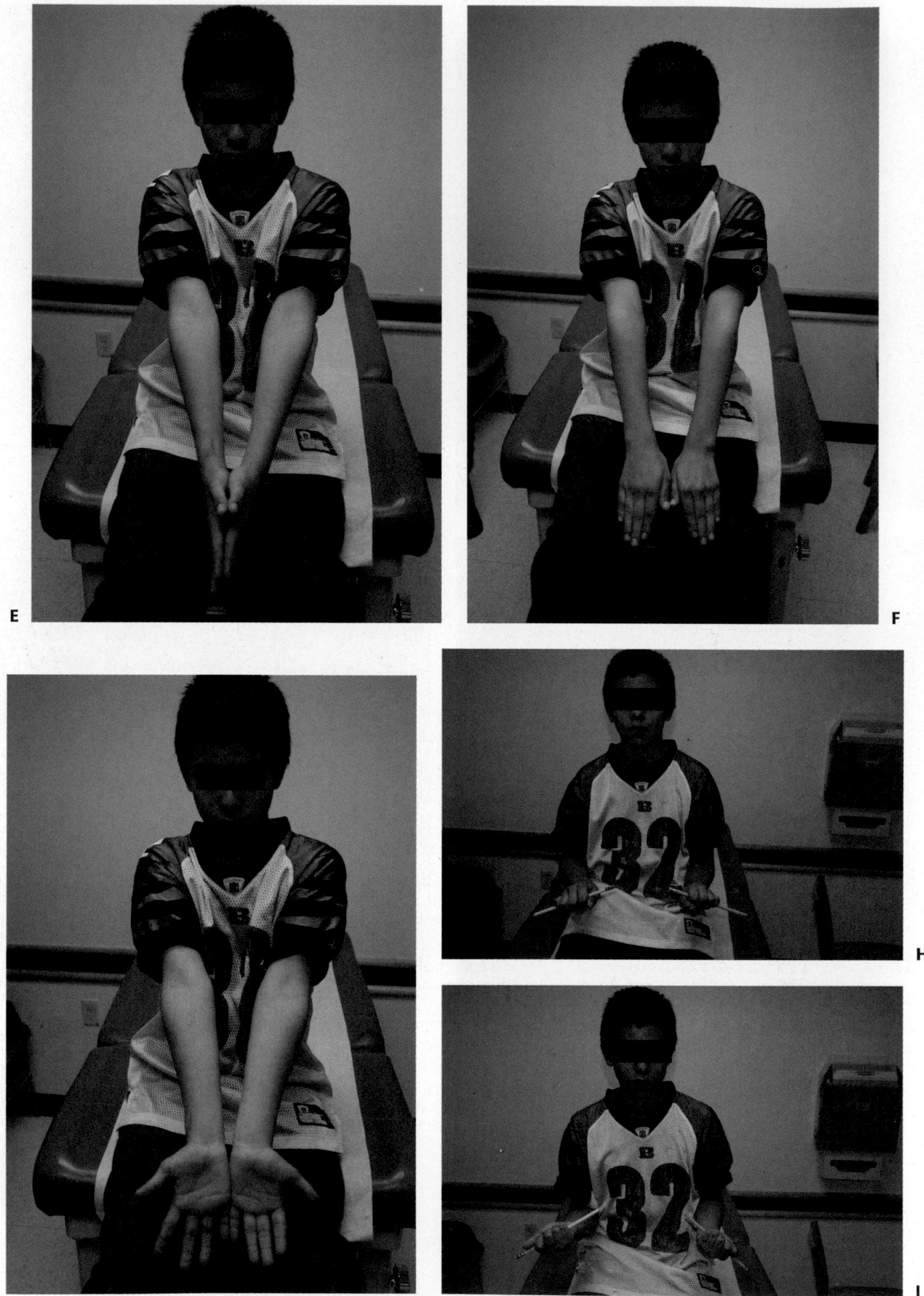

FIGURE 10-27 *(continued)* **E.** Clinical appearance with extended elbows and forearm midposition. **F.** Clinical appearance with extended elbows and pronated forearms. **G.** Clinical appearance with extended elbows and supinated forearms. **H.** Symmetrical pronation. **I.** Symmetrical supination.

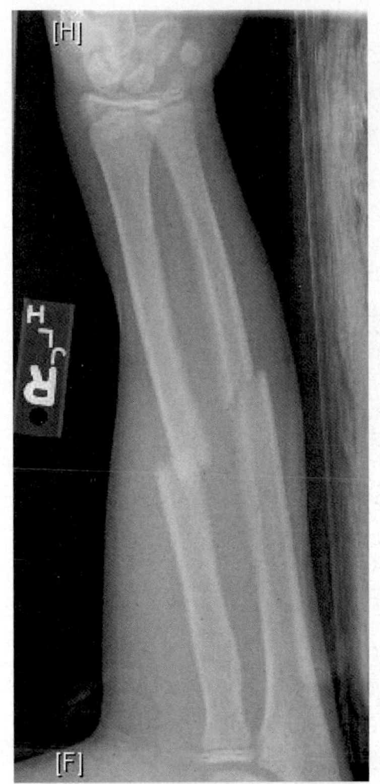

A

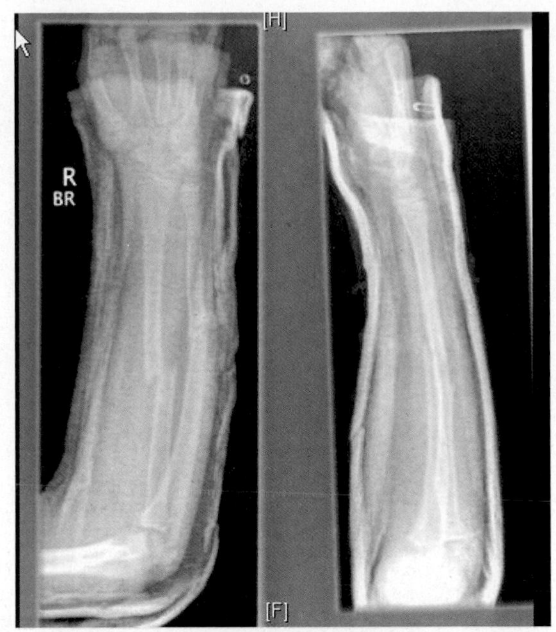

C

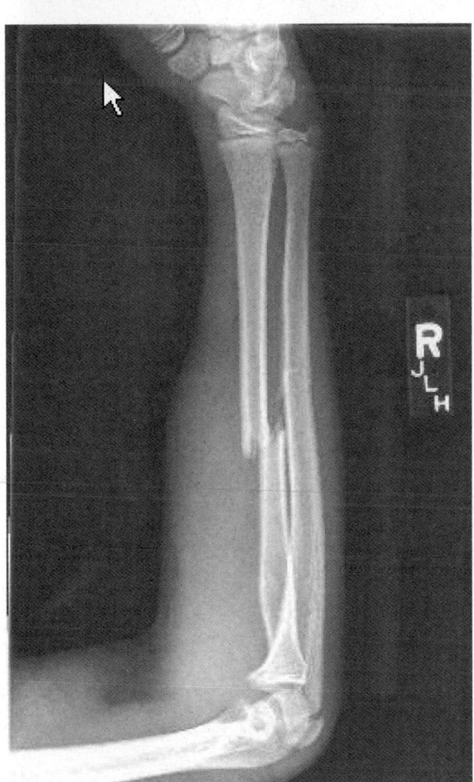

B

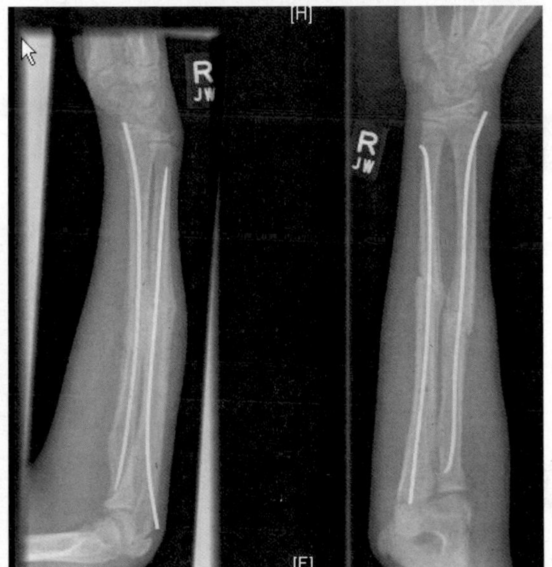

D

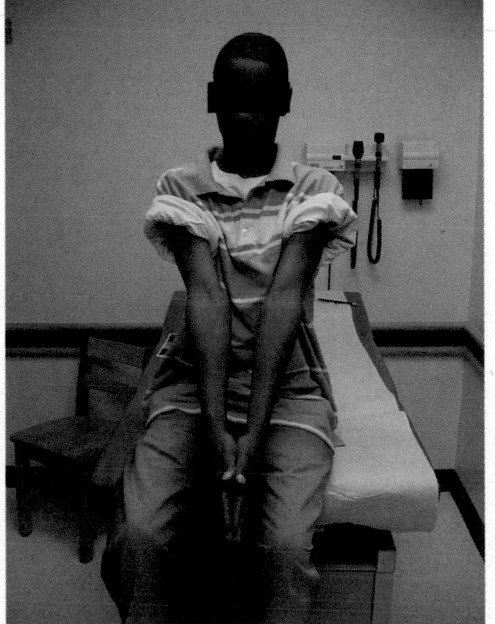

E

FIGURE 10-28 An 11-year-old male whose both-bone midshaft complete forearm shaft fracture was treated with elastic stable intramedullary nailing. **A.** Injury AP radiograph. **B.** Injury lateral radiograph. **C.** Postreduction radiographs demonstrating unacceptable angular alignment. **D.** Improved alignment status ater ESIN. **E.** Clinical appearance with extended elbows and forearm midposition. *(continues)*

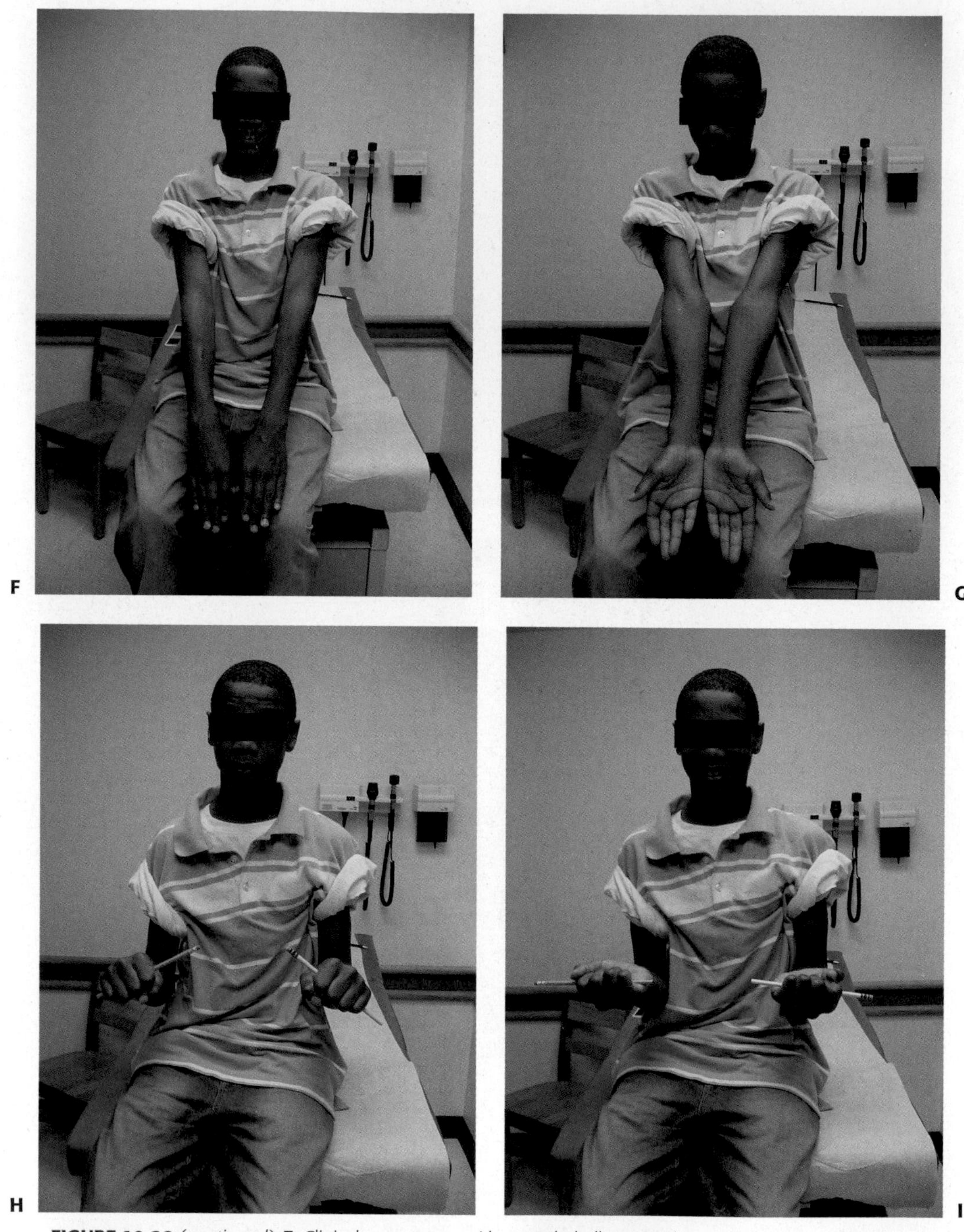

FIGURE 10-28 (*continued*) **F.** Clinical appearance with extended elbows and pronated forearms. **G.** Clinical appearance with extended elbows and supinated forearms. **H.** Symmetrical pronation. **I.** Symmetrical supination. (*continues*)

involved passage of the intramedullary nails followed by rotation of each nail until the greatest distance between the two bones was achieved in full supination.[25]

Management of Open Fractures

In one large epidemiologic study, open fractures of the shafts of the radius and ulna and open tibial shaft fractures occurred with equal frequency, making them the most common open fractures in children.[62] Although the infection rate is extremely low for open fractures, even grade I open forearm fractures in children have been associated with serious complications such as gas gangrene.[96] Early irrigation and débridement[212,302] are indicated for open forearm fractures, and care should be taken to inspect and properly clean the bone ends.[165] Roy and Crawford[275] recommended routinely inspecting both of the bone ends for the presence of intramedullary foreign material (Fig. 10-30). Once débrided, open forearm fractures can be stabilized by any of the available internal fixation methods without undue risk of infection (Fig. 10-31).[128,135,195] Open fractures tend to be more unstable than closed fractures (because of soft tissue stripping and comminution) and more commonly require internal fixation. Internal fixation also may facilitate soft tissue management and healing.[358] Professor Lim[192] and his co-authors

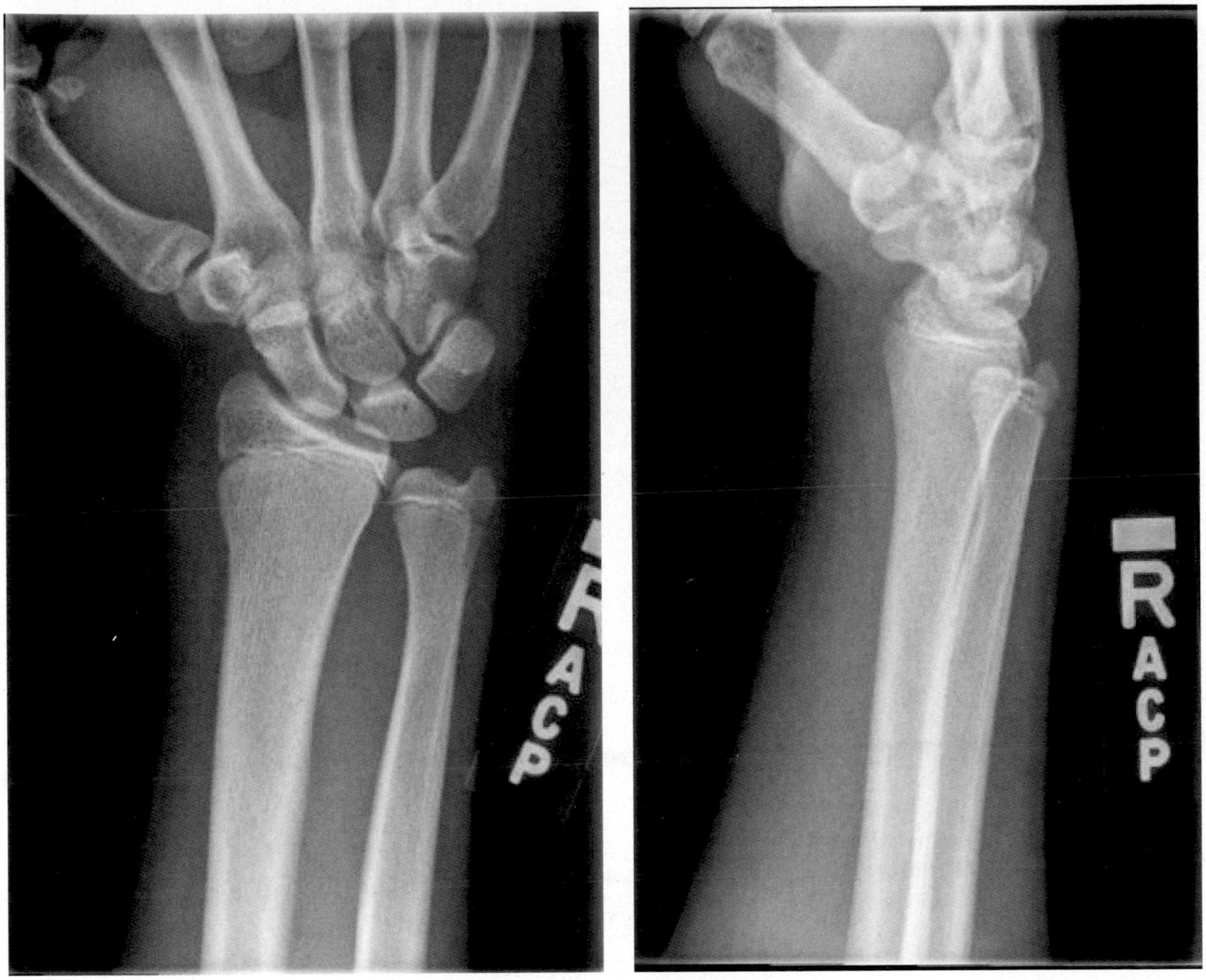

J

K

FIGURE 10-28 (*continued*) **J.** Thirty-nine month follow-up AP wrist radiograph and lateral **(K)** wrist radiograph (taken due to new trauma) demonstrating normal bony anatomy. Nails were removed 6 months postoperatively.

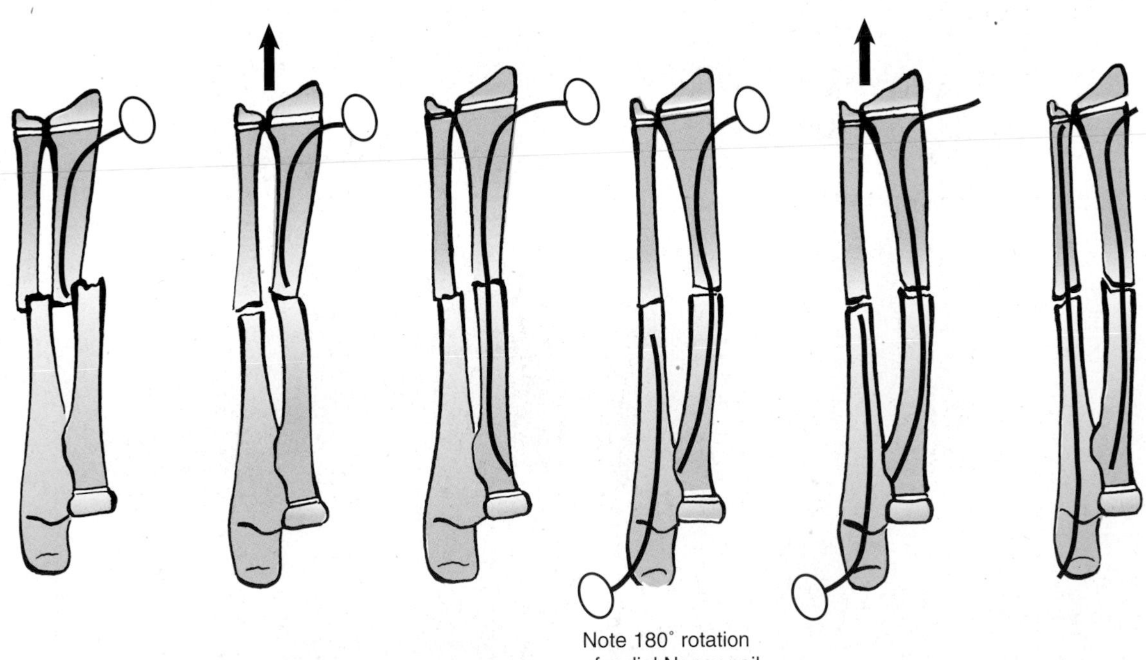
Note 180° rotation
of radial Nancy nail

FIGURE 10-29 Metaizeau elastic stable intramedullary nailing technique. The radial rod is twisted 180 degrees in step 4 to re-establish the radial bow.

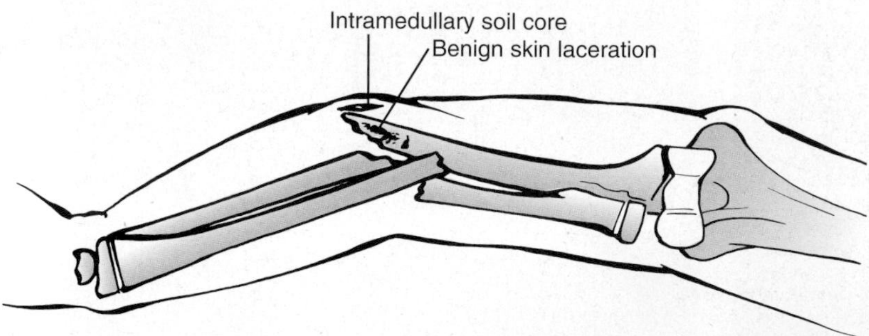

FIGURE 10-30 Intramedullary organic contamination of an open forearm fractures.

from the KK Children's Hospital in Singapore recently reminded us that internal fixation is not an absolute prerequisite and many children with such open fractures may still be successfully managed with casting alone.

The amount of periosteal stripping and possible foreign body reaction associated with open forearm fractures may produce an unusual radiographic appearance: the "ruffled border sign" (Fig. 10-32). Usually, this seems to represent a normal healing response in growing children, but occasionally it is an early sign of osteomyelitis. The infection rate ranges from 0% to 33% for open fractures in children.[128,74,128,135,179,195,230,240,255,358] Even grade I open forearm fractures in children can be complicated by gas gangrene or osteomyelitis, and therapeutic amputation has been reported.[80,96,152] Open fracture grade does not appear to correlate with the infection rate in childhood forearm fractures, with most of the serious forearm infections reported in the literature occurring after grade I fractures.

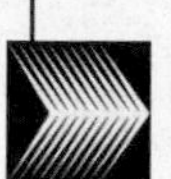

AUTHORS' PREFERRED METHOD OF TREATMENT

Closed Fracture Care

We agree with Jones and Weiner that "closed reduction still remains the gold standard for closed isolated pediatric forearm fractures."[161] Most nondisplaced and minimally displaced radial and ulnar shaft fractures can be splinted in the emergency department and referred for orthopaedic follow-up within 1 week. Radiographs are repeated at the first orthopaedic visit, and a cast is applied. During warmer weather, when fracture incidence peaks, we tend to use waterproof cast liners. We avoid flexing the elbow past 80 to 90 degrees in waterproof casts because the soft tissue crease that forms in the antecubital fossa tends to trap moisture. Because waterproof cast lining alone does not shield the skin from cast saw cuts and burns as well as traditional padding does, specialized material may be added along the anticipated

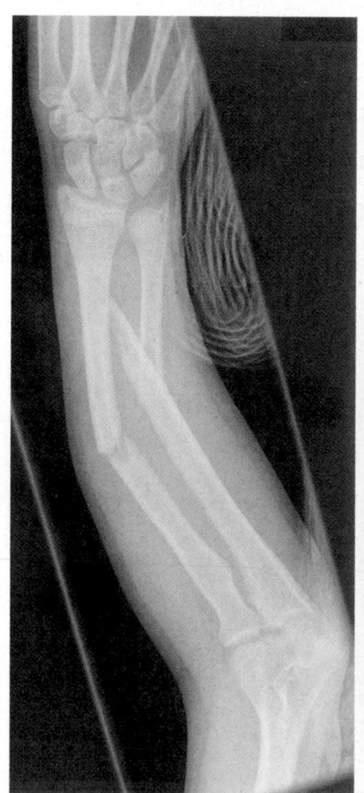
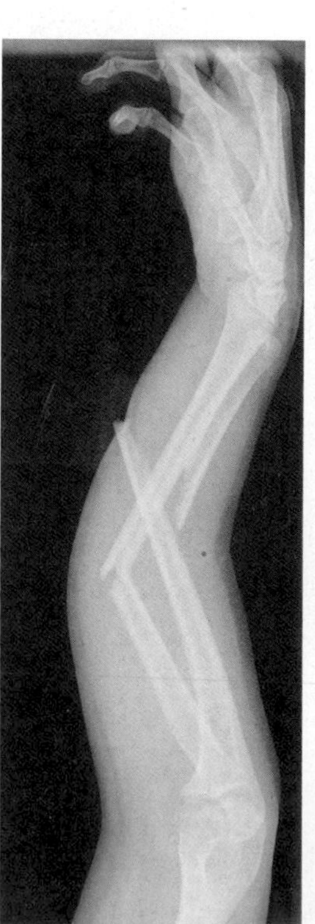
A
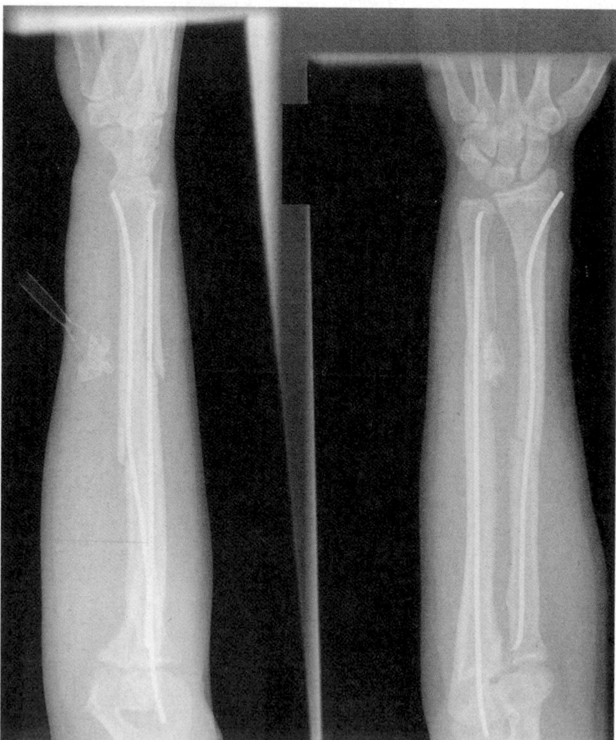
B

FIGURE 10-31 A 13-year-old female with open forearm fracture. **A.** AP and lateral radiographs; note extrusion of ulna on lateral view. **B.** After irrigation and débridement and flexible nail internal fixation. Note the Penrose drain in the ulnar wound.

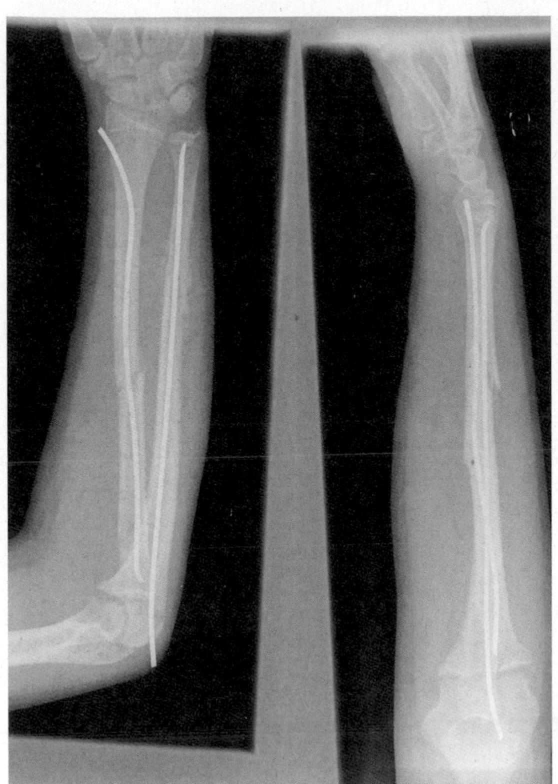

FIGURE 10-32 Ruffled border sign at the site of previous open fracture of ulna; same patient from Figure 10-28 at 1-month follow-up.

course of the cast saw to protect the skin during cast removal. Two such materials are blue cast strips (De-Flex Strip Cast Removal Aid, WL Gore & Associates, Flagstaff, AZ) and a plastic zipstrip (inserted between the skin and cast liner).

We prefer an above-elbow cast for all forearm fractures in children under the age of 4 years, because young children tend to lose or remove a below-elbow cast due to soft tissue differences (baby fat) common to the age group.[86] Most older children with forearm shaft fractures also are treated with above-elbow casting, except for those with stable distal-third fractures. Good forearm casting technique should focus on the principles outlined earlier in this chapter. Patients with nondisplaced fractures usually are re-evaluated radiographically in 1 to 2 weeks after initial immobilization to check for fracture displacement. Forearm shaft fractures heal more slowly than metaphyseal and physeal fractures of the distal radius and ulna.[15,80] The cast is removed in 6 to 8 weeks if adequate healing is present on radiographs. Because of the significant refracture rate after forearm shaft fractures, we splint these fractures for another several weeks until all transverse lucency of the original fracture disappears and all four cortices are healed. Fractures that heal in bayonet apposition (complete translation and some shortening) can take longer to heal than those with end-to-end apposition and may require prolonged splinting to prevent refracture.[86,273]

Fracture Reduction/Conscious Sedation Protocol

Significantly displaced forearm shaft fractures are usually manipulated in the emergency department using a conscious sedation protocol. After obtaining informed consent for conscious sedation and fracture manipulation, an intravenous line is started, and the child's blood pressure, pulse, respirations, electrocardiogram, and peripheral oxygen level are monitored during the procedure and for about 30 minutes after the procedure. We use ketamine and midazolam administered intravenously in divided doses. Although many children moan or cry briefly during the manipulation, very few recall pain. Reductions are done under mini-C-arm (fluoroscopy) control. The initial position of forearm rotation is based on the level of the fracture, and the final position is based on the best reduction under fluoroscopy. Small portable fluoroscopy units save time and money (estimated to be 10% of the cost of conventional radiographs) and lessen radiation dosage to patient and clinician compared to traditional fluoroscopy. Finger-trap traction with 10 to 15 pounds of counterweight frequently is used for completely displaced both-bone forearm fractures (especially those with shortening). We do not complete greenstick fractures because the partial bone continuity adds stability.

Because of concerns about soft tissue swelling, manipulated fractures are placed into a plaster sugar-tong splint (incorporating the elbow). Before manipulation, the sugar-tong splint is prepared by laying out 7 to 10 layers of appropriate-length 3-inch plaster casting material on top of a work surface. A four-layer matched length of cotton cast padding also is laid out and will form the inner padding (skin side) of the splint. A final single layer of cast padding is laid out and will form the outer layer of the splint to prevent elastic wrap adherence to the plaster. Once manipulation is completed, the plaster is dipped, wrung out, smoothed, and then sandwiched between the dry four-ply and one-ply cotton padding. This splint is then placed with the four-ply cotton side against the skin and secured with an elastic bandage. We prefer to avoid the circumferential application of cotton padding because it may limit splint expansion during follow-up swelling. If necessary, parents also can unwrap and loosen the elastic bandage at home to relieve pressure if swelling makes the splint too tight. Patients are given discharge instructions and a prescription for mild narcotic analgesics.

Patients usually return to the office within a week for repeat radiographs and clinical assessment. Provided that satisfactory alignment has been maintained, we remove the elastic wrap but leave the plaster sugar-tong splint in place. The splint is "boxed in" by applying cotton cast padding over the splint and the exposed upper arm, and by wrapping with fiberglass to convert the splint into an above-elbow cast. Follow-up radiographs are taken of manipulated fractures at about 1-week intervals for the next 2 weeks. Fractures that are losing position but are still in acceptable alignment usually require removal and remolding of a new cast to prevent further position deterioration. Minor remanipulations can be done in the office after appropriate administration of oral analgesics and anxiolytics. Major remanipulations are best done with general anesthesia. The decision regarding remanipulation may be aided by the viewing of the cosmetic deformity by the parents and physician after all splint and cast materials are removed.

By the end of the fourth week after injury, many above-elbow casts can be converted to below-elbow casts (often a waterproof cast in warm weather). This step may be omitted in younger children because of their faster healing and their minimal inconvenience from temporary elbow immobilization.[171] Patients can return to sports after conversion to a below-elbow cast as long as the cast is padded during play and league rules allow casts. Patients usually are required to have a physician's note allowing sports participation with a cast. This decision is made with the patient's and parents' understanding of potential increase in refracture risk. Adequate fracture healing (bridging callus of four cortices) usually has occurred after several more weeks of cast treatment but should be confirmed by radiographic and physical examination before unlimited athletic participation. Older children are given home elastic band strengthening exercises and allowed to participate in normal activities while they continue to be protected in either a removable Velcro fracture brace or a customized thermoplastic forearm gauntlet brace. Formal physical therapy rarely is required. This fracture protocol is aimed at minimizing refracture risk.

Acceptable Limits of Angulation

Based on available evidence in the literature, we accept approximately 20 degrees of angulation in distal-third shaft fractures of the radius and ulna, 15 degrees at the midshaft level, and 10 degrees in the proximal third (provided the child has at least 2 years of growth remaining).[361] We accept 100% translation if shortening is less than 1 cm. Although other authors recommend accepting up to 45 degrees of rotation, we find this is extremely difficult to measure accurately using the bicipital tuberosity and radial styloid as landmarks because of the lack of anatomic distinction in younger children. Plastic deformation fractures seem to have less remodeling potential than other fractures, and radiographically or cosmetically unacceptable angulation may require gradual, forceful manipulation under sedation or general anesthesia. Children approaching skeletal maturity (less than 2 years of remaining growth) should be treated using adult criteria because of their reduced remodeling potential. Parents should be cautioned that even mild angulation of the ulna, especially posterior sag, will produce an obvious deformity after cast removal because of the subcutaneous location of the bone (Fig. 10-33). This cosmetic deformity is exacerbated by abundant callus formation, but it will ultimately remodel if it falls within acceptable angulation criteria. Ulnar sag may be countered by placing the child in an extended elbow cast. Mild to moderate angulation of the radius usually produces much less cosmetic deformity but may limit motion more (Fig. 10-34).

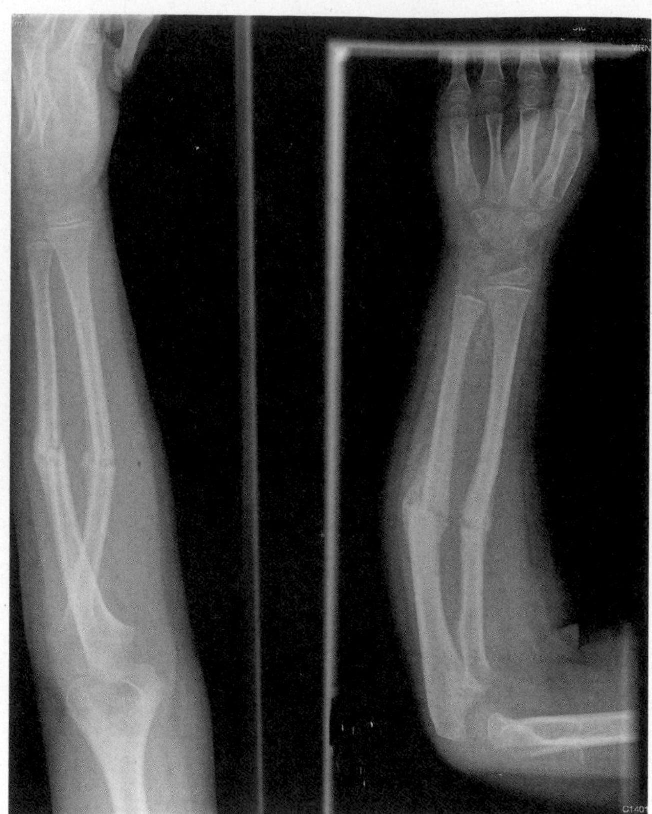

FIGURE 10-33 Ulnar sag on serial radiographs. Note the prominent ulnar fracture callus.

Surgical Treatment

Most forearm shaft fractures continue to be successfully treated with closed methods at our institution. Our top two indications for surgical treatment of these injuries are open shaft fractures and shaft fractures that exceed our stated reduction limits. If surgical treatment is deemed necessary, intramedullary fixation is preferred over plate fixation because of reduced soft tissue disruption. We occasionally fix one bone when both bones are fractured if overall forearm alignment is acceptable and stable after single-bone fixation.

If single-bone fixation is done, the ulna usually is treated first because of its more benign entry site, subcutaneous location, and relatively straight canal compared to the radius. Our preferred intramedullary ulnar entry site is just distal to the olecranon apophysis (anconeus starting point), just anterior to the subcutaneous border of the proximal ulna on its lateral side. Care is taken not to enter the ulna more than 5 mm anterior to its subcutaneous crest to avoid encroachment into the region of the proximal radioulnar joint. Pins placed directly through the tip of the olecranon apophysis have a strong tendency to cause bursitis and pain until removal. We prefer to open the cortex with an awl because it tends to wander less than motorized drills and it allows ulnar entry with little or no formal incision. The awl technique also simplifies operating room setup in that no pneumatic hose hookups or battery packs are necessary.

If dual bone fixation is elected, then the radius is fixed first as it is usually more difficult. The distal radial entry site can be either through a physeal-sparing direct lateral approach through the floor of the first dorsal compartment or dorsally near the proximal extent of the Lister tubercle between the second and third dorsal compartments. Both of these entry points are approximately 1 cm proximal to the physis of the distal radius. We insert the radial nail through a 1- to 2-cm incision, protecting the superficial radial nerve and the dorsal tendons with small blunt retractors. An awl is used to gain intramedullary access to the radius. We typically use small intramedullary nails (2.0 to 2.5 mm in diameter) to maintain some flexibility at the fracture site and stimulate appropriate callus formation. Larger nails may become incarcerated in either the narrow central canal of the radius or that of the distal third of the ulna. Care must be taken

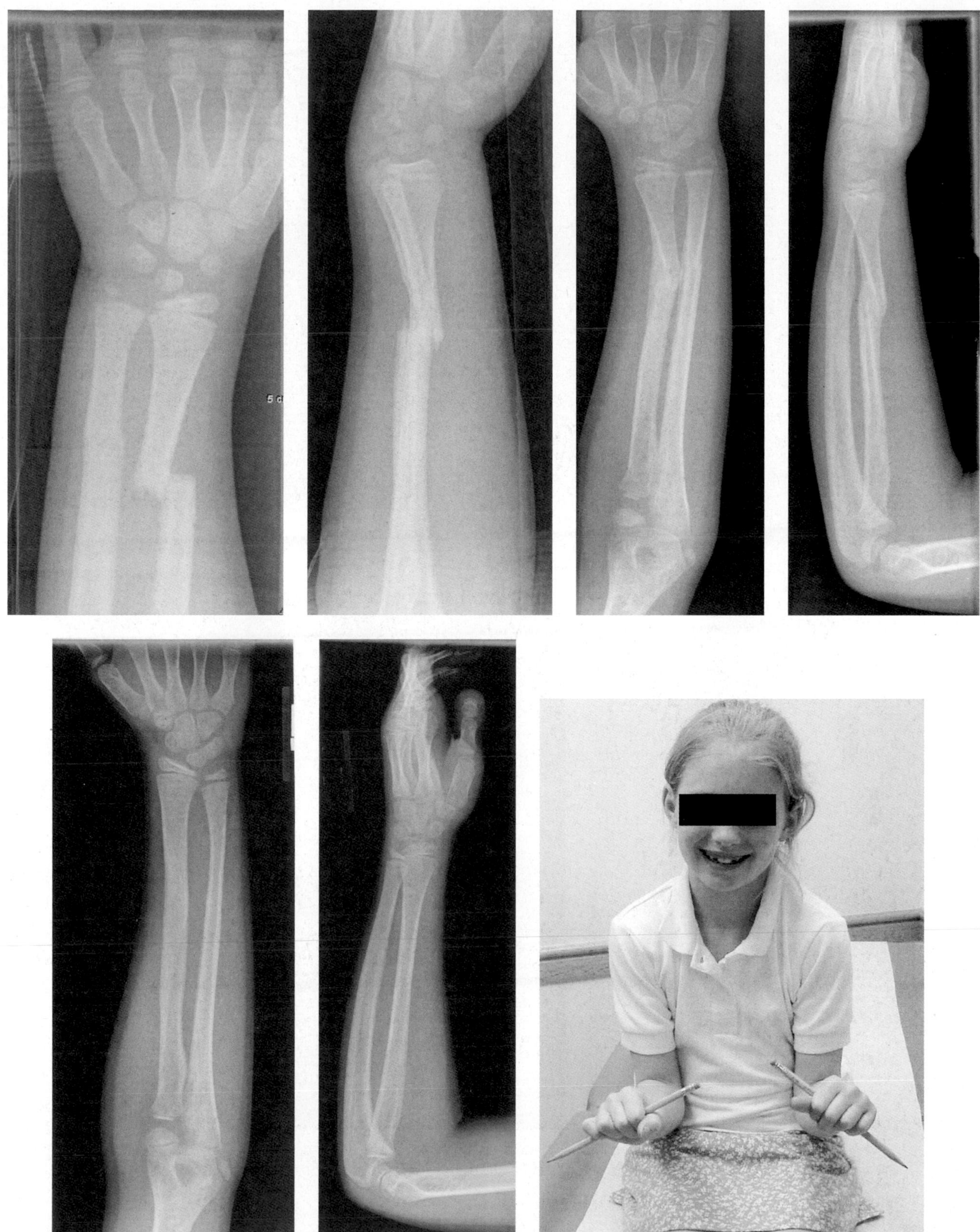

FIGURE 10-34 A 7-year-old female with left both-bone complete forearm fracture. **A.** AP and lateral injury radiographs. **B.** Two-month follow-up radiographs. **C.** Two-year follow-up radiograph shows mild residual deformity. **D.** Pronation. *(continues)*

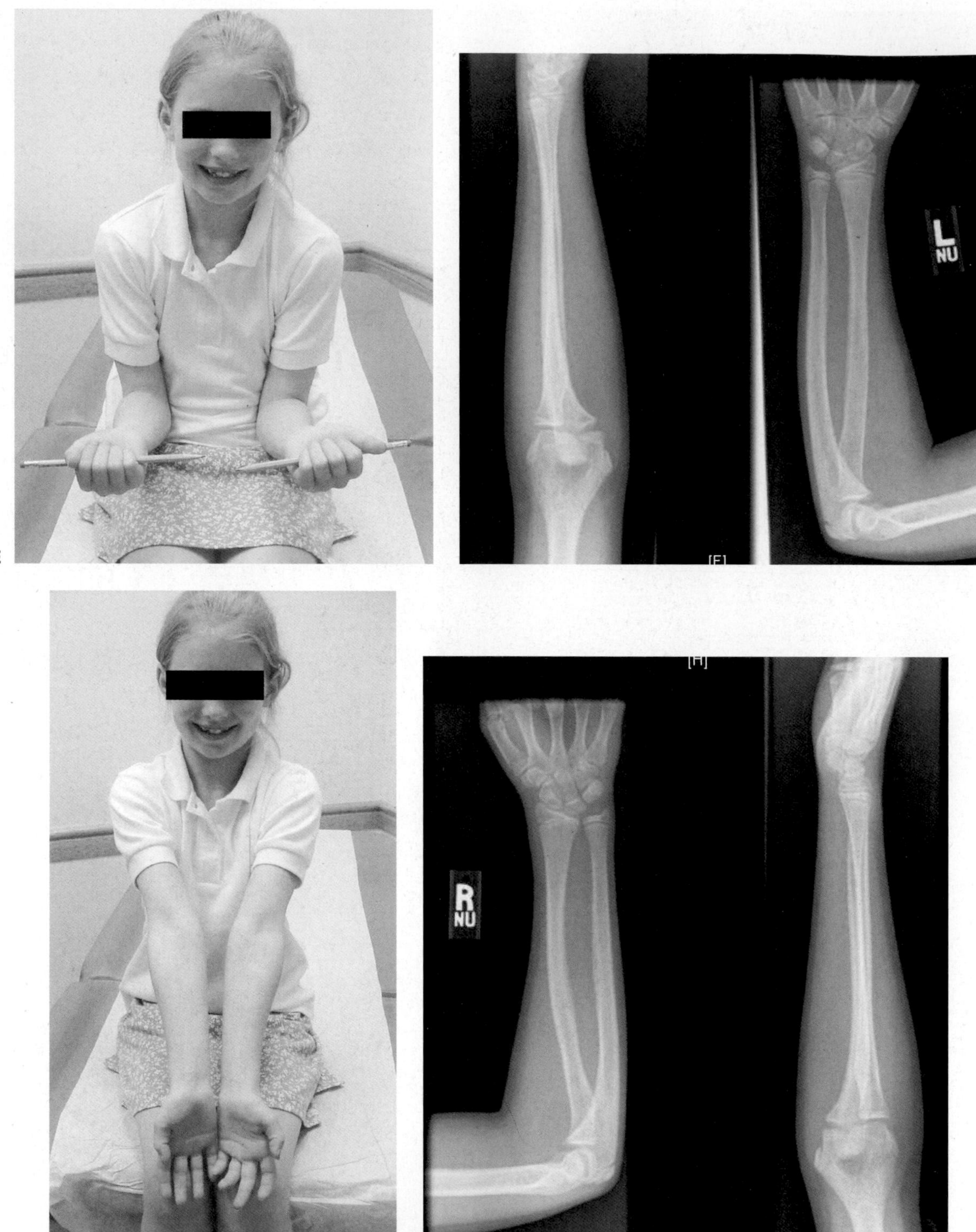

FIGURE 10-34 *(continued)* **E.** Supination. **F.** Axial alignment at 2-year follow-up. **G**. Five-year follow-up radiographs of left forearm with mild loss of radial bow. **H.** Comparison radiographs of right forearm.

(continues)

to not overbend the tip of the nail as this effectively increases the diameter of the implant and may impede its intramedullary passage. Failure to pass the intramedullary nail across the fracture site after several attempts may necessitate a limited open reduction through a 1- to 2-cm incision to directly pass the rod across the fracture site (Fig. 10-35). Persistence in attempting to achieve closed reduction and rodding has been associated with compartment syndrome.[363] We are sensitive to both time and attempts during ESIN of forearm shaft fractures in our pediatric patients and recommend adherence to the 17-minute rule (taught to us by our senior partner Alvin Crawford) and the three strikes and you are out rule. If either closed reduction attempts for a particular forearm bone exceed 17 minutes or if three low-amplitude

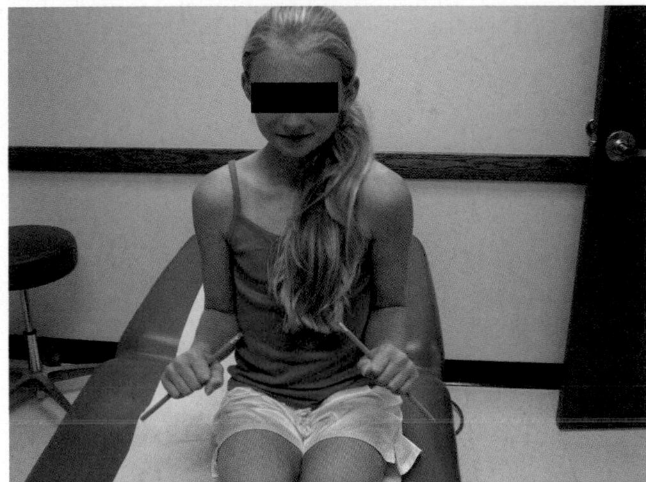

I

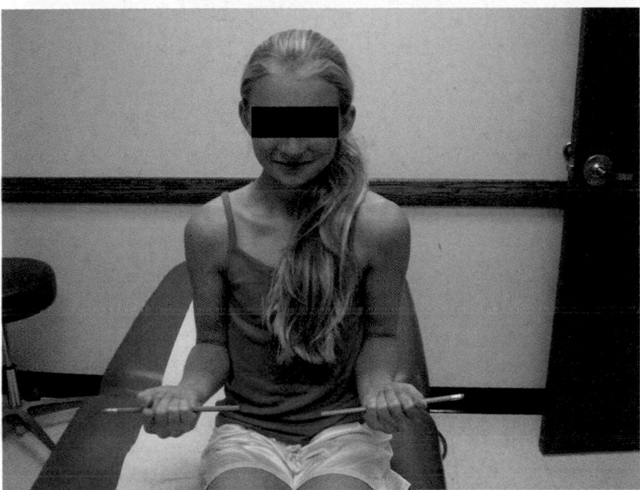

J

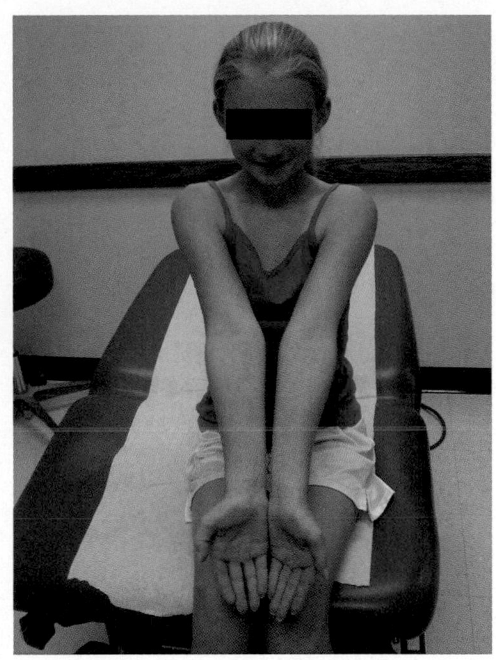

K

FIGURE 10-34 (*continued*) **I.** Pronation. **J.** Supination. **K.** Axial alignment at 5-year follow-up.

efforts to pass the intramedullary nail across the fracture site have been unsuccessful, then rapid conversion to a small open reduction is suggested.

We prefer to leave the nails buried beneath the skin because complete fracture healing takes at least 2 months, often more. Because refracture can even occur with nails in place, we protect children for at least the first month with a removable fracture brace. If a single bone of a both-bone fracture is fixed, above-elbow cast immobilization usually is necessary instead of a below-elbow cast or brace, as is used after dual-bone fixation. After the appearance of satisfactory callus, splint and activity restrictions are progressively relaxed. We recommend nail removal after complete four-cortex healing of each bone (6 to 12 months in some patients).

Plating is preferred to intramedullary nailing when early malunion is present and callus formation is noted radiographically. Plating allows open osteoclasis and reduction. The plating technique is similar to that used in adults, except that smaller plates can be used and fewer cortices (often only four cortices above and below the fracture) are required for adequate fixation. In children with both-bone forearm fractures, plating of a single bone may be adequate and reduce the morbidity associated with dual-bone plating.[26] Significant comminution of both bones also may be an indication for plate fixation.

COMPLICATIONS

Redisplacement/Malalignment

The most common short-term complication of forearm shaft fracture treatment is loss of satisfactory reduction in a previously well-reduced and well-aligned fracture, a complication that occurs in 10%[58,65,80,161,342] to 25% of patients.[58,80] Initial follow-up radiographs are a screening test aimed at identifying redisplacement. Kramhoft and Solgaard[179] recommended that children with displaced diaphyseal forearm fractures have screening radiography at 1 and 2 weeks after reduction. Voto[171] also pointed out that most fractures that redisplace do so within the first 2 weeks after injury. Inability to properly control fracture alignment with closed methods is the most commonly reported indication for operative intervention.[188,259,275,297,365]

The most common explanations for loss of fracture reduction are cast related (poor casting technique, no evidence of three-point molding).[63,342] The more experienced the surgeon, the greater the likelihood of successful reduction.[58] Other factors that have been found to be associated with forearm fracture redisplacement are quality of initial reduction,[362] missed follow-up appointments,[68] proximal-third fractures,[72] and failure of the doctor to respond to early warning signs such as slight loss of reduction at 1-week follow-up.[113] Strategies for dealing with redisplacement include allowing the deformity to remodel,[143] cast wedging,[18,152,169] rereduction and recasting,[80,342] pins and

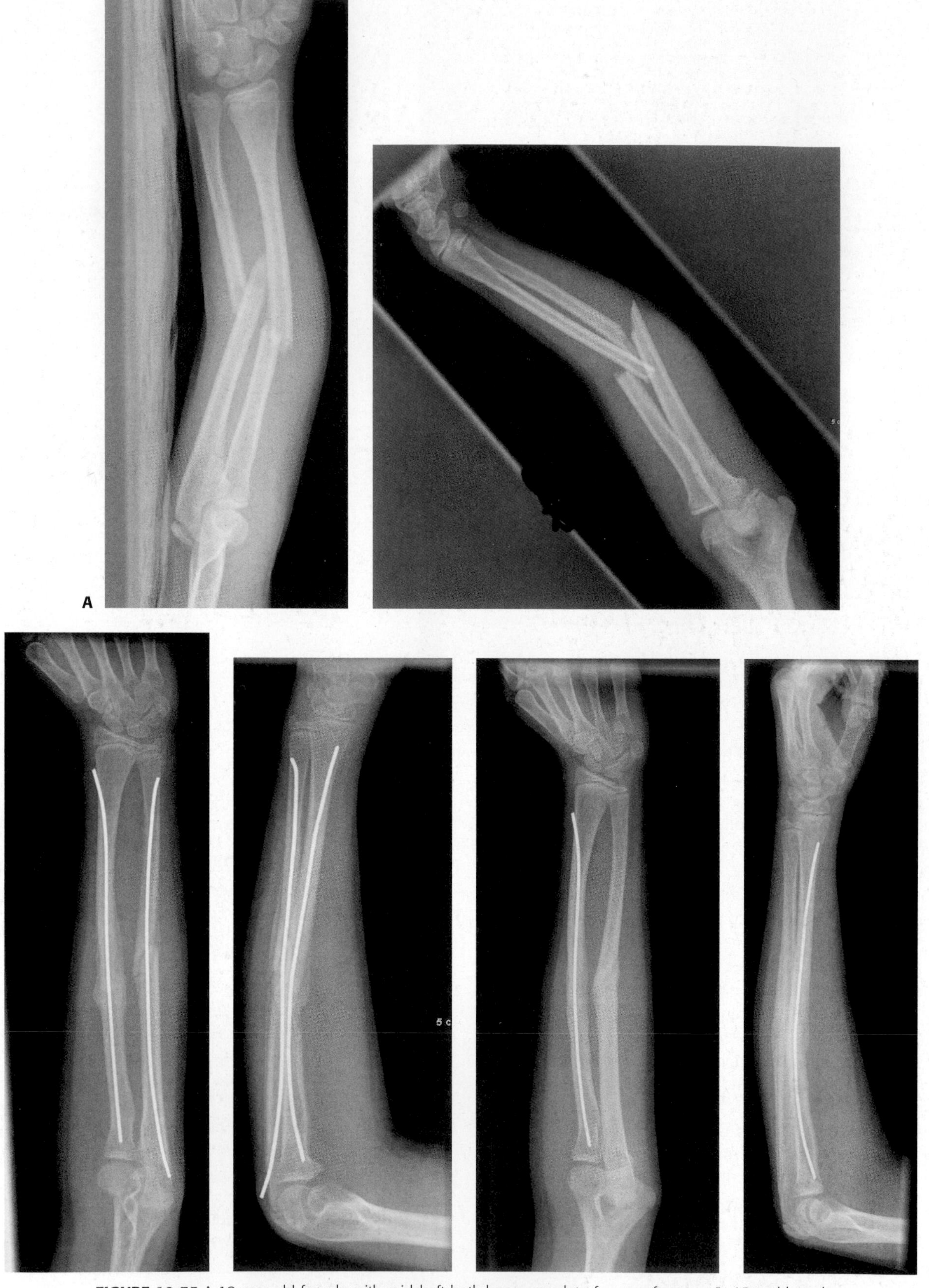

FIGURE 10-35 A 12-year-old female with midshaft both-bone complete forearm fracture. **A.** AP and lateral injury radiographs. **B.** Two-month follow-up radiographs. **C.** Six-month follow-up radiographs (ulnar nail removed).

(continues)

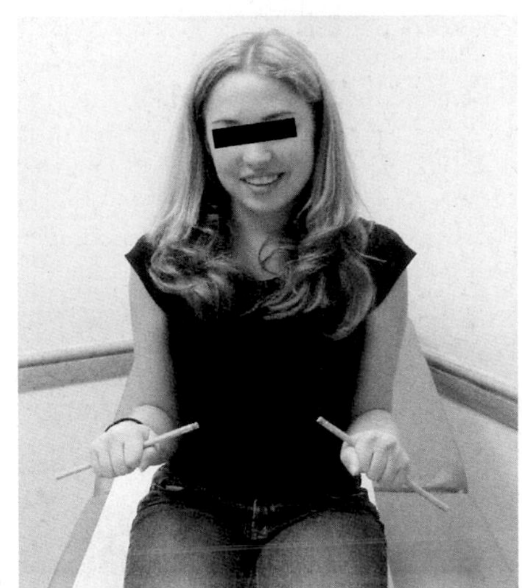
D

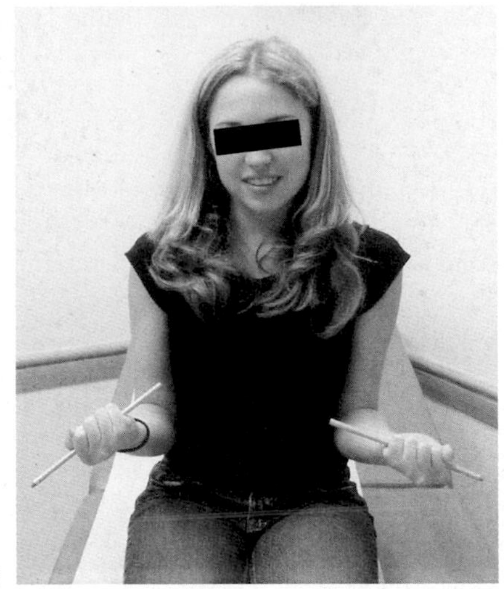
E

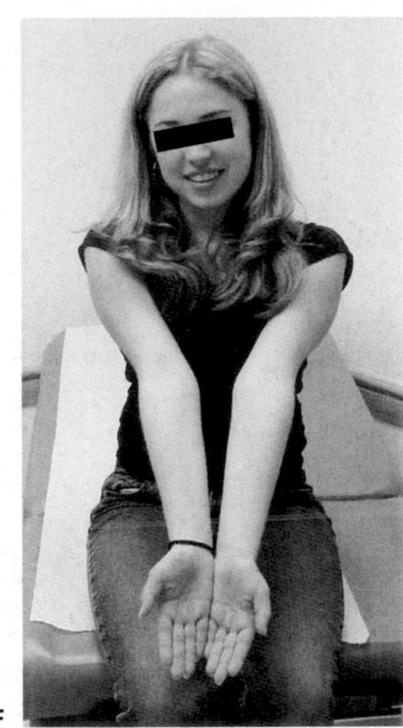
F

FIGURE 10-35 *(continued)* **D.** Pronation. **E.** Supination. **F.** Axial alignment.

plaster,[33,89,342] indirect reduction and internal fixation,[10] and open reduction and internal fixation.[358] Reports in the literature suggest that most forearm shaft fractures that redisplace can be successfully managed with repeat closed reduction and casting.[80,342]

Forearm Stiffness

The forearm is a predominantly nonsynovial joint with high-amplitude motion as its main function. The most common long-term complication of forearm shaft fracture treatment is significant forearm stiffness,[143] with pronation loss occurring almost twice as frequently as supination loss.[144] Loss of pronation or supination motion sometimes occurs despite perfectly normal-appearing radiographs.[168,229,255] Abnormal bony alignment of the forearm bones leads to predictable motion deficits.[166] Stiffness that exceeds that expected from bony malalignment alone[166] and stiffness that occurs with normal radiographs are indications of fibrosis of the interosseous membrane or contracture of the interosseous ligament.[168,255]

With focused testing of forearm motion, between 18%[52] and 72%[144] of patients show at least some minor deficits after nonsurgical treatment. Most minor deficits are not even noticed by patients and rarely are associated with functional limitations.[52,76,229] More severe losses of forearm rotation have far greater impact.[219] In their series of malunited forearm fractures (thus strongly weighted to demonstrate forearm stiffness), Price et al.[255] reported a 15% (6/39) rate of mild stiffness (up to 25-degree loss) and an 8% (3/39) rate of severe forearm stiffness (loss of 45 degrees or more of either pronation or supination). Holdsworth's[144] series of malunited pediatric forearm fractures had a similar rate (6%) of severe forearm stiffness. Holdsworth[144] told the classic story of a female whose inability to properly pronate caused her to elbow her neighbors when eating at the table. Patrick[243] pointed out that it is possible to compensate for pronation losses with shoulder abduction, but no similar compensation mechanism exists for supination losses. Such severe motion loss is a very undesirable outcome. For surgical treatment of these injuries to be a rational choice, the rates of stiffness after surgery must be lower than those after cast treatment.[130]

Bhaskar and Roberts[26] published one of the only studies of plated pediatric forearm fractures to report goniometric pronation and supination data. Both their single-bone (ulna) and both-bone plated patients showed mild forearm motion losses (maximal 18% loss of pronation).[26] Variable rates of mild forearm range-of-motion losses have been reported after intramedullary fixation. Amit et al.[10] reported a 40% rate of mild stiffness (5 to 10 degrees) in 20 pediatric patients after Rush rod fixation of forearm fractures. Combined data from five series of the flexible intramedullary nailing (Kirschner wires, Steinmann pins, Nancy nails) reveal a 1.6% rate (2/128) of mild forearm stiffness (up to a 20-degree loss) and a 0% (0/128) rate of severe motion loss (40 degrees or more loss of either pronation or supination).[10,25,98180,297,365] No published series of nonoperatively treated forearm shaft fracture patients has exceeded these results relative to preservation of forearm motion.

Refracture

Refracture occurs more often after forearm shaft fractures in children than after any other fracture.[181] Tredwell[326] found that forearm refractures occurred at an average of 6 months after original injury and were more common in males (3:1) and in older children (approximately 12 years old). Refracture rates of 4%[98] to 8%[193] have been reported in pediatric diaphyseal forearm fractures. Bould and Bannister[43] reported that diaphyseal forearm fractures were eight times more likely to refracture than metaphyseal fractures. Schwarz et al.[292] found that 84% (21/28) of the forearm refractures in their series had initially presented as greenstick fractures. Based on the stage of bony healing, refractures may occur through the original fracture site, through both the original site and partially through intact bone or completely through intact bone,[350] but most seem to occur through the original fracture site.

Several authors have suggested that internal fixation is necessary after refracture,[15,252,269] but Schwarz et al.[292] reported good results with repeat closed reduction and casting in 14 of

17 patients with refractures. Closed reduction also has been shown to be effective for forearm refractures that occur with flexible nails in place (Fig. 10-36).[222] The best treatment of refracture is prevention, and patients should be splint-protected (removable forearm splint or thermoplastic gauntlet) for a period of 2 months depending on activity after initial bone healing.[230,255] Refracture is rare during splint wear. Parents must be cautioned about the risk of refracture despite apparently adequate bone healing on radiographs.

Refracture after plate removal has been discussed frequently in the literature[103,227,254,332] and appears to be associated with decreased bone density beneath the plate.[174] This has led many authors to question the routine use of plate fixation for pediatric forearm fractures.[30,68,254,333] Refractures also have been reported after removal of intramedullary forearm fixation in children.[74,135,168,184,297,328,364] The main strategies aimed at decreasing the risk of refractures after implant removal are documentation of adequate bony healing before implant removal, and an additional period of splint protection after implant removal until the holes have filled in.

Malunion

Evaluation of pediatric forearm fracture malunion must take into account established malreduction limits and expected pedi-

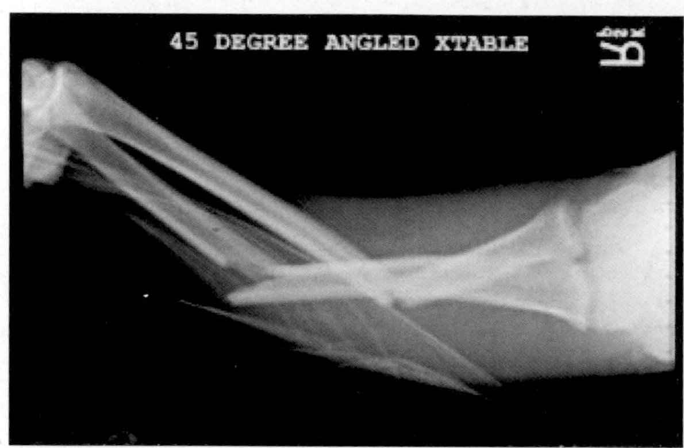

A

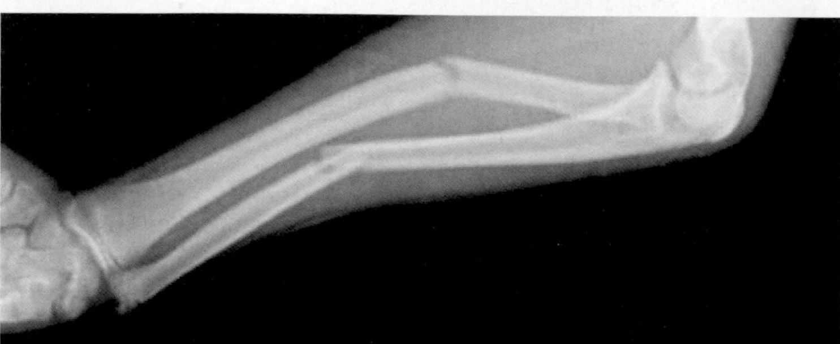

B

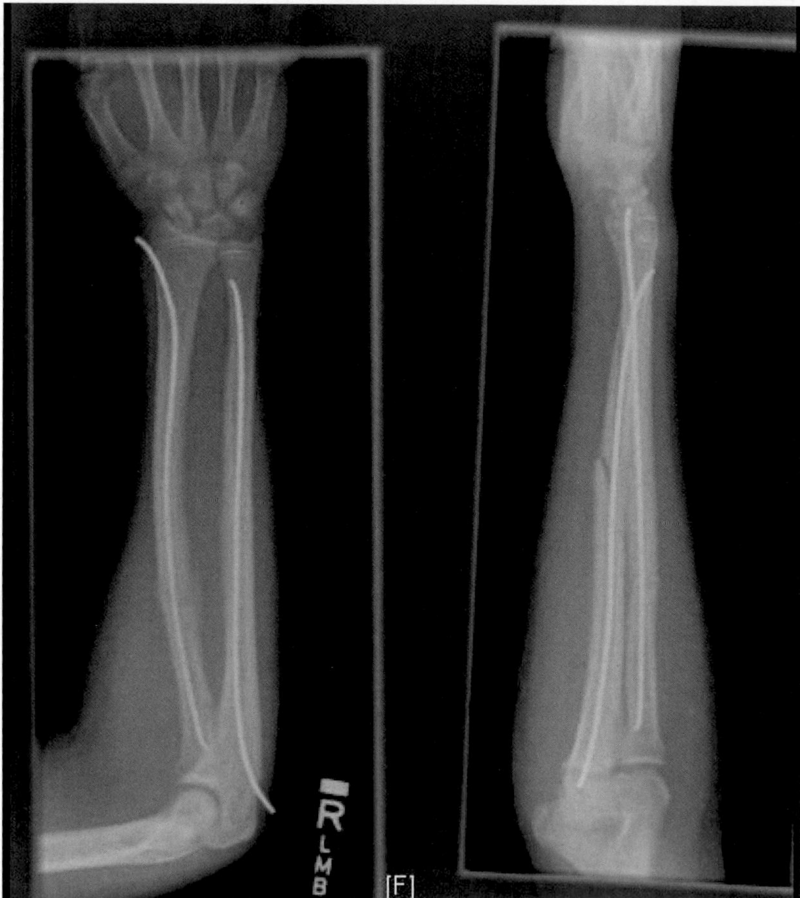

C

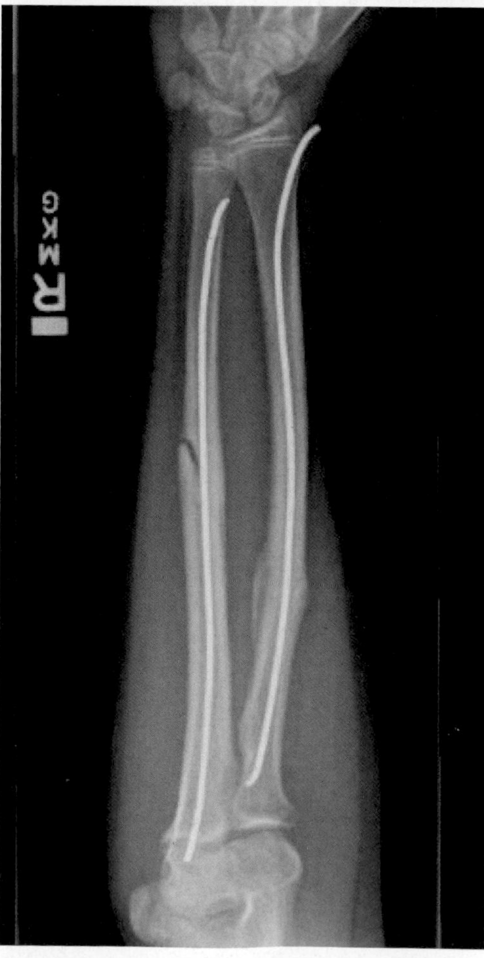

D

FIGURE 10-36 A 14-year-old ESIN patient who suffered refracture with the nails in place. **A.** Injury AP radiograph. **B.** Injury lateral radiograph. Skateboard mechanism. **C.** Early postoperative radiographs status post ESIN. **D.** Two months postoperative AP radiograph. *(continues)*

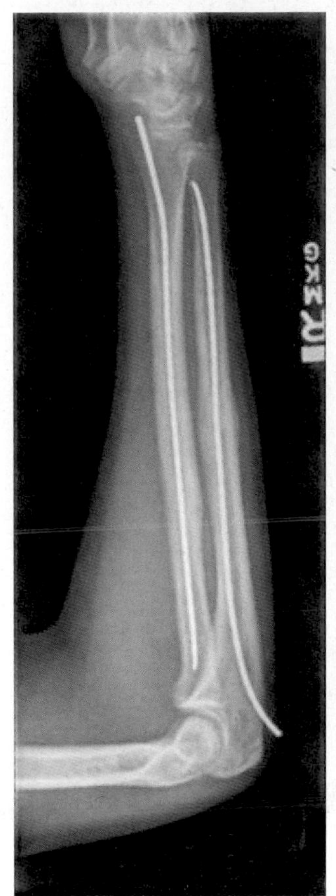

E

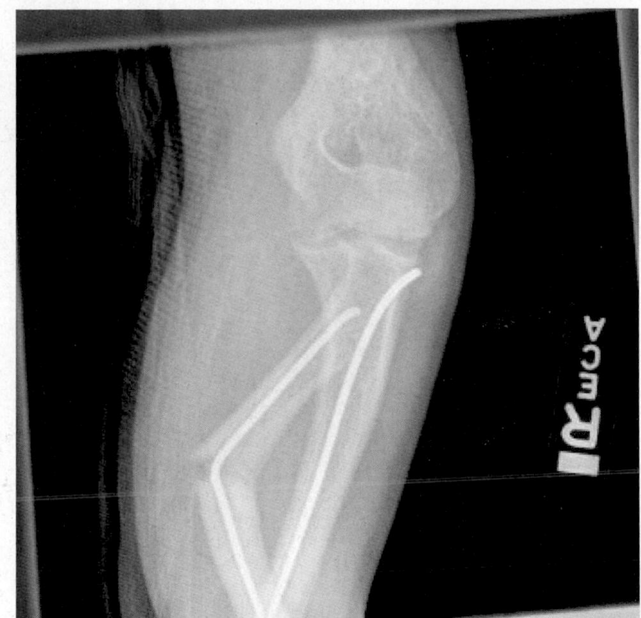

G

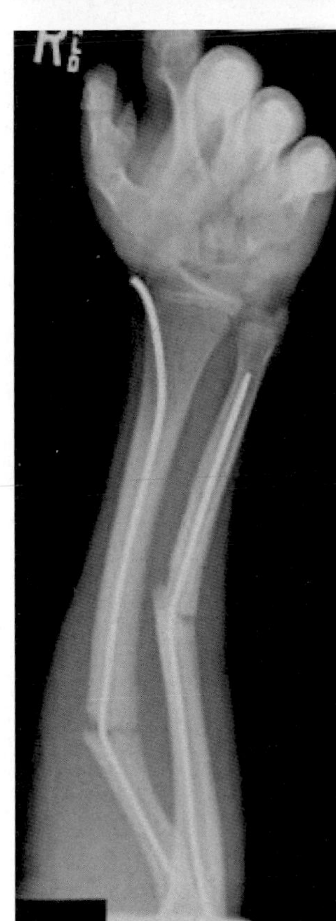

F

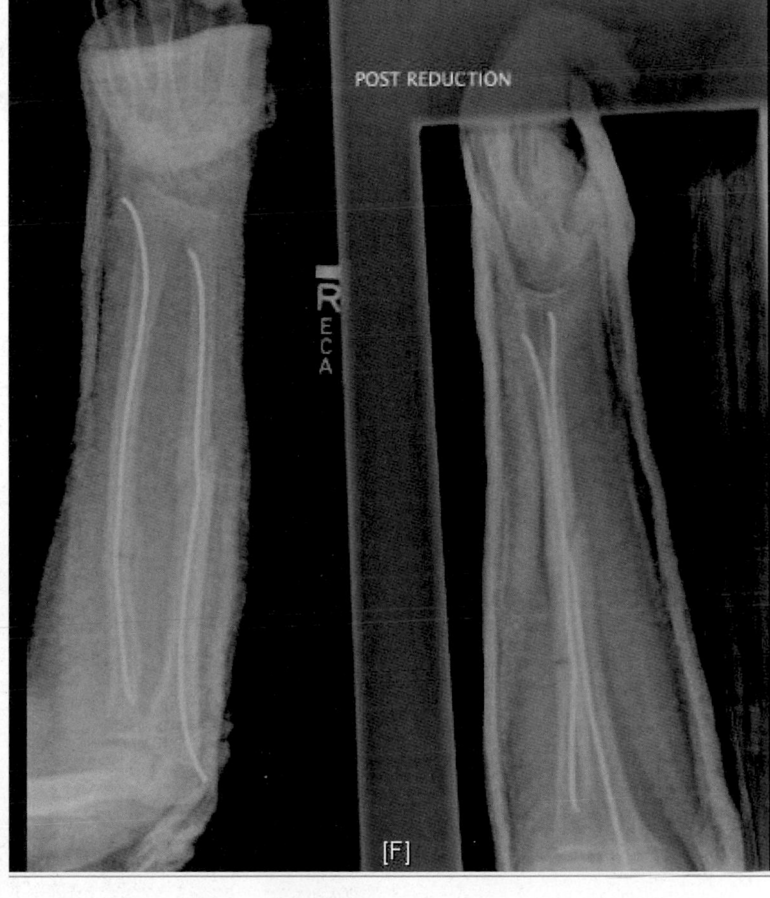

H

FIGURE 10-36 (*continued*) **E.** Two months postoperative lateral radiograph. **F.** Refracture at 2.5 months postoperative. **G.** Refracture elbow radiograph. **H.** Closed reduction of titanium nails and angulated radius and ulna fractures. (*continues*)

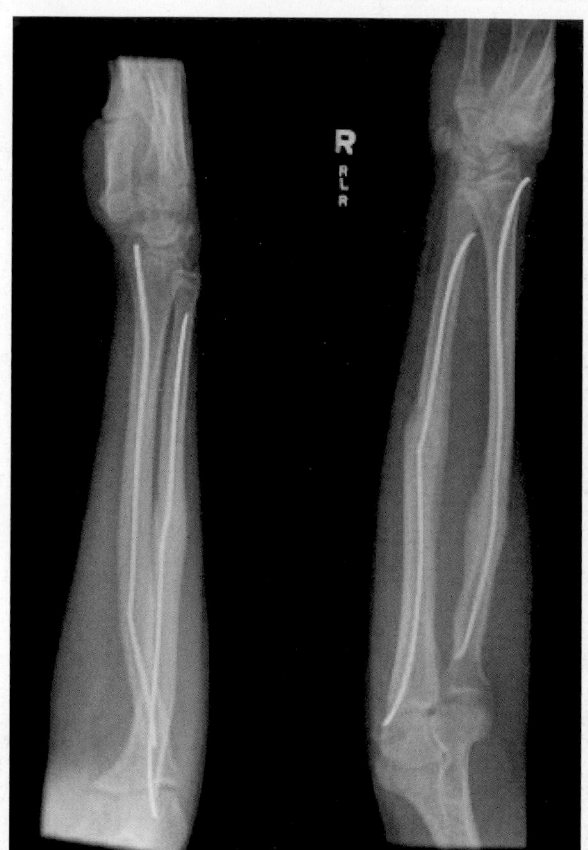

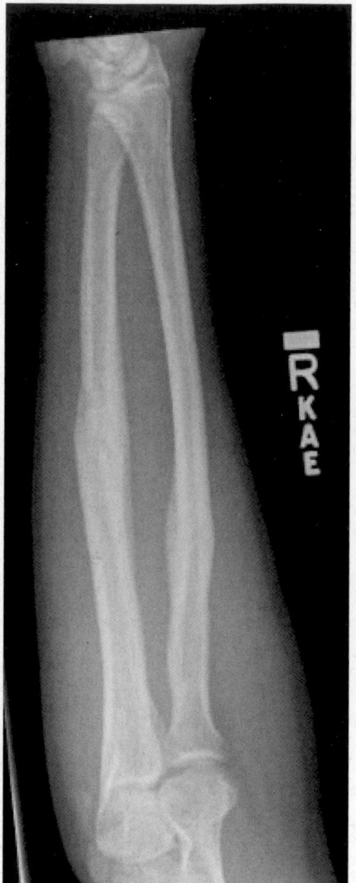

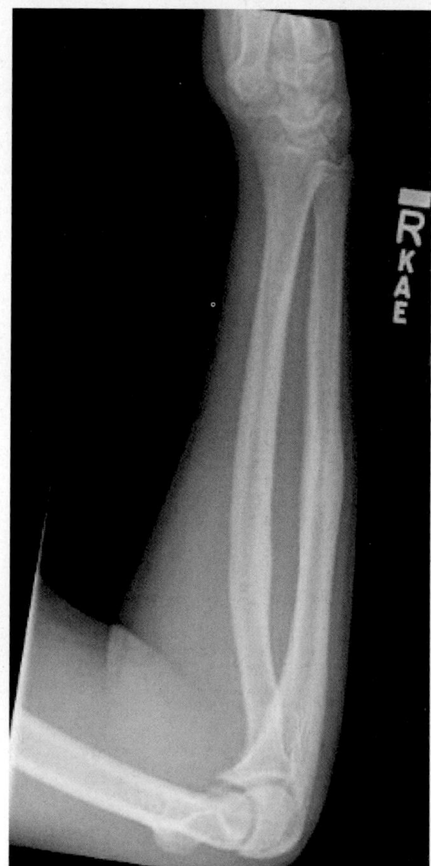

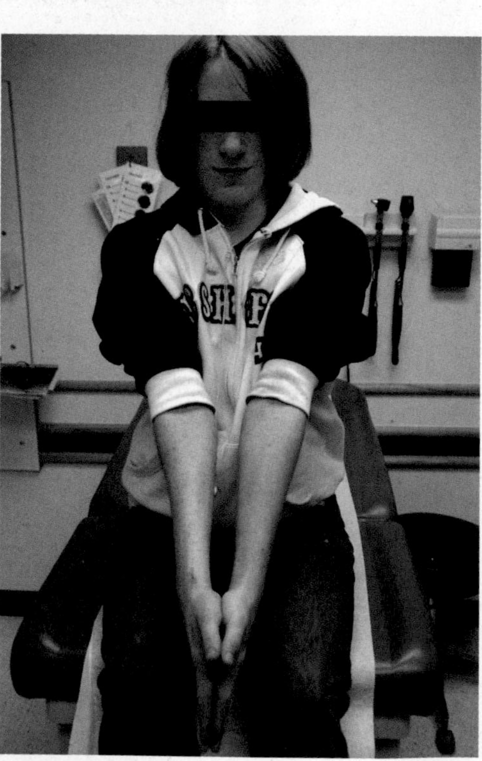

FIGURE 10-36 (*continued*) **I.** Five months after refracture. **J.** AP radiograph 1 year after refracture. **K.** Lateral radiograph 1 year after refracture. **L.** Clinical appearance with extended elbows and forearm midposition.
(*continues*)

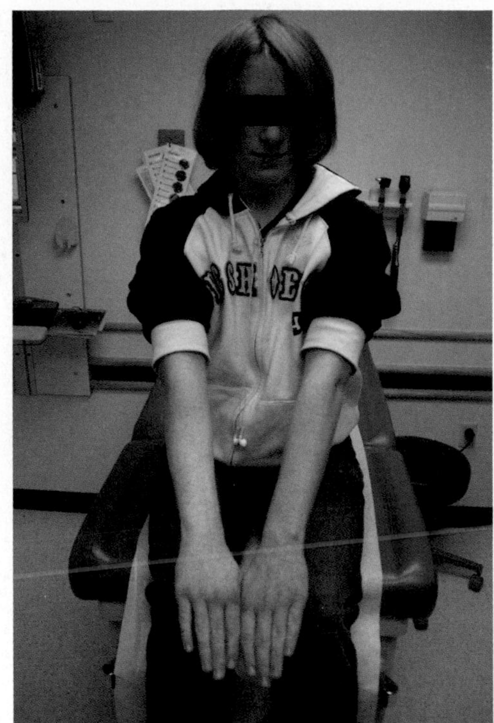
M

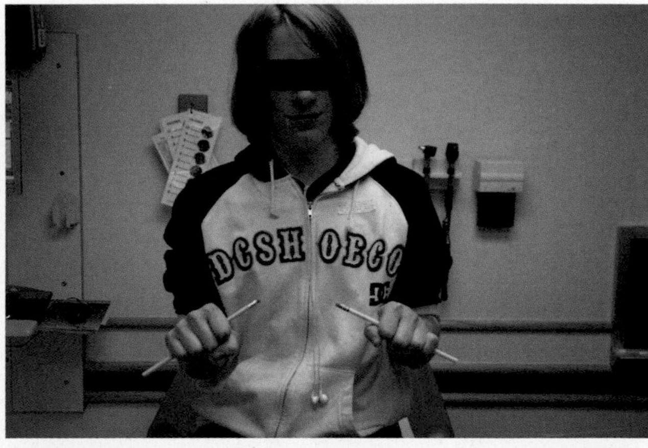
O

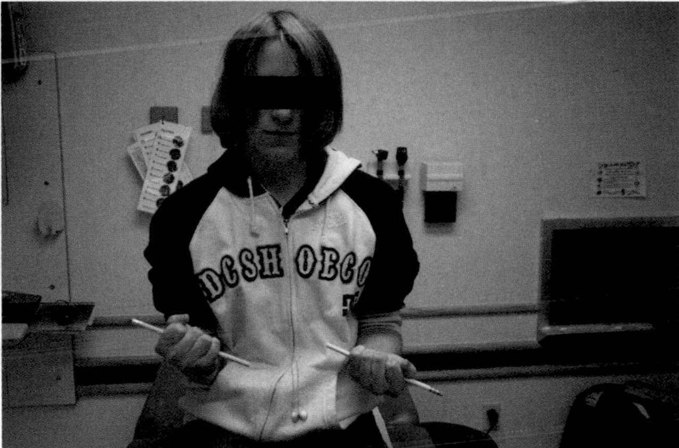
P

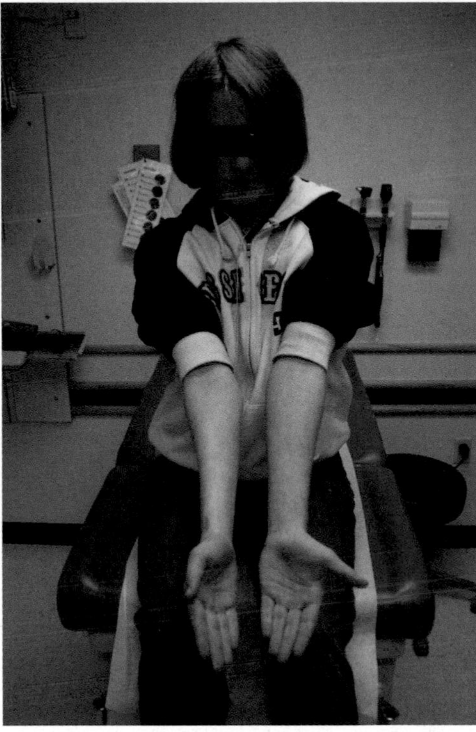
N

FIGURE 10-36 (*continued*) **M.** Clinical appearance with extended elbows and pronated forearms. **N.** Clinical appearance with extended elbows and supinated forearms. Note mild supination loss on right. **O.** Symmetrical pronation. **P.** Asymmetrical supination. Approximately 15 degree loss on right.

atric remodeling potential. Thus, a malunion of 30 degrees may become less than 10 degrees during the course of follow-up. The level of the malunited fracture also must be considered, because the consequences of malreduction vary according to level.[280,361] More deformity in the predominant plane of motion is acceptable in fractures near physes of long bones than in diaphyseal fractures. Normal motion can be preserved despite persistent radiographic abnormality (Fig. 10-37).

Malunion of radial and ulnar shaft fractures can lead to cosmetic deformity and loss of motion; however, significant loss of function occurs in only a small percentage of patients.[52,76,229] Some authors have recommended more aggressive efforts at correction of forearm fracture malunions.[214,253] Early malunions (up to 4 or 5 weeks after injury) can be treated with closed osteoclasis under anesthesia. If closed osteoclasis fails to adequately mobilize the fracture, a minimally invasive drill osteoclasis can be done.[29] A small-diameter drill (or Kirschner wire) is used to make multiple holes in the region of the mal-

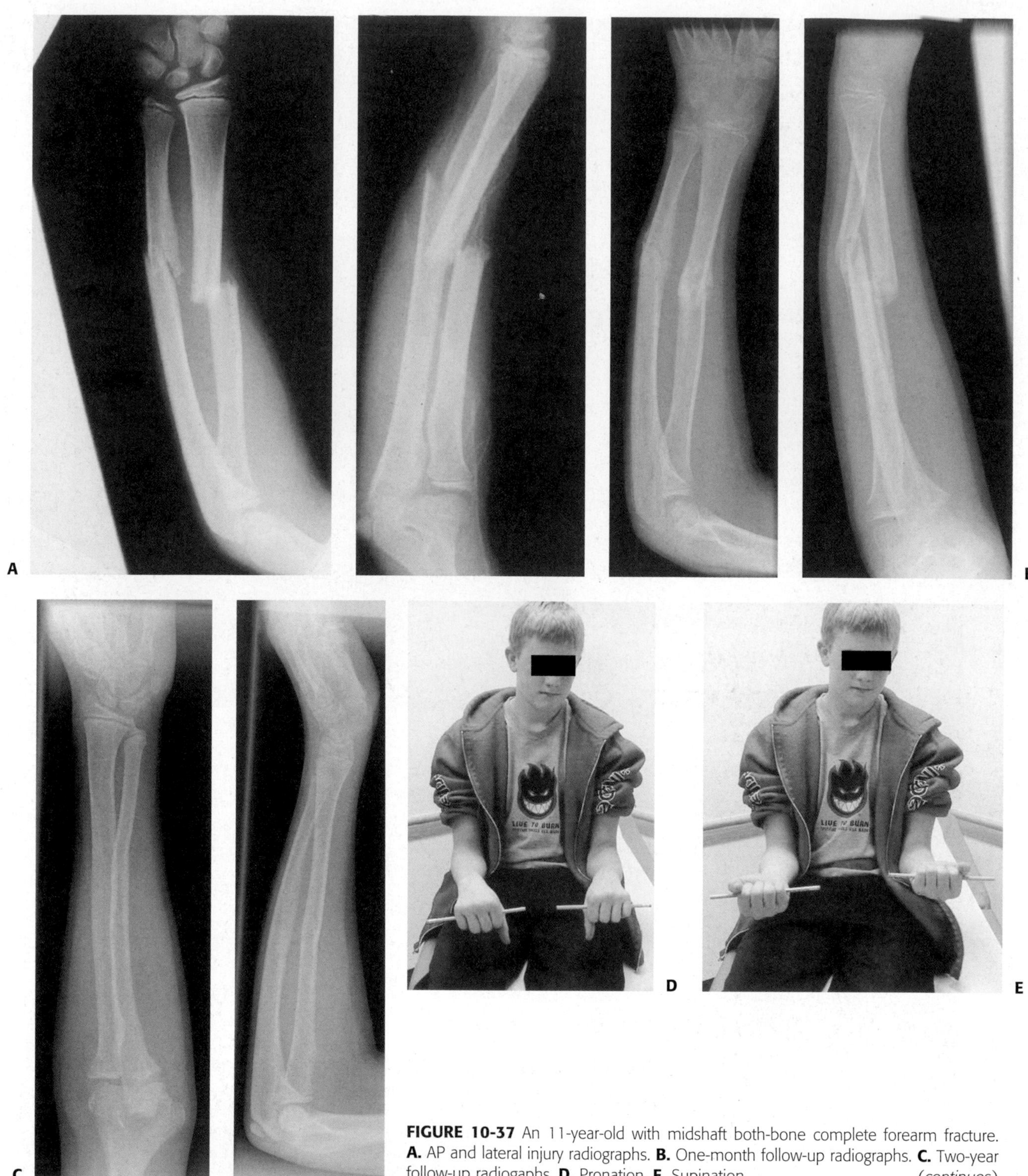

FIGURE 10-37 An 11-year-old with midshaft both-bone complete forearm fracture. **A.** AP and lateral injury radiographs. **B.** One-month follow-up radiographs. **C.** Two-year follow-up radiogaphs. **D.** Pronation. **E.** Supination. *(continues)*

union before forcefully manipulating the bone back into alignment.[29] Internal fixation is rarely, if ever, needed.

Once significant callus is present, indirect reduction and internal fixation with flexible intramedullary nails can be difficult or impossible because the fracture site is now blocked with callus. Thus, established or impending malunions that cannot be adequately controlled with a cast may require formal open reduction and plate fixation (Figs. 10-38 and 10-39). Many fractures that heal with angulation or rotation of more than the established criteria regain full motion and have an excellent cosmetic outcome. Fractures may require corrective osteotomy if they fail to remodel after an adequate period of observation or if adequate motion fails to return.[214,329] Such corrective osteotomies have been done long after injury (up to 27 years) and additional motion has still been regained.[329] There is a minor subset of malunions that

(text continues on page 396)

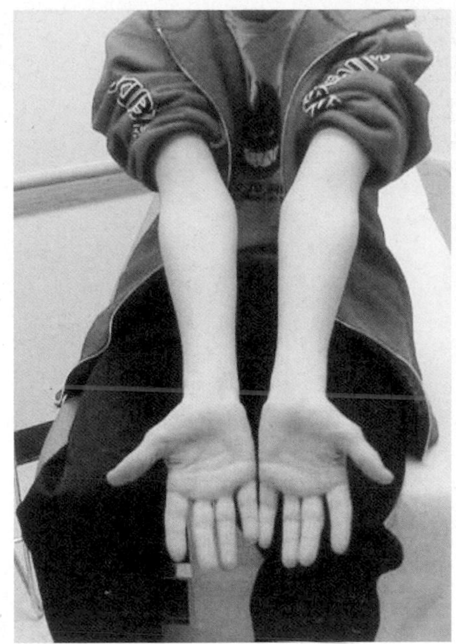

F

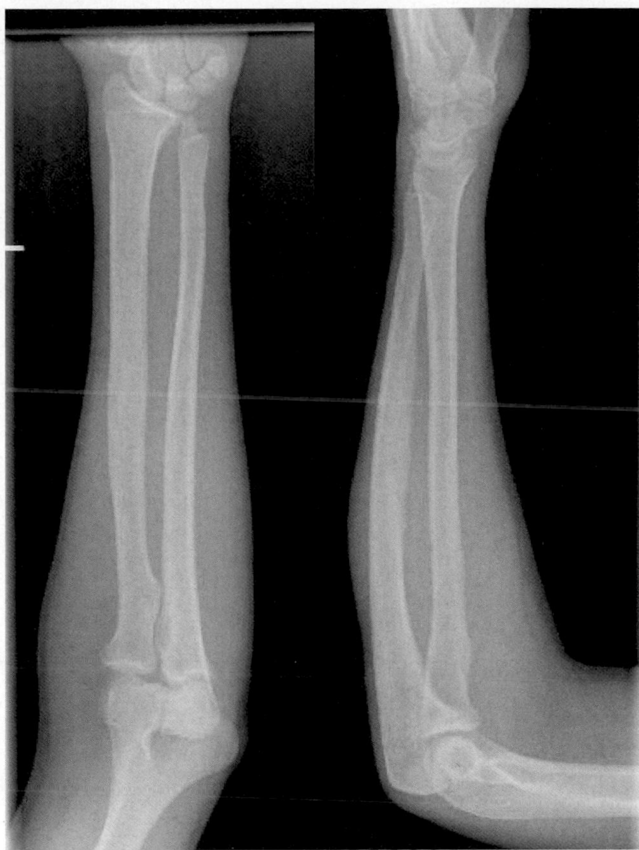

G

FIGURE 10-37 (*continued*) **F.** Axial alignment. **G.** Six-year follow-up radiographs with substantial remodeling of radius and ulna fractures.

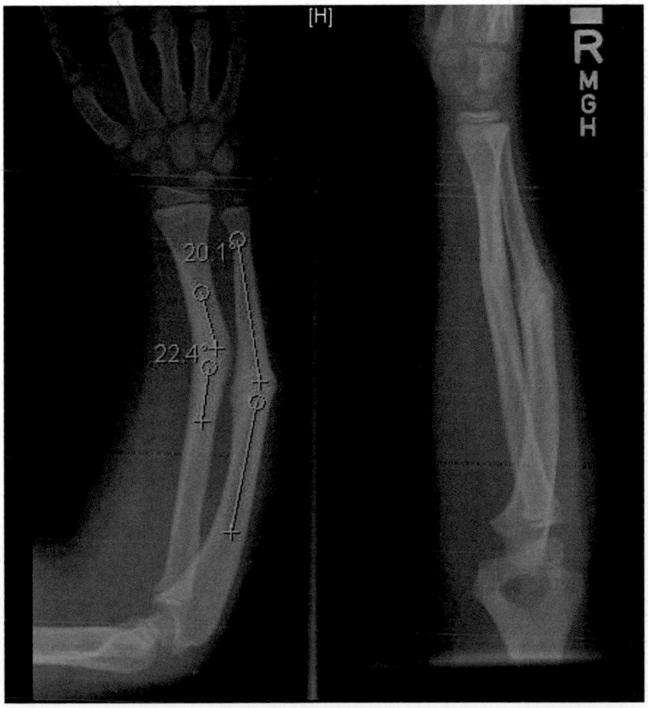

A

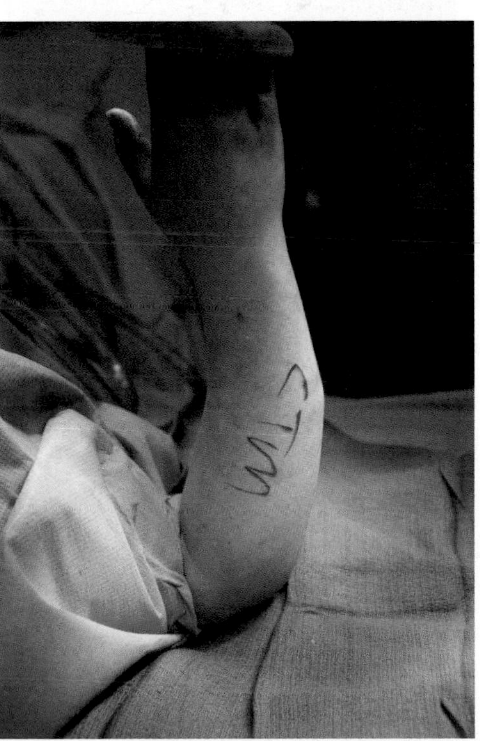

B

FIGURE 10-38 An 8-year-old male who underwent corrective osteotomy for forearm shaft malunion. **A.** Radiographs demonstrating significant angular malunion. **B.** Preoperative clinical appearance (dorsal view).

(*continues*)

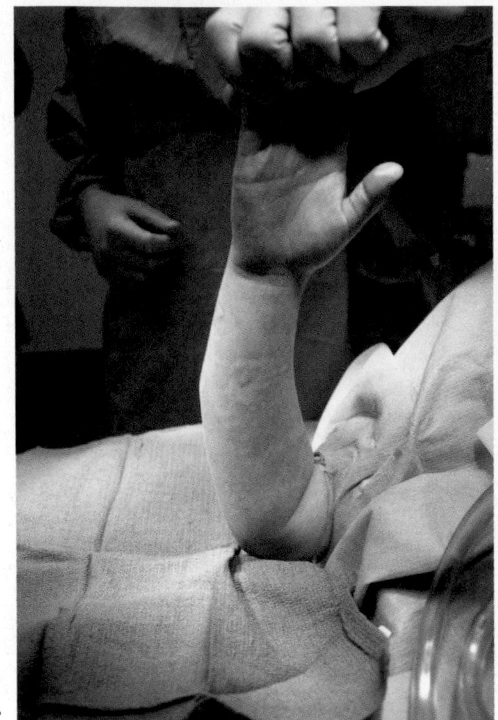

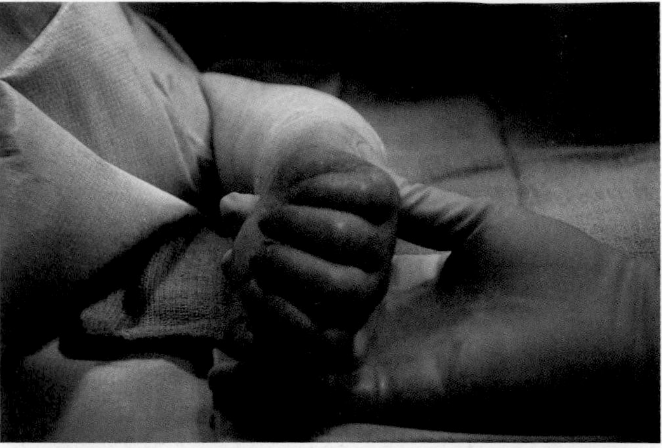

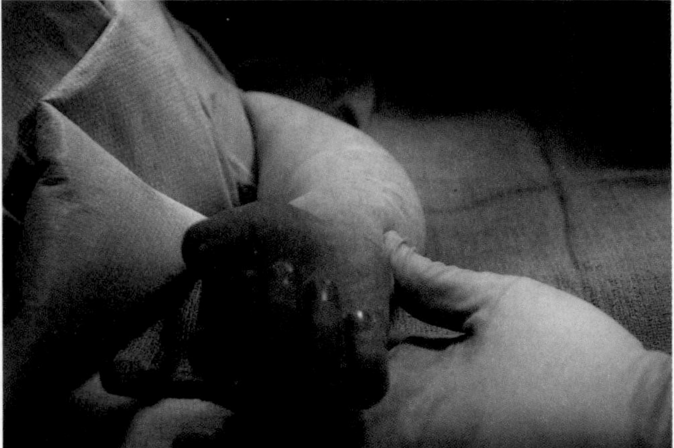

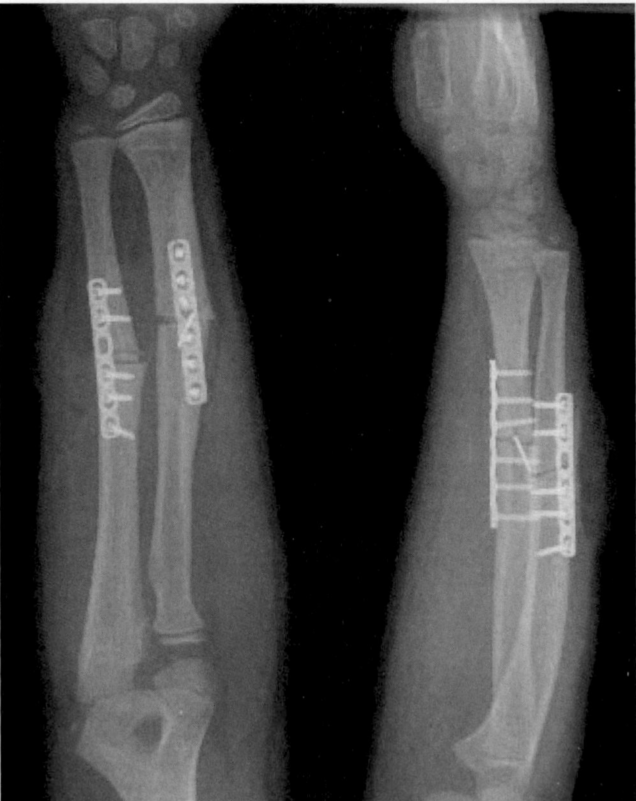

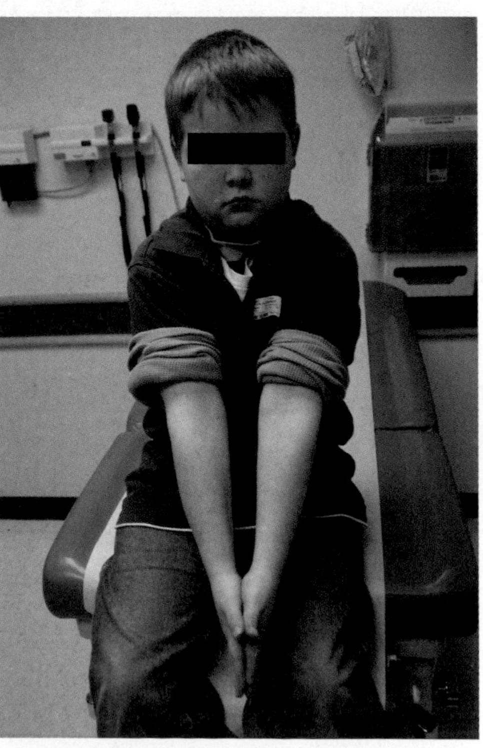

FIGURE 10-38 *(continued)* **C.** Preoperative clinical appearance (volar view). **D.** Preoperative demonstration of full passive supination. **E.** Preoperative demonstration of marked limitation in passive pronation. **F.** Early postoperative radiographs following corrective osteotomies (note intraosseous Kirschner wire tip from provisional fixation). **G.** Clinical appearance with extended elbows and forearm midposition. *(continues)*

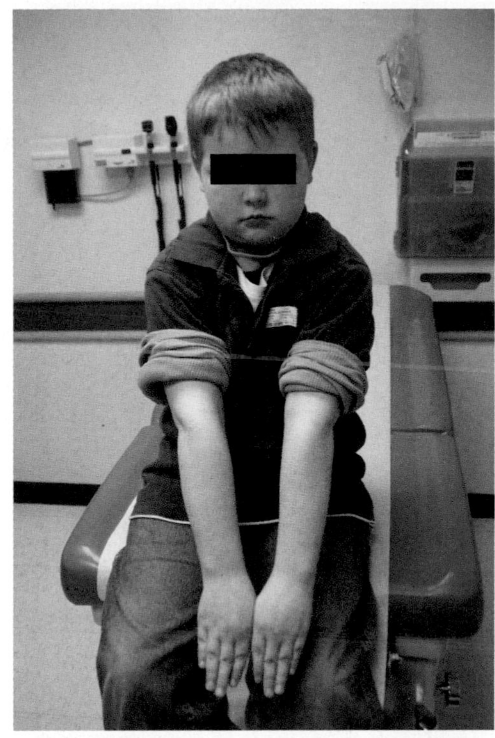

H

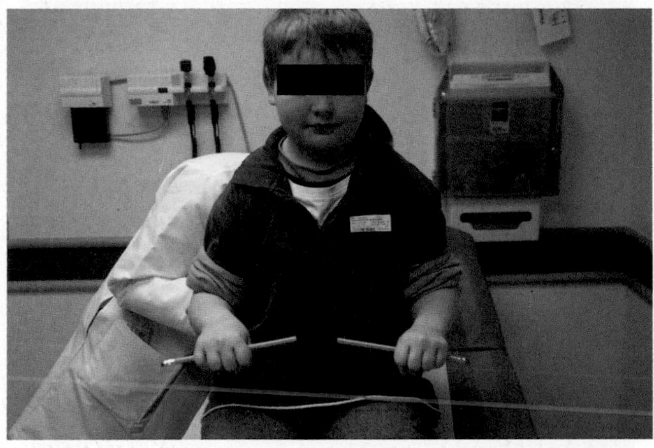

J

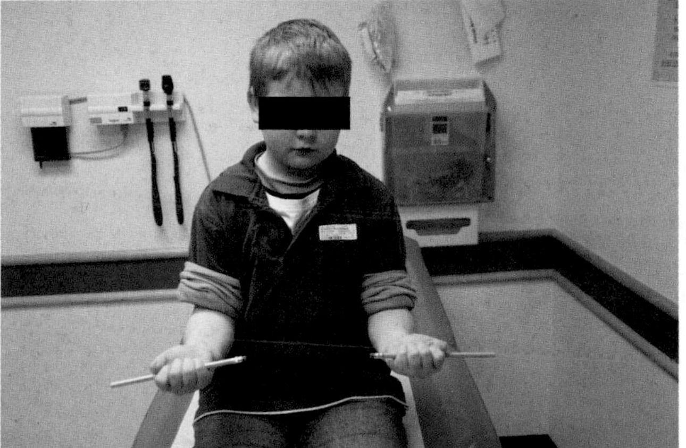

K

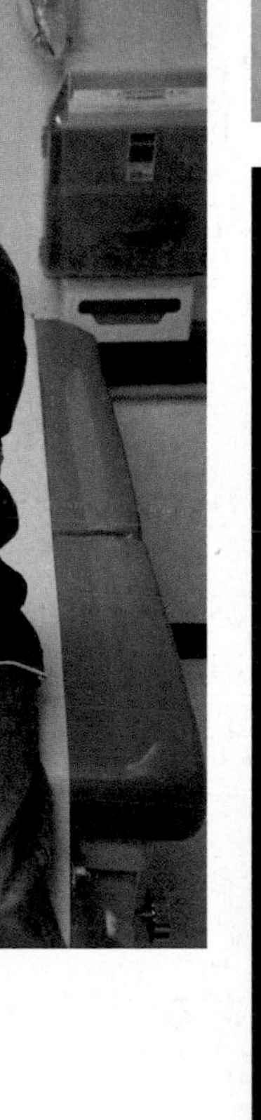

I

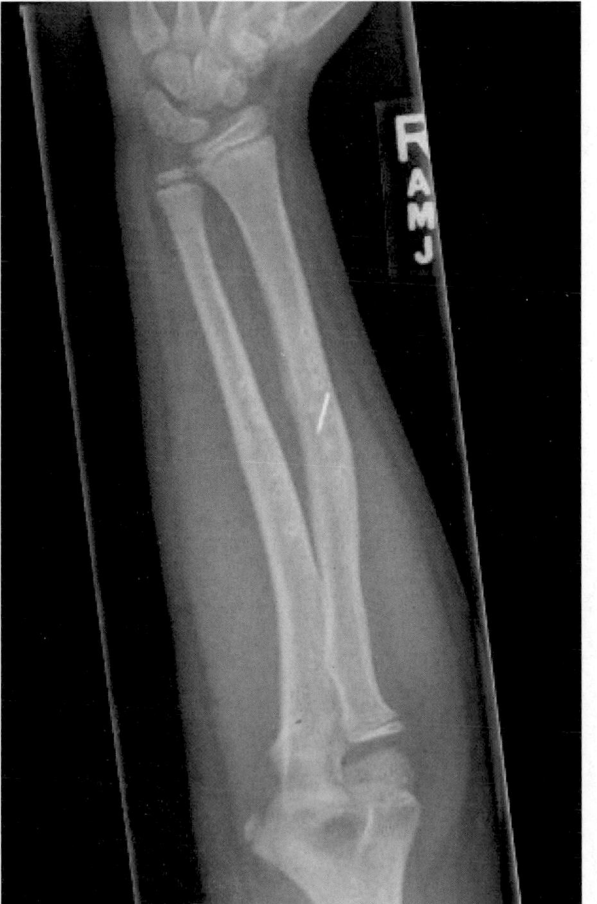

L

FIGURE 10-38 (*continued*) **H.** Clinical appearance with extended elbows and pronated forearms. **I.** Clinical appearance with extended elbows and supinated forearms. **J.** Symmetrical pronation. **K.** Symmetrical supination. **L.** AP radiograph 18 months after osteotomies (plates and screws have been removed).

(*continues*)

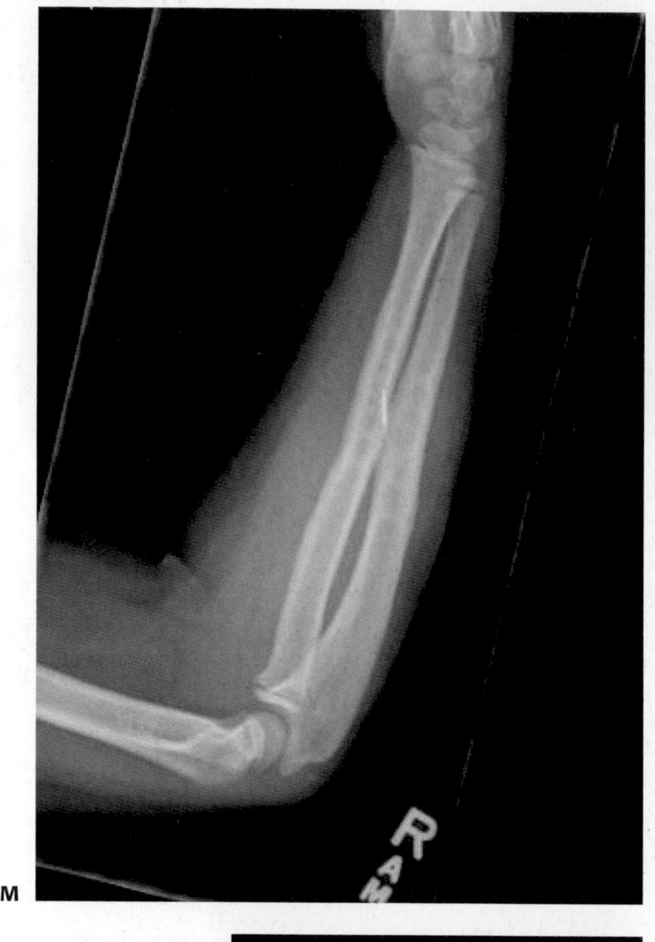

M

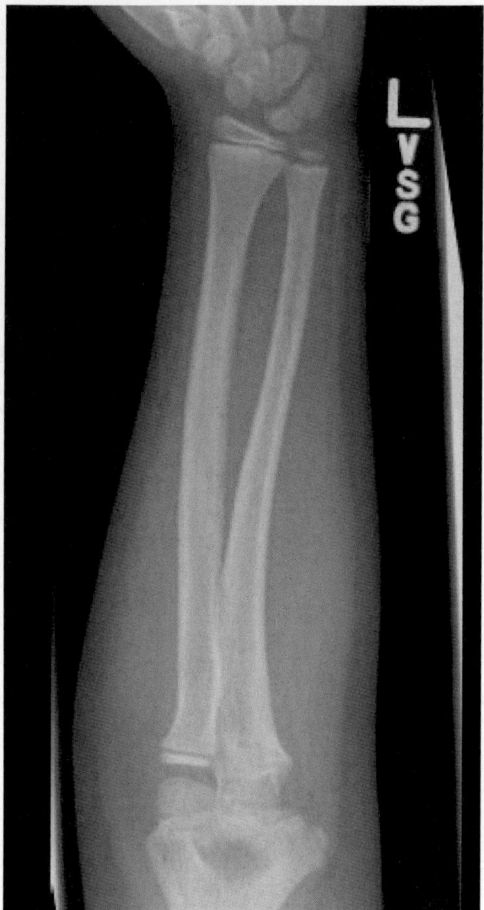

N

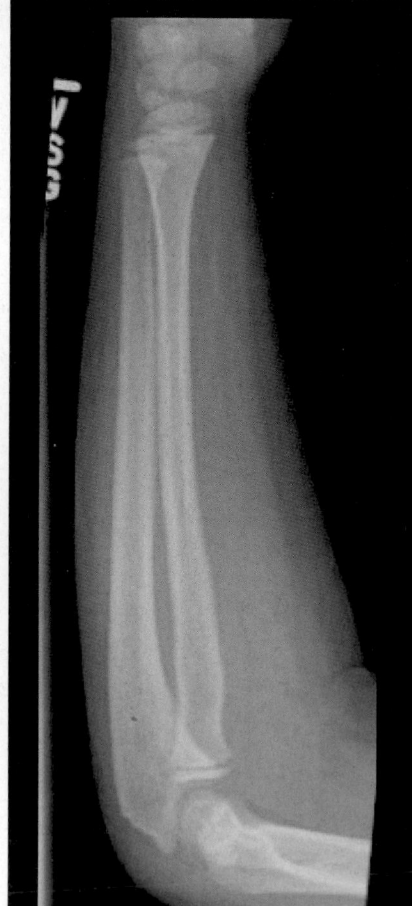

O

FIGURE 10-38 (*continued*) **M.** Lateral radiograph at 18 month follow-up. **N.** AP radiograph uninjured left forearm. **O.** Lateral radiograph uninjured left forearm.

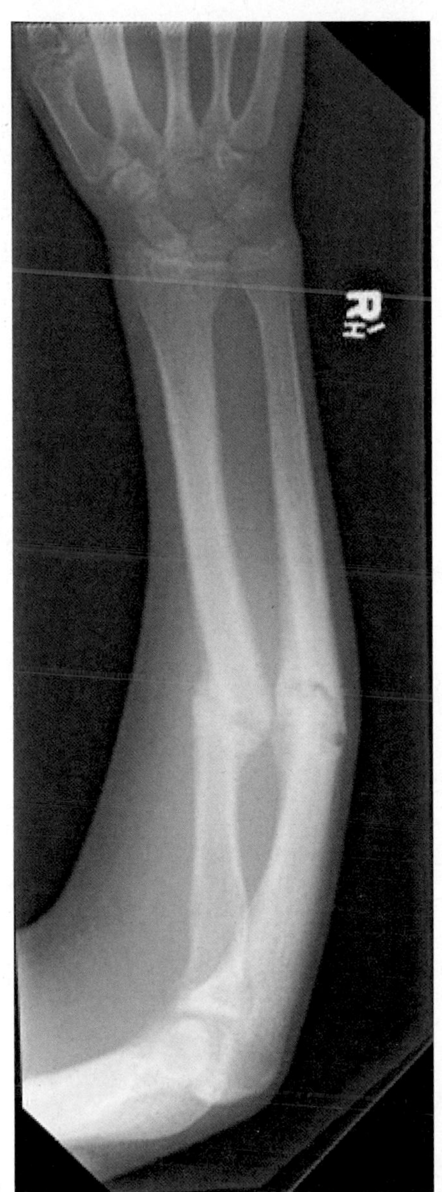

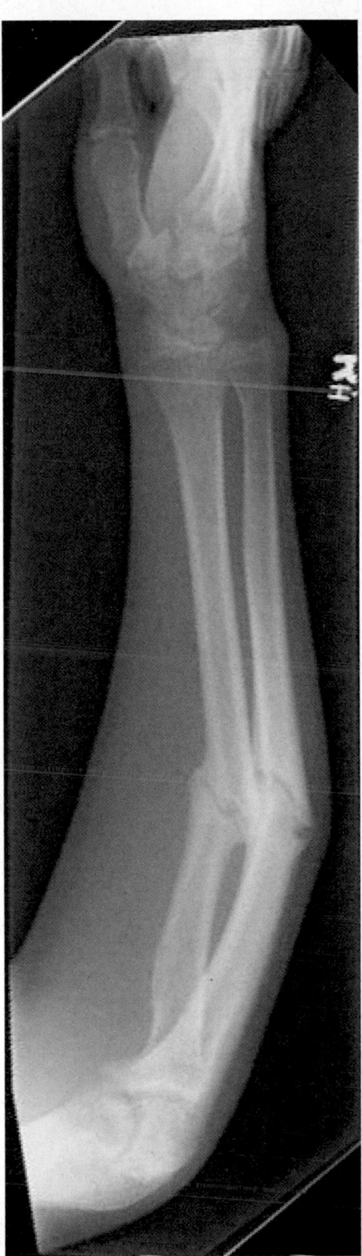

FIGURE 10-39 A 16-year-old male who underwent corrective osteotomy for forearm shaft malunion. **A.** AP radiograph at time of presentation. **B.** Lateral radiograph at time of presentation. Note rotational malunion of radius in addition to angular abnormalities of both bones. **C.** Clinical deformity (bump). **D.** Relatively symmetrical pronation noted preoperatively. *(continues)*

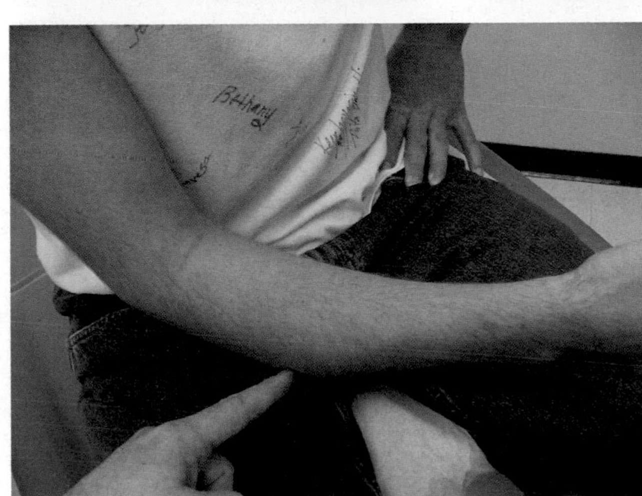

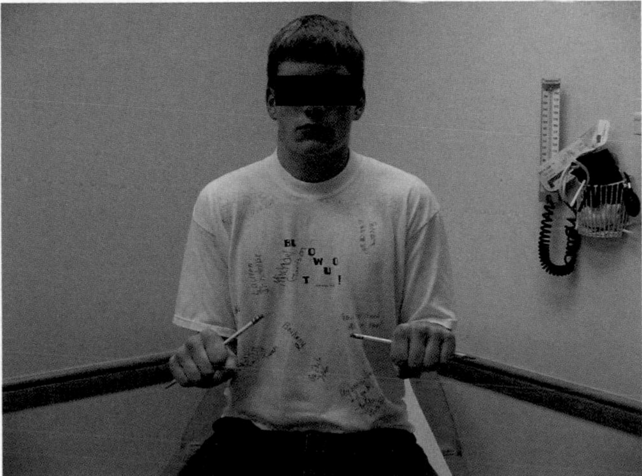

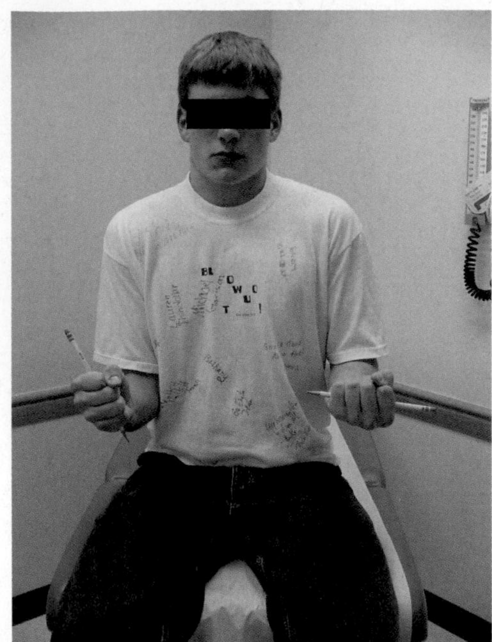

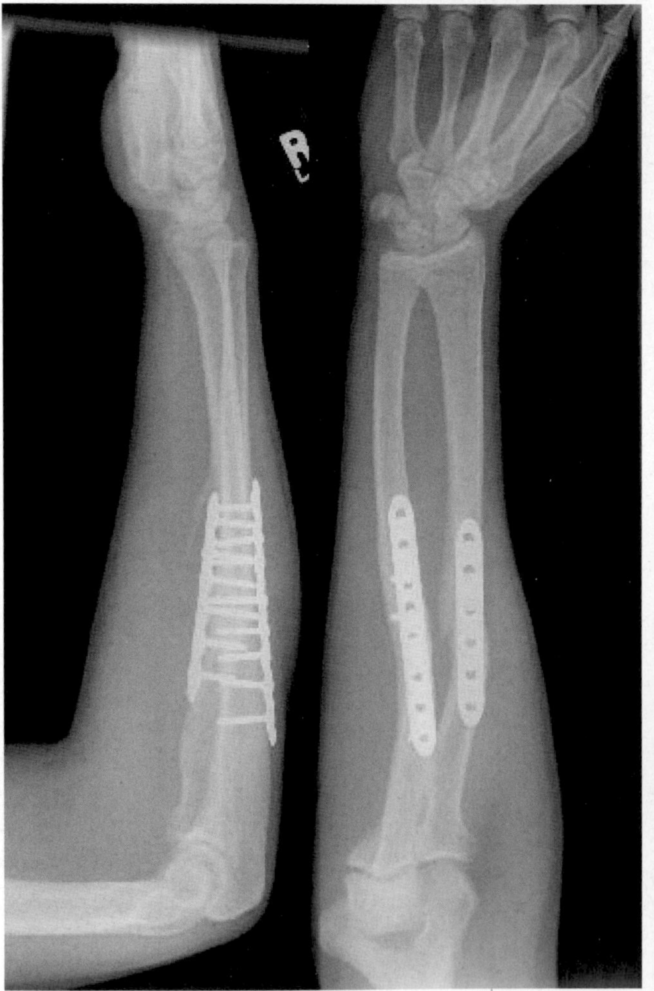

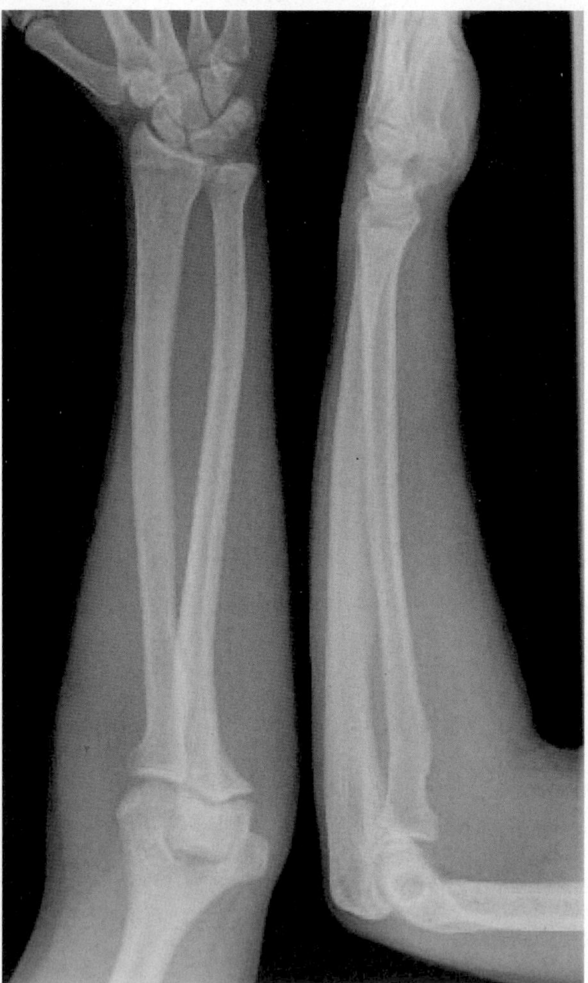

FIGURE 10-39 (*continued*) **E.** Dramatic lack of supination on the right noted preoperatively. **F.** One-year postoperative radiographs following osteotomies. Note improved rotational alignment of radius. **G.** Uninjured left forearm radiographs. (*continues*)

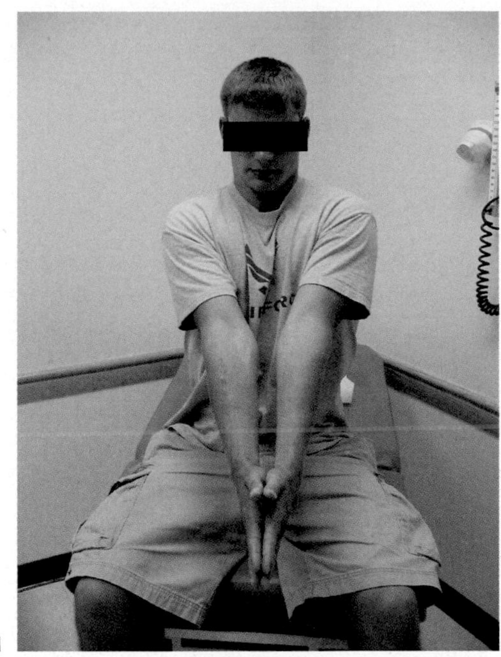
H

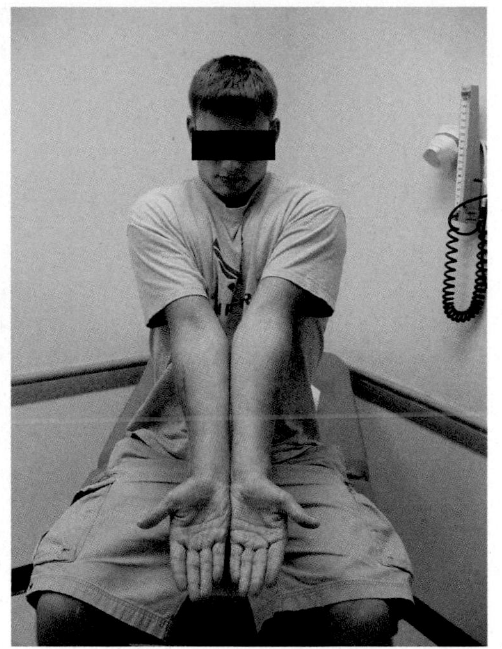

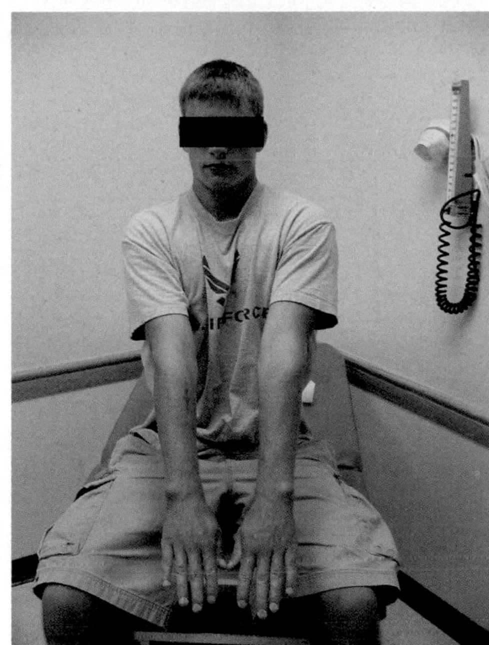
I

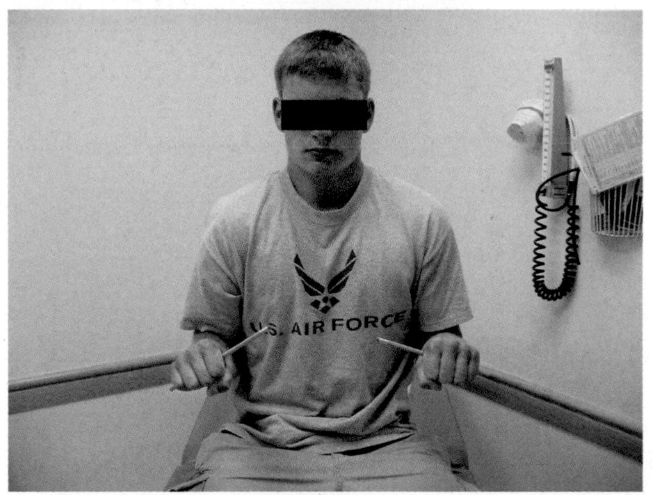

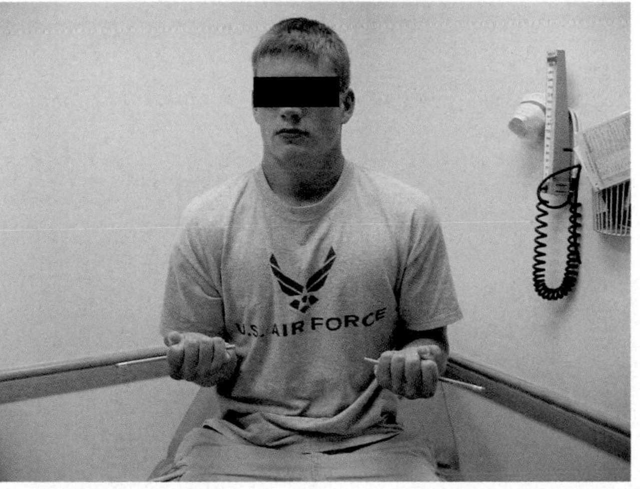

FIGURE 10-39 (*continued*) **H.** Clinical appearance with extended elbows and forearm midposition. **I.** Clinical appearance with extended elbows and pronated forearms. **J.** Clinical appearance with extended elbows and supinated forearms. **K.** Symmetrical pronation. **L.** Symmetrical supination.

do not remodel, that have functional limits (especially when there is limited supination deformity), and therefore, are candidates for osteotomy.

Delayed Union/Nonunion

The diagnosis of delayed union is based on documentation of slower-than-normal progression toward union.[189] Daruwalla[76] stated that normal healing of closed pediatric forearm shaft fractures occurs at an average of 5.5 weeks (range 2 to 8 weeks). Delayed union can be practically defined as a failure to demonstrate complete healing (four cortices) on sequential radiographs by 12 weeks after injury, which exceeds the upper limit of normal healing by about 1 month. Nonunion can be defined as absence of complete bony union by 6 months after injury, which exceeds the upper limit of normal healing by about 4 months.

Delayed unions and nonunions are rare after closed forearm shaft fractures in children.[99,189,307] In six large series of pediatric diaphyseal forearm fractures treated by closed methods, a less than 0.5% rate (1/263) of delayed union and no nonunions were reported.[255,144,76,52,168,179] Delayed unions and nonunions are more common after open reduction and internal fixation and open fractures. Particular concern has been raised about the potential of antegrade ulnar nailing (olecranon starting point) to distract the fracture site.[234] Combined data from four series of plated pediatric forearm fractures indicated a 3% (3/89) nonunion rate[26,227,333,358]; 24% (21/89) of these were open fractures and at least one[358] of the three nonunions occurred after a grade III open fracture.[227,333] Large series of open pediatric forearm fractures (treated by a variety of internal fixation methods) reported comparable numbers: 5% (8/173) delayed union rate and 1% (2/173) nonunion rate.[79,128,135] In a series of 30 nonunions in children, only 6 were in the forearm, and half of these were after open fractures.[189]

Because of the overall rarity of nonunions in children, the possibility of unusual diagnoses such as neurofibromatosis must be considered.[69,71,155,202] After open injury or surgical intervention for other reasons, the possibility of septic nonunion must be ruled out. In the absence of such extraneous factors, nonunion of pediatric forearm fractures seems to be related to surgical treatment.[69,71,155,202,307] Weber and Cech[349] divided nonunions into atrophic and hypertrophic types. Atrophic nonunions probably are best treated with bone grafting and compression plating. Compression plating or other stable internal fixation without grafting usually is sufficient for hypertrophic nonunions.[186]

Cross-Union/Synostosis

Posttraumatic radioulnar synostosis results in complete loss of forearm rotation. Most cross-unions that form after pediatric forearm shaft fractures are type II lesions (diaphyseal cross-unions), as described by Vince and Miller (Fig. 10-40).[338] Although some series of adult forearm fractures reported synostosis rates of 6% to 9%,[22,316] posttraumatic radioulnar synostosis is a rare complication of pediatric forearm shaft fractures.[338] In children, it usually is associated with high-energy injuries,[338] radial neck fractures,[274] and surgically treated forearm fractures.[74,235] Some have suggested a familial predisposition to this complication.[199] Postoperative synostosis after forearm fractures in children is almost exclusively associated with plate fixation.[354,358] The risk of cross-union is increased when open reduction and internal fixation of both-bone fractures are done through one incision.[22,68]

Both osseous and nonosseous cross-unions may form in the forearm,[11,65,343] but the more common type is osseous. After a synostosis matures (6 to 12 months), it can be excised along with any soft tissue interposition.[231,338] The results of synostosis resection may be better in adults than children,[338] perhaps be-

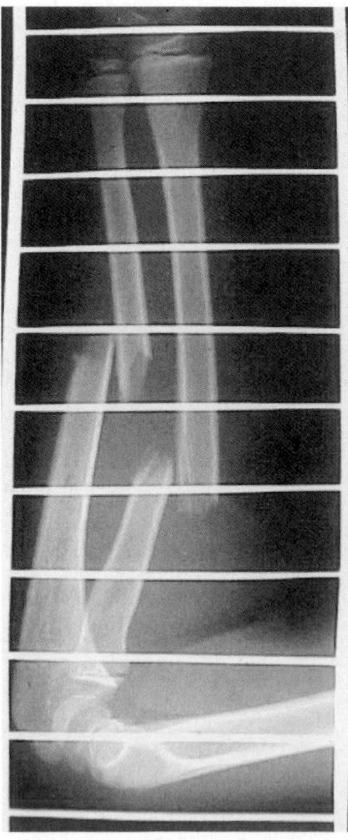

A

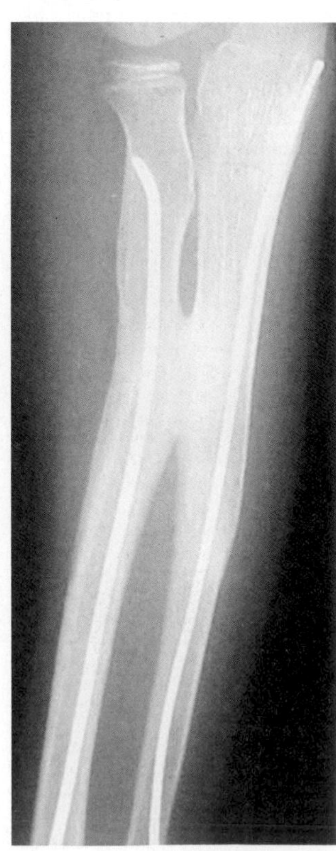

B

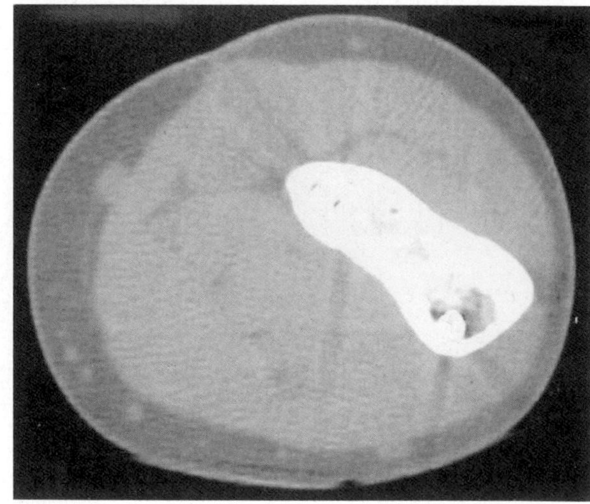

C

FIGURE 10-40 Radioulnar synostosis following closed injury. **A.** Injury radiographs. **B.** Plain radiographs showing synostosis. **C.** CT scan showing synostosis. (Courtesy of Alan Aner, MD.)

cause of the more biologically active periosteum in children.[85,338] Interposition of inert material (such as Gore-tex [W. L. Gore & Associates, Inc., Elkton, MD] or bone wax) has been used to decrease the chances of recurrent synostosis.[11,20,235,338] Nonsteroidal anti-inflammatory drugs and radiation treatment have been reported after synostosis excision in adults, but their use in children remains undefined. An alternative treatment is corrective osteotomy if the patient is synostosed in a position of either extreme pronation or supination. If the patient is stuck in a neutral position after posttraumatic synostosis, surgical intervention is usually not recommended.

Infection

Infection occurs only in surgically treated forearm shaft fractures and open fractures. Appropriately timed preoperative antibiotic prophylaxis is believed to diminish the risk of infection. Children with open forearm fractures are considered to be at high risk for infection, and early (usually less than 24 hours)[302] irrigation and débridement in the operating room is indicated.[275] Whether in the backyard, the barnyard, the football field, or the hay field, open forearm fractures that occur in organic settings are best treated with early irrigation and débridement with inspection of the intramedullary canal of both bone ends, where soil contamination tends to occur during injury (see Fig. 10-30). Soil contamination has been reported to lead to gas gangrene and subsequent upper extremity amputation in children with grade I open forearm fractures.[96] Emergency room irrigation and débridement is not recommended and is considered inadequate with increased risk of serious infection.

In four published series of plated pediatric forearm fractures (25% open fractures), deep infection (osteomyelitis) occurred in 5% (4/83).[219,227,333,358] Such deep infections usually require extensive additional surgical treatment to eradicate them. Combined data from 12 series of similar pediatric forearm fractures (15% open fractures) treated with intramedullary Kirschner wires, Steinmann pins, or Rush rods revealed a deep infection rate of 0.46% (2/437)[10,48,74,180,194,259,260,297,346,365] and a superficial infection rate of 2.5% (11/437). Six studies of ESIN fixation reported a 0.2% (1/370) deep infection rate and a 3% (12/370) superficial infection rate.[48,131,184,201,269,337] Superficial infections may require oral antibiotics, pin removal, or both.

Open forearm fractures clearly are at increased risk for infection. Most (96%) open forearm fractures in children are Gustilo and Anderson[134] grade I or II.[128,135,195] Two studies specifically investigated the relationship between the time from injury until irrigation and débridement and the risk of later infection. Luhmann et al.[195] reported on 65 fractures (52 type I, 12 type II, 1 type III) that were irrigated and débrided an average of 5.6 hours (range 1.5 to 24 hours) after injury, and Greenbaum et al.[128] reported 62 fractures (58 type I, 4 type II) that were irrigated and débrided an average of 14.6 hours (range 1.7 to 37.8 hours) after injury. No statistically significant association was found in either of these studies; however, most (87%) of these fractures were grade I injuries. Pooled data revealed an overall 1.2% rate (2/173) of deep infection and a 0.6% rate (1/173) of superficial infection after current open fracture treatment protocols.[128,135,195]

Neurapraxia

The median nerve is the most commonly injured nerve with forearm shaft fractures (whether closed or open injuries),[80,128,135,195] but any peripheral nerve and at times multiple nerves may be involved.[74] Most of these injuries are simple neurapraxias that occur at the time of injury and resolve spontaneously over weeks to months.[80,134,228] Actual nerve entrapment within or perforation by the bony fragments has been reported,[4,111,117,118,151,257,258,312] most often with greenstick fractures.[118,151,257,258] Constricting fracture callus and fibrous tissue also have been known to cause nerve palsies.[258,312] In patients who fail to recover normal nerve function within a satisfactory time period,[4] nerve exploration, decompression, and possible nerve repair should be considered. If signs of progressive nerve recovery (e.g., advancing Tinel sign, return of function) are not present by the end of the third month after injury, further diagnostic work-up (electromyography with nerve conduction studies) is indicated. Prolonged waiting can be harmful to long term outcome.

Nerve injury after internal fixation is always a concern. Operative treatment of pediatric forearm fractures by either indirect reduction and internal fixation techniques or classic open reduction and internal fixation techniques requires fracture manipulation and soft tissue retraction, which have the potential to worsen existing subclinical nerve injury or to create a new injury. Such injuries are rare and may be underreported. Nerve injury after pediatric forearm plate fixation has been alluded to but not discussed extensively.[180] Luhmann et al.[194] reported an 8% (2/25) iatrogenic nerve injury rate after fixation with intramedullary Kirschner wires or Rush rods: Both were ulnar nerve injuries that resolved in 2 to 3 weeks. Cullen et al.[74] reported one ulnar nerve injury that took 3 months to resolve in a group of 20 patients treated with Kirschner wires or Rush rods.

Certain sensory nerves also are at risk for iatrogenic damage during surgical forearm fracture treatment, especially the superficial branch of the radial nerve.[48,194,314] Pooled data from six series that included 370 ESIN procedures revealed a 2% (7/370) rate of injury to the superficial branch of the radial nerve.[48,131,184,201,269,337] The branching pattern of this sensory nerve is complex, and efforts must be taken to protect it during insertion of intramedullary nails through distal radial entry points.[1,16]

Muscle or Tendon Entrapment/Tendon Rupture

Severely displaced forearm fractures may trap portions of muscle between the fracture fragments.[146,259] Often, interposed tissue can be effectively removed during standard fracture reduction, but the muscle may become an obstacle to successful closed reduction. Much of the volar aspects of the shafts of the radius and ulna are covered by the flexor pollicis longus and flexor digitorum profundus, respectively. Many displaced forearm shaft fractures also have apex volar angulation.[230] As a result, portions of these muscles (or their tendons) are particularly prone to fracture site incarceration (Fig. 10-41). The pronator quadratus also is vulnerable to fracture site entrapment in the distal third of the radius and ulna, and it can block reduction of distal-third forearm fractures.[146]

Flexor digitorum profundus entrapment within ulnar[139,177,266,295] and radial[347] shaft fractures has been reported. Entrapment of the flexor digitorum profundus typically causes an inability to fully extend the involved finger (usually index, long, or ring fingers alone or in combination).[139,295] Even if identified early, this complication rarely responds to occupational or phys-

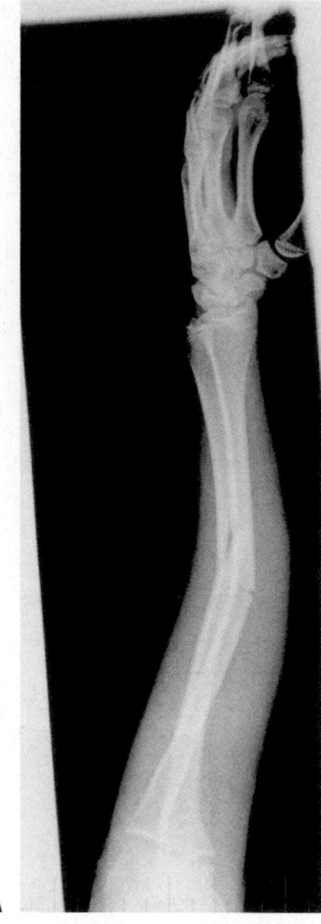

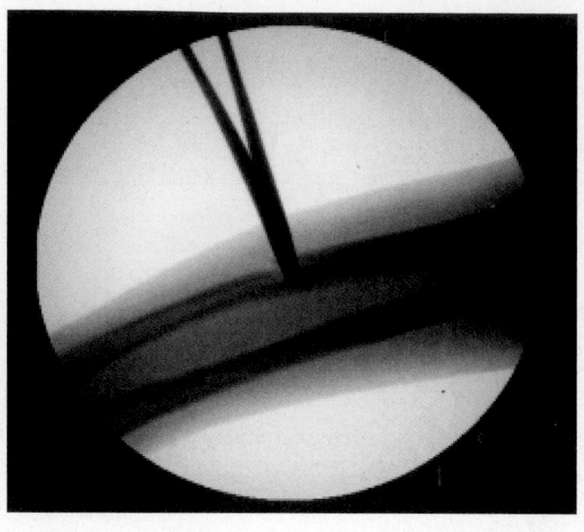

FIGURE 10-41 Muscle/tendon incarceration. **A.** Injury radiograph showing mild apex-volar fracture angulation. **B.** Flexor digitorum profundus entrapment in the ulnar fracture site required surgical extirpation.

ical therapy. Surgical intervention is the preferred treatment and requires only a small incision (usually over the ulna) through which the adherent tissue is elevated with a blunt instrument from the bone at the site of the fracture. Excellent restoration of finger motion can be achieved, even when the release is done up to 2 years after the fracture.[266]

Extensor tendon injury has been reported after intramedullary nailing of pediatric forearm shaft fractures.[131,184,248,259] Primary tendon disruption may be caused by direct trauma during either nail insertion or extraction. Delayed tendon disruption may be caused by slow erosion of the tendon as it glides past a sharp nail edge. The possibility of this complication can be minimized by using surgical incisions large enough to allow insertion of small blunt retractors to protect adjacent tendons during nail insertion and extraction. Avoidance of tendon erosion requires pin lengths that extend beyond the tendon level into either the subcutaneous tissues[74,297] or through the skin (external pins).[259] Conceivably, the pins could be buried completely within the bone, but this would require either accepting them as permanent implants (something not commonly practiced at this time) or significantly increasing the level of difficulty of nail removal. The extensor pollicis longus is more at risk near Lister's tubercle and may require a late tendon reconstruction with extensor indicis proprius transfer.

Compartment Syndrome

Compartment syndrome is rare after closed forearm fractures in children, but its consequences can be devastating. Yuan et al.[363] found no compartment syndromes in 205 closed forearm injuries, and Jones and Weiner[161] reported no compartment syndromes in their series of 730 closed forearm injuries. A single compartment syndrome that developed during cast treatment of a 12-year-old female with a closed both-bone forearm fracture was reported by Cullen et al.[74] Because the diagnosis of compartment syndrome can be difficult in children,[265] the index of suspicion must be high.

Compartment syndrome should be suspected in any child who is not reasonably comfortable 3 to 4 hours after adequate reduction and immobilization of a forearm fracture.[66] The risk of compartment syndrome is higher with open fractures[135,363] and fractures that are difficult to reduce and require extended operative efforts.[363] Yuan et al.[363] voiced concern that the 10% (3/30) rate of compartment syndrome in their patients with closed fractures might be due to multiple passes or "misses" with intramedullary devices during efforts at indirect reduction and internal fixation. Compartment syndrome was reported by Haasbeek and Cole[135] in 5 (11%) of 46 open forearm fractures in their series. The so-called floating elbow injury has been associated with a rate of compartment syndrome as high as 33%.[363] Forearm compartment syndrome is best treated with fasciotomy, releasing both the superficial and deep volar compartments and the mobile wad. Both the lacertus fibrosis and the carpal tunnel should be released as part of the procedure.

Complex Regional Pain Syndromes

Complex regional pain syndromes such as reflex sympathetic dystrophy are uncommon complications after pediatric forearm shaft fractures.[333] Paradoxically, relatively minor injuries seem to place patients at greatest risk.[315,351] The most reliable sign in children is true allodynia: significant reproducible pain with light touch on the skin. Swelling and other vasomotor changes often are accompanying signs.[187] The diagnosis in children is made based almost exclusively on the history and physical examination, with little reliance on studies such as bone scans.[315] These pain syndromes are best treated initially with physical therapy aimed at range of motion and desensitization.[315,351] Failure to respond to physical therapy may warrant a referral to a qualified pediatric pain specialist.[172,187]

CONTROVERSIES AND FUTURE DIRECTIONS

Fracture Risk/Fracture Prevention

Over the past 3 decades, the rate of forearm fractures has increased dramatically in the United States: 33% higher for males and 56% higher for females.[175] Certain risk-taking behaviors demonstrated by children, as well as increased use of motorized vehicles like all-terrain vehicles, may be at least partly to blame.[47,197] Increased general physical activity patterns and decreased calcium intake also have been suggested as explanations,[175] but gaps persist in our epidemiologic understanding. Preventing these injuries remains an admirable but elusive goal. Two main avenues of research have been explored: optimizing safety during activities known to be associated with forearm fractures, and investigating biologic mechanisms related to fracture risk.

The relationship between in-line skating (rollerblading) and pediatric forearm fractures has been shown,[218,249] with 1 in 8 children sustaining a fracture on his or her first skating attempt.[218] Prevention efforts have focused largely on protective gear. Wrist guards have been shown to decrease distal forearm bone strain[311] and injury rates.[282] Similar protective effects of wrist guards in snowboarders have been shown.[237] Trampolines are another target of injury prevention efforts aimed at a specific play activity.[91] Dramatic increases in trampoline-related injuries were reported during the 1990s, with rates doubling[305] or even tripling.[108] Safety recommendations have ranged from constant adult supervision and one-child-at-a-time use[183] to outright bans on public trampoline use.[108,305]

A variety of biologic risk factors have been studied relative to forearm fractures. Children who avoid drinking milk have been shown to have increased fracture risk,[125] as well as those who prefer to drink fruit juice and soda.[245] Several studies have shown an increased risk of fractures in females aged 3 to 15 years with low bone density.[122,124] Diet, nutrition, and exercise are being explored as causative factors, but the precise reason for the low bone density has not been confirmed. Too little physical activity (as measured by television, computer, and video viewing) has been associated with increased fracture risk, presumably because of decreased bone mineral density.[196] Caution also must be exercised when obtaining dual-energy x-ray absorptiometry data in children, as up to 88% of scans may be misinterpreted.[110] Childhood obesity is a growing problem in our society.[114,153] Increased body weight and decreased cross-sectional dimensions of the forearm bones also have been found in females who fracture their forearms.[303] Other researchers have found an increased risk of forearm fracture in obese children.[123,160]

Parental Presence during Fracture Reduction

Parental presence is becoming increasingly popular for pediatric emergency department procedures. Several studies on chest tubes, intravenous cannulation, lumbar puncture, and urethral catheterization have shown increased parental satisfaction when parents are allowed to stay for these procedures.[21,137,250] Parental presence during induction of anesthesia also has been shown to have favorable effects on children older than 4 years of age.[164] To the best of our knowledge, there are no published studies on parental presence during orthopaedic procedures performed in the emergency department setting. There also are no parental presence studies on any emergency department procedures performed on children who are under sedation, when the child is probably not aware of the parent's presence.

Certain relationships between perceived procedural invasiveness and parental presence have been borne out in the literature. Four hundred parents from the Indiana area were surveyed, and with increasing invasiveness, the parents' desire to be present decreased.[38] A survey of academic emergency medicine attendings, residents, and nurses from across the country also showed that there is an inverse relationship between increasing invasiveness and support for parental presence.[23] Boudreaux et al. published their critical review of the parental presence literature and concluded that "randomized controlled trials are mixed regarding whether family presence actually helps the patient."[12]

Extrapolation of information from the previously mentioned studies to pediatric orthopaedic settings should be done with caution. We typically allow parents to be present for the induction of sedation, and once the patient is sedated the parents are asked to wait in a designated area. If parents are allowed to be present, we strongly recommend a dedicated employee to attend to the parent or parents (a "spotter"). Several parents (typically fathers) have fainted during such orthopaedic procedures and injured themselves. Parents who stay for a reduction also should be counseled that the patient may moan or cry during reduction but will not remember it. Parents who are not present during reduction should be asked to wait far enough away from the procedure room so they cannot hear the child.

ACKNOWLEDGMENTS

The authors wish to acknowledge the priceless teaching and constructive feedback afforded us by our senior partner, Alvin H. Crawford, MD, FACS, as well as the skilled assistance of Ms. Kelli Israel and Ms. Tiffany Whatley in the preparation of this chapter.

REFERENCES

1. Abrams RA, Brown RA, Botte MJ. The superficial branch of the radial nerve: an anatomic study with surgical implications. J Hand Surg Am 1992;17:1037–1041.
2. Abrams RA, Ziets RJ, Lieber RL, et al. Anatomy of the radial nerve motor branches in the forearm. J Hand Surg Am 1997;22:232–237.
3. Aktas S, Saridogan K, Moralar U, et al. Patterns of single segment nonphyseal extremity fractures in children. Int Orthop 1999;23:345–347.
4. al-Qattan MM, Clarke HM, Zimmer P. Radiological signs of entrapment of the median nerve in forearm shaft fractures. J Hand Surg Br 1994;19:713–719.
5. Allen PE, Vickery CW, Atkins RM. A modified approach to the flexor surface of the distal radius. J Hand Surg Br 1996;21:303–304.
6. Alpar EK, Thompson K, Owen R, et al. Midshaft fractures of forearm bones in children. Injury 1981;13:153–158.
8. American Academy of Pediatrics Committee on Drugs. Guidelines for monitoring and management of pediatric patients during and after sedation for diagnostic and therapeutic procedures. Pediatrics 1992;89:1110–1115.
9. American Academy of Pediatrics Committee on Drugs. Guidelines for monitoring of pediatric patients during and after sedation for diagnostic and therapeutic procedures: addendum. Pediatrics 2002;110:836–838.

10. Amit Y, Salai M, Chechik A, et al. Closing intramedullary nailing for the treatment of diaphyseal forearm fractures in adolescence: a preliminary report. J Pediatr Orthop 1985;5:143–146.
11. Aner A, Singer M, Feldbrin Z, et al. Surgical treatment of posttraumatic radioulnar synostosis in children. J Pediatr Orthop 2002;22:598–600.
12. Anonymous. Fracture and dislocation compendium: Orthopaedic Trauma Association Committee for Coding and Classification. J Orthop Trauma 1996;10:1–153.
13. Anonymous. The treatment of forearm fractures with pins. By Georg Schöne, 1913. Clin Orthop Relat Res 1988;234:2–4.
14. Archibong AE, Onuba O. Fractures in children in south eastern Nigeria. Cent Afr J Med 1996;42:340–343.
15. Arunachalam VSP, Griffiths JC. Fracture recurrence in children. Injury 1975;7:37–40.
16. Auerbach DM, Collins ED, Kunkle KL, et al. The radial sensory nerve: an anatomic study. Clin Orthop Relat Res 1994;308:241–249.
17. Bär HF, Breitfuss H. Analysis of angular deformities on radiographs. J Bone Joint Surg Br 1989;71:710–711.
18. Bartl V, Gál P, Skotáková J, et al. Treatment of redislocated fragments of long bones using plaster cast wedging. Rozhl Chir 2002;81:415–420.
19. Bass RL, Stern PJ. Elbow and forearm anatomy and surgical approaches. Hand Clin 1994;10:343–356.
20. Bätz W, Hoffman-v Kap-herr S, Pistor G. Posttraumatic radioulnar synostoses in childhood. Aktuelle Traumatol 1986;16:13–16.
21. Bauchner H, Vinci R, Bak S, et al. Parents and procedures: a randomized controlled trial. Pediatrics 1996;98:861–867.
22. Bauer G, Arand M, Mutschler W. Posttraumatic synostosis after forearm fracture osteosynthesis. Arch Orthop Trauma Surg 1991;110:142–145.
23. Beckman AW, Sloan BK, Moore GP, et al. Should parents be present during emergency department procedures on children and who should make the decision? A survey of emergency physician and nurse attitudes. Acad Emerg Med 2002;9:154–158.
24. Beekman F, Sullivan JE. Some observations on fractures of long bones in children. Am J Surg 1941;51:722–738.
25. Bellemans M, Lamoureux J. Indications for immediate percutaneous intramedullary nailing of complete diaphyseal forearm shaft fractures in children. Acta Orthop Belg 1995;61(suppl I):169–172.
26. Bhaskar AR, Roberts JA. Treatment of unstable fractures of the forearm in children: is plating of a single bone adequate? J Bone Joint Surg Br 2001;83:253–258.
27. Biyani A, Gupta SP, Sharma JC. Ipsilateral supracondylar fractures of the humerus and forearm bone in children. Injury 1989;20:203–207.
28. Black GB, Amadeo R. Orthopedic injuries associated with backyard trampoline use in children. J Pediatr Surg 2004;39:653.
29. Blackburn N, Ziv I, Rang M. Correction of the malunited forearm fracture. Clin Orthop Relat Res 1984;188:54–57.
30. Blaisier RD, Salamon PB. Closed intramedullary rodding of pediatric adolescent forearm fractures. Oper Tech Orthop 1993;3:128–133.
31. Blakemore LC, Cooperman DR, Thompson GH, et al. Compartment syndrome in ipsilateral humerus and forearm fractures in children. Clin Orthop Relat Res 2000;376:32–38.
32. Bley L, Seitz WH Jr. Injuries about the distal ulna in children. Hand Clin 1998;14:231–237.
33. Blount WP. Forearm fractures in children. Clin Orthop Relat Res 1967;51:93–107.
34. Blount WP. Fractures in Children. Baltimore: Williams & Wilkins, 1955:78.
35. Blount WP. Osteoclasis for supination deformities in children. J Bone Joint Surg 1940;22:300–314.
36. Blount WP, Schaefer AA, Johnson JH. Fractures of the forearm in children. JAMA 1942;120:111–116.
37. Böhler L. The Treatment of Fractures. 5th ed. New York: Grune & Stratton, 1956:21–23.
38. Boie ET, Moore GP, Brummett C, et al. Do parents want to be present during invasive procedures performed on their children in the emergency department? A survey of 400 parents. Ann Emerg Med 1999;34:70–74.
39. Boone DC, Azen SP. Normal range of motion of joints in male subjects. J Bone Joint Surg Am 1979;61:756–759.
40. Borden S. Traumatic bowing of the forearm in children. J Bone Joint Surg Am 1974;56:611–616.
41. Border S. Roentgen recognition of acute plastic bowing of the forearm in children. Am J Roentgenol Radium Ther Nucl Med 1975;125:524–530.
42. Boudreaux ED, Francis JL, Loyacano T. Family presence during invasive procedures and resuscitations in the emergency department: a critical review and suggestions for future research. Ann Emerg Med 2002;40:193–205.
43. Bould M, Bannister GC. Refractures of the radius and ulna in children. Injury 1999;30:583–586.
44. Boyer BA, Overton B, Schraeder W, et al. Position of immobilization for pediatric forearm fractures. J Pediatr Orthop 2002;22:185–187.
45. Branovacki G, Hanson M, Cash R, et al. The innervation of the radial nerve at the elbow and in the forearm. J Hand Surg Br 1998;23:167–169.
46. Bratt HD, Eyres RL, Cole WG. Randomized double-blind trial of low- and moderate-dose lidocaine regional anesthesia for forearm fractures in childhood. J Pediatr Orthop 1996;16:660–663.
47. Brown RL, Koepplinger ME, Mehlman CT, et al. All-terrain vehicle and bicycle crashes in children: epidemiology and comparison of injury severity. J Pediatr Surg 2002;37:375–380.
48. Calder PR, Achan P, Barry M. Diaphyseal forearm fractures in children treated with intramedullary fixation: outcome of K-wires versus elastic stable intramedullary nail. Injury 2003;34:278–282.
49. Cameron ML, Sponseller PD, Rossberg MI. Pediatric analgesia and sedation for the management of orthopedic conditions. Am J Orthop 2000;29:665–672.
50. Campbell WC. Campbell's Operative Orthopaedics. 1st ed. St. Louis: The CV Mosby Company, 1939.
51. Campbell WC. Orthopedics of Childhood. New York: Appleton and Company, 1930:154–156.
52. Carey PJ, Alburger PD, Betz RR, et al. Both-bone forearm fractures in children. Orthopedics 1992;15:1015–1019.
53. Carsi B, Abril JC, Epeldegui T. Longitudinal growth after nonphyseal forearm fractures. J Pediatr Orthop 2003;23:203–207.
54. Carter DR, Spengler DM. Mechanical properties and composition of cortical bone. Clin Orthop Relat Res 1978;135:192–217.
55. Casey PJ, Moed BR. Greenstick fractures of the radius in adults: a report of two cases. J Orthop Trauma 1996;10:209–212.
56. Celebi L, Muratli HH, Doğan O, et al. The results of intramedullary nailing in children who developed redisplacement during cast treatment of both-bone forearm fractures. Acta Orthop Traumatol Turc 2007;41:175–182.
57. Chamay A. Mechanical and morphological aspects of experimental overload and fatigue in bone. J Biomech 1970;3:263–270.
58. Chan CF, Meads BM, Nicol RO. Remanipulation of forearm fractures in children. N Z Med J 1997;110:249–250.
59. Chantelot C, Feugas C, Guillem P, et al. Innervation of the medial epicondylar muscles: an anatomic study in 50 cases. Surg Radiol Anat 1999;21:165–168.
60. Chapman MW, Gordon JE, Zissimos AG. Compression-plate fixation of acute fractures of the diaphysis of the radius and ulna. J Bone Joint Surg Am 1989;71:159–169.
61. Charnley J. The Closed Treatment of Common Fractures. Edinburgh: Livingstone, 1957.
62. Cheng JC, Ng BK, Ying SY, et al. A 10-year study of the changes in the pattern and treatment of 6,493 fractures. J Pediatr Orthop 1999;19:344–350.
63. Chess DG, Hyndman JC, Leahey JL, et al. Short arm plaster cast for distal pediatric forearm fractures. J Pediatr Orthop 1994;14:211–213.
64. Chung KC, Spilson SV. The frequency and epidemiology of hand and forearm fractures in the United States. J Hand Surg Am 2001;26:908–915.
65. Cleary JE, Omer GE Jr. Congenital proximal radioulnar synostosis: natural history and functional assessment. J Bone Joint Surg Am 1985;76:539–545.
66. Crawford AH. Orthopedic injury in children. In: Callaham ML, ed. Current Practice of Emergency Medicine. 2nd ed. Philadelphia: BC Decker, 1991:1232–1233.
67. Crawford AH. Orthopedics. In: Rudolph CD, Rudolph AM, Hostetter MK, et al., eds. Rudolph's Pediatrics. 21st ed. New York: McGraw Hill, 2002:2451.
68. Crawford AH. Pitfalls and complications of fractures of the distal radius and ulna in childhood. Hand Clin 1988;4:403–413.
69. Crawford AH Jr, Bagamery N. Osseous manifestations of neurofibromatosis in childhood. J Pediatr Orthop 1986;6:672–688.
70. Crawford AH, Cionni AS. Management of pediatric orthopedic injuries by the emergency medicine specialist. In: Pediatric Critical Illness and Injury: Assessment and Care. Rockville: Aspen System Publications, 1984:213–225.
71. Crawford AH, Schorry EK. Neurofibromatosis in children: the role of the orthopaedist. J Am Acad Orthop Surg 1999;7:217–230.
72. Creasman C, Zaleske DJ, Ehrlich MG. Analyzing forearm fractures in children: the more subtle signs of impending problems. Clin Orthop Relat Res 1984;188:40–53.
73. Crenshaw AH Jr. Surgical approaches. In: Canale ST, ed. Campbell's Operative Orthopaedics. 10th ed. St. Louis, CV Mosby, 2003:107–109.
74. Cullen MC, Roy DR, Giza E, et al. Complications of intramedullary fixation of pediatric forearm fractures. J Pediatr Orthop 1998;18:14–21.
75. Curry JD, Butler G. The mechanical properties of bone tissue in children. J Bone Joint Surg Am 1975;57:810–814.
76. Daruwalla JS. A study of radioulnar movements following fractures of the forearm in children. Clin Orthop Relat Res 1979;139:114–120.
77. Davids JR, Frick SL, Skewes E, et al. Skin surface pressure beneath an above-the-knee cast: plaster casts compared with fiberglass casts. J Bone Joint Surg Am 1997;79:565–569.
78. Davidson AJ, Eyres RL, Cole WG. A comparison of prilocaine and lidocaine for intravenous regional anaesthesia for forearm fracture reduction in children. Paediatr Anaesth 2002;12:146–150.
79. Davidson AW. Rock, paper, scissors. Injury 2003;34:61–63.
80. Davis DR, Green DP. Forearm fractures in children: pitfalls and complications. Clin Orthop Relat Res 1976;120:172–183.
81. de Pablos J, Franzreb M, Barrios C. Longitudinal growth pattern of the radius after forearm fractures conservatively treated in children. J Pediatr Orthop 1994;14:492–495.
82. DeFrate LE, Li G, Zayontz SJ, et al. A minimally invasive method for the determination of force in the interosseous ligament. Clin Biomech 2001;16:895–900.
83. Deluca PA, Lindsey RW, Ruwe PA. Refracture of bones of the forearm after the removal of compression plates. J Bone Joint Surg Am 1988;70:1372–1376.
84. Dilberti T, Botte MJ, Abrams RA. Anatomical considerations regarding the posterior interosseous nerve during posterolateral approaches to the proximal part of the radius. J Bone Joint Surg Am 2000;82:809–813.
85. Do T. Forearm. In: Cramer KE, Scherl SA, eds. Orthopaedic Surgery Essentials. Philadelphia: Lippincott Williams & Wilkins, 2004:125–130.
86. Do TT, Strub WM, Foad SL, et al. Reduction versus remodeling in pediatric distal forearm fractures: a preliminary cost analysis. J Pediatr Orthop B 2003;12:109–115.
87. Doyle JR, Botte MJ. Surgical Anatomy of the Hand & Upper Extremity. Philadelphia: Lippincott Williams & Wilkins, 2003:34–40.
88. Dumont CE, Thalmann R, Macy JC. The effect of rotational malunion of the radius and ulna on supination and pronation. J Bone Joint Surg Br 2002;84:1070–1074.
89. Duncan J, Weiner D. Unstable pediatric forearm fractures: use of "pins and plaster." Orthopedics 2004;27:267–269.
90. Elgafy H, Ebraheim NA, Yeasting RA. Extensile posterior approach to the radius. Clin Orthop Relat Res 2000;373:252–258.
91. Esposito PW. Trampoline injuries. Clin Orthop Relat Res 2003;409:43–52.
92. Evans EM. Fractures of the radius and ulna. J Bone Joint Surg Br 1951;33:548–561.
93. Evans EM. Pronation injuries of the forearm with special reference to the anterior Monteggia fracture. J Bone Joint Surg Br 1949;31:578–588.
94. Evans EM. Rotational deformity in the treatment of fractures of both bones of the forearm. J Bone Joint Surg 1945;27:373–379.
95. Evans JK, Buckley SL, Alexander AH, et al. Analgesia for the reduction of fractures in children: a comparison of nitrous oxide with intramuscular sedation. J Pediatr Orthop 1995;15:73–77.
96. Fee NF, Dobranski A, Bisla RS. Gas gangrene complicating open forearm fractures: report of five cases. J Bone Joint Surg Am 1977;59:135–138.
97. Fernandez FF, Egenolf M, Carsten C, et al. Unstable diaphyseal fractures of both bones

of the forearm in children: plate versus intramedullary nailing. Injury 2005;36: 1210–1216.
98. Fiala M, Carey TP. Paediatric forearm fractures: an analysis of refracture rate. Orthop Trans 1994–1995;18:1265–1266.
99. Fike EA, Bartal E. Delayed union of the distal ulna in a child after both-bone forearm fracture. J South Orthop Assoc 1998;7:113–116.
100. Firl M, Wünsch L. Measurement of bowing of the radius. J Bone Joint Surg Br 2004; 86:1047–1049.
101. Fleischer H. Marrow wiring in lower-arm fractures of children. Dtsch Med Wochenschr 1975;100:1278–1279.
102. Floyd AS. Is the measurement of angles on radiographs accurate? Brief report. J Bone Joint Surg Br 1988;70:486–487.
103. Flynn JM. Pediatric forearm fractures: decision making, surgical techniques, and complications. Instr Course Lect 2002;51:355–360.
104. Flynn JM, Sarwark JF, Waters PM, et al. The surgical management of pediatric fractures of the upper extremity. Instr Course Lect 2003;52:635–645.
105. Flynn JM, Waters PM. Single-bone fixation of both-bone forearm fractures. J Pediatr Orthop 1996;16:655–659.
106. Formicola V, Pontrandolfi A, Svoboda J. The Upper Paleolithic Triple Burial of Dolní Vestonice: pathology and funerary behavior. Am J Phys Anthropol 2001;115:372–379.
107. Furia JP, Alioto RJ, Marquardt JD. The efficacy and safety of the hematoma block for fracture reduction in closed isolated fractures. Orthopedics 1997;20:423–426.
108. Furnival RA, Street KA, Schunk JE. Too many pediatric trampoline injuries. Pediatrics 1999;103:e57.
109. Gabriel MT, Pfaeffle HJ, Stabile KJ, et al. Passive strain distribution in the interosseous ligament of the forearm: implications for injury reconstruction. J Hand Surg Am 2004; 29:293–298.
110. Gafni RI, Baron J. Overdiagnosis of osteoporosis in children due to misinterpretation of dual-energy x-ray absorptiometry (DEXA). J Pediatr 2004;144:253–257.
111. Gainor BJ, Olson S. Combined entrapment of the median and anterior interosseous nerves in a pediatric both-bone forearm fracture. J Orthop Trauma 1990;4:197–199.
112. Galpin RD, Webb GR, Armstrong DG, et al. A comparison of short and long-arm plaster casts for displaced distal-third pediatric forearm fractures: a prospective randomized trial. Paper presented at: Annual Meeting of the Pediatric Orthopaedic Society of North America; April 27–May 1, 2004; St. Louis, MO.
113. Gandhi RK, Wilson P, Mason Brown JJ, et al. Spontaneous correction of deformity following fractures of the forearm in children. Br J Surg 1962;50:5–10.
114. Garcia VF, Langford L, Inge TI. Application of laparoscopy for bariatric surgery. Curr Opin Pediatr 2003;15:248–255.
115. Garg NK, Ballal MS, Malek IA, et al. Use of elastic stable intramedullary nailing for treating unstable forearm fractures in children. J Trauma 2008;65:109–115.
116. Gartland JJ. Fundamentals of Orthopaedics. 4th ed. Philadelphia: WB Saunders, 1987: 34.
117. Geissler WB, Fernandez DL, Graca R. Anterior interosseous nerve palsy complicating a forearm fracture in a child. J Hand Surg Am 1990;15:44–47.
118. Genelin F, Karlbauer AF, Gasperschitz F. Greenstick fracture of the forearm with median nerve entrapment. J Emerg Med 1988;6:381–385.
119. Giebel GD, Meyer C, Koebke J, et al. Arterial supply of forearm bones and its importance for the operative treatment of fractures. Surg Radiol Anat 1997;19:149–153.
120. Godambe SA, Elliot V, Matheny D, et al. Comparison of propofol/fentanyl versus ketamine/midazolam for brief procedural sedation in a pediatric emergency department. Pediatrics 2003;112:116–123.
121. Gonzalez MH, Lotfi P, Bendre A, et al. The ulnar nerve at the elbow and its local branching: an anatomic study. J Hand Surg Br 2001;26:142–144.
122. Goulding A, Cannan R, Williams SM, et al. Bone mineral density in girls with forearm fractures. J Bone Miner Res 1998;13:143–148.
123. Goulding A, Jones IE, Taylor RW, et al. Bone mineral density and body composition in boys with distal forearm fractures: a dual-energy x-ray absorptiometry study. J Pediatr 2001;139:509–515.
124. Goulding A, Jones IE, Taylor RW, et al. More broken bones: a 4-year double cohort study of young girls with and without distal forearm fractures. J Bone Miner Res 2000; 15:2011–2018.
125. Goulding A, Rockell JE, Black RE, et al. Children who avoid drinking cow's milk are at increased risk for prepubertal bone fractures. J Am Diet Assoc 2004;104:250–253.
126. Grauer AL, Roberts CA. Paleoepidemiology, healing, and possible treatment of trauma in the medieval cemetery population of St. Helen-on-the-Walls, York, England. Am J Phys Anthropol 1996;100:531–544.
127. Gray H. Gray's Anatomy: The Classic Collector's Edition. New York: Bounty, 1977: 152–157.
128. Greenbaum B, Zionts LE, Ebramzadeh E. Open fractures of the forearm in children. J Orthop Trauma 2001;15:111–118.
129. Gregory PR, Sullivan JA. Nitrous oxide compared with intravenous regional anesthesia in pediatric forearm fracture manipulation. J Pediatr Orthop 1996;16:187–191.
130. Greiwe RM, Mehlman CT, Moon E, et al. Stiffness following displaced pediatric both-bone forearm fractures: a meta-analysis. Paper presented at: Annual Meeting of the Orthopaedic Trauma Association; October 5–7, 2006; Phoenix, AZ.
131. Griffet J, el Hayek T, Baby M. Intramedullary nailing of forearm fractures in children. J Pediatr Orthop B 1999;8:88–89.
132. Griffin PP, Green DP. Forearm fractures in children [letter]. Clin Orthop Relat Res 1977;129:320–321.
133. Gupta RP, Danielsson LG. Dorsally angulated solitary metaphyseal greenstick fractures in the distal radius: results after immobilization in pronated, neutral, and supinated position. J Pediatr Orthop 1990;10:90–92.
134. Gustilo RB, Anderson JT. Prevention of infection in the treatment of 1025 open fractures of long bones: retrospective and prospective analyses. J Bone Joint Surg Am 1976;58: 453–458.
135. Haasbeek JF, Cole WG. Open fractures of the arm in children. J Bone Joint Surg Br 1995;77:576–581.
136. Hahn MP, Richter D, Muhr G, et al. Pediatric forearm fractures: diagnosis, therapy, and possible complications. Unfallchirurg 1997;100:760–769.
137. Haimi-Cohen Y, Amir J, Harel L, et al. Parental presence during lumbar puncture: anxiety and attitude toward the procedure. Clin Pediatr (Phila) 1996;35:2–4.
138. Harrington P, Sharif I, Fogarty EE, et al. Management of the floating elbow injury in children. Arch Orthop Trauma Surg 2000;120:205–208.
139. Hendel D, Aner A. Entrapment of the flexor digitorum profundus of the ring finger at the site of an ulnar fracture: a case report. Ital J Orthop Traumatol 1992;18:417–419.
140. Hennrikus WL, Shin AY, Klingelberger CE. Self-administered nitrous oxide and a hematoma block for analgesia in the outpatient reduction of fractures in children. J Bone Joint Surg Am 1995;77:335–339.
141. Henry AK. Extensile Exposure. 2nd ed. Edinburgh: Churchill Livingstone, 1966: 107–108.
142. Hoffman GM, Nowakowski R, Troshynski TJ, et al. Risk reduction in pediatric procedural sedation by application of an American Academy of Pediatrics/American Society of Anesthesiologists process model. Pediatrics 2002;109:236–243.
143. Högström H, Nilsson BE, Willner S. Correction with growth following diaphyseal forearm fracture. Acta Orthop Scand 1976;47:299–303.
144. Holdsworth BJ, Sloan JP. Proximal forearm fractures in children: residual disability. Injury 1982;14:174–179.
145. Hollister AM, Gellman H, Waters RL. The relationship of the interosseous membrane to the axis of rotation of the forearm. Clin Orthop Relat Res 1994;298:272–276.
146. Holmes JR, Louis DS. Entrapment of pronator quadratus in pediatric distal radius fractures: recognition and treatment. J Pediatr Orthop 1994;14:498–500.
147. Hoppenfeld S, deBoer P. Surgical Exposures in Orthopaedics. 3rd ed. Philadelphia: Lippincott Williams & Wilkins, 2003.
148. Hoppenfeld S, Zeide MS. Orthopaedic Dictionary. Philadelphia: JB Lippincott, 1994: 275.
149. Hotchkiss RN, An KN, Sowa DT, et al. An anatomic and mechanical study of the interosseous membrane of the forearm: pathomechanics of proximal migration of the radius. J Hand Surg Am 1989;14:256–261.
150. Hsu ES, Patwardhan AG, Meade KP, et al. Cross-sectional geometrical properties and bone mineral content of the human radius and ulna. J Biomech 1993;26:1307–1318.
151. Huang K, Pun WK, Coleman S. Entrapment and transection of the median nerve associated with greenstick fractures of the forearm: a case report and review of the literature. J Trauma 1998;44:1101–1102.
152. Hughston JC. Fractures of the forearm in children. J Bone Joint Surg Am 1962;44: 1678–1693.
153. Inge TH, Krebs NF, Garcia VF, et al. Bariatric surgery for severely overweight adolescents: concerns and recommendations. Pediatrics 2004;114:217–223.
154. Jacobsen FS. Periosteum: its relation to pediatric fractures. J Pediatr Orthop B 1997; 6:84–90.
155. Jacobsen FS, Crawford AH. Complications in neurofibromatosis. In: Epps CH, Bowen JR, eds. Complications in Pediatric Orthopaedic Surgery. Philadelphia: JB Lippincott, 1995:678–680.
156. Jacobsen ST, Hull CK, Crawford AH. Nutritional rickets. J Pediatr Orthop 1986;6: 713–716.
157. Johari AN, Sinha M. Remodeling of forearm fractures in children. J Pediatr Orthop B 1999;8:84–87.
158. Johnson CW, Carmichael KD, Morris RP, et al. Biomechanical study of flexible intramedullary nails. J Pediatr Orthop 2009;29:44–48.
159. Johnson PQ, Noffsinger MA. Hematoma block of distal forearm fractures: is it safe? Orthop Rev 1991;20:977–979.
160. Jones IE, Williams SM, Goulding A. Associations of birth weight and length, childhood size, and smoking with bone fractures during growth: evidence from a birth cohort study. Am J Epidemiol 2004;159:343–350.
161. Jones K, Weiner DS. The management of forearm fractures in children: a plea for conservatism. J Pediatr Orthop 1999;19:811–815.
162. Jubel A, Andermahr J, Isenberg J, et al. Outcomes and complications of elastic stable intramedullary nailing of forearm fractures in children. J Pediatr Orthop B 2005;14: 375–380.
163. Juliano PJ, Mazur JM, Cummings RJ, et al. Low-dose lidocaine intravenous regional anesthesia for forearm fractures in children. J Pediatr Orthop 1992;12:633–635.
164. Kain ZN, Mayes LC, Caramico LA, et al. Parental presence during induction of anesthesia: a randomized controlled trial. Anesthesiology 1996;84:1060–1067.
165. Kasser JR. Forearm fractures. Instr Course Lect 1992;41:391–396.
166. Kasten P, Krefft M, Hesselbach J, et al. Computer simulation of forearm rotation in angular deformities: a new therapeutic approach. Injury 2002;33:807–813.
167. Kasten P, Krefft M, Hesselbach J, et al. How does torsional deformity of the radial shaft influence the rotation of the forearm? A biomechanical study. J Orthop Trauma 2003; 17:57–60.
168. Kay S, Smith C, Oppenheim WL. Both-bone midshaft forearm fractures in children. J Pediatr Orthop 1986;6:306–310.
169. Keenan WNW, Clegg J. Intraoperative wedging of casts: correction of residual angulation after manipulation. J Pediatr Orthop 1995;15:826–829.
170. Kelly AM, Powell CV, Williams A. Parent visual analogue scale ratings of children's pain do not reliably reflect pain reported by child. Pediatr Emerg Care 2002;18:159–162.
171. Kelly JP, Zionts LE. Economic considerations in the treatment of distal forearm fractures in children. Paper presented at: Annual Meeting of the American Academy of Orthopaedic Surgeons; February 28–March 4, 2001; San Francisco, CA.
172. Kemper KJ, Sarah R, Silver-Highfield E, et al. On pins and needles? Pediatric pain patients' experience with acupuncture. Pediatrics 2000;105:941–947.
173. Kennedy RM, Porter FL, Miller JP, et al. Comparison of fentanyl/midazolam with ketamine/midazolam for pediatric orthopedic emergencies. Pediatrics 1998;102: 956–963.
174. Kettunen J, Kröger H, Bowditch M, et al. Bone mineral density after removal of rigid plates from forearm fractures: preliminary report. J Orthop Sci 2003;8:772–776.
175. Khosla S, Melton LJ III, Dekutoski MB, et al. Incidence of childhood distal forearm fractures over 30 years: a population-based study. JAMA 2003;290:1479–1485.
176. Kienitz R, Mandell R. Traumatic bowing of the forearm in children: report of a case. J Am Osteopath Assoc 1985;85:565–568.
177. Kolkman KA, Von Niekerk JL, Rieu PN, et al. A complicated forearm greenstick fracture: case report. J Trauma 1992;32:116–117.
178. Koo WW, Sherman R, Succop P, et al. Fractures and rickets in very low-birth-weight infants: conservative management and outcome. J Pediatr Orthop 1989;9:326–330.
179. Kramhøft M, Solgaard S. Displaced diaphyseal forearm fractures in children: classifica-

tion and evaluation of the early radiographic prognosis. J Pediatr Orthop 1989;9: 586–589.

180. Kucukkaya M, Kabukcuoglu Y, Tezer M, et al. The application of open intramedullary fixation in the treatment of pediatric radial and ulnar shaft fractures. J Orthop Trauma 2002;16:340–344.
181. Landin LA. Epidemiology of children's fractures. J Pediatr Orthop B 1997;6:79–83.
182. Larsen E, Vittas D, Torp-Pedersen S. Remodeling of angulated distal forearm fractures in children. Clin Orthop Relat Res 1988;237:190–195.
183. Larson BJ, Davis JW. Trampoline-related injuries. J Bone Joint Surg Am 1995;77: 1174–1178.
184. Lascombes P, Prevot J, Ligier JN, et al. Elastic stable intramedullary nailing in forearm shaft fractures in children: 85 cases. J Pediatr Orthop 1990;10:167–171.
185. Lautman S, Bergerault F, Saidani N, et al. Roentgenographic measurement of angle between shaft and distal epiphyseal growth plate of radius. J Pediatr Orthop 2002;22: 751–753.
186. Lavelle DG. Delayed union and nonunion of fractures. In: Canale ST, ed. Campbell's Operative Orthopaedics. 10th ed. St. Louis: Mosby, 2003:3125–3127.
187. Lee BH, Scharff L, Sethna NF, et al. Physical therapy and cognitive-behavioral treatment for complex regional pain syndromes. J Pediatr 2002;141:135–140.
188. Lee S, Nicol RO, Stott NS. Intramedullary fixation for pediatric unstable forearm fractures. Clin Orthop Relat Res 2002;402:245–250.
189. Lewallen RP, Peterson HA. Nonunion of long bone fractures in children: a review of 30 cases. J Pediatr Orthop 1985;5:135–142.
190. Lewis ME. Impact of industrialization: comparative study of child health in four sites from medieval and postmedieval England (A.D. 850–1859). Am J Phys Anthropol 2002;119:211–223.
191. Ligier JN, Metaizeau JP, Prévot J, et al. Elastic stable intramedullary pinning of long bone shaft fractures in children. Z Kinderchir 1985;40:209–212.
192. Lim YJ, Lam KS, Lee EH. Open Gustilo 1 and 2 midshaft fractures of the radius and ulna in children: is there a role for cast immobilization after wound débridement? J Pediatr Orthop 2007;27:540–546.
193. Litton LO, Adler F. Refracture of the forearm in children: a frequent complication. J Trauma 1963;3:41–51.
194. Luhmann SJ, Gordon JE, Schoenecker PL. Intramedullary fixation of unstable both-bone forearm fractures in children. J Pediatr Orthop 1998;18:451–456.
195. Luhmann SJ, Schootman M, Schoenecker PL, et al. Complications and outcomes of open pediatric forearm fractures. J Pediatr Orthop 2004;24:1–6.
196. Ma D, Jones G. Television, computer, and video viewing; physical activity; and upper limb fracture risk in children: a population-based case control study. J Bone Miner Res 2003;18:1970–1977.
197. Ma D, Morley R, Jones G. Risk-taking coordination and upper limb fractures in children: population-based case-control study. Osteoporos Int 2004;15:633–638.
198. Mabrey JD, Fitch RD. Plastic deformation in pediatric fractures: mechanism and treatment. J Pediatr Orthop 1989;9:310–314.
199. Maempel FZ. Posttraumatic radioulnar synostosis. A report of two cases. Clin Orthop Relat Res 1984;186:182–185.
200. Mann DC, Rajmaira S. Distribution of physeal and nonphyseal fractures in 2650 long-bone fractures in children aged 0 to 16 years. J Pediatr Orthop 1990;10:713–716.
201. Mann DC, Schnabel M, Baacke M, et al. Results of elastic stable intramedullary nailing (ESIN) in forearm fractures in childhood. Unfallchirurg 2003;106:102–109.
202. Manske PR. Forearm pseudarthrosis-neurofibromatosis: a case report. Clin Orthop Relat Res 1979;139:125–127.
203. Manson TT, Pfaeffle HJ, Herdon JH, et al. Forearm rotation alters interosseous ligament strain distribution. J Hand Surg Am 2000;25:1058–1063.
204. Markolf KL, Lamey D, Yang S, et al. Radioulnar load-sharing in the forearm: a study in cadavers. J Bone Joint Surg Am 1998;80:879–888.
205. Martin J, Marsh JL, Nepola JV, et al. Radiographic fracture assessments: which ones can we reliably make? J Orthop Trauma 2000;14:379–385.
206. Matthews LS, Kaufer H, Garver DF, et al. The effect on supination-pronation of angular malalignment of fractures of both bones of the forearm: an experimental study. J Bone Joint Surg Am 1982;64:14–17.
207. McGinley JC, Hopgood BC, Gaughan JP, et al. Forearm and elbow injury: the influence of rotational position. J Bone Joint Surg Am 2003;85:2403–2409.
208. McGinley JC, Kozin SH. Interosseous membrane anatomy and functional mechanics. Clin Orthop Relat Res 2001;383:108–122.
209. McHenry TP, Pierce WA, Lais RL, et al. Effect of displacement of ulna-shaft fractures on forearm rotation: a cadaveric model. Am J Orthop 2002;31:420–424.
210. Mehlman CT. Clinical epidemiology. In: Koval KJ, ed. Orthopaedic Knowledge Update. 7th ed. Rosemont, IL: AAOS, 2002:82.
211. Mehlman CT. Forearm, wrist, and hand trauma: pediatrics. In: JS Fischgrund, ed. Orthopaedic Knowledge Update 9. Rosemont, IL: American Academy of Orthopaedic Surgeons, 2008:669–680.
212. Mehlman CT, Crawford AH, Roy DR, et al. Undisplaced fractures of the distal radius and ulna in children: risk factors for displacement. Paper presented at: Annual Meeting of the American Academy of Orthopaedic Surgeons; February 13–17, 2001; Dallas, TX.
213. Mehlman CT, O'Brien MS, Crawford AH, et al. Irreducible fractures of the distal radius in children. Paper presented at: Annual Meeting of Pediatric Orthopaedic Society of North America; May 1–5, 2001; Cancun, MX.
214. Meier R, Prommersberger KJ, Lanz U. Surgical correction of malunited fractures of the forearm in children. Z Orthop Ihre Grenzgeb 2003;141:328–335.
215. Mekhail AO, Ebraheim NA, Jackson WT, et al. Vulnerability of the posterior interosseous nerve during proximal radius exposures. Clin Orthop Relat Res 1995;315: 199–208.
216. Metaizeau JP, Ligier JN. Surgical treatment of fractures of the long bones in children: interference between osteosynthesis and the physiological processes of consolidations: therapeutic indications. J Chir (Paris) 1984;121:527–537.
217. Milch H. Roentgenographic diagnosis of torsional deformities in tubular bones. Surgery 1944;15:440–450.
218. Mitts KG, Hennrikus WL. In-line skating fractures in children. J Pediatr Orthop 1996; 16:640–643.
219. Morrey BF, Askew LJ, Chao EY. A biomechanical study of normal functional elbow motion. J Bone Joint Surg Am 1981;63:872–877.
220. Moseley CF. Obituary: Mercer Rang, FRCSC (1933–2003). J Pediatr Orthop 2004;24: 446–447.
221. Mubarak SJ, Carroll NC. Volkmann's contracture in children: aetiology and prevention. J Bone Joint Surg Br 1979;61:285–293.
222. Muensterer OJ, Regauer MP. Closed reduction of forearm refractures with flexible intramedullary nails in situ. J Bone Joint Surg Am 2003;85:2152–2155.
223. Müller ME, Allgöwer M, Schneider R, et al. Manual of Internal Fixation: Techniques Recommended by the AO-ASIF Group. 3rd ed. Berlin: Springer-Verlag, 1991:454–467.
224. Murray WM, Delp SL, Buchanan TS. Variation of muscle moment arms with elbow and forearm position. J Biomech 1995;28:513–525.
225. Myers GJC, Gibbons PJ, Glithero PR. Nancy nailing of diaphyseal forearm fractures: single bone fixation for fractures of both bones. J Bone Joint Surg Br 2004;86:581–584.
226. Nakamura T, Yabe Y, Horiuchi Y. In vivo MR studies of dynamic changes in the interosseous membrane of the forearm during rotation. J Hand Surg Br 1999;24:245–248.
227. Nielson AB, Simonsen O. Displaced forearm fractures in children treated with AO plates. Injury 1984;15:393–396.
228. Nieman R, Maiocco B, Deeney VF. Ulnar nerve injury after closed forearm fractures in children. J Pediatr Orthop 1998;18:683–685.
229. Nilsson BE, Obrant K. The range of motion following fracture of the shaft of the forearm in children. Acta Orthop Scand 1977;48:600–602.
230. Noonan KJ, Price CT. Forearm and distal radius fractures in children. J Am Acad Orthop Surg 1998;6:146–156.
231. Ogden JA. Skeletal Injury in the Child. Philadelphia: Lea & Febiger; 1982:56–57.
232. Ogden JA. Uniqueness of growing bones. In: Rockwood CA, Wilkins KE, King RE, eds. Fractures in Children. Philadelphia: JB Lippincott, 1991:10–14.
233. Ogden JA, Beall JK, Conlogue GJ, et al. Radiology of postnatal skeletal development, IV: distal radius and ulna. Skeletal Radiol 1981;6:255–266.
234. Ogonda L, Wong-Chung J, Wray R, et al. Delayed union and nonunion of the ulna following intramedullary nailing in children. J Pediatr Orthop B 2004;13:330–333.
235. Oğün TC, Sarlak A, Arazi M, et al. Posttraumatic distal radioulnar synostosis and distal radial epiphyseal arrest. Ulus Travma Derg 2002;8:59–61.
236. OlaOlorun DA, Oladiran IO, Adeniran A. Complications of fracture treatment by traditional bonesetters in southwest Nigeria. Fam Pract 2001;18:635–637.
237. O'Neil DF. Wrist injuries in guarded versus unguarded first-time snowboarders. Clin Orthop Relat Res 2003;409:91–95.
238. Ono M, Bechtold JE, Merkow RL, et al. Rotational stability of diaphyseal fractures of the radius and ulna fixed with Rush pins and/or fracture bracing. Clin Orthop Relat Res 1989;240:236–243.
239. Oönne L, Sandblom PH. Late results in fractures of the forearm in children. Acta Chir Scand 1949;98:549–567.
240. Ortega R, Loder RT, Louis DS. Open reduction and internal fixation of forearm fractures in children. J Pediatr Orthop 1996;16:651–654.
241. Ostermann PA, Richter D, Mecklenburg K, et al. Pediatric forearm fractures: indications, technique, and limits of conservative management. J Orthop Trauma 2000;14:73.
242. Parikh SN, Brody AS, Crawford AH. Use of a picture archiving and communication system (PACS) and computed plain radiography in preoperative planning. Am J Orthop 2004;33:62–64.
243. Patrick J. A study of supination and pronation with especial reference to the treatment of forearm fractures. J Bone Joint Surg 1946;28:737–748.
244. Paul AS, Kay PR, Haines JF. Distal ulnar growth plate arrest following a diaphyseal fracture. J R Coll Surg Edinb 1992;37:347–348.
245. Petridou E, Karpathios T, Dessypris N, et al. The role of dairy products and non-alcoholic beverages in bone fractures among schoolage children. Scand J Soc Med 1997; 25:119–125.
246. Pfaeffle HJ, Kischer KJ, Manson TT, et al. Role of the forearm interosseous ligament: is it more than just longitudinal load transfer? J Hand Surg Am 2000;25:680–688.
247. Pfaeffle HJ, Tomaino MM, Grewal R, et al. Tensile properties of the interosseous membrane of the human forearm. J Orthop Res 1996;14:842–845.
248. Ponet M, Jawish R. Stable flexible nailing of fractures of both bones of the forearm in children [Article in French]. Chir Pediatr 1989;30:117–120.
249. Powell EC, Tanz RR. In-line skate and rollerskate injuries in childhood. Pediatr Emerg Care 1996;12:259–262.
250. Powers KS, Rubenstein JS. Family presence during invasive procedures in the pediatric intensive care unit: a prospective study. Arch Pediatr Adolesc Med 1999;153:955–958.
251. Prevot J, Guichet JM. Elastic stable intramedullary nailing for forearm fractures in children and adolescents. J Bone Joint Surg 1996;20:305.
252. Prevot J, Lascombes P, Guichet JM. Elastic stable intramedullary nailing for forearm fractures in children and adolescents. Orthop Trans 1996;20:305.
253. Price CT, Knapp DR. Osteotomy for malunited forearm shaft fractures in children. J Pediatr Orthop 2006;26:193–196.
254. Price CT, Mencio GA. Injuries to the shafts of the radius and ulna. In: Beaty JH, Kasser JR, eds. Rockwood & Wilkins Fractures in Children. 5th ed. Philadelphia: Lippincott Williams & Wilkins, 2001:452–460.
255. Price CT, Scott DS, Kurzner ME, et al. Malunited forearm fractures in children. J Pediatr Orthop 1990;10:705–712.
256. Pritchett JW. Does pinning cause distal radial growth plate arrest? Orthopedics 1994; 17:550–551.
257. Prosser AJ, Hooper G. Entrapment of the ulnar nerve in a greenstick fracture of the ulna. J Hand Surg Br 1986;11:211–212.
258. Proubasta IR, De Sena L, Cáceres EP. Entrapment of the median nerve in a greenstick forearm fracture: a case report and review of the literature. Bull Hosp Jt Dis 1999;58: 220–223.
259. Pugh DM, Galpin RD, Carey TP. Intramedullary Steinmann pin fixation of forearm fractures in children: long-term results. Clin Orthop Relat Res 2000;376:39–48.
260. Qidwai SA. Treatment of diaphyseal forearm fractures in children by intramedullary Kirschner wires. J Trauma 2001;50:303–307.
261. Raiss P, Rettig O, Wolf S, et al. Range of motion of shoulder and elbow in activities of daily life in 3D motion analysis. Z Orthop Unfall 2007;145:493–498.
262. Rang M. Children's Fractures. Philadelphia: JB Lippincott, 1974:126.
263. Rang M. Children's Fractures. 2nd ed. Philadelphia: JB Lippincott, 1982:203.
264. Rang M. The Story of Orthopaedics. Philadelphia: WB Saunders, 2000:472.
265. Rang M, Armstrong P, Crawford AH, et al. Symposium: management of fractures in children and adolescents, parts I & II. Contemp Orthop 1991;23:517–548, 621–644.

266. Rayan GM, Hayes M. Entrapment of the flexor digitorum profundus in the ulna with fracture of both bones of the forearm: report of a case. J Bone Joint Surg Am 1986; 68:1102–1103.
267. Reinhardt KR, Feldman DS, Green DW, et al. Comparison of intramedullary nailing to plating for both-bone forearm fractures in older children. J Pediatr Orthop 2008; 28:403–409.
268. Revol MP, Lantieri L, Loy S, et al. Vascular anatomy of the forearm muscles: a study of 50 dissections. Plast Reconstr Surg 1991;88:1026–1033.
269. Richter D, Ostermann PA, Ekkernkamp A, et al. Elastic intramedullary nailing: a minimally invasive concept in the treatment of unstable forearm fractures in children. J Pediatr Orthop 1998;18:457–461.
270. Rickert M, Bürger A, Günther CM, et al. Forearm rotation in healthy adults of all ages and both sexes. J Shoulder Elbow Surg 2008;17:271–275.
271. Ring D, Waters PM, Hotchkiss RN, et al. Pediatric floating elbow. J Pediatr Orthop 2001;21:456–459.
272. Roposch A, Reis M, Molina M, et al. Supracondylar fractures of the humerus associated with ipsilateral fractures in children: a report of forty-seven cases. J Pediatr Orthop 2001;21:307–312.
273. Roy DR. Completely displaced distal radius fractures with intact ulnas in children. Orthopedics 1989;12:1089–1092.
274. Roy DR. Radioulnar synostosis following proximal radial fracture in child. Orthop Rev 1986;15:89–94.
275. Roy DR, Crawford AH. Operative management of fractures of the shaft of the radius and ulna. Orthop Clin North Am 1990;21:245–250.
276. Rydholm U, Nilsson JE. Traumatic bowing of the forearm: a case report. Clin Orthop Relat Res 1979;139:121–124.
277. Sage FP. Medullary fixation of fractures of the forearm: a study of the medullary canal of the radius and a report of 50 fractures of the radius treated with a prebent triangular nail. J Bone Joint Surg Am 1959;41:1489–1516.
278. Sage FP, Smith H. Medullary fixation of forearm fractures. J Bone Joint Surg Am 1957; 39:91–98.
279. Sanders WE, Heckman JD. Traumatic plastic deformation of the radius and ulna: a closed method of correction of deformity. Clin Orthop Relat Res 1984;188:58–67.
280. Sarmiento A, Ebramzadeh E, Brys D, et al. Angular deformities and forearm function. J Orthop Res 1992;10:121–133.
281. Sauer HD, Mommsen U, Bethke K, et al. Fractures of the proximal and middle third of the lower arm in children. Z Kinderchir Grenzgeb 1980;29:357–363.
282. Scheiber RA, Branche-Dorsey CM, Ryan GW, et al. Risk factors for injuries from in-line skating and the effectiveness of safety gear. N Engl J Med 1996;335:1630–1635.
284. Schemitsch EH, Jones D, Henley MB, et al. A comparison of malreduction after plate and intramedullary nail fixation of forearm fractures. J Orthop Trauma 1995;9:8–16.
285. Schemitsch EH, Richards RR. The effect of malunion on functional outcome after plate fixation of fractures of both bones of the forearm in adults. J Bone Joint Surg Am 1992; 74:1068–1078.
286. Schlich T. Surgery, Science, and Industry: A Revolution in Fracture Care, 1950s–1990s. New York: Palgrave-Macmillan, 2002:21.
287. Schlickewei W, Salm R. Indications for intramedullary stabilization of shaft fractures in childhood: what is reliable and what is an assumption? Kongressbd Dtsch Ges Chir Kongr 2001;118:431–434.
288. Schmittenbecker PP, Fitze G, Gödeke J, et al. Delayed healing of forearm shaft fractures in children after intramedullary nailing. J Pediatr Orthop 2008;28:303–306.
289. Schock CC. "The crooked straight": distal radial remodeling. J Ark Med Soc 1987;84: 97–100.
290. Schranz PJ, Fagg PS. Undisplaced fractures of the distal third of the radius in children: an innocent fracture? Injury 1992;23:165–167.
291. Schranz PJ, Gultekin C, Colton CL. External fixation of fractures in children. Injury 1982;23:80–82.
292. Schwarz N, Pienaar S, Schwarz AF, et al. Refracture of the forearm in children. J Bone Joint Surg Br 1996;78:740–744.
293. Shaer JA, Smith B, Turco VJ. Midthird forearm fractures in children: an unorthodox treatment. Am J Orthop 1999;28:60–63.
294. Shah MH, Heffernan G, McGuinness AJ. Early experiences with titanium elastic nails in a trauma unit. Ir Med J 2003;96:213–214.
295. Shaw BA, Murphy KM. Flexor tendon entrapment in ulnar shaft fractures. Clin Orthop Relat Res 1996;330:181–184.
296. Shenoy RM. Biplanar exposure of the radius and ulna through a single incision. J Bone Joint Surg Br 1995;77:568–570.
297. Shoemaker SD, Comstock CP, Mubarak SJ, et al. Intramedullary Kirschner wire fixation of open or unstable forearm fractures in children. J Pediatr Orthop 1999;19:329–337.
298. Silberstein MJ, Brodeur AE, Graviss ER, et al. Some vagaries of the olecranon. J Bone Joint Surg Am 1981;63:722–725.
299. Silberstein MJ, Brodeur AE, Graviss ER. Some vagaries of the radial head and neck. J Bone Joint Surg Am 1982;64:1153–1157.
300. Simonian PT, Hanel DP. Traumatic plastic deformity of an adult forearm: case report and literature review. J Orthop Trauma 1996;10:213–215.
301. Singer AJ, Gulla J, Thode HC Jr. Parents and practitioners are poor judges of young children's pain severity. Acad Emerg Med 2002;9:609–612.
302. Skaggs DL, Kautz SM, Kay RM, et al. Effect of delay of surgical treatment on rate of infection in open fractures in children. J Pediatr Orthop 2000;20:19–22.
303. Skaggs DL, Loro ML, Pitukcheewanont P, et al. Increased body weight and decreased radial cross-sectional dimensions in girls with forearm fractures. J Bone Miner Res 2001;16:1337–1342.
304. Skahen JR III, Palmer AK, Werner FW, et al. Reconstruction of the interosseous membrane of the forearm in cadavers. J Hand Surg Am 1997;22:986–994.
305. Smith GA. Injuries to children in the United States related to trampolines 1990–1995: a national epidemic. Pediatrics 1998;101:406–412.
306. Soeur R. Intramedullary pinning of diaphyseal fractures. J Bone Joint Surg 1946;28: 309–331.
307. Song KS, Kim HK. Nonunion as a complication of an open reduction of a distal radial fracture in a healthy child: a case report. J Orthop Trauma 2003;17:231–233.
308. Soong C, Rocke LG. Clinical predictors of forearm fracture in children. Arch Emerg Med 1990;7:196–199.
309. Sop AL, Mehlman CT, Meiss L. Hyphenated history: the Böhler-Braun frame. J Orthop Trauma 2003;17:217–221.
310. Spiegel PG, Mast JW. Internal and external fixation of fractures in children. Orthop Clin North Am 1980;11:405–421.
311. Staebler MP, Moore DC, Akelman E, et al. The effect of wrist guards on bone strain in the distal forearm. Am J Sports Med 1999;27:500–506.
312. Stahl S, Rozen N, Michaelson M. Ulnar nerve injury following midshaft forearm fractures in children. J Hand Surg Br 1997;22:788–789.
313. Stanitski CL, Micheli LJ. Simultaneous ipsilateral fractures of the arm and forearm in children. Clin Orthop Relat Res 1980;153:218–222.
314. Stanley EA. Treatment of midshaft fractures of the radius and ulna utilizing percutaneous intramedullar pinning. Orthop Trans 1996;20:305.
315. Stanton RP, Malcolm JR, Wesdock KA, et al. Reflex sympathetic dystrophy in children: an orthopaedic perspective. Orthopedics 1993;16:773–780.
316. Stern PJ, Drury WJ. Complications of plate fixation of forearm fractures. Clin Orthop Relat Res 1983;175:25–29.
317. Strauch RJ, Rosenwasser MP, Glazer PA. Surgical exposure of the dorsal proximal third of the radius: how vulnerable is the posterior interosseous nerve? J Shoulder Elbow Surg 1996;5:342–346.
318. Tabak AY, Celebi L, Murath HH, et al. Closed reduction and percutaneous fixation of supracondylar fracture of the humerus and ipsilateral fracture of the forearm in children. J Bone Joint Surg Br 2003;85:1169–1172.
319. Tachakra S, Doherty S. The accuracy of length and angle measurement in videoconferencing teleradiology. J Telemed Telecare 2002;8(Suppl 2):85–87.
320. Tarr RR, Garfinkel AI, Sarmiento A. The effects of angular and rotational deformities of both bones of the forearm: an in vitro study. J Bone Joint Surg Am 1984;66:65–70.
321. Templeton PA, Graham HK. The "floating elbow" in children: simultaneous supracondylar fractures of the humerus and of the forearm in the same upper limb. J Bone Joint Surg Br 1995;77:791–796.
322. Thomas EM, Tuson KW, Browne PS. Fractures of the radius and ulna in children. Injury 1975;7:120–124.
323. Thompson GH, Wilber JH, Marcus RE. Internal fixation of fractures in children and adolescents: a comparative analysis. Clin Orthop Relat Res 1984;188:10–20.
324. Thorndike A Jr, Simmler CL Jr. Fractures of the forearm and elbow in children. N Engl J Med 1941;225:475–480.
325. Till H, Hüttl B, Knorr P, et al. Elastic stable intramedullary nailing (ESIN) provides good long-term results in pediatric long-bone fractures. Eur J Pediatr Surg 2000;10: 319–322.
326. Tredwell SJ, Van Peteghem K, Clough M. Pattern of forearm fractures in children. J Pediatr Orthop 1984;4:604–608.
327. Trinkaus E, Churchill SE. Neanderthal radial tuberosity orientation. Am J Phys Anthropol 1988;75:15–21.
328. Toussaint D, Vanderlinden C, Bremen J. Stable elastic nailing applied to diaphyseal fractures of the forearm in children. Acta Orthop Belg 1991;57:147–153.
329. Trousdale RT, Linscheid RL. Operative treatment of malunited fractures of the forearm. J Bone Joint Surg Am 1995;77:894–902.
330. Shaer JA, Smith B, Turco VJ. Midthird forearm fractures in children: an unorthodox treatment. Am J Orthop 1999;28:60–63.
331. Tynan MC, Fornalski S, McMahon PJ, et al. The effects of ulnar axial malalignment on supination and pronation. J Bone Joint Surg Am 2000;82:1726–1731.
332. Vainionpää S, Bostman O, Pätiälä H, et al. Internal fixation of forearm fractures in children. Acta Orthop Scand 1987;58:121–123.
333. Van der Reis WL, Otsuka NY, Moroz P, et al. Intramedullary nailing versus plate fixation for unstable forearm fractures in children. J Pediatr Orthop 1998;18:9–13.
334. Vanderbeek BL, Mehlman CT, Foad SL, et al. The use of conscious sedation for forearm fracture reduction in children: does race matter? Paper presented at: Annual Meeting of the American Academy of Pediatrics; October 31–November 5, 2003; New Orleans, LA.
335. Van Herpe LB. Fractures of the forearm and wrist. Orthop Clin North Am 1976;7: 543–556.
336. Verbrugge J. Clinical survey of 163 cases of internal fixation with metal in fractures in children. J Bone Joint Surg Am 1956;38:1384–1385.
337. Verstreken L, Delronge G, Lamoureux J. Shaft forearm fractures in children: intramedullary nailing with immediate motion: a preliminary report. J Pediatr Orthop 1988;8: 450–453.
338. Vince KG, Miller JE. Cross-union complication fracture of the forearm: part II, children. J Bone Joint Surg Am 1987;69:654–661.
339. Vittas D, Larsen E, Torp-Pedersen S. Angular remodeling of midshaft forearm fractures in children. Clin Orthop Relat Res 1991;265:261–264.
340. Vorlat P, De Boeck H. Bowing fractures of the forearm in children: a long-term follow-up. Clin Orthop Relat Res 2003;413:233–237.
341. Voto SJ, Weiner DS, Leighley B. Redisplacement after closed reduction of forearm fractures in children. J Pediatr Orthop 1990;10:79–84.
342. Voto SJ, Weiner DS, Leighley B. Use of pins and plaster in the treatment of unstable pediatric forearm fractures. J Pediatr Orthop 1990;10:85–89.
343. Vu L, Mehlman CT. Tarsal coalition. eMedicine Orthopaedics. Available at: http://www.emedicine.com/orthoped/topic326.htm. Accessed September 1, 2005.
344. Walker JL, Rang M. Forearm fractures in children: cast treatment with the elbow extended. J Bone Joint Surg Br 1991;73:299–301.
345. Waltzman ML, Shannon M, Bowen AP, et al. Monkeybar injuries: complications of play. Pediatrics 1999;103:e58.
346. Waseem M, Paton RW. Percutaneous intramedullary elastic wiring of displaced diaphyseal forearm fractures in children. A modified technique. Injury 1999;30:21–24.
347. Watson PA, Blair W. Entrapment of the index flexor digitorum profundus tendon after fracture of both forearm bones in a child. Iowa Orthop J 1999;19:127–128.
348. Watson-Jones R. Fractures and Other Bone and Joint Injuries, 1st ed. Edinburgh: Livingstone, 1940:379–380.
349. Weber BG, Cech O. Pseudarthrosis. Bern, Switzerland: Hans Huber, 1976.
350. White AA, Panjabi MM, Southwick WO. The four biomechanical stages of fracture repair. J Bone Joint Surg Am 1977;59:188–192.
351. Wilder RT, Berde CB, Wolohan M, et al. Reflex sympathetic dystrophy in children. J Bone Joint Surg Am 1992;74:910–919.

352. Wilkins KE. Operative management of children's fractures: is it a sign of impetuousness or do the children really benefit? J Pediatr Orthop 1998;18:1–3.
353. Williamson DM, Cole WG. Treatment of ipsilateral supracondylar and forearm fractures in children. Injury 1992;23:159–161.
354. Wilson JC Jr, Krueger JC. Fractures of the proximal and middle thirds of the radius and ulna in children: study of the end results with analysis of treatment and complications. Am J Surg 1966;112:326–332.
355. Worlock P, Stower M. Fracture patterns in Nottingham children. J Pediatr Orthop 1986;6:656–660.
356. Wright J, Rang M. Internal fixation for forearm fractures in children. Techniques Orthop 1989;4:44–47.
357. Würfel AM, Voigt A, Linke F, et al. New aspects in the treatment of complete and isolated diaphyseal fractures of the forearm in children. Unfallchirurgie 1995;21: 70–76.
358. Wyrsch B, Mencio GA, Green NE. Open reduction and internal fixation of pediatric forearm fractures. J Pediatr Orthop 1996;16:644–650.
359. Yasin MN, Talwalkar SC, Henderson JJ, et al. Segmental radius and ulna fractures with scaphocapitate fractures and bilateral multiple epiphyseal fractures. Am J Orthop 2008; 37:214–217.
360. Yasutomi T, Nakatsuchi Y, Koike H, et al. Mechanism of limitation of pronation/supination of the forearm in geometric models of deformities of the forearm bones. Clin Biomech (Bristol, Avon) 2002;17:456–463.
361. Younger AS, Tredwell SJ, Mackenzie WG, et al. Accurate prediction of outcome after pediatric forearm fracture. J Pediatr Orthop 1994;14:200–206.
362. Younger AS, Tredwell SJ, Mackenzie WG. Factors affecting fracture position at cast removal after pediatric forearm fracture. J Pediatr Orthop 1997;17:332–336.
363. Yuan PS, Pring ME, Gaynor TP, et al. Compartment syndrome following intramedullary fixation of pediatric forearm fractures. J Pediatr Orthop 2004;24:370–375.
364. Yung SH, Lam CY, Choi KY, et al. Percutaneous intramedullary Kirschner wiring for displaced diaphyseal forearm fractures in children. J Bone Joint Surg Br 1998;80:91–94.
365. Yung PS, Lam CY, Ng BK, et al. Percutaneous transphyseal intramedullary Kirschner wire pinning: a safe and effective procedure for treatment of displaced forearm fracture in children. J Pediatr Orthop 2004;24:7–12.
366. Zionts LE, Zalavras CG, Gerhardt MB. Closed treatment of displaced both-bone forearm fractures in older children and adolescents. J Pediatr Orthop 2005;25:507–512.

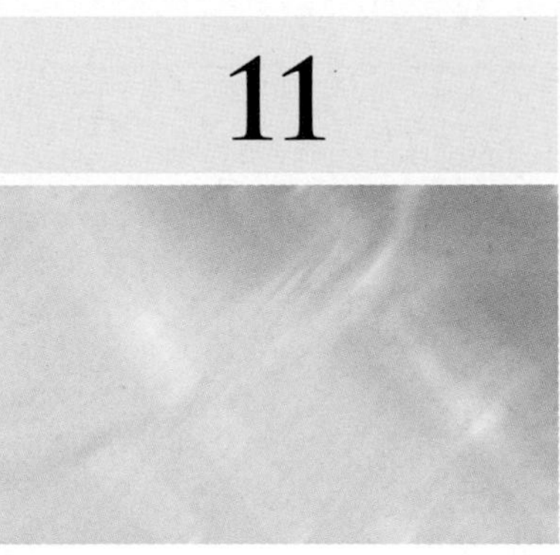

FRACTURES OF THE PROXIMAL RADIUS AND ULNA

Mark Erickson and Steven Frick

INTRODUCTION 405

FRACTURES OF THE PROXIMAL RADIUS 405
Incidence 405
Anatomy 406
Normal Angulation 406
Soft Tissue Attachments 406
The "Cam" Effect 406
Diagnosis 406
Radiographic Evaluation 407
Classification 407
Mechanisms of Injury 410

PRIMARY DISPLACEMENT OF THE RADIAL HEAD (GROUP I) 410
Valgus Injuries 410
Associated Injuries 410
Fracture Patterns in Valgus Injuries 411
Displacement Patterns 412
Neck Migration 412
During Reduction (Type D) 413
During Dislocation (Type E) 413

PRIMARY DISPLACEMENT OF THE RADIAL NECK (GROUP II) 413
Angular Forces 413
Rotational Forces 414

STRESS INJURIES (GROUP III) 414
Treatment 414
Initial Angulation and Displacement 415
Angulation and Displacement after Reduction 415
Age Effect 415
Timing 415
Outcomes 415
Associated Injuries and Complications 425
Summary 427

FRACTURES OF THE PROXIMAL ULNA (OLECRANON) 427
Fractures Involving the Proximal Apophysis 427
Associated Injuries and Complications 431
Metaphyseal Fractures of the Olecranon 431
Flexion Injuries 433
Extension Injuries 433
Shear Injuries 435
Flexion Injuries 435
Extension Injuries 438
Shear Injuries 438
Associated Injuries and Complications 439
Associated Injuries and Complications 444

INTRODUCTION

Fractures of the proximal radius in skeletally immature patients usually involve the metaphysis or physis. True isolated radial head fractures are rare. In the proximal ulna, the olecranon, which biomechanically is a metaphysis, often fails with a greenstick pattern. Fractures in this area also may involve the physis. Fractures of the olecranon associated with proximal radioulnar joint disruption are considered part of the Monteggia fracture–dislocation complex and are discussed in Chapter 12.

FRACTURES OF THE PROXIMAL RADIUS

Incidence

Fractures of the radial neck account for slightly more than 1% of all children's fractures.[48] In skeletally immature children, the radial head or epiphysis is rarely fractured, probably because of the large amount of cartilage in the radial head. If the fracture involves the epiphysis, it usually is part of a Salter-Harris type IV fracture pattern. In 90% of proximal radial fractures, the fracture line involves either the physis or the neck.[39] In six large series of elbow fractures, the incidence of fracture of the radial neck was remarkably consistent, varying only from 5% to 8.5%.[9,26,39,42,52,71] Fractures of the radial neck and head in skeletally immature patients account for only 14% to 20% of the total injuries of the proximal radius.[30,42]

In most series, the age of occurrence varies from 4 to 14 years of age, with the median age ranging from 9 to 10 years.[15,39,49,70,88,103,110,114] There is little difference in the occurrence rates between male and females[15,39,70]; however, this injury seems to occur in females approximately 2 years earlier than in males.[103]

Anatomy

Ossification Process

In the embryo, the proximal radius is well defined by 9 weeks of gestation. By 4 years of age, the radial head and neck have the same contours as in an adult.[71] Ossification of the proximal radius epiphysis begins at approximately 5 years of age as a small, flat nucleus (Fig. 11-1). This ossific nucleus can originate as a small sphere or it can be bipartite, which is a normal variation and should not be misinterpreted as a fracture.[11,60,99]

Normal Angulation

In the preossification stage, on the anteroposterior (AP) projection radiograph, the edge of the metaphysis of the proximal radius slopes distally on its lateral border. This angulation is normal and not a fracture.

In the AP view, the lateral angulation varies from 0 to 15 degrees, with the average being 12.5 degrees.[114] In the lateral view, the angulation can vary from 10 degrees anterior to 5 degrees posterior, with the average being 3.5 degrees anterior.[114]

Soft Tissue Attachments

No ligaments attach directly to the radial neck or head. The radial collateral ligaments attach to the orbicular ligament, which originates from the radial side of the ulna. The articular capsule attaches to the proximal third of the neck. Distally, the capsule protrudes from under the orbicular ligament to form a pouch (recessus sacciformis). Thus, only a small portion of the neck lies within the articular capsule.[117] Because much of the neck is extracapsular, fractures involving only the neck may not produce an intra-articular effusion, and the fat pad sign may be negative with fracture of the radial neck.[11,40,99]

The "Cam" Effect

The proximal radioulnar joint has a precise congruence. The axis of rotation of the proximal radius is a line through the center of the radial head and neck. When a displaced fracture disrupts the alignment of the radial head on the center of the radial neck, the arc of rotation changes. Instead of rotating smoothly in a pure circle, the radial head rotates with a "cam" effect. This disruption of the congruity of the proximal radioulnar joint may result in a loss of the range of motion in supination and pronation (Fig. 11-2).[120]

Diagnosis

Clinical Findings

Following a fracture, palpation over the radial head or neck is painful. The pain is usually increased more with passive forearm supination and pronation than with elbow flexion and extension. In a young child, the primary complaint may be wrist pain,[2] and pressure over the proximal radius may accentuate this referred wrist pain. The wrist pain may be secondary to radial shortening and subsequent distal radioulnar joint dysfunction. The misdirection of such a presentation reinforces the principle of obtaining radiographs of both ends of a fractured long bone.

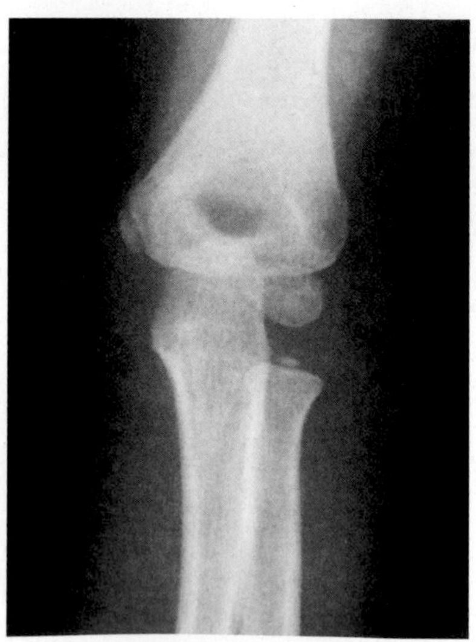

A

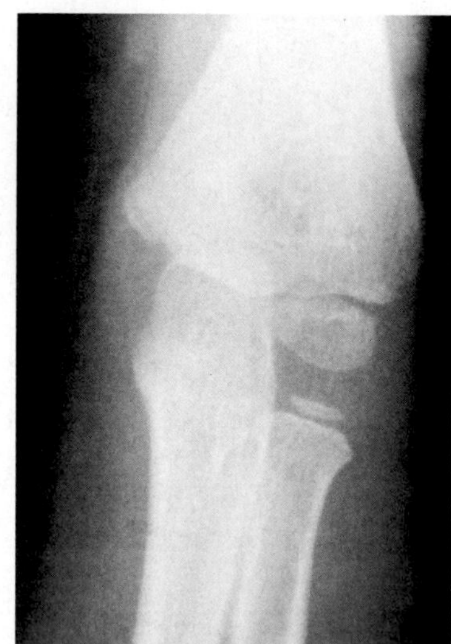

B

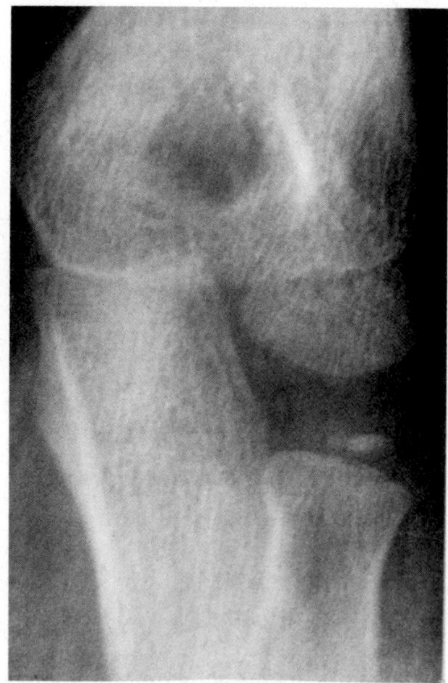

C

FIGURE 11-1 Ossification pattern. **A.** At 5 years, ossification begins as a small oval nucleus. **B.** As the head matures, the center widens but remains flat. **C.** Double ossification centers in developing proximal radial epiphysis. Reprinted with permission from Silberstein MJ, Brodeur AE, Graviss ER. Some vagaries of the radial head and neck. J Bone Joint Surgery AM 1982; 64.

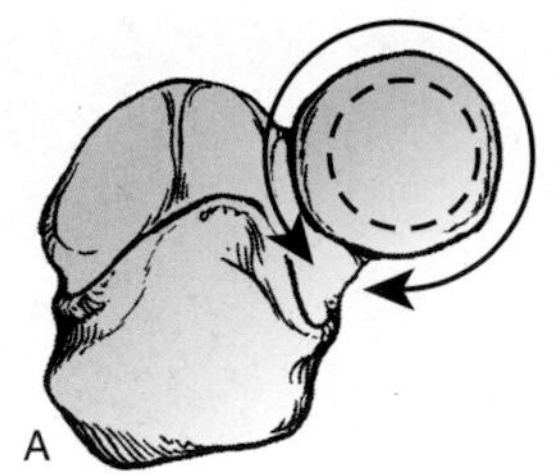

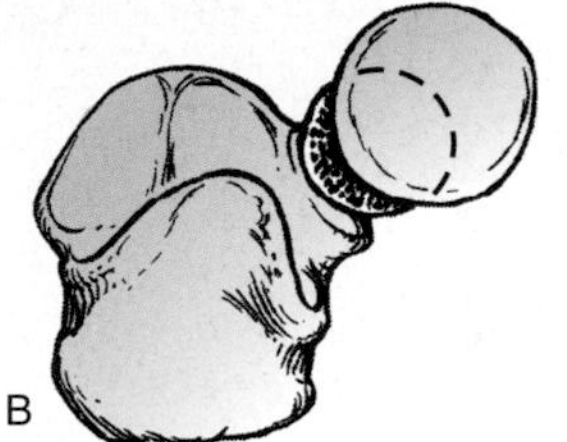

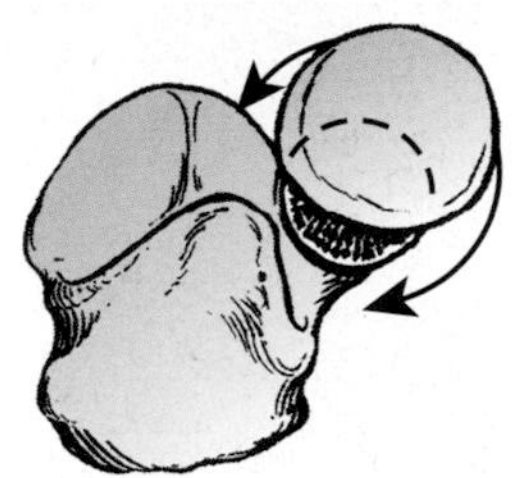

FIGURE 11-2 A. Normal rotation of the forearm causes the radial head to circumscribe an exact circle within the proximal radioulnar joint. **B.** Any translocation of the radial head limits rotation because of the "cam" effect described by Wedge and Robertson.[120]

Radiographic Evaluation

Supination–Pronation Views

The fracture is usually easy to see on both AP and lateral radiograph views. Occasionally, oblique views with the forearm both supinated and pronated will reveal the fracture line clearly.

Some variants in the ossification process can resemble a fracture. Most of these involve the radial head, although a step-off also can develop as a normal variant of the metaphysis. There may be a persistence of the secondary ossification centers of the epiphysis. Comparison views are useful for evaluation of unusual ossification centers after an acute elbow injury.

The diagnosis of a partially or completely displaced fracture of the radial neck may be difficult in children whose radial head remains unossified. The only clue may be a little irregularity in the smoothness of the proximal metaphyseal margin (Fig. 11-3). Rokito et al.[93] reported complete displacement of the radial head in a 5-year-old male, in whom the only clue on radiography was a small speck of ossification in the elbow joint. The full extent of the injury was appreciated when the radial head was outlined with magnetic resonance imaging (MRI). Javed et al.[41] suggested considering an arthrogram to assess the extent of the displacement and the accuracy of reduction in children with an unossified radial epiphysis (Fig. 11-4).

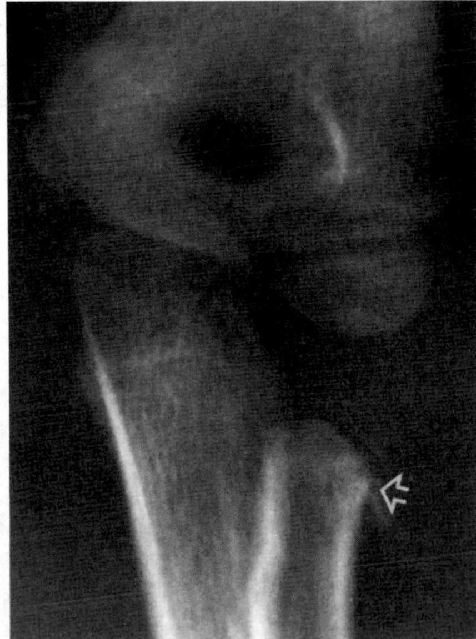

FIGURE 11-3 Preosseous fracture. The only clue to the presence of a fracture of the radial neck with displacement of the radial head was loss of smoothness of the metaphyseal margin (*arrow*).

Perpendicular Views

If the elbow cannot be extended because of pain, special views are necessary to see the elbow in full AP profile. One view is taken with the beam perpendicular to the distal humerus, and the other with the beam perpendicular to the proximal radius. A regular AP view with the elbow flexed may not show the fracture because of obliquity of the beam. The perpendicular views show the physeal line of the radius in clear profile.

With a minimally displaced fracture, the fracture line may be difficult to see because it is superimposed on the proximal ulna, and oblique views of the proximal radius may be helpful.[11,117] One oblique view that is especially helpful is the radiocapitellar view suggested by Greenspan et al.[36,37] and Hall-Craggs et al.[38] This view projects the radial head anterior to the coronoid process (Fig. 11-5) and is especially helpful if full supination and pronation views are difficult to obtain because of acute injury (Fig. 11-6).

If the epiphysis is ossified, displacement of the radial head is usually obvious on a radiograph, but a minimally displaced fracture is difficult to diagnose before ossification has begun.[90] The loss of the smoothness of the metaphyseal margin may be the only finding. Ultrasonography can be used to evaluate for hemarthrosis and displacement of the fracture and allows a dynamic range-of-motion evaluation.[50] The supinator fat pad is a small layer of fat that overlies the supinator muscle in the proximal forearm. Displacement of the supinator fat pad may indicate fracture of the proximal radius.[92] The supinator fat pad and distal humeral anterior and posterior fat pads are not always displaced with occult fractures of the radial neck or physis.[40,99,97]

If there is localized tenderness of the radial head and neck, special studies may be necessary. Arthrography, MRI, and ultrasound[50] are options for determining any displacement of the unossified radial head.

Classification

Chambers[14] classified proximal radial fractures into three major groups based on the mechanism of injury and displacement of the radial head (Table 11-1):

- Group I: The radial head is primarily displaced (most proximal radial injuries are in this group).
- Group II: The radial neck is primarily displaced.
- Group III: Stress injuries.

Head-Displaced Fractures (Group I)

To describe head-displaced fractures, Chambers[14] combined the classifications of Jeffrey[42] and Newman[70] to produce a new

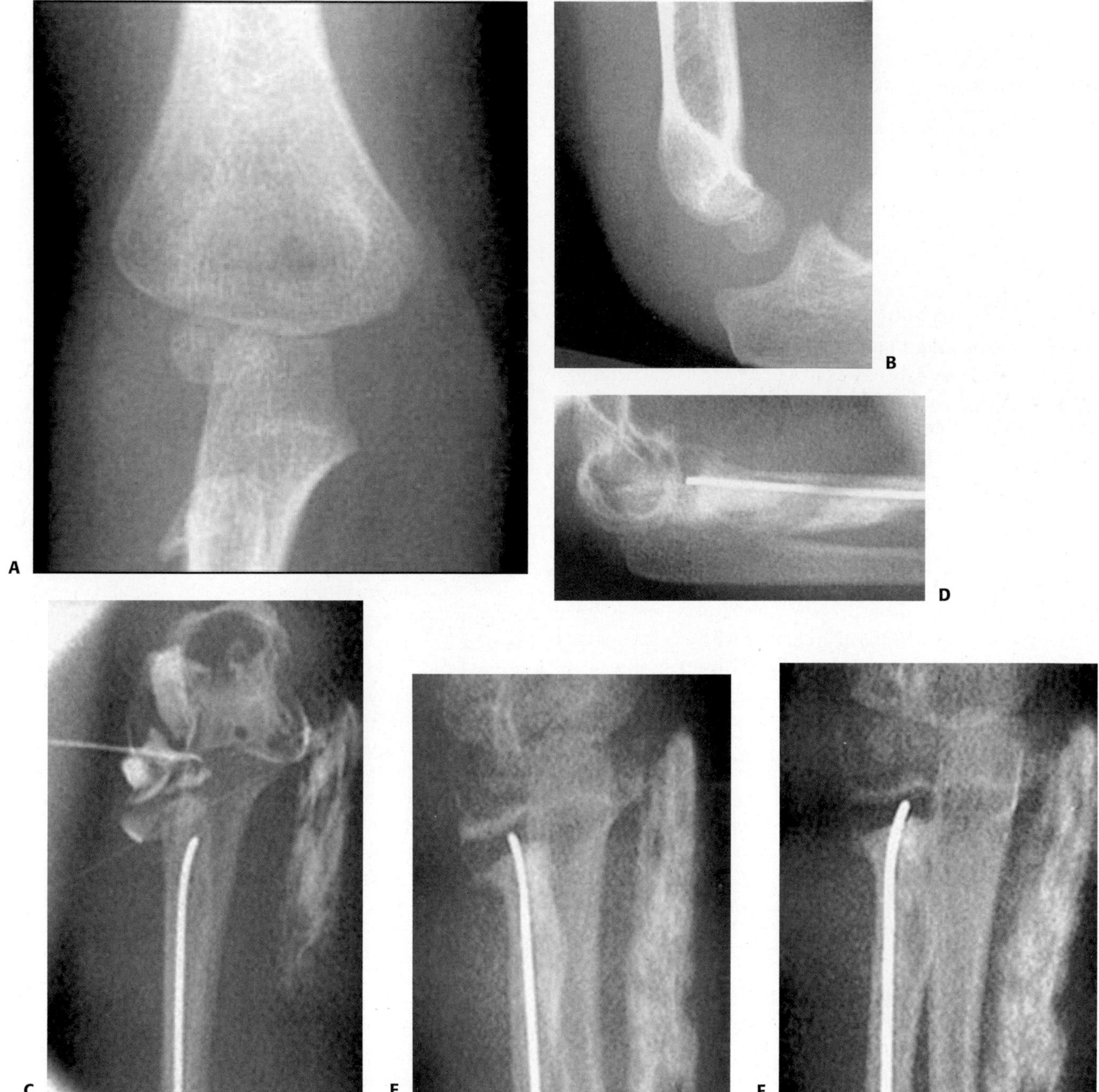
FIGURE 11-4 A,B. AP and lateral radiographs demonstrating a radial neck fracture in a patient with a nonossified proximal radial epiphysis. **C.** Arthrogram prior to reduction demonstrating location/displacement of nonossified proximal radial epiphysis. **D–F.** Arthrogram/radiographs after reduction with intramedullary technique. (From Javed A, Guichet J.M. Arthrography for reduction of a fracture of the radial neck in a child with a nonossified radial epiphysis. J Bone Joint Surg Br 2001;83-B:542–543, with permission.)

classification based primarily on the mechanism of injury. The two subclasses of fractures in group I are valgus injuries and those associated with elbow dislocations. Valgus injuries are subdivided into three types based on the location of the fracture line (Fig. 11-7). Fractures associated with an elbow dislocation are subdivided into two types. The first is based on the original concept proposed by Jeffrey[42] that the fracture occurs during spontaneous reduction (Fig. 11-8A). In this case, the radial head lies proximal to the posterior aspect of the joint. The second is based on Newman's[70] concept that the fracture and displacement occur during the process of dislocation of the elbow. In this type, the radial head lies distal to the anterior portion of the joint (see Fig. 11-8B). Most radial head fractures in children described in the literature have been Salter-Harris type IV injuries containing portions of both the epiphysis and metaphysis, and there is no need to further subclassify them.

Neck-Displaced Fractures (Group II)

For the neck-displaced fractures, there are two subgroups: angular and torsional. An angular fracture of the radial neck may be associated with a proximal ulnar fracture. This association is recognized as a Monteggia variant.

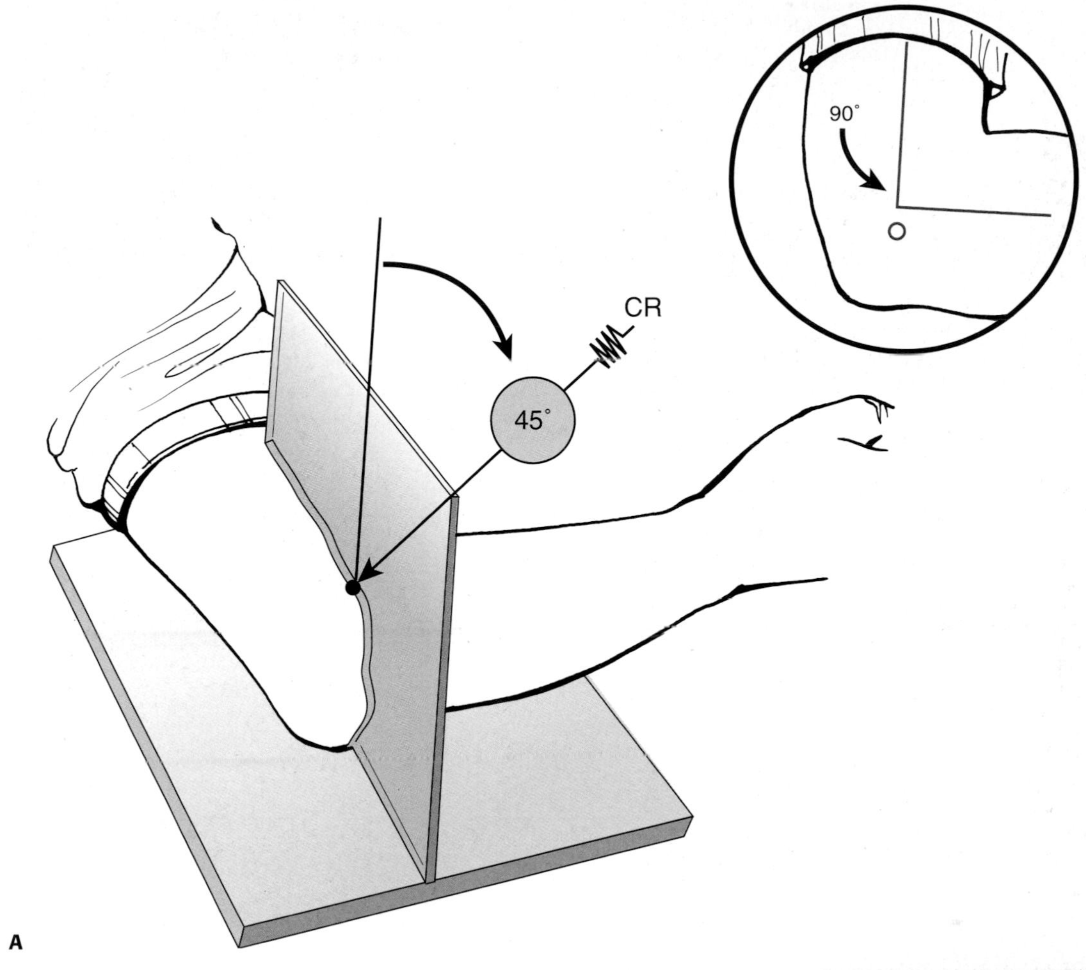

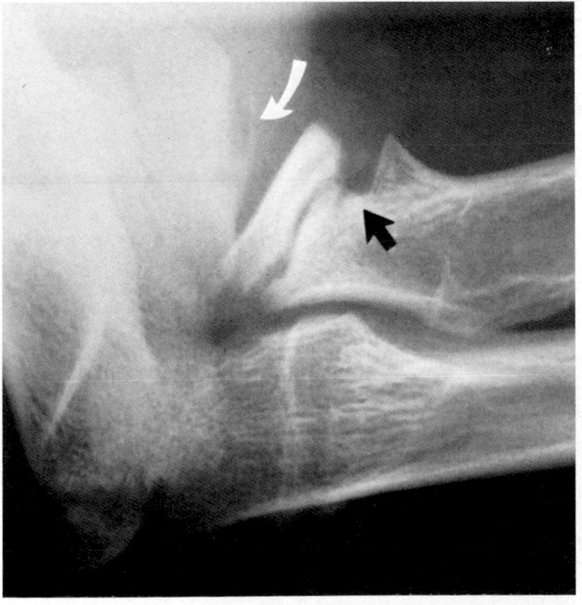

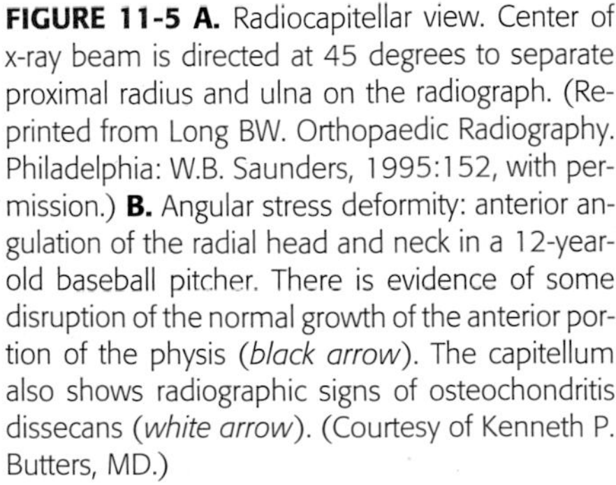

FIGURE 11-5 A. Radiocapitellar view. Center of x-ray beam is directed at 45 degrees to separate proximal radius and ulna on the radiograph. (Reprinted from Long BW. Orthopaedic Radiography. Philadelphia: W.B. Saunders, 1995:152, with permission.) **B.** Angular stress deformity: anterior angulation of the radial head and neck in a 12-year-old baseball pitcher. There is evidence of some disruption of the normal growth of the anterior portion of the physis (*black arrow*). The capitellum also shows radiographic signs of osteochondritis dissecans (*white arrow*). (Courtesy of Kenneth P. Butters, MD.)

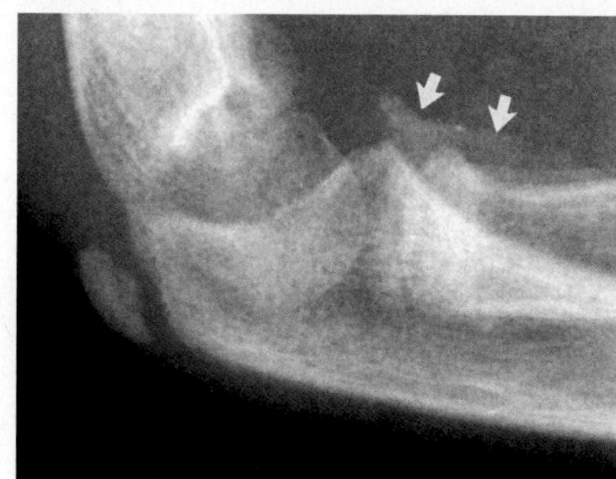

A

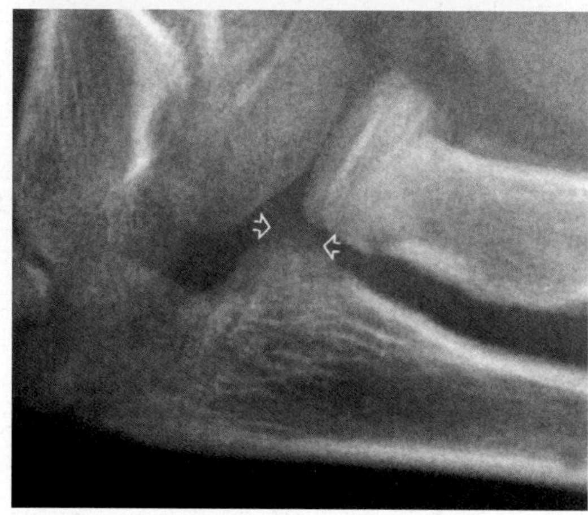

B

FIGURE 11-6 The radiocapitellar view. **A.** Radiographs of a 13-year-old female who sustained a radial neck fracture associated with an elbow dislocation. There is ectopic bone formation (*arrows*). In this view, it is difficult to tell the exact location of the ectopic bone. **B.** The radiocapitellar view separates the radial head from the coronoid process and shows that the ectopic bone is from the coronoid process (*arrows*) and not the radial neck.

TABLE 11-1 Classification of Fractures Involving the Proximal Radius

Group I: Primary displacement of the radial head
- A. Valgus fractures
  1. Type A—Salter-Harris type I and II injuries of the proximal radial physis
  2. Type B—Salter-Harris type IV injuries of the proximal radial physis
  3. Type C—Fractures involving only the proximal radial metaphysis
- B. Fractures associated with elbow dislocation
  1. Type D—Reduction injuries
  2. Type E—Dislocation injuries

Group II: Primary displacement of the radial neck
- A. Angular injuries (Monteggia type III variant)
- B. Torsional injuries

Group III: Stress injuries
- A. Osteochondritis dissecans or osteochondrosis of the radial head
- B. Physeal injuries with neck angulation

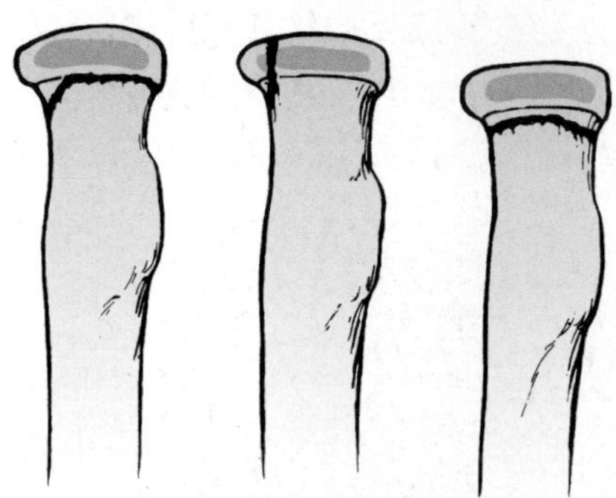

FIGURE 11-7 Types of valgus injuries. **Left.** Type A: Salter-Harris type I or II physeal injury. **Center.** Type B: Salter-Harris type IV injury. **Right.** Type C: Total metaphyseal fracture pattern.

Stress Injuries (Group III)

The final group, stress injuries, includes osteochondritis of the radial head and physeal injuries of the neck that produce angular deformities.

Mechanisms of Injury

Table 11-2 lists the proposed mechanisms for fractures of the radial head and neck in children.

PRIMARY DISPLACEMENT OF THE RADIAL HEAD (GROUP I)

In general, these fractures are caused by a force that is applied to the radial head and is secondarily transmitted to the radial neck, which fractures because it is metaphyseal bone with a thinner cortex. Angulation, rotation, translocation, or complete separation of the radial head from the neck can displace the radial head. This displacement of the radial head produces an incongruity of the proximal radioulnar joint, which is the major cause of dysfunction. For displaced radial head fractures, the treatment goal is to reduce the proximal radioulnar joint to its normal congruous position and restore range of motion.

Valgus Injuries

Angular Force on the Neck

Most of these injuries occur in a fall on the outstretched arm with the elbow in extension.[31,39,42,70,71,117] An associated valgus thrust to the forearm (Fig. 11-9) compresses the radiocapitellar joint. The cartilaginous head absorbs the force and transmits it to the weaker physis or metaphysis of the neck.[117] These fractures characteristically produce an angular deformity of the head with the neck (see Fig. 11-9A). The direction of angulation depends on whether the forearm is in a supinated, neutral, or pronated position at the time of the fall. Vostal[117] showed that in neutral, the pressure is concentrated on the lateral portion of the head and neck. In supination, the pressure is concentrated anteriorly, and in pronation it is concentrated posteriorly.

Associated Injuries

This valgus stress pattern causes associated injuries about the elbow[31,42,43,71,103] (see Fig. 11-9B,C) such as greenstick fracture of the olecranon (Fig. 11-10), which Bado[4] considered an equiv-

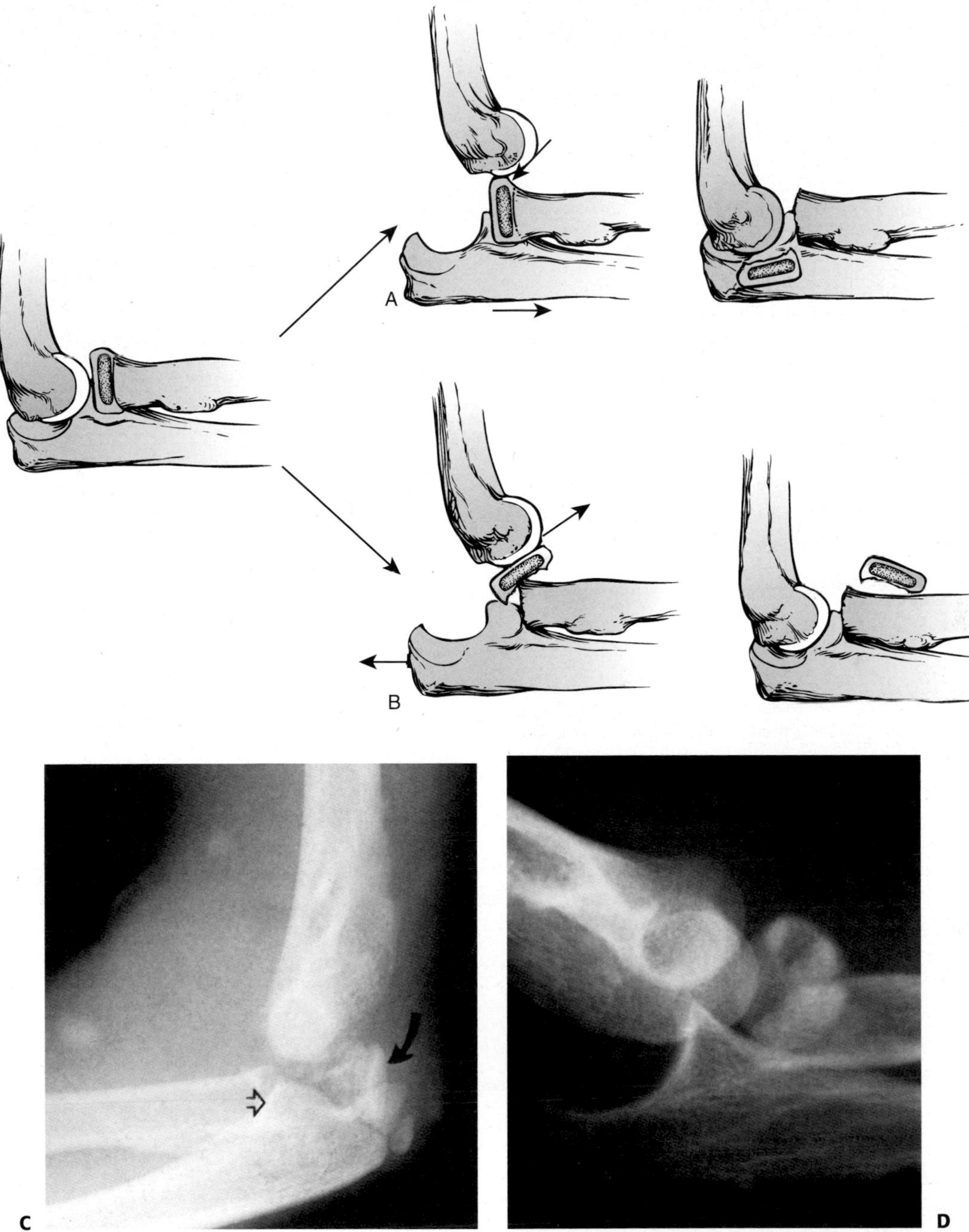

FIGURE 11-8 Dislocation fracture patterns. **A.** Type D: The radial neck is fractured during the process of reduction by the capitellum pressing against the distal lip of the radial head.[125] **B.** Type E: The radial neck is fractured during the process of dislocation by the capitellum pressing against the proximal lip of the radial head.[98] **C.** Radiographs of a radial head that was fractured during the reduction of the dislocation (type D). The radial head (*solid arrow*) lies posterior to the distal humerus, and the distal portion of the neck (*open arrow*) is anterior. (Courtesy of Richard E. King, MD.) **D.** Radiograph of the dislocated elbow in which the fracture of the radial neck occurred during the process of dislocation (type E).

alent of a type I Monteggia lesion. An avulsion fracture of the medial epicondylar apophysis also may occur.[13] In Fowles and Kassab's[26] series of patients with radial neck fractures, more than 61% had one of these associated injuries.

Children with an increased carrying angle may be predisposed to injury of the proximal radius. Henrikson[2] found that the degree of cubitus valgus in patients who sustained this injury was greater than in patients with other types of elbow fractures.

Fracture Patterns in Valgus Injuries

With valgus elbow injuries, the fracture pattern can be one of three types (A, B, or C) (Fig. 11-11). In the first two types, the fracture line involves the physis. Type A represents either a Salter-Harris type I or II physeal injury. In a Salter-Harris type II injury, the metaphyseal fragment is triangular and lies on the compression side. In type B fractures, the fracture line courses vertically through the metaphysis, physis, and epiphysis to pro-

TABLE 11-2 Fractures of the Radial Head and Neck: Proposed Mechanisms in Children

I. Primary displacement of the head (incongruous)
  A. Valgus injuries
  B. Associated with dislocation of the elbow
    1. During reduction
    2. During dislocation

II. Primary displacement of the neck
  A. Angular forces
  B. Rotational forces
  C. Chronic stress forces

duce a Salter-Harris type IV fracture pattern (see Fig. 11-11). This is the only fracture type that involves the articular surface of the radial head. In type C fractures, the fracture line lies completely within the metaphysis (Fig. 11-12), and the fracture can be transverse or oblique. Type B fractures are rare. The incidences of types A and C fractures are approximately equal.[103]

Displacement Patterns

Regardless of the type of fracture pattern, displacement can vary from minimal angulation to complete separation of the radial head from the neck (Fig. 11-13). With minimal angulation, the congruity of the proximal radioulnar joint is usually retained. If the radial head is displaced in relation to the radial neck, the congruity of the proximal radioulnar joint is lost, producing the cam effect. Completely displaced fractures are often associated with more severe injuries.

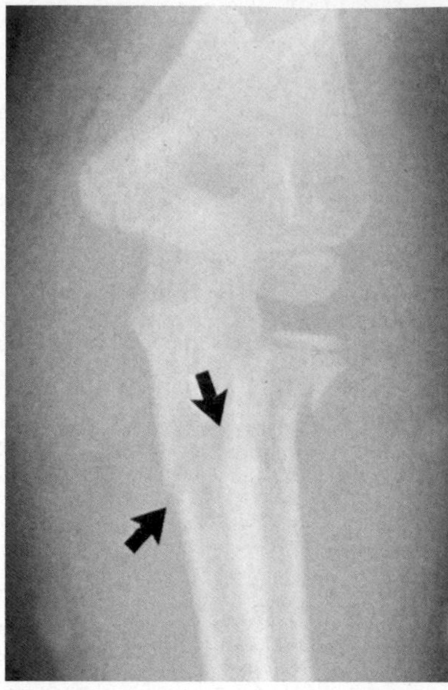

FIGURE 11-10 Associated fractures of valgus stress. Anteroposterior view of a fracture of the radial neck associated with a greenstick fracture of the olecranon (*arrows*).

Neck Migration

Patterson[75] believed that once the stabilizing effect of the radial head is lost, the radial metaphyses migrate proximally. This

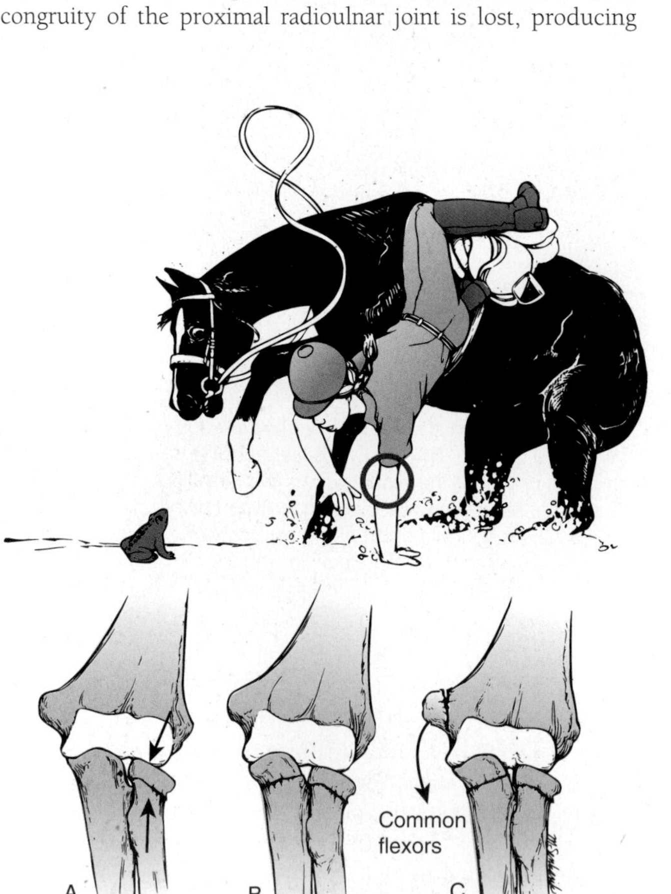

FIGURE 11-9 The most common mechanism of radial neck fractures involves a fall on the outstretched arm. This produces an angular deformity of the neck **(A)**. Further valgus forces can produce a greenstick fracture of the olecranon **(B)** or an avulsion of the medial epicondylar apophysis **(C)**. (Redrawn with permission from Jeffery CC. Fracture of the head of the radius in children. J Bone Joint Surg Br 1950;32:314–324.)

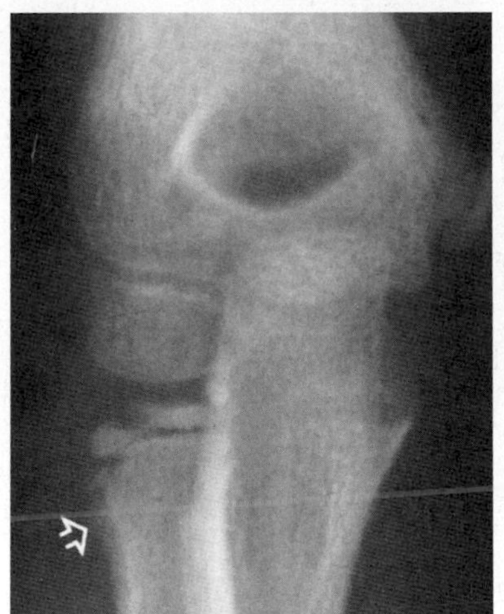

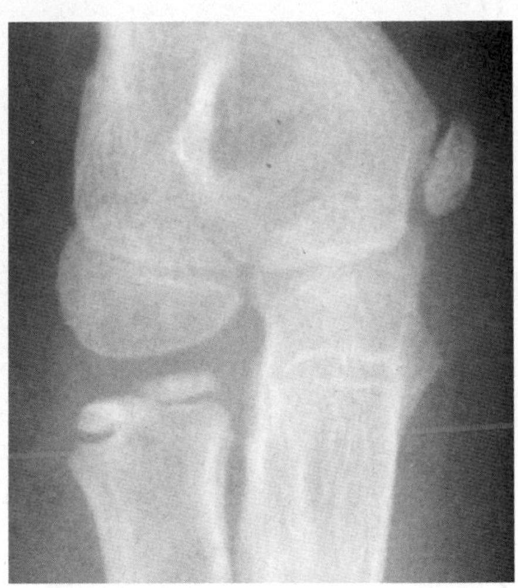

FIGURE 11-11 Valgus (type B) injury. **A.** Three weeks after the initial injury, there was evidence of distal migration of this Salter-Harris type IV fracture fragment. Periosteal new bone formation has already developed along the distal metaphyseal fragment (*arrow*). **B.** Six months after the initial injury, there is evidence of an osseous bridge formation between the metaphysis and the epiphysis. Subsequently, the patient had secondary degenerative arthritis with loss of elbow motion and forearm rotation.

proximal migration of the distal fragment tends to be ulnarward because of muscle pull by the supinator and biceps muscles (Fig. 11-14). Patterson[75] attempted to counteract these forces in his manipulative technique ("Patterson's Manipulative Technique"). When there is a strong valgus component, the proximal portion of the distal fragment of the radius can get locked medial to the coronoid process, making a closed reduction almost impossible.[24,56]

Associated with Elbow Dislocation

In two rare types of fractures of the radial neck associated with elbow dislocation, the head fragment is totally displaced from the neck.[5,13,27,42,70,118] The proposed mechanism is a fall on the hand with the elbow flexed, which causes a momentary partial dislocation of the elbow and forces the radial head posterior to the capitellum.

During Reduction (Type D)

In the original description of this injury, Jeffrey[42] suggested that displacement and fracture occurred during spontaneous reduction of the transiently dislocated elbow. During this reduction process, the capitellum applies a proximal force to the distal lip of the radial head, causing it to separate as the forearm and distal radius are reduced distally (see Fig. 11-8A). The radial neck and olecranon return to their anatomic locations while the radial head remains in the posterior aspect of the joint.[118]

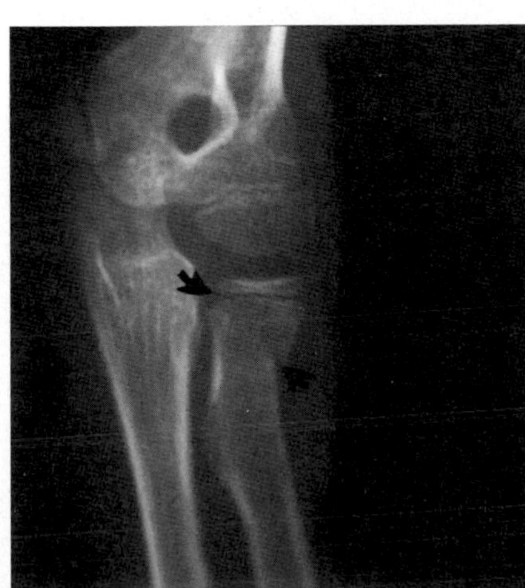

FIGURE 11-12 Valgus type C injury. The fracture line is totally metaphyseal and oblique (*arrows*).

During Dislocation (Type E)

Newman[70] described a type of radial head fracture in which the fracture occurs during the process of dislocation. In this case, the capitellum applies a distally directed force to the proximal lip of the radial head as the elbow is dislocated (see Fig. 11-8B). The elbow may remain dislocated with the radial head lying anterior and often parallel to the long axis of the neck fragment. If the dislocation is reduced, either by manipulation or spontaneously, the radial head lies free in the anterior portion of the elbow joint.[5,70,114]

PRIMARY DISPLACEMENT OF THE RADIAL NECK (GROUP II)

Rarely, angular or torsional forces cause a primary disruption or deformity of the neck while the head remains congruous within the proximal radioulnar joint. Treatment of these fractures is manipulation of the distal neck fragment to align it with the head.

Angular Forces

Angular forces always produce type III Monteggia equivalents. A Monteggia type III fracture pattern is created when a varus

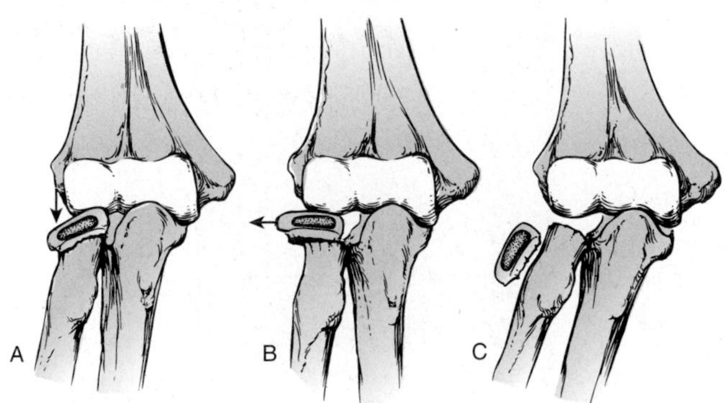

FIGURE 11-13 Displacement patterns. The radial head can be angulated **(A)**, translated **(B)**, or completely displaced **(C)**.

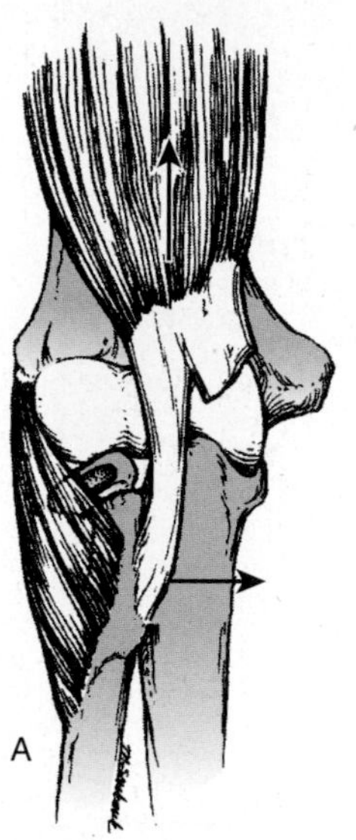

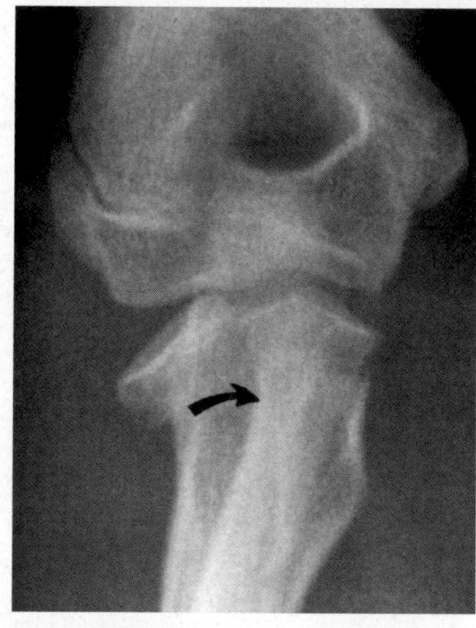

FIGURE 11-14 A. Forces producing displacement. Once the stabilizing effect of the radial head is lost, the distal fragment (radial neck and proximal shaft) is displaced ulnarward and proximally by the unopposed biceps and supinator muscles (*arrows*). (Redrawn with permission from Patterson RF. Treatment of displaced transverse fractures of the neck of the radius in children. J Bone Joint Surg 1934;16:695.) **B.** Radiograph showing proximal and medial (ulnar) displacement of distal neck fragment (*arrow*). (From Wilkins KE, ed. Operative management of upper extremity fractures in children. Rosemont, IL: American Academy of Orthopaedic Surgeons, 1994:55.)

force is applied across the extended elbow, resulting in a greenstick fracture of the olecranon or proximal ulna and a lateral dislocation of the radial head.[125] Occasionally, however, the failure occurs at the radial neck (Monteggia III equivalent) and the radial neck displaces laterally, leaving the radial head and proximal neck fragment in anatomic position under the orbicular ligament (Fig. 11-15).[72]

Rotational Forces

Rotational forces may fracture the radial neck in young children before ossification of the proximal radial epiphysis. Both reports of this injury are in the European literature,[31,39] and in both, the initial rotational force was supination. Reduction was achieved by pronation of the forearm. Diagnosis of these injuries is difficult and may require arthrography or an examination under general anesthesia. This injury should be differentiated from the more common subluxation of the radial head (pulled elbow syndrome), in which the forearm usually is held in pronation with resistance to supination. In addition, on radiography there usually are no signs of hemarthrosis, as is seen in the torsional fractures.

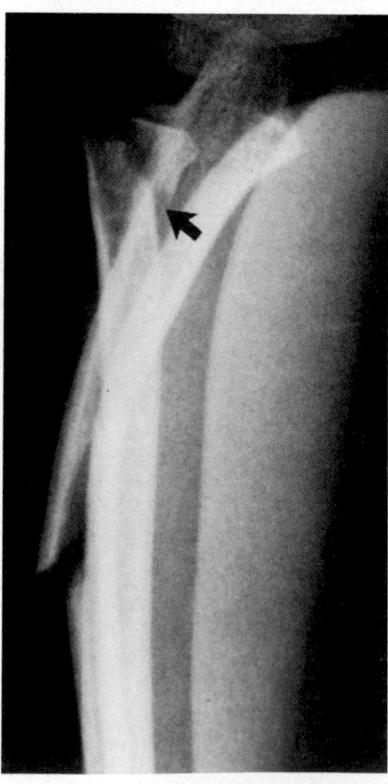

FIGURE 11-15 Angular forces. This 8-year-old sustained a type III Monteggia equivalent in which the radial neck fractured (*arrow*), leaving the radial head reduced proximally. (Courtesy of Ruben D. Pechero, MD.)

STRESS INJURIES (GROUP III)

A final mechanism of injury is chronic repetitive stress, both longitudinal and rotational, on either the head or the proximal radial physis. These injuries are usually the result of athletic activity in which the upper extremity is required to perform repetitive motions. Repetitive stresses disrupt growth of either the neck or the head with eventual deformity. A true stress fracture is not present.

In the United States, the popularity of organized sports has produced a number of unique injuries in children related to repetitive stress applied to growth centers. This is especially true in the immature elbow. Most injuries are related to throwing sports, primarily Little League baseball. Most of this "Little League pathology" involves tension injuries on the medial epicondyle. In some athletes, however, the lateral side is involved as well because of the repetitive compressive forces applied to the capitellum and radial head and neck. Athletes involved in sports requiring upper extremity weightbearing, such as gymnastics or wrestling, are also at risk. In the radial head, lytic lesions similar to osteochondritis dissecans may occur (Figs. 11-16 and 11-17).[22,112,123] Chronic compressive loading may cause an osteochondrosis of the proximal radial epiphysis, with radiographic signs of decreased size of the ossified epiphysis, increased radiographic opacity, and later fragmentation. If the stress forces are transmitted to the radial neck, the anterior portion of the physis may be injured, producing an angular deformity of the radial neck (see Fig. 11-5).[21]

Treatment

The options for treatment for radial head and neck fractures include:

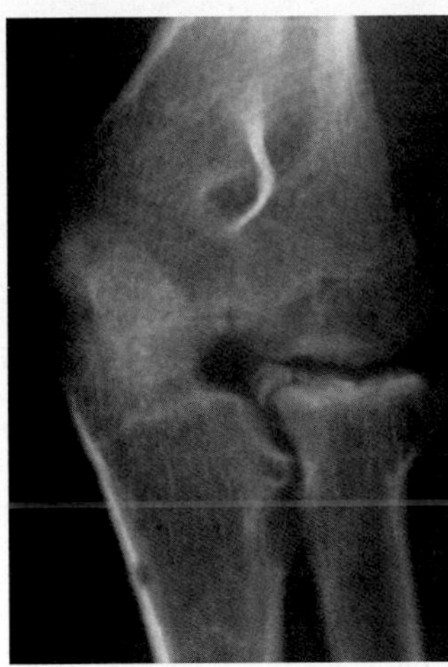

FIGURE 11-16 Osteochondritis dissecans. Radiograph of this 11-year-old Little League pitcher's elbow shows fragmentation of the subchondral surfaces of the radial head. These changes and the accelerated bone age are evidence of overuse.

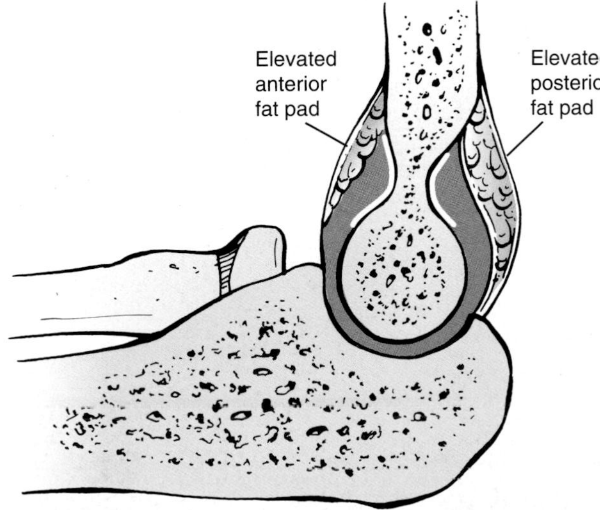

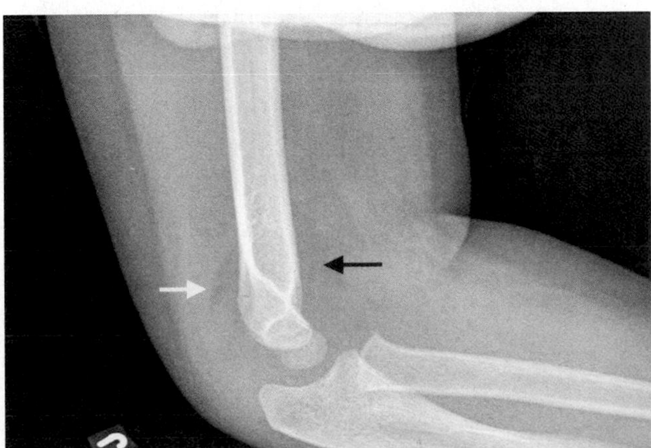

FIGURE 11-17 Elevated anterior and posterior fat pads. **A.** Illustration (adapted with permission from Skaggs DL, Mirazayan R. The posterior fat pad sign in association with occult fracture of the elbow in children. J Bone Surg AM 1999;81:1429–1433). **B.** *White arrow*: posterior fat pad sign. *Black arrow*: anterior fat pad sign.

- Immobilization with no manipulation
- Manipulative closed reduction
- Percutaneous pin reduction
- Intramedullary pin reduction
- Open reduction with or without internal fixation
- Excision of either the entire head or a small head fragment

Several factors must be considered in choosing a method of treatment, including the degree of angulation and displacement, the association of other injuries, the age of the patient, and the time elapsed since the injury.

Prognostic Factors

Some factors may be more important than the type of treatment in determining the final result. A poor result is more likely if the fracture is associated with other injuries, such as an elbow dislocation, a fracture of the olecranon, or avulsion of the medial epicondylar apophysis.[26,92] The magnitude of force to the elbow is a major factor in determining the quality of the result.[52,103]

Initial Angulation and Displacement

Tibone and Stoltz[110] reported that the number of good results decreased if the initial angulation exceeded 30 degrees or the amount of displacement exceeded 3 mm. Newman[70] found that more than 4 mm of initial displacement increased the frequency of poor results and the risk of synostosis with the proximal ulna.

Angulation and Displacement after Reduction

Residual tilt of the radial head is better tolerated than displacement. Pollen[81] believed that in older children, only 15 degrees of angulation should be accepted without attempting manipulation. The spontaneous correction that can be expected to occur with growth in younger children is approximately 10 degrees. Some clinicians accept up to 30 degrees of residual angulation,[52,60,70,84,114] whereas others believe that up to 45 degrees of residual angulation can yield a satisfactory result.[8,15,71,116]

Age Effect

It is still controversial whether age has a favorable or unfavorable effect on the outcome.[103] The cam effect will limit supination and pronation if there is significant displacement of the proximal fragment. However, adequate remodeling with a functional range of motion can occur with as much as 40% displacement (Fig. 11-18) in a young child.

Timing

Surgery should be done as soon as possible after the injury; the later the surgical intervention, the poorer the result. McBride and Monnet[59] described three patients in whom an osteotomy of the neck was done for residual angulation 3 to 5 weeks after injury. All had further loss of range of motion because of the development of a proximal cross union. Blount[8] set a limit of 5 days, after which surgical intervention is more likely to produce a poorer result than if the fracture is left untreated.

Outcomes

In general, a closed reduction will yield a better result than an open reduction. This may be true because injuries that can be managed by closed methods are the result of less severe trauma

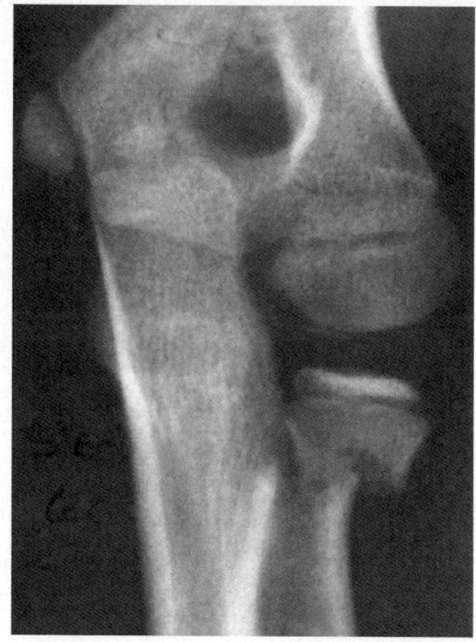

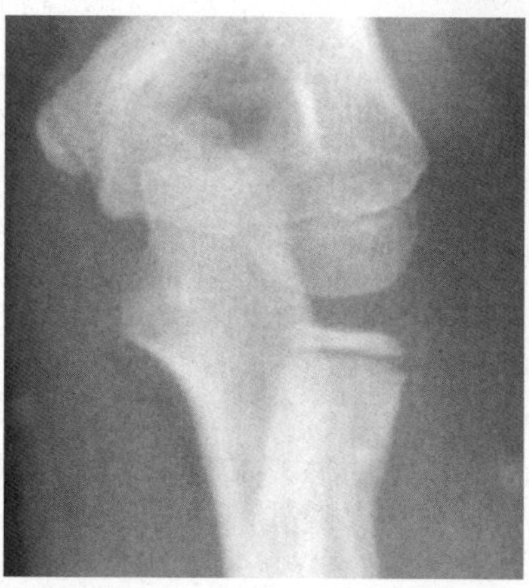

FIGURE 11-18 Translocation remodeling. **A.** Injury film of a 9-year-old who had 60 degrees of supination and pronation by clinical examination with local anesthesia into the elbow joint. Because range of motion was functional, the position was accepted. **B.** Two months after fracture, there was almost complete remodeling of the translocation. The patient's forearm rotation was 75 degrees in both directions. (Courtesy of Earl A. Stanley Jr, MD.)

than those requiring open reduction. The poor results in those managed with open methods may be due just as much to the associated soft-tissue injuries as to the surgical insult.

The overall incidence of poor results in large series varies from 15% to 33%.[26,39,43,103,114] Considering only severely displaced fractures, the incidence of poor results was as high as 50%.[103] Thus, at least one in five or six children can be expected to have a poor result despite adequate treatment. It is wise to counsel the parents before beginning treatment if poor prognostic factors are present. Very little improvement in motion occurs after 6 months. Steinberg et al.[103] found that range of motion in their patients at 6 months was almost equal to that when the patients were examined years later.

Nonoperative Methods

Immobilization (Up to 30 Degrees of Angulation). Immobilization is the treatment of choice for fractures in younger children in which the angulation of the radial head is less than 20 to 30 degrees. A collar and cuff, a posterior splint, or a light long-arm cast is sufficient to provide comfort and protection from further injury. Aspiration of the intra-articular hematoma may decrease pain.

Manipulative Closed Reduction (30 Degrees to 60 Degrees of Angulation). Although acceptable results can be obtained with angulation of up to 45 degrees, closed reduction should be attempted for fractures with more than 30 degrees of angulation. A closed reduction is usually satisfactory for fractures with angulation up to 60 degrees. The chance of achieving a satisfactory closed reduction is much less when the initial angulation exceeds 60 degrees.

Patterson's Manipulative Technique. Some authors[19,60] advocate manipulative reduction with the elbow in extension, as described by Patterson.[75] General or regional anesthesia can provide adequate relaxation. The orbicular ligament should be intact to stabilize the proximal radial head fragment.[60] In Patterson's[75] technique, an assistant grasps the arm proximal to the elbow joint with one hand (Fig. 11-19) and places the other hand medially over the distal humerus to provide a medial fulcrum for the varus stress applied across the elbow. The surgeon applies distal traction with the forearm supinated to relax the supinators and biceps. A varus force is then placed on the elbow to overcome the ulnar deviation of the distal fragment so that it can be aligned with the proximal fragment. This varus force also helps open up the lateral side of the joint, which facilitates manipulation of the head fragment.

Although forearm supination relaxes the supinator muscle, supination may not be the best position for manipulation of the head fragment. Jeffrey[42] pointed out that the tilt of the radial

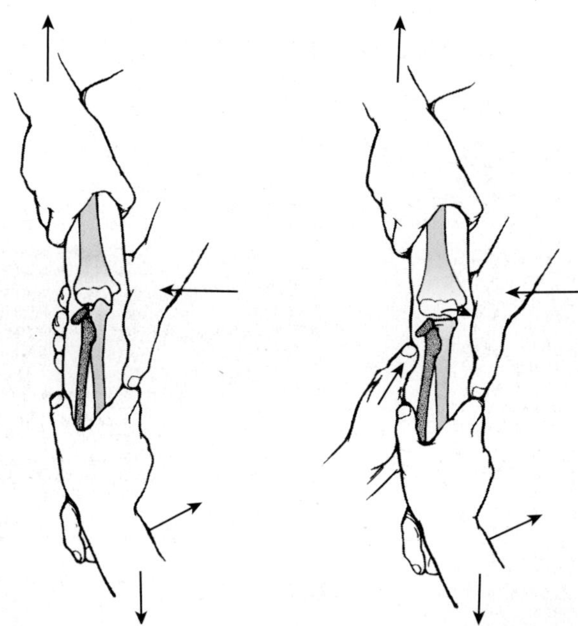

FIGURE 11-19 Patterson's manipulative technique. **Left.** An assistant grabs the arm proximally with one hand placed medially against the distal humerus. The surgeon applies distal traction with the forearm supinated and pulls the forearm into varus. **Right.** Digital pressure applied directly over the tilted radial head completes the reduction. (Redrawn with permission from Patterson RF. Treatment of displaced transverse fractures of the neck of the radius in children. J Bone Joint Surg 1934;16:696–698.)

head can be anterior or posterior depending on the position of the forearm at the time of injury. With this degree of rotation, the prominent tilt of the proximal fragment can be felt laterally. The direction of maximal tilt can be confirmed by radiograph. The best position for reduction is the degree of rotation that places the radial head most prominent laterally. If the x-ray beam is perpendicular to the head in maximal tilt, it casts an oblong or rectangular shadow; if not, the shadow is oval or almost circular.[42] With a varus force applied across the extended elbow, the maximal tilt directed laterally, and the elbow in varus, the radial head can be reduced with the pressure of a finger (see Fig. 11-19, *right*).

Neher and Torch[68] described a two-person technique for the reduction of severely displaced radial neck fractures. This technique is performed with the elbow in extension and the patient under general anesthesia. An assistant uses both thumbs to place a laterally directed force on the proximal radial shaft while the surgeon applies a varus stress to the elbow. Simultaneously, the surgeon uses his other thumb to apply a reduction force directly to the radial head (Fig. 11-20).

Kaufman et al.[45] proposed another technique in which the elbow is manipulated in the flexed position. The surgeon presses his or her thumb against the anterior surface of the radial head with the forearm in pronation.

Some authors recommend immobilization in pronation after reduction because it is the forearm motion most often restricted after fracture.[120] Some have recommended supination because they believe it is easier for the patient to regain active pronation than active supination during rehabilitation. Whether pronation or supination is chosen, they recommend 90 degrees of flexion for the elbow. Fluoroscopy can determine whether pronation or supination results in the optimal reduction of the fracture.

In uncommon circumstances, the head fragment may be completely displaced proximally, with the head perpendicular to the shaft of the radius. In four reports since 1960, closed reduction,[27,122,124] resulted in rotation of the proximal fragment180 degrees so that the articular surface of the head (concavity) was facing the fracture surface of the radial neck. Open reduction is needed to reduce the fragment, with a high risk of complications.

Operative Techniques

Although most fractures are stable after reduction, redisplacement can occur, especially if the initial tilt was more than 60 degrees.[20,43] Fractures with more than 90 degrees of angulation, especially those in which the head fragment is lying free in the joint, are almost impossible to reduce by closed methods.

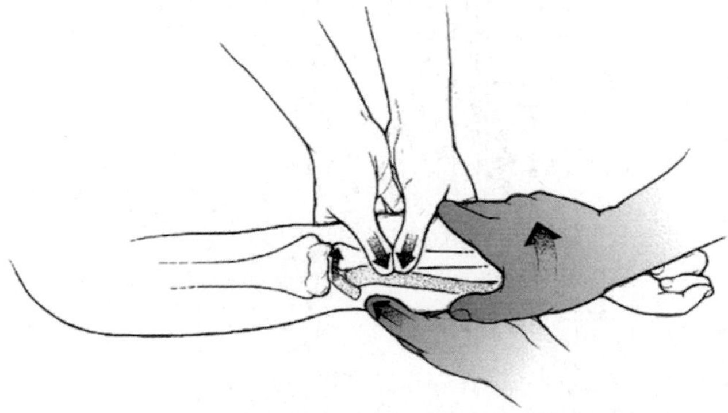

FIGURE 11-20 Neher and Torch reduction technique. (From Neher CG, Torch MA. New reduction technique for severely displaced pediatric radial neck fractures. J Pediatr Orthop 2003;23:626–628, with permission.)

Percutaneous Pin Reduction. The use of percutaneous pin reduction with an image intensifier is a popular method of satisfactorily reducing moderately to severely displaced fractures.[3,6,19,78,102] Various authors have used an awl, a Steinmann pin,[89] a periosteal elevator,[28] or a double-pointed "bident"[3] that in theory controls rotation better. Some authors describe using the pin to directly push the displaced radial head fragment back into position,[61] while others describe a pin leverage technique,[78,102] inserting the pin into the fracture site and then leveraging the radial head against the capitellum to reduce the fracture (Fig. 11-21). Pesudo et al.,[78] in their series of 22 displaced radial neck fractures, found that the results after percutaneous pin reduction were superior to those after open reduction.

Biyani et al.[7] described driving the pin used to reduce the radial head across the fracture site to stabilize it. The pin is removed and motion is allowed after 3 weeks.

Intramedullary Pin Reduction. In 1980, Metaizeau et al.[62] proposed reducing severely tilted radial neck fractures with an intramedullary wire passed from the distal metaphysis. A report 13 years later[61] demonstrated the effectiveness of this technique. A wire is inserted into the medullary canal through an entrance hole in the distal metaphysis (Fig. 11-22). Once the wire reaches the fracture site, the angulation at the tip enables it to engage the proximal fracture site at the neck. Once engaged, the wire is twisted to reduce the head and neck fragment. This technique has produced results superior to open reduction with fewer complications.[32,98]

Subsequently, multiple authors[67,83,96] have reported good to excellent results using the intramedullary pin reduction technique for severely displaced radial neck fractures. Schmittenbecher et al.[96] reported good to excellent results in 18 (78%) of 23 fractures after reduction and fixation with 2-mm elastic intramedullary nails. Other authors have recommended using Kirschner-wires for the intramedullary technique. One challenge with this technique is that oftentimes Kirschner-wires are not long enough to allow for optimal use with the intramedullary reduction method. However, the pointed tip of the Kirschner-wire is helpful in engaging the displaced radial neck fragment during this reduction maneuver. Nawabi et al.[67] reported the use of a smooth 1.8-mm Ilizarov wire in two children. The added length of the Ilizarov wire allowed sufficient wire to remain outside the skin to simplify the reduction maneuver. When using a Kirschner wire or Ilizarov wire, it is important to contour the distal 3 to 4 mm with a relatively sharp bend to allow for easier capture of the displaced radial head fragment. It remains controversial as to whether or not the intramedullary implant needs to remain in place after the fracture reduction.

Wallace Method for Reduction of Radial Neck Fracture. Fluoroscopy in an AP projection is used to determine the forearm rotation that exposes the maximum amount of deformity of the fracture, and the level of the bicipital tuberosity of the proximal radius is marked. A 1-cm dorsal skin incision is made at that level just lateral to the subcutaneous border of the ulna. A periosteal elevator is gently inserted between the ulna and the ra-

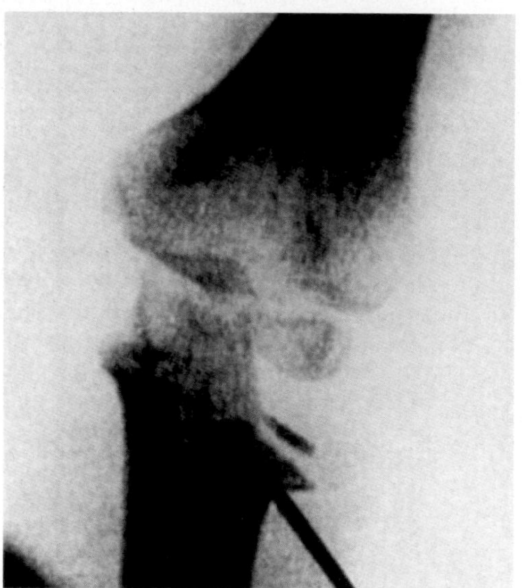

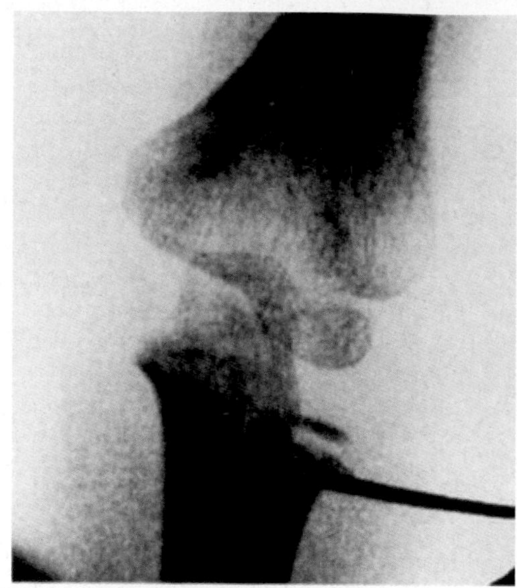

FIGURE 11-21 Radiographs demonstrating the pin leverage technique for reduction of a radial neck fracture. (From Steele JA, Graham HK. Angulated radial neck fractures in children: a prospective study of percutaneous reduction. J Bone Joint Surg Br 1992;74:760–764, with permission.)

dius, with care not to disrupt the periosteum of the radius or the ulna. The radial shaft is usually much more ulnarly displaced than expected, and the radial nerve is lateral to the radius at this level. While counterpressure is applied against the radial head, the distal fragment of the radius is levered away from the ulna. An assistant can aid in this maneuver by gently applying traction and rotating the forearm back and forth to disimpact the fracture fragments. If necessary to correct angulation, a percutaneous Kirschner-wire can be inserted into the fracture site, parallel to the radial head, to lever the physis perpendicular to the axis of the radius.

Once an adequate reduction has been obtained, an oblique Kirschner-wire is inserted to provide fracture fixation. The wire is removed 3 weeks after surgery (Figs. 11-23 and 11-24).

Open Reduction. With valgus injuries, a residual tilt of 45 degrees probably produces as good a result as trying to achieve a perfect reduction surgically. An acceptable closed reduction can produce a better result than an anatomically perfect open surgical reduction (Table 11-3).

Early reviews reported poor results with significant loss of range of motion in patients treated operatively,[9,11,14,21] but more recently Steinberg et al.[103] combined their results of open reduction of severely displaced fractures with those of five other

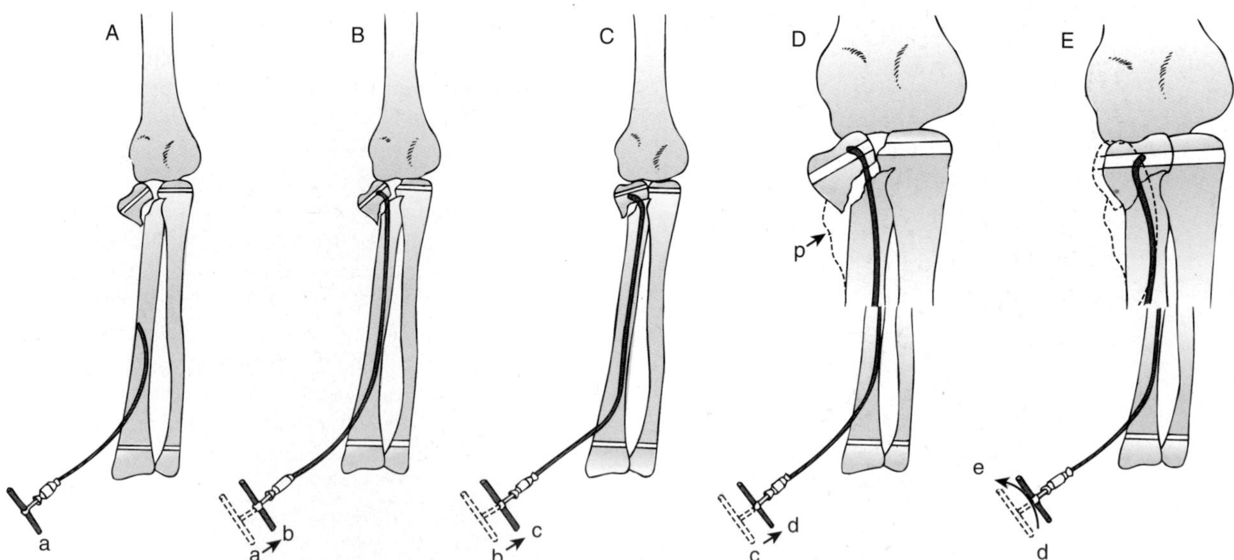

FIGURE 11-22 Intramedullary pin reduction. **A.** The insertion point for the curved flexible pin is in the metaphysis. **B.** The curved end of the rod passes in the shaft and engages the proximal fragment. **C.** Manipulation of the rod disimpacts the fracture. **D,E.** Once disimpacted, the head fragment is rotated into position with the intramedullary rod. (From Metaizeau JP, Lascombes P, Lemelle JL, et al. Reduction and fixation of displaced radial neck fractures by closed intramedullary pinning. J Pediatr Orthop 1993;13:355–356; with permission.)

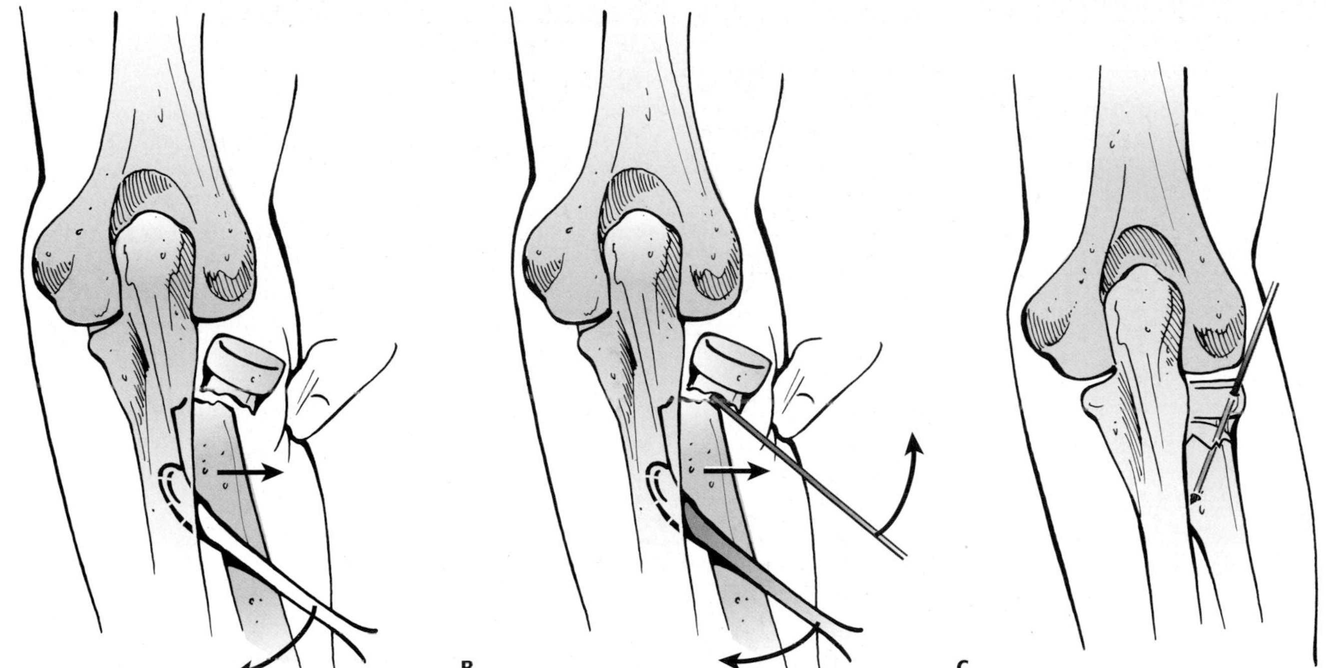

FIGURE 11-23 Wallace radial head reduction technique. **A.** A periosteal elevator is used to lever the distal fragment laterally while the thumb pushes the proximal fragment medially. **B.** Kirschner-wires are used to assist the reduction if necessary. **C.** The position of the reduction can be fixed with an oblique Kirschner-wire.

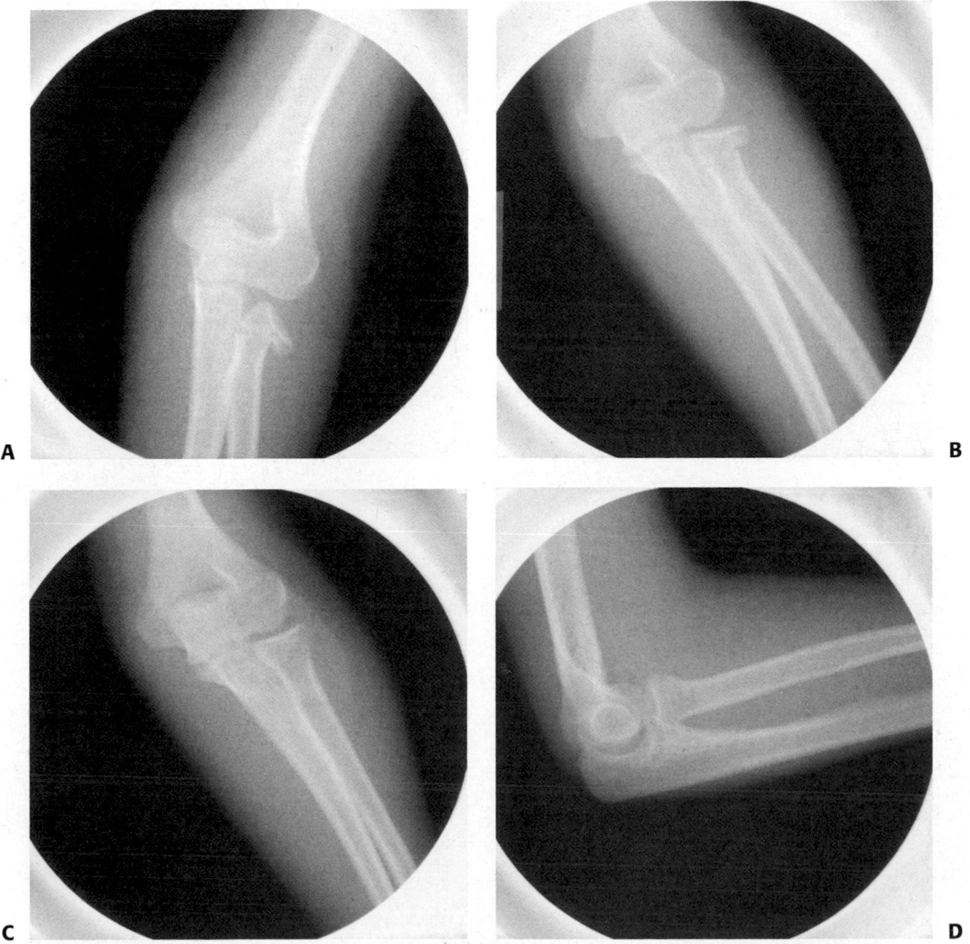

FIGURE 11-24 A. Radial neck fracture angulated 45 degrees in a 14-year-old female. **B.** Radiograph after closed reduction using thumb pressure on the radial head. **C.** Final reduction after manipulation of the distal fragment with an elevator using the Wallace technique. **D.** Lateral view of the elbow after reduction.

TABLE 11-3 Acceptable Reduction

No translation
50 to 60 degrees of pronation and supination on clinical examination

series[42,43,78,110] and reported 49% good results after operative treatment compared to 25% after nonoperative treatment. None of these authors used percutaneous pin reduction. The results of moderately displaced fractures treated operatively were equal to the results of those treated nonoperatively.

If the head of the radius is completely displaced, results are usually better with surgical intervention. Some authors have shown that a completely separated radial head remains viable if surgically replaced as late as 48 hours after injury.[30,46]

Some fractures may be irreducible by closed means because interposition of the capsule or annular ligament between the head and neck blocks reduction.[117] Strong et al.[105] described an unusual fracture pattern in which the radial head was trapped by the orbicular ligament. They found that these fractures were irreducible by closed methods and required open reduction.

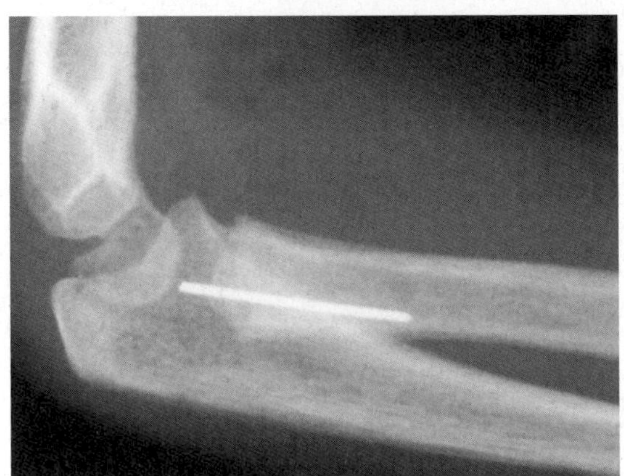

A

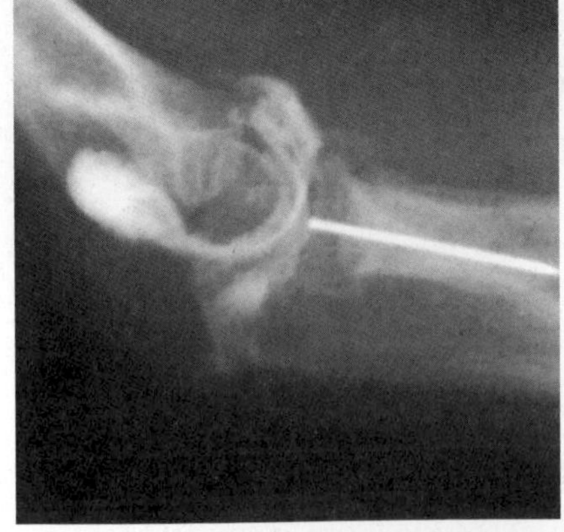

B

FIGURE 11-25 Transcapitellar pin in a 4-year-old with a completely displaced fracture of the radial neck. **A.** Three weeks after injury, when the pin was removed, it had fractured and a portion remained in the proximal radius. **B.** An arthrogram revealed that the fractured end was at the joint surface of the radial head. The piece was left in place, with subsequent resumption of normal elbow motion.

Fixation Methods

Some authors[60,89,90] have recommended inserting a small wire through the capitellum across the radial head and into the neck to fix radial head fractures, but this technique has a high incidence of complications.[26,70,97,120] Even in a long-arm cast, the elbow joint has slight motion, which can cause the pin to fatigue and break (Fig. 11-25). The retrieval of the remaining portion of the pin from the proximal radius is almost impossible without imposing considerable trauma. Even if the pin does not break, the motion of the pin may erode the joint surface and fragment the radial head.[70,120]

Other suggested methods of fixing the displaced radial neck after open reduction include intramedullary bone pegs, direct pin insertion through the head by way of an olecranon osteotomy,[55] or with a forked plate.[51]

The most common technique in current use involves placement of a pin obliquely across the fracture site into the radial head.[19,26,43] The pin can be placed either proximal to distal (Fig. 11-26) or, preferably, distal to proximal. The protruding pin is easy to remove after the fracture heals.

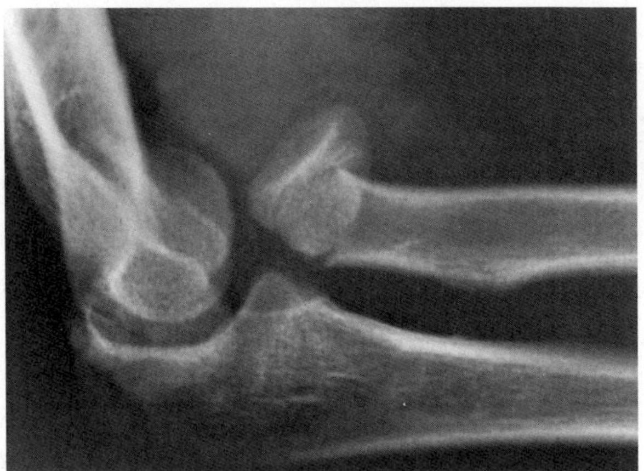

A

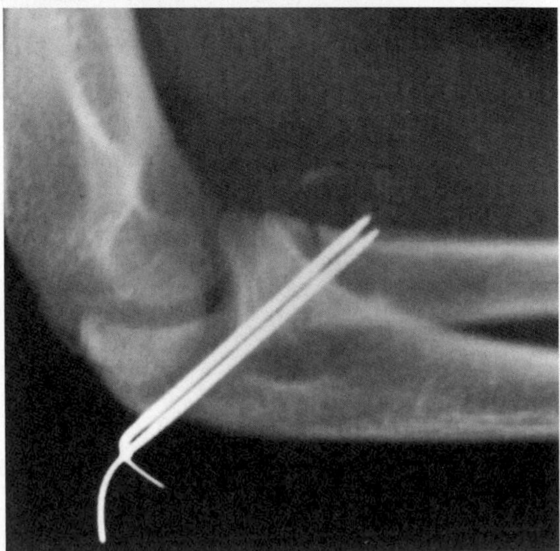

B

FIGURE 11-26 Oblique pin. **A.** Displaced fracture of the radial neck in a 10-year-old. **B.** A closed reduction was performed, and to stabilize the head fragment, two pins were placed percutaneously and obliquely across the fracture site from proximal to distal. If open reduction and pinning are done, the preferred alignment is obliquely across the fracture site from distal to proximal. (From Wilkins KE, ed. Operative Management of Upper Extremity Fractures in Children. Rosemont, IL: American Academy of Orthopaedic Surgeons, 1994:57, with permission.)

Some believe that internal fixation is unnecessary after open reduction.[8,70,120] Wedge and Robertson[120] found that patients without internal fixation had more good results than those with internal fixation. Use of internal fixation does not guarantee that the fragment will not slip. Newman[70] described two patients in whom the head slipped postoperatively despite Kirschner-wire fixation.

One complication of open reduction is injury to the posterior interosseous nerve. To avoid this complication, Jones and Esah[43] recommended identifying the nerve as it courses through the supinator muscle. Kaplan[44] and Strachan and Ellis[104] demonstrated that with the forearm in pronation, the posterior interosseous nerve displaces ulnarward, out of the way of the surgical dissection. They also recommended that the patient be prone during exploration of the proximal radius to help keep the forearm pronated.

The orbicular ligament should be left intact if possible. If dividing it is necessary for reduction, it should be repaired.[26]

Type B Injuries

For type B (Salter-Harris type IV) fractures, a small marginal fragment can be safely removed and the remaining large portion of the head reduced without internal fixation.[120]

Radial Head Fractures

Pelto et al.[77] reported good to excellent results with the use of absorbable polyglycolide pins in patients older than 13 years of age. Transient local abacterial tissue reaction occurred but did not lead to any long-term negative effects. There was no comment on the effect on the physis. To fix a large displaced head fragment in a Salter-Harris type III or IV fracture, a transepiphyseal screw is useful (Fig. 11-27).

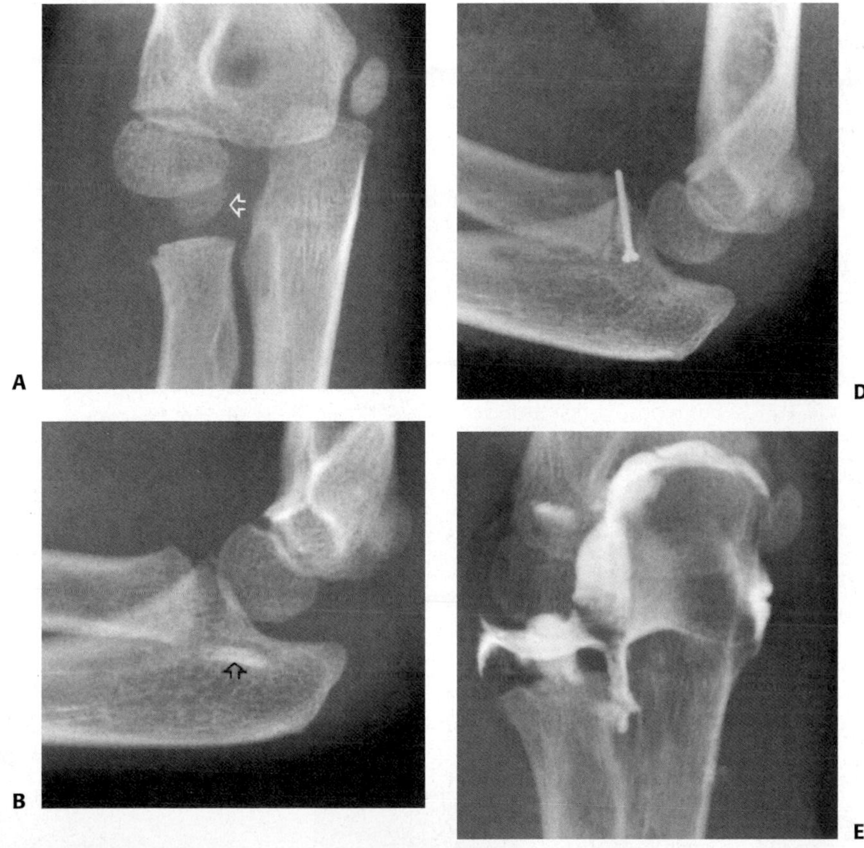

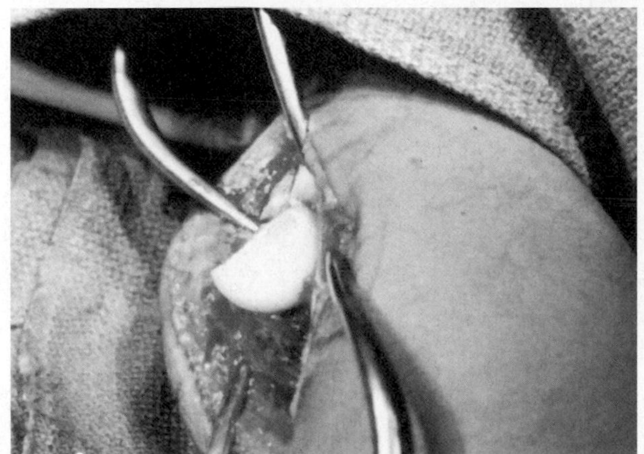

FIGURE 11-27 Miniscrew fixation. **A,B.** Anteroposterior and lateral views of the elbow of a 6-year-old male in whom the head fragment lies posterior to the capitellum (*arrows*). **C.** At the time of open reduction a Salter-Harris type III fracture through the epiphysis and proximal physis was apparent. The fragment involved 60% of the head diameter and had soft tissue attached. **D.** A screw placed through the epiphysis fixed the reduction. **E.** Six months after surgery, an arthrogram showed maintenance of the architectural structure of the medial head after screw removal. The patient had 60 degrees of supination and pronation. (From Wilkins KE, ed. Operative Management of Upper Extremity Fractures in Children. Rosemont, IL: American Academy of Orthopaedic Surgeons, 1994:58, with permission.)

TABLE 11-4 Treatment of Radial Head Fractures

Fracture Status	Treatment
Minimally displaced (<30 degrees angulation, no translation)	Long-arm cast or posterior splint (7–10 days) Early motion
Angulation >30 degrees	Closed reduction under general anesthesia using flexion–pronation (Israeli) technique, or manipulative techniques (Patterson,[75] Neher and Torch[68]) Long-arm cast (10–14 days)
Angulation >45 degrees	Elastic bandage wrap reduction Flexion–pronation (Israeli) reduction technique, or manipulative techniques (Patterson,[75] Neher and Torch[68]) Percutaneous pin reduction Long-arm cast (10–14 days)
Angulation fixed at >45 degrees, translation >3 mm	Percutaneous wire reduction Elevator reduction (Wallace) technique
Displacement, with <60 degrees supination–pronation, radial head completely displaced	Elevator reduction (Wallace) technique Open reduction (± internal fixation)

Radial Head Excision. Resection of the radial head fragment was popular in the 1920s and 1930s, but reported results have been uniformly poor.[20,39,43] Cubitus valgus and radial deviation at the wrist are common sequelae. The procedure is contraindicated in a growing child.

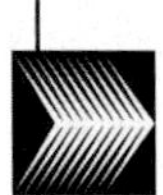

AUTHORS' PREFERRED METHOD

We tend to be as conservative as possible in treating these fractures (Table 11-4). Although they may appear reasonably minor both radiographically and clinically, we initially emphasize to the parents that some loss of motion may occur even with an anatomic reduction. The problem is usually a loss of range of motion in supination and pronation. Little pain or loss of upper extremity function occurs despite the residual loss of forearm rotation.

Nonoperative Methods

Moderate Tilt (30 to 60 Degrees)

If the radial head is tilted more than 30 degrees, we attempt a manipulative closed reduction. In adolescent patients, we may attempt a closed reduction for less than 30 degrees in an attempt to normalize the anatomy as much as possible. If there is a great amount of pain or resistance to pronation and supination, we aspirate the elbow after a sterile preparation and frequently inject 2 to 3 mL of 1% lidocaine,[18] but a general anesthetic is preferable for full relaxation. We prefer the Israeli technique for simple, moderately displaced radial head fractures (Fig. 11-28).[45] The important aspect is to ensure that the elbow is flexed at 90 degrees for the manipulation. Usually there is resistance to pronation (Fig. 11-29). With thumb pressure applied to the radial head, the opposite hand forces the forearm into full pronation (see Fig. 11-29). After reduction, the range of motion should be at least 60 degrees of supination and pronation (see Fig. 11-28B). If the range of supination and pronation is adequate, we accept the reduction regardless of the radiograph appearance. We attempt closed reduction first even with completely displaced radial neck fractures. Occasionally a surprisingly satisfactory reduction can be obtained (Fig. 11-30).

Elastic Bandage Wrap

If we cannot obtain an adequate reduction using the Patterson,[75] Israeli,[45] or Neher and Torch[68] techniques, we try some other techniques before surgical intervention. Serendipitously, Chambers[14] found that he could reduce the fracture by wrapping the extremity tightly from distal to proximal with an elastic Esmarch bandage (Fig. 11-31).

Operative Techniques

Percutaneous Pin Reduction

We try every manipulative technique before we resort to open reduction. For most moderately or severely displaced

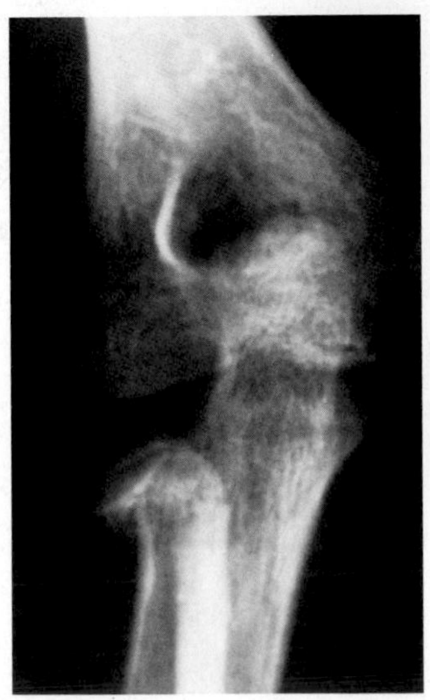

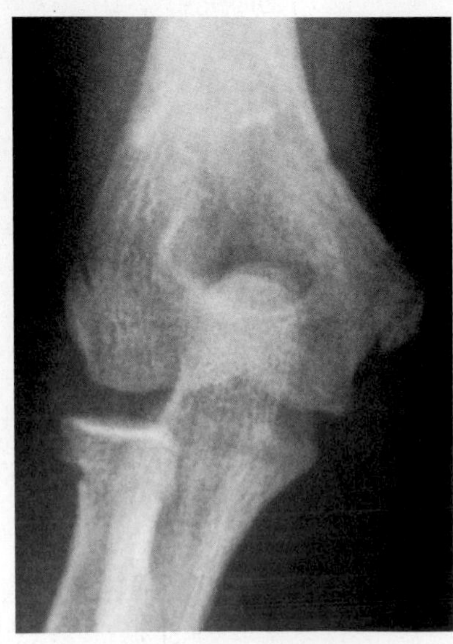

FIGURE 11-28 Flexion–pronation (Israeli) reduction technique.[45] **A.** Radiograph of the best reduction obtained by the Patterson[75] method. **B.** Position of the radial head after the flexion–pronation method. (Courtesy of Gerald R. Williams, MD.)

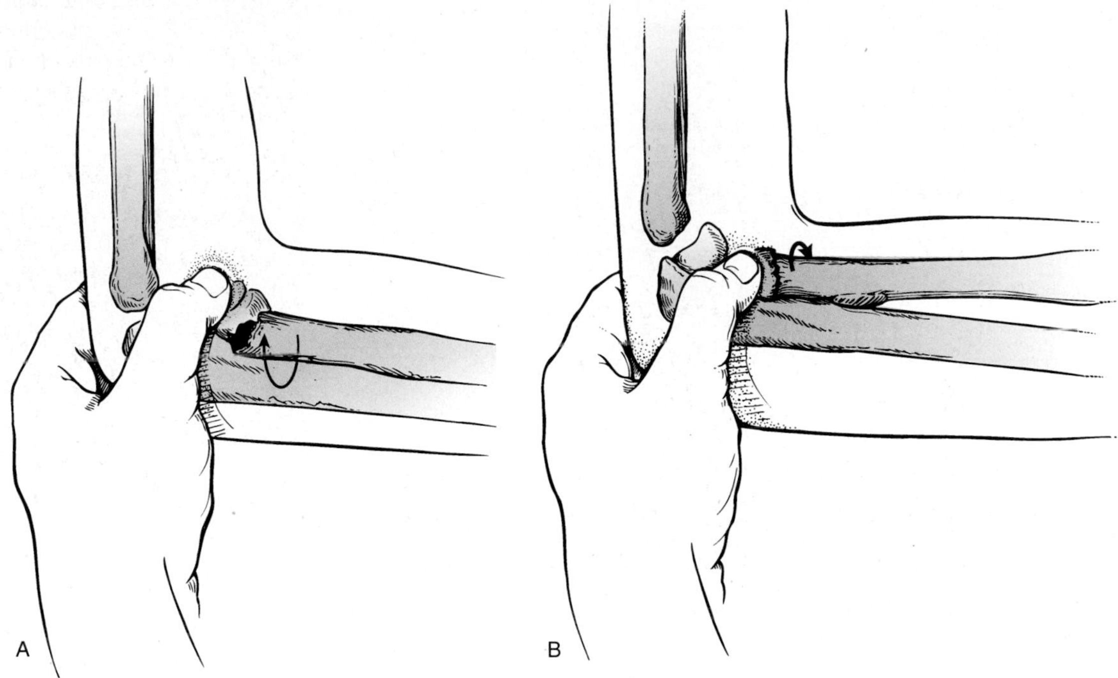

FIGURE 11-29 Flexion–pronation (Israeli) reduction technique.[45] **A.** With the elbow in 90 degrees of flexion, the thumb stabilizes the displaced radial head. Usually the distal radius is in a position of supination. The forearm is pronated to swing the shaft up into alignment with the neck (*arrow*). **B.** Movement is continued to full pronation for reduction (*arrow*) (see also Fig. 11-18).

fractures, we attempt a reduction using the percutaneous pin reduction technique (Fig. 11-32). A good image intensifier is essential. We have found that a single-point awl or the blunt end of a Steinmann pin is adequate. If the radial head is small or soft, we use a small Craig biopsy needle or the blunt end of the Steinmann pin to prevent penetration of the radial head with a sharp end of a Steinmann pin.

To avoid injury to the posterior interosseous nerve, we insert the pin as closely as possible to the lateral aspect of the olecranon (see Fig. 11-32A). The direct push technique is used initially, and if the radial head cannot be pushed into a satisfactory position, the pin leverage technique is used as described by Steele and Graham.[102] Again, we accept 45 to 60 degrees of angulation as long as the displacement is small and the patient has at least 50 to 60 degrees of supination and pronation after reduction.

Elevator Reduction Technique

We have found the Wallace method for manipulating the distal fragment useful for displaced fractures (see Figs. 11-23 and 11-24). In some instances, this technique is used in conjunction with the percutaneous pin technique. This combination is successful in obtaining a satisfactory reduction in almost all cases.

Intra-medullary Reduction Technique

We have limited use of this technique in our institution. It certainly provides a useful method for fracture reduction

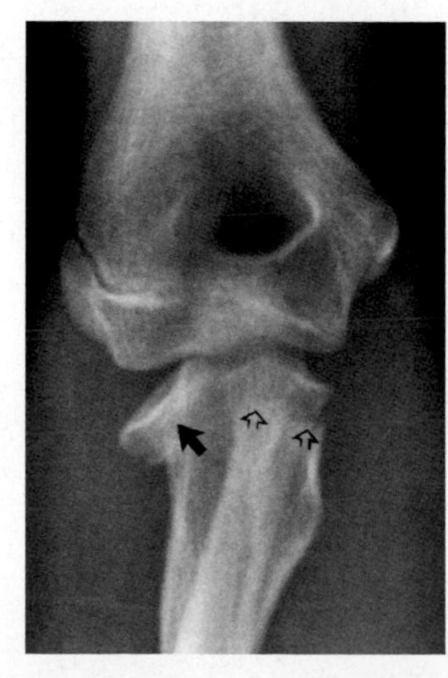

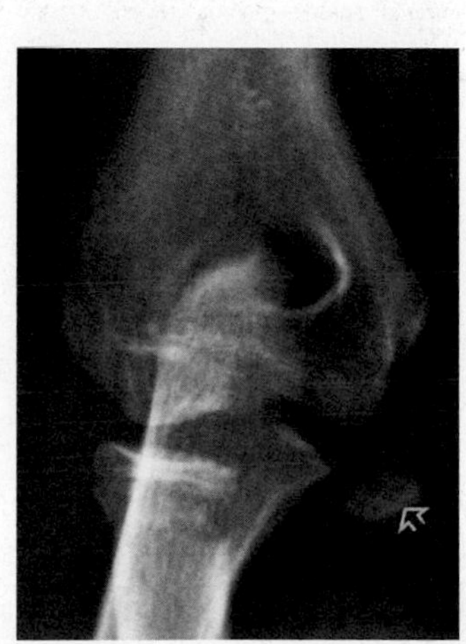

FIGURE 11-30 Widely displaced fracture of the radial head in a 9-year-old female. **A.** The neck fragment (*open arrows*) was medial and the head fragment (*closed arrow*) remained within the orbicular ligament. **B.** Reduction was satisfactory using the flexion–pronation method. The small fragment medially (*arrow*) is from the metaphysis. The patient resumed full rotation of the forearm after reduction. (From Wilkins KE, ed. Operative Management of Upper Extremity Fractures in Children. Rosemont, IL: American Academy of Orthopaedic Surgeons, 1994:55, with permission.)

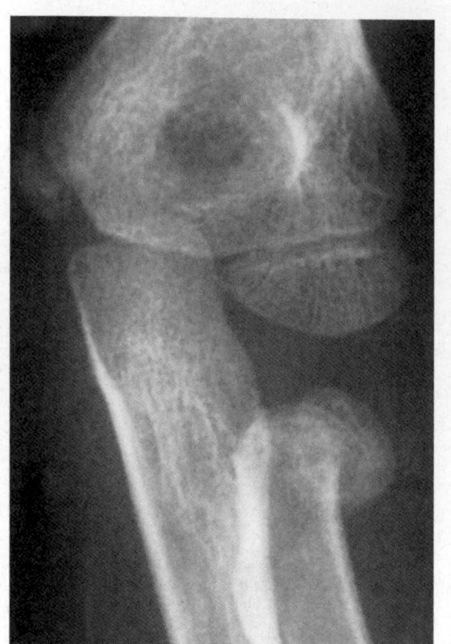

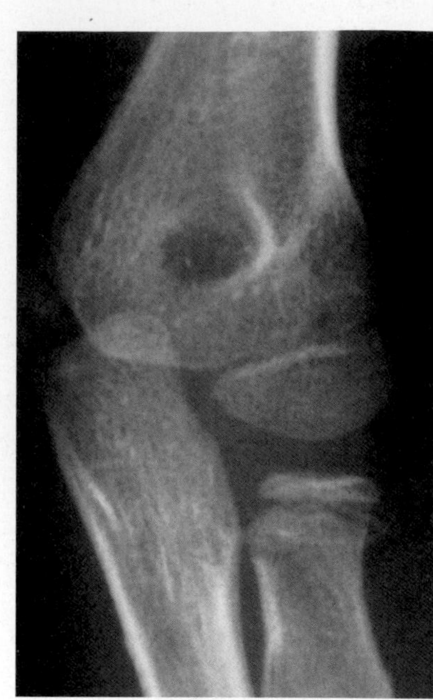

FIGURE 11-31 Elastic bandage wrap reduction. **A.** The final position achieved after manipulation by the Patterson[75] method. **B.** Position of the radial head after applying an elastic bandage to exsanguinate the extremity.

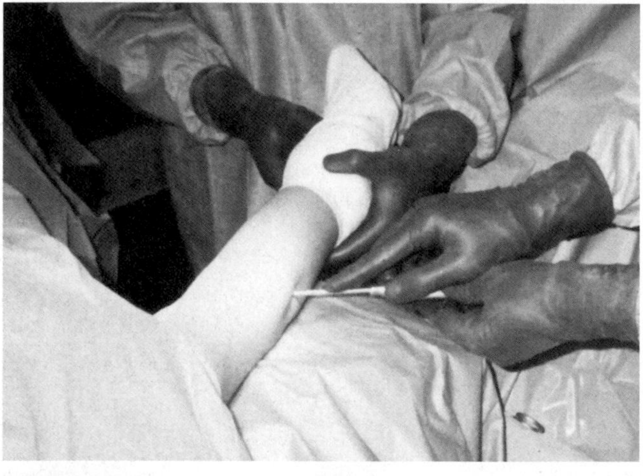

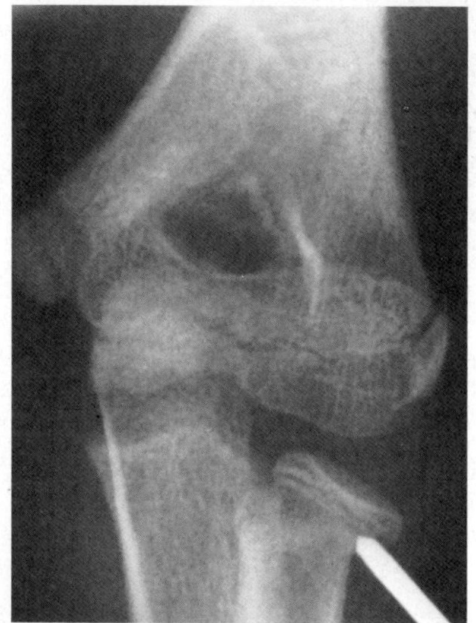

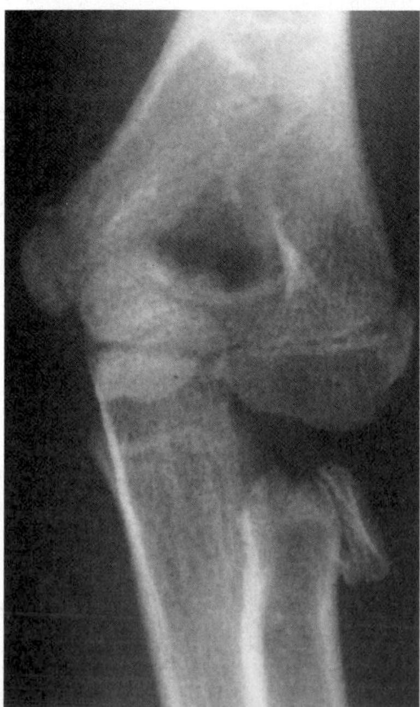

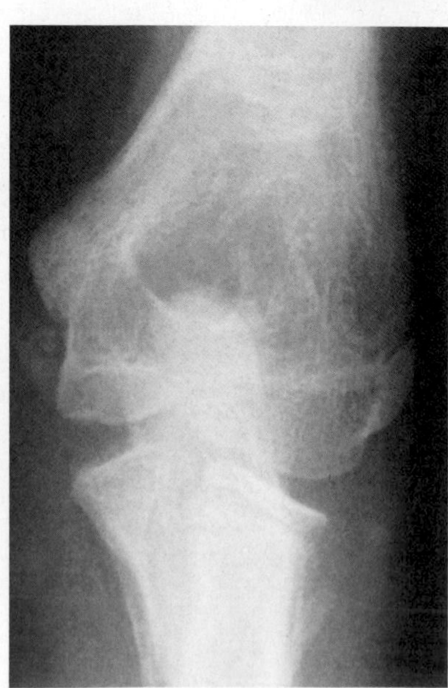

FIGURE 11-32 Percutaneous pin reduction. **A.** Image intensification shows the awl inserted next to the olecranon and directed proximally toward the radial head fragment. This is to avoid injury to the posterior interosseous nerve. **B.** Totally displaced valgus injury. **C.** Position of the Steinmann pin during reduction. **D.** Appearance 2 months after surgery. The patient has 60 degrees of supination and pronation with full elbow extension and flexion.

without the need to open the fracture. One challenge clinically with this technique is that the cut end of the pin often remains prominent at the wrist.

Open Reduction

If an adequate closed reduction is not possible and loss of motion is significant, we prefer an open reduction with as little dissection as possible. We approach the fracture with the patient prone and the forearm pronated. After making the skin incision, we dissect between the anconeus and extensor carpi ulnaris muscles to reach the orbicular ligament and reposition the head as gently as possible. Usually, the head fragment is stable after reduction. If it is not, we stabilize the reduction with a small pin placed obliquely through a separate stab incision from distal to proximal across the fracture site.

Delayed Reduction

If the fracture is more than 4 days old and there is no significant supination or pronation forearm motion, we reduce the head surgically, if reduction is not possible closed. However, we warn the patient's parents of the possibility for myositis ossificans and proximal radioulnar synostosis.

Immobilization after Reduction

After the reduction, we prefer to immobilize the upper extremity with the elbow in 90 degrees of flexion and the forearm in slight pronation. The patient starts active motion in 1 to 3 weeks. After a closed reduction, we start gradual active motion at 10 to 14 days, depending on the initial displacement and the degree of stability of reduction. We prefer to use a long-arm cast. The bivalved cast is useful as a splint during rehabilitation.

Associated Injuries and Complications

Complications of fractures of the radial neck and head, especially those associated with other fractures or a dislocation of the elbow, range from the most common problem of loss of motion to rare nerve injuries (Table 11-5). The most complete reviews of these complications are by Steinberg et al.[103] and D'Souza et al.[15]

TABLE 11-5 Complications of Radial Head and Neck Fractures

Failure to obtain acceptable reduction
Loss of motion (expected)
Radial head overgrowth
Notching of the radial neck
Premature physeal closure
Angular deformities
Nonunion
Osteonecrosis
Radioulnar synostosis
Problems with initial diagnosis

Loss of Motion

Loss of motion is secondary to a combination of loss of joint congruity and fibrous adhesions. Loss of pronation is more common than loss of supination. Flexion and extension are rarely significantly limited. Enlargement of the radial head, a common sequela, can contribute to the subsequent loss of elbow motion.[30]

Radial Head Overgrowth

Next to loss of range of motion of the elbow and forearm, radial head overgrowth is probably the most common sequela (20% to 40%).[15,114] The increased vascularity following the injury may stimulate epiphyseal growth, but the mechanisms of overgrowth following fractures are poorly understood. Radial head overgrowth usually does not compromise functional results,[19,43] but it may produce some crepitus or clicking with forearm rotation.[15]

Notching of the Radial Neck

O'Brien[71] suggested that notching of the radial head in several patients was secondary to scar tissue forming around the neck from the orbicular ligament. It did not result in any functional deficit. Notching may be a normal variant of radial head anatomy.

Premature Physeal Closure

Many series report premature physeal closure[26,30,70,71,103,120] after fractures of the radial head and neck. This complication did not appear to affect the overall results significantly, except in one patient described by Fowles and Kassab,[26] who had a severe cubitus valgus. Newman[70] found that shortening of the radius was never more than 5 mm compared with the opposite uninjured side.

Nonunion of the Radial Neck

Nonunion of the radial neck is rare; union may occur[97] after prolonged treatment (Fig. 11-33). Waters and Stewart[119] reported nine patients with radial neck nonunions, all of whom were treated with open reduction after failed attempts at closed reduction. These authors recommended observation of patients with radial neck nonunions who have limited symptoms and a functional range of motion. They suggested open reduction for displaced nonunions, patients with limited range of motion, and patients with restricting pain.

Osteonecrosis of the Radial Head

The incidence of osteonecrosis is probably higher than recognized. D'Souza et al.[15] reported the frequency to be 10% to 20% in their patients, 70% of whom had open reductions. In patients with open reduction, the overall rate of osteonecrosis was 25%. Jones and Esah[43] and Newman[70] found that patients with osteonecrosis had poor functional results. It has been our experience, however, that revascularization can occur without any significant functional loss. Only in those in whom a residual functional deficit occurs is osteonecrosis considered a problem (Fig. 11-34).

Changes in Carrying Angle (Cubitus Valgus)

In patients who have fractures of the radial neck, the carrying angle often is 10 degrees more (increased cubitus valgus) than on

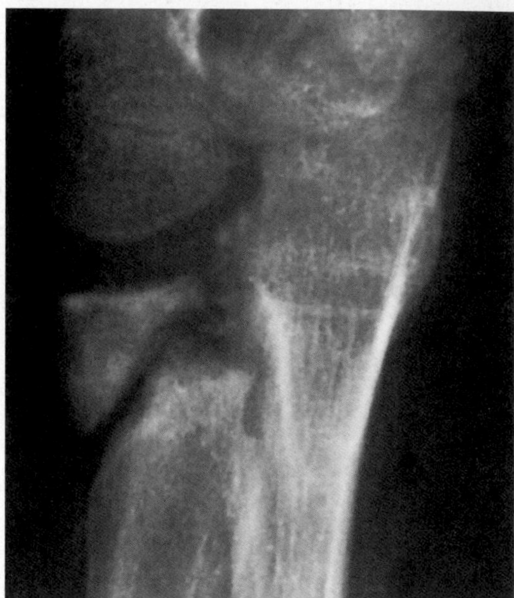
A

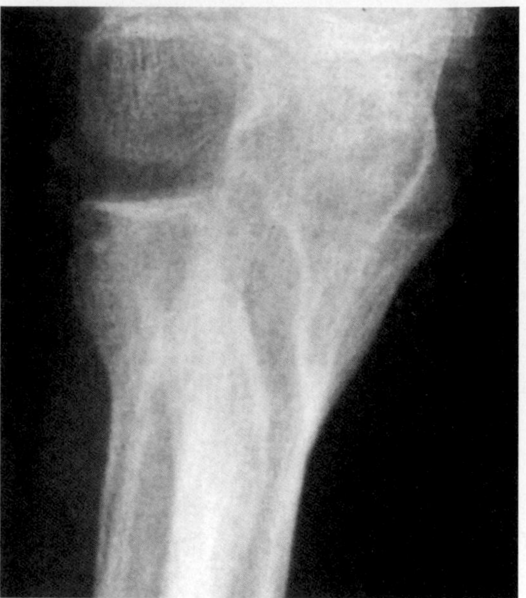
B

FIGURE 11-33 Nonunion. **A.** Eight months after radial neck fracture in an 8.5-year-old female. Patient had mild aching pain, but no loss of motion. There was some suggestion of proximal subluxation of the distal radioulnar joint. **B.** Three months later, the fracture is united after long-arm cast immobilization and external electromagnetic stimulation. (Courtesy of Charles T. Price, MD.)

FIGURE 11-34 Osteonecrosis with nonunion in a radial head 1 year after open reduction. Both nonunion and osteonecrosis of the radial neck and head are present. Severe degenerative arthritis developed subsequently. (Courtesy of Richard E. King, MD.)

the uninjured side.[15,43] The increase in carrying angle appears to produce no functional deficit and no significant deformity.

Vascular Injuries

There are no reports of major vascular injuries with isolated fractures of the proximal radius.

Nerve Injuries

Partial ulnar nerve injury[39] and posterior interosseous nerve injury may occur as a direct result of the fracture, but most injuries to the posterior interosseous nerves are caused by surgical exploration[15] or percutaneous pin reduction.[5] These posterior interosseous nerve injuries usually are transient.

Compartment Syndrome

Peters and Scott[79] described three patients with volar forearm compartment syndrome after minimally displaced or angulated fractures of the radial head. All required volar fasciotomy.

Radioulnar Synostosis

Proximal synostosis is the most serious complication that can occur after radial head fracture (Fig. 11-35). It occurs most often after open reduction of severely displaced fractures,[30,39,70,102] but it can occur after closed reduction. Delayed treatment increases the likelihood of this complication. All three patients described by Gaston et al.[30] had treatment initiated more than 5 days after injury.

Myositis Ossificans

Myositis ossificans is relatively common but usually does not impair function. Vahvanen[114] noted that some myositis ossificans occurred in 32% of his patients. In most, it was limited to the supinator muscle. If ossification was more extensive and was associated with a synostosis, the results were poor.

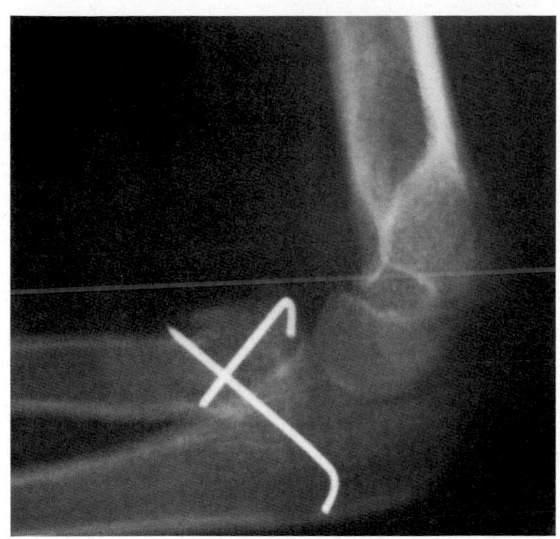
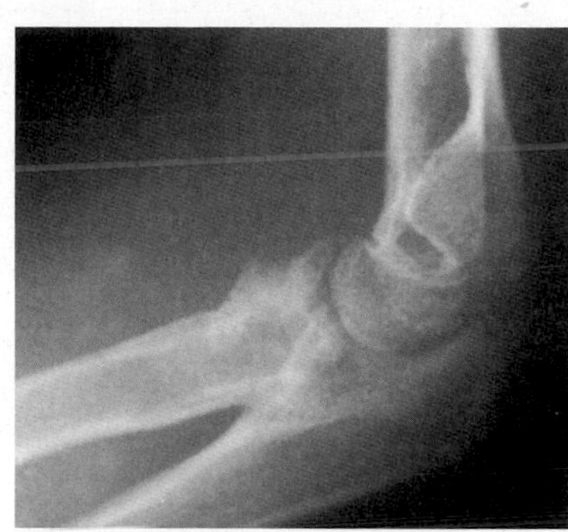
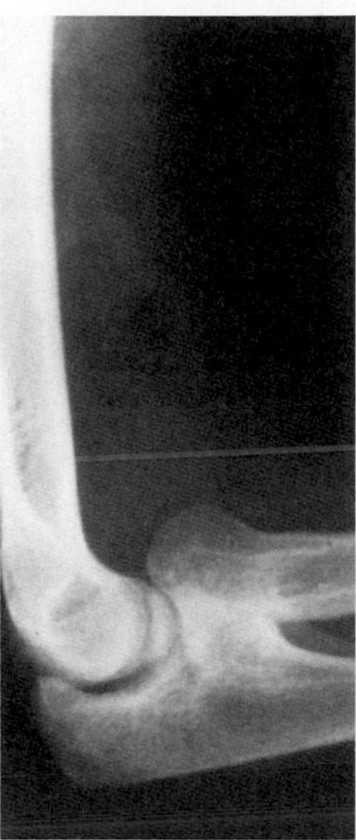

FIGURE 11-35 Radioulnar synostosis. **A.** Surgical intervention with wire fixation was necessary for a satisfactory reduction in this patient who had a totally displaced radial neck fracture. **B.** Six weeks after surgery, there was evidence of a proximal radioulnar synostosis. **C.** Radiograph taken 6 months after reduction shows a solid synostosis with anterior displacement of the proximal radius. (Courtesy of R. E. King, MD.)

Osteomyelitis

Veranis et al.[115] reported a rare case of hematogenous osteomyelitis after a closed fracture of the radial neck. The diagnosis was delayed despite the fact that the child had fever and continuous pain after the fracture.

Malunion

Failure to reduce a displaced and angulated proximal radial fracture in a young child often results in an angulated radial neck with subsequent incongruity of both the proximal radioulnar joint and the radiocapitellar joint (Fig. 11-36). Partial physeal arrest also can create this angulation (see Fig. 11-5).

In our experience, this malunion, because of the incongruity of the radiocapitellar joint, often results in erosion of the articular surface of the capitellum, with subsequent degenerative joint disease. In the English literature, there is little information about using osteotomies of the radial neck to correct this deformity.

Summary

Results after open reduction of radial head fractures are less favorable than those after closed reduction. However, fractures requiring open reduction are usually the result of a more severe injury. Closed reductions with angulations of up to 45 degrees produce clinical results as good as those with a more anatomic reduction after operation. The surgeon should warn the patient's parents of the likelihood of residual loss of motion after open reduction. Whenever possible, internal fixation should be avoided.

FRACTURES OF THE PROXIMAL ULNA (OLECRANON)

Fractures Involving the Proximal Apophysis

Incidence

"Separation of the olecranon epiphysis is the rarest form of epiphyseal detachment."[80] This quote from Poland's 1898 textbook on epiphyseal fractures is still true. Few fractures of the ulnar apophysis are described in the English literature.[34,80,95,101] In addition to acute injuries in children, some have been described in young adults with open physes.[47,76,100,111] In the French literature, Bracq[10] described 10 patients in whom the fracture extended distal and parallel to the apophyseal line and then crossed it at the articular surface. Most reports of apophyseal olecranon fractures describe patients with osteogenesis imperfecta, who seem predisposed to this injury.

Anatomy

The Ossification Process. At birth, the ossification of the metaphysis of the proximal ulna extends only to the midportion of the semilunar notch. At this age, the leading edge of the metaphysis is usually perpendicular to the long axis of the olecranon (Fig. 11-37A,B). As ossification progresses, the proximal border of the metaphysis becomes more oblique. The anterior margin extends proximally and to three fourths of the width of the semilunar notch by 6 years of age. At this age, the physis extends distally to include the coronoid process (see Fig. 11-37C). A secondary center of ossification occurs in the coronoid process. Just before the development of the secondary center of ossification in the olecranon, the leading edge of the metaphysis develops a well-defined sclerotic margin.[95] Ossification of the olecranon occurs in the area of the triceps insertion at approximately 9 years of age (see Fig. 11-37D).[95] Ossification of the coronoid process is completed about the time that the olecranon ossification center appears.[80] The term "apophysis" is usually applied to an epiphysis that is subjected to traction by a muscle insertion. "Apophysis" and "epiphysis" are used interchangeably in this chapter to describe the olecranon secondary growth center because it contributes to length and articular surface as well.

Bipartite Centers. The secondary ossification center of the olecranon may be bipartite (see Fig. 11-37E).[82] The major center

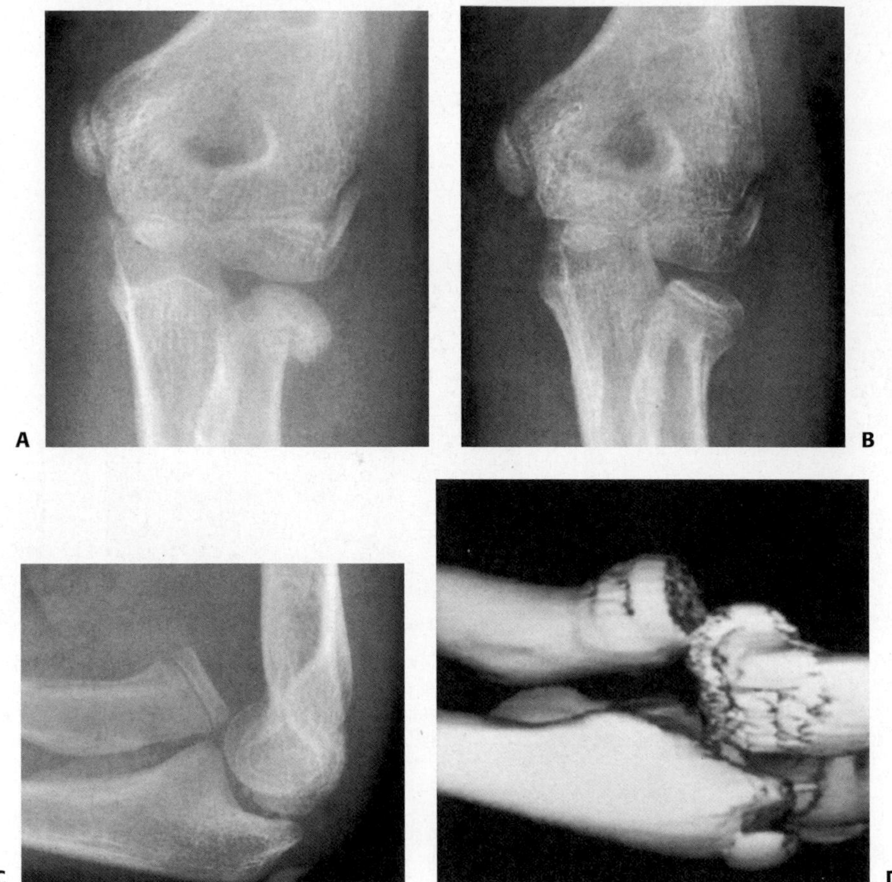

FIGURE 11-36 Angulation. **A.** Injury film showing 30 degrees of angulation and 30% lateral translocation of a radial neck fracture in a 10-year-old. **B.** Radiograph appearance of the proximal radius taken about 5 months later, showing lateral angulation of the neck. **C.** Lateral view showing the anterior relationship of the radial neck with proximal migration. At this point the patient had full supination and pronation but a clicking sensation with forearm rotation in the area of the radial head. **D.** Three-dimensional reconstruction showing the incongruity of the proximal radiocapitellar joint. (Courtesy of Vince Mosca, MD.)

within the tip of the olecranon is enveloped by the triceps insertion. This was referred to by Porteous[82] as a *traction center*. The second and smaller center, an articular center, lies under the proximal fourth of the articular surface of the semilunar notch.

Closure Process. Fusion of the olecranon epiphysis with the metaphysis, which progresses from anterior to posterior, occurs at approximately 14 years of age. The sclerotic margin that defines the edge of the metaphysis may be mistaken for a fracture (see Fig. 11-37F).[95] Rarely, the physeal line persists into adulthood,[47,76,111] usually in athletes who have used the extremity in repetitive throwing activities.[16,87,100,113,121] The chronic tension forces applied across the apophysis theoretically prevent its normal closure.

Patella Cubiti. Occasionally, a separate ossification center called a *patella cubiti* develops in the triceps tendon at its insertion on the tip of the olecranon.[109] This ossicle is completely separate and can articulate with the trochlea. It is usually unilateral, unlike other persistent secondary ossification centers, which are more likely to be bilateral and familial. Zeitlin[126] believed that the patella cubiti was a traumatic ossicle rather than a developmental variation.

Signs and Symptoms

Clinical: Swelling Plus Defect. The primary clinical findings of an olecranon fracture are tenderness and swelling. If the fragment is completely displaced, the child cannot extend the elbow. A palpable defect may be present between the apophysis and the proximal metaphysis. Poland[80] described the crepitus between the fragments as being muffled because cartilage covers the fracture surfaces.

Radiography: Proximal Metaphyseal Displacement. The radiographic diagnosis may be difficult before ossification of the olecranon apophysis. The only clue may be a displacement of the small ossified metaphyseal fragment (Fig. 11-38), and the diagnosis may be based only on the clinical sign of tenderness over the epiphyseal fragment. If there is any doubt about the degree of displacement, injection of radiopaque material into the joint may delineate the true nature of the fracture.

Mechanism of Injury

The location of the triceps expansion insertion on the metaphysis distal to the physis probably accounts for the rarity of fracture along the physeal line. Only a few reports mention the mechanism of these physeal injuries. In most of the fractures reported by Poland,[80] three of which were confirmed by amputation

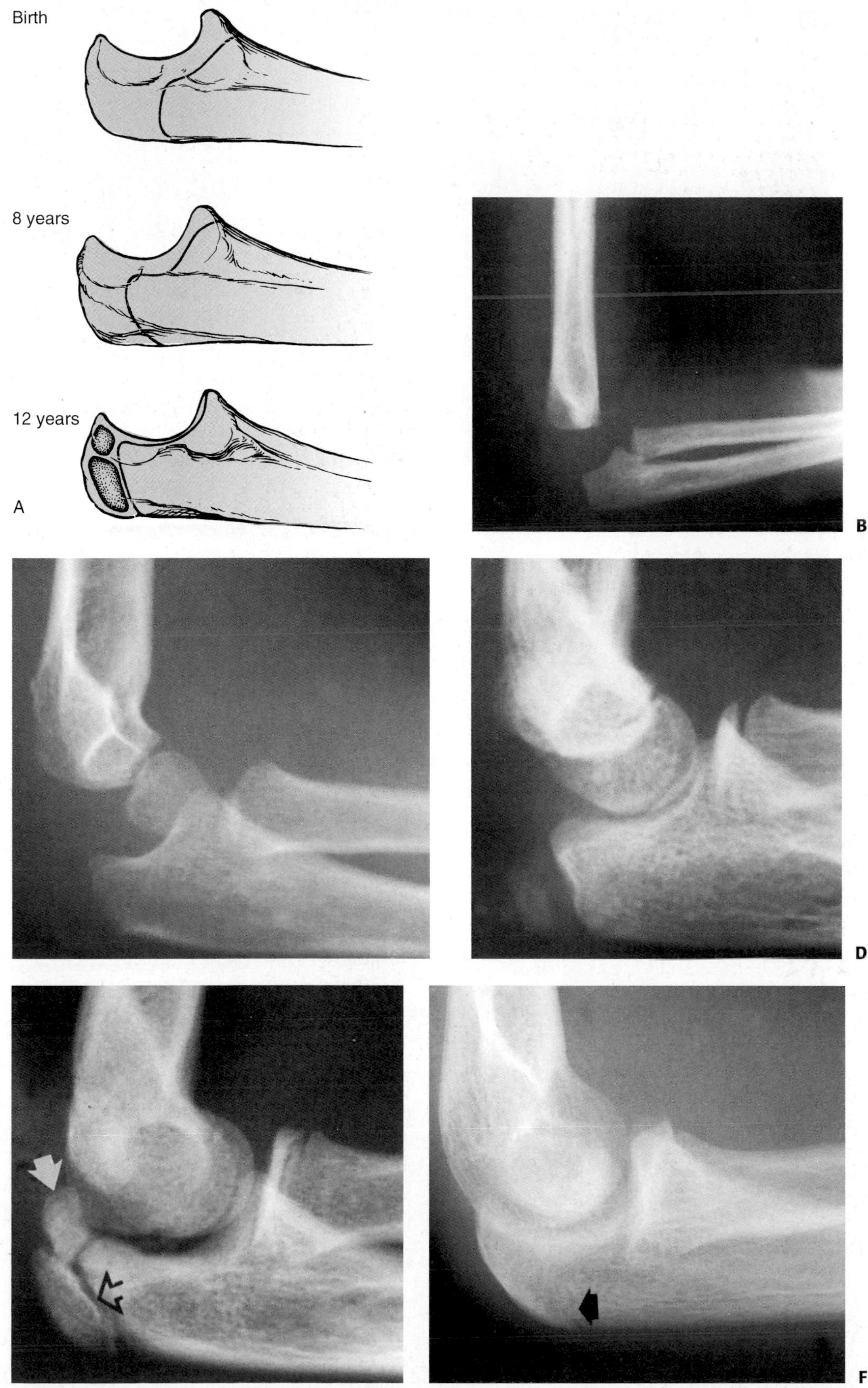

FIGURE 11-37 Olecranon ossification. **A.** Limits of the border of ossification at birth, 8 years, and 12 years. **B.** Lateral view of olecranon at 6 months of age. The proximal margin is perpendicular to the long axis of the ulna. **C.** Lateral view of the olecranon at 6 years of age. The proximal margin is oblique. **D.** Secondary ossification center developing in the olecranon in a 10-year-old. A sclerotic border has developed on the proximal metaphyseal margin. **E.** Bipartite secondary ossification center. The larger center is the traction center (*open arrow*). The smaller, more proximal center is the articular center (*white arrow*). **F.** Before complete fusion, a partial line remains (*arrow*), bordered by a sclerotic margin.

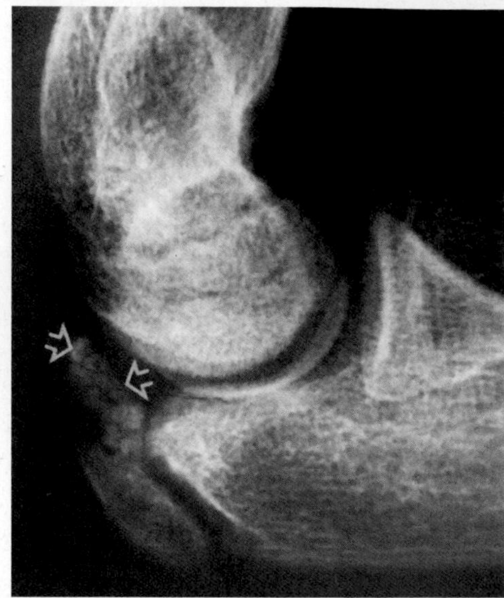

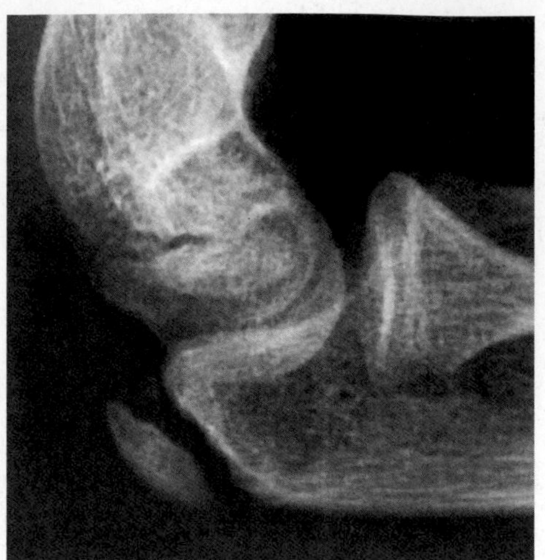

FIGURE 11-38 Apophysitis. **A.** Chronic stimulation with irregular ossification of the articular apophyseal center (*arrows*) in a basketball player who practiced dribbling 3 hours per day. **B.** Normal side for comparison.

specimens, the force of the injury was applied directly to the elbow. The force may be applied indirectly, producing an avulsion type of fracture. In our experience, this fracture is usually caused by avulsion forces across the apophysis with the elbow flexed, similar to the more common flexion metaphyseal injuries. Children with osteogenesis imperfecta (usually the tarda form) seem especially predisposed to this injury.[17,63]

Stress fractures of the olecranon apophysis can occur in athletes (especially baseball players) who place considerable recurrent tension forces on the olecranon.[74] Stress injuries also have been reported in elite gymnasts[54] and tennis players.[87] If the recurring activity persists, a symptomatic nonunion can develop.[76,87,111,113,121]

Classification

Injuries to the apophysis of the olecranon can be classified as one of three types (Table 11-6). Type I is a simple apophysitis in which there is irregularity in the secondary ossification center (Fig. 11-39A).[16,54] The apophyseal line may widen. Type II is an incomplete stress fracture that involves primarily the apophyseal line, with widening and irregularity (see Fig. 11-39B). A small adjacent cyst may form, but usually the architecture of the secondary ossification center is normal. These injuries occur primarily in sports requiring repetitive extension of the elbow, such as baseball pitching,[74] tennis,[87] or gymnastics.[54] Type III injuries involve complete avulsion of the apophysis. True apophyseal avulsions (type IIIA) occur in younger children as a fracture through the apophyseal plate (see Fig. 11-39A,B). In some of his amputation specimens, Poland[80] found that the proximal apophyseal fragment included the distal tongue, which extended up to the coronoid process. Apophyseal–metaphyseal combination fractures (type IIIB), in which metaphyseal fragments are attached to the apophysis (see Fig. 11-39C,D), usually occur in older children. Grantham and Kiernan[34] likened it to a Salter-Harris type II physeal injury. Proximal displacement of the fragment is the only clue seen on a radiograph.

TABLE 11-6 Classification of Apophyseal Injuries of the Olecranon

Type I: Apophysitis

Type II: Incomplete stress fracture

Type III: Complete fractures
- A. Pure apophyseal avulsions
- B. Apophyseal–metaphyseal combinations

Treatment

There is no standard method of treatment, because few such fractures have been described. For fractures with significant displacement, treatment is usually open reduction with internal fixation using a combination of axial pins and tension-band wiring (Fig. 11-40).[34,80,101] Gortzak et al.[33] described a technique of open reduction using percutaneously placed Kirschner-wires and absorbable sutures instead of wires for the tension band. The percutaneously placed wires are subsequently removed 4 to 5 weeks postoperatively, eliminating the need for implant removal. There has been concern that applying compressive forces across the apophysis might cause growth arrest. In our experience, fusion of the apophysis to the metaphysis is accelerated. Apophyseal fractures usually occur when the physis is near natural closure. The growth proximally is appositional rather than lengthwise across the apophyseal plate itself. As a result, we have not found any functional shortening of the olecranon because of the early fusion of the apophysis to the metaphysis (see Fig. 11-40D). In practice, the use of a compression screw across an ossified olecranon fracture causes no loss of ulnar length. Children who sustain injuries before the development of the secondary ossification center may develop a deformity that is visible on radiographs (Fig. 11-41). Although there may be shortening of the olecranon, it does not appear to produce functional problems. There are no reports of the effects of this injury in very young children or infants. Most stress injuries respond to simple rest from the offending activity.

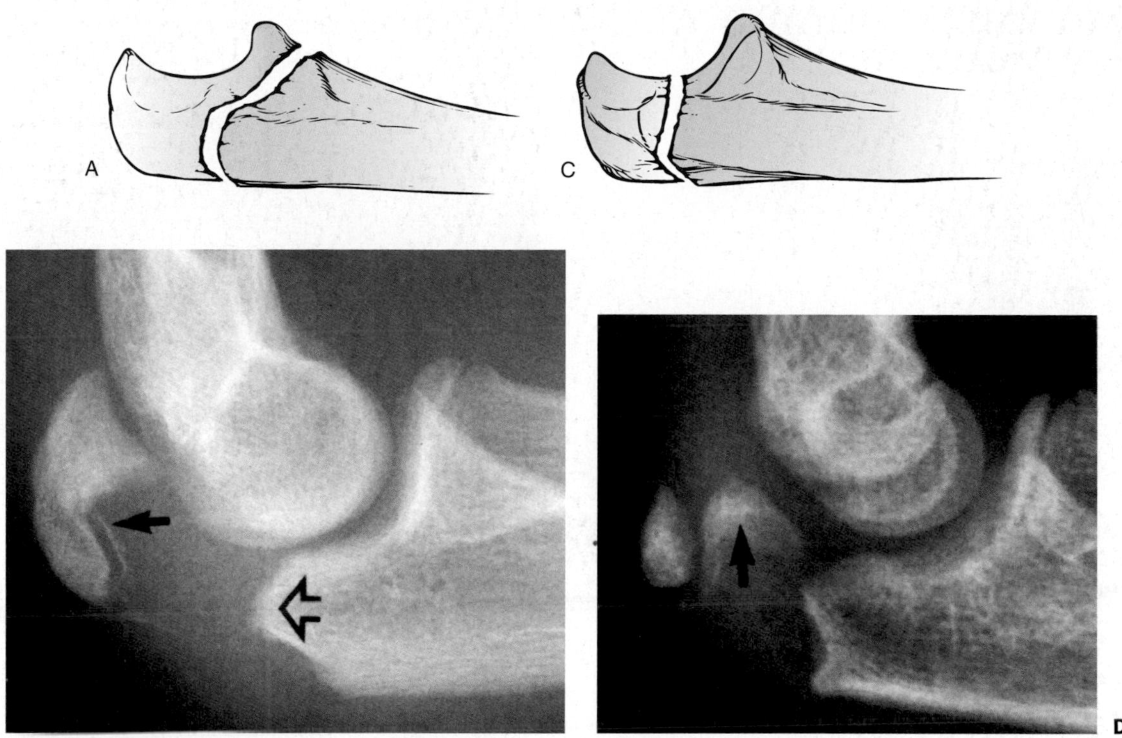

FIGURE 11-39 Apophyseal avulsions. *Pure apophyseal avulsions.* **A.** The fracture follows the contour of the apophyseal line. **B.** The distal fracture line is in the shape of the apophyseal line (*open arrow*) with a small metaphyseal flake attached to the apophysis (*solid arrow*). *Apophyseal–metaphyseal combination.* **C.** The fracture line follows the line of tension stress. **D.** A large portion of the metaphysis (*arrow*) is often with the proximal metaphyseal fragment.

However, a chronic stress fracture can result in a symptomatic nonunion. Use of a compressive screw alone across the nonunion often is sufficient,[54] but supplemental bone grafting may be necessary to achieve union.[47,76]

AUTHORS' PREFERRED METHOD

Undisplaced Fractures

For apophysitis and undisplaced stress fractures, we ask the patient to cease the offending activity. During this period of rest, the patient should maintain upper extremity strength with a selective muscle exercise program as well as maintain cardiovascular conditioning. When a persistent nonunion of the olecranon in an adolescent does not demonstrate healing after a reasonable period of simple rest, we place a cannulated compression screw across the apophysis to stimulate healing.

Displaced Fractures

With minimal displacement of the fracture, satisfactory closed reduction can be obtained with the elbow extended. We usually immobilize the elbow in a long-arm cast in extension. Percutaneous pinning will stabilize the reduction if there is any concern about loss of reduction. Completely displaced fractures are treated operatively using a tension-band technique. In young children, we use small Steinmann or Kirschner pins. The tension band is a strong absorbable suture of one of the polyglycolic acid substances. Alternatively, standard 16- to 18-gauge wire can be used in older adolescents. Patients with large ossification centers are treated with a compression screw similar to those with metaphyseal fractures.

Associated Injuries and Complications

Spur Formation

Smith[81] noted that overgrowth of the epiphysis proximally may produce a bony spur. In some patients, these proximal spurs became symptomatic and were removed.

Nonunion

The cause and treatment of nonunion are discussed in the previous section.

Apophyseal Arrest

Apophyseal arrest appears to have no significant effect on elbow function (see Fig. 11-41).

Metaphyseal Fractures of the Olecranon

Incidence

Isolated metaphyseal fractures of the olecranon are relatively rare (Table 11-7). They are often associated with other fractures about the elbow. In the combined series of 4684 elbow fractures reviewed, 230 were olecranon fractures, for an incidence of 4.9%. This agrees with the incidence of 4% to 6% in the major series reported.[25,58,73] Only 10% to 20% of the total fractures

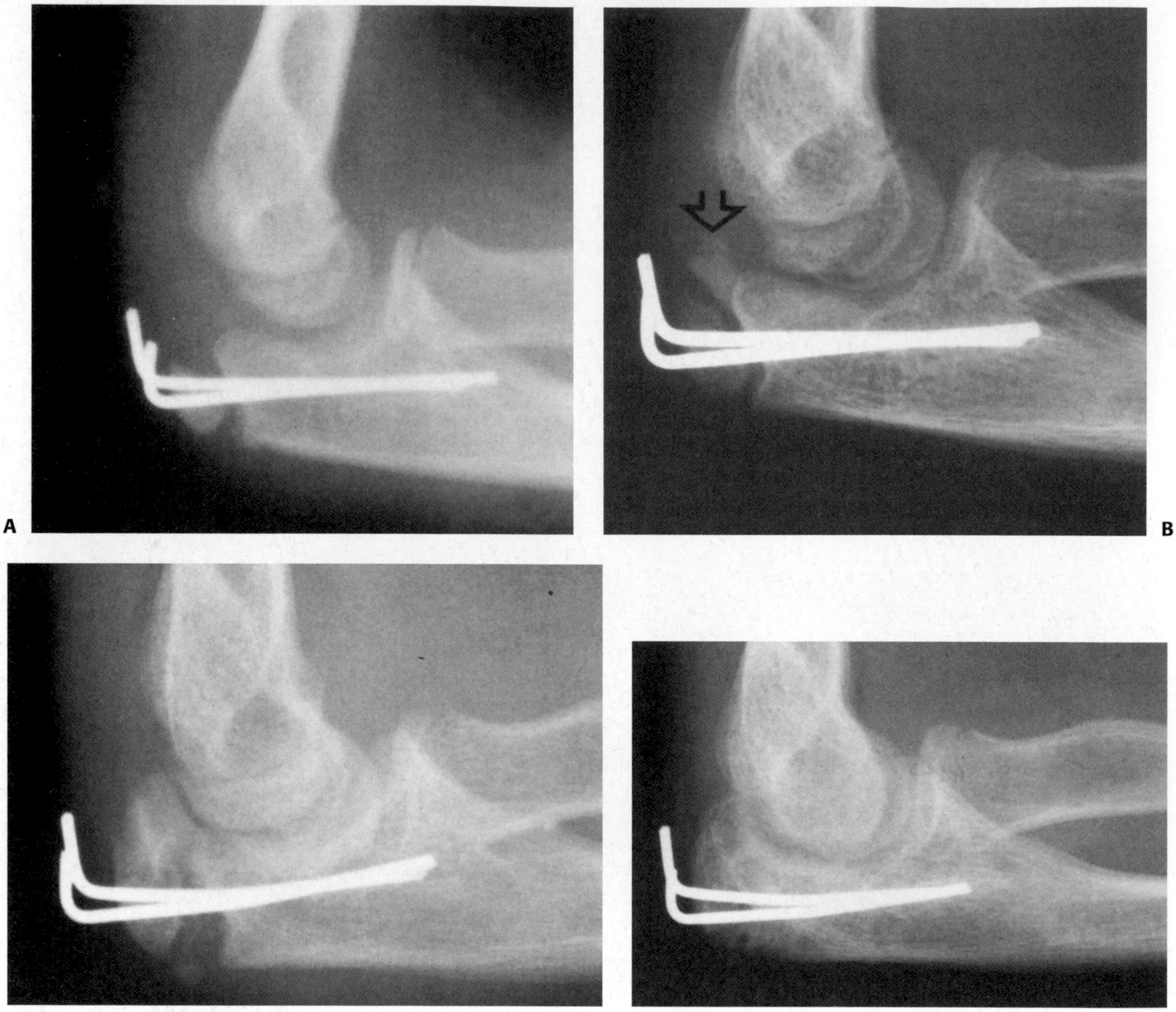

FIGURE 11-40 Operative treatment of an apophyseal fracture. **A.** Postoperative radiograph of the fracture shown in Figure 11-40D, which was stabilized with small Steinmann pins alone. **B.** Five months later, growth has continued in the traction center and the articular center is ossified (*arrow*). **C.** One year after injury, the apophysis was partially avulsed a second time. The two secondary ossification centers are now fused. **D.** Three months after the second fracture, the fracture gap has filled in, producing a normal olecranon.

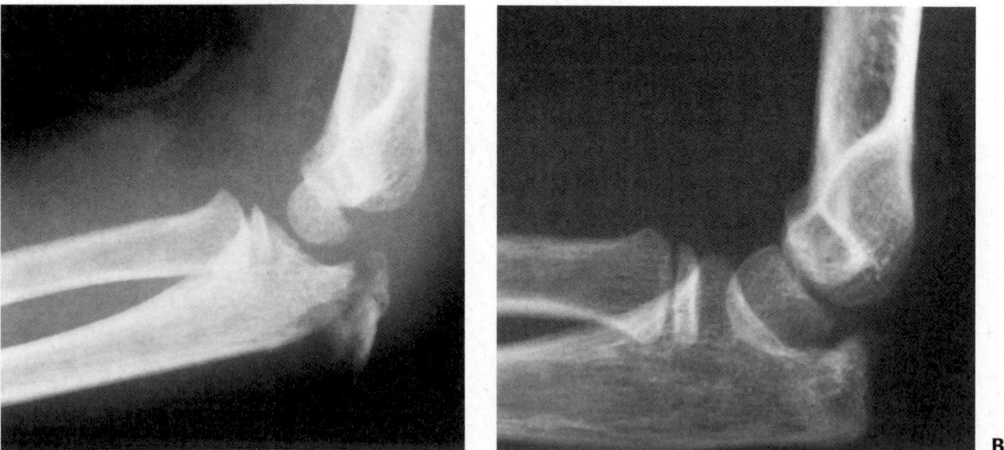

FIGURE 11-41 Preosseous apophyseal arrest. **A.** Comminuted fracture of the proximal olecranon from a direct blow to the elbow in an 8-year-old male. This fracture was treated nonoperatively. **B.** Radiograph 18 months later shows cessation of the proximal migration of the metaphyseal margin and a lack of development of a secondary ossification center. Despite this arrest of the apophysis, the patient had a full range of elbow motion.

TABLE 11-7 Incidence of Metaphyseal Fractures of the Olecranon

Age distribution: 1st decade, 25%; 2nd decade, 25%; 3rd decade, 50%

Peak age: 5–10 yr

Extremity predominance: left (55%)

Sex predominance: male (65%)

Associated elbow injuries: 20%

Requiring surgical intervention: 19%

reported in these series required an operation. Six reports totaling 302 patients with fractures of the olecranon in children are in the English literature.[29,34,58,69] Considering all age groups, 25% of olecranon fractures in these reports occurred in the first decade and another 25% in the second decade.[49] During the first decade, the peak age for olecranon fracture was between age 5 and 10 years.[35,69] Approximately 20% of patients had an associated fracture or dislocation of the elbow, most involving the proximal radius. Only 10% to 20% required an operation.

Anatomic Considerations

Because the olecranon is a metaphyseal area, the cortex is relatively thin, allowing for the development of greenstick-type fracture deformities. The periosteum is immature and thick, which may prevent the degree of separation seen in adults. Likewise, the larger amount of epiphyseal cartilage in children may serve as a cushion to lessen the effects of a direct blow to the olecranon. In the production of supracondylar fractures, ligamentous laxity in this age group tends to force the elbow into hyperextension when the child falls on the outstretched upper extremity. This puts a compressive force across the olecranon and locks it into the fossa in the distal humerus, where it is protected. An older person, whose elbow does not go into hyperextension, is more likely to fall with the elbow semiflexed. This unique biomechanical characteristic of the child's olecranon predisposes it to different fracture patterns than those in adults.

Signs and Symptoms

Flexion injuries cause soft tissue swelling over the olecranon fracture. The abrasion or contusion associated with a direct blow to the posterior aspect of the elbow provides a clue as to the mechanism the injury. If there is wide separation, a defect can be palpated between the fragments. In addition, there may be weakness or even lack of active extension of the elbow, which is difficult to evaluate in an anxious young child with a swollen elbow.

On radiograph, the fracture lines associated with flexion injuries are usually perpendicular to the long axis of the olecranon. This differentiates them from the residual physeal line, which is oblique and directed proximal and anterior.[95] In extension injuries, the longitudinally directed greenstick fracture lines may be difficult to appreciate, and radiographs should be scrutinized to detect associated fractures of the proximal radius or distal humerus.

Classification

Papavasiliou et al.[73] defined two major groups of olecranon fractures in which the fracture line is either intra-articular or

TABLE 11-8 Classification of Metaphyseal Fractures of the Olecranon

Group A: Flexion injuries

Group B: Extension injuries
1. Valgus pattern
2. Varus pattern

Group C: Shear injuries

extra-articular. The degree of displacement defines subclassifications in each group. We prefer to classify these fractures based on the mechanism of injury (Table 11-8): those associated with flexion injuries, those associated with extension injuries, and shear injuries. Extension injuries are further divided into varus and valgus patterns.

Mechanism of Injury

Three main mechanisms produce metaphyseal olecranon fractures, depending on whether the elbow is flexed or extended at the time of injury. First, in injuries occurring with the elbow flexed, posterior tension forces play an important role. Second, in injuries in which the fracture occurs with the elbow extended, the varus or valgus bending stress across the olecranon is responsible for the typical fracture pattern. Third, a less common mechanism involves a direct blow to the elbow that produces an anterior bending or shear force across the olecranon. In this type, the tension forces are concentrated on the anterior portion of the olecranon.

Flexion Injuries

A fall with the elbow semiflexed places considerable tension forces across the posterior aspect of the olecranon process. Proximally, the triceps applies a force to the tip of the olecranon process. Distally, there is some proximal pull by the insertion of the brachialis muscle. Thus, the posterior cortex is placed in tension. This tension force alone, if applied rapidly enough and with sufficient force, may cause the olecranon to fail at its midportion (Fig. 11-42). A direct blow applied to the posterior aspect of the stressed olecranon makes it more vulnerable to failure. With this type of mechanism, the fracture line is usually transverse and perpendicular to the long axis of the olecranon (Fig. 11-43). Because the fracture extends into the articular surface of the semilunar notch, it is classified as intra-articular.

The degree of separation of the fracture fragments depends on the magnitude of the forces applied versus the integrity of the soft tissues. The low incidence of displaced olecranon fractures indicates that the soft tissues are quite resistant to these avulsion forces. In flexion injuries, there are relatively few associated soft tissue injuries or other fractures.[69]

Extension Injuries

Because the ligaments are more flexible in children, the elbow tends to hyperextend when a child breaks a fall with the outstretched upper extremity. In this situation, the olecranon may be locked into the olecranon fossa. If the elbow goes into extreme hyperextension, usually the supracondylar area fails. If, however, the major direction of the force across the elbow is

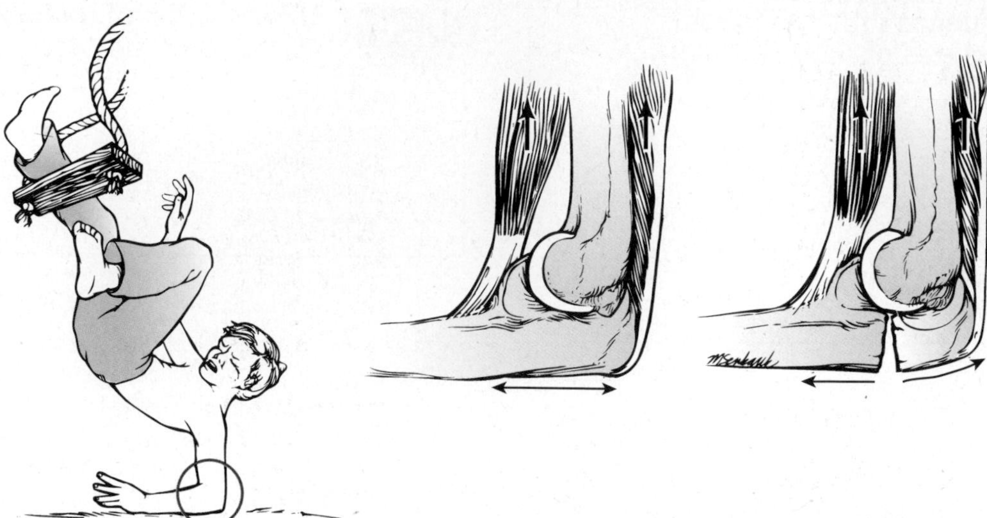

FIGURE 11-42 Mechanism of flexion injuries. **Center**. In the flexed elbow, a tension force develops on the posterior aspect of the olecranon (*small double arrow*) because of the pull of the brachialis and triceps muscles (*large arrows*). **Right**. Failure occurs on the tension side, which is posterior as a result of the muscle pull or a direct blow to the prestressed posterior olecranon.

abduction or adduction, a bending moment stresses the olecranon. Most of this force concentrates in the distal portion of the olecranon. Because the olecranon is metaphyseal bone, the force produces greenstick-type longitudinal fracture lines (Fig. 11-44). Most of these fracture lines are linear and remain extra-articular. In addition, because the fulcrum of the bending force is more distal, many of the fracture lines may extend distal to the coronoid process and into the proximal ulnar shaft regions. The major deformity of the olecranon with this type of fracture is usually an angulated greenstick type of pattern.

Many of these fractures are associated with other injuries in the elbow region, which depend on whether the bending force is directed toward varus or valgus. If a child falls with the fore-

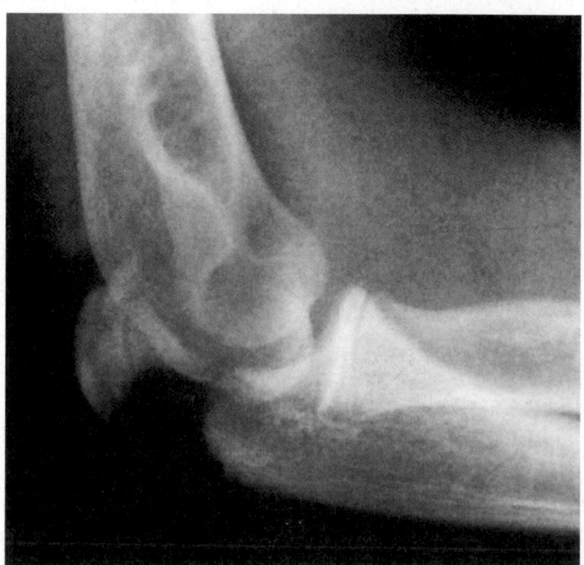

FIGURE 11-43 Radiograph of flexion injury showing greater displacement on the posterior surface.

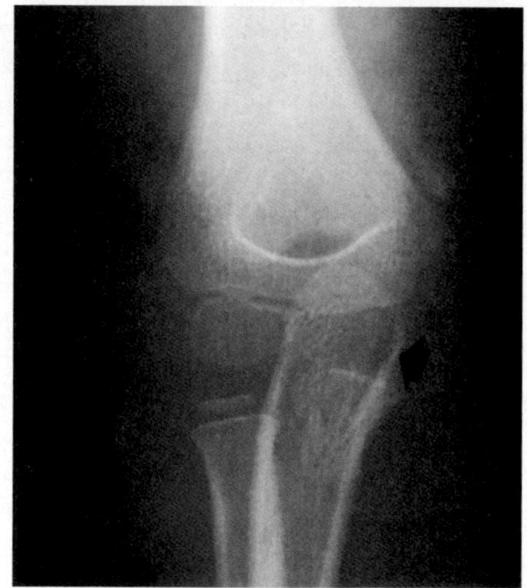

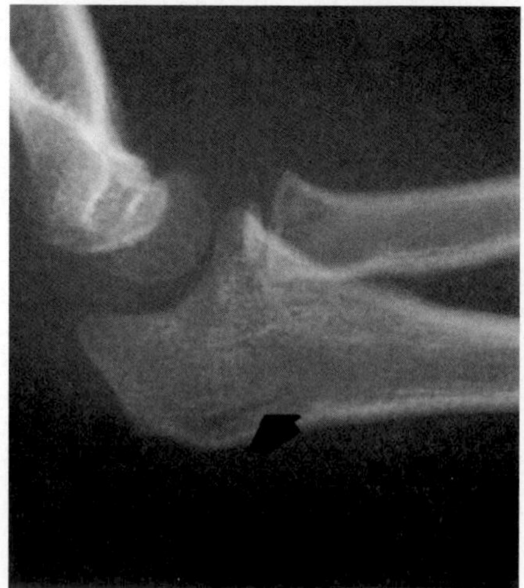

FIGURE 11-44 A. Anteroposterior view of a linear greenstick fracture line (*arrow*) in the medial aspect of the olecranon. **B.** Lateral view showing the posterior location of the fracture line (*arrow*).

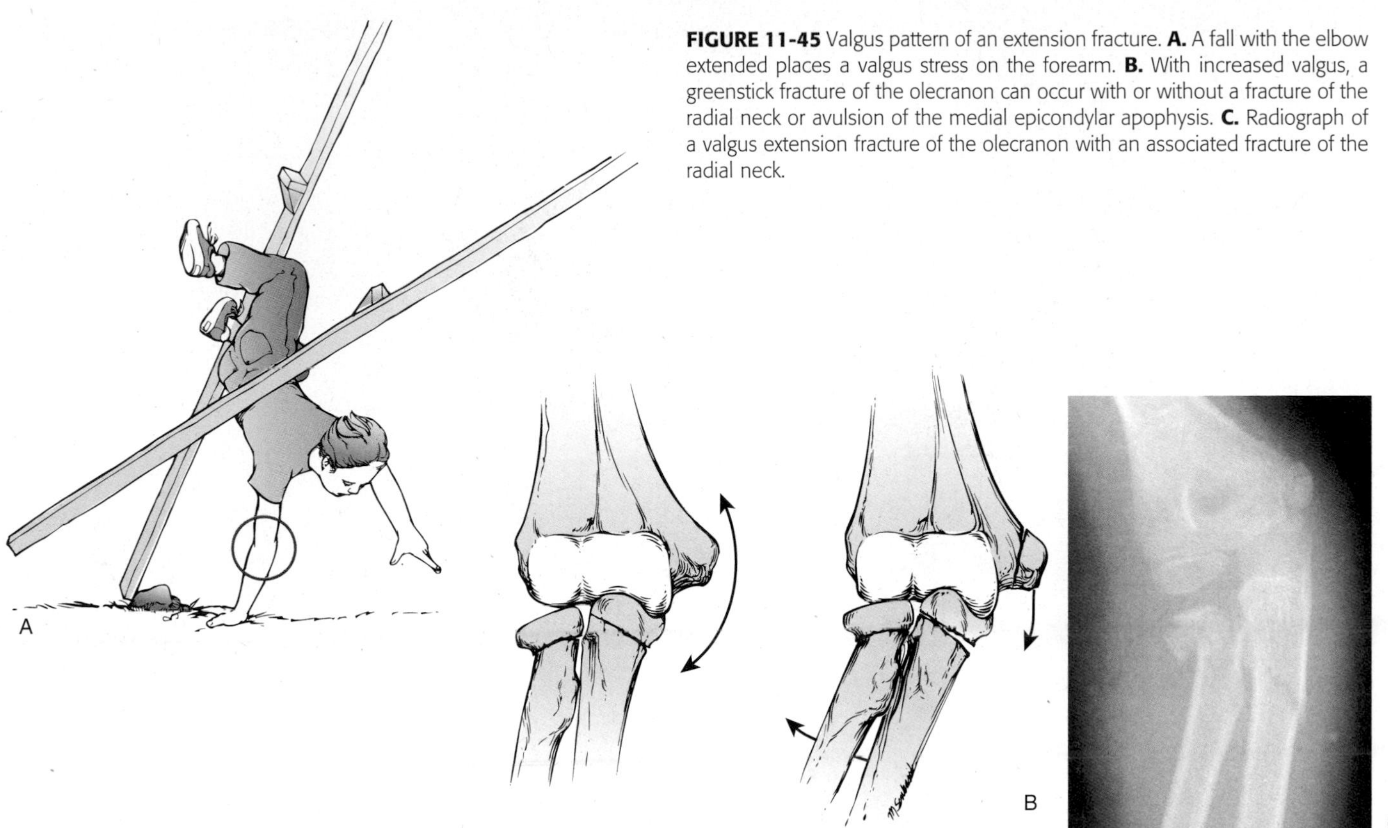

FIGURE 11-45 Valgus pattern of an extension fracture. **A.** A fall with the elbow extended places a valgus stress on the forearm. **B.** With increased valgus, a greenstick fracture of the olecranon can occur with or without a fracture of the radial neck or avulsion of the medial epicondylar apophysis. **C.** Radiograph of a valgus extension fracture of the olecranon with an associated fracture of the radial neck.

arm in supination, the carrying angle tends to place a valgus stress across the elbow. The result may be a greenstick fracture of the ulna with an associated fracture of the radial neck or avulsion of the medial epicondylar apophysis (Fig. 11-45). If the fracture involves the radial neck, Bado[35] classified it as an equivalent of the type I Monteggia lesion.

If the body falls against the inner aspect of the elbow or if the forearm is pronated, a varus force is placed across the elbow (Fig. 11-46). The major injury associated with this varus force is a partial or total lateral dislocation of the radial head. Bado[4] classified this as a type III Monteggia lesion. In this type of fracture, the posterior interosseous nerve may be injured.

Shear Injuries

Anterior tension failure is a rare injury that can occur when a direct blow to the proximal ulna causes it to fail with an anterior tension force; the proximal radioulnar joint maintains its integrity. The most common type of shear injury is caused by a shear force applied directly to the posterior aspect of the olecranon, with the distal fragment displacing anteriorly (Figs. 11-47 and 11-48). The intact proximal radioulnar joint displaces with the distal fragment. In this type of injury, the elbow may be either flexed or extended when the direct shear force impacts the posterior aspect of the olecranon. These fractures are due to a failure in tension, with the force concentrated along the anterior cortex. This is opposite to the tension failure occurring on the posterior aspect of the cortex in the more common flexion injuries. In the shear-type injury, the fracture line may be transverse or oblique. The differentiating feature from the more common flexion injury is that the thick posterior periosteum usually remains intact. The distal fragment is displaced anteriorly by the pull of the brachialis and biceps muscles. Newman[70] described one patient in whom a shear force was directed medially; the radial neck was fractured, and the radial head remained with the proximal fragment.

Associated Injuries

Associated injuries occur in 48% to 77% of patients with olecranon fractures,[12,35,73,108] especially varus and valgus greenstick extension fractures, in which the radial head and neck most commonly fracture (see Fig. 11-45). Other associated injuries include fractures of the ipsilateral radial shaft,[106] Monteggia type I lesions with fractures of both the ulnar shaft and olecranon,[72] and fractures of the lateral condyle (Fig. 11-49).[10]

Treatment

The mechanism of injury can serve as a useful guide in choosing the proper treatment method.

Flexion Injuries

Flexion injuries are the most common type of olecranon fractures. Most displace minimally and require immobilization with the elbow in no more than 75 to 80 degrees of flexion (Fig. 11-50). Even if the fracture displaces severely, immobilization in full or partial extension usually allows the olecranon to heal satisfactorily.[25,101,127]

If the fracture is significantly displaced or comminuted, open reduction with internal fixation usually is required. Recommended fixation devices vary from catgut or absorbable suture[57] to an axial screw,[55] tension-band wiring with axial

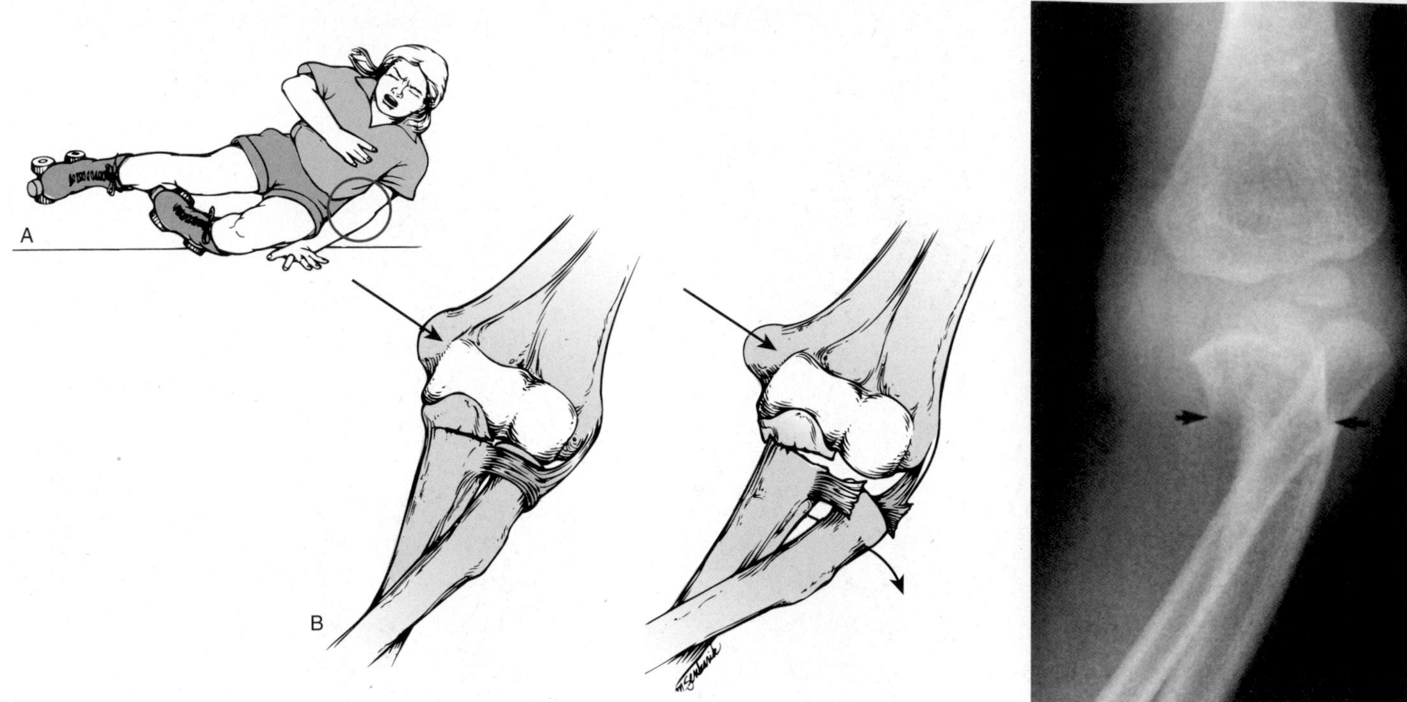

FIGURE 11-46 Varus pattern of an extension fracture. **A.** A fall against the extended elbow places a varus stress on the forearm. **B.** The result is a greenstick fracture of the olecranon with a lateral dislocation of the radial head (type III Monteggia lesion). **C.** Radiograph of a varus extension injury showing subluxation of the radial head and greenstick fracture of the ulna (*arrows*).

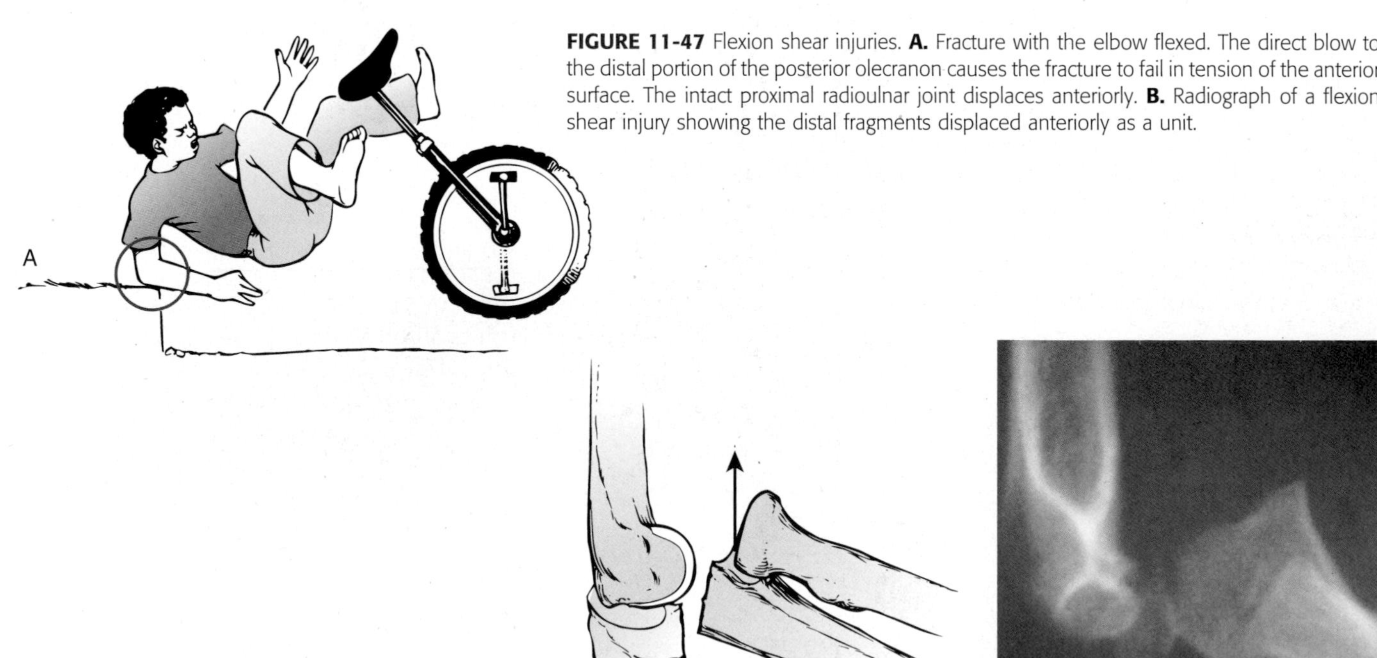

FIGURE 11-47 Flexion shear injuries. **A.** Fracture with the elbow flexed. The direct blow to the distal portion of the posterior olecranon causes the fracture to fail in tension of the anterior surface. The intact proximal radioulnar joint displaces anteriorly. **B.** Radiograph of a flexion shear injury showing the distal fragments displaced anteriorly as a unit.

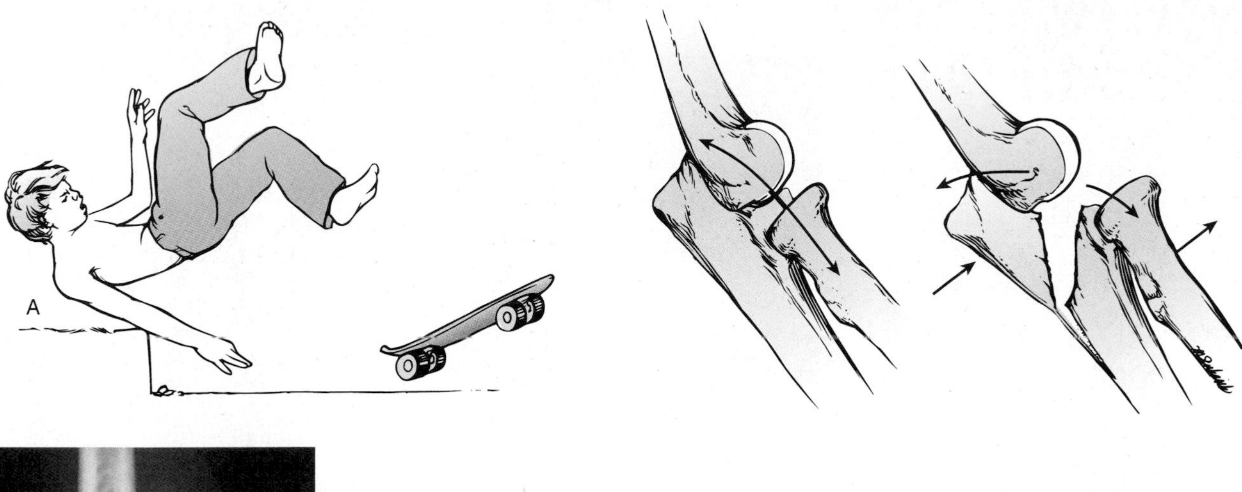

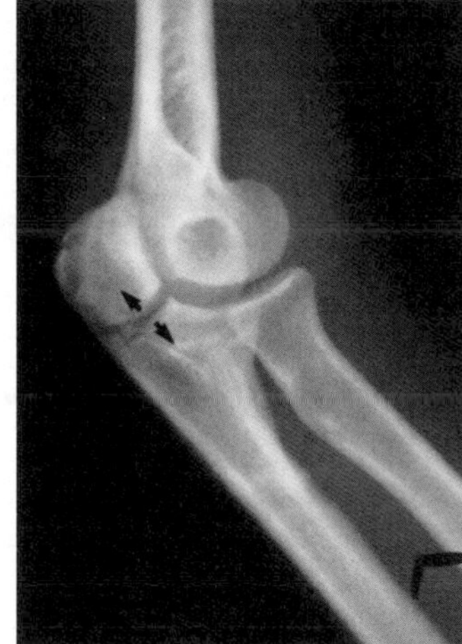

FIGURE 11-48 Extension shear injuries. **A.** Fracture with the elbow extended. If the elbow is extended when the direct blow to the posterior aspect of the elbow occurs, the olecranon fails in tension but with an oblique or transverse fracture line (*arrows*). **B.** With the elbow extended, the initial failure is in the anterior articular surface (*arrows*).

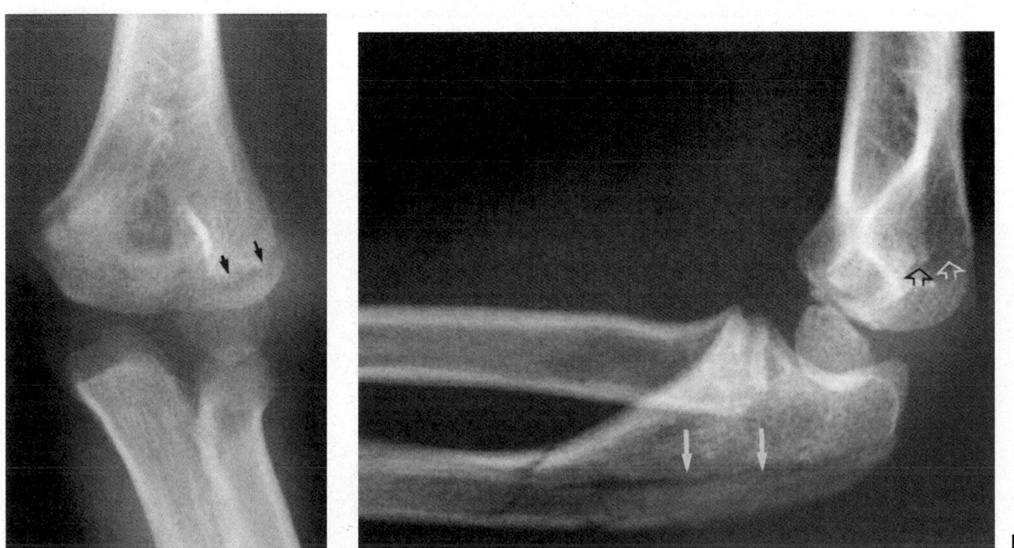

FIGURE 11-49 A. Undisplaced fracture of the lateral condyle (*arrows*) associated with a varus greenstick fracture of the olecranon. **B.** Lateral view showing greenstick fractures in the olecranon (*solid arrows*) and a nondisplaced fracture of the lateral condyle (*open arrows*).

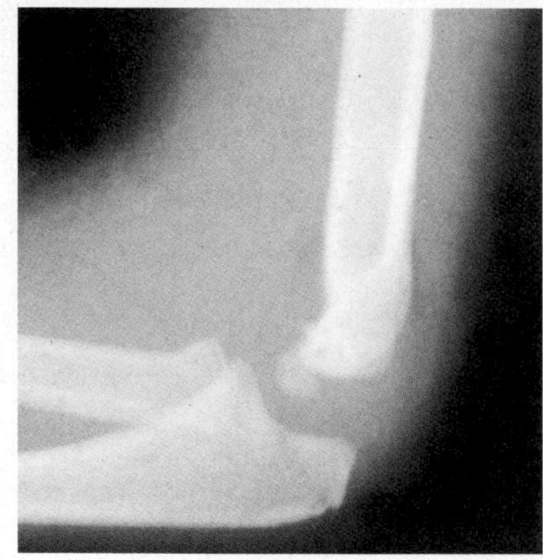

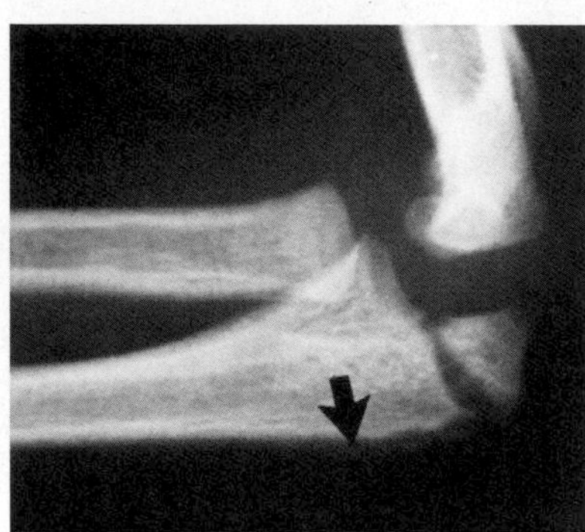

FIGURE 11-50 Simple immobilization of a flexion injury. **A.** Injury film, lateral view, showing minimal displacement. **B.** Three weeks later, the fracture has displaced further. Periosteal new bone is along the posterior border of the olecranon (*arrow*). Healing was complete with a normal range of motion. (Courtesy of Jesse C. DeLee, MD.)

pins,[23,34,57,91,94,101] or a plate.[107] Internal fixation allows early motion. No one has reported significant growth disturbances from internal fixation of metaphyseal olecranon fractures.

Murphy et al.[64] compared the failure of various fixation devices under rapid loading: (a) figure-of-eight wire alone, (b) cancellous screw alone, (c) AO tension band, and (d) cancellous screw with a figure-of-eight wire combination. The cancellous screw alone and figure-of-eight wire alone were by far the weakest. The greatest resistance to failure was found in the combination of a screw plus figure-of-eight wire, followed closely by the AO tension-band fixation. In their clinical evaluation of patients, comparing the AO tension band and combination of screw and figure-of-eight wire, they found more clinical problems associated with the AO technique.[65] The main problem with the AO technique is the subcutaneous prominence of the axial wires.[53] To prevent proximal migration of these wires, Montgomery[66] devised a method of making eyelets in the proximal end of the wires through which he passed the figure-of-eight fixation wire.

Extension Injuries

Treatment of extension injuries requires both adequate realignment of the angulation of the olecranon and treatment of the secondary injuries. Often in varus injuries, correction of the alignment of the olecranon also reduces the radial head. The olecranon angulation corrects with the elbow in extension. This locks the proximal olecranon into the olecranon fossa of the humerus so that the distal angulation can be corrected at the fracture site with a valgus force applied to the forearm. Occasionally, in extension fractures, complete separation of the fragments requires open reduction and internal fixation (Fig. 11-51).

Zimmerman[127] reported that the original angulation tends to redevelop in some fractures. If a varus force produced the fracture, the proximal ulna or olecranon may drift back into varus, which can cause a painful subluxation of the radial head. A secondary osteotomy of the proximal ulna or olecranon may be necessary if the angulation is significant.

Shear Injuries

For anterior shear fractures, the key to management is recognition that the distal fragment is displaced anteriorly and the posterior periosteum remains intact. The intact posterior periosteum can serve as an internal tension band to facilitate reduction.

Some of these fractures are reduced better in flexion, and the posterior periosteum serves as a compressive force to maintain the reduction. Smith[101] reported treatment of this fracture using an overhead sling placed to apply a posteriorly directed force against the proximal portion of the distal fragment. The weight of the arm and forearm helps supplement the tension-band effect of the posterior periosteum.

If the periosteum is torn or early motion is desirable, Zimmerman[127] advocated internal fixation of the two fragments

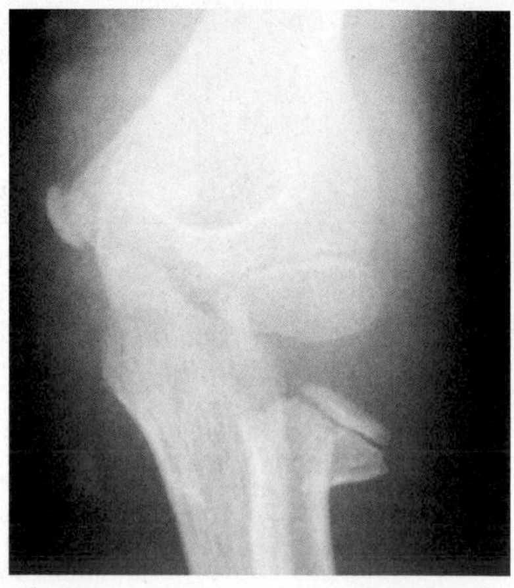

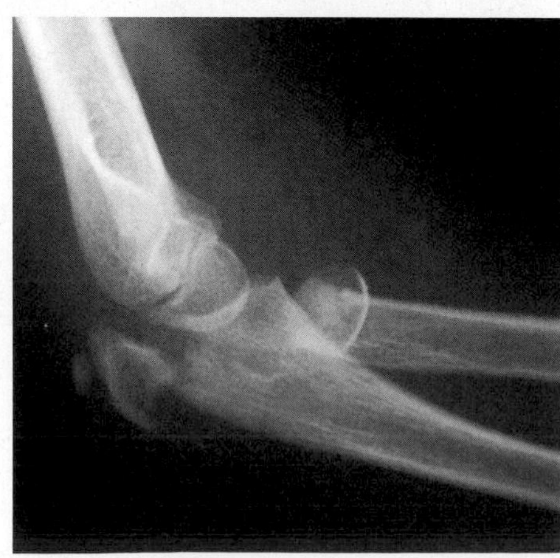

FIGURE 11-51 Open reduction of a valgus extension injury. **A.** Anteroposterior injury film shows complete displacement of the radial head. **B.** Lateral view also shows the degree of displacement of the olecranon fracture. This patient required surgical intervention with internal fixation to achieve a satisfactory reduction.

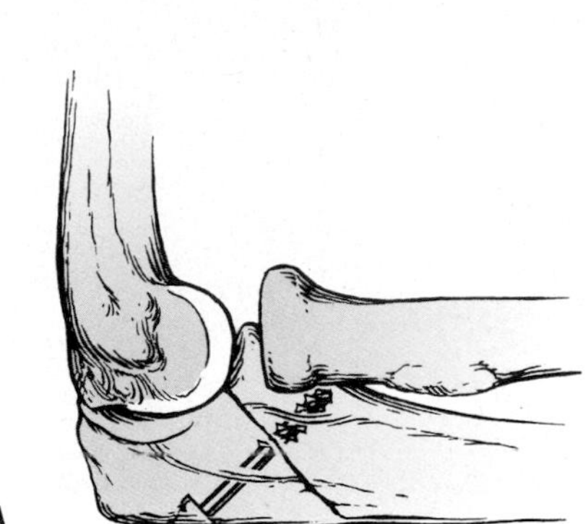
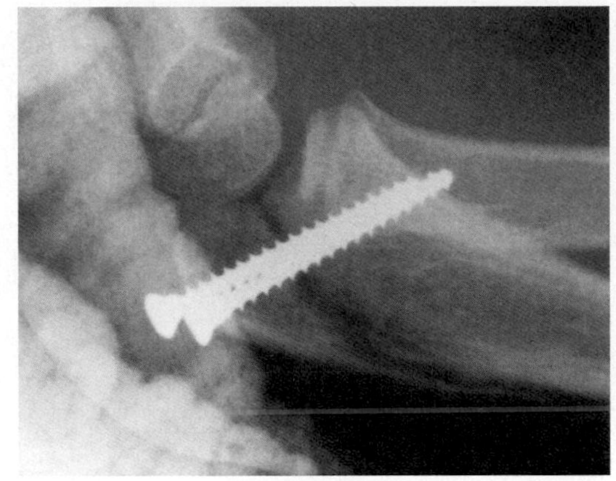

A B

FIGURE 11-52 Operative treatment of extension shear fractures. **A.** If the periosteum is insufficient to hold the fragments apposed, an interfragmentary screw can be used, as advocated by Zimmerman.[115] **B.** An extension shear type of fracture secured with two oblique interfragmentary screws.

with an oblique screw perpendicular to the fracture line (Fig. 11-52).

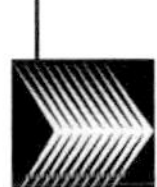

AUTHORS' PREFERRED METHOD

We use a classification based on the mechanism of injury in choosing the method of treatment (see Table 11-8).

Flexion Injuries

Nonoperative

We immobilize most nondisplaced flexion injuries with the elbow in 5 to 10 degrees of flexion for approximately 3 weeks. It is important to obtain radiographs of these fractures after approximately 5 to 7 days in the cast to ensure that there has not been any significant displacement of the fragment.

Operative: Tension Band

To determine which injuries need internal fixation, we palpate the fracture for a defect and flex the elbow to determine the integrity of the posterior periosteum. If the fragments separate with either of these maneuvers, they are unstable and are fixed internally so that active motion can be started as soon as possible.

We prefer a modification of the tension-band technique. Originally we used the standard AO technique with axial Kirschner-wires or Steinmann pins and figure-of-eight stainless steel as the tension band (Fig. 11-53A). Because removal of the wire often required reopening the entire incision, we now use an absorbable suture for the figure-of-eight tension band. Number 1 polydioxanone (PDS) suture, which is slowly absorbed over a few months, is ideal (see Fig. 11-53B). When rigid internal fixation is applied, rapid healing at the fracture site produces internal stability before the PDS absorbs. We prefer Kirschner-wires in patients who are very young and have very little ossification of the olecranon apophysis (see Fig. 11-40). If the axial wires become a problem, we remove them through a small incision. Most recently, we have used a combination of an oblique cortical screw with PDS as the tension band (see Fig. 11-53C,D) and are pleased with the results. In the past, we had to remove almost all the axial wires; very few of the screws cause enough symptoms to require removal. Occasionally, we use the tension-band wire technique with 16- or 18-gauge wire in a heavier patient.

Extension Injures

For extension injuries, we anesthetize the patient to allow a forceful manipulation of the olecranon while it is locked in its fossa in extension. Because this is a greenstick fracture, we slightly overcorrect to prevent the development of reangulation. These fractures may require manipulation/remanipulation in 1 to 2 weeks if the original angulation recurs. Associated fractures are treated as if they were isolated injuries.

Shear Injuries

Most shear fractures can be treated nonoperatively. We usually immobilize them in enough hyperflexion to hold the fragments together, if the posterior periosteum is intact (Fig. 11-54). If the periosteum is torn, an oblique screw is an excellent way to secure the fracture (see Fig. 11 52). If considerable swelling prevents the elbow from being hyperflexed enough to use the posterior periosteum as a tension band, an oblique screw is a good choice.

Postoperative Care

The elbow is placed at a 70 to 80 degrees angle and held in a long-arm cast. The cast should be bivalved if there is excessive swelling. The cast or posterior splint is worn for 3 weeks, at which time the patient begins active range of motion.

Associated Injuries and Complications

Relatively few complications arise from the olecranon fracture itself.

Irreducibility

An and Loder[1] reported inability to reduce the fracture in one of their patients because the proximal fragment was entrapped in the joint.

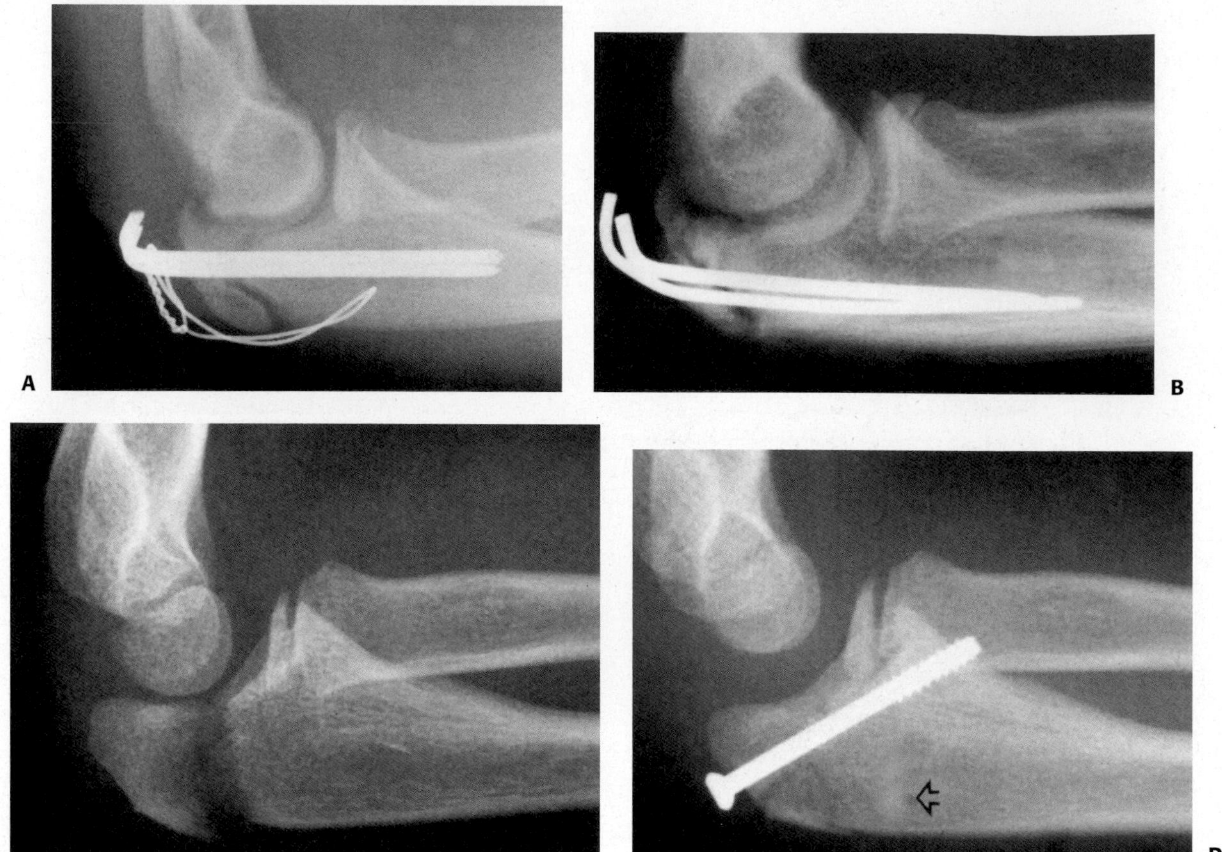

FIGURE 11-53 Internal tension-band techniques. **A.** Standard AO technique with stainless steel wire. The wire can be prominent in the subcutaneous tissues. **B.** Axial wires plus polydioxanone sutures (PDS) 6 weeks after surgery. **C.** A displaced flexion-type injury in an 11-year-old male. There is complete separation of the fracture fragments. **D.** A cancellous lag screw plus PDS. The screw engages the anterior cortex of the coronoid process. The PDS passes through a separate drill hole in the olecranon (*open arrow*) and crosses in a figure-of-eight manner over the fracture site and around the neck of the screw.

Nonunion

Nonunion is unusual and should not be confused with congenital pseudarthrosis of the ulna, which is rare (Fig. 11-55). In the latter condition, there is no antecedent trauma.

Delayed Union

Delayed radiographic union usually is asymptomatic.[57] In Mathews' series,[57] one fracture treated with suture fixation ultimately progressed to a nonunion. Despite this, the patient had only a 10 degrees extension lag and grade 4 triceps strength. An accessory ossicle, such as a patella cubiti, is not a nonunion.

Compartment Syndrome

Mathews[57] described 1 patient with Volkmann ischemic contracture after an undisplaced linear fracture in the olecranon.

Nerve Injuries

Zimmerman[127] reported ulnar nerve neurapraxia from the development of a pseudarthrosis of the olecranon where inadequate fixation was used.

Elongation

Elongation of the tip of the olecranon may complicate healing of a fracture. Figure 11-56 illustrates a delayed union in which the apophysis became elongated to the point that it limited extension. This proximal overgrowth of the tip of the apophysis has occurred in olecranon fractures after routine open reduction and internal fixation.[73]

Loss of Reduction

Apparently stable fractures treated with external immobilization may lose reduction, which results in a significant loss of elbow function (Fig. 11-57).

Fractures of the Coronoid Process

Anatomy. Up to age 6 years, the coronoid process consists of epiphyseal and physeal cartilage at the distal end of a tongue extending from the apophysis of the olecranon. The coronoid process does not develop a secondary center of ossification, but instead ossifies along with the advancing edge of the metaphysis (see Fig. 11-37).

Incidence. The incidence of fracture of the coronoid varies from less than 1% to 2% of elbow fractures.[58] Because most fractures of the coronoid process occur with dislocations of the elbow, it seems logical that they would happen in older children. However, in a review of 23 coronoid fractures in children, Bracq[10] found that the injuries occurred in 2 peak age groups: one was between 8 and 9 years of age and the other between 12 and 14 years.

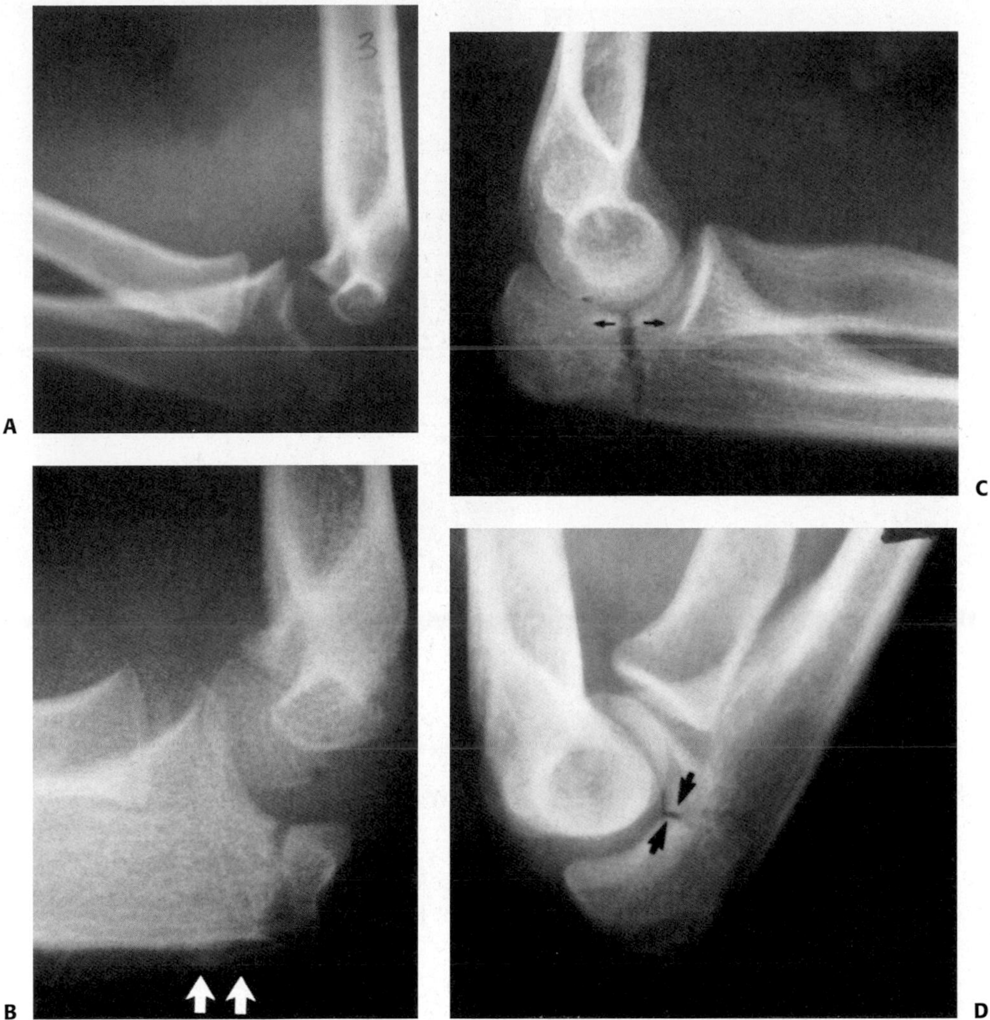

FIGURE 11-54 Shear injuries. **A.** Flexion pattern: radiograph of the patient seen in Figure 11-45A after the elbow was flexed. The intact posterior periosteum acted as a tension band and held the fracture reduced. **B.** Radiograph taken 4 weeks after surgery shows new bone formation under the intact periosteum (*arrows*) on the dorsal surface of the olecranon. **C.** Extension pattern: radiograph of patient with an extension shear injury showing an increase in the fracture gap (*arrows*) (see also Fig. 11-45B). **D.** Because the dorsal periosteum and cortex were intact, the fracture gap (*arrows*) closed with flexion of the elbow.

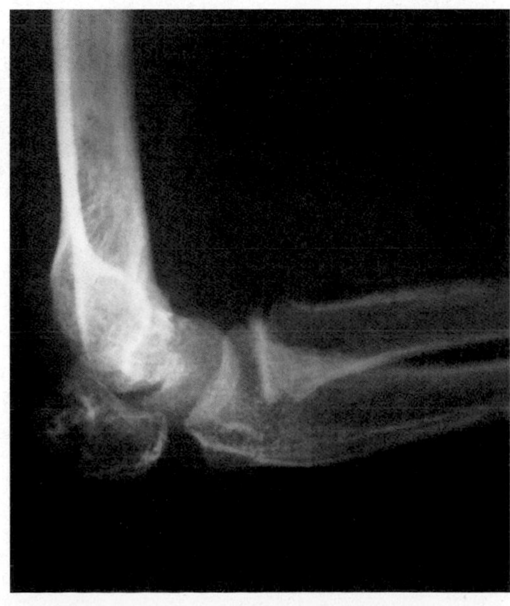

FIGURE 11-55 Congenital pseudarthrosis of the olecranon in a 9-year-old female who had limited elbow extension and no antecedent trauma. The edges of the bone were separated by thick fibrous tissue. (Courtesy of Michael J. Rogal, MD.)

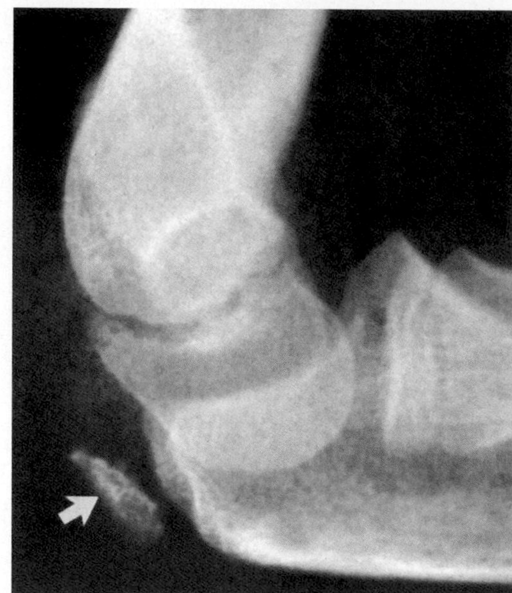
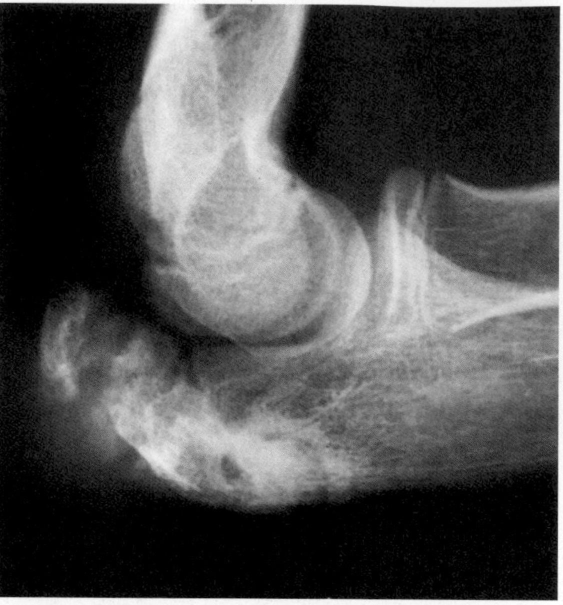

FIGURE 11-56 A. Injury film showing partial avulsion of the tip of the olecranon apophysis (*arrow*). **B.** Radiograph taken 4 years later shows a marked elongation and irregular ossification of the apophysis. (Courtesy of Joel Goldman, MD.)

Although most coronoid fractures are associated with elbow dislocations, fractures of the olecranon, medial epicondyle, and lateral condyle also can occur.[70] The fracture of the coronoid may be part of a greenstick olecranon fracture (i.e., the extension-type metaphyseal fracture; Fig. 11-58). Isolated coronoid fractures are theoretically caused by avulsion by the brachialis or secondary to an elbow dislocation that reduced spontaneously, which is usually associated with hemarthrosis and a small avulsion of the tip of the olecranon process (Fig. 11-59).

Diagnosis. The radiographic diagnosis of this fracture is often difficult because on the lateral view the radial head is superimposed over the coronoid process. Evaluation of a minimally displaced fracture may require oblique views (Fig. 11-60).[103] The radiocapitellar view (see Fig. 11-6) shows the profile of the coronoid process.

In young children, in whom the coronoid process contains mostly cartilage, an unusual flap injury may occur.[30] In this rare injury, the elbow dislocates and the articular surface flips

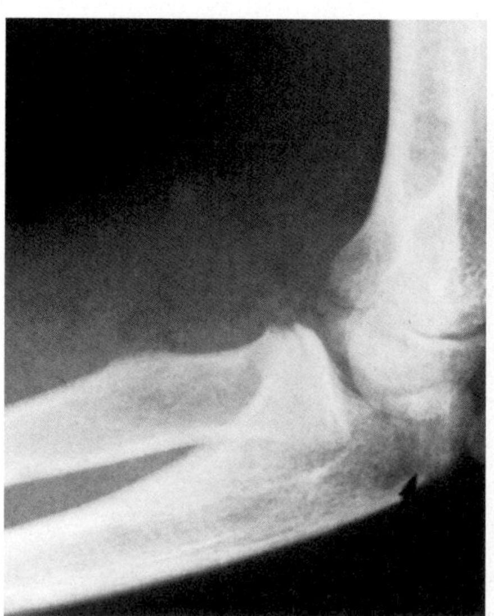
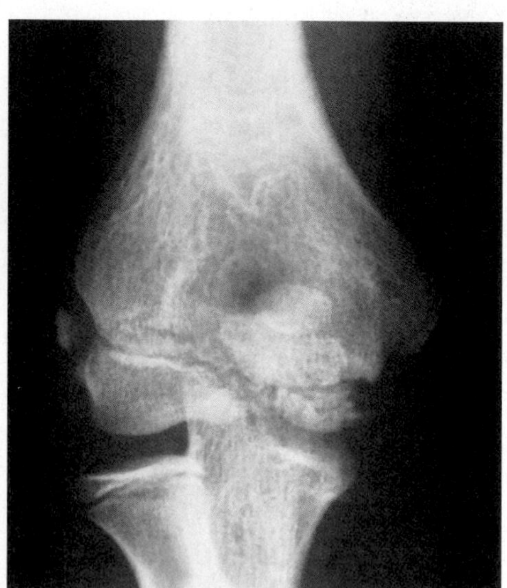
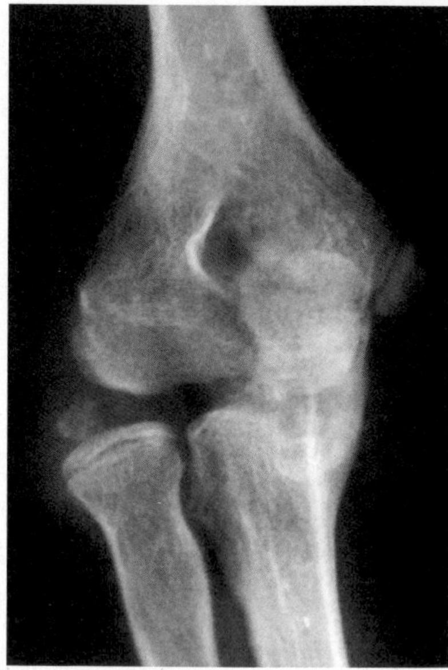

FIGURE 11-57 Loss of reduction. **A.** Lateral radiograph of what appeared to be a simple undisplaced fracture (*arrow*) of the olecranon in a 13-year-old female. **B.** On the anteroposterior film, the fracture also appears undisplaced. The mild lateral subluxation of the radial head was not recognized. **C.** Radiographs taken 5 months later showed further lateral subluxation with resultant incongruity of the elbow joint. (Courtesy of Richard W. Williamson, MD.)

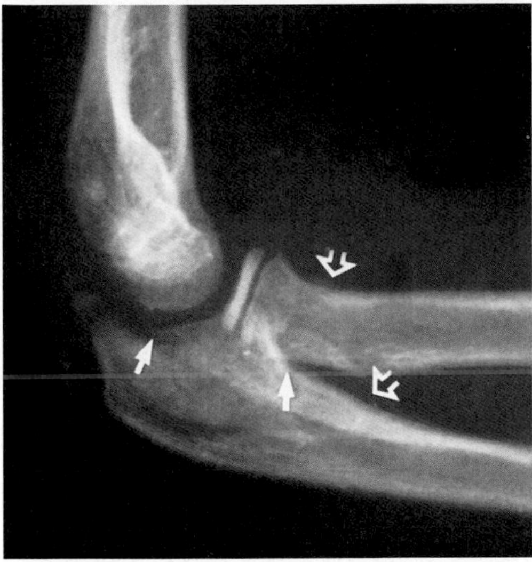

FIGURE 11-58 Fracture of the coronoid (*arrow*) as part of an extension valgus olecranon fracture pattern. There was an associated fracture of the radial neck. Both the neck fracture and the distal portion of the coronoid process show periosteal new bone formation (*open arrows*).

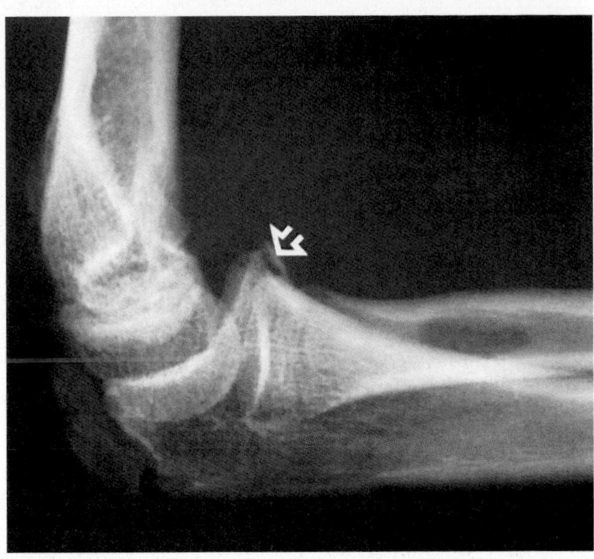

FIGURE 11-59 Lateral radiograph of an 11-year-old male who injured his left elbow. Displaced anterior and posterior fat pads, plus a small fracture of the coronoid (*arrow*), indicate a probable partially dislocated elbow as the primary injury.

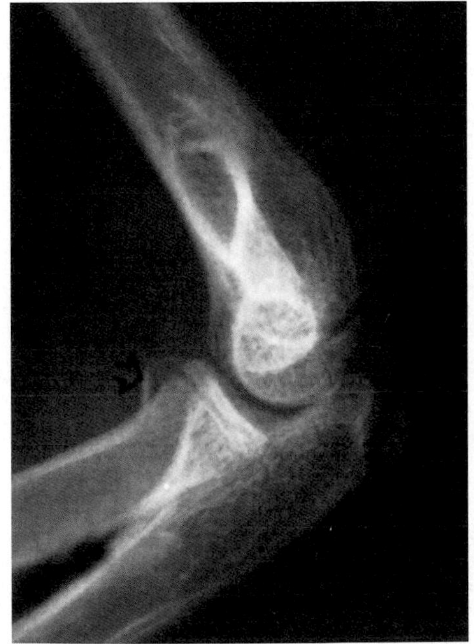

A

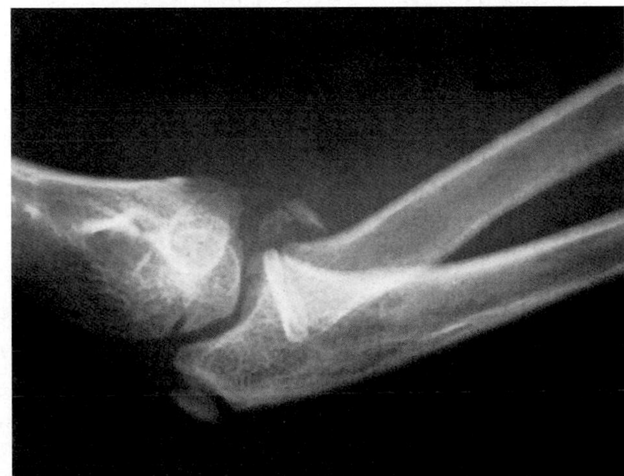

B

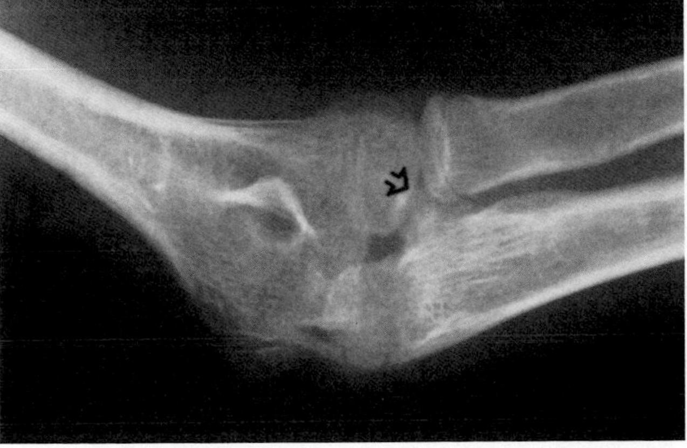

C

FIGURE 11-60 A. Based on this original lateral radiograph, a 12-year-old male with a swollen elbow was thought to have a fracture of the radial neck (*arrow*). **B.** With an oblique view, it is now obvious that the fragment is from the coronoid process. **C.** Five months later, the protuberant healed coronoid process (*arrow*) is seen on this radiocapitellar view.

TABLE 11-9 Classification of Fractures of the Coronoid Process

Type I: Involves only tip of coronoid

Type II: A single or comminuted fragment involving ≤50% of the coronoid process

Type III: A single or comminuted fragment involving >50% of the coronoid process

back into the joint. The only clue to this fracture may be the presence of a small flake of bone in the anterior part of the joint on the lateral radiograph.

Classification. Regan and Morrey[85] classified coronoid fractures into three types based on the amount of the coronoid process involved (Table 11-9). This classification is useful in predicting the outcome and in determining the treatment. Type I fractures involve only the tip of the process (see Fig. 11-59), type II fractures involve more than just the tip but less than 50% of the process (see Fig. 11-60), and type III fractures involve more than 50% of the process.

Treatment. The degree of displacement or the presence of elbow instability guides the treatment. The associated injuries also are a factor in treatment. Regan and Morrey[85,86] treated types I and II fractures with early motion if there were no contradicting associated injuries. For initial immobilization, if the fracture is associated with an elbow dislocation, the elbow is placed in approximately 100 degrees of flexion, with the forearm in full supination.[70] Occasionally, in partial avulsion fractures, the fracture reduces more easily with the elbow in extension. In these rare cases, the brachialis muscle may be an aid in reducing the fragment in extension.[69] Regan and Morrey[85] found that the elbow often was unstable in type III fractures, and they secured these fractures with internal fixation. They had satisfactory results with type I and II fractures, but in only 20% of type III fractures were the results satisfactory.

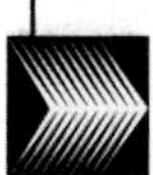

AUTHORS' PREFERRED METHOD

We usually treat coronoid fractures with early motion, much as we do elbow dislocations. The presence of a coronoid fracture alerts us to be especially thorough in looking for other injuries. In children, surgery is rarely necessary. If there is a large fragment and marked displacement, open reduction is done through a Henry anterior approach to the elbow. The fragment is fixed with a minifragment screw or sewn in place through two drill holes in the posterior aspect of the ulna.

Associated Injuries and Complications

Complications are rare. In fractures with a large fragment (type III), the elbow may be unstable and prone to recurrent dislocations. Nonunion with the production of a free fragment in the joint occurs rarely in children.[74]

REFERENCES

1. An HS, Loder RT. Intra-articular entrapment of a displaced olecranon fracture. Orthopedics 1989;12:289–291.
2. Anderson TE, Breed AL. A proximal radial metaphyseal fracture presenting as wrist pain. Orthopedics 1982;5:425–428.
3. Angelov AA. New method for treatment of the dislocated radial neck fracture in children. In: Chapchal G, ed. Fractures in Children. New York: Georg Thieme, 1981: 192–194.
4. Bado JL. The Monteggia lesion. Clin Orthop Relat Res 1967;50:71–86.
5. Baehr FH. Reduction of separated upper epiphysis of the radius. N Engl J Med 1932; 24:1263–1266.
6. Bernstein SM, McKeever P, Bernstein L. Percutaneous pinning for radial neck fractures. J Pediatr Orthop 1993;13:84–88.
7. Biyani A, Mehara A, Bhan S. Percutaneous pinning of radial neck fractures. Injury 1994;25:169–171.
8. Blount WP. Fractures in children. AAOS Instr Course Lect 1950;7:194–202.
9. Boyd HB, Altenberg AR. Fractures about the elbow in children. Arch Surg 1944;49: 213–224.
10. Bracq H. Fractures de l'olecrane. Rev Chir Orthop 1987;73:469–471.
11. Brodeur AE, Silberstein JJ, Graviss ER. Radiology of the Pediatric Elbow. Boston: GK Hall, 1981.
12. Burge P, Benson M. Bilateral congenital pseudoarthrosis of the olecranon. J Bone Joint Surg Br 1987;69:460–462.
13. Carl AL, Ain MC. Complex fracture of the radial neck in a child: an unusual case. J Orthop Trauma 1994;8:255–257.
14. Chambers HG. Fractures of the proximal radius and ulna. In: Kasser JR, Beaty JH, eds. Rockwood & Wilkins' Fractures in Children 5th ed. Philadelphia: Lippincott Williams & Wilkins, 2001:483–528.
15. D'Souza S, Vaishya R, Klenerman L. Management of radial neck fractures in children. A retrospective analysis of 100 patients. J Pediatr Orthop 1993;13:232–238.
16. Danielson LG, Hedlund ST, Henricson AS. Apophysitis of the olecranon: a report of four cases. Acta Orthop Scand 1983;54:777–778.
17. Di Cesare PE, Sew-Hoy A, Krom W. Bilateral isolated olecranon fractures in an infant as presentation of osteogenesis imperfecta. Orthopedics 1992;15:741–743.
18. Dooley JF, Angus PD. The importance of elbow aspiration when treating radial head fractures. Arch Emerg Med 1991;8:117–121.
19. Dormans JP, Rang M. Fractures of the olecranon and radial neck in children. Orthop Clin North Am 1990;21:257–268.
20. Dougall AJ. Severe fracture of the neck of the radius in children. J R Coll Surg Edinb 1969;14:220.
21. Ellman H. Anterior angulation deformity of the radial head. J Bone Joint Surg Am 1975;57:776–778.
22. Ellman H. Osteochondrosis of the radial head. J Bone Joint Surg Am 1972;54:1560.
23. Fahey JJ. Fractures of the elbow in children. AAOS Instr Course Lect 1980;17:13–46.
24. Fan G-F, Wu C-C, Shin C-H. Olecranon fractures treated with tension band wiring techniques: comparisons among three different configurations. Chang Keng I Hsueh 1993;16:231–238.
25. Fogarty EE, Blake NS, Regan BF. Fracture of the radial neck with medial displacement of the shaft of the radius. Br J Radiol 1983;56:486–487.
26. Fowles JV, Kassab MT. Observations concerning radial neck fractures in children. J Pediatr Orthop 1986;6:51–57.
27. Fraser KE. Displaced fracture of the proximal end of the radius in a child. A case report of the deceptive appearance of a fragment that had rotated 180 degrees. J Bone Joint Surg Am 1995;77:782–783.
28. Futami T, Tsukamoto Y, Itoman M. Percutaneous reduction of displaced radial neck fractures. J Shoulder Elbow Surg 1995;4:162–167.
29. Gaddy BC, Strecker WB, Schoenecker PL. Surgical treatment of displaced olecranon fractures in children. J Pediatr Orthop 1997;17:321–324.
30. Gaston SR, Smith FM, Boab OD. Epiphyseal injuries of the radial head and neck. Am J Surg 1953;85:266–276.
31. Gille P, Mourot M, Aubert F, et al. Fracture par torsion du col du radius chez l'enfant. Rev Chir Orthop 1978;64:247–248.
32. Gonzalez-Herranz P, Alvarez-Romera A, Burgos J, et al. Displaced radial neck fractures in children treated by closed intramedullary pinning (Metaizeau technique). J Pediatr Orthop 1997;17:325–331.
33. Gortzak Y, Mercado E, Atar D, et al. Pediatric olecranon fractures: open reduction and internal fixation with removable Kirschner wires and absorbable sutures. J Pediatr Orthop 2006;26:39–42.
34. Granthan SA, Kiernan HA. Displaced olecranon fractures in children. J Trauma 1975; 15:197–204.
35. Graves SC, Canale ST. Fractures of the olecranon in children: long-term follow-up. J Pediatr Orthop 1993;13:239–241.
36. Greenspan A, Norman A. The radial head-capitellum view: useful technique in elbow trauma. AJR Am J Roentgenol 1982;138:1186–1188.
37. Greenspan A, Norman A, Rosen H. Radial head-capitellum view in elbow trauma: clinical application and radiographic-anatomic correlation. AJR Am J Roentgenol 1984; 143:355–359.
38. Hall-Craggs MA, Shorvon PJ, Chapman M. Assessment of the radial head-capitellum view and the dorsal fat-pad sing in acute elbow trauma. AJR Am J Roentgenol 1985; 145:607–609.
39. Henrikson B. Isolated fracture of the proximal end of the radius in children. Acta Orthop Scand 1969;40:246–260.
40. Irshad F, Shaw NJ, Gregory RJ. Reliability of fat-pad sign in radial head/neck fractures of the elbow. Injury 1997;28:433–435.
41. Javed A, Guichet J.M. Arthrography for reduction of a fracture of the radial neck in a child with a nonossified radial epiphysis. JBJS Br 2001;83-B:542–543.
42. Jeffrey CC. Fracture of the head of the radius in children. J Bone Joint Surg Br 1950; 32:314–324.
43. Jones ERW, Esah M. Displaced fracture of the neck of the radius in children. J Bone Joint Surg Br 1971;53:429–439.

44. Kaplan EB. Surgical approach to the proximal end of the radius and its use in fractures of the head and neck of the radius. J Bone Joint Surg 1941;23:86–92.
45. Kaufman B, Rinott MG, Tanzman M. Closed reduction of fractures of the proximal radius in children. J Bone Joint Surg Br 1989;71:66–67.
46. Key AJ. Survival of the head of the radius in a child after removal and replacement. J Bone Joint Surg 1946;28:148–149.
47. Kovach JI, Baker BE, Mosher JF. Fracture-separation of the olecranon ossification center in adults. Am J Sports Med 1985;13:105–111.
48. Landin LA. Fracture patterns in children. Analysis of 8,682 fractures with special reference to incidence, etiology and secular changes in a swedish urban population. 1950–1979. Acta Orthop Scand Suppl 1983;202:1–109.
49. Landin LA, Danielsson LG. Elbow fractures in children: an epidemiological analysis of 589 cases. Acta Orthop Scand 1986;57:309.
50. Lazar RD, Waters PM, Jaramillo D. The use of ultrasonography in the diagnosis of occult fracture of the radial neck: a case report. J Bone Joint Surg Am 1998;80:1361–1364.
51. Leung KS, Tse PYT. A new method of fixing radial neck fractures: brief report. J Bone Joint Surg Br 1989;71:326–327.
52. Lindham S, Hugasson C. Significance of associated lesions including dislocation of fracture of the neck of the radius in children. Acta Orthop Scand 1979;50:79–83.
53. Macko D, Azabo RM. Complications of tension band wiring of olecranon fractures. J Bone Joint Surg Am 1985;67:1396–1401.
54. MacLennan A. Common fractures about the elbow joint in children. Surg Gynecol Obstet 1937;64:447–453.
55. Maffulli N, Chan D, Aldridge MJ. Overuse injuries of the olecranon in young gymnasts. J Bone Joint Surg [Br] 1992;74:305–308.
56. Manoli A II. Medial displacement of the shaft of the radius with a fracture of the radial neck. J Bone Joint Surg Am 1979;61:788–789.
57. Mathews JG. Fractures of the olecranon in children. Injury 1981;12:207–212.
58. Maylahn DJ, Fahey JJ. Fractures of the elbow in children. JAMA 1958;166:220–228.
59. McBride ED, Monnet JC. Epiphyseal fracture of the head of the radius in children. Clin Orthop Relat Res 1960;16:264–271.
60. McCarthy SM, Ogden JA. Radiology of postnatal skeletal development. Skeletal Radiol 1982;9:17–26.
61. Metaizeau JP, Lascombes P, Lemelle JL, et al. Reduction and fixation of displaced radial neck fractures by closed intramedullary pinning. J Pediatr Orthop 1993;13:355–360.
62. Metaizeau JP, Prevot J, Schmitt M. Reduction et fixation des fractures et decollements epiphysaires de la tete radiale par broche centromedullaire. Rev Chir Orthop 1980;66:47–49.
63. Mudgal CS. Olecranon fractures in osteogenesis imperfecta: a case report. Acta Orthop Belg 1992;58:453–456.
64. Murphy DF, Greene WB, Dameron TB. Displaced olecranon fractures in adults. Clin Orthop Relat Res 1987;224:215–223.
65. Murphy DF, Greene WB, Gilbert JA, et al. Displaced olecranon fractures in adults. Biomedical analysis of fixation methods. Clin Orthop Relat Res 1987;224:210–214.
66. Montgomery RJ. A secure method of olecranon fixation: a modification of tension band wiring technique. J R Coll Surg Edinb 1986;31:179–182.
67. Nawabi DH, Kang N, Curry S. Centromedullary pinning of radial neck fractures: length matters! J Pediatr Orthop 2006;26:278–279.
68. Neher CG, Torch MA. New reduction technique for severely displaced pediatric radial neck fractures. J Pediatr Orthop 2003;23:626–628.
69. Newell RLM. Olecranon fractures in children. Injury 1975;7:33–36.
70. Newman JH. Displaced radial neck fractures in children. Injury 1977;9:114–121.
71. O'Brien PI. Injuries involving the radial epiphysis. Clin Orthop Relat Res 1965;41:51–58.
72. Olney BW, Menelaus MB. Monteggia and equivalent lesions in childhood. J Pediatr Orthop 1989;9:219–223.
73. Papavasiliou VA, Beslikas TA, Nenopoulos S. Isolated fractures of the olecranon in children. Injury 1987;18:100–102.
74. Pappas AM. Elbow problems associated with baseball during childhood. Clin Orthop Relat Res 1982;164:30–41.
75. Patterson RF. Treatment of displaced transverse fractures of the neck of the radius in children. J Bone Joint Surg 1934,16:695–698.
76. Pavlov H, Torg JS, Jacobs B, et al. Nonunion of olecranon epiphysis: two cases in adolescent baseball pitchers. AJR Am J Roentgenol 1981;136:819–820.
77. Pelto K, Hirvensalo E, Bostman O, et al. Treatment of radial head fractures with absorbable polyglycolide pins: a study on the security of the fixation in 38 cases. J Orthop Trauma 1994;8:94–98.
78. Pesudo JV, Aracil J, Barcelo M. Leverage method in displaced fractures of the radial neck in children. Clin Orthop 1982;169:215–218.
79. Peters CL, Scott SM. Compartment syndrome in the forearm following fractures of the radial head or neck in children. J Bone Joint Surg Am 1995;77:1070–1074.
80. Poland J. A Practical Treatise on Traumatic Separation of the Epiphyses. London: Smith, Elder & Co, 1898.
81. Pollen AG. Fractures and Dislocations in Children. Baltimore: Williams & Wilkins, 1973.
82. Porteous CJ. The olecranon epiphyses. Proc J Anat 1960;94:286.
83. Prathapkumar KR, Garg NK, Bruce CE. Elastic stable intramedullary nail fixation for severely displaced fractures of the neck of the radius in children. JBJS Br 2006;88-B:358–361.
84. Radomisli TE, Rosen AL. Controversies regarding radial neck fractures in children. Clin Orthop Relat Res 1998;353:30–39.
85. Regan W, Morrey BF. Classification and treatment of coronoid process fractures. Orthopedics 1992;15:845–848.
86. Regan W, Morrey BF. Fractures of the coronoid process of the ulna. J Bone Joint Surg Am 1989;71:1348–1354.
87. Retrum RK, Wepfer JF, Olen DW, et al. Case report 355: delayed closure of the right olecranon epiphysis in a right-handed tournament-class tennis player. Skeletal Radiol 1986;15:185–187.
88. Robert M, Moulies D, Longis B, et al. Les fractures de l'extremite superieure du radius chez l'enfant. Chir Pediatr 1986;27:318–321.
89. Rodriguez-Merchan EC. Displaced fractures of the head and neck of the radius in children: open reduction and temporary transarticular internal fixation. Orthopedics 1991;14:697–700.
90. Rodriguez-Merchan EC. Percutaneous reduction of displaced radial neck fractures in children. J Trauma 1994;37:812–814.
91. Roe SC. Tension band wiring of olecranon fractures: a modification of the AO technique. Clin Orthop Relat Res 1994;308:284–286.
92. Rogers SL, Mac Ewan DW. Changes due to trauma in the fat plane overlying the supinator muscle: a radiologic sign. Radiology 1969;92:954–958.
93. Rokito SE, Anticevic D, Strongwater AM, et al. Case report and review of the literature: chronic fracture-separation of the radial head in a child. J Orthop Trauma 1995;9:259–262.
94. Rowland SA, Burkhart SS. Tension band wiring of olecranon fractures. A modification of the AO technique. Clin Orthop Relat Res 1992;277:238–242.
95. Saberstein MJ, Brodeur AE, Graviss ER, et al. Some vagaries of the olecranon. J Bone Joint Surg Am 1981;63:722–725.
96. Schmittenbecher PP, Haevernick B, Herold A, et al. Treatment decision, method of osteo synthesis, and outcome in radial neck fractures in children. A multicenter study. J Pediatr Orthop 2005;25:45–50.
97. Scullion JE, Miller JH. Fracture of the neck of the radius in children: prognostic factors and recommendations for management. J Bone Joint Surg Br 1985;67:491.
98. Sessa S, Lascombes P, Prevot J, et al. Fractures of the radial head and associated elbow injuries in children. J Pediatr Orthop B 1996;5:200–209.
99. Silberstein MJ, Brodeur AE, Graviss ER. Some vagaries of the radial head and neck. J Bone Joint Surg Am 1982;64:1153–1157.
100. Skak SV. Fracture of the olecranon through a persistent physis in an adult: a case report. J Bone Joint Surg Am 1993;75:272–275.
101. Smith FM. Surgery of the Elbow. Philadelphia: WB Saunders, 1972.
102. Steele JA, Graham HK. Angulated radial neck fractures in children: a prospective study of percutaneous reduction. J Bone Joint Surg Br 1992;74:760–764.
103. Steinberg EL, Golomb D, Salama R, et al. Radial head and neck fractures in children. J Pediatr Orthop 1988;8:35–40.
104. Strachan JCH, Ellis BW. Vulnerability of the posterior interosseous nerve during radial head resection. J Bone Joint Surg Br 1971;53:320–323.
105. Strong ML, Kropp M, Gillespie R. Fracture of the radial neck and proximal ulna with medial displacement of the radial shaft. Report of two cases. Orthopedics 1989;12:1577–1579.
106. Suprock MD, Lubahn JD. Olecranon fracture with unilateral closed radial shaft fracture in a child with open epiphysis. Orthopedics 1990;13:463–465.
107. Teasdall R, Savoie FH, Hughes JL. Comminuted fractures of the proximal radius and ulna. Clin Orthop Relat Res 1993,292:37–47
108. Theodorou SD, Ierodiaconou MN, Roussis N. Fracture of the upper end of the ulna associated with dislocation of the head of the radius in children. Clin Orthop Relat Res 1988;228:240–249.
109. Thijn CJP, van Ouwerkerk WPL, Scheele PM, et al. Unilateral patella cubiti: a probable posttraumatic disorder. Eur J Radiol 1992;14:60–62.
110. Tibone JE, Stoltz M. Fracture of the radial head and neck in children. J Bone Joint Surg Am 1981;63:100–106.
111. Torg JS, Moyer R. Nonunion of a stress fracture through the olecranon epiphyseal plate observed in an adolescent baseball pitcher. J Bone Joint Surg Am 1977;59:264–265.
112. Tullos HS, King JW. Lesions of the pitching arm in adolescents. JAMA 1972;220:264–271.
113. Turtel AH, Andrews JR, Schob CJ, et al. Fractures of unfused olecranon physis: a re-evaluation of this injury in three athletes. Orthopedics 1995;18:390–394.
114. Vahvanen V. Fracture of the radial neck in children. Acta Orthop Scand 1978;49:32–38.
115. Veranis N, Laliotis N, Vlachos E. Acute osteomyelitis complicating a closed radial fracture in a child: a case report. Acta Orthop Scand 1992;63:341–342.
116. Vocke AK, Von Laer L. Displaced fractures of the radial neck in children: long-term results and prognosis of conservative treatment. J Pediatr Orthop B 1998;7:217–222.
117. Vostal O. Fracture of the neck of the radius in children. Acta Chir Orthop Traumatol Cech 1970;37:294–301.
118. Ward WT, Williams JJ. Radial neck fracture complicating closed reduction of a posterior elbow dislocation in a child: case report. J Trauma 1991;31:1686–1688.
119. Waters P, Stewart SL. Radial neck fracture nonunion in children. J Pediatr Orthop 2001;21:570–576.
120. Wedge JH, Robertson DE. Displaced fractures of the neck of the radius. J Bone Joint Surg Br 1982;64:256.
121. Wilkerson RD, Johns JC. Nonunion of an olecranon stress fracture in an adolescent gymnast: a case report. Am J Sports Med 1990;18:432–434.
122. Woods GW, Tullos HS, King JW. The throwing arm: elbow joint injuries. J Sports Med 1973;1:43–47.
123. Wood SK. Reversal of the radial head during reduction of fractures of the neck of the radius in children. J Bone Joint Surg Br 1969;51:707–710.
124. Wray CC, Harper WM. The upside-down radial head: brief report. Injury 1989;20:241–242.
125. Wright PR. Greenstick fracture of the upper end of the ulna with dislocation of the radio-humeral joint or displacement of the superior radial epiphysis. J Bone Joint Surg Br 1963;45:727–731.
126. Zeitlin A. The traumatic origin of accessory bones at the elbow. J Bone Joint Surg 1935;17:933–938.
127. Zimmerman H. Fractures of the elbow. In: Weber BG, Brunner C, Freuler F, eds. Treatment of Fractures in Children and Adolescents. New York: Springer-Verlag, 1980.

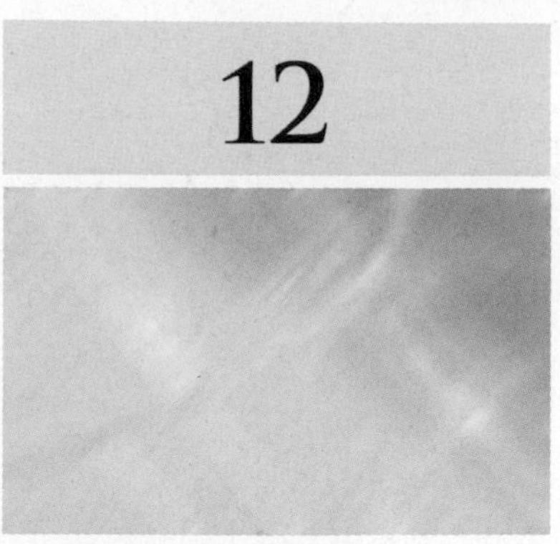

MONTEGGIA FRACTURE-DISLOCATION IN CHILDREN

Peter M. Waters

INTRODUCTION 446

HISTORICAL BACKGROUND 446

CLASSIFICATION 447
BADO CLASSIFICATION: TRUE MONTEGGIA LESIONS 447
MONTEGGIA EQUIVALENT LESIONS 447
LETTS CLASSIFICATION 448

ANATOMY AND BIOMECHANICS 448
LIGAMENTS 448
BONES AND JOINTS 449
MUSCLES 449
NERVES 450

CHARACTERISTICS AND MANAGEMENT OF MONTEGGIA LESIONS 450
TYPE I MONTEGGIA FRACTURE-DISLOCATIONS 450
TYPE II MONTEGGIA FRACTURE-DISLOCATIONS 459
TYPE III MONTEGGIA FRACTURE-DISLOCATIONS 462
TYPE IV MONTEGGIA FRACTURE-DISLOCATIONS 464
MONTEGGIA EQUIVALENT LESIONS 466

COMPLICATIONS 467
CHRONIC MONTEGGIA FRACTURE-DISLOCATIONS 467
NERVE INJURIES 472
ASSOCIATED FRACTURES AND UNUSUAL LESIONS 472

SUMMARY 473

INTRODUCTION

Monteggia fracture-dislocations are a rare but complex injury usually involving a fracture of the ulna and dislocation of the radial head. Unfortunately, despite considerable published awareness of the risk of failure to diagnose this injury,* Monteggia fracture-dislocations are still missed acutely by qualified radiologists, emergency room physicians, and orthopaedic surgeons amongst others. In addition to failure to recognize the injury pattern, undertreatment of unstable, acute injuries has also resulted in chronic Monteggia lesions.[30,34,44,53,59,67,71,74,108,110,111,144] A chronic Monteggia lesion is far more complex in terms of surgical decision making and management than an acute injury.[18,26,29,39,46,57,63,78,113,117]

*References 7,21,28–30,33,34,44,48,51,62,67,75,77,82,83,92,98,108,111,118,121,143.

HISTORICAL BACKGROUND

Giovanni Batista Monteggia, a surgical pathologist and public health official in Milan, Italy, described a variation of the injury in 1814 that now bears his name as "a traumatic lesion distinguished by a fracture of the proximal third of the ulna and an anterior dislocation of the proximal epiphysis of the radius."[106] In 1967, Jose Luis Bado,[8,9] while director of the Orthopedic and Traumatology Institute in Montevideo, Uruguay, published his classic monograph on classification of Monteggia lesions. Bado[8,9] described a Monteggia lesion as a radial head fracture or dislocation in association with a fracture of the middle or proximal ulna. For the last century, numerous authors have made significant contributions on pathoanatomy, classification, diagnosis, treatment, and complications.* Despite these advances, pediatric Monteggia lesions can still be problematic.

*References 18,38,39,44,46,57,75,78,100,111,113,118,121,139,143,147.

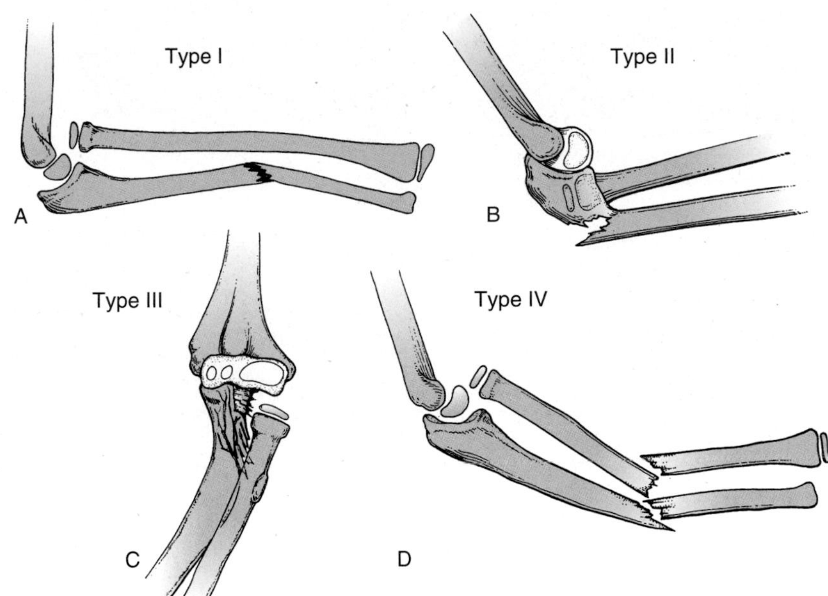

FIGURE 12-1 Bado classification. **A.** Type I (anterior dislocation): the radial head is dislocated anteriorly and the ulna has a short oblique or greenstick fracture in the diaphyseal or proximal metaphyseal area. **B.** Type II (posterior dislocation): the radial head is posteriorly and posterolaterally dislocated; the ulna is usually fractured in the metaphysis in children. **C.** Type III (lateral dislocation): there is lateral dislocation of the radial head with a greenstick metaphyseal fracture of the ulna. **D.** Type IV (anterior dislocation with radius shaft fracture): the pattern of injury is the same as with a type I injury, with the inclusion of a radius shaft fracture below the level of the ulnar fracture.

CLASSIFICATION

Bado's[8,9] original classification has stood the test of time with minimal modifications except additional equivalent lesions (Fig. 12-1). Bado's[8,9] four true Monteggia types are as follows:

Bado Classification: True Monteggia Lesions

Type I

A type I lesion is an anterior dislocation of the radial head associated with an ulnar diaphyseal fracture at any level. This is the most common Monteggia lesion in children.[34,49,75,111]

Type II

A type II lesion is a posterior dislocation of the radial head associated with an ulnar diaphyseal or metaphyseal fracture. This is the most common lesion in adults but very rare in children.[97,98,111]

Type III

A type III lesion is a lateral dislocation of the radial head associated with an ulnar metaphyseal fracture. This is the second most common pediatric Monteggia lesion.[13,44,91,95,143] When associated with an olecranon fracture and a lateral or anterolateral radiocapitellar dislocation but no radioulnar dissociation, the injury is not a true Monteggia lesion.[60,110,134]

Type IV

A type IV lesion is an anterior dislocation of the radial head associated with fractures of *both* the ulna and the radius. The original description was of a radial fracture at the same level or distal to the ulna fracture. This, too, is a relatively rare injury.

Monteggia Equivalent Lesions

Bado[8,9] classified certain injuries as equivalents to his true Monteggia lesions because of their similar mechanisms of injury, radiographic appearance, or treatment methods. Since his publication, the list of equivalent lesions has expanded case report by case report (Fig. 12-2).

Type I Equivalents

Type I equivalents include isolated anterior dislocations of the radial head without ulnar fracture. This subclassification includes a "pulled elbow" or "nursemaid's elbow" because the mechanism of longitudinal traction, pronation, and hyperextension is similar to a true type I Monteggia lesion. In this situation, the radiographs are normal. In addition, an isolated anterior dislocation of the radial head without ulnar fracture is a type I equivalent. The ulnar bow sign (Fig. 12-3) is normal. Subtle plastic deformation of the ulna will have a concave ulnar bow and could be misdiagnosed as an equivalent lesion when it is really a true type I lesion. This distinction can be critical in terms of operative decisions in that the rare but true type I equivalent lesion requires only open repair of the displaced ligament while the type I lesion with plastic deformation requires correction of the ulnar deformity. Other type I equivalencies described thus far include: anterior dislocation of the radial head with ulnar diaphyseal and radial neck fractures, anterior dislocation of the radial head with radial diaphyseal fracture more proximal to ulnar diaphyseal fracture, anterior radial head dislocation with ulnotrochlear dislocation (Fig. 12-4),[111] and anterior dislocation of the radial head with segmental ulna fracture.[2,49,60,102,115,134] More case reports will probably expand this subclassification. The type I equivalent lesions have been shown to have poorer outcomes and require more operative interventions than other Monteggia lesions.[49,91]

Type II Equivalents

Bado[8,9] described type II equivalents to include fractures of the proximal radial epiphysis or radial neck.

Type III and Type IV Equivalents

Bado[8,9] did not have equivalent lesions for his type III and type IV true Monteggia lesions. Since mechanism of injury allows

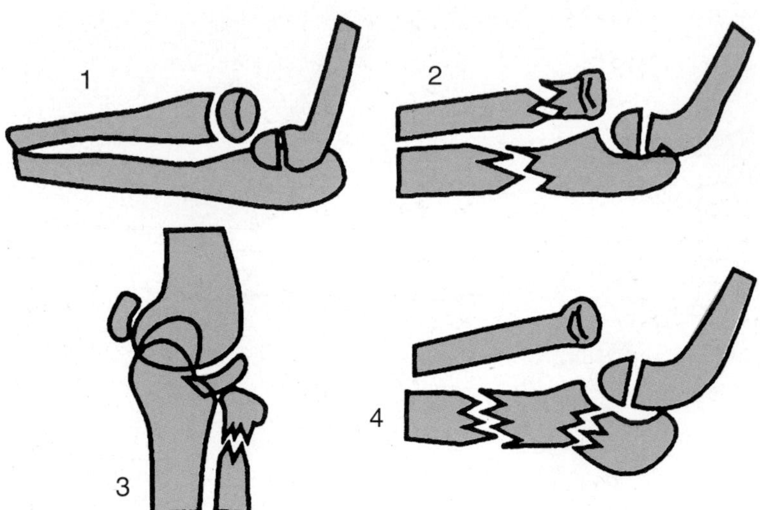

FIGURE 12-2 Type I Monteggia equivalents. **I.** Isolated anterior radial head dislocation. **II.** Ulnar fracture with fracture of the radial neck. **III.** Isolated radial neck fractures. **IV.** Elbow (ulnohumeral) dislocation with or without fracture of the proximal radius.

for subclassification, case reports have emerged over time to include fractures of the distal humerus (supracondylar, lateral condylar) in association with proximal forearm fractures (Fig. 12-5).*

Letts Classification

Letts et al.[75] classified pediatric Monteggia fracture-dislocations both on direction of radial head dislocation and type of ulnar fracture. Letts types A, B, and C were various ulnar fractures associated with anterior dislocation of the radial head, or Bado type I injuries. A type A is a plastic deformation fracture; a type B is an incomplete or greenstick fracture; a type C is a complete fracture of the ulna. Type D injuries were the same as Bado II or posterior radial head dislocation, and type E the same as Bado III or lateral radial head dislocations (Fig. 12-6).

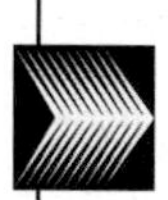

AUTHORS' PREFERRED CLASSIFICATION

Ring, Jupiter, and Waters[110,111] defined a Monteggia lesion as a proximal radioulnar joint dislocation in association with a forearm fracture. It is the character of the ulnar fracture, more so than the direction of the radial head dislocation, that is most useful in determining the optimal treatment of Monteggia fracture-dislocations in both adults and children. Stable anatomic reduction of the ulnar fracture almost always results in anatomic, stable reduction of the proximal radius, proximal radioulnar joint, and radiocapitellar joint in the acute setting. The ulnar fracture is defined similarly to all pediatric forearm fractures: plastic deformation, incomplete or greenstick fractures, and complete fractures. Complete fractures are further subdivided into transverse, short oblique, long oblique, and comminuted fractures. Treatment directly relates to the fracture type: closed reduction for plastic deformation and greenstick fractures, intramedullary fixation for transverse and short oblique fractures, and open reduction and internal fixation with plate and screws for long oblique and comminuted fractures (Table 12-1).

*References 16,17,32,42,47,49,50,80,88,102,107,112,115,119.

ANATOMY AND BIOMECHANICS

Understanding the anatomy of the proximal radioulnar joint, radiocapitellar joint, and proximal forearm is critical to understanding the treatment of acute and chronic Monteggia lesions. The ligaments, bony architecture, and joint contours provide stability to the proximal forearm and elbow. The muscle insertions and origins affect stability and determine surgical exposure along with neighboring neurovascular structures.

Ligaments

Annular Ligament

The annular ligament is one of the prime stabilizers of the proximal radioulnar joint during forearm rotation. It surrounds the radial neck from its origin and insertion on the proximal ulna (Fig. 12-7). Due to the shape of the radial head, it tightens in supination. It is part of the lateral collateral ligamentous complex that stabilizes the distal humerus and proximal forearm. Displacement of the annular ligament occurs in a Monteggia lesion.

Quadrate Ligament

The quadrate ligament[31,64] is just distal to the annular ligament and connects the proximal radius and ulna (see Fig. 12-7). It has a dense anterior portion, thinner posterior portion, and even

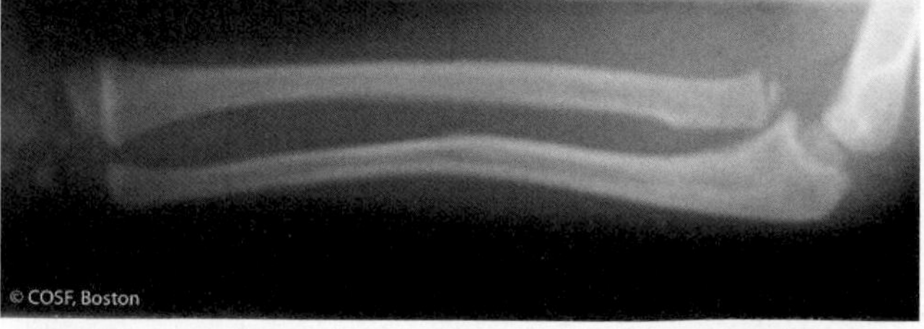

FIGURE 12-3 The ulnar bow line. This line, drawn between the distal ulna and the olecranon, defines the ulna bow. The ulnar bow sign is deviation of the ulnar border from the reference line of more than 1 mm.

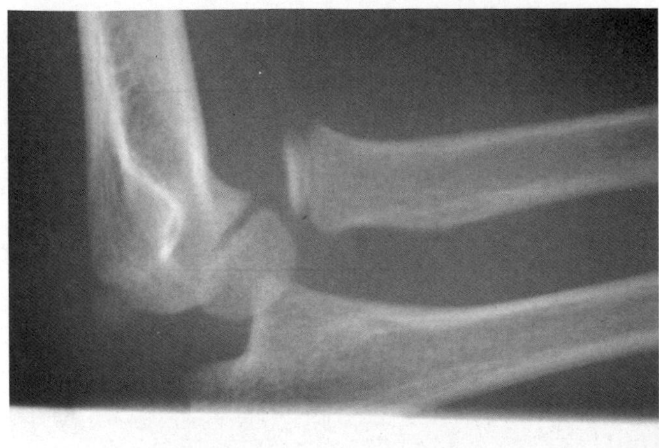

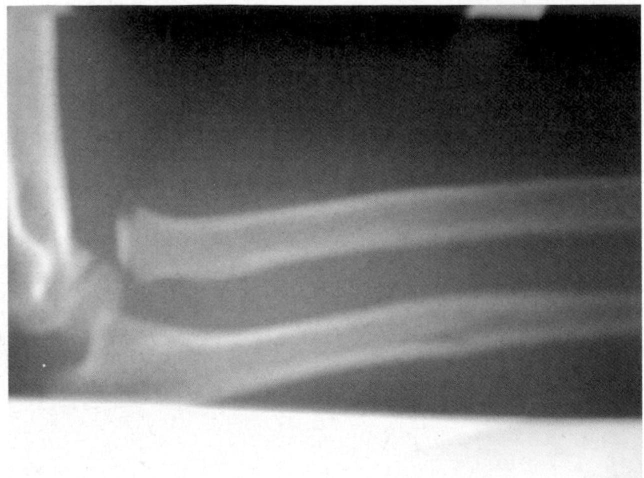

FIGURE 12-4 Type I Monteggia equivalent that includes elbow subluxation in addition to the radioulnar dislocation.

thinner central portion. The quadrate ligament also provides stability to the proximal radioulnar joint during forearm rotation. The anterior and posterior borders become taut at the extremes of supination and pronation respectively.

Oblique Ligament

The oblique ligament extends from the ulna proximally to the radius distally (Fig. 12-8). The origin of the oblique ligament is just distal to the radial notch of the ulna, and its insertion is just distal to the bicipital tuberosity of the radius. With supination, the oblique ligament tightens and provides further stability to the proximal radioulnar joint.

Interosseous Ligament

The interosseous ligament is distal to the oblique ligament with its fibers running in the opposite direction (from radius proximally to ulna distally) to the oblique ligament (see Fig. 12-8). However, similar to the oblique ligament, it tightens in supination and provides further stability to the proximal radioulnar joint.

Monteggia Equivalents

Type III

Type IV

FIGURE 12-5 Type III equivalent described by Ravessoud[107]: an oblique fracture of the ulna with varus alignment and a displaced lateral condylar fracture. Type IV equivalent described by Arazi[5]: fractures of the distal humerus, ulnar diaphysis, and radial neck.

Bones and Joints

The bony architecture provides little inherent stability to the proximal radioulnar joint.

Radius

The shape of the radial head is elliptical in cross section (Fig. 12-9). In supination, the long axis of the ellipse is perpendicular to the proximal ulna, causing the annular ligament and the anterior portion of the quadrate ligament to tighten and stabilize the proximal radioulnar joint. In addition, the contact area between the radius and the radial notch of the ulna increases in supination due to the broadened surface of the elliptical radial head proximal to distal in that position. This may provide some additional stability.

The radius "radiates" around the ulna. It must have an anatomic bow in order to achieve full forearm rotation while maintaining stability in the proximal and distal radioulnar joints (see Fig. 12-9). With the radius in supination, the bow tightens the oblique and interosseous ligaments, thereby increasing proximal radioulnar joint stability.

Muscles

Biceps

The biceps inserts into the bicipital tuberosity of the radius and acts as both a flexor of the elbow and supinator of the forearm. It is a deforming force in anterior Monteggia fracture-dislocations, pulling the radius anteriorly as the elbow is forcibly extended. In treatment, care is taken to maintain the elbow in flexion to prevent recurrent anterior subluxation of the radial head while the soft tissues heal.

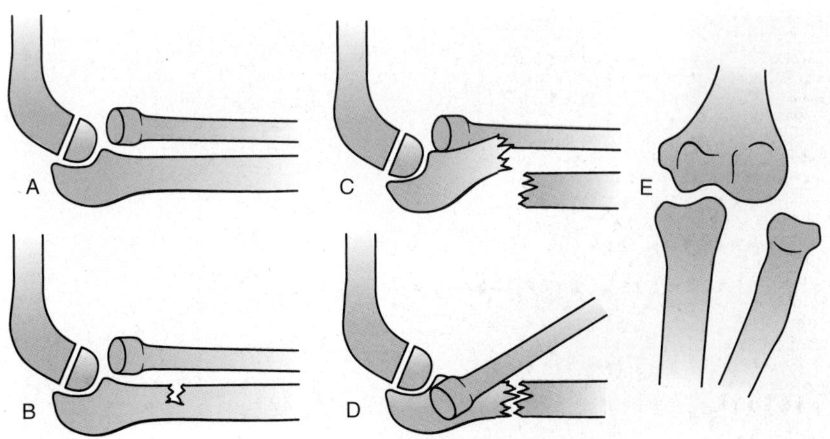

FIGURE 12-6 Pediatric Monteggia fracture classification by Letts et al.[75] **A.** Anterior dislocation of the radial head with plastic deformation of the ulna. **B.** Anterior dislocation of the radial head with greenstick fracture of the ulna. **C.** Complete fracture of the ulna with anterior dislocation of the radial head. **D.** Posterior dislocation of the radial head with fracture of the ulnar metaphysis. **E.** Lateral dislocation of the radial head and metaphyseal greenstick fracture of the ulna.

Anconeus

The anconeus may act as a dynamic stabilizer of the elbow joint by providing a valgus moment at the joint during extension and pronation.[11,139] It may also act as a deforming force, along with the forearm flexors, on complete fractures of the ulna in a Monteggia lesion. Surgical exposure of the proximal radioulnar and radiocapitellar joints is usually through the anconeus-extensor carpi ulnaris interval.

Nerves

Posterior Interosseous Branch of the Radial Nerve

The radial nerve passes the distal humerus in the brachialis-brachioradialis interval (Fig. 12-10). As it descends into the forearm, it divides into the radial sensory nerve and the posterior interosseous motor branch. The posterior interosseous nerve passes between the two heads of the supinator, when present, or beneath the supinator when there is only one head of supinator. Its close proximity to the proximal radial head and neck makes it susceptible to injury with Monteggia lesions.[67] In chronic Monteggia situations, the posterior interosseous nerve can become adherent to the dislocated head or, less commonly, entrapped in the joint.[113] Care must be taken with the nerve in surgical reconstructions of the chronic anterior dislocation.

TABLE 12-1 Author's Classification of Monteggia Fracture-Dislocations

Type	Dislocation	Fracture
True lesions		
I	Anterior	Metaphysis-diaphysis
II	Posterior	Metaphysis-diaphysis
III	Lateral	Metaphysis
IV	Anterior	Radial diaphysis, ulnar diaphysis
Hybrid lesion	Anterior, posterior, or lateral	Metaphysis or olecranon

Type	Description
Equivalent lesions	
I	Isolated dislocation of radial head
	Radial neck fracture (isolated)
	Radial neck fracture in combination with a fracture of the ulnar diaphysis
	Radial and ulnar fractures with the radial fracture above the junction of the middle and proximal thirds
	Fracture of ulnar diaphysis with anterior dislocation of radial head and an olecranon fracture
II	Posterior dislocation of the elbow
III	Ulnar fracture with displaced fracture of the lateral condyle
IV	None described

Ulnar Nerve

The ulnar nerve passes posterior to the medial intermuscular septum of the humerus, through the cubital tunnel behind the medial epicondyle, and then through the flexor carpi ulnaris into the forearm. It is at risk for injury with type II laterally displaced Monteggia lesions and with ulnar lengthening in chronic Monteggia reconstructions.

CHARACTERISTICS AND MANAGEMENT OF MONTEGGIA LESIONS

Type I Monteggia Fracture-Dislocations

Clinical Findings

Bado,[8,9] in his original description, provided an accurate clinical picture of Monteggia fracture-dislocations. In general, there is

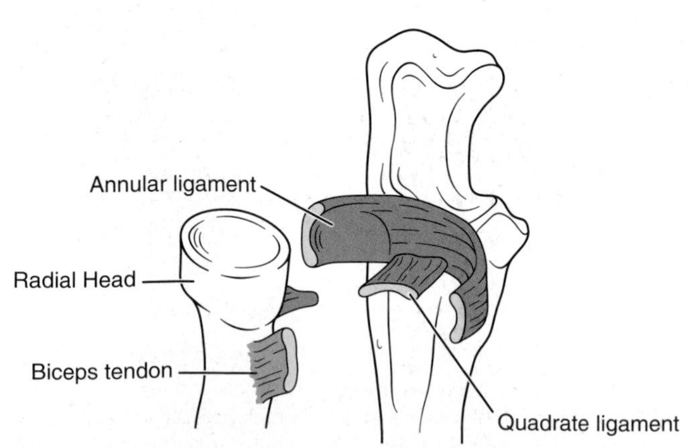

FIGURE 12-7 Ligamentous anatomy of the proximal radioulnar joint.

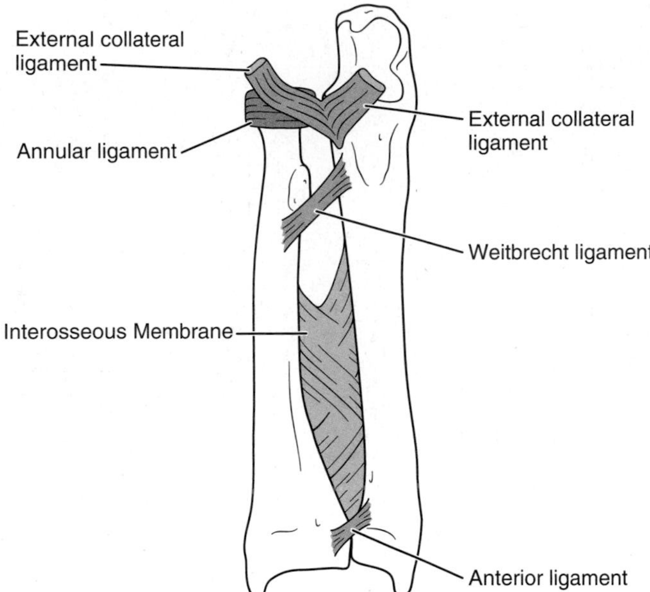

FIGURE 12-8 Ligaments of the forearm. In supination, the annular ligament, quadrate ligament, oblique ligament, and interosseous membrane are taut, stabilizing the radial head.

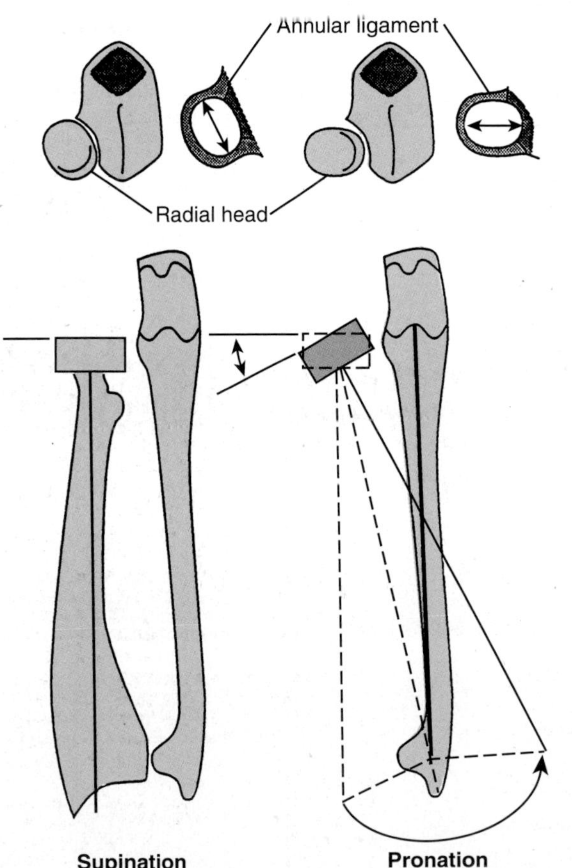

FIGURE 12-9 The radial head is an elliptical structure secured by the annular ligament, which allows movement and gives stability. Because of the shape of the radial head, the stability provided by the annular ligament is maximized in supination.

fusiform swelling about the elbow. The child has significant pain and has limitations of elbow motion in flexion and extension as well as pronation and supination. Usually, an angular change in the forearm itself is evident, with the apex shifted anteriorly and mild valgus apparent. There may be tenting of the skin or an area of ecchymosis on the volar aspect of the forearm. It is imperative to check for an open fracture wound. The child may not be able to extend the digits at the metacarpophalangeal joint or at the interphalangeal joint of the thumb because of a paresis of the posterior interosseous nerve. Later, as the swelling subsides, anterior fullness may remain in the cubital fossa for the typical Bado type I anterior dislocation. However, this may be subtle since children will usually have an elbow flexion posture postinjury. If the injury is seen late, there will be a loss of full flexion at the elbow and a palpable anterior dislocation of the radial head. The radial head-distal humerus impingement that occurs may be a source of pain with activities. There is usually loss of forearm rotation with late presentation. Progressive valgus may occur if the anterior radial head dislocation worsens. Lateral dislocations will generally have a varus bow to the forearm both with acute and chronic presentations. The laterally displaced radial head will be visible and palpable.

Radiographic Evaluation

The standard evaluation of a type I Monteggia fracture includes anteroposterior (AP) and lateral radiographs of the forearm. Any disruption of the ulna, including subtle changes in ulnar bowing, should alert the clinician to look for joint disruption at either end of the forearm.[27,28,65,67,77] Unfortunately, the dislocated radial head is all too often missed in the acute setting.

The radiographic alignment of the radial head and capitellum is particularly important and is best defined by a true lateral view of the elbow. In a type I Monteggia fracture-dislocation, the radiocapitellar relationship may appear normal on an AP radiograph despite obvious disruption on the lateral view (Fig. 12-11). If there is doubt regarding the radiocapitellar alignment, further radiographic evaluation must be obtained. Smith[118] and later Storen[128] noted that a line drawn through the center of the radial neck and head should extend directly through the center of the capitellum. This alignment should remain intact regardless of the degree of flexion or extension of the elbow (Fig. 12-12). In some instances, there is disruption of the radiocapitellar line in a normal elbow. Miles and Finlay[84] pointed out that the radiocapitellar line passes through the center of the capitellum only on a true lateral projection. They reported five patients in whom the elbow was clinically normal but the radiocapitellar line appeared disrupted. In analyzing the radiographs, they found that the radiographic projection of the elbow was usually an oblique view or that the forearm was pronated in the radiograph. If this disruption appears on radiographs in a child with an acute injury, however, it is the treating surgeon's responsibility to ensure that it is an insignificant finding. As Dr. John Hall[55] often said, "Monteggia lesions are not like throwing horse shoes; being close does not count." It is still too frequent an occurrence that a highly qualified, distraught, orthopaedic surgeon will call for referral of a chronic Monteggia lesion that was missed acutely.

With late presentation of a chronic Monteggia injury, a magnetic resonance imaging (MRI) scan may be useful to determine the congruency of the radial head and capitellum. If the radial head is no longer centrally concave or the capitellum is no

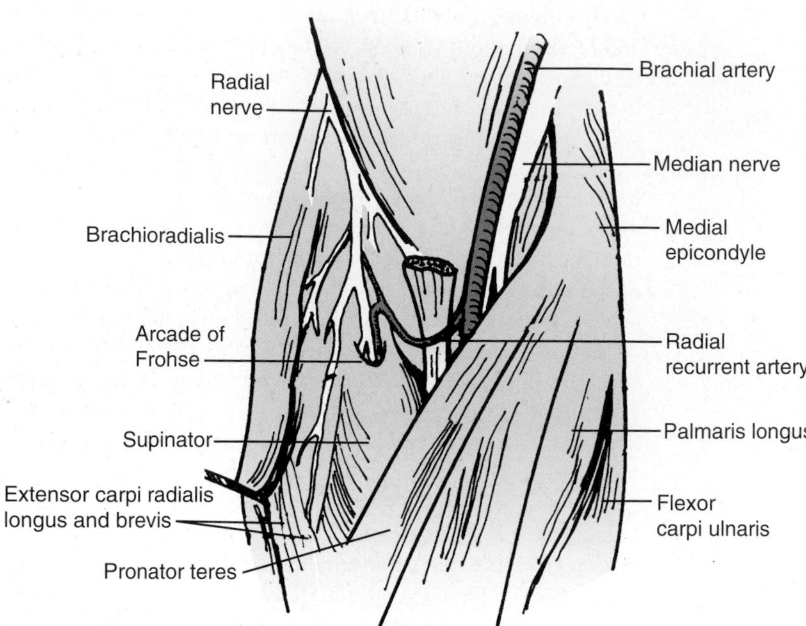

FIGURE 12-10 Dissection of the forearm at the level of the elbow.

longer symmetrically convex, surgical reduction may fail or produce pain and limited motion.

Traumatic versus Congenital Dislocation. When the radiocapitellar relation is disrupted radiographically, evaluation of the shape of the radial head and neck helps determine the cause of the disruption, especially if there is no history of trauma or the significance of the trauma is questioned. Bucknill[23] suggested that McFarland's[81] classic description of congenital radial head dislocation with an atypical deformed radial head, dysplastic capitellum, concavity of the posterior border of the proximal ulna, and periarticular ossifications probably represented old traumatic dislocations. Lloyd-Roberts and Bucknill[78] noted that many unilateral anterior dislocations were most likely old traumatic dislocations rather than congenital dislocations. Caravias[24] recognized that the existence of a congenital anterior dislocation as a separate entity was doubtful and that true anterior congenital dislocation of the radial head was rare. True congenital dislocations are usually posterior, may be bilateral, and can be associated with various syndromes such as Ehlers-Danlos, nail-patella, and Silver syndromes (Fig. 12-13).[3,78] Therefore, all isolated anterior and anterolateral dislocations of the radial head, regardless of symptoms, should be suspected as having a traumatic origin unless there is evidence of congenital or systemic differences, such as proximal radioulnar synostosis.

Mechanism of Injury

Three separate mechanisms of type I lesions have been described: direct trauma,[9,22,25,38,89,105,108,121,139] hyperpronation, and hyperextension.[22,108]

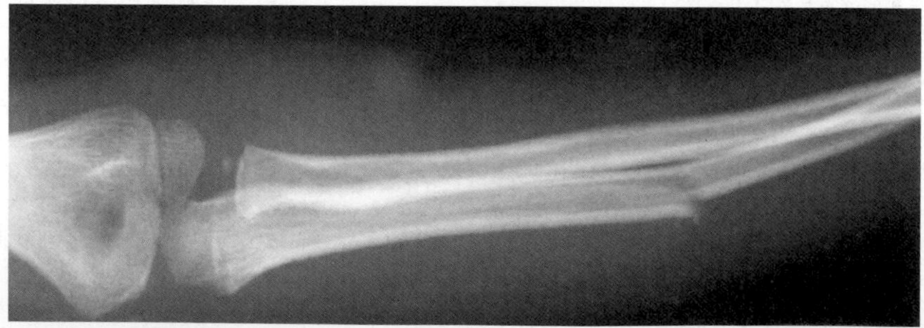

FIGURE 12-11 The AP view **(A)** demonstrates an apparently located radial head, but the lateral view **(B)** shows an anterior dislocation of the radial head. Note the disruption of the radiocapitellar line.

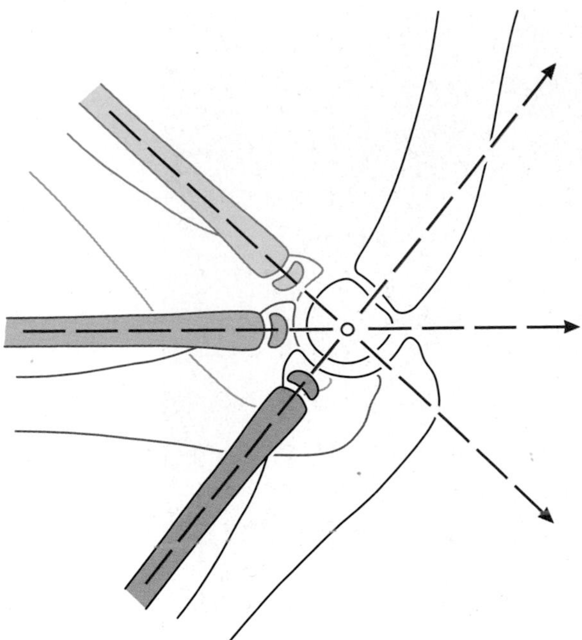

FIGURE 12-12 Composite drawing with the elbow in various degrees of flexion. A line drawn down the long axis of the radius bisects the capitellum of the humerus regardless of the degree of flexion or extension of the elbow.

Direct Blow Theory. The first theory proposed in English literature was the direct blow mechanism described by Speed and Boyd[121] and endorsed by Smith (Fig. 12-11).[118] This theory was actually proposed by Monteggia,[85] who noted that the fracture occurs when a direct blow on the posterior aspect of the forearm first produces a fracture through the ulna. Then, either by continued deformation or direct pressure, the radial head is forced anteriorly with respect to the capitellum, causing the radial head to dislocate. Monteggia[99] explained that these injuries sometimes resulted from a blow by a staff or cudgel on the forearm raised to protect the head.

The parry fracture, another eponym for the Monteggia fracture-dislocation, has been mentioned in the literature. During the American Civil War, Monteggia fractures were frequent because of direct blows on the forearm received while attempting to parry the butt of a rifle during hand-to-hand combat. The major argument against this theory as the mechanism is that in the usual clinical situation there rarely is evidence of a direct blow to the posterior aspect of the forearm, such as a contusion or laceration.[38,139]

Hyperpronation Theory. In 1949, Evans[38] published his observations regarding anterior Monteggia fractures. Previous investigators had based their direct blow theory on hypothesis and clinical observation, but Evans[38] used cadaver experiments to support his hypothesis. He demonstrated that hyperpronation of the forearm produced a fracture of the ulna with a subsequent dislocation of the radial head. He postulated that during a fall, the outstretched hand, initially in pronation, is forced into further pronation as the body twists above the planted hand and forearm (Fig. 12-15). This hyperpronation causes the radius to be crossed over the midulna, resulting in anterior dislocation of the radial head or fracture of the proximal third of the radius along with fracture of the ulna. In the patients reported in Evans'[38] article, the ulnar fractures demonstrated a pattern consistent with anterior tension and shear or longitudinal compression. His cadaver studies, however, showed the ulna fracture pattern to be consistent with a spiral or torsional force. This theory was also supported by Bado.[10]

Two arguments have been used to dispute the hyperpronation mechanism.[139] First, the ulnar fracture rarely presents clinically in a spiral pattern; it is often oblique, indicating an initial force in tension with propagation in shear rather than rotation. Second, Evans'[38] experiments, which were done on totally dissected forearms, did not take into consideration the dynamic muscle forces at play during a fall on an outstretched hand.

Hyperextension Theory. In 1971, Tompkins[139] analyzed both theories and presented good clinical evidence that type I Monteggia fractures were caused by a combination of dynamic and static forces. His study postulated three steps in the fracture mechanism: hyperextension, radial head dislocation, and ulnar fracture (Fig. 12-16). The patient falls on an outstretched arm with forward momentum, forcing the elbow joint into hyperextension. The radius is first dislocated anteriorly by the violent reflexive contracture of the biceps, forcing the radius away from the capitellum. Once the proximal radius dislocates, the weight of the body is transferred to the ulna. Because the radius is usually the main load-bearing bone in the forearm, the ulna cannot handle the transmitted longitudinal force and weight and, subsequently, fails in tension. This tension force produces an oblique fracture line or a greenstick fracture in the ulnar diaphysis or diaphyseal–metaphyseal junction. In addition to the momentum of the injury, the anterior angulation of the ulna results from the pull of the intact interosseous membrane on the distal fragment, causing it to follow the radius. The brachialis muscle causes the proximal ulnar fragment to flex at the elbow.

Summary of Mechanisms of Injury

The Monteggia lesion can probably be caused by any of the three proposed mechanisms, but the most common mechanism is a fall on an outstretched hand that forces the elbow into complete extension, locking the olecranon into the humerus. The forearm is in a rotational position of neutral to midpronation. As the proximal ulna locks into the distal humerus, the bending force stresses the proximal radioulnar joint. Because of the relatively pronated position of the joint, the ligamentous restraints are lax, providing only tenuous stability for the radial head. The anterior bending force, combined with a reflexive contraction of the biceps, violently dislocates the radial head anteriorly. The radioulnar joint and its ligamentous complex are at risk because of the ligamentous laxity and the decreased contact area between the proximal radius and ulna created by the rotation of the forearm. At midrotation, the short axis of the elliptical radial head is perpendicular to the ulna, causing the annular ligament and the dense anterior portion of the quadrate ligament to be relaxed. The contact area of the proximal radioulnar joint, because of the shape of the radial head, is also decreased, further reducing the stability of the joint. The ulna, now the main weight-bearing structure of the forearm, is loaded by a continued bending moment, causing tension on the anterior cortex and producing failure. The force at the site of failure is propagated in shear at approximately 45 degrees to the long

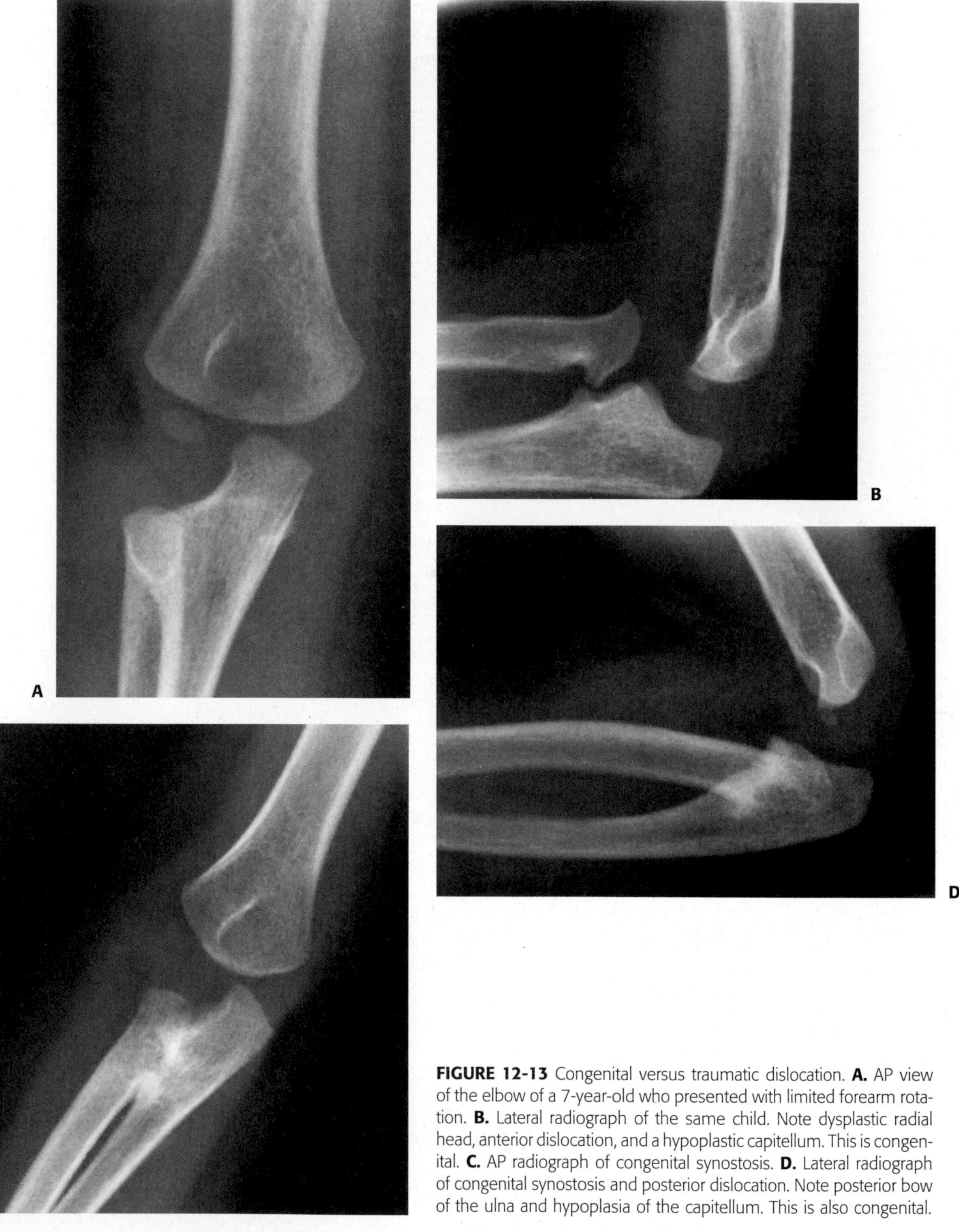

FIGURE 12-13 Congenital versus traumatic dislocation. **A.** AP view of the elbow of a 7-year-old who presented with limited forearm rotation. **B.** Lateral radiograph of the same child. Note dysplastic radial head, anterior dislocation, and a hypoplastic capitellum. This is congenital. **C.** AP radiograph of congenital synostosis. **D.** Lateral radiograph of congenital synostosis and posterior dislocation. Note posterior bow of the ulna and hypoplasia of the capitellum. This is also congenital.

axis of the ulna. This mechanism may produce plastic deformation with an anterior bow, a greenstick fracture, or an oblique fracture pattern, all of which are seen clinically. As the anterior bending movement continues, the vector of the biceps changes and acts as a tether and resists any further advance of the proximal radius. The distal fragment of the ulna continues to advance, acting as a fulcrum against the radial shaft. The anteriorly directed force of the distal ulnar fragment, combined with the retrograde resistance of the biceps, may create a fracture of the radius, or a type IV Monteggia lesion.

Treatment

Although most treatment recommendations are based on the Bado classification, Ring and Waters[111] based their treatment choices on the type of ulnar fracture rather than on the Bado type. Plastic deformation of the ulna is treated with closed reduction of the ulnar bow to obtain stable reduction of the radioulnar joint. Incomplete (greenstick or buckle) fractures of the ulna are similarly treated with closed reduction and casting. Most Monteggia injuries that are plastic deformation or greenstick fractures in children are stable when immobilized in 100

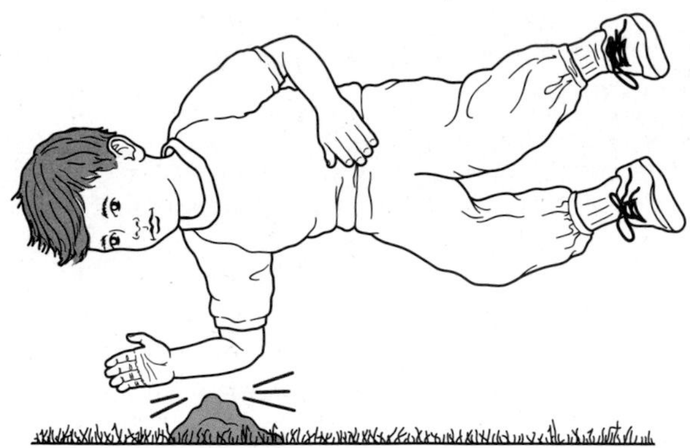

FIGURE 12-14 The fracture-dislocation is sustained by direct contact on the posterior aspect of the forearm, either by falling onto an object or by the object striking the forearm. The continued motion of the object forward dislocates the radial head after fracturing the ulna.

to 110 degrees of flexion and full supination. In all series,[4,9,21,22,34,44,75,91,108,113,118,143] anterior Monteggia lesions in children have uniformly good results when treated by manipulative closed reduction, if the radial head is properly aligned and the ulna fracture is reduced with length preserved. These results most clearly apply to plastic deformation and incomplete fractures, which make up the majority of anterior Monteggia lesions. However, complete fractures can be unstable after closed reduction. Therefore, with complete short oblique and transverse ulna fractures or ones associated with a radial fracture (type IV), intramedullary Kirschner wire (K-wire) fixation is recommended. At times, this may involve use of the intramedullary K wire in the proximal fragment to joystick the reduction under fluoroscopic guidance. Long oblique or comminuted fractures, which may develop shortening and malalignment even with intramedullary fixation, are best stabilized with plate and screw fixation. Using this treatment protocol, Ring and Waters[111] reported excellent results in all 28 patients treated within 24 hours of injury (Table 12-2). Poor results occurred in two patients who were referred late with persistent radial head dislocations.

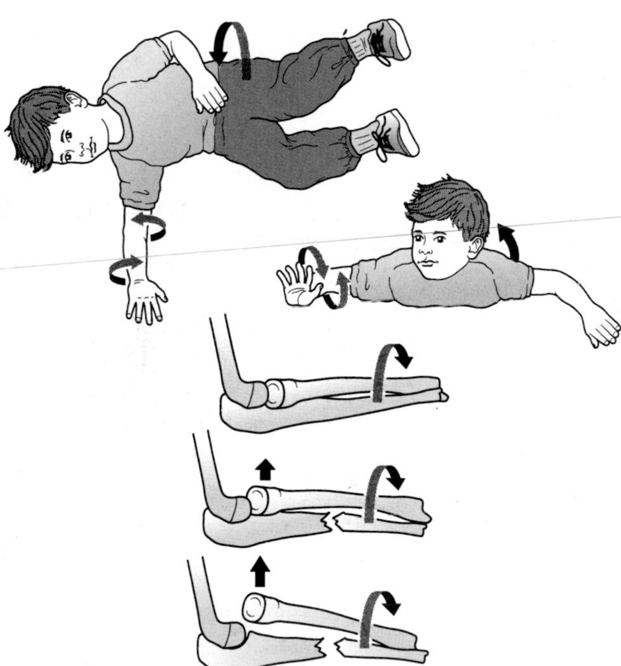

FIGURE 12-15 Hyperpronation theory (Evans).[38] Rotation of the body externally forces the forearm into pronation. The ulnar shaft fractures with further rotation, forcibly dislocating the radial head.

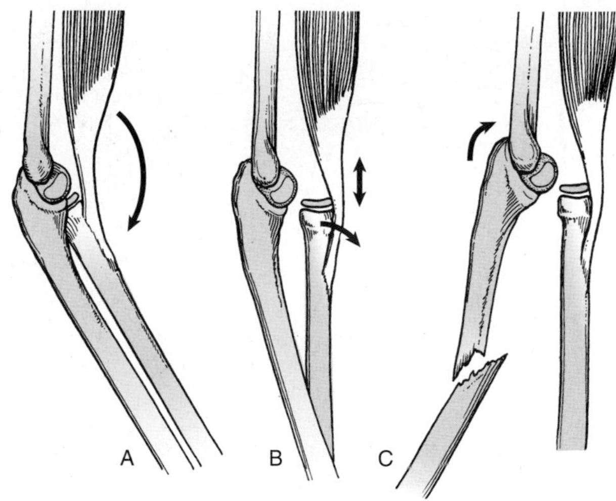

FIGURE 12-16 Hyperextension theory. **A.** Hyperextension: forward momentum caused by a fall on an outstretched hand forces the elbow into extension. **B.** Radial head dislocation: the biceps contracts, forcibly dislocating the radial head. **C.** Ulnar fracture: forward momentum causes the ulna to fracture because of tension on the anterior surface.

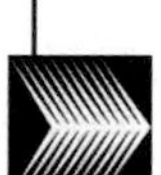

AUTHORS' PREFERRED TREATMENT

As noted above, successful treatment is dependent on three steps: correcting the ulnar deformity, providing a stable reduction of the radial head, and maintaining ulnar length and fracture stability (Fig. 12-17). For plastic deformation and incomplete fractures, this can usually be achieved with closed reduction and cast immobilization. For complete fractures, fracture instability after closed reduction may lead to

TABLE 12-2 Treatment of Monteggia Fracture-Dislocations in Children According to Ulnar Injury

Type of Ulnar Injury	Treatment
Plastic deformation	Closed reduction of the ulnar bow and cast immobilization
Incomplete (greenstick or buckle) fracture	Closed reduction and cast immobilization
Complete transverse or short oblique fracture	Closed reduction and intramedullary K-wire fixation
Long oblique or comminuted fracture	Open reduction and internal fixation with plate and screws

From Ring D, Jupiter JB, Waters PM. Monteggia fractures in children and adults. J Am Acad Orthop Surg 1998;6:215–224, with permission.

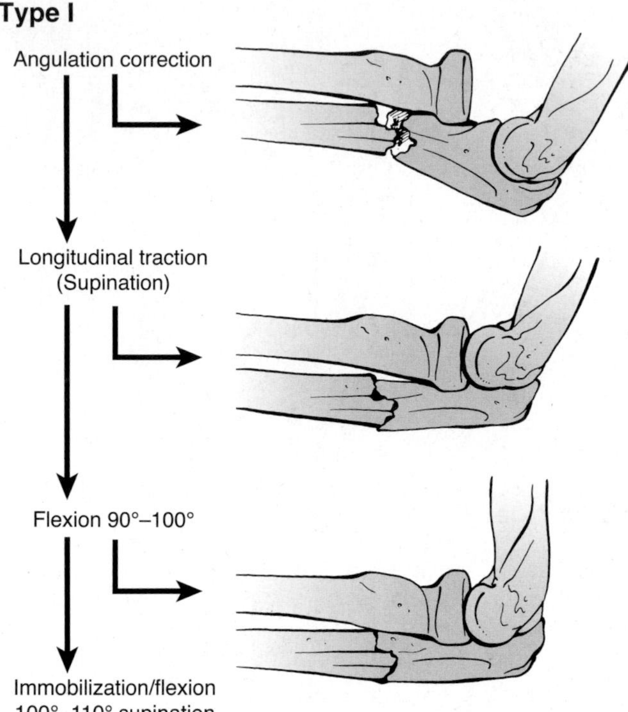

FIGURE 12-17 Reduction of a type I Monteggia fracture-dislocation.

loss of anatomic ulnar length and redislocation of the radial head.

Closed Reduction and Cast Immobilization.

Reduction of the Ulnar Fracture. The first step is to reestablish the length of the ulna by longitudinal traction and manual correction of any angular deformity. The forearm is held in relaxed supination as longitudinal traction is applied with manual pressure directed over the apex of the deformity until the malangulation is corrected clinically and radiographically (Fig. 12-18). With plastic deformation fractures, this may necessitate significant force that requires general anesthesia. With greenstick fractures, the correction of the ulnar deformity and radial head reduction can often be achieved with conscious sedation in the emergency room.

Some papers have cited successful treatment of acute Monteggia lesions (defined as maintenance of the radial head reduction) with nonanatomic alignment of the ulnar fracture (Fig. 12-19).[44,103,105] However, anatomic reduction and healing of the ulna fracture is strongly advocated.

Reduction of the Radial Head. Once ulnar length and alignment have been reestablished, the radial head can be relocated. This is often accomplished by simply flexing the elbow to 90 degrees or more, thus producing spontaneous reduction (see Fig. 12-19). Occasionally, posteriorly directed pressure over the anterior aspect of the radial head is necessary for reduction of the radial head. Flexion of the elbow to 110 to 120 degrees stabilizes the reduction. Once the radial head position is established, it should be scrutinized radiographically in numerous views to ensure a concentric reduction. With a type I fracture, the optimal radiographic view is a true lateral of the elbow with the forearm held in supination. The longitudinal axis of the radius should pass directly through the center of the capitellum (Fig. 12-20).

Alleviation of Deforming Forces. Once the concentric reduction of the radial head is confirmed, the elbow should be placed at approximately 110 to 120 degrees of flexion to alleviate the force of the biceps, which could redislocate the radial head (see Figs. 12-20 and 12-21). The forearm is placed in a position of midsupination to neutral rotation to alleviate the forces of the supinator muscle and the anconeus, as well as the forearm flexors, which tend to produce radial angulation of the ulna.

Immobilization. Once the fracture is reduced and the neutralization position is established, a molded long-arm splint or cast is applied to hold the elbow joint in the appropriate amount of flexion, usually 110 to 120 degrees. Once the cast is completed, careful radiographic assessment should establish the concentric reduction of the radial head with respect to the capitellum, as well as satisfactory alignment of the ulna.

Postreduction Care. The patient is followed at 7 to 10 day intervals to confirm continued satisfactory reduction by radiography. At 4 to 6 weeks after the initial reduction, if there is radiographic evidence of consolidation of the ulnar fracture and stability of the radial head, the long-arm cast can be removed, with progressive guarded return to full activity.

Operative Treatment.

Indications. There are two indications for operative treatment of type I fracture-dislocations: failure to obtain and maintain ulnar fracture reduction and failure of radial head reduction. The fractures most at risk are complete ulnar fractures. On rare occasions, there will be an entrapped annular ligament that prevents anatomic radial head reduction.

Failure of Ulnar Reduction. If the ulnar fracture cannot be reduced or held in satisfactory alignment by closed treatment, operative intervention is indicated. The quality of the ulnar reduction affects the ability to reduce the radial head, which is of primary importance. If the ulnar fracture can be reduced but not maintained because of the obliquity of the fracture, internal fixation is indicated.[44,91] Intramedullary fixation is standard in most series of Monteggia fracture-dislocations in children (Fig. 12-22).[8,9,34,43,44,72,74,79,91,104,111,114,128,143] This method of fixation can be accomplished percutaneously, using image intensification and flexible nails or K-wires. Entry can be through the apophysis or proximal metaphysis of the ulna, depending on the level of the fracture and surgeon's preference. Intramedullary fixation is preferred for transverse and short oblique fractures. Long oblique and comminuted fractures may redisplace even with intramedullary fixation. Plate and screw fixation is preferred with these rarer fractures.[74,96,101,136,140,145]

Failure of Radial Head Reduction. The second indication is failure to reduce the radial head satisfactorily by closed means. This is more common in type III Monteggia lesions, but it can also occur in type I lesions. It results from soft tissue interposition, including entrapped capsule or an orbicular ligament pulled over the radial head.[139,145] Interposed cartilaginous or

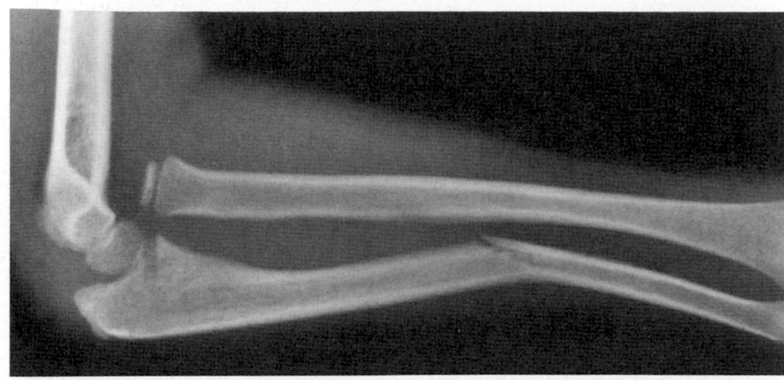
A

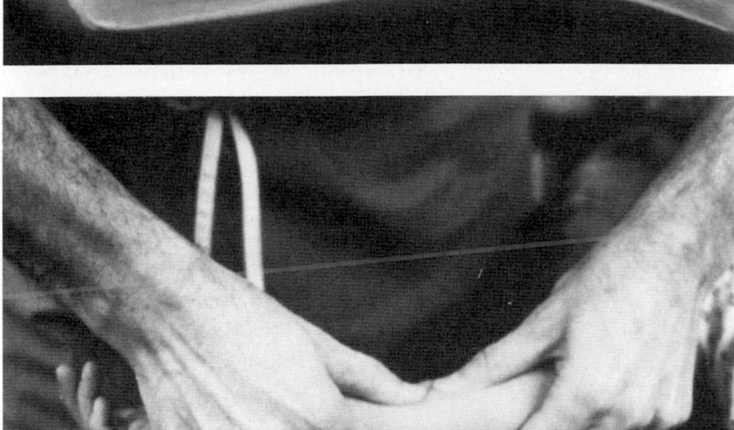
B

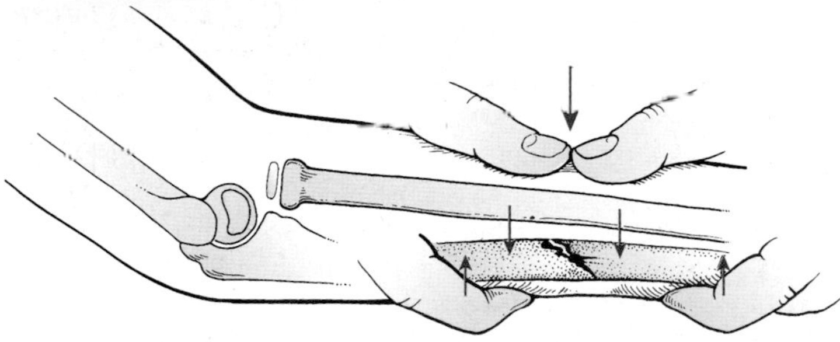
C

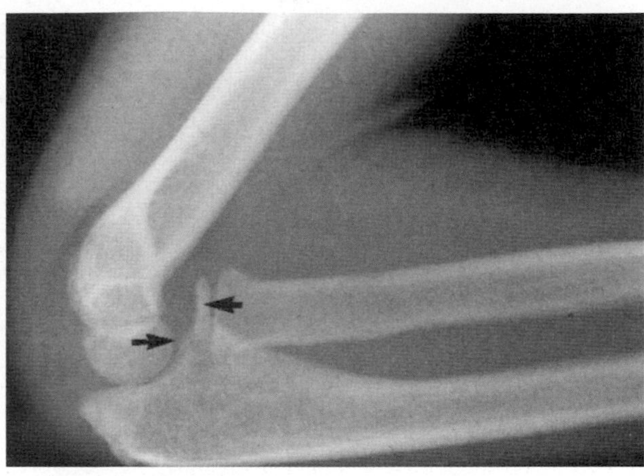
D

FIGURE 12-18 Closed reduction, type I lesion. **A.** Typical type I lesion in a 7-year-old. **B.** Correction of plastic deformation. Plastic deformation of the ulna must be corrected to prevent recurrence of the angular deformity. **C.** This allows reduction of the radial head and prevents its late subluxation. (From Wilkins KE, ed. Operative Management of Upper Extremity Fractures in Children. Rosemont, IL: American Academy of Orthopaedic Surgeons, 1994, with permission.) **D.** The deformity of the ulna is corrected first, and then the elbow is hyperflexed. However, the radial head is still anteriorly subluxed (*arrows*), and the ulna still has some anterior plastic deformation. This is not acceptable.

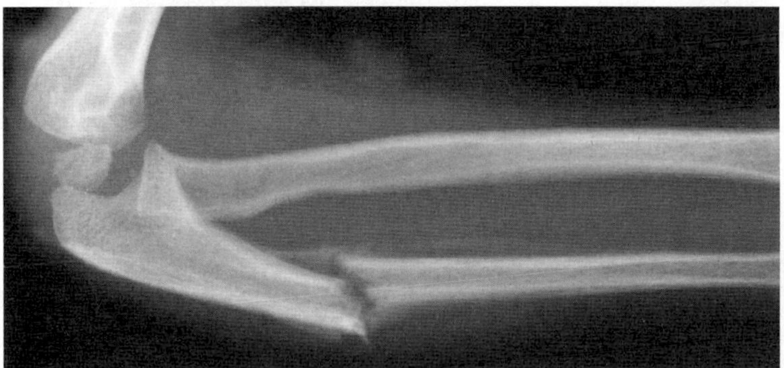
A

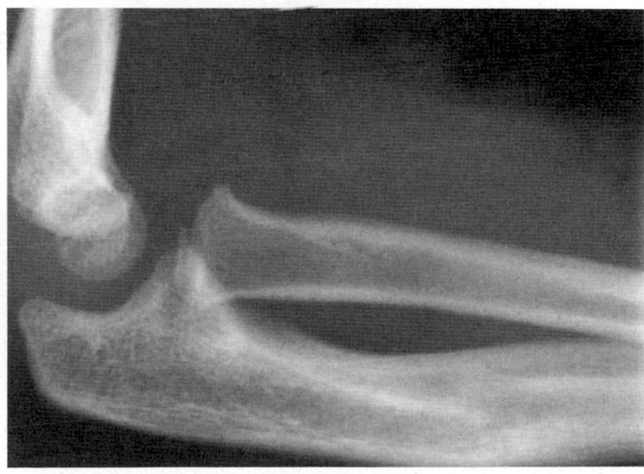
B

FIGURE 12-19 A. Malaligned ulnar fracture with radial head reduced. **B.** Subsequent apex posterior angulation healing of ulna fracture while maintaining radial head reduction.

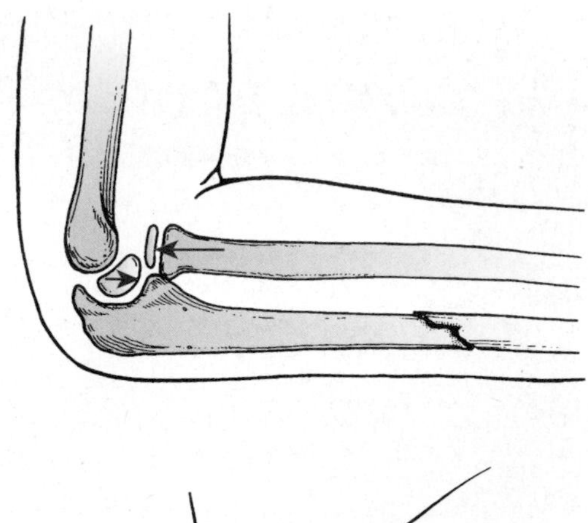

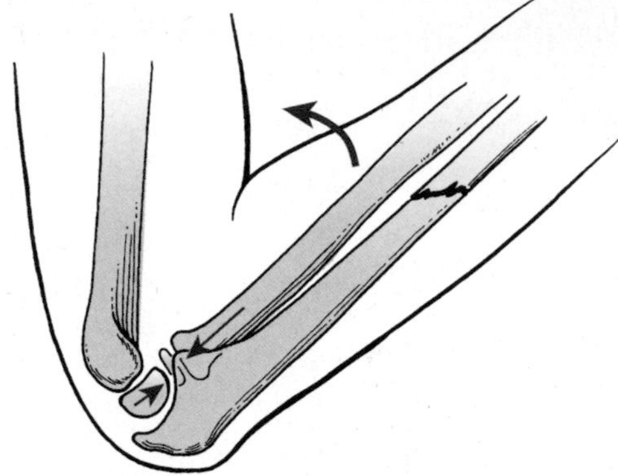

FIGURE 12-20 Reduction of the radial head. Flexing the elbow spontaneously reduces the radial head. Occasionally, manual pressure is required in combination with flexion.

osteochondral fractures (Fig. 12-23) in the radiocapitellar joint or proximal radioulnar joint may also prevent complete reduction of the radial head.[139] Morris[86] described a patient in whom reduction of the radial head was obstructed by radial nerve entrapment between the radial head and ulna.

Surgical Approach. The most direct approach to the radiocapitellar joint is from the posterolateral aspect of the elbow (Fig. 12-24). The interval between the anconeus and the extensor carpi ulnaris, using the distal portion of a Kocher incision, provides sufficient exposure of the radial head and the interposed structures.[52,129] This approach protects the posterior interosseous nerve when the forearm is pronated. A more extensile approach was described by Boyd.[20] This exposure is begun by making an incision following the lateral border of the triceps posteriorly to the lateral condyle and extending it along the radial side of the ulna (see Fig. 12-24). The incision is carried under the anconeus and extensor carpi ulnaris in an extraperiosteal manner, elevating the fibers of the supinator from the ulna. This carries the approach down to the interosseous membrane, allowing exposure of the radiocapitellar joint, excellent visualization of the orbicular ligament, access to the proximal fourth of the entire radius, and approach to the ulnar fracture all through the same incision.[20,21,121] In addition, elevation of the extensor-supinator mass from the lateral epicondyle allows more proximal exposure of the dislocated radial head if entrapped behind the capsule.

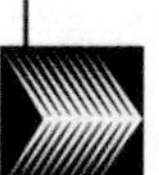

AUTHORS' PREFERRED TREATMENT

An anatomic, stable reduction of the ulnar fracture almost always leads to a stable reduction of the radial head. This in turn leads to an excellent long-term outcome. Failure to obtain and maintain ulnar fracture and radial head reduction will lead to a chronic Monteggia lesion, which is a complex clinical and surgical problem with risk of a suboptimum outcome. Therefore, I am very aggressive in my treatment of acute Monteggia fracture-dislocations. Percutaneous intramedullary fixation of complete transverse and short oblique ulna fractures is standard. Open reduction and internal fixation with plate and screws of the rarer long oblique and comminuted fracture is also standard. Any irreducible or unstable radial head after fracture reduction and stabilization is approached surgically to define and correct the cause.

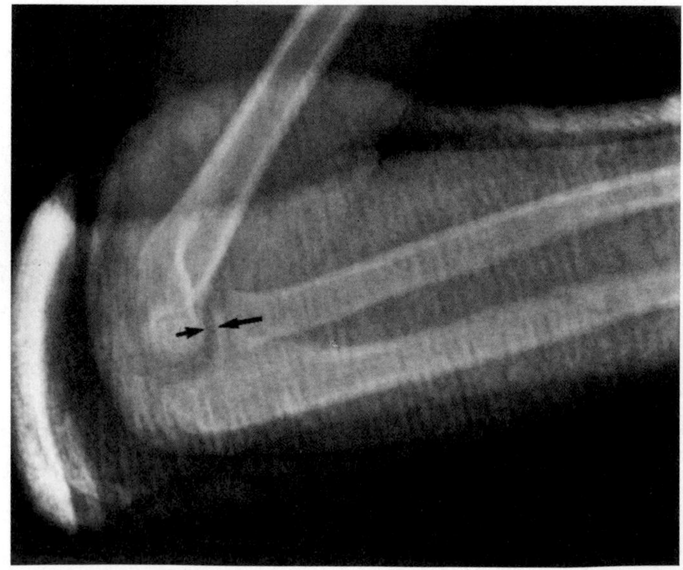

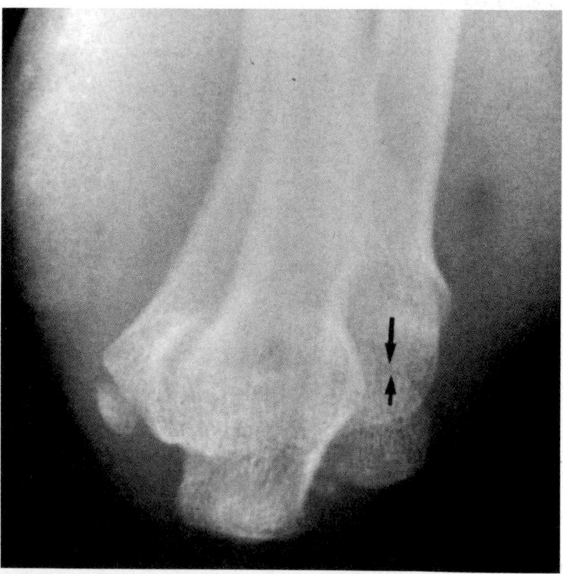

FIGURE 12-21 Once the reduction is complete, radiographs should be analyzed for re-establishment of the radiocapitellar line (*arrows*) and ulnar alignment on both the lateral **(A)** and Jones **(B)** views.

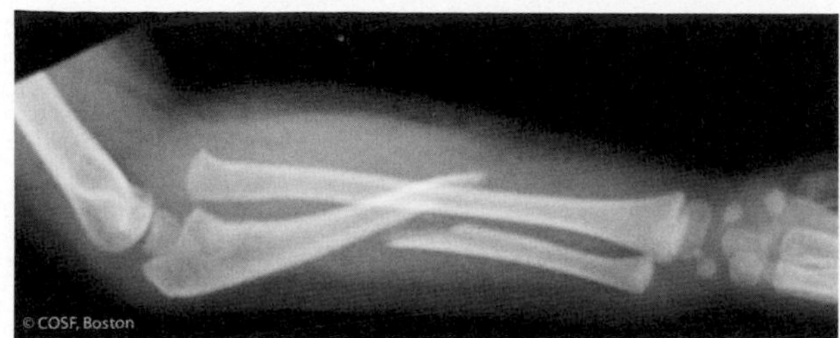

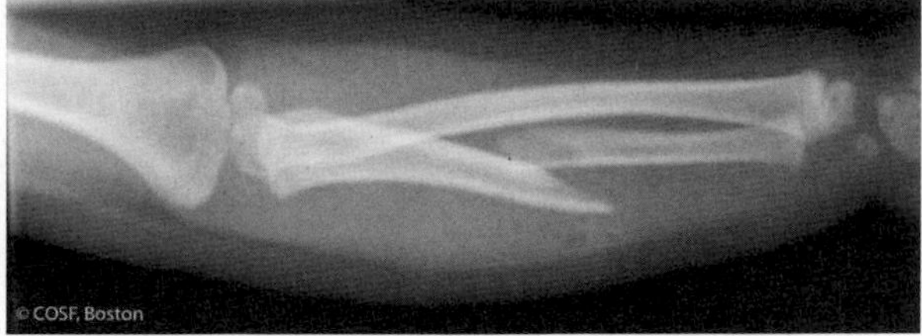

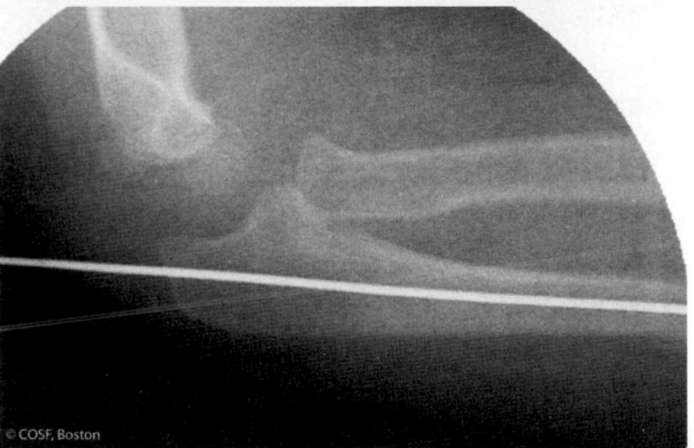

FIGURE 12-22 Lateral **(A)** and AP **(B)** views of long oblique ulnar fracture with anterior dislocated radial head. **C.** Percutaneous reduction and fixation of ulnar fracture through apophysis.

This usually involves repairing entrapped soft tissues. This aggressive approach avoids late complications.

Postoperative Care. A bivalved long-arm cast is used for 4 to 6 weeks with the forearm in slight supination and the elbow flexed 90 to 110 degrees depending on the degree of swelling. Radiographs are obtained every 1 to 2 weeks until fracture healing. Intramedullary hardware is removed with fracture healing. Plate and screw fixation is removed after 6 months only if it is irritating. Home rehabilitation is begun at 6 weeks and return-to-sports is dependent on restoration of motion and strength.

Type II Monteggia Fracture-Dislocations

Incidence

Posterior Monteggia fracture-dislocations are uncommon, accounting for 6% of Monteggia lesions in children,[73] and are usually found in older patients[97] who have sustained significant trauma.[37,108,109]

Clinical Findings

As with type I Monteggia lesions, the elbow region is swollen but exhibits posterior angulation of the proximal forearm and a marked prominence in the area posterolateral to the normal location of the radial head. The entire upper extremity should be examined because of the frequency of associated fractures.[71,97]

Radiographic Evaluation

Standard radiographic views of the forearm demonstrate the pertinent features for classifying this fracture. The typical finding is a proximal metaphyseal fracture of the ulna with possible extension into the olecranon (Fig. 12-25).[37,91,135] Midshaft fractures also occur, with an oblique fracture pattern.[8,37,91] The radial head is dislocated posteriorly or posterolaterally[9] and should be carefully examined for other injuries. Accompanying fractures of the anterior margin of the radial head have been noted.[37,97] Initially,

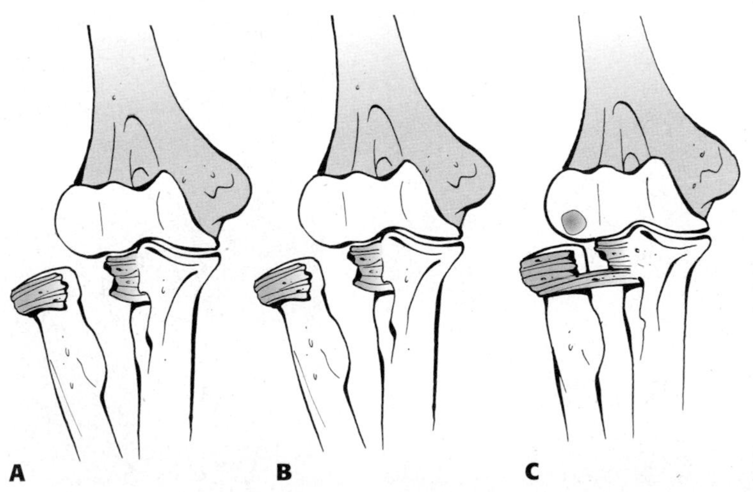

FIGURE 12-23 A. Radial head dislocation and complete annular ligament tear. **B.** Radial head dislocation and partial ligament tear. **C.** Radial head dislocation and partial or complete annular ligament tear and osteochondral fragment.

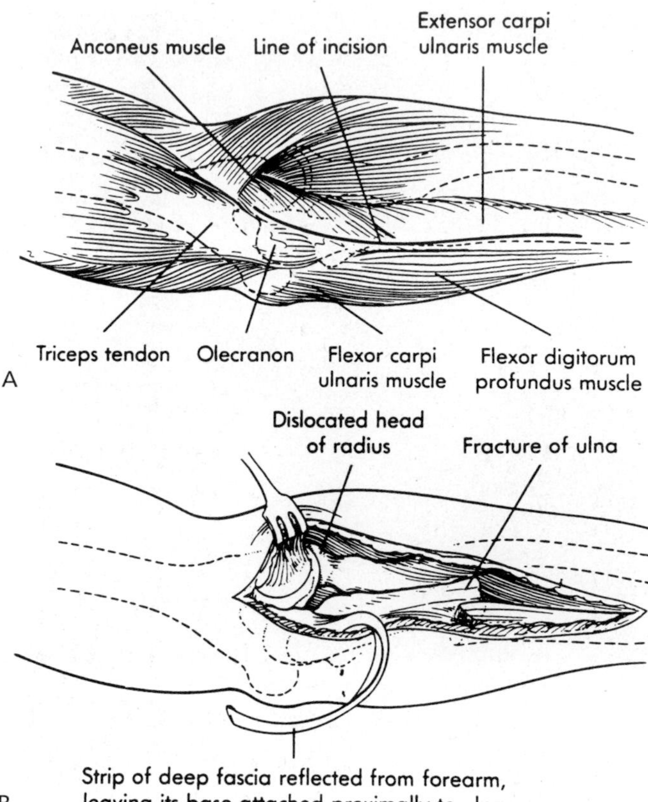

FIGURE 12-24 Surgical approach. **A.** The incision is carried under the anconeus and extensor carpi ulnaris to expose the radial head and orbicular ligament. **B.** The incision can be extended distally to allow exposure of the ulnar fracture and proximally to facilitate harvesting of the tendinous strip for orbicular ligament reconstruction, if necessary.

these are subtle in children but can lead to progressive subluxation and make late reconstruction difficult (Fig. 12-26).

Mechanism of Injury

The cause of the type II Monteggia lesion is subject to debate. Bado[9] thought the lesion was caused by direct force and sudden rotation and supination. Penrose[100] analyzed seven fractures in adults and noted that a proximal ulnar fracture was the typical pattern. He postulated that the injury occurred by longitudinal loading rather than direct trauma.[121] Olney and Menelaus[91] reported four type II lesions in their series of children's Monteggia fractures. Three of these patients had proximal ulnar

FIGURE 12-25 Type II Monteggia fracture-dislocation. The typical radiographic findings include **(A)** a posterior dislocation of the radial head (*arrows*) and **(B)** a proximal metaphyseal fracture, which may extend into the olecranon (*arrows*). The radial head also may be posterolateral (*arrows*) **(C)**.

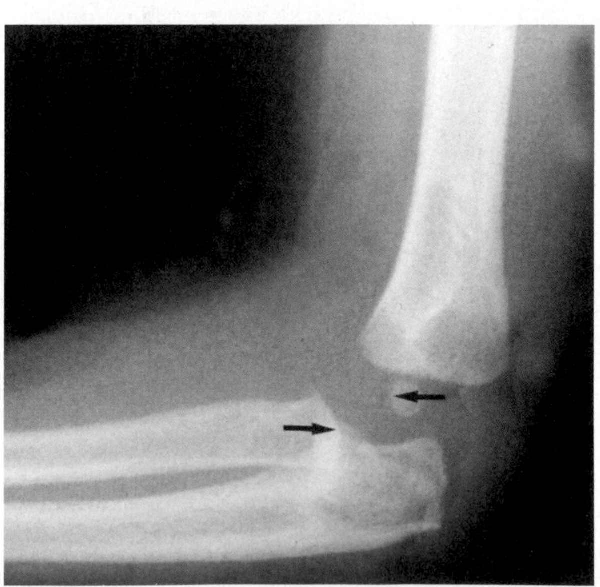

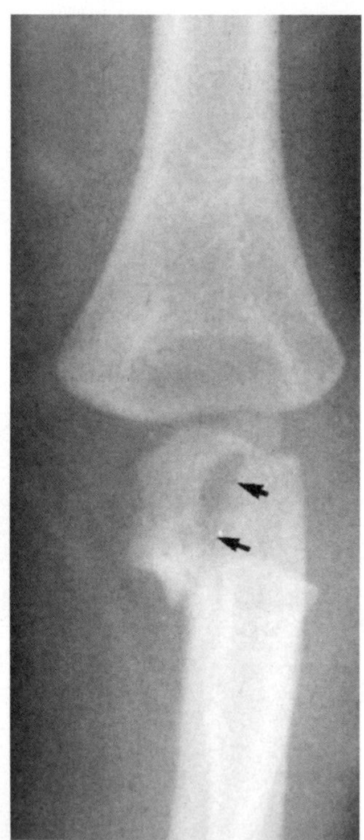

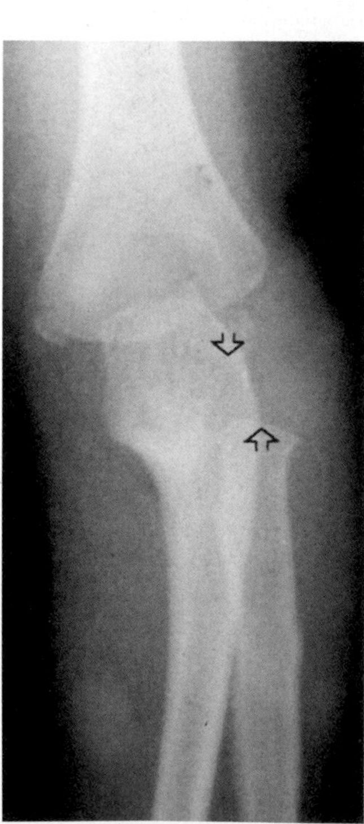

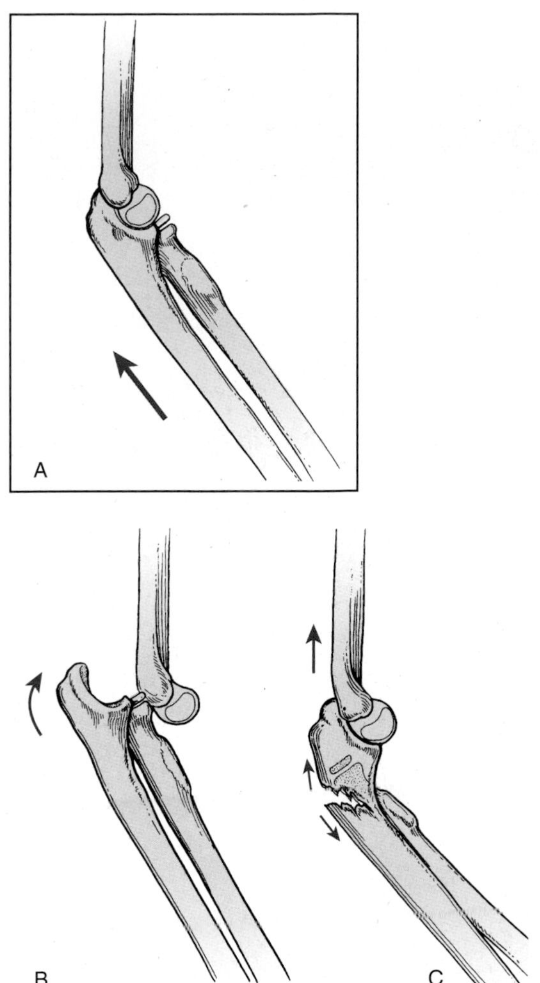

FIGURE 12-26 Mechanism of injury for type II Monteggia fracture-dislocation. **A.** The elbow is flexed approximately 60 degrees; a force is applied longitudinally, parallel to the long axis of the forearm. **B.** A posterior elbow dislocation may occur. **C.** If the integrity of the anterior cortex of the ulna is compromised, a type II fracture-dislocation occurs.

fractures and one an oblique midshaft fracture, suggesting two different mechanisms of injury.

The mechanism proposed and experimentally demonstrated by Penrose[100] was that type II lesions occur when the forearm is suddenly loaded in a longitudinal direction with the elbow flexed 60 degrees. He showed that a type II lesion occurred consistently if the ulna fractured; otherwise, a posterior elbow dislocation was produced (see Fig. 12-26). A possible difference in bony strength of the ulna suggested a reason for the high incidence of type II Monteggia fractures in older adults and their rarity in children. Penrose[100] further noted that the rotational position of the forearm did not seem to affect the type of fracture produced.

Haddad et al.[54] described type II Monteggia injuries caused by low-velocity injuries in six adults, five of whom were on long-term corticosteroid therapy. They suggested that this supports the theory that the type II (posterior) Monteggia injury is a variant of posterior elbow dislocation, in that it occurs when the ulna is weaker than the ligaments surrounding the elbow joint, resulting in an ulnar fracture before the ligament disruption associated with dislocation occurs.

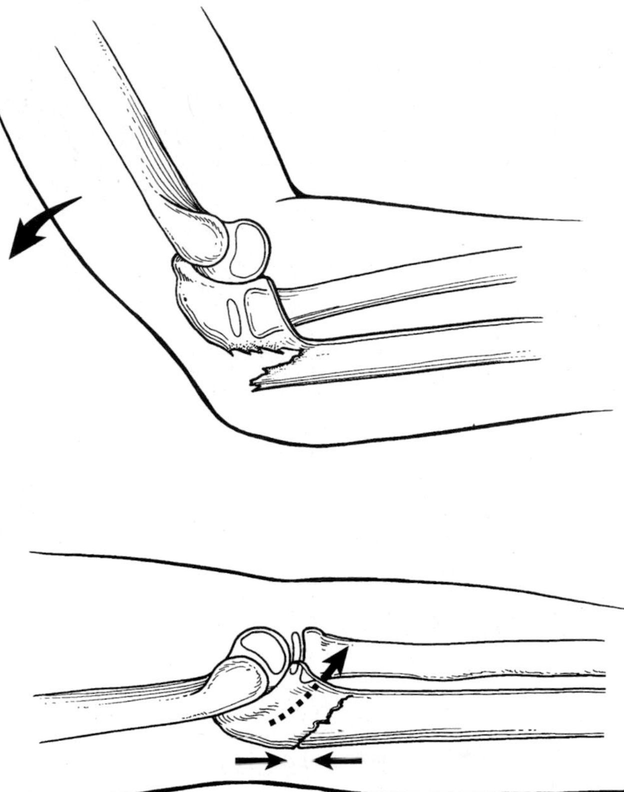

FIGURE 12-27 Longitudinal traction and pronation of the forearm and immobilization in 60 degrees flexion or complete extension.

Treatment

Nonoperative Treatment. As with type I injuries, incomplete type II fractures usually have a satisfactory result after closed reduction.[75,91,98,105,143] The ulnar fracture is reduced by longitudinal traction in line with the long axis of the forearm while the elbow is held at 60 degrees of flexion (Fig. 12-27). The radial head may reduce spontaneously or may require gentle, anteriorly directed pressure applied to its posterior aspect. The elbow is extended once the radial head is reduced and is immobilized in that position to stabilize the radial head and allow molding posteriorly to maintain the ulnar reduction.[34,98,141] If the ulnar alignment cannot be maintained, an intramedullary K-wire should be used.

Operative Treatment. Treatment goals are stable concentric reduction of the radial head and alignment of the ulnar fracture. When there is an unstable, complete ulnar fracture, percutaneous intramedullary fixation or open reduction and internal fixation with plate and screws are used similar to type I fracture-dislocations.[96,101] The radial head should be reduced by open technique if there is interposed tissue or if it is accompanied by a fractured capitellum or radial head.

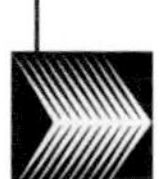

AUTHORS' PREFERRED TREATMENT

With incomplete fractures, ulnar length is re-established by applying longitudinal traction and straightening the angular deformity. The radial head may reduce spontaneously or with gentle, anteriorly directed force over the radial head. Once reduced, the position of the head can be stabilized by holding the elbow in extension. If the ulnar fracture is stable, it can be maintained by cast immobilization with the elbow in extension. However, if there is any doubt, percutaneous intramedullary fixation is preferred. Comminuted or very proximal fractures may require open reduction and internal fixation with plate and screws or tension band fixation. Postoperative radiographs are obtained approximately every 7 to 10 days to confirm continued reduction of the radial head.

The Boyd approach can be used to obtain reduction of the radial head if it cannot be obtained through closed manipulation. Management of the annular ligament is the same as described for type I Monteggia lesions.

Associated compression fractures of the radial head require early detection to avoid late loss of alignment. Open reduction and internal fixation may be required to maintain radiocapitellar joint stability. Osteonecrosis and nonunion are complications of this injury.

Cast immobilization is continued until fracture and soft tissue healing, usually 6 weeks. Home rehabilitation is performed until restoration of motion and strength.[98]

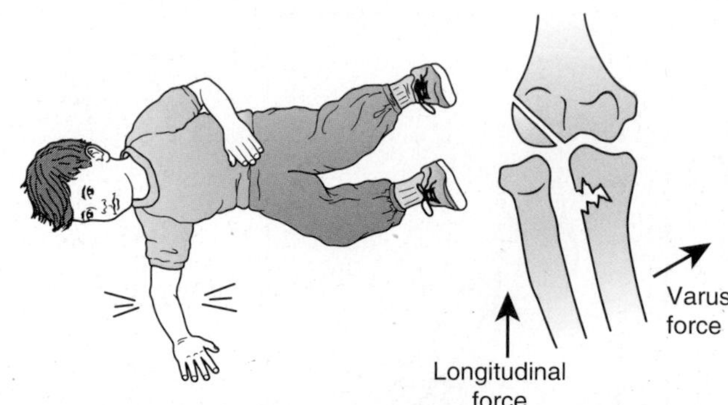

FIGURE 12-28 Mechanism of injury for type III lesions. A forced varus stress causes a greenstick fracture of the proximal ulna and a true lateral or anterolateral radial head dislocation.

Type III Monteggia Fracture-Dislocations

Clinical Findings

Lateral swelling, varus deformity of the elbow, and significant limitation of motion, especially supination, are the hallmarks of lateral (type III) Monteggia fracture-dislocations. Again, these signs can be subtle and missed by harried clinicians.

Incidence

Type III lesions are common in children, second in frequency to anterior type I Monteggia fracture-dislocations.[9,87,91,98,143] Injuries to the radial nerve, particularly the posterior interosseous branch, occur more frequently with this lesion.[13,111,124] Open reduction of the radial head may be necessary because of interposition of soft tissue between it and the ulna or capitellum.[13,60,111,133,145,147]

Radiographic Evaluation

The radial head may be displaced laterally or anterolaterally.[96,98] The ulnar fracture often is in the metaphyseal region,[9,13,60,66,86,98,111,147] but it can also occur more distally.[91,143,145] Radial angulation at the fracture site is common to all lesions, regardless of the level. Radiographs of the entire forearm should be obtained because of the association of distal radial and ulnar fractures with this complex elbow injury.[135] As with all Monteggia injuries, the acute lesion can be missed if proper radiographs are not obtained and appropriate close examination of the studies are not performed.

Mechanism of Injury

Wright[147] studied fractures of the proximal ulna with lateral and anterolateral dislocations of the radial head and concluded that the mechanism of injury was varus stress at the level of the elbow, in combination with an outstretched hand planted firmly against a fixed surface (Fig. 12-28). This usually produces a greenstick ulnar fracture with tension failure radially and compression medially. The radial head dislocates laterally, rupturing the annular ligament. Hume[60] suggested that the injury may be the result of hyperextension of the elbow combined with pronation of the forearm. Other authors confirmed the mechanism of varus force at the elbow as the cause of these injuries.[9,34,87,98,134] The direction of the radial head dislocation is probably determined by the rotation and angulation force applied simultaneously with the varus moment at the elbow.[87]

Treatment

Nonoperative Treatment. Nonoperative treatment by manipulative closed reduction is usually effective in pediatric patients with metaphyseal, incomplete, or plastic deformation fractures.[9,34,46,60,75,87,91,98,134,143,147] However, the rate of operative treatment has been reported to be as high as 12%.[91] The reduction maneuver for nonoperative type III lesions is shown in Fig.12-29.

Closed Reduction. Reduction is carried out by reversing the mechanism of injury.[34,87,98,135] The elbow is held in extension with longitudinal traction. Valgus stress is placed on the ulna at the site of the fracture, producing clinical realignment (Fig. 12-30). The radial head may spontaneously reduce or need assistance with gentle pressure applied laterally (see Fig. 12-29). Reduction sometimes produces a palpable click.[135] Ulnar length and alignment must be maintained to ensure a stable radial head. Fluoroscopic radiographs are obtained to confirm radial head reduction.[84] Any malalignment of the radiocapitellar joint in any view implies the possibility of interposed tissue or persistent malalignment of the ulna fracture. The angular alignment of the ulna must be anatomic to allow and maintain reduction of the radial head.[44]

Reduction is maintained by a long-arm cast with the elbow in flexion. The degree of flexion varies depending on the direction of the radial head dislocation. When the radius is in a straight lateral or anterolateral position, flexion to 110 to 120 degrees improves stability.[37,87,105,143] If there is a posterolateral component to the dislocation, apposition of only 70 to 80 degrees of flexion has been recommended.[135] Of note, it can be difficult to assess continued reduction of the radial head on the AP view radiographically in a cast with the elbow flexed.

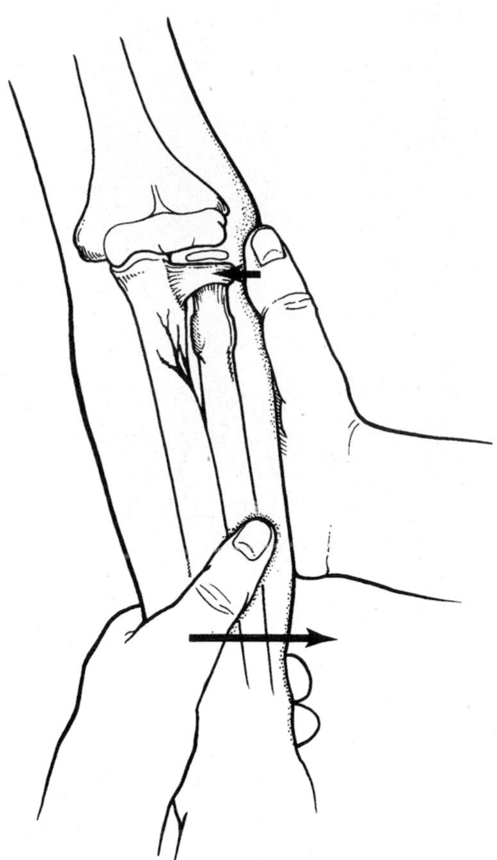

FIGURE 12-29 Reduction of type III lesion. Valgus stress is placed on the ulna at the fracture site (*arrows*), producing clinical realignment. The radial head may spontaneously reduce.

Forearm rotation in the cast is usually in supination, which tightens the interosseous membrane and further stabilizes the reduction.[9,34,87,143] Some have suggested positions of immobilization from pronation[134] to slight supination.[135] Ramsey and Pedersen[105] recommended neutral as the best position of rotation to avoid loss of motion; their patients showed no loss of reduction using this position.

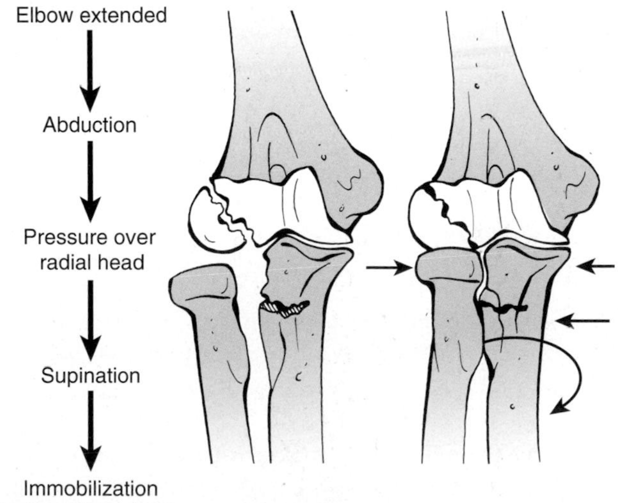

FIGURE 12-30 Schematic reduction maneuvers for type III Monteggia fracture.

Radiographic Evaluation. Radiographs are taken in the AP and lateral planes to confirm the reduction of the radial head and assess the ulnar alignment. Up to 10 degrees of ulnar angulation is acceptable in younger children, provided the radial head reduction is concentric and stable. Range-of-motion testing of stability is appropriate and necessary with plastic deformation fractures since AP radiographs in the cast will be difficult to assess.

Immobilization. A long-arm cast is applied with a valgus mold over the fracture site. Immobilization is usually in 90 to 100 degrees of flexion for lateral Monteggia lesions and 60 to 80 degrees of flexion for posterolateral dislocations. The fracture and radial head reduction need to be truly stable for cast immobilization since postreduction radiographs are hard to interpret accurately.

Postreduction Care. Cast immobilization is continued until fracture and soft tissue healing, usually by 6 weeks. Home rehabilitation is performed until restoration of motion and strength. Final radiographs are obtained with full restoration of motion and strength to be certain there is anatomic reduction of the proximal radioulnar and radiocapitellar joints.

Operative Treatment. Surgical intervention has two goals: reduction and stabilization of both the ulnar fracture and the radial head. If there is an inability to obtain and maintain anatomic alignment of the ulnar fracture, proximal radioulnar, and radiocapitellar joints, then operative treatment is indicated.

Ulnar Stabilization. Ulnar malalignment may prevent anatomic relocation of the radial head. The ulnar fracture can usually be reduced closed, but open reduction may be necessary because of interposed tissue.

Stabilization of the ulna is necessary to prevent recurrent lateral dislocation of the radial head. Persistent varus alignment or radial bow, particularly with oblique fractures, may lead to recurrent subluxation of the proximal radius (Fig. 12-31).[44,91] Anatomic reduction of the ulna and fixation with plates and screws[44] or intramedullary wires[8] will yield excellent results.

Radial Head Reduction. Failed closed reduction of the radial head with anatomic alignment of the ulna fracture implies interposition of soft tissue, which is repaired through a Boyd approach (see Fig. 12-24).[20,145] This allows removal of the interposed tissues[139,145] and repair or reconstruction of the annular ligament and the periosteum of the ulna, if necessary (Fig. 12-32).[14,23,44,46,121,133] The surgical technique is essentially the same as previously described for a type I Monteggia fracture-dislocation.

Postoperative Care. Postoperative care is the same as for a fracture treated nonoperatively.

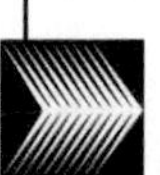

AUTHORS' PREFERRED TREATMENT

As with any Monteggia lesion, treatment is aimed at obtaining and maintaining reduction of the radial head, either by

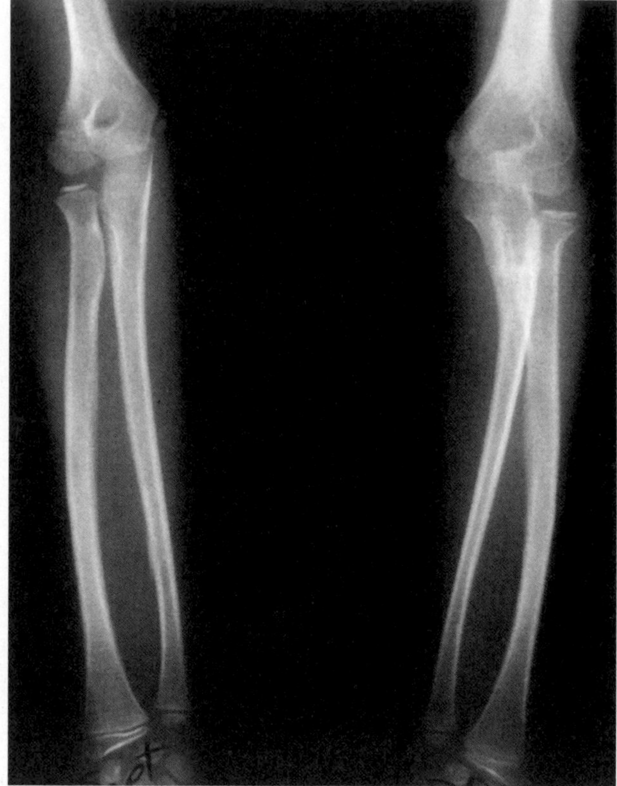

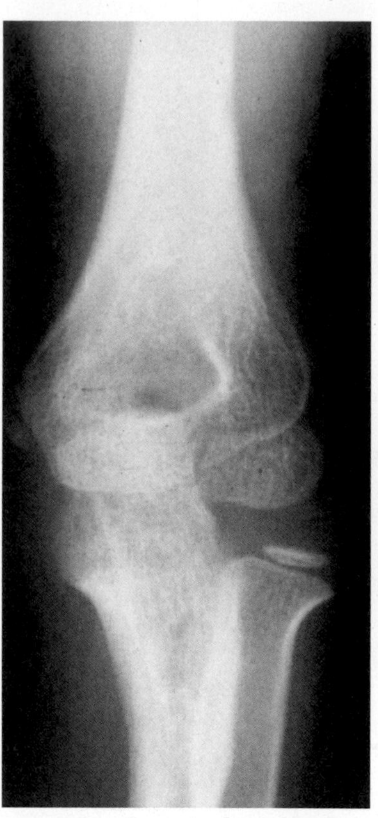

FIGURE 12-31 Varus deformity of the ulna. **A.** AP views of both elbows showing residual radial bow of the proximal ulna after an incompletely reduced Monteggia type III lesion. **B.** This bow has produced a symptomatic lateral subluxation of the radial head.

open or closed technique. This is usually performed by anatomic, stable reduction of the ulnar fracture that in turn leads to a stable reduction of the proximal radioulnar and radiocapitellar joints.

Type IV Monteggia Fracture-Dislocations

Clinical Findings

The appearance of the limb with a type IV lesion is similar to that of a type I lesion. More swelling and pain are present because of the magnitude of force required to create this complex injury. Particular attention should be given to the neurovascular status of the limb, anticipating the possible increased risk for a compartment syndrome. Although this injury is uncommon in general and rare in children, the radiocapitellar joint should be examined in all midshaft forearm fractures to avoid missing the proximal radioulnar joint disruption (Fig. 12-33). Failure to recognize the radial head dislocation is the major complication of this fracture.[12]

Radiographic Evaluation

The anterior radial head dislocation is similar to that in a type I Monteggia lesion (Fig. 12-34). The radial and ulnar fractures usually are in the middle third,[35] with the radial fracture usually distal to the ulnar injury. They may be complete or greenstick.

Mechanism of Injury

Bado[8] proposed that a type IV lesion is caused by hyperpronation. Of the case reports discussing the mechanism of injury, both hyperpronation[44] and a direct blow[112] have been postulated. Olney and Menelaus[91] reported a single type IV lesion in their series but did not discuss the mechanism. Type IV lesions appear to be caused by the mechanism described for type I lesions.

Treatment

This complex lesion has been treated by both closed[91] and open[9] techniques. Percutaneous intramedullary fixation of the radial and ulnar fractures with flexible pins and closed reduction of the radial head also have been described.[47,112]

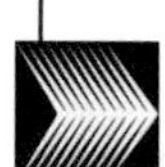

AUTHORS' PREFERRED TREATMENT

The goals of treatment for a type IV Monteggia lesion are similar to those of other types. The presence of the free-floating proximal radial fragment hampers the ability to reduce the radial head. Stabilization of the radial fracture converts a type IV lesion to a type I lesion, making treatment easier.

Nonoperative Treatment. Closed reduction should be attempted initially, with the aim of transforming the type IV lesion to a type I lesion (Fig. 12-35), especially if the radial and ulnar fractures have greenstick patterns. Use of the image intensifier allows immediate confirmation of reduction, espe-

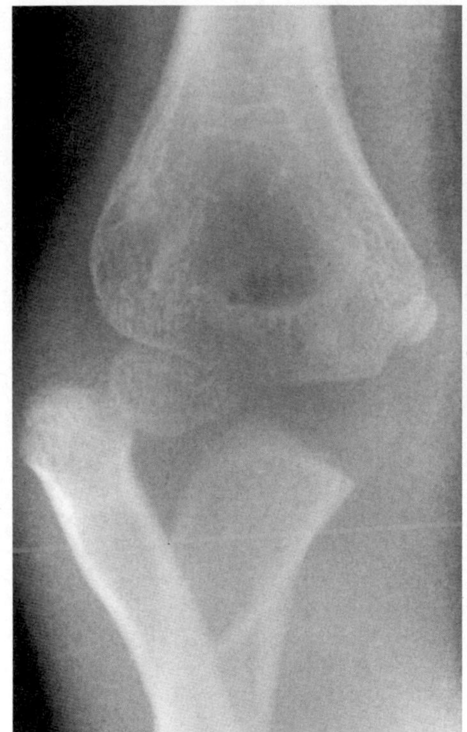

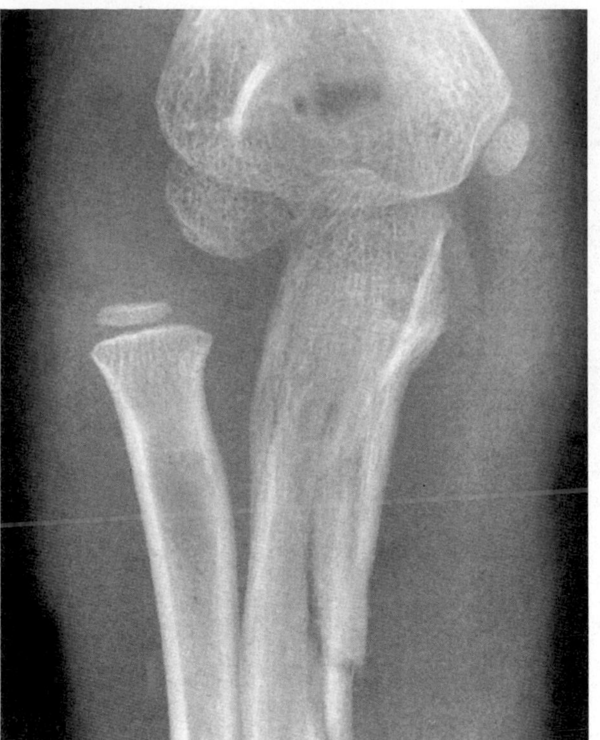

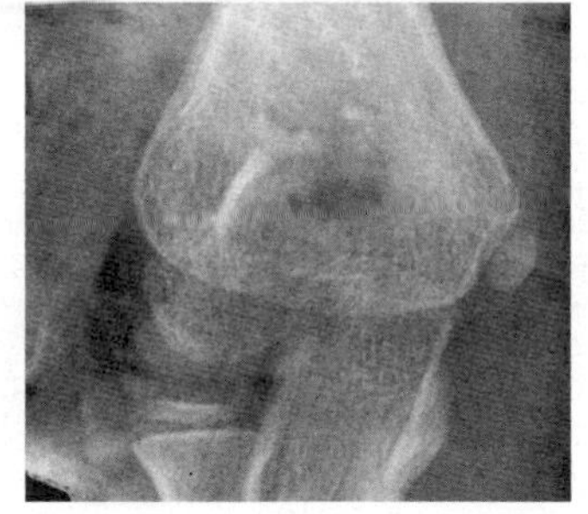

FIGURE 12-32 Irreducible type III lesion. **A.** Injury films showing typical greenstick olecranon fracture and lateral dislocation of a type III Monteggia lesion. **B.** After manipulation and correction of the ulnar deformity, the radial head still was not reduced. **C.** Open reduction was performed to extract the interposed torn orbicular ligament.

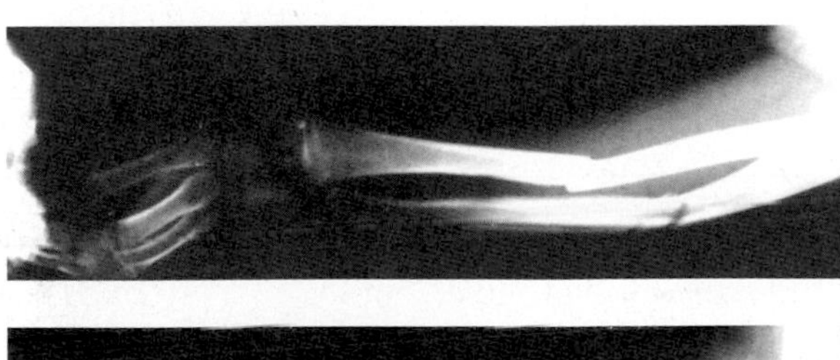

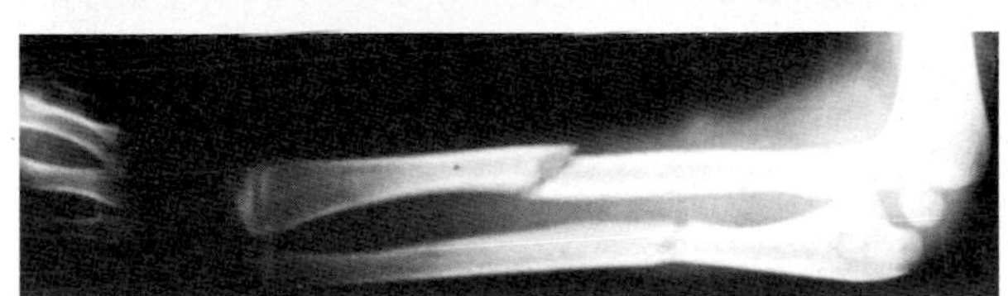

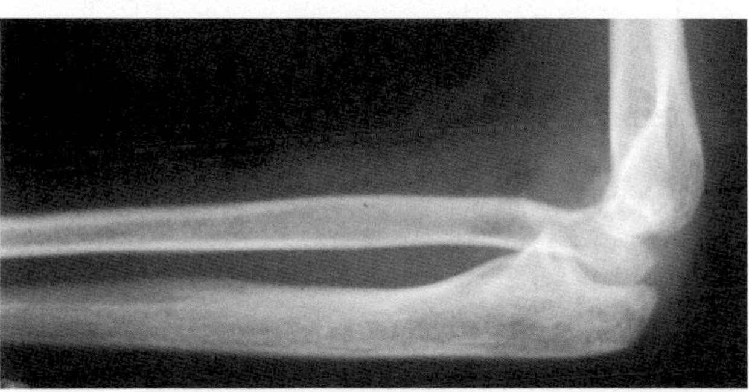

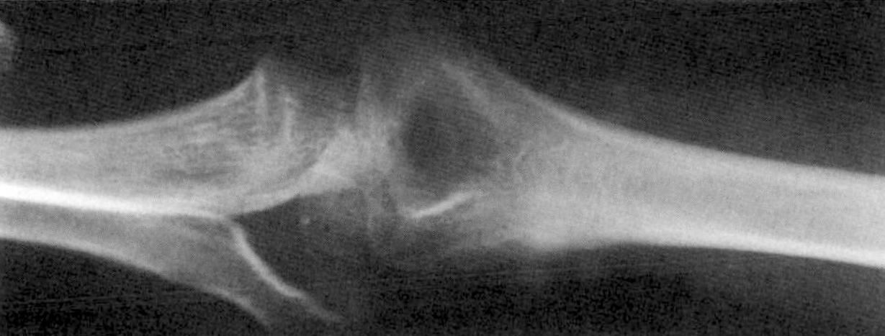

FIGURE 12-33 Type IV Monteggia lesion. **A.** Anterior dislocation of the head of the radius with fracture of the upper third of the radial shaft with the ulna fracture angulated anteriorly. The dislocation of the radial head was not recognized. **B.** Five years later, the radial head was still dislocated, misshapen, and prominent. A full range of motion was present, with the exception of a loss of 10 degrees of full supination. The patient had no pain, but generalized weakness was noted in this extremity, especially in throwing motions.

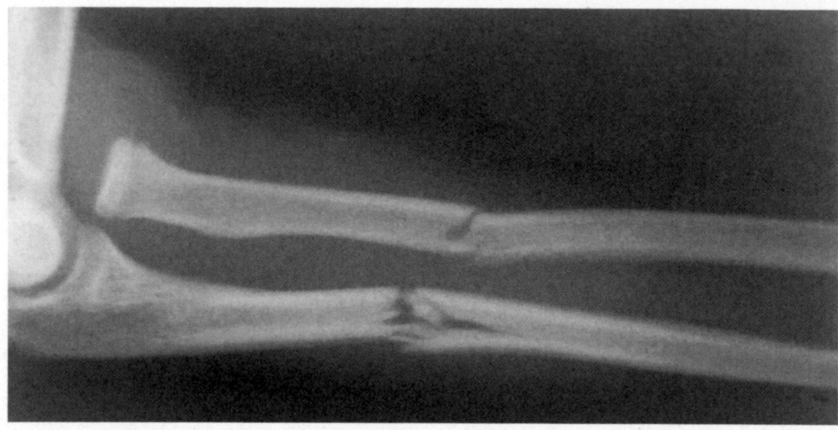

FIGURE 12-34 Type IV lesion. There is an anterior dislocation of the radial head. The radial and ulnar fractures are usually in the middle third of the shaft, with the radial fracture distal to the ulnar fracture.

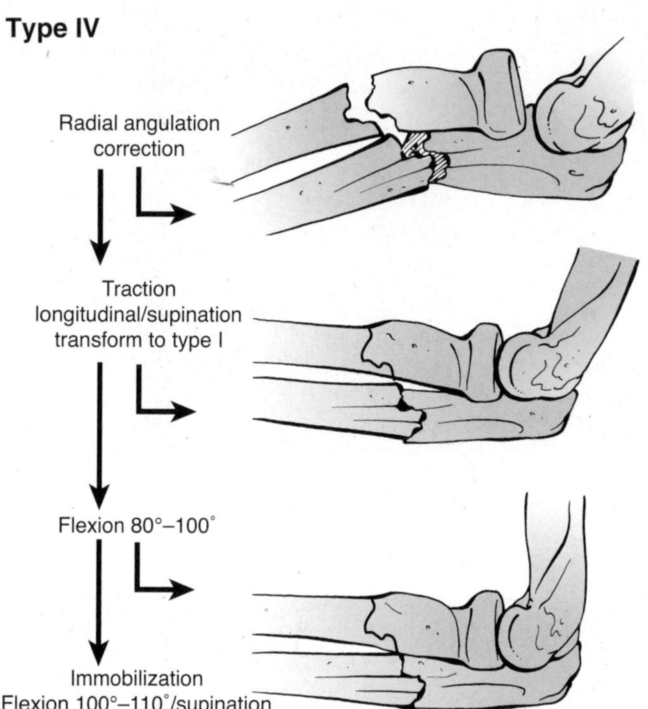

FIGURE 12-35 Reduction schematic for type IV Monteggia fracture.

cially of the radial head. Closed treatment of unstable ulnar lesions should not be attempted. If the initial reduction cannot be obtained, anatomic, stable reduction with either intramedullary or plate fixation is performed (Fig. 12-36).

Operative Treatment. Type IV fractures are usually unstable and the reduction of the radial head is easier to obtain and maintain after stable fixation of the radius. In young patients, this may be achieved by intramedullary fixation. In children older than 12 years, plating of the radius through a Henry extensile approach[56] provides more rigid stabilization (see Fig. 12-36). Once stability is achieved, a closed reduction of the radial head is attempted. This is usually successful, but any intra-articular obstruction can be removed through a Boyd approach.

Postoperative Care. The elbow is immobilized in a long-arm cast for 4 to 6 weeks in 110 to 120 degrees of flexion with the forearm in neutral rotation. A short-arm cast is used thereafter if additional fracture protection is necessary. Home rehabilitation is performed until restoration of motion and strength. Final radiographs are obtained with full restoration of motion and strength to be certain there is anatomic reduction of the proximal radioulnar and radiocapitellar joints.

Monteggia Equivalent Lesions

Clinical Findings

Clinical findings are similar to those for the corresponding Bado lesion, with the common triad of pain, swelling, and deformity.

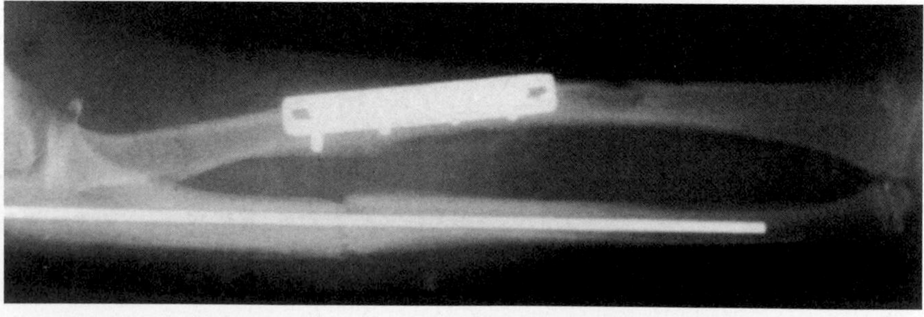

FIGURE 12-36 Operative treatment, type IV lesion. The initial goal is to stabilize the radius. In older children, a plate may be indicated. Intramedullary pinning usually is adequate.

Radiographic Evaluation

As with the Bado types, careful radiographic study should be made with at least two orthogonal views of the elbow in addition to views of the forearm. Special views such as obliques should be obtained to clearly delineate the associated injuries (e.g., radial head or neck fractures, lateral humeral condyle fractures) and allow adequate pretreatment planning.

Mechanism of Injury

The mechanism of injury by which the fracture occurs helps define its equivalent type and is discussed in the sections on the relevant Bado type.

Treatment

As with the other Bado types, treatment focuses on two general components of the lesion: ulnar fracture alignment and radial head reduction. Associated injuries must be dealt with appropriately.

Ulnar Fracture. This fracture is treated as are other Bado types. The method is dictated by the fracture pattern and location and its stability after reduction.

Associated Injury. These associated fractures and dislocations are evaluated and treated using principles based on the particular injury. They are discussed thoroughly in other sections of this chapter and book.

COMPLICATIONS

Chronic Monteggia Fracture-Dislocations

A late presenting, previously undetected dislocation of the radial head is not as uncommon as we all would prefer.[28,30,34,39,46,47,70,93,94,118,131] Isolated radial head dislocations with remote trauma have been mistaken for congenital radial head dislocations.[81] The shape of the ulna in patients with a seemingly isolated dislocation of the radial head usually indicates persistent plastic deformation or malunion of the ulna and a traumatic etiology to the radial head dislocation (see Figs. 12-3 and 12-37).[77,84,118,128] Chronic Monteggia radial head dislocations have been diagnosed as early as several weeks after injury during cast changes for a misdiagnosed, isolated ulnar fracture or years later due to pain, restriction of motion, and/or arm malalignment. Even a few weeks after injury, treatment becomes much more complicated than acute recognition and intervention. Recognition of a dislocated radial head at the time of injury can prevent the difficult problem of an untreated, chronic Monteggia lesion.

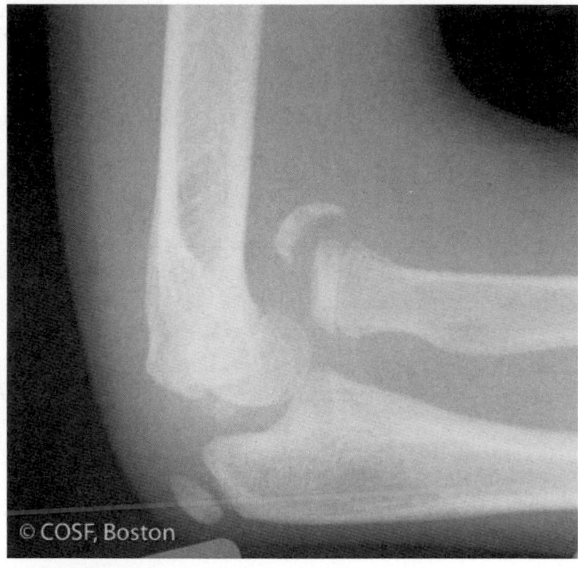

FIGURE 12-38 Late presenting anterior radial head dislocation with ossification of displaced annular ligament.

When a previously undetected proximal radioulnar and radiocapitellar dislocation is encountered (Fig. 12-38), there is controversy regarding subsequent care. At present there are limited levels of evidence and conflicting retrospective literature on this problem. Some reports indicate that the natural history of the untreated lesion is not problematic.[89,116,126] Fahey[40] suggested that, although in the short term persistent dislocations do well, they cause problems later. Other reports support the view that the natural history of persistent dislocation is not benign and is associated with restricted motion, deformity, functional impairment, pain, potential degenerative arthritis, and late neuropathy.[1,6,15,18,24,46,49,60,61,63,64,77] Kalamchi[63] re-

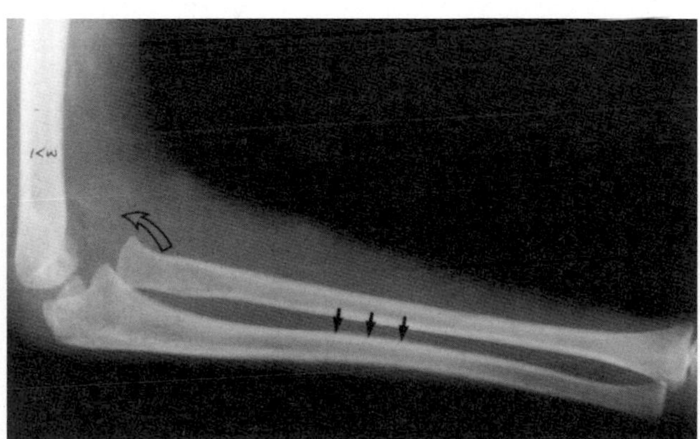

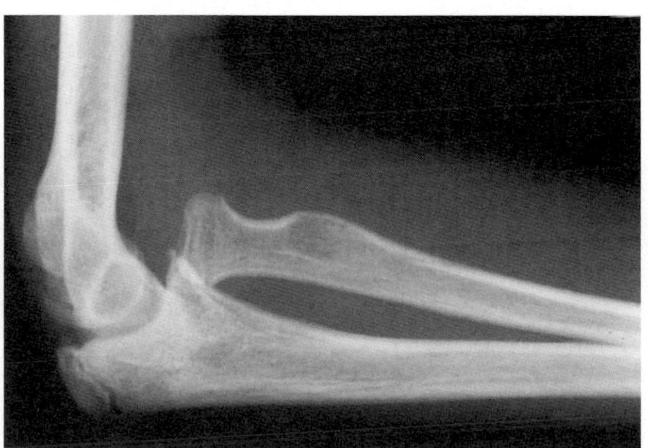

FIGURE 12-37 Ulnar bow line. **A.** The injury film of an 8-year-old girl who fell, spraining her arm. Note anterior bow of the ulna (*black arrows*) and loss of the radiocapitellar relation (*open arrow*). **B.** Film at time of diagnosis. Note the persistent ulnar bow and overgrowth of radius.

ported pain, progressive valgus deformity, and restricted motion, especially loss of forearm rotation and elbow flexion. Tardy nerve palsies have been reported subsequent to long-standing, unrecognized Monteggia lesions.[1,6,58,78]

Indications for Treatment

Treatment indications have ranged from the presence of a chronic Monteggia lesion at anytime postinjury to only when there is pain, restricted motion, and functional disability. That wide spectrum of expert opinion makes individual case decision making difficult for patients, parents, and clinicians. Blount[19] and Fowles et al.[44] suggested that reconstruction provides the best results in patients who have had a dislocation for 3 to 6 months or less. Fowles et al.[44] reported successful relocations up to 3 years after injury; Freedman et al.,[46] up to 6 years after injury. Throughout the literature, the appropriate age for radial head reduction seems to be younger than 10 years.[127] Hirayama et al.[57] suggested that the procedure not be performed if there is significant deformity of the radial head, flattening of the capitellum, or valgus deformity of the neck of the radius. Seel and Peterson[117] suggested that the age of the patient and the duration of the dislocation are unimportant. Their criteria for surgical repair were (i) normal concave radial head articular surface and (ii) normal shape and contour of the ulna and radius (deformity of either correctable by osteotomy). They treated seven patients ranging in age from 5 to 13 years for chronic dislocations that had been present from 3 months to 7 years. All seven were fully active with no elbow pain or instability at an average of 4 years after surgery.

Although they recommended surgical treatment of chronic Monteggia lesions in children because of the long-term sequelae, Rodgers et al.[112] cautioned that the results of reconstructive procedures are unpredictable and associated with a number of complications including malunion of the ulnar shaft, recurrent radiocapitellar subluxation, and radial and ulnar neuropathy.

At present, most authors advocate surgical reconstruction of a chronic Monteggia when (i) the diagnosis is made early, (ii) there is preservation of the normal concave radial head and convex capitellum, (iii) especially when there is progressive deformity (i.e., valgus), loss of motion, and pain, and, (iv) the patient and family are well aware of the concerns with operative reconstruction.

Surgical Reconstruction

Descriptions of surgical reconstruction for pediatric chronic Monteggia lesions have been variable in terms of (i) annular ligament repair or reconstruction,[53] (ii) ulnar osteotomy alone[62] or in combination with ligament reconstruction,[30,59] and (iii) radial osteotomy.[29] The technique for delayed reduction of the radial head in a Monteggia fracture-dislocation is attributed to Bell-Tawse,[14] who used the surgical approach described by Boyd.[20] Other surgical approaches have been developed.[52,129]

Annular Ligament Repair or Reconstruction. Most but not all authors advocate surgical repair or reconstruction of the annular ligament in conjunction with an ulnar osteotomy for a pediatric chronic Monteggia lesion. Ligament repair or reconstruction without an osteotomy is very rarely indicated.[146] Kalamchi[63] restored stability after open reduction and osteotomy by utilizing the native annular ligament. Bell-Tawse[14] used a strip of triceps tendon to reconstruct the annular ligament, as did Lloyd-Roberts[78] and Hurst.[61] Bell-Tawse[14] used the central portion of the triceps tendon passed through a drill hole in the ulna and around the radial neck to stabilize the reduction and immobilized the elbow in a long-arm cast in extension. Bucknill[23] and Lloyd-Roberts[78] modified the Bell-Tawse procedure by using the lateral portion of the triceps tendon, with a transcapitellar pin for stability. The elbow was immobilized in flexion. Hurst and Dubrow[61] used the central portion of the triceps tendon but carried the dissection of the periosteum distally along the ulna to the level of the radial neck, which provided more stable fixation than stopping dissection at the olecranon as described by Bell-Tawse.[14] They also used a periosteal tunnel rather than a drill hole for fixation of the tendinous strip to the ulna. Other authors have used other soft tissues for reconstruction, including the lacertus fibrous,[26] a strip of the forearm fascia,[120] palmaris longus free tendon graft,[142] and free fascia lata graft.[138] Seel and Peterson[117] described the use of two holes drilled in the proximal ulna. The holes are placed at the original attachments of the annular ligament and allow repair of the annular ligament (frequently avulsed from one attachment and trapped within the joint) or reconstruction of the annular ligament with triceps tendon. This technique secures the radial head in its normal position from any dislocated position and allows osteotomy for correction of any accompanying deformity of the ulna or radius. Seel and Peterson[117] noted that the Bell-Tawse procedure tends to pull the radius posterolaterally (Fig. 12-39) and possibly constricts the neck of the radius, thereby potentially limiting the growth of the radial neck ("notching") and reducing forearm rotation. Seel and Peterson[117] placed a single drill hole obliquely across the ulna to exit medially at the site of the medial attachment of the annular ligament on

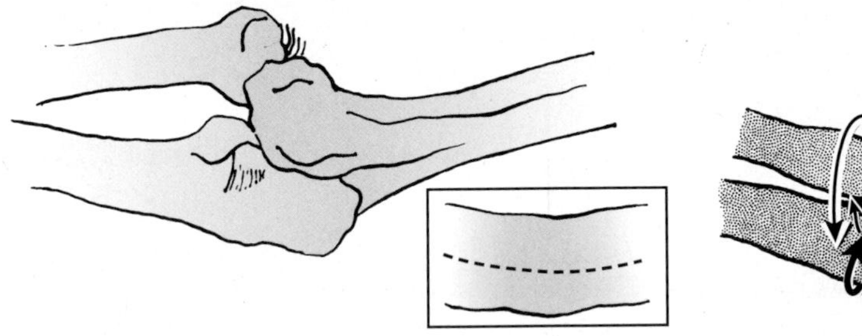

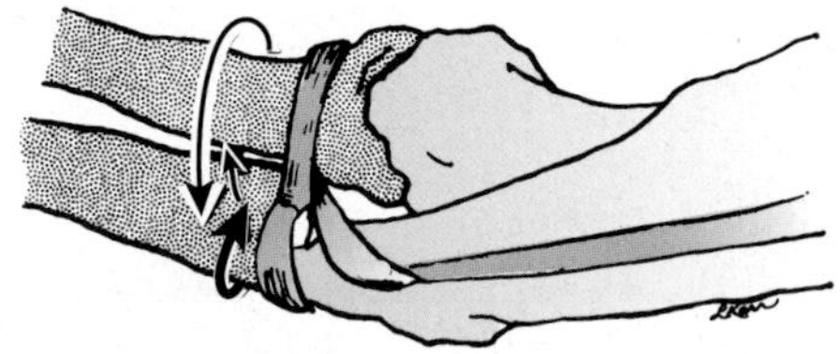

FIGURE 12-39 The central slip of the triceps is used to reconstruct an annular ligament in Bell-Tawse reconstruction. The direction of stability is posterior (*large arrow*).

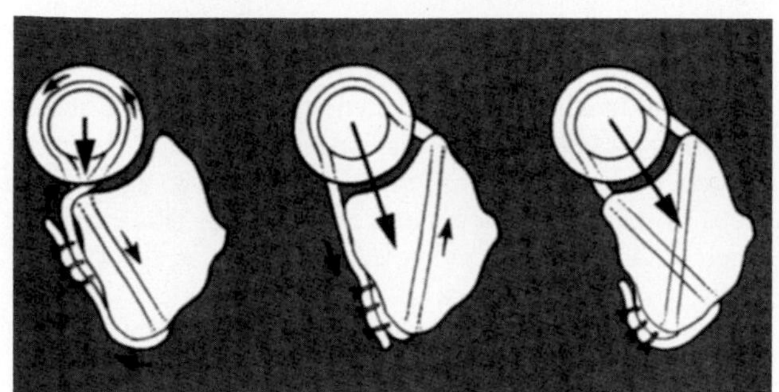

FIGURE 12-40 Drawings of transverse cuts of the proximal right radius and ulna (viewed distally) at the level of the radial head. *Left.* Route of the triceps tendon in Bell-Tawse reconstruction. The direction of stability is posterior (*large arrow*). *Center.* Drill hole placed obliquely to exit the ulna at the site of the medial annular ligament attachment. The direction of stability is posteromedial (*large arrow*). *Right.* Two drill holes exit the ulna at sites of medial and lateral annular ligament attachments. The direction of stability is anatomic (*arrow*).

the coronoid process of the ulna (Fig. 12-40). The tendon was routed through the tunnel, brought around the neck, and sutured to the lateral side of the ulna. With this construct, the direction of stability was posteromedial. The use of two drill holes to secure the annular ligament or other reconstructive tendon at both normal attachments of the annular ligament on the ulna achieved a more normal posteromedial holding force on the neck of the radius. Alternatives to holes drilled in the bone are small bone staples or bone-anchoring devices.

Osteotomy. Most surgeons advocate an ulnar osteotomy, with or without ligament repair/reconstruction, for a pediatric chronic Monteggia lesion. Various types of osteotomies have been used to facilitate reduction of the radial head and prevent recurrent subluxation after annular ligament reconstruction (Fig. 12-41). Kalamchi[63] reported using a "drill hole" ulnar osteotomy to obtain reduction of the radial head in two patients. Minimal periosteal stripping with this technique allowed the osteotomy to heal rapidly. Hirayama et al.[57] used a 1-cm distraction ulnar osteotomy approximately 5 cm distal to the tip of the olecranon with plate-and-screw fixation, but complications with loosening and plate breakage occurred. Mehta[82,83] used an osteotomy of the proximal ulna stabilized with bone graft. In neither series was annular ligament repair done. Oner and Diepstraten[92] suggested that ulnar osteotomy is not necessary in type I lesions (anterior dislocation), but in type III lesions (anterolateral dislocation) recurrent subluxation is likely without osteotomy. Freedman et al.[46] reported a delayed open reduction of a type I Monteggia lesion without annular ligament reconstruction but with ulnar osteotomy, radial shortening, and deepening of the radial notch of the ulna.

Inoue and Shionoya[62] compared the results of simple corrective ulnar osteotomy in six patients with those of posterior angular (overcorrected) osteotomy in six others, and found that better clinical outcomes were obtained with the overcorrected, angular osteotomy. Tajima and Yoshizu,[132] in a series of 23 neglected Monteggia fractures, found that the best results were obtained by opening wedge osteotomy of the proximal ulna without ligament reconstruction.

Exner[39] reported that in patients with chronic dislocation of the radial head after missed type I Monteggia lesions, reduction was successfully obtained with ulnar corticotomy and gradual lengthening and angulation of the ulna using an external fixator. Another option for type IV old Monteggia fracture is a shorten-

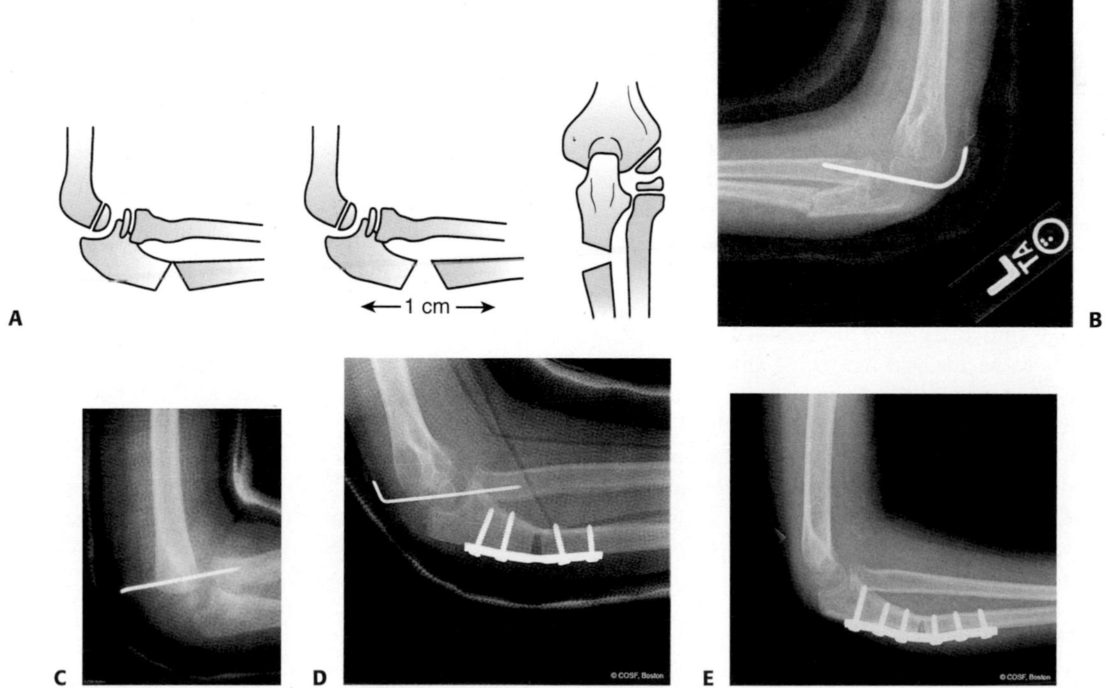

FIGURE 12-41 A. Diagram of floating open osteotomy without fixation or bone graft. **B.** Similar osteotomy with radiocapitellar pin fixation. **C.** Unfortunately in this case, the radial head was never reduced and the pin was placed without anatomic alignment. **D.** In this situation, the osteotomy was plated without bone graft, the radiocapitellar joint pinned anatomically for 4 weeks. **E.** Long-term-follow up with anatomic healing.

ing osteotomy of the radius, usually indicated for angulation of the radius without angulation of the ulna.

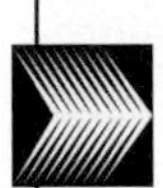

AUTHORS' PREFERRED TREATMENT

In patients younger than 12 years of age with delayed diagnosis of a Monteggia lesion, reduction and stabilization of the radial head in its appropriate relation with the capitellum are indicated. Even though the child may do well in the short term without reduction of the radial head, problems usually develop in adolescence or adulthood when progressive instability, pain, weakness of the forearm, and restriction of motion are likely to occur. There is also a risk of tardy radial or ulnar nerve palsies. The concavity of the radial head and convexity of the capitellum are assessed preoperatively, usually by MRI scan. Appropriate discussion with the patient and family regarding the risks and complications of surgery is performed. This is not an operation for the inexperienced surgeon or uninformed patient and family.

Surgical Approach

The surgical approach is extensile (Fig. 12-42). The skin incision is curvilinear to allow for proximal triceps tendon harvesting, if necessary, and distally for an ulnar opening wedge osteotomy. Initially, only the central portion is opened. The radial nerve is identified between the brachialis and brachioradialis in the distal humerus. Dissection of the nerve is performed distally to its branching into motor (posterior interosseous nerve) and sensory nerves. Generally the posterior interosseous nerve is adherent to the dislocated radial head. The nerves are mobilized and protected throughout the remainder of the reconstruction.

Next, the anconeus-extensor carpi ulnaris interval is utilized to expose the joint. The joint exposure is carried proximal with elevation of the extensor-supinator mass and capsule as a single tissue plane off the distal humerus. This gives complete exposure of the elbow joint. The radial head is usually dislocated anteriorly and superiorly with a wall of interposed capsule and ligament blocking reduction. Pulvinar and synovitis are thoroughly débrided from the elbow joint. Particular attention is paid to a thorough débridement of the proximal radioulnar joint to allow the radial head to fit anatomically into place once reduced. At this stage, a decision needs to be made if the native annular ligament can be used for reconstruction. There is usually a central perforation in the capsular wall that separates the dislocated radial head from the joint. This perforation indicates the site of the opening of the original ligament. Dilatation and radial incisions extending from the center outward are made to enlarge this opening. This usually enables the native annular ligament to be reduced over the radial neck. Capsular adhesions are removed from the radial head to assist in reduction of the radial head and neck back into the joint. The native ligament usually detaches from the ulna with a large periosteal sleeve (the site of ossification on the radiographs of a chronic Monteggia lesion), and this can be the site for suture reattachment to the ulna of the native ligament. If the native ligament cannot be used, and most of the time it can, then it is thoroughly débrided in preparation for harvesting of triceps fascia for ligament reconstruction.

Radial head reduction is then attempted. If it is accomplished, it is scrutinized for congruity between the radial head and the capitellum. If this is satisfactory, ligamentous repair or reconstruction alone can be done. This is exceedingly unusual. If the radius cannot be reduced atraumatically, an ulnar osteotomy is made at the site of maximal deformity. This involves a more distal exposure to the ulna. Subperiosteal dissection is performed with fluoroscopic assistance at the site of maximal deformity. An opening wedge osteotomy is made with a laminar spreader to allow the radial head to align itself with the capitellum without pressure. Partial overcorrection of the ulnar alignment is the goal. When reduced anatomically, the ulnar osteotomy is then fixed partially proximally and distally with a plate and screws. Further testing of a complete stable arc of rotation of the radial head is performed to be certain the correct level and degree of osteotomy were obtained to maintain radiocapitellar and radioulnar alignment. If correct, the fixation is completed. No bone graft is used, and the periosteum is repaired.

At this stage, the annular ligament repair or reconstruction is completed. If the native ligament is used, and it usually is in situations that are a year or less out from injury, then Ethibond mattress sutures (Ethicon, Somerville, NJ) are placed in the annular ligament and the ligament is repaired through ulnar periosteal tunnels. None of the radial sutures are tightened until all are placed. If reconstruction is necessary, a 6 to 8 cm strip of triceps fascia is developed from proximal to distal, carefully elevating the periosteum from the proximal ulna down to the level of the radial neck. Over the olecranon apophysis, this dissection will be delicate so as to not inadvertently amputate the fascia. The strip of tendon is then passed through the periosteum, around the radial neck, and then brought back and sutured to itself and the ulnar periosteum. The passage and securing in the periosteum is similar in design to the drill holes advocated by Seel and Peterson.[117] At this stage, the radial head and capitellum alignment should be anatomic throughout full rotation. Final closure involves repair of the capsule and extensor-supinator origin back to the lateral epicondylar region of the humerus. Final radiographs and fluoroscopic testing of a stable arc of motion in both flexion-extension and pronation-supination planes are gently tested before completion of closure. Prophylactic volar and dorsal forearm fasciotomies are carefully performed through the original incision with elevation of the skin and subcutaneous tissues and a long tenotomy scissors. Final inspection of the radial nerve is performed before subcutaneous and skin closure.

Radiocapitellar or radioulnar pin fixation is rarely needed if the osteotomy and soft tissue repair tension are correct. At times, it is used intraoperatively for temporary stability to get the osteotomy and repair right; it is then removed to test range of motion. If there is radial head deformity in very chronic reconstructions, pinning the joint is sometimes useful for 3 to 4 weeks postoperatively. In my experience, this has been occasionally necessary in repeat surgery for a chronic Monteggia lesion in which options are limited and the patient has pain and marked limitation of motion. Then, the radiocapitellar joint is secured by passing a smooth,

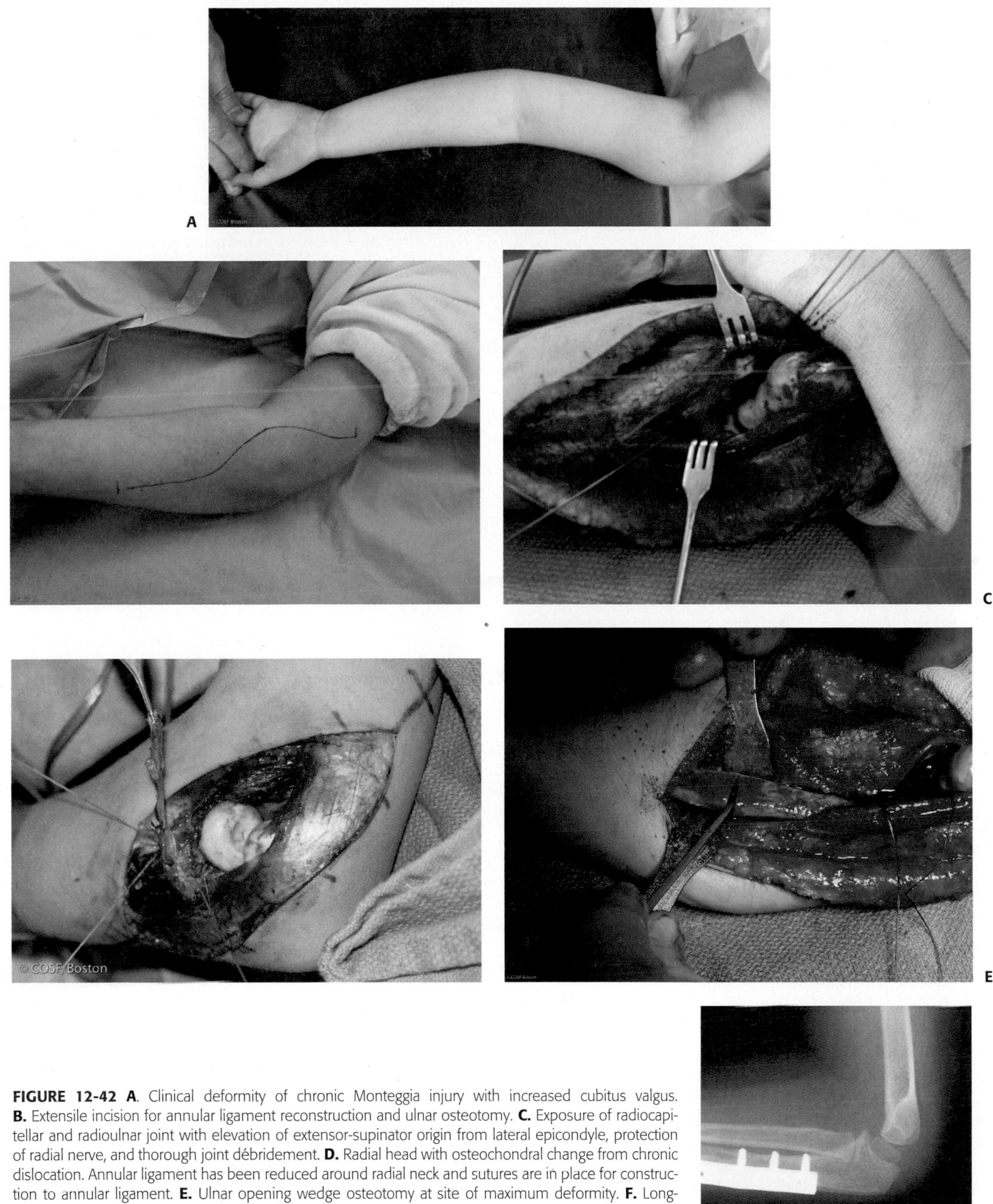

FIGURE 12-42 A. Clinical deformity of chronic Monteggia injury with increased cubitus valgus. **B.** Extensile incision for annular ligament reconstruction and ulnar osteotomy. **C.** Exposure of radiocapitellar and radioulnar joint with elevation of extensor-supinator origin from lateral epicondyle, protection of radial nerve, and thorough joint débridement. **D.** Radial head with osteochondral change from chronic dislocation. Annular ligament has been reduced around radial neck and sutures are in place for construction to annular ligament. **E.** Ulnar opening wedge osteotomy at site of maximum deformity. **F.** Long-term follow-up of ulnar osteotomy and the anatomic reduction of proximal radioulnar joint and radiocapitellar joint.

transcapitellar pin through the posterior aspect of the capitellum into the radial head and neck with the elbow at 90 degrees and the forearm in supination. A pin of sufficient size is mandatory to avoid pin failure[68]; a small pin may fatigue and break. An alternative technique to secure the reduction of the radius is transversely pinning the radius to the ulna.[75]

Postoperative Care

After wound closure, a bivalved (including Webril [Kimberly Clark, Chantilly, VA]) long-arm cast is applied with the forearm in 60 to 90 degrees of supination and the elbow flexed 80 to 90 degrees. The cast is maintained for 4 to 6 weeks and is then changed to a removable bivalve to allow active motion, especially pronation and supination. Elbow flexion and extension return more rapidly than rotary motion of the forearm which may take up to 6 months to improve, with pronation possibly limited, though minimally, permanently.[112] Final desired result is not determined until radiographs are anatomic with full restoration of motion.

Nerve Injuries

Radial Nerve

The literature reflects a 10% to 20% incidence of radial nerve injury, making it the most common complication associated with Monteggia fractures.[60] It is most commonly associated with types I and III injuries.[14,89,118] The posterior interosseous nerve is most commonly injured because of its proximity to the radial head and its intimate relation to the arcade of Frohse. The arcade may be thinner and therefore more pliable in children than in adults.[122] In addition, the periosteum is much thicker in pediatric patients. This may account in part for the rapid resolution of the nerve injury in children.

A radial nerve injury in a child is treated expectantly. Nerve function usually returns by 12 weeks after reduction, if not sooner.[123,125] A review of a series of children's Monteggia lesions[91] recommends waiting 6 months before intervention for a posterior interosseous nerve injury. Most series report 100% resolution in both fractures treated promptly and those treated late.[1,6,76]

Two reports[86,120] of irreducible Monteggia fractures caused by interposition of the radial nerve posterior to the radial head documented return of function approximately 4 months after the nerve was replaced to its normal anatomic position and the radial head was reduced. Morris,[86] in cadaver studies, showed that significant anterior dislocation of the radial head and varus angulation of the elbow allowed the radial nerve to slide posterior to the radial head and, with subsequent reduction of the radial head, become entrapped. If a chronic reconstruction is undertaken in the presence of a persistent radial nerve lesion, it is highly recommended that radial nerve exploration and decompression be performed before joint débridement. Rodgers et al.[113] cited a partial nerve injury during similar circumstances that was then microscopically repaired with full recovery. Rang[106] acknowledged the same experience to the author in an open educational forum.

Ulnar Nerve

Bryan[22] reported one adult with an ulnar nerve lesion associated with a type II Monteggia lesion, with spontaneous resolution. Stein et al.[125] reported three combined radial and ulnar nerve injuries, two of which underwent exploration and decompression for functional return of the nerve.

Median Nerve

Median nerve injuries are uncommon with Monteggia fractures, but injury to the anterior interosseous nerve has been reported.[142,143] Stein et al.,[125] in their report specifically examining nerve injuries in Monteggia lesions, reported no median nerve deficits. Watson and Singer[142] reported entrapment of the main trunk of the median nerve in a greenstick ulnar fracture in a 6-year-old girl. Completion of the fracture was necessary for release of the nerve. At 6 months after surgery, there was full motor recovery but sensation was slightly reduced in the tips of the index finger and thumb.

Tardy Nerve Palsy

Tardy radial nerve palsy associated with radial head dislocation has been infrequently reported.[1,6,58,76,148] Although reported treatment has varied, excision of the radial head with exploration and neurolysis of the nerve generally produced good results,[1,6] while exploration of the nerve alone produced variable results.[58,76] Yamamoto et al.[148] combined radial head resection and nerve exploration with tendon transfers, producing good results in two patients.

Associated Fractures and Unusual Lesions

Monteggia lesions have been associated with fractures of the wrist and the distal forearm,[9] including distal radial and ulnar metaphyseal and diaphyseal fractures.[9,61,63,112] Galeazzi fractures may also occur with Monteggia lesions.[9,25] Radial head and neck fractures are commonly associated with type II fractures[9,73] but may occur with other types.[1,41,45] With a type II lesion, the radial head fracture is usually at its anterior rim.[73] Strong et al.[130] reported two type I equivalent lesions consisting of a fractured radial neck and midshaft ulnar fracture. This injury was unique because of significant medial displacement of the distal radial fragment. Obtaining and maintaining reduction of the radius was difficult with a closed technique.

Fractures of the lateral condyle have also been associated with Monteggia fractures.[98] Ravessoud[107] reported an ipsilateral ulnar shaft lesion and a lateral condylar fracture without loss of the radiocapitellar relation, suggesting a Monteggia type II equivalent. Kloen et al.[69] reported an unusual bilateral Monteggia fracture and described the operative technique for this treatment. Despite surgical and rehabilitative challenges, excellent results were obtained in both elbows. In essence, any fracture about the elbow and forearm should be inspected for an associated Monteggia lesion.

Periarticular Ossification

Two patterns of ossification after Monteggia fracture-dislocations have been noted radiographically: around the radial head and myositis ossificans. Ossification around the radial head and neck[14,60,76,78,126,128] appears as a thin ridge of bone in a cap-like distribution and may be accompanied by other areas resembling sesamoid bones; they resorb with time. Ossification may also occur in the area of the annular ligament,[36] including in a chronic Monteggia with a displaced annular ligament. Elbow function generally is not affected by the formation of these lesions[14,60,78,126,128] as long as the radial head and neck are anatomically reduced.

The other form of ossification is true myositis ossificans, reported to occur in approximately 3% of elbow injuries and 7% of Monteggia lesions in adults and children.[90] Myositis ossificans has a good prognosis in patients younger than 15 years of age, appearing at 3 to 4 weeks after injury and resolving in 6 to 8 months. Its occurrence is related to the severity of the initial injury, association with a fractured radial head, the number of remanipulations during treatment, and passive motion of the elbow during the postoperative period.[90,137]

SUMMARY

Adherence to several fundamental principles helps ensure a good outcome after Monteggia fracture-dislocations in children:

1. Evaluation of the radial head location requires an AP view of the proximal forearm and a true lateral view of the elbow. All forearm injuries require careful inspection of the proximal radioulnar joint and the radiocapitellar joint before treatment.
2. The radiocapitellar line must be anatomic in all views.
3. If the radial head is dislocated, always look for ulnar fracture or plastic deformation. Conversely, if the ulna is fractured, always look for a radial head subluxation or dislocation.
4. Stability of the ulnar reduction is required to maintain reduction of the radial head. Stability may be inherent to the fracture pattern (plastic deformation or incomplete fractures) or achieved by internal fixation (intramedullary fixation for short oblique and transverse fractures; plate and screw fixation for long oblique and comminuted fractures).
5. Radial head reduction confirmed by an intact radiocapitellar line must be achieved by open or closed means.
6. If the radial head is irreducible or unstable, reconstruction of the annular ligament and/or removal of interposed soft tissue is required.
7. Treatment of an acute Monteggia lesion is much easier and more successful than reconstruction of a chronic Monteggia lesion.
8. Reconstruction of a chronic Monteggia lesion is not an operation for the uninitiated.

ACKNOWLEDGMENTS

The author wishes to recognize contributions of the authors of previous editions of this chapter, Drs. Earl Stanley and Jose de la Garza, as well as the outstanding assistance of Ms. Bonnie Kaufman in our hand research unit.

REFERENCES

1. Adams JR, Rizzoli HV. Tardy radial and ulnar nerve palsy: a case report. J Neurosurg 1959;16:342–344.
2. Agarwal A. Type IV Monteggia fracture in a child. Can J Surg 2008;51(2):E44–E45.
3. Almquist EE, Gordon LH, Blue AI. Congenital dislocation of the head of the radius. J Bone Joint Surg Am 1969;51:1118–1127.
4. Anderson HJ. Monteggia fractures. Adv Orthop Surg 1989;4:201–204.
5. Arazi M, Oğün TC, Kapicioğlu MI. The Monteggia lesion and ipsilateral supracondylar humerus and distal radius fractures. J Orthop Trauma 1999;13(1):60–63.
6. Austin R. Tardy palsy of the radial nerve from a Monteggia fracture. Injury 1926;7:202–204.
7. Babb A, Carlson WO. Monteggia fractures: beware! S D J Med 2005;58(7):283–285.
8. Bado JL. La lesion de Monteggia. Intermedica Sarandi 1958;328.
9. Bado JL. The Monteggia lesion. Clin Orthop Relat Res 1967;50:71–86.
10. Bado JL. The Monteggia Lesion. Springfield, IL: Charles C Thomas, 1962.
11. Basmajian JV, Griffen WR Jr. Function of anconeus muscle. An electromyographic study. J Bone Joint Surg Am 1972;54:1712–1714.
12. Beaty JH. Fractures and dislocations about the elbow in children: section on Monteggia fractures. AAOS Instr Course Lect 1991;40:373–384.
13. Beddow FH, Corkery PH. Lateral dislocation of the radiohumeral joint with greenstick fracture of the upper end of the ulna. J Bone Joint Surg Br 1960;42:782–784.
14. Bell Tawse AJ. The treatment of malunited anterior Monteggia fractures in children. J Bone Joint Surg Br 1965;47:718–723.
15. Best TN. Management of old unreduced Monteggia fracture dislocations of the elbow in children. J Pediatr Orthop 1994;14:193–199.
16. Bhandari N, Jindal P. Monteggia lesion in a child: variant of a Bado type-IV lesion. A case report. J Bone Joint Surg Am 1996;78(8):1252–1255.
17. Biyani A. Ipsilateral Monteggia equivalent injury and distal radial and ulnar fracture in a child. J Orthop Trauma 1994;8(5):431–433.
18. Blasier D, Trussell A. Ipsilateral radial head dislocation and distal fractures of both forearm bones in a child. Am J Orthop 1995;24:498–500.
19. Blount WP. Fractures in Children. Baltimore: Williams & Wilkins, 1955.
20. Boyd HB. Surgical exposure of the ulna and proximal one third of the radius through one incision. Surg Gynecol Obstet 1940;71:86–88.
21. Boyd HB, Boals JC. The Monteggia lesion: a review of 159 cases. Clin Orthop Relat Res 1969;66:94–100.
22. Bryan RS. Monteggia fracture of the forearm. J Trauma 1971;11:992–998.
23. Bucknill TM. The elbow joint. Proc R Soc Med 1977;70:620.
24. Caravias DE. Some observations on congenital dislocation of the head of the radius. J Bone Joint Surg Br 1957;39:86–90.
25. Castillo Odena I [Milch H, transl]. Bipolar fracture-dislocation of the forearm. J Bone Joint Surg Am 1952;34:968–976.
26. Corbett CH. Anterior dislocation of the radius and its recurrence. Br J Surg 1931;19:155.
27. Curry GJ. Monteggia fracture. Am J Surg 1947;123:613–617.
28. David-West KS, Wilson NI, Sherlock DA, et al. Missed Monteggia injuries. Injury 2005;36(10):1206–1209.
29. De Boeck H. Radial neck osteolysis after anular ligament reconstruction a case report. Clin Orthop Relat Res 1997;342:94–98.
30. Degreef I, De Smet L. Missed radial head dislocations in children associated with ulnar deformation: treatment by open reduction and ulnar osteotomy. J Orthop Trauma 2004;18(6):375–378.
31. Denucé P. Mémoire sun les luxations du coude. Paris, France: Thése de Paris; 1854.
32. Deshpande S, O'Doherty D. Type I Monteggia fracture dislocation associated with ipsilateral distal radial epiphyseal injury. J Orthop Trauma 2001;15(5):373–375.
33. Devnani AS. Missed Monteggia fracture dislocation in children. Injury 1997 Mar;28(2):131–133.
34. Dormans JP, Rang M. The problem of Monteggia fracture-dislocations in children. Orthop Clin North Am 1990;21:251–256.
35. Eady JL. Acute Monteggia lesions in children. J S C Med Assoc 1975;71:107–112.
36. Earwaker J. Posttraumatic calcification of the annular ligament of the radius. Skeletal Radiol 1992;21:149–154.
37. Edwards EG. The posterior Monteggia fracture. Am Surg 1952;18:323–337.
38. Evans M. Pronation injuries of the forearm. J Bone Joint Surg Br 1949;31:578–588.
39. Exner GU. Missed chronic anterior Monteggia lesion. Closed reduction by gradual lengthening and angulation of the ulna. J Bone Joint Surg Br 2001;83(4):547–550.
40. Fahey JJ. Fractures of the elbow in children: Monteggia's fracture-dislocation. AAOS Instr Course Lect 1960;17:39.
41. Fahmy NRM. Unusual Monteggia lesions in kids. Injury 1980;12:399–404.
42. Faundez AA, Ceroni D, Kaelin A. An unusual Monteggia type-I equivalent fracture in a child. J Bone Joint Surg Br 2003;85(4):584–586.
43. Fernandez FF, Egenolf M, Carsten C, et al. Unstable diaphyseal fractures of both bones of the forearm in children: plate fixation versus intramedullary nailing. Injury 2005;36(10):1210–1216.
44. Fowles JV, Sliman N, Kassah MT. The Monteggia lesion in children. Fracture of the ulna and dislocation of the radial head. J Bone Joint Surg Am 1983;65:1276–1282.
45. Frazier JL, Buschmann WR, Insler HP. Monteggia type I equivalent lesion: diaphyseal ulna and proximal radius fracture with a posterior elbow dislocation in a child. J Orthop Trauma 1991;5:373–375.
46. Freedman L, Luk K, Leong JC. Radial head reduction after a missed Monteggia fracture: brief report. J Bone Joint Surg Br 1988;70:846–847.
47. Gibson WK, Timperlake RW. Orthopedic treatment of 4 type IV Monteggia fracture-dislocations in a child. J Bone Joint Surg Br 1992;74:780–781.
48. Giustra PE, Killoran PJ, Furman RS, et al. The missed Monteggia fracture. Radiology 1974;110(1):45–47.
49. Givon U, Pritsch M, Levy O, et al. Monteggia and equivalent lesions: a study of 41 cases. Clin Orthop Relat Res 1997;337:208–215.
50. Givon U, Pritsch M, Yosepovich A. Monteggia lesion in a child: variant of a Bado type-IV lesion. A case report. J Bone Joint Surg Am 1997;79(11):1753–1754.
51. Gleeson AP, Beattie TF. Monteggia fracture-dislocation in children. J Accid Emerg Med 1994;11(3):192–194.
52. Gorden ML. Monteggia fracture: a combined surgical approach employing a single lateral incision. Clin Orthop Relat Res 1967;50:87–93.
53. Gyr BM, Stevens PM, Smith JT. Chronic Monteggia fractures in children: outcome after treatment with the Bell-Tawse procedure. J Pediatr Orthop B 2004;13(6):402–406.
54. Haddad ES, Manktelow AR, Sarkar JS. The posterior Monteggia: a pathological lesion? Injury 1996;27:101–102.
55. Hall J. Personal communication.
56. Henry AK. Extensile Exposure. Baltimore: Williams & Wilkins, 1970.
57. Hirayama T, Takemitsu Y, Yagihara K, et al. Operation for chronic dislocation of the radial head in children. J Bone Joint Surg Br 1987;69:639–642.
58. Holst-Nielson F, Jensen V. Tardy posterior interosseus nerve palsy as a result of an unreduced radial head dislocation in Monteggia fractures: a report of two cases. J Hand Surg Am 1984;9:572–575.
59. Hui JH, Sulaiman AR, Lee HC, et al. Open reduction and annular ligament reconstruc-

tion with fascia of the forearm in chronic monteggia lesions in children. J Pediatr Orthop 2005;25(4):501–506.
60. Hume AC. Anterior dislocation of the head of the radius associated with undisplaced fracture of olecranon in children. J Bone Joint Surg Br 1957;39:508–512.
61. Hurst LC, Dubrow EN. Surgical treatment of symptomatic chronic radial head dislocation: a neglected Monteggia fracture. J Pediatr Orthop 1983;3:227–230.
62. Inoue G, Shionoya K. Corrective ulnar osteotomy for malunited anterior Monteggia lesions in children: 12 patients followed for 1 to 12 years. Acta Orthop Scand 1998; 69:73–76.
63. Kalamchi A. Monteggia fracture-dislocation in children. J Bone Joint Surg Am 1986; 68:615–619.
64. Kaplan EB. The quadrate ligament of the radio-ulnar joint in the elbow. Bull Hosp Joint Dis 1964;25:126–130.
65. Karachalios T, Smith EJ, Pearse MF. Monteggia equivalent injury in a very young patient. Injury 1992;23:419–420.
66. Kay RM, Skaggs DL. The pediatric Monteggia fracture. Am J Orthop 1998;27(9): 606–609.
67. Kemnitz S, De Schrijver F, De Smet L. Radial head dislocation with plastic deformation of the ulna in children. A rare and frequently missed condition. Acta Orthop Belg 2000;66(4):359–362.
68. King RE. Treating the persistent symptomatic anterior radial head dislocation. J Pediatr Orthop 1983;3:623–624.
69. Kloen P, Rubel IF, Farley TD, et al. Bilateral Monteggia fractures. Am J Orthop 2003; 32(2):98–100.
70. Koslowsky TC, Mader K, Wulke AP, et al. Operative treatment of chronic Monteggia lesion in younger children: a report of three cases. J Shoulder Elbow Surg 2006;15(1): 119–121.
71. Kristiansen B, Eriksen AF. Simultaneous type II Monteggia lesion and fracture separation of the lower radial epiphysis. Injury 1986;17:51–62.
72. Lambrinudi C. Intramedullary Kirschner wires in the treatment of fractures. Proc R Soc Med 1940;33:153.
73. Landin LA. Fracture patterns in children. Acta Paediatr Scand Suppl 1983;54:192.
74. Lascombes P, Prevot J, Ligen JN, et al. Elastic stable intramedullary nailing in forearm shaft fractures in children: 85 cases. J Pediatr Orthop 1990;10:167–171.
75. Letts M, Locht R, Wiens J. Monteggia fracture-dislocations in children. J Bone Joint Surg Br 1985;67:724–727.
76. Lichter RL, Jacksen T. Tardy palsy of posterior interosseous nerve with Monteggia fracture. J Bone Joint Surg Am 1975;57:124–125.
77. Lincoln TL, Mubarak SJ. "Isolated" traumatic radial-head dislocation. J Pediatr Orthop 1994;14:454–457.
78. Lloyd-Roberts GC, Bucknill TM. Anterior dislocation of the radial head in children: aetiology, natural history, and management. J Bone Joint Surg Br 1977;59:402–407.
79. Luhmann SJ, Gordon JE, Schoenecker PL. Intramedullary fixation of unstable both-bone forearm fractures in children. J Pediatr Orthop 1998;18(4):451–456.
80. Maeda H, Yoshida K, Doi R, et al. Combined Monteggia and Galeazzi fractures in a child: a case report and review of the literature. J Orthop Trauma 2003;17(2):128–131.
81. McFarland B. Congenital dislocation of the head of the radius. Br J Surg 1936;24: 41–49.
82. Mehta SD. Flexion osteotomy of ulna for untreated Monteggia fracture in children. Indian J Surg 1985;47:15–19.
83. Mehta SD. Missed Monteggia fracture. J Bone Joint Surg Br 1993;75:337.
84. Miles KA, Finlay DB. Disruption of the radiocapitellar line in the normal elbow. Injury 1989;20:365–367.
85. Monteggia GB. Instituzioni Chirurgiche. Milan: Maspero, 1814.
86. Morris AH. Irreducible Monteggia lesion with radial nerve entrapment. J Bone Joint Surg Am 1974;56:1744–1746.
87. Mullick S. The lateral Monteggia fracture. J Bone Joint Surg Am 1977;57:543–545.
88. Nakashima H, Kondo K, Saka K. Type II Monteggia lesion with fracture-separation of the distal physis of the radius. Am J Orthop 2000 Sep;29(9):717–719.
89. Naylor A. Monteggia fractures. Br J Surg 1942;29:323.
90. Neviaser RJ, LeFevre GW. Irreducible isolated dislocation of the radial head: a case report. Clin Orthop Relat Res 1971;80:72–74.
91. Olney BW, Menelaus MB. Monteggia and equivalent lesions in childhood. J Pediatr Orthop 1989;9:219–223.
92. Oner FC, Diepstraten AF. Treatment of chronic posttraumatic dislocation of the radial head in children. J Bone Joint Surg Br 1993;75:577–581.
93. Osamura N, Ikeda K, Hagiwara N, et al. Posterior interosseous nerve injury complicating ulnar osteotomy for a missed Monteggia fracture. Scand J Plast Reconstr Surg Hand Surg 2004;38(6):376–378.
94. Papandrea R, Waters PM. Posttraumatic reconstruction of the elbow in the pediatric patient. Clin Orthop Relat Res 2000;(370):115–126.
95. Papavasilou VA, Nenopoulos SP. Monteggia-type elbow fracture in childhood. Clin Orthop Relat Res 1988;233:230–233.
96. Parsch KD. Die Morote-Drahtung bei proximalen und mittleren Unterarm Schaft Frakturen des Kindes. Operat Orthop Traumatol 1990;2:245–255.
97. Pavel A, Pitman JM, Lance EM, et al. The posterior Monteggia fracture: a clinical study. J Trauma 1965;5:185–199.
98. Peiró A, Andres F, Fernandez-Esteve F. Acute Monteggia lesions in children. J Bone Joint Surg Am 1977;59:92–97.
99. Peltier LF. Eponymic fractures: Giovanni Battista Monteggia and Monteggia's fracture. Surgery 1957;42:585–591.
100. Penrose JH. The Monteggia fracture with posterior dislocation of the radial head. J Bone Joint Surg Br 1951;33:65–73.
101. Pérez Sicialia JE, Morote Jurado JL, Corbach Gironés JM, et al. Osteosíntesis percutánea en fracturas diafisaris de ante brazo en niños y adolescentes. Rev Esp Cir Ost 1977; 12:321–334.
102. Powell RS, Bowe JA. Ipsilateral supracondylar humerus fracture and Monteggia lesion: a case report. J Orthop Trauma 2002;16(10):737–740.
103. Price CT, Scott DS, Kurener ME, et al. Malunited forearm fracture in children. J Pediatr Orthop 1990;10:705–712.
104. Pugh DM, Galpin RD, Carey TP. Intramedullary Steinmann pin fixation of forearm fractures in children. Long-term results. Clin Orthop Relat Res 2000;(376):39–48.
105. Ramsey RH, Pedersen HE. The Monteggia fracture–dislocation in children. Study of 15 cases of ulnar-shaft fracture with radial-head involvement. JAMA 1962;82:1091–1093.
106. Rang M. The Story of Orthopaedics. Philadelphia: Saunders, 2000.
107. Ravessoud FA. Lateral condyle fracture and ipsilateral ulnar shaft fracture: Monteggia equivalent lesions. J Pediatr Orthop 1985;5:364–366.
108. Reckling F. Unstable fracture-dislocations of the forearm (Monteggia and Galeazzi lesions). J Bone Joint Surg Am 1982;64:857–863.
109. Reckling FW, Cordell LD. Unstable fracture-dislocations of the forearm. The Monteggia and Galeazzi lesions. Arch Surg 1968;96:999–1007.
110. Ring D, Jupiter JB, Waters PM. Monteggia fractures in children and adults. J Am Acad Orthop Surg 1998;6(4):215–224.
111. Ring D, Waters PM. Operative fixation of Monteggia fractures in children. J Bone Joint Surg Br 1996;78:734–739.
112. Rodgers WB, Smith BG. A type IV Monteggia injury with a distal diaphyseal radius fracture in a child. J Orthop Trauma 1993;7:84–86.
113. Rodgers WB, Waters PM, Hall JE. Chronic Monteggia lesions in children: complications and results of reconstruction. J Bone Joint Surg Am 1996;78:1322–1329.
114. Rodríguez-Merchán EC. Pediatric fractures of the forearm. Clin Orthop Relat Res 2005; (432):65–72.
115. Ruchelsman DE, Klugman JA, Madan SS, et al. Anterior dislocation of the radial head with fractures of the olecranon and radial neck in a young child: a Monteggia equivalent fracture-dislocation variant. J Orthop Trauma 2005;19(6):425–428.
116. Salter RB, Zaltz C. Anatomic investigations of the mechanism of injury and pathologic anatomy of "pulled elbow" in young children. Clin Orthop Relat Res 1971;77:134–143.
117. Seel MJ, Peterson HA. Management of chronic posttraumatic radial head dislocation in children. J Pediatr Orthop 1999;19:306–312.
118. Smith FM. Monteggia fractures: an analysis of 25 consecutive fresh injuries. Surg Gynecol Obstet 1947;85:630–640.
119. Sood A, Khan O, Bagga T. Simultaneous monteggia type I fracture equivalent with ipsilateral fracture of the distal radius and ulna in a child: a case report. J Med Case Reports 2008;2:190.
120. Spar I. A neurologic complication following Monteggia fracture. Clin Orthop Relat Res 1977;122:207–209.
121. Speed JS, Boyd HB. Treatment of fractures of ulna with dislocation of head of radius: Monteggia fracture. JAMA 1940;125:1699.
122. Spinner M. The arcade of Frohse and its relationship to posterior interosseous nerve paralysis. J Bone Joint Surg Br 1968;50:809–812.
123. Spinner M, Freundlich BD, Teicher J. Posterior interosseous nerve palsy as a complication of Monteggia fracture in children. Clin Orthop Relat Res 1968;58:141–145.
124. Spinner M, Kaplan EB. The quadrate ligament of the elbow—its relationship to the stability of the proximal radioulnar joint. Acta Orthop Scand 1970; 41:632–647.
125. Stein F, Grabias SL, Deffer PA. Nerve injuries complicating Monteggia lesions. J Bone Joint Surg Am 1971;53:1432–1436.
126. Stelling FH, Cote RH. Traumatic dislocation of head of radius in children. JAMA 1956; 160:732–736.
127. Stoll TM, Willis RB, Paterson DC. Treatment of the missed Monteggia fracture in the child. J Bone Joint Surg Br 1992;74:436–440.
128. Storen G. Traumatic dislocation of radial head as an isolated lesion in children. Acta Chir Scand 1958–1959;116:144–147.
129. Strachen JCH, Ellis BW. Vulnerability of the posterior interosseous nerve during radial head reduction. J Bone Joint Surg Br 1971;53:320–332.
130. Strong ML, Kopp M, Gillespie R. Fracture of the radial neck and proximal ulna with medial displacement of the radial shaft. Orthopedics 1989;12:1577–1579.
131. Tait G, Sulaiman SK. Isolated dislocation of the radial head: a report of two cases. Injury 1988;19:125–126.
132. Tajima T, Yoshizu T. Treatment of long-standing dislocation of the radial head in neglected Monteggia fractures. J Hand Surg Am 1995;20:S91–S94.
133. Thakore HK. Lateral Monteggia fracture in children (case report). Ital J Orthop Traumatol 1983:55–56.
134. Theodorou SD. Dislocation of the head of the radius associated with fracture of the upper end of ulna in children. J Bone Joint Surg Br 1969;51:700–706.
135. Theodorou SD, Ierodiaconou MD, Rousis N. Fracture of the upper end of the ulna associated with dislocation of the head of the radius in children. Clin Orthop Relat Res 1988; 228:240–249.
136. Thompson GH, Wilber JH, Marcus RE. Internal fixation of fractures in children and adolescents. Clin Orthop Relat Res 1984;188:10–20.
137. Thompson HC III, Garcia A. Myositis ossificans: aftermath of elbow injuries. Clin Orthop Relat Res 1967;50:129–134.
138. Thompson JD, Lipscomb AB. Recurrent radial head subluxation treated with annular ligament reconstruction. Clin Orthop Relat Res 1989;246:131–135.
139. Tompkins DG. The anterior Monteggia fracture. J Bone Joint Surg Am 1971;53: 109–1114.
140. Verstreken L, Delronge G, Lamoureux J. Shaft forearm fractures in children. intramedullary nailing with immediate motion: a preliminary report. J Pediatr Orthop 1988;8: 450–453.
141. Walker JL, Rang M. Forearm fractures in children. Cast treatment with the elbow extended. J Bone Joint Surg Br 1991;73:299–301.
142. Watson JA, Singer GC. Irreducible Monteggia fracture: beware nerve entrapment. Injury 1994;25:325–327.
143. Wiley JJ, Galey JP. Monteggia injuries in children. J Bone Joint Surg Br 1985;67: 728–731.
144. Wilkins KE. Changes in the management of monteggia fractures. J Pediatr Orthop 2002;22(4):548–554.
145. Wise RA. Lateral dislocation of the head of radius with fracture of the ulna. J Bone Joint Surg 1941;23:379.
146. Cappellino A, Wolfe SW, Marsh JS. Use of a modified Bell Tawse procedure for chronic acquired dislocation of the radial head. J Pediatr Orthop 1998;18(3):410–414.
147. Wright PR. Greenstick fracture of the upper end of the ulna with dislocation of the radio-humeral joint or displacement of the superior radial epiphysis. J Bone Joint Surg Br 1963;45:727–731.
148. Yamamoto K, Yoshiaki Y, Tomihara M. Posterior interosseous nerve palsy as a complication of Monteggia fractures. Nippon Geka Hokan 1977;46:46–56.

13

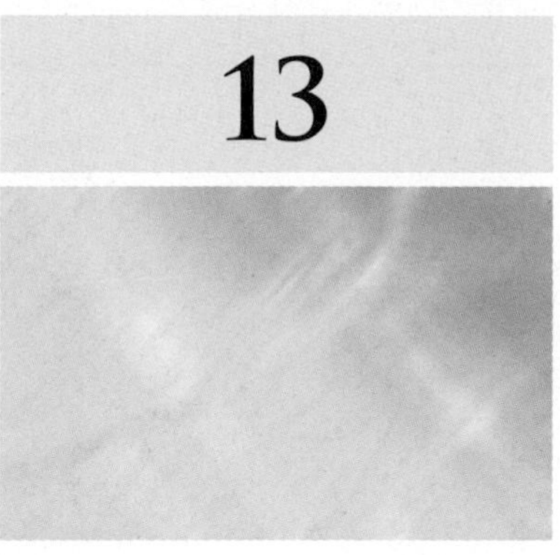

THE ELBOW REGION: GENERAL CONCEPTS IN THE PEDIATRIC PATIENT

James H. Beaty and James R. Kasser

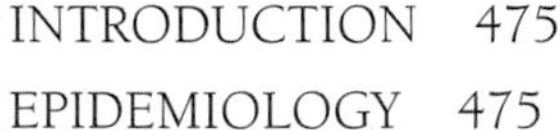

INTRODUCTION 475
EPIDEMIOLOGY 475
ANATOMY 476
The Ossification Process 476
The Fusion Process 477
Blood Supply 479
Intra-articular Structures 480
Fat Pads 481
Ligaments 481
RADIOGRAPHIC FINDINGS 481
Standard Views 481
Jones View 481
Anteroposterior Landmarks 482
Lateral Landmarks 483
Comparison Radiographs 485
Magnetic Resonance Imaging 485
Other Imaging Modalities 485

INTRODUCTION

At the turn of the century, Sir Robert Jones[29] echoed the opinion of that era about elbow injuries: "The difficulties experienced by surgeons in making an accurate diagnosis; the facility with which serious blunders can be made in prognosis and treatment; and the fear shared by so many of the subsequent limitation of function, serve to render injuries in the neighborhood of the elbow less attractive than they might otherwise have proved." These concerns are applicable even today. In other bones, good results can often be obtained with minimal treatment, but in the elbow, more aggressive treatment is often required to avoid complications. An understanding of the basic anatomy and radiographic landmarks of the elbow is essential in choosing appropriate treatment.

EPIDEMIOLOGY

Because children tend to protect themselves with their outstretched arms when they fall, upper-extremity fractures account for 65% to 75% of all fractures in children. The most common area of the upper extremity injured is the distal forearm[5,33]; 7% to 9% of upper-extremity fractures involve the elbow.

The distal humerus accounts for approximately 86% of fractures about the elbow region. Supracondylar fractures are the most frequent elbow injuries in children, reported to occur in 55% to 75% of patients with elbow fractures. Lateral condylar fractures are the second most common, followed by medial epicondylar fractures. Fractures of the olecranon, radial head, and neck and medial epicondyle and T-condylar fractures are much less common.

Elbow injuries are much more common in children and adolescents than in adults.[10,45] The peak age for fractures of the distal humerus is between 5 and 10 years old.[25] Houshian et al.[26] reported that the average age of 355 children with elbow fractures was 7.9 years (7.2 years in boys and 8.5 years in girls). Contrary to most reports, these investigators found elbow fractures more frequent in girls (54%) than in boys. In a study of 450 supracondylar humeral fractures, Cheng et al.[13] found a median age of 6 years (6.6 years in boys and 5 years in girls) and a predominance of injuries (63%) in boys.

Physeal injuries in most parts of the body occur in older children between the ages of 10 and 13; however, the peak age for injuries to the distal humeral physes is 4 to 5 years in girls and 5 to 8 years in boys. In most physeal injuries, the increased incidence with advanced age is believed to be due to weakening of the perichondrial ring as it matures (see Chapter 5). Thus, some different biomechanic forces and conditions must exist about the elbow to make the physis more vulnerable to injuries at an earlier age. (For more data on the relationship of fractures about the elbow to all types of fractures, see Chapter 1).

ANATOMY

The elbow is a complex joint composed of three individual joints contained within a common articular cavity. Several anatomic concepts are unique to the growing elbow.

The Ossification Process

The process of differentiation and maturation begins at the center of the long bones and progresses distally. The ossification process begins in the diaphyses of the humerus, radius, and ulna at the same time. By term, ossification of the humerus has extended distally to the condyles. In the ulna, it extends to more than half the distance between the coronoid process and the tip of the olecranon. The radius is ossified proximally to the level of the neck. The bicipital tuberosity remains largely unossified (Table 13-1).[20] Brodeur et al.[8] compiled a complete atlas of ossification of the structures about the elbow, and their work is an excellent reference source for finer details of the ossification process about the elbow.

Distal Humerus

Ossification of the distal humerus proceeds at a predictable rate. In general, the rate of ossification in girls exceeds that of boys.[18,19,22] In some areas, such as the olecranon and lateral epicondyle, the difference between boys and girls in ossification age may be as great as 2 years.[19] During the first 6 months, the ossification border of the distal humerus is symmetric (Fig. 13-1).

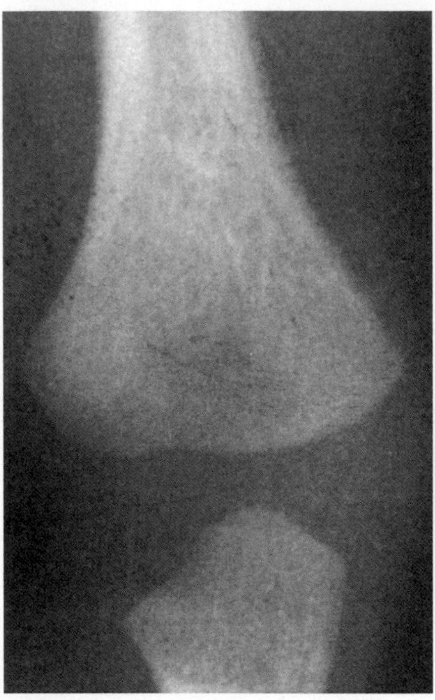

FIGURE 13-1 During the first 6 months, the advancing ossifying border of the distal humerus is symmetric.

TABLE 13-1 Sequence and Timing of Ossification in the Elbow

	Girls (y)	Boys (y)
Capitellum	1.0	1.0
Radial head	5.0	6.0
Medial epicondyle	5.0	7.5
Olecranon	8.7	10.5
Trochlea	9.0	10.7
Lateral epicondyle	10.0	12.0

Data from Cheng JC, Wing-Man K, Shen WY, et al. A new look at the sequential development of elbow-ossification centers in children. J Pediatr Orthop 1998;18: 161–167.

Lateral Condyle

On average, the ossification center of the lateral condyle appears just before 1 year of age but may be delayed as late as 18 to 24 months.[10] When the nucleus of the lateral condyle first appears, the distal humeral metaphyseal border becomes asymmetric. The lateral border slants and becomes straight to conform with the ossification center of the lateral condyle (Fig. 13-2). By the end of the second year, this border becomes well defined, possibly even slightly concave. This ossification center

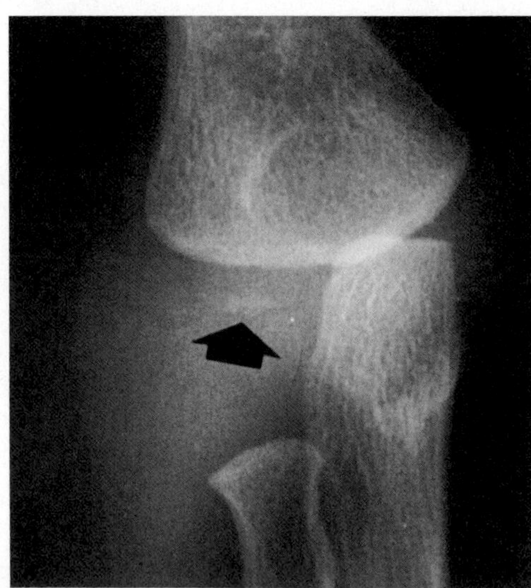

FIGURE 13-2 Ossification at 12 months. As the ossification center of the lateral condyle develops (*arrow*), the lateral border of the metaphysis becomes straighter.

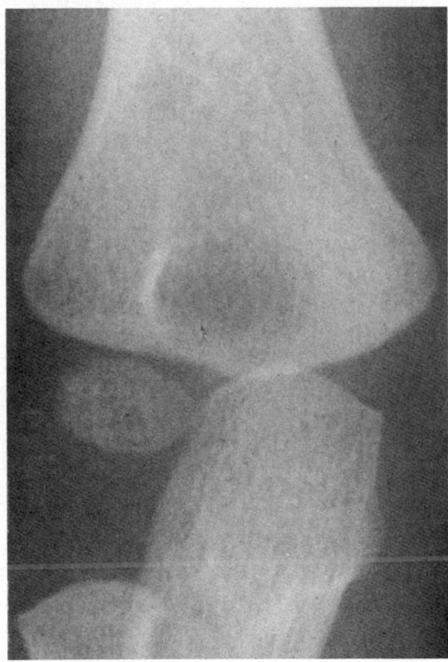

FIGURE 13-3 At 24 months, the oval-shaped secondary ossification center of the lateral condyle extends into the lateral crista of the trochlea. The lateral border of the neck (metaphysis) of the radius is normally angulated both anteriorly and laterally.

is usually spherical when it first appears. It becomes more hemispherical as the distal humerus matures,[9] and the ossific nucleus extends into the lateral ridge of the trochlea (Fig. 13-3). On the lateral view, the physis of the capitellum is wider posteriorly. This is a normal variation and should not be confused with a fracture.[9]

Medial Epicondyle

At about 5 to 6 years of age, a small concavity develops on the medial aspect of the metaphyseal ossification border. In this area, a medial epicondyle begins to ossify (Fig. 13-4).

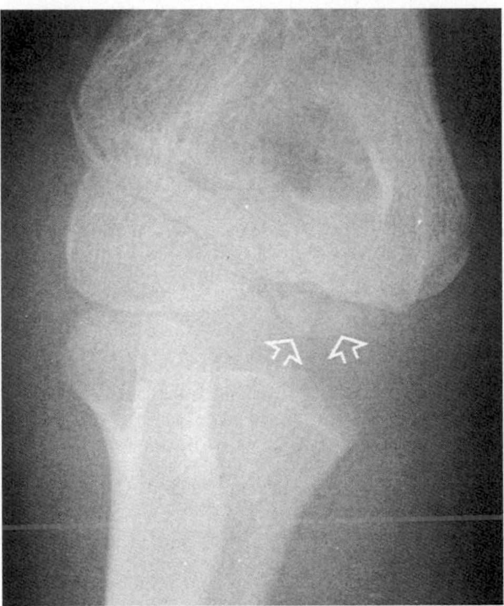

FIGURE 13-5 At about 9 years of age, the ossification of the medial crista of the trochlea may begin as two well-defined centers (*arrows*). These multiple centers can give the trochlea a fragmented appearance.

Trochlea

At about 9 to 10 years of age, the trochlea begins to ossify. Initially, it may be irregular with multiple centers (Fig. 13-5).

Lateral Epicondyle

The lateral epicondyle is last to ossify and is not always visible (Fig. 13-6). At about 10 years of age, it may begin as a small, separate oblong center, rapidly fusing with the lateral condyle.[9]

The Fusion Process

Just before completion of growth, the capitellum, lateral epicondyle, and trochlea fuse to form one epiphyseal center. Metaphy-

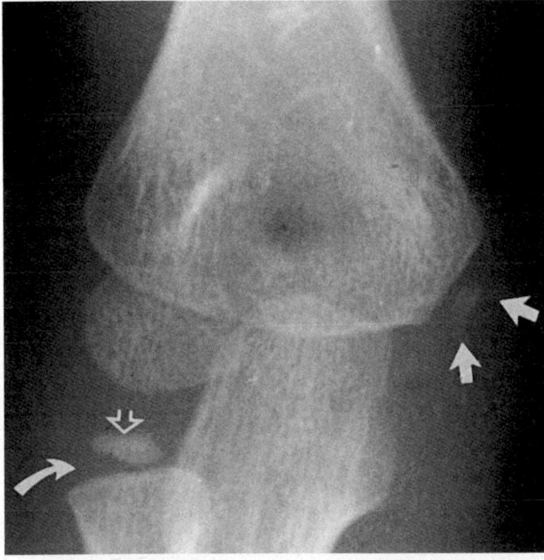

FIGURE 13-4 At about 5 or 6 years of age, a secondary center develops in the medial epicondylar apophysis (*white arrows*). At this same time, the ossification center of the radial head also develops (*open arrow*). Note that the physis of the proximal radius is widened laterally (*curved arrow*).

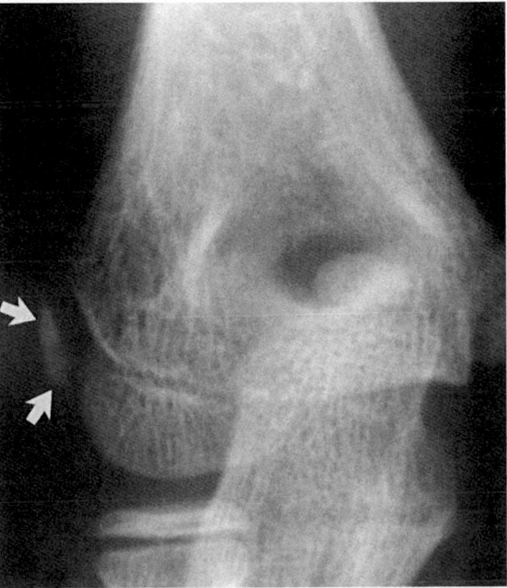

FIGURE 13-6 The apophysis of the lateral epicondyle ossifies as either an oblong or a triangular center (*arrows*). The wide separation of this center from the metaphyseal and epiphyseal borders of the lateral condyle is normal.

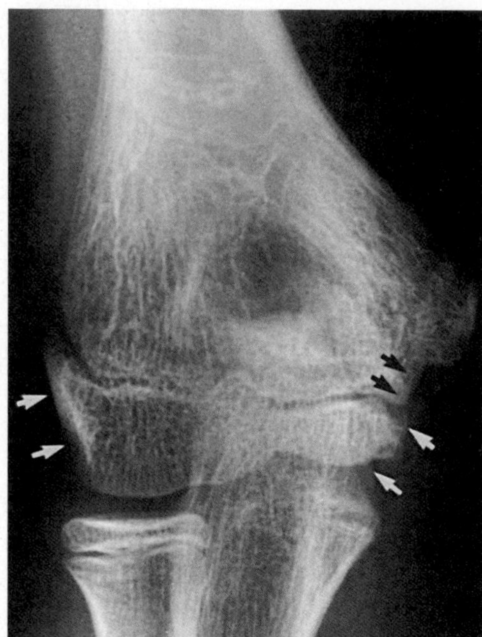

FIGURE 13-7 The secondary ossification centers of the lateral condyle, trochlea, and lateral epicondylar apophysis fuse to form one center (*white arrows*). This common center is separated from the medial epicondylar apophysis by advancing metaphyseal bone (*black arrows*).

seal bone separates the extra-articular medial epicondyle from this common humeral epiphyseal center (Fig. 13-7). The common epiphyseal center ultimately fuses with the distal humeral metaphysis. The medial epicondyle may not fuse with the metaphysis until the late teens.

Proximal Radius

The head of the radius begins to ossify at about the same time as the medial epicondyle (see Fig. 13-4). The ossification center is present in at least 50% of girls by 3.8 years of age, but may not be present in the same proportion of boys until around 4.5 years.[18] Initially, the ossification center is elliptical, and the physis is widened laterally due to the obliquity of the proximal metaphysis. The ossification center flattens as it matures. At about age 12, it develops a concavity opposite the capitellum.[9]

Ossification of the radial head may be bipartite or may produce an irregularity of the second center. These secondary or irregular ossification centers should not be interpreted as fracture fragments.

Olecranon

There is a gradual proximal progression of the proximal ulnar metaphysis. At birth, the ossification margin lies halfway between the coronoid process and the tip of the olecranon. By about 6 or 7 years of age, it appears to envelop about 66% to 75% of the capitellar surface. The final portion of the olecranon ossifies from a secondary ossification center that appears around 6.8 years of age in girls and 8.8 years in boys (Fig. 13-8A). Peterson[38] described two separate centers: one articular and the other a traction type (Fig. 13-8B). This secondary ossification center of the olecranon may persist late into adult life.[37]

Fusion of the Ossification Centers

The epiphyseal ossification centers of the distal humerus fuse as one unit and then fuse later to the metaphysis. The medial epicondyle is the last to fuse to the metaphysis. The ranges of onset of the ossification of various centers and their fusion to other centers or the metaphysis are summarized in Figure 13-9. Each center contributes to the overall architecture of the distal humerus (Fig. 13-9C).

Fusion of the proximal radial and olecranon epiphyseal centers with their respective metaphyses occurs at around the same time that the common distal humeral epiphysis fuses with its metaphysis (i.e., between 14 and 16 years of age).[6,8,42]

Noting that the pattern and ossification sequence of the six secondary ossification centers around the elbow were mainly derived from studies conducted more than 30 years ago, Cheng et al.[13] evaluated elbow radiographs of 1577 Chinese children. They found that the sequence of ossification was the same in

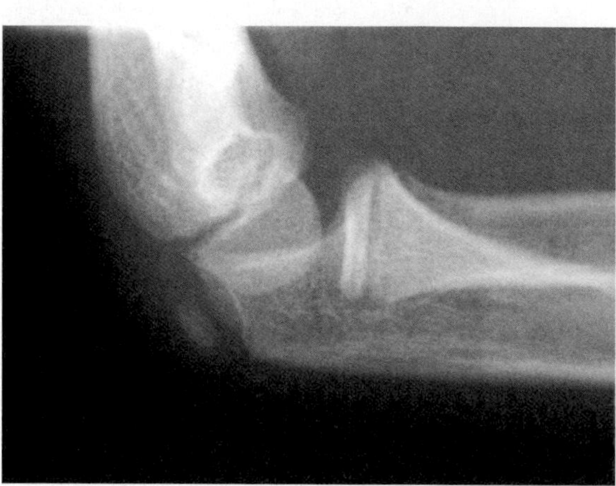

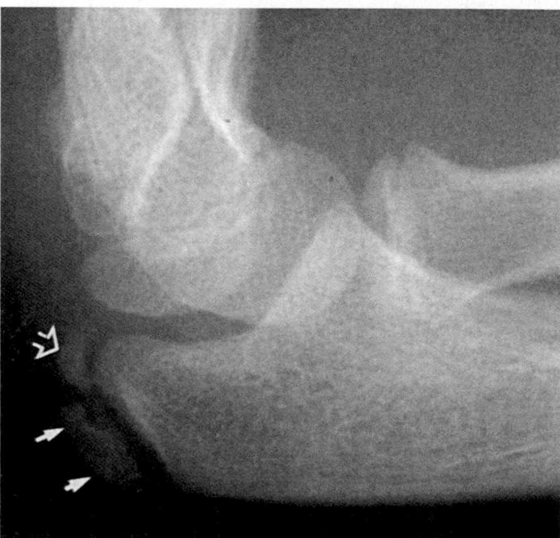

FIGURE 13-8 Ossification of the olecranon. **A.** Secondary ossification begins as an oblique oblong center at about 6 to 8 years of age. **B.** It may progress as two separate ossification centers: articular (*open arrow*) and traction (*closed arrows*).

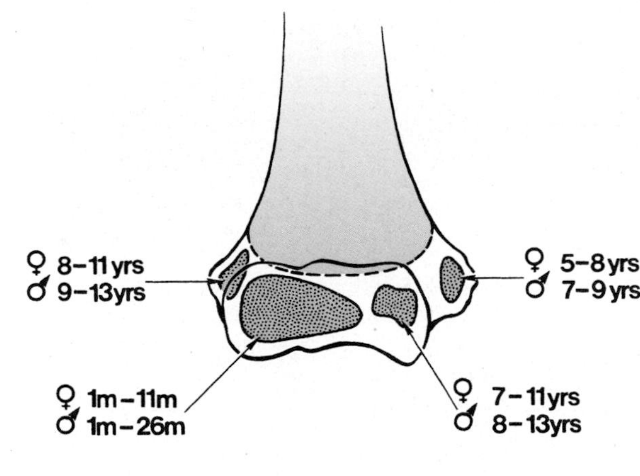

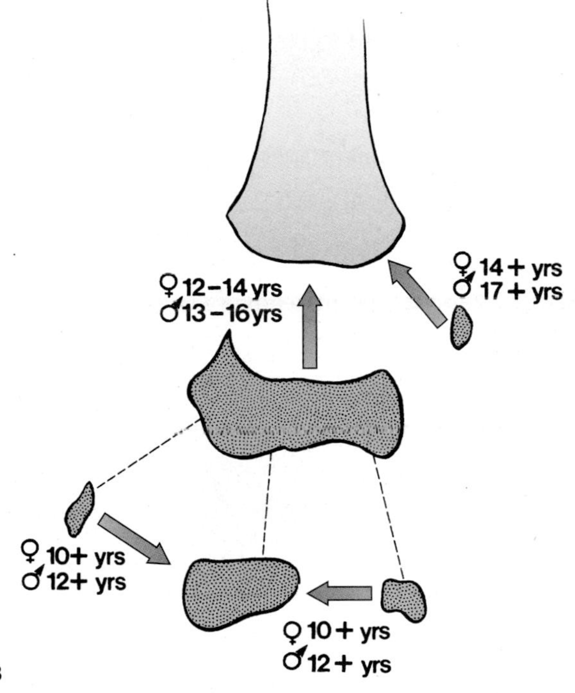

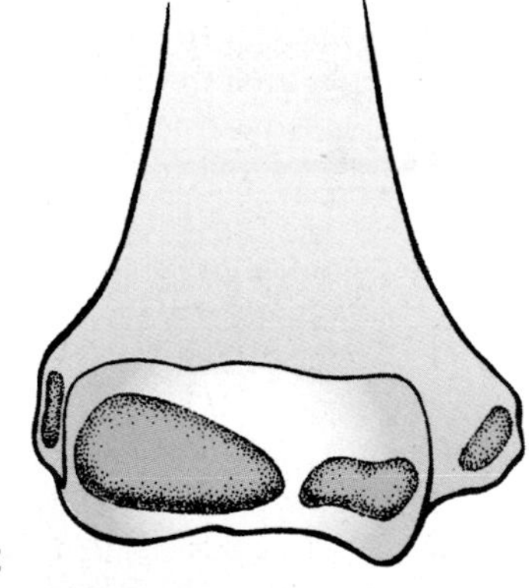

FIGURE 13-9 Ossification and fusion of the secondary centers of the distal humerus. **A.** The average ages for the onset of ossification of the various ossification centers are shown for both boys and girls. **B.** The ages at which these centers fuse with each other are shown for both boys and girls. (Modified and reprinted with permission from Haraldsson S. On osteochondrosis deformans juvenilis capituli humeri including investigation of intraosseous vasculature in distal humerus. Acta Orthop Scand 1959;Suppl 38:1–232.) **C.** The contribution of each secondary center to the overall architecture of the distal humerus is represented by the stippled areas.

boys and girls—capitellum, radial head, medial epicondyle, olecranon, trochlea, and lateral epicondyle—but ossification was delayed by about 2 years in boys in all ossification centers except the capitellum (see Table 13-1).

Blood Supply

Extraosseous

There is a rich arterial network around the elbow (Fig. 13-10).[47] The major arterial trunk, the brachial artery, lies anteriorly in the antecubital fossa. Most of the intraosseous blood supply of the distal humerus comes from the anastomotic vessels that course posteriorly.

Three structural components govern the location of the entrance of the vessels into the developing epiphysis. First, there is no communication between the intraosseous metaphyseal vasculature and the ossification centers. Second, vessels do not penetrate the articular surfaces. The lateral condyle is nonarticular only at the origin of the muscles and collateral ligaments. Third, the vessels do not penetrate the articular capsule except at the interface with the surface of the bone. Thus, only a small portion of the lateral condyle posteriorly is both nonarticular and extracapsular (Fig. 13-11).[23]

Intraosseous

The most extensive study of the intraosseous blood supply of the developing distal humerus was conducted by Haraldsson (Fig. 13-12),[22,23] who demonstrated that there are two types of vessels in the developing lateral condyle. These vessels enter the posterior portion of the condyle just lateral to the origin of the capsule and proximal to the articular cartilage near the origin of the anconeus muscle. They penetrate the nonossified cartilage and traverse it to the developing ossific nucleus. In a young child, this is a relatively long course (Fig. 13-12A). These vessels communicate with one another within the ossific nucleus but do not communicate with vessels in either the metaphysis or nonossified chondroepiphysis. Thus, for practical purposes, they are end vessels.

The ossification center of the lateral condyle extends into the lateral portion of the trochlea. Thus, the lateral crista or ridge of the trochlea derives its blood supply from these condylar vessels. The medial ridge or crista remains unossified for a longer period of time. The trochlea is covered entirely by articular cartilage and lies totally within the confines of the articular capsule. The vessels that supply the nucleus of the ossific centers of the trochlea must therefore traverse the periphery of the physis to enter the epiphysis.

Haraldsson's[23] studies have shown two sources of blood supply to the ossific nucleus of the medial portion of the trochlea (Fig. 13-12B). The lateral vessel, on the posterior surface of the distal humeral metaphysis, penetrates the periphery of the physis and terminates in the trochlear nucleus. Because this vessel supplying the trochlea is an end vessel, it is especially vulnerable to injury by a fracture that courses through either the physis or the very distal portion of the humeral metaphysis. Injury to this vessel can markedly decrease the nourishment to the developing lateral ossific nucleus of the trochlea. The medial vessel penetrates the nonarticulating portion of the medial crista of the trochlea. This multiple vascular source may account for

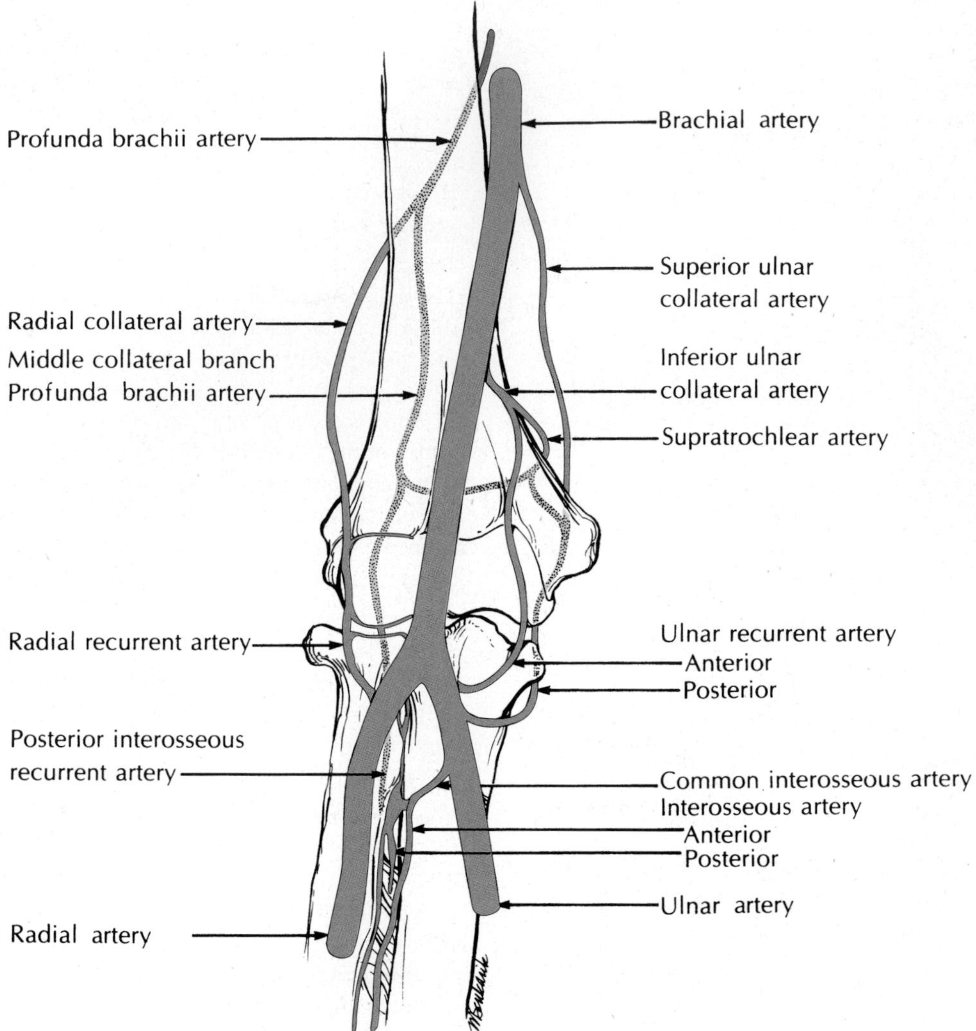

FIGURE 13-10 The major arteries about the anterior elbow.

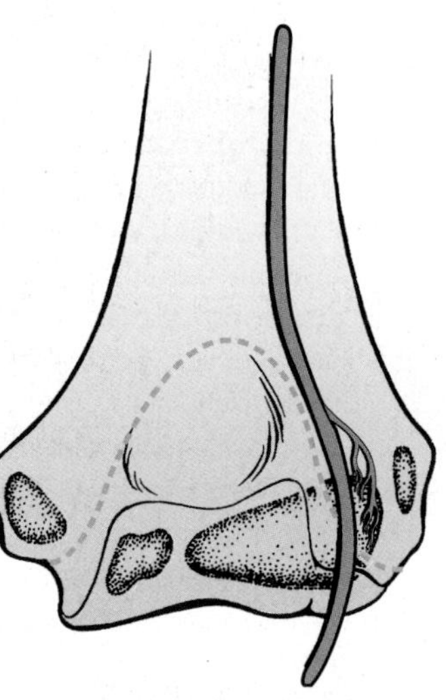

FIGURE 13-11 The vessels supplying the lateral condylar epiphysis enter the posterior aspect of the condyle, which is extra-articular. (Modified and reprinted with permission from Haraldsson S. On osteochondrosis deformans juvenilis capituli humeri including investigation of intraosseous vasculature in distal humerus. Acta Orthop Scand 1959;Suppl 38:1–232.)

the development of multiple ossification centers in the maturing trochlea, giving it a fragmented appearance (see Fig. 13-5).

When growth is complete, metaphyseal and epiphyseal vessels anastomose freely. The blood supply from the central nutrient vessel of the shaft reaches the epicondylar regions in the skeletally mature distal humerus.[31]

Intra-articular Structures

The articular surface lies within the confines of the capsule, but nonarticulating areas involving the coronoid and radial fossae anteriorly and the olecranon fossa posteriorly are also within the confines of the articular cavity.[46] The capsule attaches just distal to the coronoid and olecranon processes. Thus, these processes are intra-articular.[28] The entire radial head is intra-articular, with a recess or diverticulum of the elbow's articular cavity extending distally under the margin of the orbicular ligament. The medial and lateral epicondyles are extra-articular.

The anterior capsule is thickened anteriorly. These longitudinally directed fibers are very strong and become taut with the elbow in extension. In hyperextension, the tight anterior bands of the capsule force the ulna firmly into contact with the humerus. Thus, the fulcrum of rotation becomes transmitted proximally into the tip of the olecranon in the supracondylar area.

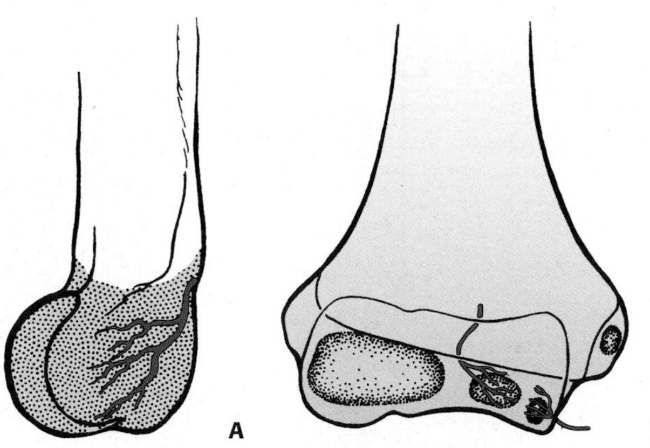

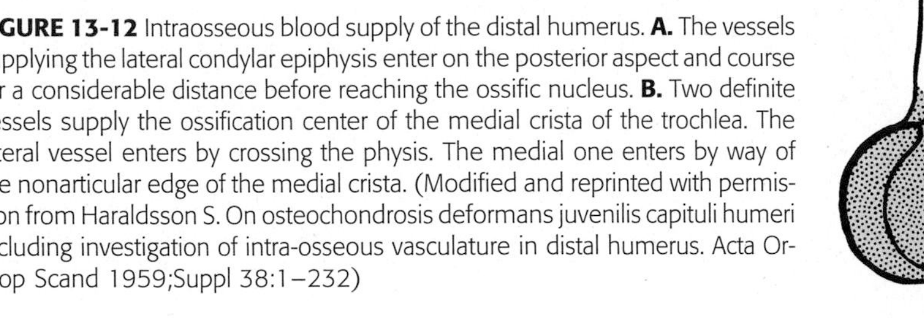

FIGURE 13-12 Intraosseous blood supply of the distal humerus. **A.** The vessels supplying the lateral condylar epiphysis enter on the posterior aspect and course for a considerable distance before reaching the ossific nucleus. **B.** Two definite vessels supply the ossification center of the medial crista of the trochlea. The lateral vessel enters by crossing the physis. The medial one enters by way of the nonarticular edge of the medial crista. (Modified and reprinted with permission from Haraldsson S. On osteochondrosis deformans juvenilis capituli humeri including investigation of intra-osseous vasculature in distal humerus. Acta Orthop Scand 1959;Suppl 38:1–232)

This is an important factor in the etiology of supracondylar fractures.

Fat Pads

At the proximal portion of the capsule, between it and the synovial layer, are two large fat pads (Fig. 13-13). The posterior fat pad lies totally within the depths of the olecranon fossa when the elbow is flexed. The anterior fat pad extends anteriorly out of the margins of the coronoid fossa. The significance of these fat pads in the interpretation of radiographs of the elbow is discussed later.

Ligaments

The pertinent ligamentous anatomy involving the orbicular and collateral ligaments is discussed in the sections on the specific injuries involving the radial neck, medial epicondyle, and elbow dislocations.

RADIOGRAPHIC FINDINGS

Because of the ever-changing ossification pattern, identification and delineation of fractures about the elbow in the immature skeleton may be subject to misinterpretation. The variables of ossification of the epiphyses should be well known to the orthopaedic surgeon who treats these injuries.

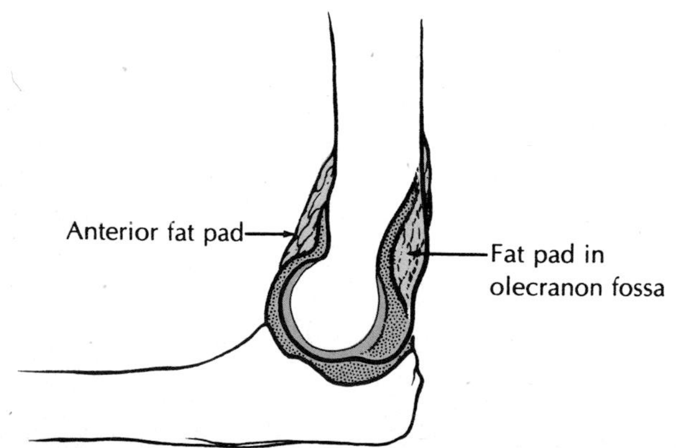

FIGURE 13-13 The elbow fat pads. Some of the coronoid fat pad lies anterior to the shallow coronoid fossa. The olecranon fat pad lies totally within the deeper olecranon fossa.

Several studies have suggested that children with a normal range of elbow motion after elbow trauma do not require immediate radiographic evaluation. In a large multicenter prospective study, Appelboam et al.[2] found that of 780 children evaluated for elbow trauma, 289 were able to fully extend their elbow; among these 12 (4%) fractures were identified, all at their first evaluation. Among the 491 children who could not fully extend their injured elbow, 210 (43%) had confirmed fractures. These authors suggested that an elbow extension test can be used to rule out the need for radiographs, provided the physician is confident that an olecranon fracture is not present and that the patient can return for re-evaluation if symptoms have not resolved in 7 to 10 days. Lennon et al.,[34] in a study involving 407 patients ranging in age from 2 to 96 years, proposed that patients aged no more than 16 years with a range of motion equal to the unaffected side do not require radiographic evaluation. Darracq et al.[15] found that limitation of active range of motion was 100% sensitive for fracture or effusion, while preservation of active range of motion was 97% specific for the absence of fracture. Other studies[16,24,32] have confirmed a high sensitivity (91% to 97%) of an inability to extend the elbow as a predictor of elbow fracture in both children and adults.

When radiographs are indicated, a number of anatomic landmarks and angles should be evaluated and measured, including any displacement of the fat pads about the elbow. It is important to be familiar with these landmarks and angles and to be aware of the significance of any deviation from normal.

Standard Views

The standard radiographs of the elbow include an anteroposterior (AP) view with the elbow extended and a lateral view with the elbow flexed to 90 degrees and the forearm neutral.

Jones View

It is often difficult for a child to extend the injured elbow, and an axial view of the elbow, the Jones view, may be helpful (Fig. 13-14). The distal humerus is normally difficult to interpret due to the superimposed proximal radius and ulna. There is often a high index of suspicion for a fracture, but none is visible on routine AP and lateral radiographs. In this case, internal and external oblique views may be helpful. This is especially true in identifying fractures of the radial head and coronoid process.

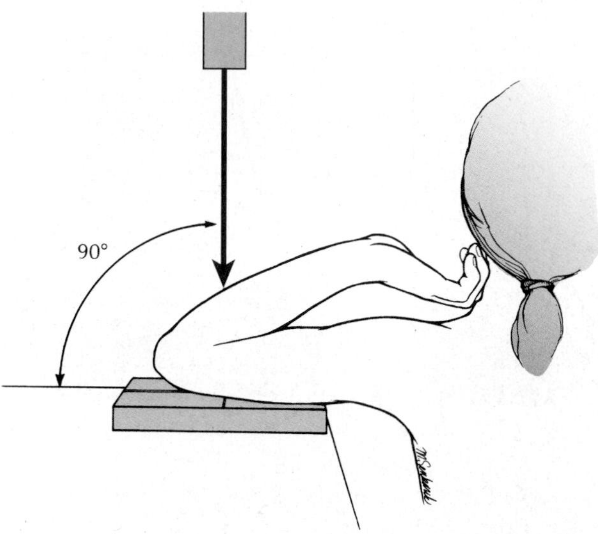

FIGURE 13-14 Jones axial radiographic view of the elbow.

Anteroposterior Landmarks

Baumann Angle

In the standard AP view, the major landmark is the angulation of the physeal line between the lateral condyle and the distal humeral metaphysis. The ossification center of the lateral condyle extends into the radial or lateral crista of the trochlea (see Fig. 13-9C). This physeal line forms an angle with the long axis of the humerus. The angle formed by this physeal line and the long axis of the humerus is the Baumann angle (Fig. 13-15A).[3] The Baumann angle is not equal to the carrying angle of the elbow in older children.[9] This is a consistent angle when both sides are compared, and the x-ray beam is directed perpendicular to the long axis of the humerus. Acton and McNally[1] reviewed the descriptions of the Baumann angle in a number of commonly used textbooks and discovered three variations of measurement technique. They recommended that the angle should always be measured between the long axis of the humerus and the inclination of the capitellar physis, as Baumann described, and that it should be called the "shaft-physeal" angle to avoid confusion.

Caudad-cephalad angulation of the x-ray tube or right or left angulation of the tube by as much as 30 degrees changes the Baumann angle by less than 5 degrees. If, however, the tube becomes angulated in a cephalad-caudad direction by more than 20 degrees, the angle is changed significantly and the measurement is inaccurate. In their cadaver studies, Camp et al.[11] found that rotation of the distal fragment or the entire reduced humerus can also alter the projection of the Baumann angle. They found that to be accurate, the humerus must be parallel to the x-ray plate, with the beam directed perpendicular to the film as well. Thus, in the routine AP radiographs of the distal humerus, including the Jones view, the Baumann angle is a good measurement of any deviation of the angulation of the distal humerus.[14]

Other Angles

Two other angles measured on AP radiographs are commonly used to determine the proper alignment of the distal humerus or carrying angle. The humeral-ulnar angle is determined by lines longitudinally bisecting the shaft of the humerus with the shaft of the ulna (Fig. 13-15B).[4,27,37] The metaphyseal-diaphyseal angle is determined by a line that longitudinally bisects the

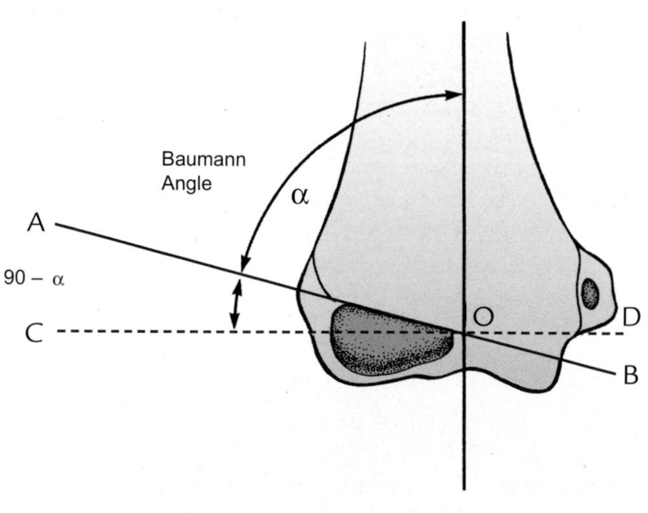

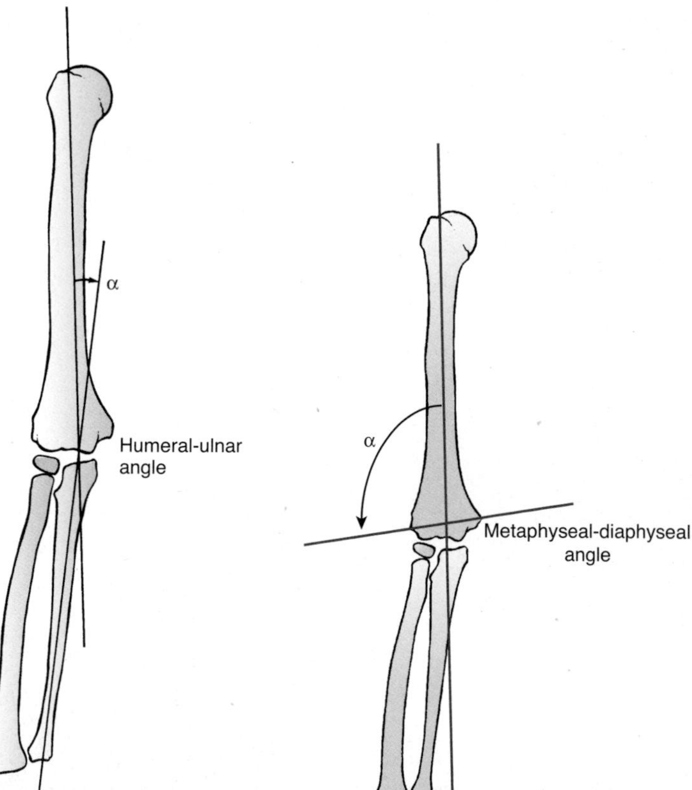

FIGURE 13-15 AP radiographic angles of the elbow. **A.** Baumann angle. **B.** The humeral-ulnar angle. **C.** The metaphyseal-diaphyseal angle. (Reprinted with permission from O'Brien WR, Eilert RE, Chang FM, et al. The metaphyseal–diaphyseal angle as a guide to treating supracondylar fractures of the humerus in children. Presented at 54th Annual Meeting of AAOS; San Francisco, CA; 1987.)

shaft of the humerus with a line that connects the widest points of the metaphysis of the distal humerus (Fig. 13-15C).[36] The humeral-ulnar angle is the most accurate in determining the true carrying angle of the elbow. The Baumann angle also has a good correlation with the clinical carrying angle, but it may be difficult to measure in adolescents in whom the ossification center of the lateral condyle is beginning to fuse with other centers. The metaphyseal-diaphyseal angle is the least accurate of the three.[44]

Lateral Landmarks

Teardrop

The lateral projection of the distal humerus presents a teardrop-like shadow above the capitellum.[42] The anterior dense line making up the teardrop represents the posterior margin of the coronoid fossa. The posterior dense line represents the anterior margin of the olecranon fossa. The inferior portion of the teardrop is the ossification center of the capitellum. On a true lateral projection, this teardrop should be well defined (Fig. 13-16A).

Shaft-Condylar Angle

On the lateral radiograph, there is an angulation of 40 degrees between the long axis of the humerus and the long axis of the lateral condyle (Fig. 13-16B). This can also be measured by the flexion angle of the distal humerus, which is calculated by measuring the angle of the lateral condylar physeal line with the long axis of the shaft of the humerus.[40]

Anterior Humeral Line

If a line is drawn along the anterior border of the distal humeral shaft, it should pass through the middle third of the ossification center of the capitellum. This is referred to as the *anterior humeral line* (Fig. 13-16C). Passage of the anterior humeral line through the anterior portion of the lateral condylar ossification center or anterior to it indicates the presence of posterior angulation of the distal humerus. In a large study of minimally displaced supracondylar fractures, Rogers et al.[41] found that this anterior humeral line was the most reliable factor in detecting the presence or absence of occult fractures.

Coronoid Line

A line directed proximally along the anterior border of the coronoid process should barely touch the anterior portion of the lateral condyle (Fig. 13-16D). Posterior displacement of the lateral condyle projects the ossification center posterior to this coronoid line.[42]

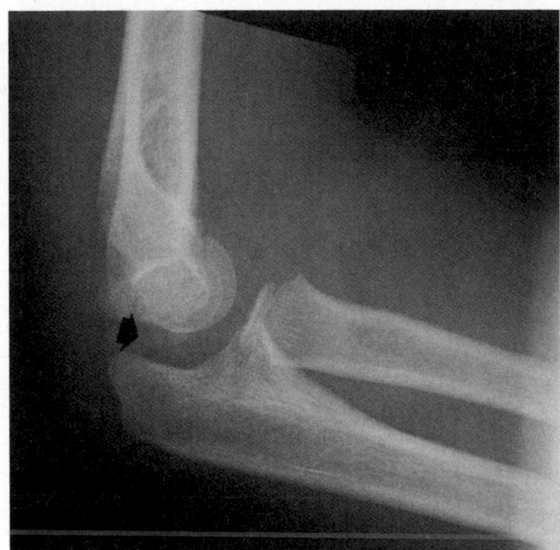

FIGURE 13-17 Pseudofracture of the elbow. The trochlea with its multiple ossification centers may be misinterpreted as fracture fragments lying between the joint surfaces (*arrow*).

Pseudofracture

Some vagaries of the ossification process about the elbow may be interpreted as a fracture.[42] For example, the ossification of the trochlea may be irregular, producing a fragmented appearance (see Fig. 13-5). This fragmentation can be misinterpreted, especially if the distal humerus is slightly oblique or tilted. These secondary ossification centers may be mistaken for fracture fragments lying between the semilunar notch and lateral condyle (Fig. 13-17).

On the lateral view, the physeal line between the lateral condyle and the distal humeral metaphysis is wider posteriorly. This appearance may give a misinterpretation that the lateral condyle is fractured and tilted.[9]

On the AP view before the radial head ossifies, there is normally some lateral angulation to the radial border of the neck of the radius that may give the appearance of subluxation (see Fig. 13-3). The true position of the radial head can be confirmed by noting the relationship of the proximal radius to the ossification center of the lateral condyle on the lateral projection.[41]

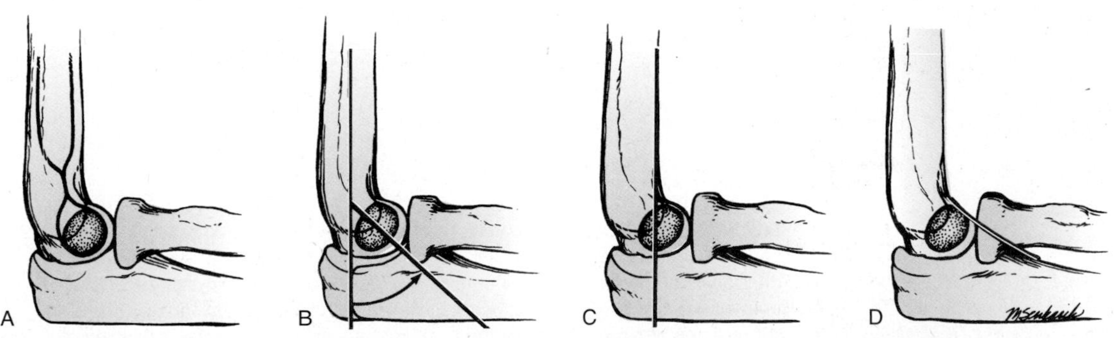

FIGURE 13-16 Lateral radiograph lines of the distal humerus. **A.** The teardrop of the distal humerus. **B.** The angulation of the lateral condyle with the shaft of the humerus. **C.** The anterior humeral line. **D.** The coronoid line.

Fat Pad Signs of the Elbow

There are three areas in which fat pads overlie the major structures of the elbow. Displacement of any of the fat pads can indicate an occult fracture. The first two areas are the fat pads that overlie the capsule in the coronoid fossa anteriorly and the olecranon fossa posteriorly. Displacement of either or both of these fat pads is usually referred to as the *classic elbow fat pad sign*. A third accumulation of fat overlies the supinator muscle as it wraps around the proximal radius.

Olecranon (Posterior) Fat Pad. Because the olecranon fossa is deep, the fat pad here is totally contained within the fossa. It is not visible on a normal lateral radiograph of the elbow flexed to 90 degrees (Fig. 13-18A).

Distention of the capsule with an effusion, as occurs with an occult intra-articular fracture, a spontaneously reduced dislocation, or even an infection, can cause the dorsal or olecranon fat pad to be visible.[48]

Coronoid (Anterior) Fat Pad. Likewise, the ventral or coronoid fat pad may be displaced anteriorly (Fig. 13-18B).[7] Because the coronoid fossa is shallow, the fat pad in this area projects anterior to the bony margins and can be seen normally as a triangular radiolucency anterior to the distal humerus. Although displacement of the classic elbow fat pads is a reliable indication of an intra-articular effusion, there may be instances in which only one of the fat pads is displaced. Brodeur et al.[9] and Kohn[31] have shown that the coronoid fat pad is more sensitive to small effusions than the olecranon fat pad. It can be displaced without a coexistent displacement of the olecranon fat pad (Fig. 13-18C).

Supinator Fat Pad. A layer of fat on the anterior aspect of the supinator muscle wraps around the proximal radius. This layer of fat or fat pad may normally bow anteriorly to some degree. Brodeur et al.[9] stated that displacement may indicate the presence of an occult fracture of the radial neck. Displacement of the fat line or pad is often difficult to interpret; in a review of fractures involving the proximal radius, Schunk et al.[42] found it to be positive only 50% of the time.

Fat Pad Variations. For the fat pads to be displaced, the capsule must be intact. This can explain why there may be no displacement of the fat pads with an elbow dislocation that has spontaneously reduced due to capsule rupture. Murphy and Siegel[36] described other variations of classic fat pad displacement. If the elbow is extended, the fat pad is normally displaced from the olecranon fossa by the olecranon (Fig. 13-18D). Distal humeral fractures may cause subperiosteal bleeding and may lift the proximal portion of the olecranon fat pad without the presence of an effusion (Fig. 13-18E). These false-negative and false-positive findings must be kept in mind when interpreting the presence or absence of a fat pad with an elbow injury.

Corbett's[14] review of elbow injuries indicated that if a displacement of the posterior fat pad existed, a fracture was almost always present. Displacement of the anterior fat pad alone, how-

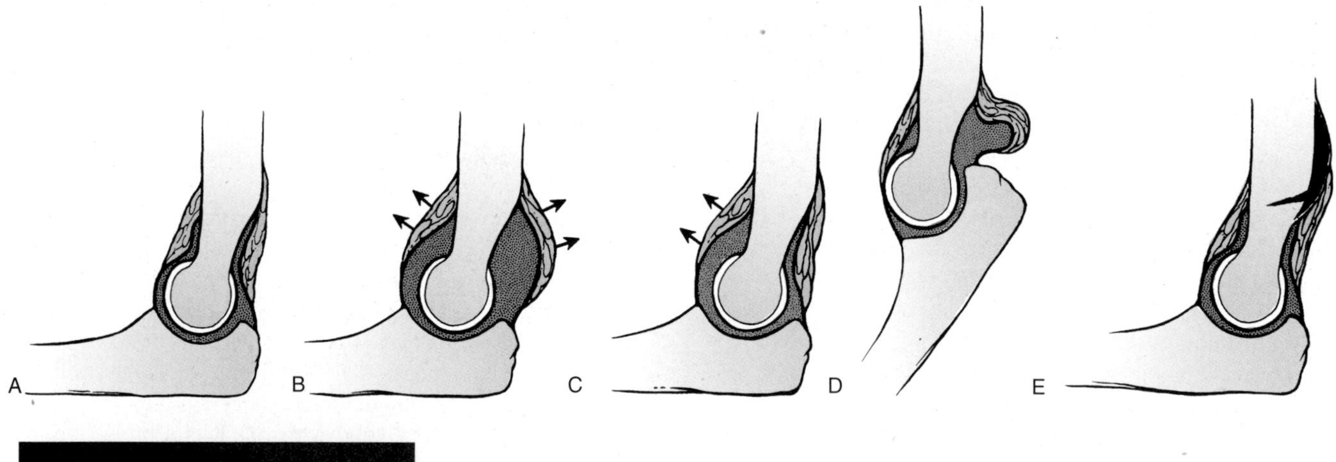

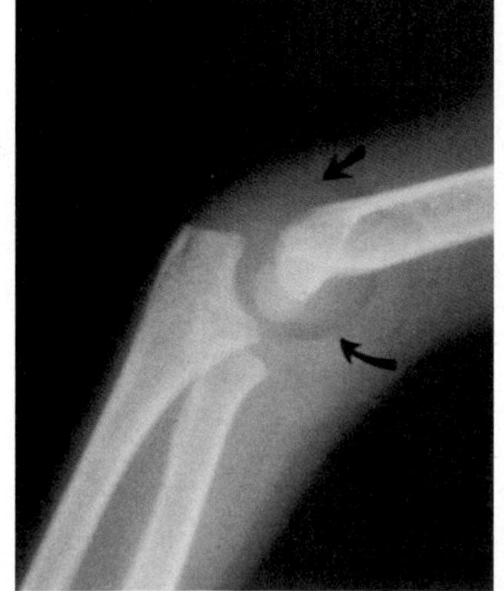

FIGURE 13-18 Radiographic variations of the elbow fat pads. **A.** Normal relationships of the two fat pads. **B.** Displacement of both fat pads (*arrows*) with an intra-articular effusion. **C.** In some cases, the effusion may displace only the anterior fat pad (*arrows*). **D.** In extension, the posterior fat pad is normally displaced by the olecranon. **E.** An extra-articular fracture may lift the distal periosteum and displace the proximal portion of the posterior fat pad. **F.** A radiograph showing displacement of both fat pads (*arrows*) from an intra-articular effusion. (Modified and reprinted with permission from Murphy WA, Siegel MJ. Elbow fat pads with new signs and extended differential diagnosis. Radiology 1977; 124:656–659.)

ever, could occur without a fracture. Corbett[14] also determined that the degree of displacement bore no relation to the size of the fracture. Skaggs and Mirzayan[43] reported that 34 of 45 children (76%) with a history of elbow trauma and an elevated posterior fat pad had radiographic evidence of elbow fractures at an average of 3 weeks after injury, although AP, lateral, and oblique radiographs at the time of injury showed no other evidence of fracture. They recommended that a child with a history of elbow trauma and an elevated fat pad should be treated as if a nondisplaced elbow fracture were present. Donnelly et al.,[17] however, found evidence of fracture in only nine of 54 children (17%) who had a history of trauma and elbow joint effusion but no identifiable fracture on initial radiographs. They concluded that joint effusion without a visible fracture on initial radiographs does not correlate with the presence of occult fracture in most patients (83%). Persistent effusion did correlate with occult fracture: 78% of those with occult fractures had persistent effusions, compared with 16% of those without fractures.

Comparison Radiographs

Although it is often tempting to order comparison radiographs in a child with an injured elbow due to the difficulty evaluating the irregularity of the ossification process, the indications for ordering comparison radiographs are rare. Kissoon et al.[30] found that using routine comparison radiographs in children with injured elbows did not significantly increase the accuracy of diagnosis, regardless of the interpreter's training. Petit et al.[39] reviewed 3128 radiographs of 2470 children admitted to a pediatric emergency department for osteoarticular trauma and found that only 22% of the radiographs revealed abnormal findings; 33.3% of elbow radiographs revealed abnormalities. Fewer than half of clinically suspected fractures were confirmed by radiograph.

Magnetic Resonance Imaging

Major and Crawford[35] used magnetic resonance imaging (MRI) to evaluate seven children who had radiographs that showed effusion but no fractures; four of the children had fractures identified by MRI. These investigators suggested that an occult fracture is usually present when effusion occurs, even if a fracture is not visible on radiograph. Griffith et al.[21] reviewed the radiographs and MRI scans of 50 children with elbow trauma. Radiographs identified effusions in 34% of the children and fractures in 52%; MRI identified effusions in 96% and fractures in 74%. Although MRI revealed a broad spectrum of bone and soft tissue injury beyond that shown on radiographs (bone bruising, muscle and ligament injuries, physeal injury, fracture), the additional information provided by MRI had little influence on patient treatment and no value in predicting clinical outcome. We have found MRI to be helpful in evaluating articular fractures to identify fracture pattern and extent, fragment position, and any interposed structure.

Other Imaging Modalities

Sonography and arthrography can be useful in examining children with posttraumatic elbow effusions, but these can be painful and invasive. The use of computed tomography (CT) in pediatric imaging has been limited by the need for sedation, but the development of multidetector CT (MDCT) technology allows examinations to be completed in seconds, eliminating the need for sedation in most cases. MDCT studies also can be reformatted and evaluated in multiple planes, reducing the manipulation necessary for a series of radiographs. Chapman et al.[12] reported that, in a series of 31 children with posttraumatic elbow effusion and normal radiographs, MDCT depicted occult injuries in 52%. They cited as additional advantages of MDCT the minimal manipulation required, making it relatively easy and pain-free, the speed with which the image is obtained, the lower radiation dose than conventional radiographs, and its sensitivity (92%), specificity (79%), and high negative predictive value (92%). A limitation of this method may be its high cost compared to standard radiographic examination.

REFERENCES

1. Acton JD, McNally MA. Baumann's confusing legacy. Injury 2001;32(1):41–43
2. Appelboam A, Reuben AD, Benger JR, et al. Elbow extension test to rule out elbow fracture: multicentre, prospective validation, and observational study of diagnostic accuracy in adults and children. Brit Med J 2008;337:a2428.
3. Baumann E. Beitrage zur Kenntnis dur Frackturen am Ellbogengelenk. Bruns Beitr F Klin Chir 1929;146:1–50.
4. Beals RK. The normal carrying angle of the elbow. Clin Orthop 1976;19:194–196.
5. Beekman F, Sullivan JE. Some observations on fractures of long bones in children. Am J Surg 1941;51:722–738.
6. Blount WP, Cassidy RH. Fractures of the elbow in children. JAMA 1951;146:699–704.
7. Bohrer SP. The fat pad sign following elbow trauma: its usefulness and reliability in suspecting "invisible" fractures. Clin Radiol 1970;21:90–94.
8. Brodeur AE, Silberstein JJ, Graviss ER. Radiology of the Pediatric Elbow. Boston: GK Hall, 1981.
9. Brodeur AE, Silberstein JJ, Graviss ER, et al. The basic tenets for appropriate evaluation of the elbow in pediatrics. Current Prob Diag Radiol 1983;12(5):1–29.
10. Buhr AJ, Cooke AM. Fracture patterns. Lancet 1959;1:531–536.
11. Camp J, Ishizue K, Gomez M, et al. Alteration of Baumann's angle by humeral position: implications for treatment of supracondylar humerus fractures. J Pediatr Orthop 1993; 13:521–555.
12. Chapman V, Grottkau B, Albright M, et al. MDCT of the elbow in pediatric patients with posttraumatic elbow effusions. Am J Roentgenol 2006;187:812-817.
13. Cheng JC, Wing-Man K, Shen WY, et al. A new look at the sequential development of elbow-ossification centers in children. J Pediatr Orthop 1998;18:161–167.
14. Corbett RH. Displaced fat pads in trauma to the elbow. Injury 1978;9:297–298.
15. Darracq MA, Vinson DR, Panacek EA. Preservation of active range of motion after acute elbow trauma predicts absence of elbow fracture. Am J Emerg Med 2008;26:779–782.
16. Docherty MA, Schwab RA, John O. Can elbow extension be used a test of clinically significant injury? South Med J 2002;95:539–541.
17. Donnelly LF, Klostermeier TT, Klosterman LA. Traumatic elbow effusions in pediatric patients: are occult fractures the rule? AJR 1998;171:243–245.
18. Elgenmark O. The normal development of the ossific centers during infancy and childhood. Acta Paediatr Scand 1946;33(Suppl 1):1–79.
19. Francis CC. The appearance of centers of ossification from 6 to 15 years. Am J Phys Anthro 1940;27:127–138.
20. Gray DJ, Gardner E. Prenatal development of the human elbow joint. Am J Anat 1951; 88:429–469.
21. Griffith JF, Roebuck DJ, Cheng JC, et al. Acute elbow trauma in children: spectrum of injury revealed by MR imaging not apparent on radiographs. AJR Am J Roentgenol 2001; 176(1):53–60.
22. Haraldsson S. The intraosseous vasculature of the distal end of the humerus with special reference to capitulum. Acta Orthop Scand 1957;27:81–93.
23. Haraldsson S. On osteochondrosis deformans juvenilis capituli humeri including investigation of intraosseous vasculature in distal humerus. Acta Orthop Scand 1959;Suppl 38:1–232.
24. Hawksworth CRE, Freeland P. Inability to fully extend the injured elbow: an indicator of significant injury. Arch Emerg Med 1991;8:253–256.
25. Henrikson B. Supracondylar fracture of the humerus in children. Acta Chir Scand 1966; 369:1–72.
26. Houshian S, Mehdi B, Larsen MS. The epidemiology of elbow fracture in children: analysis of 355 fractures, with special reference to Supracondylar humerus fractures. J Orthop Sci 2001;6(4):312–315.
27. Ippolito E, Caterini R, Scola F. Supracondylar fractures of the humerus in children. Analysis at maturity of 53 patients treated conservatively. J Bone Joint Surg Am 1986; 68:333–344.
28. Jenkins F. The functional anatomy and evolution of the mammalian humeroulnar articulation. Am J Anat 1973;137:281–298.
29. Johansson O. Capsular and ligament injuries of the elbow joint. Acta Chir Scand 1962; Suppl 287:1–159.
30. Kissoon N, Galpin R, Gayle M, et al. Evaluation of the role of comparison radiographs in the diagnosis of traumatic elbow injuries. J Pediatr Orthop 1995;15:449–453.
31. Kohn AM. Soft tissue alterations in elbow trauma. AJR 1959;82:867–874.
32. Lamprakis A, Vlasis K, Siuampou E, et al. Can elbow-extension test be used as an alternative to radiographs in primary care? Eur J Gen Pract 2007;13:221–224.
33. Landin LA, Danielsson LG. Elbow fractures in children: an epidemiological analysis of 589 cases. Acta Orthop Scand 1986;57:309.
34. Lennon RI, Riayt MS, Hilliam R, et al. Can a normal range of elbow movement predict a normal elbow x-ray? Emerg Med J 2007;24:86–88.

35. Major NM, Crawford ST. Elbow effusions in trauma in adults and children: is there an occult fracture? AJR Am J Roentgenol 2002;178(2):413–418.
36. Murphy WA, Siegel MJ. Elbow fat pad with new signs and extended differential diagnosis. Radiology 1977;124:659–665.
37. O'Brien WR, Eilert RE, Chang FM, et al. The metaphyseal diaphyseal angle as a guide to treating supracondylar fractures of the humerus in children. Presented at 54th Annual Meeting of AAOS; San Francisco, CA; 1987.
38. Peterson CA, Peterson HA. Analysis of the incidence of injuries to the epiphyseal growth plate. J Trauma 1972;12:275–281.
39. Petit P, Sapin C, Henry G, et al. Rate of abnormal osteoarticular radiographic findings in pediatric patients. AJR Am J Roentgenol 2001;176(4):987–990.
40. Porteous CJ. The olecranon epiphyses. J Anat 1960;94:286.
41. Sandegrad E. Fracture of the lower end of the humerus in children: treatment and end of the elbow in children. J Bone Joint Surg Am 1999;81:1429–1433.
42. Schunk VK, Grossholz M, Schild H. Der Supinatorfettkorper bei Frakturen des Ellbogengelenkes. ROFO 1989;150:294–296.
43. Skaggs DL, Mirzayan R. The posterior fat pad sign in association with occult fracture of the elbow in children. J Bone Joint Surg Am 1999;81:1429–1433.
44. Smith L. Deformity following supracondylar fractures of the humerus. J Bone Joint Surg Am 1960;42:235–252.
45. Wilkins KE. Fractures and dislocations of the elbow region. In: Rockwood CA Jr, Wilkins KE, Beaty JH, eds. Fractures in Children. 4th ed. Philadelphia: Lippincott-Raven, 1996: 653–904.
46. William PL, Warwick R. Gray's Anatomy. Philadelphia: WB Saunders, 1980.
47. Wilson PD. Fractures and dislocations in the region of the elbow. Surg Gynecol Obstet 1933;56:335–359.
48. Yang Z, Wang Y, Gilula LA, et al. Microcirculation of the distal humeral epiphyseal cartilage: implications for posttraumatic growth deformities. J Hand Surg Am 1998;23: 165–172.

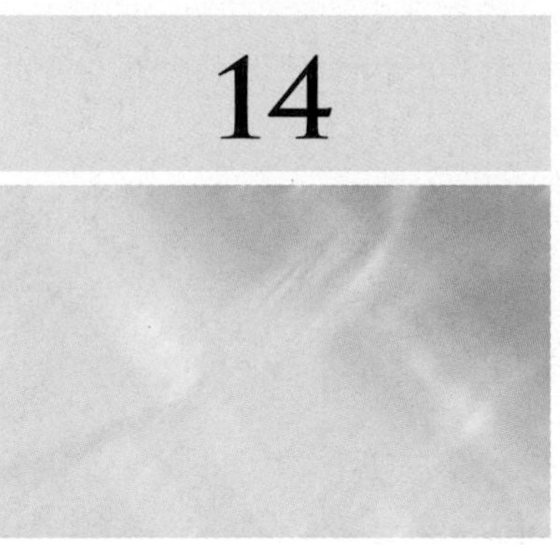

SUPRACONDYLAR FRACTURES OF THE DISTAL HUMERUS

David L. Skaggs and John M. Flynn

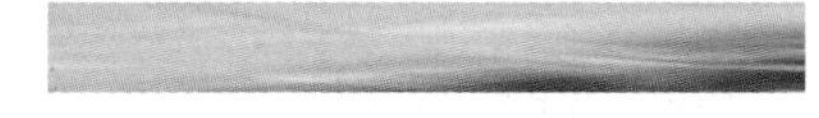

INTRODUCTION 487

PRINCIPLES OF MANAGEMENT 487
Mechanism of Injury and Anatomy 487
Posteromedial versus Posterolateral displacement of Extension-Type Supracondylar Fractures 489
Classification 490
Signs and Symptoms 490
Current Treatment Options 496
Postoperative Care 502
Complications 510
Controversies 525

FLEXION-TYPE SUPRACONDYLAR FRACTURES 526
Etiology and Pathology 526
Radiographic Findings 527
Treatment 527

INTRODUCTION

The treatment of supracondylar humeral fractures in children has been the subject of much discussion and dispute for many years. Historically, these fractures were associated with complications such as malunion that resulted in cosmetically and functionally inferior results. Results have been improved and the frequency of these complications dramatically decreased with more modern techniques of treatment.[67,110,122,127,182] With the advent of the image intensifier, which facillitates accurate pin placement, Blount's[28] caution against operative management is now of only historic interest. Controversies about the treatment of supracondylar humeral fractures in children, however, still exist: how long after injury can operative treatment be done safely and effectively, is a crossed-pin configuration better than a lateral-entry configuration, should type II supracondylar fractures be treated operatively or nonoperatively, and when does a pulseless hand require emergent treatment? In some areas of North America, the treatment of supracondylar fractures in children is shifting to pediatric subspecialists. In New England in 1991, 37% of patients were treated by pediatric orthopaedic specialists; by 1999, this figure rose to 68%.[104]

Supracondylar humeral fractures are the most common elbow fractures in children.[42,59,153] One epidemiologic study of elbow fractures in children[92] identified supracondylar fractures in 58%. The peak age range in which most supracondylar fractures occur is 5 to 6 years.[40] Although the incidence of these fractures generally has been reported to be higher in boys, more recent reports indicate that the frequencies of supracondylar humeral fractures in girls and boys seem to be equalizing, and some series actually have reported higher rates in girls.[62,92] The left or nondominant side is most frequently injured in almost all studies (Table 14-1).[41,62,92,195]

PRINCIPLES OF MANAGEMENT

Mechanism of Injury and Anatomy

Supracondylar fractures can be divided into extension and flexion types, depending on the direction of displacement of the distal fragment. Extension type fractures are the most common, accounting for approximately 97% to 99% of supracondylar humeral fractures.[128] They usually are caused by a fall onto the outstretched hand with the elbow in full extension (Fig. 14-1). Most of this chapter discusses extension-

TABLE 14-1 Overview of Supracondylar Fractures

	Percentage of Total Number of Fractures (%)
Side involved	
Right	39.2
Left	60.8
Gender incidence	
Male	59.5
Female	40.5
Ipsilateral fractures	1.0
Open fractures	1.0
Volkmann contracture	<0.5
Flexion type	2.0
Fractures with nerve injuries*	7.7
Radial nerve	41.2†
Median nerve	36.0†
Ulnar nerve	22.8†
Vascular injury	1.0

*Average age was 6.7 years.
†Percentage of total nerve injuries.
Data were compiled from 8361 fractures occurring in 64 major series.

type fractures; flexion-type fractures are discussed separately at the end of the chapter.

Between the olecranon fossa posteriorly and the coronoid fossa anteriorly, the medial and lateral columns of the distal humerus are connected by a thin segment of bone, which makes this area especially vulnerable to fracture (Fig. 14-2). Normal anatomic variants include absence of the olecranon fossa (Fig. 14-3) and presence of a supracondylar process, identified to some extent in about 1.5% of adult cadavers[56]; this should not be mistaken for pathology.

When the elbow is hyperextended, the olecranon engages the olecranon fossa and acts as a fulcrum through which the extension force can propogate a fracture across the medial and lateral columns. With the anterior capsule simultaneously providing a tensile force on the distal humerus proximal to its insertion, an extension-type supracondylar humeral fracture is created. It has been postulated that ligamentous laxity with resulting elbow hyperextension may predispose to a supracondylar humeral fracture,[147] but this association is unclear.[136]

The periosteum plays a key role in determining treatment. With extension-type injuries, although the anterior periosteum is torn, the intact posterior periosteal hinge provides stability and makes reduction easier. Abraham et al.[3] described periosteal changes with extension-type supracondylar humeral fractures in immature monkeys. With minimally angulated (<40 degrees) fractures, the periosteum was detached from the anterior humeral surface by up to 3 cm, and with more

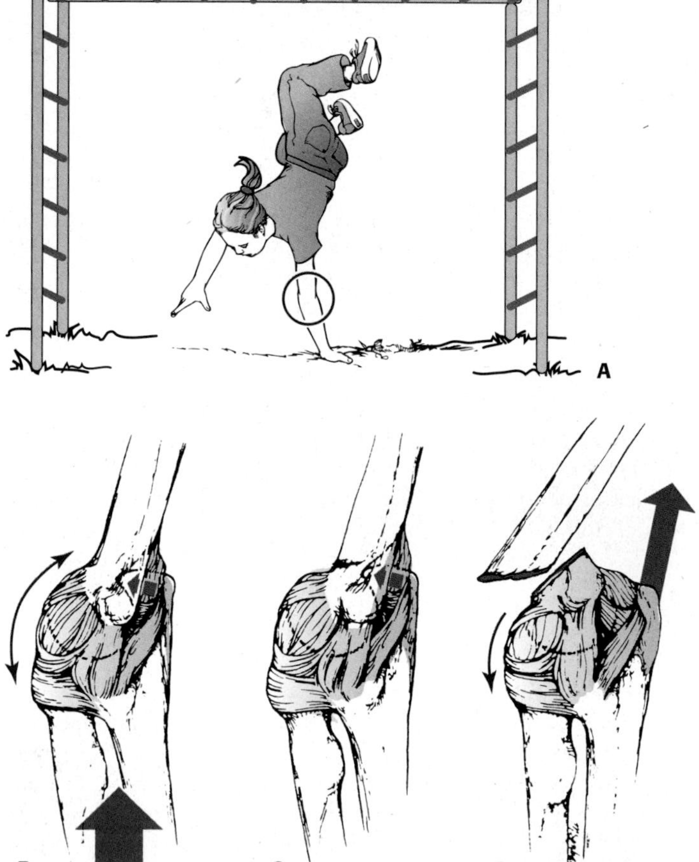

FIGURE 14-1 Mechanism of injury—elbow hyperextension. **A.** Most children attempt to break their falls with the arm extended. With hyperextension, the elbow falls into hyperextension. **B.** The linear applied force (*large arrow*) leads to an anterior tension force. Posteriorly, the olecranon is forced into the depths of the olecranon fossa (*small arrow*). **C.** As the bending force continues, the distal humerus fails anteriorly in the thin supracondylar area. **D.** When the fracture is complete, the proximal fragment can continue moving anteriorly and distally, potentially harming adjacent soft tissue structures such as the brachialis muscle, brachial artery, and median nerve.

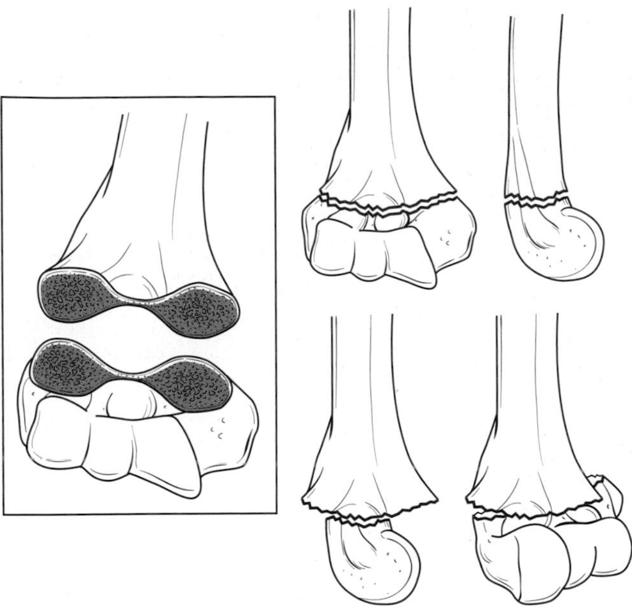

FIGURE 14-2 Supracondylar fractures occur through the thinist portion of the distal humerus in the AP plane. The thin bone makes the fracture unstable.

angulation (>40 degrees), the detached anterior periosteum was pulled distally and partially torn by the proximal fragment; in both of these situations, stable reduction was easily obtained by flexing the elbow to 90 degrees and pushing the distal fragment forward. They determined that the most stable

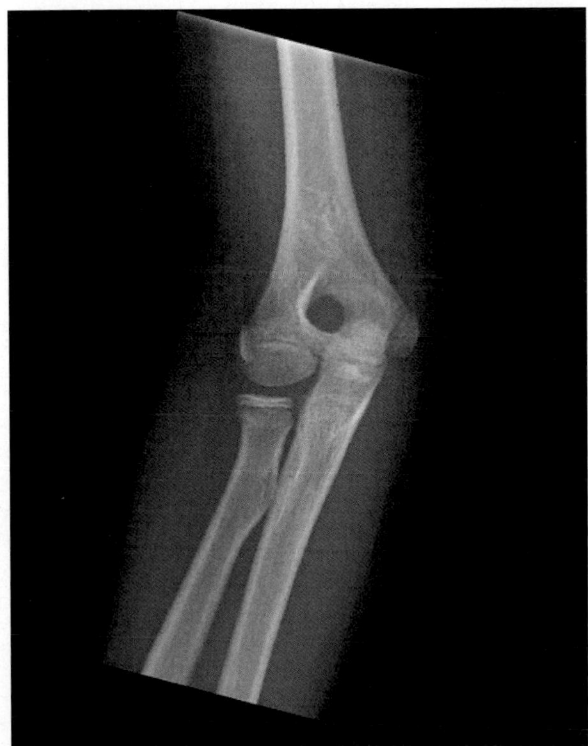

FIGURE 14-3 Normal anatomic variant in which there is no bone in the olecranon fossa. Note the minimally displaced radial neck fracture. (Reproduced with permission of Childrens Orthopaedic Center, Los Angeles, CA.)

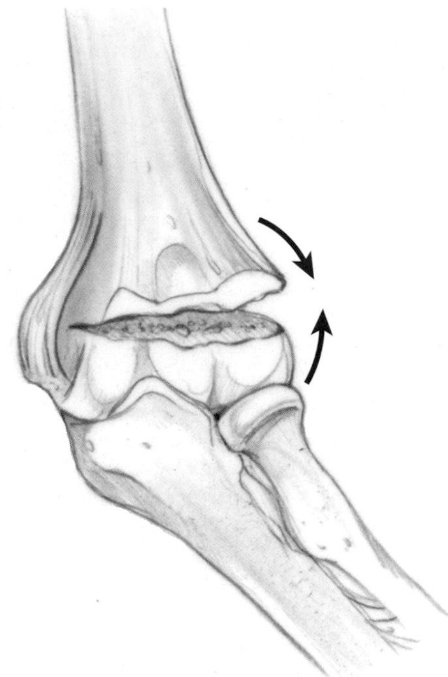

FIGURE 14-4 Laterally torn periosteum in a posteromedially displaced supracondylar humerus fracture. (From Skaggs DL. Closed reduction and pinning of supracondylar humerus fractures. In: Tolo VT, Skaggs DL, eds. Masters Techniques in Orthopaedic Surgery: Pediatric Orthopaedics. Philadelphia: Lippincott, 2007:1–15, with permission)

position of the reduced fracture was maximal elbow flexion and forearm pronation, regardless of whether the distal fragment was displaced medially or laterally; the most unstable position was full elbow extension with forearm supination. Other authors also have described using pronation to assist in reduction, but this maneuver may not be appropriate for all fractures. The integrity of the medial and lateral periosteum often can be determined by the direction of fracture displacement. In a typical posteromedially displaced fracture, the medial periosteum usually is intact. By placing the medial periosteum on tension, pronation closes the hinge and corrects varus malalignment (Fig. 14-4). In fractures with posterolateral displacement, however, the medial periosteum often is torn, making pronation counterproductive. If the lateral periosteum is intact, as usually is the case, supination may be better. Disruption of the posterior periosteal hinge makes the fracture unstable in both flexion and extension. Leitch et al.[125] described this fracture as a multidirectionally unstable, modified Gartland type IV fracture because it is less stable than a Gartland type III fracture.

Posteromedial versus Posterolateral Displacement of Extension-Type Supracondylar Fractures

Generally, medial displacement of the distal fragment is more common than lateral displacement, occurring in approximately 75% of patients in most series. Whether the displacement is medial or lateral is important because it determines which soft tissue structures are at risk from the penetrating injury of the proximal metaphyseal fragment. Medial displacement of the dis-

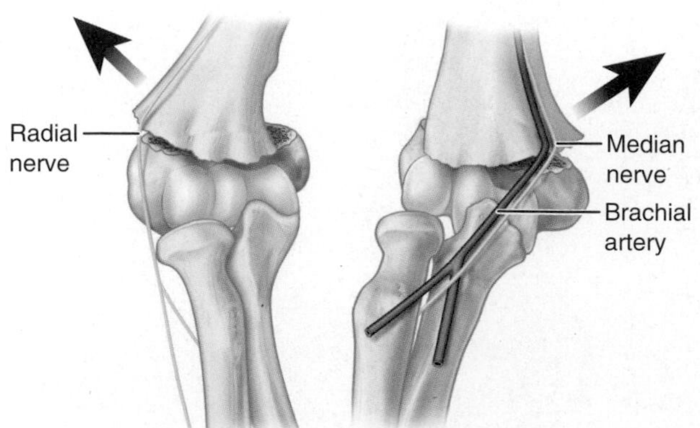

FIGURE 14-5 Relationship to neurovascular structures. The proximal metaphyseal spike penetrates laterally with posteromedially displaced fractures and places the radial nerve at risk; with posterolaterally displaced fractures, the spike penetrates medially and places the median nerve and brachial artery at risk.

tal fragment places the radial nerve at risk, and lateral displacement of the distal fragment places the median nerve and brachial artery at risk (Fig. 14-5). The brachial artery and median nerve may become entrapped in the fracture site with lateral displacement, but they are highly unlikely to become entrapped with the distal fragment displaced medially. The brachial artery is placed further at risk by the ulnar-sided tether of the supratrochlear artery (Fig. 14-6).[171]

Classification

The modified Gartland system is most often used for classification of supracondylar humeral fractures in children (Table 14-2).[73] Barton et al.[18] found that this classification had higher kappa values for intra- and interobserver variability than those reported for several other fracture classification systems.

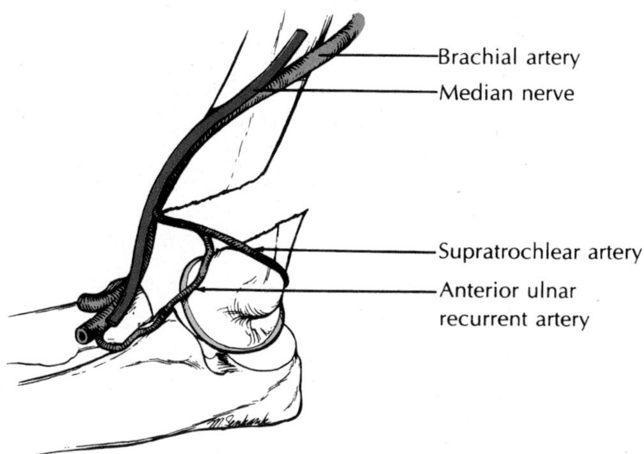

FIGURE 14-6 Arterial pathology. The supratrochlear branch that arises from the anterior ulnar recurrent artery may bind the main trunk of the brachial artery against the sharp end of the proximal fragment. (From Rowell PJW. Arterial occlusion in juvenile humeral supracondylar fracture. Injury 1974;6:254–256, with permission.)

The addition of a type IV pattern, multidirectional instability, to the original classification seems appropriate because of its treatment implications, but larger studies are needed to confirm its usefulness.

A potential pitfall is to underappreciate the extent of loss of normal alignment in fractures with comminution and collapse of the medial column (Fig. 14-7). Medial collapse signifies malrotation in the frontal plane (which defines the injury as at least a type III fracture) and is associated with a loss of the Baumann angle and varus malalignment. The lateral view (Fig. 14-8) may show reasonable alignment, which may lead to an underappreciation of the seriousness of this fracture, which requires operative reduction. Bahk et al.[16] reported that fractures with more than 10 degrees of obliquity in the coronal plane or 20 degrees in the sagittal plane were more likely than fractures with less obliquity to result in malunion.

Signs and Symptoms

An elbow or forearm fracture should be suspected in a child with elbow pain or a child who fails to use the upper extremity after a fall. Unless there is clearly localized tenderness with the remainder of the arm nontender, initial radiographs should include the entire extremity because multiple fractures may be present even with an injury that seems to be minor trauma. In children with elbow pain and failure to use the upper extremity, the differential diagnosis should include occult fracture, nursemaid's elbow, and infection. With a clear history of a "pulling type" of injury, manipulation for a nursemaid's elbow can be done before a radiograph is obtained. In general, if the history is not clear or if there is any question of a fall onto an outstretched hand as the mechanism of injury, a radiograph should be obtained before elbow manipulation. Point tenderness over the medial and lateral columns suggests a supracondylar fracture, as opposed to tenderness on only one side of the elbow, which suggests another type of injury.

With a type I supracondylar fracture, there is distal humeral tenderness and restriction of motion, particularly lack of full extension. Radiographs may be negative except for a posterior fat pad sign. In type III fractures, gross displacement of the elbow is evident (Fig. 14-9).

An anterior pucker sign may be present if the proximal fragment has penetrated the brachialis and the anterior fascia of the elbow (Fig. 14-10). Skin puckering results from the proximal segment piercing the brachialis muscle and engaging the deep dermis. This is a sign of considerable soft tissue damage. If any bleeding from a punctate wound is present, this should be considered an open fracture. When the proximal fragment is disengaged from its pucker in the skin during reduction, there is sometimes bleeding, which is a sign of a grade I open fracture.

Careful motor, sensory, and vascular examinations should be performed in all patients; this may be quite difficult in a young child but should be attempted. Sensation should be tested in discrete sensory areas of the radial nerve (dorsal first web space), medial nerve (palmar index finger), and ulnar nerve (palmar little finger). If a child is not cooperative or has altered mental status, a wet cloth can be wrapped around the hand to check for wrinkling of the skin. Motor examination should include finger, wrist, and thumb extension (radial nerve), index

TABLE 14-2 Modified Gartland Classification of Supracondylar Fractures

		Comments
Type I	Undisplaced	Fat pad present acutely
Type II	Hinged posteriorly	Anterior humeral line Anterior to capitellum
Type III	Displaced	No meaningful cortical continuity
Type IV	Displaces into extension and flexion	Usually diagnosed with manipulation under imaging.
Medial Comminution (not truly a separate type)	Collapse of medial column	Loss of Baumann anglė

distal interphalangeal flexion and thumb interphalangeal flexion (anterior interosseous nerve), thenar strength (median nerve), and interossei (ulnar nerve) muscle function. In young children, the interosseous nerve can be tested by asking the child to pinch something with his or her thumb and first finger while palpating the first dorsal interosseous for muscle contracture.

The vascular examination should include determining the presence of pulse, as well as warmth, capillary refill, and color of the hand. Assessment of the vascular status is essential, as series report up to 20% of displaced fractures present with vascular compromise.[35,157,177] The vascular status can be classified into one of three categories:

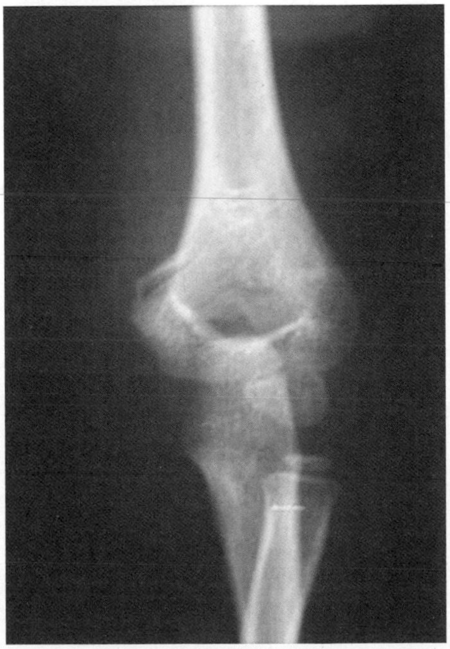

FIGURE 14-7 Medial comminution is a subtle radiographic finding and indicates a more unstable variant that may collapse into varus if not treated appropriately. (From Tolo VT, Skaggs DL, eds. Masters Techniques in Orthopaedic Surgery: Pediatric Orthopaedics. Philadelphia: Lippincott, 2007: 1–15, with permission.)

1. Hand well-perfused (warm and red), radial pulse present
2. Hand well-perfused, radial pulse absent
3. Hand poorly perfused (cool and blue or blanched), radial pulse absent

During the physical examination, a high index of suspicion is needed to recognize signs of a developing forearm compartment syndrome, such as considerable swelling or ecchymosis, anterior skin puckering, and an absent pulse. Tenseness of the volar compartment should be evaluated, and the amount of swelling about the elbow should be noted. Passive finger extension and flexion should be tested, and the findings should be accurately recorded. In the initial examination of a child with a severe supracondylar fracture with high parental and patient anxiety, it is easy to overlook vital information. Because further decision making depends on an accurate initial assessment, care should always be taken to obtain all of the previously mentioned information as accurately as possible. When the elbow injury is obvious, it is essential to evaluate the entire extremity because associated forearm fractures can occur with supracondylar fractures and substantially increase the risk of compartment syndrome (Fig. 14-11).

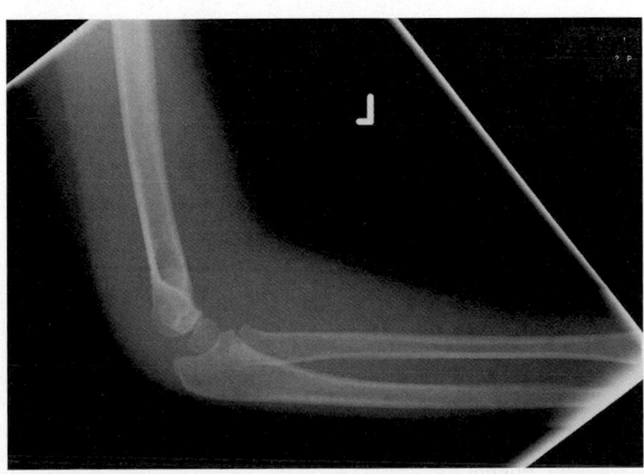

FIGURE 14-8 Note the lateral view does not show significant displacement. This view alone would suggest nonoperative treatment may be sufficient. (Reproduced with permission of Children's Orthopaedic Center, Los Angeles,CA.)

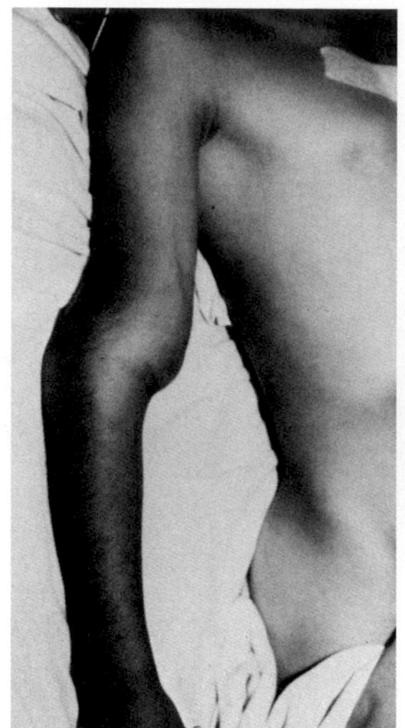

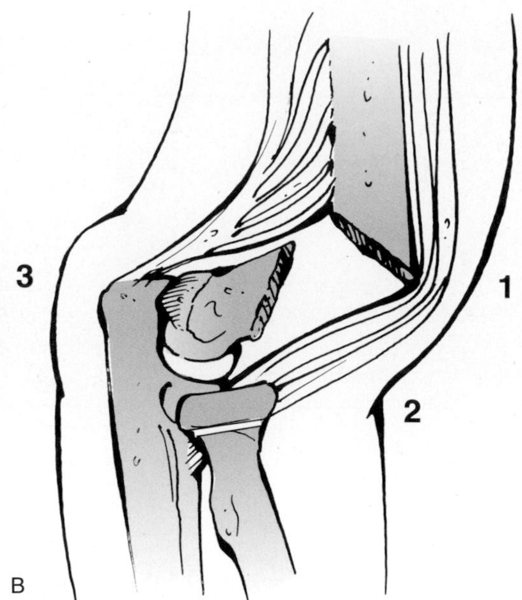

FIGURE 14-9 A. Clinical appearance. **B.** The S-shaped configuration is created by the anterior prominence of the proximal fragment's spike and extension of the distal fragment.

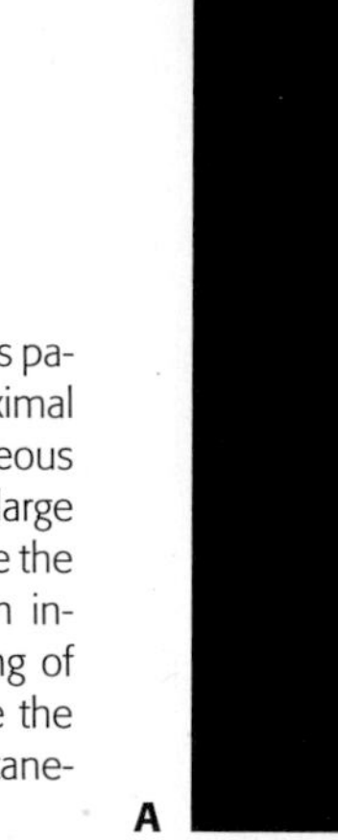

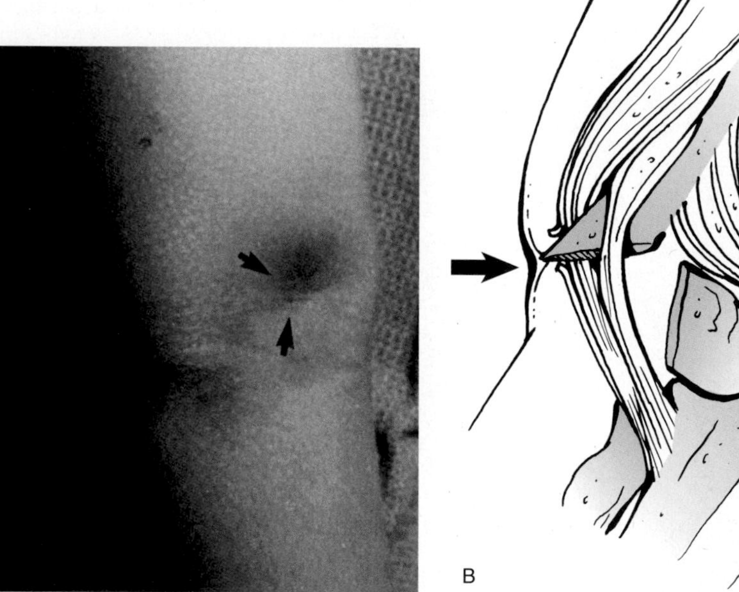

FIGURE 14-10 The pucker sign. This patient had penetration of the proximal fragment's spike into the subcutaneous tissue. **A.** In the AP view, there is a large puckering or defect in the skin where the distal fragment has pulled the skin inward. **B.** Laterally, there is puckering of the skin (*arrow*) in the area where the spike has penetrated into the subcutaneous tissue.

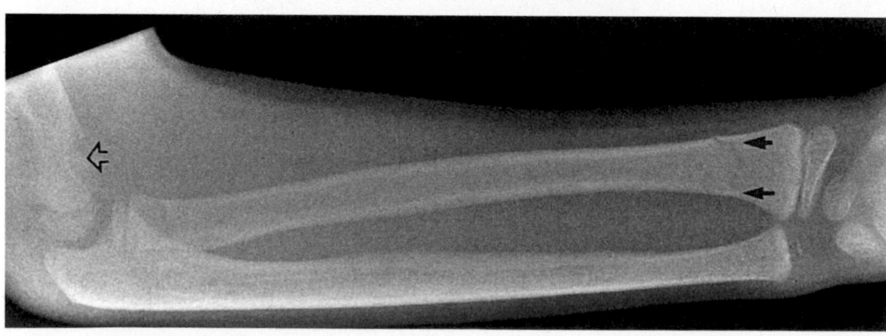

FIGURE 14-11 Occult ipsilateral fracture. Type II supracondylar fracture (*open arrow*) with an occult distal radial fracture (*solid arrows*).

Radiographic Evaluation

All patients with a history of a fall onto an outstretched hand as well as pain and inability to use the extremity should have a thorough radiographic evaluation, generally including anteroposterior (AP) and lateral views of the entire upper extremity. Comparison views rarely are required by an experienced physician, but occasionally may be needed to evaluate an ossifying epiphysis. A true AP view of the distal humerus, rather than of the elbow, allows more accurate evaluation of the distal humerus and decreases the error in determining angular malalignment in the distal humerus. The lateral film should be taken as a true lateral with the humerus held in the anatomic position and not externally rotated (Fig. 14-12). Oblique views of the distal humerus (Fig. 14-13) occasionally may be helpful when a supracondylar fracture or occult condylar fracture is suspected but not seen on standard AP and lateral views, but should not be routinely ordered to evaluate an elbow injury.

Initial radiographs may be negative except for a posterior fat pad sign. A series by Skaggs et al.[184] of 34 patients with traumatic elbow pain and a posterior fat pad sign but no visible fracture found that 18 (53%) had a supracondylar humeral fracture, 9 (26%) had a fracture of the proximal ulna, 4 (12%) had a fracture of the lateral condyle, and 3 (9%) had a fracture of the radial neck.

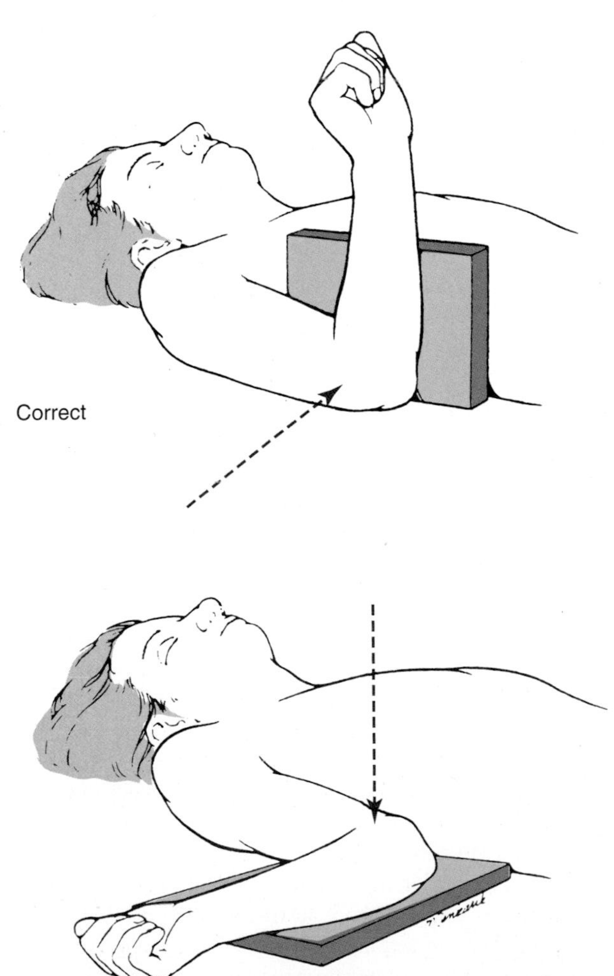

FIGURE 14-12 Radiograph positioning for taking a lateral view is with the upper extremity directed anteriorly rather than externally rotated.

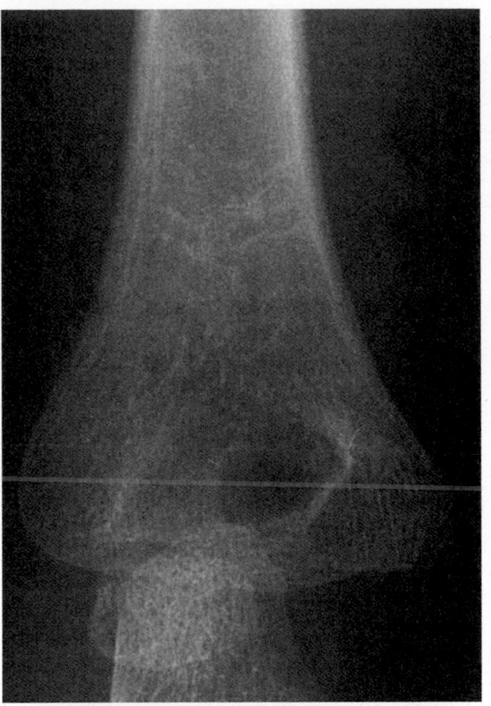

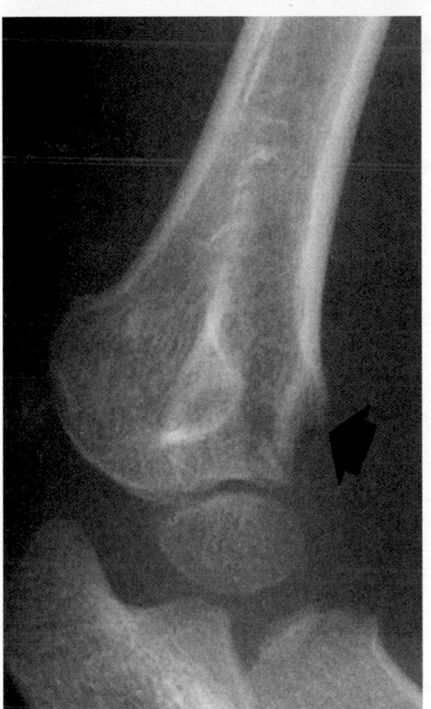

FIGURE 14-13 Oblique views. Often, the fracture line is not visualized on any of the lateral or anteroposterior views **(A)**. **B.** An oblique view of the distal humerus may demonstrate the extent of the fracture line (*arrows*).

Two main radiographic parameters are used to evaluate for the presence of a supracondylar fracture. The anterior humeral line should cross the capitellum through the middle third on a true lateral of the elbow (Fig. 14-14). In an extension-type supracondylar fracture, the capitellum is posterior to this line. The Baumann angle, also referred to as the humeral capitellar angle, is the angle between the long axis of the humeral shaft and the physeal line of the lateral condyle (normal range, about

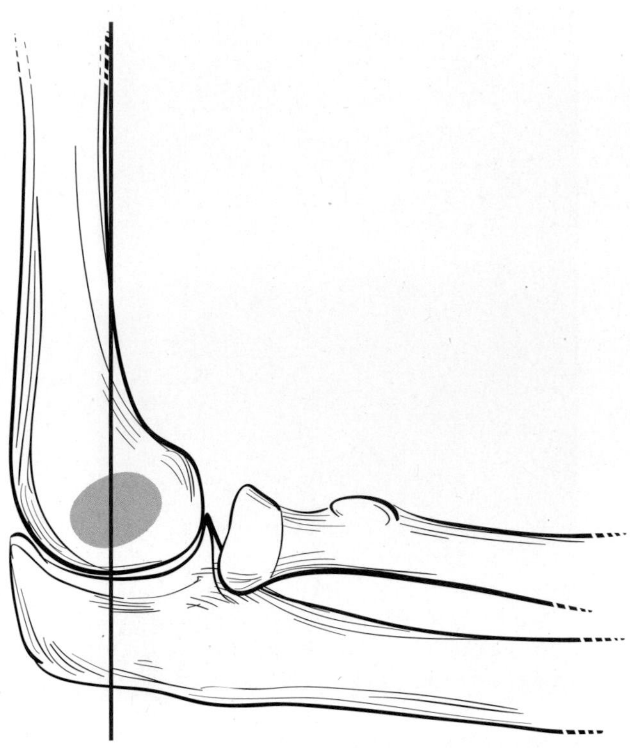

FIGURE 14-14 Anterior humeral line should cross the capitellum on a true lateral of the elbow. (From Tolo VT, Skaggs DL, eds. Master Techniques in Orthopaedic Surgery: Pediatric Orthopaedics. Philadelphia: Lippincott, 2007: 1–15, with permission.)

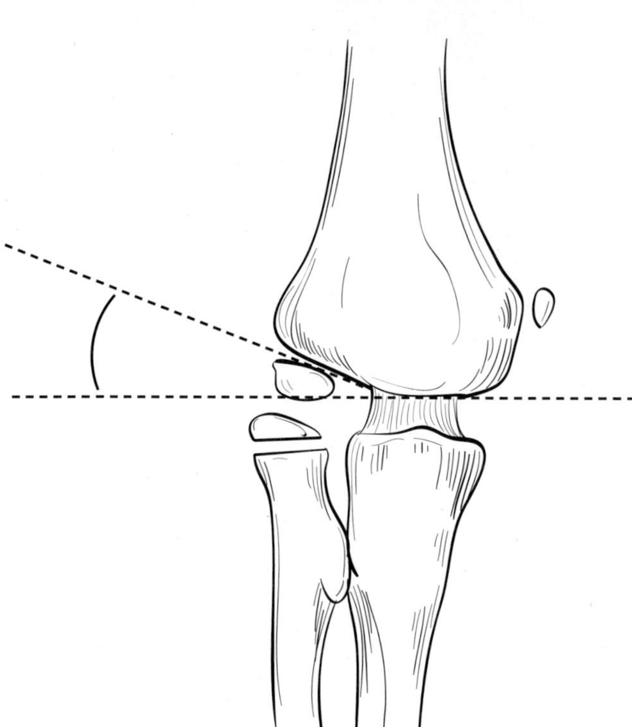

FIGURE 14-15 The Baumann angle is between the line perpendicular to the long axis of the humeral shaft and the physeal line of the lateral condyle. A decrease in the Baumann angle may indicate medial comminution. (From Tolo VT, Skaggs DL, eds. Master Techniques in Orthopaedic Surgery: Pediatric Orthopaedics. Philadelphia: Lippincott, 2007:1–15, with permission.)

9 to 26 degrees) (Fig. 14-15). A rule of thumb is that a Baumann angle of *at least* 10 degrees is acceptable; a decrease in the Baumann angle is a sign that a fracture is in varus angulation.

If the AP and lateral views show a displaced type II or III supracondylar fracture but do not show full detail of the distal humeral fragment, we usually obtain further x-ray evaluation in the operating room with the patient anesthetized. Repeat trips for radiographs evaluation in the emergency setting generally result in increased pain without significant improvement in radiographic quality. Detailed radiographs need to be obtained at some point, however, to define the fracture anatomy with particular emphasis on impaction of the medial column, supracondylar comminution, and vertical split of the epiphyseal fragment. T-condylar fractures (Fig. 14-16) can initially appear to be supracondylar fractures, but these generally occur in children over 10 years of age in whom supracondylar fractures are less likely.

In a young child, an epiphyseal separation[214] can mimic an elbow dislocation. In an epiphyseal separation, the fracture propagates through the physis without a large metaphyseal fragment. This fracture occurs in very young children with primarily chondral epiphyses. On physical examination, the patient appears to have a supracondylar fracture with gross swelling about the elbow and marked discomfort. The key to making the diagnosis and differentiating this injury from an elbow dislocation is the alignment of the capitellum with the radial head. Sometimes, a supracondylar fracture with a small metaphyseal fragment can mimic a lateral condylar fracture (Fig. 14-17). In such cases, more data are required to initiate treatment. An arthrogram may be helpful to determine the extent of the elbow injury. In selected patients, magnetic resonance imaging (MRI) or ultrasonography[214] may also aid in evaluating the injury to the unossified epiphysis.

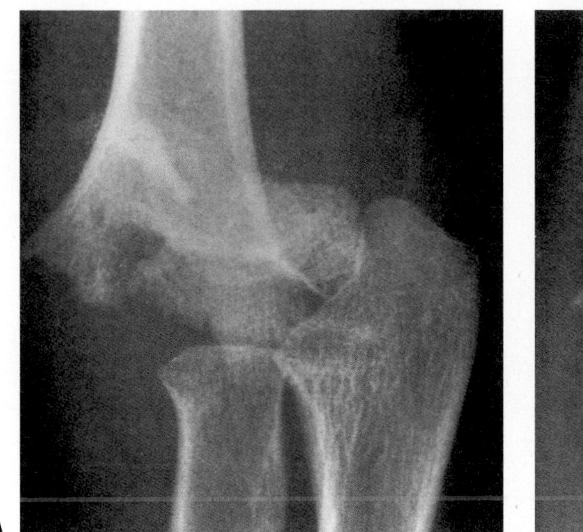

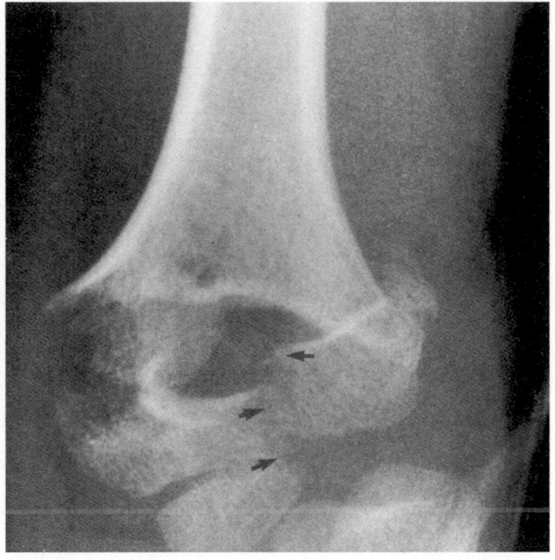

FIGURE 14-16 Occult T-condylar fracture. **A.** Original radiographs appear to show a type III posteromedial supracondylar fracture. **B.** After manipulation, the vertical intercondylar fracture line (*arrows*) was visualized.

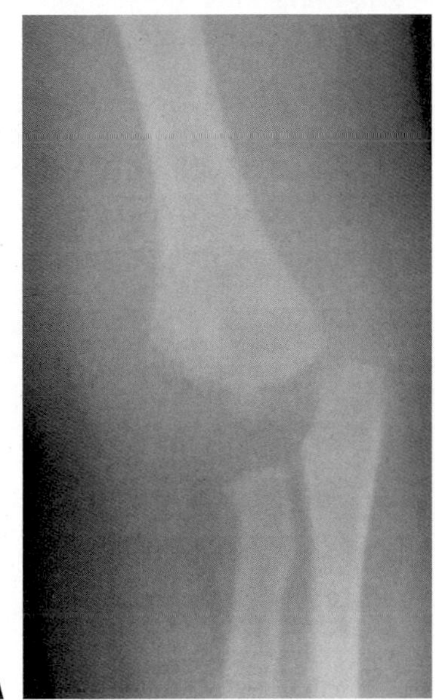

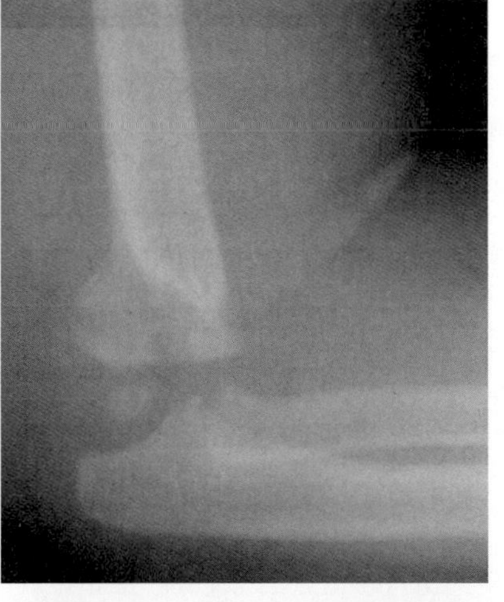

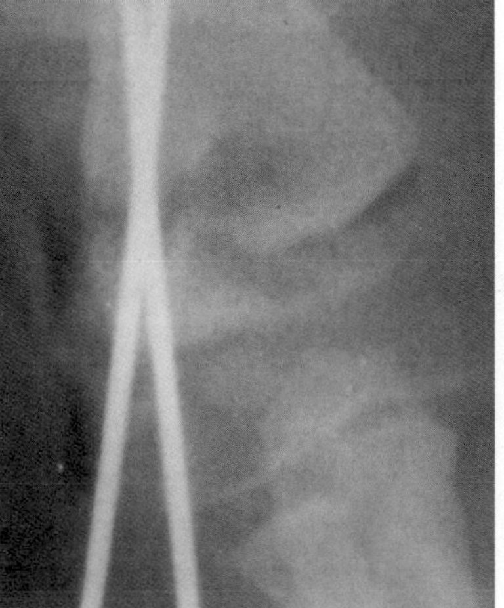

FIGURE 14-17 This 1.2-year-old girl sustained a fracture that on the anteroposterior view **(A)** appears like an elbow dislocation and on the lateral view **(B)** has the appearance of a lateral condyle fracture. **C.** Arthrography showed the outline of the entire cartilaginous epiphysis. This is an epiphyseal separation with a metaphyseal fragment (Salter-Harris type II).

Current Treatment Options

	Pro	Con
Casting in-situ	*Good for type I fractures*	*Not for displaced fractures*
Closed reduction and casting	*No surgery*	*Cannot reliably hold reduction* *Risks compartment syndrome if elbow flexed to hold reduction* *Radiographs difficult to interpret*
Closed reduction and pinning	*Predictable good outcome* *Few complications*	*Can be technically challenging to the inexperienced*
Open reduction and pinning	*Allows exposure and repair of neurovascular structures* *Removes impediments to reduction*	*Makes fracture less stable* *Scarring* *Possible stiffness*
Traction	*Salvage for rare severely comminuted fractures*	*Prolonged hospitalization* *Malunion*

Initial Management

For fractures with displacement that require reduction, initial splinting with the elbow in approximately 20 to 40 degrees of flexion provides comfort and allows further evaluation. Tight bandaging or splinting should be avoided, as should excessive flexion or extension, which may compromise the vascularity of the limb and increase compartment pressure.[19,129] The arm should then be gently elevated. A careful examination of the neurologic and vascular status is vital in all patients with a supracondylar fracture, as well as an assessment of the potential for compartment syndrome. The remainder of the limb should be assessed for other injuries, and radiographs should include any area that is tender, swollen, or lacks motion.

Closed Reduction and Pinning

Most supracondylar humeral fractures in children can be treated with closed reduction and pinning. Unless the fracture is open, a closed reduction should be initially attempted in all fractures, including type III fractures. With the patient supine and the child's arm on a radiolucent arm board, the fracture is first reduced in the frontal plane and reduction is checked with fluoroscopy. The elbow is then flexed while the olecranon is pushed anteriorly to correct the sagittal deformity. Restoration of the Baumann angle (which is generally >10 degrees) on the AP view, intact medial and lateral columns on oblique views, and the anterior humeral line passing through the middle third of the capitellum on the lateral view are indications of a successful reduction. Because of the amount of rotation present at the shoulder, some rotational malalignment in the axial plane can be tolerated at the fracture site, but any rotational malalignment can compromise fracture stability, so, if present, stability of the reduction should be carefully evaluated, and a third pin probably should be used.

Reduction is held with two or three Kirschner wires (K-wires), as discussed later in this chapter, and the elbow is immobilized in 50 to 60 degrees of flexion, depending on the amount of swelling and vascular status. A considerable gap in the fracture site or an irreducible fracture with a rubbery feeling on attempted reduction may be signs that the median nerve and/or brachial artery is trapped in the fracture site and open reduction is indicated (Fig. 14-18).

Pin Configuration Considerations: Crossed-Pins versus Lateral-Entry Pins

Clinical and X-Ray Outcomes. Good clinical outcomes in large number of patients have been reported with both pinning techniques. Although many of these reports are case series, two

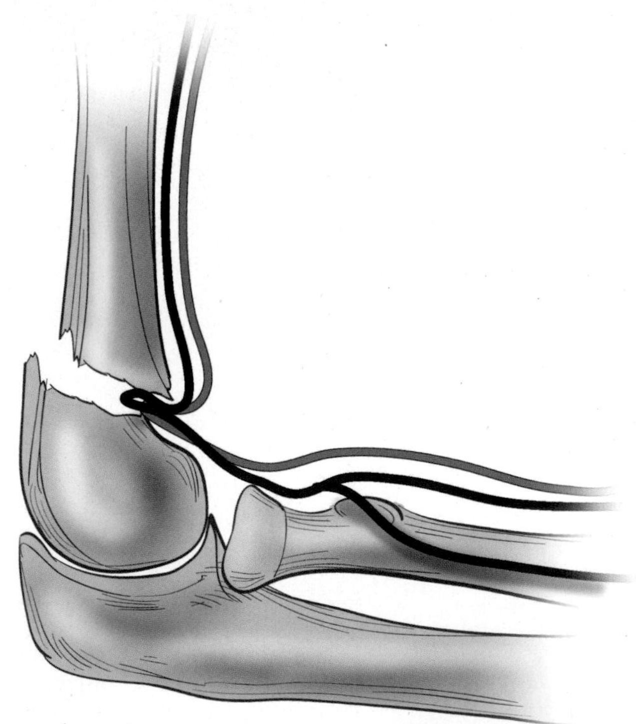

FIGURE 14-18 Brachial artery and median nerve may be trapped at the fracture site. If a reduction feels rubbery, and a gap at the fracture site is seen on imaging, entrapment is possible, especially in the setting of vascular compromise or median nerve or anterior interosseous nerve injury. (From Tolo VT, Skaggs DL, eds. Master Techniques in Orthopaedic Surgery: Pediatric Orthopaedics. Philadelphia: Lippincott, 2007:1–15, with permission.)

prospective randomized clinical trials have been reported. Kocher et al.[110] showed no statistically significant difference between the two treatment groups in any radiograph or clinical outcome measures in their prospective randomized clinical trial comparing lateral and crossed-pinning techniques in the treatment of 52 type III supracondylar humeral fractures. Another prospective randomized study by Blanco et al.[26] compared 57 patients with type III supracondylar fractures treated with lateral-entry pinning to 47 treated with crossed-pinning and found no statistically significant difference in the radiographic outcomes.

Ulnar Nerve Injury. Iatrogenic injury to the ulnar nerve with use of crossed pins has been reported to be as low as 0%; however, the two largest series of supracondylar fractures have shown the prevalence to be 5% (17 of 345) and 6% (19 of 331).[33,41,94,127,165,169,183,211] Others have reported that these iatrogenic injuries are more frequent.[169,206] In 1977, Arino et al.[12] recommended the use of two lateral pins to avoid injury to the ulnar nerve, and a recent meta-analysis seems to support this recommendation: iatrogenic ulnar nerve injury occurred in 40 of 1171 (3.4%) patients with medial and lateral crossed pins and in only 5 of 738 (0.7%) of those with lateral-entry pins. Although iatrogenic ulnar nerve injuries usually resolve, several permanent iatrogenic ulnar nerve injuries have been described.[161,165,183]

In an evaluation of 164 children (328 ulnar nerves), Zaltz et al.[211] identified a group of children who may be at particular risk of ulnar nerve injury during fracture reduction: those whose ulnar nerves sublux onto the medial epicondyler and especially those whose nerves dislocate anterior to the medial epicondyle. In 61% of children younger than 5 years of age, the ulnar nerve migrated over, or even anterior to, the medial epicondyle when the elbow was flexed more than 90 degrees.[211] Wind et al.,[206] however, identified ulnar nerve subluxation in fewer than 2% of 22 children with supracondylar fractures. Flynn et al.[65] recommended palpating the point of the medial epicondyle and inserting the pin anterior to avoid the nerve; however, Wind et al.[206] found that the location of the ulnar nerve was not determined accurately enough by palpation to allow blind medial pinning. They found an average difference of almost 2 mm between the predicted and the actual locations of the nerve. Making an incision over the medial epicondyle to make certain the ulnar nerve is not directly injured by a pin may not ensure protection of the nerve,[103] but Weiland et al.[200] reported no iatrogenic ulnar nerve injuries in 52 patients with crossed pins in whom a small medial incision was used. Green et al.[80] reported only one iatrogenic nerve injury (1.5%) in 65 patients treated with two lateral pins and one medial pin inserted with a mini-open technique. In their systematic literature review, Brauer et al.[31] found the probability of iatrogenic ulnar nerve injury to be five times higher with crossed pins than with lateral-entry pins; however, when only the two prospective studies were included there was no significant difference.

Even if the ulnar nerve is not penetrated by the pin, placement of a medial pin adjacent to the nerve can cause injury. Rasool[165] described iatrogenic ulnar nerve injuries in 6 patients in whom early exploration found direct penetration of the nerve by the pin in 2, constriction of the cubital tunnel in 3, and fixation of the nerve anterior to the medial epicondyle in 1. In a series of 345 supracondylar humeral fractures treated by percutaneous pinning, Skaggs et al.[183] found that ulnar nerve injury occurred in 4% of patients with medial pins placed without hyperflexion and in 15% of those in whom the medial pin was placed while the elbow was hyperflexed. No iatrogenic ulnar nerve injuries occurred in the 125 fractures treated with lateral-entry pins alone. These studies indicate that if a medial pin is used, the lateral pin(s) should be placed first, then the elbow should be extended and the medial pin placed without hyperflexion of the elbow. Avoidance of a medial pin is the simplest way to avoid iatrogenic ulnar nerve injury: no iatrogenic nerve injuries occurred in a series of 124 consecutive fractures stabilized with lateral-entry pins, regardless of displacement or fracture stability.[182]

Construct Stability. Another issue with pin configuration is stability, which remains somewhat unclear because some previous biomechanical studies of stability of various pin configurations have not used currently recommended configurations. For example, two studies that evaluated the torsional strength of pin configurations and found crossed-pins to be stronger than two lateral pins,[151,213] tested two lateral pins placed immediately adjacent to each other and not separated at the fracture site as is currently recommended.[174,182] Lee et al.,[123] on the other hand, found that two divergent lateral pins separated at the fracture site were stronger than crossed pins in extension loading and varus but the configurations were equal in valgus (Fig. 14-19).[123] They attributed the greater strength with lateral pins to the location of the intersection of the two pins and greater divergence between the two pins, which allowed some purchase in the medial column as well as the lateral column (see Fig. 14-6).

Intraoperative testing of the stability of lateral-entry pin fixation has been advocated. In a study of 21 children with type III fractures, two lateral-entry pins were inserted after reduction and stability was assessed by comparing lateral fluoroscopic

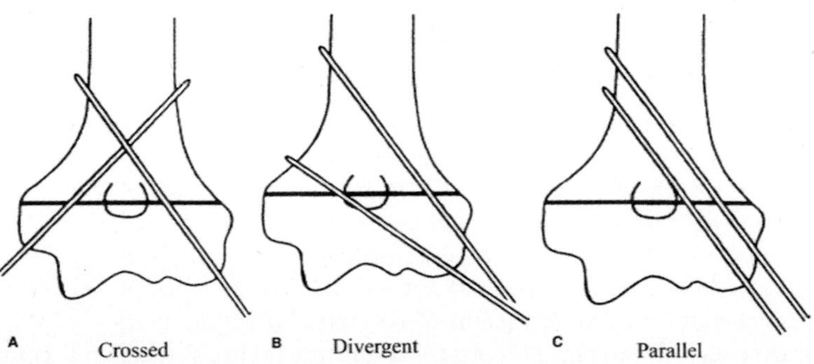

FIGURE 14-19 Three pinning techniques in study by Lee et al.[123] **A.** Crossed: one medial and one lateral pin. **B.** Divergent: two divergent lateral pins. **C.** Parallel: two parallel lateral pins.

images in internal and external rotation.[28] If the fracture remained rotationally unstable, a third lateral-entry pin was inserted and images were obtained. A medial pin was added only if instability was demonstrated after the insertion of three lateral pins. Rotational stability was achieved with two lateral-entry pins in 6 patients, with three lateral-entry pins in 10 patients, and with an additional medial pin in 5. No patient required a reoperation using this protocol. The authors concluded that supracondylar fractures that are rotationally stable intraoperatively after pin fixation are unlikely to displace postoperatively. It is notable that they found only a small proportion (26%) of these type III fractures to be rotationally stable after fixation with two lateral-entry wires.[28]

A systematic review of 35 articles reported loss of reduction in none of 849 fractures treated with crossed pins and in 4 of 606 (0.7%) of fractures treated with lateral-entry pins.[31] Deformity, defined as a carrying angle loss of more than 10 degrees or cubitus varus of more than 5 degrees, occurred in 29 (3.4%) of those with crossed pinning and 36 (5.9%) of those with lateral-entry pins. However, this article did not include the largest series in the literature that favored lateral-entry pins.[31]

Bloom et al.[27] recommended consideration of a three-pin pattern, either three laterally divergent pins or two lateral pins and one medial pin, for supracondylar humeral fractures with a less than complete anatomic reduction. In their biomechanical analysis, three lateral divergent pins were as strong as crossed-pinning and both were stronger than two lateral divergent pins.[27] Another biomechanic study of simulated fractures with medial comminution determined that three lateral divergent pins provided torsional stability equal to that of standard medial and lateral crossed-pinning.[120] These biomechanical studies support clinical recommendations that three lateral-entry pins provide the most stable fixation of type III fractures.[174,182]

Technical Points. In a series of 124 consecutive fractures treated with lateral-entry pins, Skaggs et al.[182] found no malunions or loss of fixation. From this successful series, combined with a failure analysis of eight fractures outside of this series, they concluded that the important technical points for fixation with lateral-entry pins are: (i) maximizing separation of the pins at the fracture site, (ii) engaging the medial and lateral columns proximal to the fracture, (iii) engaging sufficient bone in both the proximal segment and the distal fragment, (iv) maintaining a low threshold for use of a third lateral-entry pin if there is concern about fracture stability or the location of the first two pins, and (v) using three pins for type III fractures.[182] Gordon et al.[78] also recommended adding a third pin for type III fractures when intraoperative stress indicated lack of stability with 2 pins. Lee et al.[122] reported 92% excellent clinical results in 61 consecutive types II and II fractures treated with three lateral pins. None of their patients had loss of reduction, cubitus varus, hyperextension, loss of motion, or iatrogenic nerve injury; none required additional surgery, and only one patient had a minor pin track infection.[122]

Sankar et al.[174] studied eight supracondylar humeral fractures in which reduction was lost and determined that loss of fixation in all was due to technical errors that could have been identified on the intraoperative fluoroscopic images and could have been prevented with proper technique. Three types of pin-fixation errors were identified: (i) failure to engage both fragments with two pins or more, (ii) failure to achieve bicortical fixation with two pins or more, and (iii) failure to achieve adequate pin separation (>2 mm) at the fracture site.[174]

Open Reduction

Open reduction is indicated for open fractures, fractures in which closed reduction fails, and fractures associated with a dysvascular limb. Although earlier authors expressed concerns about elbow stiffness, myositis ossificans, ugly scarring, and iatrogenic neurovascular injury with open reduction, several more recent reports have shown low rates of complications with open reduction. Weiland et al.[200] reported that, in 52 displaced fractures treated with open reduction through a lateral approach, 10% had a moderate loss of motion but none had infection, nonunion, or myositis ossificans. Fleuriau-Chateau et al.,[63] in a series of 34 patients treated with open reduction through an anterior approach, reported a 6% (2 of 34) unsatisfactory loss of motion but no infection, myositis ossificans, malunion, or Volkmann contracture. Reitman et al.[167] reported that 78% (51) of 65 patients treated with open reduction (through either a medial or a lateral approach) had excellent or good results according to the criteria of Flynn et al.[65]; 4 patients had loss of motion. Ay et al.[14] found no loss of motion or clinical deformity in 61 patients treated with open reduction. Kaewpornsawan[99] compared closed reduction and percutaneous pin fixation with open reduction (through a lateral approach) in 28 children and found no differences in the frequency of cubitus varus, neurovascular injury, or infection; range of motion, union rate, and results according to the criteria of Flynn et al.[65] also were not significantly different.

Approach for Open Reduction. Although most orthopaedists are more familiar with lateral and medial approaches, we prefer a direct anterior approach, especially in those with neurovascular compromise. An advantage of the anterior approach is that it allows direct visualization of the brachial artery and median nerve as well as the fracture fragments. The relatively small (5 cm) transverse incision along the cubital fossa produces a scar that is much more cosmetically acceptable than that of the lateral approach, and scar contraction limiting elbow extension is not an issue. In addition, this approach does not disrupt the posterior periosteal hinge, which is useful for fracture reduction. A series of 26 patients treated with the anterior approach showed results equivalent to those of the traditional lateral or combined lateral and medial approach in terms of malunion, the criteria of Flynn et al.,[65] and range of motion.

The posterior approach is associated with high rates of loss of motion and osteonecrosis caused by disruption of the posterior end arterial supply to the trochlea of the humerus,[32,209] and it generally is not recommended for open reduction of supracondylar humeral fractures in children (Fig. 14-20).

Decreased Frequency of Complications. Open reduction has been increasingly accepted because there are relatively few complications with this method. Surgical experience[11,13,38,48,63,69,75,112,150,167,209] has dispelled the fears of infection, myositis ossificans, and neurovascular injury.[73,176,186,199] In a combined series of 470 fractures treated by open reduction, the incidence of infection was 2.5%, all of which resolved.[7,22,36,52,74,77,81,86,106,114,146,157,163,178,198,200] The incidence of neurovascular complications from the procedure itself was essentially zero.

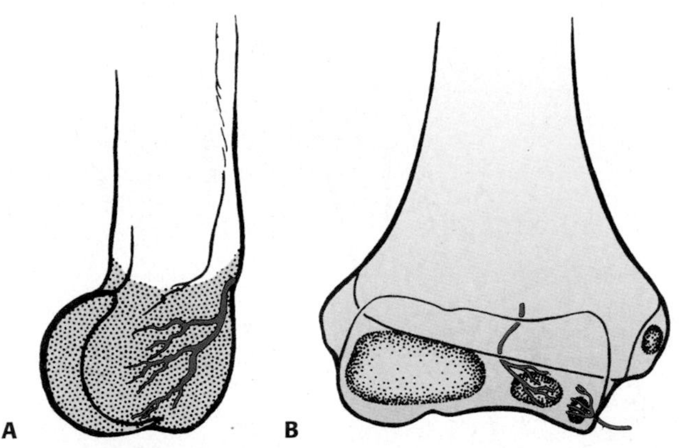

FIGURE 14-20 Intraosseous blood supply of the distal humerus. **A.** The vessels supplying the lateral condylar epiphysis enter on the posterior aspect and course for a considerable distance before reaching the ossific nucleus. **B.** Two definite vessels supply the ossification center of the medial crista of the trochlea. The lateral vessel enters by crossing the physis. The medial one enters by way of the nonarticular edge of the medial crista. (From Haraldsson S. On osteochondrosis deformans juvenilis capituli humeri including investigation of the intraosseous vasculature in the distal humerus. Acta Orthop Scand 1959;38(Suppl: 1–232, with permission.)

Four patients with myositis ossificans (1.4%) were reported, all in a single series.[77]

The most frequent complication of surgical management appears to be a loss of range of motion. One of the reasons given in the past for loss of motion was the use of a posterior approach. It has been stated that approaching the fracture through the relatively uninvolved posterior tissues induces added scarring, leading to stiffness. In earlier reported series using a posterior approach, loss of range of motion was significant. Use of the anterior approach has resulted in lower stiffness rates and complications similar to those of closed treatment. Residual cubitus varus occurred in as many as 33% of patients in some of the earlier series,[8,51,77,200] most due to inadequate surgical reduction. When good reduction was obtained, the incidence of cubitus varus deformity was low. Surgical intervention alone does not guarantee an anatomic reduction; the quality of the reduction achieved at the time of surgery is important.

Lal and Bahn[117] reported that delayed open reduction, 11 to 17 days after injury, did not increase the frequency of myositis ossificans. If a supracondylar fracture is unreduced or poorly reduced, delayed open reduction and pin fixation appear to be justified. Ağuş[4] showed that delayed open reduction and pinning can be safely accomplished after skeletal traction and malreduction.

Open supracondylar fractures generally have an anterior puncture wound where the metaphyseal spike penetrates the skin. Even if the open wound is only a small puncture in the center of an anterior pucker, open irrigation and débridement are indicated. The anterior approach, using a transverse incision with medial or lateral extension as needed, is recommended. The neurovascular bundle is directly under the skin and tented over the metaphyseal fragment, so care should be taken even as the skin is incised. The skin incision can be extended medially proximally and laterally distally. Often, only the transverse portion of the incision is required, which gives a better cosmetic result. The brachialis muscle usually is transected because its muscle belly inserts on the coronoid attachment and is highly vulnerable to trauma from the proximal metaphyseal fragment. The fracture surfaces are examined and washed, and a curette is used to remove any dirt or entrapped soft tissue. Once the débridement and washing are complete, the fracture is stabilized with K-wires. All patients with open fractures also are treated with antibiotics, generally, cephalothin for Gustilo types I, II, and IIIA injuries, with the addition of an aminoglycoside for types IIIB and IIIC fractures.

Treatment with Traction

Traction rarely is used as definitive treatment for supracondylar fractures in children in most modern centers. Indications for traction may include severe comminution, lack of anesthesia, medical conditions prohibiting anesthesia, lack of an experienced surgeon, or temporary traction to allow swelling to decrease. Devnani[58] reported using traction in the gradual reduction of 28 fractures with late presentation (mean of 5.6 days), although 18% of these children required a corrective osteotomy for malunion. Cubitus varus has been reported after traction treatment in 9% to 33% of patients in some series,[91,160] while others have reported excellent results.[51,71,187] Because of the excellent results obtained with closed reduction and pinning and the brief hospital stay required after this procedure (usually no more than one night), it is difficult to justify the 14 to 22 days of hospitalization required for traction treatment. Advocates of traction in the treatment of supracondylar fractures have reported that the use of overhead traction with use of an olecranon wing nut[15,155,208] gives superior results to sidearm traction (Fig. 14-21).

Treatment by Fracture Type

Type I Fracture (Nondisplaced). In general in a type I fracture, the periosteum is intact with significant inherent stability of the fracture. A type I fracture may become apparent only with repeat radiographs at 1- to 2-week follow-up after presentation with elbow pain and initial radiographic findings limited to a posterior fat pad sign. Periosteal reaction in the distal humerus may be all that is visible on radiograph.

Simple immobilization with a posterior splint applied at 60 to 90 degrees of elbow flexion with side supports is preferred by some.[39,203] We prefer a carefully constructed, nonconstrictive, circumferential cast to avoid skin problems, blistering, and the tourniquet effect of elastic wraps left in place for a few weeks. The arm always looks better when it comes out of an adequately-padded well-made cast than when it comes out of splint with an elastic wrap. If there is no significant swelling about the elbow, circumferential casts can be used, but the parents must be educated about elevation and the signs and symptoms of compartment syndrome. The elbow should not be flexed more than 90 degrees. Using Doppler examination of the brachial artery after supracondylar fractures, Mapes and Hennrikus[129] found that flow was decreased in the brachial artery in positions of pronation and increased flexion. Before the splint is applied, it should be confirmed that the pulse is intact and that there is good capillary refill with the amount of elbow flexion intended during immobilization. A sling helps decrease torsional forces about the fracture.

Radiographs are obtained 3 to 7 days after fracture to document lack of displacement. If there is any evidence of distal fragment extension, as judged by lack of intersection of the

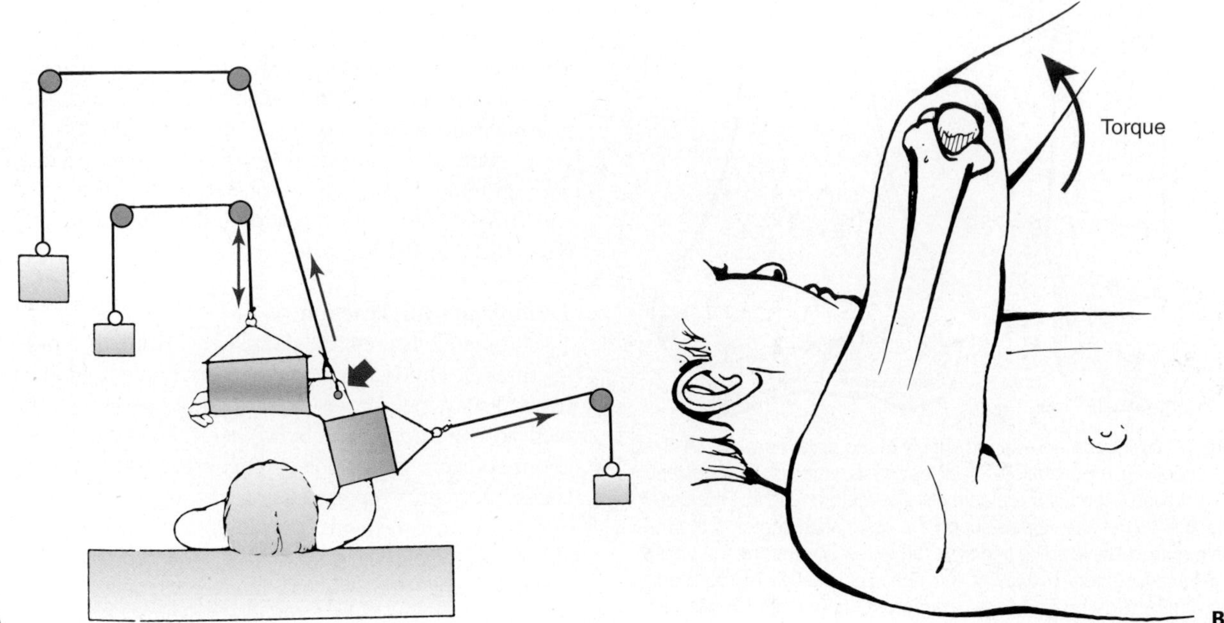

FIGURE 14-21 Overhead olecranon wing nut traction. The arm is suspended by a threaded wing nut through the olecranon (*short arrow*). The forces maintaining the reduction (*long arrows*) are exerted upward **(A)** through the pin and sideways through a counter-sling against the arm. The forearm is supported with a small sling (*double arrow*). By placing the traction rope eccentric to the axis of the screw, a torque can be created to correct varus or valgus alignment **(B)**.

anterior humeral line with the capitellum, the fracture has changed into a type II fracture and should be treated as such.

An acceptable position is determined by the anterior humeral line transecting the capitellum on the lateral radiograph, and a Baumann angle of more than 10 degrees or equal to the other side. The duration of immobilization for supracondylar fractures is 3 weeks, whether type I, II, or III. In general, no physical therapy is required after this injury. Patients may be seen 4 weeks after immobilization is removed to ensure that range of motion and strength are returning normally. Because the outcomes of type I fractures are predictably excellent if alignment is maintained at the time of early healing, follow-up visits after cast removal are optional depending on family and medical circumstances.

The initial radiograph is a static representation of the actual injury that may involve soft tissue disruption much greater than might be expected from the minimal bony abnormality. Excessive swelling, nerve or vascular disruption, and excessive pain are indicative of a more significant injury than a type I fracture, in which case periosteal disruption may render this fracture inherently unstable.

Type II Fracture (Hinged Posteriorly, with Posterior Cortex in Continuity). This fracture category encompasses a broad array of soft tissue injuries. Careful assessment of the soft tissue injury is critical in treatment decision-making. Because the posterior cortex is in continuity, good stability should be obtained with closed reduction. Significant swelling, obliteration of the pulse with flexion, neurovascular injuries, excessive angulation, and other injuries in the same extremity are indications for pin stabilization of most type II fractures.

Currently, the treatment of choice for type II fractures is operative stabilization rather than cast immobilization. The distal humerus provides only 20% of the growth of the humerus and has little remodeling potential. The upper limb grows approximately 10 cm during the first year of life, 6 cm during the second year, 5 cm during the third year, 3.5 cm during the fourth year, and 3 cm during the fifth year of life.[59] In toddlers (<3 years of age), some remodeling potential is present so nonoperative treatment may be appropriate for a type II fracture in which the capitellum abuts the anterior humeral line but does not cross it. In a child who is 8 to 10 years old, however, only 10% of growth of the distal humerus remains, so adequate reduction is essential to prevent malunion.

Two studies support the initial treatment of type II fractures with closed reduction and casting. Hadlow et al.[84] noted that if pinning of all type II fractures in their series had been done, 77% (37 of 48) of patients would have undergone an unnecessary operative procedure; however, 23% (11 of 48) of the patients required later operative reduction because they lost reduction after closed reduction; 14% (2 of 14) who were followed had poor outcomes by the Flynn criteria.[64] Parikh et al.,[64] in a retrospective review of 25 elbows treated with closed reduction and casting, found similar results: 28% (7 of 25) loss of reduction, 20% (5 of 25) delayed surgery, and 2% (2 of 25) unsatisfactory outcomes according to the Flynn criteria.

In contrast, in their consecutive series of 69 children with type II fractures treated with closed reduction and pinning, Skaggs et al.[182] found no radiographic or clinical loss of reduction, no cubitus varus, no hyperextension, and no loss of motion. No patient had an iatrogenic nerve palsy, and none required additional surgery.[182] In a review of 191 consecutive type II fractures treated with closed reduction and percutaneous pinning, there were four (2%) pin track infections, of which three were treated successfully with oral antibiotics and pin removal and one required operative irrigation and débridement for a wound infection not involving the joint. No nerve or vascular injuries, no loss of reduction, and no delayed unions or malunions were reported.[185]

Avoiding compartment syndrome is another reason for choosing operative treatment of these injuries. The amount of hyperflexion needed to maintain reduction of unpinned type II fractures predisposes these patients to increased compartment pressures.[19] Mapes et al.[129] used Doppler examination to determine that pronation and increased flexion caused decreased flow in the brachial artery, leading them to recommend a position of flexion and supination for "vascular safety." Pinning of these fractures avoids immobilization with the elbow markedly flexed. In general, for any fracture that would require elbow flexion of more than 90 degrees to hold reduction, pins should be used to hold the reduction, and the elbow should be immobilized in less flexion (usually about 45 to 70 degrees). If pinning is chosen, two lateral-entry pins[174,181,183,195] through the distal humeral fragment, engaging the opposite cortex of the proximal fragment, generally are sufficient to maintain fracture alignment (Figs. 14-22 and 14-23), although three pins can be used for added stability.[182] Because the posterior cortex and the intact periosteum provide some degree of inherent stability, crossed-pinning of type II fractures generally is not needed. The techniques for crossed and lateral pinning are described later in this chapter. If pin stabilization is used, the pins are left protruding through the skin and are removed 3 to 4 weeks after fixation, generally without the need for sedation or anesthesia.

Type III Fractures. For any child who presents to the emergency room with the elbow in either extreme flexion or extension, the arm is carefully placed in 30 degrees of flexion to minimize vascular insult and compartment pressure. In a type III fracture, the periosteum is torn, there is no cortical contact between the fragments, and soft tissue injury may accompany the fracture. Careful preoperative evaluation is mandatory. If circulatory compromise is indicated by absent pulse and a pale hand or if compartment syndrome is suspected, urgent reduction and skeletal stabilization are mandatory. Most type III fractures require operative reduction and pinning.

Cast immobilization techniques have been described as well. Because type III fractures are inherently unstable, the elbow must be held in extreme flexion to prevent the distal fragment from rotating; these fractures tend to rotate with flexion of less than 120 degrees.[141] A figure-of-eight cast (Fig. 14-24) can be used to maintain flexion of at least 120 degrees. If the arm can be flexed to 120 degrees with an intact pulse, casting can be

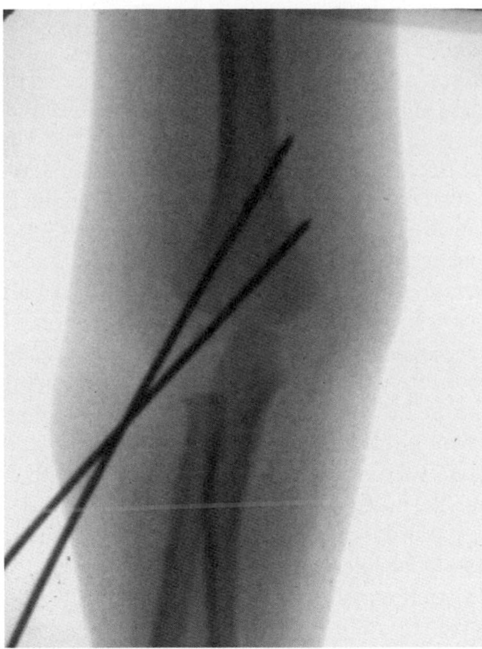

FIGURE 14-23 Intraoperative fluoroscopy of two lateral entry pins placed for a type II fracture. (Reproduced with permission from Children's Orthopaedic Center, Los Angeles, CA.)

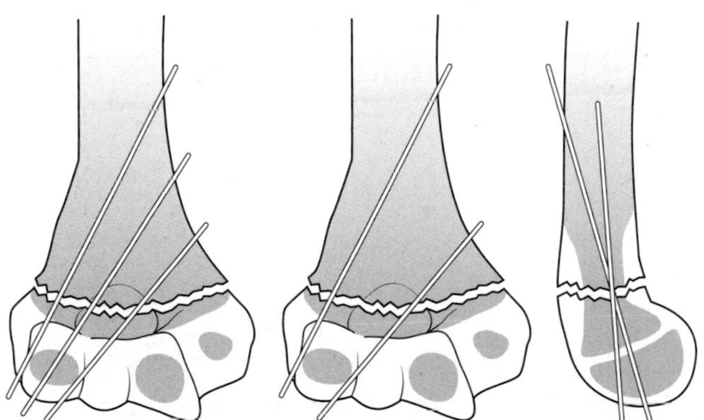

FIGURE 14-22 Properly placed divergent lateral entry pins. On the AP view, there should be maximal pin separation at the fracture site, the pins should engage both medial and lateral columns just proximal to the fracture site, and they should engage an adequate amount of bone proximal and distal to the fragments. On the lateral view, pins should incline slightly in the anterior to posterior direction in accordance with normal anatomy. (From Skaggs DL, Cluck MW, Mostofi A, et al. Lateral-entry pin fixation in the management of supracondylar fractures in children. J Bone Joint Surg Am 2004;86(4):702–707, with permission.)

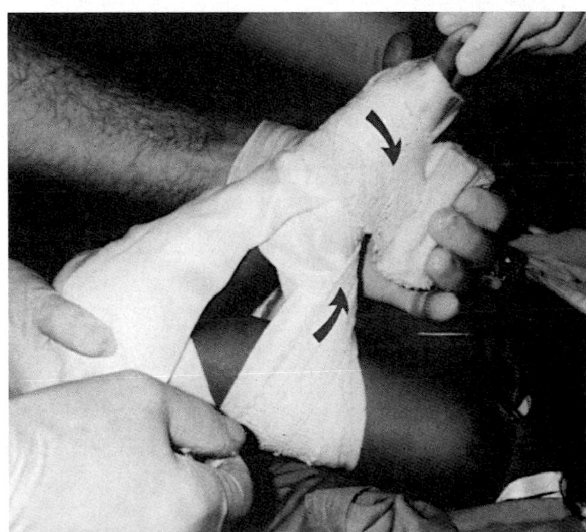

FIGURE 14-24 Figure-of-eight wrap. In the figure-of-eight cast, both the padding and the plaster are wrapped in a figure-of-eight manner (*arrows*). Flexion of a swollen elbow with a supracondylar fracture beyond 90 degrees increases the risk of compartment syndrome and is generally not recommended if operative treatment is available. (From Wilkins KE. The management of severely displaced supracondylar fractures of the humerus. Techniques Orthop 1989;4:5–24, with permission.)

used as primary treatment. Usually, however, severe swelling prevents the elbow from being kept in hyperflexion or compartment syndrome could result. Alburger et al.[6] reported that using skin traction initially until swelling decreased allowed successful casting without pinning. In most series,[48,115,158,198] the results of type III fractures treated with closed reduction and cast immobilization are not as good as the results of pinning. Hadlow et al.,[84] however, suggested that selective use of casting is beneficial, reporting that in their series, 61% of type III and 77% of type II fractures were successfully treated without pinning.

When a cast is used as primary treatment, it should be worn for 3 to 4 weeks. Although a number of historic series used casting as primary treatment, most recent reports favor pinning of this fracture because of concerns about vascular compromise, compartment syndrome, and malunion. It must be emphasized that flexion of the elbow of 90 degrees or more with a type III supracondylar fracture significantly increases the risk of compartment syndrome and should rarely, if ever, be done if modern operative facilities and an experienced surgeon are available.[19] Traction may be a safer alternative.

The Special Case of Medial Column Comminution. Although not as markedly displaced as most type III fractures, fractures with medial comminution usually require operative reduction because collapse of the medial column will lead to varus deformity in an otherwise minimally displaced supracondylar fracture (see Fig. 14-7).[55] De Boeck et al.[55] recommended closed reduction with percutaneous pinning for fractures with medial comminution even with minimal displacement to prevent cubitus varus. In their retrospective review of 13 patients with medial comminution, none of the 6 who had operative fixation had cubitus varus, while 4 of 7 treated nonoperatively developed cubitus varus.

Type IV Fractures. Open reduction has traditionally been recommended for this extremely unstable fracture, but Leitch et al.[125] described closed reduction in 9 patients. Their technique involves placing two K-wires into the distal fragment, reducing the fracture in the AP plane, and verifying the reduction with fluoroscopy. Then the fluoroscopy unit, rather than the arm, is rotated to obtain a lateral view (Fig. 14-25). The fracture is reduced in the sagittal plane, and the K-wires are driven across the fracture site. All fractures treated with this technique united with no cubitus varus, malunion, loss of motion, or additional operative treatment. Because of the limited number of these multidirectionally unstable fractures in their series, neither the need for open reduction nor the true complication rates can be determined.

Postoperative Care

For most operatively treated fractures with significant swelling, overnight observation is standard. The caregivers should be instructed about elevation and cast care and warning signs of infection and compartment syndrome. The first postoperative visit usually is 1 week after surgery, though this is not evidence-based. Ponce et al.[159] compared 52 patients with closed reduction and pinning of supracondylar fractures who had follow-up appointments 10 days or less after surgery to 52 who had follow-up visits later than 10 days. The overall complication rate was 7.7%, including four infections, three pin migrations

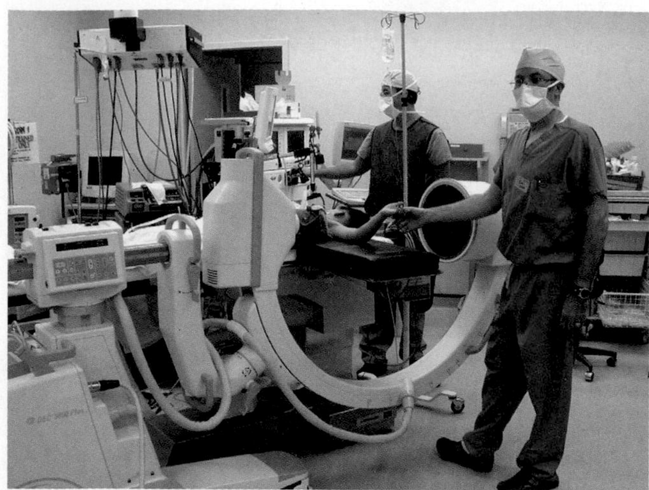

FIGURE 14-25 In very unstable fractures, rotation of the shoulder into external rotation in order to obtain a lateral image of the elbow may lead to a loss of reduction. In these rare instances, rotation of the c-arm, rather than the elbow, is a useful trick. (From Tolo VT, Skaggs DL, eds. Master Techniques in Orthopaedic Surgery: Pediatric Orthopaedics. Philadelphia: Lippincott, 2007, with permission.)

requiring surgery, and no loss of reduction. Six complications occurred in those with earlier follow-up and two in those with later follow-up. The authors concluded, and we agree, that early follow-up with radiographs after routine percutaneous pinning provides no added benefits to patient care and may unnecessarily tax the resources of the surgeon, clinic, and patient. They suggested that clinical and radiographic evaluation can be safely delayed until pin removal in most patients; however, if there is any concern about the stability of the pin configuration, we recommend early follow-up with radiographs in 5 days or less, because rereductions become increasingly more difficult beyond 1 week.[159]

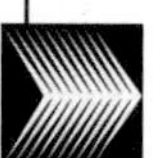

AUTHORS' PREFERRED TREATMENT

Type I Fractures

These fractures are managed in a long-arm cast with approximately 60 to 90 degrees of elbow flexion for approximately 3 weeks. Follow-up radiographic evaluation at 1 week is recommended for assessment of fracture position.

Type II Fractures

We prefer closed reduction and pinning for most type II supracondylar fractures. Two lateral pins are used for initial fixation in nearly all cases. If two lateral pins fail to provide acceptable fixation, we do not hesitate to place a third lateral pin. We believe it is safer to hold a type II fracture reduced with pins than to flex the elbow more than 90 degrees (Fig. 14-26).

Type III Fractures—Closed Reduction and Percutaneous Pinning

Once in the operating room, the patient receives a general anesthetic and prophylactic antibiotics. We prefer to have the fluoroscopy monitor opposite the surgeon for ease of viewing (Fig. 14-27).

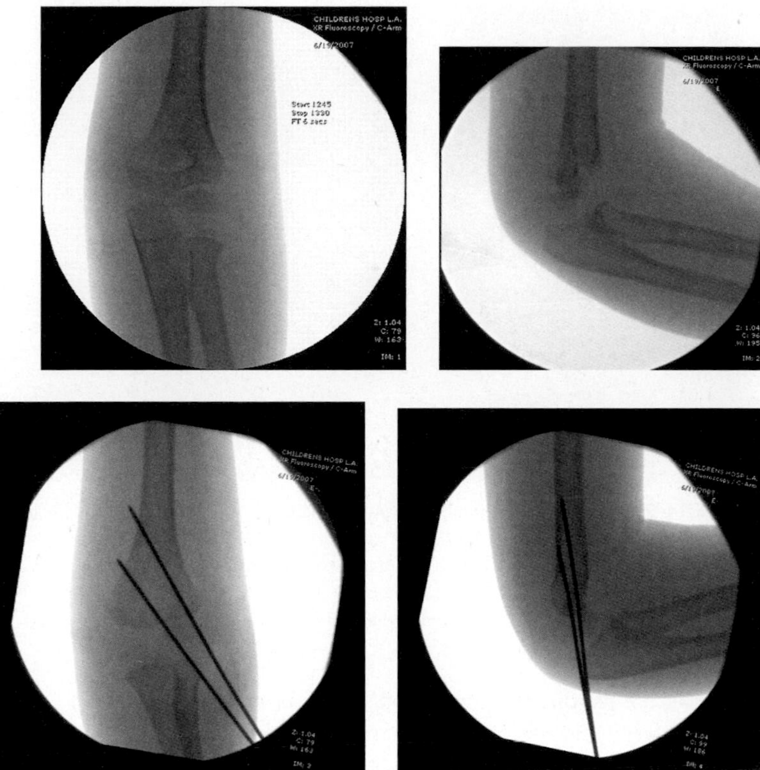

FIGURE 14-26 These intraoperative images are of a 4-year-old with a type II supracondylar humeral fracture that was closed reduced and pinned with two lateral entry pins according to the authors' preferred technique. (Reproduced with permission of Children's Orthopaedic Center, Los Angeles, CA.)

The patient is positioned supine on the operating table, with the fractured elbow on a short radiolucent arm board. Some surgeons use the wide end of the fluoroscopy unit as the table, but this does not allow rotation of the fluoroscopy unit for lateral images of the elbow in cases of unusual instability in which rotation of the arm leads to loss of reduction. It is essential that the child's arm is far enough onto the arm board that the elbow can be well visualized with fluoroscopy. In very small children, this may mean having the child's shoulder and head on the arm board (Fig. 14-28).

The patient's arm is then draped and prepared. First, traction is applied with the elbow flexed about 20 degrees to avoid tethering the neurovascular structures over an anteriorly displaced proximal fragment. For badly displaced fractures, significant traction is held for 60 seconds to allow soft tissue realignment with the surgeon grasping the forearm with both hands, and the assistant providing countertraction in the axilla (Fig. 14-29).

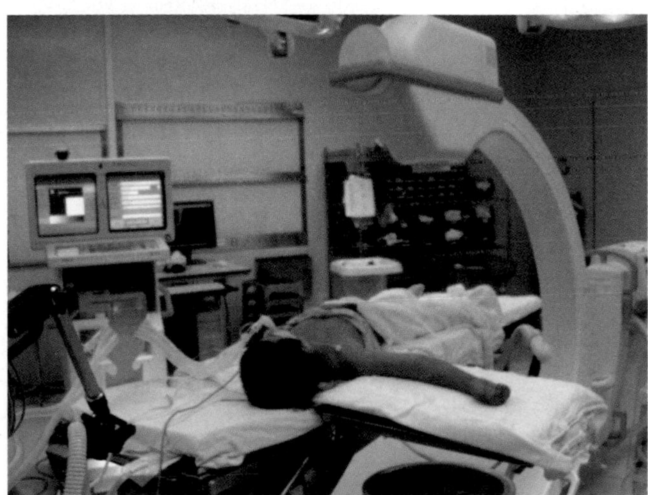

FIGURE 14-27 Positioning the fluoroscopy monitor on the opposite side of the bed allows the surgeon to easily see the images while operating. (From Tolo VT, Skaggs DL, eds. Master Techniques in Orthopaedic Surgery: Pediatric Orthopaedics. Philadelphia: Lippincott, 2007:1–15, with permission.)

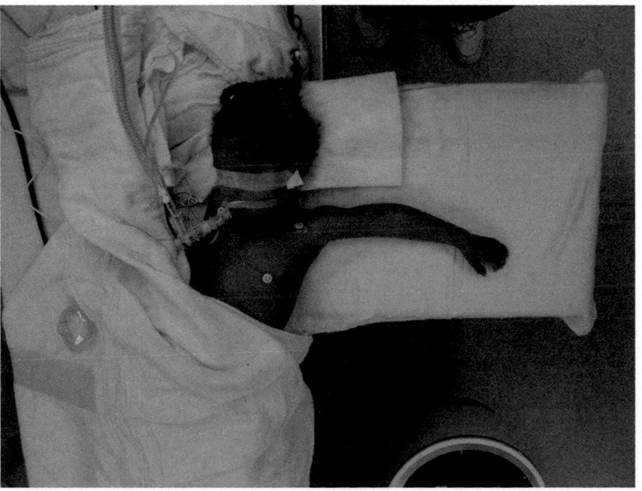

FIGURE 14-28 In small children, imaging of the elbow may be difficult if the arm is not long enough to reach the center of the fluoroscopy unit. By placing the child's head in the crack between the operating room table and the armboard, the elbow is more easily imaged, and the child's head is unlikely to be inadvertently pulled off the side of the bed during the procedure. (From Tolo VT, Skaggs DL, eds. Master Techniques in Orthopaedic Surgery: Pediatric Orthopaedics. Philadelphia: Lippincott, 2007: 1–15, with permission.)

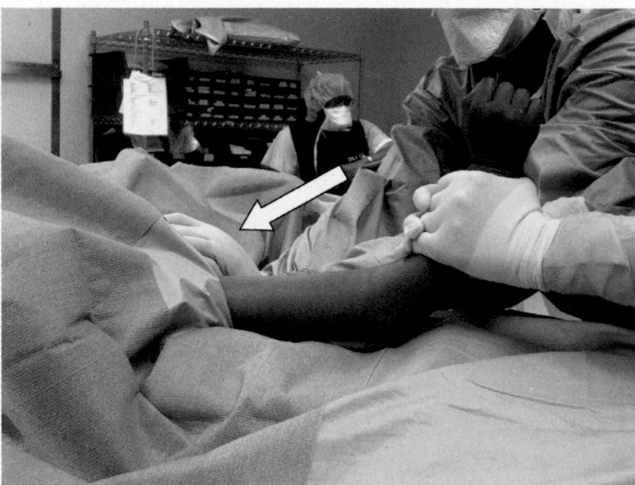

FIGURE 14-29 Reduction maneuver: traction with elbow flexed 20 to 30 degrees. Assistant provides countertraction against patient's axilla (*white arrow*) to allow for significant traction to be applied. (From Tolo VT, Skaggs DL, eds. Master Techniques in Orthopaedic Surgery: Pediatric Orthopaedics. Philadelphia: Lippincott, 2007:1–15, with permission.)

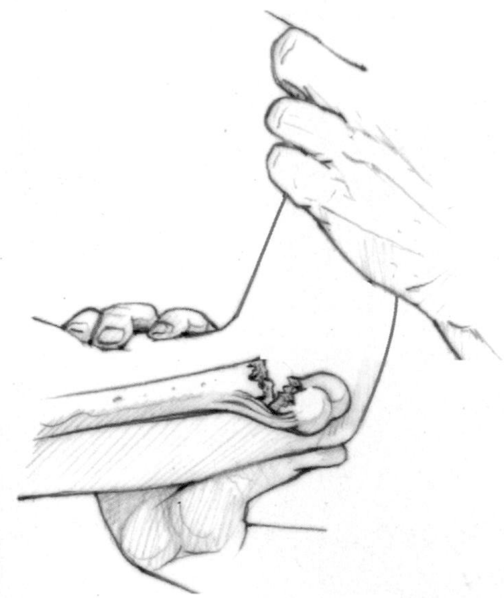

FIGURE 14-31 Reduction maneuver: flex elbow while pushing anteriorly on olecranon with the thumb(s). (From Tolo VT, Skaggs DL, eds. Master Techniques in Orthopaedic Surgery: Pediatric Orthopaedics. Philadelphia: Lippincott, 2007:1–15 with permission.)

If it the proximal fragment appears to have pierced the brachialis muscle, the "milking maneuver" is used: the biceps are forcibly "milked" in a proximal to distal direction past the proximal fragment, often culminating in a palpable release of the humerus posteriorly through the brachialis (Fig. 14-30).[156]

Next, varus and valgus angular alignment is corrected by movement of the forearm. Medial and lateral fracture translation is corrected with direct movement of the distal fragment by the surgeon's thumb(s) with image confirmation. The elbow is then slowly flexed while anterior pressure is applied to the olecranon with the surgeon's thumb(s) (Fig. 14-31).

After successful reduction, the child's elbow should sufficiently flex so that the fingers touch the shoulder. If not, the fracture likely is still not reduced and is in extension (Fig. 14-32).

If, during the reduction maneuver, the fracture does not stay reduced and a "rubbery" feeling is encountered instead of the desired "bone on bone" feeling, the median nerve or brachial artery may be trapped within the fracture site (see Fig. 14-18). If this occurs, open reduction generally is necessary to remove the neurovascular structures from the fracture site.

Although pronation can assist in reduction, this should not be done routinely. Most supracondylar humeral fractures are posterior-medially displaced with an intact medial periosteum, and pronation may aid reduction by placing tension on the medial periosteum and closing down the otherwise open lateral column (see Fig. 14-4). If the medial periosteum is torn, as it often is in a posterior-laterally displaced fracture, pronation can be counterproductive.

The reduction is checked by fluoroscopic images in AP, lateral, and oblique planes. Good reduction is indicated by (i) an anterior humeral line that intersects the capitellum, (see Fig. 14-14), (ii) a Baumann angle of more than 10 degrees (see Fig. 14-15), and (iii) intact medial and lateral columns on oblique views (Figs. 14-33 and 14-34).

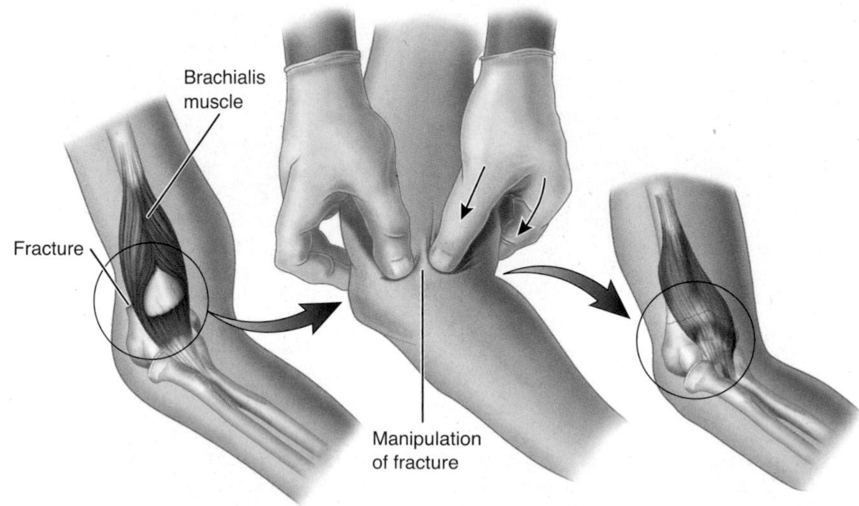

FIGURE 14-30 Brachialis muscle interposition is indicated on the left. The "milking maneuver" frees the brachialis muscle from its location in the fracture, allowing a closed reduction.

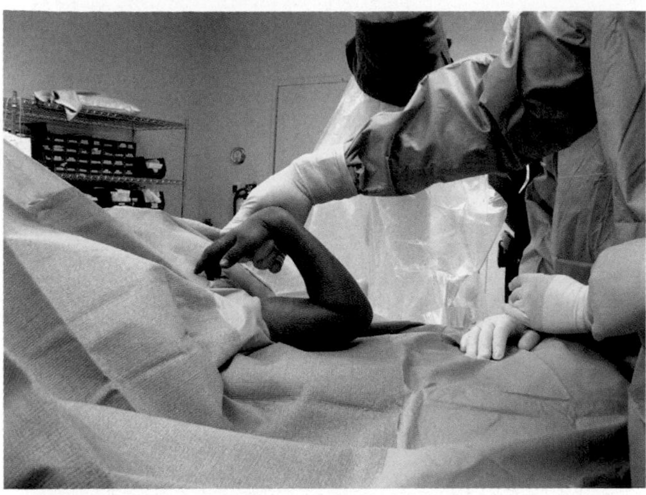

FIGURE 14-32 If fingers cannot touch shoulder, flexion deformity may not be reduced. (From Tolo VT, Skaggs DL, eds. Master Techniques in Orthopaedic Surgery: Pediatric Orthopaedics. Philadelphia: Lippincott, 2007, with permission.)

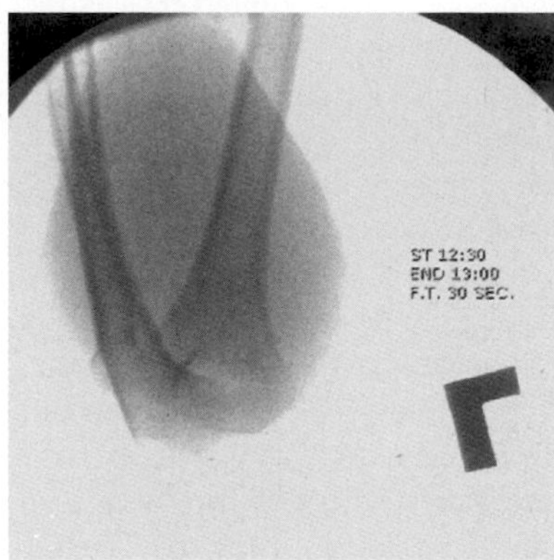

FIGURE 14-34 Demonstration of lateral column continuity. (From Tolo VT, Skaggs DL, eds. Master Techniques in Orthopaedic Surgery: Pediatric Orthopaedics. Philadelphia: Lippincott, 2007:1–15 with permission.)

If difficulty is encountered maintaining fracture reduction when eternally rotating the shoulder for a lateral view of the elbow, the C-arm can be moved instead of the patient's arm.[125]

We accept some translation of the distal fragment (up to perhaps 25%) and a moderate amount of persistent rotational malalignment, as long as the above criteria are met; the shoulder joint has so much rotation that a small amount of rotational malalignment is highly unlikely to cause a functional problem. Once reduction is satisfactory, the elbow is taped in the reduced position of elbow hyperflexion with elastic tape to prevent loss of reduction during pinning (Fig. 14-35).

The elbow is positioned on a folded towel, and the lateral humeral condyle is palpated. Most commonly, 0.062-inch smooth K-wires are used (Zimmer, Warsaw, IN), although smaller or larger sizes may be needed if the child is extremely small or large.

The aim of pin placement is to maximally separate the pins at the fracture site to engage both the medial and lateral columns (see Fig. 14-22). Whether the pins are divergent or parallel and which pin is placed first is of little importance. Care must be taken to ensure that there is sufficient bone engaged in the proximal and distal fragments. It is acceptable to cross the olecranon fossa, which adds two more cortices, to improve fixation, but this means that the elbow cannot be fully extend until the pins are removed. In the sagittal plane, to engage the most bone with the wire in the distal fragment, the wire can be passed through the capitellum. Because the reduced capitellum lies slightly anterior to the plane of the fracture, the pin can be started a bit anterior to the plane of the fracture and angulated about 10 to 15 degrees posteriorly to maximize osseous purchase. A key element to ensure a correctly placed pin is to feel the pin go through the proximal cortex. If this is not clearly appreciated,

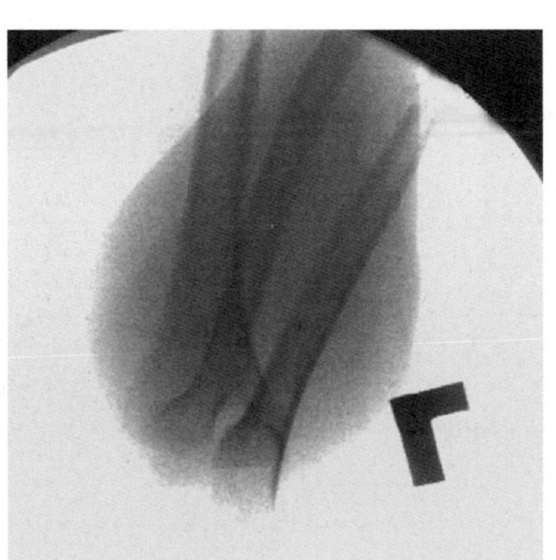

FIGURE 14-33 Oblique fluoroscopic view of the elbow demonstrating continuity of the medial column following adequate fracture reduction. (From Tolo VT, Skaggs DL, eds. Master Techniques in Orthopaedic Surgery: Pediatric Orthopaedics. Philadelphia: Lippincott, 2007:1–15, with permission.)

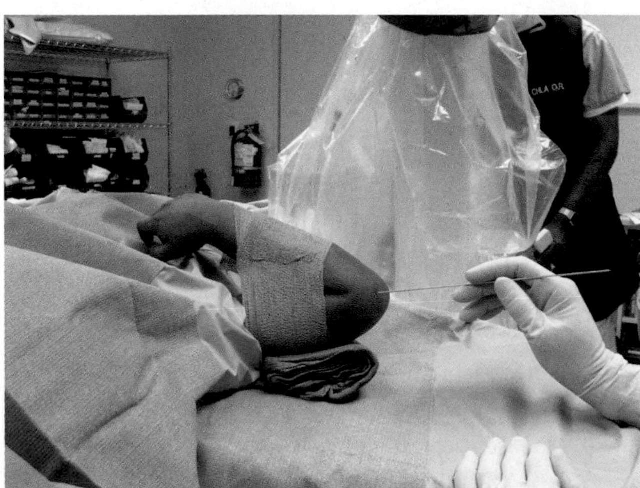

FIGURE 14-35 Fracture redcution is maintained by taping elbow in hyperflexed position. The wire may be pushed through the skin and into the cartilage, using the cartilage of the distal lateral condyle as a pincushion that will hold the K-wire in place while carefully examining the AP and lateral images. (Reproduced with permission of Children's Orthopaedic Center, Los Angeles, CA.)

careful fluoroscopic imaging often reveals that the pin did not engage the proximal fragment. As a general rule, we recommend two pins for type II fractures and three pins for type III fractures. Even though two properly placed pins probably are sufficient, placing three pins increases the odds of actually having two in proper position.

The K-wire is placed against the lateral condyle without piercing the skin, and the position is checked with an AP fluoroscopic image to assess the starting point. The K-wire is held free in the surgeon's hand at this point, not in the drill, to allow maximal control. If the starting point and trajectory are correct, the wire can be pushed through the skin and into the cartilage, using the cartilage of the distal lateral condyle as a "pincushion" (see Fig. 14-35) that will hold the K-wire in place while the AP and lateral images are carefully examined. If imaging verifies correct pin placement, then the pin is advanced with a wire driver. Precise pin placement is an important part of the procedure that should not be rushed. We believe incorrect pin placement is the cause of loss of reduction in most fractures. Whether it is important if the pins are divergent or parallel is debatable, but it is clearly important that the pins are well separated at the fracture site.

The reduction is again checked with lateral (Fig. 14-36), oblique (Fig. 14-37), and AP fluoroscopy views (Fig. 14-38). Stress should be applied in varus and valgus under fluoroscopy to ensure fracture stability, and lateral views should be obtained with the elbow flexed and extended to assess movement of the capitellum relative to the anterior humeral line. It is much better to identify any instability in the operating room rather than a week later. If there is instability, we add another lateral-entry pin.

We save the images in which the reduction looks the "worst," particularly if some translational or rotational malreduction is accepted, in order to have them for comparison during postoperative visits to determine if movement of the

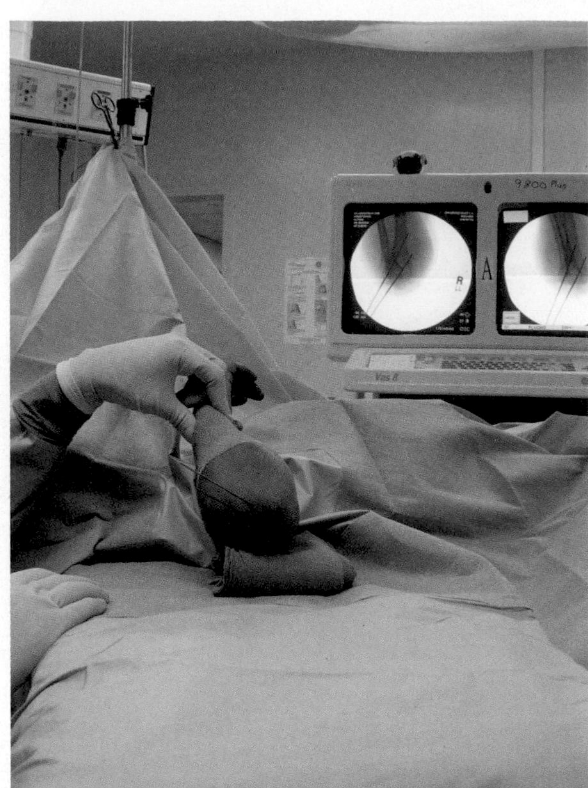

FIGURE 14-37 Both oblique views are checked to assess reduction of medial and lateral columns. (From Tolo VT, Skaggs DL, eds. Master Techniques in Orthopaedic Surgery: Pediatric Orthopaedics. Philadelphia: Lippincott, 2007:1–15, with permission.)

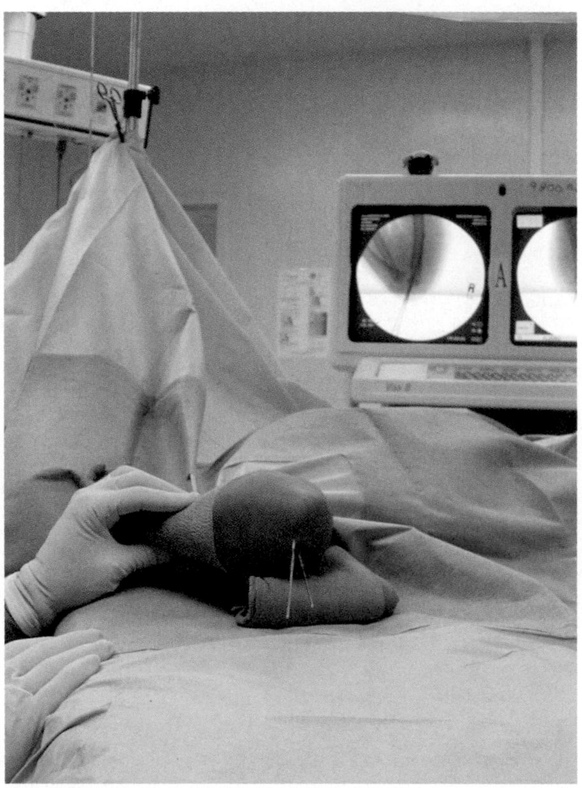

FIGURE 14-36 Assessment of sagittal alignment with lateral view. (From Tolo VT, Skaggs DL, eds. Master Techniques in Orthopaedic Surgery: Pediatric Orthopaedics. Philadelphia: Lippincott, 2007:1–15, with permission.)

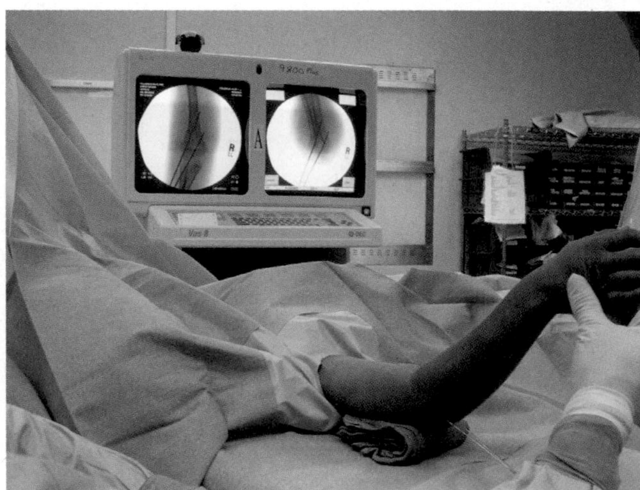

FIGURE 14-38 If the lateral and oblique views show good reduction, the tape is removed and reduction and pin placement are checked, in the AP view with elbow in relative elbow extension. (From Tolo VT, Skaggs DL, eds. Master Techniques in Orthopaedic Surgery: Pediatric Orthopaedics. Philadelphia: Lippincott, 2007:1–15, with permission.)

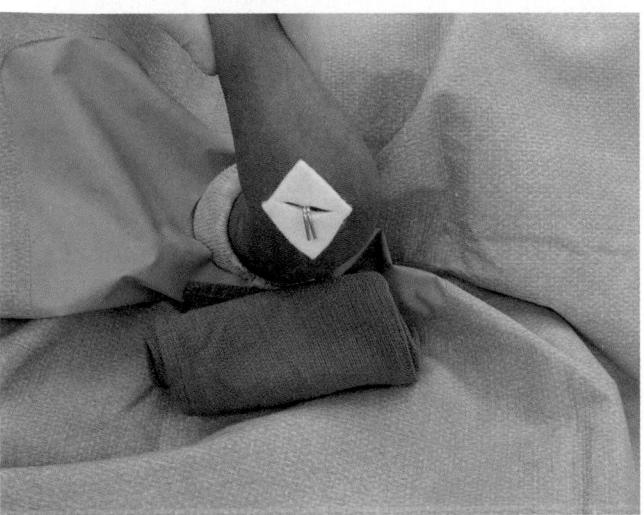

FIGURE 14-39 Skin is protected from pins with felt squares. (From Tolo VT, Skaggs DL, eds. Master Techniques in Orthopaedic Surgery: Pediatric Orthopaedics. Philadelphia: Lippincott, 2007:1–15, with permission.)

fracture has occurred. Vascular status is assessed, and the wires are bent and cut. The wires are left at least 1 to 2 cm off the skin to prevent migration of the wires under the skin. A sterile felt square with a slit cut into it is then placed around the wires to protect the skin (Fig. 14-39).

The two authors of this chapter have different casting techniques. One (David L. Skaggs) applies foam to the arm on the anterior and posterior aspects of the elbow (Fig. 14-40) before the cast is applied with the elbow flexed 45 to 70 degrees of elbow flexion, as flexion to 90 degrees may needlessly increase the risk of compartment syndrome (Fig. 14-41). The other (John M. Flynn) applies a well-padded cast that has absolutely no tightness to it, with a supracondylar mold to prevent arm rotation in the cast, with the elbow flexed about 60 or 70 degrees. It is important to remember that the pins, not the cast, are holding the fracture reduction.

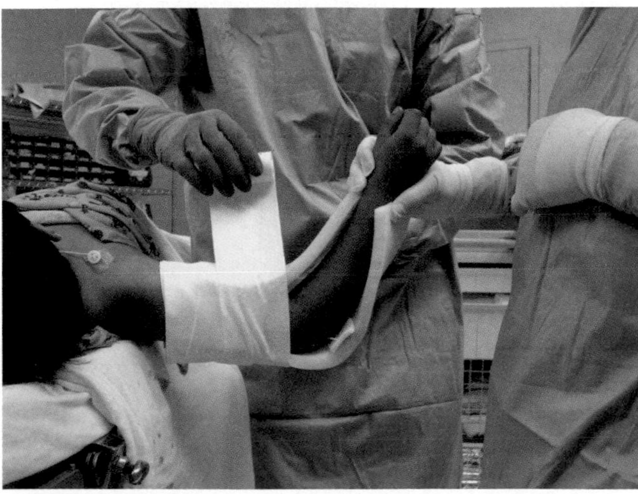

FIGURE 14-40 Sterile foam is placed directly on skin. If there is any circumferential dressing placed under the foam, it may be restricting. (From Tolo VT, Skaggs DL, eds. Master Techniques in Orthopaedic Surgery: Pediatric Orthopaedics. Philadelphia: Lippincott, 2007, with permission.)

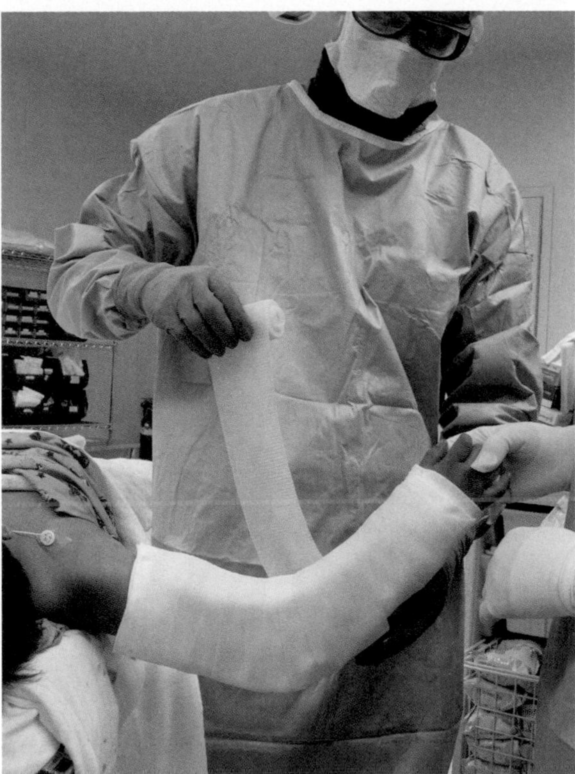

FIGURE 14-41 Cast with elbow flexion no more than 70 degrees and less flexion for very swollen elbows. (From Tolo VT, Skaggs DL, eds. Master Techniques in Orthopaedic Surgery: Pediatric Orthopaedics. Philadelphia: Lippincott, 2007:1–15, with permission.)

We use fiberglass casting material for its strength, weight, and radiolucency and believe that, when properly applied, fiberglass does not lead to a tight cast.

If there is any question of perfusion after fracture reduction in the operating room, the surgical preparation (betadine) should be removed to evaluate the skin color. In addition, Doppler evaluation can be used to assess pulse. If perfusion diminishes after reduction, the artery or adjacent tissue must be assumed to be trapped in the fracture site, and the pins should be immediately removed to allow the fracture to return to its unreduced position. If there is no pulse postoperatively in an arm that had no pulse preoperatively, but the hand is warm and well-perfused, we prefer to observe the child in the hospital for 48 hours with the arm mildly elevated. The rich collateral circulation about the elbow generally is sufficient.

Postoperative care: Patients with minimal swelling who are believed to be at little risk for compartment syndrome are discharged to home with appropriate postoperative instructions, but otherwise children generally are admitted overnight for elevation and observation. The patient customarily returns 5 to 7 days postoperatively, at which time AP and lateral radiographss are obtained. This allows rereduction if reduction has been lost; however, this is rare and this return visit probably is not necessary for most children. The cast generally is removed 3 weeks postoperatively, at which time radiographs are obtained out of the cast and the pins are removed. Range-of-motion exercises targeting gentle flexion and extension are taught to the family and are started a few days after cast removal. The child returns 6 weeks after surgery for a range-of-motion check, with no radiographs at that time.

Fractures with Medial Comminution or Multidirectional Instability

For fractures with medial comminution, significant valgus stress is applied with the elbow fully extended to reduce the varus deformity, and this is confirmed with imaging. Then standard reduction and pinning techniques are used. For type IV fractures, we use the method described by Leitch et al.[125] Neither of the authors has ever used traction or seen traction used in their centers over the last 10 years.

Pearls and Pitfalls

- Aim to separate the pins as far as possible at the fracture site—this is more important than whether the pins are divergent or parallel.
- To optimize pin placement, think of the cartilaginous distal humerus as a pincushion. With the K-wires in your fingers (not the drill) push them into the cartilage in the exact location and trajectory you want. Verify with imaging and then advance the pin with a drill.
- In general, plan on a minimum of two pins for type II fractures and three pins for type III fractures.
- If the first pin is in between the target for two pins, just leave it and place a pin on either side of it for a total of three pins.
- A small amount of translation or axial rotational malalignment can be accepted rather than doing an open reduction, but accept very little frontal plane or sagittal angular malalignment.
- After reduction and fixation, stress the fracture under live imaging to the point where there is confidence it will not fall apart postoperatively.
- Cast the elbow in significantly less than 90 degrees of flexion to avoid compartment syndrome; the pins are holding the reduction, not the cast.
- If placing a medial pin, extend the elbow when placing the pin to keep the ulnar nerve posterior and out of harm's way.

Open Reduction and Pinning

We prefer a transverse anterior incision through the antecubital fossa about 4 to 5 cm long, which allows access to the neurovascular structures and produces a better cosmetic result than a lateral or medial incision (Fig.14-42). If more

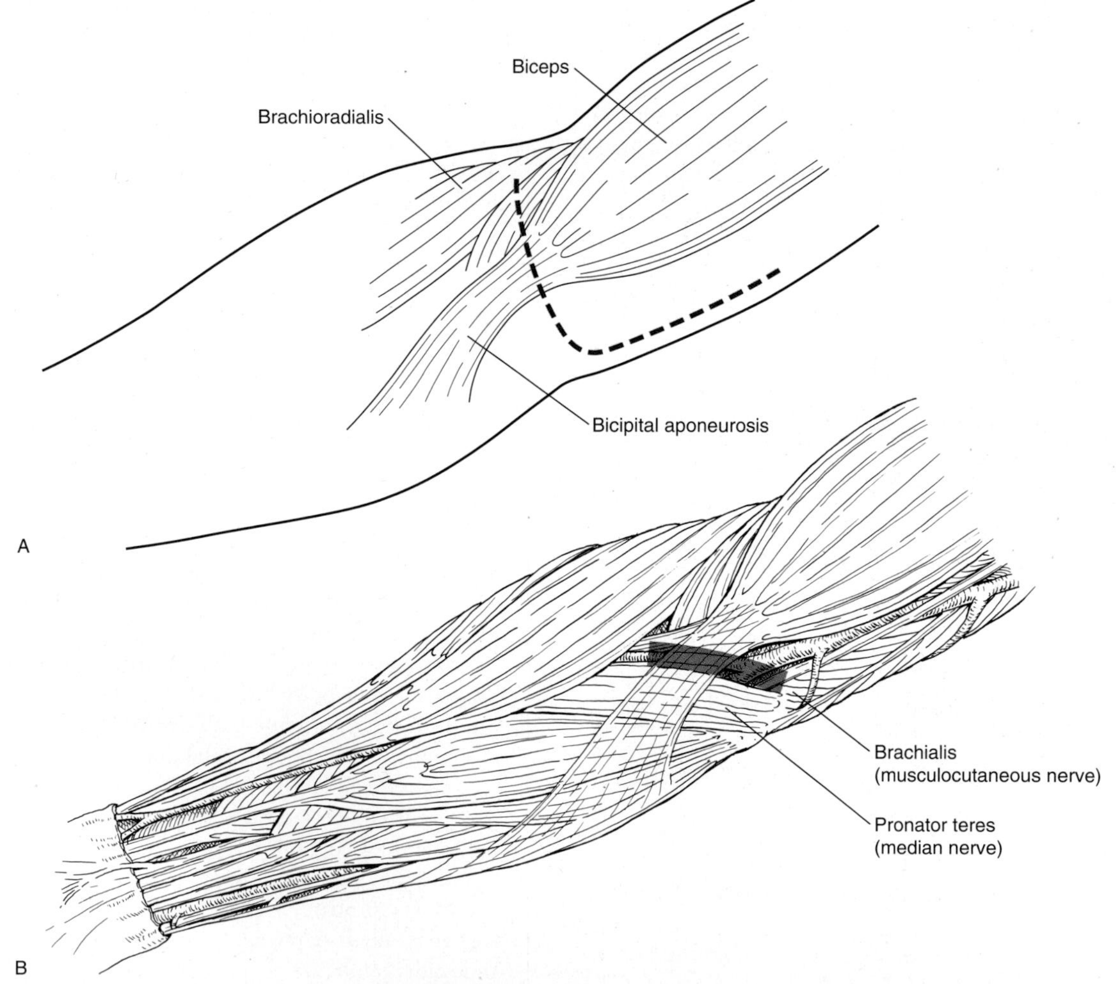

FIGURE 14-42 Anterior approach for open reduction and brachial artery and median nerve exploration. Most often, just the transverse part of the incision is needed for fracture reduction alone. *(continues)*

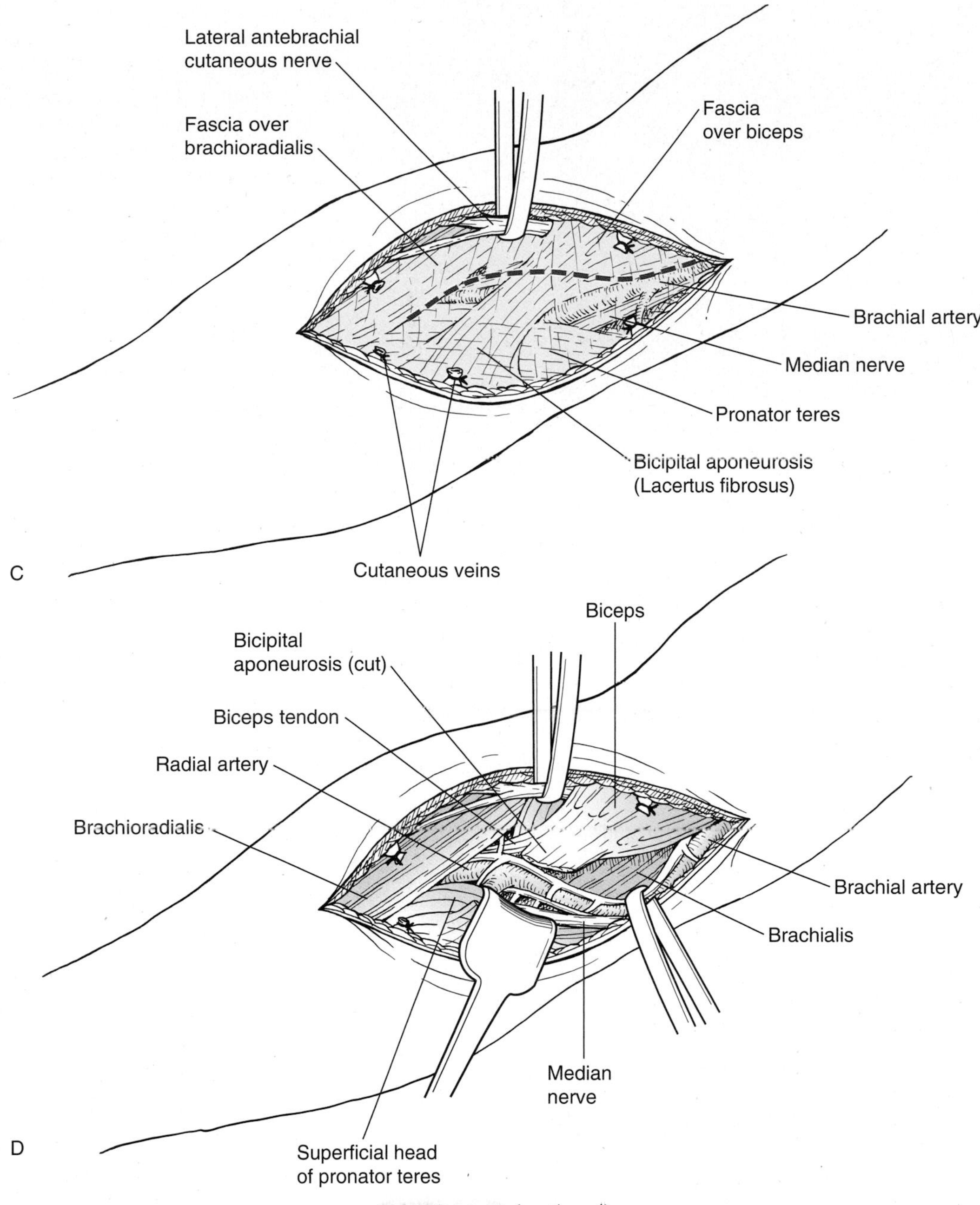

FIGURE 14-42 *(continued)*.

visualization is needed, this incision can be extended medially or laterally based on displacement. Care must be taken during dissection, because the neurovascular bundle may be immediately superficial as it is pushed against the skin by the proximal fragment (Fig. 14-43). The first major structure to be incised is the bicipital aponeurosis (lacertus fibrosus), which runs just superficial to the median nerve and brachial artery; from the biceps tendon it runs medially to the superficial flexors of the forearm. Just medial to the biceps tendon is the brachial artery, with the median nerve just medial to the artery. If the artery cannot be located in a patient with a pulseless, poorly perfused hand, the lacerated ends of the artery may have retracted (see Fig. 14-43).

Once the brachial artery and median nerve are identified, they should be retracted out of the fracture site. Identifying the distal fragment can be the most challenging aspect of the procedure. It is posterior and lateral and the periosteum is folded over its surface. Reduction is obtained by reaching into the fracture site with a hemostat and grasping the cut edge of the periosteum. This cut edge is extended with scissors to increase the size of the buttonhole and help free up the distal fragment. The fragment is then brought anteriorly and reduced. Alternatively, the surgeon can hold his thumb on the proximal fragment and push downwards while an assistant applies traction to the forearm with the elbow flexed 90 degrees. A periosteal elevator can be used as a lever to assist the reduction. Because much of the periosteum is torn, fracture reduction may be less stable after open reduction

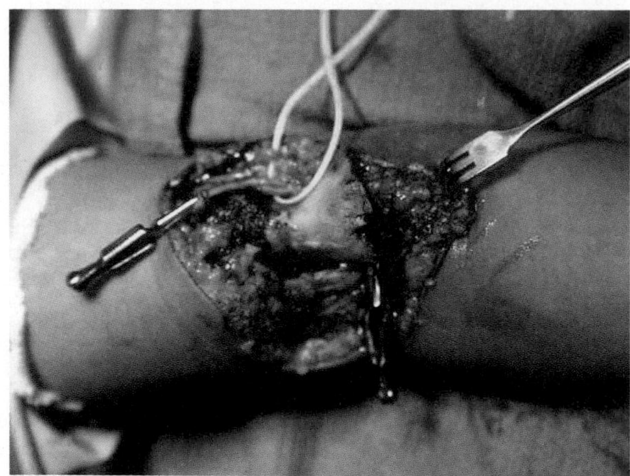

FIGURE 14-43 The brachial artery was lacerated by the proximal fragment. Bulldogs have been placed on each end of the artery to control bleeding, and the median nerve is within the vessel loop. (Reproduced with permission from Children's Orthopaedic Center, Los Angeles, CA.)

than it is after closed reduction. Once a reduction has been obtained, it must be pinned to maintain it. This is accomplished in the same manner as percutaneous pinning after closed reduction.

Complications

Vascular Injury

Approximately 10% to 20% of patients with type III supracondylar fractures present with an absent pulse.[60,157,175,177] The presence of a pulse and perfusion of the hand should be documented. Perfusion is estimated by color, warmth, and capillary refill. Capillary refill alone can be deceiving; after wrapping a rubber band around a finger, there is instant venous capillary refill, so this must be differentiated from arterial capillary refill.

A relatively recent study by Choi et al.[44] demonstrated which patients are likely to need arterial repair or to develop a compartment syndrome based on preoperative presentation. Of 1255 patients with operatively treated supracondylar humeral fractures, 33 presented with absent distal pulses. The key difference in the outcome of these patients was whether the hand was well-perfused at time of presentation. Of the 24 patients whose hands were well-perfused (but pulseless) at presentation, none required vascular repair or developed a compartment syndrome, and fracture reduction alone was effective treatment. Of the 9 patients who presented with poor distal perfusion, 4 required vascular repair, and compartment syndrome developed in 2 during the postoperative period. In 5 of these 9 patients, fracture reduction alone was definitive treatment.

Absence of the radial pulse is not an emergency because collateral circulation may keep the limb well-perfused, but timely reduction with pinning in the operating room is preferable.[172] A pulseless arm with signs of poor perfusion is an emergency. A patient with a severely displaced supracondylar fracture and compromised vascularity to the limb should have a splint applied with the elbow in approximately 20 to 40 degrees of flexion rather than extremes of flexion or extension which may compromise bloodflow.[105]

Because fracture reduction usually restores the pulse, angiographic studies should not delay fracture reduction.[44] Several reports have shown angiography to be an unnecessary test that has no bearing on treatment.[45,157,175,177] In a series of 143 type III supracondylar fractures, 17 of which had vascular compromise,[177] all had reduction and percutaneous pinning without preoperative angiogram. In 3 of the 17 patients, bloodflow to the hand was not restored after reduction and open exploration was required; in the other 14, bloodflow to the hand was restored without complications. The authors concluded that prereduction angiography would have added nothing to the management of these injuries. Another study used angiogram in 4 of 17 patients with supracondylar humeral fractures and dysvascular extremities and found that the angiogram did not alter the course of management in any.[45] Choi et al.[44] reported that of 25 patients presenting with a pulseless but well-perfused hand, all did well clinically without arterial repair—11 (52%) had a palpable pulse following surgery and 10 (48%) remained pulseless but well-perfused.

Open reduction through an anterior approach is indicated if anatomic reduction cannot be obtained by closed reduction in a patient with an absent pulse; this allows evaluation of all vital structures at risk for incarceration between the fracture fragments.[13,63] Once the artery is freed from the fracture, arterial spasm may be relieved by the application of lidocaine, warming, and 10 to 15 minutes of observation. If the pulse does not return after fracture reduction and the hand remains poorly perfused, vascular reconstruction (usually by a vascular surgeon) is indicated.

After closed reduction and stabilization, the pulse and perfusion of the hand should be evaluated. Most extension-type supracondylar fractures are reduced and pinned with the elbow in hyperflexion. With more than 120 degrees of elbow flexion, the radial pulse generally is lost, even in patients with an initially intact pulse. After pinning, when the arm is extended, the pulse frequently does not return immediately. This is presumably secondary to arterial spasm, aggravated by swelling about the artery and decreased peripheral perfusion in the anesthetized, somewhat cool intraoperative patient. Because of this phenomenon, 10 to 15 minutes should be allowed for recovery of perfusion in the operating room before any decision is made regarding the need for exploring the brachial artery and restoring flow to the distal portion of the extremity. Because most patients without a palpable pulse maintain adequate distal perfusion, the absence of a palpable pulse alone is not an indication for exploring the brachial artery.

If the pulse does not return, but the hand is well-perfused, the treatment is controversial. We prefer to admit the child to the hospital for gentle elevation and observation for at least 48 hours. Loss of perfusion or impending compartment syndrome can occur during this time and may require immediate treatment. Gillingham and Rang[76] recommended observing patients with absent pulses, because most pulses returned within 10 days. Alternatively, vascular reconstruction can be performed. However, Sabharwal et al.[172] showed that early repair of the brachial artery has a high rate of symptomatic reocclusion and residual stenosis and recommended a period of close observation with frequent neurovascular checks before more invasive correction of this problem is contemplated. Immediate rereduction, usually open reduction, is indicated in a patient in whom a pulse was present preoperatively but is absent postoperatively, because the artery or adjacent tissue is presumed to be entrapped in the fracture site.

Cold intolerance has been considered a possible long-term sequel in children without palpable distal pulses, though there is little literature on this subject. There is a single case report of a child with minor cold intolerance and decreased systolic arterial forearm blood pressure more than 1 year after a supracondyalr fracture with rupture of the median nerve and ligation of the brachial artery.[130]

The decision to explore a brachial artery should be based on objective criteria. Traditionally, the decision has been based only on whether the hand was warm and pink. The following case indicates the difficulty with these criteria. A 2-year-old girl was injured in a fall from a couch (Fig. 14-44). A type III supracondylar fracture and a pale, cool hand were documented on presentation to a local emergency department. Two hours later, the patient was brought to the operating room, where a cool, pale hand with poor capillary refill and an absent pulse

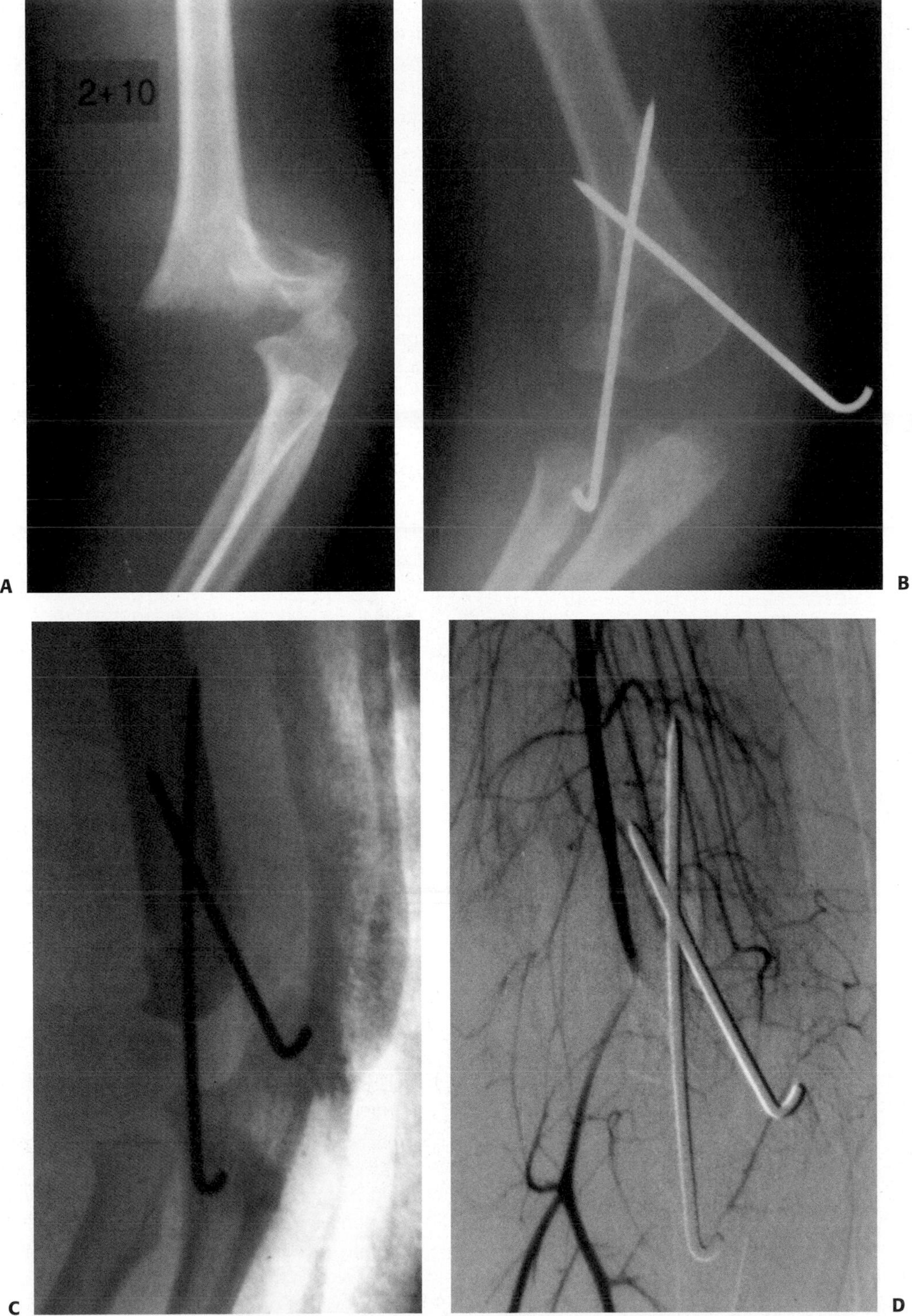

FIGURE 14-44 A. This 2-year-old patient sustained a type III supracondylar fracture with vascular compromise. **B.** Pinning was performed in a nearly anatomic position. **C,D.** Six hours postoperatively, increasing pain, a pale hand, and evolving compartment syndrome prompted arteriography, showing brachial artery occlusion.

was noted. Immediate closed reduction and pinning was done with nearly anatomic reduction. The hand felt warmer, and capillary refill was present. The pulse was not palpable, but because of the improved state of the patient's hand, the brachial artery was was not explored. During the next 4 hours, the patient was observed closely with increasing fussiness, a nonpalpable pulse, and slow capillary refill. An arteriogram showed brachial artery obstruction. Compartment pressures were measured, and increased pressure was noted in the volar compartment. A decision was made to return to the operating room for exploration, repair of the brachial artery, and forearm fasciotomy. Although the outcome in this case was satisfactory with no long-term sequelae other than scarring, the question is whether or not the low perfusion with subsequent ischemia and compartment syndrome could have been identified at the time of the closed reduction and immediate vascular repair done. What would have happened if no repair had been done in this case? Had a repair been done immediately, could the development of a compartment syndrome have been averted? What is the relationship between compartment syndrome and perfusion? Is there a more objective way to determine when flow is insufficient?

Several investigators have attempted to provide criteria for vascular repair in addition to warmth and color in the patient with absence of a palpable pulse.[175,177] In the absence of a palpable pulse, a Doppler device can be used to measure lower flow states with small-pulse amplitude. Shaw[177] found no false-positive explorations when patients with pulses that could not be palpated but were identified on Doppler evaluation were observed, and exploration was done in those in whom no pulse was found with either palpation or Doppler. The brachial artery was either transected or entrapped in all patients with surgical exploration, and none with "spasm" underwent surgery. Using the same criteria, Schoenecker et al.[175] identified 6 patients for exploration. Three had a damaged or transacted brachial artery with no flow, and 3 had an artery kinked or trapped in the fracture. At follow-up, all patients with vascular repair had a radial pulse. One patient with more than 24 hours of vascular insufficiency had an unsatisfactory outcome. Copley et al.[45] reported that of 17 patients with type III supracondylar fractures and no palpable pulse at presentation, 14 recovered pulse after reduction. The three explorations identified significant vascular injury, and the brachial artery was repaired. Most significant in their series was the finding of increasing vascular insufficiency during postoperative observation in some patients. If the hand is well-perfused despite not having a palpable pulse, close follow-up in the hospital is mandatory. The patient should be observed for increasing narcotic requirements, increasing pain, and decreased passive finger motion. A very low threshold for returning to the operating room for exploration and fasciotomy must be maintained rather than assuming that perfusion from collaterals is sufficient.

Choi et al.[44] reported that of eight patients presenting with a pulseless and poorly perfused hand, two developed compartment syndrome after operative reduction of the fracture. Perhaps the threshold for compartment release at the time of the initial surgery should be lower in this subset of patients presenting with a pulseless and poorly perfused hand.

Some surgeons recommend pulse oximetry[108,166] for evaluating postreduction circulation. We have found pulse oximetry useful for evaluating patients after vascular repair or pinning but not for intraoperative decision making.

Exploration of the Brachial Artery. Obliteration of the intact preoperative radial pulse after closed reduction and pinning is a strong indication for brachial artery exploration only when accompanied by evidence of impaired circulation to the hand. After 10 to 15 minutes is allowed for resolution of arterial spasm as a cause for loss of pulse, the brachial artery should be explored if the hand is not warm and pink. Either direct arterial entrapment at the fracture or arterial compression by a fascial band pulling across the artery may cause loss of pulse after fracture reduction. As described earlier, the other indication for brachial artery exploration is persistent vascular insufficiency after reduction and pinning.

The orthopaedic surgeon and vascular surgeon must work together to manage this problem emergently. Often, the release of a fascial band or an adventitial tether resolves the problem of obstructed flow. This is a simple procedure done at the time of exploration of the antecubital fossa and identification of the brachial artery. In some patients, however, a formal vascular repair and vein graft are required. The brachial artery should be approached through a transverse incision across the antecubital fossa, with a medial extension turning proximally at about the level of the medial epicondyle as described for open reduction (see Fig. 14-42). After reduction and pinning, care must be taken because the neurovascular bundle may be difficult to identify when it is surrounded by hematoma, and it may lie in a very superficial position. At the level of the fracture, the artery may seem to disappear into the fracture site, covered with shredded brachialis muscle. This occurs when the artery is tethered by a fascial band or arterial adventitia attached to the proximal metaphyseal spike pulling the artery in the fracture site. Dissection should occur proximally to distally, along the brachial artery, identifying both the artery and the median nerve. Arterial injury generally is at the level of the supratrochlear artery (see Fig. 14-6), which provides a tether, making the artery vulnerable at this location. Arterial transection or direct arterial injury can be identified at this level (see Fig. 14-43). Entrapment of the neurovascular bundle in the fracture is best identified by proximal to distal dissection.

The vascular surgeon generally makes the decision to repair a damaged artery or use a vein graft. If arterial spasm is the cause of inadequate flow and collateral flow is not sufficient to maintain the hand, methods to relieve the spasm can be tried. Both stellate ganglion block and application of papaverine or local anesthetic to the artery have been found to be beneficial in this situation. If these techniques do not relieve the spasm and if collateral flow is insufficient, the injured portion of the vessel is excised and a vein graft is inserted. When flow is restored, the wound is closed, and a splint is applied with the elbow flexed much less than 90 degrees and the forearm in neutral pronation and supination. Postoperative monitoring should include temperature, pulse oximetry, and frequent examinations for signs of compartment syndrome or ischemia. Although injecting urokinase has been suggested to increase flow,[34] we have had no experience with this technique.

Sabharwal et al.[172] documented that 3.2% of patients with type III supracondylar fractures have an absent pulse at presentation, for which they recommended noninvasive monitoring. MR angiography and color-flow duplex Doppler were helpful in deciding whether or not to explore the brachial artery. Although repair is technically feasible, Sabharwal et al.[172] cautioned that high rates of reocclusion and residual stenosis argued against early revascularization if not absolutely necessary. Early reocclusion, however, was not reported by Schoenecker et al.[175] or Shaw et al.[177]

The necessity of early treatment of vascular compromise was emphasized by Ottolenghi[154] who found no Volkmann ischemic contractures[143] in patients in whom vascular compromise was treated within 12 hours. The frequency of this complication increased steadily with repair between 12 and 24 hours; after 24 hours of delay in treatment, outcomes were uniformly poor. This series presents convincing evidence that prompt exploration of arterial insufficiency markedly decreases the incidence of Volkmann ischemic contracture. Note that brachial artery obstruction and compartment syndrome, although related, are not equivalent, and both are fortunately rare problems. Ischemia will lead to a compartment syndrome, but the presence of a radial pulse does not preclude it.

Compartment Syndrome

Compartment syndrome is estimated to occur in 0.1% to 0.3% of patients with supracondylar fractures.[19] Blakemore et al.[25] reported a 9% prevalence (3 of 33) of forearm compartment syndrome in patients with a supracondylar fracture and an ipsilateral radial fracture. In acute compartment syndrome,[91,143] increased pressure in a closed fascial space causes muscle ischemia. With untreated ischemia, muscle edema increases, further increasing pressure, decreasing flow, and leading to muscle necrosis, fibrosis, and death of involved muscles. A compartment syndrome of the forearm may occur with or without brachial artery injury and in the presence or absence of a radial pulse. The diagnosis of a compartment syndrome is based on resistance to passive finger movement and dramatically increasing pain after fracture. The classic five "Ps" for the diagnosis of compartment syndrome—pain, pallor, pulselessness, paresthesias, and paralysis—are poor criteria for the early detection of compartment syndrome. Special attention must be paid to supracondylar fractures with median nerve injuries because the patient will not feel pain in the volar compartment.[143]

Mubarak and Carroll[143] recommended forearm fasciotomy if clinical signs of compartment syndrome are present or if intracompartmental pressure is greater than 30 mm Hg. Heppenstall et al.[89] suggested that a difference of 30 mm Hg between diastolic blood pressure and compartment pressure should be the threshold for release. If pain is increasing and finger extension is decreasing, fasciotomy is clearly indicated. Measuring compartment pressures in a terrified, crying child is difficult, and if clinical signs of compartment syndrome are present, a trip to the operating room for evaluation and possible fasciotomy is often a better course of action than pressure measurement and observation.

Clinical conditions that contribute to the development of compartment syndrome are direct muscle trauma at the time of injury, swelling with intracompartmental fractures (associated forearm fracture), decreased arterial inflow, restricted venous outflow, and elbow position. If the mechanism of injury is high-energy, as evidenced by crushing or associated fractures, there is an increased risk for compartment syndrome. An associated forearm fracture or forearm crush injury significantly increases the likelihood of compartment syndrome.[25] An arterial injury in association with multiple injuries or crush injury further diminishes blood flow to the forearm musculature and increases the probability of a compartment syndrome. Interestingly, Battaglia et al.[19] documented the relationship between increasing elbow flexion above 90 degrees and increasing volar compartment pressure. In a patient with an evolving postoperative compartment syndrome, not only should the dressings be loosened, but the elbow should be extended to a position well below 90 degrees.

In a multicenter review, Ramachandran et al.[162] identified 11 children with supracondylar fractures who developed compartment syndrome despite presenting with closed, low-energy injuries and no associated fractures or vascular compromise. This series is disturbing because it demonstrates that compartment syndrome still occurs with modern treatment, even in children who may be thought to be at low risk. Ramachandran et al.[162] found that in 10 of 11 patients' charts, excessive swelling was noted at time of presentation, and the one child without severe swelling had arterial entrapment after reduction, with subsequent compartment syndrome requiring fasciotomy 25 hours later. The 10 children with severe elbow swelling documented at presentation had a mean delay of 22 hours before surgery. This study suggests that excessive swelling combined with delay in treatment is a risk factor for the development of compartment syndrome.

Even if a distal pulse is found by palpation or Doppler examination, an evolving compartment syndrome may be present.[161] Increased swelling over the compartment, increased pain, and decreased finger mobility are cardinal signs of an evolving compartment syndrome. Evaluation of possible compartment syndrome cannot be based on the presence or absence of a radial pulse alone. If a compartment syndrome does appear to be evolving, initial management includes removing all circumferential dressings. The volar compartment should be palpated, and the elbow should be extended. We believe that the fracture should be immediately stabilized with K-wires to allow proper management of the soft tissues.

Another factor that contributes to the development of compartment syndrome is warm ischemic time after injury. When bloodflow is compromised and the hand is pale with no arterial flow, muscle ischemia is possible, depending on the time of oxygen deprivation. After fracture reduction and flow restoration, the warm ischemic time should be noted. If this time is more than 6 hours, compartment syndrome secondary to ischemic muscle injury is likely. Prophylactic volar compartment fasciotomy can be done at the time of arterial reconstruction. The exact indication for prophylactic fasciotomy in the absence of an operative revascularization is uncertain. Even when the diagnosis is delayed or the if compartment syndrome is chronic, fasciotomy has been shown to be of some value.

Compartment syndrome is a true surgical emergency. A recent systematic review of 55 reports of 1920 fasciatomies of the upper and lower extremities found that, compared with fasciotomy before 6 hours, delayed fasciotomy beyond 12 hours was associated with a lower rate of acceptable outcome (15% for more than 12 hours versus 88% for <6 hours), a higher rate of amputation (14% versus 3.2%), and death (4.3% versus 2.0%).[87]

Technique for Volar Fasciotomy. The volar compartment of the forearm can be approached through the classic Henry ap-

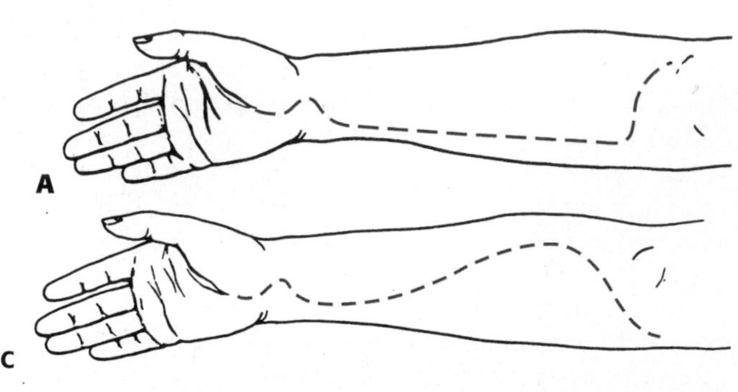

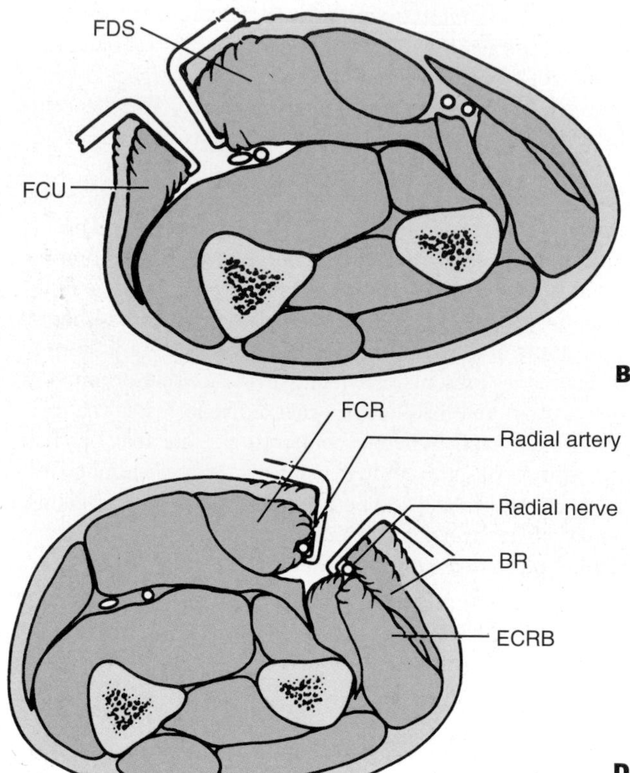

FIGURE 14-45 Surgical approach for forearm fasciotomy. **A.** Ulnar approach, skin incision. **B.** Ulnar approach, intermuscular interval. (FDS, flexor digitorum sublimis; FCU, flexor carpi ulnaris.) **C.** Henry approach, skin incision. **D.** Henry approach. (BR, brachioradialis; ECRB, extensor carpi radialis brevis; FCR, flexor carpi radialis interval.) (From Willis RB, Rorabeck CH. Treatment of compartment syndrome in children. Orthop Clin N Am 1990;21:407–408, with permission.)

proach or an ulnar approach (Fig. 14-45). If the compartment syndrome is associated with brachial artery and median nerve injuries, we generally use the Henry approach as an extension of the vascular repair. The advantage of the ulnar approach, as described by Willis and Rorabeck,[204] is that it produces a more cosmetically pleasing scar. A volar fasciotomy involves opening the volar compartment from the carpal tunnel distally to the lacertus fibrosa and antecubital fascia proximally. The fascia over the deep flexors is opened, as is the superficial fascia, to decompress the deep volar compartment of the forearm. Failure to release the deep volar fascia may cause contracture of the deep finger flexors. Generally, only the volar compartment is released, with an associated decrease in pressure in the dorsal or extensor compartment. If the volar Henry approach is used, the interval between the brachioradialis and the flexor carpi radialis is developed and the radial artery is retracted ulnarward. The deep volar compartment is exposed. The flexor digitorum profundus and flexor pollicis longus are exposed along with the pronator teres proximally and the pronator quadratus distally.

If the ulnar approach is used, as described by Willis and Rorabeck,[204] the release is done from the carpal canal to the antecubital fossa, as with the Henry approach. The skin incision begins above the elbow crease, medial to the biceps tendon (see Fig. 14-45); it crosses the elbow crease and extends distally along the ulnar border to the volar wrist, where it courses radially across the carpal canal. The fascia over the flexor carpi ulnaris is incised, and the interval between the flexor carpi ulnaris and the flexor digitorum sublimis is identified. The ulnar nerve and artery are retracted, exposing the deep flexor compartment of the forearm. The deep flexor fascia is incised. The ulnar nerve and artery, as well as the carpal tunnel, are decompressed distally.

After fasciotomy, the wound generally is left open. An effective way to manage the wound is with a criss-crossed rubber band technique, securing the rubber bands in place with skin staples. An alternative is to simply place a sterile dressing over the open wound, but this makes wound closure difficult and probably increases the need for skin grafting. Definitive closure or skin grafting generally is done within 5 to 7 days. Skeletal stabilization of the supracondylar and forearm fractures is important to properly manage compartment syndrome.

Neurologic Deficit

Neurologic injury has been reported to occur in as many as 49% of patients with supracondylar humeral fractures,[35] but in most modern series the incidence varies between 10% and 20%.[137,173] Previously, investigators believed that the radial nerve was injured most often[66,126,144,155,160]; however, as first noted by Spinner and Schreiber,[189] the anterior interosseous nerve appears to be the most commonly injured nerve with extension-type fractures.[49,60,134,161,189] The direction of fracture displacement determines the nerve most likely to be injured. If the distal fragment is displaced posteromedially, the radial nerve is more likely to be injured. Conversely, if the displacement of the distal fragment is posterolateral, the neurovascular bundle is stretched over the proximal fragment, injuring the median nerve or anterior interosseous nerve or both. In a flexion-type supracondylar fracture, which is rare, the ulnar nerve is the most likely to be injured. Injury to the anterior interosseous nerve causes paralysis of the long flexors of the thumb and index finger without sensory changes. Complete median nerve injury can be caused by contusion or transection of the nerve at the level of the fracture and causes sensory loss in the median nerve distribution as well as motor loss of all muscles innervated by the median nerve.[189,191] Nerve transections are rare and almost always involve the radial nerve.[50,17,132,134]

Open reduction and exploration of the injured nerve are not necessarily indicated for nerve injury in a closed fracture. Regardless of which nerve is injured, neural recovery generally occurs in the first 2 to 3 months, but may take up to 6 months.[33,105] Observation is indicated.

Culp et al.[50] described eight injured nerves in five patients in whom spontaneous recovery did not occur by 5 months after injury. Neurolysis was successful in restoring nerve function in all but one patient. Nerve grafting may be indicated for nerves not in continuity at the time of exploration. Neurolysis for perineural fibrosis generally is successful in restoring nerve function. There is no indication for early electromyographic analysis or treatment other than observation for nerve deficit until 4 to 6 months after fracture.

In their series of radial nerve injuries with humeral fractures, Amillo et al.[9] reported that, of 12 injuries that did not spontaneously recover within 6 months of injury, only one was associated with a supracondylar fracture. Perineural fibrosis was present in four patients, three nerves were entrapped in callus, and five were either partially or totally transected.

In the supracondylar area, perineural fibrosis appears to be the most common cause of prolonged nerve deficit. Although nerve injury is related to fracture displacement, a neural deficit can exist with even minimally displaced fractures. Sairyo et al.[173] reported one patient in whom radial nerve palsy occurred with a slightly angulated fracture that appeared to be a purely extension-type fracture on initial radiographs. Even in patients with mild injuries, a complete neurologic examination should be performed before treatment. An irreducible fracture with nerve deficit is an indication for open reduction of the fracture to ensure that there is no nerve entrapment. Chronic nerve entrapment in healed callus can give the appearance of a hole in the bone, the Metev sign.

Iatrogenic injury to the ulnar nerve has been reported to occur in 1% to 15% of patients with supracondylar fractures.[33,94,165,169,183] In a large series of type III supracondylar fractures, the rate of iatrogenic injury to the radial nerve was less than 1%. The course of the ulnar nerve through the cubital tunnel, between the medial epicondyle and the olecranon, makes it vulnerable when a medial pin is placed. Rasool[165] demonstrated with operative exploration that the pin usually did not impale the ulnar nerve, but more commonly constricted the nerve within the cubital tunnel by tethering adjacent soft tissue. These findings were later confirmed by an ultrasonographic study by Karakurt et al.[103] Zaltz et al.[211] reported that in children less than 5 years of age, when the elbow is flexed more than 90 degrees, the ulnar nerve migrated over, or even anterior to, the medial epicondyle in 61% (32/52) of children.

There is insufficient information in the literature to offer an evidence-based approach to an iatrogenic ulnar nerve injury that occurs following medial pin placement. Lyons et al.[127] reported full return of function in 17 patients with iatrogenic ulnar nerve injuries presumably caused by a medial pin, although function did not return until 4 months after surgery in several. Only 4 of the 17 (24%) had the medial pins removed, indicating that nerve function can eventually return without pin removal. Brown and Zinar[33] reported four ulnar nerve injuries associated with pinning of supracondylar fractures, all of which resolved spontaneously 2 to 4 months after pinning. Rasool[165] reported six patients with ulnar nerve injuries in whom early exploration was performed. In two patients, the nerve was penetrated, and in three, it was constricted by a retinaculum over the carpal tunnel, aggravated by the pin. In 1 patient, the nerve was subluxed and was fixed anterior to the cubital tunnel by the pin. Full recovery occurred in three patients, partial recovery in two, and no recovery in two. Royce et al.[169] reported spontaneous recovery of ulnar nerve function in three patients. One nerve that was explored had direct penetration, and the pin was replaced in the proper position. Two patients had late-onset ulnar nerve palsies discovered during healing, and the medial pin was removed.

If an immediate postoperative neural injury is documented, we prefer to replace the pin in the proper position or convert to a lateral pin construct, earlier rather than later. Routine exploration of the ulnar nerve is not recommended.[33,64,165,211]

Preventing ulnar nerve injury is more desirable than treating ulnar neuropathy. Because of the frequency of ulnar nerve injury with crossed pinning, most surgeons prefer to use two or three lateral pins if possible and no medial pin. Successful maintenance of alignment of type III supracondylar fractures with lateral pins has been reported in many series.[41,110,182,183,195] Many believe that if crossed-pinning is to be used, nerve penetration and indirect trauma to the nerve cannot be prevented by making an incision over the medial epicondyle and avoiding the nerve while placing the medial pin directly on the medial epicondyle. Skaggs et al.[183] reported that the use of crossed pins with a medial cut-down did not decrease the risk of iatrogenic ulnar nerve injuries. It is important to remember that most iatrogenic ulnar nerve injuries do not result from a pin directly penetrating the nerve, but from a pin going through adjacent tissue, resulting in pinching of the nerve. Michael and Stanislas[140] described another alternative for protecting the ulnar nerve; they attached a nerve stimulator to a needle, which was used for localizing the ulnar nerve. Once the ulnar nerve was identified, a standard pinning technique was used, placing the medial pin 0.5 to 0.75 mm anterior to the nerve. We have no experience with this technique. Some surgeons palpate the ulnar nerve and push it posteriorly. Wind et al.[206] however, showed this method to be unreliable. The only technique for avoiding iatrogenic ulnar nerve injury appears to be to use lateral-entry pins and avoid the use of crossed pins.

Elbow Stiffness

Loss of motion after extension-type supracondylar fractures is rare in children. Two series analyzed this complication in detail[47,88] and found that fractures treated closed had an average loss of motion of 4 degrees. In those treated with open reduction, the loss of flexion was 6.5 degrees and the flexion contracture was 5 degrees. In a series of 43 children with supracondylar fractures who had open reduction, about half received no physical therapy.[107] While the group with physical therapy had better motion at 12 and 18 weeks postoperatively, there was no difference in elbow motion after 1 year. The authors concluded that physical therapy is unnecessary. Loss of motion has been reported with the posterior triceps splitting incision for open reduction.[77,81,131] While most children do not require formal physical therapy, we generally teach the parents range-of-motion exercises to be done at home after pin and cast removal at about 3 weeks. A follow-up appointment to assess range of motion is scheduled about 4 to 6 weeks later, and if motion is not nearly normal at that time, physical therapy to improve elbow motion is begun.

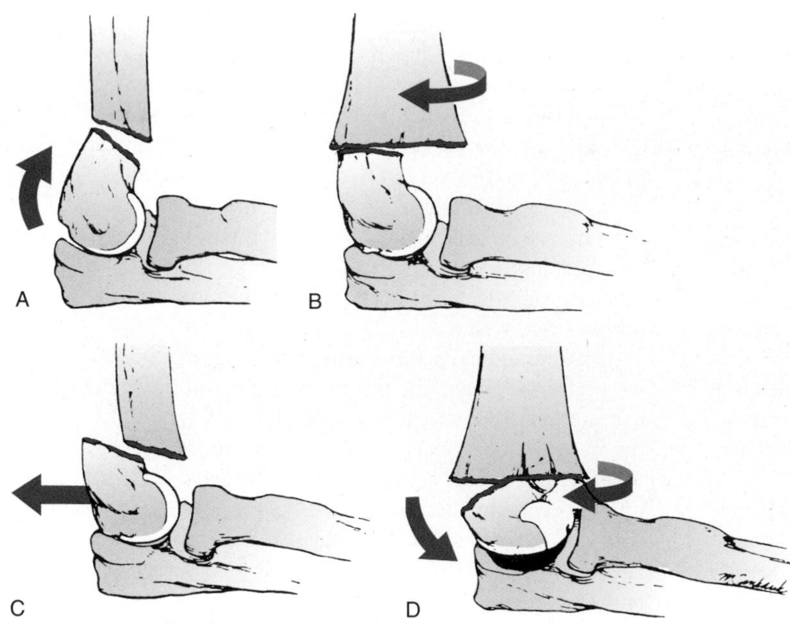

FIGURE 14-46 Distal fragment rotation. **A.** Posterior angulation only of the distal fragment. **B.** Pure horizontal rotation without angulation. **C.** Pure posterior translocation without rotation or angulation. **D.** Horizontal rotation with coronal tilting, producing a cubitus varus deformity. There is a positive crescent sign. (From Marion J, LaGrange J, Faysse R, et al. Les fractures de l'extremite inferieure de l'humerus chez l'enfant. Rev Chir Orthop 1962;48:337–413, with permission.)

Although motion loss usually is minimal, significant loss of flexion can occur. This problem generally is caused by a lack of anatomic fracture reduction: either posterior distal fragment angulation, posterior translation of the distal fragment with anterior impingement, or medial rotation of the distal fragment with a protruding medial metaphyseal spike proximally (Fig. 14-46). In young children with significant growth potential, there may be significant remodeling of anterior impingement, and any corrective surgery should be delayed at least 1 year. Although anterior impingement can significantly remodel, there is little remodeling to persistent posterior angulation or hyperextension.

Pin Track Infections

The prevalence of pin track infections in pediatric fractures treated with percutaneous K-wire fixation varies from less than 0% to 21%.[20,95] The reported prevalence of pin track infections in supracondylar humeral fractures ranges from 0% to 6.6%.[30,41,95,138,182] In a series of 202 pediatric fractures, 92.5% of which were upper extremity fractures, Battle et al.[20] reported an 8% infection rate. Twelve of the 16 infections required oral antibiotics and local pin care, one required intravenous antibiotics, and three required operative incision and débridement. In 124 supracondylar fractures, Skaggs et al.[182] noted only one pin track infection (less than 1%) which resolved with oral antibiotics and pin removal. Gupta et al.[82] also reported only one (<1%) pin track infection in 150 patients, which also resolved with oral antibiotics and pin removal. In a larger series by Mehlman et al.[138] (198 fractures), there were five (2.5%) pin track infections, which were treated with oral antibiotics and resolved without sequlae. Iobst et al.[95] reported no infections in 304 patients using a "semisterile" technique, despite the fact that only 68% of their patients received perioperative antibiotic. Their protocol involved unsterile reduction of the fracture with an assistant holding the arm in the reduced position. The surgeon then put on sterile gloves, placed sterile towels around the surgical field, and prepared the elbow locally in the anticipated area of the pin sites. There are no other reports on this technique.

Pin track infections generally resolve with pin removal and antibiotics. Fortunately, by the time a pin track infection develops the fracture usually is stable enough to remove the pin without loss of reduction. Although we have not seen this complication, an untreated pin track infection could theoretically result in a septic joint and should be treated as soon as it is recognized or suspected.

Myositis Ossificans

Myositis ossificans is a remarkably rare complication of supracondylar fractures, but it does occur (Fig. 14-47). This complication has been described after open reduction, but vigorous

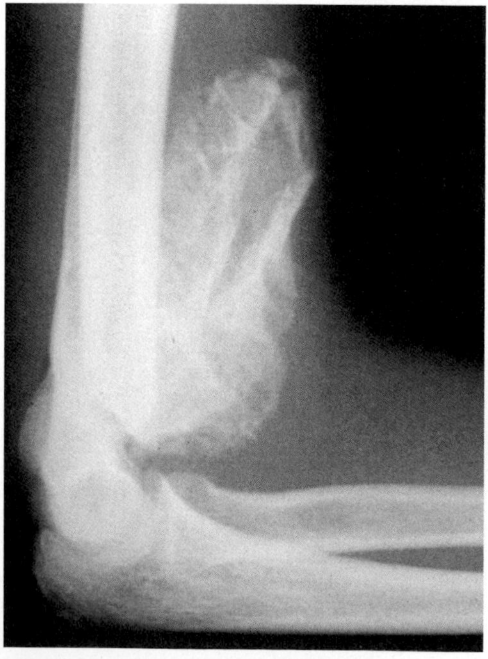

FIGURE 14-47 Myositis ossificans. Ossification of the brachialis muscle developed in this 8-year-old who had undergone multiple attempts at reduction. (Courtesy of John Schaeffer, MD.)

postoperative manipulation or physical therapy is believed to be the most commonly associated factor.[113,157]

In a report of two patients with myositis ossificans after closed reduction of supracondylar fractures, Aitken[5] noted that limitation of motion and calcification disappeared after 2 years. Postoperative myositis ossificans can be observed with the expectation of spontaneous resolution of both restricted motion and the myositis ossificans. There is no indication for early excision. Spinner[190] reported a single case of myositis ossificans associated with sudden onset of pain after trauma in which a 1-year-old lesion of myositis ossificans was fractured. With excision, the pain was relieved, and full range of motion returned.

Nonunion

The distal humeral metaphysis is a well-vascularized area with remarkably rapid healing, and nonunion of a supracondylar fracture is rare, with only a single case described by Wilkins and Beaty[202] after open reduction. We have not seen nonunion of this fracture. With infection, devascularization, and soft tissue loss, the risk of nonunion would presumably increase.

Osteonecrosis

Osteonecrosis of the trochlea after supracondylar fracture has been reported. The blood supply of the trochlea's ossification center is fragile, with two separate sources. One small artery is lateral and courses directly through the physis of the medial condyle. It provides blood to the medial crista of the trochlea. If the fracture line is very distal, this artery can be injured, producing osteonecrosis of the ossification center and resulting in a classic fishtail deformity (Fig. 14-48). Kim[109] identified 18 children with trochlear abnormalities after elbow injuries, five of which were supracondylar fractures. MRI indicated low-signal intensity on T2, indicative of cartilage necrosis. Cubitus varus

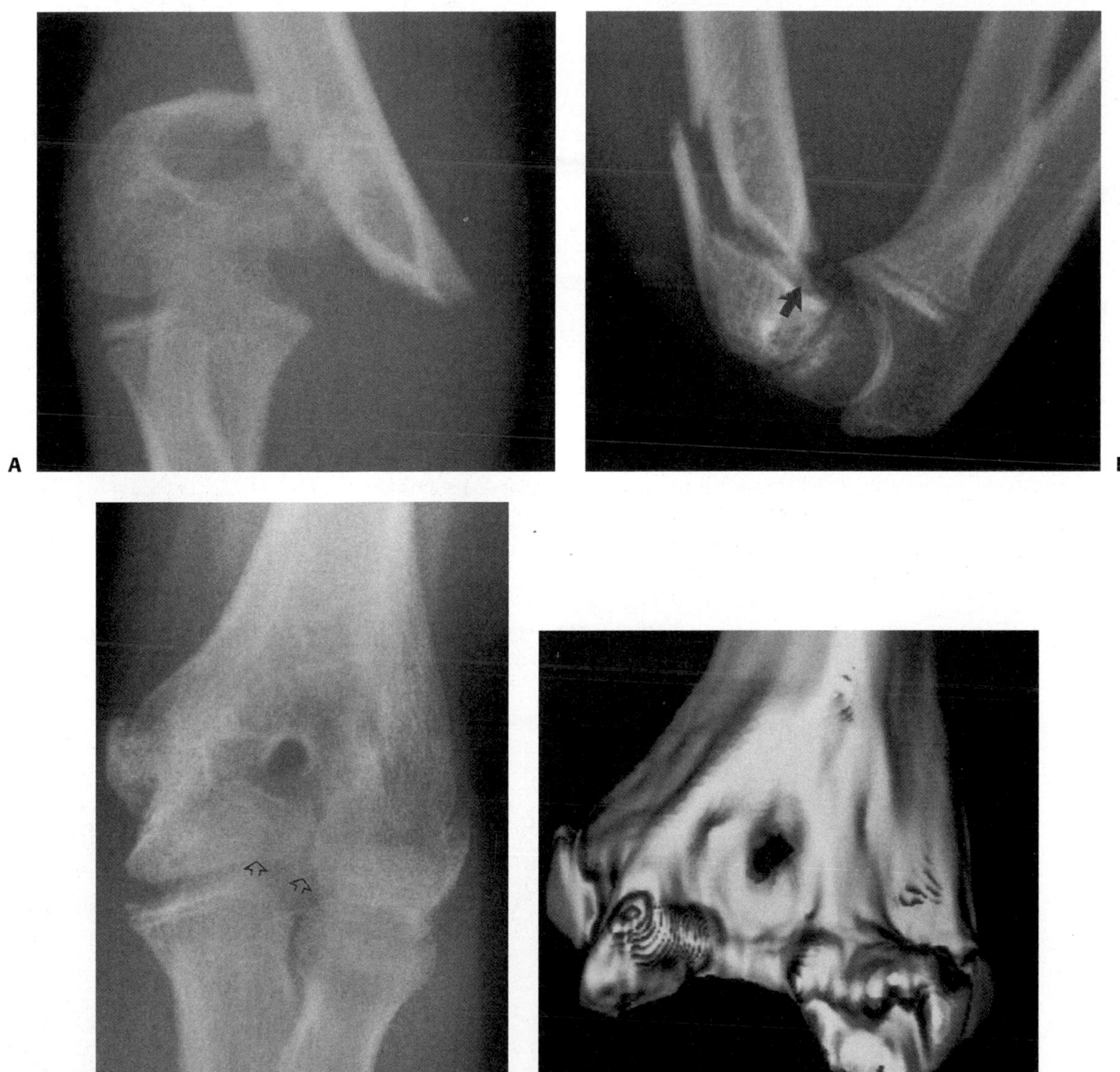

FIGURE 14-48 Osteonecrosis of the trochlea. **A.** AP injury film of an 8-year-old with a distal type III supracondylar fracture. **B.** The distal extension of the fracture (*arrow*) is best appreciated on the lateral reduction film. Postfracture, the patient was asymptomatic until 2 years later, when elbow stiffness developed. **C.** Repeat radiographs at that time showed atrophy of the trochlea (*arrows*). **D.** Three-dimensional CT reconstruction demonstrates atrophy of the trochlea.

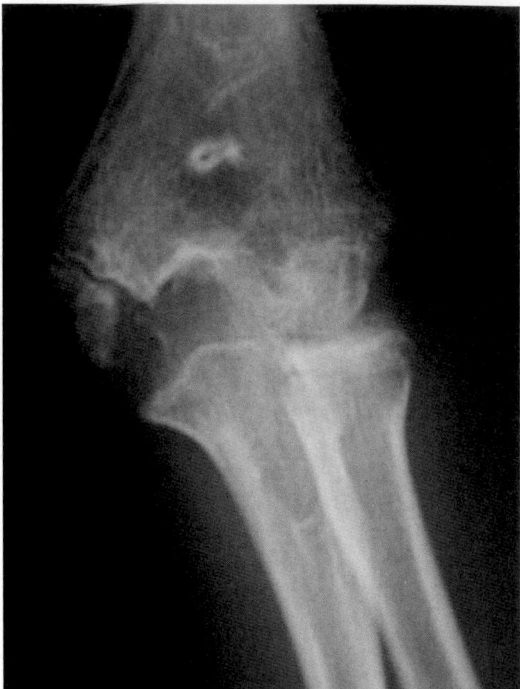

FIGURE 14-49 Osteonecrosis of the trochlea developed following open reduction through a posterior approach. The child had limited motion and symptoms of occasional catching. (Reproduced with permission from Children's Orthopaedic Center, Los Angeles, CA.)

deformity developed in all cases. Bronfen et al.[32] described six patients with severe osteonecrosis of the trochlea, which they termed "dissolution of the trochia" following closed reduction and pin fixation, indicating that open reduction is not always the cause of osteonecrosis. Five of their six patients complained of pain, crackling, and stiffness.[32]

Symptoms of osteonecrosis of the trochlea do not occur for months or years. Healing is normal, but mild pain and occasional locking develop with characteristic radiographic findings and motion may be limited depending on the extent of osteonecrosis. In our experience, the most common cause of osteonecrosis of the trochlea is open reduction of a supracondylar fracture through a posterior approach, which presumably disrupts the blood supply of the trochlea (Fig. 14-49); however, we are aware of several cases of osteonecrosis that occurred after simple closed pinning. The artery to the trochlea may be disrupted at the time of the injury.

Loss of Reduction

Clinical experience with a series of 124 consecutive supracondylar humeral fractures, including completely unstable fractures, has taught us that lateral-entry pins, when properly placed, are strong enough to maintain reduction of even the most unstable supracondylar humeral fractures.[182] In an informal collection of reports of loss of reduction of supracondylar fractures from members of the Pediatric Orthopaedic Society of North America, Skaggs et al.[182] reported only eight fractures with loss of reduction after treatment with lateral-entry pins. They identified technical points of pin placement that may be associated with loss of fracture reduction. Two lateral pins were used for all eight fractures. In five, the pins were too close together and engaged only the lateral column at the level of the fracture (Fig. 14-50). In each of these, fracture reduction was lost when the distal fragment rotated around the two pins. In another case, the two lateral pins crossed at the fracture site (Fig. 14-51). In the remaining two cases, the two lateral pins did not engage the distal fragment (Figs. 52A,B). There were no reports of loss of fixation after the use of three lateral-entry pins.

Sankar et al.,[174] in a series of 322 factures, reported that 2.9% had postoperative loss of fixation. All eight were type III fractures treated with two pins (seven lateral-entry and one crossed-pin). In all eight, loss of fixation was due to technical errors that were identifiable on the intraoperative fluoroscopic images (Fig. 14-53) and that could have been prevented with proper technique. They identified three types of pin-fixation errors: (i) failure to engage both fragments with two pins or more, (ii) failure to achieve bicortical fixation with two pins or

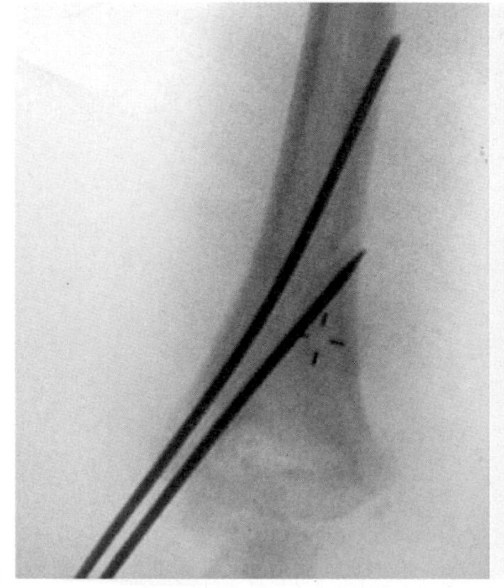

A

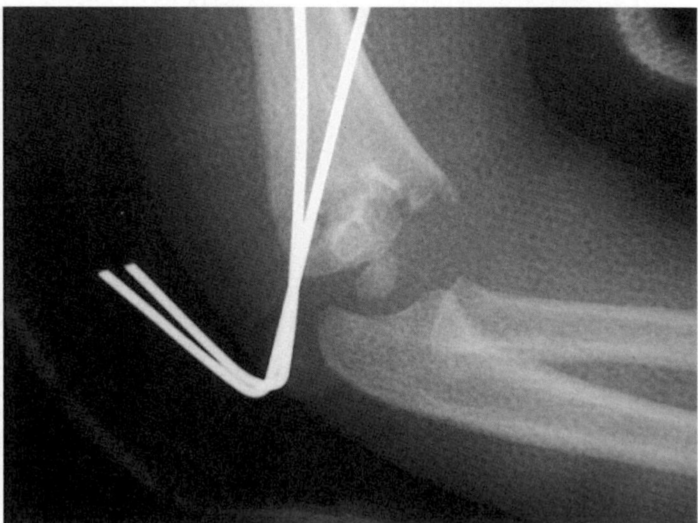

B

FIGURE 14-50 If the pins are placed too close together, they biomechanically function as one pin, and rotation around the pins is not surprising. **A.** Intraoperative radiograph. **B.** Postoperative loss of reduction in same patient. (From Skaggs DL, Cluck MW, Mostofi A, et al. Lateral-entry pin fixation in the management of supracondylar fractures in children. J Bone Joint Surg 2004;86-A(4):702–707, with permission.)

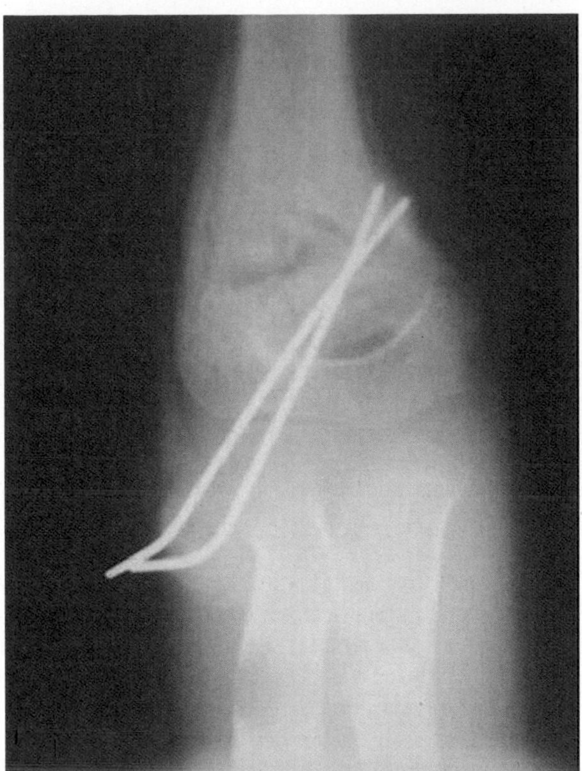

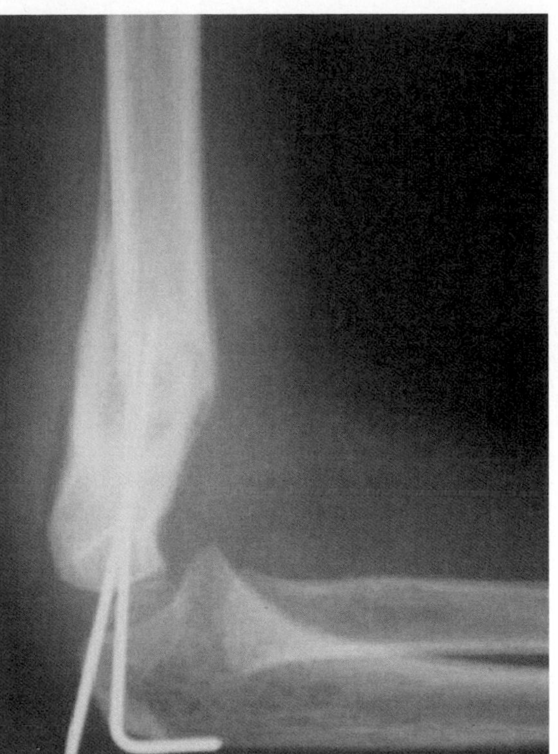

FIGURE 14-51 A,B. In accordance with standard fracture principles, pins that cross at the fracture site do not provide stability. (From Skaggs DL, Cluck MW, Mostofi A, et al. Lateral-entry pin fixation in the management of supracondylar fractures in children. J Bone Joint Surg 2004;86-A(4):702–707, with permission.)

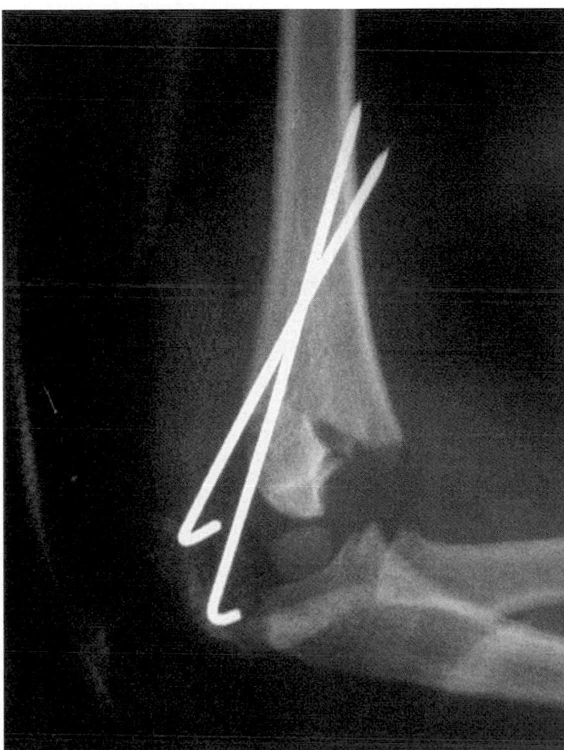

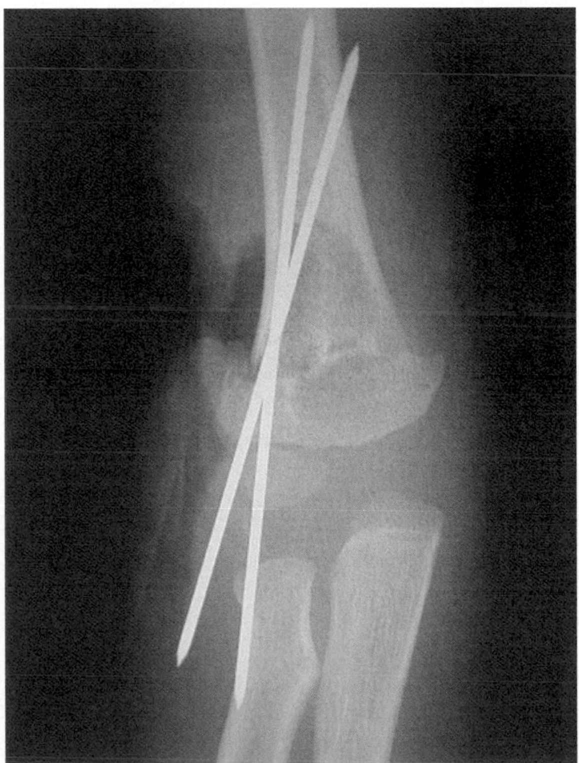

FIGURE 14-52 A,B. Insufficient bone is engaged in the distal fragments, so loss of fixation may be expected. (From Skaggs DL, Cluck MW, Mostofi A, et al. Lateral-entry pin fixation in the management of supracondylar fractures in chilren. J Bone Joint Surg 2004;86-A(4):702–707, with permission.)

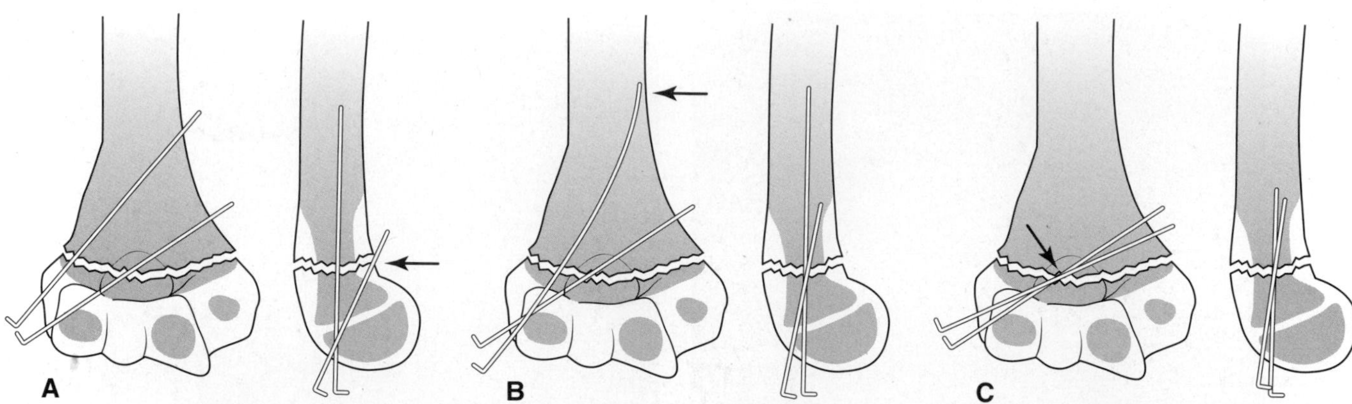

FIGURE 14-53 Illustrations depicting errors in pin-fixation technique. **A.** The black arrow demonstrates the anterior pin failing to transfix the proximal bone. **B.** The black arrow demonstrates one pin without bicortical purchase. **C.** The black arrow demonstrates pins too close together at the fracture site.

more, and (iii) failure to achieve adequate pin separation (>2 mm) at the fracture site.[174]

Hyperextension

Simanovsky et al.[180] reported 22 patients near skeletal maturity with underreduction of the extension component of the fracture. They found that 17 (77%) of the patients had radiographic abnormalities of the humerocondylar angle (a difference of 5 degrees or more compared with the uninjured side). Eleven patients (50%) had limited elbow flexion, and 7 (31%) were aware of this deficit. Patients who were left to heal with some degree of extension developed limited end-elbow flexion and were aware of it. Although only 3 patients perceived minor subjective functional disability at the last follow-up, 10 patients had unsatisfactory results according to the Flynn criteria for motion restriction.[180]

Cubitus Varus

Cubitus varus, also know as a "gunstock deformity," has a characteristic appearance in the frontal plane (Fig. 14-54). The malunion most commonly also includes hyperextension, which leads to increased elbow extension and decreased elbow flexion (Figs. 14-55 and 14-56). The appearance of cubitus varus deformity is distinctive on radiograph. On the AP view, the angle of the physis of the lateral condyle (Baumann angle) is more horizontal than normal (Fig. 14-57). On the lateral view, hyperextension of the distal fragment posterior to the anterior humeral line correlates with the clinical findings of increased extenion and decreased flexion of the elbow (Fig. 14-58).

Unequal growth in the distal humerus has been proposed as a cause of cubitus varus deformity,[93,155] though this is unlikely because not enough growth remains in this area to cause cubitus varus within the time it is recognized. A more likely reason for most cubitus varus deformities in patients with supracondylar fractures is malunion.[12,35,51,64,200] Cubitus varus can be prevented by making certain that the Baumann angle is intact at the time of reduction and remains so during healing, which generally is best assured with pin fixation. In a series of 206 patients with supracondylar humeral fractures, with ages ranging from 1.5 to 14 years (mean of 6.4 years), Pirone et al.[157] reported cubitus varus deformities in eight (7.9%) of 101 patients treated with cast immobilization compared to two (1.9%) in 105 patients treated with pin fixation. A decrease in the frequency of cubitus varus deformity after the use of percutaneous pin fixation has been reflected in other recent series.[29,30,64,65,101,139,157,158] with one large retrospective[182] and one prospective study[111] reporting no cubitus varus deformities.

The distal humeral physis provides 20% of that the overall length of the humerus. In a 5-year-old, therefore, the amount of distal humeral growth in 1 year is approximately 2 mm, making it unlikely that growth asymmetry is a significant cause of varus deformity that occurs within the first 6 to 12 months after fracture. A case report of a 4-year-old girl with progressive cubitus varus caused by a physeal bony bar demonstrated with MRI (Fig. 14-59) after cast treatment of a supracondylar fracture noted the slow progress of the deformity.[56] The Baumann angle went from 88 degrees at 6 months following injury to 92 degrees at 18 months and 96 degrees at 3 years after injury. Thus, over

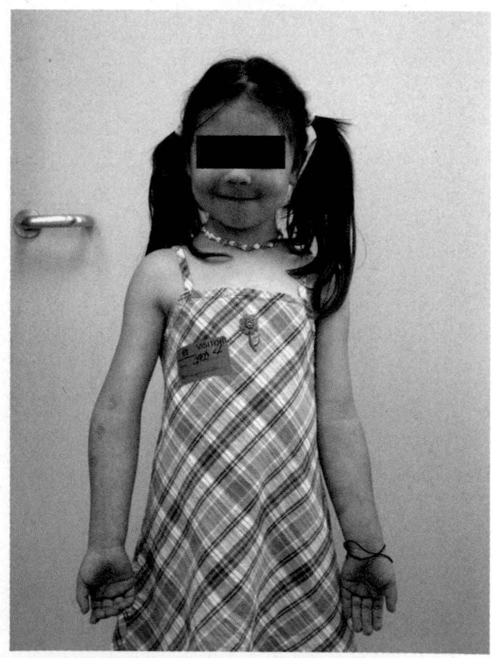

FIGURE 14-54 A 5-year-old girl with cubitus varus of right elbow following a malunion of a supracondylar humerus fracture. (Reproduced with permission of Children's Orthopaedic Center, Los Angeles, CA.)

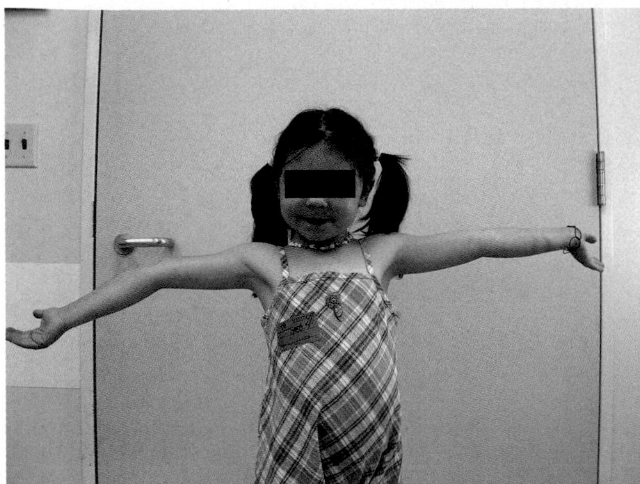

FIGURE 14-55 Hyperextension of right elbow. (Reproduced with permission of Children's Orthopaedic Center, Los Angeles, CA.)

3 years from injury, the Baumann angle changed by only 8 degrees, which we suspect is not too different from measurement variability. Osteonecrosis of the trochlea or medial portion of the distal humeral fragment can result in progressive varus deformity, however. In a series of 36 varus deformities reported by Voss et al.,[197] only 4 patients had medial growth disturbance and distal humeral osteonecrosis as a cause of progressive varus deformity.

Treatment of cubitus varus deformities has been considered a primarily cosmetic procedure, but several consequences of cubitus varus such as an increased risk of lateral condylar fractures, pain, and tardy posterolateral rotatory instability may be indications for supracondylar humeral osteotomy.[1,2,23,135,148,188] Our experience suggests that many patients have elbow discomfort with significant cubitus varus. O'Driscoll et al.[148] reported 17 patients with cubitus vars deformities after a pediatric distal humeral fracture who presented an average of 27 years following injury. The average varus deformity was 15 degrees, and all patients had tenderness over the lateral collat-

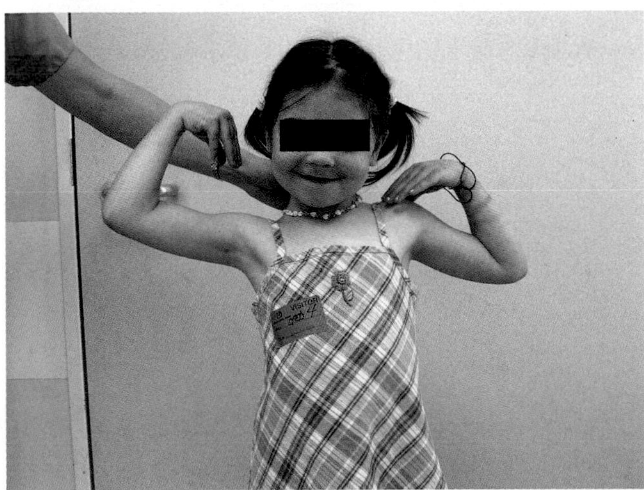

FIGURE 14-56 Decreased flexion of right elbow. (Reproduced with permission from Children's Orthopaedic Center, Los Angeles, CA.)

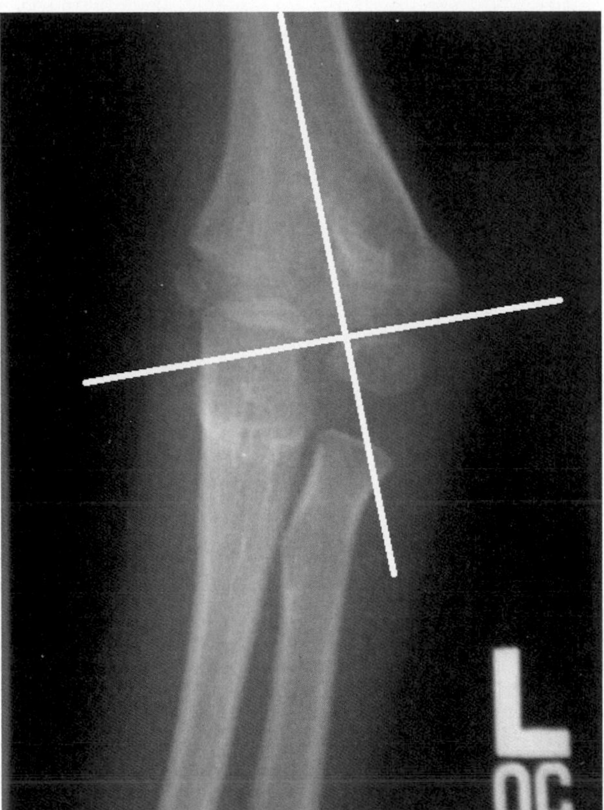

FIGURE 14-57 AP radiograph of girl in preceeding clinical photos. (Reproduced with permission from Children's Orthopaedic Center, Los Angeles, CA.)

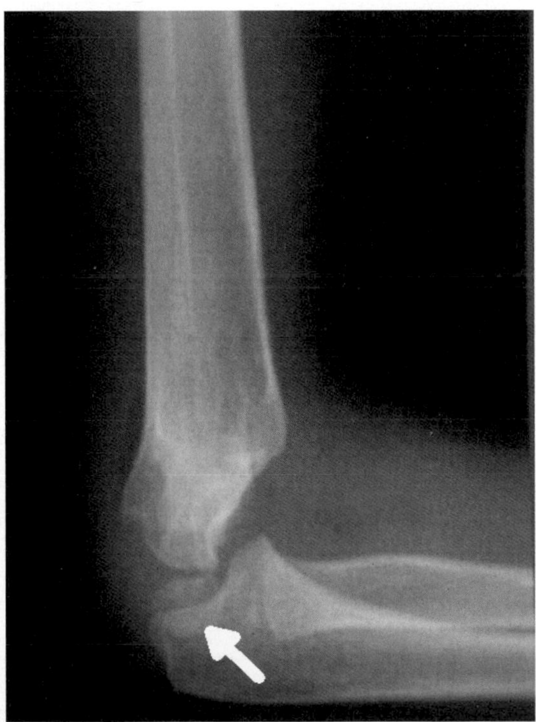

FIGURE 14-58 Lateral radiograph shows overlapping of the distal humerus with the olecranon (*arrow*) producing the typical crescent sign. Note the anterior humeral line is anterior to the capitellum. (Reproduced with permission of Children's Orthopaedic Center, Los Angeles, CA.)

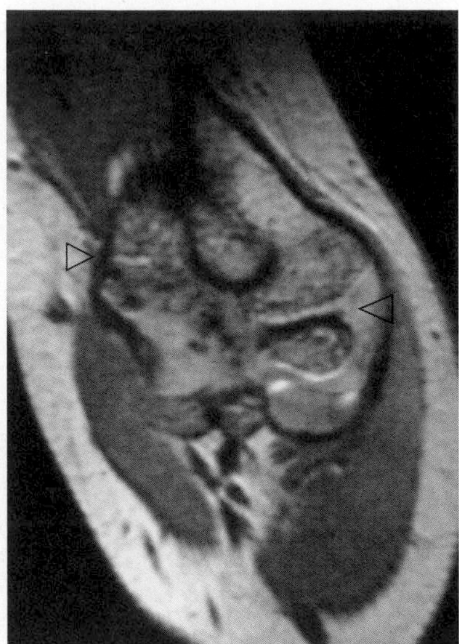

FIGURE 14-59 At 3 years postinjury, coronal dual echo steady state MRI (TR 27, TE 9) shows interruption of high signal from trochlear growth plate involving 35% of the physis. The medial epicondylar and capitellar growth plates (*arrowheads*) are preserved. (Reproduced with permission from Children's Orthopaedic Center, Los Angeles, CA.)

eral ligament complex and posterolateral rotator instability. These authors concluded that cubitus varus deformity secondary to supracondylar malunion may not always be a benign condition and may have important long-term clinical implications.[148] An increased risk of fracture,[53] especially of the lateral condyle, has been linked with cubitus varus deformity. Takahara et al.[193] reported nine patients with distal humeral fractures who deveoped varus deformities. Supracondylar fractures as well as epiphyseal separations were included in these nine fractures.

Tardy ulnar nerve palsy also has been associated with cubitus varus and internal rotational malalignment.[2,24,142,196] With a cubitus varus deformity, the olecranon fossa moves to the ulnar side of the distal humerus,[149] and the triceps shifts a bit ulnarward. Investigators theorized that this ulnar shift might compress the ulnar nerve against the medial epicondyle, narrowing the cubital tunnel and resulting in chronic neuropathy. In a recent report,[2] a fibrous band running between the heads of the flexor carpi ulnaris was thought to cause ulnar nerve compression.

Treatment of Cubitus Varus Deformity. As for the treatment of any posttraumatic malalignment, options include (i) observation with expected remodeling, (ii) hemiepiphysiodesis and growth alteration, and (iii) corrective osteotomy. Observation generally is not appropriate because, although hyperextension may remodel to some degree in a young child (Fig. 14-60), in an older child little remodeling occurs even in the plane of motion of the joint.

Hemiepiphysiodesis of the distal humerus may rarely be of value, but only to prevent cubitus varus deformity from developing in a patient with clear medial growth arrest or trochlear osteonecrosis. If untreated, medial growth disturbance will lead to lateral overgrowth and progressive deformity. Lateral epiphysiodesis will not correct the deformity, but will prevent it from increasing. Voss et al.[197] used hemiepiphysiodesis with osteotomy in two patients with growth arrest and varus deformity. The humerus varies in length by a few centimeters from one individual to another, but in general, it is about 30 cm long at skeletal maturity. Approximately 65% of the length of the humerus is achieved by age 6 years. A 6-year-old child has approximately 10 cm of growth left in the entire humerus, with

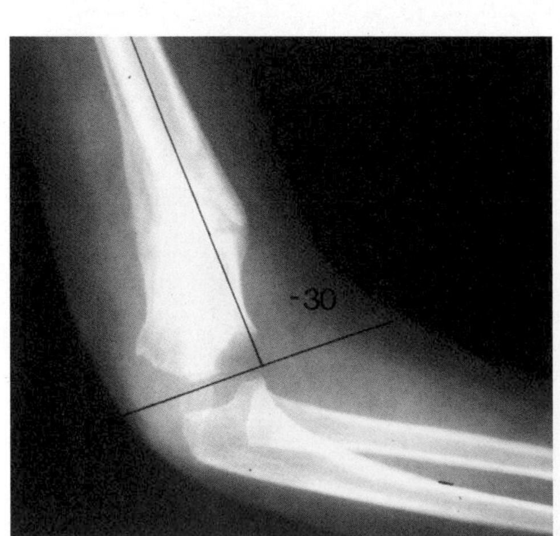

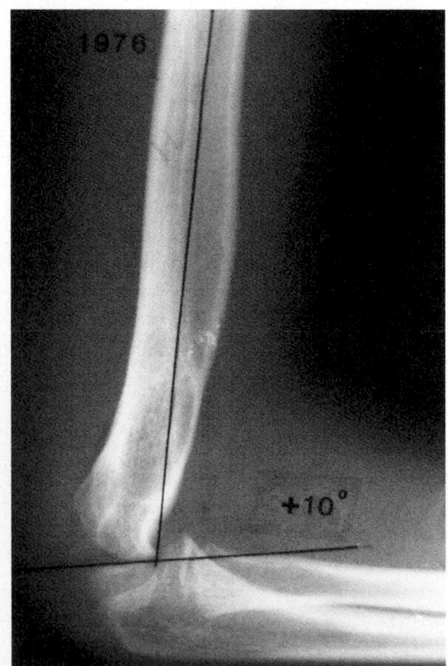

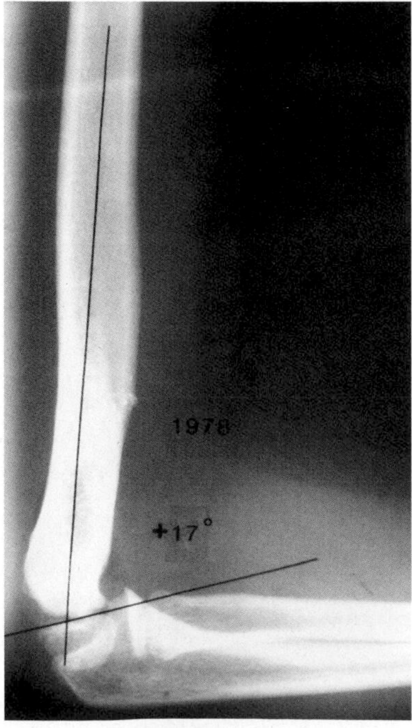

FIGURE 14-60 A hyperextension deformity in the distal humerus may remodel somewhat, whereas varus and valgus deformities do not. **A.** Hyperextension deformity in the distal humerus after fracture. **B.** Four years later, a more normal distal humeral anatomy is seen with remodeling of the hyperextension deformity; 2 years later **(C)**, a normal distal humeral anatomy is reconstituted.

only approximately 2 cm provided by the distal physis. Growth arrest, in the absence of osteonecrosis or collapse, will be a very slowly evolving phenomenon, and epiphysiodesis in a child older than 6 years will have little effect on longitudinal growth. In general, prevention of increasing deformity from medial growth arrest is the only role for lateral epiphysiodesis. Because of the slow growth rate in the distal humerus, we do not believe there is any role for lateral epiphysiodesis in correcting a varus deformity in a child with otherwise normal physis.

Osteotomy. Osteotomy is the only way to correct a cubitus varus deformity with a high probability of success. A variety of corrective osteotomies have been described, almost all with significant complications (Table 14-3). Stiffness, nerve injury,

TABLE 14-3 Results of Several Studies Using Various Osteotomies

Study (Reference)	Cases	Type Fixation	Complications
Incomplete Osteotomies			
King and Secor[168]	15	MOW, Riedel clamp, tibial graft	Three neutral Three ulnar palsies
Rang[164]	20	LCW, K-wires	One aneurysm One skin slough One nerve palsy Six varus Two stiff
Carlson et al.[37]	12	LCW, staple	None
Bellemore et al.[21]	27	LCW, K-wire, French technique	Four infections Four loss of fixation Three varus Four poor scars Five prominent condyles
Gao[72]	15	LCW, suture	Three under corrected
McCoy and Piggot[133]	20	LCW, French technique	Four neutral Two varus Two stiff One poor scar
Graham et al.[79]	16	LCW, cast	Two varus
Danielsson et al.[52]	11	LCW, staple	None
Mixed Osteotomies			
Oppenheim et al.[152]	4 incomplete, 31 complete	LCW, K-wires, French technique	Five nerve palsies Three infections Twelve varus One stiff Two poor scars
Unspecified Osteotomies			
Sweeney[192]	15	LCW, K-wires Complete osteotomies	Five varus
Langenskiöld and Kivilaakso[119]	11	LCW, unicortical plate, rot.	Two varus Two neutral Two reoperations
Labelle et al.[116]	15	LCW, K-wires, rot.	Three loss of fixation Three nerve palsies
DeRosa and Graziano[57]	11	SC, screw	One loss of fixation, varus
Kanaujia et al.[102]	11	Dome K wires	Two stiff
Laupattarakasem et al.[121]	57	SC, screws	Three loss of fixation Two reoperations Two prominent condyles
Uchida et al.[196]	12	SC, screws	None
Voss et al.[197]	34	K-wires	No nerve palsies, one loss of fixation

LCW, lateral closing wedge; MOW, medial opening wedge; rot., rotational correction; SC, step-cut osteotomy.

and recurrent deformities are the most commonly reported complications. An overall complication rate approaching 25% in many series has led to some controversy about the value of a distal humeral corrective osteotomy for cubitus varus deformity.

To choose an appropriate osteotomy, the exact location of the deformity must be determined. Because malunion is the cause of most cubitus varus deformities, the angular deformity usually occurs at the level of the fracture. Rotation and hypertension may contribute to the deformity, but varus is the most significant factor.[43] Hyperextension can produce a severe deformity in some patients. An oblique configuration (Fig. 14-61) places the center of rotation of the osteotomy as close to the actual level of the deformity as possible. On an AP radiograph of the humerus with the forearm in full supination, the size of the wedge and the angular correction needed are determined. An "incomplete" lateral closing wedge osteotomy can be done, leaving a small medial hinge of bone intact. The osteotomy usually is fixed with two K-wires placed laterally. In the absence of an intact medial hinge, two lateral wires probably are not sufficient to secure this osteotomy.[197] Wilkins and Beaty[202] recommended crossed wires in this situation. In general, a lateral closing wedge osteotomy with a medial hinge will correct the varus deformity, with minimal correction of hyperextension.[10,21,46,68,70,79,98,100,116,192,197,207] but this osteotomy tends to leave a lateral bump with poor cosmesis. Residual rotational deformity was not found to be a significant problem in studies by Voss et al.[197] and Oppenheim et al.,[152] which is logical given the amount of rotation available from the shoulder. The French osteotomy[68] aims to enable axial rotational correction as well, but does so at the expense of stability and we do not use this osteotomy.

Japanese surgeons[90] described a dome osteotomy in which a curved osteotomy is made in the supracondylar area. Proponents of this osteotomy suggest that multiplane correction is possible without inducing translation in the distal fragment and that rotation can be corrected. DeRosa and Graziano[57] described a step-cut osteotomy in which the distal fragment is slotted into the proximal fragment and the osteotomy is secured with a single screw.

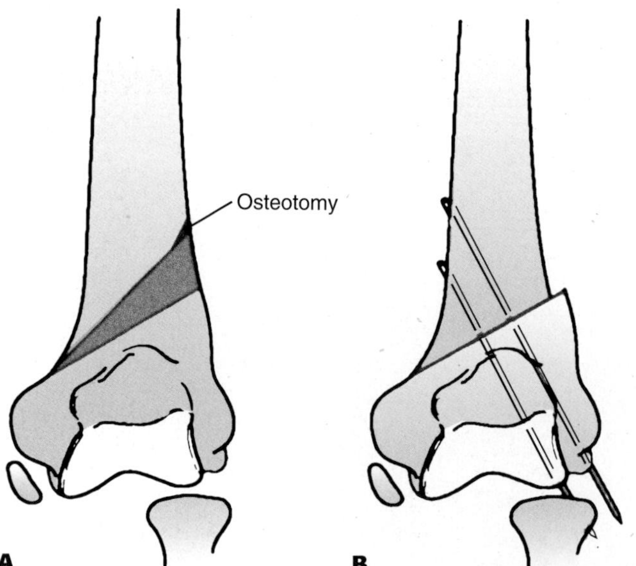

FIGURE 14-61 A. By moving the apex of the closing wedge distally, the center of rotation of the osteotomy is moved closer to the deformity. **B.** Upon closing a distally based wedge osteotomy, there is less translational effect than in a more proximally based osteotomy.

Functional outcomes generally are good, but the preoperative functional deficit is nearly always minor in patients with cubitus varus deformities. Complications of humeral osteotomy include stiffness, nerve injury, and persistent deformity (see Table 14-3); however, with a properly performed osteotomy, complications are relatively few. Ippolito et al.[96] reported long-term follow-up of patients with supracondylar osteotomies, 50% of whom had poor results. Weiss et al.[201] reported a complication rate of 16% (nine of 57 patients) with various types of osteotomies. It was notable that the authors found a complication rate of 6% (two of 34) when the surgery was done by full-time staff at a tertiary pediatric referral center, with no patient requiring additional surgery and all having excellent results. The complication rate among patients treated by non-full-time staff was 30% (seven of 23), including two transient ulnar nerve palsies, four deformity recurrences or loss of fixation requiring reoperation, and one deep infection requiring operative treatment. This can be a challenging operation, and it is not surprising that surgeons with more experience have fewer complications.

Hyperextension deformity may remodel over time (see Fig. 14-60), but correction is slow and inconsistent. In one series,[197] hyperextension deformities remodeled as much as 30 degrees in very young children, but in older children, there was no significant remodeling in the flexion–extension plane. If hyperextension appears to be a major problem, osteotomy should also be directed at this deformity rather than simple correction of the varus deformity; this situation requires a multiplane osteotomy.

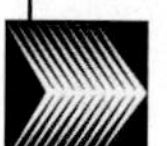

AUTHORS' PREFERRED TREATMENT

We prefer to use a Wiltse type osteotomy, similar to that described by DeRosa and Graziano,[57] but with the complete cut as distal as possible to the superior edge of the olecranon fossa to place the axis of rotation of the osteotomy as close as possible to the deformity see (Fig. 14-61). A similar technique has been described by Yun et al.[210] with good results in 22 children. Preoperative templating is used to determine the angle of correction required for correction of the varus and, if necessary, for correction of any extension deformity. Templating is based on AP radiographs of both upper extremities centered on the elbow, combined with clinical examination comparing one arm to the other in terms of frontal plane appearance and arc of motion. For example, if the affected arm has 20 degrees more extension and 20 degrees less flexion than the contralateral arm, a 20-degree wedge osteotomy is planned in the sagittal plane.

A longitudinal incision approximately 6 cm long is made over the lateral distal humerus. The antebrachial cutaneous nerve and its branches are identified and protected. The radial nerve generally is proximal to the field of dissection. Dissection is carried out in the interval between the brachioradialis and triceps. Subperiostial dissection is performed to expose the distal humerus. There is sometimes scarring from fracture healing about the area of fracture. Posterior dissection is continued to the olecranon fossa as a landmark, but not distal to it to prevent harming the blood supply to the trochlea. Chandler retractors are used for circumferential protection with special care medially near the ulnar nerve. An osteotomy is made just above the olecranon fossa perpendicular to the shaft of the humerus. The proximal humerus is delivered out of the wound to allow the more complex part of the osteotomy to be made with maximal visualization and protection. With the second cut, the osteotomy is angled correctly to account for sagittal malalignment. On average, an anterior closing wedge osteotomy of about 20 degrees is used, but this is adjusted as needed to make certain the postfixation image demonstrates the anterior humeral line through the midthird of the capitellum. A small lateral portion of the proximal fragment is left intact and a similarly shaped area with a 90-degree angle is made in the lateral portion of the distal fragment with a rongeur to allow the pieces to fit together for added stability. This technique is adapted from the osteotomy described by Wiltse[205] and prevents excessive lateral translation of the distal fragment, keeps the axis of rotation near the site of deformity, and has some inherent stability if done correctly (Fig. 14-62). Once correction is achieved, bony contact is maximized by further cuts if needed. Three 0.062-inch or 2-mm K-wires are then placed across the osteotomy from lateral to medial. A goniometer is used to measure alignment. Elbow flexion and extension are then checked to ensure that the fingers can touch the ipsilateral shoulder and full extension is achieved. The wound is irrigated, and a small amount of local bone graft from the excised wedge is packed around the osteotomy site, making certain bone graft is not in the olecranon fossa. After closure, flexion and extension are checked under live imaging to ensure that there is no motion at the osteotomy site. A long-arm cast is applied with the elbow in 60 to 80 degrees of flexion and the arm in neutral supination and pronation. The cast is removed when good callus is demonstrated on radiographs, usually approximately 4 weeks postoperatively (as opposed to 3 weeks for fractures), and the pins are removed in clinic at that time. In eight osteotomies done by one of us with this technique, there has been full frontal and sagittal plane correction with no complications (unpublished data) (Figs. 14-63 to 14-66).

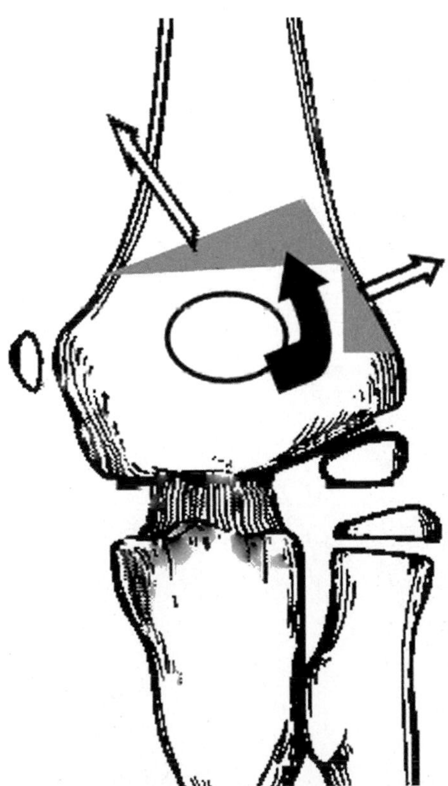

FIGURE 14-62 This osteotomy can correct frontal and sagittal plane malalignment and offer some inherent bony stability, while not producing a lateral bump that occurs with simple closing wedge osteotomies.

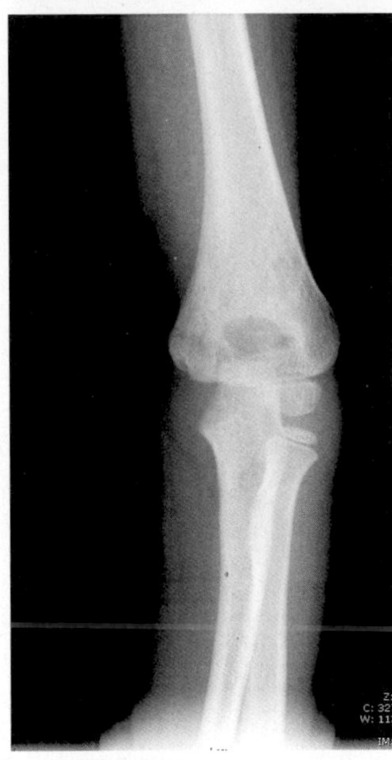

FIGURE 14-63 AP radiograph of elbow of 5-year-old girl in cubitus varus with Baumann angle about 0 degrees. (Reproduced with permission from Children's Orthopaedic Center, Los Angeles, CA.)

Controversies

In addition to questions about the number and configuration of pins used for fixation of supracondylar humeral fractures

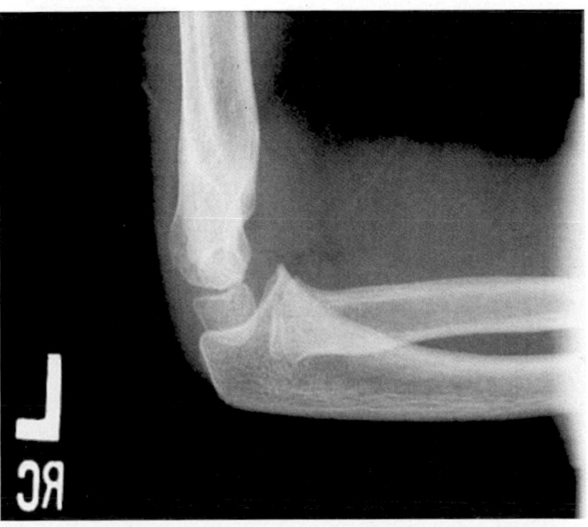

FIGURE 14-64 Lateral radiograph demonstrates capitellum posterior to the anterior humeral line. (Reproduced with permission from Children's Orthopaedic Center, Los Angeles, CA.)

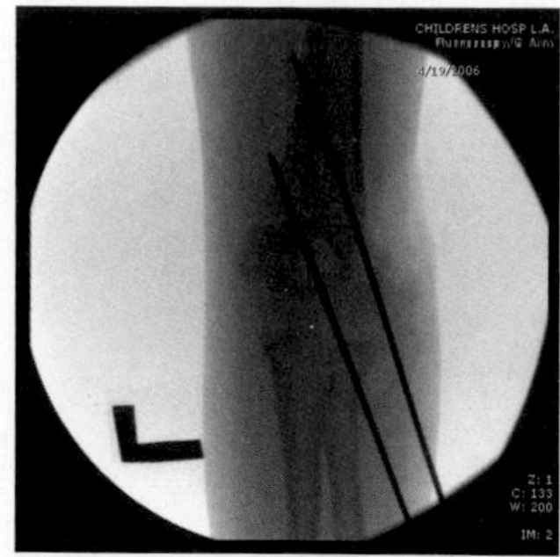

FIGURE 14-65 Intraoperative AP image demonstrates restoration of Baumann angle after Wiltse-type osteotomy. (Reproduced with permission from Children's Orthopaedic Center, Los Angeles, CA.)

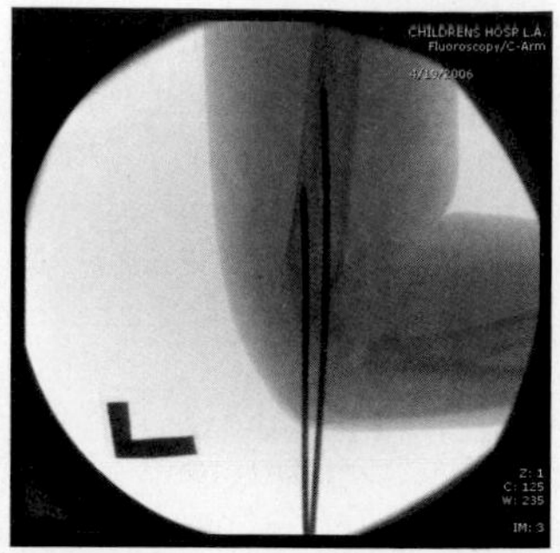

FIGURE 14-66 Lateral intraoperative image demonstrates anterior humeral line now intersecting the capitellum. Postoperatively a normal arc of elbow flexion and extension was restored. (Reproduced with permission from Children's Orthopaedic Center, Los Angeles, CA.)

(see pages 496 through 498), the effect of delaying operative treatment remains a matter of controversy, with several studies concluding that a delay of surgery of 8 to 21 hours has no deleterious effects on the outcomes[82,97,124,138,179]; however, these studies were all retrospective and their high percentage of good results may have been due to the selection bias of experienced pediatric orthopaedic surgeons who selected which fractures required urgent treatment. Although there are no high-level studies to support our opinion, we and other authorities believe[162] that urgent operative treatment is indicated for patients with poor perfusion, an associated displaced forearm fracture, firm compartments, skin puckering, antecubital ecchymosis, or very considerable swelling.

FLEXION-TYPE SUPRACONDYLAR FRACTURES

Flexion-type supracondylar humeral fractures account for about 2% of humeral fractures.[128] A flexion pattern of injury may not be recognized until reduction is attempted because initial radiographs are inadequate. A key to recognizing a flexion-type supracondylar fracture is that it is unstable in flexion, whereas extension-type fractures generally are stable in hyperflexion. A laterally displaced supracondylar fracture may actually be a flexion-type injury.

Etiology and Pathology

The mechanism of injury generally is believed to be a fall directly onto the elbow rather than a fall onto the outstretched hand with hyperextension of the elbow (Fig. 14-67). The distal fragment is displaced anteriorly and may migrate proximally in a totally displaced fracture. The ulnar nerve is vulnerable in this fracture pattern,[66,85,128,170] and it may be entrapped in the fracture or in the healing callus.[118]

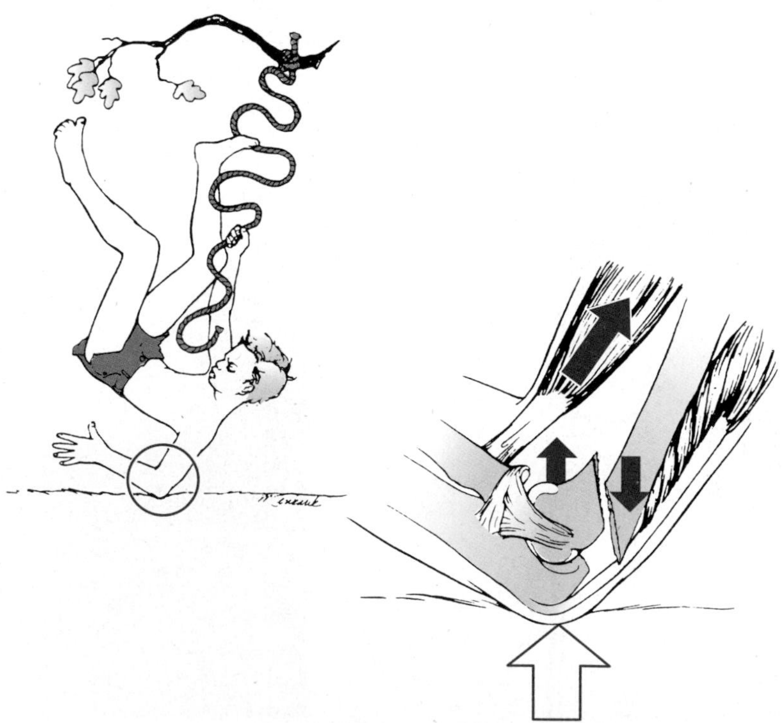

FIGURE 14-67 Flexion mechanism. Flexion-type fractures usually result from a blow to the posterior aspect of the elbow. The obliquity of the fracture line may be opposite that of an extension type. The large black arrows demonstrate the usual direction of fragment displacement.

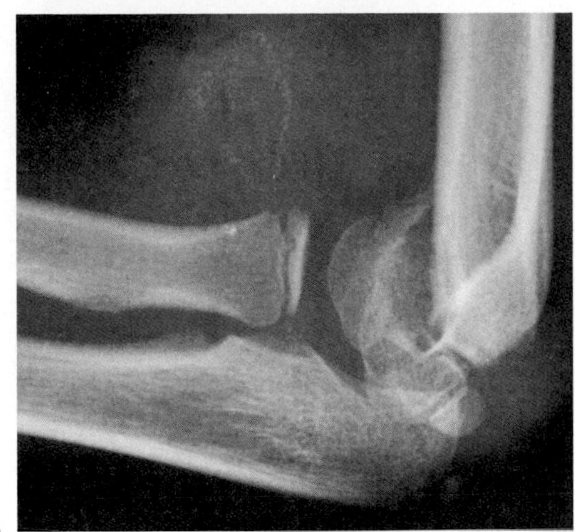

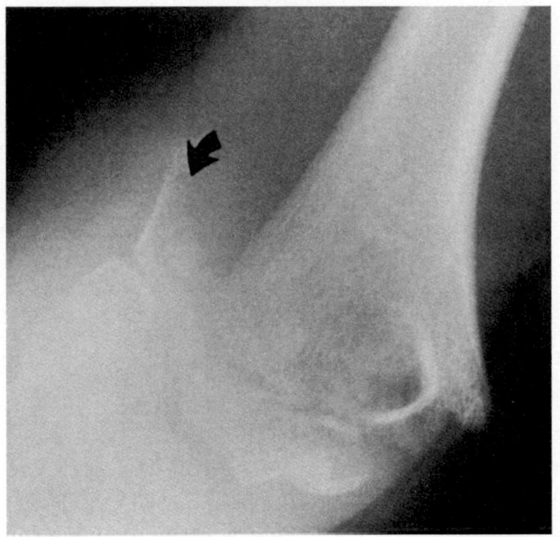

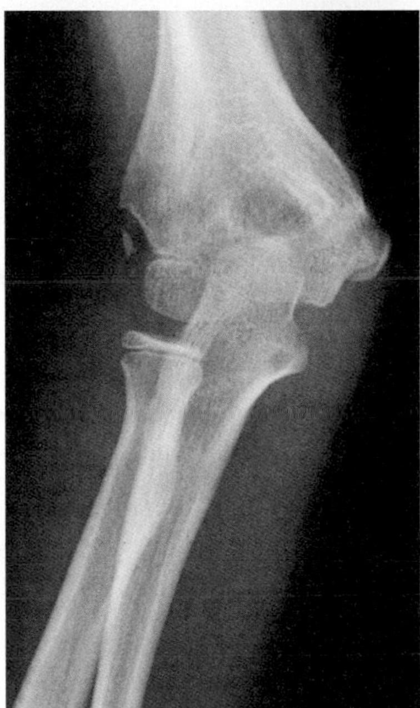

FIGURE 14-68 Flexion valgus deformity. Lateral **(A)** and AP **(B)** views of a flexion-type supracondylar fracture. The distal fragment (*arrow*) is laterally displaced in the coronal plane as well. **C.** Despite aggressive treatment, there was mild residual cubitus valgus plus a flexion contracture when the fracture healed. (From Wilkins KE. Residuals of elbow trauma in children. Orthop Clin N Am 1990;21:291–314, with permission.)

Radiographic Findings

The radiographic appearance of the distal fragment varies from mild angular deformity to complete anterior displacement. Anterior displacement often is accompanied by medial or lateral translation (Fig. 14-68). Associated fractures of the proximal humerus and radius mandate full radiographic evaluation of the upper extremity. Fracture classification is similar to extension-type supracondylar fractures[73]: type I, nondisplaced fracture; type II, minimally angulated with cortical contact; and type III, totally unstable displaced distal fracture fragment.

Treatment

In general, type I flexion-type supracondylar fractures are stable nondisplaced fractures that can simply be protected in a long-arm cast.[54,61,145,164] If mild angulation, as in a type II fracture, requires some reduction in extension, the arm can be immobilized with the elbow fully extended. Radiographic evaluation with the elbow extended is easily obtained and accurate in determining the adequacy of reduction. Reduction is assessed by evaluating the Baumann angle, the anterior humeral line intersecting the lateral condyle, and the integrity of the medial and lateral columns at the olecranon fossa. If reduction cannot be obtained, as is often the case, or if rotation persists, soft tissue interposition, possibly the ulnar nerve, should be suspected. DeBoeck[54] studied 22 flexion-type supracondylar fractures and found cast treatment satisfactory for nondisplaced fractures. In the other 15 fractures, closed reduction and percutaneous pinning were successful in most patients.

A problem with type III flexion supracondylar fractures is that reduction is not easy to achieve and when achieved, the elbow usually is in extension, making it technically challenging to stabilize the distal fragment using pins.

Types I and II fractures (Figs. 14-69 and 14-70) generally are reduced if any angular displacement is seen on fluoroscopic intraoperative evaluation. Type II fractures can be immobilized in an extension cast with the elbow fully extended (see Fig. 14-70). The cast is removed at 3 weeks. If closed reduction is done without skeletal stabilization, follow-up radiographs usually are taken at 1 week and when the cast is removed at 3 weeks. True lateral radiographs in a fully extended cast are

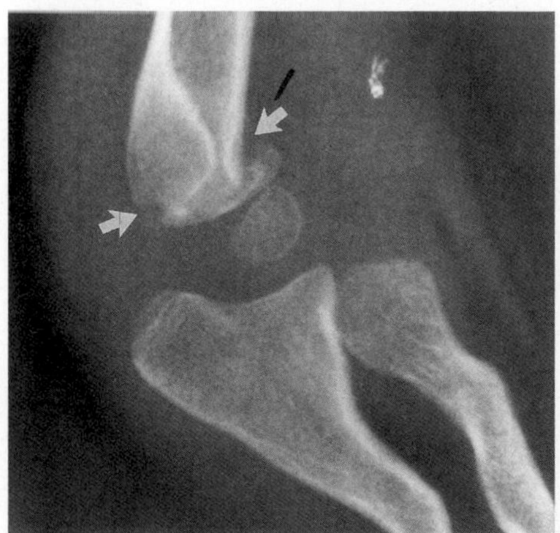

FIGURE 14-69 Type I flexion injury. A type I flexion supracondylar fracture pattern (*arrows*) in a 6-year-old below-the-elbow amputee. There is only about a 10-degree increase in the shaft condylar angle. The patient was treated with a simple posterior splint.

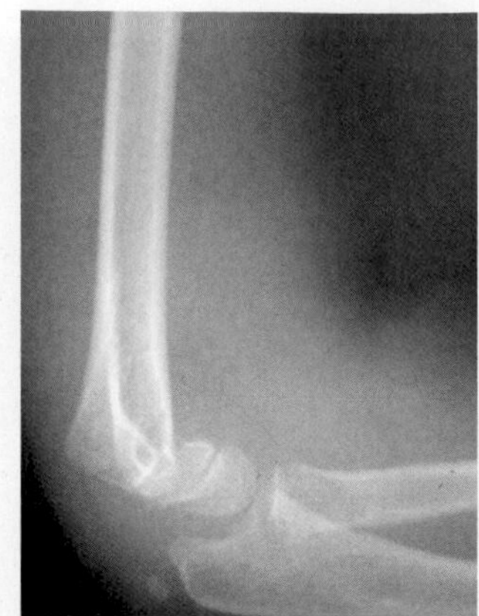

FIGURE 14-71 Lateral view of a flexion-type supracondylar fracture. The capitellum is in front of the anterior humeral line.

important and may require a few attempts or the use of live fluoroscopy.

Pinning generally is required for unstable types II and III flexion supracondylar fractures. The pinning technique de scribed for extension-type supracondylar fractures is not appropriate for this fracture because its instability in flexion precludes pinning with the elbow hyperflexed. In a flexion-type supracondylar fracture, the posterior periosteum is torn, so reduction can be obtained in extension, placing tension across the intact anterior periosteum. In general, a slightly less-than anatomic reduction can be accepted as long as (a) there is no soft tissue interposition of tissue, (b) the Baumann angle is close to that of the other side, and (c) neither flexion nor extension is seen on the lateral view. Although rotating the arm often is possible for a lateral view of an extension supracondylar fracture, the C-arm must be moved to obtain satisfactory radiographic results when pinning a flexion-type supracondylar fracture, because they often are rotationally unstable even when reduced (see Fig. 14-25).

Pinning generally is done with the elbow in approximately 30 degrees of flexion, holding the elbow in a reduced position. A roll of towels under the distal humerus at the fracture site elevates the arm and often aids in fracture reduction. If closed reduction can be obtained, pinning can be accomplished in this position. Placing two lateral-entry pins in the distal fragment first allows them to be used as a joystick to help manipulate the fracture into a reduced position, at which time the pins can be driven across the fracture site (Figs. 14-71 to 14-74).

If the fracture is held in anatomic position with pins, a flexed-arm cast can be used to provide better patient comfort, but a cast with the elbow in almost full extension is acceptable.

Open reduction may be required for flexion-type supracondylar fractures and is best done through an anteromedial or posterior approach, rather than an anterior approach as is used for extension-type supracondylar fractures. With flexion-type fractures, the brachialis remains intact and must be retracted to expose the fracture, necessitating a medial extension to the anterior approach. To ensure that the ulnar nerve is not entrapped in the fracture site, exploring the ulnar nerve or at least identifying it is probably advisable with this fracture, which is another reason for a medial approach to open reduction.

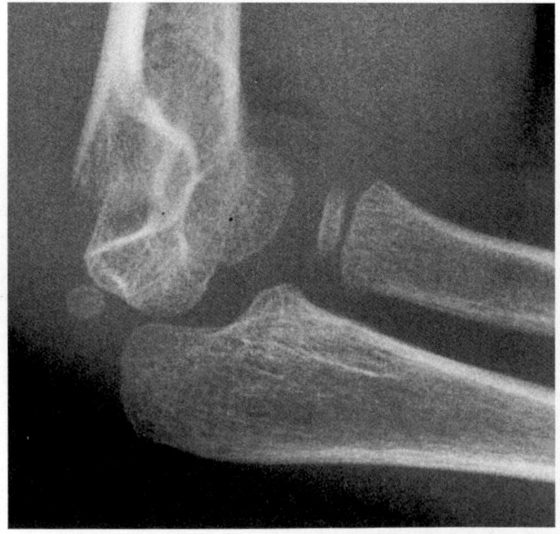

A

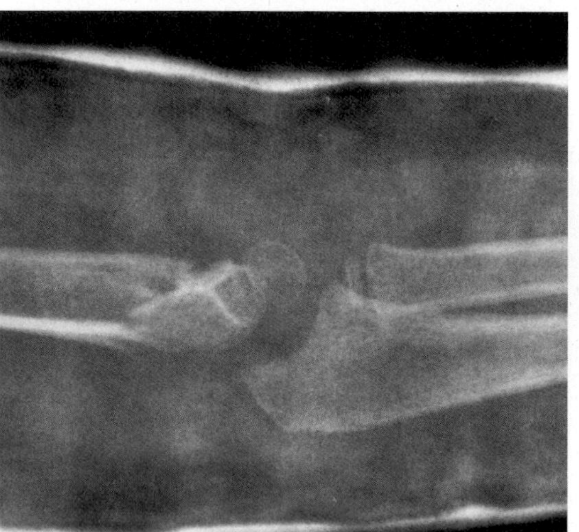

B

FIGURE 14-70 Closed reduction, extension cast. **A.** A 5-year-old girl sustained a type II flexion pattern. **B.** The fracture was manipulated into extension and found to be stable, and was maintained in a long-arm cast in extension.

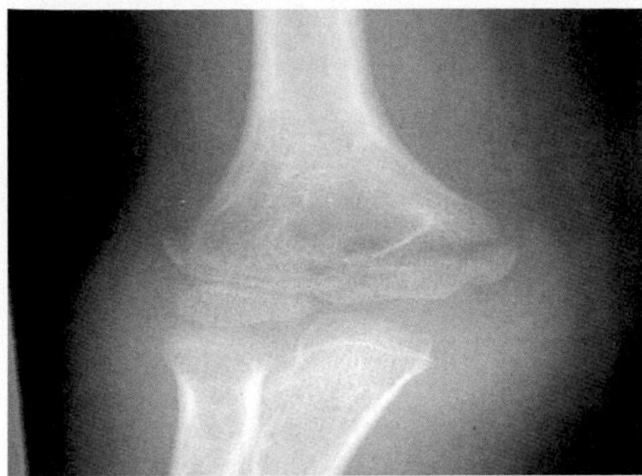

FIGURE 14-72 AP view of fracture often underestimates the amount of displacement if taken of a bent elbow rather than a true AP of the distal humerus.

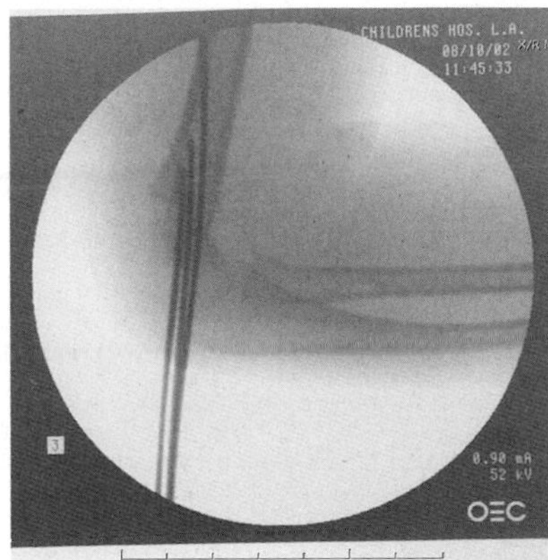

FIGURE 14-73 Intraoperative view shows anatomy has been restored, with the anterior humeral line crossing the middle third of the capitellum.

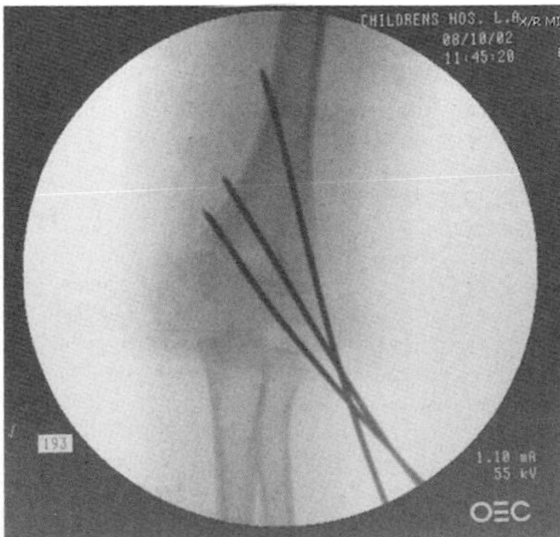

FIGURE 14-74 AP view demonstrates three well-placed lateral pins with maximal separation at fracture site, with all pins engaging solid bone.

Anteromedial Open Reduction of Flexion-Type Supracondylar Fractures

A transverse incision is made across the antecubital fossa, curving proximally posterior to the neuromuscular bundle. Dissection is carried down to the level of the superficial fascia of the forearm and antecubital fossa. The neurovascular bundle is identified and retracted medially. The brachialis and biceps tendons are retracted laterally to expose the fracture site and facilitate reduction. If there is medial soft tissue impingement or a question of ulnar nerve entrapment within the fracture, the dissection should be carried around posterior to the medial epicondyle, so the ulnar nerve and fracture can be identified.

Postoperative immobilization is maintained for 3 or 4 weeks until good callus formation is present. Pins generally are left out through the skin and removed in the office without the need for anesthetic. No formal rehabilitation is given, but the patient is encouraged to begin gentle activities with the arm and to begin regaining motion without a stressful exercise program.

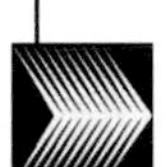

AUTHORS' PREFERRED TREATMENT

In general, we treat type I flexion supracondylar fractures with a splint or cast with the elbow flexed for comfort. Minimally displaced type II fractures that reduce in extension are treated in an extension cast. Unstable types II and III fractures are pinned. Open reduction through an anteromedial or posterior approach is used if an anatomic closed reduction cannot be obtained.

ACKNOWLEDGMENTS

The authors thank James Kasse and James Beaty for their past contributions to this chapter and Kay Daugherty for editing.

REFERENCES

1. Abe M, Ishizu T, Morikawa J. Posterolateral rotatory instability of the elbow after posttraumatic cubitus varus. J Shoulder Elbow Surg 1997;6:405–409.
2. Abe M, Ishizu T, Shirai H, et al. Tardy ulnar nerve palsy caused by cubitus varus deformity. J Hand Surg Am 1995;20(1):5–9.
3. Abraham E, Powers T, Witt P, et al. Experimental hyperextension supracondylar fractures in monkeys. Clin Orthop Relat Res 1982;171:309–318.
4. Ağuş H, Kalenderer O, Kayali C, et al. Skeletal traction and delayed percutaneous fixation of complicated supracondylar humerus fractures due to delayed or unsuccessful reductions and extensive swelling in children. J Pediatr Orthop B 200;11(2):150–154.
5. Aitken AP, Smith L, Blackette CW. Supracondylar fractures in children. Am J Surg 1943;59:161–171.
6. Alburger PD, Weidner PL, Betz RR. Supracondylar fractures of the humerus in children. J Pediatr Orthop 1992;12(1):16–19.
7. Alcott WH, Bowden BW, Miller PR. Displaced supracondylar fractures of the humerus in children: long-term follow-up of 69 patients. J Am Osteopath Assoc 1997;76(12): 910–915.
8. Alonso-Llames M. Bilaterotricipital approach to the elbow. Its application in the osteosynthesis of supracondylar fractures of the humerus in children. Acta Orthop Scand 1972;43(6):479–490.
9. Amillo S, Barrios RH, Martínez-Peric R, et al. Surgical treatment of the radial nerve lesions associated with fractures of the humerus. J Orthop Trauma 1993;7(3):211–215.
10. Amspacher JC, Messenbaugh JF Jr. Supracondylar osteotomy of the humerus for correction of rotational and angular deformities of the elbow. South Med J 1964;7:846–850.
11. Archibald DA, Roberts JA, Smith MG. Transarticular fixation for severely displaced supracondylar fractures in children. J Bone Joint Surg Br 1991;73(1):147–149.
12. Ariño VL, Lluch EE, Ramirez AM, et al. Percutaneous fixation of supracondylar fractures of the humerus in children. J Bone Joint Surg Am 1977;59(7):914–916.
13. Aronson DC, van Vollenhoven E, Meeuwis JD. K-wire fixation of supracondylar humeral fractures in children: results of open reduction via a ventral approach in comparison with closed treatment. Injury 1993;24(3):179–181.
14. Ay S, Akinci M, Kamiloglu S, et al. Open reduction of displaced pediatric supracondy-

lar humeral fractures through the anterior cubital approach. J Pediatr Orthop 2005; 25(2):149–153.
15. Badhe NP, Howard PW. Olecranon screw traction for displaced supracondylar fractures of the humerus in children. Injury 1998;29(6):457–460.
16. Bahk MS, Uma MD, Ain, MC, et al. Patterns of pediatric supracondylar humerus fractures. J Pediatr Orthop 2008;28(5):493–499.
17. Banskota A, Volz RG. Traumatic laceration of the radial nerve following supracondylar fracture of the elbow. A case report. Clin Orthop Relat Res 1984;184:150–152.
18. Barton KL, Kaminsky CK, Green DW, et al. Reliability of a modified Gartland classification of supracondylar humerus fractures. J Pediatr Orthop 2001;21(1):27–30.
19. Battaglia TC, Armstrong DG, Schwend RM. Factors affecting forearm compartment pressures in children with supracondylar fractures of the humerus. J Pediatr Orthop 2002;22(4):431–439.
20. Battle J, Carmichael KD. Incidence of pin track infections in children's fractures treated with Kirschner wire fixation. J Pediatr Orthop 2007;27(2):154–157.
21. Bellemore MC, Barrett IR, Middleton RW, et al. Supracondylar osteotomy of the humerus for correction of cubitus varus. J Bone Joint Surg Br 1984;66(4):566–572.
22. Bender J. Cubitus varus after supracondylar fracture of the humerus in children: can this deformity be prevented? Reconstr Surg Traumatol 1979;17:100–106.
23. Beuerlein MJ, Reid JT, Schemitsch EH, et al. Effect of distal humeral varus deformity on strain in the lateral ulnar collateral ligament and ulnohumeral joint stability. J Bone Joint Surg Am 2004;86(10):2235–2242.
24. Bindra RR. Brachial artery aneurysm following supracondylar fracture of the humerus. Unpublished data; 1990.
25. Blakemore LC, Cooperman DR, Thompson GH, et al. Compartment syndrome in ipsilateral humerus and forearm fractures in children. Clin Orthop Relat Res 2000;376: 32–38.
26. Blanco JS, Gaston G, Cates T, et al. Lateral pin vs crossed pin fixation in type 3 supracondylar (SC) humerus fractures: a randomized prospective study. Presented at 2007 Annual Meeting of the Pediatric Orthopaedic Society of North America, Hollywood, Floida, May 23–26, 2007.
27. Bloom T, Mahar A, Pring M, et al. Comparison of supracondylar humerus fracture pinning when the fracture is not anatomically reduced. Presented at the 34th Annual David H. Sutherland Pediatric Orthopedic Visiting Professorship; May 17–18, 2007.
28. Blount WP. Fractures in Children. Baltimore: Williams & Wilkins, 1955.
29. Bōstman O, Mâkelâ EA, Sōderĝrd J, et al. Absorbable polyglycolide pins in internal fixation of fractures in children. J Pediatr Orthop 1993;13(2):242–245.
30. Boyd DW, Aronson DD. Supracondylar fractures of the humerus: a prospective study of percutaneous pinning. J Pediatr Orthop 1992;12(6):789–794.
31. Brauer CA, Lee BM, Bae DS, et al. A systematic review of medial and lateral entry pinning versus lateral entry pinning for supracondylar fractures of the humerus. J Pediatr Orthop 2007;27(2):181–186.
32. Bronfen CE, Geffard B, Mallet JF. Dissolution of the trochlea after supracondylar fracture of the humerus in childhood: an analysis of six cases. J Pediatr Orthop 2007; 27(5):547–550.
33. Brown IC, Zinar DM. Traumatic and iatrogenic neurological complications after supracondylar humerus fractures in children. J Pediatr Orthop 1995;15(4):440–443.
34. Cairns RA, MacKenzie WG, Culham JA. Urokinase treatment of forearm ischemia complicating supracondylar fracture of the humerus in three children. Pediatr Radiol 1993; 23(5):391–394.
35. Campbell CC, Waters PM, Emans JB, et al. Neurovascular injury and displacement in type III supracondylar humerus fractures. J Pediatr Orthop 1995;15(1):47–52.
36. Carcassonne M, Bergoin M, Hornung H. Results of operative treatment of severe supracondylar fractures of the elbow in children. J Pediatr Surg 1972;7(6):676–679.
37. Carlson CS Jr, Rosman MA. Cubitus varus: a new and simple technique for correction. J Pediatric Orthop 1982;2:199–201.
38. Celiker O, Pestilci FI, Tuzuner M. Supracondylar fractures of the humerus in children: analysis of the results in 142 patients. J Orthop Trauma 1990;4(3):265–269.
39. Charnley J. Closed Treatment of Common Fractures. Edinburgh: Churchill Livingstone, 1961:105–115.
40. Cheng JC, Lam TP, Maffulli N. Epidemiological features of supracondylar fractures of the humerus in Chinese children. J Pediatr Orthop B 2001;10(1):63–67.
41. Cheng JC, Lam TP, Shen WY. Closed reduction and percutaneous pinning for type III displaced supracondylar fractures of the humerus in children. J Orthop Trauma 1995; 9(6):511–515.
42. Cheng JC, Ng BK, Ying SY, et al. A 10-year study of the changes in the pattern and treatment of 6,493 fractures. J Pediatr Orthop 1999;19(3):344–350.
43. Chess DG, Leahey JL, Hyndman JC. Cubitus varus: significant factors. J Pediatr Orthop 1994;14(2):190–192.
44. Choi PD, Melikian R, Skaggs DL. Management of vascular injuries in pediatric supracondylar humeral fractures. Presented at the Annual Meeting of American Academy of Pediatrics, Section of Orthopaedics. San Francisco, CA, 2008.
45. Copley LA, Dormans JP, Davidson RS. Vascular injuries and their sequelae in pediatric supracondylar humeral fractures: toward a goal of prevention. J Pediatr Orthop 1996; 16(1):99–103.
46. Cotton FJ. Elbow fractures in children. Ann Surg 1902;35:252–269.
47. Coventry MB, Henderson CC. Supracondylar fractures of the humerus: 49 cases in children. Rocky Mt Med J 1956;53(5):458–465.
48. Cramer KE, Devito DP, Green NE. Comparison of closed reduction and percutaneous pinning versus open reduction and percutaneous pinning in displaced supracondylar fractures of the humerus in children. J Orthop Trauma 1992;6(4):407–412.
49. Cramer KE, Green NE, Devito DP. Incidence of anterior interosseous nerve palsy in supracondylar humerus fractures in children. J Pediatr Orthop 1993;13(4):502–505.
50. Culp RW, Osterman AL, Davidson RS, et al. Neural injuries associated with supracondylar fractures of the humerus in children. J Bone Joint Surg Am 1990;72(8): 1211–1215.
51. D'Ambrosia RD. Supracondylar fractures of humerus—prevention of cubitus varus. J Bone Joint Surg Am 1972;54(1):60–66.
52. Danielsson L, Pettersson H. Open reduction and pin fixation of severely displaced supracondylar fractures of the humerus in children. Acta Orthop Scand 1980;51(2): 249–255.
53. Davids JR, Maguire MF, Mubarak SJ, et al. Lateral condylar fracture of the humerus following posttraumatic cubitus varus. J Pediatr Orthop 1994;14(4):466–470.
54. De Boeck H. Flexion-type supracondylar elbow fractures in children. J Pediatr Orthop 2001;21(4):460–463.
55. De Boeck H, De Smet P, Penders W, et al. Supracondylar elbow fractures with impaction of the medial condyle in children. J Pediatr Orthop 1995;15(4):444–448.
56. Dellon AL. Musculotendinous variations about the medial humeral epicondyle. J Hand Surg Br 1986;11(2):175–181.
57. DeRosa GP, Graziano GP. A new osteotomy for cubitus varus. Clin Orthop Relat Res 1988;236:160–165.
58. Devnani AS. Late presentation of supracondylar fracture of the humerus in children. Clin Orthop Relat Res 2005;431:36–41.
59. Dimeglio A. Growth in pediatric orthopaedics. In: Morrissy RT, Weinsten SL, eds. Lovell and Winters's Pediatric Orthopaedics. 6th ed. Philadelphia: Lippincott Williams and Wilkins, 2006:35–65.
60. Dormans JP, Squillante R, Sharf H. Acute neurovascular complications with supracondylar humerus fractures in children. J Hand Surg Am 1995;20(1):1–4.
61. el-Ahwany MD. Supracondylar fractures of the humerus in children with a note on the surgical correction of late cubitus varus. Injury 1974;6(1):45–56.
62. Farnsworth CL, Silva PD, Mubarak SJ. Etiology of supracondylar humerus fractures. J Pediatr Orthop 1998;18(1):38–42.
63. Fleuriau-Chateau P, McIntyre W, Letts M. An analysis of open reduction of irreducible supracondylar fractures of the humerus in children. Can J Surg 1998;41:112–118.
64. Flynn JC, Matthews JG, Benoit RL. Blind pinning of displaced supracondylar fractures of the humerus in children. Sixteen years' experience with long-term follow-up. J Bone Joint Surg Am 1974;56(2):263–272.
65. Flynn JC, Zink WP. Fractures and dislocations of the elbow. In: MacEwan GD, Kasser JR, Heinrich SD, eds. Pediatric Fractures: A Practical Approach to Assessment and Treatment. Baltimore: Williams & Wilkins, 1993:133–164.
66. Fowles JV, Kassab MT. Displaced supracondylar fractures of the elbow in children. A report on the fixation of extension and flexion fractures by two lateral percutaneous pins. J Bone Joint Surg Br 1974;56(3):490–500.
67. France J, Strong M. Deformity and function in supracondylar fractures of the humerus in children variously treated by closed reduction and splinting, traction, and percutaneous pinning. J Pediatr Orthop 1992;12(4):494–498.
68. French PR. Varus deformity of the elbow following supracondylar fractures of the humerus in children. Lancet 1959;2:439–441.
69. Furrer M, Mark G, Ruedi T. Management of displaced supracondylar fractures of the humerus in children. Injury 1991;22(4):259–262.
70. Gaddy BC, Manske PR, Pruitt DL, et al. Distal humeral osteotomy for correction of posttraumatic cubitus varus. J Pediatr Orthop 1994;14(2):214–219.
71. Gadgil A, Hayhurst C, Maffulli N, et al. Elevated, straight-arm traction for supracondylar fractures of the humerus in children. J Bone Joint Surg Br 2005;87(1):82–87.
72. Gao GX. A simple technique for correction of cubitus varus. Chin Med J (Engl) 1986; 99:853–854.
73. Gartland JJ. Management of supracondylar fractures of the humerus in children. Surg Gynecol Obstet 1959;109:145–154.
74. Gates DJ. Supracondylar fracture of humerus: problem in children managed with open reduction. Orthop Rev 1982;11:91–98.
75. Gehling H, Gotzen L, Giannadakis, K et al. [Treatment and outcome of supracondylar humeral fractures in childhood]. Unfallchirurg 1995;98(2):93–97.
76. Gillingham BL, Rang M. Advances in children's elbow fractures. J Pediatr Orthop 1995; 15(4):419–421.
77. Godley DR, Leong JCY, Yau A. Open reduction and internal fixation of supracondylar fractures of the humerus in children in Hong Kong: long-term results. Abbot Proc 1978;9:30–34.
78. Gordon JE, Patton CM, Luhmann SJ, et al. Fracture stability after pinning of displaced supracondylar distal humerus fractures in children. J Pediatr Orthop 2001;21(3): 313–318.
79. Graham B, Tredwell SJ, Beauchamp RD, et al. Supracondylar osteotomy of the humerus for correction of cubitus varus. J Pediatr Orthop 1990;10(2):228–231.
80. Green DW, Widmann RF, Frank JS, et al. Low incidence of ulnar nerve injury with crossed pin placement for pediatric supracondylar humerus fractures using a mini-open technique. J Orthop Trauma 2005;19(3):158–163.
81. Gruber MA, Hudson OC. Supracondylar fracture of the humerus in childhood. End result study of open reduction. J Bone Joint Surg Am 1964;46:1245–1252.
82. Gupta N, Kay RM, Leitch K, et al. Effect of surgical delay on perioperative complications and need for open reduction in supracondylar humerus fractures in children. J Pediatr Orthop 2004;24(3):245–248.
83. Gurkan I, Bayrakci K, Tasbas B, et al. Posterior instability of the shoulder after supracondylar fractures recovered with cubitus varus deformity. J Pediatr Orthop 2002;22(2): 198–202.
84. Hadlow AT, Devane P, Nicol RO. A selective treatment approach to supracondylar fracture of the humerus in children. J Pediatr Orthop 1996;16(1):104–106.
85. Hagen R. Skin-traction-treatment of supracondylar fractures of the humerus in children. A ten-year review. Acta Orthop Scand 1964;35:138–148.
86. Hart GM, Wilson DW, Arden GP. The operative management of the difficult supracondylar fracture of the humerus in the child. Injury 1977;9(1):30–34.
87. Hayakawa DJ, Aldington RA. Moore acute traumatic compartment syndrome: a systematic review of results of fasciotomy. Trauma 2009;11(1):5–35.
88. Henrikson B. Supracondylar fracture of the humerus in children. A late review of end results with special reference to the cause of deformity, disability, and complications. Acta Chir Scand 1966;369(Suppl):1–72.
89. Heppenstall RB, Sapega AA, Scott R, et al. The compartment syndrome. An experimental and clinical study of muscular energy metabolism using phosphorus nuclear magnetic resonance spectroscopy. Clin Orthop Relat Res 1988;226:138–155.
90. Higaki T, Ikuta Y. The new operation method of the domedosteotomy for four children with varus deformity of the elbow joint. J Jpn Orthop 1982;31:300–335.
91. Holden CE. The pathology and prevention of Volkmann's ischaemic contracture. J Bone Joint Surg Br 1979;61(3):296–300.
92. Houshian S, Mehdi B, Larsen MS. The epidemiology of elbow fracture in children: analysis of 355 fractures, with special reference to supracondylar humerus fractures. J Orthop Sci 2001;6:312–315.
93. Hoyer A. Treatment of supracondylar fracture of the humerus by skeletal traction in an abduction splint. J Bone Joint Surg Am 1952;34(3):623–637.

94. Ikram MA. Ulnar nerve palsy: a complication following percutaneous fixation of supracondylar fractures of the humerus in children. Injury 1996;27(5):303–305.
95. Iobst CA, Spurdle C, King WF, et al. Percutaneous pinning of pediatric supracondylar humerus fractures with the semisterile technique: the Miami experience. J Pediatr Orthop 2007;27(1):17–22.
96. Ippolito E, Moneta MR, D'Arrigo C. Posttraumatic cubitus varus. Long-term follow-up of corrective supracondylar humeral osteotomy in children. J Bone Joint Surg Am 1990;72(5):757–765.
97. Iyengar SR, Hoffinger SA, Townsend DR. Early versus delayed reduction and pinning of type III displaced supracondylar fractures of the humerus in children: a comparative study. J Orthop Trauma 1999;13(1):51–55.
98. Johnson E, Oppenheim WL. The problem: cubitus varus after elbow fracture. Orthop Consultation 1985;8–12.
99. Kaewpornsawan K. Comparison between closed reduction with percutaneous pinning and open reduction with pinning in children with closed totally displaced supracondylar humeral fractures: a randomized controlled trial. J Pediatr Orthop B 2001;10(2): 131–137.
100. Kagan N, Herold HZ. Correction of axial deviations after supracondylar fractures of the humerus in children. Int Surg 1973;58(10):735–737.
101. Kallio PE, Foster BK, Paterson DC. Difficult supracondylar elbow fractures in children: analysis of percutaneous pinning technique. J Pediatr Orthop 1992;12(1):11–15.
102. Kanaujia RR, Ikuta Y, Muneshige H, et al. Dome osteotomy for cubitus varus in children. Acta Orthop Scand 1988;59:314–317.
103. Karakurt L, Ozdemir H, Yilmaz E, et al. Morphology and dynamics of the ulnar nerve in the cubital tunnel after percutaneous cross-pinning of supracondylar fractures in children's elbows: an ultrasonographic study. J Pediatr Orthop B 2005;14(3):189–193.
104. Kasser JR. Location of treatment of supracondylar fractures of the humerus in children. Clin Orthop Relat Res 2005;434:110–113.
105. Kasser JR, Beaty JH. Supracondylar fractures of the distal humerus. In: Beaty JH, Kasser JR, eds. Rockwood and Wilkins' Fractures in Children. 6th ed. Philadelphia: Lippincott Williams and Wilkins, 2006:543–589.
106. Kekomäki M, Luoma R, Rikalainen H, et al. Operative reduction and fixation of a difficult supracondylar extension fracture of the humerus. J Pediatr Orthop 1984;4(1): 13–15.
107. Keppler P, Salem K, Schwarting B, et al. The effectiveness of physiotherapy after operative treatment of supracondylar humeral fractures in children. J Pediatr Orthop 2005; 25(3):314–316.
108. Khare GN, Gautam VK, Kochkar VL, et al. Prevention of cubitus varus deformity in supracondylar fractures of the humerus. Injury 1991;22(3):202–206.
109. Kim HT, Song MB, Conjares JN, et al. Trochlear deformity occurring after distal humeral fractures: magnetic resonance imaging and its natural progression. J Pediatr Orthop 2002;22(2):188–193.
110. Kocher MS, Kasser JR, Waters PM, et al. Lateral entry compared with medial and lateral entry pin fixation for completely displaced supracondylar humeral fractures in children. A randomized clinical trail. J Bone Joint Surg Am 2007;89(4):706–712.
111. Kocher T. Beitrage zur Kenntniss Einiger Praktisch Wichtiger Fracturformen. Basel: Carl Sallman; 1895.
112. Koudstaal MJ, De Ridder VA, De Lange S, et al. Pediatric supracondylar humerus fractures: the anterior approach. J Orthop Trauma 2002;16(6):409–412.
113. Kramhoft M, Keller IL, Solgaard S. Displaced supracondylar fractures of the humerus in children. Clin Orthop Relat Res 1987;221:215–220.
114. Krebs B. Surgical treatment of supracondylar humeral fractures in children. Ugeskr Laeger 1980;142(14):871–872.
115. Kurer MH, Regan MW. Completely displaced supracondylar fracture of the humerus in children. A review of 1708 comparable cases. Clin Orthop Relat Res 1990;256: 205–214.
116. Labelle H, Bunnell WP, Duhaime M, et al. Cubitus varus deformity following supracondylar fractures of the humerus in children. J Pediatr Orthop 1982;2(5):539–546.
117. Lal GM, Bhan S. Delayed open reduction for supracondylar fractures of the humerus. Int Orthop 1991;15(3):189–191.
118. Lalanandham T, Laurence WN. Entrapment of the ulnar nerve in the callus of a supracondylar fracture of the humerus. Injury 1984;16(2):129–130.
119. Langenskiöld A, Kivilaakso R. Varus and valgus deformity of the elbow following supracondylar fractures of the humerus. Acta Orthop Scand 1967;38:313–320.
120. Larson L, Firoozbakhsh K, Passarelli R, et al. Biomechanical analysis of pinning techniques for pediatric supracondylar humerus fractures. J Pediatr Orthop 2006;26(5): 573–578.
121. Laupattarakasem W, Mahaisavariya B, Kowsuwon W, et al. Pentalateral osteotomy for cubitus varus. Clinic experience of a new technique. J Bone Joint Surg Br 1989;71: 667–670.
122. Lee YH, Lee SK, Kim BS, et al. Three lateral divergent or parallel pin fixations for the treatment of displaced supracondylar humerus fractures in children. J Pediatr Orthop 2008;28(4):417–422.
123. Lee SS, Mahar AT, Miesen D, et al. Displaced pediatric supracondylar humerus fractures: biomechanical analysis of percutaneous pinning techniques. J Pediatr Orthop 2002;22(4):440–443.
124. Leet AI, Frisancho J, Ebramzadeh E. Delayed treatment of type 3 supracondylar humerus fractures in children. J Pediatr Orthop 2002;22(2):203–207.
125. Leitch KK, Kay RM, Femino JD, et al. Treatment of multidirectionally unstable supracondylar humeral fractures in children. A modified Gartland type-IV fracture. J Bone Joint Surg Am 2006;88(5):980–985.
126. Lipscomb PR, Burleson RJ. Vascular and neural complications in supracondylar fractures of the humerus in children. J Bone Joint Surg Am 1955;37(3):487–492.
127. Lyons JP, Ashley E, Hoffer MM. Ulnar nerve palsies after percutaneous cross-pinning of supracondylar fractures in children's elbows. J Pediatr Orthop 1998;18(1):43–45.
128. Mahan ST, May CD, Kocher MS. Operative management of displaced flexion supracondylar humerus fractures in children. J Pediatr Orthop 2007;27(5):551–556.
129. Mapes RC, Hennrikus WL. The effect of elbow position on the radial pulse measured by Doppler ultrasounography after surgical treatment of supracondylar elbow fractures in children. J Pediatr Orthop 1998;18(4):441–444.
130. Marck KW, Kooiman AM, Binnendijk B. Brachial artery rupture following supracondylar fracture of the humerus. Neth J Surg 1986;38(3):81–84.
131. Marion J, LaGrange J, Faysse R, et al. Les fractures de l'extremite inferieure de l'humerus chez enfant. Rev Chir Orthop 1962;48:337–413.
132. Martin DF, Tolo VT, Sellers DS, et al. Radial nerve laceration and retraction associated with a supracondylar fracture of the humerus. J Hand Surg 1989;14(3):542–545.
133. McCoy GF, Piggot J. Supracondylar osteotomy for cubitus varus. The value of the straight arm position. J Bone Joint Surg Br 1988;70:283–286.
134. McGraw JJ, Akbarnia BK, Hanel DP, et al. Neurological complications resulting from supracondylar fractures of the humerus in children. J Pediatr Orthop 1986;6(6): 647–650.
135. McKee MD. To the editor: progressive cubitus varus due to a bony physeal bar in a 4-year-old girl following a supracondylar fracture. A case report. J Orthop Trauma 2006;20(5):372.
136. McLauchlan GJ, Walker CR, Cowan B, et al. Extension of the elbow and supracondylar fractures in children. J Bone Joint Surg Br 1999;81(3):402–405.
137. Mehlman CT, Crawford AH, McMillion TL, et al. Operative treatment of supracondylar fractures of the humerus in children: the Cincinnati experience. Acta Orthop Belg 1996;62(Suppl 1):41–50.
138. Mehlman CT, Strub WM, Roy DR, et al. The effect of surgical timing on the perioperative complications of treatment of supracondylar humeral fractures in children. J Bone Joint Surg Am 2001;83(3):323–327.
139. Mehserle WL, Meehan PL. Treatment of the displaced supracondylar fracture of the humerus (type III) with closed reduction and percutaneous cross-pin fixation. J Pediatr Orthop 1991;11(6):705–711.
140. Michael SP, Stanislas MJ. Localization of the ulnar nerve during percutaneous wiring of supracondylar fractures in children. Injury 1996;27(5):301–302.
141. Millis MB, Singer IJ, Hall JE. Supracondylar fracture of the humerus in children. Further experience with a study in orthopaedic decision-making. Clin Orthop Relat Res 1984; 188:90–97.
142. Mitsunari A, Munishige H, Ikuta Y, et al. Internal rotation deformity and tardy ulnar nerve palsy after supracondylar humeral fracture. J Shoulder Elbow Surg 1995;4(1 Pt 1):23–29.
143. Mubarak SJ, Carroll NC. Volkmann's contracture in children: aetiology and prevention. J Bone Joint Surg Br 1979;61B(3):285–293.
144. Nacht JL, Ecker ML, Chung SM, et al. Supracondylar fractures of the humerus in children treated by closed reduction and percutaneous pinning. Clin Orthop Relat Res 1983;177:203–209.
145. Nand S. Management of supracondylar fracture of the humerus in children. Int Surg 1972;57(11):893–898.
146. Nassar A, Chater E. Open reduction and Kirschner wire fixation for supracondylar fracture of the humerus. J Bone Joint Surg Br 1976;58:135–136.
147. Nork SE, Hennrikus WL, Loncarich DP, et al. Relationship between ligamentous laxity and the site of upper extremity fractures in children: extension supracondylar fracture versus distal forearm fracture. J Pediatr Orthop B 1999;8(2):90–92.
148. O'Driscoll SW, Spinner RJ, McKee MD, et al. Tardy posterolateral rotatory instability of the elbow due to cubitus varus. J Bone Joint Surg Am 2001;83(9):1358–1369.
149. Ogino T, Minami A, Fukuda K. Tardy ulnar nerve palsy caused by cubitus varus deformity. J Hand Surg Br 1986;11(3):352–356.
150. Oh CW, Park BC, Kim PT, et al. Completely displaced supracondylar humerus fractures in children: results of open reduction versus closed reduction. J Orthop Sci 2003;8(2): 137–141.
151. Onwuanyi ON, Nwobi DG. Evaluation of the stability of pin configuration in K-wire fixation of displaced supracondylar fractures in children. Int Surg 1998;83:271–274.
152. Oppenheim WL, Clader TJ, Smith C, et al. Supracondylar humeral osteotomy for traumatic childhood cubitus varus deformity. Clin Orthop Relat Res 1984;188:34–39.
153. Otsuka NY, Kasser JR. Supracondylar fractures of the humerus in children. J Am Acad Orthop Surg 1997;5:19–26.
154. Ottolenghi CE. Acute ischemic syndrome: its treatment prophylaxis of Volkmann's syndrome. Am J Orthop 1960;2:312–316.
155. Palmer EE, Niemann KK, Vesely D, et al. Supracondylar fractures of the humerus in children. J Bone Joint Surg Am 1978;60(5):653–656.
156. Peters CL, Scott SM, Stevens PM. Closed reduction and percutaneous pinning of displaced supracondylar humerus fractures in children: description of a new closed reduction technique for fractures with brachialis muscle entrapment. J Orthop Trauma 1995; 9(5):430–434.
157. Pirone AM, Graham HK, Krajbich JI. Management of displaced extension-type supracondylar fractures of the humerus in children. J Bone Joint Surg Am 1988;70(5): 641–650.
158. Pirone AM, Krajbich JI, Graham HK. Management of displaced supracondylar fractures of the humerus in children [letter]. J Bone Joint Surg Am 1989;71:313.
159. Ponce BA, Hedequist DJ, Zurakowski D, et al. Complications and timing of follow-up after closed reduction and percutaneous pinning of supracondylar humerus fractures: follow-up after percutaneous pinning of supracondylar humerus fractures. J Pediatr Orthop 2004;24(6):610–614.
160. Prietto CA. Supracondylar fractures of the humerus. A comparative study of Dunlop's traction versus percutaneous pinning. J Bone Joint Surg Am 1979;61(3):425–428.
161. Ramachandran M, Birch R, Eastwood DM. Clinical outcome of nerve injuries associated with supracondylar fractures of the humerus in children. The experience of a specialist referral centre. J Bone Joint Surg Br 2006;88(1):90–94.
162. Ramachandran M, Skaggs DL, Crawford HA, et al. Delaying treatment of supracondylar fractures in children: Has the pendulum swung too far? J Bone Joint Surg Br 2008; 90(9):1228–1233.
163. Ramsey RH, Griz J. Immediate open reduction and internal fixation of severely displaced supracondylar fractures of the humerus in children. Clin Orthop Relat Res 1973; 90:131–132.
164. Rang M. Children's Fractures. Philadelphia: JB Lippincott, 1974.
165. Rasool MN. Ulnar nerve injury after K-wire fixation of supracondylar humerus fractures in children. J Pediatr Orthop 1998;18(5):686–690.
166. Ray SA, Ivory JP, Beavis JP. Use of pulse oximetry during manipulation of supracondylar fractures of the humerus. Injury 1991;22(2):103–104.
167. Reitman RD, Waters P, Millis M. Open reduction and internal fixation for supracondylar humerus fractures in children. J Pediatr Orthop 2001;21(2):157–161.
168. King D, Secor C. Bow elbow (cubitus varus). J Bone Joint Surg Am 1951;33:572–576.
169. Royce RO, Dutkowsky JP, Kasser JR, et al. Neurologic complications after K-wire fixa-

tion of supracondylar humerus fractures in children. J Pediatr Orthop 1991;11(2): 191–194.
170. Royle SG, Burke D. Ulna neuropathy after elbow injury in children. J Pediatr Orthop 1990;10(4):495–496.
171. Rowell PJW. Arterial occlusion in juvenile humeral supracondylar fracture. Injury 1974; 6:254–256.
172. Sabharwal S, Tredwell SJ, Beauchamp RD, et al. Management of pulseless pink hand in pediatric supracondylar fractures of humerus. J Pediatr Orthop 1997;17(3):303–310.
173. Sairyo K, Henmi T, Kanematsu Y, et al. Radial nerve palsy associated with slightly angulated pediatric supracondylar humerus fracture. J Orthop Trauma 1997;11(3): 227–229.
174. Sankar WN, Hebela NM, Skaggs DL, et al. Loss of pin fixation in displaced supracondylar humeral fractures in children: causes and prevention. J Bone Joint Surg Am 2007; 89(4):713–717.
175. Schonenecker PL, Delgado E, Rotman M, et al. Pulseless arm in association with totally displaced supracondylar fracture. J Orthop Trauma 1996;10(6):410–415.
176. Sharrad WJW. Pediatric Orthopaedics and Fractures. Oxford: Blackwell Scientific, 1971.
177. Shaw BA, Kasser JR, Emans JB, et al. Management of vascular injuries in displaced supracondylar humerus fractures without arteriography. J Orthop Trauma 1990;4(1): 25–29.
178. Shifrin PG, Gehring HW, Iglesias LJ. Open reduction and internal fixation of displaced supracondylar fractures of the humerus in children. Orthop Clin N Am 1976;7(3): 573–581.
179. Sibinski M, Sharma H, Bennet GC. Early versus delayed treatment of extension type-3 supracondylar fractures of the humerus in children. J Bone Joint Surg Br 2006;88(3): 380–381.
180. Simanovsky N, Lamdan R, Mosheiff R. Underreduced supracondylar fracture of the humerus in children: clinical significance at skeletal maturity. J Pediatr Orthop 2007; 27(7):733–738.
181. Skaggs DL. Closed reduction and pinning of supracondylar humerus fractures. In Tolo VT, Skaggs DL, eds. Masters Techniques in Orthopaedic Surgery: Pediatric Orthopaedics. Philadelphia: Lippincott, 2007: 1–15.
182. Skaggs DL, Cluck MW, Mostofi A, et al. Lateral-entry pin fixation in the management of supracondylar fractures in children. J Bone Joint Surg Am 2004;86A(4):702–707.
183. Skaggs DL, Hale JM, Bassett J, et al. Operative treatment of supracondylar fractures of the humerus in children. The consequence of pin placement. J Bone Joint Surg Am 2001;83(5):735–740.
184. Skaggs DL, Mirzayan R. The posterior fat pad sign in association with occult fracture of the elbow in children. J Bone Joint Surg Am 1999;81(10):1429–1433.
185. Skaggs DL, Sankar WN, Albrektson J, et al. How safe is the operative treatment of Gartland type 2 supracondylar humerus fractures in children? J Pediatr Orthop 2008; 28(2):139–141.
186. Smith FM. Surgery of the Elbow. Philadelphia: WB Saunders, 1972.
187. Smith L. Supracondylar fractures of the humerus treated by direct observation. Clin Orthop Relat Res 1967;50:37–42.
188. Spinner RJ, O'Driscoll SW, Davids JR, et al. Cubitus varus associated with dislocation of both the medial portion of the triceps and the ulnar nerve. J Hand Surg Am 1999; 24(4):718–726.
189. Spinner M, Schreiber SN. Anterior interosseous-nerve paralysis as a complication of supracondylar fractures of the humerus in children. J Bone Joint Surg Am 1969;51(8): 1584–1590.
190. Spinner RJ, Jacobson SR, Nunley JA. Fracture of a supracondylar humeral myositis ossificans. J Orthop Trauma 1995;9(3):263–265.
191. Sunderland S. The intraneural topography of the radial, median, and ulnar nerves. Brain 1945;68(4):243–298.
192. Sweeney JG. Osteotomy of the humerus for malunion of supracondylar fractures. J Bone Joint Surg Br 1975;57:117.
193. Takahara M, Sasaki I, Kimura T, et al. Second fracture of the distal humerus after varus malunion of a supracondylar fracture in children. J Bone Joint Surg Br 1998;80(5): 791–797.
194. Theruvil B, Kapoor V, Fairhurst J, et al. Progressive cubitus varus due to a bony physeal bar in a 4-year-old girl following a supracondylar fracture: a case report. J Orthop Trauma 2005;19(9):669–672.
195. Topping RE, Blanco JS, Davis TJ. Clinical evaluation of crossed-pin versus lateral-pin fixation in displaced supracondylar humerus fractures. J Pediatr Orthop 1995;15(4): 435–439.
196. Uchida Y, Sugioka Y. Ulnar nerve palsy after supracondylar humerus fracture. Acta Orthop Scand 1990;61(2):118–119.
197. Voss FR, Kasser JR, Trepman E, et al. Uniplanar supracondylar humeral osteotomy with preset Kirschner wires for posttraumatic cubitus varus. J Pediatr Orthop 1994; 14(4):471–478.
198. Walloe A, Egund N, Eikelund L. Supracondylar fracture of the humerus in children: review of closed and open reduction leading to a proposal for treatment. Injury 1985; 16(5):296–299.
199. Watson-Jones R. Fractures and Joint Injuries. Edinburgh: ES Livingstone, 1956.
200. Weiland AJ, Meyer S, Tolo VT, et al. Surgical treatment of displaced supracondylar fractures of the humerus in children. Analysis of fifty-two cases followed for five to fifteen years. J Bone Joint Surg Am 1978;60:657–661.
201. Weiss JM, Kay RM, Waters P. Distal humeral osteotomy for supracondylar fracture malunion in children: a study of perioperative complications. To be published in Am J Orthop Surg, January 2010.
202. Wilkins KE, Beaty J. Fractures in Children. Philadelphia: Lippincott-Raven, 1966.
203. Williamson DM, Cole WG. Treatment of selected extension supracondylar fractures of the humerus by manipulation and strapping in flexion. Injury 1993;24(4):249–252.
204. Willis RB, Rorabeck CH. Treatment of compartment syndrome in children. Orthop Clin N Am 1990;21(2):401–412.
205. Wiltse LL. Valgus deformity of the ankle: a sequel to acquired or congenital abnormalities of the fibula. J Bone Joint Surg Am 1972;54(3):595–606.
206. Wind WM, Schwend RM, Armstrong DG. Predicting ulnar nerve location in pinning of supracondylar humerus fractures. J Pediatr Orthop 2002;22(4):444–447.
207. Wong HK, Balasubramaniam P. Humeral torsional deformity after supracondylar osteotomy for cubitus varus: its influence on the postosteotomy carrying angle. J Pediatr Orthop 1992;12(4):490–493.
208. Worlock PH, Colton C. Severely displaced supracondylar fractures of the humerus in children: a simple method of treatment. J Pediatr Orthop 1987;7(1):49–53.
209. Yang Z, Wang Y, Gilula LA, et al. Microcirculation of the distal humeral epiphyseal cartilage: implications for posttraumatic growth deformities. J Hand Surg Am 1998; 23(1):165–172.
210. Yun YH, Shin SJ, Moon JG. Reverse V osteotomy of the distal humerus for the correction of cubitus varus. J Bone Joint Surg Br 2007;89(4):527–531.
211. Zaltz I, Waters PM, Kasser JR. Ulnar nerve instability in children. J Pediatr Orthop 1996;16(5):567–569.
212. Zenios M, Ramachandran M, Milne B, et al. Intraoperative stability testing of lateral-entry pin fixation of pediatric supracondylar humeral fractures. J Pediatr Orthop 2007; 27(6):695–702.
213. Zionts LE, McKellop HA, Hathaway R. Torsional strength of pin configurations used to fix supracondylar fractures of the humerus in children. J Bone Joint Surg Am 1994; 76(2):253–256.
214. Ziv N, Litwin A, Katz K, et al. Definitive diagnosis of fracture-separation of the distal humeral epiphysis in neonates by ultrasonography. Pediatr Radiol 1996;26(7): 493–496.

15

THE ELBOW: PHYSEAL FRACTURES, APOPHYSEAL INJURIES OF THE DISTAL HUMERUS, OSTEONECROSIS OF THE TROCHLEA, AND T-CONDYLAR FRACTURES

James H. Beaty and James R. Kasser

PHYSEAL FRACTURES 533
Fractures Involving the Lateral Condylar Physis 534
Fractures of the Capitellum 551
Fractures Involving the Medial Condylar Physis 554
Fractures of the Trochlea 561
Fractures Involving the Entire Distal Humeral Physis 561

APOPHYSEAL INJURIES OF THE DISTAL HUMERUS 566
Fractures Involving the Medial Epicondylar Apophysis 566
Fractures through the Epicondylar Apophysis 572
Fractures Involving the Lateral Epicondylar Apophysis 577
Fractures Involving the Olecranon Apophysis 578
Chronic Tension Stress Injuries (Little League Elbow) 580

OSTEONECROSIS OF THE TROCHLEA 580
Vascular Anatomy 580
Patterns of Osteonecrosis 581
Treatment 581

T-CONDYLAR FRACTURES 584
Incidence 584
Mechanism of Injury 584
Fracture Patterns 584
Classification 584
Diagnosis 584
Treatment 585
Complications 589

PHYSEAL FRACTURES

All the physes of the distal humerus are vulnerable to injury, each with a distinct fracture pattern. The vulnerability of the various physes to injury is altered by age and injury mechanism. Next to those of the distal radius, injuries to the distal humeral physes are the most common physeal injuries. In general, the physes of the major long bones are most vulnerable to fracture just before puberty, when the perichondral ring is weakest.[142] Fractures involving the medial epicondylar apophysis are most common in preadolescents (peak ages: 11 to 15 years), probably because many avulsions of this apophysis are associated with posterolateral dislocations, which are also common in this age group. Fractures involving the lateral condylar physis occur early, with the average age around 6 years.[59,73,83,98,142] Fractures concerning the medial condylar physis are rare and occur most often in children 8 to 12 years of age.[59,83,98] Fractures involving the total distal humeral physis may occur in neonates or within the first 2 to 3 years of life.[40,127]

The specific fracture patterns, incidence, and mechanism of injury are discussed in detail in the following sections dealing with these specific fractures.

Fractures Involving the Lateral Condylar Physis

Incidence and Outcome

Fractures involving the lateral condylar region in the immature skeleton either cross the physis or follow it for a short distance into the trochlea. Fractures of the lateral condylar physis constitute 16.9% of distal humeral fractures.

Fractures of the lateral condylar physis are only occasionally associated with injuries outside the elbow region.[67,78,117] Within the elbow region, the associated injuries that can occur with this fracture include dislocation of the elbow (which may be a result of the injury to the lateral condylar physis rather than a separate injury), radial head fractures, and fractures of the olecranon, which are often greenstick fractures. Acute fractures involving only the anatomic capitellum are rare in the immature skeleton.

The diagnosis of lateral condylar physeal injuries may be less obvious both clinically and on radiograph than that of supracondylar fractures, especially if the fracture is minimally displaced. Functional loss of range of motion in the elbow is much more frequent with lateral condylar physis fractures because the fracture line often extends into the articular surface. Malunion of a supracondylar fracture that results in cubitus varus is likely to result in a surgically correctable cosmetic deformity with an essentially normal range of motion in the elbow. A poorly treated lateral condylar physeal injury, however, is likely to result in a significant loss of range of motion that is not as responsive to surgical correction. The complications of supracondylar fractures are usually evident in the immediate postinjury period. The poor outcome of a lateral condylar physeal fracture may not be obvious until months or even years later.[84,172,179] Ippolito et al.[84] evaluated 49 individuals with humeral condylar fractures 18 to 45 years after the injury. Twenty fractures with displacement of 2 mm to 10 mm with no tilting of the osteochondral fragment had been treated without reduction, and 16 fractures with marked displacement and fragment tilting had been treated surgically; all 36 had good results. All 13 patients treated operatively or nonoperatively for old, displaced fractures had poor results. Nonunion developed in four patients, and osteonecrosis occurred in six. Arthrosis of the elbow was found in fractures complicated by osteonecrosis and nonunion and in old fractures when the humeral condyle was resected, but it was not observed in uncomplicated fractures.

Fracture Anatomy and Classification

Milch[119] defined fractures that exited through the trochleocapitellar groove as type I and those that exited through the trochlea as type II. Around the same time, Cotton[35] described more details of the various subluxations of both the fragment and elbow joint that occurred with this type of fracture. He noted that because the fragment was usually still attached to the proximal radius, both the radius and ulna were subluxed. The most common displacement was "outward and backward"; "inward and forward" displacement was rare. Cotton[35] also noted that the main pathology was associated with condylar fragment rotation. He observed that this fracture often resulted in limited extension, had some local lateral outgrowth at the fracture site, and rarely resulted in axial deviation of the elbow unless there was a resultant nonunion. More recent investigators have added little to his description of this lesion's pathology.

Lateral condylar physeal fractures can be classified by either the fracture line's anatomic location or by the stage of displacement, as described by Wilkins.[199]

Anatomic Location. Salter and Harris[160] classified lateral condylar physeal injuries as type IV injuries in their classification of physeal fractures. A true Salter-Harris type IV injury through the ossific nucleus of the lateral condyle is rare. Although lateral condylar fractures are similar to Salter-Harris type II and IV fractures, treatment guidelines follow those of a type IV injury: open reduction and internal fixation of displaced intra-articular fractures, with the potential for mild growth disturbance of the distal humeral physis. There is no contact between the trochlea's ossification center and the exposed bone in the metaphyseal fragment.

Because the fracture line starts in the metaphysis and then courses along the physeal cartilage, it has some of the characteristics of both type II and IV injuries according to the Salter-Harris classification. This fracture classification is debatable, because the fracture exits the joint in the not-yet-ossified cartilage of the trochlea.

Mirsky, Karas, and Weiner[122] compared intraoperative findings to preoperative radiographic classification in 25 displaced fractures of the lateral condyle and found that in 13 (52%), the Milch classification did not correlate with intraoperative findings. Eight of 17 fractures (47%) classified preoperatively as Milch type I fractures (Fig. 15-1) were unstable, and five of eight fractures classified preoperatively as Milch type II fractures (Fig. 15-2) were extra-articular, extending across the distal humeral physis medially. Mirsky et al.[122] identified three distinct fracture patterns: nine fractures exited the distal humeral epiphysis just medial to the capitellum, 11 exited through the trochlear epiphysis, and five extended across the physis medially. No fracture appeared to traverse the ossified portion of the capitellum (Milch type I).

Stages of Displacement

Displacement has been described as occurring in three stages (Fig. 15-3).[85,193] In the first stage, the fracture is relatively undisplaced, and the articular surface is intact (Fig. 15-3A,B). Because the trochlea is intact, there is no lateral shift of the olecranon.

In the second stage, the fracture extends completely through the articular surface (Fig. 15-3C,D). This allows the proximal fragment to become more displaced and can allow lateral displacement of the olecranon. In the third stage, the condylar fragment is rotated and totally displaced laterally and proximally, which allows translocation of both the olecranon and the radial head (Fig. 15-3E,F).

Badelon et al.[8] modified the description of stage I displacement to include fractures with less than 2 mm of displacement seen on the anteroposterior (AP) or lateral radiograph only or seen on both views.

Soft Tissue Injuries

The fracture line usually begins in the posterolateral metaphysis, with a soft tissue tear in the area between the origins of the

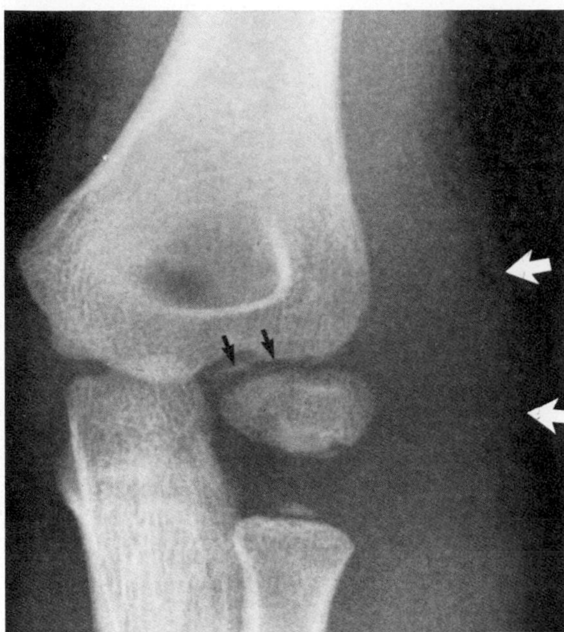
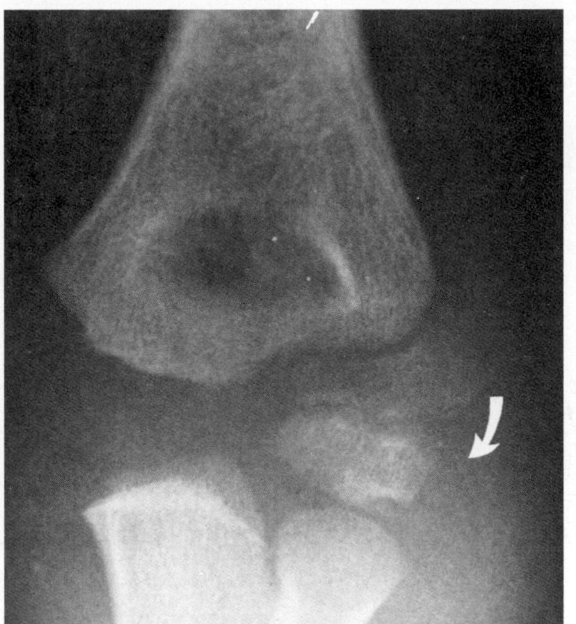

FIGURE 15-1 A. Injury film of a 7-year-old with an undisplaced fracture of the lateral condyle (*small arrows*). Attention was drawn to the location of the fracture because of extensive soft tissue swelling on the lateral aspect (*white arrows*). **B.** Because of the extensive soft tissue injury, there was little intrinsic stability, allowing the fracture to become displaced at 7 days (*arrow*).

extensor carpi radialis longus and the brachioradialis muscle. The extensor carpi radialis longus and brevis muscles remain attached to the free distal fragment, along with the lateral collateral ligaments of the elbow. If there is much displacement, both the anterior and posterior aspects of the elbow capsule are usually torn. This soft tissue injury, however, is usually localized to the lateral side and may help identify a minimally displaced fracture. More extensive soft tissue swelling at the fracture site may indicate more severe soft tissue injury,[106,143] which may indicate that the fracture is prone to late displacement.

Displacement of the Fracture and Elbow Joint. The degree of displacement varies according to the magnitude of the force applied and whether the cartilaginous hinge of the articular surface remains intact. If the articular surface is intact, the resultant displacement of the condylar fragment is simply a lateral tilt hinging on the intact medial articular surface. Horn et al.[82] studied 16 lateral humeral condylar fractures with radiographs and magnetic resonance imaging (MRI) and determined that all fractures unstable on radiograph had disruption of the cartilage hinge on MRI, confirming the relation of the cartilage hinge on fracture stability. If the fracture is complete, the fragment can be rotated and displaced varying degrees; in the most severe fractures, rotation is almost the full 180 degrees, so that the lateral condylar articular surface opposes the denuded metaphyseal fracture surface. Wilson[203] showed that in addition to this coronal rotation of the distal fragment, rotation can also occur in the horizontal plane. The lateral margin is carried posteriorly, and the medial portion of the distal fragment rotates anteriorly.

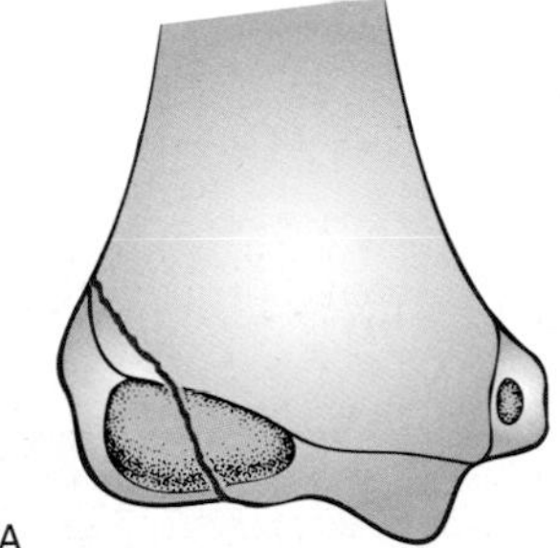
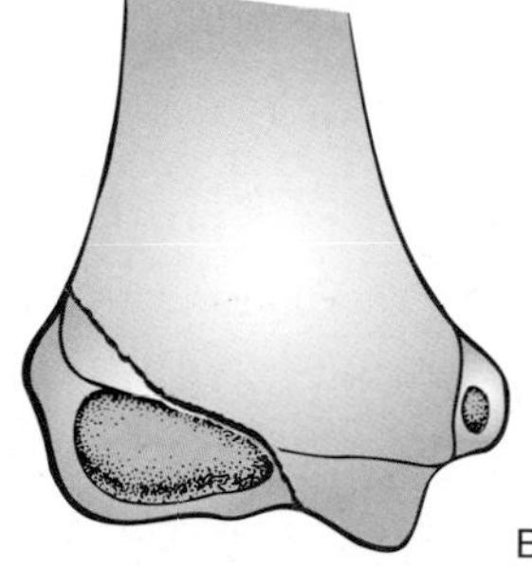

FIGURE 15-2 Physeal fractures of the lateral condyle. **A.** Physeal injury (Milch type II) through the nonossified trochlea. **B.** Physeal injury (Milch type I) through the ossific nucleus of the lateral condyle. (Adapted and reprinted with permission from Milch HE. Fractures and fracture–dislocations of the humeral condyles. J Trauma 1964;4:592–607.)

Because the usual fracture line disrupts the lateral crista of the trochlea, the elbow joint is unstable, creating the possibility of posterolateral subluxation of the proximal radius and ulna. Thus, the forearm rotates along the coronal plane into valgus, and there may also be lateral translocation of the lateral condyle with the radius and ulna (Fig. 15-4). This concept of lateral translocation is important in the late reconstruction of untreated fractures.

In physeal fractures, where the fracture line traverses the lateral condylar epiphysis, the elbow remains reasonably stable because the trochlea remains intact. Total coronal rotation of the condylar fragment can occur with this injury. The axial deformity that results is pure valgus without translocation (see Fig. 15-4).

This posterolateral elbow instability with the lateral condylar physeal injury has led to the mistaken concept that this injury is associated with a primary dislocation of the elbow,[32] which is rarely the case. The posterolateral instability of the elbow is usually a result of the injury, not a cause of it.[156]

Mechanism of Injury. As Heyl[79] stated, the local biomechanics of the distal humerus must be different in children because this

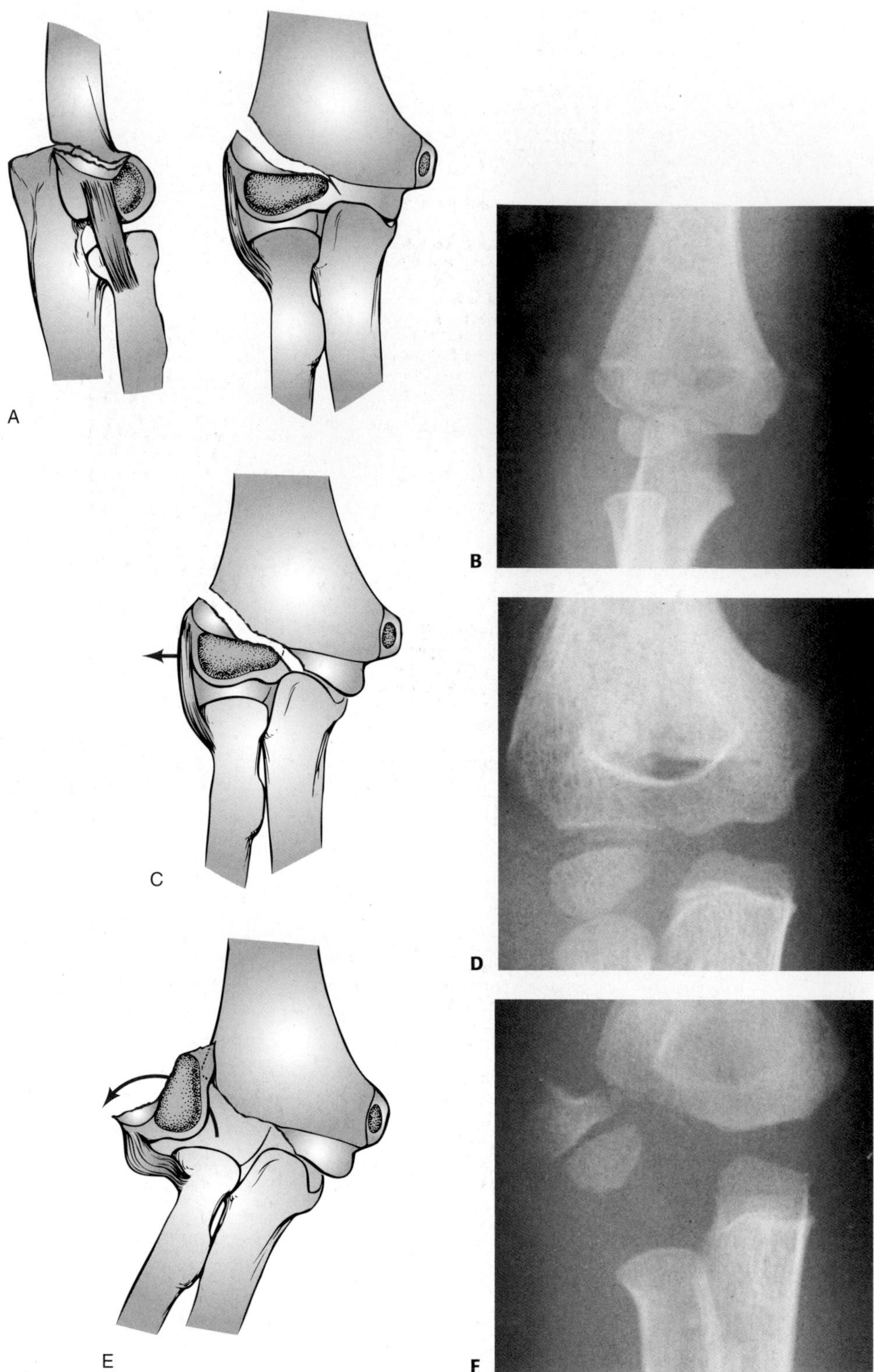

FIGURE 15-3 Stages of displacement. **A,B.** Stage I displacement—articular surface intact. **C,D.** Stage II displacement—articular surface disrupted. **E,F.** Stage III displacement—fragment rotated. (A, C, and E: Reprinted with permission from Jakob R, Fowles JV, Rang M, et al. Observations concerning fractures of the lateral humeral condyle in children. J Bone Joint Surg Br 1975;57:430–436.)

injury is rare in adults. Two mechanisms have been suggested: "push-off" and "pull-off." The pull-off or avulsion theory has more advocates than the push-off mechanism.[85,181] In early studies,[181] this injury was consistently produced in young cadavers by adducting the forearm with the elbow extended and the forearm supinated. The work of Jakob and Fowles[85] confirmed the results of these studies. Some of Stimson's[181] work strengthens the push-off theory. In his cadaver studies, he produced the injury by applying a sharp blow to the palm when the elbow was flexed[35]; other investigators have speculated that because the forearm goes into valgus when extended, the radial head can push off the lateral condyle or that the injury can result from a direct blow to the olecranon.

It is likely that both mechanisms can produce this injury. The more common type of fracture, which extends to the apex of the trochlea, is probably a result of avulsion forces on the condyle, with the olecranon's sharp articular surface serving to direct the force along the physeal line into the trochlea. When a child falls forward on his or her palm with the elbow flexed, the radial head is forced against the capitellum and may cause

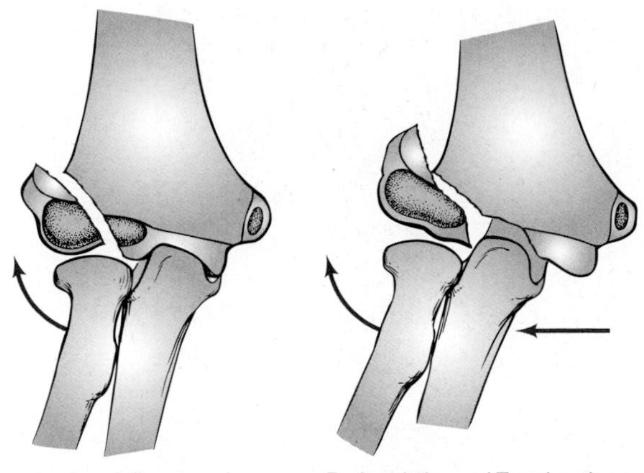

FIGURE 15-4 Angular deformities. **A.** Milch type I fractures tend only to angulate. **B.** Milch type II fractures are unstable with lateral translocation in addition to angulation. (Adapted and reprinted with permission from Milch HE. Fractures and fracture–dislocations of the humeral condyles. J Trauma 1964;4:592–607.)

the less common Milch type I physeal fracture that courses through the ossific nucleus of the capitellum.

Signs and Symptoms. Compared with the marked distortion of the elbow that occurs with displaced supracondylar fractures, little distortion of the elbow, other than that produced by the fracture hematoma, may be present with lateral condylar fractures. The key to the clinical evaluation of this fracture is the location of soft tissue swelling concentrated over the lateral aspect of the distal humerus.[106] Stage I displacement may produce only local tenderness at the condylar fracture site, which may be increased by forcibly flexing the wrist. Stage II or III displacement may result in some local crepitus with motion of the lateral condylar fragment. The benign appearance of the elbow with some stage I and II displacements may account for the delay of parents seeking treatment for a child with a minimally displaced fracture.

Radiographic Findings. The radiographic appearance varies according to the fracture line's anatomic location and the displacement stage. In the AP view, the metaphyseal flake may be small and seemingly minimally displaced. The degree of displacement can often be better appreciated on the true lateral view. In determining whether the articular hinge is intact (i.e., stage I vs. stage II), the relationship of the proximal ulna to the distal humerus is evaluated for the presence of lateral translocation. Oblique views are especially helpful in patients in whom a stage I displacement is suspected.

In a prospective study of 112 children with nondisplaced and minimally displaced fractures of the lateral condyle, Finnbogason et al.[54] identified three groups of fractures: stable fractures, fractures with an undefinable risk, and fractures with a high risk of later displacement. Stable fractures had no gap or a small gap and did not extend all the way to the epiphyseal cartilage; most of these 65 fractures were in younger children and none had later displacement. Fractures with undefinable risk of displacement were the same type as stable fractures, but the fracture could be clearly observed extending all the way to the epiphyseal cartilage; displacement occurred in 6 (17%) of these 35 fractures. High-risk fractures had a gap that was as wide or almost as wide laterally as medially; displacement occurred in five of 12 (42%) of these fractures.

Kamegaya et al.[90] reported that MRI evaluation of 12 minimally displaced (less than 2 mm on radiograph) lateral condylar fractures identified five fractures that crossed the physis into the joint space and were unstable fractures. One of five fractures with 1-mm displacement was unstable, and four fractures of seven with 2-mm displacement were unstable. These investigators suggested that MRI evaluation might prevent late displacement or delayed union by identifying those minimally displaced fractures that required percutaneous pin fixation rather than cast immobilization.

To determine the importance of the internal oblique view in the radiographic evaluation of nondisplaced or minimally displaced lateral condylar fractures, Song et al.[177] compared the oblique view to standard anteroposterior views in 54 children. They found that 38 fractures (70%) had different amounts of displacement on the two views; 30 of these had more displacement on the oblique view than on the AP view and eight had more displacement on the AP view. Fracture patterns differed between the two views in 75%. These authors recommended routine use of an internal oblique view if a lateral condylar fracture is suspected to evaluate the amount of fracture displacement and to assess stability.

A major diagnostic difficulty lies in differentiating this fracture from a fracture of the entire distal humeral physis. In a young child in whom the condyle is unossified, an arthrogram or MRI may be helpful (Figs. 15-5, 15-6, and 15-7).[67] Potter[31] recommended MRI with thin (1.5-mm to 2-mm) sections and appropriate pulse sequencing to provide differential contrast between subchondral bone, cartilage, and joint fluid. Chapman et al.[29] recommended multidetector computed tomography (MDCT) for the evaluation of pediatric lateral condylar fractures because it is painless and fast, usually requiring no sedation even in very young children, and is highly reproducible. They compared MDCT to standard radiographs in 10 children with lateral condylar fractures and found that interobserver agreement was better with MDCT than with radiographs regarding fracture displacement and fracture classification. Based on MDCT, fracture management was altered in two patients with displacement near the surgical threshold of 2 mm. Their study also suggested that cartilage integrity can be assessed on MDCT in patients with fracture displacement of more than 2 mm. Because of its relatively high cost compared to standard radiographs, MDCT probably should be reserved for evaluation of fractures in which displacement is near 2 mm so that appropriate surgical or conservative treatment can be chosen.

In fractures of the entire distal humeral physis, the proximal radius and ulna are usually displaced posteromedially (Fig. 15-8A). The relationship of the lateral condylar ossification center to the proximal radius remains intact. In true fractures involving only the lateral condylar physis, the relationship of the condylar ossification center to the proximal radius is lost (Fig. 15-8B). In addition, any displacement of the proximal radius and ulna is more likely to be lateral due to the loss of stability provided by the lateral crista of the distal humerus.

Treatment Methods. Fractures involving the lateral condylar physis can be treated with simple immobilization alone,

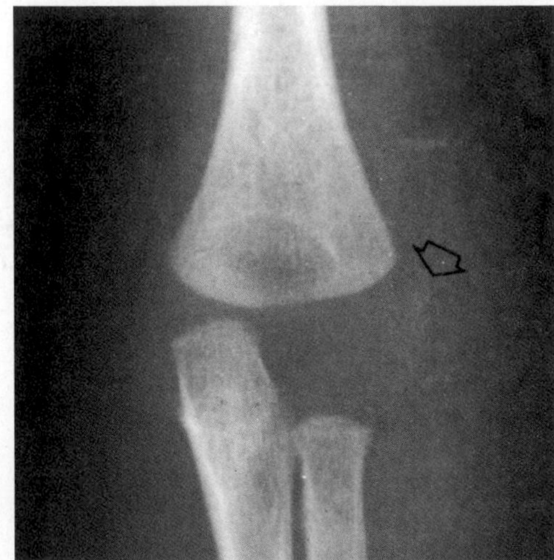

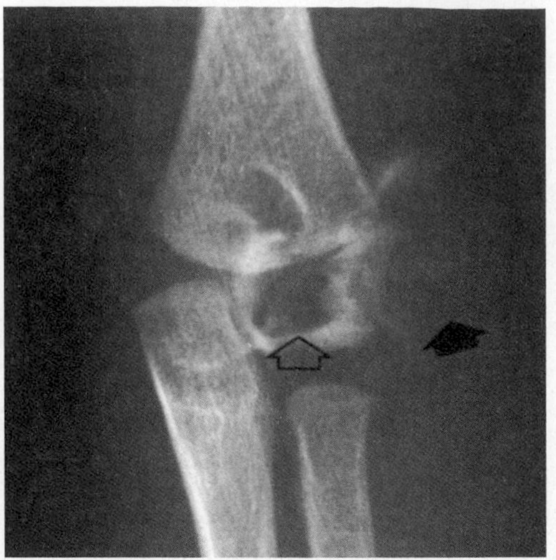

FIGURE 15-5 Unossified lateral condyle. **A.** AP view. A small ossific nucleus can barely be seen (*arrow*) in the swollen lateral soft tissues. **B.** An arthrogram shows the defect left by the displaced lateral condyle (*open arrow*). The displaced condyle is outlined in the soft tissues (*solid arrow*).

closed reduction and percutaneous pinning, or open surgical reduction.

Immobilization

Minimally displaced fractures are stable and have considerable intrinsic soft tissue attachments that prevent displacement of the distal fragment. About 40% of lateral condylar physeal fractures are sufficiently undisplaced so that they can be treated by simple immobilization without surgical intervention.[85] If the fracture line is barely perceptible on the original radiograph (stage I displacement), the degree of displacement is usually minimal and the chance for subsequent displacement is low. Radiographs should be obtained weekly for the first 3 weeks after injury to ensure that late displacement does not occur.

Undisplaced fractures can usually be treated via simple immobilization with good results. Speed and Macey[178] reported uniformly excellent results both anatomically and functionally in patients with undisplaced fractures, none of whom had any abnormalities of growth or premature physeal fusion. Simple immobilization of nondisplaced or minimally displaced (less than 2 mm) fractures in a sling, collar and cuff, or posterior splint appears adequate.[8,10,11,20,178] Close follow-up and repeat radiographs to detect any late displacement are mandatory if this method is used.

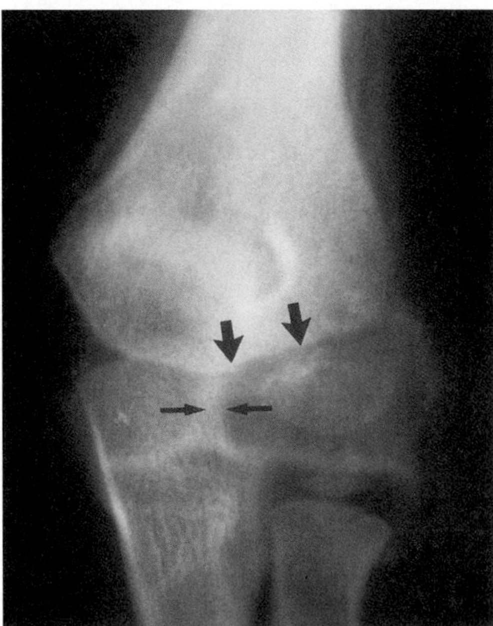

FIGURE 15-6 Arthrogram of stage I fracture of the lateral condyle (*large arrows*). Articular surface is intact with no displacement (*small arrows*).

In their long-term study of fractures treated nonoperatively, Badelon et al.[8] determined that only fractures with type I displacement (i.e., the fracture line is seen on only one radiographic view) can be safely treated nonoperatively. In their experience, any fracture with displacement, even of less than 2 mm, can displace later in the cast or splint. In a review of 57 fractures of the lateral condyle, Beaty and Wood[11] found that two of 24 fractures with stage I displacement displaced late. Bast, Hoffer, and Aval[10] reported a union rate of 98% after nonoperative treatment of 95 nondisplaced or minimally displaced fractures of the lateral humeral condyle. Their criteria for nonoperative treatment were acute fracture (less than 24 hours at initial evaluation) and displacement of less than 2 mm in three radiographic planes (AP, lateral, and internal oblique). Two fractures that displaced 6 and 9 days after closed reduction required open reduction and internal fixation before they united without complications.

Late Displacement

Careful clinical examination is important in predicting which fractures will displace later. The potential to displace often depends more on the degree of associated soft tissue injury and whether the articular cartilage of the trochlea is intact, rather than on the amount of initial displacement. Considerable soft tissue swelling on the lateral aspect of the distal humerus, which can be appreciated both clinically and on radiographs, should alert the physician to the fact that the fracture may be unstable and has the potential to displace. If crepitus between the fragments is detected with motion of the forearm or elbow, significant loss of soft tissue attachments and a potentially unstable fracture should be suspected.[35]

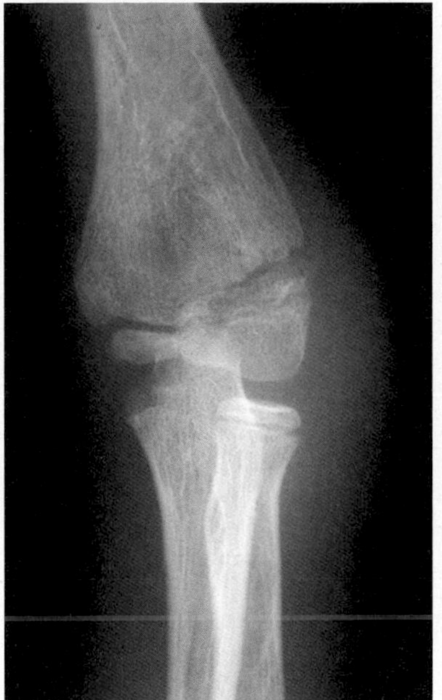
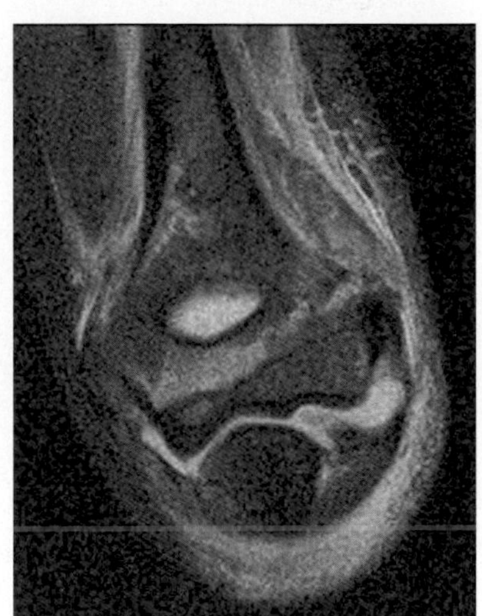

FIGURE 15-7 A. Radiograph of a stable type II fracture of the lateral condyle in a 10-year-old child. **B.** Gradient-echo MRI clearly differentiates this fracture from a fracture of the entire distal humeral physis.

Closed Reduction and Percutaneous Pinning

Several techniques have been described for initial reduction, with the recommended elbow position ranging from hyperflexion to full extension; however, it appears from clinical experience and experimental studies that reduction is best achieved with the forearm supinated and the elbow extended. Placing a varus stress on the extended elbow allows further room for manipulation of the fragment. Unfortunately, it is difficult to maintain reduction of a displaced lateral condylar fracture with closed techniques, and closed reduction is not recommended for treating stage III displaced lateral condylar fractures. Minimally displaced fractures can be stabilized with percutaneous pins across the fracture. In lateral condylar physeal fractures with moderate displacement, confirmation of fracture stability by stress testing and arthrography may precede percutaneous pin fixation. Mintzer et al.[121] reported good results after percutaneous pin fixation of 12 lateral condylar fractures with displacement of more than 2 mm. They believed this method is

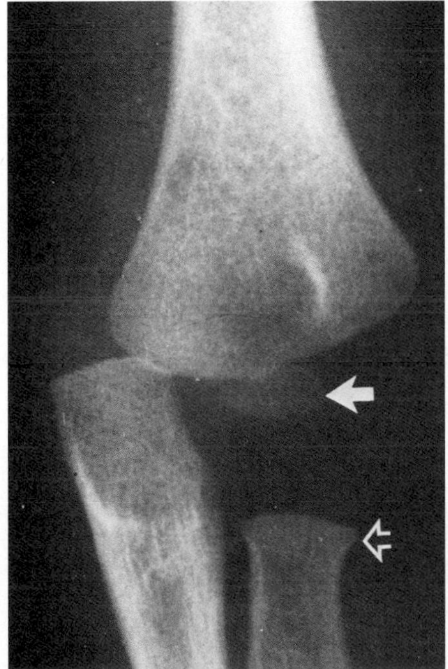
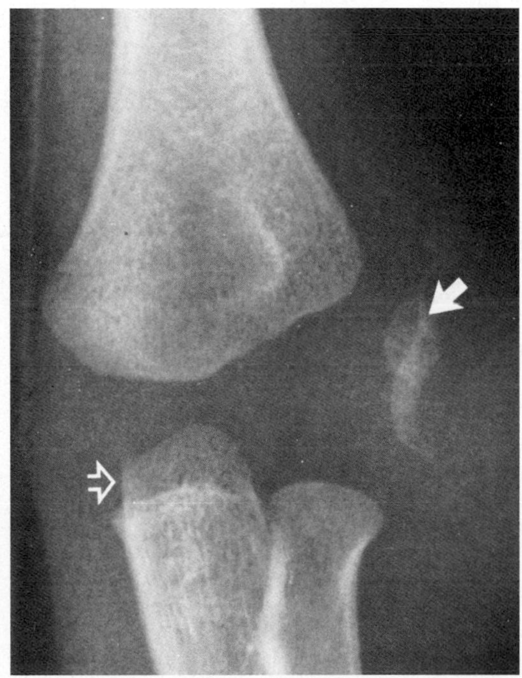

FIGURE 15-8 A. Total distal humeral physeal fracture in a 2-year-old. The lateral condyle (*closed arrow*) has remained in line with the proximal radius. The proximal radius, ulna, and lateral condyle have all shifted medially (*open arrow*). **B.** Displaced fracture of the lateral condyle in a 2-year-old. The relationship of the lateral condyle (*closed arrow*) to the proximal radius is lost. Both the proximal radius and ulna (*open arrow*) have shifted slightly laterally.

appropriate for selected fractures with 2 mm to 4 mm of displacement and an arthrographically demonstrated congruent joint surface. If a satisfactory reduction cannot be obtained, then reduction should be achieved and maintained by open reduction and internal fixation.

More recently, Song et al.[177] reported good results in 46 (73%) of 63 unstable lateral condylar fractures, 53 of which were treated with closed reduction and percutaneous pinning. They formulated a treatment algorithm based on a five-stage classification system that considered degree of displacement and fracture pattern. Closed reduction was attempted in all fractures, regardless of the amount of displacement. If closed reduction up to 2 mm failed, open reduction and internal fixation were performed. These authors suggested that open reduction is not necessary for all lateral condylar fractures with no less than 2 mm of displacement and rotation of the fragment (stage V in their classification), noting excellent results in three such fractures treated with closed reduction and pinning. They listed three elements as essential to obtaining good results with this treatment protocol: (i) accurate interpretation of the direction of fracture displacement (mainly posterolaterally, not purely laterally) and the amount of displacement of the fracture fragment, (ii) routine intraoperative confirmation of the reduction on both anteroposterior and internal oblique radiographs, and (iii) maintenance of the reduction with two parallel percutaneous Kirschner wires (K-wires).

Arthroscopically-Assisted Reduction and Percutaneous Pinning. To avoid the dissection required for open reduction and anatomic reduction, arthroscopic techniques have been used to reduce the lateral condylar fracture before the insertion of percutaneous pins.[26,76] Micheli et al.,[118] in an earlier study, established the safety and efficacy of elbow arthroscopy in pediatric and adolescent patients with osteochondrosis dissecans, arthrofibrosis, synovitis, acute trauma, and posterior olecranon impingement syndrome. None of their 47 patients had nerve injury, infection, or loss of elbow motion after arthroscopy. Hausman et al.[76] reported arthroscopic reduction and percutaneous pinning of six fractures of the lateral humeral condyle in patients ranging from 2 to 6 years old. All fractures healed within 4 weeks, and all patients had full active and passive ranges of motion and were pain-free at latest evaluation (average 8 months). These authors[76] cited as advantages to the arthroscopic technique improved visualization of the fracture reduction over uniplanar arthrography, the ability to remove fragments from the fracture site, more direct assistance in fracture reduction than that provided by closed reduction, and less dissection than with open reduction. Standard anterolateral and anteromedial arthroscopic portals are used, and K-wires are used as joysticks to reduce the fracture. A 2.5-mm wrist arthroscope may be needed in small patients (usually younger than 3 years), but in older children and adolescents, a standard 4.5-mm arthroscope can be used.

Open Reduction and Internal Fixation

Because of the high incidence of poor functional and cosmetic results with closed reduction methods, open reduction has become the most widely advocated method for unstable fractures with stage II displacement and fractures with stage III displacement.[6,19,20,32,73,85,87,113,125,174,193,201,208] In a study of 97 children with minimally displaced lateral condylar fractures, Launay et al.[99] found that immobilization alone resulted in additional displacement and more nonunions than did operative treatment. About 60% of all fractures involving the lateral condylar physis require open reduction and internal fixation.[85] There is uniform agreement regarding the need for open reduction of displaced fractures of the lateral condylar physis. Most investigators recommend fixation with smooth K-wires in children or screws in adolescents nearing skeletal maturity. Parent et al.,[139] in a biomechanical study, compared compression and stability in simulated lateral condylar fractures fixed with a tension band technique using wire or bioabsorbable sutures. Although the suture tension bands had lower ultimate failure loads and less compression at the fracture site, the authors suggested that fixation with bioabsorbable sutures might be appropriate for small children to avoid the need for surgery to remove fixation materials.[139]

Pin and Screw Fixation. Smooth pins are the most frequently used method of fragment fixation.[11,57,85,178,193,201,208] Blount et al.[19] believed that at least two pins were necessary to prevent rotation. The passage of a smooth wire through the physis does not result in any growth disturbance,[51,105] which is of note because only 20% of the humerus' growth occurs through the distal humeral physis. It also appears that the wires can be placed either parallel or crossed in the distal fragments.

The ideal place for the pins is in the metaphyseal fragment. They should cross at the lateral aspect of the metaphysis and diverge as much as possible to enhance the stability of fixation. If there is only a small metaphyseal fragment, the pins can be placed across the physis without concern.

When adequate reduction and internal fixation are carried out early (i.e., within the first few days after the injury), the results are uniformly good. The key, however, is to be sure that the reduction is adequate. Hardacre et al.[73] found that poor results after open reduction occurred when the reduction was incomplete. Surgery alone does not ensure a good result unless the reduction is nearly anatomic and the fixation is secure.

Early surgical intervention is essential, because organization of the clot with early fibrin development makes it difficult to achieve a reduction without extensive soft tissue dissection in fractures that are treated late. The pins can be buried or left protruding through the skin with a low incidence of infection. Leaving pins buried requires a second operative procedure, even though it usually can be accomplished with a local anesthetic. The fracture generally is sufficiently stable to allow pin removal by 3 to 4 weeks and to allow the patient to begin protected active range of elbow motion at 2 to 3 weeks.

Screw fixation has been used less frequently in children, although Jeffrey[87] recommended it in 1958. Sharma et al.[165] reported painless, full range of elbow motion in 36 of 37 children who had displaced (more than 2 mm in any direction) lateral condylar fractures fixed with partially threaded 4-mm AO cancellous screws. One patient had delayed union, with loss of 10 degrees of elbow motion.

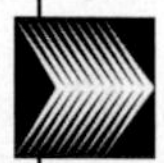

AUTHORS' PREFERRED TREATMENT

Immobilization

If the fracture is minimally displaced on radiograph (i.e., the metaphyseal fragment is less than 2 mm from the proximal fragment on AP and lateral views) and the clinical signs also indicate there is reasonable soft tissue integrity, we simply immobilize the elbow in a long-arm cast with the forearm in neutral rotation and the elbow flexed 60 to 90 degrees. Radiographs are taken within the first 3 to 5 days after the fracture with the cast removed and the elbow comfortably extended. If there is no displacement, the radiographs are repeated in another 3 to 5 days. If the radiographs again show no displacement, then another long-arm cast is applied and is worn for about 3 to 5 weeks, or until fracture union is apparent.

In some fractures with more than the allowable 2 mm of displacement (type II injury), the fracture pattern is such that the articular cartilage appears intact. If there is any question about the stability at the time of the fracture, MRI can be obtained or the extremity can be examined with the patient under general anesthesia. Gentle varus stress views with the forearm supinated and the elbow extended should be taken to determine if the fracture displaces significantly. Preoperative MRI or intraoperative arthrography can be used to determine the stability of the nonossified articular cartilage of the trochlea.

Percutaneous Pins

For fractures with stage II displacement (2 to 4 mm), varus stress views should be obtained and arthrography should be done with the patient under anesthesia. If the fracture is stable, percutaneous pinning is indicated (Fig. 15-9).

Open Reduction

If the fracture is grossly unstable, open reduction and internal fixation are indicated. We prefer open reduction and internal fixation of all fractures with stage III displacement. It is important that open reduction is performed as soon as possible after the injury. The standard lateral Kocher approach provides sufficient exposure of the fragment. Often, a tear in the aponeurosis of the brachioradialis muscle laterally leads directly to the fracture site. Extreme care must be taken to avoid dissecting near the posterior portion of the fragment because this is the entrance of the blood supply of the lateral condylar epiphysis.

Mohan, Hunter, and Colton[124] recommended a posterolateral approach because of the excellent exposure it provides with minimal dissection. Another suggested advantage is the improved cosmetic results by more posterior placement of the surgical scar. Mohan et al.[124] reported no complications in 20 patients in whom this approach was used.

The quality of the reduction is determined by evaluating the fracture line along the anterior aspect of the articular surfaces. This usually can be determined either by direct vision or by digital palpation. We prefer to use smooth K-wires that cross just medial to the condylar fragment to maintain the reduction (Fig. 15-10). The wires penetrate the skin through a separate stab incision posterior to the main incision. A long-arm cast is applied with the elbow flexed 60 to 90 degrees and the forearm in neutral or slight pronation. The cast and pins are removed in 3 weeks if there is adequate healing on radiographs. Early active motion is started at that time. If necessary, pin removal can be delayed 1 to 2 weeks to allow further healing in older children.

Technique of Open Reduction and Internal Fixation of Lateral Humeral Condylar Fractures

The elbow is exposed through a 5- to 6-cm lateral approach, placing two thirds of the incision above the joint and one

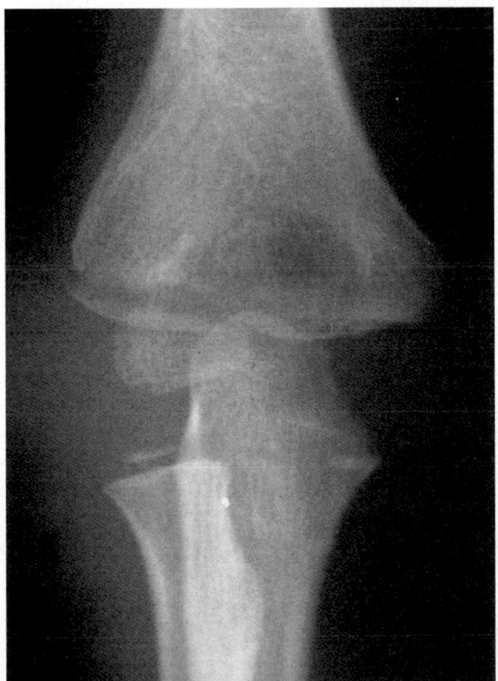
A

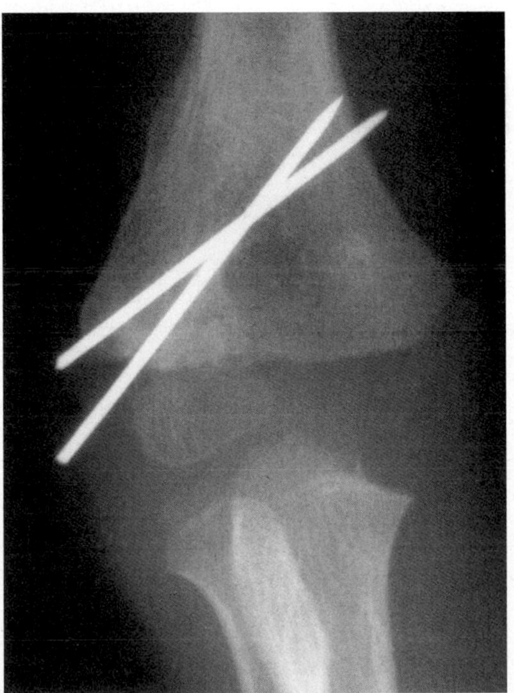
B

FIGURE 15-9 Stage II fracture of the lateral condyle. **A.** AP radiograph shows 4 mm of displacement of the metaphyseal segment; however, the fracture was stable by stress examination and arthrography. **B.** Four weeks after percutaneous pinning, the fracture is healed.

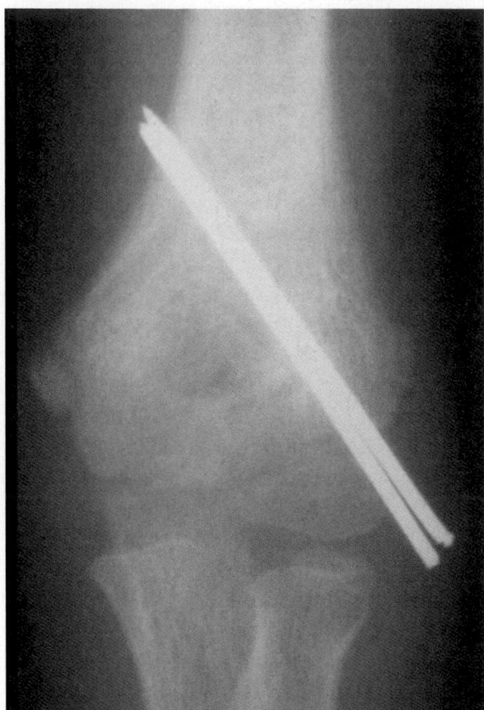

FIGURE 15-10 Fixation of lateral condylar fracture with two smooth K-wires, crossing just medial to the condylar fragment.

third distal (Fig. 15-11). In the interval between the brachioradialis and the triceps, the dissection is carried down to the lateral humeral condyle. The joint's anterior surfaces are exposed by separating the fibers of the common extensor muscle mass. Soft tissue detachment is limited to only that necessary to expose the fragment, the fracture, and the joint; the posterior soft tissues are left intact. Retracting the antecubital structures exposes the anterior joint surface. The trochlea and the more medial entry point of the condylar fracture are inspected. The displacement and the size of the fragment are always greater than is apparent on the radiographs because much of the fragment is cartilaginous. The fragment usually is rotated as well as displaced. The joint is irrigated to remove blood clots and debris, the articular surface and the metaphyseal fragment are reduced accurately, and the reduction is confirmed by observing the articular surface, particularly at the trochlea. The position is held with a small tenaculum, bone holder, or towel clip. When a large metaphyseal fragment is present, two smooth K-wires are inserted across it into the medial portion of the metaphysis. When the epiphyseal portion is small, as is more common, two smooth K-wires are inserted through the condyle, across the physis, and into the humeral metaphysis, penetrating the medial cortex of the humerus. The wires are directed 45 to 60 degrees; the reduction and the position of the internal fixation are checked by AP and lateral radiographs before closing the wound. The ends of the wires are cut off beneath the skin but are left long enough to allow easy removal. The arm is placed in a posterior plaster splint with the elbow flexed 60 to 90 degrees.

The splint is worn for 2 to 3 weeks after surgery. The pins can be removed at 3 weeks if union is progressing. Gentle active motion of the elbow is then usually resumed and continued until full range of motion returns.

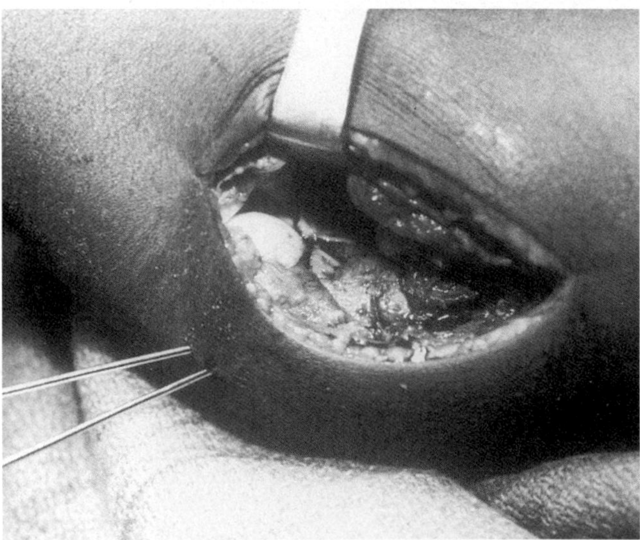

FIGURE 15-11 Lateral approach for open reduction and internal fixation of a lateral humeral condylar fracture of the left elbow. The approach is made through the brachioradialis–triceps interval; an anterior retractor is used to expose the joint surfaces, and the fracture is reduced and pinned percutaneously posterior to the incision.

Delayed Union and Nonunion

If sophisticated surgical treatment is unavailable, these fractures may go untreated or unrecognized for a prolonged period. Even in modern medical settings, elbow injuries may be treated as "sprains," and the diagnosis of a displaced lateral condylar fracture is not made. Thus, patients often present months or even years later with a nonunited or malunited fracture fragment.

Delayed Union. Delayed union, in contrast to nonunion or malunion, occurs in a fracture in which the fracture fragments are in satisfactory position but union of the lateral condylar fragment to the metaphysis is delayed. Various reasons have been suggested for delayed union of lateral condylar fractures. Flynn and Richards[56] speculated that it was caused by poor circulation to the metaphyseal fragment. Hardacre et al.[73] believed that bathing the fracture site by articular fluid inhibited fibrin formation and subsequent callus formation. It is most likely that a combination of these two factors, in addition to the constant tension forces exerted by the muscle arising from the condylar fragment, is responsible for delayed union.

This complication is most common in patients treated nonoperatively. The symptoms and clinical examination determine the aggressiveness of treatment. The fragment is usually stable during clinical examination, the elbow is nontender, and the range of elbow motion increases progressively. On radiographs, the position of the fragment remains unchanged. With time, these fractures usually heal (Fig. 15-12). Lateral spur formation or cubitus varus is relatively common with these fractures. The need for further treatment depends on the presence of significant symptoms or further displacement that may disrupt the joint surface and cause functional impairment. If neither of these conditions is present, the radiographic persistence of the fracture line requires only follow-up observation. If there is any question as to the integrity of the joint surface, an MRI may

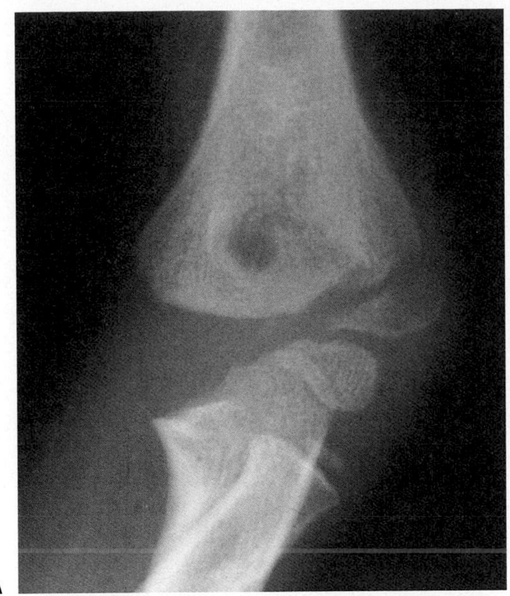

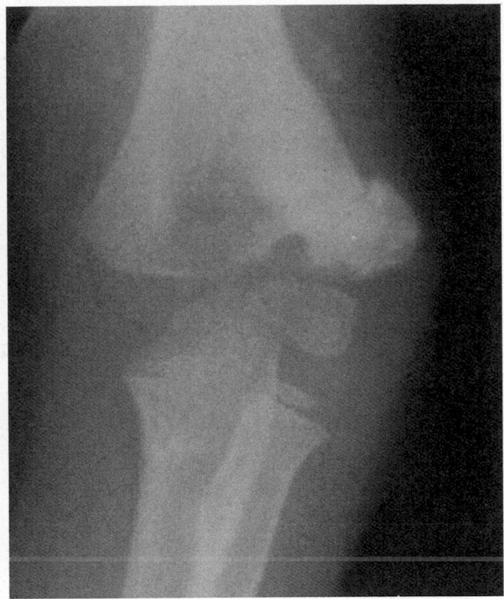

FIGURE 15-12 Delayed union and cubitus varus. **A.** Stage III lateral condylar fracture in a 7-year-old boy was treated in a cast. **B.** Seven months later, delayed union with malunion of the fracture and cubitus varus deformity was present.

help determine any loss of continuity and the need for surgical treatment as a nonunion rather than a simple delayed union.

Flynn and Richards[55] recommended long-term immobilization for minimally displaced fractures with delayed union. They found that 70% of minimally displaced fractures had united by 12 weeks. Jeffrey[87] recommended screw fixation with bone grafting. Hardacre et al.,[73] however, found that minimally displaced fractures with delayed union ultimately united if there was no significant displacement of the condylar fragment.

Controversy exists as to whether elbow function can be improved by a late open reduction and internal fixation of the fracture fragment. Delayed open reduction has been complicated by osteonecrosis and further loss of elbow motion. Speed and Macey[178] were among the first investigators to question whether patients treated with late surgery did better than those not treated. In patients with malunion who were treated late, they found a high incidence of poor results due to "epiphyseal changes" that probably represented osteonecrosis. There have been many subsequent reports of osteonecrosis occurring after late open reduction. The high incidence of osteonecrosis of the fragment is believed to be due to the extensive soft tissue dissection necessary to replace the fragment (Fig. 15-13). Böhler,[20] on the other hand, had good results in his patients with delayed treatment. He avoided extensive soft tissue dissection by approaching the fragment transarticularly after performing an osteotomy of the olecranon. Yang et al.[205] used Böhler's technique in six children with Milch type II lateral condylar fractures with displacement of more than 10 mm, rotation of the fragments, and abundant callus formation. The delay from injury to surgery averaged 4 months and ranged from 2 to 5 months. All fractures and osteotomies united within 3 months of surgery. Four children had excellent functional results and two had good results; all were pain-free.

The key to preventing osteonecrosis is to recognize the course of the blood supply to the lateral condyle. Only a small portion of the condyle is extra-articular. In his studies, Haraldsson[71] found that the vessels that supply the lateral condylar epiphysis penetrate the condyle in a small posterior nonarticular area (Fig. 15-14).

Jakob and Fowles[85] reported that patients treated later than 3 weeks after the fracture did no better than those who received no treatment at all. They found that early callus and fibrous tissue made it extremely difficult to obtain a satisfactory open reduction without performing considerable soft tissue dissection. All their patients treated after 3 weeks lost range of motion (at least 34 degrees on average), and osteonecrosis, premature physeal closure, as well as valgus deformity were common. In patients who received no treatment, valgus deformity due to nonunion and malunion was frequent, but no osteonecrosis of the lateral condylar epiphysis occurred. These investigators recommended that no open reduction should be performed for fractures older than 3 weeks, but that early ulnar nerve transposition should be performed to eliminate the possibility of late ulnar nerve symptoms that occur with cubitus valgus deformity after nonunion. Dhillon et al.[41] and Zionts and Stolz[211] also reported that osteonecrosis was frequent after late open reduction and recommended no treatment for these fractures.

Nonunion. In 1932, Cooper[33] drew attention to the development of nonunion after lateral humeral condylar fractures when he described his findings in two cadaver specimens. He pointed out that there was absolutely no bony continuity between the distal humerus and the condylar fragment. True nonunion with significant deformity is rare because it usually is the result of a nontreated displaced fracture of the lateral condylar physis.[19,113]

True nonunion occurs in patients with progressive displacement of the fragment. The mobile fragment can be palpated, or the patient has weakness or pain in the elbow. According to the criteria of Flynn et al.,[55] if the fracture has not united by 12 weeks, it is classified as a nonunion.

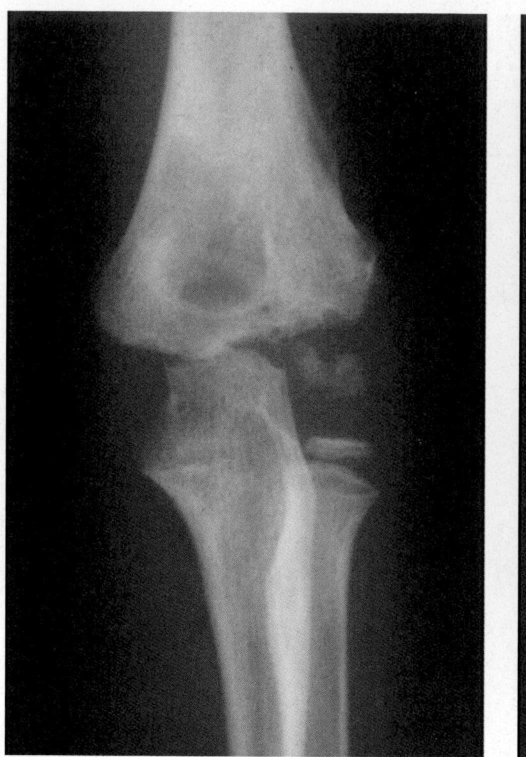

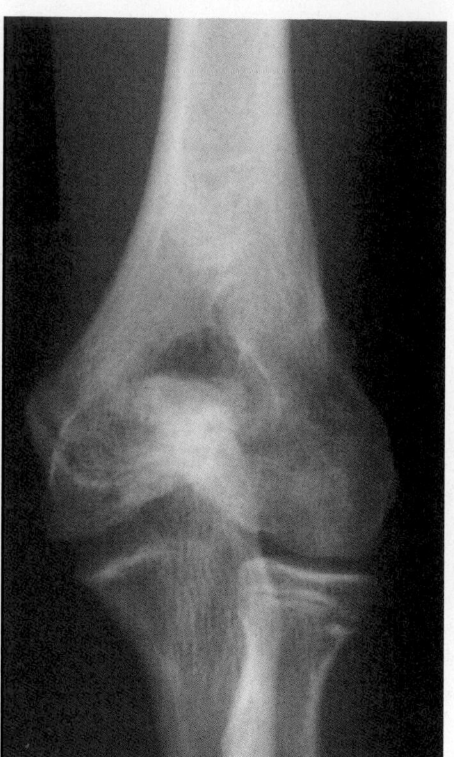

FIGURE 15-13 Osteonecrosis of the lateral condyle after lateral condylar fracture in a 10-year-old boy. AP **(A)** and lateral **(B)** radiographs.

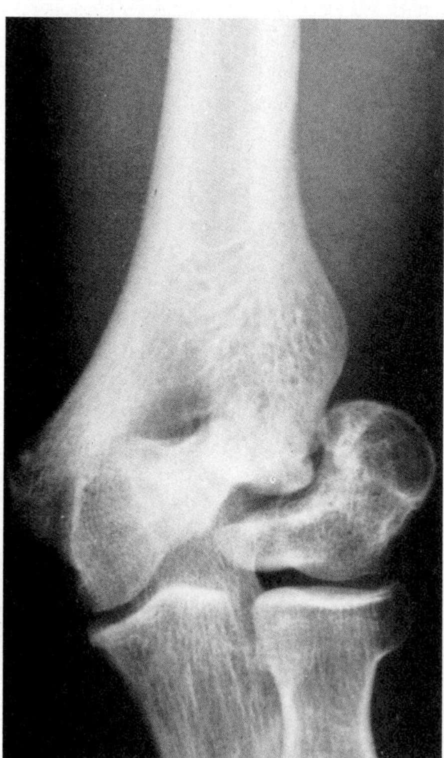

FIGURE 15-14 Asymptomatic nonunion of a lateral condyle in a 19-year-old military recruit. Because the patient had a completely normal and asymptomatic range of motion in his nondominant extremity, operative stabilization was not thought to be necessary.

Nonunion can occur with or without angular deformity. Many patients with nonunions and minimal fragment displacement have no angulation and remain relatively asymptomatic for normal activities (see Fig. 15-14). Others have weakness or symptoms when the arm is used for high-performance activities. Because they are not significantly displaced, these fractures can often be stabilized with minimal extra-articular dissection using a combination of screw fixation and a laterally placed bone graft.

Nonunion with subsequent fragment displacement is more common after unstable fractures with stage II and III displacement. If the fragment becomes free, it tends to migrate proximally with a subsequent valgus elbow deformity. Nonunion can lead to a cubitus valgus deformity, which in turn, is associated with the development of a tardy ulnar nerve palsy.

Nonunion seems to occur when the distal fragment is displaced enough to allow the condylar fragment's cartilaginous articular surface to oppose the bony surface of the humeral metaphysis. In such a situation, union is impossible. Flynn and Richards[55] reported successful treatment of nonunion 9 months to 3 years after fracture and strongly advised early surgery for established nonunion when the condylar fragment is in "good position" in a child with open physes. Papandrea and Waters[133] recommended stable internal fixation with percutaneously placed pins or cannulated screws for early (less than 12 weeks), minimally displaced nonunions. For late displaced nonunions, they recommended staged procedures: ulnar nerve transposition and bone grafting and fixation in situ of the lateral condyle followed by osteotomy to correct angulation once the nonunion is healed and elbow range of motion is regained.

The most common sequela of nonunion with displacement is the development of a progressive cubitus valgus deformity.

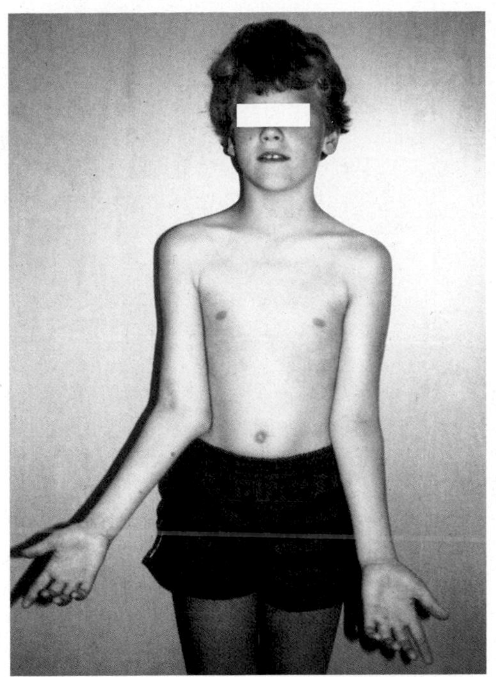

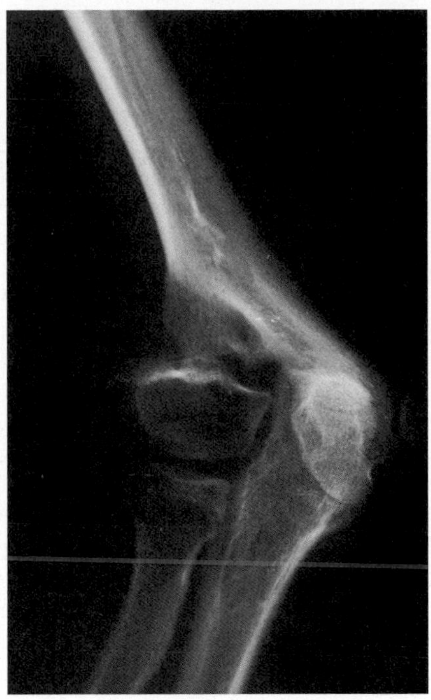

FIGURE 15-15 A. A 10-year-old boy with cubitus valgus resulting from a fracture of the lateral condylar physis with nonunion. **B.** Nonunion with cubitus valgus. Radiograph showing both angulation and translocation secondary to nonunion of the condylar fragment.

The fragment migrates both proximally and laterally, giving not only an angular deformity but also lateral translocation of the proximal radius and ulna (Fig. 15-15). Milch[119] noted that lateral translocation is not as likely to develop in the more lateral type of these fractures (Milch type I) because the lateral crista of the trochlea is intact (Fig. 15-16).

FIGURE 15-16 Nonunion without translocation. Milch type I fracture pattern. Despite nonunion, elbow stability was maintained because the lateral crista of the trochlea had remained intact (*arrow*). Valgus angulation also developed.

Surgical treatment of the nonunion deformity of the lateral condylar fragment is difficult and requires correcting two problems. First, articular cartilage may be opposing the distal humeral metaphysis, and union seldom can be obtained without mobilizing the fragments and applying an internal compressive device. The second problem is correcting the angular deformity (Fig. 15-17).

Shimada et al.[166] reported excellent or good results in 15 of 16 patients at an average follow-up of 11 years after osteosynthesis for nonunion of fractures of the lateral humeral condyle. The one patient with a poor result had evidence of osteonecrosis

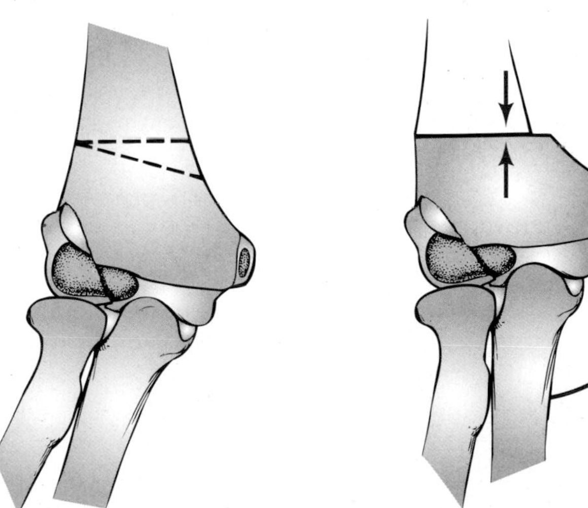

FIGURE 15-17 In the Milch type I fracture pattern, there is only an angular deformity that can be easily corrected with a closing wedge osteotomy. (Adapted and reprinted with permission from Milch HE. Fractures and fracture–dislocations of the humeral condyles. J Trauma 1964;4:592–607.)

of the fragment. The average interval between injury and osteosynthesis was 5 years (range, 5 months to 10 years). To prevent progression of cubitus valgus deformity and subsequent ulnar nerve dysfunction, Shimada et al.[166] recommended osteosynthesis for nonunion of lateral humeral condylar fractures in children because union is easily achieved, the range of motion is maintained, ulnar nerve function usually returns, and remodeling of the articular surfaces can be expected. They noted that bone grafting is essential to bridge the defect, to obtain congruity of the joint, and to promote union; damage to the blood supply should be avoided to prevent osteonecrosis. Wattenbarger et al.[196] described late (>3 weeks) open reduction and internal fixation of lateral condylar fractures in 11 children, 10 of whom had nonunions and one a malunion. Of the nine children available for follow-up, seven had good results and two had fair results. To avoid the development of osteonecrosis, the authors accepted malreduction rather than stripping the soft tissue off the lateral condylar fragment to achieve a more anatomic reduction. For fractures with more than 1 cm of displacement, the position of the fragment often was improved very little by surgery, but all fractures united, alignment of the arm was good, and no child had developed osteonecrosis at an average 6-year follow-up.

Tien et al.[187] described a technique that includes in situ compression fixation of the lateral condylar nonunion and a dome-shaped supracondylar osteotomy of the distal humerus through a single posterior incision. In their eight patients (average age: 8.6 years), the average interval between fracture and surgery was 5 years. All eight nonunions healed within 3 months, as did all of the supracondylar dome osteotomies. At 4.5-year follow-up, results were excellent in two patients, good in four, and fair in two. The authors recommended this procedure for minimally displaced, established lateral condylar nonunions with a cubitus valgus deformity of 20 degrees or more, especially when the deformity is progressing or is complicated by a concurrent ulnar neuropathy or is in patients with elbow instability or elbow pain during sports activities. They listed as a contraindication to the procedure a lateral condylar nonunion associated with radiographic evidence of prominent displacement and rotation. In situ fixation of the nonunion is recommended because the extensive soft tissue stripping required for mobilization and reduction of the fracture fragments results in devascularization of the fragment, which can cause osteonecrosis, loss of motion, and persistent nonunion.

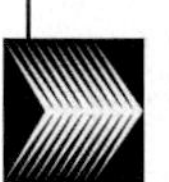

AUTHORS' PREFERRED TREATMENT

We distinguish between fractures seen late (more than 7 to 14 days after injury) and established nonunions (usually from 3 months to several years after injury). If we believe that we can obtain fracture union without loss of elbow motion and avoid osteonecrosis of the lateral condyle, then we recommend surgery for selected patients.

Treating an established nonunion of a lateral humeral condylar fracture poses a difficult dilemma. If no treatment is rendered, a progressive cubitus valgus deformity may occur with growth. Patients are usually asymptomatic except for those with high-demand athletic or labor activities. A mild flexion contracture of the elbow is present, but the cubitus valgus deformity is more cosmetic than functional. The danger in this approach is failure to recognize and treat early a tardy ulnar nerve palsy. If surgery is performed for an established nonunion, the potential risks of osteonecrosis and loss of elbow motion must be carefully considered.

We believe the criteria outlined by Flynn et al.[55,56] are helpful in determining if surgical treatment is appropriate for an established nonunion:

- A large metaphyseal fragment
- Displacement of less than 1 cm from the joint surface
- An open, viable lateral condylar physis

It is also helpful to distinguish between three distinct clinical situations. First, for an established nonunion with a large metaphyseal fragment, minimal migration, and an open lateral condylar physis, we recommend modified open reduction, screw fixation, and a lateral extra-articular iliac crest bone graft. This technique is markedly different from the surgical treatment of an acute lateral condylar fracture. The metaphyseal fragment of the lateral condyle and the distal humeral metaphysis are exposed, but no attempt is made to realign the articular surface. Intra-articular dissection should be avoided to help prevent any further loss of elbow motion. The metaphyseal fragments are débrided by gently removing any interposed fibrous tissue. The lateral condylar fragment can usually be moved distally a small distance. The metaphyseal fragments are firmly apposed, and a cancellous or cortical screw is used to fix the fragments with interfragmentary compression. Iliac crest bone graft can be placed between the metaphyseal fragments and laterally. The elbow is immobilized in 80 to 90 degrees of flexion for 3 to 4 weeks (Fig. 15-18).

Second, in patients with a nonunion who have cosmetic concerns but no functional complaints, treatment is similar to that for cubitus varus deformity after a supracondylar humeral fracture. If the patient and family desire, a supracondylar osteotomy can be performed.[110] Rigid internal fixation should be used to allow early motion. Late osteosynthesis of the lateral condyle is rarely indicated in an adolescent or young adult with high functional demands and symptoms of instability.

Third, patients with asymptomatic nonunion, cubitus valgus deformity, and symptomatic tardy ulnar nerve palsy should be treated with anterior transposition of the ulnar nerve.

Complications

If an adequate reduction is obtained promptly and maintained with solid fixation, results are uniformly good. In supracondylar fractures, an incomplete reduction may result in a cosmetic deformity, but functional results are generally good. In displaced fractures of the lateral condylar physis, a marginal reduction can result in both cosmetic deformities and functional loss of motion.[179] The complications that affect the outcome can be classified as either biologic or technical. Biologic problems occur as a result of the healing process, even if a perfect reduction is obtained. These problems include spur formation with pseudocubitus varus or a true cubitus varus. The technical problems usually arise from management errors and result in nonunion or malunion with or without valgus angulation and osteonecrosis.

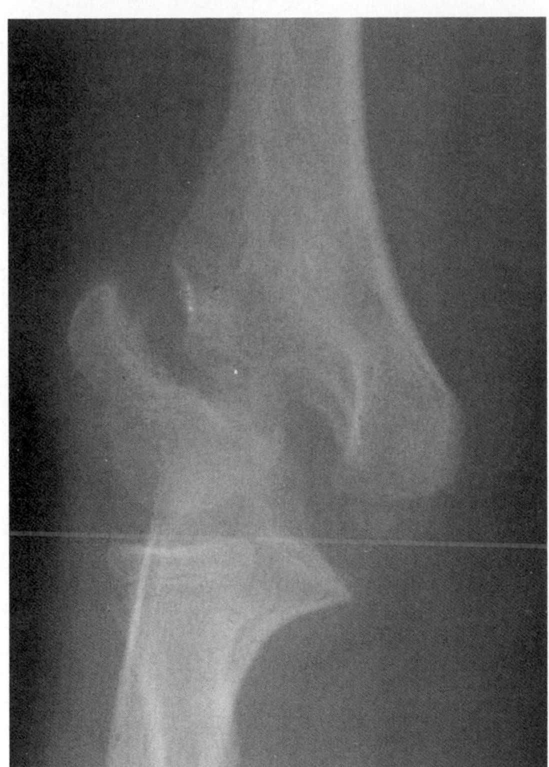

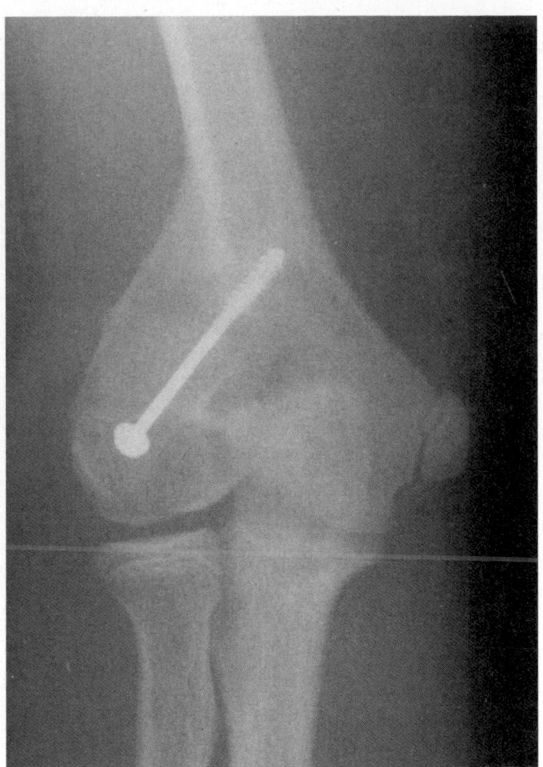

FIGURE 15-18 A. Established nonunion with a large metaphyseal fragment. **B.** After fixation with a cancellous screw and bone grafting of the metaphyseal fragment.

Other technical problems can arise from the injury itself, including neurologic injuries and myositis ossificans.

Lateral Spur Formation. Lateral condylar spur formation is one of the most common deformities after a fracture involving the lateral condylar physis. Cotton[35] believed that it is caused by coronal rotation of the distal fragment, which tends to displace the flap of periosteum associated with the distal fragment laterally. This periosteum then produces new bone formation in the form of a spur.

The spur occurs after both nonoperative and operative treatment. After nonoperative treatment, it results from the minimal displacement of the metaphyseal fragment and usually has a smooth outline. In patients with no real change in carrying angle, the lateral prominence of the spur may produce an appearance of mild cubitus varus (pseudovarus). In patients in whom a true cubitus varus develops, the presence of the lateral spur accentuates the varus alignment (Fig. 15-19A,B). The spur that occurs after operative treatment has a more irregular outline and is usually the result of hypertrophic bone formation from extensive dissection at the time of open reduction and internal fixation. During open reduction, care should be taken to limit the aggressiveness of the dissection and to carefully replace the lateral periosteal flap of the metaphyseal fragment.

Before treatment of lateral condylar fractures, the parents may be told that either lateral overgrowth with mild cubitus varus or lateral spur may develop, regardless of the treatment method. They should be told that this mild deformity is usually not of cosmetic or functional significance.

Cubitus Varus. Reviews of lateral condylar fractures show that a surprising number heal with some residual cubitus varus angulation.[58,78,113,126,158,171,175,191] In some series, the incidence of cubitus varus is as high as 40%,[58,175] and the deformity seems to be as frequent after operative treatment as after nonoperative treatment.[158,175] Skak et al.[171] reported visible varus deformities in six and valgus deformities in three of 28 children with displaced lateral condylar fractures. All patients with a valgus tilt of the joint surface were younger than 9 years of age at the time of injury. These investigators concluded that reduced growth potential at the trochlear groove is a regular complication of Milch type III fractures. The exact cause is not completely understood. In some instances, it is probably a combination of both an inadequate reduction and growth stimulation of the lateral condylar physis from the fracture insult (Fig. 15-20).[175]

The cubitus varus deformity is rarely severe enough to cause concern or require further treatment. This is probably because it is a pure coronal varus angulation and does not have the horizontal anterior rotation of the lateral condyle along with the sagittal extension that makes the cubitus varus that occurs after supracondylar fractures such an unacceptable deformity. Some investigators have noted that children with cubitus varus deformities have pain, decreased range of motion, epicondylitis, and problems with sports such as sidearm pitching, swimming, judo, and pushups. Davids et al.[37] reported lateral condylar fractures in six children with pre-existing cubitus varus deformities from previous elbow fractures, usually supracondylar humeral fractures. They concluded that posttraumatic cubitus varus deformity may predispose a child to subsequent lateral condylar fracture and should be viewed as more than just a cosmetic deformity. They recommended valgus supracondylar osteotomy of the distal humerus.

Cubitus Valgus. Cubitus valgus is much less common after united lateral condylar fractures than cubitus varus. It has rarely

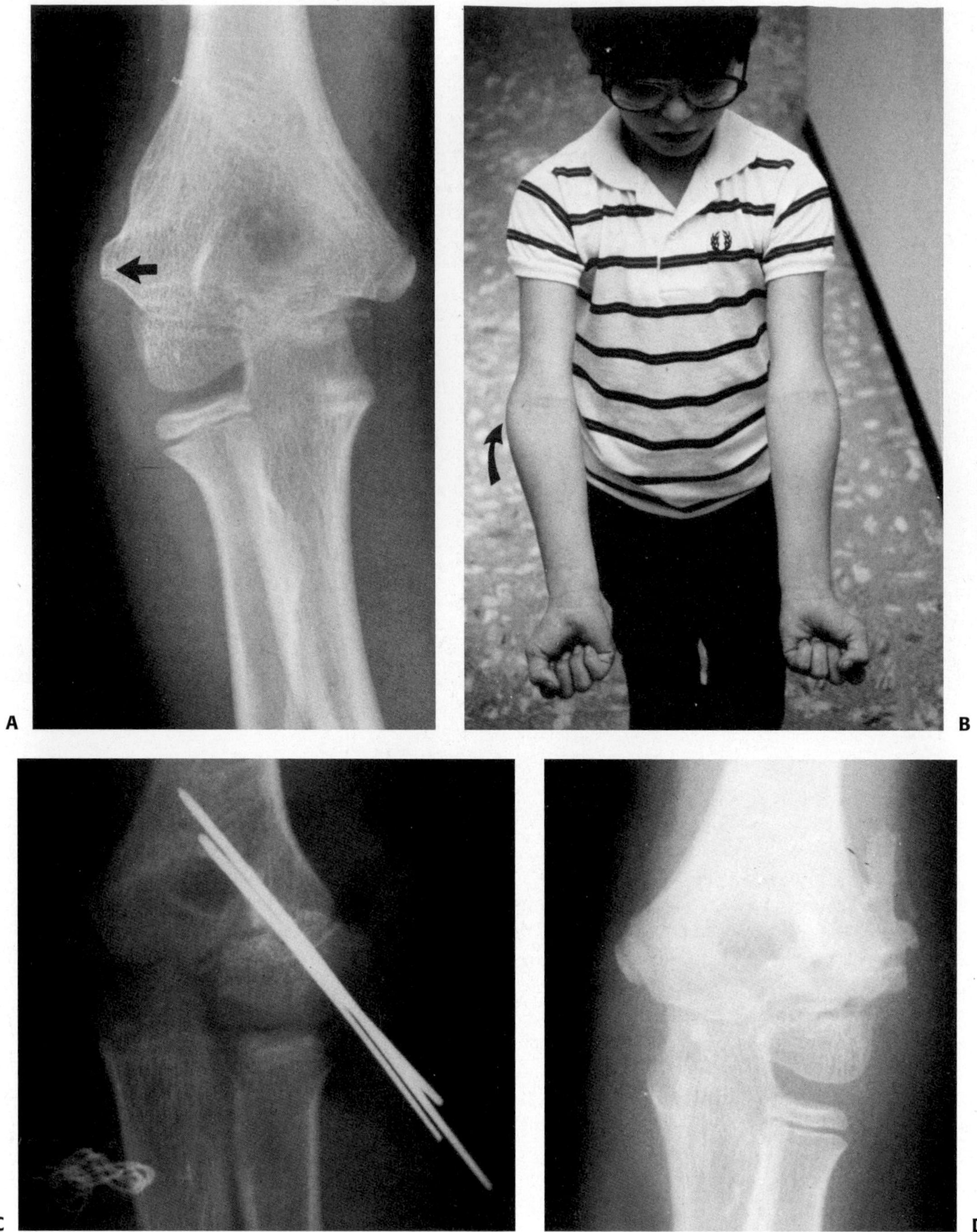

FIGURE 15-19 Spur formation. **A.** Follow-up radiograph of a boy whose lateral condylar fracture was treated nonoperatively. The periosteal flap produced a spur on the lateral aspect of the metaphysis (*arrow*). This fracture healed with a mild varus angulation as well. **B.** Clinically, the spur accentuated the lateral prominence (*arrow*) of the elbow, which in turn accentuated the mild valgus angulation. **C.** Considerable soft tissue dissection was performed in the process of open reduction of this lateral condylar fracture. **D.** At 2 months postsurgery, there is a large irregular spur formation secondary to periosteal new bone formation from the extensive dissection. (From Wilkins KE. Residuals of elbow fractures. Orthop Clin N Am 1990;21:289–312, with permission.)

been reported to result from premature epiphysiodesis of the lateral condylar physis.[193] As with cubitus varus, it is usually minimal and is rarely of clinical or functional significance. Piskin et al.,[145] however, described cubitus valgus deformity after lateral condylar fractures in eight adolescent patients who were treated with osteotomy and gradual distraction using the Ilizarov method. They cited as advantages to this method an ability to adjust the position of the distal fragment in all planes, immediate mobilization, which prevents elbow stiffness, and avoidance of an unsightly scar. Two patients with tardy ulnar nerve palsies did not have anterior nerve transposition before frame application and the ulnar nerve palsy persisted despite correction of the deformity, leading the authors to recommend routine nerve transposition before frame application.

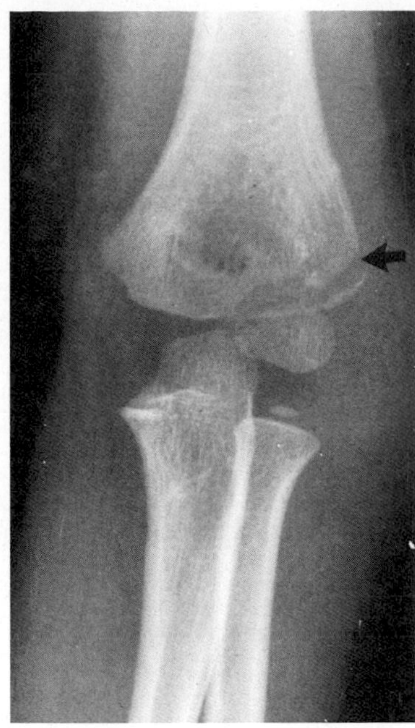

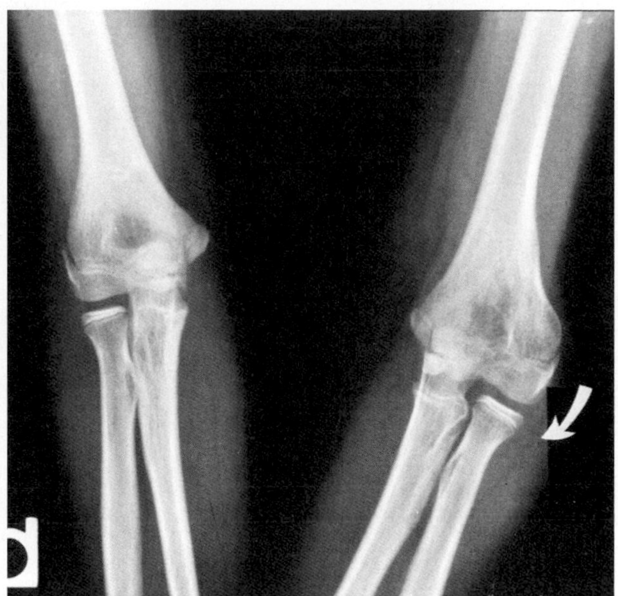

FIGURE 15-20 True varus. **A.** The injury film with a minimally displaced fracture (*arrow*). This 5-year-old child was treated with simple immobilization until the fracture was healed. **B.** Five years later, the patient had a persistent cubitus varus (*arrow*) that remained clinically apparent. The carrying angle of the uninjured right elbow measured 5 degrees of valgus; the injured elbow had 10 degrees of varus. (From Wilkins KE. Residuals of elbow trauma in children. Orthop Clin N Am 1990;21:289–312, with permission.)

The more difficult type of cubitus valgus associated with nonunions was discussed in the preceding section on nonunions.

Growth Disturbance: Fishtail Deformity. Two types of "fishtail deformity" of the distal humerus may occur. The first, a sharp-angled wedge, commonly occurs after fractures of the lateral condyle (Fig. 15-21). It is believed that this type of malformation is caused by persistence of a gap between the lateral condylar physis ossification center and the medial ossification of the trochlea.[193,201] Because of this gap, the lateral crista of the trochlea may be underdeveloped, which may represent a small "bony bar" in the distal humeral physis.[78] Despite some reports of loss of elbow motion with this type of fishtail deformity,[193] most investigators[8,11,41,58] have not found this type of radiographic deformity to produce any functional deficiency. Nwakama et al.[130] reported four patients (average age: 5 years) with fishtail deformities accompanied by premature closure of a portion of the distal humeral physis with resultant deformity, length retardation, decreased elbow motion, and functional impairment. Kim et al.[95] reviewed the records of 18 children in whom trochlear deformities developed after distal humeral fractures (12 transcondylar or transphyseal, five supracondylar, one lateral condylar) and found that 17 of the 18 had cubitus varus deformities (varus angulation from 2 to 18 degrees). Bony defects in the medial and central trochlea were evident on radiographs as early as 1 month after injury (average: 3.4 months). At intermediate follow-up, eight of 10 patients evaluated had no progression of their deformities, and none of the five patients seen at long-term follow-up (more than 10 years) had progression.

The second type of fishtail deformity is a gentler, smooth curve. It is usually believed to be associated with osteonecrosis of the lateral part of the medial crista of the trochlea.[126] The mechanisms of the development of this type of deformity are discussed in the section on osteonecrosis of the trochlea.

Neurologic Complications

The neurologic complications can be divided into two categories: acute nerve problems at the time of the injury and delayed

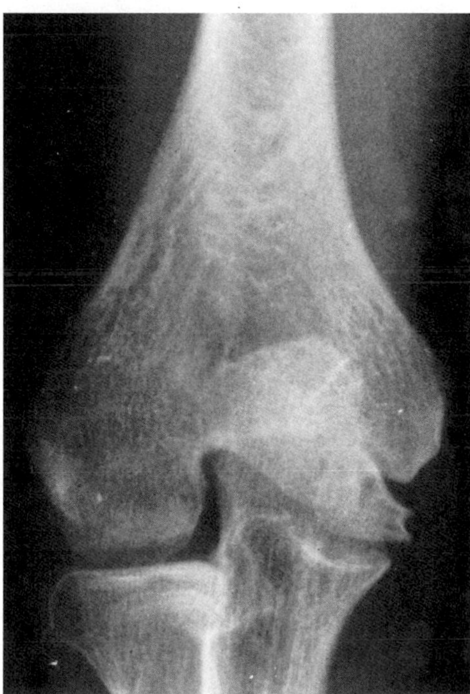

FIGURE 15-21 An angular "fishtail" deformity that persisted in this 14-year-old boy after operative treatment of a lateral condylar fracture, which occured 6 years previously.

neuropathy involving the ulnar nerve (the so-called tardy ulnar nerve palsy).

Acute Nerve Injuries. Reports of acute nerve injuries associated with this injury are rare. Smith and Joyce,[174] reported two patients with posterior interosseous nerve injury after open reductions of the lateral condylar fragment, both of whom recovered spontaneously. McDonnell and Wilson[113] reported a case of transient radial nerve paralysis after an acute injury.

Friedman and Smith[64] reported a delayed radial nerve laceration from the tip of the screw that was used to stabilize a lateral condylar fracture 26 years earlier. This occurred when the patient sustained a hyperextension injury to the elbow.

Tardy Ulnar Nerve Palsy. Tardy ulnar nerve palsy as a late complication of fractures of the lateral condylar physis is well known, especially after the development of cubitus valgus from malunion or nonunion of fractures of the lateral condylar physis.[65] The symptoms are usually gradual in onset. Motor loss occurs first, with sensory changes developing somewhat later.[65] In Gay and Love's[65] series of 100 patients, the average interval of onset was 22 years.

Various treatment methods have been advocated, ranging from anterior transposition of the ulnar nerve (originally the most commonly used procedure) to simple relief of the cubital tunnel. We prefer simple subcutaneous anterior transposition of the nerve.

Physeal Arrest

Physeal arrest may be manifest by no more than premature fusion of the various secondary ossification centers to each other, with little or no deformity. Such a situation occurs much later than the original fracture. This phenomenon probably occurs because the fracture stimulates the ossification centers to grow more rapidly, and thus they reach maturity sooner; it is rarely caused by inadvertent dissection in the lateral condylar physis. Because only 20% of humeral growth occurs in the distal physis, physeal arrest seldom causes any significant angular or length deformities.

Malunion

The fragment rarely unites in an undesirable position. Cubitus valgus has been reported to occur as a result of malunion of the fracture fragments.[193] Malunion of a Milch type I fracture pattern can result in the development of a bifid lateral condyle (Fig. 15-22). No reliable operative treatment has been described to re-establish the congruity of the articular surfaces in condylar malunions, and they are probably best left untreated. We have seen several patients with malunions in which the lateral condyle rotates in the coronal plane, with subsequent cubitus varus deformity.

Osteonecrosis

Osteonecrosis of the condylar fragment may be iatrogenic and is most commonly associated with the extensive dissection necessary to effect a late reduction or from loss of the blood supply at the time of injury.[73,85,113] Wilson,[201] however, described partial osteonecrosis in an essentially nondisplaced fracture of the lateral condylar physis that had a radiographic appearance and clinical course similar to those of osteochondritis dissecans. Osteonecrosis is rare in fractures of the lateral condylar physis that receive little or no initial treatment and result in nonunion.[85,203]

Overly vigorous dissection of fresh fractures can result in osteonecrosis of either the lateral condylar ossification center[58,135] or, rarely, the metaphyseal portion of the fragment, leading to nonunion (Fig. 15-23). If the fracture unites, osteonecrosis of the lateral condyle reossifies over many years,

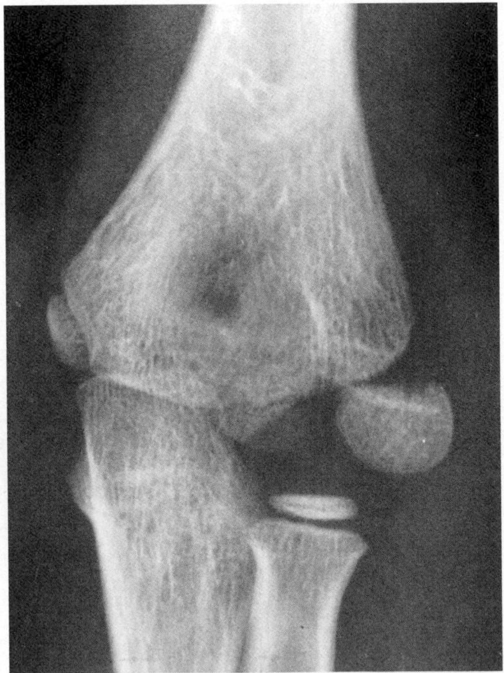

A

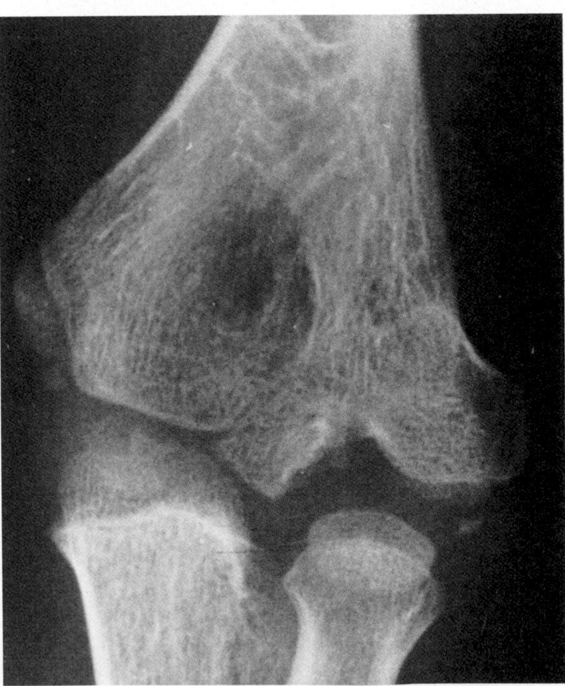

B

FIGURE 15-22 A. Injury film of a 7-year-old who sustained a Milch type I lateral condylar fracture. This patient was treated with cast immobilization alone. **B.** Radiograph taken 2 years later showed complete fusion of the condylar epiphysis to the metaphysis, with the development of a "bifid" condyle.

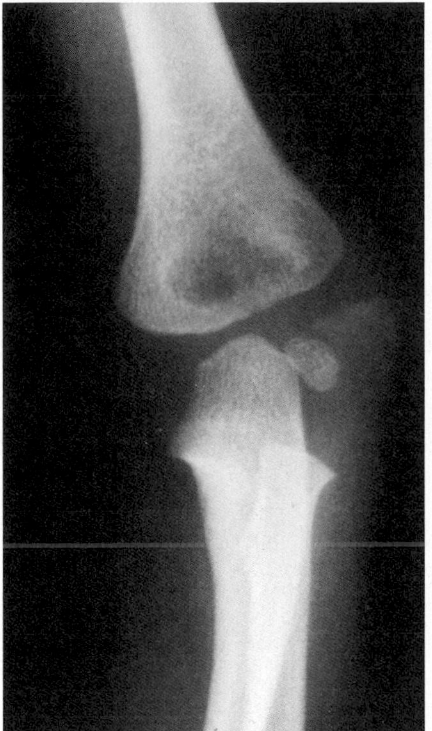
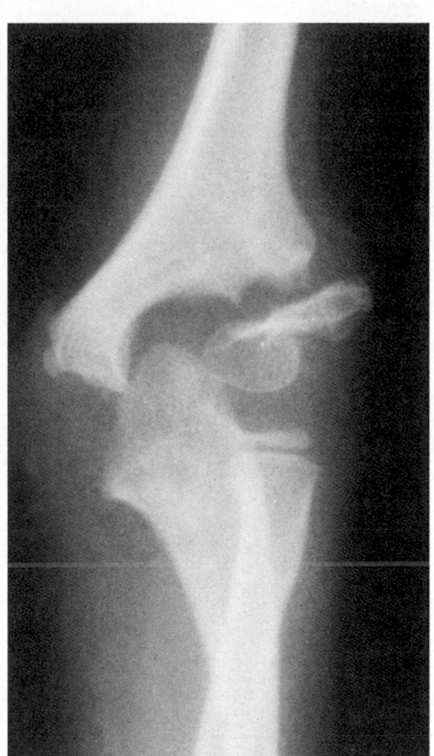

FIGURE 15-23 Osteonecrosis and nonunion developed in this child after extensive dissection and difficulty in obtaining a primary open reduction. **A.** Injury film. **B.** Two years later, there was extensive bone loss in the metaphysis and a nonunion of the condyle.

much like Legg-Calveé-Perthes disease in the hip. Any residual deformity is usually related to loss of motion.

Ipsilateral Injuries

Fractures of the lateral condyle have been associated with elbow dislocations,[20] ulnar shaft fractures,[117,149] and fractures of the medial epicondyle. Often, an elbow dislocation is misdiagnosed in a patient with a lateral condylar fracture. Loss of the lateral crista can make the elbow unstable and allow the proximal radius or ulna to translocate laterally. This is a part of a normal pathologic condition associated with completely displaced lateral condylar fractures. In a true elbow dislocation, the proximal radius and ulna are displaced not only medially or laterally but also proximally (Fig. 15-24).

Fractures of the Capitellum

Fractures of the capitellum involve only the true articular surface of the lateral condyle. This includes, in some instances, the

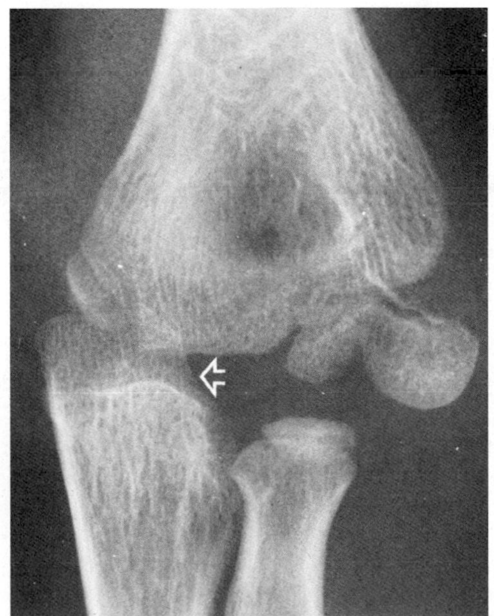
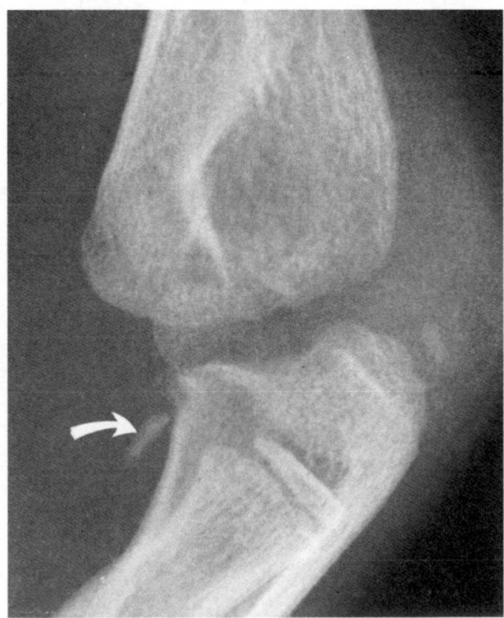

FIGURE 15-24 Ipsilateral injury. **A.** AP radiograph of an 8-year-old boy with a true posteromedial elbow dislocation (*open arrow*) and a Milch type I lateral condylar fracture. **B.** A small fracture of the coronoid process of the ulna (*closed arrow*) confirms the primary nature of the elbow dislocation on the lateral radiograph.

articular surface of the lateral crista of the trochlea. Generally, this fragment comes from the anterior portion of the distal articular surface. In adults, these fractures are not uncommon, but they are rare in children. In their review of 2000 elbow fractures in children, Marion and Faysse[108] found only one fracture of the capitellum. Since then, this fracture has been frequently reported in older adolescents.[60,88,105,108,132] Marion and Faysse[108] pointed out that verified fractures of the capitellum have not been described in children under 12 years of age. There have been two reports,[3,46] however, of so-called anterior sleeve fractures of the lateral condyles, both in 8-year-olds (Fig. 15-25). These fractures involved a good portion of the anterior articular surface, although technically they could not be classified as pure capitellar fractures because they contained nonarticular epicondylar and metaphyseal portions in the fragment. Sodl et al.[176] described an acute osteochondral shear fracture (Kocher-Lorenz) of the capitellum in a 12-year-old boy.

This fracture is often difficult to diagnose because there is little ossified tissue. It is composed mainly of pure articular surface from the capitellum and essentially nonossified cartilage from the secondary ossification center of the lateral condyle.

Classification

Two fracture patterns have been described. The first is the more common Hahn-Steinthal type,[180] which usually contains a rather large portion of cancellous bone of the lateral condyle. The lateral crista of the trochlea is often also included (Fig. 15-26). The second, or Kocher-Lorenz, type is more of a pure articular fracture with little if any subchondral bone attached and may represent a piece of articular cartilage from an underly-

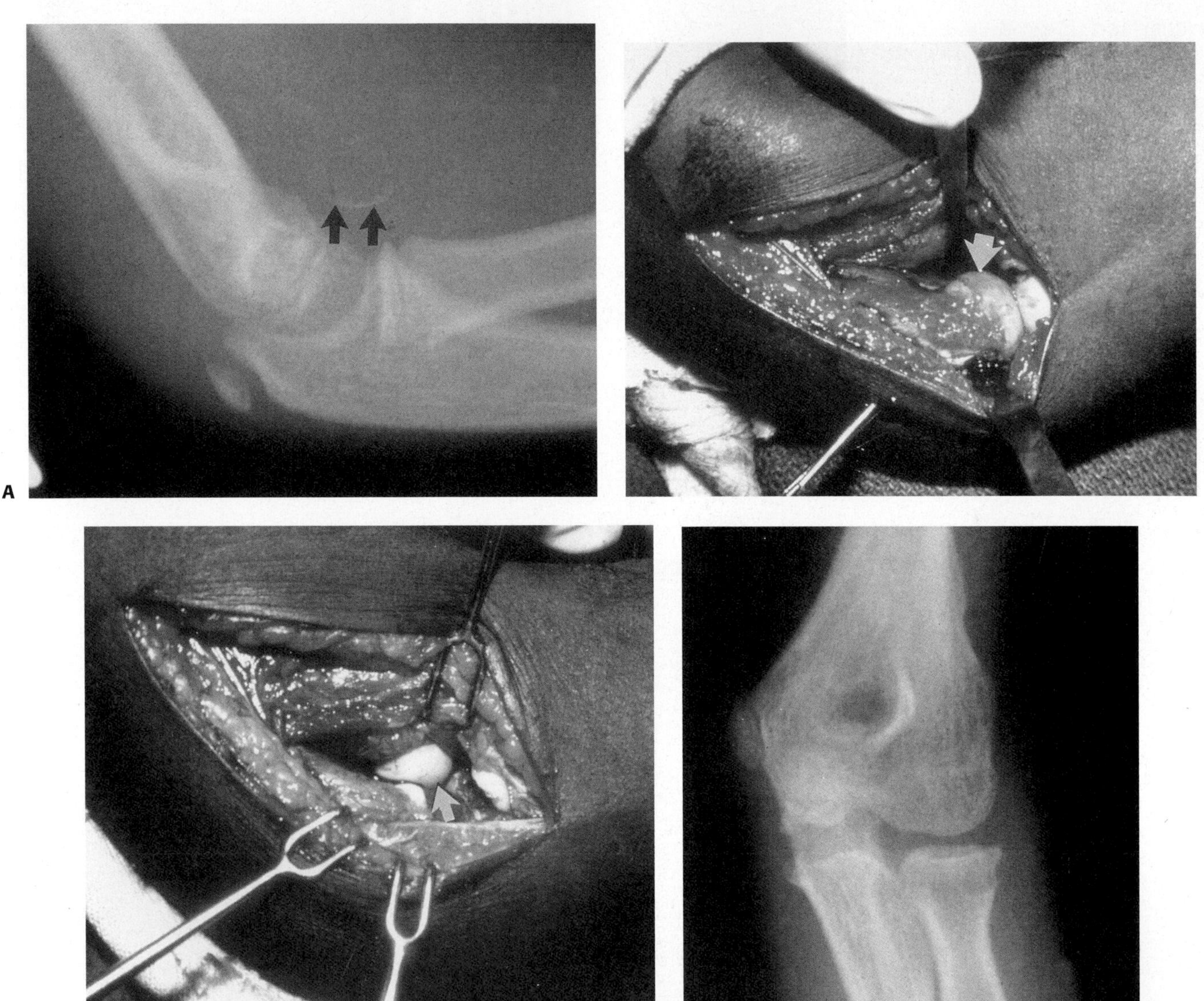

FIGURE 15-25 Fracture of the capitellum. **A.** Osteochondral fracture of the capitellum in an 8-year-old girl. Note the small fleck of bone (*arrow*), which indicates possible osteochondral fragment. **B.** Intraoperative photograph shows the size and origin of the fracture fragment from the lateral humeral epiphysis. **C.** Intraoperative photograph after fragment reduction into the bed of the capitellum. **D.** Healed fracture with articular congruity, restoration of cartilage space, and no osteonecrosis. (From Drvaric DM, Rooks MD. Case report. Anterior sleeve fracture of the capitellum. J Orthop Trauma 1990;4:188, with permission.)

these often are called *trochlear fractures*. For purposes of description in this chapter, fractures of the trochlea are those that include only the articular surface.

Incidence

Fractures involving the medial condylar physis are rare in skeletally immature children, accounting for less than 1% of fractures involving the distal humerus.[40]

Many of the large series of elbow fractures in the literature and early fracture texts do not mention these fractures as a separate entity. Blount[18] described only one such fracture in his classic text. In Faysse and Marion's[53] review of more than 2000 fractures of the distal humerus in children, only 10 fractures involved the medial condylar physis. Although it has been reported in a child as young as 2 years of age,[7] this fracture pattern is generally considered to occur during later childhood.

Most series[53,137] show medial condylar fractures occurring somewhat later than lateral condylar fractures. A review of 38 patients in nine series[7,28,34,47,51,53,70,137,147,192] in which the specific ages were given showed that 37 patients were in the age range of 8 to 14 years. Thus, this fracture seems to occur after the ossification centers of the medial condylar epiphysis begin to appear. This fracture can occur as early as 6 months of age, however, before any ossification of the distal humerus has appeared,[14,38] making the diagnosis extremely difficult.

Surgical Anatomy and Pathology

Fractures of the medial condylar physis involve both intra- and extra-articular components. They behave as Salter-Harris type IV physeal injuries, but not enough fractures have been described to show whether the fracture line courses through the secondary ossification center of the medial condylar epiphysis or whether it enters the common physeal line separating the lateral condylar ossification center from the medial condylar ossification center. This common physeal line terminates in the notch of the trochlea. The trochlea's lateral crista is ossified from the lateral condylar epiphysis. Only the medial crista is ossified by the secondary ossification centers of the medial condylar epiphysis. We believe that this fracture is a "mirror image" of the lateral condylar physeal injury and thus has characteristics of Salter-Harris type IV physeal injuries (Fig. 15-28). The deformity that develops if the fracture is untreated is nonunion, similar to that after lateral condylar physeal fracture, rather than physeal fusion, as occurs after a typical Salter-Harris type IV injury. The resultant deformity is cubitus varus instead of the cubitus valgus deformity that occurs with nonunion of the lateral condyle.

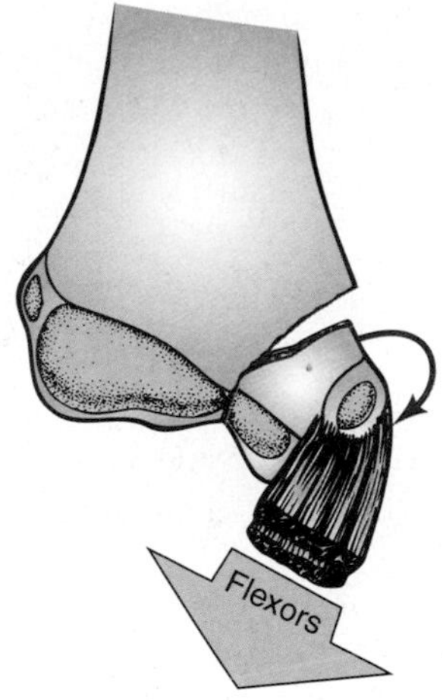

FIGURE 15-29 Displacement of the medial condyle. The pull of the forearm flexor muscles rotates the fragment so that the fracture surface is facing anteromedially and the articular surface is posterolateral. (Adapted and reprinted with permission from Chacha PB. Fractures of the medial condyle of the humerus with rotational displacement. J Bone Joint Surg Am 1970;52:1453–1458.)

Characteristically, the metaphyseal fragment includes the intact medial epicondyle along with the common flexor origin of the muscles of the forearm. These flexor muscles cause the loosened fragment to rotate so that the fracture surface is facing anteriorly and medially and the articular surface is facing posteriorly and laterally (Fig. 15-29).[7,28] Rotation of the fragment is especially accentuated when the elbow is extended. Chacha[28] also noted that often the lateral aspect of the common flexor origin and the anterior capsule of the joint were torn and the fracture surface could usually be reached through this anterior opening into the joint.

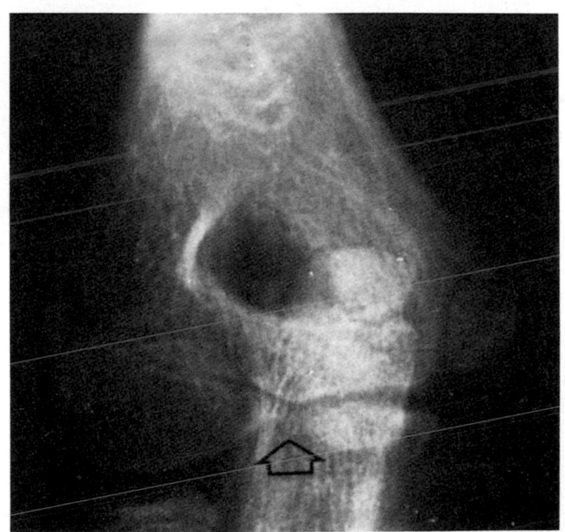

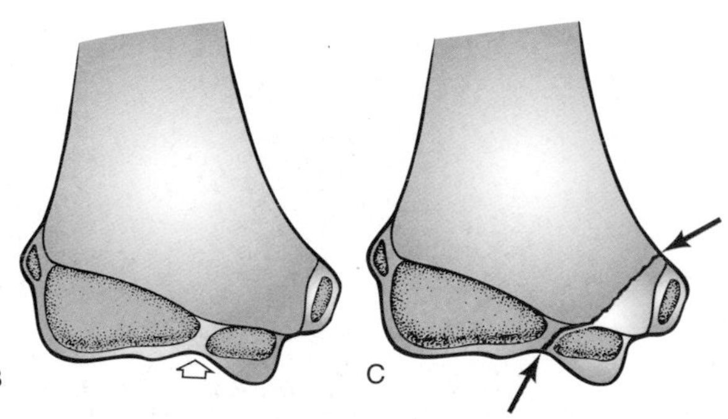

FIGURE 15-28 A. The AP radiograph of a 9-year-old boy demonstrates the location of the ossification centers. A common physeal line (*arrow*) separates the medial and lateral condylar physes. **B.** Relationship of the ossification centers to the articular surface. The common physis terminates in the trochlear notch (*arrow*). **C.** Location of the usual fracture line involving the medial condylar physis (*arrows*).

The blood supply to the medial epicondyle and medial metaphysis courses extra-articularly along with the medial flexor muscle groups. The blood supply to the lateral ossification center of the medial crista of the trochlea, however, must traverse the surface of the medial condylar physis. If the fracture line disrupts these small intra-articular vessels, disruption and subsequent circulation loss to the lateral portion of the medial crista can result, leading to the development of a fishtail deformity.

Mechanism of Injury

Two separate mechanisms can produce physeal fractures of the medial condyle. Ashurst's[7] patients described falling directly on the point of the flexed elbow. This mechanism was also implicated in other reports.[14,28,74,147] In this mechanism, it is speculated that the semilunar notch's sharp edge of the olecranon splits the trochlea directly (Fig. 15-30A). In three more recent series,[27,47,59] many patients sustained this injury when they fell on their outstretched arms. The theory is that this is an avulsion injury caused by a valgus strain at the elbow (Fig. 15-30B). Fowles and Kassab[59] reported a patient with a concomitant valgus greenstick fracture of the olecranon associated with a fracture of the medial condylar physis. They believed this fracture provided further evidence that this was a valgus avulsion type of injury. Once the fragment becomes disassociated from

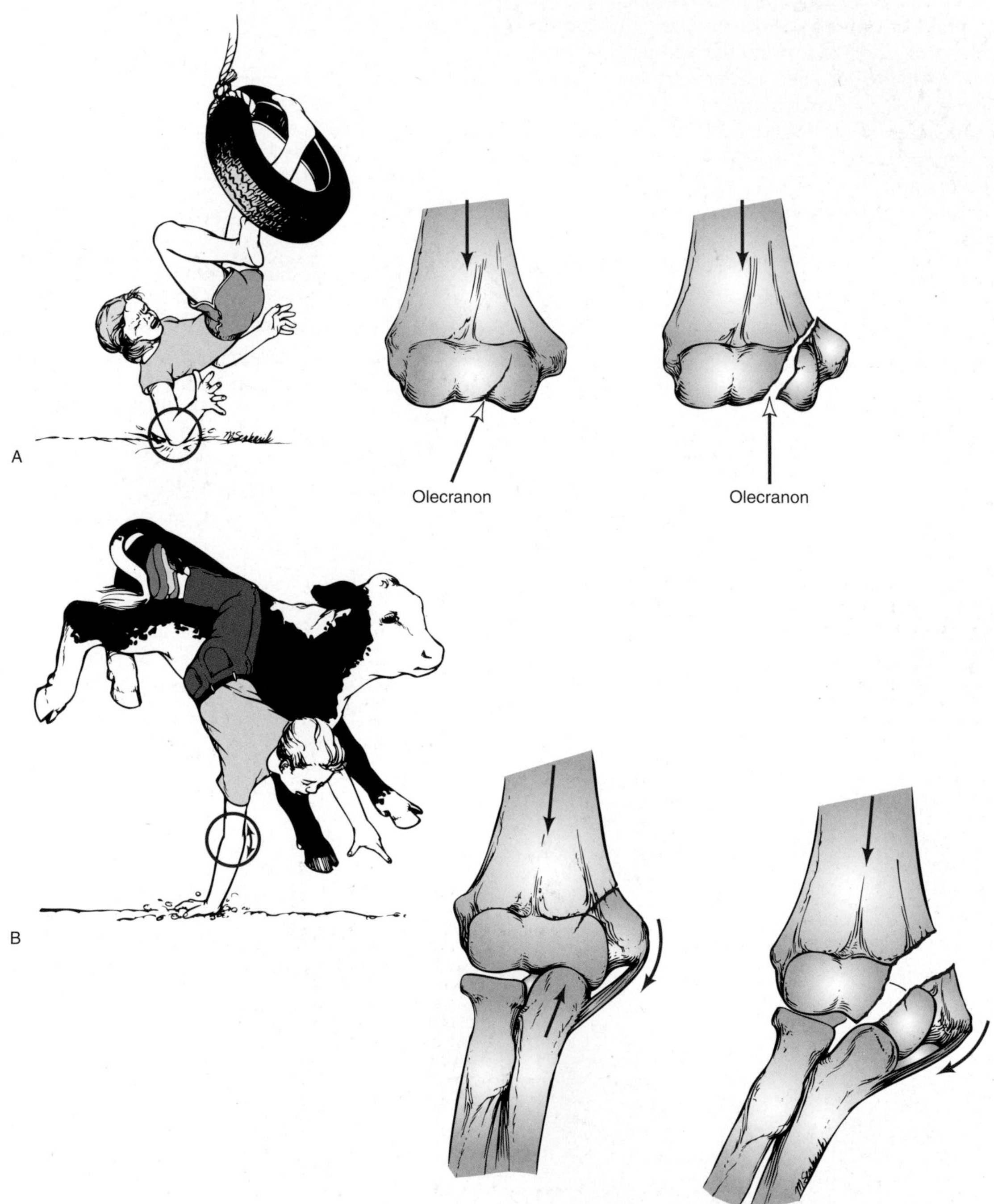

FIGURE 15-30 Medial condylar fracture mechanisms of injury. **A.** A direct force applied to the posterior aspect of the elbow causes the sharp articular margin of the olecranon to wedge the medial condyle from the distal humerus. **B.** Falling on the outstretched arm with the elbow extended and the wrist dorsiflexed causes the medial condyle to be avulsed by both ligamentous and muscular forces.

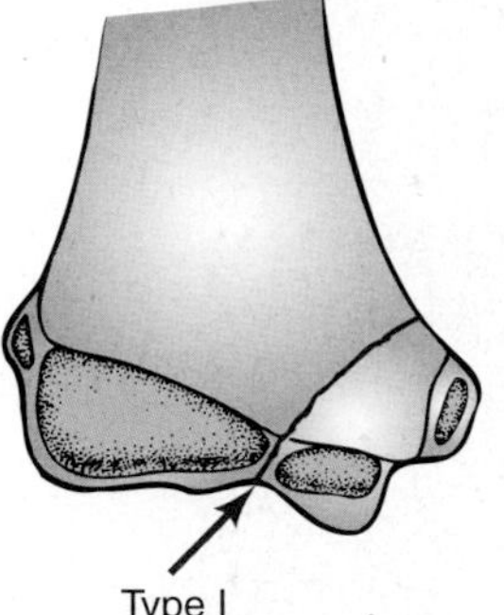

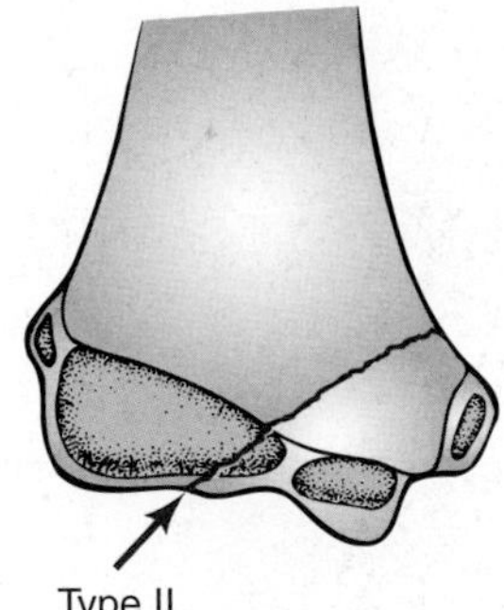

FIGURE 15-31 Medial condylar fracture patterns. In the Milch type I injury, the fracture line terminates in the trochlear notch (left, *arrow*). In the Milch type II injury, the fracture line terminates more laterally in the capitulotrochlear groove (right, *arrow*). (Adapted and reprinted with permission from Milch H. Fractures and fracture–dislocations of the humeral condyles. J Trauma 1964;4:592–607.)

the distal humerus, the forearm flexor muscles produce a sagittal anterior rotation of the fragment.

Classification

Classification, as with fractures of the lateral condylar physis, is based on the fracture line's location and the degree of the fracture's displacement.

Location of the Fracture Line. Milch[119] classified fractures of the medial condylar physis in adults into two types. In type I fractures, the fracture line traverses the apex of the trochlea. In type II fractures, it traverses the capitulotrochlear groove. He believed that the origin of the fracture line depended on whether the radial head, as in type II, or the semilunar notch of the olecranon, as in type I, served as the impinging force for the abduction injury. Both fracture patterns occur in children (Fig. 15-31), but type I fractures seem to be more common because the common physeal line, which serves as a point of weakness, ends in the apex of the trochlea.

Displacement of the Fracture. Kilfoyle[94] described three fracture displacement patterns that can be helpful in determining appropriate treatment (Fig. 15-32). In type I, the fracture line in the medial condylar metaphysis extends down to the physis. He noted that some of these might represent incomplete supracondylar fractures. Unless there is a greenstick crushing of the medial supracondylar column, these fractures are usually of no clinical significance. In type II, the fracture line extends into the medial condylar physis. The intra-articular portion, as it is in preosseous cartilage, is often not recognized. In this second type, the medial condylar fragment usually remains undisplaced. In type III, the condylar fragment is both rotated and displaced.

Bensahel et al.[14] and Papavasiliou et al.[137] found that type III displacement fractures, which accounted for only 25%, were more likely to occur in older adolescents, and type I fractures were more common in younger children. These studies also confirmed the correlation between the type of displacement and the treatment method.

Medial condylar physeal fractures have been reported in association with greenstick fractures of the olecranon and with true posterolateral elbow dislocations (Fig. 15-33).[14,162] Some investigators[14,38] found that child abuse was more common in their younger patients with these fractures than with other elbow fractures.

Diagnosis

Clinically and on radiographs, a fracture of the medial condylar physis is most often confused with a fracture of the medial epicondyle.[100] In both types of intra- and extra-articular fractures, swelling is concentrated medially, and there may be valgus instability of the elbow joint. In a true intra-articular fracture, however, there is varus instability as well. Such is usually not the case with an isolated extra-articular fracture of the medial epicondyle. Ulnar nerve paresthesia may be present with both types of fractures.

In older children with a large metaphyseal fragment, involvement of the entire condyle is usually obvious on radiographs; in younger children, in whom only the epicondyle is ossified, fracture of the medial condylar physis may be erroneously diagnosed as an isolated fracture of the medial epicondyle (Fig. 15-34).[34,51,59]

In differentiating these two fractures, it is helpful to remember that medial epicondylar fractures are often associated with elbow dislocations, usually posterolateral, and that elbow dislocations are rare before ossification of the medial condylar epiphysis begins. With medial condylar physeal fractures, the

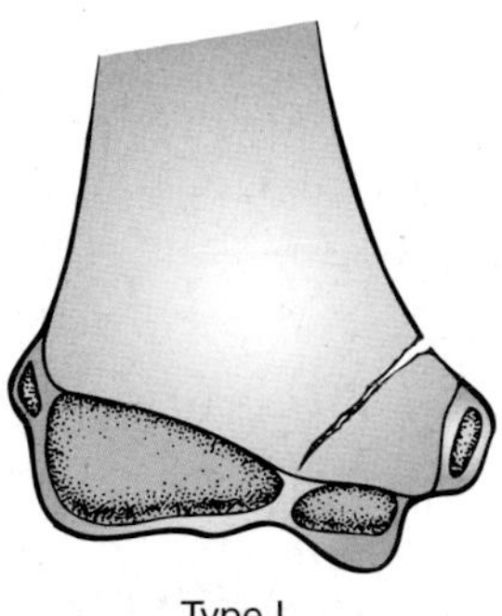

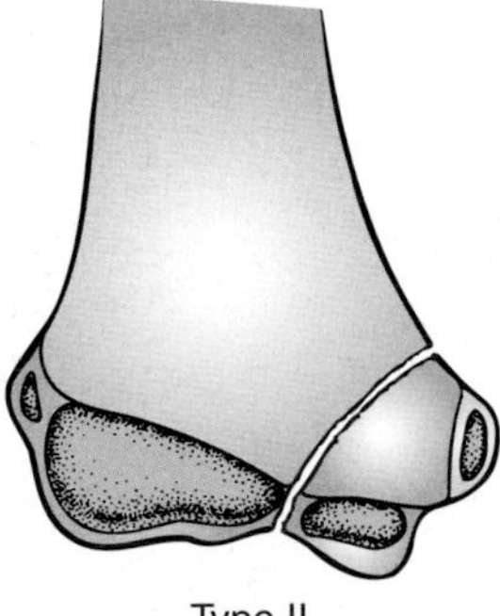

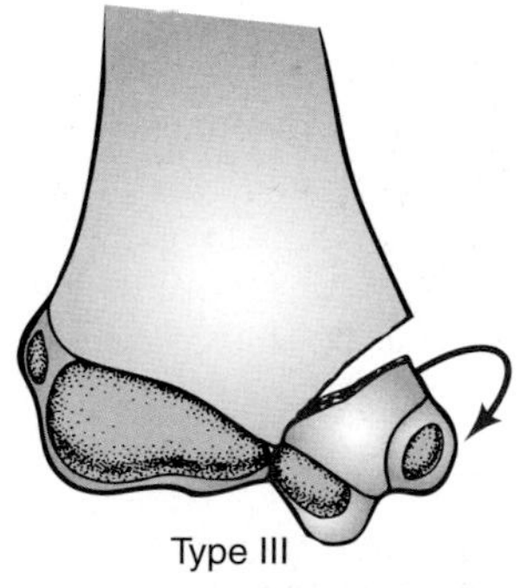

FIGURE 15-32 Kilfoyle classification of displacement patterns. (Adapted and reprinted with permission from Kilfoyle RM. Fractures of the medial condyle and epicondyle of the elbow in children. Clin Orthop 1965;41: 43–50.)

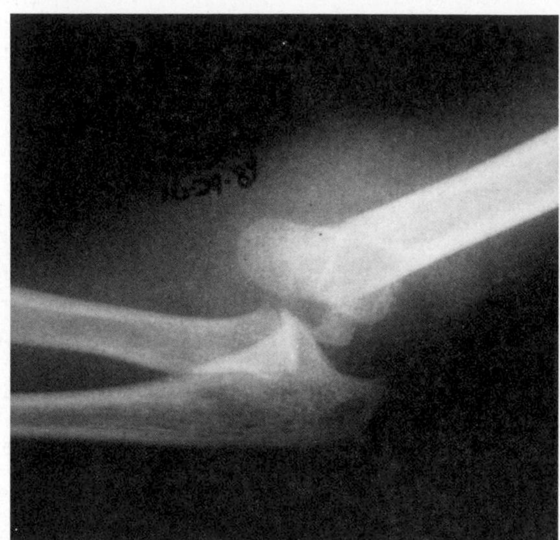

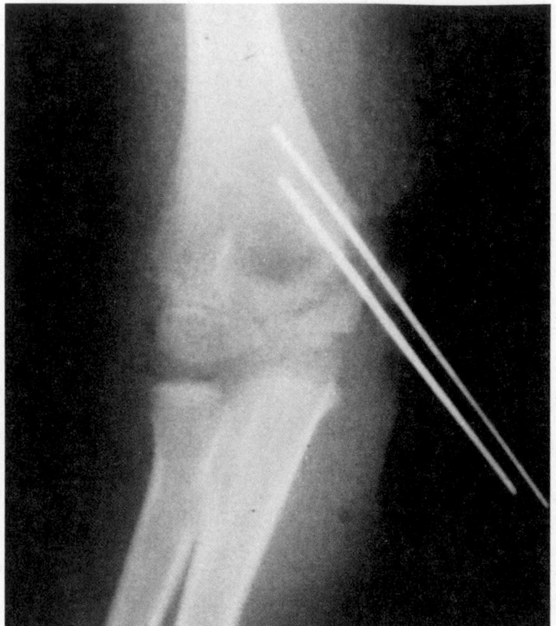

FIGURE 15-33 A. Injury film of a 10-year-old girl who sustained a type III displaced fracture of the medial condyle associated with a posterolateral elbow dislocation. **B.** After open reduction and K-wire fixation through an anteromedial approach. (Courtesy of Elizabeth A. Szalay, MD.)

elbow tends to subluxate posteromedially[34] due to the loss of trochlear stability.

Any metaphyseal ossification with the epicondylar fragment suggests the presence of an intra-articular fracture of the medial condyle and is an indication for further evaluation. Often, the medial condyle and the medial epicondyle are markedly displaced as a unit. A positive fat pad sign indicates that the injury has entered the elbow joint and a fracture of the medial condyle is likely.[74,170] Isolated fractures of the medial epicondyle are extra-articular and usually do not have positive fat pad signs.

If the true location of the fracture line is questionable in a child younger than 8 to 10 years of age with significant medial elbow ecchymosis, arthrography or MRI of the elbow should be performed.

Treatment

For displaced fractures, open reduction with internal fixation is the most often used treatment method.[14,27,47,59,94,134,144,147] The fracture fragment can be approached by a posteromedial incision that allows good exposure of both the fracture site and the ulnar nerve. Fixation is easily achieved with smooth K-wires (see Fig. 15-33) or with screws in older adolescents. Two wires are necessary because of the sagittal rotation forces exerted on the fracture fragment by the common flexor muscles. El Ghawabi[47] reported frequent delayed union and nonunion in fractures that were not rigidly stabilized.

In Kilfoyle's displacement types I and II fracture patterns, enough residual internal stability is usually present to allow the fracture to be simply immobilized in a cast or posterior splint.[14,47,53,94,137] As with fractures of the lateral condylar physis, union may be slow. In fractures treated promptly, results have been satisfactory.[28,51,59] Because there usually is more displacement in older children, the results in this age group are not as satisfactory as those in younger children, who tend to have relatively nondisplaced fractures.[14]

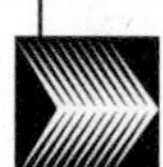

AUTHORS' PREFERRED TREATMENT

We generally treat type I nondisplaced fractures with simple observation and a posterior splint. Follow-up radiographs at weekly intervals are taken to ensure there is no late displacement. When there is good callus at the metaphyseal portion of the fracture line by 3 to 4 weeks, the splint is removed and early active motion is initiated. We continue to follow the patient until there is a full range of motion and obliteration of the fracture line.

Types II and III displaced fractures must be reduced and stabilized. This is usually difficult to do by closed methods because the swelling associated with this injury makes it hard to accurately identify the landmarks for pin placement. We proceed with an open reduction through a medial approach with identification and protection of the ulnar nerve. The posterior surface of the condylar fragment and the medial aspect of the medial crista of the trochlea should be avoided in the dissection because these are the blood supply sources to the ossific nuclei of the trochlea. Fixation with two parallel pins should be in the metaphyseal segment if possible (Fig. 15-35). Cannulated screw fixation can be used in adolescents near skeletal maturity.

Complications

The major complication is failure to make the proper diagnosis. This is especially true in younger children, in whom a medial condylar fracture can be confused with a displaced fracture of the medial epicondyle (see Fig. 15-34). When the diagnosis is a real possibility, especially in a child with no ossification of the trochlea, examination with anesthesia, arthrography, or MRI may be helpful. Leet, Young, and Hoffer[101] reported complica-

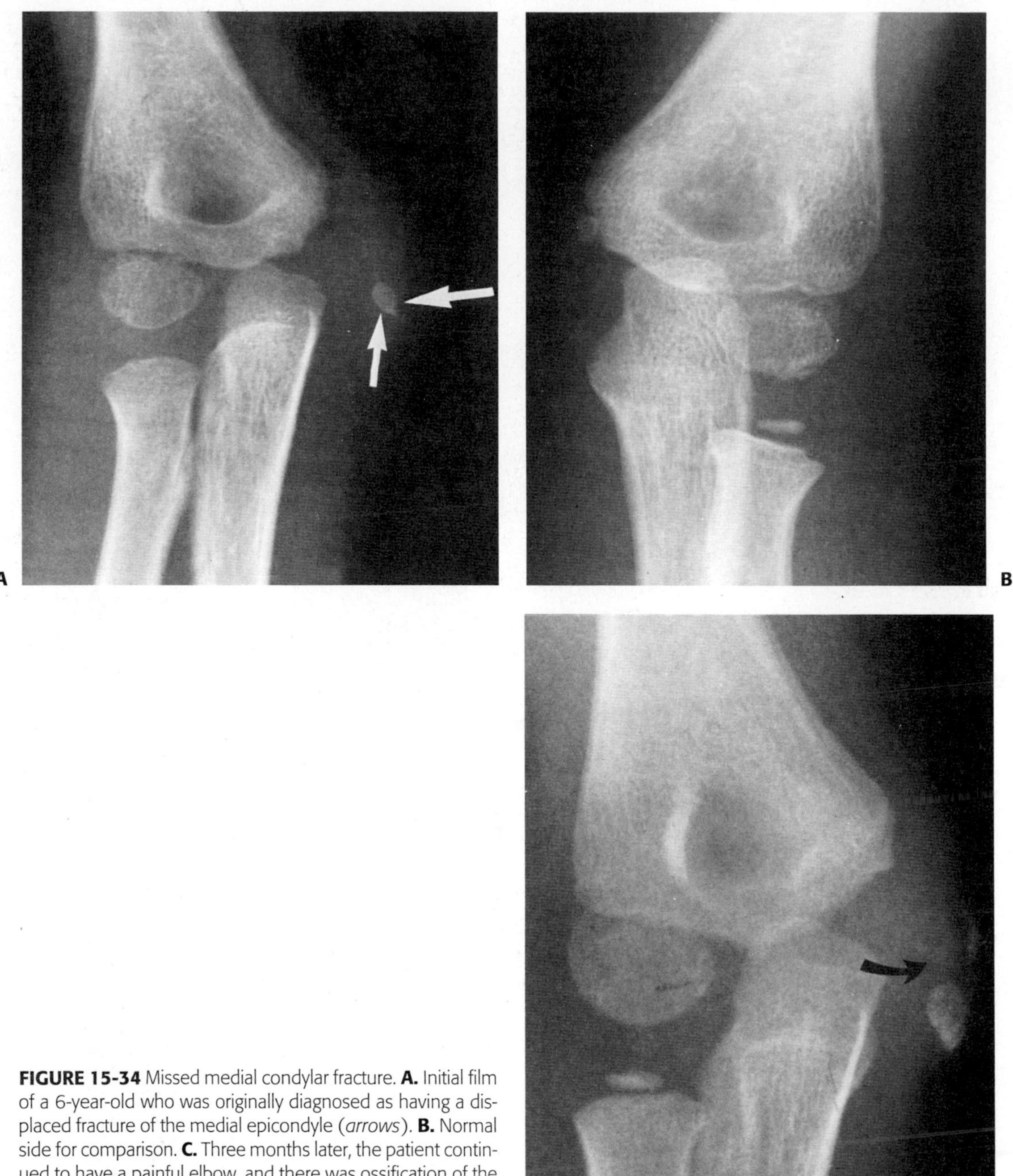

FIGURE 15-34 Missed medial condylar fracture. **A.** Initial film of a 6-year-old who was originally diagnosed as having a displaced fracture of the medial epicondyle (*arrows*). **B.** Normal side for comparison. **C.** Three months later, the patient continued to have a painful elbow, and there was ossification of the metaphysis (*arrow*) adjacent to the epicondyle.

tions after 33% of 21 medial condylar fractures, including osteonecrosis of the trochlea, nonunion, and loss of reduction. Untreated displaced fractures usually result in nonunion with cubitus varus deformity (Fig. 15-36).[59,192] Ryu et al.[159] described a painful nonunion of the medial condyle in an adolescent that apparently resulted from a fracture when he was 3 years old. An osteotomy was made to remove the ununited section of bone, and an iliac bone graft was inserted and fixed with two malleolar screws. Union was obtained, and the patient was able to participate in sports without pain. We have seen one nonunion after a fracture of the medial condyle. Delayed union has been reported in patients treated with insecure fixation or simply placed in a cast.[47,94]

Some disturbance of the vascular supply to the medial condylar fragment may occur during open reduction and internal fixation or at the time of initial injury. Several investigators have reported subsequent avascular changes in the medial crista of the trochlea.[47,59,94,137] Hanspal[70] reviewed Cothay's original patient[34] 18 years after delayed open reduction and found that despite some minimal loss of motion, the patient was asymptomatic. Radiographs, however, showed changes compatible with osteonecrosis of the medial condyle.

Both cubitus varus and valgus deformities have been reported in patients whose fractures united uneventfully. The valgus deformity appears to be caused by secondary stimulation or overgrowth of the medial condylar fragment. Some simple stimulation of the medial epicondyle's prominence may also produce the false appearance of a cubitus valgus deformity. Cubitus varus appears to result from decreased growth of the trochlea, possibly caused by a vascular insult. Principles for

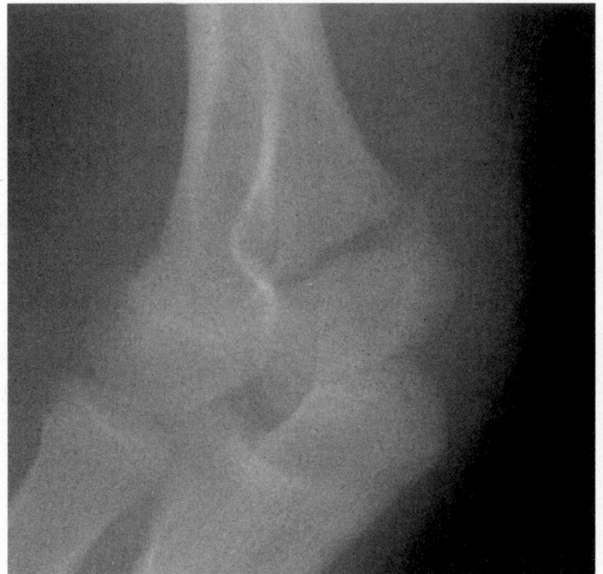

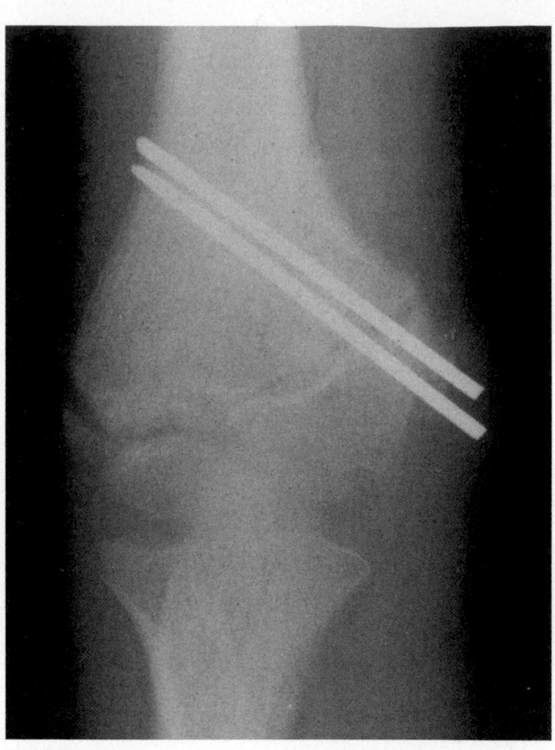

FIGURE 15-35 A. Stage II fracture of the medial condyle in a 10-year-old girl. **B.** After open reduction and K-wire fixation through a medial approach

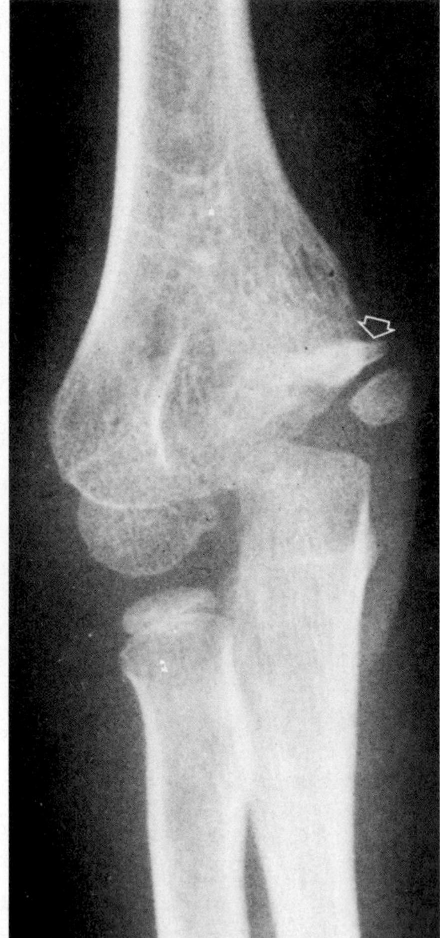

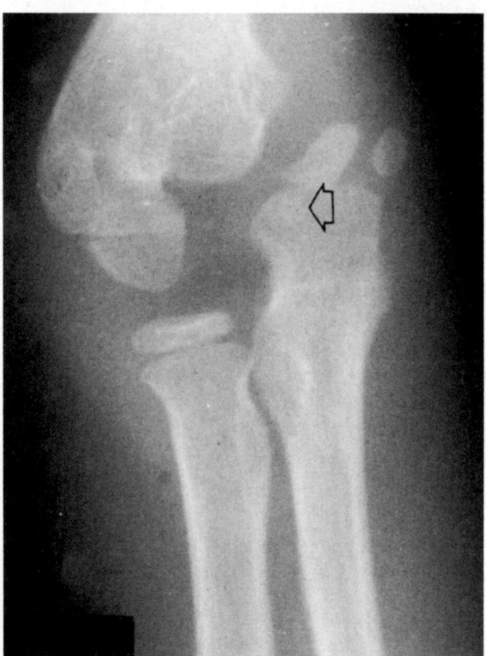

FIGURE 15-36 Nonunion in addition to cubitus varus deformity. **A.** Original film of a 5-year-old girl who sustained an injury 1 year previously. The metaphyseal fragment (*arrow*) is attached to the medial epicondyle. **B.** Film taken 2 years later. Some ossification has developed in the medial condylar epiphysis (*arrow*). (Courtesy of Roy N. Davis, MD.)

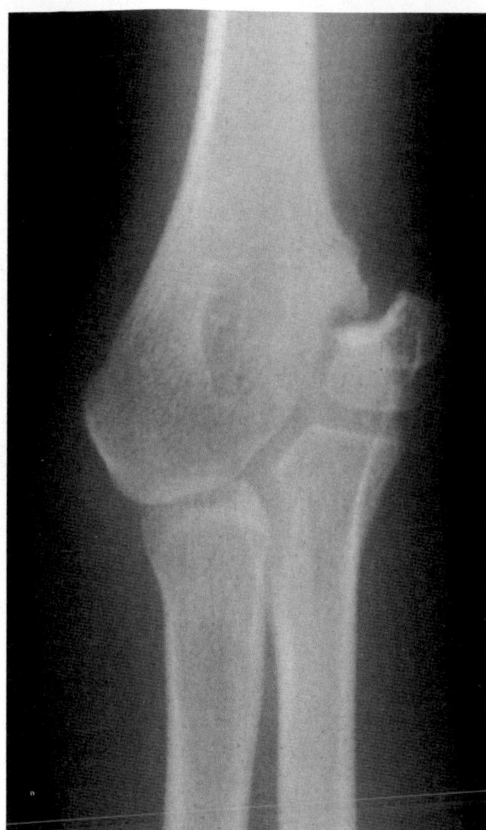

FIGURE 15-37 Nonunion of a medial condylar fracture in a 10-year-old girl. Note medial subluxation of the radius and ulna.

treating nonunion of lateral condylar fractures are generally applicable to nonunions of the medial condyle (Fig. 15-37).

El Ghawabi[47] described one partial ulnar neuropathy occurring after this type of injury. The neuropathy almost completely recovered after anterior transposition of the ulnar nerve.

Fractures of the Trochlea

Osteochondral fractures involving only the articular portion of the trochlea are extremely rare in skeletally immature children. Grant and Miller[66] reported a 13-year-old boy who had a posterolateral dislocation of the elbow with marked valgus instability and fractures of the medial epicondyle and radial neck. When the elbow was explored to secure the epicondyle, a large osteochondral fragment from the medial crista of the trochlea was found lying between the two articular surfaces. The fragment was replaced and fixed, and a satisfactory result was obtained, although the presence of the fragment was not detected preoperatively.

Patel and Weiner[139] described osteochondritis dissecans (OCD) in two patients (three elbows) aged 12 and 14 years. In one patient, open biopsy was done because the osteochondral lesion was thought to be a neoplastic lesion. The other patient with bilateral lesions was treated conservatively with good results. Matsuura et al.[111] evaluated 1802 young baseball players, 717 (40%) of whom had elbow pain. Of the 150 who had bilateral elbow radiographic examination, osteochondral lesions of the elbow were identified in 121 (81%); trochlear lesions accounted for 0.5% of these. More recently, Marshall et al.[109] reported osteochondral lesions of the trochlea in 18 young athletes ranging in age from 6 to 17 years; 10 of the 18 were throwing athletes and two were gymnasts. Based on MRI and MR arthrogram findings, injuries were classified as chondral/osteochondral injury/OCD lesions (13 patients) or trochlear osteonecrosis (five patients). Ten of the 13 osteochondral lesions involved the lateral trochlea and were described as classic OCD; the three medial trochlear lesions were small (<6 mm) and were located on the posterior articular surface of the medial trochlea. Trochlear osteonecrosis in five patients was characterized by growth disturbance involving the ossification centers of the trochlea. The affected trochleas were misshapen and underdeveloped, and radiographs showed the secondary ossification centers to be fragmented, small, and sclerotic, or absent entirely. All five of the patients with osteonecrosis had histories of distal humeral fractures treated with K-wire fixation earlier in childhood (two lateral condylar fractures and one each supracondylar, medial epicondylar, and medial condylar fracture). The authors suggested that the athletic demands placed on the adolescent elbow revealed osteonecrosis from these earlier fractures.[109] The OCD lesions consistently occurred in the posteroinferior aspect of the lateral trochlea corresponding to a watershed zone of diminished vascularity, and the authors hypothesized that the lesions were caused by repeated forced elbow extension/hyperextension that led to impingement of the normal blood supply.[109] Small osteochondral lesions on the posteromedial trochlea were suggested to result from olecranon abutment occurring in an elbow with collateral ligament laxity or insufficiency.

In an older child who sustains an elbow dislocation and in whom there is some widening of the joint after reduction, an intra-articular fracture of the trochlea or capitellum should be suspected. Arthrography, MRI, or computed tomography-arthrography, should be used for confirmation.

Fractures Involving the Entire Distal Humeral Physis

Incidence

From 1960 to 1978, many individual patients were reported.[92,154,167,184] Once the presence of this injury became recognized, larger series appeared. Seven separate series reported a total of 45 fractures,[4,3940,,81,114,123,141] and Abe et al.[1] reported a series of 21 fractures. Originally thought to be a rare injury, it appears that fractures involving the entire distal humeral physis occur frequently in children. The major problem is the initial recognition of this injury.

Surgical Anatomy

The distal humeral epiphysis extends across to include the secondary ossification of the medial epicondyle until about 6 to 7 years of age in girls and 8 to 9 years in boys. Thus, fractures involving the entire physeal line include the medial epicondyle up to this age. In older children, only the lateral and medial condylar physeal lines are included.

Most fractures involving the entire distal humeral physis occur before the age of 6 or 7. The younger the child is, the greater the volume of the distal humerus that is occupied by the distal epiphysis will be. As the humerus matures, the physeal line progresses more distally, with a central V forming between the medial and lateral condylar physes (Fig. 15-38). Ashhurst[7] believed that this V-shaped configuration of the physeal line helps protect the more mature distal humerus from physeal fractures.

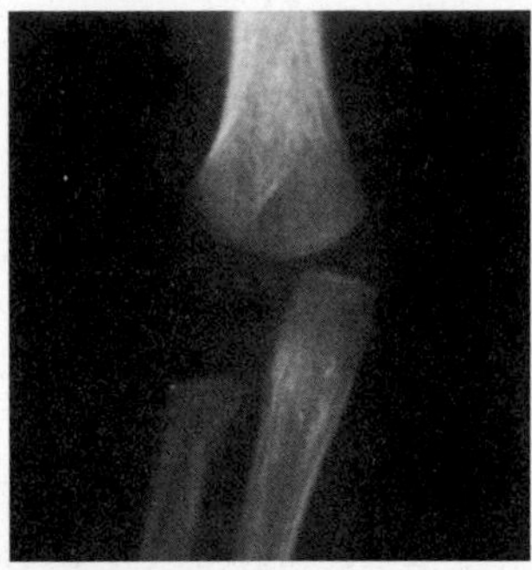
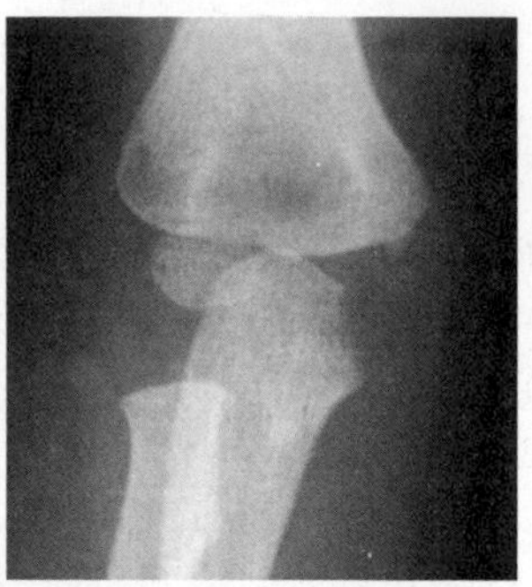

FIGURE 15-38 A. At 5 months of age, the metaphysis has advanced only to the supracondylar ridges. **B.** By 4 years of age, the edge of the metaphysis has advanced well into the area of the epicondyles

Because fractures coursing along the distal humeral physis traverse the anatomic centers of the condyles, they are the pediatric counterparts of the adult bicondylar fracture. Because the fracture is distal, the fracture surfaces are broader than those proximally through the supracondylar fractures. This broader surface area of the fracture line may help prevent tilting of the distal fragment. Because the fracture lines do not involve the articular surface, development of joint incongruity with resultant loss of elbow motion is unlikely if malunion occurs.

Finally, part of the blood supply to the medial crista of the trochlea courses directly through the physis. The blood supply to this area is vulnerable to injury, which may cause osteonecrosis in this part of the trochlea.

Because the physeal line is more proximal in young infants, it is nearer the center of the olecranon fossa (see Fig. 15-38). A hyperextension injury in this age group is more likely to result in a physeal separation than a bony supracondylar fracture.[36]

Mechanism of Injury

The exact mechanism of this injury is unknown and probably varies with the age group involved. A few consistent factors are evident.

First, many fractures of the entire distal humeral physis have occurred as birth injuries associated with difficult deliveries.[4,9,15,45,167] Siffert[167] noted that the clinical appearance of these injured elbows at the time of delivery was not especially impressive. There was only moderate swelling and some crepitus.

Second, DeLee et al.[40] noted a high incidence of confirmed or suspected child abuse in their very young patients. Other reports[4,39,200] have confirmed the frequency of child abuse in infants and young children with these fractures.

Bright[22] showed that a physis is more likely to fail with rotary shear forces than with pure bending or tension forces. Young infants have some residual flexion contractures of the elbow from intrauterine positioning; this prevents the hyperextension injury that results in supracondylar elbow fractures in older children. Rotary forces on the elbow, which can be caused by child abuse or birth trauma in young infants, are probably more responsible for this injury than hyperextension or varus or valgus forces, which produce other fracture patterns in older children.

Abe et al.[1] reported 21 children, ranging in age from 1 to 11 years (average: 5 years), with fracture separations of the distal humeral epiphysis, all of which were sustained in falls.

Classification

DeLee et al.[40] classified fractures of the entire distal humeral physis into three groups based on the degree of ossification of the lateral condylar epiphysis (Fig. 15-39). Group A fractures occur in infants up to 12 months of age, before the secondary ossification center of the lateral condylar epiphysis appears (Fig. 15-39A,B). They are usually Salter-Harris type I physeal injuries. This injury is often not diagnosed due to the lack of an ossification center in the lateral condylar epiphysis. Group B fractures occur most often in children 12 months to 3 years of age in whom there is definite ossification of the lateral condylar epiphysis (Fig. 15-39C). Although there may be a small flake of metaphyseal bone, this is also essentially a type I Salter-Harris physeal injury. Group C fractures occur in older children, from 3 to 7 years of age and result in a large metaphyseal fragment that is most commonly lateral but can be medial or posterior (Fig. 15-39D,E).

These fractures are almost always extension-type injuries with the distal epiphyseal fragment posterior to the metaphysis. A rare flexion type of injury can occur in which the epiphyseal fragment is displaced anteriorly.[15] Stricker et al.[183] reported a coronal plane transcondylar (Salter-Harris type IV) fracture in a 3-year-old child that was initially diagnosed as a fracture of the lateral humeral condyle. No growth disturbance was evident 3 years after open reduction and pin fixation.

Clinical Signs and Symptoms

In an infant less than 18 months of age, whose elbow is swollen secondary to trauma or suspected trauma, a fracture involving the entire distal humeral physis should be considered. In a young infant or newborn, swelling may be minimal with little crepitus. Poland[146] described the crepitus as "muffled" crepitus because the fracture ends are covered with softer cartilage than the firm osseous tissue in other fractures about the elbow. The relationship between the epicondyles and the olecranon is maintained. Because of the large, wide fracture surfaces, there are fewer tendencies for tilting with distal fragment rotation, and the angular deformity is less severe than that with supracondylar fractures. In older children, the elbow is often so swollen that a clinical assessment of the bony landmarks is impossible, and radiographic evaluation must provide confirmation of the diagnosis (see Fig. 15-39A,B).

Radiographic Findings

Radiographic diagnosis can be difficult, especially if the ossification center of the lateral condyle is not visible in an infant. The only relationship that can be determined is that of the primary ossification centers of the distal humerus to the proximal radius and ulna. The proximal radius and ulna maintain an anatomic relationship to each other but are displaced posteriorly and medially in relation to the distal humerus. This posteromedial relationship is diagnostic. Although theoretically, the distal fragment can be displaced in any direction, with rare exceptions[15] most fractures reported have been displaced posteromedially. Comparison views of the opposite uninjured elbow may be helpful to determine the presence of posteromedial displacement (see Fig. 15-39A,B).

Once the lateral condylar epiphysis becomes ossified, displacement of the entire distal epiphysis is much more obvious. The anatomic relationship of the lateral condylar epiphysis with the radial head is maintained, even though the distal humeral

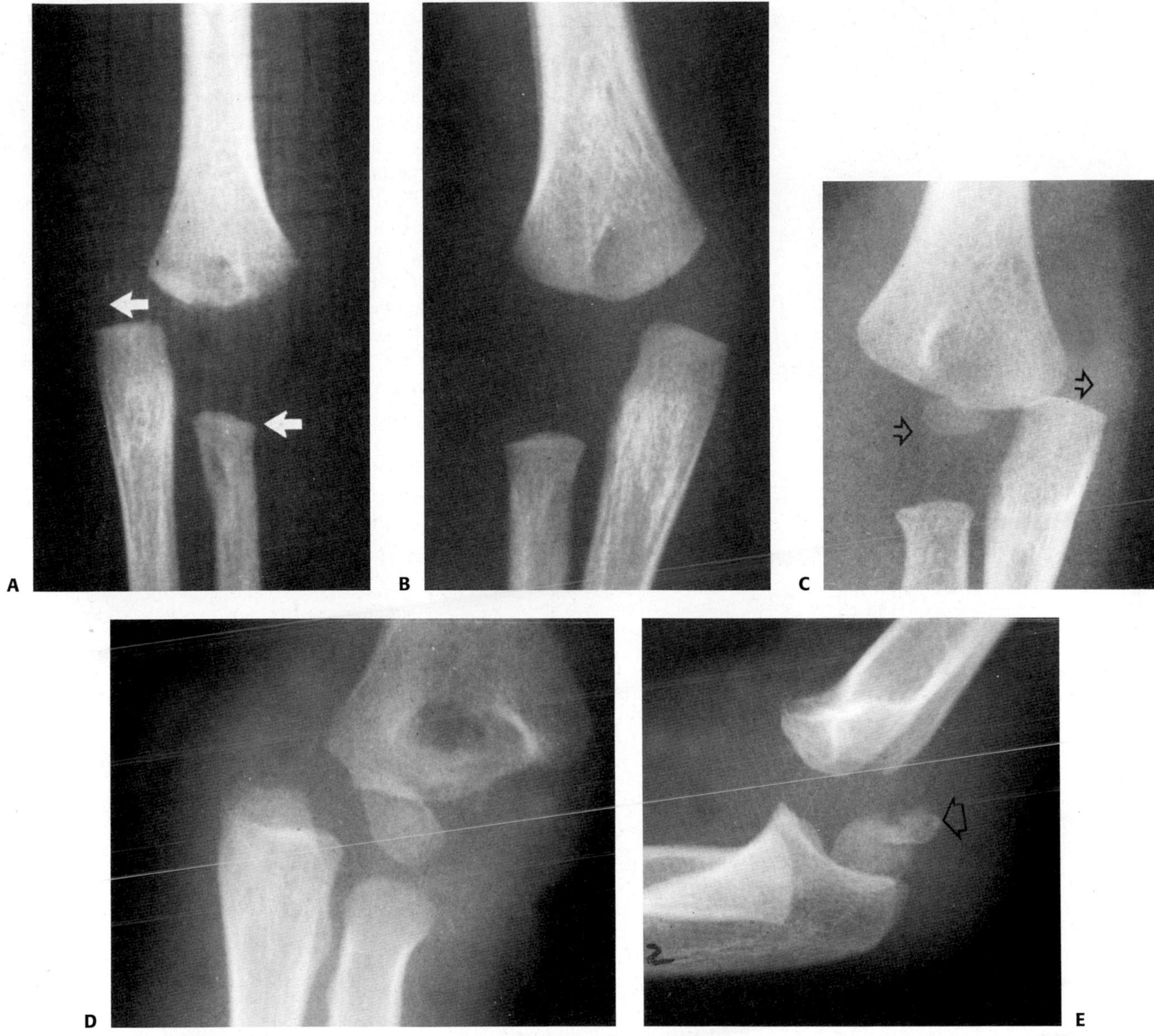

FIGURE 15-39 A. Group A—AP view of a small infant who had a swollen left elbow after a difficult delivery. The displacement medially of the proximal radius and ulna (*arrows*) helps to make the diagnosis of a displaced total distal humeral physis. **B.** Normal elbow for comparison. **C.** Group B—AP view showing the posteromedial displacement of the distal fragment (*arrows*). The relationship between the ossification center of the lateral condyle and the proximal radius has been maintained. **D.** Group C—AP view with marked medial displacement of the distal fragment. **E.** Group C—lateral view of the same patient showing posterior displacement of the distal fragment. There is also a large metaphyseal fragment associated with the distal fragment (*arrow*).

epiphysis is displaced posterior and medial in relation to the metaphysis of the humerus (see Fig. 15-39C,D).

Because they have a large metaphyseal fragment, type C fractures may be confused with either a low supracondylar fracture or a fracture of the lateral condylar physis. The key diagnostic point is the smooth outline of the distal metaphysis in fractures involving the total distal physis. With supracondylar fractures, the distal portion of the distal fragment has a more irregular border.

Differentiation from a fracture of the lateral condylar physis and the rare elbow dislocation in an infant can be made on radiograph. With a displaced fracture of the lateral condylar physis, the relationship between the lateral condylar epiphysis and the proximal radius is usually disrupted (see Fig. 15-8B). If the lateral crista of the trochlea is involved, the proximal radius and ulna may be displaced posterolaterally.

Elbow dislocations are rare in the peak age group for fractures of the entire distal humeral physis. With elbow dislocations, the displacement of the proximal radius and ulna is almost always posterolateral, and the relationship between the proximal radius and lateral condylar epiphysis is disrupted.

If differentiation of this injury from an intra-articular fracture is uncertain, arthrography or MRI may be helpful (see Fig. 15-5).[4,9,69,123]

In neonates and infants in whom ossification has not begun, ultrasonography can be used to outline the epiphysis of the humerus.[43] Comparison with the opposite uninjured humeral epiphysis may help determine the presence of a separation.

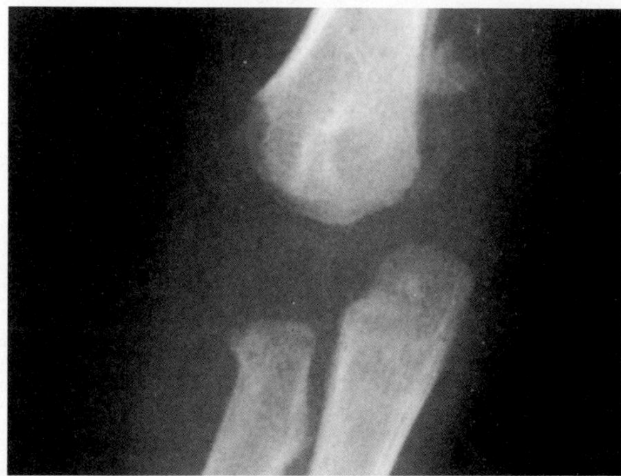

FIGURE 15-40 The true nature of this injury as involving the entire distal humeral physis was not appreciated until periosteal new bone became visible 3 weeks after injury.

If the diagnosis is delayed, new periosteal bone forms around the distal humerus, and the whole epiphysis may remain displaced posteriorly and medially (Fig. 15-40).

Treatment

Treatment is first directed toward prompt injury recognition. Because this damage may be associated with child abuse, the parents may delay seeking treatment.

De Jager and Hoffman[39] reported 12 fracture separations of the distal humeral epiphysis, three of which were initially diagnosed as fractures of the lateral condyle and one as an elbow dislocation. Due to the frequency of cubitus varus after this injury in young children, they recommended closed reduction and percutaneous pinning in children younger than 2 years of age so that the carrying angle can be evaluated immediately after reduction and corrected if necessary.

Several investigators have reported open reduction, usually performed owing to misdiagnosis as a displaced fracture of the lateral humeral condyle.[4,81,154,200] Mizuno et al.,[123] however, recommended primary open reduction because of his poor results with closed reduction. They approached the fracture posteriorly by removing the triceps insertion from the olecranon with a small piece of cartilage. If the fracture is old (more than 5 to 6 days) and the epiphysis is no longer mobile, manipulation should not be attempted, and the elbow should be splinted for comfort. Many essentially untreated fractures remodel completely without any residual deformity if the distal fragment is only medially translocated and not tilted (Fig. 15-41).

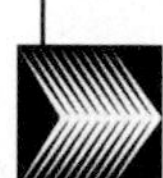

AUTHORS' PREFERRED TREATMENT

We usually first attempt a manipulative closed reduction of fresh fractures. The elbow is initially manipulated into extension to correct the medial displacement, and then the fragment is stabilized by flexing the elbow and pronating the forearm. The distal epiphysis is more securely held with the elbow flexed and the forearm pronated. When the forearm is supinated with the elbow flexed, the distal fragment tends to displace medially. This displacement is usually a pure medial horizontal translocation without mediolateral coronal tilting.

In neonates and very small infants in whom general anesthesia or percutaneous pin fixation may be difficult, we typically simply immobilize the extremity in 90 degrees of flex-

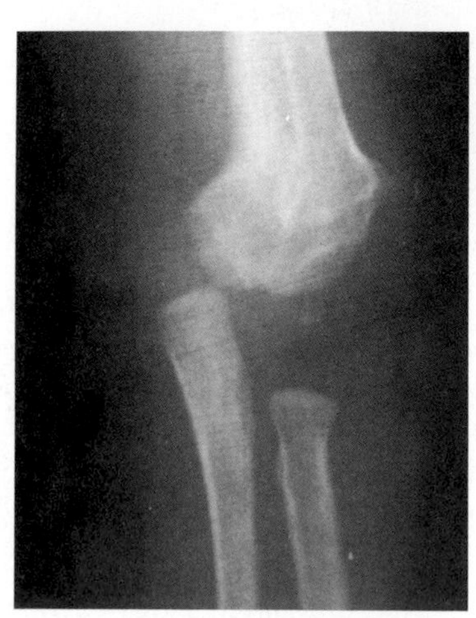

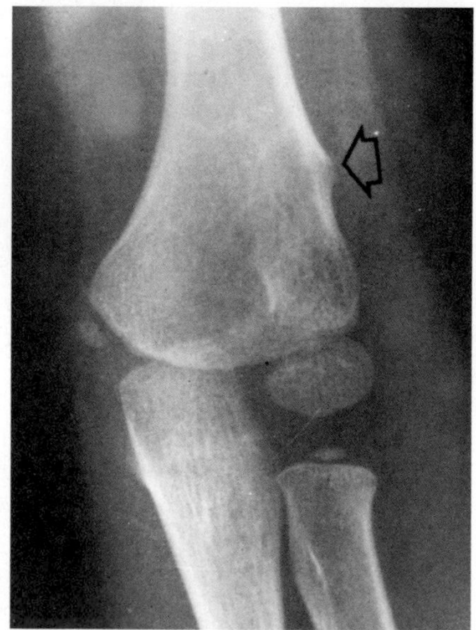

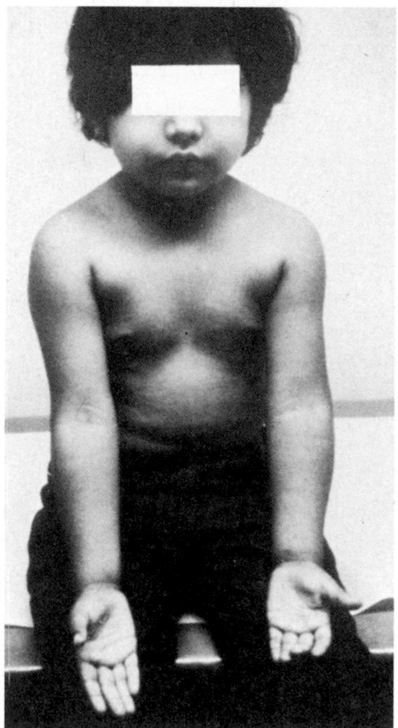

A B C

FIGURE 15-41 Remodeling of untreated fractures. **A.** AP view of a 2-year-old who had an unrecognized and untreated fracture of the distal humeral physis. The medial translocation is apparent. There was no varus or valgus tilting. **B.** Four years later, there had been almost complete remodeling of the distal humerus. A small supracondylar prominence (*arrow*) remains as a scar from the original injury. **C.** Clinical appearance 4 years after injury shows no difference in elbow alignment.

ion with the forearm pronated. The extremity is then externally stabilized with a figure-of-eight splint.

In most older infants and young children, external immobilization is usually not dependable in maintaining the reduction. As a rule, in these patients, we perform the manipulation with the patient under general anesthesia and secure the fragment with two lateral pins (Fig. 15-42). Due to the swelling and immaturity of the distal humerus, the medial epicondyle is difficult to define as a distinct landmark, making it risky to attempt the percutaneous placement of a medial pin. If a medial pin is necessary for stable fracture fixation, a small medial incision can be made to allow direct observation of the medial epicondyle. In small infants and young children with minimal ossification of the epiphyseal fragment, an intraoperative arthrogram may be obtained to help determine the quality of the reduction.

The cast or splint and pins are removed in 3 weeks to allow active elbow motion to resume. The patient is then followed until full motion is regained and until there is radiographic evidence of normal physeal and epiphyseal growth. Usually, 3 weeks of immobilization is sufficient.

If treatment is delayed more than 3 to 5 days and if the epiphysis is not freely movable, the elbow is simply immobilized in a splint or cast. It is probably better to treat any resulting deformity later with a supracondylar osteotomy rather than risk the complication of physeal injury or osteonecrosis of the epiphysis by performing a delayed open reduction. Only occasionally does an untreated patient have a deformity severe enough to require surgical correction at a later date. Because the articular surface is intact, complete functional recovery can usually be expected.

Child Abuse

Child abuse should always be considered in children with this injury, especially a type A fracture pattern, unless it occurs at birth. A young infant is unlikely to incur this type of injury spontaneously from the usual falls that occur during the first year of life. Of the 16 fractures reported by DeLee et al.,[40] six resulted from documented or highly suspected child abuse, all in children younger than 2 years of age.

Complications

Neurovascular Injuries. Neurovascular injuries, either transient or permanent, are rare with this fracture, probably because the fracture fragments are covered with physeal cartilage and do not have sharp edges as do other fractures in this area. In addition, the fracture fragments are usually not markedly displaced.

Nonunion. Only one nonunion after this fracture has been reported; it occurred in a patient seen 3 months after the initial injury.[123] Because of the extreme vascularity and propensity for osteogenesis in this area, union is rapid even in patients who receive essentially no treatment.

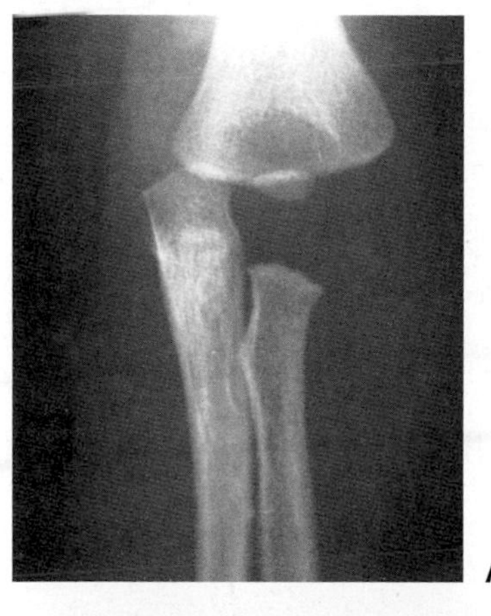

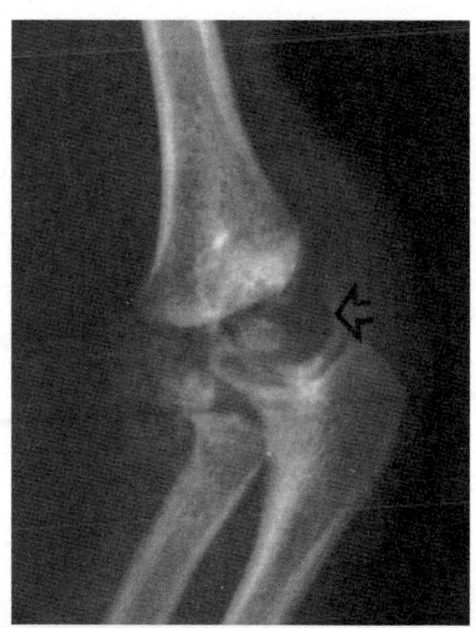

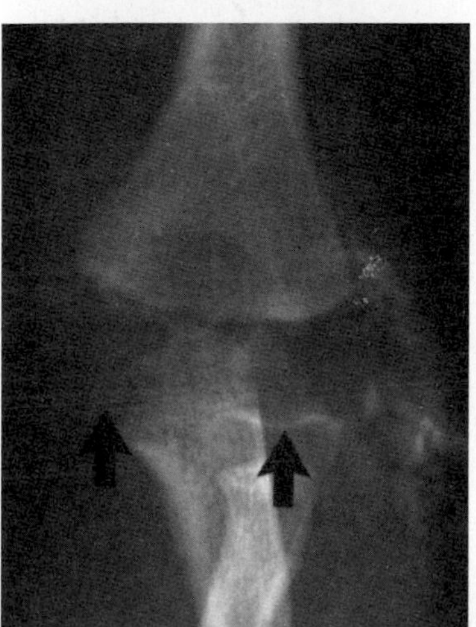

D

FIGURE 15-42 A. Injury film of a 20-month-old showing medial displacement of the distal fragment. **B,C.** The medial and posterior displacement of the condylar fragment (*arrow*) is better defined after an arthrogram. **D.** Fixation is achieved by two lateral pins placed percutaneously

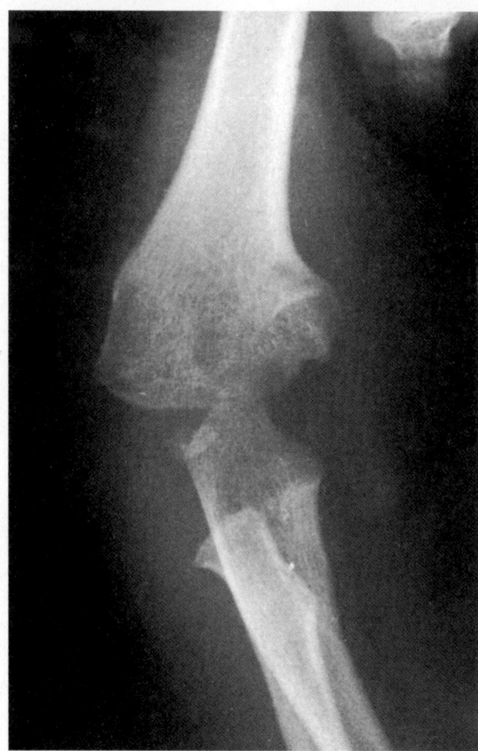

FIGURE 15-43 An AP view of a residual cubitus varus in a 2-year-old 6 months after physeal fracture of the distal humerus. This patient was treated initially with simple immobilization.

Malunion. Significant cubitus varus deformity is common after this injury (Fig. 15-43).[114,118] Because the fracture surfaces are wider with this injury than with supracondylar fractures, the distal fragment tends to tilt less, which seems to account for the lower incidence of cubitus varus after this injury than after untreated supracondylar fractures (see Fig. 15-43); however, reduction and percutaneous pinning are recommended for acute fractures with displacement.

Osteonecrosis. Osteonecrosis of the epiphysis of the lateral condyle or the trochlear epiphysis has rarely been reported after fractures of the entire distal humeral physis. Yoo et al.[207] reported eight patients with osteonecrosis of the trochlea after fracture separations of the distal end of the humerus. Six of the eight fractures were diagnosed initially as medial condylar fractures, lateral condylar fractures, or traumatic elbow dislocation. All eight patients had rapid dissolution of the trochlea within 3 to 6 weeks after injury, followed by the development of a medial or central condylar fishtail defect. We have noted osteonecrosis of the trochlea after three fractures of the entire humeral physis, two of which were inadequately reduced and one of which was anatomically reduced by closed methods (Fig. 15-44). All three had marked displacement of the distal epiphyseal fragment. In one, the osteonecrosis of the trochlea produced a secondary cubitus varus deformity that continued to progress with growth and a significant loss of elbow motion. The etiology of this complication was discussed in the section on osteonecrosis of the trochlea.

APOPHYSEAL INJURIES OF THE DISTAL HUMERUS

Fractures Involving the Medial Epicondylar Apophysis

In the early 1900s, it was recognized that this fracture was often associated with elbow dislocation and the apophyseal fragment could become entrapped within the joint.[194] Much of the discussion during that era centered on the manipulative techniques used to extract the fragment from the joint. In recent years, the proponents of uniform nonoperative management[89,134,202] have outnumbered the proponents of uniform operative management.[80] In the interval since the third edition of this volume, little has been written about the treatment of this injury; most of the focus has been on the increased recognition of this injury occurring during sports.[103,104,131]

Incidence

Fractures involving the medial epicondylar apophysis constitute approximately 14.1% of fractures involving the distal humerus and 11.5% of all fractures in the elbow region.[12,16,31]

Fractures involving the epicondylar apophysis have a later peak age, similar to fractures involving the medial condylar physis. The youngest reported patient with this injury was 3.9 years.[31] In the large series of fractures of the medial epicondylar

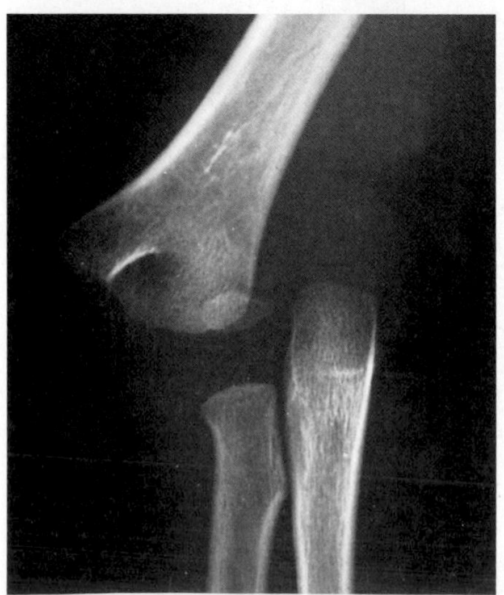

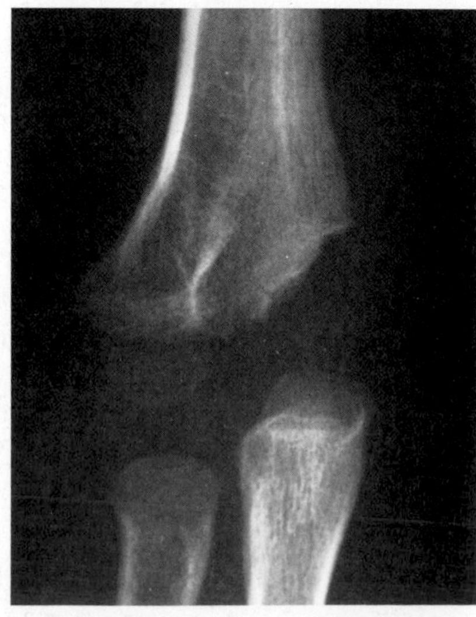

FIGURE 15-44 Osteonecrosis. **A.** Injury film in a 5-year-old with marked displacement of the distal epiphysis. Closed reduction was followed by lateral pin fixation. **B.** Nevertheless, radiographs taken 14 months later showed early evidence of osteonecrosis of the medial condyle. (Courtesy of Salvador J. Mendez, MD.)

TABLE 15-1 Fractures of the Medial Epicondylar Apophysis: Incidence

Overall incidence: Fractures of the elbow region, 11.5%

Age: peak, 11–12 years

Sex: males, 79% (4:1, male:female)

Association with elbow dislocation: Approximately 50% (15% to 18% of these involve incarceration of the epicondylar apophysis)

apophysis, most occurred between ages 9 and 14, and the peak age incidence was 11 to 12 years.[12,62,80,94,129,134,173,202] Fractures of the epicondylar apophysis affect boys by a ratio of almost 4 to 1. In six large series in the literature, boys constituted 79% of the patients.[62,63,107,155,194,202]

Association with Elbow Dislocation

The reported incidence of association with dislocation of the elbow has varied from as low as 30% to as high as 55% in many of the reported series.[12,202] Two bilateral injuries associated with bilateral elbow dislocations have been reported.[16,52] Both patients sustained their injuries while participating in gymnastics.

In summary, the peak age for fractures of the epicondylar apophysis is 9 to 12 years. The injury occurs in boys four times more often than in girls. About 50% of such injuries are associated with elbow dislocations. In at least 15% to 18% of patients, the fragment is incarcerated in the joint (Table 15-1).

Surgical Anatomy

The medial epicondyle is a traction apophysis, so the term *apophysis* rather than *physis* is used throughout the description of this injury. The forces across its physis are tension rather than the compressive forces present across the condylar physes of the distal humerus. Because it is an apophysis, it does not contribute to the overall length of the distal humerus.

In the early ossification process, the medial epicondylar apophysis is part of the entire distal humeral epiphysis. With growth and maturity, it becomes separated from the entire distal humeral epiphysis by intervening metaphyseal bone. In younger children, when there is a separation of the distal humeral epiphysis, the medial epicondylar apophysis is included as part of the distal fragment.

Posteromedial Location

The medial epicondylar apophysis actually arises from the posterior surface of the medial distal humeral metaphysis. As was mentioned in Chapter 14, this posterior location is important when percutaneous pin fixation is used. Likewise, this posterior position affects the image of the apophysis on radiographs (Fig. 15-45).

Ossification Sequence

Silberstein et al.[169] described various unique aspects of the ossification process of the medial epicondylar apophysis. The following discussion is paraphrased from their work.

Ossification begins from 4 to 6 years of age, with fusion

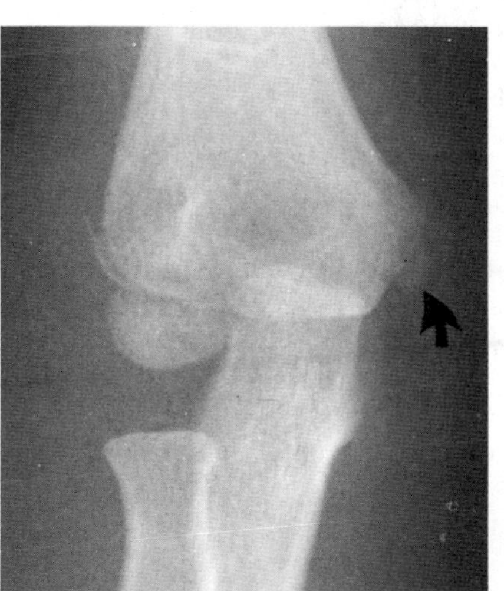

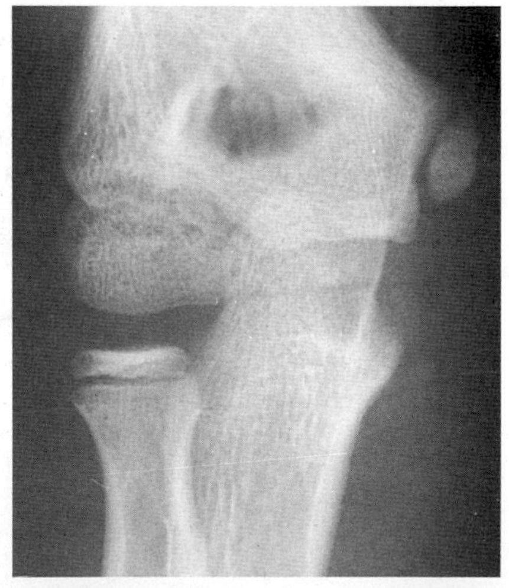

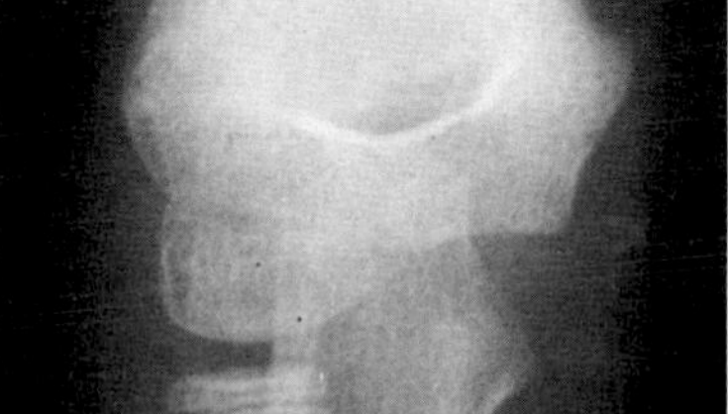

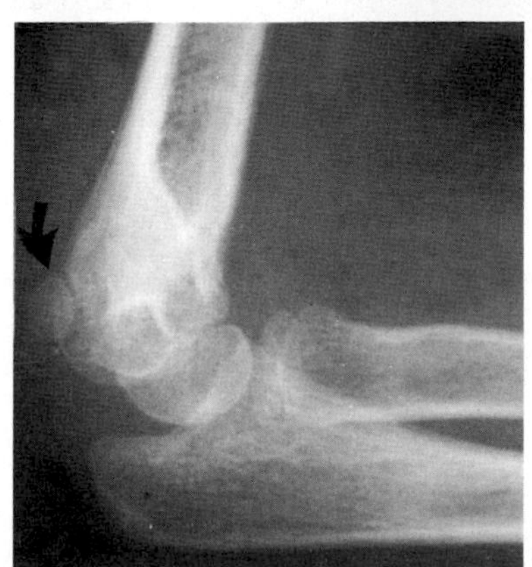

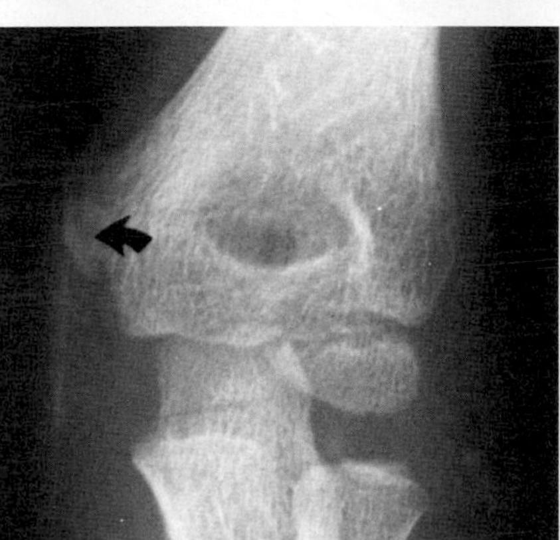

FIGURE 15-45 Ossification of the medial epicondyle. **A.** The concentric oval nucleus of ossification of the medial epicondylar apophysis (*arrow*). **B.** As ossification progresses, parallel smooth sclerotic margins develop in each side of the physis. **C.** Because it is somewhat posterior, on a slightly oblique anteroposterior view the apophysis may be hidden behind the distal metaphysis. **D.** The posterior location of the apophysis (*arrow*) is appreciated on this slightly oblique lateral view. **E.** On the anteroposterior view, the line created by the overlapping of the metaphysis (*arrow*) can be misinterpreted as a fracture line (pseudofracture).

occurring at about 15 years of age. It is the last secondary ossification center to fuse with the distal humeral metaphysis. The ossification center starts as a small eccentric oval nucleus (Fig. 15-45A). As it matures, parallel sclerotic margins develop along both sides of the physis (Fig. 15-45B). There may be some irregularity of the ossification process, which gives the ossific nucleus a fragmented appearance. This fragmentation may be falsely interpreted as a fracture.

Because the apophysis is posteromedial, the ossification center may be difficult to see on an AP radiograph, especially if the elbow is slightly oblique (Fig. 15-45C). The posterior position of the apophysis is best appreciated on a lateral radiograph. If the elbow is slightly oblique, the outline of the epicondyle may be better appreciated (Fig. 15-45D). Because of this posterior location on AP radiographs, the distal medial metaphyseal border may overlap the ossific nucleus of the apophysis. This overlapping may appear as a lucent line that can be misinterpreted as a fracture (Fig. 15-45E).

Soft Tissue Attachments

Flexor Mass. The flexor mass, which includes the origin of the flexor carpi radialis, flexor carpi ulnaris, flexor digitorum superficialis, palmaris longus, and part of the pronator teres, originates from the anterior aspect of the apophysis (Fig. 15-46).[169] Part of the flexor carpi ulnaris also originates on the posterior aspect of the epicondyle.

Capsule. In younger children, some of the capsule's origin extends up to the physeal line of the epicondyle. In older children and adolescents, as the epicondyle migrates more proximally, the capsule is attached only to the medial crista of the trochlea.[7] Thus, in younger children, a fracture line involving the medial epicondylar apophysis can enter the joint because part of the capsule is attached to the epicondylar fragment. In older children, however, if there is a pure avulsion force on the epicondyle, the capsule may remain attached to the trochlea's outer border. In this age group, the fracture may be totally extra-articular.

Ligamentous Structures. The two major medial collateral ligaments originate from this apophysis. The ulnar collateral ligament is composed of three separate bands (Fig. 15-47).[204] Woods and Tullos[204] pointed out that the major stabilizing ligamentous structure in the elbow is the anterior band of the ulnar collateral ligament. The band's anterior portion is taut in extension, and the posterior fibers are taut in flexion. The fibers of the posterior band of the ulnar collateral ligament are relaxed in extension and are taut in flexion (see Fig. 15-47). Thus, this posterior band provides stability only in flexion. Because the radial collateral ligaments do not attach directly to the ulna or radius, but instead attach to the orbicular ligament, they provide only minimal stability to the elbow joint.

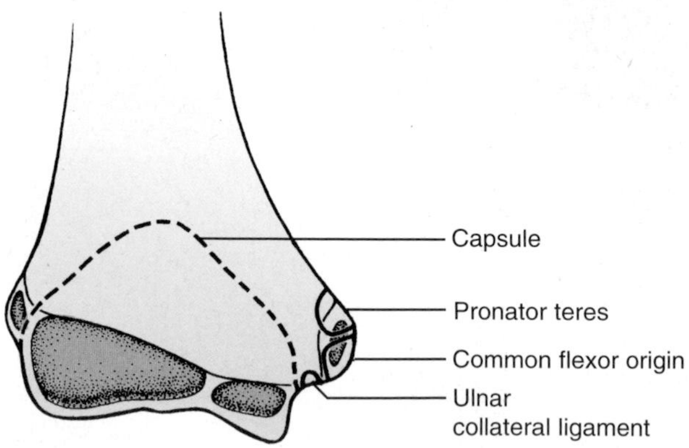

FIGURE 15-46 Soft tissue attachments. The AP view of the distal humerus demonstrates the relationship of the apophysis to the origins of the medial forearm muscles. The origin of the ulnar collateral ligament lies outside the elbow capsule. The margin of the capsule is outlined by the dotted line.

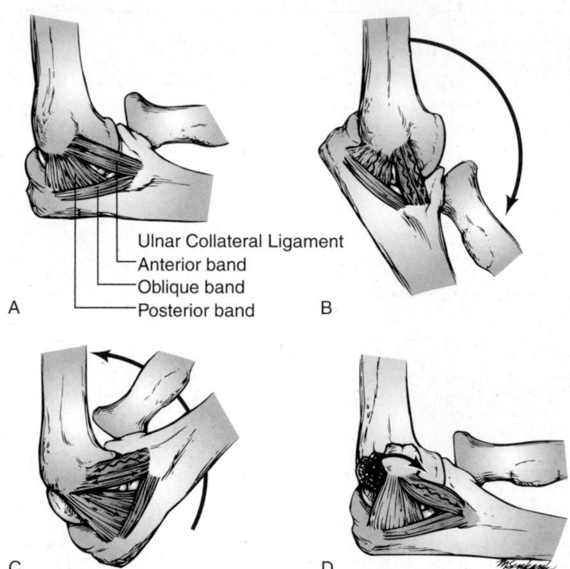

FIGURE 15-47 Ligamentous structures. **A.** The ulnar collateral ligament is divided into anterior, posterior, and oblique bands. **B.** On extension, the anterior fibers of the anterior band are taut. The posterior fibers of the anterior band and the entire posterior band are loose in this position. **C.** In flexion, the posterior fibers of the anterior bands and posterior band become taut. The anterior fibers of the anterior band become loose. **D.** When the epicondyle is rotated anteriorly, the entire anterior band can become loose. (From Woods WG, Tullos HS. Elbow instability and medial epicondyle fractures. Am J Sports Med 1977;5:23–30, with permission.)

Mechanism of Injury

Injuries to the medial epicondylar apophysis most commonly occur as acute injuries in which a distinct event produces a partial or a complete separation of the apophyseal fragment. Three theories have been proposed about the mechanism of acute medial epicondylar apophyseal injuries: a direct blow, avulsion mechanisms, and association with elbow dislocation (Table 15-2).

Direct Blow. Stimson[181] speculated that this type of injury could occur as a result of a direct blow on the posterior aspect of the epicondyle. Among more recent investigators, however, only Watson-Jones[195] described this injury as being associated with a direct blow to the posterior medial aspect of the elbow. In rare patients in whom the fragment is produced by a direct blow to the medial aspect of the joint, the medial epicondylar fragment is often fragmented (Fig. 15-48). In these injuries, there may also be more superficial ecchymosis in the skin.

Avulsion Mechanisms. Various investigators have suggested that some of these injuries are due to a pure avulsion of the

TABLE 15-2 Fractures of Medial Condylar Apophysis: Mechanism of Injury

Acute injuries
Direct blow
Avulsion mechanisms
Avulsion in elbow extension (valgus stress)
Avulsion with elbow flexed (pure muscle forces)
Associated with elbow dislocation
Chronic tension stress injuries

epicondyle by the flexor muscles of the forearm.[94,140] This muscle avulsion force can occur in combination with a valgus stress in which the elbow is locked in extension, or as a pure musculature contraction that may occur with the elbow partially flexed.

Avulsion and Extension (Valgus Stress). Smith[173] proposed that when a child falls on his outstretched upper extremity with the elbow in extension, the wrist and fingers are often hyperextended as well, placing an added tension force on the epicondyle by the forearm flexor muscles (Fig. 15-49). The normal valgus carrying angle tends to accentuate these avulsion forces when the elbow is in extension. Many proponents of this theory point to the other associated elbow fractures that have been seen with this injury as evidence to confirm that a valgus force is applied across the elbow at the time of the injury. These associated injuries include radial neck fractures with valgus angulation and greenstick valgus fractures of the olecranon.[94]

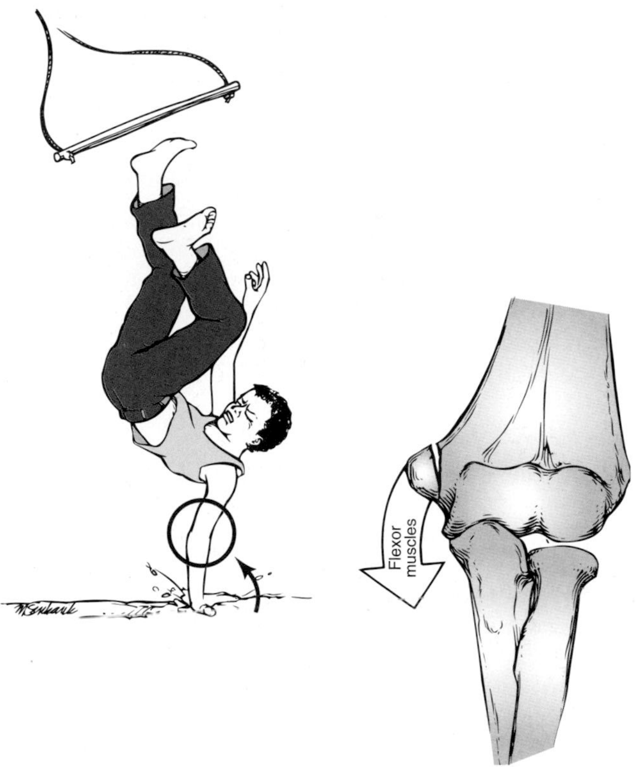

FIGURE 15-49 Hyperextension forces. When a person falls on the outstretched upper extremity, the wrist and fingers are forced into hyperextension (*solid arrow*), which places tension on the forearm flexor muscles. This sudden tension along with the normal valgus carrying angle tends to place a strong avulsion force on the medial epicondyle (*open arrow*).

Isolated Muscle Avulsions. Isolated avulsion can also occur in adolescents with the simple act of throwing a baseball. In this instance, the sudden contracture of the forearm flexor muscles may be sufficient to cause the epicondyle to fail (Fig. 15-50). The literature has reflected a high incidence of medial epi-

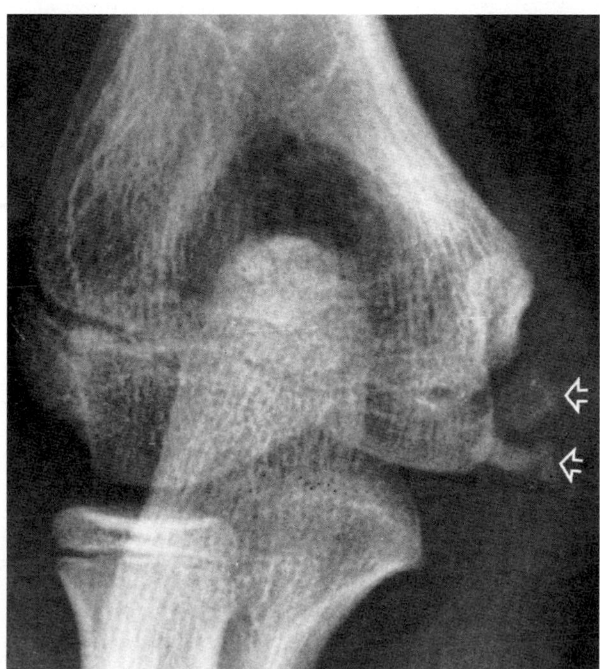

FIGURE 15-48 Direct fragmentation. The fragmented appearance of the medial epicondyle (*arrows*) in a 13-year-old who sustained a direct blow to the medial aspect of the elbow. (From Wilkins KE. Fractures of the medial epicondyle in children. Instr Course Lect 1991;40:1–8, with permission.)

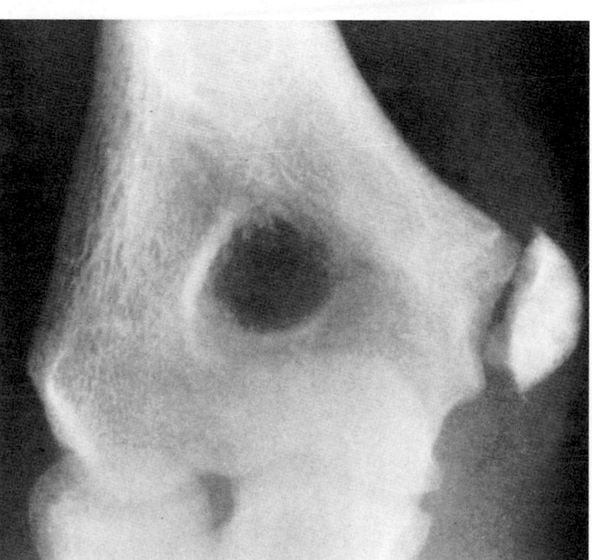

FIGURE 15-50 Muscle avulsion. Isolated avulsion of the medial epicondyle occurred suddenly in this 14-year-old Little League pitcher after throwing a curve ball. (From Wilkins KE. Fracture of the medial epicondyle in children. Instr Course Lect 1991;40:1–8, with permission.)

condylar apophyseal avulsions occurring with arm wrestling in patients near skeletal maturity.[104,131] The largest series, reported by Nyska et al.[131] from Israel, involved eight boys 13 to 15 years of age, all of whom were treated conservatively with good results.

Associated with Elbow Dislocations. The final mechanism proposed is that this injury is associated with elbow dislocation in which the ulnar collateral ligament provides the avulsion force. If the elbow is dislocated when the patient is initially seen, there is no doubt that this is a major factor in the cause of this fracture. The question of whether this fracture is caused by an occult or partial elbow dislocation that has reduced spontaneously is often raised. Some investigators[12,16,62] have noticed calcification development in the lateral collateral ligaments and adjacent lateral periosteum after fracture. They believed this calcification was evidence that this ligament had been stretched during the process of elbow dislocation. Marion and Faysse[107] found that most elbow dislocations associated with this injury were posterolateral, but some pure lateral, posterior, and posteromedial dislocations were also observed.

The question arises as to whether incarceration of the epicondylar fragment into the joint can occur without a dislocation. Patrick[140] believed that when an extreme valgus stress was applied to the joint, a vacuum was created within the joint that "sucked in" the avulsed epicondylar fragment.

It appears that any of these mechanisms can produce an acute apophyseal injury of the distal humerus. The direct blow mechanism appears to occur only rarely. Many of these injuries may be associated with an elbow dislocation that may or may not have reduced spontaneously.

Acute Fractures. Usually, the epicondyle is displaced distally. Avulsion generally involves only the apophysis, but a small flake of metaphyseal bone is occasionally attached to the apophyseal fragment. The fracture line rarely passes through the apophysis, and only part of the apophysis is avulsed.[169] Although these partial avulsions may appear as only minor injuries, the partial fragment can be incarcerated within the joint just as easily as the full apophysis (Fig. 15-51).

Chronic Incarceration. When the fragment becomes incarcerated into the joint, the raw bone surface may become adherent to the coronoid process of the ulna.[155] In late cases, the union of the fragment to the coronoid process may make extraction difficult. A universal finding when the fragment is incarcerated within the joint is a thick fascial band that binds the ulnar nerve to the underlying muscle.[7,140] The constriction that this band creates is believed to be responsible for either the immediate or late dysfunction of the ulnar nerve.

Associated Injuries. Other elbow fractures that can be associated with this injury include fracture of the radial neck, olecranon, or coronoid process. If the epicondyle fragment is only rotated on its axis, the anterior band of the ulnar collateral ligament can become lax. This laxity can produce some medial elbow instability during extension.[204]

Classification

The various classifications proposed for this injury[12,107] are similar. We have combined them to form a comprehensive classification (Table 15-3) that can be useful in determining the proper treatment method. In the discussion of this classification, the clinical and radiographic findings are delineated for each type

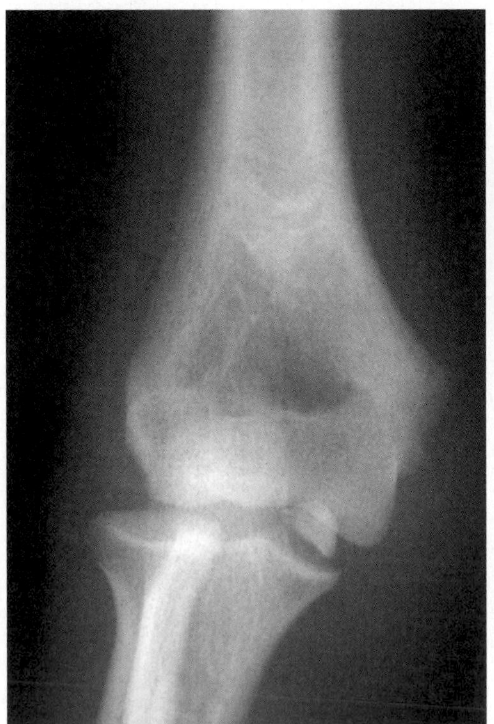

A

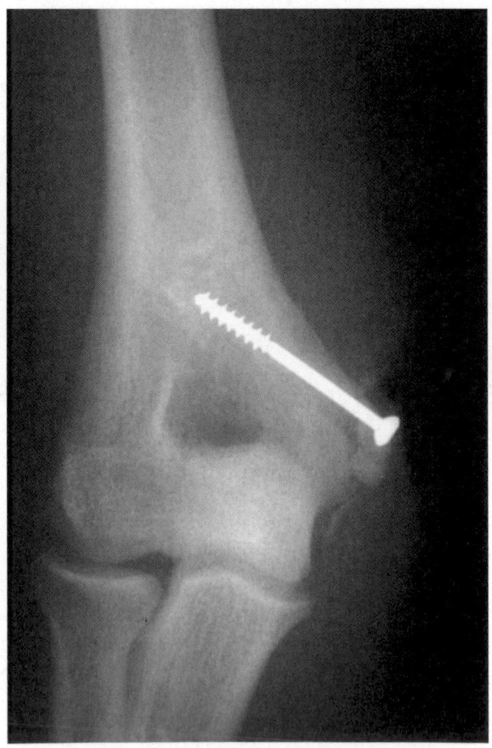

B

FIGURE 15-51 A. Entrapment of fracture fragment in medial epicondylar fracture with posterolateral elbow dislocation. **B.** After fragment extraction, open reduction, and screw fixation.

TABLE 15-3 Fractures of the Medial Epicondyle Apophysis: Classification

Acute injuries
Undisplaced or minimally displaced
Displaced fractures
Incarcerated fractures (without elbow dislocation)
Incarcerated fractures (with elbow dislocation)
Chronic tension (stress) injuries

of fracture pattern. Initially, we have separated these injuries into two primary categories based on whether the injuries are acute or chronic.

Acute Injuries.

Undisplaced or Minimally Displaced Fractures. In undisplaced fractures, the physeal line remains intact. The clinical manifestations usually consist only of swelling and local tenderness over the medial epicondyle. Crepitus and motion of the epicondyle are usually not present. On radiograph, the smoothness of the edge of the physeal line remains intact. Although there may be some loss of soft tissue planes medially on the radiograph, displacement of the elbow fat pads may not be present because the pathology is extra-articular.[74]

Minimally displaced fractures usually result from a stronger avulsion force, so there is often more soft tissue swelling. Palpating the fragment may elicit crepitus because the increased displacement allows motion of the fragment. On radiograph, there is a loss of parallelism of the smooth sclerotic margins of the physis (Fig. 15-52).[169] The radiolucency in the area of the apophyseal line is usually increased in width.

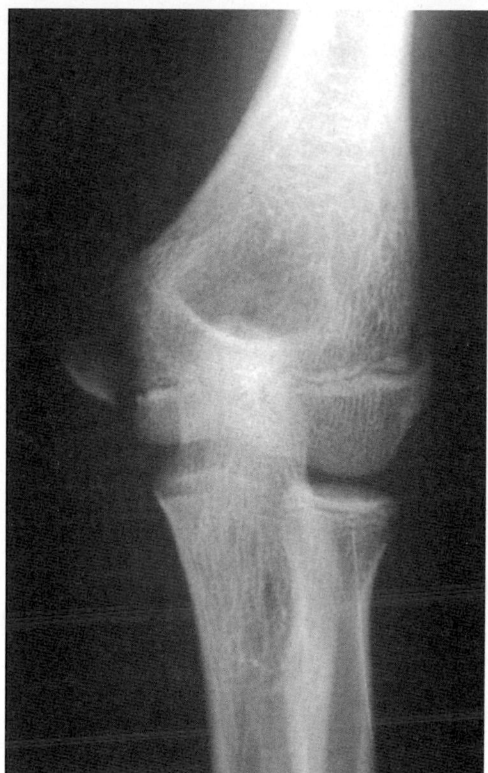

FIGURE 15-52 AP radiograph shows loss of normal smooth margins of the physis after type II medial epicondylar fracture.

Significantly Displaced Fractures. In significantly displaced fractures, there is no question as to whether the fragment is displaced, as it may be palpable and freely movable. Because it is displaced a considerable distance from the distal humerus, crepitus between the fragments may not be present. There may have been an elbow dislocation that reduced spontaneously or by manipulation. On the other hand, there may have been no documentation of the original dislocation. On radiograph, the long axis of the epicondylar epiphysis is rotated medially (Fig. 15-53). The displacement usually exceeds 5 mm, but the fragment remains proximal to the true joint surface. This fragment may contain a metaphyseal fragment.

Entrapment of the Epicondylar Fragment Into the Joint.
Without Elbow Dislocation. In many instances, the elbow appears reduced. The key clinical finding is a block to motion, especially extension. The epicondylar fragment is usually between the joint surfaces of the trochlea and the semilunar notch of the olecranon. On radiograph, any time the fragment appears at the level of the joint, it must be considered to be totally or partially within the elbow joint until proven otherwise.[140] If the radiograph is examined carefully, the elbow is usually still found to be incompletely reduced. Due to an impingement of the fragment within the joint, a good AP view may be difficult to obtain because of the inability to extend the elbow fully. If the fracture is old and if the fragment is fused to the coronoid process, widening of the medial joint space may be the only clue that the fragment is lying in the joint. The epicondylar ossification center may become fragmented and mistaken for the fragmented appearance of the medial crista of the trochlea.[31,155] Absence of the apophyseal center on radiograph may be further

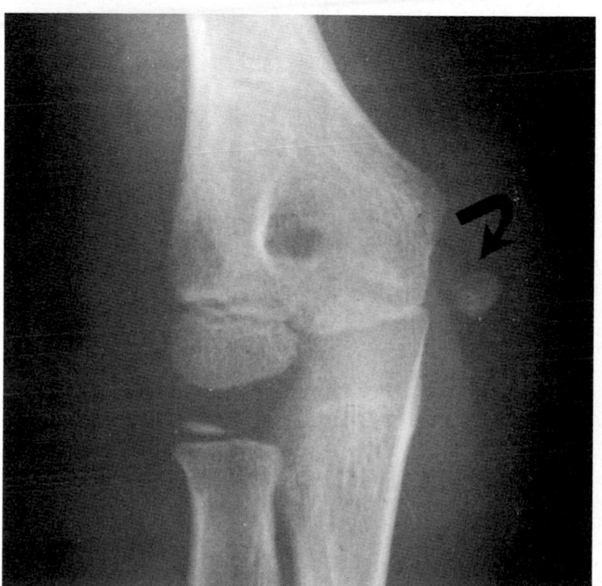

FIGURE 15-53 Type III displaced medial epicondylar fracture. AP view of an elbow in which the epicondyle (*arrow*) is significantly displaced both distally and medially. In addition, the fragment is rotated medially.

confirmatory evidence that the fragment is within the joint. Comparison radiographs of the opposite elbow may be necessary to delineate the true pathology.

With Elbow Dislocation. Even if the elbow is dislocated, the fragment can still lie within the joint and prevent reduction. Recognition of this fragment as being within the joint before a manipulation should alert the physician of the possible need for open reduction. There should be adequate relaxation during the manipulative process. An initial manipulation to extract the fragment from the elbow joint may need to be accomplished before a satisfactory closed reduction of the elbow joint can be obtained (Fig. 15-54).

Fractures through the Epicondylar Apophysis

Fractures through the body of the epicondyle can result from either a direct blow or avulsion of only part of the apophysis. In either case, the fragments may or may not be displaced. The normal lucent line formed by the overlying metaphyseal border should not be confused with this injury. Although described by Silberstein et al.,[169] this intrafragment fracture is a rare presentation.

Clinical Findings

Valgus Stress Test. Because many of the clinical diagnostic points have been discussed in the previous section on the classification of this injury, much of the emphasis in this section is on the determination of elbow instability. Because the anterior oblique band of the ulnar collateral ligament may be attached to the medial epicondylar apophysis, the elbow may exhibit some instability after injury. To evaluate the medial stability of the elbow, Woods and Tullos[204] and Schwab et al.[164] advocated a simple valgus stress test. This test is performed with the patient supine and the arm abducted 90 degrees. The shoulder and arm are externally rotated 90 degrees. The elbow must be flexed at least 15 degrees to eliminate the stabilizing force of the olecranon. If the elbow is unstable, simple gravity forces will open the medial side. A small additional weight or sedation may be necessary to acquire an accurate assessment of the medial stability with this test.

Evaluating the Ulnar Nerve. The function of the ulnar nerve must be carefully assessed. It is especially wise to document the presence or absence of an ulnar nerve injury before instituting therapy.

Radiographic Findings

Widening or irregularity of the apophyseal line may be the only clue in fractures that are only slightly displaced or nondisplaced. If the fragment is significantly displaced, the radiographic diagnosis is usually obvious. If the fragment is totally incarcerated in the joint, however, it may be hidden by the overlying ulnar or distal humerus. The clue here is the total absence of the epicondyle from its normal position just medial and posterior to the medial metaphysis.

Potter[148] suggested that properly performed MRI might disclose acute or chronic injury to the medial epicondylar apophysis. Recommended pulse sequences for evaluating the apophysis include fat-suppressed gradient echo imaging. On MRI, increased signal intensity and abnormal widening of the medial epicondylar physis are seen, typically with surrounding soft tissue edema.

Fractures of the medial epicondyle, even if displaced, may not produce positive fat pad signs.[74,169] If the fracture is only minimally displaced and if it is the result of an avulsion injury, there may be no effusion because all the injured tissues remain extra-articular. In fractures associated with elbow dislocation, there is rupture of the capsule, so its ability to confine the hemarthrosis is lost. In minimally displaced fractures of the medial

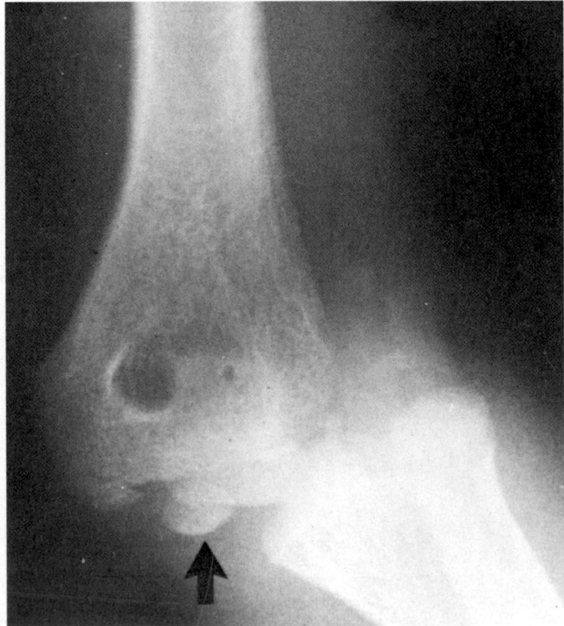

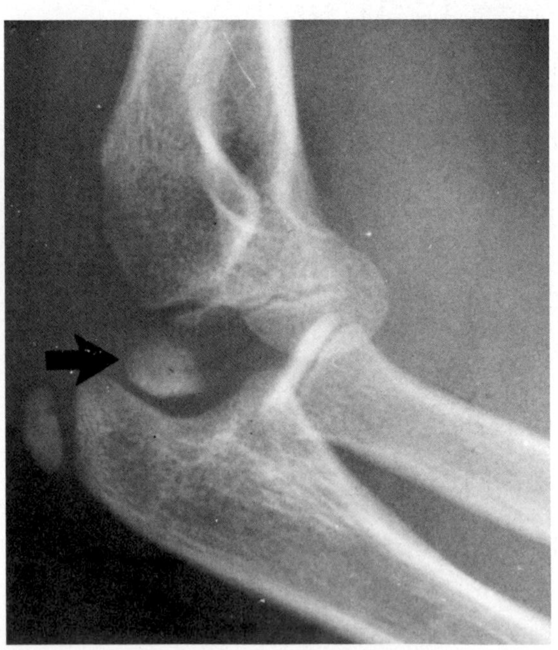

FIGURE 15-54 Dislocation with incarceration. **A.** AP view showing a posterolateral elbow dislocation. The presence of the medial epicondyle within the elbow joint (*arrow*) prevented a closed reduction. **B.** The lateral view of the same elbow demonstrates the fragment (*arrow*) between the humerus and olecranon.

epicondyle with significant hemarthrosis, the evaluation must be especially thorough to ensure that an unrecognized fracture involving the medial condylar physis or an associated elbow dislocation is not present.

Differential Diagnosis

The major injury to differentiate involves the medial condylar physis. This is especially true if the secondary ossification centers are not present (see "Fractures Involving the Medial Condylar Physis"). If there is a significant hemarthrosis or a significant piece of metaphyseal bone accompanying the medial epicondylar fragment, arthrography or MRI may be indicated to determine if there is an intra-articular component to the fracture (Fig. 15-55).

Treatment

Areas of General Agreement. There seems to be universal agreement as to the proper method of treating fractures that are undisplaced or only minimally displaced. These first two types are easily treated with simple immobilization for comfort. Some investigators have recommended initiation of motion early to prevent stiffness, which is the most common complication of this injury.[16,173] Likewise, if the fragment is incarcerated in the joint, the accepted treatment is to extract the fragment from the joint by manipulation or surgical intervention.

The controversy seems to be in determining the proper treatment method for patients with significant displacement (fragment displacement more than 5 mm).

Nonoperative Management. In reports in which only one method (i.e., operative or nonoperative) of treatment of all displaced fractures was used, results tend to support that method. The best argument for surgical management comes from Hines et al.[80] whose practice was to surgically repair all fractures displaced more than 2 mm. They found that 96% of their patients had good to excellent results. Bad results were attributed mainly to technical errors. Josefsson and Danielsson[89] obtained equal results and treated all of these injuries nonoperatively. Although more than 60% of their patients demonstrated nonunion on radiograph, these investigators had an equal number of good results at a mean follow-up of 11 years. Other reports in the literature[5,134,202] also demonstrated the overall good results with nonoperative management.

The best comparison of operative and nonoperative treatment results comes from reports in which both methods were used in the same institution. Bede et al.[12] had superior results in patients treated nonoperatively compared with those treated operatively. This same superiority of nonoperative management has been found in subsequent reports as well.[16,62,202]

The results of fractures associated with a documented elbow dislocation are poorer[12,62] for patients treated operatively and nonoperatively. Fowles et al.[62] reported that surgical intervention only added to the original trauma produced by the dislocation, increasing the residual loss of motion.

Indications for Operative Intervention. The indications for operative intervention in acute injuries are divided into two categories: absolute and relative. The single absolute indication is incarceration of the epicondylar fragment within the joint. The relative indications include ulnar nerve dysfunction and a need for elbow stability.

Incarceration in the Joint—Absolute. If the fragment is found in the joint acutely, it must be removed. There are proponents and techniques of both nonoperative and operative extraction of the fragment.

Nonoperative Extraction—Various methods of extracting the fragment by nonoperative methods have been proposed. The success rate of extracting the fragment successfully from the joint by manipulation alone is only about 40%.[140] All the nonoperative methods require either heavy sedation or light general anesthesia.

Roberts' Manipulative Technique—The manipulative technique most commonly used is the method popularized by Roberts.[52,153] It involves placing a valgus stress on the elbow while supinating the forearm and simultaneously dorsiflexing the wrist and fingers to place the forearm muscles on stretch; theoretically, this maneuver should extract the fragment from the

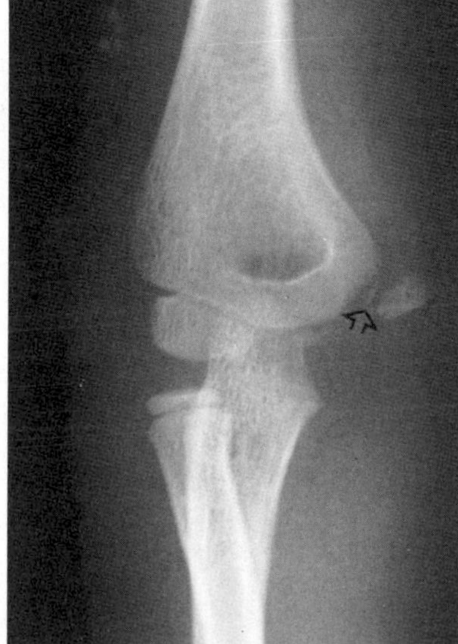

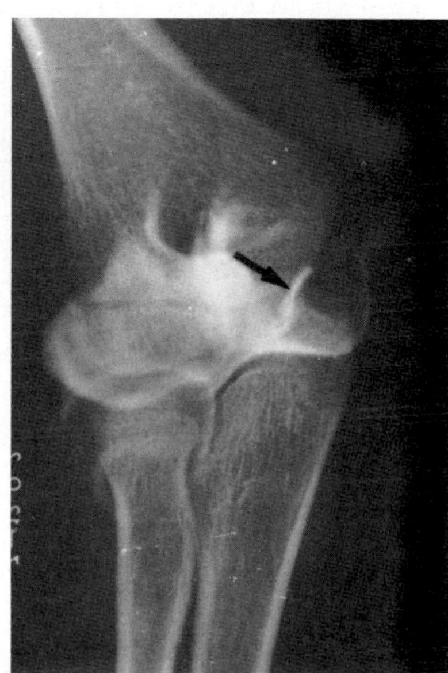

FIGURE 15-55 Intra-articular extension. **A.** Injury film in a 7-year-old girl who was initially suspected of having only a fracture of the medial epicondyle. In addition to moderate displacement, there was a significant metaphyseal fragment (*arrow*). **B.** An arthrogram revealed intra-articular components (*arrow*), which defined this injury instead as a fracture involving the medial condylar physis. (Courtesy of Carl McGarey, MD.)

joint. To be effective, this procedure should be carried out within the first 24 hours after injury.

Operative Extraction—Failure to extract the fragment by manipulative techniques is an indication to proceed with open surgical extraction. Once open extraction and reduction have been performed, many methods have been advocated to stabilize the fragment, including screw fixation or sutures in the comminuted fracture. Excision has also been advocated, especially if the fragment is comminuted.

Incarceration Discovered Late—Fowles et al.[61] challenged the opinion that surgery is detrimental in patients with late incarceration, and the idea remains controversial. In their patients in whom the fragment was surgically extracted an average of 14 weeks after injury, 80% more elbow motion was regained. In addition, the patients' preoperative pain was relieved, and the ulnar dysfunction resolved. On a long-term basis, intra-articular retention of the fragment may not be all that disabling. Rosendahl[155] reported an 8-year follow-up of a fragment retained within the joint. The epicondyle had fused to the semilunar surface of the ulna, producing a large bony prominence clinically. There was only minor loss of elbow motion, with little functional disability.

Ulnar Nerve Dysfunction—Relative. Ulnar nerve dysfunction is a relative indication for operative intervention. If there are mild-to-moderate ulnar nerve symptoms at the time of the injury, there is usually no need to explore the nerve, because most of these mild symptoms resolve spontaneously.[16,42] If the dysfunction is complete, then the ulnar nerve is probably wrapped around the fragment and should be explored surgically. One of the original fears was that the raw surface of the fracture fragment would create scar tissue around or adjacent to the nerve and cause continued dysfunction. Thus, it was originally recommended that the ulnar nerve should be transposed at the time of open reduction.[195] Subsequent reports have not found this step to be necessary.[186]

There is some question as to whether delayed ulnar nerve symptoms can even occur after fractures of the epicondyle that are not associated with elbow dislocation. In a review of more than 100 patients with uncomplicated fractures involving the medial epicondylar apophysis, Patrick[140] could not find any instance in which a delayed ulnar neuritis developed. He found some patients with late ulnar neuritis after fractures that were associated with elbow dislocation. Bernstein et al.[16] found that their patients with initial ulnar nerve symptoms all did well when treated nonoperatively. Thus, the original fear of delayed ulnar nerve dysfunction has been dispelled.

Joint Stability—Relative. Woods and Tullos[204] suggested that even minor forms of valgus instability after elbow injuries involving the medial epicondylar apophysis can cause significant disability in athletes. This condition is especially true in athletes who must have a stable upper extremity, such as baseball pitchers, gymnasts, or wrestlers. In younger adolescents (younger than 14 years of age), the anterior band of the ulnar collateral ligament often displaces with the apophyseal fragment. In older individuals (15 years or older), large fragments may be avulsed without a ligamentous injury. Rather than depending on arbitrary measurements of fracture displacement, Woods and Tullos[204] recommended using the gravity valgus stress test to determine the presence or absence of valgus instability. They believed that demonstration of a significant valgus instability, using this simple gravity test, was an indication for surgical intervention in patients who require a stable elbow for their athletic activities. Pimpalnerkar et al.[144] also suggested that clinical evidence of instability, as shown by gravity valgus stress testing, is an indication for operative fixation.

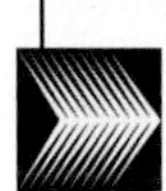

AUTHORS' PREFERRED TREATMENT

We use the classification scheme (see Table 15-3) as a rough guide to treatment. We also strongly consider the expected activity of the involved extremity in deciding on nonoperative or operative treatment (Table 15-4).

For most uncomplicated fractures, regardless of the number of millimeters of displacement, we prefer nonoperative management (Fig. 15-56), including fractures associated with elbow dislocations. The parents are warned that no matter which type of treatment is provided, some loss of elbow extension may occur. They should be reassured, however, that this loss of motion, if it does occur, is not usually of any functional or cosmetic significance. The elbow is immobilized initially with a removable posterior splint, used mainly for comfort and some support.

Because stiffness is the most common complication of this injury, we promote early active motion. The patient is encouraged to remove the splint and start active motion as soon as 3 to 4 days after injury. The splint is exchanged for a sling as soon as the patient feels he or she no longer needs it for support. The same instructions apply to the sling: it is also discarded when it is no longer needed. This regimen of early motion is also used in fractures associated with a documented dislocation. Redislocation after elbow dislocation is rare, but elbow stiffness is common, so it is more important to initiate motion as soon as possible after reduction of the elbow. Due to the greater amount of soft tissue injury associated with an elbow dislocation, the patient may not feel comfortable initiating early motion until about 5 to 7 days after reduction. Physical therapy should be used only if voluntary active motion is difficult to obtain. The therapist should emphasize modalities designed to decrease swelling and pain and re-establish strength. Range of motion should be achieved only by active means, not by passive stretching.

Operative Indications

Our indications for operative intervention are basically twofold. First and foremost are fractures in which the fragments

TABLE 15-4 Authors' Preferred Treatment

Nonoperative treatment indications

Nondisplaced or minimally displaced
- Significantly displaced in patients with low-demand upper-extremity function

Operative treatment Indications:
- Absolute: Irreducible incarcerated fragment in the elbow joint
- Relative: Ulnar nerve dysfunction
- Relative: Patient with high-demand upper extremity-function

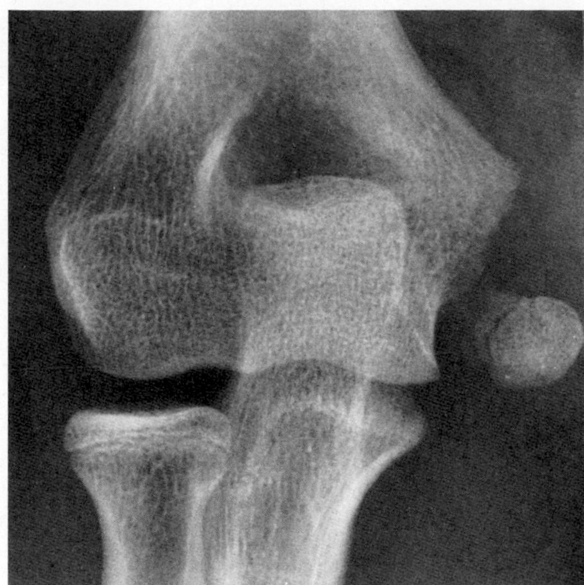
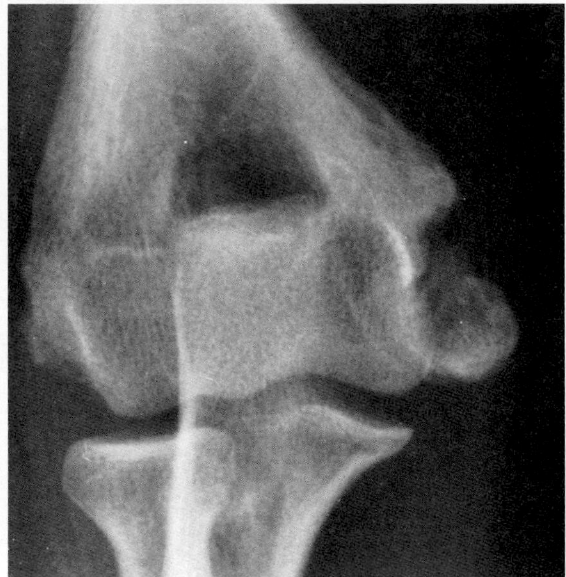

FIGURE 15-56 Nonoperative management. **A.** Postreduction film of a 13-year-old girl who sustained a displaced medial epicondyle following an acute elbow dislocation in her nondominant extremity. She was treated nonoperatively. **B.** One year later, the fragment has remained distally displaced with an apparent fibrous union. The patient, however, had a full painless range of elbow motion. (From Wilkins KE. Fractures of the medial epicondyle in children. Instr Course Lect 1991;40:1–8, with permission.)

cannot be extracted by manipulative means from within the elbow joint. Second, we stabilize the epicondyles operatively in patients whose expected high level physical activity requires a stable elbow. We realize, however, that it is difficult to predict the athletic potential of a young child.

Acute Incarceration in the Joint

If the elbow is reduced and if the ulnar nerve is intact, we use Roberts' manipulative technique[153] to attempt to extract the fragment before reduction. If this technique fails to remove the fragment or if there is any ulnar nerve dysfunction, we proceed directly with an open procedure. The fragment is then extracted under direct vision just before reducing the elbow dislocation. If the elbow is reduced and if the fragment is incarcerated, we avoid the initial manipulation and proceed directly with an open extraction. We usually stabilize these fractures with a single cannulated screw, which allows almost immediate motion, rather than wires or pins.

Follow-up is essentially the same as after closed treatment. Active motion is initiated 5 to 10 days postoperatively.

Prevention of Valgus Instability

Currently, our most common indication for operative intervention is to ensure a stable elbow in patients participating in high-demand activities with their upper extremity (Fig. 15-57). This usually involves the dominant extremity of baseball pitchers, tennis players, or football quarterbacks. In wrestlers and gymnasts, the stability of the nondominant extremity also must be considered, which is best achieved with operative fixation.

We have not found the valgus stress test to be helpful in deciding on the need for operative stabilization of an athlete's medial epicondyle. Almost all of these patients with any significant displacement have a positive valgus stress test. Our decision is based primarily on the patient's need to have a very stable elbow for his or her athletic or work activity.

Fixation must be stable enough to allow early motion. Pins provide stability but do not allow early motion. Fortunately, most patients are mature enough so that the fragment can be secured with a cannulated screw.

Operative Technique

Our operative technique involves a direct medial approach to the fracture site. We make a longitudinal incision just anterior to the medial epicondyle. The fragment is usually displaced distally and anteriorly. The periosteum is removed from the fracture site, and the clot is extracted by irrigation. It is important to identify and protect the ulnar nerve, but a complete dissection of the nerve is usually unnecessary. A small towel clip is used to reduce the fracture while the elbow is flexed and the forearm is pronated. Again, the medial epicondyle is normally situated posteriorly. The fragment is reduced and stabilized temporarily with one or two small K-wires. The final fixation is achieved using a screw, either partially threaded and overdrilled, in the epicondylar fragment to compress it against the metaphysis or a cannulated 4.0-mm screw. After removal of the K-wires, the elbow is checked to ensure valgus stability and re-establishment of a full range of motion. After the surgical incision is closed, the extremity is placed in a long-arm cast, which is bivalved at 5 to 10 days, and active motion is initiated.

Fragmented Apophysis

If the epicondyle is fragmented and if there is a need to achieve elbow stability, an American Society for Internal Fixation spiked washer can be used to secure the multiple pieces to the metaphysis. If the washer is used, a second procedure may be necessary

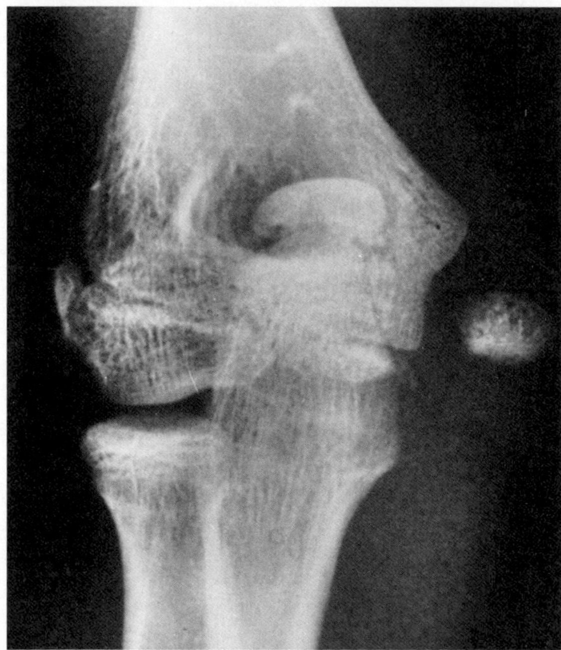

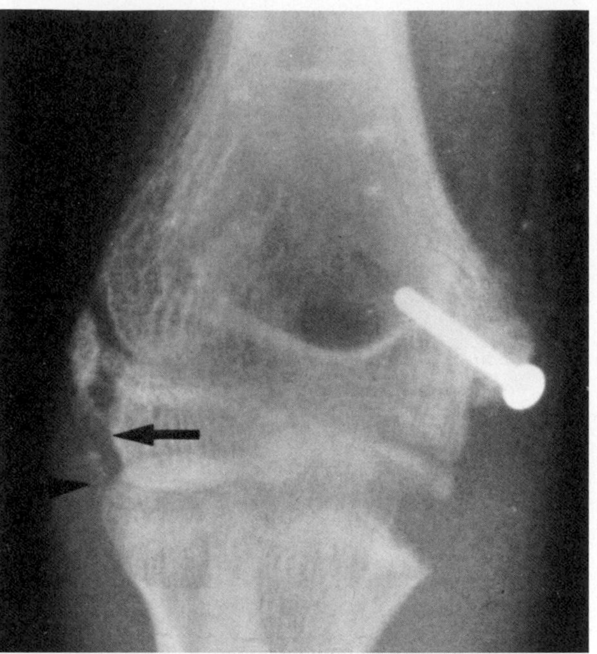

FIGURE 15-57 Operative stabilization. **A.** Injury film in a 12-year-old gymnast. Although this was a nondominant extremity, it was thought that both elbows needed stability. **B.** Radiographs taken 4 weeks postoperatively show stabilization of the fragment with a single screw. There was also calcification of the lateral ligaments (*arrows*), confirming that the elbow was probably originally dislocated as well. (From Wilkins KE. Fractures of the medial epicondyle in children. Instr Course Lect 1991;40:1–8, with permission.)

to remove the spike washer once the epicondyle is securely united to the metaphysis. If removal is impossible, we simply excise the fragments and reattach the ligament to the bone and periosteum at the base of the epicondylar defect.

Complications

Although much has been written about fractures involving the medial epicondylar apophysis, few complications are attributed to the fracture itself. The major complications that result in loss of function are failure to recognize incarceration in the joint and ulnar or medial nerve dysfunction. Most of the other complications are minor and result in only minimal functional or cosmetic sequelae (Table 15-5).

TABLE 15-5 Fractures of the Medial Epicondylar Apophysis: Complications

Major
Failure to recognize incarceration in the elbow
Ulnar nerve dysfunction
Minor
Loss of elbow extension
Myositis ossificans
Calcification of the collateral ligaments
Loss of motion
Cosmetic effects
Nonunion in the high-performance athlete

Major Complications.

Failure to Recognize Incarceration. Failure to recognize incarceration of the epicondylar fragment into the joint can result in significant loss of elbow motion, especially if it remains incarcerated for any length of time. The management for late incarceration was detailed in the previous section on treatment.

Ulnar Nerve Dysfunction. The other major complication associated with this injury is the development of ulnar nerve dysfunction. The incidence of ulnar nerve dysfunction varies from 10% to 16%.[12,107] If the fragment is entrapped in the joint, the incidence of ulnar nerve dysfunction may be as high as 50%.[12,52]

The incidence of delayed ulnar nerve neuritis is low. More profound ulnar nerve injury has been reported after manipulative procedures.[140] Thus, in patients with fragments incarcerated in the joint, manipulation may not be the procedure of choice if a primary ulnar nerve dysfunction is present. Patients in whom the fragment was left incarcerated in the joint for a significant time have experienced poor recovery of the primary ulnar nerve injury.[107]

Dysfunction. Although the ulnar nerve is the major nerve injured, the median nerve may be trapped between a bony fragment and the distal humerus.[133] It is speculated that the nerve can be entrapped between the apophyseal fragment and the distal humerus at the time of the original injury. This type of injury is described in greater detail in the section on complications of elbow dislocations.

Minor Complications. Other complications are minimal. Nonunion of the fragment with the distal metaphysis occurs in up to 50% of fractures with significant displacement.[12] This appears to be more of a radiographic problem than a functional problem.

Another common problem is loss of the final degrees of elbow extension. A loss of 5% to 10% can be expected to develop in about 20% of these fractures. Little functional deficit is attributed to this loss of elbow dysfunction. Prolonged immobilization seems to be the key factor in loss of elbow extension. Again, it is important to emphasize before treatment is begun that loss of motion is common after this injury, regardless of the treatment method used.

Myositis ossificans is a rare occurrence following vigorous and repeated manipulation to extract the fragment from the joint. As with many other elbow injuries, myositis may be a result of the treatment rather than the injury itself. Myositis ossificans must be differentiated from ectopic calcification of the collateral ligaments, which involves only the ligamentous structures. This condition may occur after repeated injuries to the epicondyle and ligamentous structures (Fig. 15-58). Often, this calcified ligament is asymptomatic and does not seem to create functional disability. The cosmetic effects are minimal. In some patients, an accentuation of the medial prominence of the epicondyle creates a false appearance of an increased carrying angle of the elbow. In his extensive review, Smith[173] recognized only a slight decrease in the carrying angle in two patients.

Nonunion in a high-performance athlete may be difficult to treat. One of the authors has treated a high-performance adolescent baseball pitcher who had to stop pitching after nonoperative management of a medial epicondylar fracture. The patient had developed a fibrous nonunion (Fig. 15-59). Attempts to establish union surgically were unsuccessful. The patient continued playing baseball, but had to change to another position.

Fractures Involving the Lateral Epicondylar Apophysis

Incidence

Fracture of the lateral epicondylar apophysis is a rare injury, with only a few isolated injuries described, mostly in textbooks.

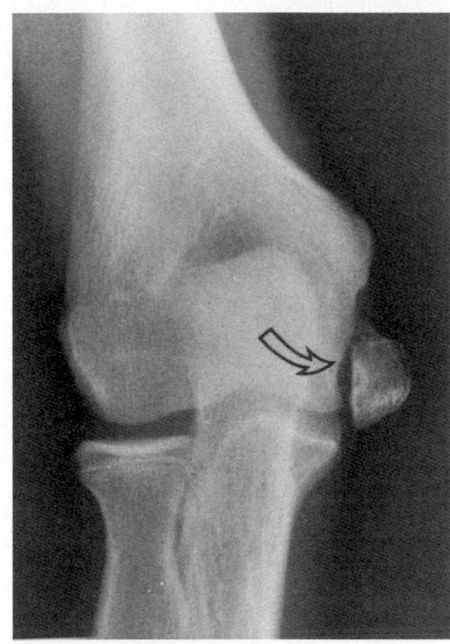

FIGURE 15-59 Nonunion in an athlete. This 15-year-old baseball pitcher had an untreated medial epicondyle fracture 1 year before this radiograph He developed a fibrous union, but the epicondyle was shifted distally (*arrow*). His elbow was unstable enough to prevent him from pitching.

Anatomic Considerations

Because the presence of this apophysis is often misinterpreted as a small chip fracture, a thorough understanding of the anatomy and ossification process is essential for evaluating injuries in this area.

Late Ossification. The lateral epicondylar apophysis is present for a considerable period but does not become ossified until the second decade. The best discussion of the anatomy of the ossification process is in a report by Silberstein et al.,[168] and much of the following discussion is paraphrased from their

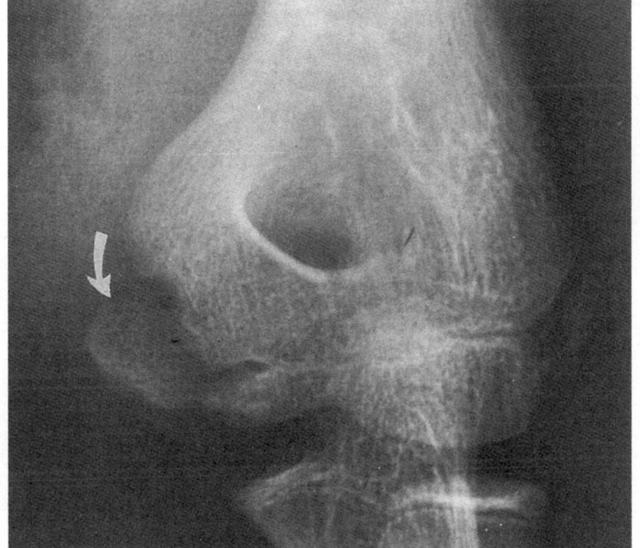

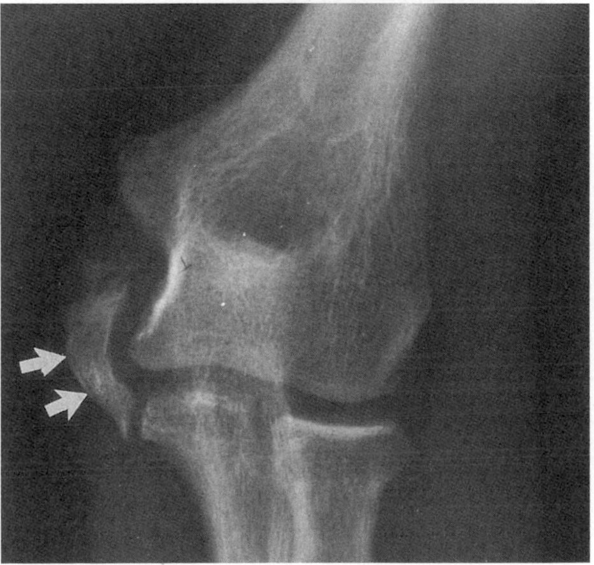

FIGURE 15-58 Heterotopic calcification. **A.** Injury to an 11-year-old who had moderate displacement of the medial epicondyle (*arrow*). **B.** One year later, she had considerable calcification of the ulnar collateral ligament (*arrows*). Other than mild instability with valgus stress, the patient had full range of motion and was asymptomatic. (Courtesy of Mark R. Christofersen, MD.)

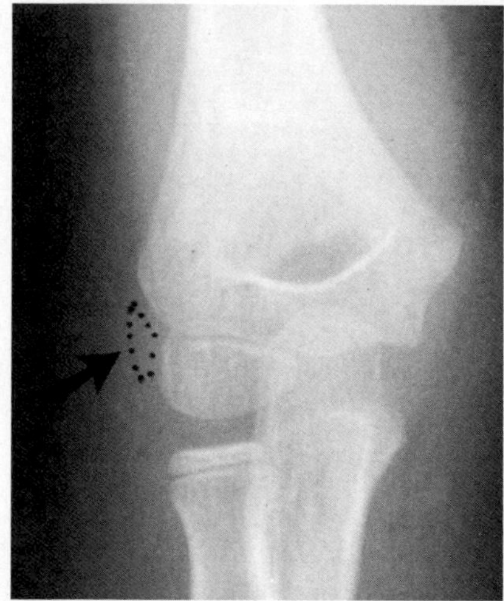

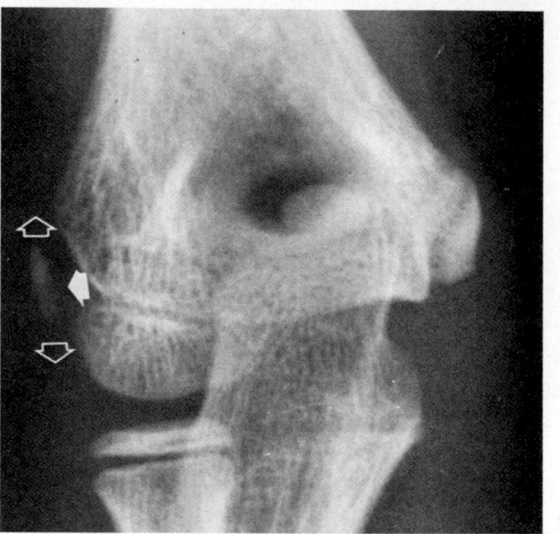

FIGURE 15-60 Lateral epicondylar apophysis. **A.** The cartilaginous apophysis occupies the wedge-shaped defect at the margin of the lateral condyle and metaphysis (*arrow*). The dotted line shows the margin of the cartilaginous apophysis. **B.** Ossification of the apophysis begins at the central portion of the wedge defect (*solid arrow*) and progresses both proximally and distally (*open arrows*) to form a triangular center.

work. Just before ossification of the apophysis, the ossification margin of the lateral supracondylar ridge of the distal metaphysis curves abruptly medially toward the lateral condylar physis (Fig. 15-60). This process causes the osseous borders on the lateral aspect of the distal humerus to take the shape of the number 3. The central wedge of this defect contains the cartilaginous lateral epicondylar apophysis, which begins to ossify around 10 to 11 years of age. Ossification begins at the level of the lateral condylar physeal line and proceeds proximally and distally to form a triangle, with the apex directed toward the physeal line. The shape of the epicondylar apophyseal ossification center may also be in the form of a long sliver of bone with an irregular ossification pattern. Silberstein et al.[168] noted that the fracture line involving the lateral condylar physis often involves the proximal physeal line of the lateral epicondylar apophysis. Thus, this apophysis is almost always included with the lateral condylar fragment.

Mechanism of Injury

In adults, the most common etiology is that of a direct blow to the lateral side of the elbow. In children, because the forearm extensor muscles originate from this area, it is believed that avulsion forces from these muscles can be responsible for some of these injuries. Hasner and Husby[75] suggested that the location of the fracture line in relation to the origins of the various extensor muscles determines the degree of displacement that can occur (Fig. 15-61). If the proximal part of the fracture line lies between the origin of the common extensors and the extensor carpi radialis longus, there is usually little displacement. If the fracture lines enter the area of origin of the extensor carpi radialis longus, then considerable displacement can occur.

Radiographic Findings

Because the ossification process starts on the external surface of the apophysis and proceeds centrally, the ossification center often appears separated from the lateral metaphysis and lateral condylar epiphysis. This natural separation can be confused with an avulsion fracture. The key to determining true separation is looking beyond the osseous tissues for the presence of associated soft tissue swelling (Fig. 15-62). If the ossification center lies distal to the osteochondral border of the lateral condylar epiphysis, it should be considered displaced (Fig. 15-63).

Treatment

Unless the fragment is incarcerated within the joint,[115] treatment usually consists of simple immobilization for comfort. Although nonunion of the fragment can occur, this radiographic finding usually does not affect elbow function.

Complications

Only one rare major complication has been described with fractures involving the lateral epicondylar apophysis: entrapment of the fragment, either within the elbow joint[115] or between the capitellum and the radial head.[59]

Fractures Involving the Olecranon Apophysis

Fractures involving the olecranon apophysis are believed to be caused by avulsion forces on the proximal ulna that occur with

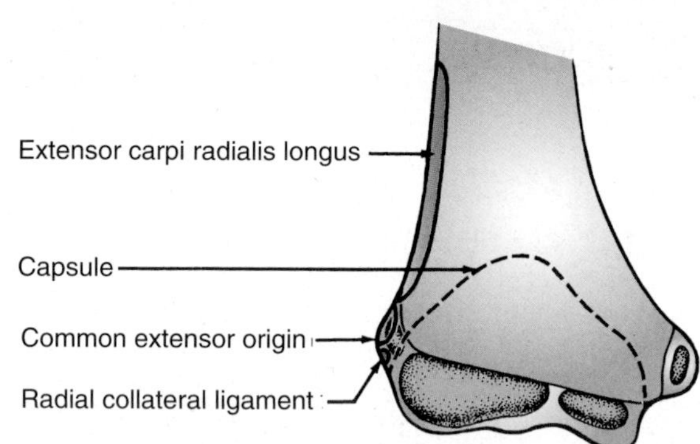

FIGURE 15-61 Soft tissue attachments. The origins of the forearm and wrist extensor muscles, radial collateral ligament, and outline of the capsule are shown in relation to the lateral epicondylar apophysis. (From Hasner E, Husby J. Fracture of the epicondyle and condyle of humerus. Acta Chir Scand 1951;101:195–202, with permission.)

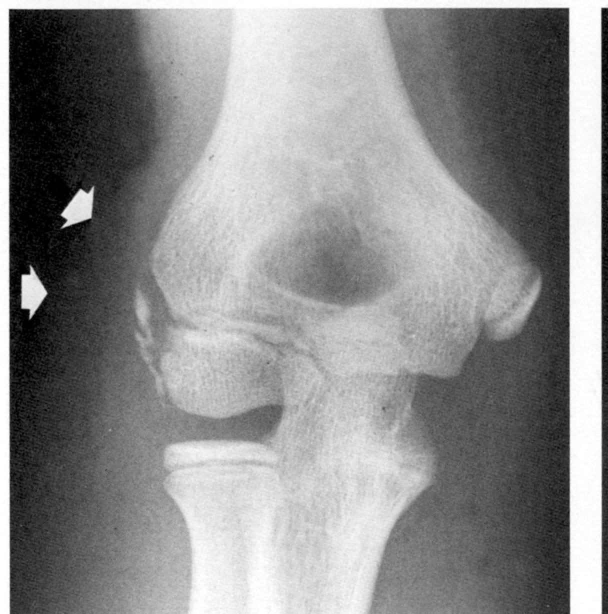

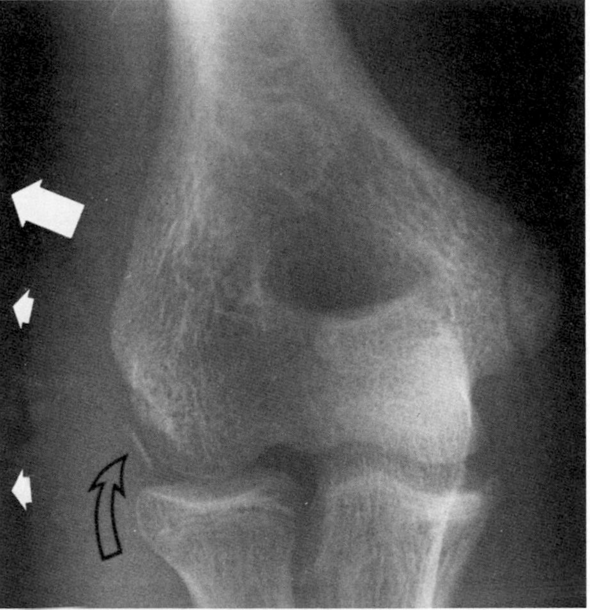

FIGURE 15-62 Lateral swelling. **A.** Soft tissue swelling in the area of the lateral epicondylar apophysis (*arrows*) suggests an undisplaced fracture involving the apophysis. The fragmentation of the apophysis is caused by irregular ossification. **B.** A small avulsion of the lateral epicondyle (*open arrow*) in an adolescent who is almost skeletally mature. There was considerable soft tissue swelling in this area (*solid arrows*).

the elbow flexed.[210] This injury is rare in normal children because an avulsion force generated through the expansion of the triceps tendon inserting on the metaphysis distal to the physis usually results in a fracture through the more distal metaphysis. Carney et al.[25] described a healthy 11-year-old boy who sustained a displaced apophyseal olecranon fracture in a fall. Bracq[21] noted that fractures of the olecranon apophysis appeared to occur more often in children with osteogenesis imperfecta (OI), and several reports since that time have confirmed his observation.[44,68,97,182,210] Why children with OI may be predisposed to this injury is unknown. Zionts and Moon[210] suggested that a combination of weakness of the subchondral bone adjacent to the physis of the proximal olecranon and increased laxity of the triceps expansion might make the olecranon apophysis more vulnerable to injury in children with OI. Because OI was not recognized in half of their patients, they suggested that OI should be considered in any child who has an isolated, displaced fracture of the olecranon apophysis, especially when the injury results from relatively minor trauma.[210]

Undisplaced fractures can be treated with cast immobilization. Operative treatment is usually recommended for displaced fractures of the olecranon apophysis in all children, although the amount of "acceptable" displacement ranges from 3 to 5 mm. Fixation is with two smooth intramedullary K-wires and

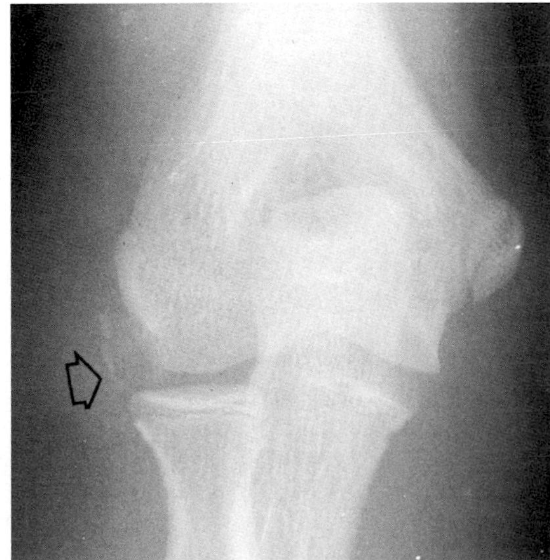

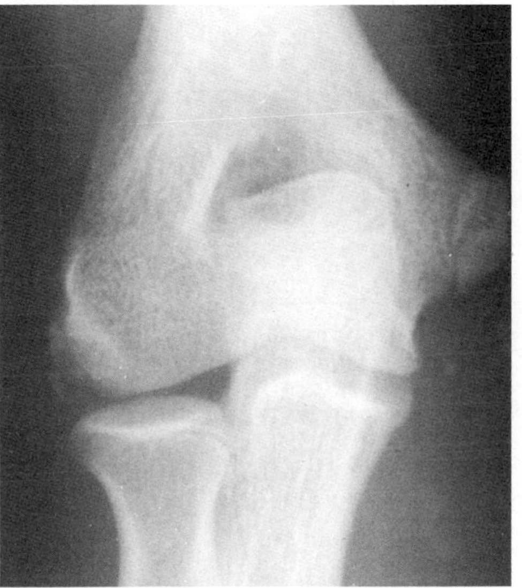

FIGURE 15-63 Avulsion injury. **A.** Avulsion of a portion of the lateral epicondyle in an adolescent (*arrow*). The fragment is at the level of the joint. Most of the epicondyle has fused to the condyle. **B.** The appearance 9 months later shows fragmentation and partial union of the fragment. (Courtesy of R. Chandrasekharan, MD.)

a tension band of either stainless-steel wire or absorbable suture. Problems with the K-wires backing out and refracture after hardware removal have been reported in children with OI[50,68,128,210]; Gwynne-Jones[68] suggested that retaining the hardware or using nonabsorbable sutures might decrease the risk of refracture.

Reports in the literature indicate that approximately 70% of children with OI who sustain an olecranon apophyseal fracture later have a fracture of the contralateral olecranon apophysis; the mean time to second fracture reported by Gwynne-Jones[68] and by Zionts and Moon[210] was 7 months. Parents should be advised of this possibility, and the child's high-risk activities should be avoided.

Nonunions of stress fractures of the olecranon apophysis have been described in adolescent baseball pitchers[30,190] and gymnasts.[198] Painful nonunion of the physis appears on clinical and radiographic examinations as a persistent physis.[151] Rettig et al.[151] reported 5 adolescent baseball pitchers with chronic elbow pain and radiographic evidence of olecranon nonunions; the patients ranged in age from 13 to 17 years (average age: 15 years) and had symptoms for 1 week to 18 months before operative treatment. All five had open reduction and internal fixation with cannulated compression screws, and four had additional figure-of-eight tension band wiring. Bone grafting was done in four, using cancellous bone from the starting hole of the cannulated screw. All returned to their previous activity levels at an average of 30 weeks.

Chronic Tension Stress Injuries (Little League Elbow)

This chronic injury is related to overuse in skeletally immature baseball pitchers. Brogdon and Crow[23] described the original radiographic findings in 1960. Later, Adams[2] demonstrated that the radiographic changes were due to excessive throwing and emphasized the need for preventive programs. This injury is thought to be due to excessive tension on the medial epicondyle with secondary tendinitis. There can also be a repeated compression on the lateral condyle, producing an osteochondritis.

Studies have shown that as long as the rules outlined by the Little League are followed (i.e., pitch counts of 50 to 75 pitches per game depending on age), the incidence of these chronic tension stress injuries is fairly low.[63] Most of the problems arise when overzealous parents and coaches require excessive pitching preseason and at home between practices. Albright[5] found a greater incidence in pitchers who had improper pitching techniques. The spectrum of these chronic injuries is outlined in Table 15-6.

TABLE 15-6 Spectrum of Chronic Tension Stress Injuries of Medial Elbow Epicondylar Apophysis

Stress fracture of the epicondylar physis
Calcification of the ulnar collateral ligaments
Hypertrophy of the medial epicondyle
Acceleration of growth maturity with generalized synovitis and stiffness
Osteochondritis of the lateral condyle

In chronic tension stress injuries (Little League Elbow Syndrome), the history is usually quite characteristic. It is found in young baseball pitchers who are throwing an excessive number of pitches or who are just starting to throw curve pitches.[63] Clinically, this syndrome is manifested by a decrease in elbow extension. Medial epicondylar pain is accentuated by a valgus stress to the elbow in extension. There is usually significant local tenderness and swelling over the medial epicondyle.

On radiographs, the density of the bone of the distal humerus is increased due to the chronicity of the stress. The physeal line is irregular and widened. If the stress has been going on for a prolonged period, there may be hypertrophy of the distal humerus with accelerated bone growth. The bone age of the elbow is greater than the patient's chronologic age (Fig. 15-64).

We use a multifaceted approach that involves educating the parents, coaches, and player. Once symptoms develop, all pitching activity must cease until the epicondyle and adjacent flexor muscle origins become nontender. In addition, local and systemic measures to decrease the inflammatory response are used. Once the initial pain and inflammation have decreased, a program of forearm and arm muscle strengthening is initiated. The pitching technique is also examined to see if any corrections need to be made. Once strength has been re-established in the muscles in the upper extremity and motion has been fully re-established, the patient is gradually returned to pitching with careful monitoring of the number of innings and pitches within a specified time period.

OSTEONECROSIS OF THE TROCHLEA

Three theories have been proposed to account for the posttraumatic changes that occur in the distal humerus after fractures in the vicinity of the trochlea: malunion, partial growth arrest, and vascular injury. The most common form follows some type of elbow trauma. In some cases, the trauma is occult or poorly defined.[17,85,113,116,126,207] This form results in a spectrum from simply a small defect of the trochlea (fishtail deformity) to complete destruction of the medial aspect of the distal humerus with a progressive varus deformity, decreased range of motion, and associated instability of the elbow. Because it is seldom reported in the literature, the exact incidence is unknown. Toniolo and Wilkins[188] reported a series of 30 cases collected over the past 20 years from various sources and suggested that osteonecrosis of the trochlea is probably one of the most unrecognized sequela of injuries to the distal humerus.

Vascular Anatomy

In Haraldsson's classic studies[71,72] of the blood supply of the distal humerus, it was demonstrated that the medial crista of the trochlea had two separate blood supply sources (Fig. 15-65). Neither has anastomoses with each other or with the other metaphyseal vessels. In the young infant, the vessels are small and lie on the surface of the perichondrium.

The lateral vessels supply the apex of the trochlea and the lateral aspect of the medial crista. These vessels cross the physis to enter the posterior aspect of the lateral trochlear ossification center. Their terminal branches lie just under the articular surface. Thus, they are particularly vulnerable to injury when the fracture line occurs through this area, as is typical in fractures of the medial condylar physis, lateral condyle, or a T-condylar

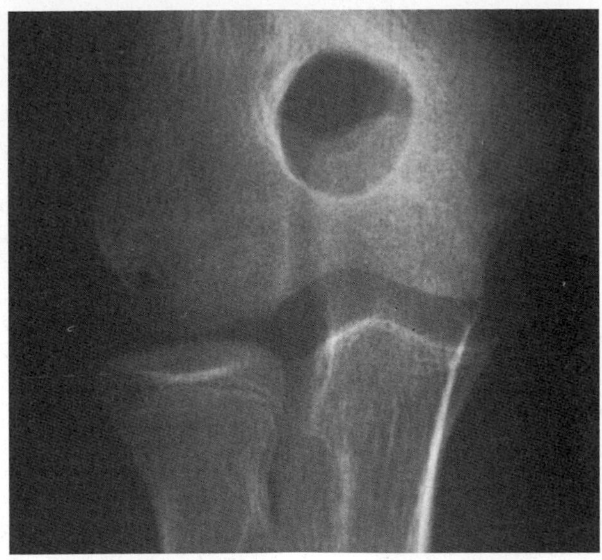

A

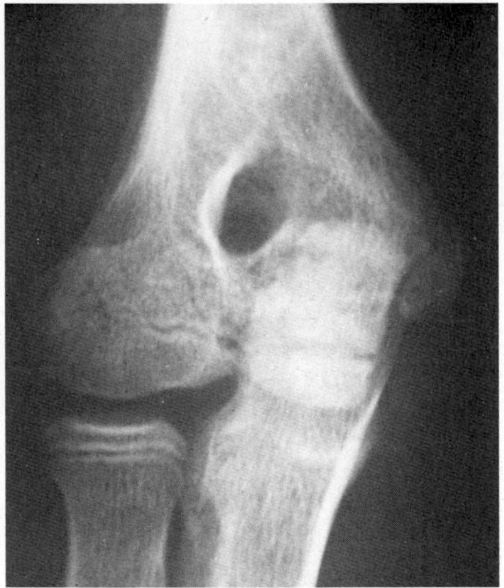

B

FIGURE 15-64 Chronic tension stress. **A.** AP view of a 13-year-old pitcher with chronic pain and significant loss of elbow motion. The bone age is around 15 years. **B.** Same view of the opposite elbow with a bone age of 13 years.

fracture. By the same token, a fracture in the supracondylar area in which the fracture line is very distal or a total distal humeral physeal displacement can also disrupt the lateral trochlear epiphyseal vessels as they course along the surface of the metaphysis or at their entrance into the physeal plate.

Another set of vessels enters medially through the nonarticulating surface of the trochlea. This set of vessels supplies the most medial aspect of the medial crista or the medial portion of the trochlear epiphysis. As shown in Haraldsson's[71,72] studies, there appear to be no anastomoses between the two sets of vessels supplying the trochlear epiphysis.

Ossification centers need blood supply for their appearance and development. Before these centers appear, the vessels are more superficial and less well defined. It is speculated that a lesion in these immature vessels in children leads only to a delay in the appearance of the centers. In older children, where there is already a well-defined ossification center, disruption produces a true bony osteonecrosis of one or both of the trochlea's ossification centers. This can result in a partial or total absence of further epiphyseal ossification, leading to hypoplasia of the central or whole medial aspect of the trochlea.

Patterns of Osteonecrosis

Osteonecrosis of the trochlea can appear as either a central defect (type A) or total hypoplasia manifest by complete absence of the trochlea (type B), depending on the extent of the vascular injury.

Type A—Fishtail Deformity

In the type A deformity, only the lateral portion of the medial crista or apex of the trochlea becomes involved in the necrotic process, which produces the typical fishtail deformity (Fig. 15-66). This more common pattern of necrosis seems to occur with very distal supracondylar fractures or with fractures involving the lateral condylar physis.

Type B—Malignant Varus Deformity

The type B deformity involves osteonecrosis of the entire trochlea and sometimes part of the metaphysis (Fig. 15-67). This type of necrosis has occurred as a sequela of fractures involving the entire distal humeral physis or fractures of the medial condylar physis[192] and can lead to a cubitus varus deformity in which the angulation progresses as the child matures.

The clinical signs and symptoms differ considerably between the two patterns of necrosis. Patients who have the type A or fishtail deformity usually do not develop any angular deformities. The severity of the fishtail deformity is related to the degree of necrosis and seems to dictate the severity of the symptoms. In children who have a pattern of total osteonecrosis of the trochlea, including part of the nonarticular surface, a progressive varus deformity usually develops. Because the total medial trochlear surface is disrupted, significant loss of range of motion also develops. These deformities usually worsen cosmetically and functionally as the child matures. Early degenerative joint disease with a loss of range of motion is the most common sequela in severe cases.

Some children with osteonecrosis of the trochlea develop late-onset ulnar neuropathy,[120,157,185,206] thought to be due to a multiplicity of factors, including joint malalignment, abnormal position of the ulnar nerve and triceps tendon, loss of protection by a deep ulnar groove, and the acute angle of entrance of the two heads of the flexor carpi ulnaris.

Treatment

Because the osteonecrosis of the trochlea is a direct consequence of trauma to the vessels at the time of injury, there is no effective prevention or treatment of the primary necrosis. Treatment is aimed at only the sequelae of the osteonecrosis of the trochlea. If a loss of range of motion is due to a significant disruption of the articular surface itself, there does not appear to be any good operative or nonoperative method that significantly improves elbow function. If the osteonecrosis of the trochlea has resulted in a varus deformity of the elbow, this deformity can be corrected by a supracondylar osteotomy with ulnar nerve transposition. The correction of the carrying angle is mostly cosmetic, with little functional improvement. Surgical treatment carries the risk of increased stiffness to the already limited elbow.

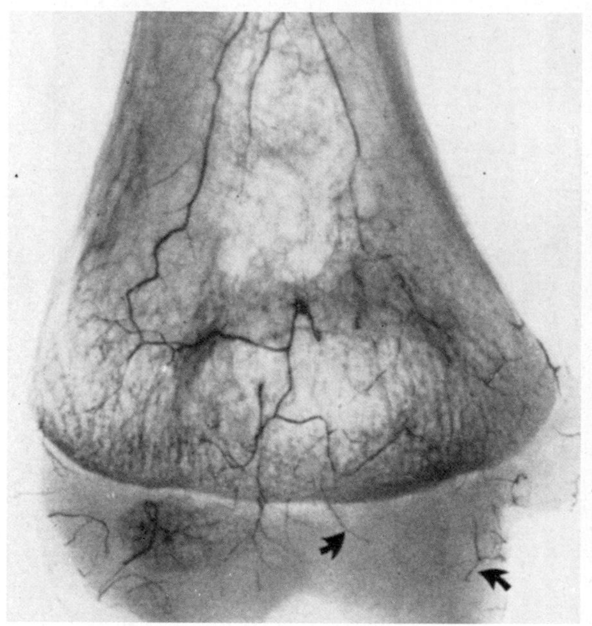

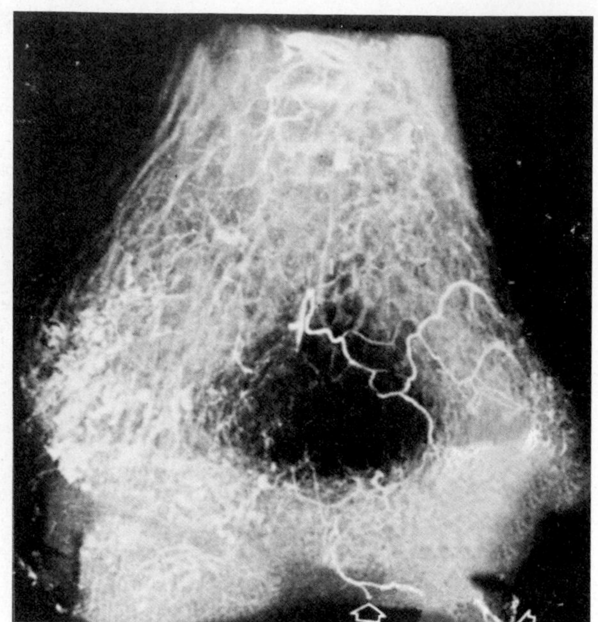

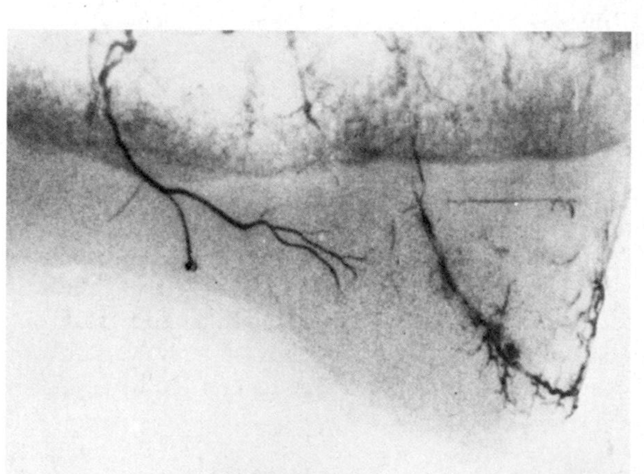

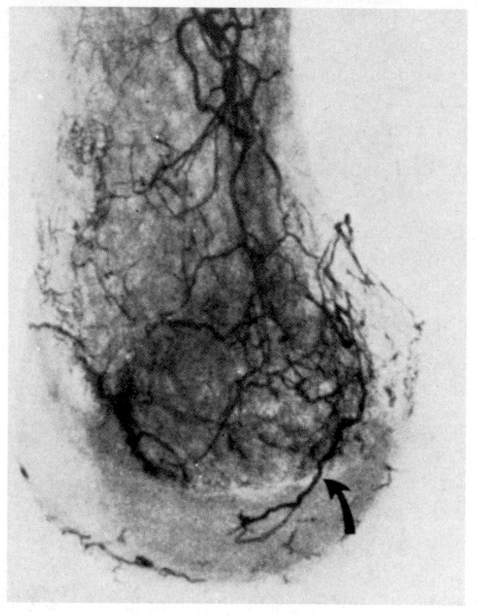

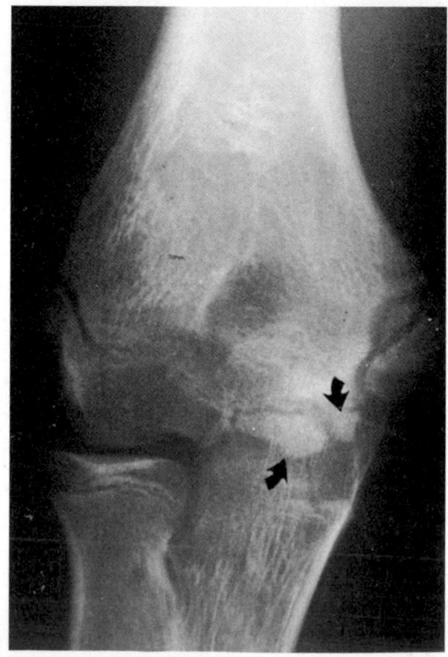

FIGURE 15-65 Blood supply of the trochlea. **A.** Intraosseus vasculature in a 3-year-old boy. Only two small vessels supply the medial crista of the trochlea (*arrows*). The central portion of the crista appears avascular. **B.** In the lateral view through the medial crista of the trochlea, note that the vessels penetrate the physis posteriorly (*arrow*) to enter the epiphyseal cartilage. **C**. Close-up view showing the extent of the vascular supply of the trochlea. Note that no anastamoses are seen between these medial and lateral vessels. **D.** Lateral view through the medial crista of the trochlea. Note that the vessels penetrate the physis posteriorly (*arrow*) to enter the epiphyseal cartilage. (A–D: reprinted from Haraldsson S. On osteochondritis deformans juvenilis capituli humeri including investigation of intraosseous vasculature in distal humerus. *Acta Orthop Scand* Suppl 1959;38:1–232, with permission.) **E.** Radiograph of a 12-year-old boy. The persistence of the two separate ossification centers (*arrows*) of the media crista is seen. The area supplied by the lateral vessel is larger than that supplied by the medial vessel.

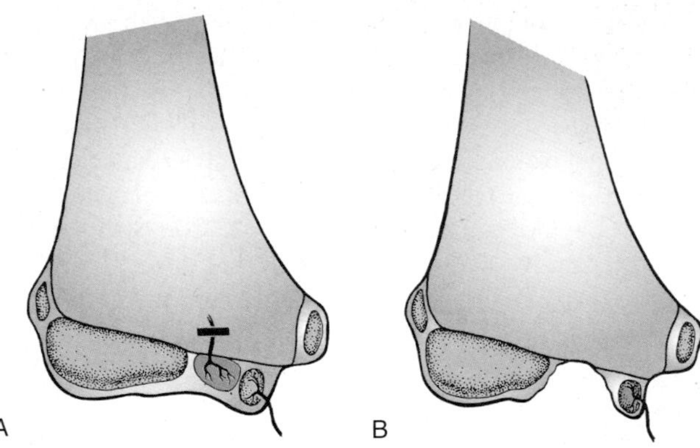

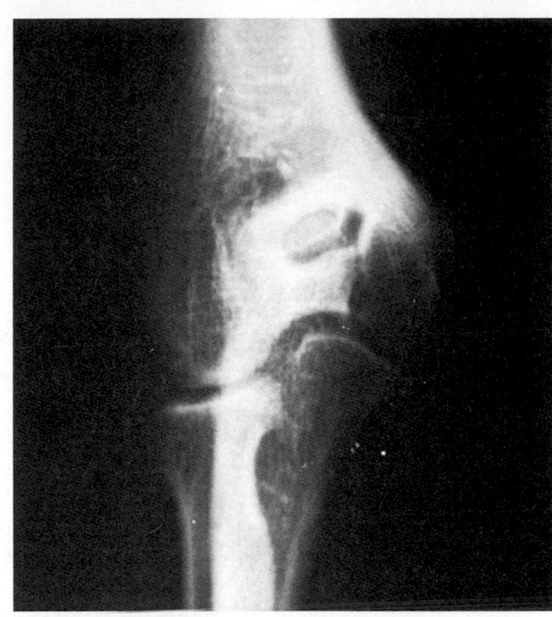

FIGURE 15-66 Fishtail deformity. **A,B.** Type A deformity. Osteonecrosis of only the lateral ossification center creates a defect in the apex of the trochlear groove. **C.** The typical fishtail deformity is seen in a radiograph of a 14-year-old boy who sustained an undisplaced distal supracondylar fracture 5 years previously.

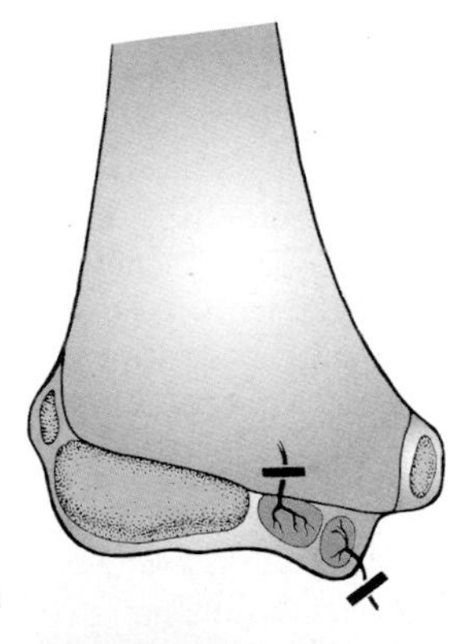

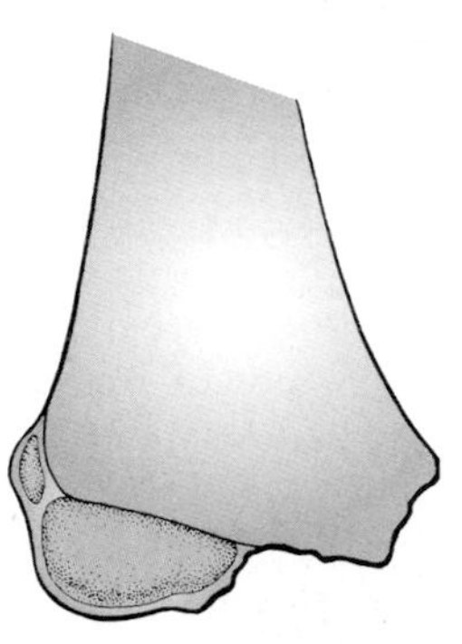

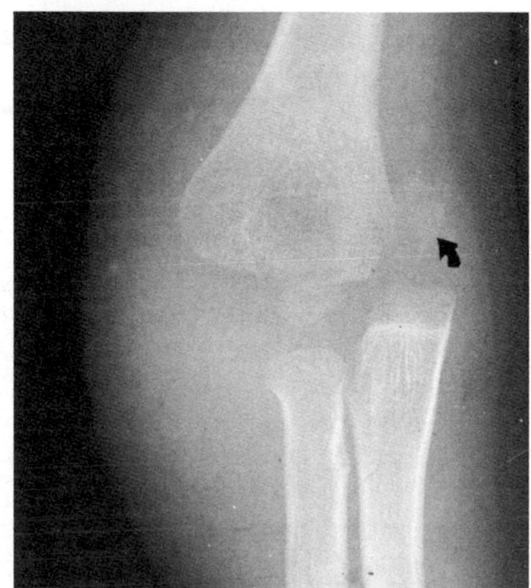

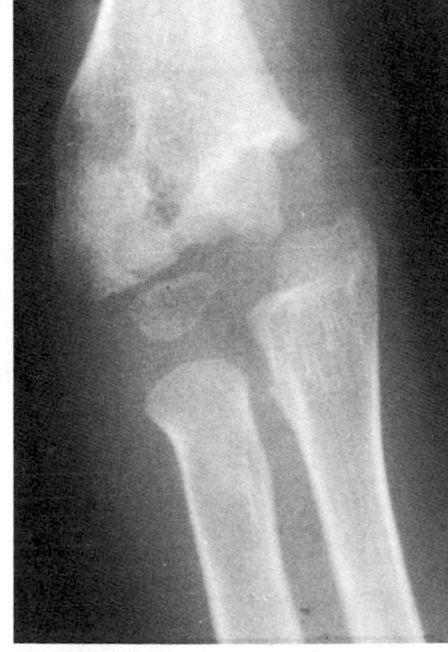

FIGURE 15-67 Osteonecrosis of the entire trochlea. **A.** In this type B deformity, loss of blood supply from both the medial and lateral vessels results in osteonecrosis of the entire medial crista along with a portion of the metaphysis. **B.** Radiograph of a 4-year-old boy who sustained a type II physeal fracture involving the entire distal humeral physis. In this injury film, there is a large metaphyseal fragment on the medial side (*arrow*). **C.** As shown by the appearance 5 months later, a mild varus deformity present is due to an incomplete reduction. The ossification in the medial metaphyseal fragment has disappeared.

T-CONDYLAR FRACTURES

In T-condylar fractures, the fracture line originates in the central groove of the trochlea and courses proximal to the olecranon and the coronoid fossae, where it divides and separates the medial and lateral bony columns of the distal humerus. If the proximal fracture lines are oblique, the fracture may be termed *Y-condylar*. This injury is rare in skeletally immature children.

Incidence

The early modern literature reflects only reports by Blount[18] and Zimmerman,[209] who each described a case in an 11-year-old patient. The average age of patients reported in three major series[86,93,136] was 12.6 years. Thus, Maylahn and Fahey,[112] who reported 6 patients near skeletal maturity, were accurate when they said, "the fractures [T-condylar] take on the characteristics of an adult fracture and should be treated as such."

The actual incidence in younger children is certainly low, but it may be underdiagnosed because it is often confused with other fractures, such as those involving the lateral condylar physis or total distal physis. Special imaging studies such as arthrograms or MRI may be necessary to demonstrate the intracondylar aspect in young children. The combination of an increased awareness of the possibility of this injury and a more aggressive diagnostic approach may result in more cases being uncovered in this younger age group.

Mechanism of Injury

The primary mechanism of this injury is the direct wedge effect of the articular surface of the olecranon on the distal end of the humerus. The sharp edge of the semilunar notch or coronoid process acts as a wedge to break the trochlea and split the condyles, which in turn separates the two columns of the distal humerus. Flexion and extension types of injuries have been described.

The most common mechanism producing a flexion injury is a direct blow to the posterior aspect of the elbow, usually when the child falls directly on the flexed elbow. This flexion mechanism in young children contributes to its rarity because most upper-extremity injuries in children have a component of elbow hyperextension. In these flexion injuries, the wedge effect is produced at the apex of the trochlea by the central portion of the trochlear notch. The condylar fragments usually lie anterior to the shaft in these flexion injuries (Fig. 15-68A,B).

A T-condylar fracture may be caused by a fall on the outstretched arm with the elbow in only slight flexion. This extension mechanism has been suggested by patients in their description of the dynamics of the fall and indirectly by the position of the distal fragments in relation to the diaphyses of the humerus—in other words, lying posterior (Fig. 15-68C,D). In the extension type of injury, the coronoid portion of the semilunar notch produces the wedge effect.

It has been suggested that contraction of the elbow flexor and extensor muscles may play a role in the displacement pattern of this fracture. Because of their origins on the epicondyles, they accentuate both the separation in the coronal plane and the forward displacement in the sagittal plane. This displacement pattern is often evident on the injury films (see Fig. 15-68C,D).

Fracture Patterns

The fracture pattern in adolescents is similar to that in adults. The condylar fragments are often separated, with the articular surface completely disrupted. In addition to separation of the condylar fragments by the force of the original injury, the muscles that originate on these condylar fragments rotate them in both the coronal and sagittal planes (see Fig. 15-68C,D). In the sagittal plane, the position of the condylar fragments in relation to the humeral shaft and metaphysis can either be anterior (flexor mechanism; see Fig. 15-68B) or posterior (extension mechanism; see Fig. 15-68D).

In skeletally immature patients, the central portions of the condylar fragments are usually separated, but the articular surface may remain intact because of its large cartilage component (Fig. 15-69).[136] Thus, the disruption and displacement are primarily in the osseous supracondylar area. The elasticity of the cartilage of the distal end of the humerus often protects the articular surface from being completely disrupted.

Classification

Various classifications[86,152] for adult T-condylar fractures have been proposed, but there are problems with applying these classifications to children's injuries. For example, the number of children with this fracture is so small that no clinician can include all types of fracture patterns in his or her own experience. In addition, there is no useful classification for younger patients, in whom the unossified intact articular cartilage is not visible on radiograph. Toniolo and Wilkins[189] proposed a simple classification based on the degree of displacement and comminution of the fracture fragments. Type I fractures are minimally displaced (Fig. 15-70A,B). Type II fractures are displaced but do not have comminution of the metaphyseal fragments (Fig. 15-70C). Type III fractures are displaced fractures with comminution of the metaphyseal fragments (Fig. 15-70D,E).

In a child, the integrity of the articular surface may be difficult to determine without using arthrography or MRI. Because the initial integrity of the articular surface may not be that important to the prognosis, this factor was not believed to significantly contribute to a general classification scheme.

In adolescents aged 12 years or older, classification and treatment are as those in adults (see Chapter 28).

Diagnosis

Clinically, these fractures are most often confused with extension-type supracondylar fractures. The extended position of the elbow, along with the massive swelling, is almost identical to that of the displaced extension type of supracondylar fracture.

Plain radiographs are the cornerstone to the diagnosis. In older children, the differentiation must be made from that of a comminuted supracondylar fracture. Sometimes, the diagnosis is not obvious until the fragments have been partially reduced, which allows the vertical fracture lines splitting the trochlea to become more evident. In younger children, the diagnosis is much more difficult because the articular surface is not visible. In addition, because of its rarity, the possibility of a T-condylar fracture may not be considered in this age group.

The diagnosis must exclude common fracture patterns of either the isolated lateral or medial condyles and complete separation of the distal humeral physis. In these latter fractures, an important sign is the presence of a medial or lateral Thurstan-Holland fragment in the metaphysis.[13] The key differential for the T-condylar fracture is the presence of a vertical fracture line extending down to the apex of the trochlea.

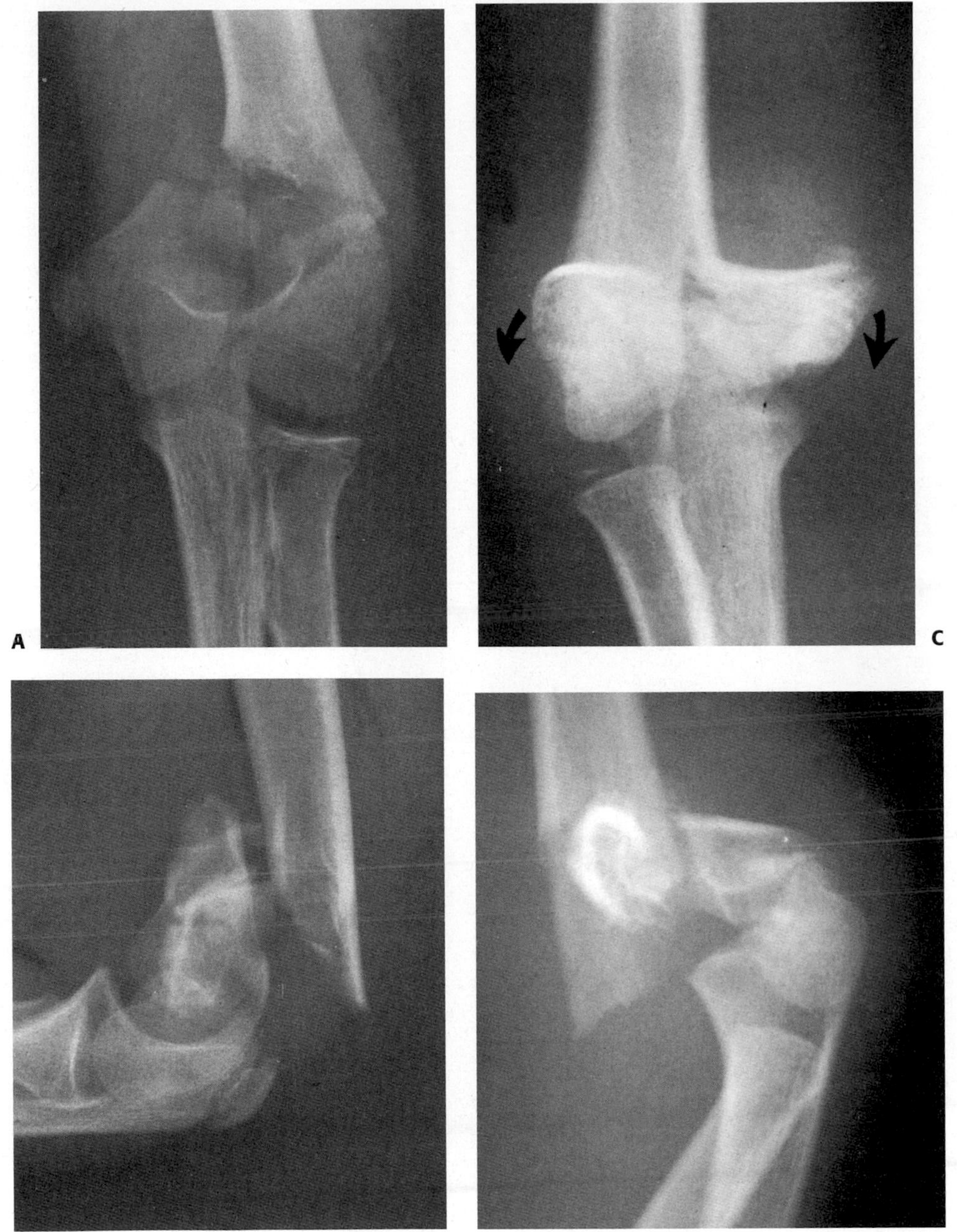

FIGURE 15-68 Mechanism patterns. **A,B.** The more common flexion pattern in which the condylar fragments are situated anterior to the distal shaft. **C,D.** An extensor pattern in which the condylar fragments are situated posterior to the distal shaft. The muscle origins on the respective condyles cause them to diverge in the coronal plane (*arrows*) and flex in the sagittal plane.

If the diagnosis is suspected after a careful evaluation of the static radiographs, it can be confirmed with varus or valgus stress films made while the patient is under general anesthesia.[13] The use of contrast medium in the form of an arthrogram also is helpful.

Treatment

Because of the rarity of this injury, treatment recommendations cannot be based on multiple case experiences. Most of the experience has been based on isolated cases or small series.[13,86,93,136] Regardless of the treatment method, certain basic principles must be considered in dealing with these fractures.

A treatment plan must be individualized for the specific fracture and the surgeon's level of expertise and experience. The following principles must be considered in planning a treatment method:

- Elbow articular mobility depends on articular congruity, correct alignment of the axis of motion, and debris- and bone-free fossae.
- The stability depends on the integrity of the lateral and medial supracondylar columns.
- The T-condylar fracture is an articular fracture, so the first goal is to restore and stabilize the joint surface.
- Closed methods alone usually cannot produce an acceptable result because of the muscle forces applied to the fragments.
- Most patients are adolescents with minimal potential for bone remodeling.

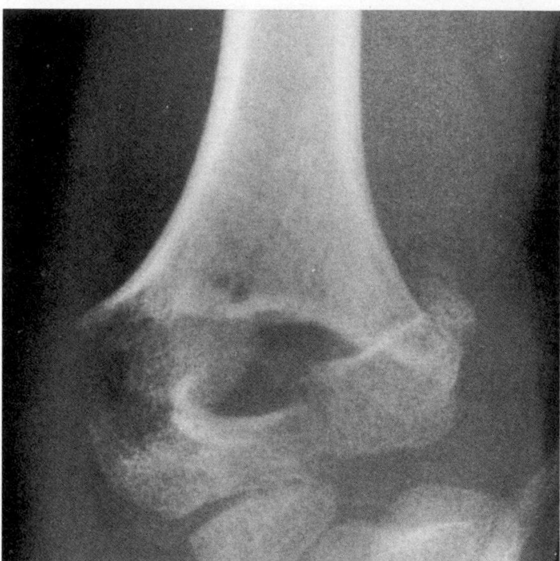

FIGURE 15-69 Intact articular surface. In this T-condylar fracture in a 7-year-old boy, the thick articular cartilage remains essentially intact, preventing separation of the condylar fragments. This fracture was secured with simple percutaneous pins.

- Although surgical reduction may produce an acceptable reduction on radiograph, it may add to the already extensive damage to soft tissues; this in turn can contribute to postoperative stiffness.

The literature reflects good results with surgical management. Zimmerman[209] advocated establishing an anatomic reduction with internal fixation so that early motion could facilitate a more rapid rehabilitation. In the two young children described by Beghin et al.,[13] operative intervention was necessary to achieve a satisfactory reduction. A review of three series[86,93,136] supports surgical management: 29 of the 31 elbows in these combined series were treated operatively. The investigators of these series maintained that open reduction and internal fixation was the best way to restore the integrity of the articular surface and stabilize the fracture sufficiently to allow early mobilization. All but one of the patients in this combined series who were treated surgically had good or very good results at follow-up.

Kanellopoulus and Yiannakopoulos[91] described closed reduction of the intra-articular component, with fixation by partially threaded pins for interfragmentary compression. Two elastic titanium intramedullary nails were used for stabilizing the supracondylar component. T-condylar fractures in two adolescents healed without complications after using this technique. Both patients returned to sports with full elbow range of motion at 6 weeks after surgery.

The surgical approach most widely accepted is the posterior longitudinal splitting of the triceps without an osteotomy of the olecranon. This approach gives adequate exposure of the fracture and the articular surface and does not seem to produce any loss of strength from splitting the triceps.[93] Although one reported patient had radiographic evidence of osteonecrosis of the trochlea,[136] another had a nonunion,[93] and many had some loss of range of motion, none of these surgically treated patients demonstrated any significant loss of elbow function or discomfort.

Bryan and Morrey[24] described a triceps-sparing approach in which the extensor mechanism is reflected laterally, exposing the whole distal humerus. Remia et al.[150] evaluated triceps function and elbow motion in nine patients with T-condylar fractures treated with open reduction through a triceps-sparing approach and compared them to those reported after a triceps-splitting approach. No statistically significant differences were found in function or range or motion.

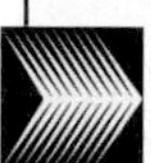

AUTHORS' PREFERRED TREATMENT

Because this fracture is rare in children, there is no standard recommended treatment. Our suggestions are based on a combination of our clinical experience and the experience of others in a few series.[86,93,136] Our first consideration in these fractures is to re-establish the integrity of the articular surface to maintain the congruity of the joint. Usually, this cannot be achieved adequately by closed methods, so we proceed with an open surgical technique. We have found the simple classification into three types based on the degree of displacement or comminution to be helpful in guiding the aggressiveness of our treatment.

Type I (Undisplaced or Minimally Displaced)

In type I injuries, there is little displacement of the bony supracondylar columns. In children, the periosteum is often intact and can provide some intrinsic stability. In addition, the thicker articular and epiphyseal cartilage in skeletally immature children may still be intact, even if the bony epiphysis appears severed by a vertical fracture line. Because of this condition, we have found two methods to be successful for these types of fractures.

Closed Reduction—Percutaneous Pin Fixation

These fractures require minimal manipulation under general anesthesia and radiographic control to re-establish the supracondylar columns. If there is anterior or posterior rotation in the sagittal plane of the metaphyseal portion of the column, a pin placed into that column can be used as a "joystick" to manipulate the fragment into a satisfactory position. Once a satisfactory reduction is achieved, the pin can then be advanced across the fracture site for fixation. These fractures usually require multiple pins placed percutaneously, such as those used in comminuted supracondylar fractures (Fig. 15-71). Because of the rapid healing, the pins can be removed at 3 weeks to allow early active motion.

Traction

If the articular cartilage is intact, it may close as a hinge with traction. The rotational displacement of the condyles created by the origins of the forearm muscles can be neutralized with olecranon traction, in which the elbow is suspended at 90 degrees of flexion. There is usually adequate stability from the callus around the fracture site at 2 to 3 weeks to discontinue the traction. The elbow is then immobilized in a hinged cast brace for an additional 2 to 3 weeks. This immobilization allows the initiation of protected active motion. With the present emphasis on short hospitalization, however, we find that skeletal traction is less acceptable for both social and financial reasons. Skeletal traction may be the only acceptable method of treatment in patients seen on a delayed basis with extensive skin abrasions, severe soft

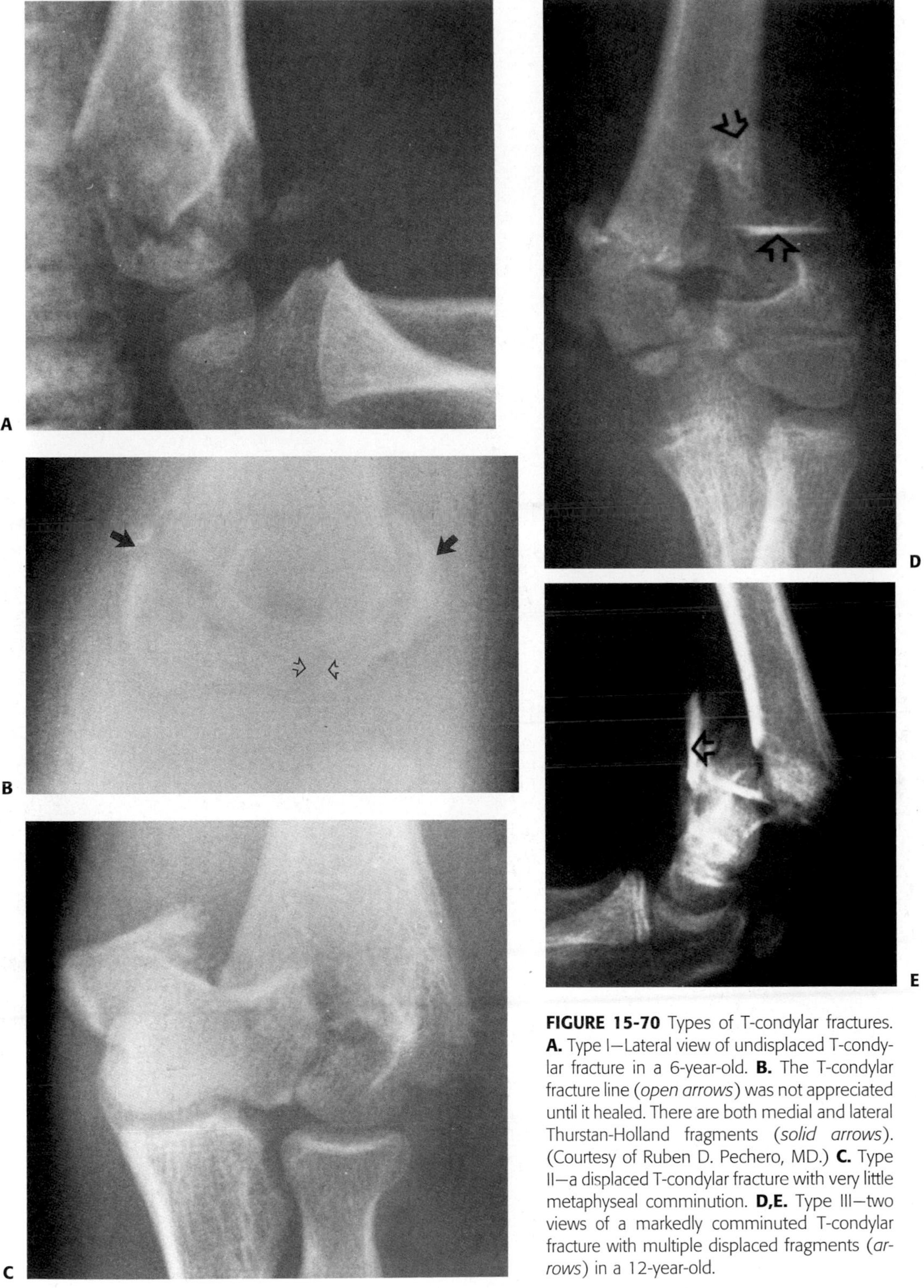

FIGURE 15-70 Types of T-condylar fractures. **A.** Type I—Lateral view of undisplaced T-condylar fracture in a 6-year-old. **B.** The T-condylar fracture line (*open arrows*) was not appreciated until it healed. There are both medial and lateral Thurstan-Holland fragments (*solid arrows*). (Courtesy of Ruben D. Pechero, MD.) **C.** Type II—a displaced T-condylar fracture with very little metaphyseal comminution. **D,E.** Type III—two views of a markedly comminuted T-condylar fracture with multiple displaced fragments (*arrows*) in a 12-year-old.

tissue injury, or gross comminution, in which cast application or other operative interventions might carry a high risk of infection.

Type II (Displaced without Comminution)

Open Reduction and Internal Fixation

If there is wide separation of the condylar fragments with marked disruption of the articular surface, stability and articular congruity can be established only with an open surgical procedure. We prefer the Bryan-Morrey posterior triceps-sparing approach.[24] The patient is placed prone on the operating table with the arm supported on a pillow and the forearm hanging down off the edge of the operating table. This position provides the best approach for direct observation of the posterior surface of the distal humerus. Olecranon osteotomy is reserved for severely comminuted articular fractures in adolescents.

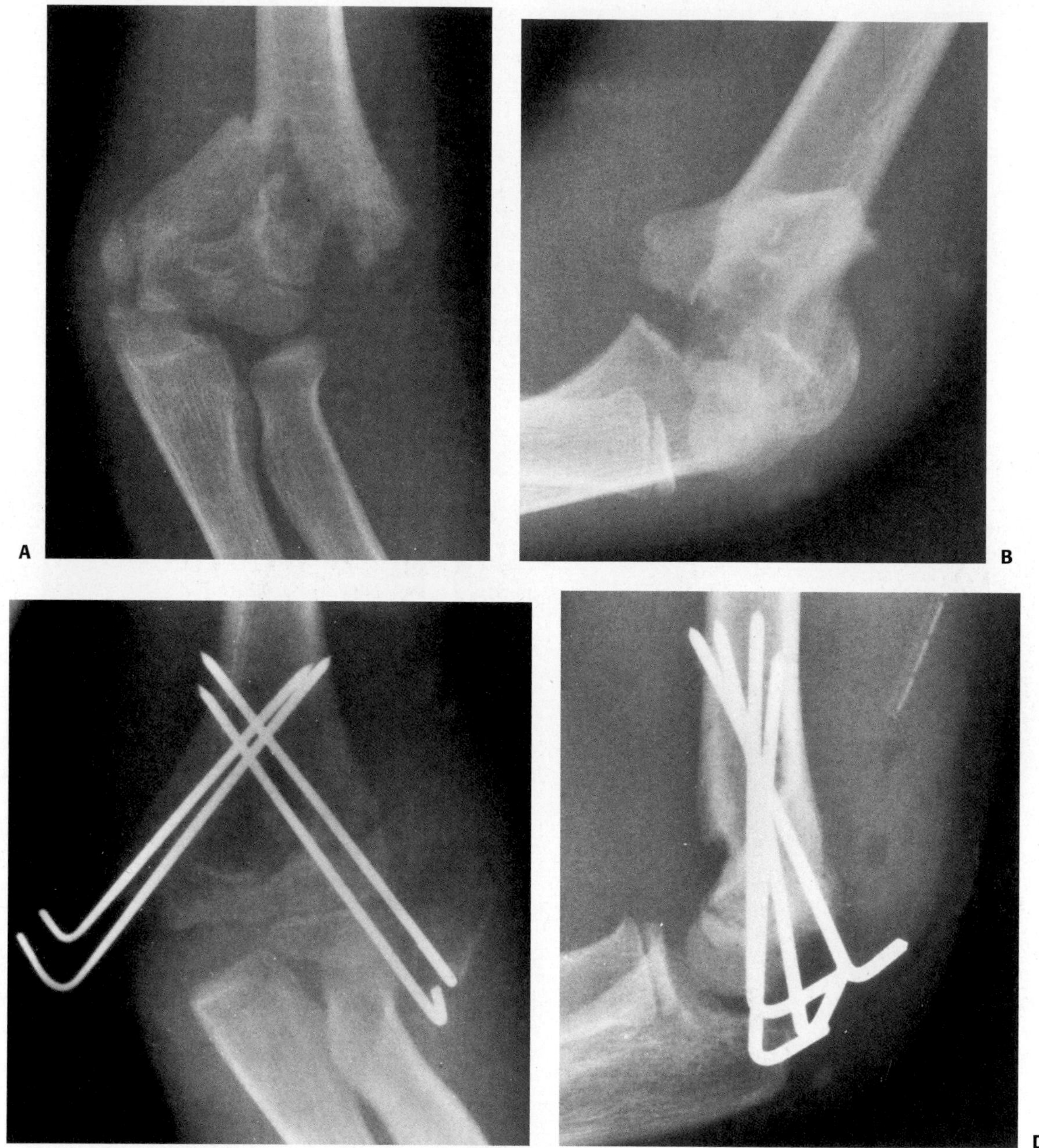

FIGURE 15-71 Closed reduction and pin fixation. **A,B.** Two views of a type II T-condylar fracture in a 15-year-old. **C,D.** Because an anatomic reduction was achieved by manipulative closed reduction, it was secured with simple multiple pin fixation placed percutaneously. The articular surface was minimally displaced. The pins were removed at 3 weeks. At this age, healing was rapid enough to pull the pins at 3 weeks to allow active motion. Ultimately, the patient was deficient only 10 degrees from achieving full extension.

Reconstruction of the Articular Surface

Our first priority is to re-establish the integrity of the articular fragments—in other words, to convert it to a supracondylar fracture (Fig. 15-72A–C). The olecranon and coronoid fossae must be cleared of bony fragments or debris to eliminate the chance of bony impingement with their respective processes. The best way to stabilize the condyles is with a screw passed transversely through the center of the axis of rotation in such a manner as to apply transverse compression. This stabilization method may require a small temporary secondary transverse pin proximal to the screw to prevent rotation of the fragments as the guide hole is drilled or when the compression screw is being applied. This pin can be removed after the fragments are secured.

Stabilization of the Supracondylar Columns

Once the condylar and articular integrity has been re-established, the distal fragments must be secured to the proximal fragment by stabilizing the supracondylar fragment columns. The decision here is how important it is to initiate early motion. In a younger child with rapid bony healing, pin fixation is often satisfactory; the pins can be removed after 3 weeks in order to start protected motion. In an older adolescent nearer to skeletal maturity, we prefer fixation—

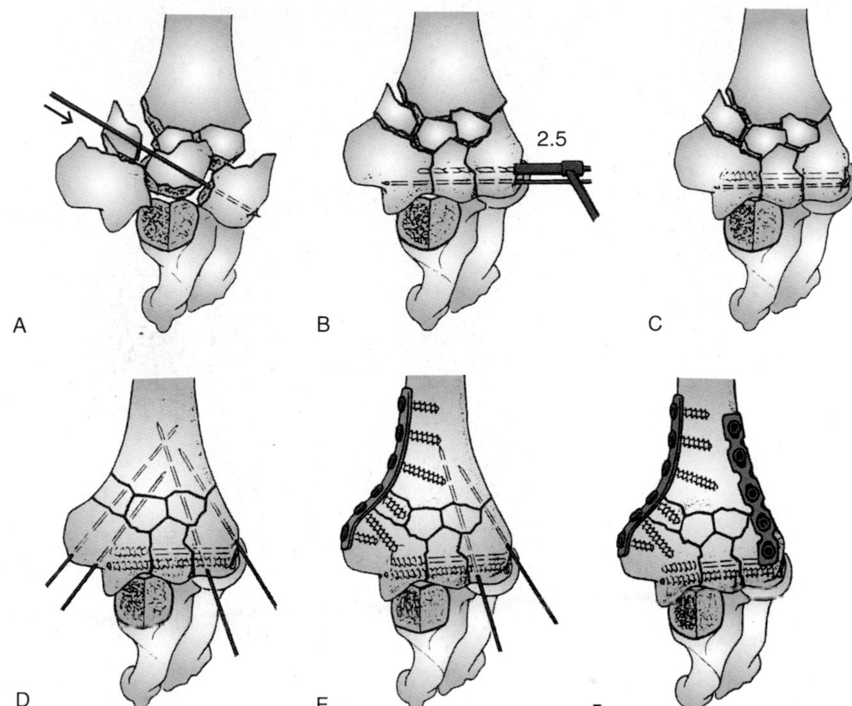

FIGURE 15-72 Sequence of distal humerus reconstruction. **A–C.** First, the articular portions are reassembled with provisional K-wire fixation, followed by screw fixation. **D.** K-wires can then also be used to provide temporary fixation of the distal humerus. **E.** A one-third tubular plate is attached to the medial side. **F.** A 3.5 pelvic reconstruction plate was attached to the posterolateral border. (From Heim U, Pfeiffer KM. Internal Fixation of Small Fractures. 3rd ed. Berlin: Springer-Verlag, 1988, with permission.)

usually plates or screws—that allows early motion (Figs. 15-72E,F and 15-73). Before applying the plates, the supracondylar columns can be stabilized temporarily with pin fixation (Fig. 15-73D).

Principles of Plate Fixation

The plates must be strong; thin semitubular plates are inadequate and may break.[197] The reinforced malleable reconstructive type of plates used for fixation of pelvic fractures provide very secure fixation. A J-type of plate can also provide rigid fixation when used to stabilize the lateral column.[163] It is best to place the plates at 90 degrees to each other, which provides for a more stable construct.[77,96,161]

In most adolescents, this is essentially an adult type of fracture pattern. The reader is therefore referred to *Fractures in Adults* for a more detailed description of the various techniques used in treating adults with this type of fracture.

Postoperative Care

If plate fixation is used, we place the extremity in a supporting posterior splint for 5 to 7 days to allow the soft tissue swelling to decrease and the incisions to heal. At this time, active flexion and extension are initiated and the arm is protected with a removable cast brace.

Type III (Displaced with Comminution)

Limited Open Reduction Followed by Traction

Sometimes, the supracondylar columns are too fragmented to allow adequate fixation. In such cases, we have found that the best initial treatment method in children involves reestablishing the articular surface and joint congruity with a limited open reduction. The separated condyles are secured with a transverse screw providing compression through the axis of rotation. This procedure can usually be done with minimal soft tissue dissection. Once this is stabilized, the supracondylar columns are then re-established by placing the extremity in olecranon traction and allowing them to reconstitute with callus formation. Traction must be maintained until there appears to be good osseous tissue formed in the supracondylar areas. While in traction, motion can be initiated. This technique can also be used in patients seen late with contaminated soft tissue abrasions or severe soft tissue problems. In selected patients, such as an adolescent with severe bone loss, plating followed by bone grafting may be indicated.

Complications

It is important to emphasize to the parents initially that this is a serious fracture. Because of the considerable soft tissue injury and the involvement of the articular surface of the distal humerus, stiffness and loss of motion of the elbow can be expected regardless of the treatment mode.[86,112,136] In adolescents, failure to provide solid internal fixation that facilitates early motion (i.e., using only pin fixation) can result in a satisfactory radiographic appearance but considerable dysfunction due to residual loss of elbow motion.

Although neurovascular complications have not been mentioned in the few cases reported in the literature, the incidence is probably about equal to that of supracondylar fractures. Because these fractures occur late in the growth process, partial or total growth arrest due to internal fixation is not thought to be a major complication. Likewise, because these are older children, little remodeling can be expected. Nonunion,[93] osteonecrosis of the trochlea,[136] and failure of internal fixation have also been reported as complications.

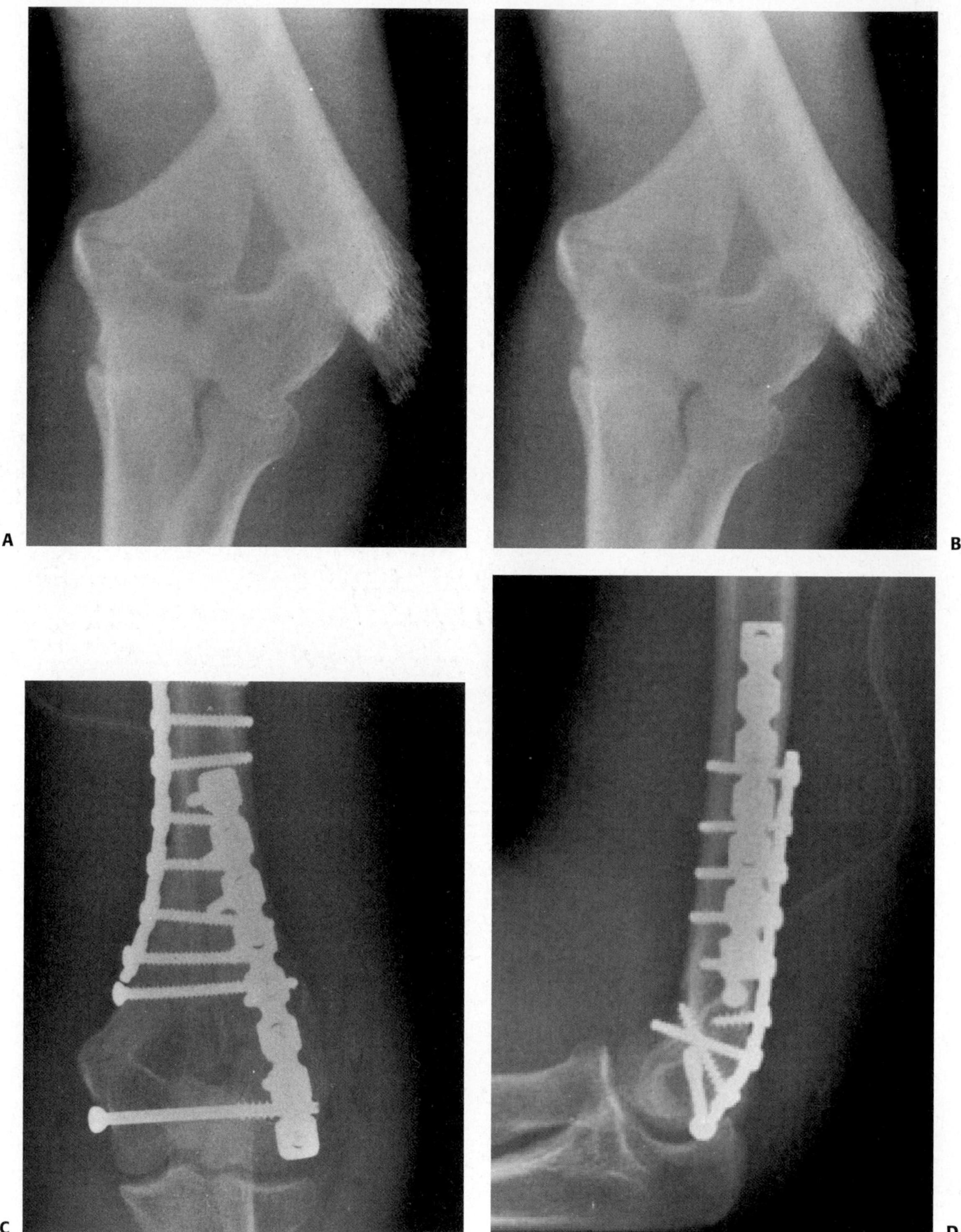

FIGURE 15-73 T-condylar numeral fractures with plate and screw fixation. **A,B.** Injury films of a type II flexion pattern in a 16-year-old boy. **C,D.** Articular integrity was first restored with a transcondylar compression screw. The condyles were secured to the metaphysis and distal shaft using pelvic reconstruction plates placed at 90 degrees to each other.

REFERENCES

1. Abe M, Ishizu T, Nagaoka T, et al. Epiphyseal separation of the distal end of the humeral epiphysis: a follow up note. J Pediatr Orthop 1995;15:426–434.
2. Adams JE. Injury to the throwing arm. A study of traumatic changes in the elbow joints of boy baseball players. Calif Med 1965;102:127–132.
3. Agins HJ, Marcus NW. Articular cartilage sleeve fracture of the lateral humeral condyle capitellum: a previously undescribed entity. J Pediatr Orthop 1984;4:620–622.
4. Akbarnia BA, Silberstein MJ, Rende RJ, et al. Arthrography in the diagnosis of fractures of the distal end of the humerus in infants. J Bone Joint Surg Am 1986;68:599–602.
5. Albright JA, Jokl P, Shaw R, et al. Clinical studies of baseball players: correlation of injury to throwing arm with method of delivery. Am J Sports Med 1978;6:15–21.
6. Rutherford, AJ. Fractures of the lateral humeral condyle in children. J Bone Joint Surg Am 1985;67:851–856.
7. Ashurst APC. An Anatomical and Surgical Study of Fractures of the Lower End of the Humerus. Philadelphia: Lea & Febiger, 1910.
8. Badelon O, Bensahel H, Mazda K, et al. Lateral humeral condylar fractures in children: a report of 47 cases. J Pediatr Orthop 1988;8:31–34.
9. Barrett WP, Almquist EA, Staheli LT. Fracture separation of the distal humeral physis in the newborn. J Pediatr Orthop 1984;4:617–619.
10. Bast SC, Hoffer MM, Aval S. Nonoperative treatment for minimally and nondisplaced lateral humeral condyle fractures in children. J Pediatr Orthop 1998;18:448–450.
11. Beaty JH, Wood AB. Fractures of the lateral humeral condyle in children. Paper presented at the annual meeting of the American Academy of Orthopedic Surgeons, January 18, 1985; Las Vegas, NV.
12. Bede WB, Lefebure AR, Rosmon MA. Fractures of the medial humeral epicondyle in children. Can J Surg 1975;18:137–142.
13. Beghin JL, Bucholz RW, Wenger DR. Intercondylar fractures of the humerus in young children. J Bone Joint Surg Am 1982;64A:1083–1087.
14. Bensahel H, Csukonyi Z, Badelon O, et al. Fractures of the medial condyle of the humerus in children. J Pediatr Orthop 1986;6:430–433.
15. Berman JM, Weiner DS. Neonatal fracture separation of the distal humeral chondroepiphysis: a case report. Orthopedics 1980;3:875–879.
16. Bernstein SM, King JD, Sanderson RA. Fractures of the medial epicondyle of the humerus. Contemp Orthop 1981;12:637–641.
17. Beyer WF, Heppt P, Glückert K, et al. Aseptic osteonecrosis of the humeral trochlea (Hegemann's disease). Arch Orthop Trauma Surg 1990;110:45–48.
18. Blount WP. Fractures in children. Baltimore: Williams & Wilkins, 1955.
19. Blount WP, Schulz I, Cassidy RH. Fractures of the elbow in children. JAMA 1951;146: 699–704.
20. Böhler L. The Treatment of Fractures. Vol. 1. New York: Grune & Stratton, 1956.
21. Bracq H. Fractures of the olecranon. Rev Chir Orthop Reparatrice Appar Mot 1987; 73:469–471.
22. Bright RW, Burstein AH, Elmore SM. Epiphyseal-plate cartilage. A biomechanical and histological analysis of failure modes. J Bone Joint Surg Am 1974;56:688–703.
23. Brogdon BJ, Crow NE. Little leaguer's elbow. AJR Am J Roentgenol 1960;83:671–675.
24. Bryan RS, Morrey BF. Extensive posterior exposure of the elbow. A triceps sparing approach. Clin Orthop Relat Res 1982;166:188–192.
25. Carney JR, Fox D, Mazurek MT. Displaced apophyseal olecranon fracture in a healthy child. Mil Med 2007;172:1225–1227.
26. Carro LP, Golano P, Vega J. Arthroscopic-assisted reduction and percutaneous external fixation of lateral condyle fractures of the humerus. Arthroscopy 2007;23:1131–1134.
27. Case SL, Hennrikus WL. Surgical treatment of displaced medial epicondyle fractures in adolescent athletes. Am J Sports Med 1997;25:682–686.
28. Chacha PB. Fractures of the medial condyle of the humerus with rotational displacement. J Bone Joint Surg Am 1970;52:1453–1458.
29. Chapman VM, Grottkau BE, Albright M, et al. Multidector computed tomography of pediatric lateral condylar fractures. Comput Assist Tomogr 2005;29:842–846.
30. Charlton WP, Chandler RW. Persistence of the olecranon physis in baseball players: results following operative management. J Shoulder Elbow Surg 2003;12:59–62.
31. Chessare JW, Rogers LF, White H, et al. Injuries of the medial epicondyle ossification center of the humerus. AJR Am J Roentgenol 1977;129:49–55.
32. Conner A, Smith MGH. Displaced fracture of lateral humeral condyle in children. J Bone Joint Surg 1970;52:460–464.
33. Cooper AP. A Treatise on Dislocations and Fractures of the Joints. Boston: Lilly, Wait, Carter, and Hendee, 1932.
34. Cothay DM. Injury to the lower medial epiphysis of the humerus before development of the ossific centre. Report of a case. J Bone Joint Surg Br 1967;49:766–767.
35. Cotton FJ. Elbow fractures in children. Fractures of the lower end of the humerus; lesions and end results, and their bearing upon treatment. Ann Surg 1902;35:75–104.
36. Dameron TB Jr. Transverse fractures of distal humerus in children. Instr Course Lect 1981;30:224–235.
37. Davids JR, Maguire MF, Mubarak SJ, et al. Lateral condylar fracture of the humerus following posttraumatic cubitus varus. J Pediatr Orthop 1994;14:466–470.
38. De Boeck H, Casteleyn PP, Opdecam P. Fracture of the medial humeral condyle. J Bone Joint Surg Am 1987;69:1442–1444.
39. de Jager LT, Hoffman EB. Fracture-separation of the distal humeral epiphysis. J Bone Joint Surg Br 1991;73B:143–146.
40. DeLee JC, Wilkins KE, Rogers LF, et al. Fracture separation of the distal humeral epiphysis. J Bone Joint Surg Am 1980;67:46–51.
41. Dhillon KS, Sengupta S, Singh BJ. Delayed management of fracture of the lateral humeral condyle in children. Acta Orthop Scand 1988;59:419–424.
42. Dias JJ, Johnson GV, Hoskinson J, et al. Management of severely displaced medial epicondyle fractures. J Orthop Trauma 1987;1:59–62.
43. Dias JJ, Lamont AC, Jones JM. Ultrasonic diagnosis of neonatal separation of the distal humeral epiphysis. J Bone Joint Surg Br 1988;70:825–828.
44. DiCesare PE, Sew-Hoy A, Krom W. Bilateral isolated fractures in an infant as presentation of osteogenesis imperfecta. Orthopedics 1992;15:741–743.
45. Downs DM, Wirth CR. Fracture of the distal humeral chondroepiphysis in the neonate. A case report. Clin Orthop Relat Res 1982;169:155–158.
46. Drvaric DM, Rooks MD. Anterior sleeve fracture of the capitellum. J Orthop Trauma 1990;4:188–192.
47. El Ghawabi MH. Fracture of the medial condyle of the humerus. J Bone Joint Surg Am 1975;57:677–680.
48. Elkowitz SJ, Kubiak EN, Polatsch D, et al. Comparison of two headless screw designs for fixation of capitellum fractures. Bull Hosp Jt Dis 2003;61:123–126.
49. Elkowitz SJ, Polatsch DB, Egol KA, et al. Capitellum fractures: a biomechanical evaluation of three fixation methods. J Orthop Trauma 2002;16:503–506.
50. Fabry J, De Smet L, Fabry G. Consequences of a fracture through a minimally ossified apophysis of the olecranon. J Pediatr Orthop B 2000;9:212–214.
51. Fahey JJ, O'Brien ET. Fracture-separation of the medial humeral condyle in a child confused with fracture of the medial epicondyle. J Bone Joint Surg Am 1971;53: 1102–1104.
52. Fairbank HAT, Buxton JD. Displacement of the internal epicondyle into the elbow joint. Lancet 1934;2:218.
53. Faysse R, Marion J. Fractures du condyle interne. Rev Chir Orthop 1962;48:473–477.
54. Finnbogason T, Karlsson G, Lindberg L, et al. Nondisplaced and minimally displaced fractures of the lateral humeral condyle in children: a prospective radiographic investigation of fracture stability. J Pediatr Orthop 1995;15:422–425.
55. Flynn JC, Richards JF Jr. Nonunion of minimally displaced fractures of the lateral condyle of humerus in children. J Bone Joint Surg Am 1971;53:1096–1101.
56. Flynn JC, Richards JF Jr, Saltzman RI. Prevention and treatment of nonunion of slightly displaced fractures of the lateral humeral condyle in children. J Bone Joint Surg Am 1975;57:1087–1092.
57. Fontanetta P, Mackenzie DA, Rosman M. Missed, maluniting, and malunited fractures of the lateral humeral condyle in children. J Trauma 1978;18:329–335.
58. Foster DE, Sullivan JA, Gross RH. Lateral humeral condylar fractures in children. J Pediatr Orthop 1985;5:16–22.
59. Fowles JV, Kassab MT. Displaced fracture of medial humeral condyle in children. J Bone Joint Surg 1980;62:1159–1163.
60. Fowles JV, Kassab MT. Fracture of the capitulum humeri, treatment by excision. J Bone Joint Surg Am 1974;56:794.
61. Fowles JV, Kassab MT, Moula T. Untreated intra-articular entrapment of the medial humeral epicondyle. J Bone Joint Surg Br 1984;60:562–565.
62. Fowles JV, Slimane N, Kassab MT. Elbow dislocation with avulsion of the medial humeral epicondyle. J Bone Joint Surg Br 1990;72B:102–104.
63. Frances R, Bunch T, Chandler B. Little league elbow: a decade later. Phys Sports Med 1978;88–94.
64. Friedman RJ, Smith RJ. Radial nerve laceration 26 years after screw fixation of a humeral fracture. J Bone Joint Surg Am 1984;66:959–960.
65. Gay JR, Love JG. Diagnosis and treatment of tardy paralysis of the ulnar nerve. J Bone Joint Surg 1947;29:1087–1097.
66. Grant IR, Miller JH. Osteochondral fracture of the trochlea associated with fracture-dislocation of the elbow. Injury 1975;6:257–260.
67. Griffith JF, Roebuck DJ, Cheng JC, et al. Acute elbow trauma in children: spectrum of injury revealed by MR imaging not apparent on radiographs. AJR Am J Roentgenol 2001;176:53–60.
68. Gwynne-Jones DP. Displaced olecranon apophyseal fractures in children with osteogenesis imperfecta. J Pediatr Orthop 2005;25:154–157.
69. Hansen PE, Barnes DA, Tullos HS. Case report—arthrographic diagnosis of an injury pattern in the distal humerus of an infant. J Pediatr Orthop 1982;2:569–572.
70. Hanspal RS. Injury to the medial humeral condyle in a child reviewed after 18 years. Report of a case. J Bone Joint Surg Br 1985;67:638–639.
71. Haraldsson S. Osteochondrosis deformans juvenilis capituli humeri including investigation of intra osseous vasculature in distal humerus. Acta Orthop Scand Suppl 1959; 38:1–232.
72. Haraldsson S. The interosseous vasculature of the distal end of the humerus with special reference to capitulum. Acta Orthop Scand 1957;27:81–93.
73. Hardacre JA, Nahigian SH, Froimson AI, et al. Fracture of the lateral condyle of humerus in children. J Bone Joint Surg Am 1971;53:1083–1095.
74. Harrison RB, Keats TE, Frankel CJ, et al. Radiographic clues to fractures of the unossified medial humeral condyle in young children. Skeletal Radiol 1984;11:209–212.
75. Hasner E, Husby J. Fracture of the epicondyle and condyle of the humerus. Acta Chir Scand 1951;101:195–202.
76. Hausman MR, Qureshi S, Goldstein R, et al. Arthroscopically-assisted treatment of pediatric lateral humeral condyle fractures. J Pediatr Orthop 2007;27:739–742.
77. Helfet DL, Hotchkiss RN. Internal fixation of the humerus: a biomechanical comparison of methods. J Orthop Trauma 1990;4:260–264.
78. Herring JA, Fitch RD. Lateral condylar fracture of the elbow. J Pediatr Orthop 1986; 6:724–727.
79. Heyl JH. Fractures of the external condyle of the humerus in children. Ann Surg 1935; 101:1069–1077.
80. Hines RF, Herndon WA, Evans JP. Operative treatment of medial epicondyle fractures in children. Clin Orthop Relat Res 1987;221:170–174.
81. Holda ME, Manoli A II, LaMont RL. Epiphyseal separation of the distal end of the humerus with medial displacement. J Bone Joint Surg Am 1980;62:52–57.
82. Horn BD, Herman MJ, Crisci K, et al. Fractures of the lateral humeral condyle: role of the cartilage hinge in fracture stability. J Pediatr Orthop 2002;22:8–11.
83. Houshian S, Mehdi B, Larsen MS. The epidemiology of elbow fracture in children: analysis of 355 fractures, with special reference to supracondylar humerus fractures. J Orthop Sci 2001;6:312–315.
84. Ippolito E, Tudisco C, Farsetti P, et al. Fracture of the humeral condyles in children: 49 cases evaluated after 18 to 45 years. Acta Orthop Scand 1996;67:173–178.
85. Jakob R, Fowles JV, Rang M, et al. Observations concerning fractures of the lateral humeral condyles in children. J Bone Joint Surg Br 1975;57(4):430–436.
86. Jarvis JG, D'Astous JL. The pediatric T-supracondylar fracture. J Pediatr Orthop 1984; 4:697–699.
87. Jeffrey CC. Nonunion of epiphysis of the lateral condyle of the humerus. J Bone Joint Surg Br 1958;40:396–405.
88. Johansson J, Rosman M. Fracture of the capitulum humeri in children: a rare injury, often misdiagnosed. Clin Orthop Relat Res 1980;146:157–160.
89. Josefsson PO, Danielsson LG. Epicondylar elbow fracture in children: 35-year follow-up of 56 unreduced cases. Acta Orthop Scand 1986;57:313–315.

90. Kamegaya M, Shinohara Y, Kurokawa M, et al. Assessment of stability in children's minimally displaced lateral humeral condyle fracture by magnetic resonance imaging. J Pediatr Orthop 1999;19:570–572.
91. Kanellopoulos AD, Yiannakopoulos CK. Closed reduction and percutaneous stabilization of pediatric T-condylar fractures of the humerus. J Pediatr Orthop 2004;24:13–16.
92. Kaplan SS, Reckling FW. Fracture separation of lower humeral epiphysis with medial displacement. J Bone Joint Surg 1971;53:1105–1108.
93. Kasser JR, Richards K, Millis M. The triceps dividing approach to open reduction of complex distal humerus fractures in adolescents: a cybex evaluation of triceps function and motion. J Pediatr Orthop 1990;10:93–96.
94. Kilfoyle RM. Fractures of the medial condyle and epicondyle of the elbow in children. Clin Orthop Relat Res 1965;41:43–50.
95. Kim HT, Song MB, Conjares JN, et al. Trochlear deformity occurring after distal humeral fractures: magnetic resonance imagines and its natural progression. J Pediatr Orthop 2002;22:188–193.
96. Kirk P, Goulet JA, Freiberg A, et al. A biomechanical evaluation of fixation methods for fractures of the distal humerus. Orthop Trans 1990;14:674.
97. Kocher MS, Shapiro F. Osteogenesis imperfecta. J Am Acad Orthop Surg 1998;6: 225–236.
98. Landin LA, Danielsson LG. Elbow fractures in children. An epidemiological analysis of 589 cases. Acta Orthop Scand 1986;57:309–312.
99. Launay F, Leet AI, Jacopin S, et al. Lateral humeral condyle fractures in children: a comparison of two approaches to treatment. J Pediatr Orthop 2004;24:385–391.
100. Lee HH, Shen HC, Chang JH, et al. Operative treatment of displaced medial epicondyle fractures in children and adolescents. J Shoulder Elbow Surg 2005;14:178–185.
101. Leet AI, Young C, Hoffer MM. Medial condyle fractures of the humerus in children. J Pediatr Orthop 2002;22:2–7.
102. Letts M, Rumball K, Bauermeister S, et al. Fractures of the capitellum in adolescents. J Pediatr Orthop 1997;17:315–320.
103. Lokiec F, Velkes S, Engel J. Avulsion of the medial epicondyle of the humerus in arm wrestlers: a report of five cases and a review of the literature. Injury 1991;22:69–70.
104. Low BY, Lim J. Fracture of humerus during arm wrestling: report of five cases. Singapore Med J 1991;32:47–49.
105. Ma YZ, Zheng CB, Zhou TL, et al. Percutaneous probe reduction of frontal fractures of the humeral capitellum. Clin Orthop Relat Res 1984;183:17–21.
106. Major NM, Crawford ST. Elbow effusions in trauma in adults and children: is there an occult fracture? AJR Am J Roentgenol 2002;178:413–418.
107. Marion J, Faysse R. Fraclures de l'epitrochlea. Rev Chir Orthop 1962;48:447–469.
108. Marion J, Faysse R. Fracture du capitellum. Rev Chir Orthop 1962;48:484–490.
109. Marshall KW, Marshall DL, Busch MT, Williams JP. Osteochondral lesions of the humeral trochlea in the young athlete. Skeletal Radiol 2009;38:479–491.
110. Masada K, Kawai H, Kawabata H, et al. Osteosynthesis for old, established nonunion of the lateral condyle of the humerus. J Bone Joint Surg (Am) 1990;72:32–40.
111. Matsuura T, Kashiwaguchi S, Iwase T, et al. Epidemiology of elbow osteochondral lesions in young baseball players. Presented at the 75th Annual Meeting of the American Academy of Orthopaedic Surgeons, San Francisco, California, February, 2008.
112. Maylahn DJ, Fahey JJ. Fracture of the elbow in children. J Am Med Assoc 1958;166: 220–228.
113. McDonnell DP, Wilson JC. Fracture of the lower end of the humerus in children. J Bone Joint Surg Am 1948;30:347–358.
114. McIntyre WM, Wiley JJ, Charette RJ. Fracture-separation of the distal humeral epiphysis. Clin Orthop Relat Res 1984;188:98–102.
115. McLeod GG, Gray AJ, Turner MS. Elbow dislocation with intra articular entrapment of the lateral epicondyle. J R Coll Surg Edinb 1993;38:112–113.
116. Mead CA, Martin M. Aplasia of the trochlea—an original mutation. J Bone Joint Surg Am 1963;45:379–383.
117. Menkowitz M, Flynn JM. Floating elbow in an infant. Orthopedics 2002;25:185–186.
118. Micheli LJ, Santore R, Stanitski CL. Epiphyseal fractures of the elbow in children. Am Fam Physician 1980;22:107–116.
119. Milch H. Fractures and fracture dislocations of humeral condyles. J Trauma 1964;4: 592–607.
120. Minami A, Sugawara J. Humeral trochlear hypoplasia secondary to epiphyseal injuries as a cause of ulnar nerve palsy. Clin Orthop Relat Res 1988;221:225–230.
121. Mintzer CM, Water PM, Brown DJ, et al. Percutaneous pinning in the treatment of displaced lateral condyle fractures. J Pediatr Orthop 1994;14:462–465.
122. Mirsky EC, Karas EH, Weiner LS. Lateral condyle fractures in children: evaluation of classification and treatment. J Orthop Trauma 1997;11:117–120.
123. Mizuno K, Hirohata K, Kashiwagi D. Fracture-separation of distal humeral epiphysis in young children. J Bone Joint Surg 1979;61:570–573.
124. Mohan N, Hunter JB, Colton CL. The posterolateral approach to the distal humerus for open reduction and internal fixation of fractures of the lateral condyle in children. J Bone Joint Surg Br 2000;82:643–645.
125. Morin B, Fassier F, Poitras B, et al. Results of early surgical treatment of fractures of the lateral humeral condyle in children. Rev Chir Orthop Reparatrice Appar Mot 1988; 74:129–131.
126. Morrissey RT, Wilkins KE. Deformity following distal humeral fracture in childhood. J Bone Joint Surg Am 1984;66A:557–562.
127. Moucha CS, Mason DE. Distal humeral epiphyseal separation. Am J Orthop 2003;32: 497–500.
128. Mudgal CS. Olecranon fracture in osteogenesis imperfecta: a case report. Acta Orthop Belg 1992;58:453–456.
129. Murakami Y, Komiyama Y. Hypoplasia of the trochlea and the medial epicondyle of the humerus associated with ulnar neuropathy—report of two cases. J Bone Joint Surg Br 1978;60:225–227.
130. Nwakama AC, Peterson HA, Shaughnessy WJ. Fishtail deformity following fracture of the distal humerus in children: historical review, case presentations, discussion of etiology, and thoughts on treatment. J Pediatr Orthop B 2000;9:309–318.
131. Nyska M, Peiser J, Lukiec F, et al. Avulsion fracture of the medial epicondyle caused by arm wrestling. Am J Sports Med 1992;20:347–350.
132. Palmer I. Open treatment of transcondylar T fracture of the humerus. Acta Chir Scand 1961;121:486–490.
133. Papandrea R, Waters PM. Posttraumatic reconstruction of the elbow in the pediatric patient. Clin Orthop Relat Res 2000;370:115–126.
134. Papavasilou VA. Fracture–separation of the medial epicondylar epiphysis of the elbow joint. Clin Orthop Relat Res 1982;171:172–174.
135. Papavasiliou VA, Beslikas TA. Fractures of the lateral humeral condyle in children—an analysis of 39 cases. Injury 1985;16:364–366
136. Papvasilious VA, Beslikas TA. T-condylar fractures of the distal humeral condyles during childhood: an analysis of six cases. J Pediatr Orthop 1986;6:302–305.
137. Papavasiliou VA, Nenopoulos S, Venturis T. Fractures of the medial condyle of the humerus in childhood. J Pediatr Orthop 1987;7:421–423.
138. Parent S, Wedemeyer M, Mahar AT, et al. Displaced olecranon fractures in children: a biomechanical analysis of fixation methods. J Pediatr Orthop 2008;28:147–151.
139. Patel N, Weiner SD. Osteochondritis dissecans involving the trochlea: report of two patients (three elbows) and review of the literature. J Pediatr Orthop 2002;22:48–51.
140. Patrick J. Fracture of the medial epicondyle with displacement into the elbow joint. J Bone Joint Surg 1946;28:143–147.
141. Peiro A, Mut T, Aracil J, et al. Fracture-separation of the lower humeral epiphysis in young children. Acta Orthop Scand 1981;52:295–298.
142. Peterson CA, Peterson HA. Analysis of the incidence of injuries to the epiphyseal growth plate. J Trauma 1972;12:275–281.
143. Petit P, Sapin C, Henry G, et al. Rate of abnormal osteoarticular radiographic findings in pediatric patients. Am J Roentgenol 2001;176:987–990.
144. Pimpalnerkar AL, Balasubramaniam G, Young SK, et al. Type four fractures of the medial epicondyle: a true indication for surgical intervention. Injury 1998;29:751–756.
145. Piskin A, Tomak Y, Sen C, Tomak L. The management of cubitus varus and valgus using the Ilizarov method. J Bone Joint Surg Br 2007;89:1615–1619.
146. Poland J. A Practical Treatise on Traumatic Separation of the Epiphyses. London: Smith, Elder & Co., 1898.
147. Potter CM. Fracture-dislocation of the trochlea. J Bone Joint Surg 1954;36:250–253.
148. Potter HG. Imaging of posttraumatic and soft tissue dysfunction of the elbow. Clin Orthop Relat Res 2000;370:9–18.
149. Ravessoud FA. Lateral condylar fracture and ipsilateral ulnar shaft fracture: Monteggia equivalent lesions? J Pediatr Orthop 1985;5:364–366.
150. Remia LF, Richards K, Waters PM. The Bryan-Morrey triceps-sparing approach to open reduction of T-condylar humeral fractures in adolescents: cybex evaluation of triceps function and elbow motion. J Pediatr Orthop 2004;24:615–619.
151. Rettig AC, Wurth TR, Mieling P. Nonunion of olecranon stress fractures in adolescent baseball pitchers. A case series of 5 athletes. Am J Sports Med 2006;34:653–656.
152. Riseborough EJ, Radin EL. Intercondylar T fracture of the humerus in the adult. A comparison of operative and nonoperative treatment in 29 cases. J Bone Joint Surg Am 1969;51A:130–141.
153. Roberts NW. Displacement of the internal epicondyle into the joint. Lancet 1934;2: 78–79.
154. Rogers LF, Rockwood CA. Separation of entire distal humeral epiphysis. Radiology 1973;106:393–400.
155. Rosendahl B. Displacement of the medial epicondyle into the elbow joint: the final result in a case where the fragment has not been removed. Acta Orthop Scand 1959; 28:212–219.
156. Rovinsky D, Ferguson C, Younis A, et al. Pediatric elbow dislocations associated with a Milch type I lateral condyle fracture of the humerus. J Orthop Trauma 1999;13: 458–460.
157. Royle SG, Burke D. Ulna neuropathy after elbow injury in children. J Pediatr Orthop 1990;10:495–496.
158. Rutherford AJ. Fractures of the lateral humeral condyle in children. J Bone Joint Surg Am 1985;67:851–856.
159. Ryu K, Nagaoka M, Ryu J. Osteosynthesis for nonunion of the medial humeral condyle in an adolescent: a case report. J Shoulder Elbow Surg 2007;26:e8–e12.
160. Salter RB, Harris WR. Injuries involving the epiphyseal plate. J Bone Joint Surg 1963; 45:587–632.
161. Sanders RA, Raney EM, Pipkin S. Operative treatment of bicondylar intraarticular fractures of the distal humerus, original research. Orthopedics 1992;15:159–163.
162. Saraf SK, Tuli SM. Concomitant medial condyle fracture of the humerus in a childhood posterolateral dislocation of the elbow. J Orthop Trauma 1989;3:352–354.
163. Schemitsch EH, Tencer AF, Henley MB. Biomechanical evaluation of methods of internal fixation of the distal humerus. J Orthop Trauma 1994;8:468–475.
164. Schwab GH, Bennett JB, Woods GW, et al. Biomechanics of elbow instability: the role of the medial collateral ligament. Clin Orthop Relat Res 1980;146:42–52.
165. Sharma JC, Arora A, Mathur NC, et al. Lateral condylar fractures of the humerus in children: fixation with partially threaded 4.0-mm AO cancellous screws. J Trauma 1995;39:1129–1133.
166. Shimada K, Masada K, Tada K, et al. Osteosynthesis for the treatment of nonunion of the lateral humeral condyle in children. J Bone Joint Surg Am 1997;79:234–240.
167. Siffert RS. Displacement of distal humeral epiphysis in newborn infant. J Bone Joint Surg 1963;45:165–169.
168. Silberstein MJ, Brodeur AE, Graviss ER. Some vagaries of the lateral epicondyle. J Bone Joint Surg Am 1982;64:444–448.
169. Silberstein JJ, Brodeur AE, Graviss ER, et al. Some vagaries of the medial epicondyle. J Bone Joint Surg Am 1981;63:524–528.
170. Skaggs DL, Mirzayan R. The posterior fat pad sign in association with occult fracture of the elbow in children. J Bone Joint Surg Am 1999;81:1429–1433.
171. Skak SV, Olsen SD, Smaabrekke A. Deformity after fracture of the lateral humeral condyle in children. J Pediatr Orthop B 2001;10:142–152.
172. Smith FM. An 84-year follow-up on a patient with ununited fracture of the lateral condyle of humerus. A case report. J Bone Joint Surg Am 1973;55:378–380.
173. Smith FM. Medial epicondyle injuries. J Am Med Assoc 1950;142:396–402.
174. Smith FM, Joyce JJ III. Fracture of lateral condyle of humerus in children. Am J Surg 1954;87:324–329.
175. So YC, Fang D, Orth MC, et al. Varus deformity following lateral humeral condylar fracture in children. J Pediatr Orthop 1985;5:569–572.
176. Sodl JF, Ricchetti ET, Huffman GR. Acute osteochondral shear fracture of the capitellum in a twelve-year-old patient. A case report. J Bone Joint Surg Am 2008;90:629–633.
177. Song KS, Kang CH, Min BW, et al. Closed reduction and internal fixation of displaced unstable lateral condylar fracture of the humerus. J Bone Joint Surg Am 2008;90: 2673–2681.

178. Speed JS, Macey HB. Fracture of humeral condyles in children. J Bone Joint Surg 1933; 15:903–919.
179. Stans AA, Maritz NG, O'Driscoll SW, et al. Operative treatment of elbow contracture in patients 21 years of age or younger. J Bone Joint Surg Am 2002;84A:382–387.
180. Steinthal D. Die Isolirte Fraktur der Eminentia Capitata im Ellenbogengelenk. Zentralbl F Chir 1898;15:17–20.
181. Stimson LA. A Practical Treatise on Fractures and Dislocations. Philadelphia: Lea Brothers & Co., 1900.
182. Stott NS, Zionts LE. Displaced fractures of the apophysis of the olecranon in children who have osteogenesis imperfecta. J Bone Joint Surg Am 1993;75:1026–1033.
183. Stricker SJ, Thomson JD, Kelly RA. Coronal plane transcondylar fracture of the humerus in a child. Clin Orthop Relat Res 1993;292:308–311.
184. Sutherland DH. Displacement of the entire distal humeral epiphysis. J Bone Joint Surg 1974;56:206.
185. Tanabu S, Yamauchi T, Fukushima M. Hypoplasia of the trochlea of the humerus as a cause of ulnar nerve palsy. Report of two cases. J Bone Joint Surg Am 1985;67: 151–154.
186. Tayob AA, Shively RA. Bilateral elbow dislocations with intra articular displacement of medial epicondyles. J Trauma 1980;20:332–335.
187. Tien YC, Chen JC, Fu YC, et al. Supracondylar dome osteotomy for cubitus valgus deformity associated with a lateral condylar nonunion in children. Surgical technique. J Bone Joint Surg Am 2006;88 Suppl 1 Pt 2:191–201.
188. Toniolo RM, Wilkins KE. Avascular necrosis of the trochlea. Paper presented at the 15th Annual Meeting of European Orthopaedic Society, April 13, 1996; Prague, Czech Republic.
189. Toniolo RM, Wilkins KE. Part VI: T-condylar fractures. Fractures and dislocations of the elbow region. In: Rockwood CA Jr, Wilkins KE, Beaty JH, eds. Fractures in Children. 4th ed. Philadelphia: Lippincott-Raven, 1996.
190. Torg JS, Moyer RA. Nonunion of a stress fracture through the olecranon epiphyseal plate observed in an adolescent baseball pitcher. J Bone Joint Surg Am 1977;59:264–265.
191. van Vugt AB, Severijnen RV, Festern C. Fractures of the lateral humeral condyle in children: late results. Arch Orthop Trauma Surg 1988;107:206–209.
192. Varma BP, Srivastava TP. Fractures of the medial condyle of the humerus in children: a report of four cases including the late sequelae. Injury 1972;4:171–174.
193. Wadsworth TG. Premature epiphyseal fusion after injury of capitulum. J Bone Joint Surg Br 1964;46:46–49.
194. Walker HB. A case of dislocation of the elbow with separation of the internal epicondyle and displacement of the latter into the joint. Br J Surg 1928;15:667–679.
195. Watson-Jones R. Primary nerve lesions in injuries of the elbow and wrist. J Bone Joint Surg 1930;12:121–140.
196. Wattenbarger JM, Gerardi J, Johnson CE. Late open reduction internal fixation of lateral condyle fractures. J Pediatr Orthop 2002;22:394–398.
197. Wildburger R, Mähring M, Hofer HP. Supraintercondylar fractures of the distal humerus: results of internal fixation. Review of two consecutive series. J Orthop Trauma 1991;5:301–307.
198. Wilkerson RD, Johns JC. Nonunion of an olecranon stress fracture in an adolescent gymnast: a case report. Am J Sports Med 1990;18:432–434.
199. Wilkins KE. Fractures and dislocation of the elbow region. In: Rockwood CA Jr, Wilkins KE, King RE, editors: Fractures in Children, 3rd edition. Philadelphia, JB Lippincott, 1991:509–828.
200. Willems B, Stuyck J, Hoogmartens M, et al. Fracture-separation of the distal humeral epiphysis. Acta Orthop Belg 1987;53:109–111.
201. Wilson JN. Fracture of external condyle of humerus in children. Br J Surg 1936;18: 299–316.
202. Wilson NIL, Ingran R, Rymaszewski L, et al. Treatment of fractures of the medial epicondyle of the humerus. Injury 1988;19:342–344.
203. Wilson PD. Fracture of the lateral condyle of humerus in children. J Bone Joint Surg 1936;18:299–316.
204. Woods GM, Tullos HB. Elbow stability and medial epicondyle fracture. Am J Sports Med 1977;5:23–30.
205. Yang WE, Shih CH, Lee ZL, et al. Anatomic reduction of old displaced lateral condylar fractures of the humerus in children via a posterior approach with olecranon osteotomy. J Trauma 2008;64:1281–1289.
206. Yngve DA. Distal humeral epiphyseal separation. Orthopaedics 1985;8:100,102–103.
207. Yoo CI, Suh JT, Suh KT, et al. Avascular necrosis after fracture-separation of the distal end of the humerus in children. Orthopedics 1992;15:959–963.
208. Zeir FG. Lateral condylar fracture and its many complications. Orthop Rev 1981;10: 49–55.
209. Zimmerman H. Fractures of the elbow. In: Weber BG, Brunner C, Freuler F, eds. Treatment of fractures in children and adolescents. New York: Springer-Verlag, 1980.
210. Zionts LE, Moon CN. Olecranon apophysis fractures in children with osteogenesis imperfecta revisited. J Pediatr Orthop 2002;22:745–750.
211. Zionts LE, Stolz MR. Late fracture of the lateral condyle of the humerus. Orthopedics 1984;7:541–545.

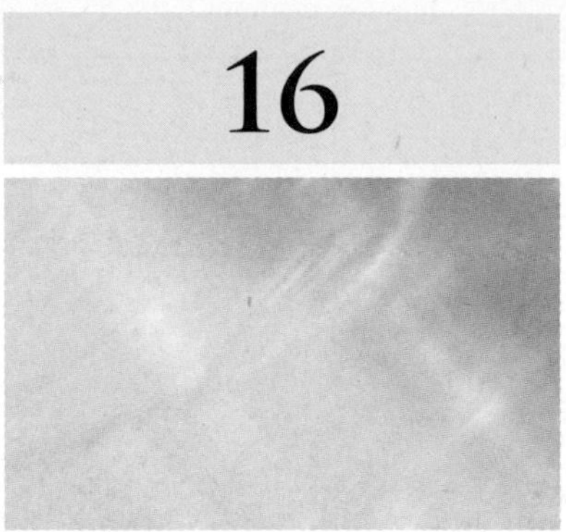

16

DISLOCATIONS OF THE ELBOW

Anthony A. Stans

INTRODUCTION 594

SURGICAL AND APPLIED ANATOMY 594

CLASSIFICATION 595

POSTERIOR ELBOW DISLOCATIONS 595
Principles of Management 595
Treatment Options 597
Complications 602
Recurrent Posterior Dislocations 605
Unreduced Posterior Elbow Dislocations 609
Congenital Elbow Dislocations 610

ANTERIOR ELBOW DISLOCATIONS 610
Principles of Management 610
Treatment Options 610
Complications 611

MEDIAL AND LATERAL ELBOW DISLOCATIONS 611
Signs and Symptoms 611
X-ray and Other Imaging Studies 612
Treatment Options 612

DIVERGENT ELBOW DISLOCATION 612
Treatment Options 613

PROXIMAL RADIOULNAR TRANSLOCATION 613
Principles of Management 613
Current Treatment Options 614

PULLED ELBOW SYNDROME (NURSEMAID'S ELBOW) 614
Principles of Management 615
Current Treatment Options 616
Complications 617

INTRODUCTION

Disruptions of the elbow joint represent a spectrum of injuries involving three separate articulations: the radiocapitellar, the ulnohumeral, and the proximal radioulnar joints. Dislocations of the elbow joint in children are not common. Henrikson[52] studied 1579 injuries about the elbow in skeletally immature patients in Gothenburg, Sweden, in 1966, and found only 45 dislocations, for an overall incidence of 3%. Peak incidence of pediatric elbow dislocations typically occurred in the second decade of life, usually between 13 and 14 years of age when the physes begin to close. The same second-decade peak incidence was reported by Josefsson and Nilsson[64] in 1986. In their series, most elbow dislocations occurred in conjunction with sports activities.

SURGICAL AND APPLIED ANATOMY

Constraints about the elbow preventing dislocation can be considered as either dynamic or static. Dynamic elbow stabilizers consist of the elbow musculature, over which the patient has conscious control, which changes depending on the degree of muscular contraction. Unlike the shoulder, dynamic stabilizers play only a modest role in elbow stability. One indirect but important role of the elbow musculature related to elbow stability is determining elbow position in space at the time of injury. In general, flexion and supination are positions of stability, while extension and pronation are positions of relative instability.

Static constraints are of greater importance and can be divided into osseous and ligamentous restraints (Figs. 16-1 to 16-3). The bone geometry of the elbow creates a relatively constrained hinge. The coronoid and olecranon form a semicircle of approximately 180 degrees into which the trochlea of the humerus securely articulates. The concave surface of the radial head matches the convex capitellum and provides stability to the lateral aspect of the elbow joint. The bony configuration of the medial and lateral aspects of the elbow complement each other with the ulnohumeral articulation providing stability

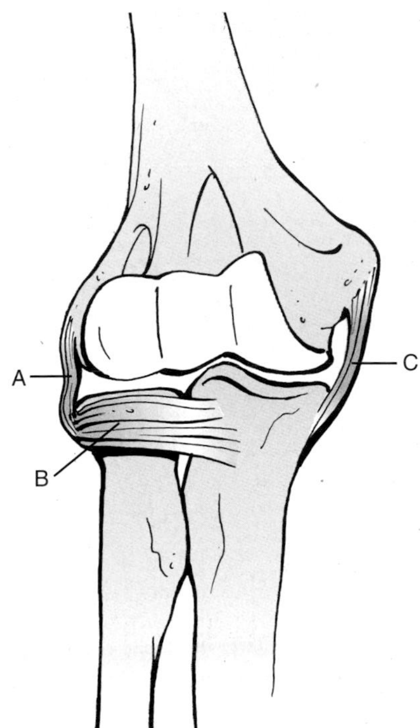

FIGURE 16-1 Anteroposterior view of the elbow illustrates the bone and ligamentous structures which contribute to elbow stability. (A, lateral collateral ligament; B, annular ligament; C, medial collateral ligament.)

against medial-lateral or longitudinal translation, while the radiocapitellar joint provides resistance to axial compression.

Ligamentous constraints include the annular ligament which encircles the radial neck and head, having its origin and insertion on the proximal ulna. Radial (lateral) collateral ligaments originate from the lateral epicondyle and insert into the annular ligament and lateral aspect of the proximal ulna. The primary role of the annular ligament and lateral collateral ligament complex is to provide stability to the proximal radiocapitellar and proximal radioulnar joints and to resist varus stress. The ulnar (medial) collateral ligament resists opening of the medial aspect of the elbow with valgus stress. Having its origin from the medial epicondyle, the medial collateral ligament has two primary components that contribute to elbow stability. The primary stabilizing segment courses from the medial epicondyle to the coronoid process. A fan-shaped posterior oblique ligament inserts on the olecranon and functions mainly in flexion. A small transverse ligament runs from the olecranon to the coronoid but has little functional importance.

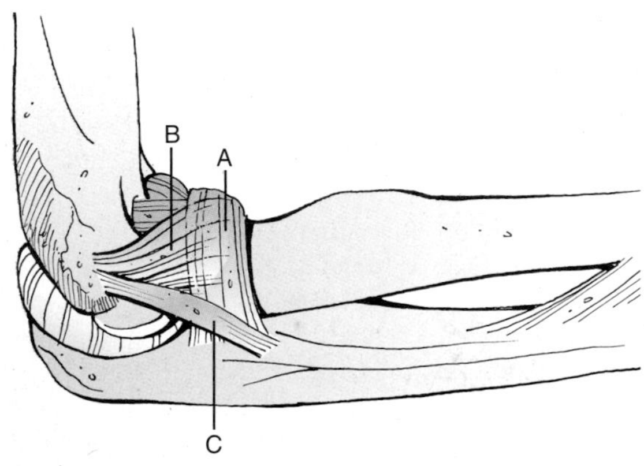

FIGURE 16-2 The annular ligament and lateral collateral ligament complex provides stability to the proximal radioulnar joint and radial capitellar articulation. (A, annular ligament; B, lateral collateral ligament insertion on annular ligament; C, lateral collateral ligament inserting on ulna.)

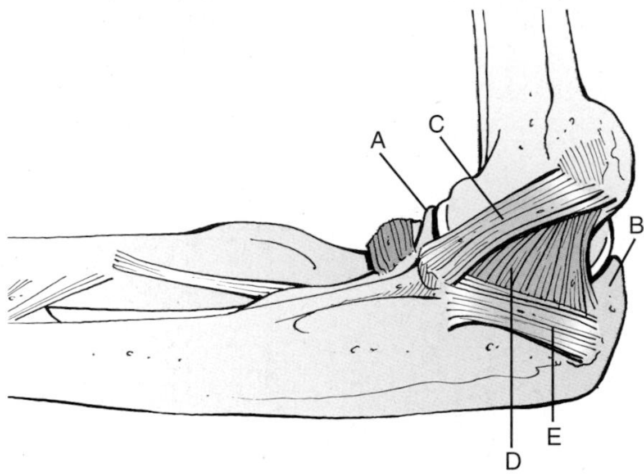

FIGURE 16-3 The medial elbow is stabilized by the hinge articulation between the proximal ulna and the humerus. Three components of the ulnar collateral ligament provide additional elbow stability. (A, coronoid process; B, olecranon process; C, anterior oblique medial collateral ligament; D, posterior oblique medial collateral ligament; E, transverse medial collateral ligament.)

CLASSIFICATION

Elbow dislocations are described by the position of the proximal radioulnar joint relative to the distal humerus: posterior, anterior, medial, or lateral. Posterior dislocations are further subdivided into posterolateral and posteromedial displacement. Occasionally, the proximal radioulnar joint is disrupted. When this happens, the radius and ulna can diverge from each other. Rarely, the radius and ulna translocate, with the radius medial and the ulna lateral. Isolated dislocations of the radial head must be differentiated from congenital dislocations. Isolated dislocations of the proximal ulna are exceedingly rare and have not been reported in children. Included in this chapter is a discussion of the commonly occurring subluxation of the radial head, or "nursemaid's elbow." This is not a true subluxation but rather a partial entrapment of the annular ligament in the radiocapitellar joint.

POSTERIOR ELBOW DISLOCATIONS

Principles of Management

Posterior dislocation is the most common type of elbow dislocation. The general principles of management include promptly obtaining a concentric reduction of the elbow joint while identifying and treating all associated injuries, allowing timely motion and rehabilitation with the goal of restoring full-elbow motion without recurrent instability.

Mechanism of Injury

The first stage in a posterior or posterolateral dislocation is a disruption of the ulnar collateral ligaments or failure of the medial epicondyle apophysis. This produces valgus instability.

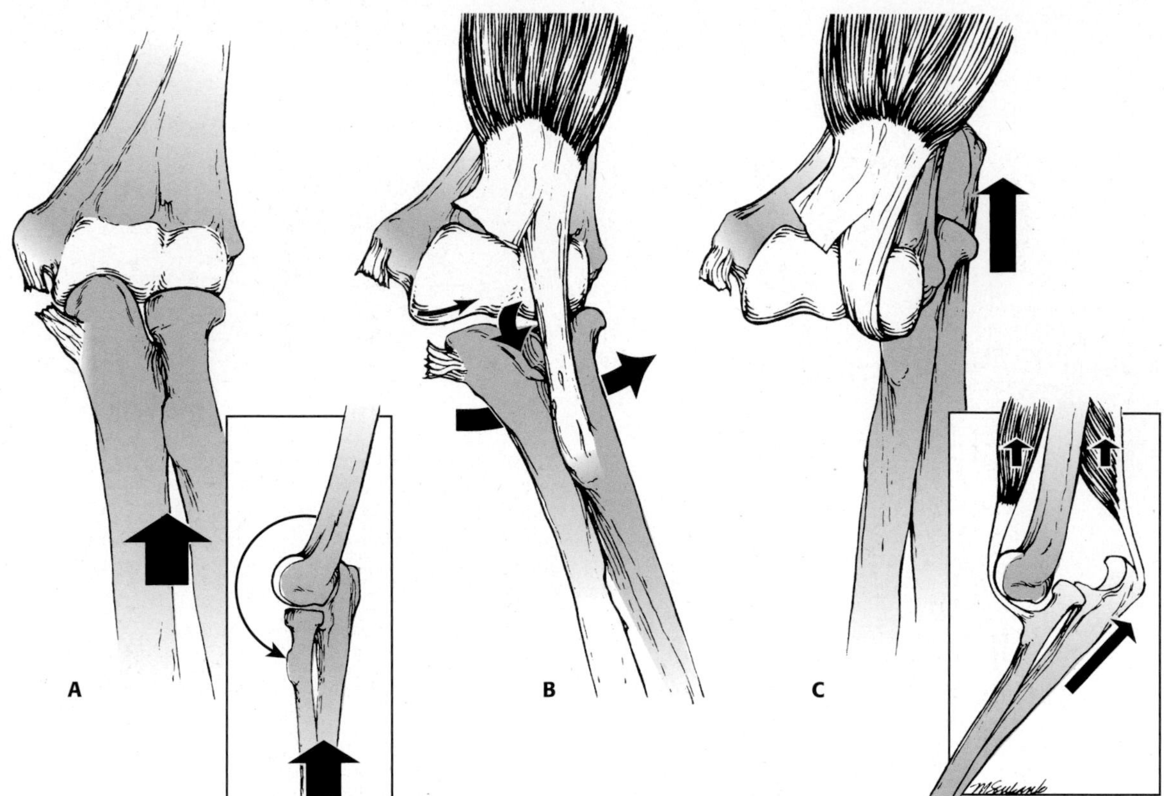

FIGURE 16-4 Mechanism of injury producing a posterior elbow dislocation. **A.** The elbow is forced into extension that ruptures the medial collateral ligaments. The normal valgus alignment of the elbow accentuates the valgus force at the elbow. **B.** The lateral slope of the medial crista of the trochlea forces the proximal ulna posterolaterally (*small arrow*). The biceps tendon serves as a fulcrum for rotation (*medium arrow*) leading to valgus hinging (*large arrow*) of the forearm. **C.** The proximal ulna and radius are then impacted posteriorly and held against the distal articular surface by the contraction of the biceps and triceps (*arrows*).

The proximal radius and ulna displace laterally with the intact biceps tendon acting as the center of rotation for the displaced forearm (Fig. 16-4). Application of both abduction and extension forces with anterior soft tissue disruption results in a posterior or posterolateral elbow dislocation.[100,128]

Signs and Symptoms

Posterior elbow dislocation must be differentiated from extension-type supracondylar fracture of the distal humerus. With both injuries, the elbow is held semiflexed, and swelling may be considerable. Swelling initially is usually less with a dislocation than with a type III supracondylar humeral fracture. Crepitus is usually absent in children with a dislocation and the forearm appears shortened. The prominence produced by the distal humeral articular surface is more distal and is palpable as a blunt articular surface. The tip of the olecranon is displaced posteriorly and proximally so that its triangular relationship with the epicondyles is lost. The skin may have a dimpled appearance over the olecranon fossa. If the dislocation is posterolateral, the radial head also may be prominent and easily palpable in the subcutaneous tissues.

Associated Fractures

Concomitant fractures occur in over one half of posterior elbow dislocations.[72,97,114,116] Fractures involving the medial epicondyle, radial head and neck, and coronoid process are most common. Fractures involving the lateral epicondyle, lateral condyle, olecranon, capitellum, and trochlea occur less frequently.[21]

Soft Tissue Injury

Posterior dislocations normally produce moderate soft tissue injury and can be associated with neurovascular injuries and concomitant fractures (Fig. 16-5). The anterior capsule fails in tension, opening the joint cavity. Radial head displacement strips the capsule from the posterolateral aspect of the lateral condyle with the adjacent periosteum. Because of the large amount of cartilage on the posterolateral aspect of the lateral condyle, the posterior capsule may not reattach firmly with healing. This lack of a strong reattachment is believed to be a factor in recurrent elbow dislocations.[101] In a series of 62 adults and adolescents with elbow dislocations requiring surgical treatment, McKee et al.[87] reported that disruption of the lateral collateral ligament complex occurred in all 62 elbows.

Medially, the ulnar collateral ligament complex is disrupted either by an avulsion of the medial epicondyle or a direct tear of the ligament.[123,128] Cromack[23] found that with medial epicondylar fractures, the origins of the ulnar collateral ligaments and the medial forearm flexor muscles remain as a unit, along with most of the pronator teres, which is stripped from its humeral origin proximal to the epicondyle. These structures are then displaced posterior to the medial aspect of the distal humerus. The ulnar collateral ligaments and the muscular origins of the common flexor muscles tear if the epicondyle remains

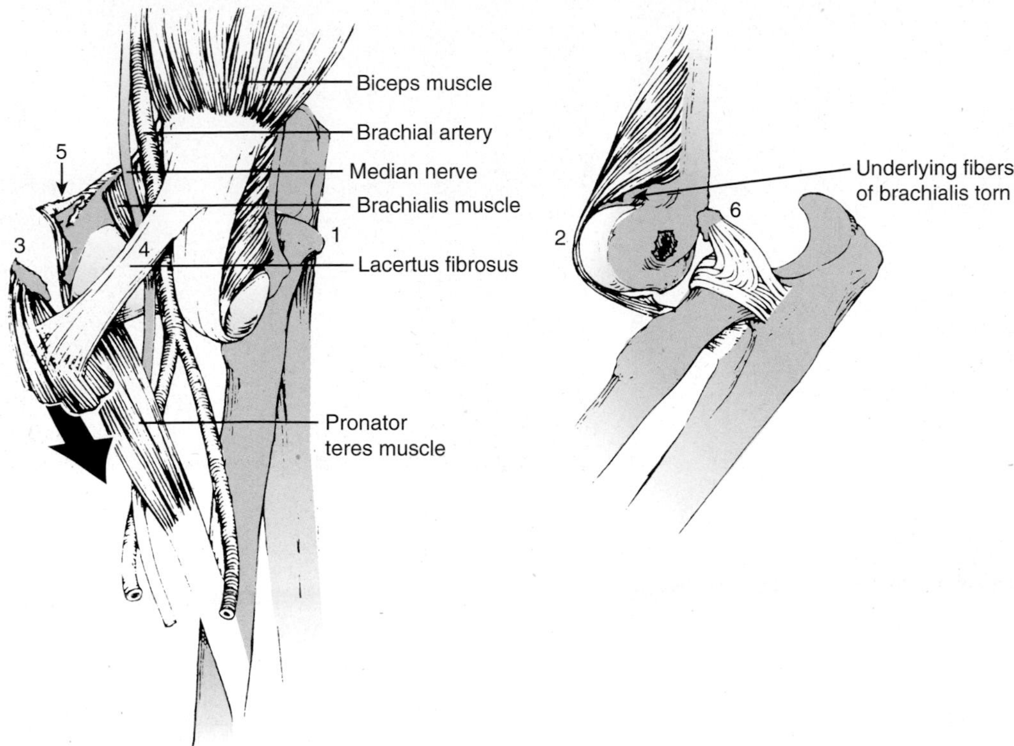

FIGURE 16-5 Injuries associated with elbow dislocation. **1.** The radial head and olecranon are displaced posterolaterally. **2.** The brachialis muscle is stretched across the articular surface of the distal humerus. **3.** The origins of the medial forearm flexion muscles are either torn or avulsed with the medial epicondyle from the medial condyle. **4.** The median nerve and brachial artery are stretched across the medial condyle and held firmly by the lacertus fibrosus. **5.** The medial condyle lies in the subcutaneous tissue between the brachialis anteriorly and the pronator teres posteriorly. **6.** The lateral (radial) collateral ligaments often avulse a piece of cartilage or bone from the lateral condyle.

attached to the humerus. With posterolateral displacement of the forearm, the medial aspect of the distal humerus most often passes into the intermuscular space between the pronator teres posteriorly and the brachialis anteriorly. The brachialis, because it has little distal tendon, is easily ruptured. The rent in the anterior capsule usually is in this same area.

The structure most commonly torn on the lateral aspect of the elbow is the annular ligament.[128] On occasion, the lateral collateral ligament either avulses a small osteochondral fragment from the lateral epicondyle or tears completely within its substance.

Neurovascular Injuries

When the elbow is dislocated, the medial aspect of the distal humerus lies subcutaneously between the pronator teres posteriorly and the brachialis anteriorly. The median nerve and brachial artery lie directly over the distal humerus in the subcutaneous tissues. In a cadaver and clinical study by Louis et al.,[74] there was a consistent pattern of disruption of the anastomosis between the inferior ulnar collateral artery and the anterior ulnar recurrent artery. If the main brachial arterial trunk also is compromised, the loss of this collateral system can result in the loss of circulation to the forearm and hand.

The ulnar nerve is also at risk in posterior elbow dislocation because of its position posterior to the medial epicondyle.

X-ray and Other Imaging

Anteroposterior and lateral x-rays usually are diagnostic of a posterior elbow dislocation. There is a greater superimposition of the distal humerus on the proximal radius and ulna in the anteroposterior view. The radial head may be proximally and laterally displaced, or it may be directly behind the middistal humerus, depending on whether the dislocation is posterolateral, posterior, or posteromedial (Fig. 16-6). The normal valgus angulation between the forearm and the arm usually is increased. On the lateral view, the coronoid process lies posterior to the condyles. The x-rays must be examined closely for associated fractures. Subtle osteochondral fracture fragments can become entrapped in the joint. If anatomic, congruent reduction is not feasible, and further evaluation with computerized tomography or magnetic resonance imaging is utilized to further define complex injury patterns.

Rationale

If untreated, elbow dislocation predictably results in dramatic loss of elbow function characterized by loss of motion and eventually pain (Fig. 16-7). In comparison, reduction of the dislocated elbow usually achieves marked improvement of acute pain as well as restoration of long-term function.

Treatment Options

Closed Reduction

Closed reduction of posterior elbow dislocations is successful in most cases. In the combined series of 317 dislocations,[72,97,114,116] only two cases[72] could not be reduced by closed methods. In the Carlioz and Abols[21] series, two disloca-

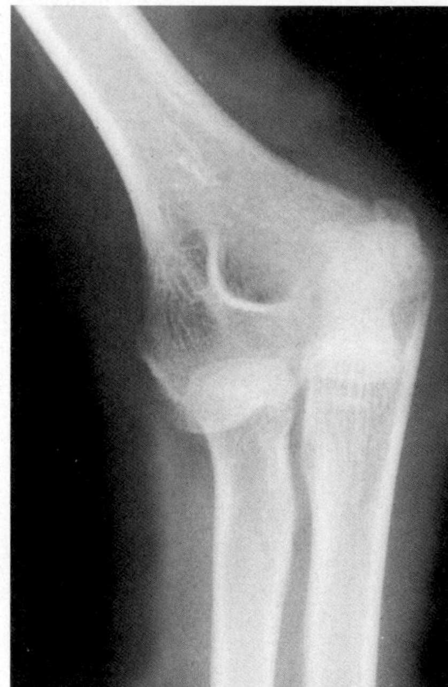

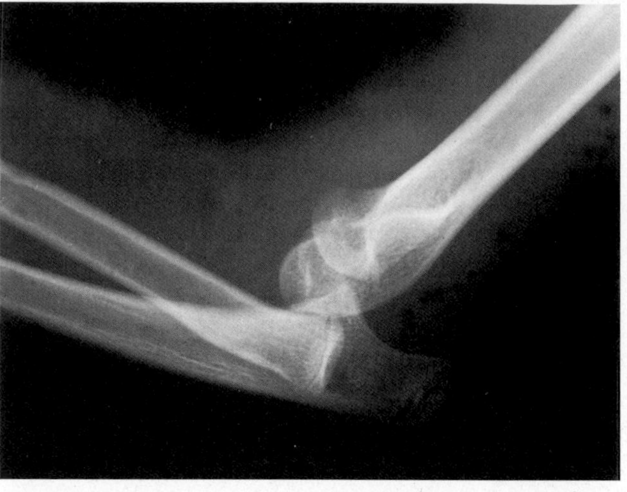

FIGURE 16-6 Radiographic findings. **A.** Anteroposterior radiograph. The radial head is superimposed behind the distal humerus. There is increased cubitus valgus. The medial epicondyle has not been avulsed. **B.** Lateral radiograph demonstrating that the proximal radius and ulna are both displaced posteriorly to the distal humerus.

tions reduced spontaneously and closed reduction was successful in 50 cases, but failed in 6 cases (10%). Josefsson et al.[63] reported that all 25 dislocations without associated fractures were successfully reduced.

Progressive elbow swelling secondary to the soft tissue injury associated with an elbow dislocation makes it imperative that the joint be promptly reduced. Royle[116] found that dislocations reduced soon after the injury had better outcomes than those in which reduction was delayed.

All methods of closed reduction must overcome the deforming muscle forces so that the coronoid process and the radial head can slip past the distal end of the humerus. Adequate sedation or anesthesia is necessary to permit muscle relaxation. Before the primary reduction forces are applied, the forearm is hypersupinated to dislodge the coronoid process and radial head from their position behind the distal humerus and to reduce tension on the biceps tendon.[101] The reducing forces are applied in two major directions (Fig. 16-8). The first reducing force must be along the long axis of the humerus to overcome the contractions of the biceps and brachialis anteriorly and the triceps posteriorly. Once these forces are neutralized, the proximal ulna and radius must be passed from posterior to anterior.

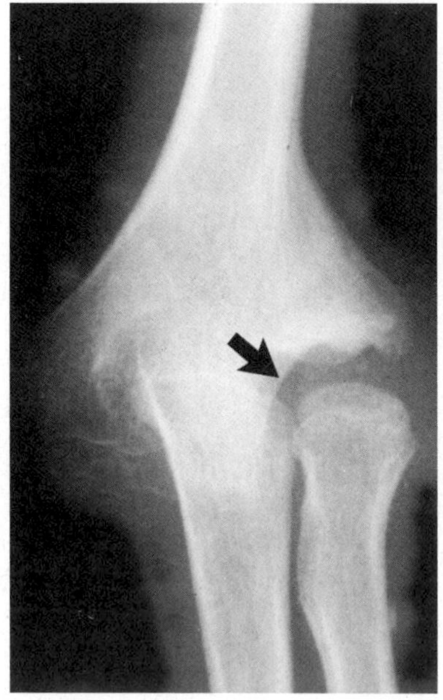

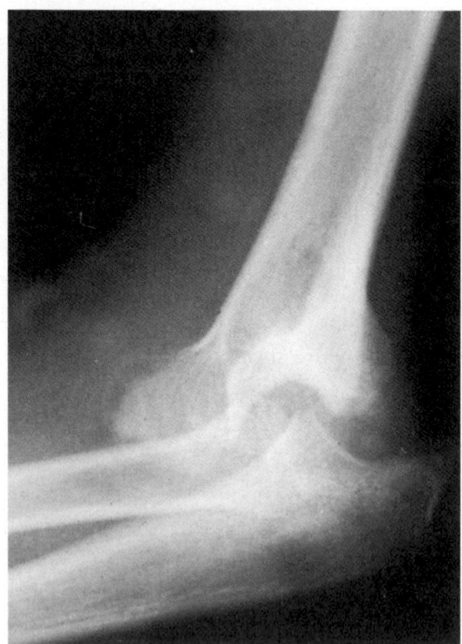

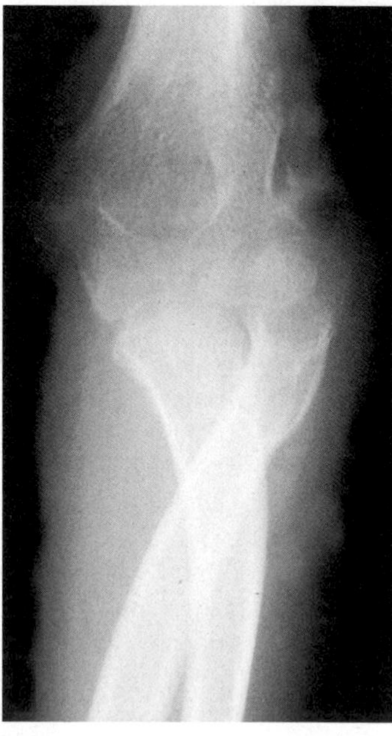

FIGURE 16-7 Unreduced dislocation. **A.** Preoperative anteroposterior radiograph. The elbow sustained an injury 3 years before surgery. Elbow motion was extremely limited and painful. The lateral supracondylar ridge had been eroded by the radial head (*arrow*). **B.** Lateral radiograph. The posterior position of the olecranon is apparent. **C.** Anteroposterior radiograph 3 months postoperatively. Total elbow motion was 30 degrees, but there was less pain and more stability.

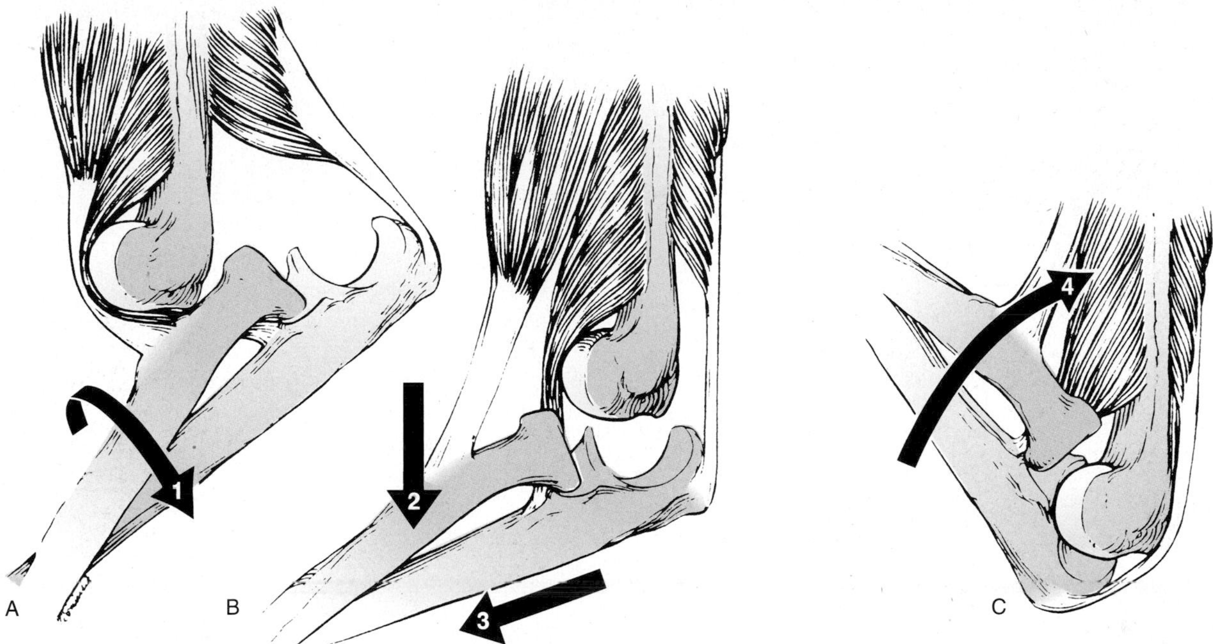

FIGURE 16-8 Forces required to reduce posterior elbow dislocations. **A.** The forearm is hypersupinated (*arrow 1*) to unlock the radial head. **B.** Simultaneous forces are applied to the proximal forearm along the axis of the humerus (*arrow 2*) and distally along the axis of the forearm (*arrow 3*). **C.** The elbow is then flexed (*arrow 4*) to stabilize the reduction once the coronoid is manipulated distal to the humerus.

This requires a second force along the long axis of the forearm. There appears to be two main philosophies as to the best method of applying force to counteract the muscles of the arm: the "pullers"[10,24,103] (Figs. 16-9 to 16-11) and the "pushers"[71,91,93] (Fig. 16-12). There also are combined unassisted pusher-puller techniques.[46,70]

Previous authors[72,141] have strongly advised against initial hyperextension before reduction forces are applied to the elbow. Loomis[73] demonstrated that when the coronoid process is locked against the posterior aspect of the humerus and the elbow is extended, the force applied to the anterior muscles is multiplied by as much as five times because of the increased

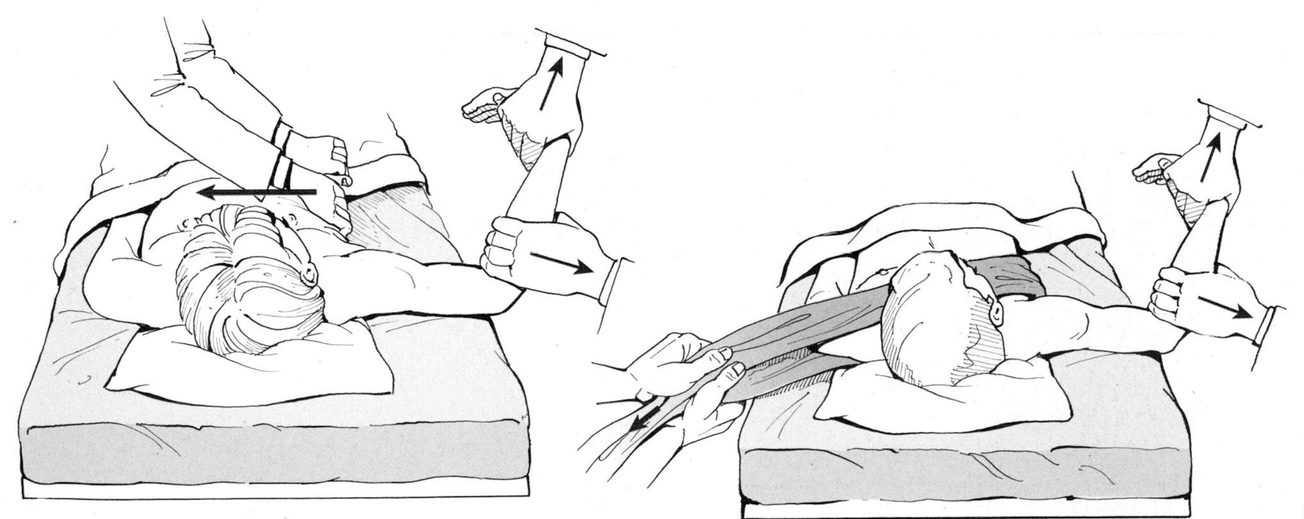

FIGURE 16-9 Reduction by "puller" techniques in a supine position. **A.** With the elbow flexed to almost 90 degrees, a force is applied to the anterior portion of the forearm with one hand while the other hand pulls distally along the forearm. A counterforce is applied to offset the manipulating forces by direct stabilization of the patient by a second medical person. **B.** The counterforce is applied with a sheet around the chest in the ipsilateral axilla. (Redrawn from Parvin RW. Closed reduction of common shoulder and elbow dislocations without anesthesia. Arch Surg 1957;75:972–975, with permission. Copyright 1957, American Medical Association.)[15]

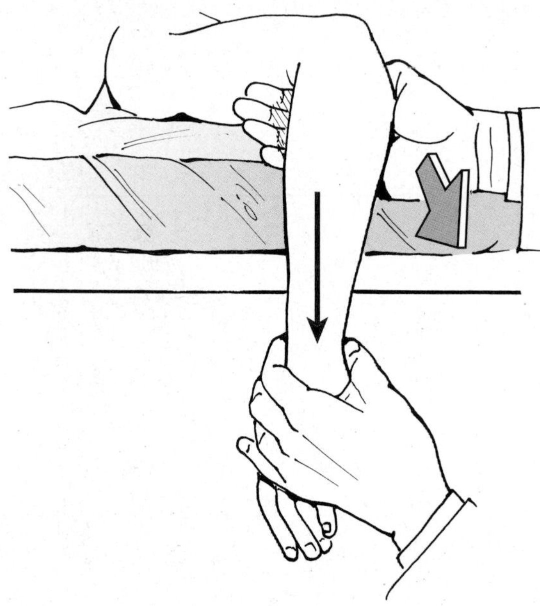

FIGURE 16-10 Reduction by "puller" technique in a prone position. The same forces are applied to the proximal portion of the anterior forearm and distal forearm as in the supine position. The table provides a counterforce against the anterior portion of the distal humerus when the patient is prone.

leverage. This places a marked strain on the injured anterior capsule and the brachialis muscle (Fig. 16-13). By contrast, when the distal force is applied to the proximal forearm with the elbow flexed, the force exerted against the muscles across the elbow is equal to the distracting force. For patients with posterolateral dislocations, the lateral displacement of the proximal radius and ulna must first be corrected to prevent the median nerve from being entrapped or injured during reduction.[11,16] Hyperextension reduction puts the median nerve more at risk for entrapment.

Postreduction Care. After reduction, the surgeon should determine and document the stability of the elbow by examination while the patient is under sedation. A concentric reduction must be documented in all cases. Some type of immobilization, usually a posterior splint, is advocated by most investigators. A frequently recommended period of immobilization is 3 weeks,[72,73,103,125] although some have advocated early motion.[115,116,147] In a recent study of 42 adult patients comparing 2 weeks of cast immobilization with the use of a simple arm sling and early motion, Maripuri et al.[83] demonstrated improved early and final functional outcomes in the early mobilization group compared to the group placed in a cast following reduction. O'Driscoll et al.[100] suggested that if the elbow was stable in response to valgus stress with the forearm pronated then the anterior portion of the medial collateral ligament was intact and the patient could begin early motion. Ninety degrees of elbow flexion appears to be the standard position of immobilization.

Surgical Treatment

Indications for primary open reduction include an inability to obtain a concentric closed reduction, an open dislocation, and a displaced osteochondral fracture.

Primary ligament repair is not routinely indicated. Adults with posterior elbow dislocations without concomitant fracture have no better function or stability following a primary ligamentous repair than those treated nonoperatively.[61,62] Excellent results have been reported by Josefsson et al.[63] in 28 children and adolescents with simple posterior dislocations treated nonoperatively.

Open Posterior Dislocations. Open dislocations have a high incidence of associated arterial injury.[50,66,72,74] Operative intervention is necessary in open posterior dislocations to irrigate and débride the open wound and elbow and to evaluate the brachial artery. If there is vascular disruption, most advocate vascular repair or reconstruction with a vein graft even in the presence of adequate capillary refill. This lessens the risk of late cold intolerance, dysesthesias, or dysvascularity.

Associated Fractures. Children with an elbow dislocation can have an associated fracture of the coronoid, lateral condyle, olecranon (Fig. 16-14), or medial epicondyle (Fig. 16-15). Recently, fracture of the anteromedial facet of the coronoid has been recognized as an important injury associated with elbow dislocations in adolescents and adults.[31,32] The presence of a concomitant displaced fracture is a common indication for surgical intervention.[21,38,142] Surgery for associated fractures produced better results than nonoperative treatment in the series of Carlioz and Abols,[21] and similar results were reported by Wheeler and Linscheid.[142] Repair of an associated medial epicondylar fracture may also improve elbow stability in throwing athletes when the injury is in the dominant arm.[123,147] Entrapment of a displaced medial epicondylae fracture within the joint after reduction is an absolute indication for surgical treatment (see Fig. 16-15). Ultimately, the of surgical treatment for fractures associated with an elbow dislocation is based on the circumstances surrounding each individual patient. Factors favoring operative treatment include older patient age, instability of the elbow during examination under sedation at the time of reduction, the presence of a displaced intra-articular fracture, injury to multiple elbow stabilizers, injury to the patient's dominant arm, and anticipated significant sports or activity demands on the elbow.

Postoperative Care. Immobilization after surgery depends on the procedure performed. After open reduction, management is similar to that after satisfactory closed reduction. The length of immobilization for fractures is up to 3 to 4 weeks. Protected arc of motion with a hinged brace or intermittent splinting is utilized frequently to lessen the risk of posttraumatic contracture.

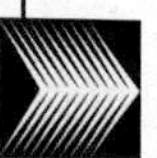

AUTHORS' PREFERRED METHOD OF TREATMENT: POSTERIOR ELBOW DISLOCATION

The "pusher" technique of reduction of an elbow dislocation is preferred in children 9 years of age or younger. In this age group, the child often can be seated comfortably in the parent's lap (see Fig. 16-12). Hanging the arm over the back of a well-padded chair may provide some stabilization.

For a child 9 years of age and older, the puller technique advocated by Parvin[103] is used (see Figs. 16-9 and 16-10).

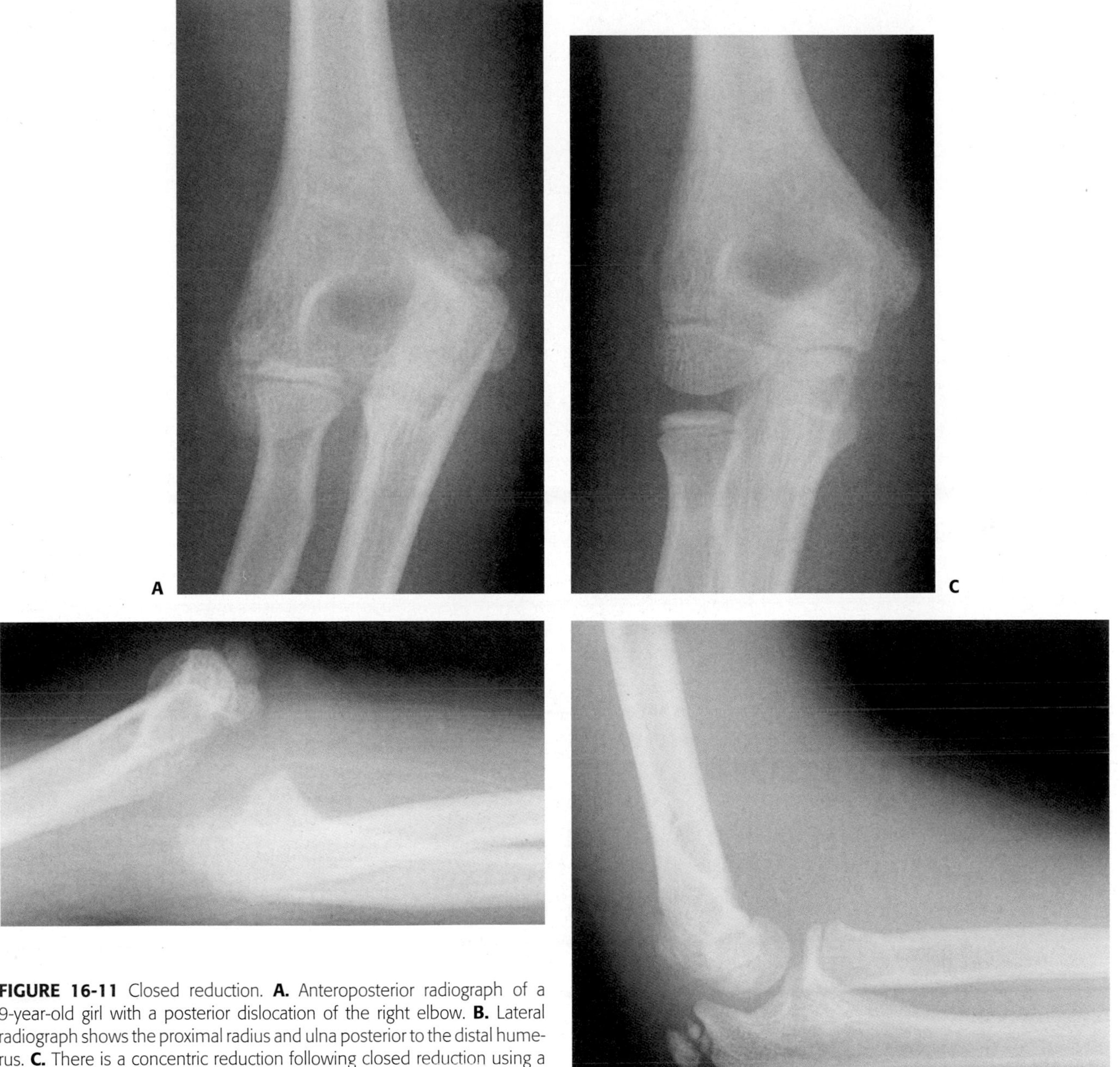

FIGURE 16-11 Closed reduction. **A.** Anteroposterior radiograph of a 9-year-old girl with a posterior dislocation of the right elbow. **B.** Lateral radiograph shows the proximal radius and ulna posterior to the distal humerus. **C.** There is a concentric reduction following closed reduction using a puller technique. **D.** Lateral radiograph.

The forearm must remain supinated during the process of reduction. Occasionally, it is necessary to hypersupinate the forearm to unlock the coronoid process and radial head before reduction. Closed reduction is done with either heavy sedation or general anesthesia. X-rays are obtained after the manipulation to assess the adequacy of the reduction (see Fig. 16-11) and to be certain the joint is congruently reduced. The elbow is immobilized in a posterior splint with the elbow flexed 90 degrees. If there is a question of persistent instability, the forearm is held in full supination. If the elbow is absolutely stable following reduction, the forearm can be immobilized in midpronation to allow the patient to be more functional in the splint.

Because the major complication of elbow dislocations is stiffness, the splint is removed after approximately 1 week and the patient begins intermittent active elbow motion. The patient can discard the splint and use a sling after 10 to 14 days. The emphasis is on early active motion to prevent stiffness that often occurs after this injury. Before reduction, it is important to emphasize to the parents that there may be some loss of motion, especially extension, regardless of the treatment. This is usually less than 30 degrees and not of functional or cosmetic significance.

A careful neurologic examination must be done before and after the reduction with special attention to the median nerve in terms of entrapment. This same careful examination must be made at all follow-up evaluations. Persistent median nerve motor-sensory loss associated with severe pain and resistance with elbow flexion-extension arc of motion may be indicative of entrapment. Of note, ulnar neuropathy is not uncommon and usually resolves spontaneously.

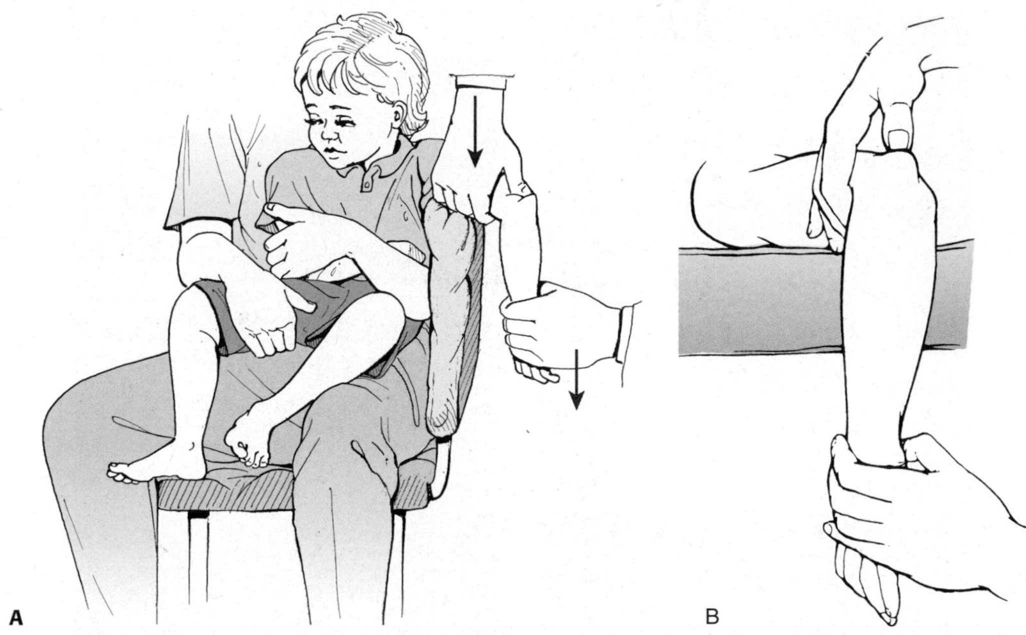

FIGURE 16-12 Reduction by "pusher" techniques. **A.** Lavine's method. The child is held by the parent while the elbow is draped over the edge of the chair. The olecranon is pushed distally past the humerus by the thumb of the physician while the other arm pulls distally along the axis of the forearm. **B.** Meyn's technique with patient lying prone on the table. (Redrawn from Meyn MA, Quigley TB. Reduction of posterior dislocation of the elbow by traction on the dangling arm. Clin Orthop 1974;103:106–107, with permission.)

Pearls and Pitfalls

Closed reduction of pediatric elbow dislocations should always be done with adequate analgesia, sedation, or anesthesia. In addition to making the experience much less frightening and traumatic for the child, adequate analgesia, sedation, or anesthesia will achieve sufficient muscle relaxation for the reduction to be obtained more effectively with less force, thereby reducing the risk of creating an iatrogenic fracture (such as fracture of the radial neck) during reduction.

Complications

Complications associated with posterior elbow dislocations can be divided into those occurring early and those occurring later. Early complications include neurologic and vascular injuries. Late complications include loss of motion, myositis ossificans, recurrent dislocations, radioulnar synostosis, and cubitus recurvatum. The special problems of chronic, unreduced dislocations are not considered complications of treatment.

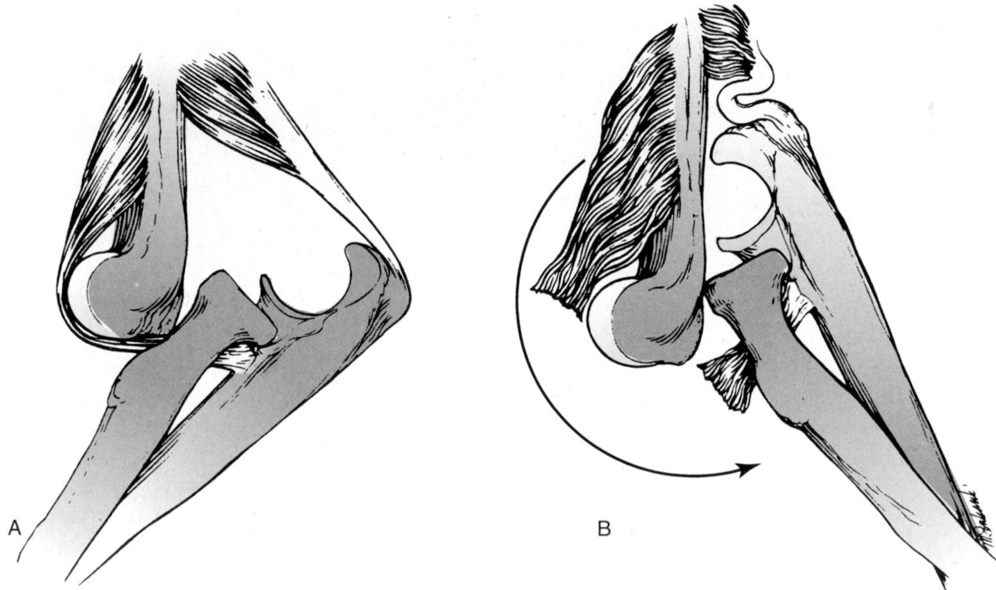

FIGURE 16-13 Hyperextension forces. **A.** The brachialis is stretched across the distal humerus. **B.** Hyperextending the elbow before it is reduced greatly increases the arc of motion and leverage placed across the brachialis. This can result in rupture of large portions of the muscle. (Reprinted from Loomis LK. Reduction and aftertreatment of posterior dislocation of the elbow. Am J Surg 1944;63:56–60, with permission.)

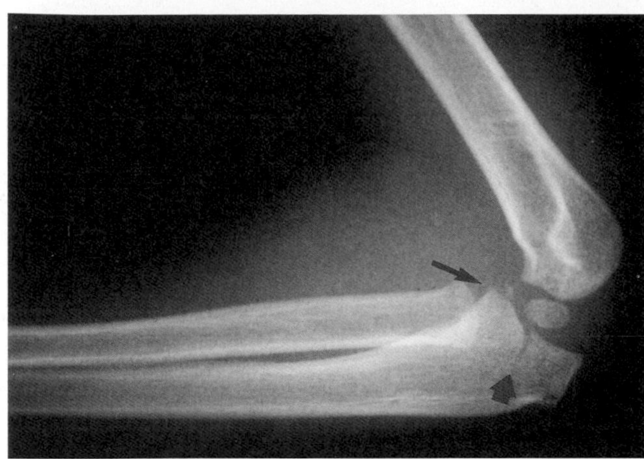

FIGURE 16-14 Lateral radiograph of a 4-year-old child who sustained an elbow dislocation with a concomitant olecranon fracture (*large arrow*) and a coronoid fracture (*small arrow*).

Neurologic Injuries

Ulnar Nerve Lesions. In a combined series of 317 patients,[72,97,114,116] the most commonly injured nerve was the ulnar nerve. Of the 32 patients (10%) who had nerve symptoms after reduction, 21 had isolated ulnar nerve injuries, 7 had isolated median nerve injuries, and in 4 patients both the median and ulnar nerves were involved. Linscheid and Wheeler[72] recommended ulnar nerve transposition if ulnar nerve symptoms were present in a patient undergoing open reduction and internal fixation of a displaced medial epicondylar fracture. Except for the one patient described by Linscheid and Wheeler,[72] the reported ulnar nerve injuries were transient and resolved completely.

Radial Nerve Lesions. Radial nerve injury with posterior elbow dislocation is very rare. Watson-Jones[141] reported two radial nerve injuries associated with elbow dislocation; in both the symptoms rapidly resolved after reduction. Rasool[111] reported a third case.

Median Nerve Lesions. The most serious neurologic injury involves the median nerve, which can be damaged directly by the dislocation or can be entrapped within the joint. Median nerve injuries occur most commonly in children 5 to 12 years of age. There were seven median and four median-ulnar nerve injuries (3%) in the combined series.[72,97,114,116]

Types of Median Nerve Entrapment. Fourrier et al.,[36] in 1977, delineated three types of medial nerve entrapment (Fig. 16-16).

A

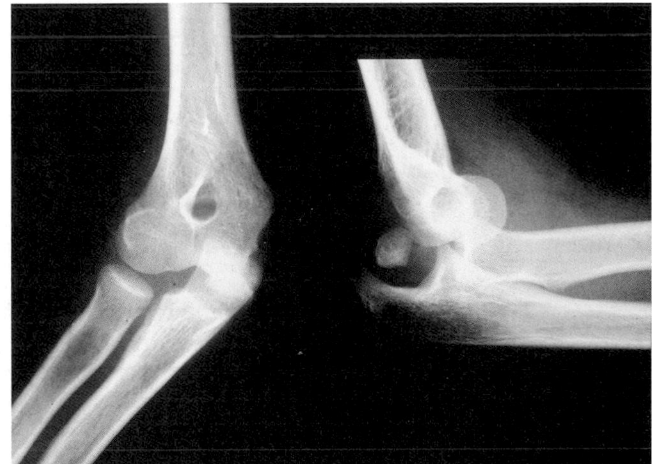

B

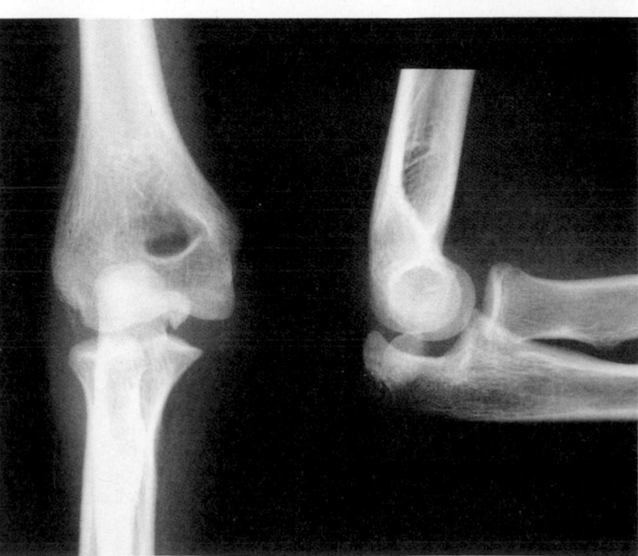

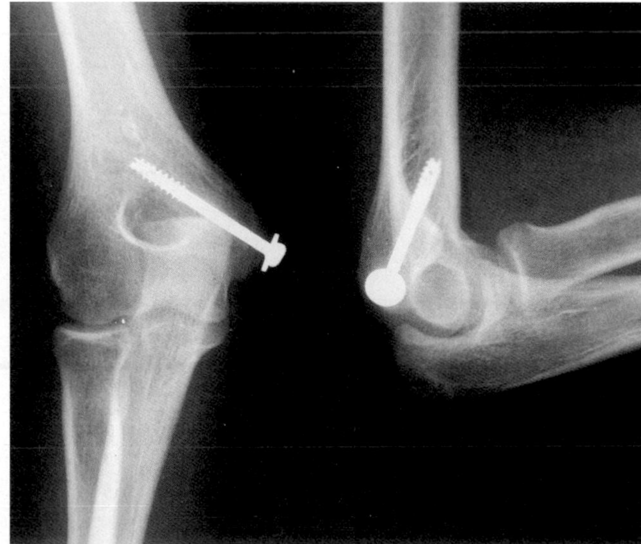

C

FIGURE 16-15 A. Anteroposterior and lateral radiograph of a 14-year-old male who sustained an elbow dislocation with an ipsilateral medial epicondyle fracture. **B.** Anteroposterior radiographs after a closed reduction. Note the entrapment of the medial epicondyle in the joint. **C.** This patient was treated with an open reduction to extract the medial epicondyle from the joint and an internal fixation using a cannulated screw that allowed rapid mobilization of his elbow.

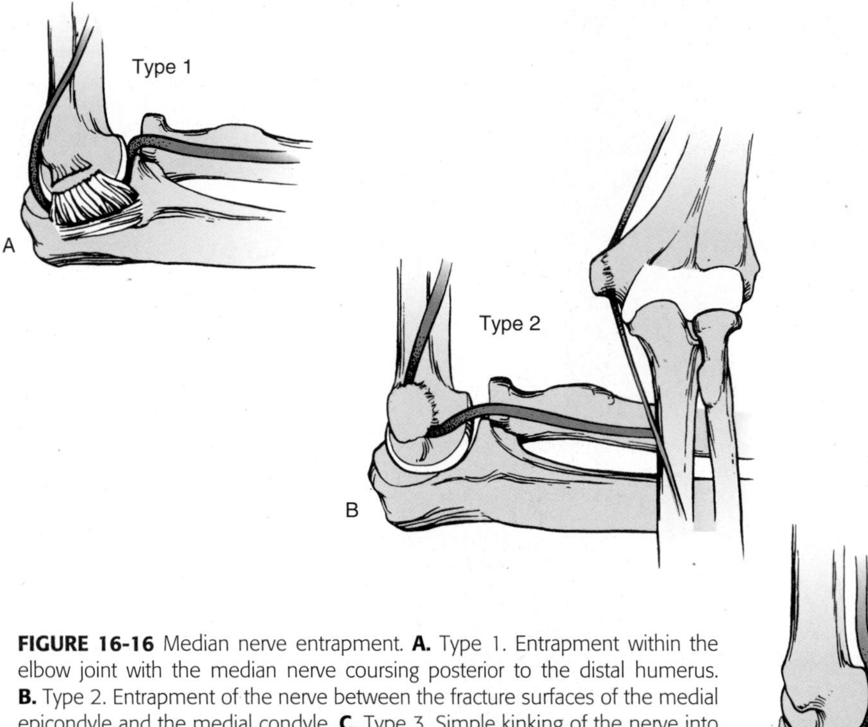

FIGURE 16-16 Median nerve entrapment. **A.** Type 1. Entrapment within the elbow joint with the median nerve coursing posterior to the distal humerus. **B.** Type 2. Entrapment of the nerve between the fracture surfaces of the medial epicondyle and the medial condyle. **C.** Type 3. Simple kinking of the nerve into the anterior portion of the elbow joint. (Redrawn from Hallett J. Entrapment of the median nerve after dislocation of the elbow. J Bone Joint Surg Br 1981;63: 408–412, with permission.)

Type 1. The child has an avulsion of the medial epicondyle or has a rupture of the medial muscles at their origin and the ulnar collateral ligaments (see Fig. 16-16A). This allows the median nerve, with or without the brachial artery, to displace posteriorly. The nerve is especially prone to being entrapped between the trochlea and the olecranon during the process of reduction if the lateral displacement of the proximal radius and ulna is not corrected before reduction. Hallett[45] demonstrated in cadavers that pronation of the forearm while the elbow is hyperextended forces the median nerve posteriorly during the process of reduction making it vulnerable to entrapment. This type of entrapment also has been reported by other authors.[8,11,16,36,42,84,107,110,132] Delay in diagnosis is common. In some patients with an associated medial epicondylae fracture, the nerve can be so severely damaged after being entrapped that neuroma resection and either nerve transposition and direct repair or grafting is necessary.[11,42,84] Good recovery of nerve function has been reported.

If the nerve has been entrapped for a considerable period, the Matev sign may be present on the x-rays.[84] This represents a depression on the posterior surface of the medial epicondylar ridge where the nerve has been pressed against the bone.[8,25,42,45,107,110,132] This groove is seen on x-ray as two sclerotic lines parallel to the nerve (Fig. 16-17). This sign disappears when the nerve has been decompressed.

Type 2. The nerve is entrapped between the fracture surfaces of the medial epicondyle and the distal humerus (see Fig. 16-16B). The fracture heals and the nerve is surrounded by bone, forming a neuroforamen.[107,113,132] This may or may not be visible on x-ray. The medial epicondyle is osteomized to free the nerve. Again, decompression alone may be adequate treatment, although neuroma resection and repair or reconstruction with nerve grafts may be necessary.

Type 3. The nerve is kinked and entrapped between the distal humerus and the olecranon (see Fig. 16-16C). Only three injuries of this type have been reported.[8,106,109] Decompression, neuroma resection, and repair resulted in return of good function over 6 to 24 months.

Al Qattan et al.[3] described a fourth type of median nerve entrapment in a 14-year-old boy who had a posterior elbow dislocation with a medial epicondylar fracture. The median

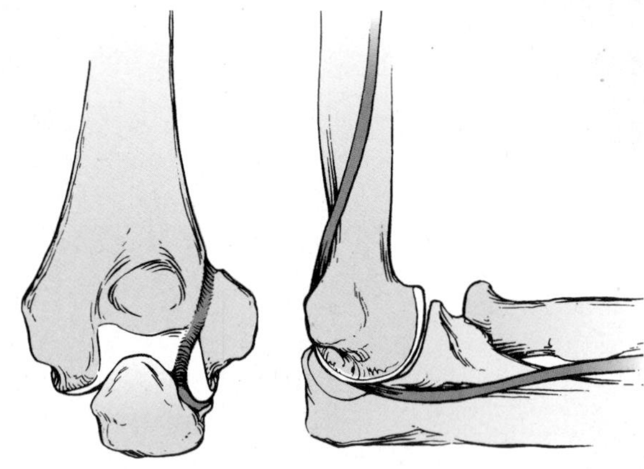

FIGURE 16-17 The Matev sign suggesting entrapment of the median nerve in the elbow joint and impingement of the nerve against the posterior surface of the medial condyle. This produces a depression with sclerotic margins. (Redrawn from Matev I. A radiographic sign of entrapment of the median nerve in the elbow joint after posterior dislocation. J Bone Joint Surg Br 1976;58:353–355, with permission.)

nerve was found entrapped in a healed medial epicondylar fracture (type 2) in an anterior to posterior direction 18 months after injury. The nerve then passed through the elbow joint in a posterior to anterior direction (type 1). The nerve was so severely damaged that it had to be resected and repaired with sural nerve grafts. A second type 4 median nerve entrapment also requiring nerve segment resection and grafting was reported by Ozkoc et al.[102]

The combination of an associated fracture of the medial epicondyle and significant median nerve dysfunction was cited by Rao and Crawford[110] as an absolute indication for surgical exploration of the nerve because of the frequency of median nerve entrapment with fractures of the medial epicondyle (types 1 and 2). Magnetic resonance imaging (MRI) may be helpful in defining the course of the median nerve if entrapment is suspected.[2] Electromyography and nerve conduction studies have been utilized to assist in operative decision making. Painful dysesthesias with arc of motion is usually indicative of entrapment. Once the entrapped nerve is removed from the joint, neurologic function typically improves. Resection and repair or nerve grafting are may be necessary.

Arterial Injuries

Arterial injuries are uncommon with posterior elbow dislocations in children and adolescents with only eight vascular injuries (3%) reported in the combined series of 317 patients.[72,97,114,116] However, Carlioz and Abols[21] reported 4 patients with diminished radial pulses that resolved after reduction. Arterial injuries have been associated with open dislocations in which collateral circulation is disrupted.[50,66,74,117] In these situations, usually the brachial artery is ruptured,[44,50,54,66,74,81] but it also can be thrombosed[144] as well as entrapped in the elbow joint.[51,104,144] Pearce[104] reported an entrapped radial artery in which there was a high bifurcation of the brachial artery. When there is a complete rupture, there usually is evidence of ischemia distally. However, the presence of good capillary circulation to the hand or a Doppler pulse at the wrist does not always mean the artery is intact.[44,54] Arteriograms usually are not necessary because the arterial injury is at the site of the dislocation. If imaging is indicated to evaluate possible arterial injury, its minimal risk and invasiveness make vascular ultrasound an attractive initial imaging choice.

Treatment usually consists of relocation of the elbow dislocation which returns the displaced brachial vessels to their normal position[51,144] and operative repair of those that are ruptured or severely damaged. Ligation of the ends has been done in the past with adults, especially if there was good capillary circulation distally,[50,66] but this may predispose to late ischemic changes such as claudication, cold sensitivity, or even late amputation. Most investigators recommend direct arterial repair or a vein graft.[44,54,74,81,117] Louis et al.[74] recommended arterial repair because their cadaver studies demonstrated that a posterior elbow dislocation usually disrupted the collateral circulation necessary to maintain distal blood flow.

Loss of Motion

Almost all patients with elbow dislocations lose some range of elbow motion.[21,38,61–63] This loss is less in children than in adults[63] and usually is no more than 10 degrees of extension. This rarely is of functional or cosmetic significance. However, this potential for loss of motion must be explained to the parents before reduction and may be an indication for a supervised rehabilitation program. If there is displaced medial epicondylar nonunion, the loss of major range of motion can be severe and limiting. Similarly, an incongruent elbow joint will have marked limitations of motion.

Myositis Ossificans versus Heterotopic Calcification

True myositis ossificans should be differentiated from heterotopic calcification, which is a dystrophic process. Myositis ossificans involves ossification within the muscle sheath that can lead to a significant loss of range of motion of the elbow. Disruption of the brachialis muscle is believed to be a contributory factor.[73] Fortunately, myositis ossificans is rare in children.[63,136] Although heterotopic calcification in the ligaments and capsule of the elbow is common,[63,114] it rarely results in loss of elbow function (Fig. 16-18).

In Neviaser and Wickstrom's[97] series of 115 patients, 10 had x-ray evidence of myositis ossificans; all, however, were asymptomatic. Roberts[114] differentiated true myositis ossificans from heterotopic calcification in his series of 60 elbow dislocations, and noted that only 3 patients had true myositis ossificans. Linscheid and Wheeler[72] reported that the incidence of some type of heterotopic calcification was 28%, which was most common around the condyles. Only in five patients was it anterior to the capsule (which probably represented true myositis ossificans in the brachialis muscle). Four of these patients had some decrease in elbow function. Josefsson et al.[63] reported that 61% of 28 children with posterior dislocations had periarticular calcification, but this did not appear to be functionally significant.

Radioulnar Synostosis

In dislocations with an associated fracture of the radial neck, the incidence of a secondary proximal radioulnar synostosis is increased (Fig. 16-19). This can occur regardless of whether the radial neck fracture is treated operatively or nonoperatively.[16,21,100] Carlioz and Abols[21] reported a synostosis in 1 of 3 patients with posterior elbow dislocations associated with radial neck fractures.

Cubitus Recurvatum

Occasionally, a severe elbow dislocation results in significant tearing of the anterior capsule. As a result, after reduction, when all the stiffness created by the dislocation has subsided, the patient may have some hyperextension (cubitus recurvatum) of the elbow. This usually is minimally symptomatic but if asymmetric, may be cosmetically disturbing to the parents and adolescent.

Recurrent Posterior Dislocations

Recurrent posterior elbow dislocation is rare. In the combined series of dislocations, only 2 of 317 patients (0.6%) experienced recurrent dislocations.[72,97,114,116] Approximately 80% of recurrent dislocations are in males. Three investigators have reported bilateral cases.[65,92,112]

Mechanism of Injury

The pathology of recurrent dislocation involves any or all of collateral ligament instability, capsular laxity, and bone and articular cartilage defects.

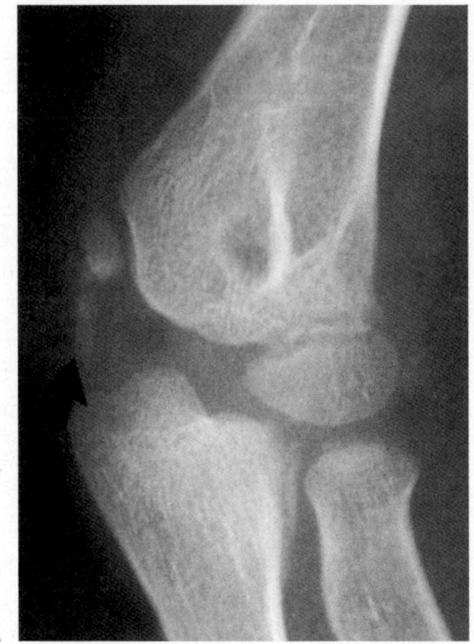

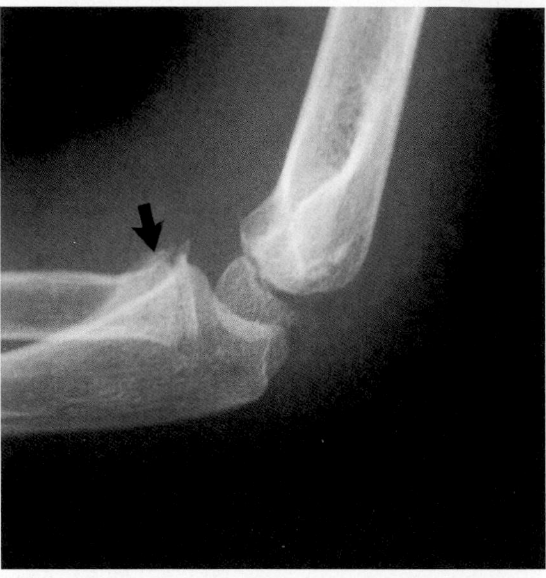

FIGURE 16-18 A. Heterotopic calcification of the ulnar collateral ligaments in an elbow that had been dislocated for 2 months (*arrow*). **B.** Lateral view of the same elbow. Some myositis ossification has occurred where the brachialis inserts into the coronoid process (*arrow*).

Ligamentous and Capsular Laxity. Osborne and Cotterill[101] suggested that articular changes are secondary and that the primary defect is a failure of the posterolateral ligamentous and capsular structures to become reattached after reduction (Fig. 16-20). Osborne and Cotterill[101] proposed that the extensive articular cartilage covering the surface of the distal humerus leaves little surface area for soft tissue reattachment and the presence of synovial fluid further inhibits soft tissue healing. With recurrent dislocations, the radial head impinges against the posterolateral margin of the capitellum, creating an osteochondral defect (Fig. 16-21). In addition to the defect in the capitellar articular surface, a similar defect develops in the anterior articular margin of the radial head. When these two defects oppose each other, recurrence of the dislocation is more likely. Subsequent studies have confirmed these findings in almost all recurrent dislocations, especially in children.[33,49,99,133,138,146]

O'Driscoll et al.[99] described posterolateral instability in 5 patients, including 2 children, in whom laxity of the ulnar part of the radial collateral ligament allowed a transitory rotary subluxation of the ulnohumeral joint and a secondary dislocation of the radiohumeral joint. Patients with posterolateral instability often describe a history of recurrent temporary dislocation of the elbow but, when examined, exhibit no unusual clinical findings. The instability is diagnosed with a posterolateral rotary instability test. In some patients, posterolateral rotary instability can be detected only with the patient completely relaxed under general

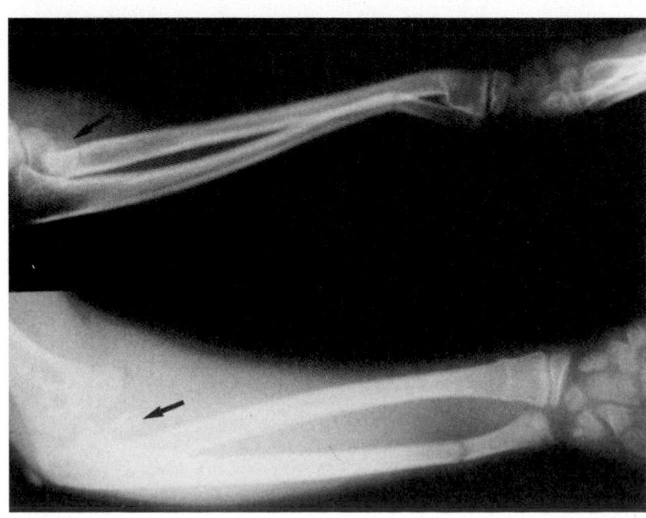

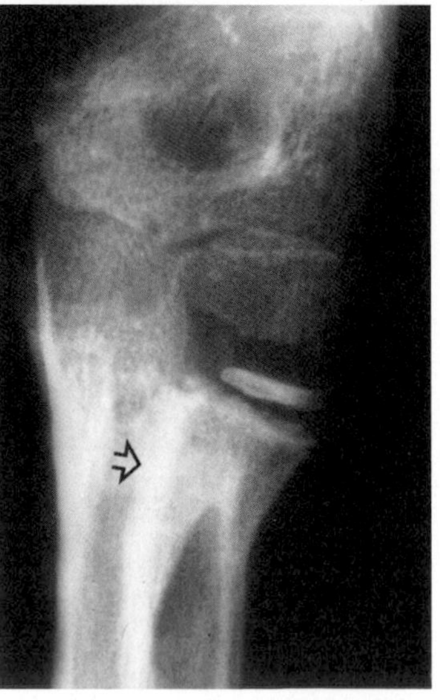

FIGURE 16-19 Radioulnar synostosis. **A.** Injury radiographs demonstrating a posterolateral dislocation associated with a Salter-Harris type II proximal radius fracture (*arrow*). Open reduction of the proximal radial fracture was performed. **B.** Six months later, the patient developed a proximal radioulnar synostosis (*arrow*). (Courtesy of Ruben Pachero, MD.)

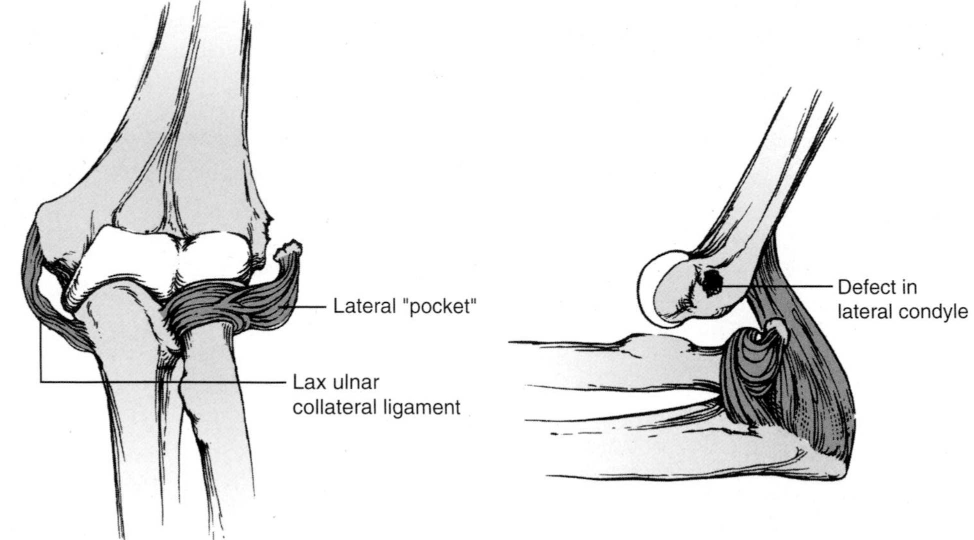

FIGURE 16-20 Pathology associated with recurrent elbow dislocations. The three components that allow the elbow to dislocate: a lax ulnar collateral ligament, a "pocket" in the radial collateral ligament, and a defect in the lateral condyle. (Reprinted from Osborne G, Cotterill P. Recurrent dislocation of the elbow. J Bone Joint Surg Br 1966;48: 340–346, with permission.)

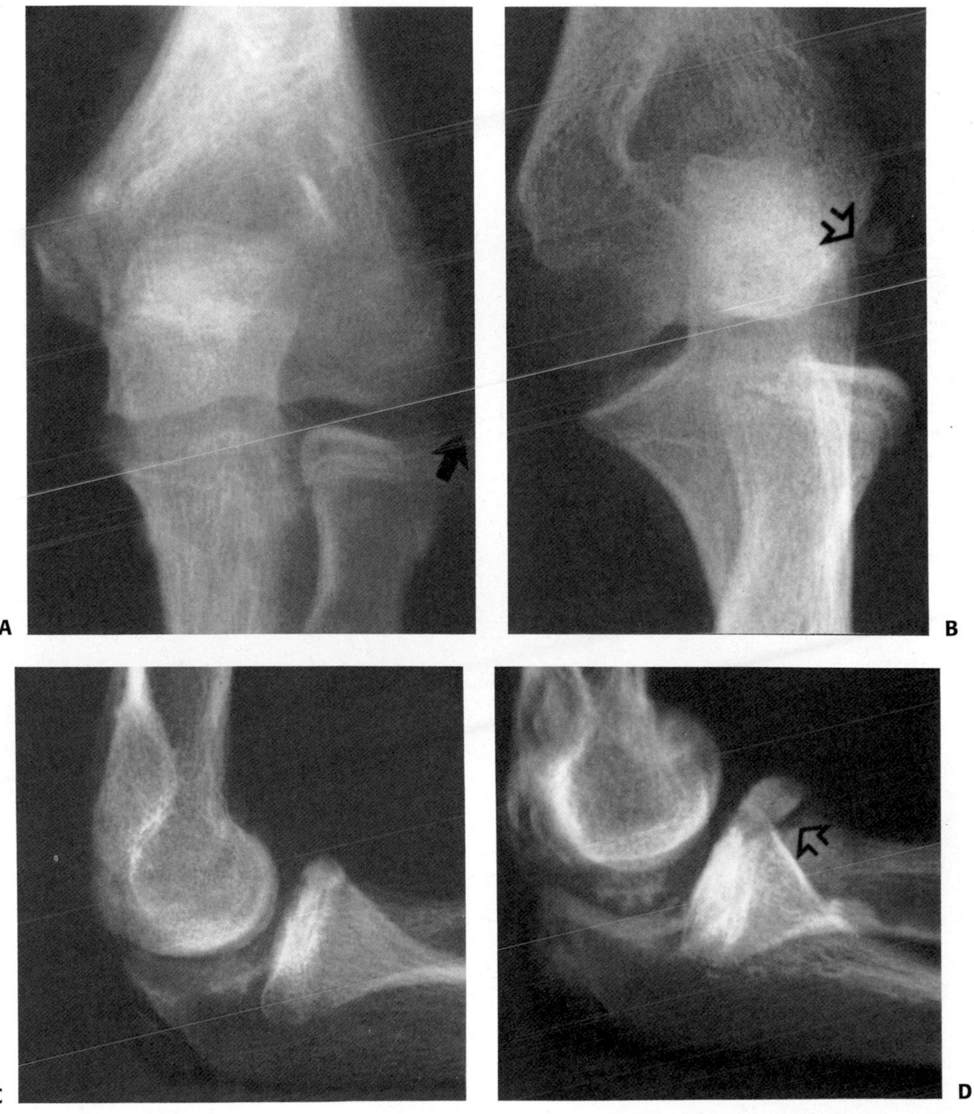

FIGURE 16-21 Radiographic changes associated with recurrent elbow dislocation. **A.** Anteroposterior radiograph of a 13-year-old who had recurrent dislocations. An osteochondral fragment (*arrow*) is attached to the lateral ligament. **B.** An oblique radiograph shows the defect (*arrow*) in the posterolateral condylar surface. **C.** Radiographs of an 11-year-old after his first dislocation. **D.** One year later, after recurrent dislocation and subluxations, blunting of the radial head has developed (*arrow*). (Courtesy of Marvin E. Mumme, MD.)

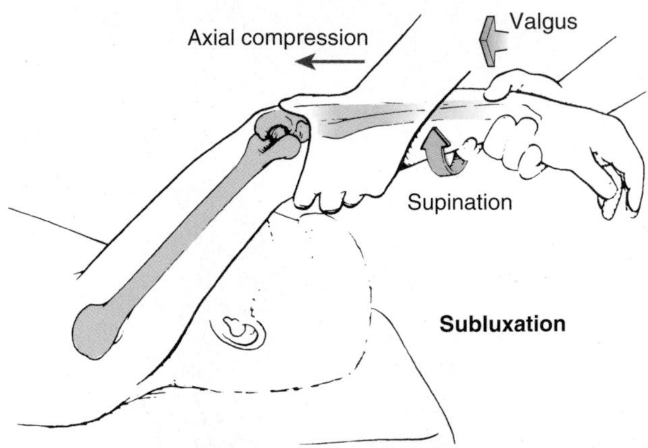

FIGURE 16-22 Posterolateral rotary instability. Posterolateral rotational instability is best demonstrated with the upper extremity over the head with the patient supine. The radial head can be subluxated or dislocated by applying a valgus and supination force to the forearm at the same time proximal axial compression is applied along the forearm. (Reprinted from O'Driscoll SW, Bell DF, Morrey BF. Posterolateral rotary instability of the elbow. J Bone Joint Surg Am 1991;73:441, with permission.)

anesthesia. This test is done by holding the patient's arm over the head while applying proximal axial compression plus a valgus and supination force to the forearm with the elbow flexed to 20 to 30 degrees (Fig. 16-22). O'Driscoll et al.[99] reported that surgical repair of the lax ulnar portion of the radial collateral ligament eliminated the posterolateral rotary instability. In children and adolescents, the same instability can occur from cartilage nonunion of the origin of the radial collateral ligament.

Bone Defects. In addition to the osteochondral defects in the capitellum and radial head, bone defects may include a shallow semilunar notch resulting from a coronoid fossa process fracture or multiple recurrent dislocations.

Treatment Options

Nonoperative. There is only one report of successful nonsurgical management of recurrent elbow dislocations. Herring[53] used an orthosis that blocked the last 15 degrees of extension. After his patient wore this orthosis constantly for 2 years and with vigorous activities for another 6 months, there were no further dislocations, but the follow-up period was only 1 year. Beaty and Donati[9] emphasized that physical therapy and the use of an orthosis should be tried before surgery is considered.

Surgical Procedures. The treatment of recurrent posterior elbow dislocations is predominately surgical. Various surgical procedures have been described to correct bone and soft tissue abnormalities (Fig. 16-23).

Bone Procedures. These are directed toward correcting dysplasia of the semilunar notch of the olecranon. Milch[92] inserted a boomerang-shaped bone block. Others[41,88,140] found that a simple bone block was all that was necessary (Fig. 16-23A). Mantle[82] increased the slope of the semilunar notch in two patients with an opening wedge osteotomy of the coronoid process (Fig. 16-23B).

Soft Tissue Procedures. Reichenheim[112] and King[67] transferred the biceps tendon just distal to the coronoid process to

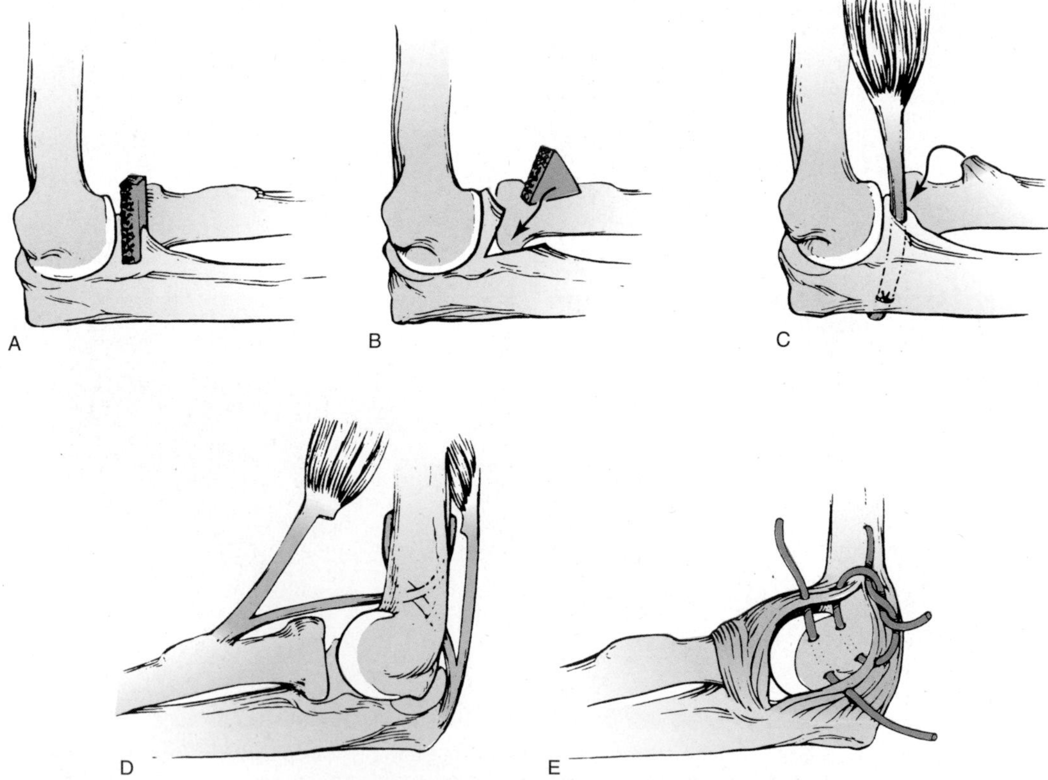

FIGURE 16-23 Surgical procedures for recurrent dislocation. **A.** Simple coronoid bone block. **B.** Open wedge coronoid osteotomy. **C.** Biceps tendon transfer to coronoid process. **D.** Cruciate ligament reconstruction. **E.** Lateral capsular reattachment of Osborne and Cotterill.[101]

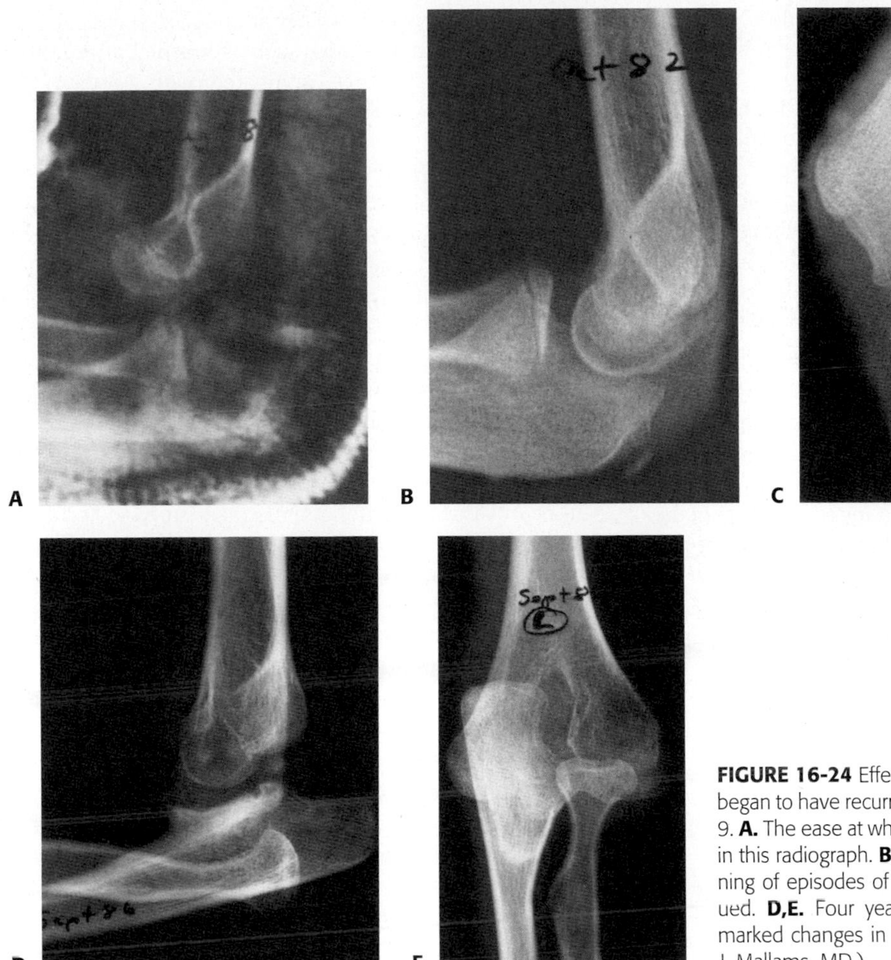

FIGURE 16-24 Effects of recurrent dislocation. This girl began to have recurrent dislocations of her elbow at age 9. **A.** The ease at which the elbow redislocates is shown in this radiograph. **B,C.** Radiographs taken at the beginning of episodes of dislocation. Her dislocation continued. **D,E.** Four years later, the elbow demonstrated marked changes in its architecture. (Courtesy of David J. Mallams, MD.)

reinforce it (Fig. 16-23C). Kapel[65] developed a cruciate ligament reconstruction in which distally based strips of the biceps and triceps tendon were passed through the distal humerus (Fig. 16-23D). Beaty and Donati[9] modified this technique by transferring a central slip of the triceps through the humerus posterior to anterior and attaching it to the proximal ulna.

The most widely accepted technique is that described by Osborne and Cotterill,[101] in which the lateral capsule is reattached to the posterolateral aspect of the capitellum with sutures passing through holes drilled in the bone (Fig. 16-23E). The joint should be inspected at surgery because osteocartilaginous loose bodies may be present.[49,80,133] Since Osborne and Cotterill's[101] initial report of eight patients, successful use of this technique has been reported in numerous others.[33,49,80,99,133,138,146] Zeier[148] and O'Driscoll et al.[99] reinforced the lateral repair with strips of fascia lata, triceps fascia, or palmaris longus tendon.

Posttreatment Care

Postoperatively, especially after the repair described by Osborne and Cotterill,[101] the arm is immobilized in a long arm cast with the elbow flexed 90 degrees for 4 to 6 weeks. Protected active range of motion exercises are performed for an additional 4 to 6 weeks. Strenuous activities are avoided for 12 weeks postoperative.

Complications

Major complications after correction of recurrent dislocations include loose osteocartilaginous fragments and destruction of the articular surface of the joint (Fig. 16-24), elbow stiffness, or recurrent instability.

Unreduced Posterior Elbow Dislocations

Untreated posterior dislocations of the elbow in children are extremely rare in North America. Most reported series are from other countries.[37]

Diagnosis

Children with untreated dislocations typically have pain and limited mid-range of motion (see Fig. 16-7). Pathologically, there is usually subperiosteal new bone formation that produces a radiohumeral horn, myositis ossificans of the brachialis muscle, capsular contractures, shortening of the triceps muscle, contractures of the medial and lateral collateral ligaments, and compression of the ulnar nerve.[36,37] These factors have to be considered when planning treatment.

Treatment Options. Closed reduction of dislocations recognized within 3 weeks of injury may be possible.[4,37] If this fails or if the dislocation is of longer duration, open reduction is necessary.

Surgical Procedures. Open reduction through a posterior approach, as described by Speed,[131] involves lengthening of the triceps muscle and release or transposition of the ulnar nerve.[37] Satisfactory results usually can be obtained if a stable concentric reduction is achieved within 3 months of the initial dislocation.[4] Results after surgical reconstruction decline thereafter but still may produce some improvement in function.[30,37,78,90,94] Fixation of the elbow joint to maintain reduction with one or two large smooth pins for 2 to 4 weeks followed by vigorous but protected physical therapy has been recommended.[37,94]

Mahaisavariya et al.[79] reported improved extension and better functional results 1 to 3 months after injury in 34 patients with chronic elbow dislocation reconstruction in whom the triceps tendon was not lengthened compared with 38 patients who had the triceps lengthened at surgery.

Congenital Elbow Dislocations

Chronic elbow dislocation may be congenital in origin. Altered anatomy and limited motion predispose these patients to injury. The key to differentiating a congenital from an acute traumatic elbow dislocation is examination of the x-ray architecture of the articulating surfaces. In a congenitally dislocated elbow, there is atrophy of the humeral condyles and the semilunar notch of the olecranon. The radial head and neck may be hypoplastic, and the articular surface of the radial head may be dome-shaped instead of concave. Unfortunately, these same changes can result from chronic recurrent dislocation after trauma, making the differentiation between congenital and chronic traumatic dislocation difficult. If other congenital anomalies are present or the child has an underlying syndrome, such as Ehlers-Danlos or Larsen syndrome, the dislocation is likely to be congenital. Obtaining comparison x-rays of the asymptomatic, contralateral elbow often reveals identical anatomy, confirming the etiology of the dislocation as congenital.

ANTERIOR ELBOW DISLOCATIONS

Principles of Management

Anterior elbow dislocations are rare. Of the 317 elbows in the combined series,[72,97,114,116] only five were anterior, for an incidence of slightly over 1%. They are associated with an increased incidence of complications, such as brachial artery disruption and associated fractures, compared with posterior dislocations.[59,143]

Mechanism of Injury

Anterior elbow dislocations usually are caused by a direct blow to the posterior aspect of the flexed elbow.[57] Hyperextension of the elbow also has been implicated in one study.[143] Twisting of the forearm on the elbow commonly occurs.

Signs and Symptoms

The elbow is held in extension upon presentation. There is a fullness in the antecubital fossa. Swelling usually is marked because of the soft tissue disruption associated with this type of dislocation. There is severe pain with attempted motion. A careful neurovascular examination is mandatory.

X-ray and Other Imaging Studies

Routine anteroposterior and lateral x-rays are diagnostic. In most cases, the proximal radius and ulna dislocate in an anteromedial direction (Fig. 16-25). Associated fractures are common. In children, the triceps insertion may be avulsed from the olecranon with a small piece of cortical bone.[145] This fragment usually reduces to the olecranon after reduction. Wilkerson[143] reported an anterior dislocation associated with a displaced olecranon fracture in a 7-year-old boy. Inoue and Horii[57] reported an 11-year-old girl with an anterior elbow dislocation with displaced fractures of the trochlea, capitellum, and lateral epicondyle. These were repaired with open reduction and internal fixation using Herbert bone screws.

Treatment Options

Closed Reduction

Reduction usually is accomplished by flexing the elbow and pushing the forearm proximally and downward at the same

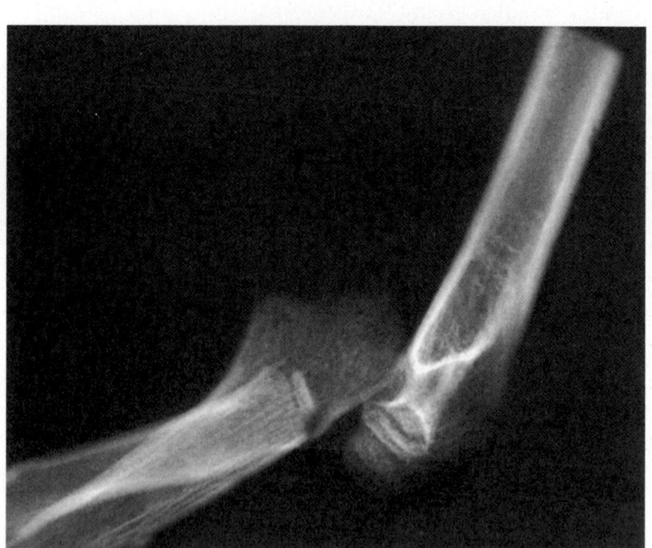

A

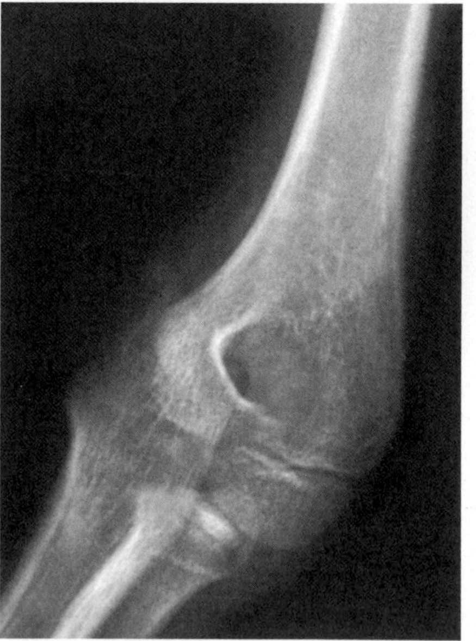

B

FIGURE 16-25 Anterior dislocation of the elbow. **A.** Initial anteroposterior radiograph. The olecranon lies anterior to the distal humerus. **B.** Initial lateral radiograph. The proximal ulna and radial head lie anteromedial, and the elbow carrying angle is in varus. (Courtesy of Hilario Trevino, MD.)

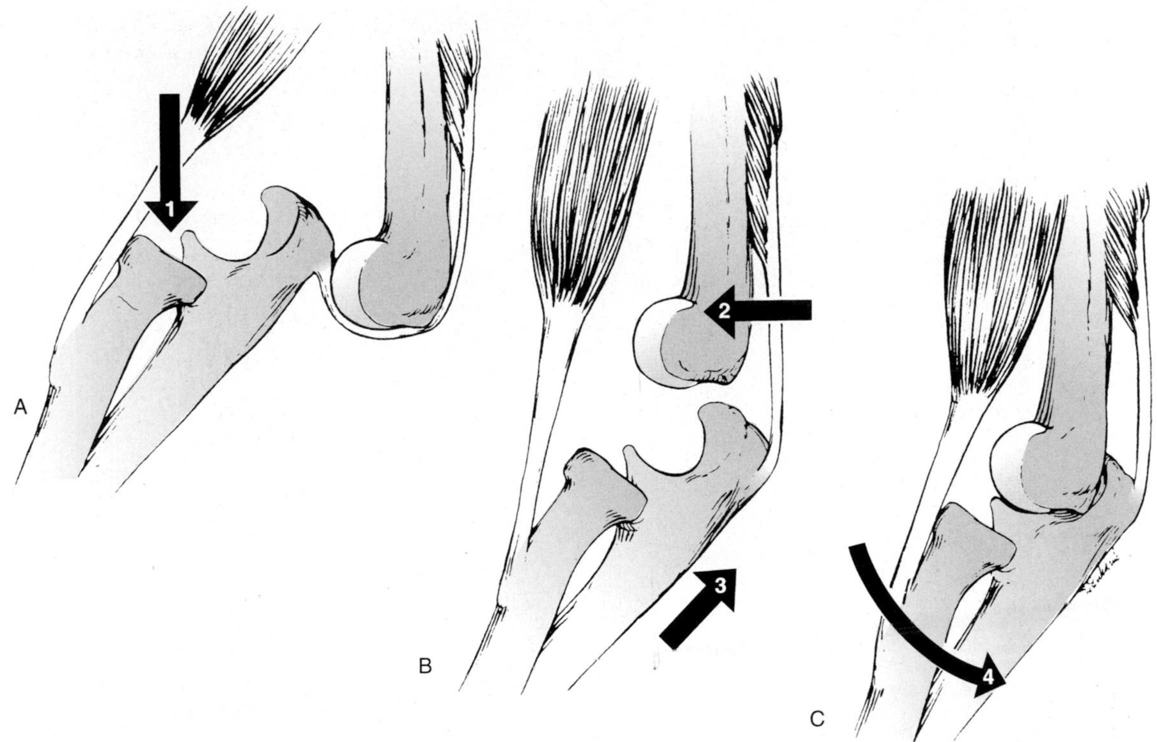

FIGURE 16-26 Reduction of anterior dislocation. **A.** With the elbow semiflexed, a longitudinal force is applied along the long axis of the humerus (*arrow 1*). Pulling distally on the forearm may be necessary to initially dislodge the olecranon. **B.** Once the olecranon is distal to the humerus, the distal humerus is pushed anteriorly (*arrow 2*) while a proximally directed force is applied along the long axis of the forearm (*arrow 3*). **C.** Finally, the elbow is immobilized in some extension (*arrow 4*).

time.[145] As with posterior dislocations, a force must first be applied longitudinally along the axis of the humerus with the elbow semiflexed to overcome the forces of the biceps and triceps. The longitudinal force along the axis of the forearm is directed toward the elbow (Fig. 16-26). To make reduction easier, the distal humerus can be forced in an anterior direction by pushing on the posterior aspect of the distal arm.

Surgical Procedures

Surgery usually is not required unless the dislocation is open, there is a brachial artery injury, or there is an associated fracture that does not realign satisfactorily after closed reduction. Open reduction and internal fixation of the fracture may then be necessary.[57,143]

Postreduction Care

Because most anterior dislocations occur in flexion, the elbow should be immobilized in some extension for 1 to 3 weeks, followed by protected active range-of-motion exercises. Early motion after open reduction and internal fixation of an associated olecranon fracture usually can be allowed.[57,143]

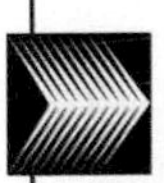

AUTHORS' PREFERRED METHOD OF TREATMENT: ANTERIOR ELBOW DISLOCATION

Closed reduction (see Fig. 16-26) is the initial procedure of choice. A distal force must be applied in line with and parallel to the long axis of the humerus first. Once the length has been re-established, a posteriorly directed force along the axis of the forearm is applied until the elbow is reduced.

Complications

There appears to be an increased incidence of brachial artery rupture or thrombosis associated with anterior elbow dislocations.[59,130] When present, prompt arterial repair or reconstruction with grafting is necessary.

MEDIAL AND LATERAL ELBOW DISLOCATIONS

These are rare dislocations. Lateral dislocations, either incomplete or complete, are more common than medial dislocations in adults. There are no recent reports of medial dislocations in children.

Signs and Symptoms

In an incomplete lateral dislocation, the semilunar notch articulates with the captilulo-trochlear groove, and the radial head appears more prominent laterally. There often is good flexion and extension of the elbow, increasing the likelihood that a lateral dislocation will be overlooked. In a complete lateral dislocation, the olecranon is displaced lateral to the capitellum. This gives the elbow a markedly widened appearance.

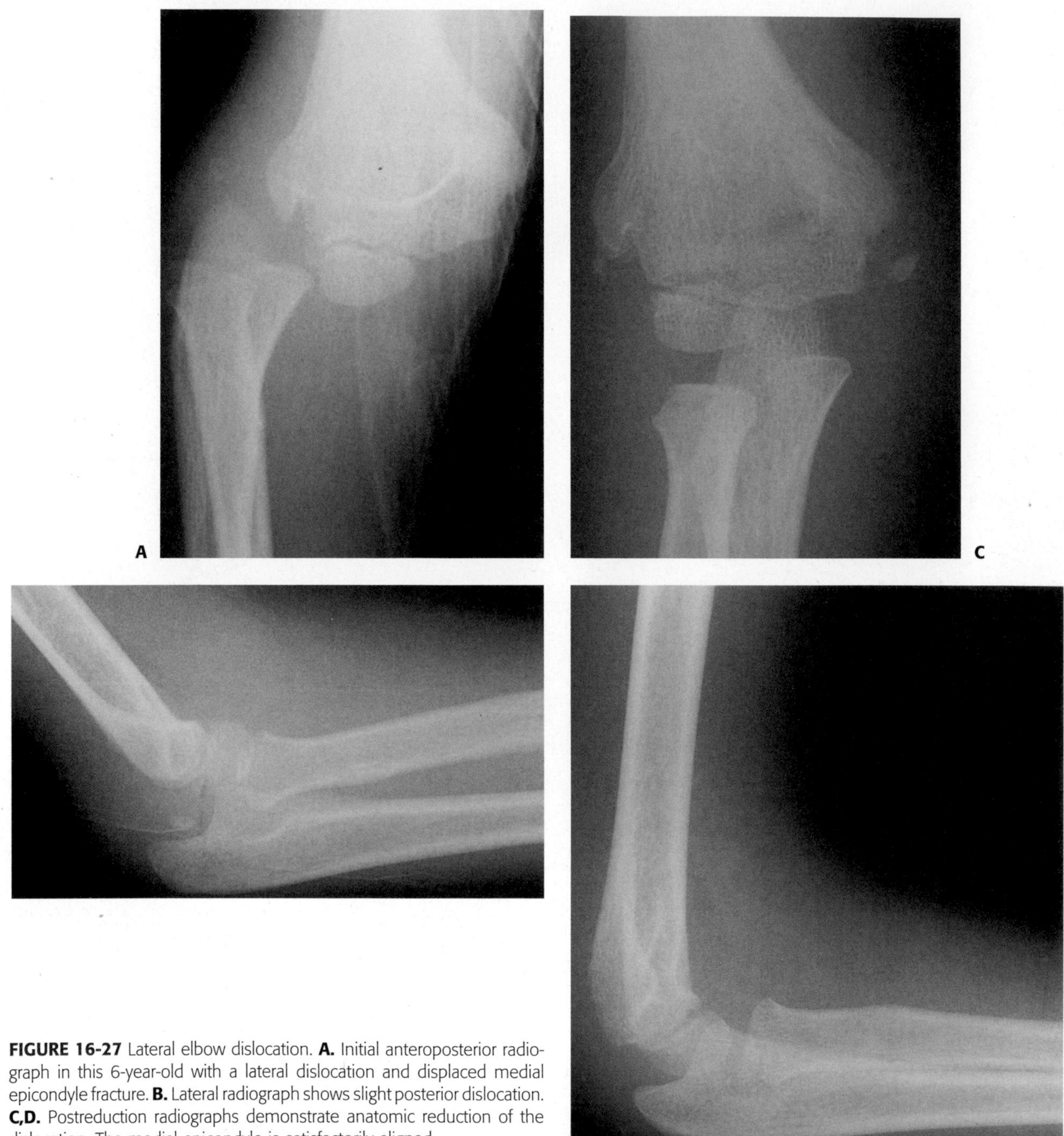

FIGURE 16-27 Lateral elbow dislocation. **A.** Initial anteroposterior radiograph in this 6-year-old with a lateral dislocation and displaced medial epicondyle fracture. **B.** Lateral radiograph shows slight posterior dislocation. **C,D.** Postreduction radiographs demonstrate anatomic reduction of the dislocation. The medial epicondyle is satisfactorily aligned.

X-ray and Other Imaging Studies

Anteroposterior x-rays of the elbow usually are diagnostic. On the lateral view, the elbow may appear reduced.

Treatment Options

These rare dislocations are treated by closed reduction. A longitudinal force is applied along the axis of the humerus to distract the elbow, and then direct medial or lateral pressure (opposite the direction of the dislocation) is applied over the proximal forearm (Fig. 16-27).

DIVERGENT ELBOW DISLOCATION

Divergent dislocation represents a posterior elbow dislocation with disruption of the interosseous membrane between the proximal radius and ulna with the radial head displaced laterally and the proximal ulna medially (Fig. 16-28). These dislocations are extremely rare.[7,19,29,56,55,86,95,125,129,139]

Divergent dislocations usually are caused by high-energy trauma. Associated fractures of the radial neck, proximal ulna, and coronoid process are common.[1,19,35,139] It has been speculated that, in addition to the hyperextension of the elbow that produces the dislocation, a strong proximally directed force is applied parallel to the long axis of the forearm, disrupting the annular ligament and interosseous membrane and allowing the divergence of the proximal radius and ulna. In a cadaveric study, Altuntas et al.[5] confirmed that only after release of all the ligamentous stabilizers of the elbow and release of the intraosseous membrane from the elbow to the distal third of the forearm could a divergent dislocation be replicated.

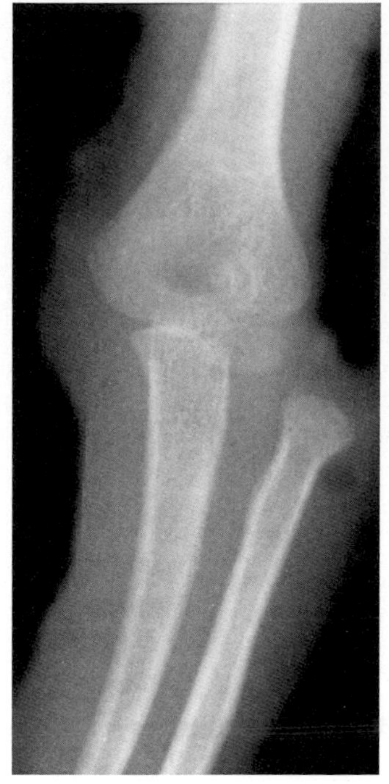
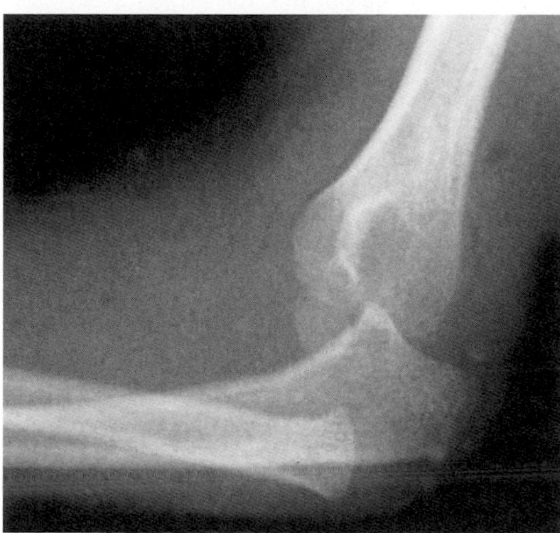
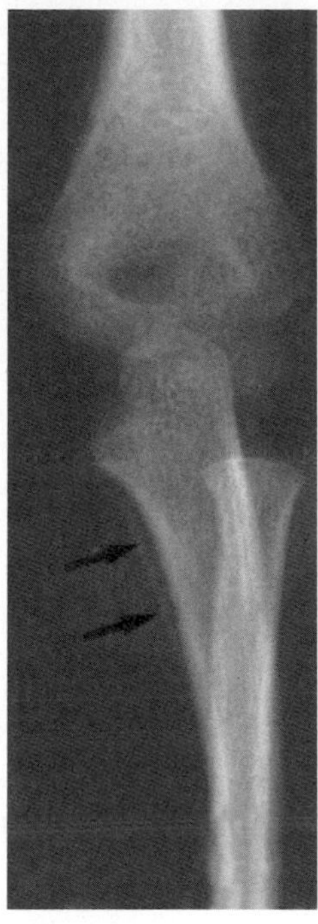

FIGURE 16-28 Medial-lateral divergent dislocation. **A.** Anteroposterior view demonstrating disruption of the proximal radioulnar joint with the radius lateral and the ulna medial. **B.** Lateral radiograph confirms that the radius and ulna are both posterior to the distal humerus. **C.** A radiograph taken 4 weeks after injury shows periosteal new bone formation (*arrows*), indicating where the soft tissues were extensively torn away from the proximal ulna.

Treatment Options

Closed Reduction

Divergent dislocations are typically easily reduced using closed reduction under general anesthesia. Reduction is achieved by applying longitudinal traction with the elbow semiextended and at the same time compressing the proximal radius and ulna together.

Open Reduction

This is rarely indicated. There have been only three divergent dislocations reported that required open reduction.[35,86,96] Closed reduction failed in one child,[86] and another had a displaced fracture of the proximal ulna.[35] In the third child, after attempted closed reduction was unsuccessful, surgical exploration found the avulsed anterior band of the medial collateral ligament complex of the elbow was found to be interposed between the medial condyle of the humerus and the olecranon.[96] After removing and repairing the interposed ligament, stable reduction was achieved.

Postreduction Care

After successful closed reduction, the elbow is immobilized in 90 degrees of flexion and the forearm in neutral for approximately 1 to 3 weeks. Active range-of-motion exercises are then begun. Most patients typically regain full elbow motion, including forearm pronation and supination.

PROXIMAL RADIOULNAR TRANSLOCATION

Principles of Management

Translocation of the proximal radius and ulna is an extremely rare injury with fewer than 10 cases having been reported in the English literature.[19,20,34,40,47,58,76] Radioulnar translocation is commonly missed on the anteroposterior x-ray unless the proximal radius and ulna are noted to be completely reversed in relation to the distal humerus.

Mechanism of Injury

Translocations are believed to be caused by a fall onto the pronated hand with the elbow in full or nearly full extension, producing an axial force on the proximal radius. The anterior radial head dislocation occurs first, followed by the posterior dislocation of the olecranon. The radial head, depending on the degree of pronation, can be lodged in the coronoid fossa or dislocated posteriorly. As a consequence, fractures of the radial head, radial neck, or coronoid process may occur.[19,20,34,76] Harvey and Tchelebi [47] reported a case in which the cause of radioulnar translocation may have been iatrogenic: the result of inappropriate technique used to reduce a posterior elbow dislocation.

Signs and Symptoms

Swelling and pain may obscure the initial examination, and minimal deformity may be apparent. Once pain has been adequately managed with analgesics, the most consistent finding on clinical examination is limited elbow range of motion, especially in supination.

Associated Injuries

Radial neck fracture is the most common fracture associated with proximal radioulnar translocation.[20,34,58,76] Eklöf et al.[34] also reported one patient who sustained a fracture of the tip of the coronoid. Proposed soft tissue injuries include radial collateral ligament, medial collateral ligament, annular ligament, and interosseous ligament injury.[34,58] Isbister[58] described transient ulnar nerve paresthesia that resolved after reduction of the translocation. Osteonecrosis of the radial head was noted in one patient after open reduction of a proximal radioulnar translocation.[47]

Current Treatment Options

Nonoperative Treatment: Closed Reduction

Successful closed reduction of proximal radioulnar translocation has been reported.[58,76] The patient must be completely relaxed under general anesthesia, as sedation or regional anesthesia is unlikely to provide sufficient relaxation. With the elbow flexed approximately 90 degrees, longitudinal traction is applied to the elbow while the forearm is supinated (Fig. 16-29). If the radial head can be palpated, gentle anterior-directed pressure may help slide the radial head and neck over the coronoid process, allowing the proximal radius and ulna to resume their normal configuration. As always, just the right amount of force should be used; excessive force risks iatrogenic fracture to the proximal radius. Successful closed reduction should be confirmed on x-ray, and the elbow should be immobilized for approximately 3 to 4 weeks with the forearm supinated and the elbow flexed 90 to 100 degrees.

Surgical Treatment: Open Reduction

Most reported cases of radioulnar translocations have required open reduction.[19,20,34,40,47,58] A lateral approach provides adequate exposure to the translocation and radial neck fracture if present. At surgery, the radial head and neck are typically found trapped beneath the trochlea of the distal humerus. Elbow extension tightens the biceps tendon, making reduction more difficult. With the elbow flexed, a freer or joker elevator can be placed beneath the radial head and neck facilitating delivery over the coronoid process as the forearm is supinated. If present, a radial neck fracture may now be treated in standard fashion. Internal fixation also may be necessary for an unstable displaced fracture.

Harvey and Tchelebi[47] used an osteotomy of the proximal ulna to expose and reduce the radius that was complicated by a postoperative ulnar nerve paralysis that recovered completely over 2 months.

After successful closed or open reduction, the forearm is immobilized for approximately 3 to 4 weeks with the forearm supinated and the elbow flexed 90 to 100 degrees, followed by active elbow range-of-motion exercises.

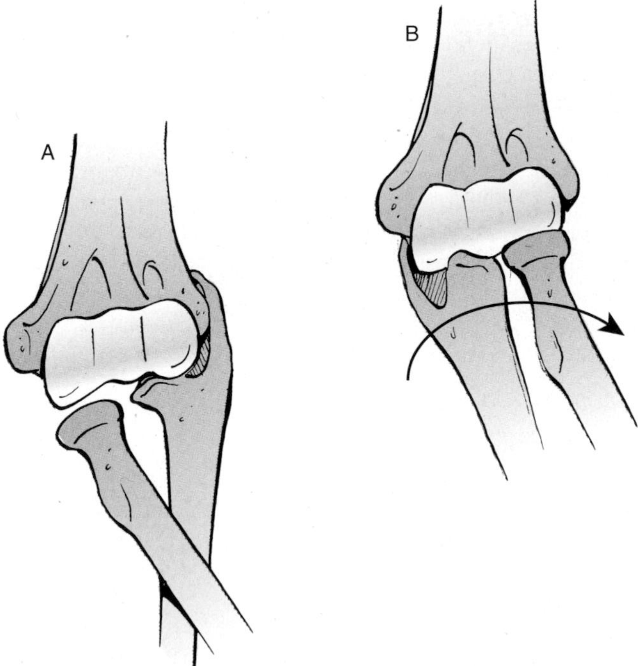

FIGURE 16-29 Proximal radioulnar translocation. **A.** Position of the proximal radius and ulna with a proximal radioulnar translocation. **B.** Closed reduction is rarely successful, but may be attempted under general anesthesia using gentle longitudinal traction while supinating the forearm. (Redrawn from Harvey S, Tchelebi H. Proximal radioulnar translocation. J Bone Joint Surg 1979;61:447–449, with permission.)

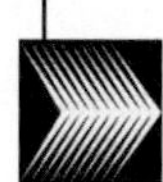

AUTHORS' PREFERRED TREATMENT: PROXIMAL RADIOULNAR TRANSLOCATION

Closed versus Open Reduction

Within 24 hours of injury, before swelling and contracture impede reduction, the patient is brought to the operating room where as little as possible but as much as necessary is done to obtain and maintain a stable reduction of the elbow. With the patient completely relaxed under general anesthesia and pharmacologic paralysis, closed reduction is attempted by applying longitudinal traction to the flexed elbow while the forearm is gently but firmly supinated. If the radial head can be palpated, gentle anterior-directed pressure may help slide the radial head and neck over the coronoid process, allowing the proximal radius and ulna to resume their normal configuration.

If closed reduction cannot be achieved, then open reduction is done through a lateral approach as described above. Once closed or open reduction is achieved, stability of the elbow is assessed. The elbow is immobilized in the position of maximal stability, which typically involves flexion of 90 to 100 degrees and forearm supination. If the elbow remains unstable, radiocapitellar pin placement may be considered. A pin of adequate size must be selected and the elbow must be immobilized the entire time the pin is in place (typically 3 weeks) to avoid pin breakage. Annular ligament reconstruction or ulnar osteotomy has not been necessary, but might be considered if a stable reduction can not be achieved by other means.

PULLED ELBOW SYNDROME (NURSEMAID'S ELBOW)

Subluxation of the annular ligament, or pulled elbow syndrome, is a common elbow injury in young children.[6,22,56,60,126] The term "nursemaid's elbow" and other synonyms have been used to describe this condition. The demographics associated with subluxation of the radial head have been well described.[6,22,56,60,126] The mean age at injury is 2 to 3 years, with the youngest reported patient 2 months of age. It rarely occurs after 7 years of age. Sixty to 65% of the children affected are girls, and the left elbow is involved in approximately 70%. It is difficult to determine the actual incidence because many subluxations are treated in primary care physician's offices, by parents, or resolve spontaneously before being seen by a physician.

Principles of Management

Mechanism of Injury

Longitudinal traction on the extended elbow is the usual mechanism of injury (Fig. 16-30). Cadaver studies have shown that longitudinal traction on the extended elbow can produce a partial slippage of the annular ligament over the head of the radius and into the radiocapitellar joint, sometimes tearing the subannular membrane. Displacement of the annular ligament occurs most easily with the forearm in pronation. In this position, the lateral edge of the radial head, which opposes the main portion of the annular ligament, is narrow and round at its margin.[77,85] In supination, the lateral edge of the radial head is wider and more square at its margin, thereby restricting slippage of the annular ligament. McRae and Freeman[89] demonstrated that forearm pronation maintained the displacement of the annular ligament.

Presumably, the annular ligament displaces proximally, partially over the radial head in this condition. This anatomic finding has been confirmed in numerous cadaver experiments.[85,89,120] After 5 years of age, the distal attachments of the subannular membrane and annular ligament to the neck of the radius have strengthened sufficiently to prevent its tearing and subsequent displacement.[120] Previously, the theory was proposed that the radial head diameter was less in children than in adults and this contributed to subluxation of the annular ligament. However, cadaver studies of infants, children, and adults have shown that the ratio of the head and neck diameters is essentially the same.[118,120] Griffin[43] suggested that the lack of ossification of the proximal radial epiphysis in children less than 5 years of age made it more pliable, thereby facilitating slippage of the annular ligament.

Amir et al.[6] performed a controlled study comparing 30 normal children with 100 who had pulled elbow syndrome. They found an increased frequency of hypermobility or ligamentous laxity among children with pulled elbows. Also, there was an increased frequency of hypermobility in one or both parents of the involved children compared with noninvolved children, suggesting that hypermobility could be a factor predisposing children to this condition.

Thus, the most widely accepted mechanism is that the injury occurs when the forearm is pronated, the elbow extended, and longitudinal traction is applied to the patient's wrist or hand (see Fig. 16-30).[85,89,122] Such an injury typically occurs when a young child is lifted or swung by the forearm or when the child suddenly steps down from a step or off a curb while one of the parents is holding the hand or wrist.

Unusual Mechanisms. Newman[98] reported that 5 of 6 infants under 6 months of age with a pulled elbow sustained the injury when rolling over in bed with the extended elbow trapped under the body. It was believed that this maneuver, especially if the infant was given a quick push to turn over by an older sibling or a parent, provided enough longitudinal traction to displace the annular ligament proximally.

Signs and Symptoms

The history is usually that of an episode of a longitudinal pull on the elbow of the young child. The initial pain usually subsides rapidly, and the child does not appear to be in distress except that he or she is reluctant to use the involved extremity. The upper extremity is typically held at the side with the forearm pronated. A limited painless arc of flexion and extension may be present; however, any attempt to supinate the forearm produces

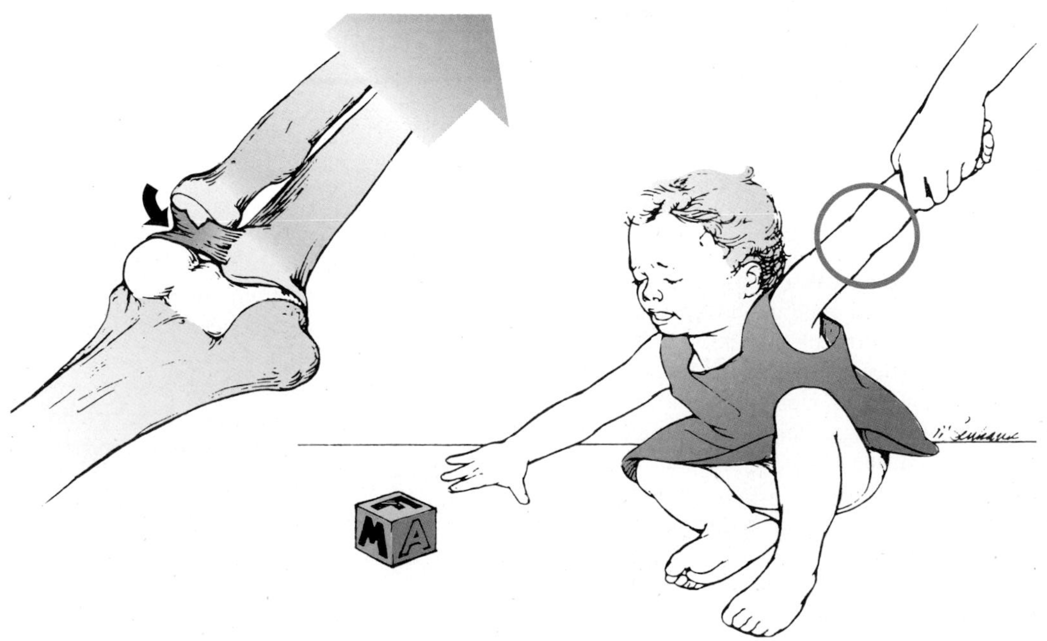

FIGURE 16-30 The injury most commonly occurs when a longitudinal pull is applied to the upper extremity. Usually the forearm is pronated. There may be a partial tear in the subannular membrane, allowing the annular ligament to subluxate into the radiocapitellar joint.

pain and is met with resistance. Although there is no evidence of an elbow effusion, local tenderness may be present over the radial head and annular ligament. In some patients, the pain may be referred proximally to the shoulder but most complain of pain distally toward the wrist.[6,56]

Unfortunately, the classic history is not always present.[22,105,108,119,122] In some studies 33% to 49% of patients had no clear history of longitudinal traction to the elbow.[119,122] In patients without a witnessed longitudinal traction injury, other causes, such as occult fracture or early septic arthritis, must be carefully ruled out.

Associated Injuries

No other associated injuries have consistently been linked with pulled elbow syndrome.

Diagnosis and Classification

There is no commonly used classification system for this condition because there is essentially only one type of pulled elbow syndrome.

Imaging

Should x-rays be taken of every child before manipulation is attempted? If there is a reliable history of traction to the elbow, the child is 5 years of age or younger, and the clinical findings strongly support the diagnosis, x-rays are not necessary.[6,22,108,120,137] If, however, there is an atypical history or clinical examination, x-rays should be obtained to be certain there is not a fracture before manipulation is attempted.

Anteroposterior and lateral x-rays usually are normal,[14,22,43,108,120,122,127] but subtle abnormalities may be present. Normally, the line down the center of the proximal radial shaft should pass through the center of the ossification center of the capitellum (radiocapitellar line).[39,127] Careful review of x-rays may demonstrate the radial capitellar line to be lateral to the center of the capitellum in up to 25% of patients.[39,127] Determination of this subtle change requires a direct measurement on the x-ray. Interestingly, the pulled elbow can be reduced by the radiology technician because the elbow x-rays are usually taken with the forearm supinated. The subluxation is reduced inadvertently when the technician places the forearm into supination to position it for the x-ray. Bretland[13] suggested that if the best x-ray that can be obtained is an oblique view with the forearm in pronation, pulled elbow syndrome is the likely diagnosis.

Ultrasonography. When the diagnosis is not evident, ultrasonography may be helpful,[69,77] although not always reliable.[121] The diagnosis is made by demonstrating an increase in the echonegative area between the articular surfaces of the capitellum and the radial head and increased radial capitellar distance. Kosuwon et al.[118] found that this distance is normally about 3.8 mm with forearm pronated. With a subluxated radial head, this measured 7.2 mm. A difference of 3 mm between the normal and affected sides, therefore, suggests radial head subluxation.

Current Treatment Options

Nonoperative Treatment: Closed Reduction

Virtually all annular ligament subluxations are successfully treated by closed reduction. This is usually best done by forearm supination.[22,43,56,75,108,122,126] Some have recommended that supination be done with the elbow flexed, and others have found that supination alone with the elbow extended can effect a reduction. In many patients, a snapping sensation can be both heard and palpated when the annular ligament reduces (Fig. 16-31). Macias et al.[75] reported that hyperpronation was more successful than supination in a randomized study. Reduction was successful in 40 of 41 patients (98%) in the hyperpronation group, compared with 38 of 44 patients (86%) in the supination group. They concluded that the hyperpronation technique was more successful, required fewer attempts, and was often successful when supination failed. Generally, a full arc of supination to pronation of the forearm, with elbow flexion and extension, will reduce all pulled elbows.

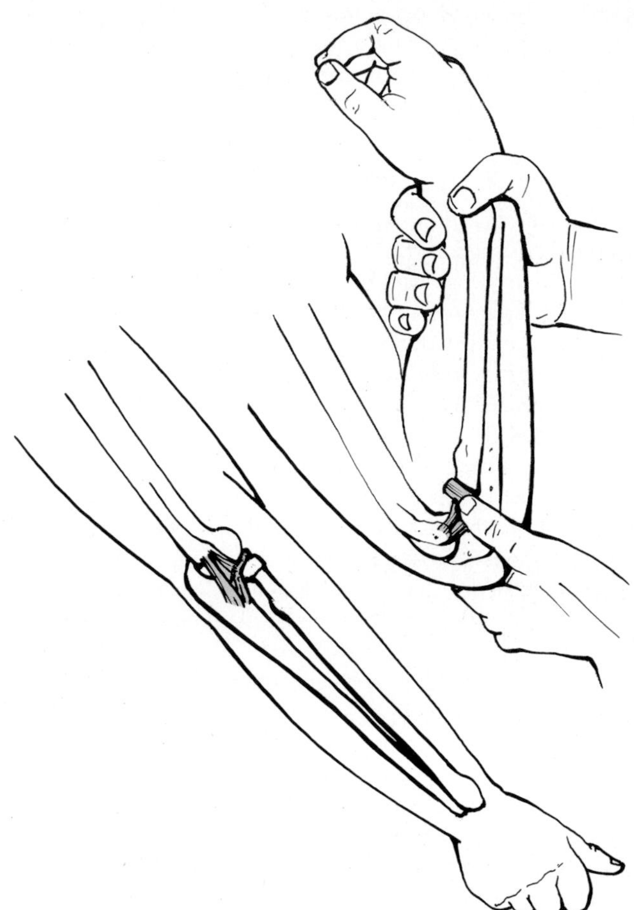

FIGURE 16-31 Reduction technique for nursemaid's elbow. **Left:** The forearm is first supinated. **Right:** The elbow is then hyperflexed. The surgeon's thumb is placed laterally over the radial head to feel the characteristic snapping as the ligament is reduced.

The value of immobilizing the elbow following reduction has been debated. Taha[134] reported a decreased rate of recurrence during the 10 days following reduction if the elbow was splinted in a flexed supinated position for 2 days following reduction. Salter and Zaltz[120] recommended the use of a sling, mainly to prevent the elbow from being pulled a second time. Kohlhaas and Roeder[68] recommended a T-shirt technique for flexed elbow stabilization in very young children. This provided adequate immobilization without the use of a sling by pinning the sleeve of the long sleeve T-shirt to the opposite chest. In general, after a successful closed reduction of a first time annular ligament subluxation, immobilization of the extremity is not necessary if the child is comfortable and using the arm normally. After the reduction, it is important to explain to the parents the mechanism of injury and to emphasize the need to prevent longitudinal pulling on the upper extremities. Picking the child up under the axillae and avoiding games such as "ring around the roses" and involve longitudinal traction to the arm are stressed. However, recurrence rate is high even with the most diligent parents. Therefore, instruction in home reduction of the pulled elbow is very useful and lessens visits to the emergency room and primary care physician.

Surgical Treatment

Even if untreated, most annular ligament subluxations reduce spontaneously. There are no reported cases of long-term sequelae of untreated annular ligament subluxation. Therefore, open reduction is rarely if ever indicated for annular ligament subluxation. An indication for surgery might be the chronic, symptomatic, irreducible subluxation.[137] In such a circumstance, the annular ligament must be partially transected to achieve reduction.

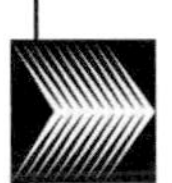

AUTHORS' PREFERRED TREATMENT: PULLED ELBOW SYNDROME—CLOSED REDUCTION

It is important to elicit a reliable history as to whether or not the child had a traction force applied across the extended elbow. The entire extremity is then carefully examined. Focal tenderness should be present directly over the radiocapitellar joint. If the history or physical examination is not entirely consistent with annular ligament subluxation, then x-rays of the upper extremity are obtained to assess for other injuries before manipulating the elbow.

Once the diagnosis of annular ligament subluxation is clearly established, manipulation is performed. It is first explained to the parents that there will be a brief episode of pain followed by relief of the symptoms. The patient usually is seated on the parent's lap. The patient's forearm is grasped with the elbow semiflexed while the thumb of the surgeon's opposite hand is placed over the lateral aspect of the elbow. The forearm is first supinated. If this fails to produce the characteristic snap of reduction, then the elbow is gently flexed maximally until the snap occurs (see Fig. 16-31). Just before reaching maximal flexion, there often is an increase in the resistance to flexion. At this point, a little extra pressure toward flexion is applied, which usually produces the characteristic snap as the annular ligament suddenly returns to its normal position. If this fails, then the hyperpronation technique of Macias et al.[75] is used. Full flexion-extension elbow motion and forearm pronation-supination motion is performed to the extremes, and this usually resolves the "outliers" which do not reduce with the usual mechanisms.

What should be done if a definite snap or pop is not felt or if the patient fails to use the extremity after manipulation? In a few patients, discomfort may persist despite successful annular ligament reduction. If the subluxation has occurred more than 12 to 24 hours before the child is seen, there often is a mild secondary synovitis, and recovery may not be immediate and dramatic. One must confirm that the initial diagnosis was correct. If not taken before the manipulation, x-rays should be obtained and the entire extremity careful re-examined. If the x-ray results are normal and the elbow can be fully flexed with free supination and pronation, the physician can be assured that the subluxated annular ligament has been reduced. In this circumstance, the patient's arm may be placed in a splint or sling for a few days to 1 week and re-examined clinically and by x-ray if needed.

Pearls and Pitfalls

It should never be assumed that an unwitnessed fall has resulted in annular ligament subluxation. Such an injury mechanism is much more likely to result in a fracture (possibly occult) about the elbow.

Complications

There are no reports of long-term sequelae from unrecognized and unreduced subluxations. Almost all subluxations reduce spontaneously. The only problem seems to be discomfort to the patient until the annular ligament reduces.

Recurrent Subluxations

The reported incidence of recurrent subluxation has varied from 5% to 39%.[22,43,56,108,122,126,135] Children 2 years of age or younger appear to be at greatest risk for recurrence.[122,137] Recurrent subluxations usually respond to the same manipulative procedure as the initial injury. They eventually cease after 4 to 5 years when the annular ligament strengthens and ligament laxity lessens. Recurrences do not lead to any long-term sequelae. If recurrent annular ligament subluxation significantly impacts a patient's quality of life because of pain or limited activity, immobilization in an above-elbow cast with the forearm in supination or neutral position for 2 to 3 weeks is usually effective at preventing recurrence.

ACKNOWLEDGMENTS

We thank Stephen D. Heinrich, Kaye Wilkins, and George Thompson for their contributions to this chapter. The information presented in this chapter is based on their efforts in previous editions.

REFERENCES

1. Afshar A. Divergent dislocation of the elbow in an 11-year-old child. Arch Iranian Med 2007;10:413–416.
2. Akansel G, Dalbayrak S, Yilmaz M, et al. MRI demonstration of intra-articular median nerve entrapment after elbow dislocation. Skeletal Radiol 2003;32:537–541.
3. al-Qattan MM, Zuker RM, Weinberg MJ. Type 4 median nerve entrapment after elbow dislocation. J Hand Surg 1994;19(5):613–615.
4. Allende G, Freytes M. Old dislocation of the elbow. J Bone Joint Surg Am 1944;26: 692–706.
5. Altuntas AO, Balakumar J, Howells RJ, et al. Posterior divergent dislocation of the elbow in children and adolescents: a report of three cases and review of the literature. J Pediatr Orthop 2005;25:317–321.
6. Amir D, Frankl U, Pogrund H. Pulled elbow and hypermobility of joints. Clin Orthop Relat Res 1990;257:94–99.
7. Andersen K, Mortensen AC, Gron P. Transverse divergent dislocation of the elbow. A report of two cases. Acta Orthop Scand 1985;56:442–443.
8. Ayala H, De Pablos J, Gonzalez J, et al. Entrapment of the median nerve after posterior dislocation of the elbow. Microsurgery 1983;4:215–220.
9. Beaty JH, Donati NL. Recurrent dislocation of the elbow in a child. A case report and review of the literature. J Pediatr Orthop 1991;11:392–396.
10. Bhan S, Mehara AK. A method of closed reduction of posterior dislocation of the elbow. Int Orthop 1994;18:271–272.
11. Boe S, Holst-Nielsen F. Intra-articular entrapment of the median nerve after dislocation of the elbow. J Hand Surg Br 1897;12(3):356–358.
12. Bouyala JM, Bollini G, Jacquemrier M, et al. The treatment of old dislocations of the

radial head in children by osteotomy of the upper end of the ulna. Apropos of 15 cases [Article in French]. Rev Chir Orthop Reparatrice Appar Mot 1988;74:173–182.
13. Bretland PM. Pulled elbow in childhood. Br J Radiol 1994;67:1176–1185.
14. Broadhurst BW, Buhr AJ. The pulled elbow. Br Med J 1959;1:1018–1019.
15. Bucknill TM. Anterior dislocation of the radial head in children. Proc R Soc Med 1977; 70:620–624.
16. Capo SR, Tito AV, Cuesta FJG, et al. Median nerve paralysis following elbow fractures and dislocations. Apropos of a series of 12 cases [Article in French]. Ann Chir 1984; 38:270–273.
17. Cappellino A, Wolfe SW, Marsh JS. Use of a modified Bell Tawse procedure for chronic acquired dislocation of the radial head. J Pediatr Orthop 1998;18:410–414.
18. Caravias DE. Some observations on congenital dislocation of the head of the radius. J Bone Joint Surg 1957;39B:86–90.
19. Carey RPL. Simultaneous dislocation of the elbow and the proximal radioulnar joint. J Bone Joint Surg Br 1984;66B:254–256.
20. Carl A, Prada S, Teixeira K. Case report and review of the literature. Proximal radioulnar transposition in an elbow dislocation. J Orthop Trauma 1992;6:106–109.
21. Carlioz H, Abols Y. Posterior dislocation of the elbow in children. J Pediatr Orthop 1984;4:8–12.
22. Choung W, Heinrich SD. Acute annular ligament interposition into the radiocapitellar joint in children (nursemaid's elbow). J Pediatr Orthop 1995;15:454–456.
23. Cromack PI. The mechanism and nature of the injury in dislocations of the elbow and a method of treatment. Aust N Z J Surg 1960;30:212–216.
24. Crosby EH. Dislocation of the elbow reduced by means of traction in four directions. J Bone Joint Surg Am 1936;18:1077.
25. Danielsson LG. Median nerve entrapment and elbow dislocation. A case report. Acta Orthop Scand 1986;57:450–452.
26. Danielsson LG, Theander G. Traumatic dislocation of the radial head at birth. Acta Radiol Diagn (Stockh) 1981;22:279–382.
27. De Boeck H. Radial neck osteolysis after annular ligament reconstruction. A case report. Clin Orthop Relat Res 1997;342:94–98.
28. De Boeck H. Treatment of chronic isolated radial head dislocation in children. Clin Orthop Relat Res 2000;380:215–219.
29. DeLee JC. Transverse divergent dislocation of the elbow in a child. Case report. J Bone Joint Surg Am 1981;63(2):322–323.
30. Devnani AS. Outcome of longstanding dislocated elbows treated by open reduction and excision of collateral ligaments. Singapore Med J 2004;45:14–19.
31. Doornberg JN, Ring D. Coronoid fracture patterns. J Hand Surg Am 2006;31(1):45–52.
32. Doornberg JN, Ring DC. Fracture of the anteromedial facet of the coronoid process. Surgical Technique. J Bone Joint Surg Am 2007;89(Suppl 2):267–283.
33. Durig M, Gauer EF, Muller W. Die Operative Behandlung der Rezidivierenden und Traumatischen Luxation des Ellenbogengelenkes nach Osborne une Cotterill. Arch Orthop Unfall Chir 1976;86:141–156.
34. Eklöf O, Nybonde T, Karlsson G. Luxation of the elbow complicated by proximal radio ulnar translocation. Acta Radiol 1990;31:145–146.
35. el Bardouni A, Mahfoud M, Ouadghiri M, et al. Divergent dislocation of the elbow. A case report [Article in French]. Rev Chir Orthop Reparatrice Appar Mot 1994;80: 150–152.
36. Fourrier P, Levai JP, Collin JPH. Median nerve entrapment in elbow dislocation [Article in French]. Rev Chir Orthop Reparatrice Appar Mot 1977;63:13–16.
37. Fowles JV, Kassab MT, Douik M. Untreated posterior dislocation of the elbow in children. J Bone Joint Surg Am 1984;66(6):921–926.
38. Fowles JV, Slimane N, Kassab MT. Elbow dislocation with avulsion of the medial humeral epicondyle. J Bone Joint Surg Br 1990;72(1):102–104.
39. Frumkin K. Nursemaid's elbow. A radiographic demonstration. Ann Emerg Med 1985; 14:690–693.
40. Gillingham Bl, Wright JG. Convergent dislocation of the elbow. Clin Orthop Relat Res 1997;340:198–201.
41. Gosman JA. Recurrent dislocation of the ulna at the elbow. J Bone Joint Surg 1943; 25:44.
42. Green NE. Case report. Entrapment of the median nerve following elbow dislocation. J Pediatr Orthop 1983;3:384–386.
43. Griffin ME. Review article. Subluxation of the head of the radius in children. Pediatrics 1955;15:103–106.
44. Grimer RJ, Brooks S. Brachial artery damage accompanying closed posterior dislocation of the elbow. J Bone Joint Surg Br 1985;67(3):378–381.
45. Hallett H. Entrapment of the median nerve after dislocation of the elbow. A case report. J Bone Joint Surg Br 1981;63B(3):408–412.
46. Hankin FM. Posterior dislocation of the elbow. A simplified method of closed reduction. Clin Orthop Relat Res 1984;190:254–256.
47. Harvey S, Tchélébi H. Proximal radio-ulnar translocation. A case report. J Bone Joint Surg Am 1979;61(3):447–449.
48. Hasler CC, Von Laer L, Hell AK. Open reduction, ulnar osteotomy and external fixation for chronic anterior dislocation of the head of the radius. J Bone Joint Surg Br 2005; 87(1):88–94.
49. Hassmann GC, Brunn F, Neer CS. Recurrent dislocation of the elbow. J Bone Joint Surg Am 1975;57(8):1080–1084.
50. Henderson RS, Roberston IM. Open dislocation of the elbow with rupture of the brachial artery. J Bone Joint Surg Br 1952;34B(4):636–637.
51. Hennig K, Franke D. Posterior displacement of brachial artery following closed elbow dislocation. J Trauma 1980;20:96–98.
52. Henrikson B. Supracondylar fractures of the humerus in children. Acta Chir Scand Suppl 1966;369:1–72.
53. Herring JA. Instructional case. Recurrent dislocation of the elbow. J Pediatr Orthop 1989;9:483–484.
54. Hofammann III KE, Moneim MS, Omer GE, et al. Brachial artery disruption following closed posterior elbow dislocation in a child. A case report with review of the literature. Clin Orthop Relat Res 1984;184:145–149.
55. Holbrook Jl, Green NE. Divergent pediatric elbow dislocation. A case report. Clin Orthop Relat Res 1988;234:72–74.
56. Illingsworth CM. Pulled elbow: a study of 100 patients. Br Med J 1975;2:672–674.
57. Inoue G, Horii E. Case report. Combined shear fractures of the trochlea and capitellum associated with the anterior fracture–dislocation of the elbow. J Orthop Trauma 1992; 6:373–375.
58. Isbister ES. Proximal radioulnar translocation in association with posterior dislocation of the elbow. Injury 1991;22:479–482.
59. Jackson JA. Simple anterior dislocation of the elbow joint with rupture of the brachial artery. Case report. Am J Surg 1940;47:479–486.
60. Jongschaap HCN, Youngson GG, Beattie TF. The epidemiology of radial head subluxation ("pulled elbow") in the Aberdeen City area. Health Bull (Edinb) 1990;48:58–61.
61. Josefsson P, Gentz CF, Johnell O, et al. Surgical versus nonsurgical treatment of ligamentous injuries following dislocations of the elbow joint. Clin Orthop Relat Res 1987; 214:165–169.
62. Josefsson PO, Gentz CF, Johnell O, et al. Surgical versus nonsurgical treatment of ligamentous injuries following dislocations of the elbow joint. A prospective randomized study. J Bone Joint Surg Am 1987;69(4):605–608.
63. Josefsson PO, Johnell O, Gentz CF. Long-term sequelae of simple dislocation of the elbow. J Bone Joint Surg Am 1984;66(6):927–930.
64. Josefsson PO, Nilsson BE. Incidence of elbow dislocation. Acta Orthop Scand 1986; 57(6):537–538.
65. Kapel O. Operation for habitual dislocation of the elbow. J Bone Joint Surg Am 1951; 33-A(3):707–710.
66. Kilburn P, Sweeney JG, Silk FF. Three cases of compound posterior dislocation of the elbow with rupture of the brachial artery. J Bone Joint Surg Br 1962;44B:119–121.
67. King T. Recurrent dislocation of the elbow. J Bone Joint Surg Br 1953;35-B(1):50–54.
68. Kohlhaas AR, Roeder J. Tee shirt management of nursemaid's elbow. Am J Orthop 1995;24:74.
69. Kosuwon W, Mahaisavariya B, Saengnipanthkul S, et al. Ultrasonography of pulled elbow. J Bone Joint Surg Br 1993;75(3):421–422.
70. Kumar A, Ahmed M. Technical tricks. Closed reduction of posterior dislocation of the elbow: a simple technique. J Orthop Trauma 1999;13:58–59.
71. Lavine LS. A simple method of reducing dislocations of the elbow joint. J Bone Joint Surg Am 1953;35-A(3):785–786.
72. Linscheid Rl, Wheeler DK. Elbow dislocations. JAMA 19865;194:113–118.
73. Loomis LK. Reeducation and after–treatment of posterior dislocation of the elbow. With special attention to the brachialis muscle and myositis ossificans. Am J Surg. 1944;63:56–60.
74. Louis DS, Ricciardi JE, Spengler DM. Arterial injury: a complication of posterior elbow dislocation. A clinical and anatomical study. J Bone Joint Surg Am 1974;56(8): 1631–1636.
75. Macias CG, Bothner J, Wiebe R. A comparison of supination/flexion to hyperpronation in the reduction of radial head subluxations. Pediatrics 1998;102:10.
76. MacSween WA. Transposition of radius and ulna associated with dislocation of the elbow in a child. Injury 1978;10:314–316.
77. Magill HK, Aitken AP. Pulled elbow. Surg Gynecol Obstet 1954;98:753–756.
78. Mahaisavariya B, Laupattarakasem W. Neglected dislocation of the elbow. Clin Orthop Relat Res 2005;431:21–25.
79. Mahaisavariya B, Laupattarakasem W, Supachutikul A, et al. Late reduction of dislocated elbow. Need triceps be lengthened? J Bone Joint Surg Br 1992;75(3):426–428.
80. Malkawi H. Recurrent dislocation of the elbow accompanied by ulnar neuropathy. A case report and review of the literature. Clin Orthop Relat Res 1981;161:270–274.
81. Manouel M, Minkowitz B, Shimotsu G, et al. Brachial artery laceration with closed posterior elbow dislocation in an eight-year-old. Clin Orthop Relat Res 1993;296: 109–112.
82. Mantle JA. Recurrent posterior dislocation of the elbow. J Bone Joint Surg Br 1966; 48B:590.
83. Maripuri SN, Debnath UK, Rao P, Mohanty K. Simple elbow dislocation among adults: A comparative study of two different methods of treatment. Injury 2007;38: 1254–1258.
84. Matev I. A radiological sign of entrapment of the median nerve in the elbow joint after posterior dislocation. A report of two cases. J Bone Joint Surg Br 1976;58(3):353–355.
85. Matles A, Eliopoulos K. Internal derangement of the elbow in children. Int Surg 1967; 48:259–263.
86. McAuliffe TB, Williams D. Transverse divergent dislocation of the elbow. Injury 1988; 19:279–280.
87. McKee MD, Schemitsch EH, Sala MJ, et al. The pathoanatomy of lateral ligamentous disruption in complex elbow instability. J Shoulder Elbow Surg 2003;12:391–396.
88. McKellar Hall R. Recurrent posterior dislocation of the elbow joint in a boy. Report of a case. J Bone Joint Surg Br 1953;35B:56.
89. McRae R, Freeman PA. The lesion of pulled elbow. J Bone Joint Surg Br 1965;47B: 808.
90. Mehta S, Sud A, Tiwari A, et al. Open reduction for late-presenting posterior dislocation of the elbow. J Orthop Surg 2007;15:15–21.
91. Meyn MA, Quigley TB. Reduction of posterior dislocation of the elbow by traction on the dangling arm. Clin Orthop Relat Res 1974;103:106–108.
92. Milch H. Bilateral recurrent dislocation of the ulna at the elbow. J Bone Joint Surg Am 1936;18:777–780.
93. Minford EJ, Beattie TF. Hanging arm method for reduction of dislocated elbow. J Emerg Med 1993;11:161–162.
94. Naidoo KS. Unreduced posterior dislocations of the elbow. J Bone Joint Surg Br 1982; 64(5):603–606.
95. Nakano A, Tanaka S, Hirofuji E, et al. Transverse divergent dislocation of the elbow in a six-year-old boy: case report. J Trauma 1992;32:118–119.
96. Nanno M, Sawaizumi T, Ito H. Transverse divergent dislocation of the elbow with ipsilateral distal radius fracture in a child. J Orthop Trauma 2007;21:145–149.
97. Neviaser JS, Wickstrom JK. Dislocation of the elbow: a retrospective study of 115 patients. South Med J 1977;70:172–173.
98. Newman J. "Nursemaid's elbow' in infants 6 months and under. J Emerg Med 1985; 2:403–404.
99. O'Driscoll SW, Bell DF, Morrey BF. Posterolateral rotatory instability of the elbow. J Bone Joint Surg Am 1991;73A:440–446.
100. O'Driscoll SW, Morrey BF, Korinek S, et al. Elbow subluxation and dislocation. A spectrum of instability. Clin Orthop Relat Res 1992;280:186–197.
101. Osborne G, Cotterill P. Recurrent dislocation of the elbow. J Bone Joint Surg Br 1966; 48B:340–346.

102. Ozkoc G, Akpinar S, Hersekli MA, et al. Type 4 median nerve entrapment in a child after elbow dislocation. Arch Orthop Trauma Surg 2003;123:555–557.
103. Parvin RW. Closed reduction of common shoulder and elbow dislocations without anesthesia. AMA Arch Surg 1957;75:972–975.
104. Pearce MS. Radial artery entrapment. A rare complication of posterior dislocation of the elbow. Int Orthop 1993;17:127–182.
105. Piroth P, Gharib M. Traumatic subluxation of the head of the radius [Article in German]. Deutsch Med Wochenschr 1976;101:1520–1523.
106. Pritchard DJ, Linscheid RL, Svien HJ. Intra-articular median nerve entrapment with dislocation of the elbow. Clin Orthop Relat Res 1973;90:100–103.
107. Pritchett JW. Case report. Entrapment of the median nerve after dislocation of the elbow. J Pediatr Orthop 1984;4:752–753.
108. Quan L, Marcuse EK. The epidemiology and treatment of radial head subluxation. Am J Dis Child 1985;139:1194–1197.
109. Rana NA, Kenwright J, Taylor RG, et al. Complete lesion of the median nerve associated with dislocation of the elbow. Acta Orthop Scand 1974;45:365–369.
110. Rao SB, Crawford AH. Median nerve entrapment after dislocation of the elbow in children. A report of 2 cases and review of the literature. Clin Orthop Relat Res 1995; 312:232–237.
111. Rasool MN. Dislocations of the elbow in children. J Bone Joint Surg Br 2004;86(7): 1050–1058.
112. Reichenheim PP. Transplantation of the biceps tendon as a treatment for recurrent dislocation of the elbow. Br J Surg 1947;35:201–204.
113. Roaf R. Foramen in the humerus caused by the median nerve. J Bone Joint Surg Br 1957;39-B(4):748–749.
114. Roberts PH. Dislocation of the elbow. Br J Surg 1969;56:806–815.
115. Ross G, McDevitt ER, Chronister R, et al. Treatment of simple elbow dislocation using an immediate motion protocol. Am J Sports Med 1999;27:308–311.
116. Royle SG. Posterior dislocation of the elbow. Clin Orthop Relat Res1991;269:201–204.
117. Rubens MK, Auliciano PL. Open elbow dislocation with brachial artery disruption: case report and review of the literature. Orthopedics 1986;9:539–542.
118. Ryan JR. The relationship of the radial head to radial neck diameters in fetuses and adults with reference to radial head subluxation in children. J Bone Joint Surg Am 1969;51(4):781–783.
119. Sacchetti A, Ramoska EE, Glascow C. Nonclassic history in children with radial head subluxations. J Emerg Med 1990;8:151–153.
120. Salter RB, Zaltz C. Anatomic investigations of the mechanism of injury and pathologic anatomy of pulled elbow in young children. Clin Orthop Relat Res 1971;77:134–143.
121. Scapinelli R, Borgo A. Pulled elbow in infancy: Diagnostic role of imaging. Radiologia Medica 2005;110:655–664.
122. Schunk JE. Radial head subluxation: epidemiology and treatment of 87 episodes. Ann Emerg Med 1990;19:1019–1023.
123. Schwab GH, Bennett JB, Woods GW, et al. A biomechanics of elbow instability: the role of the medial collateral ligament. Clin Orthop Relat Res 1980;146:42–52.
124. Seel MJ, Peterson HA. Management of chronic posttraumatic radial head dislocation in children. J Pediatr Orthop 1999;19:306–312.
125. Shankarappa YK, Tello E, D. FB. Transverse divergent dislocation of the elbow with ipsilateral distal radius epiphyseal injury in a seven-year-old. Injury 1998;29:798–802.
126. Snellman O. Subluxation of the head of the radius in children. Acta Orthop Scand 1959;28:311–315.
127. Snyder HS. Radiographic changes with radial head subluxation in children. J Emerg Med. 1990;8:265–269.
128. Sojbjerg JO, Helmig P, Kjaersgaard-Andersen P. Dislocation of the elbow: an experimental study of the ligamentous injuries. Orthopedics 1987;12:461–463.
129. Sovio OM, Tredwell SJ. Case report. Divergent dislocation of the elbow in a child. J Pediatr Orthop 1986;6:96–97.
130. Spear HC, Jones JM. Rupture of the brachial artery accompanying dislocation of the elbow or supracondylar fracture. J Bone Joint Surg Am 1951;33A:889–894.
131. Speed JS. An operation for unreduced posterior dislocation of the elbow. South Med J 1925;18:193–197.
132. Steiger RN, Larrick RB, Meyer TL. Median nerve entrapment following elbow dislocation in children. A report of two cases. J Bone Joint Surg Am 1969;51(2):381–385.
133. Symeonides PO, Paschaloglou C, Stavrou Z, et al. Recurrent dislocation of the elbow. Report of three cases. J Bone Joint Surg Am 1975;57A:1084–1086.
134. Taha AM. The treatment of pulled elbow: a prospective randomized study. Arch Orthop Trauma Surg 2000;120:336–337.
135. Teach SJ, Schutzman SA. Prospective study of recurrent radial head subluxation. Arch Pediatr Adolesc Med 1986;150:164–166.
136. Thompson HC, Garcia A. Myositis ossificans after elbow injuries. Clin Orthop Relat Res 1967;50:129–134.
137. Triantafyllou SJ, Wilson SC, Rychak J. Irreducible pulled elbow in a child. A case report. Clin Orthop Relat Res 1992;284:153–155.
138. Trias A, Comeau Y. Recurrent dislocation of the elbow in children. Clin Orthop Relat Res 1974;100:74–77.
139. Vicente P, Orduna M. Transverse divergent dislocation of the elbow in a child. A case report. Clin Orthop Relat Res 1993;294:312–313.
140. Wainwright D. Recurrent dislocation of the elbow joint. Proc R Soc Med 1947;40: 88–886.
141. Watson-Jones R. Primary nerve lesions in injuries of the elbow and wrist. J Bone Joint Surg Am 1930;12:121–140.
142. Wheeler DK, Linscheid RL. Fracture-dislocations of the elbow. Clin Orthop Relat Res 1967;50:95–106.
143. Wilkerson RD. Anterior elbow dislocation associated with olecranon fractures. Review of the literature and case report. Iowa Orthop J 1993;13:223–225.
144. Wilmshurst AD, Millner PA, Batchelor AG. Brachial artery entrapment in closed elbow dislocation. Injury 1989;20:240–241.
145. Winslow R. A case of complete anterior dislocation of both bones of the forearm at the elbow. Surg Gynecol Obstet 1913;16:570–571.
146. Witvoet J, Tayon B. Recurrent dislocation of the elbow. Apropos of 6 cases [Article in French]. Rev Chir Orthop Reparatrice Appar Mot 1974;60:485–495.
147. Woods GW, Tullos HS. Elbow instability and medial epicondyle fracture. Am J Sports Med 1977;5:23–30.
148. Zeier FG. Recurrent traumatic elbow dislocation. Clin Orthop Relat Res 1982;169: 211–214.

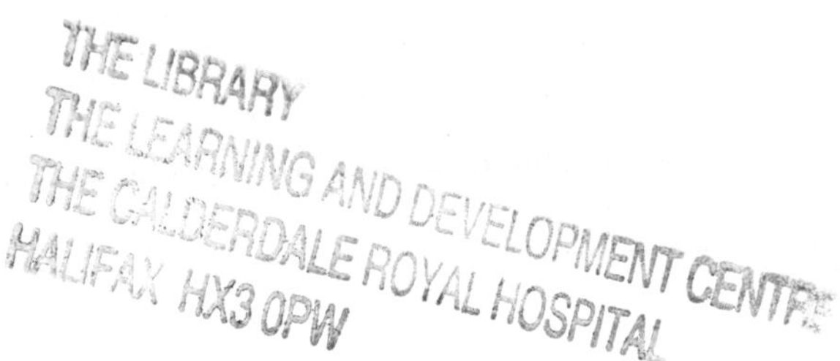

17

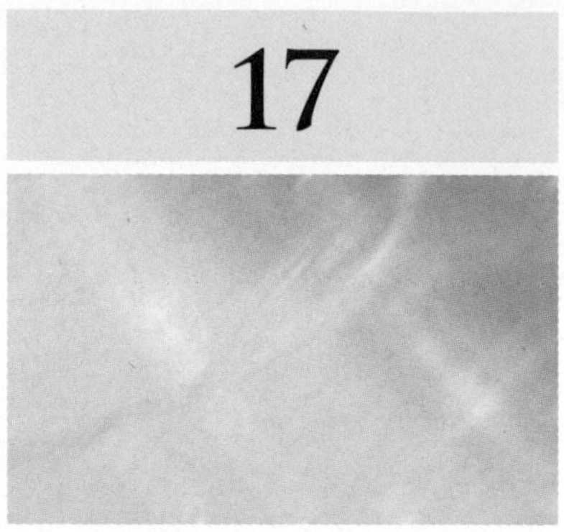

PROXIMAL HUMERUS, SCAPULA, AND CLAVICLE

John F. Sarwark, Erik C. King, and Joseph A. Janicki

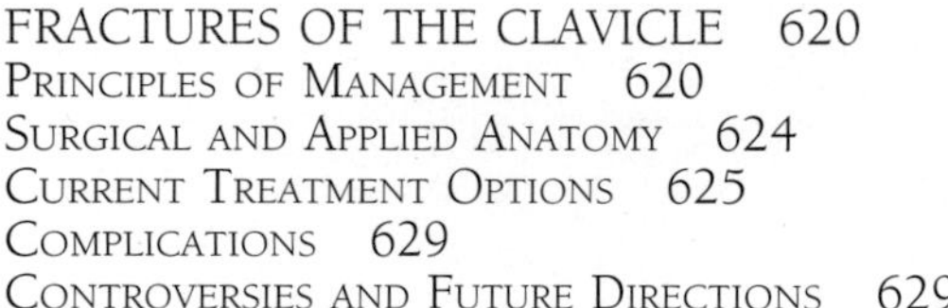

FRACTURES OF THE CLAVICLE 620
Principles of Management 620
Surgical and Applied Anatomy 624
Current Treatment Options 625
Complications 629
Controversies and Future Directions 629

FRACTURES OF THE SCAPULA 629
Principles of Management 629
Surgical and Applied Anatomy 632
Current Treatment Options 633
Complications 634

GLENOHUMERAL SUBLUXATION AND DISLOCATION 634
Principles of Management 635
Surgical and Applied Anatomy 640
Current Treatment Options 642
Complications 644
Controversies and Future Directions 644

FRACTURES OF THE PROXIMAL HUMERUS 644
Principles of Management 644
Surgical and Applied Anatomy 647
Current Treatment Options 649
Complications 654
Controversies and Future Directions 655

FRACTURES OF THE HUMERAL SHAFT 656
Principles of Management 656
Surgical and Applied Anatomy 657
Current Treament Options 658
Complications 667

DISTAL HUMERAL DIAPHYSEAL FRACTURES 667
Principles of Management 668
Current Treatment Options 668

SUPRACONDYLOID PROCESS FRACTURES 672
Principles of Management 674
Current Treatment Options 674

FRACTURES OF THE CLAVICLE

The clavicle has the important function of linking, as a strut, the axial skeleton to the upper extremity (Fig. 17-1). Through its sternoclavicular and the acromioclavicular (AC) joints, the clavicle contributes to the overall motion of the upper extremity. The clavicle can protract and retract.[394] It also rotates and elevates to contribute to shoulder abduction.[2,263,394] In addition, the clavicle provides the attachment site for the two predominant mobilizers of the upper extremity: the pectoralis major and the deltoid muscles. The integrity of the clavicle, therefore, is crucial to the optimal functioning of the entire upper extremity.

As a result of two factors, the clavicle is one of the most frequently fractured bones in the body. First, the clavicle is subcutaneous throughout most of its span, being situated on the anterosuperior aspect of the thorax. Second, nearly all of the forces imparted onto the upper extremity are transmitted through the clavicle to the trunk. The clavicle is the bone most commonly injured during labor and delivery, occurring in 0.5% of all deliveries and accounting for nearly 90% of all obstetrical fractures.[40,106,160,474] Congenital pseudarthrosis of the clavicle, usually right-sided, needs to be distinguished from birth-related fractures. In older children, clavicular fractures occur frequently, with the reported rates ranging between 8% and 15% of all pediatric fractures.[314,336,412]

Principles of Management

Mechanism of Injury

The clavicle is the most common site of all obstetrical fractures, with an incidence of 1% to 13% of all births.[83,106,160,192,194,272,

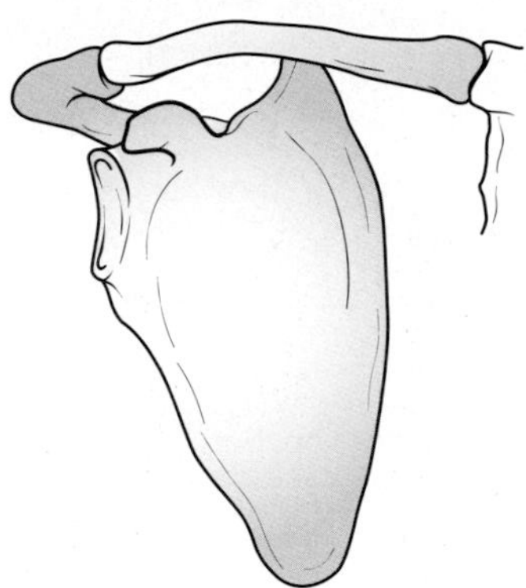

FIGURE 17-1 Relationship between the scapula, clavicle, and sternum.

[427,474,480,567] The incidence of obstetrical clavicle fractures is increased for larger-birth weight infants.[40,106,272,332] In addition, deliveries requiring the use of instruments or specialized obstetric maneuvers are more likely to result in clavicular fractures.[106,194,272,332] Based on these findings, it has been postulated that fractures in these difficult deliveries result from lateral to medial pressure on the shoulders during passage through the narrow birth canal. However, despite the above trends, the majority of birth-related clavicular fractures occur in deliveries of average-birth weight infants who receive routine and otherwise uneventful obstetrical care. Thus, on the whole, obstetrical clavicle fractures are sometimes unavoidable consequences of vaginal deliveries for anatomic or physiologic reasons that may not be evident before or even after delivery.

The most common mechanism of clavicular fractures in children is a fall onto the shoulder.[302,412,525] Other mechanisms include accidents where the traumatic insult is applied directly to the clavicle.[525] Indirect applications of force, typically falling onto an outstretched hand, are much less likely to result in clavicular fractures.[525] Clavicular fractures may also occur in children victimized by child abuse, but no pathognomonic pattern for isolated clavicular fractures resulting from child abuse has been described.[238,293]

A significant amount of energy can be applied directly to the clavicle during athletic activities such as football or indirectly through athletic activities such as gymnastics. Most commonly, the direct mechanism is responsible for clavicle fractures, AC joint injuries, or sternoclavicular joint injuries.[314,412] A large proportion of these sports injuries may be preventable with the use of protective equipment and adequate padding.[512] Although rare, stress fractures of the clavicle have been reported.[2,593]

Signs and Symptoms

Clavicular fractures in newborns may be difficult to identify. The presence of generalized edema may prevent the palpation of normal clavicular margins.[196] To minimize pain, newborns with clavicular fractures demonstrate pseudoparalysis of the affected arm, characterized by voluntary splinting or immobilization of the ipsilateral arm.[125,374] This pseudoparalysis is similar in presentation to a brachial plexus birth injury. To reduce the pull of the sternocleidomastoid muscle across the fracture site, affected infants turn their head toward the side of the fracture. In addition, infants with acute clavicular fractures typically exhibit an asymmetric Moro reflex.[443,485] In the absence of radiographic confirmation, the diagnosis of clavicle fracture may be suspected and later confirmed after a mass is noticed in the affected clavicle. This mass represents a healing fracture callus that forms 7 to 10 days after the initial trauma. Often by this point, the fracture is sufficiently stabilized by fracture callus that it causes little discomfort to the infant. At this stage of healing, the pseudoparalysis will resolve. If there is an associated, unresolved birth palsy, neurologic limitations would persist.

Diagnosis of clavicular fractures in older children is usually straightforward. Children have moderate to severe pain around the area of the fracture and voluntarily immobilize and stop using the affected arm. Tenderness, ecchymosis, and edema are invariably present; in fractures with large displacement, a bony prominence or deformity may be noted. Most children with clavicular fractures keep their heads turned to the side of the fracture to relax the sternocleidomastoid muscle.[196]

Swelling, tenderness, and ecchymosis may be detected over the affected joints in children with either AC or sternoclavicular joint injuries. The children usually self-protect against painful motion of the limb. True dislocations of the AC joint or the sternoclavicular joint are rare. Injuries to the medial and lateral end of the clavicle in children are more commonly physeal fractures.

Associated Injuries

Atlantoaxial (C1–C2) rotatory displacement (subluxation) and clavicular fracture occur together on rare occasions. Attributing acute torticollis entirely to the clavicular fracture may delay the diagnosis of atlantoaxial displacement, and delayed diagnosis of atlantoaxial displacement increases the risk of permanent atlantoaxial rotatory fixation.[3,57] When present, the child's head will be laterally bent toward and rotated away from the fractured clavicle. The diagnosis of C1–C2 subluxation is best confirmed by dynamic computed tomography (CT).

Posterior fracture–dislocations of the medial clavicle are particularly worrisome for associated injury or compression of the great vessels, the esophagus, or the trachea.[184,591] Suspicion of these injuries is further increased in children who have difficulty speaking, breathing, or swallowing. Pulses in the ipsilateral upper extremity may be diminished or absent, and the neck veins may be distended if there is vascular compromise from the displaced medial clavicle. Any of these injuries associated with posterior sternoclavicular joint dislocations can be life-threatening, and precautionary diagnostic and treatment steps should be taken at the onset of treatment. If available, a thoracic or vascular surgeon should be consulted or notified prior to reduction attempts.

Diagnosis and Classification

Imaging Studies. An anteroposterior (AP) radiograph of the clavicle is the standard study for a clavicular fracture. In addition, ultrasonography has been a valuable supplement in establishing the diagnosis of clavicular fractures in neonates.[230,285,287] Ultrasonography can be used to detect occult clavicular fractures.[203,442] Bone healing may be detected on ultrasound 1 week before on radiographs.

For older children, other radiographic studies may be necessary to supplement the AP radiograph in evaluating the clavicular fracture. For fractures in the middle third of the clavicle, several views may be beneficial: cephalad-directed views, the apical oblique view, and the apical lordotic view. The cephalad-directed views are helpful in illustrating the degree of fracture displacement. These views are taken with the x-ray beam 20 to

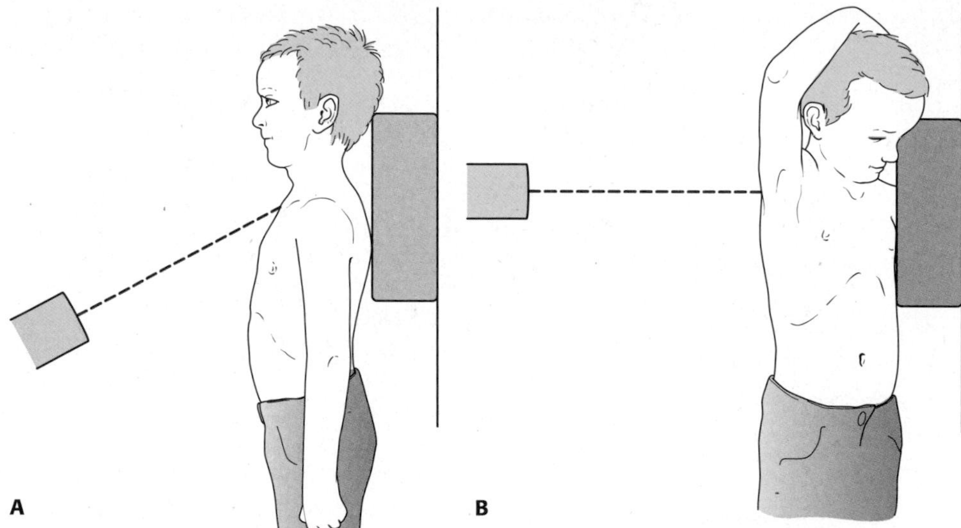

FIGURE 17-2 A. Cephalad-directed views. **B.** Apical lordotic view.

40 degrees cephalad to the clavicle (Fig. 17-2A). The apical oblique view is taken with the x-ray beam 45 degrees lateral to the axial axis of the body and 20 degrees cephalad to the clavicle. This view is better suited to identify fractures in the middle third of the clavicle, where significant curvature is present in the bone.[574] The apical lordotic view is a perpendicular view of the AP radiograph. It is taken laterally with the shoulder abducted more than 130 degrees (Fig.17-2B). This degree of shoulder abduction, however, can cause significant discomfort in children with acute clavicular fractures. Therefore, this radiographic view may be better suited for evaluating the healing of the clavicular fracture rather than for the initial assessment of the fracture.[456]

Fractures in the lateral aspect of the clavicle may require additional radiographic views for full assessment. In addition to the views mentioned above, an axillary lateral view is helpful in evaluating the fracture and its displacement. If the injury to the lateral clavicle or the AC joint is not obvious on the radiographs, a radiographic stress view with the child holding 5 to 10 pounds of weight with his or her hand or having an assistant gently pull on the arm downward is helpful. The stress view may show subtle injuries to the distal clavicle or the degree of instability with ligamentous injuries to AC joint. If enhanced evaluation of the AC joint is desired, a CT scan should be performed.

Additional radiographic views are usually necessary to characterize fractures of the medial third of the clavicle and sternoclavicular injuries. The "serendipity" view, where a broad x-ray beam with 40 degrees of cephalic tilt projects both clavicles on the same film, is helpful for evaluating fractures in this portion of the clavicle (Fig. 17-3).[459] By comparing with the uninjured contralateral side, the location of injury and the degree of displacement often can be determined. However, this view can be difficult to interpret, especially for mild injuries. Currently, CT is the best method for evaluating injuries in the medial third of the clavicle. Thin slice CT provides detailed information about the morphology of the medial clavicle, the medial physis, the degree of displacement, and possible injury to the underlying intrathoracic structures (Fig. 17-4). Virtually every acute injury of the medial end of the clavicle should be evaluated with CT, and it also is useful for follow-up of chronic injuries.

Classification. Because of differences in the mechanism and rate of injury, prognosis, and treatment options, clavicular fractures

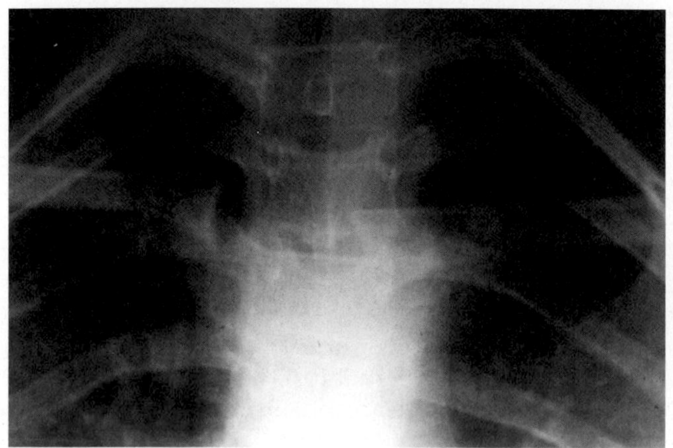

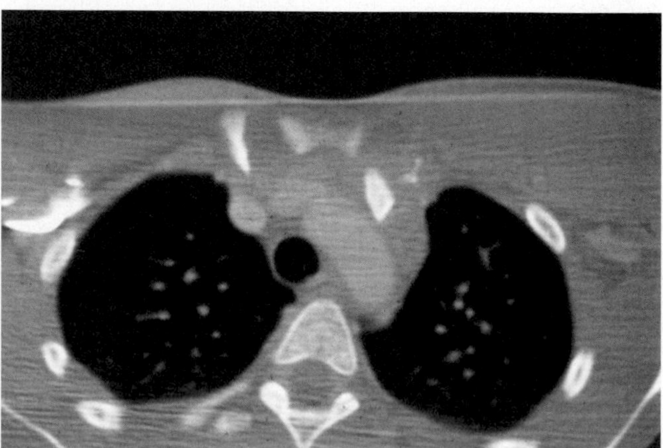

FIGURE 17-3 A. Serendipity view of the medial clavicle. Note inferior displacement of medial end of left clavicle. **B.** CT confirmed left sternoclavicular posterior dislocation.

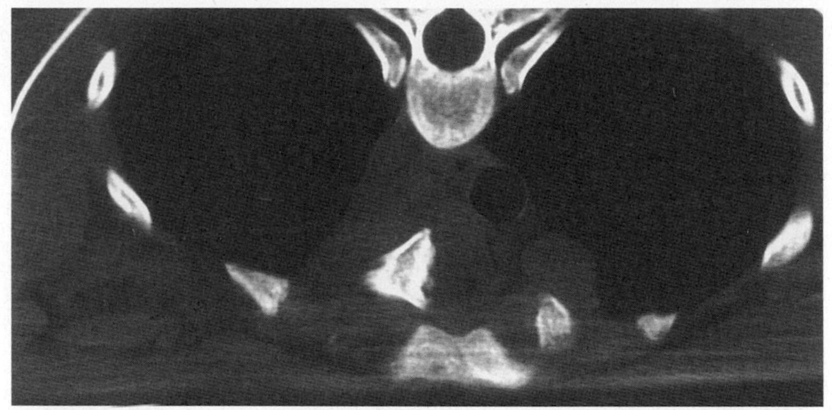

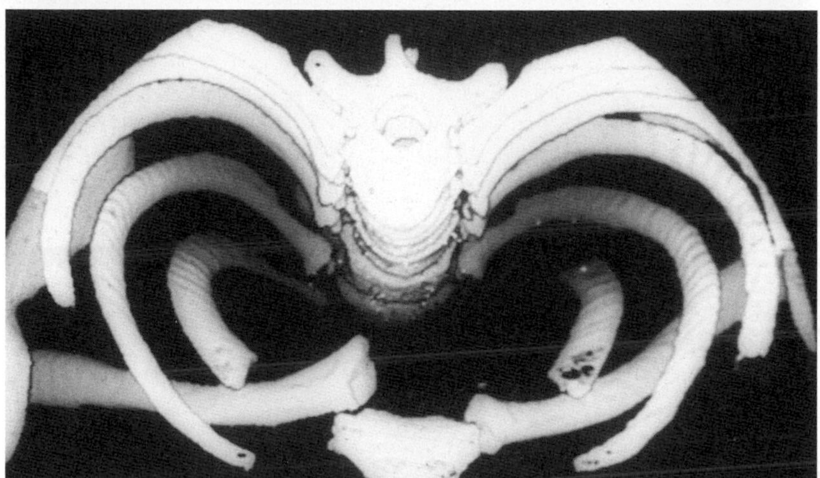

FIGURE 17-4 A. CT image of the clavicle showing posterior retrosternal dislocation of the medial end of the clavicle. **B.** Three-dimensional reconstruction of image shown in **A**.

are broadly categorized by their anatomic location: medial third, middle third, and distal third (Fig. 17-5). Most clavicular fractures occur at the middle third, with the reported rates ranging from 76% to 85%.[386,412] The second most common site of clavicular injury is the distal third, with the reported rates between 10% and 21%.[386,412,451,469] Fractures in the medial third of the clavicle are relatively uncommon and represent only 3% to 5% of all clavicular fractures.[412,469]

The commonly used classification for clavicular fracture is based on the anatomic location of the fracture (see Fig. 17-5).[8] Type I fractures occur in the middle third of the clavicle and generally include all fractures lateral to the sternocleidomastoid muscle and medial to the coracoclavicular ligament. Type II fractures are in the distal clavicle, including all injuries lateral to the coracoclavicular ligament. Type III fractures are medial to the sternocleidomastoid muscle. Within this general framework, further classifications exist for injuries to the distal and medial ends of the clavicle.

Distal Clavicular Injuries. Distal clavicular fractures lateral to the coracoclavicular ligament and injuries to the AC joint are categorized by a system proposed by Dameron and Rockwood

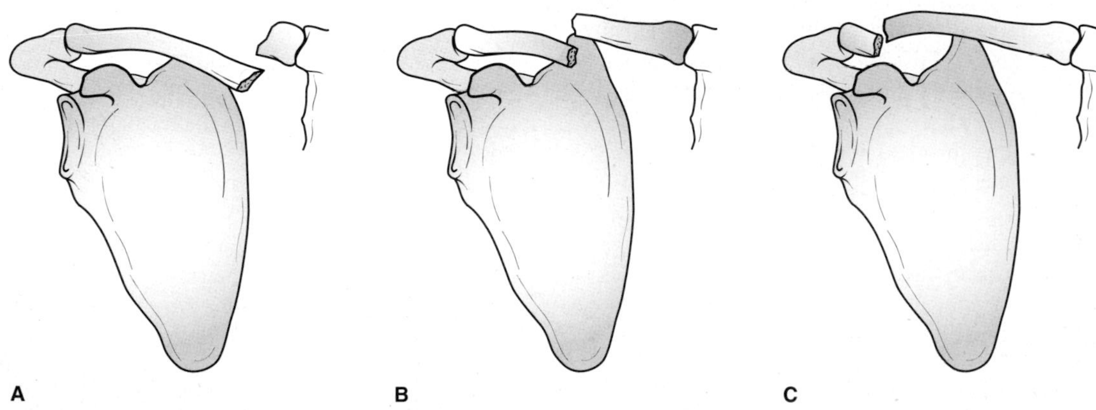

FIGURE 17-5 A. Fracture of the medial third of the clavicle. **B.** Fracture of the middle third of the clavicle. **C.** Fracture of the lateral third of the clavicle.

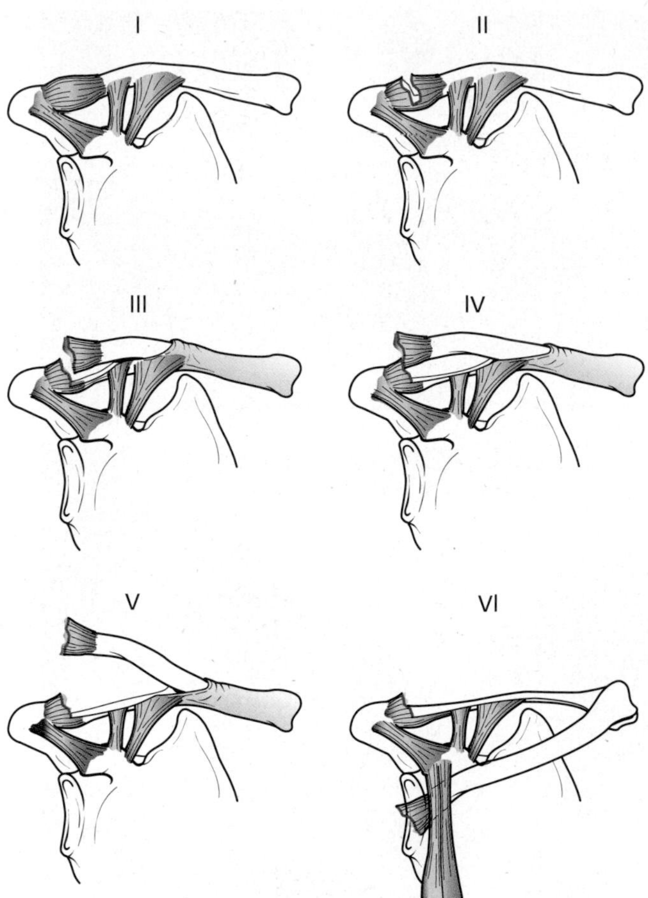

FIGURE 17-6 Dameron and Rockwood[125] classification of distal/lateral fractures.

(Fig. 17-6).[125] Although derived from the system for adult distal clavicular injuries, this classification system incorporates the observation that the distal clavicle displaces through a disruption in its periosteal sleeve rather than by true disruption of the coracoclavicular ligaments. Also, true AC dislocations rarely occur in children. Most injuries in this region are either metaphyseal or physeal fractures.[159,420] However, because distal clavicular epiphyseal ossification does not occur until age 18 or 19, these injuries may have the radiographic appearance of an AC dislocation rather than a fracture (pseudodislocation).[159,420,543]

Type I AC injuries are caused by low-energy trauma and are characterized by mild strains of the ligaments or periosteal tears. No gross changes are seen on radiographs. Type II injury includes complete disruption of the AC ligaments or lateral periosteal attachment, with mild damage to the superolateral aspect of the periosteal sleeve. Mild instability of the distal clavicle results from this type of injury, and minimal widening of the AC joint may be seen on a radiograph. In type III injury, complete disruption of the AC ligaments or periosteal attachment occurs in addition to a large disruption in the superolateral periosteal sleeve. Noticeable superior displacement of the distal clavicle is seen on an AP radiograph, and the coracoid–clavicle interval is 25% to 100% greater than on the contralateral uninjured side.[73,126] Similar soft tissue disruptions are seen in type IV injuries. The distal clavicle, however, is displaced posteriorly and is often embedded in the trapezius muscle.[31] Minimal changes may be noted on an AP radiograph, and an axillary lateral radiograph may be required to identify the posterior clavicular displacement. Type V injuries are similar to type III injuries; the difference lies in the fact that the superior aspect of the periosteal sleeve is completely disrupted in type V injuries. This allows displacement of the distal clavicle into the subcutaneous tissues, occasionally splitting the deltoid and the trapezius muscles. On an AP radiograph, the coracoid–clavicle interval is more than 100% greater than on the contralateral uninjured side. In type VI injuries, the distal clavicle is displaced inferiorly, with its distal end located inferior to the coracoid process.[188]

Medial Clavicular Injuries. The medial physis of the clavicle is the last physis in the body to close, and the fusion of this epiphysis to the shaft occurs as late as 23 to 25 years of age.[274,572] The sternoclavicular ligaments attach primarily to the epiphysis, leaving the physis unprotected outside the capsule.[296] Because of its unique anatomy, traumatic insults to the medial end of the clavicle in children usually result in fractures through the physis rather than dislocations through the sternoclavicular joint. Therefore, these injuries are categorized most appropriately in the Salter-Harris classification system.[481]Most fractures at the medial end of the clavicle are Salter-Harris type I or II fractures. These injuries are further subdivided by the direction of the clavicular displacement, either anterior or posterior. Although anterior displacement of the clavicle occurs more frequently, more attention is given to fractures with posterior displacement due to the possibility of concomitant mediastinal injuries requiring emergent intervention. Many anterior instability patients have ligamentous laxity and no significant traumatic history. Posterior fracture–dislocations are usually secondary to an adduction force, such as a soccer goalie fall on the ground.

Surgical and Applied Anatomy

The clavicle is an S-shaped bone whose medial end is connected to the axial skeleton through the sternoclavicular joint. The medial two thirds of the bone are tubular, whereas the lateral end is flatter and is stabilized in its position by the two coracoclavicular ligaments. The clavicle appears early during embryonic development. By the fifth or sixth week of gestation, it begins ossification at two separate centers: medial and lateral.[183,394,418] By the seventh or eighth week of gestation, its overall contour and shape are already formed.[183] During childhood, approximately 80% of clavicular growth and longitudinal growth occur at the medial physis.[423] Despite this early ossification and growth, complete growth of the clavicle does not occur until early adulthood. The lateral physis continues to proliferate until 18 to 19 years of age, and the medial physis does not close until 23 to 25 years of age.[274,543,572]

The distal clavicle articulates with the scapula through the AC joint, a joint that lacks inherent structural stability. It is held together in part by the AC ligaments, which are relatively weak secondary stabilizers. The primary stabilizers of the joint are the two coracoclavicular ligaments, the conoid and the trapezoid, which stabilize the lateral end of the clavicle next to the acromion. Although the distal clavicle and the coracoid process usually do not articulate, a coracoclavicular joint has been reported in adults.[286] In children, the distal clavicle and the acromion are surrounded by thick periosteum that forms a protective tube

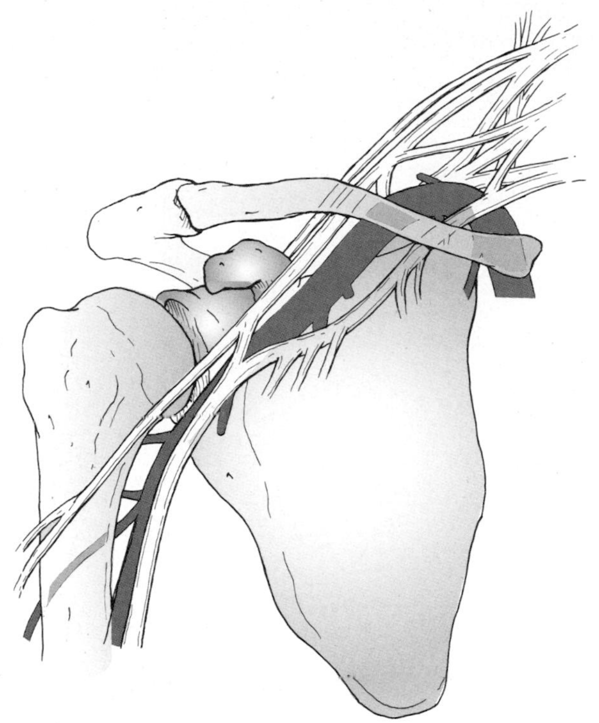

FIGURE 17-7 Relationship of the brachial plexus and artery to the proximal humerus and the scapula.

around the bony structures. The coracoclavicular ligaments are attached to the periosteum on the inferior surface of the distal clavicle. Because these ligament attachments are stronger than the periosteum, displacement of the distal clavicle occurs through a disruption in the periosteum rather than by detachment of the ligaments. In fact, displacement of the distal clavicle through this periosteum in children has been likened to having "a banana being peeled out of its skin." As mentioned above, the distal clavicular physis does not completely ossify until late adolescence.[543] Therefore, fractures through the distal clavicular physis or metaphysis may be mistakenly identified as AC joint dislocations.

Medially, the clavicle articulates with the sternum and the first rib through the sternoclavicular joint. Similar to the AC joint, this joint also lacks inherent structural stability. It is held together by a series of strong ligaments, including the intra-articular disc ligament, the anterior and posterior capsular ligaments, the interclavicular ligament, and the costoclavicular ligament.[41] In children, the medial physis of the clavicle is still open, and the capsular ligaments attach primarily to the epiphysis.[41,274,572] Therefore, injuries to the medial clavicle typically result in physeal fractures with the epiphysis attached to the sternum.

The clavicle also serves as attachment sites for a number of different muscles. On its superior surface, the clavicular head of the sternocleidomastoid muscle is attached. On the posterior surface, the trapezius muscle is attached, whereas the pectoralis major and the deltoid muscles are attached on the anterior surface. Inferiorly, the clavicle provides attachment sites for the subclavius muscle as well as the clavipectoral fascia.

The clavicle provides protection for the subclavian vessels and the brachial plexus. These vital structures are located posterior to the clavicle, crossing the clavicle at the junction between the medial two thirds and lateral one third of the bone (Fig. 17-7). Due to this close proximity, the neurovascular status of the ipsilateral upper extremity may be jeopardized in children with displaced clavicular shaft fractures. In addition, as discussed above, posterior dislocation of the sternoclavicular joint can lead to compression or injuries of the great vessels within the mediastinum. Therefore, the neurovascular status of the ipsilateral upper extremity must be documented before the initiation of treatment for any clavicular injury.

The clavicle contributes significantly to the overall motion and optimal function of the upper extremity. In the anterior to posterior direction, the clavicle can protract and retract approximately 35 degrees.[394] Laterally, it can rotate and elevate to contribute approximately 30 degrees to shoulder abduction.[263,394] The clavicle provides the attachment sites for the major mobilizers of the upper arm, the pectoralis major, and the deltoid muscles. Finally, together with the scapula, the distal clavicle forms the superior shoulder suspensory complex (SSSC, described in the scapula section). As proposed by Goss,[202] the SSSC provides a scaffold from which the upper extremity suspends and articulates in order to function.

Current Treatment Options

Treatment options are listed in Tables 17-1 and 17-2 as well as in the following text.

Middle Third Fractures

Treatment of the birth-related clavicle fracture is nonoperative. If the infant appears to be in significant discomfort, the affected arm can be immobilized to the body for a short period of time, typically less than 2 weeks. Immobilization of the affected arm can be easily and effectively accomplished by using a safety pin

TABLE 17-1 Interventions for Clavicle Fractures

	Immobilization	Closed Reduction and Immobilization	Operative Reduction and Internal Fixation
Middle third	X		X (adolescent and young adults)
Distal third	X		Rare
Medial third	X		X
Sternoclavicular dislocation, anterior	X	X	
Sternoclavicular dislocation, posterior		X—Urgent	X—Urgent

TABLE 17-2 Treatment Pros and Cons: Clavicle Fractures

	Pros	Cons
No reduction (sling or shoulder immobilizer)	1. No anesthesia/sedation 2. Sling/shoulder immobilizer well tolerated	1. No improvement of fracture alignment 2. Functional loss of shoulder range of motion (rare)
Reduction and internal fixation	1. Improves fracture alignment 2. Direct rigid fixation of fracture 3. Improved patient comfort due to rigid fracture fixation 4. No cumbersome cast or splint 5. Lower rate of malunion and nonunion in adults 6. Potentially improved shoulder function	1. General anesthesia 2. Minimal increased risk of infection 3. Implant concerns 4. Potential implant removal

to attach the long shirt sleeve to the shirt or simple stockinette sling.[279,361,484] The parents should be warned not to disturb the upper extremity by unnecessary movements in the acute period. In addition, they should be informed that the infant will develop a noticeable mass over the fracture site that will typically resolve within 6 months.[443]

In older children, good to excellent results also can be expected from nonoperative treatment with a sling or figure-of-eight splint. This is particularly true in younger children. Furthermore, reduction of a clavicle fracture is seldom necessary because of the great potential for remodeling these fractures.[422]

A sling to support the weight of the arm is sufficient treatment in most cases of diaphyseal clavicle fractures. Use of a sling is typically well tolerated by children and is not associated with any of the difficulties of the figure-of-eight splint. Treatment of both nondisplaced and displaced clavicular fractures with a sling has shown remarkably good results. In fact, in comparison with a figure-of-eight splint, treatment of clavicular fractures with a sling resulted in similar final outcomes.[13,273,524] One review found that complications such as nonunion, malunion, and neurovascular problems were so rare in pediatric clavicle fractures that follow-up beyond the initial visit was not necessary.[81]

Nonoperative treatment with a figure-of-eight splint has also produced successful outcomes.[273,398,443,486] Although reduction of the fracture is not required for a successful outcome, correct application of the figure-of-eight splint retracts the shoulders and may achieve improved alignment of the fracture.[422] However, the figure-of-eight splint can be difficult to keep in proper alignment and sometimes is poorly tolerated because of discomfort. Caution must be exercised when using the figure-of-eight splint in order to avoid known complications, such as edema, compression of the axillary vessels, and brachial plexopathy.[171,324,398]

Historically, indications for operative treatment of middle third clavicular fractures include severely displaced and irreducible fractures that threaten skin integrity, concomitant vascular injury requiring repair, irreducible compression of the subclavian vessels, compromise of the brachial plexus, and open fractures.[252,267,396,439,598] In addition, as discussed separately in this chapter, concomitant displaced fractures in various regions of the scapula, including the acromion, the coracoid, and the scapular neck, may compromise the SSSC and require operative repair.[202] However, a prospective, randomized study reported that operatively treated adult clavicle fractures had improved functional outcomes, decreased time to union, and fewer symptomatic malunions and nonunions than those treated nonoperatively with a sling.[84] While the patients treated operatively also had more hardware-related complications, the study supported primary plate fixation of midshaft clavicle fractures in adults. Therefore, internal fixation can be offered to active, skeletally mature adolescents and young adults with displaced diaphyseal clavicle fractures (Fig. 17-8).

For the surgical case, either plating or intramedullary fixation

A
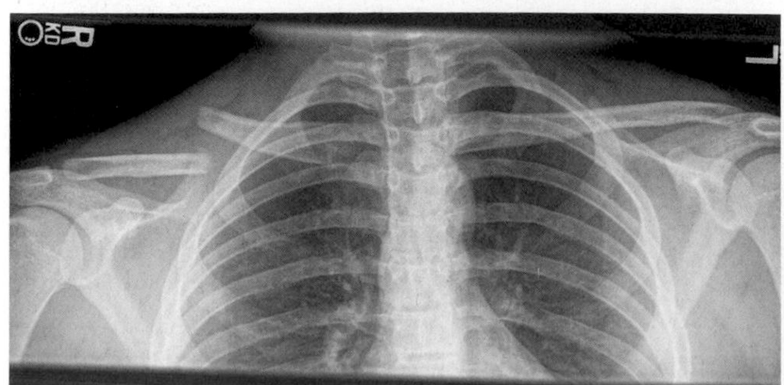

B
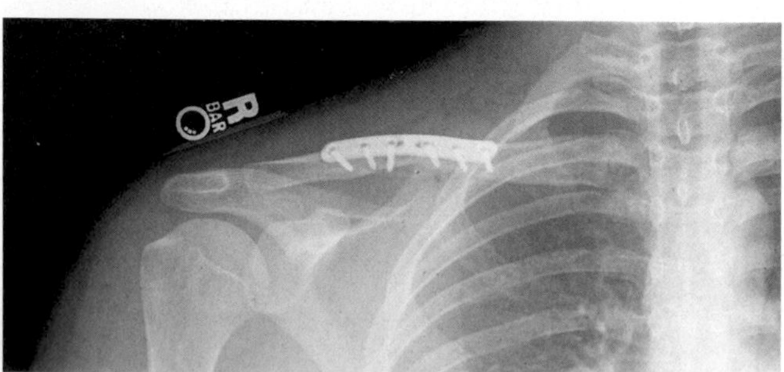

FIGURE 17-8 A. Radiograph of displaced midshaft clavicle fracture of the dominant upper extremity of a throwing athlete. **B.** Surgical fixation was performed with a contoured plate and screws.

can be performed. Various precontoured clavicle plates are available. Intramedullary stabilization with elastic nails or screws is a less invasive procedure.[280,304] Because of the subcutaneous location of the clavicle, implant prominence can be expected and may lead to soft tissue irritation.[84]

Distal Third Fractures

Injuries to the distal clavicle in the pediatric population typically are pseudodislocations of the AC joint, with fractures through the metaphysis or the physis and fracture displacement through the torn periosteum.[152,420] The AC joint and the coracoclavicular ligaments usually are undamaged. Therefore, exceptional remodeling potential exists for these fractures, allowing successful nonoperative treatment for most injuries to the distal clavicle.

Most investigators agree that nondisplaced or minimally displaced injuries of the distal clavicle (types I, II, and III) are treated without surgery.[50,125,223,420,460] These injuries are managed with a sling immobilization followed by early rehabilitation with range-of-motion exercises. Most children treated with nonoperative management have no significant long-term functional or cosmetic deficits.

The treatment of displaced types IV, V, and VI distal clavicle fractures remains controversial. Some investigators report that most children experience no functional deficits regardless of the method of treatment.[50,223] Others report that distal clavicular injuries with either fixed or gross displacement should be treated with open reduction. In the young, this involves periosteal repair and internal fixation in the older patient to prevent permanent deformity.[28,73,125,127,159,223,420,466] One report suggested that although displaced distal clavicular injuries in children under 13 years of age can be treated nonoperatively, those in children over 13 years of age should be treated with open reduction and internal fixation.[152] Any intra-articular fracture fragment displacement, similar to an adult injury, requires anatomic reduction and fixation.

Although no clear consensus exists for the treatment of grossly displaced distal clavicular fractures in children, as long as the integrity of the SSSC is maintained, it appears that neither nonoperative nor operative management results in long-term deficit in the normal function of the shoulder. Treatment options, therefore, should be individualized for each child and his or her family based on compliance as well as acceptance of the possible cosmetic deformity.

Medial Third Clavicular Injuries

Most pediatric injuries in the medial clavicle are fractures through the physis. Similar to distal clavicular injuries, there is debate regarding the remodeling potential of these fractures. Acute posteriorly displaced injuries are more commonly treated with operative reduction and repair now.[198,569]

Nondisplaced fractures of the medial physis do not require active intervention. Symptomatic treatment is all that is required for these stable fractures. In fact, nondisplaced fractures often are missed during initial examination and are only discovered after a mass or bump is noted over the medial clavicle and periosteal healing is seen on the radiograph. The patient and parents should be informed that the mass is a healing callus surrounding the fracture and that it should remodel and disappear in 4 to 8 months.

Most anterior displaced sternoclavicular dislocations are associated with atraumatic, generalized ligamentous laxity, similar to multidirectional instability of the shoulder. These will spontaneously reduce with shoulder motion and do not require emergency room or acute operative care. Appropriate physical therapy and patience is recommended. Late reconstruction for chronic, symptomatic instability has variable results.[27] There are rare acute, anterior traumatic dislocations. In adults, this has been seen in power weightlifters with disruption of the anterior ligaments. Closed reduction can be performed by longitudinal traction to the affected upper extremity while the shoulder is abducted to 90 degrees.[484] Gentle posterior pressure also should be applied over the fracture for reduction. After the reduction is accomplished, the clavicle should be immobilized with a figure-of-eight splint.[484] However, anteriorly displaced sternoclavicular dislocations do not pose a risk to the underlying mediastinal structures, and once achieved, maintenance of reduction can be difficult to maintain. Moreover, while a cosmetic deformity exists, there is no evidence that there is a decrease in shoulder function.[48] Therefore, management without reduction and with a sling or figure-of-eight sling is acceptable. With the rare, anteriorly displaced physeal fracture, remodeling may occur in the young.

Posteriorly displaced medial clavicular fractures and sternoclavicular dislocations require immediate evaluation for the presence of concomitant injuries of the airway and/or great vessels. CT scans are mandatory to assess the degree of displacement. Nondisplaced and minimally displaced fractures can be treated without reduction. These mild injuries can be expected to remodel without significant residual deformity or pain. For fractures and dislocations with significant posterior displacement or those associated with compromise of the airway or great vessels, reduction should be performed. The timing of this is based on whether the underlying structures are compressed and whether the compression is causing respiratory or hemodynamic compromise. Under general anesthesia, closed reduction has been recommended, followed by open reduction if necessary. It is advisable to notify thoracic surgery before beginning reduction in the operating room in case of a mediastinal emergency and surgical instruments should be prepared for a possible open reduction. Excellent results have been reported with open reduction and stabilization with either nonabsorbable or wire suture, and many centers now utilize this as primary, definitive treatment for posterior fracture–dislocations of the medial clavicle.[198,569]

Technique of Closed Reduction. After induction of general anesthesia, a bolster is placed in the midline between the scapulae with the patient in the supine position. This positioning alone may cause reduction. Gentle longitudinal traction through the ipsilateral arm is then applied if necessary. If these reduction maneuvers are unsuccessful, direct reduction using a sterile towel clip is then attempted. After sterile preparation of the skin, the surgeon pierces the skin with the towel clip and grasps the medial end of the clavicle while an assistant applies longitudinal traction to the ipsilateral upper arm. The clavicle is then manipulated into a reduced position.[484] If the above reduction techniques are unsuccessful or the reduction is unstable, then open reduction is performed. In many centers, closed reduction is no longer attempted and open repair is primary treatment due to loss of reduction by closed treatment.

Technique of Open Reduction. The entire ipsilateral chest, clavicle, and mediastinum to opposite anterior chest is prepped in case of a surgical mediastinal emergency with reduction. An anterior incision is utilized from the midportion of the clavicle to the sternum. Dissection is carried through the platysma and fascia to the periosteum while protecting the sensory nerves. Anterior periosteal incision is started laterally to safely identify the bone. Care is taken in dissection medially as the clavicle is displaced into the mediastinum. Anterior dissection is completed to the sternum while protecting the intact soft tissue attachments medially from the sternum to the epiphysis in the posteriorly displaced, physeal fractures. A bone-holding clamp is applied to the clavicle, and the anesthesiologist is notified that reduction is to be performed. Reduction to anatomic location is achieved. Careful hemodynamic monitoring is observed. If all is well, then repair is performed. In the situation of a fracture, nonabsorbable sutures are passed from the anterior medial metaphysis to the epiphysis through drill holes. In the less common posterior dislocation, the sutures are passed from the anterior sternum to the epiphysis. Periosteal repair is then performed and this provides anatomic reduction and stability. Internal fixation with metal implants is contraindicated because of the possibility of implant migration with resulting potential serious or fatal consequences.[103]

A figure-of-eight harness or sling-and-swathe is used for postoperative immobilization for 4 to 6 weeks, followed by range-of-motion and strengthening rehabilitation. Return to sports is delayed until 3 months.

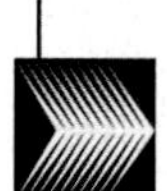

AUTHORS' PREFERRED TREATMENT

The approach to neonatal or birth injuries is one of diagnosis and reassurance and education of the parents. The family is told that a bump will develop over the fracture site and that the fracture will heal uneventfully. If the infant initially demonstrates discomfort with the fracture, the long arm sleeve of the infant's shirt can be pinned to the shirt for 7 to 10 days to provide adequate immobilization.

Older children who present to the emergency room generally have a significant level of pain and discomfort. We usually prefer a sling for relief of pain through immobilization. Occasionally, we use a figure-of-eight harness to provide retraction of the shoulder to gain length at the level of the fracture and to reduce pain. With the use of the figure-of-eight harness, it is important to inspect the skin on weekly follow-ups for 3 weeks to ensure that no unusual sharp bone fragments create any skin problems at the site of passage of the figure-of-eight harness over the fracture. Despite this intervention, the parents are still informed that the fracture will take a couple of months to remodel and that there may be a bump for up to a year after the fracture.

Operative management of clavicular fractures in skeletally immature children is rarely indicated. The indications for surgery are fractures that have the potential to develop full-thickness skin loss over the apex of a fracture and fractures that cause clavicular impingement on either the brachial plexus or the subclavian vessels. Even with these fractures, gentle manipulation and closed reduction should be attempted. Open fractures require open surgery. If open repair is done, the fractured clavicle generally can be placed into the periosteal sleeve and the periosteal sleeve can be repaired over the fractured clavicle without the need for additional internal fixation in the young. In the active, skeletally mature patient, operative management and stabilization with a plate, intramedullary screw, or flexible nail can be considered (see Fig 17-8). The possible earlier union time by surgical stabilization and improved function should be balanced against the potential for implant-related complication, such as implant prominence.

Most fractures of the medial end of the clavicle are treated nonoperatively by our team. A CT study is performed acutely on every posterior displaced fracture or dislocation and on the majority of injuries with anterior displacement as well. Anterior displacements of the medial end of the clavicle generally are associated with ligamentous laxity and usually treated nonoperatively. If a decision is made to treat an anterior displaced physeal fracture with closed reduction, longitudinal traction is applied to the upper extremity with moderate abduction of the humerus, and general pressure is applied over the sternoclavicular joint. Persistent instability with anterior displacement of the sternoclavicular joint from laxity is acceptable. With anterior physeal fractures, there may be remodeling. With or without a reduction, after 2 to 4 weeks of immobilization, a program of progressive rehabilitation can begin.

Posterior dislocations of the medial end at the clavicle of the sternoclavicular joint may be either joint dislocations or a physeal disruption. This injury may be acute and life-threatening. If posterior displacement causes impingement of posterior vital structures, closed reduction is performed under general anesthesia in the operating room followed by open reduction if closed techniques are unsuccessful. Some of these injuries can be treated successfully with closed reduction with general anesthesia and stand-by support of the cardiovascular service. Our current preference is to perform open reduction in most cases.

The technique for the closed reduction is quite specific and involves the placement of a bolster in the midline along the level of the spine and spinous processes. Both humeri are adducted to the level of the chest, and anterior pressure is placed over the deltoid and humeral head toward the table with a downward pressure over both proximal humeri. This is generally sufficient to provide adequate retraction of the shoulder and restore the length of the clavicle at the level of the sternoclavicular joint. Further downward pressure to the level of the table provides a fulcrum force to reduce the medial end of the clavicle anteriorly into the sternoclavicular joint. A towel clip may be required to assist the reduction in difficult cases. When performed, the towel clip is placed subcutaneously and grasps the medial third of the clavicle to aid in the reduction process. It is usually difficult to confirm reduction given the overlying soft tissue swelling and technical difficulty in obtaining adequate confirmatory radiographs, so a small incision is helpful in confirming reduction. Furthermore, open reduction of the medial end of the sternoclavicular joint is indicated when closed reduction fails or results in an unstable retrosternal displacement. If the dislocation is unstable, generally repair of the capsule with a nonabsorbable suture through the capsule of the joint at the level of the sternum through holes drilled into the medial end of the clavicle is sufficient to provide anterior stability of the dislocation. Internal fixation is not recommended in this location. Postoperatively, we place the patient in a figure-of-eight harness for 3 to 6 weeks after a closed reduction or a sling after an open reduction and suture stabilization.

Most injuries to the distal end of the clavicle in children and adolescents are treated nonoperatively. These fractures heal rapidly because of the early deposition of periosteal new bone and remodeling. Generally, patients can be treated with a sling and pain management with appropriate oral analgesics and ice to control swelling. Early range-of-motion therapy is recommended at approximately 10 days to 2 weeks. Clinical union is generally seen by 4 to 6 weeks.

For the rare type IV, V, or VI displaced distal clavicular injury, an open approach can be useful in replacing the distal clavicle in its periosteal sleeve, and repair of the periosteal sleeve may be sufficient to provide adequate fixation.

Pearls and Pitfalls

- Every newborn with a delivery-related clavicle fracture should be evaluated for concurrent brachial plexus palsy.
- Obtain a CT scan for posterior displaced medial clavicle fractures and posterior displaced sternoclavicular dislocations.
- When performing reduction of posterior displaced clavicles with a towel clip, grasp the clavicle in the central portion of the middle third. This enables better mobilization than grasping near the medial end. If adequate closed reduction is uncertain or unstable, an open reduction and suture stabilization is a safe and effective procedure.

Complications

Early Complications

Serious vascular injuries also have been described in association with clavicular fractures, including subclavian and axillary artery disruption, subclavian vessel compression, and the development of a arteriovenous fistula.[37,252,276,387,547] In addition, displaced fractures of the medial clavicle may result in compression or injury of the great vessels within the mediastinum.[184,591] Occasionally, these compressions can be relieved nonoperatively by reducing the fracture and eliminating the excessive pressure on the vessels.[252,387] However, if nonoperative treatment does not alleviate the vascular compromise, operative reduction of the fracture and possible vascular repair may be required. Certainly, if the structural integrity of the vessels is compromised, operative repair by an experienced vascular or thoracic surgeon is necessary.

In addition to the compression of the great vessels, displaced medial clavicular fractures can result in compression of the trachea and esophagus, causing difficulty with speech, the airway, or with swallowing (dysphonia or dysphagia).[184,591] Clavicular fractures resulting from severe trauma can be associated with pneumothorax.[146,382] Rarely, a pneumothorax results from obstetrical clavicular fractures.[350]

Neurologic deficits of the brachial plexus have been reported in association with both birth-related and traumatic clavicular fractures. Brachial plexus palsy may present early or late after the traumatic insult and occasionally requires operative reduction of the fracture.[37,131,132,252,268] Rarely, nerve deficits can result from inappropriate use of the figure-of-eight splints.[324,398] Although permanent nerve deficits have been reported, most brachial plexus injuries resolve spontaneously.[268,277]

Late Complications

Open reduction and internal fixation devices for clavicular fractures have been associated with numerous complications, including hardware irritation, migration, infection, and nonunion.[103,170,373,374,408,493,494] Although most of these complications can be adequately treated, there have been serious, even fatal, results from hardware migration.[103] Therefore, whenever possible, fixation of pediatric clavicular fractures should use nonmigratory, low-profile hardware. If plate fixation is utilized, implant removal may be necessary and carries with it the risk of refracture.

Malunions are common after initial fracture healing, but most children experience no long-term deformities because of their tremendous potential for remodeling. Older patients with segmental or marked fracture displacement may have symptomatic malunions. Exostectomy or osteotomy have been performed in these circumstances. Refracture does occur in less than 3% of clavicle fractures. Return to contact sports should take this risk into consideration. Rare cases of clavicular reduplication and cleidoscapular synostosis have been reported.[420,452] These unusual complications may require additional intervention.

Nonunions following traumatic clavicular fractures should be distinguished from congenital pseudarthrosis and pseudarthrosis secondary to other pathologic processes.[72,77,408,429,451,566,584] Operative indications for posttraumatic clavicle fracture pseudarthroses are unacceptable cosmetic deformity and pain.[55,77,364,584] However, operative repair with grafting and internal fixation of the pseudarthroses have been associated with additional iatrogenic complications, such as pneumothorax, subclavian vessel damage, air embolism, and brachial plexus deficit.[157]

Controversies and Future Directions

Whether internal fixation of clavicle fractures with titanium elastic nails will take hold for severely displaced fractures remains to be seen. There may be greater use of open reduction and plate or intramedullary screw fixation of midshaft clavicle fracture in the active, skeletally mature patient. Operative indications for midshaft clavicular fractures without skin or neurovascular compromise in adolescents remains debatable at this time.

FRACTURES OF THE SCAPULA

Injury to the scapula is rare because it is well protected by multiple layers of muscle and other soft tissue. Only 1% of all fractures involve the scapula.[202,221] However, when scapular injuries occur, they are almost certainly a result of high-energy trauma and may be associated with significant injuries to other major organ systems.[377,540,583] Therefore, all children with apparently isolated scapular fractures should be meticulously evaluated on the secondary trauma survey for the presence of potentially life-threatening visceral injuries that require further intervention.

Principles of Management

Mechanism of Injury

Glenoid. Fractures of the glenoid typically occur in a fall onto an upper extremity. This is believed to drive the humeral head into the glenoid fossa, which in turn results in the fracture. Depending on the direction of the force, the fracture may injure the rim of the glenoid or the entire glenoid fossa. Less commonly, fractures may result from direct trauma to the glenoid.

Body of Scapula. Fractures to the body of the scapula occur via direct impact or avulsion mechanisms. The direct impact mechanism is typically of high-energy and rarely is an isolated injury. As with all other high-energy injuries, child abuse must be excluded as a cause for scapular injury when no clear traumatic cause is evident.[296] The avulsion-type fractures may occur at any of the several muscle attachments on the scapula.

Signs and Symptoms

Children with scapular fractures have significant pain and tenderness around the shoulder girdle and resist movement of the affected arm. Localized edema may obscure the overall shoulder contour, which may be more evident by comparison with the contralateral shoulder. The diagnosis of scapular fractures is frequently missed because of the attention required by more significant injuries.

Associated Injuries

Greater than 75% of patients with scapular fractures have associated injuries,[4,261,471,540] many of which are life-threatening. In one reported series, the rate of death among patients with scapular fractures exceeded 14%.[540]

Because of the proximity of the scapula to the axillary artery and the brachial plexus, fractures of the scapula often are associated with neurovascular injury.[540] The ipsilateral arm must be carefully examined to document arterial or neurologic deficits before the initiation of treatment. When injury to axillary or distal vasculature is suspected, an angiogram may be performed to examine the integrity of the vessels.

Scapular fractures also are associated with several life-threatening injuries, such as hemothorax, pneumothorax, cardiac contusions, as well as fractures of the spine, clavicle, rib, and humerus.[377,540]

Diagnosis and Classification

Scapular fractures typically are discovered during the evaluation of the multiply injured patient. In the rare case where the scapular fracture is the initially identified fracture, a complete trauma evaluation should be undertaken for head, chest, abdominal, and retroperitoneal injuries. If suspicion is high, a general trauma evaluation may be requested. Conversely, scrutiny for fractures of the scapula should be included in the evaluation of the multiply traumatized child.

Imaging Studies. Most scapular injuries are identified initially on the AP chest radiograph from a trauma series. However, AP and lateral radiographs of the scapula will facilitate detection of fractures not evident on the AP chest view, as well as allowing better description of the fracture pattern. In addition to these, other special radiographic views can aid in fracture characterization. The Stryker notch view, for example, better reveals coracoid fractures, whereas the axillary lateral view is better suited to identify glenoid fractures. The axillary lateral view also is helpful in confirming the location of the humeral head with the glenoid. When available, CT with three-dimensional reconstruction provides the most detailed representation of scapular anatomy. In addition, CT is essential in characterizing intra-articular injuries of the glenoid.

In high-energy trauma, the AP chest radiograph should also be scrutinized for evidence of scapulothoracic dissociation. Scapulothoracic dissociation typically occurs in patients with massive, direct trauma to the chest or proximal upper extremity and is highly associated with ipsilateral neurovascular injury.[150,471] This devastating injury should be suspected if the medial border of the scapula is displaced laterally, if there is a clavicular fracture with a large displacement, or if there is a complete AC joint separation with large displacement.[11,428]

Developmental variations in scapular anatomy may confuse radiographic interpretation. For example, os acromiale is commonly mistaken for an acute fracture. This variation occurs when the centers of ossification in the acromion fail to unite.[99] Os acromiale is considered a normal variant, is present in 10% of normal shoulders, and is bilateral in 60% of affected individuals.[11,335] Typically, os acromiale is located in the anterior and inferior aspect of the distal acromion and has a smooth and uniform appearance on radiographs. Occasionally os acromiale is symptomatic. If radiographic studies and clinical examination cannot distinguish between a fracture and a developmental variation, further evaluation with a bone scan may clarify the diagnosis.[150] Other variants in scapular anatomy include Sprengel's anomaly, absent acromion, bipartite or tripartite acromion, bipartite coracoid, and coracoid duplication.[99,290,375,430,483]

Classification. Multiple classification systems for scapular fractures have been reported. Many are descriptive and based primarily on the anatomic location of fracture. Ada and Miller[4] divided scapular fractures into categories of acromion, spine, coracoid, neck, glenoid, and body. In their series of children and adults, fractures occurred most often in the body (35%), followed by the neck (27%); fractures of the coracoid were least common (7%).[4] Thompson et al.[540] classified scapular fractures into three broad anatomic locations: fractures of the glenoid and the glenoid neck, fractures of the acromion and the coracoid, and fractures of the body (Fig 17-9). Other anatomic location-based scapular classifications have been reported by Imatani[261] and by Wilbur and Evans.[583]

The classification described below is also based on the anatomic location of the fracture, with additional subclassifications based on multiple reported studies (see Fig. 17-9 and Table 17-3). However, most of these studies are not specific for pediatric scapular fractures, so application of this classification system and its supportive studies to pediatric scapular fractures should be individualized to each child. The fracture should be adequately evaluated for its anatomic location, displacement, comminution, and articular involvement. In addition, ipsilateral neurovascular status, the overall status of the patient, and other concomitant injuries should be fully characterized.

Fractures of the body and the spine of the scapula, which make up nearly 50% of all scapular fractures, are broadly categorized into those with and without displacement. Although an isolated fracture of the scapular neck is believed to be a stable bony construct, ipsilateral fractures to both the scapular neck and the clavicle may lead to disruption of the suspensory mechanism of the shoulder.[202,330] Therefore, fractures of the scapular neck are categorized into those with and without concomitant

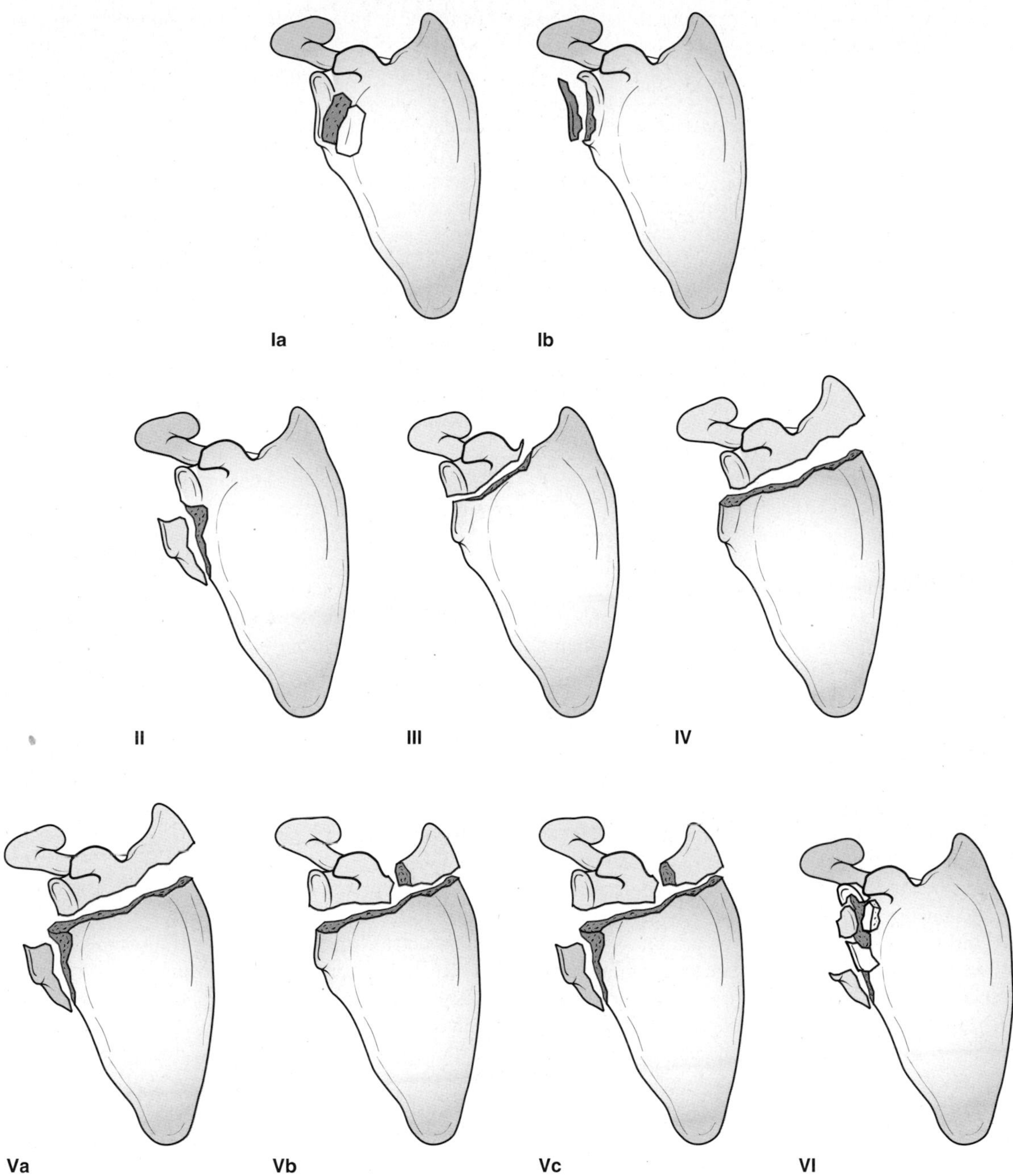

FIGURE 17-9 General classification of scapular/glenoid fractures.

TABLE 17-3 Interventions for Scapular Fractures

	Immobilization	Operative Reduction and Immobilization	Operative Reduction and Internal Fixation
Body of scapula	X		
Acromion	X		X
Glenoid rim/fossa	X		X
Scapula–thoracic dissociation	X	X	

injury to the clavicle. For similar considerations, fractures of the coracoid process are categorized into those with and without concomitant injury to the AC joint.

Fractures of the acromion are categorized into those with and without displacement. Displaced fractures are further subclassified based on the presence or absence of subacromial narrowing. Subacromial space narrowing may occur after inferior displacement of the acromion or after superior displacement of an ipsilateral glenoid fracture. When treated conservatively, these fracture patterns often lead to subacromial impingement in adults and result in decreased range of shoulder motion and increased shoulder pain.[305] Although its applicability to acromial fractures in younger children is still debated, this finding significantly affects the treatment options for acromial fractures in older children.

Fractures of the glenoid typically occur when the humeral head is driven onto the glenoid fossa. Depending on the direction of the force applied to the humeral head, the fracture may involve the entire fossa or just the rim. If the entire fossa is involved, the fracture line may then exit in multiple locations about the scapula. Hence, fractures of the glenoid are classified into five distinct groups based on their anatomic location and course of the fracture. This system was initially proposed by Ideberg[257,258] and later expanded by Goss.[201] Type I fractures are isolated glenoid rim fractures, with Ia involving the anterior rim and Ib involving the posterior rim. Type II, III, and IV fractures are glenoid fractures with fracture lines exiting through lateral, superior, and medial aspects of the scapula, respectively. Type V fractures are various combinations of type II, III, and IV fractures. Type Va, for example, is a combination of types II and IV. Type Vb is a combination of types III and IV, whereas type Vc is a combination of types II, III, and IV. Type VI fractures are comminuted fractures of the glenoid fossa. These various types of glenoid fractures are associated with distinct patterns of morbidity and treatment options.

Scapulothoracic dissociation occurs when all attachments or articulations between the thorax and the scapula are completely severed. When there is an ipsilateral neurovascular injury, it is sometimes referred to as a forequarter amputation. This is in contrast to scapulothoracic dislocation, where only the inferior scapulothoracic articulation is displaced.[150] Although intrathoracic dissociations have been reported,[406] scapulothoracic dissociations are typically laterally displaced. These injuries are categorized as open or closed with intact or compromised neurovascular status.

Surgical and Applied Anatomy

During development, the scapula forms in the first trimester of gestation. It first appears near the level of lower cervical spine, C4–C7, and then descends to its final position on the lateral aspect of the upper thorax during development. Most of the scapula is formed by intramembranous ossification. Numerous centers of ossification exist for the scapula: three for the body, two for the coracoid process, two to five for the acromion,[99] and one for the glenoid. These ossification centers during childhood are often mistakenly identified as fractures. In some developmental anomalies, distinct ossification centers fail to fuse and persist into adulthood.[375] These conditions are also frequently characterized as fractures. With few exceptions, however, a developmental variation and a fracture can be distinguished by clinical history, physical examination, and radiographic appearance.

The scapula is roughly triangular and has a complex three-dimensional structure. It is responsible for linking the upper extremity to the axial skeleton and contains attachments to 17 distinct muscles. The anterior aspect of the scapular body is a relatively flat surface, most of which is covered by the subscapularis muscle. The posterior aspect of the scapula is divided into two fossae by the scapular spine. These superior and inferior scapula fossae are mostly covered by the supraspinatus and the infraspinatus muscles, respectively. The anteromedial border of the scapular body provides attachment to the serratus anterior muscle. The posteromedial border contains the attachment sites of the levator scapulae, rhomboideus major and minor, and latissimus dorsi muscles. The omohyoid muscle attaches to the superior aspect of the scapular body, whereas the teres minor and major muscles and the triceps muscle attach to the lateral border. The scapular spine provides attachments to the trapezius and deltoid muscles, and the long head of the biceps muscle originates from the superior rim of the glenoid. Finally, the pectoralis minor muscle, as well as the conjoined tendon of the coracobrachialis and short head of the biceps muscles, attach to the coracoid process.

In addition to these muscle attachments, the scapula participates in the formation of both glenohumeral and AC joints. The glenohumeral joint is stabilized by multiple dynamic and static forces about the joint, which are discussed separately. The AC joint is stabilized in part by the presence of two coracoclavicular ligaments that position the distal clavicle immediately medial to the acromion. The two ligaments are the conoid and the trapezoid ligaments, with the conoid being the more medial of the two.

In close proximity to the scapula are a number of neurovascular structures that can be injured during a scapular fracture. Most notable are the brachial plexus and the axillary artery, which course across the anterosuperior aspect of the scapula. They are immediately posterior and inferior to the tip of the coracoid process. Medial to the base of the coracoid process is the scapular notch with the overlying transverse scapular ligament. The suprascapular nerve and artery pass under and over the ligament, respectively, in the scapular notch and are susceptible to injury with nearby fractures. The axillary nerve travels within an intermuscular interval immediately inferior to the glenoid and is also susceptible to injury with displaced fractures of the glenoid neck.[376]

A traumatic insult may cause fractures in multiple locations about the scapula, with one fracture influencing the stability of another. Goss[202] proposed this and subsequently introduced the concept of a SSSC. The SSSC is a set of bony struts attached to a circular complex of structures at the lateral end of the scapula (Fig. 17-10). The superior and inferior bony struts are the middle clavicle and the lateral scapula body/spine, respectively. The circular complex is composed of the AC ligament, acromion, glenoid process, coracoid process, coracoclavicular ligament, and distal clavicle. As a whole, the SSSC is responsible for linking the upper extremity to the axial skeleton. Traumatic injury to any single component of the SSSC may result in a minimally displaced fracture because the inherent stability of the circular complex is still intact. However, when multiple structures of the circular complex are injured, a double disruption to the circle occurs. This, in turn, results in significant

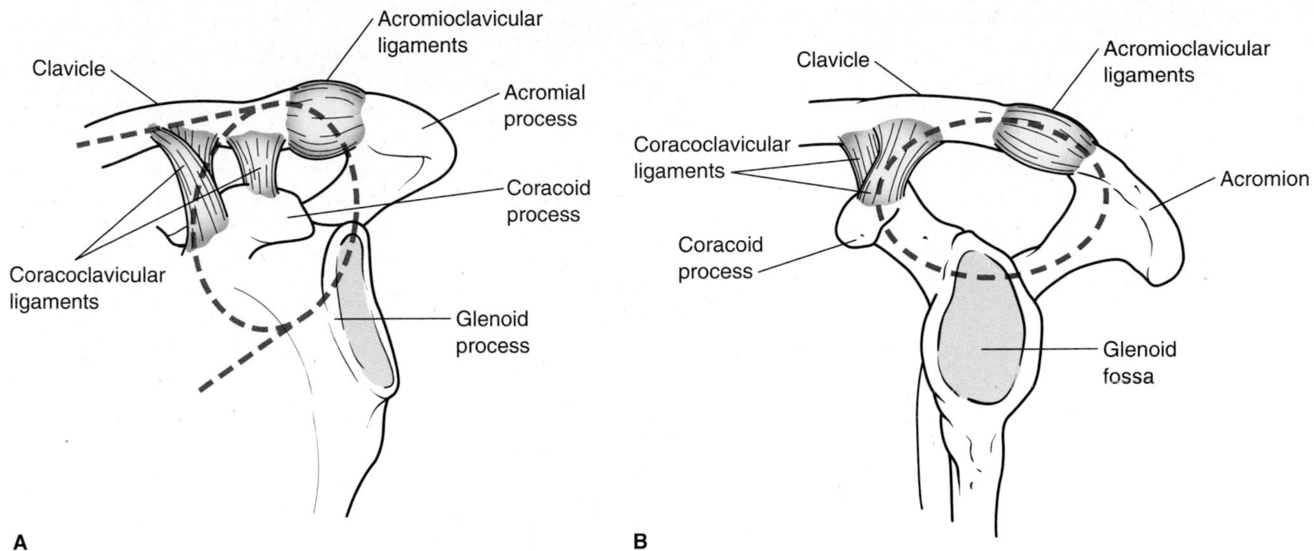

FIGURE 17-10 Superior shoulder suspensory complex. **A.** AP view of the bone–soft tissue ring and superior and inferior bone struts. **B.** Lateral view of the bone–soft tissue ring.

instability. Similarly, injury to one of the structures of the ring complex with a concomitant injury to a bony strut also may create an unstable construct. Goss[202] proposed that the treatment decisions for scapular injuries should be based on the maintenance of SSSC integrity.

Current Treatment Options

There are few published studies to provide evidence-based recommendations regarding current treatment options for scapular fractures in children. Therefore, most of the following comments are inferred from studies of adult populations.

Isolated fractures of the scapular body do not affect the integrity of the SSSC. In addition, because of the numerous muscle attachments, fractures of the scapular body are quite stable and can be treated conservatively in most cases (see Table 17-3). Several studies have shown that conservative treatment of nondisplaced or minimally displaced scapular body fractures in adults is generally associated with excellent results. Based on these studies, similar treatment is recommended for equivalent fractures in the pediatric population.[261,410,471,488] In adults, conservative treatment of scapular body fractures with significant displacement of more than 10 mm, however, resulted in unfavorable outcomes.[410] Since a comparable study of pediatric scapular body fractures has not yet been reported, we can only assume that widely displaced fractures in children would have a similarly poor long-term outcome. The threshold for acceptable displacement has not been described. A closed reduction of an angulated, greenstick fracture of the scapula mimicking scapular winging has been reported which yielded satisfactory results.[58]

Nondisplaced or mildly displaced scapular neck fractures without concomitant injury to the clavicle can be treated conservatively.[341] However, if there is also ipsilateral clavicular injury, surgical intervention generally is recommended to re-establish the SSSC.[4,240,330,401] Whether open reduction and fixation of the clavicle is sufficient to stabilize the fracture[240] or whether the neck fracture also must be reduced in addition to the clavicle[330] is debatable. For patients in whom surgical intervention is not possible, external fixation or traction may be an acceptable option.[134]

Fractures of the coracoid process typically occur at the base. Isolated fractures of the coracoid process usually are nondisplaced and can be treated conservatively with a sling and mobilization as tolerated. Displaced coracoid fractures occur with ipsilateral injury to the distal clavicle or the AC joint. Most investigators favor open reduction and internal fixation of these fractures to restore the integrity of the SSSC.[390,471,583] Displaced coracoid fractures near the suprascapular notch with injury to the suprascapular nerve also have been described, with some investigators advocating early exploration.[402]

Isolated fractures of the acromion in children are typically nondisplaced. In adults, acromial fractures with subacromial narrowing are associated with subsequent development of subacromial impingement when treated nonsurgically.[305] Therefore, most investigators recommend open reduction and internal fixation for displaced acromial fractures where the subacromial space has been compromised,[305] or with another disruption in the SSSC.[202]

Fractures of the glenoid neck typically are nondisplaced unless other elements of the SSSC are disrupted. These fractures generally have excellent outcomes with nonsurgical treatment. Significant displacement or angulation, however, may limit glenohumeral motion.[134,410] In adults, glenoid neck fractures with more than 10 mm of displacement or 40 degrees of angulation result in poor outcomes when treated without surgical reduction.[4] Therefore, it is reasonable to infer that pediatric glenoid neck fractures with significant displacement or angulation also require surgical intervention.

Treatment of glenoid rim fractures (types I and II) is based on the presence or absence of shoulder instability. Immobilization treatment of asymptomatic glenoid rim fractures rarely results in long-term morbidity.[601] For glenoid rim fractures with resulting shoulder subluxation or instability, however, operative reduction and fixation are recommended to prevent permanent or recurrent dislocations.[134,214,221] In adults, shoulder instability occurs when the fracture was displaced more than 10 mm or when the fracture involved more than either 25% of the anterior or 33% of the posterior aspects of the glenoid.[134] Anterior and posterior approaches to the glenoid generally are recommended for open reduction and internal fixation of anterior and posterior rim fractures, respectively.[202]

Nondisplaced glenoid fossa fractures (types III through VI) also can be successfully treated nonsurgically.[202] Displaced fractures, on the other hand, are associated with significant morbidity (pain, stiffness, and limited range of motion) when treated without surgical reduction. Patients with intra-articular displacement greater than 5 mm should be considered for surgical reduction and fixation.[134,323,519] In type IV glenoid fractures, where significant comminution is present, acceptable operative reduction and fixation may be difficult to achieve, and these fractures may be better treated with nonsurgical options.[202,258] For open reduction and internal fixation of these fractures, a posterior approach generally provides the most acceptable exposure.[202]

Initial treatment of scapulothoracic dissociations generally focuses on stabilization and repair of the neurovascular injury. If the axillary artery and the brachial plexus are not salvageable, an early amputation should be considered.[428] Limb salvage is usually attempted if limb viability cannot be determined. Immediate exploration of the brachial plexus is warranted when a concomitant vascular injury requires an operative repair. If a vascular injury is not present, the brachial plexus need not be explored acutely. After a period of 4 to 6 weeks, the extent of the brachial plexus injury should be documented (physical examination, electromyography/nerve conduction velocity, magnetic resonance imaging [MRI]) prior to surgical reconstruction, such as nerve repair or musculotendinous transfer.[202,428] Immediate operative stabilization of an ipsilateral clavicular fracture generally is necessary only if the bony instability compromises the integrity of the neurovascular structures.

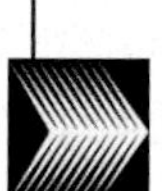

AUTHORS' PREFERRED TREATMENT

Once the patient is stabilized, the approach to the scapula or glenoid fractures can be undertaken more thoroughly. With rare exception, scapula fractures are treated without surgery. Fractures of the glenoid generally are treated with observation and follow-up, including physical therapy and rehabilitation. For the rare displaced glenoid intra-articular and highly displaced fractures, open reduction with internal fixation is recommended.[108] This is generally performed via an anterior deltopectoral approach, but posterior approaches to the scapula and glenoid may be necessary depending on the fracture type.

Intrathoracic dislocation is rare. Most can be reduced by closed manipulative methods. In those associated with residual scapular deformity, an open approach may be required. With scapulothoracic disassociation, it is important to attend to the priorities of trauma care, including an appropriate and detailed neurovascular examination. Vascular consultation or evaluation may be required, given the potential for massive injury to the brachial artery or plexus. In these instances, early or late amputation should be considered.

Pearls and Pitfalls

- Suspect scapula fractures in patients with multiple trauma and scrutinize the radiographs.
- Maintain a high index of suspicion for visceral injuries when a scapula body fracture presents as an isolated injury.
- Be aware of normal variants in scapular anatomy, such as os acromiale. Review radiographs of the contralateral scapula if necessary.
- Look for radiographic evidence of scapulothoracic dissociation.
- Most scapula fractures are managed without surgery.
- Highly displaced scapula body fractures and glenoid fossa fractures require open reduction and internal fixation.

Complications

Early Complications

Complications of scapular fractures are rare. The concomitant injuries frequently associated with scapular fractures were discussed throughout this section.[11,261,471,540] Due to their proximity, the axillary and the suprascapular nerves may be injured in association with glenoid and coracoid fractures, respectively.[376,402] In addition, the energy required to create scapular fractures likely results in other injuries, such as rib fractures, pneumothorax, and vascular avulsions. All or portions of the lower brachial plexus are susceptible to injury with scapulothoracic dissociations.[150,428,483] This devastating injury also has been associated with the development of compartment syndrome in the upper arm.[588] The presence of a complete brachial plexus avulsion is predictive of a poor functional outcome with a scapulothoracic dissociation.[597]

Late Complications

Late complications associated with scapular fractures generally involve improper functioning of the upper extremity. Displaced fractures of the scapular body and spine, for example, infrequently result in upper extremity weakness and pain with movement.[4] Similarly, fractures of the acromion can result in pain and decreased range of upper extremity motion secondary to subacromial impingement.[305] Displaced intra-articular fractures of the glenoid are associated with glenohumeral subluxation or dislocation, as well as early progression of degenerative arthritis.[134,214,202,221]

Symptomatic nonunion of scapula body fractures has been reported.[163,282] Most problems related to injuries of the scapula are not necessarily related to treatment but are more often related to failure to accurately evaluate associated major systems injuries.

GLENOHUMERAL SUBLUXATION AND DISLOCATION

Dislocation of the glenohumeral joint in healthy, skeletally immature children is rare. None of the ancient writings of Hippocrates (460–375 B.C.), Galen (A.D. 131–201), and Paul of Aegena (A.D. 625–690) made specific mention of this injury in children.[460] Most textbooks that address children's shoulder problems do not even discuss dislocations of the glenohumeral joint, and others merely touch on the subject.[54,440,453,504,537,573]

A review of the literature would suggest that traumatic glenohumeral dislocations in children less than 12 years of age are rare. Although several case reports have been presented, no large series of this entity are available.[227,237,337,565] In Rowe's[472] review of 500 dislocated shoulders, only 8 patients were under 10 years of age. In this same series, 99 patients were 10 to 20 years of age, but no details on skeletal maturity were given.[470,472] Rockwood[460] reported a series of 44 patients with shoulder dislocations, predominantly adolescents. Many articles have been published on adolescent patients without discussing their skeletal maturity.[197,371,389,416] As the child reaches adolescence, the incidence of shoulder instability increases, but in the skeletally immature patient, this injury can still be considered rare. However, Marans et al.,[365] in 1992, presented a series of 21 patients with open physes from two major trauma centers. The recent trend in highly competitive, organized youth sports may be a reason for the change. In addition, generalized ligamentous laxity is clearly an associative causative factor for glenohumeral instability in the young.

Principles of Management

Mechanism of Injury

Traumatic Dislocations. Significant evidence of trauma should be present to assign patients to this group, whereas patients who dislocate with relatively minor trauma should be assigned to the atraumatic group. The vast majority of traumatic dislocations are anterior. The mechanism of injury is similar to that observed in the adult. Typically, a force applied to the outstretched hand forces the arm and shoulder into a maximally abducted, externally rotated position. At this point, the humeral head is levered out of the glenoid process anteriorly, with the head lodging against the anterior neck of the glenoid. This occurs commonly in contact sports, falls, fights, and motor vehicle accidents.[51,247,392] A labral tear (Bankart lesion) and/or capsular stretch injury occurs, potentially with a compression injury to the humeral head (Hill-Sachs lesion).

Posterior dislocations are rare. In reported series of all age groups, posterior dislocations represent only 2% to 4% of all traumatic dislocations. The history for posterior dislocations is one of violent trauma with the arm in a position of flexion, internal rotation, and adduction. This can occur in falls and in motor vehicle accidents as the arm braces the body against impact. Other common mechanisms that produce posterior dislocations include convulsions and electroshock. In these cases, the shoulder is dislocated posteriorly by the violent contraction of the shoulder internal rotators, which normally are stronger than the shoulder external rotators. The history of the mechanism of injury and a high index of suspicion are necessary to avoid missing a posterior dislocation.[138,142,225,414,557]

In neonates, pseudodislocation of the shoulder can occur.[218] This problem represents traumatic epiphyseal separation of the proximal humerus, which is certainly much more common than a true traumatic dislocation of the shoulder in this age group. Most true traumatic dislocations of the shoulder in the neonatal period occur in babies with underlying birth trauma to the brachial plexus or central nervous system.

Laskin and Sedlin[320] reported on a 3-month-old infant with Erb-Duchenne palsy who sustained a traumatic luxatio erecta of the shoulder during a planned shoulder manipulation. Posterior dislocation of the shoulder also can occur as a secondary traumatic phenomenon in unrecognized brachial plexus injuries of the upper trunk at delivery.[23,339,581,582] Green and Wheelhouse[205] reported a dislocation in a 7.5-month-old infant that was secondary to a septic brain injury. Progressive posterior dislocation and glenohumeral deformity is extremely common in infants and children with chronic birth brachial plexopathy.

Atraumatic Dislocations. Atraumatic shoulder instability is common in children and adolescents. The child who presents with shoulder dislocation without a clear history of trauma should arouse suspicion that atraumatic instability may be present. These patients have inherent joint laxity that allows the shoulder to be dislocated either voluntarily or involuntarily as the result of a minimal traumatic event (Fig. 17-11).[87] For example, throwing, hitting an overhead tennis shot, or pushing the body up when in bed would not constitute significant trauma. These patients have multidirectional instability. In the individual who dislocates voluntarily, conscious selective firing of muscles while antagonists are inhibited, combined with arm positioning, allows the shoulder to dislocate. A key to the diagnosis is that atraumatic instability, whether voluntary or involuntary, is not associated with much pain. Even if reduction is necessary, the pain usually disappears rapidly. In most instances, spontaneous reduction occurs without manipulation.[460] In these cases, the use of conscious sedation or general anesthesia will often lead to reduction without manipulation.

Other causes of atraumatic shoulder instability, in addition to multidirectional joint laxity, include Ehlers-Danlos and Marfan's syndrome, congenital glenoid and/or humeral deformities, and emotional and psychiatric instability. True congenital dislocations of the shoulder are most commonly associated with developmental defects and multiple congenital abnormalities.[99,114,187,208,436] Arthrogryposis, neglected septic arthritis, and neurologic defects also have been implicated in atraumatic dislocations in the young child.[23,197,205,232,528,581]

Signs and Symptoms

Traumatic Dislocations. The patient with a traumatic anterior dislocation presents with a painful, swollen shoulder. Obvious deformity is present with a prominent acromion and flattening of the contour of the lateral upper arm. The arm is often supported by the contralateral hand and held in a slightly abducted and externally rotated position. Despite swelling, the humeral head can usually be palpated in a position anterior to the glenoid.

Careful examination of the neurologic and vascular status should be performed. The axillary nerve is the most commonly injured with anterior dislocation, and special attention to its function should be included in the physical examination.[53] The sensory distribution of the axillary nerve is along the upper lateral arm, and motor innervation is to the deltoid and teres minor muscles. Light touch is adequate for sensory testing in the upper arm region. A convenient way to test deltoid function is to support the involved elbow in one of the examiner's hands while using the examiner's opposite hand to palpate the muscle belly of the deltoid. The patient is asked to abduct the arm against resistance for about 1 inch so that deltoid firing is initiated. This examination confirms the motor function of the axillary nerve (Fig. 17-12).

In recurrent anterior dislocation or subluxation that has spontaneously reduced, the arm is well located with an overall normal appearance of the shoulder. The shoulder demonstrates a full range of motion, although the patient avoids the cocking position in abduction, external rotation. The apprehension test

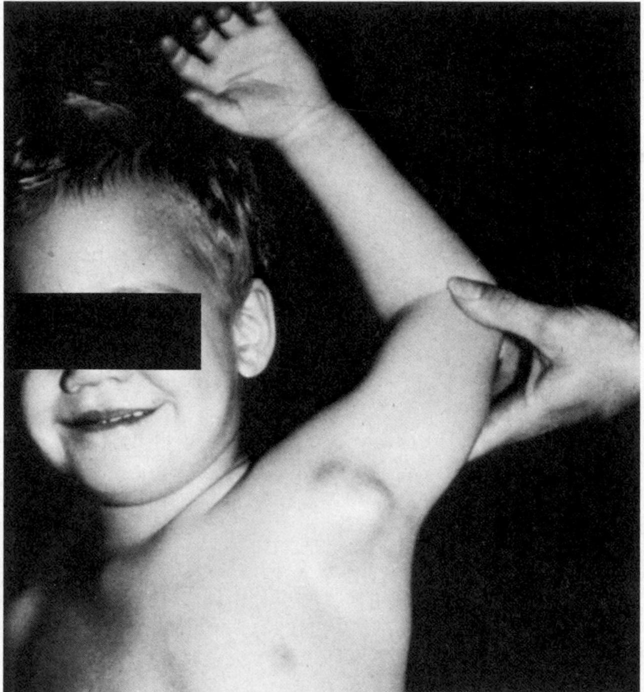

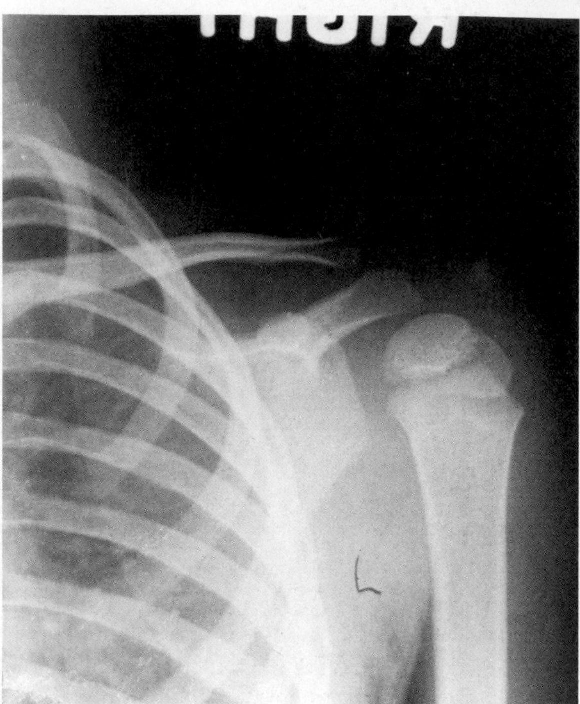

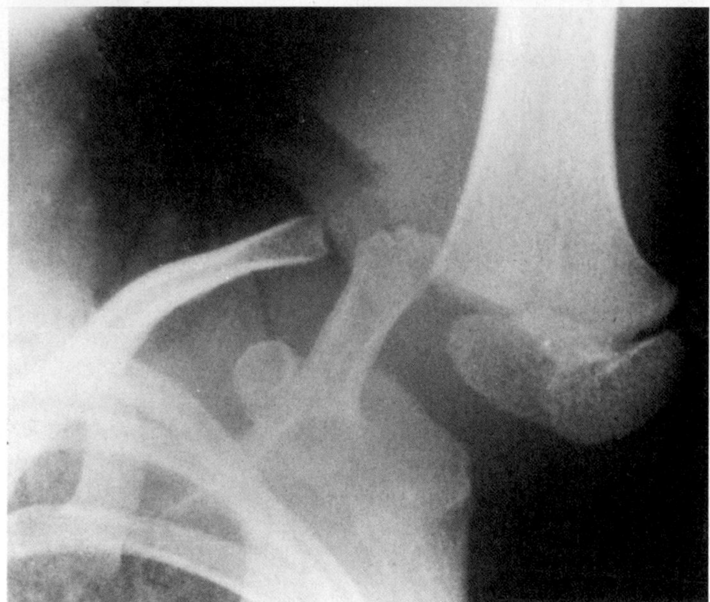

FIGURE 17-11 Congenital laxity of the left shoulder in a 4-year-old boy who is totally asymptomatic and has full range of motion of the left shoulder. **A.** With abduction and extension, the head subluxates anteriorly and inferiorly. **B.** An AP radiograph shows some lateral displacement of the humeral head. **C.** With overhead elevation, the humeral head is noted to displace anteriorly, laterally, and inferiorly. (Courtesy of Don Jones, MD.)

with the arm abducted above 90 degrees is positive. A positive apprehension test, along with a suggestive history, is a very diagnostic physical sign for recurrent anterior instability.

For the much less common traumatic posterior dislocation, an affected patient presents with flattening of the anterior aspect of the shoulder and posterior fullness. The arm is held at the side with the forearm internally rotated across the chest. A Putti sign with superior scapular winging is present. The patient resists any attempt at motion. Although difficult to elicit in the acute situation because of pain, hallmark findings of posterior dislocation are lack of shoulder external rotation and inability to supinate the forearm. It is advantageous to examine the shoulder with the patient seated so that the examiner can visualize the shoulders from above. From this perspective, posterior fullness and anterior flattening can be better visualized. As for anterior dislocations, the neurovascular status should be evaluated meticulously. A history of convulsion or electrical shock should raise the index of suspicion for posterior dislocation.

In neonates, traumatic separation of the upper humeral physis, the so-called pseudodislocation of the shoulder, can mimic an anterior dislocation. As is the case for true dislocations, the child is irritable and holds the affected arm abducted and externally rotated. There is resistance to any type of motion.

Atraumatic Dislocations. The most notable finding in patients with atraumatic shoulder instability is the relative lack of pain associated with the subluxation or dislocation.[15,128,288,321,362,473,511] Even in cases of involuntary atraumatic dislocation, the minor pain associated with the dislocation itself subsides rapidly after reduction. Episodes of atraumatic subluxation and disloca-

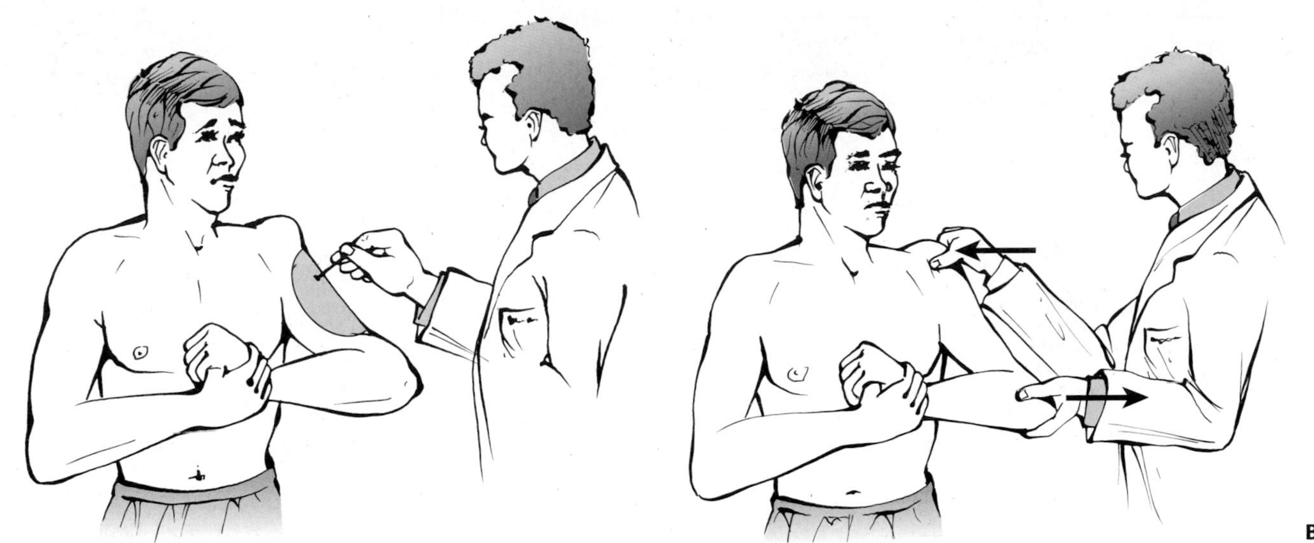

FIGURE 17-12 A. Sensory distribution for the axillary nerve important in anterior dislocation. **B.** Deltoid muscle can be tested in acute anterior dislocation by grabbing the muscle belly with the right hand while supporting the elbow with the left. The patient then can actively contract the deltoid by pushing the elbow against the examiner's hand while the examiner feels the muscle contraction.

tion occur much more frequently than traumatic dislocations, and in almost all cases spontaneous reduction is the rule.

On clinical examination, multidirectional laxity or instability of the contralateral shoulder is usually present.[416,460,461] In addition, there is evidence of laxity of multiple joints.[403] Characteristics of multiple joint laxity include hyperextension at the elbows, knees, and metacarpophalangeal joints along with pes planus. Striae of the skin can be present. Skin hyperelasticity is a noted characteristic of Ehlers-Danlos syndrome.

Multidirectional laxity of the shoulder is characterized by a positive sulcus sign and significant translation on an anterior and posterior drawer test. The sulcus sign is a dimpling of the skin below the acromion when manual longitudinal traction is applied to the arm (Fig. 17-13). This produces an inferior subluxation of the humeral head away from the acromion that enlarges the subacromial space and causes dimpling of the skin. The drawer or shift and load test is performed with the examiner seated behind the patient. The scapula is stabilized with one hand and forearm while the humeral head is manually translated anteriorly and posteriorly by the examiner's opposite hand (Fig. 17-14). Although some translation within the glenohumeral joint is expected in all patients, those with multidirectional laxity demonstrate translation of greater than 5 mm anteriorly and posteriorly from a neutral position.

In atraumatic dislocation, the shoulder often dislocates anteriorly, posteriorly, or inferiorly. The most common direction of dislocation in voluntary instability is posterior or inferior. The patient who can voluntarily dislocate the shoulder can force the humeral head posteriorly by contracting the anterior deltoid and internal rotators while inhibiting the antagonistic muscles (Fig. 17-15). The elbow is positioned in horizontal adduction, and the head is dislocated. The arm can then be abducted, and the shoulder reduces, often with an audible clunk.

Associated Injuries

Although any of the nerves that traverse the axilla may be injured at the time of a shoulder dislocation, the axillary nerve is the most common associated nerve injury. Fortunately, most axillary nerve injuries associated with dislocations are neurapraxic and recover spontaneously with time and observation. In the event of complete, unresolved axillary nerve palsy, significant disability can result due to the lack of deltoid function.[35,53,105,116,153,353]

Vascular injuries are rare, but either the axillary artery or vein can be traumatized. Morrison and Egan[393] reported an axillary artery and a brachial plexus injury in a luxatio erecta dislocation in an 11-year-old child. The artery was repaired with a vein graft and the brachial plexus injury fully recovered.

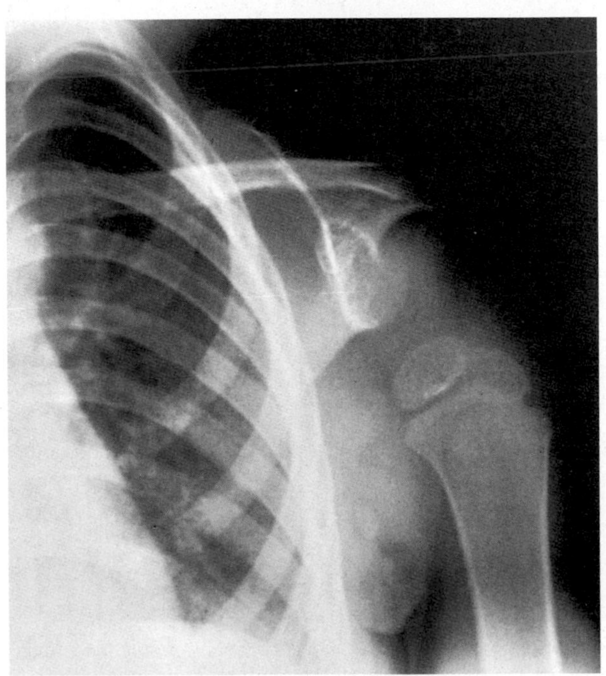

FIGURE 17-13 Dramatic demonstration of inferior subluxation of the glenohumeral joint in a patient with multidirectional instability. The clinical correlate is the sulcus sign.

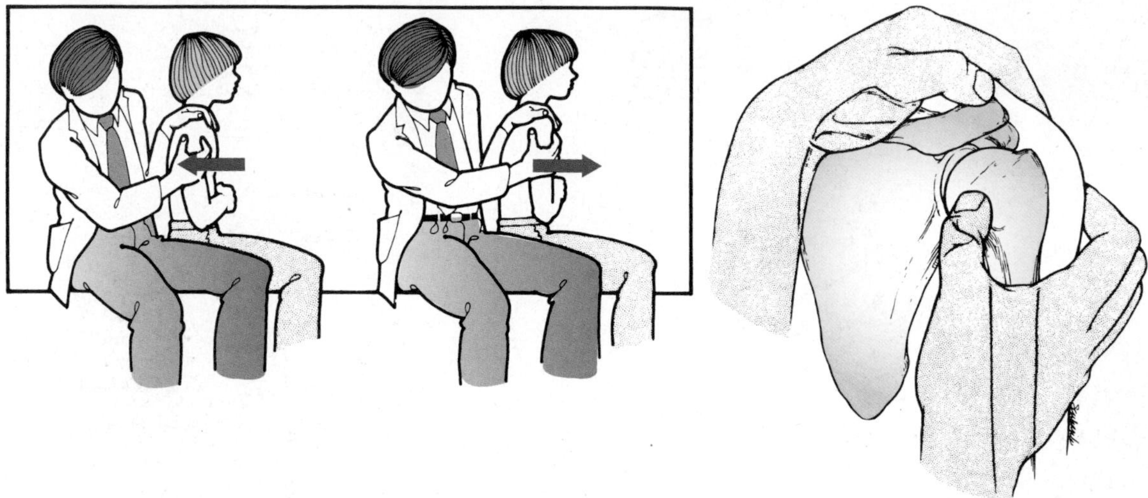

FIGURE 17-14 Drawer test. This technique is used to subluxate the shoulder manually both anteriorly and posteriorly to demonstrate multidirectional laxity.

Diagnosis and Classification

Radiographic Studies. Children and adolescents with open growth plates have a low incidence of true traumatic dislocation of the shoulder. Traumatic lesions on plain radiographs are similar to those found in adults (Fig. 17-16). On the AP or internally rotated views of the proximal humerus, the Hill-Sachs compression lesion on the posterolateral aspect of the humeral head is commonly found. This injury to the proximal humerus occurs as the humeral head is impacted against the anterior rim of the glenoid during a dislocation (Fig. 17-17). Bony injury to the anterior glenoid rim can occur with dislocation as well. Injury to the glenoid ranges from small avulsion-type fractures to substantial bony fractures. Anterior glenoid rim injuries are best seen as a double density on the AP view of the shoulder or as a separate fragment on the axillary and West Point lateral views. The West Point lateral view projects the anteroinferior glenoid rim and most clearly shows this lesion when it is present. In traumatic posterior dislocation, the reverse Hill-Sachs lesion can be seen on the anterior part of the humeral head and in some cases will be seen in conjunction with fracture of the posterior rim of the glenoid.

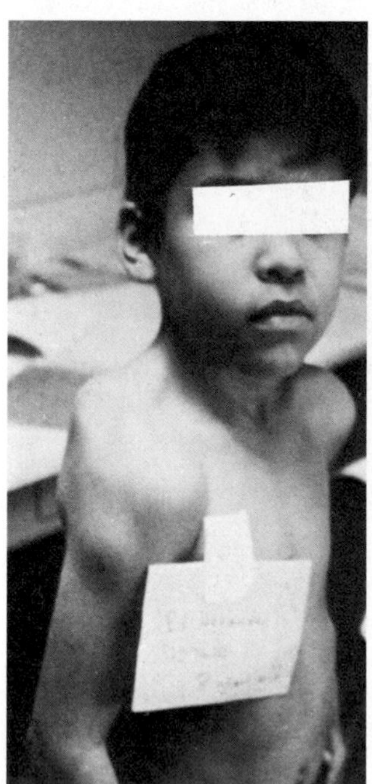

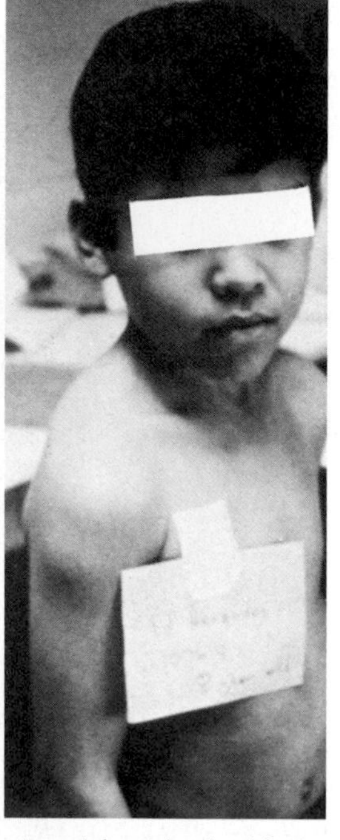

FIGURE 17-15 Voluntary anterior dislocation of the right shoulder in an 8-year-old boy. **A.** The patient voluntarily has dislocated the right shoulder anteriorly. **B.** The shoulder voluntarily reduced. The patient explained that he was taught to do this by an older brother who also had voluntary dislocation of the shoulders.

In cases of traumatic subluxation of the shoulder in which the diagnosis may be unclear clinically, an arthrogram with CT scan can sometimes better delineate the extent of capsular stripping from the anterior glenoid rim. More recently, saline arthrograms and contrast MRI scans have enhanced our ability to define the degree of injury to the labrum, capsule, and articular surfaces.[210,461] CT scanning and MRI are useful for analyzing the significance of fractures of the glenoid rim (Figs. 17-18 and 17-19). In addition, the size of the reverse Hill-Sachs lesion of the humeral head in posterior dislocations is best analyzed with a CT scan.[309,578]

With atraumatic dislocations in patients who do not have congenital or developmental defects, radiographs are usually normal. Among patients who do have congenital defects, the most common abnormality seen on radiographs is hypoplasia or aplasia of the glenoid. In patients with multidirectional laxity and atraumatic dislocation, stress radiographs can usually show instability in anterior, posterior, and inferior directions. The inferior component of multidirectional instability can be demonstrated by applying weights to the arm in an AP film. If laxity is present, this stress view will show the humeral head subluxating inferiorly in its relation to the glenoid.[269] In diagnostic dilemmas, contrast-injected MRI scans can define the presence of labral pathology which will aid in surgical decisions.

Classification. The following scheme is useful for the classification of shoulder dislocation based on etiology:

1. Traumatic dislocations.
   a. Primary trauma to the shoulder itself

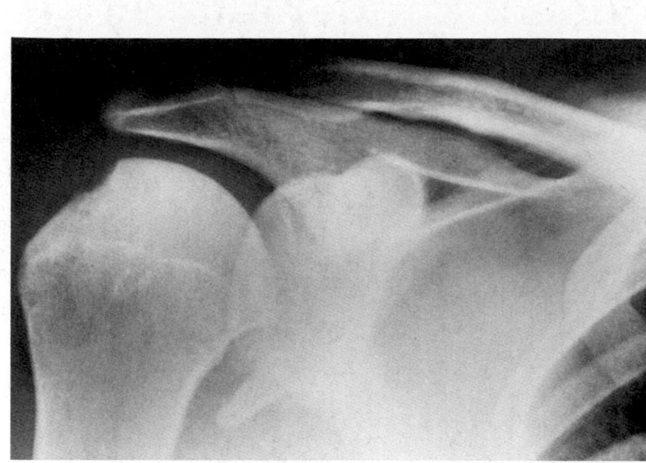

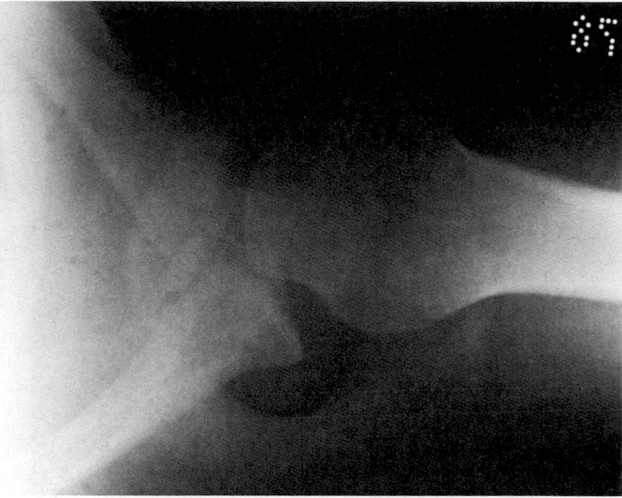

FIGURE 17-16 Traumatic anterior dislocation of the right shoulder in a 15-year-old boy. **A.** On the AP view, note the Hill-Sachs lesion as well as the anteroinferior bony fragment off the glenoid rim. **B.** Axillary radiograph made with the arm in 90 degrees of abduction demonstrates the anterior subluxation as well as the deficiency of the anterior glenoid rim.

   b. Secondary to birth trauma of the brachial plexus or central nervous system
2. Atraumatic dislocations—voluntary or involuntary
   a. Congenital abnormalities or deficiencies of bone or soft tissue
   b. Hereditary joint laxity problems, such as Ehlers-Danlos syndrome
   c. Developmental joint laxity problems
   d. Emotional and psychiatric disturbances

The above etiologic classification is commonly used in adults, but no consensus exists as to a classification scheme in children and adolescents.

Shoulder instability can be classified as to direction, degree, and chronicity. Two basic schemes have been used to classify shoulder dislocations in children and adolescents. The more common of these is based on the direction or location of the dislocation. Although this scheme is useful in describing the clinical and radiographic features of the injury, it does not address the underlying pathology in children and adolescents.[460] Therefore, a second classification scheme describing the etiology of the dislocation is also useful when considering treatment options for this injury in children. This second system is similar to that used for adults but takes into account the rare congenital and developmental problems unique to children. As discussed later in the section on treatment of this problem, accurate classification is important in selecting the appropriate conservative versus surgical options.[21,125,421]

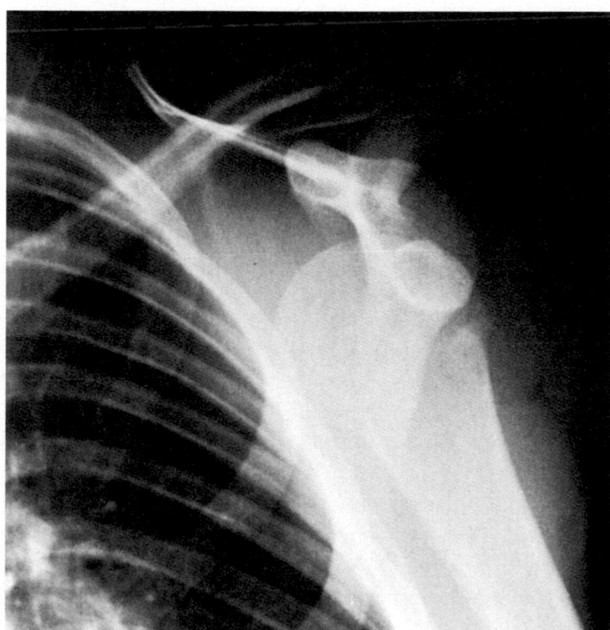

FIGURE 17-17 AP radiograph of anterior shoulder dislocation in a skeletally immature adolescent patient.

The directional classification has four categories: anterior, posterior, inferior (luxatio erecta), and multidirectional. As in adults, anterior dislocation in children and adolescents is the most common, constituting at least 90% of glenohumeral dislocations (Fig. 17-20). Several isolated reports of posterior dislocation in children and adolescents have been documented, but traumatic posterior dislocation is rare in children, as in adults.[60,168,237,372] Luxatio erecta or an inferior locked dislocation is uncommon but has been reported in children.[174,320,380] Multidirectional luxatio of the shoulder has been well described as a distinct clinical entity by Burkhead and Rockwood,[80] O'Driscoll and Evans,[416] and Rockwood.[460,461]

The degree of instability can be classified as a subluxation or a dislocation. A subluxation is an incomplete dislocation characterized by pain, a feeling of slipping, or a dead feeling in the arm. A complete dislocation of the humeral head out of the glenoid fossa is characterized by a displacement and locking of the head on the rim of the glenoid.

The chronicity of instability can be classified as acute, recurrent, or chronic. A single episode of instability can be described as an acute injury. As in the skeletally mature patient, an acute injury can lead to a recurrent instability, depending on the damage to the labral, capsule and ligaments, and bony restraints of the joint. A chronic instability exists when an acute dislocation

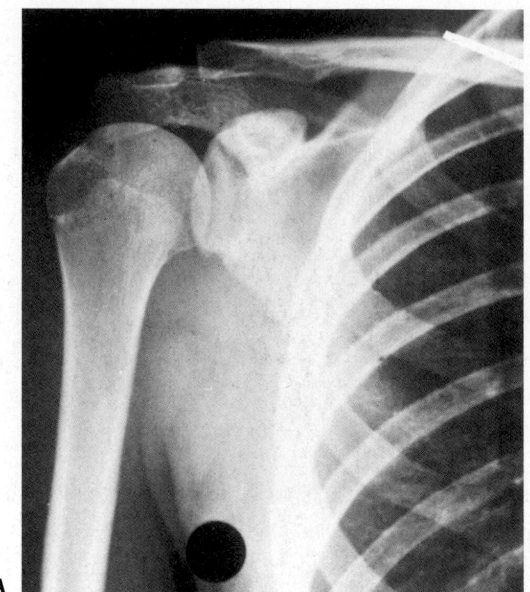

A

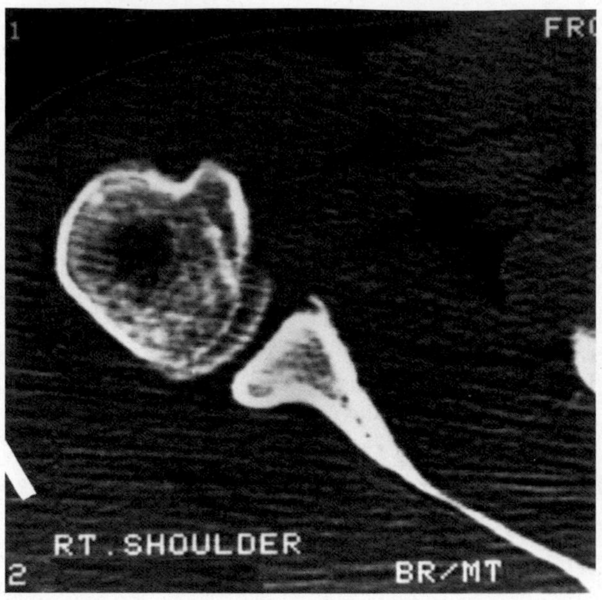

B

FIGURE 17-18 A. AP radiograph of a 14-year-old boy with recurrent anterior subluxation. Notice the presence of a Hill-Sachs compression fracture on the humeral head and a subtle double density at the anteroinferior glenoid rim. **B.** CT scan shows this to be an avulsion-type bony injury of the anterior glenoid.

is not reduced, and in children, is usually associated with congenital or neuropathic dislocations.

Surgical and Applied Anatomy

Developmental bony and physeal anatomy is discussed in the section on fractures of the proximal humerus. The glenohumeral joint consists of the articulation between the large convex humeral head and the relatively flat, concave glenoid fossa. Since there is very little bony constraint inherent to the glenohumeral joint, this joint is anatomically suited to accommodate the wide range of motion necessary to perform upper extremity function. The articular surface area and radius of curvature of the humeral head are about three times that of the relatively flat glenoid surface. Although the glenoid fossa is deepened by the labrum, the mismatch in the surface area and the radius of curvature explains the relative lack of joint stability.

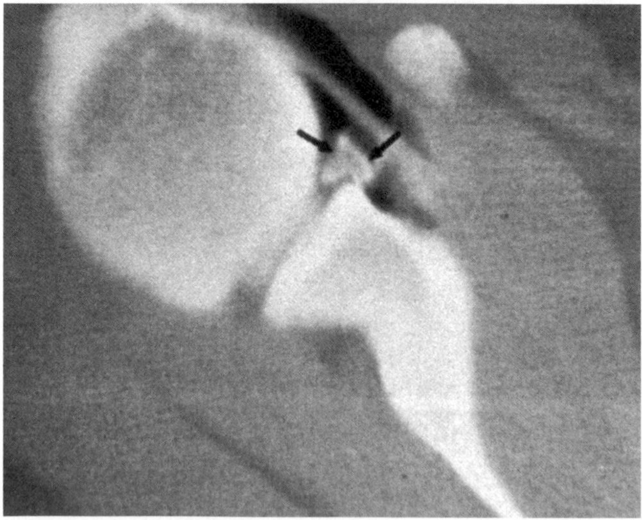

FIGURE 17-19 MRI in a patient with recurrent anterior instability of the shoulder. The arrows demonstrate a calcified bony Bankart lesion.

The primary constraint for the glenohumeral joint is the capsular/ligamentous complex. The capsule on its inner surface is reinforced by thickened areas known as the anterior glenohumeral ligaments. This complex capsular/ligamentous structure must provide stability against abnormal translation while allowing a wide range of motion. With the arm abducted, the inferior capsule is highly redundant. The most important ligament is the anteroinferior glenohumeral ligament, located within the inferior redundant area. It is mechanically designed to tighten as the arm is abducted and externally rotated, much like the effect of wringing out a washcloth. This structure becomes the primary site of pathology in anterior shoulder instability, either when the anteroinferior glenohumeral ligament attachment to the glenoid and labrum is stripped from the anterior neck of the glenoid or as these ligaments are disrupted in midsubstance (Fig. 17-21). Disruption of the capsular labral attachment is known as a Perthes or Bankart lesion.

The humeral attachment of the capsule of the glenohumeral joint is along the anatomic neck of the humerus except medially, where the attachment is more distal along the shaft. The physis, therefore, lies in an extracapsular position except on the medial side. As in most pediatric joint injuries, the strong capsular attachment to the epiphysis makes failure through the physis a much more common injury than true capsular/ligamentous injury.[125,293,551] Therefore, fracture through the physis is more common than a dislocation in the skeletally immature patient.

The rotator cuff muscles consist of the subscapularis, supraspinatus, infraspinatus, and teres minor. These muscle–tendon units surround the joint anteriorly, superiorly, and posteriorly. They serve an important function as dynamic secondary stabilizers of the joint by forming a force-couple with the large shoulder muscles (deltoid, pectoralis major, teres major, and latissimus dorsi). As the glenohumeral joint moves through its range of motion, the cuff provides a dynamic stabilizing effect, prevent-

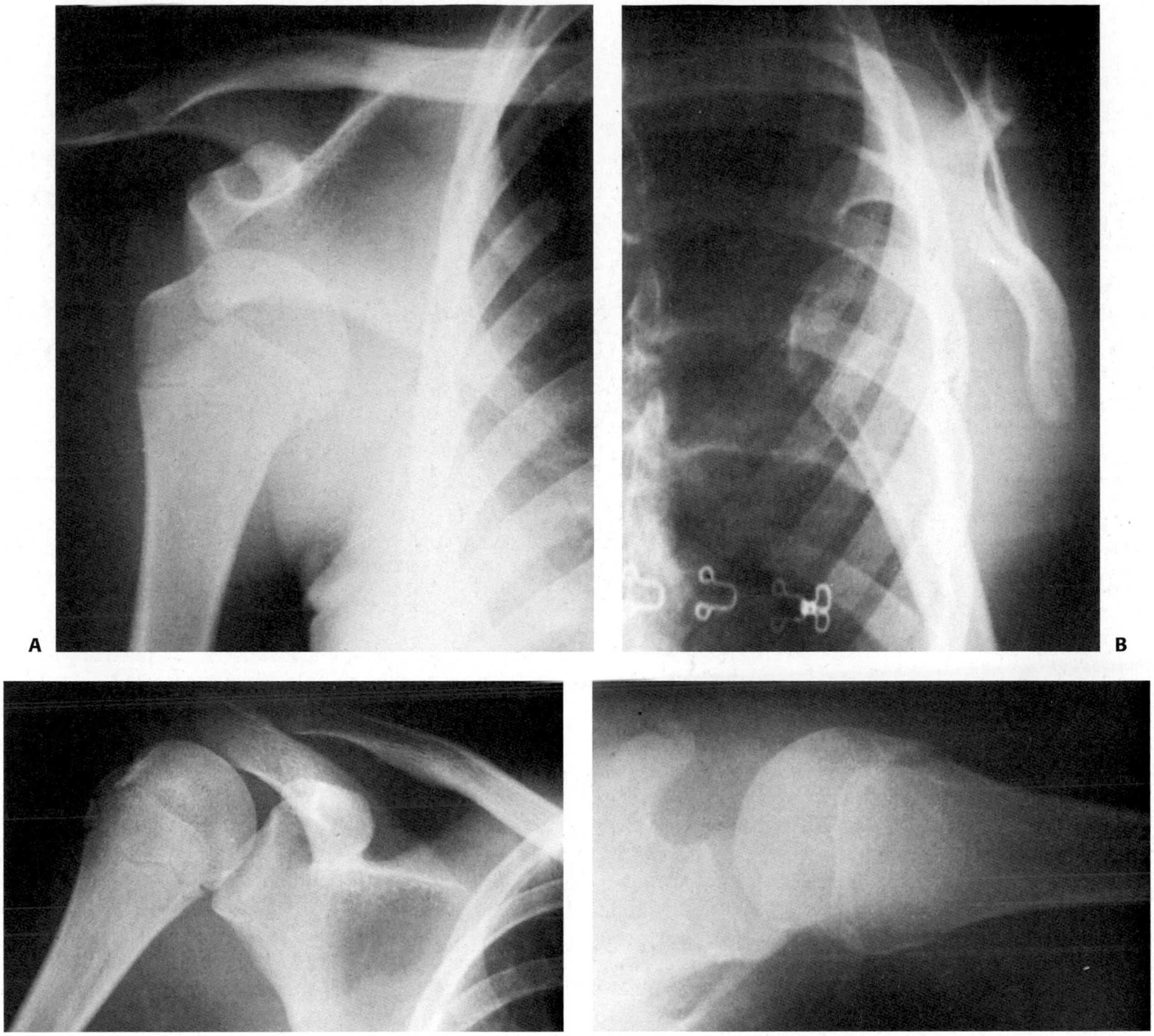

FIGURE 17-20 Anterior dislocation of the right shoulder in a 15-year-old girl. **A.** Note the typical subcoracoid position on the AP film. **B.** On a true scapular lateral film, note the anterior displacement of the humeral head. **C.** Postreduction film demonstrates a Hill-Sachs compression fracture in the posterolateral aspect of the humeral head. **D.** On the postreduction axillary film, note the posterolateral compression fracture of the humeral head.

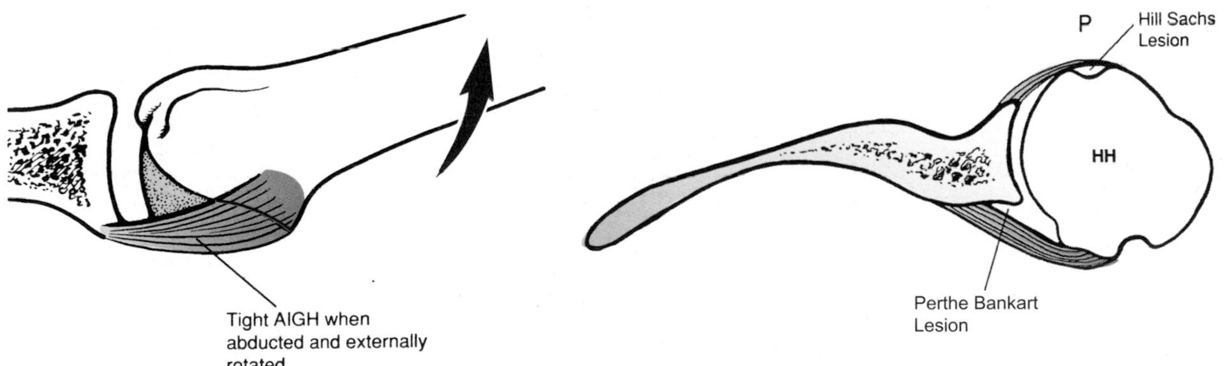

FIGURE 17-21 A. The tight anteroinferior glenohumeral ligament complex with the arm abducted and externally rotated. This ligament sling is the primary restraint against anterior instability of the shoulder. **B.** A cross-section in the transverse plane through the glenohumeral joint demonstrates the common lesions associated with anterior instability of the shoulder: Hill-Sachs lesion, Perthes-Bankart lesion, and redundant anteroinferior glenohumeral ligaments. (HH, humeral head; P, posterior.)

ing excessive translation of the humeral head on the glenoid. In addition, the biceps and triceps as well as parascapular muscles are important dynamic stabilizers of the shoulder. This is important when addressing rehabilitation of acute and recurrent glenohumeral dislocation.

Current Treatment Options

Treatment options are listed in Table 17-4 as well as in the following text.

Traumatic Instability

The literature on the specific treatment of shoulder instability in skeletally immature children is limited.[21,104,453,537] Most clinicians make the same treatment recommendations based on the sustained injury, regardless of the patient's age.[1,18,36,51,136,284] The majority of treatment recommendations presented in this section are extrapolated from the adult and adolescent literature, as well as from the experience of Dameron and Rockwood.[125]

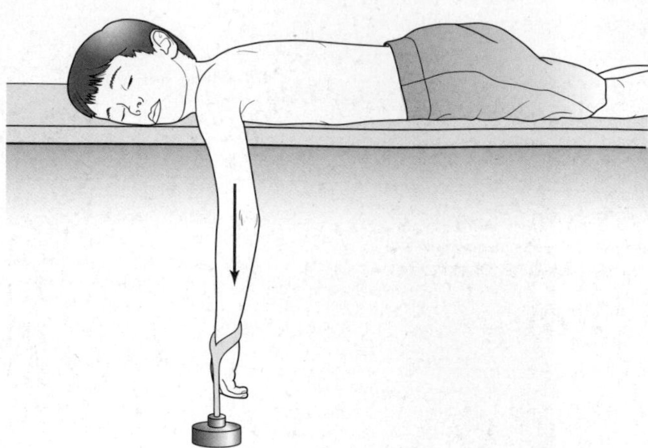

FIGURE 17-22 The Stimson technique for closed shoulder reduction. With the patient in prone position, weight is hung from the wrist to distract the shoulder joint. Eventually, with sufficient fatigue in the shoulder musculature, the joint can be easily reduced.

Acute Dislocation

Patients with acute dislocations of the shoulder should undergo closed reduction by one of the standard techniques. For anterior dislocation, many reduction techniques have been described. Most clinicians prefer light sedation with intravenous or intramuscular injection. The traction/countertraction method is believed to be the most gentle. A bed sheet placed in the axilla of the affected shoulder passes above and below the patient so that countertraction can be applied to the body while longitudinal traction in line with the deformity is applied to the arm. Steady, continuous traction fatigues the muscles that lock the dislocation, and eventually reduction is accomplished by disimpacting the humerus from the glenoid.

The Stimson maneuver is equally effective. In this technique, the patient is placed prone on the examination table. A weight is applied to the affected arm. As the shoulder girdle muscles relax, reduction is achieved atraumatically (Fig. 17-22).[389] Another less-often-practiced technique is scapular manipulation. Kothari and Dronen[301] and McNamara[379] report that this latter technique is a safe, effective way to reduce glenohumeral dislocations.

Postreduction immobilization remains a subject for debate. The adult literature suggests that the period of immobilization may not be truly important in predicting recurrent dislocation.

TABLE 17-4 Interventions for Glenohumeral Subluxation and Dislocation

	Closed Reduction and Immobilization	Operative Reconstruction
Traumatic—acute, anterior	X	X (less common)
Traumatic—acute, posterior	X	
Atraumatic	X	
Atraumatic—multidirectional	X	X—with caution, see text

A sling or a sling-and-swathe with the arm internally rotated is the most common method of immobilization.[18,135] However, a recent randomized trial noted that immobilization in external rotation may decrease the risk of recurrence when compared to immobilization in internal rotation.[265]

Closed reduction for acute posterior dislocations is somewhat similar to that for anterior dislocations. Traction/countertraction is the most effective method. Traction is applied in line with the deformity, and the humeral head is gently lifted back into its normal relationship with the glenoid. Most clinicians agree that immobilization should be with the arm in neutral rotation or slight external rotation at the shoulder. This may require the use of a spica cast or modified shoulder spica cast, as described by Dameron and Rockwood.[125]

Recurrent Dislocation

The true incidence of recurrent dislocation after traumatic shoulder dislocation in children is understandably poorly defined, given the rarity of reports in the pediatric orthopaedic literature.[187,249] In 1963, Rowe[470] reported a 100% incidence of recurrence in children 1 to 10 years of age with anterior dislocation. He also reported a 94% incidence of recurrence in adolescents and young adults (ages 11 to 20).[470] Elbaum et al.[153] reported a recurrence rate of 71% in 9 pediatric patients with traumatic anterior dislocations. The average age was 9 years. After reduction, they were immobilized for 3 weeks and then were treated with rehabilitation. However, Rockwood[460] reported a recurrence rate of only 50% in a series of adolescents and young adults 13.8 to 15.8 years of age. Hovelius et al.[249] reported a 47% recurrence rate in patients less than 20 years of age. In the 25 years following, it was found that half of the primary dislocations that had been treated nonoperatively in patients from 12 to 25 years old had not recurred or had surgical stabilization.[248,250] Furthermore, recurrent dislocation necessitating operative treatment had developed in 38% of shoulders in patients who were 12 to 25 years of age at the time of initial dislocation, compared with 18% in patients who were 26 to 40 years old. The type and duration of the initial treatment had no effect on the rate of recurrence. Vermeiren et al.[558] reported a recurrence rate of 68% in patients younger than 20 years of age. Younger patients involved in contact sports or who require overhead occupational use of the arm are more likely to have a redislocation when compared to older less active peers.[477] They reported a better prognosis if the dislocation was associated with a fracture of the joint. Heck[227] reported a case of traumatic anterior dislocation in a 7-year-old boy who remained stable at a 5-year follow-up. Endo et al.[155] reported no recurrence in 2 patients, ages 3 and 9, with traumatic anterior dislocation. However, the follow-up was only 2 years in the 3-year-old and 1 year in the 9-year-old. Wagner and Lyne[565] reported an 80% recurrence rate in 10 patients with clearly open proximal humeral epiphyses. Marans et al.[365] reported the fate of traumatic anterior dislocations of the shoulder in 21 children (15 boys, 6 girls) in what may be the largest documented series to date. All the children had one or more documented anterior dislocation(s) after the initial injury. Some of the children had been immobilized in a sling-and-swathe for 6 weeks. The literature reflects that the natural history of shoulder dislocations in adolescents and young adults demonstrates recurrence rates for dislocation of 50% to 90% despite the treatment program used after the initial dislocation.

Multiple surgical procedures have been described for the treatment of anterior shoulder instability. Once again, specific results for procedures such as the Putti-Platt, Bankart, and Magnuson-Stack have not been documented for children. Barry et al.[36] described the effective use of the coracoid transfer for recurrent anterior instability in adolescents. Capsular procedures that specifically address the capsular pathology have been described by Neer,[403] Jobe,[349] and Rockwood et al.,[461] but results in specifically in children's dislocations were not documented. Goldberg et al.[197] and Jones et al.[278] have reported on the use of arthroscopic techniques for capsular repair in adolescents. A meta-analysis at that time comparing open and arthroscopic repairs in the treatment of anterior shoulder instability found a significantly higher risk of recurrent instability, recurrent dislocation, and reoperation for arthroscopic repairs. However, arthroscopic repairs appeared to have a better functional result.[326] The keys to any surgical procedure is labral repair and appropriate capsular tightening. The trend is towards more arthroscopic repairs of the labrum and capsule.

Atraumatic Instability

Treatment of patients with atraumatic dislocations of the shoulder appears more difficult than treatment for true traumatic dislocations. Emphasis should be placed on careful diagnosis in these cases. Specific congenital bony or neurologic deficits should be recognized. The sequelae of Ehlers-Danlos syndrome or other collagen deficiency syndromes should be noted.

In patients with multidirectional laxity and voluntary or involuntary dislocations, a significant history of trauma is usually lacking. These patients have minimal pain associated with the dislocation and on clinical examination usually have other signs of multidirectional laxity of the opposite shoulder. Most of these dislocations reduce spontaneously and are associated with little pain. Rowe et al.,[473] Neer,[403] and Burkhead and Rockwood[80,460,461] have described the use of a vigorous rehabilitation program involving strengthening of the rotator cuff as the treatment of choice for these patients. Most patients who do not have significant emotional and psychiatric problems are reasonably successful over time in improving their shoulder stability with a program of scapular stabilization with dynamic muscle rebalancing and strengthening.

Most clinicians would agree that surgical intervention is considered only if a strict 6- to 12-month rehabilitation program fails. Shoulder reconstructions involving subscapularis shortening, including the Magnuson-Stack and Putti-Platt procedures, or "bone blocks" such as the Bristow are not sufficient for preventing future instability, and are rarely performed. Neer[403] described the inferior capsular shift reconstruction specifically for patients with multidirectional laxity of the shoulder with atraumatic instability. This procedure attempts to eliminate the overall capsular laxity and is used only after rehabilitation has failed. Huber and Gerber[254] reported on 25 consecutive children with 36 involved shoulders with voluntary subluxation of the shoulder. The children managed by "skillful neglect" had a satisfactory outcome, but only 50% of those treated with an operative procedure to prevent later degenerative arthritis had good results. They concluded that voluntary subluxation of the shoulder has a favorable result and that there is no indication for surgery with this problem in children.

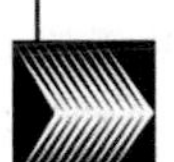

AUTHORS' PREFERRED TREATMENT

The initial challenge in managing shoulder dislocations in children is to establish whether the dislocation is traumatic or atraumatic in nature. A careful history of the mechanism of injury and physical examination designed to elicit evidence of multidirectional instability of the opposite shoulder, generalized joint laxity, or a congenital or developmental problem will facilitate this distinction. Care should be taken to identify the voluntary dislocator, who should be treated nonoperatively in all cases, with rare exceptions.

For all acute traumatic dislocations, gentle closed reduction with analgesia or anesthesia should be performed. Prereduction and postreduction radiographs are taken, and neurologic and vascular examinations are performed before and after reduction. We generally perform the traction/countertraction method under light sedation. For an anterior traumatic dislocation, we immobilize the shoulder in internal rotation for 4 weeks. For a posterior dislocation, we immobilize the shoulder for 4 weeks in a prefabricated commercially available splint or a modified spica cast with the shoulder in neutral rotation. After the 4 weeks of immobilization, we institute a rehabilitation program stressing rotator cuff strengthening.

The recurrence rate after a traumatic anterior dislocation is 50% or higher. Although we hesitate to intervene surgically after the initial dislocation, the patient and parents should be counseled regarding the high recurrence rate, in some cases even after compliance to rehabilitation program. With a second dislocation, the patient should be considered a recurrent dislocator, and surgical intervention should be considered. If present, a Bankart lesion is repaired anatomically to the anterior glenoid rim. A stable, healed labrum in anatomic location is the key to surgical success either open or arthroscopically. In cases without a Bankart lesion, we use the capsular shift procedure as described by Rockwood.[461] A capsular shift may also be used in conjunction with a Bankart repair to tighten the redundant anteroinferior capsule. Care must be taken not to overtighten the capsule by either open or arthroscopic technique.

A 6-month course of rehabilitation follows surgical intervention. For the first month, pendulum exercises and gentle elevation exercises are performed. The shoulder is protected in a sling, especially at night. The second and third months are used to regain range of motion, including protected external rotation. This procedure is designed to address the pathology without limiting motion. The fourth through sixth months are used for a progressive strengthening program, which includes strengthening of the rotator cuff and deltoid. At 6 months, the reconstruction is mature enough to release the child to a full activity level.

For atraumatic dislocation, reduction can be accomplished if necessary after an acute dislocation in a fashion similar to that described for traumatic dislocations. Again, attention should be focused on confirming the diagnosis of atraumatic dislocation. Patients with voluntary dislocation and their families should be counseled that the dislocations can be harmful to the joint and should be discouraged.

Patients with atraumatic instability should be treated with a vigorous rehabilitation program. Only in the face of recurrence after 6 to 12 months of supervised rehabilitation should surgical intervention be considered. Great care should be taken to exclude the voluntary dislocator as a surgical candidate. Psychiatric evaluation is instituted if necessary. A capsular procedure as described by Neer or the capsular shift technique described by Rockwood can be used to eliminate laxity of the joint capsule in a circumferential manner.[403,460,461] Surgical management of the atraumatic dislocator is difficult and requires meticulous attention to detail during both the surgical procedure and the postoperative rehabilitation program. Recurrence rate is much higher in the atraumatic patient treated surgically.

Rehabilitation

The importance of an extensive rehabilitation program for instability about the shoulder for both traumatic and atraumatic problems is emphasized.[18,125] Specific exercises are used to strengthen the rotator cuff and deltoid muscles. The scapular stabilizers are also strengthened. Three-inch wide strips of rubber (Thera-Bands, The Hygenic Corporation, Akron, OH) are used to strengthen the cuff and deltoid muscles; Theratubes (The Hygenic Corporation, Akron, OH) are used later if necessary.

The amount of weight or Theraband resistance for progressive resistive strengthening varies depending on the extent of the problem as well as the patient's age, size, and baseline strength. Exercises are performed four to six times a day. After basic strengthening has been accomplished, isokinetic exercises using the flexion/extension plane and the internal and external rotation plane are effective for maximizing endurance and strength in the shoulder girdle musculature.

Complications

Any of the neurologic or vascular injuries can occur at the time of dislocation or during relocation. Although rare, axillary or brachial plexus neurapraxia that does not spontaneously recover requires neurodiagnostic evaluation and possibly surgical reconstruction. Vascular injury should be evaluated immediately for repair.

Little information is available in the literature about the success or failure rates of surgical reconstruction of the shoulder for recurrent dislocation in children. As discussed, traumatic dislocation in a child or adolescent can progress to recurrent dislocation in 50% to 100% of cases. Rockwood et al.[80,460,461] have shown that more than 85% of atraumatic dislocators can be managed with a vigorous rehabilitation program and do not require surgery. Surgical treatment of these problems in children could be expected to have a success rate at least equal to that in adults. Greater than 90% success in stopping traumatic dislocations would be expected with surgical reconstruction.[1,36,284]

Complications of surgical reconstruction of the shoulder include recurrent dislocation, recurrent subluxation, painfully restricted motion, problems with anchor migration or impingement about the shoulder, and neurologic injury. Perhaps the most common problem associated with the standard reconstructions about the shoulder that include subscapularis tendon-shortening procedures (Magnuson-Stack and Putti-Platt) is loss of external rotation. This loss in adults has been associated in some patients with a more rapid progression to glenohumeral arthritis.[224,355] It is no longer recommended.

Procedures that use metallic implants about the shoulder, including the Bristow and the DuToit stapling procedures, have been associated with complications of metal impingement on the humeral head or encroachment on the articular surface. Both problems can lead to pain and eventual arthritic change.[26,54,417,603] More recent osseous suture anchors may extrude into the joint and cause articular damage.

Controversies and Future Directions

The role of primary capsular and/or labral repair (Bankart repair) for the acute first-time traumatic dislocator remains to be seen and played out in research of this injury. Initial indications seem to suggest that the procedure has value for the very active individual with a high likelihood of recurrent dislocation. Arthroscopic results continue to improve as these techniques become more disseminated. In the future, long-term studies will provide for further comparison with open repair procedures.

FRACTURES OF THE PROXIMAL HUMERUS

Fractures of the proximal humerus are relatively uncommon injuries of childhood, with an incidence of 1.2 to 4.4 per 1000 per year,[45,313,590] fewer than 5% of all pediatric fractures.[242,264,313,314,467] Fractures in this region have enormous potential to heal and remodel, perhaps more so than anywhere else in the body, mainly due to the thick periosteum of the proximal humerus, the proximity to the physis, the near universal motion of the joint, and the fact that 80% of humeral growth is proximal. Thus, proximal humeral fractures in children with sufficient growth remaining can be expected to heal without significant residual functional or cosmetic deficits in most cases.

Principles of Management

Mechanism of Injury

Fractures of the proximal humerus can occur rarely during birth.[325,509] As an infant is passing through the birth canal, the

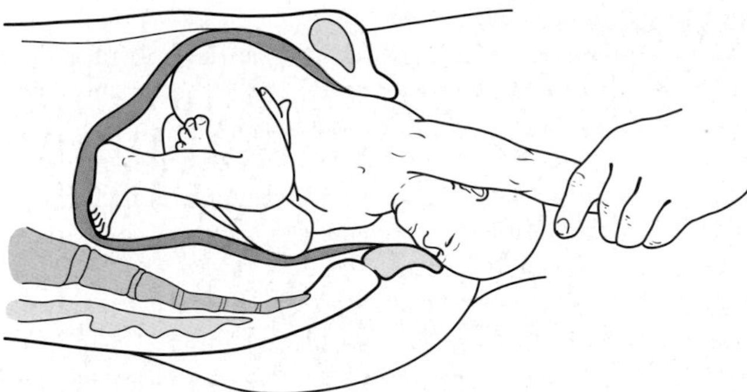

FIGURE 17-23 Hyperextension or rotation of the ipsilateral arm may result in a proximal humeral or physeal injury during birth.

arm may be stressed such that a separation through the physis of the proximal humerus can occur.[124,209,218,222,325,361,509] These fractures are generally believed to result from hyperextension and/or rotation of the arm during the passage through the birth canal (Fig. 17-23).[124,209,218,222,325,361,509] As might be expected, obstetric proximal humeral fractures occur most frequently during vaginal deliveries of infants with larger size or breech presentation.[83,177,271,509] Prenatal size and presentation, however, have not been accurate predictive factors for these fractures because proximal humeral fractures may occur during vaginal deliveries of infants of all sizes and weights. Hence, other infant and maternal factors play a role.[83,177,271]

In older children, the predominant cause of fractures in the proximal humerus is trauma, both direct and indirect. In this age group, these fractures can involve the metaphysis, the physis, or both. The trauma can be a direct blow to the shoulder area, especially to the posterior aspect,[124,404,515] or indirect, as in a fall onto an outstretched hand that transmits the force through the arm to the proximal humerus.[6,67,271] Indirect trauma can result in forced or nonphysiologic positioning of the upper extremity, which in turn may cause a fracture of the proximal humerus. Specifically, six potential mechanisms of upper extremity positioning have been proposed to explain the resulting proximal humeral fractures: forced extension, forced flexion, forced extension with lateral or medial rotation, and forced flexion with lateral or medial rotation.[585] Although trauma has been acknowledged as the most common mechanism of pediatric proximal humeral fractures, it is still controversial whether a fall or a direct blow is the more common etiology of the fracture.

Proximal humeral fractures are typically moderate- to higher-energy injuries and are frequently seen in motor vehicle crashes and sporting activities (Figs. 17-24 and 17-25).[30,298] Approximately 50% of shoulder girdle fractures in children have been reported to be associated with sports and play activities.[411] Athletic activities associated with proximal humeral fractures include contact sports (football, hockey), horseback riding (fall from horses), gymnastics (upper extremity impact and weight bearing), and baseball (repetitive throwing).[121,314,345,548]

Less often, pediatric proximal humeral fractures can be pathologic and result from other conditions such as malignant or benign tumors and pituitary gigantism.[5,308,458,484] They also can be a complication of radiation therapy to the shoulder region.[151] In addition, shoulder joint neuropathy secondary to Arnold-Chiari malformation, myelomeningocele, or syringomyelia has been implicated as an etiologic factor in proximal humeral fractures.[30,346] An unknown percentage of pediatric proximal humeral fractures are part of the injuries associated with child abuse (Fig. 17-26).[175] Because no clear fracture pattern in the proximal humerus is suggestive of abuse, an index of suspicion must remain high when evaluating infants or young children with humeral fractures.[505]

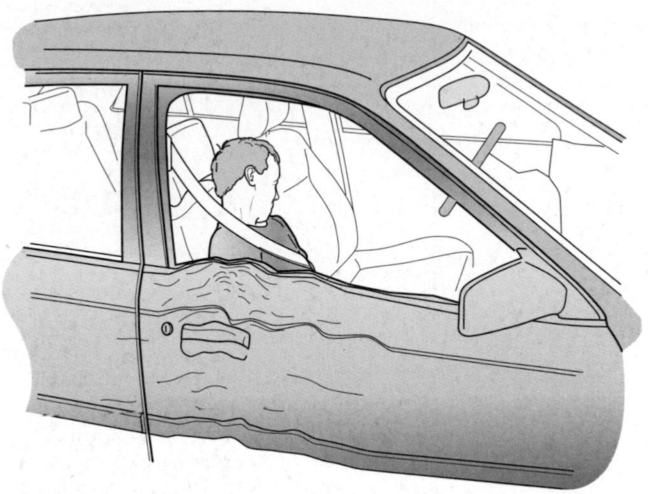

FIGURE 17-24 Motor vehicle crashes may result in proximal humeral fracture due to blunt trauma to the shoulder region.

Signs and Symptoms

Clinical features of proximal humeral fractures in newborns may be subtle and not readily identified. For example, the infant may be irritable when handled by caregivers or when there is movement of the upper extremity. The infant may refuse to move the arm, giving the appearance of paralysis, called "pseudoparalysis." Infants exhibiting upper extremity paralysis also may be suffering from posterior humeral head dislocation.[544]

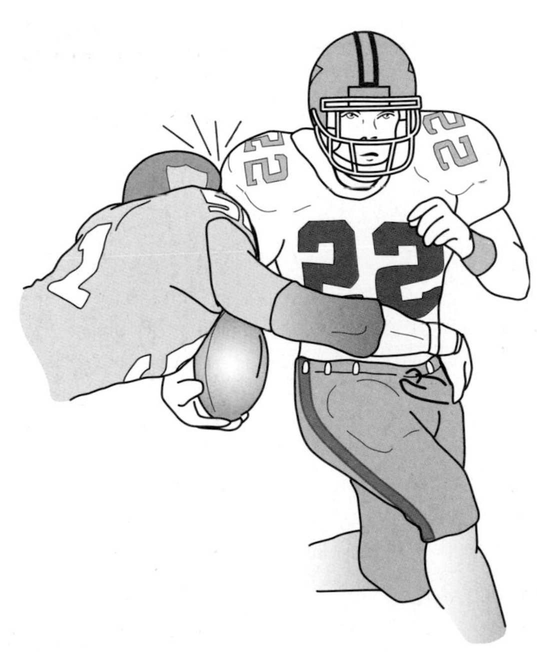

FIGURE 17-25 Blunt trauma from contact sports may result in fracture of the proximal humerus in children.

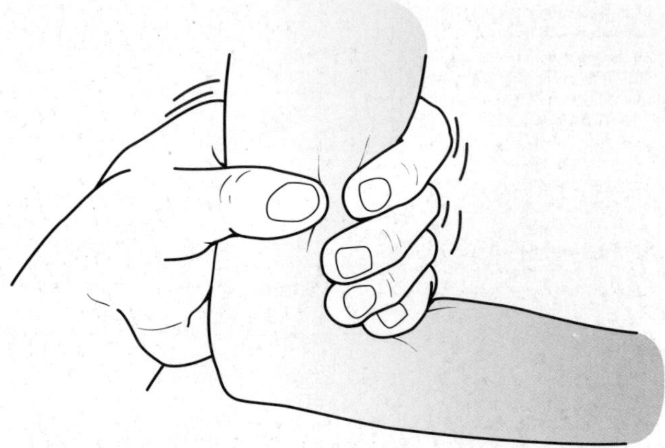

FIGURE 17-26 Although the exact mechanism of injury may vary in child abuse, fracture of the proximal humerus may result from twisting at the elbow or forearm.

Older children typically report a history consistent with a proximal humeral fracture: a traumatic injury with the immediate development of moderate to severe global shoulder pain exacerbated by motion of the arm. They often present with an obvious deformity, or fullness, in the anterior shoulder region, with the overall contour of the shoulder altered in comparison with the contralateral uninjured shoulder. The arm is internally rotated against the abdomen and the patient usually refuses to use the involved arm. Pain, swelling, and ecchymosis are invariably present to some degree.

The internally rotated position of the injured extremity is due to the pull of the pectoralis major muscle on the distal fragment. With posterior fracture dislocations, children demonstrate limited and extremely painful external rotation. Some children with fractures of the greater tuberosity have an unusual presentation of luxatio erecta where the involved shoulder is positioned in extreme abduction.[174] This position reduces the displacement across the fracture as the greater tuberosity is pulled superiorly by the supraspinatus muscle. The elbow is typically flexed in luxatio erecta, allowing the hand to be near or above the head.[174,300] Fractures of the lesser tuberosity affect the function of the inserting subscapularis muscle; hence, abduction and external rotation of the shoulder will be limited and painful.[292,468,564]

Associated Injuries

In high-energy trauma, fractures of the proximal humerus may be associated with concomitant dislocations of the glenohumeral joint. The direction of the dislocation may be anterior, posterior, or inferior.[107,174,175,207,300,416,557] Neurologic injury to the brachial plexus can result from fractures and fracture–dislocations of the proximal humerus.[19,144,174,557,561] The fracture can be displaced into the axilla and may have vascular compromise requiring emergent reduction. Typically, these nerve deficits are transient, and full function returns in 6 to 12 months.[268,306] There may be an associated pain syndrome that lasts for months in these rare situations of proximal humerus fracture associated with brachial plexopathy. Fractures of the proximal humerus in children also can be associated with other injuries, including rib fractures and pneumothorax.[484]

Diagnosis and Classification

The proximal humeral epiphysis is not visible on plain radiographs until about 6 months of age,[268,306,424] and plain radiographs are of limited value in evaluation of proximal humeral fractures in infants. On an AP radiograph, a change in the positional relationship between the proximal humeral metaphysis and the scapula and acromion often is visible. A comparison with the uninjured contralateral shoulder may reveal this alteration more clearly. A "vanishing epiphysis" sign also has been reported to describe posteriorly displaced physeal fractures of the proximal humerus (Fig. 17-27).[294,491] On an AP radiograph, the epiphysis appears to vanish when it is displaced posteriorly. For complete evaluation of proximal humeral fractures in newborns and infants, ultrasonographic studies can be diagnostic and informative.[71,164,251,553] MRI will reveal the injury pattern clearly but requires conscious sedation or general anesthesia in infants for accurate analysis. In addition to proximal humeral fractures, the differential diagnosis for such "paralysis" in infants includes brachial plexus injury, septic shoulder, and clavicular fractures.

For evaluation of proximal humeral fractures in older children, two radiographs in perpendicular views can be diagnostic.[536] Ideally, a true AP view of the shoulder and an axillary lateral view provide the most information about the fracture. Because some lesser tuberosity fractures may be visible only on an axillary lateral view, this radiograph should be included whenever possible.[252] Ideally, a properly positioned axillary view should position the normal humeral head between the acromion and the coracoid. Often, however, an axillary lateral view is difficult to obtain in a child with an acutely fractured proximal humerus. In these instances, transthoracic axillary view or scapular-Y views can be obtained. In obese patients, transthoracic views are difficult to interpret. In addition, an apical oblique view, an AP radiograph with the x-ray beam at 45 degrees of caudal tilt, also can provide significant informa-

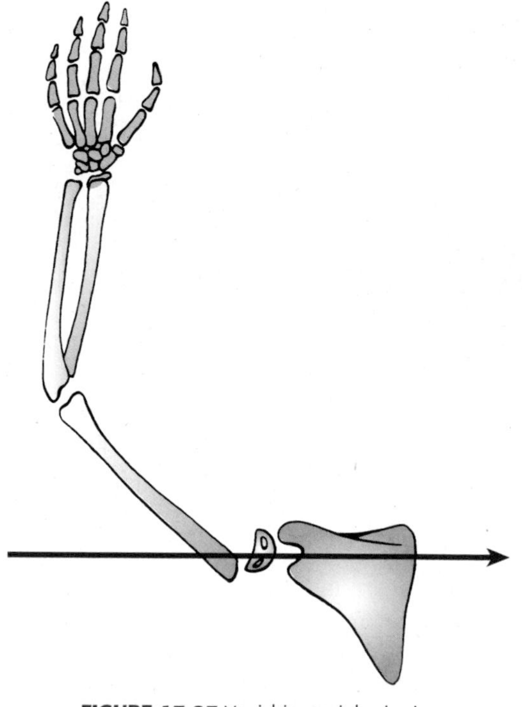

FIGURE 17-27 Vanishing epiphysis sign.

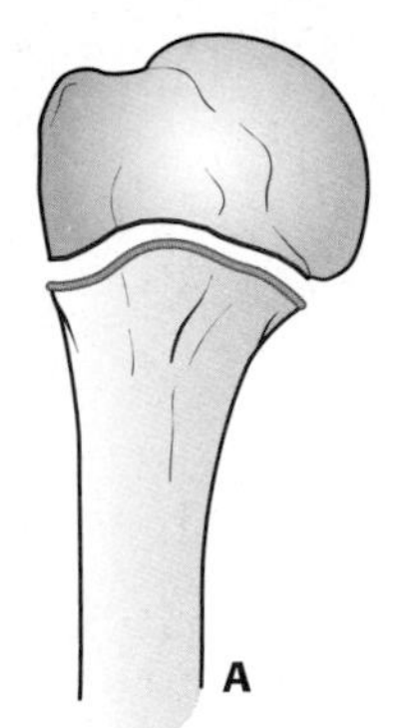

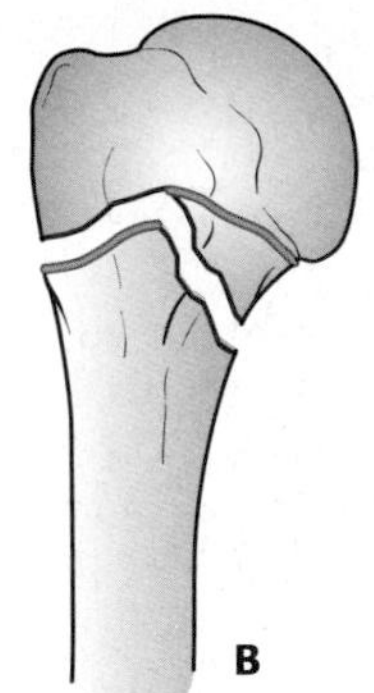

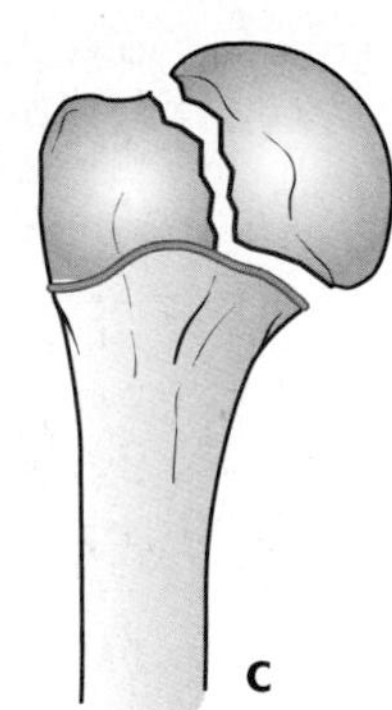

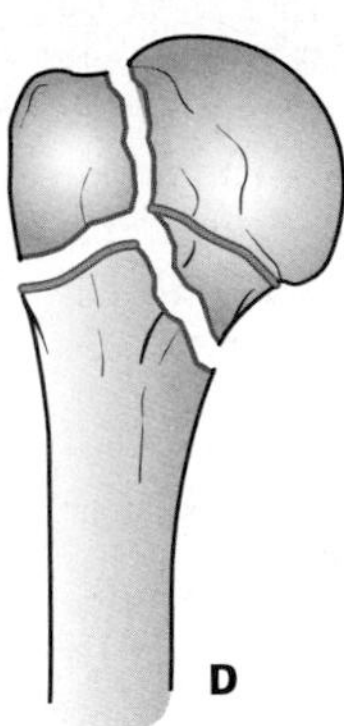

FIGURE 17-28 Physeal fractures of the proximal humerus. **A.** Salter-Harris type I. **B.** Salter-Harris type II. **C.** Salter-Harris type III. **D.** Salter-Harris type IV.

tion about the proximal humerus.[513] In fact, some authors report that most shoulder trauma can be evaluated with AP and apical oblique radiographs and that a lateral view (axillary lateral or scapular-Y view) can be obtained if a humeral fracture is suspected.[61]

When adequate radiographs cannot be obtained, CT is useful in evaluating proximal humeral fractures. CT may be especially useful in characterizing posterior fracture–dislocations.[207,545,564] If the child continues to report shoulder pain despite negative radiographic and CT results, an occult fracture must be ruled out. For this purpose, MRI can be diagnostic, due to its ability to identify the intramedullary signal change of edema and the fracture plane.[45,476,541]

Fractures of the proximal humerus in the pediatric population are broadly categorized by their anatomic location. The fractures may involve the physis, the metaphysis, the lesser tuberosity, or the greater tuberosity. In addition, the degree of fracture deformity (angulation and translation) plays an important role in the overall treatment option. Other fracture characteristics that must be evaluated include the presence or absence of open fractures, concomitant glenohumeral dislocations, and fracture stability.

Fractures involving the physis are classified according to the Salter-Harris classification (Fig. 17-28).[481] Salter-Harris type I injuries with fractures through the physis occur mostly in patients under 5 years of age.[124,435] After 11 years of age, most fractures of the proximal humerus are Salter-Harris type II injuries, with the fracture line exiting through the metaphysis,[79,124,164,435] and they occasionally are associated with an additional anterolateral bony fragment.[79] Salter-Harris type III injuries with the fracture line exiting through the epiphysis rarely occur in the proximal humerus of children[124,435] and have been reported with and without concomitant glenohumeral dislocation.[107,207,538,568,589] Salter-Harris type IV injuries involving both the metaphysis and the epiphysis of the proximal humerus have not been reported in children.

Fractures of the metaphysis occur mostly in children 5 to 12 years of age (Fig. 17-29) and are categorized by their anatomic location and degree of displacement.[124] This rather unexpected finding has been attributed to the rapid metaphyseal growth that occurs during this age, which in turn results in a relative structural weakness of the metaphysis.[124] The anatomic location is described in relation to the major deforming forces in the region, namely the insertions of the pectoralis major and the deltoid muscles. Presence or absence of other fractures in the ipsilateral upper extremity also must be documented, because segmental fractures may require alternative treatments.[270,357,425] Other isolated fractures of the proximal humerus may include the greater and the lesser tuberosities.[174,292,300,468,577]

In the Neer classification, the degree of displacement in proximal humerus fractures is classified with respect to the shaft diameter of the humerus.[404] In grade I injuries, there is up to 5 mm of displacement. In grade II and III injuries, fractures are displaced by up to one third and two thirds of the humeral shaft diameter, respectively. Displacement of greater than two thirds of the shaft diameter is classified as a grade IV injury. In addition to degree of displacement, fractures in this region typically demonstrate concomitant angular deformities.

Surgical and Applied Anatomy

The proximal humeral ossification center cannot be seen on plain radiographs until about 6 months of age.[268,306,424] In addition to the proximal humerus, both the greater and lesser tuberosities contain their own separate ossification centers. The ossification center for the greater tuberosity appears at around 1 to 3 years of age, while the ossification center for the lesser tuberosity takes form at 4 to 5 years of age.[424,483] The two tuberosities

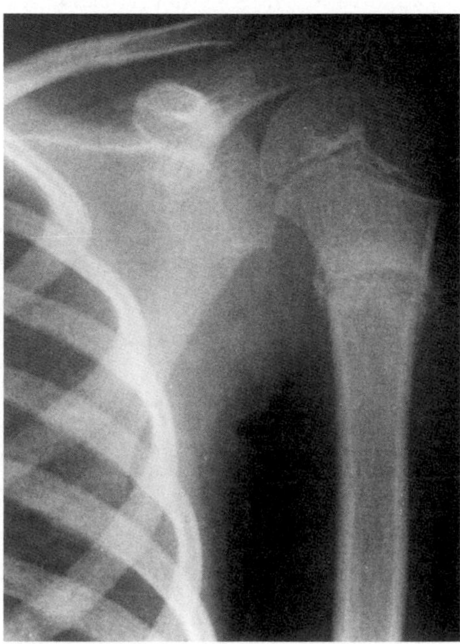

FIGURE 17-29 Healing undisplaced fracture of the proximal humerus in a 5-year-old child. Note the absence of a physeal injury.

typically coalesce between 5 and 7 years of age and subsequently fuse with the humeral head at 7 to 13 years of age.[424,483]

The proximal physis of the humerus continues to be active well into the teenage years and is ultimately responsible for approximately 80% of the overall humeral growth.[56,447,448,522] Interestingly, longitudinal growth at the proximal humeral physis changes during development, such that it is responsible for only 75% of humeral growth before age 2 but up to 90% of growth after age 11.[56,447,448] For girls, this growth continues until around 14 years of age, with subsequent fusion of the epiphysis to the shaft at 14 to 17 years of age.[56,118,522] For boys, growth continues until about age 16, when closure of the physis begins.[56,447,448] For most boys, the proximal humeral physis is closed by about 18 years of age.[118] The extracapsular location of the proximal humeral physis makes this structure susceptible to injury. Physeal fractures are thought to occur through the zone of hypertrophy and provisional calcification while relatively sparing the cells in the resting and proliferative zones.[481] Salter-Harris type I or II fractures in children have high remodeling potential and rarely result in growth arrest.[38,124]

The articular surface of the proximal humerus covers most of the medial aspect of the epiphysis as well as the proximal medial corner of the metaphysis (Fig. 17-30). The glenohumeral joint capsule surrounds the articular surface such that most of the medial epiphysis and the proximal medial corner of the metaphysis are intra-articular (Fig. 17-31). Conversely, a predominant proportion of the physis is extracapsular and remains susceptible to injury. Most fractures of the pediatric proximal humerus involve the physis.[79,124,435] The periosteum is quite strong in the posteromedial aspect of the proximal humerus, but the periosteum in the anterolateral aspect is relatively weak, occasionally allowing the fractured fragment to displace. The interposed periosteum can prevent reduction.[124]

The proximal humerus is the site of insertion for a number of different muscles that can influence the pattern of fracture displacement. These muscles and their attachments form early during development and are grossly similar to those of an adult shoulder by the time of birth. The four muscles of the rotator cuff insert onto the epiphysis. The subscapularis muscle inserts on the anterior aspect of the epiphysis on the lesser tuberosity,

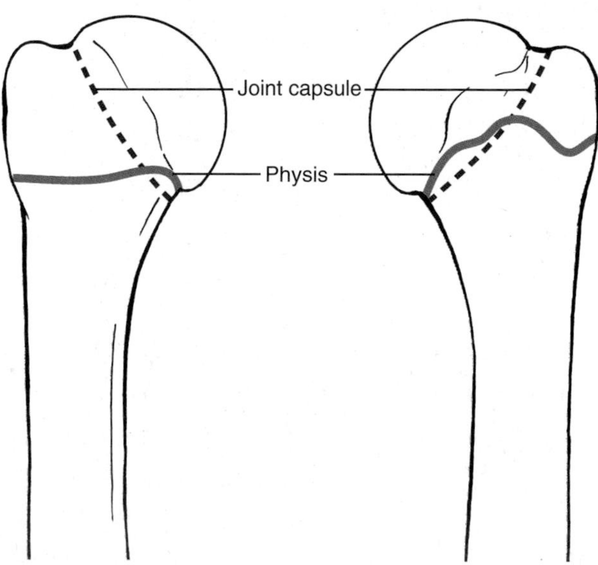

FIGURE 17-30 The anatomy of the proximal humerus.

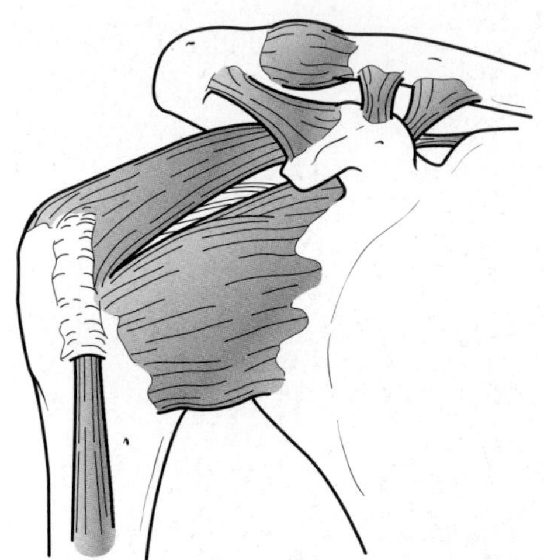

FIGURE 17-31 Glenohumeral joint capsule.

whereas the teres minor, the infraspinatus, and the supraspinatus muscles insert onto the superior and posterior aspect of the epiphysis near the greater tuberosity (Fig. 17-32). In addition to the rotator cuff muscles, the deltoid and pectoralis major muscles can also affect fracture displacement. The deltoid muscle attaches in the lateral aspect of the humeral shaft, whereas the pectoralis major muscle attaches to the anteromedial aspect of the metaphysis.

The muscular attachments to the proximal humerus contribute to the degree and the overall pattern of fracture displacement. With fractures of the physis (Salter-Harris types I, II, and III) and metaphyseal fractures proximal to the insertion of the pectoralis major muscle, the rotator cuff muscles displace the epiphysis into abduction, flexion, and slight external rotation. The distal fragment is displaced proximally by the deltoid muscle, whereas the pectoralis major muscle displaces the fragment anteriorly and medially. If the metaphyseal fracture occurs between the insertions of the deltoid and the pectoralis major muscles, the proximal fragment is adducted by the pull of the pectoralis major muscle, and the distal fragment is pulled proximally and abducted by the deltoid muscle. If the fracture occurs distal to the deltoid muscle insertion, the proximal fragment is abducted by the deltoid muscle and displaced anteriorly by the pectoralis major muscle. The distal fragment is pulled proximally and medially by the biceps and the triceps muscles.[123]

The vascular supply to the proximal humerus arises from the axillary artery. Distal to the pectoralis minor muscle, three different arterial branches arise from the axillary artery before it becomes the brachial artery to supply the upper extremity and hand. One of these branches is the subscapular artery, which runs with the subscapular nerve to supply the rotator cuff muscles. The remaining two branches, the anterior and the posterior humeral circumflex arteries, supply the proximal humerus. Most of the humeral head vascularity is from the arcuate artery, which in turn is from the ascending branch of the anterior humeral circumflex artery.[189,312] The posterior humeral circumflex artery is a less dominant vascular supplier of the proximal humerus because it supplies a small portion of the greater tuberosity and posteroinferior portion of the humeral head (Fig. 17-33).[189]

The close proximity of the axillary nerve to the proximal humerus makes this neural structure susceptible to injury dur-

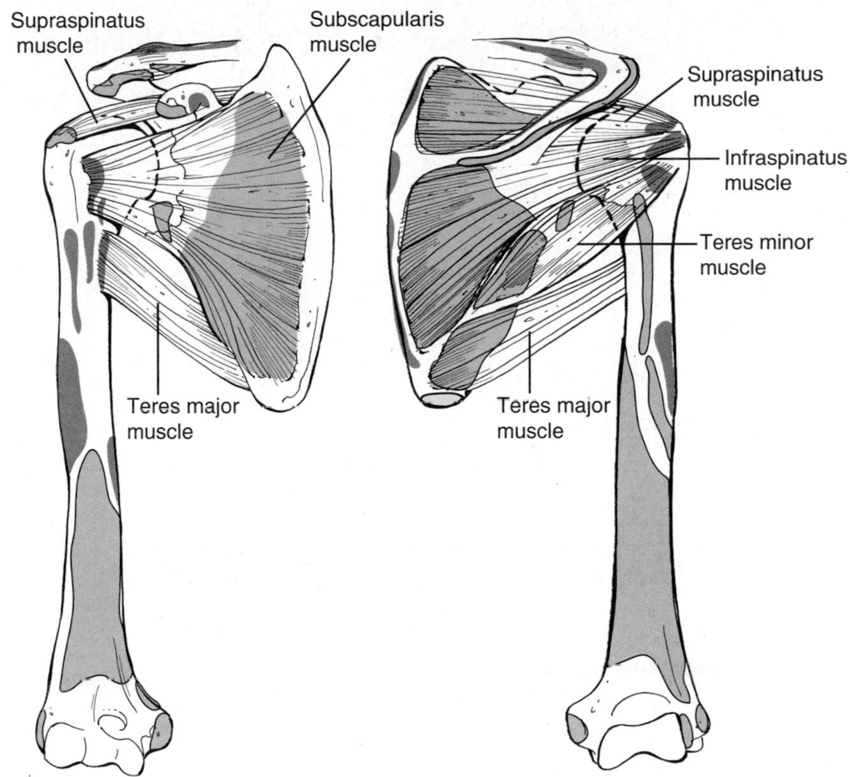

FIGURE 17-32 Origins and insertions of the cuff muscles in a child: subscapularis, teres minor, infraspinatus, and supraspinatus.

ing fracture and fracture–dislocations of the proximal humerus.[19,174,557] The axillary nerve is a branch of the posterior cord of the brachial plexus. It traverses the anterior aspect of the subscapularis muscle before passing inferior to the glenohumeral joint to the posterior aspect of the proximal humerus (see Fig. 17-7). The axillary nerve provides innervation to the deltoid and teres minor muscles as well as cutaneous sensation over the lateral aspect of the shoulder. Documentation of the normal motor and sensory function of this nerve at the initial evaluation and prior to treatment is essential.

Current Treatment Options

Because of their tremendous potential for healing and remodeling, fractures of the proximal humerus in children infrequently require operative reduction and fixation (Table 17-5). This is especially true for obstetric proximal humeral fractures in infants. If needed, these fractures are amenable to gentle reduction with minimal anesthesia or sedation. If desired, the adequacy of the reduction can be evaluated via ultrasonography in infants, but due to the incredible remodeling capability in this age group, this is not routine. With or without anatomic reduction, the affected upper extremity can be immobilized to the body by using a safety pin to attach the shirt sleeve to the shirt or stockinette sling-and-swathe that is age and size appropriate.[484] Proximal humeral fractures in this age group heal quite rapidly, typically within 1 to 3 weeks, and result in no residual functional or cosmetic deficits.[124,218,271,327,509,579]

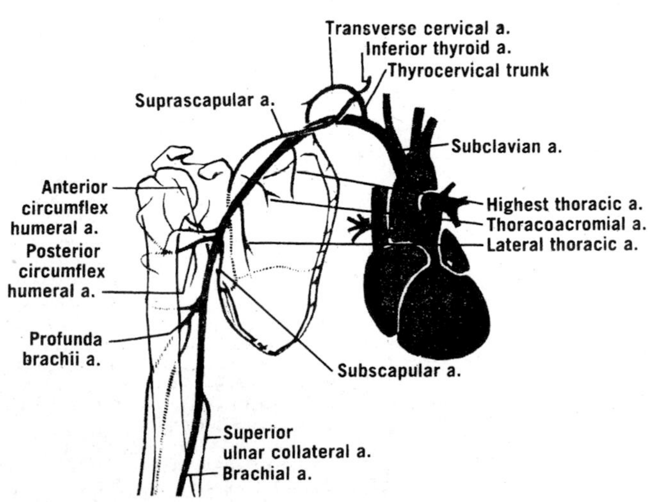

FIGURE 17-33 The arterial anatomy of the shoulder region.

Nondisplaced or minimally displaced proximal humeral fractures (Neer grades I and II) in older children and adolescents also should be treated nonoperatively. Initial management of these fractures involves sling-and-swathe immobilization (Fig. 17-34) followed by protected motion. Overall, nonoperative treatment provides excellent long-term results.[82,124,174]

The remodeling potential of the fracture in young children is significant but decreases with the increasing age of the child; hence, the degree of acceptable displacement and angulation also changes with the age of the child. Generally, relative greater displacement and angulation can be accepted in younger children. For fractures in children under the age of 11, good to excellent long-term outcomes have been reported regardless of the fracture displacement.[124,318,404,515] Various types of shoulder immobilization to maintain reduction have been advocated and include sling-and-swathe, thoracobrachial bandage (Velpeau), hanging arm cast, shoulder spica cast, salute position shoulder spica cast, and "Statue of Liberty" cast.[82,124,218,318,404]

Grossly displaced or angulated proximal humeral fractures (Neer grades III and IV) in children over 11 are managed with

TABLE 17-5 Interventions for Proximal Humerus Fractures

	Immobilization	Operative Reduction and Immobilization	Operative Reduction and Internal Fixation
Birth fractures	X		
Chronic slipped proximal humeral epiphysis	X		
Metaphyseal fractures	X	X	X
Salter-Harris type I before age 11 years	X	X	X (rarely)
Salter-Harris type I after age 11 years	X		X

fracture reduction and sometimes with specialized immobilization.[124,319,404,507] Multiple maneuvers exist for the reduction of pediatric proximal humeral fractures. Most fractures can be reduced by applying longitudinal traction to the arm while positioning it in abduction, flexion, and external rotation. If this maneuver does not sufficiently reduce the fracture, better reduction can be obtained by moderate abduction, flexion to 90 degrees, and external rotation.[404] Alternatively, the fracture can be reduced by direct manual manipulation of the fragments while the arm is placed in marked abduction (about 135 degrees), slight flexion (about 30 degrees), and longitudinal traction.[67,271,579] Despite significant efforts, however, some fractures cannot be adequately reduced because of a barrier at the fracture site. Anatomic structures that can prevent reduction of proximal humeral fractures include the periosteum, the shoulder joint capsule, and the biceps tendon.[42,173,266,322,327,562] In these situations, open reduction through a small deltopectoral incision is needed to remove the obstacles to reduction. Good glenohumeral motion and function have been reported when severely displaced (Neer III and IV) fractures were reduced to Neer grade I or II displacement followed by immobilization or fixation.[143]

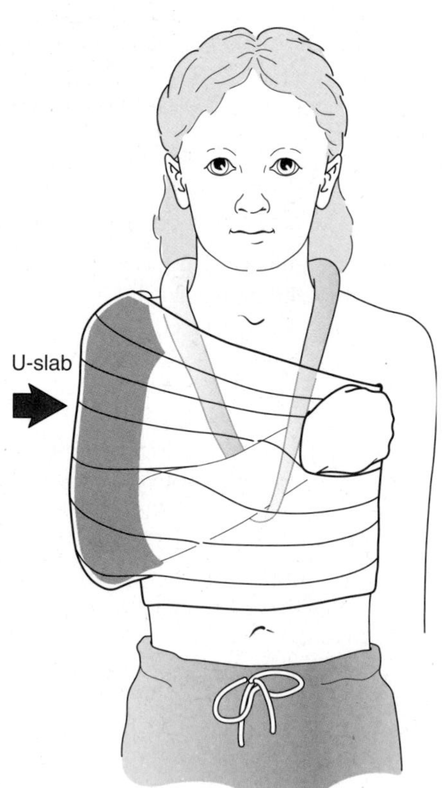

FIGURE 17-34 Sling-and-swathe for immobilization of proximal humeral fracture.

In children over 11 years old, gentle reduction of Salter-Harris type I and II fractures with greater than 50% displacement, followed by immobilization with a thoracobrachial bandage (Velpeau) or shoulder spica cast is usually sufficient (Fig. 17-34).[124] An acceptable reduction of proximal humeral fractures in children over 11 years of age has been proposed by some to be less than 50% displacement and 20 degrees of angulation.[507] However, there have been no comparative outcome studies. Traditional thinking has been that nonoperative treatment of pediatric proximal humeral fractures has produced good to excellent results in all age groups.[124,318,404] Because of this, the reported indications for operative treatment of pediatric proximal humeral fractures have been limited to include open fractures, fractures associated with neurovascular injury, fractures associated with multiple trauma, displaced intra-articular fractures (i.e., Salter-Harris type III fractures), irreducible fractures, and significantly displaced fractures in older adolescents.[30,117,242,322,347,367,397,435,500,530,568]

Interestingly, the cited literature that has been reported to support nonoperative treatment regimens for all patients actually supports this method for children less than 11 years of age and in fractures with no to minimal displacement.[124,318,404] These classic references identified fractures in older children (11 years of age or older) and those with Neer grades III and IV displacements at increased risk for less-than-optimal outcome.[124,318,404] Minimal remodeling, specifically angular correction, occurs in the older child and adolescent, which can lead to limitation of glenohumeral motion (abduction) and pain.[124,318] Case by case decisions regarding acceptable angulation and displacement should be based on age since older patients have less capacity for remodeling.[42,143] Achieving acceptable fracture alignment can typically be accomplished with closed manipulation of the fracture and only infrequently requires an open reduction to remove obstructions. Immobilization of the reduced fracture comes in two types: specialized casts or splints, or internal fixation. Various types of external immobilization have been reported to maintain reduc-

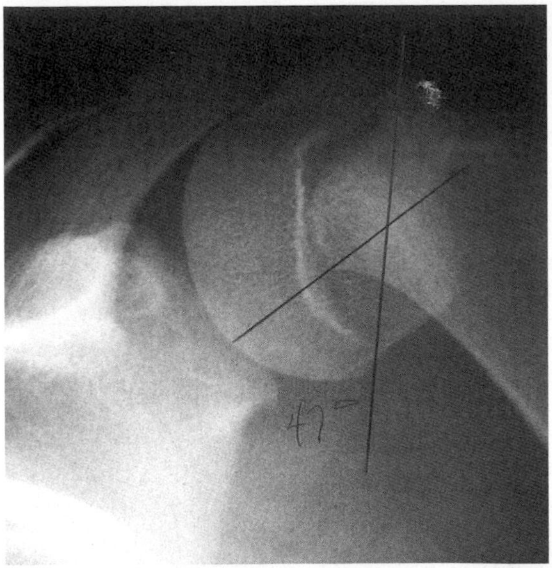

FIGURE 17-35 A. Salter-Harris type I fracture of proximal humerus. **B.** Intraoperative pinning through the metaphysis. **C.** Postoperative view. **D.** Healed physeal fracture.

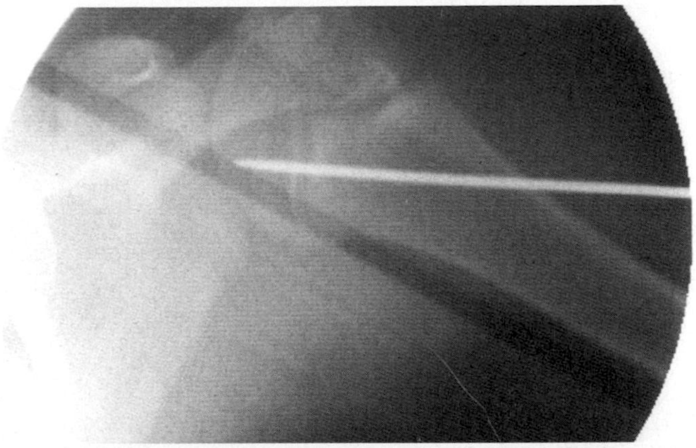

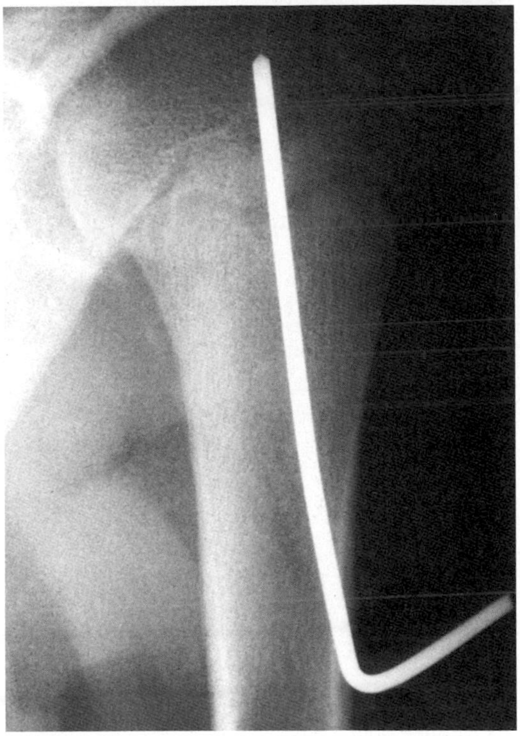

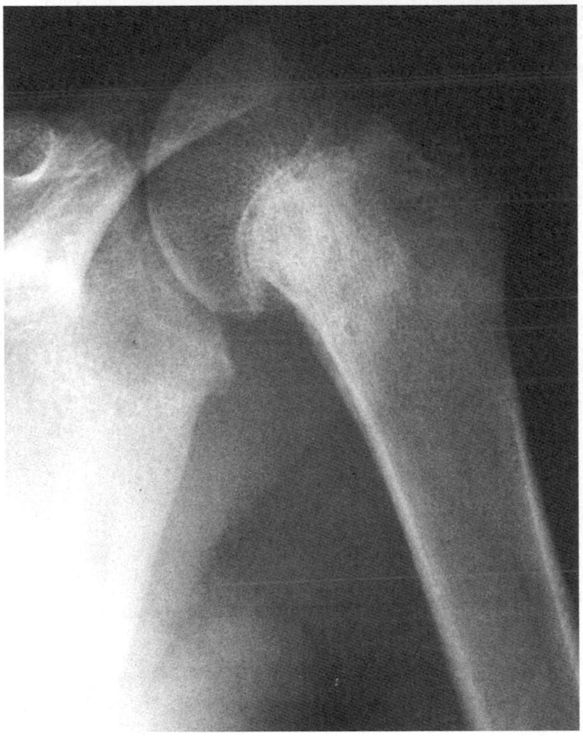

tion.[82,124,218,318,404] Loss of reduction has been reported to be as high as 50% in one older series in which only external immobilization was used.[404] Internal fixation with plates and screws, percutaneous cannulated screws, or more commonly smooth or threaded wires (Figs. 17-35 and 17-36) can be used to stabilize the reduction, which obviates the need for cumbersome immobilization such as a Velpeau bandage or spica cast.[30] Intramedullary fixation from distal to proximal insertion is also a viable option for stabilizing displaced proximal metaphyseal fractures (Fig. 17-37).[95]

A stress fracture of the metaphysis or a slipped epiphysis can be produced by chronic or repetitive trauma, such as repetitive throwing, gymnastics with humeral weight bearing, or trauma after localized radiation therapy.[59,121,151,345,548,549] Because of the tremendous healing and remodeling potential in the pediatric proximal humerus, these injuries can be successfully treated with nonsurgical therapy.

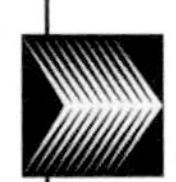

AUTHORS' PREFERRED TREATMENT

Surgical Procedure

Proximal humeral fractures that have significant displacement (Neer grades III and IV) and angulation in patients over 11 years of age are the fractures that typically undergo reduction to improve fracture alignment. General anesthesia is typically necessary for patient comfort and for adequate muscle relaxation due to the difficulties that can be encoun-

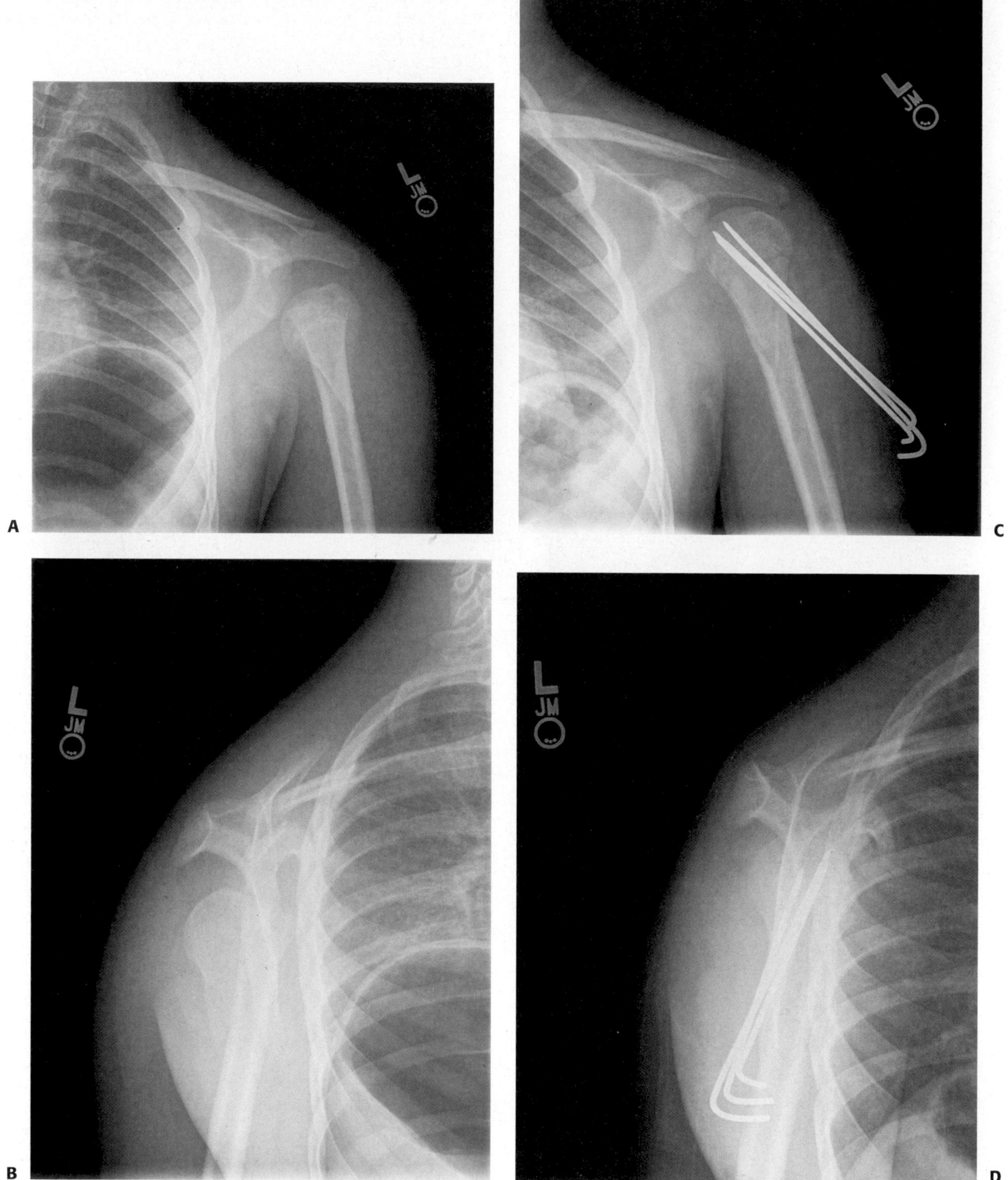

FIGURE 17-36 A. AP radiograph of displaced fracture of the proximal humeral metaphysis with shortening with inferior subluxation of the humeral head with respect to the glenoid. **B.** Scapular Y-view. **C,D.** Postoperative films after open reduction and fixation. The inferior subluxation has resolved.

tered in obtaining and maintaining an acceptable reduction. A radiolucent operating table is optimal, but a regular operating room table can be used if the patient's torso is moved as far lateral as possible and supported by a radiolucent arm table or an additional piece of radiolucent Plexiglas. Adequate fluoroscopic imaging is essential for a successful intervention, and the fluoroscope is set up in the AP projection; it is not routinely moved during the procedure. A small towel bump is placed under the medial border of the ipsilateral scapula to elevate the shoulder away from the table to allow adequate circumferential access to the shoulder. The sterile preparation should be medial enough to allow the surgeon

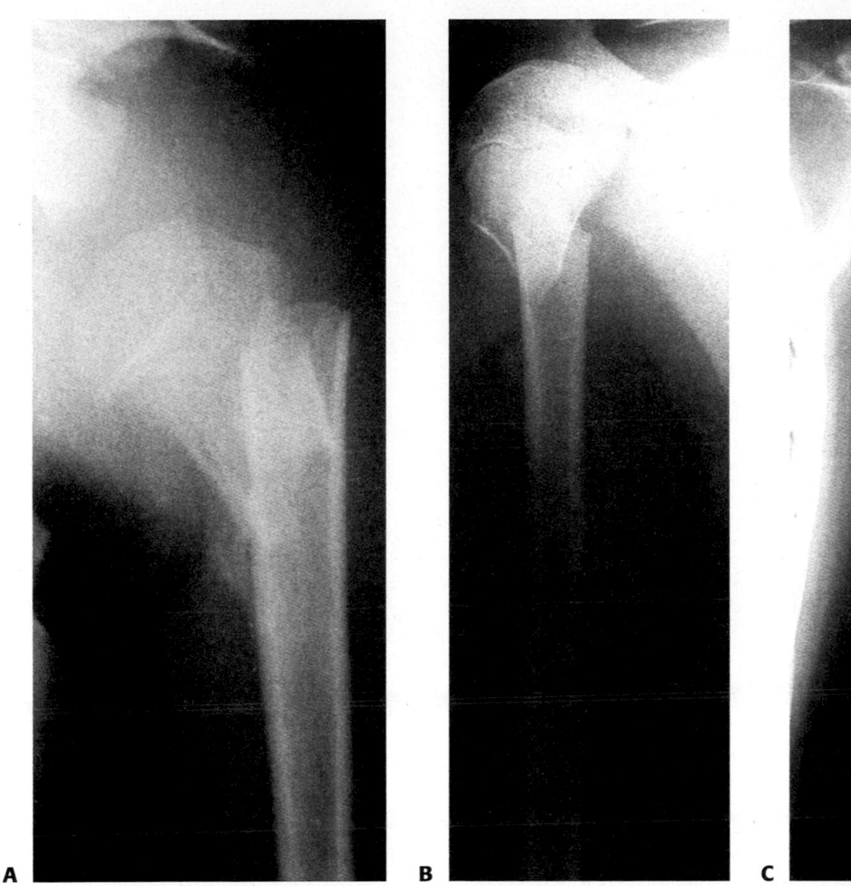
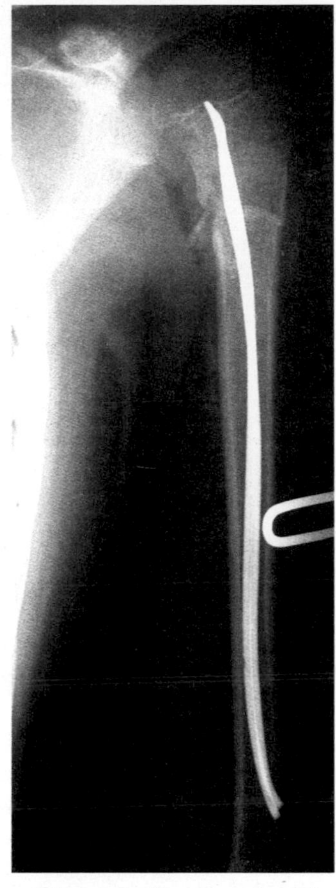
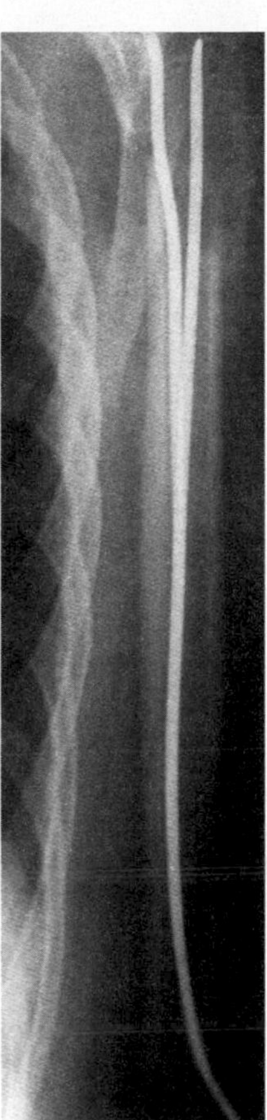

FIGURE 17-37 A. AP radiograph of displaced, shortened fracture of the proximal humerus. **B.** Axillary image of same. **C.** Intramedullary fixation using retrograde technique. Note the satisfactory restoration of alignment. **D.** Postoperative lateral view.

the option of performing a low deltopectoral or axillary approach to the shoulder should closed reduction be inadequate. Reduction is performed with longitudinal traction on the injured limb while the arm is placed in abduction, external rotation, and flexion to align the distal fragment with the epiphysis. Increasing the abduction (up to 90 degrees) and flexion (up to 90 degrees) of the distal fragment may be necessary to reduce the fracture. For fractures requiring operative reduction, percutaneous smooth or threaded wire stabilization is used routinely (see Fig. 17-36). The starting point for percutaneously placed implants is at the lateral cortex of the distal fragment, near the insertion of the deltoid muscle, and aimed obliquely into the humeral epiphysis. By measuring the articular cartilage height, entry can be two times the height to safely avoid injury to the axillary nerve. Care must be taken not to penetrate the humeral head into the joint or enter the axilla and injure the neurovascular structures. At least two pins (0.062 or 5/64 inches), and preferentially three pins, are used and typically allow adequate stabilization. The Kirschner-wires may be cut beneath the level of the skin or may be left through the skin and protected with Jergens balls (Jergens, Inc., Cleveland, OH). The arm is placed into a shoulder immobilizer, with the arm at the patient's side, while the patient is under general anesthesia. The implants can usually be removed as early as 4 weeks after surgery after documenting healing on radiograph. Figure 17-38 from Dobbs et al.[143] summarizes our approach.

Pearls and Pitfalls

- Most fractures of the proximal humeral physis are managed nonoperatively. This includes nondisplaced and most minimally to moderately displaced physeal injuries of the proximal humerus, which are treated with a shoulder sling or immobilizer. Range-of-motion exercises (pendulum) are initiated as soon as tolerated, and the immobilization is discontinued when healing is confirmed by radiographs and clinical examination. The great majority of metaphyseal fractures are also treated nonoperatively, with only a few requiring closed reduction. Because of the tremendous remodeling potential of metaphyseal fractures in children, up to 1 cm of displacement is acceptable if the fracture is in bayonet apposition.
- Due to the significant instability after reduction of displaced fractures involving the humeral epiphysis or metaphysis, we prefer to percutaneously pin the unstable fractures, particularly those in children over 11 years of age (see Fig. 17-36). The rationale behind reduction and percutaneous pinning of proximal humeral physeal fractures is a more rapid return of normal active and passive range of motion, improved patient comfort, and easier care of the patient. There is a minimally increased, but acceptable, risk of infection. In our opinion, this approach is more acceptable than leaving the fracture unreduced and risking a decrease in shoulder range of motion due to impingement with secondary shoulder pain. We prefer to place the pin percutaneously through the metaphyseal fragment up into the physis, similar conceptually to the pinning of a slipped capital femoral epiphysis in the hip (see Fig.17-35). One drawback of Kirschner-wire fixation is that if the

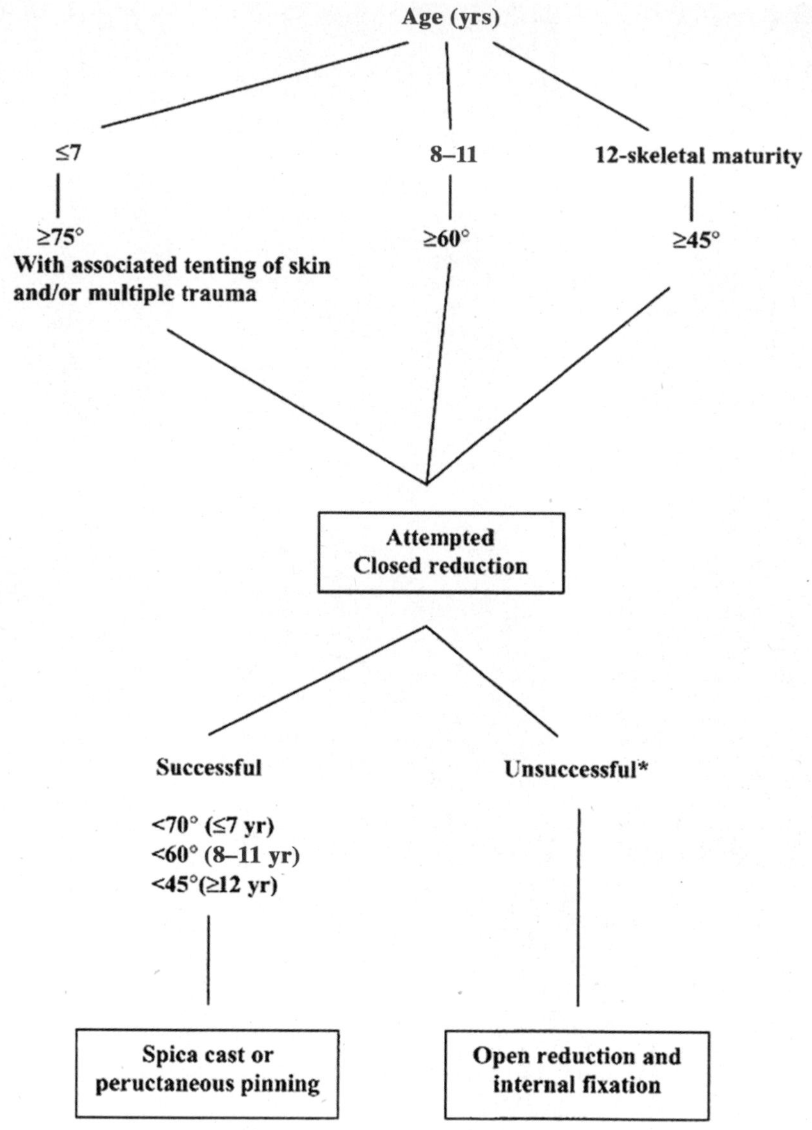

***An interposed long head of biceps tendon is often the culprit preventing a successful closed reduction**

FIGURE 17-38 Algorithm for closed epiphyseal fractures of the proximal humerus. Assumed Neer Grade III or IV.

wires are left under the skin, another general anesthetic is needed to remove the implants. In metaphyseal fractures, if the fracture is more distal, it may not be technically feasible to place a percutaneously placed Kirschner-wire obliquely into the epiphysis. In this situation, distal to proximal intramedullary fixation with flexible nails is an effective method (see Fig.17-37). Occasionally a fracture is irreducible, requiring open reduction. Generally, the biceps is the offending structure. An anterior deltopectoral exposure is used.

- Fracture–dislocations of the shoulder require closed reduction of the glenohumeral joint dislocation with appropriate anesthesia. After reduction of the glenohumeral dislocation, radiographic confirmation of the reduction and re-evaluation of the physeal or metaphyseal fracture is essential. If the dislocation does not concentrically reduce or the fracture is in unacceptable alignment, open reduction is generally done through a low anterior or axillary approach to the proximal humerus.
- Displaced fractures of the lesser tuberosity generally are treated with open reduction to restore the subscapularis tendon and anterior capsule. Lag screws or suture anchors are very useful in this region, particularly for injuries with small bony fragments. Fractures of the greater tuberosity generally are associated with acute dislocations of the shoulder and are typically treated nonoperatively after closed reduction of the shoulder dislocation. Rarely, after closed reduction of the shoulder dislocation, the greater tuberosity fracture reduction is unacceptable, and an open approach to repair the tuberosity fracture along with the rotator cuff is required.

Complications

Early Complications

Diagnosis of a proximal humeral fracture can be delayed in a child who is asymptomatic or minimally symptomatic. This is usually not a problem as the fracture can heal well and remodel minor displacement with growth. In children with multiple trauma, the diagnosis can be delayed due to the need to focus on more life- or limb-threatening problems and the absence of any dramatic limb malalignment. Even after the diagnosis of proximal humeral fracture is made, full evaluation and characterization of the fracture pattern can remain incomplete because of inadequate radiographic studies. A high index of suspicion, thorough physical examination, and insistence on high-quality radiographs must all be present to ensure prompt diagnosis and treatment of proximal humeral fractures.

Neurologic injury to the brachial plexus can result from fractures and fracture–dislocations of the proximal humerus.[19,144,174,557,561] Most nerve deficits can be diagnosed immediately because the clinical signs are readily apparent. Often, the distal fracture fragment is displaced into the axilla, with resulting adduction and valgus malalignment and nerve compression or traction injury. There may be an associated vascular compromise that requires emergent reduction of the fracture to restore blood supply to the distal arm and hand.[256] Rarely, however, nerve deficits from proximal humeral fractures can evolve slowly and delay the diagnosis.[144] Typically, these nerve deficits are transient, and full function typically returns in 3 to 12 months.[256,268,306] If the neurologic deficit persists longer than 3 to 6 months, further evaluation with electromyography is warranted. If no evidence of nerve recovery or regeneration is present, nerve exploration, repair, and grafting can be considered.[19,105] Salvage operations for permanent nerve deficits include proximal humeral osteotomy and muscle or tendon transfers.[7,113,241,291,437]

Fractures of the proximal humerus in children also can be associated with other injuries, including rib fractures and pneumothorax.[484] These fractures have been associated with disruptions and thrombosis of the axillary vessels as well in children[575] and adults.[344,499,533,602] Operative fixation of proximal humeral fractures with pins and wires has been associated with hardware migration, which can be fatal.[338,356] Therefore, serial radiographic monitoring of the hardware after shoulder operations is essential.

Late Complications

Humerus varus after trauma is a rare complication that typically affects neonates and children under 5 years of age.[154,317,352,517,546] Children with humerus varus have a significant decrease in the humeral neck–shaft angle and shortening of the upper extremity. Although shoulder abduction may be moderately limited, most children with humerus varus have only mild functional deficits and do not require surgical correction of the deformity.[154,317,352,546] If, however, active abduction and flexion are severely limited and corrective growth is not possible, corrective osteotomy of the proximal humerus can produce good results.[193,517]

Hypertrophic scarring can occur after surgical reduction of proximal humeral fractures. When the scarring is present in the anterior shoulder region after an anterior deltopectoral incision, the cosmetic deformity may be significant and psychologically damaging, especially for girls.[173,191] Therefore, many investigators have argued for the more cosmetically appealing axillary or anterior axillary incision.[211,328]

Limb length inequality after proximal humeral fractures occurs more frequently in children treated with surgical intervention than in those treated nonoperatively.[38,124,478] This is likely due to the degree of damage to the physis at the time of injury and not iatrogenically induced due to the surgical reduction. The inequality is not significantly affected by the quality of initial fracture reduction and may be more pronounced in older children (1 to 3 cm).[38,404] Despite this inequality, however, these children rarely develop any functional deficits to warrant surgical intervention. Full arrest of physeal growth after traumatic proximal humeral fractures is extremely uncommon.[124] Although still quite rare, it does occur more frequently in children with pathologic fractures through unicameral bone cysts.[239,388,413] If the functional or cosmetic deficit is significant, a limb-lengthening procedure may be of benefit for these children.[492]

Osteonecrosis of the humeral head after proximal humeral fractures occurs frequently in adults but is rare in children.[368,594] Even after acute disruption of the vascular supply to the proximal humeral epiphysis, subsequent remodeling and revascularization usually occur in children and lead to excellent clinical results.[568] Similarly, glenohumeral subluxation after proximal humeral fractures is a rare complication in the pediatric population that typically results in good clinical outcomes.[594] These children are best treated with a short period of immobilization followed by early physical therapy and rehabilitation.[484]

Controversies and Future Directions

Little controversy exists in the treatment of minimally displaced fractures and fractures in children 11 years old and younger; the main area of controversy is in the treatment of displaced fractures in the patient older than 11 years old. Two main areas of controversy are the amount of acceptable displacement (angulation and translation) and the optimal method of stabilization. The Neer classification is currently the most widely accepted method for the radiographic classification of proximal humeral fractures, but it has not been validated as a guide for treatment.[404] This system defines the fractures based on the bony translation at the fracture site but does not integrate fracture angulation into the schema. Multiple published reports document a high percentage of good and excellent outcomes in Neer grade III and IV fractures.[124,318,404,507] It is likely that fracture angulation, and not translation, is the more important factor in the overall outcome of these fractures. Unfortunately, due to the anatomy of the proximal humerus and epiphysis, plain radiographic assessment of fracture angulation can be very imprecise, especially in physeal fractures. This makes preoperative and postoperative analysis of the fracture alignment difficult, if not impossible. Further study into the role of fracture angulation, and the ability to quantify angulation, is likely to shed new light onto this topic by improving treatment algorithms and patient outcomes. In addition, applying validated outcome assessments to postfracture patients would help determine which fractures are clinically acceptable.

The classic treatment method for stabilization of the reduced proximal humerus fracture has been a specialized cast or splint designed to position the distal fracture fragment in alignment with the proximal fragment. Improvements in intraoperative imaging and equipment have permitted an evolution in pediatric fracture care to more widespread use of percutaneously placed Kirschner-wires, cannulated screws, or intramedullary fixation. Hence, external immobilization is rarely used. Both methods, external immobilization and internal fixation, have their advantages and disadvantages in proximal humerus frac-

TABLE 17-6 Treatment Pros and Cons: Proximal Humerus Fractures

	Pros	Cons
No reduction (sling or shoulder immobilizer)	1. No anesthesia/sedation 2. Sling/shoulder immobilizer well tolerated	1. No improvement of fracture alignment 2. Possible loss of shoulder range of motion
Reduction and external immobilization	1. Improves fracture alignment 2. No implant concerns (infection, migration, malposition, etc.) 3. No need for secondary anesthesia for implant removal	1. Need general anesthesia 2. Cumbersome cast/splint 3. No direct rigid fixation of fracture (potential for loss of reduction)
Reduction and internal fixation	1. Improves fracture alignment 2. Semirigid fixation of fracture 3. Improved patient comfort (due to fracture fixation) 4. No cumbersome cast or splint	1. Need general anesthesia 2. Minimal increased risk of infection 3. Implant concerns 4. Need for implant removal

tures (Table 17-6), but direct comparison of the techniques has not been performed to date.

FRACTURES OF THE HUMERAL SHAFT

Fractures of the humeral shaft represent 10% or less of humerus fractures in children[96,264,336] and 2% to 5.4% of all children's fractures.[96,571] They are most common in children under 3 and over 12 years of age.[42] The incidence is greater in children with more severe trauma.[482] The incidence is 12 to 30 per 100,000 per year.[314,571,590] Birth injuries to the humerus have a reported incidence ranging from 0.035% to 0.34%.[83,361]

Principles of Management

Mechanisms of Injury

Birth Injuries. Humeral fractures are more common in breech presentations and with macrosomic infants. The most difficult position is when the child's arms have gone above the head with maneuvers to bring the arm down after version and extraction.[361]

Child Abuse. Humeral fractures in child abuse represent 61% of all new fractures and 12% of all fractures in these unfortunate children.[348,505] Shaw et al.,[505] in a retrospective review of 34 humeral shaft fractures in children under 3 years of age, found that most occurred accidentally: only 6 were classified as caused by probable abuse. Child abuse must be part of the differential diagnosis in children with humeral diaphyseal fractures.[426] The fractures may be spiral from a twisting injury or transverse from a direct blow.

Older Children. Older children sustain primarily transverse fractures from direct blows to the arm, frequently from falls, pedestrian/vehicle accidents, gunshot wounds, and machinery. Sports injuries are direct from contact sports or indirect from throwing. Throwing injuries occur as a stress injury from overuse or acutely during the throwing cycle from poor mechanics.[9,76,186,200,206,235,343,321,527,548,576] A stress fracture also has been reported in an adolescent tennis player.[454] Acute throwing fractures result from a sudden external rotation torque developed on the distal humerus with concomitant proximal internal rotation from the pectoralis major between the cocking and acceleration phases[141] as shoulder external rotation and elbow flexion suddenly changes to shoulder internal rotation and elbow extension. Humeral fractures may occur from arm wrestling in older adolescents.[39,351,391] Some humeral fractures are pathologic through benign lesions such as simple bone cysts or through dysplastic bones from osteogenesis imperfecta or fibrous dysplasia. Occasionally, pathologic fractures occur from malignant tumors.

Signs and Symptoms

History. The infant who does not move the shoulder poses a diagnostic challenge. Establishing and evaluating a differential diagnosis is the first concern. According to the history, was the delivery normal? When was the problem noticed? Does the child move any part of the extremity? Was there a history of maternal gestational diabetes or of fetal macrosomia? Does the child nurse from each breast? A broad, useful differential diagnosis consists of clavicle fracture, proximal humeral physeal fracture, humeral shaft fracture, shoulder dislocation, brachial plexus palsy, septic shoulder, osteomyelitis, hemiplegia, stroke, and child abuse.

Examination. Initially, the child should be observed for spontaneous motion of the upper extremity. Is there any hand or elbow motion? Are there any areas of swelling, ecchymosis, or increased warmth? Does the child move the ipsilateral lower extremity? The clinician should carefully palpate each area of the upper extremity, starting with the clavicle and comparing it carefully with the opposite side for any change in soft tissue contour or tenderness. The upper arms and shoulders should then be examined, looking for any tenderness in the supraclavicular fossa. Lastly, the spine should be examined for tenderness or swelling.

Birth Fractures of the Humerus. In the newborn, a humeral fracture can simulate a brachial plexus palsy with pseudoparalysis and an asymmetric Moro reflex. The fracture site is tender and may have swelling or ecchymosis. The diagnosis is confirmed by plain radiography.[253,361]

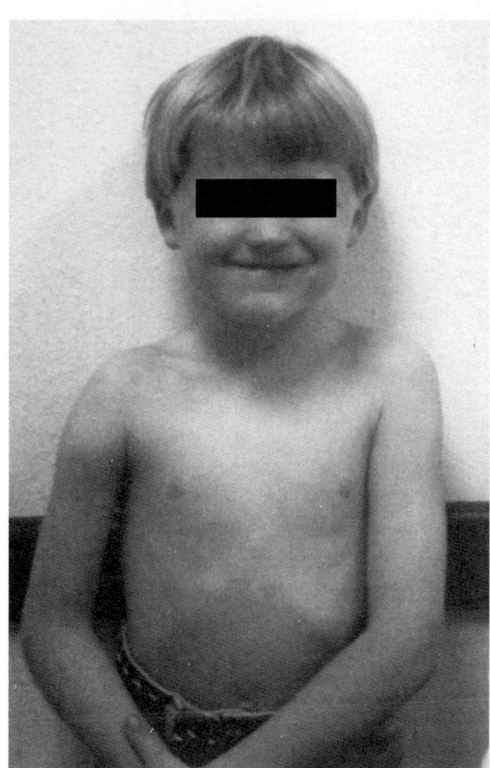

FIGURE 17-39 A young patient with a humeral shaft fracture holding the arm tightly to his side.

Older Children. In older children, the diagnosis is usually evident with pain, swelling, and unwillingness to move the arm. The arm is often supported by the opposite hand and is held tightly to the body (Fig. 17-39). It is essential to perform a complete neurologic and vascular examination of the extremity before any treatment except emergency splinting.

Children with torus or greenstick fractures may have localized tenderness but no deformity. In multiple-trauma victims, careful evaluation should be made of the arm because the diagnosis can be missed, especially if the patient is medically unstable.[316] Humeral fractures should be sought in patients with massive upper extremity trauma.

Diagnosis and Classification

The simplest classification for humeral diaphyseal fractures describes the location (proximal third, middle third, or distal third, or the diaphyseal–metaphyseal junction), the pattern (spiral, short oblique, or transverse), the direction of displacement, and any tissue damage. Anatomically, the location is noted as proximal to the pectoralis major insertion, between the pectoralis major and deltoid insertions, below the deltoid insertion, or at the distal metaphyseal–diaphyseal junction.[123] Humeral shaft fractures may be segmental, with fractures of the shaft and neck,[526,539] or associated with shoulder dislocation.[17,34] If they are associated with fractures of the ipsilateral forearm, they result in the so-called floating elbow.[69,523]

The Association for the Study of Internal Fixation has a classification for humeral shaft fractures designed for adults,[245,397] but it is not as helpful in the evaluation and treatment of most children's humeral fractures, and like most classifications, it is subject to some interobserver variability.[182,275]

Imaging Studies. Radiographs may be needed of the shoulder, clavicle, humerus, and cervical spine. Often the shoulder, clavicle, and humerus can be seen on a single AP view of both upper extremities and the chest. Ultrasonography can be used to identify a fracture of the clavicle or the proximal humeral epiphysis, a shoulder dislocation, or a shoulder effusion by a skilled radiologist. A CT and MRI scan may be necessary to evaluate a pathologic fracture. The radiographic findings for each fracture are discussed in the particular anatomic sections.

AP and lateral radiographs are sufficient and complete in most instances of humeral shaft fractures. In the occasional case where the diagnosis is suspect but not readily apparent on these views, oblique views may be useful.

Radiographic Findings. Fractures of the humerus are usually quite apparent on AP and lateral radiographs of the humerus. Radiographs should be taken in both the AP and lateral planes to obtain two films perpendicular to each other to assess displacement. A true lateral view of the distal humerus is noted by superimposition of the posterior supracondylar ridges of the medial and lateral epicondyles.[204,518] A supracondylar process of the humerus, when present, is best seen on an oblique radiograph showing the anterior medial aspect of the distal humerus.

Displaced fractures above the pectoralis major have marked abduction of the proximal fragment with external rotation by the rotator cuff attachment.[118,123] The distal fragment is pulled proximally by the deltoid and medially by the pectoralis major. Displaced fractures between the pectoralis major and deltoid insertions show adduction of the proximal fragment from the pectoralis major and shortening by pull of the deltoid on the distal fragment. Fractures below the deltoid insertion have abduction of the long proximal fragment by the deltoid, but with shortening and medial displacement of the distal fragment by the pull of the biceps and triceps.[123]

Pathologic bone may be evident.[526,539] Simple bone cysts are a common cause of fractures. Periostitis or periosteal reaction of the humerus necessitates differentiating osteomyelitis or Ewing sarcoma from a stress fracture; every effort must be made to identify a cortical fissure using other imaging techniques.[17,34,69,523]

Holstein and Lewis[245] described a short oblique fracture of the distal third of the humerus with risk of radial nerve palsy.[397] This has been called the Holstein-Lewis fracture.

Surgical and Applied Anatomy

Embryology and Development

The end of the embryonic period is marked by vascular invasion of the humerus at age 8 weeks. During the subsequent fetal period, the humerus resembles the adult bone in both form and muscular relationships.[182,204,275,518] A bony collar is present very early with subsequent enchondral bone formation. The secondary ossification centers at the ends are not generally ossified radiographically until after birth.[204,518]

Osseous

The proximal metaphysis of the humerus is wider than the thinner, triangular shaft. Distally, this flattens and widens to form the condylar region of the elbow. The deltoid inserts into a protuberance midway down the shaft known as the deltoid tuberosity. Distal to the tuberosity, the muscular spinal groove

TABLE 17-7 Interventions for Fractures of the Humeral Shaft and Distal Humeral Diaphyseal Fractures

	Nonoperative (sling-and-swathe; U plaster; hanging arm cast)	Functional Bracing	Operative Reduction and Internal Fixation
Birth fractures, humeral shaft	X		
Humeral shaft	X	X	
Distal humeral diaphyseal	X	X	X

wraps posteriorly around the humerus. The groove gives origin to the uppermost fibers of the brachialis. The periosteum of the humeral diaphysis is thick and provides good remodeling potential.[118,122] The main vascular foramen is at midshaft, but accessory foramina are common—most enter the anterior surface usually below the main foramen, but many are posterior.[86,204,518]

Nerves

The radial nerve ordinarily lies close to the inferior lip of the spiral groove but not directly in it.[580] The profunda artery either accompanies the radial nerve or passes in a second narrower groove. The nerve is protected from the humerus by a layer of either the triceps or the brachialis until the lower margin of the spiral groove near the lateral intermuscular septum.[580] The ulnar nerve passes from anterior to posterior just distal to the humeral midshaft. A well-formed arcade (arcade of Struthers) covers the ulnar nerve as it passes distally.[283] This arcade is always posterior to the medial intermuscular septum and subsequently joins the medial intermuscular septum proximal to the medial epicondyle. A few patients with a modified arcade have only superficial fibers of the triceps medial head passing superficial to the ulnar nerve and none deep to the nerve, making the nerve very close to the bone and vulnerable during a fracture.[283]

Muscles

Several major muscle attachments occur throughout the metaphyseal and diaphyseal regions of the humerus. The pectoralis major muscle inserts laterally and distal to the bicipital groove along the anterior aspect of the humerus. The latissimus dorsi and teres major insert on the upper medial aspect of the humerus medial to the bicipital groove. The deltoid originates from the clavicle, acromion, and scapular spine to insert over a broad area of the deltoid tuberosity. The coracobrachialis arises from the coracoid process and inserts on the anterior medial aspect of the humerus at the junction of the middle and lower thirds. The brachialis originates from the anterior humerus about midway down the shaft. Knowledge of these muscles and their orientation is essential to understand fracture displacement and treatment.[118,243]

Current Treatment Options

Treatment options are listed in Tables 17-7 and 17-8 as well as in the following text.

Birth Injuries

Neonatal humeral shaft fractures heal and remodel quite well, with 40% to 50% remodeling within 2 years (Fig. 17-40).[47] Reported treatments include a sling-and-swathe[244] or a traction device using the von Rosen splint.[22] The primary potential com-

TABLE 17-8 Treatment Pros and Cons: Fractures of the Humeral Shaft and Distal Humeral Diaphyseal Fractures

	Pros	Cons
No reduction (sling or shoulder immobilizer)	1. No anesthesia/sedation 2. Sling/shoulder immobilizer well tolerated	1. No improvement of fracture alignment 2. Possible loss of shoulder range of motion
Reduction and external immobilization	1. Improves fracture alignment 2. No implant concerns (infection, migration, malposition, etc.) 3. No need for secondary anesthesia for implant removal	1. Need general anesthesia 2. Cumbersome cast/splint 3. No direct rigid fixation of fracture (potential for loss of reduction)
Reduction and internal fixation	1. Improves fracture alignment 2. Direct rigid fixation of fracture 3. Improved patient comfort (due to rigid fracture fixation) 4. No cumbersome cast or splint	1. Need general anesthesia 2. Minimal increased risk of infection 3. Implant concerns 4. Possible need for implant removal

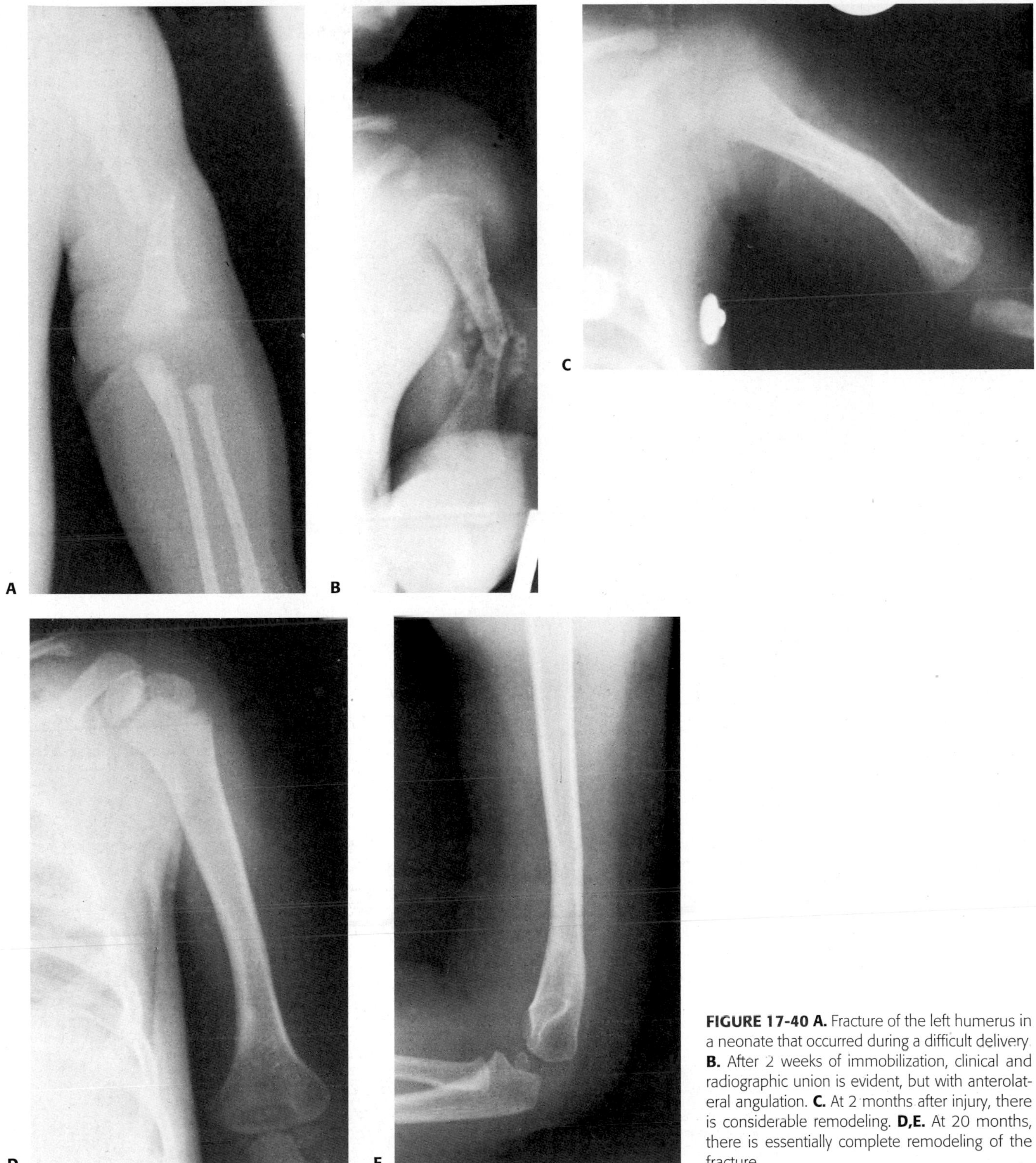

FIGURE 17-40 A. Fracture of the left humerus in a neonate that occurred during a difficult delivery. **B.** After 2 weeks of immobilization, clinical and radiographic union is evident, but with anterolateral angulation. **C.** At 2 months after injury, there is considerable remodeling. **D,E.** At 20 months, there is essentially complete remodeling of the fracture

plication of birth injuries is an internal rotation deformity. Therefore, the fracture can be stabilized by splinting the arm in extension. The long-term, resultant angulation of the healed fracture is minimal due to the child's tremendous capacity of remodeling. Attempts at anatomic reduction are not necessary.[255] If the parents will be moving the child, the splinted arm can be bound to the chest with a soft wrap. These fractures usually heal with some varus and overlap that remodels. Children with arthrogryposis and brachial plexus palsies are prone to internal rotation contractures of the shoulder; these can be exacerbated if the birth fracture's rotation is not controlled.

Stress Fractures

Virtually all nondisplaced stress injuries heal well with temporary rest and immobilization.[9,139,186,200,343,454,527,550,576] They can displace if athletic participation continues without protected rest and healing.[9] Displaced stress fractures should be treated like other humerus fractures.

Acceptable Alignment

Because the humerus is not a weight-bearing bone, it does not require the precise mechanical alignment of the lower extremity. The marked mobility of the shoulder also allows some axial and rotational deviation without functional problems. Severe internal rotation contractures can cause difficulties in some overhead activities such as ball throwing and facial hygiene. Varus of 20 to 30 degrees is necessary before becoming clinically apparent (Fig. 17-41).[123,295,453] Anterior bowing may be appar-

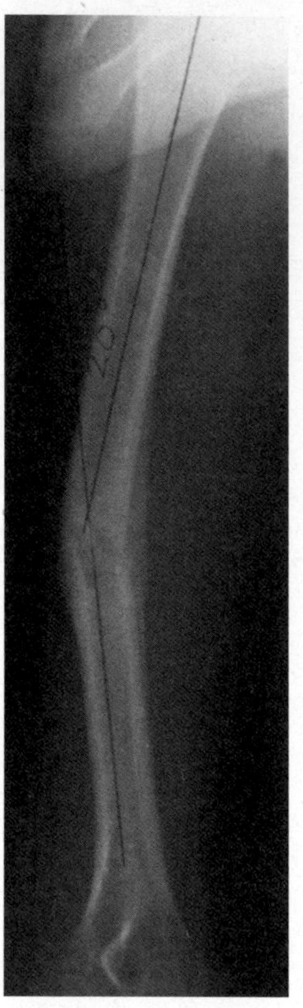

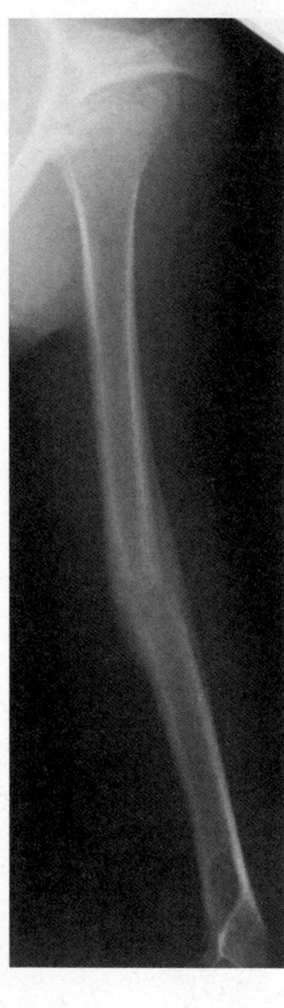

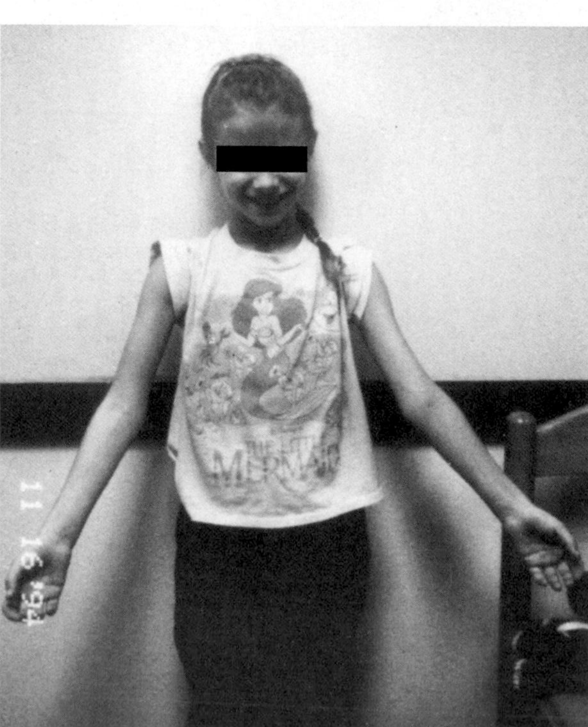

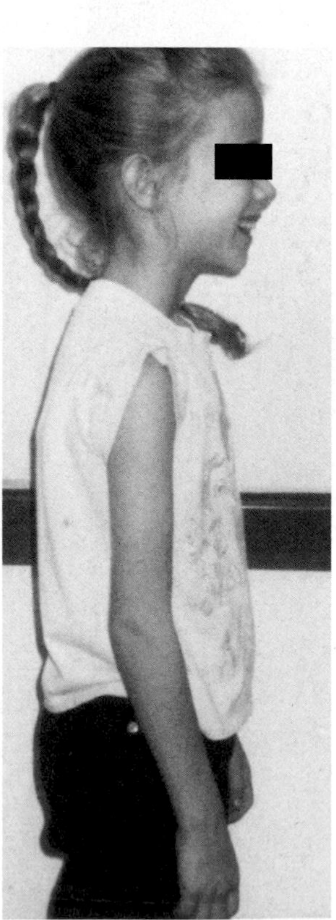

FIGURE 17-41 A,B. Radiographic appearance of a malunited humerus fracture showing 20 degrees of varus. **C,D.** The same patient with no clinical deformity or disability, despite her thin extremities.

ent with 20 degrees of angulation.[295] Functional impairment does not occur with 15 degrees or less of internal rotation deformity.[123] Even adolescents can correct up to 30 degrees spontaneously.[123] Beaty[42] gives guidelines based on the patient's age: children under 5 years of age tolerate 70 degrees angulation and total displacement, children 5 to 12 tolerate 40 to 70 degrees angulation, and children over 12 tolerate 40 degrees and 50% apposition. While not based on a study, these numbers underscore the tremendous remodeling potential of the humerus and the ability to functionally compensate for angulation. Bayonet apposition is acceptable,[171,324,422] with 1 to 2 cm of shortening well-tolerated (Fig. 17-42). Clinical appearance is more important than radiographic alignment.

Nonoperative Treatment

Nonoperative treatment often increases internal rotation by 3 to 12 degrees at the expense of external rotation.[123] This rarely is a functional problem. Nonoperative methods include a sling-and-swathe, the U plaster, a hanging arm cast, a thoracobrachial cast or dressing, a coaptation splint, functional bracing, and traction.

Sling-and-Swathe. The simplest form of treatment for fractures is a sling-and-swathe. It is sufficient for patients with minimally displaced greenstick and torus fractures.[228,453] Although this treatment may yield good results in displaced fractures,[520] it can be quite difficult to control anterior angulation,[246] varus in an obese patient, and may be uncomfortable.

U Plaster-Sugartong or Coaptation Splint. Böhler[63] described a U plaster similar to the sugartong splint used on forearms. Plaster of appropriate width for the upper arm is formed from over the shoulder along the lateral aspect of the arm, underneath the olecranon, and along the medial aspect of the arm to the axilla. Cotton webbing is placed between the plaster and the skin, and the plaster is secured using a wrap (Fig. 17-43). Results have been quite good,[123] particularly in children.[297] Holm[244] suggested applying benzoin before the cotton webbing and using a collar-and-cuff sling about the wrist. To prevent slippage, Shantharam[502] suggested applying the splint from the base of the neck, over the shoulder, and around to the axillary fold, with a strap securing the proximal end to the chest. The U plaster may not control alignment satisfactorily in more displaced fractures, which may require a thoracobrachial cast[62,244,453] or internal fixation if better alignment is necessary. Böhler[62,64] actually abandoned the immediate use of the U plaster for a thoracobrachial cast because of problems with early swelling.

Hanging Arm Cast. The hanging arm cast, described by Caldwell[82] as a technique already in use, consists of a long-arm cast with a sling around the neck tied to the cast along the forearm. The weight of the cast and arm provides longitudinal traction. The position of the sling is modified to correct anterior or posterior angulation and varus or valgus. Rotation is difficult to control. Stewart and Hundley[530] suggested not using it in children under age 12 because children cannot keep their arms in a

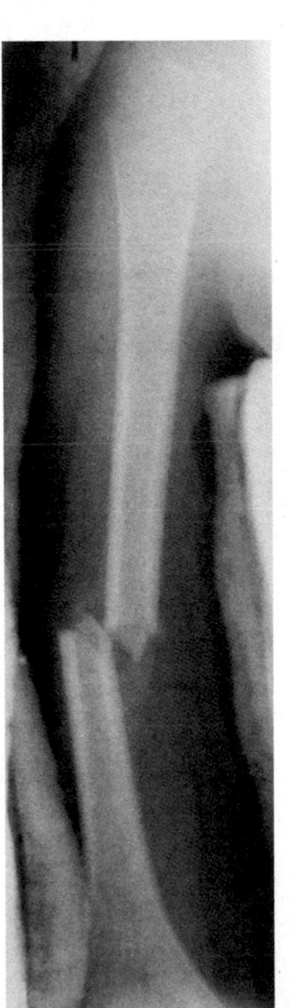

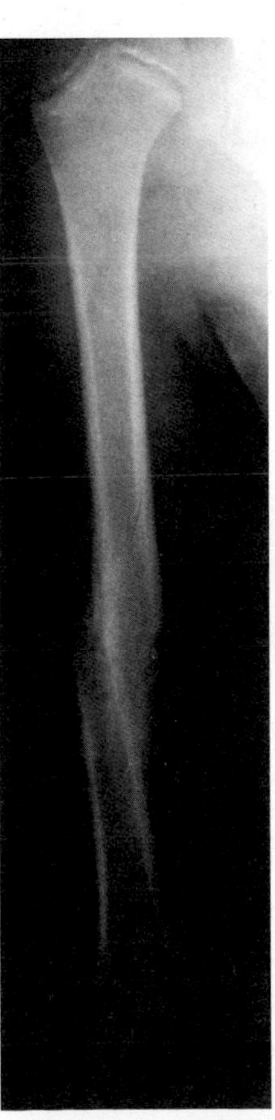

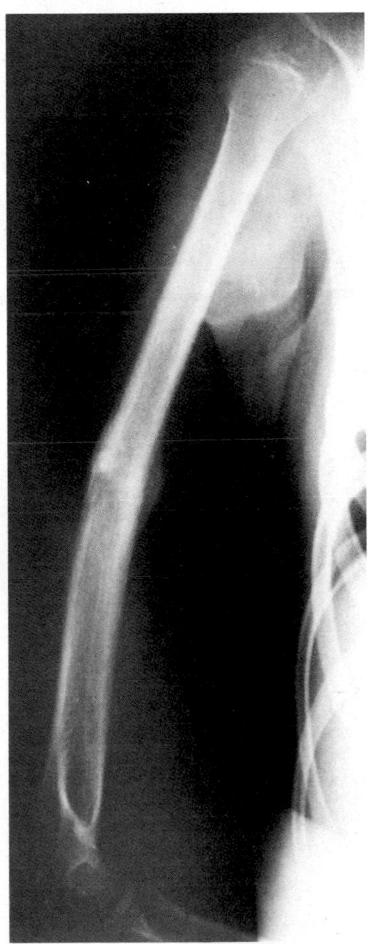

FIGURE 17-42 A. Humerus fracture allowed to heal in slight varus and bayonet apposition. **B,C.** The ultimate result with essentially normal alignment.

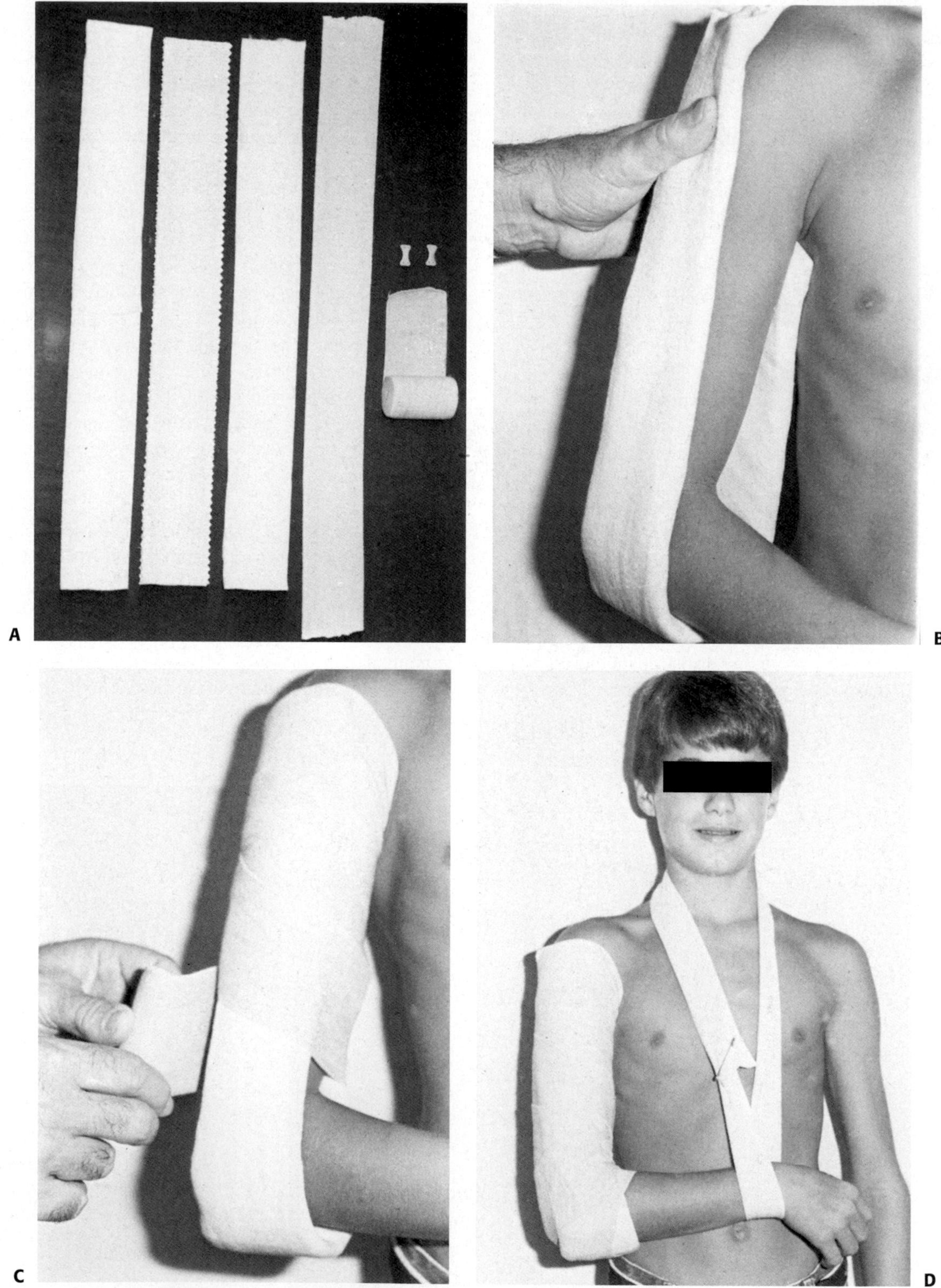

FIGURE 17-43 Coaptation splints with collar and cuff. **A.** The material used for a sugartong arm splint is two pieces of cast padding rolled out to the length of the plaster-of-paris splint and applied to each side of the splint after it is wet. The splint is then brought into the tubular stockinette of the same width but 4 in longer than the splint. **B.** The plaster splint is applied to the arm from the axilla up to the tip of the acromion. **C.** As the plaster is setting, the splint is molded to the arm. An elastic bandage holds the splint in place. **D.** Stockinette is applied and attached to the wrist to form a collar-and-cuff sling.

dependent position during sleep and often keep the arm supported rather than hanging while awake. However, excellent results are reported in patients under age 10.[586] This is probably due to the marked remodeling and potential for good results regardless of treatment in children. Possible complications of the hanging cast include inferior shoulder subluxation,[101] decreased external rotation,[101] and shoulder stiffness,[25] but these are rarely significant in children.

Thoracobrachial Immobilization. Severely unstable fractures uncontrollable in a hanging cast or U plaster may necessitate extending the cast to the chest as a thoracobrachial cast or splint.[62,64,244,246,453] Various types of thoracobrachial dressings are often described as a Velpeau, but technically this is incorrect: Velpeau described a thoracobrachial bandage with acute elbow flexion. If a thoracobrachial cast or splint is used for a grossly unstable fracture, usually only a few degrees of abduction is necessary.[244] Distal diaphyseal fractures rarely require extension to the chest.

Functional Bracing. Functional bracing, as described by Sarmiento,[489] has been quite effective in adults.[29,145,179,217,329,385,400] It may be difficult to use in children because size differences require a customized brace for each patient or a large supply of braces; however, modern thermoplastics can keep this economical (Fig. 17-44).[43] A prefabricated brace is placed on the initial visit if possible or on subsequent visits after placement of a U plaster or sling-and-swathe at the initial evaluation.[595] The patient must be followed closely and the splint tightened as needed. It should not be used in bedridden patients because of loss of gravity support.[29] Sarmiento[487–489] noted difficulty in controlling anterior angulation and indicated that patients should not lean on the elbow. The results in adults may be functionally superior to those of the U plaster.[503]

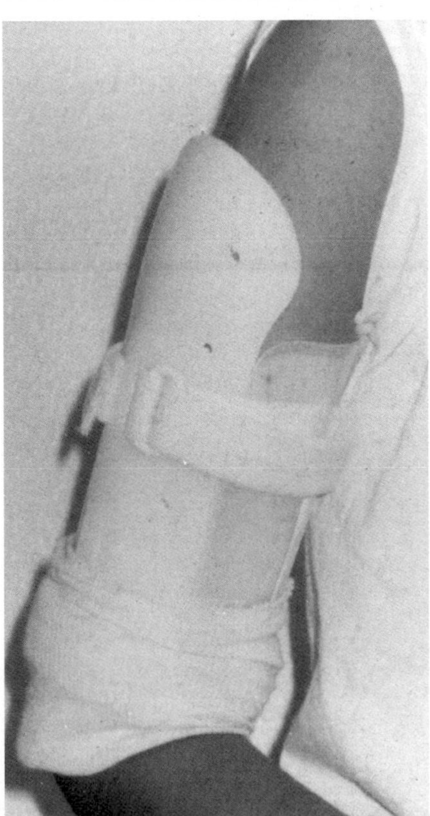

FIGURE 17-44 Light plastic functional braces are useful to maintain alignment and allow early restoration of motion, particularly in older children and adolescents.

Traction. Side-arm and overhead skin and skeletal forms of traction have been described.[20,244,453,559] If olecranon skeletal traction is used, the AO method of an eye screw in the olecranon is less likely to produce ulnar nerve irritation than is a transolecranon pin.[275,453] Excessive traction can lead to nonunion in adults[236] and elbow dislocation in children.[229] This technique is rarely utilized now due to economic and family considerations.

Operative Treatment

There are several surgical alternatives for humeral diaphyseal fractures: pinning, external fixation, intramedullary rodding, screw fixation, and compression plating. Biomechanically, interlocking rods are the stiffest in bending, and dynamic compression plating is stiffest in torsion. Flexible intramedullary rods are not as stiff as intact bone.[233]

Open Reduction and Internal Reduction. Open reduction and internal reduction can be performed through either a posterior triceps-splitting approach, as advocated by the AO group,[275,475] or through an anterior lateral approach between the brachialis and brachioradialis with extension proximally between the deltoid and pectoralis.[44,166] The normal 4.5-mm dynamic compression plate does not provide adequate stability for the adult humerus shaft. The broad 4.5-mm dynamic compression plate is designed to allow compact screw placement without causing excessive stress on the humerus in adults.[275] At least six cortices of screw fixation proximal and distal to the fracture site are needed. In children, smaller plates can be used, such as small pelvic reconstruction plates and double stacked semitubular plates depending on the size of the child. With either the anterolateral or posterior approach, the lateral intermuscular septum should be split in the distal third to release the tether of the radial nerve. Interfragmentary lag screws should be used when possible. The plate should be slipped underneath the radial nerve and vessels and some muscle placed between the plate and the nerve. Multiple screws in oblique fractures without a compression plate are unsatisfactory in adults[475] but may be sufficient in children. Extensively comminuted fractures may require bone graft.

Generally, the results are good,[44,230,231,399,587,600] and plating is particularly advocated in multiple-trauma patients to facilitate nursing care and management of other injuries.[44] Potential complications include radial nerve palsy, infection, delayed union, nonunion, and failure of fixation.[600]

Intramedullary Rodding. Several types of intramedullary rods are available. Currently, there are no indications for reamed intramedullary nailing in children because of potential proximal physeal damage and the small diaphyseal diameter. However, they may be used in skeletally mature adolescents if the canal has sufficient diameter.[457] Reamed nailing has been reported in patients as young as 16.[115,149] The results are generally good,[115,141,219,262,299,369,450,465,554,556,596] with a low risk of nonunion and infection.[24]

Unreamed nails, such as Ender nails, Rush rods, or flexible titanium rods, have been used most extensively in adults with multitrauma. Nails or rods can be inserted via a posterior triceps-splitting approach through a hole just above the olecranon fossa. This can be useful for rapid management of fractures, including open fractures in patients with multiple trauma.[76,93,110,133,220] Rods should not be inserted through the greater tuberosity in children (except under extenuating circumstances) because of risk of injury to the proximal humeral physis and the potential for shoulder impingement.[359,467,529] Inserting these relatively large rods through the epicondyles results in a high incidence of nail back-out.[220]

There are two techniques of using small, flexible, smooth wires. In the Hackethal technique,[216] fluoroscopy is used with a tourniquet placed on the upper arm. A hole is made just proximal to the olecranon fossa using a triceps-splitting approach. Smooth, blunt-tipped Steinmann pins are placed up the canal of the humerus, progressively filling the canal with smaller and smaller pins as needed (Fig. 17-45). Results are generally good,[92,137,147,234,383,433,599] although pin back-out can be a problem and care must be taken not to distract the fracture site. The rods should be bent 90 degrees at the cortical window.[433] This technique may be useful for segmental and pathologic fractures.[342]

The other technique consists of using small smooth rods or Steinmann pins placed through the epicondyles.[340,384] The tips of the rods should be blunt and slightly bent. These are placed through the lateral epicondyle or through both the medial and lateral epicondyles. A hole is made in the epicondyle, and a blunt-tipped Steinmann pin is tapped up the diaphysis using a mallet or passed by hand, with a drill chuck holding the pin.

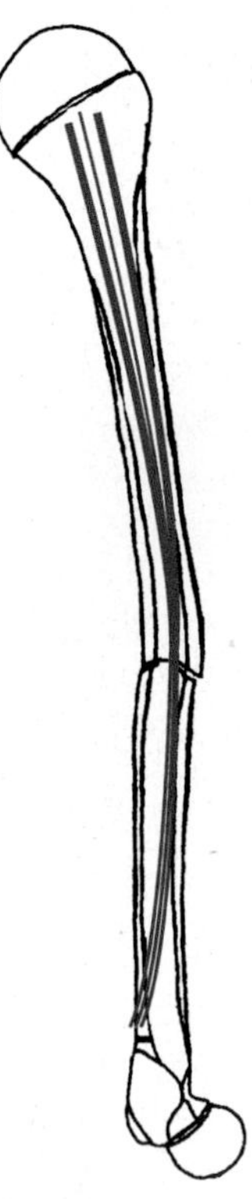

FIGURE 17-45 The Hackethal technique involves multiple smooth pins placed up the humeral shaft through a cortical window just above the olecranon fossa. The pins are placed until the canal is filled.

The bend on the tip of the rods facilitates crossing the fracture site and manipulating the fracture reduction. A splint is necessary postoperatively. Alignment need be only within the tolerances for a closed reduction (Fig. 17-46). The use of flexible intramedullary nailing has also been described with good success in children and adolescents.[319]

External Fixation. Both unilateral and multiplanar external fixation techniques are occasionally useful for humeral shaft fractures.[20,129,281,289] External fixators are primarily useful for severe open fractures or as an alternative to internal fixation. In patients with open fractures, immediate external fixation with subsequent bone grafting yields good results.[449,514] External fixation can be combined with internal fixation for immediate stability[112] and early rehabilitation. Severe open fractures with bone loss can be treated with primary shortening followed by callus distraction[479] to provide early soft tissue coverage and subsequent restoration of humeral length. Care must be taken during pin placement to avoid radial nerve injury. If screws are used, limited open screw placement can prevent this injury.[449] Ring fixators may be useful for reconstructing the injured humerus.[78,89,90,102,259,260,508,510]

Operative versus Conservative Treatment

Because most humeral fractures are controllable nonoperatively, there are few surgical indications.[46] Potential operative indications include open fractures, multiple trauma, bilateral injuries, arterial injuries, compartment syndromes, pathologic fractures, significant nerve injuries, inadequate closed reduction, and ipsilateral upper extremity injuries or paralysis.

Preadolescents can almost always be managed nonoperatively, except those with severe soft tissue injury. If fracture reduction cannot obtain less than 30 degrees varus and 20 degrees anterior angulation in older children and adolescents—or more importantly, if the arm appears deformed—alternatives such as internal fixation, intramedullary rodding, external fixation, or a thoracobrachial cast should be considered. Inadequate closed reduction is most common in obese patients and in thin women with large breasts.[475] However, obesity tends to hide the deformity of the fracture, and large breasts are seldom encountered in thin children.

Open fractures may require fixation. Small, stable grade 1 wounds can still be managed using coaptation splints or other closed methods. Unstable open fractures should be stabilized with internal or external fixation to protect soft tissues.[98,133,331,358,475,560]

Multiple-trauma victims are often best treated with internal or external fixation for more rapid mobilization.[42,76,44,66,347,366] This is particularly true in patients with chest injuries, where thoracobrachial immobilization would compromise pulmonary care.[133,347,358] Excellent results have been reported with external fixation[98,281,449,514]; retrograde rodding using titanium, Ender, or Rush rods[76]; and internal fixation.[44] In older adolescents, more rigid locked or unlocked intramedullary rodding can be used for patients requiring their upper extremities for mobility.[166] However, this luxury does not exist for younger children.

Arterial injury and compartment syndromes requiring fasciotomy are potential indications for internal fixation.[178,445,455,516] Continued fracture mobility can damage a vascular anastomosis,[180,378,455,516] and fasciotomy can make the fracture less sta-

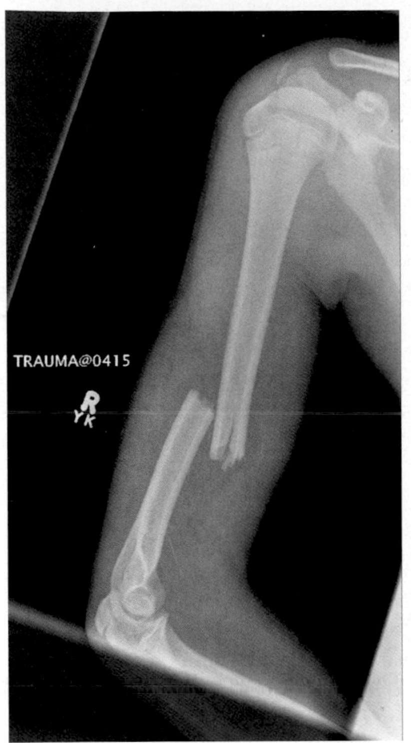

A

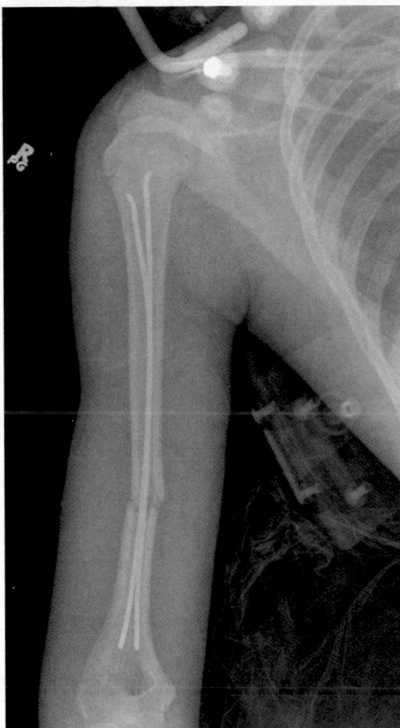

B

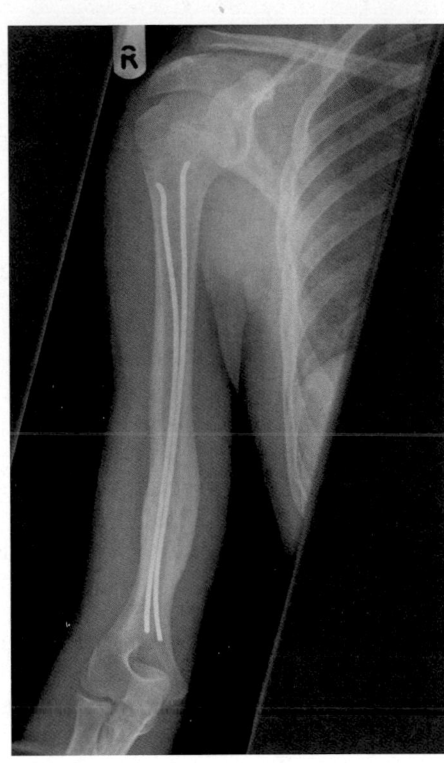

C

FIGURE 17-46 A. Displaced fracture difficult to align with nonoperative methods. **B.** Surgical treatment with tow intramedullary rods. Alignment need be only within the same tolerances as closed reduction. **C.** Healed fracture.

ble. Temporary vascular shunting before internal fixation allows the orthopaedist and the vascular surgeon to work under optimal conditions.[97]

Most pathologic fractures in children, including those from malignancy,[462] fibrous dysplasia,[190,526,539] osteogenesis imperfecta, and simple bone cysts, can be treated nonoperatively. Simple bone cysts are discussed in the section on proximal humerus fractures. A report of a 6-year-old with progressive ossifying fibrodysplasia suggests that internal fixation may prevent stiffness after fractures in this condition.[405] In fractures secondary to malignancy, intramedullary rodding is necessary if extensive cortical loss causes instability.[109,149,334,529,552] Spontaneous fracture in a severely brain-injured or unresponsive cerebral palsy patient is best treated nonoperatively.[557]

Ipsilateral injuries, particularly fractures of the proximal or distal humerus and of the forearm, can be difficult to control. In adults with a floating elbow, internal fixation or elastic nailing of the humeral fracture provides optimal results.[76,315,463] This is also true for supracondylar humeral fractures in children but is not documented in diaphyseal fractures.[69,523] The floating elbow is often associated with other organ system injuries; nerve injury occurs in up to 50% of these patients.[438]

Humeral shaft fractures with ipsilateral brachial plexus palsies in adults heal best with open reduction and internal fixation.[70] The same is true with spinal cord injuries.[185] Functional bracing is precluded in these patients because the muscles do not function and sensation is altered. Because of the excellent healing potential in children, they may be treated nonoperatively if satisfactory alignment can be maintained. Older adolescents should be treated like adults.

Radial Nerve Palsies

Radial nerve palsies with humeral shaft fractures have been reported in children (Fig. 17-47).[94,358] Primary radial nerve palsies occur at the time of the fracture; secondary radial nerve palsies occur after manipulation of the fracture. Many clinicians recommend exploration of secondary radial nerve palsies[42,123,181,431,444,506,555,571] and a few do for primary nerve injuries.[10,119,181,245,307,311,397,431,444,464,542] The incidence of concomitant radial nerve palsy with a humeral shaft fracture

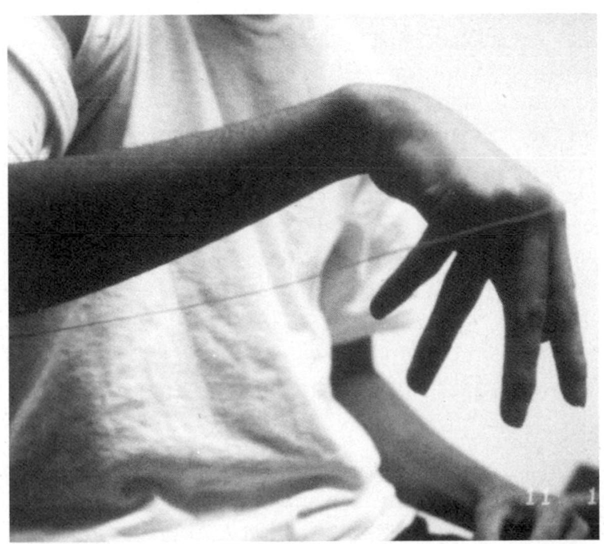

FIGURE 17-47 Radial nerve palsy secondary to a humeral shaft fracture from a low-velocity gunshot wound.

ranges from 2.4% to 20.6%[24,52,181,358,370,441,464,501,563] and has been reported in 4.4% of children's humeral shaft fractures.[358] Most occur with middle and distal humeral shaft fractures, but they may occur with more proximal fractures as well.[370] In explored primary radial nerve palsies, the incidence of complete nerve laceration is small.[204,358,431,501,518,563] Commonly, the nerve is tented over the bone, trapped in the fracture site, or contused. The natural history is excellent, with recovery ranging from 78% to 100%.[12,52,65,66,140,181,195,431,441,444,482,501,563] Therefore, most clinicians recommend observation rather than early exploration.[52,140,181,195,431,441,444,482,501,563] This is especially true in children where the periosteum can be protective against entrapment and the nerves can recovery quickly from contusion and traction ischemia. Open fractures resulting in severe soft tissue injury requiring débridement should have the radial nerve identified. If lacerated, exploration and tagging for later repair,[535] or preferably, primary repair is performed.[167] More severe open fractures should be stabilized using either intramedullary rodding, internal or external fixation to provide stability for soft tissue healing, or radial nerve recovery. Early repair of the nerve provides the best anatomic results.[49] Bostman et al.[66] recommended exploration and internal fixation in patients with bayonet apposition because the abundant callus may endanger nerve recovery. The recommended waiting time before radial nerve exploration ranges from 8 weeks to 6 months.[10,12,123,140,246,370,441,444,453,506,571] Nerve grafting up to 18 months after the injury can provide good function.[49,165] Ogawa[419] reported a complete radial nerve division which was repaired with a sural nerve graft resulting in full function. Seddon[495] suggested a physiologic time of allowing 1 mm per day after the 1 to 2 months of Wallerian degeneration and nerve growth through the neuroma. Nerves grow 1 to 3 mm per day,[495,496,534] and this rate has been used clinically with good success.[199,535] In children, healing is usually faster and signs of spontaneous recovery are usually present by 3 months. This is noted by an advancing Tinel sign, radial wrist extension recovery followed by central wrist extension, digital metacarpophalangeal extension, and then thumb retropulsion and ipsilateral extension.

In secondary radial nerve palsies, the surgeon may feel compelled to explore the nerve because he or she "caused" the radial nerve injury. However, natural history studies of observed secondary radial nerve palsies show recovery rates of 80% to 100% with nonoperative treatment.[66,181] Secondary palsies occurring after manipulation may be observed.[52,140,310,432,501] If the palsy occurs after a considerable time, the nerve is probably encased in callus and further investigation, including exploration, is warranted.[148,531] Late presentation may result in an osseous foramen containing the nerve and requiring decompression.[148] Again, in children, there should be signs of recovery by 3 months, and no later than 6 months, if natural history is chosen.

AUTHORS' PREFERRED TREATMENT

Birth fractures have a very good prognosis for full recovery. To prevent an internal rotation contracture, we place the arm in either a U plaster or a plaster coaptation splint with the palm facing anteriorly. A soft wrap holds the arm to the body so the child can be carried. The splint can be removed in 2 weeks. On healing, the radiographic angulation can be quite worrisome to the parents. We like to show them radiographs of other infants with marked remodeling, and we keep photographs handy for this purpose.

Most humeral diaphyseal fractures in children are treated nonoperatively. Torus fractures are treated with a commercial shoulder immobilizer or a sling. Greenstick fractures and displaced fractures in younger children are treated with a U plaster or a plaster coaptation splint; these are usually applied in the emergency department with mild sedation. We prefer general anesthesia if more manipulation is needed. A careful neurologic and vascular evaluation is performed before and after manipulation. We place a U plaster with Webril (Covidien, Mansfield, MA) padding extending from over the deltoid, around the olecranon, and up to the axillary fold, and secure it with a gauze wrap followed by an elastic bandage. We have had similar results applying plaster coaptation splints on the medial and lateral aspects of the arm and rewrapping frequently with an elastic wrap. We carefully pad all bony prominences and neurovascular prominences, especially the ulnar nerve. The patient is placed in a collar-and-cuff sling for forearm support. If alignment is unsatisfactory, a new splint is reapplied and molded.

In those rare fractures uncontrollable by closed means, we prefer smooth intramedullary rodding using two 2-mm rods placed retrograde through the epicondyles. For unstable fractures with extensive comminution, we prefer to use a unilateral external fixator, with small incisions made during screw placement to avoid the radial nerve. Open fractures are treated in a similar manner. Significant bone loss can be treated using bone transport techniques. We avoid plate fixation because it creates a stress riser, particularly in growing children. If a fracture occurs distal or proximal to the plate, it must be re-explored for plate removal, necessitating re-exploration of the radial nerve and potential nerve damage. We observe both primary and early secondary radial nerve palsies, exploring them only after 3 months of observation, failure of anticipated recovery of at least 1 mm per day, and if electromyography shows no return.

Rehabilitation

Patients treated with closed manipulation should be followed weekly for the first few weeks to ensure that alignment is maintained. The coaptation splint or long-arm cast should be replaced as needed. Patients with radial nerve palsies must be instructed in finger motion to keep the fingers supple and prevent contractures. Noncompliance requires formal hand therapy or a radial nerve outrigger. Long-term stiffness of the shoulder and elbow is uncommon in children, but pendulum exercises are started at 3 to 4 weeks in older children and adolescents. Some form of immobilization is generally continued for 6 weeks. Patients should not return to contact sports until there is adequate healing, and the family should be cautioned that refracture may occur during the first 6 months after injury.

The prognosis for healing and remodeling of humeral shaft fractures in children is excellent. Internal rotation deformity is usually minimal, and the outlook for radial nerve palsies is good. Loss of shoulder motion may occur but is more common in older patients.[453]

Complications

Early Complications

Nerve Palsies. Radial nerve palsies were discussed previously. They may occur immediately after operative treatment,[130] or may be delayed and occur many years after internal fixation.[176] Ulnar nerve paralysis has been reported from entrapment of the nerve in the fracture site.[283] A few people have an abnormal arcade of Struthers in which only superficial fibers of the triceps medial head pass superficial to the ulnar nerve and none pass deep to the nerve, making the nerve extremely close to the bone and vulnerable to an abduction extension mechanism of fracture, which opens the anterior medial aspect of the humerus.[283] In about 10% of the population, the median nerve crosses posterior to the brachial artery rather than anterior, placing it closer to the humerus. Median nerve palsy has been reported from an apex anterior middiaphyseal fracture.[360] After an easy fracture reduction, the median nerve was caught in the fracture between the coracobrachialis and brachialis muscles, where the nerve crossed anteriorly. Anterior interosseous nerve palsies have not been reported in fractures above the supracondylar region.

Compartment Syndrome. The fascia of the upper arm is not as strong as it is in the lower arm, making compartment syndrome less common. Mubarak and Carroll[395] reported a dorsal forearm compartment syndrome in a 9-year-old boy with a humerus shaft fracture. Gupta and Sharma[212] described an adult with a triceps compartment syndrome from a middle third minimally displaced fracture; this fracture did not disrupt the intercompartmental boundaries.

Vascular Injuries. Vascular injuries require a high index of suspicion and rapid treatment.[74,130,363,381] The fracture should be stabilized sufficiently to prevent disruption of the vascular repair.

Infection. Infections have been reported in patients undergoing surgery. They have not been reported in closed fractures of the humerus in children, but have been reported in closed fractures elsewhere.[85,570]

Late Complications

Malunion. Malunion is uncommon in children's humeral diaphyseal fractures. Varus of 20 to 30 degrees can be accepted (see Fig. 17-41),[69,123,154,453,523] but anterior bowing of 20 degrees may be apparent.[295] An internal rotation deformity of 15 degrees causes no functional impairment.[123] Most patients under 6 years of age grow out of angular deformities.[246] Children 6 to 13 years of age may not, although some remodeling is possible even in adolescents.[246,409] Obese patients are more prone to malunion, but they also hide their deformity better.[475] Green and Gibbs[333] noted that the deformity visible on the AP and lateral radiographs is generally not the maximum deformity, which is the vector sum of the two deformities. This can be appreciated by obtaining a radiograph perpendicular to the plane of the deformity, similar to the Stagnara view for scoliosis.

Nonunion. Primarily a problem in adults and occasionally in older adolescents, there are few reports of humeral nonunion in children: one in a child with progeria at age 4,[172] four in children with osteogenesis imperfecta,[180] and three from severe trauma.[97] In adults, numerous treatments have been used successfully. These include reamed nails[100] and modified flexible nails.[213,446] However, the best results appear to be from ASIF techniques with the broad dynamic compression plate and autogenous bone grafting.[33,91,161,226,245,397,592] Currently, treatment in children and adolescents must be extrapolated from adult treatment. In general, the atrophic ends of the nonunion are taken back to bleeding surfaces and apposed, a compression plate is applied with fixation of at least six cortical screws proximally and distally, and bone grafting is performed.[226] The Ilizarov technique also reportedly produces good results.[17,34,78,89,259,260,508] Electrical stimulation also has been used with success.[111,156,158,497,498,532] Children with dysplastic bone, such as those with osteogenesis imperfecta, are best treated with intramedullary rodding and bone grafting.[180]

Loss of Motion. Loss of shoulder and elbow motion is more common in older patients.[14,246] The joint affected is usually the one closest to the fracture site.

Upper Extremity Limb-Length Discrepancy. Overgrowth after humeral fracture occurs in about 81% of patients but is generally minimal (<1 cm).[228] Some generalized stimulus to the extremity is evident, with overgrowth of the carpals as well.[490] Lengthening is rarely indicated as the humerus can tolerate 5 to 8 cm of shortening without functional loss due to shoulder and truncal compensation. However, lengthening has been performed in patients with limb-length discrepancy of 3 cm or more at maturity.[120,434] Unilateral or ring fixators may be used with Ilizarov's principles.[89,90]

Other Complications. Uncommon complications include reflex sympathetic dystrophy[169] and fat embolism.[303] Late refracture may occur from retained internal fixation.[68]

DISTAL HUMERAL DIAPHYSEAL FRACTURES

Little has been written about distal humeral diaphyseal or metaphyseal–diaphyseal junction fractures. These injures are much less common than supracondylar humeral fractures occurring in about 3% of displaced fractures of the distal humerus.[162] Fractures in this region should not be confused with supracondylar humeral fractures. The distal diaphysis is more triangular and the periosteum is thinner than in the supracondylar region,[118,122] making these fractures generally less stable than supracondylar fractures. The cortical bone also heals more slowly than metaphyseal bone, requiring longer immobilization. The mobile wad, anconeus, and flexor pronator mass originate off the epicondyles; the biceps, brachialis, and triceps all insert distally. Therefore, forearm position greatly affects the fracture position. Because the brachial artery is tethered by the lacertus fibrosus, injury to the artery is more likely than with more proximal fractures.

Distal humeral diaphyseal–metaphyseal junction fractures may be caused by transverse or longitudinal loading, torsion, or moments generated by the forearm about the elbow. They

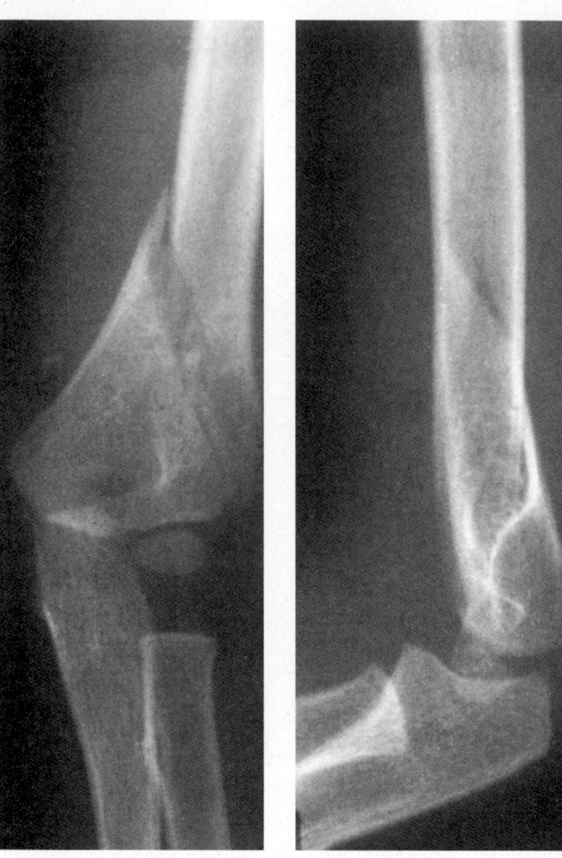

FIGURE 17-48 Distal humeral diaphyseal fracture extending to the epicondyles. This fracture was treated by casting with the forearm in pronation.

are caused by direct blows and twisting more often than ulnar leverage in the olecranon fossa. The diagnosis, made on plain radiographs, must be differentiated from a supracondylar humerus fracture.

Principles of Management

Diagnosis and Classification

Most distal humeral diaphyseal fractures are transverse, spiral, or short oblique. Occasionally, an oblique or spiral fracture extends distally toward or beyond the epicondyles (Fig. 17-48). The description must include the direction of displacement, the neurologic and vascular status, and the degree of comminution. Medial column comminution predisposes to varus malunion.

Current Treatment Options

Nonoperative

Closed treatment usually is possible because acute flexion of the elbow, with potential vascular compromise, is not required to maintain reduction. These fractures tend toward varus malunion (Fig. 17-49),[75] which may be cosmetically unacceptable, particularly in more distal fractures. With 20% or less of humeral growth occurring distally,[56,447,448] significant remodeling may not occur. Because of the proximity to the epicondyles with their muscular origins, supination and pronation affect fracture reduction. If one cortex is open, then the muscles originating on that side should be tightened to reduce the fracture.[16] Because of the varus tendency, this is usually by pronation.[63,64,516] However, this is best checked radiographically (Figs. 17-50 and 17-51).

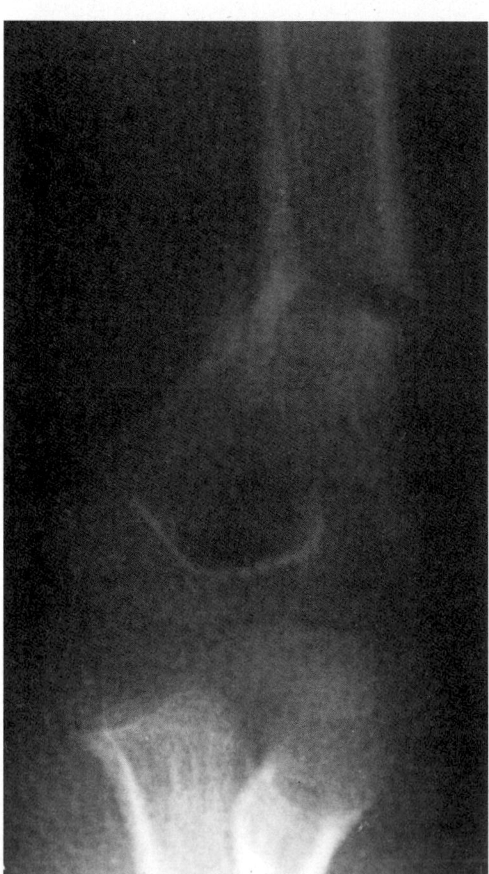

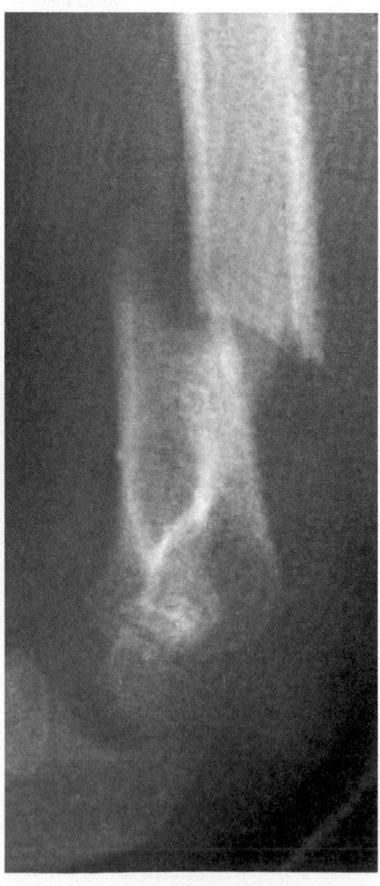

FIGURE 17-49 Radiographs showing the tendency of distal humeral diaphyseal fractures toward varus malunion. The fracture required remanipulation.

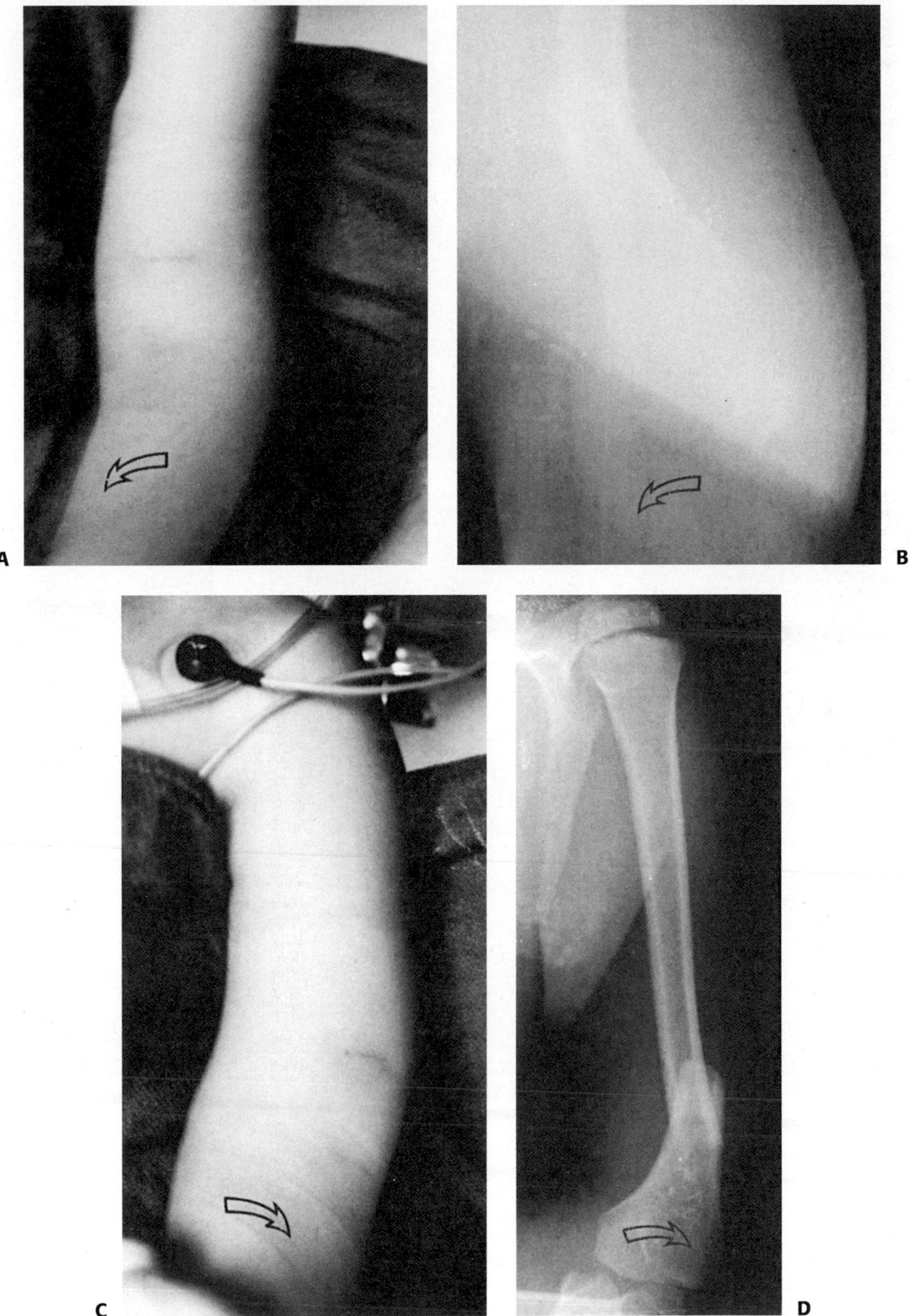

FIGURE 17-50 Influence of forearm rotation. Pronation **(A,B)** of the forearm produces a valgus angulation at the fracture site (*arrows*). Supination **(C,D)** creates a varus angulation (*arrows*).

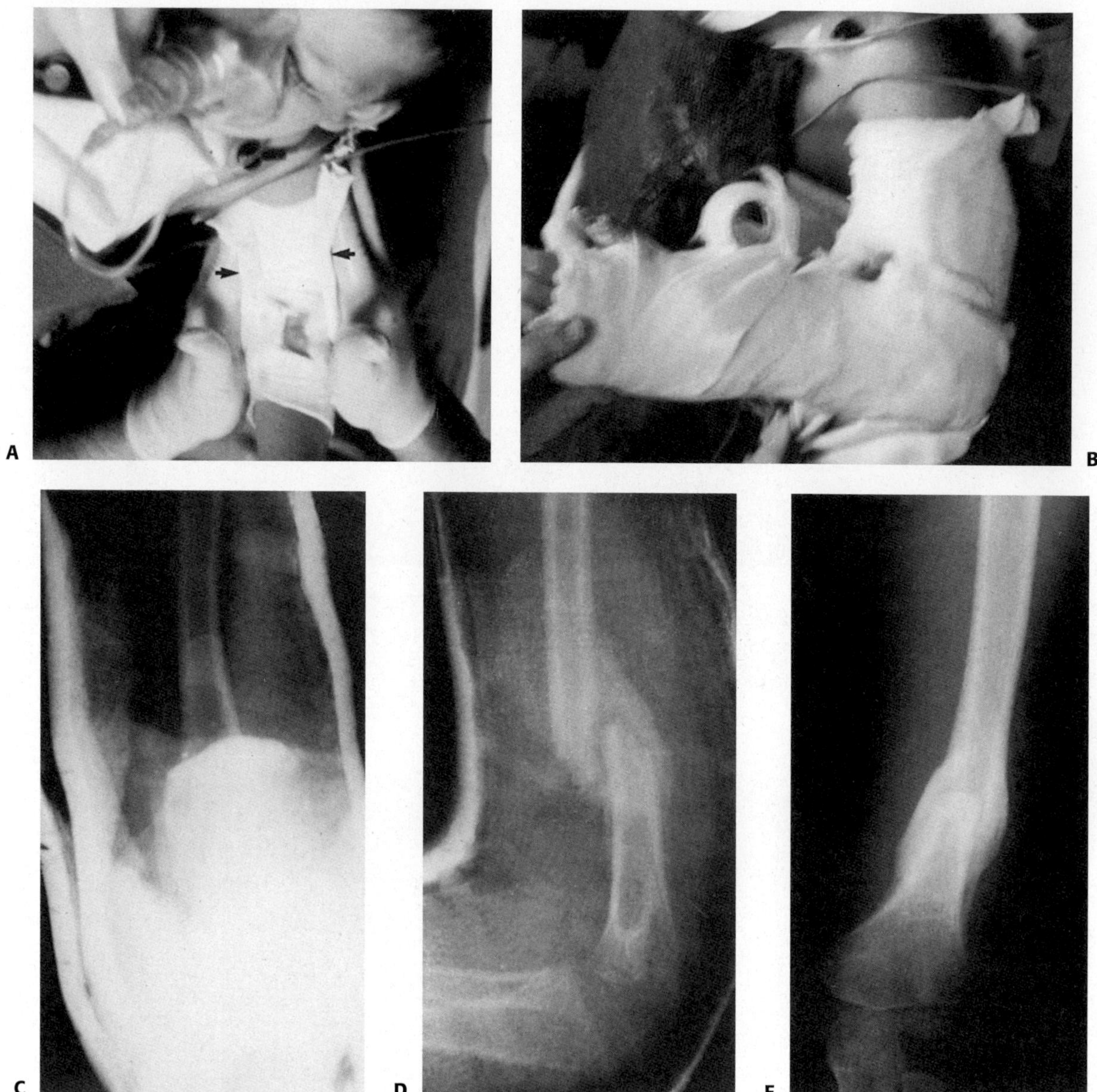

FIGURE 17-51 The same patient shown in Figure 17-50. **A.** The humeral coaptation splint is molded (*arrows*) with the forearm in neutral. **B.** A second forearm coaptation splint is added, and the extremity is suspended with a loop. **C.** Radiographs show satisfactory linear alignment. **D,E.** The fracture healed in bayonet apposition but with satisfactory alignment.

Operative Treatment

Unstable fractures may require fixation[75,453] and possibly open reduction. Closed reduction and percutaneous pinning should be performed in a similar fashion to supracondylar humerus fractures. However, because the fracture is more proximal, it is difficult to get the pins into the diaphysis without crossing them at the fracture site (Fig. 17-52). The difficulty in stabilizing these fractures has been demonstrated by a longer operative time when compared to standard supracondylar fractures.[162] In addition, transverse fractures in this region have a high incidence of loss of fixation, reoperation, pin migration, cubitus varus deformity, and prolonged loss of motion.[162] Attempts can be made to pass the wires in intramedullary fashion up the lateral or medial and lateral columns separately to provide stability (Fig. 17-53).[453] This can be done by drilling the wires, but it is easier to create a starting site at the epicondyles and pass blunt-tipped wires up the columns. Holding the wires with a drill chuck helps, too. Because of the bony anatomy and the ulnar nerve, lateral wires are easier to place, particularly in younger children (Fig. 17-54). However, unilateral intramedullary fixation may lead to bowing. Alternatively, the fracture can be managed with skeletal traction until callus forms; then either

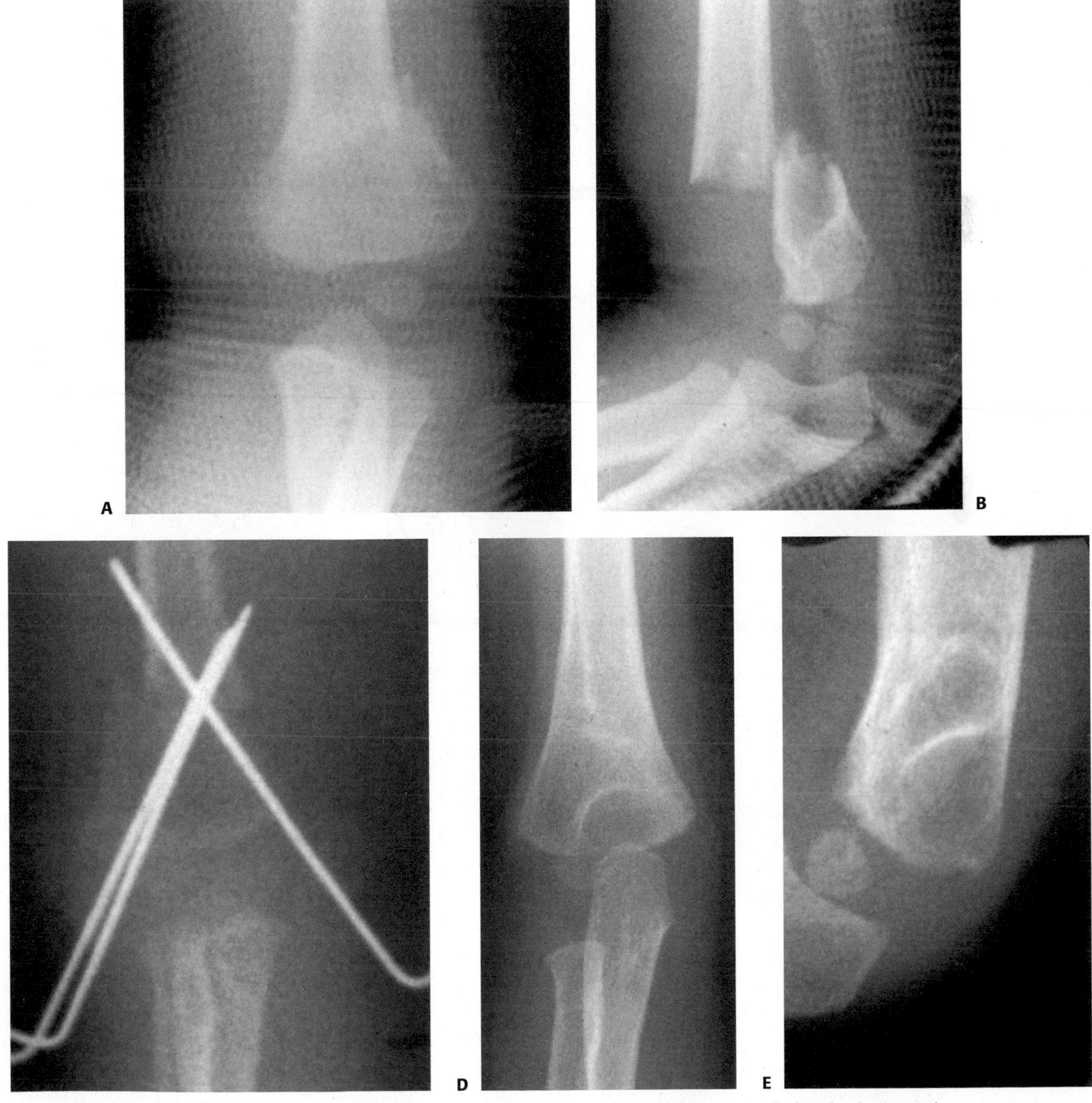

FIGURE 17-52 A,B. Distal humeral diaphyseal fracture in an 18-month-old treated with closed reduction and percutaneous pinning. **C.** The pins cross at the fracture site with decreased stability and some loss of position. **D,E.** The ultimate outcome was good.

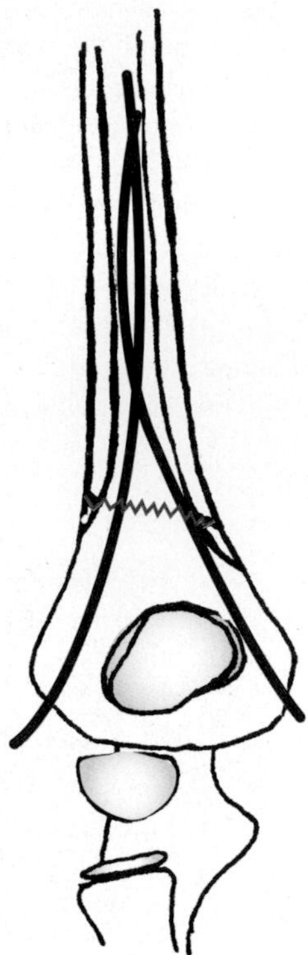

FIGURE 17-53 Ideally, pin fixation for distal humeral diaphyseal–metaphyseal junction fractures involves pins placed in intramedullary fashion up the medial and lateral columns.

a U plaster splint or a long-arm cast can be applied (Fig. 17-55). Brug et al.[75] reported the best results with flexible intramedullary rodding. If internal fixation with a plate is chosen, both columns need to be stabilized.

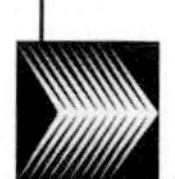

AUTHORS' PREFERRED TREATMENT

For distal humeral diaphyseal–metaphyseal junction fractures, we prefer closed treatment. Nondisplaced fractures are treated with a long-arm cast split to allow for swelling. A double sugartong splint is used if swelling is severe. We reduce displaced fractures under general anesthesia. Because supination and pronation of the forearm can affect the position, we use the image intensifier to determine the position best for maintaining the reduction; this is usually pronation. If the reduction obtained is unstable and cannot be held with a cast, we do not hesitate to treat it by percutaneous pinning with small Steinmann pins placed through the medial and lateral epicondyles and up their respective columns, keeping the pins as divergent as possible at the fracture site or with lateral column pins. It is helpful to introduce them through the epicondyle and then tap rather than drill them up the column to prevent convergence at the fracture site. The pins are removed once good callus forms.

SUPRACONDYLOID PROCESS FRACTURES

Occasionally, a proboscis-like supracondyloid process extends from a few centimeters above the medial epicondyle. The

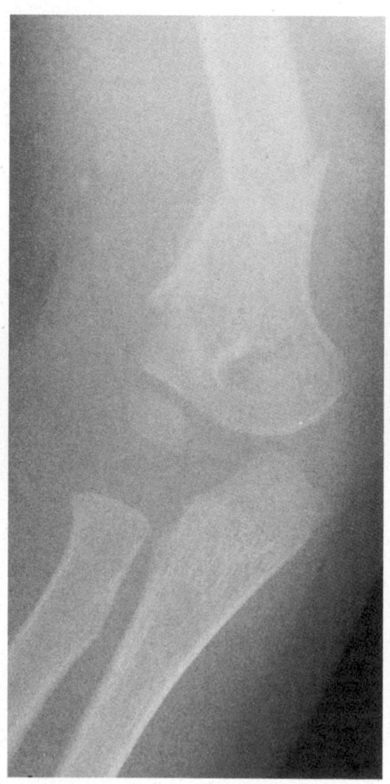

A

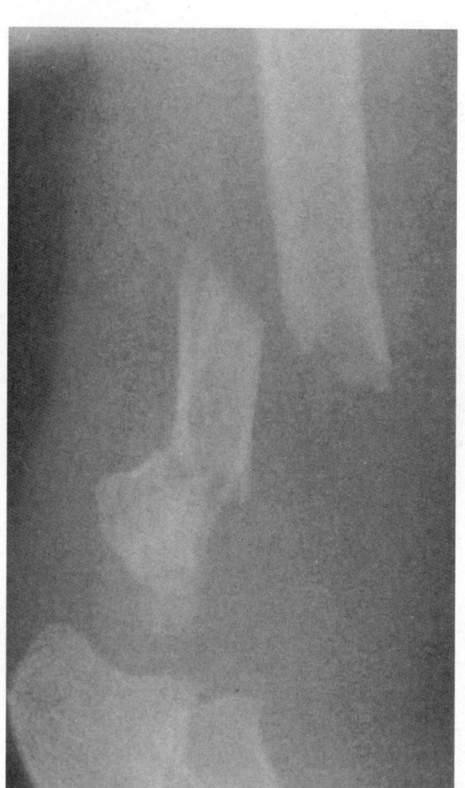

B

FIGURE 17-54 Segmental distal humeral diaphyseal and supracondylar fracture in a 4-year-old boy. **A,B.** Both fractures could not be controlled by closed means. *(continues)*

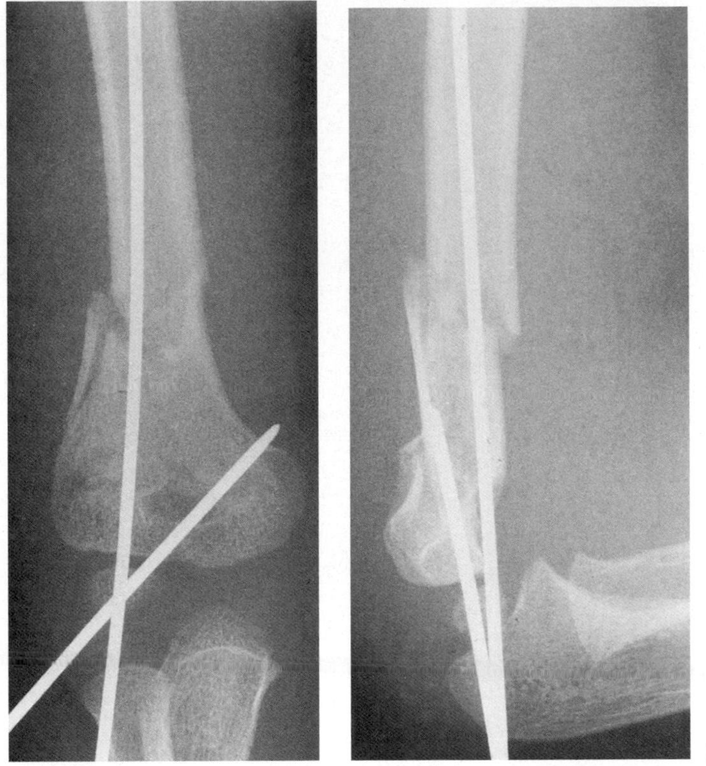

FIGURE 17-54 (*continued*) **C,D.** A lateral column pin acting as an internal splint is technically easier than medial column pins.

incidence of this process ranges from 0.1% to 2.7%, with the lower percentages in Blacks and the higher percentages in Whites.[32,354,407] The process extends obliquely downward and may be connected with the medial epicondyle by a tough fibrous band.[32,88,281,354,407] Frequently, the foramen formed between the fibrous band and the humerus is traversed by the median nerve and the brachial artery. They may be entrapped by the fibrous band or the fracture. Anomalous attachments of the coracobrachialis and the pronator teres may occur on the process (Fig. 17-56).[215,299]

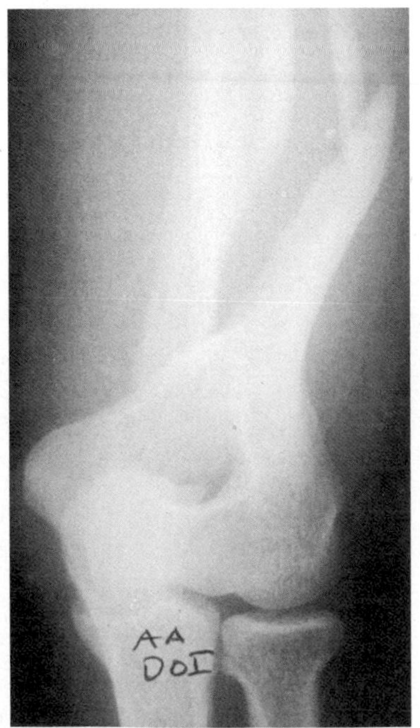

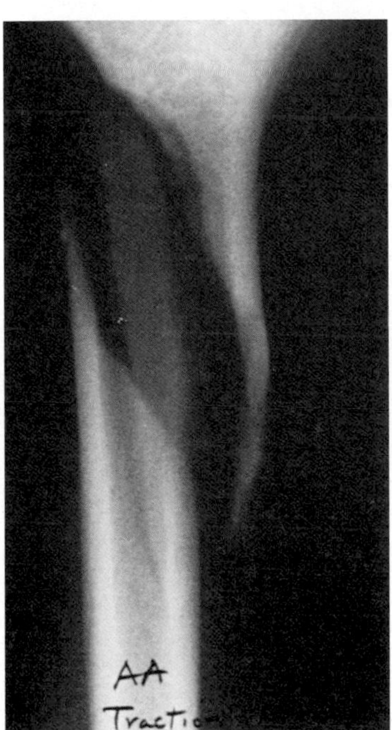

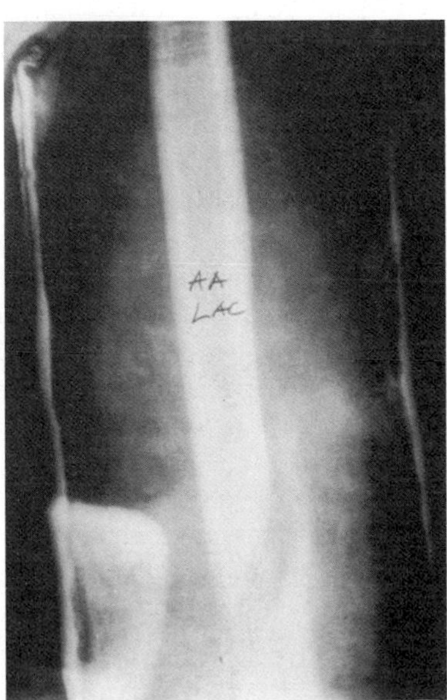

FIGURE 17-55 A comminuted distal humeral metaphyseal–diaphyseal fracture in a 14-year-old boy. Injury films **(A)** show multiple fragments in the metaphyseal–diaphyseal area. **B.** The patient was placed in traction for 2 weeks until callus appeared and then was transferred to a long-arm cast **(C)**.

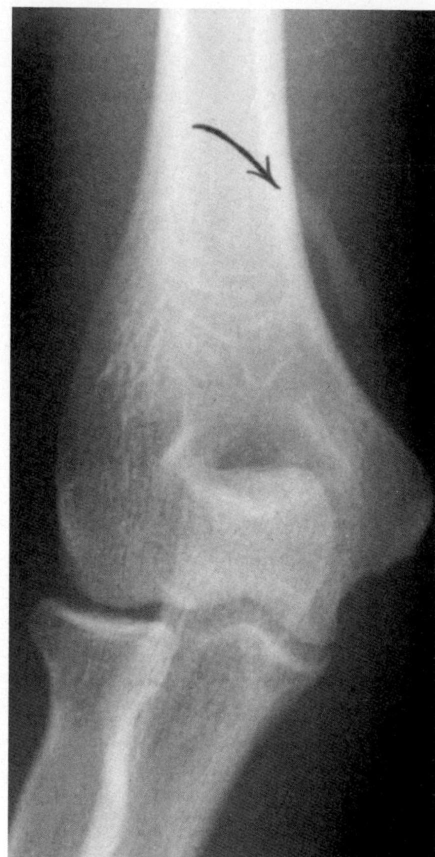

FIGURE 17-56 Radiographic appearance of a supracondylar process (*arrow*).

Principles of Management

Supracondyloid process fractures are the result of direct blows. There are no reports of avulsion from the anomalous muscle attachments.

Diagnosis and Classification

Supracondyloid process fractures are classified as displaced or nondisplaced, with notation of median nerve or brachial artery compromise.

Current Treatment Options

Supracondyloid process fractures have been reported in children[299] and usually are caused by direct blows to the distal humeral area. They may be quite painful and result in compression of the brachial artery or median nerve.[32,88,215,299,354,407] The process is best seen on oblique views.[407] If there are no symptoms of median nerve or brachial artery compression, they are treated by elevation, ice, and temporary immobilization for comfort. However, if a painful nonunion or neurovascular symptoms develop, the fragment should be excised.[407] Fractures with neurologic signs or symptoms are treated by fragment excision and nerve and artery decompression.

REFERENCES

1. Aamoth GM, O'Phelan EM. Recurrent anterior dislocation of the shoulder: a review of 40 athletes treated by subscapularis transfer (modified Magnuson-Stack procedure). Am J Sports Med 1977;5:188–190.
2. Abbott AE, Hannafin JA. Stress fracture of the clavicle in a female lightweight rower. A case report and review of the literature. Am J Sports Med 2001;29(3):370–372.
3. Abbott LC, Lucas DB. The function of the clavicle; its surgical significance. Ann Surg 1954;140:583–599.
4. Ada JR, Miller ME. Scapular fractures. Analysis of 113 cases. Clin Orthop Relat Res 1991;269:174–180.
5. Ahn JI, Park JS. Pathological fractures secondary to unicameral bone cysts. Int Orthop 1994;18:20–22.
6. Aitken AP. End results of fractures of the proximal humeral epiphysis. J Bone Joint Surg Am 1936;18:1036–1041.
7. al Zahrani S. Modified rotational osteotomy of the humerus for Erb's palsy. Int Orthop 1993;17:202–204.
8. Al-Etani H, D'Astous J, Letts J, et al. Masked rotatory subluxation of the atlas associated with fracture of the clavicle: a clinical and biomechanical analysis. J Bone Joint Surg Am 1998;27(5):375–380.
9. Allen ME. Stress fracture of the humerus. A case study. Am J Sports Med 1984;12: 244–245.
10. Alnot JY, Le Reun D. Traumatic lesions of the radial nerve of the arm. Rev Chir Orthop Reparatrice Appar Mot 1989;75:433–442.
11. Althausen PL, Lee MA, Finemeier CG. Scapulothoracic dissociation: diagnosis and treatment. Clin Orthop Relat Res 2003;416:237–244.
12. Amillo S, Barrios RH, Martínez-Peric R, et al. Surgical treatment of the radial nerve lesions associated with fractures of the humerus. J Orthop Trauma 1993;7:211–215.
13. Andersen K, Jensen PO, Lauritzen J. Treatment of clavicular fractures. Figure-of-eight bandage versus a simple sling. Acta Orthop Scand 1987;58:71–74.
14. André S, Feuilhade de Chauvin P, Camilleri A, et al. Recent fractures of the humeral diaphysis in adults-comparison of orthopedic and surgical treatment apropos of 252 cases [in French]. Rev Chir Orthop Reparatrice Appar Mot 1984;70:49–61.
15. Anonymous. Editorial: voluntary dislocation of the shoulder. Br Med J 1973;4:505.
16. Arnold JA, Nasca RJ, Nelson CL. Supracondylar fractures of the humerus. The role of dynamic factors in prevention of deformity. J Bone Joint Surg Am 1977;59:589–595.
17. Arrivé L, Sellier N, Kalifa G, et al. Diagnostic difficulties of isolated symptomatic unilamellar periosteal appositions. Uncommon form of fatigue fracture in children [in French]. J Radiol 1988;69:351–356.
18. Aronen JG, Regan K. Decreasing the incidence of recurrence of first-time anterior shoulder dislocation with rehabilitation. Am J Sports Med 1984;12:283–291.
19. Artico M, Salvati M, D'Andrea V, et al. Isolated lesion of the axillary nerve: surgical treatment and outcome in 12 cases. Neurosurgery 1991;29:697–700.
20. Asche G. Use of external fixation in pediatric fractures [article in German]. Zentralbl Chir 1986;111:391–397.
21. Asher MA. Dislocations of the upper extremity in children. Orthop Clin North Am 1976;7:583–591.
22. Astedt B. A method for the treatment of humerus fractures in the newborn using the S. von Rosen splint. Acta Orthop Scand 1969;40:234–236.
23. Babbitt DP, Cassidy RH. Obstetrical paralysis and dislocation of the shoulder in infancy. J Bone Joint Surg Am 1968;50:1447–1452.
24. Babin SR, Graf P, Vidal P, et al. The risk of nonunion following closed-focus nailing and reaming. Results of 1059 interventions using the Kuntscher method. Int Orthop 1983;7:133–143.
25. Babin SR, Steinmetz A, Wuyts JL, et al. A reliable orthopedic technic in the treatment of humeral diaphyseal fractures in the adult: the hanging plaster. Report of a series of 74 cases [in French]. J Chir (Paris) 1978;115:653–658.
26. Bach BR Jr, O'Brien SJ, Warren RF, et al. An unusual neurological complication of the Bristow procedure: a case report. J Bone Joint Surg Am 1988;70:458–460.
27. Bae DS, Kocher MS, Waters PM, et al. Chronic recurrent anterior sternoclavicular joint instability: results of surgical management. J Pediatr Orthop 2006;26(1):71–74.
28. Bakalim G, Wilpulla E. Surgical or conservative treatment of total dislocation of the acromioclavicular joint. Acta Chir Scand 1975;141:43–47.
29. Balfour GW, Mooney V, Ashby ME. Diaphyseal fractures of the humerus treated with a ready-made fracture brace. J Bone Joint Surg Am 1982;64:11–13.
30. Barber DB, Janus RB, Wade WH. Neuroarthropathy: an overuse injury of the shoulder in quadriplegia. J Spinal Cord Med 1996;19:9–11.
31. Barber FA. Complete posterior acromioclavicular dislocation. Orthopaedics 1987;10: 493–496.
32. Barnard BB, McCoy SM. The supracondyloid process of the humerus. J Bone Joint Surg Am 1946;28:845–850.
33. Barquet A, Fernandez A, Luvizio J, et al. A combined therapeutic protocol for aseptic nonunion of the humeral shaft: a report of 25 cases. J Trauma 1989;29:95–98.
34. Barquet A, Schimchak M, Carreras O, et al. Dislocation of the shoulder with fracture of the ipsilateral shaft of the humerus. Injury 1985;16:300–302.
35. Barratta JB, Lim V, Mastromonaco E, et al. Axillary artery disruption secondary to anterior dislocation of the shoulder. J Trauma 1983;23:1009–1011.
36. Barry TP, Lombardo SJ, Kerlan RK, et al. The coracoid transfer for recurrent anterior instability of the shoulder in adolescents. J Bone Joint Surg Am 1985;67:383–387.
37. Bateman JE. Neurovascular syndromes related to the clavicle. Clin Orthop Relat Res 1968;58:75–82.
38. Baxter MP, Wiley JJ. Fractures of the proximal humeral epiphysis. Their influence on humeral growth. J Bone Joint Surg Br 1986;68:570–573.
39. Bay BH, Sit KH, Lee ST. Mechanisms of humoral fractures in arm-wrestlers. Br J Clin Pract 1993;47(5):279-80.
40. Beall MH, Ross MG. Clavicle fracture in labor: risk factors and associated morbidities. J Perinatol 2001;21(8):513–515.
41. Bearn JG. Direct observations on the function of the capsule of the sternoclavicular support. J Anat 1967;101:159–170.
42. Beaty JH. Fractures of the proximalhumerus and shaft in children. Instr Course Lect 1992:41:369–372.
43. Bell CH. Construction of orthoplast splints for humeral shaft fractures. Am J Occup Ther 1979;33:114–115.
44. Bell MJ, Beauchamp CG, Kellam JK, et al. The results of plating humeral shaft fractures in patients with multiple injuries. The Sunnybrook experience. J Bone Joint Surg Br 1985;67:293–296.
45. Berger PE, Ofstein RA, Jackson DW, et al. MRI demonstration of radiographically occult fractures: what have we been missing? Radiographics 1989;9:407–436.

46. Beringer DC, Weiner DS, Noble JS, et al. Severely displaced proximal humeral epiphyseal fractures: a follow-up study. J Pediatr Orthop 1998;18:31–37.
47. Bianco AJ, Schlein AP, Kruse RL, et al. Birth fractures. Minn Med 1972;55:471–474.
48. Bicos J, Nicholson GP. Treatment and results of sternoclavicular joint injuries. Clin Sports Med 2003;22(2):359–370.
49. Birch R. Lesions of peripheral nerves: the present position. J Bone Joint Surg Br 1986; 68:2–8.
50. Black GH, McPherson JA, Reed MH. Traumatic pseudodislocation of the acromioclavicular joint in children. A 15-year review. Am J Sports Med 1991;19:644–646.
51. Blazina ME, Satzman JS. Recurrent anterior subluxation of the shoulder in athletics-a distinct entity (proceedings). J Bone Joint Surg Am 1969;51:1037–1038.
52. Bleeker WA, Nijsten MW, ten Duis HJ. Treatment of humeral shaft fractures related to associated injuries. A retrospective study of 237 patients. Acta Orthop Scand 1991; 62:148–153.
53. Blom S, Dahlback LO. Nerve injuries in dislocations of the shoulder joint and fractures of the neck of the humerus. Acta Chir Scand 1970;136:461–466.
54. Blount WP. Fractures in Children. Baltimore: Williams & Wilkins, 1955.
55. Boehme D, Curtis RJ Jr, DeHaan JT, et al. Nonunion of fractures of the midshaft of the clavicle. Treatment with a modified Hagie intramedullary pin and autogenous bone grafting. J Bone Joint Surg Am 1991;73:1219–1226.
56. Bortel DT, Pritchett JW. Straight-line graphs for the predictions of growth of the upper extremities. J Bone Joint Surg Am 1993;75:885–892.
57. Bowen RE, Mah JY, Otsuka NY. Midshaft clavicle fractures associated with atlantoaxial rotatory displacement: a report of two cases. J Orthop Trauma 2003;17(6):444–447.
58. Bowen TR, Miller F. Greenstick fracture of the scapula: a cause of scapular winging. J Orthop Trauma 2006;20(2):147–149.
59. Boyd KT, Batt ME. Stress fracture of the proximal humeral epiphysis in an elite junior badminton player. Br J Sports Med 1997;31:252–253.
60. Boyd HB, Sisk TD. Recurrent posterior dislocation of the shoulder. J Bone Joint Surg Am 1972;54:779–786.
61. Brems-Dalgaard E, Davidsen E, Sloth C. Radiographic examination of the acute shoulder. Eur J Radiol 1990;11:10–14.
62. Böhler L. Conservative treatment of fresh closed fractures of the shaft of the humerus. J Trauma 1965;5:464.
63. Böhler L. The Treatment of Fractures. New York: Grune & Stratton, 1956:618–694.
64. Böhler L. The Treatment of Fractures-Supplement. New York: Grune & Stratton, 1966.
65. Böstman O, Bakalim G, Vainionpää S, et al. Immediate radial nerve palsy complicating fracture of the shaft of the humerus: when is early exploration justified? Injury 1985; 16:499–502.
66. Böstman O, Bakalim G, Vainionpää S, et al. Radial palsy in shaft fracture of the humerus. Acta Orthop Scand 1986;57:316–319.
67. Bourdillan JF. Fracture-separation of the proximal epiphysis of the humerus. J Bone Joint Surg Br 1950;32:35–37.
68. Bransby-Zachary MA, MacDonald DA, Singh I, et al. Late fracture associated with retained internal fixation. J Bone Joint Surg Br 1989;71:539.
69. Bretagne MC, Mouton JN, Pierson M, et al. [Periostitis or, rather, periosteal appositions in paediatrics (author's translation).] J Radiol Electrol Med Nucl 1977;58(2):119–123.
70. Brien WW, Gellman H, Becker V, et al. Management of fractures of the humerus in patients who have an injury of the ipsilateral brachial plexus. J Bone Joint Surg Am 1990;72:1208–1210.
71. Broker FH, Burbach T. Ultrasonic diagnosis of separation of the proximal humeral epiphysis in the newborn. J Bone Joint Surg Am 1990;72:187–191.
72. Brooks S. Bilateral congenital pseudarthrosis of the clavicles? Case report and review of the literature. Br J Clin Pract 1984;38:432–433.
73. Browne JE, Stanley RF, Tullos HS, et al. Acromioclavicular joint dislocations: comparative results following operative treatment with and without primary distal clavisectomy. Am J Sports Med 1977;5:258–263.
74. Broyn T, Bie K. Peripheral arterial occlusion following traumatic intimal rupture. Acta Chir Scand 1966;131:167–170.
75. Brug E, Winckler S, Klein W. Distal diaphyseal fracture of the humerus. Unfallchirurgie 1994;97:74–77.
76. Brumback RJ, Bosse MJ, Poka A, et al. Intramedullary stabilization of humeral shaft fractures in patients with multiple trauma. J Bone Joint Surg Am 1986;68:960–970.
77. Brunner C, Morger R. Congenital nonunion of the clavicle. Pediatr Padol 1981;16: 137–141.
78. Buachidze OS, Onoprienko GA, Shternberg AA, et al. Treatment of diaphyseal pseudarthrosis with transosseous osteosynthesis [in Russian]. Vestn Khir Im I I Grek 1977; 119:84–87.
79. Burgos-Flores J, Gonzales-Herranz P, Lopez-Mondejar JA, et al. Fractures of the proximal humeral epiphysis. Int Orthop 1993;17:16–19.
80. Burkhead WZ Jr, Rockwood CA Jr. Treatment of instability of the shoulder with an exercise program. J Bone Joint Surg Am 1993;75:311–312.
81. Calder JD, Solan M, Gidwani S, et al. Management of paediatric clavicle fractures—is follow-up necessary? An audit of 346 cases. Ann R Coll Surg Engl 2002;84(5):331–333.
82. Caldwell JA. Treatment of fractures in the Cincinnati General Hospital. Ann Surg 1933; 97:161–176.
83. Camus M, Lefebvre G, Veron P, et al. Obstetrical injuries of the newborn infant. Retrospective study apropos of 20,409 births [in Russian]. J Gynecol Obstet Biol Reprod (Paris) 1985;14:1033–1043.
84. Canadian Orthopaedic Trauma Society. Nonoperative treatment compared with plate fixation of displaced midshaft clavicular fractures. A multicenter, randomized clinical trial. J Bone Joint Surg Am 2007;89(1):1–10.
85. Canale ST, Puhl J, Watson FM, et al. Acute osteomyelitis following closed fractures. Report of three cases. J Bone Joint Surg Am 1975;57:415–418.
86. Carroll SE. A study of the nutrient foramina of the humeral diaphysis. J Bone Joint Surg Br 1963;45:176–181.
87. Carter C, Sweetnam R. Recurrent dislocation of the patella and of the shoulder: their association with familial joint laxity. J Bone Joint Surg Br 1960;42:721–727.
88. Casadei R, Ferraro A, Ferruzzi A, et al. Supracondylar process of the humerus: four cases. Chir Organi Mov 1990;75:265–277.
89. Cattaneo R, Catagni MA, Guerreschi F. Applications of the Ilizarov method in the humerus. Lengthenings and nonunions. Hand Clin 1993;9:729–739.
90. Cattaneo R, Villa A, Catagni MA, et al. Lengthening of the humerus using the Ilizarov technique. Description of the method and report of 43 cases. Clin Orthop Relat Res 1990;250:117–124.
91. Chacha PB. Compression plating without bone grafts for delayed and nonunion of humeral shaft fractures. Injury 1973;5:283–290.
92. Champetier J, Brabant A, Charignon G, et al. Treatment of fractures of the humerus by intramedullary fixation. J Chir (Paris) 1975;109:75–82.
93. Chapman MW. Closed intramedullary nailing of the humerus. AAOS Instr Course Lect 1983;32:324–328.
94. Chan D, Petricciuolo F, Maffulli N. Fracture of the humeral diaphysis with extreme rotation. Acta Orthop Belg 1991;57:427–429.
95. Chee Y, Agorastides I, Garg N, et al. Treatment of severely displaced proximal humeral fractures in children with elastic stable intramedullary nailing. J Pediatr Orthop B 2006; 15(1):45–50.
96. Cheng JC, Shen WY. Limb fracture pattern in different pediatric age groups: a study of 3,350 children. J Orthop Trauma 1993;7:15–22.
97. Chitwood WR Jr, Rankin JS, Bollinger RR, et al. Brachial artery reconstruction using the heparin-bonded Sundt shunt. Surgery 1981;89:355–358.
98. Choong PF, Griffiths JD. External fixation of complex open humeral fractures. Aust NZ J Surg 1988;58:137–142.
99. Chung SM, Nissenbaum MM. Congenital and developmental defects of the shoulder. Orthop Clin North Am 1975;6:381–392.
100. Christensen NO. Kuntscher intramedullary reaming and nail fixation for nonunion of the humerus. Clin Orthop Relat Res 1976;116:222–225.
101. Ciernik IF, Meier L, Hollinger A. Humeral mobility after treatment with hanging cast. J Trauma.1991;31:230–233.
102. Ciuccarelli C, Cervelalti C, Montanari G, et al. The Ilizarov method for the treatment of nonunion in the humerus. Chir Organi Mov 1990;75:115–120.
103. Clark RL, Milgram JW, Yawn DH. Fatal aortic perforation and cardiac tamponade due to a Kirschner wire migrating from the right sternoclavicular joint. South Med J 1974; 67:316–318.
104. Cleeman E, Flatow EL. Shoulder dislocations in the young patient. Orthop Clin North Am 2000;31:217–229.
105. Coene LN, Narakas AO. Operative management of lesions of the axillary nerve, isolated or combined with other nerve lesions. Clin Neurol Neurosurg 1992;94(suppl): S64–S66.
106. Cohen AW, Otto SR. Obstetric clavicular fractures: a 3-year analysis. J Reprod Med 1980;25:119–122.
107. Cohn BT, Froimson AI. Salter 3 fracture dislocation of glenohumeral joint in a 10-year-old. Orthop Rev 1986;15:403–404.
108. Cole PA. Scapula fractures. Orthop Clin North Am 2002;33(1):1–18.
109. Colyer RA. Surgical stabilization of pathological neoplastic fractures. Curr Probl Cancer 1986;10:117–168.
110. Confalonieri N, Simonatti R, Ramondetta V, et al. Intramedullary nailing with a rush pin in the treatment of diaphyseal humeral fractures [in Italian]. Arch Putti Chir Organi Mov 1990;38:395–403.
111. Connolly JF. Selection, evaluation, and indications for electrical stimulation of ununited fractures. Clin Orthop Relat Res 1981;161:39–53.
112. Costa P, Giancecchi F, Cavazzuti A. Internal and external fixation in complex diaphyseal and metaphyseal fractures of the humerus. Ital J Orthop Traumatol 1991;17:87–94.
113. Covey DC, Riordan DC, Milstead ME, et al. Modification of the L'Episcopo procedure for brachial plexus birth palsies. J Bone Joint Surg Br 1992;74:897–901.
114. Cozen L. Congenital dislocation of the shoulder and other anomalies. Arch Surg 1937; 35:956–966.
115. Crolla RM, de Vries LS, Clevers GJ. Locked intramedullary nailing of humeral fractures. Injury 1993;24:403–406.
116. Curr JF. Rupture of the axillary artery complicating dislocation of the shoulder: report of a case. J Bone Joint Surg Br 1970;52:313–317.
117. Curtis RJ Jr. Operative management of children's fracture of the shoulder region. Orthop Clin North Am 1990;21:315–324.
118. Curtis RJ Jr, Dameron TB Jr, Rockwood CA Jr, et al., eds. Fractures and Dislocations of the Shoulder in Children. 3rd ed. Philadelphia: JB Lippincott, 1991:829–919.
119. Dabezies EJ, Banta CJ II, Murphy CP, et al. Plate fixation of the humeral shaft for acute fractures, with and without radial nerve injuries. J Orthop Trauma 1992;6:10–13.
120. Dal Monte A, Andrisano A, Manfrini M, et al. Humeral lengthening in hypoplasia of the upper limb. J Pediatr Orthop 1985;5:202–207.
121. Dalldorf PG, Bryan WJ. Displaced Salter-Harris type I injury in a gymnast. A slipped capital humeral epiphysis? Orthop Rev 1994;23:538–541.
122. Dameron TB Jr. Transverse fractures of distal humerus in children. AAOS Instr Course Lect 1981;30:224–235.
123. Dameron TB Jr, Grubb SA. Humeral shaft fractures in adults. South Med J 1981;74: 1461–1467.
124. Dameron TB Jr, Reibel DB. Fractures involving the proximal humeral epiphyseal plate. J Bone Joint Surg Am 1969;51:289–297.
125. Dameron TB, Rockwood CA. Fractures and dislocations of the shoulder. In: Rockwood CA, Wilkins KE, King RE, eds. Fractures in Children. Philadelphia: JB Lippincott, 1984: 624–676.
126. Darrow JC Jr, Smith JA, Lockwood RC. A new conservative method for the treatment of type III acromioclavicular separations. Orthop Clin North Am 1980;11:727–733.
127. Dartoy C, Fenoll B, Le Nen D, et al. Epiphyseal fracture-avulsion of the distal extremity of the clavicle. Ann Radiol (Paris) 1993;36:125–128.
128. Davis AG. A conservative treatment for habitual dislocations of the shoulder. JAMA 1936;107:1012–1015.
129. De Bastiani G, Aldegheri R, Renzi Brivio L. The treatment of fractures with a dynamic axial fixator. J Bone Joint Surg Br 1984;66:538–545.
130. de Mourgues G, Fischer LP, Gillet JP, et al. Arterial intraosseous vascularization of the humerus [Recent fractures of the humeral diaphysis apropos of a continuous series of 200 cases, of which 107 were treated with a hanging cast alone]. Rev Chir Orthop Reparatrice Appar Mot 1975;61:191–207.
131. Della Santa DR, Narakas AO. Fractures of the clavicle and secondary lesions of the brachial plexus [in French]. Z Unfallchir Versicherungsmed 1992;85:58–65.
132. Della Santa DR, Narakas AO, Bonnard C. Late lesions of the brachial plexus after fracture of the clavicle. Ann Chir Main Memb Super 1991;10:531–540.

133. DeLong WG Jr, Born CT, Marcelli E, et al. Ender nail fixation in long bone fractures: experience in a level I trauma center. J Trauma 1989;29:571–576.
134. DePalma AF, ed. Surgery of the Shoulder. 3rd ed. Philadelphia: JB Lippincott, 1983.
135. DePalma AF, Cooke AJ, Probhakar M. The role of the subscapularis in recurrent anterior dislocations of the shoulder. Clin Orthop Relat Res 1967;54:35–49.
136. DePalma AF, Silverstein CE. Results following a modified Magnuson procedure in recurrent dislocation of the shoulder. Surg Clin North Am 1963;43:1651–1653.
137. Destree C, Safary A. The treatment of fractures of the neck and diaphysis of the humerus by Hackethal's bundle nailing. Acta Orthop Belg 1979;45:666–677.
138. Detenbeck LC. Posterior dislocations of the shoulder. J Trauma 1972;12:183–192.
139. Devas MB. Stress fractures in athletes. Proc R Soc Med 1969;62:933–937.
140. Di Filippo P, Mancini GB, Gillio A. Humeral fractures with paralysis of the radial nerve. Arch Putti Chir Organi Mov 1990;38:405–409.
141. DiCicco JD, Mehlman CT, Urse JS. Fracture of the shaft of the humerus secondary to muscular violence. J Orthop Trauma 1993;7:90–93.
142. Dimon JH III. Posterior dislocation and posterior fracture dislocation of the shoulder: a report of 25 cases. South Med J 1967;60:661–666.
143. Dobbs MB, Luhmann SL, Gordon JE, et al. Severely displaced proximal humeral epiphyseal fractures. J Pediatr Orthop 2003;23(2):208–215.
144. Drew SJ, Giddins GE, Birch R. A slowly evolving brachial plexus injury following a proximal humerus fractures in a child. J Hand Surg Br 1995;20:24–25.
145. Dufour O, Beaufils P, Ouaknine M, et al. Functional treatment of recent fractures of the humeral shaft using the Sarmiento method [in French]. Rev Chir Orthop Reparatrice Appar Mot 1989;75:292–300.
146. Dugdale TW, Fulkerson JP. Pneumothorax complicating a closed fracture of the clavicle. A case report. Clin Orthop Relat Res 1987;221:212–214.
147. Durbin RA, Gottesman MJ, Saunders KC. Hackethal stacked nailing of humeral shaft fractures. Experience with 30 patients. Clin Orthop Relat Res 1983;179:168–174.
148. Duthie HL. Radial nerve in osseous tunnel at humeral fracture site diagnosed radiographically. J Bone Joint Surg Br 1957;39:746–747.
149. D'Ythurbide B, Augereau B, Asselineau A, et al. Closed intramedullary nailing of fractures of the shaft of the humerus. Int Orthop 1983;7:195–203.
150. Ebraheim NA, An HS, Jackson WT, et al. Scapulothoracic dissociation. J Bone Joint Surg Am 1988;70:428–432.
151. Edeiken BS, Libshitz HI, Cohen MA. Slipped proximal humeral epiphysis: a complication of radiotherapy to the shoulder in children. Skeletal Radiol 1982;9:123–125.
152. Eidman DK, Siff SJ, Tullos HS. Acromioclavicular lesions in children. Am J Sports Med 1981;9:150–154.
153. Elbaum R, Parent H, Zeller R, et al. Traumatic scapulohumeral dislocation in children and adolescents. Apropos of nine patients [in French]. Acta Orthop Belg 1994;60: 204–209.
154. Ellefsen BK, Frierson MA, Raney EM, et al. Humerus varus: a complication of neonatal, infantile, and childhood injury and infection. J Pediatr Orthop 1994;14:479–486.
155. Endo S, Kasai T, Fujii N, et al. Traumatic anterior dislocation of the shoulder in a child. Arch Orthop Trauma Surg 1993;112: 201–202.
156. Epps CH. Nonunion of the humerus. AAOS Instr Course Lect 1988;37:161–166.
157. Eskola A, Vainionpaa S, Myllynen P, et al. Surgery for ununited clavicular fracture. Acta Orthop Scand 1986;57:366–367.
158. Esterhai JL Jr, Brighton CT, Heppenstall RB, et al. Nonunion of the humerus. Clinical, roentgenographic, scintigraphic, and response characteristics to treatment with constant direct current stimulation of osteogenesis. Clin Orthop Relat Res 1986;211: 228–234.
159. Falstie-Jensen S, Mikkelsen P. Pseudodislocation of the acromioclavicular joint. J Bone Joint Surg Br 1982;64:368–369.
160. Farkas R, Levine S. X-ray incidence of fractured clavicle in vertex presentation. Am J Obstet Gynecol 1950;59:204–206.
161. Fattah HA, Halawa EE, Shafy TH. Nonunion of the humeral shaft: a report on 25 cases. Injury 1982;14:255–262.
162. Fayssoux RS, Stankovits L, Domzalski ME, et al. Fractures of the distal humeral metaphyseal-diaphyseal junction in children. J Pediatr Orthop 2008;28(2):142–146.
163. Ferraz IC, Papadimitriou NG, Sotreanos DG. Scapular body nonunion: a case report. J Shoulder Elbow Surg 2002;11(1):98–100.
164. Fisher NA, Newman B, Lloyd J, et al. Ultrasonographic evaluation of birth injury to the shoulder. J Perinatol 1995;15:398–400.
165. Fisher TR, McGeorch CM. Severe injuries of the radial nerve treated by sural nerve grafting. Injury 1985;16:411–412.
166. Foster RJ, Dixon GL Jr, Bach AW, et al. Internal fixation of fractures and nonunions of the humeral shaft. Indications and results in a multicenter study. J Bone Joint Surg Am 1985;67:857–864.
167. Foster RJ, Swiontkowski MF, Back AW, et al. Radial nerve palsy caused by open humeral shaft fractures. J Hand Surg Am 1993;18:121–124.
168. Foster WS, Ford TB, Drez D. Isolated posterior shoulder dislocation in a child. Am J Sports Med 1985;13:198–200.
169. Fourastier J, Pialoux B, Bracq H, et al. Posttraumatic algodystrophy in children [in French]. Chir Pediatr 1986;27:313–317.
170. Fowler AW. Migration of a wire from the sternoclavicular joint to the pericardial cavity. Injury 1981;13:261–262.
171. Fowler AW. Treatment of fractured clavicle. Lancet 1968;1:46–47.
172. Franklyn PP. Progeria in siblings. Clin Radiol 1976;27:327–333.
173. Fraser RL, Haliburton RA, Barber JR. Displaced epiphyseal fractures of the proximal humerus. Can J Surg 1967;10:427–430.
174. Freundlich BD. Luxatio erecta. J Trauma 1983;23:434–436.
175. Friedlander HL. Separation of the proximal humeral epiphysis: a case report. Clin Orthop Relat Res 1964;35:163–170.
176. Friedman RJ, Smith RJ. Radial nerve laceration 26 years after screw fixation of a humeral fracture-a case report. J Bone Joint Surg Am 1984;66:959–960.
177. Gagnaire JC, Thoulon JM, Chappuis JP, et al. Injuries to the upper extremities in the newborn diagnosed at birth [in French]. J Gynecol Obstet Biol Reprod (Paris) 1975; 4:245–254.
178. Gainor BJ, Metzler M. Humeral shaft fracture with brachial artery injury. Clin Orthop Relat Res 1986;204:154–161.
179. Galasko CS. The fate of simple bone cysts which fracture. Clin Orthop Relat Res 1974; 101:302–304.
180. Gamble JG, Rinsky LA, Strudwick J, et al. Nonunion of fractures in children who have osteogenesis imperfecta. J Bone Joint Surg Am 1988;70:439–443.
181. Garcia A, Maeck BH. Radial nerve injuries in fractures of the shaft of the humerus. Am J Surg 1960;99:625–627.
182. Gardner E. Prenatal development of the human shoulder joint. Surg Clin North Am 1953;92:219–276.
183. Gardner E. The embryology of the clavicle. Clin Orthop Relat Res 1968;58:9–16.
184. Gardner MA, Bidstrup BP. Intrathoracic great vessel injury resulting from blunt chest trauma associated with posterior dislocation of the sternoclavicular joint. Aust N Z J Surg 1983;53:427–430.
185. Garland DE, Jones RC, Kunkle RW. Upper extremity fractures in the acute spinal cord injured patient. Clin Orthop Relat Res 1988;233:110–115.
186. Garth WP Jr, Leberte MA, Cool TA. Recurrent fractures of the humerus in a baseball pitcher—a case report. J Bone Joint Surg Am 1988;70:305–306.
187. Gartland JJ, Dowling JJ. Recurrent anterior dislocation of the shoulder joint. Clin Orthop Relat Res 1954;3:86–91.
188. Gerber C, Rockwood CA Jr. Subcoracoid dislocation of the lateral end of the clavicle. A report of three cases. J Bone Joint Surg Am 1987;69:924–927.
189. Gerber C, Schneeberger AG, Vinh TS. The arterial vascularization of the humeral head. An anatomical study. J Bone Joint Surg Am 1990;72:1486–1494.
190. Gibson MJ, Middlemiss JH. Fibrous dysplasia of bone. Br J Radiol 1971;44:1–13.
191. Giebel G, Suren EG. Injuries of the proximal humeral epiphysis. Indications for surgical therapy and results. Chirurgie 1983;54:406–410.
192. Gilbert WM, Tchabo JG. Fractured clavicle in newborns. Int Surg 1988;73:123–125.
193. Gill TJ, Waters P. Valgus osteotomy of the humeral neck: a technique for the treatment of humerus varus. J Shoulder Elbow Surg 1997;6:306–310.
194. Gitch G, Schatten C. Incidence and potential factors in the genesis of birth injury induced clavicular fractures [in German]. Zentralbl Gynakol 1987;109:909–912.
195. Gjengedal E, Slungaard U. Treatment of humeral fractures with and without injury to the radial nerve-a follow-up study. Tidsskr Nor Laegeforen 1981;101:1746–1749.
196. Goddard NJ, Stabler J, Albert JS. Atlantoaxial rotatory fixation and fracture of the clavicle: an association and classification. J Bone Joint Surg Br 1990;72:72–75.
197. Goldberg BJ, Nirschl RP, McConnell JP, et al. Arthroscopic transglenoid suture capsulolabral repairs: preliminary results. Am J Sports Med 1993;21:656–665.
198. Goldfarb CA, Bassett GS, Sullivan S, et al. Retrosternal displacement after physeal fracture of the medial clavicle in children treatment by open reduction and internal fixation. J Bone Joint Surg Br 2001;83(8):1168–1172.
199. Goodsell JO. The resilient radial nerve. Mich Med 1965;64:756–758.
200. Gore RM, Rogers LF, Bowerman J, et al. Osseous manifestations of elbow stress associated with sports activities. AJR Am J Roentgenol 1980;134:971–977.
201. Goss TP. Current concepts review: fractures of the glenoid cavity. J Bone Joint Surg Am 1992;72:299–305.
202. Goss TP. Scapular fracture and dislocations: diagnosis and treatment. J Am Acad Orthop Surg 1995;3:22–33.
203. Graif M, Stahl-Kent V, Ben-Ami T, et al. Sonographic detection of occult bone fractures. Pediatr Radiol 1988;18:383–385.
204. Gray DJ, Gardner E. The prenatal development of the human humerus. Am J Anat 1969;124:431–434.
205. Green NE, Wheelhouse WW. Anterior subglenoid dislocation of the shoulder in an infant following pneumococcal meningitis. Clin Orthop Relat Res 1978;135:125–127.
206. Gregersen HN. Fractures of the humerus from muscular violence. Acta Orthop Scand 1971;42:506–512.
207. Gregg-Smith SJ, White SH. Salter-Harris III fracture-dislocation of the proximal humeral epiphysis. Injury 1992;23:199–200.
208. Grieg DM. On true congenital dislocation of the shoulder. Edinb Med J 1923;30: 157–175.
209. Gross SJ, Shime J, Farine D. Shoulder dystocia: predictors and outcome. A 5-year review. Am J Obstet Gynecol 1987;156:334–336.
210. Gudinchet F, Naggar L, Ginalski JM, et al. Magnetic resonance imaging of nontraumatic shoulder instability in children. Skeletal Radiol 1992;21:19–21.
211. Guibert L, Allouis M, Bourdelat D, et al. Fractures and slipped epiphysis of the proximal humerus in children. Place and methods of surgical treatment. Chir Pediatr 1983;24: 197–200.
212. Gupta A, Sharma S. Volar compartment syndrome of the arm complicating a fracture of the humeral shaft—a case report. Acta Orthop Scand 1991;62:77–78.
213. Gupta RC, Gaur SC, Tiwari RC, et al. Treatment of ununited fractures of the shaft of the humerus with bent nail. Injury 1985;16:276–280.
214. Guttentag IJ, Rechtine GR. Fractures of the scapula: a review of the literature. Orthop Rev 1988;17:147–158.
215. Haagedoorn EL. Fracture of the supracondylar humeral process [in Dutch]. Ned Tijdschr Geneeskd 1968;112:313–316.
216. Hackethal KH. Die Bundel-Nagelung. Berlin: Springer-Verlag, 1961.
217. Hackstock H. Functional bracing of fractures. Orthopadie 1988;17:41–51.
218. Haliburton RA, Barber JR, Fraser RL. Pseudodislocation: an unusual birth injury. Can J Surg 1967;10:455–462.
219. Hall RF Jr. Closed intramedullary fixation of humeral shaft fractures. AAOS Instr Course Lect 1987;36:349–358.
220. Hall RF Jr, Pankovich AM. Ender nailing of acute fractures of the humerus. A study of closed fixation by intramedullary nails without reaming. J Bone Joint Surg Am 1987; 69:558–567.
221. Hardegger FH, Simpson LA, Weber BG. The operative treatment of scapula fractures. J Bone Joint Surg Br 1984;66:725–731.
222. Harris BA Jr. Shoulder dystocia. Clin Obstet Gynecol 1984;27:106–111.
223. Havranek P. Injuries of distal clavicular physis in children. J Pediatr Orthop 1989;9: 213–215.
224. Hawkins RJ, Angelo RL. Glenohumeral osteoarthritis: acute complications of the Putti-Platt repair. J Bone Joint Surg Am 1990;72:1193–1197.
225. Hawkins RJ, Koppert G, Johnston G. Recurrent posterior instability (subluxation) of the shoulder. J Bone Joint Surg Am 1984;66:169–174.
226. Healy WL, White GM, Mick CA, et al. Nonunion of the humeral shaft. Clin Orthop Relat Res 1987;219:206–213.
227. Heck CC. Anterior dislocation of the glenohumeral joint in a child. J Trauma 1981; 21:174–175.

228. Hedstrom O. Growth stimulation of long bones after fracture or similar trauma. A clinical and experimental study. Acta Orthop Scand Suppl 1969;122:1–134.
229. Heilbronner DM, Manoli A II, Little RE. Elbow dislocation during overhead skeletal traction therapy: a case report. Clin Orthop Relat Res 1981;154:185–187.
230. Heim D, Herkert R, Hess P, et al. Can humerus shaft fractures be treated with osteosynthesis? Helv Chir Acta 1992;58:673–678.
231. Heim D, Heckert F, Hess P, et al. Surgical treatment of humeral shaft fractures-the Basel experience. J Trauma 1993;35:226–232.
232. Heim M, Horoszowski H. Martinowitz U. Hemophilic arthropathy resulting in a locked shoulder. Clin Orthop Relat Res 1986;202:169–172.
233. Henley MB, Monroe M, Tencer AF. Biomechanical comparison of methods of fixation of a midshaft osteotomy of the humerus. J Orthop Trauma 1991;5:14–20.
234. Hennig F, Link W, Wofel R. Bundle nailing—an evaluation after 27 years. Aktuel Traumatol 1988;18:117–119.
235. Hennigan SP, Bush-Joseph CA, Kuo KN, et al. Throwing-induced humeral shaft fracture in skeletally immature adolescents. Orthopedics 1999;22:621–622.
236. Hermichen HG, Pfister U, Weller S. Influence of the treatment of fractures on the development of pseudoarthroses of the humerus shaft. Aktuel Traumatol 1980;10: 137–142.
237. Hernandez A, Drez D. Operative treatment of posterior shoulder dislocations by posterior glenoidplasty, capsulorrhaphy, and infraspinatus advancement. Am J Sports Med 1986;14:187–191.
238. Herndon WA. Child abuse in a military population. J Pediatr Orthop 1983;3:73–76.
239. Herring JA, Peterson HA. Simple bone cyst with growth arrest. J Pediatr Orthop 1987; 7:231–235.
240. Herscovici D Jr, Fiennes AG, Allgöwer M, et al. The floating shoulder: ipsilateral clavicle and scapular neck fractures. J Bone Joint Surg Br 1992;74:362–364.
241. Hoffer MM, Phipps GJ. Closed reduction and tendon transfer for treatment of dislocations of the glenohumeral joint secondary to brachial plexus birth palsy. J Bone Joint Surg Am 1998;80:997–1001.
242. Hohl JC. Fractures of the humerus in children. Orthop Clin North Am 1976;7: 557–571.
243. Hollingshead WH. Anatomy for Surgeons: the Back and Limbs. New York: Harper & Row, 1982.
244. Holm CL. Management of humeral shaft fractures. Fundamental nonoperative technics. Clin Orthop Relat Res 1970;71:132–139.
245. Holstein A, Lewis GB. Fractures of the humerus with radial nerve paralysis. J Bone Joint Surg Am 1963;45:1382–1388.
246. Hosner W. Fractures of the shaft of the humerus: an analysis of 100 consecutive cases. Reconstr Surg Traumatol 1974;14:38–64.
247. Hovelius L. Anterior dislocation of the shoulder in teenagers and young adults. J Bone Joint Surg Am 1987;69A:393–399.
248. Hovelius L, Augustini BG, Fredin H, et al. Primary anterior dislocation of the shoulder in young patients: a 10-year prospective study. J Bone Joint Surg Am 1996;78: 1677–1684.
249. Hovelius L, Eriksson K, Fredin H, et al. Recurrences after initial dislocation of the shoulder. J Bone Joint Surg 1983;65: 343–349.
250. Hovelius L, Olofsson A, Sandström B, et al. Nonoperative treatment of primary anterior shoulder dislocation in patients 40 years of age and younger. a prospective 25-year follow-up. J Bone Joint Surg Am 2008;90(5):945–952.
251. Howard CB, Shinwell E, Nyska M, et al. Ultrasound diagnosis of neonatal fracture separation of the upper humeral epiphysis. J Bone Joint Surg Br 1992;74:471–472.
252. Howard FM, Shafer SJ. Injuries to the clavicle with neurovascular complications. A study of fourteen cases. J Bone Joint Surg Am 1965;47:1335–1346.
253. Howard NJ, Eloesser L. Treatment of fracture of the upper end of the humerus: an experimental and clinical study. J Bone Joint Surg Am 1934;16:1–29.
254. Huber H, Gerber C. Voluntary subluxation of the shoulder in children. A long-term follow up study of 36 shoulders. J Bone Joint Surg Am 1994;76:118–122.
255. Husain SN, King EC, Young JL, et al. Remodeling of birth fractures of the humeral diaphysis. J Pediatr Orthop 2008;28(1):10–13.
256. Hwang RW, Bae DS, Waters PM. Brachial plexus palsy following proximal humerus fracture in patients who are skeletally immature. J Orthop Trauma 2008;22(4): 286–290.
257. Ideberg R. Fractures of the scapula involving the glenoid fossa. In: Bateman JE, Walsh RD, eds. Surgery of the Shoulder. Toronto: BC Decker, 1984:63–66.
258. Ideberg R. Unusual glenoid fractures: a report on 92 cases. Acta Orthop Scand 1987; 58:191–192.
259. Ilizarov GA. Transosseous Osteosynthesis. Berlin: Springer-Verlag, 1992.
260. Ilizarov GA, Shevtsov VI. Bloodless compression-distraction osteosynthesis in the treatment of pseudarthroses of the humerus [in Russian]. Voen Med Zh 1974;6:27–31.
261. Imatani RJ. Fractures of the scapulae: a review of 53 fractures. J Trauma 1975;15: 473–478.
262. Ingman AM, Waters DA. Locked intramedullary nailing of humeral shaft fractures. Implant design, surgical technique, and clinical results. J Bone Joint Surg Br 1994,76: 23–29.
263. Inman VT, Saunders JB, Abbott LC. Observations on the function of the shoulder joint. J Bone Joint Surg 1944;26:1–30.
264. Iqbal QM. Long bone fractures among children in Malaysia. Int Surg 1974;59:410–415.
265. Itoi E, Hatakeyama Y, Sato T, et al. Immobilization in external rotation after shoulder dislocation reduces the risk of recurrence. A randomized controlled trial. J Bone Joint Surg Am 2007;89(10):2124–2131.
266. Jaberg H, Warner JJ, Jakob RP. Percutaneous stabilization of unstable fractures of the humerus. J Bone Joint Surg Am 1992;74:508–515.
267. Jablon M, Sutker A, Post M. Irreducible fracture of the middle third of the clavicle. Report of a case. J Bone Joint Surg Am 1979;61:296–298.
268. Jackson ST, Hoffer MM, Parrish N. Brachial plexus palsy in the newborn. J Bone Joint Surg Am 1988;70:1217–1220.
269. Jalovaara P, Myllyla V, Paivansalo M. Autotraction stress roentgenography for demonstration of anterior and inferior instability of the shoulder joint. Clin Orthop Relat Res 1992;284:136–143.
270. James P, Heinrich SD. Ipsilateral proximal metaphyseal and flexion supracondylar humerus fractures with an associated olecranon avulsion fracture. Orthopedics 1991;14: 713–716.
271. Jeffery CC. Fracture separation of the upper humeral epiphysis. Surg Gynecol Obstet 1953;96:205–209.
272. Jelić A, Marin L, Pracny M, et al. Fractures of the clavicle in neonates [in Croatian]. Lijec Vjesn 1992;114:32–35.
273. Jensen PO, Andersen K, Lauritzen J. Treatment of midclavicular fractures. A prospective randomized trial comparing treatment with a figure-of-eight dressing and a simple arm sling [in Danish]. Ugeskr Laeger 1985;147:1986–1988.
274. Jit I, Kulkarni M. Times of appearance and fusion of epiphysis at the medial end of the clavicle. Ind J Med Res 1976;64:773–782.
275. Johnstone DJ, Radford WJ, Parnel EJ. Interobserver variation using the AO/ASIF classification of long-bone fractures. Injury 1993;24:163–165.
276. Jójárt G, Nagy G. Ultrasonographic screening of neonatal adrenal apoplexy. Int Urol Nephrol 1992;24:591–596.
277. Jójárt G, Zubek L, Toth G. Clavicle fractures in the newborn [in Hungarian]. Orv Hetil 1991;132:2655–2657.
278. Jones KJ, Wiesel B, Ganley TJ, et al. Functional outcomes of early arthroscopic bankart repair in adolescents aged 11 to 18 years. J Pediatr Orthop 2007;27(2):209–213. Erratum in: J Pediatr Orthop 2007;27(4):483.
279. Joseph PR, Rosenfeld W. Clavicular fractures in neonates. Am J Dis Child 1990;144: 165–167.
280. Jubel A, Andermahr J, Schiffer G, et al. Elastic stable intramedullary nailing of midclavicular fractures with a titanium nail. Clin Orthop Relat Res 2003;408:279–285.
281. Kamhin M, Michaelson M, Waisbrod H. The use of external skeletal fixation in the treatment of fractures of the humeral shaft. Injury 1978;9:245–248.
282. Kaminsky SB, Pierce VD. Nonunion of a scapula body fracture in a high school football player. Am J Orthop 2002;31(8):456–457.
283. Kane E, Kaplan EB, Spinner M. Observations of the course of the ulnar nerve in the arm. Ann Chir 1973;27:487–496.
284. Karadimas J, Rentis G, Varouchas G. Repair of anterior dislocation of the shoulder using transfer of the subscapularis tendon. J Bone Joint Surg Am 1980;62:1147–1149.
285. Katz R, Landman J, Dulitzky F, et al. Fracture of the clavicle in the newborn. An ultrasound diagnosis. J Ultrasound Med 1988;7:21–23.
286. Kaur H, Jit I. Brief communication: coracoclavicular joint in northwest Indians. Am J Phys Anthropol 1991;85:457–460.
287. Kayser R, Mahlfeld K, Heyde C, et al. Ultrasonographic imaging of fractures of the clavicle in newborn infants. J Bone Joint Surg Br 2003;85(1):115–116.
288. Keiser RP, Wilson CL. Bilateral recurrent dislocation of the shoulder (atraumatic) in a 13-year-old girl. J Bone Joint Surg Am 1961;43:553–554.
289. Kim NH, Hahn SB, Park HW, et al. The Orthofix external fixator for fractures of long bones. Int Orthop 1994;18:42–46.
290. Kim SJ, Min BH. Congenital bilateral absence of the acromion: a case report. Clin Orthop Relat Res 1994;300:117–119.
291. Kirkos JM, Papadopoulos IA. Late treatment of brachial plexus palsy secondary to birth injuries: rotational osteotomy of the proximal part of the humerus. J Bone Joint Surg Am 1998;80:1477–1483.
292. Klasson SC, Vander Schilden JL, Park JP. Late effect of isolated avulsion fractures of the lesser tubercle of the humerus in children. Report of two cases. J Bone Joint Surg Am 1993;75:1691–1694.
293. Kleinman PK, Goss TP, Aappas A. Injuries of the glenoid labrum in athletic teenagers [Abstract]. Pediatr Radiol 1985;15:71.
294. Kleinman PK, Akins CM. The "vanishing" epiphysis: sign of Salter type I fracture of the proximal humerus in infancy. Br J Radiol 1982;55:865–867.
295. Klenerman L. Fractures of the shaft of the humerus. J Bone Joint Surg Br 1966;48: 105–111.
296. Kogutt MS, Swischuk LE, Fagan CJ. Patterns of injury and significance of uncommon fractures in the battered child syndrome. Am J Roentgenol Radium Ther Nucl Med 1974;121:143–149.
297. Koch G. Treatment of humeral fractures using the U splint. Chirurgie, 1971;42: 327 329.
298. Kohler R, Trillaud JM. Fracture and fracture separation of the proximal humerus in children: report of 136 cases. J Pediatr Orthop 1983;3:326–332.
299. Kolb LW, Moore RD. Fractures of the supracondylar process of the humerus. Report of two cases. J Bone Joint Surg Am 1967;49:532–534.
300. Kothari K, Bernstein RM, Griffiths HJ, et al. Luxatio erecta. Skeletal Radiol 1984;11: 47–49.
301. Kothari RU, Dronen SC. Prospective evaluation of the scapular manipulation technique in reducing anterior shoulder dislocations. Ann Emerg Med 1992;21:1349–1352.
302. Kreisinger V. Sur le traitement des fractures de la clavicule. Rev Chir 1927;65:396–407.
303. Kretzschmar HJ. [Posttraumatic fat embolism in a 13-year-old girl]. Zentralbl Chir 1970;95:1223–1225.
304. Kubiak R, Slongo T. Operative treatment of clavicle fractures in children: a review of 21 years. J Pediatr Orthop 2002;22(6):736–739.
305. Kuhn JE, Blasier RB, Carpenter JE. Fractures of the acromion process: a proposed classification system. J Orthop Trauma 1994;8:6–13.
306. Kuhns LR, Sherman MP, Poznanski AK, et al. Humeral head and coracoid ossification in the newborn. Radiology 1973;107:145–149.
307. Kulenkampff HA, Rustemeier M. Clinical experiences in the treatment of humeral shaft fractures with the Sarmiento brace. Unfallchirurgie 1988;14:191–198.
308. Kumar R, Cornah MS, Morris DL. Hydatid cyst—a rare cause of pathological fracture: a case report. Injury 1984;15:284–285.
309. Kummel BM. Arthrography in anterior capsular derangements of the shoulder. Clin Orthop Relat Res 1972;83:170–176.
310. Kwasny O, Maier R, Kutscha-Lissberg F, et al. Treatment procedure in humeral shaft fractures with primary or secondary radial nerve damage. Unfallchirurgie 1992;18: 168–173.
311. Kwasny O, Maier R, Scharf W. The surgical treatment of humeral shaft fractures. Aktuel Traumatol 1990;20:87–92.
312. Laing PG. The arterial supply of the adult humerus. J Bone Joint Surg Am 1956;38: 1105–1116.
313. Landin LA. Epidemiology of children's fractures. J Pediatr Orthop B 1997;6:79–83.
314. Landin LA. Fracture patterns in children. Analysis of 8682 fractures with special reference to incidence, etiology, and secular changes in Swedish urban population 1950–1979. Acta Orthop Scand Suppl 1983;202:1–109.

315. Lange RH, Foster RJ. Skeletal management of humeral shaft fractures associated with forearm fractures. Clin Orthop Relat Res 1985;195:173–177.
316. Langenberg R. Missed humeral fracture in multiple injury of the arm. Zentralbl Chir 1986;111:1536–1539.
317. Langenskiöld A. Adolescent humerus varus. Acta Chir Scand 1953;105:353–362.
318. Larsen CF, Kiaer T, Lindequist S. Fractures of the proximal humerus in children: 9-year follow-up of 64 unoperated on cases. Acta Orthop Scand 1990;61:255–257.
319. Lascombes P, Haumont T, Journeau P. Use and abuse of flexible intramedullary nailing in children and adolescents. J Pediatr Orthop 2006;26(6):827–834.
320. Laskin RS, Sedlin ED. Luxatio erecta in infancy. Clin Orthop Relat Res 1971;80: 126–129.
321. Lawhon SM, Peoples AB, MacEwen GD. Voluntary dislocation of the shoulder. J Pediatr Orthop 1982;2:590.
322. Lee HG. Operative reduction of an unusual fracture of the upper epiphyseal plate of the humerus. J Bone Joint Surg 1944;26:401–404.
323. Lee SJ, Meinhard BP, Schultz E, et al. Open reduction and internal fixation of a glenoid fossa fracture in a child: a case report and review of the literature. J Orthop Trauma 1997;11(6):452–454.
324. Leffert RD. Brachial plexus injuries. N Engl J Med 1974;291:1059–1067.
325. Lemperg R, Liliequist B. Dislocation of the proximal epiphysis of the humerus in newborns. Acta Paediatr Scand 1970;59:377–380.
326. Lenters TR, Franta AK, Wolf FM, et al. Arthroscopic compared with open repairs for recurrent anterior shoulder instability. A systematic review and meta-analysis of the literature. J Bone Joint Surg Am 2007;89(2):244–254.
327. Lentz W, Meuser P. The treatment of fractures of the proximal humerus. Arch Orthop Trauma Surg 1980;96:283–285.
328. Leslie JT, Ryan TJ. The anterior axillary incision to approach the shoulder joint. J Bone Joint Surg Am 1962;44:1193–1196.
329. Leung KS, Kwan M, Wong J, et al. Therapeutic functional bracing in upper limb fracture-dislocations. J Orthop Trauma 1999;2:308–313.
330. Leung KS, Lam TP. Open reduction and internal fixation of ipsilateral fractures of the scapular neck and clavicle. J Bone Joint Surg Am 1993;75:1015–1018.
331. Levin LS, Goldner RD, Urbaniak JR, et al. Management of severe musculoskeletal injuries of the upper extremity. J Orthop Trauma 1990;4:432–440.
332. Levine MG, Holroyde J, Woods JR Jr, et al. Birth trauma: incidence and predisposing factors. Obstet Gynecol 1984;63:792–795.
333. Green SA, Gibbs P. The relationship of antigulation to translation in fracture deformities. J Bone Joint Surg Am 1994;76:390–397.
334. Lewallen RP, Pritchard DJ, Sim FH. Treatment of pathologic fractures or impending fractures of the humerus with rush rods and methylmethacrylate. Experience with 55 cases in 54 patients, 1968–1977. Clin Orthop Relat Res 1982;166:193–198.
335. Liberson F. Os acromiale? A contested anomaly. J Bone Joint Surg 1937;19:683–689.
336. Lichtenberg RP. A study of 2532 fractures in children. Am J Surg 1954;87:330–338.
337. Lichtblau PD. Shoulder dislocation in the infant. Case report and discussion. J Fla Med Assoc 1977;64:313–320.
338. Liebling G, Bartel HG. Unusual migration of a Kirschner wire following drill wire fixation of a subcapital humerus fracture [in German]. Beitr Orthop Traumatol 1987; 34:585–587.
339. Liebolt FL, Furey JG. Obstetrical paralysis with dislocation of the shoulder: a case report. J Bone Joint Surg Am 1953;35:227–230.
340. Ligier JN, Metaizeau JP, Prevot J. Closed flexible medullary nailing in pediatric traumatology. Chir Pediatr 1983;24:383–385.
341. Lindblom A, Levén H. Prognosis in fractures of body and neck of the scapula. Acta Chir Scand 1974;140:33–36.
342. Link W, Herzog T, Hoffmann A. Bundle wire nailing in pathological upper arm fractures. Zentralbl Chir 1990;115:665–670.
343. Linn RM, Kerigshauser LA. Ball-thrower's fracture of the humerus-a case report. Am J Sports Med; 1991;19:194–197.
344. Linson MA. Axillary artery thrombosis after fracture of the humerus. A case report. J Bone Joint Surg Am 1980;62:1214–1215.
345. Lipscomb AB. Baseball pitching injuries in growing athletes. J Sports Med 1975;3: 25–34.
346. Lock TR, Aronson DD. Fractures in patients who have myelomeningocele. J Bone Joint Surg Am 1989;71:1153–1157.
347. Loder RT. Pediatric polytrauma: orthopaedic care and hospital course. J Orthop Trauma 1987;1:48–54.
348. Loder RT, Bookout C. Fracture patterns in battered children. J Orthop Trauma 1991; 5:428–433.
349. Lombardo SJ, Kerlan RK, Jobe FW, et al. The modified Bristow procedure for recurrent dislocation of the shoulder. J Bone Joint Surg Am 1976;58:256–261.
350. Longo R, Ruggiero L. Left pneumothorax with subcutaneous emphysema secondary to left clavicular fracture and homolateral obstetrical paralysis of the arm. Minerva Pediatr 1982;34:273–276.
351. Low BY, Lim J. Fracture of humerus during arm-wrestling: report of five cases. Singapore Med J 1991;32:47–49.
352. Lucas LS, Gill JH. Humerus varus following birth injury to the proximal humeral epiphysis. J Bone Joint Surg 1947;29:367–369.
353. Lucas GL, Peterson MD. Open anterior dislocation of the shoulder: case report. J Trauma 1977;17:883–884.
354. Lund HJ. Fracture of the supracondyloid process of the humerus. Report of a case. J Bone Joint Surg Am 1930;12:925–928.
355. Lusardi DA, With MA, Wurtz D, et al. Loss of external rotation following anterior capsulorrhaphy of the shoulder. J Bone Joint Surg Am 1993;75:1185–1192.
356. Lyons FA, Rockwood CA Jr. Current concepts review. Migration of pins used in operations on the shoulder. J Bone Joint Surg Am 1990;72:1262–1267.
357. Macfarlane I, Mushayt K. Double closed fractures of the humerus in a child. A case report. J Bone Joint Surg Am 1990;72:443.
358. Machan FG, Vinz H. Humeral shaft fracture in childhood. Unfallchirurgie 1993;19: 166–174.
359. Mackay I. Closed Rush pinning of fractures of the humeral shaft. Injury 1984;16: 178–181.
360. Macnicol MF. Roentgenographic evidence of median-nerve entrapment in a greenstick humeral fracture. J Bone Joint Surg Am 1978;60:998–1000.
361. Madsen ET. Fractures of the extremities in the newborn. Acta Obstet Gynecol Scand 1955;34:41–74.
362. Magnuson PB, Stack JK. Bilateral habitual dislocation of the shoulders in twins: a familial tendency. JAMA 1940;114:2103.
363. Makin GS, Howard JM, Green RL. Arterial injuries complicating fractures or dislocations: the necessity for a more aggressive approach. Surgery 1966;59:203–209.
364. Manske DJ, Szabo RM. The operative treatment of midshaft clavicular nonunions. J Bone Joint Surg Am 1985;67:1367–1371.
365. Marans HJ, Angel KR, Schemitsch EH, et al. The fate of traumatic anterior dislocation of the shoulder in children. J Bone Joint Surg Am 1992;74:1242–1244.
366. Marcus RE, Mills MF, Thompson GH. Multiple injury in children. J Bone Joint Surg Am 1983;65:1290–1294.
367. Markel DC, Donley BG, Blasier RB. Percutaneous intramedullary pinning of proximal humeral fractures. Orthop Rev 1994;23:667–671.
368. Martin RP, Parsons DL. Avascular necrosis of the proximal humeral epiphysis after physeal fracture. A case report. J Bone Joint Surg Am 1997;79:760–762.
369. Marty B, Käch K, Candinas D, et al. Results of intramedullary nailing in humerus shaft fractures. Helv Chir Acta 1993;59:681–685.
370. Mast JW, Spiegel PG, Harvey JP Jr, et al. Fractures of the humeral shaft. A retrospective study of 240 adult fractures. Clin Orthop Relat Res 1975;112:254–262.
371. Matton D, Van Looy F, Geens S. Recurrent anterior dislocations of the shoulder joint treated by the Bristow-Latarjet procedure. Acta Orthop Belg 1992;58:16–22.
372. May VR Jr. Posterior dislocation of the shoulder: habitual, traumatic, and obstetrical. Orthop Clin North Am 1980;11:271–285.
373. Mazet R Jr. Migration of a Kirschner wire from the shoulder region into the lung: a report of two cases. J Bone Joint Surg Am 1943;25:477–483.
374. McCaughan JS Jr, Miller PR. Migration of Steinmann pin from shoulder to lung [Letter]. JAMA 1969;207:1917.
375. McClure JG, Raney RB. Anomalies of the scapula. Clin Orthop Relat Res 1975;110: 22–31.
376. McGahan JP, Rab GT. Fracture of the acromion associated with an axillary nerve deficit: a case report and review of the literature. Clin Orthop Relat Res 1980;147:216–218.
377. McGahan JP, Rab GT, Dublin A. Fractures of the scapula. J Trauma 1980;20:880–883.
378. McNamara JJ, Brief DK, Stremple JF, et al. Management of fractures with associated arterial injury in combat casualties. J Trauma 1973;13:17–19.
379. McNamara RM. Reduction of anterior shoulder dislocations by scapular manipulation. Ann Emerg Med 1993;22:1140–1144.
380. McNeil EL. Luxatio erecta [Letter]. Ann Emerg Med 1984;13:490–491.
381. McQuillan WM, Nolan B. Ischemia complicating injury. J Bone Joint Surg Am 1968; 50:482–492.
382. Meeks RJ, Riebel GD. Isolated clavicle fracture with associated pneumothorax. A case report. Am J Emerg Med 1991;9:555–556.
383. Menger DM, Gauger JU, Schmitt-Koppler A. Experiences with cluster nailing of humeral shaft fractures. Unfallchirurgie 1985;11:70–75.
384. Metaizeau JP, Ligier JN. Surgical treatment of fractures of the long bones in children. Interference between osteosynthesis and the physiological processes of consolidation. Therapeutic indications. J Chir (Paris) 1984;121:527–537.
385. Michiels I, Broos P, Gruwez JA. The operative treatment of humeral shaft fractures. Acta Chir Belg 1986;86:147–152.
386. Miller DS, Boswick JA Jr. Lesions of the brachial plexus associated with fractures of the clavicle. Clin Orthop Relat Res 1969;64:144–149.
387. Mital MA, Aufranc OE. Venous occlusion following greenstick fracture of clavicle. JAMA 1968;206:1301–1302.
388. Moed BR, LaMont RL. Unicameral bone cyst complicated by growth retardation. J Bone Joint Surg Am 1982;64:1379–1381.
389. Montgomery SP, Loyd RD. Avulsion fracture of the coracoid epiphysis with acromioclavicular separation. Report of two casesin adolescents and review of the literature. J Bone Joint Surg Am 1977;59:963–965.
390. Montgomery WH III, Jobe FW. Functional outcomes in athletes after modified anterior capsulolabral reconstruction. Am J Sports Med 1994;22:352–358.
391. Moon MS, Kim I, Suh KH, et al. Arm-wrestler's injury: report of seven cases. Clin Orthop Relat Res 1980;147:219–221.
392. Morrey BF, Janes JM. Recurrent anterior dislocation of the shoulder. J Bone Joint Surg Am 1976;58:252–256.
393. Morrison PD, Egan TJ. Axillary artery injury in erect dislocation of the shoulder (luxatio erecta): a case report. J Ir Orthop 1983:260–261.
394. Moseley HF. The clavicle: its anatomy and function. Clin Orthop Relat Res 1968;58: 17–27.
395. Mubarak SJ, Carroll NC. Volkmann's contracture in children: aetiology and prevention. J Bone Joint Surg Br 1979;61:285–293.
396. Mullaji AB, Jupiter JB. Low contact dynamic compression plating of the clavicle. Injury 1994;25:41–45.
397. Müller ME, Allgower M, Schneider R, et al. Manual of Internal Fixation. Techniques Recommended by the AO-ASIF Group. 3rd ed. Berlin: Springer-Verlag, 1991.
398. Mullick S. Treatment of midclavicular fractures. Lancet 1967;1:499.
399. Nast-Kolb D, Knoefel WT, Schweiberer L. The treatment of humeral shaft fractures. Results of a prospective AO multicenter study. Unfallchirurgie 1991;94:447–454.
400. Naver L, Aalberg JR. Humeral shaft fractures treated with a ready-made fracture brace. Arch Orthop Trauma Surg 1986;106:20–22.
401. Neer CS II. Fractures. Shoulder Reconstruction. Philadelphia: WB Saunders, 1990:412
402. Neer CS II. Fractures about the Shoulder. In: Wood CA, Green DP, eds. Fractures. Philadelphia: JB Lippincott, 1984:713–721.
403. Neer CS II. Involuntary inferior and multidirectional instability of the shoulder: etiology, recognition, and treatment. AAOS Instr Course Lect 1985;34:232–238.
404. Neer CS II, Horwitz BS. Fractures of the proximal humeral epiphysial plate. Clin Orthop Relat Res 1965;41:24–31.
405. Nerubay J, Horoszowski H, Goodman RM. Fracture in progressive ossifying fibrodysplasia—a case report. Acta Orthop Scand 1987;58:289–291.
406. Nettrour LF, Krufky EL, Mueller RE, et al. Locked scapula: intrathoracic dislocation of the inferior angle. A case report. J Bone Joint Surg Am 1972;54(2):413–416.
407. Newman A. The supracondylar process and its fracture. Am J Roentgenol Radium Ther Nucl Med 1969;105:844–849.

408. Nogi J, Heckman JD, Hakala M, et al. Nonunion of the clavicle in a child. A case report. Clin Orthop Relat Res 1975;110:19–21.
409. Nonnemann HC. Limits of spontaneous correction of incorrectly healed fractures in adolescence. Langenbecks Arch Chir 1969;324:78–86.
410. Nordqvist A, Petersson C. Fracture of the body, neck, or spine of the scapula. A long-term follow-up study. Clin Orthop Relat Res 1992;283:139–144.
411. Nordqvist A, Petersson CJ. Incidence and causes of shoulder girdle injuries in an urban population. J Shoulder Elbow Surg 1995;4:107–112.
412. Nordqvist A, Petersson C. The incidence of fractures of the clavicle. Clin Orthop Relat Res 1994;300:127–132.
413. Norman A, Schiffman M. Simple bone cysts: factors of age dependency. Radiology 1977;124:779–782.
414. Norwood L, Terry GC. Shoulder posterior subluxation. Am J Sports Med 1984;12: 25–30.
415. Obremskey W, Routt ML Jr. Fracture-dislocation of the shoulder in a child: case report. J Trauma 1994;36:137–140.
416. O'Driscoll SW, Evans DC. Contralateral shoulder instability following anterior repair. An epidemiological investigation. J Bone Joint Surg Br 1991;73:941–946.
417. O'Driscoll SW, Evans DC. Long-term results of staple capsulorrhaphy for anterior instability of the shoulder. J Bone Joint Surg Am 1993;75:249–258.
418. Ogata S, Uhthoff HK. The early development and ossification of the human clavicle. An embryologic study. Acta Orthop Scand 1990;61:330–334.
419. Ogawa BK, Kay RM, Choi PD, et al. Complete division of the radial nerve associated with a closed fracture of the humeral shaft in a child. J Bone Joint Surg Br 2007;89(6): 821–824.
420. Ogden JA. Distal clavicular physeal injury. Clin Orthop Relat Res 1984;188:68–73.
421. Ogden JA. Skeletal Injury in the Child. Philadelphia: Lea & Febiger, 1982:227–228.
422. Ogden JA, ed. Skeletal Injury in the Child. 2nd ed. Philadelphia: WB Saunders, 1990.
423. Ogden JA, Conlogue GJ, Bronson ML. Radiology of postnatal skeletal development. III. The clavicle. Skeletal Radiol 1979;4:196–203.
424. Ogden JA, Conlogue GJ, Jensen P. Radiology of postnatal skeletal development: the proximal humerus. Skeletal Radiol 1978;2:153–160.
425. Olszewski W, Popiński M. Fractures of the neck and shaft of the humerus as a rare form of double fractures in children [in Polish]. Chir Narzadow Ruchu Ortop Pol 1974; 39:121–123.
426. O'Neill JA Jr, Meacham WF, Griffin JP, et al. Patterns of injury in the battered child syndrome. J Trauma 1973;13:332–339.
427. Oppenheim WL, Davis A, Growdon WA, et al. Clavicle fractures in the newborn. Clin Orthop Relat Res 1990;250:176–180.
428. Oreck SL, Burgess A, Levine AM. Traumatic lateral displacement of the scapula: a radiographic sign of neurovascular disease. J Bone Joint Surg Am 1984;66:758–763.
429. O'Rourke IC, Middleton RW. The place and efficacy of operative management of fractured clavicle. Injury 1975;6:236–240.
430. Orrell KG, Bell DF. Structural abnormality of the clavicle associated with Sprengel's deformity: a case report. Clin Orthop Relat Res 1990;258:157–159.
431. Packer JW, Foster RR, Garcia A, et al. The humeral fracture with radial nerve palsy: is exploration warranted? Clin Orthop Relat Res 1972;88:34–38.
432. Peeters PM, Oostvogel HJ, Bongers KJ, et al. Early functional treatment of humerus shaft fractures by the Sarmiento method [in German]. Aktuel Traumatol 1987;17: 150–152.
433. Peter RE, Hoffmeyer P, Henley MB. Treatment of humeral diaphyseal fractures with Hackethal stacked nailing: a report of 33 cases. J Orthop Trauma 1992;6:14–17.
434. Peterson HA. Surgical lengthening of the humerus: case report and review. J Pediatr Orthop 1989;9:596–601.
435. Peterson HA, Madhok R, Benson JT, et al. Physeal fractures: Part 1. Epidemiology in Olmsted County, Minnesota, 1979–1988. J Pediatr Orthop 1994;14:423–430.
436. Pettersson H. Bilateral dysplasia of the neck of the scapula and associated anomalies. Acta Radiol Diagn (Stockh) 1981;22:81–84.
437. Phipps GJ, Hoffer MM. Latissimus dorsi and teres major transfer to rotator cuff for Erb's palsy. J Shoulder Elbow Surg 1995;4:124–129.
438. Pierce RO Jr, Hodurski DF. Fractures of the humerus, radius, and ulna in the same extremity. J Trauma 1979;19:182–185.
439. Poigenfurst J, Rappold G, Fischer W. Plating of fresh clavicular fractures: results of 122 operations. Injury 1992;23:237–241.
440. Pollen AG. Fractures and Dislocations in Children. Baltimore: Williams & Wilkins, 1973.
441. Pollock FH, Drake D, Bovill EG, et al. Treatment of radial neuropathy associated with fractures of the humerus. J Bone Joint Surg Am 1981;63:239–243.
442. Pollock RC, Bankes MJ, Emery RJ. Diagnosis of retrosternal dislocation of the clavicle with ultrasound. Injury 1996;27:670–671.
443. Post M. Current concepts in the treatment of fractures of the clavicle. Clin Orthop Relat Res 1989;245:89–101.
444. Postacchini F, Morace GB. Fractures of the humerus associated with paralysis of the radial nerve. Ital J Orthop Traumatol 1988;14:455–465.
445. Pradhan DJ, Juanteguy JM, Wilder RJ, et al. Arterial injuries of the extremities associated with fractures. Arch Surg 1972;105:582–585.
446. Pritchett JW. Delayed union of humeral shaft fractures treated by closed flexible intramedullary nailing. J Bone Joint Surg Br 1985;67:715–718.
447. Pritchett JW. Growth and predictions of growth in the upper extremity. J Bone Joint Surg Am 1988;70:520–525.
448. Pritchett JW. Growth plate activity in the upper extremity. Clin Orthop Relat Res 1991; 268:235–242.
449. Putnam MD, Walsh TM. External fixation for open fractures of the upper extremity. Hand Clin 1993;9:613–623.
450. Putz P, Lusi K, Baillon JM, et al. The treatment of fractures of the humeral diaphysis with fasciculated intramedullary pins by the Hackethal method apropos of 194 cases [in French]. Acta Orthop Belg 1984;50:521–538.
451. Pyper JB. Nonunion of fractures of the clavicle. Injury 1978;9:268–270.
452. Qureshi AA, Kuo KN. Posttraumatic cleidoscapular synostosis following a fracture of the clavicle. J Bone Joint Surg Am 1999;81:256–258.
453. Rang M. Children's Fractures. 2nd ed. Philadelphia: JB Lippincott, 1983.
454. Rettig AC, Beltz HF. Stress fracture in the humerus in an adolescent tennis tournament player. Am J Sports Med 1985;13:55–58.
455. Rich NM, Metz CW Jr, Hutton JE Jr, et al. Internal versus external fixation of fractures with concomitant vascular injuries in Vietnam. J Trauma 1971;11:463–473.
456. Riemer BL, Buterfield SL, Daffner RH, et al. The abduction lordotic view of the clavicle: a new technique for radiographic visualization. J Orthop Trauma 1991;5:392–394.
457. Riemer BL, Foglesong ME, Burke CJ III, et al. Complications of Seidel intramedullary nailing of narrow-diameter humeral diaphyseal fractures. Orthopaedics 1994;17: 19–29.
458. Robin GC, Kedar SS. Separation of the upper humeral epiphysis in pituitary gigantism. J Bone Joint Surg Am 1962;44:189–192.
459. Rockwood CA Jr. Dislocations of the sternoclavicular joint. AAOS Instr Course Lect 1975;24:144–159.
460. Rockwood CA Jr. The shoulder: facts, confusion, and myths. Int Orthop 1991;15: 401–405.
461. Rockwood CA Jr, Matsen FA, Thomas SC. Anterior glenohumeral instability. In: CA Rockwood, FA Matsen III, eds. The Shoulder. Philadelphia: WB Saunders, 1990: 592–598.
462. Rogalsky RJ, Black GR, Reed MH. Orthopaedic manifestations of leukemia. J Bone Joint Surg Am 1986;68:494–501.
463. Rogers JF, Bennett JB, Tullos HS. Management of concomitant ipsilateral fractures of the humerus and forearm. J Bone Joint Surg Am 1984;66:552–556.
464. Rommens PM, Vansteenkiste F, Stappaerts KH, et al. Indications, dangers, and results of surgical treatment of humeral shaft fractures [in German]. Unfallchirurg 1989;92: 565–570.
465. Rommens PM, Vergruggen J, Broos PL. Retrograde locked nailing of humeral shaft fractures. J Bone Joint Surg Br 1995;77:84–89.
466. Roper BA, Levack B. The surgical treatment of acromioclavicular dislocations. J Bone Joint Surg Am 1982;69:1045–1051.
467. Rose SH, Melton LJ III, Morrey BF, et al. Epidemiologic features of humeral fractures. Clin Orthop Relat Res 1982;168:24–30.
468. Ross GJ, Love MB. Isolated avulsion fracture of the lesser tuberosity of the humerus: report of two cases. Radiology 1989;172:833–834.
469. Rowe CR. An atlas of anatomy and treatment of midclavicular fractures. Clin Orthop Relat Res 1968;58:29–42.
470. Rowe CR. Anterior dislocation of the shoulder: prognosis and treatment. Surg Clin North Am 1963;43:1609–1614.
471. Rowe CR. Fractures of the scapula. Surg Clin North Am 1963;43:1565–1571.
472. Rowe CR. Prognosis in dislocation of the shoulder. J Bone Joint Surg Am 1956;38: 957–977.
473. Rowe CR, Pierce DS, Clark JG. Voluntary dislocation of the shoulder. J Bone Joint Surg Am 1973;55:445–459.
474. Rubin A. Birth injuries: incidence, mechanisms, and end results. Obstet Gynecol 1964; 23:218–221.
475. Rüedi T, Moshfegh A, Pfeiffer KM, et al. Fresh fractures of the shaft of the humerus-conservative or operative treatment? Reconstr Surg Traumatol 1974;14:65–74.
476. Runkel M, Kreitner KF, Wenda K, et al. Nuclear magnetic tomography in shoulder dislocation. Unfallchirurgie 1993;96:124–128.
477. Sachs RA, Lin D, Stone ML, et al. Can the need for future surgery for acute traumatic anterior shoulder dislocation be predicted? J Bone Joint Surg Am 2007;89(8): 1665–1674.
478. Sakakida K. Clinical observations on the epiphysial separation of long bones. Clin Orthop Relat Res 1964;34:119–141.
479. Sales de Gauzy J, Vidal H, Cahuzac JP. Primary shortening followed by callus distraction for the treatment of a posttraumatic bone defect: case report. J Trauma 1993;34: 461–463.
480. Salonen IS, Uusitalo R. Birth injuries: incidence and predisposing factors. Z Kinderchir 1990;45:133–135.
481. Salter RB, Harris WR. Injuries involving the epiphyseal plate. J Bone Joint Surg Am 1963;45:587–622.
482. Samardzic M, Grujicic D, Milinkovic ZB. Radial nerve lesions associated with fractures of the humeral shaft. Injury 1990;21:220–222.
483. Samilson RL. Congenital and developmental anomalies of the shoulder girdle. Orthop Clin North Am 1980;11:219–231.
484. Sanders JO, Rockwood CA Jr, Curtis RJ. Fractures and dislocations of the humeral shaft and shoulder. In: Rockwood CA Jr, Wilkins KE, Beaty JH, eds. Fractures in Children. Philadelphia: Lippincott-Raven, 1996:905–1021.
485. Sanford HN. The Moro reflex as a diagnostic aid in fracture of the clavicle in the newborn infant. Am J Dis Child 1931;41:1304–1306.
486. Sankarankutty M, Turner BW. Fractures of the clavicle. Injury 1975;7:101–106.
487. Sarmiento A. Functional fracture bracing: an update. AAOS Instr Course Lect 1987; 36:371–376.
488. Sarmiento A, Horowitch A, Aboulafia A, et al. Functional bracing for comminuted extra-articular fractures of the distal third of the humerus. J Bone Joint Surg Br 1990; 72:283–287.
489. Sarmiento A, Kinman PB, Galvin EG, et al. Functional bracing of fractures of the shaft of the humerus. J Bone Joint Surg Am 1977;59:596–601.
490. Sattel W. [Effect of dia- and pericondylar humeral fractures on the growth of the carpal bones in children.] Handchir Mikrochir Plast Chir 1982;14:103–105.
491. Scaglietti O. The obstetrical shoulder trauma. Surg Gynecol Obstet 1938;66:866–877.
492. Schopler SA, Lawrence JF, Johnson MK. Lengthening of the humerus for upper extremity limb length discrepancy. J Pediatr Orthop 1986;6:477–480.
493. Schwarz N, Höcker K. Osteosynthesis of irreducible fractures of the clavicle with 2.7-mm ASIF plates. J Trauma 1992;33:179–183.
494. Schwarz N, Leixnering M. Technique and results of clavicular medullary wiring. Zentralbl Chir 1986;111:640–647.
495. Seddon HJ. Nerve lesions complicating certain closed bone injuries. JAMA 1947;135: 691–694.
496. Seddon HJ, Medawar PB, Smith H. Rate of regeneration of peripheral nerves in man. J Physiol (Paris) 1943;102:191–215.
497. Sedel L, Christel P, Duriez J, et al. Acceleration of repair of nonunions by electromagnetic fields. Rev Chir Orthop Reparatrice Appar Mot 1981;67:11–23.
498. Sedel L, Christel P, Duriez R, et al. Results of nonunions treatment by pulsed electromagnetic field stimulation. Acta Orthop Scand Suppl 1982;196:81–91.
499. Seitz J, Valdés F, Kramer A. Acute ischemia of the upper extremity caused by axillary

contused trauma. Report of three cases [in Spanish]. Rev Med Child 1991;119: 567–571.
500. Sessa S, Lascombes P, Prevot J, et al. Centromedullary nailing in fractures of the upper end of the humerus in children and adolescents. Chir Pediatr 1990;31:43–46.
501. Shah JJ, Bhatti NA. Radial nerve paralysis associated with fractures of the humerus: a review of 62 cases. Clin Orthop Relat Res 1983;172:171–176.
502. Shantharam SS. Tips of the trade: 41. Modified coaptation splint for humeral shaft fractures. Orthop Rev 1991;20:1033–1039.
503. Sharma VK, Jain Ak, Gupta RK, et al. Nonoperative treatment of fractures of the humeral shaft: a comparative study. J Indian Med Assoc 1991;89:157–160.
504. Sharrard WJW. Paediatric Orthopaedics and Fractures. Oxford: Blackwell, 1971.
505. Shaw BA, Murphy KM, Shaw A, et al. Humerus shaft fractures in young children: accident or abuse? J Pediatr Orthop 1997;17:293–297.
506. Shaw JL, Sakellarides H. Radial nerve paralysis associated with fractures of the humerus. A review of 45 cases. J Bone Joint Surg Am 1967;49:899–902.
507. Sherk HH, Probst C. Fractures of the proximal humeral epiphysis. Orthop Clin North Am 1975;6:401–413.
508. Shevtsov VI. Outcome of treatment of pseudarthroses of the humerus by methods of closed perosseous osteosynthesis by the Ilizarov technic. Sov Med 1977;10:75–79.
509. Shulman BH, Terhune CB. Epiphyseal injuries in breech delivery. Pediatrics 1951;8: 693–700.
510. Shumada IV, Zhila IS, Rybachuk OI. Compression-distraction osteosynthesis in pseudarthroses of long tubular bones. Vestn Khir Im I I Grek 1976;116:90–94.
511. Shvartzman P, Guy N. Voluntary dislocation of shoulder. Postgrad Med 1988;84: 265–271.
512. Silloway KA, McLaughlin RE, Edlich RC, et al. Clavicular fractures and acromioclavicular joint dislocations in lacrosse: preventable injuries. J Emerg Med 1985;3:117–121.
513. Sloth C, Just SL. The apical oblique radiograph in examination of acute shoulder trauma. Eur J Radiol 1989;9:147–151.
514. Smith DK, Cooney WP. External fixation of high-energy upper extremity injuries. J Orthop Trauma 1990;4:7–18.
515. Smith FM. Fracture-separation of the proximal humeral epiphysis: a study of cases seen at the Presbyterian Hospital from 1929–1953. Am J Surg 1956;91:627–635.
516. Smith RF, Szilagyi E, Elliott JP Jr. Fracture of long bones with arterial injury due to blunt trauma. Principles of management. Arch Surg 1969;99:315–324.
517. Solonen KA, Vastamaki M. Osteotomy of the neck of the humerus for traumatic varus deformity. Acta Orthop Scand 1985;56:79–80.
518. Sonneveld GJ, Patka P, van Mourik JC, et al. Treatment of fractures of the shaft of the humerus accompanied by paralysis of the radial nerve. Injury 1987;18:404–406.
519. Soslowsky LJ, Flatow EL, Bigliani LU, et al. Articular geometry of the glenohumeral joint. Clin Orthop Relat Res 1992;285:181–190.
520. Spak I. Humeral shaft fractures. Treatment with a simple hand sling. Acta Orthop Scand 1978;49:234–239.
521. Sprenger TR. Fracture of humerus from muscular violence: case report. J Fla Med Assoc 1985;72:101–103.
522. Stahl EJ, Karpman R. Normal growth and growth predictions in the upper extremity. J Hand Surg Am 1986;11:593–596.
523. Stanitski CL, Micheli LJ. Simultaneous ipsilateral fractures of the arm and forearm in children. Clin Orthop Relat Res 1980;153:218–222.
524. Stanley D, Norris SH. Recovery following fractures of the clavicle treated conservatively. Injury 1988;19:162–164.
525. Stanley D, Trowbridge EA, Norris SH. The mechanism of clavicular fractures. A clinical and biomechanical analysis. J Bone Joint Surg Br 1988;70:461–464.
526. Stephenson RB, London MD, Hankin FM, et al. Fibrous dysplasia: an analysis of options for treatment. J Bone Joint Surg Am 1987;69:400–409.
527. Sterling JC, Calvo RD, Holden SC. An unusual stress fracture in a multiple sport athlete. Med Sci Sports Exerc 1991;23:298–303.
528. Stern WA. Arthrogryposis multiplex congenity. JAMA 1923;81:1507–1510.
529. Stern PJ, Mattingly DA, Pomeroy DL, et al. Intramedullary fixation of humeral shaft fractures. J Bone Joint Surg Am 1984;66:639–646.
530. Stewart MJ, Hundley JM. Fractures of the humerus: a comparative study in methods of treatment. J Bone Joint Surg Am 1955;37:681–692.
531. Stimson LA. A practical treatise on fractures and dislocations. 3rd ed. New York: Lea Brothers & Co; 1900.
532. Sturmer KM, Schmit-Neuerburg KP. Indications and clinical results of electromagnetically induced alternating current stimulation of poorly reacting pseudarthroses. Unfallchirurgie 1985;11:197–203.
533. Strömqvist B, Lidgren L, Norgren L, et al. Neurovascular injury complicating displaced proximal fractures of the humerus. Injury 1987;18:423–425.
534. Sunderland S. Rate of regeneration in human peripheral nerves. Arch Neurol Psych 1947;58:251–295.
535. Szalay EA, Rockwood CA Jr. Fractures of the distal shaft of the humerus associated with radial nerve palsy. Orthop Trans 1982;6:455.
536. Szalay EA, Rockwood CA Jr. Injuries of the shoulder and arm. Emerg Med Clin North Am 1984;2:279–294.
537. Tachdjian MO. Paediatric Orthopaedics. Philadelphia: WB Saunders, 1990.
538. te Slaa RL, Nollen AJ. A Salter type 3 fracture of the proximal epiphysis of the humerus. Injury 1987;18:429–431.
539. Thomas IH, Chow CW, Cole WG. Giant cell reparative granuloma of the humerus. J Pediatr Orthop 1988;8:596–598.
540. Thompson DA, Flynn TC, Miller PW, et al. The significance of scapular fractures. J Trauma 1985;25:974–977.
541. Tirman PF, Stauffer AE, Crues JV III, et al. Saline magnetic resonance arthrogaphy in the evaluation of glenohumeral instability. Arthroscopy 1993;9:550–559.
542. Titze A. The operative treatment of fractures of the shaft of the humerus. Reconstr Surg Traumatol 1974;14:75–83.
543. Todd TW, D'Errico J Jr. The clavicular epiphyses. Am J Anat 1928;41:25–50.
544. Torode I, Donnan L. Posterior dislocation of the humeral head in association with obstetric paralysis. J Pediatr Orthop 1998;18:611–615.
545. Troum S, Floyd WE III, Waters PM. Posterior dislocation of the humeral head in infancy associated with obstetrical paralysis. A case report. J Bone Joint Surg Am 1993; 75:1370–1375.
546. Trueta J. Studies of the Development and Decay of the Human Frame. Philadelphia: WB Saunders, 1968.
547. Tse DH, Slabaugh PB, Carlson PA. Injury to the axillary artery by a closed fracture of the clavicle. A case report. J Bone Joint Surg Am 1980;62:1372–1374.
548. Tullos HS, Erwin WD, Woods GW, et al. Unusual lesions of the pitching arm. Clin Orthop Relat Res 1972;88:169–182.
549. Tullos HS, Fain RH. Little league shoulder: rotational stress fracture of proximal epiphysis. J Sports Med 1974;2:152–153.
550. Tullos HS, King JW. Lesions of the pitching arm in adolescents. JAMA 1972;220: 264–271.
551. Uhthoff HK, Piscopo M. Anterior capsular redundancy of the shoulder: congenital or traumatic? An embryological study. J Bone Joint Surg Br 1985;67:363–366.
552. Vail TP, Harrelson JM. Treatment of pathologic fracture of the humerus. Clin Orthop Relat Res 1991;268:197–202.
553. van den Broek JA, Vegter J. Echography in the diagnosis of epiphysiolysis of the proximal humerus in a newborn infant [in Dutch]. Ned Tijdscr Geneeskd 1988;132: 1015–1017.
554. van der Ghinst M, De Geeter L, Thiry A. Treatment of collum and diaphyseal fractures of the humerus using Kirschner wire nailing. Acta Chir Belg 1972;Suppl 2:105–116.
555. Vander Griend RA, Tomasin J, Ward EF. Open reduction and internal fixation of humeral shaft fractures. Results using AO plating techniques. J Bone Joint Surg Am 1986;68:430–433.
556. Vander Griend RA, Ward EF, Tomasin J. Closed Kuntscher nailing of humeral shaft fractures. J Trauma 1985;25:1167–1169.
557. Vastamäki M, Solonen KA. Posterior dislocation and fracture-dislocation of the shoulder. Acta Orthop Scand 1980;51:479–484.
558. Vermeiren J, Handelberg F, Casteleyn PP, et al. The rate of recurrence of traumatic anterior dislocation of the shoulder. Int Orthop 1993;17:337–341.
559. Vichare NA. Fractures of the humeral shaft associated with multiple injuries. Injury 1974;5:279–282.
560. Vinz H. Treatment of open fractures in children. Zentralbl Chir 1980;105:1483–1493.
561. Visser CP, Coene LN, Brand R, et al. Nerve lesions in proximal humeral fractures. J Shoulder Elbow Surg 2001;10:421–427.
562. Visser JD, Rietberg M. Interposition of the tendon of the long head of biceps in fracture separation of the proximal humeral epiphysis. Neth J Surg 1980;32:12–15.
563. Vukadinovic S, Mikic Z, Lartey J. Humeral fractures complicated by radial nerve lesions. Acta Chir Iugosl 1981;28:211–217.
564. Wadlington VR, Hendrix RW, Rogers LF. Computed tomography of posterior fracture-dislocations of the shoulder: case reports. J Trauma 1992;32:113–115.
565. Wagner KT, Lyne ED. Adolescent traumatic dislocations of the shoulder with open epiphysis. J Pediatr Orthop 1983;3:61–62.
566. Wall JJ. Congenital pseudarthrosis of the clavicle. J Bone Joint Surg Am 1970;52: 1003–1009.
567. Walle T, Hartikainen-Sorri AL. Obstetric shoulder injury: associated risk factors, prediction, and prognosis. Acta Obstet Gynecol Scand 1993;72:450–454.
568. Wang P Jr, Koval KJ, Lehman W, et al. Salter-Harris type III fracture-dislocation of the proximal humerus. J Pediatr Orthop 1997;6:219–222.
569. Waters P, Bae D, Kadiyala R. Short-term outcomes after surgical treatment of traumatic posterior sternoclavicular fracture-dislocations in children and adolescents. J Pediatr Orthop 2003;23(4):464–469.
570. Watson FM, Whitesides TE Jr. Acute hematogenous osteomyelitis complicating closed fractures. Clin Orthop Relat Res 1976;117:296–302.
571. Webb LX, Green NE, Swiontkowski MF, eds. Skeletal Trauma in Children. Philadelphia: WB Saunders, 1993:257–281.
572. Webb PA, Suchey JM. Epiphyseal union of the anterior iliac crest and medial clavicle in a modern multiracial sample of American males and females. Am J Phys Anthropol 1985;68:457–466.
573. Weber BG, Brunner C, Freuler F. Treatment of fractures in children and adolescents. Berlin: Springer-Verlag; 1980:94–95.
574. Weinberg B, Seife B, Alonso P. The apical oblique view of the clavicle: its usefulness in neonatal and childhood trauma. Skeletal Radiol 1991;20:201–203.
575. Wera GD, Friess DM, Getty PO, et al. Fracture of the proximal humerus with injury to the axillary artery in a boy aged 13 years. J Bone Joint Surg Br 2006;88(11):1521–1523.
576. Weseley MS, Barenfeld PA. Ball throwers' fracture of the humerus. Clin Orthop Relat Res 1969;64:153–156.
577. White GM, Riley LH Jr.,Isolated avulsion of the subscapularis insertion in a child. A case report. J Bone Joint Surg Am 1985;67:635–636.
578. White SJ, Blance CE, DiPietro MA, et al. Arthrography in evaluation of birth injuries of the shoulder. J Can Assoc Radiol J 1987;38:113–115.
579. Whitman RA. Treatment of epiphyseal displacement and fractures of the upper extremity of the humerus designed to assure deficit adjustment and fixation of the fragments. Ann Surg 1908;47:706–708.
580. Whitson RO. Relation of the radial nerve to the shaft of the humerus. J Bone Joint Surg Am 1954;36:85–88.
581. Wickstrom J. Birth injuries of the brachial plexus treatment defects in the shoulder. Clin Orthop Relat Res 1962;23:187–196.
582. Wickstrom J, Haslam ET, Hutchinson RH. The surgical management of residual deformities of the shoulder following birth injuries of the brachial plexus. J Bone Joint Surg Am 1955;37:27–36.
583. Wilber MC, Evans EB. Fractures of the scapula: an analysis of 40 cases and a review of literature. J Bone Joint Surg Am 1977;59:358–362.
584. Wilkins RM, Johnston RM. Ununited fractures of the clavicle. J Bone Joint Surg Am 1983;65:773–778.
585. Williams DJ. The mechanisms producing fracture-separation of the proximal humeral epiphysis. J Bone Joint Surg Br 1981;63B:102–107.
586. Winfield JM, Miller H, LaFerte AD. Evaluation of the "hanging cast" as a method of treating fractures of the humerus. Am J Surg 1942;55:228–249.
587. Winker H, Vosberg W, Cyris A. Results of treatment of humerus shaft fractures. Aktuel Traumatol 1993;23(suppl):36–41.
588. Wippermann B, Schmidt U, Nerlich M. Results of treatment of compartment syndrome of the upper arm [in German]. Unfallchirurg 1991;94:231–235.
589. Wong-Chung J, O'Brien T. Salter-Harris type III fracture of the proximal humeral physis. Injury 1988;19:453–454.

590. Worlock P, Stower M. Fracture patterns in Nottingham children. J Pediatr Orthop 1986;6:656–660.
591. Worman LW, Leagus C. Intrathoracic injury following retrosternal dislocation of the clavicle. J Trauma 1967;7:416–423.
592. Wright TW, Miller GJ, Vander Griend RA, et al. Reconstruction of the humerus with an intramedullary fibular graft. A clinical and biomechanical study. J Bone Joint Surg Br 1993;75:804–807.
593. Wu CD, Chen YC. Stress fracture of the clavicle in a professional baseball player. J Shoulder Elbow Surg 1998;7(2):164–167.
594. Yosipovitch Z, Goldberg I. Inferior subluxation of the humeral head after injury to the shoulder. A brief note. J Bone Joint Surg Am 1989;71:751–753.
595. Zagorski JB, Latta LL, Zych GA, et al. Diaphyseal fractures of the humerus. Treatment with prefabricated braces. J Bone Joint Surg Am 1988;70:607–610.
596. Zanasi R, Romano P, Rotolo F, et al. Intramedullary osteosynthesis: 3. Kuntscher nailing in the humerus. Ital J Orthop Traumatol 1990;16:311–322.
597. Zella BA, Pape HC, Gerich TG, et al. Functional outcome following scapulothoracic dissociation. J Bone Joint Surg Am 2004;86A:2–8.
598. Zenni EJ Jr, Krieg JK, Rosen MJ. Open reduction and internal fixation of clavicular fractures. J Bone Joint Surg Am 1981;63:147–151.
599. Zifko B, Poigenfurst J. Treatment of unstable fractures of the proximal end of the humerus using elastic curved intramedullary wires [in German]. Unfallchirurgie 1987; 13:72–81.
600. Zinghi GF, Sabetta E, Bungaro P, et al. The role of osteosynthesis in the treatment of fractures of the humerus. Ital J Orthop Traumatol 1988;14:67–75.
601. Zravkovic D, Damholt VV. Comminuted and severely displaced fractures of the scapula. Acta Orthop Scand 1974;45:60–65.
602. Zuckerman JD, Flugstad DL, Teitz CC, et al. Axillary artery injury as a complication of proximal humerus fractures. Two case reports and a review of the literature. Clin Orthop Relat Res 1984;189:234–237.
603. Zuckerman JD, Matsen FA. Complications about the glenohumeral joint related to the use of screws and staples. J Bone Joint Surg Am 1984;66:175–180.

SECTION

THREE

SPINE

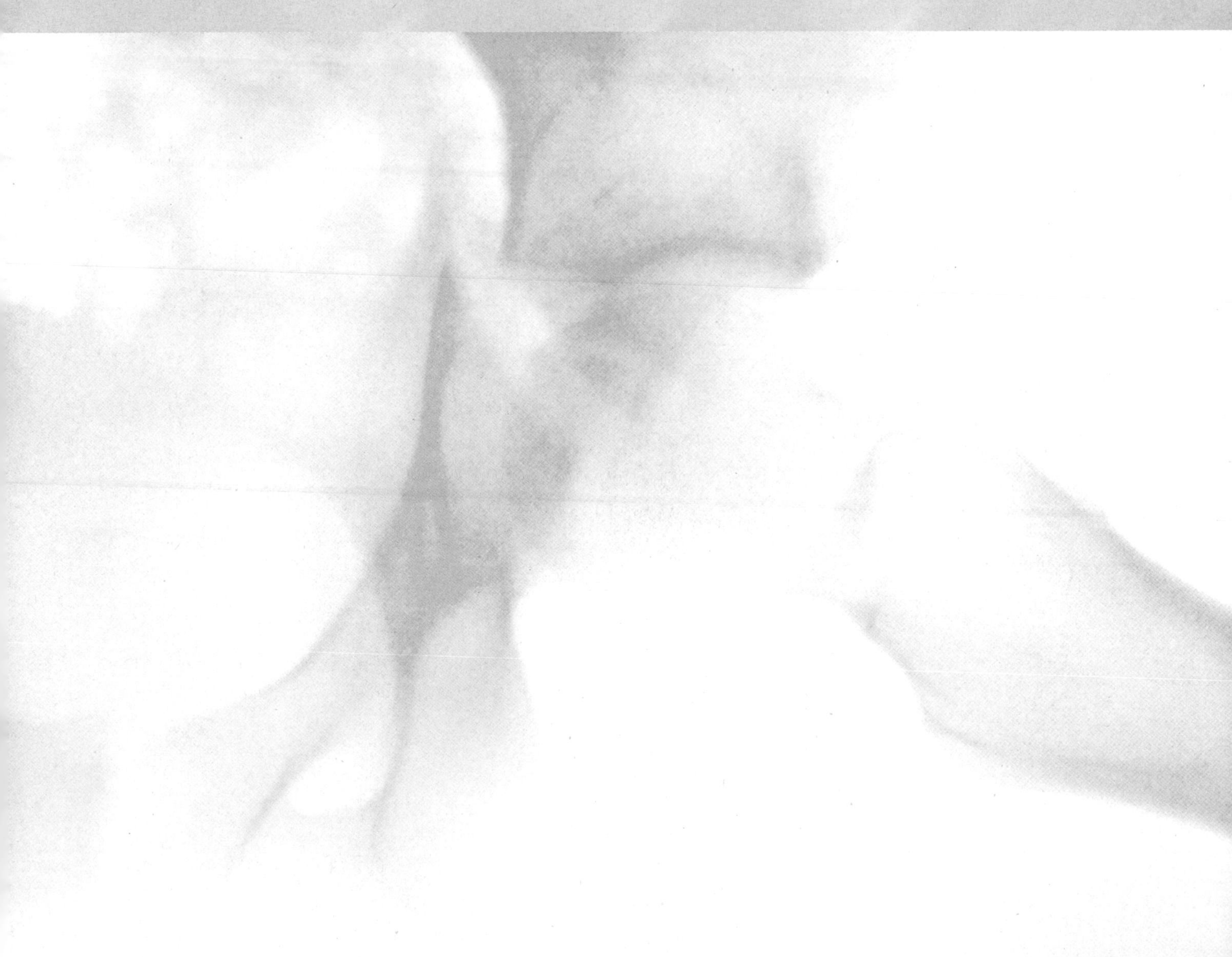

18

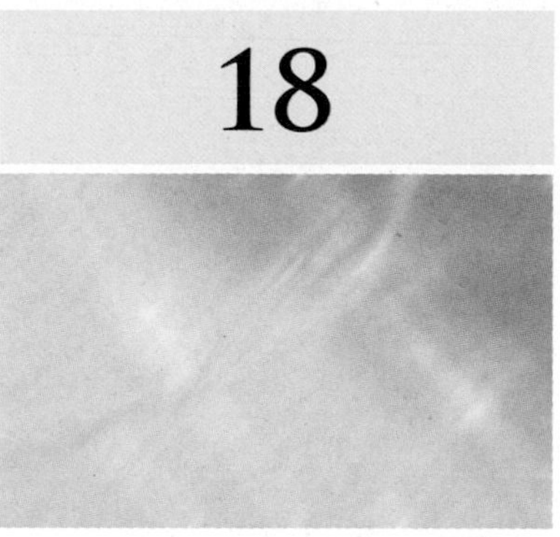

CERVICAL SPINE INJURIES IN CHILDREN

William C. Warner Jr. and Daniel J. Hedequist

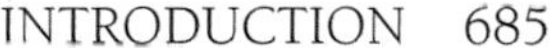

INTRODUCTION 685

ANATOMY 686
Upper Cervical Spine 686
Lower Cervical Spine 688

HISTORY 688

SYMPTOMS 689

EVALUATION 689

RADIOGRAPHIC EVALUATION 689
Plain Radiographs 689
Radiographic Evaluation of Specific Areas of the Spine 690
Special Imaging Studies 692

INITIAL MANAGEMENT OF CERVICAL SPINE INJURIES 693
Technique of Halo Application 695

SPINAL CORD INJURY WITHOUT RADIOGRAPHIC ABNORMALITIES 696

SPINAL CORD INJURY IN CHILDREN 696

NEONATAL INJURY 697

OCCIPITAL CONDYLAR FRACTURE 697

ATLANTO-OCCIPITAL INSTABILITY 698
Operative Treatment 699

FRACTURES OF THE ATLAS 703

ATLANTOAXIAL INJURIES 704
Odontoid Fractures 704
Os Odontoideum 706
Traumatic Ligamentous Disruption 707

OPERATIVE TREATMENT 707
Atlantoaxial Arthrodesis 707
Atlantoaxial Instability Associated with Congenital Anomalies and Syndromes 710
Atlantoaxial Rotatory Subluxation 711
Hangman's Fracture 713

SUBAXIAL INJURIES 714
Posterior Ligamentous Disruption 714
Compression Fractures 715
Unilateral and Bilateral Facet Dislocations 715
Burst Fractures 716
Spondylolysis and Spondylolisthesis 716
Operative Treatment 716

INTRODUCTION

Cervical spine fractures in children are rare, accounting for only 1% of pediatric fractures and 2% of all spinal injuries.[7,9,87,88,102,108,119,132,164,189,212] The incidence is estimated to be 7.41 in 100,000 per year[145]; however, that may be misleading because some injuries are not detected or are detected only at autopsy. Aufdermaur[13] examined the autopsied spines of 12 juveniles who had spinal injuries. All 12 had cartilage endplates that were separated from the vertebral bodies in the zone of columnar and calcified cartilage, similar to a Salter-Harris type I fracture, although clinically and radiographically, a fracture was suggested in only one patient. Only radiographs at autopsy showed the disruption, represented by a small gap apparent widening of the intervertebral space.[13]

Cervical spine injuries in children younger than 8 years age occur in the upper cervical spine, while older children and adolescents tend to have fractures involving either the upper or lower cervical spine.[163] The upper cervical spine in children is more prone to injury because of the anatomic and biomechanical properties of the immature spine. The immature spine is hypermobile because of ligamentous laxity, and the facet joints are oriented in a more horizontal position; both of these properties predispose children to more forward translation. Younger children also have a relatively large head compared to the body, which changes the fulcrum of motion of the upper cervical spine. All of these factors predispose younger children to injuries of the upper cervical spine; with age, the anatomic changes lead to an increased prevalence of lower cervical spine injuries.

The mechanism of injury in pediatric patients also is age-related. Infants with cervical spine injuries should be evaluated for abuse.[81] In children up to 9 years of age, the most common mechanism of injury is related to motor vehicle accidents; the second most common mechanism in this age group is falls.[33,243] In older children and adolescents, the most common mechanism of cervical spine injuries is sporting activities, followed by motor vehicle accidents.[13,224]

Cervical spine injuries associated with neurologic deficits are infrequent in children, and when incomplete there tends to be a better prognosis for recovery in children than in adults.[21,59] Complete neurologic deficits, regardless of patient age, tend to have a poor prognosis for any recovery and may be indicative of the severity and magnitude of injury.[58,120,155,171] Death from cervical spine injuries tends to be related to the level of injury and the associated injuries. Higher cervical spine injuries (i.e., atlanto-occipital dislocation) in younger children are associated with the highest mortality rate.[161,162] Children with significant cervical spine injuries also may have associated severe head injuries, leading to an increase in mortality. In a study of 61 pediatric deaths related to spinal cord injuries, 89% of fatalities occurred at the scene, and most were related to high cervical cord injuries in patients who had sustained multiple injuries.[90]

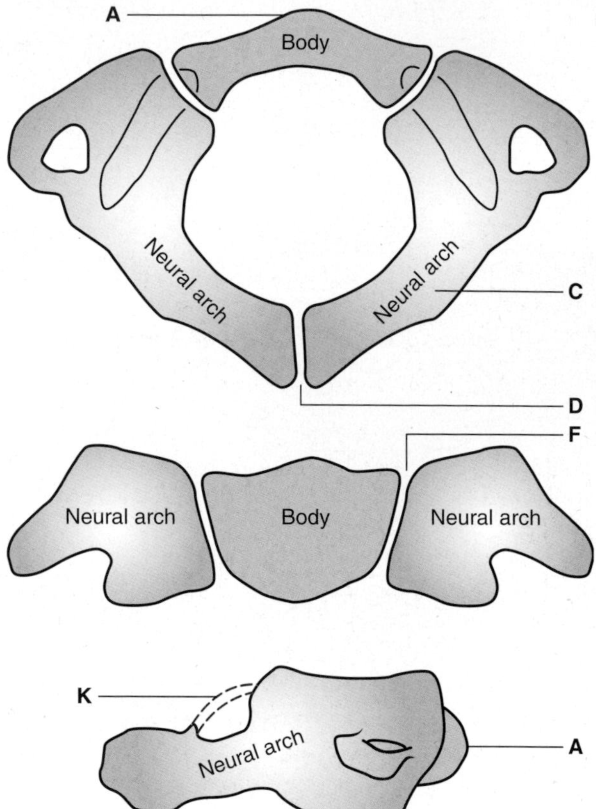

FIGURE 18-1 Diagram of C1 (atlas). The body (*A*) is not ossified at birth, and its ossification center appears during the first year of life. The body may fail to develop, and forward extension of neural arches (*C*) may take its place. Neural arches appear bilaterally about the seventh week (*D*), and the most anterior portion of the superior articulating surface usually is formed by the body. The synchondrosis of the spinous processes unites by the third year. Union rarely is preceded by the appearance of the secondary center within the synchondrosis. Neurocentral synchondrosis (*F*) fuses about the seventh year. The ligament surrounding the superior vertebral notch (*K*) may ossify, especially in later life. (From Bailey DK. Normal cervical spine in infants and children. Radiology 1952;59: 713–714, with permission.)

ANATOMY

Understanding the normal growth and development of the cervical spine is essential when treating a child with a suspected cervical spine injury. This will allow the physician to differentiate normal physes or synchondroses from pathologic fractures or ligamentous disruptions and will alert the physician to any possible congenital anomalies that may be mistaken for a fracture.

Upper Cervical Spine

At birth, the atlas is composed of three ossification centers, one for the body and one for each of the neural arches (Fig. 18-1). The ossification center for the anterior arch is present in approximately 20% of individuals at birth, appearing in the remainder during the first year of life. Occasionally, the anterior arch is bifid, and the body may be formed from two centers or may fail to completely appear. The posterior arches usually fuse by the age of 3 years; however, occasionally the posterior synchondrosis between the two fails to fuse, resulting in a bifid arch. The neurocentral synchondroses that link the neural arches to the body are best seen on an open-mouth odontoid view. These synchondroses close by 7 years of age and should not be mistaken for fractures.[41] The canal of the atlas is large to allow for the amount of rotation that occurs at this joint as well as some forward translation.[43] The vertebral arteries are about 2 cm from the midline and run in a groove on the superior surface of the atlas. This must be remembered during lateral dissection at the occipital cervical junction. Because the ring of C1 reaches about normal adult size by 4 years of age, arthrodesis after this time should not cause spinal canal stenosis.

The axis develops from at least four separate ossification centers: one for the dens, one for the body, and two for the neural arches (Fig. 18-2). Between the odontoid and the body of the axis is a synchondrosis or vestigial disk space that often is mistaken for a fracture line. This synchondrosis runs well below the level of the articular processes of the axis and usually fuses at 6 to 7 years of age, although it may persist as a sclerotic line until 11 years of age.[43] The most common odontoid fracture pattern in adults and adolescents is transverse and at the level of the articular processes. The normal synchondrosis should not be confused with this fracture; the synchondrosis is more cup-shaped and below the level of the articular processes. After 7 years of age, the synchondrosis should not be present on an open-mouth odontoid view; a fracture should be considered if a lucent line is present after this age. The neural arches of C2 fuse at 3 to 6 years of age; these are seen as vertical lucent lines on the open-mouth odontoid view. Occasionally, the tip of the odontoid is V-shaped (dens bicornum), or a small separate sum-

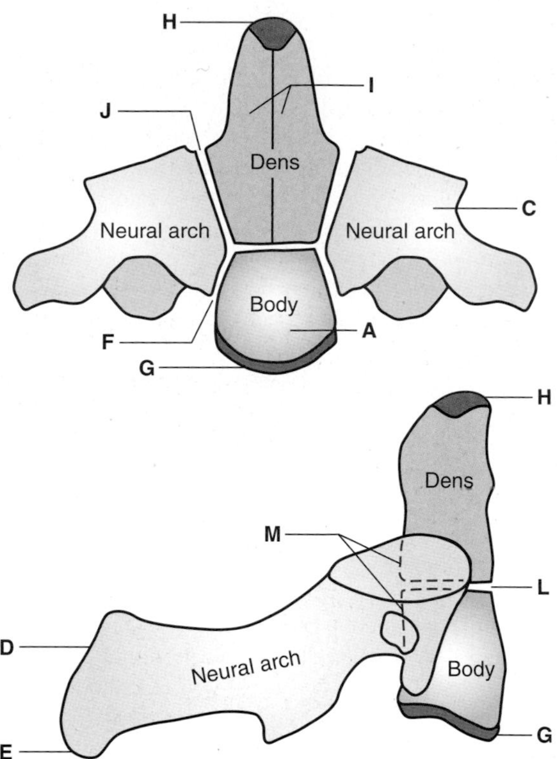

FIGURE 10-2 Diagram of C2 (axis). The body (*A*) in which one center (occasionally two) appears by the fifth fetal month. Neural arches (*C*) appear bilaterally by the seventh fetal month. Neural arches fuse (*D*) posteriorly by the second or third year. Bifid tip (*E*) of spinous process (occasionally a secondary center is present in each tip). Neurocentral synchondrosis (*F*) fuses at 3 to 6 years. The inferior epiphyseal ring (*G*) appears at puberty and fuses at about 25 years of age. The summit ossification center (*H*) for the odontoid appears at 3 to 6 years and fuses with the odontoid by 12 years. Odontoid (dens) (*I*). Two separate centers appear by the fifth fetal month and fuse with each other by the seventh fetal month. The synchondrosis between the odontoid and neural arch (*I*) fuses at 3 to 6 years. Synchondrosis between the odontoid and body (*L*) fuses at 3 to 6 years. Posterior surface of the body and odontoid (*M*). (From: Bailey DK. Normal cervical spine in infants and children. Radiology 1952;59:713–714, with permission.)

mit ossification center may be present at the tip of the odontoid (ossiculum terminale). An os odontoideum is believed to result from a history of unrecognized trauma. The differentiation between an os odontoideum and the synchondrosis of the body is relatively easy because of their relationships to the level of the C1–C2 facet (Fig. 18-3).

The arterial supply to the odontoid is derived from the vertebral and carotid arteries. The anterior and posterior ascending arteries arise from the vertebral artery at the level of C3 and ascend anterior and posterior to the odontoid, meeting superiorly to form an apical arcade. These arteries supply small penetrating branches to the body of the axis and the odontoid process. The internal carotid artery gives off cleft perforators that supply the superior portion of the odontoid. This arrangement of arteries and vessels is necessary for embryologic development and anatomic function of the odontoid. The synchondrosis prevents direct vascularization of the odontoid from C2, and vascularization from the blood supply of C1 is not possible because the synovial joint cavity surrounds the odontoid. The formation of an os odontoideum after cervical trauma may be related to this peculiar blood supply (Fig. 18-4).

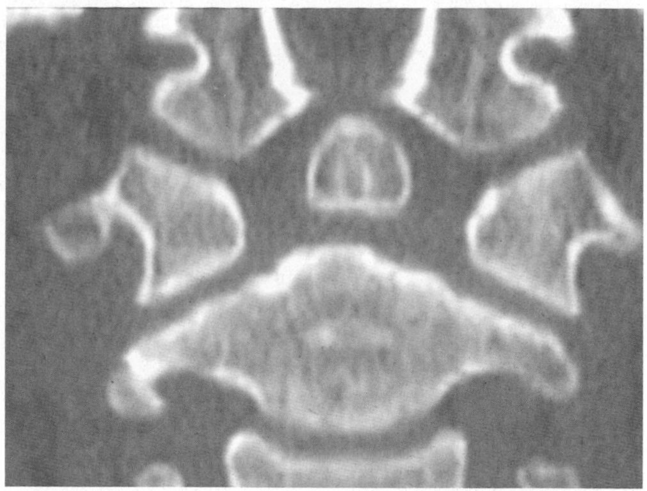

FIGURE 18-3 CT scan showing presence of an os odontoideum. Note the position of the os well above the C1–C2 facets. The scan also shows the vestigial scar of the synchondrosis between the dens and the body below the C1–C2 facet.

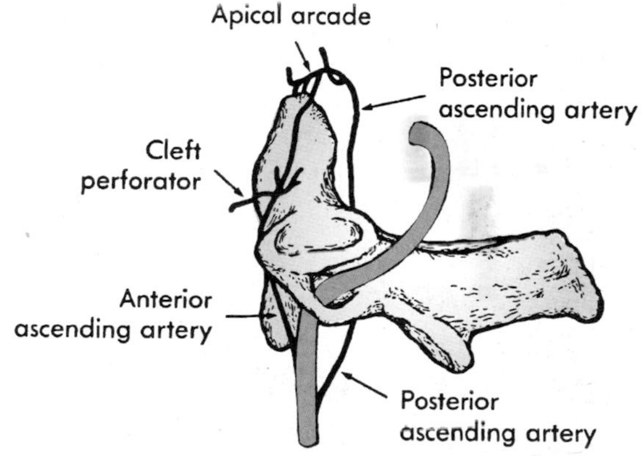

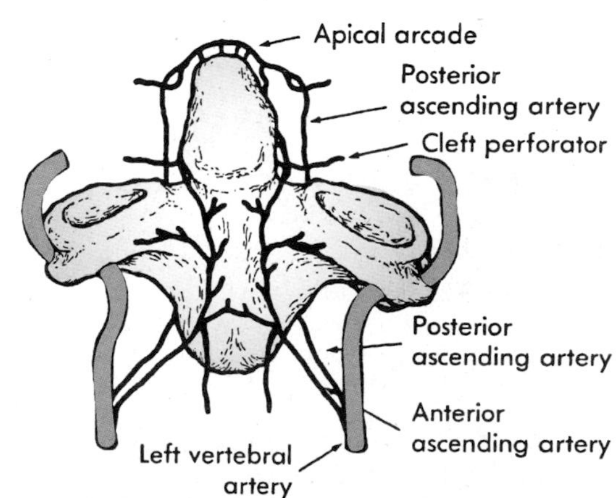

FIGURE 18-4 Blood supply to odontoid: posterior and anterior ascending arteries and apical arcade. (From Schiff DC, Parke WW. The arterial supply of the odontoid process. J Bone Joint Surg Am 1973;55:1450–1464, with permission.)

Lower Cervical Spine

The third through seventh cervical vertebrae share a similar ossification pattern: a single ossification center for the vertebral body and an ossification center for each neural arch (Fig. 18-5). The neural arch fuses posteriorly between the second and third years, and the neurocentral synchondroses between the neural arches and the vertebral body fuse by 3 to 6 years of age. These vertebrae normally are wedge-shaped until 7 to 8 years of age.[13,131,179] The vertebral bodies, neural arches, and pedicles enlarge by periosteal appositional growth, similar to that seen in long bones. By 8 to 10 years of age, a child's spine usually reaches near adult size and characteristics. There are five secondary ossification centers that can remain open until 25 years of age.[131] These include one each for the spinous processes, transverse processes, and the ring apophyses about the vertebral endplates. These should not be confused with fractures.

The superior and inferior endplates are firmly bound to the adjacent disk. The junction between the vertebral body and the endplate is similar to a physis of a long bone. The vertebral body is analogous to the metaphysis and the endplate to the physis, where longitudinal growth occurs. The junction between the vertebral body and the endplate has been shown to be weaker than the adjacent vertebral body or disk, which can result in a fracture at the endplate in the area of columnar and calcified cartilage of the growth zone, similar to a Salter-Harris type I fracture of a long bone.[13] The inferior end plate may be more susceptible to this injury than the superior endplate because of the mechanical protection afforded by the developing uncinate processes.[24]

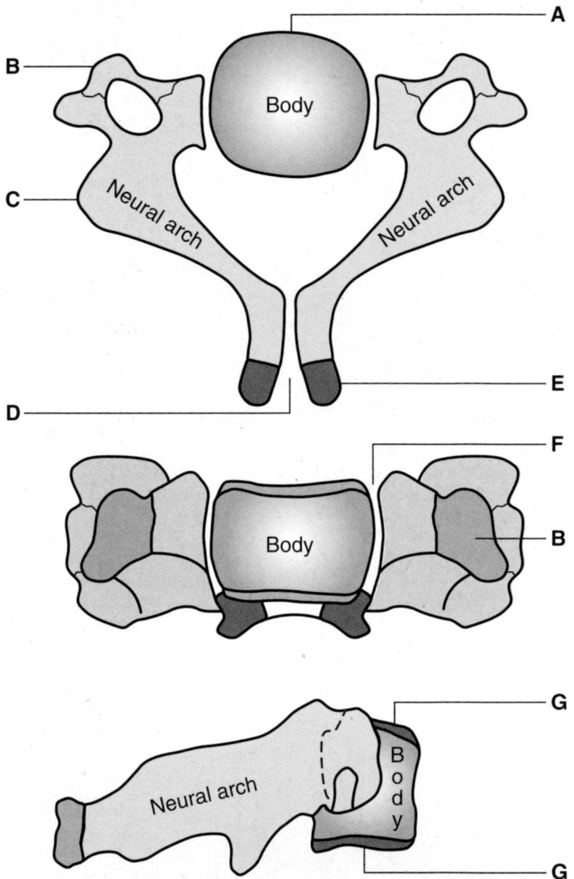

FIGURE 18-5 Diagram of typical cervical vertebrae, C3 to C7. The body (*A*) appears by the fifth fetal month. The anterior (costal) portion of the transverse process (*B*) may develop from a separate center that appears by the sixth fetal month and joins the arch by the sixth year. Neural arches (*C*) appear by the seventh to ninth fetal week. The synchondrosis between spinous processes (*D*) usually unites by the second or third year. Secondary centers for bifid spine (*E*) appear at puberty and unite with spinous process at 25 years. Neurocentral synchondrosis (*F*) fuses at 3 to 6 years. Superior and inferior epiphyseal rings (*G*) appear at puberty and unite with the body at about 25 years. The seventh cervical vertebra differs slightly because of a long, powerful, nonbifid spinous process. (From: Bailey DK. Normal cervical spine in infants and children. Radiology 1952; 59:713–714, with permission.)

The facet joints of the cervical spine change in orientation with age. The angle of the C1–C2 facet is 55 degrees in newborns and increases to 70 degrees at maturity. In the lower cervical spine, the angle of the facet joints is 30 degrees at birth and 60 to 70 degrees at maturity. This may explain why the pediatric cervical spine may be more susceptible to injury from the increased motion or translation allowed by the facet joint orientation.

Increased ligamentous laxity in young children allows a greater degree of spinal mobility than in adults. Flexion and extension of the spine at C2–C3 are 50% greater in children between the ages of 3 and 8 years than in adults. The level of the greatest mobility in the cervical spine descends with increasing age. Between 3 and 8 years of age, the most mobile segment is C3–C4; from 9 to 11 years, C4–C5 is the most mobile segment, and from 12 to 15 years, C5–C6 is the most mobile segment.[4,172] This explains the tendency for craniocervical injuries in young children.

Several anomalies of the cervical spine may influence treatment recommendations. The atlas can fail to segment from the skull, a condition called occipitalization of the atlas, and can lead to narrowing of the foramen magnum, neurologic symptoms, and increased stresses to the atlantoaxial articulation, which often causes instability. Failure of fusion of the posterior arch of C1 is not uncommon and should be sought before any procedure that involves C1. Wedge-shaped vertebrae, bifid vertebrae, or a combination of these also can occur. Klippel-Feil syndrome consists of the classic triad of a short neck, low posterior hairline, and severe restriction of motion of the neck from fusion of the cervical vertebrae.[101,122] Congenital fusion of the cervical spine may predispose a child to injury from trauma by concentrating stresses in the remaining mobile segments.

Hensinger et al.[100] reported congenital anomalies of the odontoid, including aplasia (complete absence), hypoplasia (partial absence in which there is a stubby piece at the base of the odontoid located above the C1 articulation), and os odontoideum. Os odontoideum consists of a separate ossicle of the odontoid with no connection to the body of C2. The cause may be traumatic. These anomalies also may predispose a child to injury or instability.

HISTORY

Most cervical spine injuries in young children are the result of motor vehicle accidents, sporting injuries, or pedestrian injuries.[124] Infants are at risk for cervical spine injuries during the obstetric period as well as during early development because of their lack of head control; however, most cervical spine injuries in infants are spinal cord injury without radiologic abnormality (SCIWORA) and are related to child abuse.[13] Younger children may sustain injuries to their neck from seemingly low-energy falls of less than 5 feet; however, most of their cervical spine injuries are sustained as a result of motor vehicle accidents.[109,195] As children become adolescents, the prevalence of sporting injuries increases, as does the prevalence of athletic-related SCIWORA.[33,124] Regardless of the cause, an adequate history may be difficult to obtain at the initial evaluation, and repeat evaluations may be needed.

SYMPTOMS

The most common presenting symptom in patients with cervical spine injuries is pain localized to the cervical region. Other complaints, such as headache, inability to move the neck, subjective feelings of instability, and neurologic symptoms, all warrant complete evaluation. Infants may present with unexplained respiratory distress, motor weakness, or hypotonia, which warrant further evaluation. Patients with head and neck trauma, distracting injuries, or altered levels of consciousness are at high risk for a cervical spine injury and need to be thoroughly evaluated before obtaining cervical spine clearance.[33] The presence of an occult cervical spine injury in an uncooperative or obtunded patient needs to be considered because of the frequency of SCIWORA in the pediatric population.[164,189]

EVALUATION

The evaluation of any patient with a suspected cervical spine injury should begin with inspection. Head and neck trauma is associated with a high incidence of cervical spine injuries.[4,13] Soft tissue abrasions or shoulder-harness marks on the neck from a seatbelt are clues to an underlying cervical spine injury (Fig. 18-6).[72,81,107] Unconscious patients should be treated as if they have a cervical spine injury until further evaluation proves otherwise. The next step in the evaluation is palpation of the cervical spine for tenderness, muscle spasm, and overall alignment. The most prominent levels should be the spinous processes at C2, C3, and C7. Anterior palpation should focus on the presence of tenderness or swelling. The entire spine should be palpated and thoroughly examined because 20% of patients with cervical spine injuries have other spinal fractures.

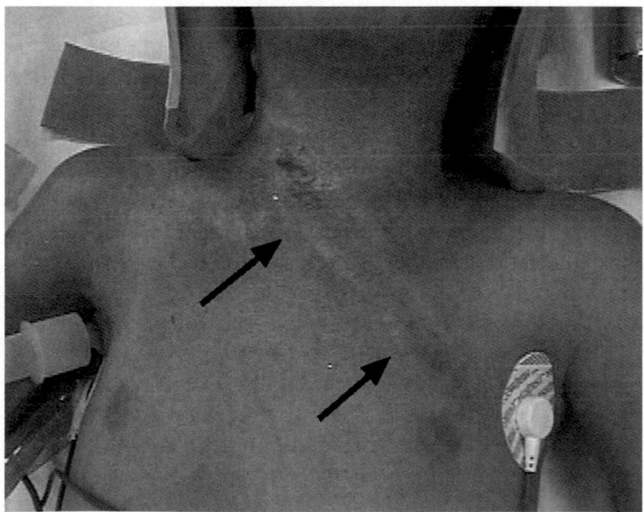

FIGURE 18-6 Clinical photograph of a patient with a cervical spine injury resulting from impact with the shoulder harness of a seat belt. Note location of skin contusions from the seatbelt.

A thorough neurologic examination should be done, which can be difficult in pediatric patients. Strength, sensation, reflexes, and proprioception should be documented. In patients who are uncooperative because of age or altered mental status, repeat examinations are important; however, the initial neurovascular examination should be documented even it if entails only gross movements of the extremities. The evaluation of rectal sphincter tone, bulbocavernosus reflex, and perianal sensation are important, especially in obtunded patients and patients with partial or complete neurologic injuries, regardless of age. Patients who are cooperative and awake can be asked to perform supervised flexion, extension, lateral rotation, and lateral tilt. Uncooperative or obtunded patients should not have any manipulation of the neck.

RADIOGRAPHIC EVALUATION

Plain Radiographs

Plain radiographs remain the standard for evaluating the cervical spine in children. There currently is no consensus regarding whether or not all pediatric trauma patients require cervical spine films. The presence of tenderness and a distracting injury are the most common clinical presentations of a cervical spine injury.[230] While some studies have shown that plain radiographs are of low yield in patients without evidence of specific physical findings, the burden remains on the treating physician to clear the cervical spine.[8,53,130,134] Clearly, patients with tenderness, distracting injuries, neurologic deficits, head and neck trauma, and altered levels of consciousness need to have a complete set of cervical spine radiographs. Initial radiographs should include an anteroposterior view, open-mouth odontoid view, and lateral view of the cervical spine. Patients who are deemed unstable in the emergency room and are not able to tolerate multiple radiographs should have a cross-table lateral view of the cervical spine until further radiographs can be taken. The false-negative rates for a single cross-table radiograph have been reported to be 23% to 26%, indicating that complete radiographs are necessary when the patient is stable.[15,200]

Flexion and extension radiographs may further aid the evaluation of the cervical spine, but these views are unlikely to be abnormal when standard views show no abnormalities. These views are helpful, however, in ruling out acute ligamentous injury.[180] We recommend flexion and extension views in an alert patient with midline tenderness who has normal plain films of the cervical spine. These views must be taken only with a cooperative and alert child; they should not be used in obtunded or uncooperative patients, nor should they be done by manually placing the child in a position of flexion and extension.

Evaluation of cervical spine radiographs should proceed with a knowledge of the anatomic ossification centers and variations that occur in children. Each vertebral level should be systematically evaluated, as should the overall alignment of the cervical spine with respect to the anterior and posterior aspects of the vertebral bodies, the spinolaminar line, and the interspinous distances. The absence of cervicallordosis, an increase in the

TABLE 18-1 Normal Ossification Centers and Anomalies Frequently Confused with Injury

Avulsion fracture
- Apical ossification center of the odontoid. Secondary ossification centers at the tips of the transverse and spinous processes

Fracture
- Persistence of the synchondrosis at the base of the odontoid
- Apparent anterior wedging of a young child's vertebral body
- Normal posterior angulation of the odontoid seen in 4% of normal children

Instability
- Pseudosubluxation of C2 to C3
- Incomplete ossification, especially of the odontoid process, with apparent superior subluxation of the anterior arch of C1
- Absence of the ossification center of the anterior arch of C1 in the first year of life may suggest posterior displacement of C1 on the odontoid
- Increase in the atlanto–dens interval of up to 4.5 mm

Miscellaneous
- Physiologic variations in the width of the prevertebral soft tissue due to crying misinterpreted as swelling due to edema or hemorrhage
- Overlying structures such as ears, braided hair, teeth, or hyoid bone. Plastic rivets used in modern emergency cervical immobilization collars can simulate fracture line
- Horizontally placed facets in the younger child, creating the illusion of a pillar fracture
- Congenital anomalies such as os odontoideum, spina bifida, and congenital fusion or hemivertebrae

prevertebral soft tissue space, and subluxation of C2 on C3 are all anatomic variations that may be normal in children.[41] Ossification centers also may be confused with fractures, most commonly in evaluation of the dens. The presence of a synchondrosis at the base of the odontoid can be distinguished from a fracture based on the age of the patient and the location of synchondrosis well below the facet joints. Knowledge of these normal variants is useful in evaluating plain radiographs of the cervical spine in children (Table 18-1).

Radiographic Evaluation of Specific Areas of the Spine

Atlanto-Occipital Junction

The atlanto-occipital interval remains the most difficult to assess for abnormalities, partly because of the difficulty in obtaining quality radiographs and partly because of the lack of discrete and reproducible landmarks. The distance between the occipital condyles and the facet joints of the atlas should be less than 5 mm; any distance of more than this suggests an atlanto-occipital disruption.[54,172] The foramen magnum and its relationship to the atlas also are useful in detecting injuries of the atlanto-occipital region. The anterior cortical margin of the foramen magnum is termed the basion, while the posterior cortical margin of the foramen magnum is termed the opisthion. The distance between the basion and the tip of the dens should be less than 12 mm as measured on a lateral radiograph.[35] The Powers ratio (Fig. 18-7) is used to assess the position of the skull base relative to the atlas and is another way of evaluating the atlanto-

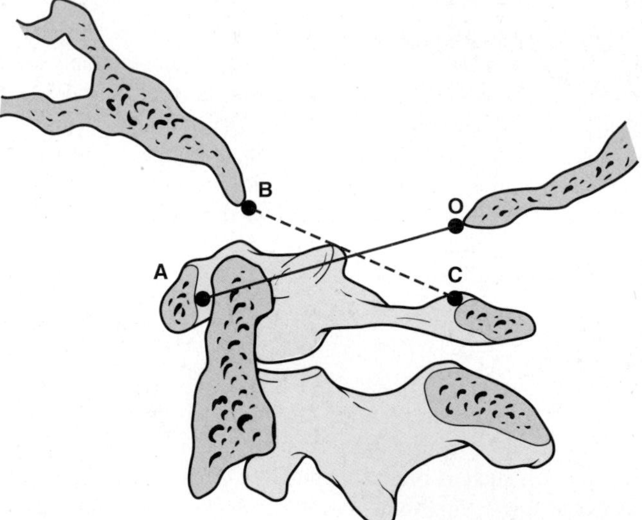

FIGURE 18-7 The Powers ratio is determined by drawing a line from the basion (*B*) to the posterior arch of the atlas (*C*) and a second line from the opisthion (*O*) to the anterior arch of the atlas (*A*). The length of the line BC is divided by the length of the line OA, producing the Powers ratio. (From Lebwohl NH, Eismont FJ. Cervical spine injuries in children. In: Weinstein SL, ed. The Pediatric Spine: Principles and Practice. New York: Raven, 1994,with permission.)

occipital region. To determine this ratio, a line is drawn from the basion to the anterior cortex of the posterior arch of C1, and this distance is divided by the distance of a line drawn from the opisthion to the posterior cortex of the anterior arch of C1. The value should be between 0.7 and 1; a higher value indicates anterior subluxation of the atlanto-occipital joint and a lower value indicates a posterior subluxation. The problem lies in the fact that the basion is not always visible on plain radiographs. The Wackenheim line, which is drawn along the posterior aspect of the clivus, probably is the most easily identified line to determine disruption of the atlanto-occipital joint. If the line does not intersect the tip of the odontoid tangentially and if this line is displaced anteriorly or posteriorly, disruption or increased laxity about the atlanto-occipital joint should be suspected.

Atlantoaxial Joint

The atlanto–dens interval (ADI) and the space available for the spinal canal are two useful measurements for evaluation of the atlantoaxial joint (Fig. 18-8). The ADI in a child is considered normal up to 4.5 mm, partly because the unossified cartilage of the odontoid, which is not seen on plain films, gives an apparent increase in the interval. At the level of the atlantoaxial joint, the space taken up is broken into Steel's rule of thirds: one third is taken up by the odontoid, one third by the spinal cord, and one third is space available for the cord. These intervals also are easily measured on flexion and extension views and are helpful in determining instability. In children, extension views give the appearance of subluxation of the anterior portion of the atlas over the unossified dens, but this represents a pseudosubluxation and not instability.[43,51]

Upper Cervical Spine

Anterior displacement of one vertebral body on another may or may not indicate a true bony or ligamentous injury. Displace-

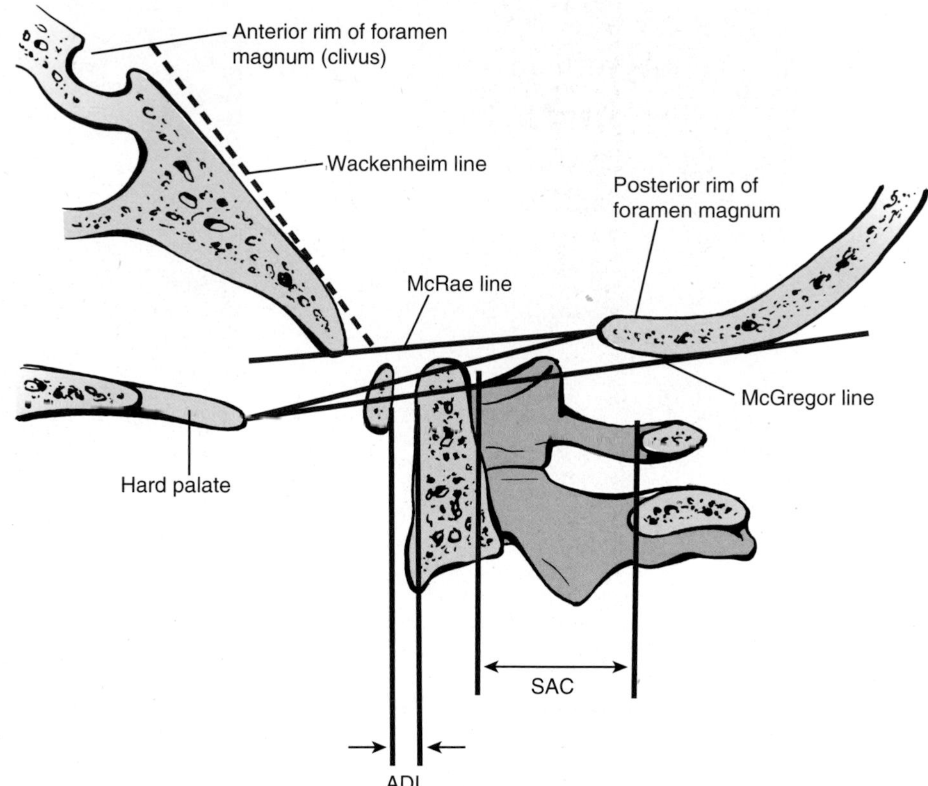

FIGURE 18-8 The ADI and the space available for cord are used in determining atlantoaxial instability. The Wackenheim clivus-canal line is used to determine atlanto-occipital injury, while the McRae and McGregor lines are used in the measurement of basilar impression. (From Copley LA, Dormans JP. Cervical spine disorders in infants and children. J Am Acad Orthop Surg 1998;6:204–214, with permission.)

ment of less than 3 mm at one level is a common anatomic variant in children at the levels of C2–C3 and C3–C4. This displacement is seen on flexion radiographs and reduces in extension. The posterior line of Swischuk[218] has been described to differentiate pathologic subluxation from normal anatomic variation; this line is drawn from the anterior cortex of the spinous process of C1 to the spinous process of C3 (Fig. 18-9). The anterior cortex of the spinous process of C2 should lie within 3 mm of this line; if the distance is more than this, a true subluxation should be suspected (Fig. 18-10). Widening of the spinous processes between C1 and C2 of more than 10 mm also is indicative of a ligamentous injury and should be evaluated by further imaging studies.[3]

Lower Cervical Spine

Lateral radiographs of the cervical spine should be evaluated for overall alignment as well as at each level. The overall alignment can be evaluated by the continuous lines formed by the line adjoining the spinous processes, the spinolaminar line, and the lines adjoining the posterior and anterior vertebral bodies (Fig. 18-11). These lines should all be smooth and continuous with no evidence of vertebral translation at any level. Loss of normal cervical lordosis may be normal in children, but there should be no associated translation at any level.[231] The interspinous distance at each level should be evaluated and should be no more than 1.5 times the distance at adjacent levels; if this ratio is greater, an injury should be suspected. There are calculated norms for the interspinous distances in children, and any value greater than two standard deviations above normal is indicative of a ligamentous injury.[129] The measurement of soft tissue spaces is important in evaluating any evidence of swelling or hemorrhage, which may be associated with an occult injury. The normal retropharyngeal soft tissue space should be less than 6 mm at C3 and less than 14 mm at C6. These spaces may be increased in children without an injury who are crying at the time of the radiograph, because the attachment of the pharynx to the hyoid bone results in its forward displacement

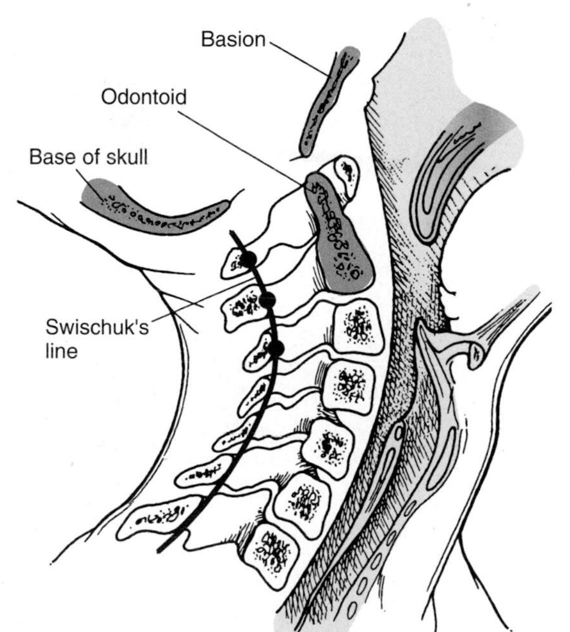

FIGURE 18-9 The spinolaminar line (Swischuk line) is used to determine the presence of pseudosubluxation of C2 on C3. (From Copley LA, Dormans JP. Cervical spine disorders in infants and children. J Am Acad Orthop Surg 1998;6:201–214, with permission.)

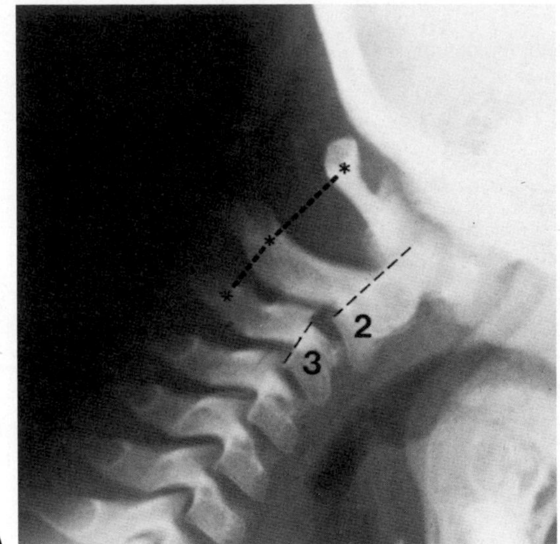

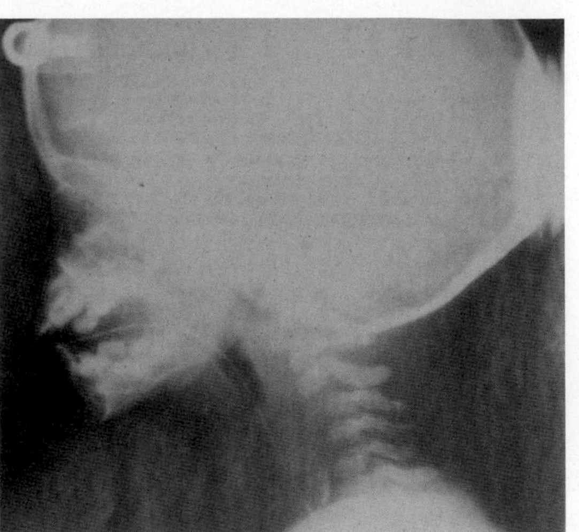

FIGURE 18-10 A. Pseudosubluxation of C2 on C3. In flexion, the posterior element of C2 should normally align itself with the posterior elements C1 and C3. The relationship of the body of C2 with the body of C3 gives the appearance of subluxation; however, the alignment of the posterior elements of C1–C3 confirms pseudosubluxation. **B.** True subluxation.

with crying, producing an apparent increase in the width of these spaces. These radiographs must be taken with the patient quiet and repeated if there is any doubt.

Special Imaging Studies

Most cervical spine injuries in children are detected by plain radiographs.[9] Most ligamentous injuries can be identified on flexion and extension views of the cervical spine in a cooperative and alert patient. The roles of computed tomography (CT) scanning and magnetic resonance imaging (MRI) continue to evolve in the evaluation of trauma patients.

When CT scanning is used in children, a few salient points should be kept in mind. First, the proportion of a child's head to his or her body is greater than that of an adult, so care must be taken not to position the head in flexion to obtain the scan. Inadvertent flexion may potentiate any occult fracture not seen on plain films. Second, the radiation doses for CT scanning are significantly higher than for plain radiographs. CT protocols for children should be used to limit the amount of radiation that the head and neck receive during scanning of the cervical spine. While axial views are standard, coronal and sagittal formatted images and three-dimensional reconstruction views provide improved anatomic details of the spine and can be obtained without any additional radiation to the patient.[96] In patients with head injuries, CT scanning of the cervical spine can be done at the time of CT scanning of the head to reduce the number of plain films that may be required to document that there is not a neck injury.[117] However, plain radiographs remain the standard for initial evaluation of the pediatric cervical spine; CT scanning as an initial imaging study is associated with an increase in radiation with no demonstrable benefit over plain films.[2]

MRI has become increasingly useful in evaluating pediatric patients with suspected cervical spine injuries (Fig. 18-12), especially for ruling out ligamentous injuries in patients who cannot cooperate with flexion and extension views.[70] The advantages of an early MRI are the ability to allow mobilization if no injury is present and the early detection of an unrecognized spinal fracture to allow proper treatment. MRI also is useful in evaluating patients with SCIWORA. MR angiography (MRA) has replaced standard arteriography for evaluation of the vertebral arteries in patients with upper cervical spine injuries who have suspected arterial injuries.[168] MRI also remains the best imaging modality for evaluating injuries of the intervertebral disks and is especially useful to detect disk herniation in adolescent

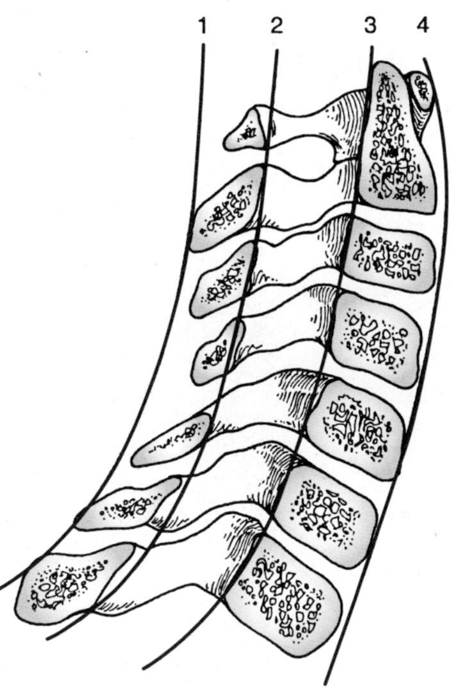

FIGURE 18-11 Normal relationships in the lateral cervical spine: *1*, spinous processes; *2*, spinolaminar line; *3*, posterior vertebral body line; *4*, anterior vertebral body line. (From Copley LA, Dormans JP. Cervical spine disorders in infants and children. J Am Acad Orthop Surg 1998;6:204–214, with permission.)

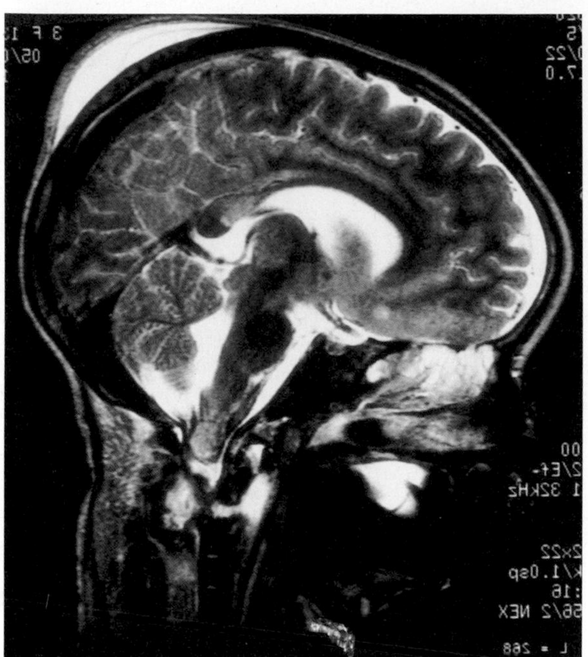

FIGURE 18-12 MRI depicts injury to the cervical cord and upper cervical spine.

patients with facet joint injuries that may require operative reduction.

INITIAL MANAGEMENT OF CERVICAL SPINE INJURIES

The initial management of any child suspected of having a cervical spine injury starts with immobilization in the field. Extraction from an automobile or transport to the hospital may cause damage to the spinal cord in a child with an unstable cervical spine injury if care is not taken to properly immobilize the neck. The immobilization device should allow access to the patient's oropharynx and anterior neck if intubation or tracheostomy becomes necessary. The device should allow splintage of the head and neck to the thorax to minimize further movement.

The use of backboards in pediatric trauma patients deserves special attention because of the anatomic differences between children and adults. Compared to adults, children have a disproportionately larger head with respect to the body. This anatomic relationship causes a child's cervical spine to be placed in flexion if immobilization is done on a standard backboard. Herzenberg et al.[103] reported 10 children under the age of 7 years whose cervical spines had anterior angulation or translation on radiograph when they were placed on a standard backboard. The use of a backboard with a recess so that the head can be lowered into it to obtain a neutral position of the cervical spine is one way to avoid unnecessary flexion. Another is a split-mattress technique in which the body is supported by two mattresses and the head is supported by one mattress, allowing the cervical spine to assume a neutral position. Children younger than 8 years of age should be immobilized on a backboard using one of these techniques (Figs. 18-13 and 18-14).[159]

Cervical collars supplement backboards for immobilization in the trauma setting. While soft collars tend to be more comfortable and cause less soft tissue irritation, rigid collars are preferred for patients with acute injuries because they provide better immobilization. Even rigid collars may allow up to 17 degrees of flexion, 19 degrees of extension, 4 degrees of rotation, and 6 degrees of lateral motion[48,150] Supplemental sandbags and taping on either side of the head are recommended in all children and have been shown to limit the amount of spinal motion to 3 degrees in any plane.[109]

Further displacement of an unstable cervical injury may occur if resuscitation is required. The placement of pediatric patients on an appropriate board with the neck in a neutral position makes recognition of some fractures difficult because positional reduction may have occurred, especially with ligamentous injuries or endplate fractures. An apparently normal lateral radiograph in a patient with altered mental status or multiple injuries does not rule out a cervical spine injury. A study of 4 patients with unstable cervical spine injuries who had attempted resuscitation in the emergency department showed that axial traction actually increased the deformity.[24] Any manipulation of the cervical spine, even during intubation, must be done with caution and with the assumption that the patient has an unstable cervical spine injury until proven otherwise.

Immobilization of the cervical spine may continue after the emergency setting if there is an injury that requires treatment. Specific injuries and their treatment are described later in this chapter. Further immobilization of some cervical spine injuries requires a cervical collar. A rigid collar can be used for immobilization if it is an appropriately fitting device with more padding than a standard cervical collar placed in the emergency depart-

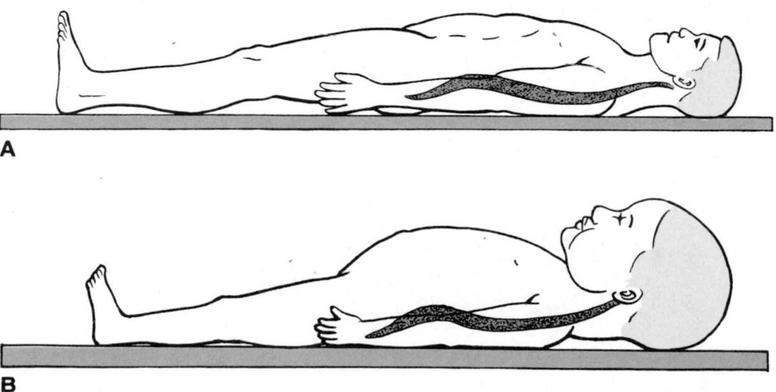

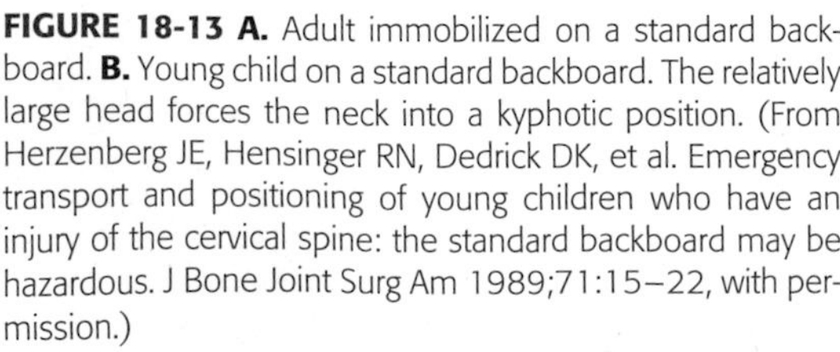

FIGURE 18-13 A. Adult immobilized on a standard backboard. **B.** Young child on a standard backboard. The relatively large head forces the neck into a kyphotic position. (From Herzenberg JE, Hensinger RN, Dedrick DK, et al. Emergency transport and positioning of young children who have an injury of the cervical spine: the standard backboard may be hazardous. J Bone Joint Surg Am 1989;71:15–22, with permission.)

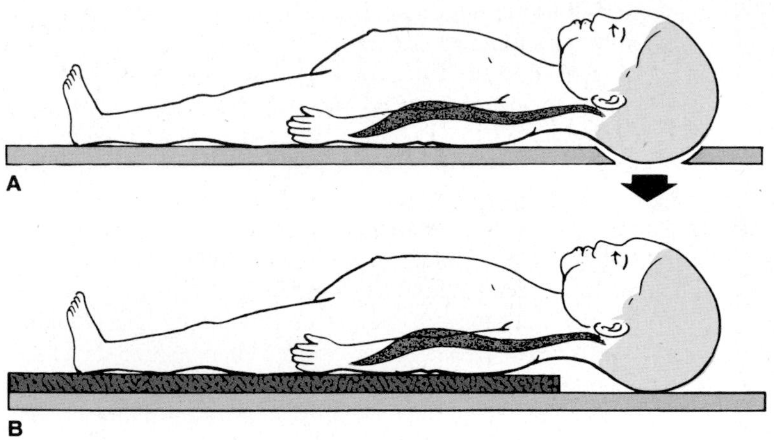

FIGURE 18-14 A. Young child on a modified backboard that has a cutout to the recess of the occiput, obtaining better supine cervical alignment. **B.** Young child on modified backboard that has a double-mattress pad to raise the chest, obtaining better supine cervical alignment. (From Herzenberg JE, Hensinger RN, Dedrick DK, et al. Emergency transport and positioning of young children who have an injury of the cervical spine: the standard backboard may be hazardous. J Bone Joint Surg Am 1989;71:15–22, with permission.)

ment. More unstable or significant injuries can be treated with a custom orthosis, a Minerva cast, or a halo device. An advantage of custom devices is the ability to use lightweight thermoplastic materials that can be molded better to each patient's anatomy and can be extended to the thorax (Fig. 18-15). These devices must be properly applied for effective immobilization, and skin breakdown, especially over the chin region, needs to be carefully monitored. Minerva casts tend to provide more immobilization than thermoplastic devices, but their use is not as common and their application requires attention to detail.

A halo device can be used for the treatment of cervical spine injuries even in children as young as 1 year old. The halo can be used as either a ring alone to apply traction or with a vest for definitive immobilization of an unstable cervical spine injury. The complication rate related to the use of a halo in one series of patients was 68%; however, all patients were able to wear the halo until fracture healing occurred or arthrodesis.[55] The most common complications in this series were superficial pin track infection and pin loosening. Other complications that occur less frequently include dural penetration, supraorbital nerve injury, unsightly pin scars, and deep infection.[17,55] Prefabricated halo vests are used in adults and are easily fitted to older adolescents. Because of the age and size ranges of children, however, a custom vest or even a cast vest may be needed. Prefabricated vests are available in sizes for infants, toddlers, and children, with measurements based on the circumference of the chest at the xiphoid process. Improper fitting of a vest may allow unwanted movement of the neck despite the halo, and any size mismatch requires a custom vest or cast vest (Fig. 18-16).

The fabrication of a halo for any patient needs to consider both the size of the ring and the size of the vest. Prefabricated rings and prefabricated vests are available for even for the smallest of patients and are based on circumferential measurements at the crown and at the xiphoid process. If the size of the patient or the anatomy of the patient does not fit within these standard sizes, the fabrication of a custom halo may be necessary. Mubarak et al.[154] recommended the following steps in the fabrication of a custom halo for a child: (a) the size and configuration

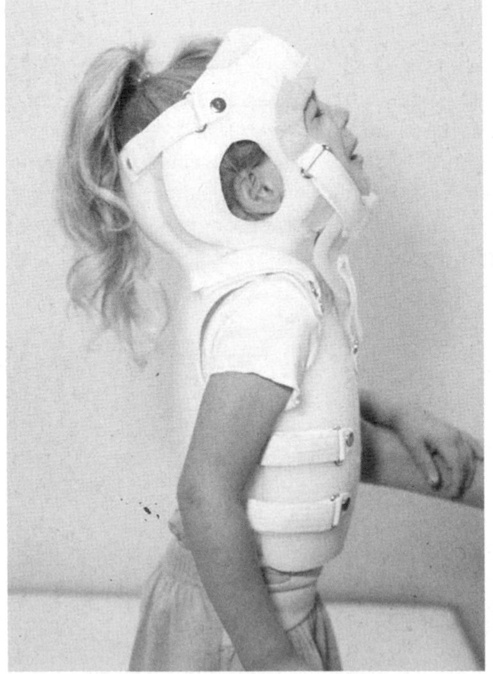

FIGURE 18-15 Custom-made cervicothoracic brace used to treat a C2 fracture that reduced in extension.

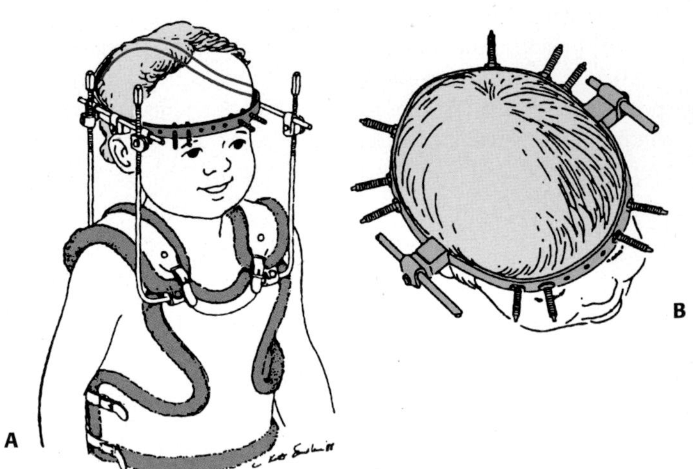

FIGURE 18-16 A. Custom halo vest and superstructure. **B.** In the multiple-pin, low-torque technique, 10 pins are used for an infant halo ring attachment. Usually, four pins are placed anteriorly, avoiding the temporal region, and the remaining six pins are placed in the occipital area. (From Mubarak SJ, Camp JF, Fuletich W, et al. Halo application in the infant. J Pediatr Orthop 1989;9:612–613, with permission.)

of the head are obtained with the use of the flexible lead wire placed around the head, (b) the halo ring is fabricated by constructing a ring 2 cm larger in diameter than the wire model, (c) a plaster mold of the trunk is obtained for the manufacture of a custom bivalved polypropylene vest, and (d) linear measurements are made to ensure appropriate length of the superstructure.

The placement of pins into an immature skull deserves special attention because of the dangers of inadvertent skull penetration with a pin. CT scanning before halo application aids in determining bone structure and skull thickness. It also aids in determining whether or not cranial suture interdigitation is complete and if the fontanels are closed. The thickness of the skull varies greatly up to 6 years of age and is not similar to that of adults until the age of 16 years.[134] Garfin et al.[74] evaluated the pediatric cranium by CT and determined that the skull is thickest anterolaterally and posterolaterally, making these the optimal sites for pin placement.

The number of pins used for placement of a ring and the insertion torques used in younger children also deserve special mention. The placement of pins at the torque pressures used in adults will lead to penetration during insertion.[134] Pins should be inserted at torques of 2- to 4-inch pounds; however, the variability and reliability of pressures found with various torque wrenches during cadaver testing are great, and each pin must be inserted cautiously.[46] The use of 8 to 12 pins inserted at lower torque pressures aids in obtaining a stable ring with less chance of inadvertent penetration (Fig. 18-17). The insertion of each pin perpendicular to the skull also improves the pin–bone interface and the overall strength of the construct.[47] We have had success using halo vests even in children younger than 2 years of age by using multiple pins inserted to finger-tightness rather than relying on torque wrenches.

Technique of Halo Application

A halo can be applied in older children and adolescents with a local anesthetic; however, in most younger children a general anesthetic should be used. The patient is positioned on the operating table in a position that prevents unwanted flexion of the neck and maintains the proper relationship of the head and neck with the trunk. The area of skin in the region of pin insertion is cleaned with antiseptic solution and appropriate areas are shaved as needed for pin placement posteriorly. The ring is placed while an assistant holds the patient's head; it should be placed just below the greatest circumference of the skull, which corresponds to just above the eyebrows anteriorly and 1 cm above the tips of the earlobes laterally. We recommend injection of local anesthetic into the skin and periosteum through the ring holes in which the pins will be placed. The pins are placed with sterile technique.

To optimize pin placement, a few points should be kept in mind. The thickest area of the skull is anterolaterally and posterolaterally, and pins inserted at right angles to the bone have greater force distribution and strength.[47,74] Anterior pins should be placed to avoid the anterior position of the supraorbital and supratrochlear nerves (Fig. 18-18). Placement of the anterior pins too far laterally will lead to penetration of the temporalis muscle, which can lead to pain with mastication and talking, as well as early pin loosening. The optimal position for the anterior pins is in the anterolateral skull, just above the lateral two thirds of the orbit and just below the greatest circumference of the skull. The posterior pins are best placed posterolaterally directly diagonal from the anterior pins. We also recom-

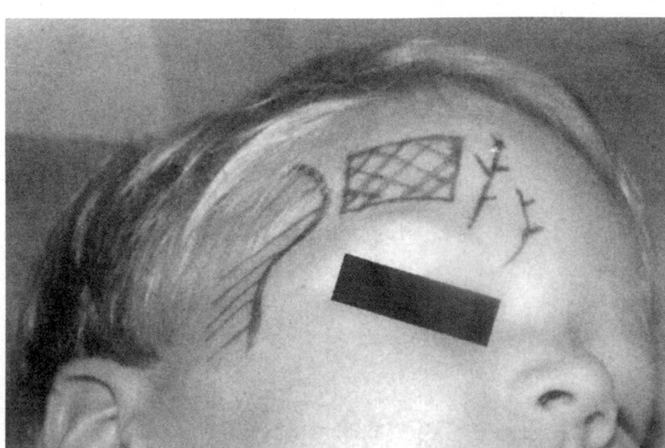

FIGURE 18-17 Shaded area represents the "safe zone" for pin placement, avoiding the supraorbital and supratrochlear nerves anteriorly and the temporalis posteriorly. (From Crawford H. Traction. In: Weinstein SL, ed. Pediatric Spine Surgery. 2nd ed. Philadelphia: Lippincott Williams & Wilkins, 2001, with permission.)

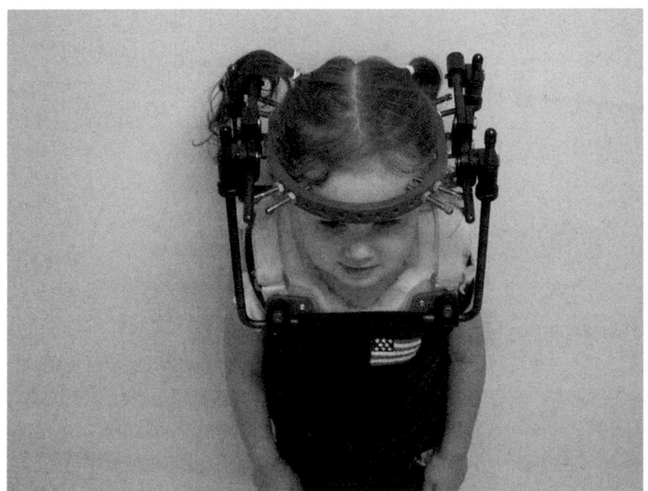

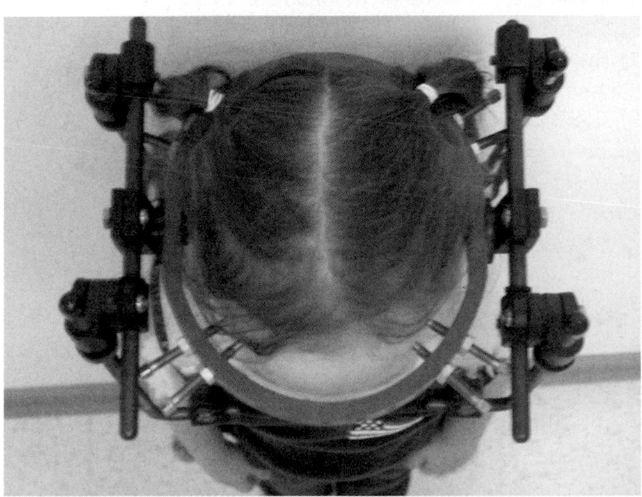

FIGURE 18-18 Child immobilized in a halo for C1 to C2 rotary subluxation. Note the position of the anterior pins, as well as the placement of the posterior pins at 180 degrees opposite the anterior pins.

mend placing the pins to finger-tightness originally and tightening two directly opposing pins simultaneously. During placement of the pins, meticulous attention should be paid to the position of the ring in order to have a circumferential fit on the patient's skull and to avoid any pressure of the ring on the scalp, especially posteriorly.

The number of pins used and the torque pressures applied vary according to the age of the patient. In infants and younger children, we recommend the placement of multiple pins (8 to 12) tightened to finger-tightness or 2 to 4 inch-pounds to avoid unwanted skull penetration. In older children, six to eight pins are used and tightened to 4-inch pounds. In adolescents, four to eight pins can be tightened with a standard torque wrench to 6 to 8 inch-pounds. Once the pins are tightened, they must be fastened to the ring by the appropriate lock nuts or set screws. The halo vest and superstructure are then applied, with care to maintain the position of the head and neck. Appropriate positioning of the head and neck can be done by adjusting the superstructure (see Fig. 18-18).

Daily pin care should consist of hydrogen peroxide/saline cleaning at the pin–skin interface. Retightening of pins at 48 hours should be avoided in infants and children to prevent skull penetration; however, in adolescents, the pins can be retightened at 48 hours with a standard torque wrench. Local erythema or drainage may occur about the pins and can be managed with oral antibiotics and continued pin site care. If significant loosening occurs or the infection is more serious, the pin or pins should be removed. Occasionally, a dural puncture occurs during pin insertion or during the course of treatment. This necessitates pin removal and prophylactic antibiotics until the tear heals, usually at 4 to 5 days.

SPINAL CORD INJURY WITHOUT RADIOGRAPHIC ABNORMALITIES

SCIWORA, a syndrome first brought to the attention of the medical community by Pang and Wilberger,[164] is unique to children. This condition is defined as a spinal cord injury in a patient with no visible fracture or dislocation on plain radiographs, tomograms, or CT scans.

A complete or incomplete spinal cord lesion may be present, and the injury usually results from severe flexion or distraction of the cervical spine. SCIWORA is believed to occur because the spinal column (vertebrae and disk space) in children is more elastic than the spinal cord and can undergo considerable deformation without being disrupted.[37,221] The spinal column can elongate up to 2 inches without disruption, whereas the spinal cord ruptures with only a quarter-inch of elongation.

SCIWORA also may represent an ischemic injury in some patients, although most are believed to be due to a distraction-type injury in which the spinal cord has not tolerated the degree of distraction but the bony ligamentous elements have not failed. Aufdermaur[13] suggested another possibility: a fracture through a pediatric vertebral endplate reduces spontaneously (much like a Salter-Harris type I fracture), giving a normal radiograph appearance, although the initial displacement could have caused spinal cord injury.

SCIWORA abnormalities are more common in children under 8 years of age than in older children,[164,170,189,231] perhaps because of predisposing factors such as cervical spine hypermobility, ligamentous laxity, and an immature vascular supply to the spinal cord. The reported incidence of this condition varies from 7% to 66% of patients with cervical spine injuries.[163,164,242]

Delayed onset of neurologic symptoms has been reported in as many as 52% of patients in some series.[148,164] Pang and Pollock[163] reported 15 patients who had delayed paralysis after their injuries. Nine had transient warning signs such as paresthesia or subjective paralysis. In all patients with delayed onset of paralysis, the spine had not been immobilized after the initial trauma, and all were neurologically normal before the second event. This underlines the importance of diligent immobilization of a suspected spinal cord injury in a child. Approximately half of the young children with SCIWORA in reported series had complete spinal cord injuries, whereas the older children usually had incomplete neurologic deficit injuries that involved the subaxial cervical spine.[10,13,92,148]

Careful radiographic evaluation is helpful in the workup of these patients, but MRI will show a spinal cord lesion that often is some distance from the vertebral column injury. As many as 5% to 10% of children with spinal cord injuries have normal radiographic results.[87,99]

SPINAL CORD INJURY IN CHILDREN

Spinal cord injuries are still rare in children. Rang[181] reviewed spinal injuries at the Toronto Hospital for Sick Children over 15 years and found that children constituted a small percentage of the patients with acquired quadriplegia or paraplegia. He found that paraplegia was three times more common than quadriplegia. When a spinal cord injury is suspected, the neurologic examination must be complete and meticulous and may take several examinations of sensory and motor function. If an acute spinal cord injury is documented by examination, the administration of methylprednisolone within the first 8 hours after injury has been shown to improve the chances of neurologic recovery.[25–28] Methylprednisolone in the treatment of acute spinal cord injuries has been shown to improve motor and sensory recovery when evaluated 6 weeks and 6 months after injury[28]; however, this positive effect on neurologic recovery is limited to those treated within the first 8 hours of injury. The initial loading dose of methylprednisolone is 30 mg/kg body weight. If the loading dose is given within 3 hours after injury, then a maintenance infusion of 5.4 mg/kg is given for 24 hours after injury. If the loading dose is given between 3 and 8 hours after injury, then a maintenance infusion of 5.4 mg/kg is given for 48 hours after injury. Methylprednisolone decreases edema, has an anti-inflammatory effect, and protects the cell membranes from scavenging oxygen-free radicals.[25–28]

In several series,[25–28] there was a slight increase in the incidence of wound infections but no significant increase in gastrointestinal bleeding. All of these studies involved patients 13 years or older, so no documentation of the efficacy in young children exists. A combination of methylprednisolone and GM1-ganglioside (GM1) is being studied for its possible beneficial effect on an injured spinal cord.[76–79] GM1 is a complex acid-like lipid found at high levels in the cell membrane of the central nervous system that is thought to have a neuroprotective and neurofunctional restorative potential. Early studies have shown that patients given both drugs had improved recovery over those who had received just methylprednisolone.

Once spinal cord injury is documented, routine care includes prophylaxis for stress ulcers, routine skin care to prevent pressure sores, and initial Foley catheterization followed by intermittent catheterization and a bowel training program. With incomplete lesions, children have a better chance than adults for useful recovery. Hadley et al.[87] noted that 89% of pediatric patients with incomplete spinal cord lesions improved, whereas only 20% of patients with complete injuries had evidence of significant recovery. Laminectomy has not been shown to be beneficial and can actually be harmful[204,241] because it increases instability in the cervical spine; for example, it can cause a swan-neck deformity or progressive kyphotic deformity.[142,207] The risk of spinal deformity after spinal cord injury has been investigated by several researchers.[16,19,38,63,120,142] Mayfield et al.[142] found that patients who had a spinal cord injury before their growth spurt all developed spinal deformities, 80% of which were progressive. Ninety-three percent developed scoliosis, 57% kyphosis, and 18% lordosis. Sixty-one percent of these patients required spinal arthrodesis for stabilization of their curves. Orthotic management usually is unsuccessful, but in some patients it delays the age at which arthrodesis is necessary. Lower extremity deformities also may occur, such as subluxations and dislocations about the hip. Pelvic obliquity can be a significant problem and may result in pressure sores and difficulty in seating in a wheelchair.

NEONATAL INJURY

Spinal column injury and spinal cord injury can occur during birth, especially during a breech delivery.[158,220] Injuries associated with breech delivery usually are in the lower cervical spine or upper thoracic spine and are thought to result from traction, whereas injuries associated with cephalic delivery usually occur in the upper cervical spine and are thought to result from rotation. It is unclear whether cesarean section reduces spinal injury in neonates[137]; however, Bresnan and Abroms[30] noted that neck hyperextension in utero (star-gazing fetus) in breech presentations is likely to result in an estimated 25% incidence of spinal cord injury with vaginal delivery and can be prevented by delivering by cesarean section.

Distraction-type injuries to the upper cervical spine have been reported in infants in forward-facing car seats. Because infants have poor head control and muscular development, if they are placed in a forward-facing car seat and a sudden deceleration occurs, the head continues forward while the remainder of the body is strapped in the car seat, resulting in a distraction-type injury.[45,83]

Neuromuscular control of the cervical spine in neonates and infants is underdeveloped, and a normal infant cannot adequately support his or her head until about 3 months of age. Infants, therefore, cannot protect their spines against excessive forces that may occur during delivery or during the months after birth. Skeletal injuries from obstetric trauma are probably underreported because the infantile spine is largely cartilaginous and difficult to evaluate with radiographs, especially if the injury is through the cartilage or cartilage–bone interface.[13] A cervical spine lesion should be considered in an infant who is floppy at birth, especially after a difficult delivery. Flaccid paralysis with areflexia usually is followed by a typical pattern of hyperreflexia once spinal cord shock is over. Brachial plexus palsies also warrant cervical spine radiographs. MRI can sometimes be helpful in this diagnosis.

Shulman et al.[206] found atlanto-occipital and axial dislocations at autopsy, and Tawbin[220] found a 10% incidence of brain and spinal injuries at autopsy.

Treatment of neonatal cervical spine injuries is nonoperative and should consist of careful realignment and positioning of the child on a bed with neck support or a custom cervical thoracic orthosis. Healing of bony injuries usually is rapid and complete.[212]

Caffey[41] in 1974 and Swischuk[219] in 1969 described a child abuse syndrome called the shaken infant syndrome. Children have weak and immature neck musculature and cannot support their heads when they are subjected to whiplash stresses. Intercranial and interocular hemorrhages can occur. This injury can result in death or cerebral injury with retardation and permanent visual and hearing defects. Fractures of the spinal column and spinal cord injuries can occur during violent shaking of a child. Swischuk[219] reported a spinal cord injury in a 2-year-old that was the result of violent shaking that produced a cervical fracture–dislocation that spontaneously reduced.

OCCIPITAL CONDYLAR FRACTURE

Occipital condylar fractures are rare, and their diagnosis requires a high index of suspicion.[152,156] Most patients with occipital condylar fractures have associated head injuries.[152] Plain radiographs often do not clearly show occipital condylar fractures, and CT with multiplanar reconstruction usually is necessary to establish the diagnosis.[14,42] Tuli et al.[225] recommended that a CT scan be obtained in the following circumstances: presence of lower cranial nerve deficits, associated head injury or basal skull fracture, or persistent neck pain despite normal radiographs. Reports of associated cranial nerve deficits vary from 53% to 31% of patients with occipital condylar fractures.[9,92,225] Anderson and Montesano[9] described three types of occipital condylar fractures (Table 18-2, Fig. 18-19): type I, impaction fracture; type II, basilar skull fracture extending into the condyle; and type III, avulsion fractures. An avulsion fracture is the only type of occipital condylar fracture that is unstable. Type I injuries are the result of axial compression with a component of ipsilateral flexion. Type II injuries are basilar skull fractures that extend to involve the occipital condyle and usually are caused by a direct blow. Type III injuries are avulsion fractures of the inferomedial portion of the condyle that is attached to the alar ligament. Types I and II occipital condylar fractures usually are stable and can be treated with a cervical orthosis. Type III or avulsion fractures can be unstable and may require halo immobilization or occipitocervical arthrodesis.[6]

Tuli et al.[225] also classified occipital condylar fractures based on displacement and stability of the occiput/C1–C2 complex (Table 18-3). In their classification, type 1 fractures are nondisplaced and type 2 are displaced. They further subdivided type 2 fractures into type 2A, displaced but stable, and type 2B, displaced and unstable. Most occipital condylar fractures are stable and can be treated with a cervical orthosis or halo immobilization. The decision for surgery is based on cranial cervical instability. Bilateral occipital condylar fractures usually are unstable and require occipital cervical fusion.[92]

TABLE 18-2 Anderson and Montesano Classification of Occipital Condylar Fractures

Type	Description	Biomechanics
I	Impaction	Results from axial loading; ipsilateral alar ligament may be compromised, but stability is maintained by contralateral alar ligament and tectorial membrane.
II	Skull base extension	Extends from occipital bone via condyle to enter foramen magnum; stability is maintained by intact alar ligaments and tectorial membrane.
III	Avulsion	Mediated via alar ligament tension; associated disruption of tectorial membrane and contralateral alar ligament may cause instability.

From Hanson JA, Deliganis AV, Baxter AB, et al. Radiologic and clinical spectrum of occipital condyle fractures: retrospective review of 107 consecutive patients in 95 patients. AJR Am J Roentgenol 2002;178:1261–1268.

TABLE 18-3 Classification of Occipital Condylar Fractures[225]

Type	Description	Biomechanics
1	Nondisplaced	Stable
2A	Displaced*	Stable; no radiographic, CT, or MRI evidence of occipitoatlantoaxial instability of ligamentous disruption
2B	Displaced*	Unstable; positive radiographic, CT, or MRI evidence of occipitoatlantoaxial instability or ligamentous disruption

*At least 2 mm of osseous separation.
From Hanson JA, Deliganis AV, Baxter AB, et al. Radiologic and clinical spectrum of occipital condyle fractures: retrospective review of 107 consecutive patients in 95 patients. AJR Am J Roentgenol 2002;178:1261–1268.

ATLANTO-OCCIPITAL INSTABILITY

Atlanto-occipital dislocation was once thought to be a rare fatal injury found only at the time of autopsy (Fig. 18-20).[13,23,26,34,206] This injury is now being recognized more often, and children are surviving.[55,60,167,211] Bulas et al.[35] reported 11 atlanto-occipital dislocations in 1600 pediatric trauma patients (a 0.7% prevalence) seen over a 5-year period; six children died with severe neurologic deficits, but five patients survived with minimal or no neurologic sequela. This increase in the survival rate may be due to increased awareness and improved emergency care with resuscitation and spinal immobilization by emergency personnel. Atlanto-occipital dislocation occurs in sudden deceleration accidents, such as motor vehicle or pedestrian–vehicle accidents. The head is thrown forward, and this can cause sudden craniovertebral separation.

The atlanto-occipital joint is a condylar joint that has little inherent bony stability. Stability is provided by the ligaments about the joint. The primary stabilizers are the paired alar ligaments, the articular capsule, and the tectorial membrane (a continuation of the posterior longitudinal ligament and the major stabilizer of the atlanto-occipital joint). In children, this articulation is not as well formed as in adults and it is less cup-shaped. Therefore, there is less resistance to translational forces.[13,20,23,34,35,206]

Diagnosis may be difficult because atlanto-occipital dislocation is a ligamentous injury. Although patients with this injury have a history of trauma, some may have no neurologic findings. Others, however, may have symptoms such as cranial nerve injury, vomiting, headache, torticollis, or motor or sensory deficits.[34,40,44,93,105,167] Brain stem symptoms, such as ataxia and vertigo, may be caused by vertebrobasilar vascular insufficiency. There is a high association of closed head injures that may mask other physical findings. Unexplained weakness or difficulty in weaning off a ventilator after a closed head injury may be a sign of this injury.

The treating physician must have a high index of suspicion in children with closed head injuries or associated facial trauma and must be aware of the radiographic findings associated with atlanto-occipital dislocation. A significant amount of anterior soft tissue swelling usually can be seen on a lateral cervical spine radiograph. This increased anterior soft tissue swelling should be a warning sign that an atlanto-occipital dislocation may have occurred.

Radiographic findings that aid in the diagnosis of atlanto-occipital dislocation are the Wackenheim line, Powers ratio, dens–basion interval, and occipital condylar distance. The

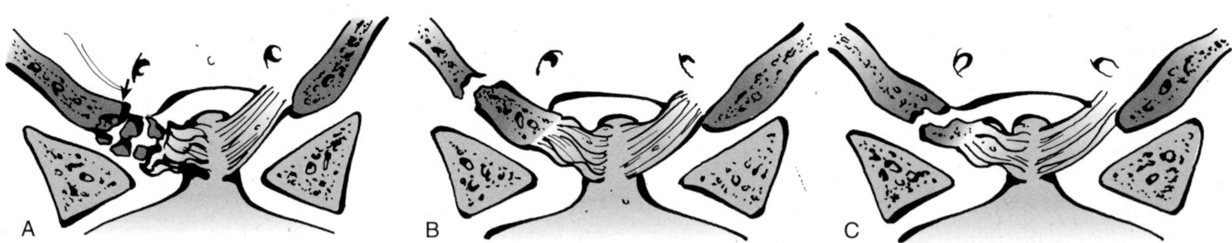

FIGURE 18-19 Classification of occipital condylar fractures according to Anderson and Monsanto.[9] **A.** Type I fractures can occur with axial loading. **B.** Type II fractures are extensions of basilar cranial fractures. **C.** Type III fractures can result from an avulsion of the condyle during rotation, lateral bending, or a combination of mechanisms. (From Hadley MN. Occipital condyle fractures. Neurosurgery 2002;50[Suppl]:S114–S119, with permission.)

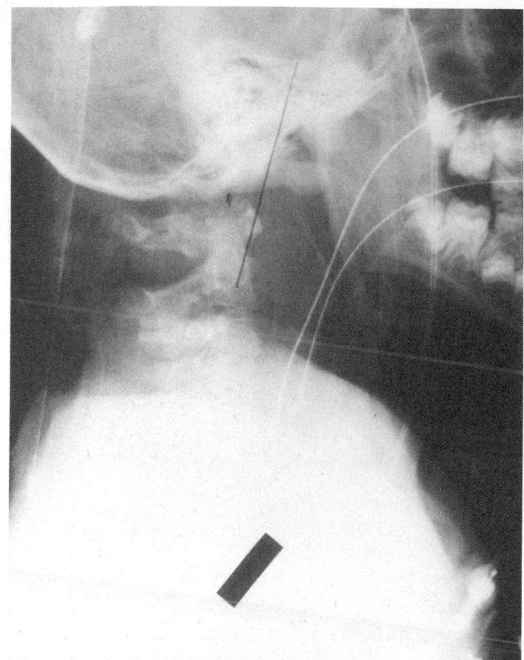

FIGURE 18-20 Patient with atlanto-occipital dislocation. Note the forward displacement of the Wackenheim line and the significant anterior soft tissue swelling.

Wackenheim line is drawn along the clivus and should intersect tangentially the tip of the odontoid. A shift anterior or posterior of this line represents either an anterior or posterior displacement of the occiput on the atlas (Fig.18-21). This line is probably the most helpful because it is reproducible and easy to identify on a lateral radiograph. The Powers ratio (see Fig. 18-7) is determined by drawing a line from the basion to the posterior arch of the atlas (BC) and a second line from the opisthion to the anterior arch of the atlas (OA). The length of line BC is divided by the length of the line OA, producing the Powers ratio. A ratio of more than 1.0 is diagnostic of anterior atlanto-occipital dislocation. A ratio of less than 0.7 is diagnostic of posterior atlanto-occipital dislocation. Values between 1.0 and 0.7 are considered normal.[118] The Powers ratio has the advantage of not being affected by magnification of the radiograph, but the landmarks may be difficult to define. Another radiographic measurement is the dens–basion interval. If the interval measures more than 1.2 cm, then disruption of the atlanto-occipital joint has occurred.[35,175] Kaufman et al.[115] described an occipital condylar facet distance of more than 5 mm from the occipital condyle to the C1 facet as indicative of atlanto-occipital injury. They recommended measuring this distance from five reference points along the occipital condyle and the C1 facet (Fig. 18-22).

MRI is useful in diagnosing atlanto-occipital dislocation by showing soft tissue edema around the tectorial membranes and lateral masses and ligament injury or disruption.[36] Steinmetz et al.[214] and Sun et al.[217] suggested that the disruption of the tectorial membrane is the critical threshold for instability of the occipitoatlanal joint. Disruption of the tectorial membrane can best be identified by MRI.

Operative Treatment

Because atlanto-occipital dislocation is a ligamentous injury, nonoperative treatment usually is unsuccessful. Although Farley et al.[62] reported successful stabilization in a halo, Georgopoulos et al.[80] found persistent atlanto-occipital instability after halo immobilization. Immobilization in a halo should be used with caution: if the vest or cast portion is not fitted properly, displacement can increase (Fig. 18-23) because the head is fixed in the halo but movement occurs because of inadequate immobilization of the trunk in the brace or cast. Traction should be avoided because it can cause distraction of the skull from the atlas. Surgical stabilization is the recommended treatment.[136] Posterior arthrodesis can be performed in situ, with wire fixation or fixation with a contoured Luque rod and wires or contoured rod and

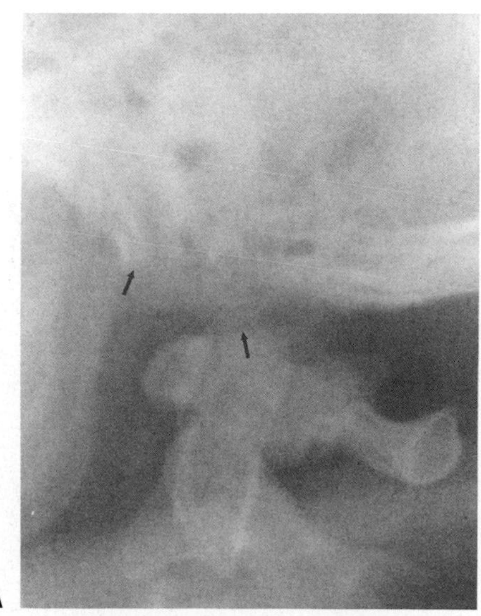

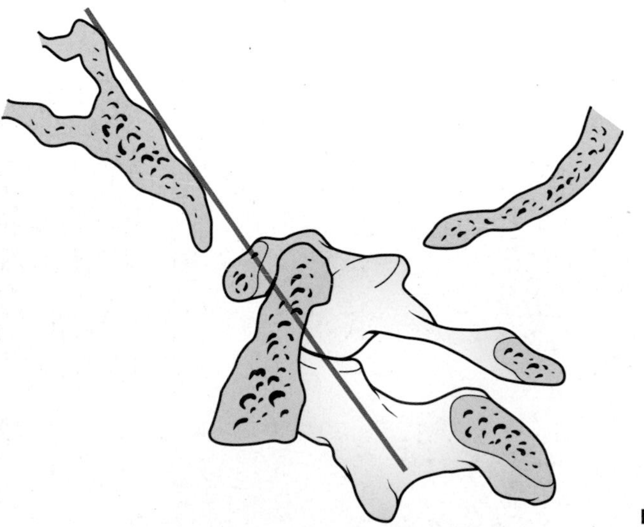

FIGURE 18-21 Craniovertebral dislocation. **A.** Lateral view shows extensive soft tissue swelling. The distance between the basion and the dens is 2.4 cm (*arrows*) (normal is <1 cm). **B.** Line drawing shows the abnormal relationship between the occiput and the upper cervical spine. (From El-Khoury GY, Kathol MH. Radiographic evaluation of cervical trauma. Semin Spine Surg 1991;3:3–23, with permission.)

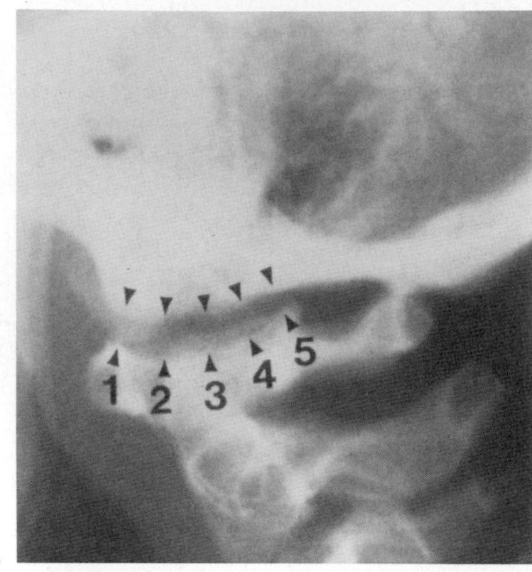

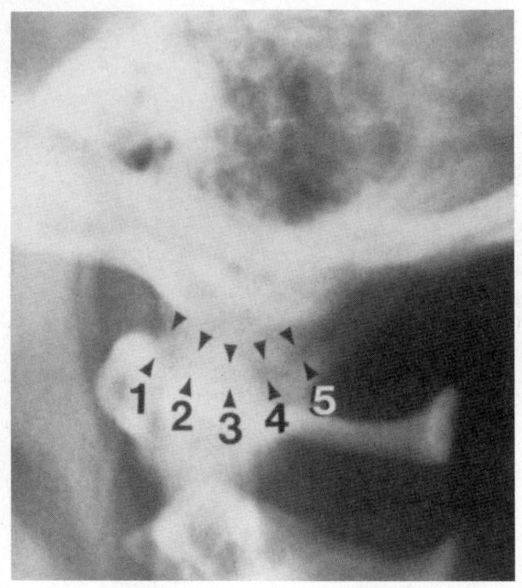

FIGURE 18-22 Atlanto-occipital joint measurement points 1 through 5 demonstrated on a normal crosstable lateral skull radiograph in an 8-year-old **(A)** and a 14-year-old **(B)**. (From: Kaufman RA, Carroll CD, Buncher CR. Atlantooccipital junction: standards for measurement in normal children. AJNR Am J Neuroradiol 1987; 8:995–999, with permission.)

screw fixation.[12,97,147] If the C1–C2 articulation is stable, arthrodesis should be only from the occiput to C1 so that C1–C2 motion is preserved.[210] Some researchers have expressed reservations about the chance of obtaining fusion in the narrow atlanto-occipital interval and have recommended arthrodesis from the occiput to C2. If stability of the C1–C2 articulation is questionable, arthrodesis should extend to C2.[114] Acute hydrocephalus can occur after this injury or in the early postoperative period because of changes in cerebrospinal fluid flow at the cranial cervical junction.

For a patient who presents very late with an unreduced dislocation, an in situ arthrodesis is recommended. DiBenedetto and Lee[52] recommended arthrodesis in situ with a suboccipital craniectomy to relieve posterior impingement.

Instability at the atlanto-occipital joint is increased in patients with Down syndrome as well as in those with a high cervical arthrodesis below the axis. These patients may be at risk of developing chronic instability patterns and are at higher risk of having instability after trauma.

Occiput to C2 Arthrodesis

Arthrodesis Without Internal Fixation. In younger children in whom the posterior elements are absent at C1 or separation is extensive in the bifid part of C1 posteriorly, posterior cervical arthrodesis from the occiput to C2 with iliac crest bone graft is performed using a periosteal flap from the occiput to provide an osteogenic tissue layer for the bone graft (Fig. 18-24).[125]

A halo is applied after the patient is anesthetized, endotracheal intubation is obtained, and all anesthesia lines are in place. For younger children, 8 to 12 pins with lower-pressure torque are used in the halo (see Fig. 18-17); in older children, 4 pins can be used.

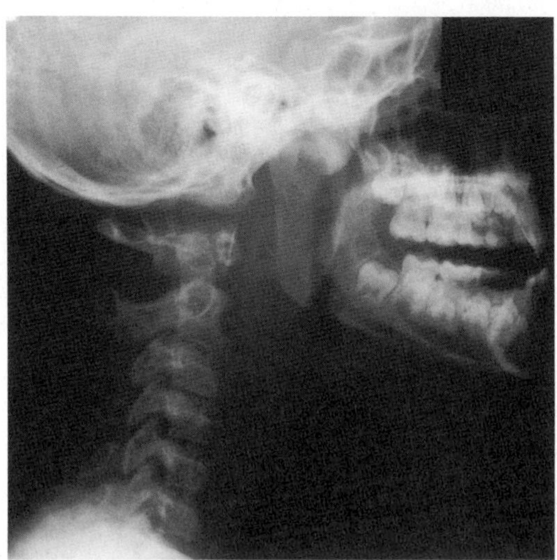

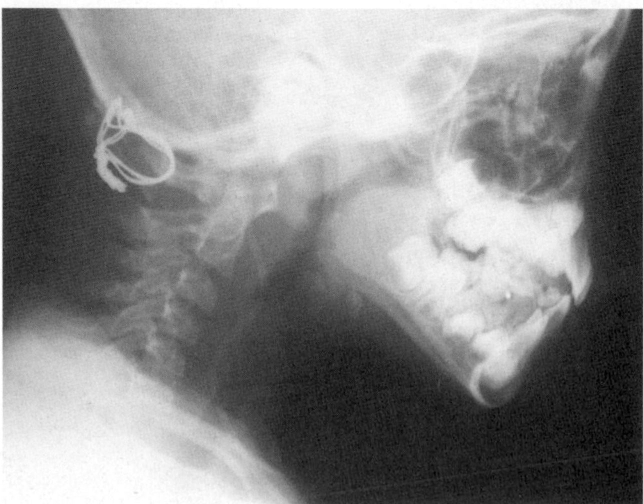

FIGURE 18-23 A. Lateral radiograph of a patient with atlanto-occipital dislocation. Note the increase in the facet condylar distance. **B.** Lateral radiograph after occipital C1 arthrodesis.

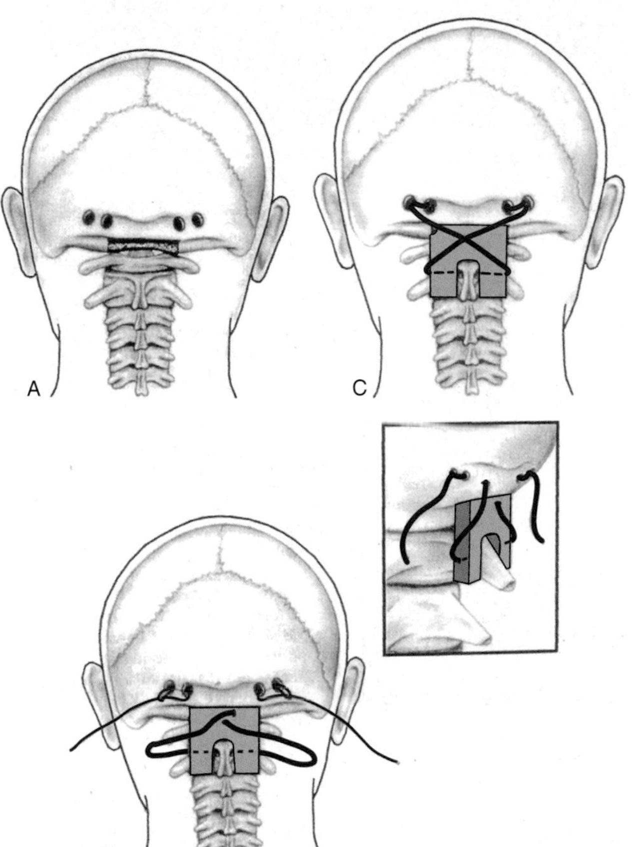

FIGURE 18-26 Occipitocervical arthrodesis. **A.** Four burr holes are placed into the occiput in transverse alignment, with two on each side of the midline, leaving a 1-cm osseous bridge between the two holes of each pair. A trough is fashioned into the base of the occiput. **B.** Sixteen- or 18-gauge Luque wires are passed through the burr holes and looped on themselves. Wisconsin button wires are passed through the base of the spinous process of either the second or third cervical vertebra. The graft is positioned into the occipital trough and spinous process of the cervical vertebra at the caudal extent of the arthrodesis. The graft is locked into place by the precise contouring of the bone. **C.** The wires are crossed, twisted, and cut. The extension of the cervical spine can be controlled by positioning of the head with the halo frame, by adjustment of the size and shape of the bone graft, and to a lesser extent by tightening of the wires. (From Dormans JP, Drummond DS, Sutton LN, et al. Occipitocervical arthrodesis in children. J Bone Joint Surg Am 1995;77:1234–1240, with permission.)

the ring of C1 is exposed and the periosteum of the skull is elevated so that it forms a flap from the foramen magnum located posteriorly–superiorly. The ring of C1 is carefully exposed, with care taken not to dissect more than 1 cm to either side of the midline to protect the vertebral arteries. Care also is taken not to expose any portion of C2 to prevent bridging of the fusion. The dissection of C1 should be done gently. A trough for the iliac crest bone graft is made in the occiput at a level directly cranial to the ring of C1. This trough is unicortical only and extends the width of the exposed portion of C1. Superior to this, two holes are drilled through the occiput as close to the trough as possible to avoid an anteriorly translating vector on the skull when tightening it down to C1. One 22-gauge wire is passed through the holes and another is placed around the ring of C1. The periosteal flap is turned down to bridge the occiput–C1 interval. A small, rectangular, bicortical, iliac crest bone graft approximately 1.5 cm wide and 1 cm high is shaped to fit the trough in the occiput; the graft is contoured to fit the individual patient's occiput–C1 interval. The inferior surface of the bone graft is contoured to fit snugly around the ring of C1 to keep it from migrating anteriorly into the epidural space. Two holes are drilled directly above the distal end of the graft, and the wire around C1 is passed through these holes, forming two distal strands; the wire passed through the occiput forms two proximal strands. These are twisted together and sequentially tightened to apply slight compression to the bone graft. This keeps the graft in the occipital trough and prevents migration into the canal by the occiput. Additional cancellous bone is added to any available space.

The halo vest is kept in place for 6 to 8 weeks in a young child and for as long as 12 weeks in an older child or adolescent. Union is confirmed by a coned, lateral radiograph of the posterior occiput–C1 interval and by flexion–extension lateral views. A rigid cervical collar is used for an additional 2 to 4 weeks to protect the fusion and support the patient's cervical muscles while motion is regained.

Occipitocervical Arthrodesis with Contoured Rod and Segmental Wire

Occipitocervical arthrodesis using a contoured rod and segmental wire has the advantage of achieving immediate stability of the occipitocervical junction (Fig. 18-27), which allows the patient to be immobilized in a cervical collar after surgery, avoiding the need for halo immobilization.

The base of the occiput and the spinous processes of the upper cervical vertebrae are approached through a longitudinal midline incision, which extends deep within the relatively avascular intermuscular septum. The entire field is exposed subperiosteally. A template of the intended shape of the stainless steel rod is made with the appropriate length of Luque wire. Two burr holes are made on each side, about 2 cm lateral to the midline and 2.5 cm above the foramen magnum. Care should be taken to avoid the transverse and sigmoid sinus when making these burr holes. At least 10 mm of intact cortical bone should be left between the burr holes to ensure solid fixation. Luque wires or Songer cables are passed in an extradural plane through the two burr holes on each side of the midline. The wires or cables are passed sublaminar in the upper cervical spine. The rod is bent to match the template; this usually will have a head–neck angle of about 135 degrees and slight cervical lordosis. A Bend Meister (Sofamor/Danek, Memphis, TN) may be helpful in bending the rod. The wires or cables are secured to the rod. The spine and occiput are decorticated, and autogenous cancellous bone grafting is performed.

FRACTURES OF THE ATLAS

Fracture of the ring of C1 (Jefferson fracture) is caused by an axial load applied to the head and is not a common injury in children.[22,112,114,140,149,184,223] This rare injury accounts for less than 5% of all cervical spine fractures in children.[11,21] The force is transmitted through the occipital condyles to the lateral masses of C1, causing a disruption in the ring of C1, usually in two places, with fractures occurring in both the anterior and posterior rings. In children, an isolated single fracture of the ring can occur with the remaining fracture hinging on a syn-

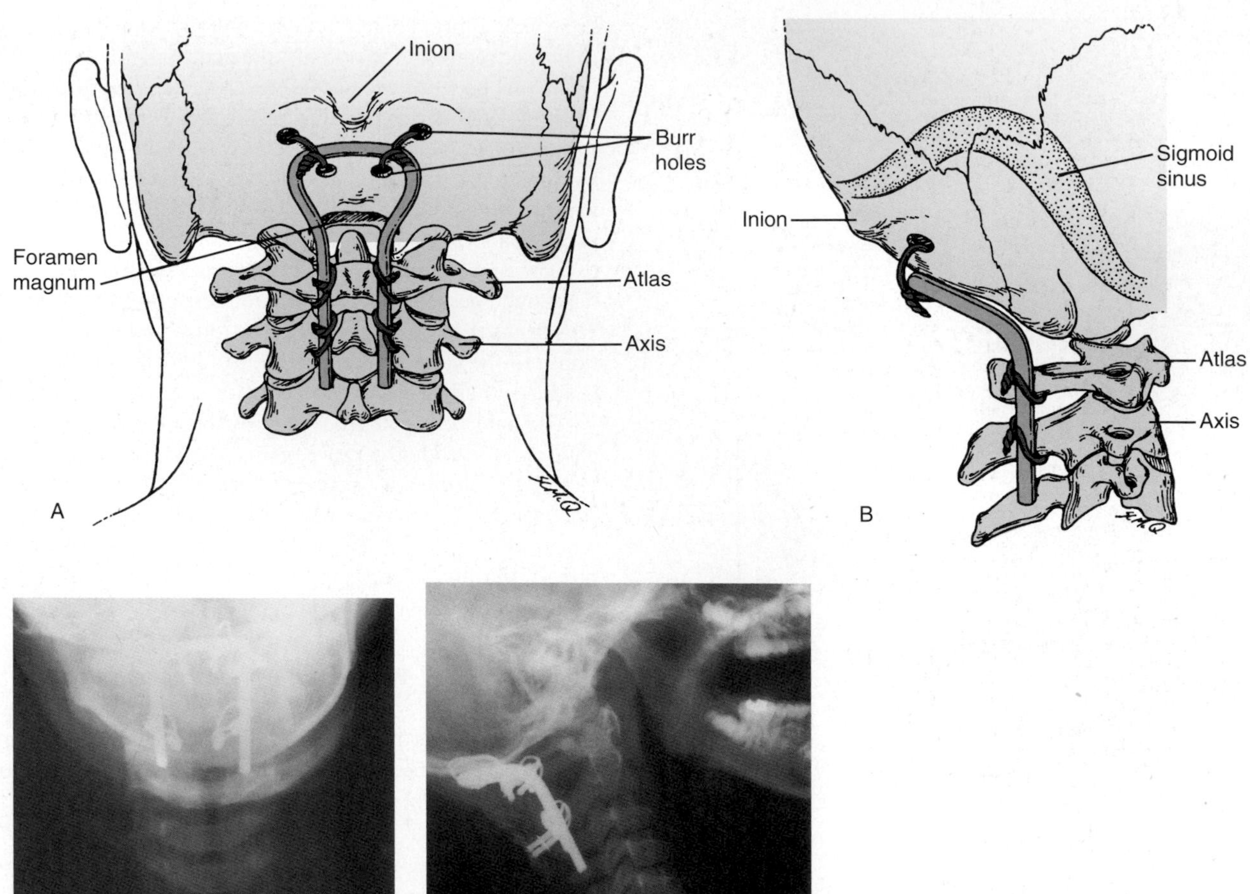

FIGURE 18-27 Occipitocervical arthrodesis using a contoured rod and segmental wire or cable fixation. (**A,B** reprinted from Warner WC. Pediatric cervical spine. In: Canale ST, ed. *Campbell's operative orthopaedics*. St. Louis: Mosby, 1998; with permission.)

chondrosis.[18] This is an important distinction in children because often fractures occur through a normal synchondrosis and there can be plastic deformation of the ring with no evidence of a fracture.[114,222] This distinction can be seen on plain radiographs and CT scan, with fractures appearing through what appears to be normal physes. As the lateral masses separate, the transverse ligament may be ruptured or avulsed, resulting in C1 and C2 instability.[149] If the two lateral masses are widened more than 7 mm beyond the borders of the axis on an anteroposterior radiograph, then an injury to the transverse ligament is presumed. Injury to the transverse ligament may be from a rupture of the ligament or an avulsion of the ligament attachment to C1. Jefferson fractures may be evident on plain radiographs, but CT scans are superior at showing this injury (Fig 18-28). CT scans also can be used to follow the progress of healing. MRI is useful in determining the integrity of the transverse atlantal ligament and detecting fractures through the normal synchondroses of the atlas. With a fracture through a synchondrosis, associated edema and hemorrhage are seen on MRI.[126] Other cervical spine fractures may be present with an atlas fractures, and MRIs should be carefully scrutinized to identify other fractures.[143] The classic signs of an atlas fracture in a child are neck pain, cervical muscle spasm, decreased range of motion, and head tilt.[114]

Treatment consists of immobilization in an orthosis (rigid collar or sternal occipital mandibular immobilizer), Minerva cast, or halo brace. The extent of this immobilization is debatable and should consider the patients age and cooperation.[126] If there is excessive widening (>7 mm), halo traction followed by halo brace or cast immobilization is recommended. Stablility of C1–C2 must be documented on flexion and extension lateral radiographs once the fracture is healed. Surgery rarely is necessary to stabilize these fractures (Fig. 18-29).

ATLANTOAXIAL INJURIES

Odontoid Fractures

Odontoid fractures are one of the most common fractures of the cervical spine in children,[85] occurring at an average age of 4 years.[56,86,198] This fracture accounts for approximately 10% of all cervical spine fractures and dislocations in children. The unique feature of odontoid fractures in children is that the fracture most commonly occurs through the synchondrosis of C2

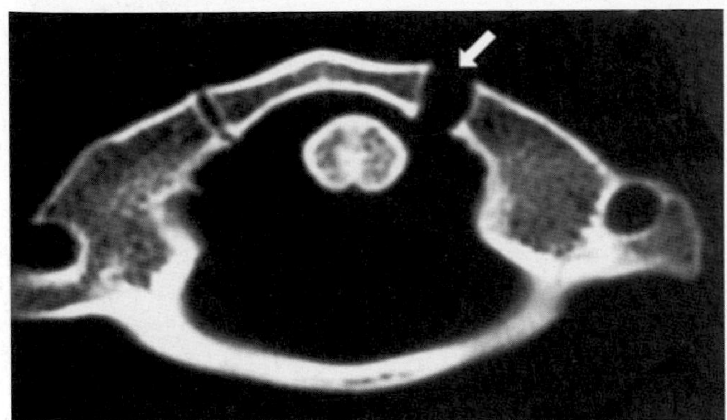

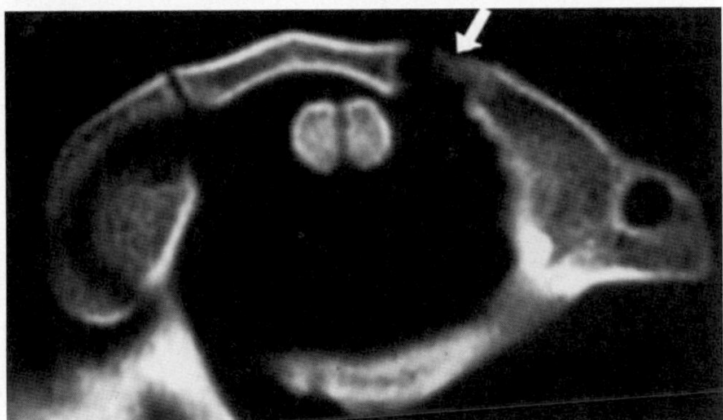

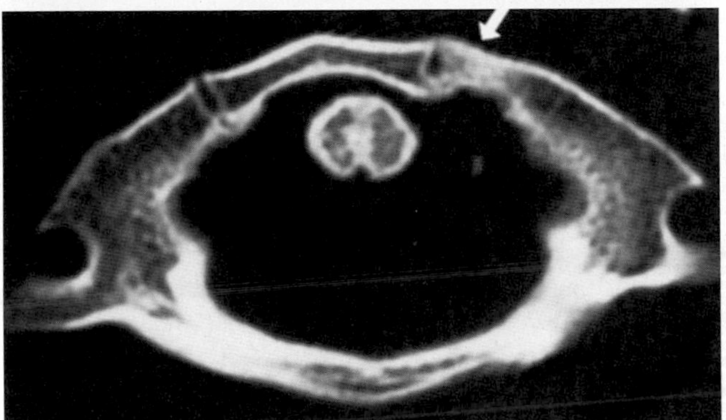

FIGURE 18-28 A. Initial CT scan through the atlas, demonstrating left anterior synchondrosis diastasis *(arrow)*. **B.** CT scan 1 month after presentation with callus formation at the synchondrosis, demonstrating healing at the fracture site. **C.** CT scan 4 months after presentation, showing bony bridging across the fracture site. (From Judd D, Liem LK, Petermann G. Pediatric atlas fracture: a case of fracture through a synchondrosis and review of the literature. Neurosurgery 2000;46:991–994, with permission.)

distally at the base of the odontoid. This synchondrosis is a cartilage line at the base of the odontoid and looks like a physeal or Salter-Harris type I injury.

A fracture of the odontoid usually is associated with head trauma from a motor vehicle accident or a fall from a height, although it also can occur after trivial head trauma. Radiographs should be obtained in any child complaining of neck pain. Clinically, children with odontoid fractures complain of neck pain and resist attempts to extend the neck. Odent et al.[160] reported that 8 of 15 odontoid fractures in children were the result of motor vehicle accidents, with the child fastened in a forward-facing seat. The sudden deceleration of the body as it is strapped into the car seat while the head continues to travel forward causes this fracture.

FIGURE 18-29 CT scan of an atlas fracture.

Most odontoid injuries are anteriorly displaced and usually have an intact anterior periosteal sleeve that provides some stability to the fracture when immobilized in extension and allows excellent healing of the fracture.[11,185,192,201] Growth disturbances are uncommon after this type of fracture. This synchondrosis normally closes at about 3 to 6 years of age and adds little to the longitudinal growth of C2.

Most often, the diagnosis can be ascertained by viewing the plain radiographs. Anteroposterior views usually appear normal, and the diagnosis must be made from lateral views because displacement of the odontoid usually occurs anteriorly. Plain radiographs sometimes can be misleading when the fracture occurs through the synchondrosis and has spontaneously reduced. When this occurs, the fracture has the appearance of a nondisplaced Salter-Harris type I fracture. CT scans with three-dimensional reconstruction views may be needed to fully delineate the injury.[202] MRI also may be useful in nondisplaced fractures by detecting edema around the injured area, indicating that a fracture may have occurred. Dynamic flexion and extension views to demonstrate instability may be obtained in a cooperative child if a nondisplaced fracture is suspected. These studies should be done only in a cooperative child and under the direct supervision of the treating physician.

Odontoid fractures in children generally heal uneventfully and rarely have complications. Neurologic deficits rarely have been reported after this injury.[160,215] Odent et al.[160] described neurologic injuries in 8 of 15 patients, although most were stretch injuries to the spinal cord at the cervical thoracic junction and not at the level of the odontoid fracture.

Treatment of odontoid fractures is by closed reduction (usually extension or slight hyperextension of the neck), although complete reduction of the translation is not necessary. At least 50% apposition should be obtained to provide adequate cervical alignment, and then the patient should be immobilized in a Minerva or halo cast or custom orthosis. This fracture will heal in about 6 to 8 weeks. After bony healing, stability should be documented by flexion–extension lateral radiographs. Once the Minerva cast or halo is removed, a soft collar is worn for 1 to 2 weeks. If an adequate reduction cannot be obtained by recumbency and hyperextension, then a head halter or halo traction is needed. Rarely, manipulation under general anesthesia is needed for irreducible fractures (Fig. 18-30). Surgery with internal fixation rarely has been reported due to the good results that are achieved with conservative treatment in children.[84,176,193,200,226]

Os Odontoideum

Os odontoideum consists of a round ossicle that is separated from the axis by a transverse gap, which leaves the apical segment without support. Fielding et al.[64–68] suggested that this was an unrecognized fracture at the base of the odontoid. Some studies have documented normal radiographs of the dens with abnormal radiographs after trivial trauma. This can be explained by a distraction force being applied by the alar ligaments, which pulls the tip of the fractured odontoid away from the base and produces a nonunion.[95,110,128,183,194,216,229] Other authors believe this to be of congenital origin because of its association with other congenital anomalies and syndromes.[82,203,240]. Sankar et al.[190] reported that 6 of their 16 patients had associated congenital anomalies in the cervical spine and only 8 of the 16 reported any previous trauma.

The presentation of an os odontoideum can be variable. Signs and symptoms can range from a minor to a frank compressive myelopathy or vertebral artery compression. Presenting symptoms may be neck pain, torticollis, or headaches caused by local irritation of the atlantoaxial joint. Neurologic symptoms can be transient or episodic after trauma to complete myelopathy caused by cord compression.[57] Symptoms may consist of weakness and loss of balance with upper motor neuron signs, although upper motor neuron signs may be completely absent. Proprioceptive and sphincter dysfunctions also are common. Cerebellar infarctions due to vertebrobasilar artery insufficiency caused by an unstable os odontoideum were described by Sasaki et al.[191]

Os odontoideum usually can be diagnosed on routine cervical spine radiographs, which include an open-mouth odontoid view (Fig. 18-31). Lateral flexion and extension views should be obtained to determine if any instability is present. With os odontoideum, there is a space between the body of the axis and a bony ossicle. The free ossicle of the os odontoideum usually is half the size of a normal odontoid and is oval or round, with smooth sclerotic borders. The space differs from that of an acute fracture, in which the space is thin and irregular instead of wide and smooth. The amount of instability should be documented on lateral flexion and extension plain radiographs that allow measurement of both the anterior and posterior displacement of the atlas on the axis. Because the ossicle is fixed to the anterior arch of C1 and moves with the anterior arch of C1 both in flexion and extension, measurement of the relationship of C1 to the free ossicle is of little value because they move as a unit. A more meaningful measurement is made by projecting lines superiorly from the body of the axis to a line projected inferiorly from the posterior border of the anterior arch of the atlas. This gives more information as to the stability of C1–C2. Another measurement that is very helpful is space available for the cord, which is the distance from the back of the dens to the anterior border of the posterior arch of C1.

Recommended treatment is posterior arthrodesis of C1 to C2. Before arthrodesis is attempted, the integrity of the arch of C1 must be documented by CT scan. Incomplete development of the posterior arch of C1 is uncommon but has been reported to occur with increased frequency in patients with os odontoideum. This may necessitate an occiput to C2 arthrodesis for stability. If a C1–C2 arthrodesis is done, one must be careful not to overreduce the odontoid and cause posterior translation.

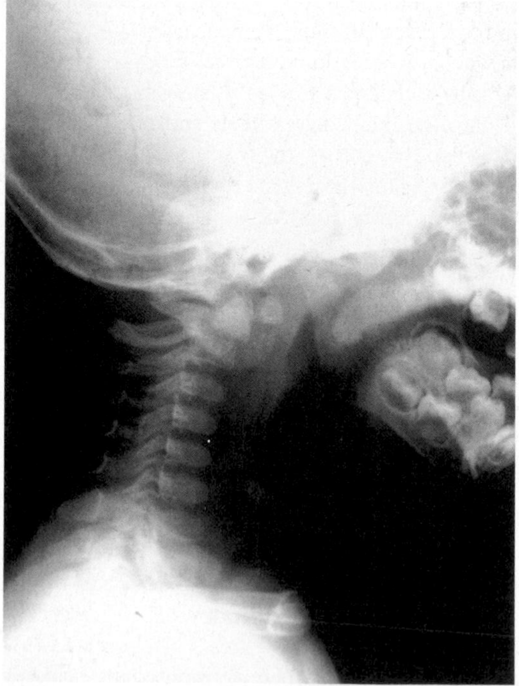

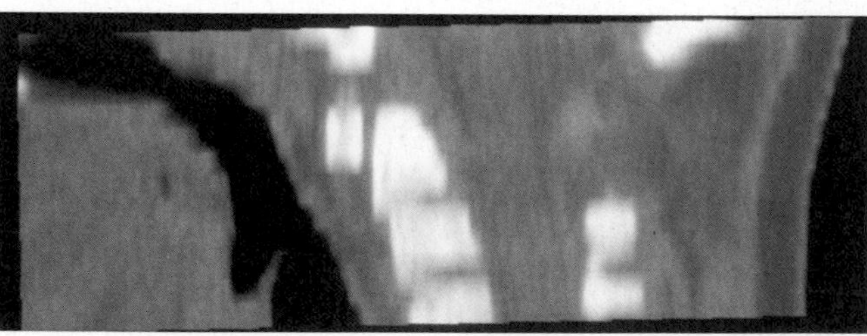

FIGURE 18-30 Lateral radiograph and CT reconstruction view of odontoid fracture through the synchondrosis of C2. Note the anterior displacement.

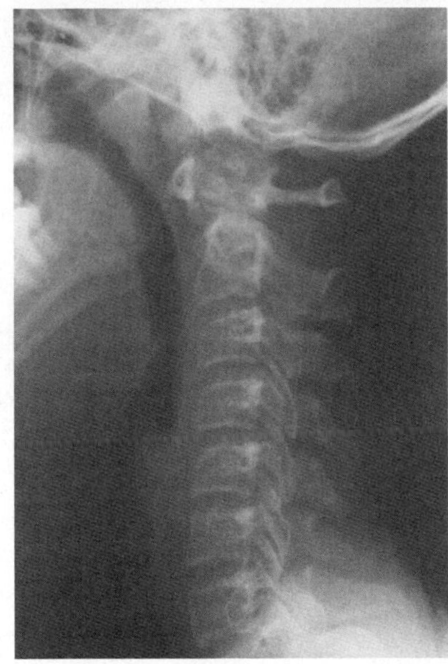

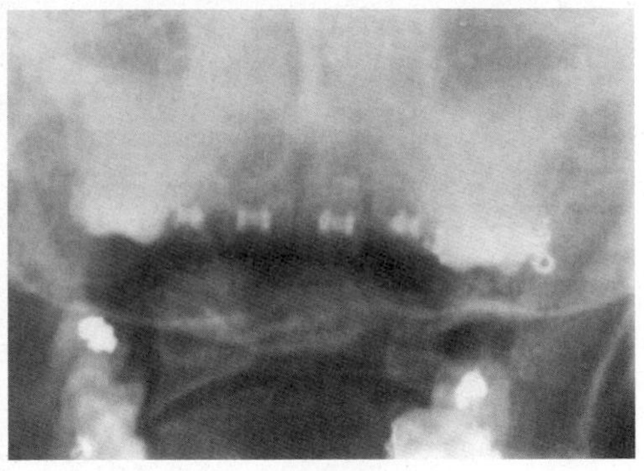

FIGURE 18-31 Lateral radiograph **(A)** and open-mouth odontoid radiograph **(B)** showing os odontoideum. (From Warner WC. Pediatric cervical spine. In: Canale ST, ed. Campbell's Operative Orthopaedics. St. Louis: Mosby Year Book, 1999:2817, with permission.)

Care also must be taken in positioning the neck at the time of arthrodesis and when tightening the wires if a Gallie or Brooks arthrodesis is performed to prevent posterior translation (Figs. 18-32 and 18-33). Brockmeyer et al.[32] and Wang et al.[232] both reported good results with transarticular screw fixation and fusion in the treatment of children with os odontoideum (Fig. 18-34). Wang et al.[232] reported the use of this technique in children as young as 3 years of age. This technique may be preferred depending on the patient's anatomy and the surgeon's experience. Harms et al.[94] and Brecknell et al.[29] reported that a high-riding vertebral artery may make transarticular screw placement impossible in about 20% of patients.

Traumatic Ligamentous Disruption

The transverse ligament is the primary stabilizer of an intact odontoid against forward displacement. Secondary stabilizers consist of the apical and alar ligaments, which arise from the tip of the odontoid and pass to the base of the skull. These also stabilize the atlanto-occipital joint indirectly.[85] The normal distance from the anterior cortex of the dens to the posterior cortex of the anterior ring of C1 is 3 mm in adults and 4.5 mm in children. In children, if the distance is more than 4.5 mm, disruption of the transverse ligament is presumed. The spinal canal at C1 is large compared with other cervical segments and accommodates a large degree of rotation and some degree of pathologic displacement without compromising the spinal cord. Steel[213] expressed this as a rule of thirds: the spinal canal at C1 is occupied equally by the spinal cord, odontoid, and a free space, which provides a buffer zone to prevent neurologic injury. Steel[213] found that anterior displacement of the atlas that exceeds a distance equal to the width of the odontoid may place the spinal cord at risk.

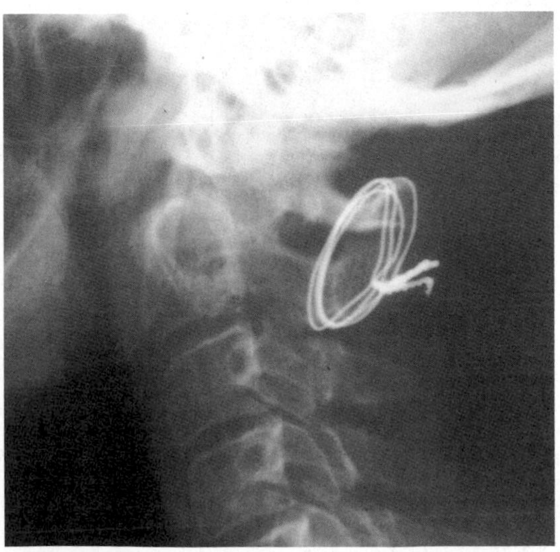

FIGURE 18-32 Posterior translation of atlas after C1–C2 posterior arthrodesis.

Acute rupture of the transverse ligament is rare and reportedly occurs in fewer than 10% of pediatric cervical spine injuries.[135,145] However, avulsion of the attachment of the transverse ligament to C1 may occur instead of rupture of the transverse ligament.

A patient with disruption of the transverse ligament usually has a history of cervical spine trauma and complains of neck pain, often with notable muscle spasms. Diagnosis is confirmed on lateral radiographs that show an increased atlanto–dens interval. An active flexion view may be required to show instability in cooperative patients with unexplained neck pain or neurologic findings. CT scans are useful to demonstrate avulsion of the transverse ligament from its origins to the bony ring of C1.

Although rarely used, conservative treatment of acute transverse ligament injuries has been reported. For acute injuries, reduction in extension is recommended, followed by surgical stabilization of C1 and C2 and immobilization for 8 to 12 weeks in a Minerva cast, a halo brace, or a cervical orthosis. Flexion and extension views should be obtained after stabilization to document stability.

OPERATIVE TREATMENT

Atlantoaxial Arthrodesis

Technique of Brooks and Jenkins

The supine patient is intubated in the supine position while still on a stretcher and is then placed prone on the operating

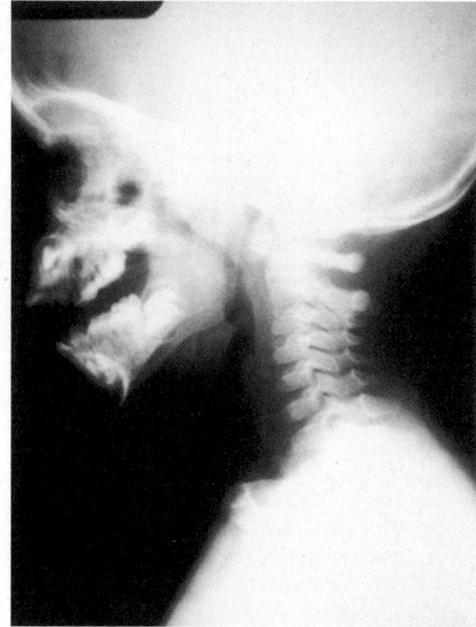

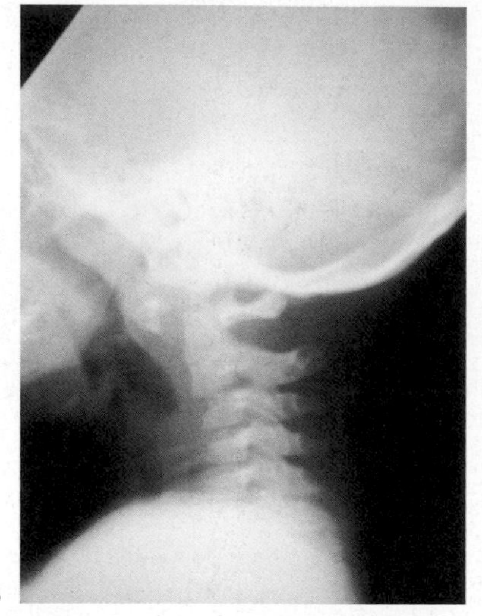

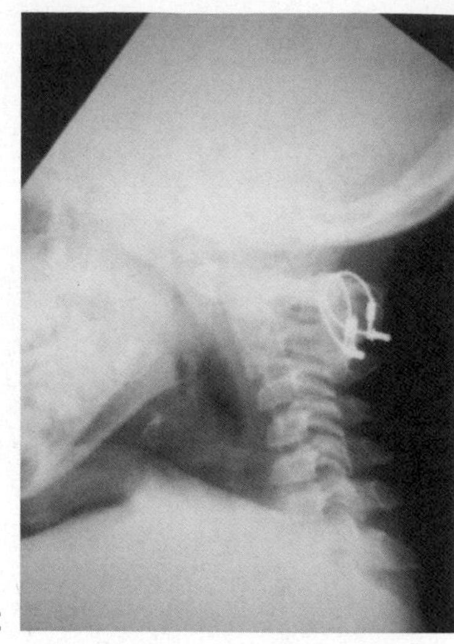

FIGURE 18-33 A. Lateral radiograph of traumatic C1–C2 instability. **B.** Note the increase in the atlanto–dens interval. **C.** Lateral radiograph after C1–C2 posterior arthrodesis.

table, with the head supported by traction; the head–thorax relationship is maintained at all times during turning (Fig. 18-35).[33] A lateral cervical spine radiograph is obtained to ensure proper alignment before surgery. The skin is prepared and draped in a sterile fashion and a solution of epinephrine (1:500,000) is injected intradermally to aid hemostasis.

C1 and C2 are exposed through a midline incision. With an aneurysm needle, a Mersiline suture is passed from cephalad to caudad on each side of the midline under the arch of the atlas and then beneath the lamina of C2. These serve as guides to introduce two doubled 20-gauge wires. The size of the wire used varies depending on the size and age of the patient. Two full-thickness bone grafts, approximately 1.25 × 3.5 cm, are harvested from the iliac crest and beveled so that the apex of the graft fits in the interval between the arch of the atlas and the lamina of the axis. Notches are fashioned in the upper and lower cortical surfaces to hold the circumferential wires and prevent them from slipping. The doubled wires are tightened over the graft and twisted on each side. The wound is irrigated and closed in layers over suction drains.

Technique of Gallie

The supine patient is intubated while on a stretcher (Fig. 18-36).[73] The prone patient then is placed on the operating table with the head supported by traction, maintaining the head–thorax relationship during turning. A lateral cervical spine radiograph is obtained to ensure proper alignment before surgery. The skin is prepared and draped in a sterile fashion, and a solution of epinephrine (1:500,000) is injected intradermally to aid hemostasis.

A midline incision is made from the lower occiput to the level of the lower end of the fusion, extending deeply within

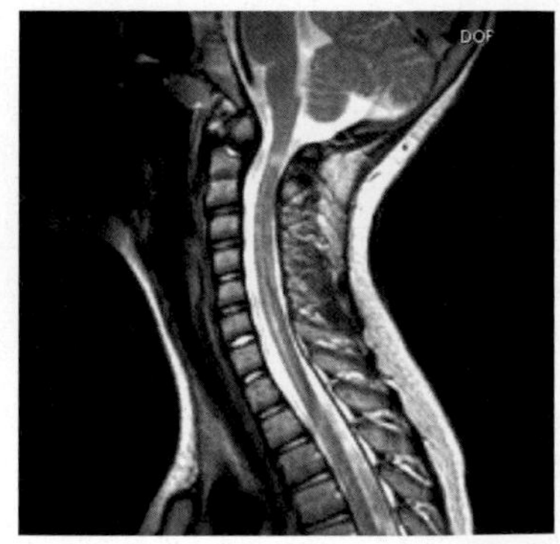

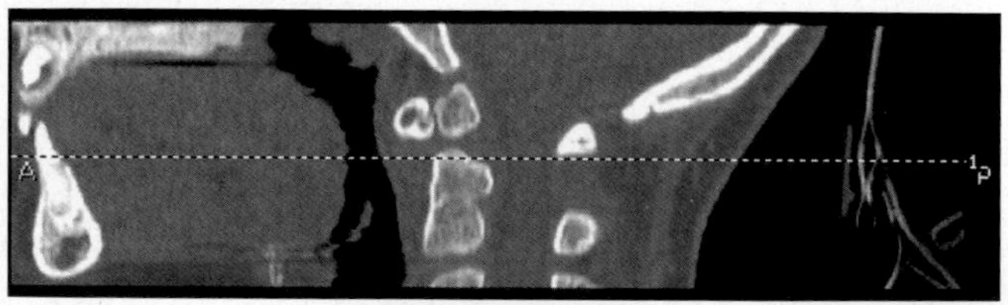

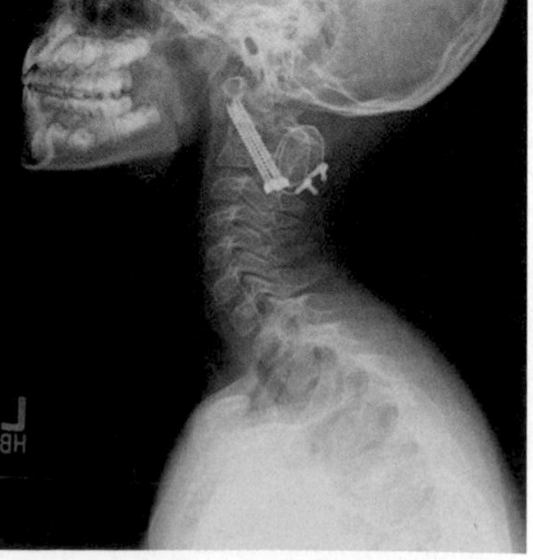

FIGURE 18-34 MRI **(A)** and CT scan **(B)** of 9-year-old girl with os odontodeium. **C.** After Brooks posterior fusion and transarticular screw fixation.

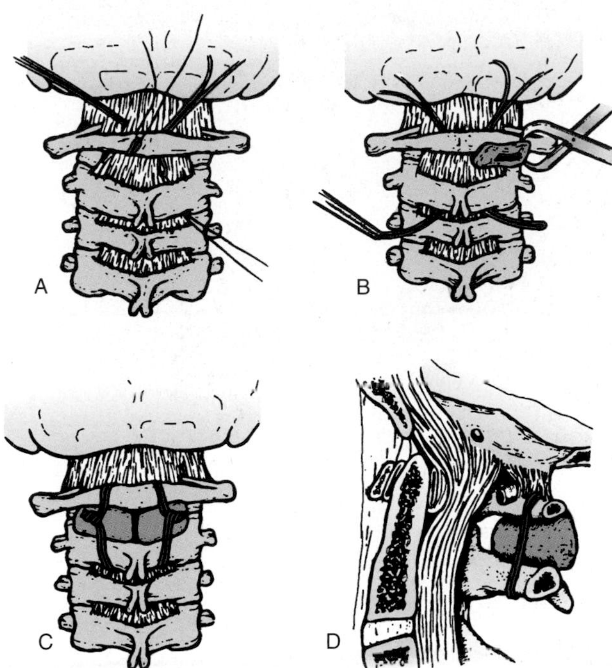

FIGURE 18-35 Technique of atlantoaxial arthrodesis (Brooks-Jenkins). **A.** Wires are inserted under the atlas and axis. **B.** Full-thickness bone grafts from the iliac crest are placed between the arch of the atlas and the lamina of the axis. **C,D.** The wires are tightened over the graft and twisted on each side. (From Brooks AL, Jenkins EB. Atlantoaxial arthrodesis by the wedge compression method. J Bone Joint Surg Am 1978;60:279, with permission.)

the relatively avascular midline structures, the intermuscular septum, or ligamentum nuchae. Care should be taken not to expose any more than the area to be fused to decrease the chance of spontaneous extension of the fusion. By subperiosteal dissection, the posterior arch of the atlas and the lamina of C2 are exposed. The muscular and ligamentous attachments from C2 are removed with a curet. Care should be taken to dissect laterally along the atlas to prevent injury to the vertebral arteries and vertebral venous plexus that lie on the superior aspect of the ring of C1, less than 2 cm lateral to the midline. The upper surface of C1 is exposed no farther laterally than 1.5 cm from the midline in adults and 1 cm in children. Decortication of

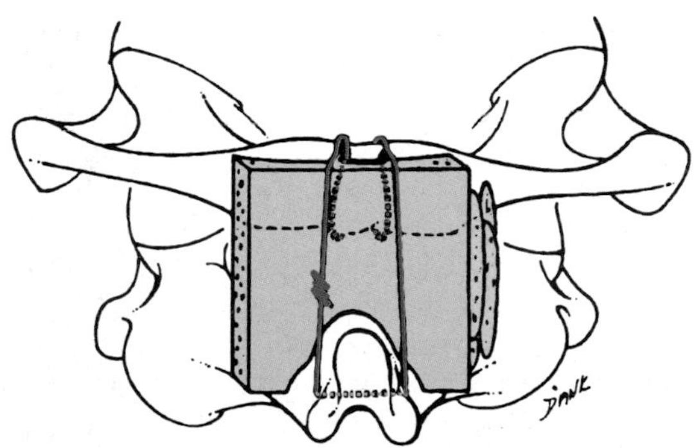

FIGURE 18-36 Wires are passed under the lamina of the atlas and through the spine of the axis and tied over the graft. This method is used most frequently. (From Fielding JW, Hawkins RJ, Ratzan SA. Spine fusion for atlanto-axial instability. J Bone Joint Surg Am 1976;58:400, with permission.)

C1 and C2 generally is not necessary. From below, a wire loop of appropriate size is passed upward under the arch of the atlas either directly or with the aid of a Mersiline suture. The Mersiline suture can be passed with an aneurysm needle. The free ends of the wire are passed through the loop, grasping the arch of C1 in the loop.

A corticocancellous graft is taken from the iliac crest and placed against the lamina of C2 and the arch of C1 beneath the wire. One end of the wire is passed through the spinous process of C2, and the wire is twisted on itself to secure the graft in place. The wound is irrigated and closed in layers with suction drainage tubes.

Posterior C1–C2 Transarticular Screw Fixation

Posterior C1–C2 transarticular screw fixation can be used to stabilize the atlantoaxial joint. This technique has the advantage of being biomechanically superior to posterior wiring techniques,[98] and postoperative halo vest immobilization usually is not required. The disadvantages of this technique are potential injury to the vertebral artery, its technical difficulty, and the requirement for sublaminar wire and fusion (Brooks or Gallie technique). Preoperative imaging should include plain radiographs, CT scan, MRI, and MRA of the cervical spine. Supervised dynamic lateral flexion and extension views must determine the reducibility of the atlantoaxial joint.[147] If an anatomic reduction cannot be obtained, transarticular screws cannot be safely used. MRA can delineate the course of the vertebral artery through the foramen transversarium and its relationship to the surrounding bony architecture. Approximately 20% of patients show anatomic variations in the path of the vertebral artery and osseous anatomy that would preclude transarticular screw placement.[1,29,94]

The patient is placed prone with the head held in a Mayfield skull clamp or with a halo ring attached to the Mayfield attachment. Under fluoroscopic guidance, proper alignment of the atlantoaxial joint is confirmed. The spine is prepared and draped from the occiput to the upper thoracic spine. The upper thoracic spine must be included in the surgical field to allow percutaneous placement of the transarticular screw. Percutaneous screw placement may be necessary because of the cephalad orientation of the C1–C2 transarticular screw.

A midline posterior cervical exposure is made from C1 to C3. The C2 inferior facet is used as the landmark for screw entry: the entry point is 2 mm lateral to the medial edge and 2 mm above the inferior border of the C2 facet (Fig. 18-37A). The drill trajectory is angled medially 5 to 10 degrees. On the lateral fluoroscopic radiograph, the drill trajectory is adjusted toward the posterior cortex of the anterior arch of C1. Percutaneous placement of the C1–C2 facet screws may be necessary if the intraoperative atlantoaxial alignment precludes drilling or placement of screws through the operative incision. After tapping, a 3.5-mm lag screw is placed across the C1–C2 joint (Fig. 18-37B). Another screw is then placed in exactly the same way on the other side. After placement of the C1–C2 transarticular screw, a bone graft is harvested from the posterior iliac crest. A traditional posterior C1–C2 fusion is done using either the Gallie or the Brooks technique (Fig 18-38).

The patient is immobilized in a hard cervical collar only; no halo or Minerva cast is used postoperatively.

Posterior C1–C2 Polyaxial Screw and Rod Fixation

Harms and Melcher[94] described a technique of atlantoaxial stabilization using fixation of the C1 lateral mass and the C2 pedi-

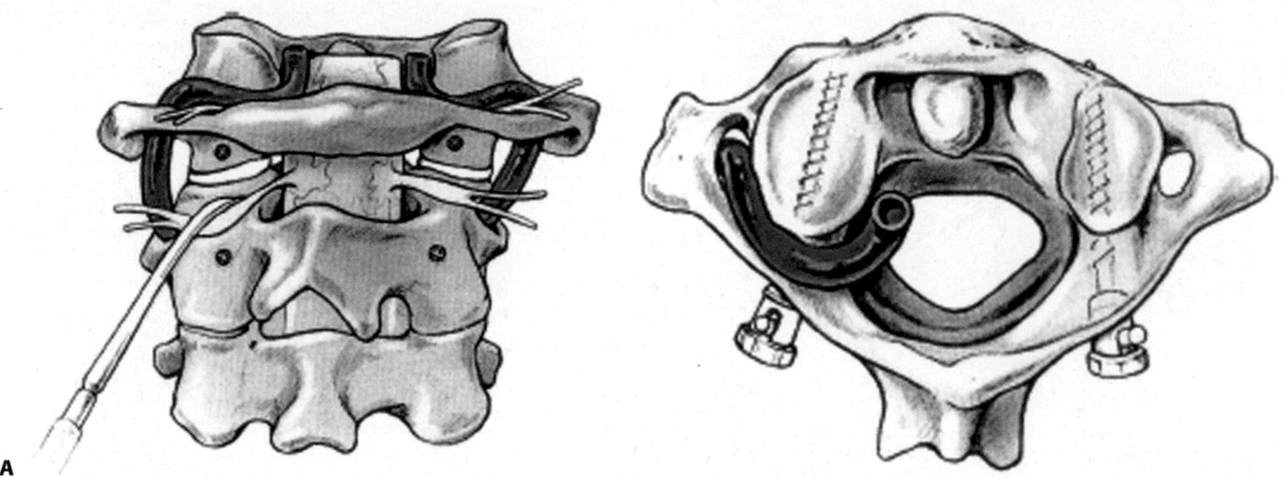

FIGURE 18-37 Posterior C1–C2 transarticular screw fixation. **A.** Location of entry points in C1 and C2 for screw placement. **B.** Polyaxial screws placed bicortically into the lateral mass. (From Harms J, Melcher RP. Posterior C1–C2 fusion with polyaxial screw and rod fixation. Spine 2001;26:2467–2471, with permission.)

cle with polyaxial screws and rods (Fig. 18-39). This technique has the advantages of minimizing the risk of vertebral artery injury, does not require the use of sublaminar wires, and does not require an intact posterior arch of C1. Disadvantages are the anatomic limitations of the C1 lateral mass, which may prevent the use of a 3.5-mm screw, and the potential risk of irritation or injury of the C2 ganglion.

The patient is placed prone with the head held in a Mayfield skull clamp or with a halo ring attached to the Mayfield attachment. Under fluoroscopic guidance, proper alignment of the atlantoaxial joint is confirmed. The cervical spine is exposed from the occiput to C3. The C1–C2 complex is exposed to the lateral border of the C1–C2 articulation. The C1–C2 joint is exposed and opened by dissection over the superior surface of the C2 pars interarticularis. The dorsal root ganglion of C2 is retracted in a caudal direction to expose the entry point for the C1 screw. This entry point is at the midpoint of the C1 lateral mass at its junction with the posterior arch of C1. A 2-mm high-speed burr is used to mark the starting point for the drill. The drill bit is directed in a straight to slightly convergent trajectory in the anteroposterior plane, and parallel to the posterior arch of C1 in the sagittal plane. After determining the appropriate screw length, the drill hole is tapped and a 3.5-mm polyaxial screw is inserted. A number 4 Penfield elevator is used to define the medial border of the C2 isthmus or pedicle. The starting point for the C2 pedicle screw is in the superior and medial quadrant of the C2 lateral mass. A C2 pedicle pilot hole is drilled with a 2-mm drill in a 20 to 30 degree convergent and cephalad trajectory, using the superior and medial surface of the C2 pedicle as a guide. The hole is tapped, and a 3.5-mm polyaxial screw of appropriate length is inserted. Fixation of the rods to the polyaxial screws is obtained with locking nuts (Fig. 18-40). C1 and C2 are decorticated posteriorly and cancellous bone from the posterior iliac crest is used for bone graft. Rigid cervical collar immobilization is used postoperatively.

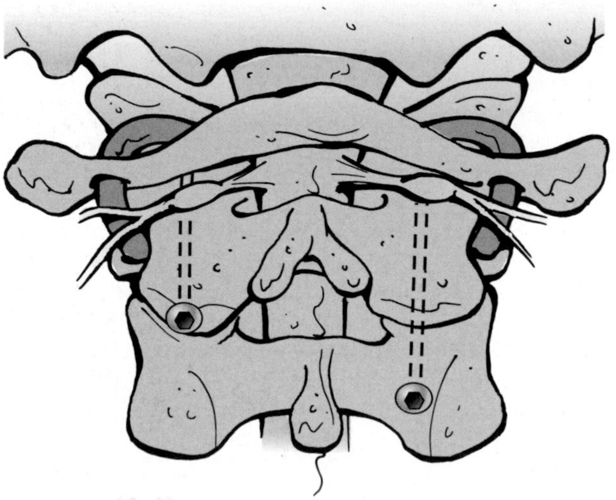

FIGURE 18-38 Position of vertebral arteries and position of screws across atlantoaxial joint. (From Menezes AH. Surgical approaches to the craniocervical junction. In: Weinstein SL, ed. Pediatric Spine Surgery. 2nd ed. Philadelphia: Lippincott Williams & Wilkins, 2001.)

Atlantoaxial Instability Associated with Congenital Anomalies and Syndromes

Although acute atlantoaxial instability in children is rare, chronic atlantoaxial instability occurs in certain conditions such as juvenile rheumatoid arthritis, Reiter syndrome, Down syndrome, and Larsen syndrome. Bone dysplasia—such as Morquio polysaccharidosis, spondyloepiphyseal dysplasia, and Kniest syndrome—also may be associated with atlantoaxial instability, as well as os odontoideum, Klippel-Feil syndrome, and occipitalization of the atlas.[39,50,91,99,123,127,151]

Certain cranial facialmal formations have high incidences of associated anomalies of the cervical spine, such as Apert syndrome, hemifacial microsomy, and Goldenhar syndrome.[205] Treatment recommendations are individualized based on the natural history of the disorder and future risk to the patient. Although there is little literature on cervical spine instability in each of these syndromes, there has been considerable interest in the incidence and treatment of atlantoaxial instability in children with Down syndrome.[5,49,177,178,227,238]

Some Down syndrome patients have C1–C2 instability of

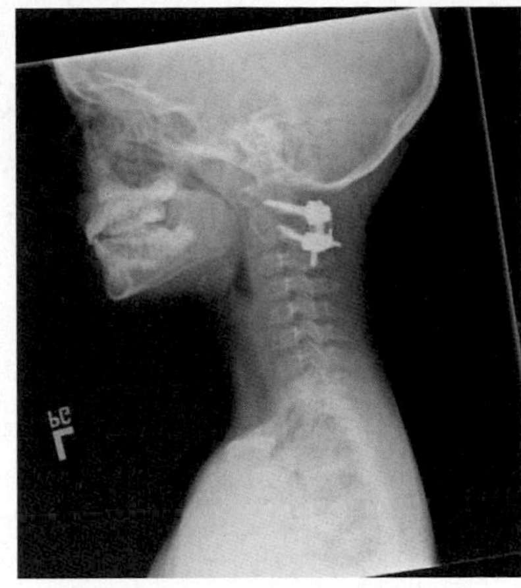

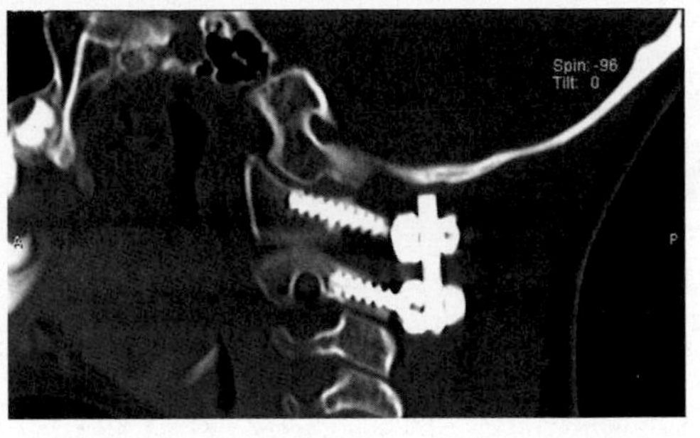

FIGURE 18-39 Radiograph **(A)** and MRI **(B)** after fixation with polyaxial screws and rods.

more than 5 mm. The Committee on Sports Medicine of the American Academy of Pediatrics (AAP) issued a policy statement in 1984[5] asserting that Down syndrome patients with 5 to 6 mm of instability should be restricted from participating in sports that carry a risk of stress to the head and neck. In 1995, the AAP retired this recommendation and issued the following statement: "From the available scientific evidence, it is reasonable to conclude that lateral plain x-rays of the cervical spine are of potential but unproven value in detecting patients at risk for developing spinal cord injury during sports participation."[6] Current opinion is that in asymptomatic children, yearly examinations to detect any neurologic symptoms or signs of myelopathy are more predictive of progressive myelopathy or neurologic injury than are screening radiographs.[49] Evaluation of lateral cervical spine radiographs in full flexion and full extension is still required before participation in sports considered by the Special Olympics to have potential risk: certain activities that axially load the head in flexion, such as gymnastics, diving, and soccer.[209] Davidson[49] found that neurologic signs were more predictive of impending dislocation than the radiograph criteria. Studies have shown that by adolescence, the frequency of atlantoaxial instability approaches 10% to 30%.[6,39,178,197,239] It also appears that 12%[39] to 16%[177] of children with Down syndrome who have instability develop neurologic signs and symptoms.

Surgical stabilization is indicated for patients with translation of more than 10 mm. In patients with less than 10 mm of translation and a neurologic deficit or history of neurologic symptoms, surgical stabilization also may be indicated. Once surgical stabilization is needed, the treating physician must understand the increased risk of complications (i.e., pseudarthrosis) in this patient population. Segal et al.[197] reported a high complication rate after posterior arthrodesis of the cervical spine in patients with Down syndrome. Six of 10 patients developed resorption of the bone graft and associated pseudarthrosis. Other complications in this patient population after attempted posterior arthrodesis were wound infection, dehiscence of the operative site, instability of adjacent motion segments, and neurologic sequelae.[205]

Atlantoaxial Rotatory Subluxation

Atlantoaxial rotatory subluxation is a common cause of childhood torticollis. This condition is known by several names, such as rotatory dislocation, rotatory displacement, rotatory subluxation, and rotatory fixation. Atlantoaxial rotatory subluxation probably is the most accepted term used, except for long-standing cases (3 months), which are called rotatory fixation.

A significant amount of motion occurs at the atlantoaxial joint; half of the rotation of the cervical spine occurs there. Through this range of motion at the C1–C2 articulation, some children develop atlantoaxial rotatory subluxation. The two most common causes are trauma and infection; the most common cause is an upper respiratory infection (Grisel syndrome).[234] Subluxation also can occur after a retropharyngeal abscess, tonsillectomy, pharyngoplasty, or trivial trauma. There is free blood flow between the veins and lymphatics draining the pharynx and the periodontoid plexus.[170] Any inflammation

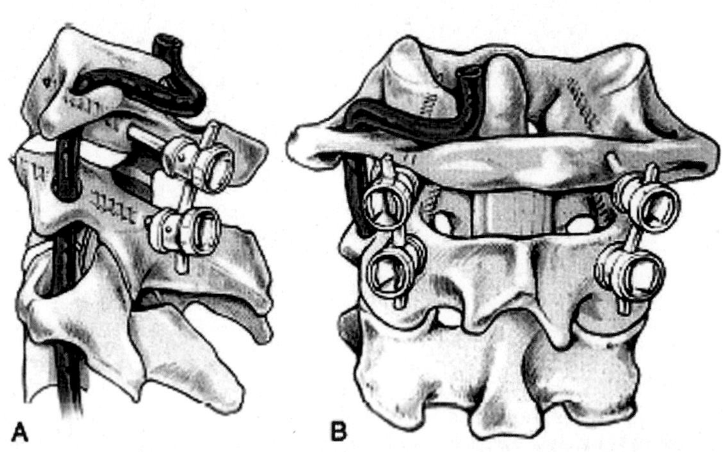

FIGURE 18-40 Lateral **(A)** and posterior **(B)** views after C1–C2 fixation by the polyaxial screw and rod technique. (From Harms J, Melcher RP. Posterior C1–C2 fusion with polyaxial screw and rod fixation. Spine 2001;26:2467–2471, with permission.)

of these structures can lead to attenuation of the synovial capsule or transverse ligament or both, with resulting instability. Another potential etiologic factor is the shape of the superior facets of the axis in children. Kawabe et al.[116] showed that the facets are smaller and more steeply inclined in children than in adults. A meniscus-like synovial fold was found between C1 and C2 that could prohibit reduction after displacement has occurred. Although atlantoaxial rotatory subluxation is most commonly seen from inflammatory syndromes, it also can occur after trauma.

Classification

Fielding and Hawkins[66] classified atlantoaxial rotatory displacements into four types based on the direction and degree of rotation and translation (Fig. 18-41). Type 1 is a unilateral facet subluxation with an intact transverse ligament. This is the most common and benign type. Type 2 is a unilateral facet subluxation with anterior displacement of 3 to 5 mm. The unilateral anterior displacement of one of the lateral masses may indicate an incompetent transverse ligament with potential instability. Type 3 is bilateral anterior facet displacement with more than 5 mm of anterior displacement. This type is associated with deficiencies of the transverse and secondary ligaments, which can result in significant narrowing of the space available for the cord at the atlantoaxial level. Type 4 is an unusual type in which the atlas is displaced posteriorly. This usually is associated with a deficient dens. Although types 3 and 4 are rare, neurologic involvement may be present or instantaneous death can occur. Both types must be managed with great care.

Signs and Symptoms

Clinical findings include neck pain, headache, and a cock-robin position of rotating to one side, as well as lateral flexion to the other (Fig. 18-42). When rotatory subluxation is acute, the child resists attempts to move the head and has pain with any attempts at correction. Usually, the child is able to make the deformity worse but cannot correct it. Associated muscle spasms of the sternocleidomastoid muscle occur predominantly on the side of the long sternocleidomastoid muscle in an attempt to correct the deformity. If the deformity becomes fixed, the pain subsides but the torticollis and the decreased range of motion will persist.[66] If rotatory fixation has been present for a long time in a small child, plagiocephaly is sometimes noted. Neurologic abnormalities are extremely rare, although a few cases have been reported.

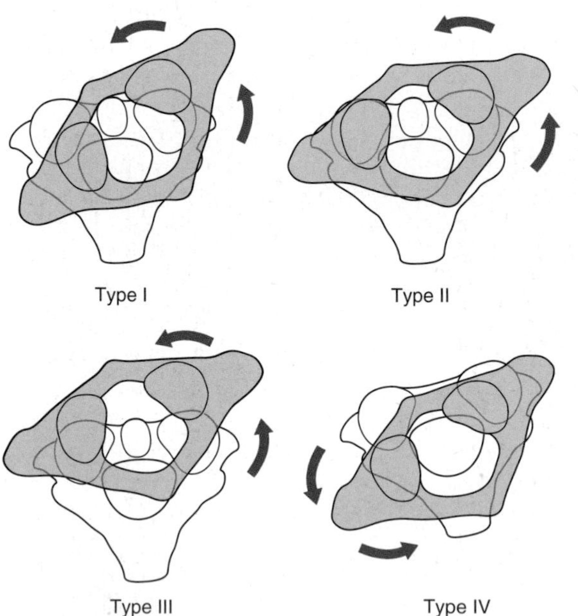

FIGURE 18-41 Classification of rotary displacement. (From Fielding JW, Hawkins RJ. Atlantoaxial rotary fixation. J Bone Joint Surg Am 1977;59: 37, with permission.)

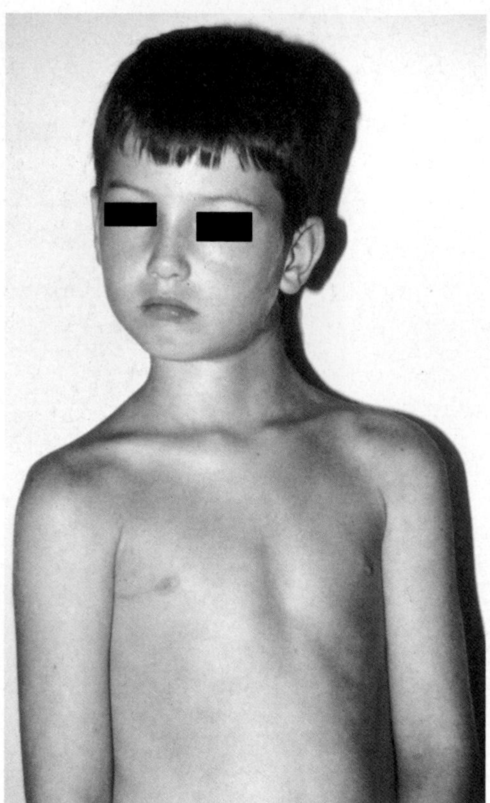

FIGURE 18-42 Child with rotary subluxation of C1 on C2. Note the direction of head tilt and rotation of the neck.

Radiographic Findings

Adequate radiographs may be difficult to obtain because of the associated torticollis and difficulty in positioning the head and neck. Anteroposterior and open-mouth odontoid views should be taken with the shoulders flat and the head in as neutral a position as possible.[139] Lateral masses that have rotated forward appear wider and closer to the midline, whereas the opposite lateral mass appears narrower and farther away from the midline on this view. One of the facet joints may be obscured because of apparent overlapping. The distance between the lateral mass and the dens also will be asymmetric. On the lateral view, the lateral facet appears anterior and usually appears wedge-shaped instead of the normal oval shape. The posterior arches of the atlas may fail to superimpose because of head tilt, giving the appearance of fusion of C1 to the occiput (occipitalization). Flexion and extension lateral views are recommended to exclude instability.

Cineradiography has been used for the evaluation of atlantoaxial rotatory subluxation.[64,68,104] This technique is limited in the acute stage because pain restricts the motion necessary for a satisfactory study. With atlantoaxial rotatory fixation, cine-

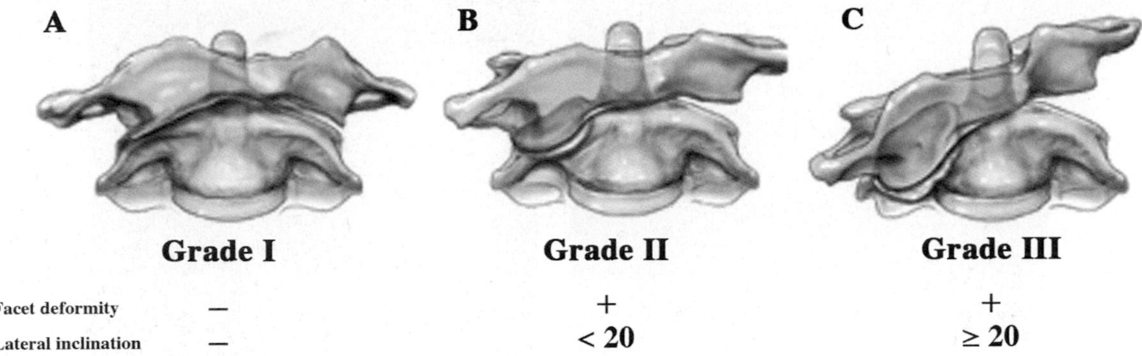

FIGURE 18-43 Classification of chronic atlantoaxial rotatory fixation: grade I, no lateral inclination; grade II, <20 degrees; grade III, >20 degrees. (From Ishii K, Chiba K, Maruiwa H, et al. Pathognomonic radiological signs for predicting prognosis in patients with chronic atlantoaxial rotatory fixation. J Neurosurg Spine 2006; 5:385–391, with permission.)

radiography may be helpful in confirming the diagnosis by showing that the atlas and axis are rotating as a unit. However, this technique requires high radiation exposure and generally has been replaced by CT scanning.[11,56,68,75,174] CT should be performed with the head and body positioned as close to neutral as possible. This will show a superimposition of C1 on C2 in a rotated position and will allow the degree and amount of malrotation to be quantified. Some researchers have recommended dynamic CT scans taken with the patient looking to the right and the left to diagnose rotatory fixation.[173] McGuire et al.[146] classified findings on dynamic CT scans into three stages: stage 0, torticollis but a normal dynamic CT scan; stage 1, limitation of motion with less than 15 degrees difference between C1 and C2, but with C1 crossing the midline; and stage 2, fixed with C1 not crossing the midline. Duration of treatment and intensity of treatment were greater the higher the stage. Three-dimensional CT scans also are helpful in identifying rotatory subluxation.[192] Ishii et al.[111] reported the use of the lateral inclination angle to grade the severity of subluxation: grade 1, no lateral inclination; grade 2, less than 20 degrees; and grade 3, more 20 degrees (Fig.18-43). They also noted adaptive changes in the superior facet joint of C2 in grade 3 subluxations and reported that grade 3 subluxations were more commonly irreducible. MRI demonstrates more soft tissue detail, such as associated spinal cord compression and underlying vertebral or soft tissue infections (Fig. 18-44).[186]

Differential Diagnoses

Differential diagnoses include torticollis caused by ophthalmologic problems, sternocleidomastoid tightness from muscular torticollis, brain stem or posterior fossa tumors or abnormalities, congenital vertebral anomalies, and infections of the vertebral column.

Treatment

Treatment depends on the duration of the symptoms.[173] Many patients probably never receive medical treatment because symptoms may be mild and the subluxation may reduce spontaneously over a few days before medical attention is sought. If rotatory subluxation has been present for a week or less, a soft collar, anti-inflammatory medication, and an exercise program are indicated. If this fails to produce improvement and the symptoms persist for more than a week, head halter traction should be initiated. This can be done either at home or in the hospital, depending on the social situation and the severity of symptoms. Muscle relaxants and analgesics also may be needed. Phillips and Hensinger[173] found that if rotatory subluxation was present for less than 1 month, head halter traction and bedrest were usually sufficient to relieve symptoms. If the subluxation has been present for longer than a month, successful reduction is not very likely.[40] However, halo traction can still be used to try to reduce the subluxation. The halo allows increased traction weight to be applied without interfering with opening of the jaw or causing skin pressure on the mandible. While the traction is being applied, active rotation to the right and left should be encouraged. Once the atlantoaxial rotatory subluxation has been reduced, motion has been restored, and the reduction is documented by CT scan, the patient is maintained in a halo vest for 6 weeks. If reduction cannot be maintained, posterior atlantoaxial arthrodesis is recommended. Even though internal rotation and alignment of the atlas and axis may not be restored, successful fusion should result in the appearance of normal head alignment by relieving the muscle spasms that occurred in response to the malrotation. Posterior arthrodesis also is recommended if any signs of instability or neurologic deficits secondary to the subluxation are present, if the deformity has been present for more than 3 months, or if conservative treatment of 6 weeks of immobilization has failed.

Hangman's Fracture

Bilateral spondylolisthesis of C2, or hangman's fractures, also may occur in children.[174] The mechanism of injury is forced hyperextension and axial loading. Most reports of this injury have been in children under the age of 2 years.[61,71,106,121,169,174,182,188] This injury probably occurs more frequently in this age group because of the disproportionately large head, poor muscle control, and hypermobility. The possibility of child abuse also must be considered.[121,181,228] Patients present with neck pain and resist any movement of the head and neck. There should be a positive history of trauma (Fig. 18-45).

Radiographs reveal a lucency anterior to the pedicles of the axis, usually with some forward subluxation of C2 on C3. One must be sure this is a fracture and not a persistent synchondrosis of the axis.[141,157,208,228,237] Differentiating a persistent synchondrosis from a fracture may be difficult. Several radiographic

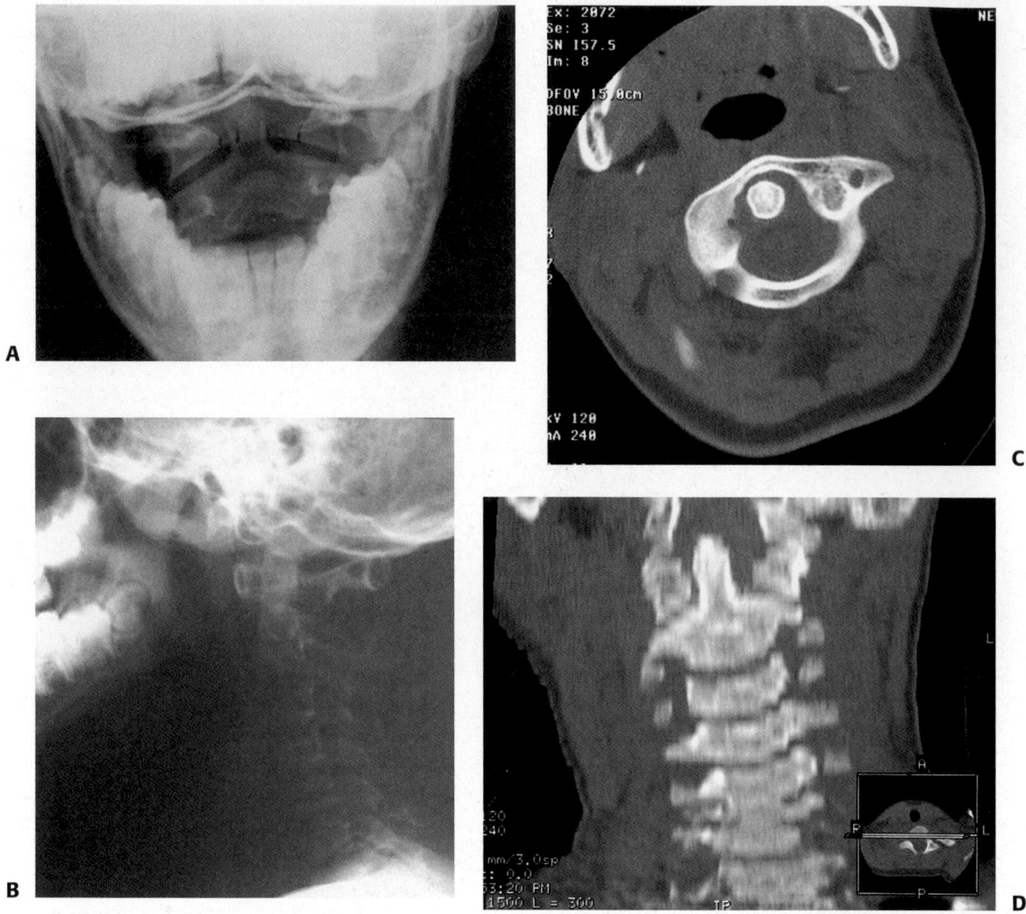

FIGURE 18-44 A,B. Odontoid view and lateral cervical spine radiograph of rotary subluxation of C1 on C2. **C.** Note the asymmetry on the open-mouth odontoid view. **D.** CT and CT reconstruction documenting rotary subluxation.

findings can help distinguish congenital spondylolysis from a hangman's fracture. With congenital spondylolysis, there should be a symmetrical osseous gap with smooth, clearly defined cortical margins; no prevertebral soft tissue swelling should be observed; and there should be no signs of instability. Often, small foci of ossification are seen in the defect. CT scans show the defect to be at the level of the neurocentral chondrosis. MRI does not show any edema or soft tissue swelling that typically is present with a fracture.[153,228]

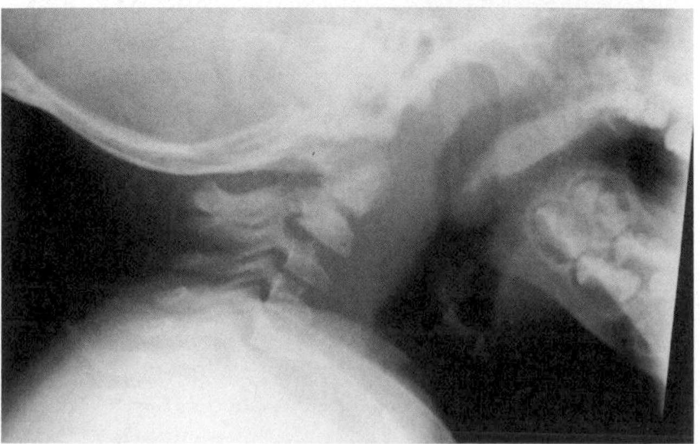

FIGURE 18-45 Lateral radiograph of patient with traumatic C2 spondylolisthesis (hangman's fracture).

Treatment of hangman's fractures should be with immobilization in a Minerva cast, halo, or cervical orthosis for 8 to 12 weeks. Pizzutillo et al.[174] reported that 4 of 5 patients healed with immobilization. If union does not occur or there is documented instability, a posterior or anterior arthrodesis can be done to stabilize this fracture.

SUBAXIAL INJURIES

Fractures and dislocations involving C3 through C7 are rare in children and infants.[69,113,144,204] and usually occur in teenagers or older children. Lower cervical spine injuries in children as opposed to those in adults can occur through the cartilaginous endplate.[52] The endplate may break completely through the cartilaginous portion (Salter-Harris type I) or may exit through the bony edge (Salter-Harris type II). Usually, the inferior endplate fractures because of the protective effect of the uncinate processes of the superior endplate.[13]

Posterior Ligamentous Disruption

Posterior ligamentous disruption can occur with a flexion or distraction injury to the cervical spine. The patient usually has point tenderness at the injury site and complains of neck pain. Initial radiographs may be normal except for loss of normal cervical lordosis. This may be a normal finding in young children but should be evaluated for possible ligamentous injury in an adolescent. Widening of the posterior interspinous distance is suggestive of this injury. MRI may be helpful in documenting ligamentous damage.

With posterior ligamentous disruption, gradual displacement of one segment on the other can occur, and secondary adaptive changes in the growing spine may make reduction difficult. Posterior ligamentous injuries should be protected with an extension orthosis, and patients should be followed closely for the development of instability. If signs of instability are present, then a posterior arthrodesis should be performed. Guidelines for instability in children have not been fully developed. Instability in adults has been defined as angulation between adjacent vertebrae in the sagittal plane of 22 degrees more than the adjacent normal segment or translation in the sagittal plane of 3.5 mm or more.[165,166,235,236]

Compression Fractures

Compression fractures, the most common fractures of the subaxial spine in children, are caused by flexion and axial loading that results in loss of vertebral body height. This can be detected on a lateral radiograph. Because the vertebral disks in children are more resilient than the vertebral bodies, the bone is more likely to be injured. Compression fractures are stable injuries and heal in children in 3 to 6 weeks. Many compression fractures may be overlooked because of the normal wedge shape of the vertebral bodies in young children. Immobilization in a cervical collar is recommended for 3 to 6 weeks. Flexion and extension films to confirm stability should be obtained 2 to 4 weeks after injury. In children under 8 years of age, the vertebral body may reconstitute itself with growth, although Schwarz et al.[196] reported that kyphosis of more than 20 degrees may not correct with growth. Associated injuries can include anterior teardrop, laminar, and spinous process fractures.

Unilateral and Bilateral Facet Dislocations

Unilateral facet dislocations and bilateral facet dislocations are the second most common injuries in the subaxial spine in children. Most occur in adolescents and are similar to adult injuries. The diagnosis usually can be made on anteroposterior and lateral radiographs. In children, the so-called perched facet is a true dislocation. The cartilaginous components are overlapped and locked. On the radiograph, the facet appears perched because the overlapped cartilage cannot be seen. Unilateral facet dislocation is treated with traction and reduction. If reduction cannot be easily obtained, open reduction and arthrodesis are indicated. Complete bilateral facet dislocation, although rare, is more unstable and has a higher incidence of neurologic deficit (Fig. 18-46). Treatment consists of reduction and stabilization with a posterior arthrodesis.

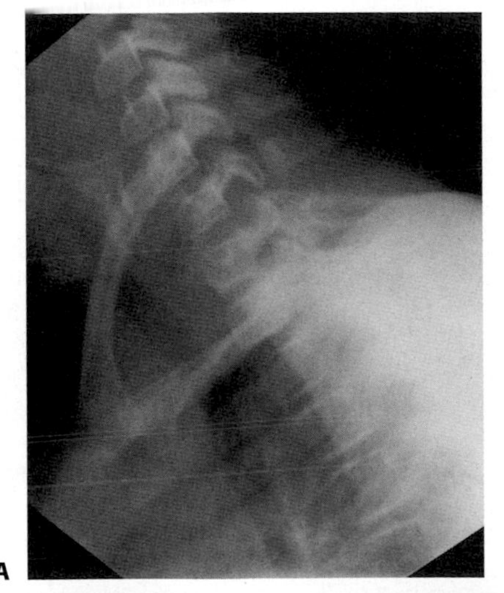
A

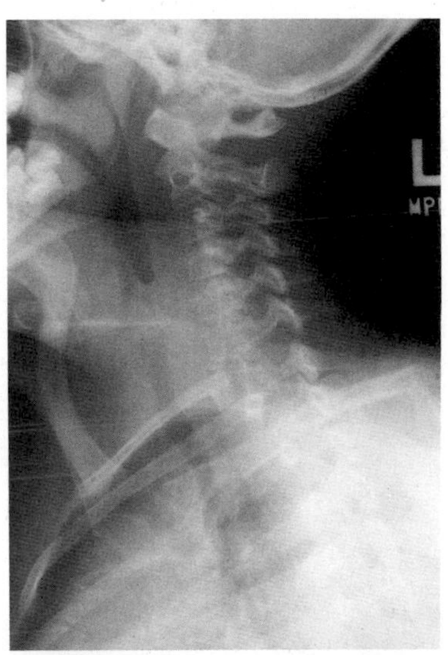
B

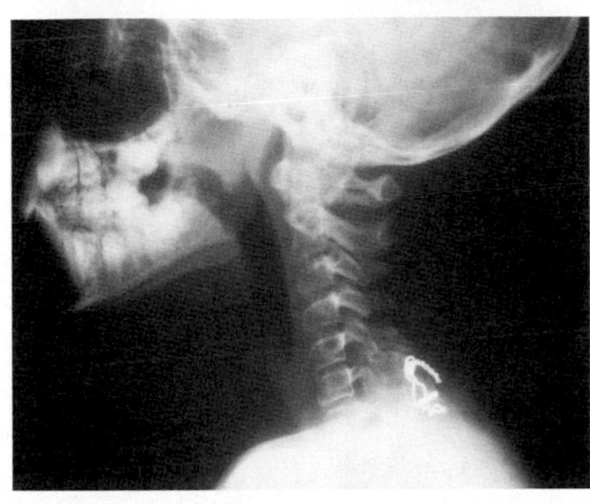
C

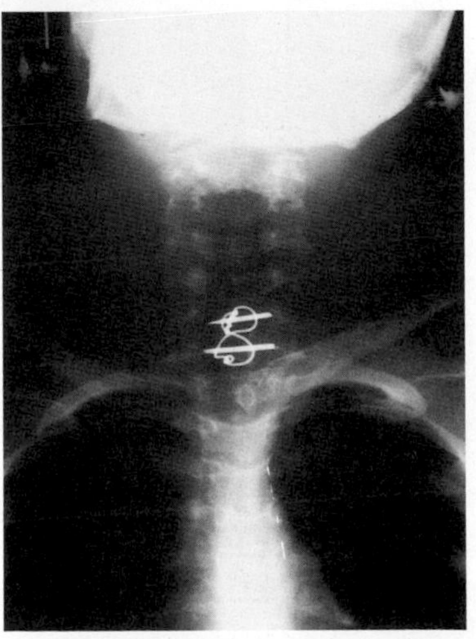
D

FIGURE 18-46 A,B. Lateral radiograph of a patient with so-called perched facets, demonstrating a facet dislocation. **C,D.** Lateral and anteroposterior radiographs after reduction and posterior arthrodesis.

Burst Fractures

Although rare, burst fractures can occur in children. These injuries are caused by an axial load. Radiographic evaluation should consist of anteroposterior and lateral views. CT scans aid in detecting any spinal canal compromise from retropulsed fracture fragments and occult laminar fractures. The posterior aspect of the vertebral body can displace posteriorly, causing canal compromise and neurologic deficit. If no neurologic deficit or significant canal compromise is present, then treatment consists of traction followed by halo immobilization. Anterior arthrodesis rarely is recommended in pediatric patients, except in a patient with a burst fracture and significant canal compromise.[199] Anterior arthrodesis destroys the anterior growth potential; as posterior growth continues, a kyphotic deformity may occur (Fig. 18-47). In older children and adolescents, anterior instrumentation can be used for stabilization (Fig. 18-48).

Spondylolysis and Spondylolisthesis

Spondylolysis and spondylolisthesis of C2 through C6 have been reported. These injuries can occur from either a hyperextension or flexion axial loading injury. Associated anterosuperior avulsion or compression fractures of the vertebral body may occur. The diagnosis usually is made on plain radiographs that show a fracture line through the pedicles. Oblique views may be necessary to better identify the fracture line. CT scanning may be useful in differentiating an acute fracture from a normal synchondrosis. Treatment consists of immobilization in a cervical orthosis or halo brace. Surgical stabilization is recommended only for truly unstable fractures or nonunions. Neurologic involvement is rare.

Operative Treatment

Posterior Arthrodesis

General anesthesia is administered with the patient supine (Fig. 18-49). The patient is turned prone on the operating table, with care taken to maintain traction and proper alignment of the head and neck. The head may be positioned in a head rest or maintained in skeletal traction. Radiographs are obtained to confirm adequate alignment of the vertebrae and to localize the vertebrae to be exposed. Extension of the fusion mass can occur when extra vertebrae or spinous processes are exposed in the cervical spine. A midline incision is made over the chosen spinous processes, and the spinous process and lamina are exposed subperiosteally to the facet joints. If the spinous process is large enough, a hole is made in the base of the spinous process with a towel clip or Lewin clamp. An 18-gauge wire is passed through this hole, looped over the spinous process, and passed through the hole again. A similar hole is made in the base of the spinous process of the inferior vertebra to be fused, and the wire is passed through this vertebra. The wire is then passed through this hole, looped under the inferior aspect of the spinous process, and then passed back through the same hole. The wire is tightened and corticocancellous bone grafts are placed along the exposed lamina and spinous processes. The wound is closed in layers. If the spinous process is too small to pass wires, then an in situ arthrodesis can be performed and external immobilization used.

Hall et al.[89] used a 16-gauge wire and threaded Kirschner wires. The threaded Kirschner wires are passed through the bases of the spinous processes of the vertebrae to be fused. This is followed by a figure-of-eight wiring with a 16-gauge wire (Fig. 18-50). After tightening the wire about the Kirschner wires, strips of corticocancellous and cancellous bone are packed over the posterior arches of the vertebrae to be fused.

In older children and adolescents, lateral mass plates or screw-and-rod systems can be used in the lower cervical spine. The instrumentation should be of appropriate size to match the size of the child's cervical spine.

Posterior Arthrodesis with Lateral Mass Screw Fixation

Several techniques of lateral mass screw fixation for the lower cervical spine have been described. They differ primarily in the entry points for the screws and in the trajectory of screw placement, which yield different exit points.[138,187]

Roy-Camille Technique. The entry point for the screw is at the center of the rectangular posterior face of the lateral mass or can be measured 5 mm medial to the lateral edge and midway between the facet joints (Fig. 18-51A). The drill is directed perpendicular to the posterior wall of the vertebral body with a 10-degree lateral angle (Fig. 18-51B). This trajectory establishes an exit point slightly lateral to the vertebral artery and below the exiting nerve root. The lateral mass depth from C3

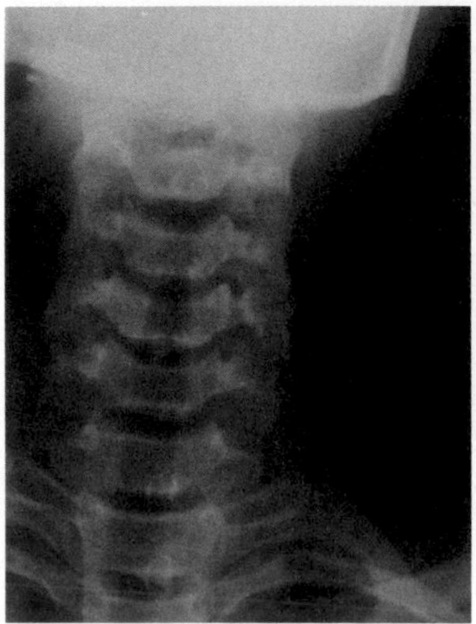
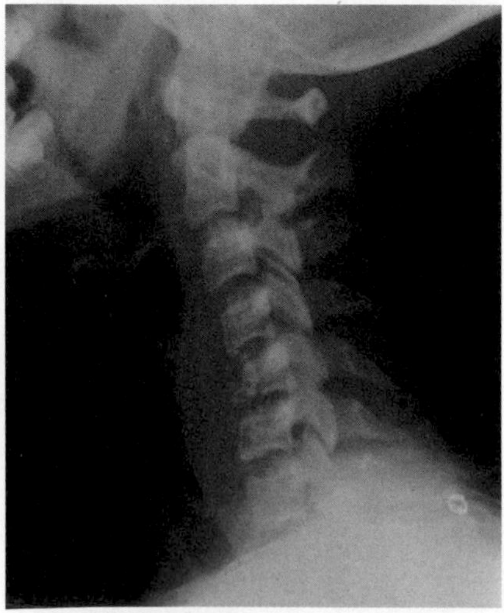
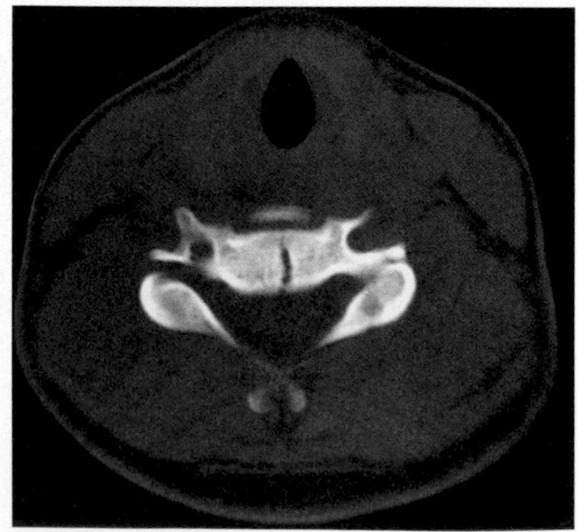

FIGURE 18-47 Anteroposterior and lateral radiographs and CT scan of patient with a minimally displaced burst fracture of C5.

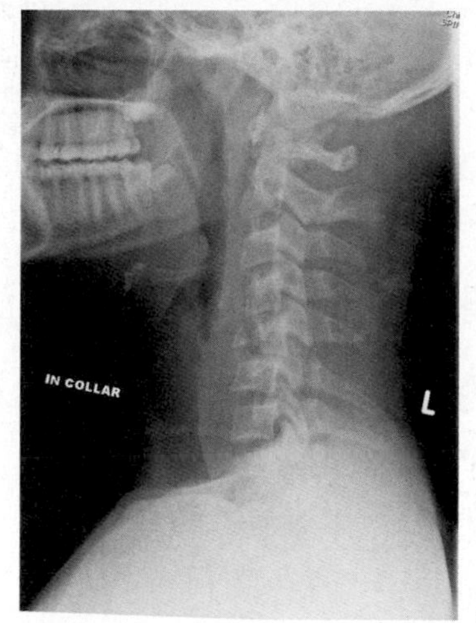

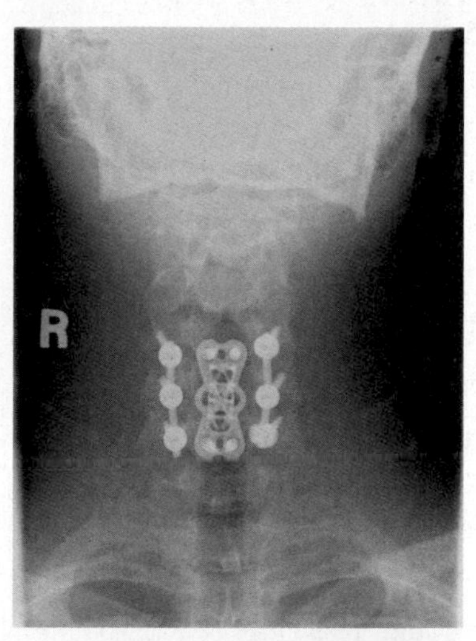

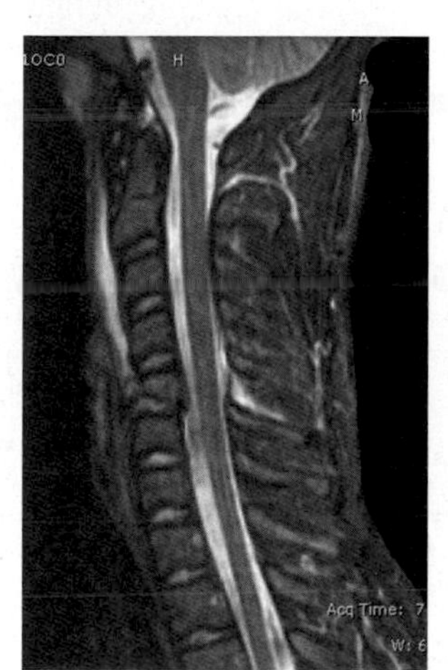

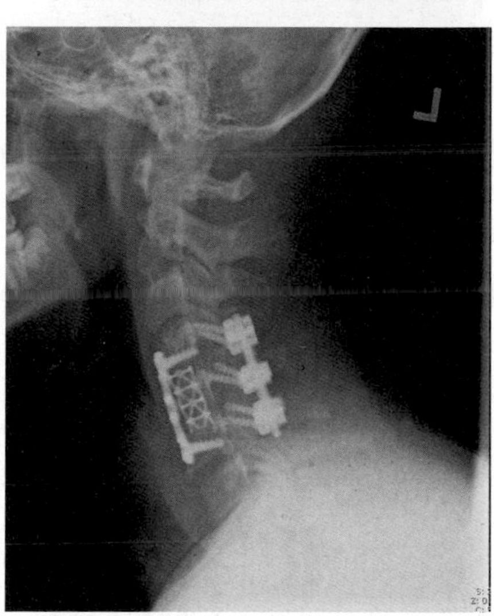

FIGURE 18-48 Radiograph **(A)** and MRI **(B)** of 12-year-old boy with three-column injury sustained during football game. **C,D.** After anterior and posterior fusion and fixation with anterior plate and screws and posterior instrumentation.

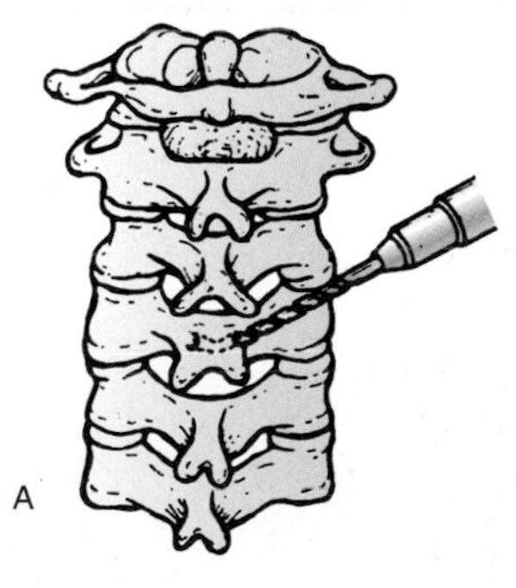

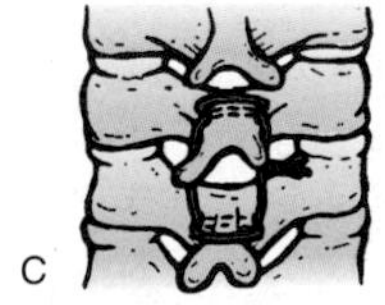

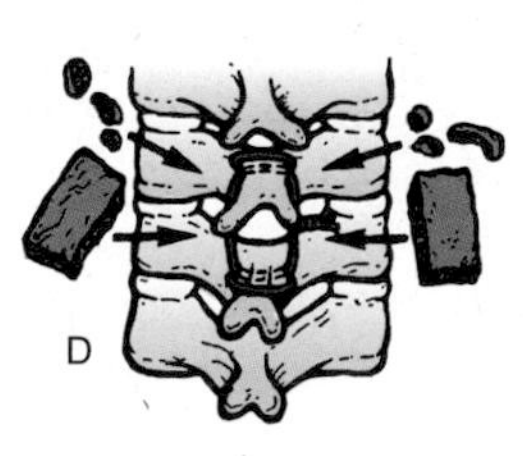

FIGURE 18-49 Technique of posterior arthrodesis in subaxial spine levels C3–C7. **A.** A hole is made in the spinous process of the vertebrae to be fused. **B.** An 18-gauge wire is passed through both holes and around the spinous processes. **C.** The wire is tightened. **D.** Corticocancellous bone grafts are placed. (From Murphy MJ, Southwick WO. Posterior approaches and fusions. In: Cervical Spine Research Society. The Cervical Spine. Philadelphia: JB Lippincott, 1983:506–507, with permission.)

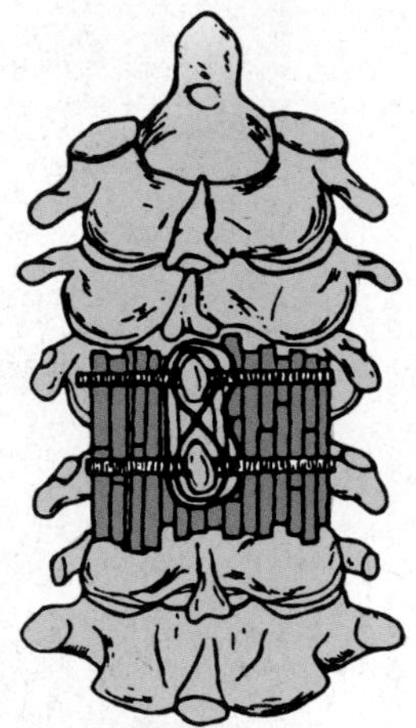

FIGURE 18-50 Alternative fixation method for posterior arthrodesis of C3–C7. A 16-gauge wire is placed in a figure-of-eight pattern around two threaded Kirschner wires passed through the bases of the spinous processes of the vertebrae to be fused. (From Hall JE, Simmons ED, Danylchuk K, et al. Instability of the cervical spine and neurological involvement in Klippel-Feil syndrome: a case report. J Bone Joint Surg Am 1990; 72:460, with permission.)

to C6 ranges from 6 to 14 mm in men (average 8.7 mm) and 6 to 11 mm in women (average 7.9 mm). An adjustable drill guide set to a depth of 10 to 12 mm is used to prevent penetration beyond the anterior cortex. The depth can be gradually and safely increased if local anatomy permits. If the additional 20% of pullout strength with bicortical fixation is desired, the exit point should be at the junction of the lateral mass and the transverse process. Lateral fluoroscopic imaging makes it easier to choose the optimal trajectory and avoid penetration of the subjacent facet joint (Fig. 18-51C), which is especially important at the caudal level of fixation because this joint should be included in the fusion.

Magerl Technique. The entry point for the screw is 1 mm medial and rostral (proximal) to the center point of the posterior surface of the lateral mass (Fig. 18-52A). It is oriented at a 45- to 60-degree rostral angle, parallel to the adjacent facet joint articular surface, and at a 25-degree lateral angle (Fig. 18-52B). This trajectory establishes an exit point lateral to the vertebral artery and above the exiting nerve root while engaging the lateral portion of the ventral cortex of the superior articular facet (Fig. 18-52C). The proper trajectory for this technique is more difficult to achieve that in the Roy-Camille technique. The prominence of the thorax can impede proper alignment of the drill and guide, risking injury to the nerve root if the second cortex is penetrated. The depth of penetration at this angle is approximately 18 mm, compared to 14 mm with the Roy-Camille technique, which has some implications for purchase strength and mode of screw failure.

Crossing Translaminar Screw Fixation of C2

The patient is placed prone with the head maintained in the neutral position in a Mayfield head holder. The posterior arch of C1 and the spinous process, laminae, and medial-lateral masses of C2 are exposed. A high-speed drill is used to open a small cortical window at the junction of the C2 spinous pro-

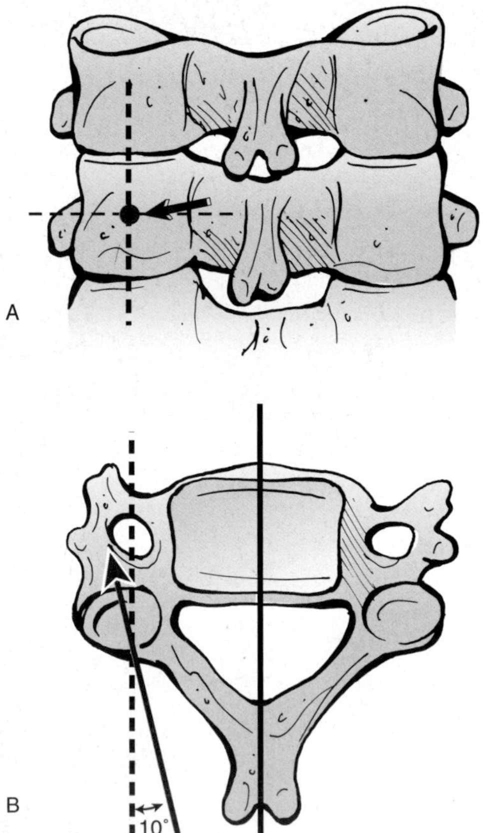

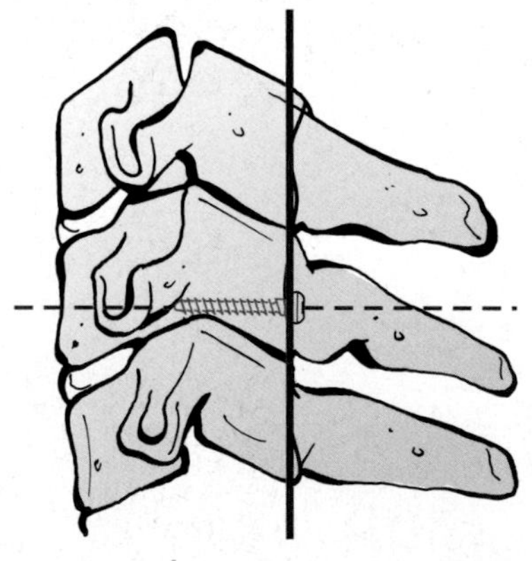

FIGURE 18-51 Roy-Camille technique of lateral mass screw insertion. **A.** Entry point for screw insertion. **B.** Drill is directed perpendicular to posterior wall of vertebral body with a 10-degree lateral angle. **C.** Final screw position. (From Heller JG, Jeffords P. Internal fixation of the cervical spine. Posterior instrumentation of the lower cervical spine. In: Frymoyer JW, Wiesel SW, eds. The Adult and Pediatric Spine. 3rd ed. Philadelphia: Lippincott Williams & Wilkins, 2004, with permission.)

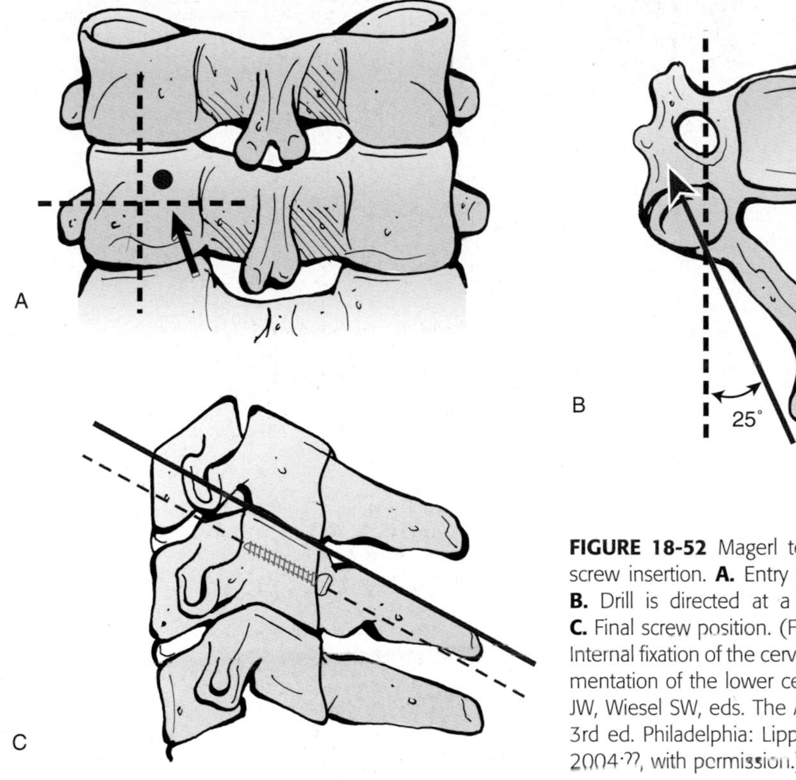

FIGURE 18-52 Magerl technique of lateral mass screw insertion. **A.** Entry point for screw insertion. **B.** Drill is directed at a 25-degree lateral angle. **C.** Final screw position. (From Heller JG, Jeffords P. Internal fixation of the cervical spine. Posterior instrumentation of the lower cervical spine. In: Frymoyer JW, Wiesel SW, eds. The Adult and Pediatric Spine. 3rd ed. Philadelphia: Lippincott Williams & Wilkins, 2004:??, with permission.)

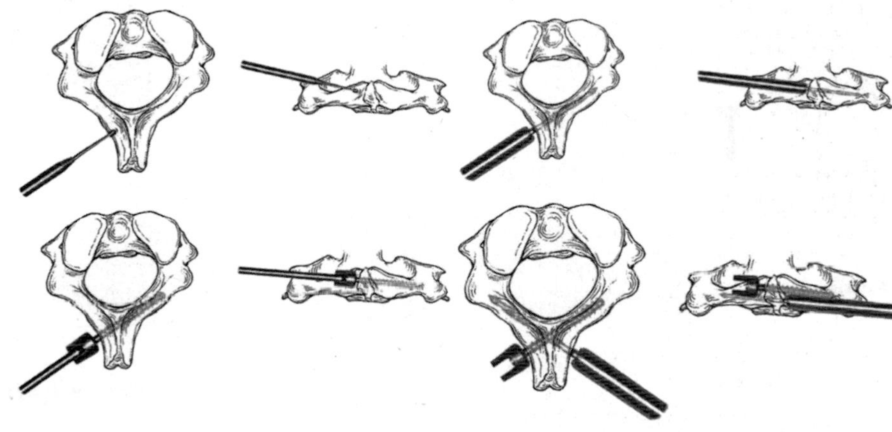

FIGURE 18-53 C2 translaminar screw placement (see text). (From Leonard JR, Wright NM. Pediatric atlantoaxial fixation with bilateral, crossing C2 translaminar screws. Technical note. J Neurosurg: Pediatrics 2006;104:59–63, with permission.)

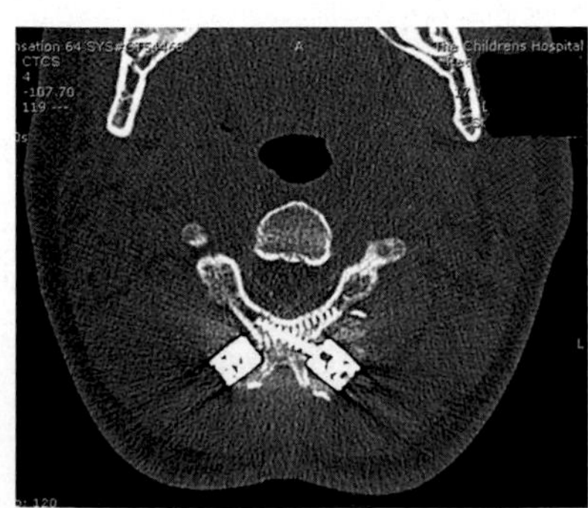

FIGURE 18-54 CT shows placement of screws.

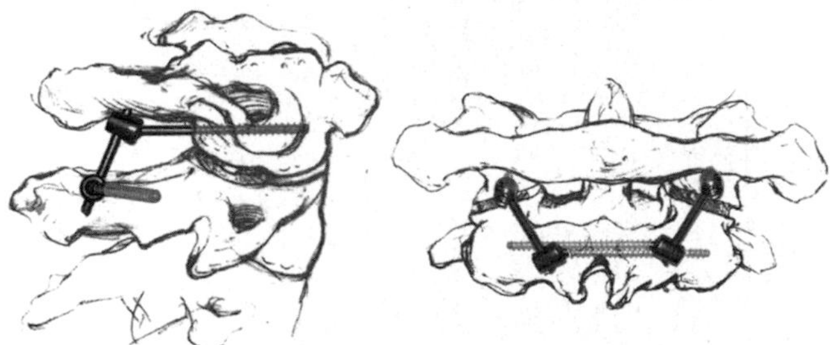

FIGURE 18-55 Lateral (*left*) and anteroposterior (*right*) views of completed C1–C2 fixation with C1 lateral mass screws connected to C2 laminar screws (*lateral view*). (From Leonard JR, Wright NM. Pediatric atlantoaxial fixation with bilateral, crossing C2 translaminar screws. Technical note. J Neurosurg: Pediatrics 2006;104:59–63, with permission.)

cess and the lamina on the left, close to the rostral margin of the C2 lamina (Fig. 18-53). With a hand drill, the contralateral (right) lamina is carefully drilled along its length, with the drill visually aligned along the angle of the exposed contralateral laminar surface. A small ball probe is used to palpate the length of the drill hole and verify that no cortical breakthrough into the spinal canal has occurred. A 4-mm diameter polyaxial screw is inserted along the same trajectory. In the final position, the screw head remains at the junction of the spinous process and lamina on the left, with the length of the screw within the right lamina. Next, a small cortical window is made at the junction of the spinous process and lamina of C2 on the right, close to the caudal aspect of the lamina. Using the same technique, a 4-mm diameter screw is placed into the left lamina, with the screw head remaining on the right side of the spinous process (Fig. 18-54). Appropriate rods are then placed into the screw heads and attached to C1 screws or lateral mass screws below C2 (Fig. 18-55).[133]

REFERENCES

1. Abou Madawi A, Solanki G, Casey AT, et al. Variation of the groove in the axis vertebra for the vertebral artery. Implications for instrumentation. J Bone Joint Surg Br 1997; 79:820–823.
2. Adlegais KM, Grossman DC, Langer SC, et al. Use of helical computed tomography for imaging the pediatric cervical spine. Acad Emerg Med 2004;11:228–236.
3. Allington JJ, Zembo M, Nadell J, et al. C1–C2 posterior soft tissue injuries with neurologic impairment in children. J Pediatr Orthop 1990;10:596–601.
4. American Academy of Orthopaedic Surgeons, Committee on Pediatric Orthopaedics. Trauma of the Cervical Spine. Position Statement. Rosemont, IL: Author; 1990.
5. American Academy of Pediatrics. Committee on Sports Medicine. Atlantoaxial instability in Down syndrome. Pediatrics 1984;74:152–154.
6. American Academy of Pediatrics Committee on Sports Medicine and Fitness. Atlantoaxial instability in Down syndrome: subject review. Pediatrics 1995;96(1 Pt 1): 151–154.
7. Anderson JM, Schutt AH. Spinal injury in children: a review of 156 cases seen from 1950 through 1978. Mayo Clin Proc 1980;55:499–504.
8. Anderson LD, Smith BL Jr, DeTorre J, et al. The role of polytomography in the diagnosis and treatment of cervical spine injuries. Clin Orthop Relat Res 1982;165:64–68.
9. Anderson PA, Montesano PX. Morphology and treatment of occipital condyle fractures. Spine 1988;13:731–736.
10. Annis JA, Finlay DB, Allen MJ, et al. A review of cervical-spine radiographs in casualty patients. Br J Radiol 1987;60:1059–1061.
11. Apple JS, Kirks DR, Merten DF, et al. Cervical spine fractures and dislocations in children. Pediatr Radiol 1987;17:45–49.
12. Arlet V, Aebi M. Anterior and posterior cervical spine fusion and instrumentation. In: Weinstein SL, ed. Pediatric Spine Surgery. 2nd ed. Philadelphia: Lippincott Williams & Wilkins, 2001:209–226.
13. Aufdermaur M. Spinal injuries in juveniles: necropsy findings in 12 cases. J Bone Joint Surg Br 1974;56:513–519.
14. Aulino JM, Tutt LK, Kaye JJ, et al. Occipital condyle fractures: clinical presentation and imaging findings in 76 patients. Emerg Radiol 2005;11:342–347.
15. Bachulis BL, Long WB, Hynes GD, et al. Clinical indications for cervical spine radiographs in the traumatized patient. Am J Surg 1987;153:473–477.
16. Banniza von Bazan UK, Paeslack V. Scoliotic growth in children with acquired paraplegia. Paraplegia 1977;15:65–73.
17. Baum JA, Hanley EN Jr, Pullekines J. Comparison of halo complications in adults and children. Spine 1989;14:251–252.
18. Bayar MA, Erdem Y, Ozturk K, et al. Isolated anterior arch fracture of the atlas: child case report. Spine 2002;27:E47–E49.
19. Bedbrook GM. Correction of scoliosis due to paraplegia sustained in pediatric age group. Paraplegia 1977;15:90–96.
20. Bernini EP, Elefante R, Smaltino F, et al. Angiographic study on the vertebral artery in cases of deformities of the occipitocervical joint. AJR Am J Roentgenol 1969;107: 526–529.
21. Birney TJ, Hanley EN Jr. Traumatic cervical spine injuries in childhood and adolescence. Spine 1989;14:1277–1282.
22. Bivins HG, Ford S, Bezmalnovic Z, et al. The effect of axial traction during orotracheal intubation of the trauma victim with an unstable cervical spine. Ann Emerg Med 1988; 17:25–29.
23. Bohlman HH. Acute fractures and dislocations of the cervical spine. J Bone Joint Surg Am 1969;61:1119–1142.
24. Bohn D, Armstrong D, Becker L, et al. Cervical spine injuries in children. J Trauma 1990;30:463–469.
25. Bracken MB. Pharmacological treatment of acute spinal cord injury: current status and future projects. J Emerg Med 1993;11(Suppl 1):43–48.
26. Bracken MB. Treatment of acute spinal cord injury with methylprednisolone: results of a multicenter randomized clinical trial. J Neurotrauma 1991;8(Suppl 1):47–50.
27. Bracken MB, Shepard MJ, Collins WF Jr, et al. Methylprednisolone or naloxone treatment after acute spinal cord injury: 1-year follow-up data. Results of the Second National Acute Spinal Cord Injury Study. J Neurosurg 1992;76:23–31.
28. Bracken MB, Shepard MJ, Collins WF Jr, et al. A randomized controlled trial of methylprednisolone or naloxone in the treatment of acute spinal cord injury: results of the Second National Spinal Cord Injury Study. N Engl J Med 1990;322:1405–1411.
29. Brecknell JE, Malham GM. Os odontoideum: report of three cases. J Clin Neurosci 2008;15:295–301.
30. Bresnan MJ, Abroms IF. Neonatal spinal cord transection secondary to intrauterine hyperextension of neck in breech presentation. J Pediatr 1974;84:734–737.
31. Brockmeyer DL, Apfelbaum RI. A new occipitocervical fusion constuct in pediatric patients with occipitocervical instability. Technical note. J Neurosurg 1999;90(Suppl 2):271–275.
32. Brockmeyer DL, York JE, Apfelbaum RI. Anatomic suitability of C1–C2 transarticular screw placement in pediatric patients. J Neurosurg 2000;92(Suppl 1):7–11.
33. Brooks AL, Jenkins EB. Atlantoaxial arthrodesis by the wedge compression method. J Bone Joint Surg Am 1978;60:279–290.
34. Bucholz RW, Burkhead WZ. The pathological anatomy of fatal atlanto-occipital dislocations. J Bone Joint Surg Am 1979;61:248–250.
35. Bulas DI, Fitz CR, Johnson DL. Traumatic atlanto-occipital dislocation in children. Radiology 1993;188:155–158.
36. Bundschuh CV, Alley JB, Ross M, et al. Magnetic resonance imaging of suspected atlanto-occipital dislocation. Spine 1992;17:245–248.
37. Burke DC. Spinal cord trauma in children. Paraplegia 1971;9:1–14.
38. Burke DC. Traumatic spinal paralysis in children. Paraplegia 1971;9:268–276.
39. Burke SW, French HG, Roberts JM, et al. Chronic atlanto-axial instability in Down syndrome. J Bone Joint Surg Am 1985;67:1356–1360.
40. Burkus JK, Deponte RJ. Chronic atlantoaxial rotatory fixation: correction by cervical traction, manipulation, and branching. J Pediatr Orthop 1986;6:631–635.
41. Caffey J. The whiplash shaken infant syndrome. Pediatrics 1974;54:396–403.
42. Capuano C, Costagliola C, Shamsaldin M, et al. Occipital condyle fractures: a hidden nosological entity. An experience with 10 cases. Acta Neurochir (Wien) 2004;146: 779–784.
43. Cattell HS, Filtzer DL. Pseudosubluxation and other normal variations in the cervical spine in children. J Bone Joint Surg Am 1965;47:1295–1309.
44. Collalto PM, DeMuth WW, Schwentker EP, et al. Traumatic atlanto-occipital dislocation. J Bone Joint Surg Am 1986;68:1106–1109.
45. Conry BG, Hall CM. Cervical spine fractures and rear car seat restraints. Arch Dis Child 1987;62:1267–1268.
46. Copley LA, Dormans JP, Pepe MD, et al. Accuracy and reliability of torque wrenches used for halo application in children. J Bone Joint Surg Am 2003;85:2199–2204.
47. Copley LA, Pepe MD, Tan V, et al. A comparison of various angles of halo pin insertion in an immature skull model. Spine 1999;24:1777–1780.
48. Curran C, Dietrich AM, Bowman MJ, et al. Pediatric cervical-spine immobilization: achieving neutral position? J J Trauma 1995;39:729–732.
49. Davidson RG. Atlantoaxial instability in individuals with Down syndrome: a fresh look at the evidence. Pediatrics 1988;81:857–865.
50. Dawson EG, Smith L. Atlanto-axial subluxation in children due to vertebral anomalies. J Bone Joint Surg Am 1979;61:582–587.
51. de Beer JD, Hoffman EB, Kieck CF. Traumatic atlantoaxial subluxation in children. J Pediatr Orthop 1990;10:397–400.
52. DiBenedetto T, Lee CK. Traumatic atlanto-occipital instability: a case report with follow-up and a new diagnostic technique. Spine 1990;15:595–597.
53. Dietrich AM, Ginn-Pease ME, Bartkowski HM, et al. Pediatric cervical spine fractures: predominately subtle presentation. J Pediatr Surg 1991;26:995–1000.
54. Donahue D, Maulbauer MS, Kaufman RA, et al. Childhood survival of atlanto-occipital dislocation: underdiagnosis, recognition, treatment, and review of the literature. Pediatr Neurosurg 1994;21:105–111.
55. Dormans JP, Criscitiello AA, Drummond DS, et al. Complications in children managed with immobilization in a halo vest. J Bone Joint Surg Am 1995;77:1370–1373.
56. Dvorak J, Panjabi M, Gerber M, et al. CT-functional diagnostics of the rotatory instability of the cervical spine: 1. An experimental study on cadavers. Spine 1987;12: 197–205.
57. Dyck P. Os odontoideum in children: neurological manifestations and surgical management. Neurosurgery 1978;2:93–99.
58. Eleraky MA, Theodore N, Adams M, et al. Pediatric cervical spine injuries: report of 102 cases and review of the literature. J Neurosurg 2000;92(1 Suppl):12–17.
59. Evans DL, Bethem D. Cervical spine injuries in children. J Pediatr Orthop 1989;9: 563–568.
60. Evarts CM. Traumatic occipito-atlanto dislocation. J Bone Joint Surg Am 1970;52: 1653–1660.
61. Fardon DF, Fielding JW. Defects of the pedicle and spondylolisthesis of the second cervical vertebra. J Bone Joint Surg Br 1981;63:526–528.
62. Farley FA, Graziano GP, Hensinger RN. Traumatic atlanto-occipital dislocation in a child. Spine 1992;17:1539–1541.
63. Farley FA, Hensinger RN, Herzenberg JE Cervical spinal cord injury in children. J Spinal Disord 1992;5:410–416.
64. Fielding JW. Cineroentgenography of the normal cervical spine. J Bone Joint Surg Am 1957;39:1280–1288.
65. Fielding JW, Griffin PP. Os odontoideum: an acquired lesion. J Bone Joint Surg Am 1974;56:187–190.
66. Fielding JW, Hawkins RJ. Atlanto-axial rotary fixation (fixed rotary subluxation of the atlanto-axial joint). J Bone Joint Surg Am 1977;59:37–44.
67. Fielding JW, Hensinger RN, Hawkins RJ. Os odontoideum. J Bone Joint Surg Am 1980; 62:376–383.
68. Fielding JW, Stillwell WT, Chynn KY, et al. Use of computed tomography for the diagnosis of atlanto-axial rotatory fixation. A case report. J Bone Joint Surg Am 1978; 60:1102–1104.
69. Finch GD, Barnes MJ. Major cervical spine injuries in children and adolescents. J Pediatr Orthop 1998;18:811–814.
70. Flynn JM, Closkey RF, Mahboubi S, et al. Role of magnetic resonance imaging in the assessment of pediatric cervical spine injuries. J Pediatr Orthop 2002;22:573–577.
71. Francis WR, Fielding JW, Hawkins RJ, et al. Traumatic spondylolisthesis of the axis. J Bone Joint Surg Br 1981;63:313–318.
72. Fuchs S, Barthel MJ, Flannery AM, et al. Cervical spine fractures sustained by young children in forward-facing car seats. Pediatrics 1989;84:348–354.

73. Gallie WE. Fractures and dislocations of the cervical spine. Am J Surg 1939;46: 495–499.
74. Garfin SR, Roux R, Botte MJ, et al. Skull osteology as it affects halo pin placement in children. J Pediatr Orthop 1986;6:434–436.
75. Geehr RB, Rothman SLG, Kier EL. The role of computed tomography in the evaluation of upper cervical spine pathology. Comput Tomogr 1978;2:79–97.
76. Geisler FH, Dorsey FC, Coleman WP. GM-1 ganglioside in human spinal cord injury. J Neurotrauma 1992;9(Suppl1):407–416.
77. Geisler FH, Dorsey FC, Coleman WP. Past and current clinical studies with GM-1 ganglioside in acute spinal cord injury. Rev Ann Emerg Med 1993;22:1041–1047.
78. Geisler FH, Dorsey FC, Coleman WP. Recovery of motor function after spinal cord injury—a randomized, placebo-controlled trial with GM-1 ganglioside. N Engl J Med 1991;324:1829–1838.
79. Geisler FH, Dorsey FC, Coleman WP. Recovery of motor function after spinal cord injury—a randomized, placebo-controlled trial with GM-1 ganglioside [erratum]. N Engl J Med 1991;325:1669–1670.
80. Georgopoulos G, Pizzutillo PD, Lee MS. Occipito-atlanto instability in children. A report of five cases and review of the literature. J Bone Joint Surg Am 1987;69:429–436.
81. Ghatan S, Ellenbogen RG. Pediatric spine and spinal cord injury after inflicted trauma. Neurosurg Clin North Am 2002;13:227–233.
82. Giannestras NJ, Mayfield FH, Maurer J. Congenital absence of the odontoid process. J Bone Joint Surg Am 1964;46:839–843.
83. Givens T, Polley KA, Smith GF, et al. Pediatric cervical spine injury: a 3-year experience. J Trauma 1996;41:310–314.
84. Godard J, Hadji M, Raul JS. Odontoid fractures in the child with neurologic injury. Direct osteosynthesis with a cortico-spongious screw and literature review. Childs Nerv Syst 1997;13:105–107.
85. Grantham SA, Dick HM, Thompson RC, et al. Occipitocervical arthrodesis: indications, technique, and results. Clin Orthop Relat Res 1969;65:118–129.
86. Griffiths SC. Fracture of the odontoid process in children. J Pediatr Surg 1972;7: 680–683.
87. Hadley MN, Zabramski JM, Browner CM, et al. Pediatric spinal trauma: review of 122 cases of spinal cord vertebral column injuries. J Neurosurg 1988;68:18–24.
88. Haffner DL, Hoffer MM, Wiedebusch R. Etiology of children's spinal injuries at Rancho Los Amigos. Spine 1993;18:679–684.
89. Hall JE, Denis F, Murray J. Exposure of the upper cervical spine for spinal decompression by a mandible and tongue-splitting approach. Case report. J Bone Joint Surg Am 1977;59:121–125.
90. Hamilton MG, Myles ST. Pediatric spinal injury. Review of 61 deaths. J Neurosurg 1988;77:705–708.
91. Hammerschlag W, Ziv I, Wald U, et al. Cervical instability in an achondroplastic infant. J Pediatr Orthop 1988;8:481–484.
92. Hanson JA, Deliganis AV, Baxter AB, et al. Radiologic and clinical spectrum of occipital condyle fractures: retrospective review of 107 consecutive fractures in 95 patients. AJR Am J Roentgenol 2002;178:1261–1268.
93. Harmanli O, Kaufman Y. Traumatic atlanto-occipital dislocation with survival. Surg Neurol 1993;39:324–330.
94. Harms J, Melcher RP. Posterior C1–C2 fusion with polyaxial screw and rod fixation. Spine 2001;26:2467–2471.
95. Hawkins RJ, Fielding JW, Thompson WJ. Os odontoideum: congenital or acquired. J Bone Joint Surg Am 1976;58:413.
96. Hedequist DJ, Emans JB. The correlation of preoperative three-dimensional computed tomography reconstructions with operative findings in congenital scoliosis. Spine 2003; 28:2531–2534.
97. Heller JG, Jeffords P. Internal fixation of the cervical spine. C. Posterior instrumentation of the lower cervical spine. In: Frymoyer JW, Wiesel SW, eds. The Adult and Pediatric Spine. Philadelphia: Lippincott Williams & Wilkins, 2004:803–816.
98. Henriques T, Cunningham BW, Olerud C, et al. Biomechanical comparison of five different atlantoaxial posterior fixation techniques. Spine 2000;25:2877–2883.
99. Hensinger RN, DeVito PD, Ragsdale CG. Changes in the cervical spine in juvenile rheumatoid arthritis. J Bone Joint Surg Am 1986;68:189–198.
100. Hensinger RN, Fielding JW, Hawkins RJ. Congenital anomalies of the odontoid process. Orthop Clin North Am 1978;9:901–912.
101. Hensinger RN, Lang JE, MacEwen GD. Klippel-Feil syndrome: a constellation of associated anomalies. J Bone Joint Surg Am 1974;56:1246–1252.
102. Herzenberg JE, Hensinger RN. Pediatric cervical spine injuries. Trauma Q 1989;5: 73–81.
103. Herzenberg JE, Hensinger RN, Dedrick DK, et al. Emergency transport and positioning of young children who have an injury of the cervical spine: the standard backboard may be hazardous. J Bone Joint Surg Am 1989;71:15–22.
104. Hohl M, Baker HR. The atlanto-axial joint: roentgenographic and anatomical study of normal and abnormal motion. J Bone Joint Surg Am 1964;46:1739–1752.
105. Hosono N, Yonenobu K, Kawagoe K, et al. Traumatic anterior atlanto-occipital dislocation. Spine 1993;18:786–790.
106. Howard AW, Letts RM. Cervical spondylolysis in children: is it posttraumatic? J Pediatr Orthop 2000;20:677–681.
107. Hoy GA, Cole WG. The paediatric cervical seat belt syndrome. Injury 1993;24: 297–299.
108. Hubbard DD. Injuries of the spine in children and adolescents. Clin Orthop Relat Res 1974;100:56–65.
109. Huerta C, Griffith R, Joyce SM. Cervical spine stabilization in pediatric patients. Evaluation of current techniques. Ann Emerg Med 1987;16:1121–1126.
110. Hukda S, Ota H, Okabe N, et al. Traumatic atlantoaxial dislocation causing os odontoideum in infants. Spine 1980;5:207–210.
111. Ishii K, Chiba K, Maruiwa H, et al. Pathognomonic radiological signs for predicting prognosis in patients with chronic atlantoaxial rotatory fixation. J Neurosurg Spine 2006;5:385–391.
112. Jefferson G. Fracture of the atlas vertebra: report of four cases and a review of those previously recorded. Br J Surg 1920;7:407–422.
113. Jones ET, Hensinger RN. Cervical spine injuries in children. Contemp Orthop 1982; 5:17–23.
114. Judd DB, Liem LK, Petermann G. Pediatric atlas fracture: a case of fracture through a synchondrosis and review of the literature. Neurosurgery 2000;46:991–995.
115. Kaufman RA, Carroll CD, Buncher CR. Atlanto-occipital junction: standards for measurement in normal children. AJNR Am J Neuroradiol 1987;8:995–999.
116. Kawabe N, Hirotoni H, Tanaka O. Pathomechanism of atlanto-axial rotatory fixation in children. J Pediatr Orthop 1989;9:569–574.
117. Keenan HT, Hollingshead MC, Chung CJ, et al. Using CT of the cervical spine for early evaluation of pediatric patients with head trauma. AJR Am J Roentgenol 2001;177: 1405–1409.
118. Kenter K, Worley G, Griffin T, et al. Pediatric traumatic atlanto-occipital dislocation: five cases and a review. J Pediatr Orthop 2001;21:585–589.
119. Kewalramani LS, Kraus JF, Sterling HM. Acute spinal-cord lesions in a pediatric population: epidemiological and clinical features. Paraplegia 1980;18:206–219.
120. Kilfoyle RM, Foley JJ, Norton PL. Spine and pelvic deformity in childhood and adolescent paraplegia. J Bone Joint Surg Am 1965;47:659–682.
121. Kleinman PK, Shelton YA. Hangman's fracture in an abused infant: imaging. Pediatr Radiol 1997;27:776–777.
122. Klippel M, Feil A. Anomalies de la collone vertebrale par absence des vertebres cervicales; avec cage thoraque remontant jusqu'ala bas du crane. Bull Soc Anat Paris 1912; 87:185.
123. Kobori M, Takahashi H, Mikawa Y. Atlanto-axial dislocation in Down syndrome: report of two cases requiring surgical correction. Spine 1986;11:195–200.
124. Kokoska ER, Keller MS, Rallo MC, et al. Characteristics of pediatric cervical spine injuries. J Pediatr Surg 2001;36:100–105.
125. Koop SE, Winter RB, Lonstein JE. The surgical treatment of instability of the upper part of the cervical spine in children and adolescents. J Bone Joint Surg Am 1984;66: 403–411.
126. Korinth MC, Kapser A, Weinzierl MR. Jefferson fracture in a child—illustrative case report. Pediatr Neurosurg 2007;43:526–530.
127. Kransdorf MJ, Wherle PA, Moser RP Jr. Atlantoaxial subluxation in Reiter syndrome. Spine 1988;13:12–14.
128. Kuhns LR, Loder RT, Farley FA, et al. Nuchal cord changes in children with os odontoideum: evidence for associated trauma. J Pediatr Orthop 1998;18:815–819.
129. Kuhns LR, Strouse PJ. Cervical spine standards for flexion radiograph interspinous distance ratios in children. Acta Radiol 2000;7:615–619.
130. Lally KP, Senac M, Hardin WD Jr, et al. Utility of the cervical spine radiograph in pediatric trauma. Am J Surg 1989;158:540–542.
131. Lawson JP, Ogden JA, Bucholz RW, et al. Physeal injuries of the cervical spine. J Pediatr Orthop 1987;7:428–435.
132. Lebwohl NH, Eismont FJ. Cervical spine injuries in children. In: Weinstein SL, ed. The Pediatric Spine: Principles and Practice. Philadelphia: Lippincott Williams & Wilkins, 2001:553–566.
133. Leonard JR, Wright NM. Pediatric atlantoaxial fixation with bilateral, crossing C2 translaminar screws. Technical note. J Neurosurg:Pediatrics 2006;104:59–63.
134. Letts M, Kaylor D, Gouw G. A biomechanical study of halo fixation in children. J Bone Joint Surg Br 1987;70:277–279.
135. Lui TN, Lee ST, Wong CW, et al. C1–C2 fracture-dislocations in children and adolescents. J Trauma 1996;40:408–411.
136. Lynch JM, Meza MP, Pollack IF, et al. Direct injury to the cervical spine of a child by a lap-shoulder belt resulting in quadriplegia: case report. J Trauma 1996;41:747–749.
137. Maekawa K, Masaki T, Kokubun Y. Fetal spinal cord injury secondary to hyperextension of the neck: no effect of caesarean section. Dev Med Child Neurol 1976;18: 228–232.
138. Magerl F, Seeman P. Stable posterior fusion of the atlas and axis by transarticular screw fixation. In: Kehr P, Weidner A, eds. Cervical Spine. Vienna: Springer-Verlag, 1985: 322–327.
139. Maheshwaran S, Sgouros S, Jeyapalan K, et al. Imaging of childhood torticollis due to atlanto-axial rotatory fixation. Childs Nerv Syst 1995;11:667–671.
140. Marlin AE, Gayle RW, Lee JF. Jefferson fractures in children. J Neurosurg 1983;58: 277–279.
141. Matthews LS, Vetter LW, Tolo VT. Cervical anomaly stimulating hangman's fracture in a child. J Bone Joint Surg Am 1982;64:299–300.
142. Mayfield JK, Erkkila JC, Winter RB. Spine deformities subsequent to acquired childhood spinal cord injury. Orthop Trans 1979;3:281–282.
143. Mazur JM, Loveless EA, Cummings RJ. Combined odontoid and Jefferson fracture in a child: a case report. Spine 2002;27:E197–E199.
144. McClain RF, Clark CR, El-Khoury GY. C6–C7 dislocation in a neurologically intact neonate: a case report. Spine 1989;14:125–126.
145. McGrory BJ, Klassen RA, Chao EY, et al. Acute fracture and dislocations of the cervical spine in children and adolescents. J Bone Joint Surg Am 1993;75:988–995.
146. McGuire KJ, Silber J, Flynn JM, et al. Torticollis in children: can dynamic computed tomography help determine severity and treatment? J Pediatr Orthop 2002;22: 766–770.
147. Menezes AH. Surgical approaches to the craniocervical junction. In: Weinstein SL, ed. Pediatric Spine Surgery. 2nd ed. Philadelphia: Lippincott Williams & Wilkins, 2001: 127–148.
148. Menezes AH, Ryken JC. Craniovertebral junction abnormalities. In: Weinsten SL, ed. The Pediatric Spine: Principles and Practice. 2nd ed. Philadelphia: Lippincott Williams & Wilkins, 2001:219–238.
149. Mikawa Y, Watanabe R, Yamano Y, et al. Fractures through a synchondrosis of the anterior arch of the atlas. J Bone Joint Surg Br 1987;69:483.
150. Millington PJ, Ellingsen JM, Hauswirth BE, et al. Thermoplastic Minerva body jacket—a practical alternative to current methods of cervical spine stabilization. Phys Ther 1987; 67:223–225.
151. Miz GS, Engler GL. Atlanto-axial subluxation in Larsen's syndrome: a case report. Spine 1987;12:411–412.
152. Momjian S, Dehdashti AR, Kehrli P, et al. Occipital condyle fractures in children: case report and review of the literature. Pediatr Neurosurg 2003;38:265–270.
153. Mondschein J, Karasick D. Spondylolysis of the axis vertebra: a rare anomaly simulating hangman's fracture. AJR Am J Roentgenol 1999;172:556–557.
154. Mubarak SJ, Camp JF, Vuletich W, et al. Halo application in the infant. J Pediatr Orthop 1989;9:612–614.

155. Nitecki S, Moir CR. Predictive factors of the outcome of traumatic cervical spine fracture in children. J Pediatr Surg 1994;29:1409–1411.
156. Noble ER, Smoker WRK. The forgotten condyle: the appearance, morphology, and classification of occipital condyle fractures. AJNR Am J Neuroradiol 1996;17:507–513.
157. Nordström RE, Lahrendanta TV, Kaitila II, et al. Familial spondylolisthesis of the axis is vertebra. J Bone Joint Surg Br 1986;68:704–706.
158. Norman MG, Wedderburn LC. Fetal spinal cord injury with cephalic delivery. Obstet Gynecol 1973;42:355–358.
159. Nypaver M, Treloar D. Neutral cervical spine positioning in children. Ann Emerg Med 1994;23:208–211.
160. Odent T, Langlais J, Glorion C, et al. Fractures of the odontoid process: a report of 15 cases in children younger than 6 years. J Pediatr Orthop 1999;19:51–54.
161. Orenstein JB, Klein BL, Gotschall CS, et al. Age and outcome in pediatric cervical spine injury: 11-year experience. Pediatr Emerg Care 1994;10:132–137.
162. Orenstein JB, Klein BL, Oschensclager DW. Delayed diagnosis of pediatric cervical spine injury. Pediatrics 1992;89:1185–1188.
163. Pang D, Pollack IF. Spinal cord injury without radiologic abnormality in children: the SCIWORA syndrome. J Trauma 1989;29:654–664.
164. Pang D, Wilberger JE. Spinal cord injury without radiologic abnormalities in children. J Neurosurg 1982;57:114–129.
165. Panjabi MM, White AA III, Johnson RM. Cervical spine mechanics as a function of transection of components. J Biomech 1975;8(5):327–336.
166. Panjabi MM, White AA III, Keller D, et al. Stability of the cervical spine under tension. J Biomech 1978;11:189–197.
167. Papadopoulos SM, Dickman CA, Sonntag VK, et al. Traumatic atlanto-occipital dislocation with survival. Neurosurgery 1991;28:574–579.
168. Parbhoo AH, Govender S, Corr P. Vertebral artery injury in cervical spine trauma. Injury 2001;32:565–568.
169. Parisi M, Lieberson R, Shatsky S. Hangman's fracture or primary spondylolysis: a patient and a brief review. Pediatr Radiol 1991;21:367–368.
170. Parke WW, Rothman RH, Brown MD. The pharyngovertebral veins: an anatomical rationale for Grisel syndrome. J Bone Joint Surg Am 1984;66:568–574.
171. Patel JC, Tepas JJ 3rd, Mollitt DL, et al. Pediatric cervical spine injuries: defining the disease. J Pediatr Surg 2001;36:373–376.
172. Pennecot GF, Gourard D, Hardy JR, et al. Roentgenographical study of the stability of the cervical spine in children. J Pediatr Orthop 1984;4:346–352.
173. Phillips WA, Hensinger RN. The management of rotatory atlantoaxial subluxation in children. J Bone Joint Surg Am 1989;71:664–668.
174. Pizzutillo PD, Rocha EF, D'Astous J, et al. Bilateral fractures of the pedicle of the second cervical vertebra in the young child. J Bone Joint Surg Am 1986;68:892–896.
175. Powers B, Miller MD, Kramer RS, et al. Traumatic anterior occipital dislocation. Neurosurgery 1979;4:12–17.
176. Price E. Fractured odontoid process with anterior dislocation. J Bone Joint Surg Br 1960;42:410–413.
177. Pueschel SM. Atlantoaxial subluxation in Down syndrome. Lancet 1983;1:980.
178. Pueschel SM, Scolia FH. Atlantoaxial instability in individuals with Down syndrome: epidemiologic, radiographic, and clinical studies. Pediatrics 1987;4:555–560.
179. Rachesky I, Boyce WT, Duncan B, et al. Clinical prediction of cervical spine injuries in children: radiographic abnormalities. Am J Dis Child 1987;141:199–201.
180. Ralston ME, Chung K, Barnes PD, et al. Role of flexion-extension radiographs in blunt pediatric cervical spine injury. Acad Emerg Med 2001;8:237–245.
181. Ranjith RK, Mullett JH, Burke TE. Hangman's fracture cause by suspected child abuse. A case report. J Pediatr Orthop B 2002;11:329–332.
182. Reinges MH, Mayfrank L, Rohde V, et al. Surgically treated traumatic synchondrotic disruption of the odontoid process in a 15-month-old girl. Childs Nerv Syst 1998;14:85–87.
183. Ricciardi JE, Kaufer H, Louis DS. Acquired os odontoideum following acute ligament injury. J Bone Joint Surg Am 1976;58:410–412.
184. Richards PG. Stable fractures of the atlas and axis in children. J Neurol Neurosurg Psychiatry 1984;47:781–783.
185. Ries MD, Ray S. Posterior displacement of an odontoid fracture in a child. Spine 1986;11:1043–1044.
186. Roche CJ, O'Malley M, Dorgan JC, et al. A pictorial review of atlantoaxial rotatory fixation: key points for the radiology. Clin Radiol 2001;56:947–958.
187. Roy-Camille R, Saillant G, Mazel C. Internal fixation of the unstable cervical spine by posterior osteosynthesis with plates and screws. In: Sherk HH, ed. The Cervical Spine. 2nd ed. Philadelphia: JB Lippincott, 1989:390–412.
188. Ruff SJ, Taylor TKF. Hangman's fracture in an infant. J Bone Joint Surg Br 1986;68:702–703.
189. Ruge JR, Sinson GP, McLone DG, et al. Pediatric spinal injury: the very young. J Neurosurg 1988;68:25–30.
190. Sankar WN, Wills BPD, Dormans JP, et al. Os odontoideum revisited: the case for a multifactorial etiology. Spine 2006;31:979–984.
191. Sasaki H, Itoh T, Takei H, et al. Os odontoideum with cerebellar infarction. A case report. Spine 2000;25:1178–1181.
192. Scapinelli R. Three-dimensional computed tomography in infantile atlantoaxial rotatory fixation. J Bone Joint Surg Br 1994;76:367–370.
193. Schippers N, Könings P, Hassler W, et al. Typical and atypical fractures of the odontoid process in young children. Report of two cases and a review of the literature. Acta Neurochir (Wien) 1996;138:524–530.
194. Schuler TC, Kurz L, Thompson DE, et al. Natural history of os odontoideum. J Pediatr Orthop 1991;11:222–225.
195. Schwartz GR, Wright SW, Fein JA, et al. Pediatric cervical spine injury sustained in falls from low heights. Ann Emerg Med 1997;30:249–252.
196. Schwarz N, Genelin F, Schwarz AF. Posttraumatic cervical kyphosis in children cannot be prevented by nonoperative methods. Injury 1994;25:173–175.
197. Segal LS, Drummond DS, Zanotti RM, et al. Complications of posterior arthrodesis of the cervical spine in patients who have Down syndrome. J Bone Joint Surg Am 1991;73:1547–1560.
198. Seimon LP. Fracture of the odontoid process in young children. J Bone Joint Surg Am 1977;59:943–948.
199. Shacked I, Ram Z, Hadani M. The anterior cervical approach for traumatic injuries to the cervical spine. Clin Orthop Relat Res 1993;292:144–150.
200. Shaffer MA, Doris PE. Limitation of the cross-table lateral view in detecting cervical spine injuries: a retrospective review. Ann Emerg Med 1981;10:508–513.
201. Shaw BA, Murphy KM. Displaced odontoid fracture in a 9-month-old child. Am J Emerg Med 1999;1:73–75.
202. Sherburn EW, Day RA, Kaufman BA, et al. Subdental synchondrosis fracture in children: the value of three-dimensional computerized tomography. Pediatr Neurosurg 1996;25:256–259.
203. Sherk HH, Dawoud S Congenital os odontoideum with Klippel-Feil anomaly and fatal atlantoaxial instability. Spine 1981;6:42–45.
204. Sherk HH, Schut L, Lane J. Fractures and dislocations of the cervical spine in children. Orthop Clin North Am 1976;7:593–604.
205. Sherk HH, Whitaker LA, Pasquariello PS. Fascial malformations and spinal anomalies: a predictable relationship. Spine 1982;7:526–531.
206. Shulman ST, Madden JD, Esterly JR, et al. Transection of the spinal cord. A rare obstetrical complication of cephalic delivery. Arch Dis Child 1971;46:291–294.
207. Sim F, Svien HJ, Bickel WH, et al. Swan neck deformity following extensive cervical laminectomy. J Bone Joint Surg Am 1974;56:564–580.
208. Smith T, Skinner SR, Shonnard NH. Persistent synchondrosis of the second cervical vertebra simulating a hangman's fracture in a child. J Bone Joint Surg Am 1993;75:1228–1230.
209. Special Olympics, Inc. Participation by individuals with DS who suffer from atlantoaxial dislocation. Washington, DC: Author; 1983.
210. Sponseller PD, Cass J. Atlanto-occipital arthrodesis for instability with neurologic preservation. Spine 1997;22:344–347.
211. Sponseller PD, Herzenberg JE. Cervical spine injuries in children. In: Clark CR, Dvorak J, Ducker TB, et al, eds. The Cervical Spine. Philadelphia: Lippincott-Raven, 1998:357–371.
212. Stauffer ES, Mazur JM. Cervical spine injuries in children. Pediatr Ann 1982;11:502–511.
213. Steel HH. Anatomical and mechanical consideration of the atlantoaxial articulation. J Bone Joint Surg Am 1968;50:1481–1482.
214. Steinmetz MP, Lechner RM, Anderson JS. Atlantooccipital dislocation in children: presentation, diagnosis, and management. Neurosurg Focus 2003;14:1–7.
215. Stevens JM, Chong WK, Barber C, et al. A new appraisal of abnormalities of the odontoid process associated with atlantoaxial subluxation and neurological disability. Brain 1994;117:133–148.
216. Stillwell WT, Fielding W. Acquired os odontoideum. Clin Orthop Relat Res 1978;135:71–73.
217. Sun PP, Poffenbarger GJ, Durham S, et al. Spectrum of occipitoatlantoaxial injury in young children. J Neurosurg 2000;93(1 Suppl):28–39.
218. Swischuk EH Jr, Rowe ML. The upper cervical spine in health and disease. Pediatrics 1952;10:567–572.
219. Swischuk LE. Spine and spinal cord trauma in the battered child syndrome. Radiology 1969;92:733–738.
220. Tawbin A. CNS damage in the human fetus and newborn infant. Am J Dis Child 1951;33:543–547.
221. Taylor AR, The mechanism of injury to the spinal cord in the neck without damage to the vertebral column. J Bone Joint Surg Br 1951;33:453–547.
222. Thakar C, Harish S, Saifuddin A, et al. Displaced fracture through the anterior atlantal synchondrosis. Skeletal Radiol 2005;34:547–549.
223. Tolo VT, Weiland AJ. Unsuspected atlas fractures and instability associated with oropharyngeal injury: case report. J Trauma 1979;19:278–280.
224. Torg B, Das M. Trampoline and minitrampoline injuries to the cervical spine. Clin Sports Med 1985;4:45–60.
225. Tuli S, Tator CH, Fehlings MG, et al. Occipital condyle fractures. Neurosurgery 1997;41:368–377.
226. Uchiyama T, Kawaji Y, Moriya K, et al. Two cases of odontoid fracture in preschool children. J Spinal Disord Tech 2006;19:204–207.
227. Van Dyke DC, Gahagan CA. Down syndrome: cervical spine abnormalities and problems. Clin Pediatr 1988;27:415–418.
228. van Rijn RR, Kool DR, de Witt Hamer PC, et al. An abused 5-month-old girl: hangman's fracture or congenital arch defect? J Emerg Med 2005;29:61–65.
229. Verska JM, Anderson PA. Os odontoideum. A case report of one identical twin. Spine 1997;22:706–709.
230. Viccellio P, Simon H, Pressman BD, et al. A prospective multicenter study of cervical spine injury in children. Pediatrics 2001;108:E20.
231. Walsh JW, Stevens DB, Young AB. Traumatic paraplegia in children without contiguous spinal fracture or dislocation. Neurosurgery 1983;12:439–445.
232. Wang J, Vokshoor A, Kim S, et al. Pediatric atlantoaxial instability: management with screw fixation. Pediatr Neurosurg 1999;30:70–78.
233. Wertheim SB, Bohlman HH. Occipitocervical fusion: indications, technique, and long-term results. J Bone Joint Surg Am 1987;69:833–836.
234. Wetzel FT, Larocca H. Grisel syndrome. A review. Clin Orthop Relat Res 1989;240:141–152.
235. White AA III, Johnson RM, Panjabi MM, et al. Biomechanical analysis of clinical stability in the cervical spine. Clin Orthop Relat Res 1975;109:85–96.
236. White AA III, Panjabi MM. The basic kinematics of the human spine. A review of past and current knowledge. Spine 1978;3:12–20.
237. Williams JP III, Baker DH, Miller WA. CT appearance of congenital defect resembling the hangman's fracture. Pediatr Radiol 1999;29:549–550.
238. Wind WM, Schwend RM, Larson J. Sports for the physically challenged child. J Am Acad Orthop Surg 2004;12:126–137.
239. Windell J, Burke SW. Sports participation of children with Down syndrome. Orthop Clin North Am 2003;34:439–443.
240. Wollin DG. The os odontoideum. J Bone Joint Surg Am 1971;45:1459–1471.
241. Yasuoko F, Peterson H, MacCarty C. Incidence of spinal column deformity after multiple level laminectomy in children and adults. J Neurosurg 1982;57:441–445.
242. Yngve DA, Harris WP, Herndon WA, et al. Spinal cord injury without osseous spine fracture. J Pediatr Orthop 1988;8:153–159.
243. Zuckerbraun BS, Morrison K, Gaines B, et al. Effect of age on cervical spine injuries in children after motor vehicle collisions: effectiveness of restraint devices. J Pediatr Surg 2004;39:483–486.

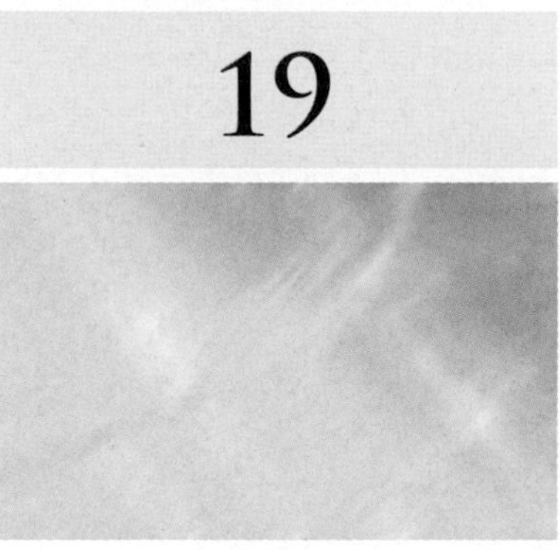

19

THORACOLUMBAR SPINE FRACTURES

Peter O. Newton and Scott J. Luhmann

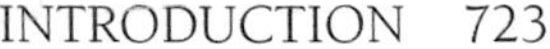

INTRODUCTION 723

PRINCIPLES OF MANAGEMENT 723
MECHANISM OF INJURY 723
SIGNS AND SYMPTOMS 724
ASSOCIATED INJURIES 724
RATIONALE OF TREATMENT 725
CLASSIFICATION 725
RADIOGRAPHIC EVALUATION 728

SURGICAL AND APPLIED ANATOMY 729

CURRENT TREATMENT OPTIONS 730
COMPRESSION FRACTURES 730
BURST FRACTURES 730
FLEXION-DISTRACTION INJURIES (CHANCE FRACTURES) 733
FRACTURE-DISLOCATIONS 734

CONTROVERSIES AND FUTURE DIRECTIONS 736

INTRODUCTION

Fractures of the thoracic and lumbar spine in pediatric patients are relatively uncommon compared to those in adult patients.[29,57] Although cervical spine injuries outnumber thoracic and lumbar spinal column injuries, fractures of the thoracolumbar region are certainly not rare. The mechanisms of injury vary with age,[13,58] while the classification of these injury patterns follow adult spine fracture guidelines. These fractures can be broadly grouped as compression, burst, flexion-distraction, and fracture-dislocations. The treatment principles are based on the mechanism of injury and the "stability" of the fracture

Clarifying the stability of any given fracture can be challenging, and controversy remains as to how to establish which fractures require surgical stabilization. The status of the neurological system is an important variable in treatment.[2,21] In addition, other associated injuries are common,[4] particularly with flexion-distraction "lap belt" injuries.[27,32,40,44,55] Understanding the mechanism of injury, the neurologic status and associated injuries will allow logical decision-making about the treatment approach to a pediatric patient with thoracolumbar spinal injury.

PRINCIPLES OF MANAGEMENT

Mechanism of Injury

One of the most important aspects of treating thoracolumbar spinal fractures is understanding the mechanism of injury. In general, the mechanism of injury correlates with the age of the patient.[13] Spine trauma, just like appendicular trauma, should generate concern for nonaccidental injury in infants and young children.[9,15,35] Levin et al.[41] reported on seven unstable thoracolumbar spinal fractures in abused children.

Motor vehicle accidents may be the most common cause of spinal column injury in all age groups.[4] The type of seatbelt restraint has clear implications in the mechanism of forced transfer to the spine, with the lap belt a common cause of both intra-abdominal and spinal injury.[27,40,55,59,65] The lap belt has been long known to create hyperflexion of the trunk over the belt with the spine pinching the intra-abdominal organs anteriorly. The point of flexion is anterior to the spine leading to anterior compression combined with posterior column distraction (Fig. 19-1). Addition of a shoulder strap or child seat with a full frontal harness limits flexion with frontal impact accidents and protects the spine (and other parts of the body) from injury.

Falls from a height generally result in axial loading of the spine, which may result in a "burst" fracture or wedge compression fracture, depending on the degree of flexion of the trunk at the time of impact. These fracture patterns are possible with any mechanism associated with axial compression and can occur with motor vehicle accidents and sporting injuries.[13] Compression of the vertebra with the trunk flexed creates the greatest forces in the anterior aspect of the vertebra, leading more commonly to anterior column wedging. This is in contrast

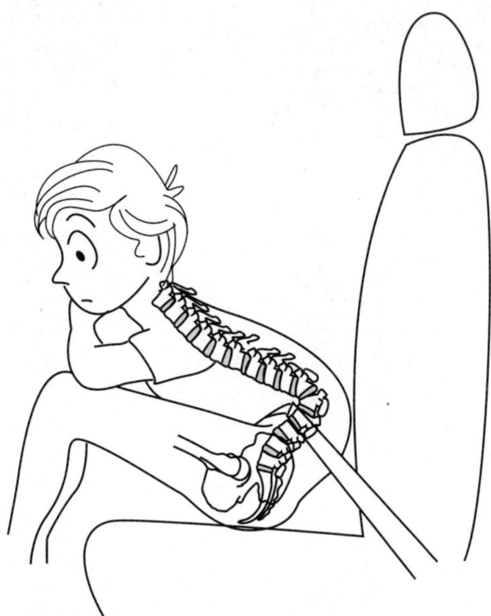

FIGURE 19-1 A lap belt used for a child can create a point of rotation about which the spine is flexed with an abrupt stop. This is a common mechanism for creating both intra-abdominal and flexion-distraction spinal injuries.

to the trunk in an extended position, which loads the vertebral body more symmetrically. Fractures in this case often collapse with radial expansion or "bursting." Displacement of the posterior vertebral body fragments into the spinal canal may cause injury or compression of the neurologic elements (spinal cord or cauda equina).[30]

If the magnitude of injury sustained seems out of proportion to the force applied, the possibility of an insufficiency fracture due to weak bone should be considered. Osteoporotic insufficiency fractures, common in the elderly, are rare in children; however, several disease states may predispose children to these fractures. Steroid use frequent in the management of many pediatric diseases often leads to osteoporosis when taken chronically.[68] In addition, primary lesions of the bone, such as Langerhans histiocytosis, often affects thoracic vertebrae.[3,22] Other tumors and infections warrant consideration when nontraumatic compression fractures are identified.[47,56]

Signs and Symptoms

Careful evaluation of a patient with a potential traumatic spinal injury begins as with any serious trauma victim. The ABCs of resuscitation are performed while maintaining cervical and thoracolumbar spinal precautions. The frequency of spinal injuries in the setting of major trauma (motor vehicle accident, fall, etc.) is particularly high. After stabilizing the cardiorespiratory systems, symptoms of pain, numbness, and tingling should be sought if the patient is old enough and alert enough to cooperate. Pain in the back is often not appreciated when other distracting injuries exist and the patient is immobilized on a backboard. Examination of the back must not be forgotten and is performed by logrolling the patient. Visual inspection, along with palpation, should seek areas of swelling, deformity, ecchymosis, and/or tenderness that may provide a clue to the presence of an injury. In trauma patients, thoracolumbar fractures are more common in older children and adolescents, and there is a low mortality rate and infrequent need for operative stabilization.[60]

Neurologic examination provides information on the integrity of the spinal cord. The age of the patient may limit the thoroughness of this assessment, but some indication of sensory and motor function should be sought. In cases of spinal cord deficit, a detailed examination of the strength of each muscle group, sensory levels, and rectal tone will need to be serially compared over time and the quality of the documentation cannot be over emphasized. The prognosis for recovery is significantly better if the spinal cord injury (SCI) is incomplete.[10,28,71] The status of the neurologic function over time may lead to important treatment decisions regarding the necessity and timing of surgical intervention. A progressive neurologic deficit warrants immediate surgical attention, while an improving status may suggest a less urgent approach. Overall, the physical examination has a sensitivity of 87% in identifying thoracolumbar fractures.[60]

Associated Injuries

Just as the mechanism of injury should raise suspicion of a particular injury (e.g., lap belt injury and flexion-distraction lumbar fracture pattern), so should the presence of one injury raise suspicion of a concomitant associated injury. First, any spinal fracture should be considered a significant risk factor for a spinal fracture at another level. The traumatic force required to create one fracture is often enough to result in one or more additional fractures at other locations. Similarly, a cervical injury is frequently associated with closed head injury and vice versa.

The lap belt mechanism of injury is well known to create flexion-distraction injuries of the spine, but also is associated with intra-abdominal injury.[55] Compressed between the seatbelt and the spinal column, the aorta, intestinal viscera, and abdominal wall musculature are at risk for laceration. Abdominal injuries are present in almost 50% of pediatric patients with Chance fractures.[49] Ecchymosis on the anterior abdomen is suggestive of intra-abdominal injury that warrants further evaluation with laparoscopy, laparotomy, or additional imaging by computed tomography (CT).[4,65] A high index of suspicion is required, because missed injuries may be life threatening.[40]

Associated injury to the spinal cord has obvious significance and may be present with many fracture patterns. Disruption of the stability of the spinal column or bony intrusion into the spinal canal may result in compromise of neurologic function. All patients with a known spinal column fracture or dislocation warrant a careful neurologic examination. Overall, most pediatric patients with thoracolumbar fractures are neurologically intact (85%), and less commonly present with SCIs (incomplete in 5% and complete in 10%).[17] Similarly, patients with a traumatic neurologic deficit require a careful evaluation of the spinal column integrity. There are, however, a subset of patients who present with SCI without radiographic abnormality.[50,51] This scenario has been termed SCIWORA, a phenomenon much more common in children than adults. It is thought that the flexibility of the immature spine allows spinal column segmental displacements great enough to lead to SCI without mechanically disrupting the bony and/or ligamentous elements.[50] Although these injuries may not be visible on plain radiographs, nearly all will have some evidence of soft tissue injury of the spine on more sensitive magnetic resonance imaging (MRI) studies.[25] The term SCIWORA is less relevant in the era of routine MRI, which is now routinely obtained in all patients with possible spinal cord injury.[33]

Rationale of Treatment

The goals of treatment for all spinal injuries is to maximize the potential for recovery of spinal cord function if an SCI was present and/or to provide skeletal stability to the spinal column to protect against future SCI. These two goals may be analyzed separately when both instability and SCI exist. Optimizing return of any lost spinal cord function is paramount, and the potential for recovery of spinal cord function in general is greater in children than in adults.[21,71]

SCIs in children have remarkable potential for recovery. In a study from a major metropolitan trauma center, complete SCIs were associated with fatal injuries in one third and no neurologic recovery in another third, while most of the remaining one-third of patients made improvements that ultimately allowed functional ambulation. Less surprisingly, nearly all patients with incomplete SCI made some improvement over time as well.[71] This ability to recover, even from complete injuries, has led some to suggest more aggressive attempts at spinal cord decompression in the early course of treatment,[20,52] while others have suggested a period of "spinal cord rest" with observation.[42] There is certainly no controlled series of patients treated by both approaches to support either hypothesis. The data do, however, suggest a more optimistic view regarding the potential recovery of traumatic SCIs in children compared with adults.

Spinal column structural integrity should be assessed in all cases of injury because the functional capacity of the vertebral elements to protect the spinal cord will continue to be required. This evaluation may be performed with functional radiographs, such as flexion-extension views (much more common in the cervical spine) or with an MRI evaluation of associated soft tissue injuries that may coexist with more obvious bony fractures. Several methods of estimating spinal column stability have been proposed including the three-column concept of Denis.[14] Based on division into anterior, middle, and posterior columns, injuries to two and certainly three of these sagittal columns may be associated with an unstable injury pattern. Plain radiography with a CT scan is appropriate for evaluating the bony elements. An MRI is often required to elucidate the nature of the disc and ligamentous injuries.[26,33,67] MRI is extremely sensitive and, given the brightness of edema fluid on T2 images, may be overinterpreted. A study correlating MRI and intraoperative surgical findings, however, demonstrated high levels of both sensitivity and specificity in the MRI evaluation of posterior soft-tissue injuries (Fig. 19-2).[39]

The final treatment goal is a stable spinal column. This often requires surgical treatment in unstable fracture patterns. In contrast, most stable injuries can be managed nonoperatively. There are particular exceptions to these generalizations, of course. At times the associated SCI or a substantial associated deformity may alter the treatment approach to an otherwise mechanically stable injury. The presence of a complete SCI in a child younger than 10 years is also a determinant that may affect treatment strategies. The incidence of paralytic spinal deformity (scoliosis) is nearly 100% in such cases,[38,53] and a long instrumented fusion will likely be required at some point. Depending on the fracture pattern and age of the patient, it may be prudent to include much of the thoracic and lumbar spine in the initial instrumented fusion.[45]

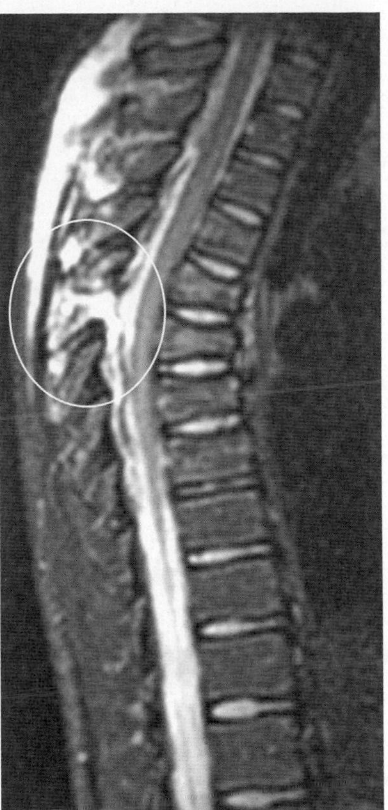

FIGURE 19-2 This sagittal MRI demonstrates marked increased signal in the posterior ligamentous complex. Anteriorly a loss of height at the vertebra can be seen, suggesting a three-column spinal injury.

Classification

There are several methods of classifying thoracolumbar fractures (Holdsworth—two column, Denis—three column,[14] McCormack—load sharing,[46] Gertzbein—comprehensive[24]), each with purported advantages. Designed primarily with the adult spine fracture patterns in mind, the Denis classification translates well for the categorization of most pediatric thoracolumbar injuries.[37] Based on theories of stability related to the three-column biomechanical concept of the spine (anterior, middle, posterior columns), the Denis classification in its simplest form includes compression, burst, flexion-distraction, and fracture-dislocations (Fig. 19-3).

Compression fractures are the most common thoracolumbar spine fracture pattern.[8,31] The vertebral body loses height anteriorly compared to the posterior wall. Axial load with flexion is the common mechanism. Depending on the degree and direction of flexion, the wedging may vary between the coronal and sagittal planes (Fig 19-4). The percentage of lost height defines the severity of compression fractures, which rarely have an associated neurologic deficit. However, the fractures are often associated with similar or occasionally more severe fractures at adjacent or distant levels. Contiguous compression fractures, each of a modest degree, together may result in a substantial kyphotic deformity. Because the cause of these injuries, such as a fall, are fairly common, it is at times necessary to determine if a

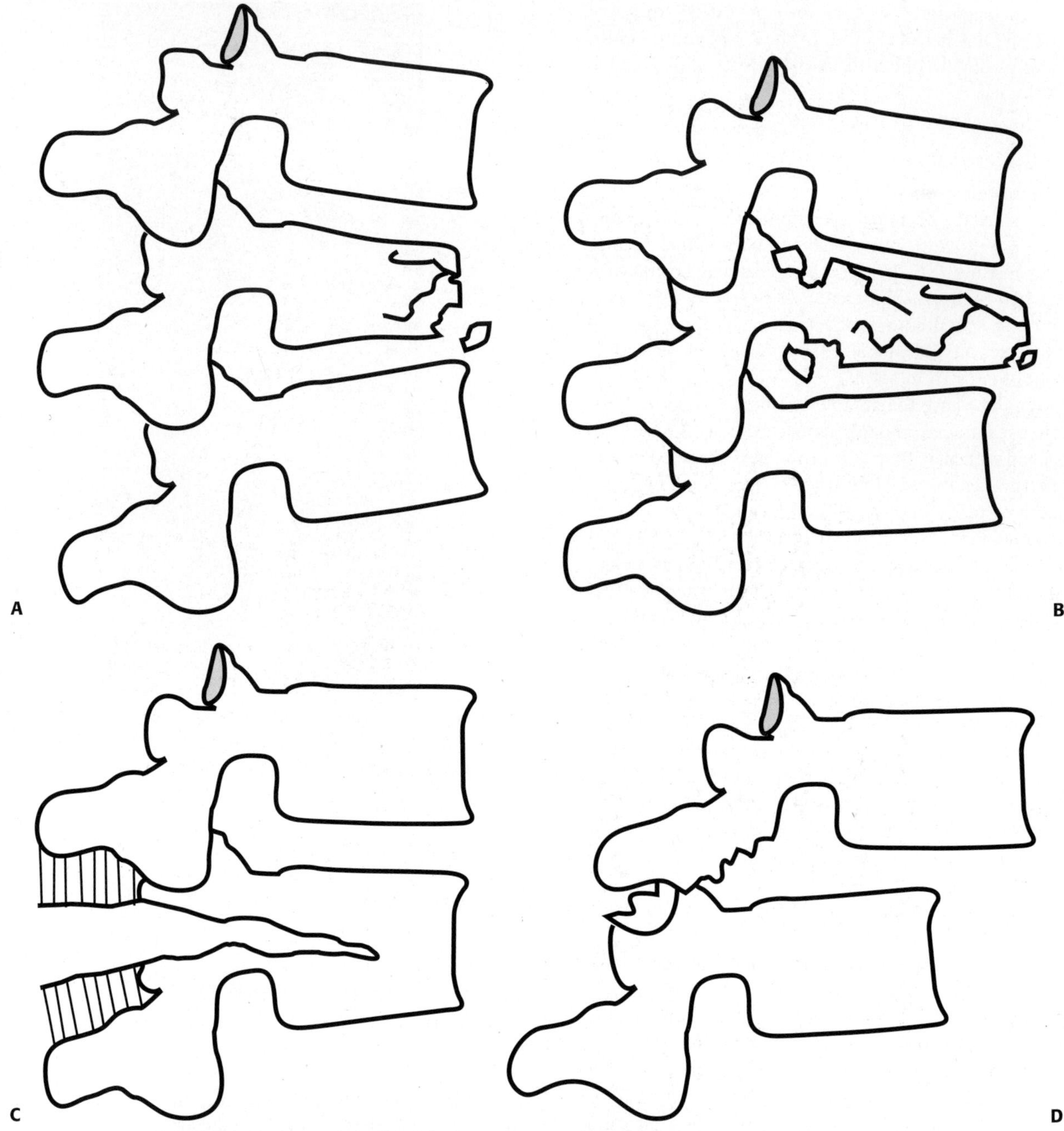

FIGURE 19-3 Denis classification of thoracolumbar fractures. **A.** Compression fracture: This injury results in mild wedging of the vertebra primarily involving the anterior aspects of the vertebral body. The posterior vertebral height and posterior cortex remain intact. **B.** Burst fracture: A burst fracture involves both the anterior and middle columns with loss of height throughout the vertebral body. There may be substantial retropulsion of the posterior aspect of the vertebra into the spinal canal. In addition, posterior vertebral fractures and/or ligamentous injury may occur. **C.** Flexion distraction injuries: This fracture, which occurs commonly with a seatbelt injury mechanism, results in posterior distraction with disruption of the ligaments and bony elements of the posterior column, commonly extending into the anterior columns with or without compression of the most anterior aspects of the vertebra. **D.** Fracture dislocation: These complex injuries involve marked translation of one vertebra on another with frequently associated SCI as a result of translations through the spinal canal.

wedged vertebra seen radiographically represents an acute compression fracture, sequelae of Scheuermann kyphosis, or a remote injury. Clinical examination can localize pain to the site of the fracture in acute injuries; however, MRI or bone scanning can confirm acute fracture based on signal changes and increased isotope uptake.

Burst fractures likely represent a more severe form of compression fracture that extends posteriorly in the vertebral body to include the posterior wall (middle column). Axial compression is the primary mechanism, although posterior ligamentous injury and/or posterior element fractures may also occur. Laminar fractures have been known to entrap the dural contents. The fractures are most common in the lower thoracic and upper lumbar levels. Associated neurologic injury is related

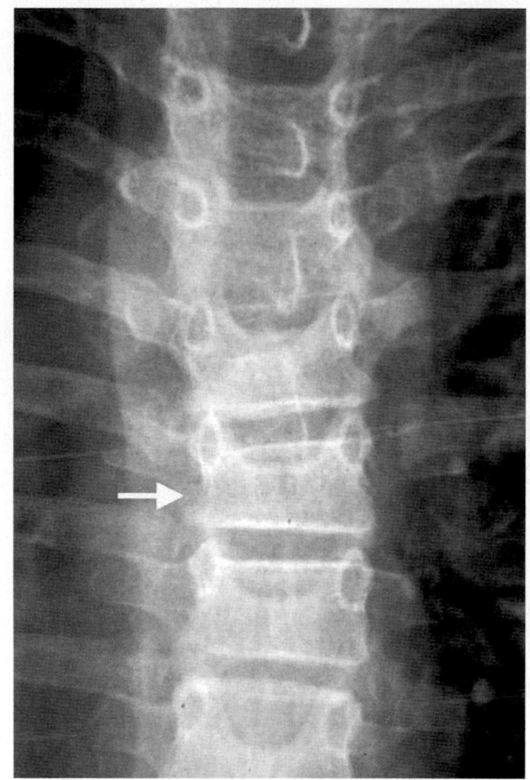

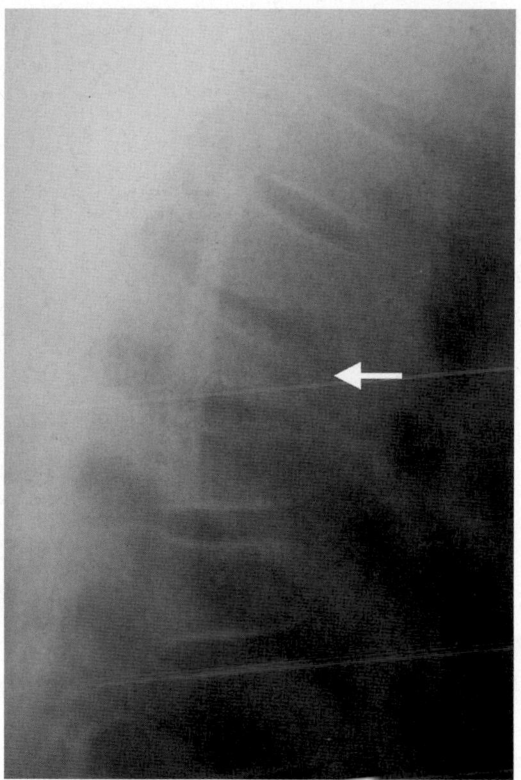

FIGURE 19-4 Compression fractures. **A.** This PA view demonstrates wedging in the coronal plane. **B.** The more commonly recognized compression fractures involve wedging primarily in the sagittal plane with loss of anterior vertebral height.

to the severity of injury (greater injury index scores correlate with greater frequency of spinal cord injury[42]) and the degree of spinal canal encroachment by retropulsed bony fragments.[30] SCI at the thoracolumbar junction may result in conus medullaris syndrome or cauda equina syndrome. Careful examination of the perineal area is required to identify these spinal lesions.

Flexion-distraction injuries are especially relevant to the pediatric population because this classic lap belt injury is more frequent in back seat passengers, particularly when a shoulder strap is lacking. Motor vehicle accidents are the primary cause of this injury. The lap belt, which restrains the pelvis in adults, may ride up onto the abdomen in children. Chance, and later Smith, described how with a frontal impact, the weight of the torso is driven forward, flexing over the restraining belt. With the axis of rotation in front of the spine, distractive forces are placed on the posterior elements, with variable degrees of anterior vertebral compression. This three-column injury is generally unstable. The disruption of the posterior elements may occur entirely through the bony (Chance) or ligamentous (Smith) elements, although many times the fracture propagates through both soft and hard tissues.

The injury is most obvious on lateral radiographs; however, if no fracture exists, widening of the intraspinous distance may be the only finding on an anteroposterior (AP) radiograph. Standard transverse plain CT imaging may also miss this injury because the plane of injury lies within the plane of imaging. One classic finding in ligamentous flexion-distraction injuries is the "empty facet" sign. When the inferior articular process of the superior vertebra is no longer in contact with the superior articular process of the inferior vertebra, the facet appears empty in the transverse CT image.[23] Sagittal reconstructions are most revealing and MRI will provide information about the integrity of the posterior ligamentous complex. Identification of a purely intravertebral flexion-distraction fracture is important, because this may alter the treatment in patients with these injuries compared to those with severe ligamentous injury.

Fracture dislocations of the spinal column result from complex severe loading mechanisms. These are by definition unstable injuries with a component of shearing and/or rotational displacement. A special note in the pediatric population is the documentation of this injury pattern in young patients exposed to nonaccidental trauma.[15,35]

Injury patterns specific to the pediatric population that do not fit the Denis classification include apophyseal avulsion fractures and SCIWORA. Apophyseal injuries, typically of the lumbar spine, occur in adolescents as a result of trauma. The mechanism is thought to be related to flexion with a portion of the posterior corner of the vertebral body (ring apophysis) fracturing and displacing posteriorly into the spinal canal. Symptoms may mimic disc herniation, although the offending structure is bone and cartilage rather than disc material (Fig. 19-5).[16,18]

The concept of SCIWORA was popularized by Pang and Wilberger[51] who described their experience at the University of Pittsburgh. They noted a series of patients presenting with traumatic SCIs that were not evident on plain radiographs or tomograms. Several mechanisms to explain these findings have been proposed, including spinal cord stretch and vascular disruption/infarction. MRI studies have confirmed patterns of both cord edema and hemorrhage in such cases.[25] Important additional facts about SCIWORA include the finding that some

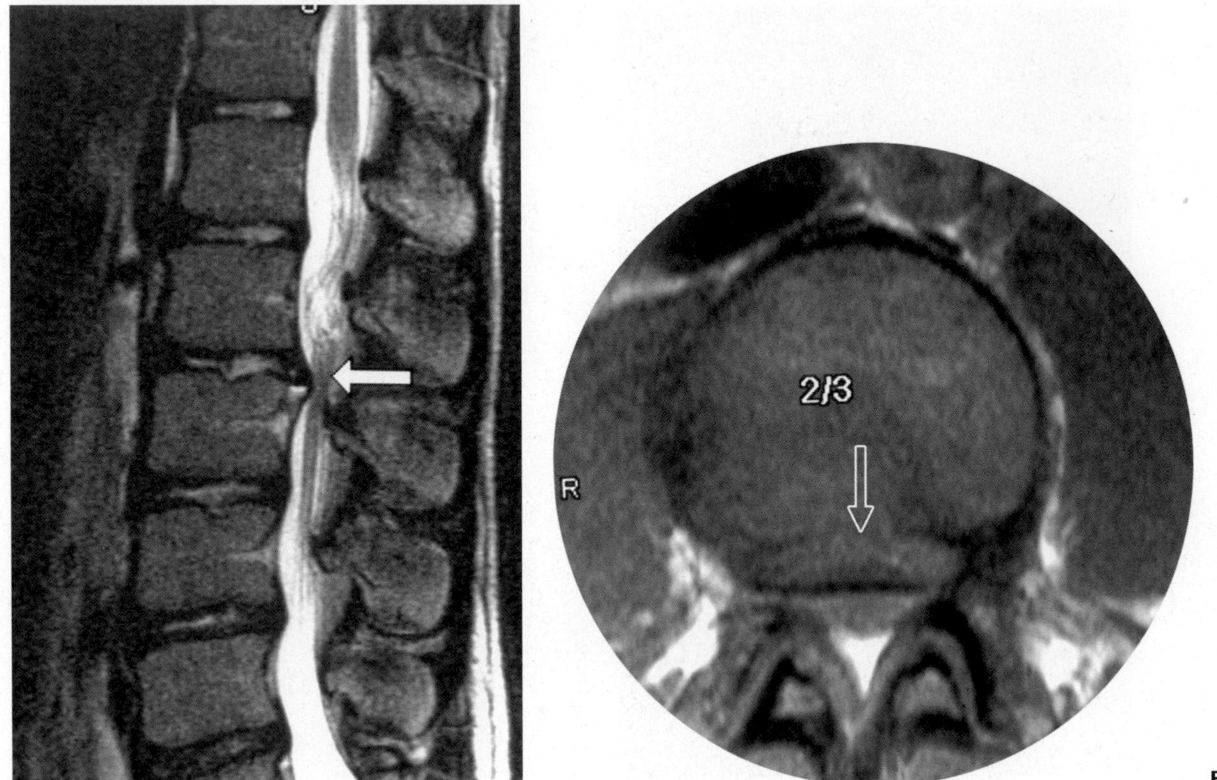

FIGURE 19-5 Ring apophyseal avulsion injuries. **A.** This lateral MRI image demonstrates displacement of the ring apophysis, which functionally acts as a disc herniation. This, however, represents largely a bony and cartilaginous fragment, which results in neural element compression. **B.** Transverse image demonstrating canal stenosis associated with this injury.

patients had a delayed onset of their neurologic deficits. Transient neurologic symptoms were persistent in many who later developed a lasting deficit. Additionally, the younger patients (less than 8 years old) had more severe neurologic involvement.[5,50,51]

Radiographic Evaluation

Following a careful clinical examination of all patients with a suspected spinal injury, plain radiographs are usually valuable. An alert, cooperative patient without pain or tenderness in the back can be cleared without radiographs. However, any patient with a significant mechanism or associated injury (motor vehicle accident, fall from greater than 10 feet, major long bone fracture, cervical or head injury) requires thoracolumbar spine radiographs if they have spinal tenderness, are obtunded, or have a distracting injury. Initial films should include supine AP and lateral views of the thoracic and lumbar spine. In addition, due to the strong association between cervical spine fractures and thoracolumbar spine fractures after blunt vehicular trauma, routine imaging of the complete spine when a cervical fracture is identified is indicated.[75]

Plain radiographs often show with relatively subtle findings that should be sought in all cases. On AP radiographs, soft tissue shadows may be widened by paravertebral hematoma. The bony anatomy is viewed to evaluate for loss of height of the vertebral body as compared to adjacent levels. Similar comparisons can be made with regard to pedicle width and interspinous spacing. The lateral radiographs give important information about the sagittal plane: anterior vertebral wedging or collapse or posterior element distraction or fracture. Careful scrutiny of the plain radiographs is always prudent; however, the CT scan will nearly always be used to clarify any suspected fractures. Antevil et al.[1] reported the sensitivity of plain radiographs to be 70% (14 of 20 patients) for spine trauma, while the sensitivity was 100% for CT scanning (34 of 34 patients).

CT is now a standard component of the evaluation of many trauma patients. Multidetector scanners allow rapid assessment with axial, coronal, and sagittal images for patients with plain radiographic abnormalities. The axial images are best for evaluating the integrity of the spinal canal in cases of a burst fracture, while the sagittal views will demonstrate vertebral body compression as well as posterior element distraction or fracture. In addition, major dislocations easily seen on plain radiographs will be better understood with regard to the space left in the spinal canal for the neurologic elements. The amount of spinal canal compromise has been correlated with the probability of neurological deficit.[48]

MRI is the modality of choice for evaluating the discs, spinal cord, and posterior ligamentous structures.[33,39,66] Although more difficult to obtain in a multiply injured patient, this study is mandatory in patients with a neurologic deficit in order to assess the potential cause of cord dysfunction. The MRI is able to distinguish areas of spinal cord hemorrhage and edema. Assessment of the posterior ligamentous complex it critical in differentiating stable and unstable burst fractures, as well as compression fractures and flexion-distraction injuries. Although subject to overinterpretation, MRI has been shown to correlate very well with intraoperative findings of the structural integrity of the posterior soft tissues.[39]

SURGICAL AND APPLIED ANATOMY

The thoracic and lumbar spine link the upper and lower extremities through the torso. The twelve thoracic and five lumbar vertebrae are joined by intravertebral discs and strong ligaments, both anteriorly and posteriorly. The bony architecture of the vertebrae varies, with the smaller thoracic vertebrae having a more shingled overlapping configuration compared to the lumbar segments. The thoracic facets are oriented in the sagittal plane while those in the lumbar spine lie nearly in the sagittal plane (Fig. 19-6).

Mobility is less in the thoracic spine owing both to the adjacent and linked rib cage, as well as the smaller intervertebral discs. The ribs make an important connection between the vertebra with each rib head articulating across a given disc's space. This is in contrast to the relatively mobile lumbar segments, which have thick intravertebral discs that permit substantial flexion-extension, lateral bending, and axial rotation motion. The junction between the stiffer thoracic spine and more flexible lumbar spine is a region of frequent injury because of this transition between these two regions, which have differing inherent regional stability.

Ligamentous components include the anterior and posterior longitudinal ligaments, facet capsules, ligamentum flavum, and interspinous and supraspinous ligaments. Together, these structures limit the motion between vertebrae to protect the neuro-

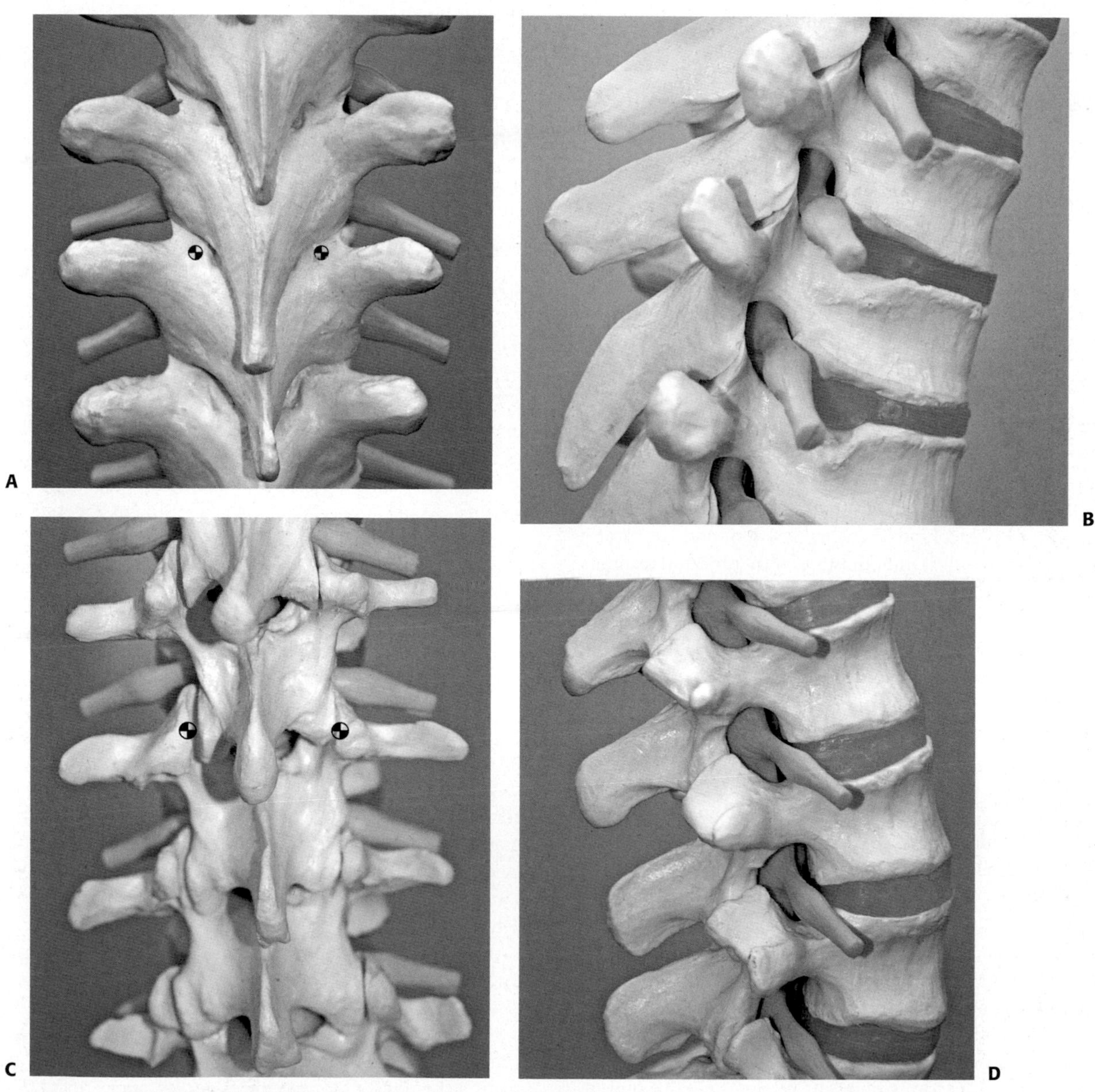

FIGURE 19-6 A,B. Thoracic spine posterior and lateral views demonstrating the overlapping lamina and spinous processes present in this region. The circles mark the location of the thoracic pedicles, which may be important in surgical reconstruction. **C,D.** Lumbar spine posterior and lateral projections demonstrating the differences in lumbar spine anatomy. Again, the circles mark locations of the lumbar pedicles relative to the facets and transverse processes.

logic elements. The anterior longitudinal ligament is rarely disrupted in flexion injuries but may be rendered incompetent by extension loading or a severe fracture dislocation. On the contrary, flexion is the primary mechanism of injury to the posterior ligaments—supraspinous and interspinous, facet capsule, and ligamentum flavum. The healing capacity of the completely torn posterior ligamentous complex is limited, whereas bony fractures are more likely to heal with resultant stability.

The neural anatomy varies over the length of the thoracolumbar spine as well. The space within the canal is largest in the lumbar spine. The spinal cord traverses the entirety of the thoracic spine and typically terminates as the conus medullaris at the L-1 or L-2 level. The cauda equina occupies the dural tube below this level, and injuries below L-1 are generally less likely to lead to permanent neurologic deficit. This is not to say that compression at this level cannot be serious, and careful examination of the perineum for sensation as well as rectal tone is important in the evaluation of potential conus medullaris and cauda equina syndromes.

CURRENT TREAMENT OPTIONS

Compression Fractures

Anterior vertebral body compression fractures are the most likely fractures to occur in the thoracic spine secondary to axial compression and flexion loading. The anterior aspect of the vertebral body is involved, but the posterior wall of the vertebral body is by definition intact. The degree of wedging is variable, as is the loss of anterior height. These are nearly always stable injuries, although examination of the posterior soft tissues is required to rule out any more severe flexion-distraction injury, and a CT scan is required to rule out a burst fracture (Fig. 19-7).

An isolated fracture without neurologic involvement is the most common thoracolumbar fracture pattern and can nearly always be treated with immobilization with a brace that limits flexion, provides pain relief, and reduces further loading of the fracture. Most fractures heal in 4 to 6 weeks without significant additional collapse; however, radiographs in the first several weeks should be obtained to follow the sagittal alignment. Long-term studies have suggested modest remodeling capacity of compression fractures occurring in childhood.[43,54] Asymmetric growth at the endplates seems to allow some correction in the wedged alignment over time in the skeletally immature patient. Long-term results of compression fractures have been generally favorable, although fractures of the endplates are associated with later disc degeneration.[34]

If the kyphosis associated with a fracture is initially more than 40 degrees or markedly alters the local sagittal alignment, surgical treatment may be considered. This is most frequent in multiple adjacent compression fractures that together create unacceptable kyphosis. The preferred surgical treatment of such fractures is generally a posterior compression instrumentation construct that spans one or two levels above and below the affected vertebrae. Anterior surgical treatment is rarely required. The intact posterior vertebral wall provides a fulcrum to achieve kyphosis correction. The method of posterior fixation may be either hooks or pedicle screws. A posterior fusion over the instrumented segments ensures a lasting stable correction. Cadaver studies and clinical studies on the use of balloon vertebroplasty with calcium phosphate cement in adult patients are encouraging, as this technique may be a potentially viable option to treat compression fractures with significant angulation.[36,69,70]

Osteoporosis of a variety of etiologies may affect children and adolescents to a degree that predisposes them to insufficiency fractures that are most often compression fractures (Fig. 19-8). Multiple-level fractures are more frequent in this setting, and problematic kyphosis may develop. Differentiating new from old fractures can be difficult if serial radiographs are not available. A thoracolumbosacral orthosis (TLSO) for a period of time longer than typically used for simple compression fracture healing may be necessary to prevent progressive kyphosis, though treating the primary cause of the osteopenia is critical to maintaining normal alignment in such cases. An endocrinologic evaluation and assessment of bone density by dual energy x-ray absorptiometry are advised.

Burst Fractures

Axial compression injuries that are more severe and extend into the posterior wall of the vertebral body are labeled as burst fractures. The treatment and classification of this fracture pattern are controversial areas of spinal trauma management. There are clearly some burst fractures that can be easily managed nonoperatively in a brace and others that collapse further, resulting in increased deformity unless surgically stabilized. Defining the characteristics of stable and unstable burst fractures has been attempted by several authors.[14,24,46] An additional compounding variable in the treatment algorithm is SCI, which is more frequent with burst fractures than with compression fractures.

Assuming an intact neurologic system, defining stable and unstable burst fractures has been attempted based on the degree of comminution, loss of vertebral height, kyphotic wedging, and integrity of the posterior ligamentous complex. A load-sharing classification system assigns points based on comminution, fragment apposition, and kyphosis.[46] Although the Denis classification suggests that all burst fractures are unstable because of the involvement of at least two columns, it is clear that in many cases the addition of a third-column injury (posterior ligamentous complex) is required to result in a truly unstable condition. Some advocate differentiating stable and unstable burst fractures solely on the integrity of the posterior ligamentous complex.[63,76] When a burst fracture is deemed stable, it must be done so on a presumptive basis. Treatment is then based on an extension molded cast or TLSO with the goal of allowing an upright position and ambulation.[64] Frequent radiographic and neurologic follow-up is necessary to identify early failures. Depending on the age of the patient and severity of the fracture, immobilization is suggested for a duration of 2 to 4 months.

Studies of immature patients treated for burst fractures are uncommon,[37] yet much of the adult literature provides valuable information about the outcomes to expect following nonoperative treatment. Most of these fractures in adults heal with little change in kyphosis and function and minimal, if any, residual pain.[73] It is reasonable to expect adolescent patients to heal at least as well and probably even faster. Wood et al.[76] compared operative and nonoperative treatment in a prospective randomized study of patients with burst fractures who were neurologically intact with a normal posterior ligamentous complex. The

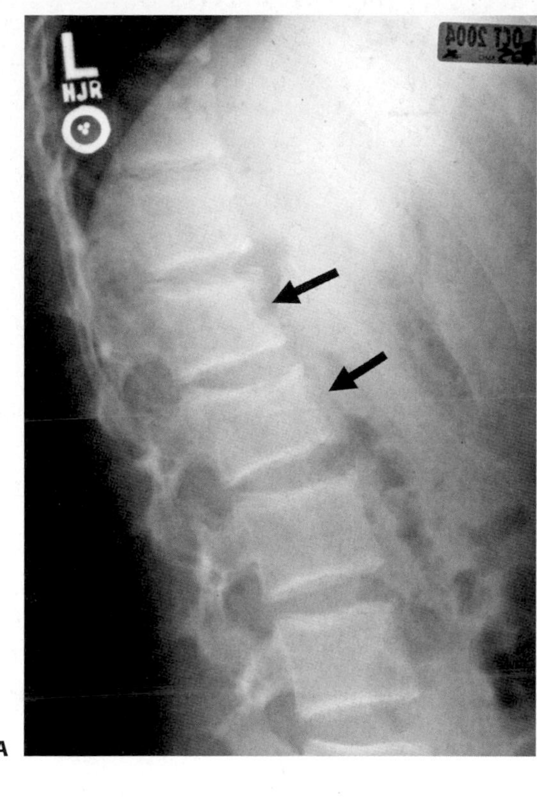

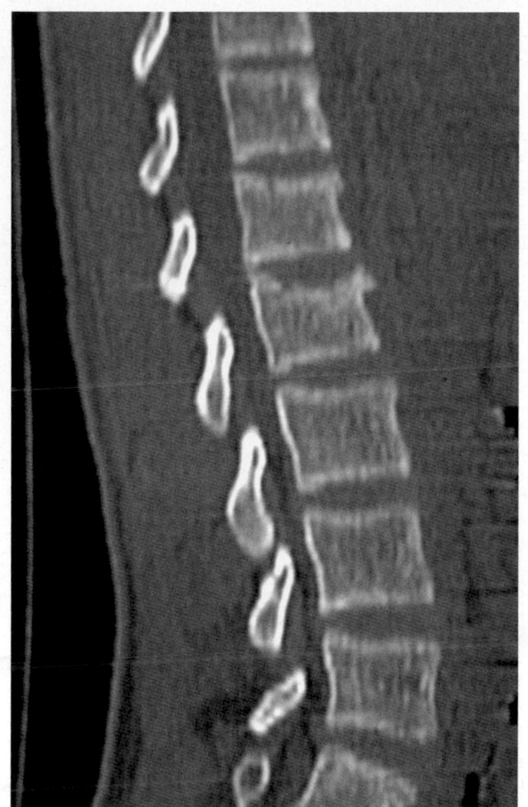

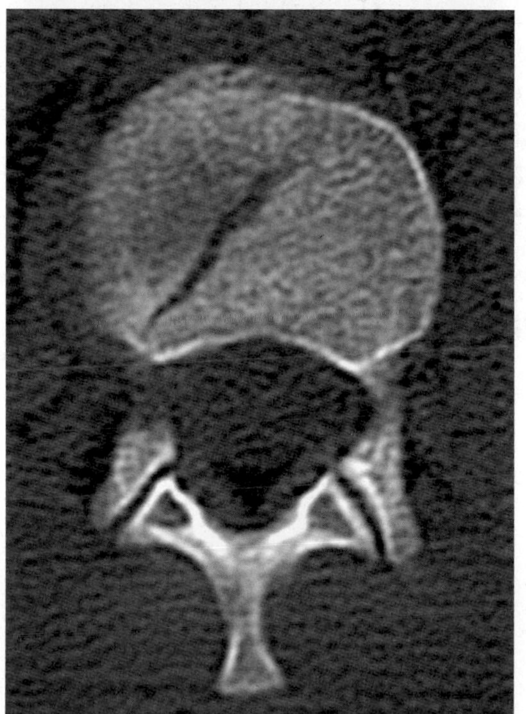

FIGURE 19-7 A. This lateral radiograph demonstrates two upper lumbar vertebrae with slight loss of height suggestive of compression fractures. **B,C.** The CT images confirm an intact posterior vertebral body wall. This injury, therefore, represents a compression fracture rather than a burst fracture injury.

radiologic and functional outcomes were not substantially different, and these authors concluded that nonoperative treatment should be considered when the posterior ligamentous complex and neurologic function are intact.[76] Functional outcome does not appear to correlate with the degree of spinal kyphosis, although long-term studies of scoliosis treatment do suggest that an alteration of sagittal alignment may be detrimental (flat back syndrome) in the long term.

Even some fractures with posterior ligamentous complex disruption have been successfully treated nonoperatively[12]; however, these three-column injuries are often operatively stabilized. When surgical treatment is selected, either an anterior or posterior approach can be used, although this also remains controversial. Anterior stabilization generally involves discectomy and strut grafting that spans the fractured vertebra. Stabilization with a plate or dual-rod system is appropriate. Posterior

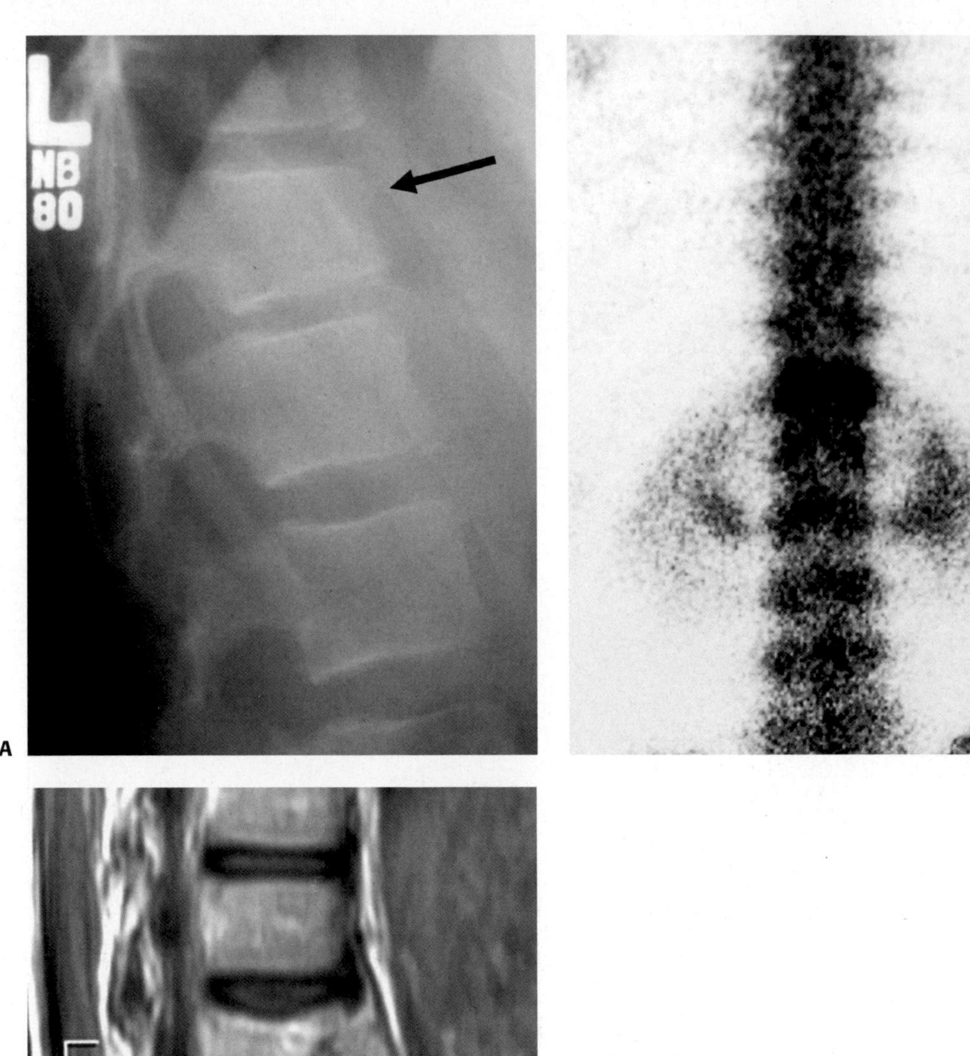

FIGURE 19-8 A. Lateral radiograph demonstrating what appears to be a routine compression fracture. The patient did not have a significant history of trauma; however, pain was present and a bone scan was obtained to further evaluate this site. **B.** The bone scan demonstrated markedly increased uptake, confirming an acute process and prompting additional study. **C.** An MRI was obtained, which demonstrated loss of height and a lesion within the anterior aspect of the vertebral body, which was later confirmed to be an infectious process.

options include pedicle screw fixation one or two levels above and below the fractured vertebra. Advances in the application of posterior instrumentation for thoracolumbar fractures has demonstrated encouraging, early outcomes with fracture stabilization without fusion and in minimally invasive surgical techniques.[72,74]

The decision to proceed anteriorly or posteriorly for the surgical treatment of a burst fracture is largely dictated by surgeon preference and, to some degree, the features of the fracture. Posterior approaches are familiar to all surgeons and can easily be extended over many levels. Decompression of the spinal cord can be achieved by indirect or direct methods. Restoration of the sagittal alignment frequently leads to spontaneous repositioning of the posteriorly displaced vertebral body fracture fragments. If additional reduction of posterior wall fragments is required, direct fracture reduction can be accomplished with a posterolateral or transpedicular decompression.[20] This also allows additional anterior column bone grafting that may add structural integrity and speed fracture healing.

The anterior approach allows direct canal decompression

through a corpectomy of the fractured vertebra. Structural strut grafting restores the integrity of the anterior column. With this graft, a load-sharing anterior plate or rod system completes the reconstruction. This approach deals most directly with the pathology, which in a burst fractures lies within the anterior and middle vertebral columns (Fig. 19-9). Proponents of the anterior approach cite better biomechanical stabilization of the unstable spine, better correction of segmental kyphosis, and less loss of correction postoperatively.[61,62,77]

Flexion-Distraction Injuries (Chance Fractures)

The treatment of flexion-distraction injuries is dictated by the particular injury pattern and the associated abdominal injuries. In general, these fractures are reduced by an extension moment that can be maintained with either a cast or internal fixation. A hyperextension cast is idea for younger patients (less than approximately 10 years) with a primary bony injury pattern and no significant intra-abdominal injuries. As described above, the posterior disruption may pass through ligaments or joint

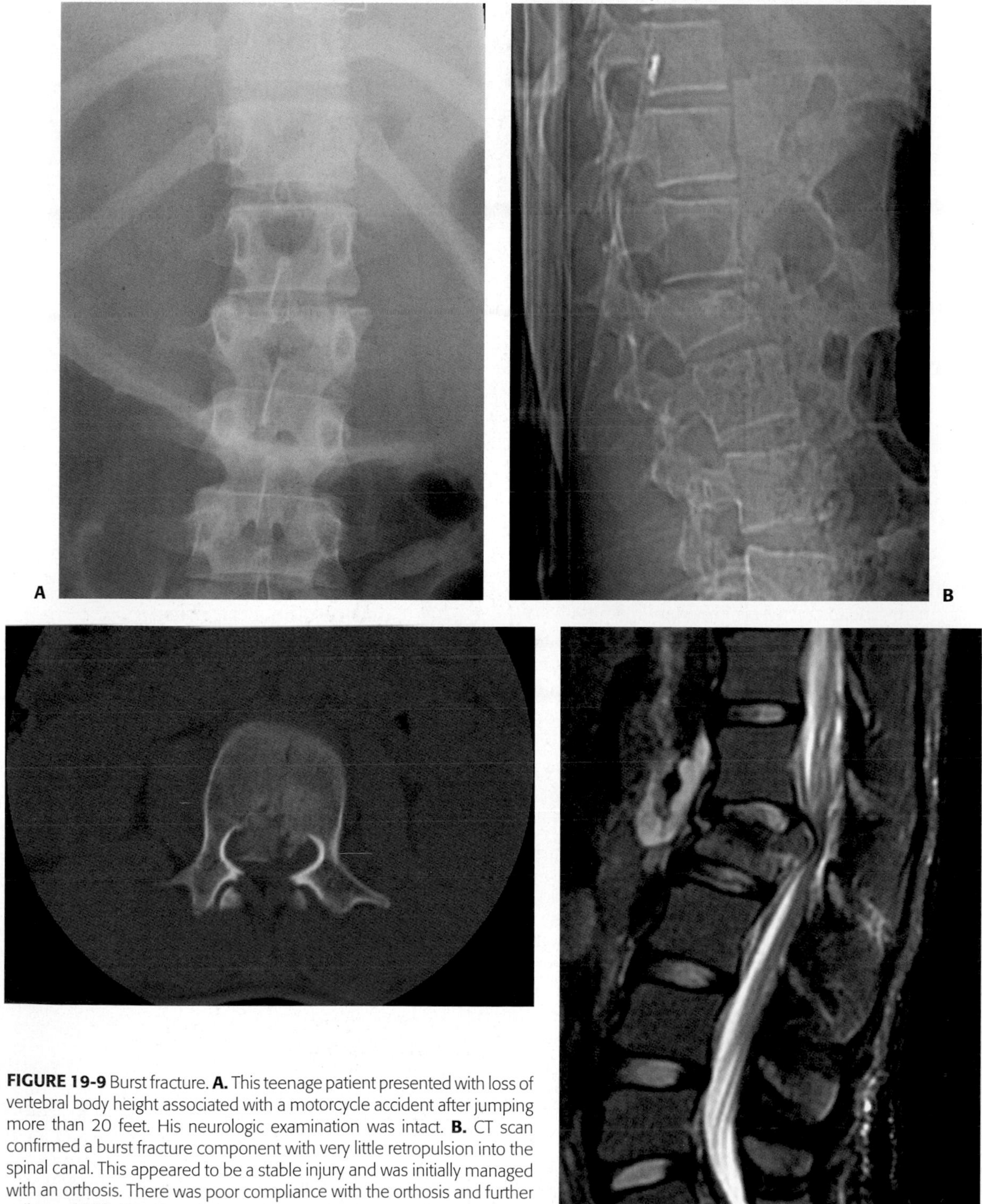

FIGURE 19-9 Burst fracture. **A.** This teenage patient presented with loss of vertebral body height associated with a motorcycle accident after jumping more than 20 feet. His neurologic examination was intact. **B.** CT scan confirmed a burst fracture component with very little retropulsion into the spinal canal. This appeared to be a stable injury and was initially managed with an orthosis. There was poor compliance with the orthosis and further collapse **(C,D)**. *(continues)*

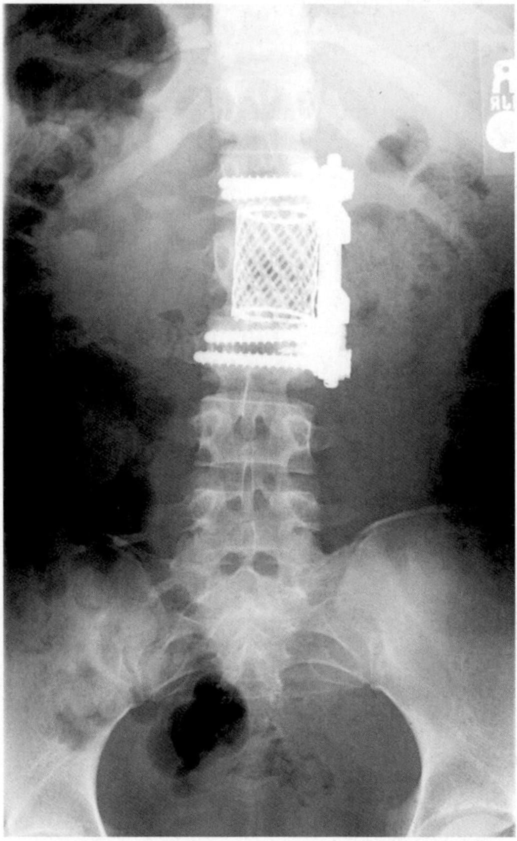

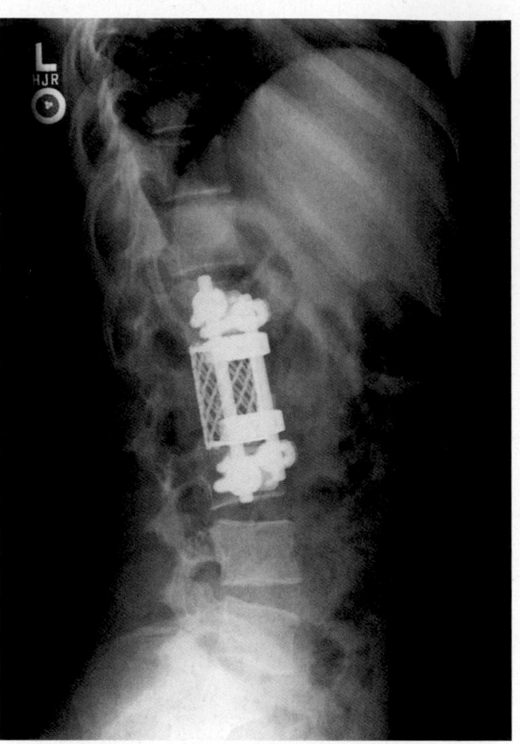

FIGURE 19-9 (*Continued*) Given the lack of compliance and progressive kyphosis, the patient underwent anterior reconstruction with an iliac crest strut graft and plating **(E,F)**.

capsules in a purely soft tissue plane of injury or traverse an entirely bony path. The distinction is important, because bony fractures have the potential for primary bony union, while the severe ligamentous injuries are less likely to heal with lasting stability without surgical intervention. As such, the greater the degree of ligamentous/facet disruption, the more likely the need for stabilization with an arthrodesis of the injured motion segment. Options for internal fixation include posterior wiring in young children (supplemented with a cast) and segmental fixation in a primarily compressive mode (Fig. 19-10).

Fracture-Dislocations

These highly unstable injuries nearly always require surgical stabilization. When the spinal cord function remains intact, instrumented fusion gives the greatest chance for maintaining cord function. On the other hand, if a complete SCI has occurred, internal fixation will aid in the rehabilitation process, allowing early transfers and upright sitting. At least two levels above and below the level of injury should be instrumented to ensure restoration of stability. In cases of SCI below the age of 10 years, a longer fusion may be considered to reduce the incidence and severity of subsequent paralytic scoliosis. Those injured after the adolescent growth spurt are at low risk for late deformity if the fracture is well aligned at the time of initial fixation (Fig. 19-11).

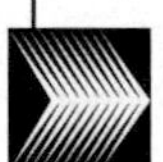

AUTHORS' PREFERRED TREATMENT

Compression Fractures

Nearly all are managed nonoperatively in an off-the-shelf Jewitt brace. Occasionally, a fracture is too proximal for such an orthosis and an extension to the chin/occiput is required. For fractures proximal to T6, a Minerva brace is used. These fractures typically heal within 4 to 6 weeks, when the immobilization can be discontinued. Activities should be limited for an additional 6 weeks. Compression fractures with more than 50% loss of anterior vertebral height are considered for either a closed reduction in an extension molded body cast or surgical correction with posterior instrumentation. The determination of which of these two approaches to choose is based on associated injuries and a discussion with the family. Compression fractures associated with neurological injury are managed surgically.

Burst Fractures

Our preferred approach to neurologically intact patients with burst fractures is nonoperative approach in light of recent studies. If the neurologic status is normal and the posterior soft tissues are intact, a TLSO or cast is used for 3 months. A cast is used when local kyphosis is more than 20 degrees, and the cast is placed in a hyperextension position in an

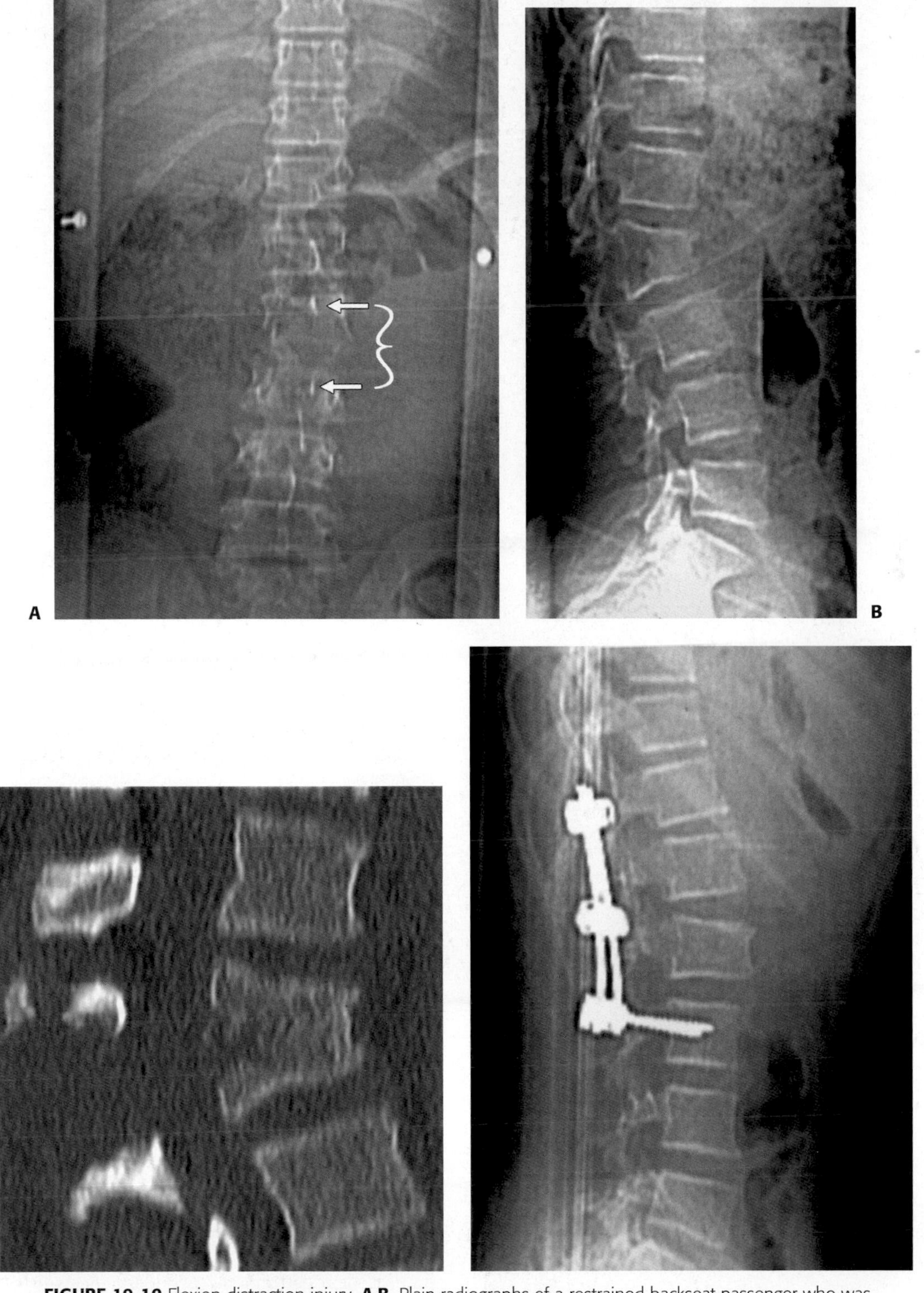

FIGURE 19-10 Flexion-distraction injury. **A,B.** Plain radiographs of a restrained backseat passenger who was involved in a motor vehicle accident. The wedging of L2 with posterior distraction is visible on the lateral radiograph. The intraspinous widening is noted on the AP radiograph as well (*arrows*). **C.** Sagittal CT images confirm the injury pattern. **D.** Lateral radiographs following reconstruction with posterior spinal instrumentation.

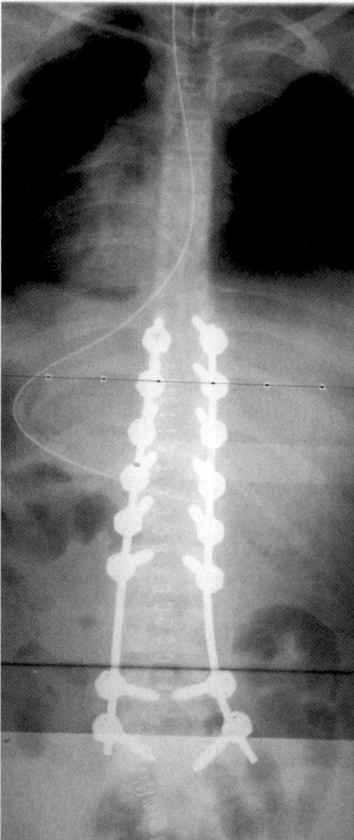
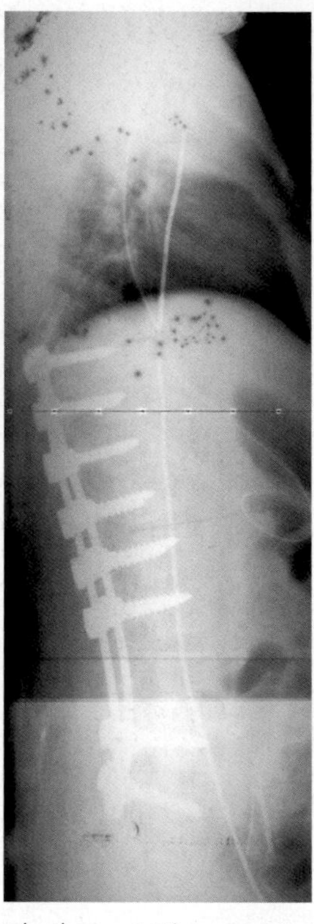

FIGURE 19-11 A,B. AP and lateral radiographs demonstrating reconstruction after a lower thoracic level complete SCI associated with fracture-dislocation in the lumbar spine combined with a burst fracture in the lower thoracic spine. Given the complete paraplegia present, a relatively long instrumentation construct was selected to provide a stable foundation in this skeletally immature patient. Four years postoperatively, the patient has no evidence of progressive spinal deformity; however, there is certainly some risk remaining of developing pelvic obliquity and upper thoracic deformity given the paraplegia.

attempt to restore sagittal alignment. If the posterior soft tissues are disrupted (and the patient is neurologically intact), posterior surgical stabilization is preferred. An anterior decompression is used in patients with SCI if canal compromise is more than 50%.

Flexion-Distraction Injuries

Our treatment of Chance fractures is based on two findings: associated abdominal injuries and the presence of a ligamentous component to the fracture. If either exists, surgical treatment is the preferred approach. Casting in extension is appropriate for fractures that transverse an entirely bony plane without intra-abdominal pathology. A thigh is incorporated into the cast for greater control of lumbar lordosis. Surgical treatment is by a posterior approach and includes only the involved vertebrae. Monosegmental pedicle screw fixation is generally preferred.

Fracture-Dislocation

Posterior surgery is the treatment of choice for all fracture-dislocations with or without neurologic injury (Fig. 19-12). The timing of such intervention depends on the associated injuries and the ability of the patient to tolerate surgical intervention; however, stabilization as early as possible is preferred. SCI nearly always complicates the management of these injuries, and a deteriorating neurologic examination makes surgical treatment of the spine an emergency that should be treated as quickly as possible.

Steroid Treatment

Despite the controversies, we continue to follow the recommendations of the Third National Acute Spinal Cord Injury Study and prescribe methylprednisolone if it can be given within 8 hours of the time of injury. We are skeptical that this provides significant benefit, but we believe this remains the current medical and legal standard.

PEARLS AND PITFALLS

Pearls:

- Do not hesitate to get advanced imaging, especially CT scanning.
- Understand the mechanics of the injury to develop a rational treatment plan.
- Always seek to identify additional levels of spinal injury when one is discovered.
- Document the neurologic examination precisely and repeat it often.

Pitfalls:

- Watch for associated injuries, both musculoskeletal and others.
- Do not let MRI/CT findings replace a careful examination of the back.
- Monitor neurologic status carefully because an unrecognized change may limit the ability to intervene early and prevent permanent sequelae.

CONTROVERSIES AND FUTURE DIRECTIONS

Several areas of controversy remain with regards to the management of acute SCI associated with thoracolumbar fractures. These include both nonoperative and operative methods of treatment. Investigations into the benefits of steroids in mitigating the effects of the secondary phase of SCI that follows the acute trauma have been mixed, although clinical trials have suggested benefit in specific instances.

SCI that results from direct trauma may acutely disrupt the neural tissue, possibly with compression remaining from fracture fragments or displacement. Once the initial injury occurs, biochemical cascades are set into motion, resulting in further injury of spinal cord tissue. Experimental studies have suggested that steroids administered early in the postinjury period could limit of these detrimental secondary effects. Based on randomized clinical trails of methylprednisolone administration after acute spinal cord injury,[6,7] current recommendations for steroid use are dependent on the timing of administration relative to the occurrence of the injury. If the time lapse is less than 3 hours, a bolus of 30 mg/kg of methylprednisolone is followed by an hourly infusion of 5.4 mg/kg for 24 hours duration. If the lapse between injury and treatment is 3 to 8 hours, an infusion of the same dose is continued for 48 hours. More importantly, if more than 8 hours have passed following the SCI, no steroids are recommended.[7]

The benefit of steroids with regard to functional levels of recovery has been questioned, and in all studies of high-dose

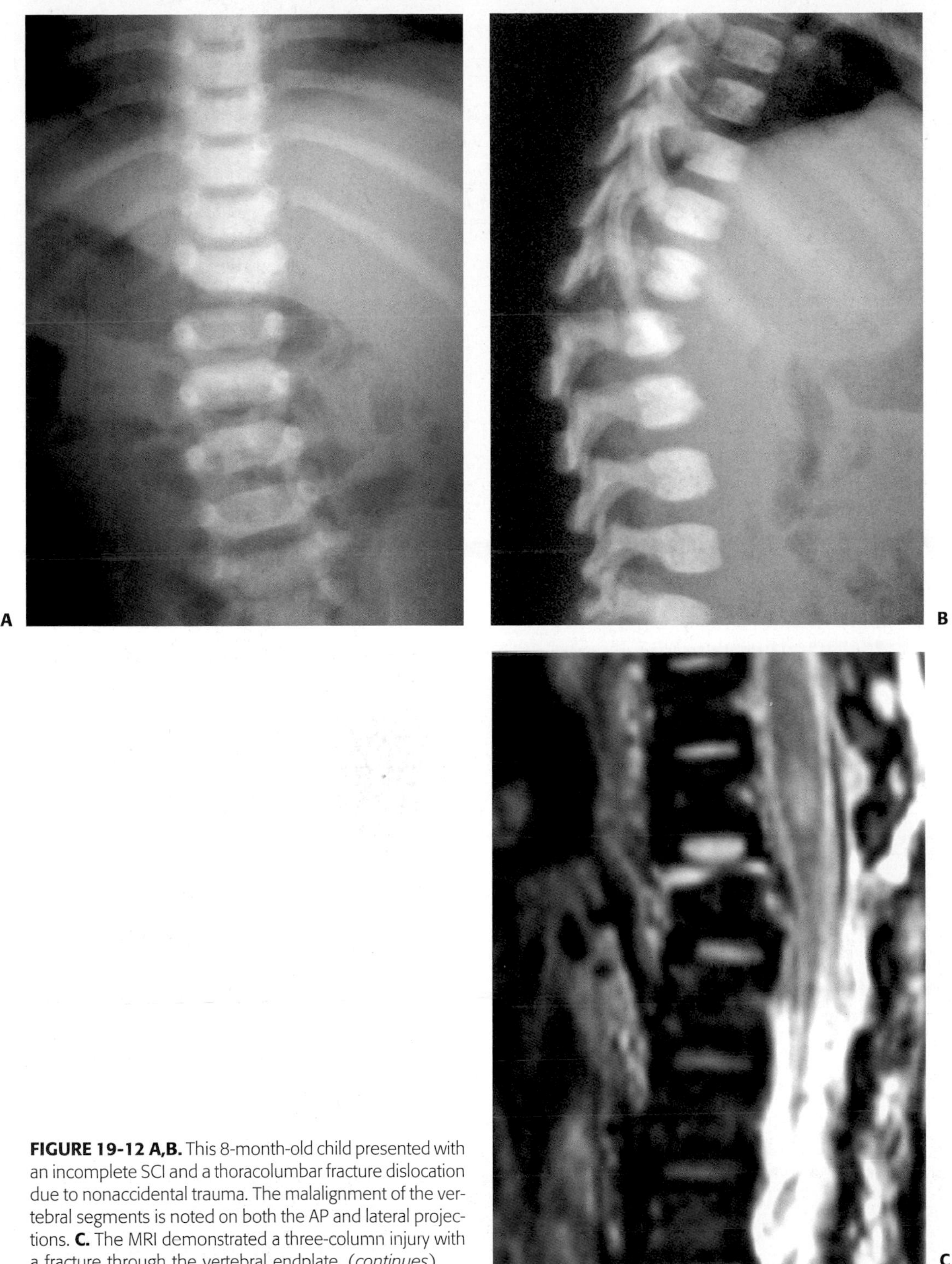

FIGURE 19-12 A,B. This 8-month-old child presented with an incomplete SCI and a thoracolumbar fracture dislocation due to nonaccidental trauma. The malalignment of the vertebral segments is noted on both the AP and lateral projections. **C.** The MRI demonstrated a three-column injury with a fracture through the vertebral endplate. (*continues*)

steroid use, there has been an increased complication rate. Infection is the most common with both pneumonia and sepsis occurring. Steroids are known to depress the immune response.[19] These issues have resulted in an inconsistent adoption of the National Acute Spinal Cord Injury Study recommendations.

The timing and necessity of spinal decompression for an SCI also remains debated. Traditional teaching suggests no benefit to decompression when a complete SCI exists. This may be true, but if early decompression of an incomplete SCI is beneficial, and there are experimental data to suggest it is, then it may be impossible to determine early on if the patient has an incomplete injury but remains in spinal shock. Spinal shock may last for 24 hours, leaving an incomplete SCI patient completely unresponsive with regard to spinal cord function. The data to suggest a benefit to early decompression are largely experimental; however, a clinical study also reported a benefit. In a series of 91 pediatric patients, 66 with immediate decompression were compared to 25 with whom decompression was delayed. Improvement of at least one Frankel grade occurred in one half of the early decompression patients compared to

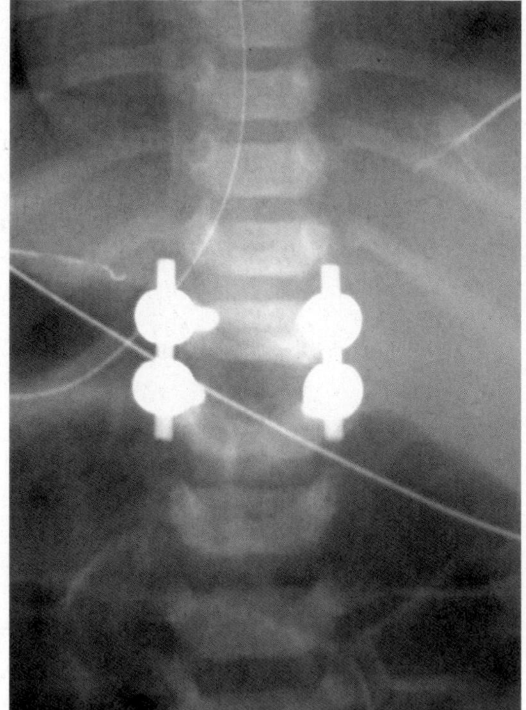

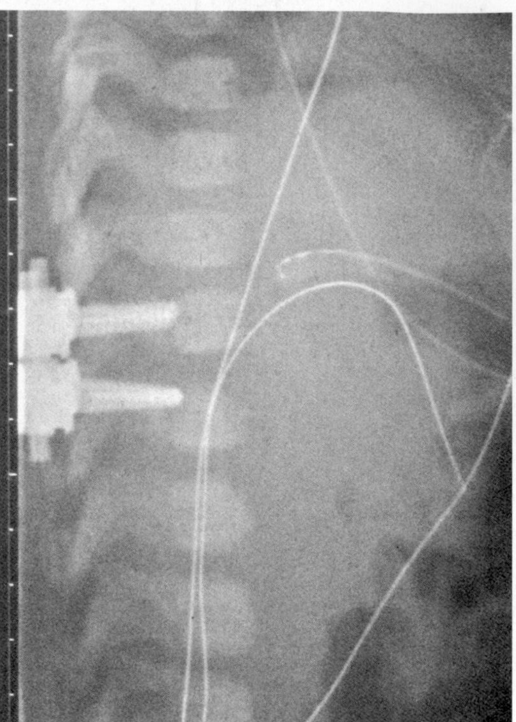

FIGURE 19-12 (*Continued*) **D,E.** The patient had an open reduction and instrumentation with pedicle screw fixation using a 3.5-mm cervical system.

one quarter of those that who had delayed decompression.[52] Early surgery has been documented to shorten the intensive care unit stays and length of hospitalizations, shorten time on mechanical ventilation support, and lower overall complication rates in patients with thoracolumbar spine injuries.[11]

In pediatric patients with SCI, it is difficult to argue against spinal cord decompression if the MRI documents persistent compression in the setting of an SCI. Pediatric patients have a substantial potential for recovery, and reducing pressure on the neural elements may be important in maximizing functional recovery. There is little controversy if spinal cord function is deteriorating in a patient with a known compressive lesion. This is an emergency that warrants decompression by either an anterior or posterior approach. Realignment of the spinal column and removal of fragments from the canal are required. The exact surgical approach depends on the location of offending structures and the nature of the instability.

REFERENCES

1. Antevil JL, Sise MJ, Sack DI, et al. Spiral computed tomography for the initial evaluation of spine trauma: a new standard of care? J Trauma 2006:61:382–387.
2. Augutis M, Levi R. Pediatric spinal cord injury in Sweden: incidence, etiology, and outcome. Spinal Cord 2003;41:328–336.
3. Baghaie M, Gillet P, Dondelinger RF, et al. Vertebra plana: benign or malignant lesion? Pediatr Radiol 1996;26:431–433.
4. Beaunoyer M, St-Vil D, Lallier M, et al. Abdominal injuries associated with thoracolumbar fractures after motor vehicle collision. Pediatr Surg 2001;36:760–762.
5. Bosch PP, Vogt MT, Ward WT. Pediatric spinal cord injury without radiographic abnormality (SCIWORA): the absence of occult instability and lack of indication for bracing. Spine 2002;27:2788–2800.
6. Bracken MB. Methylprednisolone in the management of acute spinal cord injuries. Med J Aust 1990;153:368.
7. Bracken MB, Shepard MJ, Holford TR, et al. Administration of methylprednisolone for 24 or 48 hours or tirilazad mesylate for 48 hours in the treatment of acute spinal cord injury. Results of the Third National Acute Spinal Cord Injury Randomized Controlled Trial. National Acute Spinal Cord Injury Study. JAMA 1997;277:1597–1604.
8. Carreon LY, Glassman SD, Campbell MJ. Pediatric Spine fractures: a review of 137 hospital admissions. J Spinal Disord 2004;17:477–482.
9. Carrion WV, Dormans JP, Drummond DS, et al. Circumferential growth plate fracture of the thoracolumbar spine from child abuse. J Pediatr Orthop 1996;16:210–214.
10. Catz A, Thaleisnik M, Fishel B, et al. Recovery of neurologic function after spinal cord injury in Israel. Spine 2002;27:1733–1735.
11. Chipman JG, Deuser WE, Beilman GJ. Early surgery for thoracolumbar spine injuries decreases complications. J Trauma 2004;56:52–57.
12. Chow GH, Nelson BJ, Beghard JS, et al. Functional outcome of thoracolumbar burst fractures managed with hyperextension casting or bracing and early mobilization. Spine 1996;21:2170–2175.
13. Cirak B, Ziegfeld S, Knight VM, et al. Spinal injuries in children. Pediatr Surg 2004; 39:607–612.
14. Denis F. The three-column spine and its significance in the classification of acute thoracolumbar spinal injuries. Spine 1983;8:817–831.
15. Diamond P, Hansen CM, Christofersen MR. Child abuse presenting as a thoracolumbar spinal fracture dislocation: a case report. Pediatr Emerg Care 1994;10:83–86.
16. Dietemann JL, Runge M, Badoz A, et al. Radiology of posterior lumbar apophyseal ring fractures: report of 13 cases. Neuroradiology 1988;30:337–344.
17. Dogan S, Safavi-Abbasi S, Theodore N, et al. Thoracolumbar and sacral spinal injuries in children and adolescents: a review of 89 cases. J Neurosurg 2007;106:426–433.
18. Epstein NE, Epstein JA. Limbus lumbar vertebral fractures in 27 adolescents and adults. Spine 1991;16:962–966.
19. Galandiuk S, Raque G, Appel S, et al. The two-edged sword of large-dose steroids for spinal cord trauma. Ann Surg 1993;218:419–425.
20. Gambardella G, Coman TC, Zaccone C, et al. Posterolateral approach in the treatment of unstable vertebral body fractures of the thoracic-lumbar junction with incomplete spinal cord injury in the paediatric age group. Childs Nerv Syst 2003;19:35–41.
21. Garcia RA, Gaebler-Spira D, Sisung C, et al. Functional improvement after pediatric spinal cord injury. Am J Phys Med Rehabil 2002;81:458–463.
22. Garg S, Mehta S, Dormans JP. Langerhans cell histiocytosis of the spine in children. Long-term follow-up. J Bone Joint Surg Am 2004;86-A:1740–1750.
23. Gellad FE, Levine AM, Joslyn JN, et al. Pure thoracolumbar facet dislocation: clinical features and CT appearance. Radiology 1986;161:505–508.
24. Gertzbein SD, Court-Brown CM. Rationale for the management of flexion-distraction injuries of the thoracolumbar spine based on a new classification. J Spinal Disord 1989; 2:176–183.
25. Grabb PA, Pang D. Magnetic resonance imaging in the evaluation of spinal cord injury without radiographic abnormality in children. Neurosurgery 1994;35:406–414.
26. Green RA, Saifuddin A. Whole spine MRI in the assessment of acute vertebral body trauma. Skeletal Radiol 2004;33:129–135.
27. Griffet J, Bastiani-Griffet F, El-Hayek T, et al. Management of seat-belt syndrome in children. Gravity of 2-point seat-belt. Eur J Pediatr Surg 2002;12:63–66.
28. Hadley MN, Zabramski JM, Browner CM, et al. Pediatric spinal trauma. Review of 122 cases of spinal cord and vertebral column injuries. Neurosurg Clin N Am 1988;68: 18–24.
29. Haffner DL, Hoffer MM, Wiedebusch R. Etiology of Children's Spinal Injuries at Rancho Los Amigos. Spine 1993;18:679–684.
30. Hashimoto T, Kanada K, Abumi K. Relationship between traumatic spinal canal stenosis and neurologic deficits in thoracolumbar burst fractures. Spine 1988;13:1268–1272.

31. Holmes JF, Miller PQ, Panacek EA, et al. Epidemiology of thoracolumbar spine injury in blunt trauma. Acad Emerg Med 2001;8:866–872.
32. Inaba K, Kirkpatrick AW, Finkelstein J, et al. Blunt abdominal aortic trauma in association with thoracolumbar spine fractures. Injury 2001;32:201–207.
33. Kerslake RW, Jaspan T, Worthington BS. Magnetic resonance imaging of spinal trauma. Br J Radiol 1991;64:386–402.
34. Kerttula LI, Serlo WS, Tervonen OA, et al. Posttraumatic findings of the spine after earlier vertebral fracture in young patients: clinical and MRI study. Spine 2000;25: 1104–1108.
35. Kleinman PK, Marks SC. Vertebral body fractures in child abuse. Radiologic-histopathologic correlates. Invest Radiol 1992;27:715–722.
36. Korovessis P, Repantis T, Petsinis G, et al. Direct reduction of thoracolumbar burst fractures by means of balloon kyphoplasty with calcium phosphate and stabilization with pedicle-screw instrumentation and fusion. Spine 2008;33:E100–E108.
37. Lalonde F, Letts M, Yang YP, et al. An analysis of burst fractures of the spine in adolescents. Am J Orthop 2001;30:115–120.
38. Lancourt JE, Dickson JH, Carter RE. Paralytic spinal deformity following traumatic spinal-cord injury in children and adolescents. J Bone Joint Surg Am 1981;63:47–53.
39. Lee HM, Kim HS, Kim DJ, et al. Reliability of magnetic resonance imaging in detecting posterior ligament complex injury in thoracolumbar spinal fractures. Spine 2000;25: 2079–2084.
40. Letts M, Davidson D, Fleuriau-Chateau P, et al. Seat belt fracture with late development of an enterocolic fistula in a child. A case report. Spine 1999;24:1151–1155.
41. Levin TL, Berdon WE, Cassell I, et al. Thoracolumbar fracture with listhesis—an uncommon manifestation of child abuse. Pediatric Radiology 2003;33:305–310.
42. Limb D, Shaw DL, Dickson RA. Neurological injury in thoracolumbar burst fractures. J Bone Joint Surg Br 1995;77:774–777.
43. Mangus KK, Anders M, Ralph H, et al. A modeling capacity of vertebral fractures exists during growth—an up to 47-year follow-up. Spine 2003;28:2087–2092.
44. Mann DC, Dodds JA. Spinal injuries in 57 patients 17 years or younger. Orthopedics 1993;16:159–64.
45. Mayfield JK, Erkkila JC, Winter RB. Spine deformity subsequent to acquired childhood spinal cord injury. J Bone Joint Surg Am 1981;63:1401–411.
46. McCormack T, Karaikovic E, Gaines RW. The load sharing classification of spine fractures. Spine 1994;19:1741–1744.
47. Meehan PL, Viroslav S, Jr EWS. Vertebral collapse in childhood leukemia. J Pediatr Orthop 1995;15:592–595.
48. Meves R, Avanzi O. Correlation between neurologic deficit and spinal canal compromise in 198 patients with thoracolumbar and lumbar fractures. Spine 2005;30:787–791.
49. Mulpuri K, Reilly CW, Perdios A, et al. The spectrum of adominal injuries associated with chance fractures in pediatric patients. Eur J Pediatr Surg 2007;17:322–327.
50. Pang D, Pollack IF. Spinal cord injury without radiographic abnormalityin children—the SCIWORA syndrome. Trauma 1989;29:654–664.
51. Pang D, Wilberger JE. Spinal cord injury without radiographic abnormalities in children. Neurosurg 1982;57:114–129.
52. Papadopoulos SM, Selden NR, Quint DJ, et al. Immediate spinal cord decompression for cervical spinal cord injury: feasibility and outcome. Trauma 2002;52:323–332.
53. Parisini P, DiSilvestre M, Greggi T. Treatment of spinal fractures in children and adolescents: long-term results in 44 patients. Spine 2002;27:1989–1994.
54. Pouliquen JC, Kassis B, Glorion C, et al. Vertebral growth after thoracic or lumbar fracture of the spine in children. J Pediatr Orthop 1997;17:115–120.
55. Reid AB, Letts RM, Black GB. Pediatric Chance fractures: association with intra-abdominal injuries and seatbelt use. Trauma 1990;30:384–391.
56. Ribeiro RC, Pui CH, Schell MJ. Vertebral compression fracture as a presenting feature of acute lymphoblastic leukemia in children. Cancer 1988;61:589–592.
57. Roche C, Carty H. Spine trauma in children. Pediatric Radiology 2001;31:677–700.
58. Ruge JR, Sinson GP, McLeon DG, et al. Pediatric spinal injury: the very young. Neurosurgery 1988;68:25–30.
59. Rumball K, Jarvis J. Seat-belt injuries of the spine in young children. J Bone Joint Surg Br 1992;74:571–574.
60. Santiago R, Guenther E, Carroll K, et al. The clinical presentation of pediatric thoracolumbar fractures. J Trauma 2006;60:187–192.
61. Sasso RC, Best NM, Reilly TM, et al. Anterior-only stabilization of three-column thoracolumbar injuries. J Spinal Disord Tech 2005;18:S7–S14.
62. Sasso RC, Renkens K, Hanson D, et al. Unstable thoracolumbar burst fractures : anterior-only versus short-segment posterior fixation. J Spinal Disord Tech 2006;19:242–248.
63. Shen WJ, Liu TJ, Shen YS. Nonoperative treatment versus posterior fixation for thoracolumbar junction burst fractures without neurologic deficit. Spine 2001;26:1038–1045.
64. Shen WJ, Shen YS. Nonsurgical treatment of three-column thoracolumbar junction burst fractures without neurologic deficit. Spine 1999;24:412–415.
65. Sivit CJ, Taylor GA, Newman KD, et al. Safety-belt injuries in children with lap-belt ecchymosis: CT findings in 61 patients. AJR Am J Roentgenol 1991;157:111–114.
66. Sledge JB, Allred D, Hyman J. Use of magnetic resonance imaging in evaluating injuries to the pediatric thoracolumbar spine. J Pediatr Orthop 2001;21:288–293.
67. Smith AD, Koreska J, Moseley CF. Progression of scoliosis in Duchenne muscular dystrophy. J Bone Joint Surg Am 1989;71:1066–1074.
68. Varonos S, Ansell BM, Reeve J. Vertebral collapse in juvenile chronic arthritis: its relationship with glucocorticoid therapy. Calcif Tissue Int 1987;41:75–78.
69. Verlaan JJ, van de Kraats EB, Oner FC, et al. Bone displacement and the role of longtudinal ligaments during balloon vertebroplasty in traumatic thoracolumbar fractures. Spine 2005;30:1832–1839.
70. Verlaan JJ, van de Kraats EB, Oner Fc, et al. The reduction of endplate fractures during balloon vertebroplasty: a detailed radiological analysis of the treatment of burst fractures using pedicle screws, balloon vertebroplasty, and calcium phosphate cement. Spine 2005;30:1840–1845.
71. Wang MY, Hoh DJ, Leary SP, et al. High rates of neurological improvement following severe traumatic pediatric spinal cord injury. Spine 2004;29:1493–1497.
72. Wang ST, Ma HL, Liu CL, et al. Is fusion necessary for surgically treated burst fractures of the thoracolumbar and lumbar spine? A prospective, randomized study. Spine 2006; 31:2646–2652.
73. Weinstein JN, Collalto P, Lehmann TR. Thoracolumbar "burst" fractures treated conservatively: a long-term follow-up. Spine 1988;13:33–38.
74. Wild MH, Glees M, Plieschnegger C, et al. Five-year follow-up examination after purely minimally invasive posterior stabilization of thoracolumbar fractures: a comparison of minimally invasive percutaneously and conventionally open treated patients. Arch Orthop Trauma Surg 2007;127:335–343.
75. Winslow JE, Hensberry R, Bozeman WP, et al. Risk of thoracolumbar fractures doubled in victims of motor vehicle collisions with cervical spine fractures. J Trauma 2006;61: 686–687.
76. Wood K, Butterman G, Mehbod A, et al. Operative compared with nonoperative treatment of a thoracolumbar burst fracture without neurological deficit. J Bone Joint Surg 2003;85:773–781.
77. Wood KB, Bohn D, Mehbod A. Anterior versus posterior treatment of stable thoracolumbar burst fractures without neurologic deficit: a prospective, randomized study. J Spinal Disord Tech 2005;18:S15–823.

SECTION

FOUR

LOWER EXTREMITY

20

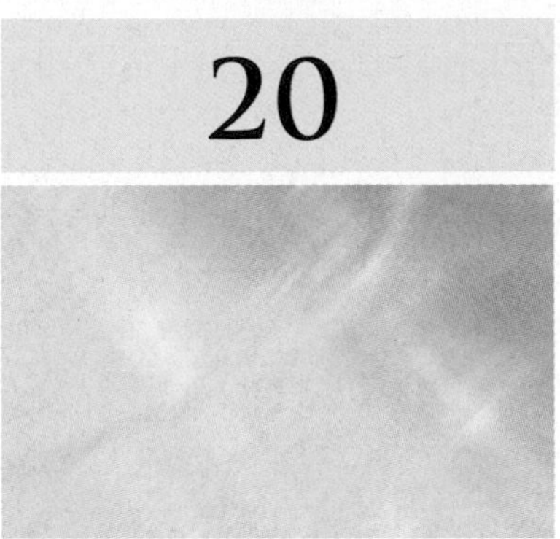

FRACTURES OF THE PELVIS

Ernest L. Sink and Dale Blaiser

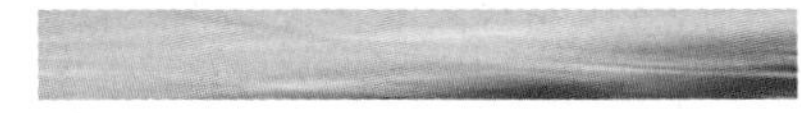

INTRODUCTION 743

PRINCIPLES OF MANAGEMENT 744
Mechanisms of Injury 744
Associated Injuries 744
Signs and Symptoms 745
Imaging and Other Diagnostic Studies 745
Classification 746

APPLIED ANATOMY 747
Ossification Centers 747

CURRENT TREATMENT OPTIONS: STABLE PELVIC FRACTURES 748
Avulsion Fractures (Torode and Zeig Type I) 748
Iliac Wing Fractures (Torode and Zeig Type II) 749
Simple Fractures of the Pubis or Ischium (Torode and Zieg Type III) 750
Ring Disruption: Unstable Fracture Patterns (Torode and Zieg Type IV) 753
Fractures of the Sacrum 759
Fractures of the Coccyx 759

ACETABULAR FRACTURES 760
Classification 760
Radiographic Evaluation 761
Treatment 761
Surgical Treatment 765
Postoperative Management 767

COMPLICATIONS 767

INTRODUCTION

Pelvic fractures comprise less than 0.2% of all pediatric fractures,[14,96] but pelvic fractures constitute between 1% and 5% of admissions to level 1 pediatric trauma centers.[7,15,19,29,37] This chapter includes simple apophyseal avulsion fractures, stable and unstable pelvic ring fractures, and acetabular and triradiate fractures. The nature and treatment of pediatric pelvic fractures are challenging to describe and summarize, as they are dependent on changing anatomy and bone structure with age.

The most important aspect of treatment is the appreciation of the high-energy mechanism of injury and the associated injuries to other systems including the neurovascular structures, abdominal viscera, genitourinary system, musculoskeletal system, and central nervous system. The rate of concomitant injury to peripelvic soft tissues is between 58% and 87%.[15,24,29,69,80] The mortality rate in children with pelvic fractures ranged from 2.4% to 14.8% in a large series collected from level 1 pediatric trauma centers.[7,15,19,29,37,52,55,67,69,80,92,94] In a recent study comparing pelvic fractures in adults and children, there was no difference in mortality or injury to concomitant peripelvic soft tissues between the groups.[32] The authors found no difference in the trauma severity as expressed by the Injury Severity Score between children and adults.[32] Central nervous system head injury was cited as the most common cause of death in two recent large single-institution retrospective studies of pediatric pelvic fractures.[15,80] Other causes of death include multiorgan failure and visceral injuries.[15,37,52,80] In children, hemorrhage from pelvic fracture-related vascular injury was the cause of death in only 0.3% to 0.7% compared with 3.4% in adults.[37] Thus, the majority of deaths are not directly linked to the pelvic injury itself in children and adults.[32]

Historically, treatment of pediatric pelvic fractures has been nonoperative based on the concept that the growing pelvis is likely to remodel and anatomic reduction and fixation are therefore not required. There is a trend toward operative treatment of unstable fractures as new retrospective reviews have revealed significant long term morbidity from malunion associated with nonoperative management.[42,93] In addition, disruption of the immature pelvis may injure the triradiate cartilage. Damage to the triradiate cartilage has the potential to cause acetabular deformity because of growth derangement.[42] Long-term studies suggest a need for operative anatomic reduction to lessen the chance of late deformity due to malunion, instability, or growth disturbance.

In this chapter, we will aim to increase the understanding of pediatric pelvic fractures, the natural history, and recommended treatments.

PRINCIPLES OF MANAGEMENT

Mechanisms of Injury

Between 75% and 95% of pelvic fractures in children result from motor vehicle-related accidents.[7,15,45,52,55,65,67–69,80,92] In the largest consecutive series of pediatric pelvic fractures from a single urban level 1 trauma center, the most common mechanism of injury was pedestrian struck by a motor vehicle (60%), followed by passenger in a motor vehicle (22%), and falls (13%).[80] Sporting activities account for between 4% and 11% of pelvic fractures in other series.[69,92] Child abuse is a rare cause of pelvic fracture, but isolated fracture of the pelvis may be the only skeletal manifestation of child abuse.[64] Radiographs of the pelvis should be included in any skeletal survey for child abuse.[1] Avulsion injuries most commonly occur secondary to athletic injuries, especially soccer, gymnastics, and track.

Associated Injuries

Because children's bones have a lower modulus of elasticity, they deform more and absorb more energy than adult bones before fracture.[18] In addition, there is greater elasticity in the sacroiliac joints and symphysis pubis in children, and greater energy is required to cause a fracture in an immature pelvis than in an adult pelvis.[80] Thus, the presence of a pelvic fracture in a child is a marker of severe injury that should alert the clinician to search actively for other injuries including abdominal, genitourinary, neurologic, and other fractures.[15]

Because most pelvic fractures in children result from high-energy trauma, multisystem injuries are common. Between 58% and 87% of pelvic fractures have at least one and often several associated injuries.[15,24,29,69,80] Of the 57 consecutive children with pelvic fractures reported by Grisoni et al.,[29] 58% had one or more other body area injuries in addition to the pelvic fracture. This included nonpelvic fractures (49%), neurologic injury (26%), significant hemorrhage requiring transfusion (21%), abdominal injury (14%), thoracic injury (7%), and genitourinary injury (4%). The incidence of associated injuries increases with the severity of the pelvic fracture. Bond et al.[7] noted that the location and number of pelvic fractures were strongly associated with the probability of abdominal injury: 1% for isolated pubic fractures, 15% for iliac or sacral fractures, and 60% for multiple fractures of the pelvic ring. However, a study by Grisoni et al.[29] found no association between multiple pelvic fractures and associated abdominal injuries. Almost all authors agree that the outcome of patients with pelvic fractures is largely determined by the associated injuries rather than the pelvic fracture itself.[7,15,24,29,37,52,69,80,91,94]

The incidence of head injury in association with pelvic fracture is between 9% and 48% in retrospective studies.[7,15,29,52,55,67,69,80,89] Rieger and Brug[69] reported the highest incidence of head injuries in 48% of the 54 patients in their series, ranging from mild concussion to brain death. The two largest single institution studies of pediatric pelvic fractures reported closed head injuries in 39%[15] and 44% of patients.[80] The correlation of pelvic fractures with head injury has been noted by others as well.[92] Brain injury merits the highest priority because it is the leading cause of death and major cause of long-term morbidity in patients with pelvic fracture.

Although children with high-energy pelvic fractures often require blood transfusions, exsanguination is rarely the primary cause of death, which is distinctly different from the adult situation. In three recent studies, each with between 57 and 166 patients, the incidence of transfusion was between 20% and 30%[15,19,29] and similar to adult rates of transfusions.[19] In none of these studies did children die of an exsanguinating pelvic fracture or associated vascular injury. In a recent study, only one pediatric patient (0.7%) had mortality directly related to exsanguination from the pelvic injury.[32] Direct vascular injury with marked superior displacement of the hemipelvis can injure the superior and inferior gluteal arteries at the sciatic notch. Other studies of pelvic fractures in children have documented retroperitoneal hemorrhage from disruption of branches of the iliac artery adjacent to a grossly disrupted sacroiliac joint in children.[52,65] Children are thought to have lower incidence of exsanguinating hemorrhage compared with adults because of a more effective vasoconstrictive response in younger patients with nonatherosclerotic blood vessels.[37] The study by McIntyre et al.[52] was the only study of pelvic fractures in children that correlated the risk of life-threatening hemorrhage to pelvic fracture complexity. In children with unstable fracture patterns or uncontrolled hypotension in spite of adequate resuscitation and transfusion, external fixation, angiography, and selective embolization may be indicated. In 90% of studied cases, the pelvic bleeding is venous thus directly proceeding to arteriography will not usually be helpful. A simple external wrapping may reduce pelvic volume enough to tamponade bleeding and preclude or delay the need for operative measures. When the abdomen is opened either surgically or traumatically, direct packing of the retroperitoneum may arrest life-threatening hemorrhage.[82]

Children with pelvic fractures should be specifically examined for vaginal and rectal lacerations. The incidence of these injuries is between 2% and 18% in children with pelvic fractures,[6,55,68,87] and early detection and repair or diversion may prevent pelvic infection or abscess formation.[56] The incidence of injury to the lower urinary tract (47%), vaginal laceration (33%), and rectal laceration (66%) is significantly increased in open fractures.[54] Some studies warn of a high rate of association of urogenital injury with multiple pelvic fractures and anterior pelvic fractures,[7,91] but the largest series to address this issue found no association between pelvic fracture type or instability and urinary tract injury.[87] Hematuria is noted on initial urinalysis in 14% to 52% of children with pelvic fractures.[15,67,87] The incidence of significant lower urinary tract injuries including bladder rupture or urethral tear has been between 4% and 15% in retrospective studies.[7,44,55,67–69] The two largest single-center retrospective studies of pediatric pelvic fractures reported a 1% incidence of lower urinary tract injury in association with pelvic fracture.[80,87] Although controversial, most authors agree that microhematuria can be followed expectantly, whereas patients with gross hematuria or significant local findings on physical examination should undergo formal urologic assessment.

This assessment should include abdominopelvic computed tomography (CT), retrograde urography, and cystography.[87]

The incidence of abdominal injuries to solid organs injury and hollow viscera is between 14% and 21% in children with pelvic fractures.[7,15,19,55,80] Rapid diagnosis and treatment of severe abdominal injury is important because abdominal injury ranks second to head injury as the cause of death in children with pelvic fractures.[15] The presence of extremity fracture concomitant with pelvic fracture is associated with increased risk of abdominal injury.[94] CT scan best demonstrates injury to organs, viscera, and mesentery after blunt injury to the abdomen.[15] The incidence of abdominal injury with pelvic fracture is similar in children (13.7%) and adults (16.7%).[19] Ultrasonography and diagnostic peritoneal lavage may be helpful in the diagnosis of intra-abdominal injury and vascular injury.[76]

Fractures of other bones are present in 40% to 50% of children with pelvic fractures.[15,24,29,52,69,80] The most frequently fractured bone is the femur followed by the tibia and fibula. Vazquez and Garcia,[94] in a study of 79 children with pelvic fractures, found that the presence of any additional fracture was a significant indication that head or abdominal injury was also present and that transfusion would be required in the first 24 hours after injury. The patients with an additional fracture had twice the frequency of death, thorax injury, laparotomy, and other nonorthopaedic procedures compared with the group with pelvic fractures alone. Vazquez and Garcia[94] suggested that this easily identifiable risk factor can help identify patients at risk who may benefit from early transfer to a regional pediatric trauma center.

Pelvic fractures with posterior displacement of a hemipelvis or iliac wing may result in damage to the lumbosacral plexus or sciatic nerve. The incidence of lumbosacral plexus injury is low, between 1% and 3%.[24,68,91] Myelography with computed axial tomography or magnetic resonance imaging (MRI) can be helpful in assessing plexus injury or root avulsion. Complete neurologic examination of the extremities, sphincter tone, and perianal sensation should be routine and documented.

Signs and Symptoms

The evaluation of a child with a pelvic fracture begins with a thorough history and physical examination. Dangerous associated injuries to the head injury, chest, abdomen, and genitourinary tract take precedence over the pelvic fracture in evaluation and treatment. The examination of the pelvic area begins with a visual inspection. Areas of contusion, abrasion, laceration, ecchymosis, or hematoma, especially in the perineal and pelvic areas, should be recorded.

Pelvic landmarks including the anterior superior iliac spine, crest of the ilium, sacroiliac joints, and symphysis pubis should be palpated. Pushing posteriorly on the anterior superior iliac crest produces pain at the fracture site as the pelvic ring is opened. Compressing the pelvic ring by squeezing the right and left iliac wings together also causes pain, and crepitation may be felt if a pelvic fracture is present. Pressure downward on the symphysis pubis and posteriorly on the sacroiliac joints causes pain and possibly motion if there is a disruption. Pain with range of motion of the extremities, especially the hip joint, may indicate articular involvement. Careful examination of the head, neck, and spine should be performed to assess for spinal injury and closed head injury. A complete neurovascular examination including peripheral pulses should be part of the initial survey. A careful genitourinary evaluation must be performed because of the intimate relationship between the pelvis and the bladder and urethra. Rectal exam is indicated in significantly displaced fractures or if there is any blood in the perineal area, but recent studies have found a poor sensitivity for diagnosing injury with a routine rectal exam in pediatric patients.[77]

Imaging and Other Diagnostic Studies

Emergency assessment and stabilization of the child with pelvic trauma should be performed before obtaining survey radiographs. If the patient is stable, scout views of the cervical spine, chest, and pelvis should be obtained quickly. Once the primary survey is completed and the patient is stable, region-specific radiographs should be obtained of any area with signs of trauma on secondary assessment.

In a child with a pelvic fracture, unless there is a significant fracture–dislocation, multiple radiographic views can be deferred. A single anteroposterior radiograph will provide a lot of information about pelvic ring stability in the acute situation.[90] The presence of sacroiliac displacement on the anteroposterior view indicates instability and the possibility of associated major hemorrhage. If there is an indication of an unstable injury on the anteroposterior view, two other views, the inlet and outlet views, should be obtained. These evaluate the pelvic ring by taking views that are approximately at right angles to each other.[90] The inlet view is obtained by directing the x-ray beam caudally at an angle of 60 degrees to the x-ray plate. The inlet view is best for the determination of posterior displacement of a hemipelvis. The outlet view is obtained by directing the x-ray beam in a cephalad direction at an angle of 45 degrees to the x-ray plate. The outlet view best demonstrates superior displacement of the hemi pelvis or vertical shifting of the anterior pelvis.[90] Internal and external rotation (Judet or oblique) are reserved for fractures of the acetabulum. Comparison views of the contralateral apophysis may be helpful in evaluating avulsion fractures.

CT scanning is the best modality to evaluate the bony pelvis, especially at the sacroiliac joint, sacrum, and acetabulum. Most authors agree that CT scanning is indicated if there is doubt about the diagnosis on plain radiograph or if operative intervention is planned.[81] It has been shown that plain films alone could reliably predict the need for operative intervention, but the addition of CT scanning changed the injury classification in 15% and the management in 3% of patients.[11] Some of the advantages of CT over plain radiographs include optimized imaging with CT reconstruction and improved fracture definition. This aids in decision making between conservative and operative treatment and improves the selection of operative approach.[49] Others have noted that CT scans of the pelvis are more sensitive than plain radiographs in all anatomic areas including the iliac region, pubis, sacroiliac joint, hip, sacrum, and soft tissues.[30] Many trauma centers routinely obtain CT scans of the abdomen and pelvis looking for visceral injury. Including CT cuts through the bony pelvis may obviate the need for dedicated pelvic screeing radiographs. MRI offers similar benefits, with the advantages over CT in delineating soft tissue injuries, absence of ionizing radiation, and fractures of cartilaginous structures such as posterior wall fractures associated with hip dislocations.[71] Rarely, a radioisotope bone scan is useful for the diagnosis of nondis-

TABLE 20-1 Torode and Zieg Classification of Pelvic Fractures in Children

1. Avulsion fractures
2. Iliac wing fractures
   a. Separation of the iliac apophysis
   b. Fracture of the bony iliac wing
3. Simple ring fractures
   a. Fractures of the pubis and disruption of the pubic symphysis
   b. Fractures involving the acetabulum, without a concomitant ring fracture
4. Fractures producing an unstable segment (ring disruption fracture)
   a. "Straddle" fractures, characterized by bilateral inferior and superior pubic rami fractures
   b. Fractures involving the anterior pubic rami or pubic symphysis and the posterior elements (e.g., sacroiliac joint, sacral ala)
   c. Fractures that create an unstable segment between the anterior ring of the pelvis and the acetabulum

TABLE 20-2 Tile and Pennal Classification of Pelvic Fractures

A. Stable fractures
   A1. Avulsion fractures
   A2. Undisplaced pelvic ring or iliac wing fractures
   A3. Transverse fractures of the sacrum and coccyx
B. Partially unstable fractures
   B1. Open-book fractures
   B2. Lateral compression injuries (includes triradiate injury)
   B3. Bilateral type B injuries
C. Unstable fractures of the pelvic ring
   C1. Unilateral fractures
      C1-1. Fractures of the ilium
      C1-2. Dislocation or fracture–dislocation of the sacroiliac joint
      C1-3. Fractures of the sacrum
   C2. Bilateral fractures, one type B and one type C
   C3. Bilateral type C fractures

placed pelvic fractures and in the identification of acute injuries in children and adults with head injuries or multiple-system injuries.[35,90]

Classification

The multitude of classification systems and the changes in the anatomy with age makes the comparison of incidence, mechanism of injury, morbidity and mortality, and outcome difficult among studies using different systems. In addition, many of the classifications do not include triradiate cartilage injury, which may be associated with the pelvic fracture. Although many recent studies of children's fractures use the Torode and Zieg[92] (Table 20-1 and Fig. 20-1) or Tile et al.[90] classifications (Table 20-2) or both, the basic classifications, (a) mature or immature pelvis and (b) stable or unstable fracture, are very useful information for making treatment decisions. Regardless of the classification system that is used, if there is a break in the anterior and posterior pelvic ring, an extremely misshapen pelvis, a displaced posterior ring injury, or a displaced triradiate fracture, the pelvis is unstable.

Silber and Flynn[79] reviewed radiographs of 133 children and adolescents with pelvic fractures and classified them into two groups: immature (Risser 0 and all physes open) and mature (closed triradiate cartilage). They suggested that in the immature group, management should focus on the associated injuries because the pelvic fractures in this group rarely required surgical intervention.[79] Fractures in the mature group were best classified and treated according to adult pelvic fracture classification

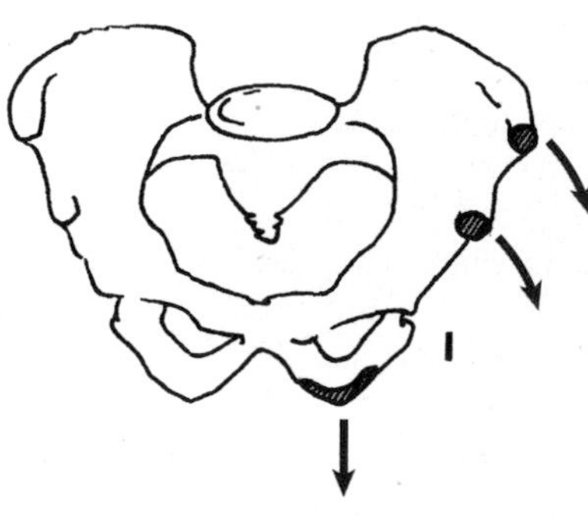

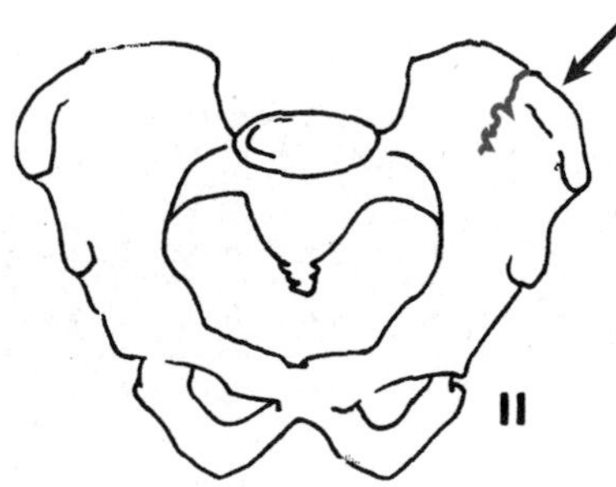

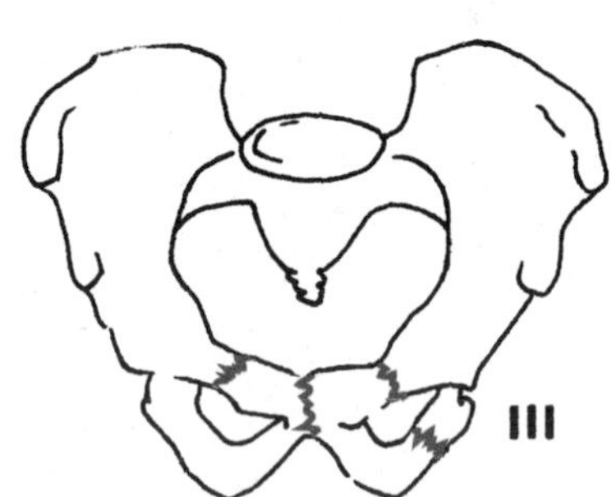

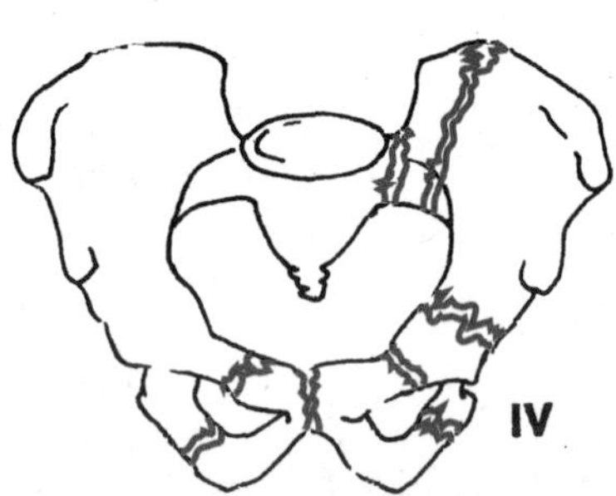

FIGURE 20-1 Torode and Zieg[92] classification of pelvic fractures in children: type I, avulsion fractures; type II, iliac wing fractures; type III, simple ring fractures; type IV, ring disruption fractures.

and management principles. Thus, pelvic fractures in patients with closed triradiate cartilage should follow adult fracture classifications and treatment protocols.[11,62,90] Torode and Zieg[92] retrospectively reviewed 141 children with pelvic fractures and classified the injuries on the basis of the severity of the fractures as well as associated prognosis. Their classification does not include acetabular fractures (see Table 20-1 and Fig. 20-1). The morbidity, mortality, and complications were greatest in the type IV group with segmental instability of the pelvis.

Quinby[65] and Rang[66] classified pelvic fractures in children into three categories: (i) uncomplicated or mild fractures, (ii) fractures with visceral injury requiring surgical exploration, and (iii) fractures with immediate, massive hemorrhage often associated with multiple and severe pelvic fractures. This classification system emphasizes the importance of the associated soft tissue injuries, but does not account for the mechanism of injury or the prognosis of the pelvic fracture itself. Watts[95] classified pediatric pelvic fractures according to the severity of skeletal injury: (a) avulsion, caused by violent muscular contraction across the unfused apophysis; (b) fractures of the pelvic ring (secondary to crushing injuries), stable and unstable; and (c) acetabular fracture associated with hip dislocation.

Pennal et al.[59] classified pelvic fractures according to the direction of force producing the injury: (a) anteroposterior compression, (b) lateral compression with or without rotation, and (c) vertical shear. This classification was modified and expanded by Tile et al. (see Table 20-2).[90] Burgess et al.[11] further modified the Pennal system and incorporated subsets to the lateral compression and anteroposterior compression groups to quantify the amount of force applied to the pelvic ring. They also created a fourth category, combined mechanical injury, to include injuries resulting from combined forces that may not be strictly categorized according to the classification scheme of Pennal.

The Tile classification has been incorporated into the Orthopaedic Trauma Association/AO classification, which is divided into bone segments, type, and groups (Table 20-3).[62] The Orthopaedic Trauma Association/AO system classifies pelvic fractures on the basis of stability versus instability, and surgical indications are based on the fracture types. Surgery is rarely indicated for type A fractures, whereas anterior or posterior surgical stabilization or both may be indicated for types B and C. Numerous subtypes are included, and further details are described in the chapter on adult pelvic fractures.

TABLE 20-3 AO/Association for the Study of Internal Fixation Classification of Pelvic Fractures

A. Stable fractures

B. Rotationally unstable fractures, vertically stable

C. Rotationally and vertically unstable fractures
- C1. Unilateral posterior arch disruption
  - C1-1. Iliac fracture
  - C1-2. Sacroiliac fracture–dislocation
  - C1-3. Sacral fracture
- C2. Bilateral posterior arch disruption, one side vertically unstable
- C3. Bilateral injury, both unstable

APPLIED ANATOMY

There are several important anatomic differences between the pelvis of a child and that of an adult. First, a child's pelvis is more malleable because of the bone is more elastic and less brittle, the joints are more elastic, more of the pelvis is cartilaginous rather than bony, and the cartilaginous structures are better able to absorb energy than bone.[58] Second, the elasticity of the joints may allow significant displacement and resultant fracture in only one area rather than the traditional concept of a mandatory "double break" in the ring for a displaced fracture.[58,66] Third, avulsion fractures of an apophysis occur more often in children and adolescents than in adults because cartilage is weaker in tension and shear compared with bone. Fractures of the acetabulum through the triradiate cartilage also occur more often for the same reason.[66,94] Fourth, fractures through physeal cartilage in children can result in late growth arrest, leg-length discrepancy, and late deformity (e.g., a fracture through the triradiate cartilage with resultant "bony bar" formation and ultimately a deficient and dysplastic acetabulum).[58]

Ossification Centers

The pelvis of a child arises from three primary ossification centers: the ilium, ischium, and pubis. The three centers meet at the triradiate cartilage and fuse at approximately 16 to 18 years of age (Fig. 20-2).[58] The pubis and ischium fuse inferiorly at the pubic ramus at 6 or 7 years of age. Occasionally, at approximately the time of fusion of the ischium to the pubis, an asymptomatic lucent area is noted on radiographs in the midportion of the inferior pubic ramus. This, termed ischiopubic synchondrosis, is a normal variant with a benign natural history. It is often bilateral and does not require treatment. The condition is often confused with a fracture of the pelvis.

Secondary centers of ossification arise in the iliac crest, ischial apophysis, anterior inferior iliac spine, pubic tubercle, angle of the pubis, ischial spine, and lateral wing of the sacrum. Secondary ossification of the iliac crest is first seen at 13 to 15 years and fuses to the ilium at 15 to 17 years of age. The secondary ossification center of the ischium is first seen at 15 to 17 years and fuses at 19 years of age, although sometimes as late as 25 years of age. A center of ossification may be present at the anterior inferior iliac spine at approximately 14 years, fusing at 16 years of age.[58,95] Knowledge about the location, age of appearance, and fusion of the secondary centers is important in differentiating them from true fractures.

The acetabulum contains the shared physes of the ilium, ischium, and pubis that merge to become the triradiate cartilage. Interstitial growth in the triradiate part of the cartilage complex causes the acetabulum to expand during growth and causes the pubis, ischium, and ilium to enlarge as well. The concavity of the acetabulum develops in response to the presence of a spherical head. The depth of the acetabulum increases during development as the result of interstitial growth in the acetabular cartilage, appositional growth of the periphery of this cartilage, and periosteal new bone formation at the acetabular margin.[63] At puberty, three secondary centers of ossification appear in the hyaline cartilage surrounding the acetabular cavity. The os acetabuli, which is the epiphysis of the pubis, forms the anterior wall of the acetabulum. The epiphysis of the ilium, the acetabular epiphysis,[63,95] forms a large part of the superior wall of the acetabulum. The small secondary center of the ischium is rarely

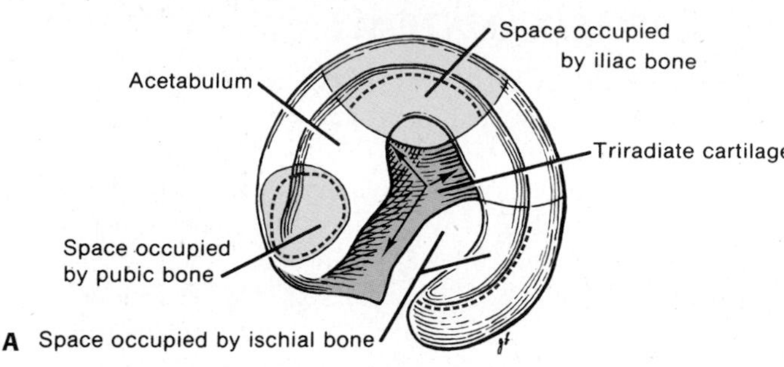

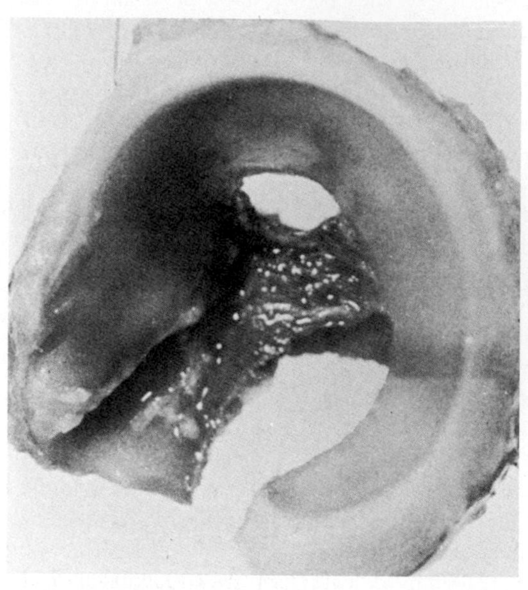

FIGURE 20-2 A. Triradiate-acetabular cartilage complex viewed from the lateral side, showing the sites occupied by the iliac, ischial, and pubic bones. **B.** Normal acetabular cartilage complex of a 1-day-old infant. The ilium, ischium, and pubis have been removed with a curet. The lateral view shows the cup-shaped acetabulum. (From Ponseti IV. Growth and development of the acetabulum in the normal child. Anatomical, histological, and roentgenographic studies. J Bone Joint Surg Am 1978;60(5): 575–585, with permission.)

seen. The os acetabuli, the largest part, starts to develop at approximately 8 years of age and expands to form the major portion of the anterior wall of the acetabulum; it unites with the pubis at approximately 18 years of age. The acetabular epiphysis develops in the iliac acetabular cartilage at approximately 8 years and fuses with the ilium at 18 years of age, forming a substantial part of the superior acetabular joint surface (Fig. 20-3). The secondary center of the ischium, the smallest of the three, develops in the ninth year, unites with the acetabulum at 17 years, and contributes very little to acetabular development. These secondary centers should not be confused with avulsion fractures or loose bodies in the hip joint.

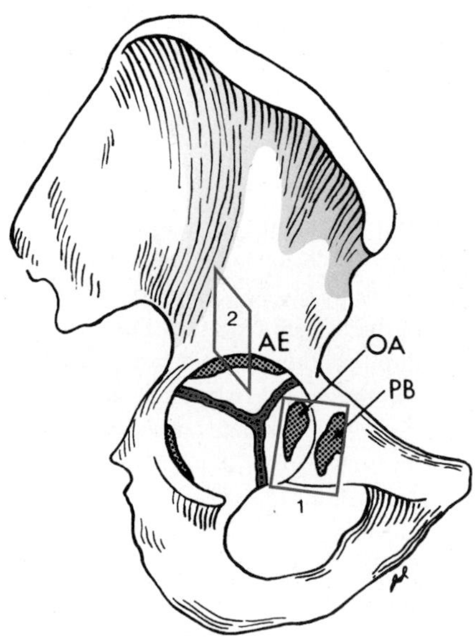

FIGURE 20-3 Right innominate bone of an adolescent. The os acetabuli (OA) is shown within the acetabular cartilage adjoining the pubic bone (PB); the acetabular epiphysis (AE), within the acetabular cartilage adjoining the iliac bone; and another small epiphysis (not labeled), within the acetabular cartilage adjoining the ischium (*left*). (From Ponseti IV. Growth and development of the acetabulum in the normal child. Anatomical, histological, and roentgenographic studies. J Bone Joint Surg Am 1978; 60(5):575–585, with permission.)

CURRENT TREATMENT OPTIONS: STABLE PELVIC FRACTURES

Avulsion Fractures (Torode and Zeig Type I)

Avulsion fractures of the pelvis usually occur in adolescent athletes as a result of forceful contraction of the attached muscle while the athlete is actively engaged in activities such as kicking, running, or jumping.[23,53,70] As these injuries are painful, but not disabling, the incidence of avulsion fractures is most certainly underrepresented in large hospital-based clinical series because most of these injuries are never seen in the emergency room. The incidence in two large recent series was approximately 4%.[67,69] Chronic repetitive traction on the developing iliac apophysis may result in an incomplete avulsion fracture or apophysitis without a history of acute trauma.[16,26] The sartorius muscle originates at the anterior superior iliac spine, the direct head of the rectus femoris at the anterior inferior iliac spine, and the hamstrings and adductors from the ischial tuberosity (Fig. 20-4).

Of the 268 pelvic avulsion fractures reported in the four largest series,[23,53,70,86] 50% were ischial avulsions, 23% were avulsions of the anterior superior iliac spine, and 22% were avulsions of the anterior inferior iliac spine. Avulsions of the lesser trochanter (3%) (Fig. 20-5) and iliac apophysis (2%) accounted for the rest.

Mechanism of Injury

The mechanism of injury is sudden forceful traction through large muscles, which have their origins on the pelvic apophyses. This may be active contraction as in sprinting or jumping, or avulsion may result from sudden passive traction such as performing splits in gymnastics or dance.[53] The distribution of fracture patterns with respect to sporting activity reveals that gymnastics are responsible for the greatest number of acute ischial tuberosity avulsion fractures, whereas soccer is responsible for the greatest numbers of anterior superior and anterior inferior iliac spine avulsion fractures.[70] Iliac apophysitis is most frequently associated with long distance running and thought to result from either repetitive muscle traction injury or stress fractures of the apophysis.[16]

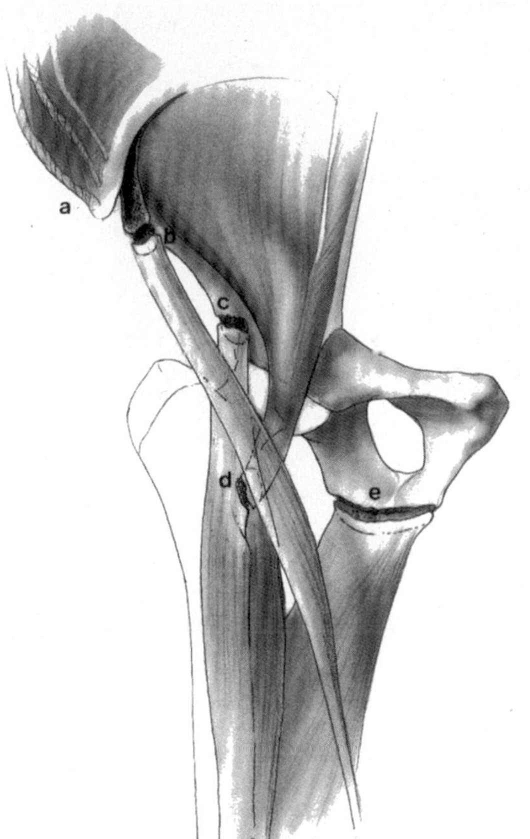

FIGURE 20-4 Locations for pelvis apophyseal fractures. **A.** Iliac apophysis from external oblique. **B.** Anterior superior iliac spine avulsion attached to sartorius. **C.** Anterior inferior iliac spine avulsion from recuts; femoris attachment. **D.** Lesser trochanter avulsion from iliopsoas attachment. **E.** Ishial tuberosity avulsion from hamstring muscles.

Diagnosis

Symptoms usually include localized swelling and tenderness at the site of the avulsion fracture. Motion is limited due to guarding, and pain may be mild or marked. In the case of repetitive stress injury, pain and limitation of motion usually are gradually progressive. In patients with ischial avulsions, pain at the ischial tuberosity can be elicited by flexing the hip and extending the knee (straight-leg raising). In this position, as the hip is moved into abduction, the pain increases. Patients may also have pain while sitting or moving on the involved tuberosity.

In patients with avulsion of the anterior superior iliac spine, radiographs show displacement of the apophysis. In patients with anterior inferior iliac spine avulsions, radiographs show minimal distal displacement of the fragment. Further displacement is probably prevented because of tethering by the conjoined tendon, as the reflected head of the rectus femoris muscle is intact. Contralateral views can be obtained and compared to ensure that this fragment is not actually a secondary center of ossification, either the os acetabuli or acetabular epiphysis. In the case of ischial tuberosity avulsion, radiographs typically reveal a semilunar fragment displaced distally compared with the opposite ischial tuberosity. The intact sacrotuberous ligament resists significant displacement.

Because these avulsion injuries affect secondary centers of ossification before the center is fused with the pelvis, primarily in children ages 11 to 17 years,[23,53,86] comparison views of the contralateral apophysis should be obtained to ensure that what appears to be an avulsion fracture is not in reality a normal adolescent variant. Later, exuberant callus formation can occasionally mimic a malignant neoplasm.[4] Recognition of the initial fracture is important to avoid unnecessary evaluations such as CT, MRI, and radionuclide scans, and inappropriate biopsy.

Treatment and Prognosis

Most pelvic avulsion fractures in children heal satisfactorily with conservative nonoperative management including rest, partial weight bearing on crutches for 2 or more weeks, and extremity positioning to minimize muscle stretch. Two small series of adolescents with pelvic avulsion fractures treated conservatively concluded that nonsurgical treatment was successful in all patients, and all patients returned to preinjury activity levels.[23,53] Others have suggested that conservative nonoperative treatment is associated with a significantly higher incidence of functional disability and inability to return to competitive athletic activity.[86] On long-term follow-up of 12 patients with ischial avulsions, 8 reported significant reduction in athletic ability and 5 had persistent local symptoms.[86] In the largest series published to date, only 3 of 198 competitive adolescent athletes with pelvic avulsion fractures were treated operatively.[70] Anecdotally, long-term functional disability and inability to return to preinjury activity levels have been reported in the setting of conservatively managed ischial avulsion fractures.[73,86] Controversy exists surrounding the acute management of ischial avulsion fractures, but most agree that excision of the ischial apophysis is indicated in the setting of chronic pain and disability. Some authors recommend open reduction and internal fixation of those rare acute pelvic avulsion fragments displaced more than 1 to 2 cm (Fig. 20-6).[48]

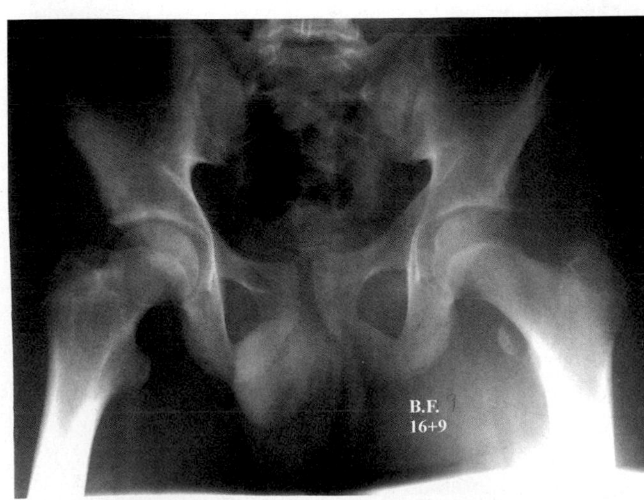

FIGURE 20-5 Avulsion fracture of the lesser trochanter.

Iliac Wing Fractures (Torode and Zeig Type II)

Direct trauma may fracture the wing of the ilium, but isolated iliac wing fractures are relatively rare. Reed[67] reported an incidence of 12% in children with fractures of the pelvis. Rieger and Brug[69] reported iliac wing fractures in only 3 (5.6%) of their patients, and McIntyre et al.[52] reported only 7 (12%) in 57 fractures. However, this fracture often occurs in conjunction with other fractures of the pelvis, and thus the overall incidence

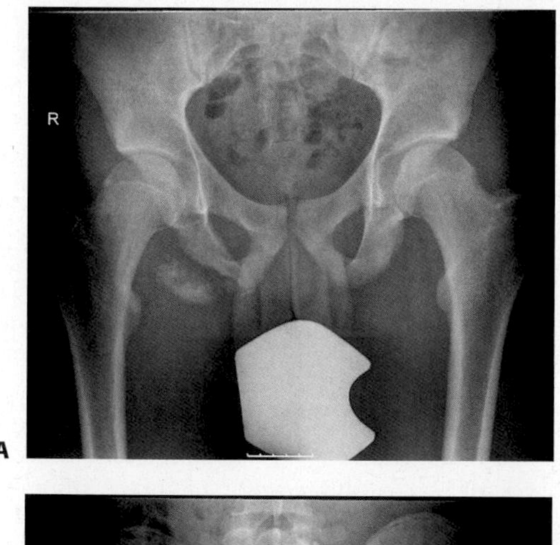

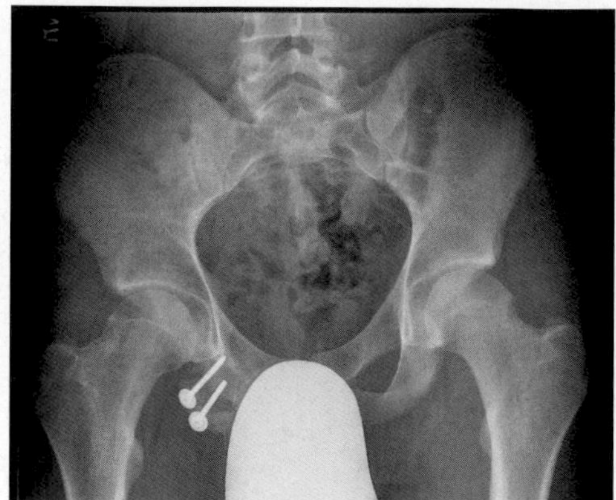

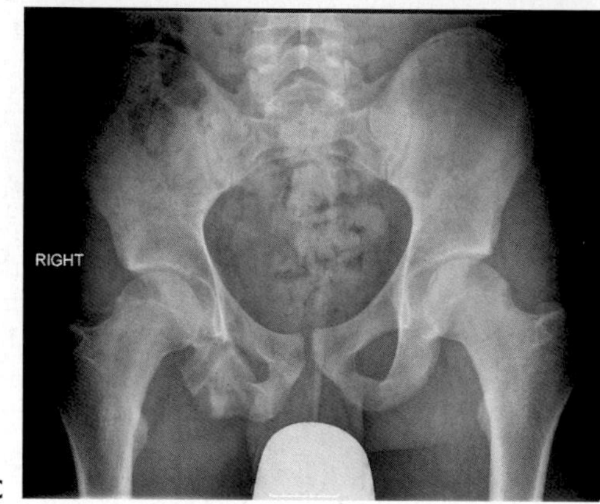

FIGURE 20-6 A. A painful ischial apophyseal nonunion in an athlete. **B.** Fixation of the apophysis. **C.** Healed apophysis after implant removal. (Courtesy of Dr. David Scher, Hospital for Special Surgery, NY.)

of iliac wing fractures is probably significantly higher than the incidence of isolated iliac wing fractures.

Displacement of the fracture usually occurs laterally, but it can occur medially or proximally. Severe displacement is rare as the iliac wing is tethered by the abdominal muscles and the hip abductors. Pain is located over the wing of the ilium, and motion at the fracture site may be noted. A painful Trendelenburg gait may be present because of spasm of the hip abductor muscles. A fracture of the wing of the ilium may be overlooked on an underexposed radiograph of the pelvis where the ilium is poorly seen as a large area of radiolucency.

Treatment of an iliac wing fracture usually is dictated by the associated injuries. Symptomatic treatment is all that is necessary for treatment of the fracture itself. This should be followed by partial weight bearing on crutches until the symptoms are completely resolved. Regardless of comminution or displacement, these fractures usually unite without complications or sequelae (Fig. 20-7).

Simple Fractures of the Pubis or Ischium (Torode and Zieg Type III)

In children, pelvic ramus fractures are usually caused by high-energy trauma and frequently have associated injuries. Reed[67] reported that 45% of the pelvic fractures in children in his series were pubic ramus fractures. Reiger[69] reported that 37% of their series of 54 pelvic fractures in children were "simple ring fractures," and McIntyre et al.[52] reported that 40% of 57 pelvic fractures were "type I" (unilateral anterior) fractures. Silber et al.[80] reported that 56% of pelvic fractures in their series of 166 consecutive pediatric pelvic fractures were simple ring fractures (excluding acetabular fractures) and were caused by a motor vehicle striking a pedestrian in 60%. Single ramus fractures are more common than multiple ramus fractures, and the superior ramus is fractured more often than the inferior ramus (Fig. 20-8).[67]

In patients with isolated pubic ramus fractures, clinical examination reveals tenderness and sometimes crepitus at the fracture site. CT scanning or inlet and outlet radiographic views are helpful in determining whether there are any other pelvic fractures presenting in the pelvic ring. If there is significant displacement of the pubic rami, a second fracture through the pelvic ring should be suspected. However, because of the plasticity of bone and elasticity of the symphysis and sacroiliac joints in children, more displacement can be expected than in adults

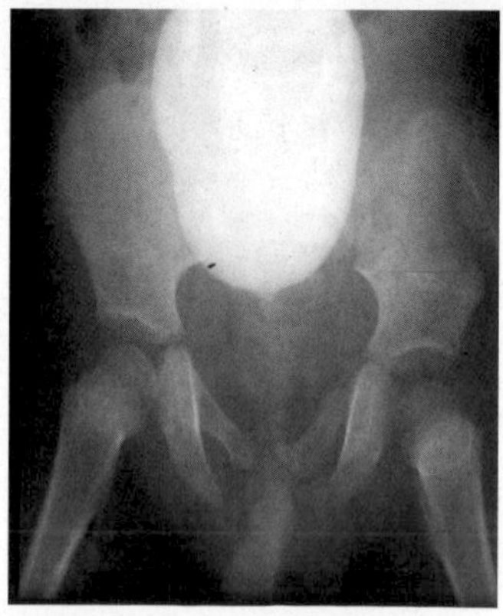

FIGURE 20-7 Stable fracture of the iliac wing.

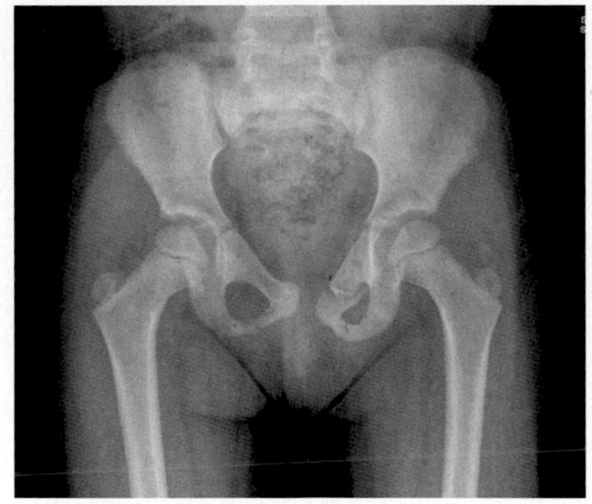
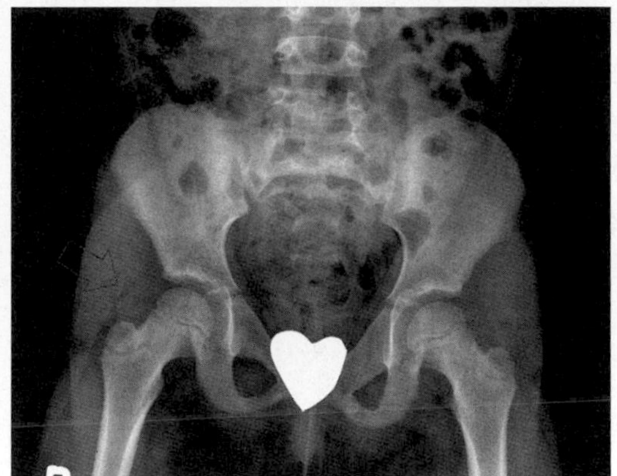

FIGURE 20-8 A. Stable superior pubic ramus fracture. The patient was allowed full weight bearing as tolerated. **B.** Radiographs show complete fracture union and remodelling.

with a similar injury. In the immature pelvis, ramus fractures may extend into the triradiate cartilage. Treatment of theses patients is usually symptomatic, and progressive weight bearing is allowed. These are stable injuries and do not require surgery.

Fractures of the Two Ipsilateral Rami

Fractures of the ipsilateral superior and inferior pubic rami comprised 18% of pediatric pelvic fractures in the series of 120 pediatric pelvic fractures reviewed.[15] Although these fractures are generally stable, they may be associated with injuries of the abdominal viscera, especially the genitourinary system (e.g., bladder rupture).[22] There is a high incidence of associated head injury, which correlates with the mechanism of injury, which is very often a motor vehicle–pedestrian incident.[92]

Considerable force is necessary to cause this fracture pattern, and other associated fractures should be expected. A general evaluation should be followed by examination of the pelvis and lower extremities, with special attention to abrasions, contusions, lacerations, and ecchymosis about the pelvis. Palpation reveals discomfort anteriorly, and crepitus at the fracture site may be noted.

Various methods of treatment have been advocated for adults. However, in children, the fracture almost always unites with adequate remodeling of even the most displaced fractures. For this reason, symptomatic treatment and progressive weight bearing on the involved side is all that is necessary.

Fractures of the Body of the Ischium

Fracture of the body of the ischium near the acetabulum is extremely rare in children. The fracture occurs from external force to the ischium, most commonly in a fall from a considerable height. The fracture usually is minimally displaced, and treatment consists of symptomatic treatment and progressive weight bearing (Fig. 20-9).

Stress Fractures of the Pubis or Ischium

Stress fractures are rare in small children, but they do occur in adolescents and young adults from chronic, repetitive stress to a bony area or during the last trimester of pregnancy. Stress fractures of the pubis are likewise uncommon, but a small series of stress fractures, primarily in the inferior pubic rami, has been reported. Chronic symptoms and pain increased by stress may be noted in the inferior pubic area. Radiographs may show no evidence of fracture for as long as 4 to 6 weeks, and then only faint callus formation may be visible; however, MRI or a technetium bone scan may reveal increased uptake early.[35] Treatment should consist of avoiding the stressful activity and limited weight bearing for 4 to 6 weeks.

The ischiopubic synchondrosis usually closes between 4 and 8 years of age.[41] The radiographic appearance of the synchondrosis at the ischiopubic junction may be misinterpreted as a fracture. Caffey and Ross[12,43] noted that bilateral fusion of the ischiopubic synchondrosis is complete in 6% of children at 4 years of age and in 83% of children at 12 years of age. The presence of the synchondrosis itself is common and usually asymptomatic. Bilateral swelling of the synchondrosis was also noted in 47% of children at age 7 years. Irregular ossification and clinical swelling at the ischiopubic synchondrosis has been called ischiopubic osteochondritis or van Neck disease. If this

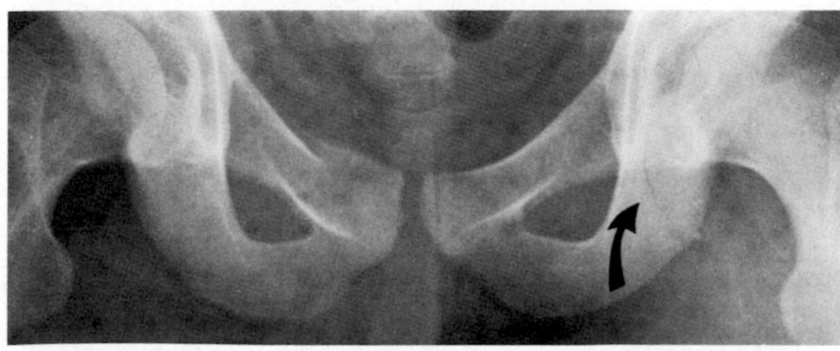
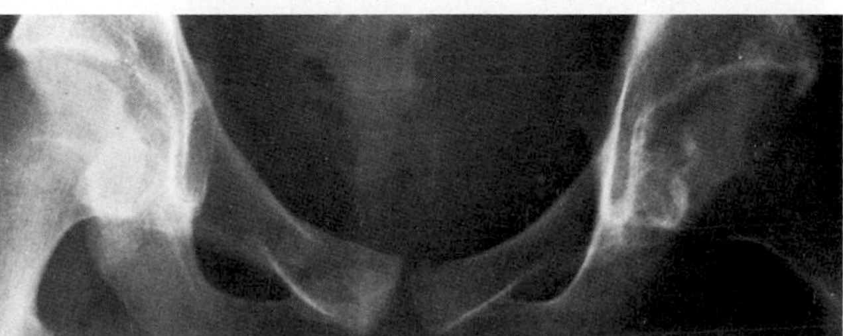

FIGURE 20-9 A. Nondisplaced fracture through the left ischium and contralateral pubic ramus fracture. **B.** Follow-up radiograph shows mild displacement and incongruity of the acetabulum and complete healing of the superior pubic ramus fracture. Either displacement of the fracture fragments or premature closure of the triradiate cartilage could have contributed to the incongruity of the femoral head in the acetabulum.

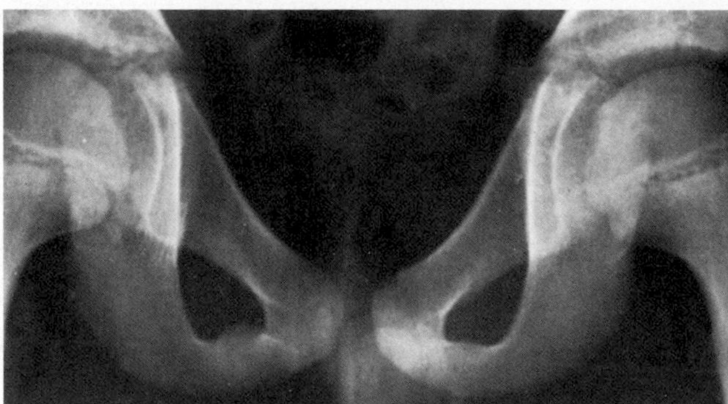

FIGURE 20-10 Radiograph of the pelvis of a 9-year-old child. Although the differentiation could not be made between a fracture and fusion of the right ischiopubic ossification at the time of radiograph, the patient was asymptomatic and the mass was considered a variant of normal development.

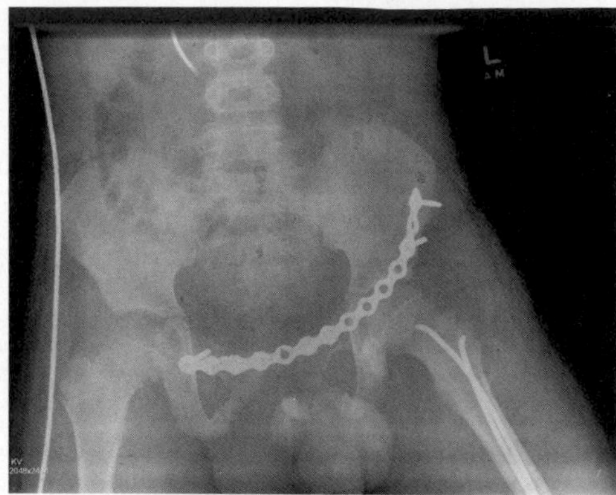

FIGURE 20-12 Radiograph of the pelvis after plating of the pubic symphysis that also includes acetabular fixation.

syndrome is noted in a child older than 10 years of age, it should be treated as a repetitive stress injury (Fig. 20-10).

Fractures Near or Subluxation of the Symphysis Pubis (May Be Unstable Fractures)

Isolated injuries in the symphysis pubis area are rare because they usually occur in association with disruption of the posterior ring near the sacroiliac joint. Although significant force appears to be necessary to disrupt or fracture the symphysis pubis, isolated disruption of the symphysis pubis can occur.[95] There is normally some elasticity at the symphysis, even in adults (0.5 mm in men, 1.5 mm in women), and there is probably even more in children, depending on maturity. In children and adolescents, diastasis greater than or equal to 2.5 cm or rotational deformity greater than 15 degrees suggests significant instability and the need for reduction.[27]

Clinically, exquisite pain is present anteriorly at the symphysis; the legs are externally rotated and often pain is worse in the supine position than in the side-lying position.[95] Motion of the hips in flexion, abduction, external rotation, and extension is restricted and painful (fabere sign).

Radiographs may reveal subluxation or widening of the symphysis, as if opening a book.[88] The two sides may be offset vertically or front-to-back. Disruption may occur near or through the symphysis pubis. Because of normal variation of the width of the symphysis in children, the extent of traumatic separation may be difficult to evaluate. Watts[95] suggested radiographs with and without lateral compression of the pelvis. More than 1 cm of difference in the width of the symphysis pubis between the two views suggests a symphyseal separation. Radiographic evaluation including CT should be performed to specifically exclude sacroiliac joint disruption and triradiate cartilage fracture because both of these injuries may occur in association with symphysis pubis separation (Fig. 20-11).[58]

Treatment of isolated injury symphysis pubis without significant displacement (2 cm) or posterior injury should be symptomatic. If there is wide diastasis, reduction and external fixation with an anterior frame will provide immediate stability and allow early mobilization.[2] Open reduction and internal fixation with a plate may be considered if a fixator is too bulky or restricts access to the abdomen (Fig. 20-12).

Isolated Fractures Near or Subluxation of the Sacroiliac Joint (May Be Unstable)

Isolated ring disruption near or through the sacroiliac joint are rare, probably even less common than isolated fractures at the weaker symphysis pubis. More commonly, posterior disruptions of the pelvic ring require a concomitant disruption of the anterior pelvis. These double-ring disruptions are considered unstable. Sacroiliac dislocations differ from those in adults in several ways. In children, disruptions tend to be incomplete

A 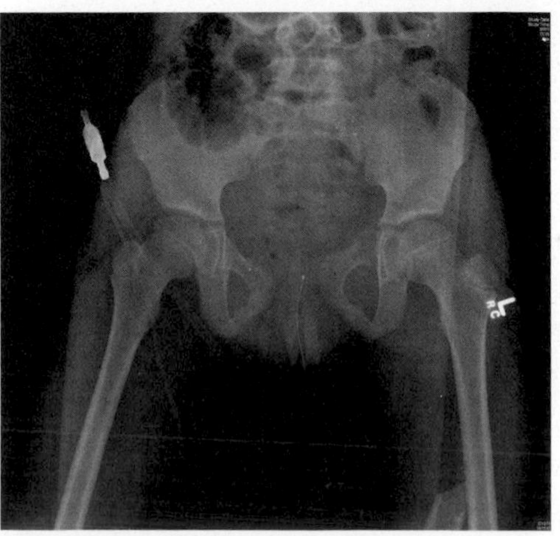

B 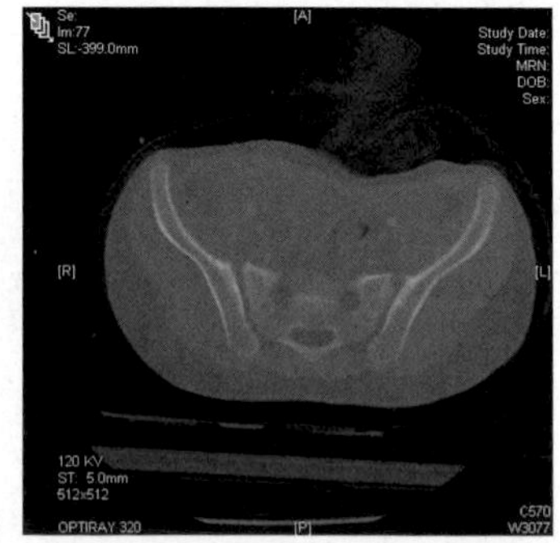

FIGURE 20-11 A. Fracture adjacent to the symphysis pubis with symphysis pubis separation. **B.** CT scan showing no posterior instability.

because the anterior sacroiliac ligaments tend to tear incompletely. The sacroiliac joint may also fail through the epiphysis of the ilium adjacent to the joint.[58] A fracture through the relatively weak physeal cartilage may leave the sacroiliac joint technically intact.[20] Associated vascular and neurologic injuries may occur. Lumbosacral nerve root avulsions have been described in children with this fracture.[76] Derangement of the sacroiliac joint should be suspected after high-velocity trauma with impact to the posterior pelvis. In patients with these injuries, the fabere sign is markedly positive on the ipsilateral side.[20,33] Comparison views of both sacroiliac joints should be carefully evaluated looking for asymmetry of the iliac wings or the clear space at the sacroiliac joint. Offset of the distal articular surface is an indication of sacroiliac joint disruption. Because it is rare to have an isolated posterior injury, in the case of a seemingly isolated sacroiliac disruption, special views including inlet and outlet, or axial, CT scan are indicated to look for anterior ring fracture (Fig. 20-13).

Symptomatic treatment and limited weight bearing on crutches are sufficient treatment for isolated subluxations or fractures. Heeg and Klasen[33] reported sacroiliac joint dislocations in 18 children, 10 of whom had extensive degloving injuries of the posterior pelvis. Ten were treated nonoperatively, six with open reduction and internal fixation, one with open reduction but no internal fixation, and one with external fixation. Long-term sequelae included occasional back pain in six, daily back pain in three, and incomplete neurologic recovery in six.

Ring Disruption: Unstable Fracture Patterns (Torode and Zieg Type IV)

Unstable pelvic fracture combinations usually fall into three types:

1. Double anterior injury with bilateral pubic rami fractures (the straddle or floating injury) or disruptions of the pubis with an associated second break in the anterior ring
2. Double fractures in the pelvic ring with anterior and posterior, disruptions through the bony pelvis, sacroiliac joint, or symphysis pubis (Malgaigne fractures)
3. Multiple crushing injuries that produce at least two severely comminuted fractures in the pelvic ring

Bilateral Fractures of the Inferior and Superior Pubic Rami

Bilateral fractures of the inferior and superior pubic rami (straddle fractures) cause a floating anterior arch of the pelvic ring that is inherently unstable (Fig. 20-14). Disruption of the symphysis pubis with unilateral fractures of the rami causes similar instability. This fracture pattern frequently is associated with bladder or urethral disruption.[58]

Bilateral fractures of the inferior and superior pubic rami can occur in a fall while straddling a hard object, by lateral compression of the pelvis, or by sudden impact while riding a motorized cycle. The floating fragment usually is displaced superiorly, being pulled in this direction by the rectus abdominis muscles.[95] Radiographically, an inlet view most accurately determines the amount of true displacement of the floating fragment.

If there is no posterior ring injury and the fractures are not grossly displaced, these injuries should heal and remodel without any orthopaedic intervention. Because these injuries do not involve the weight-bearing portion of the pelvis, there is no residual leg-length discrepancy. Skeletal traction is unnecessary, and a pelvic sling is contraindicated because of the possibility that compression will cause medial displacement of the ilium.[58,95]

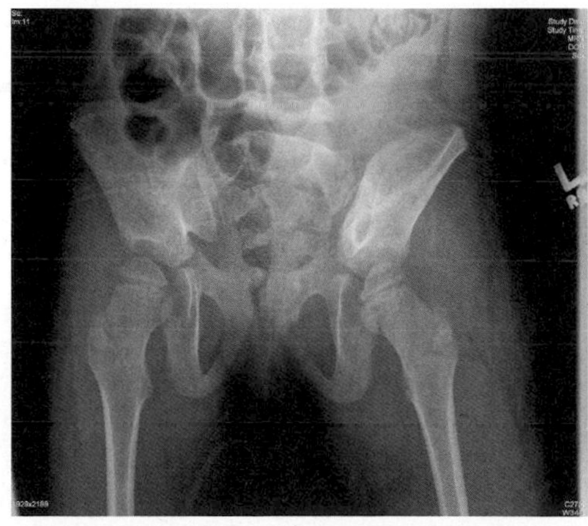

A

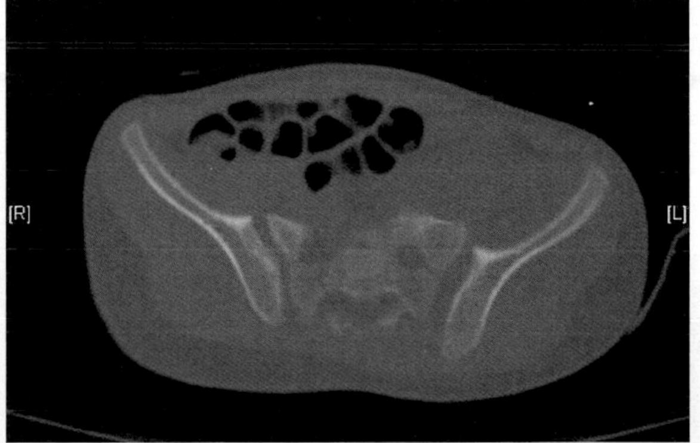

B

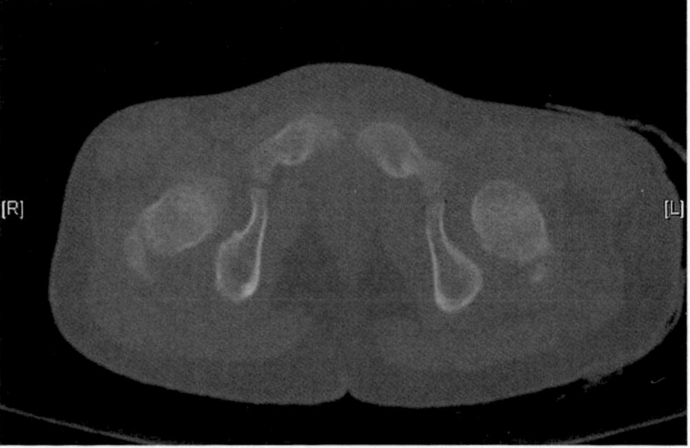

C

FIGURE 20-13 A 4-year-old with a pelvic fracture primarily with posterior involvement. **A.** Pelvic outlet radiograph showing a posterior injury at the sacroiliac joint. **B.** CT scan showing the minimal posterior SI widening. **C.** CT scan showing no anterior ring injury.

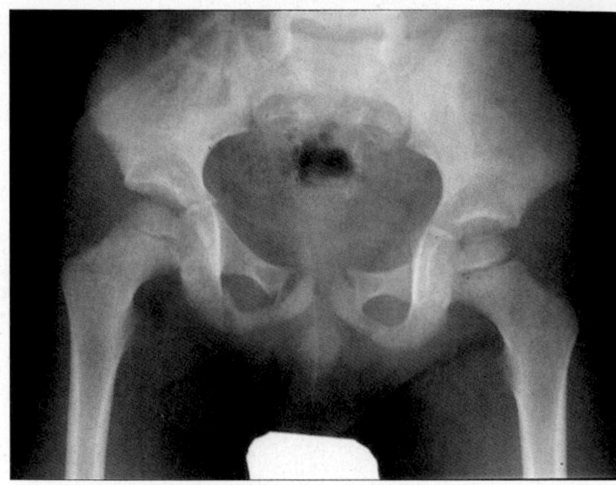

FIGURE 20-14 Example of a straddle fracture.

Treatment should consist of management of symptoms and associated soft tissue injuries.

Complex Fracture Patterns

Double breaks in the pelvic ring (anterior and posterior to the acetabulum) (Fig. 20-15) result in instability of the hemipelvis. These unstable fractures are often accompanied by retroperitoneal and intraperitoneal bleeding. There has been a 35% to 60% incidence of concomitant abdominal injury in these unstable pelvic fractures versus 11% to 18% in more stable pelvic fractures.[7,93] Bilateral anterior and posterior fractures are the most likely fracture pattern to cause severe hemorrhage. Initial treatment involves resuscitation with fluids and blood and stabilization of the child's overall condition before treatment of the pelvic fractures.[91]

These injuries may result from a variety of mechanisms: Silber et al.[80] implied that the majority were from anteroposterior compression forces. Other possibilities are direct lateral compression force and indirect forces transmitted proximally along the femoral shaft with the hip fixed in extension and abduction.

Aside from the physical signs usually associated with pelvic fractures, leg-length discrepancy and asymmetry of the pelvis also may be present because of displacement of the hemipelvis. Inlet and outlet radiographs and CT scan reveal the amount of pelvic displacement. The degree of residual pelvic asymmetry can be described by the method of Keshishyan.[42] With this method, pelvic asymmetry is determined by the difference in length (in centimeters) between two diagonal lines drawn from the border of the sacroiliac joint to the contralateral triradiate cartilage.

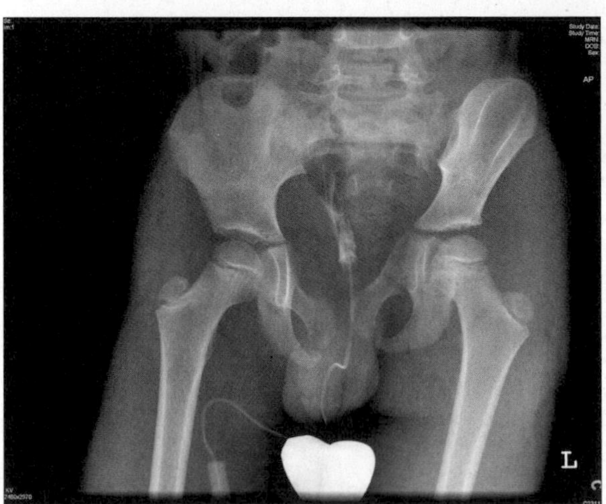

FIGURE 20-15 An unstable pelvis fracture with fractures in both the anterior and posterior ring of the pelvis. The left hemipelvis is displaced and rotated.

Numerous treatment regimens have been successful, depending on the type of fracture and the amount of displacement. For fractures with minimal displacement, symptomatic treatment, weight-bearing restrictions, and close follow-up for displacement are suggested (Fig. 20-16). Spica casting can be used in the younger child.

Displaced and unstable fractures require more thought. Historically and in general, operative treatment of pelvic fractures in children has not been routinely recommended because of the following: (a) exsanguinating hemorrhage is unusual in children, so operative pelvic stabilization to control bleeding rarely is necessary[5,55]; (b) pseudarthrosis is rare in children and fixation is not necessary to promote healing; (c) the thick periosteum in children tends to help stabilize the fracture, so surgery usually is not necessary to obtain stability[67]; (d) prolonged immobilization is not necessary for fracture healing[57]; (e) significant remodeling may occur in skeletally immature patients; and (f) long-term morbidity after pelvic fracture is rare in children.[29,39,55] Many of these assumptions are correct and some have proven to be untrue.

There has been a trend toward operative treatment in the unstable displaced fracture to prevent long-term morbidity. There are several reasons for advocating more aggressive treatment for unstable pelvic fractures in children. The ability of the immature pelvis to remodel has been overestimated in the past. Residual pelvic and acetabular deformity may have a poor long-term outcome.[82] The long-term musculoskeletal morbidities include leg-length discrepancy, back pain, scoliosis, pelvic asymmetry, and sacroiliac arthrosis.[82,83] The short-term morbidity of pelvic fracture in children centers on pain, immobility, loss of independence, and effects of associated injuries. Signorino et al.[78] studied short-term outcome parameters after pelvic fracture in children. They found that in three important domains—self-care, mobility, and cognition—children tended to return to near normal status by 6 months postinjury.

Long-term morbidities of pelvic fracture relate to persistent obliquity of the pelvis and damage to the pelvic floor. Smith et al.[83] followed 20 patients with open triradiate cartilages and unstable pelvic fracture for a mean of 6.5 years. They were evaluated using the Short Musculoskeletal Function Assessment (SMFA) questionnaire, physical exam, and radiographs. Pelvic asymmetry did not remodel even in younger patients. Eighteen patients were treated operatively with external fixation, internal fixation, or a combination of both, and pelvic asymmetry of no more than 1 cm was achieved in 10 of them. Patients who had no more than 1 cm of pelvic asymmetry had no lumbar or sacroiliac pain, no or mild sacroiliac tenderness, no Trendelenburg sign, no lumbar scoliosis, and lower (better) bother and dysfunction scores on the SMFA compared with patients with more pelvic asymmetry. All patients with greater than 1.1 cm of pelvic asymmetry had three or more of the following: nonstructural scoliosis, lumbar pain, a Trendelenburg sign, or sacro-

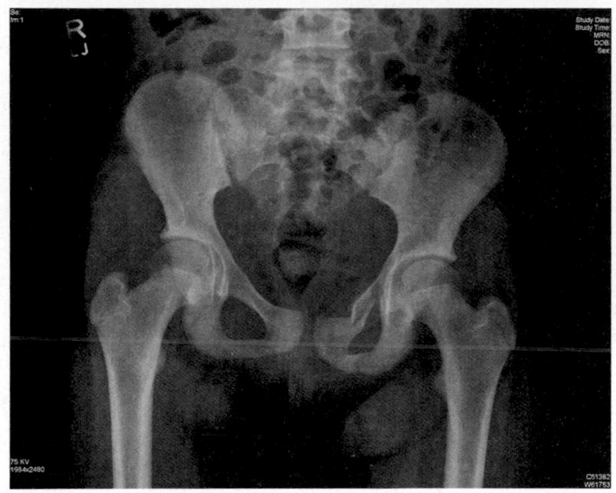

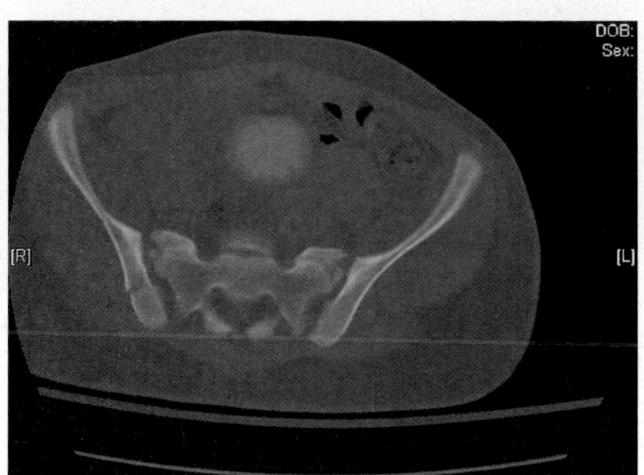

FIGURE 20-16 A potentially unstable pelvic fracture with anterior and posterior injury. **A.** The radiograph shows a left superior and inferior rami fractures. **B.** The CT scan shows a minimally displaced fracture adjacent to the sacroiliac joint. This is also an example where both CT and plan radiographs can be used to evaluate the injury and help decide on displacement and treatment. This patient was treated nonoperatively with follow-up making sure there was no displacement.

iliac joint tenderness and pain. Patients with fewer associated injuries and pelvic asymmetry of no more than 1 cm had better clinical results. They concluded that fractures associated with at least 1.1 cm of pelvic asymmetry following closed reduction should be treated with open reduction and internal or external fixation in order to improve alignment and the long-term functional outcome.[83]

Schwarz et al.,[74] in a long-term (2 to 25 years) follow-up of 17 children with nonoperatively treated unstable pelvic fractures, reported moderate to severe pelvic asymmetry in eight patients. Measured leg-length discrepancies between 2 and 5 cm were reported in 5 patients. These authors emphasized that reduction of the pelvic ring fractures should be as anatomic as possible because healing in malposition resulted in unsatisfactory results in half of the cases. McDonald[51] found that that one third of 15 skeletally immature patients with unstable fractures treated nonoperatively had residual pain. Heeg and Klasen[7] retrospectively followed 18 children at an average of 14 years after injury. Ten were treated with bedrest and 8 surgically. Nine patients had a leg-length discrepancy of greater then 1.0 cm and 3 patients reported daily back pain.[7] Rieger and Brug[69] concluded that the principles of operative management should not differ much between children and adults due to their review of long-term morbidity in unstable fractures. Nierenberg et al.,[57] however, reported excellent or good results after conservative treatment of 20 unstable pelvic fractures in children despite radiographic evidence of deformity. They suggested that treatment guidelines for unstable pelvic fractures are not the same for children as for adults, and recommended that external or internal fixation should be used only when conservative methods fail.[57] Silber and Flynn,[79] in a retrospective review of 166 consecutive children with pelvic fractures, found that all 4 patients who required open reduction and internal fixation had a mature pelvis with a closed triradiate cartilage. The average age of the children that required operative fixation was 14.3 years versus 8.7 years in those children that did not require operative fixation. These reviews suggest that younger children with an immature pelvis are unlikely to require operative intervention; however, treatment of children with unstable pelvic fractures and treatment of adolescents with a "mature" pelvis should follow adult treatment guidelines.

Subasi[85] studied 58 patients treated nonoperatively for unstable pelvic fractures. At 7.4 years follow-up, in addition to various orthopaedic complaints, 23 patients had genitourinary dysfunction including urethral stricture, urinary incontinence, and erectile dysfunction. Thirty-one patients were diagnosed with 41 psychiatric illnesses, including dysthymic disorder, social phobia, posttraumatic stress disorder, and major depression. They suggested that long hospital stays and urologic complications are associated with serious psychologic problems, and thus should be considered during selection of treatment modality. Baessler et al.[3] studied symptoms of pelvic floor dysfunction after pelvic trauma. Twenty-four women who had sustained AO type B and C fractures completed questionnaires at a median age of 24 years. Sixteen women reported new symptoms. Bladder symptoms occurred in 12, bowel problems in 11, and sexual dysfunction in 7 of 17 sexually active women. They concluded that pelvic fracture is a risk factor for pelvic floor dysfunction.[3]

The principles of fracture care are first obtaining and then maintaining reduction until healing. Reductive maneuvers may include manipulation, traction, or open reduction. After successful reduction is obtained, casting, traction, external fixation, or internal fixation can be used to maintain the reduction. Spica casting is most suited to small children. Skeletal traction may be suited to children who can tolerate prolonged recumbency or who are unable to tolerate internal fixation. Anterior external fixation is achieved by placing one or two pins in the supra-acetabular bone on each side (Fig. 20-17).[72] Pins can be placed open or percutaneously. External fixation has been advocated to stabilize an unstable fracture, maintain accurate reduction, achieve earlier ambulation, and decrease pain secondary to instability. Keshishyan et al.[42] advocated external fixation of complex pelvic fractures, especially in children with polytrauma, and Gordon et al.[27] suggested external fixation or open reduction and internal fixation in children older than 8 years of age because spica casting is poorly tolerated in older children. Symphysis plating via a Pfannenstiel approach is a good alternative for anterior ring external fixation. It is less bulky then external

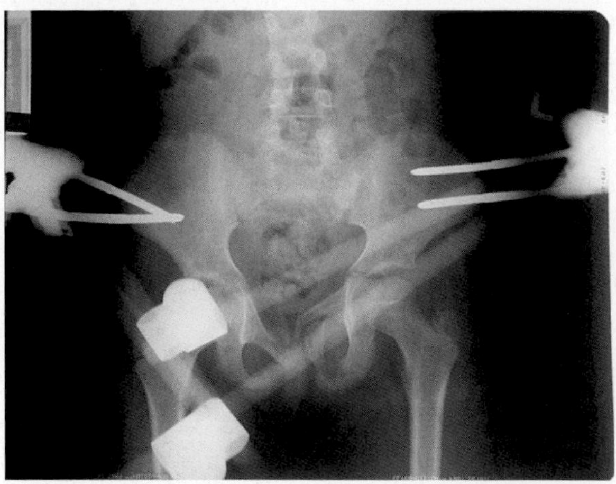

FIGURE 20-17 Fixation of an unstable pelvic fracture with external fixation. One or two pins are placed in the iliac wing. The starting point is 1 to 2 cm posterior to the anterior superior iliac spine. An anterior to posterior supra-acetabular pin may also be used.

fixation and can often be performed when the surgeons are repairing the bladder or laparotomy, which is not uncommon with a widely displaced symphysis.

External fixation may not be effective in controlling the posterior ring.[50] For this reason, separate fixation of the sacroiliac joint through an anterior or posterior approach may be needed (Fig. 20-18). Open reduction can be achieved through an anterior retroperitoneal approach in the iliac fossa in the supine position. Fixation is by small screws or plate. Alternatively, reduction and fixation can be done with the patient prone through a posterior approach. Holden et al.[36] determined after a review of the literature that fractures with at least 2 cm of displacement must be reduced and stabilized. They suggested that external fixation is not ideal for vertical shear injuries, but it is appropriate when emergent stabilization is needed to control blood loss.[36] Internal fixation with anterior pubic symphysis plating and percutaneous sacroiliac screw fixation may be required.[36] Stiletto[84] (Fig. 20-19) reported good results after open reduction and internal fixation of unstable pelvic fractures in two toddlers. AO small-fragment instrumentation was used in both. During a 7-year period, Karunaker et al.[40] operatively treated 18 unstable pelvic and acetabular fractures in children. Their results suggest that unstable pelvic and acetabular fractures in the skeletally mature patient should be managed by the same principles used in the adult population. Clinical and radiographic follow-up at a mean of 2 years in their group showed that adolescents recover full function with minimal deficits and residual pain if anatomic or near-anatomic reductions are achieved. Unstable pelvic and acetabular fractures in skeletally immature patient were also successfully managed operatively with a low incidence of complications. No sacroiliac or triradiate growth arrests were identified at 3 years of follow-up. They recommended operative intervention in skeletally immature patients with significant deformity of the pelvis at the time of injury to prevent late morbidities.[40]

Optimal fixation of the sacroiliac joint is by sacroiliac screws. Insertion of sacroiliac screws requires expertise and image guidance. The patient is placed prone on a radiolucent table. A lateral image of S1 can find the starting point for the guidewire. Then a fluoroscopic 40-degree pelvic inlet and 40-degree pelvic

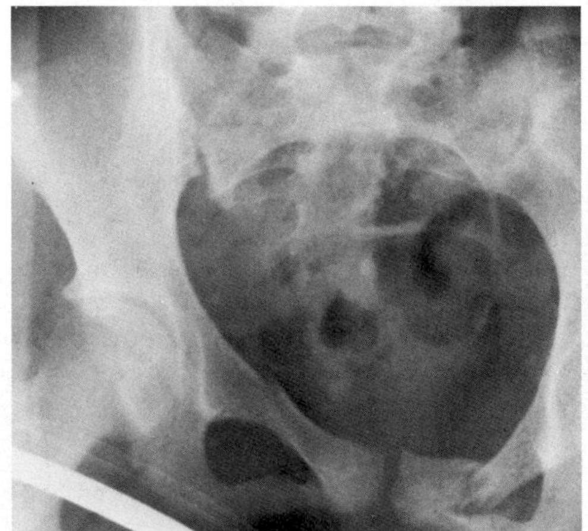

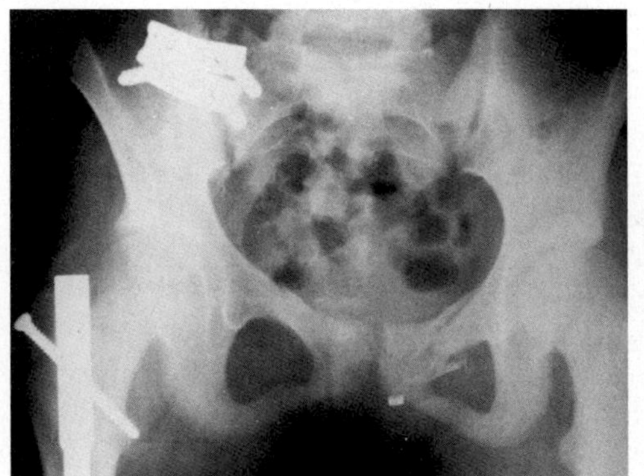

FIGURE 20-18 A. Multiple trauma in this 12-year-old child included three fractures of the pubic rami, disruption and fracture of the sacroiliac joint on the right, and a femoral shaft fracture on the right. **B.** CT shows fracture of the ilium and disruption of the sacroiliac joint. **C.** After open reduction and internal fixation of the sacroiliac joint and closed intramedullary nailing of the femoral shaft fracture. Note femoral nail inserted through the tip of the greater trochanter.

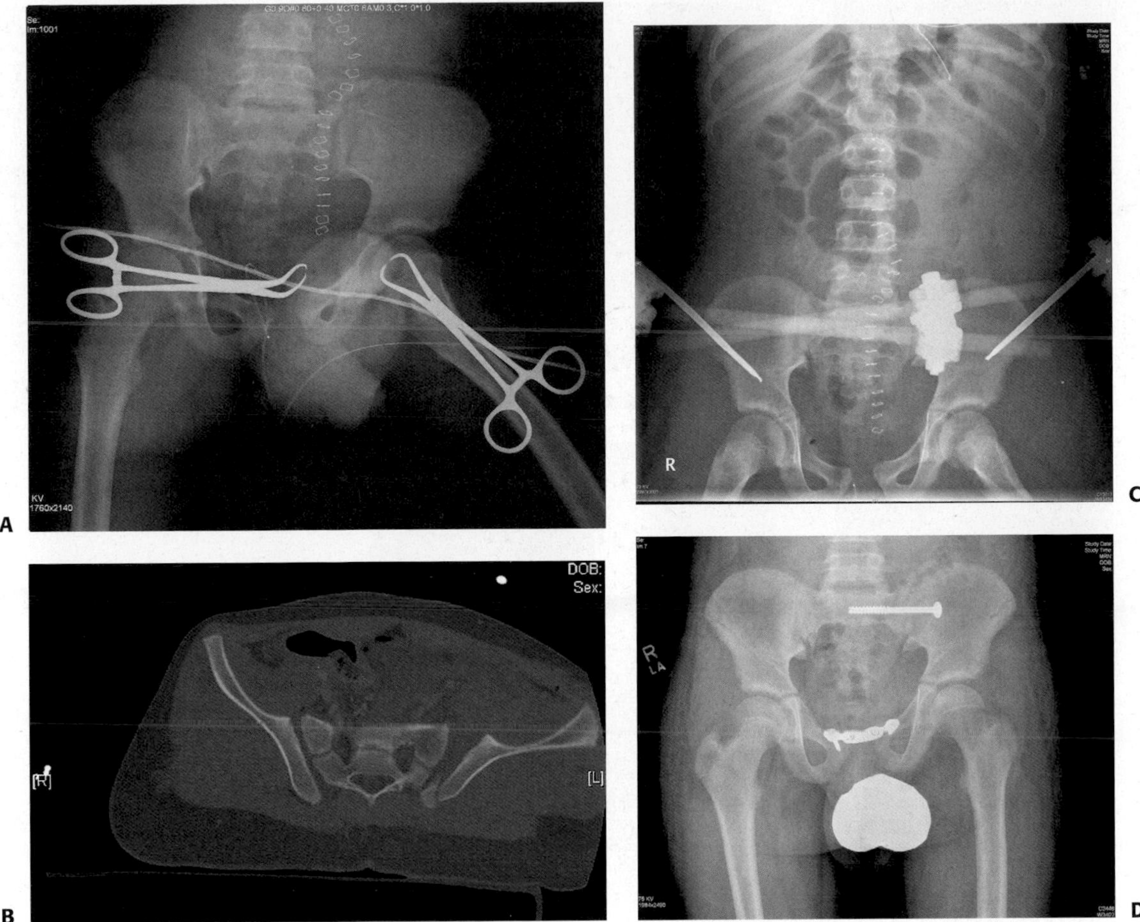

FIGURE 20-19 This radiographic series highlights treatment of an unstable pelvic fracture with hemodynamic instability. **A.** Anteroposterior pelvic radiograph of a 12-year-old boy who was a pedestrian hit by a car. There is a wide symphysis and a displaced fracture adjacent to the left sacroiliac joint. The towel clips seen on radiograph are to hold a sheet (sling) around the pelvis to help temporarily control hemorrhage. **B.** CT scan showing the displaced posterior injury. **C.** Pelvic radiograph after an anterior external fixation was placed urgently to stabilize the pelvis. This along with resuscitation stabilized the hemodynamic status. **D.** Once the patient had stabilized, the external fixation was converted to anterior internal fixation with a plate on the symphysis pubis and the posterior instability was treated with a sacroiliac screw.

outlet views are obtained to direct the guidewire across the sacroiliac joint into the body of S1(Fig. 20-20). One 6.5-mm cannulated screw is optimal. In the pediatric patient, the narrow corridor for safe screw placement makes the procedure difficult.[83] In the patient with a small corridor, the use of screw placement with CT guidance has been described.[97] The use of cannulated screws facilitates accurate placement.

To summarize, most pelvic fractures in skeletally immature patients do not need operative intervention. When the pelvis is more mature, adult guidelines should be followed. There is data to suggest that significant residual deformity may lead to a poor outcomes so unstable fracture patterns may benefit from operative reduction. The following are indications for operative fixation of pelvic fractures in children: (i) severe instability for which the goals are to control pain associated with motion of fragments, to control bleeding, and to facilitate mobility and patient transfer; (ii) associated visceral or soft tissue injuries that could not be managed without a stable skeleton; and (iii) a displaced (>1 cm) unstable fracture that is likely to lead to long-term mechanical problems.

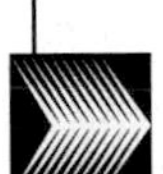

AUTHORS' PREFERRED TREATMENT

A multispecialty approach has improved the outcome of adult pelvic fractures and should be part of pediatric pelvic fracture treatment. The team should be aware of the large incidence of concomitant injuries to the head, thorax, and abdomen. The urogenital system should be carefully evaluated specifically evaluating for open fractures. If there is hemodynamic instability, the trauma surgeon, orthopaedic surgeon, radiologist, and blood bank should work together to stabilize the patient. The orthopaedic surgeon can provide temporary relief with pelvic wrapping, external fixation, or wound packing depending on the treatment of other injuries. If needed, operative fixation can be done in the same session as surgery for associated injuries or it can be timed later when the patient is stabilized.

Treatment is more likely to be conservative in children with an immature pelvis and operative in children with an unstable fracture pattern and a mature pelvis or closed tria-

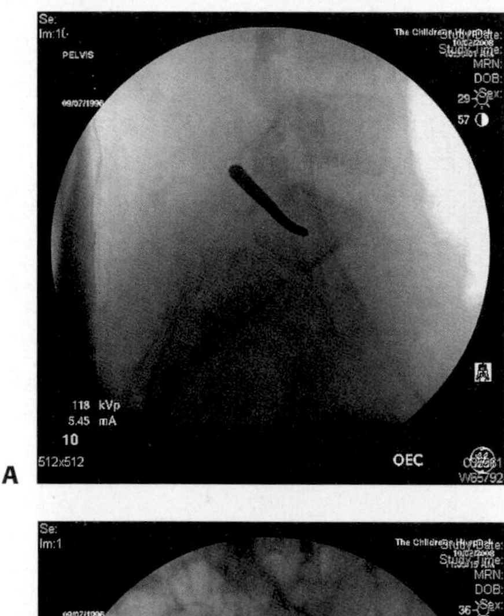

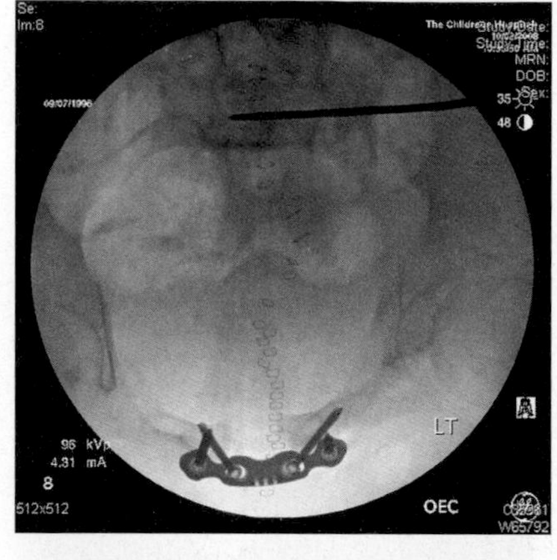

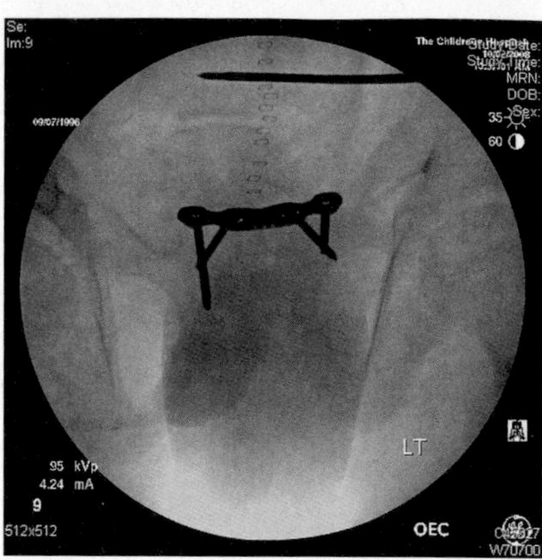

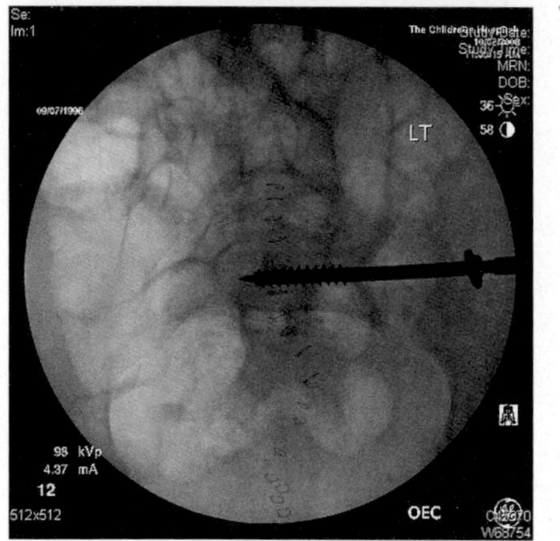

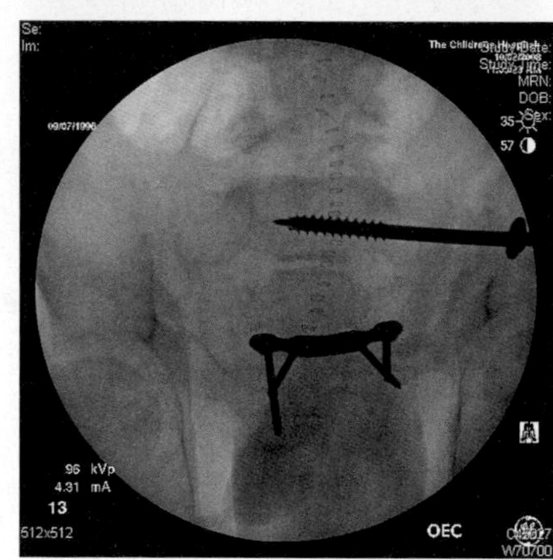

FIGURE 20-20 Placement of a sacroiliac screw. **A.** Fluoroscopic lateral image of S1 to percutaneously localize the starting point for the guidewire. **B.** Fluoroscopic 40-degree inlet view showing the direction of the guidewire for anterior and posterior placement in the sacroiliac body. **C.** Fluoroscopic 40-degree outlet view showing location of the guidewire in relation to the S1 foramen. **D.** Inlet view after screw placement. **E.** Outlet view showing screw placement in the body of S1.

diate cartilage.[79] For toddlers, we prefer symptomatic treatment that may include a spica cast for immobilization and comfort. In the younger child with severe displacement, femoral traction on the displaced side of the hemipelvis may be indicated if operative reduction with implants may not be technically feasible. There is growing body of evidence that unstable pelvic fractures treated nonoperatively have poor results. Fracture reduction is indicated in unstable fractures. The challenge is deciding what is unstable, the uncommon incidence of these fractures, and the methods of fixation. The technical principles are identical to those used for unstable pelvic fractures in adults. Torode and Zieg class IV injuries with displacement and/or pelvic ring fractures with displacement of more than 1 cm and anterior and posterior ring fractures should have reduction and fixation. Open reduction of the sacroiliac joint or a posterior iliac injury can be performed with a combination of plate and/or screws. The approach can be anterior in the iliac fossa or posterior depending on the fracture characteristics. Sacroiliac screws can be used in the immature pelvis. The anatomy and size of S1 must be adequate for screw placement. Imaging, including the use of fluoroscopy for placement of the screws, is necessary. In older adolescents, treatment should follow the guidelines for the treatment of adult fractures, including a combination of internal and external fixation for fracture stabilization and early mobilization. With a widened symphysis, anterior external fixation or plating is recommended along with posterior stabilization.

Severe Multiple or Open Fractures

In patients with crushing injuries, distortion of the pelvis is severe and, in addition to multiple breaks in the pelvic ring, apparent or occult fractures of the sacrum may be present, with or without neurologic involvement (Fig. 20-21). Massive hem-

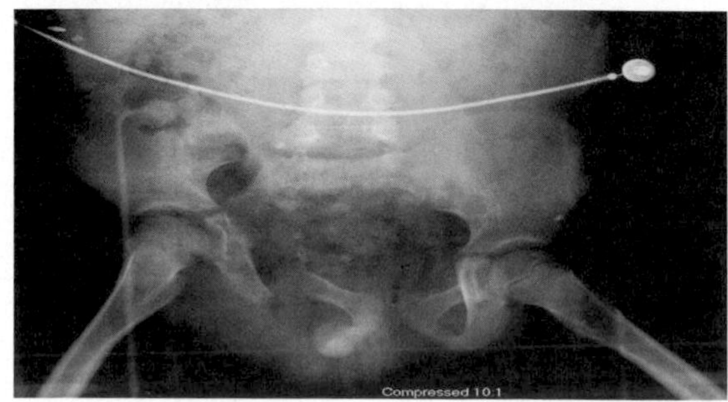

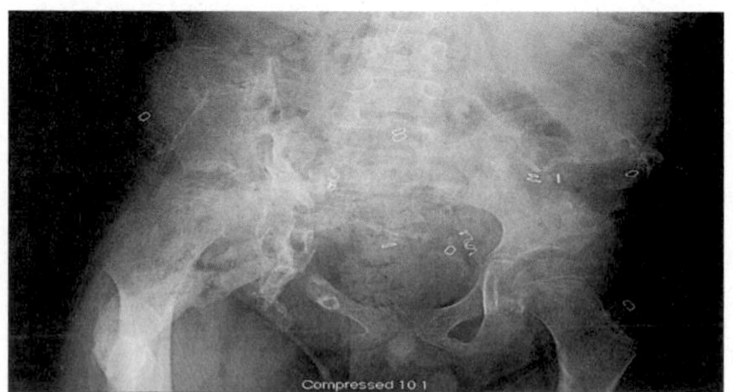

FIGURE 20-21 A. Open pelvic fracture with severe displacement. **B.** The soft tissue injury precluded pelvic reduction and fixation. This radiograph shows remarkable late deformity.

orrhage, although common in adults with severe pelvic fractures,[19] is much less common in children with pelvic fractures.[79] Nevertheless, up to 20% of children with crushed open pelvic fractures in one series died within hours of admission secondary to uncontrolled hemorrhage.[54] The overall need for blood transfusion in two large retrospective series including all types of pediatric pelvic fractures was between 21% and 33%.[19,29] In the setting of hypovolemic shock, however, emergency measures may be necessary.

The patient should be stable without evidence of ongoing blood loss before operative intervention. Occasionally, an external fixator will be applied spanning the iliac crests in order to limit the pelvic volume and thereby tamponade persistent bleeding. The rare patient may also require arterial embolization and placement of an inferior vena cava filter before operative intervention. It is important to recognize injuries with marked comminution because mobile fracture fragments may penetrate viscera (e.g., the bladder or abdominal viscera) or lacerate the vagina or rectum.

Open pelvic fractures are rare in children. Mosheiff et al.[54] reported that 13% of 116 pediatric pelvic fractures seen over a 12-year period were open injuries. Fourteen of the 15 children were struck by motor vehicles, and one sustained a gunshot wound. Five children with stable fractures were treated nonoperatively, and 10 with unstable fractures were treated operatively: external fixation alone (8 patients), combined external fixation and internal fixation (3 patients), and internal fixation alone (2 patients). Three of the children died secondary to uncontrollable hemorrhage (2 patients) and chest injury (1 patient). Eleven of the 12 surviving children had deep wound infection or sepsis, and 3 had premature physeal closure. Mosheiff and colleagues[54] emphasized that the treatment of the soft tissue injuries depends on stabilization of the pelvis and that external fixation is often insufficient, and posterior internal fixation and stabilization are often necessary.

Fractures of the Sacrum

Sacral fractures constitute a small fraction of pelvic fractures reported in children. Rieger and Brug[69] reported two sacral fractures and seven sacroiliac fracture–dislocations in their 54 patients. Sacral fractures are probably more common than reported, but because they are obscured by the bony pelvis and the soft tissue shadows of the abdominal viscera, and because they are rarely displaced, they may be overlooked. Nine of 166 patients (5.4%) with pelvic fractures in the series by Silber et al.[80] had associated sacral fractures, none with nerve root involvement. There are two general types of sacral injuries. Spinal type injuries may present as crush injury with vertical foreshortening of the sacrum or horizontal fractures across the sacrum. These fractures may be significant because they may damage the sacral nerves, resulting in loss of bowel and bladder function. Alar type injuries are generally vertical fractures through the ala or foramina. There fractures are significant in that they may represent the posterior break of the double ring fracture.

The presence of sacral fractures may be suggested clinically. Pain and swelling may be present, usually over the sacrum. Rectal examination elicits pain on palpation. Occasionally, the fracture fragments may be felt. Manual attempts at reduction should be avoided because of the risk of rectal tear.

Sacral fractures are difficult to see on plain radiographs. The fracture can be oblique, but most are transverse with minimal displacement and occur through a sacral foramen, which is the weakest part of the body of the sacrum. Minimal offset of the foramen or offset of the lateral edge of the body of the sacrum is an indication of sacral fracture. Lateral views are helpful only if there is anterior displacement, which is rare. A 35-degree caudad view of the pelvis may reveal a fracture of the body of the sacrum. CT and MRI scans are best in the identification of sacral fractures missed on plain radiographic images.[28,30,75] In one study comparing radiographs with CT scans in a consecutive series of 103 pediatric trauma patients with pelvic radiographs and pelvic CT scans, only three sacral fractures were identified with plain radiographs whereas nine sacral fractures were identified with CT (Fig. 20-22).[30] Sacral fractures are generally managed expectantly and treated symptomatically. In rare cases, pinched sacral nerve roots may need to be decompressed.

Fractures of the Coccyx

Many children fall on the tailbone and have subsequent pain. The possibility of fracture must be entertained. Because the coccyx is made up of multiple small segments, is obscured by soft tissue, and naturally has a crook in it, it is difficult to determine

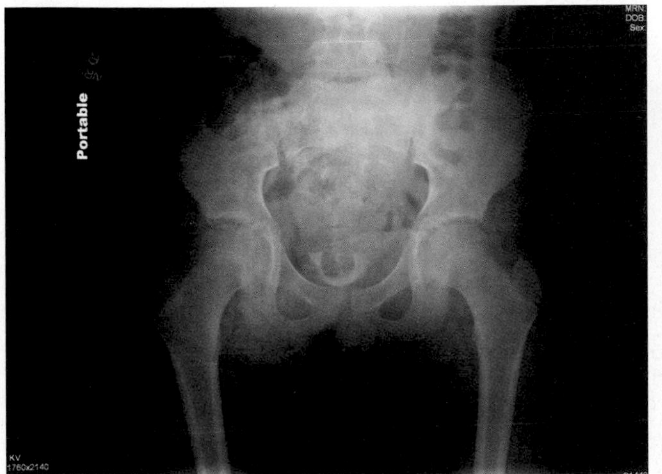

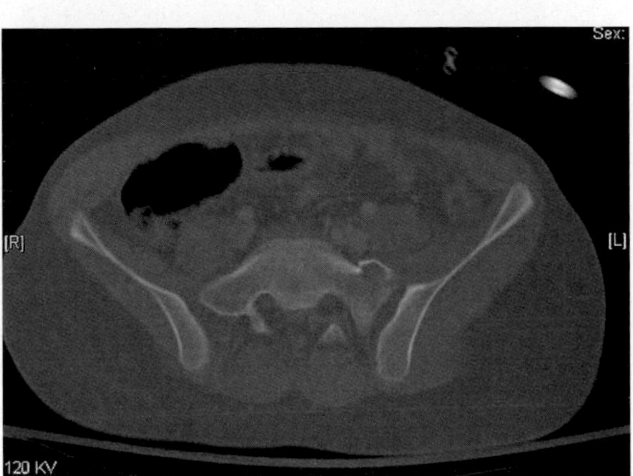

FIGURE 20-22 A. An example of an anterior posterior pelvic radiograph where the sacral fracture is not well visualized. **B.** CT scan of the patient showing the sacral fracture.

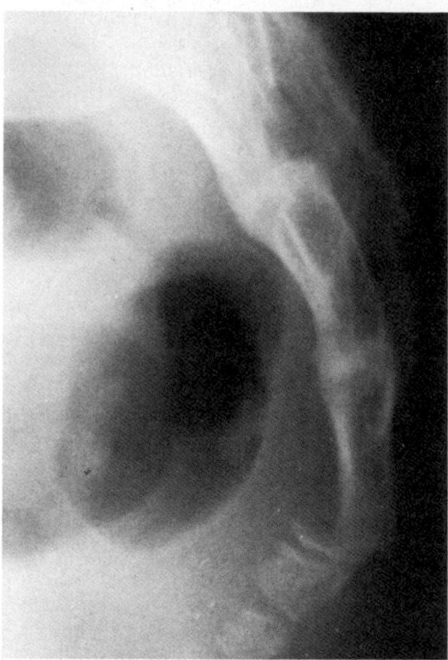

FIGURE 20-23 Lateral radiograph with the hips maximally flexed reveals displaced coccygeal fracture in a 14-year-old boy.

on radiographs whether a coccygeal fracture has occurred, especially in a child. These fractures rarely have associated injuries. Clinically, patients describe immediate, severe pain in the area of the coccyx. Pain on defecation may be present as well as pain on rectal examination. Because radiographic identification is difficult, the diagnosis should be made clinically by digital rectal examination. Exquisite pain may be elicited, and an abnormal mobility of the coccygeal fragments may be noted. Acute symptoms may abate in 1 to 2 weeks, but may be remarkably persistent. The differential diagnosis is between fracture and coccydynia. Lateral radiographs of the coccyx with the hips flexed maximally may reveal a fracture (Fig. 20-23). Apex posterior angulation of the coccyx is normal variant, and should not be falsely interpreted as a fracture or dislocation. CT and MRI scanning may be helpful in differentiating between physeal plates and fracture lines.[8] Treatment is symptomatic only and consists of activity restriction and pressure-relieving doughnut cushion for sitting with an expectation of resolution in 4 to 6 weeks.

ACETABULAR FRACTURES

Acetabular fractures constitute only 6% to 17% of pediatric pelvic fractures, making them very uncommon.[29,54,79] The remarkable difference between acetabular fractures in children and adults is the presence of the triradiate cartilage in growing children. This critical physeal area is responsible for acetabular growth and development, acts as a stress riser in the pelvic ring, and is susceptible to permanent damage. The mechanism of injury of acetabular fractures in children is similar to that in adults: The fracture occurs from a force transmitted through the femoral head. The position of the leg with respect to the pelvis and the location of the impact determine the fracture pattern; the magnitude of the force determines the severity of the fracture or fracture–dislocation. Patients with high-energy injuries usually have major associated injuries. Fractures of the acetabulum are intimately associated with pelvic fractures. Some acetabular fractures involve only the hip socket. Others represent the exit point of a fracture of the pelvic ring. Pelvic fractures, particularly ramus fractures, may propagate into the triradiate cartilage (Fig. 20-24).

Classification

Bucholz et al.[10] classified pediatric acetabular fractures based on the Salter-Harris classification (Fig. 20-25). Their classification system is used to help determine the prognosis of a triradiate cartilage injury that may result in a deformity of the acetabulum with growth. The anatomy of the triradiate is such that the superior weight-bearing portion of the acetabulum is separated from the inferior third by the superior arms of the triradiate cartilage. These superior arms are usually the ones involved in a fracture. In the Bucholz classification, a type I or II injury occurs from a traumatic force to the ischial ramus, pubic ramus, or proximal femur resulting in a shearing force through the to superior arms of the triradiate cartilage. If there is a metaphyseal bone fragment, this is a type II fracture. A type V injury is a crush injury to the physis.[10,47] Watts[95] described four types of acetabular fractures in children: (i) small fragments that most often occur with dislocation of the hip, (ii) linear fractures that occur in association with pelvic fractures without displacement and usually are stable, (iii) linear fractures with hip joint insta-

A

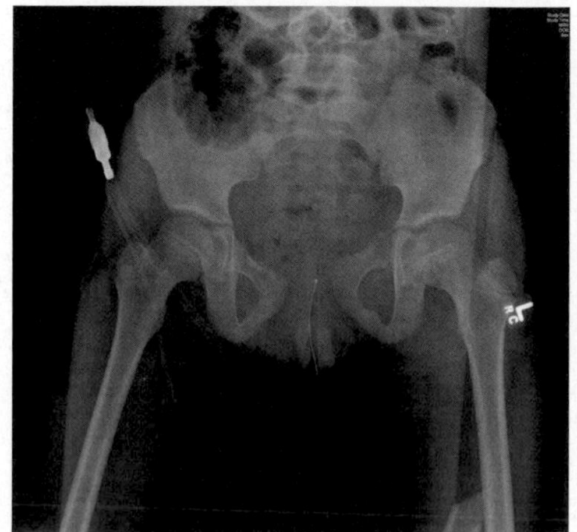

B

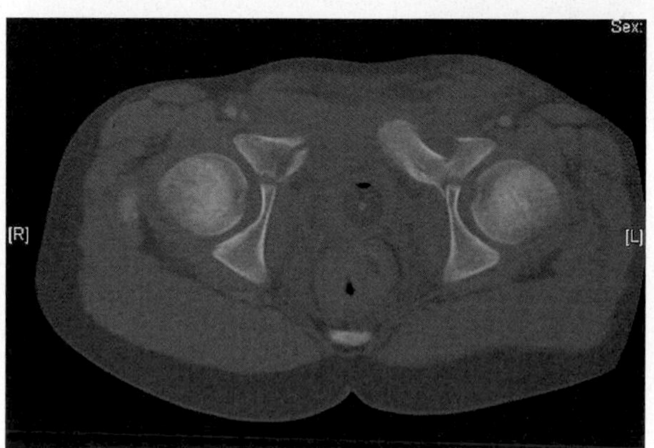

FIGURE 20-24 A. Pelvic radiograph showing a pelvic fracture with the left superior rami injury propagating towards the triradiate cartilage. **B.** CT scan showing the rami fractures propagating into the triradiate cartilage.

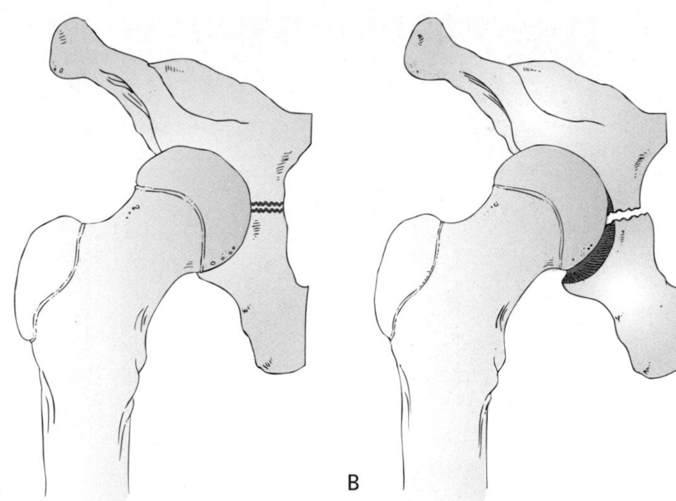

FIGURE 20-25 Types of triradiate cartilage fractures. **A.** Normal triradiate cartilage. **B.** Salter-Harris type I fracture.

bility, and (iv) fractures secondary to central fracture–dislocation of the hip.

Acetabular fractures in children can also be described similarly to those in adults which are usually classified by the system of Judet et al.[38] and Letournel and Judet.[46] A more comprehensive system is the AO comprehensive fracture classification, which groups all fractures into A, B, and C types with increasing severity. Type A acetabular fractures involve a single wall or column; type B fractures involve both columns (transverse or T-types) and a portion of the dome remains attached to the intact ilium; and type C fractures involve both columns and separate the dome fragment from the axial skeleton by a fracture through the ilium. Both of these classification systems are discussed in more detail in Rockwood and Green's, Fractures in Adults, Chapter 36, Volume 2, of this series in relation to adult fractures.

Radiographic Evaluation

Anteroposterior views may not be adequate to show the displacement of acetabular fragments after fracture. Inlet, outlet, and 45-degree oblique (Judet) views often are often needed to show displacement. CT scanning is even better to show displacement and can detect retained intra-articular fragments which can prevent concentric reduction (Fig. 20-26).[13] Three-dimensional CT reconstructions can give an excellent view of the overall bony fracture pattern but often underestimate the magnitude of cartilaginous fragments, especially of posterior wall fractures in children.[71] Rubel et al.[71] recommend MRI as an adjunctive imaging study for all pediatric acetabular fractures because MRI discloses the true size of largely cartilaginous posterior wall fragments in children (Fig. 20-27).

Treatment

The goals of treatment for acetabular fractures in children are two. The first is to restore the mechanics of the hip. The second is restoring alignment of the triradiate cartilage in hopes of ensuring normal growth. The mechanical goals of treatment for acetabular fractures in children are the same as for adults: to restore joint congruity and hip stability. Schlickewei et al.[72] noted that there are a variety of injury patterns and limited evidence of outcomes for any specific treatment. Thus, each fracture should be evaluated on an individual basis with the following guidelines: (i) anatomic reduction will likely result in a good long-term outcome; (ii) MRI is the best tool for identifying closure of the triradiate cartilage; and (iii) patients should be informed on the possible growth arrest and secondary associated problems such as joint subluxation or dysplasia.[72]

Treatment guidelines in general follow those for adults. Non–weight-bearing ambulation with crutches can be used for nondisplaced or minimally (≤1 mm) displaced fractures. Because weight-bearing forces must not be transmitted across the fracture, crutch ambulation is appropriate only for older children

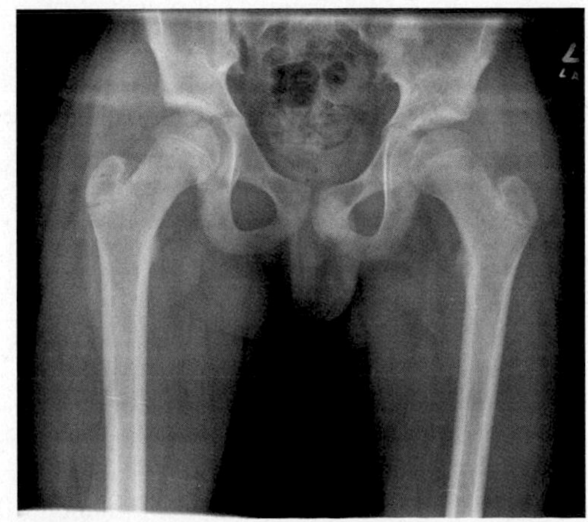

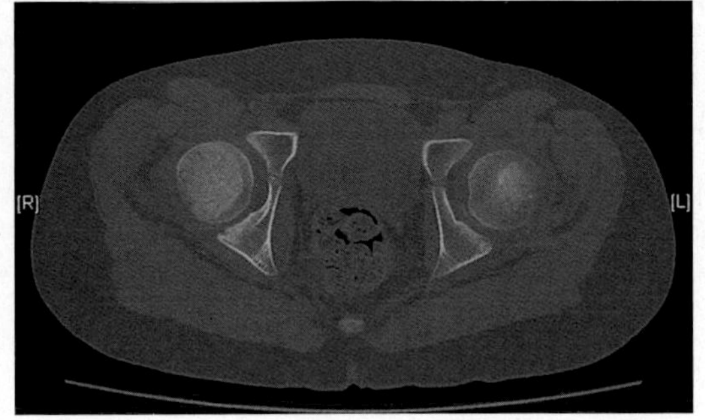

FIGURE 20-26 A. Postreduction anteroposterior pelvis radiograph of a 12-year-old with the left hip appearing nonconcentric. **B.** CT scan showing a bony fragment from the posterior wall impeding reduction.

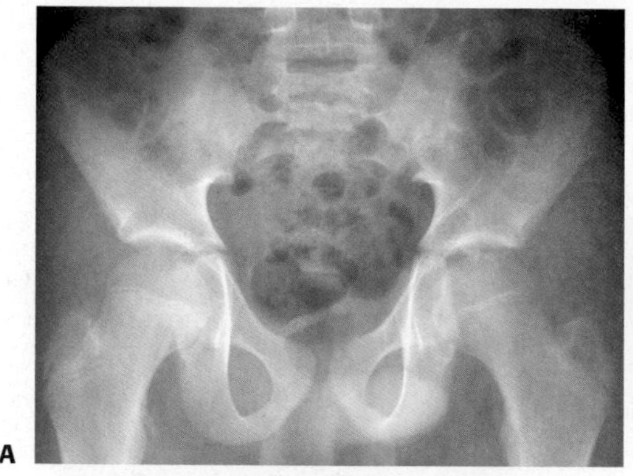

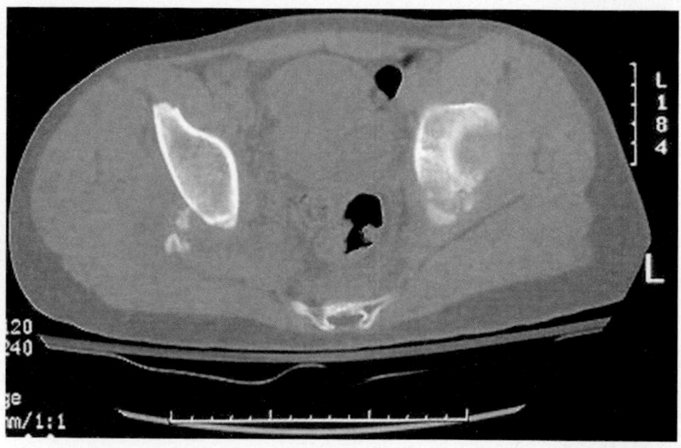

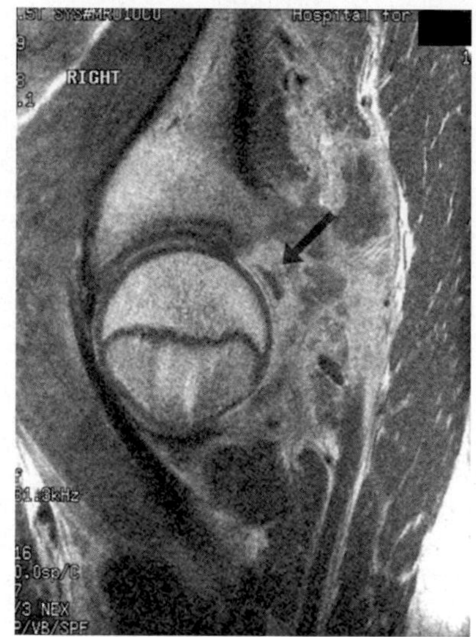

FIGURE 20-27 A. Postreduction radiograph of a left hip dislocation in a 12-year-old boy. **B.** CT scan demonstrates small ossified posterior wall fragments. **C.** Sagittal MRI demonstrates 90% posterior wall involvement with intra-articular step-off (*black arrow*). (From Rubel IF, Kloen P, Potter HG, Helfet DL. MRI assessment of the posterior acetabular wall fracture in traumatic dislocation of the hip in children. Pediatr Radiol 2002;32(6):435–439, with permission.)

who can reliably avoid weight bearing on the injured limb. Non–weight bearing usually is continued for 6 to 8 weeks. In younger children, this may be shortened to 5 to 6 weeks.

Gordon et al.[27] recommended accurate reduction and internal fixation of any displaced acetabular fracture in a child. They noted that the presence of incomplete fractures and plastic deformation may make accurate reduction difficult or impossible; they recommended that incomplete fractures be completed and that osteotomies of the pubis, ilium, or ischium be made if necessary for accurate reduction of the acetabulum.[27] In children with open physes, all periacetabular metallic implants should be removed 6 to 18 months after surgery. Improved outcomes with early (<24 hours) fixation of acetabular fractures in adults have been reported,[61] and Gordon et al.[27] noted that early fixation (before callus formation) is especially important to prevent malunion in young patients in whom healing is rapid (Fig. 20-28).

Anatomic alignment of the triradiate cartilage should be obtained in children (Fig. 20-29). Linear growth of the acetabulum occurs by interstitial growth in the triradiate part of the cartilage complex, causing the pubis, ischium, and ilium to enlarge. The depth of the acetabulum develops in response to the presence of a spherical femoral head and interstitial growth of the acetabular cartilage. Growth derangement of all or part of the triradiate cartilage as a result of fracture and a triradiate physeal bar may result in a dysplastic acetabulum. Since the ilioischial limb of the triradiate contributes the most to acetabular growth, injury to the ilioischial limb of the triradiate cartilage has a greater potential for late acetabular deformity that an anterior iliopubic limb injury.[25]

Acetabular dysplasia secondary to growth arrest (bony bridge) of the triradiate cartilage has been reported after trauma to the acetabulum. Heeg[34] reported acetabular deformity and subluxation of the hip in 2 of 3 patients with premature fusion of the triradiate cartilage. Peterson and Robertson[60] reported formation of a physeal osseous bar in a 7-year-old boy 2 years after fracture of the lateral portion of the superior ramus at the junction with the triradiate cartilage. After excision of the osseous bridge, the physis remained open. Although the injured physis closed earlier than the contralateral side, there was only a slight increase in the thickness of the acetabular wall and lateral displacement of the femoral head. Peterson and Robertson[60] emphasized that early recognition and treatment are essential before premature closure of the entire physis and development of permanent osseous deformity (Fig. 20-30).[60] The typical dysplastic changes seen after trauma to the triradiate cartilage differ significantly from developmental dysplasia and include both lateralization of the hip joint and acetabular retroversion.[21]

Bucholz et al.[10] noted two main patterns of physeal injury in nine patients with triradiate cartilage injury: a Salter-Harris type I or II injury, which had a favorable prognosis for continued normal acetabular growth, and a crush injury (Salter-Harris V), which had a poor prognosis with premature closure of the

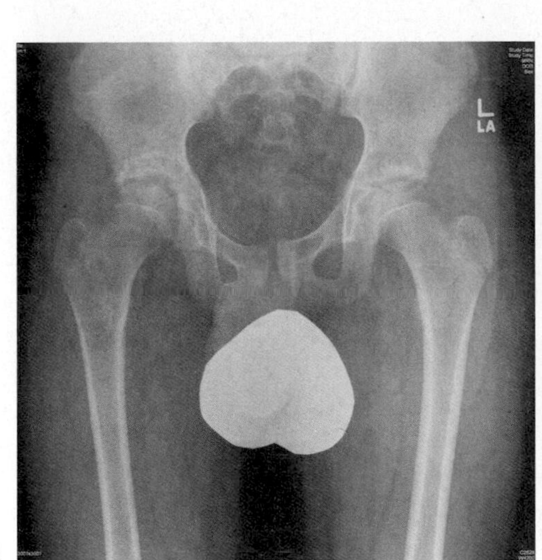

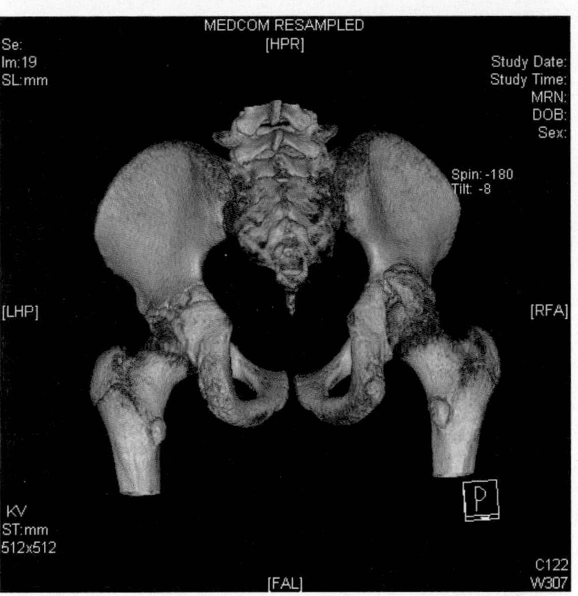

FIGURE 20-28 A. Pelvic radiograph of a 12-year-old 1 year after an acetabular fracture. The fracture is a malunion with subluxation of the hip joint. **B.** Three-dimensional CT scan showing the malunited fragment.

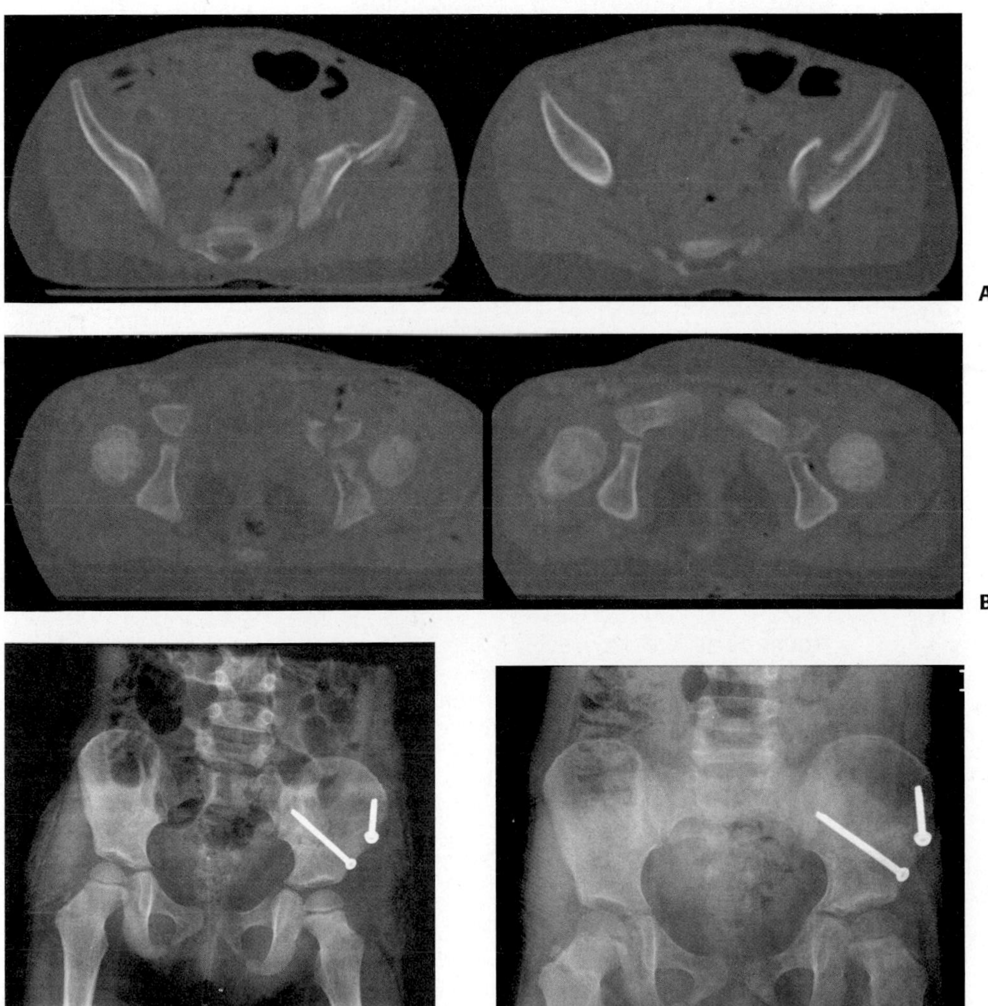

FIGURE 20-29 A. CT scan of a 7-year-old with a displaced pelvic wing fracture **B.** CT scan showing the fracture propagation into the triradiate cartilage. **C.** Anatomic reduction of the triradiate cartilage with open reduction and internal fixation. **D.** Despite anatomic reduction, a medial osseous bar spans the triradiate cartilage.

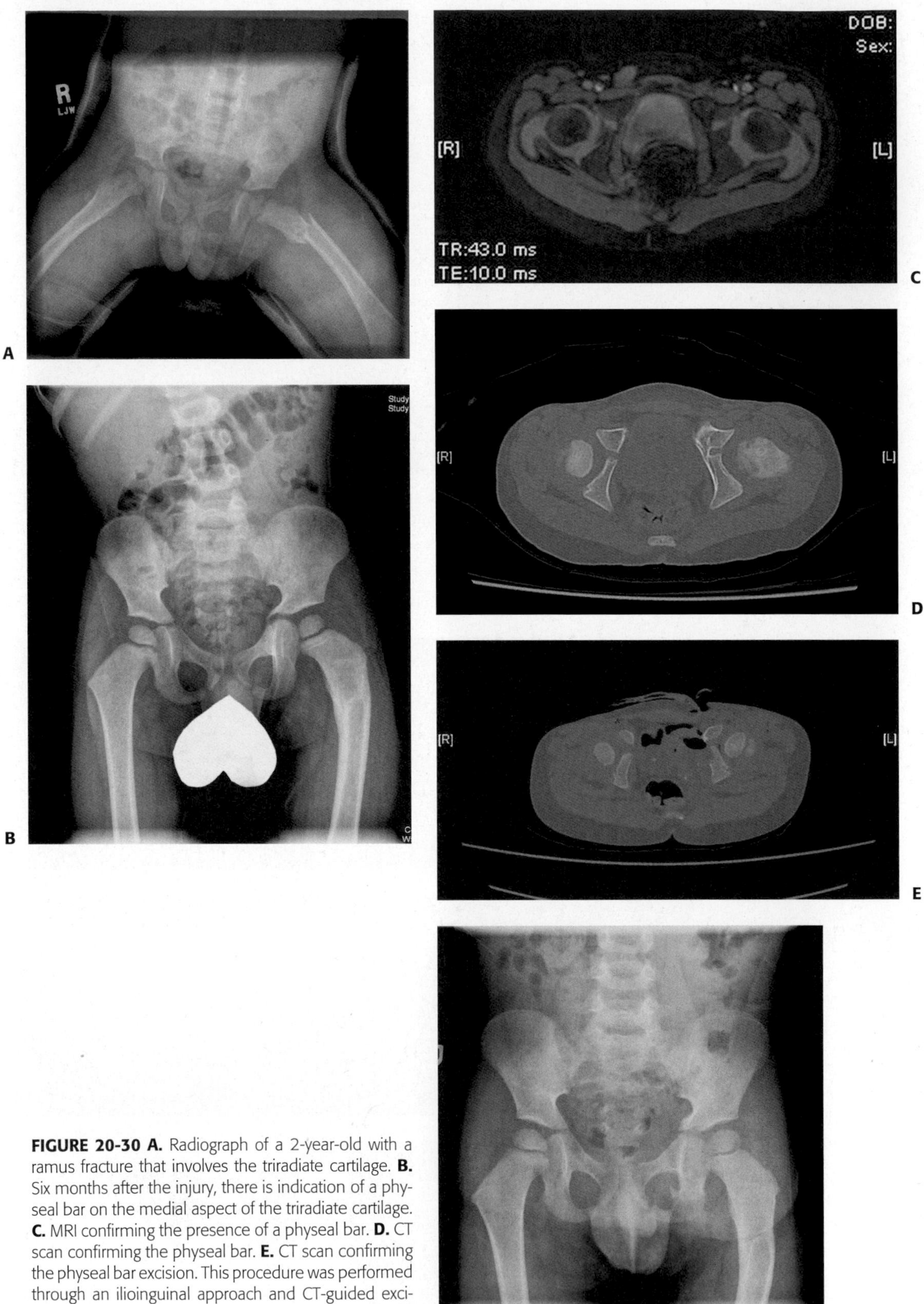

FIGURE 20-30 A. Radiograph of a 2-year-old with a ramus fracture that involves the triradiate cartilage. **B.** Six months after the injury, there is indication of a physeal bar on the medial aspect of the triradiate cartilage. **C.** MRI confirming the presence of a physeal bar. **D.** CT scan confirming the physeal bar. **E.** CT scan confirming the physeal bar excision. This procedure was performed through an ilioinguinal approach and CT-guided excision. **F.** Radiograph of the pelvis after bar excision.

triradiate cartilage caused by formation of a medial osseous bridge. In either pattern, the prognosis depended on the child's age at the time of injury. In young children, especially those younger than 10 years of age, acetabular growth abnormality was common and resulted in a dysplastic acetabulum. By the time of skeletal maturity, disparate growth increased the incongruity of the hip joint and led to progressive subluxation. These authors found that acetabular reconstruction was frequently necessary to correct the gradual subluxation of the femoral head.[10]

TABLE 20-4 Surgical Exposure for Operative Fixation of Acetabular Fractures

Fracture Type	Exposure
Anterior column or wall	Ilioinguinal
Posterior column or wall	Kocher-Langenbeck
Transverse	Ilioinguinal (or extended lateral)
T-shaped	Ilioinguinal and Kocher-Langenbeck (or extended lateral)
Anterior column and posterior hemitransverse	Ilioinguinal
Both columns	Ilioinguinal (or extended lateral)

From Gordon RG, Karpik K, Hardy Sea. Techniques of operative reduction and fixation of pediatric and adolescent pelvic fractures. Oper Tech Orthop 1995;5: 95–114, with permission.

Surgical Treatment

The surgical treatment varies according to the pattern of the fracture and the direction of the displacement as determined on the preoperative radiographs and CT scans (Table 20-4).[27] Fractures of the posterior wall or posterior column can be approached through a Kocher-Langenbeck approach with the patient either in the lateral decubitus position (isolated posterior wall fracture) or supine (associated posterior column fracture) (Fig. 20-31). Anterior column injuries can be approached through an ilioinguinal approach. Some transverse fractures may require an extended iliofemoral approach.[17] The extended lateral approaches, which include the extended iliofemoral and triradiate approaches, should be avoided as much as possible because of the risk of devascularization of the ilium and heterotopic bone formation.[31]

The surgeon should be familiar with the treatise by Judet et al.[38] on the operative reduction of acetabular fractures and with Letournel and Judet's[46] work before performing this surgery. For smaller children and smaller fragments, Watts[95] recommended threaded Kirschner-wires for fixation. In larger children, cannulated screws can provide secure fixation (Figs. 20-32 and 20-33). Small-fragment reconstruction plates, appropriately contoured, also can be used. Gordon et al.[27] described the addition of a small (two- or three-hole) "hook plate" for small or comminuted fragments (Fig. 20-34). Because future operative procedures about the hip may be necessary, the hardware should probably be removed after healing.

Brown et al.[9] described the use of CT image-guided fixation of acetabular fractures in 10 patients, including bilateral posterior wall fractures in a 14-year-old girl. They cite as advantages of image-guided surgery reduced operating time (~20% reduction), less extensive surgical dissection, reduced fluoroscopic time, and compatibility with traditional fixation techniques. Most important, it allows accurate and safe placement of screws

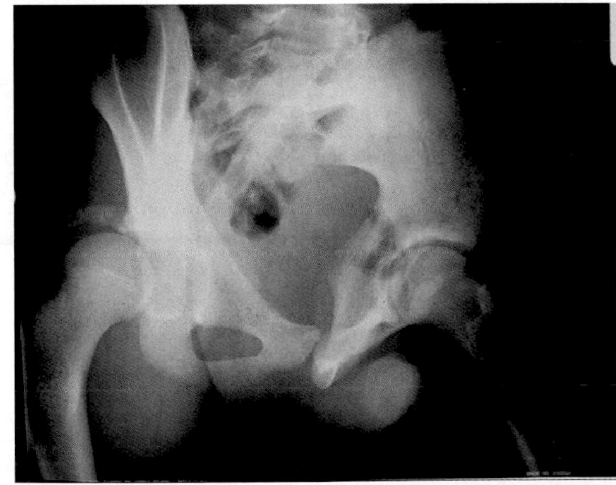

A

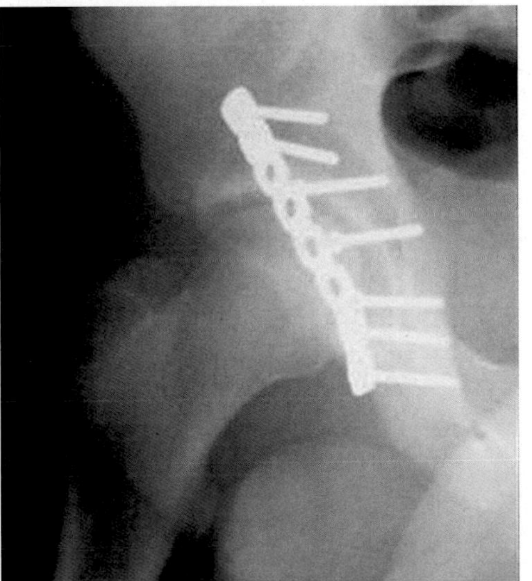

B

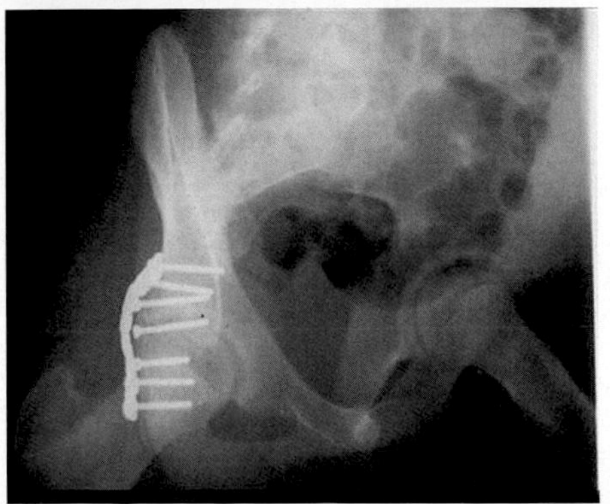

C

FIGURE 20-31 A. Radiograph of a football injury with posterior acetabular fracture and dislocation. **B,C.** Postoperative radiographs after a posterior approach and plating.

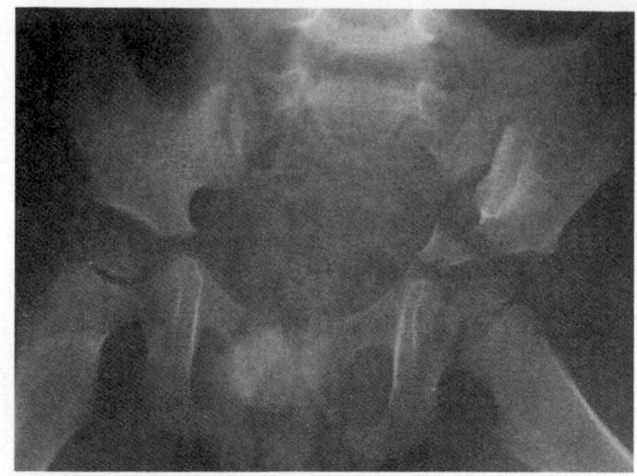

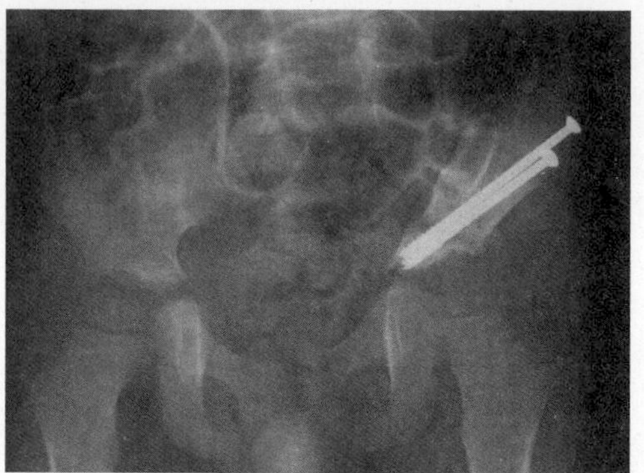

FIGURE 20-32 A. Fracture of the wing of the ilium with extension into the dome of the acetabulum in a 3-year-old boy. **B.** After reduction and fixation with two cannulated screws. (From Habacker TA, Heinrich SD, Dehne R. Fracture of the superior pelvic quadrant in a child. J Pediatr Orthop 1995;15(1):69–72, with permission.)

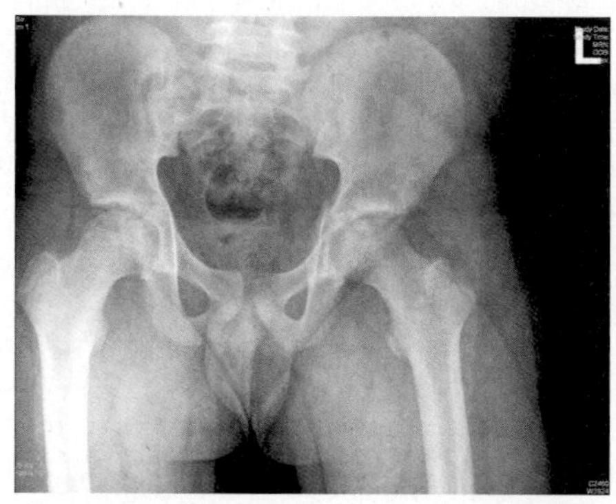

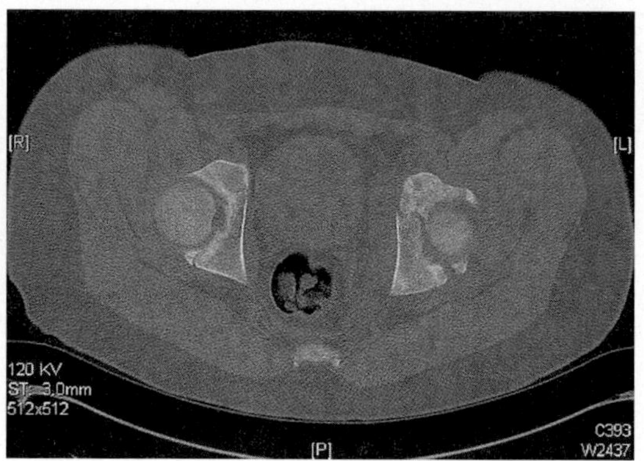

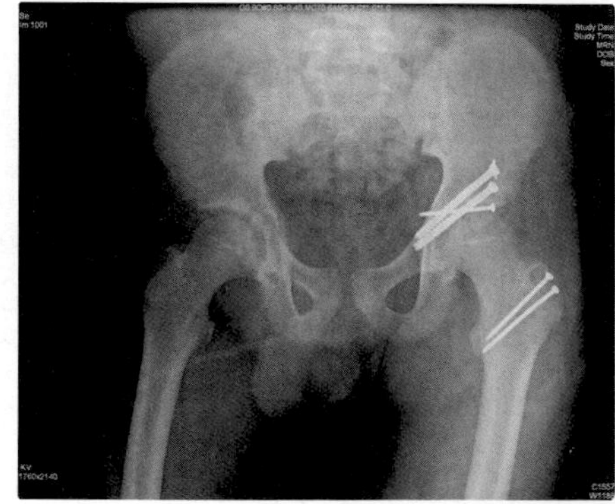

FIGURE 20-33 A. Radiograph of a 13-year-old with an acetabular fracture though the closing triradiate cartilage. **B.** CT scan showing the fracture in the region of the triradiate and posterior wall. **C.** Postoperative radiograph of the fracture fixed with cannulated screws via a surgical hip dislocation approach.

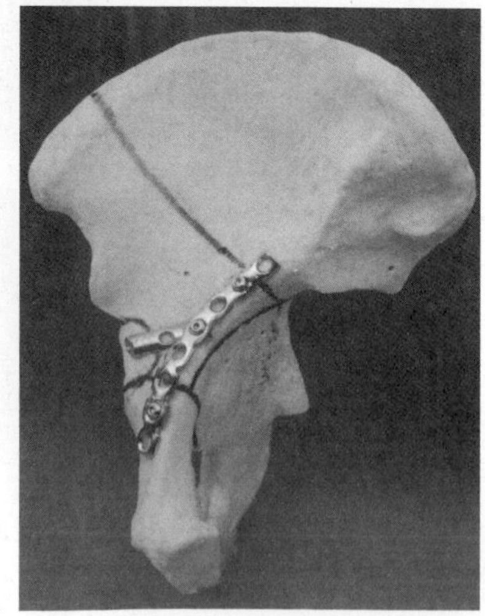

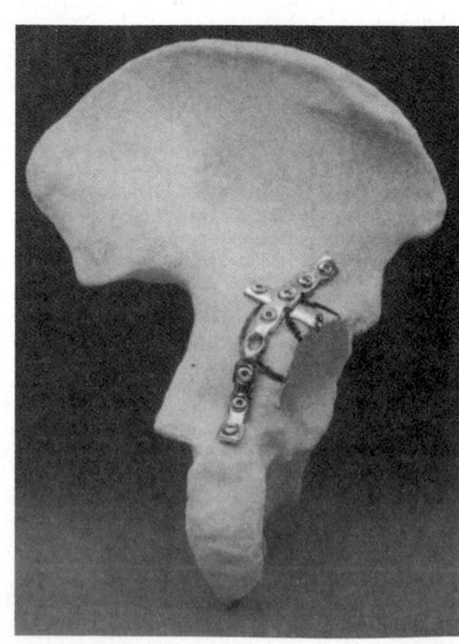

FIGURE 20-34 A. Anterior column plate and additional wall "hook" plate. **B.** Posterior wall buttress plate and hook plate. (From Gordon RG, Karpik K, Hardy SEA. Techniques of operative reduction and fixation of pediatric and adolescent pelvic fractures. Oper Tech Orthop 1995;5:95–114, with permission.)

and pins for acetabular fixation. This technology is attractive, but anatomic reduction of the joint surface and secure fixation outweigh the benefits of surgical convenience.

Postoperative Management

Small children can be immobilized in a spica cast for 6 weeks. If radiographs show adequate healing at that time, the cast is removed and free mobility is allowed. In an older child with stable fixation, crutches are used for protected weight bearing for 6 to 8 weeks. If radiographs show satisfactory healing, weight bearing is progressed as tolerated. Return to vigorous activities, especially competitive sports is delayed for at least 3 months.

Pelvic radiographs should be obtained for 2 years after an acetabular fracture looking for a triradiate closure. If the radiographs indicate a physeal bar, CT and MRI can be obtained to confirm the diagnosis. If the patient is less than 10 years of age, a triradiate bar excision should be performed.

COMPLICATIONS

The major complications are malunion of the pelvic fracture leading to long-term morbidity and premature triradiate closure after acetabular fracture. Because of the rapid healing in young children, loss of reduction and nonunion usually are not problems. Other reported complications include osteonecrosis, traumatic arthritis, sciatic nerve palsy, heterotopic ossification, and stenosis of the birth canal in female patients. Because of the possibility dystocia during childbirth, pelvimetry is recommended before pregnancy. Rieger and Brug[69] reported one female patient who required cesarean section because of ossification of the symphysis pubis after nonoperative treatment of an open-book fracture. Schwarz et al.[74] reported leg-length discrepancies of 1 to 5 cm in 10 of 17 patients after nonoperative treatment of unstable pelvic fractures; 5 had low back pain at long-term follow-up. Nine of 10 patients with lumbar scoliosis had low back pain. McDonald[51] reported that one third of 15 skeletally immature patients treated nonoperatively with unstable pelvic fractures had residual pain. Heeg and Klassen[33] reviewed 18 children with unstable pelvic fractures and reported that 9 had a leg-length discrepancy greater the 1 cm and 3 had back pain.

In summary, the major complication of pelvic fracture in children is residual deformity, which may lead to leg-length discrepancy, sacroiliac joint arthrosis, back pain, lumbar scoliosis, incompetency of the pelvic floor, and distortion of the birth canal. The complications of acetabular fracture include late hip instability, hip arthrosis, and triradiate growth that may lead to joint subluxation or dysplasia.

REFERENCES

1. Ablin DS, Greenspan A, Reinhart MA. Pelvic injuries in child abuse. Pediatr Radiol 1992; 22(6):454–457.
2. Alonso JE, Horowitz M. Use of the AO/ASIF external fixator in children. J Pediatr Orthop 1987;7(5):594–600.
3. Baessler K, Bircher MD, Stanton SL. Pelvic floor dysfunction in women after pelvic trauma. Br. J Obster Gynecol 2004;111:499–502.
4. Barnes ST, Hinds RB. Pseudotumor of the ischium. A late manifestation of avulsion of the ischial epiphysis. J Bone Joint Surg Am 1972;54(3):645–647.
5. Blasier RD, McAtee J, White R, et al. Disruption of the pelvic ring in pediatric patients. Clin Orthop Relat Res 2000;376:87–95.
6. Blount WP. Fractures in Children. Huntington, NY: Robert E. Krieger Publishing Company, 1977.
7. Bond SJ, Gotschall SC, Eichelberger MR. Predictors of abdominal injury in children with pelvic fracture. J Trauma 1991;31(8):1169–1173.
8. Broome DR, Hayman LA, Herrick RC, et al. Postnatal maturation of the sacrum and coccyx: MR imaging, helical CT, and conventional radiography. AJR Am J Roentgenol 1998;170(4):1061–1066.
9. Brown GA, Willis MC, Firoozbakhsh K, et al. Computed tomography image-guided surgery in complex acetabular fractures. Clin Orthop Relat Res 2000;370:219–226.
10. Bucholz RW, Ezaki M, Ogden JA. Injury to the acetabular triradiate physeal cartilage. J Bone Joint Surg Am 1982;64(4):600–609.
11. Burgess AR, Eastridge BJ, Young JW, et al. Pelvic ring disruptions: effective classification system and treatment protocols. J Trauma 1990;30(7):848–856.
12. Caffey J, Ross SE. The ischiopubic synchondrosis in healthy children: some normal roentgenologic findings. Am J Roentgenol Radium Ther Nucl Med 1956;76(3):488–494.
13. Canale ST, Manugian AH. Irreducible traumatic dislocations of the hip. J Bone Joint Surg Am 1979;61(1):7–14.
14. ChengJC, Ng BK, Ying SY, et al. A 10-year study of the changes in the pattern and treatment of 6493 fractures. J Pediatr Orthop 1999;19(3):344–350.
15. Chia JP, Holland AJ, Little D, et al. Pelvic fractures and associated injuries in children. J Trauma 2004;56(1):83–88.
16. Clancy WG Jr, Foltz AS. Iliac apophysitis and stress fractures in adolescent runners. Am J Sports Med 1976;4(5):214–218.
17. Crenshaw AH. Extensile acetabular approaches. In Canale ST, ed. Campbell's Operative Orthopaedics. Vol. 1. 10th ed. St. Louis: Mosby, 2003:77–86.
18. Currey JD, Butler G The mechanical properties of bone tissue in children. J Bone Joint Surg Am 1975;57(6):810–814.
19. Demetriades D, Karaiskakis M, Velmahos GC, et al. Pelvic fractures in pediatric and adult trauma patients: are they different injuries? J Trauma 2003;54(6):1146–1151.
20. Donoghue V, Daneman A, Krajbich I, et al. CT appearance of sacroiliac joint trauma in children. J Comput Assist Tomogr 1985;9(2):352–356.
21. Dora C, Zurbach J, Hersche O, et al. Pathomorphologic characteristics of posttraumatic acetabular dysplasia. J Orthop Trauma 2000;14(7):483–489.
22. Dunn AW, Morris HD. Fractures and dislocations of the pelvis. J Bone Joint Surg Am 1968;50(8):1639–1648.
23. Fernbach SK, Wilkinson RH. Avulsion injuries of the pelvis and proximal femur. AJR Am J Roentgenol 1981;137(3):581–584.
24. Garvin KL, McCarthy RE, Barnes CL, et al. Pediatric pelvic ring fractures. J Pediatr Orthop 1990;10(5):577–582.
25. Gepstein R, Weiss R, Hallel T. Acetabaular dyspasia and hip dislocation after selective premature fusion of the triradiate cartilage. J Bone Joint Surg Br 1984;66(3):334–336.
26. Godshall RW, Hansen CA. Incomplete avulsion of a portion of the iliac epiphysis: an injury of young athletes. J Bone Joint Surg Am 1973;55(6):1301–1302.
27. Gordon RG, Karpik K, Hardy S.Techniques of operative reduction and fixation of pediatric and adolescent pelvic fractures. Oper Tech Orthop 1995;5:95–114.
28. Grier D, Wardell S, Sarwark S, et al. Fatigue fractures of the sacrum in children: two case reports and a review of the literature. Skeletal Radiol 1993;22(7):515–518.
29. Grisoni N, Connor S, Marsh E, et al. Pelvic fractures in a pediatric level I trauma center. J Orthop Trauma 2002;16(7):458–463.
30. Guillamondegui OD, Mahboubi S, Stafford PW,et al. The utility of the pelvic radiograph in the assessment of pediatric pelvic fractures. J Trauma 2003;55(2):236–239.
31. Hall BB, Klassen RA, Ilstrup DM. Pelvic fractures in children: a long-term follow-up study.
32. Hauschild O, Strohm PC, Culemann U, et al. Mortality in patients with pelvic fractures: results from the German pelvic injury register. J Trauma 2008;64(2):449–455.
33. Heeg M, Klasen HJ. Long-term outcome of sacroiliac disruptions in children. J Pediatr Orthop 1997;17(3):337–341.
34. Heeg M, Visser JD, Oostvogel HJ. Injuries of the acetabular triradiate cartilage and sacroiliac joint. J Bone Joint Surg Br 1988;70(1):34–37.
35. Heinrich SD, Gallagher D, Harris M, et al. Undiagnosed fractures in severely injured children and young adults. Identification with technetium imaging. J Bone Joint Surg Am 1994;76(4):561–572.
36. Holden C, Holman J, Herman MJ. Pediatric pelvic fractures. J Am Acad Orthop Surg 2007;15(3):172–177.
37. Ismail N, Bellemare JF, Mollitt DL, et al. Death from pelvic fracture: children are different. J Pediatr Surg 1996;31(1):82–85.
38. Judet R, Judet J, Letournel E. Fractures of the acetabulum: classification and surgical approaches for open reduction. Preliminary report. J Bone Joint Surg Am,1964;46: 1615–1646.
39. Junkins EP Jr, Nelson DS, Carroll KL, et al. A prospective evaluation of the clinical presentation of pediatric pelvic fractures. J Trauma 2001;51(1):64–68.
40. Karunaker M, Goulet JA, Mueller KL, et al. Operative treatment of unstable pediatric pelvis and acetabular fractures. J Pediatr Orthop 2005;25(1):34–38.
41. Keats TE, Anderson MW. Atlas of Normal Roentgen Variants That May Simulate Disease. St. Louis: Mosby, 2001:371.
42. Keshishyan RA, Rozinov VM, Malakhov OA, et al. Pelvic polyfractures in children. Radiographic diagnosis and treatment. Clin Orthop Relat Res 1995;320:28–33.
43. Kuhn JP, Slovis TL, Haller JA, eds. Caffey's Pediatric Diagnostic Imaging. Philadelphia: Mosby, 2004.
44. Landin LA. Epidemiology of children's fractures. J Pediatr Orthop B 1997;6(2):79–83.
45. Lane-O'Kelly A, Fogarty E, Dowling F. The pelvic fracture in childhood: a report supporting nonoperative management. Injury 1995;26(5):327–329.
46. Letournel E, Judet R, eds. Fractures of the Acetabulum. 2nd ed. New York: Springer-Verlag, 1993.
47. Liporace F, Ong B, Mohaideen A, et al. Development and injury of the triradiate cartilage with its effects on acetabular development: review of the literature. J Trauma 2003; 54(6):1245–1249.
48. Lynch SA, Renstrom PA. Groin injuries in sport: treatment strategies. Sports Med 1999; 28(2):137–144.
49. Magid D, Fishman EK, Ney DR, et al. Acetabular and pelvic fractures in the pediatric patient: value of two- and three-dimensional imaging. J Pediatr Orthop 1992;12(5): 621–625.
50. Matta J, Saucedo T. Internal fixation of pelvic ring fractures. Clin Orthop Relat Res 1989; 242:83–97.
51. McDonald G. Pelvic disruptions in children. Clin Orthop Relat Res 1980;151:130–134.

52. McIntyre RC Jr, Bensard DD, Moore EE, et al. Pelvic fracture geometry predicts risk of life-threatening hemorrhage in children. J Trauma 1993;35(3):423–429.
53. Metzmaker JN, Pappas AM. Avulsion fractures of the pelvis. Am J Sports Med 1985; 13(5):349–358.
54. Mosheiff R, Suchar A, Porat S, et al. The "crushed open pelvis" in children. Injury 1999; 30(Suppl 2):B14–18.
55. Musemeche CA, Fischer RP, Cotler HB, et al. Selective management of pediatric pelvic fractures: a conservative approach. J Pediatr Surg 1987;22(6):538–540.
56. Niemi TA, Norton LW. Vaginal injuries in patients with pelvic fractures. J Trauma 1985; 25(6):547–551.
57. Nierenberg G, Volpin G, Bialik V. Pelvic fractures in children: a follow-up in 20 children treated conservatively. J Pediatr Orthop B 1993;1:140–142.
58. Ogden JA, ed. Skeletal Injury in the Child. 3rd ed. New York: Springer-Verlag, 2000.
59. Pennal GF, Tile M, Waddell JP, et al. Pelvic disruption: assessment and classification. Clin Orthop Relat Res 1980;151:12–21.
60. Peterson HA, Robertson, RC. Premature partial closure of the triradiate cartilage treated with excision of a physical osseous bar. Case report with a 14-year follow-up. J Bone Joint Surg Am 1997;79(5):767–770.
61. Plaisier BR, Meldon SW, Super DM, et al. Improved outcome after early fixation of acetabular fractures. Injury 2000;31(2):81–84.
62. Pohlemann T. Pelvic ring injuries: assessment and concepts of surgical management. In: Ruedi TP, Murphy W, eds. AO Principles of Fracture Management. New York: Thieme, 2000:391–439.
63. Ponseti IV. Growth and development of the acetabulum in the normal child. Anatomical, histological, and roentgenographic studies. J Bone Joint Surg Am 1978;60(5):575–585.
64. Prendergast NC, deRoux SJ, Adsay NV. Nonaccidental pediatric pelvic fracture: a case report. Pediatr Radiol 1998;28(5):344–346.
65. Quinby WC Jr. Fractures of the pelvis and associated injuries in children. J Pediatr Surg 1966;1(4):353–364.
66. Rang M, ed. Children's Fractures. 2nd ed. Philadelphia: J.B. Lippincott Company, 1983.
67. Reed MH. Pelvic fractures in children. J Can Assoc Radiol 1976;27(4):255–261.
68. Reichard SA, Helikson MA, Shorter N, et al. Pelvic fractures in children-review of 120 patients with a new look at general management. J Pediatr Surg 1980;15(6):727–734.
69. Rieger H, Brug E. Fractures of the pelvis in children. Clin Orthop Relat Res 1997;336: 226–239.
70. Rossi F, Dragoni S. Acute avulsion fractures of the pelvis in adolescent competitive athletes: prevalence, location, and sports distribution of 203 cases collected. Skeletal Radiol 2001;30(3):127–131.
71. Rubel IF, Kloen P, Potter HG, et al. MRI assessment of the posterior acetabular wall fracture in traumatic dislocation of the hip in children. Pediatr Radiol 2002;32(6): 435–439.
72. Schlickewei W, Keck T. Pelvic and acetabular fractures in childhood. Injury 2005; 36(Suppl 1):A57–63.
73. Schlonsky J, Olix ML. Functional disability following avulsion fracture of the ischial epiphysis. Report of two cases. J Bone Joint Surg Am 1972;54(3):641–644.
74. Schwarz N, Posch E, Mayr J, et al. Long-term results of unstable pelvic ring fractures in children. Injury 1998;29(6):431–433.
75. Shah MK, Stewart GW. Sacral stress fractures: an unusual cause of low back pain in an athlete. Spine 2002;27(4): E104–108.
76. Shaw BA, Holman M. Traumatic lumbosacral nerve root avulsions in a pediatric patient. Orthopedics 2003;26(1):89–90.
77. Shlamovitz G, Mower WR, Bergman J, et al. Poor test characteristics for the digital rectal examination in trauma patients. Ann Emerg Med 2007;50(1):25–33.
78. Signorino P, Densmore J, Werner M, et al. Pediatric pelvic injury: functional outcome at 6-month follow-up. J Pediatr Surg 2005;40(1):107–112.
79. Silber JS, Flynn JM. Changing patterns of pediatric pelvic fractures with skeletal maturation: implications for classification and management. J Pediatr Orthop 2002;22(1): 22–26.
80. Silber J, Flynn JM, Koffler KM, et al. Analysis of the causes, classification, and associated injuries of 166 consecutive pediatric pelvic fractures. J Pediatr Orthop 2001;21(4): 446–450.
81. Silber JS, Flynn JM, Katz AM, et al. Role of computed tomography in the classification and management of pediatric pelvic fractures. J Pediatr Orthop 2001;21(2):148–151.
82. Smith W, Oakley M, Morgan SJ. Pediatric pelvic fractures. J Pediatri Orthop 2004;24: 130–135.
83. Smith W, Shurnas P, Morgan S, et al. Clinical outcomes of unstable pelvic fractures in skeletally immature patients. J Bone Joint Surg Am 2005;87(11):2423–2431.
84. Stiletto RJ, Baacke M, Gotzen L. Comminuted pelvic ring disruption in toddlers: management of a rare injury. J Trauma 2000;48(1):161–164.
85. Subasi M, Arslan H, Necmioglu S, et al. Long-term outcomes of conservatively treated pediatric pelvic fractures. Injury 2004;35(8):771–781.
86. Sundar M, Carty H. Avulsion fractures of the pelvis in children: a report of 32 fractures and their outcome. Skeletal Radiol 1994;23(2):85–90.
87. Tarman GJ, Kaplan GW, Lerman SL, et al. Lower genitourinary injury and pelvic fractures in pediatric patients. Urology 2002;59(1):123–126.
88. Tile M. Pelvic fractures: operative versus nonoperative treatment. Orthop Clin North Am 1980;11(3):423–464.
89. Tile M. Pelvic ring fractures: should they be fixed? J Bone Joint Surg Br 1988;70(1): 1–12.
90. Tile M, Helfet DL, Kellam J, eds. Fractures of the Pelvis and Acetabulum. 3rd ed. Baltimore: Lippincott Williams & Wilkins, 2003.
91. Tolo VT. Orthopaedic treatment of fractures of the long bones and pelvis in children who have multiple injuries. Instr Course Lect 2000;49:415–423.
92. Torode I, Zieg D. Pelvic fractures in children. J Pediatr Orthop 1985;5(1):76–84.
93. Upperman J, Gardner M, Gaines B, et al. Early functional outcomes in children with pelvic fractures. J Pediatr Surg 2000;35(6):1002–1005.
94. Vazquez WD, Garcia, VF. Pediatric pelvic fractures combined with an additional skeletal injury is an indicator of significant injury. Surg Gynecol Obstet 1993;177(5):468–472.
95. Watts HG. Fractures of the pelvis in children. Orthop Clin North Am 1976;7(3): 615–624.
96. Worlock P, Stower M. Fracture patterns in Nottingham children. J Pediatr Orthop 1986; 6(6):656–660.
97. Ziran B, Smith WR, Towers J, et al. Iliosacral screw fixation of the posterior pelvic ring using local anaesthesia and computerised tomography. J Bone Joint Surg Br 2003;85(3): 411–418.

21

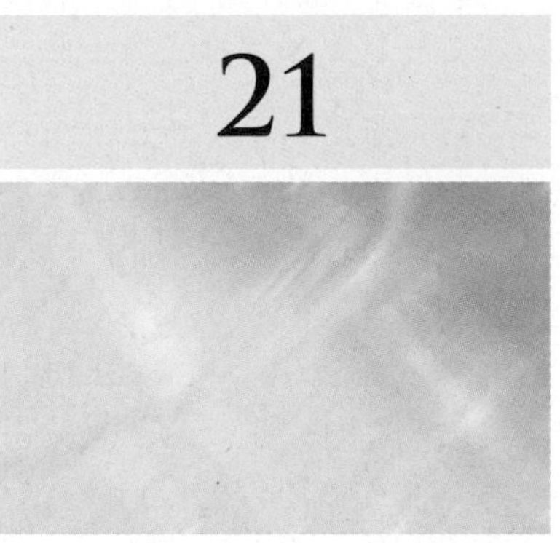

FRACTURES AND TRAUMATIC DISLOCATIONS OF THE HIP IN CHILDREN

James McCarthy and Kenneth Noonan

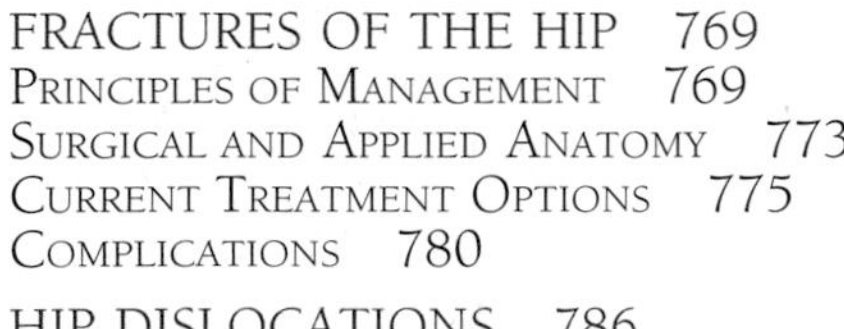

FRACTURES OF THE HIP 769
Principles of Management 769
Surgical and Applied Anatomy 773
Current Treatment Options 775
Complications 780
HIP DISLOCATIONS 786
Principles of Management 786
Surgical and Applied Anatomy 789
Current Treatment Options 791
Complications 793
CONCLUSION 794

FRACTURES OF THE HIP

Hip fractures are very common in adults, but are rare in children, comprising less than 1% of all pediatric fractures.[11,84] Pediatric hip fractures typically result from high-energy mechanisms that can result in other extremity, visceral, or head injuries in 30% of patients, unlike low-energy adult hip fractures common in elderly patients (whose fractures are typically associated with osteoporosis). Occasionally, pediatric hip fractures result from minor trauma superimposed upon bone that is weakened by tumor or metabolic bone disease. These fractures can occur through the physis, but more commonly occur through the femoral neck and the intertrochanteric region.

The presence of the proximal femoral physis presents many important considerations when treating pediatric femoral neck fractures. Injury to the greater trochanter apophysis following an intertrochanteric fracture can lead to coxa valga.[17] Damage to the physis of the femoral neck from fracture, necrosis, or from implant use can result in limb length discrepancies or coxa breva or vara. The surgeon should generally place fixation across the physis in older children with poor bone quality and in adolescents who have little growth potential remaining. If fixation is not placed across the physis; it may be less robust and the surgeon has to be cognizant how to guide weight-bearing status and provide further immobilization. Most importantly, the physis is a significant barrier to interosseous blood supply for the femoral head. Because of this, and the fact that there is little blood supply to the femoral head from the ligamentum teres, an increased risk of necrosis is present following fracture and injury to the important retinacular vessels.

These fractures deserve focused study because of the high rate of complications and the important lifetime morbidity that may result from complications. Potential complications from the fracture and its treatment include chondrolysis osteonecrosis (ON), varus malunion, nonunion, delayed physiolysis, and growth abnormalities leading to length discrepancy or angular deformities.[17] Because the hip is developing in the growing child, deformities can progress with age. In addition, review of more recent publications is important because it has been suggested that outcome can be significantly improved if certain treatment principles are consistently followed.[34,96]

Principles of Management

Mechanism of Injury

Hip fractures in children can be caused by axial loading, torsion, hyperabduction, or a direct blow to the hip. Almost all hip fractures in children are caused by severe, high-energy trauma.[33,90,102] Except for the physis, the proximal femur in children is extremely strong, and high-energy forces, such as from motor vehicle accidents and high falls, are necessary to

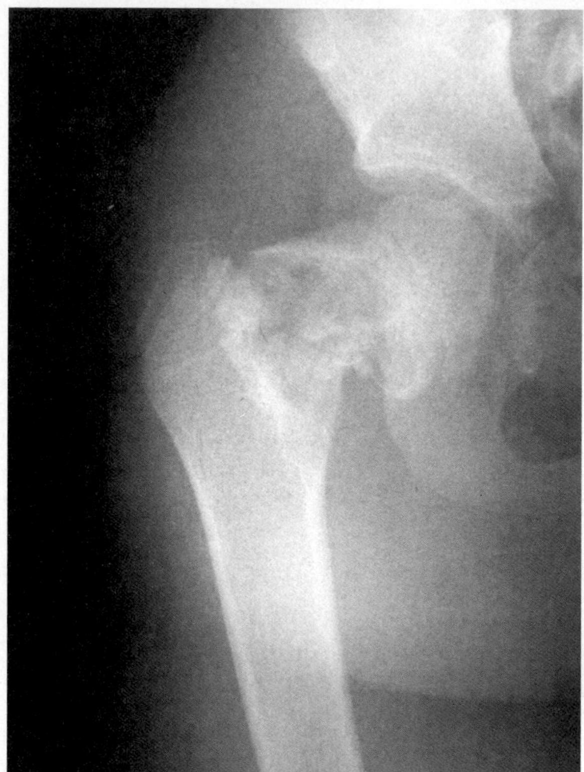

FIGURE 21-1 A 10-year-old boy with a fracture through a unicameral bone cyst sustained while running for a soccer ball.

cause fracture.[26] If a child suffers a fracture as a result of insignificant trauma, then one should suspect an underlying etiology such as prior injury or surgery,[20] metabolic bone disease, or pathologic processes of the proximal femur (Fig. 21-1).

Signs and Symptoms

Clinical examination is usually obvious, and a patient with a complete fracture is unable to ambulate due to severe pain in the hip and has a shortened, externally rotated extremity. With an incomplete or stress fracture of the femoral neck, the patient may be able to bear weight with a limp and may demonstrate hip or knee pain only with extremes of range of motion, especially internal rotation. An infant with a hip fracture holds the extremity flexed, abducted, and externally rotated. Infants and newborns with limited ossification of the proximal femur can be challenging patients to diagnose with hip fractures as the differential diagnosis can include infection and congenital dislocation of the hip. In the absence of infection symptoms, pseudoparalysis, shortening, and a strong suspicion are the keys to a fracture diagnosis in this age group.

Associated Injuries

Because these fractures are caused by high-energy trauma, they frequently are accompanied by associated injuries that can affect the patient's overall outcome. Pape et al.,[78] in a series of 28 patients with a mean follow-up of 11 years, found favorable outcomes in types II, III, and IV fractures according to Ratliff's criteria.[84] Poor functional outcomes were attributed to head trauma, amputation, or peripheral neurologic damage.[78] In a series of 14 patients with hip fractures, all of which were caused by vehicular accidents or falls from heights, 12 patients had associated injuries including head and facial injury, other fractures, as well as visceral injury.[67] In a series of fractures from high-energy trauma, Bagatur and Zorer[6] similarly found associated injuries in 4 of their 17 patients. Infants with hip fractures and without a plausible cause for fracture should be studied for other signs of nonaccidental trauma by carefully examining the other extremities, trunk, and head. Careful evaluation by a child protective team is required to diagnose life-threatening head and visceral injuries that can be easily missed in this group.

Rationale for Management

Much of the early, classic literature on hip fractures in children documented high rates of coxa vara, delayed union, and nonunion in patients treated without internal fixation.[57,84] Canale and Bourland[18] noted that fractures treated by spica casting alone had a greater incidence of coxa vara. They attributed a lower rate of coxa vara and nonunion in some of their patients to the use of internal fixation for all transcervical fractures.[18] More recent literature supports the concept that attempted conservative treatment can result in unacceptably high rates of coxa vara.[102] These high rates of complications may be due to an underappreciation of the uniqueness of this injury and its requisite necessity for operative treatment in most patients, which is in contrast to other pediatric injuries.[102] Subsequent authors have documented lower rates of ON, coxa vara, and nonunion in patients who were aggressively treated with anatomic reduction (open or closed) and internal fixation (with or without supplemental casting) within 24 hours of injury.[6,21,33,70,74,90] Therefore, contemporary management is directed at early, anatomic reduction of these fractures with stable internal fixation and selective use of supplemental external stabilization (casting), with the goal of minimizing devastating late complications.[21,84,96]

Diagnosis

The diagnosis of hip fracture in a child is based on the history of high-energy trauma and the typical signs and symptoms of the shortened, externally rotated, and painful lower extremity.

A good-quality anteroposterior (AP) pelvic radiograph will provide a comparison view of the opposite hip if a displaced fracture is suspected. For the pelvic radiograph, the leg should be held in extension and in as much internal rotation as possible without causing extreme pain to the patient. A cross-table lateral radiograph should be considered to avoid further displacement and unnecessary discomfort to the patient from an attempt at a frog-leg lateral view. Any break or offset of the bony trabeculae near Ward's triangle is evidence of a nondisplaced or impacted fracture. Nondisplaced fracture or stress fractures may be difficult to detect on radiographs. Special studies may be required to reveal an occult fracture as case examples of further displacement of nondisplaced fracture have been reported.[35] Adjunctive studies for stress fracture diagnosis may include a computed tomography (CT) scan or a technetium bone scan which can demonstrate increased uptake at the fracture site. The typical magnetic resonance imaging (MRI) appearance of a fracture is a linear black line (low signal) on all sequences surrounded by a high-signal band of bone marrow edema and hemorrhage. The low signal represents trabeculae impaction. MRI may detect an occult hip fracture within the first 24 hours after injury.[51] In addition, pathologic fractures may require special imaging to aid diagnosis or to fully appreciate bone quality which would impact implant placement. MRI is also a useful test in planning treatment for a pathologic fracture; this test will delineate soft tissues in and around the fracture which can provide insight into diagnosis and delineate high-yield areas for biopsy.

In infants, an ultrasound can be used to detect epiphyseal separation. Additionally, an ultrasound can determine if the patient's epiphysis is located and the presence of an effusion which may be aspirated to confirm diagnosis of sepsis. A bloody aspirate establishes the diagnosis of fracture, whereas a serous or purulent aspirate suggests synovitis or infection, respectively. If performed in the operating room, an aspiration and confirmatory arthrogram of the hip can also be useful, especially if closed reductions and cast immobilization is chosen for the newborn with physiolysis.

In a patient with posttraumatic hip pain without evidence of a fracture, other diagnoses must be considered, including Perthes Disease, synovitis, spontaneous hemarthrosis, and infection. A complete blood count, erythrocyte sedimentation rate, C-reactive protein, and temperature are helpful to evaluate for infection. MRI scan is a useful test to diagnose aseptic ON as a result of Perthes disease or more remote causes of necrosis. In children under 5 years of age, developmental coxa vara can be confused with an old hip fracture.[17]

Classification

Pediatric hip fractures generally are classified by the method of Delbet (Fig. 21-2).[24] This classification system is one that has stood the test of time because it is not only descriptive but also has prognostic significance.[68] In general, more significant rates of ON and growth arrest are noted in type I and type II injuries; while lower rates of osteonecrosis are noted in type III and type IV injuries. Conversely, the latter two groups tend to have higher rates of significant varus malunion if not treated appropriately. Subtrochanteric fractures have been included by some in the discussion of proximal femoral fractures but they are not included in the Delbet classification and are discussed elsewhere.

Type I Transphyseal fractures occur through the proximal femoral physis, with (type IA) or without (type IB) dislocation

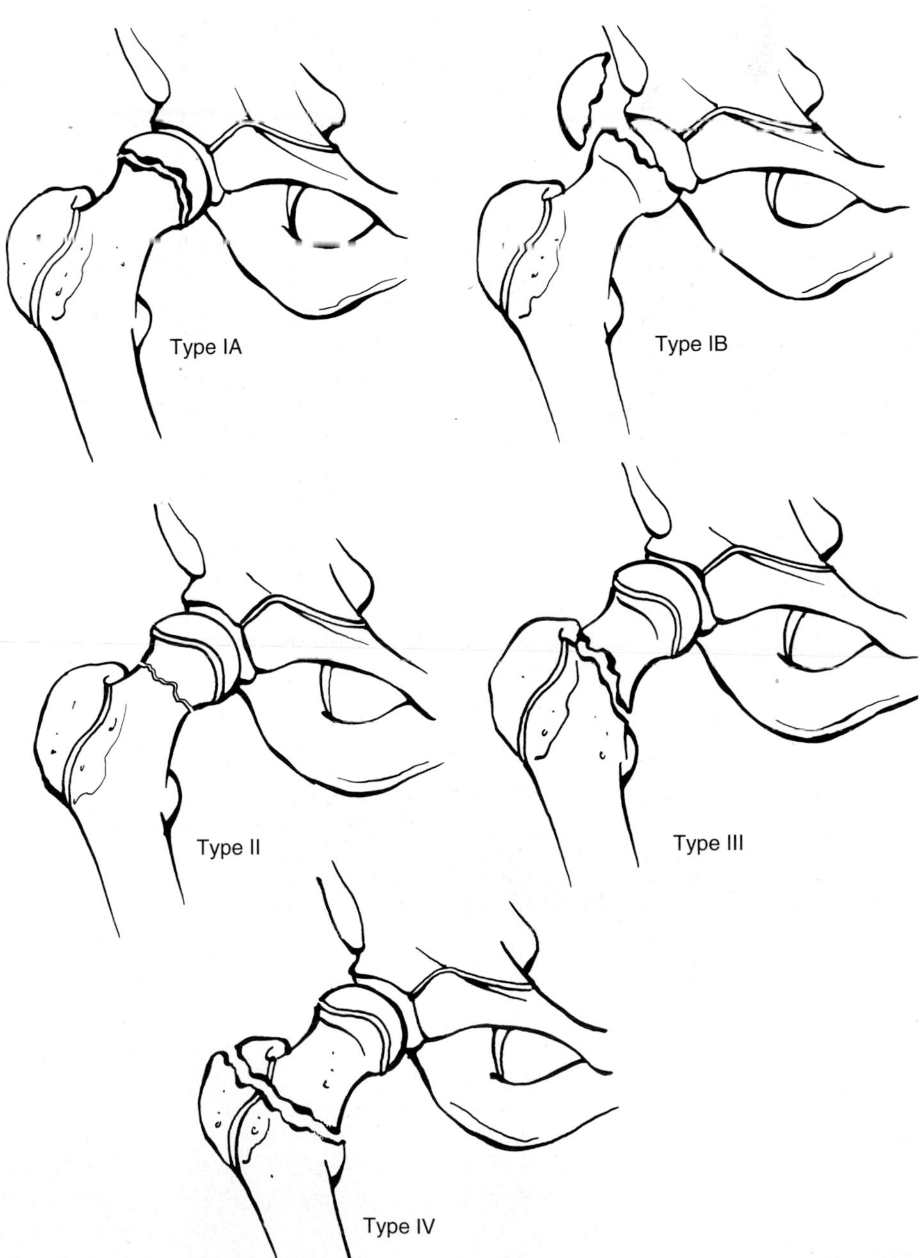

FIGURE 21-2 Delbet classification of hip fractures in children. I, transepiphyseal with (IB) or without (IA) dislocation from the acetabulum; II, transcervical; III, cervicotrochanteric; and IV, intertrochanteric.

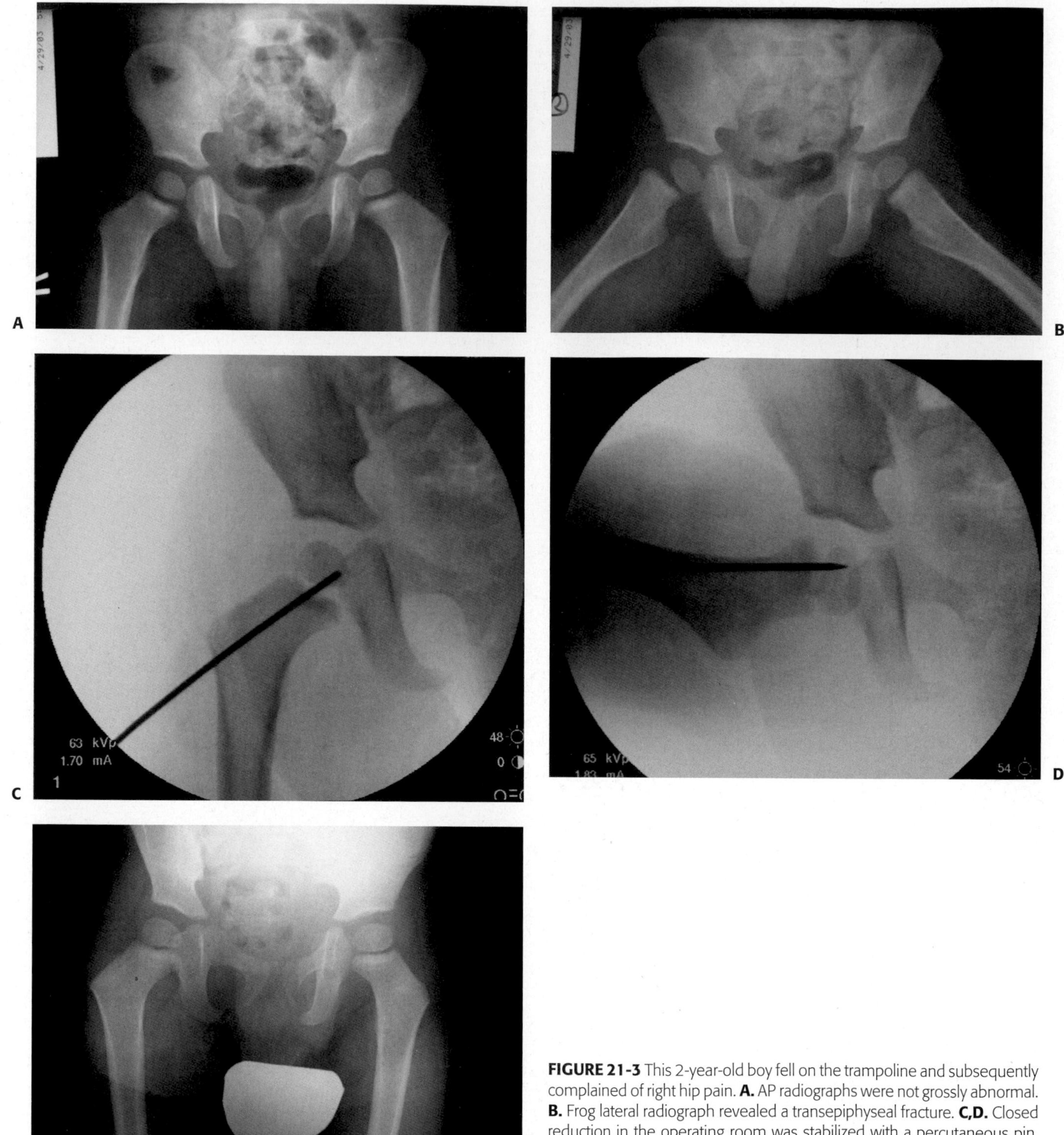

FIGURE 21-3 This 2-year-old boy fell on the trampoline and subsequently complained of right hip pain. **A.** AP radiographs were not grossly abnormal. **B.** Frog lateral radiograph revealed a transepiphyseal fracture. **C,D.** Closed reduction in the operating room was stabilized with a percutaneous pin. **E.** At 8 months, he was asymptomatic and there was no evidence of ON.

of the femoral head from the acetabulum (Fig. 21-3). Such fractures are rare, constituting 8% of femoral neck fractures in children.[50]

Type II Transcervical fractures are the most common fracture type (45% to 50% of all femoral neck fractures),[50] occur between the physis and are above the intertrochanteric line, and by definition are consider intracapsular femoral neck fractures.

Type III Cervicotrochanteric fractures are, by definition, located at or slightly above the anterior intertrochanteric line and are the second most common type of hip fracture in children, representing about 34% of fractures.[50] It is conceivable that a certain portion of these fractures may be intra- and extracapsular as a result of anatomic differences in capsule insertion.

Type IV Intertrochanteric fractures account for only 12% of fractures of the head and neck of the femur in children.[50]

Type I. Approximately half of type I fractures are associated with a dislocation of the capital femoral epiphysis. True transphyseal fractures tend to occur in young children after high-energy trauma[18,30] and are different from unstable slipped capital femoral epiphysis (SCFE) of the preadolescent, which usually follows a prodrome of activity-related hip or knee pain. Unstable SCFE differs from traumatic separation as it occurs following minor trauma which is superimposed on a weakened physis from a combination of multiple factors including obesity and subtle endocrinopathy.

Iatrogenic fracture of the physis in children and adolescents may occur during reduction of a hip dislocation.[14,48] It is possible that these patients had unrecognized physeal injury at the time of dislocation or, alternatively, the epiphysis may be displaced with vigorous reduction methods.

Transphyseal fractures without femoral head dislocation have a better prognosis then those with dislocation. Similarly, in children under 2 or 3 years of age, a better prognosis exists than in older children. ON in younger children is unlikely, although coxa vara, coxa breva, and premature physeal closure can cause subsequent leg length discrepancy.[17,20] In cases of femoral head dislocation, the outcome is dismal because of ON and premature physeal closure in virtually 100% of patients.[18,30]

Type II. Nondisplaced transcervical fractures have a better prognosis and a lower rate of ON than displaced fractures, regardless of treatment.[18,68,84] Necrosis can still occur in minimally displaced fractures, and this may be due to the fact that it is difficult to document how much displacement occurs at the time of trauma. Moon and Mehlman[68] performed a meta-analysis of available literature and documented a 28% incidence of ON in type II fractures. The occurrence of ON is thought by these and other investigators to be directly related to fracture displacement, which may lead to disruption or kinking of the blood supply to the femoral head. In addition, the meta-analysis demonstrated higher rates of ON in children older than 10 years of age at the time of their injury.[68] Because the pediatric hip capsule is tough and less likely to tear, some have hypothesized that a possible etiology of vascular impairment in minimally displaced fractures is a result of intra-articular hemarthrosis leading to vessel compression from tamponade.[18,50]

Type III. Nondisplaced type III fractures also have a much lower complication rate than displaced fractures. Displaced type III fractures are similar to type II fractures in regard to the type of complications that can occur. For instance, the incidence of ON is 18% and is slightly less than in type II fractures[68]; the risk of ON is directly related to the degree of displacement at the time of injury.[14] Premature physeal closure occurs in 25% of patients, and coxa vara in can also occur in approximately 14% of patients.[50]

Type IV. This fracture is completely extracapsular and has the lowest complication rate of all four types. Nonunion in this fracture is rare, and Moon and Mehlman[68] documented a rate of ON of only 5%, which is much lower than in intracapsular fractures. Coxa vara and premature physeal closure have occasionally been reported.[18,50,57,83,84]

Unusual Fracture Patterns

Rarely, proximal femoral physiolysis occurs during a difficult delivery and can be confused on radiographs with congenital dislocation of the hip. Type I fracture in a neonate deserves special attention. This injury is exceedingly rare and, because the femoral head is not visible on plain radiographs, the index of suspicion must be high. The differential diagnosis includes septic arthritis and hip dislocation. Plain radiographs may show a high-riding proximal femoral metaphysis on the involved side, thus mimicking a congenital hip dislocation.

Ultrasonography is useful in diagnosis of neonatal physiolysis; with this test, the cartilaginous head remains in the acetabulum but its dissociation from the femoral shaft can be appreciated. The diagnosis can be missed if there is no history of trauma (such as in child abuse) or if there is an ipsilateral fracture of the femoral shaft.[2] In the absence of a history of significant trauma in a young child, battered child syndrome should be suspected.[100]

Stress fractures are caused by repetitive injury and result in hip or knee pain and a limp. Pain associated with long-distance running, marching, or a recent increase in physical activity is suggestive of stress fracture. Close scrutiny of high-quality radiographs may identify sclerosis, cortical thickening, or new bone formation. Undisplaced fractures may appear as faint radiolucencies. If radiographs are inconclusive, adjunctive tests such as MRI, CT or bone scintigraphy may be helpful.

On radiographs, acute unstable SCFE can be indistinguishable from a traumatic type I fracture; however, SCFE is caused by an underlying abnormality of the physis and occurs after trivial trauma, usually in preadolescents, whereas type I fractures usually occur in young children.

Fracture after minor trauma suggests weakened bone possibly from systemic disease, tumors, cysts, and infections. If the physical and radiographic evidence of trauma is significant but the history is not consistent, nonaccidental trauma must always be considered.[4,100]

In the multiply traumatized patient, it is easy to miss hip fractures that are overshadowed by more dramatic or painful injuries. Radiographs of the proximal femur should be examined carefully in patients with femoral shaft fractures because ipsilateral fracture or dislocation of the hip is not unusual.[2]

Surgical and Applied Anatomy

Ossification of the femur begins in the seventh fetal week.[30] In early childhood, only a single proximal femoral chondroepiphysis exists. During the first year of life, the medial portion of this physis grows faster than the lateral, creating an elongated femoral neck by 1 year of age. The capital femoral epiphysis begins to ossify at approximately 4 months in girls and 5 to 6 months in boys. The ossification center of the trochanteric apophysis appears at 4 years in boys and girls.[50] The proximal femoral physis is responsible for the metaphyseal growth in the femoral neck, whereas the trochanteric apophysis contributes to the appositional growth of the greater trochanter and less to the metaphyseal growth of the femur.[58] Fusion of the proximal femoral and trochanteric physes occurs at about the age of 14 in girls and 16 in boys.[46] The confluence of the greater trochanteric physis with the capital femoral physis along the superior femoral neck and the unique vascular supply to the capital femoral epiphysis make the immature hip vulnerable to growth derangement and subsequent deformity after a fracture (Fig. 21-4).

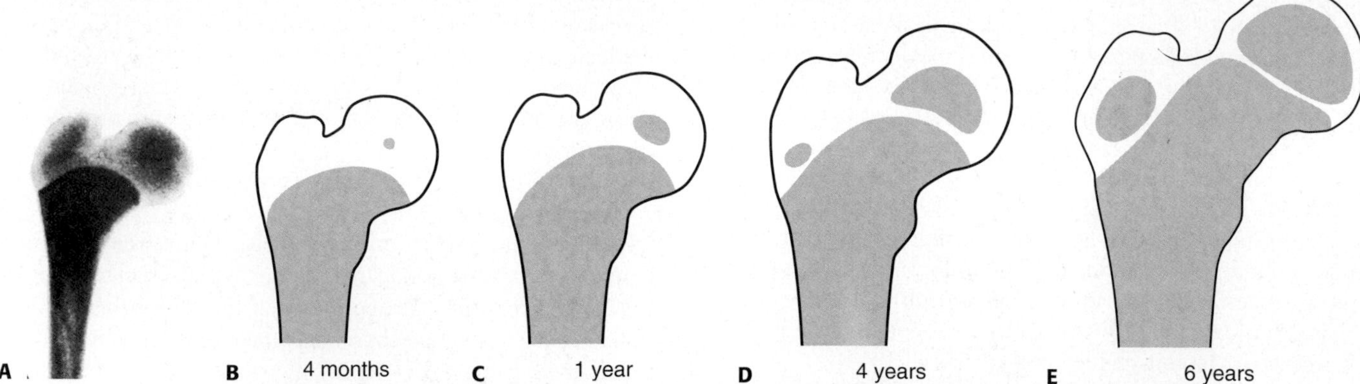

FIGURE 21-4 The transformation of the preplate to separate growth zones for the femoral head and greater trochanter. The diagram shows development of the epiphyseal nucleus. **A.** Radiograph of the proximal end of the femur of a stillborn girl, weight 325 g. **B–E.** Drawings made on the basis of radiographs. (Reprinted from Edgren W. Coxa plana. A clinical and radiological investigation with particular reference to the importance of the metaphyseal changes for the final shape of the proximal part of the femur. Acta Orthop Scand 1965: 84(suppl):24, with permission.)

Vascular Anatomy

Because of the frequency and sequelae of ON of the hip in children, the blood supply has been studied extensively.[23,76,103,104] Postmortem injection and microangiographic studies have provided clues to the vascular changes with age. These observations are as follows:

- At birth, interosseous continuation of branches of the medial and lateral circumflex arteries (metaphyseal vessels) traversing the femoral neck predominately supply the femoral head. These arteries gradually diminish in size as the cartilaginous physis develops and forms a barrier thus preventing transphyseal continuity of these vessels into the femoral head. Thus metaphyseal blood supply to the femoral head is virtually nonexistent by age 4.
- When the metaphyseal vessels diminish, the intracapsular lateral epiphyseal vessels predominate and the femoral head is primarily supplied by these vessels, which extend superiorly on the exterior of the neck, bypassing the physeal barrier and then continuing into the epiphysis.
- Ogden[76] noted that the lateral epiphyseal vessels consist of two branches: the posterosuperior and posteroinferior branches of the medial circumflex artery (Fig. 21-5). At the level of the intertrochanteric groove, the medial circumflex artery branches into a retinacular arterial system (the posterosuperior and posteroinferior arteries). These arteries penetrate the capsule and traverse proximally (covered by the retinacular folds) along the neck of the femur to supply the femoral head peripherally and proximally to the physis. The posteroinferior and posterosuperior arteries persist throughout life and supply the femoral head. At about 3 to 4 years of age, the lateral posterosuperior vessels appear to predominate and supply the entire anterior lateral portion of the capital femoral epiphysis.
- The vessels of the ligamentum teres are of virtually no importance. They contribute little blood supply to the femoral head until age 8, and then only about 20% as an adult.

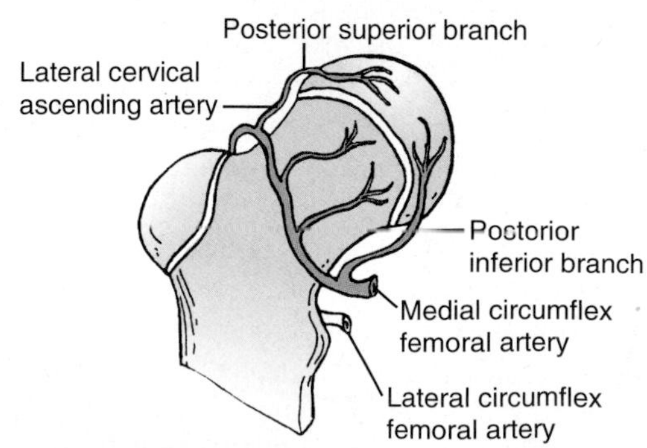

FIGURE 21-5 Arterial supply of the proximal femur. The capital femoral epiphysis and physis are supplied by the medial circumflex artery through two retinacular systems: the posterosuperior and posteroinferior. The lateral circumflex artery supplies the greater trochanter and the lateral portion of the proximal femoral physis and a small area of the anteromedial metaphysis.

The above information has clinical importance. For instance, the multiple small vessels of the young coalesce with age to a limited number of larger vessels. As a result, damage to a single vessel can have serious consequences; for example, occlusion of the posterosuperior branch of the medial circumflex artery can cause ON of the anterior lateral portion of the femoral head.[17]

It is also important for surgeons to recognize where capsulotomy should be performed in order to decrease iatrogenic injury to existing blood supply (Fig. 21-6A,B). It is suspected that anterior capsulotomy does not damage the blood supply to the femoral head as long as the intertrochanteric notch and the superior lateral ascending cervical vessels are avoided.

Soft Tissue Anatomy

The hip joint is enclosed by a thick fibrous capsule that is considered less likely to tear than in adult hip fractures. Bleeding within an intact capsule may lead to a tense hemarthrosis after intracapsular fracture which can tamponade the ascending cervical vessels and may have implications in the development of ON. The hip joint is surrounded on all sides by a protective cuff of musculature; as such, open hip fracture is rare. In the absence of associated hip dislocation, neurovascular injuries are rare.

The sciatic nerve emerges from the sciatic notch beneath the piriformis and courses superficial to the external rotators and

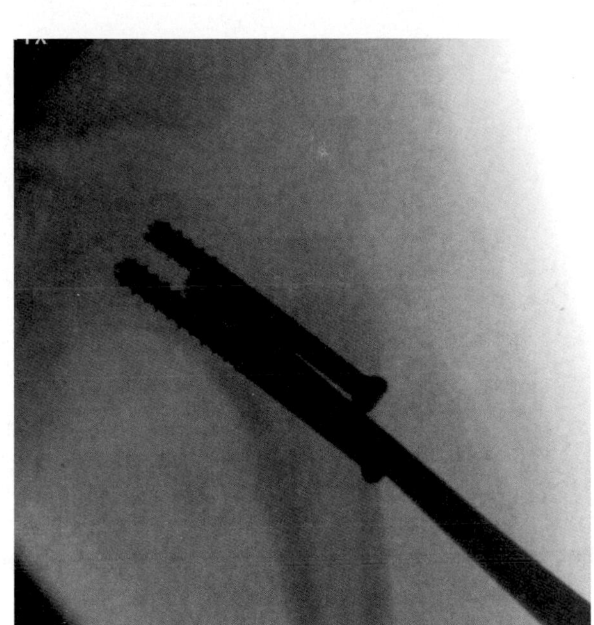
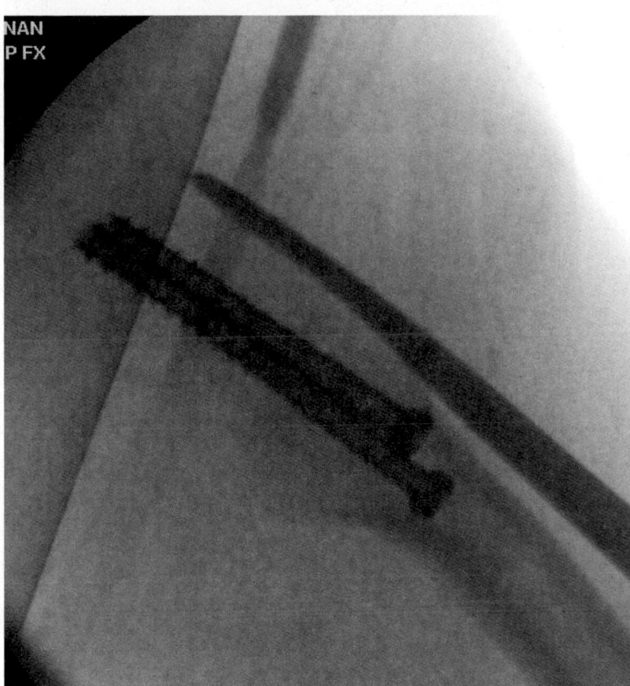

FIGURE 21-6 A,B. Percutaneous placement of a periosteal elevator along the anterior femoral neck should allow fenestration of the capsule while protecting the posterior and superior blood supply.

the quadratus medial to the greater trochanter. The lateral femoral cutaneous nerve lies in the interval between the tensor and sartorius muscles and supplies sensation to the lateral thigh. This nerve must be identified and preserved during an anterolateral approach to the hip. The femoral neurovascular bundle is separated from the anterior hip joint by the iliopsoas. Thus, any retractor placed on the anterior acetabular rim should be carefully placed deep to the iliopsoas to protect the femoral bundle. Inferior and medial to the hip capsule, coursing from the deep femoral artery toward the posterior hip joint, is the medial femoral circumflex artery. Placement of a distal Hohmann retractor too deeply can tear this artery, and control of the bleeding may be difficult.

Preferred Approaches

The Watson-Jones Approach. If open reduction is necessary, the Watson-Jones approach is a useful and direct approach to the femoral neck. A lateral incision is made over the proximal femur, slightly anterior to the greater trochanter (Fig. 21-7A). The fascia lata is incised longitudinally (Fig. 21-7B). The innervation of the tensor muscle by the superior gluteal nerve is 2 to 5 cm above the greater trochanter, and care should be taken not to damage this structure. The tensor muscle is reflected anteriorly. The interval between the gluteus medius and the tensor muscles will be used (Fig. 21-7C). The plane is developed between the muscles and the underlying hip capsule (Fig. 21-7D). If necessary, the anterior-most fibers of the gluteus medius tendon can be detached from the trochanter for wider exposure. After clearing the anterior hip capsule, longitudinal capsulotomy is made along the anterosuperior femoral neck. A transverse incision can be added superiorly for wider exposure (Fig. 21-7E). Once the hip fracture is reduced, guide wires for cannulated screws can be passed perpendicular to the fracture along the femoral neck from the base of the greater trochanter.

The Smith-Peterson Approach. Alternatively, a bikini approach can be used through the Smith-Peterson interval (Fig. 21-8). Care should be taken to identify and protect the lateral femoral cutaneous nerve. The sartorius and rectus muscles can be detached to expose the hip capsule. Medial and inferior retractors should be carefully placed to avoid damage to the femoral neurovascular bundle and medial femoral circumflex artery, respectively. Care must be taken not to violate the intertrochanteric notch and the lateral ascending vessels. Because the lateral aspect of the greater trochanter is not exposed, wires must be passed percutaneously once the hip fracture is reduced.

Lateral Approach for Decompression. In many cases, an adequate closed reduction can be obtained thus avoiding the need to open the hip joint for reduction purposes. However, the surgeon may decide to perform a capsulotomy to decompress the hip joint. The authors prefer to do this from a lateral approach. With this method, a 4-cm incision is made distal and lateral to the greater trochanter. From this incision, the fascia lata is incised and guide pins for cannulated screws are placed and screws are inserted in the standard manner. The anterior fibers of the gluteus medius are elevated allowing incision of the anterior capsule with a Cobb elevator, knife, or osteotome.

Current Treatment Options

Type I

Fracture treatment is based on the age of the child, presence of femoral head dislocation, and fracture stability after reduction. In toddlers under 2 years of age with nondisplaced or minimally displaced fractures, simple spica cast immobilization is likely to be successful. Because the fracture tends to displace into varus and external rotation, the limb should be casted in

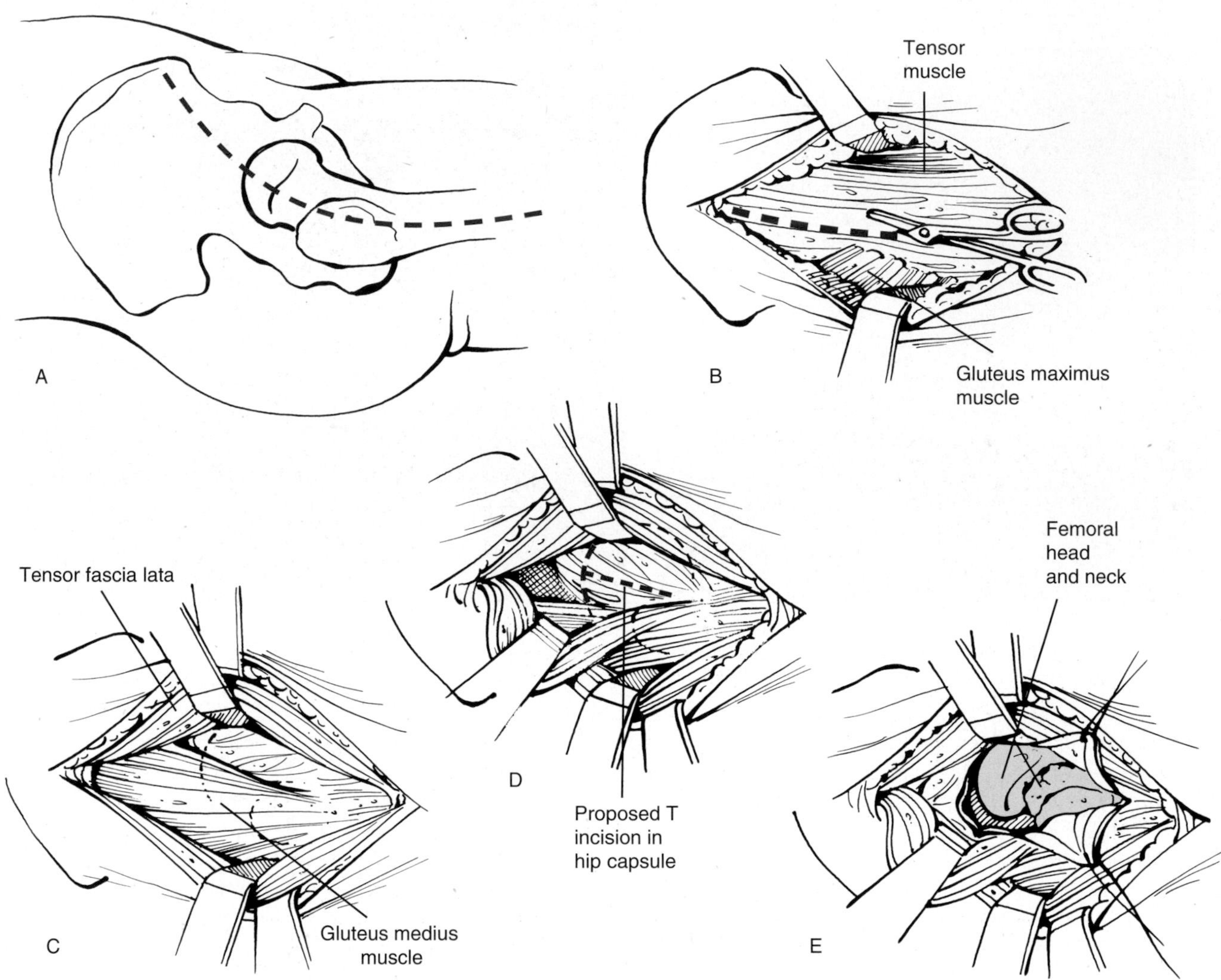

FIGURE 21-7 Watson-Jones lateral approach to the hip joint for open reduction of femoral neck fractures in children. **A.** Skin incision. **B.** Incision of the fascia lata between the tensor muscle (anterior) and gluteus maximus (posterior). **C.** Exposure of the interval between the gluteus medius and tensor fascia lata (retracted anteriorly). Development of the interval will reveal the underlying hip capsule. **D.** Exposure of the hip capsule. **E.** Exposure of the femoral neck after T-incision of the capsule.

mild abduction and neutral rotation to prevent displacement. Close follow up in the early postinjury period is critical. Displaced fractures in toddlers should be reduced closed by gentle traction, abduction, and internal rotation. If the fracture "locks on" and is stable, casting without fixation is indicated. If casting without fixation is done, repeat radiographs should be taken within days to look for displacement because the likelihood of successful repeat reduction decreases rapidly with time and healing in a young child.

If the fracture is not stable, it should be fixed with small-diameter (2-mm) smooth pins that cross the femoral neck and into the physeal. Use of smooth pins will theoretically decrease risk of physis injury in younger patients with a transphyseal fracture. An arthrogram *after* reduction and stabilization of the fracture may be indicated to insure alignment is anatomic. An arthrogram *prior* to reduction and pinning may obscure bony detail and hinder assessment during reduction.

Children older than 2 years should have operative fixation, even if the fracture is nondisplaced; because the complications of late displacement may be great, fixation should cross the physis into the capital femoral epiphysis. Smooth pins can be used in young children, but cannulated screws are better for older, larger children and adolescents. In this older group (>10 years of age) the effect of eventual limb length discrepancy is small and is a reasonable tradeoff for the superior fixation and stabilization needed to avoid complications in larger and older children.

Closed reduction of type IB fracture-dislocations may be attempted, but immediate open reduction is necessary if a single attempt at closed reduction is unsuccessful. Internal fixation is mandatory. The surgical approach should be from the side to which the head is dislocated, generally posterolateral. Parents must be advised in advance about the risk of ON.

Postoperative spica cast immobilization is mandatory in all but the oldest and most reliable adolescents who have large threaded screws crossing the physis. Fixation may be removed shortly after fracture healing to enable further growth in patients.

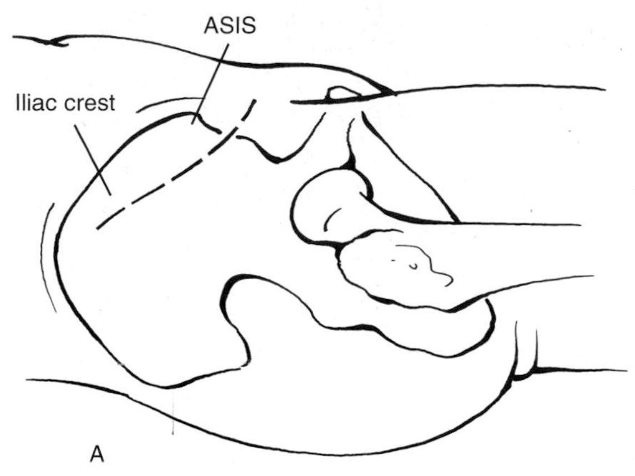

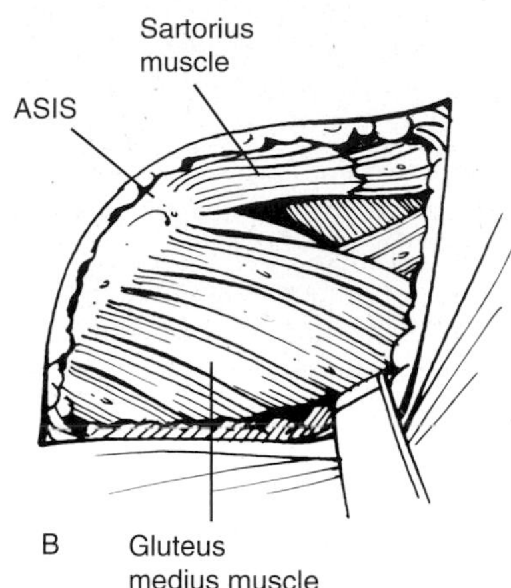

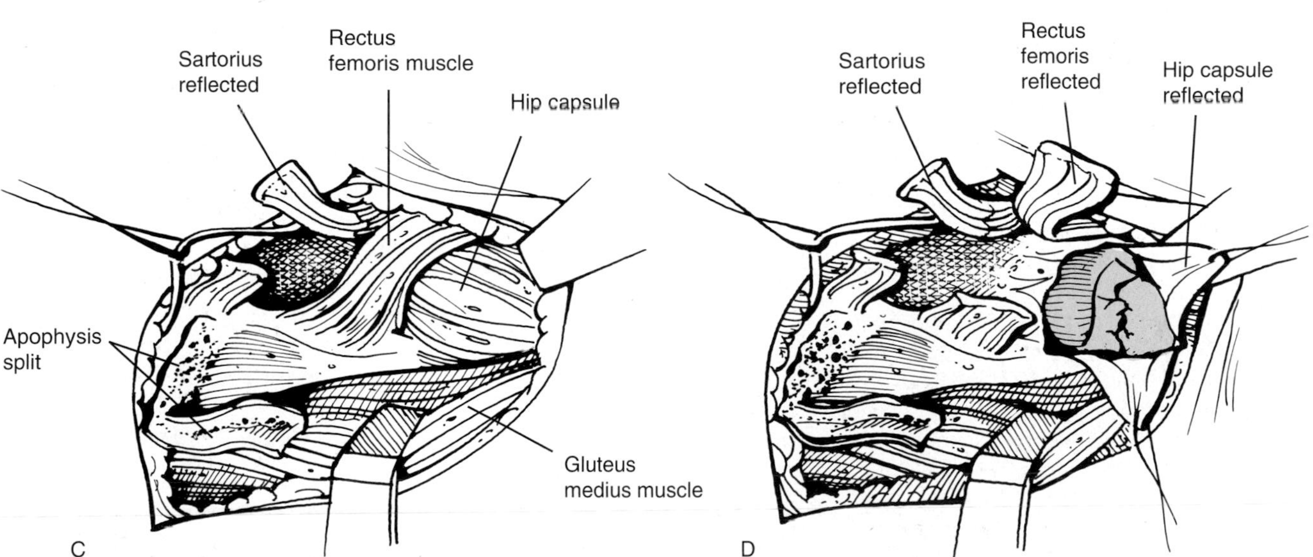

FIGURE 21-8 Smith-Petersen anterolateral approach to the hip joint. **A.** Skin incision. Incision is 1 cm below the iliac crest and extends just medial to the anterior superior iliac spine. **B.** Skin is retracted, exposing the fascia overlying the anterior superior iliac spine. The interval between the sartorius and the tensor fascia lata is identifiable by palpation. **C.** The sartorius is detached from the anterior superior iliac spine. Splitting of the iliac crest apophysis and detachment of the rectus femoris (shown attached to anterior inferior iliac spine) will facilitate exposure of the hip capsule. **D.** The hip capsule is exposed. A T incision is made to reveal the femoral head and neck.

Type II and Type III

Intracapsular femoral neck fractures mandate anatomic reduction and, in most cases, internal fixation. In rare cases, children under 5 years of age with nondisplaced and completely stable type II and cervicotrochanteric fractures can be managed with spica casting and close follow-up to detect varus displacement in the cast.[27,50,57] However, in almost all cases, internal fixation is recommended by most investigators for nondisplaced transcervical fractures[35,50] because the risk of late displacement in such fractures far outweighs the risk of percutaneous screw fixation, especially in young children.[15]

Displaced neck fractures should be treated with anatomic reduction and stable internal fixation to minimize the risk of late complications. Coxa vara and nonunion were frequent in several large series of displaced transcervical fractures treated with immobilization but without internal fixation.[18,57,102] However, when an anatomic closed or open reduction and internal fixation was used, the rates of these complications were much lower.[18,33,70,96]

Gentle closed reduction of displaced fractures is accomplished with the use of longitudinal traction, abduction, and internal rotation. Open reduction frequently is necessary for displaced fractures and should be done through a Watson-Jones surgical approach.

Internal fixation with cannulated screws is done through a small lateral incision with planned entry above the level of the lesser trochanter. Two to three screws should be placed; if possible, the most inferior screw will skirt along the calcar with the remaining screws spaced as widely as possible.[15] Usually, the small size of the child's femoral neck will accommodate only two screws. Care should be taken to minimize unnecessary drill holes in the subtrochanteric region because they increase the risk of subtrochanteric fracture.

In type II fractures, physeal penetration may be necessary for purchase[50,70]; the sequelae of premature physeal closure and trochanteric overgrowth are much less than those of nonunion, pin breakage, and ON. Treatment of the fracture is the first priority, and any subsequent growth disturbance and leg length discrepancy are secondary. Consideration may be given to simultaneous capsulotomy or aspiration of the joint to eliminate pressure from a hemarthrosis at the time of surgery.

Displaced cervicotrochanteric fractures have been shown to have a complication rate similar to that for type II fractures and should be treated similarly. If possible, screws should be inserted short of the physis in type III fractures. Fixation generally does not need to cross the physis in type III fractures. Alternatively, a pediatric hip compression screw can be used for more secure fixation of distal cervicotrochanteric fractures in a child over 5 years of age. Spica casting is routine in most type II and III fractures, except in older reliable children where the screws cross the physis.[33]

Type IV

Good results can be obtained after closed treatment of most intertrochanteric fractures, regardless of displacement. Traction and spica cast immobilization are effective.[14] Instability or failure to maintain adequate reduction and polytrauma are indications for internal fixation. Children old enough to use crutches or those with multiple injuries can be treated with open reduction and internal fixation (Fig. 21-9). A pediatric hip screw provides the most rigid internal fixation for this purpose.

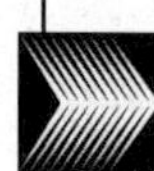

AUTHORS' PREFERRED TREATMENT

Type I

Nondisplaced or minimally displaced stable fractures in toddlers up to age 2 should be treated in a spica cast without internal fixation. The limb should be casted in a position of abduction and neutral rotation to prevent displacement into varus. If the fracture requires reduction or moves significantly during reduction or casting maneuvers, then internal fixation is mandatory. Two millimeter smooth Kirschner-wires are inserted percutaneously to cross the physis. We recommend two or three wires. Wires should be cut off and bent below the skin for retrieval under a brief general anesthetic when the fractures healed. We do not recommend leaving the wires outside the skin. Frequent radiographs are necessary to check for migration of the pins into the joint space. A spica cast is always applied in this age group and should remain in place for at least 6 weeks.[33] Even if type I fractures in children older than 2 years are anatomically reduced, these patients should always have stabilization with internal fixation. While Kirschner-wires are appropriate for small children, 4.0- to 4.5-mm cannulated screws crossing the physis can be considered in older, larger children after closed reduction. Fluoroscopically placing a guide-pin across the femoral head and neck allows one to locate the proper site for a small incision overlying the lateral femur in line with the femoral neck. Two guide pins are placed into the epiphysis, and the wires are overdrilled to the level of the physis (but not across in order to avoid growth arrest as much as possible). The hard metaphysis and lateral femoral cortex are tapped (in contrast to elderly patients with osteoporosis) to the level of the physis and stainless steel screws are placed.

If gentle closed reduction cannot be achieved, a Watson-

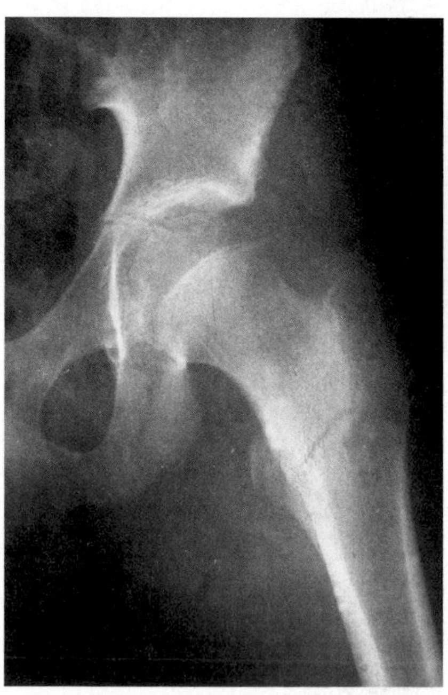
A

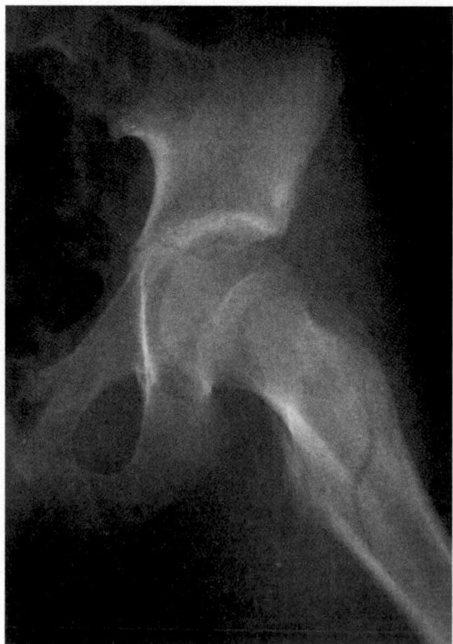
B

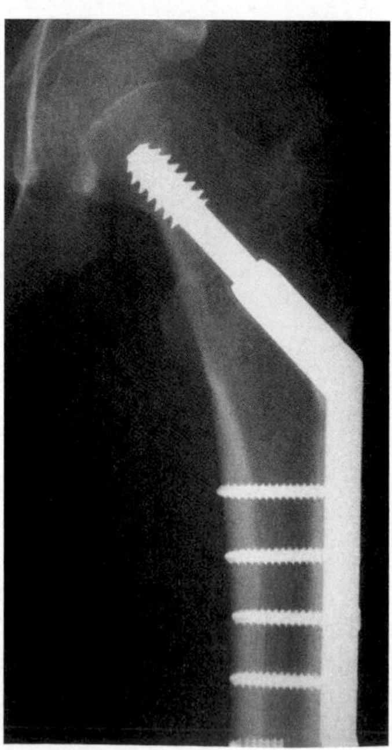
C

FIGURE 21-9 A. A 14-year-old boy who fell from a tree swing sustained this nondisplaced left intertrochanteric hip fracture. **B.** Lateral radiograph shows the long spiral fracture. **C.** Three months after fixation with an adult sliding hip screw.

Jones approach is preferred for type IA fractures. For type IB fractures, the choice of approach is dictated by the position of the femoral epiphysis. If it is anterior or inferior, a Watson-Jones approach should be used. On the other hand, most type IB fractures are displaced posteriorly, in which case a posterior approach should be selected. Under direct vision, the fracture is reduced and guide wires are passed from the lateral aspect of the proximal femur up the neck perpendicular to the fracture; predrilling and tapping are necessary before the insertion of screws. All children are immobilized in a spica cast.

Older children and adolescents will usually require similar reduction methods on a fracture table, and the fracture is stabilized after closed or, if needed, open reduction. Larger 6.5- or 7.3-mm screws are needed and are placed after predrilling and tapping over the guide pins. Through a lateral incision, the screws are placed, and an anterior capsulotomy is performed. Such stout fixation usually obviates the need for spica casting in an adolescent but, if future patient compliance or fracture stability is in doubt, a spica cast is used.

Types II and III

In all cases, we attempt a closed reduction. If unsuccessful, we prefer reduction through a Watson-Jones approach because it provides the most direct exposure of the femoral neck for gentle fracture reduction. This approach allows the fracture to be anatomically reduced under direct vision. Guide wires are then placed up the femoral neck perpendicular to the fracture. If possible, penetration of the physis should be avoided.[20,32] However, in most unstable Type II fractures, penetration of the physis may be necessary to achieve stability and avoid the complications associated with late displacement.[14,70] Good fixation of type III fractures generally is possible without penetration of the physis. Type II and III fractures should be stabilized with 4.0- to 4.5-mm cannulated screws in small children up to age 8 years. After the age of 8 years, fixation with 6.5-mm cannulated screws is appropriate. Two or three appropriately sized screws should be used, depending on the size of the child's femoral neck. As in type I fractures, we recommend placing at least two guide pins, and predrilling and tapping of the femoral neck is necessary to avoid displacement of the fracture while advancing the screws. Finally, we believe that if the physis is not crossed with implants, supplementary spica casting is needed to prevent malunion or nonunion.

Type IV

Undisplaced type IV fractures in children younger than 3 to 4 years are treated without internal fixation with immobilization in a spica cast for 12 weeks. Great care is needed to cast the limb in a position that best aligns the bone (Fig. 21-10A,B). Frequent radiographic examination is necessary to assess for late displacement, particularly into varus. In some cases, it may be difficult to assess reduction in a spica cast so that alternative testing such as a limited CT scan may be useful to compare to intraoperative positioning (Fig. 21-10C,D). Displaced type IV fractures in all children more than 3 years of age should be treated with internal fixation with a pediatric or juvenile compression hip screw placed into femoral neck short of the physis. It is important to place an antirotation wire before drilling and tapping the neck for the dynamic hip screw. Closed reduction often is possible with a combination of traction and internal rotation of the limb. If open reduction is necessary, a lateral approach with anterior extension to close reduce the fracture is preferred.

Postoperative Fracture Care

In general, we believe supplementary casting should be considered for the majority of patients with proximal femoral fractures. For instance, casting is indicated in all type I fractures except in the rare adolescents who have been treated with two to three large screws that cross the physis and who will be obviously compliant with restricted weight bearing. For type II and III fractures, we recommend a hip spica cast to be used for at least 6 weeks in all patients whose implants do not cross the femoral physis. This recommendation makes sense when one considers that in children younger than 10, we try to avoid crossing the physis, and these patients usually do well with these casts. On the other hand, children older than 12 years of age can be treated with transphyseal fixation that will be stable enough to avoid cast fixation and which coincidently also tends to be poorly tolerated in this age group. For children 10 to 12 years of age, the use of a postoperative cast depends on the stability of fracture fixation and the patient's compliance; if either is in doubt, a single hip spica cast is used.

Type IV fractures treated with a hip screw and side plate do not require cast immobilization. Formal rehabilitation usually is unnecessary unless there is a severe persistent limp, which may be due to abductor weakness. Stiffness is rarely a problem in the absence of ON.

Pearls and Pitfalls

- Table 21-1 summarizes the pearls of surgical stabilization of pediatric hip fractures, including recommended choices of implants for internal fixation.
- For young, small patients, the operation should be done on a radiolucent operating table rather than on a fracture table, which is more appropriate for older and larger adolescents.
- Because the femoral bone in children is harder than the osteoporotic bone in elderly patients, predrilling and pretapping are necessary for insertion of all screws.
- Multiple attempts at wire placement should be avoided because they result in empty holes in the subtrochanteric region of the femur. This predisposes to late subtrochanteric fracture below or at the level of the screw heads after removal of the spica cast.
- A hip spica cast must be used to supplement internal fixation in all patients who are younger than 10 years. For older patients, if the stability of the fracture is questionable or if the child's compliance is doubtful, the surgeon should not hesitate to apply a hip spica cast. The quality of reduction and the stability of the fixation have a direct impact on the occurrence of nonunion.[33,57,70,84]
- Growth of the femur and the contribution of the proximal femoral physis are important; however, this physeal contribution to growth is only 13% of the entire extremity, or 3 to 4 mm per year on average. Once the decision for internal fixation of a fracture of the head or neck of the femur is made, stable fixation of the fracture is a higher priority than preservation of the physis. If stability is questionable, the internal fixation device should extend into the femoral head for rigid, stable fixation, regardless of the type of fracture or the age of the child.

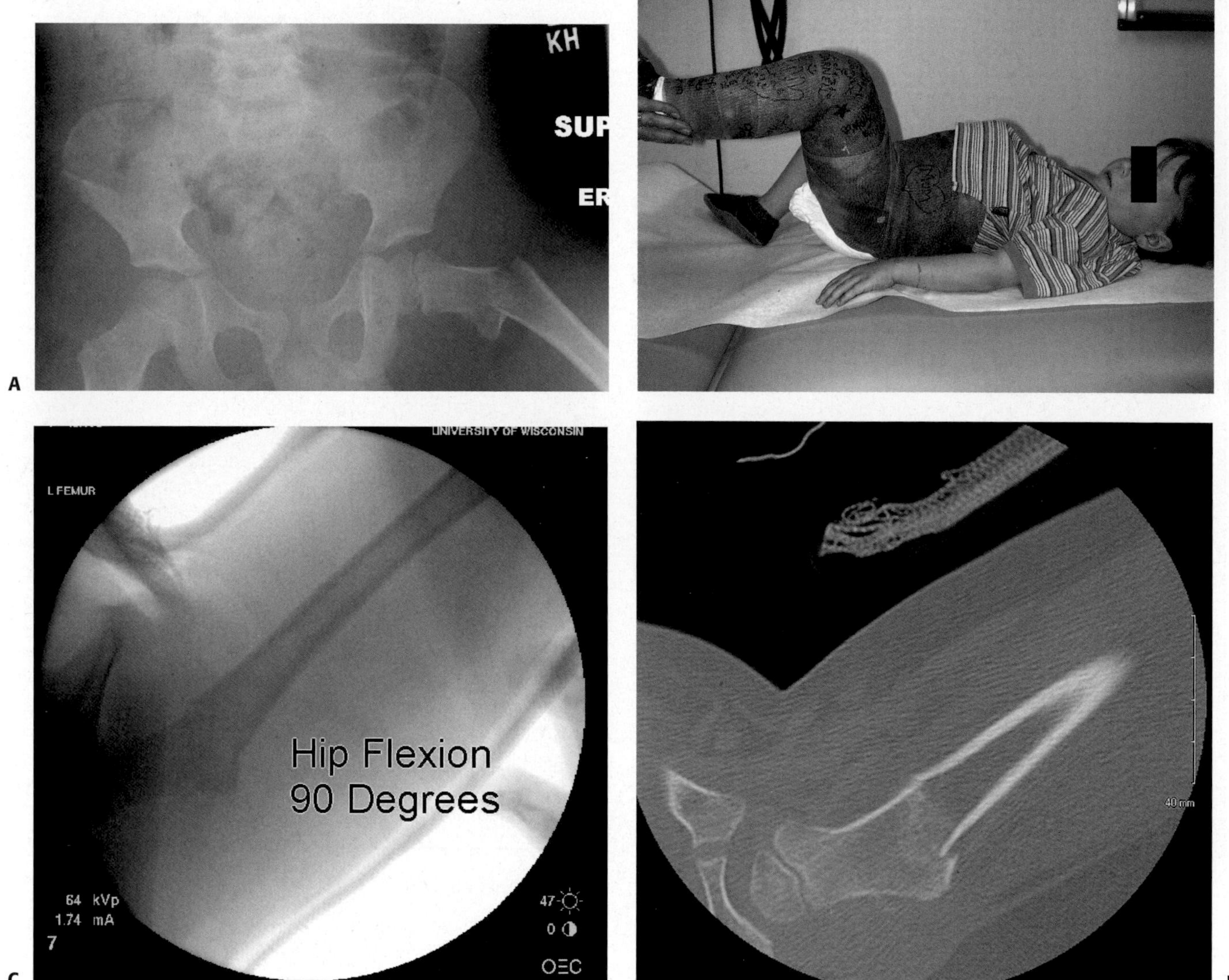

FIGURE 21-10 A. A 4-year-old boy fell from his window, causing a displaced type IV fracture. **B.** Positioning of the hip in a spica cast is usually in hip flexion and confirmed under fluoroscopy. **C.** Fluoroscopic radiographs in 90 degrees of hip flexion insure anatomic correctness. **D.** At 1-week follow-up, radiographs were inconclusive; a CT scan assists in confirming location.

TABLE 21-1 Surgical Tips and Pearls for Hip Fractures in Children

- Anterolateral approach
- Age 0–3 years: smooth pins, 5/64-inch or 3/32-inch
- Age 3–8 years: cannulated 4.0-mm screws
- Age 8+ years: 6.5- or 7.0-mm cannulated screws
- Type IV fractures
  - Age <8 years: pediatric hip compression screw
  - Age >8 years: juvenile or adult hip compression screw
- Always predrill and tap before inserting screws.
- Avoid crossing physis if possible, but cross physis if necessary for stability.
- Age <10 years: hip spica for 6–12 weeks

Complications

Osteonecrosis is the most serious and frequent complication of hip fractures in children and is the primary cause of poor results after fractures of the hip in children. Its overall prevalence is approximately 30%, based on the literature.[21,50,71] The risk of ON is highest after displaced type IB, II, and III fractures (Fig. 21-11).[14] In the meta-analysis by Moon and Mehlman,[68] the incidence of ON in type I through type IV is 38%, 28%, 18%, and 5%, respectively. In addition to location of the fracture (via Delbet classification), ON is believed to be increased with increased fracture displacement and older age at the time of injury.[61] Several studies report lower rates of ON in their series of patients treated within 24 hours of injury with prompt reduction and internal fixation.[21,33,96] This approach to early reduction and stabilization may decrease ON by preventing further injury to the tenuous blood supply, and open reduction or cap-

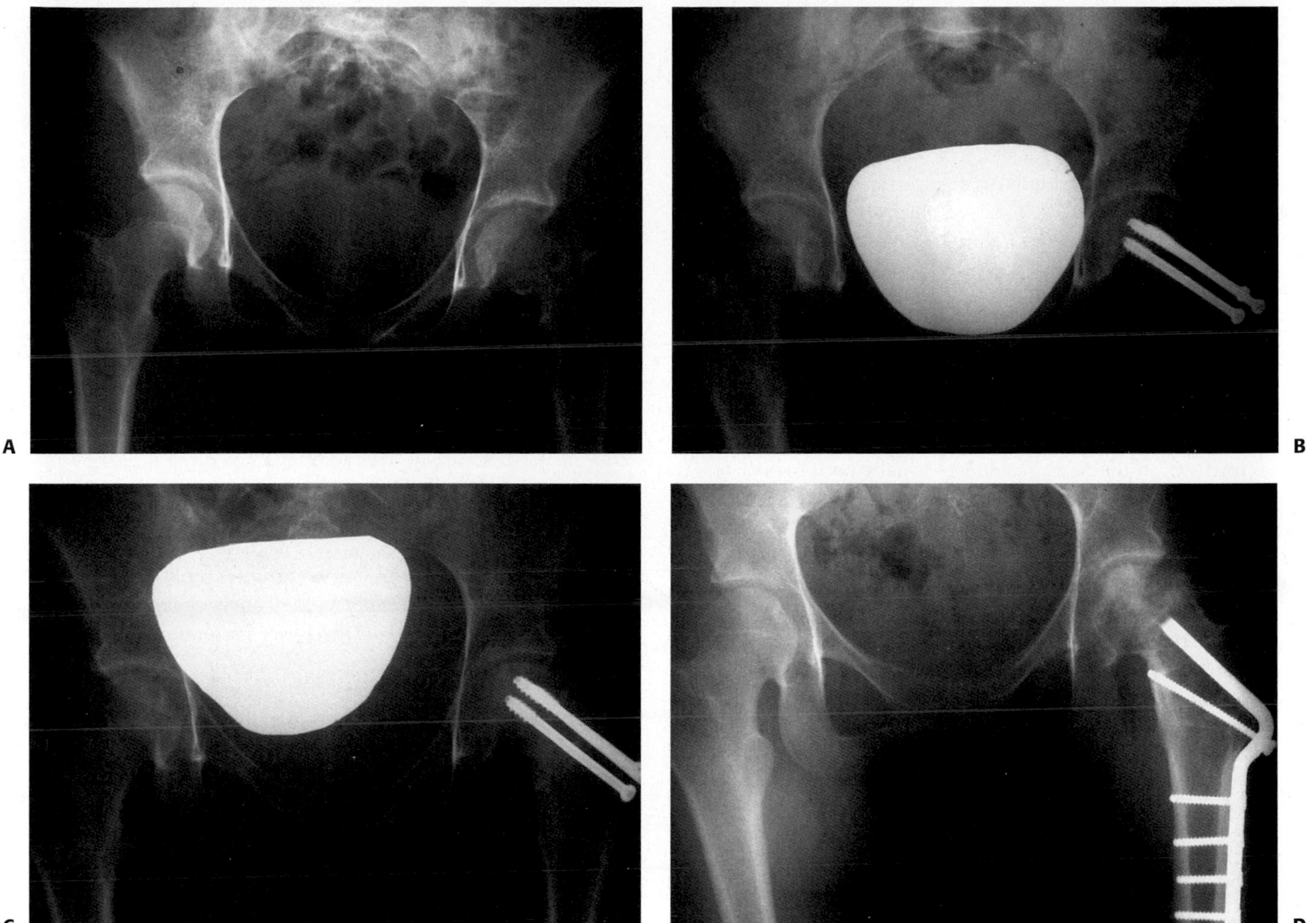

FIGURE 21-11 A. A 14-year-old girl with a type II fracture of the left femoral neck. **B.** After fixation with three cannulated screws. **C.** ON with collapse of the superolateral portion of the femoral head. **D.** After treatment with valgus osteotomy.

sulotomy may decrease intra-articular pressure caused by fracture hematoma.[50,71,97] The later concept has equivocal support in the literature with some papers reporting that aspirating the hematoma may decrease the intracapsular pressure and increase blood flow to the femoral head[21,71]; others suggest that this may have little effect.[50,64,78]A final important factor that may reduce ON is stability and quality of reduction: this is highlighted in a recent 30-year experience of hip fractures from Mayo Clinic.[90] In this paper, ON was associated with inadequate reduction and use of older implant styles. In our institution, we recognize that the die may already be cast at the time of injury, but we still advocate emergent anatomic reduction and stabilization of the fracture in order to reduce risk of ON. ON has been classified by Ratliff as follows: type I, involvement of the whole head; type II, partial involvement of the head; and type III, an area of necrosis of the femoral neck from the fracture line to the physis (Fig. 21-12).[84] Type I is the most severe and most common form and has the poorest prognosis. Type I probably results from damage to all of the retinacular epiphyseal vessels, type II from localized damage to one or more of the

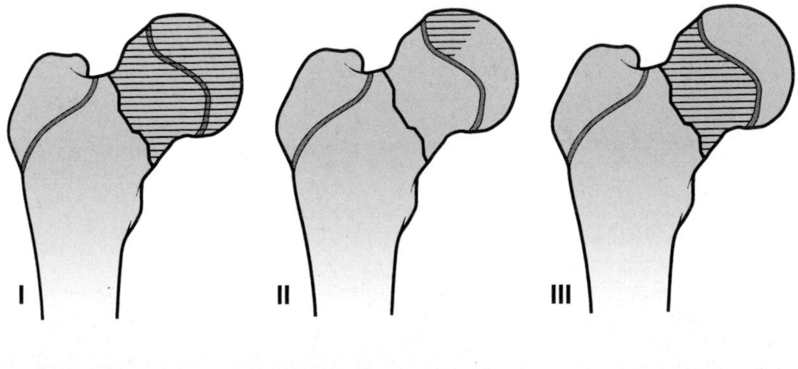

FIGURE 21-12 The three types of ON. Type I, whole head; type II, partial head; and type III, femoral neck. (Reprinted from Ratliff AHC. Fractures of the neck of the femur in children. J. Bone Joint Surg Br 1962:44:528, with permission.)

I II III

lateral epiphyseal vessels near their insertion into the anterolateral aspect of the femoral head, and type III from damage to the superior metaphyseal vessels. Type III is rare but has a good prognosis provided the fracture goes on to heal.[84] Signs and symptoms of ON usually develop within the first year after injury, but many patients may not become symptomatic for up to 2 years.[50,83]Some authors have utilized bone scanning for early detection of ON as further collapse may be prevented with use of bisphosphonate therapy. Little and his colleagues[82] treated 17 children and adolescents with early bone scan changes of ON from slipped capital femoral epiphysis or femoral neck fracture. The group was treated with an intravenous bisphosphonate (pamidronate or zolendronate) for an average of 20 months, which greatly improved the outcome at 3 year follow-up.[82] The long-term results of established ON are likely related to age of the patient and extent and location of the necrosis within the head; results are usually poor in over 60% of patients.[18,27,34,74] There is no clearly effective treatment for established posttraumatic ON in children.[50,83] Older children (more than 10 years of age) tend to have worse outcomes than younger children. Treatment of ON is controversial and inconclusive and is beyond the scope of this text. Ongoing research includes the role of redirectional osteotomy,[62] distraction arthroplasty with external fixation, core decompression, vascularized fibular grafting (Fig. 21-13), and direct bone grafting.

Coxa Vara

The prevalence of coxa vara has been reported to be approximately 20% to 30% in nine series[50]; although it is significantly lower in series in which internal fixation was used after reduction of displaced fractures.[18] Coxa vara may be caused by malunion, ON of the femoral neck, premature physeal closure, or a combination of these problems (Fig. 21-14). Severe coxa vara raises the greater trochanter in relation to the femoral head, causing shortening of the extremity and leading to inefficiency of the abductors. Remodeling of an established malunion may occur if the child is less than 8 years of age, or with a neck–shaft angle greater than 110 degrees. Older patients with progressive deformity may not remodel and subtrochanteric valgus osteotomy may be considered to heal nonunion, and restore limb length and the abductor moment arm (Fig. 21-15).[50]

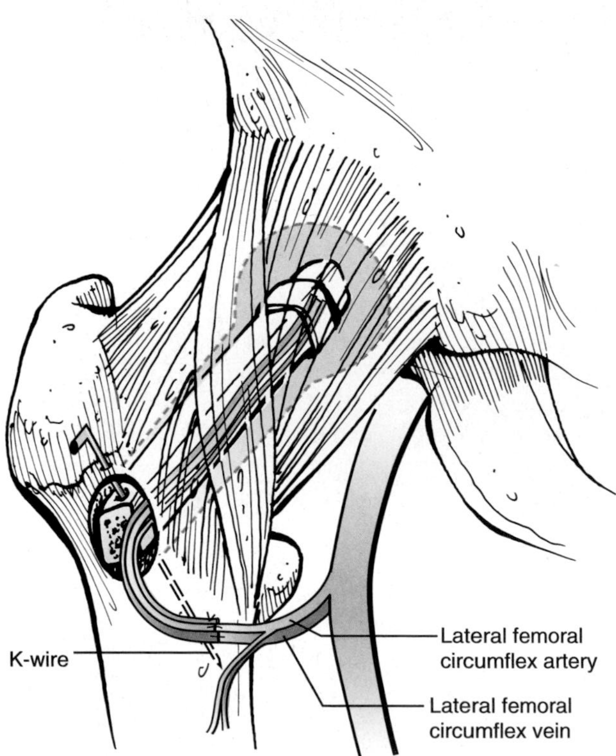

FIGURE 21-13 Vascularized fibular grafting for osteonecrosis of the femoral head. (Redrawn after Aldrich JM III, Berend KR, Gunneson EE, et al. Free vascularized fibular grafting for the treatment of postcollapse osteonecrosis of the femoral head. J Bone Joint Surg Am 2004;86:87–101, with permission).

Premature Physeal Closure

Premature physeal closure has occurred after approximately 28% of fractures.[50] The risk of premature physeal closure increases with penetration by fixation devices or when ON is present. It is most common in patients who have type II or III ON (see Fig. 21-14).[83,84]

The capital femoral physis contributes only 13% of the growth of the entire extremity and normally closes earlier than most of the other physes in the lower extremity. As a result, shortening due to premature physeal closure is not significant except in very young children.[14,52] Treatment for leg length discrepancy is indicated only for significant discrepancy (2.5 cm or more projected at maturity).[50] If femoral growth arrest is expected due to the implant use or injury to the physis, the surgeon may consider concomitant greater trochanteric epiphysiodesis to maintain a more normal articular trochanteric relationship (Fig. 21-16).

Nonunion

Nonunion occurs infrequently, with an overall incidence of 7% of hip fractures in children.[50] Nonunion is a complication seen in types II and III fractures and is not generally seen after type I or type IV fractures. The primary cause of nonunion is failure to obtain or maintain an anatomic reduction.[14,16] After femoral neck fracture in a child, pain should be gone and bridging new bone should be seen at the fracture site by 3 months after injury. A CT scan may be helpful to look for bridging bone. If no or minimal healing is seen by 3 to 6 months, the diagnosis of nonunion is established. Nonunion should be treated operatively as soon as possible. Either rigid internal fixation or subtrochanteric valgus osteotomy should be performed to allow compression across the fracture (Fig. 21-17).[58] Because the approach necessary for bone grafting is extensive, it should be reserved for persistent nonunion. Internal fixation should extend across the site of the nonunion, and spica cast immobilization should be used in all but the most mature and cooperative adolescents.

Other Complications

Infection is uncommon after hip fractures in children. The reported incidence of 1%[1,8,10] is consistent with the expected infection rate in any closed fracture treated surgically with open reduction and internal fixation. Chondrolysis is exceedingly rare and has been reported only in two series.[6,34] Care must be taken to avoid persistent penetration of hardware into the joint, which can cause chondrolysis in conditions such as SCFE. Finally,

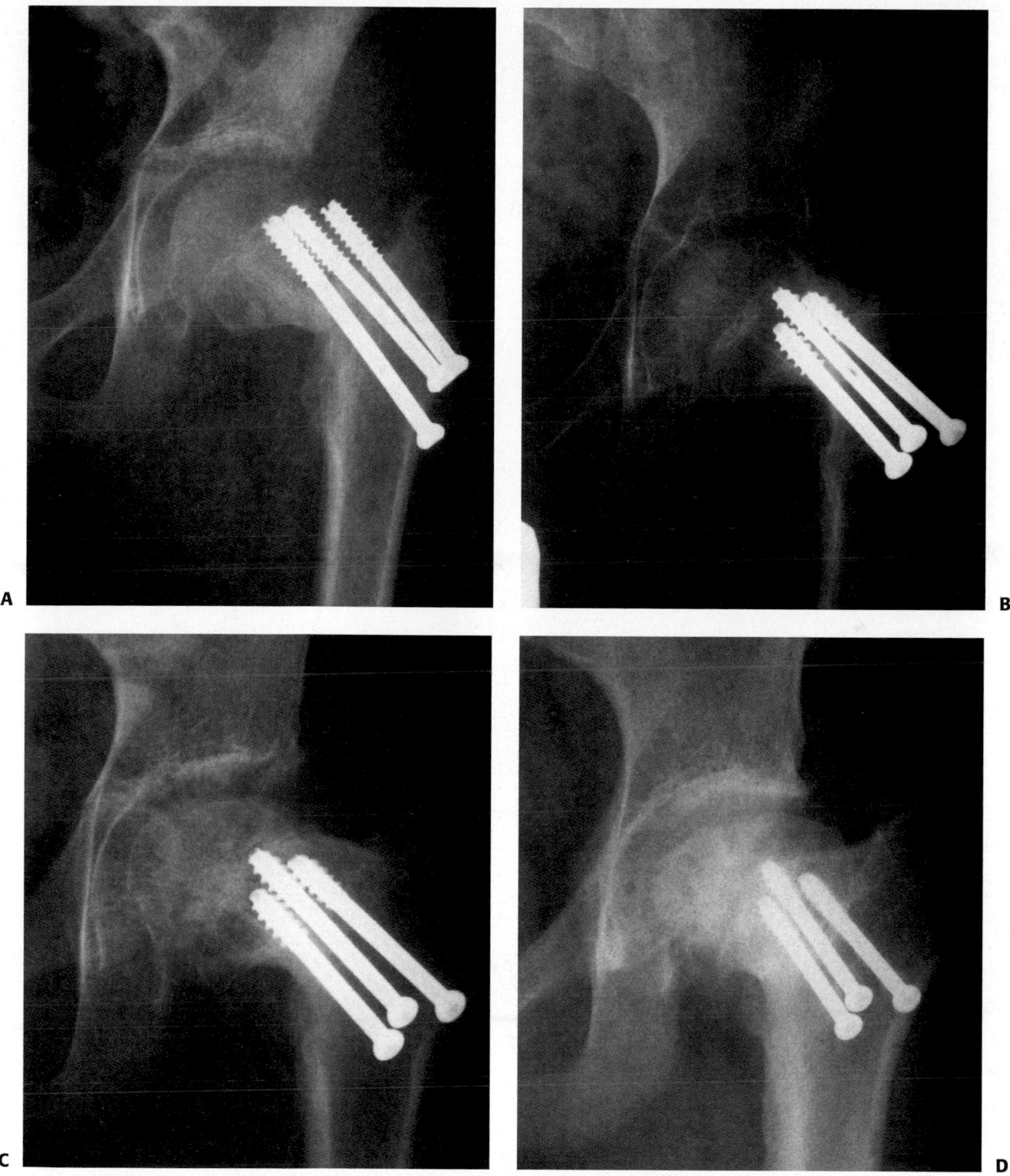

FIGURE 21-14 A. A 12-year-old boy with a type III left hip fracture. Poor pin placement and varus malposition are evident. **B.** The fracture united in mild varus after hardware revision. **C.** Fourteen months after injury, collapse of the weight-bearing segment is evident. **D.** Six years after injury, coxa breva and trochanteric overgrowth are seen secondary to osteonecrosis, nonunion, and premature physeal closure.

SCFE has been reported after fixation of an ipsilateral femoral neck fracture.[51]

Stress Fractures. Stress fractures of the femoral neck are extremely uncommon in children, and only a few cases have been published in the English-language literature. In one study of 40 stress fractures in children, there was only one femoral neck stress fracture.[28] The rarity of such fractures underscores the need for a high index of suspicion when a child has unexplained hip pain. The differential can be long for hip pain in children, and early diagnosis and treatment are essential to avoid complete fracture with displacement.

Mechanism. Stress fractures of the femoral neck in children usually result from repetitive cyclic loading of the hip, such as that produced by a new or increased activity. A recent increase in the repetitive activity is highly suggestive of the diagnosis. An increase in intensity of soccer,[12] and an increase in distance running are examples of such activities. Younger children often present with a limp or knee pain and may not have a clear history of increased activity.[65] Underlying metabolic disorders or immobilizations that weaken the bone may predispose to stress fracture. In adolescent female athletes, amenorrhea, anorexia nervosa, and osteoporosis have been implicated in the development of stress fractures of the femoral neck.[44]

FIGURE 21-15 A. A 10-year-old boy with a type III fracture treated without cast immobilization develops progressive varus deformity 4 months after surgery. Inset CT scan demonstrates delayed union. Valgus osteotomy is indicated for his progressive varus deformity and delayed healing. **B.** Three years after valgus osteotomy, the fracture is healed and the deformity corrected.

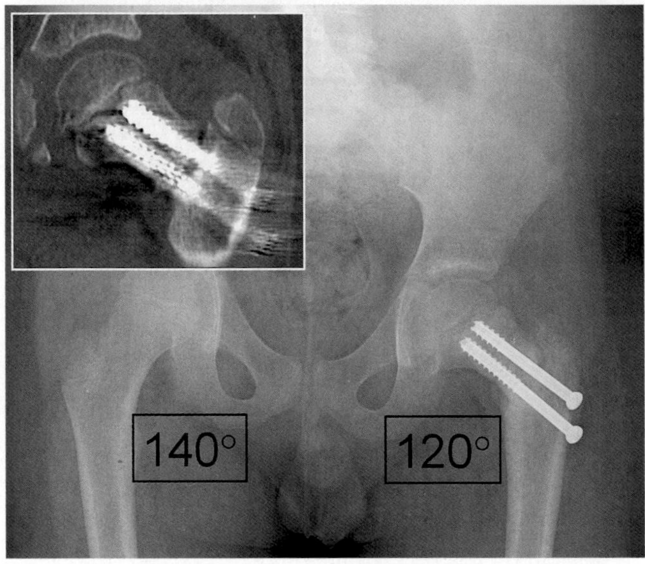

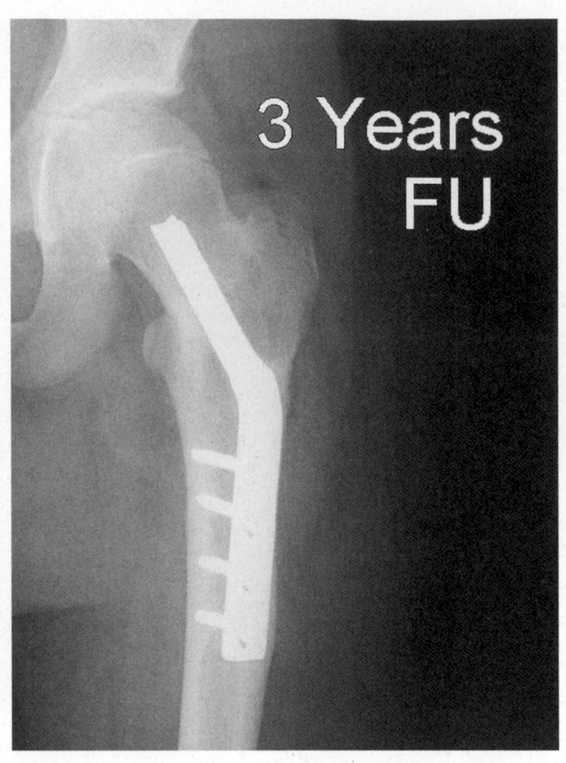

The usual presentation is that of progressive hip or groin pain with or without a limp. The pain may be perceived in the thigh or knee and may be mild enough so that it does not significantly limit activities. In the absence of displacement, examination typically reveals slight limitation of hip motion with increased pain, especially with internal rotation. Usually plain radiographs reveal the fracture, but in the first 4 to 6 weeks after presentation, plain films may be negative. If there are no changes or only linear sclerosis, a bone scan will help identify the fracture. MRI has been documented as a sensitive test for undisplaced fractures of the femoral neck. If a sclerotic lesion is seen on plain radiographs, the differential diagnosis should include osteoid osteoma, chronic sclerosing osteomyelitis, bone infarct, and osteosarcoma. Other causes of hip pain, include slipped capital femoral epiphysis, Legg-Calvé-Perthes disease, infection, avulsion injuries of the pelvis, eosinophilic granu-

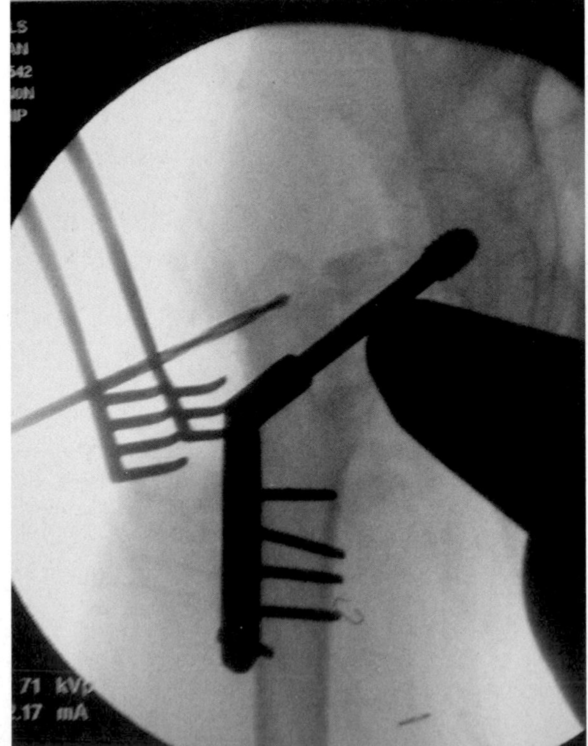

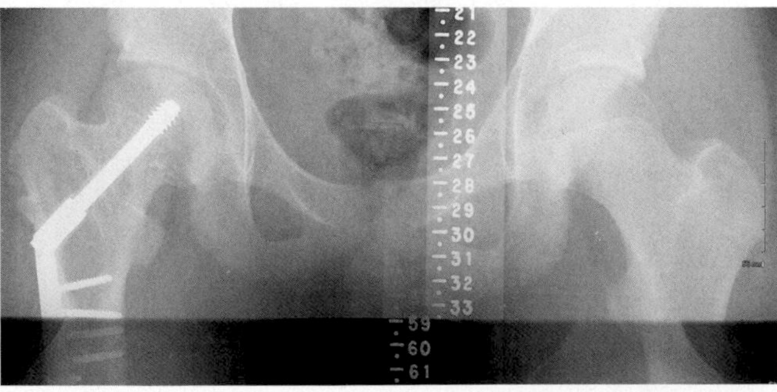

FIGURE 21-16 A. Greater trochanteric epiphysiodesis was performed at time of open reduction and internal fixation of a pathologic femoral neck fracture (see Fig. 21-1) in 10-year-old boy. Because the implant crosses the physis, growth arrest is expected and trochanteric arrest may minimize trochanteric overgrowth. **B.** Seven-year follow-up shows that growth arrest occurred and some trochanteric mismatch is present despite prior epiphysiodesis.

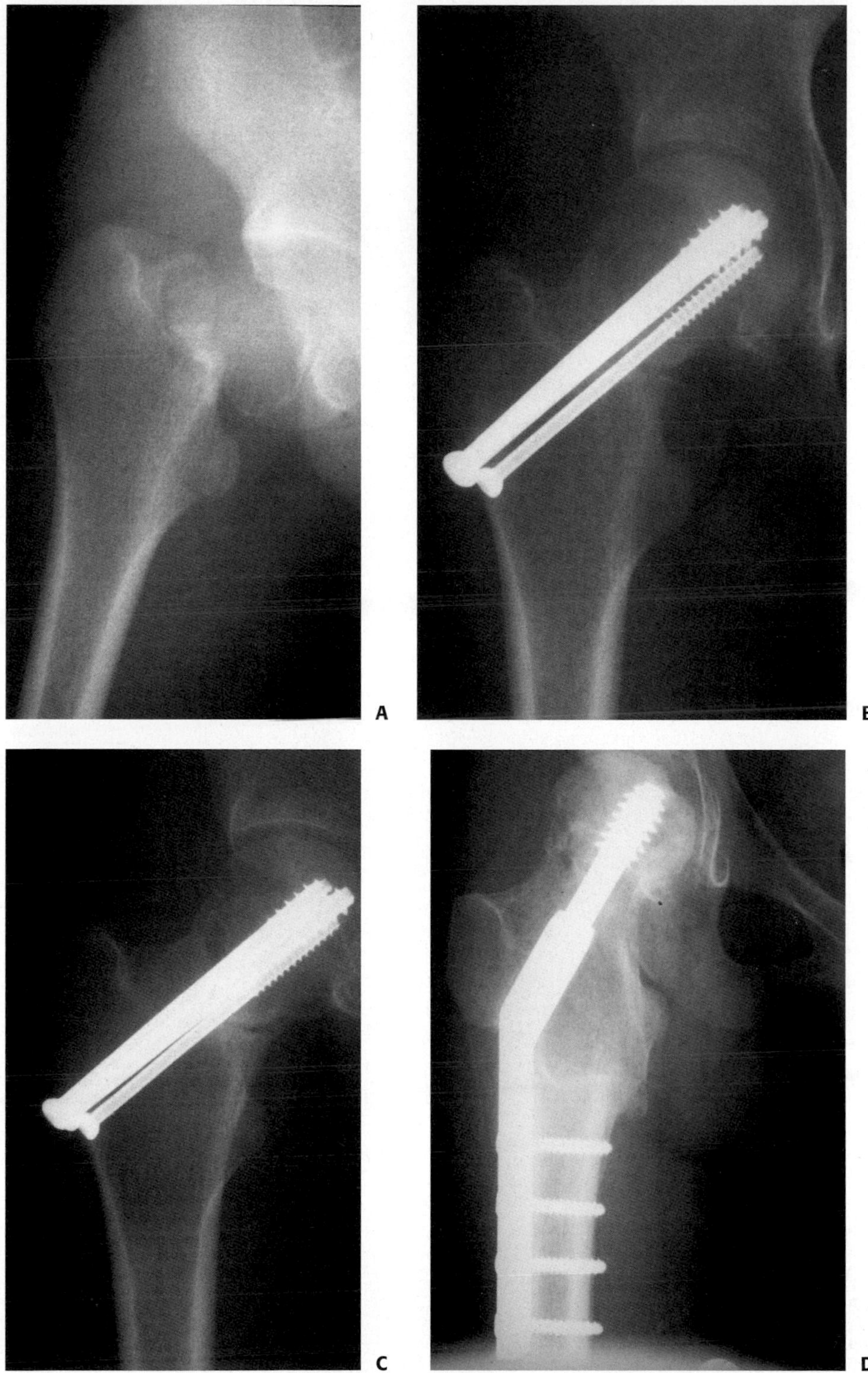

FIGURE 21-17 A. A 15-year-old girl with a markedly displaced type II femoral neck fracture. **B.** She underwent open reduction and internal fixation with two 7.3-mm cannulated screws and one 4.5-mm cannulated screw. Primary bone grafting of a large defect in the superior neck was also performed. **C.** Radiograph at 5 months showing a persistent fracture line **D.** Six weeks after valgus intertrochanteric osteotomy. The fracture is healing.

loma, and bony malignancies. Stress fractures unrelieved by rest or treatment may progress with activity to complete fracture with displacement.[98] For this reason, prompt diagnosis and treatment are important.

Classification. Femoral neck stress fractures have been classified into two types: compression fractures and tension fractures.[28] The compression type appears as reactive bone formation on the inferior cortex without cortical disruption. This type rarely becomes completely displaced but may collapse into a mild varus deformity,[29] and compression types have been reported to progress to complete fracture without early treatment (Fig. 21-18).[98] The tension type is a transverse fracture line appearing on the superior portion of the femoral neck. This type is inherently unstable because the fracture line is perpendicular to the lines of tension. Tension stress fractures have not been reported in children but may occur in skeletally mature teenagers.[98]

Treatment. Compression-type fractures generally can be treated with a period of nonweight bearing on crutches. Partial weight bearing can be allowed at 6 weeks with progression to

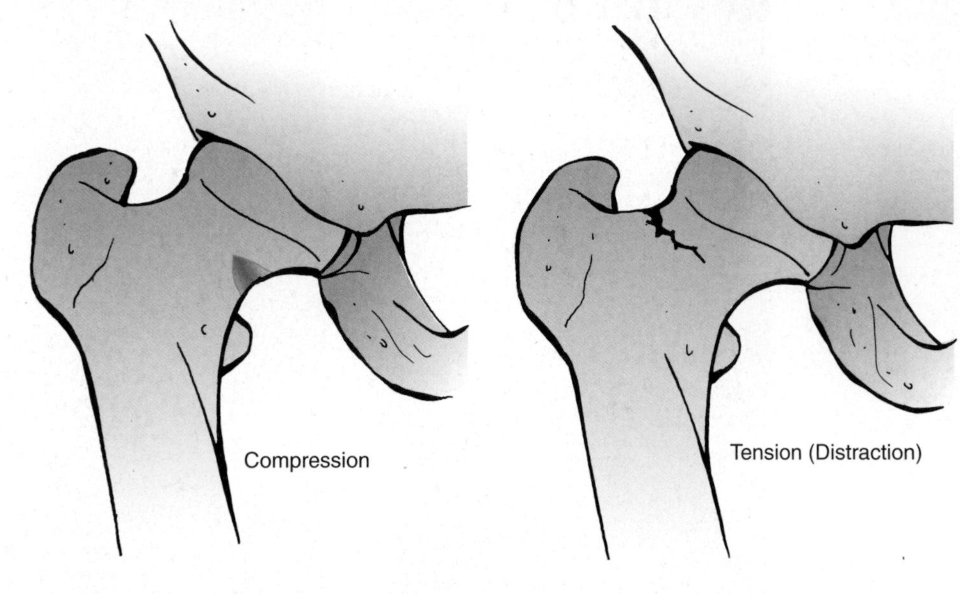

FIGURE 21-18 A line drawing of stress fractures, comparing compression **(A)** and tension **(B)** types.

full weight bearing at 12 weeks provided that the pain is resolved and there is radiographic evidence of healing. Close follow-up and careful evaluation is mandatory to insure that the fracture heals without propagation. Underlying conditions should be evaluated and addressed. In small or uncooperative children, spica casting may be necessary. Displacement into varus, however minimal, mandates internal fixation. Tension fractures are at high risk for displacement and should be treated with in situ compression fixation using cannulated screws.

Complications. Coxa vara is the most common complication of untreated compression-type fractures. Acute displacement of this type also has been described.[108] Once displaced, the stress fracture is subject to all the complications of Type II and Type III displaced femoral neck fractures.

HIP DISLOCATIONS IN CHILDREN

Traumatic hip dislocations are uncommon injuries in children, constituting less than 5% of pediatric dislocations.[60] In one study, the author identified only 15 cases over a 20-year period at a large trauma center.[5] The character of the injury tends to vary in that children under age 6 commonly suffer isolated hip dislocation from a low-energy injury, whereas older children require a high-energy mechanism to dislocate the hip, and these injuries are often associated with more severe trauma.[5,10,36,43,75,88] Most hip dislocations in children can be reduced easily, and long-term outcome is generally good with prompt and complete reduction. Delay in reduction or neglected dislocations routinely do poorly, with a high incidence of AVN.[7,8] Incomplete reductions can occur from interposed soft tissue or bony fragments, and postoperative imaging is mandatory to insure complete reduction.[22,106] Difficult reductions or those that occur during the early teenage years (with a widened proximal femoral physis) should be performed with anesthesia, muscle relaxation, and the use of fluoroscopy to ensure that physeal separation does not occur.[48,74] Open reduction may be needed if the hip cannot be reduced or if there is a femoral head fracture or an incarcerated fragment. Incomplete reductions may be treated open or arthroscopically.[54] Complications, although uncommon, may occur, and these patients should be closely followed for recurrent subluxation, dislocation, and AVN.[5,46,88]

Principles of Management

Mechanism of Injury

The mechanism of injury in children with hip dislocation varies. Posterior hip dislocations are the most common[10,88,91] and generally occur when a force is applied to the leg with the hip flexed and slightly adducted (Fig. 21-19). Anterior dislocations comprise fewer than 10% of hip dislocations (Fig. 21-20).[5,88] Anterior dislocations can occur superiorly or inferiorly and result from forced abduction and external rotation. If the hip is extended while undergoing forced abduction and external rotation, it will dislocate anteriorly and superiorly; if the hip is flexed while abducted and externally rotated, the femoral head

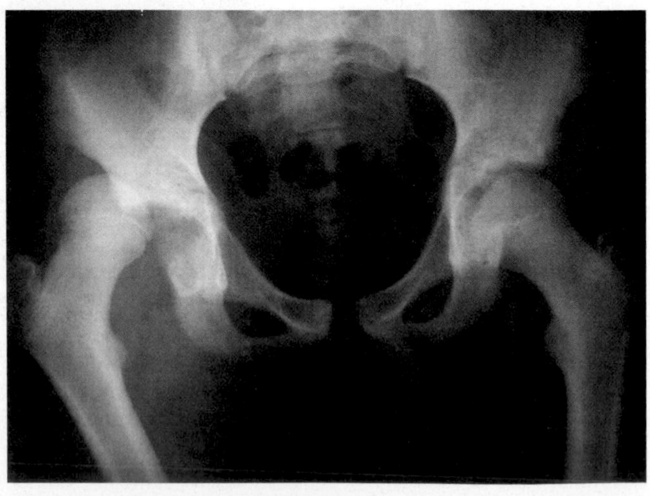

FIGURE 21-19 A typical posterior dislocation of the hip.

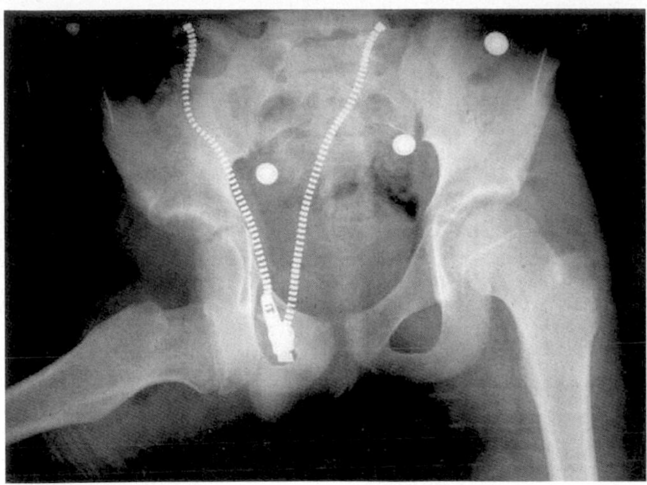

FIGURE 21-20 An anterior (inferior) dislocation of the hip.

tends to dislocate anteriorly and inferiorly. In very rare cases, the femoral head may dislocate directly inferiorly, a condition known as luxatio erecta femoris or infracotyloid dislocation. Although this condition is extremely rare, it tends to occurs more commonly in children than adults.[87]

In younger children, hip dislocations can occur with surprisingly little force, such as a fall while at play. The mechanism for hip dislocations in older children and adolescents is similar to that of adults in that significant trauma is needed. In a recent French study,[5] the authors assessed children with hip dislocations and divided them into two groups by age: those under 6 years old (seven patients) and those age 6 and older (seven patients). All the children in the under age 6 group had low-energy mechanisms and isolated hip dislocations without other injuries, but often had predisposing factors, such as hyperlaxity, coxa valga, or decreased acetabular coverage (Fig. 21-21). In the over 6-year-old group, all the dislocations were a result of higher-energy injuries and often had associated injuries.[5] Football and motor vehicle accidents are the most common etiology,

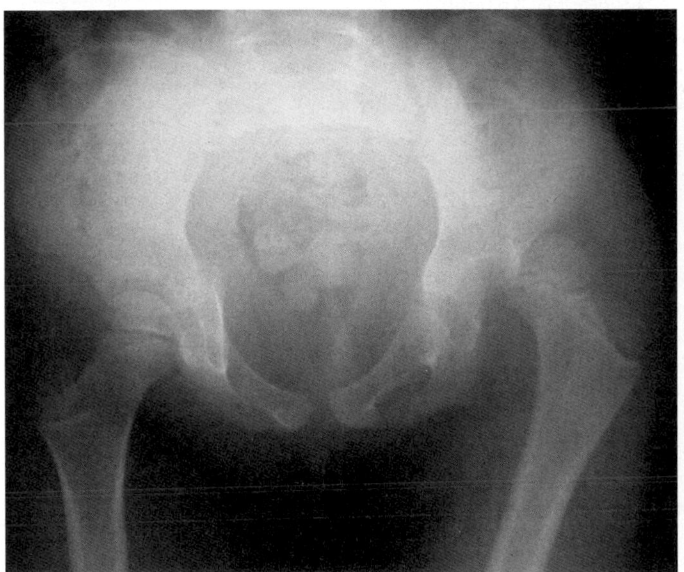

A

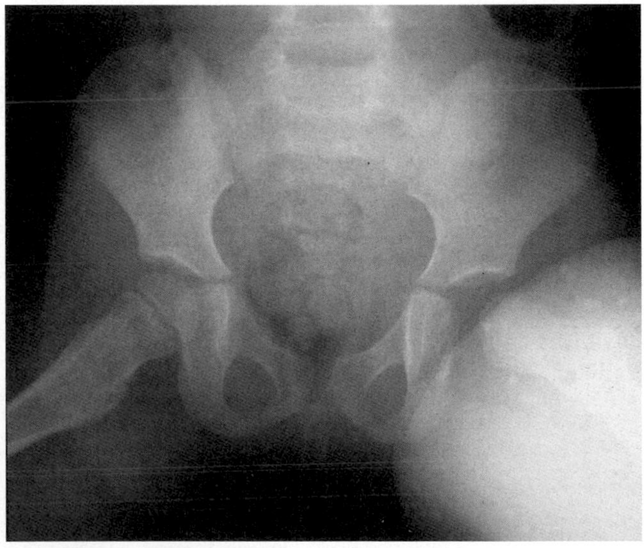

B

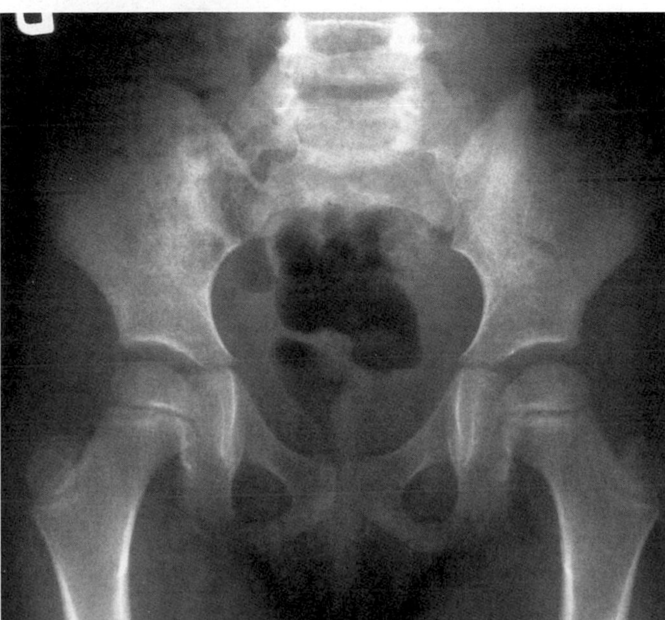

C

FIGURE 21-21 A. A girl age 4 years and 7 months presented with a posterior dislocation of the left hip. This is often the result of a low-energy injury, such as a fall from play. **B.** Frog-leg lateral radiograph at injury. **C.** Eight months after successful closed reduction, radiographic appearance is normal.

combining for over 50% of the dislocations in older children and adolescents.[66]

Signs and Symptoms

The injured child has pain and inability to ambulate. Children sometimes feel the pain in the knee rather than in the hip. The hallmark of the clinical diagnosis of dislocation of the hip is abnormal positioning of the limb, which is not seen in fracture of the femur. Dislocations may spontaneously reduce, leaving the child with an incompletely reduced hip that is commonly misdiagnosed. Price et al.[81] reported on 3 children who presented with a history of trauma and an incongruous hip. In all cases, the diagnosis was originally missed.[81]

Associated Injuries

Older children with dislocations due to a high-energy mechanism of injury often present with associated injuries. In one study of 42 patients, there were 17 fractures in 9 patients and 1 closed head injury. Of the 17 fractures, 6 were posterior acetabular wall factures and 1 required open reduction and internal fixation.[66] Careful evaluation of this injury in younger children with MRI is important because standard radiographic assessments and CT may underestimate the size of the fragment.[86] Posterior dislocations of the femoral head can result in injury to the sciatic nerve in about 10% of adults and 5% of children. Partial recovery occurs in 60% to 70% of patients.[25] The function of the sciatic nerve should be specifically tested at the time of the initial assessment and after reduction.

Anterior dislocations can damage the femoral neurovascular bundle, and femoral nerve function and perfusion of the limb should be assessed. Tears of the capsule or acetabular labrum occur and prevent concentric reduction of the hip. Postreduction imaging must be carefully evaluated to insure that there is not interposed soft tissue, such as the labrum or capsule, or osteochondral fragments (Fig. 21-22). Rupture of the ligament teres is common in hip dislocations and can rarely be a cause of residual pain in some patients.[16]

In addition, ipsilateral knee injuries commonly occur in high-energy injuries. One study evaluated the ipsilateral knees in 28 adults who had a traumatic hip dislocation and found that 75% had knee pain and 93% had MRI evidence of a knee injury; effusion, bone bruise, and meniscal tears were the most common findings.[89]

Diagnosis

Plain radiographs combined with the physical exam as described above usually confirm the diagnosis of a dislocated hip.

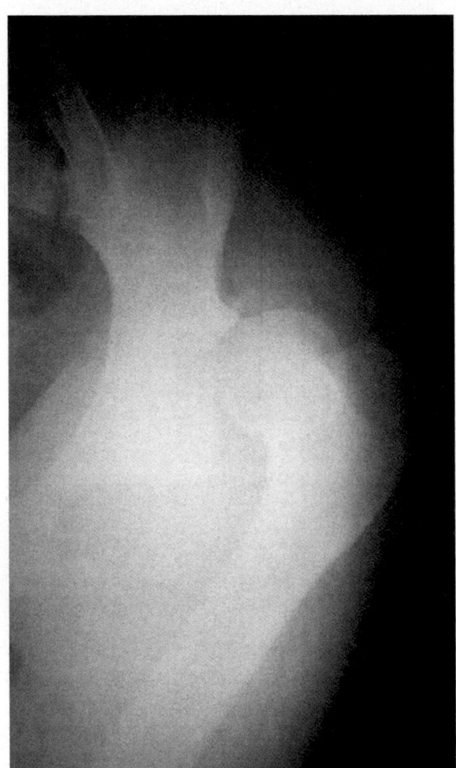

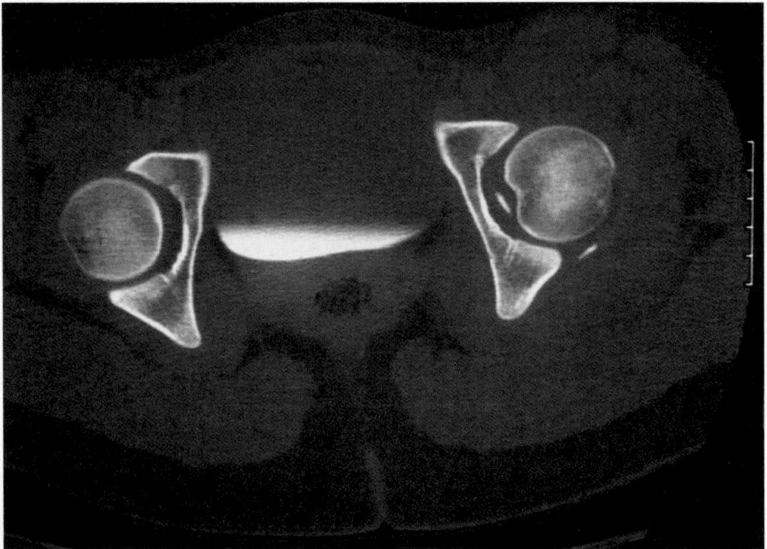

FIGURE 21-22 A. A girl aged 13 years and 11 months sustained a left posterior hip dislocation in a motor vehicle accident. **B.** CT scan after reduction showed intra-articular bony fragments. **C.** At open reduction and capsulorrhaphy, the bony fragments were removed. Suture anchors were used to reattach capsule to bone. Ten months after injury, there is no sign of ON. Heterotopic ossification is seen. Bony fragments can also be removed arthroscopically.

Traumatic dislocations with spontaneous reductions may be more subtle and are often missed. Radiographs should be examined for fracture of the acetabular rim and proximal femur, which may be associated with dislocation. Any asymmetry of the joint space, as compared to the contralateral hip, is a common finding with interposed tissue. MRI or CT scanning is useful for evaluating the acetabulum and may be useful in localizing intra-articular bony fragments or soft tissue interposition after reduction.[47,66,106] The identification of nonbony fragments is difficult by CT without the use of concomitant arthrography.[47] MRI is useful for evaluating soft tissues that may be interposed between the femoral head and acetabulum. MRI is especially helpful in nonconcentric reductions when the initial direction of dislocation is unknown, and in younger children with less boney ossification (Fig. 21-23).[86,106]

Spontaneous reduction may occur after hip dislocation,[69,77,81] and the diagnosis is commonly missed if it is not considered. The presence of air in the hip joint, which may be detectable on CT scan of the pelvis, is evidence that a hip dislocation has occurred.[32] Dislocation and spontaneous reduction with interposed tissue can occur and lead to late arthropathy if untreated.[77] Widening of the joint space on plain radiographs suggests the diagnosis. In patients with hip pain, a history of trauma, and widening of the joint space, consideration should be given to MRI or arthrography to rule out dislocation with spontaneous relocation incarcerating soft tissue. If incarcerated soft tissues or osseous cartilage fragments are found, open or arthroscopic removal is required to obtain concentric reduction of the hip.[54]

Classification

Hip dislocations in children are generally classified depending on where the femoral head lies in relation to the pelvis, namely posterior, anterior superior, anterior inferior, or infracotyloid.[105] The dislocation is posterior more than 90% of the time. The Stewart-Milford classification is based on associated fractures. Grade I is defined as dislocation without an associated fracture or only a small bony avulsion of the acetabular rim, grade II is a posterior rim fracture with a stable hip after reduction, grade III is a posterior rim fracture with an unstable hip (Fig. 21-24), and grade IV is a dislocation that has an associated fracture of the femoral head or neck.

Fracture-dislocation of the hip involving the femoral head or the acetabulum is much more unusual in children than in adults. Older adolescents may sustain adult-type fracture-dislocations of the hip, and these are most commonly classified by the methods of Pipkin.[79] He classified the head fractures as occurring either caudal to the fovea with a resultant small fragment (type 1) (Fig. 21-25), cranial to the fovea with a resultant large fragment (type 2), any combined femoral head and neck fracture (type 3), and any femoral neck fracture with an acetabular fracture (type 4). The youngest patient in his series from 1957 was 20, and most of these fractures were due to the relatively new phenomena of traffic accidents.

Habitual dislocation of the hip has been described in children. In this condition, the child can actually voluntarily dislocate the hip. Many factors may contribute to this ability, including generalized ligamentous laxity or hyperlaxity disorders, excessive anteversion of the femur and acetabulum, and coxa valga.[95] A commonly confused condition is snapping of the iliotibial band over the greater trochanter, and often the patient will describe this as "dislocating their hip." Yet, the hip remains well seated both before and after the snap, which can be quite dramatic. The more common iliotibial band snapping can usually be differentiated from a true hip dislocation by exam, or if needed, radiographs with the hip "in" versus "out." A snapping iliotibial band will demonstrate a well seated hip on both radiographs.

Surgical and Applied Anatomy

The hip joint is a synovial ball and socket joint formed by the articulation of the rounded head of the femur and the cup-like acetabulum of the pelvis. If this is injured early in childhood, the growth of the acetabulum can be affected and result in acetabular dysplasia[13,93] or impingement.[37,42,73]

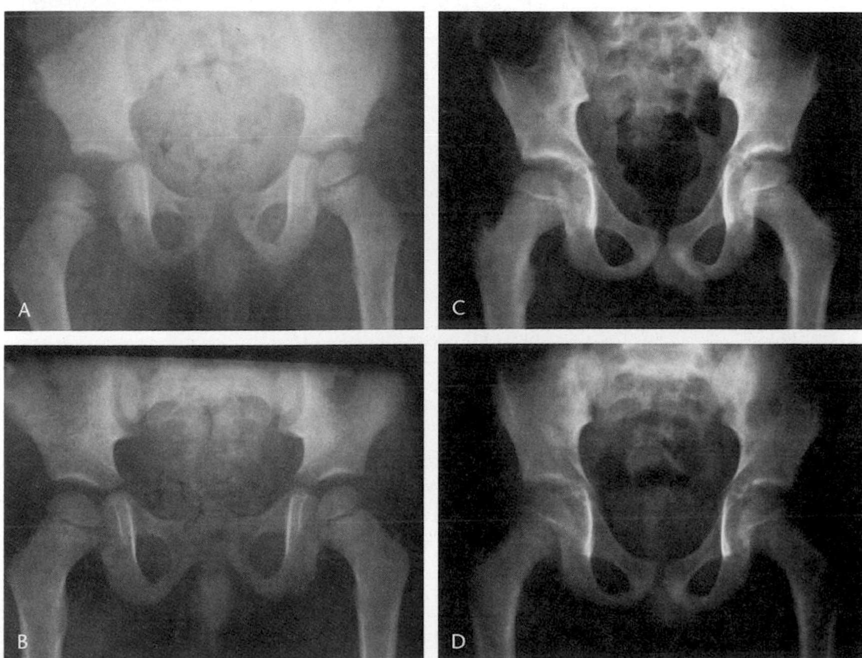

FIGURE 21-23 Two examples of partial reduction after reduction of a dislocated hip. In the first case the asymmetry is well visualized **(A)**, labral entrapment was identified and removed and complete reduction was achieved **(B)**. The asymmetry is less obvious in the second case **(C)**, yet arthrotomy was still needed to remove an osteochondral fragment and achieve complete reduction **(D)**.

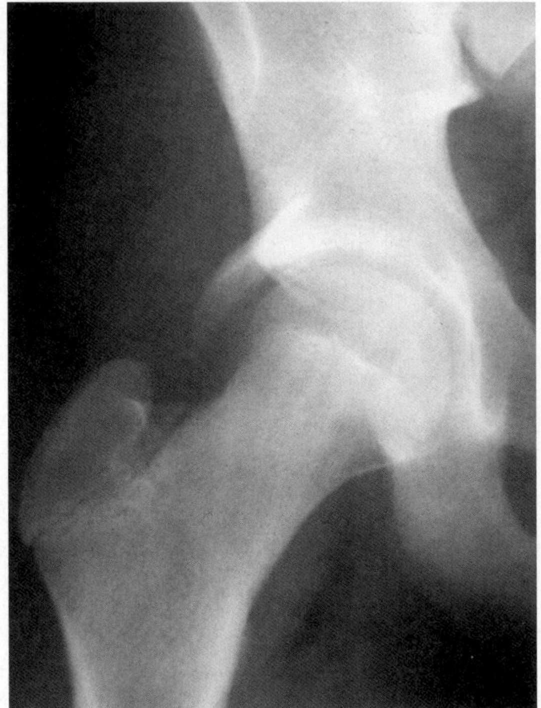

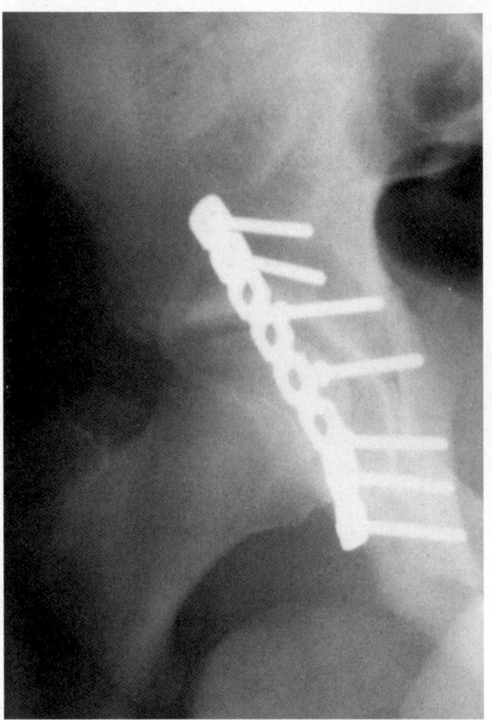

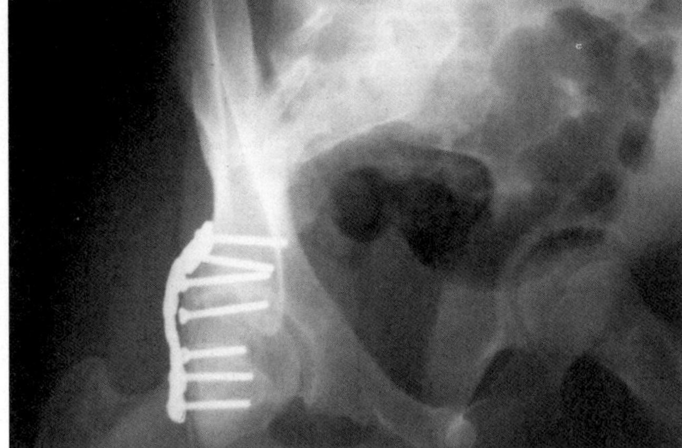

FIGURE 21-24 A. A 12-year-old boy was tackled from behind in football. The right hip was dislocated. Reduction was easily achieved, but the hip was unstable posteriorly as a result of fracture of the posterior rim of the acetabulum. This is the most common fracture, occuring with hip dislocation. **B.** The fracture and capsule were fixed via a posterior approach. **C.** Oblique view shows reconstitution of the posterior rim.

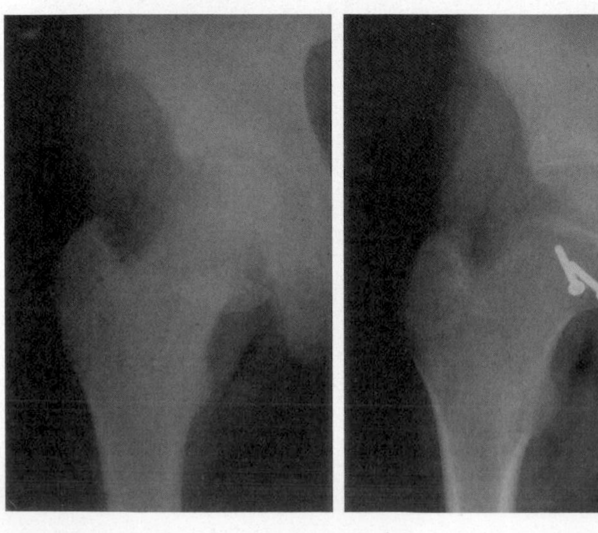

FIGURE 21-25 A. A posterior dislocation associated after reduction with a femoral head fracture caudal to the ligamentum teres (Pipkin type 2). This is uncommon in children. This was treated with open reduction and internal fixation, with follow-up radiographs taken 1 year after the injury **(B)**.

Current Treatment Options

The immediate goal in the treatment of a dislocated hip is to obtain concentric reduction as soon as possible. Reduction of a pediatric or adolescent hip dislocation should be considered an orthopaedic emergency. Generally, closed reduction should be attempted initially. Successful closed reduction can be achieved with intravenous or intramuscular sedation in the emergency room in many patients.[85] Complete muscle relaxation is required for others, and this is best provided in the operating room with a general anesthetic. Open reduction is indicated if closed reduction is unsuccessful or incomplete. In children, especially in their early teenage years, cases of proximal physeal separation with attempted closed reduction have been reported, and therefore the uses of fluoroscopy to assess the stability of the proximal femoral physis is highly recommended.[48,74]

Several methods of closed reduction have been described for reduction of posterior dislocations. With any type of dislocation, traction along the axis of the thigh coupled with gentle manipulation of the hip often affects reduction after satisfactory relaxation of the surrounding muscles.

Allis[3] described a maneuver in which the patient is placed supine and the surgeon stands above the patient. For this reason, either the patient must be placed on the floor or the surgeon must climb onto the operating table. The knee is flexed to relax the hamstrings. While an assistant stabilizes the pelvis, the surgeon applies longitudinal traction along the axis of the femur and gently manipulates the femoral head over the rim of the acetabulum and back into the acetabulum.

Bigelow described a technique similar to the Allis method but after traction the femoral head is levered into the acetabulum by abducting, externally rotating, and extending the hips. This is a more forceful maneuver and may cause damage to the articular surfaces of hip or even fracture the femoral neck; this technique is not therefore recommended and must be performed with caution, especially in children.

The gravity method of Stimson[99] entails placing the patient prone with the lower limbs hanging over the edge of a table. An assistant stabilizes the patient while the surgeon applies gentle downward pressure with the knee and hip flexed 90 degrees, in an attempt to pull the femoral head anteriorly over the posterior rim of the acetabulum and back into the socket. Gentle internal and external rotation may assist in the reduction.

If satisfactory closed reduction cannot be obtained using reasonable measures, it is appropriate to proceed with open reduction and inspection of the joint, to remove any obstructing soft tissues, and identify intra-articular osteochondral fragments. Imaging can be performed prior to reduction but it should not delay treatment.

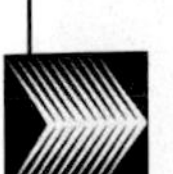

AUTHORS' PREFERRED TREATMENT

Urgent closed reduction by applying traction in line with the femur and gently manipulating the femoral head back into the acetabulum should be performed. A controlled reduction with sedation or general anesthesia and muscle relaxation is preferable, and aggressive techniques should not be attempted without muscle relaxant. The use of fluoroscopy to monitor the reduction, especially in children over 12 with open physis, is important to insure that proximal femoral epiphysiolysis does not occur. Surgery is indicated for dislocations that are irreducible or for nonconcentric reductions. More advanced imaging (CT or MRI) should be considered after reduction to assess for interposing fragments of bone, cartilage, or soft tissue.

Surgical Procedures

Open reduction of a posterior dislocation should be performed through a posterolateral (Kocher-Langenbeck) approach. The patient is positioned in the lateral decubitus position with the dislocated side facing up. The incision is centered on and just posterior to the greater trochanter and goes up into the buttock. Generally, a straight incision can be made with the hip flexed approximately 90 degrees. Once the fascia lata is incised, the femoral head can be palpated beneath or within the substance of the gluteus maximus muscle. The fibers of the gluteus maximus can then be divided by blunt dissection, exposing the dislocated femoral head. The path of dislocation is followed through the short external rotator muscles and capsule down to the acetabulum. The sciatic nerve lies on the short external rotators and should be identified and inspected. The piriformis may be draped across the acetabulum, obstructing the view of the reduction. It may be necessary to detach the short external rotators to see inside the joint. After the joint is inspected, repair of the fracture of the posterior acetabular rim can be performed in the standard fashion.

Anterior dislocations should be approached through an anterior approach. This can be done through a bikini incision that uses the interval between the sartorius and the tensor fascia lata. The deep dissection follows the defect created by the femoral head down to the level of the acetabulum.

At the time of open reduction, the femoral head and acetabulum should be inspected for damage. Any intra-articular fragments should be removed. The labrum and capsule should be inspected for repairable tears. Labral fragments that cannot be securely replaced should be excised, but repair should be attempted. Frequently, the labrum or hip capsule is entrapped in the joint. The femoral head should be dislocated and any interposed soft tissue extracted. A headlight may be needed for visualization, and a Schanz screw or bone hook may be needed to displace the femur enough to see inside the joint.

Obstacles to reduction should be teased out of the way and the traumatic defect enlarged if necessary. The hip joint is then reduced under direct vision. Postreduction radiographs should be taken to confirm concentric reduction. If the joint appears slightly widened, repeat investigation is indicated to rule out interposed tissue. Slight widening may be due to fluid in the hip joint or decreased muscle tone, and this may improve over the next few days. The capsule is repaired if possible.

Open injuries should be treated with immediate irrigation and débridement. The surgical incision should incorporate and enlarge the traumatic wound. Inspection should proceed as detailed above. Capsular repair should be attempted if the hip joint is not contaminated. The wound should be left open or should be well drained to prevent invasive infection.

As in all open fractures, intravenous antibiotics should be administered and patients should be screened for tetanus.

After reduction, a short period of immobilization should be instituted. In younger children, a spica cast can be used for 4 to 6 weeks; older cooperative children can be treated with hip abduction orthosis, total hip precautions and gradually return to ambulation with crutches.[45,88,91]

Pearls and Pitfalls

- Reduce the hip urgently. The most devastating outcome is ON, and prolonged time to reduction (more than 6 hours) appears to be the greatest risk factor. In multitrauma patients, this concept needs to be expressed to the trauma team so that it can be prioritized properly.
- Look for associated fractures and other injuries. In older children, it is important to evaluate the posterior rim of the acetabulum after posterior dislocation to rule out fracture. Relying on plain radiographs and CT may underestimate the extent of damage to the posterior wall of the acetabulum in children due to the incomplete ossification of the pediatric bone. MRI may be required to adequately assess the posterior wall of the acetabulum in children.[86]
- Fractures at other sites in the femur must be considered. It is important to obtain radiographs that show the entire femur to rule out ipsilateral fracture. Careful evaluation of the entire patient is needed especially for high-energy injuries that result in a hip dislocation in older children and adults.
- Separation of the capital femoral epiphysis and femoral neck fracture has been reported in association with dislocation of the hip and the attempted reduction. Children in their early teenage years, aged 12 to 16, should have reduction performed with fluoroscopy under general anesthesia when possible. This strategy may avoid the possibility of displacing the proximal femoral epiphysis (with attendant increased ON risk) during attempted closed reduction (Fig. 21-26).
- Spontaneous relocation of a dislocation of the hip may occur with subsequent soft tissue or osteocartilaginous interposition. Failure to appreciate the presence of hip dislocation may lead to inadequate treatment. Traumatic hip subluxation may go undetected or may be treated as a sprain or strain if the diagnosis is not considered.[69,81] After dislocation and spontaneous reduction, soft tissue may become interposed in the hip joint potentially resulting chronic arthropathy. In a child with posttraumatic hip pain without obvious deformity, the possibility of dislocation-relocation must be considered.
- Always image the hip for evaluation of interposed tissue after reduction. The incidence of widened joint space after hip reductions is as high as 26%.[106] After reduction, hemarthrosis may initially cause the hip joint to appear slightly wider on the affected side, but this should decrease after a few days. If the hip fails to appear concentric, the possibility of interposed soft tissue must be considered and MRI or CT scan should be performed.[39,45,77,85,94]

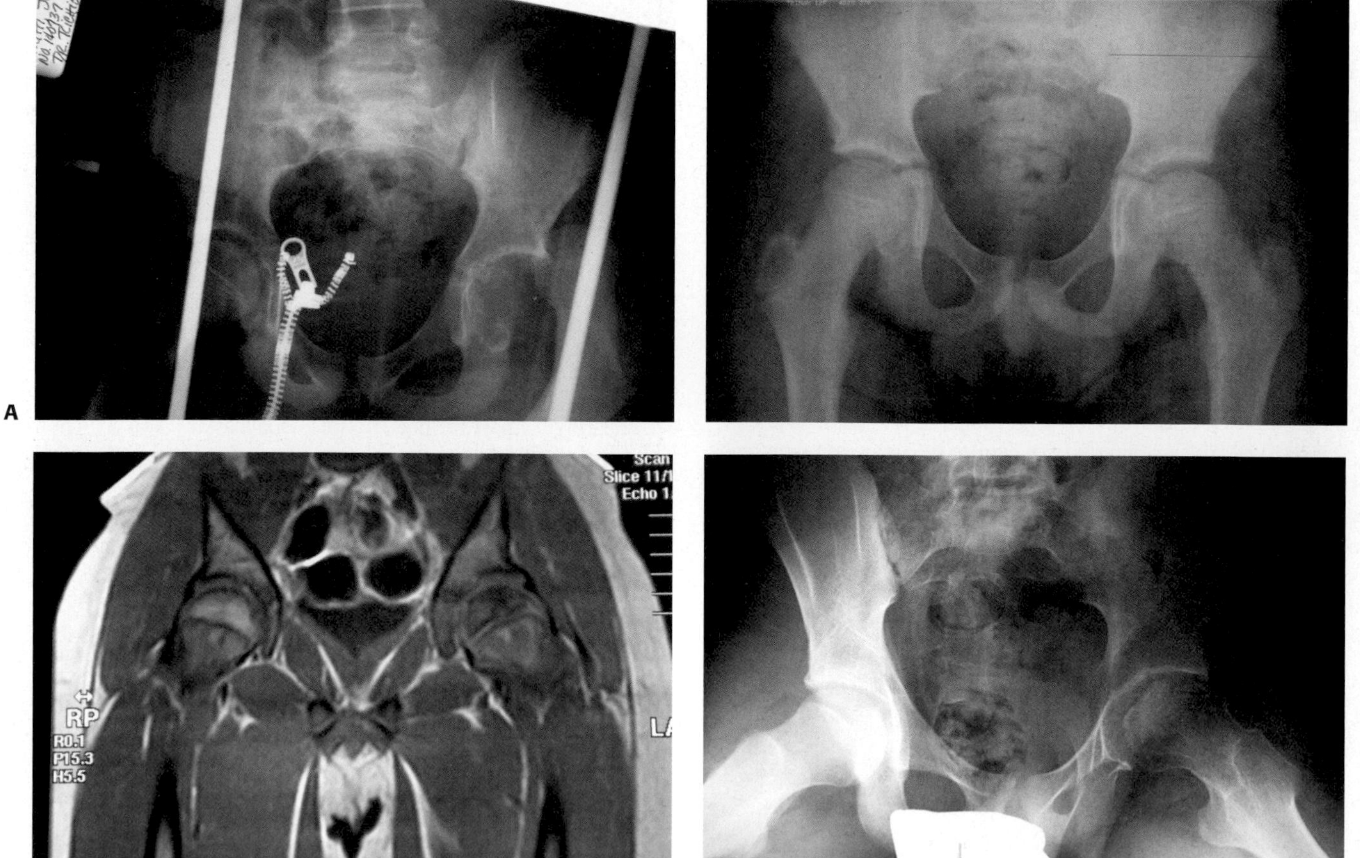

FIGURE 21-26 A. An 11-year-old boy dislocated his left hip while wrestling. **B.** The hip was easily reduced. **C.** After 5 months, hip pain led to an MRI, which shows ON of the capital femoral epiphysis. **D.** At 10 months after injury, there are typical changes of ON despite non–weight bearing.

- Long-term follow-up is important in children who undergo hip dislocation. Injury to the triradiate cartilage may cause acetabular dysplasia with growth. ON, although uncommon, may lead to early arthrosis, and this may not be identified radiographically for several years. If there has been a significant delay in time to reduction or the patient is otherwise at higher risk for ON, then consideration of a bone scan or MRI to evaluate for ON may be warranted, especially if early treatment with bisphosphonates is considered.

Complications

Osteonecrosis occurs in about 10% of hip dislocations in children (Fig. 21-27).[40,66,72,91] Urgent relocation may decrease the incidence of this complication.[36,66,91] The risk of ON is probably also related to the severity of initial trauma.[91] If the force of hip dislocation is so strong as to disrupt the obturator externus muscle, the posterior ascending vessels may be torn.[72] In the rare case of dislocation with an intact capsule, increased intracapsular pressure as a result of hemarthrosis may have a role in developing ON.[85] The type of postreduction care has not been shown to influence the rate of ON.

Early technetium bone scanning with pinhole collimated images detects ON as an area of decreased uptake. Findings on T2-weighted images are abnormal but of variable signal intensity. MRI may be falsely negative if performed within a few days of injury[80]; conversely, many perfusion defects seen on MRI spontaneously resolve after several months.[41,80] As treatment for early ON develops this algorithm may change, and early assessment maybe considered for those at high risk of ON. If hips are followed by serial radiographs for ON, it is recommended that they be studied for at least 2 years after dislocation, because radiographic changes may appear late.[10]

If ON develops, pain, loss of motion, and deformity of the femoral head are likely.[8] ON in a young child resembles Perthes disease and may be treated like Perthes disease.[8] Priorities are to maintain mobility and containment of the femoral head to maximize congruity after resolution. ON in older children should be treated as in adults and may require hip fusion, osteotomy, or reconstruction. If identified early, medical treatment with bisphosphonates or revascularization techniques, such as a vascularized fibular bone graft, can be considered.[1,92]

Chondrolysis

Chondrolysis has been reported after hip dislocation in up to 6% of children[40,45,49,75] and probably occurs as a result of articular damage at the time of dislocation. Chondrolysis cannot be re-

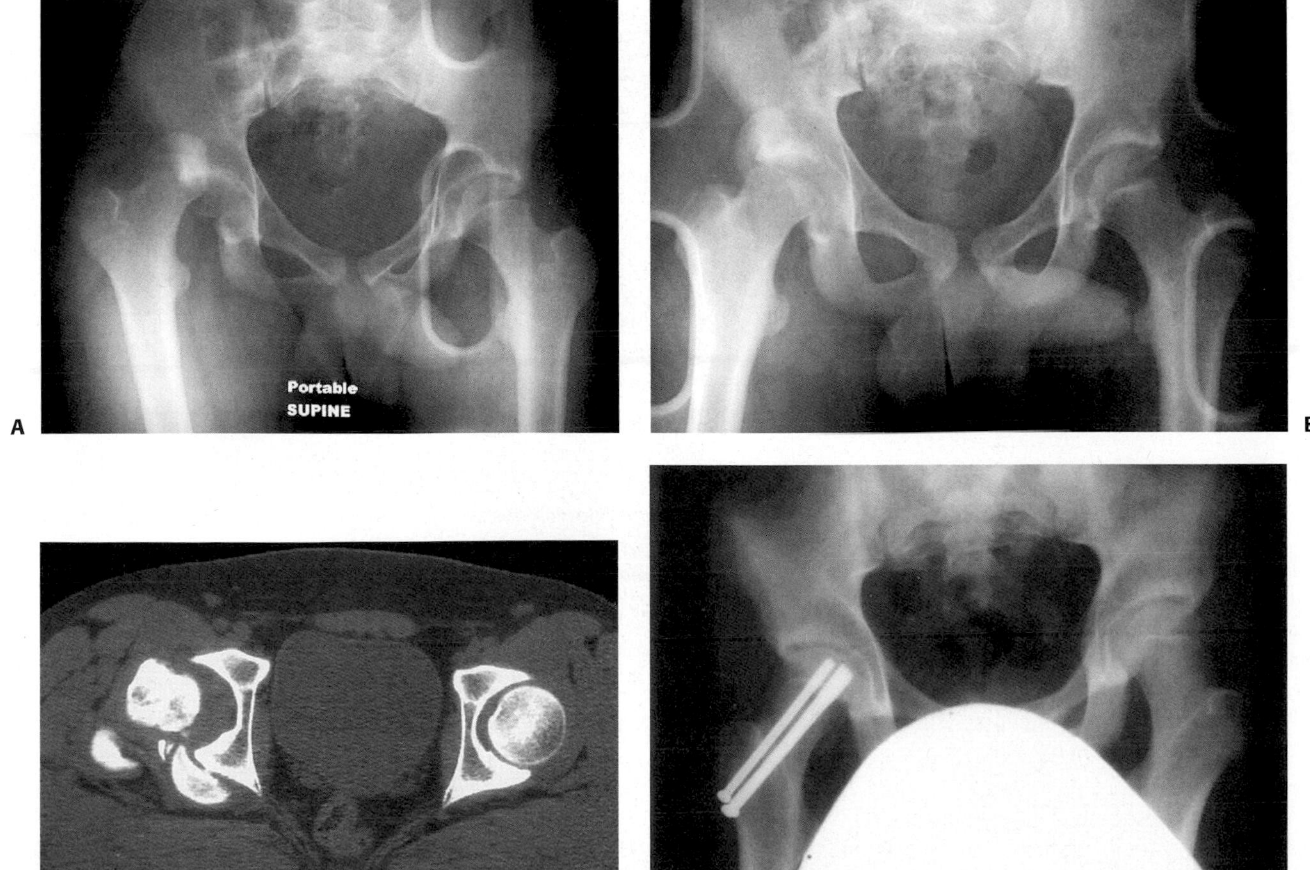

FIGURE 21-27 A. A 15-year-old boy who was involved in a motor vehicle accident sustained a right posterior hip dislocation. **B.** After attempted closed reduction under conscious sedation in the emergency department. The proximal femoral epiphysis remains displaced posterior to the acetabulum while the neck is reduced into the acetabulum. **C.** A CT scan showing the posteriorly displaced proximal femoral epiphysis. **D.** AP radiograph after open reduction and internal fixation of the proximal femur with three cannulated screws.

versed by medical means, and treatment should be symptomatic. Anti-inflammatory medicines and weight-relieving devices should be used as needed. Hip joint distraction with a hinged external fixator may improve range of motion and decrease pain.[101] If the joint fails to reconstitute, fusion or reconstruction should be considered.

Coxa Magna

Coxa magna occasionally occurs after hip dislocation. The reported incidence ranges from 0% to 47%.[40,49,75] It is believed to occur as a result of posttraumatic hyperemia.[75] In most children, this condition is asymptomatic and does not require any treatment.[75] There is no intervention that will prevent coxa magna.

Habitual Dislocation

Habitual or voluntary dislocation of the hip usually is unrelated to trauma. Many factors may contribute to this ability, including generalized ligamentous laxity, excessive anteversion of the femur and acetabulum, and coxa valga. Initial management should include counseling the child to cease the activity (with or without psychiatric counseling) and observation. If episodes of dislocation persist, permanent changes such as secondary capsular laxity or osteocartilaginous deformation of the hip may occur. These changes may lead to pain, residual subluxation, or degenerative joint disease. Conservative treatment should be initially attempted and may include simple observation with or without psychiatric counseling or immobilization with cast or brace. Hip stabilization by surgical means may be indicated for persistent painful episodes of hip despite conservative treatment.[55,95] Corrective surgery, if considered, should be performed only to correct specific anatomic abnormality and may include capsular plication, redirectional pelvic osteotomy, or osteotomy of the proximal femur.[95]

Heterotopic Ossification

Heterotopic ossification can result after closed reduction of hip dislocations in children. In one study, three children (all under 16 years of age) developed heterotopic ossification, one of which required surgical excision.[66]

Interposed Soft Tissue

Interposed tissues may cause nonconcentric reduction or result in complete failure of closed reduction. Muscle, bone, articular cartilage, and labrum have been implicated.[19,36,39,45,81,94] CT arthrography or MRI provide information on obstacles to complete reduction and the direction of the initial dislocation.[39,94] Open reduction generally is necessary to clear impeding tissues from the joint.[19,39,45,75,81,94] Untreated nonconcentric reduction may lead to permanent degenerative arthropathy.[77]

Late Presentation

Not all hip dislocations in children cause severe or incapacitating symptoms. Ambulation may even be possible. As a result, treatment may be delayed or the diagnosis missed until shortening of the limb and contracture are well established, making reduction difficult. Nearly all patients with a delayed treatment of traumatic hip dislocation develop ON.[7,56] Prolonged heavy traction may be considered as method to effect reduction.[43] If this fails, preoperative traction, extensive soft tissue release, or primary femoral shortening should be considered if open reduction is required. Open reduction will likely be difficult and will not always be successful. Even if the hip stays reduced, progressive arthropathy may lead to a stiff and painful hip. The likelihood of a good result decreases with the duration of dislocation.

Nerve Injury

The sciatic nerve may be directly compressed by the femoral head after a posterior dislocation of the hip in 2% to 13% of patients.[31,88,91] If the hip is expediently reduced, nerve function returns spontaneously in most patients.[31,45] If the sciatic palsy is present prior to reduction, the nerve does not need to be explored unless open reduction is required for other reasons. If sciatic nerve function is shown to be intact and is lost during the reduction maneuver, the nerve should be explored to ensure that it has not displaced into the joint. Other nerves around the hip joint are rarely injured at dislocation. Treatment is generally expectant unless laceration or incarceration is suspected; if so, exploration is indicated.

Recurrent Dislocation

Recurrence after traumatic hip dislocation is rare but occurs most frequently after posterior dislocation in children under 8 years of age[7,38] or in children with known hyperlaxity (Down syndrome, Ehlers-Danlos disease). The incidence of recurrence is estimated to be less than 3%.[75] Recurrence can be quite disabling, and in the long-term may result in damage to the articular surfaces as a result of shear damage to the cartilaginous hip. Prolonged spica casting (at least 3 months) may be effective.[107] Surgical exploration with capsulorrhaphy can be performed if conservative treatment fails.[7,38,105] Prior to hip reconstruction, arthrography is recommended to identify a capsular defect or redundancy.[7] In older children, recurrent dislocation can occur as a result of a bony defect in the posterior rim of the acetabulum similar to that in adults and may require posterior acetabular reconstruction.

Vascular Injury

Impingement on the femoral neurovascular bundle has been described after anterior hip dislocation in children, and this may occur in 25% of patients.[91] The hip should be relocated as soon as possible to remove the offending pressure from the femoral vessels. If relocation of the hip fails to restore perfusion, immediate exploration of the femoral vessels is indicated.

CONCLUSION

The treatment for hip disorders is evolving. We now have new surgical and medical treatments options for hip disorders. Although most do not directly apply to the urgent reduction of hip dislocations, they are applicable to the sequelae that occur. The use of bisphosphonates and other medications that inhibit bone resorption is an active area of research and may have direct affects on limiting collapse of the femoral head if ON occurs.[1] This could soon change our paradigm for the evaluation of a hip after reduction of a dislocation, and early MRI or bone scans may be indicated.

A host of surgical methods are available to manage deformity as a result of necrosis or hip instability. Techniques to increase vascularity, such as vascularized bone grafting, remain a controversial method to improve the natural history. Hinged distraction across the hip is now more commonly performed and much easier technically, given the newer generation of external fixation devices designed just for this purpose. Hinged distraction may play a role as a primary treatment (i.e., for chondrolysis) or as an adjunct to other techniques.[101] Hip arthroscopy is much more commonly performed and allows for a much less invasive approach to removing loose bodies in the hip and assessing and treating soft tissue injuries.[15,54] Together, these new techniques offer future opportunities to decrease the severity of known complications and potentially improve functional outcomes. Time and follow-up will be required to determine if these methods improve the natural history of these post traumatic sequelae.

REFERENCES

1. Agarwala S, Jain D, Joshi VR, et al. Efficacy of alendronate, a bisphosphonate, in the treatment of AVN of the hip. A prospective open-label study. Rheumatology (Oxford) 2005;44(3):352–359.
2. Alho A. Concurrent ipsilateral fractures of the hip and femoral shaft. Acta Orthop Scand 1996;67:19–28.
3. De Yoe LE. A Suggested Improvement to the Allis' Method of Reduction of Posterior Dislocation of the Hip. Ann Surg 1940;112(1):127–9.
4. Ashwood N, Wojcik AS. Traumatic separation of the upper femoral epiphysis in a 15-month-old girl: an unusual mechanism of injury. Injury 1995;26:695–696.
5. Avadi K, Trigui M, Gdoura F, et al. Traumatic hip dislocations in children. Rev Chir Orthop Reparatrice Appar Mot 2008;94(1):19–25.
6. Bagatur AE, Zorer G. Complications associated with surgically treated hip fractures in children. J Pediatr Orthop B 2002;11:219–228.
7. Banskota AK, Spiegel DA, Shrestha S, et al. Open reduction for neglected traumatic hip dislocation in children and adolescents. J Pediatr Orthop 2007;27(2):187–191.
8. Barquet A. Natural history of avascular necrosis following traumatic hip dislocation in childhood: a review of 145 cases. Acta Orthop Scand 1982;53:815–820.
9. Barquet A. Recurrent traumatic dislocation of the hip in childhood. J Trauma 1980; 20(11):1003–1006.
10. Barquet A. Traumatic hip dislocation in childhood. A report of 26 cases and review of the literature. Acta Orthop Scand 1979;50:549–553.
11. Beaty JH. Fractures of the hip in children. Orthop Clin North Am 2006:223–232.
12. Bettin D, Pankalla T, Böhm H, et al. Hip pain related to femoral neck stress fracture in a 12-year-old boy performing intensive soccer playing activities—a case report. Int J Sports Med 2003;24:593–596.
13. Blair W, Hanson C. Traumatic closure of the triradiate cartilage. J Bone Joint Surg Am 1979;61:144–145.
14. Boardman MJ, Herman MJ, Buck B, et al. Hip fractures in children. J Am Acad Orthop Surg 2009;17(3):162–173.
15. Bray TJ. Femoral neck fracture fixation. Clinical decision making. Clin Orthop Relat Res 1997;339:20–31.
16. Byrd JW, Jones KS. Traumatic rupture of the ligamentum teres as a source of hip pain. Arthroscopy 2004;20(4):385–391.
17. Canale ST, Beaty JH. Pelvic and hip fractures. In: Rockwood CA Jr, Wilkins KE, Beaty JH, eds. Fractures in Children, 4th ed. Philadelphia: Lippincott-Raven; 1996: 1109–1193.
18. Canale ST, Bourland WL. Fracture of the neck and intertrochanteric region of the femur in children. J Bone Joint Surg Am 1977;59(4):431–443.
19. Canale ST, Casillas M, Banta JV. Displaced femoral neck fractures at the bone-screw interface after in situ fixation of slipped capital femoral epiphysis. J Pediatr Orthop 1997;17(2):212–215.
20. Canale ST, Manugian AH. Irreducible traumatic dislocations of the hip. J Bone Joint Surg Am 1979;61:7–14.
21. Cheng JC, Tang N. Decompression and stable internal fixation of femoral neck fractures in children can affect the outcome. J Pediatr Orthop 1999;19:338–343.
22. Chun KA, Morcuende J, El-Khoury GY. Entrapment of the acetabular labrum following reduction of traumatic hip dislocation in a child. Skeletal Radiol 2004;33(12):728–731.
23. Chung SM. The arterial supply of the developing proximal end of the human femur. J Bone Joint Surg Am 1976;58:961–970.
24. Colonna PC. Fracture of the neck of the femur in childhood: a report of six cases. Ann Surg 1928;88:902–907.
25. Cornawall R, Radomisli TE. Nerve injury in traumatic dislocation of the hip. Clin Orthop Relat Res 2000;377:84–91.
26. Currey JD, Butler G. The mechanical properties of bone tissue in children. J Bone Joint Surg Am 1975;57:810–814.
27. Davison BL, Weinstein SL. Hip fractures in children: a long-term follow-up study. J Pediatr Orthop 1992;12:355–358.
28. Devas MB. Stress fractures in children. J Bone Joint Surg Br 1963;45:528–541.
29. Devas MB. Stress fractures of the femoral neck. J Bone Joint Surg Br 1965;47:728–738.
30. Edgren W. Coxa plana. A clinical and radiological investigation with particular reference to the importance of the metaphyseal changes for the final shape of the proximal part of the femur. Acta Orthop Scand Suppl 1965;84:1–129.
31. Epstein HC. Traumatic dislocations of the hip. Clin Orthop Relat Res 1973;92: 116–142.
32. Fairbairn KJ, Mulligan ME, Murphey MD, et al. Gas bubbles in the hip joint on CT: an indication of recent dislocation. AJR Am J Roentgenol 1995;164(4):931–934. Comment in AJR Am J Roentgenol 1996;166:472–473.
33. Flynn JM, Wong KL, Yeh GL, et al. Displaced fractures of the hip in children. Management by early operation and immobilization in a hip spica cast. J Bone Joint Surg Br 2002;84:108–112.
34. Forlin E, Guille JT, Kumar SJ, et al. Transepiphyseal fractures of the neck of the femur in very young children. J Pediatr Orthop 1992;12:164–168.
35. Forster N, Ramseier LE, Exner GU. Undisplaced femoral neck fractures in children have a high risk of secondary displacement. J Pediatr Orthop B 2006;15(2):131–133.
36. Funk FJ. Traumatic dislocation of the hip in children. J Bone Joint Surg Am 1962;44: 1135–1145.
37. Ganz R, Parvizi J, Beck M, et al. Femoroacetabular impingement: a cause for early osteoarthritis of the hip. Clin Orthop Relat Res 2003;417:112–120.
38. Gaul RW. Recurrent traumatic dislocation of the hip in children. Clin Orthop Relat Res 1973;90:107–109.
39. Gennari JM, Merrot T, Bergoin V, et al. X-ray transparency interpositions after reduction of traumatic dislocations of the hip in children. Eur J Pediatr Surg 1996;6:288–293.
40. Glass A, Powell HDW. Traumatic dislocation of the hip in children. An analysis of 47 patients. J Bone Joint Surg Br 1961;43:29–37.
41. Godley DR, Williams RA. Traumatic dislocation of the hip in a child: usefulness of MRI. Orthopedics 1993;16:1145–1147.
42. Guevara CJ, Pietrobon R, Carothers JT, et al. Comprehensive morphologic evaluation of the hip in patients with symptomatic labral tear. Clin Orthop Relat Res 2006;453: 277–285.
43. Gupta RC, Shravat BP. Reduction of neglected traumatic dislocation of the hip by heavy traction. J Bone Joint Surg Am 1977;59:249–251.
44. Haddad FS, Bann S, Hill RA, et al. Displaced stress fracture of the femoral neck in an active amenorrhoeic adolescent. Br J Sports Med 1997;31:70–72.
45. Hamilton PR, Broughton NS. Traumatic hip dislocation in childhood. J Pediatr Orthop 1989;18:691–694.
46. Hansman CF. Appearance and fusion of ossification centers in the human skeleton. AJR Am J Roentgenol Radium Ther Nucl Med 1962;88:476–482.
47. Hernandez RJ, Poznanski AK. CT evaluation of pediatric hip disorders. Orthop Clin North Am 1985;16:513–541.
48. Herrera-Soto JA, Price CT, Reuss BL, et al. Proximal femoral epiphysiolysis during reduction of hip dislocation in adolescents. J Pediatr Orthop 2006;26(3):371–374.
49. Hougard K, Thomsen PB. Traumatic hip dislocation in children. Follow-up of 13 cases. Orthopedics 1989;12:375–378.
50. Hughes LO, Beaty JH. Current concepts review: fractures of the head and neck of the femur in children. J Bone Joint Surg Am 1994;76:283–292.
51. Ingari JV, Smith DK, Aufdemorte TB, et al. Anatomic significance of magnetic resonance imaging findings in hip fracture. Clin Orthop Relat Res 1996;332:209–214.
52. Jerre R, Karlsson J. Outcome after transphyseal hip fractures. Four children followed 34 to 48 years. Acta Orthop Scand 1997;68:235–238.
53. Joseph, B, Mulpuri K. Delayed separation of the capital femoral epiphysis after an ipsilateral transcervical fracture of the femoral neck. J Orthop Trauma 2000;14(6): 446–448.
54. Kashiwagi N, Suzuki S, Seto Y. Arthroscopic treatment for traumatic hip dislocation with avulsion fracture of the ligamentum teres. Arthroscopy 2001;17(1):67–69.
55. Kirkos JM, Papavasiliou KA, Kyrkos MJ, et al. Multidirectional habitual bilateral hip dislocation in a patient with Down syndrome. Clin Orthop Relat Res 2005;(435): 263–266.
56. Kumar S, Jain AK. Neglected traumatic hip dislocation in children. Clin Orthop Relat Res 2005;431:9–13.
57. Lam SF. Fractures of the neck of the femur in children. J Bone Joint Surg Am 1971; 53:1165–1179.
58. Langenskiöld A, Salenius P. Epiphyseodesis of the greater trochanter. Acta Orthop Scand 1967;38:199–219.
59. Ramachandran M, Ward K, Brown RR, Munns CF, Cowell CT, Little DG. Intravenous bisphosphonate therapy for traumatic osteonecrosis of the femoral head in adolescents. J Bone Joint Surg Am 2007;89(8):1727–34.
60. Macfarlane I, King D. Traumatic dislocation of the hip joint in children. Aust N Z J Surg 1976;46(3):227–231.
61. Maeda S, Kita A, Fujii G, et al. Avascular necrosis associated with fractures of the femoral neck in children: histological evaluation of core biopsies of the femoral head. Injury 2003;34:283–286.
62. Magu NK, Singh R, Sharma AK, et al. Modified Pauwels intertrochanteric osteotomy in neglected femoral neck fractures in children: a report of 10 cases followed for a minimum of 5 years. J Orthop Trauma 2007;21(4):237–243.
63. Magu NK, Singh R, Sharma A, et al. Treatment of pathologic femoral neck fractures with modified Pauwel osteotomy. Clin Orthop Relat Res 2005;437:229–235.
64. Maruenda JI, Barrios C, Gomar-Sancho F. Intracapsular hip pressure after femoral neck fracture. Clin Orthop Relat Res 1997;340:172–180.
65. Meaney JEM, Carty H. Femoral stress fractures in children. Skeletal Radiol 1992;21: 173–176.
66. Mehlman CT, Hubbard GW, Crawford AH, et al. Traumatic hip dislocation in children. Clin Orthop Relat Res 2000;376:68–79.
67. Mirdad T. Fractures of the neck of the femur in children: an experience at the Aseer Central Hospital, Abha, Saudi Arabia. Injury Int J Care Injured 2002;33:823–827.
68. Moon ES, Mehlman CT. Risk factors for avascular necrosis after femoral neck fractures in children: 25 Cincinnati cases and meta-analysis of 360 cases. J Orthop Trauma 2006;20(5):323–329.
69. Moorman CT 3rd, Warren RF, Hershman EB, et al. Traumatic posterior hip subluxation in American football. J Bone Joint Surg Am 2003;85:1190–1196.
70. Morsy HA. Complications of fracture of the neck of the femur in children. A long-term follow-up study. Injury 2001;32:45–51.
71. Ng GP, Cole WG. Effect of early hip decompression on the frequency of avascular necrosis in children with fractures of the neck of the femur. Injury 1996;27:419–421.
72. Nötzli HP, Siebenrock KA, Hempfing A, et al. Perfusion of the femoral head during

surgical dislocation of the hip. Monitoring by laser Doppler flowmetry. J Bone Joint Surg Br 2002;84:300–304.
73. Nötzli HP, Wyss TF, Stoecklin CH, et al. The contour of the femoral head-neck junction as a predictor for the risk of anterior impingement. J Bone Joint Surg Br 2002;84(4): 556–560
74. Odent T, Glorion C, Pannier S, et al. Traumatic dislocation of the hip with separation of the capital epiphysis: 5 adolescent patients with 3 to 9 years of follow-up. Acta Orthop Scand 2003;74(1):49–52
75. Offierski CM. Traumatic dislocation of the hip in children. J Bone Joint Surg Br 1981; 63:194–197.
76. Ogden JA. Changing patterns of proximal femoral vascularity. J Bone Joint Surg Am 1974;56:941–950.
77. Olsson O, Landin LA, Johansson A. Traumatic hip dislocation with spontaneous reduction and capsular interposition. Acta Orthop Scand 1994;65:476–479.
78. Pape H, Krettek C, Friedrich A, et al. Long-term outcome in children with fractures of the proximal femur after high-energy trauma. J Trauma 1999;46:58–64.
79. Pipkin G. Treatment of Grade IV Fracture-Dislocation of the Hip. A review. J Bone Joint Surg 1957;(39-A):1027–1042.
80. Poggi JJ, Callaghan JJ, Spritzer CE, et al. Changes on magnetic resonance images after traumatic hip dislocation. Clin Orthop Relat Res 1995;319:249–259.
81. Price CT, Pyevich MT, Knapp DR, et al. Traumatic hip dislocation with spontaneous incomplete reduction: a diagnostic trap. J Orthop Trauma 2002;16:730–735.
82. Ramachandran M, Ward K, Brown RR, et al. Intravenous biphosphonate therapy for traumatic osteonecrosis of the femoral head in adolescents. J Bone Joint Surg Am 2007; 89:1727–1734.
83. Ratliff AH. Complications after fractures of the femoral neck in children and their treatment. J Bone Joint Surg Br 1970;52:175.
84. Ratliff AH. Fractures of the neck of the femur in children. J Bone Joint Surg Br 1962; 44:528–542.
85. Rieger H, Pennig D, Klein W, et al. Traumatic dislocation of the hip in young children. Arch Orthop Trauma Surg 1991;110:114–117.
86. Rubel IF, Kloen P, Potter HG, et al. MRI assessment of the posterior acetabular wall fracture in traumatic dislocation of the hip in children. Pediatr Radiol 2002;32: 435–439.
87. Salisbury RD, Eastwood DM. Traumatic dislocation of the hip in children. Clin Orthop Rel Res 2000;377:106–111.
88. Schlonsky J, Miller PR. Traumatic hip dislocations in children. J Bone Joint Surg Am 1973;55:1057–1063.
89. Schmidt GL, Sciulli R, Altman GT. Knee injury inpatients experiencing a high-energy traumatic ipsilateral hip dislocation. J Bone Joint Surg Am 2005:87:1200–1204.
90. Schrader MW, Jacofsky DJ, Stans AA, et al. Femoral neck fractures in pediatric patients. Clin Orthop Relat Res 2006;454:169–173.
91. Scientific Research Committee of the Pennsylvania Orthopaedic Society. Traumatic dislocation of the hip in children. Final report. J Bone Joint Surg Am 1968;50:79–88.
92. Scully SP, Aaron RK, Urbaniak JR. Survival analysis of hips treated with core decompression or vascularized fibular grafting because of avascular necrosis. J Bone Joint Surg Am 1998;80(9):1270–1275.
93. Sener M, Karapinar H, Kazimoglu C, et al. Fracture dislocation of sacroiliac joint associated with triradiate cartilage injury in a child: a case report. J Pediatr Orthop Br 2008; 17(2):65–68.
94. Shea KP, Kalamachi A, Thompson GH. Acetabular epiphysis–labrum entrapment following traumatic anterior dislocation of the hip in children. J Pediatr Orthop 1986;6: 215–219.
95. Song KS, Choi IH, Sohn YJ, et al. Habitual dislocation of the hip in children: a report of eight additional cases and literature review. J Pediatr Orthop 2003;23:178–183.
96. Song KS, Kim YS, Sohn SW, et al. Arthrotomy and open reduction of the displaced fracture of the femoral neck in children. J Ped Orthop Br 2001;10:205–210.
97. Soto-Hall R, Johnson LH, Johnson RA. Variations in the intra-articular pressure of the hip joint in injury and disease. J Bone Joint Surg Am 1964;46:509–516.
98. St. Pierre P, Staheli LT, Smith JB, et al. Femoral neck stress fractures in children and adolescents. J Pediatr Orthop 1995;15:470–473.
99. Stimson LA. An easy method of reduction dislocation of the shoulder and hip. Med Record 1900;57:356.
100. Swischuk LE. Irritable infant and left lower extremity pain. Pediatr Emerg Care 1997; 13:147–148.
101. Thacker MM, Feldman DS, Madan SS, et al. Hinged distraction of the adolescent arthritic hip. J Pediatr Orthop 2005;25(2):178–182.
102. Togrul E, Bayram H, Gulsen M, et al. Fractures of the femoral neck in children: long-term follow-up in 62 hip fractures. Injury 2005;36:123–130.
103. Trueta J. The normal vascular anatomy of the human femoral head during growth. J Bone Joint Surg Br 1957;39:358–393.
104. Trueta J, Morgan JD. The vascular contribution to osteogenesis. J Bone Joint Surg Br 1960;42:97–109.
105. Vialle R, Odent T, Pannier S, et al. Traumatic Hip dislocation in childhood. J Pediatric Orthop 2005;25(2):140–141.
106. Vialle R, Pannier S, Odent T, et al. Imaging of traumatic dislocation of the hip in childhood. Pediatr Radiol 2004;34(12):970–979.
107. Wilchinsky ME, Pappas AM. Unusual complications in traumatic dislocation of the hip in children. J Pediatr Orthop 1985;5:534–539.
108. Egol KA, Koval KJ, Kummer F, Frankel VH. Stress fractures of the femoral neck. Clin Orthop Relat Res 1998;348:72–8.

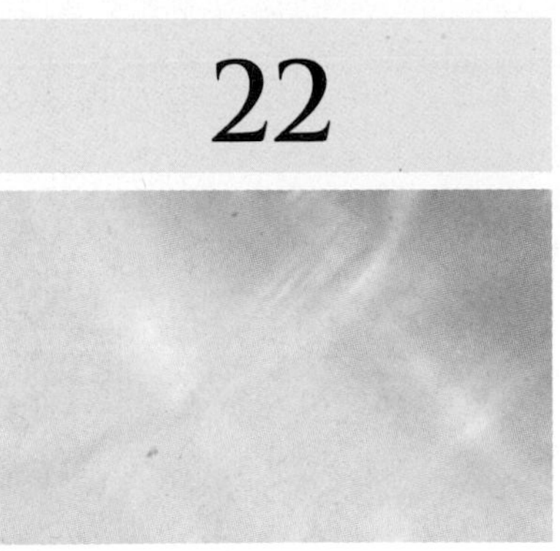

22

FEMORAL SHAFT FRACTURES

John M. Flynn and David L. Skaggs

INTRODUCTION 797

ANATOMY 798

MECHANISM OF INJURY 798

DIAGNOSIS 798

X-RAY FINDINGS 799

CLASSIFICATION 799

TREATMENT 800
Treatment Variation with Age 800
Treatment Options 803
Spica Cast Application: Technique 805
Traction Pin Insertion: Technique 807
Postoperative Care 808
Results of Traction and Casting 808
Complications of Spica Casting 809
Flexible Intramedullary Nail Fixation 809
Fixation with Flexible Intramedullary Nails: Technique 811
External Fixation 815
Fixator Design 816
Frame Application: Technique 817
Complications of External Fixation 818
Rigid Intramedullary Rod Fixation 818
Antegrade Transtrochanteric Intramedullary Nailing: Technique 819
Plate Fixation 823
Standard Compression Plating: Technique 824
Submuscular Bridge Plating 824
Submuscular Bridge Plating: Technique 824
Complications of Plate Fixation 827

COMPLICATIONS OF FEMORAL SHAFT FRACTURES 827
Leg-Length Discrepancy 827
Angular Deformity 829
Rotational Deformity 830
Delayed Union 830
Nonunion 830
Muscle Weakness 831
Infection 831
Neurovascular Injury 832
Compartment Syndrome 832

SPECIAL FRACTURES OF THE FEMORAL SHAFT 832
Subtrochanteric Fractures 832
Supracondylar Fractures 832
Open Femoral Fractures 834
Femoral Fractures in Patients with Metabolic or Neuromuscular Disorders 835
Floating Knee Injuries 838
Fractures in the Multiple-System Trauma Patient 838

INTRODUCTION

A femoral shaft fracture is the most common major pediatric orthopaedic injury that most orthopaedists will treat routinely and is the most common pediatric orthopaedic injury requiring hospitalization.[64,125] When subtrochanteric and supracondylar fractures are included, the femoral shaft represents about 1.6% of all bony injuries in children. Fractures are more common in boys (2.6:1), and occur in an interesting bimodal distribution with a peak during the toddler years (usually from simple falls) and then again in early adolescence (usually from higher-energy injury).[66,84,92,117]

Although pediatric femoral shaft fractures create substantial short-term disability, these injuries can generally be treated successfully with few long-term sequelae. For generations, traction and casting were standard treatment for all femoral shaft fractures in children, and femoral fractures ranked high in duration of hospitalization for a single diagnosis.[87] Over the past 20 years, however, there has been a dramatic and sustained trend towards the operative stabilization of femoral shaft fractures in school-aged children using flexible intramedullary nails, external fixation, locked intramedullary nails, and more recently, submuscular plates. These advances have decreased the substantial early disability for the children, as well as the family's burden of care during the recovery period.

ANATOMY

Through remodeling during childhood, a child's bone changes from primarily weak woven bone to stronger lamellar bone.[179] Strength also is increased by a change in geometry (Fig. 22-1). The increasing diameter and area of bone result in a markedly increased area moment of inertia, leading to an increase in strength. This progressive increase in bone strength helps explain the bimodal distribution of femoral fractures. In early childhood, the femur is relatively weak and breaks under load conditions reached in normal play. In adolescence, high-velocity trauma is required to reach the stresses necessary for fracture.

MECHANISM OF INJURY

The etiology of femoral fractures in children varies with the age of the child. Before walking age, up to 80% of femoral fractures may be caused by abuse.[10,18,74,183] In a study of over 5000 children at a trauma center, Coffey et al.[39] found that abuse was the cause of only 1% of lower extremity fractures in children older than 18 months, but 67% of lower extremity fractures in children younger than 18 months.

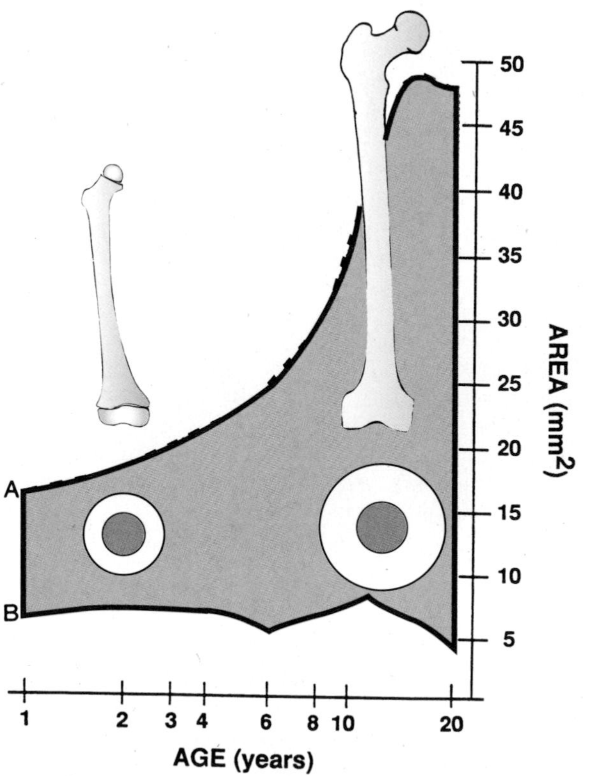

FIGURE 22-1 The shaded area represents cortical thickness by age group. This rapid increase in cortical thickness may contribute to the diminishing incidence of femoral fractures during late childhood. (From Netter FH. The Ciba collection of medical illustrations. Vol. 8. Musculoskeletal System. I. Anatomy, Physiology, and Metabolic Disorders. Summit, NJ: Ciba-Geigy, 1987, with permission.)

An unusual femoral fracture reported in infants is a greenstick fracture of the medial distal femoral metaphysis that occurs when the parent falls on a child who is straddling the parent's hip. It is important to recognize this fracture because it occurs in infants at an age when abuse is the leading cause of femoral fracture. The fracture is caused by bending of the femur, which produces a compression injury to the medial cortex. This injury is not consistent with abuse and may confirm a parent's description of a fall as the cause.

Older children are unlikely to have a femoral shaft fracture caused by abuse because their bone is sufficiently strong to tolerate forceful blows and is able to resist torque without fracture. In older children, femoral fractures are most likely to be caused by high-energy injuries; motor vehicle accidents account for over 90% of femoral fractures in this age-group.[44,84,124] Pathologic femoral fractures are relatively rare in children, but may occur because of generalized osteopenia in infants or young children with osteogenesis imperfecta. Osteogenesis imperfecta should be considered when a young child, with no history suggestive of abuse or significant trauma, presents with a femoral shaft fracture.[116] X-ray evaluation is often insufficient to diagnose osteogenesis imperfecta; skin biopsy, collagen analysis, and bone biopsy may be required to make a definitive diagnosis. Generalized osteopenia also may accompany neurologic diseases, such as cerebral palsy or myelomeningocele, leading to fracture with minor trauma in osteopenic bone.[66,111,116] Pathologic fractures may occur in patients with neoplasms, most often benign lesions such as nonossifying fibroma, aneurysmal bone cyst, unicameral cyst, or eosinophilic granuloma. Although pathologic femoral fractures are rare in children, it is essential that the orthopaedist and radiologist study the initial injury films closely for the subtle signs of primary lesions predisposing to fracture, particularly in cases of low-energy injury from running or tripping. X-ray signs of a pathologic fracture may include mixed lytic-blastic areas disrupting trabecular architecture, a break in the cortex and periosteal reaction in malignant lesions such as osteosarcoma, or better-defined sclerotic borders with an intact cortex seen in benign lesions such as nonossifying fibroma (Fig. 22-2).

Stress fractures can occur in any location in the femoral shaft.[29,106,139] In this era of high intensity, year-round youth sports, orthopaedists are encountering more adolescents with femoral stress fractures from running, soccer, and basketball.[24] Although uncommon (4% of all stress fractures in children), femoral shaft or femoral neck stress fractures should be considered in a child with thigh pain because an unrecognized stress fracture may progress to a displaced femoral fracture. A high index of suspicion is important, because even nontraditional sports can lead to stress fractures with extreme overuse; bilateral femoral stress fractures were reported in a rollerblade enthusiast.[199]

DIAGNOSIS

The diagnosis of pediatric femoral shaft fractures is usually not subtle: there is a clear mechanism of injury, a deformity and

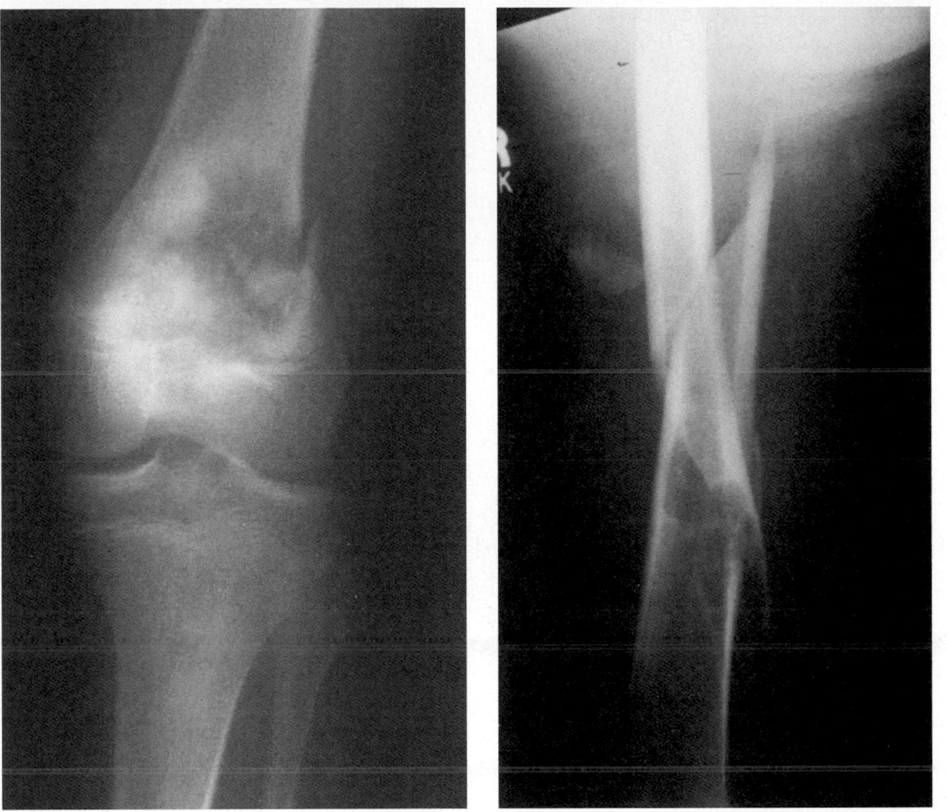

FIGURE 22-2 A. Femoral fracture through a poorly demarcated mixed, osteoblastic, osteolytic lesion—an osteosarcoma. **B.** Sclerotic borders of this lesion in the distal femur are typical of a pathologic fracture through a nonossifying fibroma.

swelling of the thigh, and obvious localized pain. The diagnosis is more difficult in patients with multiple trauma or head injury and in nonambulatory, severely disabled children. A physical examination usually is sufficient to document the presence of a femoral fracture. In patients lacking sensation (myelomeningocele), swelling and redness may simulate infection.

The entire child must be carefully examined. Hypotension rarely results from an isolated femoral fracture. The Waddell triad of femoral fracture, intra-abdominal or intrathoracic injury, and head injury are associated with high-velocity automobile injuries. Multiple trauma may necessitate rapid stabilization of femoral shaft fractures[124,165] to facilitate overall care. This is particularly true with head injury and vascular disruption.

The hemodynamic significance of femoral fracture has been studied by two groups.[37,127] Hematocrit levels below 30% rarely occur without multisystem injury. A declining hematocrit should not be attributed to closed femoral fracture until other sources of blood loss have been eliminated.[37,127]

X-RAY FINDINGS

X-ray evaluation should include the entire femur, including the hip and knee, because injury of the adjacent joints is common. An anteroposterior (AP) pelvic x-ray is a valuable supplement to standard femoral shaft views, because there may be an associated intertrochanteric fracture of the hip, fracture of the femoral neck, or physeal injuries of the proximal femur.[13,31] Distal femoral fractures may be associated with physeal injury about the knee, knee ligament injury, meniscal tears,[202] and tibial fractures.[121]

Plain radiographs generally are sufficient for making the diagnosis. In rare circumstances, bone scanning and magnetic resonance imaging (MRI) may be helpful in the diagnosis of small buckle fractures in limping children or stress fractures in athletes. The orthopaedist should carefully evaluate x-rays for comminution or nondisplaced "butterfly" fragments, second fractures, joint dislocations, and pathologic fractures, as these findings can substantially alter the treatment plan.

CLASSIFICATION

Femoral fractures are classified as transverse, spiral, or short oblique; comminuted or noncomminuted; and open or closed. Open fractures are classified according to Gustilo's system.[87] The presence or absence of vascular and neurologic injury is documented and is part of the description of the fracture. The most common femoral fracture in children (over 50%) is a simple transverse, closed, noncomminuted injury.

The level of the fracture (Fig. 22-3) leads to characteristic displacement of the fragments based on the attached muscles. With subtrochanteric fractures, the proximal fragment lies in abduction, flexion, and external rotation. The pull of the gastrocnemius on the distal fragment in a supracondylar fracture produces an extension deformity (posterior angulation of the femoral shaft), which may make the femur difficult to align.

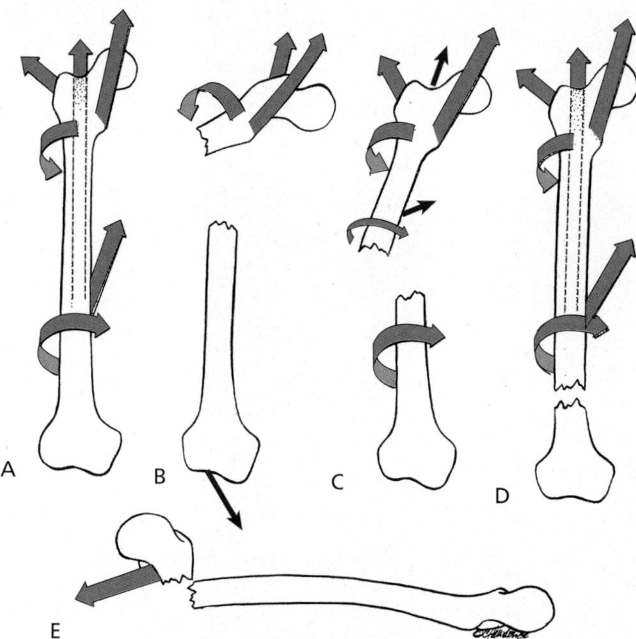

FIGURE 22-3 The relationship of fracture level and position of the proximal fragment. **A.** In the resting unfractured state, the position of the femur is relatively neutral because of balanced muscle pull. **B.** In proximal shaft fractures, the proximal fragment assumes a position of flexion (iliopsoas), abduction (abductor muscle group), and lateral rotation (short external rotators). **C.** In midshaft fractures, the effect is less extreme because there is compensation by the adductors and extensor attachments on the proximal fragment. **D.** Distal shaft fractures produce little alteration in the proximal fragment position because most muscles are attached to the same fragment, providing balance. **E.** Supracondylar fractures often assume a position of hyperextension of the distal fragment due to the pull of the gastrocnemius.

TABLE 22-1 Treatment Options for Isolated Femoral Shaft Fractures in Children and Adolescents

Age	Treatment
Birth to 24 mo	Pavlik harness (newborn to 6 mo) Early spica cast Traction → spica cast (very rare)
24 mo to 5 yr	Early spica cast Traction → spica cast External fixation (rare) Flexible intramedullary nails (rare)
6–11 yr	Flexible intramedullary nails Traction → spica cast Submuscular plate External fixation
12 yr to maturity	Trochanteric-entry intramedullary rod Flexible intramedullary nails Submuscular plate External fixation (rare)

Treatment choices are influenced by fracture pattern, the child's weight, the presence of other injuries (head, chest, abdominal, etc.), and associated soft tissue trauma.

TREATMENT

Treatment of femoral shaft fractures in children is age dependent, with considerable overlap between age groups (Table 22-1). In addition to age, the orthopaedic surgeon should consider the child's weight, associated injuries, fracture pattern, and mechanism of injury. Economic concerns, the family's ability to care for a child in a spica cast or external fixator, and the advantages and disadvantages of any operative procedure also are important factors.

The comparative economics of nonoperative and operative treatment of femoral shaft fractures have been evaluated by several researchers, but no clear consensus has been reached, as charge data are not always an accurate reflection of true costs to the patient, the family unit, and the healthcare system. In a prospective comparative study of 83 consecutive children and adolescents treated with either traction and casting or titanium elastic nailing, Flynn et al.[63] showed no significant difference in charges between the two methods. Newton and Mubarak[154] analyzed the financial aspects of femoral shaft fracture treatment in 58 children and adolescents and determined that total charges were lowest for those treated with early spica casting and highest for those treated with skeletal traction or intramedullary nailing. Similarly, Coyte et al.[42] found the cost of surgical treatment (external fixation) to exceed that of early spica casting in all cases. Stans and Morrissy,[193] in evaluating the cost of treating femoral fractures in children 6 to 16 years of age, found that all surgical treatments cost approximately the same. Nork and Hoffinger[157] showed that hospital profit was highest in the traction group, despite charges being equivalent to the surgical group, because the actual hospital resources required were significantly less. Wright,[211] in an extensive review of the literature and meta-analysis, concluded that immediate spica casting had a lower cost and lower malunion rate than traction. Hedin et al.,[82] in a cost analysis comparing three methods of treating femoral shaft fracture, found that the major determinant of cost was length of hospital stay. Certainly, cost is a factor, but it should not be the overriding consideration in discussions of treatment options with the family. In addition to monetary cost to the medical system, the treatment's social cost to the family can vary significantly. This social cost includes disruption of schedules, lost work, and time out of school.

Treatment Variation with Age

Infants

Because their periosteum is thick, infants usually sustain stable femoral fractures. In fractures occurring in infancy, management should include evaluation for underlying metabolic bone abnormality or abuse. Once these have been ruled out, most infants with a proximal or midshaft femoral fracture are comfortably and successfully treated with simple splinting, with or without a Pavlik harness. For the rare unstable fracture, the Pavlik harness may not offer sufficient stabilization. Morris et al.[150] reported a group of 8 birth-related femoral fractures in 55,296 live births. Twin pregnancies, breech presentation, and prematurity were associated with birth-related femoral fractures. The typical fracture is a spiral fracture of the proximal femur with flexion of the proximal fragment. With thick periosteum and remarkable remodeling potential, newborns rarely need a formal reduction of their fracture or rigid external immobilization. For femoral fractures with excessive shortening (>1 to 2 cm) or angulation (>30 degrees), spica casting can be used. Traction rarely is necessary in this age group.

Preschool Children

In children 6 months to 5 years of age, early spica casting (Fig. 22-4) is the treatment of choice for isolated femoral fractures with less than 2 cm of initial shortening (Fig. 22-5). In low-energy fractures, a "walking spica" is ideal (Fig. 22-6). Femoral fractures with more than 2 cm of initial shortening or marked instability and fractures that cannot be reduced with early spica casting require 3 to 10 days of skin or skeletal traction. In this age group, skeletal stabilization by external fixation generally is reserved for children with open fractures or multiple trauma. Intramedullary fixation is used in children with metabolic bone disease that predisposes to fracture or after multiple fractures, such as in osteogenesis imperfecta, or following multitrauma. Flexible nailing can be used in the normal-sized preschool child[21] but is rarely necessary. Larger children (in whom reduction cannot be maintained with a spica cast) occasionally may

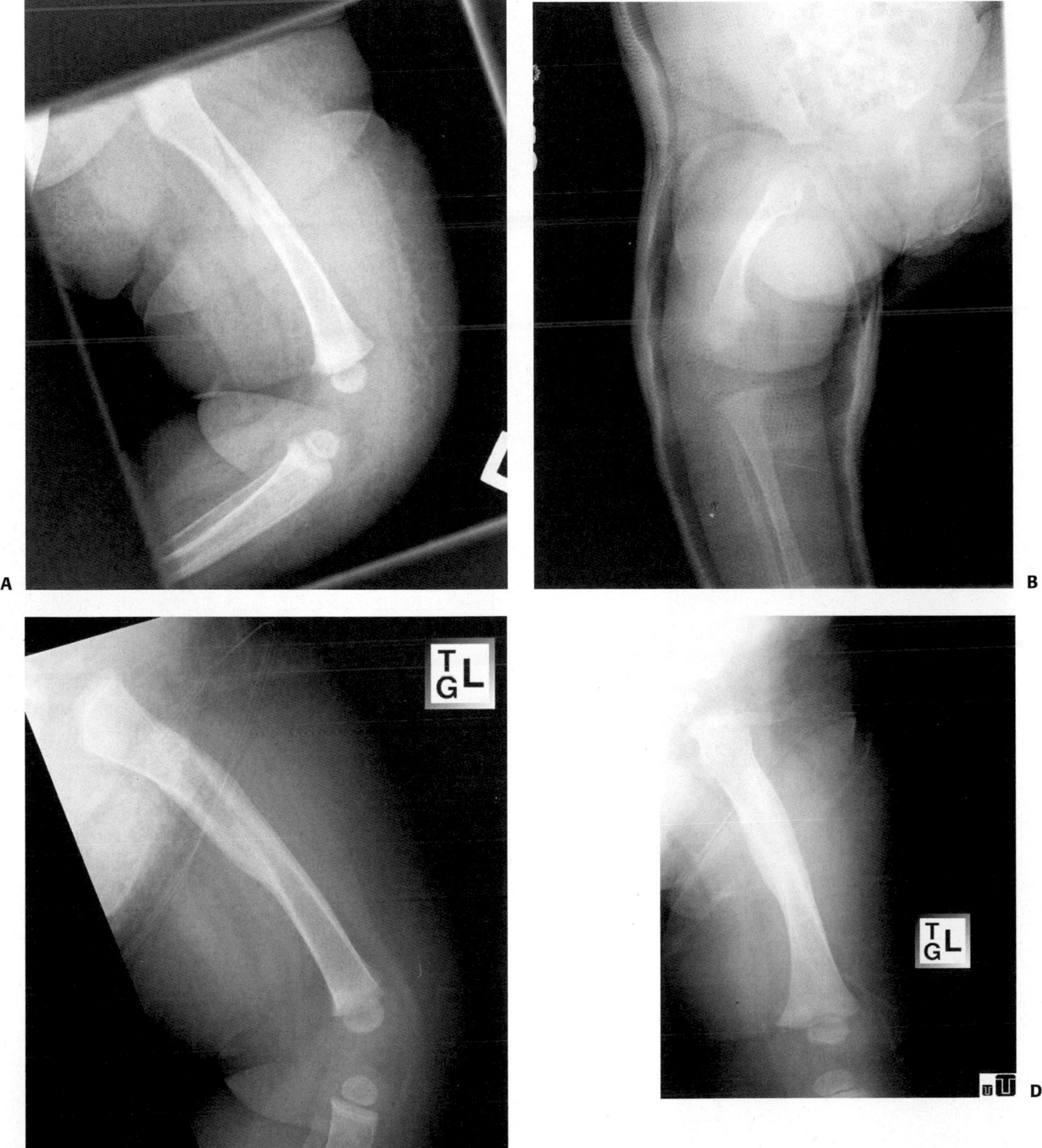

FIGURE 22-4 A. This 7-month-old sustained a low-energy spiral femoral shaft fracture. **B.** Treatment was in a spica cast. **C,D.** Excellent healing with abundant callus at only 4 weeks after injury.

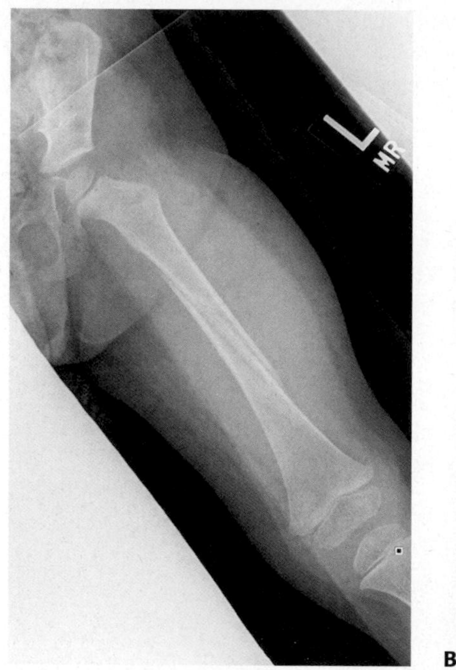

A

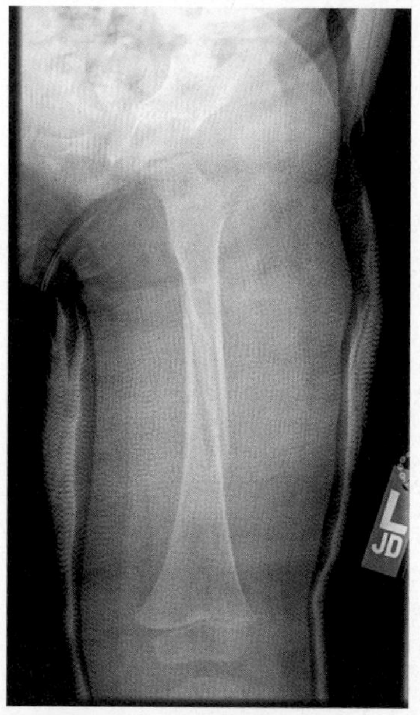

B

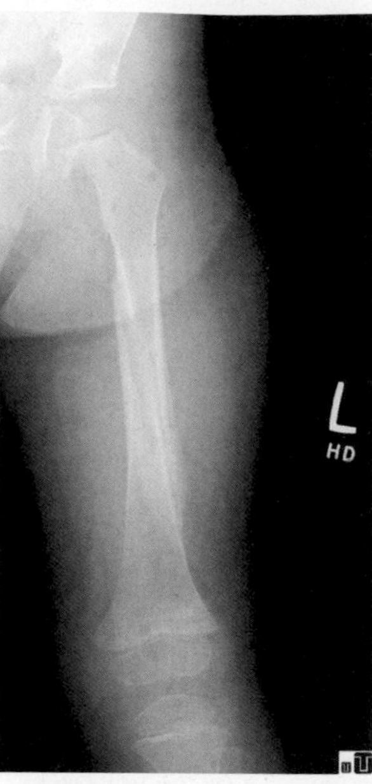

C

FIGURE 22-5 A. This 2-year-old sustained a low-energy spiral femoral shaft fracture, ideal for walking spica treatment. **B.** Immediately after reduction; note the lateral mold at the fracture site. **C.** Six weeks after injury, there is anatomic alignment, minimal shortening, and good callus formation.

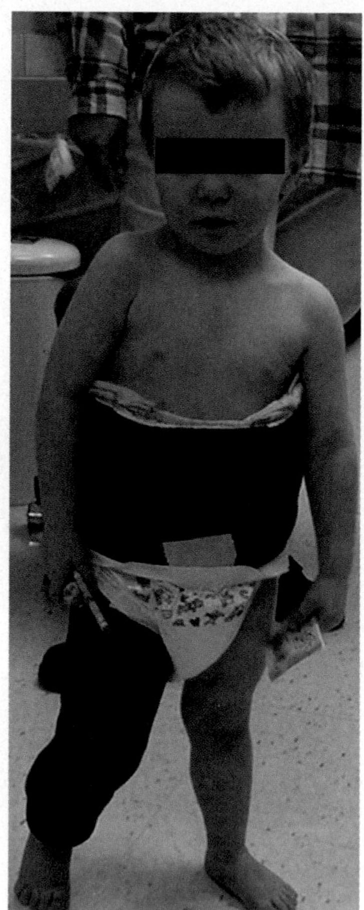

FIGURE 22-6 A 3-year-old standing in his walking spica cast (Courtesy of Howard Epps, MD.)

benefit from flexible intramedullary nailing, traction, or in rare cases, submuscular plating.

Children 5 to 11 Years of Age

In children 5 to 11 years of age, many different methods can be used successfully, depending on the fracture type, patient characteristics, and surgeon skill and experience.[64] For the rare, minimally displaced fracture, early spica casting usually produces satisfactory results, although cast wedging or a cast change may be necessary to avoid excessive shortening and angulation. In children with unstable, comminuted fractures, traction may be necessary before cast application. Although traction and casting is still a very acceptable and successful method of managing femoral fractures in young school-age children, the cost and the social problems related to school-age children in casts has resulted in a strong trend towards fracture fixation. Spica cast management is generally not used for children with multiple trauma, head injury, vascular compromise, floating knee injuries, significant skin problems, or multiple fractures. Flexible intramedullary nails are the predominant treatment for femoral fractures in 5 to 11 year olds, although submuscular plating and external fixation have their place, especially in length-unstable fractures or fractures in the proximal and distal third of the femoral shaft.

Children Age 12 to Skeletal Maturity

Refined indications and technological advances have led to the increasing use of trochanteric entry, locked intramedullary nailing for femoral fractures in the preadolescent and adolescent age groups. Several studies designed to refine the indications for flexible intramedullary nailing have concluded that although most results are excellent or satisfactory in children older than 11, complications rise significantly when this popular technique is used for bigger and older children. In an international multi-

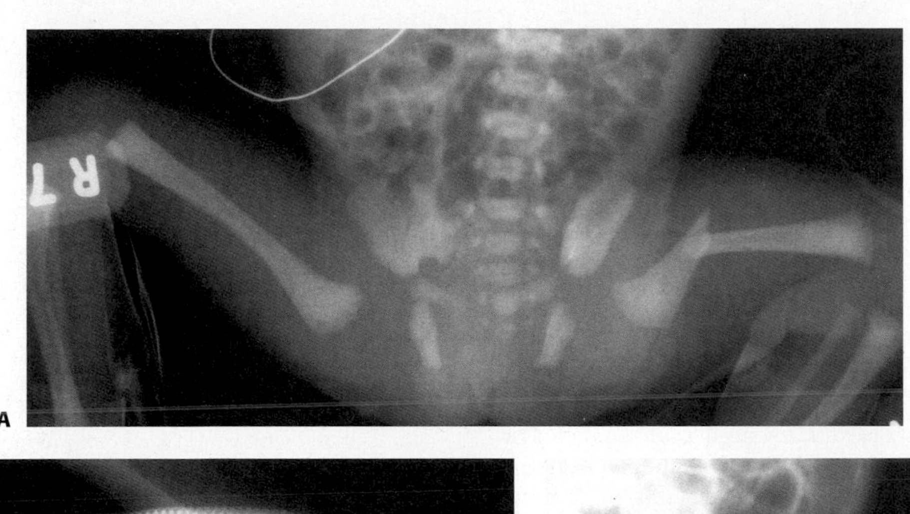

A

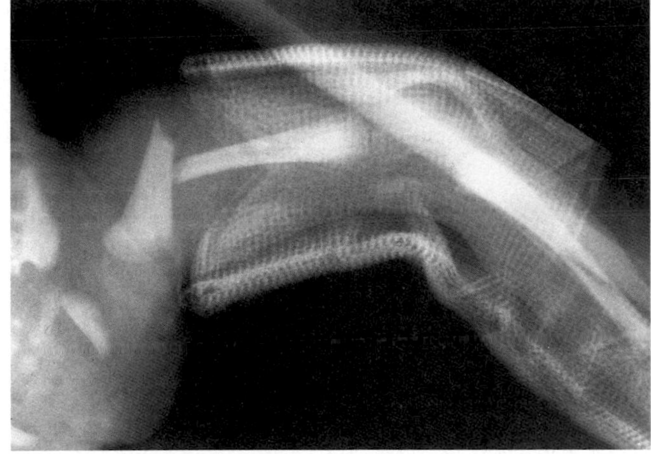

B

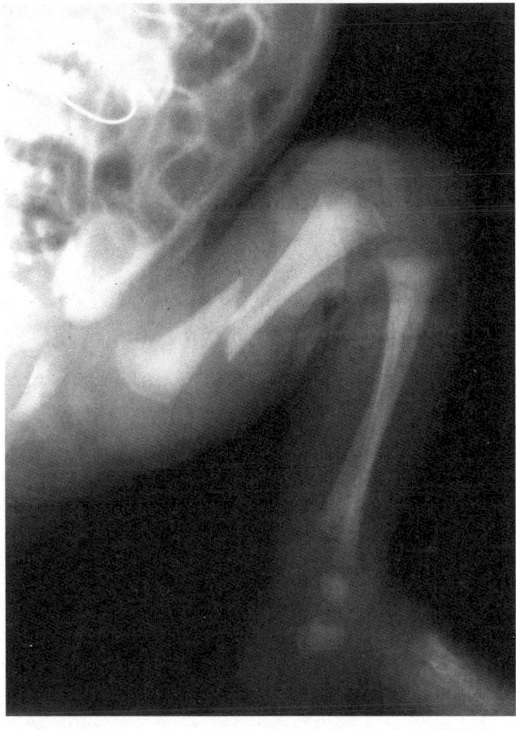

C

FIGURE 22-7 A. This infant had a birth-related left femoral fracture. **B.** An AP splint was used but ended at the fracture site, only increasing the angulation. **C.** A Pavlik harness reduced the fracture by flexing the distal fragment.

center, retrospective study, Moroz et al.[149] found a statistically significant relationship between age and outcome, with children older than 11 years or heavier than 49 kg faring worse. Sink et al.[185] found a much higher rate of complications in length-unstable fractures. Fortunately, surgeons can now select from several different trochanteric-entry nails that allow a relatively safe, lateral entry point, with the stability of proximal and distal locking. With this new information and technology, locked intramedullary nailing is used commonly for obese children ages 10 to 12 and most femoral shaft fractures in children aged 13 to skeletal maturity.

Treatment Options for Femoral Shaft Fractures

Pavlik Harness

Stannard et al.[192] popularized the use of the Pavlik harness for femoral fractures in infants. This treatment is ideal for a proximal or midshaft femoral fracture that occurs as a birth-related injury. Reduction can be aided by a wrap around the thigh if greater stability is needed. In a newborn infant in whom a femoral fracture is noted in the intensive care unit or nursery, the femur is immobilized with simple padding or a soft splint. For a stable fracture, this approach may be sufficient and will allow intravenous access to the feet if needed. The Pavlik harness can be applied with the hip in moderate flexion and abduction. This often helps align the distal fragment with the proximal fragment (Fig. 22-7). Evaluation of angulation in the coronal plane (varus-valgus) is difficult because of hyperflexion. Stannard et al.[192] reported acceptable alignment in all patients with less than 1 cm of shortening. Morris et al.[150] showed that all treatments, including traction, spica cast, and Pavlik harness, are effective and resulted in satisfactory outcome in all patients regardless of treatment.

Even unstable fractures can be managed using a Pavlik harness and a small wrap around the thigh; immediate spica or traction is reserved for the rare fracture that cannot be managed with simpler means because of failure to align the fracture or excessive shortening of more than 2 cm. Podeszwa et al.[163] reported that infants treated with a Pavlik harness had higher pain scores when compared to those treated with immediate spica casting; however, none of the Pavlik patients had skin problems but one third of the spica patients did. For this reason, some pediatric orthopaedists prefer a single-leg Gore-tex (Gore,

Newark, DE) spica cast, which protects the fracture site better than a Pavlik harness and allows reasonably easy bathing and infant care.

Early Spica Casting

Early spica casting, popularized by Irani et al.[102] and Staheli et al.,[190] is usually the best treatment option for isolated femoral shaft fractures in children under 6 years of age, unless there is shortening of more than 2 cm, massive swelling of the thigh, or an associated injury that precludes cast treatment. The word "early" is used to imply that the cast is placed in the first few days after injury, as opposed to the word "immediate," which implies that the cast is placed within minutes of the patient's presentation to the orthopaedist. Cassinelli et al.[35] reported on true "immediate" spica cast application, with the cast being applied upon arrival in the emergency department. Over an 8-year period, their group treated 145 femoral fractures, all in children younger than 7 years of age, with immediate spica cast application in the emergency department; 33% of the children were discharged from the emergency department (no hospital admission). All children younger than 2 years of age and 86.5% of children aged 2 to 5 years met acceptable alignment parameters on final x-rays. Rereduction in the operating room was needed in 11 patients. The investigators concluded that initial shortening was the only independent risk factor associated with lost reduction. They concluded that if there was no associated factor requiring admission, spica casting in the emergency department followed by immediate discharge is safe, with a low complication rate in children younger than 6 years of age, nearly eliminating the need for general anesthesia.

The advantages of a spica cast include low cost, excellent safety profile, and a very high rate of good results, with acceptable leg length equality, healing time, and motion.[59,101] Hughes et al.[95] evaluated 23 children ranging in age from 2 through 10 years who had femoral fractures treated with early spica casting to determine the impact of treatment on the patients and their families. The greatest problems encountered by the family in caring for a child in a spica cast were transportation, cast intolerance by the child, and hygiene. Although most children did not attend school while in the cast, no child was required to repeat a grade and no permanent psychologic effects were reported by the parents. The researchers found that overall treatment in a spica cast was much easier for families of preschool children than for those with school-age children. In a similar study, Kocher[114] used a validated questionnaire for assessing the impact of medical conditions on families demonstrated that for the family having a child in a spica cast is similar to having a child on renal dialysis. They found that the impact was greatest for children older than 5 years and when both parents are working. Such data should inform the decisions of orthopaedic surgeons and families who are trying to choose among the many options for young school-age children.

Illgen et al.,[100] in a series of 114 isolated femoral fractures in children under 6 years of age, found that 90/90 spica casting was successful in 86% without cast change or wedging, based on tolerance of shortening less than 1.5 cm and angulation less than 10 degrees. Of the 20 patients requiring a cast change, only 2 healed with unacceptable position (>2 cm of leg length discrepancy). One of these overgrew by 1.5 cm, and the other was lost to follow-up. Illgen et al.[100] used an immediate spica regardless of initial shortening and placed the child in traction only if unacceptable shortening occurred. Shortening requiring spica cast change was associated with a knee flexion angle of less than 50 degrees. Similar excellent results have been reported by Czertak and Hennrikus[43] using the 90/90 spica cast. Ferguson and Nicol[59] conducted a prospective study of early spica casting in children less than 10 years of age including 101 fractures in a 30-month period. Only four spica casts had to be removed for unacceptable position. Age greater than 7 years was a variable predictive of a higher risk of failure of this technique to achieve satisfactory alignment.

Thompson et al.[195] described the telescope test in which patients were examined with fluoroscopy at the time of reduction and casting. If more than 3 cm of shortening could be demonstrated with gentle axial compression, traction was used rather than immediate spica casting. By using the telescope test, these researchers decreased unacceptable results (>2.5 cm of shortening) from 18% to 5%. Martinez et al.[131] reported excessive shortening and angular deformity in 26 of 51 patients after immediate spica casting, especially in comminuted fractures. Although shortening and angulation can occur in a spica cast, excessive deformity can be detected with weekly radiograph and clinical evaluations during the first 2 to 3 weeks after injury. Shortening is acceptable, but should not exceed 2 cm. This is best measured on a lateral radiograph taken through the cast. If follow-up radiographs reveal significant varus (>10 degrees) or anterior angulation (>30 degrees), the cast may be wedged. However, Weiss et al.[209] noted that wedging of 90/90 spica casts can cause peroneal nerve palsy, especially during correction of valgus angulation (a problem that rarely occurs). For unacceptable position, the fracture can be manipulated and a new cast applied, or the cast can be removed and the patient placed in traction to regain or maintain length. Angular deformity of up to 15 degrees in the coronal plane and up to 30 degrees in the sagittal plane may be acceptable, depending on the patient's age (Table 22-2). Finally, if shortening exceeds 2 cm, traction or an external fixator can be used (Fig. 22-8).

Shortening and angulation occur most often in fractures associated with polytrauma and those with loss of the periosteal sleeve.[44,66] Fry et al.[66] found that 50% (12 of 23) of closed femoral shaft fractures caused by high-energy trauma in children under 10 years of age required repeat reduction or other treatment to correct excessive shortening or angulation that occurred after initial reduction; only 8% (2 of 24) of low-energy fractures required repeat closed reduction. Wright[211] showed that limb-length discrepancy and angular deformity were lower with spica treatment than with traction treatment. The lower

TABLE 22-2 Acceptable Angulation

Age	Varus/ Valgus (degrees)	Anterior/ Posterior (degrees)	Shortening (mm)
Birth to 2 yr	30	30	15
2–5 yr	15	20	20
6–10 yr	10	15	15
11 yr to maturity	5	10	10

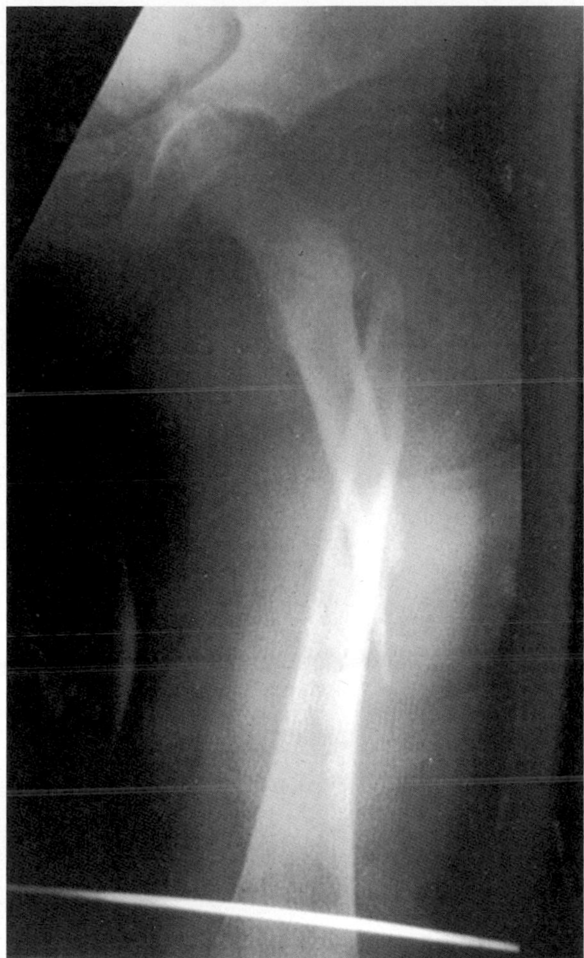

A

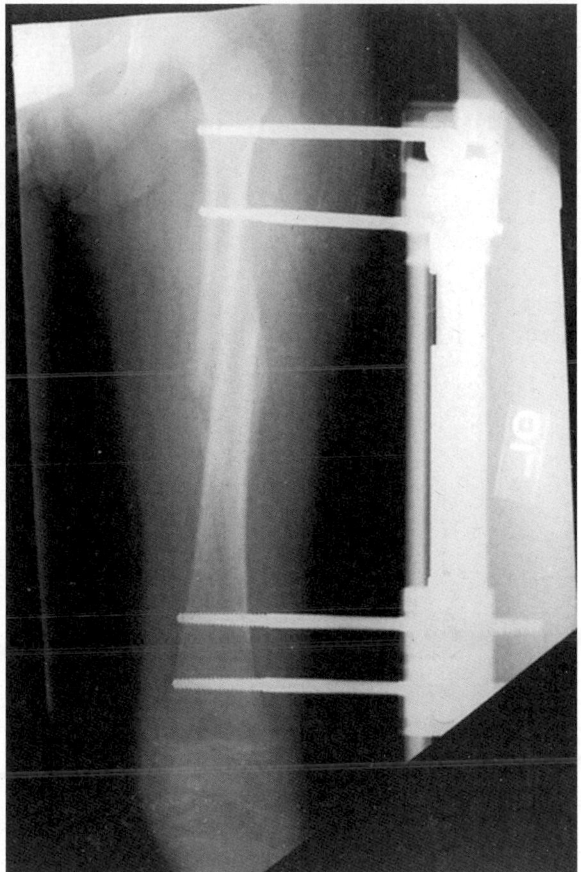

B

FIGURE 22-8 A. A proximal spiral femur fracture, which failed treatment with pins and plaster. **B.** Salvaged with an external fixator.

cost of spica management is an added reason to pursue this method of management.

The position of the hips and knees in the spica cast is controversial. Some centers prefer a spica cast with the hip and knee extended and the bottom of the foot cut out to prevent excessive shortening.[136] Varying the amounts of hip and knee flexion in the spica cast based on the position of the fracture also has been recommended: the more proximal the fracture, the more flexed the hip should be.[190]

Many orthopaedic surgeons trained over the last two decades were taught to place children in the sitting position, with the hips and knees set in about 90 degrees of flexion. Studies have shown that the results from the sitting spica cast are good.[135,145] The child is placed in a sitting position with the legs abducted about 30 degrees on either side. The synthetic material used for the cast gives it sufficient strength so that no bar is required between the legs. This not only allows the child to be carried on the parent's hip but also aids in toiletry needs, making bedpans unnecessary. Also, a child who can sit upright during the day can attend school in a wheelchair.

Recently, there has been a resurgence of interest in the "walking spica cast" (see Fig. 22-6). Epps et al.[55] reported immediate single leg spica cast for pediatric femoral diaphyseal fractures. In a series of 45 children, 90% pulled to stand and 62% walked independently by the end of treatment; 50% of patients were able to return to school or daycare while in the cast. Only two children had unacceptable shortening, and two required repeat reduction. Five children broke the cast at the hip joint. There was one rotational malunion. The authors found that the single-leg technique effectively treated the fracture and addressed some of the social concerns of spica casting. Practitioners of the single-leg or walking spica have learned to use the technique primarily on toddlers with very stable, low-energy fractures. The cast must be extensively reinforced at the hip. With the hip and knee much more extended, the single leg spica not only improves function and ease of care, but also avoids a technique that has been associated with compartment syndrome in several children (see below).[118,152]

Spica Cast Application: Technique

In most centers, the cast is applied in the operating room or sedation unit. For the sitting spica cast technique, a long leg cast is placed with the knee and ankle flexed at 90 degrees (Fig. 22-9A). Knee flexion of more than 60 degrees improved maintenance of length and reduction.[100] However, if one applies excessive traction to maintain length (Fig. 22-10), the risk of compartment syndrome is unacceptably high. Less traction, less knee flexion, and accepting slightly more shortening is a reasonable compromise. Extra padding, or a felt pad, is placed in the area of the popliteal fossa. The knee should not be flexed after padding because this may create vascular obstruction by producing a lump of material in the popliteal fossa (Fig. 22-9B). Because most diaphyseal fractures tend to fall into varus angula-

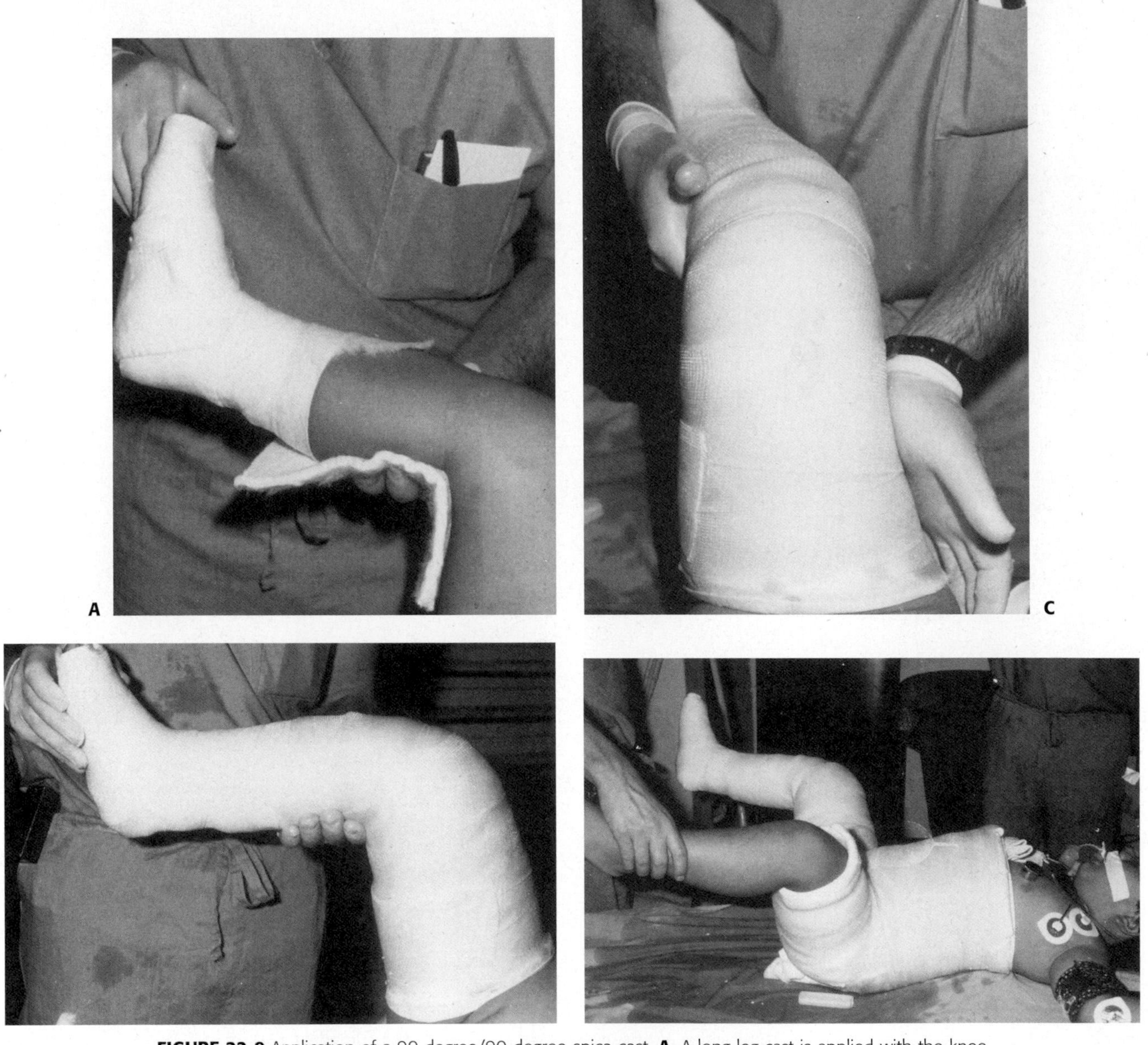

FIGURE 22-9 Application of a 90 degree/90 degree spica cast. **A.** A long leg cast is applied with the knee flexed 90 degrees. **B.** Generous padding is applied over the foot, and a pad is placed on the popliteal fossa to prevent injury to the peroneal nerve and popliteal vessels. **C.** A mold is placed over the apex of the fracture, generally correcting a varus deformity into slight valgus. **D.** Using a standard spica table, a one and a half leg spica cast is applied with the hip flexed 90 degrees and abducted 30 degrees.

tion while in a spica cast, a valgus mold is necessary (Fig. 22-9C). The patient is then placed on a spica table, supporting the weight of the legs with manual traction, and the remainder of the cast is applied with the hips in 90 degrees of flexion and 30 degrees of abduction, holding the fracture out to length (Fig. 22-9D). It is mandatory to avoid excessive traction because compartment syndromes and skin sloughs have been reported. The leg should be placed in 15 degrees of external rotation to align the distal fragment with the external rotation of the proximal fragment. After the spica cast is in place, AP and lateral radiographs are obtained to ensure that length and angular and rotational alignment are maintained. We observe all patients for 24 hours after spica application to be sure that the child is not at risk for neurovascular compromise or compartment syndrome. Gore-tex liners can be used to decrease the skin problems of diaper rash and superficial infection. Several centers have found that this has been beneficial, justifying the cost of a Gore-tex liner.

For the single-leg spica or walking spica technique, the long-leg cast is applied with approximately 50 degrees of knee flexion, and when the remainder the cast is placed, the hip is flexed 45 degrees and externally rotated 15 degrees. The hip should be reinforced anteriorly with multiple layers of extra fiberglass. The pelvic band should be fairly wide so that the hip is controlled as well as possible. A substantial valgus mold is important to prevent varus malangulation. Increasingly, we have been leaving the foot out, stopping the distal end of the cast in the supramalleolar area, which is protected with plenty of extra

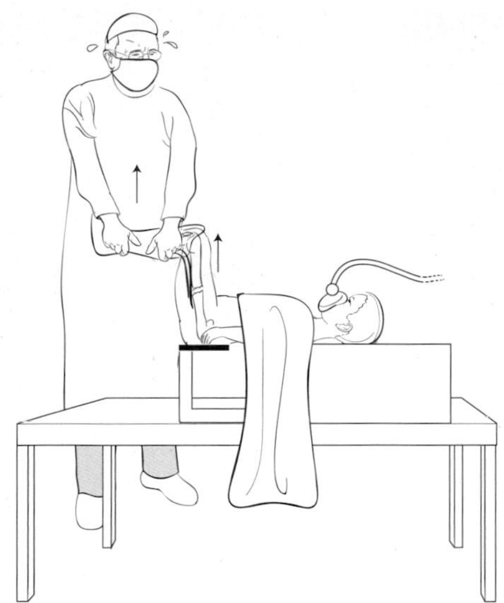

FIGURE 22-10 The dangers of pulling upward on the calf when applying a popliteal: this upward pull, which is used to reduce the fracture, can be dangerous, because it puts pressure on the gastrocnemius muscle and the other posterior leg structures, such as the popliteal artery and vein. (From Skaggs D, Flynn J.Trauma about the pelvis/hip/femur. Staying Out of Trouble in Pediatric Orthopaedics. Philadelphia: Lippincott Williams & Wilkins, 2006:105.)

padding. Seven to 10 days after injury is the perfect window of time to wedge the cast and correct small amounts of shortening and varus angulation which commonly occur. Most toddlers pull to a stand and begin walking in their walking cast about 2 to 3 weeks after injury.

If excessive angulation occurs, the cast should be changed with manipulation in the operating room. Casts can be wedged for less than 15 degrees of angulation. If shortening of more than 2 cm is documented, the child should be treated with cast change, traction, or conversion to external fixation, using lengthening techniques if the shortening is not detected until the fracture callus has developed. When conversion to external fixation is required, we recommend osteoclasis (either closed or open if needed) at the time of the application of the external fixator, with slow lengthening over a period of several weeks (1 mm per day) to re-establish acceptable length (see Fig. 22-8).

Generally, the spica cast is worn for 4 to 8 weeks, depending on the age of the child and the severity of the soft tissue damage accompanying the fracture. Typically, an infant's femoral shaft fracture will heal in 3 to 4 weeks; and a toddler's fracture will heal in 6 weeks. After the cast hass been removed, parents are encouraged allow their child to stand and walk whenever the child is comfortable; most children will need to be carried or pushed in a stroller for a few days until hip and knee stiffness gradually results. Most joint stiffness resolves spontaneously in children after a few weeks. It is unusual to need formal physical therapy. In fact, aggressive joint range-of-motion exercises with the therapist immediately after cast removal makes children anxious and may prolong rather then hasten recovery. A few follow-up visits are recommended in the first year after femoral fracture, analyzing gait, joint range of motion, and leg lengths.

Traction and Casting

Since as early as the eighteenth century, traction has been used for management of femoral fractures. Vertical overhead traction with the hip flexed 90 degrees and the knee straight was introduced by Bryant in 1873,[26,41] but this often resulted in vascular insufficiency[155] and is now rarely used for treatment of femoral fractures. Modified Bryant's traction, in which the knee is flexed 45 degrees, increases the safety of overhead skin traction.[60]

Traction before spica casting is indicated when the fracture is length unstable and the family and surgeon agree that nonoperative measures are preferred. Rapid shortening in an early spica cast can be salvaged with cast removal and subsequent traction. The limit of skin traction is the interface between skin and tape or skin and foam traction boot. Skin complications, such as slough and blistering, usually occur when more than 5 pounds of traction is applied. When more than 5 pounds of traction is required, or simply for ease in patient management, skeletal traction can be used to maintain alignment.[5] Casas et al.[34] studied a group of 41 patients between the ages of 4 and 10 years treated with skin traction followed by spica casting. Spica casts were applied at an average of 20.7 days. No leg-length difference or deformity resulted. In this situation, hospital length of stay was not thought to be a reason to reject this conservative yet clearly effective method of management. Abandonment of traction and casting in children younger than 10 years in many centers is in reaction to costs and burden on the family, not because of poor outcomes.

Skeletal traction also can be used in adolescents with comminuted proximal femoral shaft and intertrochanteric fractures where secure fixation cannot be obtained without risk of vascular compromise to the proximal femur. In general, however, skeletal traction then spica casting is not recommended for children 12 years of age or older because of significant incidences of shortening and angular malunion.

The distal femur is the location of choice for a traction pin.[5,51,178] Although proximal tibial traction pins have been recommended by some clinicians,[97] growth arrest in the proximal tibial physis and subsequent recurvatum deformity have been associated with their use (Fig. 22-11). Also, knee ligament and meniscal injuries that sometimes accompany femoral fractures may be aggravated by the chronic pull of traction across the knee. The rare indication for a tibial traction pin is a child in whom fracture configuration or skin problems prevent placement of a femoral traction wire and in whom no knee injury is present.

Traction Pin Insertion: Technique

After preparation of the thigh circumferentially from the knee to the midthigh, the limb is draped in a sterile manner. The knee is held in the position in which it will remain during traction; that is, if 90/90 traction is being used, the traction pin should be inserted with the knee bent 90 degrees. The patient should be sedated and the wound treated with a local anesthetic, or general anesthesia should be given before the traction pin is inserted. The location of pin insertion is one finger breadth above the patella with the knee extended or just above the flare of the distal femur. A small puncture wound is made over the medial side of the femur. A medial-to-lateral approach is used so that the traction pin does not migrate into the area of the femoral artery that runs through Hunter's canal on the medial side of the femur. A traction pin between 3/32 inch and 3/16 inch is chosen depending on the size of the child. The pin is placed parallel to the joint surface[5] to help maintain alignment

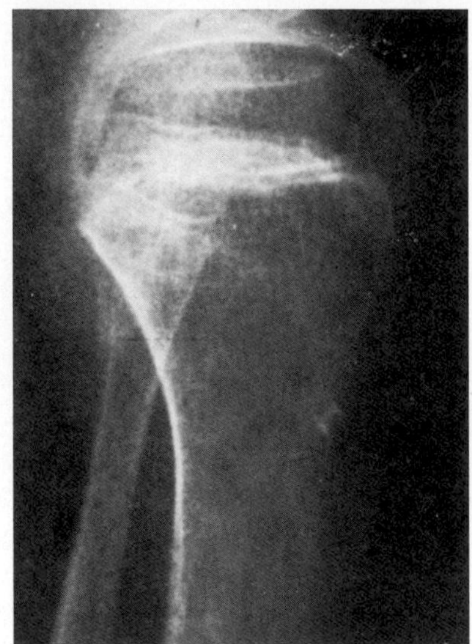
A

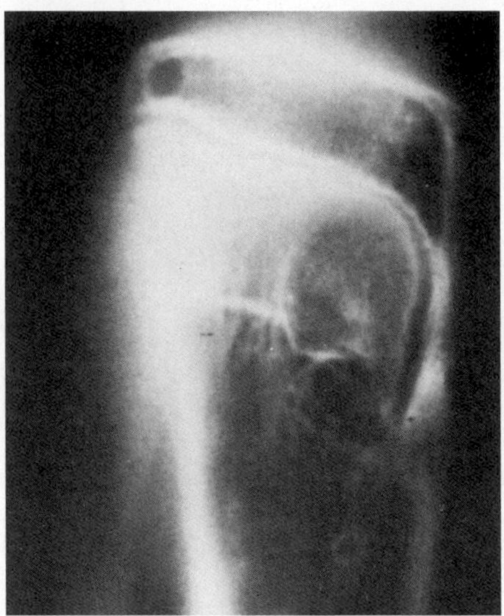
B

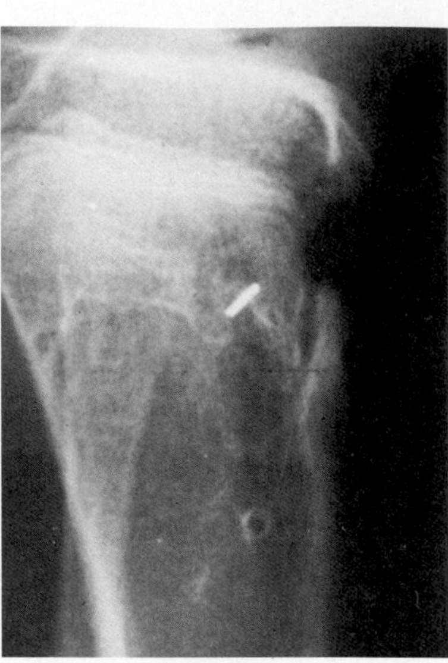
C

FIGURE 22-11 Tibial epiphyseal injury in association with tibial pin traction treatment for a femoral fracture. A 14-year-old boy sustained a femoral fracture that was treated by tibial skeletal traction. Two years later, the fracture was well healed but 2.5 cm short. A recurvatum deformity of the same side was apparent. **A**. An apparent fusion of the tibial tubercle. **B**. The bridge was confirmed by tomography. **C**. Bridge resection was performed with free fat interposition. A marker was placed to facilitate subsequent evaluation of growth. A tibial pin, if used, should be inserted posterior to the anterior aspect of the tibial tubercle.

while in traction. After the pin protrudes through the lateral cortex of the femur, a small incision is made over the tip of the pin. The pin is then driven far enough through the skin to allow fixation with a traction bow. If 90/90 traction is used, a short leg cast is placed with a ring through its midportion to support the leg. Alternatively, a sling to support the calf can be used. If a sling is used, heel cord stretching should be done while the patient is in traction.

After the skeletal traction pin has been placed in the distal femur, traction is applied in a 90/90 position (the hip and knee flexed 90 degrees) (Fig. 22-12) or in an oblique position (the hip flexed 20 to 60 degrees). If the oblique position is chosen, a Thomas splint or sling is necessary to support the leg. The fracture may be allowed to begin healing in traction, and radiographs should be obtained once or twice a week to monitor

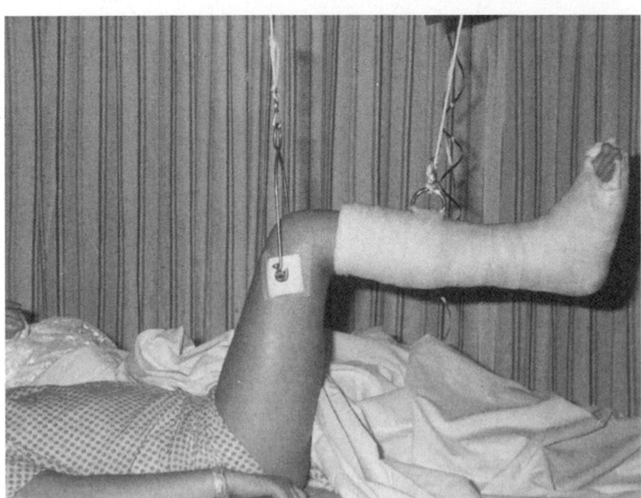

FIGURE 22-12 In 90/90 traction, a femoral pin is used and the lower leg and foot are supported with a short leg cast or a sling.

alignment and length. In preschool-age children, traction will be necessary for 2 to 3 weeks; in school-age children, a full 3 weeks of traction usually are necessary before the fracture is stable enough to permit casting. In a child under 10 years of age, the ideal fracture position in traction should be less than 1 cm of shortening and slight valgus alignment to counteract the tendency to angulate into varus in the cast and the eventual overgrowth that may occur (average 0.9 cm). If this method is used for adolescents (11 years or older), normal length should be maintained.

Technique Tips

Threaded traction pins, although more difficult to remove, are preferable to smooth pins because of their secure fixation within the bone without side-to-side movement; however, they have a slightly higher incidence of skin interface complications.

Aronson et al.[5] found that obliquely placed femoral traction pins were associated with an increased incidence of varus or valgus angulation. Pins for skeletal traction should be placed parallel to the axis of the knee joint or the articular surface, and in children over 11 years of age the fracture should be reduced without shortening.

Postoperative Care

Traction of 3 weeks or more followed by immobilization in a spica cast is well tolerated by young children. In older children, maintaining the knee in 90 degrees of flexion for a prolonged period may lead to knee stiffness and a difficult period of rehabilitation.[97]

Results of Traction and Casting

In a study by Gross et al.,[73] 72 children with femoral fractures were treated with early cast brace/traction management. In this technique, a traction pin is placed in the distal femur and then incorporated in a cast brace. The traction pin is left long enough to be used for maintaining traction while the patient is in the cast brace or traction is applied directly to the cast. The patient is allowed to ambulate in the cast brace starting 3 days after application. Radiographs are taken of the fracture in the cast brace to document that excessive shortening is not occurring. The patient is then returned to traction in the cast brace until satisfactory callus is present to prevent shortening or angular deformity with weight bearing. The technique was not effective in older adolescents with midshaft fractures but achieved excellent results in children 5 to 12 years of age. The average hospital stay was 17 days.

Complications of Spica Casting

Comparative studies and retrospective reviews have demonstrated unsatisfactory results in a small, yet significant, percentage of patients treated with skeletal traction.[90,97,113,170] Recently, increased attention has been focused on the risk of compartment syndrome in children treated in 90/90 spica cast.[152] Mubarak et al.[152] presented a multicenter series of 9 children with an average age of 3.5 years who developed compartment syndrome of the leg after treatment of a low-energy femoral fracture in a 90/90 spica cast. These children had extensive muscle damage and the skin loss around the ankle (Fig 22-13). The authors emphasized the risk in placing an initial below-knee cast, then using that cast to apply traction while immobilizing the child in the 90/90 position. The authors recommended avoiding traction on a short leg cast, leaving the foot out, and using less hip and knee flexion (Fig 22-14).

Flexible Intramedullary Nail Fixation

Flexible intramedullary nailing of pediatric femoral fractures, a dominant technique in Europe since the 1970s, has been rapidly adopted throughout North America as the most popular method of fixation for midshaft femoral fractures in children between the ages of 5 and 11 years. The flexible intramedullary nailing technique can be done with either stainless steel nails[169] or titanium elastic nails.

The popularity of flexible intramedullary nailing is a result of safety and efficacy. Safety and complications were a concern with two methods of rigid fixation: solid antegrade nailing (osteonecrosis) and external fixation (pin site infection, refracture after external fixator removal). The flexible nailing technique offered satisfactory fixation, enough stress at the fracture site to allow abundant callus formation, and relatively easy insertion and removal. The implants are inexpensive and the technique has a short learning curve. The primary limitation of flexible nailing is the lack of rigid fixation. Length-unstable fractures can shorten and angulate, especially in older and heavier children. Compared to children with rigid fixation, children who have their femoral fracture treated with flexible nailing clearly have more pain and muscle spasm in the early postoperative period. The surgeon should take this into consideration in planning the early rehabilitation.

As the flexible nailing technique has become more popular, there have been many studies to refine the technique and indications and to elucidate the inherent limitations of fixation with flexible implants. Mechanical testing of femoral fracture fixation systems showed that the greatest rigidity is provided by an external fixation device and the least by flexible intramedullary rodding.[120] Stainless steel rods are stiffer than titanium in bending tests. A study comparing steel to titanium flexible nails found a higher complication rate in the titanium group.[206] They reported that a typical 3.5-mm stainless steel nail has the same strength as a 4.0-mm titanium nail. Lee et al.[120] analyzed a group of synthetic fractured femurs instrumented with Enders rods and determined that there was sufficient axial and torsional stiffness to allow "touch down weight-bearing" despite fracture type. Gwyn et al.[76] similarly showed that 4-mm titanium rods imparted satisfactory torsional stability regardless of fracture pattern. Recognizing this flexibility, the French pioneers[119,123] of elastic nailing stressed the critical importance of proper implant technique, including prebending the nails so that the apex of the bend was at the fracture site, and so that the two implants balance one another to prevent bending and control rotation. Frick et al.[65] found greater stiffness and resistance to torsional deformation when retrograde nails were contoured into a double C pattern than with the antegrade C and S configuration.

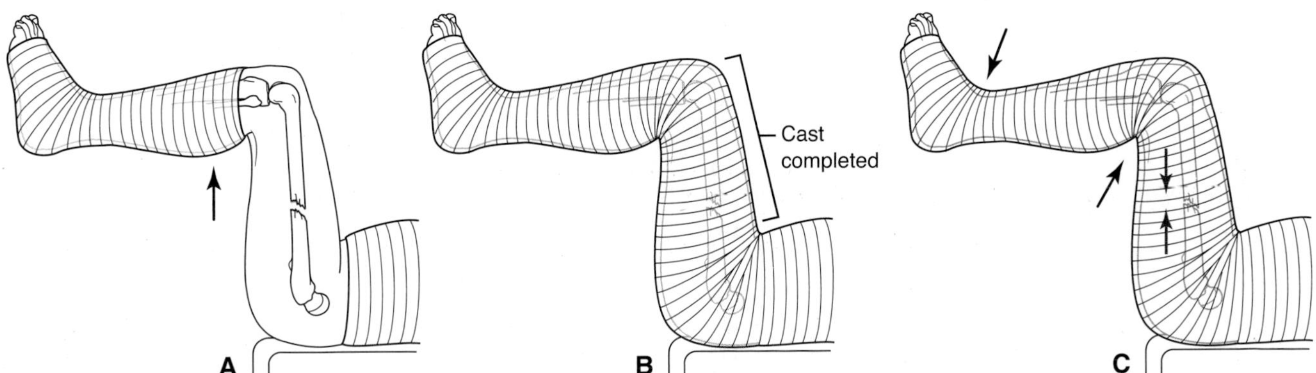

FIGURE 22-13 Application of the 90/90 spica and pathogenesis of the resulting problem. **A.** Below-knee cast is applied with the patient is on the spica frame. **B.** Next, traction is applied to the below-knee cast to produce distraction at the fracture site. The remainder of the cast is applied, fixing the relative distance between the leg and the torso. **C.** After the child awakens from general anesthesia, there is a shortening of the femur from muscular contraction which causes the thigh and leg to slip somewhat back into the spica. This causes pressure to occur at the corners of cast (*arrows*, proximal posterior calf and anterior ankle). (From Mubarak SJ, Frick S, Rathjen K, et al. Volkmann contracture and compartment syndromes after femur fractures in children treated with 90/90 spica casts. J Pediatr Orthop 2006;26(5):570.)

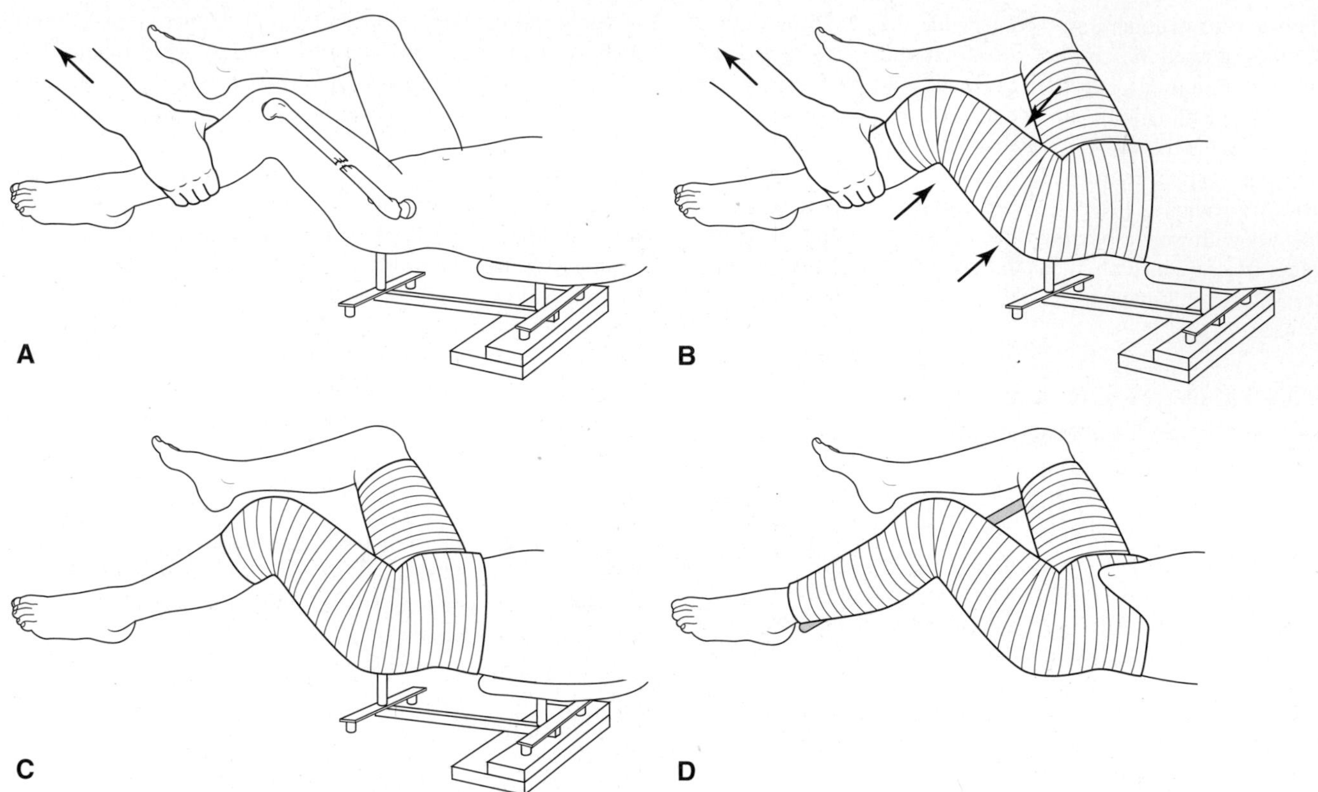

FIGURE 22-14 Authors' recommended technique of spica cast application. **A.** The patient is placed on a child's fracture table. The leg is held in about 45-degree angle of flexion at the hip and knee with traction applied to the proximal calf. **B.** The one and a half leg spica cast is then applied down to the proximal calf. Molding of the thigh is accomplished during this phase. **C.** The x-rays of the femur are obtained and any wedging of the cast that is necessary can be done at this time. **D.** The leg portion of the cast and the cross bar are applied. The belly portion of the spica is trimmed to the umbilicus. (From Mubarak SJ, Frick S, Rathjen K, et al. Volkmann contracture and compartment syndromes after femur fractures in children treated with 90/90 spica casts. J Pediatr Orthop 2006;26(5):571.)

The prevailing technique for flexible nail insertion at most centers throughout the world has been retrograde, with small medial and lateral incisions just above the distal femoral physis; however, some prefer an antegrade technique, with entry in the subtrochanteric area. The primary advantages of a proximal insertion site are a fewer knee symptoms postoperatively. Bourdela[22] compared retrograde and antegrade (ascending and descending) flexible intramedullary rodding in a group of 73 femoral fractures. Sixty-one fractures were treated with antegrade nails and 12 with retrograde nails. All children with antegrade nailing had good clinical and x-ray results; all 12 children with retrograde nails had knee pain that impaired knee motion until the nails were removed. An antegrade transtrochanteric approach was recommended by Carey and Galpin,[32] who reported excellent results in 25 patients without growth arrest of the upper femur and no osteonecrosis. Satisfactory alignment and fracture healing were obtained in all patients.

Retrograde intramedullary nailing with Ender nails or titanium nails has been reported by Ligier et al.,[123] Mann et al.,[130] Heinrich et al.,[86] Herscovici et al.,[91] and others.[32,110,137] Heinrich et al.[86] recommended a 3.5-mm Ender nail in children 6 to 10 years of age and a 4.0-mm nail in children over 10 years of age. Ligier et al.[123] used titanium nails ranging from 3 to 4 mm inserted primarily in a retrograde fashion. Heinrich et al.[91] recommended flexible intramedullary nails for fixation of diaphyseal femoral fractures in children with multiple system injury, head injury, spasticity, or multiple long bone fractures. Flynn et al.[62] published the first North American experience with titanium elastic nails in 2001. In this multicenter study, 57 of 58 patients had an excellent or satisfactory result and there was no loss of rotational alignment, but 4 patients healed with an angular malunion of more than 10 degrees. Narayanan et al.[153] looked at one center's learning curve with titanium elastic nails, studying the complications of 79 patients over a 5-year period. Nails that were bent excessively away from the bone led to irritation at the insertion site in 41. The center also had eight malunions and two refractures. They noted that complications could be diminished by using rods with similar diameter and contour and by avoiding bending the distal end of the nail way from the bone. Luhmann et al.[126] reported 21 complications in 43 patients with titanium elastic nails. Most of the problems were minor, but a hypertrophic nonunion and a septic joint occurred in their cohort. They suggested that problems could be minimized by using the largest nail possible and leaving only 2.5 cm out of the femoral cortex.

Flexible nails are removed after fracture union at most centers; however, some surgeons choose to leave the implants permanently. There is a theoretical concern that if flexible nails are left in young children, they will come to lie in the distal diaphysis as the child grows older. This may create a stress riser in the distal diaphysis, leading to a theoretical risk of fracture (Fig. 22-15). Morshed et al.[151] performed a retrospective analysis of

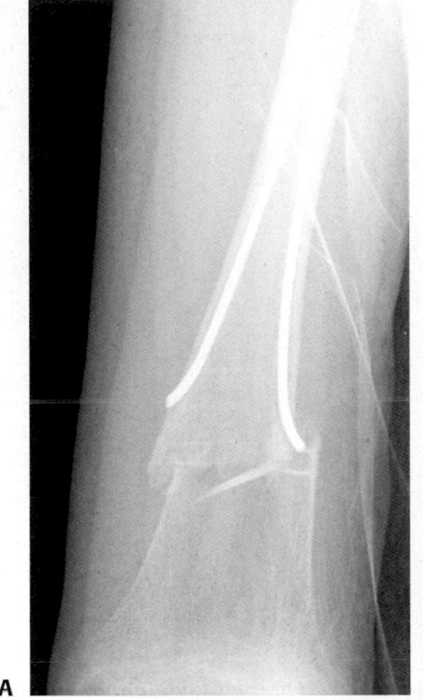

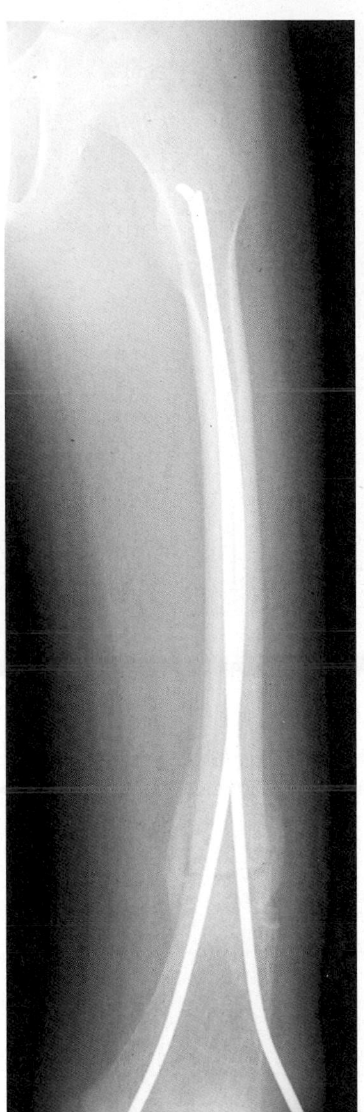

FIGURE 22-15 A. A few years after titanium elastic nailing, the nails have migrated proximally with growth, creating a stress riser and the subsequent insufficiency fracture. **B.** The refracture was treated with removal of the old nails and replacement with longer implants.

24 children treated with titanium elastic nails and followed for an average of 3.6 years. The original plan with these children was to retain their implants, but about 25% of the children had their nails removed because of persistent discomfort.

Fixation with Flexible Intramedullary Nails: Technique

Preoperative Planning

The ideal patient for flexible intramedullary nailing is a child between the ages of 5 and 11 years with a length-stable femoral fracture in the mid-80% of the diaphysis (Fig. 22-16), who has a body weight less than 50 kg.[149] Unstable fracture patterns can also be treated with flexible nailing, but the risk of shortening and angular malunion is greater,[185] and supplemental immobilization during the early healing phase may be valuable.

Initial x-rays should be studied carefully for fracture lines that propagate proximally and distally and might be otherwise unnoticed (Fig. 22-17). Although it is technically difficult to obtain satisfactory fixation with a retrograde technique when the fracture is near the distal metaphysis, a 2006 biomechanical study[140] demonstrated that retrograde insertion provides better stability than antegrade insertion for distal femoral shaft fractures. Nail size is determined by measuring the minimal diameter of the diaphysis, then multiplying by 0.4 to get nail diameter. For instance, if the minimal diameter of the diaphyseal canal is 1.0 cm, 4-mm nails are used. The largest possible nail size that permits two nails to fit into the medullary canal should be chosen.

Flexible nailing is most effectively done on a fracture table, with a fracture reduced to near anatomic position before incisions are made. Alternatively, a fluoroscopic table can be used, but the surgeon should assure that a reduction can be obtained before the start of the procedure, and extra assistance may be necessary.

The procedure described is with titanium elastic rods, but other devices are available and can be used with slight variations in procedure.

Rod Bending

The distance from the top of the inserted rod to the level of the fracture site is measured, and a gentle 30-degree bend is placed

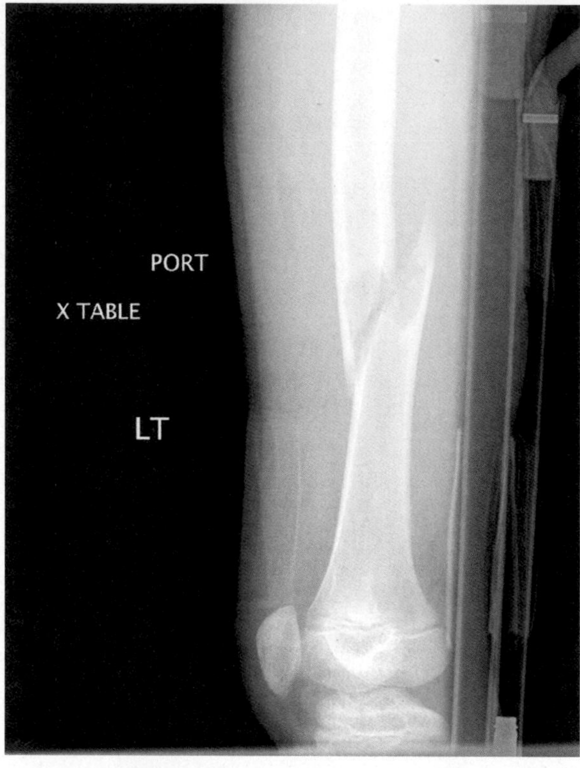

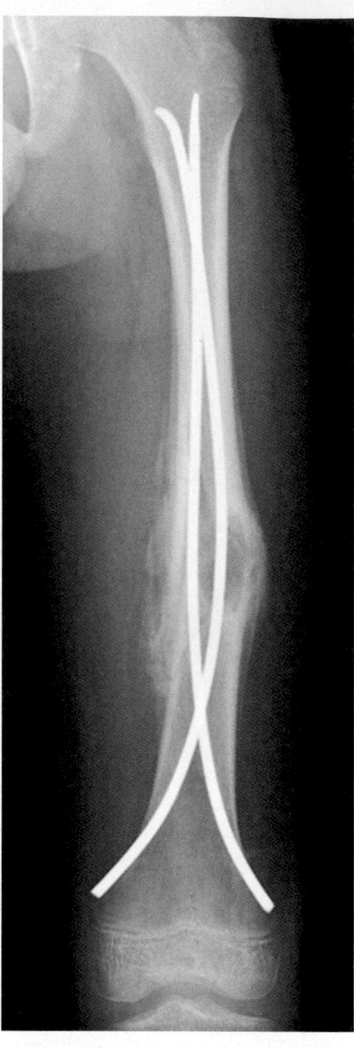

FIGURE 22-16 Titanium elastic nailing of a midshaft femur fractures through a benign lytic defect.

in the nail. The technique of elastic fixation of femoral fractures as described by Ligier et al.[123] requires that a bend be placed in the midportion of the rod at the level of the fracture site. This produces a spring effect (Fig. 22-18) that adds to the rigidity of the fracture fixation. The spread of the rods in opposite directions provides a "prestressed" fixation that increases resistance to bending. The opposite bends of the two rods at the level of the fracture significantly increase resistance to varus and valgus stress, as well as torsion. A second bend is sometimes helpful near the entering tip of the nail to facilitate clearance of the opposite cortex during initial insertion.

The nails used generally are 3.5 to 4.0 mm in diameter. Two nails of similar size should be used, and they should be as large as possible. Using nails that are too small or mismatched in size increases the rate of complications.[153] It is very unusual to use nails smaller than 3.5 mm, except in the very youngest, smallest children.

Retrograde Insertion

After the child is placed on the fracture table, the leg is prepared and draped with the thigh (hip to knee) exposed. The image intensifier is used to localize the placement of skin incisions by viewing the distal femur in the AP and lateral planes. Incisions are made on the medial and lateral sides distal to the insertion site in the bone. The proximal end of the 2- to 3-cm incision should be at or just distal to the level of the insertion site, which is about 2.5 to 3 cm proximal to the distal femoral physis (Fig. 22-19). A 4.5-mm drill bit or awl is used to make a hole in the cortex of the bone. The distal femoral metaphysis is opened 2.5 cm proximal to the distal femoral physis using a drill or awl. The drill is then steeply angled in the frontal plane to facilitate passage of the nail through the dense metaphyseal bone.

Rods are inserted from the medial and lateral sides and driven up to the level of the fracture. Upon insertion, the rod glances off the cortex as it advances toward the fracture site. Both medial and lateral rods are inserted to the level of the fracture. At this point, the fracture is reduced using longitudinal traction and a fracture reduction tool. This tool is radiolucent and holds the unstable femoral fracture in the appropriate position to allow fixation. The surgeon should select the nail that is most difficult to pass, and pass this one first. If the easier nail is passed first, it may stabilize the two fragments such that the second, more difficult nail cannot be passed easily. The two nails then are driven into the proximal end of the femur, with one driven toward the femoral neck and the other toward the greater trochanter. When passing the second nail across the fracture site and rotating it, care must be taken not to wind one rod around the other. After the nails are driven across the fracture and before they are seated, fluoroscopy is used to confirm satisfactory reduction of the fracture and to ensure that the nails did not comminute the fracture as they were driven into the proximal fragment.

The nails are pulled back approximately 2 cm, and the end

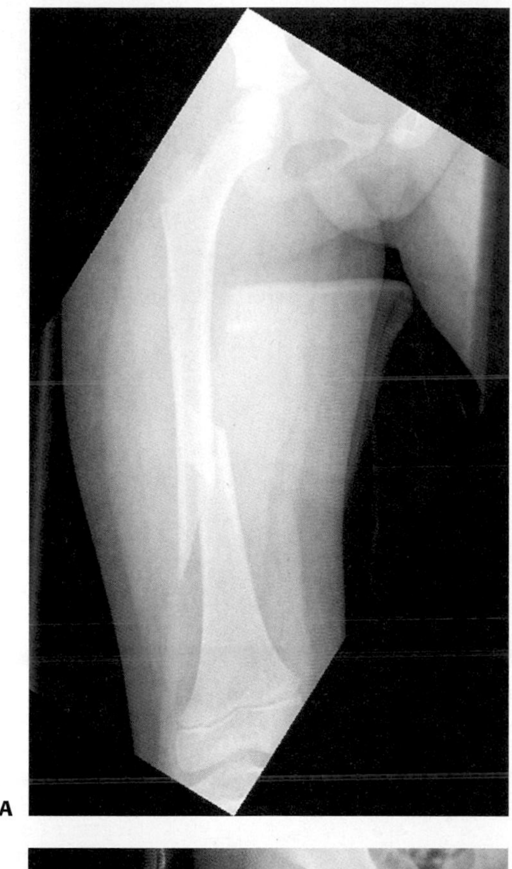

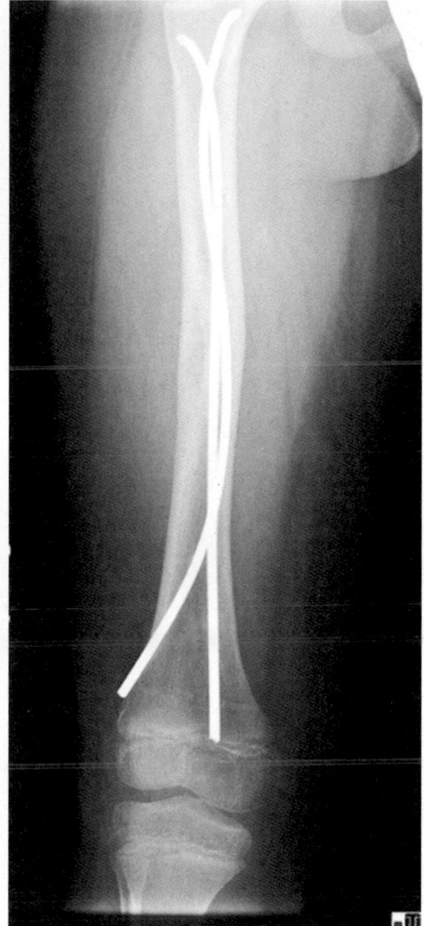

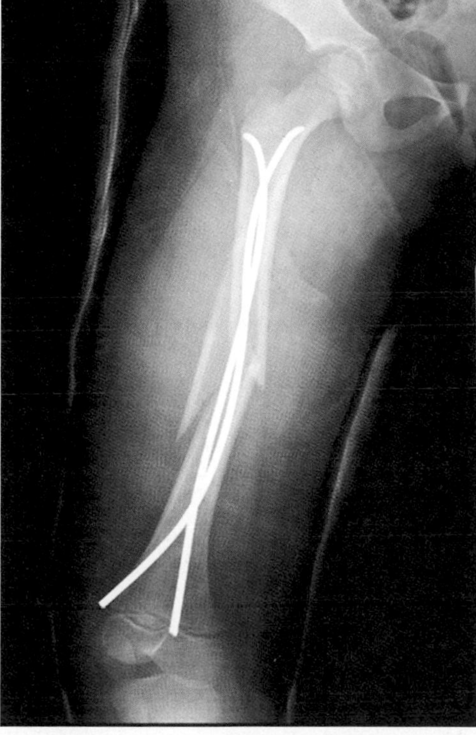

FIGURE 22-17 A. This high-energy, midshaft femur fracture was treated with titanium nails. **B.** A large butterfly fragment was dislodged during nail insertion. Because the fracture is now length-unstable, the surgeon wisely chose to protect the child for a few weeks in a one leg spica cast. **C.** The fracture healed in excellent alignment. Note how the nails have wound around each other. This can make nail removal more difficult.

of each nail is cut and driven back securely into the femur. The end of the nail should lie adjacent to the bone of the distal femoral metaphysis, exposed just enough to allow easy removal once the fracture is healed. The exposed to distal tip of the nail should not be bent away from the femoral metaphysis because this will irritate surrounding tissues.

A proximal insertion site can also be used. An insertion site through the lateral border of the trochanter avoids creating the stress riser that results from subtrochanteric entry.

Technique Tip

Mazda et al.[134] emphasized that for insertion of titanium elastic nails, the nails have to be bent into an even curve over the entire length, and the summit of the curve must be at the level

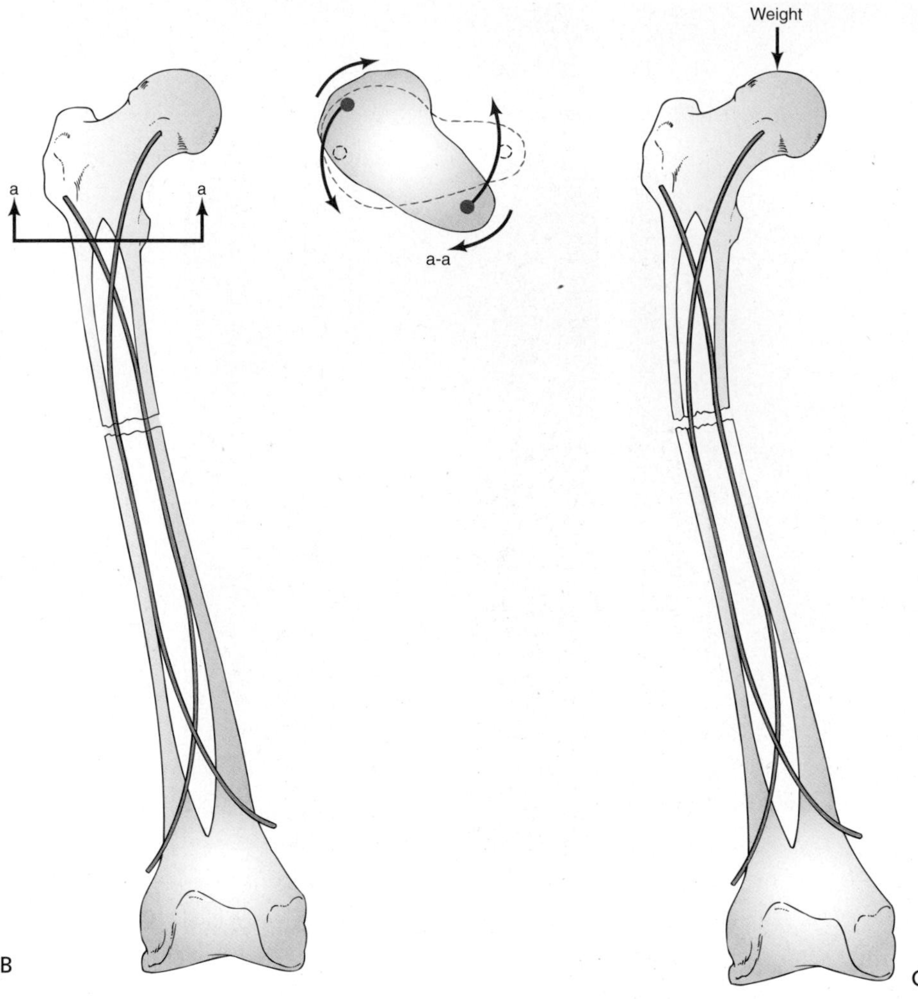

FIGURE 22-18 A. Stability from flexible rods comes from proper technique. **B.** Torsional stability results from divergence of the rods in the metaphysis. **C.** Resistance to sagittal and coronal bending results from spreading of the prebent rods through the diaphysis, as well as the size and material properties of the rods. Elastic rods return to their predetermined alignment when loaded unless plastic deformation occurs.

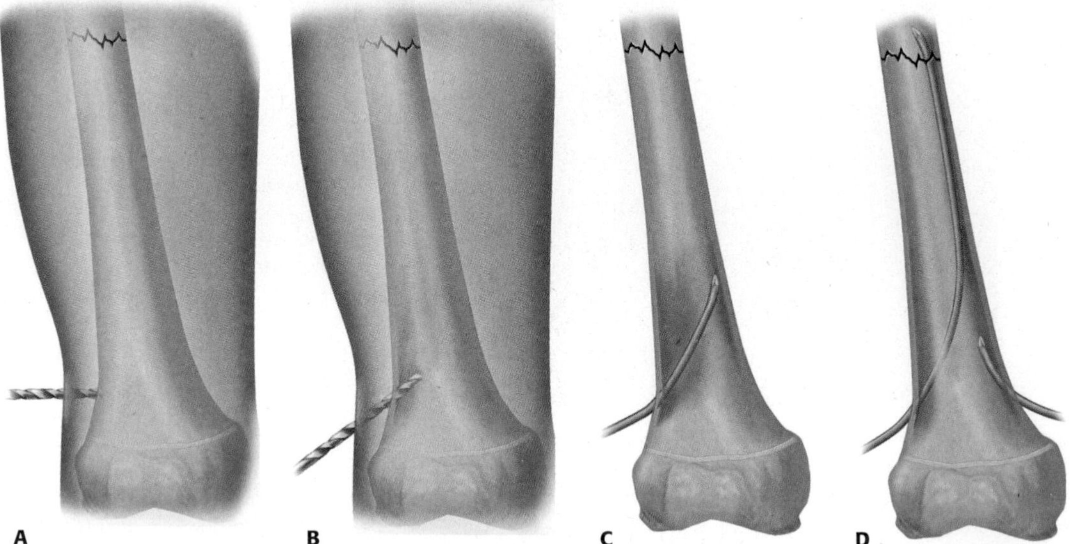

FIGURE 22-19 A. Once the incision has been made, the entry point for the nail is identified 2 cm superior to the growth plate at the midpoint of the femur anteroposteriorly. A 4.5-mm drill bit is used to make the starting point. **B.** Once the cortex has been entered the drill is angled obliquely to fashion a tract. **C.** The first nail is inserted until it reaches the fracture line. **D.** Once the first nail has reached the fracture line, the second nail is inserted in the same fashion.

of the fracture or very close to it in comminuted fractures. The depth of curvature should be about three times the diameter of the femoral canal. Flynn et al.[62] also stressed the importance of contouring both nails with similar gentle curvatures, choosing nails that are 40% of the narrowest diaphyseal diameter, and using medial and lateral starting points that are at the same level in the metaphysis.

Postoperative Management

A knee immobilizer is beneficial in the early postoperative course to decrease knee pain and quadriceps spasm. When the flexible nailing technique is used for length-unstable fractures, a walking (or one leg) spica is recommended, generally for about 4 to 6 weeks until callus is visible on x-rays. For length-stable fractures, touchdown weight bearing can begin as soon as the patient is comfortable. Gentle knee exercises and quadriceps strengthening can be begun, but there should be no aggressive-passive motion of the knee, which increases the motion at the fracture site and increases quadriceps spasm. Postoperative knee motion does return to normal, but this requires time. Full weight bearing generally is tolerated by 6 weeks. Ozdemir et al.[162] recommended the use of postoperative functional bracing, demonstrating its effectiveness in a group of patients treated with elastic rodding. Such postoperative support may occasionally be required, but in most cases it appears not to be needed.

The nails can be removed 6 to 12 months after injury when the fracture is fully healed, usually as an outpatient procedure.

Complications of Flexible Intramedullary Nailing

Complications are relatively infrequent after flexible intramedullary nailing. In 351 fractures reported in seven studies,[9,32,58,85,123,126,134] one nonunion, one infection, and no occurrence of osteonecrosis were reported. Approximately 12% of patients had malunions, most often mild varus deformities, and approximately 3% had clinically significant leg-length discrepancies from either overgrowth or shortening. A 2007 study noted overgrowth of more than 1 cm in 8.2% of preschool children treated with titanium elastic nailing.[21] This is a much higher rate of overgrowth than seen in older children, suggesting the technique should be used infrequently in preschool children. Mazda et al.[134] pointed out a technique-related complication that occurred in 10 of their 34 patients: rods were left too long and caused painful bursae and limited knee flexion. All 10 patients had the nails removed 2 to 5 months after surgery. Flexible nails inserted in a retrograde fashion may also penetrate into the knee joint, causing an acute synovitis.[175] In a multicenter study[62] that included 58 femoral fractures stabilized with titanium elastic nails, irritation of the soft tissue near the knee by the nail tip occurred in 4 patients (7%), leading to a deeper infection in 2 patients. This study also reported one refracture after premature nail removal, leading to a recommendation that nail removal be delayed until callus is solid around all cortices and the fracture line is no longer visible. Ozdemir et al.[162] measured overgrowth with a scanogram and found that the average increase in length was 1.8 mm, suggesting that significant femoral overgrowth is not seen with this method of treatment.

Flynn et al.[63] compared traction and spica casting with titanium elastic nails for treatment of femoral fractures in 83 consecutive school-aged children. The three unsatisfactory results were treated with traction followed by casting. The overall complication rate was 34% in the traction group and 21% in the elastic nail group.

An international multicenter study focused on factors that predict a higher rate of complications after flexible nailing of pediatric femoral shaft fractures.[149] Analyzing 234 fractures in 229 patients from six different Level 1 trauma centers, the authors found significantly more problems in older, heavier children. A poor outcome was 5 times more likely in patients who weighed more than 108.5 pounds. A poor outcome was also almost four times more likely in patients older than 11 years old. The authors concluded that results were generally excellent for titanium elastic nailing, but poor results were more likely in children older than 11 and heavier than 50 kg. Ho et al.[93] reported a 34% complication rate in patients 10 years old and older, but only a 9% complication rate in patients younger than 10 years, emphasizing the concept that complications of flexible nailing are higher in older, heavier children.

External Fixation

External fixation of femoral shaft fractures offers an efficient, convenient method to align and stabilize the fractured pediatric femur. It is the method of choice when severe soft tissue injury is present, and may be considered in any patient where traditional closed methods of management are not appropriate.[116] In head-injured or multiply-injured patients and those with open fractures, external fixation offers an excellent method of rapid fracture stabilization. It is also valuable for very proximal or distal fractures, where options for flexible nailing, plating, or casting are limited. External fixation is particularly valuable for benign pathologic fractures (e.g., through a nonossifying fibroma) at the distal metaphyseal–diaphyseal junction (Fig. 22-20), where the fracture will heal rapidly, but minimal angular malunion can be tolerated.

Aronson and Tursky[6] reported their early experience with 44 femoral fractures treated with primary external fixation and early weight bearing. Most patients returned to school by 4 weeks after fracture and had full knee motion by 6 weeks after the fixator was removed. In this early study, end-on alignment was the goal and overgrowth was minimal. More recently, Matzkin et al.[133] reported a series of 40 pediatric femoral fractures treated with external fixation; 72% of the fixators were dynamized before removal, and their refracture rate was only 2.5%. They had no overgrowth, but one patient ended up 5 cm short.

Following early enthusiasm for the use of external devices, the 1990s saw waning interest in their use because of complications with pin track infections, pin site scarring, delayed union, and refracture. These complications, coupled with the very low complication rate from flexible nailing, led to a decline of external fixation for pediatric femoral shaft fractures. Data from comparison studies also contributed to the change. Bar-On et al.[9] compared external fixation with flexible intramedullary rodding in a prospective randomized study. They found that the early postoperative course was similar but that the time to return to school and to resume full activity was less with intramedullary fixation. Muscle strength was better in the flexible intramedullary fixation group at 14 months after fracture. Parental satisfaction was also significantly better in the flexible intramedullary rodding group. Bar-On et al.[9] recommended that external fixation be reserved for open or severely comminuted fractures.

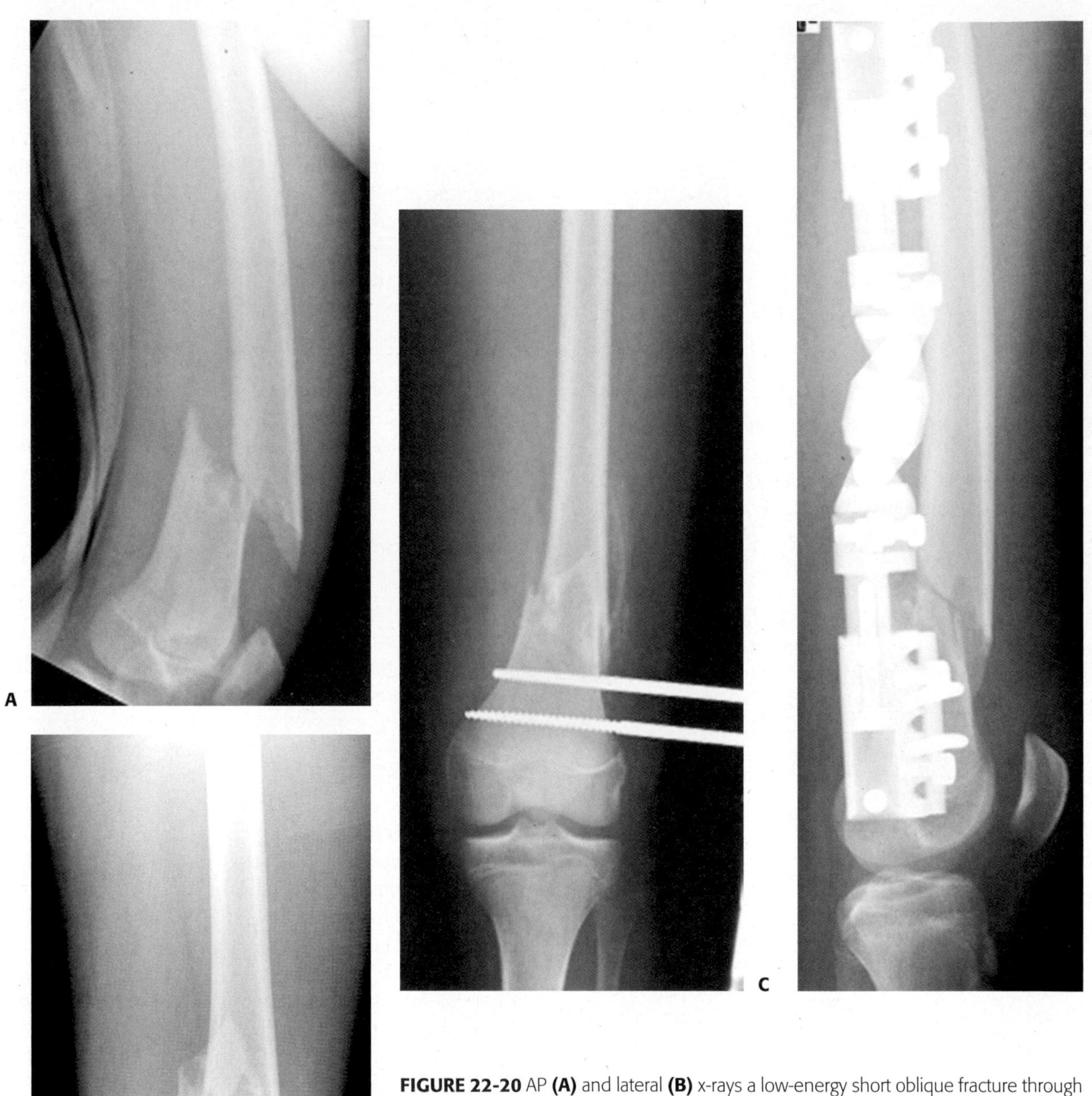

FIGURE 22-20 AP **(A)** and lateral **(B)** x-rays a low-energy short oblique fracture through a fibrous cortical defect in the distal femur; this type of fracture is not unusual. The surgeon judged that there was enough distance between the fracture site and the growth plate to allow external fixation. AP **(C)** and lateral **(D)** x-rays 3 weeks after external fixation shows early callus and good alignment. The external fixation was removed shortly after this x-ray and the child was placed in a long leg cast, with weight bearing as tolerated.

Fixator Design

In general, circular fixation devices are rarely, if ever, indicated for femoral fractures in young children. One of two types of monolateral devices are typically used. The AO system, in which pins can be placed at any point along a bar, with a special clamp holding the pins at a variable angle to the bar has been used at many centers. The advantage of this system is that the stability of fixation is increased if the two pins on each side of the fracture are spread widely, with one pin close to the fracture and one quite distant from it. A second longitudinal rod can be added to this system to increase its rigidity. A second type of external fixation system has pin clamps at the end of a telescopic tube. The pin clamps provide easy application, but the stability of the fixation device is decreased because the pins are widely separated from the fracture. The pin clamps may be constrained to rotation only (Wagner) or attached with a universal joint to the barrel of the device (Orthofix, EBI) (Fig. 22-21). The telescoping barrel provides lengthening or "dynamization," and the universal joints provide adjustment. Dynamization refers to the amount of longitudinal motion allowed by a given frame or construct. A fracture can be dynamized before frame removal to increase strength of healing callus. Different external fixation devices allow for varying amounts of dynamization. Excessive rigidity is thought to relate to poor bone healing and strength. For this reason, many pediatric trauma experts purposely build a less stable frame to increase the forces on the fracture site. Pins are more closely clustered and placed farther from the fracture site, and the frame itself is placed more laterally away

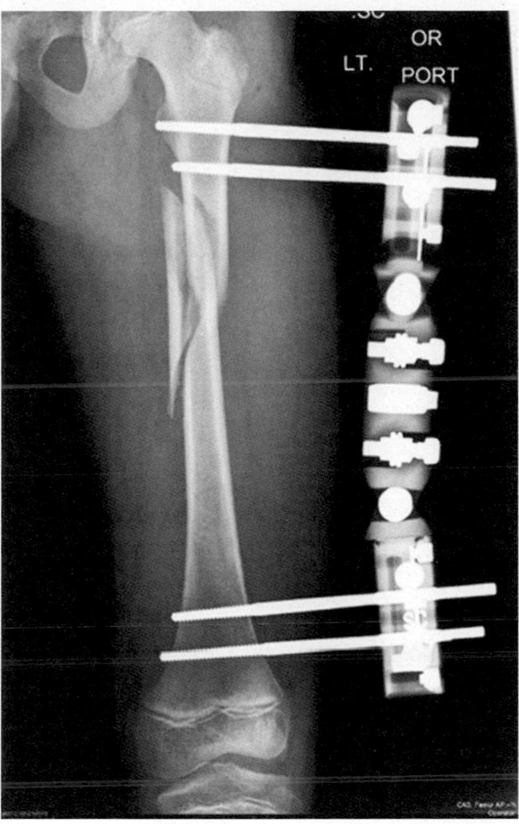

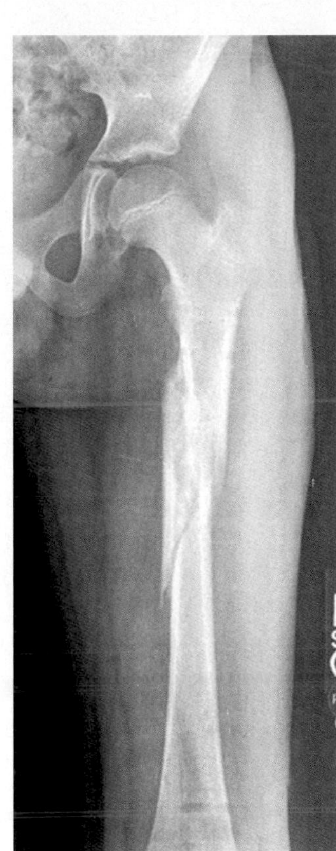

FIGURE 22-21 A. This proximal spiral femur fracture was deemed length-unstable and a poor candidate for titanium elastic nails. The surgeon chose an external fixator, rather than a plate. **B.** Eight weeks after injury, the fracture is healing in excellent alignment and there is good early callus. Fixator removal is easier than plate removal.

from the femur. Domb et al.[52] compared static to dynamic external fixation in pediatric femoral fractures. Average time to early callus formation was similar, and the average time to complete healing was 70.1 days in the dynamic group and 63.1 days in the static group. The assumption that less rigid frames decrease fracture healing remains unproven. The problem may be that smaller, lighter children simply do not place enough force across the dynamized fracture to stimulate callus production.

The ease and speed with which an external fixation device can be applied make it ideal for management of a polytrauma victim who cannot tolerate extended anesthesia. Nowotarski et al.,[158] in a review of 1507 femoral fractures at a trauma center, found 59 (4%) that were managed with urgent external fixation followed by intramedullary rodding. The average time to rodding was 7 days, and the infection rate was 1.7% (1 patient). They concluded that emergent external fixation followed by early intramedullary rodding was safe.

Frame Application: Technique

During preoperative planning, the fracture should be studied carefully for comminution or fracture lines that propagate proximally or distally. The surgeon should assure that the fixator devices available are long enough to span the distance between the optimal proximal and distal pin insertion sites.

As in the elastic nailing technique, either a fracture table or radiolucent table can be used, although a fracture table is much more efficient because an anatomic reduction can be obtained before preparation and draping. First, the fracture is reduced both in length and alignment. If the fracture is open, it should be irrigated and débrided before application of the external fixation device. With the fracture optimally aligned, fixation is begun. The minimal and maximal length constraints characteristic of all external fixation systems must be kept in mind, and the angular adjustment intrinsic to the fixation device should be determined. Rotation is constrained with all external fixation systems once the first pins are placed. That is, if parallel pins are placed with the fracture in 40 degrees of malrotation, a 40-degree malalignment will exist. Rotational correction must be obtained before placing the pins in the proximal and distal shafts of the femur.

Application of the fixator is similar no matter what device is chosen. One pin is placed proximally in the shaft, and another pin is placed distally perpendicular to the long axis of the shaft. Alignment is based on the long axis of the shaft, rather than the joint surface. Rotation should be checked before the second pin is placed because it constrains rotation but not angulation or length. After pins are correctly placed, all fixation nuts are secured and sterile dressings are applied to pins.

Technique Tips

Pin sizes vary with manufacturers, as do drill sizes. In general, the pins are placed through predrilled holes to avoid thermal necrosis of bone. Sharp drills should be used. The manufacturer's recommendation for drill and screw sizes should be checked before starting the procedure. Some self-drilling and self-tapping pins are available. At least two pins should be placed proximally and two distally. An intermediate or auxiliary pin may be beneficial.

Postoperative Care

The key to preventing pin site irritation is avoiding tension at the skin–pin interface. We recommend that our patients clean their pin sites daily with soap and water, perhaps as part of regular bath or shower. Showering is allowed once the wound is stable and there is no communication between the pin and the fracture hematoma. Antibiotics are commonly used at some point while the fixator is in place, because pin site infections are common and easily resolved with antibiotic treatment, usually cephalosporin.

There are two general strategies regarding fixator removal. The external fixation device can be used as "portable traction." With this strategy, the fixator is left in place until early callus stabilizes the fracture. At this point, usually 6 to 8 weeks after injury, the fixator device is removed and a walking spica cast is placed. This minimizes stress shielding from the fixator and allows time for the pin holes to fill in while the cast is on. The alternative, classic strategy involves using the fixator until the fracture is completely healed. Fixator dynamization, which is difficult in small, young children, is essential for this strategy. The device should not be removed until three or four cortices show bridging bone continuous on AP and lateral radiographs, typically 3 to 4 months after injury.

Complications of External Fixation

The most common complication of external fixation is pin track irritation or infection, which has been reported to occur in up to 72% of patients.[147] This problem generally is easily treated with oral antibiotics and local pin site care. Sola et al.[189] reported a decreased number of pin track infections after changing their pin care protocol from cleansing with peroxide to simply having the patient shower daily. Superficial infections should be treated aggressively with pin track releases and antibiotics. Deep infections are rare, but if present, surgical débridement and antibiotic therapy are usually effective. Any skin tenting over the pins should be released at the time of application or at follow-up.

In a study of complications of external fixators for femoral fractures, Gregory et al.[70] reported a 30% major complication rate and a high minor complication rate. Among the major complications were five refractures or fractures through pin sites. Another comprehensive study of external fixation complications[33] found an overall rate of refracture of 4.7%, with a pin track infection rate of 33.1%. Skaggs et al.[187] reviewed the use of external fixation devices for femoral fractures and found a 12% rate of secondary fractures in 66 patients. Multivariate linear regression analysis showed no correlation between the incidence of refracture and the fracture pattern, percentage of bone contact after fixator application, type of external fixator used, or dynamization of the fracture. A statistically significant association was found between the number of cortices demonstrating bridging callus on both the AP and lateral views at the time of fixator removal and refracture. Fractures with fewer than three cortices with bridging callus at the time of fixator removal had a 33% risk of refracture, whereas those with three or four cortices showing bridging callus had only a 4% rate of refracture. Other reports in the literature with smaller numbers, but still substantial experience, document refracture rates as high as 21.6% with more significant complications.[47,48,71,96,147,167,184] In 1997, in a follow-up of the original article by Aronson and Tursky,[6] Blasier et al.[19] reported 139 femoral fractures treated with external fixation; they found that pin track infection was common and there was a 2% incidence of fracture after removal of the device. El Hayek et al.[54] demonstrated the benefit of modern techniques of external fixation in a series of 28 fractures in 21 children. Despite the complications, patients and treating physicians have found wound care and ability to lengthen through the fracture to be of great benefit with this technique.

Although joint stiffness has been noted in older patients treated with external fixation, it is relatively uncommon in children with femoral fractures unless major soft tissue injury is present.[57]

Rigid Intramedullary Rod Fixation

With reports by Beaty et al.[11] and others in the early 1990s alerting surgeons that antegrade intramedullary nailing can be complicated by osteonecrosis of the proximal femur, flexible nailing (either antegrade or retrograde) quickly became more popular than standard locked, antegrade rigid intramedullary nailing. Recently, however, locked antegrade femoral nailing for pediatric femoral fractures has enjoyed a resurgence of interest with the introduction of newer generation implants that allow a very lateral trochanteric entry point. These newer implant systems avoid a piriformis entry site, reducing (but perhaps not completely eliminating) the risk of osteonecrosis. Others have adapted humeral nails for pediatric femoral fractures.[16] Antegrade locked intramedullary fixation is particularly valuable for femoral fractures in adolescents. Comparative studies by Reeves et al.[170] and Kirby et al.,[113] as well as retrospective reviews of traction and casting, suggest that femoral fractures in adolescents are better treated with intramedullary fixation[11,30,47,68,69,73,90,108,113,123,197,210,212] than with traditional traction and casting (Table 22-3). Kanellopoulos et al.[107] reported excellent results in 20 skeletally immature patients, ranging in age from 11 to 16 years, treated with closed, locked intramedullary nailing through the tip of the greater trochanter. There were no complications, including no osteonecrosis, with an average follow-up of 29 months.

Length-unstable adolescent femoral fractures benefit from interlocking proximally and distally to maintain length and rotational alignment.[12,25,78] Beaty et al.[11] reported the use of interlocking intramedullary nails for the treatment of 31 femoral shaft fractures in 30 patients 10 to 15 years of age. All fractures united, and the average leg length discrepancy was 0.51 cm. No angular or rotational malunions occurred. All nails were removed at an average of 14 months after injury; no refracture or femoral neck fracture occurred after nail removal. One case of osteonecrosis of the femoral head occurred, which was thought to be secondary to injury to the ascending cervical artery during nail insertion.

Reamed antegrade nailing in children with an open proximal femoral physis must absolutely avoid the piriformis fossa, due to the risk of proximal femoral growth abnormalities,[168] the risk of osteonecrosis of the femoral head,[11,143,166,194] the size of the proximal femur, and the relative success of other treatment methods. However, Maruenda-Paulino et al.[131] reported good results using 9-mm Kuntscher rods in children 7 to 12 years of age, and Beaty et al.[11] reported the use of pediatric "intermediate" interlocking nails for femoral canals with diameters as small as 8 mm. Townsend and Hoffinger[200] and Momberger et al.[148] published reviews of trochanteric nailing in adolescents with very good results. The combined series included 82 patients aged 10 to 17 with follow-up of 6 years with no reported

TABLE 22-3 Results of Treatment of Femoral Shaft Fractures in Adolescents

Series	Number of Patients	Average Age (Range) in Years	Treatment	Results and Complications (n)
Kirby et al.[113]	13	12 + 7 (10 + 11 − 15 + 6)	Traction + cast	Short >2.5 cm (2) Significant residual angulation (4)
	12	12 + 0 (10 − 10 − 15 + 7)	Intramedullary nailing	No overgrowth No significant residual angulation
Ziv et al.[212]	17	8 + 3 (6 − 12)	Intramedullary nailing (9 Rush pins, 9 Kuntscher nails)	No leg length discrepancy >1 cm Change in ATD 0.5–1 cm = 3 with Kuntscher nails
Reeves et al.[170]	41	12 + 4 (9 + 9 − 16 + 4)	Traction + cast	Delayed union (4) Malunion (5) Growth disturbance (4) Psychotic episodes (2)
	49	14 + 11 (11 − 16 + 10)	Intramedullary nailing	No infection, nonunion, or malunion
Beaty et al.[11]	30	12 + 3 (10 − 15)	Intramedullary nailing	Overgrowth >2.5 cm (2) Osteonecrosis femoral head (1)
Aronson et al.[5]	42	9 + 7 (2 + 5 − 17 + 8)	External fixation	8.5% pin infection 10% cast or reapplication
Ligier et al.[123]	123	10 (5 − 16)	Flexible intramedullary rods	1 infection 13 wound ulcerations 2 LLD >2 cm
Mazda et al.[134]	34	9.5 (6 − 17)	Flexible intramedullary rods	1.0 to 1.5 cm overgrowth (3) 1.0 to 15 degrees malalignment (2)

cases of osteonecrosis and no significant alteration in proximal femoral anatomy.

Open fractures in older adolescents can be effectively treated with intramedullary rodding, either as delayed or primary treatment, including those caused by gunshot wounds and high-velocity injuries.[15,198] Antegrade intramedullary rod insertion maintains length, prevents angular malunion and nonunion, and allows the patient to be rapidly mobilized and discharged from the hospital. However, other techniques with fewer potential risks should be considered.

Retrograde rodding of the femur has become an accepted procedure in adults.[161,172] In a large patient approaching skeletal maturity (bone age >16 years) but with an open proximal femoral physis and an unstable fracture pattern, this treatment might be considered as a way to avoid the risk of osteonecrosis yet stabilize the fracture (Fig. 22-22). If growth from the distal femur is predicted to be less than 1 cm, leg length inequality should not be a problem. Ricci et al.[172] have shown that the complication rate with this technique compares favorably to that of antegrade nailing, with a higher rate of knee pain but a lower rate of hip pain. The malunion rate was slightly lower with retrograde rodding than with antegrade rodding of the femur.

Antegrade Transtrochanteric Intramedullary Nailing: Technique

The patient is placed either supine or in the lateral decubitus position on a fracture table. The upper end of the femur is approached through a 3-cm longitudinal incision proximal that allows access to the lateral trochanteric entry point. The skin incision can be precisely placed after localization on both the AP and lateral views. Dissection should be limited to the lateral aspect of the greater trochanter, avoiding the piriformis fossa. This prevents dissection near the origin of the lateral ascending cervical artery medial to the piriformis fossa. The rod should be inserted through the lateral aspect of the greater trochanter. In children and adolescents, it is preferable to choose the smallest implant with the smallest diameter reaming to avoid damage to the proximal femoral insertion area.

The technique for reaming and nail insertion varies according to the specifics of the implant chosen. In general, the smallest rod that maintains contact with the femoral cortices is used (generally 9 mm or less) and is locked proximally and distally (Fig. 22-23). Only one distal locking screw is necessary, but two can be used.[112] Rods that have an expanded proximal cross-section should be avoided, because they require excessive removal of bone from the child's proximal femur. The proximal end of the nail should be left slightly long (up to 1 cm) to make later removal easier. The rod chosen should be angled proximally and specifically designed for transtrochanteric insertion (Fig. 22-24).

Technique Tips

Dissection should be limited to the lateral aspect of the greater trochanter (Fig. 22-25), without extending to the capsule or midportion of the femoral neck. Some systems provide a small diameter, semiflexible tube that can be inserted up to the fracture site after initial entry-site reaming. This tube is extremely helpful in manipulating a flexed, abducted proximal fragment in proximal third femoral fractures.

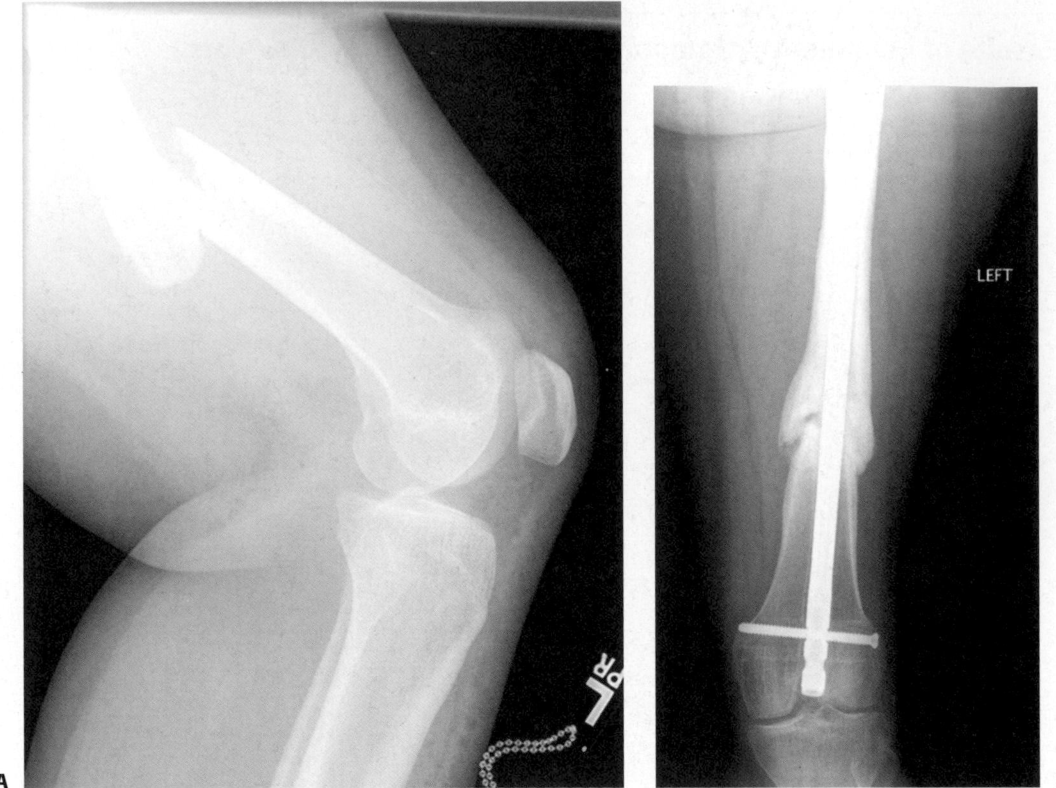

FIGURE 22-22 A. This distal femoral shaft fracture in a skeletally mature girl was treated with retrograde femoral nailing. **B.** There is a delayed union.

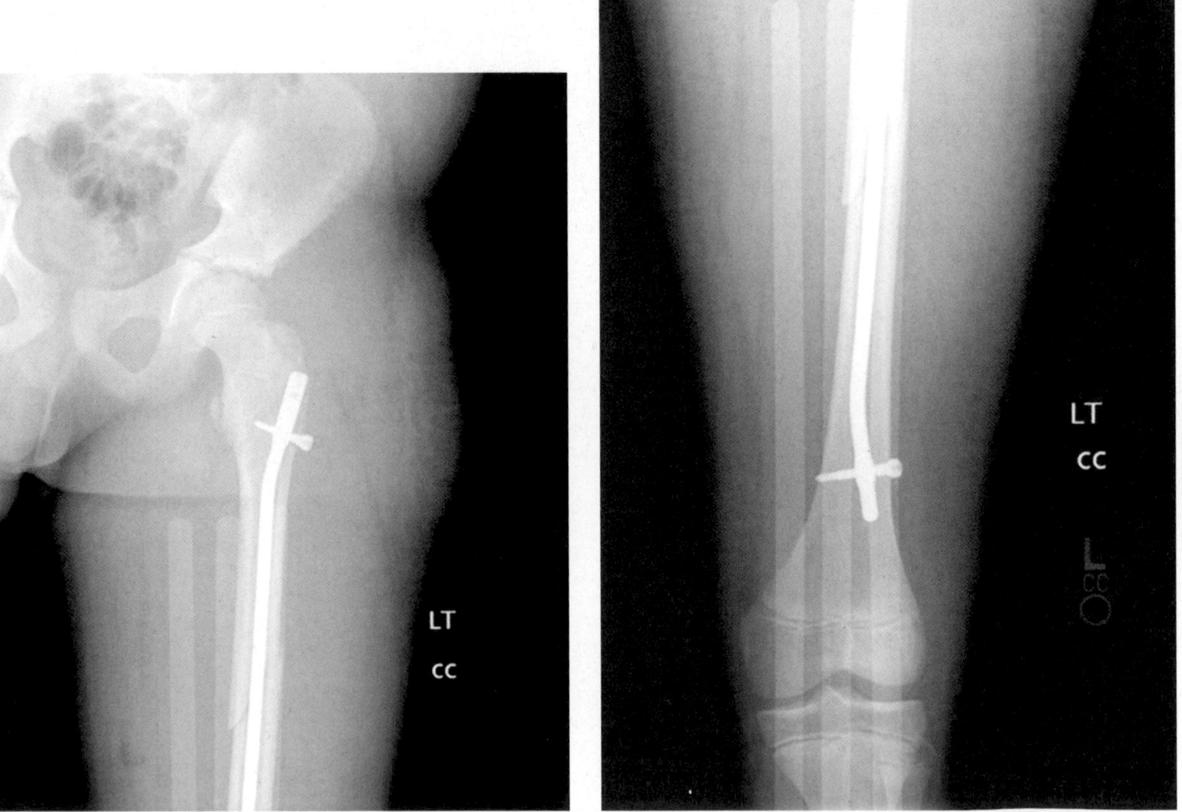

FIGURE 22-23 AP **(A)** and lateral **(B)** x-rays immediately after internal fixation of the midshaft femur fracture in a 13-year-old with a pediatric locking nail that permits easy lateral entry and requires minimal reaming of the child's proximal femur.

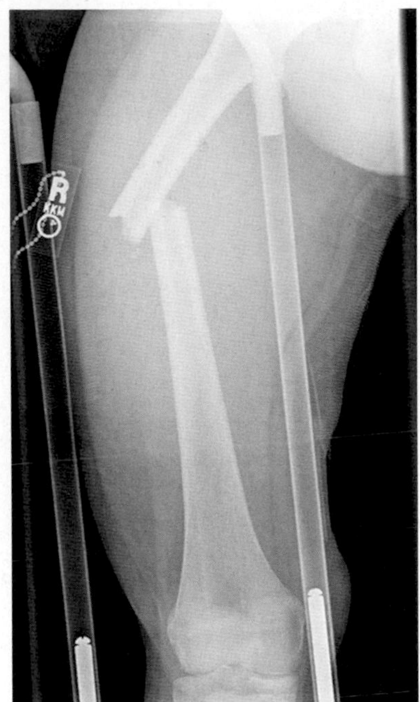

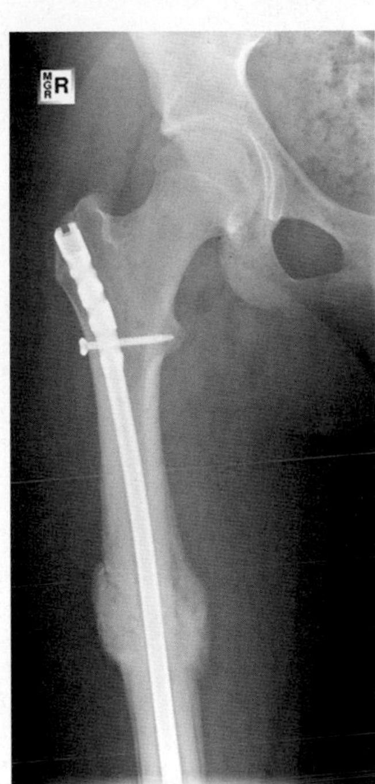

FIGURE 22-24 Preoperative **(A)** and postoperative **(B)** images showing the use of a newer generation lateral entry nail to treat a proximal third femur fracture in a 14-year-old girl.

Postoperative Management

Nails can be removed 9 to 18 months after x-ray union to prevent bony overgrowth over the proximal tip of the nail. We do not routinely remove locked antegrade nails from our teenage patients unless they are symptomatic or request removal for another reason. Dynamization with removal of the proximal or distal screw generally is not necessary.

Complications of Locked Intramedullary Nailing

Although good results have been reported with this technique and patient satisfaction is high, problems with proximal femoral growth, osteonecrosis, and leg-length discrepancy cannot be ignored.

In a series of intramedullary nailing of 31 fractures, Beaty et al.[11] reported 1 patient with segmental osteonecrosis of the femoral head (Fig. 22-26), which was not seen on radiograph until 15 months after injury. Kaweblum et al.[112] reported a patient with osteonecrosis of the proximal femoral epiphysis after a greater trochanteric fracture, suggesting that the blood supply to the proximal femur may have been compromised by vascular disruption at the level of the greater trochanter during rod insertion. Other researchers have reported single patients

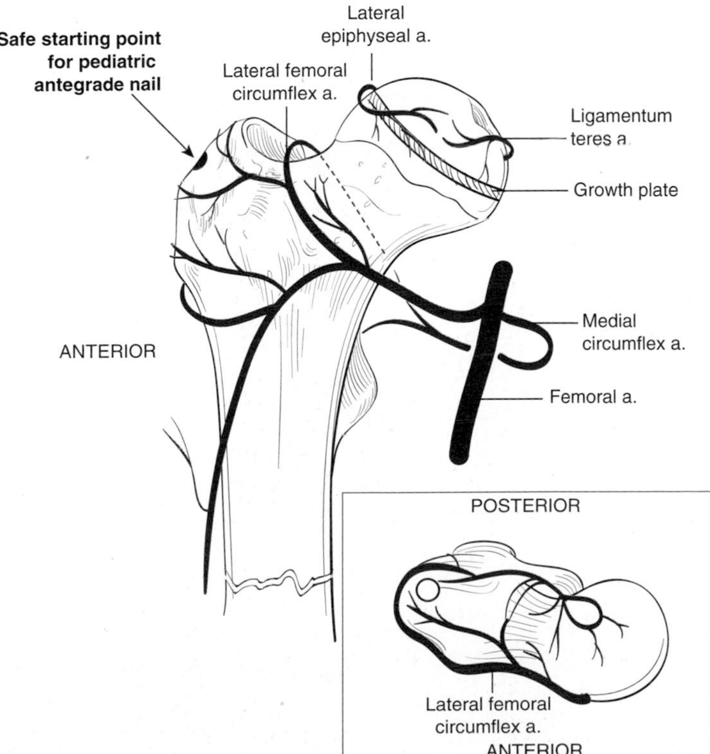

FIGURE 22-25 Trochanteric entry point for intramedullary nail indicated with *arrow*. Entry here with smaller diameter nails limits the risk of avascular necrosis and ensures no awl in the piriformis fossa. (From Skaggs D, Flynn J. Trauma about the pelvis/hip/femur. Staying Out of Trouble in Pediatric Orthopaedics. Philadelphia: Lippincott Williams & Wilkins, 2006:109.)

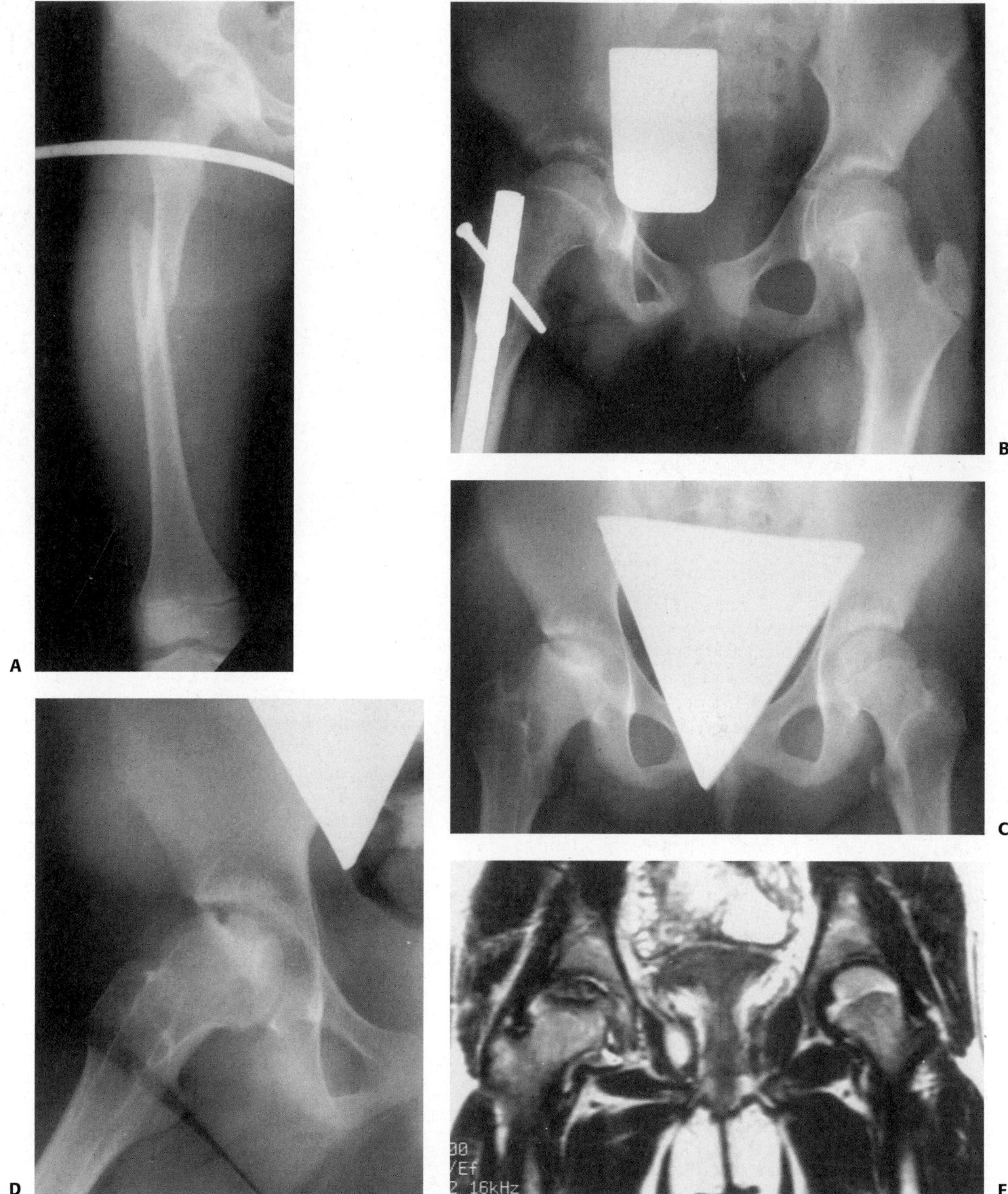

FIGURE 22-26 A. Isolated femoral shaft fracture in an 11-year-old. **B.** After fixation with an intramedullary nail, femoral head appears normal. **C.** Eight months after injury, fracture is healed; note early signs of osteonecrosis of right femoral head. **D.** Fifteen months after injury, segmental osteonecrosis of the femoral head is evident on x-rays. **E.** MRI shows extent of osteonecrosis of right femoral head. (**D.** reprinted from Beaty JH, Austin SM, Warner WC, et al. Interlocking intramedullary nailing of femoral-shaft fractures in adolescents: preliminary results and complications. J Pediatr Orthop 1994;14:178–183, with permission.)

with osteonecrosis of the femoral head after intramedullary nailing.[143,160,194] A poll of the members of the Pediatric Orthopaedic Society disclosed 14 patients with osteonecrosis in approximately 1600 femoral fractures. Despite the use of a "safe" transtrochanteric insertion site for antegrade femoral rodding, a case of osteonecrosis has been reported. Buford et al.[28] showed in their MRI study of hips after antegrade rodding that subclinical osteonecrosis may be present. Antegrade rodding through the trochanter or the upper end of the femur appears to be associated with a risk of osteonecrosis in children with open physes, regardless of chronologic age. Chung[36] noted the absence of transphyseal vessels to the proximal femoral epiphysis and demonstrated that the singular lateral ascending cervical artery predominantly supplies blood to the capital femoral epiphysis (Fig. 22-27). He stated that all of the epiphyseal and metaphyseal branches of the lateral ascending cervical artery originate from a single stem that crosses the capsule at the trochanteric notch. Because the space between the trochanter and the femoral head is extremely narrow, this single artery is vulnerable to injury and appears to be so until skeletal maturity, regardless of chronologic age.

Townsend and Hoffinger[200] reported no ostonecrosis in 34 patients in whom a trochanteric tip starting point was used. Simonian et al.,[184] in a long-term study of 52 children and adolescents with femoral fractures treated with plating and intramedullary rodding, found that excessive overgrowth was less common with nailing than with plating. Three patients had moderate valgus deformities of the hip and one had late arthrosis after intramedullary rodding despite using a transtrochanteric approach. Simonian et al.[184] concluded that open physes were a contraindication to antegrade rodding even with a transtrochanteric approach. Thometz and Lamdan[194] also documented an association between osteonecrosis and antegrade rodding in an adolescent.

Growth abnormality in the proximal femur may occur with arrest of the greater trochanteric physis. Although most growth from the greater trochanter after 8 years of age is appositional, Raney et al.[168] reported 5 patients who developed coxa valga and mild hip subluxation from trochanteric physeal arrest after antegrade nailing. These patients ranged in age from 9 to 13 years, suggesting that even in older children greater trochanteric physeal arrest occasionally can produce clinical problems. Beaty et al.[11] reported 2 patients, boys age 13 years, with overgrowth of more than 2.5 cm that required epiphysiodesis because of leg length discrepancy. Gordon et al.,[69] in a study of the effect of trochanteric nailing on proximal femoral anatomy, found no significant changes in the articulotrochanteric distance, the neck-shaft angle, or the width of the femoral neck after trochanteric antegrade nailing. They also found no incidence of osteonecrosis.

The proximal femoral physis is a continuous cartilaginous plate between the greater trochanter and the proximal femur in young children. Interference with the physis may result in abnormal growth of the femoral neck, placing the child at a small risk for subsequent femoral neck fracture.[184] Antegrade nailing with reaming of a large defect also may result in growth disturbance in the proximal femur as well as femoral neck fracture (Fig. 22-28). Beaty et al.[11] reported no "thinning" of the femoral neck in their patients, which they attributed to an older patient group (10 to 15 years of age) and design changes in the femoral nail that allowed a decrease in the cross sectional diameter of the proximal portion of the femoral rods.

Plate Fixation

Open Reduction and Compression Plate Fixation

With the trend towards submuscular plating, there remain few

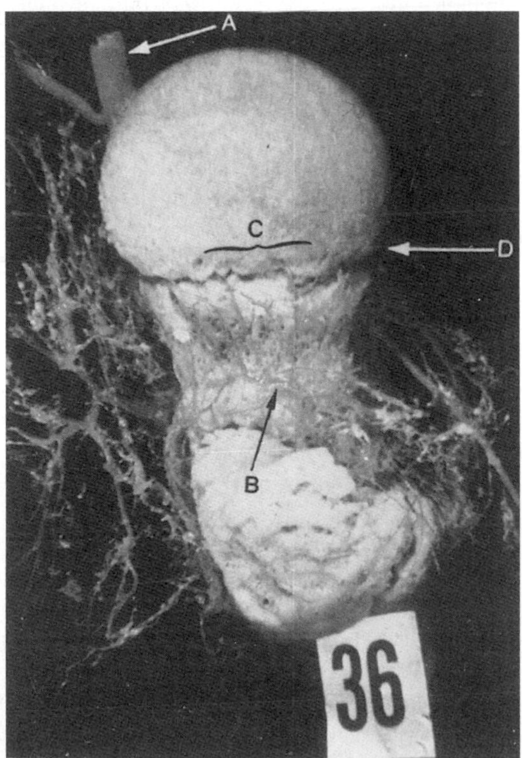

FIGURE 22-27 The single ascending cervical artery (*A*) is the predominant blood supply to the femoral head. The vessel is at risk during antegrade insertion of an intramedullary rod. (From Chung S. The arterial supply of the developing proximal end of the femur. J Bone Joint Surg Am 1976;58:961, with permission.)

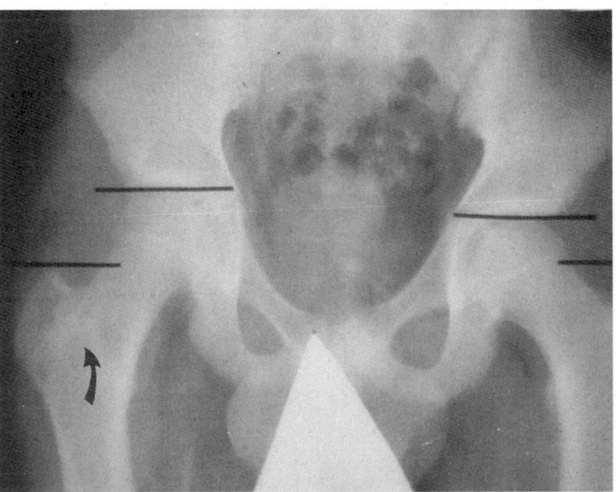

FIGURE 22-28 Fifteen-year-old boy 3 years after intramedullary nailing of the right femur. Articulotrochanteric distance increased by 1.5 cm; note partial trochanteric epiphysiodesis (*arrow*) with mild overgrowth of the femoral neck. (From Beaty JH, Austin SM, Warner WC, et al. Interlocking intramedullary nailing of femoral-shaft fractures in adolescents: preliminary results and complications. Pediatr Orthop 1994;14:178–183, with permission.)

indications for traditional open reduction and plate fixation (i.e., full length incision, subperiosteal dissection and plate fixation, filling most or all screw holes), except perhaps with extensile exposure to repair an arterial injury. Ward et al.,[208] Kregor et al.,[115] Fyodorov et al.,[67] and Hansen[79] recommended open compression plate fixation in selected femoral fractures. Ward et al.[208] reported the use of AO compression plates for the treatment of femoral shaft fractures in 25 children 6 to 16 years of age, 22 of whom had associated fractures or multisystem injuries. They recommended plate fixation for children under 11 years of age with closed-head injuries or multiple trauma. Disadvantages of plate fixation include the long incision necessary and the risks of plate breakage and stress fracture after plate removal. All the patients reported by Kregor et al.[115] had multiple trauma, and this form of treatment was selected to stabilize the femoral fracture quickly and mobilize the patient. Fyodorov et al.[67] reviewed 21 patients in whom 4.5-mm dynamic compression plates (DCPs) were used for fixation. Patients were kept nonweight bearing on crutches for 8 weeks. There were two plate breakages requiring revision and one requiring spica casting to achieve healing.

Standard Compression Plating: Technique

The injured thigh is prepared and draped on a radiolucent operating table. The femur is approached laterally. The vastus lateralis is retracted anteriorly to expose the femur. Soft tissue attachments to the bone are preserved to the extent possible. Fragments are lagged into place and secured with a DCP. A 4.5-mm or larger compression plate is used in children. If the fracture is at either end of the bone, leaving insufficient bone for cortical fixation, fully threaded cancellous screws add to the stability of fixation and are preferable to either cortical or partially threaded cancellous screws. Both interfragmentary compression and dynamic compression techniques can be used to achieve stability and anatomic alignment. Locking screws are rarely necessary and may be difficult to remove if they "cold-weld" to the plate.

Technique Tips

A long and strong plate should be used. Soft tissue stripping should be limited, and three screws should be used proximal and distal to the fracture site.

Postoperative Management

Protected weight bearing is progressed to weight bearing to tolerance. Active range-of-motion exercise of the hip and knee is encouraged.

Submuscular Bridge Plating

Submuscular bridge plating[81,109] allows stable internal fixation with maintenance of vascularity to small fragments of bone, facilitating early healing (Fig 22-29).

Modern techniques of femoral plating,[177] limiting incisions, maintaining the periosteum, using long plates, and filling only a few selected screw holes, are being adopted by an increasing number of pediatric orthopaedic trauma surgeons as a valuable tool to manage length-unstable femoral fractures. Pathologic fractures, especially in the distal femoral metaphysis, create large areas of bone loss that can be treated with open biopsy, plate fixation, and immediate bone grafting.

Kanlic et al.[108] reported a series of 51 patients with submuscular bridge plating with up to 10 year follow-up; 55% had unstable fracture patterns. There were two significant complications: one plate breakage (3.5 mm) and one fracture after plate removal. Functional outcome was excellent, with 8% significant leg-length discrepancy. Hedequist et al.[80] reported 32 patients aged 6 to 15 years old, most of whom had fractures that were comminuted, pathologic, osteopenic, or in a difficult location. Rozbruch et al.[177] described modern techniques of plate fixation popularized by the AO Association for the Study of InternalFixation that include indirect reduction, biologic approaches to internal fixation, and greater use of blade plates and locked plates (Fig. 22-30).

In very rare situations, such as when there is limited bone for fixation between the fracture and the physes, locked plating techniques may be valuable. This technique provides greater stability by securing the plate with a fixed-angle screw in which the threads lock to the plate, as well as in the bone. This effectively converts the screw–plate to a fixed-angle blade plate device. In using this type of device, one should lock first, then compress, and finally lock the plate on the opposite side of the fracture. The locked plate can be used with an extensile exposure or with a submuscular plating technique, but the latter is more difficult and should be attempted only when the technique is mastered.

We do not routinely use locking plates unless a pathologic lesion, severe osteopenia, or severe comminution is present. Locking screws can cold-weld to the plate, later turning a simple implant removal into a very difficult procedure involving large exposures, cutting of the implant, and possible locally destructive maneuvers to remove the screws.

Submuscular Bridge Plating: Technique

The technique for submuscular bridge plating of pediatric femoral fractures has been well described in recent publications.[108,185,186] The patient is positioned on a fracture table, and a provisional reduction is obtained with gentle traction. In most cases, a 4.5-mm narrow, low-contact DCP plate is used. In osteopenic patients or when there is a proximal or distal fracture, locking plates may be used. A very long plate, with 10 to 16 holes, is preferred; the plate selection is finalized by obtaining an image with the plate over the anterior thigh, assuring that there are six screw holes proximal and distal to the fracture (although in some more proximal and distal fractures, only three holes will be available). Depending on the fracture location and thus the position of the plate, the plate will need to be contoured to accommodate the proximal or distal femur. The table-top plate bender is used to create a small flare proximally for the plate to accommodate the contour of the greater trochanter or a larger flare to accommodate the distal femoral metaphysis. The plate must be contoured anatomically because the fixed femur will come to assume the shape of the plate after screw fixation. A 2- to 3-cm incision is made over the distal femur, just above the level of the physis. Exposure of the periosteum just below the vastus lateralis facilitates the submuscular passage of the plate. A Cobb elevator is used to dissect the plane

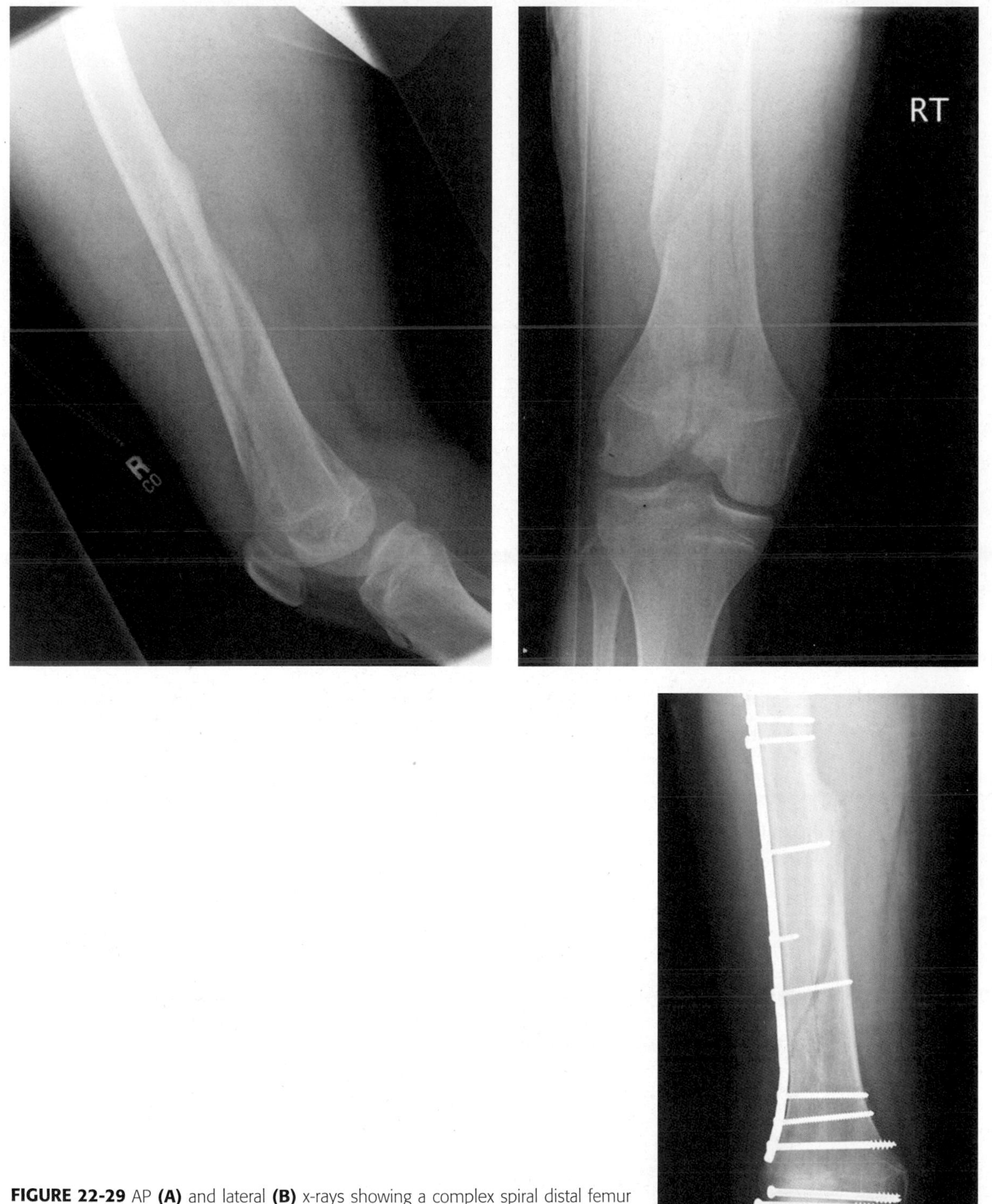

FIGURE 22-29 AP **(A)** and lateral **(B)** x-rays showing a complex spiral distal femur fracture that extends into the joint. This is a variation of Salter-Harris type IV fracture. **C.** Ihe fracture was managed with submuscular plating and percutaneous lag screw fixation of the distal femoral condyle fractures.

between the periosteum and the vastus lateralis. The fracture site is not exposed, and, in general, a proximal incision is not required. The plate is inserted underneath the vastus lateralis, and the femoral shaft is held to length by traction. The plate is advanced slowly, allowing the surgeon to feel the bone against the tip of the plate. Fluoroscopy is helpful in determining proper positioning of the plate. A bolster is placed under the thigh to help maintain sagittal alignment. Once the plate is in position and the femur is out to length, Kirschner wires are placed in the most proximal and most distal holes of the plate to maintain length (Fig. 22-31). Fluoroscopy is used to check the AP and lateral views and to be sure the bone is at appropriate length at this point. A third Kirschner wire can be used to provide a more stable reduction of the femoral shaft. Although screws can be used to facilitate angular reduction to the plate, length must be achieved before the initiation of fixation.

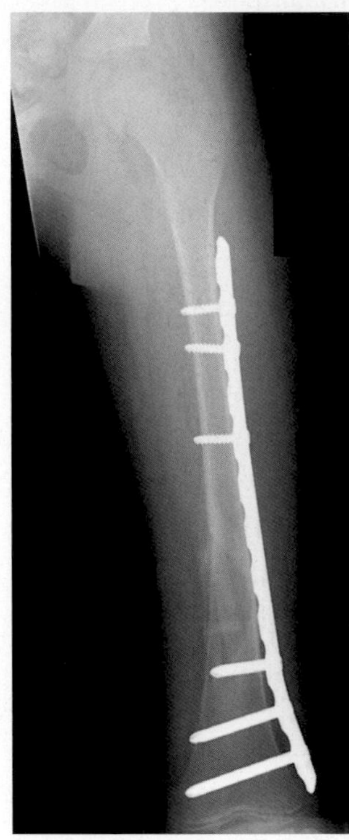

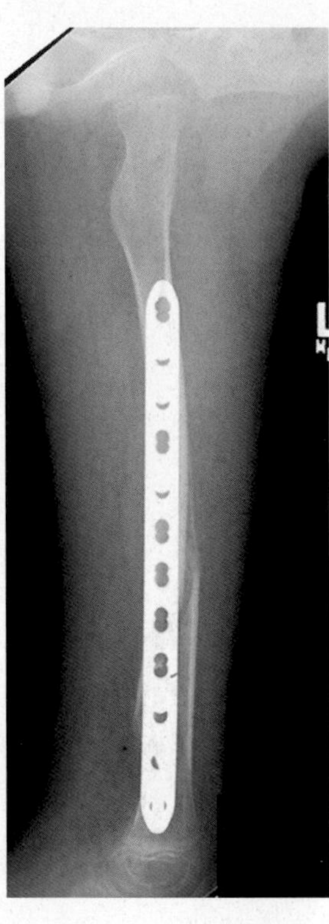

A B

FIGURE 22-30 A. This child with an unstable femoral fracture in osteopenic bone was managed with a submuscular locking plate providing alignment and stability. **B.** The lateral bow of the femur may be partially preserved despite a straight plate.

The principles of external fixation are used in choosing sites for screw fixation. Greater spread of screws increases the stability of fracture fixation. We generally place one screw through the distal incision under direct observation. At the opposite end of the femur, the next most proximal screw is placed to fix length and provisionally improve alignment. Central screws are then placed, using a free-hand technique with the "perfect circle" alignment of the plate over the fracture fragments. Stab holes are made centrally for drill and screw insertion. Rather than using a depth gauge directly, because the bone will be pulled to the plate, the depth gauge is placed over the thigh itself to measure appropriate length of the screw. When screws are inserted, a Vicryl (Ethicon, Inc., Somerville, NJ) tie is placed around the shank to avoid losing the screw during percutaneous placement. Self-tapping screws are required for this procedure. Six cortices are sought on either side of the fracture.

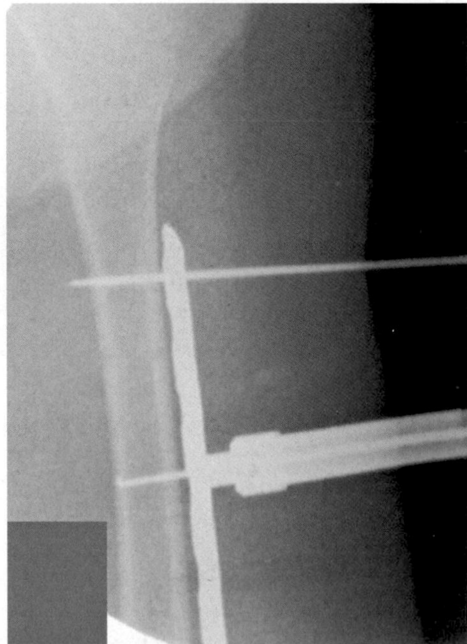

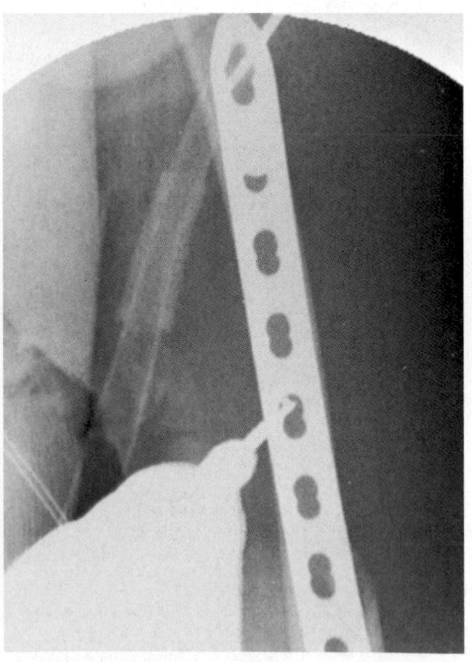

A B

FIGURE 22-31 A. A Kirschner wire is inserted in the end holes of the plate to maintain length. **B.** Drill holes and screws are placed with fluoroscope imaging.

The postoperative management includes protected weight bearing on crutches with no need for cast immobilization, as long as stable fixation is achieved. At times, there is benefit to a knee immobilizer; however, in general, this is not required. Early weight bearing in some series of plate fixation has resulted in a low but significant incidence of plate breakage and nonunion. These complications should be decreased by a cautious period of postoperative management.

There are occasional cases with sufficient osteopenia or comminution to require a locked plate to provide secure fixation. In using a locked plate submuscularly, a large enough incision must be used to be sure the bone is against the plate when it is locked. The articular fragment is fixed first to ensure that the angular relationship between the joint surface and the shaft is perfect.

Complications of Plate Fixation

Extensive dissection and periosteal stripping during traditional compression plate application may lead to overgrowth. Overgrowth was not a significant problem in the series of Kregor et al.,[115] with an average increase in length of 0.9 cm (range 0.5 to 1.5 cm), but Ward et al.[208] reported several patients with considerable overgrowth (approximately 1 inch), and Hansen[79] reported overgrowth of an inch in a 12-year-old boy, suggesting that overgrowth is possible in children over 10 years of age. Eren et al.[56] reported a series of 40 children aged 4 to 10 years with significant lengthening on the operated side in 40% of patients, averaging 1.2 cm (0.4 to 1.8 cm).

Fyodorov et al.[67] reported implant failure in 2 of 23 femoral shaft fractures treated with DCPs. One was treated with revision plating and the other with spica casting; both fractures healed uneventfully. No other complications were noted in their patients.

Refracture is rare at the end of the plate or through screw holes, and whether bone atrophy under a plate is caused by stress shielding or by avascularity of the cortex is unknown. Although still somewhat controversial, the plate and screws can be removed at 1 year after fracture to avoid fracture at the end of the plate.

Quadriceps strength after plate fixation appears not to be compromised[61] relative to intramedullary fixation or cast immobilization.

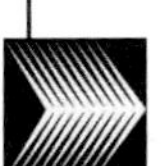

AUTHORS' PREFERRED TREATMENT

For stable femoral fractures in children under 6 months of age, we use a Pavlik harness. One of us gently wraps the thigh in Webril (Kendall Health Care Products, Mansfield, MA) before placing the harness. If the fracture is unstable, usually the proximal fragment is flexed and a Pavlik harness is the ideal device for reducing and holding the fracture. The use of a Pavlik harness requires an attentive and compliant caregiver. A Gore-tex lined spica is an alternative, especially for bigger, older babies. Traction with a spica cast is rarely if ever needed in this group.

For children 6 months to 5 years of age with an isolated femoral fracture, an early spica cast is usually the treatment of choice. In a typical low-energy toddler femoral fracture, we have noted similar clinical results but much happier families and children when we use a one-leg walking spica, so this has become our choice for this age group. Some children with a walking spica benefit from cast wedging 1 to 2 weeks after injury, so we prepare families for this possibility. A Gore-tex liner, if available, markedly improves skin care. If length or alignment cannot be maintained in an early spica cast (this is rare in low-energy fractures), traction followed by casting can be used. We typically use a distal femoral traction pin and place the child in a 90/90 or oblique position in the bed for traction. We must emphasize that over 95% of infants and toddlers can be managed without traction with a low complication rate and low cost. In children with multiple-system trauma, either flexible intramedullary nailing or external fixation is often a better choice, based on the fracture anatomy and the soft-tissue injury. Traction is rarely used in patients with multiple-system trauma.

In children 5 to 11 years of age, retrograde flexible intramedullary nailing is generally the safest and best option for length-stable fractures (and many length-unstable) fractures. Submuscular bridge plating or external fixation is used for unstable fracture patterns, comminuted fractures, and fractures with severe soft tissue injury. Early spica casting can be used for nondisplaced or minimally displaced fractures in this age group. In certain situations, the family and surgeon prefer a nonsurgical option; in such cases, spica casting, usually with traction, can be used in school-aged children.

In children 11 years to maturity, we generally prefer a trochanteric-entry locked intramedullary nail or submuscular bridge plating. Flexible intramedullary rods are also effective in this age group (Fig. 22-32), especially for midshaft transverse fractures in smaller children. The surgeon should be aware that the complication rate rises with flexible nailing in this older group.[149] External fixation is occasionally valuable in the 11- to 16-year-old group, particularly in complex proximal or distal fractures. Healing is slow, however, and the full treatment course may take 4 months or more. Locked plating can be used for subtrochanteric and supracondylar fractures of the femur, whereas intramedullary nails are ideal for midshaft fractures. If antegrade rodding is chosen, a transtrochanteric approach is used. There is a limited role for retrograde locked intramedullary nailing in adolescents approaching skeletal maturity.

COMPLICATIONS OF FEMORAL SHAFT FRACTURES

Leg-Length Discrepancy

The most common sequela after femoral shaft fractures in children is leg-length discrepancy. The fractured femur may be initially short from overriding of the fragments at union; growth acceleration occurs to "make up" the difference, but often this acceleration continues and the injured leg ends up being longer. The potential for growth stimulation from femoral fractures has long been recognized, but the exact cause of this phenomenon is still unknown. Growth acceleration has been attributed to age,

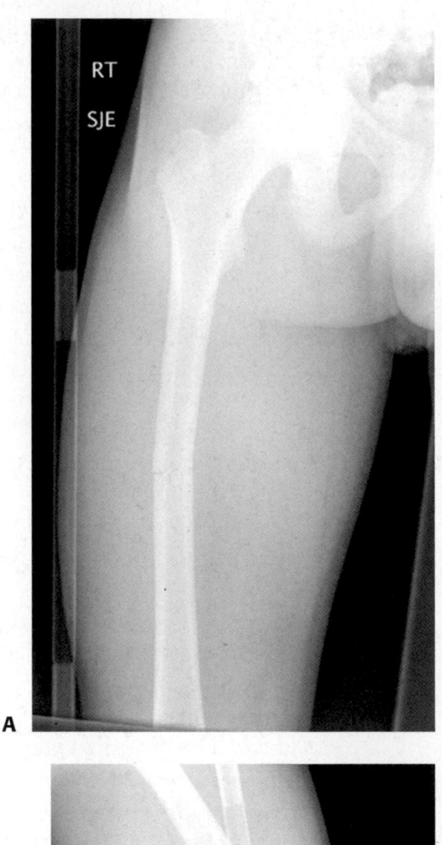

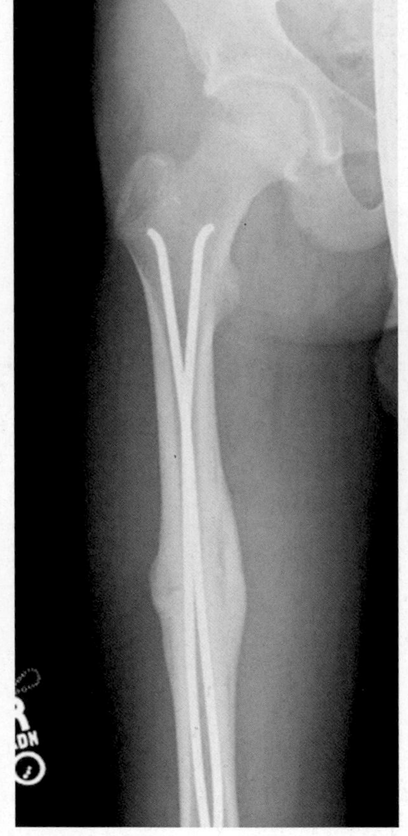

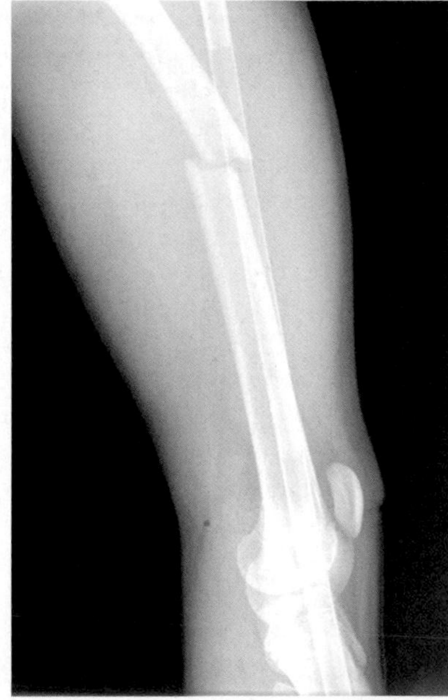

FIGURE 22-32 Successful use of titanium elastic nails in older teenager. This 15-year-old sustained a minimally displaced midshaft femur fracture AP **(A)** and lateral **(B)** views at presentation. **C.** This x-ray, taken 3 months after injury, shows that the fracture healed in perfect alignment with abundant callus.

sex, fracture type, fracture level, handedness, and the amount of overriding of the fracture fragments. Age seems to be the most constant factor, but fractures in the proximal third of the femur and oblique comminuted fractures also have been associated with relatively greater growth acceleration

Shortening

Because the average overgrowth after femoral fracture is approximately 1.5 cm, shortening of 2 to 3 cm in the cast is the maximal acceptable amount. The maximal acceptable shortening depends on the age of the child; for example, in a 6-year-old child, 2.5 cm may be acceptable, whereas only 1 to 2 cm should be accepted in a 14-year-old approaching skeletal maturity.

Overgrowth

Overgrowth after femoral fracture is most common in children 2 to 10 years of age. The average overgrowth is 0.9 cm, with a range of 0.4 to 2.5 cm.[182] Overgrowth occurs whether the fracture is short, at length, or overpulled in traction at the time of healing. In general, overgrowth occurs most rapidly during the first 2 years after fracture and to a much lesser degree for the next year or so.[72]

Truesdell[201] first reported the phenomenon of overgrowth in 1921, and many researchers since have verified the existence of growth stimulation after fracture.[1,2,4,8,38,40,53,129,138,168] The relationship of the location of the fracture to growth is somewhat controversial. Staheli[190] and Malkawi et al.[129] reported that overgrowth was greatest if the fracture occurred in the proximal third of the femur, whereas Henry[89] stated that the most overgrowth occurred in fractures in the distal third of the femur. Other investigators have found no relationship between fracture location and growth stimulation.[53,89,171,182] The relationship between fracture type and overgrowth also is controversial. In general, most researchers believe that no specific relationship exists between fracture type and overgrowth, but some have reported overgrowth to be more frequent after spiral, oblique, and comminuted fractures associated with greater trauma.

Angular Deformity

Some degree of angular deformity is frequent after femoral shaft fractures in children, but this usually remodels with growth. Angular remodeling occurs at the site of fracture, with appositional new bone formation in the concavity of the long bone. Differential physeal growth also occurs in response to diaphyseal angular deformity. Wallace and Hoffman[207] stated that 74% of the remodeling that occurs is physeal, and appositional remodeling at the fracture site occurs to a much lesser degree. However, this appears to be somewhat age dependent. It is clear that angular remodeling occurs best in the direction of motion at the adjacent joint.[207] That is, anterior and posterior remodeling in the femur occurs rapidly and with little residual deformity. In contrast, remodeling of a varus or valgus deformity occurs more slowly. The differential physeal growth in a varus or valgus direction in the distal femur causes compensatory deformity, which is usually insignificant. In severe varus bowing, however, a hypoplastic lateral condyle results, which may cause a distal femoral valgus deformity if the varus bow is corrected.

Guidelines for acceptable alignment vary widely. The range of acceptable anterior and posterior angulation varies from 30 to 40 degrees in children up to 2 years of age (Fig. 22-33), decreasing to 10 degrees in older children and adolescents.[128] The range of acceptable varus and valgus angulation also becomes smaller with age. Varus angulation in infants and children should be between 10 and 15 degrees, although greater degrees of angulation may have a satisfactory outcome. Acceptable valgus angulation is 20 to 30 degrees in infants, 15 to 20 degrees in children up to 5 years of age, and 10 degrees in older children and adolescents. Compensation for deformity around the knee is limited, so guidelines for the distal femoral fractures should be stricter than for proximal femoral fractures.

Late development of genu recurvatum deformity of the proximal tibia after femoral shaft fracture has been most often reported as a complication of traction pin or wire placement through or near the anterior aspect of the proximal tibial physis, excessive traction, pin track infection, or prolonged cast immobilization.[203] However, proximal tibial growth arrest may complicate femoral shaft fracture, presumably as a result of occult

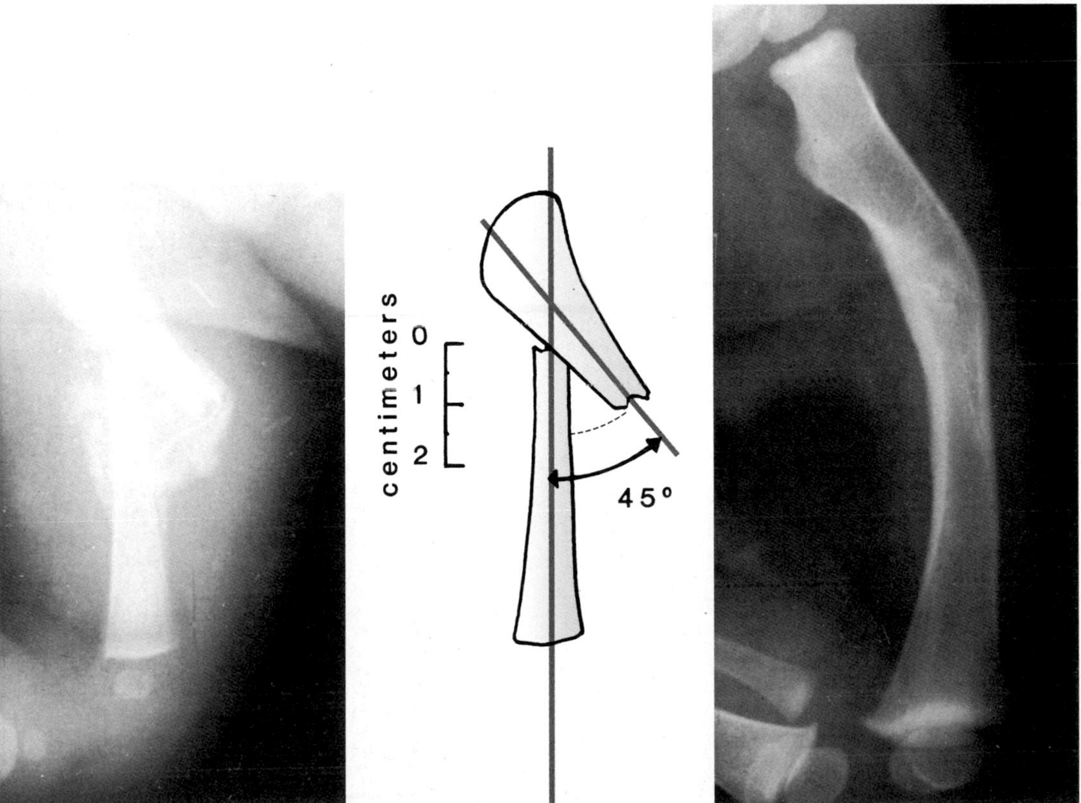

FIGURE 22-33 Remodeling potential of the femur during infancy. This infant sustained a femoral fracture during a breech delivery and was placed in a spica cast but with insufficient flexion of the hip. **Left:** At 3 weeks, union is evident with about 45 degrees of angulation in the sagittal plane and 1.5 cm of overriding. **Center:** Line drawing demonstrating true angulation. **Right:** Twelve months later, the anterior angulation has reduced to a level such that it was not apparent to the family, and the shortening has reduced to less than 1 cm.

injury.[94] Femoral pins are preferred for traction, but if tibial pins are required, the proximal anterior tibial physis must be avoided.[146] Femoral traction pins should be placed one or two fingerbreadths proximal to the superior pole of the patella to avoid the distal femoral physis.

If significant angular deformity is present after fracture union, corrective osteotomy should be delayed for at least a year unless the deformity is severe enough to markedly impair function. This will allow determination of remodeling potential before deciding that surgical correction is necessary. The ideal osteotomy corrects the deformity at the site of fracture. In juvenile patients, however, metaphyseal osteotomy of the proximal or distal femur may be necessary. In adolescents with midshaft deformities, diaphyseal osteotomy and fixation with an interlocking intramedullary nail are often preferable.

Rotational Deformity

According to Verbeek,[204] rotational deformities of 10 degrees to more than 30 degrees occur in one third of children after conservative treatment of femoral shaft fractures. Malkawi et al.[129] found asymptomatic rotational deformities of less than 10 degrees in two thirds of their 31 patients. Torsional deformity usually is expressed as increased femoral anteversion on the fractured side compared with the opposite side, as demonstrated by physical exam; a difference of more than 10 degrees has been the criterion of significant deformity. However, Brouwer et al.[24] challenged this criterion, citing differences of 0 to 15 degrees in a control group of 100 normal volunteers. The accuracy of measurements from plain radiographs also has been disputed, and Norbeck et al.[156] suggested the use of computed tomographic (CT) scanning for greater accuracy.

Rotational remodeling in childhood femoral fractures is another controversy in the search for criteria on which to base therapeutic judgments. According to Davids[46] and Braten et al.,[23] up to 25 degrees of rotational malalignment at the time of healing of femoral fractures appears to be well-tolerated in children. In their patients with more than 25 degrees of rotational malalignment, however, deformity caused clinical complaints. Davids[46] found no spontaneous correction in his study of malunions based on CT measurements, but the length of follow-up is insufficient to state that no rotational remodeling occurs. Brouwer et al.[24] and others[14,77,159,204] reported slow rotational correction over time. Buchholz et al.[27] documented 5 children between 3 and 6 years old with increased femoral anteversion of 10 degrees or more after fracture healing. In 3 of the 5 children, there was full correction of the rotational deformity but the oldest of the children the deformity failed to correct spontaneously.

Certainly, in older adolescents, no significant rotational remodeling will occur. In infants and juveniles, some rotational deformity can be accepted[60] because either true rotational remodeling or functional adaptation allows resumption of normal gait. Up to 30 degrees of malrotation in the femur should result in no functional impairment unless there is pre-existing rotational malalignment. The goal, however, should be to reduce a rotational deformity to 10 degrees, based on alignment of the proximal and distal femur on x-ray, interpretation of skin and soft tissue envelope alignment, and correct positioning within a cast, based on the muscle pull on the proximal fragment. The distal fragment should be lined up with the position of the proximal fragment determined by the muscles inserted on it (see Fig. 22-3).

Delayed Union

Delayed union of femoral shaft fractures is uncommon in children. The rate of healing also is related to soft-tissue injury and type of treatment. The time to fracture union in most children is rapid and age dependent. In infants, the fracture can be healed in 2 to 3 weeks. In children under 5 years of age, healing usually occurs in 4 to 6 weeks. In children 5 to 10 years of age, fracture healing is somewhat slower, requiring 8 to 10 weeks. Throughout adolescence, the time to healing continues to lengthen. By the age of 15 years, the mean time to healing is about 13 weeks, with a range from 10 to 15 weeks (Fig. 22-34). Application of an external fixation device appears to delay callus formation and slow the rate of healing. Flexible nailing allows some motion at the fracture site, promoting extensive callus formation. In adults, there is an association between nonunion and the use of nonsteroidal anti-inflammatory drugs (NSAIDs) after injury and delayed fracture healing,[1,60] which is very significant. Although there is not similar data for children, perhaps patients with risk factors for delayed healing should avoid NSAIDs.

Bone grafting and internal fixation with either a compression plate or locked intramedullary nail are the usual treatment for delayed union in older children and adolescents. Delayed union of a femoral fracture treated with casting in a child 1 to 6 years of age is probably best treated by continuing cast immobilization until bridging callus forms or (rarely) by additional bone grafting.

Nonunion

Nonunions of pediatric femoral fractures are rare.[122] They tend to occur in adolescents, in infected fractures, or in fractures with segmental bone loss or severe soft tissue loss. Tibial fractures

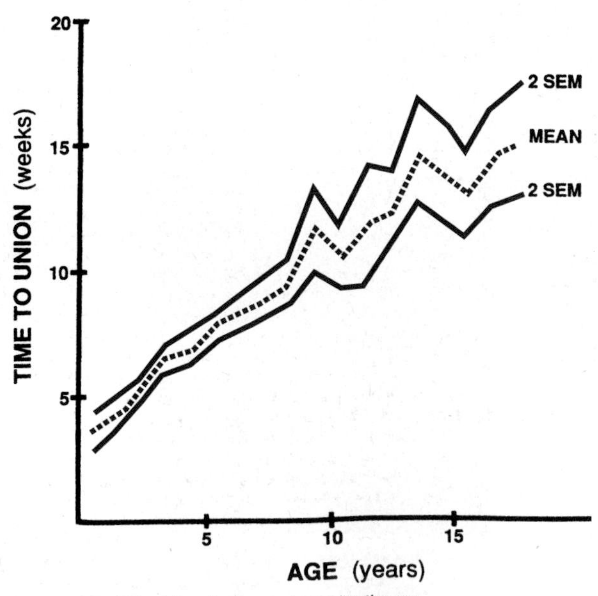

FIGURE 22-34 Time required for union of femoral shaft fractures in childhood and adolescence. (From Skak SV, Jensen TT. Femoral shaft fracture in 265 children. Acta Orthop Scand 1988;59:704–707, with permission.)

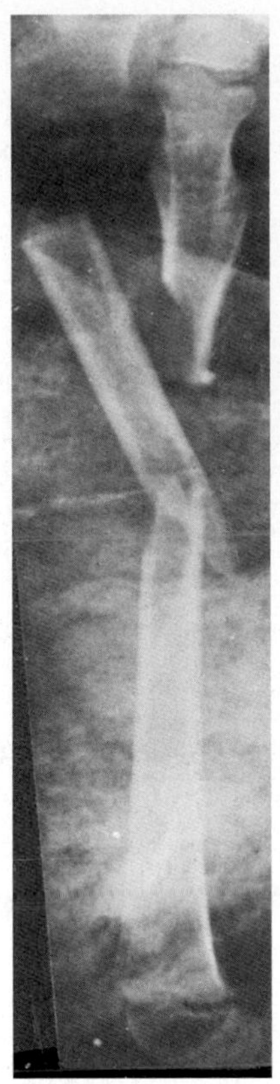
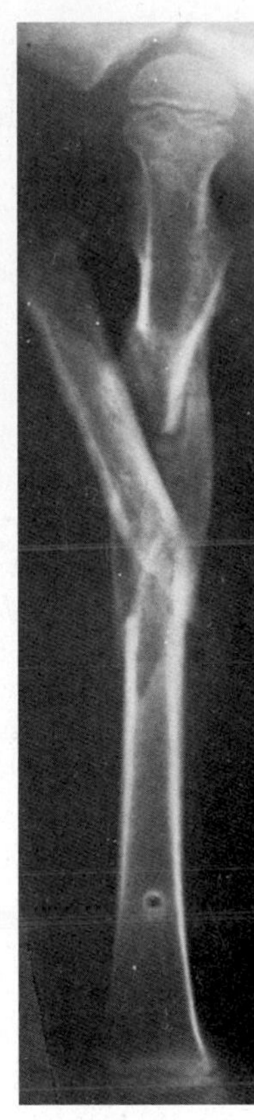
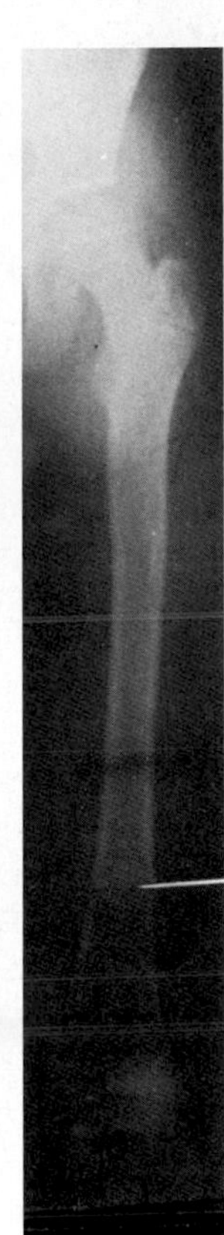

FIGURE 22-35 The effectiveness of remodeling of the femur in a child. **Left:** Comminuted fracture in an 8-year-old child managed with a femoral pin incorporated in a spica cast. The midfragment is markedly angulated. **Center:** Fracture after union 12 weeks later with filling in of the defect and early absorption of the protruding fragment. **Right:** Appearance at age 12 with only a minimal degree of irregularity of the upper femur remaining.

are the most common source of pediatric nonunions; femoral fractures account for only 15% of nonunions in children. Even in segmental fractures with bone loss, young children may have sufficient osteogenic potential to fill in a significant fracture gap (Fig. 22-35).[142] For the rare femoral shaft nonunion in a child 5 to 10 years of age, bone grafting and plate-and-screw fixation have been traditional treatment methods, but more recently insertion of an interlocking intramedullary nail and bone grafting have been preferred, especially in children over 10 to 12 years of age. Aksoy et al.[3] reported a small series of nonunions and malunions salvaged with titanium elastic nails. Union was achieved in 6 to 9 months in most cases.

Robertson et al.[174] reported the use of external fixators in 11 open femoral fractures. The time to union was delayed, but a satisfactory outcome occurred without subsequent procedures. This supports the belief that the rates of delayed union and nonunion are low in pediatric femoral fractures, because open fractures would have the highest rates of delayed union.

Muscle Weakness

Weakness after femoral fracture has been described in the hip abductor musculature, quadriceps, and hamstrings, but persistent weakness in some or all of these muscle groups seldom causes a long-term functional problem. Hennrikus et al.[88] found that quadriceps strength was decreased in 30% of his patients and 18% had a significant decrease demonstrated by a one-leg hop test. Thigh atrophy of 1 cm was present in 42% of patients. These deficits appeared to be primarily related to the degree of initial displacement of the fracture. Finsen et al.[61] found hamstring and quadriceps deficits in patients with femoral shaft fractures treated with either rods or plates.

Damholt and Zdravkovic[45] documented quadriceps weakness in approximately one third of patients with femoral fractures, and Viljanto et al.[205] reported that this weakness was present whether patients were treated operatively or nonoperatively. Biyani et al.[17] found that hip abductor weakness was related to ipsilateral fracture magnitude, long intramedullary rods, and, to a lesser degree, heterotopic ossification from intramedullary rodding. Hedin and Larsson[83] found no significant weakness in any of 31 patients treated with external fixation for femoral fractures based on either Cybex testing (Cybex International, Inc., Medway, MA) or a one-leg hop test. They suggested that the weakness seen in other studies may be related to prolonged immobilization.

Injury to the quadriceps muscle probably occurs at the time of femoral fracture, and long-term muscle deficits may persist in some patients regardless of treatment. Severe scarring and contracture of the quadriceps occasionally require quadricepsplasty.[99]

Infection

Infection may rarely complicate a closed femoral shaft fracture, with hematogenous seeding of the hematoma and subsequent osteomyelitis. Fever is commonly associated with femoral fractures during the first week after injury,[191] but persistent fever or fever that spikes exceedingly high may be an indication of infection. One should have a high index of suspicion for infection in type III open femoral fractures. A series of 44 open femoral fractures[98] reported no infection in types I and II fractures, but a 50% (5 of 10) of type III fractures developed osteomyelitis. Presumably, this occurs because of the massive soft tissue damage accompanying this injury.

Pin track infections occasionally occur with the use of skeletal traction, but most are superficial infections that resolve with local wound care and antibiotic therapy. Occasionally, however, the infections may lead to osteomyelitis of the femoral metaphysis or a ring sequestrum that requires surgical débridement.

Neurovascular Injury

Nerve and vascular injuries are uncommonly associated with femoral fractures in children.[49,104,176,191] An estimated 1.3% of femoral fractures in children are accompanied by vascular injury[49,104,176,191] such as intimal tears, total disruptions, or injuries resulting in the formation of pseudoaneurysms.[180] Vascular injury occurs most frequently with displaced Salter-Harris physeal fractures of the distal femur and distal femoral metaphyseal fractures. If arteriography indicates that vascular repair is necessary after femoral shaft fracture, open reduction with internal fixation or external fixation of the fracture is usually recommended first to stablize the fracture and prevent injury of the repair. Secondary limb ischemia also has been reported after the use of both skin and skeletal traction. Documentation of peripheral pulses at the time of presentation, as well as throughout treatment, is necessary.

Nerve abnormalities reported with femoral fractures in children include those caused by direct trauma to the sciatic or femoral nerve at the time of fracture and injuries to the peroneal nerve during treatment. Weiss et al.[209] reported peroneal nerve palsies in 4 of 110 children with femoral fractures treated with early 90/90 hip spica casting. They recommended extending the initial short-leg portion of the cast above the knee to decrease tension on the peroneal nerve.

Riew et al.[173] reported eight nerve palsies in 35 consecutive patients treated with locked intramedullary rodding. The nerve injuries were associated with delay in treatment, preoperative shortening, and boot traction. Resolution occurred in less than 1 week in 6 of 8 patients.

Many peroneal nerve deficits after pediatric femoral shaft fractures will resolve with time. In infants, however, the development of an early contracture of the Achilles tendon is more likely. Because of the rapid growth in younger children, this contracture can develop quite early; if peroneal nerve injury is suspected, an ankle-foot orthosis should be used until the peroneal nerve recovers. If peroneal, femoral, or sciatic nerve deficit is present at initial evaluation of a closed fracture, no exploration is indicated. If a nerve deficit occurs during reduction or treatment, the nerve should be explored. Persistent nerve loss without recovery over a 4- to 6-month period is an indication for exploration.

Compartment Syndrome

Compartment syndromes of the thigh musculature are rare, but have been reported in patients with massive thigh swelling after femoral fracture and in patients treated with intramedullary rod fixation.[144] If massive swelling of thigh musculature occurs and pain is out of proportion to that expected from a femoral fracture, compartment pressure measurements should be obtained and decompression by fasciotomy should be considered. It is probable that some patients with quadriceps fibrosis[171] and quadriceps weakness[43,196] after femoral fracture had intracompartmental pressure phenomenon. Mathews et al.[132] reported two compartment syndromes in the "well leg" occurring when the patient was positioned for femoral nailing in the hemilithotomy position. Vascular insufficiency related to Bryant traction may produce signs of compartment syndrome with muscle ischemia.[38] Janzing et al.[105] reported the occurrence of compartment syndrome when skin traction was used for treatment of femoral fractures. Skin traction has been associated with compartment syndrome in the lower leg in both the fractured and nonfractured side. It is important to realize that in a traumatized limb, circumferential traction needs to be monitored closely and is contraindicated in the multiply injured or head-injured child. As noted in the spica cast section, several cases of leg compartment syndrome have been reported after spica cast treatment in younger children with femoral fractures.

SPECIAL FRACTURES OF THE FEMORAL SHAFT

Subtrochanteric Fractures

Subtrochanteric fractures generally heal slowly, angulate into varus, and are more prone to overgrowth. These fractures offer a challenge, as the bone available between the fracture site and the femoral neck limits internal fixation options. In younger children, traction and casting can be successful.[50] Three weeks of traction is usually necessary. The cast should have a good valgus mold at the fracture site, and the fracture should be monitored closely in the first 2 weeks after casting. When the patient returns for follow-up, if the subtrochanteric fracture has slipped into varus malangulation, the cast can be wedged in clinic (Fig. 22-36) or casting can be abandoned for another method. Parents should be warned that loss of reduction in the cast is quite common, and wedging in clinic is a routine step in management. An external fixation strategy can be quite successful if there is satisfactory room proximally to place pins. Once there is satisfactory callus (about 6 weeks), the fixator can be removed and weight bearing allowed in a walking spica (long leg cast with a pelvic band and a valgus mold to stabilize fracture in the first few weeks after external fixator removal). Flexible nailing can be used, with a proximal and distal entry strategy (Fig. 22-37). A pitfall in this fracture is thinking that the proximal fragment appears too short to use flexible intramedullary nails on the AP x-ray because the proximal fragment is pulled into flexion by the unopposed psoas muscle. Pombo et al.[164] reported a series of 13 children, average 8 years old, with subtrochanteric fractures treated with flexible nailing. Results were excellent or satisfactory in all cases. Submuscular plating can also produce satisfactory results.[103] In adolescents, there is insufficient experience with this fracture to determine at what age intramedullary fixation with a reconstruction-type nail and an angled transfixion screw into the femoral neck is indicated. Antegrade intramedullary nail systems place significant holes in the upper femoral neck and should be avoided. Unlike subtrochanteric fractures in adults, nonunions are rare in children with any treatment method.

Supracondylar Fractures

Supracondylar fractures represent as many as 12% of femoral shaft fractures[188] and are difficult to treat because the gastrocnemius muscle inserts just above the femoral condyles and pulls the distal fragment into a position of extension (Fig. 22-38),[75] making alignment difficult (see Fig. 22-3). The traditional methods of casting and single-pin traction may be satisfactory in

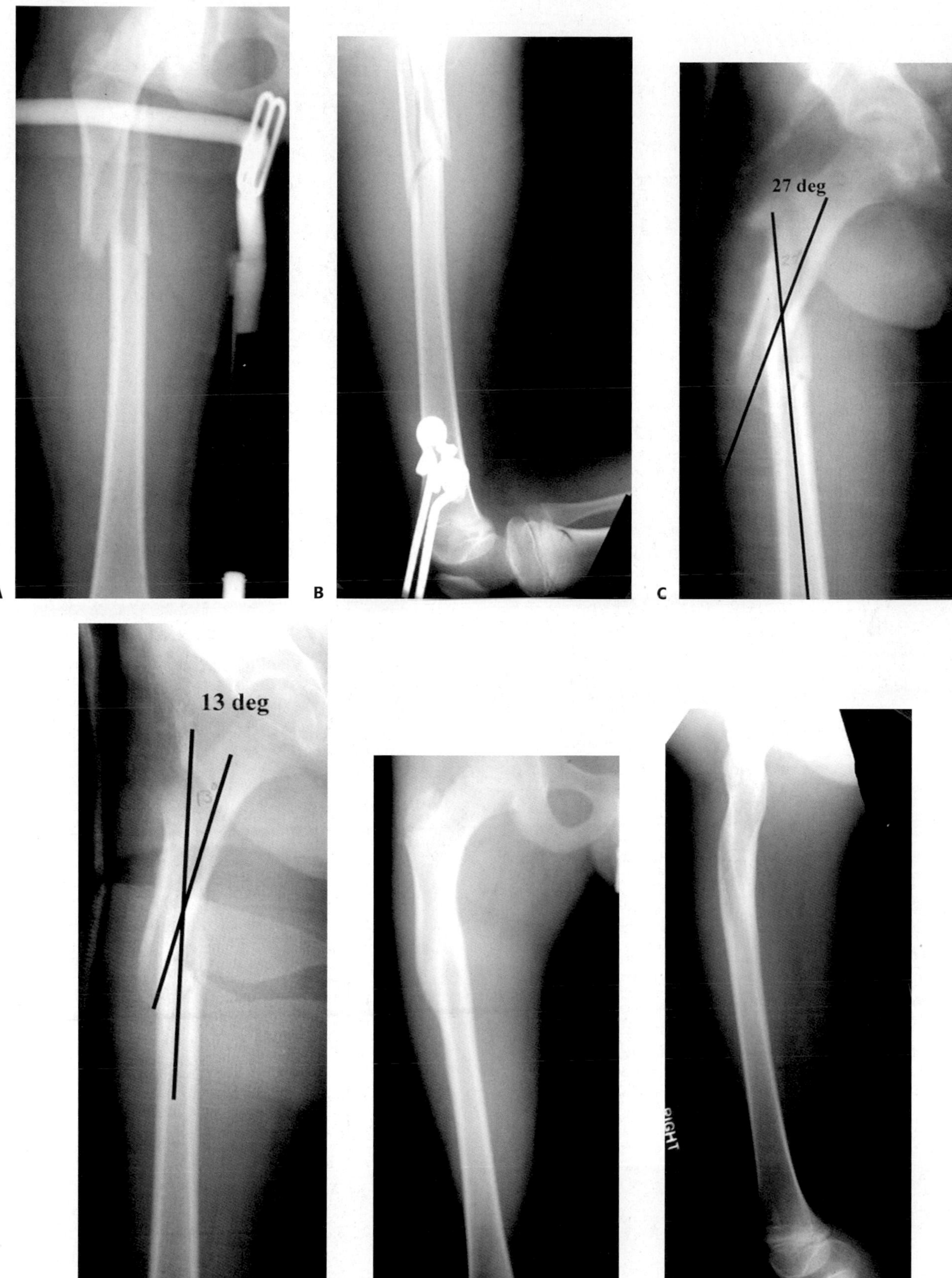

FIGURE 22-36 Comminuted spiral femur fracture in a 12-year-old treated with traction and casting. **A.** This 12-year-old was struck by a car, sustaining this length-unstable proximal femur fracture. The family wanted nonoperative management. X-ray at presentation shows a subtrochanteric spiral fracture with an intact, large butterfly fragment. **B.** The fracture is out to length in traction. The traction pin was removed and a cast was placed about 3 weeks after injury. **C.** The child returns 1 week after casting (4 weeks after injury) with 27 degrees of proximal femoral varus angulation. **D.** The cast was wedged, correcting the deformity to 13 degrees, which was deemed acceptable. **E,F.** This AP and lateral view, 6 months after injury, shows quite satisfactory alignment. There was no significant limb-length inequality or deformity on physical examination.

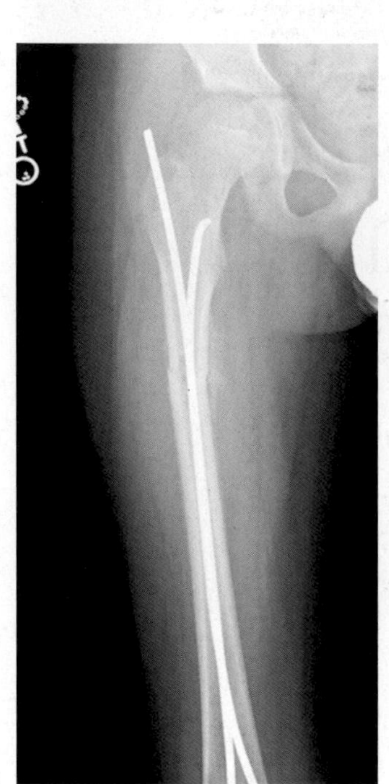
A

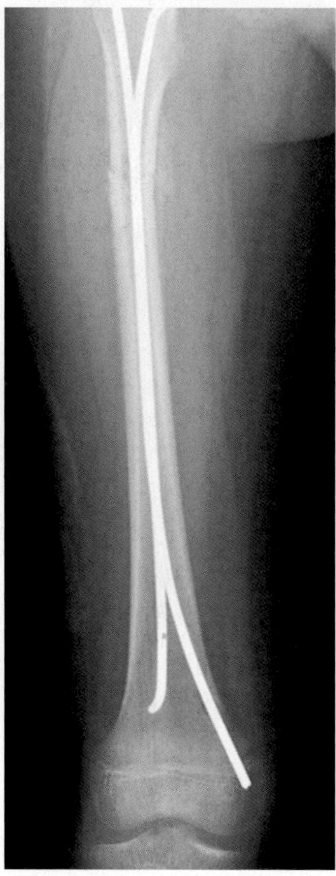
B

FIGURE 22-37 A,B. The combination of anterograde and retrograde titanium elastic nail insertion is a good solution for the proximal femur fracture.

young children (Fig. 22-39). As mentioned in the external fixation section, supracondylar fractures through a benign lesion are safely and efficiently treated with a brief period (4 to 6 weeks) of external fixation (Fig. 22-40), followed by a walking cast until the callus is solid and the pin sites are healed. In other cases, internal fixation is preferable, either with submuscular plating (see Figs. 22-29 and 22-41) and fully threaded cancellous screws (if there is sufficient metaphyseal length) or with crossed smooth Kirschner-wires transfixing the fracture from the epiphysis to the metaphysis, as described for distal femoral physeal separations.[181] If there is sufficient metaphyseal length, flexible nailing can be used so long as fixation is satisfactory. The flexible nails can be placed antegrade as originally described or retrograde if there is satisfactory distal bone for fixation near the nail entry site. Biomechanically, retrograde insertion is superior.[140] Pathologic fractures in this area are common, and an underlying lesion should always be sought.

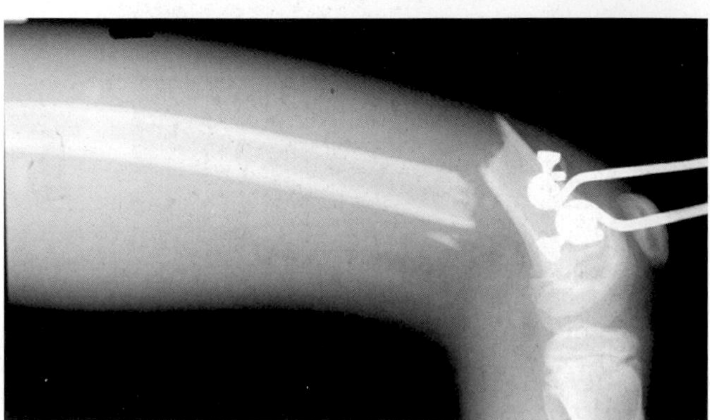

FIGURE 22-38 Treating distal femoral fractures in traction can be very difficult.

Open Femoral Fractures

Open femoral fractures are uncommon in children because of the large soft tissue compartment around the femur. Proper wound care, débridement, stabilization, and antibiotic therapy are required to reduce the chance of infection.[75] In a study by Hutchins et al.,[98] 70% of children with open femoral fractures had associated injuries and 90% were automobile related. The average time to healing was 17 weeks, and 50% of the Gustilo type III injuries developed osteomyelitis.

External fixation of open femoral shaft fractures simplifies wound care and allows early mobilization. The configuration of the external fixator is determined by the child's size and the fracture pattern. Generally, monolateral half-pin frames are satisfactory, but thin-wire circular frames may be necessary if bone loss is extensive. External fixation provides good fracture control, but, as always, family cooperation is required to manage pin and fixator care.

Plate fixation also allows early mobilization, as well as anatomic reduction of the femoral fracture. Wound care and treatment of other injuries are made easier in children with multiple trauma. However, this is an invasive technique with the potential for infection and additional injury to the already traumatized soft tissues in the area of the fracture. In emergency situations, plate fixation or intramedullary fixation can be used for Gustilo-Anderson types I and II fractures; type III fractures in older adolescents are better suited for external fixation or intramedul-

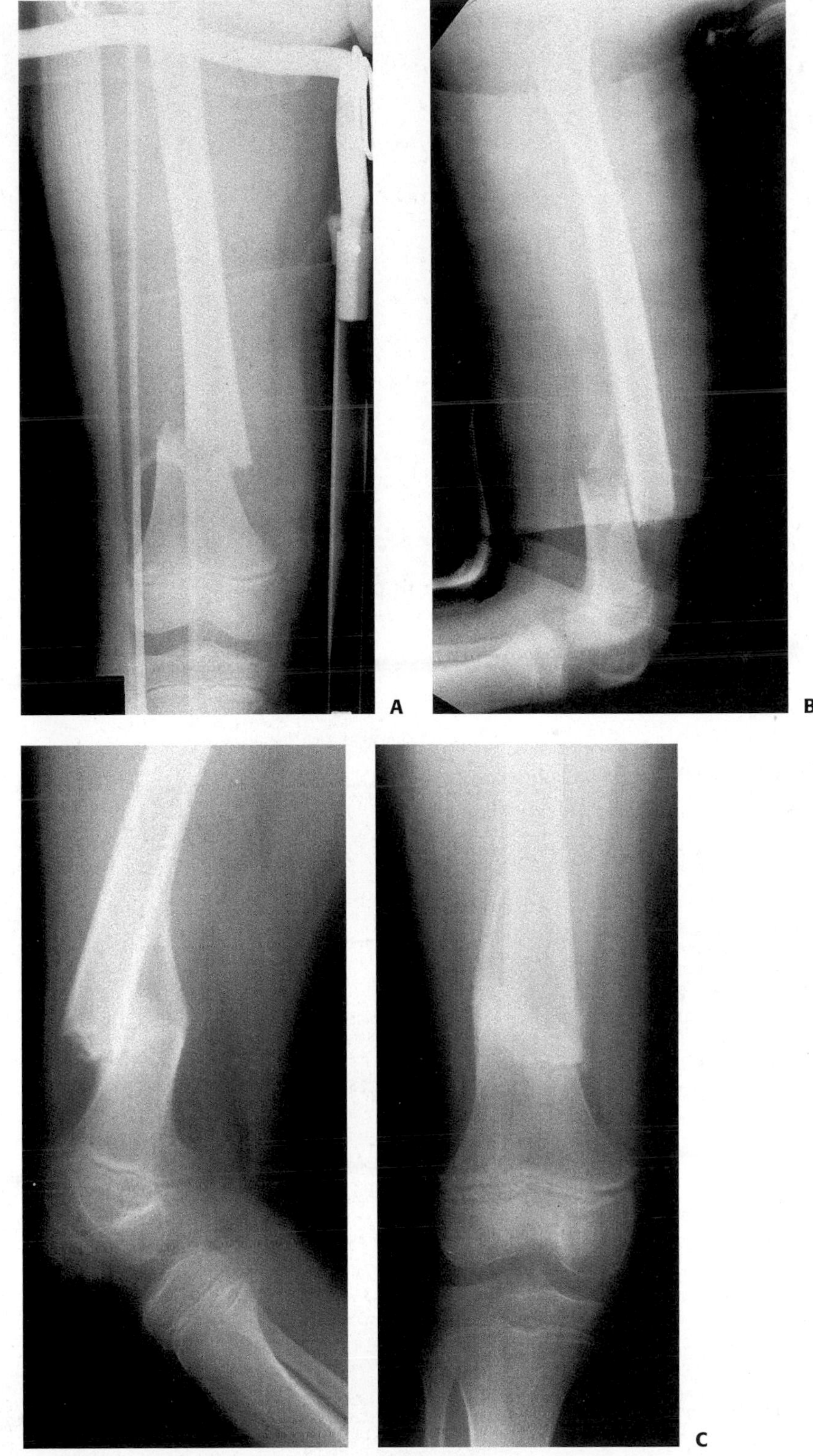

FIGURE 22-39 A. This 6-year-old patient sustained an unstable supracondylar fracture of the femur. **B.** The fracture was managed with immediate spica casting with the knee in 90 degrees of flexion, mandatory in such a case to prevent posterior angulation. **C.** Bayonet apposition is acceptable in a child this age.

lary nailing. Plate breakage can occur if bone grafting is not used for severe medial cortex comminution.

In older adolescents, submuscular plating or trochanteric-entry nailing is often the optimal treatment choice. Closed nailing after irrigation and drainage of the fracture allows early mobilization and easy wound care in patients with Gustilo-Anderson types I, II, IIIA, and IIIB injuries, but the risk of osteonecrosis must be recognized.

Femoral Fractures in Patients with Metabolic or Neuromuscular Disorders

For patients with osteogenesis imperfecta who have potential for ambulation, surgical treatment with Rush, Bailey-Dubow, or Fassier rods (see Chapter 6) is recommended for repeated fractures or angular deformity. Cast immobilization is minimized in patients with myelomeningocele or cerebral palsy because of the frequency of osteoporosis and refracture in these

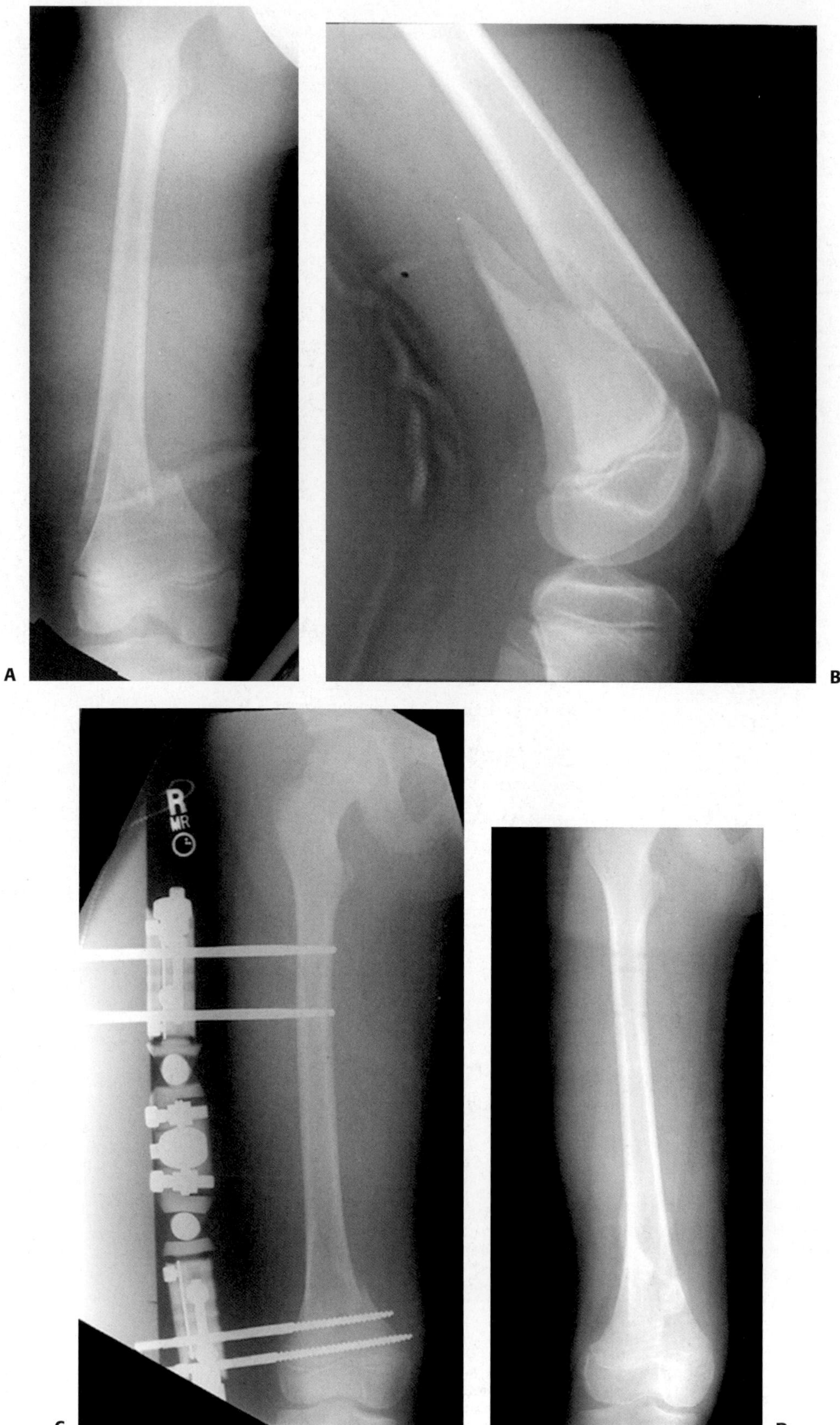

FIGURE 22-40 AP **(A)** and lateral **(B)** x-rays showing a fracture at the junction of the distal femoral metaphysis and diaphysis. **C.** The fractures reduced into near anatomic alignment, and an external fixator was used to control the distal fragment. **D.** The fixator was removed 8 weeks after injury, and after a brief period of weight bearing is tolerated in a long leg cast, the fracture has healed in anatomic alignment with no shortening.

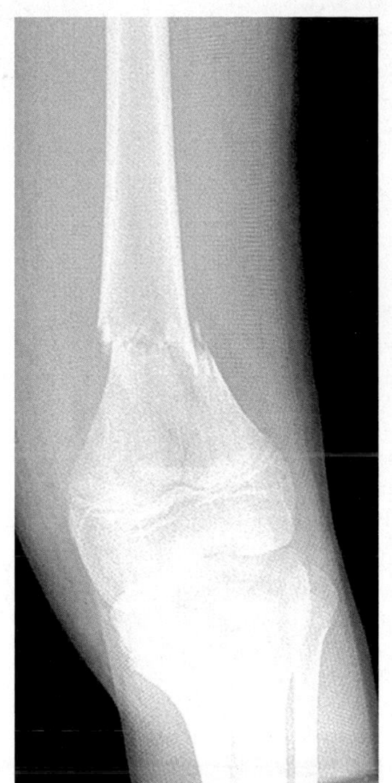

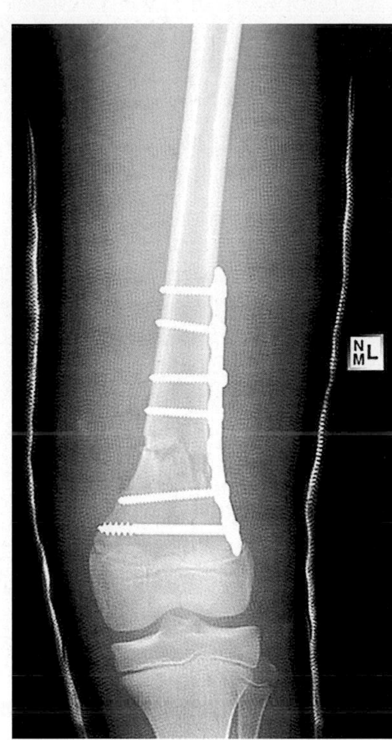

FIGURE 22-41 Preoperative **(A)** and postoperative **(B)** x-rays showing a fracture at the junction of the distal femoral metaphysis and diaphysis treated with plate fixation.

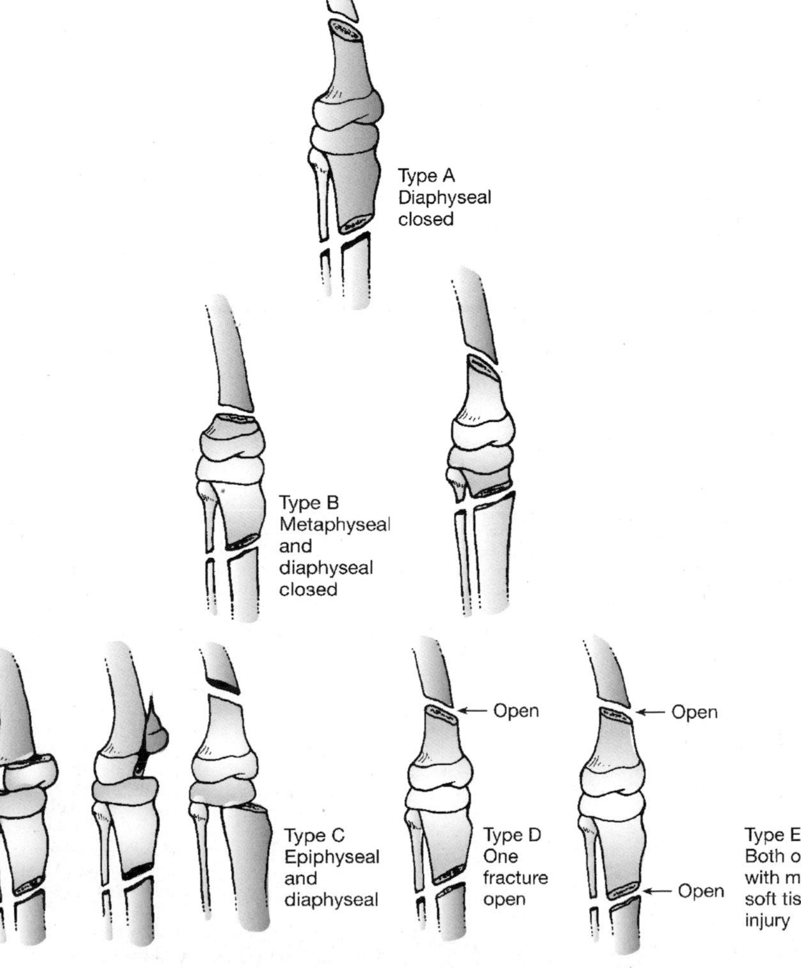

FIGURE 22-42 Classification of floating knee injuries in children. (From Letts M, Vincent N, Gouw G. The "floating knee" in children. J Bone Joint Surg Br 1986;68:442, with permission.)

patients. If possible, existing leg braces are modified for treatment of the femoral fracture. In nonambulatory patients, a simple pillow splint is used.

Floating Knee Injuries

These rare injuries occur when ipsilateral fractures of the femoral and tibial shafts leave the knee joint "floating" without distal or proximal bony attachments. They are high-velocity injuries, usually resulting from collision between a child pedestrian or cyclist and a motor vehicle. Most children with floating knee injuries have multiple-system trauma, including severe soft tissue damage, open fractures, and head, chest, or abdominal injuries.

Except in very young children, it is usually best to fix both fractures. If both fractures are open, external fixation of both the tibial and femoral fractures may be appropriate. If immediate mobilization is necessary, fixation of both fractures with external fixation, intramedullary nails, compression plates, or any combination of these may be indicated.

Letts et al.[121] described five patterns of ipsilateral tibial and femoral fractures and made treatment recommendations based on those patterns (Fig. 22-42). Because of the high prevalence of complications after closed treatment, Bohn and Durbin[20] recommended open or closed reduction and internal fixation of the femoral fracture in older children. Arslan et al.[7] evaluated the treatment of the "floating knee" in 29 consecutive cases, finding that those treated operatively had a shorter hospital stay, decreased time to weight bearing, and fewer complications than those managed with splinting casting or traction. Arslan et al.[7] demonstrated that open knee fracture rather than ligamentous injury was a risk factor for poor outcome and that angulation was a predictor of future compromise of function.

Bohn and Durbin[20] reported that of 19 patients with floating knee injuries, at long-term follow-up 11 had limb-length discrepancy secondary to either overgrowth of the bone after the fracture or premature closure of the ipsilateral physis (7 patients), genu valgum associated with fracture of the proximal tibial metaphysis (3 patients), or physeal arrest (1 patient). Four patients had late diagnosis of ligamentous laxity of the knee that required operation. Other complications included peroneal nerve palsy, infection, nonunion, malunion, and refracture.

Fractures in the Multiple-System Trauma Patient

In a study of 387 previously healthy children with femoral fractures, the authors evaluated the effect of stabilization on pulmonary function. Patients with severe head trauma or cervical spine trauma are at greatest risk for pulmonary complications. Timing of treatment of femoral fractures appears to not affect the prevalence of pulmonary complications in children. Mendelson et al.[141] similarly showed no effect of timing of femoral fixation on long-term outcome, but early fracture fixation did decrease hospital stay without increasing the risk of central nervous system or pulmonary complications.

ACKNOWLEDGMENTS

The authors thank James Kasser and James Beaty for their past contributions to this chapter.

REFERENCES

1. Aitken AP. Overgrowth of the femoral shaft following fracture in children. Am J Surg 1948;49:147–148.
2. Aitken AP, Blackett CW, Cincotti JJ. Overgrowth of the femoral shaft following fracture in childhood. J Bone Joint Surg Am 1939;21:334–338.
3. Aksoy MC, Caglar O, Ayvaz M, et al. Treatment of complicated pediatric femoral fractures with titanium elastic nail. J Pediatr Orthop B 2008;17(1):7–10.
4. Anderson M, Green WT. Lengths of the femur and the tibia: norms derived from orthoroentgenograms of children from five years of age until epiphyseal closure. Am J Dis Child 1948;75:279–290.
5. Aronson DD, Singer RM, Higgins RF. Skeletal traction for fractures of the femoral shaft in children. A long-term study. J Bone Joint Surg Am 1987;69(9):1435–1439.
6. Aronson J, Tursky EA. External fixation of femur fractures in children. J Pediatr Orthop 1992;12(2):157–163.
7. Arslan H, Kapukaya A, Kesemenli C, et al. Floating knee in children. J Pediatr Orthop 2003;23(4):458–463.
8. Barfod B, Christensen J. Fractures of the femoral shaft in children with special reference to subsequent overgrowth. Acta Chir Scand 1959;116(3):235–250.
9. Bar-On E, Sagiv S, Porat S. External fixation or flexible intramedullary nailing for femoral shaft fractures in children. A prospective, randomised study. J Bone Joint Surg Br 1997;79(6):975–978.
10. Beals RK, Tufts E. Fractured femur in infancy: the role of child abuse. J Pediatr Orthop 1983;3(5):583–586.
11. Beaty JH, Austin SM, Warner WC, et al. Interlocking intramedullary nailing of femoral-shaft fractures in adolescents: preliminary results and complications. J Pediatr Orthop 1994;14(2):178–183.
12. Benirschke SK, Melder I, Henley MB, et al. Closed interlocking nailing of femoral shaft fractures: assessment of technical complications and functional outcomes by comparison of a prospective database with retrospective review. J Orthop Trauma 1993;7(2):118–122.
13. Bennett FS, Zinar DM, Kilgus DJ. Ipsilateral hip and femoral shaft fractures. Clin Orthop Relat Res 1993;296:168–177.
14. Benum P, Ertresvag K, Hoiseth K. Torsion deformities after traction treatment of femoral fractures in children. Acta Orthop Scand 1979;50(1):87–91.
15. Bergman M, Tornetta P, Kerina M, et al. Femur fractures caused by gunshots: treatment by immediate reamed intramedullary nailing. J Trauma 1993;34(6):783–785.
16. Bienkowski P, Harvey EJ, Reindl R, et al. The locked flexible intramedullary humerus nail in pediatric femur and tibia shaft fractures: a feasibility study. J Pediatr Orthop 2004;24(6):634–637.
17. Biyani A, Jones DA, Daniel CL, et al. Assessment of hip abductor function in relation to peritrochanteric heterotopic ossification after closed femoral nailing. Injury 1993; 24(2):97–100.
18. Blakemore LC, Loder RT, Hensinger RN. Role of intentional abuse in children 1 to 5 years old with isolated femoral shaft fractures. J Pediatr Orthop 1996;16(5):585–588.
19. Blasier RD, Aronson J, Tursky EA. External fixation of pediatric femur fractures. J Pediatr Orthop 1997;17(3):342–346.
20. Bohn WW, Durbin RA. Ipsilateral fractures of the femur and tibia in children and adolescents. J Bone Joint Surg Am 1991;73(3):429–439.
21. Bopst L, Reinberg O, Lutz N. Femur fracture in preschool children: experience with flexible intramedullary nailing in 72 children. J Pediatr Orthop 2007;27(3):299–303.
22. Bourdelat D. Fracture of the femoral shaft in children: advantages of the descending medullary nailing. J Pediatr Orthop B 1996;5:110–114.
23. Braten M, Terjesen T, Rossvoll I. Torsional deformity after intramedullary nailing of femoral shaft fractures. Measurement of anteversion angles in 110 patients. J Bone Joint Surg Br 1993;75(5):799–803.
24. Brouwer KJ, Molenaar JC, van Linge B. Rotational deformities after femoral shaft fractures in childhood. A retrospective study 27–32 years after the accident. Acta Orthop Scand 1981;52(1):81–89.
25. Brumback RJ, Ellison TS, Poka A, et al. Intramedullary nailing of femoral shaft fractures: long term effects of static interlocking fixation. J Bone Joint Surg Am 1922;74:106–112.
26. Bryant T. The Practice of Surgery. Philadelphia: American Publishing Co.; 1873.
27. Buchholz IM, Bolhuis HW, Broker FH, et al. Overgrowth and correction of rotational deformity in 12 femoral shaft fractures in 3–6-year-old children treated with an external fixator. Acta Orthop Scand 2002;73(2):170–174.
28. Buford D Jr, Christensen K, Weatherall P. Intramedullary nailing of femoral fractures in adolescents. Clin Orthop Relat Res 1998;350:85–89.
29. Burks RT, Sutherland DH. Stress fracture of the femoral shaft in children: report of two cases and discussion. J Pediatr Orthop 1984;4(5):614–616.
30. Cameron CD, Meek RN, Blachut PA, et al. Intramedullary nailing of the femoral shaft: a prospective, randomized study. J Orthop Trauma 1992;6(4):448–451.
31. Cannon SR, Pool CJ. Traumatic separation of the proximal femoral epiphysis and fracture of the mid-shaft of the ipsilateral femur in a child. A case report and review of the literature. Injury 1983;15(3):156–158.
32. Carey TP, Galpin RD. Flexible intramedullary nail fixation of pediatric femoral fractures. Clin Orthop Relat Res 1996;332:110–118.
33. Carmichael KD, Bynum J, Goucher N. Rates of refracture associated with external fixation in pediatric femur fractures. Am J Orthop 2005;34(9):439–444; discussion 444.
34. Casas J, Gonzalez-Moran G, Albinana J. Femoral fractures in children from 4 years to 10 years: conservative treatment. J Pediatr Orthop B 2001;10(1):56–62.
35. Cassinelli EH, Young B, Vogt M, et al. Spica cast application in the emergency room for select pediatric femur fractures. J Orthop Trauma 2005;19(10):709–716.
36. Chung SM. The arterial supply of the developing proximal end of the human femur. J Bone Joint Surg Am 1976;58(7):961–970.
37. Ciarallo L, Fleisher G. Femoral fractures: are children at risk for significant blood loss? Pediatr Emerg Care 1996;12(5):343–346.
38. Clark MW, D'Ambrosia RD, Roberts JM. Equinus contracture following Bryant's traction. Orthopedics 1978;1(4):311–312.
39. Coffey C, Haley K, Hayes J, et al. The risk of child abuse in infants and toddlers with lower extremity injuries. J Pediatr Surg 2005;40(1):120–123.

40. Cole WH. Compensatory lengthening of the femur in children after fracture. Ann Surg 1925;82(4):609–616.
41. Cole WH. Results of treatment of fractured femurs in children with special reference to Bryant's overhead traction. Arch Surg 1922;5:702–716.
42. Coyte PC, Bronskill SE, Hirji ZZ, et al. Economic evaluation of 2 treatments for pediatric femoral shaft fractures. Clin Orthop Relat Res 1997;336:205–215.
43. Czertak DJ, Hennrikus WL. The treatment of pediatric femur fractures with early 90-90 spica casting. J Pediatr Orthop 1999;19(2):229–232.
44. Daly KE, Calvert PT. Accidental femoral fracture in infants. Injury 1991;22(4): 337–338.
45. Damholt B, Zdravkovic D. Quadriceps function following fractures of the femoral shaft in children. Acta Orthop Scand 1974;45:756.
46. Davids JR. Rotational deformity and remodeling after fracture of the femur in children. Clin Orthop Relat Res 1994;302:27–35.
47. Davis TJ, Topping RE, Blanco JS. External fixation of pediatric femoral fractures. Clin Orthop Relat Res 1995;318:191–198.
48. de Sanctis N, Gambardella A, Pempinello C, et al. The use of external fixators in femur fractures in children. J Pediatr Orthop 1996;16(5):613–620.
49. Dehne E, Kriz FK Jr. Slow arterial leak consequent to unrecognized arterial laceration. Report of five cases. J Bone Joint Surg Am 1967;49(2):372–376.
50. DeLee JC, Clanton TO, Rockwood CA Jr. Closed treatment of subtrochanteric fractures of the femur in a modified cast-brace. J Bone Joint Surg Am 1981;63(5):773–779.
51. Dencker H. Wire traction complications associated with treatment of femoral shaft fractures. Acta Orthop Scand 1964;35:158–163.
52. Domb BG, Sponseller PD, Ain M, et al. Comparison of dynamic versus static external fixation for pediatric femur fractures. J Pediatr Orthop 2002;22(4):428–430.
53. Edvardsen P, Syversen SM. Overgrowth of the femur after fracture of the shaft in childhood. J Bone Joint Surg Br 1976;58(3):339–342.
54. El Hayek T, Daher AA, Meouchy W, et al. External fixators in the treatment of fractures in children. J Pediatr Orthop B 2004;13(2):103–109.
55. Epps HR, Molenaar E, O'Connor D P. Immediate single-leg spica cast for pediatric femoral diaphysis fractures. J Pediatr Orthop 2006;26(4):491–496.
56. Eren OT, Kucukkaya M, Kockesen C, et al. Open reduction and plate fixation of femoral shaft fractures in children aged 4 to 10. J Pediatr Orthop 2003;23(2):190–193.
57. Evanoff M, Strong ML, MacIntosh R. External fixation maintained until fracture consolidation in the skeletally immature. J Pediatr Orthop 1993;13(1):98–101.
58. Fein LH, Pankovich AM, Spero CM, et al. Closed flexible intramedullary nailing of adolescent femoral shaft fractures. J Orthop Trauma 1989;3(2):133–141.
59. Ferguson J, Nicol RO. Early spica treatment of pediatric femoral shaft fractures. J Pediatr Orthop 2000;20(2):189–192.
60. Ferry AM, Edgar MS Jr. Modified Bryant's traction. J Bone Joint Surg Am 1966;48(3): 533–536.
61. Finsen V, Harnes OB, Nesse O, et al. Muscle function after plated and nailed femoral shaft fractures. Injury 1993;24(8):531–534.
62. Flynn JM, Hresko T, Reynolds RA, et al. Titanium elastic nails for pediatric femur fractures: a multicenter study of early results with analysis of complications. J Pediatr Orthop 2001;21(1):4–8.
63. Flynn JM, Luedtke LM, Ganley TJ, et al. Comparison of titanium elastic nails with traction and a spica cast to treat femoral fractures in children. J Bone Joint Surg Am 2004;86-A(4):770–777.
64. Flynn JM, Schwend RM. Management of pediatric femoral shaft fractures. J Am Acad Orthop Surg 2004;12(5):347–359.
65. Fricka KB, Mahar AT, Lee SS, et al. Biomechanical analysis of antegrade and retrograde flexible intramedullary nail fixation of pediatric femoral fractures using a synthetic bone model. J Pediatr Orthop 2004;24:167–171.
66. Fry K, Hoffer MM, Brink J. Femoral shaft fractures in brain-injured children. J Trauma 1976;16(5):371–373.
67. Fyodorov I, Sturm PF, Robertson WW Jr. Compression-plate fixation of femoral shaft fractures in children aged 8 to 12 years. J Pediatr Orthop 1999;19(5):578–581.
68. Galpin RD, Willis RB, Sabano N. Intramedullary nailing of pediatric femoral fractures. J Pediatr Orthop 1994;14(2):184–189.
69. Gordon JE, Swenning TA, Burd TA, et al. Proximal femoral radiographic changes after lateral transtrochanteric intramedullary nail placement in children. J Bone Joint Surg Am 2003;85-A(7):1295–1301.
70. Gregory P, Pevny T, Teague D. Early complications with external fixation of pediatric femoral shaft fractures. J Orthop Trauma 1996;10(3):191–198.
71. Gregory P, Sullivan JA, Herndon WA. Adolescent femoral shaft fractures: rigid versus flexible nails. Orthopedics 1995;18(7):645–649.
72. Griffin PP, Green WT. Fractures of the shaft of the femur in children: treatment and results. Orthop Clin North Am 1972;3(1):213–224.
73. Gross RH, Davidson R, Sullivan JA, et al. Cast brace management of the femoral shaft fracture in children and young adults. J Pediatr Orthop 1983;3(5):572–582.
74. Gross RH, Stranger M. Causative factors responsible for femoral fractures in infants and young children. J Pediatr Orthop 1983;3(3):341–343.
75. Gustilo RB. Current concepts in the management of open fractures. Instr Course Lect 1987;36:359–366.
76. Gwyn DT, Olney BW, Dart BR, et al. Rotational control of various pediatric femur fractures stabilized with titanium elastic intramedullary nails. J Pediatr Orthop 2004; 24(2):172–177.
77. Hagglund G, Hansson LI, Norman O. Correction by growth of rotational deformity after femoral fracture in children. Acta Orthop Scand 1983;54(6):858–861.
78. Hajek PD, Bicknell HR Jr, Bronson WE, et al. The use of one compared with two distal screws in the treatment of femoral shaft fractures with interlocking intramedullary nailing. A clinical and biomechanical analysis. J Bone Joint Surg Am 1993;75(4): 519–525.
79. Hansen TB. Fractures of the femoral shaft in children treated with an AO-compression plate. Report of 12 cases followed until adulthood. Acta Orthop Scand 1992;63(1): 50–52.
80. Hedequist D, Bishop J, Hresko T. Locking plate fixation for pediatric femur fractures. J Pediatr Orthop 2008;28(1):6–9.
81. Hedequist DJ, Sink E. Technical aspects of bridge plating for pediatric femur fractures. J Orthop Trauma 2005;19(4):276–279.
82. Hedin H, Borgquist L, Larsson S. A cost analysis of three methods of treating femoral shaft fractures in children: a comparison of traction in hospital, traction in hospital/home and external fixation. Acta Orthop Scand 2004;75(3):241–248.
83. Hedin H, Larsson S. Muscle strength in children treated for displaced femoral fractures by external fixation: 31 patients compared with 31 matched controls. Acta Orthop Scand. 2003;74(3):305–311.
84. Hedlund R, Lindgren U. The incidence of femoral shaft fractures in children and adolescents. J Pediatr Orthop 1986;6(1):47–50.
85. Heinrich SD, Drvaric DM, Darr K, et al. The operative stabilization of pediatric diaphyseal femur fractures with flexible intramedullary nails: a prospective analysis. J Pediatr Orthop 1994;14(4):501–507.
86. Heinrich SD, Drvaric D, Darr K, et al. Stabilization of pediatric diaphyseal femur fractures with flexible intramedullary nails (a technique paper). J Orthop Trauma 1992; 6(4):452–459.
87. Henderson J, Goldacre MJ, Fairweather JM, et al. Conditions accounting for substantial time spent in hospital in children aged 1–14 years. Arch Dis Child 1992;67(1):83–86.
88. Hennrikus WL, Kasser JR, Rand F, et al. The function of the quadriceps muscle after a fracture of the femur in patients who are less than seventeen years old. J Bone Joint Surg Am 1993;75(4):508–513.
89. Henry AN. Overgrowth after femoral shaft fractures in children. J Bone Joint Surg Br 1963;45:222.
90. Herndon WA, Mahnken RF, Yngve DA, et al. Management of femoral shaft fractures in the adolescent. J Pediatr Orthop 1989;9(1):29–32.
91. Herscovici D Jr, Scott DM, Behrens F, et al. The use of Ender nails in femoral shaft fractures: what are the remaining indications? J Orthop Trauma 1992;6(3):314–317.
92. Hinton RY, Lincoln A, Crockett MM, et al. Fractures of the femoral shaft in children. Incidence, mechanisms, and sociodemographic risk factors. J Bone Joint Surg Am 1999; 81(4):500–509.
93. Ho CA, Skaggs DL, Tang CW, et al. Use of flexible intramedullary nails in pediatric femur fractures. J Pediatr Orthop 2006;26(4):497–504.
94. Hresko MT, Kasser JR. Physeal arrest about the knee associated with non-physeal fractures in the lower extremity. J Bone Joint Surg Am 1989;71(5):698–703.
95. Hughes BF, Sponseller PD, Thompson JD. Pediatric femur fractures: effects of spica cast treatment on family and community. J Pediatr Orthop 1995;15(4):457–460.
96. Hull JB, Sanderson PL, Rickman M, et al. External fixation of children's fractures: use of the Orthofix Dynamic Axial Fixator. J Pediatr Orthop B 1997;6(3):203–206.
97. Humberger FW, Eyring EJ. Proximal tibial 90-90 traction in treatment of children with femoral-shaft fractures. J Bone Joint Surg Am 1969;51(3):499–504.
98. Hutchins CM, Sponseller PD, Sturm P, et al. Open femur fractures in children: treatment, complications, and results. J Pediatr Orthop 2000;20(2):183–188.
99. Ikpeme JO. Quadricepsplasty following femoral shaft fractures. Injury 1993;24(2): 104–108.
100. Illgen R 2nd, Rodgers WB, Hresko MT, et al. Femur fractures in children: treatment with early sitting spica casting. J Pediatr Orthop 1998;18(4):481–487.
101. Infante AF Jr, Albert MC, Jennings WB, et al. Immediate hip spica casting for femur fractures in pediatric patients. A review of 175 patients. Clin Orthop Relat Res 2000; 376:106–112.
102. Irani RN, Nicholson JT, Chung SM. Long-term results in the treatment of femoral-shaft fractures in young children by immediate spica immobilization. J Bone Joint Surg Am 1976;58(7):945–951.
103. Ireland DC, Fisher RL. Subtrochanteric fractures of the femur in children. Clin Orthop Relat Res 1975;110:157–166.
104. Isaacson J, Louis DS, Costenbader JM. Arterial injury associated with closed femoral-shaft fracture. Report of five cases. J Bone Joint Surg Am 1975;57(8):1147–1150.
105. Janzing H, Broos P, Rommens P. Compartment syndrome as a complication of skin traction in children with femoral fractures. J Trauma 1996;41(1):156–158.
106. Johnson AW, Weiss CB Jr, Wheeler DL. Stress fractures of the femoral shaft in athletes—more common than expected. A new clinical test. Am J Sports Med 1994;22(2): 248–256.
107. Kanellopoulos AD, Yiannakopoulos CK, Soucacos PN. Closed, locked intramedullary nailing of pediatric femoral shaft fractures through the tip of the greater trochanter. J Trauma 2006;60(1):217–222; discussion 222–213.
108. Kanlic EM, Anglen JO, Smith DG, et al. Advantages of submuscular bridge plating for complex pediatric femur fractures. Clin Orthop Relat Res 2004;426:244–251.
109. Kanlic E, Cruz M. Current concepts in pediatric femur fracture treatment. Orthopedics 2007;30(12):1015–1019.
110. Karaoğlu S, Baktir A, Tuncel M, et al. Closed Ender nailing of adolescent femoral shaft fractures. Injury 1994;25(8):501–506.
111. Katz JF. Spontaneous fractures in paraplegic children. J Bone Joint Surg Am 1953;35-A(1):220–226.
112. Kaweblum M, Lehman WB, Grant AD, et al. Avascular necrosis of the femoral head as sequela of fracture of the greater trochanter. A case report and review of the literature. Clin Orthop Relat Res 1993;294:193–195.
113. Kirby RM, Winquist RA, Hansen ST Jr. Femoral shaft fractures in adolescents: a comparison between traction plus cast treatment and closed intramedullary nailing. J Pediatr Orthop 1981;1(2):193–197.
114. Kocher M. American Academy of Orthopaedic Surgeons Specialty Day; 2004.
115. Kregor PJ, Song KM, Routt ML Jr, et al. Plate fixation of femoral shaft fractures in multiply injured children. J Bone Joint Surg Am 1993;75(12):1774–1780.
116. Krettek C, Haas N, Walker J, et al. Treatment of femoral shaft fractures in children by external fixation. Injury 1991;22(4):263–266.
117. Landin LA. Fracture patterns in children: analysis of 8,682 fractures with special reference to incidence, etiology and secular changes in a Swedish urban population 1950–1979. Acta Orthop Scand Suppl 1983;202:1–109.
118. Large TM, Frick SL. Compartment syndrome of the leg after treatment of a femoral fracture with an early sitting spica cast. A report of two cases. J Bone Joint Surg Am 2003;85-A(11):2207–2210.
119. Lascombes P, Haumont T, Journeau P. Use and abuse of flexible intramedullary nailing in children and adolescents. J Pediatr Orthop 2006;26(6):827–834.
120. Lee SS, Mahar AT, Newton PO. Ender nail fixation of pediatric femur fractures: a biomechanical analysis. J Pediatr Orthop 2001;21(4):442–445.
121. Letts M, Vincent N, Gouw G. The "floating knee" in children. J Bone Joint Surg Br 1986;68(3):442–446.

122. Lewallen RP, Peterson HA. Nonunion of long bone fractures in children: a review of 30 cases. J Pediatr Orthop 1985;5(2):135–142.
123. Ligier JN, Metaizeau JP, Prevot J, et al. Elastic stable intramedullary nailing of femoral shaft fractures in children. J Bone Joint Surg Br 1988;70(1):74–77.
124. Loder RT. Pediatric polytrauma: orthopaedic care and hospital course. J Orthop Trauma 1987;1(1):48–54.
125. Loder RT, O'Donnell PW, Feinberg JR. Epidemiology and mechanisms of femur fractures in children. J Pediatr Orthop 2006;26(5):561–566.
126. Luhmann SJ, Schootman M, Schoenecker PL, et al. Complications of titanium elastic nails for pediatric femoral shaft fractures. J Pediatr Orthop 2003;23(4):443–447.
127. Lynch JM, Gardner MJ, Gains B. Hemodynamic significance of pediatric femur fractures. J Pediatr Surg 1996;31(10):1358–1361.
128. MacEwen GD, Kasser JR, Heinrich SD. Pediatric Fractures. Baltimore: Williams & Wilkins; 1993.
129. Malkawi H, Shannak A, Hadidi S. Remodeling after femoral shaft fractures in children treated by the modified blount method. J Pediatr Orthop 1986;6(4):421–429.
130. Mann DC, Weddington J, Davenport K. Closed Ender nailing of femoral shaft fractures in adolescents. J Pediatr Orthop 1986;6(6):651–655.
131. Maruenda-Paulino JI, Sanchis-Alfonso V, Gomar-Sancho F, et al. Kuntscher nailing of femoral shaft fractures in children and adolescents. Int Orthop 1993;17(3):158–161.
132. Mathews PV, Perry JJ, Murray PC. Compartment syndrome of the well leg as a result of the hemilithotomy position: a report of two cases and review of literature. J Orthop Trauma 2001;15(8):580–583.
133. Matzkin EG, Smith EL, Wilson A, et al. External fixation of pediatric femur fractures with cortical contact. Am J Orthop 2006;35(11):498–501.
134. Mazda K, Khairouni A, Pennecot GF, et al. Closed flexible intramedullary nailing of the femoral shaft fractures in children. J Pediatr Orthop B 1997;6(3):198–202.
135. McCarthy RE. A method for early spica cast application in treatment of pediatric femoral shaft fractures. J Pediatr Orthop 1986;6(1):89–91.
136. McCollough NC 3rd, Vinsant JE Jr, Sarmiento A. Functional fracture-bracing of long-bone fractures of the lower extremity in children. J Bone Joint Surg Am 1978;60(3): 314–319.
137. McGraw JJ, Gregory SK. Ender nails: an alternative for intramedullary fixation of femoral shaft fractures in children and adolescents. South Med J 1997;90(7):694–696.
138. Meals RA. Overgrowth of the femur following fractures in children: influence of handedness. J Bone Joint Surg Am 1979;61(3):381–384.
139. Meaney JE, Carty H. Femoral stress fractures in children. Skeletal Radiol 1992;21(3): 173–176.
140. Mehlman CT, Nemeth NM, Glos DL. Antegrade versus retrograde titanium elastic nail fixation of pediatric distal-third femoral-shaft fractures: a mechanical study. J Orthop Trauma 2006;20(9):608–612.
141. Mendelson SA, Dominick TS, Tyler-Kabara E, et al. Early versus late femoral fracture stabilization in multiply injured pediatric patients with closed head injury. J Pediatr Orthop 2001;21(5):594–599.
142. Mesko JW, DeRosa GP, Lindseth RE. Segmental femur loss in children. J Pediatr Orthop 1985;5(4):471–474.
143. Mileski RA, Garvin KL, Huurman WW. Avascular necrosis of the femoral head after closed intramedullary shortening in an adolescent. J Pediatr Orthop 1995;15(1):24–26.
144. Miller DS, Markin L, Grossman E. Ischemic fibrosis of the lower extremity in children. Am J Surg 1952;84(3):317–322.
145. Miller ME, Bramlett KW, Kissell EU, et al. Improved treatment of femoral shaft fractures in children. The "pontoon" 90-90 spica cast. Clin Orthop Relat Res 1987;219:140–146.
146. Miller PR, Welch MC. The hazards of tibial pin replacement in 90-90 skeletal traction. Clin Orthop Relat Res 1978;135:97–100.
147. Miner T, Carroll KL. Outcomes of external fixation of pediatric femoral shaft fractures. J Pediatr Orthop 2000;20(3):405–410.
148. Momberger N, Stevens P, Smith J, et al. Intramedullary nailing of femoral fractures in adolescents. J Pediatr Orthop 2000;20(4):482–484.
149. Moroz LA, Launay F, Kocher MS, et al. Titanium elastic nailing of fractures of the femur in children. Predictors of complications and poor outcome. J Bone Joint Surg Br 2006;88(10):1361–1366.
150. Morris S, Cassidy N, Stephens M, et al. Birth-associated femoral fractures: incidence and outcome. J Pediatr Orthop 2002;22(1):27–30.
151. Morshed S, Humphrey M, Corrales LA, et al. Retention of flexible intramedullary nails following treatment of pediatric femur fractures. Arch Orthop Trauma Surg 2007; 127(7):509–514.
152. Mubarak SJ, Frick S, Sink E, et al. Volkmann contracture and compartment syndromes after femur fractures in children treated with 90/90 spica casts. J Pediatr Orthop 2006; 26(5):567–572.
153. Narayanan UG, Hyman JE, Wainwright AM, et al. Complications of elastic stable intramedullary nail fixation of pediatric femoral fractures, and how to avoid them. J Pediatr Orthop 2004;24(4):363–369.
154. Newton PO, Mubarak SJ. Financial aspects of femoral shaft fracture treatment in children and adolescents. J Pediatr Orthop 1994;14(4):508–512.
155. Nicholson JT, Foster RM, Heath RD. Bryant's traction; a provocative cause of circulatory complications. J Am Med Assoc 1955;157(5):415–418.
156. Norbeck DE Jr, Asselmeier M, Pinzur MS. Torsional malunion of a femur fracture: diagnosis and treatment. Orthop Rev 1990;19(7):625–629.
157. Nork SE, Hoffinger SA. Skeletal traction versus external fixation for pediatric femoral shaft fractures: a comparison of hospital costs and charges. J Orthop Trauma 1998; 12(8):563–568.
158. Nowotarski PJ, Turen CH, Brumback RJ, et al. Conversion of external fixation to intramedullary nailing for fractures of the shaft of the femur in multiply injured patients. J Bone Joint Surg Am 2000;82(6):781–788.
159. Oberhammer J. Degree and frequency of rotational deformities after infant femoral fractures and their spontaneous correction. Arch Orthop Trauma Surg 1980;97(4): 249–255.
160. O'Malley DE, Mazur JM, Cummings RJ. Femoral head avascular necrosis associated with intramedullary nailing in an adolescent. J Pediatr Orthop 1995;15(1):21–23.
161. Ostrum RF, DiCicco J, Lakatos R, et al. Retrograde intramedullary nailing of femoral diaphyseal fractures. J Orthop Trauma 1998;12(7):464–468.
162. Ozdemir HM, Yensel U, Senaran H, et al. Immediate percutaneous intramedullary fixation and functional bracing for the treatment of pediatric femoral shaft fracture. J Pediatr Orthop 2003;23(4):453–457.
163. Podeszwa DA, Mooney JF 3rd, Cramer KE, et al. Comparison of Pavlik harness application and immediate spica casting for femur fractures in infants. J Pediatr Orthop 2004; 24(5):460–462.
164. Pombo MW, Shilt JS. The definition and treatment of pediatric subtrochanteric femur fractures with titanium elastic nails. J Pediatr Orthop 2006;26(3):364–370.
165. Porat S, Milgrom C, Nyska M, et al. Femoral fracture treatment in head-injured children: use of external fixation. J Trauma 1986;26(1):81–84.
166. Pott P. Some Few General Remarks on Fractures and Dislocations. London: Howes, Clark, and Collins; 1769.
167. Probe R, Lindsey RW, Hadley NA, et al. Refracture of adolescent femoral shaft fractures: a complication of external fixation. A report of two cases. J Pediatr Orthop 1993;13(1): 102–105.
168. Raney EM, Ogden JA, Grogan DP. Premature greater trochanteric epiphysiodesis secondary to intramedullary femoral rodding. J Pediatr Orthop 1993;13(4):516–520.
169. Rathjen KE, Riccio AI, De La Garza D. Stainless steel flexible intramedullary fixation of unstable femoral shaft fractures in children. J Pediatr Orthop 2007;27(4):432–441.
170. Reeves RB, Ballard RI, Hughes JL. Internal fixation versus traction and casting of adolescent femoral shaft fractures. J Pediatr Orthop 1990;10(5):592–595.
171. Reynolds DA. Growth changes in fractured long-bones: a study of 126 children. J Bone Joint Surg Br 1981;63-B(1):83–88.
172. Ricci WM, Bellabarba C, Evanoff B, et al. Retrograde versus antegrade nailing of femoral shaft fractures. J Orthop Trauma 2001;15(3):161–169.
173. Riew KD, Sturm PF, Rosenbaum D, et al. Neurologic complications of pediatric femoral nailing. J Pediatr Orthop 1996;16(5):606–612.
174. Robertson P, Karol LA, Rab GT. Open fractures of the tibia and femur in children. J Pediatr Orthop 1996;16(5):621–626.
175. Rohde RS, Mendelson SA, Grudziak JS. Acute synovitis of the knee resulting from intra-articular knee penetration as a complication of flexible intramedullary nailing of pediatric femur fractures: report of two cases. J Pediatr Orthop 2003;23(5):635–638.
176. Rosental JJ, Gaspar MR, Gjerdrum TC, et al. Vascular injuries associated with fractures of the femur. Arch Surg 1975;110(5):494–499.
177. Rozbruch SR, Muller U, Gautier E, et al. The evolution of femoral shaft plating technique. Clin Orthop Relat Res 1998;354:195–208.
178. Ryan JR. 90-90 skeletal femoral traction for femoral shaft fractures in children. J Trauma 1981;21(1):46–48.
179. Schenck RC Jr. Basic Histomorphology and Physiology of Skeletal Growth. New York: Springer-Verlag; 1980.
180. Shah A, Ellis RD. False aneurysm complicating closed femoral fracture in a child. Orthop Rev 1993;22(11):1265–1267.
181. Shahcheraghi GH, Doroodchi HR. Supracondylar fracture of the femur: closed or open reduction? J Trauma 1993;34(4):499–502.
182. Shapiro F. Fractures of the femoral shaft in children. The overgrowth phenomenon. Acta Orthop Scand 1981;52(6):649–655.
183. Silverman FN. Radiological Aspects of the Battered Child Syndrome. Chicago: University of Chicago Press; 1987.
184. Simonian PT, Chapman JR, Selznick HS, et al. Iatrogenic fractures of the femoral neck during closed nailing of the femoral shaft. J Bone Joint Surg Br 1994;76(2):293–296.
185. Sink EL, Gralla J, Repine M. Complications of pediatric femur fractures treated with titanium elastic nails: a comparison of fracture types. J Pediatr Orthop 2005;25(5): 577–580.
186. Sink EL, Hedequist D, Morgan SJ, et al. Results and technique of unstable pediatric femoral fractures treated with submuscular bridge plating. J Pediatr Orthop 2006; 26(2):177–181.
187. Skaggs DL, Leet AI, Money MD, et al. Secondary fractures associated with external fixation in pediatric femur fractures. J Pediatr Orthop 1999;19(5):582–586.
188. Smith NC, Parker D, McNicol D. Supracondylar fractures of the femur in children. J Pediatr Orthop 2001;21(5):600–603.
189. Sola J, Schoenecker PL, Gordon JE. External fixation of femoral shaft fractures in children: enhanced stability with the use of an auxiliary pin. J Pediatr Orthop 1999;19(5): 587–591.
190. Staheli LT. Femoral and tibial growth following femoral shaft fracture in childhood. Clin Orthop Relat Res 1967;55:159–163.
191. Staheli LT. Fever following trauma in childhood. JAMA 1967;199(7):503–504.
192. Stannard JP, Christensen KP, Wilkins KE. Femur fractures in infants: a new therapeutic approach. J Pediatr Orthop 1995;15(4):461–466.
193. Stans AA, Morrissy RT, Renwick SE. Femoral shaft fracture treatment in patients age 6 to 16 years. J Pediatr Orthop 1999;19(2):222–228.
194. Thometz JG, Lamdan R. Osteonecrosis of the femoral head after intramedullary nailing of a fracture of the femoral shaft in an adolescent. A case report. J Bone Joint Surg Am 1995;77(9):1423–1426.
195. Thompson JD, Buehler KC, Sponseller PD, et al. Shortening in femoral shaft fractures in children treated with spica cast. Clin Orthop Relat Res 1997;338:74–78.
196. Thomson SA, Mahoney LJ. Volkmann's ischaemic contracture and its relationship to fracture of the femur. J Bone Joint Surg Br 1951;33-B(3):336–347.
197. Timmerman LA, Rab GT. Intramedullary nailing of femoral shaft fractures in adolescents. J Orthop Trauma 1993;7(4):331–337.
198. Tolo VT. External fixation in multiply injured children. Orthop Clin North Am 1990; 21(2):393–400.
199. Toren A, Goshen E, Katz M, et al. Bilateral femoral stress fractures in a child due to in-line (roller) skating. Acta Paediatr 1997;86(3):332–333.
200. Townsend DR, Hoffinger S. Intramedullary nailing of femoral shaft fractures in children via the trochanter tip. Clin Orthop Relat Res 2000;376:113–118.
201. Truesdell ED. Inequality of the lower extremities following fracture of the shaft of the femur in children. Ann Surg 1921;74(4):498–500.
202. Vangsness CT Jr, DeCampos J, Merritt PO, et al. Meniscal injury associated with femoral shaft fractures. An arthroscopic evaluation of incidence. J Bone Joint Surg Br 1993; 75(2):207–209.
203. Van Meter JW, Branick RI. Bilateral genu recurvatum after skeletal traction. A case report. J Bone Joint Surg Am 1980;62(5):837–839.
204. Verbeek HO. Does rotation deformity, following femur shaft fracture, correct during growth? Reconstr Surg Traumatol 1979;17:75–81.

205. Viljanto J, Kiviluoto H, Paananen M. Remodelling after femoral shaft fracture in children. Acta Chir Scand 1975;141(5):360–365.
206. Wall EJ, Jain V, Vora V, et al. Complications of titanium and stainless steel elastic nail fixation of pediatric femoral fractures. J Bone Joint Surg Am 2008;90(6):1305–1313.
207. Wallace ME, Hoffman EB. Remodelling of angular deformity after femoral shaft fractures in children. J Bone Joint Surg Br 1992;74(5):765–769.
208. Ward WT, Levy J, Kaye A. Compression plating for child and adolescent femur fractures. J Pediatr Orthop 1992;12(5):626–632.
209. Weiss AP, Schenck RC Jr, Sponseller PD, et al. Peroneal nerve palsy after early cast application for femoral fractures in children. J Pediatr Orthop 1992;12(1):25–28.
210. Winquist RA, Hansen ST Jr, Clawson DK. Closed intramedullary nailing of femoral fractures. A report of five hundred and twenty cases. J Bone Joint Surg Am 1984;66(4):529–539.
211. Wright JG. The treatment of femoral shaft fractures in children: a systematic overview and critical appraisal of the literature. Can J Surg 2000;43(3):180–189.
212. Ziv I, Blackburn N, Rang M. Femoral intramedullary nailing in the growing child. J Trauma 1984;24(5):432–434.

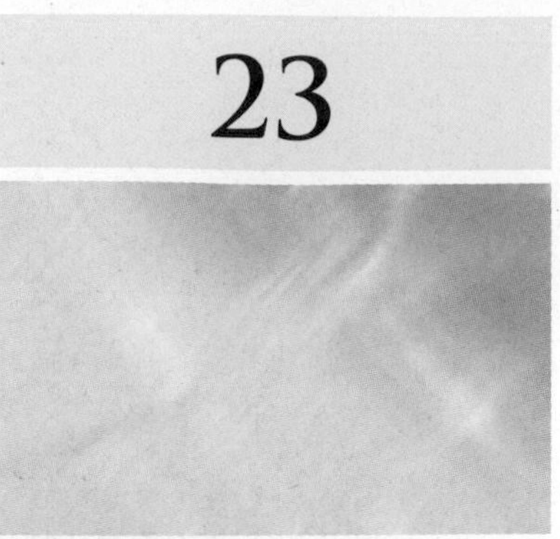

23

EXTRA-ARTICULAR INJURIES OF THE KNEE

Charles T. Price and Jose Herrera-Soto

INTRODUCTION 842

FRACTURES OF THE DISTAL FEMORAL PHYSIS 842
Mechanism of Injury 843
Signs and Symptoms 845
Associated Injuries 845
Diagnosis and Classification 847
Surgical and Applied Anatomy 852
Current Treatment Options 854
Complications 860
Controversies 862

FRACTURES OF THE PROXIMAL TIBIAL PHYSIS 862
Mechanism of Injury 862
Signs and Symptoms 862
Associated Injuries 862
Diagnosis and Classification 863
Surgical and Applied Anatomy 866
Current Treatment Options 866
Complications 869

AVULSION OF THE TIBIAL TUBEROSITY 870
Mechanism of Injury 870
Signs and Symptoms 870
Associated Injuries 871
Diagnosis and Classification 871
Surgical and Applied Anatomy 872
Current Treatment Options 873
Complications 875

FRACTURES OF THE PATELLA 876
Mechanism of Injury 876
Signs and Symptoms 876
Associated Injuries 877
Diagnosis and Classification 877
Surgical and Applied Anatomy 880
Current Treatment Options 880
Complications 883

INTRODUCTION

Extra-articular injuries of the knee principally involve the patella and the physes of the distal femur and proximal tibia. Great force generally is required to disrupt these structures in children and adolescents. This leads to increased risks of associated injuries and growth arrest. Neurovascular structures are also at increased risk because of close proximity to the distal femur and proximal tibia. Growth disturbances may have severe consequences due to rapid growth around the knee. Accurate reduction is critical for proper knee function. Therefore, careful assessment and anatomic alignment with stable fixation are generally recommended for extra-articular injuries of the knee. Parents should be advised that x-ray follow-up is essential for early detection and treatment of growth disturbances from these injuries.

FRACTURES OF THE DISTAL FEMORAL PHYSIS

Distal femoral physeal injuries are uncommon, accounting for fewer than 2% of all physeal injuries.[78,96,124] However, complications requiring additional surgery occur after approximately 40% to 60% of these injuries.[3,44,53,71,89,133,154,159] The most common complication is growth disturbance with angular deformity and/or shortening; this has been reported in 35% to 50% of patients regardless of anatomic reduction.[3,44,53,71,89,154,159] The prognosis is better for very young children and nondisplaced fractures, but complications are frequent and may occur with any distal femoral physeal injury. Careful assessment, anatomic reduction, and secure immobilization or fixation are recommended for most injuries. Follow-up for many months is recommended for early detection of growth disturbances.

Mechanism of Injury

In the days of horse-drawn wagons, this injury was termed "wagon-wheel injury" or "cartwheel injury" because it occurred when boys attempted to jump onto a moving wagon and the leg became entrapped between the spokes of the moving wheel. This often led to amputation because of associated neurovascular trauma.[70] Today, most distal femoral fracture separations are the result of motor vehicle or sports-related trauma (Table 23-1).[3] Underlying conditions such as neuromuscular disorders, joint contractures, difficult deliveries, or nutritional deficiencies may predispose some children to separation of the distal femoral epiphysis.[4,5,7,94,121] The principles of management for pathologic fractures may vary from those for fractures in otherwise healthy children because severe trauma is generally necessary to separate the distal femoral epiphysis in healthy children. This is especially true between the ages of 2 to 11 years. Less force is required for physeal disruption in infants and adolescents.[133] Child abuse should be suspected in infants and toddlers when a small peripheral metaphyseal fragment of bone, also called a "corner fracture," is identified in association with a nondisplaced distal femoral epiphyseal fracture (Fig 23-1).[87] In the adolescent age group, valgus and torsional injury during sports are a common cause of distal femoral epiphyseal separation (Fig 23-2).

The most common mechanism of injury is a varus or valgus stress across the knee joint. In skeletally mature individuals, this mechanism of injury can cause ligamentous disruption because ligaments commonly fail before bone fails when a bending stress is applied across the knee joint (Fig. 23-3A). However, loading to failure across the immature knee is more likely to lead to physeal failure due to tensile stresses that are transmitted through the ligaments to the adjacent physis (Fig. 23-3B).[45] Bending creates tension on one side of the physis and compression on the opposite side. This leads to disruption of the periosteum and perichondrial ring on the tension side, followed by a fracture plane that begins in the hypertrophic zone and proceeds in an irregular manner through the physis.[21] Salter-Harris type I fractures generally extend through the hypertrophic zone and the zone of provisional calcification without traversing the germinal layers. Salter-Harris type II fractures exit through the

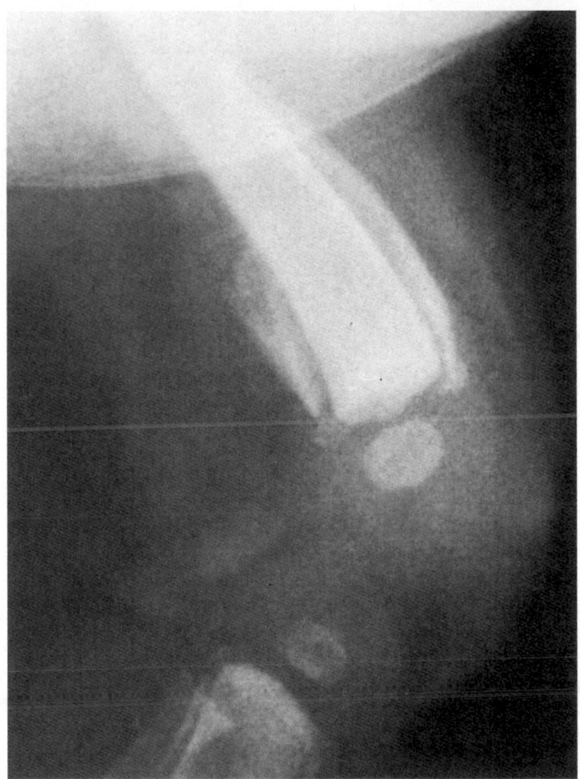

FIGURE 23-1 Lateral radiograph of a swollen knee in a 3-month-old girl who reportedly fell out of her crib 8 days earlier. Subperiosteal ossification along the distal femoral shaft indicates separation of the distal femoral epiphysis. Note evidence of fracture-separation of the proximal tibial epiphysis as well. Final diagnosis: abused child.

TABLE 23-1 Mechanism of Injury in Clinical Reviews of Separation of the Distal Femoral Epiphysis

	Neer*	Bassett†	Roberts‡	Stephens**	Total
Sports injury	5	4	64	8	81 (49%)
Hit by automobile	9	8	15	10	42 (25%)
Falls	3	3	12	1	19 (12%)
Auto accident	—	3	5	1	9 (5%)
Other	4	7	4	—	15 (9%)

*Neer CS II. Separation of the lower femoral epiphyses. Am J Surg 1960;99:756–761.
†Bassett FH III, Goldner JL. Fractures involving the distal femoral epiphyseal growth line. South Med J 1962;55:545–557.
‡Roberts JM. Fracture separation of the distal femoral epiphysis. J Bone Joint Surg Am 1973;55A:1324.
**Stephens DC, Louis DS, Louis E. Traumatic separation of the distal femoral epiphyseal cartilage plate. J Bone Joint Surg Am 1974;56:1383–1390.

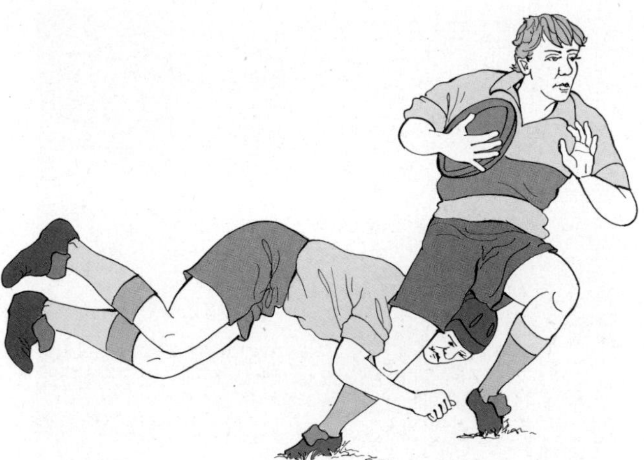

FIGURE 23-2 Valgus and torsional stress across the knee may cause a ligament injury or physeal separation.

metaphysis with a spike of metaphyseal bone attached to the epiphysis on the compression side (Thurstan-Holland fragment) (Fig. 23-4A). Salter-Harris type III and IV fractures cross the entire physis vertically and enter the joint through the articular cartilage. Bright et al.[21] demonstrated that male and prepubescent animals are less resistant to epiphyseal separation when various loads are applied, and that the growth plate is also weakest in torsion. Direction of force determines direction of displacement of the distal fragment. When the knee is hyperextended, the distal fragment is displaced anteriorly. Pure compression force also can cause distal femoral physeal damage (Salter-Harris type V). Premature growth arrest has been reported after pure compression injuries and also in association with nonphyseal fractures of the femoral and tibial shafts.[10,]

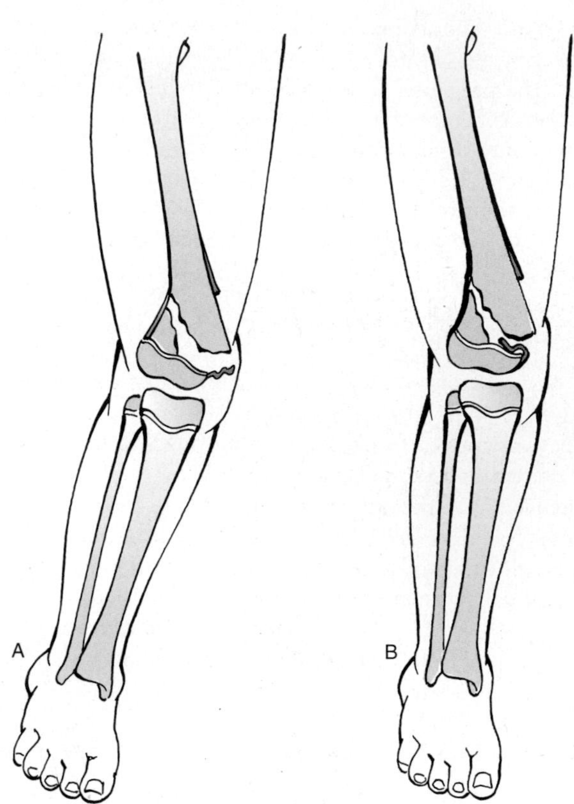

FIGURE 23-4 A. In a Salter-Harris type II fracture, the side where the fracture occurred through the physis fails in tension, with disruption of the periosteum. The side of the fracture with the Thurstan-Holland fragment failed in compression, with the periosteum usually intact. The intact periosteum can be used for fracture reduction. **B.** With fracture reduction, the periosteum may become interposed within the fracture site, preventing an anatomic reduction

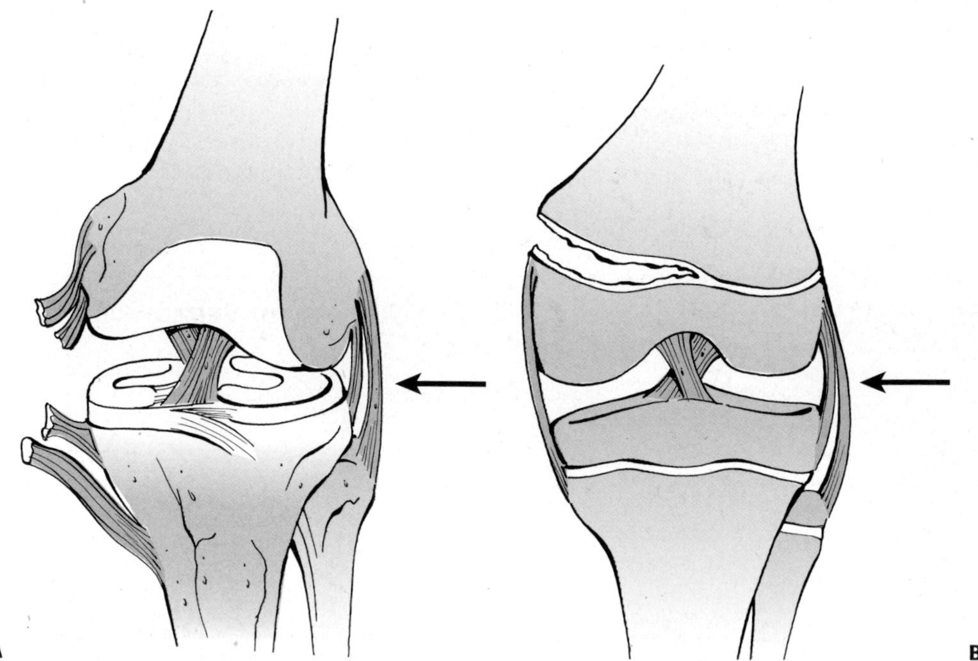

FIGURE 23-3 A. In a skeletally mature patient with closed physis, tensile failure usually occurs across the ligament. **B.** In a skeletally immature patient with open physis, failure usually occurs across the physis. (Reprinted with permission from Skaggs DL, Flynn JF. Trauma about the knee, tibia, and foot. In Skaggs DL, Flynn JF, eds. Staying out of Trouble in Pediatric Orthopaedics. Philadelphia: Lippincott Williams & Wilkins; 2006.)

[66,107,142] Salter-Harris type III fractures of the distal medial femoral condyle result from the same mechanism of injury that produces medial collateral and cruciate ligament disruption in skeletally mature patients. The pull of the medial collateral ligament (MCL) results in condylar separation instead of MCL disruption. Salter-Harris type III fractures of the medial femoral condyle are frequently associated with cruciate ligament injuries.[22,98,130,162] This pattern of fracture occurs near skeletal maturity when the central portion of the distal femoral physis begins to close before the medial and lateral physis. Thus the mechanism of this injury is similar to that of the juvenile Tillaux fracture in the adolescent ankle.[98]

Signs and Symptoms

The clinical diagnosis of distal femoral epiphyseal separation is usually obvious, but minor degrees of displacement may require careful examination and x-ray interpretation. The patient is in pain and cannot walk or bear weight on the injured limb immediately after sustaining a displaced separation of the distal femoral epiphysis. Most often, these injuries result from significant force causing visible malalignment of the limb, swelling, and/or ecchymosis that make the diagnosis of a fracture obvious (Fig. 23-5). Abrasion or laceration of the overlying soft tissues may be a clue to the mechanism of injury or to an open fracture. More swelling and prominence may be noted on the side that opened in tension. On this side, the periosteum is usually ruptured and the metaphyseal fragment may buttonhole through the quadriceps muscle. On the opposite side, in the direction of displacement, the periosteum is usually intact and may help guide reduction. If a fracture is suspected, it is better to obtain x-rays before any manipulation. When muscle spasm can be relaxed, instability just above the knee joint may be felt. Fracture crepitus sometimes may be absent if the periosteum is interposed between the metaphysis and the epiphysis. Whenever epiphyseal separation is suspected, careful neurovascular examination of the lower leg and foot should be performed, including pulses, color, temperature, and motor and sensory status. The extremity may become cyanotic if venous return is impaired. The use of Doppler ultrasound may be helpful in evaluating circulation distal to the injury. Compartmental pressure recordings should be obtained if there are clinical findings of compartment syndrome. Extravasation of blood into the soft tissues of the distal thigh and popliteal fossa produces ecchymosis that may become more apparent within 72 hours after injury.

Occasionally, with a nondisplaced separation the patient is able to bear some weight on the limb and it may be possible to localize tenderness to the level of the physis rather than the joint line where ligament disruptions are more frequent. Abnormal laxity may be perceived on clinical examination but can be the result of physeal instability rather than a ligamentous tear. In an adolescent or child with a knee injury and swelling, occult physeal instability should be suspected. Stress x-rays or magnetic resonance imaging (MRI) may be indicated when doubt exists.[98,147,162] MRI may be tolerated better by patients and provides the advantage of evaluating possible ligament injuries. Ultrasonography may be used as a diagnostic tool in infants and toddlers.[68]

Associated Injuries

Ligamentous Injuries

Symptomatic knee joint instability may persist after the epiphyseal separation has healed. This finding at follow-up implies

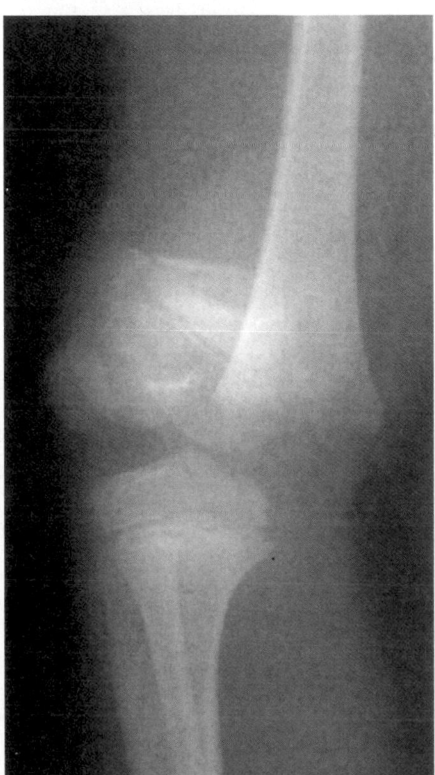

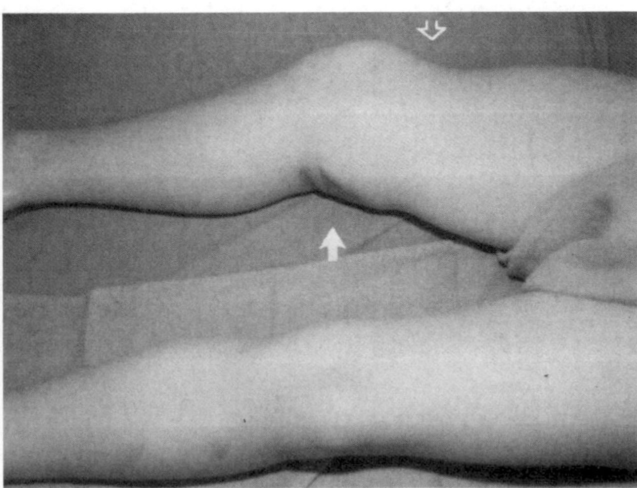

FIGURE 23-5 A. Completely displaced Salter-Harris type II fracture of the distal femur in a 6-year-old girl whose foot was on the back of the driver's headrest when the automobile in which she was riding was involved in an accident. **B.** Ecchymosis in the popliteal fossa and anterior displacement of the distal femur are evident. Clinical examination revealed absence of peroneal nerve function and a cold, pulseless foot. *(continues)*

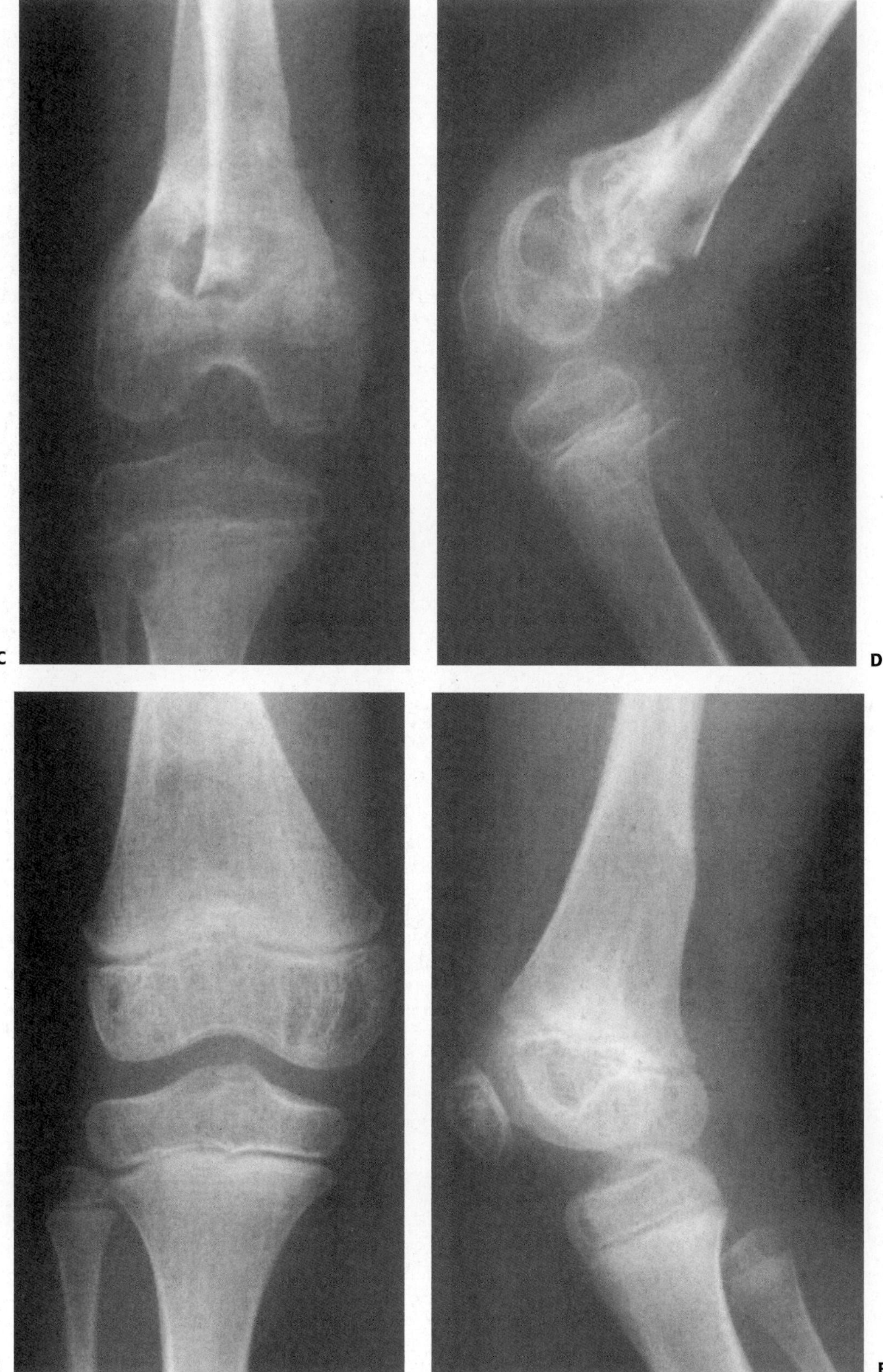

FIGURE 23-5 (*continued*) The fracture was irreducible by closed methods and required open reduction, internal fixation, and repair of a popliteal artery laceration. **C,D.** Incomplete reduction Salter-Harris type II fracture in a 6-year-old girl with 25 degrees of posterior angulation and abundant callus formation. **E,F.** Four years later, remodeling has occurred and no growth disturbance is noted. Results such as this cannot be relied upon, and early anatomic reduction is recommended.

concomitant injury to knee ligaments that may be present at the time of initial management of the epiphyseal separation. Bertin and Goble[15] found that six of 16 patients seen in follow-up for distal femoral physeal fractures had ligamentous instability. A review of 151 children with distal femoral physeal fractures found symptomatic knee ligamentous laxity in 12 patients (8%).[44] Salter-Harris type III fractures of the medial femoral condyle are frequently associated with cruciate ligament injuries.[22,98,130,162] For this reason, an MRI, instead of stress x-rays, may provide more information about Salter-Harris type III fractures to help diagnose ligamentous injury. Early diagnosis of injury to the ligaments or menisci can facilitate early management.[15] In general, fracture stabilization is the first step with ligament reconstruction or meniscal repair done after physeal healing. If there is no meniscal injury, a rehabilitation program is indicated initially. If there is a reparable meniscal tear, cruciate reconstruction can be done at the time of meniscal repair depending on the patient's age and activity level.

Vascular Impairment

Vascular injuries are uncommon with this fracture, with most series reporting no vascular injuries.[44,89,133,159] However, compartment syndrome has been reported and should be suspected when pain is severe.[44] Intimal tear and thrombosis in the popliteal artery may be caused by trauma from the distal end of the metaphysis when the epiphysis is displaced anteriorly during a hyperextension injury.[11,44,140] In patients with known vascular injury, vascular repair should be carried out immediately after fracture stabilization. If vascular impingement occurs but is relieved by prompt reduction of the displaced epiphysis, the patient should still be closely observed for the classic signs of vascular impairment or compartment syndrome. Arteriography and vascular consultation should be considered when perfusion is less than normal. If there is an associated fracture of the pelvis or femoral shaft, arteriography may be necessary to localize the vascular injury. Vascular impairment may develop slowly from increasing compartmental pressure. If the patient has inordinate persistent pain or a cool and pale foot, a femoral arteriogram and compartment pressure measurement should be considered even when peripheral pulses are present.

For known vascular injuries associated with fracture, it is unclear whether vascular repair or fracture stabilization should be carried out first.[20,26,153] Most distal femoral epiphyseal separations can be stabilized rapidly with screw or pin fixation before vascular repair. Ischemia time may be increased when prolonged fracture stabilization is performed first, but vascular repair is at risk for avulsion when it is done before manipulations necessary for fracture stabilization.

Peroneal Nerve Injury

The peroneal nerve is the only nerve injured with any frequency in this type of fracture.[44] It may be stretched by anterior or medial displacement of the epiphysis with resulting neurapraxia. Spontaneous recovery can be expected following reduction and fixation of the fracture.[44,149] The exception to this is a transected nerve in association with an open injury, which can be treated with repair or grafting. Persistent neurologic deficit after 6 months warrants electromyographic examination. If the conduction time is prolonged and fibrillation or denervation is present in distal muscles, exploration and microneural reanastomosis or resection of any neuroma may be indicated.

Diagnosis and Classification

Separations of the distal femoral epiphysis have been classified according to the pattern of fracture, the direction and magnitude of displacement, and the age of the patient. The Salter-Harris classification[140] is useful for description and treatment planning. Classification by direction and degree of displacement may help plan the reduction and predict the risk of complications.[3,71] Classification by age may help identify the mechanism of injury and the implications for growth disturbance.

Classification by Fracture Pattern

The Salter-Harris classification is useful for fracture description and treatment planning (Fig. 23-6). This classification is also a good indicator of the mechanism of injury.[36] Posttraumatic growth arrest is common after all types of distal femoral epiphyseal fractures[89,154] and opinions vary as to whether or not this classification system helps predict potential complications in-

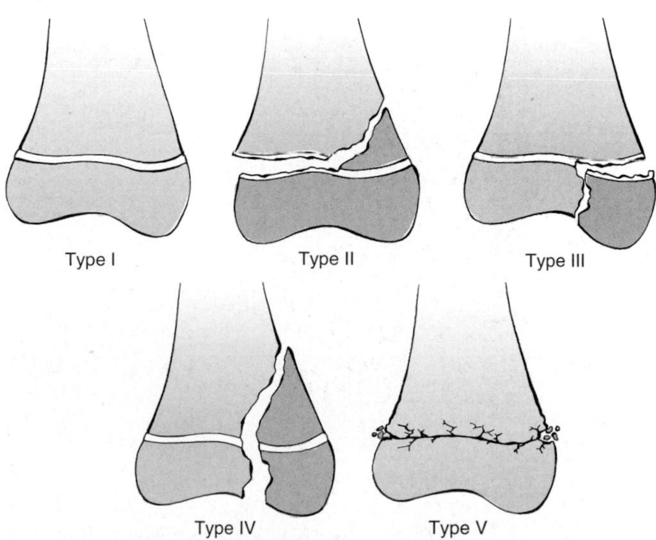

FIGURE 23-6 The Salter-Harris classification of fractures involving the distal femoral physis.

cluding growth disturbance.[3,36,44,89,133] Salter-Harris type I and II fractures in other areas of the body usually have a low risk of growth arrest, even minimally displaced Salter-Harris type I and II fractures of the distal femur should be followed closely for physeal injury. Growth disturbance is uncommon in patients younger than 2 years of age,[133] but these fractures in older children lead to growth arrest in 40% to 50% of patients.[71,133]

The Salter-Harris type I pattern is a separation through the distal femoral physis, without fracture through the adjacent epiphysis or metaphysis (Fig. 23-7). It occurs in infants as a birth injury or abuse and in adolescents, often as a nondisplaced separation. This type of fracture may go undetected. Sometimes, the diagnosis is made only in retrospect, when subperiosteal new bone formation occurs along the adjacent metaphysis. When displacement is present before the age of 2 years, it is usually in the sagittal plane.

The Salter-Harris type II pattern is the most common type of separation of the distal femoral epiphysis (Fig. 23-8). This pattern is characterized by an oblique extension of the fracture across one corner of the adjacent metaphysis. The metaphyseal

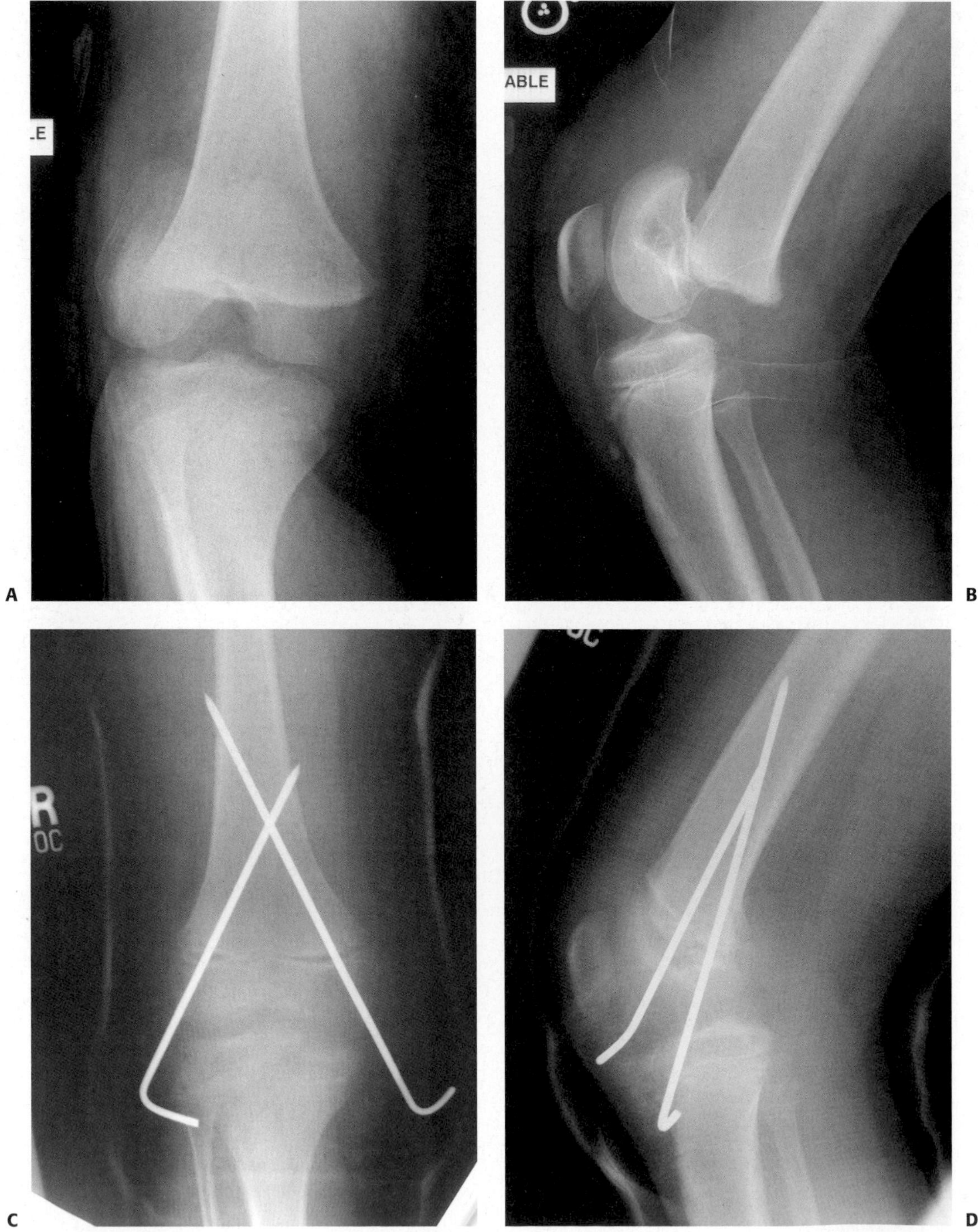

FIGURE 23-7 A. Salter-Harris type I fracture of the distal femur in an 8-year-old. **B.** Lateral view shows hyperextension. **C.** Fixation following closed reduction under general anesthesia. Note that pins are widely separated at the fracture site. **D.** Lateral view of fixation.

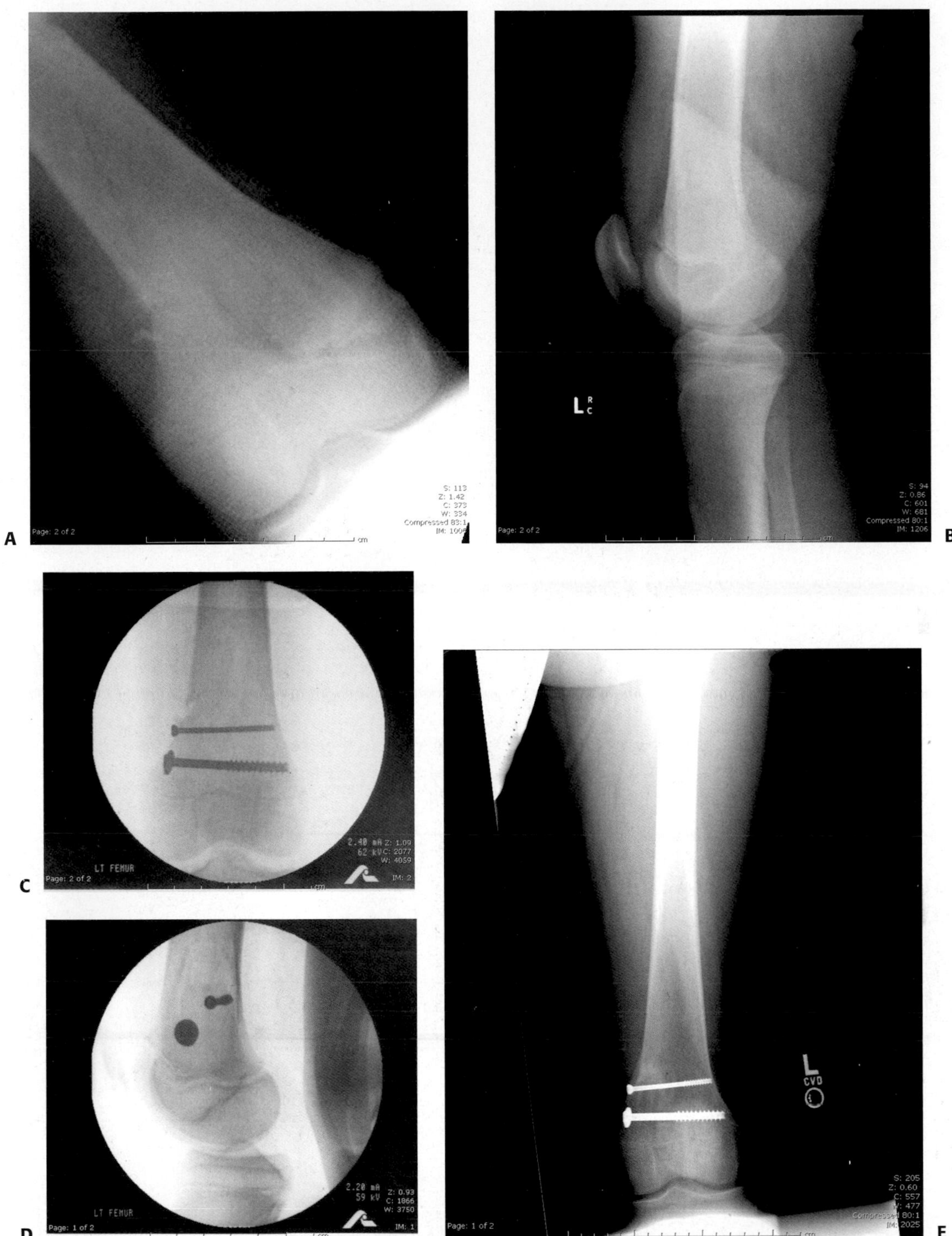

FIGURE 23-8 A. Salter-Harris type II fracture in a 12-year-old boy. **B.** Lateral view. **C.** AP view after closed reduction and fixation. Note that screws function in compression with threads across fracture line. **D.** Lateral view. **E.** Six months after injury, this plain radiograph and clinical picture was suspicious of increased valgus. Note that the radiograph is not centered on the distal physis, and thus the physis is difficult to visualize.

corner that remains attached to the epiphysis is called the Thurston-Holland fragment. Displacement is usually toward the side of the metaphyseal fragment.

The Salter-Harris type III injury is a separation of a portion of the epiphysis, with a vertical fracture line extending from the physis down to or through the articular surface of the epiphysis (Fig. 23-9). Salter-Harris type III injuries of the distal femur usually involve the medial condyle. These injuries are produced by valgus stress during sports activity and may have an associated injury to the cruciate ligaments.[22,125] Nondisplaced fractures may only be detectable with a stress x-ray or MRI.[98] McKissick et al.[98] noted that the Salter-Harris type III fracture pattern may be related to the sequence of closure of the distal femoral physis, similar to a juvenile Tillaux fracture of the distal tibia.[98]

Occasionally, a type III fracture may be in the coronal plane

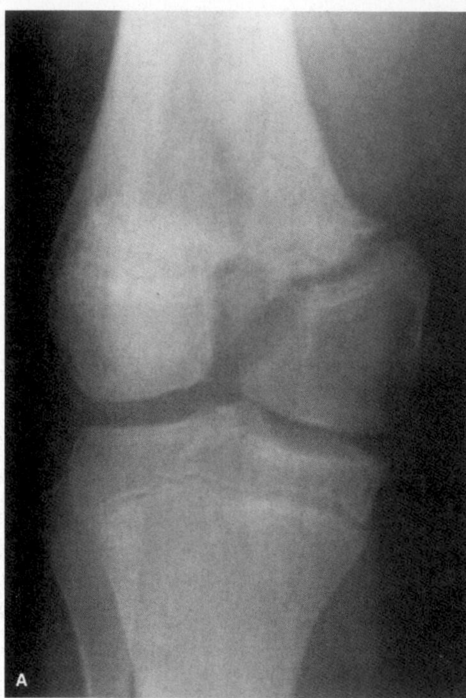

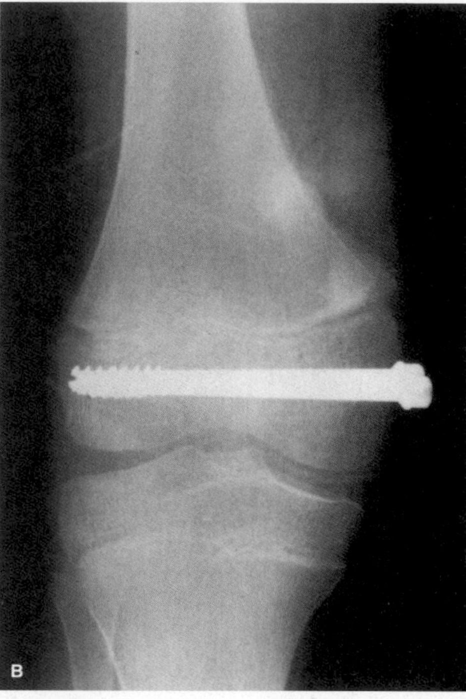

FIGURE 23-9 A. Salter-Harris type III fracture–separation of the distal femur. Note the vertical fracture line extending from the physis distally into the intercondylar notch with displacement. **B.** After reduction and fixation with two compression screws extending transversely across the epiphyseal fragments. Note closure and healing of the vertical fracture line in the epiphysis, with restoration of the articular surface.

of the condyle similar to the "Hoffa fracture" of the posterior condyle seen in adults.[85,110] This fracture is very difficult to diagnose with standard x-rays.[138]

Salter-Harris type IV injuries of the distal femur are uncommon. The fracture line extends vertically through the metaphyseal cortex, across the physis, and exits through the articular surface of the epiphysis (Fig. 23-10). Even slight displacement of a Salter-Harris type IV fracture may produce a bony bridge from the displaced epiphysis to the metaphysis. Therefore, anatomic reduction and internal fixation are essential for type IV fractures.

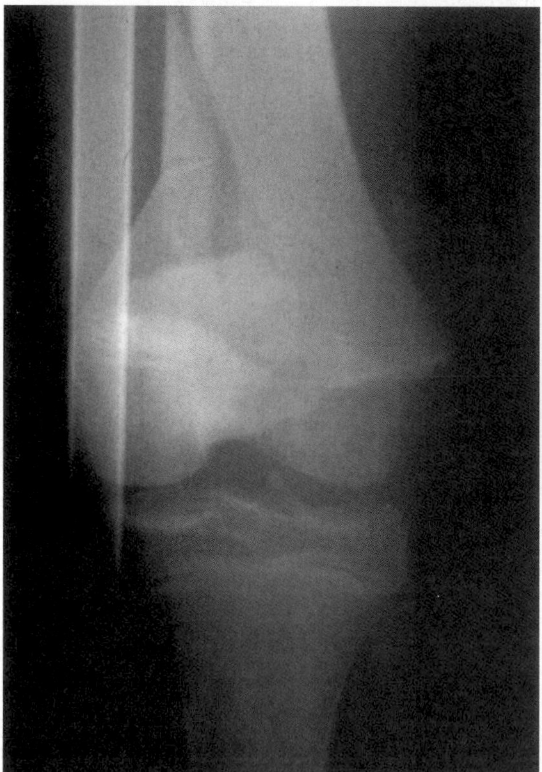

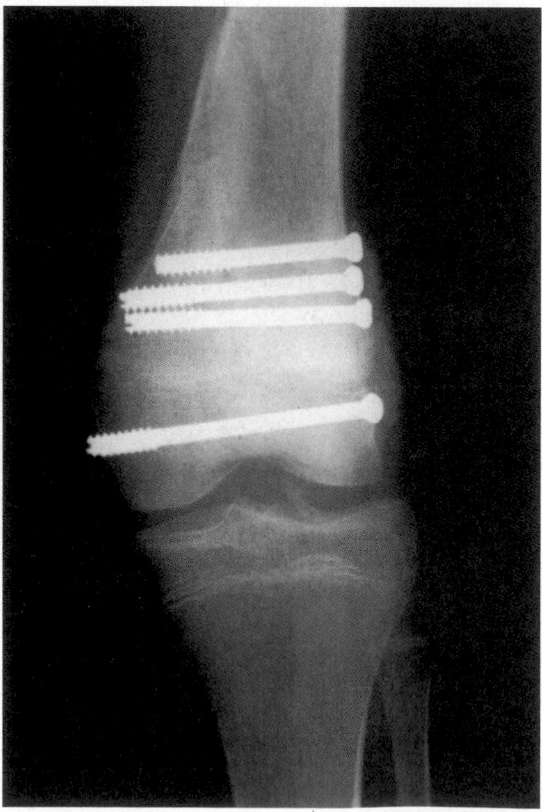

FIGURE 23-10 A. Comminuted Salter-Harris type IV fracture of the distal femur in a 14-year-old boy involved in a motor vehicle accident. **B.** Six months after open reduction and internal fixation with cannulated screws in the metaphysis and epiphysis

Salter-Harris type V injury occurs when the physis is crushed without displacement. This injury is rare and often diagnosed retrospectively when growth disturbance is observed following an injury to the knee.[148] When a type V injury is suspected, an MRI may identify bone contusion on both sides of the growth plate, suggesting compression damage of the growth plate.[142]

Other patterns of epiphyseal injury can occur that do not fit into the original Salter-Harris classification. A type VI injury has been proposed and is occasionally identified following femoral epiphyseal trauma.[113,131] A type VI injury is an avulsion of the periphery of the physis with a fragment of metaphyseal and epiphyseal bone attached. This small fragment, including a portion of the perichondrium and underlying bone, may be torn off when the proximal attachment of the collateral ligament is avulsed.

Classification by Displacement

Several authors have evaluated magnitude and direction of displacement to predict final outcome.[3,71,89,159] Direction of displacement may guide treatment but does not predict the frequency of poor outcomes in general.[3,71,149] Anterior displacement of the epiphysis results from hyperextension of the knee and has an increased risk of neurovascular damage,[36,149] but *direction* of displacement does not correlate with other complications such as angular deformity, growth disturbance, or loss of motion. In contrast, *severity* of displacement does predict final outcome and complications.[3,71,159] Amount of displacement has been evaluated by several different methods, but displacement of more than one third of bone width correlates with higher-energy trauma and more frequent complications.[3,71,89,159] Metaphyseal comminution which may indicate higher-energy trauma has also been correlated with an increased risk of complications.[71]

Classification According to Age

Age at time of injury correlates with frequency and severity of complications.[133] Distal femoral epiphyseal fractures in children aged 2 to 11 years are caused by more severe trauma and have the worst prognosis.[44,133] In adolescents, low-energy sports injuries are the most frequent cause of epiphyseal separation. Because adolescents have little growth, remaining severe growth retardation is uncommon. Separations of the distal femoral epiphysis before the age of 2 years generally have satisfactory outcomes,[95,133,159] possibly because epiphyseal undulations and the central peak are not as prominent in infants as in older children (Fig. 23-11A).[111] In juveniles and adolescents, the fracture may pass through the central prominence and lead to central growth arrest due to interference with vascularity in this region or due to the fracture plane exiting and re-entering the central physis (Fig.23-11B).[111,133,151]

Imaging

Because the physis normally is radiolucent, injury is diagnosed by widening, displacement of the epiphysis, or adjacent bony disruption; however, a nondisplaced Salter-Harris type I or III fracture without separation can be easily overlooked.[7,138,162] Oblique views of the distal femur may reveal an occult fracture through the epiphysis or metaphysis (Table 23-2). It has been suggested that stress views should be considered if multiple plain films are negative in a patient with an effusion or tenderness localized to the physis;[147] however, when a fracture is not visible on standard x-rays, immobilization in a cast may be preferable because stress x-rays may be painful or further disrupt alignment. Also, there is no urgent reason to repair ligamentous injuries, so 2 weeks of immobilization will usually define the injury as accurately as stress radiographs.[151] Another option for early diagnosis of occult injury is MRI, which should be diagnostic for fracture and/or associated soft tissue injuries.[98] A computed tomography (CT) scan may be preferable for evaluating fractures with metaphyseal comminution or determining fracture geometry for fixation purposes.

Standard x-rays are sufficient for initial evaluation of most distal femoral epiphyseal fractures. The magnitude and direction of displacement along with the fracture pattern are used to guide treatment. Medial or lateral displacement or a vertical epiphyseal fracture line is best seen on an anteroposterior (AP) view. This view allows differentiation of Salter-Harris types III and IV injuries from other types. Minor degrees of displacement may be difficult to measure on plain films unless the x-ray projection is precisely in line with the plane of fracture. Even small amounts of displacement are significant.[71,89] Anterior or posterior displacement of the epiphysis is best appreciated on the

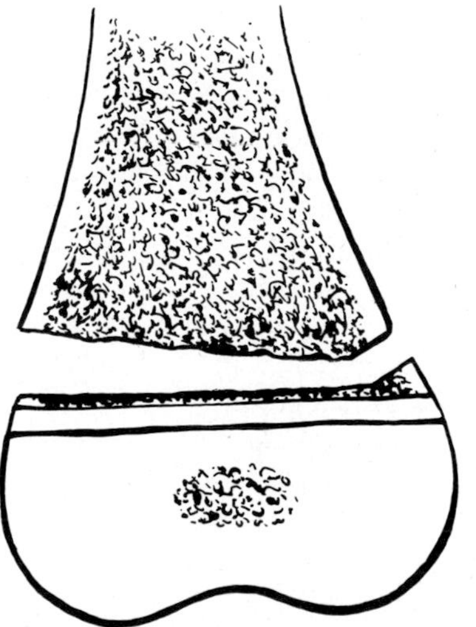

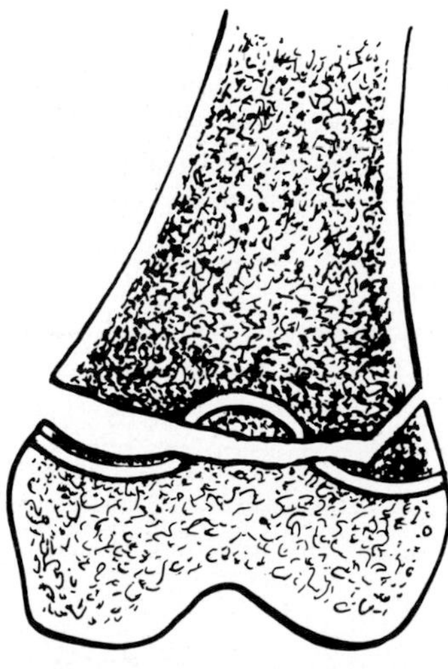

FIGURE 23-11 A. Distal femoral physeal separation prior to the age of 2 years may not disrupt growth because the physis is flat. **B.** After the age of 2 years, a central ridge and four quadrants of undulation develop in the distal femur. Fractures in this age group are more likely to cross multiple planes of bone and cartilage.

TABLE 23-2 Imaging Studies in the Evaluation of Distal Femoral Physeal Fractures

Study	Indications	Limitations
Standard radiographs	First study, often sufficient.	May miss nondisplaced Salter-Harris type I or III fractures or underestimate fracture displacement.
CT scan	Best defines fracture pattern and amount of displacement. Useful for planning surgery, especially for metaphyseal comminution.	Poor cartilage visualization. Less useful than MRI in evaluating for occult Salter-Harris type I or III fractures.
MRI	Evaluation of occult Salter-Harris type I fracture, especially in infants with little epiphyseal ossification. Identifies associated soft tissue injuries, especially with Salter-Harris type III fractures.	Availability, cost, duration of procedure. Fracture geometry less clear than with CT scans.
Stress views	Differentiate occult Salter-Harris fracture from ligament injury.	Painful, muscle spasm may not permit opening of fracture if patient awake. Unclear that study changes initial treatment.
Contralateral radiographs	Infants, or to assess physeal width. Follow-up to compare growth.	Usually not helpful in acute fractures.
Ultrasonography arthrography	Infants to assess swelling and displacement of epiphysis.	Not useful after infancy.

lateral projection. The anteriorly displaced epiphysis is usually tilted so that the distal articular surface faces anteriorly (hyperextension). The posteriorly displaced epiphysis is rotated so that the distal articular surface faces the popliteal fossa. Separation of the distal femoral epiphysis in an infant is difficult to see on initial x-rays unless there is displacement because only the center of the epiphysis is ossified at birth. This ossification center should be in line with the axis of the femoral shaft on both AP and lateral views. Comparison views of the opposite knee may be helpful. Ultrasonography, arthrography, or MRI of the knee may help to identify a separation of the relatively unossified femoral epiphysis.[69,173]

MRI may be helpful for accurate diagnosis of fracture in adolescent knee injuries. In a review of MRI scans of 315 adolescents with traumatic knee injuries, physeal injuries of the distal femur were diagnosed in seven patients and of the proximal tibia in two patients. Plain films available on eight patients showed signs of fracture in seven patients, but the fracture was clearly delineated in only one patient.[32] For evaluation of the physis with MRI, fat-suppressed three-dimensional spoiled gradient-recalled echo sequences reportedly provide the best information.[41]

Impending growth disturbance can be identified early with MRI[41,46] and MR or CT imaging can be useful to evaluate growth arrest before excision of a bony bar.[41,88]

Surgical and Applied Anatomy

The epiphysis of the distal femur is the first epiphysis to ossify and is present at birth. From birth to skeletal maturity, the distal femoral physis contributes 70% of the growth of the femur and 37% of the growth of the lower extremity. The annual rate of growth is approximately three eighths of an inch or 9 to 10 mm. The growth ceases at a mean skeletal age of 14 years in girls and 16 years in boys.[2,172]

Physeal Anatomy

At birth, the distal femoral physis is flat. With maturation, the physis assumes an undulating and convoluted shape.[86] An intercondylar groove develops along with medial and lateral sulci. This divides the physis into four quadrants of concave configuration that match the four convex surfaces of the distal femoral metaphysis. This complex geometry may help resist shear and torsional forces and also the large cross-sectional area of the distal femoral physis contributes to stability. The perichondral ring and ligamentous structures provide additional resistance to disruption of the physis, but these structures become thinner during the adolescent growth period.[30,103] Thus, substantial force is required to disrupt the distal femoral physis in juveniles, but less force may produce separation in infants and adolescents. When fractures do occur in the distal femur, the irregular configuration of the physis may predispose to crack lines that extend through multiple regions of the physis regardless of fracture type (see Fig. 23-11).[133] During reduction of displaced fractures, epiphyseal ridges may grind against the metaphyseal projections and damage germinal cells. Gentle, anatomic reduction is recommended, but reduction under general anesthesia does not correlate with reduced risk of growth disturbance.[159] Salter-Harris type I fractures generally extend through the hypertrophic zone and the zone of provisional calcification without traversing the germinal layers. Salter-Harris type II fractures exit through the metaphysis with a spike of metaphyseal bone attached to the epiphysis on the compression side (Thurston-Holland fragment) (see Fig. 23-4A). In any type of epiphyseal fracture, a flap of torn periosteum may become interposed between the fragments and prevent reduction (see Fig. 23-4B). Salter-Harris types III and IV fractures cross the entire physis vertically and enter the joint through articular cartilage.

Bony Anatomy

Immediately above the medial border of the medial condyle, the metaphysis of the distal femur widens sharply to the adductor tubercle. In contrast, the metaphysis flares minimally on the lateral side to produce the lateral epicondyle. The mechanical axis of the femur is formed by a line between the centers of the hip and knee joints (Fig. 23-12). A line tangential to the distal surfaces of the two condyles (the joint line) is in approximately 3 degrees of valgus relative to the mechanical axis. The longitudinal axis of the diaphysis of the femur inclines medially in a distal direction at an angle of 6 degrees relative to the mechanical axis and an angle of 9 degrees relative to the distal articular plane.[67]

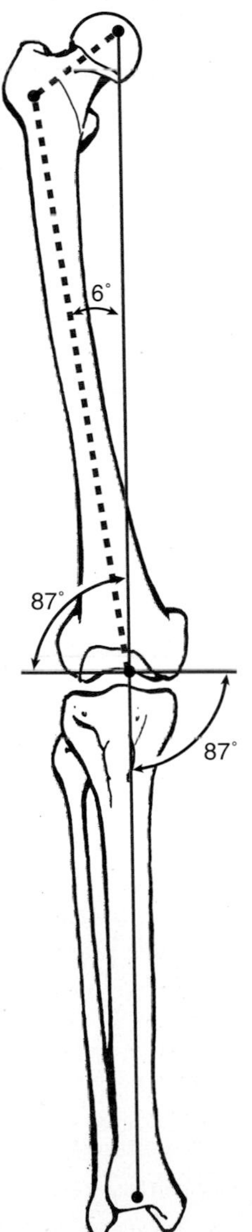

FIGURE 23-12 The mechanical and anatomic axis of the lower extremity. Note that the knee joint is in a mean of 3 degrees of valgus. The femoral shaft intersects the transverse plane of the distal femoral articular surface at an angle of 87 degrees.

A large part of the surface of the distal femoral epiphysis is covered by cartilage for articulation with the proximal tibia and patella. The anterior or patellar surface has a shallow midline concavity to accommodate the longitudinal ridge on the undersurface of the patella. The distal or tibial surface of each condyle extends on either side of the intercondylar notch far around onto the posterior surface. Here, the articular cartilage nearly reaches the posterior margin of the physis.

Soft Tissue Anatomy

The distal femoral physis is completely extra-articular. Anteriorly and posteriorly, the synovial membrane and joint capsule of the knee attach to the femoral epiphysis close to the distal femoral physis. Anteriorly, the suprapatellar pouch balloons proximally over the anterior surface of the metaphysis. On the medial and lateral surfaces of the epiphysis, the proximal attachment of the synovium and capsule is below the physis and separated from the physis by the insertions of the collateral ligaments. The strong posterior capsule and all major supporting ligaments of the knee are attached to the epiphysis of the femur distal to the physis. Both cruciate ligaments originate in the upward-sloping roof of the intercondylar notch distal to the physis. Compression and tension forces can be transmitted across the extended knee to the epiphysis of the femur by taut ligaments.

The medial and lateral head of the gastrocnemius originate from the distal femur, proximal to the joint capsule. Thus, fractures due to forces transmitted through the muscles and tendons do not seem to be as much of a factor as forces transmitted through the ligaments and capsule.

Neurovascular Anatomy

The popliteal artery is separated from the posterior surface of the distal femur by only a thin layer of fat. Directly proximal to the femoral condyles, the superior geniculate arteries pass medially and laterally to lie between the femoral metaphysis and the overlying muscles. As the popliteal artery continues distally, it lies on the posterior capsule of the knee joint between the femoral condyles. At this level, the middle geniculate artery branches anteriorly to enter the posterior aspect of the distal femoral epiphysis. The popliteal artery and its branches are vulnerable to injury from the distal femoral metaphysis at the time of hyperextension injury.

The sciatic nerve divides into the peroneal and tibial nerves proximal to the popliteal space. The peroneal nerve descends posteriorly between the biceps femoris muscle and the lateral head of the gastrocnemius muscle to a point just distal to the head of the fibula. Thus, there is interposed muscle protecting the nerve from the potentially sharp edges of a physeal fracture. The nerve is subject to stretch if the distal femoral epiphysis is tilted into varus or rotated medially.

The distal femoral epiphysis receives its blood supply from a rich anastomosis of vessels. It is unlikely that the distal femoral epiphysis would be completely shorn of its blood supply unless an articular fragment is extruded or completely stripped of its soft tissue attachments. Clinically, osteonecrosis of the epiphysis is not a commonly recognized sequela of distal femoral epiphyseal fractures.

Current Treatment Options

Rationale

The most common complication of distal femoral physeal fractures is growth disturbance with angular deformity and/or limb length discrepancy.[3,36,44,89] Ligamentous instability and loss of knee motion are also frequently reported long-term sequelae. Completely nondisplaced fractures can be managed with cast immobilization, but close follow-up is recommended to detect and treat any displacement (Table 23-3).[3,71] Closed reduction can be attempted for Salter-Harris types I and II fractures, but subsequent displacement is frequent when patients are immobilized in long-leg casts without internal fixation.[44,53,159] Anything less than anatomic reduction increases the risk of growth disturbance.[44,51,89,133] Fracture remodeling is unpredictable when small degrees of malalignment are accepted in patients older than 2 years of age.[133] For these reasons, anatomic reduction, stable fixation, and careful follow-up are the basis of treatment of physeal fractures of the distal femur.

Closed Reduction and Cast Immobilization

Nondisplaced Fractures (≤2 mm). Nondisplaced fractures of the distal femoral epiphysis are uncommon. Outcomes with cast immobilization are usually satisfactory,[89,159] but displacement can occur even with cast immobilization.[3,44] A well-molded long-leg cast is applied with the knee in approximately 15 degrees to 20 degrees of flexion with the intact periosteal hinge tightened. Thus, if the metaphyseal fragment of a nondisplaced Salter-Harris type II separation is on the lateral side of the metaphysis, the cast is applied with three-point molding into slight varus. Alternative methods of immobilization include a posterior splint, cylinder cast from proximal thigh to ankle, and a single hip spica cast. The more secure form of immobilization or internal fixation should be considered if the patient is obese or potentially unreliable.

Displaced Fractures (>2 mm). Displaced Salter-Harris types III and IV fractures are managed by open reduction and stable fixation, which are discussed later in this section. Closed reduction can be attempted up to 10 days after injury for Salter-Harris types I and II fractures, but these fractures are inherently unstable when immobilized without restricting motion of the hip. Anatomic reduction is recommended, with less than a 2-mm gap following reduction.[44,71] Redisplacement in long-leg casts has been reported in 30% to 70% of patients treated without internal fixation.[44,53,133,159] Minor degrees of displacement may increase the risk of angular deformity or growth disturbance. Gentle reduction has been recommended by some authors.[133,159] General anesthesia often is helpful to decrease associated muscle spasm and diminish the risk of further injury to the physis, but Thomson et al.[159] observed that while reduction under general anesthesia was more likely to be associated with anatomic alignment it did not reduce the risk of premature physeal arrest. One cause of failure of reduction is interposed periosteum which may become entrapped in the fracture (see Fig. 23-4B). Although the alignment may be acceptable, the interposed periosteum, increases the risk of premature growth arrest.[126]

The technique of closed reduction depends on the direction and degree of displacement of the epiphysis (Fig. 23-13A,B). Joint aspiration may precede manipulation. The periosteum is usually intact in the direction of displacement of the distal fragment, which is on the side of the metaphyseal fragment in a Salter-Harris type II fracture. The first principle for reduction is to avoid harm to the physis. The maneuver should be 90% traction and 10% leverage. The first maneuver increases the deformity slightly while traction is applied. The proximal edge of the displaced epiphysis can then be aligned with the edge of the metaphysis on the same side as the periosteal tether. Reduction is then completed by correcting angular deformity and

TABLE 23-3 Methods of Treatment for Distal Femoral Physeal Fractures

Treatment	Pros	Cons	Indications
Closed reduction and immobilization	Avoids anesthesia	High risk of loss of reduction	Nondisplaced, stable fractures
Closed reduction and screw fixation	Minimal dissection	Only in reducible fractures	Reducible Salter-Harris type II fractures Nondisplaced Salter-Harris type III and IV fractures
Closed reduction and smooth pinning	Minimal dissection	Pins may lead to joint infection or require later removal	Reducible Salter-Harris type I fractures, and Salter-Harris type II fractures with small metaphyseal fragment
Open reduction and screws and/or pins	Anatomic reduction	Stiffness	Irreducible Salter-Harris type I and II fractures, displaced Salter-Harris type III and IV fractures
External fixation	Allows soft tissue access	Pin site (joint) infection	Severe soft tissue injury
Rigid plate crossing physis	Rigid fixation	Can stop future growth when spans physis	Adolescents near the end of growth Severe injuries with severe disturbance inevitable Possible temporary fixation with extraperiosteal locked plating removed soon after union

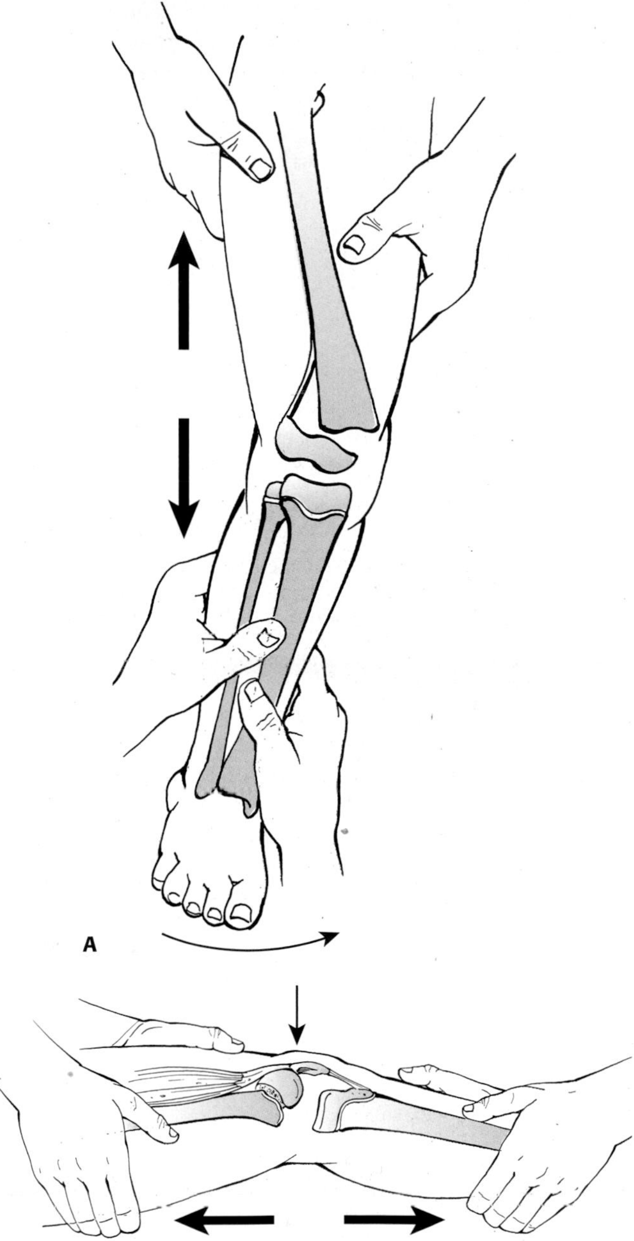

FIGURE 23-13 Closed reduction and stabilization of a Salter-Harris type I or II fracture. **A.** With medial or lateral displacement, traction is applied longitudinally along the axis of the deformity to bring the fragments back to length. **B.** For anterior displacement, the reduction can be done with the patient prone or supine. Length is gained first, then a flexion moment is added.

closing the fracture gap without sliding the distal fragment over the corner of the femoral metaphysis. The sequence of events is to pull, tip, and close the separation. Multiple attempts at closed manipulation are not warranted and may increase the risk of growth disturbance.

Medial or Lateral Displacement. With patient supine, the leg is grasped with the knee in extension and the hip in slight flexion. The thigh is held by an assistant as moderate longitudinal traction is exerted by a handhold on the leg above the ankle. If the displacement of the epiphysis is medial, varus is increased gently and cautiously to avoid stretching the peroneal nerve. With one hand holding traction on the leg, the palm of the other hand is placed against the concave surface of the angulated distal femur. The epiphysis is pushed toward the metaphysis as the leg is realigned with the thigh. Once reduction is obtained, longitudinal traction is released.

Anterior Displacement. Anterior displacement of the epiphysis can be reduced with the patient either supine or prone. With the patient supine, the hip is flexed approximately 60 degrees and the thigh is held by an assistant. Longitudinal traction is applied with the knee in partial flexion. Posterior pressure on the epiphysis is exerted manually. With continuing traction on the leg, the knee is flexed 45 to 90 degrees. Prone reduction requires fewer assistants. If the reduction is done with the patient prone, traction is applied to the limb, an assistant pushes down on the posterior aspect of the proximal femur, and the knee is flexed approximately 110 degrees. This sequence is similar to that for reduction of a supracondylar humeral fracture. After reduction of an anteriorly displaced epiphysis, it is important to check the pulses in the foot and ankle. Maintaining reduction in a cast may be problematic following reduction of this type of fracture. Immobilization of a swollen knee in flexion of more than 90 degrees may compromise the popliteal vessels and interfere with circulation to the leg, and regaining extension of the knee may be difficult after prolonged immobilization in flexion.[55] In addition, judgment of frontal plane alignment is difficult in the flexed knee. For this reason, casting in mild knee flexion of 20 to 30 degrees may be preferable.

Posterior Displacement. For reduction of posterior displacement of the distal femoral epiphysis, the patient is placed supine and the surgeon grasps the leg and exerts downward longitudinal traction while the knee is held partly flexed. Longitudinal traction is continued as the leg is brought up to extend the knee. An assistant pulls up directly under the distal femoral epiphysis with one hand and pushes down on the distal metaphysis of the femur with the other. Such flexion type injuries can be immobilized in extension.[36]

Postreduction Management. X-ray and clinical follow-up is recommended 5 to 7 days after immobilization to detect any subsequent displacement. Union is normally rapid because the distal femoral physis is a metabolically active area of bone formation. Partial weight-bearing on crutches with touchdown gait can be started 2 to 3 weeks after injury. Cast immobilization is continued for approximately 4 weeks in most cases, and this can be followed by a removable knee immobilizer and gentle range-of-motion exercises. Full weight-bearing is generally permitted 6 weeks after initial injury. X-ray and clinical follow-ups at 6 and 12 months after injury are recommended to detect early growth disturbances. Even nondisplaced fractures should be followed until normal resumption of growth can be determined.

Closed Reduction and Percutaneous Fixation

Salter-Harris Types I and II Fractures. Most displaced Salter-Harris types I and II epiphyseal fractures of the distal femur can be reduced by closed manipulation and stabilized with percutaneous pins or screws under fluoroscopic control. Internal fixation maintains anatomic reduction better than cast immobilization and is recommended by most of the more recent authors on this subject.[3,44,53,133,157,159,179] A basic principle is that fixation devices should avoid crossing the physis if adequate fixation can be achieved without doing so.[3] In Salter-Harris type I fractures as well as type II fractures with small metaphyseal fragments, crossing the physis is necessary but fracture stabilization is important to avoid loss of reduction during the postoperative period. When traversing the physis is unavoidable, smooth pins are recommended. Although it may not be possible to tell with complete certainty whether a subsequent growth disturbance arose from the injury or pins crossing the physis, clinical experience suggests smooth pins crossing a physis are unlikely to cause a growth disturbance. Studies in the rabbit model have determined that drill holes of 2 to 2.5 mm (3% to 5% of physeal area) do not cause growth disturbance.[73,93] Thus, it is unlikely that a 3 to 3.5 mm (one eighth of an inch) smooth pin would contribute to growth disturbance following fixation of a distal femoral epiphyseal fracture. Pins should be widely separated at the fracture site (see Fig. 23-7C), which is generally easiest to achieve by inserting the pins at a high angle so they cross proximal to the physis. Pins can be inserted from each condyle across the fracture and into the femoral metaphysis, or both pins can be inserted laterally with one entering the lateral femoral shaft and proceeding distally and medially. The other pin then enters the distal femoral epiphysis and proceeds proximally and medially to engage the opposite cortex. The pins can be cut off under the skin before application of a long-leg cast or left percutaneous. Infection is frequent if pins in this region are left out through the skin for longer than 4 weeks, and intra-articular pins may lead to a septic knee. If the metaphyseal fragment is large enough, cannulated screws can be directed transversely across the metaphysis after reduction (Fig. 23-14; see also Fig. 23-8C). Stability should be gently tested because the metaphyseal spike may not be firmly attached to the epiphysis in high-energy injuries with comminution. After stabilization with pins or screws, the lower extremity is immobilized in a long-leg cast. Postoperative management is similar to that after closed reduction without fixation. Pins are generally removed 2 to 3 weeks after fracture, with continued cast immobilization for a total of 4 weeks.

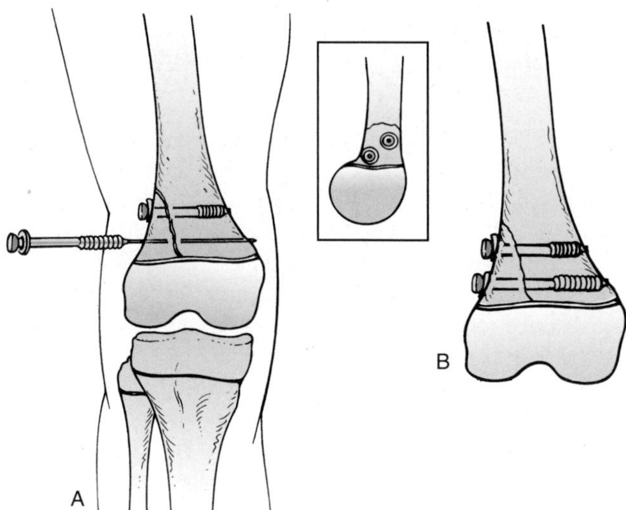

FIGURE 23-14 Screw fixation following closed oropen reduction of Salter-Harris type II fracture with a large metaphyseal fragment. **A.** When using cannulated screws, place both guidewires before screw placement to avoid rotation of the fragment while drilling or inserting screw. Screw threads should be past the fracture site to enable compression. Washers help increase compression. Screws may be placed anterior and posterir to each other, which is particularly helpful when trying to fit multiple screws in a small metaphyseal fragment. **B.** This form of fixation is locally "rigid," but must be protected with long-leg immobilization or long lever arm.

Salter-Harris types III and IV separations generally require open reduction to obtain anatomic alignment, although arthroscopic-assisted reduction and percutaneous fixation of a Salter-Harris type IV fracture have been described.[83]

Open Reduction of Physeal Fractures

Salter-Harris Types I and II Fractures. Open reduction is indicated for irreducible Salter-Harris types I and II fractures and for most displaced Salter-Harris types III and IV fractures. Open reduction is also appropriate for open fractures or when associated injuries mandate it (i.e., vascular or ligament injury). A tourniquet around the proximal thigh can be used for temporary hemostasis if it is placed proximally enough to avoid binding the thigh muscles under the inflated tourniquet. How much of a "fracture gap" of a type II fracture is acceptable is open to debate. Interposed periosteum may contribute to growth arrest[125,126] and has been identified as a possible cause of growth arrest in distal tibial physeal fractures. [8] Anatomic reduction is recommended, with less than 2-mm gap following reduction.[44,71]

Surgical approach is determined by the direction of fracture displacement because the apex of deformity is the most likely location of any obstacles to reduction. For a Salter-Harris type II separation in the coronal plane, a longitudinal incision over the distal femoral metaphyseal fragment gives direct exposure of any obstacles to reduction and avoids disruption of the periosteal hinge. If the displacement is anterior, exposure is best obtained with a standard medial approach at the anterior border of the sartorius because this can be extended to expose the popliteal artery if necessary. After exposure of the fracture, irrigation and removal of clotted blood permit better inspection of the separation. Interposed muscle or a flap of periosteum may be identified and removed between the epiphysis and metaphysis. Special care is taken to avoid any additional damage to the physis. Once the muscle and periosteal flap are removed, reduction is carried out primarily with traction and gentle realignment. To avoid damage to the physis, instruments should not be placed in the physeal interval. Fixation should be performed as described previously. After closure of the wound, a long-leg or hip spica cast is applied.

Salter-Harris Types III and IV Fractures. Open reduction with internal fixation is almost always necessary for displaced Salter-Harris types III and IV fractures of the distal femur. Precise reduction and rigid internal fixation restore articular congruity and can reduce the risk of growth arrest.[51] An anteromedial or anterolateral longitudinal incision is used (Fig. 23-15). For severely comminuted fractures, an anterior approach may be chosen with a future total knee replacement in mind. The anterior physeal and articular margins of the fracture are exposed. Reduction is checked by noting the apposition of the articular surfaces, the physeal line anteriorly, and the fracture configuration (see Fig. 23-15). Final reduction can be confirmed with fluoroscopy. The gastrocnemius has been reported as an obsta-

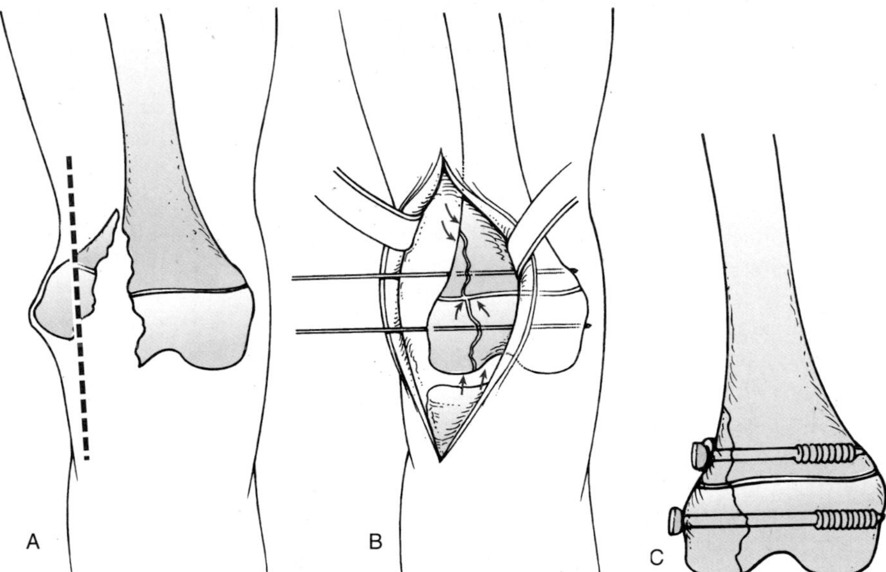

FIGURE 23-15 Open reduction of displaced lateral Salter-Harris type IV fracture of the distal femur. **A.** A longitudinal skin incision, cheating anteriorly if fracture severity raises concern of needing total knee replacement in future. **B.** Alignment of joint and physis are used to judge reduction. Guidewires for cannulated screws placed above and below physis, parallel to physis. **C.** Screws inserted in compression with washer on metaphyseal fragment. Washer is optional in epiphyseal fragment if later prominence is of more concern than need for additional compression.

cle to reduction in a Salter-Harris type III fracture of the medial femoral epiphysis.[1] Provisional stabilization is obtained with Kirschner-wires (K-wires). When reduction is accomplished, screws are directed transversely across the epiphysis in Salter-Harris type III separations or across the metaphysis and epiphysis in Salter-Harris type IV injuries (see Figs. 23-10, 23-14, and 23-15). If crossing the physis with fixation is unavoidable, smooth pins should be used. A coronal plane fracture, or Hoffa fracture, usually involves the lateral condyle and is approached through an anterolateral incision except for the unusual medial condyle coronal plane fracture, which the approach is anteromedial.[110] Fixation is generally a lag screw inserted from anterior to posterior. It may be possible to use an extra-articular starting point.[138] Otherwise, the screw can be placed perpendicularly through the articular surface with the screw head or headless screw slightly buried beneath the articular surface. Alternatively, Jarit et al.[74] demonstrated in cadavers that posterior to anterior stabilization is more stable, but a small posterolateral exposure is required for screw insertion. After reduction and fixation, the knee joint is thoroughly irrigated and inspected for other fractures and ligament disruption. The limb is immobilized in a long-leg cast in addition to the internal fixation. Postoperative management is as described on page 873.

The use of indomethacin to reduce the incidence of growth disturbance in a rabbit distal femoral fracture model has been reported with equivocal results.[149] Although nonsteroidal anti-inflammatory medications have been shown to inhibit callus formation, recommendations for this treatment to prevent growth arrest are premature.

Surgery for Associated Injuries

If an associated collateral ligament injury is identified with preoperative imaging or at the time of surgery, it can be repaired at the time of open reduction. Otherwise, internal fixation is used to allow early mobilization and rehabilitation of both the physeal separation and the ligamentous injury. As noted previously, a rehabilitation program is initiated following union of the fracture when there is a cruciate ligament tear without meniscal injury. If there is a repairable meniscal tear and a cruciate ligament tear, then cruciate ligament reconstruction can be done at the time of meniscal repair depending on the patient's age and activity level (see Chapter 24).

If vascular repair is indicated, a posterior modified S-shaped incision or medial approach is used to follow the course of the femoral artery. The medial incision is usually preferred because it provides adequate exposure of the fracture and the artery. Care should be taken during the incision because the vessel may be superficial beneath the skin, particularly in an anteriorly displaced fracture. The hamstring tendons may be "bowstrung" around the femoral metaphysis. The artery may be in spasm, occluded by intimal tear, or disrupted. After the vascular structures are identified, the fracture is reduced and stabilized rapidly before vascular repair, except as noted earlier on page 847.

External Fixation

When access is needed for treatment of severe soft-tissue injuries or staged surgeries are planned, external fixation may be indicated. Spanning external fixation may also be indicated in combination with limited internal fixation for severely comminuted fractures or other special circumstances. Because of the risks of secondary knee joint infection and loss of motion, external fixation is not indicated for most distal femoral physeal fractures.[161]

Rigid Plate Fixation

Rigid compression plate fixation across the physis will stop all remaining growth while the plate is in place. Standard screw fixation of the plate to bone may crush the perichondral ring and contribute to growth arrest; however, more modern periarticular locking compression plates may allow fixation with the plate slightly elevated from the physis and bone. Also, unicortical fixation is sufficient in some fracture segments. These plates may eventually provide a method of temporary fixation of some epiphyseal fractures to reduce damage to the physis. After bone union, the plates need to be removed so that growth can resume in a manner similar to temporary staples for guided growth. At the time of this writing, this option is reserved for adolescents near the end of growth and children with severe injuries in which severe growth disturbance is believed to be inevitable.

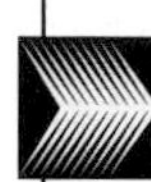

AUTHORS' PREFERRED TREATMENT

Guiding principles. The age of the patient is useful information for advising parents about the types and severity of potential complications, but management is primarily based on the fracture pattern and amount of displacement. The amount of displacement guides treatment only to the extent that the fracture is nondisplaced or displaced more than 2 mm. Only nondisplaced fractures are managed closed with cast immobilization. Special imaging studies are indicated whenever doubt exists about minor displacement and for assessment of unusual fracture patterns. MRI is recommended for type III fractures before surgery. Increasing amounts of displacement indicate more severe trauma and greater potential for complications, but the treatment of all displaced fractures is reduction and surgical stabilization, regardless of the amount of displacement.

The fracture pattern helps guide treatment to the extent that types III and IV fractures almost always require open reduction, and there is a higher frequency of ligamentous injury associated with type III fractures. Types I and II fractures can usually be managed with closed reduction and percutaneous fixation as the primary treatment. The possibility of child abuse in infants or presence of compartment syndrome, coronal plane fractures of the condyle, ligament damage, and neurologic injury should be kept in mind. The need for follow-up for at least a year should be emphasized to parents at the time of the initial encounter. The opportunity for early intervention for growth disturbance is frequently missed because parents believe their asymptomatic child has fully recovered.

Surgical Procedures

Nondisplaced Fractures

Cast immobilization without reduction is reserved for minimally displaced fractures that are barely visible on standard x-rays (Fig. 23-16). We believe that even 1 or 2 mm of displacement is cause for concern about increased risk for growth arrest and also for further displacement in the cast. A long-leg cast is applied for fractures with no more than 2 mm or less displacement and less than 3 degrees of angulation. The cast is applied as closely towards the groin as possible with firm triangular molding of the shape of the proximal thigh to aid rotational control. Clinical and x-ray follow-up is strongly recommended 5 to 7 days after initial treatment to assess maintenance of reduction. Limited weight-bearing is recommended for 6 weeks, but the cast is removed at 4 weeks. A knee immobilizer is then provided for 2 more

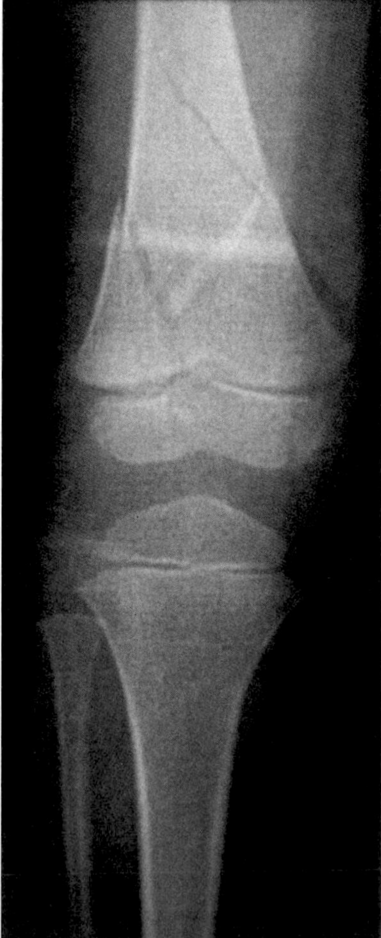
A

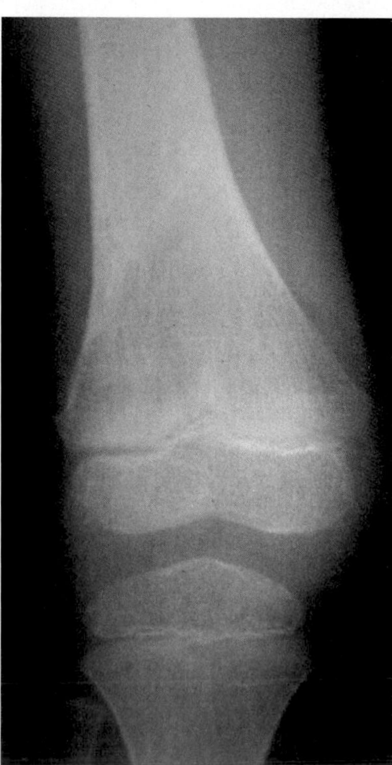
B

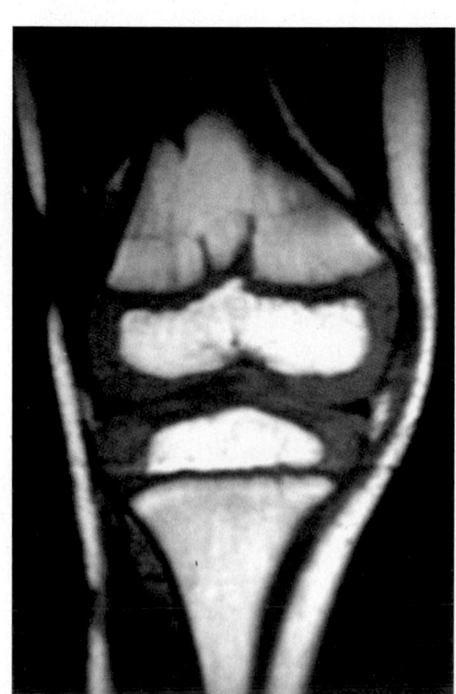
C

FIGURE 23-16 Five-year-old boy hit by car with fracture of the distal femur. **A.** AP radiograph of minimally displaced Salter-Harris type IV fracture of the distal femur. **B.** AP radiograph of healed fracture. From this view, it is difficult to determine if injury to the physis has occurred, though a central growth arrest was suspected. **C.** MRI shows a central growth plate injury probably did occur, although this did not result in formation of a bony bar or growth arrest. (Courtesy of Robert Kay, MD, Los Angeles, CA.)

weeks along with gentle range-of-motion exercises to reduce the risk of loss of knee motion. X-ray follow-up is continued until resumption of normal growth is documented.

Displaced Salter-Harris Types I and II Fractures

Alignment is generally deemed unacceptable when displacement is more than 2 mm or angulation is more than 3 degrees. In all age groups, these fractures are reduced under general anesthesia and stabilized with percutaneous crossed pins or metaphyseal screws. If the displacement is anterior, we perform the reduction with the patient supine. Otherwise, reductions are performed as described earlier in this chapter. Open reduction is done when anatomic reduction better than the above criteria cannot be achieved by closed manipulation. For Salter-Harris type I fractures, smooth 2.0- to 3.2-mm pins are used in a crossed configuration. Pins are bent to prevent migration, and the skin is protected by sterile quarter-inch thick felt (see Fig. 23-7C). We attempt to maximally separate the pins at the fracture site for stability. Pin insertion sites should avoid the synovial cavity of the knee. One pin can be inserted from the lateral thigh proximal to the fracture, across the physis medially, and into the epiphysis. Pins are removed in 2 to 3 weeks to reduce the risk of pin track infection, but cast immobilization is continued for 4 weeks after injury.

For Salter-Harris type II fractures with a large metaphyseal fragment, one or two cannulated cancellous screws are placed across the metaphyseal spike and into the femur proximal to the physis (see Figs. 23-8 and 23-14). At least two guidewires are placed before drilling and tapping to prevent rotation of the fragment. Different sized screws, such as a 6.5-mm or 7.3-mm screw in the base of the metaphyseal fragment and a 4.5-mm screw in the smaller upper portion, can be used (see Fig. 23-8E).

Salter-Harris Types III and IV Fractures

The amount of displacement can be difficult to evaluate for some of these fractures. Also, there may be additional fracture planes that are difficult to detect with standard x-rays. When possible, an MRI is recommended preoperatively for types III fractures. An MRI or CT scan is also useful for Salter-Harris type IV fractures when there is concern about amount of displacement or fracture pattern.

We prefer open or arthroscopically-guided anatomic reduction for all displaced type III and IV fractures to reduce the risk of growth disturbance and to restore anatomic congruity of the articular surface of the knee. Anecdotally, we have noted that significant joint incongruity can be present even with apparently anatomic fluoroscopic films intraoperatively. X-rays should be scrutinized for rotational deformity of individual fragments. For a truly nondisplaced type III fracture, percutaneous screw fixation is adequate. Medial condylar type III fractures are more common than lateral condylar fractures, but an anteromedial or anterolateral approach is used based on the location of the fracture. The fracture line, the physis, and the joint surface are observed to confirm anatomic reduction. Cannulated screws are then inserted with either an open technique or percutaneously with the aid of image intensification. Insertion through articular cartilage is rarely necessary, but large osteochondral fragments can be fixed with headless screws countersunk below the articular surface in the unusual instance where extra-articular fixation is not possible. Every effort is made to achieve rigid fixation to allow early motion approximately 4 weeks after injury. A long-leg fiberglass cast is placed with the knee in 10 to 30 degrees of flexion.

X-Ray Management

X-ray and clinical follow-up is recommended 5 to 7 days after initial treatment to detect any subsequent redisplacement. Partial weight-bearing is allowed 2 weeks after injury. Cast immobilization is continued for approximately 4 weeks in most cases, and this is followed by a removable knee immobilizer and gentle range-of-motion exercises for 2 more weeks. Full weight-bearing is generally permitted 6 weeks after initial injury. When smooth pins have been used, these are removed 2 to 3 weeks postoperatively to reduce the risk of infection, but cast immobilization is continued until approximately 4 weeks postoperatively. Cannulated screws can be removed as early as 3 to 4 months after injury if MRI is necessary to evaluate potential growth arrest. A full-length standing x-ray of both lower extremities is recommended in the early postoperative period to document limb lengths and alignment. A scanogram may also be obtained, but we prefer a full-length standing x-ray.[139] Repeat full-length x-rays are recommended 6 and 12 months after injury, regardless of fracture type or initial displacement. Early detection of complete or partial growth arrest is essential because any growth disturbance is rapidly progressive and should be treated as soon as it is detected.

Pearls and Pitfalls

- When the knee is swollen in infants and children, distal femoral epiphyseal separation associated with difficult deliveries, child abuse, myelodysplasia, or other pathologic conditions should be suspected.
- Minimally displaced fractures of the distal femoral epiphysis are at risk for further displacement.
- A significantly painful knee examination with normal x-rays warrants stress x-rays or MRI to detect obscure distal femoral or proximal tibial epiphyseal fractures.
  - Stable fixation with pins or cannulated screws is recommended for all fractures that require reduction.
  - When a cast is used, it should be extended as far proximally as possible and molded at the proximal thigh into a triangular shape to provide a small amount of rotational support.
  - Repeat x-rays are obtained 5 to 7 days after injury and treatment.
- Growth disturbance is frequent and troublesome, especially between the ages of 2 and 12 years.
  - Reduction is 90% traction and 10% leverage.
  - Multiple closed reduction attempts should be avoided.
  - Follow-up with full-length x-rays of both legs at 3, 6, and 12 months after injury is essential.
- Associated ligamentous injuries may be present.
  - Joint stability should be checked following union.
  - MRI should be considered, especially for type III injuries.

TABLE 23-4 Distal Femoral Physeal Fractures: Pitfalls and Prevention

Pitfall	Preventative Strategy
Missed diagnosis	Immobilize and re-examine if uncertain, or MRI Be cognizant of nondisplaced injury in infants, pathologic conditions, multitrauma, or unresponsive patients
Redisplacement of fracture	Pin or screw fixation for all fractures that require reduction Radiographs at 5–7 days postinjury High long-leg cast with triangular molding proximally or spica cast
Growth disturbance	Minimize trauma at reduction Follow-up at 6, 12, and possibly 24 months with full-length radiographs of both lower extremities
Knee joint instability	Check ligaments when fracture stabilized or healed Consider MRI, especially for type III fractures
Stiffness	Avoid prolonged immobilization Remove casts in 4 weeks and apply knee immobilizer with gentle range of motion in most cases Avoid manipulation due to risk of added injury

- Stiffness is not uncommon.
  - The cast is removed at 4 weeks and a knee immobilizer is applied for most cases.
  - Gentle range of motion is begun early, but forceful manipulation must be avoided because of the risk of added injury (Table 23-4).

Complications

Complications of fractures of the distal femoral epiphysis are listed in Table 23-5.

Recurrent Displacement and Late Reduction

Redisplacement has been reported in 30% to 70% of patients immobilized in a long-leg cast following reduction of displaced fractures without internal fixation.[44,53,133,159] Eid et al.[44] reported that a hip spica cast reduced the risk of redisplacement, but loss of reduction still occurred in 10% of their patients treated in a spica cast. Late reductions may be problematic whether performed for redisplacement or for initial treatment. Rang and Wenger[131] advised that multiple attempts at closed reduction, or reductions more than 7 to 10 days after fracture, may do more damage to the physis. An experimental study in rats did not demonstrated increased risk of growth disturbance associated with physeal fractures reduced at the human equivalent of 7 days after injury; however, attempts at reduction at the equivalent of 10 days resulted in diaphyseal fracture rather than reduction of the epiphysis.[42] Based on this study and opinions of others, it seems reasonable to attempt closed reduction

TABLE 23-5 Complications of Fractures of the Distal Femoral Epiphysis

	Number of Patients	Ligamentous Injury	Neurovascular Problems	Angular Deformity	Shortening	Stiffness
Stephens[154]	20	25%	5%	25%	40%	25%
Lombardo[89]	34	23%	3%	33%	36%	33%
Czitrom[36]	41	0	2.5%	41%	14% clinical 68% radiographic	22%
Riseborough[133]*	66		4%	25%	56%	23%
Robert	41	18%		32%	36%	30%
Thomson[159]	30	Two anterior cruciate ligament injuries		18%	47%	18%
Eid[44]	151	8% symptomatic 14% asymptomatic	10%	51%	38%	29%
Ilharreborde[71]†	20	0%		65%	40%	25%
Arkader[3]	73		1%	12%	12%	4%

*Series contains referred patients and may not represent true incidence.
†Salter-Harris type II fractures only.

before fixation up to 10 days following initial distal femoral epiphyseal separation.[64,131] After 10 days, open reduction may be required to re-establish alignment. When fractures are treated more than 10 days after initial injury, it may be better to observe Salter-Harris types I and II fractures for possible remodeling or to perform later osteotomies rather than perform open reduction. For displaced Salter-Harris types III and IV fractures that are treated late, open reduction is recommended as soon as possible to restore articular congruity.[102]

Physeal Injury

The most common complication of distal femoral epiphyseal fracture is growth disturbance with angular deformity or shortening. This has been reported in 35% to 50% of patients regardless of anatomic reduction.[3,44,53,71,89,154,159] Salter-Harris types I and II fractures in other areas of the body usually have a low risk of growth arrest, but even minimally displaced fractures in the distal femur should be followed closely for growth arrest (see Fig. 23-16) Growth disturbance is uncommon in patients younger than 2 years of age due to the flat shape of the physis in this age group.[133] In juveniles, more energy is required to disrupt the physis and the complex shape of the physis may predispose to fracture lines that extend through multiple regions of the physis regardless of fracture type.[133] In adolescents, less force is required to disrupt the physis, but the consequences of growth arrest are not as severe as in patients between the ages of 2 and 12 years.

When growth arrest occurs, it usually is evident by 6 months after distal femoral epiphyseal fracture. The distal femur grows approximately 1 cm a year and growth should resume within this time frame. Full-length standing x-rays of both lower extremities are recommended as soon as possible following the initial injury. These are repeated approximately 6 months later to identify early angular deformity or increasing length discrepancy. Bilateral AP and lateral femoral x-ryas 6 months after injury should demonstrate growth arrest lines (Park-Harris lines) that can be examined for symmetry and alignment. Growth arrest lines develop when there is a temporary slowing of growth during periods of malnutrition, trauma, chemotherapy, or alcohol consumption.[52,61,112,120] The normal longitudinal orientation of the zone of provisional calcification becomes dense and interconnected, forming a transverse line in the metaphysis. After growth resumes, this dense layer moves away from the physis and is visible on x-rays as a radiodense line of bone in the metaphysis.[112] If the line is growing symmetrically away from the physis, then normal growth has resumed. Failure of a Park-Harris line to appear is evidence of premature growth arrest when a line is visible in the uninjured distal femoral metaphysis. An oblique Park-Harris line that converges toward the physis indicates asymmetrical growth caused by a bone bridge across the physis that is preventing growth of one side of the physis. When there is doubt about premature physeal closure, screw removal is recommended before an MRI study. Growth disturbance can be detected by MRI as early as 2 months after injury.[41] Fat-suppressed three-dimensional spoiled gradient-recalled echo sequence MRI technique has been described as the best method for diagnosis and follow-up of premature physeal arrest.[41]

Physeal Arrest with Progressive Angulation

Early recognition and management of progressive angulation can reduce the need for osteotomy if diagnosis is made before a clinically significant deformity develops. After deformity has developed, an osteotomy is generally required whether bar excision is performed or not. The risk of significant angular disturbance is greatest in patients with significant growth remaining. When asymmetric growth follows a type II separation, the portion of the physis protected by the Thurston-Holland fragment is usually spared. The localized area of growth inhibition occurs in that portion of the physis not protected by the metaphyseal fragment. Therefore, if the metaphyseal spike is medial, deformity is more likely to be valgus due to lateral growth arrest.

If a localized area of premature arrest constitutes less than 50% of the total area of the physis and at least 2 years of growth remains, excision of the bony bridge has been recommended.[80,123] Although Langenskiöld[82] reported normal resumption of growth in 80% of patients, others have reported normal growth in only 25% to 50% of patients.[16,23,62,174] Therefore, bilateral epiphysiodesis should be considered when there is less than 3 to 4 cm of growth remaining and deformity is minor. Hemiepiphysiodesis alone is not an option for correcting deformity when a bone bridge already exists on one side of the physis. However, ipsilateral hemiepiphysiodesis combined with contralateral total epiphysiodesis can maintain the current status of length and alignment when growth arrests are diagnosed early in adolescent patients. We recommend bar excision without osteotomy in an attempt to restore growth when angular deformity is 5 to 20 degrees, there are more than 2 years of growth remaining, and the area of bar is less than 33% of the area of the physis. Osteotomy at the time of physeal resection is recommended when angular deformity exceeds 20 degrees.[80,123] For bone bridges larger than 33% of the area of the physis or when angulation is more than 20 degrees, we recommend osteotomy with bilateral epiphysiodesis or ipsilateral lengthening depending on the extent of growth remaining and current amount of discrepancy. Descriptions of techniques for bar excision, epiphysiodesis, osteotomy, or lengthening are beyond the scope of this text and are well-described in other textbooks or periodicals.

Physeal Injury with Leg-Length Discrepancy

Limb-length discrepancy is a frequently reported complication of distal femoral physeal fractures,[3,44,71,133,159] but the amount of discrepancy may not be clinically relevant.[3,71] Up to 2 cm of limb-length inequality does not cause significant gait disturbance or clinical symptoms in adulthood.[50,57,150] The distal femoral epiphysis grows at a rate of approximately 1 cm per year until skeletal maturity.[2,172] Thus, when the patient is within 2 years of skeletal maturity at the time of injury, the shortening probably will be insignificant. Serial scanograms for calculation and timing of epiphysiodesis are not helpful following posttraumatic distal femoral growth arrest. When complete distal femoral arrest is diagnosed, the only method to prevent progressive discrepancy is immediate epiphysiodesis of the contralateral distal femur. Thus, the only decision following diagnosis is whether to close the opposite physis, allow the discrepancy to increase within physiological limits, or plan for limb lengthening.

Stiffness

Limitation of knee motion after separation of the distal femoral epiphysis may be caused by intra-articular adhesions, capsular contracture, or muscular contracture. This should be treated with active and active-assistive range-of-motion exercises. Following prolonged immobilization and osteoporosis, periarticular fractures from overzealous manipulation for knee contracture has been reported.[30] Drop-out casts and dynamic braces may be of benefit for persistent stiffness. For patients with stiff knees in whom conservative treatment has failed, surgical release of contractures and adhesions, followed by continuous passive motion, may regain significant motion.[146]

Controversies

Stress X-rays

Stanitski[152] presented a cogent argument against the use of stress views to differentiate between a collateral ligament injury and a physeal fracture of the distal femur. He reported that this test may have been needed in the past, when the treatment of a collateral ligament injury was operative and the treatment of a nondisplaced physeal fracture was immobilization. Stanitski[152] argued that, because the current initial treatment of both a collateral ligament injury and a nondisplaced femoral fracture is immobilization, the need for an immediate diagnosis and stress views is no longer valid.

Special Imaging Studies

When to obtain an MRI or CT scan is also controversial. There is no clear answer at the current time. Some prefer an MRI for diagnosis of obscure injuries because of comfort to the patient along with the potential to diagnose associated ligamentous or chondral injuries and bone contusions.[98,151] An MRI should always be considered for evaluation of type III fractures of the medial condyle because the mechanism of injury is similar to the "triad" injury associated with anterior cruciate ligament and meniscal disruption.[98] Also, MRI is preferred for evaluation of partial or complete growth arrest.[41] A CT scan is preferred to assess fracture patterns for surgical fixation, especially when there is metaphyseal comminution and intra-articular involvement.

FRACTURES OF THE PROXIMAL TIBIAL EPIPHYSIS

Proximal tibial physeal injuries account for less than 1% of all physeal separations.[96,124] In contrast to the distal femoral physis, the proximal tibial physis has intrinsic anatomic stability.[25] For this reason, separation of the proximal tibial epiphysis requires significant force. The collateral ligaments provide some protection from epiphyseal disruption. On the lateral side, the fibula also provides a buttress for the proximal tibial epiphysis. Anteriorly, the tibial tubercle projects distally from the epiphysis and overhangs the adjacent metaphysis. This provides some stability for anterior and posterior translational forces. Avulsion injuries of the tibial tuberosity are discussed in the next section. These are very rare prior to adolescence. Perhaps the most critical feature of fractures of the proximal tibial epiphysis is the proximity and tethering of the popliteal artery to the posterior tibia. This increases the risk for associated vascular injury. Treatment consists of careful observation and management of associated injuries along with anatomic reduction and stable fixation of displaced fractures.

Mechanism of Injury

These injuries are usually due to motor vehicle trauma, sports activities, or other traumatic events such as lawn mower accidents. Child abuse has been reported to cause a Salter-Harris type II fracture.[158] Separations of this epiphysis can also occur during passive manipulation of the lower limbs in infants with arthrogryposis.[39] Hyperextension force is a common mechanism, with the metaphyseal fragment displacing posteriorly. Valgus stress can open the physis medially with the fibula acting as a lateral resistance force.[176] Rarely, a flexion force can cause a Salter-Harris type II or III fracture. This flexion fracture pattern has a mechanism similar to that of tibial tuberosity avulsion injuries.

Signs and Symptoms

Physical Examination

A patient with a separation of the proximal tibial epiphysis usually presents with pain, knee swelling, and a hemarthrosis. Limb deformity may or may not be present. Extension is limited because of hamstring spasm. Pain is present over the proximal tibial physis distal to the joint line. When the proximal metaphysis of the tibia is displaced posteriorly, a concavity is seen clinically and can be palpated anteriorly at the level of the tibial tubercle. If the metaphysis is displaced medially, a valgus deformity is present. There may be tenderness or angulation of the proximal fibula as well. When the proximal end of the metaphysis protrudes under the subcutaneous tissues on the medial aspect of the knee, a tear of the distal end of the MCL should be suspected. Vascular status should be carefully evaluated, including distal pulses and warmth and color of extremity should be noted. Compartments should be assessed by palpation and by assessment of sensation plus passive and active ankle and toe motion, especially active dorsiflexion.

X-ray Findings

Nondisplaced separations may not be visible on x-ray. An associated hemarthrosis may be identified as an increased distance between the patella and distal femur on a lateral view. Small fracture lines may be seen extending proximally through the epiphysis or distally through the metaphysis. A tiny bony fragment at the periphery of the metaphysis may be the only clue to the diagnosis. Other fracture lines may be visible only on oblique views. Differentiating a proximal tibial physeal fracture from a ligament injury should be attempted at time of presentation, and stress views may be warranted. However, the same concerns regarding stress films are present with proximal tibial epiphyseal fractures as with distal femoral epiphyseal fractures. MRI is a safe, accurate, and more comfortable method for diagnosis of obscure fractures or ligamentous injuries.[151] CT scans may be helpful to determine treatment for Salter-Harris types III and IV injuries because it provides better identification of the fracture pattern, articular incongruity, and metaphyseal comminution.

Associated Injuries

Ligamentous Injuries

Internal derangement of the knee joint may occur with separation of the proximal tibial epiphysis and may be unrecognized. One series reported concomitant avulsion of the tibial eminence in 40% of patients with types III and IV fractures.[128]

Vascular Injuries

The most serious injury associated with proximal tibial physeal fracture is vascular compromise.[25,144,177] The popliteal artery is tethered by its major branches near the posterior surface of the proximal tibial epiphysis. The posterior tibial branch passes under the arching fibers of the soleus. The anterior tibial artery travels anteriorly over an aperture above the proximal border of the interosseous membrane. A hyperextension injury that results in posterior displacement of the proximal tibial metaphysis may stretch and tear the tethered popliteal artery (Figs. 23-17 and 23-18).

Routine angiography is not mandatory because ischemia usually resolves following reduction, but motor function, pulses, warmth, and color should be checked frequently during the initial 48 to 72 hours. It is important to remember that even a fracture that appears minimally displaced at presentation in an emergency department may have had significant displacement at the time of injury, particularly in motor vehicle accidents (see Fig. 23-18).[160] Careful attention to evaluating and monitoring the arterial status is particularly warranted for proximal tibial physeal fractures. Arterial insufficiency may result from either a tear in the popliteal artery at the time of epiphyseal separation or from a compartment syndrome. Delay in recognition results in delay of treatment, which is potentially catastrophic. Arteriography for isolated injuries but may be helpful when vascularity is questionable. Fracture fixation is generally recommended before vascular repair, as discussed for distal femoral epiphyseal fractures. The extended medial approach usually provides the best approach for fracture and vessel management, but the posterior approach provides easier access to the popliteal space and can be used with percutaneous fixation of the fracture. The lateral approach is rarely used for vascular access except for localized injuries to the bifurcation of the popliteal artery.

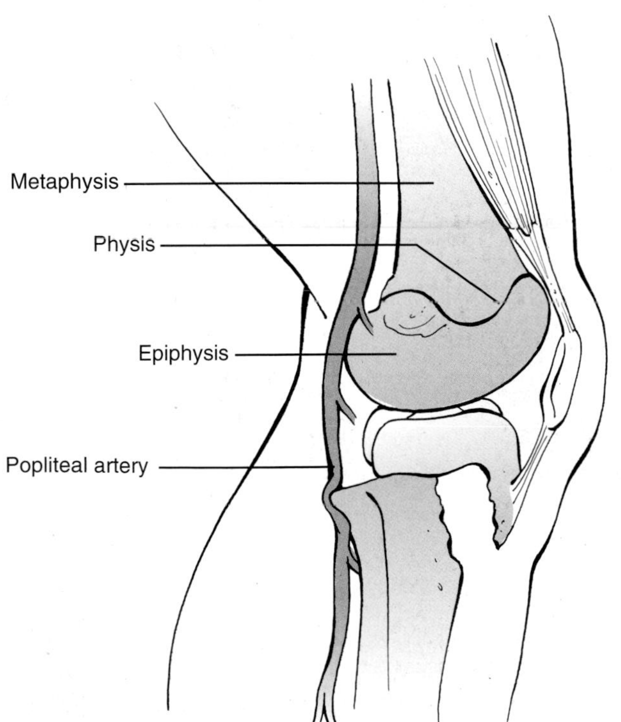

FIGURE 23-17 Posterior displacement of the epiphysis following fracture–separation at the time of injury can cause arterial injury. In addition, a posteriorly displaced fragment can cause persistent arterial occlusion by direct pressure. (Reprinted with permission from Skaggs DL, Flynn JF. Trauma about the knee, tibia, and foot. In Skaggs DL, Flynn JF, eds. Staying out of Trouble in Pediatric Orthopaedics. Philadelphia: Lippincott Williams & Wilkins; 2006.)

Nerve Injuries. Peroneal neuropathy associated with a separation of the proximal tibial epiphysis usually recovers spontaneously with time. Therefore, observation is recommended unless there is an open wound with possible sharp trauma to the nerve.

Diagnosis and Classification

Proximal tibial epiphyseal separations are usually described by Salter-Harris type along with direction and amount of displacement (Table 23-6). A specific classification for these fractures has not been proposed. Most separations of the proximal tibial epiphysis are Salter-Harris types I and II injuries. The frequency of Salter-Harris type III injuries may be skewed by the inclusion of displaced avulsion fractures of the tibial tubercle. The incidence of Salter-Harris type IV injuries depends on whether certain open injuries to the knee are included (i.e., lawnmower injuries).[25] Fifty percent of Salter-Harris type I separations of the proximal tibia are nondisplaced. When these fractures are displaced, the metaphysis is usually medial or posterior relative to the epiphysis.

Presumably, the overhanging tubercle prevents anterior displacement and the fibula prevents lateral displacement of the metaphysis. There may be an associated fracture of the proximal diaphysis of the fibula or a separation of the proximal fibular epiphysis. Two thirds of Salter-Harris type II fracture–separations of the proximal tibial are displaced. Displacement of the tibial metaphysis usually is medial (Fig. 23-19), and the associated metaphyseal fracture usually is lateral, resulting in valgus deformity. The proximal fibula may also be fractured. Salter-Harris type III separations have a vertical fracture line through the proximal epiphysis into the articular surface to the physis. There is some controversy about whether intra-articular tibial tubercle avulsion fractures should be included as a type III proximal tibial physeal fracture.[144] Generally, this fracture is not included in series of tibial epiphyseal fractures. When the fracture line of a tibial tubercle avulsion fracture is visible on the AP view, we consider it a proximal tibial epiphyseal fracture. If, on the other hand, the fracture line is visible only on the lateral film, then we consider it as a tibial tubercle fracture (see Fig. 23-26). When avulsion fractures of the tibial tubercle are excluded from Salter-Harris type III injuries, the most common fracture involves the lateral epiphysis, and this is frequently accompanied by a tear of the ligament. This lateral fragment usually requires internal fixation, and the ligament may need surgical repair. Triplane and coronal split fractures of the proximal tibial epiphysis have also been described. These occur through a partially closed physis during the normal sequence of physeal closure.[34,63,122]

Salter-Harris type IV injuries can involve the medial or lateral tibial plateau. Salter-Harris type V injuries are rare but have been reported in the proximal tibia.[79] Usually, the diagnosis of a type V injury is made in retrospect when progressive angulation or leg-length discrepancy is noted. Another type of proxi-

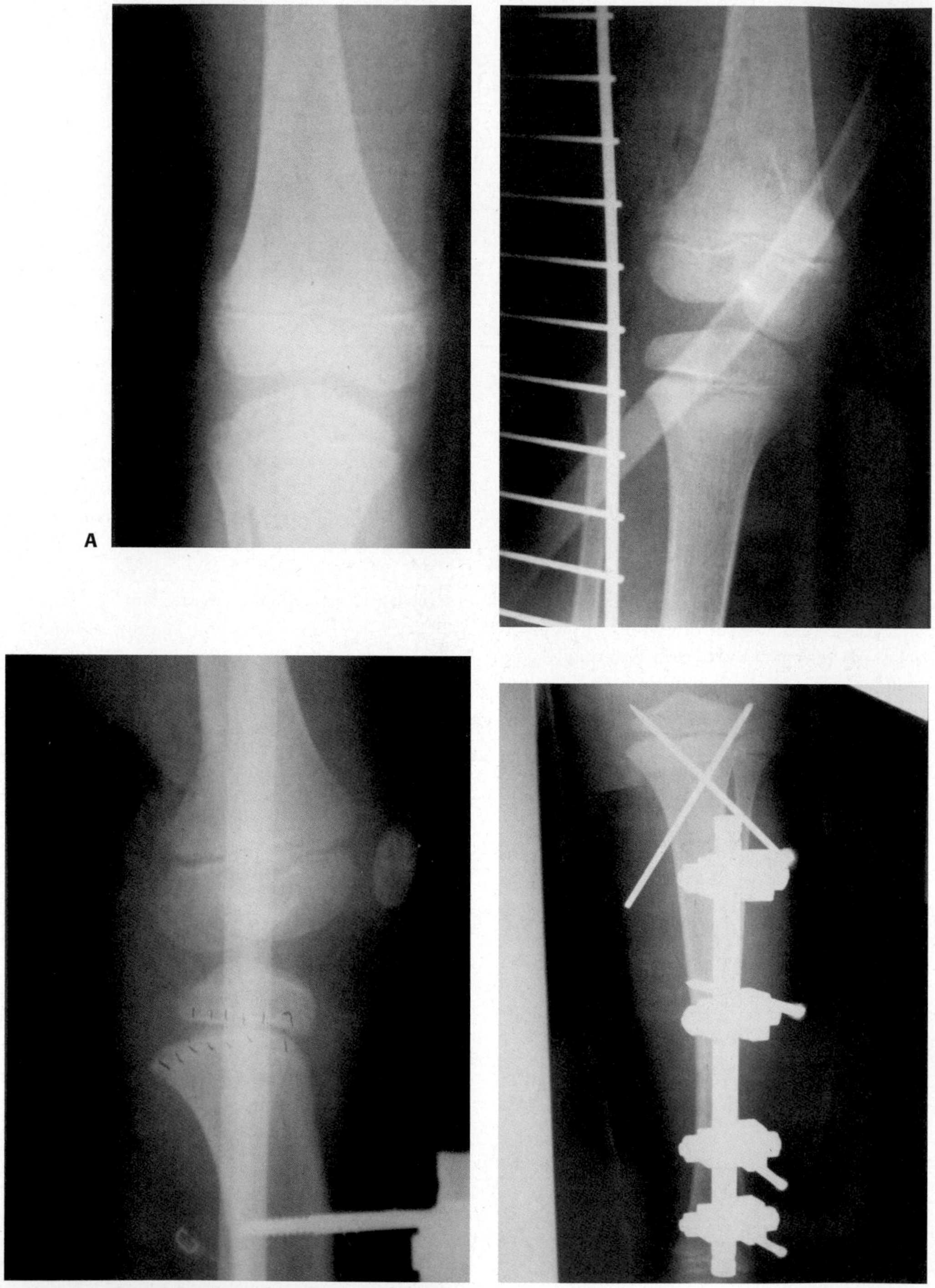

A

B

C

D

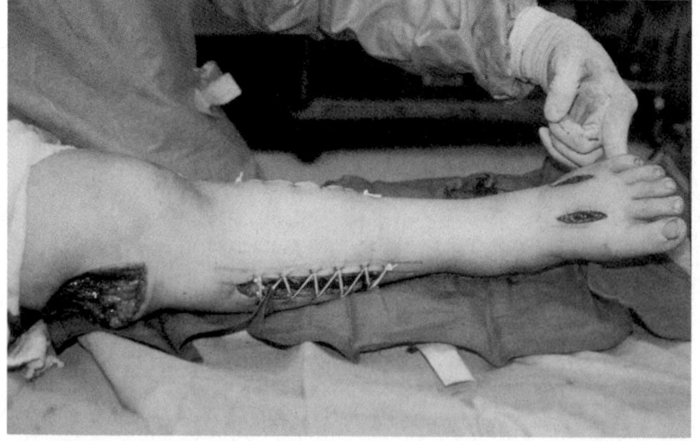

E

FIGURE 23-18 Child on back of bicycle struck by car sustained ipsilateral proximal femoral and tibial shaft fracture. **A,B.** Proximal tibial physeal fracture on initial radiographs were not appreciated. **C.** Following external fixation of the tibial diaphyseal fracture, a Salter-Harris type I fracture of the proximal tibial physeal is evident. **D.** Closed reduction and K-wire fixation were used to treat the proximal tibial physeal fracture. **E.** Compartment syndrome occurred, which is associated with proximal physeal fractures of the tibia. In this case, the contribution of concomitant injuries to the compartment syndrome is difficult to discern. (**A** and **E** reprinted with permission from Skaggs DL, Flynn JF. Trauma about the knee, tibia, and foot. In Skaggs DL, Flynn JF, eds. Staying out of Trouble in Pediatric Orthopaedics. Philadelphia: Lippincott Williams & Wilkins; 2006.)

TABLE 23-6 Classifications and Implications of Proximal Tibial Physeal Fractures

Classification	Implications
Mechanism of injury	
I. Hyperextension	Risk of vascular disturbance
II. Varus/valgus	Usually results from jumping; very near maturity
III. Flexion	See tibial tubercle fractures, type IV, in the next section
Salter-Harris pattern	
I	Fifty percent nondisplaced
II	Thirty percent nondisplaced
III	Associated collateral ligament injury possible
IV	Rare
V	Has been reported; diagnosis usually late

mal tibial epiphyseal fracture is of an avulsion of lateral tibial condyle. Sferopoulos et al.[143] described seven patients with either a fracture of Gerdy's tubercle or a Segond fracture. All were sustained during a sporting event, and all were treated nonoperatively in a cylinder cast for 6 weeks. All of the patients returned to sports between 3 and 4 months after injury. Of note, two patients also had a concomitant and ipsilateral fractures of the anterior intercondylar eminence.

Proximal tibial epiphyseal fractures also can be classified by the direction of deformity (Fig. 23-20). This classification may help recognize potential complications and plan the reduction

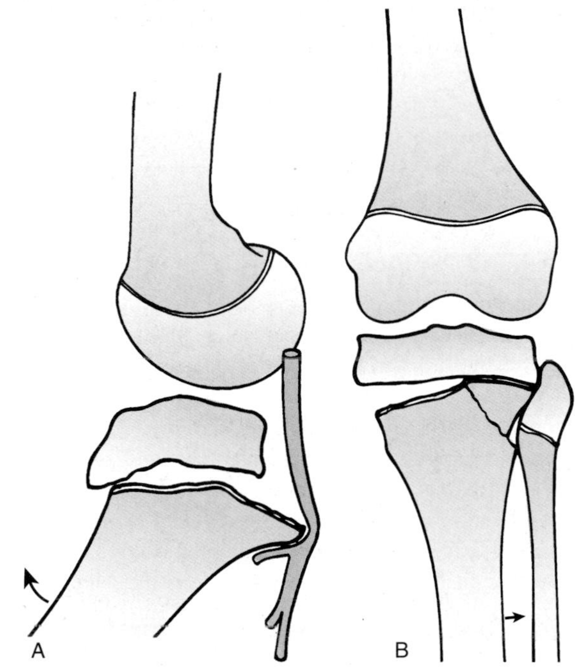

FIGURE 23-20 Classification of proximal tibial physeal fractures by direction of displacement. **A.** Type I: hyperextension type usually caused by direct force. Risk of vascular damage exists. **B.** Type II: varus or valgus type. Vascular injury is uncommon. Reduction may be inhibited by interposition of pes anserinus or periosteum.

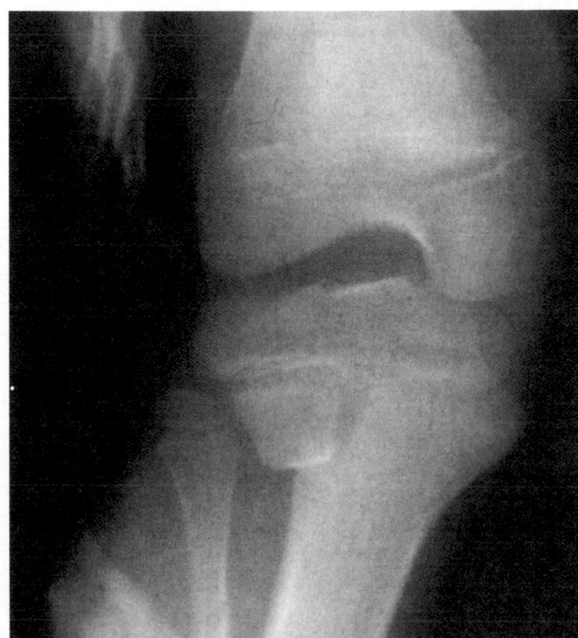

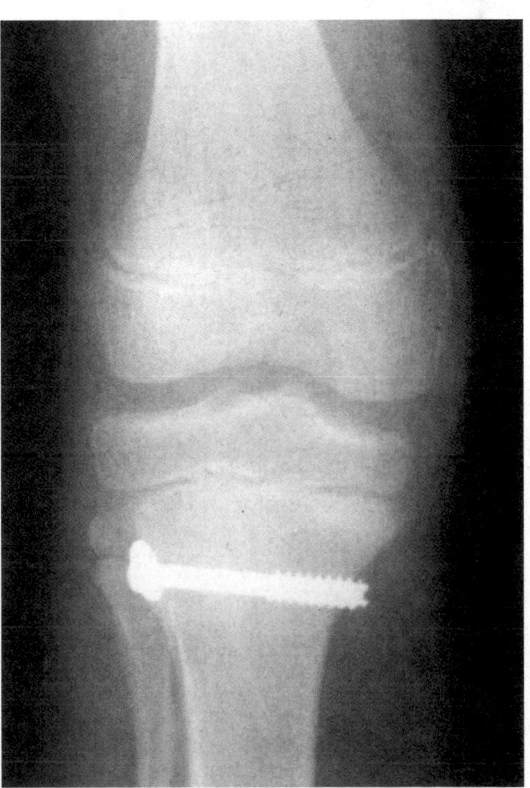

FIGURE 23-19 A. Salter-Harris type II separation of the proximal tibial metaphysis, with medial displacement of the proximal tibial metaphysis and complete fracture of the upper third of the fibula. **B.** After reduction and percutaneous fixation with a 4.5-mm cannulated screw.

technique. The classic hyperextension type has an apex-posterior angulation and results from forced hyperextension. Varus and valgus types result from abduction or adduction forces. A flexion type injury may separate the entire proximal tibial epiphysis in a manner similar to avulsion of the tibial tubercle except that the epiphysis stays intact as it separates from the metaphysis.[72,137]

Surgical and Applied Anatomy

Bony Anatomy

The ossific nucleus of the proximal tibial epiphysis is normally present at birth. It lies in the center of the cartilaginous anlage, somewhat closer to the metaphysis than to the articular surface. Occasionally, the ossification center is double. The secondary center in the tubercle appears between the ages of 9 and 14 years. The proximal epiphyseal ossification center unites with the tubercle and is almost completely ossified by age 15.

The lateral edge of the physis is separated from the proximal tibiofibular joint by a thin layer of joint capsule. Hemorrhage from an epiphyseal separation may extend into the adjacent tibiofibular joint cavity and through it into the knee joint itself. The physis closes from central to anteromedially followed by posteromedial closure.[72,116]

Soft Tissue Anatomy

The collateral ligaments provide some protection from epiphyseal disruption. The superficial portion of the MCL extends distal to the physis inserting into the medial metaphysis of the tibia. The lateral collateral ligament inserts on the proximal pole of the fibula. The patellar ligament attaches to the secondary ossification center of the tibial tuberosity that forms the anterior extension of the physis. This attachment can lead to avulsion injuries of the anterior epiphysis, but these are uncommon until adolescence when the quadriceps becomes stronger and the physis weaker. Also, some fibers extend distal to the physis into the anterior aspect of the upper tibial diaphysis. The synovium and the capsule of the knee joint insert into the proximal tibial epiphysis proximal to the physis. There is a defect in the capsule where the popliteus tendon runs over the posterolateral corner of the tibia. The capsular ligament anchors the menisci to the tibial epiphysis medially and laterally.

Vascular Anatomy

The distal portion of the popliteal artery lies close to the posterior aspect of the proximal tibia. Firm connective tissue septa hold the vessel against the knee capsule. The popliteus muscle intervenes between the artery and bone (Fig. 23-21). The lateral inferior geniculate artery runs across the surface of the popliteus muscle, anterior to the lateral head of the gastrocnemius, and turns forward underneath the lateral collateral ligament. The medial inferior geniculate artery passes along the proximal border of the popliteus muscle, anterior to the medial head of the gastrocnemius, and extends anterior along the medial aspect of the proximal tibia. The popliteal artery divides into the anterior tibial and posterior tibial branches beneath the arch of the soleus muscle.

The proximal tibial epiphysis derives much of its blood supply from an anastomosis between the geniculate arteries. The lateral tibial condyle derives its blood supply anteriorly from the anterior tibial recurrent artery and posteriorly from branches

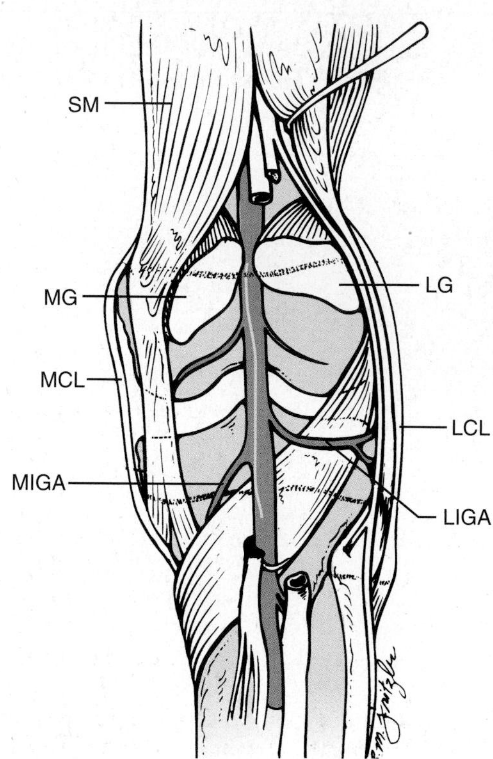

FIGURE 23-21 Posterior anatomy of the right popliteal region. Note that the popliteal vessels are protected from bone (especially the tibia) only by the popliteus muscle. The vessels are tethered by the geniculate branches and by the trifurcation of the popliteal artery into the peroneal, posterior tibial, and anterior tibial arteries. Note that the anterior tibial artery passes anteriorly between the proximal tibia and fibula, thus causing the popliteal artery to press against a posteriorly displaced tibial metaphysis. ATA, anterior tibial artery; LCL, lateral collateral ligament; LG, lateral gastrocnemius head; LIGA, lateral inferior geniculate artery; MCL, medial collateral ligament; MG, medial gastrocnemius head; MIGA, medial inferior geniculate artery; SM, semimembranosus.

of the inferior lateral geniculate artery.[35,60] Hannouche et.al.[60] suggested that the standard anterolateral approach to the lateral tibial condyle with submeniscal arthrotomy may damage the epiphyseal vascularity.

Current Treatment Options

Closed Reduction and Immobilization

Types I and II fractures usually can be treated with closed reduction (Table 23-7). Traction is important during reduction to minimize the risk of damage to the physis. Hyperextension fractures are reduced with traction in combination with gentle flexion. A fracture with valgus angulation can usually be reduced by adducting the leg into varus with the knee extended. This should be done with gentle manipulation to decrease the risk of injury to the peroneal nerve. After reduction, a long-leg cast with varus molding is applied with the knee in slight flexion.

Closed Reduction and Fixation

Separations of the proximal tibial epiphysis may be surprisingly unstable. Reducible but unstable types I and II fractures can be stabilized with smooth pins inserted percutaneously. Salter-Harris type II fractures with a large metaphyseal spike can be stabilized with compression screws that fix the spike to the metaphysis without crossing the physis (see Fig. 23-19).

TABLE 23-7 Methods of Treatment for Proximal Tibial Epiphyseal Fractures

	Pros	Cons	Indications
Closed reduction and immobilization	Avoids anesthesia	High risk of loss of reduction. May require significant knee flexion for hyperextension injuries.	Nondisplaced, stable fractures
Closed reduction and smooth pin or screw fixation	Minimal dissection	Intra-articular pins may lead to joint infection or require later removal.	Reducible Salter-Harris type I and II fractures
Open reduction and screw or pin fixation	Anatomic reduction	Stiffness	Nonreducible Salter-Harris type I and II fractures, displaced Salter-Harris type III and IV fractures

Open Reduction

Salter-Harris II fractures that cannot be anatomically reduced require open reduction for removal of soft tissue interposition. The pes anserinus and periosteum have been reported as obstructions to reduction of Salter-Harris type II fractures.[31,158,176] Operative fixation of a Salter-Harris type I or II hyperextension injury is recommended to facilitate wound management when vascular repair is necessary. Pin or screw fixation in an expeditious manner is generally recommended before vascular repair.

Open reduction is indicated for displaced Salter-Harris types III and IV injuries. An anterior incision is used to allow inspection of the articular surface. Anatomic reduction is performed, using the joint surface as a guide. A pin can be inserted in the displaced fragment as a joystick to assist reduction if needed. Smooth pins or screws are then inserted horizontally across the epiphysis in type III fractures. Metaphyseal and epiphyseal screws parallel to the physis are recommended for Salter-Harris type IV fractures to avoid physeal damage and allow growth to resume. A torn meniscus should be repaired if possible.

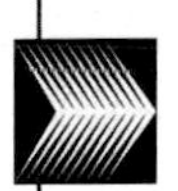

AUTHORS' PREFERRED TREATMENT

Closed Treatment

Tense painful knee effusions can be aspirated using sterile precautions. Injection of 2 to 5 cc of 0.5% bupivacaine can help relieve pain and allow better examination. Conscious sedation or general anesthesia can be used for additional pain relief and muscle relaxation. Patients with a nondisplaced (2 mm or less) proximal tibial epiphyseal fracture are placed in a long-leg cast with the knee flexed 20 to 30 degrees. One-half-inch thick foam is placed along the popliteal fossa and calf and/or the cast is bivalved to permit swelling. In most instances, the child is admitted to the hospital for observation and gentle elevation because of the high incidence of vascular injury and the possibility of developing a compartment syndrome. AP and lateral x-rays are repeated 1 week after the injury to confirm maintenance of reduction. The cast is removed 4 to 6 weeks after injury if the fracture is radiographically and clinically healed. Return to normal activities is generally permitted in 3 to 6 weeks following cast removal.

Before reducing a Salter-Harris type I hyperextension injury, we check for signs of neurologic or circulatory impairment. If there are signs of poor circulation, the child is brought urgently to the operating room for reduction under general anesthesia. When this is not possible, a closed reduction can be done in the emergency department with conscious sedation. For all closed reductions of physeal fractures, the principle of 90% traction and 10% leverage is used. The patient is positioned supine. The hip and knee are flexed to 45 degrees while an assistant provides countertraction by stabilizing the thigh. The surgeon grasps the proximal leg and applies traction while displacing the metaphysis anteriorly. Further flexion of the knee is rarely necessary, but may aid initial reduction. Reduction is confirmed with fluoroscopy or standard x-rays. When the reduction is stable through a gentle range of knee motion, a bivalved cast is applied. If the reduction is not stable, percutaneous smooth pin fixation is used to avoid excessive knee flexion. With or without internal fixation, a long-leg cast is applied with the knee in 20 to 30 degrees of flexion. The child is admitted for observation and elevation. For an abduction injury with valgus angulation, the reduction is done with the knee in full extension, followed by immobilization in almost full extension with varus molding.

Surgical Treatment

Percutaneous smooth-pin fixation with 2 to 2.5 mm diameter Kirschner-wires is used for Salter-Harris types I and II fractures. These are inserted in a crossing manner through the tibial metaphysis and across the physis to stabilize the epiphysis (Fig. 23-22). The leg is immobilized in a bivalved cast with the knee in 20–30 degrees of flexion. Three weeks after fixation, the pins are removed, but cast immobilization is continued for up to 3 more weeks. Return to normal activities is generally permitted in 4 to 8 weeks following cast removal.

Open reduction with surgical stabilization is performed when reduction is incomplete. Most Salter-Harris types III and IV fractures should be stabilized with smooth Kirschner-wires or with cannulated screws. We prefer cannulated screws inserted parallel to the physis. After internal fixation, the knee is carefully stressed into valgus to verify if the MCL is intact. Similarly, a gentle Lachman test is performed to ensure anterior cruciate ligament/tibial spine integrity. An MCL injury should heal with immobilization of the fracture but, an anterior cruciate ligament/tibial spine injury may require reconstruction and/or fixation (see Chapter 24).

If a Salter-Harris type IV fracture is open and the fragment is devitalized (i.e., lawn mower injury), the avascular piece

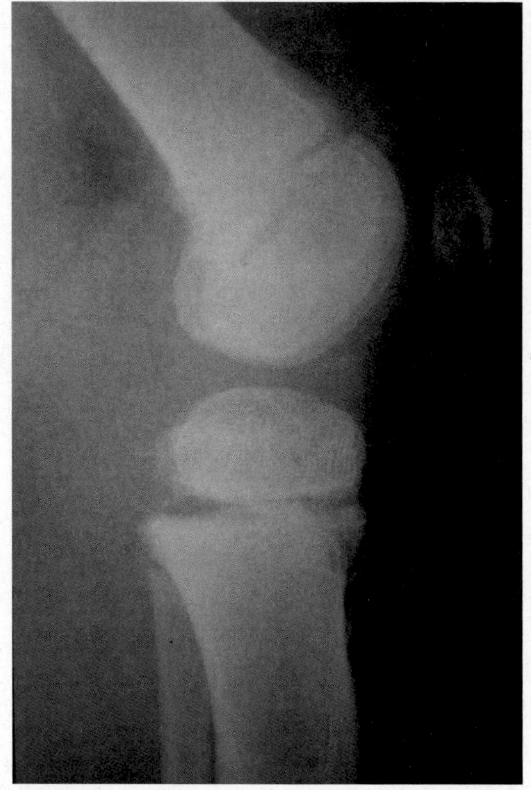

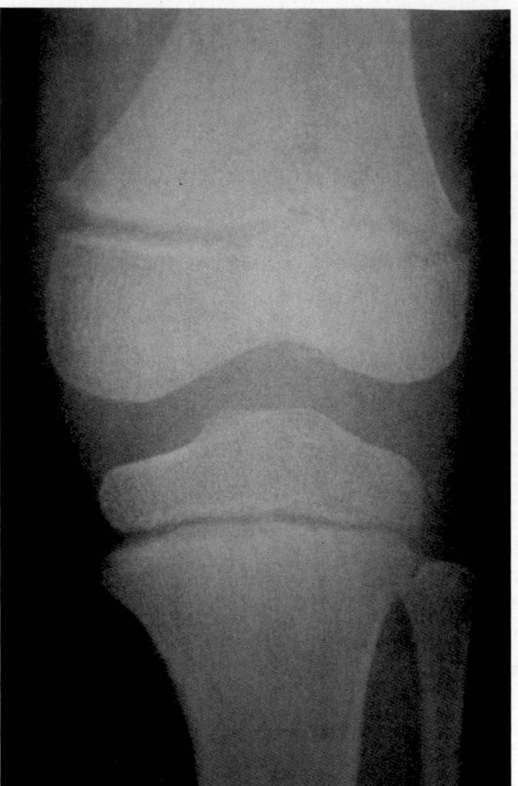

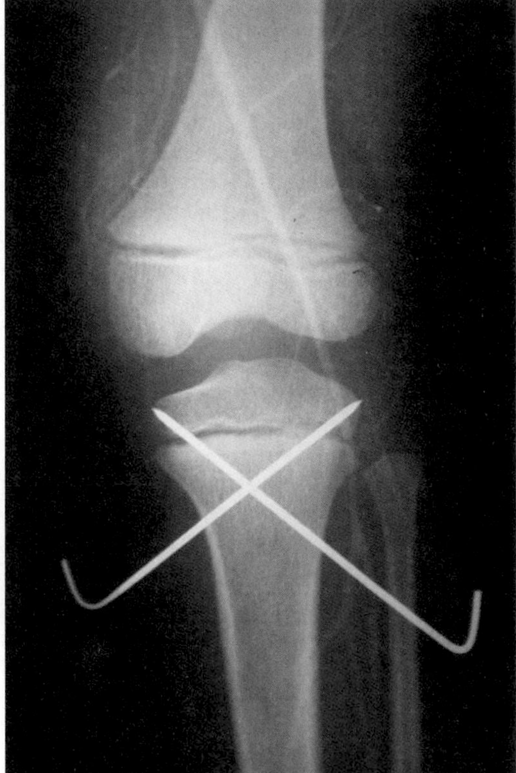

FIGURE 23-22 A. Lateral radiograph demonstrating minimal posterior displacement of a Salter-Harris type I fracture of the proximal tibia. **B.** No significant displacement is noted on the AP radiograph. **C.** Although angiogram demonstrates good flow past the fracture site, a compartment syndrome developed. (**A** reprinted with permission from Skaggs DL, Flynn JF. Trauma about the knee, tibia, and foot. In Skaggs DL, Flynn JF, eds. Staying out of Trouble in Pediatric Orthopaedics. Philadelphia: Lippincott Williams & Wilkins; 2006.)

is removed. Non–weight-bearing is recommended during early healing of Salter-Harris types III and IV injuries to reduce the risk of displacement.

Pearls and Pitfalls

- X-rays should be scrutinized for nondisplaced proximal tibial fractures especially for
  - children with knee pain following trauma.
  - patients with polytrauma.[58,143]
- Observation in the hospital is recommended for all fractures of the proximal tibia because of the risk of vascular injury or development of compartment syndrome.
- All casts should be bivalved or nonconstricting splints should be used for early immobilization.
- Unrecognized or late presentation of arterial injury.
  - Even minimally displaced fractures may have arterial injury from displacement at time of injury.
- Compartment syndrome.
- Nondisplaced fractures can be misdiagnosed as medial collateral ligament injuries.[169] Stress x rays or MRI can help make the correct diagnosis.
- Proximal tibial growth disturbance can occur following diaphyseal fractures.[66,107]
  - This may be due to unrecognized trauma or generalized response to injury.
  - Recurvatum is the most common deformity and must be carefully assessed on lateral x-rays with comparison to the contralateral side. Osteotomy may be necessary for correction.[119]
- Intra-articular pin placement can lead to a septic joint.
- An unrecognized anterior cruciate ligament/tibial spine avulsion can cause late instability.

Complications

Complications reported in three series of proximal tibial epiphyseal injuries are summarized in Table 23-8.[25,144,177]

Loss of Reduction

Separations of the proximal tibial epiphysis can be unstable, regardless of the Salter-Harris type. It is wise to obtain x-rays 1 week after injury to verify alignment. At that point, it is still possible to remanipulate if necessary. This complication can usually be avoided by using screw or smooth pin fixation following fracture reduction.

Compartment Syndrome

Compartment syndrome may occur following proximal tibial physeal fractures because of mechanical blockage of the vascular structures by a displaced fracture, damage to the popliteal artery, or collateral damage to soft tissues at time of a large force injury. It is important to remember in this injury that even a small posterior displacement of the metaphysis may obstruct popliteal blood flow as the artery is tethered anteriorly against the metaphysis by the anterior tibial artery (see Fig. 23-17) Burkhart and Peterson[25] reported a 12-year-old hurdler who sustained a closed Salter-Harris type III injury that was treated with closed reduction and a long leg cast. Increased pressure in both the anterior and posterior muscle compartments caused narrowing of the terminal branches of the popliteal artery, although arteriography showed that the popliteal artery itself remained patent. Fasciotomies and a sympathectomy failed to save the leg.

Growth Disturbance and Leg-Length Discrepancy

Similar to separations of the distal femoral epiphysis, injuries to the proximal tibial epiphysis may cause shortening or angulation from subsequent growth inhibition. This inhibition can occur after all types of proximal tibial epiphyseal injuries. Anatomic reduction with internal fixation reduces the risk of growth disturbance.[140] The amount of angulation depends on the proximity of the area of growth arrest to the periphery of the physis and the years left for growth after injury. When partial or complete growth arrest is diagnosed, the only methods to prevent progressive deformity are excision of an epiphyseal bar or bilateral epiphysiodesis. Hemiepiphysiodesis will not correct angular deformity when that deformity is caused by a bone bridge. Early recognition and treatment of growth disturbance following fracture may prevent the need for osteotomy. The proximal tibial physis grows approximately 6 mm per year and growth ceases at approximately age 14 in girls and 16 in boys.[2,172] If complete growth arrest follows an epiphyseal separation at this level and the patient is within 3 years of the end of growth, an equalization procedure may be unnecessary. If more years of growth remain, immediate epiphysiodesis of the opposite extremity may be considered, or leg lengthening at a later stage may be indicated depending on the expected final leg length discrepancy.

Knee Instability/Degenerative Changes

In a series of 10 patients with Salter-Harris types III and IV injuries, Poulsen et al.[55] reported that two patients had symp-

TABLE 23-8 Complications of Proximal Tibial Physeal Fractures*

	Patients	Neurovascular	Ligamentous Instability	Growth Disturbance
Burkhart[25]	28	3	Not reported	9
Shelton[144]	34	5	3	10
Wozasek[177]	16	3	1	4
Totals	78	14%	5%	29%

*Includes 10 cases of tibial tubercle avulsion with intra-articular extension as type III fractures.
See section on associated injuries for discussion of vascular and nerve injuries.

tomatic instability and two additional patients had asymptomatic anterior laxity. In the same series, degenerative changes were noted on x-rays in two patients with varus deformity. Bertin and Goble[15] reported eight cases of ligamentous laxity in 13 patients with proximal tibial physeal fractures. Most other series do not report late instability or degenerative changes, but this may be underreported for type III and IV fractures.

AVULSION OF THE TIBIAL TUBEROSITY

Avulsion fracture of the tibial tuberosity is an uncommon injury accounting for less than 1% of all epiphyseal injuries and approximately 3% of all proximal tibial fractures in adults and children.[18,96,124] This injury is most commonly sustained by adolescents during sports activity.

Mechanism of Injury

Most acute traumatic avulsions of the tibial tubercle occur in adolescents during jumping activities such as basketball, when jumping is resisted, or during eccentric loading while landing.[18,28,29,59,104,116] Tibial tuberosity fractures are reported almost exclusively in males.[18,28,29,59,104,116] Avulsion of the tibial tubercle occurs when the patellar ligament traction exceeds the combined strength of the physis and the supporting soft tissues. During adolescence, quadriceps strength increases and physeal stability decreases.[21,91] There are two mechanisms of injury: violent contraction of the quadriceps muscle against a fixed tibia, as occurs in resisted jumping, and acute passive flexion of the knee against the contracted quadriceps. A study of two adolescent gymnasts with tibial tuberosity fractures found extension strength of the contralateral and injured knee was greater than nonathletic controls and their gymnastic peers. The authors hypothesized that the greater-than-usual strength of the quadriceps was able to overcome the strength of the tibial tuberosity or the physis.[91]

Signs and Symptoms

Swelling and tenderness are centered over the anterior aspect of the proximal tibia. Joint effusion and tense hemarthrosis may be present. A freely movable triangular fragment of bone may be palpated subcutaneously between the proximal tibia and the femoral condyles. This fragment may have rotated so that the distal end projects forward, tenting the overlying skin. The bed from which the fragment was avulsed may be identified by a palpable defect on the anterior aspect of the proximal tibia.

The amount of patella alta is proportional to the severity of displacement of the tibial tubercle and may be as much as 10 cm. With a type I avulsion, the patient may be able to partially extend the knee actively through the remaining soft tissue attachments. Active extension is very impaired or impossible with types II and type III injuries.

Radiographic Findings

Most patients with tibial tubercle fractures are adolescents in whom the secondary ossification of the tibial tubercle has developed. The best x-ray view to demonstrate displacement is a lateral projection with the tibia rotated slightly internally because the tubercle lies just lateral to the midline of the tibia. In this projection, the size and degree of displacement of the fragment can be identified more clearly. Two nondisplaced fragments may represent normal ossification of the tibial tubercle since two or more secondary ossification centers can be present as the tibial tubercle matures. A smooth, horizontal nondisplaced radiolucent line through the tubercle should not be confused with an epiphyseal fracture. Patella alta is absent in normal knees and can indicate a displaced tibial tuberosity avulsion fracture or distal pole patella sleeve fracture. The patella will displace proximally the same distance as the tibial tuberosity is displaced (Fig. 23-23). Patella alta[17,165] may also help diagnose sleeve avulsion fractures of the tibial tubercle, or patellar tendon ruptures, which have also been reported in children.[38,106]

A
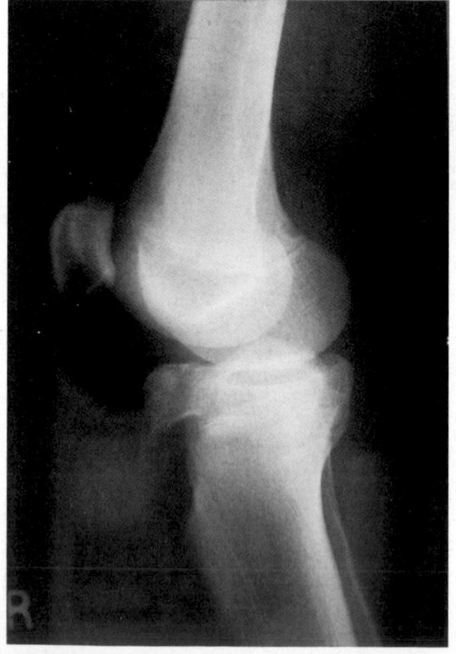

B
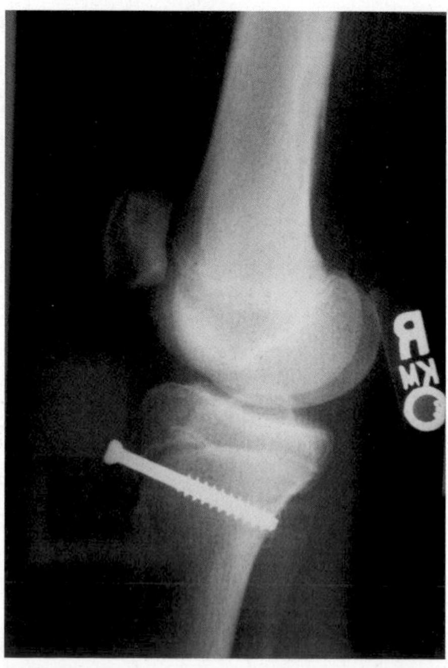

FIGURE 23-23 Type III tibial fracture with intra-articular extension. **A.** Lateral view demonstrates fracture and patella alta. **B.** Fracture was treated with open reduction and internal fixation with one 7.3-mm cannulated screw. Alternatively, multiple smaller screws could have been used.

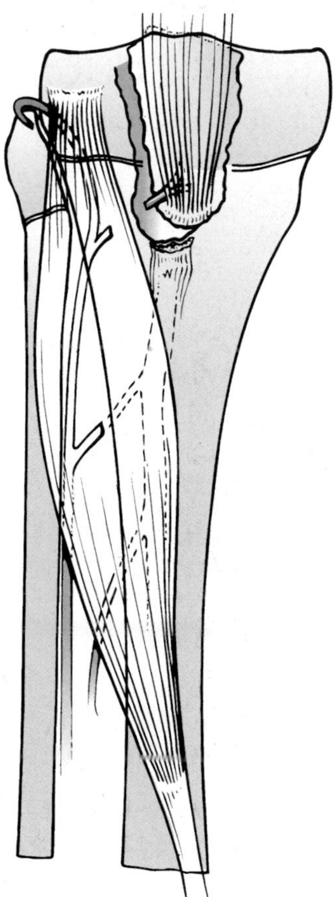

FIGURE 23-24 Probable mechanism of development of compartment syndrome after tibial tubercle avulsion. The anterior tibial recurrent artery, and possibly its branches, is torn and retracts into the anterior compartment musculature.

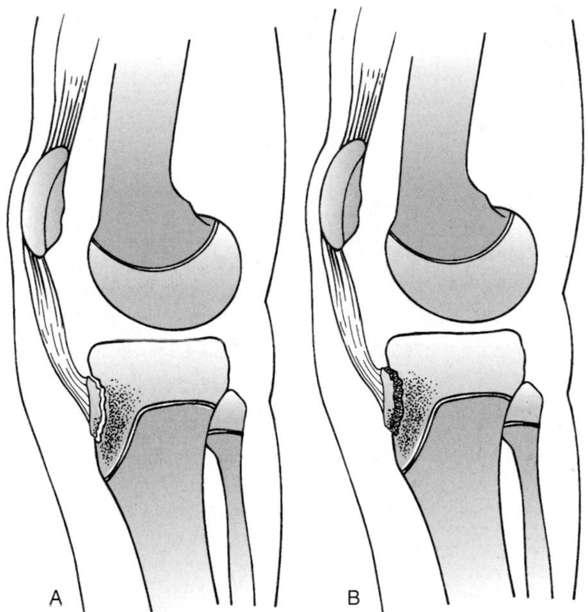

FIGURE 23-25 Development of Osgood-Schlatter lesion. **A.** Avulsion of osteochondral fragment that includes anterior surface cartilage and a portion of the secondary ossification center of the tibial tubercle. This may be clearly differentiated from a tibial tuberosity fracture, which occurs along the apophysial cartilage. **B.** New bone fills in the gap between the avulsed osteochondral fragment and the tibial tubercle but does not disrupt the physis.

Associated Injuries

Proximal tibial tubercle avulsion fractures are predisposed to development of compartment syndrome. The anterior tibial recurrent artery near the base of the tibial tubercle may be avulsed and bleed into the anterior compartment of the leg (Fig. 23-24).[118] Severe pain greater than expected from this injury alone should raise suspicion of impending compartment syndrome.

Associated soft tissue injuries that have been reported include patellar ligament and quadriceps tendon avulsions, collateral and cruciate ligament tears, meniscal damage, and a lateral plateau rim fracture.[18,99,104,117] Avulsion of the anterior tibialis muscle has also been reported.[76,175]

Diagnosis and Classification

Avulsion fractures of the tibial tuberosity are differentiated from Osgood-Schlatter disease by anatomic pathology and clinical presentation. Osgood-Schlatter disease is a chronic traction injury of the anterior ossicle of the tuberosity with no involvement of the physis (Fig. 23-25). Ogden and Southwick[116] observed new bone formation anterior to the secondary ossification center in Osgood-Schlatter disease and concluded that the weak link in Osgood-Schlatter disease is the attachment of the tendon to the anterior surface of the tibial tubercle. In contrast, tibial tubercle avulsions fail through the underlying physis, which is the posterior surface of the tibial tubercle. A prospective study of Osgood-Schlatter lesions evaluated with serial MRI, CT, and bone scans showed that the most striking feature was soft tissue inflammation, not bony avulsion.[135] An ossicle was seen anterior to the tibial tubercle in only one third of the patients. There are clear differences in presentation as well. Avulsion of the tibial tubercle occurs acutely with a specific injury, whereas the patient with an Osgood-Schlatter lesion usually presents with a gradual onset of symptoms characteristic of an overuse injury. An adolescent with a displaced acute avulsion of the tibial tubercle is immediately unable to stand or walk; however, an adolescent with Osgood-Schlatter disease often tries to continue athletic activities despite discomfort. There are several reports of acute tibial tubercle avulsions patients with pre-existing Osgood-Schlatter disease,[33,104,109,116] which has led to speculation that Osgood-Schlatter disorder may predispose children to tibial tuberosity avulsion, but convincing scientific evidence is absent and both conditions are prevalent in adolescent male athletes.

There is some overlap in reporting of tibial tuberosity fractures that extend into the joint with Salter-Harris type III separations of the anterior tibial epiphysis. For example, Shelton and Canale[144] and Burkhart and Peterson[25] included tubercle avulsions in their reviews of proximal tibial physeal separations, because the mechanism of injury, associated injuries, and treatment of tibial tubercle avulsions with intra-articular extension are more similar to tibial avulsion fractures than proximal tibial epiphyseal fractures, we consider this type of fracture a tibial tuberosity fracture.

Watson-Jones[166] described three types of avulsion fractures of the tibial tubercle, with subsequent modifications by Ogden and associates[116] who noted that the degree of displacement depends on the severity of injury to adjacent soft tissue attachments (Fig. 23-26). Ryu[137] and Inoue[72] proposed a type IV

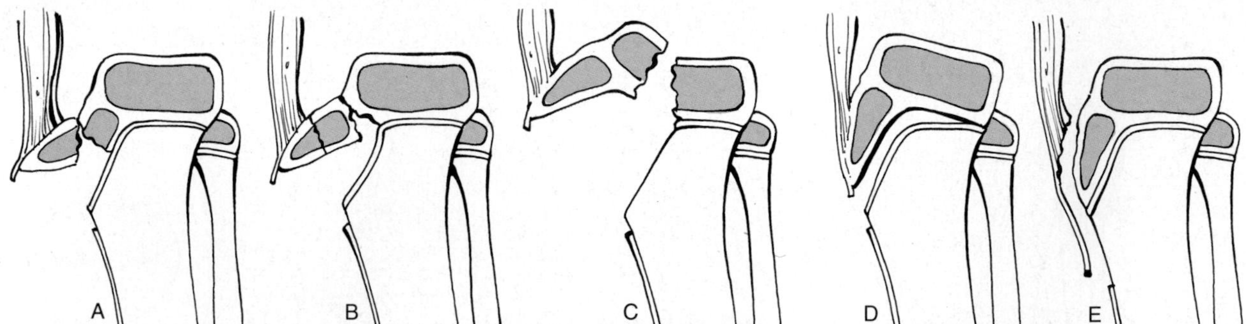

FIGURE 23-26 A. Type I—the physeal separation occurs through the tubercle apophysis. The fracture of tubercle is distal to the junction of the ossification centers of the tibial tubercle and the proximal tibial epiphysis. **B.** Type II—the physeal separation occurs through the tubercle apophysis. The fracture extends anteriorly through the area bridging the ossification centers of the tibial tubercle and the proximal tibial epiphysis. **C.** Type III—the physeal separation occurs through the tubercle apophysis. The fracture propagates through the proximal tibial epiphysis into the knee joint under the anterior attachments of the menisci. **D.** Type IV—the physeal separation occurs through the tubercle apophysis and propagates posteriorly through the horizontal proximal tibial epiphysis. The fracture may exit posteriorly through the physis, as a Salter-Harris type I equivalent, or through the metaphyseal, as a Salter-Harris type II equivalent. **E.** Type V—avulsion of a large area of periosteal attachment of the patellar tendon associated with small subchondral fragments of bone. Not a true physeal fracture.

fracture in which the physeal separation occurs through the tibial tuberosity and extends posteriorly into the horizontal tibial physis. Sleeve avulsion fractures of the tibial tuberosity extending over the anterior metaphyseal area of the tibia have been described in four children, aged 10 to 15 years.[24,38] These injuries are similar to patellar sleeve fractures in that initial x-rays may show no more than small subchondral fragments of bone. Open reduction and fixation were recommended. We follow Davidson and Letts'[38] recommendation that sleeve avulsion injuries of the tibial tubercle can be added to the Watson-Jones system as a type V. Fractures may be comminuted or have multiple fracture lines not easily classifiable

Surgical and Applied Anatomy

Bony Anatomy

In its final adult form, the tibial tubercle is a bony prominence on the anterior aspect of the proximal tibia. It lies approximately one to two fingerbreadths distal to the proximal articular surface of the tibia and forward of the anterior rim of the proximal articular surface.

Ehrenborg[43] divided the postnatal development of the tibial tubercle into four stages. The cartilaginous stage occurs before the secondary ossification center appears and persists in girls until approximately 9 years of age and in boys until 10 years of age. The apophyseal stage, in which the ossification center appears in the tongue of cartilage, occurs between 8 and 12 years in girls and between 9 and 14 years of age in boys. The epiphyseal stage, in which the secondary ossification centers coalesce to form a tongue of bone continuous with the proximal tibial epiphysis, occurs in girls between 10 and 15 years and in boys between 11 and 17 years of age. In the final bony stage, the epiphyseal line is closed between the fully ossified tuberosity and the tibial metaphysis.

Soft Tissue Anatomy

The patellar ligament, which lies between the distal pole of the patella and the tibial tubercle, is the terminal portion of the powerful quadriceps muscle. During the apophyseal stage of development of the tubercle, the patellar ligament inserts into an area of cartilage proximal and anterior to the secondary ossification center of the tubercle. The main attachment is in the proximal area of this insertion zone between the secondary ossification centers of the tubercle and the proximal tibial epiphysis. The fibrocartilaginous tissue lying anterior to the secondary ossification center receives only the distal part of the insertion. During the epiphyseal stage, the patellar ligament inserts through fibrocartilage on the anterior aspect of the downward-projecting tongue of the proximal tibial epiphysis. The inserting fibers merge distally into deep fascia after spanning the physis. With traumatic avulsion of the tibial tubercle in this stage of development, a broad flap of adjacent periosteum is attached to the displaced fragment. In the final bony stage, the tendon fibers insert directly into bone. After physiologic epiphysiodesis has occurred, the tibial tubercle rarely is avulsed if the patient has normal bone.

Although the patellar ligament represents the main insertion of the quadriceps muscle onto the leg beyond the knee joint, it is reinforced by retinacular fibers radiating from the medial and lateral margins of the patella obliquely down to the respective tibial condyles. After traumatic avulsion of the tibial tuberosity, a limited amount of active extension of the knee still is possible through the retinacular extensions of the extensor mechanism. However, patella alta and an extensor lag are present. The anatomic position of the tibial tubercle is biomechanically important in terms of patellar tracking and patellofemoral forces.

Vascular Anatomy

The tibial tubercle receives its main blood supply from a plexus of arteries behind the patellar ligament at the level of the attachment to the tibial tubercle.[35] This vascular anastomosis arises from the anterior tibial recurrent artery and may be torn with this fracture.[118,175] Several small branches extend down into the secondary ossification center. A smaller part of the blood supply enters the superficial surface of the tubercle from adjacent periosteal vessels.

Current Treatment Options

Nonoperative Treatment

Closed treatment is primarily reserved for nondisplaced type I fractures. Persistence of even a small gap between the distal end of the tubercle and the adjacent metaphysis may indicate an interposed flap of periosteum.[29,59] Minimally displaced, small avulsion fragments have been treated successfully with immobilization in a cylinder cast or long-leg cast.[28,29,104,116] The leg is positioned with the knee extended, but even with a long-leg cast, a straight leg raise can place tension on the fracture. Molding above the proximal pole of the patella has been suggested to help maintain reduction.

Operative Treatment

Open reduction with fixation is recommended for tibial tubercle avulsions that are intra-articular or displaced more than 2 to 3 mm.[18,28,59,109] Residual displacement may lead to extensor lag and quadriceps weakness. It may also be difficult to maintain reduction following closed reduction.

All type III fractures are intra-articular. For these fractures, anatomic reduction with stable fixation is recommended by several authors.[28,29,104,116]

A midline longitudinal incision is recommended to facilitate any possible knee surgery in the future. The fracture bed is carefully cleared of debris. A periosteal flap is frequently an impediment to reduction.[29,59] This is extracted and the fragment is reduced with the knee extended. Screw fixation is used when the tuberosity fragment is large enough for this type of fixation. The screw is inserted from anterior to posterior but does not need to engage the posterior cortex when cancellous lag screws are used. When there are 3 or more years of growth remaining or when the fragment is too small for screw fixation, transfixing pins can be used instead of screw fixation. Alternatively, a tension band can be passed around the fragment or through the patellar ligament and fixed through a drill hole across the anterior tibia distal to the attachment of the tuberosity. Tension band wiring has also been reported as a method to facilitate rapid rehabilitation in athletes.[109] The wire is driven around the proximal pole of the patella or through a drill hole in the distal pole and then looped distally through a cannulated cortical screw that is inserted across the anterior tibia distal to the patellar tendon insertion. This method may also be useful when the fracture fragments are comminuted or too small for secure fixation to the tibial metaphysis.

Sleeve avulsion fractures of the tuberosity can be challenging to stabilize because there is not a bone fragment for fixation.[38] Davidson and Letts[38] recommended fixation with small cancellous screws and heavy nonabsorbable sutures to repair the torn retinaculum and periosteum. Protection in a cast is recommended for 6 weeks because fixation depends on soft-tissue stability.

Postoperative Management

Immobilization in a long-leg cast with the knee in 5 to 10 degrees of flexion is recommended for a period of 4 to 6 weeks. Shorter periods of immobilization are used in younger adolescents when fixation is secure. For large fragments that are securely fixed with two or more screws, a knee immobilizer can be substituted for cast immobilization. Range of motion and quadriceps strengthening are initiated 6 weeks following injury.

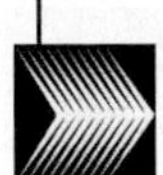

AUTHORS' PREFERRED TREATMENT

Closed Reduction and Immobilization

Closed treatment is used only for extra-articular fractures that are displaced less than 2 mm and are stable enough for the patient to actively fully extend the knee against gravity. A long-leg cast is applied, and straight leg raising is discouraged. Lateral x-rays are repeated at 1 week to verify anatomic alignment. Postreduction treatment is as described after operative treatment.

Operative Treatment

Open reduction with secure internal fixation is recommended for all tibial tuberosity avulsion fractures that are displaced or intra-articular (Fig. 23-27). Even when closed reduction is successful, percutaneous surgical stabilization is recommended. For open reduction, a longitudinal incision just lateral to the tibial tubercle is preferred to minimize the potential for scar discomfort over prominent bone. The gap between the displaced fragment and its bed is cleared of any soft tissue interposition. A tourniquet can be used high on the thigh, but may need to be released if it is hindering reduction of a displaced fracture due to constriction of the quadriceps muscle. If the reduced fragment is large enough, we prefer to use cancellous screws in compression, extending through the tubercle and parallel to the joint into the metaphysis. Fixation across the posterior cortex is not essential, because the cortex is quite thin at this level. If large screw heads are a concern for later discomfort in thin patients or if bone fragments are small and/or comminuted, multiple 4.5-mm screws are used (Fig. 23-28) instead of a larger 6.5 or 7.3-mm screw. If the patient is more than 3 years from skeletal maturity, which is uncommon for this fracture, smooth pins are used. Alternatively, a tension band technique can be used to prevent fixation across the distal tibial physis. A number 1 braided polyester nonabsorbable suture (Ticron, Kendall Company, Mansfield, MA, or Ethibond, Johnson & Johnson, Langhorne, PA) can be used for this repair. The suture is passed through the distal patellar ligament and looped through a cancellous screw that has been inserted through a drill hole across the anterior tibial cortex. Sutures are also used to repair the periosteum to add stability. During an open reduction, the anterior compartment fascia is released when there is early swelling of the anterior compartment. Following wound closure, a long-leg or cylinder cast is applied in full knee extension and the patient is observed in the hospital with elevation overnight.

For fractures with intra-articular extension, the articular surface is used as a guide to fracture reduction, and the menisci should be inspected for tears.

Pearls and Pitfalls

- Open reduction with internal fixation is recommended for almost all tibial tuberosity avulsion fractures.
- There is an increased risk of compartment syndrome due to bleeding of the recurrent anterior tibial artery.
- Recognition of sleeve avulsion fractures without bone may be difficult.

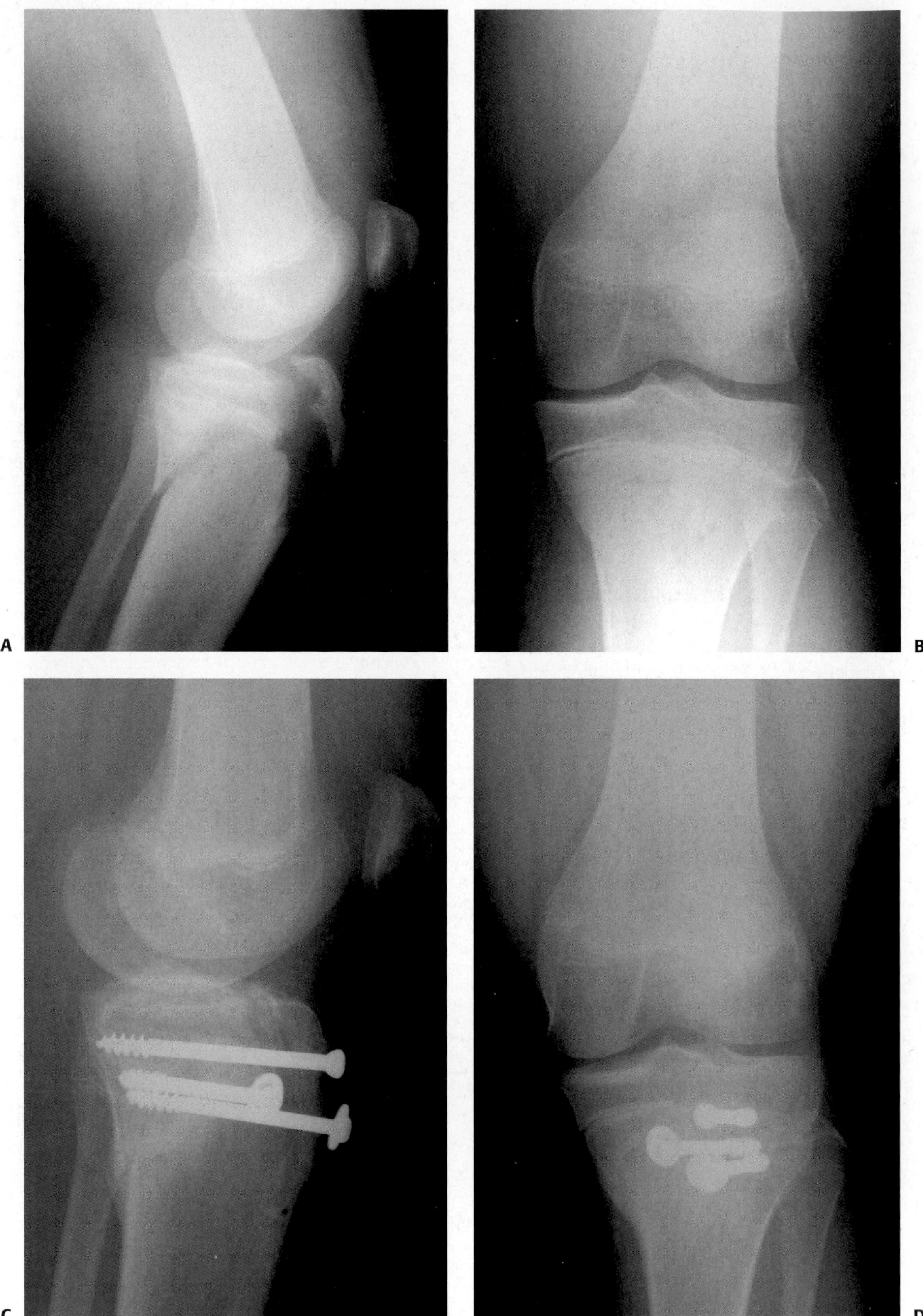

FIGURE 23-27 A. Lateral radiograph demonstrating a complex tibial tuberosity fracture extending into the joint, as seen in a type III fracture, as well as posterior along the physis and out the epiphysis. **B.** AP radiograph. **C.** Lateral view 3 months after surgery. **D.** AP view 3 months after surgery. (Courtesy of Robert Kay, MD.)

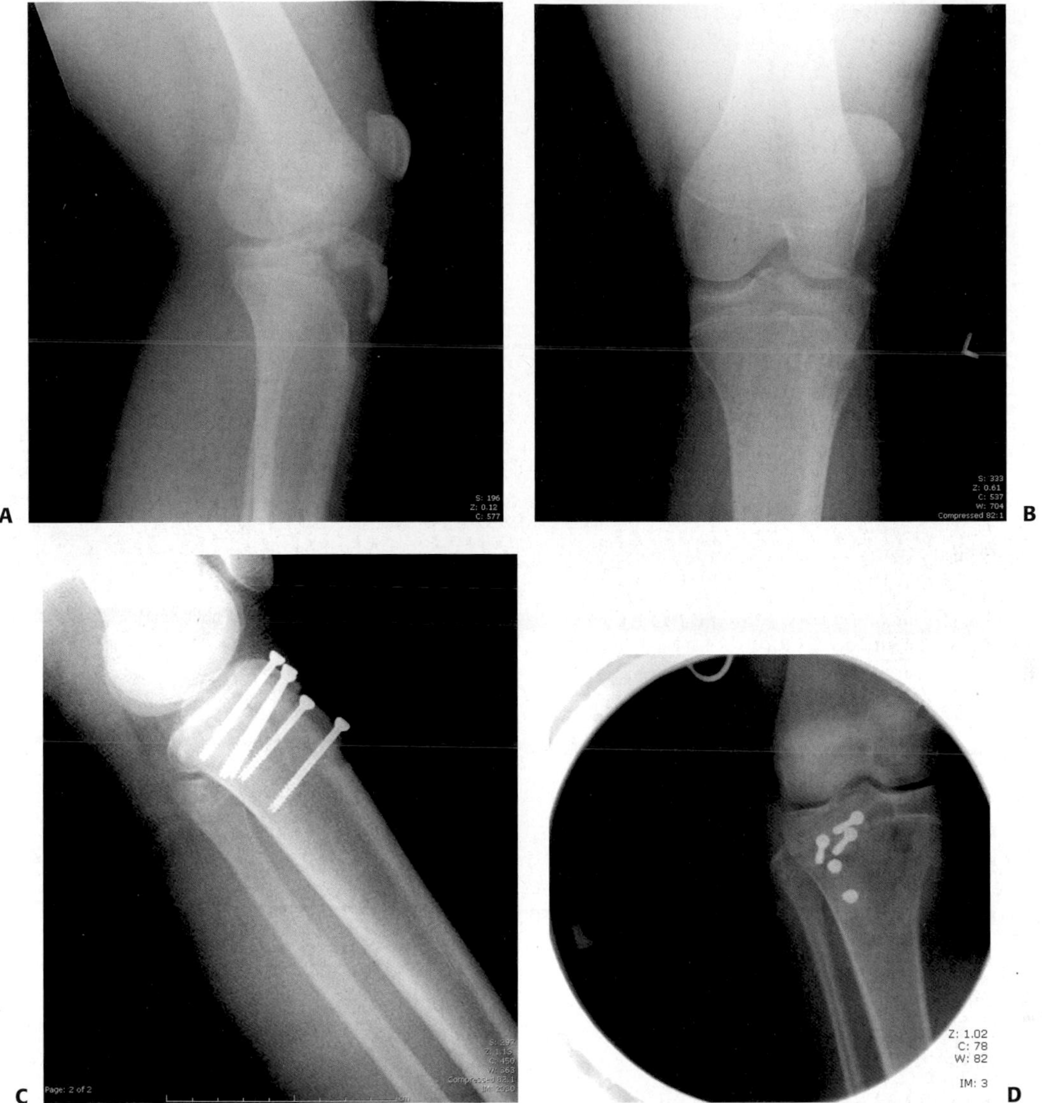

FIGURE 23-28 Type III tibial tuberosity avulsion in a 14-year-old girl sustained while landing after a jump in basketball. This is a very common mechanism of injury. **A.** Lateral view at injury. **B.** AP view at injury. **C.** Lateral view following open reduction and internal fixation with cannulated 4.5-mm screws. Note that screws are in compression with threads not crossing the fracture site. There is no significant growth left in this patient, so screw placement relative to the proximal tibial physis was not of concern. **D.** AP view of fixation. Note that screws are placed perpendicular to the plane of the fracture, which often leads to the screws directed laterally.

- Use of a tourniquet may bind the quadriceps and hinder reduction of a displaced fracture.
- Premature anterior physeal growth arrest may cause genu recurvatum that requires osteotomy for correction.[119]

Complications

Tibial tuberosity fractures have an excellent prognosis, with few complications after reduction and surgical stabilization of displaced fractures and closed management of nondisplaced extra-articular fractures (Table 23-9). When fractures unite in anatomic position, many series report no complications other than prominent screws. Most patients return to full athletic activity without residual sequelae within 3 to 6 months.[42,52,61,64,120,176]

Growth Disturbance

Premature closure of the tibial tubercle may lead to genu recurvatum in a growing child. However, this complication is rare because most of these injuries occur near the end of growth. If this complication occurs, we recommend a proximal tibial osteotomy as described by Pappas et al.[119]

Compartment Syndrome

Compartment syndrome has been reported in seven patients with displaced fractures, presumably because of tearing of the

TABLE 23-9 Complications of Tibial Tubercle Avulsion Fracture

Common	Screw prominence
Uncommon	Compartment syndrome
Rare	Genu recurvatum, stiffness, refracture, thrombophlebitis

anterior tibial recurrent vessels, which fan out at the tubercle but retract into the anterior compartment when torn.[118,175] Close monitoring is recommended for all patients with displaced tibial tuberosity avulsion fractures. Prophylactic anterior compartment fasciotomy should be considered at the time of open reduction when the anterior compartment is already swollen.[18]

Prominent Screw Heads

Deep screw insertion or countersinking the screw heads may be impossible without risking fracture of a tuberosity fragment. Wiss et al.[175] reported five of 15 patients with bursitis over prominent screw heads, four of whom had 6.5-mm screws. Overall, eight of the 15 patients underwent screw removal. Fixation with small screws or use of a tension band may be an alternative, but we recommend secure fixation even if prominent screws may require secondary procedures for removal.

Other Complications

Loss of fixation can occur if the tuberosity fragment fractures in the postoperative period. Cast immobilization is recommended to reduce this risk unless fixation is securely placed into a large tuberosity fracture fragment. Wiss et al.[175] reported one refracture in a child who returned to sports 4 weeks after injury. In one patient, a transverse proximal tibial fracture occurred 7 months postoperatively at the level of the retained screws.[18] Recovery of motion and strength is rarely problematic. Christie and Dvonch[29] reported a patient with persistent loss of 25 degrees of knee flexion 19 months after a type III injury. Patella alta can be expected if a displaced tibial tubercle is not reduced adequately. Thrombophlebitis has also been reported.[116]

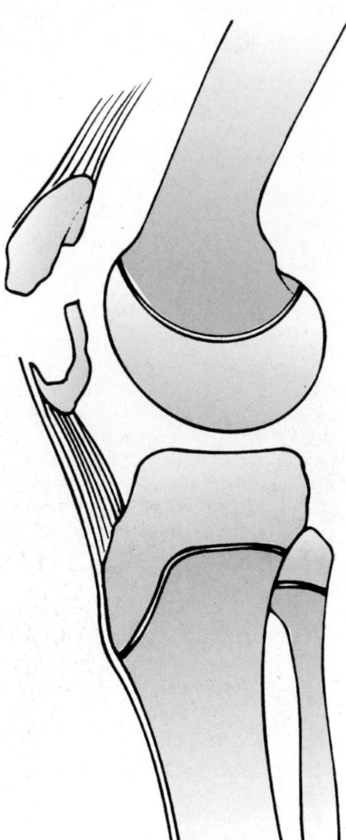

FIGURE 23-29 Sleeve fracture of the patella. A small segment of the distal pole of the patella is avulsed with a relatively large portion of the articular surface.

FRACTURES OF THE PATELLA

Patellar fractures are much less common in children than in adults, with estimates ranging from 1% to 6% of all patellar fractures.[92,132] Avulsion fractures of the patella are more common in children and may be difficult to diagnose.[56,92] The sleeve fracture is unique to children and consists of a large chondral fragment pulled from the ossification center with only a small rim of bone attached (Fig. 23-29).[47,65] In general, the treatment of patellar fractures in children is similar to treatment in adults.[92,132]

Mechanism of Injury

Fractures of the patella result from either a direct blow, sudden contraction of the extensor mechanism, or a combination of these direct and indirect forces. The patella is primarily in tension when the quadriceps contracts with the knee in extension. However, flexion produces compression and three-point bending forces on the patella with the distal femur acting as a fulcrum (Fig. 23-30). The bending moment increases with increasing knee flexion.[27] Thus, a direct blow with the knee in flexion is the most common mechanism for patellar fracture.[27] A typical history is that the patient fell with the knee flexed or the knee was struck while it was in a flexed position with the quadriceps under tension. Fractures of the patella may also occur without a direct blow when the quadriceps forcefully contracts with the knee flexed. This is a more likely mechanism during jumping or other sports activities,[27,37] and injury is most likely to produce a transverse, sleeve, or other avulsion fracture.[27,56] Comminuted fractures are most often the result of a high-energy direct blow such as motor vehicle trauma.[27,37] In a young child, the patella is more flexible and adapts to three-point bending or compression forces without breaking. The patellar ossification center appears between the ages of 3 to 6 years,[114,115] and patellar fractures have rarely been reported in patients younger than 8 years of age.

Another common mechanism of patellar fracture is avulsion of medial osteochondral fragments in association with acute patellar dislocation.[108] This injury and its treatment are discussed in Chapter 24. Stress fractures of the patella have also been reported in children, but are rare.[48] Grogan et.al.[56] cautioned that avulsion fractures of the inferior pole of the patella may be confused with Sindig-Larsen-Johanssen lesion, but acute onset or separation of the distal fragment is more likely to indicate fracture.

Signs and Symptoms

The injured knee is swollen and tender, often with tense hemarthrosis. Active knee extension is impaired and may be painful, and weight-bearing is often impossible. Palpation may reveal a high-riding patella or a palpable defect in the extensor mechanism. If the distal pole is avulsed, voluntary contraction of the quadriceps muscle draws the patella upward, but the patellar ligament remains lax. With marginal avulsion fractures, there may be little more than tenderness and localized swelling over the lateral or medial margin of the patella, and a straight-leg

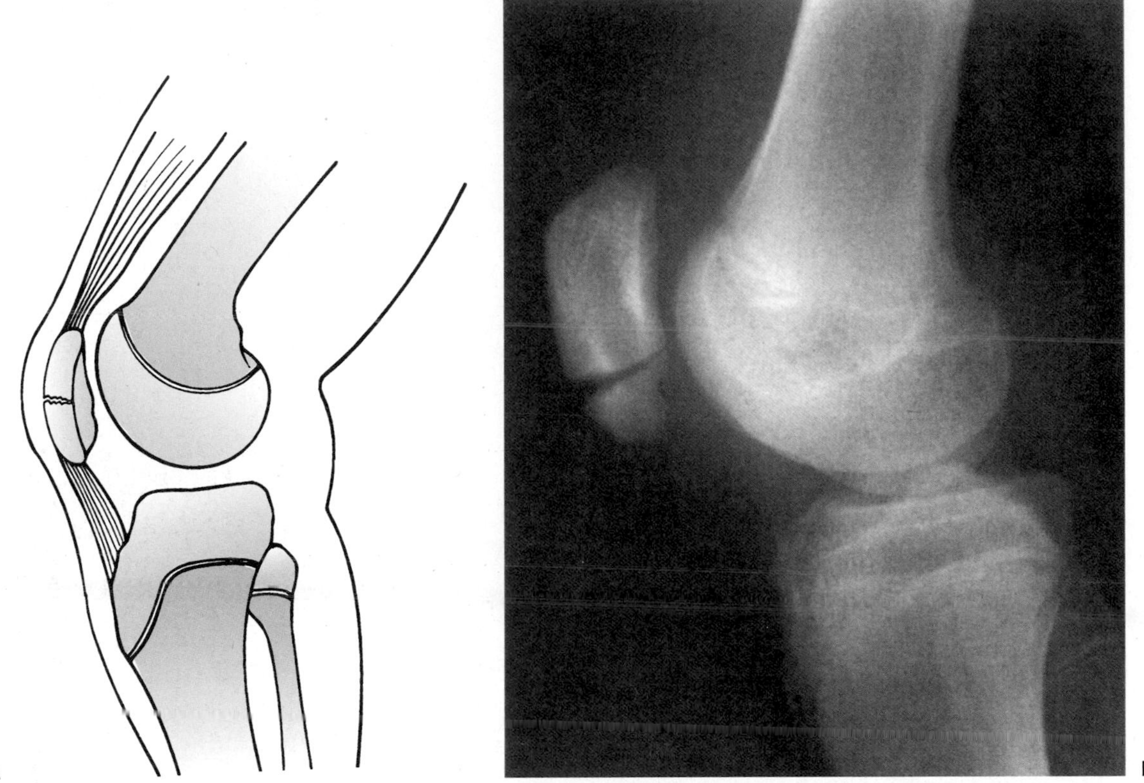

FIGURE 23-30 A. Incomplete transverse fracture of the patella. The articular cartilage of the patella remains intact, but the fracture gaps anteriorly. **B.** Lateral radiograph shows incomplete transverse fracture of the patella.

raise may be possible. An avulsion fragment adjacent to the medial margin of the patella may indicate that an acute lateral dislocation of the patella has occurred. The patella may have reduced spontaneously after the injury. If dislocation has occurred, the apprehension test is positive when the patient either resists passive manipulation by contracting the quadriceps or may even grasp the examiner's hand to prevent further passive displacement. Pain at the lateral-superior margin of the patella along with radiographic findings of a nondisplaced fracture most likely represents a bipartite patella rather than an acute fracture.[54,115]

X-ray Findings

Standard x-rays are usually sufficient to diagnose and plan treatment for patellar fractures in children, but careful attention should be paid to small flakes of bone that could represent larger osteochondral avulsion fragments (see Fig. 23-29).[9,81,170,171] When in doubt, MRI can help determine the nature and extent of injury.[9] Transverse fractures are best seen on the lateral view. In a child, the major fragments may tilt away from one another, with the maximal separation anteriorly and minimal separation posteriorly.[12] This may signify that the articular cartilage remains intact, even with a complete fracture through the bony portion of the patella. The extent of displacement may not be fully appreciated unless the knee is flexed to 30 degrees when the x-ray is made.

Small flecks of bone adjacent to the distal pole may be noteworthy. A symptomatic, small, visible radiodensity on the inferior pole of the patella may represent a Sindig-Larsen–Johanssen lesion. Displacement is more likely to indicate an acute fracture.[49,56] Fragmentation or elongation of the distal pole associated with patella alta in a child with cerebral palsy indicates long-standing extensor mechanism stress.

The x-ray appearance of a sleeve fracture is often not appreciated at first presentation to an emergency room. A barely visible fleck of bone proximal to the patella may be the only x-ray abnormality seen with a superior patellar sleeve fracture (Fig. 23-31). In an inferior patellar sleeve fracture, there may be patella alta in addition to a fleck of bone distal to the patella (Fig. 23-32).

Longitudinally oriented marginal fractures are best seen on axial or skyline views. It is important to differentiate a medial marginal fracture that traverses the entire thickness of the bone from a medial tangential osteochondral fracture. CT scan may help differentiate the two. An osteochondral fracture may include a substantial amount of cartilage not visible on plain x-rays.

A bipartite patella is best seen on an AP x-ray, which shows a crescent-shaped radiolucent line in the superolateral quadrant of the patella and rounded margins of the accessory ossicle. If symptoms are confusing, comparison x-rays of the opposite knee may be helpful. A similar x-ray appearance of the contralateral patella supports the diagnosis of bipartite patella.

Associated Injuries

Medial avulsion fractures of the patella may be associated with lateral dislocation of the patella. Comminuted fractures are more likely to be caused by high-energy trauma with associated fractures of the tibia, femur, or pelvis.

Diagnosis and Classification

Diagnosis

The greatest difficulty with fractures of the patella in children is diagnosis of avulsion fractures with very small flakes of bone

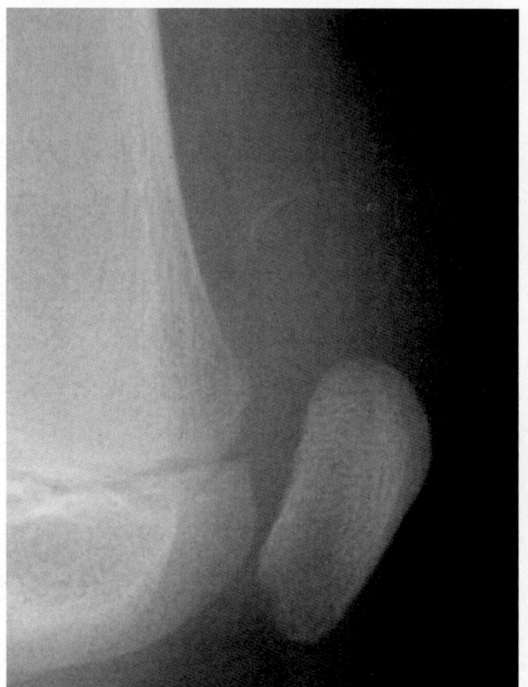

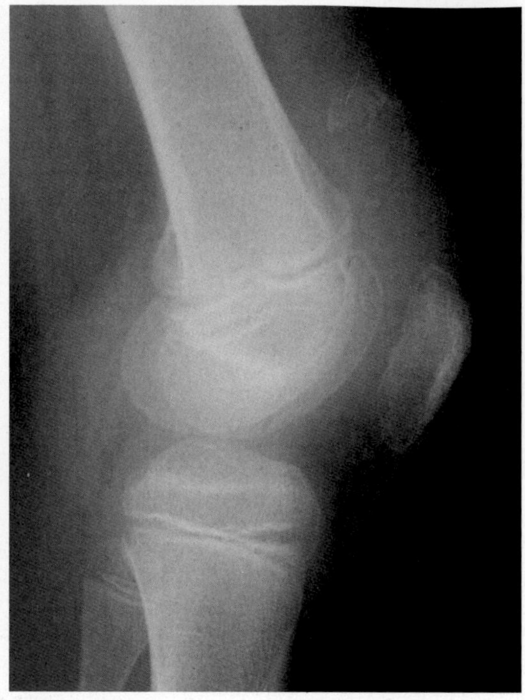

FIGURE 23-31 A. Lateral view of a child's knee with a superior patella sleeve fracture. The fracture was initially unrecognized at presentation. **B.** Two weeks later, ossification of the fracture is evident. Open reduction was necessary.

attached. Signs and symptoms of acute traumatic injury to the knee in the presence of a flake of bone on standard x-rays generally indicate an avulsion injury of some type. A high-riding patella without evidence of bony fragments suggests a sleeve fracture of the inferior patella or tibial tubercle. A palpable defect along the extensor mechanism or inability to actively extend the knee is consistent with a patellar fracture. Developmental anomalies may also be confused with fractures especially when bipartite patellae are symptomatic. Bipartite patellae are generally tender near the proximal lateral pole, which is the most common location of an extra ossification center. Also, bipartite patella is generally nondisplaced and is not associated with hemarthrosis or loss of active knee extension. Sindig-Larsen–Johanssen lesions may also be confused with distal pole avulsion injuries, but these are chronic repetitive injuries with point tenderness as the principle clinical finding.[49,100] Acute injuries are more likely to demonstrate swelling and slight displacement of fragments on x-rays. Rosenthal and Levine[136] found fragmentation of the distal pole of the patella in seven patients with spastic cerebral palsy involving the lower extremities. They believed that the fragmentation represented stress fractures caused by excessive tension in the muscle associated with a flexed-knee gait. Three of the fragmented patellae healed after hamstring lengthening.

Classification

Patellar fractures are usually classified according to morphology of the fracture pattern. Common categories of morphologic classification are transverse, vertical, comminuted, osteochondral, and sleeve.[27] Grogan et al.[56] classified avulsion fractures according to location of the avulsed fragment into four categories: superior, inferior, medial, and lateral.

Classification for Management

We believe it is more useful to classify fractures as nondisplaced and displaced. Other classifications may help understand the fracture mechanism and diagnostic challenges, but nondisplaced fractures are treated nonoperatively regardless of fracture pattern, and displaced fractures require accurate reduction and stable fixation regardless of fracture pattern.

Classification by Mechanism of Injury

Fracture pattern is influenced by the mechanism of injury to some extent and may provide a more useful classification than just description of the fracture morphology.[27] The following classification is recommended for consideration as a combination of mechanism of injury and fracture pattern:

1. *Comminuted Fractures* are more likely to be caused by direct trauma.[27] These are often nondisplaced, but direct trauma can produce damage to the articular contact area with poor outcomes.[92] Direct impact with comminution is also more likely to be present with open wounds or associated fractures of the femur, tibia, or pelvis.[27,132]
2. *Transverse Fractures* and *Sleeve Fractures* are the result of a combination of tension and three-point bend. This may occur during forceful contraction of the quadriceps with the knee flexed or with a blow to the patella with the knee flexed during quadriceps contraction. When the patella has a large ossification center, a transverse fracture through bone is more likely to occur from this mechanism; before the age of 13 years, sleeve fractures have been reported as the most common fracture pattern.[37,47,132] In this juvenile age group, the patella bends with transverse fracture of the cartilage followed by avulsion of the cartilage from the ossific nucleus. Thus, the outer shell is pulled off the ossification center like

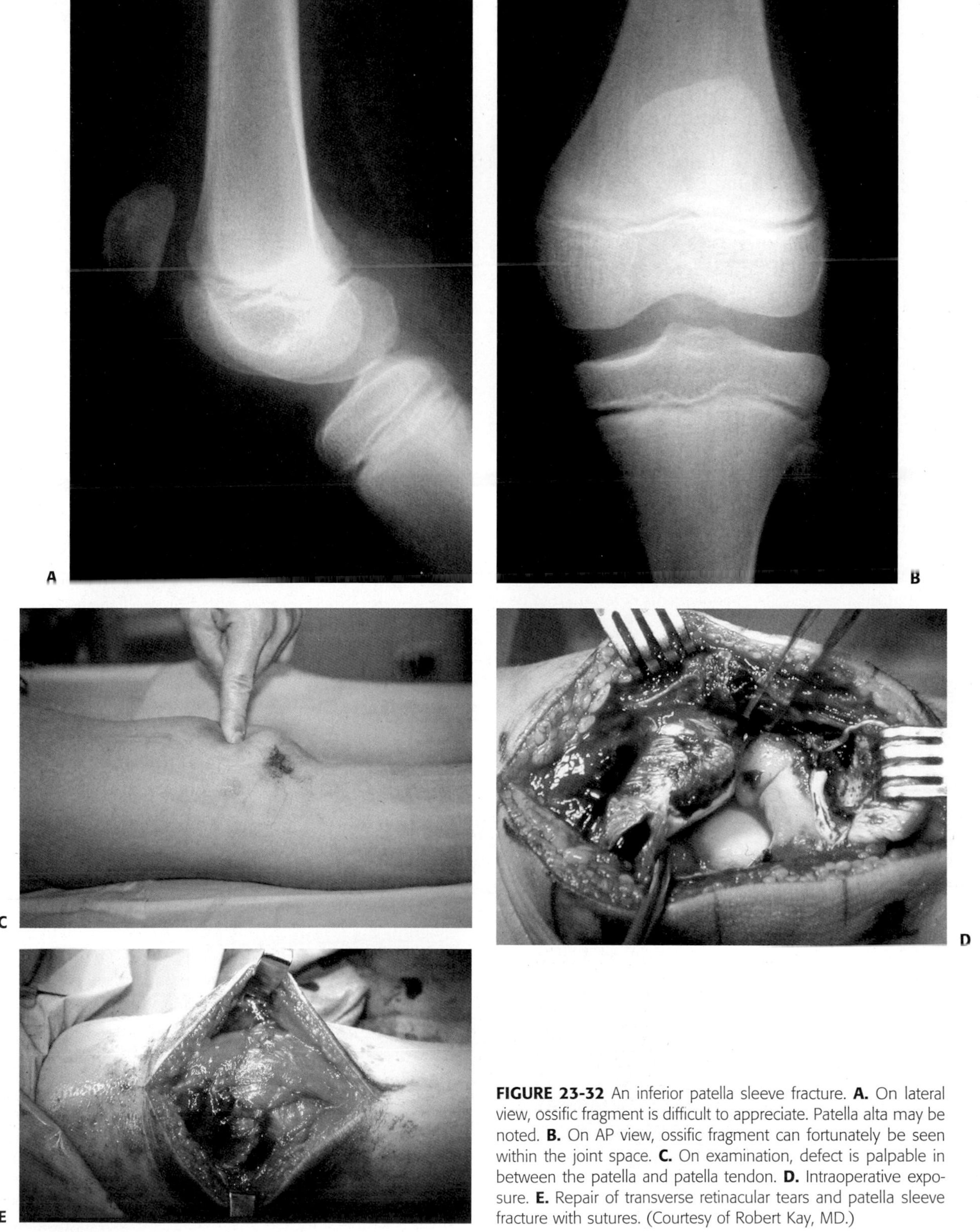

FIGURE 23-32 An inferior patella sleeve fracture. **A.** On lateral view, ossific fragment is difficult to appreciate. Patella alta may be noted. **B.** On AP view, ossific fragment can fortunately be seen within the joint space. **C.** On examination, defect is palpable in between the patella and patella tendon. **D.** Intraoperative exposure. **E.** Repair of transverse retinacular tears and patella sleeve fracture with sutures. (Courtesy of Robert Kay, MD.)

the shell of a nut that is cracked transversely and pulled off the seed that remains inside the opposite half of the shell (see Figs. 23-29 and 23-32) A small bone fragment from the ossification center remains attached to the inside of the avulsed cartilage sleeve. The extent of injury is often not appreciated on initial x-rays. Inferior pole avulsion is the most common type.[47,56,164,178] Superior pole avulsions are rare and more likely to be nondisplaced.[56,164,178] Small traumatic fractures of the superior and inferior poles of the patella should be distinguished from chronic repetitive stress injuries

3. *Medial Avulsion Fractures* are associated with lateral dislocation of the patella and are discussed in Chapter 24. These are best seen on axial x-rays of the patella such as the Mer-

chant view with the knee flexed 45 degrees and the x-ray beam angled distally to intersect the knee at an angle of 30 degrees to the long axis of the femur.[101] Most medial avulsion fractures consist of small osteochondral fragments, but large vertical sleeve fractures or vertical fractures of the patella may also occur.[56]

Surgical and Applied Anatomy

Bony Anatomy

At birth, the shape of the patella is well defined in cartilage form. Ossification of the cartilaginous anlage begins between 3 and 6 years of age.[114,115] Often, there is more than one central ossicle, and there may be as many as six irregular centers. Gradually, the ossicles coalesce and ossification proceeds peripherally until all cartilage except the articular surface is replaced by bone. Until ossification is complete, the edges of the enlarging ossific nucleus may appear irregular. The pattern of bony development is similar in this respect to the growing epiphysis of the distal femur (Fig. 23-33). Ossification of the patella usually is complete by the beginning of the second decade. Internal fixation of the patella at any age does not retard growth because the patella enlarges by appositional growth through intramembranous ossification without a discrete physis.

The patella may be bipartite or multipartite.[115,180] The overall incidence of bipartite patella in adolescents is reported to be 2% to 15%, but that may include accessory ossification centers instead of discrete bipartite patella in older adolescents.[115] The true incidence of well-formed bipartite patella is probably much lower than 2%. The most common location of the bipartite segment is the superolateral pole of the patella.[54,115]

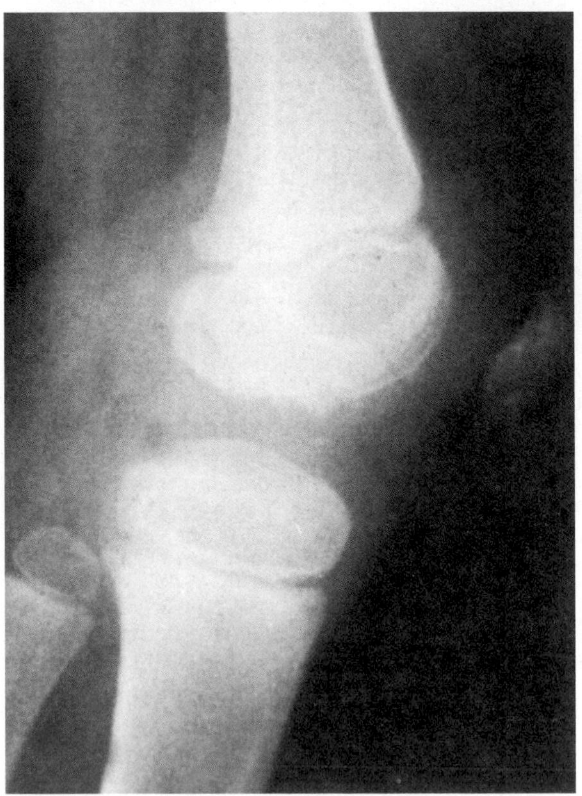

FIGURE 23-33 Normal knee in a 6-year-old child. Note irregular ossification of the patella and the distal femoral condyle.

Congenital absence[14] and congenital hypoplasia[6] of the patella are uncommon. Although these variations in development have been reported as isolated findings, they can also occur as part of the hereditary symptom complex onycho-osteodysplasia or nail-patella syndrome.[6,19]

Vascular Anatomy

Scapinelli[141] studied the blood supply to the human patella in specimens ranging from birth to old age. Neither he[141] nor Crock[35] noted differences between immature and mature specimens except for the intraosseous arborization that occurs in the ossification center. An anastomotic circle surrounds the patella with contributions from the paired superior and inferior geniculate arteries, as well as the anterior tibial recurrent artery. From the anastomotic ring, branches converge centripetally toward the anterior surface of the patella and enter through foramina in the middle third of this surface. Additional blood supply to the patella enters the distal pole behind the patellar ligament. Thus, virtually the entire blood supply to the patella comes from the anterior surface or distal pole, with essentially no penetration of vessels from the medial, proximal, or lateral margins of the patella. Scapinelli[141] noted that these findings correlate with the fact that marginal fractures of the patella are more likely to progress to nonunion. Also, injury to blood vessels entering the anterior aspect of the patella may lead to osteonecrosis of the proximal pole.[141] Also, osteochondrosis and posttraumatic disturbance of ossification have been reported that may indicate ischemia following trauma.[105,127]

Current Treatment Options

Rationale

Closed treatment is recommended for nondisplaced fractures. Aspiration of a tense hemarthrosis may relieve pain. A cylinder cast in extension is applied, and progressive weight-bearing is permitted. Immobilization may be continued for 6 weeks.

Indications for surgical stabilization of patellar fractures in children are essentially the same as for patellar fractures in adults.[37,92,132] Restoration of the extensor function and articular congruity is essential. This requires accurate reduction and stabilization of fracture fragments. Repair of torn retinaculum is also recommended,[168] although percutaneous fixation with excellent outcomes has been reported in adults.[90,156,163] An inability to actively extend the knee fully suggests major disruption of the retinaculum and may be an indication for open repair.

Operative Repair

Fixation techniques include a circumferential wire loop, nonabsorbable sutures through longitudinally drilled holes or cannulated screws, the tension-band technique, and screws or pins without tension band fixation. Choice of fixation is determined by the fracture pattern. Displaced transverse fractures, including sleeve fractures, are the most common type requiring internal fixation. An experimental study by Weber et al.[168] supported fixation by modified tension-band wiring. The method tested by Weber et al.[168] consisted of a wire loop passed transversely behind the tips of two longitudinal fixation wires and then tensioned as a longitudinal oval over the anterior surface of the patella. The AO group popularized a variation by crossing the tension band in a longitudinal figure-of-eight on the anterior surface of the patella (Fig. 23-34) Carpenter et al.[27] studied

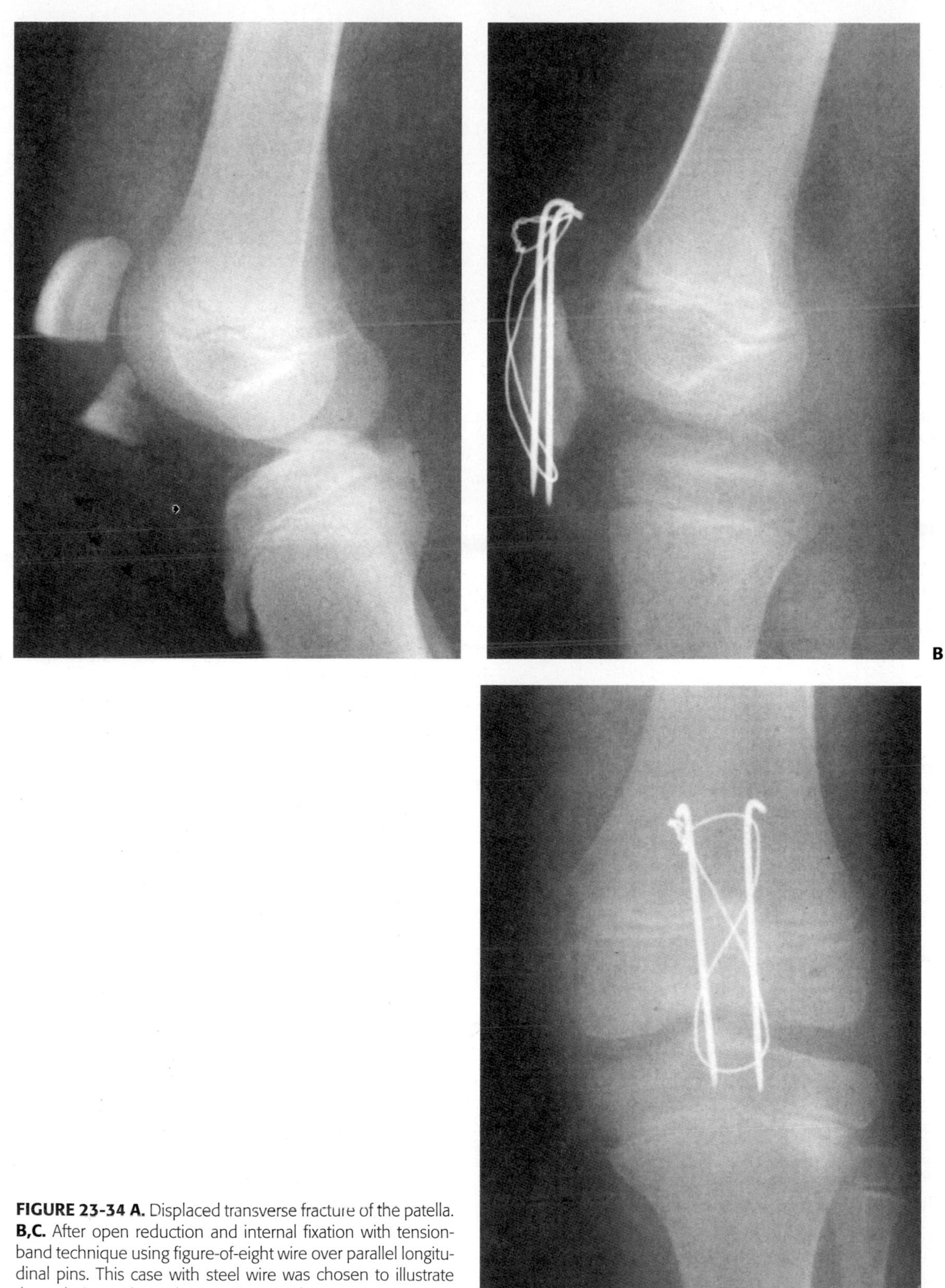

FIGURE 23-34 A. Displaced transverse fracture of the patella. **B,C.** After open reduction and internal fixation with tension-band technique using figure-of-eight wire over parallel longitudinal pins. This case with steel wire was chosen to illustrate the technique. The authors prefer using heavy suture to possibly avoid the need for future hardware removal.

several methods of fixation and determined that the strongest repair was provided by two longitudinal cannulated screws with a tension band wire passed through the central holes and twisted in a figure-of-eight over the anterior surface of the patella. This forms a horizontal figure-of-eight instead of a vertical figure-of-eight. In 2007, John et al.[75] tested different orientations of the figure-of-eight and determined that the horizontal figure-of-eight with two twists of wire at adjacent corners provided the greatest interfragmentary compression and stability (Fig. 23-35). Braided wire or braided polyester suture can also be used instead of stainless steel wire. Absorbable suture has also been successfully used in a child.[155] Fortunately, children heal rap-

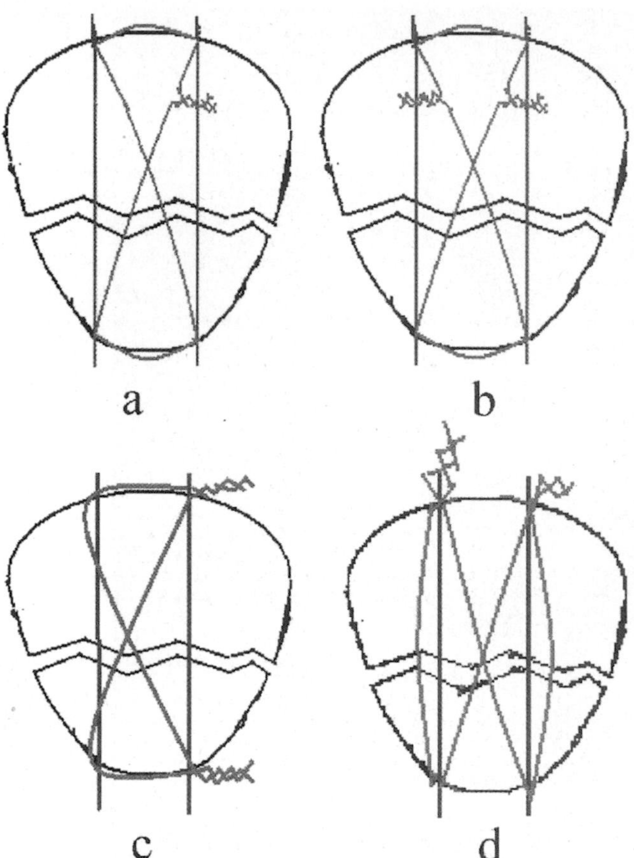

FIGURE 23-35 Four configurations of tension band loops. When stainless steel wire is used, configuration "D" provides greater interfragmentary compression and stability. **A.** Vertical figure-of-eight with one wire twist. **B.** Vertical figure-of-eight with two wire twists. **C.** Vertical figure-of-eight with two wire twists placed at adjacent corners. **D.** Horizontal figure-of-eight with two wire twists placed at adjacent corners. Method "D" can be achieved with two cannulated compression screws for added stability. (Reprinted with permission from John J, Wagner WW, and Kuiper JH. Tension-band wiring of transverse fractures of the patella. Intl Orthop 2007;31:703–707.)

idly and tolerate immobilization, so the technique of wiring may not be as important in children as it is in adults.

Medial avulsion fractures associated with acute patellar dislocation should be repaired to reduce the risk of recurrent instability.[56,134] The osteochondral fragment is either removed or repaired depending primarily on the size of the avulsed fragment.[56,129] When larger than 1 cm, the fragment can usually be securely replaced and fixed with pins, headless screws, sutures, or resorbable fixation devices.[13,56,97,129] Rorabeck and Bobechko[134] advised repairing the extensor apparatus in children when osteochondral fractures are associated with patellar dislocation. Repair was successful with or without excision of the osteochondral fragment.[134] A more detailed discussion of this injury can be found in Chapter 24.

Comminuted fractures may be difficult to reduce and stabilize. Comminution may produce fragments that are small or detached. Cerclage wiring with small fragment fixation may allow restoration of extensor function and articular congruity. Partial patellectomy may be necessary, but total patellectomy should be avoided if at all possible.[27,37,92,132] Preservation of some of the articular surface is preferred to total patellectomy. When partial patellectomy is necessary, the quadriceps tendon or patellar tendon is pulled to the remnant of patella and sutured as close as possible to the articular surface through drill holes to minimize the step-off between the tendon and articular margin of the patellar fragment. On the rare occasion when total patellectomy is unavoidable, transverse closure is preferred to longitudinal closure of the defect in the extensor mechanism.[77]

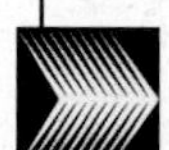

AUTHORS' PREFERRED TREATMENT

We advise closed treatment for nondisplaced fractures of the patella. A long-leg cast is applied with the knee in slightly less than full extension. Partial weight-bearing is allowed as soon as symptoms permit, usually within the first several days.

Open reduction and internal fixation are recommended for fractures that are displaced more than 2 to 3 mm. Surgery for transverse fractures including sleeve fractures is different from surgery for comminuted fractures. For transverse fractures, percutaneous fixation with arthroscopic control is an alternative, but open reduction allows repair of any torn patellar retinaculum. We prefer a longitudinal midline incision to facilitate possible future surgery about the knee. Following irrigation and débridement of the fracture, reduction is performed and evaluated. Visualization of the articular surface should be possible through the retinacular tear. If not, a small medial capsular incision can be made to expose the articular surface of the patella. Then the fracture surfaces are examined and a 2.0 or 2.5-mm Kirschner wire or guidewire is placed through the fracture surface into the proximal or distal pole of the patella. The wire is advanced until it is flush with the fracture surface. Then provisional fixation is obtained with one or two bone reduction forceps or towel clamps. The Kirschner-wire or guidewire is then advanced into the opposite fragment until it exits the pole of the patella. The wires can be left in place for tension band wiring or cannulated lag screws can be inserted over the guidewires. Two wires or screws in a parallel longitudinal orientation are recommended. Final fixation is achieved with a tension band looped around the protruding tips of the wires proximally and distally. The loop crosses in the middle of the patella to form a figure-of-eight. Recently, it has been demonstrated that the horizontal configuration of the tension band wire with two twist points provides stronger fixation and greater compression at the fracture site (see Fig. 23-35).[75] When screws are used, they should be stopped a few millimeters short of the margin of the patella to avoid irritation or stress points on the tension band. Lag screws with the tension band through the center holes with two twist points is the strongest configuration for fixation of transverse fractures.[27,75] We have found that steel wire frequently causes irritation and requires further surgery, where strong suture is less irritating and provides sufficient fixation. In most children, due to rapid fracture healing, we prefer internal fixation using the horizontal figure-of-eight tension-band technique with a strong suture such as FiberWire braided polyblend suture with Kevlar woven into it, size no. 2 (Arthrex, Naples, FL) or size no. 2 braided polyester suture instead of wire. When a vertical figure-of-eight is used, it is important to fit the transverse limbs underneath the wires and directly against the superior and inferior poles of the patella without any interposed soft tissue that may allow relaxation of tension in the postoperative period. The retinaculum on both the medial and lateral sides is repaired meticulously from outward in toward the margins of the patella.

For comminuted fractures, a circular tension band is used to gather all the fragments together. Small pins or small fragment screws are used to approximate fragments that have soft-tissue attachments. Devitalized or free, fragments may need to be discarded. Every attempt should be made to avoid patellectomy, but partial patellectomy may be necessary. When part of the patella remains, the patellar tendon or quadriceps tendon is sutured to the remaining portion of the patella with heavy no. 2 braided polyester sutures that are attached to parallel drill holes placed in the bone as close as possible to the articular surface of the remaining patella. A figure-of-eight tension band can then be passed through the patellar remnant and looped distally to the tibial tubercle or proximally into the quadriceps tendon to protect the repair. This loop should not be tightened so much that the remaining patella is displaced too far distally or proximally.

Medial osteochondral avulsion fractures are repaired with screws or sutures if large enough for fixation. Small fragments are excised with repair of the retinaculum. This is described in more detail in the next chapter.

Postoperative and Postfracture Care

Immobilization in a cast or knee immobilizer is recommended for children because stiffness is not as much of a concern as it is in adults. Approximately 4 weeks after repair, gentle range of motion is initiated. This is followed with strengthening exercises 6 to 8 weeks following injury and repair.

Pearls and Pitfalls

- Late recognition of patellar sleeve fractures is not uncommon—this diagnosis should be considered in any patient who does not have full active extension of the knee.
- When repairing the retinaculum, all the sutures are placed first without tying them. If the sutures are tied as they are placed, it becomes increasingly difficult to visualize the torn retinaculum and fracture.
- If closing the gap of the extensor mechanism is difficult:
    - The tourniquet, which may be tethering the quadriceps, can be released.
    - If the fracture is not acute, quadriceps contraction may have occurred, in which case judicious musculotendinous lengthening of the quadriceps complex may be needed.

Complications

Early complications include fracture displacement and wound complications. These may be due to the magnitude of the initial trauma, technical deficiencies, or patient noncompliance. Repeat fixation is recommended when secondary displacement is more than 3 to 4-mm of gap or more than 2 mm of step-off of the articular surface.

Late complications include joint stiffness, patellofemoral pain, and weakness. Fortunately, these are rare in children when accurate reduction of the fracture is obtained and maintained until union. Early gentle motion beginning 4 weeks after surgery, with later strengthening exercises, can diminish the risk of weakness or limited motion. Delayed diagnosis of sleeve fractures of the patella is not uncommon.[47,65,178] Repair with débridement and approximation of the fracture fragments has been reported as late as 2 months, although loss of knee flexion may be a result.[178] It is best to avoid quadriceps lengthening at the time of repair even if knee extension is required to approximate the fragments. Quadriceps lengthening can be done at a later time if satisfactory flexion cannot be achieved. Manipulation should be avoided because of the risk of distal femoral physeal separation during manipulation under anesthesia.

In particular, sleeve fractures if unrecognized or inadequately reduced and fixed can lead to extensor lag.[84,116]

REFERENCES

1. Abraham E, Ansari A, Huang TL. Fracture of the distal medial femoral epiphysis with subluxation of the knee joint. J Trauma 1980;20:339–341.
2. Anderson M, Green WT, Messner MB. Growth and predictions of growth in the lower extremities. J Bone Joint Surg Am 1963;45A:1–14.
3. Arkader A, Warner WC Jr, Horn BD, et al. Predicting the outcome of physeal fractures of the distal femur. J Pediatr Orthop 2007;27:703–708.
4. Aroojis AJ, Gajjar SM, Johari AN. Epiphyseal separations in spastic cerebral palsy. J Pediatr Orthop B 2007;16:170–174.
5. Aroojis AJ, Johari AN. Epiphyseal separations after neonatal osteomyelitis and septic arthritis. J Pediatr Orthop 2000;20:544–549.
6. Azouz EM, Kozlowski K. Small patella syndrome: a bone dysplasia to recognize and differentiate from the nail-patella syndrome. Pediatr Radiol 1997;27:432–435.
7. Banagale RC, Kuhns LR. Traumatic separation of the distal femoral epiphysis in the newborn. J Pediatr Orthop 1983;3:396–398.
8. Barmada A, Gaynor T, Mubarak SJ. Premature physeal closure following distal tibia physeal fractures: a new radiographic predictor. J Pediatr Orthop 2003;23:733–739.
9. Bates DG, Hresko MT, Jaramillo D. Patellar sleeve fracture: demonstration with MR imaging. Radiology 1994;193:825–827.
10. Beals RK. Premature closure of the physis following diaphyseal fractures. J Pediatr Orthop 1990;10(6):717–720.
11. Beaty JH, Kumar A. Fractures about the knee in children. J Bone Joint Surg Am 1994; 76:1870–1880.
12. Belman DA, Neviaser RJ. Transverse fracture of the patella in a child. J Trauma 1973; 13:917–918.
13. Benz G, Kallieris D, Seeböck T, et al. Bioresorbable pins and screws in paediatric traumatology. Eur J Pediatr Surg 1993;4:103–107.
14. Bernhang A, Levine S. Familial absence of the patella. J Bone Joint Surg Am 1973; 55(5):1088–1090.
15. Bertin KC, Goble EM. Ligament injuries associated with physeal fractures about the knee. Clin Orthop Relat Res 1983;177:188–195.
16. Birch JG. Surgical treatment of physeal bar resection. In: Eilert RE, ed. Instructional Course Lectures. Rosemont: Amer Acad Orthop Surg; 1992:445–450.
17. Blackburne JS, Peel TE. A new method of measuring patellar height. J Bone Joint Surg Br 1977;59(2):241–242.
18. Bolesta MJ, Fitch RD. Tibial tubercle avulsions. J Pediatr Orthop 1986;6(2):186–192.
19. Bongers EM, Van Bokhoven H, Van Thiensen MN, et al. The small patella syndrome: description of five cases from three families and examination of possible allelism with familial patella aplasia-hypoplasis syndrome. J Med Genetics 2001;38:209–214.
20. Braten M, Helland P, Myhre HO, et al. 11 femoral fractures with vascular injury: good outcome with early vascular repair and internal fixation. Acta Orthop Scand 1996;67: 161–164.
21. Bright RW, Burstein AH, Elmore SM. Epiphyseal-plate cartilage. A biomechanical and histological analysis of failure modes. J Bone Joint Surg Am 1974;56(4):688–703.
22. Brone LA, Wroble RR. Salter-Harris type III fracture of the medial femoral condyle associated with an anterior cruciate ligament tear. Report of three cases and review of the literature. Am J Sports Med 1998;26(4):581–586.
23. Broughton NS, et al. Epiphyseolysis for partial growth plate arrest. Results after four years or at maturity. J Bone Joint Surg Br 1989;71(1):13–16.
24. Bruijn JD, Sanders RJ, Jansen BR. Ossification in the patellar tendon and patella alta following sports injuries in children. Complications of sleeve fractures after conservative treatment. Arch Orthop Trauma Surg 1993;112:157–158.
25. Burkhart SS, Peterson HA. Fractures of the proximal tibial epiphysis. J Bone Joint Surg Am 1979;61(7):996–1002.
26. Cakir O, Subari M, Erdem K, et al. Treatment of vascular injuries associated with limb fractures. Ann R Coll Surg Engl 2005;87:348–352.
27. Carpenter JE, Kasman R, Matthews LS. Fractures of the patella. J Bone Joint Surg Am 1993;75A:1550–1561.
28. Chow SP, Lam JJ, Leong JCY. Fracture of the tibial tubercle in the adolescent. J Bone Joint Surg Am 1990;72B:231–234.
29. Christie MJ, Dvonch VM. Tibial tuberosity avulsion fracture in adolescents. J Pediatr Orthop 1981;1:391–394.

30. Chung SM, Batterman SC, Brighton CT. Shear strength of the human femoral capital epiphyseal plate. J Bone Joint Surg Am 1976;58(1):94–103.
31. Ciszewski WA, Buschman WR, Rudolph CN. Irreducible fracture of the proximal tibial physis in an adolescent. Orthop Rev 1989;18:891–893.
32. Close BJ, Strouse PJ. MR of physeal fractures of the adolescent knee. Pediatr Radiol 2000;30:756–762.
33. Cohen DA, Hinton RY. Bilateral tibial tubercle avulsion fractures associated with Osgood-Schlatter's disease. Am J Orthop 2008;37:92–93.
34. Conroy J, Cohen A, Smith RM, et al. Triplane fractures of the proximal tibia. Injury 2000;31:546–548.
35. Crock HV. An Atlas of Vascular Anatomy of the Skeleton and Spinal Cord. London: Martin Dunitz; 1996.
36. Czitrom AA, Salter RB, Willis RB. Fractures involving the distal epiphyseal plate of the femur. Intl Orthop 1981;4:269–77.
37. Dai LY, Zhang WM. Fractures of the patella in children. Knee Surg Sports Traumatol Arthrosc 1999;7:243–245.
38. Davidson D, Letts M. Partial sleeve fractures of the tibia in children: an unusual fracture pattern. J Pediatr Orthop 2002;22:36–40.
39. Diamond LS, Alegardo R. Perinatal fractures in arthrogryposis multiplex congenita. J Pediatr Orthop 1981;1:189–192.
40. Dvonch VM, Bunch WH. Pattern of closure of the proximal femoral and tibial epiphyses in man. J Pediatr Orthop 1983;3:498–501.
41. Ecklund K, Jaramillo D. Patterns of premature physeal arrest: MR imaging of 111 children. Am J Roentgenol 2002;178:967–972.
42. Egol KA, Karunakar M, Phieffer L, et al. Early versus late reduction of a physeal fracture in an animal model. J Pediatr Orthop 2002;22:208–211.
43. Ehrenborg G. The Osgood-Schlatter lesion: a clinical and experimental study. Acta Chir Scand Suppl 1962;288:1–36.
44. Eid AM, Hafez MA. Traumatic injuries of the distal femoral physis. A retrospective study on 151 cases. Injury 2002;33:251–255.
45. El-Zawawy HB, Silva MJ, Sandell LJ, et al. Ligamentous versus physeal failure in murine medial collateral ligament biomechanical testing. J Biomech 2005;38:703–706.
46. Gabel GT, Peterson HA, Berquist TH. Premature partial physeal arrest. Diagnosis by magnetic resonance imaging in two cases. Clin Orthop Relat Res 1991;272:242–247.
47. Gao GX, Mahadev A, Lee EH. Sleeve fracture of the patella in children. J Orthop Surg 2008;16:43–46.
48. García Mata S, Hidalgo Ovejero A, Martinez Grande M. Transverse stress fracture of the patella in a child. J Pediatr Orthop 1999;8(3):208–211.
49. Gardiner JS, McInernay VK, Avella DG, et al. Injuries to the inferior pole of the patella in children. Orthop Rev 1990;7:643–649.
50. Gibson PH, Papaioannou T, Kenwright J. The influence on the spine of leg-length discrepancy after femoral fracture. J Bone Joint Surg Br 1983;65(5):584–587.
51. Gomes LS, Volpon JB. Experimental physeal fracture-separations treated with rigid internal fixation. J Bone Joint Surg Am 1993;75A:1756–1764.
52. González-Reimers E, Pérez-Ramírez A, Santolaria-Fernández F, et al. Association of Harris lines and shorter stature with ethanol consumption during growth. Alcohol 2007;41:511–515.
53. Graham JM, Gross RH. Distal femoral physeal problem fractures. Clin Orthop Relat Res 1990;255:51–53.
54. Green WT Jr. Painful bipartite patella. Clin Orthop Relat Res 1975;110:197–200.
55. Griswold A. Early motion in the treatment of separation of the lower femoral epiphysis. J Bone Joint Surg Am 1928;10:75–77.
56. Grogan DP, Carey TP, Leffers D, et al. Avulsion fractures of the patella. J Pediatr Orthop 1990;10(6):721–730.
57. Gross RH. Leg length discrepancy: how much is too much? Orthopedics 1978;1: 307–310.
58. Gupta SP, Agarwal A. Concomitant double epiphyseal injuries of the tibia with vascular compromise: a case report. J Orthop Sci 2004;9:526–528.
59. Hand WL, Hand CR, Dunn AW. Avulsion fractures of the tibial tubercle. J Bone Joint Surg Am 1971;53(8):1579–1583.
60. Hannouche D, Duparc F, Beaufils P. The arterial vascularization of the lateral tibial condyle: anatomy and surgical applications. Surg Radiol Anat 2006;28:38–40.
61. Harris HA. The growth of the long bones in childhood with special reference to certain bony striations of the metaphysis and to the role of vitamins. Arch Int Med 1926;38: 785–806.
62. Hasler CC, Foster BK. Secondary tethers after physeal bar excision. a common source of failure? Clin Orthop Relat Res 2002;405:242–249.
63. Hermus JP, Driessen MJ, Mulder H, et al. The triplane variant of the tibial apophyseal fracture: a case report and review of the literature. J Pediatr Orthop B 2003;12: 406–408.
64. Herring JA. General principles for managing orthopedic injuries. In: Herring JA, ed. Tachdjian's Pediatric Orthopedics. Philadelphia: WB Saunders; 2002:2059–2086.
65. Houghton GR, Ackroyd CE. Sleeve fractures of the patella in children: a report of three cases. J Bone Joint Surg Br 1979;61-B(2):165–168.
66. Hresko MT, Kasser JR. Physeal arrest about the knee associated with non-physeal fractures in the lower extremity. J Bone Joint Surg Am 1989;71(5):698–703.
67. Hsu RW, Himeno S, Coventry MB, et al. Normal axial alignment of the lower extremity and load-bearing distribution at the knee. Clin Orthop Relat Res 1990;255:215–227.
68. Hübner U, Schlicht W, Outzen S, et al. Ultrasound in the diagnosis of fractures in children. J Bone Joint Surg Br 2000;82:1170–113.
69. Hughes LO, Beaty JH. Fractures of the head and neck of the femur in children. J Bone Joint Surg Am 1994;76(2):283–292.
70. Hutchinson JJ. Lectures on injuries to the epiphysis and their results. Br Med J 1894; 1:669–673.
71. Ilharreborde B, Raquillet C, Morel E, et al. Long-term prognosis of Salter-Harris type 2 injuries of the distal femoral physis. J Pediatr Orthop B 2006;15:433–438.
72. Inoue G, Kubboyama K, Shido T. Avulsion fractures of the proximal tibial epiphysis. Br J Sports Med 1991;25:52–56.
73. Janarv PM, Wikstrom B, Hirsch G. The influence of transphyseal drilling and tendon grafting on bone growth: an experimental study in the rabbit. J Pediatr Orthop 1998; 18(2):149–154.
74. Jarit GJ, Kummer FJ, Gibber MJ, et al. A mechanical evaluation of two fixation methods using cancellous screws for coronal fractures of the lateral condyle of the distal femur (OTA type 33B). J Orthop Trauma 2006;20:273–276.
75. John J, Wagner WW, Kuiper JH. Tension-band wiring of transverse fractures of patella. The effect of site of wire twists and orientation of stainless steel wire loop: a biomechanical investigation. Intl Orthop 2007;31:703–707.
76. Kaneko K, Matsuda T, Mogami A, et al. Type III fracture of the tibial tubercle with avulsion of the tibialis anterior muscle in the adolescent male athlete. Injury 2004;35: 919–921.
77. Kaufer H. Mechanical function of the patella. J Bone Joint Surg Am 1971;53(8): 1551–1560.
78. Kawamoto K, Kim WC, Tsuchida Y, et al. Incidence of physeal injuries in Japanese children. J Pediatr Orthop B 2006;15:126–130.
79. Keret D, Mendez AA, Harcke HT. Type V physeal injury: a case report. J Pediatr Orthop 1990;10:545–548.
80. Khoshhal KI, Kiefer GN. Physeal bridge resection. J Am Acad Orthop Surg 2005;13: 47–58.
81. King SJ. Magnetic resonance imaging of knee injuries in children. Eur Radiol 1997;7: 1245–1251.
82. Langenskiöld A. Surgical treatment of partial closure of the growth plate. J Pediatr Orthop 1981;1(1):3–11.
83. Lee YS, Jung YB, Ahn JH, et al. Arthroscopic assisted reduction and internal fixation of lateral femoral epiphyseal injury in an adolescent soccer player: report of one case. Knee Surg Sports Traumatol Arthrosc 2007;15:744–746.
84. Levi JH, Coleman CR. Fracture of the tibial tubercle. Am J Sports Med 1976;4:254–263.
85. Lewis SL, Pozo JL, Muirhead-Allwood WFG. Coronal fractures of the lateral femoral condyle. J Bone Joint Surg Br 1989;71(1):118–120.
86. Lippiello L, Bass R, Connolly JF. Stereological study of the developing distal femoral growth plate. J Orthop Res 1989;7:868–875.
87. Loder RT, Bookout C. Fracture patterns in battered children. J Orthop Trauma 1991; 5:428–433.
88. Loder RT, Swinford A, Kuhns L. The use of helical computed tomographic scan to assess bony physeal bridges. J Pediatr Orthop 1977;17:356–359.
89. Lombardo SJ, Harvey JP Jr. Fractures of the distal femoral epiphyses. Factors influencing prognosis: a review of thirty-four cases. J Bone Joint Surg Am 1977;59(6):742–51.
90. Luna-Pizarro D, Amato D, Arellano F, et al. Comparison of a technique using a new percutaneous osteosynthesis device with conventional open surgery for displaced patella fractures in a randomized controlled trial. J Orthop Trauma 2006;20:529–535.
91. Maffulli J, Grewal R. Avulsion of the tibial tuberosity: muscles too strong for a growth plate. Clin J Sports Med 1997;7:129–133.
92. Maguire JK, Canale ST. Fractures of the patella in children and adolescents. J Pediatr Orthop 1993;13(5):567–571.
93. Mäkelä EA, Vainionpää S, Vihtonen K, et al. The effect of trauma to the lower femoral epiphyseal plate. An experimental study in rabbits. J Bone Joint Surg Br 1988;70(2): 187–191.
94. Mangurten HH, Puppala G, Knuth A. Neonatal distal femoral physeal fracture requiring closed reduction and pinning. J Perinatol 2005;25:216–219.
95. Mani GV, Hui PW, Cheng JC. Translation of the radius as a predictor of outcome in distal radial fractures of children. J Bone Joint Surg Br 1993;75(5):808–811.
96. Mann DC, Rajmaira S. Distribution of physeal and nonphyseal fractures in 2,650 long-bone fractures in children aged 0-16 years. J Pediatr Orthop1990;10(6):713–716.
97. Matsusue Y, Nakamura T, Suzuki R, et al. Biodegradable pin fixation of osteochondral fragments of the knee. Clin Orthop Relat Res 1996;322:166–173.
98. McKissick RC, Gilley JS, DeLee JC. Salter-Harris Type III fractures of the medial distal femoral physis—a fracture pattern related to the closure of the growth plate: report of 3 cases and discussion of pathogenesis. Am J Sports Med 2008;36:572–576.
99. McKoy BE, Stanitski CL. Acute tibial tubercle avulsion fractures. Orthop Clin North Am 2003;34:397–403.
100. Medlar RC, Lyne ED. Sinding-Larsen-Johansson disease. Its etiology and natural history. J Bone Joint Surg Am 1978;60(8):1113–1116.
101. Merchant AC, Mercer RL, Jacobsen RH, et al. Roentgenographic analysis of patellofemoral congruence. J Bone Joint Surg Am 1974;56(7):1391–1396.
102. Meyers RA, Calvo RD, Sterling JC, et al. Delayed treatment of a malreduced distal femoral epiphyseal plate fracture. Med Sci Sports Exerc 1992;24:1311–1315.
103. Morscher E. Strength and morphology of growth cartilage under hormonal influence of puberty. Reconstr Surg Traumatol 1978;10:3–104.
104. Mosier SM, Stanitski CL. Acute tibial tubercle avulsion fractures. J Pediatr Orthop 2004;24:181–184.
105. Muller U. Posttraumatic disturbance of the ossification of the patella. Arch Orthop Trauma Surg 1979;94:151–153.
106. Muratli HH, Celebil L, Hapa O, et al. Bilateral patellar tendon rupture in a child: a case report. Knee Surg Sports Traumatol Arthrosc 2005;13:677–682.
107. Navascués JA, González-López JL, López-Valverde S, et al. Premature physeal closure after tibial diaphyseal fractures in adolescents. J Pediatr Orthop 2000;20:193–196.
108. Nietosvaara Y, Aalto K, Kallio PE. Acute patellar dislocation in children: incidence and associated osteochondral fractures. J Pediatr Orthop 1994;14:513–515.
109. Nikiforidis PA, Babis GC, Triantafillopolos IK, et al. Avulsion fractures of the tibial tuberosity in adolescent athletes treated by internal fixation and tension band wiring. Knee Surg Sports Traumatol Arthrosc 2004;12:271–276.
110. Nork SE, Segina DN, Aflatoon K, et al. The association between supracondylar-intercondylar distal femoral fractures and coronal plane fractures. J Bone Joint Surg Am 2005;87(3):564–569.
111. Ogden JA. Distal Femoral epiphyseal injuries. In: Ogden JA, ed. Skeletal Injury in the Child. New York: Springer, 2000:896–912.
112. Ogden JA. Growth slowdown and arrest lines. J Pediatr Orthop 1984;4:409–415.
113. Ogden JA. Injury to the growth mechanisms of the immature skeleton. Skeletal Radiol 1981;6:237–253.
114. Ogden JA. Radiology of postnatal skeletal development. X. Patella and tibial tuberosity. Skeletal Radiol 1984;11:246–257.
115. Ogden JA, McCarthy SM, Jokl P. The painful bipartite patella. J Pediatr Orthop 1982; 2:263–269.
116. Ogden JA, Tross RB, Murphy MJ. Fractures of the tibial tuberosity in adolescents. J Bone Joint Surg Am 1980;62(2):205–215.

117. Ozer H, Turanli S, Baltaci G, et al. Avulsion of the tibial tuberosity with a lateral plateau rim fracture. Knee Surg Sports Traumatol Arthrosc 2002;10:310–312.
118. Pape JM, Goulet JA, Hensinger RN. Compartment syndrome complicating tibial tubercle avulsion. Clin Orthop Relat Res 1993;295:201–204.
119. Pappas AM, Anas P, Toczylowski HM. Asymmetrical arrest of the proximal tibial physis and genu recurvatum deformity. J Bone Joint Surg Am 1984;66(4):575–581.
120. Park EA. The imprinting of nutritional disturbances on the growing bone. Pediatrics 1964;33:815–862.
121. Parsch K. Origin and treatment of fractures in spina bifida. Eur J Pediatr Surg 1991; 1:298–305.
122. Patari SK, Lee FY, Behrens FF. Coronal split fracture of the proximal tibial epiphysis through a partially closed physis: a new fracture pattern. J Pediatr Orthop 2001;21: 451–455.
123. Peterson HA. Partial growth plate arrest and its treatment. J Pediatr Orthop 1984;4(2): 246–258.
124. Peterson HA, Madhok R, Benson JT, et al. Physeal fractures: Part 1. Epidemiology in Olmsted County, Minnesota, 1979-1988. J Pediatr Orthop 1994;14(4): 423–430.
125. Petrin M, Weber E, Stauffer UG. Interposition of periosteum in joint fractures in adolescents; comparison of operative and conservative treatment [article in German]. Z Kinderchir 1981;33:84–88.
126. Phieffer LS, Meyer RA Jr, Gruber HE, et al. Effect of interposed periosteum in an animal physeal fracture model. Clin Orthop Relat Res 2000;376:15–25.
127. Pinar H, Gul O, Boya H, et al. Osteochondrosis of the primary ossification center of the patella (Kohler's disease of the patella). Report of three cases. Knee Surg Sports Traumatol Arthrosc 2002;10:141–143.
128. Poulsen TD, Skak SV, Jensen TT. Epiphyseal fractures of the proximal tibia. Injury 1989;20:111–113.
129. Pritsch M, Velkes S, Levy O, et al. Suture fixation of osteochondral fractures of the patella. J Bone Joint Surg Br 1995;77(1):154–155.
130. Rafee A, Kumar A, Shah SV. Salter-Harris type III fracture of the lateral femoral condyle with a ruptured posterior cruciate ligament: an uncommon injury pattern. Arch Orthop Trauma Surg 2007;127:29–31.
131. Rang M, Wenger DR. The physis and skeletal injury. In: Wenger DR, Pring ME, eds. Rang's Children's Fractures. Philadelphia: Lippincott Williams & Wilkins; 2005: 11–25.
132. Ray JM, Hendrix J. Incidence, mechanism of injury, and treatment of fractures of the patella in children. J Trauma 1992;32:464–467.
133. Riseborough EJ, Barrett IR, Shapiro F. Growth disturbances following distal femoral physeal fracture-separations. J Bone Joint Surg Am 1983;65(7):885–893.
134. Rorabeck CH, Bobechko WP. Acute dislocation of the patella with osteochondral fracture. J Bone Joint Surg Br 1976;58(2):237–240.
135. Rosenberg ZS, Kwelblum M, Cheung YY, et al. Osgood-Schlatter lesion: fracture or tendinitis? Scintigraphic, CT, and MR Imaging features. Radiol 1992;185:853–858.
136. Rosenthal R, Levine DB. Fragmentation of the distal pole of the patella in spastic cerebral palsy. J Bone Joint Surg Am 1977;59(7):934–939.
137. Ryu RKN, Debenham JO. An unusual avulsion fracture of the proximal tibial epiphysis. Clin Orthop Relat Res 1985;194:181–184.
138. Sabharwal S, Henry P, Behrens F. Two cases of missed Salter-Harris III coronal plane fracture of the lateral femoral condyle. Am J Orthop 2008;37:100–103.
139. Sabharwal S, Zhao C, McKeon JJ, et al. Computed radiographic measurement of limb-length discrepancy. Full-length standing anteroposterior radiograph compared with scanogram. J Bone Joint Surg Am 2006;88(10):2243–2251.
140. Salter R, Harris WR. Injuries involving the epiphysial plate. J Bone Joint Surg Am 1963; 45:587.
141. Scapinelli R. Blood supply of the human patella: its relation to ischaemic necrosis after fracture. J Bone Joint Surg Br 1967;49(3):563–570.
142. Sferopoulos NK. Type v physeal injury. J Trauma 2007;63:E121–123.
143. Sferopoulos NK, Rafailidis D, Traios S, et al. Avulsion fractures of the lateral tibial condyle in children. Injury 2006;37:57–60.
144. Shelton WR, Canale ST. Fractures of the tibia through the proximal tibial epiphyseal cartilage. J Bone Joint Surg Am 1979;61(2):167–173.
145. Shindell R, Lippiello L, Connolly JF. Uncertain effect of indomethacin on physeal growth injury. Experiments in rabbits. Acta Orthop Scand 1988;59:46–49.
146. Simonian PT, Staheli LT. Periarticular fractures after manipulation for knee contractures in children. J Pediatr Orthop 1995;15:288–291.
147. Simpson WC Jr, Fardon DF. Obscure distal femoral epiphyseal injury. South Med J 1976;69:1338–1340.
148. Skak SV. A case of partial physeal closure following compression injury. Arch Orthop Trauma Surg 1989;108:185–188.
149. Sloboda JF, Benfanti PL, McGuigan JJ, et al. Distal femoral physeal fractures and peroneal palsy: outcome and review of the literature. Am J Orthop 2007;36:E43–45.
150. Song KM, Halliday SE, Little DG. The effect of limb-length discrepancy on gait. J Bone Joint Surg Am 1997;79(11):1690–1698.
151. Stanitski CL. Stress view radiographs of the skeletally immature knee: a different view. J Pediatr Orthop 2002;24:342.
152. Stanitski CL, Harvell JC, Fu F. Observations on acute knee hemarthrosis in children and adolescents. J Pediatr Orthop 1993;13(4):506–510.
153. Starr AJ, Hunt JL, Reinert CM. Treatment of femur fracture with associated vascular injury. J Trauma 1996;40:17–21.
154. Stephens DC, Louns DS. Traumatic separation of the distal femoral epiphyseal cartilage. J Bone Joint Surg Am 1974;66A:1383–190.
155. Sturdee SW, Templeton PA, Oxborrow NJ. Internal fixation of a patella fracture using an absorbable suture. J Orthop Trauma 2002;16:272–273.
156. Tandogan RN, Demirors H, Tuncay CI, et al. Arthroscopic-assisted percutaneous screw fixation of select patellar fractures. Arthroscopy 2002;18:156–162.
157. Tepper KB, Ireland ML. Fracture patterns and treatment in the skeletally immature knee. AAOS Instr Course Lect 2003;52:667–676.
158. Thompson GA, Gesler JW. Proximal tibial epiphyseal fracture in an infant. J Pediatr Orthop 1984;4:114–117.
159. Thomson JD, Stricker SJ, Williams MM. Fractures of the distal femoral epiphyseal plate. J Pediatr Orthop 1995;15(4):474–478.
160. Tjoumakaris FP, Wells L. Popliteal artery transection complicating a non-displaced proximal tibial epiphyseal fracture. Orthopedics 2007;30:876–7.
161. Tolo VT. External skeletal fixation for children's fractures. J Pediatr Orthop 1983;3: 435–442.
162. Torg JS, Pavlov H, Morris VB. Salter-Harris type-III fracture of the medial femoral condyle occurring in the adolescent athlete. J Bone Joint Surg Am 1981;63(4):586–591.
163. Turgut A, Gunal I, Acar S, et al. Arthroscopic-assisted percutaneous stabilization of patellar fractures. Clin Orthop Relat Res 2001;389:57–61.
164. Van Isacker T, De Boeck H. Sleeve fracture of the upper pole of the patella: a case report. Acta Orthop Belg 2007;73:114–117.
165. Walker P, Harris I, Leicester A. Patellar tendon-to-patella ratio in children. J Pediatr Orthop 1998;18:129–131.
166. Watson-Jones R. Fractures and Joint Injuries. 5th ed. Baltimore: Williams and Wilkins; 1976.
167. Wattenbarger JM, Gruber HE, Phieffer LS. Physeal Fractures, part I: histologic features of bone, cartilage, and bar formation in a small animal model. J Pediatr Orthop 2002; 22:703–709.
168. Weber MJ, Janecki CJ, McLeod P, et al. Efficacy of various forms of fixation of transverse fractures of the patella. J Bone Joint Surg Am 1980;62(2):215–220.
169. Welch P, Wynne GJ. Proximal tibial epiphyseal fracture-separation: case report. J Bone Joint Surg Am 1963;45:782–784.
170. Wessel LM, Scholz S, Rusch M. Characteristic patterns and management of intra-articular knee lesions in different pediatric age groups. J Pediatr Orthop 2001;21:14–19.
171. Wessel LM, Scholz S, Rusch M, et al. Hemarthrosis after trauma to the pediatric knee joint: what is the value of magnetic resonance imaging in the diagnostic algorithm? J Pediatr Orthop 2001;21:338–342.
172. Westh R, Menelaus M. A simple calculation for the timing of epiphysial arrest: a further report. J Bone Joint Surg Br 1981;63B:117–119.
173. White PG, Mah JY, Friedman L. Magnetic resonance imaging in acute physeal injuries. Skeletal Radiol 1994;23:627–631.
174. Williamson RV, Staheli LT. Partial physeal growth arrest: treatment by bridge resection and fat interposition. J Pediatric Orthop 1990;10(6):769–776.
175. Wiss DA, Schilz JL, Zionts L. Type III fractures of the tibial tubercle in adolescents. J Trauma 1991;5:475–479.
176. Wood KB, Bradley JP, Ward WT. Pes anserinus interposition in a proximal tibial physeal fracture. Clin Orthop Relat Res 1991;264:239–242.
177. Wozasek GE, Moser KD, Haller H, et al. Trauma involving the proximal tibial epiphysis. Arch Orthop Trauma Surg 1991;110:301–306
178. Wu CD, Huang SC, Liu TK. Sleeve fracture of the patella in children: a report of five cases. Am J Sports Med 1991;19:525–528.
179. Zionts LE. Fractures around the knee in children. J Am Acad Orthop Surg 2002;10: 345–355.
180. Zumstein M, Sukthankar A, Exner GU. Tripartite patella: late appearance of a third ossification center in childhood. J Pediatr Orthop B 2006;15:75–76.

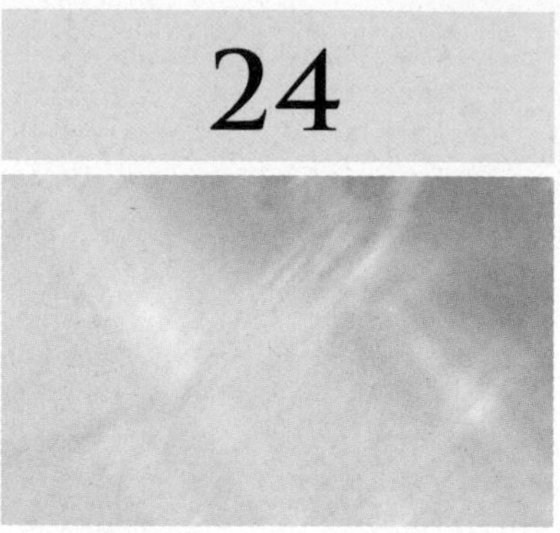

24

INTRA-ARTICULAR INJURIES OF THE KNEE

Mininder S. Kocher

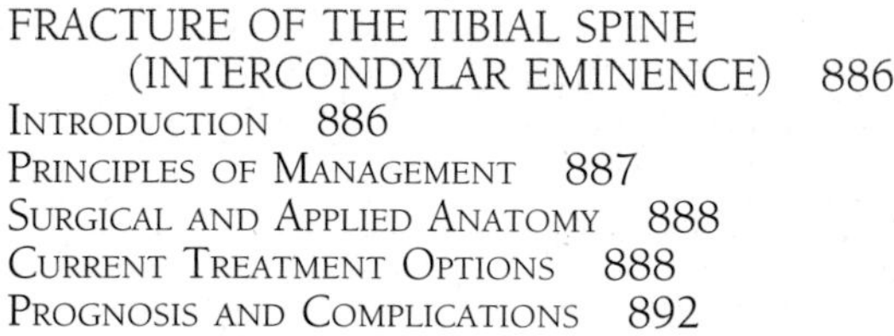

FRACTURE OF THE TIBIAL SPINE (INTERCONDYLAR EMINENCE) 886
Introduction 886
Principles of Management 887
Surgical and Applied Anatomy 888
Current Treatment Options 888
Prognosis and Complications 892

OSTEOCHONDRAL FRACTURES 895
Introduction 895
Principles of Management 895
Surgical and Applied Anatomy 896
Current Treatment Options 897
Prognosis and Complications 898

PATELLAR DISLOCATION 900
Introduction 900
Principles of Management 900
Surgical and Applied Anatomy 902
Current Treatment Options 902
Prognosis and Complications 904

MENISCAL INJURIES 904
Introduction 904
Principles of Management 905
Surgical and Applied Anatomy 906
Current Treatment Options 907
Prognosis and Complications 910

LIGAMENT INJURIES 911
Introduction 911
Principles of Management 911
Surgical and Applied Anatomy 915
Current Treatment Options 916
Prognosis and Complications 925

FRACTURE OF THE TIBIAL SPINE (INTERCONDYLAR EMINENCE)

Introduction

Fractures of the tibial eminence occur due to chondroepiphyseal avulsion of the anterior cruciate ligament (ACL) insertion on the anteromedial tibial eminence.[232,311] Tibial eminence fractures were once thought to be the pediatric equivalent of midsubstance ACL tears in adults.[30,36,61,120,148,176,188,200,201,236,240,307,308]

Avulsion fracture of the tibial spine is a relatively uncommon injury in children: Skak et al.[273] reported that it occurred in 3 per 100,000 children each year. The most common causes of these fractures are bicycle accidents and athletic activities.[217]

Historically, treatment has evolved from closed treatment of all fractures to operative treatment of certain fractures. Garcia and Neer[107] reported 42 fractures of the tibial spine in patients ranging in age from 7 to 60 years, 6 of whom had positive anterior drawer signs indicating associated collateral ligament injuries. They reported successful closed management in half their patients. Meyers and McKeever,[216] however, recommended arthrotomy and open reduction for all displaced fractures, followed by cast immobilization with the knee in 20 degrees of flexion rather than hyperextension, believing that hyperextension aggravated the injury in one of their patients. Gronkvist et al.[120] reported late instability in 16 of 32 children with tibial spine fractures, and recommended surgery for all displaced tibial spine fractures, especially in children older than 10 years because "the older the patient, the more the demand on the anterior cruciate ligament–tibial spine complex."[120] Baxter and Wiley[30] noted mild to moderate knee laxity at follow-up in 45 patients, even after anatomic reduction of the tibial spine. McLennan[212] reported 10 patients with type III intercondylar eminence fractures treated with closed reduction and with arthroscopic reduction with or without internal fixation. At second-look arthroscopy 6 years after the initial injury, those treated with closed reduction had more knee laxity than those treated arthroscopically.

Modern treatment is based on fracture type. Nondisplaced fractures and hinged or displaced fractures which are able to be reduced can be treated closed. Hinged and displaced fractures which do not reduce require open or arthroscopic reduction with internal fixation. A variety of treatment options have been reported including cast immobilization,[188,223] closed reduction with immobilization,[236,308] open reduction with immobilization,[223] open reduction with internal fixation,[225,236] arthroscopic reduction with immobilization,[212] arthroscopic reduction with suture fixation,[49,137,155,188,200,201] and arthroscopic reduction with wire,[27] screw fixation,[36,188,212] anchor fixation,[298] and bioabsorbable fixation.[264]

The prognosis for closed treatment of nondisplaced and reduced tibial spine fractures and for operative treatment of displaced fractures is good. Most series report healing with an excellent functional outcome despite some residual knee laxity.[27,30,36,155,170,188,195,200,201,211,212,223,225,276,307,308] Potential complications include nonunion, malunion, arthrofibrosis, residual knee laxity, and growth disturbance.[27,30,36,155,170,188,200,201,211,212,223,225,276,296,308]

Principles of Management

Mechanism of Injury

Historically, the most common mechanism of tibial eminence fracture in children has been a fall from a bicycle.[216,251] However, with increased participation in youth sports at earlier ages and at higher competitive levels, tibial spine fractures resulting from sporting activities are being seen with increased frequency. The most common mechanism of tibial eminence fracture is forced valgus and external rotation of the tibia, although tibial spine avulsion fractures can also occur from hyperflexion, hyperextension, or tibial internal rotation. As with ACL injury, tibial eminence fractures in sport may result from both contact and noncontact injuries.

Tibial eminence fractures occur due to chondroepiphyseal avulsion of the ACL insertion on the anteromedial tibial eminence. In a cadaver study by Roberts and Lovell,[250,251] fracture of the anterior intercondylar eminence was simulated by oblique osteotomy beneath the eminence and traction on the ACL. In each specimen, the displaced fragment could be reduced into its bed by extension of the knee. In adults, the same stress might cause an isolated tear of the ACL, but in children the incompletely ossified tibial spine is generally weaker to tensile stress than the ligament, so failure occurs through the cancellous bone beneath the subchondral bone of the tibial spine. In addition, loading conditions may result in differential injury patterns. In experimental models, midsubstance ACL injuries tend to occur under rapid loading rates, whereas tibial eminence avulsion fractures tend to occur under slower loading rates in cadaveric and animal models.[232,311]

Intercondylar notch morphology may also influence injury patterns. In a retrospective case-control study of 25 skeletally immature patients with tibial spine fractures compared to 25 age- and sex-matched skeletally immature patients with midsubstance ACL injuries, Kocher et al.[175] found narrower intercondylar notches in those patients sustaining midsubstance ACL injuries.

Signs and Symptoms

Patients typically present with a painful swollen knee after an acute traumatic event. They are unable to bear weight on their affected extremity.

On physical examination, there is often a large hemarthrosis because of the intra-articular fracture and limited motion due to effusion. Sagittal plane laxity is often present, but the contralateral knee should be assessed for physiologic laxity. Gentle stress testing should be performed to detect any tear of the medial collateral ligament (MCL) or lateral collateral ligament (LCL) or physeal fracture of the distal femur or proximal tibia.

Patients with late malunion of a displaced tibial spine fracture may lack full extension because of a mechanical bony block. Patients with late nonunion of a displaced tibial spine fracture may have increased knee laxity, with a positive Lachman examination and pivot-shift examination.

Imaging

Roentgenograms typically demonstrate the fracture, seen best on the lateral and tunnel views. The lateral radiograph is most useful in fracture classification. Radiographs should be carefully scrutinized as the avulsed fragment may be mostly nonossified cartilage with only a small, thin ossified portion visible on the lateral view.

In order to guide treatment, important information to ascertain from the radiographs includes the classification type, amount of displacement, size of the fracture fragment, comminution of the fracture fragment, and status of the physes.

Magnetic resonance imaging (MRI) is not always needed in the diagnosis and management of tibial eminence fractures in children. MRI may be helpful to confirm the diagnosis in cases with a very thin ossified portion of the avulsed fragment or define adequacy of closed redcution. MRI may also be useful to evaluate for associated collateral ligament or distal femoral physeal injury; however, these are uncommon.

Associated Injuries

Associated intra-articular injuries are uncommon. In a series of 80 skeletally immature patients who underwent surgical fixation of tibial eminence fractures, Kocher et al.[177] found no associated chondral injuries and associated meniscal tear in only 3.8% (3/80) of patients (Fig. 24-1). Associated collateral ligament in-

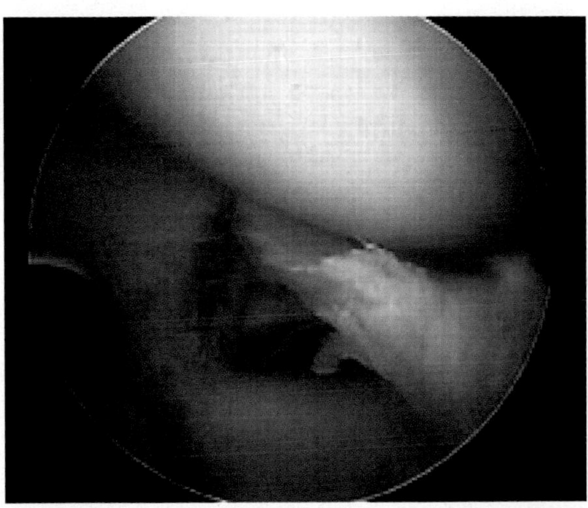

FIGURE 24-1 Longitudinal meniscus tear associated with tibial eminence fracture.

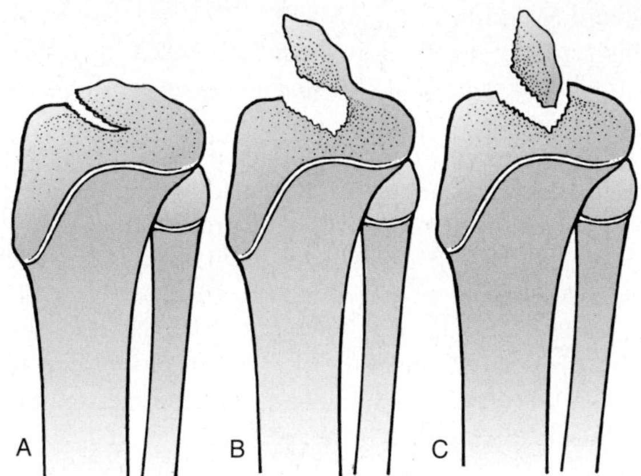

FIGURE 24-2 Classification of tibial spine fractures. **A.** Type I, minimal displacement. **B.** Type II, hinged posteriorly. **C.** Type III, complete separation.

jury or proximal ACL avulsion are uncommon, but have been reported.[131,252]

Classification

The classification system of Meyers and McKeever,[216] based on the degree of displacement, is widely used to classify fractures and to guide treatment (Fig. 24-2):

1. Type 1—minimal displacement of the fragment from the rest of the proximal tibial epiphysis
2. Type 2—displacement of the anterior third to half of the avulsed fragment, which is lifted upward but remains hinged on its posterior border in contact with the proximal tibial epiphysis
3. Type 3—complete separation of the avulsed fragment from the proximal tibial epiphysis, with upward displacement and rotation

Radiographs of these fracture types are shown in Figure 24-3. The interobserver reliability between type 1 and types 2 and 3 fractures is good; however, differentiation between types 2 and 3 fractures may be difficult.[175]

Zaricznyj[317] further classified a type 4 fracture to describe comminution of the tibial eminence fragment.

Surgical and Applied Anatomy

The intercondylar eminence is that part of the tibial plateau lying between the anterior poles of the menisci forward to the anterior tibial spine. It is triangular, with its base at the anterior border of the proximal tibia. In the immature skeleton, the proximal surface of the eminence is covered entirely with cartilage. The ACL attaches distally to the anterior tibial spine with separate slips anterior and lateral as well (Fig. 24-4). The ligament originates off the posterior margin of the lateral aspect of the intercondylar notch. The anterior horn of the lateral meniscus is typically attached in the region of the intercondylar eminence at the ACL insertion. In 12 patients with displaced tibial spine fractures which did not reduce closed, Lowe et al.[196] reported that the anterior horn of the lateral meniscus consistently remained attached to the tibial eminence fracture fragment. The posterior cruciate ligament (PCL) originates off the medial aspect of the intercondylar notch and inserts on the posterior aspect of the proximal tibia, distal to the joint line.

Meniscal or intermeniscal ligament entrapment under the displaced tibial eminence fragment has been reported and may be a rationale for considering arthroscopic or open reduction of displaced tibial spine fractures (Fig. 24-5).[54,59,94,177] Meniscal entrapment prevents anatomic reduction of the tibial spine fragment, which may result in increased anterior laxity or a block to extension.[120,148,211,236,240] Furthermore, meniscal entrapment itself may cause knee pain after fracture healing.[59] Falstie-Jensen and Sondergard Petersen,[94] Burstein and colleagues,[54] and Chandler and Miller[59] have all reported cases of meniscal incarceration blocking reduction of type 2 or 3 tibial spine fractures in children. The prevalence of meniscal entrapment in tibial spine fractures may be common for displaced fractures. As aforementioned, the anterior horn of the lateral meniscus typically remains attached to the tibial eminence fracture fragment. However, the anterior horn of the medial meniscus or the intermeniscal ligament may become incarcerated. Mah and colleagues[200] found medial meniscal entrapment preventing reduction in 8 of 10 children with type 3 fractures undergoing arthroscopic management. In a consecutive series of 80 skeletally immature patients who underwent surgical fixation of hinged or displaced tibial eminence fractures which did not reduce in extension, Kocher et al.[177] found entrapment of the anterior horn of the medial meniscus (n = 36), intermeniscal ligament (n = 6), or anterior horn of the lateral meniscus (n = 1) in 26% (6/23) of hinged (type 2) fractures and 65% (37/57) of displaced (type 3) fractures. The entrapped meniscus can typically be extracted with an arthroscopic probe and retracted with a retaining suture (Fig. 24-6).

Current Treatment Options

Treatment options include cast immobilization,[188,223] closed reduction with immobilization,[236,308] open reduction with immobilization,[223] open reduction with internal fixation,[225,308] arthroscopic reduction with immobilization,[212] arthroscopic reduction with suture fixation,[137,155,188,200,201] and arthroscopic reduction with wire,[27] screw fixation,[36,188,212] anchor fixation,[298] and bioabsorbable fixation.[264] Studies of the biomechanical strength of internal fixation suggest similar fixation strength between bioabsorbable and metallic internal fixation[202] and increased fixation strength of suture fixation over screw fixation.[87,202]

Closed treatment is typically used for type 1 fractures and for type 2 or 3 fractures that reduce closed. Closed reduction is usually performed after aspiration of the hematoma with placement of the knee in full extension or 20 to 30 degrees of flexion. Radiographs are used to assess adequacy of reduction. If the fracture fragment extends into the medial or lateral tibial plateaus, extension may effect a reduction through pressure applied by medial or lateral femoral condyle congruence (Fig. 24-7). Fractures confined within the intercondylar notch, however, will not reduce in this manner. Portions of the ACL are tight in all knee flexion positions; therefore, there may not be any one position without traction being applied by the ACL. Interposition of the anterior horn of the medial meniscus or intermeniscal ligament may further block reduction.

Closed reduction can be successful for some type 2 fractures, but is infrequently successful in type 3 fractures. Kocher et al.[177] reported successful closed reduction in approximately 50% of type 2 fractures (26/49). However, no type 3 fractures could

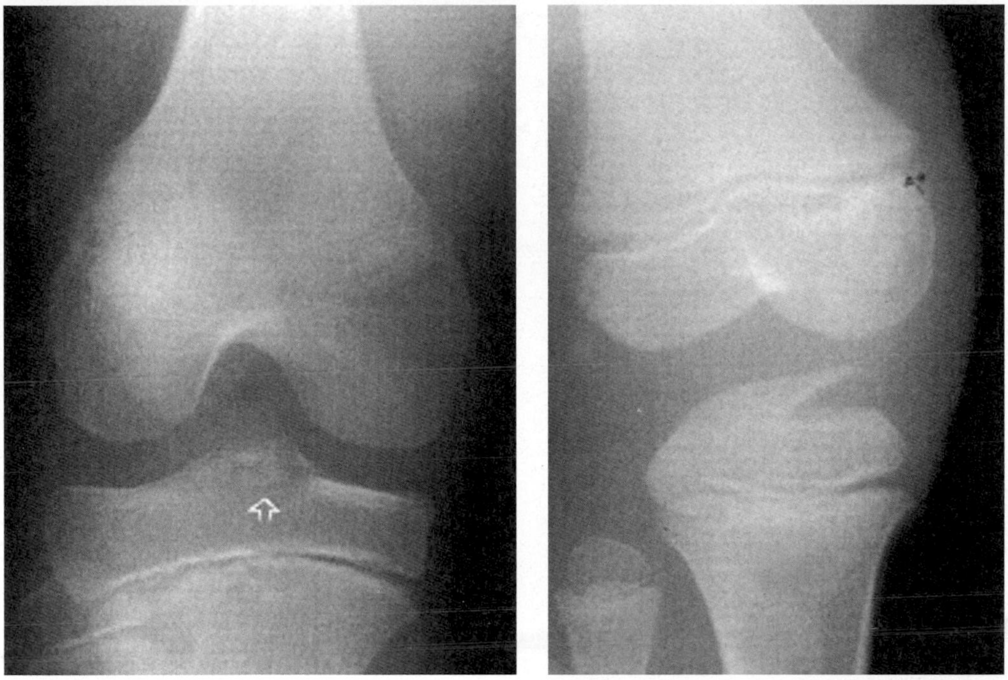

FIGURE 24-3 Stages of displacement of tibial spine fractures. **A.** Type 1 fracture, minimal displacement (*open arrow*). **B.** Type 2 fracture, posterior hinge intact. **C.** Type 3 fracture, complete displacement and proximal migration.

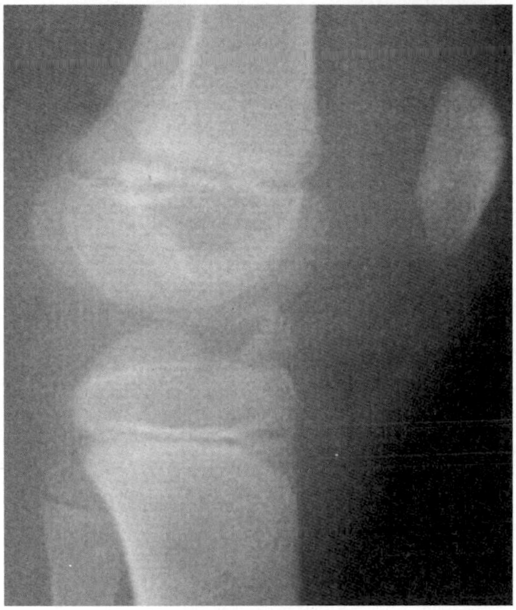

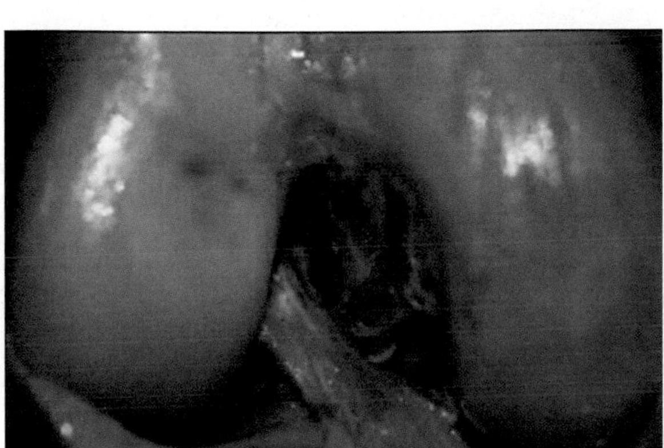

FIGURE 24-4 ACL insertion on the tibial eminence.

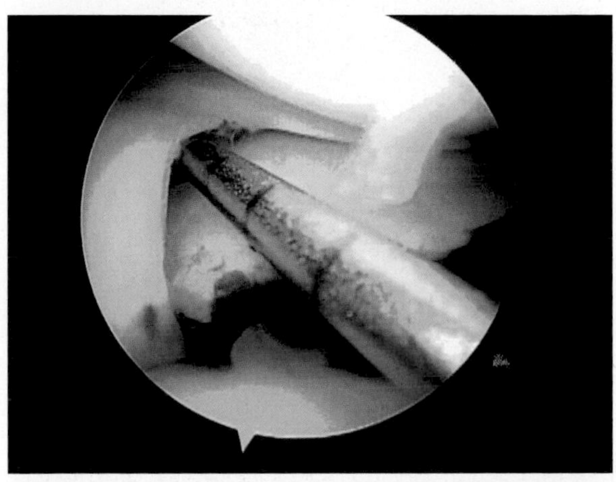

FIGURE 24-5 Meniscal entrapment under a tibial eminence fracture.

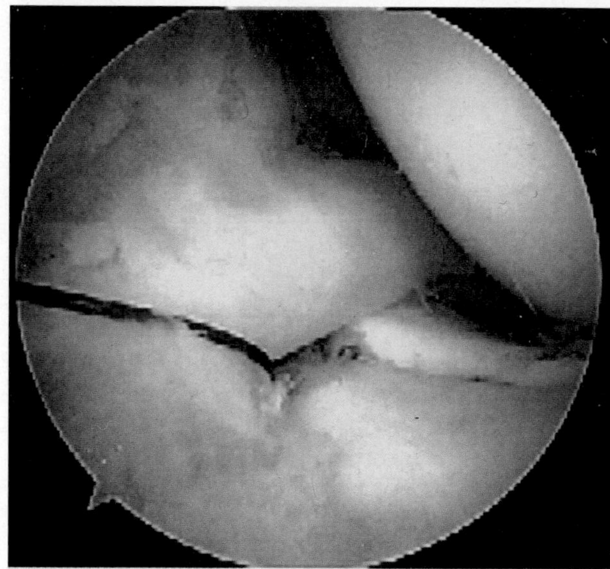

FIGURE 24-6 Retraction of an entrapped anterior horn medial meniscus using a retaining suture.

to be close reduced (0/57). Bakalim and Wilpulla[26] reported successful closed reduction in 10 patients. Smillie[275] suggested that closed reduction by hyperextension can be accomplished only with a large fragment. Meyers and McKeever[216] recommended cast immobilization with the knee in 20 degrees of flexion for all type I and II fractures and open reduction or arthroscopic treatment of all type III fractures.

Arthroscopic or open reduction with internal fixation of type 2 and 3 tibial eminence fractures which do not reduce has been advocated because of the potential for meniscal entrapment under the fractured tibial eminence preventing anatomic closed reduction,[54,59,94,200] the potential for instability and loss of extension associated with closed reduction and immobilization,[120,148,211,236] the ability to evaluate and treat associated intra-articular meniscal or osteochondral injuries, and the opportunity for early mobilization. For displaced fractures, Wiley and Baxter[307] found a correlation between fracture displacement at healing with knee laxity and functional outcome.

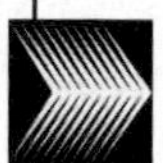

AUTHORS' PREFERRED TREATMENT

The author's algorithm to decision making is shown in Figure 24-8.

Type 1 fractures are treated with cast immobilization. Aspiration of hematoma and injection of local anesthetic is performed under sterile conditions if the patient is in severe pain. A long-leg cast is applied in 0 to 20 degrees of flexion. The patient and family are cautioned to elevate the leg to avoid swelling. Radiographs are repeated in 1 to 2 weeks to ensure that the fragment has not displaced. The cast is removed 6 weeks after injury. A hinged knee brace is then used and physical therapy initiated to regain motion and strength. Patients are typically allowed to return to sports at 3 months after injury if they demonstrate fracture healing and adequate motion and strength.

Type 2 fractures are treated with attempted closed reduction. The hematoma is aspirated and local anesthetic is injected into the knee under sterile conditions. Reduction is attempted at both full extension and 20 degrees of flexion.

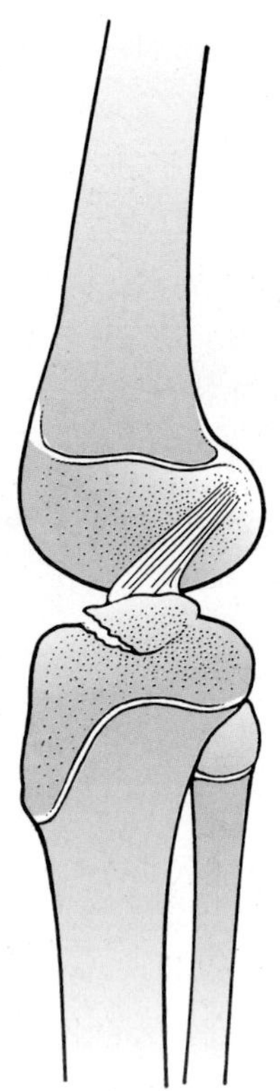

FIGURE 24-7 Reduction of type II tibial fracture with knee in 10 to 20 degrees of flexion.

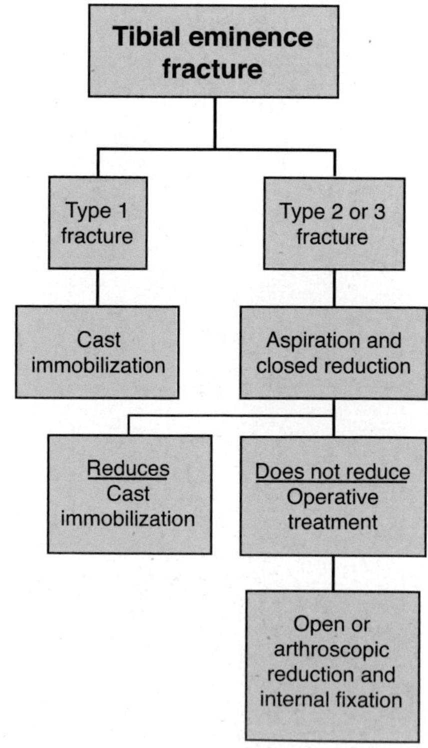

FIGURE 24-8 Algorithm for the management of tibial eminence fractures in children.

Radiographs are taken to assess reduction. If anatomic reduction is obtained, a long-leg cast is applied in the position of reduction. Follow-up radiographs are performed at 1 and 2 weeks postreduction to ensure maintenance of reduction. Length of casting and postcasting management is similar to type 1 fractures. If the fracture does not reduce anatomically or if the fracture later displaces, operative treatment is performed.

Type 3 fractures may be treated with attempted closed reduction; however, this is usually unsuccessful. Operative treatment is typically performed.

The author's preferred operative treatment is arthroscopic reduction and internal fixation. However, open reduction through a medial parapatellar incision can also be performed per surgeon preference/experience or if arthroscopic visualization is difficult. The author's preferred fixation is epiphyseal cannulated screws if the fragment is large or suture fixation if the fragment is small or comminuted.

Arthroscopic Reduction and Internal Fixation with Epiphyseal Cannulated Screws

General anesthesia is typically used. The patient is positioned supine on the operating room table. A lateral breakaway post is used. Alternatively, a circumferential post can be utilized. A standard arthroscope is used in most patients. A small (2.7-mm) arthroscope is used in younger children. An arthroscopic fluid pump is used at 35 torr. A tourniquet is routinely used. Standard anteromedial and anterolateral portals are used. Accessory superomedial and superolateral portals are used for screw insertion. Prior to insertion of the arthroscope through the arthroscopic cannula, the large hematoma is evacuated.

Thorough arthroscopic examination of the patellofemoral joint, medial compartment, and lateral compartment are essential to evaluate for concomitant injuries. Usually, some anterior fat pad must be excised with an arthroscopic shaver for complete visualization of the intercondylar eminence fragment. Entrapped medial meniscus or intermeniscal ligament is extracted with an arthroscopic probe and retracted with a retention suture (see Fig. 24-5). The base of the tibial eminence fragment is elevated (Fig. 24-9A) and the fracture bed débrided with an arthroscopic shaver and hand curette (Fig. 24-9B). Anatomic reduction is obtained using an arthroscopic probe or microfracture pick with the knee in 30 to 90 degrees of flexion (Fig. 24-9C). Cannulated guidewires are placed through portals just off the superomedial and superolateral borders of the patella. A spinal needle can be helpful for the localization of these portals. The guidewires are placed into the intercondylar eminence at the base of the ACL. Fluoroscopic assistance is utilized to confirm anatomic reduction, to guide correct wire orientation, and to avoid guidewire protrusion across the proximal tibial physis. A cannulated drill is used over the guidewires and one or two screws are placed based on the size of the tibial eminence fragment (Fig. 24-9D). Partially threaded 3.5-mm diameter screws (Fig. 24-9E) are used in children and 4.5-mm diameter screws are used in adolescents. The knee is brought through a range of motion to ensure rigid fixation without fracture displacement and to evaluate for impingement of the screw heads in extension.

Postoperatively, patients are placed in a postoperative hinged knee brace and maintain touch-down weight bearing for 6 weeks postoperatively. Motion is restricted to 0 to 30 degrees for the first 2 weeks, 0 to 90 degrees for the next 2 weeks, and then full range of motion. The brace is kept locked in extension at night. Radiographs are obtained to evaluate maintainance of reduction and fracture healing (Fig. 24-10). Cast immobilization for 4 weeks postoperatively may be necessary in younger children unable to comply with protected weight bearing and brace immobilization. Physical therapy is routinely utilized to achieve motion, strength, and sport-specific training. Patients are typically allowed to return to sports at 12 to 16 weeks postoperatively depending on knee function. Screws are not routinely removed. Functional ACL bracing is utilized if there is residual knee laxity.

Arthroscopic Reduction and Internal Fixation with Suture

Arthroscopic set-up and examination is similar to the technique described for epiphyseal screw fixation. Accessory superomedial and superolateral portals are not used. The fracture is elevated (Fig. 24-11A) and the fracture base débrided (Fig. 24-11B). The fracture is reduced. A suture is passed through the base of the ACL using a suture punch (Fig. 24-11C) or a suture passer. Two guidewires are placed using the tibial ACL guide system from a small incision made just below the tibial tubercle. The guidewires are placed through the base of the intercondylar eminence fragment (Fig. 24-11D). Suture retrievers are placed through the guidewire tracts, the sutures are retrieved (Fig. 24-11E), and the sutures are tied down onto the tibia (Fig. 24-11F). The procedure may be repeated for additional sutures. Heavy nonabsorbable braided sutures or fiberwire is used. Although these sutures traverse the proximal tibial physis, the risk of growth disturbance is minimal given the small diameter of the guide wire holes.

Pearls and Pitfalls

- In the closed management of tibial eminence fractures, follow-up radiographs must be obtained at 1 and 2 weeks postinjury to verify maintenance of reduction. Late displacement and malunion can occur, particularly for type 2 fractures.
- Aspiration of hemarthrosis and injection of local anesthetic under sterile conditions can be helpful to minimize pain and allow for full knee extension for attempted closed reduction.
- During arthroscopic reduction and fixation of tibial spine fractures, arthroscopic visualization can be difficult unless the large hematoma is evacuated prior to introduction of the arthroscope. Adequate inflow and outflow is essential for proper visualization.
- Careful attention to preparation of the fracture bed is important to provide optimal conditions for bony healing.
- Attempted epiphyseal cannulated screw fixation of small or comminuted tibial eminence fragments can fail as the screw may further comminute the fragment. In these cases, suture fixation is a better method.
- If epiphyseal cannulated screw fixation is used, fluoroscopy is necessary to ensure that the screw does not traverse the proximal tibial physis, which may result in a proximal tibial physeal growth arrest.

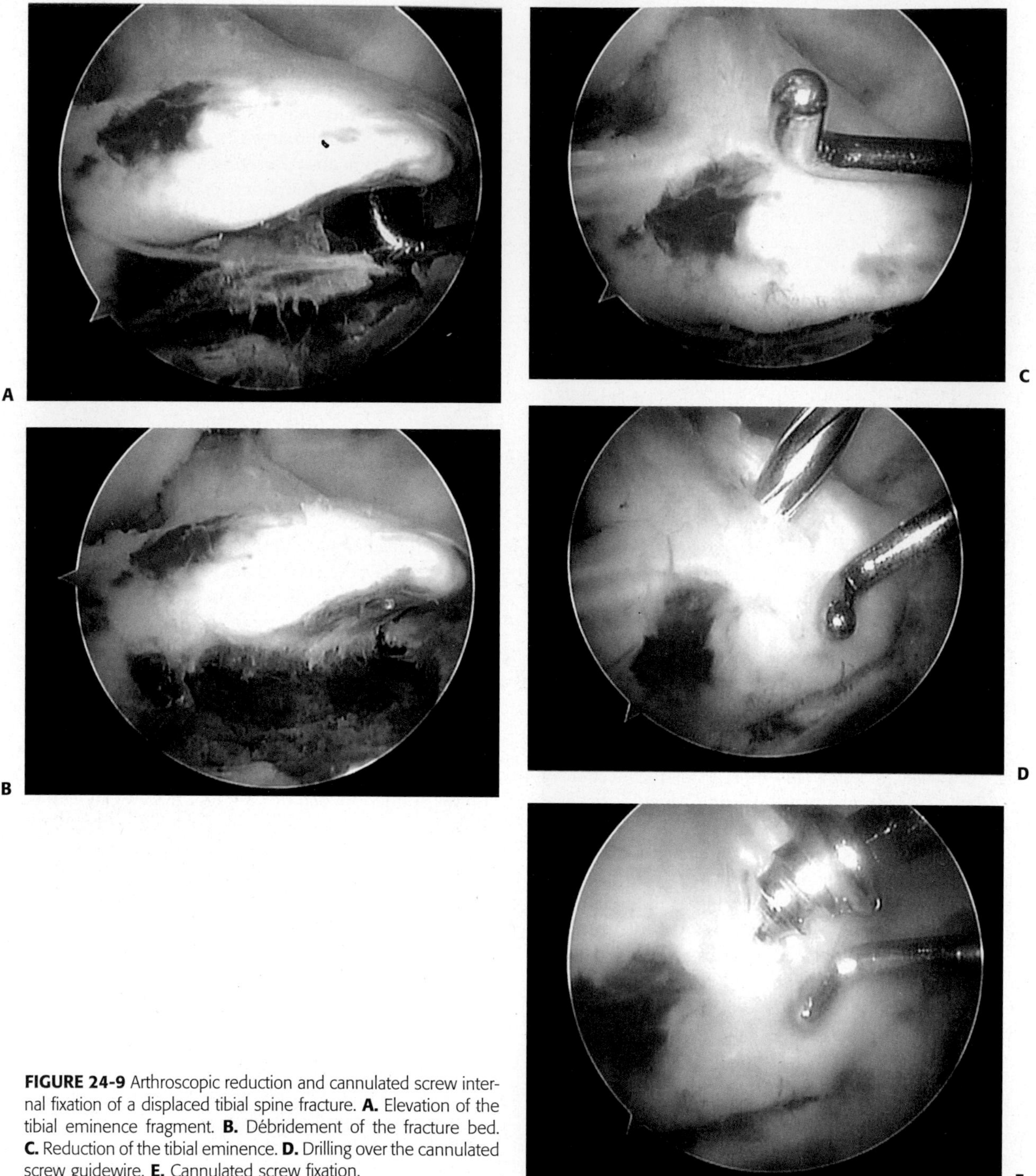

FIGURE 24-9 Arthroscopic reduction and cannulated screw internal fixation of a displaced tibial spine fracture. **A.** Elevation of the tibial eminence fragment. **B.** Débridement of the fracture bed. **C.** Reduction of the tibial eminence. **D.** Drilling over the cannulated screw guidewire. **E.** Cannulated screw fixation.

- Early mobilization is helpful to avoid arthrofibrosis which can occur with immobilization. However, in younger children (less than 7 years old), compliance with protected weight bearing and brace use can be problematic.

Prognosis and Complications

The prognosis for closed treatment of nondisplaced and reduced tibial spine fractures and for operative treatment of displaced fractures is good. Most series report healing with an excellent functional outcome despite some residual knee laxity.[27,30,36,170,188,200,201,211,212,223,225,276,307,308] Potential complications include nonunion, malunion, arthrofibrosis, residual knee laxity, and growth disturbance.[27,30,36,170,188,200,201,211,212,223,225,276,307,308]

Mild residual knee laxity is seen frequently, even after anatomic reduction and healing of tibial eminence fractures. Baxter and Wiley[30,307] found excellent functional results without symptomatic instability in 17 pediatric knees with displaced tibial spine fractures, despite a positive Lachman examination in 51% of patients and increased mean instrumented knee laxity of 3.5 mm. After open reduction and internal fixation of type III fractures in 13 pediatric knees, Smith[276] found instability symptoms in only 2 patients despite a positive Lachman exam in 87% of patients. In a group of 50 children after closed or

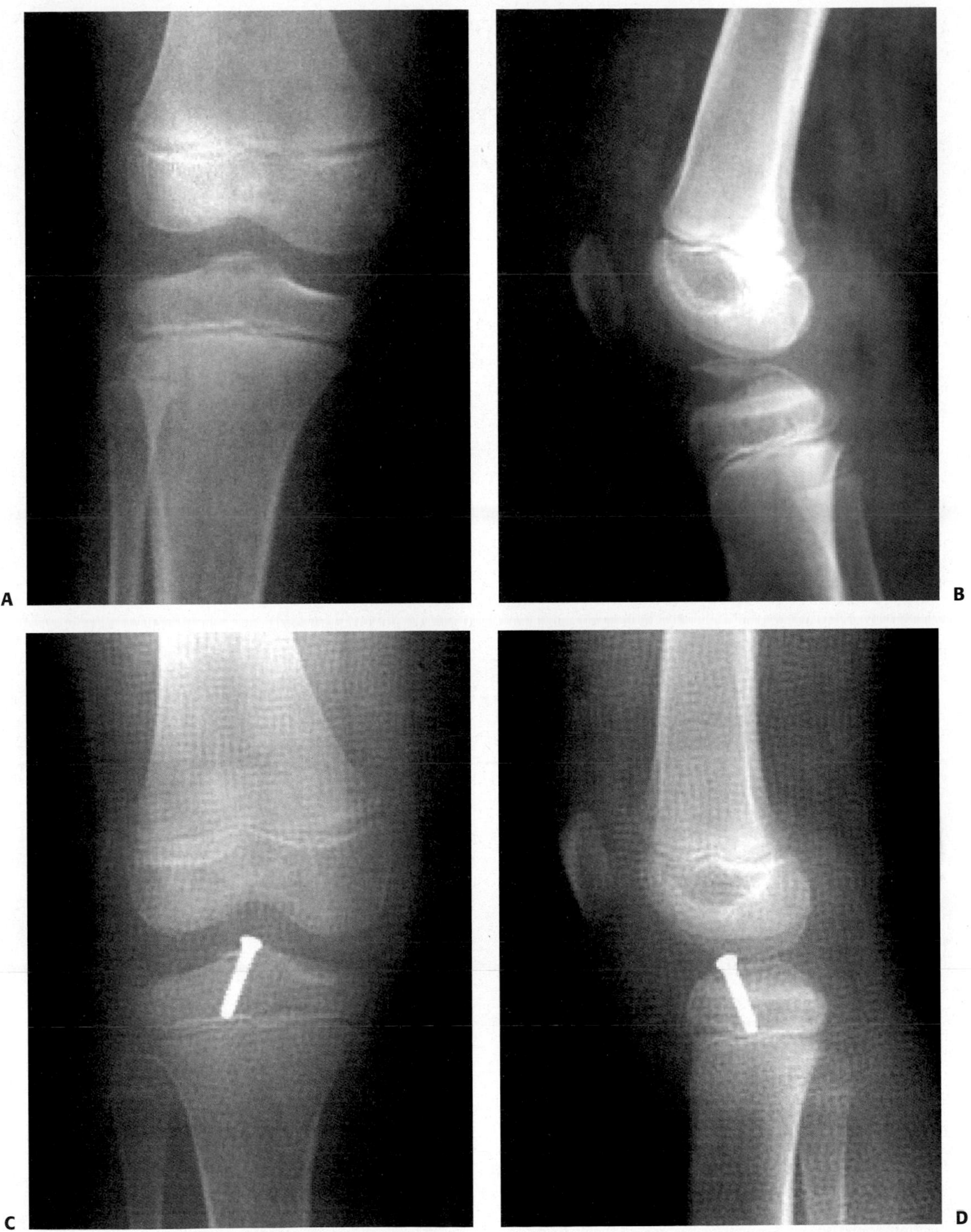

FIGURE 24-10 Type III tibial spine fracture in an 11-year-old male child treated with arthroscopic reduction and 3.5-mm cannulated screw fixation. Preoperative anteroposterior **(A)** and lateral **(B)** radiographs. Postoperative anteroposterior **(C)** and lateral **(D)** radiographs.

open treatment, Willis and coworkers[308] found excellent clinical results despite a positive Lachman exam in 64% of patients and instrumented knee laxity of 3.5 mm for type II fractures and 4.5 mm for type III fractures. Similarly, Janarv et al.[148] and Kocher et al.[170] found excellent functional results despite persistent laxity even in anatomically healed fractures.

Persistent laxity despite anatomic reduction and healing of tibial spine fractures in children is likely related to plastic deformation of the ACL with tibial spine fracture. At the time of tibial spine fixation, the ACL often appears hemorrhagic within its sheath, but grossly intact and in continuity. In a primate animal model, Noyes and coworkers[232] found frequent elongation and disruption of ligament architecture despite gross ligament continuity in experimentally produced tibial spine fractures at both slow and fasting loading rates. This persistent anteroposterior laxity despite anatomic reduction may be avoided by countersinking the tibial spine fragment within the epiphysis at the time of reduction and fixation. However, ACL injury after previous tibial spine fracture is rare.

Poor results may occur after type 3 eminence fractures asso-

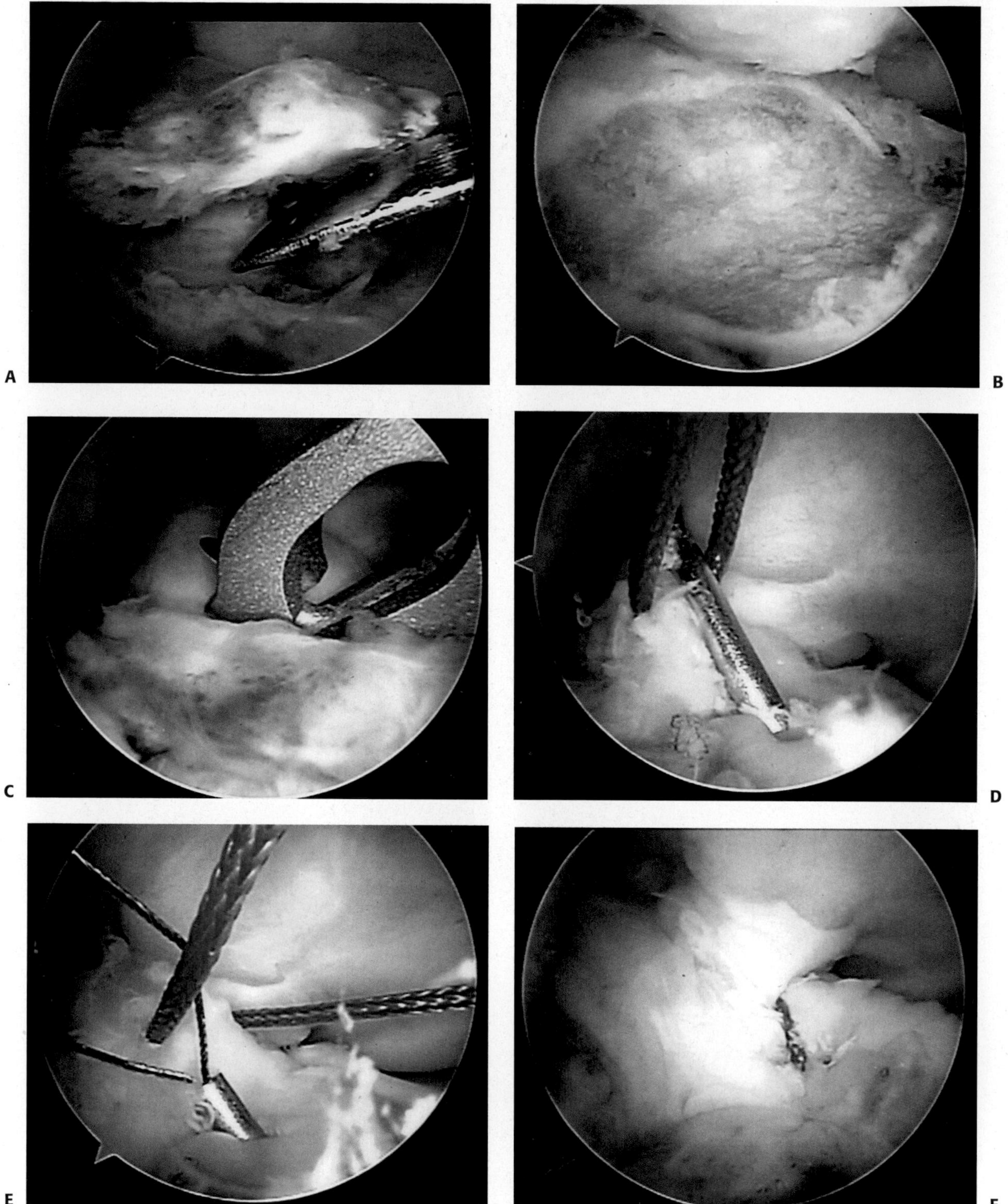

FIGURE 24-11 Arthroscopic reduction and suture fixation of a displaced tibial spine fracture. **A.** Elevation of the tibial eminence. **B.** Débridement of the fracture bed. **C.** Suture passing through the base of the ACL using a suture punch. **D.** Drilling of a tibial tunnel into the tibial eminence fragment using the ACL tibial guide. **E.** Retrieval of sutures using a suture passer. **F.** Appearance after suture fixation.

ciated with unrecognized injuries of the collateral ligaments or complications from associated physeal fracture.[215,276,286] In addition, hardware across the proximal tibial physis may result in growth disturbance with recurvatum deformity or shortening.[226]

Malunion of type 2 and 3 fractures may cause mechanical impingement of the knee during full extension (Fig. 24-12).[106,200,201] For symptomatic patients, this can be corrected by excision of the manumitted fragment and anatomic reinsertion of the ACL. Alternatively, excision of the fragment and ACL reconstruction can be considered in adults and older adolescents.

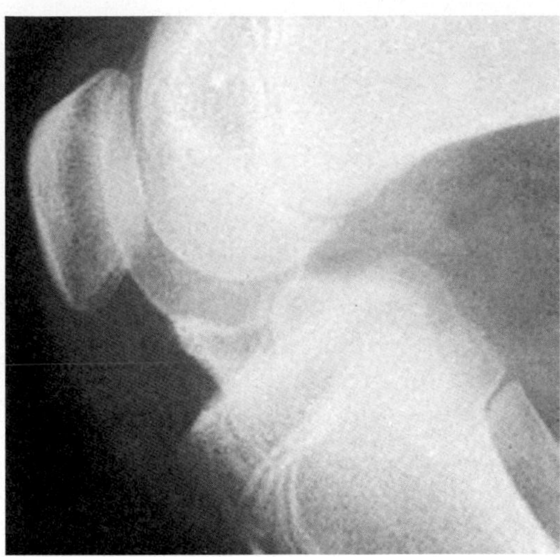

FIGURE 24-12 Lateral radiograph of a malunited displaced fracture of the intercondylar eminence of the tibia with an extension block.

Nonunion of type 2 and 3 tibial spine fractures treated closed can usually be managed by arthroscopic or open reduction with internal fixation.[161,194,296] Technically, débridement of the fracture bed and the fracture fragment to fresh, bleeding bone is essential to optimize bony healing. Bone graft may be required in cases of chronic nonunion. Again, excision of the fragment and ACL reconstruction can be alternatively be considered in adults and older adolescents.

Stiffness and arthrofibrosis can be a challenging problem after both nonoperative and operative management of tibial eminence fractures. The milieu of a major traumatic intra-articular injury, a large hemarthrosis, and immobilization can predispose to arthrofibrosis. Avoidance of cast immobilization with early mobilization and physical therapy can minimize the risk of arthrofibrosis. Dynamic splinting and aggressive physical therapy can be used during the first 3 months after fracture if stiffness is present. If significant stiffness remains after 3 months, patients should be managed with manipulation under anesthesia and arthroscopy with lyses of adhesions. Overly vigorous manipulation should be avoided to prevent iatrogenic proximal tibial or distal femoral physeal fracture.

OSTEOCHONDRAL FRACTURES

Introduction

Osteochondral fractures in skeletally immature patients are more common than once thought. They are typically associated with acute lateral patellar dislocations. The most common locations for these fractures are the medial patellar facet and the lateral femoral condyle (Fig. 24-13). The osteochondral fracture fragments may range from small incidental loose bodies to large portions of the entire articular surface. The prevalence of osteochondral fractures associated with acute patella dislocation ranges from 25% to 50%.[13,43,95,206,229,282] Matelic et al.[206] found 67% of children presenting with an acute hemarthrosis of the knee had an osteochondral fracture.

The diagnosis can be difficult because even a large osteochondral fragment may contain only a small ossified portion that is visible on plain radiographs. MRI may be useful in identifying associated osteochondral fractures in cases of traumatic patellar dislocation. Acute osteochondral fractures must be differentiated from acute chondral injuries, which do not involve subchondral bone, and osteochondritis dissecans,[100,178] which is a repetitive overuse lesion of the subchondral bone that may result in a nonhealing stress fracture that can progress to fragment dissection.

Treatment of osteochondral fractures includes removal of small loose bodies and fixation of larger osteochondral fragments. In cases associated with patellar dislocation, lateral retinacular release, medial retinacular repair, and medial patellofemoral ligament repair may be performed adjunctively.

Principles of Management

Mechanism of Injury

There are two primary mechanisms for production of an osteochondral fracture.[13,43,63,95,98,160,206,213,229,282] First, a direct blow to the knee with a shearing force applied to either the medial or lateral femoral condyle can create an osteochondral fracture. The second mechanism involves a flexion–rotation injury of the knee in which an internal rotation force is placed on a fixed foot, usually coupled with a strong quadriceps contraction. The subsequent contact between the tibia and femur or patella and lateral femoral condyle causes the fracture. This occurs during an acute patellar dislocation. As the patella dislocates, the medial retinaculum tears but the remaining quadriceps muscle–patellar ligament complex still applies significant compressive forces as the patella dislocates laterally and shears across the lateral femoral condyle. The medial border of the patella then temporarily becomes impacted on the prominent edge of the lateral femoral condyle before it slides back tangentially over the surface of the lateral femoral condyle due to pull of the quadriceps. Either the dislocation or the relocation phase of this injury can cause an osteochondral fracture to the lateral femoral condyle, the medial facet of the patella, or both (Fig. 24-14). Interestingly, osteochondral fractures are uncommon with chronic, recurrent subluxation or dislocation of the patella. In this situation, the laxity of the medial knee tissues and decreased compressive forces between the patella and the lateral femoral condyle prevents development of excessive shear forces.

Ahstrom[8] reported 18 osteochondral fractures; 14 occurred

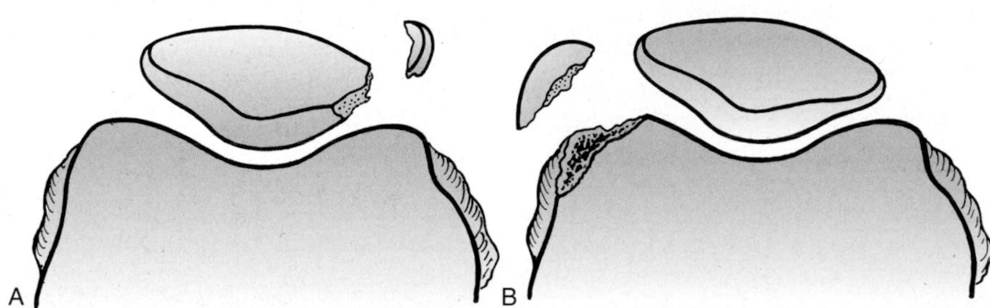

FIGURE 24-13 Osteochondral fractures associated with dislocation of the right patella. **A.** Medial facet. **B.** Lateral femoral condyle.

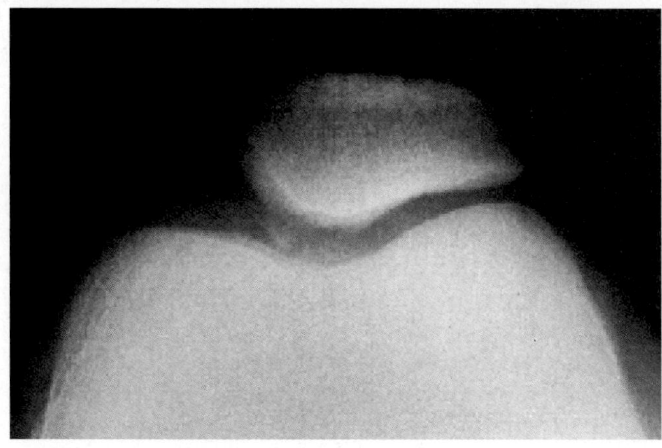

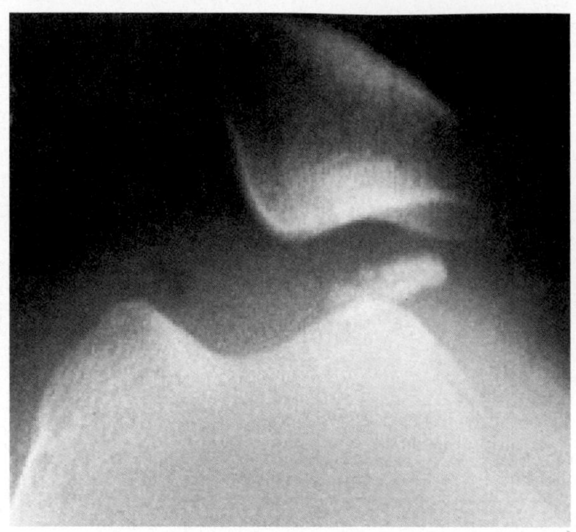

FIGURE 24-14 Osteochondral fractures associated with dislocation of the patella. **A.** Medial facet of patella. **B.** Lateral femoral condyle.

during sports-related activities. Most patients give a history of a twisting injury consistent with acute patellar dislocation, but a few report a direct blow to the lateral or medial femoral condyle, accounting for a shear injury. The prevalence of osteochondral fractures associated with acute patella dislocation ranges from 25% to 50% in the literature.[13,43,95,206,229,282] Matelic et al.[206] found 67% of children presenting with an acute hemarthrosis of the knee had an osteochondral fracture. Nietosvaara et al.[229] reported that of 69 acute patellar dislocations in children and adolescents, 62 (90%) occurred in falls; 39% also had osteochondral fractures.

Signs and Symptoms

Acutely, osteochondral fractures present with severe pain, swelling, and difficulty weight bearing.* On exam, tenderness to palpation over the medial femoral condyle, lateral femoral condyle, or medial patella is exhibited. The patient will usually resist attempts to flex or extend the knee and may hold the knee in 15 to 20 degrees of flexion for comfort. The large hemarthrosis is due to an intra-articular fracture of the highly vascular subchondral bone. Joint aspiration may reveal a supernatant layer of fat if allowed to stand for 15 minutes indicating an intra-articular fracture. Late exam findings may be similar to those of a loose body with intermittent locking or catching of the knee.

Imaging

Radiographic visualization of the osteochondral fracture should begin with anteroposterior, lateral, and skyline plain radiographs. However, a roentgenographic diagnosis can be difficult because even a large osteochondral fragment may contain only a small ossified portion that is visible on plain radiographs. A tunnel view may help locate a fragment in the region of the intercondylar notch. Because the osteochondral fragment may be difficult to see on plain radiographs, radiographs must be carefully assessed for even the smallest ossified fragment (Fig. 24-15).

Matelic et al.[206] reported that standard radiographs failed to identify the osteochondral fracture in 36% of children who had an osteochondral fracture found during arthroscopy. For this reason, supplemental studies such as MRI or computed tomography (CT) arthrography may be necessary in cases where there is high suspicion of osteochondral fracture despite negative radiographs.[48,169,305] Such cases would include an acute traumatic patellar dislocation in a patient with a large hemarthrosis. Ligamentously lax patients with chronic, recurrent, atraumatic patellar instability are less likely to sustain osteochondral fractures. A high-riding patella may also have a protective effect against associated intra-articular osteochondral fractures. Patients with an Insall index greater than 1.3 have a decreased chance of sustaining an osteochondral fracture compared with patients that have an Insall index within normal limits.[48] An arthrogram effect is usually present during MRI given the large hemarthrosis. Arthroscopic examination can also be done as the definitive diagnostic (and potentially therapeutic) test.

Classification

The classification of osteochondral fractures of the knee is based on the site, the type, and the mechanism of injury. The classification outlined in Table 24-1 is based on the descriptions of osteochondral fractures by Kennedy[160] and Smillie.[275]

Surgical and Applied Anatomy

The patella tracks in the intercondylar notch between the medial and lateral femoral condyles during flexion and extension of the knee.[113,142] With increasing knee flexion, the contact area on the articular surface of the patella moves to the proximal patella. Between 90 and 135 degrees of flexion, the patella glides into the intercondylar notch between the femoral condyles. The two primary areas of contact are the medial patellar facet with the medial femoral condyle and the superolateral quadrant of the lateral patellar facet with the lateral femoral condyle. Soft tissue support for the patellofemoral joint includes the quadriceps muscle, the medial patellofemoral ligament, the patellar tendon, and the vastus medialis and lateralis muscles.

Dislocation of the patella may tear the medial retinaculum,

*References 8,9,25,29,35,63,64,84,113,133,141,142,149,160,190,213, 229,234,253,254,263,275,280,309,310.

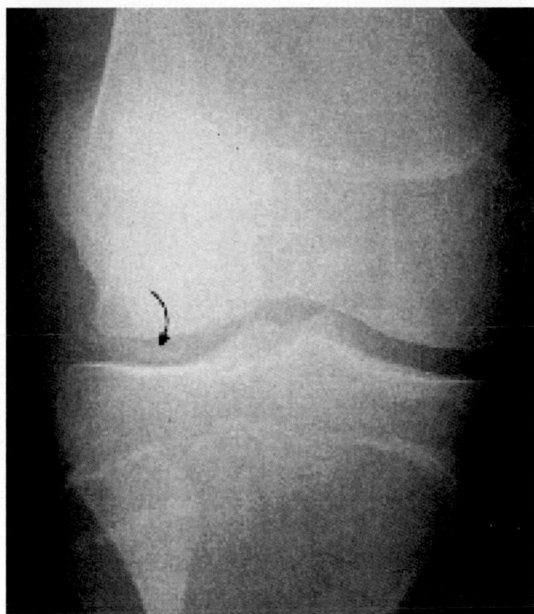

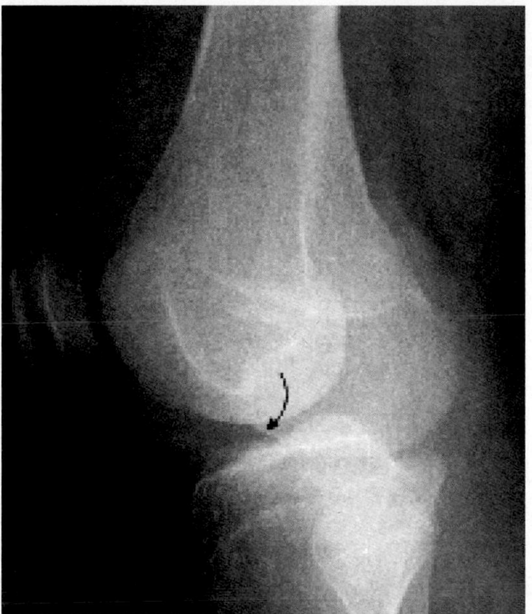

FIGURE 24-15 Osteochondral fracture of lateral femoral condyle after patellar dislocation. **A.** Fragment seen in lateral joint space. **B.** Lateral view.

but the rest of the quadriceps muscle–patellar ligament complex continues to apply significant compression forces as the patella dislocates laterally. These forces are believed to cause fracture of the medial patellar facet, the lateral femoral condyle articular rim, or both (see Fig. 24-13).[160,234,254] Osteochondral fractures are uncommon with chronic recurrent subluxation or dislocation of the patella because of laxity of the medial retinaculum and lesser compressive forces on the patella and the lateral femoral condyle.

A histopathologic study by Flachsmann et al.[98] helped to explain the occurrence of osteochondral fractures in the skeletally immature at a ultrastructural level. They noted that in the joint of a juvenile, interdigitating fingers of uncalcified cartilage penetrate deep into the subchondral bone providing a relatively strong bond between the articular cartilage and the subchondral bone. In the adult, the articular cartilage is bonded to the subchondral bone by the well-defined calcified cartilage layer, the cement line. When shear stress is applied to the juvenile joint, the forces are transmitted into the subchondral bone by the interdigitating cartilage with the resultant bending forces causing the open pore structure of the trabecular bone to fail. In mature tissue, the plane of failure occurs between the deep and calcified layers of the cartilage, the tidemark, leaving the osteochondral junction undisturbed. Although the juvenile and adult tissue patterns are different, they both provide adequate fracture toughness to the osteochondral region. As the tissue transitions, however, from the juvenile to the adult pattern during adolescence, the fracture toughness is lost. The calcified cartilage layer is only partially formed and the interdigitating cartilage fingers are progressively replaced with calcified matrix. Consequently, the interface between the articular cartilage and the subchondral bone becomes a zone of potential weakness in the joint which may explain why osteochondral fractures are seen frequently in adolescents and young adults.

TABLE 24-1 Mechanism of Osteochondral Fractures

Site	Mechanism
Medial femoral condyle	Direct blow (fall) Compression and rotation (tibiofemoral)
Lateral condyle	Direct blow (kick) Compression and rotation (tibiofemoral) Acute patellar dislocation
Patella (medial margin)	Acute patellar dislocation

Current Treatment Options

The recommended management of acute osteochondral fractures of the knee is either surgical removal of the fragment or fixation of the fragment.[176]

If the lesion is large (>1 cm), easily accessible, involves a weight-bearing area, and has adequate cortical bone attached to the chondral surface, then fixation should be attempted.[113,160,276,281,310,311] This can be done via arthroscopy or arthrotomy. Fixation options include Kirschner wires, Steinmann pins, cannulated screws, and variable pitch headless screws. Hardware removal is typically performed after fracture healing. Lewis and Foster[190] reported good results in eight osteochondral fractures after fixation with Herbert bone screws without need for hardware removal. More recently, bioabsorbable fixation devices are available which may eliminate the need for hardware removal.

If the fracture fragment is small (<1 cm), chronic, or from a non–weight-bearing region of the knee, then removal of loose bodies is recommended.[9,141,149,254,263] The fragment's crater should be débrided to stable edges, and the underlying subchondral bone should be perforated to encourage fibrocartilage formation.

In patients with an osteochondral fracture after acute patellar dislocation, concomitant repair of the medial retinaculum and medial patellofemoral ligament at the time of fragment excision or fixation may decrease the risk of recurrent patellar instability.[64,253]

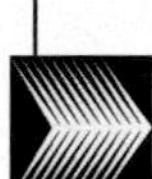

AUTHORS' PREFERRED METHOD OF TREATMENT

The author's algorithm to decision making is shown in Figure 24-16.

In patients with an acute, traumatic patellar dislocation with a large hemarthrosis, MRI is performed if initial radiographs do not show any associated osteochondral fracture. If MRI does not reveal any associated osteochondral fracture, these patients are treated with a brief (1 to 2 weeks) period of immobilization, followed by patellofemoral bracing and physical therapy emphasizing patellar mobilization, straight-leg raises, progressive resistance exercises, and vastus medialis strengthening. Routine diagnostic arthroscopy and routine medial patellofemoral ligament repair are not performed on initial patellofemoral dislocators. Patients are allowed to return to sports 6 to 12 weeks after dislocation depending on their patellar alignment and rehabilitation.

Patients with small (<1 cm) osteochondral fractures, chronic loose bodies, and fractures involving nonweight-bearing areas are treated with arthroscopic removal of loose bodies. The fragment's crater is débrided to stable edges to prevent further loose bodies and the underlying subchondral bone should be perforated to encourage fibrocartilage formation. Lateral retinacular release with medial retinacular/patellofemoral ligament repair is performed adjunctively in cases of traumatic patellofemoral dislocation to decrease the risk of recurrent patellofemoral instability.

Patients with large (>1 cm) osteochondral fractures involving weight-bearing areas with adequate subchondral bone are treated with fragment fixation. At times, these osteochondral fracture fragments can be very large, involving nearly the entire weight-bearing surface of the medial patellar facet (Fig. 24-17) or lateral femoral condyle (Fig. 24-18). Medial patellar facet osteochondral fractures can be fixed through an open lateral retinacular release by manually tilting the patella (see Fig. 24-17). Lateral femoral condyle osteochondral fractures typically require an oblique lateral arthrotomy for fragment fixation (see Fig. 24-18). Z-knee retractors are helpful for exposure, and the knee is flexed or extended to optimize visualization of the fracture bed. The osteochondral fracture fragment and the fracture bed are débrided of fibrous tissue to healthy bone. The fragment is replaced anatomically. Countersunk cannulated screws (3.5- or 4.5-mm) or Herbert screws are preferred for fixation because of the strength of fixation that allows for fragment compression and early mobilization. Lateral retinacular release with medial retinacular/patellofemoral ligament repair is performed adjunctively in cases of traumatic patellofemoral dislocation to decrease the risk of recurrent patellofemoral instability.

Postoperatively, patients treated by excision of the fragment can begin range-of-motion exercises immediately. Crutches may be necessary in the immediate postoperative period but patients can progress to weight bearing as tolerated. After osteochondral fracture fixation, patients are treated with touch-down weight bearing in a postoperative brace until fracture healing. Range of motion is allowed from 0 to 30 degrees for the first 2 weeks, followed by 0 to 90 degrees until fracture healing. The fracture is typically healed by 6 to 8 weeks postoperatively, and arthroscopy is then performed to confirm fragment healing, remove hardware, and assess the integrity of the articular surface. Return to athletic activities is permitted when full range of motion is recovered and strength is symmetric.

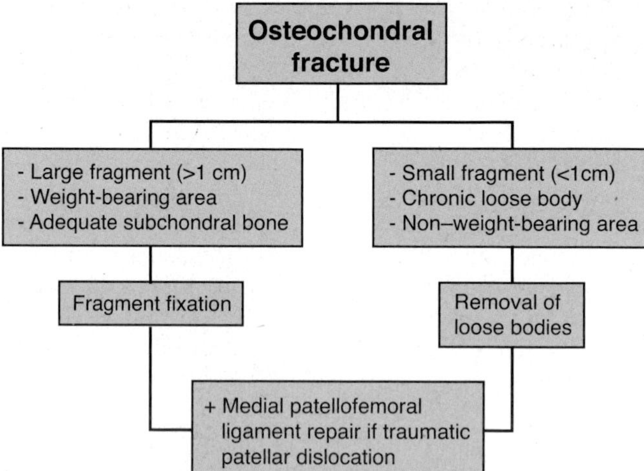

FIGURE 24-16 Algorithm for the management of osteochondral fracture in children.

Pearls and Pitfalls

- An important pitfall to avoid is the failure to diagnose osteochondral fractures associated with acute, traumatic patellar dislocations. Radiographs should be scrutinized for small osseous fragments, and MRI should be obtained in cases with negative radiographs despite a high clinical suspicion for osteochondral fracture.
- In cases of arthroscopic removal of loose bodies associated with acute, traumatic patellar dislocation, strong consideration should be given to repair of the medial structures (medial retinaculum and medial patellofemoral ligament) in order to decrease the risk of recurrent patellar instability.
- In cases of osteochondral fracture fixation, adequate internal fixation must be obtained to allow for early motion.
- Screw heads should be countersunk or headless, variable pitch screws should be used in order to avoid scuffing of articular surfaces.
- In children or adolescents with growth remaining, care must be taken to prevent crossing the distal femoral physis with hardware.

Prognosis and Complications

Osteochondral fractures with small fragments not involving the weight-bearing portion of the joint usually have a good prognosis after removal of loose bodies.

The prognosis for larger osteochondral fractures involving the weight-bearing surfaces is more variable. Excision of large fragments involving the weight-bearing articular surfaces predictably leads to the development of degenerative changes.[16]

FIGURE 24-17 Fixation of a medial patellar facet osteochondral fracture in an adolescent male athlete. **A.** Skyline radiograph demonstrating a fracture of the medial patellar facet with the fragment in the lateral recess. **B.** Axial MRI demonstrating medial facet fracture and loose fragment. **C.** Arthroscopic view of osteochondral fragment in the lateral recess. **D.** Open view of patella. **E.** Open view of osteochondral fragment. **F.** Open view of reduction and cannulated screw fixation of medial patellar facet. *(continues)*

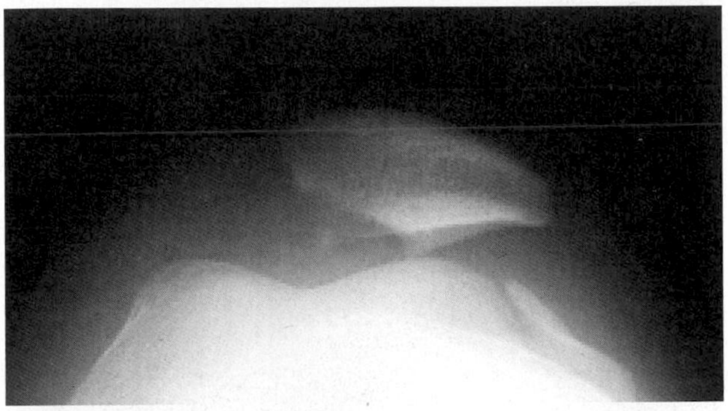

A

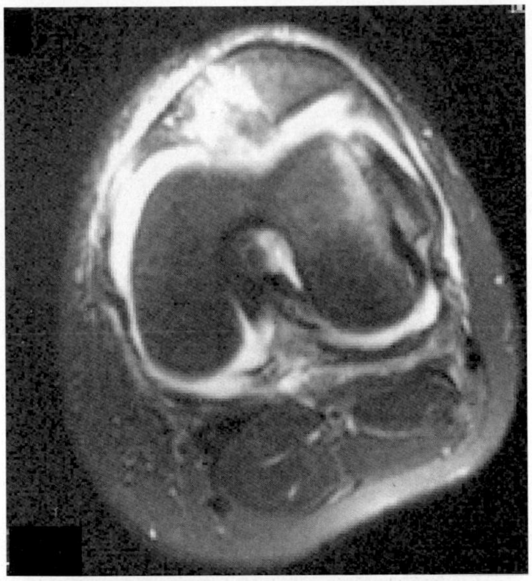

B

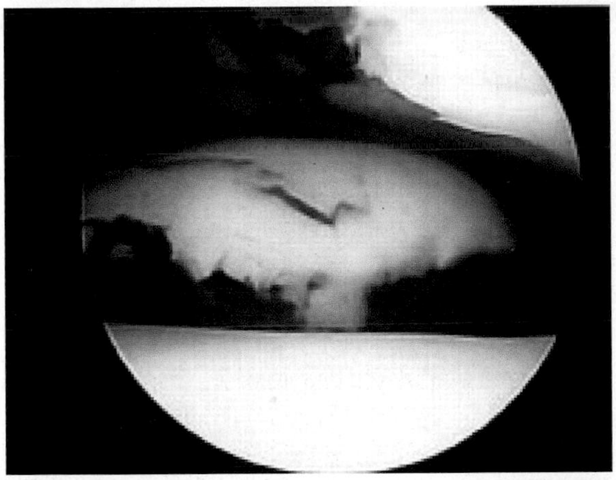

C

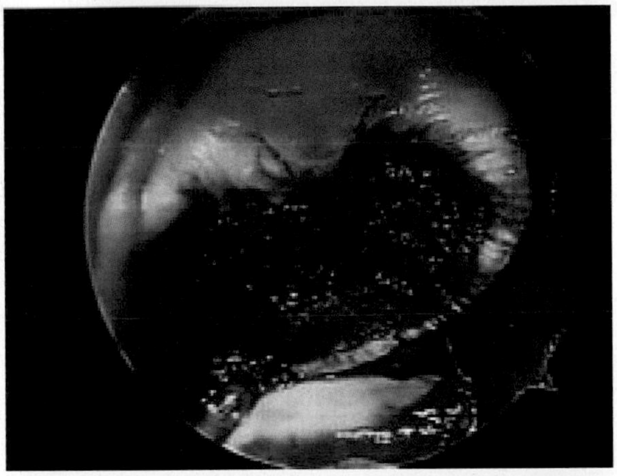

D

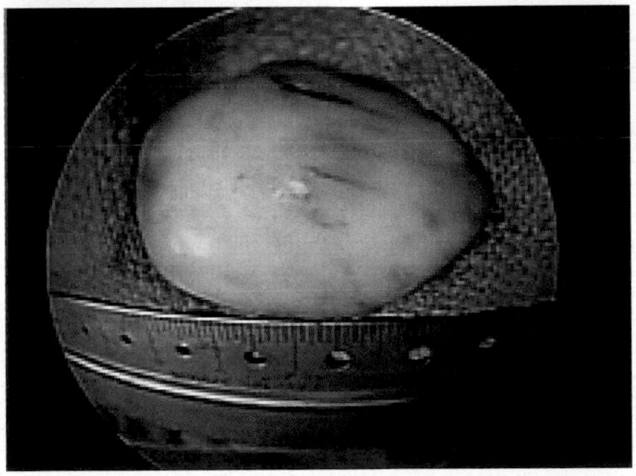

E

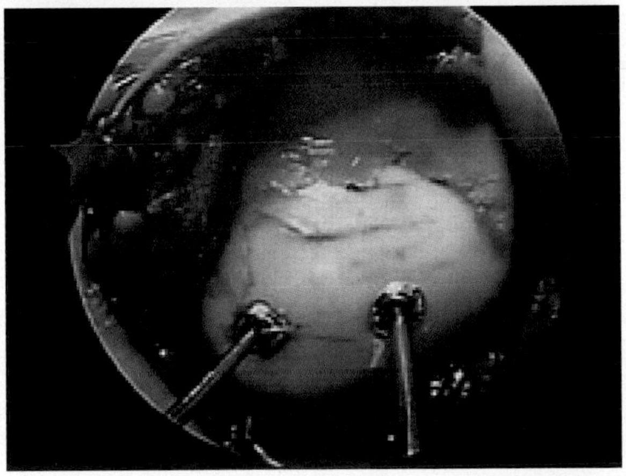

F

Fracture fixation resulting in fragment healing with a congruous articular surface offers the best long-term prognosis; however, even these cases may develop crepitus, stiffness, and degenerative changes.[8]

Complications include recurrent patellar instability with further osteochondral injury after both excision of loose bodies and fracture fixation. Concomitant medial patellofemoral ligament repair appears to decrease the risk of recurrent instability.[29,253] Stiffness may occur, particularly after fracture fixation. Adequate internal fixation is necessary to allow for early motion, which decreases the risk of loss of motion. Stiffness may be treated with aggressive therapy and dynamic splinting during the first 3 to 4 months after injury. Beyond this time frame, manipulation under anesthesia with arthroscopic lysis of adhesions is typically required. Nonunion after fragment fixation may also occur, necessitating further attempts at fracture fixation or fracture excision. Excision of larger osteochondral fractures involving the weight-bearing articular surfaces requires associated chondral resurfacing, such as marrow stimulation procedures (microfracture), osteochondral grafting (mosaic-

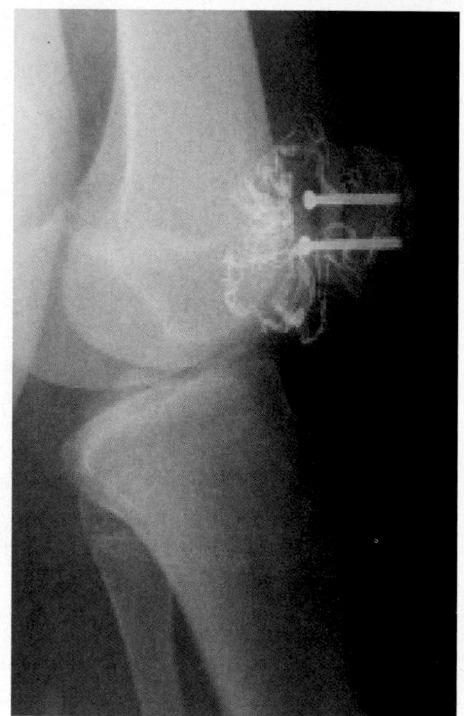

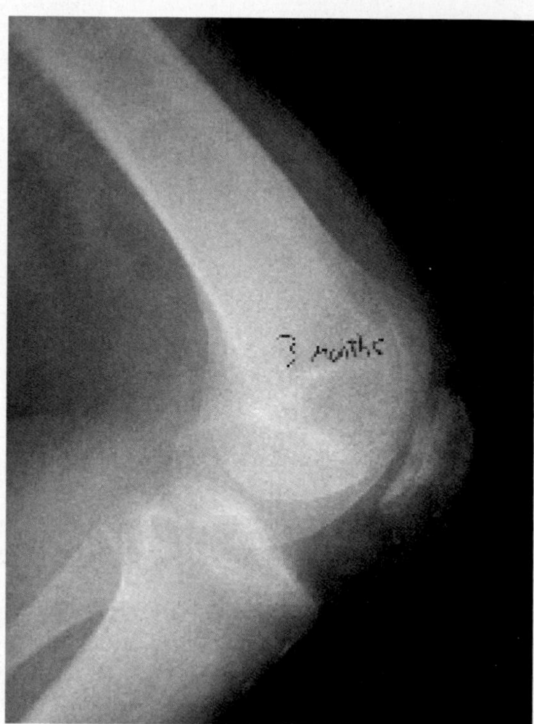

G H

FIGURE 24-17 *(continued)* **G.** Intraoperative lateral radiograph after fracture fixation. **H.** Lateral radiograph 3 months after fracture fixation and 6 weeks after screw removal demonstrating healing.

plasty), or autologous chondrocyte implantation.[34,38,242,283] Complications related to hardware for fracture fixation may also occur. Proud screw heads may scuff articular surfaces. Bioabsorbable implants may result in synovitis with sterile effusions.

PATELLAR DISLOCATION

Introduction

Patellar instability is relatively common in children if all subluxations and dislocations from varying causes are considered. Patellar instability involves cases ranging from acute, traumatic patellar dislocation to chronic, recurrent patellar subluxation in a patient with ligamentous laxity.

Acute, traumatic patellar dislocation typically occurs in adolescents. Acute patellar dislocations in younger children usually occur in the context underlying patellofemoral dysplasia.[213] Chronic, atraumatic, recurrent patellofemoral instability occurs most often in adolescent females, with underlying laxity and alignment risk factors.

Acute, traumatic patellar dislocations without associated osteochondral fracture are treated with a short period of immobilization followed by patellofemoral bracing and rehabilitation. Acute, traumatic patellar dislocations with osteochondral fractures are treated as discussed in the previous section with removal of loose bodies or fracture fixation. Chronic, recurrent, atraumatic patellofemoral instability is typically treated with patellofemoral bracing, rehabilitation, and orthotics if needed. Recurrent patellofemoral instability which has been recalcitrant to nonoperative treatment can be managed with a variety of proximal and distal realignment procedures.

Principles of Management

Mechanism of Injury

Patellar dislocations usually occur because of a flexion–rotation injury of the knee in which an internal rotation force is placed on a fixed foot, usually coupled with a strong quadriceps contraction. As the patella dislocates, the medial retinaculum and medial patellofemoral ligament tear but the remaining quadriceps muscle–patellar ligament complex still applies significant compressive forces as the patella dislocates laterally and shears across the lateral femoral condyle. This may result in associated osteochondral fracture.

Less commonly, patellar dislocation can be caused by a direct blow to the medial aspect of the patella. Larsen and Lauridsen[185] found that a direct blow accounted for only 10% of the acute patellar dislocations in their series.

Spontaneous reduction often occurs as the knee is extended. Patellar dislocations are likely to be caused by falls, gymnastics, dancing, cheerleading, and a wide variety of other activities. Acute patellar dislocation also should be considered in the evaluation of all athletic knee injuries in adolescents and young adults.

Signs and Symptoms

Patients with an acute, traumatic patellar dislocation often give a history of a twisting injury. Patients may remember feeling or seeing the patella in a laterally displaced position. Most acute patellar dislocations spontaneously reduce or reduce with incidental knee extension. It is more unusual to see a patient with a patellar dislocation which is unreduced (Fig. 24-19). Patients may report a "pop" associated with dislocation and a second "pop" associated with spontaneous reduction.

Symptoms include diffuse parapatellar tenderness and pain

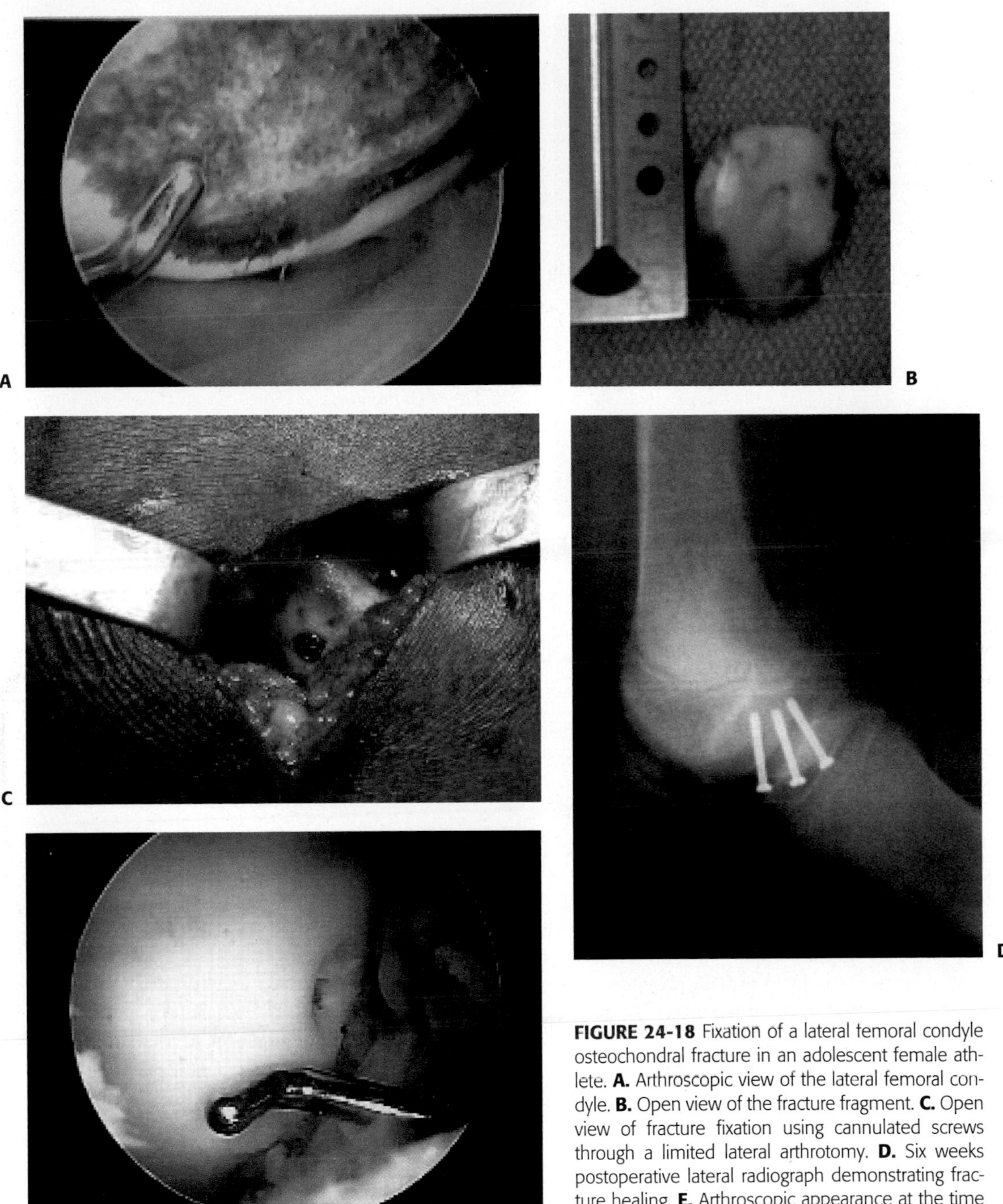

FIGURE 24-18 Fixation of a lateral femoral condyle osteochondral fracture in an adolescent female athlete. **A.** Arthroscopic view of the lateral femoral condyle. **B.** Open view of the fracture fragment. **C.** Open view of fracture fixation using cannulated screws through a limited lateral arthrotomy. **D.** Six weeks postoperative lateral radiograph demonstrating fracture healing. **E.** Arthroscopic appearance at the time of screw removal 6 weeks postoperatively.

with any attempt passively to displace the patella. Patients may have a positive apprehension test with lateral translation of the patella. A defect may be palpable in the medial attachment of the vastus medialis obliqus to the patella if the medial retinaculum is completely avulsed. Tenderness on the lateral aspect of the knee usually is not as severe as on the medial side. Hemorrhage into the joint may cause hemarthrosis, and severe hemarthrosis should suggest the possibility of an osteochondral fracture.[253] Nietosvaara et al.[229] reported that of 72 patients with acute patellar dislocations, 28 (39%) had associated osteochondral fractures. These fractures included 15 capsular avulsions of the medial patellar margin and 15 loose intra-articular fragments detached from the patella, the lateral femoral condyle, or both. All knee ligaments should be carefully evaluated because the mechanism of patellar dislocation may cause associated ligamentous injuries.

Imaging

Radiographs after acute dislocation are obtained primarily to detect any associated osteochondral fracture. Occasionally, an osteochondral fragment from the medial aspect of the patella or the lateral femoral condyle is visible on the anteroposterior or lateral view. The classic "sunrise" view is difficult to obtain in a child after acute dislocation because the required positioning of the knee causes pain. Rarely, stress radiographs may be obtained for evaluation of suspected physeal fracture or ligamentous injury. CT or MRI may be valuable to check for an osteochondral fracture.

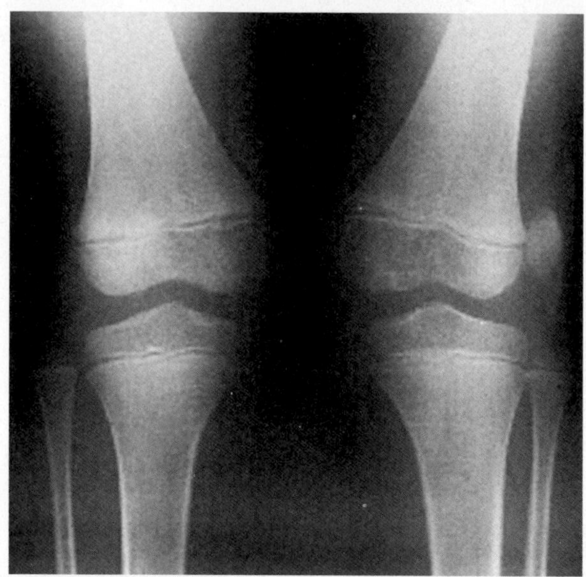

FIGURE 24-19 Acute dislocation of the left patella in a 6-year-old boy.

Classification

Although there is no specific classification of patellar dislocations in children, acute dislocation should be distinguished clinically from chronic patellar subluxation or dislocation.[51,81,103,112] Approximately 15% of children with acute patellar dislocations experience recurrent dislocations. Cash and Hughston[58] reported a 60% incidence of redislocation in patients 11 to 14 years of age, 30% in patients 19 to 28 years of age, and in only one patient older than 28 years of age.

Surgical and Applied Anatomy

The patella is a sesamoid bone in the quadriceps mechanism. As the insertion site of all muscle components of the quadriceps complex, it serves biomechanically to provide an extension moment during range of motion of the knee joint. The trochlear shape of the distal femur stabilizes the patella as it tracks through a range of motion. The hyaline cartilage of the patella is the thickest in the body.

At 20 degrees of knee flexion, the inferior pole of the patella contacts a relatively small area of the femoral groove. With further flexion, the contact area moves superiorly and increases in size. The medial facet of the patella comes in contact with the femoral groove only when flexion reaches 90 to 130 degrees.

The average adult trochlear femoral groove height is 5.2 mm and lateral femoral condyle height is 3.4 mm. The patellar articular cartilage is 6 to 7 mm deep, the thickest articular cartilage in the body and a reflection of the joint's inherent incongruity. The usual normal lateral alignment of the patella is checked by the medial quadriceps expansion and focal thickening of the capsule in the areas of the medial patellofemoral and medial meniscopatellar ligaments.[78] Dynamic stability depends on muscle forces, primarily the quadriceps and hamstrings acting through an elegant lower extremity articulated lever system that creates and modulates forces during gait. The quadriceps blends with the joint capsule to provide a combination of dynamic and static balance. Tightness or laxity of any of the factors involved with maintenance of the balance leads to varying levels of instability. Acute patellar dislocation almost always is in a lateral direction unless it is due to a medially oriented direct blow or follows over vigorous lateral retinacular release. Sallay et al.[259] demonstrated avulsions of the medial patellofemoral ligament from the femur in 94% (15 of 16) of patients during surgical exploration after acute patellar dislocation. Desio et al.,[78] using a cadaveric serial cutting model, found that the medial patellofemoral ligament provided 60% of the resistance to lateral patellar translation at 20 degrees of knee flexion. The medial patellomeniscal ligament accounted for an additional 13% of the medial quadrant restraining force. If the deficit produced by attenuation of the medial vectors after acute dislocation is not eliminated, patellofemoral balance is lost, resulting in feelings of giving way and recurrent dislocation.

The patella is under significant biomechanical compressive load during activity. It has been estimated that at 60 degrees of knee flexion, the forces across the patellofemoral articulation are three times the body weight and increase to over seven times the body weight during full knee flexion with weight-bearing.

The quadriceps mechanism is aligned in a slightly valgus position in relation to the patellar tendon. This alignment can be approximated by a line drawn from the anterosuperior iliac spine to the center of the patella. The force of the patellar tendon is indicated by a line drawn from the center of the patella to the tibial tubercle. The angle formed by these two lines is called the *quadriceps angle* or *Q angle* (Fig. 24-20). As this angle increases, the pull of the extensor mechanism tends to sublux the patella laterally. Recurrent patellar dislocation is most likely associated with some congenital or developmental deficiency of the extensor mechanism, such as patellofemoral dysplasia, deficiency of the vastus medialis obliquus, or an increased Q angle with valgus malalignment of the quadriceps–patellar tendon complex.

Current Treatment Options

Most acute patellar dislocations in children reduce spontaneously; if not, reduction usually can be easily obtained. After

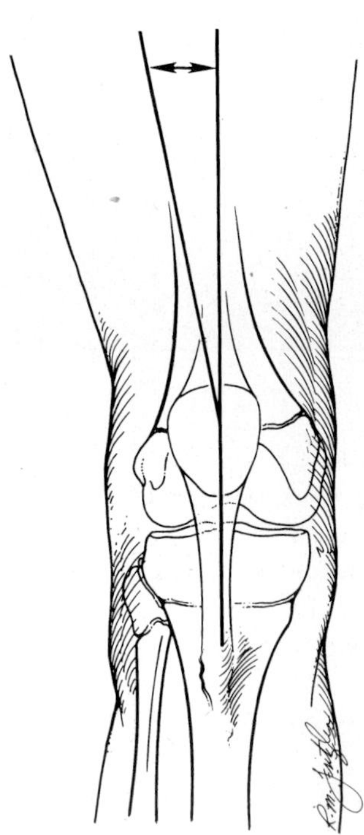

FIGURE 24-20 The Q angle. Normal valgus alignment of the quadriceps mechanism: line drawn from the anterosuperior iliac spine to center of the patella, line drawn from center of the patella to tibial spine.

appropriate sedation, reduction is done by flexing the hip to relax the quadratus femoris, gradually extending the knee, and gently pushing the patella medially back into its normal position. Gentle reduction should be emphasized to avoid the risk of osteochondral fracture associated with patellar relocation.

Surgery is usually not indicated for acute patellar dislocations in children.[29,63,169] Most patellar dislocations are treated nonoperatively with immobilization, followed by patellofemoral bracing and rehabilitation. Surgical repair may be indicated if the vastus medialis obliquus and/or medial patellofemoral ligament is completely torn from the medial aspect of the patella, leaving a large, palpable soft tissue gap. If osteochondral fracture has occurred, arthroscopy/arthrotomy may be indicated for removal or repair of an osteochondral loose body as discussed in the previous section.

Recurrent instability of the patella which has been recalcitrant to nonoperative treatment is typically managed through various proximal/distal patellofemoral realignment procedures. Surgical options include isolated or combination procedures including lateral retinacular release, medial retinacular plication, extensor mechanism realignment, Galeazzi semitendinosis tenodesis, patellar tendon hemitransfer, and tibial tunbercle osteotomy. Tibial tubercle osteotomy is contraindicated in patients with an open tibial tubercle apophysis due to the risk of a growth arrest resulting in recurvatum deformity. Recently, increased attention has been paid to medial patellofemoral ligament reconstruction.[31,53,74]

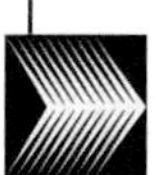

AUTHORS' PREFERRED METHOD OF TREATMENT

Most acute patellar dislocations in children without osteochondral fracture are treated by closed methods with satisfactory results. A cylinder cast or knee immobilizer is used for 2 weeks. Patients are allowed full weight bearing as tolerated. After immobilization, the patient is placed in a patellofemoral brace with a lateral bolster. Physical therapy is begun, emphasizing straight-leg raises, progressive resistance exercises, patellar mobilization, and vastus medialis strengthening. Structural risk factors such as lateral patellar tightness and pes planus with pronation are addressed. Patients are allowed to return to sports 6 to 12 weeks after injury, depending on their patellofemoral mechanics and rehabilitation.

Acute surgical intervention is indicated most commonly for an associated osteochondral fracture, as described in the previous section. Removal of loose bodies or fracture fixation is performed. Adjunctive medial retinacular repair and medial patellofemoral ligament repair is usually also performed to reduce the risk of recurrent patellar instability.

Chronic patellar subluxation or dislocation is common in adolescents, especially girls. Several risk factors have been identified in children likely to have chronic subluxation or dislocation, including age younger than 16 years, radiographic evidence of dysplasia of the patella or lateral femoral condyle, significant atrophy of the vastus medialis obliquus, hypermobility of the patella, and multiple previous dislocations (Fig. 24-21). Initial treatment of chronic patellar subluxation or dislocation in adolescents is immobilization followed by aggressive physical therapy for rehabilitation of the vastus medialis obliquus and quadriceps muscles. Surgical intervention is warranted in children with several risk factors who do not respond to this treatment regimen and continue to have subluxation or dislocation.[40,132,186,199] Micheli and Stanitski[219] reviewed 33 skeletally immature patients with lateral retinacular releases and found that the procedure did not interfere with permanent alignment of the extensor mechanism. They recommended the technique for children who do not respond to an aggressive physical therapy program. The author usually performs medial retinaculum/medial patellofemoral ligament repair with lateral retinacular release for cases of patellar instability (Fig. 24-22A).

If subluxation or dislocation persists after adequate lateral release and medial repair, further correction of the medial deficiency is indicated. Galeazzi transfer of the semitendinosis through the inferior pole of the patella also has been reported in skeletally immature patients (Fig. 22-22B).[125] This may be indicated in adolescents with continued instability after lateral release and medial realignment, or in children with associated connective tissue disorders. In lieu of Galeazzi transfer, medial patellofemoral ligament reconstruction may be considered.[31,53,74] In skeletally mature patients with a significantly abnormal Q angle, tibial tubercle osteotomy usually achieves good results. This technique displaces the anterior tibial tubercle medially to decrease the Q angle and anteriorly to reduce the patellofemoral contact forces (Fig. 24-22C). Tibial tubercle osteotomy is contraindicated in patients with open physes because of the possibility of growth disturbance of the anterior tibial tubercle, with resulting genu recurvatum.

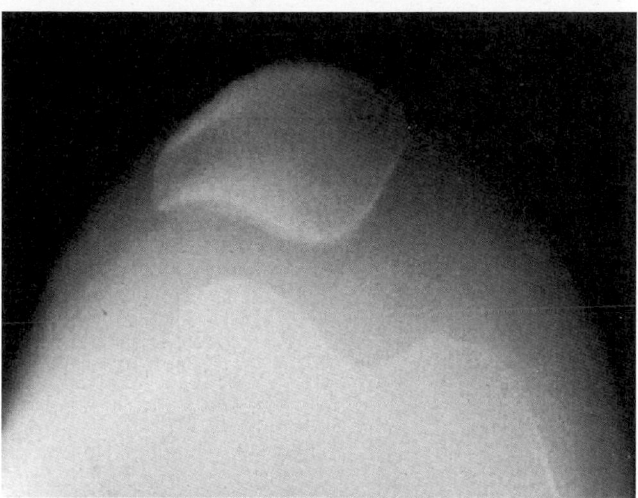

FIGURE 24-21 Chronic lateral patellar subluxation in a 13-year-old girl.

Pearls and Pitfalls

- Unrecognized associated osteochondral fractures may present later as loose bodies.
- Unrecognized associated ligamentous injury can present later as knee instability.
- Aggressive nonoperative treatment should be pursued for cases of patellofemoral instability before considering surgical management.
- Patients with recurrent patellar instability, particularly children, should be evaluated for underlying patellofemoral dysplasia.

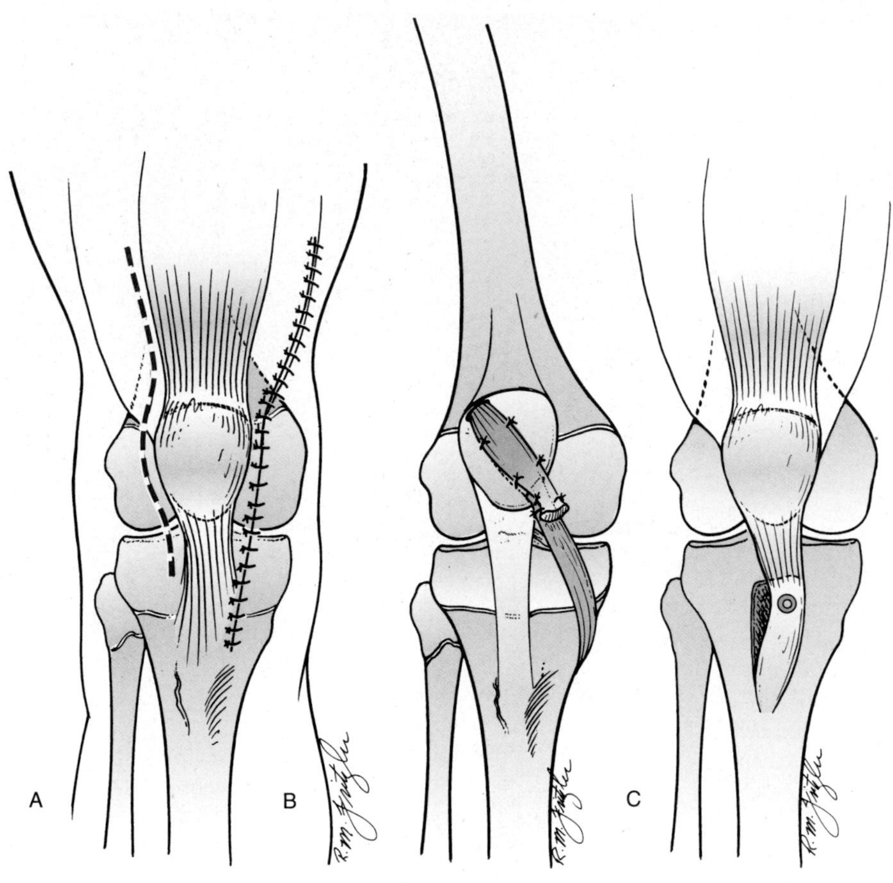

FIGURE 24-22 Surgical technique for treatment of chronic patellar subluxation or dislocation. **A.** Lateral retinacular release and medial imbrication. **B.** Semitendinosis tenodesis. **C.** Elmslie-Trillat procedure.

- Overzealous and injudicious use of lateral retinacular release may result in iatrogenic medial patellar instability.

Prognosis and Complications

The prognosis of patellar dislocations in children is generally good. Approximately 1 in 6 children with acute patellar dislocations experiences recurrent dislocations. Patients with a younger age at first dislocation are at higher risk for recurrent instability. Cash and Hughston[58] noted 75% satisfactory results after nonoperative treatment in carefully selected patients.

Recurrent patellar dislocations with associated osteochondral injuries may lead to osteoarthritis of the patellofemoral joint.

Complications may occur after surgery for patellar instability. Lateral release alone without medial retinaculum/medial patellofemoral ligament repair may not adequately prevent recurrent dislocation. Stiffness, with lack of knee flexion, may occur after Galeazzi tenodesis, if the graft is overly tensioned. After tibial tubercle osteotomy, nonunion, hardware failure, neurovascular injury, and compartment syndrome have been reported.

MENISCAL INJURIES

Introduction

Meniscal injuries in the pediatric athlete are being seen with increased frequency.[†] Meniscal disorders include meniscal tears, discoid meniscus, and meniscal cysts. The exact incidence of meniscal injuries in children and adolescents is unknown. King[164] reported 52 patients younger than 15 years of age who had undergone arthrotomy because of suspected meniscal injuries, and Fowler[102] reported 117 meniscectomies in patients 12 to 16 years of age. Meniscal injuries under the age of 10 are rare, unless associated with a discoid meniscus.[‡] The incidence of meniscal, as well as other intra-articular disorders, increases with age.[73] With adolescence, increased size and speed, and increased athletic demands, come higher-energy injuries and an increase of intra-articular lesions.

Meniscal injury patterns differ in children compared to adults. It is estimated that longitudinal tears comprise 50% to 90% of meniscal tears in children and adolescents.[176] Bucket-handle displaced tears are not uncommon (see Fig. 24-1). Also in these age groups, meniscal injuries are commonly associated with ACL injuries.[57,88,177,203] Cannon[57] estimated that repairable meniscal tears occur in 30% of all knees with acute ACL rupture and in 30% of patients under 20 years old. Approximately two thirds of repairable meniscal tears are associated with ACL rupture, with the majority of these tears limited to the posterior horn.

The incidence of medial meniscal tears is greater than lateral meniscal tears in the pediatric and especially the adolescent age group.[281] There appears to be a relatively increased incidence

[†]References 1,2,18,19,42,55,62,102,128,154,164,174,176,203,214, 221,224,230,258,294,299,313,316.

[‡]References 5,10,12,33,68,79,80,99,102,105,126,130,144,151,152, 157,158,167,176,227,228,233,239,241,246,261,275,284,285,295, 303,312,315.

of lateral tears in the preadolescent age group, which may be due to the existence of lateral discoid menisci.[176]

Principles of Management

Mechanism of Injury

Injury to the nondiscoid meniscus is virtually always traumatic in nature in children and adolescents. Multiple studies have shown that between 80% to 90% of meniscal injuries in children and adolescents are sustained during sporting activities.[5,117,118,203,282] These numbers may be lower in the preadolescent age group. Meniscal tears most commonly occur with twisting motions, associated frequently with football, soccer, and basketball.

Meniscal tears are most commonly produced by rotation as the flexed knee moves toward extension. This rotational force with the knee partially flexed changes the relation of the femoral condyles to the menisci, and forces the menisci toward the center of the joint, where they are likely to be injured. These twisting mechanisms occur primarily in sports and may cause associated ligamentous injuries. Meniscal injuries also may be associated with degenerative changes, cyst formation, or congenital anomalies.[102]

Signs and Symptoms

Pain and swelling are the most common chief complaint. Other complaints include mechanical symptoms such as snapping, catching, and locking. A bucket-handle tear that is displaced into the intercondylar notch may present with a locked knee or a knee unable to fully extend.

The differential diagnosis of acute meniscal tear in the pediatric patient includes conditions resulting in a traumatic effusion such as as ligamentous injury, osteochondral fracture, chondral injury, and patellofemoral dislocation. In addition, conditions causing joint line pain must be distinguished from meniscal tears, such as plica syndrome, iliotibial friction band syndrome, osteochondritis dissecans, and bone bruises.[176]

The diagnosis of meniscal tear in children and adolescents can be difficult to make. Due to the diversity of pathology and the difficulty of examination of children, diagnostic accuracy of clinical exam for meniscus tear has been shown to be as low as 29% to 59%.[169,176] An accurate history may be difficult to obtain in a very young child. The older the patient, the more likely a history of specific injury. The patient usually relates feeling or hearing a "pop" at the time of injury, with frequent popping and giving way after injury. Pain is reported by approximately 85% of patients, with tenderness over the affected joint line. More than half report giving way and effusion of the knee joint. McMurray's and Apley's tests may be helpful in the diagnosis of a chronic lesion, but with acute injury the knee usually is too painful to allow these maneuvers.[69]

The most common findings, similar to adults, are joint line tenderness and effusion.[19,214] However, some patients may have minimal findings on physical examination. In Vahvanen and Aalto's[297] series of patients with documented meniscal tears, almost one third of the patients had no significant findings on physical examination. The classic McMurray test may be of little value in this age group whose tears are peripheral and not degenerative posterior horn lesions.[176] The most accurate physical findings are joint line tenderness (especially middle to posterior) and exacerbation of the pain with varus (medial), valgus (lateral), and rotation stress (internal, medial; external, lateral) at 30 to 40 degrees of knee flexion. Two recent studies, by examiners with pediatric sports medicine experience, have shown the diagnostic accuracy of clinical exam to be 86.3% and 93.5% overall.[169,280] When medial meniscus tears were looked at alone, the sensitivity and specificity of clinical exam were 62.1% and 80.7%, respectively.[169] The sensitivity and specificity for lateral meniscal tears were 50% and 89.2%, respectively.[169]

Imaging

Routine radiographs are obtained primarily to eliminate other sources of knee pain. Arthrography[66] may help delineate meniscal tears, but has been used less frequently since the advent of arthroscopy and MRI.[224,231]

MRI is the preferred imaging method for evaluating meniscal injuries in children. MRI accuracy rates reportedly range from 45% to 90% in the diagnosis of meniscal tears.[47,146,243,269] Sensitivity and specificity of 83% and 95%, respectively, has been shown in skeletally immature patients.[169,279] Kocher et al.[169] showed that for medial meniscal tears, the sensitivity and specificity for MRI diagnosis was 79% and 92%, respectively. For lateral meniscal tears, these numbers were 67% and 83%, respectively.[169]

MRI should not be used as a screening procedure because of significant limitations of the technique in this age group.[46,184,243,279] Only the specificity for medial meniscal tears was significantly higher with MRI as compared to clinical exam.[169] The sensitivity and specificity of MRI decrease in younger children compared with older adolescents.[169,280] In recent studies that compared the diagnostic accuracy of physical exam versus MRI, clinical exam rates were equivalent or superior to MRI.[152,169] These authors recommended judicious use of MRI in evaluating intra-articular knee disorders.

Normal MRI signal changes exist in the posterior horn of the medial and lateral meniscus in children and adolescents.[152,166,169,318] These signal changes do not extend to the superior or inferior articular surfaces of the meniscus and likely represent vascular developmental changes.[176] Takeda et al.[288] reviewed the MRI signal intensity and pattern in the menisci of 108 knees in 80 normal children 8 to 15 (average 12.2) years of age using the classification of Zobal et al.,[318] which allows for equivocation for type III signals. Using tibial tubercle maturity as a definition of skeletal maturity, Takeda et al.[288] found signal intensity to be proportional to age, with high signal (grades III and III) evident in 80% of patients 10 years of age or younger, 65% by 13 years of age, and 33% at 15 years of age, similar to the false-positive rate of 29% reported in asymptomatic adults.[111,184] Overall, two thirds of the patients had positive findings (grades II or III), often grade III-A, which is equivocal extension through the surface of the meniscus. Takeda et al.[288] suggested that the decrease in signal intensity was proportional to diminution of peripheral vascularity, especially in the posterior horn of the meniscus. These investigators cautioned against misinterpretation of pediatric knee MRI and emphasized the necessity for correlation of the clinical findings with any imaging study results. When interpreting an MRI of the developing knee, care must be taken to identify a meniscal tear only when linear signal changes extend to the articular surface. As with any test, clinical correlation is mandatory before treatment decisions are made.

Classification

Classification is based on the meniscus involved (medial versus lateral), the location of the tear (posterior horn, body, anterior

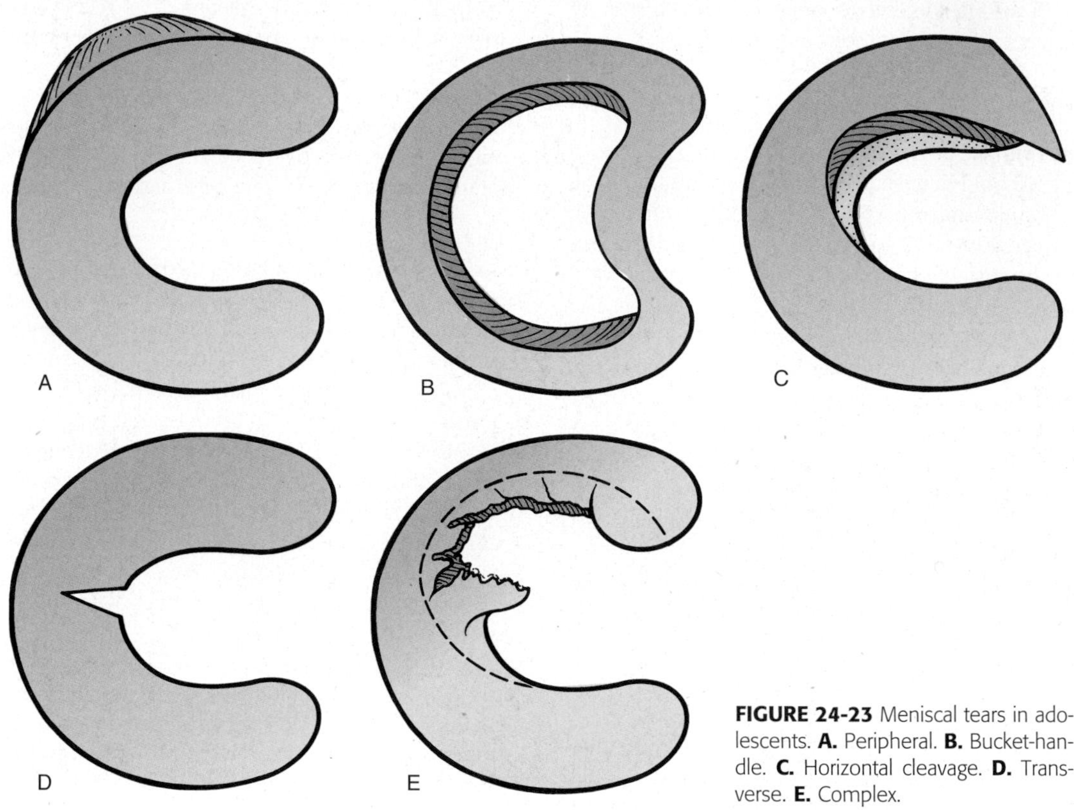

FIGURE 24-23 Meniscal tears in adolescents. **A.** Peripheral. **B.** Bucket-handle. **C.** Horizontal cleavage. **D.** Transverse. **E.** Complex.

horn), the chronicity of the tear (acute (<3 weeks), chronic (>3 weeks), and the tear pattern (peripheral, bucket-handle, horizontal cleavage, transverse, or complex) (Fig. 24-23). Other important factors include site of the tear (outer third, middle third, inner third), stability, and associated ligamentous and chondral injuries.

Surgical and Applied Anatomy

The menisci become clearly defined by as early as 8 weeks of embryologic development.[157] By week 14, they assume the normal mature anatomic relationships. At no point during their embryology are the menisci discoid in morphology.[157] Thus, the discoid meniscus represents an anatomic variant, not a vestigial remnant. The developmental vasculature of the menisci has been studied extensively by Clark.[62] The blood supply arises from the periphery and supplies the entire meniscus. This vascular pattern persists through birth. During postpartum development, the vasculature begins to recede and, by the ninth month, the central third is avascular. This decrease in vasculature continues until approximately age 10, when the menisci attain their adult vascular patter. Injection dye studies by Arnoczky and Warren[22] have shown that only the peripheral 10% to 30% of the medial and 10% to 25% of the lateral meniscus receive vascular nourishment.

The medial meniscus is C-shaped. The posterior horn is larger in anterior–posterior width than the anterior horn. The medial meniscus covers approximately 50% of the medial tibial plateau. The medial meniscus is attached firmly to the medial joint capsule through the meniscotibial or coronary ligaments. There is a discrete capsular thickening at its midportion which constitutes the deep MCL. The inferior surface is flat and the superior surface concave so that the meniscus conforms to its respective tibial and femoral articulations. To maintain this conforming relationship, the medial meniscus translates 2.5 mm posteriorly on the tibia as the femoral condyle rolls backward during knee flexion.[117,118]

The lateral meniscus is more circular in shape and covers a larger portion, approximately 70%, of the lateral tibial plateau. The lateral meniscus is more loosely connected to the lateral joint capsule. There are no attachments in the area of the popliteal hiatus and the fibular collateral ligament does not attach to the lateral meniscus. Accessory meniscofemoral ligaments exist in up to one third of cases. These arise from the posterior meniscus. If this ligament inserts anterior to the PCL, it is known as the ligament of Humphrey; if it inserts posterior to the PCL, it is known as the ligament of Wrisberg. Due to the lack of restraining forces, the lateral meniscus is able to translate 9 to 11 mm on the tibia with knee flexion. This may account for the lower incidence of lateral meniscal tears. Both menisci are attached anteriorly via the anterior transverse meniscal ligament.[117,118]

The blood supply arises from the superior and inferior, medial and lateral geniculate arteries. These vessels form a perimeniscal synovial plexus. There may be some contribution from the middle geniculate artery. King,[165] in the 1930s, published classic research indicating that the peripheral meniscus did communicate with the vascular supply and thus was capable of healing. It is believed that the inner two thirds of the meniscus receives its nutrition through diffusion and mechanical pumping.

The menisci are composed primarily of type I collagen (60% to 70% is dry weight). Lesser amounts of types II, III, and

VI collagen are also present. The collagen fibers are oriented primarily in a circumferential pattern, parallel with the long access of the meniscus.[117,118] There are also radial, oblique, and vertically oriented fibers. Proteoglycans and glycoproteins are present in smaller concentrations than in articular cartilage. The menisci also contain neural elements including mechanoreceptors and type I and II sensory fibers. In a sensory mapping study, Dye[82] demonstrated that the probing of the peripheral meniscus led to pain where as stimulation of the central meniscus elicited little or no discomfort.

Our understanding of the functional importance of the meniscus has evolved. In 1897, Bland-Sutton[45] characterized the menisci as "functionless remnants of intra-articular leg muscles." The sentiment was held onto through the 1970s, when menisci were routinely excised. Fairbanks,[93] in 1948, published the first long-term follow-up of patients after total menisectomy. His article warned that degenerative changes followed menisectomy in a substantial proportion of patients. Now, several reports have established the deleterious consequences of total and even partial meniscectomy.[5,71,88,176,203,214,246,248,295,303,313] Nowhere are these facts more important than in children and adolescents, in whom the long-term effects of menisectomy will be magnified by the activity level and longevity.

It is now realized that the menisci have many functions. The menisci serve to increase contact area and congruency of the femoral tibial articulation. This allows the menisci to participate in load sharing and reduces the contact stresses across the knee joint. It is estimated that the menisci transmit up to 50% to 70% of the load in extension and 85% of the load in 90 degrees of flexion.[6] Baratz and Fu[28] showed that after total meniscectomy, contact area may decrease by 75% and contact stresses increase by 235%. They also documented the deleterious effects of partial menisectomy, demonstrating that the contact stresses increased in proportion to the amount of meniscus removed. Excision of small bucket-handle tears of the medial meniscus increased contact stress by 65%, and resecting 75% of the posterior horn increased contact stresses equivalent to that after total meniscectomy.[28] Repair of meniscal tears, by either arthroscopic or open techniques, reduced the contact stresses to normal. Multiple other studies have corroborated the mechanical importance of the meniscus.[117,118]

Meniscal tissue is about half as stiff as articular cartilage, allowing it to participate in shock absorption. Shock absorption capacity in the normal knee is 20% higher than in the menisectomized knee.[189,300] The menisci also have a role in joint stability. In the ACL deficient knee, the posterior horn of the medial meniscus plays a very important passive stabilizing role. In the ACL deficient knee, medial menisectomy leads to a 58% increase in anterior translation at 90 degrees of flexion.[189,267] Given the presence of neural elements with in their substance, it is also theorized that the menisci may have a role in proprioception.

Current Treatment Options

Some small, nondisplaced meniscal tears in the outer vascular region of the meniscus may heal nonoperatively or may become asymptomatic.[117,118,176] Nonoperative treatment usually consists of rehabilitation of the injured knee with the avoidance of pivoting and sports for 12 weeks.

However, the majority of meniscal tears in pediatric patients are larger and require surgical treatment.[117,118,176] Arthroscopic management is standard, with either partial menisectomy using motorized shavers and baskets or meniscal repairs using outside-in, all-inside, or inside-out techniques.[155,225,308]

The traditional treatment of a torn meniscus has been menisectomy, but numerous reports[5,21,42,88,138,164,176,183,203,214,246,247,290,295,303,313] indicating the poor long-term results of menisectomy in children have made this less common. Up to 60% to 75% of patients have degenerative changes after menisectomy. Manzione et al.[203] reported 60% poor results in 20 children and adolescents after menisectomy. In cadaver studies, Baratz et al.[28] showed that the contact stresses on the tibiofemoral articulation increase in proportion to the amount of the meniscus removed and the degree of disruption of the meniscal structure. Clearly, as much of the meniscus should be preserved as possible.

The exact meniscal injury and potential for repair can be determined arthroscopically to help formulate treatment plans. Zaman and Leonard[316] recommended observation of small peripheral tears, repair of larger peripheral tears, and, when necessary, partial menisectomy, leaving as much of the meniscus as possible; they concluded that total menisectomy is contraindicated in young patients. In general, peripheral tears, which are most common in children, and longitudinal tears are good candidates for repair, with success rates of up to 90% reported.[70,127,134,224]

Although King[157] suggested over six decades ago that, based on experimental evidence in dogs, longitudinal meniscal tears could heal if communication with peripheral blood supply existed, it was not until the work of Arnoczky and Warren[23] in the 1980s that meniscal repairs were begun based on documentation of the meniscal blood supply. They believed that tears within 3 mm of the meniscosynovial junction were vascularized, and ones more than 5 mm away were avascular unless bleeding was seen at surgery. Tears in the 3- to 5-mm range had inconsistent vascularity. Children and adolescents may have greater healing potential for meniscal repair. In adults, meniscal repair is indicated for tears involving the outer third. In children and adolescents, repair of tears in the middle third zone typically heal as well.[70,127,134,224]

Discoid Lateral Meniscus

Meniscal tears may be seen with an underlying discoid lateral meniscus, particularly in younger children. The discoid lateral meniscus represents an anatomic variant of meniscal morphology. The incidence is thought to be 3% to 5% in the general population[80,151,152,176] and slightly higher in Asian populations.[99,151,152,176] Discoid morphology almost exclusively occurs within the lateral meniscus, but medial discoid menisci have also been reported.[99,151,152,176] The incidence of bilateral abnormality has been reported to be as high as 20%.[10,33,241,274]

Discoid menisci are classified based on the system of Watanabe[304]: complete morphology (type I), incomplete morphology (type II), and any morphology that lack peripheral attachments (type III). Although often synonymous with so-called "snapping knee syndrome," discoid lateral menisci may manifest in a variety of ways. Symptoms are often related to the type of discoid present, peripheral stability of the meniscus, and the presence or absence of an associated meniscal tear.[12,80,99,151,228,255,312] Stable discoid menisci without associated tears will often remain asymptomatic, identified only as incidental findings during MRI or arthroscopy.[163] Unstable discoid menisci more commonly present in younger children and often produce the snapping knee syndrome. In such instances, a painless and palpable, audible or visible snap is produced with knee range of motion, especially near terminal extension. Discoid menisci with posterior instability and a redundant anterior segment may limit knee extension.[314] In children with stable discoid lateral menisci, symptoms often present when an associated tear is present. Unlike acute meniscal tears, such symptoms may present insidiously without previous trauma. Signs and symptoms of a meniscal tear may exist including pain, swelling, catching, locking, and limited motion. On physical examination, there may be joint line tenderness, popping, limited motion, effusion, terminal motion pain, and positive provocative tests (McMurray maneuvers, Apley test). Degenerative horizontal cleavage tears are the most common type of tear seen, reported in the largest series to occur in 58% to 98% of symptomatic discoid menisci.[6,33,241]

Several treatment options exist if the diagnosis of a discoid lateral meniscus is confirmed. For asymptomatic discoid lateral menisci, even if found incidentally on arthroscopy, conservative treatment is indicated. For stable, complete or incomplete discoid menisci, partial menisectomy, "saucerization," is the treatment of choice (Fig. 24-24). If meniscal instability with detachment also exists, meniscal repair can also be performed. Traditionally, complete menisectomy via open or arthroscopic means was suggested for such lesions. However, the long-term results of complete menisectomy and near-total menisectomy in children are poor with early degenerative changes.[5,7,88,124,176,187,203,214,235,246,248,294,295,303,313] Although there may be a rare instance where salvage of a discoid meniscus may seem unobtainable, better arthroscopic technology and techniques have made meniscal preservation the ideal treatment through saucerization and repair.[4] Osteochondritis dissecans has been described associated with discoid lateral meniscus or after saucerization.[41,75,129]

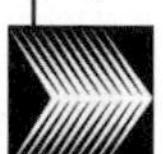

AUTHORS' PREFERRED METHOD OF TREATMENT

The author's treatment algorithm is shown in Figure 24-25. Treatment is based on size, site, shape, and stability of the tear, acuity of the lesion, and knee stability.

In a stable knee with an acute, arthroscopically documented outer third peripheral tear that is less than 1 cm long and cannot be displaced more than 3 mm, the tear is allowed to heal. For a similar tear in a chronic setting, we

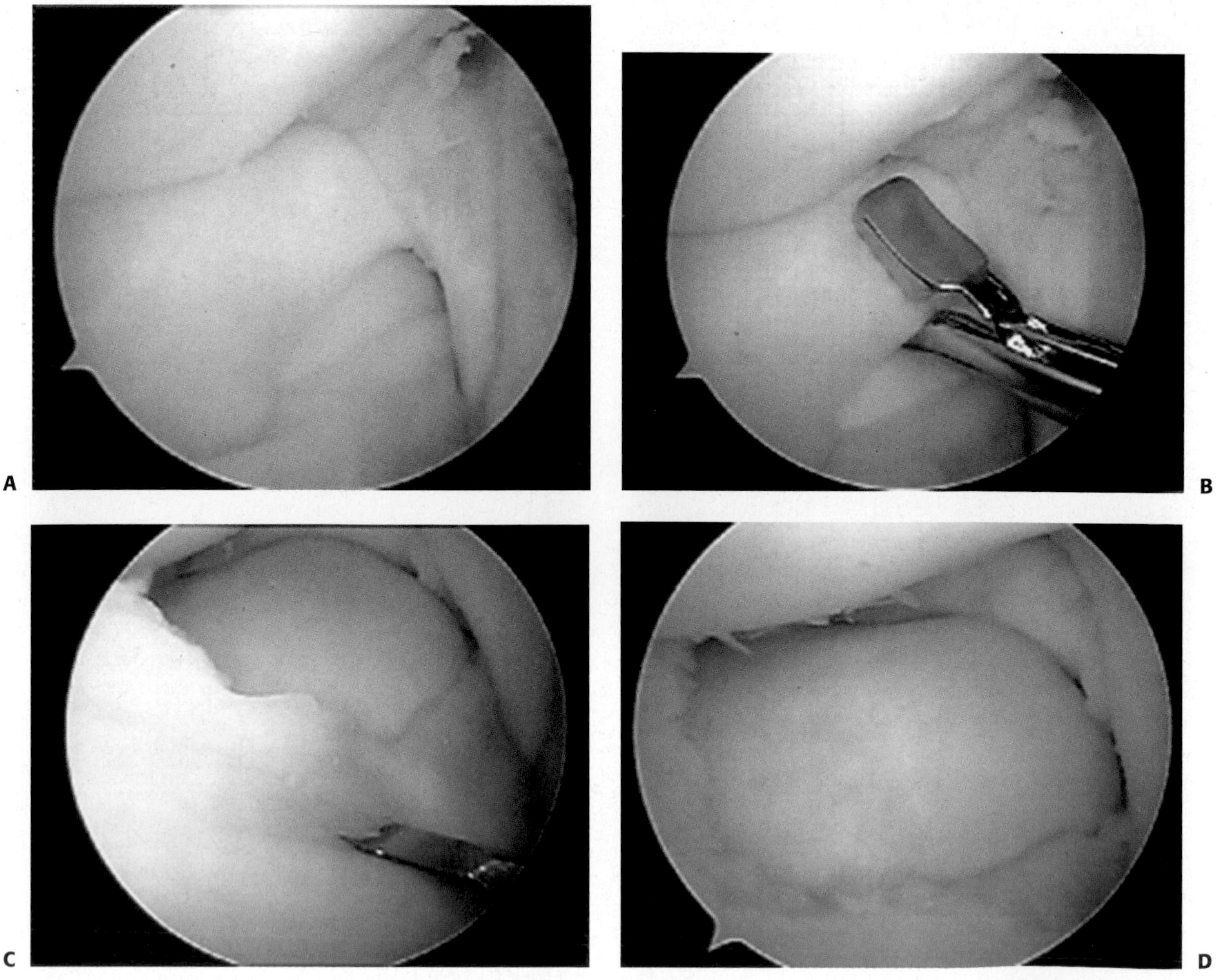

A B C D

FIGURE 24-24 Discoid lateral meniscus saucerization. **A.** Complete type discoid lateral meniscus extending into the intercondylar notch. **B.** Excision of the central portion of the discoid meniscus. **C.** Excision of the anterior portion of the discoid meniscus. **D.** Appearance after saucerization.

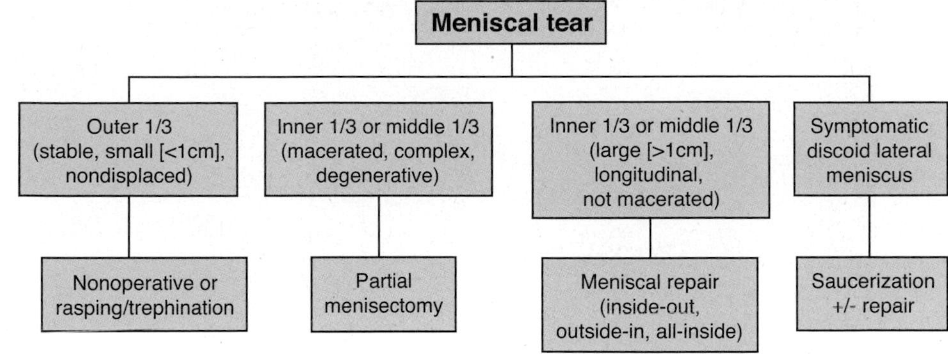

FIGURE 24-25 Algorithm for the management of meniscal tears in children and adolescents.

arthroscopically rasp or trephinate the interface between the meniscal edges and allow the tear to heal. Protected weight bearing and limitation of flexion beyond 90 degrees is prescribed for 4 weeks. Healing can be assessed based on physical examination. Return to sports and activities are based on the absence of physical examination findings and adequate rehabilitation, usually at 2 to 3 months postoperatively.

For larger tears involving the outer third or middle third, which are longitudinal with a noncomminuted inner segment that can be reduced anatomically, meniscal repair is performed. In the chronic setting, rasping of the fragment edge, trephination, and use of a fibrin clot may enhance healing. Patients are protected postoperatively to allow for meniscal healing. Our postoperative protocol for isolated meniscal repair involves touchdown weight bearing for 6 weeks postoperatively. Range of motion is restricted to 0 to 30 degrees for the first 2 weeks followed by 0 to 90 degrees for the next 6 weeks. Progressive mobilization, strengthening, and sports-specific therapy is performed under the direction of a physical therapy protocol. Return to sports is allowed at 3 months postoperatively if there is full range of motion, adequate strength, no symptoms (pain, swelling, locking), and resolution of physical examination findings (joint line tenderness, McMurray maneuvers, terminal range joint line pain). Follow-up MRI is performed only in patients with persistent symptoms or physical examination findings. Return to sports is typically 3 to 4 months after meniscal repair.

Partial menisectomy is performed for tears involving the inner third or middle third tears that are macerated, horizontal, degenerative, or complex. Care should be taken to preserve as much tissue as possible (Fig. 24-26). With horizontal tears, the smaller of the two leaves is resected. Rehabilitation after partial menisectomy includes weight bearing as tolerated, range of motion, and strengthening. Return to sports and activities is based on the absence of physical examination findings and adequate rehabilitation, usually at 2 to 3 months postoperatively. Patients who have undergone complete or near-total meniscectomy should be followed longer term to assess the development of degenerative changes. In symptomatic patients or those developing degenerative changes, replacement with an allograft meniscus or synthetic scaffold may be considered.

In children and adolescents, the emphasis should be on meniscal repair over menisectomy whenever possible because of greater healing potential in this age group, the long life span of these patients, the poor results of total and near-total menisectomy, and the lack of longer-term results of partial menisectomy. Meniscal repair techniques include inside-out techniques, outside-in techniques, and all-inside techniques. Outside-in techniques can be useful for anterior horn medial or lateral meniscal tears. For body and posterior horn tears, the traditional technique of meniscal repair has been inside-out repair with vertical or horizontal sutures (Fig. 24-27). Zone-specific cannulae are helpful to direct the flexible suture needles to the appropriate position to avoid neurovascular structures. In addition, we routinely make an incision posteromedially or posterolaterally to retrieve the suture needles and tie the sutures onto the joint capsule,

A

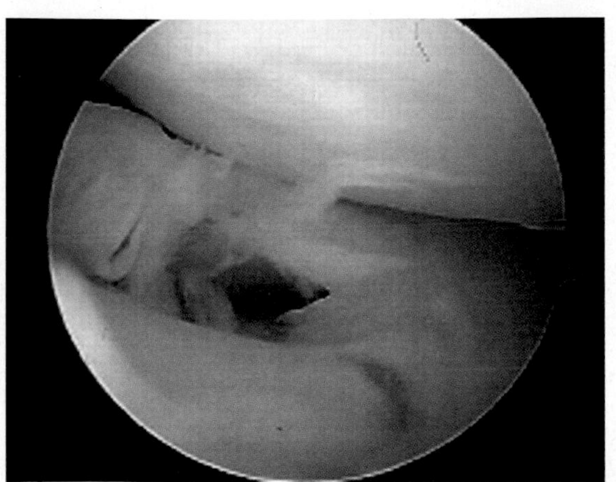

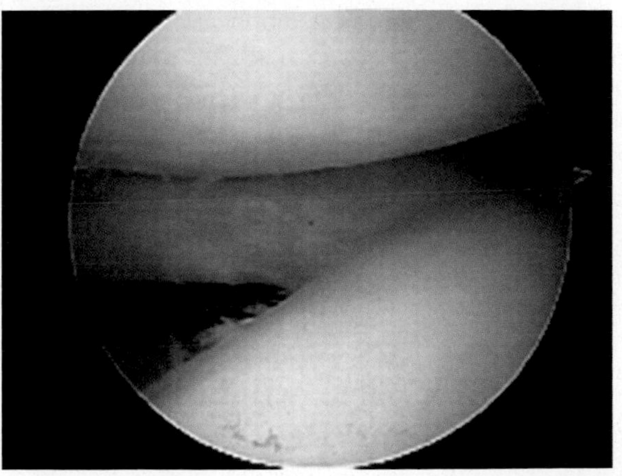

B

FIGURE 24-26 Complex inner third tear of the meniscus **(A)** treated with partial menisectomy **(B)**.

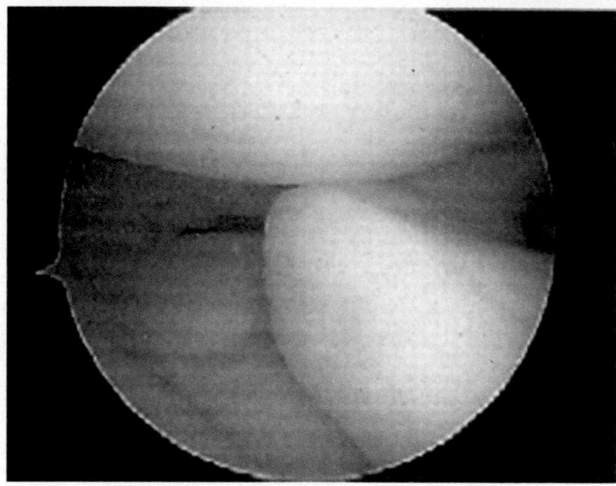

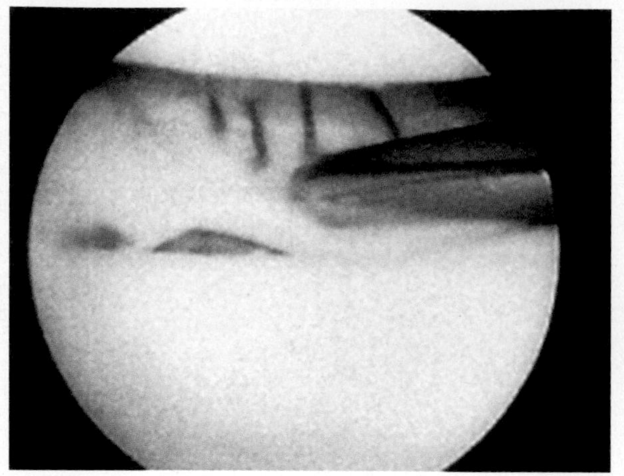

FIGURE 24-27 Longitudinal middle third tear of the meniscus **(A)** treated with inside-out meniscal repair **(B)**.

thus protecting the saphenous nerve and vein medially and the peroneal nerve laterally. Newer all-inside devices have eased the technique of meniscal repair (Fig. 24-28). However, reports of articular cartilage damage from the heads of bioabsorbable arrows and darts exist.[117,118] In addition, many of the available devices extend too far through the capsule in the small pediatric knee, with potential for neurovascular injury. The author prefers more recent all-inside suture devices with a low profile in the joint. The author tends to use these for posterior horn tears in adolescent knees. For smaller tears without substantial displacement, the author uses these alone. For larger tears with displacement such as displaced bucket-handle tears, the author uses these in a hybrid manner with inside-out sutures.

Bucket-handle displaced tears with a locked knee are treated urgently to allow for reduction and meniscal repair and to avoid further injury to the meniscus. Meniscal tears in association with ACL injuries are usually treated concurrently with ACL reconstruction. ACL reconstruction is essential to provide a stable environment for meniscal healing and prevention of further meniscal tears. Healing rates are high with concurrent ACL reconstruction, perhaps due to the healing environment of the associated postoperative hemarthrosis. For meniscal repair in association with ACL reconstruction, return to sports is dictated by the ACL reconstruction, usually at 6 months postoperatively. For large, unstable meniscus tears requiring a more involved meniscus repair, staging of the ACL reconstruction approximately 3 months after meniscal repair can be considered. This may result in a lower risk of arthrofibrosis, rehabilitation focused on meniscal repair, and arthroscopic assessment of meniscal healing at the time of ACL reconstruction.

Pearls and Pitfalls

- Making the diagnosis of a meniscal tear can be difficult in the child or adolescent. The differential diagnosis is varied and includes other injuries and disorders that cause pain and swelling or that cause joint line pain. Physical examination findings are variable. MRI scans must be carefully scrutinized by the orthopaedist because of the relatively high prevalence of normal signal changes in the posterior horns. Extension of the meniscal signal to the superior or inferior edge of the meniscus must be confirmed before considering the MRI diagnostic of a meniscal tear.
- Total or near-total menisectomy should be avoided in children and adolescents if at all possible to avoid the development of degenerative changes. Patients who have had near total or total menisectomy should be counseled regarding the risk of arthritis and the potential for meniscus replacement with allograft or synthetic scaffolds.
- Several technical pitfalls exist during meniscal repair. During inside-out meniscal repair, a posterolateral incision should be made for lateral meniscus repair to avoid iatrogenic injury to the peroneal nerve and a posteromedial incision should be made for medial meniscus repair to avoid iatrogenic injury to the saphenous vein or nerve. During all-inside repair with meniscal repair devices, consideration must be given to the size of the implant relative to the pediatric knee. Implants that protrude too far may injure neurovascular structures or cause local irritation or cysts. Implants that are high-profile or protrude may damage the articular surface of the femoral condyle. Sterile effusions and synovitis may occur with bioabsorbable implants.

Prognosis and Complications

The prognosis after complete or near-total menisectomy is poor with numerous reports* indicating poor long-term results with degenerative changes.

The prognosis of meniscus repair in appropriately selected cases is good. Mintzer and Richmond[221] reported on meniscal repair in 29 patients under the age of 18 (25 had closed physes and 17 underwent concomitant ACL reconstruction). They reported 100% clinical healing at an average follow up of 5 years.[221] Noyes and Barber-Westin[229] looked at meniscal tears extending into the avascular zone in patients younger than 20 years old.[91] Skeletal maturity had been reached in 88%. Their success rate in this group was 75%. This study showed a higher rate of healing with concomitant ACL reconstruction. Eggli et al.[88] found an overall healing rate for repair of isolated meniscal tears of 88% in patients younger than 30, compared to 67% in patients over age 30. Johnson et al.[150] showed a 76% healing rate at an average follow-up of greater than 10 years in a popula-

*References 5,21,42,88,138,164,176,183,203,214,246,248,290,294, 295,303,313.

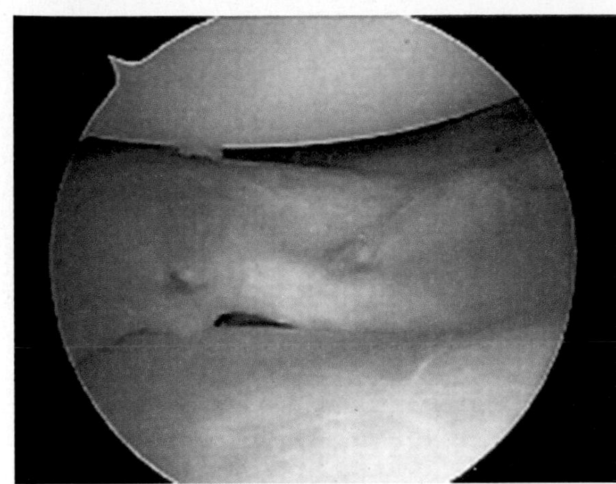

FIGURE 24-28 Longitudinal tear of the outer third of the posterior horn meniscus treated with all-inside fixation devices.

tion that averaged 20 years old at the time of surgery. Factors that have been shown to correlate with increased healing of meniscal repairs include younger age, decreased rim width (peripheral tears), repairs of the lateral meniscus, concomitant ACL reconstruction, time from injury to surgery of less than 8 weeks, and tear length of less than 2.5 cm.[3,56,57,88,117,118,150,291]

Complications after either arthroscopic or open repair may include hemorrhage, infection, persistent effusion, stiffness, and neuropathy. Both the popliteal artery and inferior geniculate branches are close to the posterior capsule and are easily lacerated. Postoperative infection should be suspected if swelling or pain persists with an elevated temperature. Swelling is best treated with external compression dressings, and stiffness is best prevented by appropriate postoperative rehabilitation. Neuroma formation rarely causes significant symptoms, but occasionally persistent localized tenderness may warrant excision.

LIGAMENT INJURIES

Introduction

Ligamentous injuries of the knee in children and adolescents were once considered rare.[65,247] Tibial eminence avulsion fractures were considered the pediatric ACL injury equivalent.[170,175,177,247] However, major ligamentous injuries are being seen with increased frequency and have received increased attention.[†] The increased frequency of diagnosis of knee ligament injuries in children is likely related to increased participation in youth sports at higher competitive levels, the advent of arthroscopy and MRI, and an increased awareness of injuries in this age group.

ACL injury has been reported in 10% to 65% of pediatric knees with acute traumatic hemarthroses in series ranging from 35 to 138 patients.[91,168,179,197,281,293] Stanitski et al.[278] reported 70 children and adolescents with acute traumatic knee hemarthroses; arthroscopic examination revealed ACL injuries in 47% of those 7 to 12 years of age and in 65% of those 13 to 18 years of age. They determined that boys 16 to 18 years of age engaged in organized sports and girls 13 to 15 years of age engaged in unorganized sports had the highest risk for complete ACL tears; 60% of these patients had isolated ACL tears.

Injury patterns in the skeletally immature knee are dependent on the loading conditions and the developmental anatomy. Fractures of the epiphyses or physes about the knee are more common than ligamentous injuries alone. Isolated knee ligament injury in children younger than 14 years of age tends to be rare because of the relative strength of the ligaments compared to the physes.[83,153,208,302] The inherent ligamentous laxity in children also may offer some protection against ligament injury, but this decreases as the adolescent approaches skeletal maturity. Faster loading conditions favor ligamentous injuries, whereas slower loading conditions favor fracture. Narrowing of the intercondylar notch during skeletal development may also predispose to ligamentous injury.[175] Fractures and ligamentous injuries may occur concurrently. Bertin and Goble,[39] after reviewing 29 fractures, concluded that physeal fractures about the knee are associated with a higher incidence of ligamentous injury than physeal fractures around other joints. In addition, tibial eminence fractures, even after anatomic fixation and healing, tend to demonstrate persistent ACL laxity.[170]

Before the 1990s, reports of ligamentous injuries in children were isolated case reports, and most recommendations were for conservative treatment. More recent reports have indicated an increased awareness of ligament injury in association with physeal fractures,[65] as well as isolated ligament injuries, and a more aggressive approach, especially in adolescents approaching skeletal maturity.[37,89,90,224,268,287] Management of some of these injuries, particularly ACL injuries in skeletally immature patients, is controversial. Nonreconstructive treatment of complete tears typically results in recurrent functional instability with risk of injury to meniscal and articular cartilage. A variety of reconstructive techniques have been utilized, including physeal sparing, partial transphyseal, and transphyseal methods using various grafts. Conventional adult ACL reconstruction techniques risk potential iatrogenic growth disturbance due to physeal violation. Growth disturbances after ACL reconstruction in skeletally immature patients have been reported.

Principles of Management

Mechanism of Injury

The mechanism of ligamentous injury varies with the child's age. In younger children, ligamentous injury typically is associated with significant polytrauma. Clanton et al.[61] reported that 5 of 9 children with acute knee ligament injuries were struck by automobiles. In contrast, adolescents are more likely to sustain ligamentous injury during contact sports or sports that require "cutting" maneuvers while running.[273] As exact a description as possible of the mechanism of injury should be obtained, including the position of the knee at the time of injury, the weight-supporting status of the injured knee, whether the force applied was direct or indirect (generated by the patient's own momentum), and the position of the extremity after injury. Older adolescents may describe the knee as buckling or "jumping out of place" and can usually relate the location and severity of their pain as well as the time between injury and onset of pain and swelling. Rapid intraarticular effusion within 2 hours of injury suggests hemarthrosis, usually from injury to the ACL.

†References 11,14,17,20,24,32,37,39,44,50,52,61,77,85,86,89–92, 104,115,121–123,136,143,147,153,156,162,168,179,180,182,192, 193,197,205,207–210,218,220,222,224,238,244,249,260,266,268, 270,271,277,278,281,287,293,301,302,306.

Palmer[237] described four mechanisms capable of producing disruption of the ligamentous structures about the knee: abduction, flexion, and internal rotation of the femur on the tibia; adduction, flexion, and external rotation of the femur on the tibia; hyperextension; and anterior–posterior displacement. The most common mechanism in adolescents is abduction, flexion, and internal rotation of the femur on the tibia occurring during athletic competition when the weight-bearing extremity is struck from the lateral side. The classic abduction, flexion, and internal rotation injury in the adolescent may cause the "unhappy triad" of O'Donoghue: tears of the MCL and ACL and injury to the medial meniscus.

Isolated injury of the LCL is rare in children, but a direct blow to the medial aspect of the knee may tear the LCL, usually with avulsion from the fibula or a physeal injury through the distal femur.[145] Isolated injuries of the ACL and PCL have been reported.[140,208,260] Disruption of the ACL with minimal injury to other supporting structures may be caused by hyperextension, marked internal rotation of the tibia on the femur, and pure deceleration. In contrast, isolated injury of the PCL most often is caused by a direct blow to the front of the tibia with the knee in flexion.

Signs and Symptoms

Both lower extremities are examined for comparison. Large areas of ecchymosis and extensive effusion are easily identified, but smaller areas may require careful palpation. In general, acute hemarthrosis suggests rupture of a cruciate ligament, an osteochondral fracture, a peripheral tear in the vascular portion of a meniscus, or a tear in the deep portion of the joint capsule.[69,72] The absence of hemarthrosis is not, however, an indication of a less severe ligament injury, because with complete disruption the blood in the knee joint may escape into the soft tissues rather than distend the joint. The range of motion of the injured knee, especially extension, is compared with that of the uninjured knee. If significant effusion prevents full extension, sterile aspiration can be performed. If complete knee extension is impossible after aspiration, the diagnosis of an entrapped meniscus should be considered.

Palpation of the collateral ligaments and their bony origins and insertions should locate tenderness at the site of the ligament injury. A defect in the collateral ligaments often can be felt if the MCL is avulsed from its insertion on the tibia or if the LCL is avulsed from the fibular head. If the neurovascular status is normal, stability should be evaluated by stress testing.

Stress testing for ligament injury in children,[96,97] with or without concomitant fracture, is very subjective, and its usefulness depends on the knowledge and experience of the examiner. Stress testing may be done immediately after injury in cooperative adolescents who do not have other significant injuries, but sedation or general anesthesia may be required for accurate diagnosis. In nonemergent situations, beginning the examination by testing the uninjured knee often calms patients and makes them more cooperative; it also establishes a baseline for assessing the ligamentous stability of the injured knee as knee laxity varies during childhood.[135] In the standard stress tests of specific collateral and cruciate ligaments of the knee described in the following sections, the uninjured knee should be examined first.

Valgus Stress Test of the Medial Collateral Ligament. The valgus or abduction stress test is done with the child supine on the examining table and the knee to be examined on the side of the table closest to the examiner. The extremity is abducted off the side of the table and the knee is flexed approximately 20 degrees (Fig. 24-29). With one hand about the lateral aspect of the knee and the other supporting the ankle, the examiner applies gentle abduction or valgus stress to the knee while the hand at the ankle gently externally rotates the leg. Stability of the knee is noted at 20 degrees of flexion and again at neutral.

Varus or Adduction Stress Test of the Lateral Collateral Ligament. The varus or adduction stress test is done in a manner similar to the valgus stress test. It should be done with the

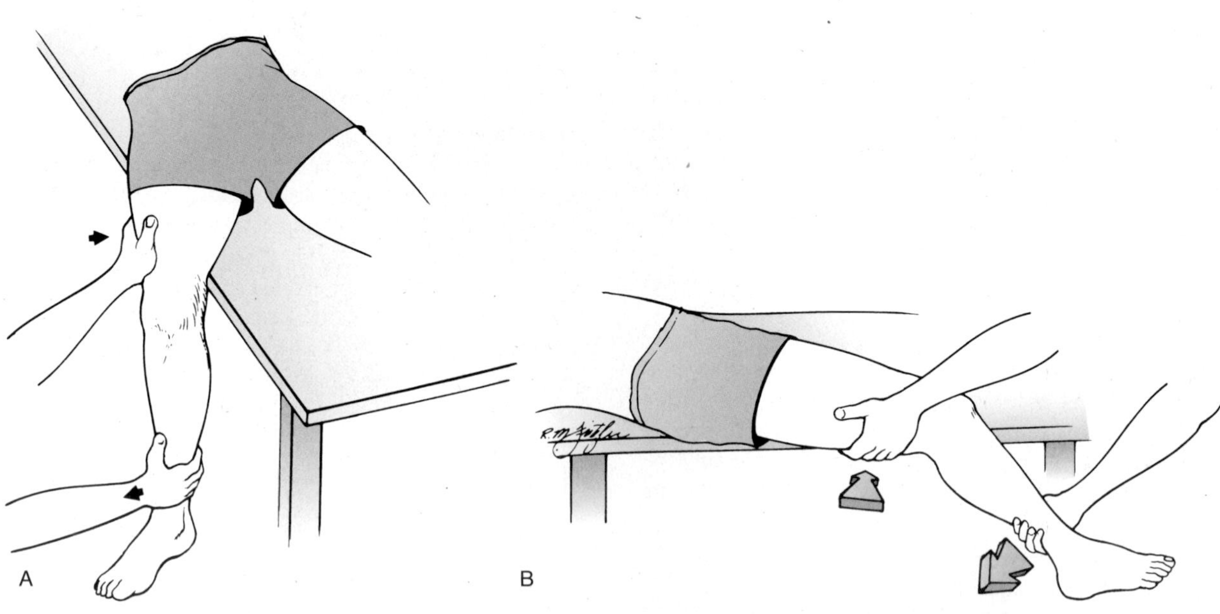

FIGURE 24-29 Valgus stress test of MCL. Extremity is abducted off table, knee is flexed to 20 degrees, and valgus stress is applied. **A.** Frontal view. **B.** Lateral view.

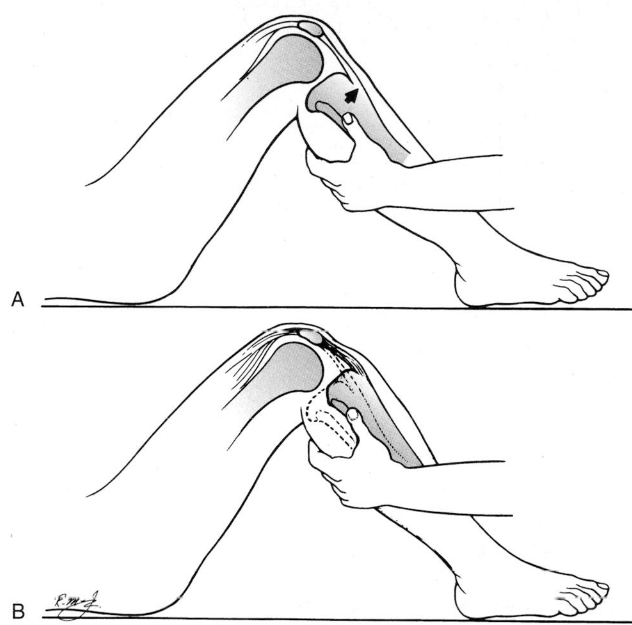

FIGURE 24-30 Anterior drawer test of ACL. Foot is positioned in internal, external, and neutral rotation during examination. With anterior cruciate insufficiency, an anterior force **(A)** displaces the tibia forward **(B)**.

knee in full extension and in 20 degrees of flexion. The LCL may be palpable as a taut structure on the lateral aspect of the knee.

The stability of the collateral ligaments may be different when tested in extension and in flexion. If a collateral ligament is torn but the cruciate ligaments and posterior capsule are intact, little instability can be detected with the knee extended. Flexion of the knee relaxes the capsule and more instability is evident with the same degree of ligamentous injury. Significant instability with varus or valgus stress testing with the knee in full extension usually indicates a cruciate as well as a collateral ligament disruption.

Stress Testing of the Anterior Cruciate Ligament. The anterior drawer test, as described by Slocum, is the classic maneuver for testing the stability of the ACL (Fig. 24-30). The Lachman and pivot-shift tests, however, are considered more sensitive for evaluating ACL injury when the examination can be done in a relaxed, cooperative adolescent (Fig. 24-31). To perform the Lachman test, the examiner firmly stabilizes the femur with one hand while using the other hand to grip the proximal tibia, with the thumb placed on the anteromedial joint margin. An anteriorly directed lifting force applied by the palm and fingers causes anterior translation of the tibia in relation to the femur that can be palpated by the thumb; a soft or mushy end point indicates a positive test. When the ACL is disrupted, the normal patellar ligament slope is obliterated.

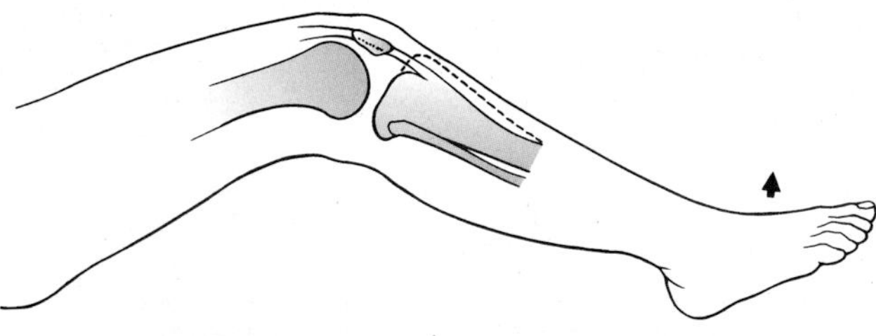

FIGURE 24-31 Lateral pivot-shift test of ACL.

Stress Testing of the Posterior Cruciate Ligament. The posterior drawer test for evaluation of the PCL is done with the patient supine. With the patient's foot secured to the table and the hip flexed, a posterior force is applied to the proximal tibia. Posterior movement of the tibia on the femur greater than in the uninjured extremity indicates posterior instability (Fig. 24-32).

Imaging

Anteroposterior and lateral radiographs are obtained when any ligament injury of the knee is suspected in children. The radiographs are carefully inspected for evidence of occult epiphyseal or physeal fractures or bony avulsions. The intercondylar notch, especially, is inspected to detect a tibial spine fracture, which is confirmed by anterior or posterior instability on physical examination. Occasionally, a small fragment of bone avulsed from the medial femur or proximal tibia indicates injury to the MCL. Similarly, avulsion of a small fragment of bone from the proximal fibular epiphysis or the lateral aspect of the distal femur may indicate LCL injury.

In children with open physes, stress radiographs may be helpful to evaluate medial and lateral instability associated with physeal fractures. Gentle stress views may be obtained with sedation, but general anesthesia may be required if the diagnosis is unclear. Stress must be performed carefully to avoid further physeal injury, which may lead to physeal arrest. There are no accepted guidelines correlating joint space widening medially or laterally with knee joint instability in children, and stress views of the opposite knee may be required for comparison. If plain radiographs show a fracture of the distal femoral or proximal tibial physis, stress views may be obtained only to evaluate suspected ligamentous instability. Conversely, if the initial radiographs appear normal but there is significant effusion about the knee, stress views or MRI may be obtained to rule out a fracture of the physis of the distal femur or proximal tibia.

Other radiographic findings include avulsion of the anterior or posterior tibial spine indicative of injury to the ACL or PCL, widening of the joint space, and posterior subluxation of the tibia on the femur. Clanton et al.[61] considered a joint space of 8 mm or wider to be a definitive indication of ligament injury. Sanders et al.[260] reported 1.8 cm of posterior subluxation of the tibia on the anteroposterior stress view in a 6-year-old child with complete PCL disruption.

MRI is frequently used to further delineate ligamentous injuries in the knee. MRI should be used to confirm an uncertain diagnosis or to gain further information that may affect treatment. Conventional MRI can give information regarding MCL injury, LCL injury, ACL injury, PCL injury, posterolateral corner injury, bone bruising, chondral injury, and meniscal injury.

Classification

Classification of knee ligament injuries is based on the severity of the injury, the specific anatomic location of the injury, and the direction of the subsequent instability caused by an isolated ligament injury or combination of ligament injuries.

A first-degree ligament sprain is a tear of a minimal number of fibers of the ligament with localized tenderness but no insta-

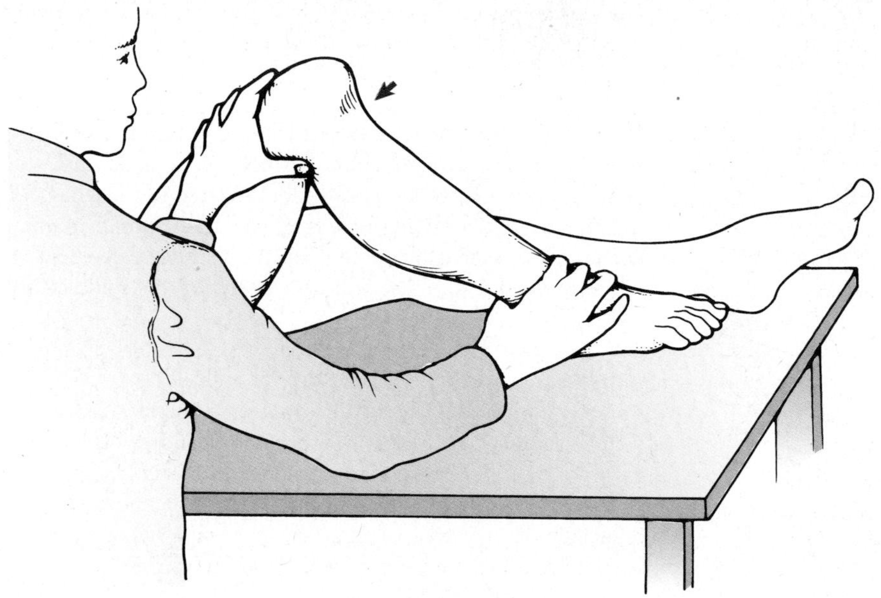

FIGURE 24-32 PCL injury. Note posterior sagging of the tibia with posterior cruciate injury.

bility. A second-degree sprain is disruption of more ligamentous fibers, causing loss of function and more joint reaction but no significant instability. A third-degree sprain is complete disruption of the ligament, resulting in instability. Although difficult to assess clinically, the degree of sprain also is determined during stress testing by the amount of separation of the joint surfaces: first-degree sprain, 5 mm or less; second-degree sprain, 5 to 10 mm; and third-degree sprain, more than 10 mm.

The anatomic classification of ligament injuries describes the exact location of the disruption[101]:

A. MCL insufficiency (Fig. 24-33)
   1. Femoral origin
   2. Middle portion
   3. Tibial insertion
B. ACL insufficiency
   1. Femoral origin
   2. Interstitial
   3. Tibial insertion
      a. Without avulsion of the intercondylar eminence
      b. With avulsion of the intercondylar eminence
C. LCL insufficiency (Fig. 24-34)
   1. Femoral origin
   2. Middle portion
   3. Fibular insertion
D. PCL insufficiency
   1. Femoral origin
   2. Interstitial
   3. Tibial insertion

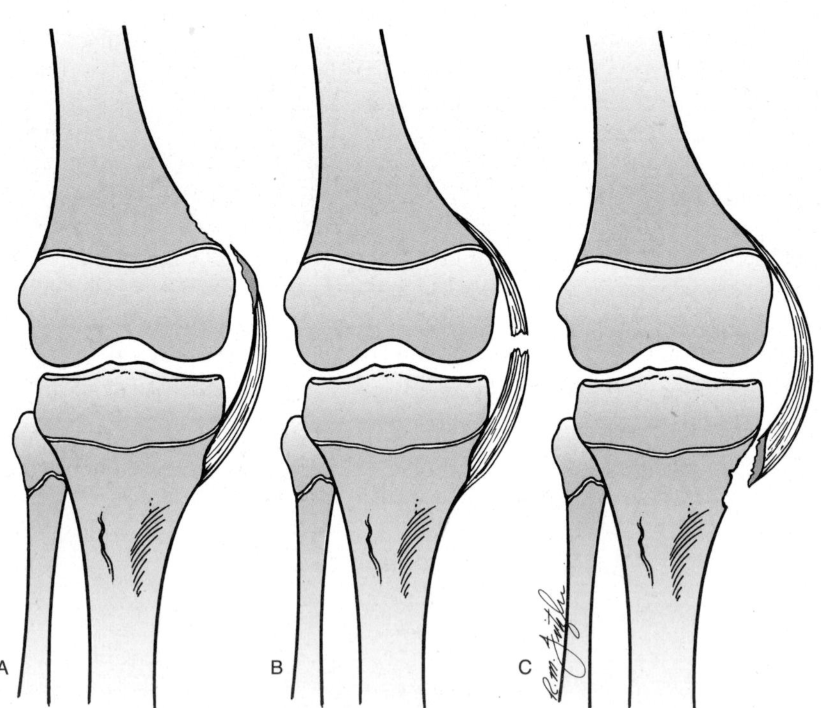

FIGURE 24-33 MCL injury. **A.** Femoral origin. **B.** Middle portion. **C.** Tibial insertion.

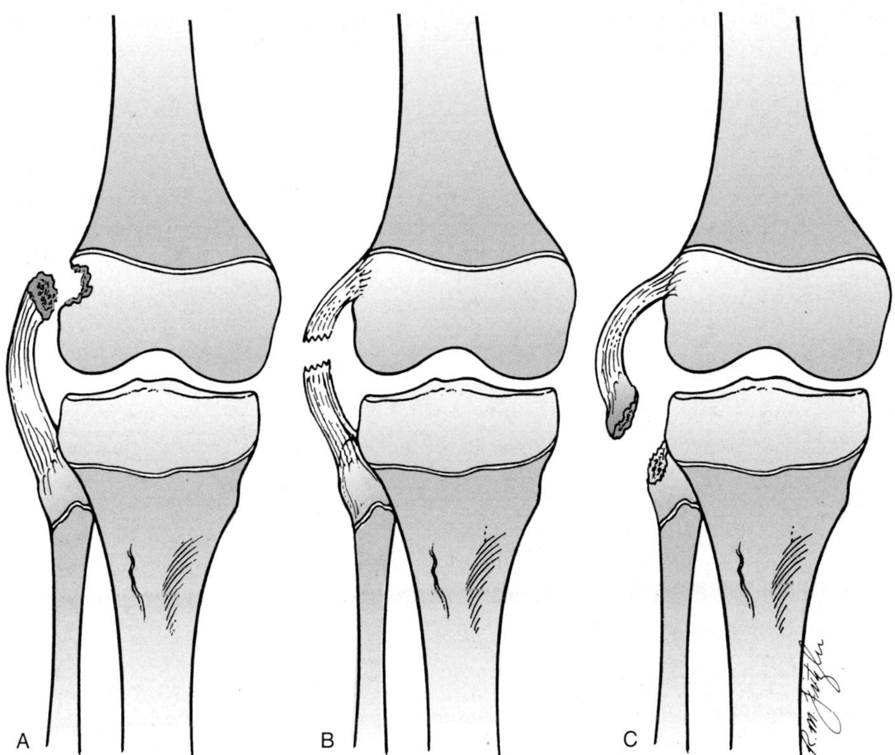

FIGURE 24-34 LCL injury. **A.** Femoral origin. **B.** Middle portion. **C.** Fibular insertion.

a. Without avulsion of the proximal tibia
b. With avulsion of the proximal tibia

Finally, the instability of the knee joint caused by the ligament disruption is classified as follows[139,272]:

A. One-plane instability (simple or straight)
  1. One-plane medial
  2. One-plane lateral
  3. One-plane posterior
  4. One-plane anterior
B. Rotary instability
  1. Anteromedial
  2. Anterolateral
    a. In flexion
    b. Approaching extension
  3. Posterolateral
  4. Posteromedial
C. Combined instability
  1. Anterolateral–posterolateral
  2. Anterolateral–anteromedial
  3. Anteromedial–posteromedial

Using this classification, one-plane medial instability, for example, means that the tibia moves abnormally away from the femur on the medial side. In anteromedial rotary instability, the tibia rotates anteriorly and externally and moves away from the femur on the medial side. The classification becomes more complex as more significant ligamentous injuries involving more anatomic locations are included, but determining the type of instability resulting from the injury is helpful in planning treatment.

Surgical and Applied Anatomy

The MCL and LCL of the knee originate from the distal femoral epiphysis and insert into the proximal tibial and fibular epiphyses, except for the superficial portion of the MCL, which inserts into the proximal tibial metaphysis distal to the physis (Fig. 24-35). In children, these ligaments are stronger than the physes, and significant tensile stresses usually produce epiphyseal or physeal fractures rather than ligamentous injury. The ACL originates from the posterolateral intercondylar notch and

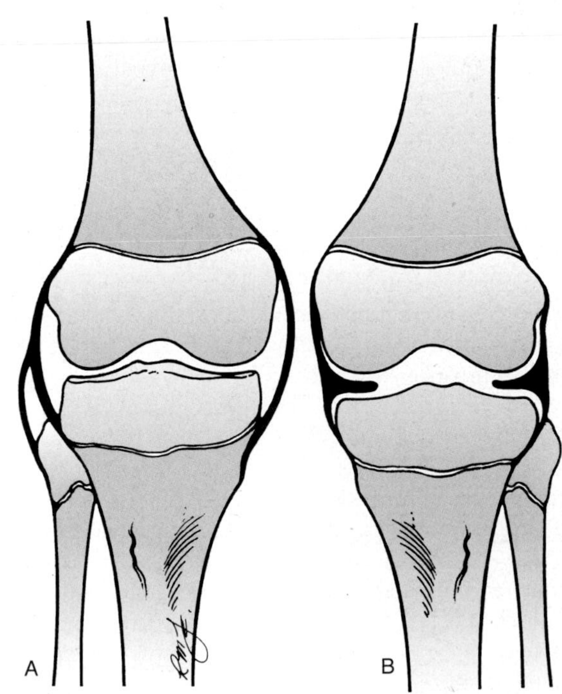

FIGURE 24-35 Anatomy of medial and collateral ligaments of the knee in the adolescent. **A.** Superficial origins and insertions. **B.** Capsular and meniscal attachments.

inserts into the tibia slightly anterior to the intercondylar eminence. The PCL originates from the posteromedial aspect of the intercondylar notch and attaches on the posterior aspect of the proximal tibial epiphysis. The ACL in children has collagen fibers continuous with the perichondrium of the tibial epiphyseal cartilage; in adults, the ligament inserts directly into the proximal tibia by way of Sharpey's fibers. This anatomic difference probably accounts for the fact that fracture of the anterior tibial spine occurs more frequently in children than does ACL injury.

Current Treatment Options

Isolated collateral ligament injuries are usually successfully treated with bracing and rehabilitation.

Controversy exists regarding the management of ACL injuries in patients with open physes. Nonoperative management of partial tears may be successful in some patients.[179] However, nonoperative management of complete tears in skeletally immature patients generally has a poor prognosis with recurrent instability leading to further meniscal and chondral injury, which has implications in terms of development of degenerative joint disease.[11,115,147,209,220,222,244] Graf et al.,[115] Mizuta et al.,[222] and Janarv et al.[147] have reported instability symptoms, subsequent meniscal tears, decreased activity level, and need for ACL reconstruction in the majority of skeletally immature patients treated nonoperatively in series of 8, 18, and 23 patients, respectively. Similarly, when comparing the results of operative versus nonoperative management of complete ACL injuries in adolescents, McCarroll et al.[209] and Pressman et al.[244] found that those managed by ACL reconstruction had less instability, higher activity and return to sport levels, and lower rates of subsequent reinjury and meniscal tears.

Conventional surgical reconstruction techniques risk potential iatrogenic growth disturbance due to physeal violation. Cases of growth disturbance have been reported in animal models[86,121,136] and clinical series.[180,182,192] Animal models have demonstrated mixed results regarding growth disturbances from soft tissue grafts across the physes. In a canine model with iliotibial band grafts through 5/32 inch tunnels, Stadelmeier et al.[277] found no evidence of growth arrest in the four animals with soft tissue graft across the physis, whereas the four animals with drill holes and no graft demonstrated physeal arrest. In a sheep model of transphyseal reconstruction, Seil et al.[262] did not find clinically relevant growth disturbances despite consistent physeal damage. In a rabbit model using a semitendinosis graft through 2-mm tunnels, Guzzanti et al.[121] did have cases of growth disturbance; however, these were not common: 5% shortening (1/21) and 10% distal femoral valgus deformity (2/21). Examining the effect of a tensioned soft tissue graft across the physis, Edwards et al.[86] found a substantial rate of deformity. In a canine model with iliotibial band graft tensioned to 80 N, these investigators found significant increases, compared to the nonoperated control limb, in distal femoral valgus deformity and proximal tibial varus deformity despite no evidence of a bony bar.[86] Similarly, Houle et al.[136] reported growth disturbance after a tensioned tendon graft in a bone tunnel across the rabbit physis.

Clinical reports of growth deformity after ACL reconstruction are unusual. Lipscomb and Anderson[192] reported one case of 20 mm shortening in a series of 24 skeletally immature patients reconstructed with transphyseal semitendinosis and gracilis grafts. This was associated with staple graft fixation across the physis. Koman and Sanders[182] reported a case of distal femoral valgus deformity requiring osteotomy and contralateral epiphyseodesis after transphyseal reconstruction with a doubled semitendinosis graft. This case was also associated with fixation across the distal femoral physis. Kocher et al.[180] reported an additional 15 cases of growth disturbances gleaned from a questionnaire of expert experience, including 8 cases of distal femoral valgus deformity with an arrest of the lateral distal femoral physis, 3 cases of tibial recurvatum with an arrest of the tibial tubercle apophysis, 2 cases of genu valgum without arrest due to a lateral extra-articular tether, and 2 cases of leg-length discrepancy (one shortening and one overgrowth). Associated factors included fixation hardware across the lateral distal femoral physis in three cases, bone plugs of a patellar tendon graft across the distal femoral physis in three cases, large (12-mm) tunnels in two cases, lateral extra-articular tenodesis in two cases, fixation hardware across the tibial tubercle apophysis in two cases, over-the-top femoral position in one case, and suturing near the tibial tubercle apophysis in one case.[180]

Surgical techniques to address ACL insufficiency in skeletally immature patients include primary repair, extra-articular tenodesis, transphyseal reconstruction, partial transphyseal reconstruction, and physeal sparing reconstruction. Primary ligament repair[61,92] and extra-articular tenodesis alone[115,209] have had poor results in children and adolescents, similar to adults. Transphyseal reconstructions with tunnels that violate both the distal femoral and proximal tibial physes have been performed with hamstrings autograft, patellar tendon autograft, and allograft tissue.[11,181,191,209] Partial transphyseal reconstructions violate only one physis with a tunnel through the proximal tibial physis and over-the-top positioning on the femur or a tunnel through the distal femoral physis with an epiphyseal tunnel in the tibia.[17,44,123] A variety of physeal-sparing reconstructions have been described to avoid tunnels across either the distal femoral or proximal tibial physis.[14,52,77,122,138,162,171,172,218,293]

In prepubescent patients, physeal sparing techniques have been described that utilize hamstrings tendons under the intermeniscal ligament and over-the-top on the femur, through all-epiphyseal femoral and tibial tunnels, and with a femoral epiphyseal staple.[14,52,77,122,162,218,238,293] In adolescent patients with growth remaining, transphyseal reconstructions have been performed with hamstrings autograft, patellar tendon autograft, quadriceps tendon autograft, and allograft tissue.[11,20,24,85,104,109,110,205,209,210,266,270,278,301] In addition, partial transphyseal reconstructions have been described with a tunnel through the proximal tibial physis and over-the-top positioning on the femur or a tunnel through the distal femoral physis with an epiphyseal tunnel in the tibia.[17,44,123,193]

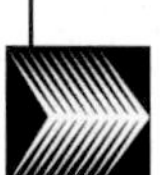

AUTHORS' PREFERRED METHOD OF TREATMENT

Medial Collateral Ligament

Isolated grade I or II sprains of the MCL are treated with crutches or a hinged knee brace for 1 to 3 weeks, depending on resolution of symptoms. Return to athletic activities is allowed when a full, painless range of motion is achieved and the patient can run and cut without pain. Isolated complete (grade III) disruption of the MCL can be treated with 6 weeks of immobilization in a hinged knee brace followed by rehabilitation of the quadriceps muscles and knee motion provided this is an isolated injury. The physician must ensure that there is no associated injury to the ACL before using nonoperative treatment for a grade III MCL injury. Grade III disruptions of the MCL in adolescents associated with injury of the ACL are usually treated with ACL reconstruction without formal MCL repair. The MCL is protected with a hinged knee brace and allowed to heal.

Anterior Cruciate Ligament

A torn ACL does not constitute a surgical emergency, despite the image projected by celebrity athletes and their urgent care. A frank discussion must be held with the parents and the patient concerning future vocation, sport demands, treatment options, outcomes, and risks involved with return to current sport activity. The orthopaedic surgeon must assume the role of a "knee counselor," particularly with patients with a history of chronic knee abuse. All treatment algorithms are based on an accurate and complete diagnosis, which is achieved by clinical, imaging, and, if necessary, arthroscopic means. The treatment goal is a functional knee without progressive intra-articular damage or predisposition to premature osteoarthrosis.

All skeletally immature patients are not the same. Some have a tremendous amount of growth remaining, while others are essentially done growing. The consequences of growth disturbance in the former group would be severe, requiring osteotomy and/or limb lengthening. However, the consequences of growth disturbance in the latter group would be minimal. When treating a skeletally immature athlete with an ACL injury, it is important to know their chronologic age, their skeletal age, and their physiologic age. Skeletal age can be determined from an anteroposterior radiograph of the left hand and wrist per the atlas of Greulich and Pyle.[119] Alternatively, skeletal age can be estimated from knee radiographs per the atlas of Pyle and Hoerr.[245] Physiologic age is established using the Tanner staging system (Table 24-2).[289] In the office, the patient can be informally staged by questioning. In the operating room, after the induction of anesthesia, Tanner staging can be confirmed. The vast majority of ACL injuries in skeletally immature patients occur in adolescents. The management of these injuries in preadolescent children is particularly vexing, given the poor prognosis with nonoperative management, the substantial growth remaining, and the consequences of potential growth disturbance.

Nonsurgical treatment does not indicate nontreatment. The goal of this program is defined from the outset: it is a temporizing measure until the patient becomes mature enough for an adult type ACL reconstruction, or it is the definitive choice for a patient willing to accept the functional limitations. The author uses a three-phase approach. Phase one begins shortly after injury and lasts 7 to 10 days. Brief immobilization (3 to 5 days) with a knee immobilizer for comfort is followed by daily out-of-brace exercises with active knee flexion and passive knee extension. Ambulation is with crutch-protected partial weight bearing. During this time, the author reinforces patient education on the consequences of imprudent return to high-level sports. Phase two focuses on rehabilitation of the lower extremity and lasts

TABLE 24-2 Tanner Staging Classification of Secondary Sexual Characteristics

Tanner Stage		Male	Female
Stage 1 (Prepubertal)	**Growth** **Development**	5–6 cm/yr Testes <4 mLor <2.5 cm No pubic hair	5–6 cm/yr No breast development No pubic hair
Stage 2	**Growth** **Development**	5–6 cm/yr Testes 4 mL or 2.5–3.2 cm Minimal pubic hair at base of penis	7–8 cm/yr Breast buds Minimal pubic hair on labia
Stage 3	**Growth** **Development**	7–8 cm/yr Testes 12 mL or 3.6 cm. Pubic hair over pubis Voice changes Muscle mass increases	8 cm/yr Elevation of breast; areolae enlarge Pubic hair of mons pubis Axillary hair Acne
Stage 4	**Growth** **Development**	10 cm/yr Testes 4.1–4.5 cm Pubic hair as adult Axillary hair Acne	7 cm/yr Areolae enlarge Pubic hair as adult
Stage 5	**Growth** **Development**	No growth Testes as adult Pubic hair as adult Facial hair as adult Mature physique	No growth Adult breast contour Pubic hair as adult
Other		Peak height velocity: 13.5 years	Adrenarche: 6–8 years Menarche: 12.7 years Peak height velocity: 11.5 years

approximately 6 weeks. Emphasis is placed on restoration of full knee motion, flexibility, strength, and endurance with particular attention to regaining the normal quadriceps/hamstring strength ratio. As the ratio is normalized, crutch use is decreased and then eliminated. The role of functional bracing has not been defined in children and issues of fit, size, and cost need to be considered. Phase three continues the rehabilitation, incorporates the use of a functional brace for sports, and allows return to low- and moderate-demand sports when quadriceps and hamstring strength and endurance are equal to those of the opposite, noninjured side as determined by isokinetic testing at functional speeds (>260 degrees/second). In the final part of this phase, sports readiness tasks are done at less than full speed. Monthly follow-up evaluates program compliance and rules out any further knee changes in function. Compliance with a nonoperative program designed to be a temporizing measure often is quite difficult for an emerging athlete who is surrounded by peer, coaching, and, often, parental pressures to return to high-demand sports.

The author's algorithm to ACL reconstruction in the skeletally immature patient is based on physiologic age (Fig. 24-36). In prepubescent patients, the author performs a physeal-sparing, combined intra-articular and extra-articular reconstruction utilizing autogenous iliotibial band.[171,172] In adolescent patients with significant growth remaining, the author performs transphyseal ACL reconstruction with autogenous hamstrings tendons with fixation away from the physes.[181] In older adolescent patients approaching skeletal maturity, the author performs conventional adult ACL reconstruction with interference screw fixation using either autogenous central third patellar tendon or autogenous hamstrings.

In skeletally immature patients as in adult patients, acute ACL reconstruction is not performed within the first 3 weeks after injury to minimize the risk of arthrofibrosis. Prereconstructive rehabilitation is performed to regain range of motion, decrease swelling, and resolve the reflex inhibition of the quadriceps. ACL reconstruction may be staged in some cases if there is a displaced, bucket-handle tear of the meniscus that requires extensive repair in order to protect the meniscal repair from the early mobilization prescribed by ACL reconstruction. Skeletally immature patients must be emotionally mature enough to actively participate in the extensive rehabilitation required after ACL reconstruction.

Prepubescent Patient: Physeal-Sparing Anterior Cruciate Ligament Reconstruction

In the prepubescent patient with a complete ACL tear without concurrent chondral or repairable meniscal injury, the author first attempts nonreconstructive treatment with a program of rehabilitation, functional bracing, and return to non-high-risk activities. Although the results of nonreconstructive treatment are generally poor with subsequent functional instability and risk of injury to meniscal and articular cartilage, surgical reconstruction poses the risk of growth disturbance. Furthermore, some patients are able to cope with their ACL insufficiency or modify their activities, allowing for further growth and aging such that an adolescent-type reconstruction can be performed with transphyseal hamstrings tendons in a more anatomic manner.

For those prepubescent patients with concurrent chondral or repairable meniscal injury or those with functional instability after nonreconstructive treatment, the author performs a physeal-sparing, combined intra-articular and extra-articular reconstruction utilizing autogenous iliotibial band (Fig. 24-37).[171,172] This procedure is a modification of the combined intra-articular and extra-articular reconstruction described by MacIntosh and Darby.[198] The author's rationale for utilization of this technique is to provide knee stability and improve function in prepubescent skeletally immature patients with complete intrasubstance ACL injuries while

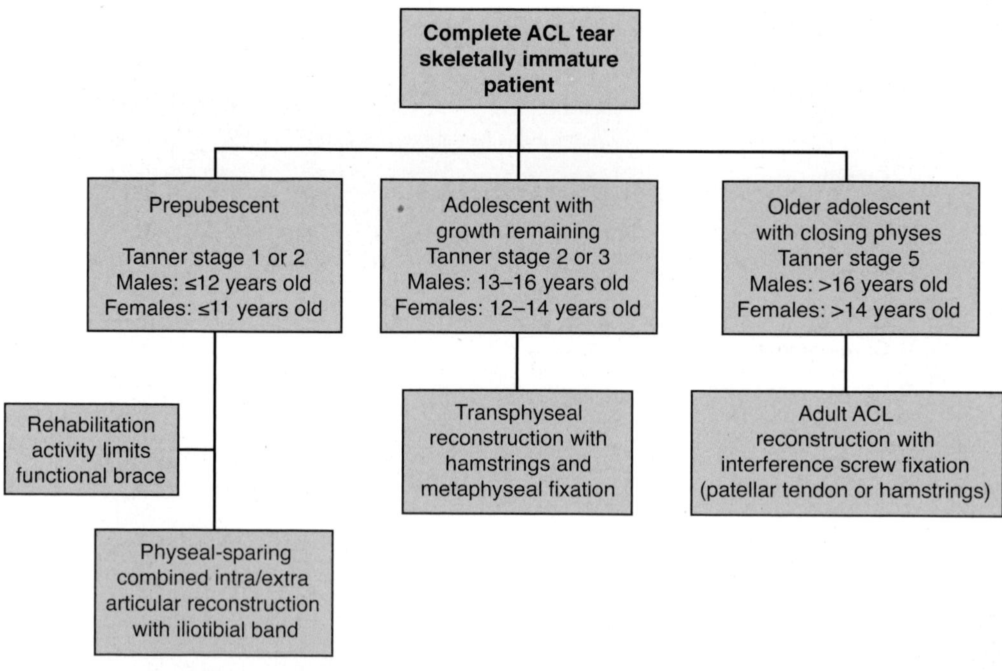

FIGURE 24-36 Algorithm for ACL reconstruction in skeletally immature patients.

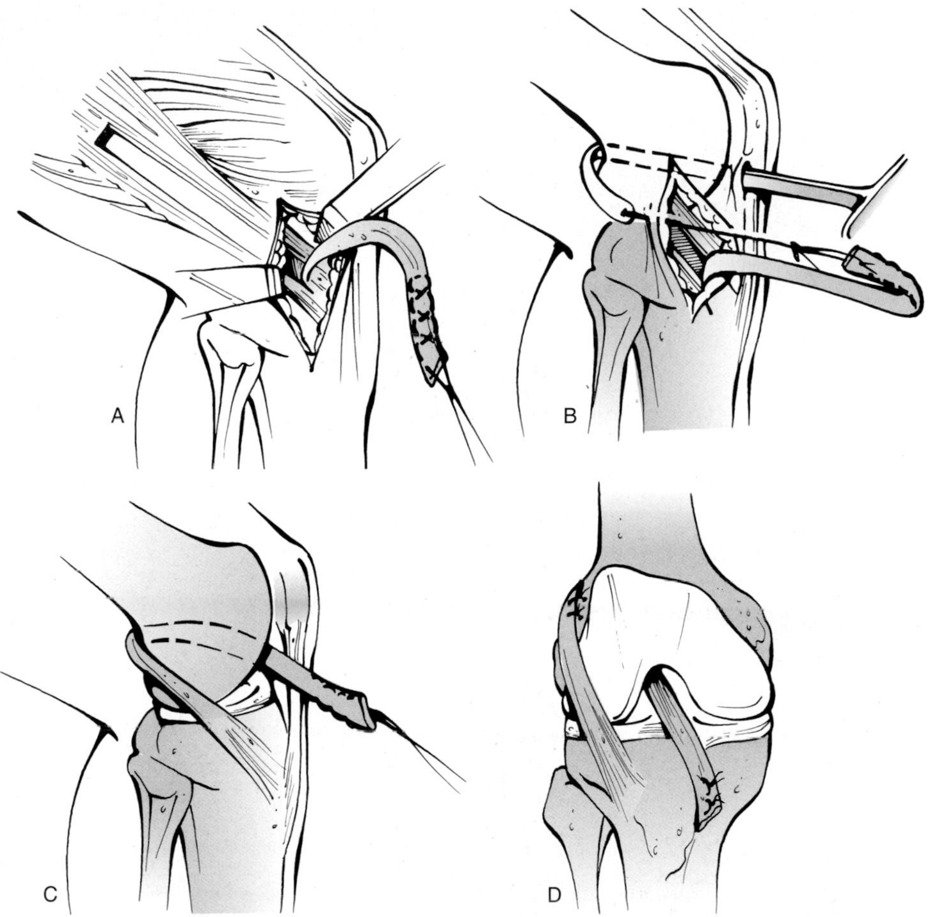

FIGURE 24-37 Physeal-sparing, combined intra-articular and extra-articular reconstruction utilizing autogenous iliotibial band for prepubescents. **A.** The iliotibial band graft is harvested free proximally and left attached to the Gerdy tubercle distally. **B.** The graft is brought through the knee in the over-the-top position posteriorly. **C.** The graft is brought through the knee and under the intermeniscal ligament anteriorly. **D.** Resulting intra-articular and extra-articular reconstruction.

avoiding the risk of iatrogenic growth disturbance by violating the distal femoral and/or proximal tibial physes. In the author's opinion, the consequences of potential iatrogenic growth disturbance caused by transphyseal reconstruction in these young patients is prohibitive. Recognizing that this reconstruction is nonanatomic, the author counsels patients and families that they may require revision reconstruction if they develop recurrent instability, but that this procedure may temporize for further growth such that they may then undergo a more conventional reconstruction with drill holes.

The procedure is performed under general anesthesia as an overnight observation procedure. Local anesthesia with sedation may not be reliable in prepubescent children with the potential for a paradoxical effect of sedation. The child is positioned supine on the operating table with a pneumatic tourniquet about the upper thigh which is used routinely. Examination under anesthesia is performed to confirm ACL insufficiency.

First, the iliotibial band graft is obtained. An incision of approximately 6 cm is made obliquely from the lateral joint line to the superior border of the iliotibial band (Fig. 24-38A). Proximally, the iliotibial band is separated from subcutaneous tissue using an periosteal elevator under the skin of the lateral thigh. The anterior and posterior borders of the iliotibial band are incised and the incisions carried proximally under the skin using curved meniscotomes (see Fig. 24-38A). The iliotibial band is detached proximally under the skin using a curved meniscotome or an open tendon stripper. Alternatively, a counterincision can be made at the upper thigh to release the tendon. The iliotibial band is left attached distally at the Gerdy tubercle. Dissection is performed distally to separate the iliotibial band from the joint capsule and from the lateral patellar retinaculum (Fig. 24-38B). The free proximal end of the iliotibial band is then tubularized with a no. 5 ethibond whip stitch.

Arthroscopy of the knee is then performed through standard anterolateral viewing and anteromedial working portals. Management of meniscal injury or chondral injury is performed if present. The ACL remnant is excised. The over-the-top position on the femur and the over-the-front position under the intermeniscal ligament are identified. Minimal notchplasty is performed to avoid iatrogenic injury to the perichondrial ring of the distal femoral physis which is in very close proximity to the over-the-top position.[32] The free end of the iliotibial band graft is brought through the over-the-top position using a full-length clamp (Fig. 24-38C) or a two-incision rear-entry guide (see Fig. 24-37) and out the anteromedial portal (Fig. 24-38D).

A second incision of approximately 4.5 cm is made over the proximal medial tibia in the region of the pes anserinus insertion. Dissection is carried through the subcutaneous tissue to the periosteum. A curved clamp is placed from this incision into the joint under the intermeniscal ligament (Fig. 24-38E). A small groove is made in the anteromedial proximal tibial epiphysis under the intermeniscal ligament using a curved rat-tail rasp to bring the tibial graft placement more posterior. The free end of the graft is then brought through the joint (Fig. 24-38F), under the intermeniscal ligament in

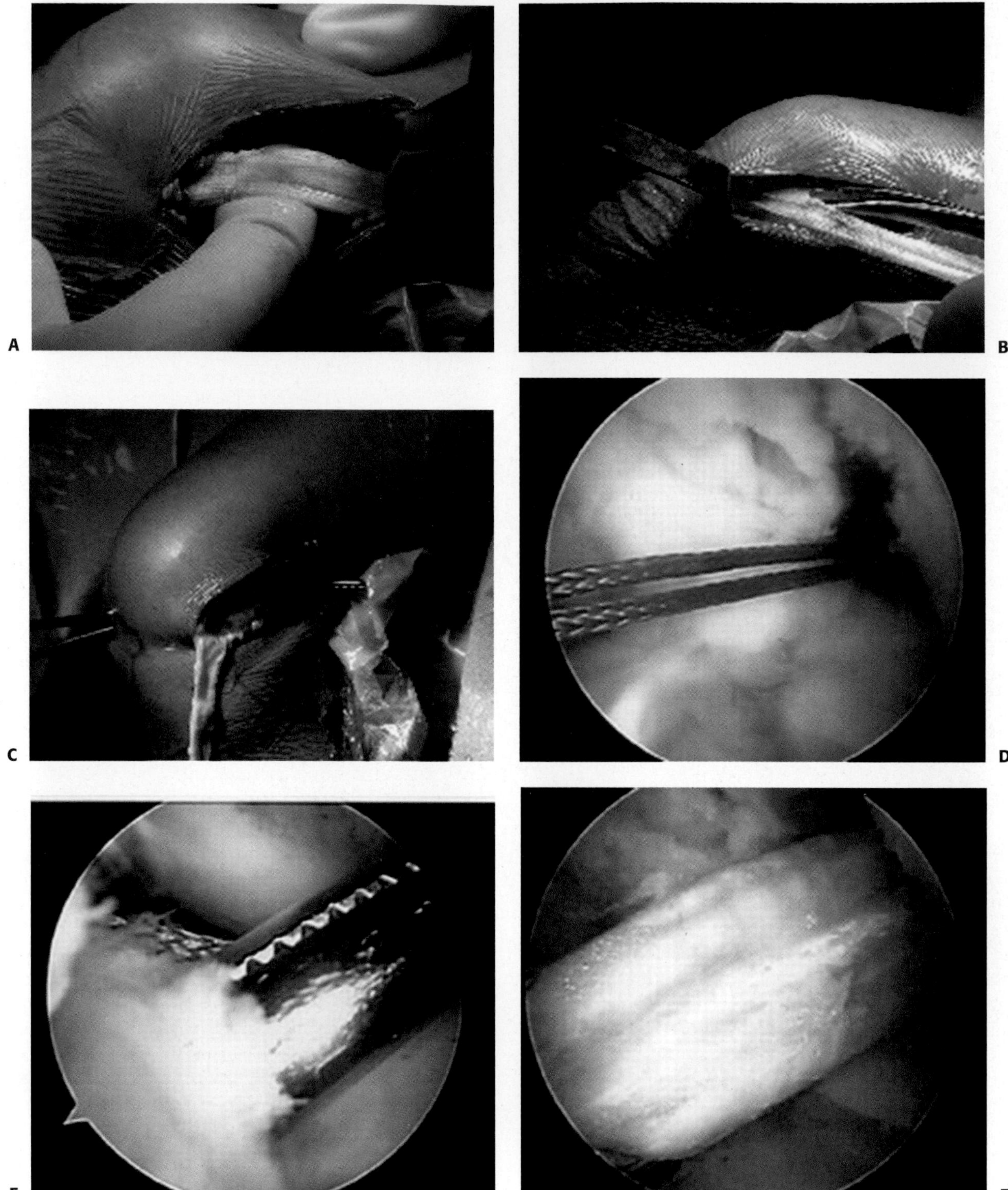

FIGURE 24-38 Technique of physeal sparing combined intra-articular and extra-articular ACL reconstruction using iliotibial band. **A.** The iliotibial band is harvested through an oblique lateral knee incision. **B.** The iliotibial band graft is detached proximally, left attached distally, and dissected free from the lateral patellar retinaculum. **C.** The iliotibial band graft is brought through the knee using a full-length clamp placed from the anteromedial portal through the over-the-top position into the lateral incision. **D.** The graft is then brought through the over-the-top position. **E.** A clamp is placed from a proximal medial leg incision under the intermeniscal ligament. A groove is made in the anteromedial tibial epiphysis using a rasp. **F.** The graft is brought through the knee in the over-the-top position and under the intermeniscal ligament. *(continues)*

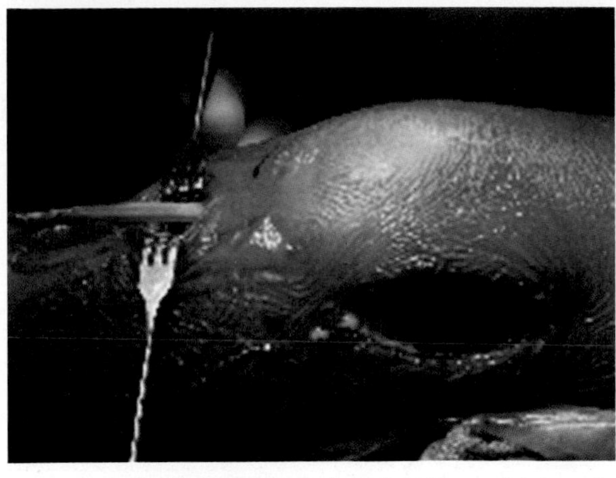

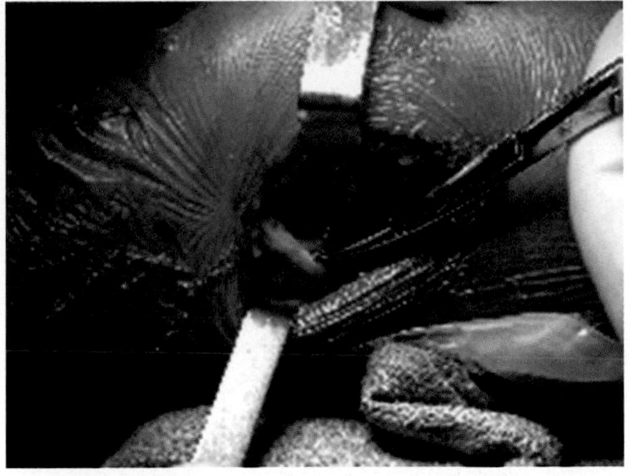

FIGURE 24-38 *(continued)* **G.** The graft is brought out the proximal medial leg incision. **H.** It is sutured to the intermuscular septum and periosteum of the lateral femoral condyle through the lateral knee incision, and it is sutured in a trough to the periosteum of the proximal medial tibial metaphysis.

the anteromedial epiphyseal groove, and out the medial tibial incision (Fig. 24-38G). The graft is fixed on the femoral side through the lateral incision with the knee at 90 degrees flexion and 15 degrees external rotation using mattress sutures to the lateral femoral condyle at the insertion of the lateral intermuscular septum to effect an extra-articular reconstruction (Fig. 24-38H). The tibial side is then fixed through the medial incision with the knee flexed 20 degrees and tension applied to the graft. A periosteal incision is made distal to the proximal tibial physis as checked with fluoroscopic imaging. A trough is made in the proximal tibial medial metaphyseal cortex and the graft is sutured to the periosteum at the rough margins with mattress sutures (see Fig. 24-37).

Postoperatively, the patient is maintained touchdown weight bearing for 6 weeks. Range of motion is limited from 0 to 90 degrees for the first 2 weeks, followed by progressive full range of motion. A continuous passive motion from 0 to 90 degrees and cryotherapy are used for 2 weeks postoperatively. A protective postoperative brace is used for 6 weeks.

Skeletally Immature Adolescent Patient: Transphyseal Anterior Cruciate Ligament Reconstruction

For adolescent patients with growth remaining who have a complete ACL tear, the author does not advocate initial nonreconstructive treatment since the risk of functional instability with injury to the meniscal and articular cartilage is high, the risk and consequences of growth disturbance from ACL reconstruction are less, and the author's transphyseal technique is an anatomic reconstruction. In these patients, the author performs transphyseal ACL reconstruction with autogenous hamstrings tendons with fixation away from the physes.[181]

The procedure is performed under general anesthesia as an overnight observation procedure. Local anesthesia with sedation may be performed in the emotionally mature adolescent child. The patient is positioned supine on the operating table with a pneumatic tourniquet about the upper thigh which is not used routinely. Examination under anesthesia is performed to confirm ACL insufficiency.

First, the hamstrings tendons are harvested. If the diagnosis is in doubt, arthroscopy can be performed first to confirm ACL tear. A 4-cm incision is made over the palpable pes anserinus tendons on the medial side of the upper tibia (Fig. 24-39A). Dissection is carried through skin to the sartorius fascia. Care is taken to protect superficial sensory nerves. The sartorius tendon is incised longitudinally and the gracilis and semitendinosis tendons are identified. The tendons are dissected free distally and their free ends whip-stitched with no. 2 or no. 5 ethibond suture. They are dissected proximally using sharp and blunt dissection. Fibrous bands to the medial head of gastrocnemius should be sought and released. A closed tendon stripper is used to dissect the tendons free proximally. Alternatively, the tendons can be left attached distally, and an open tendon stripper used to release the tendons proximally. The tendons are taken to the back table, where excess muscle is removed and the remaining ends are whip-stitched with no. 2 or no. 5 ethibond sutures. The tendons are folded over a closed loop endobutton. The graft diameter is sized and the graft is placed under tension.

Arthroscopy of the knee is then performed through standard anterolateral viewing and anteromedial working portals. Management of meniscal injury or chondral injury is performed if present. The ACL remnant is excised. The over-the-top position on the femur is identified. Minimal notch-plasty is performed to avoid iatrogenic injury to the perichondrial ring of the distal femoral physis, which is in very close proximity to the over-the-top position.[32]

A tibial tunnel guide (set at 55 degrees) is used through the anteromedial portal (Fig. 24-39B). A guidewire is drilled through the hamstrings harvest incision into the posterior aspect of the ACL tibial footprint. The guidewire entry point on the tibia should be kept medial to avoid injury to the tibial tubercle apophysis. The guidewire is reamed with the appropriate diameter reamer. Excess soft tissue at the tibial tunnel is excised to avoid arthrofibrosis. The transtibial over-the-top guide of the appropriate offset to ensure a 1-mm or 2-mm back wall is used to pass the femoral guide pin (Fig. 24-39C). The femoral guide pin is overdrilled with the endobutton reamer. Both are removed in order to use the depth gauge to measure the femoral tunnel length. The guide pin is replaced and brought through the distal lateral thigh. The

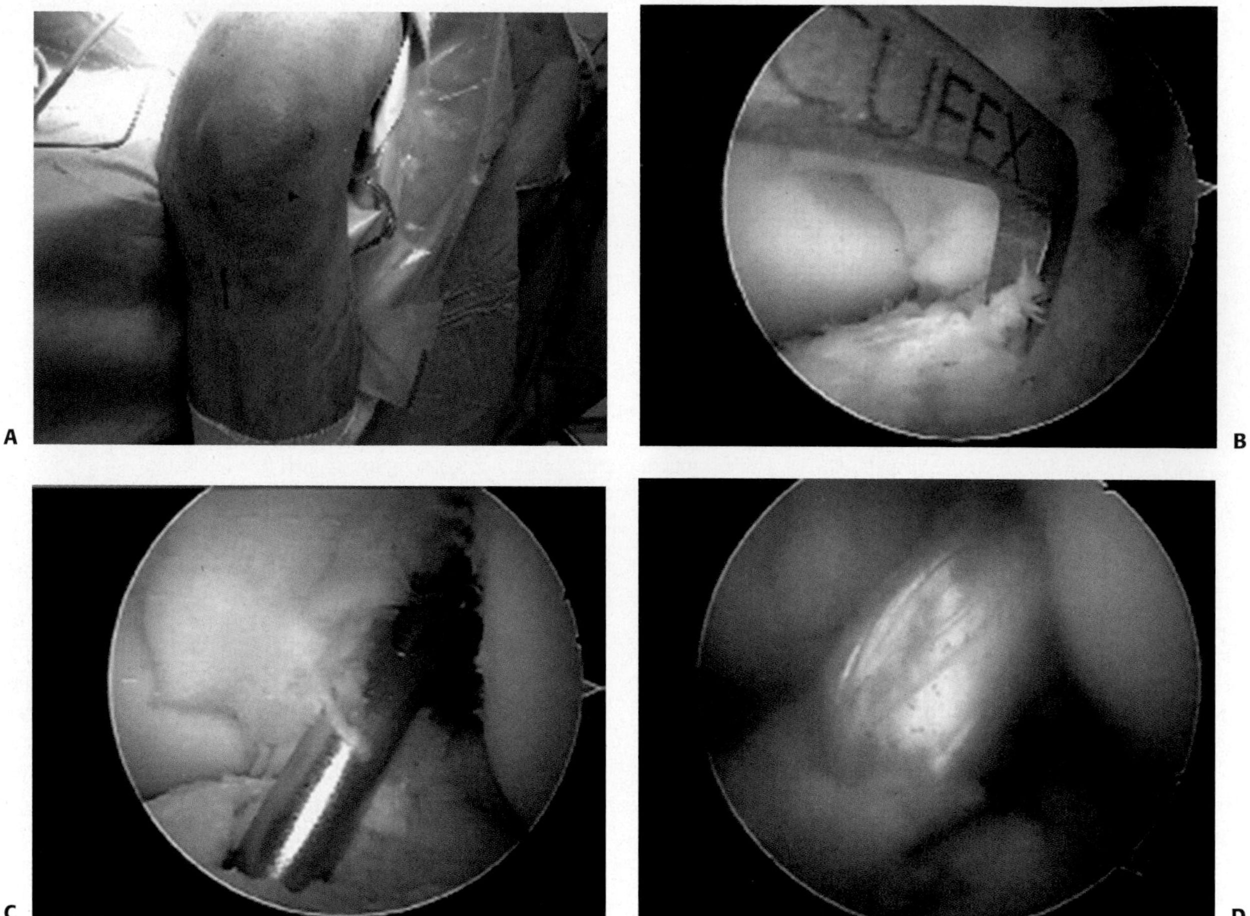

FIGURE 24-39 Transphyseal reconstruction with autogenous hamstrings for adolescents with growth remaining. **A.**The gracilis and semitendinosis tendons are harvested through an incision over the proximal medial tibia. **B.** The tibial guide is used to drill the tibial tunnel. **C.** The transtibial over-the-top offset guide is used to drill the femoral tunnel. **D.** Hamstrings graft after fixation.

femur is reamed to the appropriate depth (femoral tunnel length – endobutton length + 8 mm to flip the endobutton).

The no. 5 ethibond sutures on the endobutton are placed in slot of the guidewire and pulled through the tibial tunnel, through the femoral tunnel, and out the lateral thigh. These are then pulled to bring the endobutton and graft through the tibial tunnel and into the femoral tunnel. One set of sutures is used to "lead" the endobutton, while the other set of sutures is used to "follow." Once the graft is fully seated in the femoral tunnel, the "follow" sutures are pulled to flip the endobutton (Fig. 24-39D). The flip can be palpated in the thigh and tension is applied to the graft to endure no graft slippage. The knee is then extended to ensure no graft impingement. The knee is then cycled approximately 10 times with tension applied to the graft. The graft is fixed on the tibial side with the knee in 20 to 30 degrees of flexion, tension applied to the graft, and a posterior force placed on the tibia. On the tibial side, the graft is either fixed with a soft tissue interference screw if there is adequate tunnel distance (at least 30-mm) below the physis to ensure metaphyseal placement of the screw or with a post and spiked washer. Fluoroscopy can be used to ensure that the fixation is away from the physes. Postoperative radiographs are shown in Figure 24-40.

Postoperatively, the patient is maintained touchdown weightbearing for 2 weeks. Range of motion is limited from 0 to 90 degrees for the first 2 weeks, followed by progressive full range of motion. A continuous passive motion from 0 to 90 degrees and cryotherapy are used for 2 weeks postoperatively. A protective postoperative brace is used for 6 weeks.

Lateral Collateral Ligament

Grade III injuries of the LCL are rare in children. Occasionally, the lateral capsular sign is seen on radiographs obtained for evaluation of knee injury. Most often, the LCL is avulsed from the proximal fibular epiphysis; proximal and midsubstance tears are uncommon. This injury is treated in the same manner as injury to the MCL. For isolated grade III injuries, a 6-week period of immobilization in a hinged knee brace is recommended. If ACL injury is associated with LCL injury, treatment is as described for combined injuries of the MCL and ACL. In young children, the LCL is repaired and the ACL is left untreated. If instability persists as the adolescent nears skeletal maturity, intra-articular reconstruction can be done at that time. In adolescents near skeletal maturity at the time of injury, the author prefers to repair both the ACL and LCL.

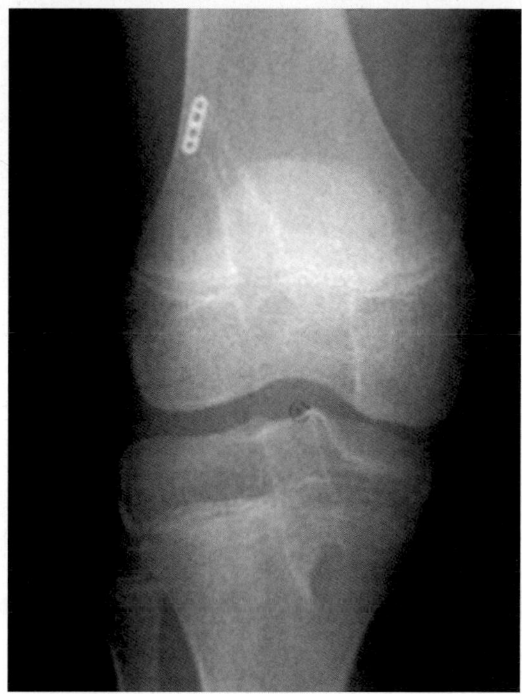
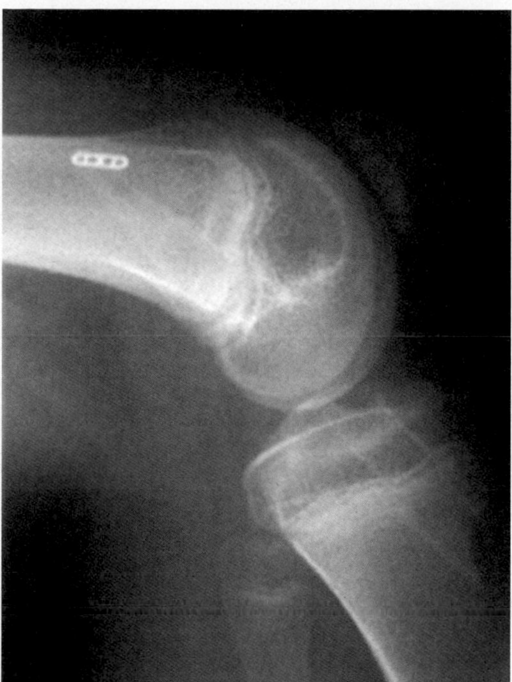

FIGURE 24-40 Transphyseal reconstruction with autogenous hamstrings for adolescents with growth remaining. Postoperative anteroposterior **(A)** and lateral **(B)** radiographs.

Posterior Cruciate Ligament

In general, PCL injuries in children are associated with a bony avulsion.[114,256,292] If nondisplaced, they should be treated with immobilization; if displaced, they should be treated with open reduction and internal fixation.

Isolated grade III injury of the PCL in children and adolescents can be treated with 6 weeks of immobilization in a cast-brace or hinged knee brace. If significant functional symptoms persist in an adolescent, the PCL can be reconstructed at or near skeletal maturity. In a young child with grade III MCL or LCL injury in addition to PCL injury, the collateral ligament can be surgically repaired to convert the multiplane instability to single-plane instability. PCL injury may be associated with ACL injury, primarily in knee dislocations, and surgical intervention usually is appropriate for this combination of injuries, especially in patients nearing skeletal maturity.[60]

Knee Dislocation

Acute dislocations of the knee are uncommon in children because the forces required to produce dislocation are more likely to fracture the distal femoral or proximal tibial epiphysis.[108] Acute knee dislocation usually involves major injuries of associated soft tissues and ligaments and often neurovascular injuries. Injuries typically occur in older skeletally mature adolescents from high-energy trauma, such as motor vehicle injuries, pedestrian versus motor vehicle injury, bicycle versus motor vehicle injury, trampoline injuries, and high-energy contact sports.

Adequate follow-up studies of acute knee dislocations in children younger than 10 years of age are few,[76] and most information has been obtained from reports of knee dislocations in adults. Because of the potential for associated vascular injury, acute knee dislocations in children may be emergent situations. The dislocation causes obvious deformity about the knee. With anterior dislocation, the tibia is prominent in an abnormal anterior position (Fig. 24-41). With posterior dislocation, the femoral condyles are abnormally prominent anteriorly.

After the dislocation is reduced, the stability of the knee should be evaluated with gentle stress testing. For isolated anterior or posterior dislocations, the integrity of the collateral ligaments should be carefully evaluated. Some knees may spontaneously reduce after dislocation or reduce with manipulation of the leg for transport.

The neurovascular status of the extremity should be carefully evaluated both before and after reduction, especially the dorsalis pedis and posterior tibial pulses and peroneal nerve function. Any abnormal vascular findings, either before or after reduction, require arteriography.[67,76,108,116,159] Arteriography is unnecessary when pulses are normal before and after reduction; however, the vascular status should be carefully monitored for 48 to 72 hours after reduction. Vascular status may also be assessed with ultrasonography or MR angiography. Abnormalities in the sensory or motor function of the foot and distribution of the peroneal nerve function should be noted. Peroneal nerve injury has been reported in 16% to 40% of cases.[67,76,108,116,159] MRI is usually performed to assess the integrity of the cruciate and collateral ligaments, the posterolateral and posteromedial corners, the menisci, and the articular surfaces.

Knee dislocation usually occurs with disruption of both cruciate ligaments. With direct anterior or posterior dislocation, the collateral ligaments and the soft tissues may be retained because the femoral condyles are stripped out of their capsular and collateral ligament attachments and when reduced slip back inside them. Associated medial displace-

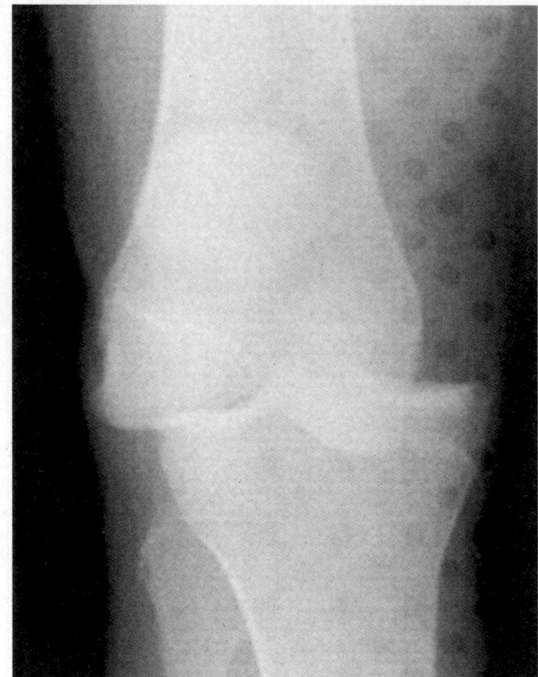
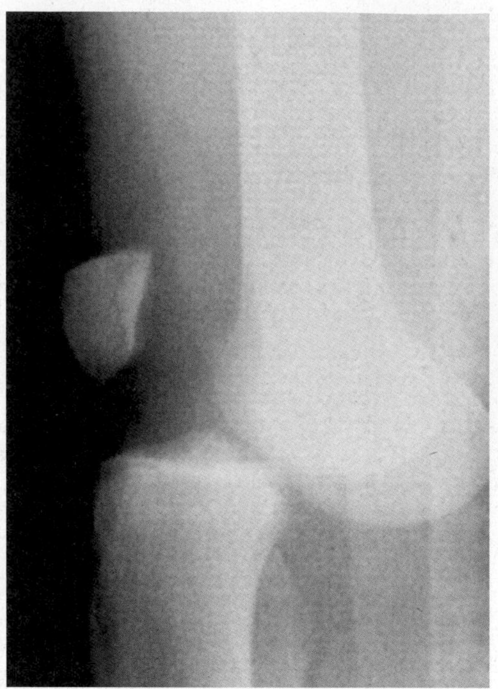

FIGURE 24-41 Dislocation of the knee. **A,B.** Anteromedial dislocation of the knee in a 14-year-old girl.

ment is often accompanied by LCL disruption. Associated lateral displacement is often accompanied by MCL disruption. Knee dislocations in adolescents have been associated with tibial spine fractures, osteochondral fractures of the femur or tibia, meniscal injuries, and peroneal nerve injuries.[67]

Treatment of knee dislocations includes both acute and reconstructive management. Acutely, the knee is reduced under anesthesia. The knee should then be examined to assess the ligamentous injuries. The neurovascular status of the extremity is carefully assessed pre- and postreduction. Vascular imaging is performed if indicated. Arterial exploration and repair or bypass grafting is performed by a vascular surgeon if indicated. If emergent vascular repair is performed, fasciotomies are usually also performed however ligamentous reconstruction is typically delayed. An MRI is obtained to document the injured structures. The knee is braced with protected weight bearing and limited motion.

Reconstruction is delayed approximately 2 to 3 weeks after injury. Primary ligament repairs become more difficult after this period of time because of scarring and lack of definition of tissues. Reconstructions may be staged or at one setting. Surgery often combines arthroscopic and open techniques. General principles include ligament repair for collateral ligament injuries, ligament repair for cruciate ligament avulsions, ligament reconstruction for midsubstance cruciate ligament injuries, and meniscal repair. Allograft tissue is often used because of the multiligamentous nature of the injury. PCL reconstruction can be performed with tibial inlay techniques or arthroscopic techniques with a tibial tunnel and one or two femoral tunnels. Medially, the MCL can be primarily repaired or reattached if avulsed. The medial meniscus may be torn if the MCL is torn in its midsubstance. Laterally, the LCL, popliteofibular ligament, popliteus, and posterolateral capsule may need to be repaired. The peroneal nerve should be decompressed and protected during repair.

Prolonged immobilization should be avoided because of the substantial risk of stiffness after knee dislocation surgery. Limited motion in a hinged knee brace and protected weight bearing are utilized, followed by mobilization and strengthening.

Pearls and Pitfalls

- With nonoperative treatment of complete ACL tears in children and adolescents, sufficient counseling must be performed so that the patient and the family understand the relative risks and benefits of nonoperative treatment versus ACL reconstruction. Compliance with bracing and activity restriction must be monitored. Careful regular follow-up is necessary to evaluate for instability episodes and further meniscal/chondral injury. Once further meniscal or chondral injury occurs, ACL reconstruction should be advised because of the risk of degenerative joint disease associated with injury episodes.
- Pitfalls to avoid with the physeal-sparing iliotibial band reconstruction in prepubescents include harvesting a short graft insufficient to reach the medial tibial incision, difficulty passing the graft through the posterior joint capsule, and difficulty passing the graft under the intermeniscal ligament.
- Pitfalls to avoid with the transphyseal hamstrings reconstruction in adolescents with growth remaining include amputation of the hamstring grafts, poor tunnel placement, and graft impingement.
- Based on the 15 cases of growth disturbance after ACL reconstruction in skeletally immature patients reported, the author recommends careful attention to technical details during ACL reconstruction in skeletally immature patients, particularly the avoidance of fixation hardware across the lateral distal femoral epiphyseal plate.[180] Care should also be taken to avoid injury to the vulnerable tibial tubercle apophysis.[173,265] Given the cases of growth disturbances associated with transphyseal placement of patellar tendon graft bone blocks, the author recommends the use of soft tissue grafts. Large tunnels should likely be avoided as likelihood of arrest is associated with greater violation of epiphyseal plate

cross-sectional area. The two cases of genu valgum without arrest associated with lateral extra-articular tenodesis raise additional concerns about the effect of tension on physeal growth. Finally, care should be taken to avoid dissection or notching around the posterolateral aspect of the physis during over-the-top nonphyseal femoral placement to avoid potential injury to the very close perichondrial ring and subsequent deformity.[173]

Prognosis and Complications

The prognosis of nonoperative management of complete tears in skeletally immature patients is generally poor with recurrent instability leading to further meniscal and chondral injury which has implications in terms of development of degenerative joint disease.[11,115,121,147,209,220,222,244]

The prognosis of ACL reconstruction depends on the surgical procedure. Several case series exist regarding ACL reconstruction in skeletally immature patients. However, most series are small and variably report the patients' skeletal age and growth remaining. Primary ligament repair[61,92] and extra-articular tenodesis alone[158,209] have had poor results in children and adolescents, similar to adults. Transphyseal reconstructions with tunnels that violate both the distal femoral and proximal tibial physes have been performed with hamstrings autograft, patellar tendon autograft, and allograft tissue.[11,20,24,85,104,205,209,210,266,270,278,301] These anatomic ACL reconstruction procedures have high success rates as in adult patients; however, there is risk injury to the physis, particularly in prepubescent patients. In a follow-up outcome study of 61 knees in 59 skeletally immature Tanner stage 3 adolescents with growth remaining (mean chronologic age: 14.7 years old, range: 11.6 to 16.9 years old) who underwent transphyseal reconstruction with autogenous hamstrings graft and metaphyseal fixation, a revision rate of 3% with excellent functional outcome, return to competitive sports, and no cases of growth disturbance was found.[181] Partial transphyseal reconstructions violate only one physis with a tunnel through the proximal tibial physis and over-the-top positioning on the femur or a tunnel through the distal femoral physis with an epiphyseal tunnel in the tibia.[17,44,123] These procedures are also near anatomic with good clinical results; however, the potential for growth disturbance exists.

A variety of physeal-sparing reconstructions have been described to avoid tunnels across either the distal femoral or proximal tibial physis.[14,52,77,122,162,218,238,293] In general, these procedures are nonanatomic and have some persistent knee laxity; however, they avoid physeal violation. In a follow-up outcome study of 44 skeletally immature prepubescent children who were Tanner stage 1 or 2 (mean chronologic age: 10.3 years old; range: 3.6–14 years old) who underwent the physeal sparing combined intra-articular and extra-articular ACL reconstruction technique using autogenous iliotibial band that were described above, a revision ACL reconstruction rate of 4.5% with excellent functional outcome, return to competitive sports,

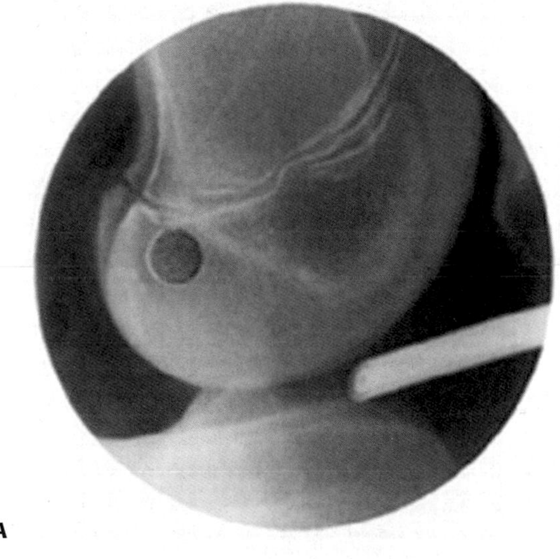
A

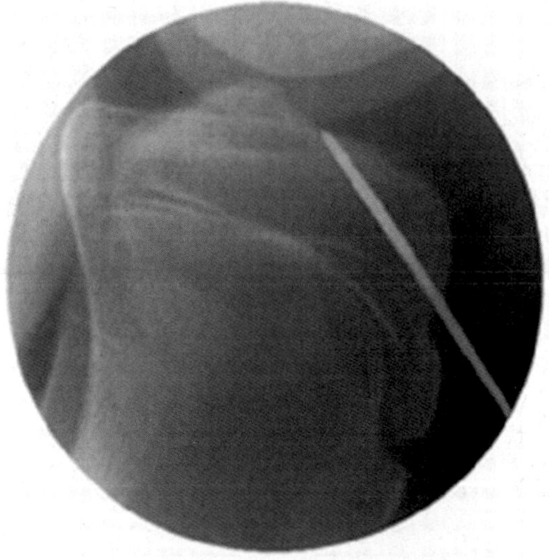
B

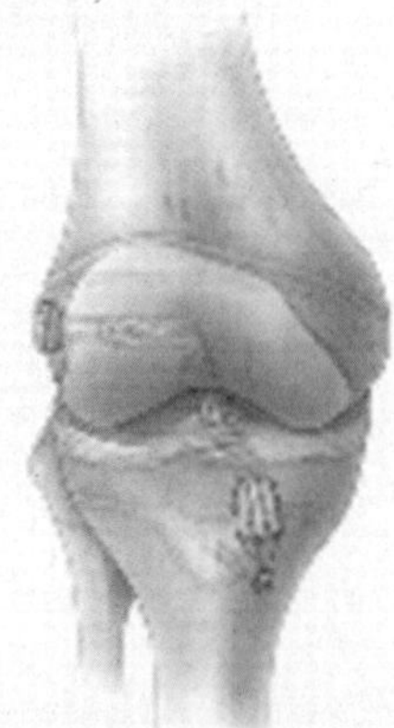
C

FIGURE 24-42 Physeal-sparing epiphyseal ACL reconstruction with autogenous hamstrings for prepubescents with growth remaining. **A.** Femoral tunnel placement within the epiphysis. **B.** Tibial tunnel placement within the epiphysis. **C.** Appearance after epiphyseal graft fixation.

and no cases of growth disturbance was found.[171,172] Anderson[14,15] described a more anatomic physeal-sparing reconstruction in prepubescent children by utilizing carefully placed epiphyseal femoral and tibial tunnels with an autogenous hamstrings graft and epiphyseal fixation (Fig. 24-42). In 12 skeletally immature patients with mean age 13.3 years old (SD: 1.4), he found excellent functional outcome without growth disturbance.[14,15]

Complications after ligament injury in children are similar to adults: arthrofibrosis, persistent instability, unrecognized concomitant injury, infection, graft failure, neurovascular injury, and donor site morbidity. In skeletally immature patients, growth disturbance can occur from iatrogenic physeal injury as previously discussed.

REFERENCES

1. Abdou P, Bauer M. Incidence of meniscal lesions in children. Acta Orthop Scand 1989; 60:710–711.
2. Abrams RC. Meniscus lesions in the knee in young children. J Bone Joint Surg Am 1957;39:194–195.
3. Accadbled F, Cassard X, Sales de Gauzy J, et al. Meniscal tears in children and adolescents: results of operative treatment. J Pediatr Orthop B 2007;16(1):56–60.
4. Adachi N, Ochi M, Uchio Y, et al. Torn discoid lateral meniscus treated using partial central meniscectomy and suture of the peripheral tear. Arthroscopy 2004;20(5): 536–542.
5. Aglietti P, Bertini FA, Buzzi R, et al. Arthroscopic meniscectomy for discoid lateral meniscus in children and adolescence: a 10-year follow-up. Am J Knee Surg 1999;12: 83–87.
6. Ahmed AM, Burke DL. In-vitro measurement of static pressure distribution in synovial joints. Part I: tibial surface of the knee. J Biomech Eng 1983;105:216–225.
7. Ahn JH, Lee SH, Yoo JC, et al. Arthroscopic partial meniscectomy with repair of the peripheral tear for symptomatic discoid lateral meniscus in children: results of minimum 2 years of follow-up. Arthroscopy 2008;24(8):888–898.
8. Ahstrom JP. Osteochondral fracture in the knee joint associated with hypermobility and dislocation of the patella: report of 18 cases. J Bone Joint Surg Am 1965;47: 1491–1502.
9. Aichroth PM. Osteochondral fractures and osteochondritis dissecans in sportsmen's knee injuries. J Bone Joint Surg Br 1977;59:108.
10. Aichroth PM, Patel DV, Marx CI. Congenital discoid lateral meniscus in children: a followup study and evaluation of management. J Bone Joint Surg Br 1991;73:932–939.
11. Aichroth PM, Patel DV, Zorrilla P. The natural history and treatment of rupture of the anterior cruciate ligament in children and adolescents. A prospective review. J Bone Joint Surg Br 2002;84(1):618–619.
12. Albertsson M, Gillquist S. Discoid lateral meniscus: a report of 29 cases. Arthroscopy 1998;4:211–214.
13. Alleyne KR, Galloway MT. Management of osteochondral injuries of the knee. Clin Sports Med 2001;20:343–363.
14. Anderson AF. Transepiphyseal replacement of the anterior cruciate ligament in skeletally immature patients. A preliminary report. J Bone Joint Surg Am 2003;85-A(7): 1255–1263.
15. Anderson AF. Transepiphyseal replacement of the anterior cruciate ligament using quadruple hamstring grafts in skeletally immature patients. J Bone Joint Surg Am 2004; 86-A(Suppl 1 Pt 2):201–209.
16. Anderson AF, Pagnani MJ. Osteochondritis dissecans of the femoral condyles: long-term results of excision of the fragment. Am J Sports Med 1997;25: 830–834.
17. Andrews M, Noyes FR, Barber-Westin SD. Anterior cruciate ligament allograft reconstruction in the skeletally immature athlete. Am J Sports Med 1994;22(1):48–54.
18. Andrish J. The diagnosis and management of meniscus injuries in skeletally immature athlete. Oper Tech Sports Med 1998;6:186–196.
19. Andrish JT. Meniscal injuries in children and adolescents: diagnosis and management. J Am Acad Orthop Surg 1996;4:231–237.
20. Angel KR, Hall DJ. Anterior cruciate ligament injury in children and adolescents. Arthroscopy 1989;5(3):197–200.
21. Appel H. Late results after meniscectomy in the knee joint: a clinical and roentgenologic follow-up investigation. Acta Orthop Scand Suppl 1970;133:1–111.
22. Arnoczky SP, Warren RF. Microvasculature of the human meniscus. Am J Sports Med 1982;2:90–95.
23. Arnoczky SP, Warren RF, Spivak JM. Meniscal repair using an exogenous fibrin clot: an experimental study in dogs. J Bone Joint Surg Am 1988;70:1209–1217.
24. Aronowitz ER, Ganley TJ, Goode JR, et al. Anterior cruciate ligament reconstruction in adolescents with open physes. Am J Sports Med 2000;28(2):168–175.
25. Bailey WH, Blundell GE. An unusual abnormality affecting both knee joints in a child. J Bone Joint Surg Am 1974;56:814–816.
26. Bakalim G, Wilpulla E. Closed treatment of fracture of the tibial spines. Injury 1974; 5:210–212.
27. Bale RS, Banks AJ. Arthroscopically guided Kirschner wire fixation for fractures of the intercondylar eminence of the tibia. J R Coll Surg Edinb1995;40:260–262.
28. Baratz ME, Fu FH, Mentago R. Meniscal tears: the effect of menisectomy and of repair on intraarticular contact areas and stress in the human knee. Am J Sports Med 1986; 14:270–274.
29. Bassett FH. III. Acute dislocation of the patella, osteochondral fractures, and injuries to the extensor mechanism of the knee. Instr Course Lect 1976;25:40–49.
30. Baxter MP, Wiley JJ. Fractures of the tibial spine in children. An evaluation of knee stability. J Bone Joint Surg Br 1988;70B:228–230.
31. Beasley LS, Vidal AF. Traumatic patellar dislocation in children and adolescents: treatment update and literature review. Curr Opin Pediatr 2004;16(1):29–36.
32. Behr CT, Potter HG, Paletta GA Jr. The relationship of the femoral origin of the anterior cruciate ligament and the distal femoral physeal plate in the skeletally immature knee. An anatomic study. Am J Sports Med 2001;29:781–787.
33. Bellier G, Dupont JY, Larrain M, et al. Lateral discoid meniscus in children. Arthroscopy 1989;5:52–56.
34. Bentley G, Biant LC, Carrington RW, et al. A prospective, randomized comparison of autologous chondrocyte implantation versus mosaicplasty for osteochondral defects in the knee. J Bone Joint Surg Br 2003;85(2):223–230.
35. Benz G, Roth H, Zachariou Z. Fractures and cartilage injuries of the knee joint in children. Z Kinderchir 1986;41:219–226.
36. Berg EE. Pediatric tibial eminence fractures: arthroscopic cannulated screw fixation. Arthroscopy 1995;11:328–331.
37. Bergstrom R, Gillquist J, Lysholm J, et al. Arthroscopy of the knee in children. J Pediatr Orthop 1984;4:542–545.
38. Berlet GC, Mascia A, Miniaci A. Treatment of unstable osteochondritis dissecans lesions of the knee using autogenous osteochondral grafts mosaicplasty. Arthroscopy 1999; 15:312–316.
39. Bertin KC, Goble EM. Ligament injuries associated with physeal fractures about the knee. Clin Orthop Relat Res 1983;177:188–195.
40. Betz RR, Longergan R, Patterson R, et al. The percutaneous lateral retinacular release. Orthopaedics 1982;5:57–62.
41. Beyzadeoglu T, Gokce A, Bekler H. Osteochondritis dissecans of the medial femoral condyle associated with malformation of the menisci. Orthopedics 2008;31(5):504.
42. Bhaduri T, Glass A. Meniscectomy in children. Injury 1972;3:176–178.
43. Birk GT, DeLee JC. Osteochondral injuries. Clin Sports Med 2001;20:279–287.
44. Bisson LJ, Wickiewicz T, Levinson M, et al. ACL reconstruction in children with open physes. Orthopedics 1998;21(6):659–663.
45. Bland-Sutton J, ed. Ligaments: Their Nature and Morphology. 2nd ed. London, UK: JK Lewis, 1897.
46. Boden S, Davis D, Dina T, et al. A prospective and blinded investigation of magnetic resonance imaging of the knee: abnormal findings in asymptomatic subjects. Clin Orthop Relat Res 1992;282:177–185.
47. Boger DC, Kingston S. MRI of the normal knee. Am J Knee Surg 1988;1:99–103.
48. Bohndorf K. Imaging of acute injuries of the articular surfaces (chondral, osteochondral, and subchondral fractures). Skeletal Radiol 1999;28:545–560.
49. Bong MR, Romero A, Kubiak E, et al. Suture versus screw fixation of displaced tibial eminence fractures: a biomechanical comparison. Arthroscopy 2005;21(10): 1172–1176
50. Bradley GW, Shives TC, Samuelson KM. Ligament injuries in the knees of children. J Bone Joint Surg Am 1979;61:588–591.
51. Brady TA, Russell D. Interarticular horizontal dislocation of the patella: a case report. J Bone Joint Surg Am 1965;47:1393–1396.
52. Brief LB. Anterior cruciate ligament reconstruction without drill holes. Arthroscopy 1991;7:350-357.
53. Brown GD, Ahmad CS. Combined medial patellofemoral ligament and medial patellotibial ligament reconstruction in skeletally immature patients. J Knee Surg 2008;21(4): 328–332.
54. Burstein DB, Viola A, Fulkerson JP. Entrapment of the medial meniscus in a fracture of the tibial eminence arthroscopy. Arthroscopy 1988;4:47–50.
55. Busch MT. Meniscal injuries in children and adolescents. Clin Sports Med 1990;9: 661–680.
56. Busek MS, Noyes FR. Arthroscopic evaluation of meniscal repairs after anterior cruciate ligament reconstruction and immediate motion. Am J Sports Med 1991;19:489–494.
57. Cannon WD, Vittori JM. The incidence of healing in arthroscopic meniscal repairs in the anterior cruciate ligament-reconstructed knee versus stable knees. Am J Sports Med 1992;20:176–181.
58. Cash JD, Hughston JC. Treatment of acute patellar dislocation. Am J Sports Med 1988; 16:244–249.
59. Chandler JP, Miller TK. Tibial eminence fracture with meniscal entrapment. Arthroscopy 1995;11:499–502.
60. Clancy WG, Shelbourne KD, Zoellner GB, et al. Treatment of knee joint instability secondary to rupture of the posterior cruciate ligament: report of a new procedure. J Bone Joint Surg Am 1983;65:310–322.
61. Clanton TO, DeLee JC, Sanders B, et al. Knee ligament injuries in children. J Bone Joint Surg Am 1979;61:1195–1201.
62. Clark CR, Ogden JA. Development of the menisci of the human knee joint: morphological changes and their potential role in childhood meniscal injury. J Bone Joint Surg Am 1983;65:538–547.
63. Cofield RH, Bryan RS. Acute dislocations of the patella: results of conservative treatment. J Trauma 1977;17:526–531.
64. Coleman HM. Recurrent osteochondral fracture of the patella. J Bone Joint Surg Br 1948;30:153–157.
65. Crawford AH. Fractures about the knee in children. Orthop Clin North Am 1976;7: 639–656.
66. Dalinka MK, Brennan RE, Canino C. Double-contrast knee arthrography in children. Clin Orthop Relat Res 1977;125:88–93.
67. Dart CH Jr, Braitman HE. Popliteal artery injury following fracture or dislocation at the knee: diagnosis and management. Arch Surg 1977;112:969–973.
68. Dashefsky JH. Discoid lateral meniscus in three members of a family. J Bone Joint Surg Am 1971;53:1208–1210.
69. DeHaven KE. Diagnosis of acute knee injuries with hemarthrosis. Am J Sports Med 1980;8:9–14.
70. DeHaven KE. Meniscus repair in the athlete. Clin Orthop Relat Res 1985;98:31–35.
71. DeHaven KE, Arnoczky SP. Meniscus repair: basic science, indications for repair, and open repair. Instr Course Lect 1994;43:65–74.
72. DeHaven KE, Collins HR. Diagnosis of internal derangement of the knee. J Bone Joint Surg Am 1975;57:802–810.

73. DeHaven KE, Linter DM. Athletic injuries: comparison by age, sport, gender. Am J Sports Med 1986;14:218–224.
74. Deie M, Ochi M, Sumen Y, et al. Reconstruction of the medial patellofemoral ligament for the treatment of habitual or recurrent dislocation of the patella in children. J Bone Joint Surg Br 2003;85(6):887–890.
75. Deie M, Ochi M, Sumen Y, et al. Relationship between osteochondritis dissecans of the lateral femoral condyle and lateral menisci types. J Pediatr Orthop 2006;26(1): 79–82.
76. DeLee JC. Complete dislocation of the knee in a 9-year-old. Contemp Orthop 1979; 1:29–32.
77. DeLee JC, Curtis R. Anterior cruciate ligament insufficiency in children. Clin Orthop Relat Res 1983;172:112–118.
78. Desio S, Burks R, Bachus K. Soft tissue restraints to lateral patellar translation in the human knee. Am J Sports Med 1998;26:59–65.
79. Dickason JM, del Pizzo W, Blazina ME, et al. A series of 10 discoid medial menisci. Clin Orthop Relat Res 1982;168:75–79.
80. Dickhaut SC, DeLee JC. The discoid lateral meniscus syndrome. J Bone Joint Surg Am 1982;64:1068–1073.
81. Donelson RG, Tomaiuoli M. Intra-articular dislocation of the patella. J Bone Joint Surg Am 1979;61:615–616.
82. Dye SF, Vaupel GL, Dye CC. Conscious neurosensory mapping of the internal structures of the human knee without intraarticular anesthesia. Am J Sports Med 1998;26: 773–777.
83. Eady JL, Cardenas CD, Sopa D. Avulsion of the femoral attachment of the anterior cruciate ligament in a 7-year-old child. J Bone Joint Surg Am 1982;64:1376–1378.
84. Edwards DH, Bentley G. Osteochondritis dissecans patellae. J Bone Joint Surg Br 1977; 59:58–63.
85. Edwards PH, Grana WA. Anterior cruciate ligament reconstruction in the immature athlete: long-term results of intra-articular reconstruction. Am J Knee Surg 2001;14: 232–237.
86. Edwards TB, Greene CC, Baratta RV, et al. The effect of placing a tensioned graft across open growth plates. A gross and histologic analysis. J Bone Joint Surg Am 2001;83-A(5):725–734.
87. Eggers AK, Becker C, Weimann A, et al. Biomechanical evaluation of different fixation methods for tibial eminence fractures. Am J Sports Med 2007;35(3):404–410.
88. Eggli S. Long-term results of arthroscopic meniscal repair: an analysis of isolated tears. Am J Sports Med 1995;23:715–720.
89. Eilert R. Arthroscopy of the knee joint in children. Orthop Rev 1976;5(9):61–65.
90. Eiskjaer S, Larsen ST. Arthroscopy of the knee in children. Acta Orthop Scand 1987; 58:273–276.
91. Eiskjaer S, Larsen ST, Schmidt MB. The significance of hemarthrosis of the knee in children. Arch Orthop Trauma Surg 1988;107(2):96–98.
92. Engebretsen L, Svenningsen S, Benum P. Poor results of anterior cruciate ligament repair in adolescents. Acta Orthop Scand 1988;59:684–686.
93. Fairbank TJ. Knee joint changes after menisectomy. J Bone Joint Surg 1948;30B: 664–670.
94. Falstie-Jensen S, Sondergard Petersen PE. Incarceration of the meniscus in fractures of the intercondylar eminence of the tibia in children. Injury 1974;15:236–238.
95. Farmer JM, Martin DF, Boles CA, et al. Chondral and osteochondral injuries. Clin Sports Med 2001;20:299–319.
96. Fetto JF, Marshall JL. Injury to the anterior cruciate ligament producing the pivot-shift sign. J Bone Joint Surg Am 1979;61:710–714.
97. Fetto JF, Marshall JL. The natural history and diagnosis of anterior cruciate ligament insufficiency. Clin Orthop Relat Res 1980;147:29–38.
98. Flachsmann R, Broom ND, Hardy AE, et al. Why is the adolescent joint particularly susceptible to osteochondral shear fracture? Clin Orthop Rel Res 2000;381:212–221.
99. Fleissner PR, Eilert RF. Discoid lateral meniscus. Am J Knee Surg 1999;12:125–131.
100. Flynn JM, Kocher MS, Ganley T. Osteochondritis dissecans of the knee. J Pediatr Orthop 2004;24(4):434-443.
101. Fowler PJ. The classification and early diagnosis of knee joint instability. Clin Orthop Relat Res 1980;147:15–21.
102. Fowler PJ. Meniscal lesions in the adolescent: the role of arthroscopy in the management of adolescent knee problems. In: Kennedy JC, ed. The Injured Adolescent Knee. Baltimore: Williams & Wilkins, 1979:43–76.
103. Frangakis EK. Intra-articular dislocation of the patella: a case report. J Bone Joint Surg Am 1974;56:423–424.
104. Fuchs R, Wheatley W, Uribe JW, et al. Intra-articular anterior cruciate ligament reconstruction using patellar tendon allograft in the skeletally immature patient. Arthroscopy 2002;18(8):824–828.
105. Fujikawa K, Iseki F, Mikura Y. Partial resection of the discoid meniscus in the child's knee. J Bone Joint Surg Br 1981;63:391–395.
106. Fyfe IS, Jackson JP. Tibial intercondylar fractures in children: a review of the classification and the treatment of malunion. Injury 1981;13:165–169.
107. Garcia A, Neer CS II. Isolated fractures of the intercondylar eminence of the tibia. Am J Surg 1958;95:593–598.
108. Gartland JJ, Brenner JH. Traumatic dislocations in the lower extremity in children. Orthop Clin North Am 1976;7:687–700.
109. Gaulrapp HM, Haus J. Intraarticular stabilization after anterior cruciate ligament tear in children and adolescents: results 6 years after surgery. Knee Surg Sports Traumatol Arthrosc 2006;14(5):417–424.
110. Gebhard F, Ellermann A, Hoffmann F, et al. Multicenter-study of operative treatment of intraligamentous tears of the anterior cruciate ligament in children and adolescents: comparison of four different techniques. Knee Surg Sports Traumatol Arthrosc 2006; 14(9):797–803.
111. Gelb H, Glasgow S, Sapega A, et al. Magnetic resonance imaging of knee disorders: clinical value and cost effectiveness in a sports medicine practice. Am J Sports Med 1996;24:99–103.
112. Goletz TH, Brodhead WT. Intra-articular dislocation of the patella: a case report. Orthopaedics 1981;4:1022–1024.
113. Goodfellow J, Hungerford DS, Zindel M. Patellofemoral joint mechanics and pathology: I. Functional anatomy of the patellofemoral joint. J Bone Joint Surg Br 1976;58: 287–290.
114. Goodrich A, Ballard A. Posterior cruciate ligament avulsion associated with ipsilateral femur fracture in a 10-year-old child. J Trauma 1988;28:1393–1396.
115. Graf BK, Lange RH, Fujisaki CK, et al. Anterior cruciate ligament tears in skeletally immature patients: meniscal pathology at presentation and after attempted conservative treatment. Arthroscopy 1992;8(2):229–233.
116. Green NE, Allen BL. Vascular injuries associated with dislocation of the knee. J Bone Joint Surg Am 1977;59:236–239.
117. Greis PE, Bardana DD, Holstrom MC, et al. Meniscal injury: basic science and evaluation. J Am Acad Orthop Surg 2002;10:168–176.
118. Greis PE, Holstrom MC, Bardana DD, et al. Meniscal injury: II. Management. J Am Acad Orthop Surg 2002;10:177–187.
119. Greulich WW, Pysle SI, eds. Radiographic Atlas of Skeletal Development of the Hand and Wrist. 2nd ed. Stanford: Stanford University Press, 1959.
120. Gronkvist H, Hirsch G, Johansson L. Fracture of the anterior tibial spine in children. J Pediatr Orthop 1984;4:465–468.
121. Guzzanti V, Falciglia F, Gigante A, et al. The effect of intra-articular ACL reconstruction on the growth plates of rabbits. J Bone Joint Surg Br 1994;76(6):960–963.
122. Guzzanti V, Falciglia F, Stanitski CL. Physeal-sparing intraarticular anterior cruciate ligament reconstruction in preadolescents. Am J Sports Med 2003;31(6):949–953.
123. Guzzanti V, Falciglia F, Stanitski CL. Preoperative evaluation and anterior cruciate ligament reconstruction technique for skeletally immature patients in Tanner stages 2 and 3. Am J Sports Med 2003;31(6):941–948.
124. Habata T, Uematsu K, Kasanami R, et al. Long-term clinical and radiographic follow-up of total resection for discoid lateral meniscus. Arthroscopy 2006;22(12):1339–1343.
125. Hall JE, Micheli LJ, McManana GB. Semitendinosus tenodesis for recurrent subluxation or dislocation of the patella. Clin Orthop Relat Res 1979;144:31–35.
126. Hamada M, Shino K, Kawano K, et al. Usefulness of MRI for detecting intrasubstance tear and/or degeneration of lateral discoid meniscus. Arthroscopy 1994;10:645–653.
127. Hamberg P, Gillquist J, Lysholm J. Suture of new and old peripheral meniscus tears. J Bone Joint Surg Am 1983;65:193–197.
128. Harway RA, Handler S. Internal derangement of the knee in an infant. Contemp Orthop 1988;17:49–51.
129. Hashimoto Y, Yoshida G, Tomihara T, et al. Bilateral osteochondritis dissecans of the lateral femoral condyle following bilateral total removal of lateral discoid meniscus: a case report. Arch Orthop Trauma Surg 2008;128(11):1265–1268.
130. Hayashi LK, Yamaga H, Ida K, et al. Arthroscopic meniscectomy for discoid lateral meniscus in children. J Bone Joint Surg Am 1988;70:1495–1500.
131. Hayes JM, Masear VR. Avulsion fracture of the tibial eminence associated with severe medial ligamentous injury in an adolescent: a case report and review of the literature. Am J Sports Med 1984;12:330–333.
132. Hejgaard N, Skive L, Perrild C. Recurrent dislocation of the patella. Acta Orthop Scand 1980;51:673–678.
133. Henderson NJ, Houghton GR. Osteochondral fractures of the knee in children. In: Houghton GR, Thompson GH, eds. Problematic Musculoskeletal Injuries in Children. London: Butterworths, 1983.
134. Henning CE, Lynch MA, Clark JR. Vascularity for healing of meniscus repairs. Arthroscopy 1987;3:13–18.
135. Hinton RY, Rivera VR, Pautz MJ, et al. Ligamentous laxity of the knee during childhood and adolescence. J Pediatr Orthop 2008;28(2):184–187.
136. Houle JB, Letts M, Yang J. Effects of a tensioned tendon graft in a bone tunnel across the rabbit physis. Clin Orthop Relat Res 2001;391:275–281.
137. Huang TW, Hsu KY, Cheng CY, et al. Arthroscopic suture fixation of tibial eminence avulsion fractures. Arthroscopy 2008;24(11):1232–1238.
138. Huckell JR. Is meniscectomy a benign procedure? A long-term follow-up study. Can J Surg 1965;8:254–260.
139. Hughston JC, Andrews JR, Cross MJ, et al. Classification of knee ligament instabilities: part I. The medial compartment and cruciate ligaments. J Bone Joint Surg Am 1976; 58:159–172.
140. Hughston JC, Bowden JA, Andrews JR, et al. Acute tears of the posterior cruciate ligament. J Bone Joint Surg Am 1980;62:438–450.
141. Hughston JC, Hergenroeder PT, Courtenay BG. Osteochondritis dissecans of the femoral condyles. J Bone Joint Surg Am 1984;66:1340–1348.
142. Hungerford DS, Barry M. Biomechanics of the patellofemoral joint. Clin Orthop Relat Res 1979;144:9–15.
143. Hyndman JC, Brown JC. Major ligamentous injuries of the knee in children. J Bone Joint Surg Br 1979;61:245.
144. Ikeuchi H. Arthroscopic treatment of lateral discoid meniscus: technique and long-term results. Clin Orthop Relat Res 1982;167:19–28.
145. Indelicato PA. Nonoperative treatment of complete tears of the medial collateral ligaments of the knee. J Bone Joint Surg Am 1983;65:323–329.
146. Jackson DW, Jennings LD, Maywood RM, et al. MRI of the knee. Am J Sports Med 1988;16:29–38.
147. Janarv PM, Nystrom A, Werner S, et al. Anterior cruciate ligament injuries in skeletally immature patients. J Pediatr Orthop 1996;16(5):673–677.
148. Janarv PM, Westblad P, Johansson C, et al. Long-term follow-up of anterior tibial spine fractures in children. J Pediatr Orthop 1995;15:63–68.
149. Johnson EW, McLeod TL. Osteochondral fragments of the distal end of the femur fixed with bone pegs: report of two cases. J Bone Joint Surg Am 1977;59:677–679.
150. Johnson MJ, Lucas GL, Dusek JK, et al. Isolated arthroscopic meniscal repair: a long-term outcome study (more than 10 years). Am J Sports Med 1999;27:44–49.
151. Jordan M. Lateral meniscal variants: evaluation and treatment. J Am Acad Orthop Surg 1996;4:191–200.
152. Jordan M, Duncan J, Bertrand S. Discoid lateral meniscus: a review. South Orthop J 1993;2:239–253.
153. Joseph KN, Pogrund H. Traumatic rupture of the medial ligament of the knee in a 4-year-old boy: a case report and review of the literature. J Bone Joint Surg Am 1978; 60:402–403.
154. Juhl M, Boe S. Arthroscopy in children, with special emphasis on meniscal lesions. Injury 1986;17:171–173.
155. Jung YB, Yum JK, Koo BH. A new method for arthroscopic treatment of tibial eminence fractures with eyed Steinmann pins. Arthroscopy 1999;15:672–675.
156. Kannus P, Järvinen M. Knee ligament injuries in adolescents: 8-year follow-up of conservative management. J Bone Joint Surg Br 1988;70:772–776.

157. Kaplan EB. Discoid lateral meniscus of the knee joint. Bull Hosp Joint Dis 1955;16: 111–124.
158. Kaplan EB. Discoid lateral meniscus of the knee joint. nature, mechanism, and operative treatment. J Bone Joint Surg Am 1957;39:77–87.
159. Kennedy JC. Complete dislocation of the knee joint. J Bone Joint Surg Am 1963;45: 889–904.
160. Kennedy JC. The Injured Adolescent Knee. Baltimore: Williams & Wilkins, 1979.
161. Keys GW, Walters J. Nonunion of intercondylar eminence fracture of the tibia. J Trauma 1988;28:870–871.
162. Kim SH, Ha KI, Ahn JH, et al. Anterior cruciate ligament reconstruction in the young patient without violation of the epiphyseal plate. Arthroscopy 1999;15(7):792–795.
163. Kim YG, Ihn JC, Park SK, et al. An arthroscopic analysis of lateral meniscal variants and a comparison with MRI findings. Knee Surg Sports Traumatol Arthrosc 2006; 14(1):20–26.
164. King AG. Meniscal lesions in children and adolescents: a review of the pathology and clinical presentation. Injury 1983;15:105–108.
165. King D. The healing of semilunar cartilage. J Bone Joint Surg 1936;18:333–342.
166. King SL, Carty HML, Brady O. Magnetic resonance imaging of knee injuries in children. Pediatr Radiol 1996;26:287–290.
167. Klingele KE, Kocher MS, Hresko MT, et al. Discoid lateral meniscus: prevalence of peripheral rim instability. J Pediatr Orthop 2004;24:79–82.
168. Kloeppel-Wirth S, Koltai JL, Dittmer H. Significance of arthroscopy in children with knee joint injuries. Eur J Pediatr Surg 1992;2(3):169–172.
169. Kocher MS, DiCanzio J, Zurakowski D, et al. Diagnostic performance of clinical examination and selective magnetic resonance imaging in the evaluation of intraarticular knee disorders in children and adolescents. Am J Sports Med 2001;29:292–296.
170. Kocher MS, Foreman ES, Micheli LJ. Laxity and functional outcome after arthroscopic reduction and internal fixation of displaced tibial spine fractures in children. Arthroscopy 2003;19:1085–1090.
171. Kocher MS, Garg S, Micheli LJ. Physeal sparing reconstruction of the anterior cruciate ligament in skeletally immature prepubescent children and adolescents. J Bone Joint Surg Am 2005;87(11):2371–2379.
172. Kocher MS, Garg S, Micheli LJ. Physeal sparing reconstruction of the anterior cruciate ligament in skeletally immature prepubescent children and adolescents. Surgical technique. J Bone Joint Surg Am 2006;88(Suppl 1 Pt 2):283–293.
173. Kocher MS, Hovis WD, Curtin MJ, et al. Anterior cruciate ligament reconstruction in skeletally immature knees: an anatomical study. Am J Orthop 2005;34(6):285–290.
174. Kocher MS, Klingele KE, Rassman S. Meniscal disorders: normal, discoid, and cysts. Ortho Clin N Am 2003;34:329–340.
175. Kocher MS, Mandiga R, Klingele KE, et al. Anterior cruciate ligament injury versus tibial spine fracture in the skeletally immature knee: a comparison of skeletal maturation and notch width index. J Pediatr Orthop 2004;24(2):185–188.
176. Kocher MS, Micheli LJ. The pediatric knee: evaluation and treatment. In Insall JN, Scott WN, eds. Surgery of the Knee. 3rd ed. New York: Churchill-Livingstone, 2001: 1356–1397.
177. Kocher MS, Micheli LJ, Gerbino PG, et al. Tibial eminence fractures in children: prevalence of meniscal entrapment. Am J Sports Med 2003;31(3):404–407.
178. Kocher MS, Micheli LJ, Yaniv M, et al. Functional and radiographic outcome of juvenile osteochondritis dissecans of the knee treated with transarticular drilling. Am J Sports Med 2001;29(5):562–566.
179. Kocher MS, Micheli LJ, Zurakowski D, et al. Partial tears of the anterior cruciate ligament in children and adolescents. Am J Sports Med 2002;30(5):697–703.
180. Kocher MS, Saxon HS, Hovis WD, et al. Management and complications of anterior cruciate ligament injuries in skeletally immature patients: survey of the Herodicus Society and the ACL Study Group. J Pediatr Orthop 2002;22(4):452–457.
181. Kocher MS, Smith JT, Zoric BJ, et al. Transphyseal anterior cruciate ligament reconstruction in skeletally immature pubescent adolescents. J Bone Joint Surg Am 2007; 89(12):2632–2639.
182. Koman JD, Sanders JO. Valgus deformity after reconstruction of the anterior cruciate ligament in a skeletally immature patient. A case report. J Bone Joint Surg
183. Krause WR, Pope MH, Johnson RJ, et al. Mechanical changes in the knee after meniscectomy. J Bone Joint Surg Am 1976;58:599–604.
184. LaPrade R, Burnett Q, Veenstra M, et al. The prevalence of abnormal magnetic resonance imaging findings in asymptomatic knees: with correlation of magnetic resonance imaging arthroscopic findings in symptomatic knees. Am J Sports Med 1994;22: 739–745.
185. Larsen E, Lauridsen F. Conservative treatment of patellar dislocations. Clin Orthop Relat Res 1982;171:131–136.
186. Larson RL. The unstable patella in the adolescent and preadolescent. Orthop Rev 1985; 14:156–162.
187. Lee DH, Kim TH, Kim JM, et al. Results of subtotal/total or partial meniscectomy for discoid lateral meniscus in children. Arthroscopy 2009;25(5):496–503.
188. Lee YH, Chin LS, Wang NH, et al. Anterior tibial spine fracture in children: follow-up evaluation by biomechanical studies. Chung Hua I Hsueh Tsa Chih 1996;58:183–189.
189. Levy IM, Torzilli PA, Warren RF. The effect of medial menisectomy on anterior-posterior motion of the knee. J Bone Joint Surg Am 1982;64:883–888.
190. Lewis PC, Foster BK. Herbert screw fixation of osteochondral fractures about the knee. Aust N Z J Surg 1990;60:511–513.
191. Liddle AD, Imbuldeniya AM, Hunt DM. Transphyseal reconstruction of the anterior cruciate ligament in prepubescent children. J Bone Joint Surg Br 2008;90(10): 1317–1322.
192. Lipscomb AB, Anderson AF. Tears of the anterior cruciate ligament in adolescents. J Bone Joint Surg Am 1986;68(1):19–28.
193. Lo IK, Kirkley A, Fowler PJ, et al. The outcome of operatively treated anterior cruciate ligament disruptions in the skeletally immature child. Arthroscopy 1997;13(5): 627–634.
194. Lombardo SJ. Avulsion of a fibrous union of the intercondylar eminence of the tibia: a case report. J Bone Joint Surg Am 1994;76:1565–1567.
195. Louis ML, Guillaume JM, Launay F, et al. Surgical management of type II tibial intercondylar eminence fractures in children. J Pediatr Orthop B 2008;17(5):231–235.
196. Lowe J, Chaimsky G, Freedman A, et al. The anatomy of tibial eminence fractures: arthroscopic observations following failed closed reduction. J Bone Joint Surg Am 2002; 84-A(11):1933–1938.
197. Luhmann SJ. Acute traumatic knee effusions in children and adolescents. J Pediatr Orthop 2003;23(2):199–202.
198. MacIntosh DL, Darby TA. Lateral substitution reconstruction. J Bone Joint Surg Br 1976;58:142.
199. Madigan R, Wissinger AH, Donaldson WF. Preliminary experience with a method of quadricepsplasty in recurrent subluxation of the patella. J Bone Joint Surg Am 1975; 57:600–607.
200. Mah JY, Adili A, Otsuka NY, et al. Follow-up study of arthroscopic reduction and fixation of type III tibial eminence fractures. J Pediatr Orthop 1998;18:475–477.
201. Mah JY, Otsuka NY, McLean J. An arthroscopic technique for the reduction and fixation of tibial-eminence fractures. J Pediatr Orthop 1996;16:119–121.
202. Mahar AT, Duncan D, Oka R, et al. Biomechanical comparison of four different fixation techniques for pediatric tibial eminence avulsion fractures. J Pediatr Orthop 2008; 28(2):159–162.
203. Manzione M, Pizzutillo PD, Peoples AB, et al. Menisectomy in children: a long-term follow-up study. Am J Sports Med 1983;11:111–115.
204. Marshall SC. Combined arthroscopic/open repair of meniscal injuries. Contemp Orthop 1987;14(6):15–24.
205. Matava MJ, Siegel MG. Arthroscopic reconstruction of the ACL with semitendinosis-gracilis autograft in skeletally immature adolescent patients. Am J Knee Surg 1997; 10(2):60–69.
206. Matelic TM, Aronsson DD, Boyd DW, et al. Acute hemarthrosis of the knee in children. Am J Sports Med 1995;23:668–671.
207. Matz SO, Jackson DW. Anterior cruciate ligament injury in children. Am J Knee Surg 1988;1:59–63.
208. Mayer PJ, Micheli LJ. Avulsion of the femoral attachment of the posterior cruciate ligament in an 11-year-old boy: a case report. J Bone Joint Surg Am 1979;61:431–432.
209. McCarroll JR, Rettig AC, Shelbourne KD. Anterior cruciate ligament injuries in the young athlete with open physes. Am J Sports Med 1988;16(1):44–47.
210. McCarroll JR, Shelbourne KD, Porter DA, et al. Patellar tendon graft reconstruction for midsubstance anterior cruciate ligament rupture in junior high school athletes: an algorithm for management. Am J Sports Med 1994;22:478–484.
211. McLennan JG. Lessons learned after second-look arthroscopy in type III fractures of the tibial spine. J Pediatr Orthop 1995;15:59–62.
212. McLennan JG. The role of arthroscopic surgery in the treatment of fractures of the intercondylar eminence of the tibia. J Bone Joint Surg Br 1982;64B:477–480.
213. McManus F, Rang M, Heslin DJ. Acute dislocation of the patella in children: the natural history. Clin Orthop Relat Res 1979;139:88–91.
214. Medlar RC, Manidberg JJ, Lyne ED. Menisectomies in children—report of long-term results. Am J Sports Med 1980;8:87–92.
215. Meyers MH. Isolated avulsion of the tibial attachment of the posterior cruciate ligament of the knee. J Bone Joint Surg Am 1975;57:669–672.
216. Meyers MH, McKeever FM. Follow-up notes. fracture of the intercondylar eminence of the tibia. J Bone Joint Surg Am 1970;52:1677–1684.
217. Meyers MH, McKeever FM. Fracture of the intercondylar eminence of the tibia. J Bone Joint Surg Am 1959;41:209–222.
218. Micheli LJ, Rask B, Gerberg L. Anterior cruciate ligament reconstruction in patients who are prepubescent. Clin Orthop Relat Res 1999;364:40–47.
219. Micheli LJ, Stanitski CL. Lateral patellar retinacular release. Am J Sports Med 1981;9: 330–336.
220. Millett PJ, Willis AA, Warren RF. Associated injuries in pediatric and adolescent anterior cruciate ligament tears: does a delay in treatment increase the risk of meniscal tear? Arthroscopy 2002;18(9):955–999.
221. Mintzer CM, Richmond JC, Taylor J. Meniscal repair in the young athlete. Am J Sports Med 1998;26:630–633.
222. Mizuta H, Kubota K, Shiraishi M, et al. The conservative treatment of complete tears of the anterior cruciate ligament in skeletally immature patients. J Bone Joint Surg Br 1995;77(6):890–894.
223. Molander ML, Wallin G, Wikstad I. Fractures of the intercondylar eminence of the tibia. A review of 35 patients. J Bone Joint Surg Br 1981;63B:89–91.
224. Morrissy RT, Eubanks RG, Park JP, et al. Arthroscopy of the knee in children. Clin Orthop Relat Res 1982;162:103–107.
225. Mulhall KJ, Dowdall J, Grannell M, et al. Tibial spine fractures. An analysis of outcome in surgically treated type III injuries. Injury 1999;30:289–292.
226. Mylle J, Reynders R, Broos P. Transepiphyseal fixation of anterior cruciate avulsion in a child: report of a complication and review of the literature. Arch Orthop Trauma Surg 1993;112:101–103.
227. Nathan PA, Cole SC. Discoid meniscus: a clinical and pathological study. Clin Orthop Relat Res 1969;64:107–113.
228. Neuschwander DC, Drez D, Finney TP. Lateral meniscal variant with absence of posterior coronary ligament. J Bone Joint Surg Am 1992;74:1186–1190.
229. Nietosvaara Y, Aalto K, Kallio PE. Acute patellar dislocation in children: incidence and associated osteochondral fractures. J Pediatr Orthop 1994;14:513–515.
230. Noyes FR, Barber-Westin SD. Arthroscopic repair of meniscal tears extending into the avascular zone in patients younger than 20 years of age. Am J Sports Med 2002;30: 589–600.
231. Noyes FR, Bassett RW, Grood ES, et al. Arthroscopy in acute traumatic hemarthrosis of the knee: incidence of anterior cruciate tears and other injuries. J Bone Joint Surg Am 1980;62:687–695.
232. Noyes FR, Delucas JL, Torvik PJ. Biomechanics of ACL failure: an analysis of strain-rate sensitivity and mechanisms of failure in primates. J Bone Joint Surg Am 1974; 56A: 236–253.
233. Ogata K. Arthroscopic technique: two-piece excision of discoid meniscus. Arthroscopy 1997;13(5):666–670.
234. Ogden JA. Skeletal Injury in the Child. 2nd ed. Philadelphia: Lea & Febiger, 1989.
235. Okazaki K, Miura H, Matsuda S, et al. Arthroscopic resection of the discoid lateral meniscus: long-term follow-up for 16 years. Arthroscopy 2006;22(9):967–971.
236. Oostvogel HJ, Klasen HJ, Reddingius RE. Fractures of the intercondylar eminenece in children and adolescents. Arch Orthop Trauma Surg 1988;107:242–247.
237. Palmer L. On the injuries to the ligaments of the knee: a clinical study. Acta Chir Scand Suppl 1938;81:53.
238. Parker AW, Drez D, Cooper JL. Anterior cruciate ligament injuries in patients with open physes. Am J Sports Med 1994;22(1):44–47.

239. Patel D, Dimakopoulos P, Penoncourt P. Bucket handle tear of a discoid meniscus: arthroscopic diagnosis and partial excision. Orthopaedics 1986;9:607–608.
240. Pellaci F, Mignani G, Valdiserri L. Fractures of the intercondylar eminence of the tibia in children. Ital J Orthop Traumatol 1986;12:441–446.
241. Pellacci F, Montanari G, Prosperi P, et al. Lateral discoid meniscus: treatment and results. Arthroscopy 1992;8:526–530.
242. Peterson L, Minas T, Brittberg M, et al. Treatment of osteochondritis dissecans of the knee with autologous chondrocyte transplantation: results at 2 to 10 years. J Bone Joint Surg Am 2003;85-A(Suppl 2):17–24.
243. Polly DW, Callaghan JJ, Sikes RA, et al. The accuracy of selective MRI compared to the findings of arthroscopy of the knee. J Bone Joint Surg Am 1988;70:192–198.
244. Pressman AE, Letts RM, Jarvis JG. Anterior cruciate ligament tears in children: an analysis of operative versus nonoperative treatment. J Pediatr Orthop 1997;17(4): 505–511.
245. Pyle SI, Hoerr NL. A Radiographic Standard of Reference the Growing Knee. Springfield, IL: Charles Thomas, 1969.
246. Raber DA, Friederich NF, Buzzi R, et al. Discoid lateral meniscus in children: long-term follow-up after total meniscectomy. J Bone Joint Surg Am 1998;8:1579–1586.
247. Rang M. Children's Fractures. 2nd ed. Philadelphia: Lippincott, 1983.
248. Rangger C, Klesti T, Gloetzer W, et al. Osteoarthritis after arthroscopic partial menisectomy. Am J Sports Med 1995;23:230–244.
249. Ritter G, Neugebauer H. Ligament lesions of the knee in childhood. Z Kinderchir 1989; 44:94–96.
250. Roberts JM. Fractures of the condyles of the tibia: an anatomical and clinical end-result study of 100 cases. J Bone Joint Surg Am 1968;50:1505–1521.
251. Roberts JM, Lovell WW. Fractures of the intercondylar eminence of the tibia. J Bone Joint Surg Am 1970;52:827.
252. Robinson SC, Driscoll SE. Simultaneous osteochondral avulsion of the femoral and tibial insertion of the anterior cruciate ligament: report of a case in a 13-year-old boy. J Bone Joint Surg Am 1981;63:1342–1343.
253. Rorabeck CH, Bobechko WP. Acute dislocation of the patella with osteochondral fracture. J Bone Joint Surg Br 1976;58:237–240.
254. Rosenberg NJ. Osteochondral fractures of the lateral femoral condyle. J Bone Joint Surg Am 1964;46:1013–1026.
255. Rosenberg TD, Paulos LE, Parker RD, et al. Discoid lateral meniscus: case report of arthroscopic attachment of a symptomatic Wrisberg-ligament type. Arthroscopy 1987; 3:277–282.
256. Ross AC, Chesterman PJ. Isolated avulsion of the tibial attachment of the posterior cruciate ligament in childhood. J Bone Joint Surg Br 1986;68:747.
257. Rubman MH, Noyes FR, Barber-Westin SD. Arthroscopic repair of meniscal tears that extend into the avascular zone. A review of 198 single and complex tears. Am J Sports Med 1998;26:87–95.
258. Saddawi ND, Hoffman BK. Tear of the attachment of a normal meniscus of the knee in a 4-year-old child. J Bone Joint Surg Am 1970;52:809–811.
259. Sallay P, Poggi J, Speer K, et al. Acute dislocation of the patella. Am J Sports Med 1996;24:52–60.
260. Sanders WE, Wilkins KE, Neidre A. Acute insufficiency of the posterior cruciate ligament in children. J Bone Joint Surg Am 1980;62:129–130.
261. Schlonsky J, Eyring EJ. Lateral meniscus tears in young children. Clin Orthop Relat Res 1973;97:117–118.
262. Seil R, Pape D, Kohn D. The risk of growth changes during transphyseal drilling in sheep with open physes. Arthroscopy 2008;24(7):824–833.
263. Seitz WH Jr, Bibliani LU, Andrews DL, et al. Osteochondritis dissecans of the knee: a surgical approach. Orthop Rev 1985;14(2):56–63.
264. Sharma A, Lakshmanan P, Peehal J, et al. An analysis of different types of surgical fixation for avulsion fractures of the anterior tibial spine. Acta Orthop Belg 2008;74(1): 90–97.
265. Shea KG, Apel PJ, Pfeiffer RP, et al. The anatomy of the proximal tibia in pediatric and adolescent patients: implications for ACL reconstruction and prevention of physeal arrest. Knee Surg Sports Traumatol Arthrosc 2007;15(4):320–327.
266. Shelbourne KD, Gray T, Wiley BV. Results of transphyseal anterior cruciate ligament reconstruction using patellar tendon autograft in Tanner stage 3 or 4 adolescents with clearly open growth plates. Am J Sports Med 2004;32(5):1218–1222.
267. Shoemaker SC, Markolf KL. The role of the meniscus in the anterior-posterior stability of the loaded cruciate deficient knee: effect of partial versus total excision. J Bone Joint Surg Am 1988;68:71–79.
268. Sigge W, Ellebrecht T. Arthroscopy of the injured knee in children. Z Kinderchir 1988; 43(Suppl 1):68–70.
269. Silva I, Silver DM. Tears of the meniscus as revealed by MRI. J Bone Joint Surg Am 1988;70:199–202.
270. Simonian PT, Metcalf MH, Larson RV. Anterior cruciate ligament injuries in the skeletally immature patient. Am J Orthop 1999;28(11):624–628.
271. Singer KM, Henry J. Knee problems in children and adolescents. Clin Sports Med 1985;4:385–397.
272. Sisk TD. Knee injuries. In: Crenshaw AH, ed. Campbell's Operative Orthopaedics. 7th ed. St. Louis: CV Mosby, 1987:2336–2338.
273. Skak SV, Jensen TT, Poulsen TD, et al. Epidemiology of knee injuries in children. Acta Orthop Scand 1987;58:78–81.
274. Smillie I. The congenital discoid meniscus. J Bone Joint Surg Br 1948;30:671–682.
275. Smillie IS. Injuries of the Knee Joint. 5th ed. Edinburgh: Churchill-Livingstone, 1978.
276. Smith JB. Knee instability after fractures of the intercondylar eminence of the tibia. J Ped Orthop 1984;4:462–464.
277. Stadelmaier DM, Arnoczky SP, Dodds J, et al. The effect of drilling and soft tissue grafting across open growth plates. A histologic study. Am J Sports Med 1995;23(4): 431–435.
278. Stanitski CL. Anterior cruciate ligament injury in the skeletally immature patient: diagnosis and treatment. J Am Acad Orthop Surg 1995;3(3):146–158.
279. Stantiski CL. Correlation of arthroscopic and clinical examinations with magnetic resonance imaging findings of injured knees in children. Am J Sports Med 1998;26:2–6.
280. Stanitski CL. Patellar instability in the school-age athlete. Instr Course Lect 1998;47: 345–350.
281. Stanitski CL, Harvell JC, Fu F. Observations on acute knee hemarthrosis in children and adolescents. J Pediatr Orthop 1993;13(4):506–510.
282. Stanitski CL, Paletta GA. Articular cartilage injury with acute patellar dislocation in adolescents. Am J Sports Med 1998;26(1):52–55.
283. Steadman JR, Briggs KK, Rodrigo JJ, et al. Outcomes of microfracture for traumatic chondral defects of the knee: average 11-year follow-up. Arthroscopy 2003;19(5): 477–484.
284. Stilli S, DiGennaro GL, Marchiodi L, et al. Arthroscopic surgery of the discoid meniscus during childhood. Chir Degli Org Mov 1997;82:335–339.
285. Sugawara O, Miyatsu M, Yamashita I, et al. Problems with repeated arthroscopic surgery in the discoid meniscus. Arthroscopy 1991;7:68–71.
286. Sullivan DJ, Dines DM, Hershon SJ, et al. Natural history of a type III fracture of the intercondylar eminence of the tibia in an adult: a case report. Am J Sports Med 1989; 17:132–133.
287. Suman RK, Stother IG, Illingworth G. Diagnostic arthroscopy of the knee in children. J Bone Joint Surg Br 1984;66:535–537.
288. Takeda Y, Ikata T, Yoshida S, et al. MRI high signal intensity in the menisci of asymptomatic children. J Bone Joint Surg Br 1998;80:463–467.
289. Tanner JM, Whitehouse RH. Clinical longitudinal standards for height, weight, height velocity, and stages of puberty. Arch Dis Child 1976;51:170–179.
290. Tapper EM, Hoover NW. Late results after meniscectomy. J Bone Joint Surg Am 1969; 51:517–526.
291. Tenuta JJ, Arciero RA. Arthroscopic evaluation of meniscal repairs: factors that affect healing. Am J Sports Med 1994;22:797–802.
292. Torisu T. Isolated avulsion fracture of the tibial attachment of the posterior cruciate ligament. J Bone Joint Surg Am 1977;59:68–72.
293. Vahasarja V, Kinnuen P, Serlo W. Arthroscopy of the acute traumatic knee in children. Prospective study of 138 cases. Acta Orthop Scand 1993;64(5):580–582.
294. Vahvanen V, Aolto K. Menisecetomy in children. Acta Orthop Scand 1979;50: 791–795.
295. Vandermeer R, Cunningham F. Arthroscopic treatment of the discoid lateral meniscus: Results of long term followup. Arthroscopy 1989;5:101–109.
296. Vargas B, Lutz N, Dutoit M, et al. Nonunion after fracture of the anterior tibial spine: case report and review of the literature. J Pediatr Orthop B 2009;18(2):90–92.
297. Vedi V, Williams A, Tennant SJ, et al. Meniscal movement: an in-vivo study using dynamic MRI. J Bone Joint Surg Br 1999;81:37–41.
298. Vega JR, Irribarra LA, Baar AK, et al. Arthroscopic fixation of displaced tibial eminence fractures: a new growth plate-sparing method. Arthroscopy 2008;24(11):1239–1243.
299. Volk H, Smith FM. "Bucket-handle" tear of the medial meniscus in a 5-year-old boy. J Bone Joint Surg Am 1953;35:234–236.
300. Voloshin As, Wosk J. Shock absorption of the menisectomized and painful knees: a comparative in vivo study. J Biomed Eng 1983;5:157–161.
301. Volpi P, Galli M, Bait C, et al. Surgical treatment of anterior cruciate ligament injuries in adolescents using double-looped semitendinosis and gracilis tendons: supraepiphysary femoral and tibial fixation. Arthroscopy 2004;20(4):447–449.
302. Waldrop JI, Broussard TS. Disruption of the anterior cruciate ligament in a 3-year-old child. J Bone Joint Surg Am 1984;66:1113–1114.
303. Washington ER, Root L, Lierner U, et al. Discoid lateral meniscus in children—long-term follow-up after excision. J Bone Joint Surg Am 1995;77(9):1357–1361.
304. Watanabe M, Takada S, Ikeuchi H. Atlas of Arthroscopy. Tokyo: Igaku-Shoin, 1969.
305. Wessel LM, Scholz S, Rusch M, et al. Hemarthrosis after trauma to the pediatric knee joint: what is the value of magnetic resonance imaging in the diagnostic algorithm? J Pediatr Orthop 2001;21(3):338–342.
306. Wester W, Canale ST, Dutkowsky JP, et al. Prediction of angular deformity and leg-length discrepancy after anterior cruciate ligament reconstruction in skeletally immature patients. J Pediatr Orthop 1994;14:516–521.
307. Wiley JJ, Baxter MP. Tibial spine fractures in children. Clin Orthop Relat Res 1990; 255:54–60.
308. Willis RB, Blokker C, Stoll TM, et al. Long-term follow-up of anterior tibial eminence fractures. J Pediatr Orthop 1993;13:361–364.
309. Wombwell JH, Nunley JA. Compressive fixation of osteochondritis dissecans fragments with Herbert screws. J Orthop Trauma 1987;1:74–77.
310. Woo R, Busch M. Management of patellar instability in children. Oper Tech Sports Med 1998;6:247–258.
311. Woo SL-Y, Hollis JM, Adams DJ, et al. Tensile properties of the human femur-anterior cruciate ligament-tibia complex: the effects of specimen age and orientation. Am J Sports Med 1991;19:217–225.
312. Woods GW, Whelan JM. Discoid meniscus. Clin Sports Med 199;9(3):695–706.
313. Wroble RR, Henderson RC, Campion ER, et al. Menisectomy in children and asolescents: a long term follow-up study. Clin Orthop Relat Res 1992;279:180–189.
314. Yoo WJ, Choi IH, Chung CY, et al. Discoid lateral meniscus in children: limited knee extension and meniscal instability in the posterior segment. J Pediatr Orthop 2008; 28(5):544–548.
315. Young RB. The external semilunar cartilage as a complete disc. In: Cleland J, Mackey JY, Young RB, eds. Memoirs and Memoranda in Anatomy. London: Williams and Norgate, 1889:179.
316. Zaman M, Leonard MA. Meniscectomy in children: a study of 59 knees. J Bone Joint Surg Br 1978;60:436–437.
317. Zaricznyj B. Avulsion fracture of the tibial eminence: treatment by open reduction and pinning. J Bone Joint Surg Am 1977;59:1111–1114.
318. Zobel MS, Borrello JA, Siegel MJ et al. Pediatric knee MR imaging: pattern of injury in the immature skeleton. Radiology 1994;190:397–401.

25

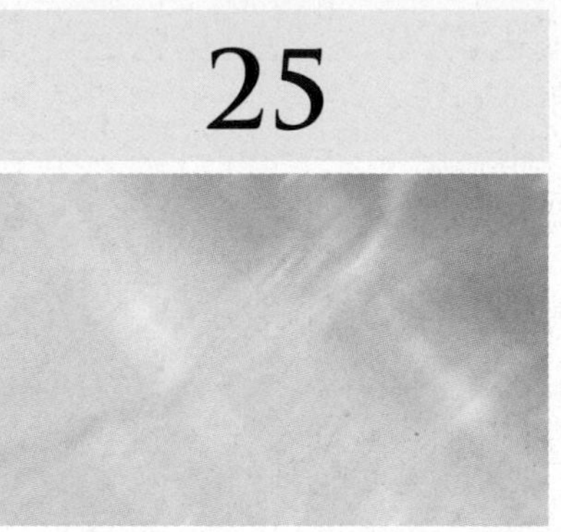

FRACTURES OF THE SHAFT OF THE TIBIA AND FIBULA

Stephen D. Heinrich and James F. Mooney

EPIDEMIOLOGY 930
Classification 931

SURGICAL ANATOMY 931
Bony Structure 931

VASCULAR ANATOMY 931
Nerves 932
Fascial Compartments 932

FRACTURES OF THE PROXIMAL TIBIAL METAPHYSIS 933

DIAPHYSEAL FRACTURES OF THE TIBIA AND FIBULA 936
Signs and Symptoms 939
Radiographic Evaluation 939
Treatment 940

OPEN FRACTURES OF THE TIBIA 944
Treatment Principles 944
Open Tibia Fractures—Associated Issues 946
Immobilization 952
Rehabilitation 952

FRACTURES OF THE DISTAL TIBIAL METAPHYSIS 952

COMPLICATIONS ASSOCIATED WITH DIAPHYSEAL TIBIAL AND FIBULAR FRACTURES 954
Compartment Syndrome 954
Vascular Injuries 955
Angular Deformity 955
Malrotation 956
Leg-Length Discrepancy 956
Anterior Tibial Physeal Closure 957
Delayed Union and Nonunion 957

SPECIAL FRACTURES 957
Toddler's Fractures 957
Bicycle Spoke Injuries 959
Floating Knee 959
Tibial Fracture in Paraplegic Children 959
Stress Fractures of the Tibia and Fibula 961

EPIDEMIOLOGY

Tibial and fibular fractures are the third most common pediatric long bone injuries (15%) after radial/ulnar and femoral fractures.[133,142] The prevalence of tibial fractures in both boys and girls has increased since 1950.[79] The average age of occurrence is 8 years, and the frequency of occurrence does not change significantly with age.[61] Seventy percent of pediatric tibial fractures are isolated injuries; ipsilateral fibular fractures occur with 30% of tibial fractures.[18,142,151] Fifty to 70% of tibial fractures occur in the distal third, and 19% to 39% in the middle third. The least commonly affected portion of the tibia is the proximal third, yet these may be the most problematic. Thirty-five percent of pediatric tibial fractures are oblique, 32% comminuted, 20% transverse, and 13% spiral.[133] Tibial fractures in children under 4 years of age usually are isolated spiral or short oblique fractures in the distal and the middle one third of the bone. Most tibial fractures in older children and adolescents are in the distal third.

Rotational forces produce an oblique or a spiral fracture, and are responsible for approximately 81% of all tibial fractures that present without an associated fibular fracture.[10,18,51,100,133] Tibial fractures due to bicycle spoke injuries occur almost exclusively in children 1 to 4 years of age, whereas most tibial fractures in children 4 to 14 years of age are the result of sporting or traffic accidents.[10,18,61,79,100,133] More than 50% of ipsilateral tibial and fibular fractures result from vehicular trauma. Most isolated fibular fractures result from a direct blow.[61,133] The tibia is the second most commonly fractured bone in abused children. Approximately 16% to 26% of all abused children with a fracture have an injured tibia.[82,95] Nine percent of pediatric tibial fractures are open. Concomitant fractures of the ankle and foot are the most common injuries associated with fractures of the tibia and fibula, followed by humeral, femoral, and radial/ulnar fractures.[13] In a 1994 report, the average Injury Severity Score of a child with a tibial fracture was 10 (range, 0 to 45) with an average hospital stay of 6.5 days (range, 1 to 50 days).[13] There have been no updates of this information in the recent English literature; however, it would seem certain that the current average hospital stay is less in 2008.

Classification

Nonphyseal injuries of the tibia and the fibula can be classified into three major categories based on the combination of bones fractured and the location of the injuries.

TABLE 25-1 Muscle Origins and Insertions on the Tibia

Semimembranosus	Inserts on inner tuberosity of the proximal tibia
Tibialis anterior, extensor digitorum longus, biceps femoris	Attaches to the lateral condyle of the tibia
Sartorius, gracilis, semitendinosus	Inserts on the proximal medial surface of the tibial metaphysis
Tibialis anterior	Arises on the lateral surface of the tibial diaphysis
Popliteus, soleus, flexor digitorum longus, tibialis posterior	Attaches to the posterior diaphysis of the tibia
Patellar tendon	Inserts into the tibial tubercle
Tensor fascia lata	Attaches to the Gerdy tubercle, the lateral aspect of the proximal tibial metaphysis
Secondary slip of fascia lata	Occasionally inserts into the tibial tubercle

From Gray H. Anatomy: descriptive and surgical. In: Pick TP, Howden R, eds. Anatomy: Descriptive and Surgical. New York: Bounty Books, 1977:182, with permission.

SURGICAL ANATOMY

Bony Structure

The tibia ("flute") is the second largest bone in the body. There are two concave condyles at the proximal aspect of the tibia. The medial condyle is larger, deeper, and narrower than the lateral condyle. An elevated process, the tibial tubercle, located between the two condyles, is the site of attachment of the patellar tendon. The shaft of the tibia is prismoid, with a broad proximal extent that decreases in size until the distal third, where it gradually increases again in size. The tibial crest is prominent medially from the tibial tubercle to the tibial plafond and is subcutaneous without any overlying muscles.[51]

The tibia develops from three ossification centers: one in the shaft and one in each epiphysis. The tibial diaphysis ossifies at 7 weeks of gestation and expands both proximally and distally. The proximal epiphyseal center appears shortly after birth and unites with the shaft between 14 and 16 years of age. The distal epiphyseal ossification center appears in the second year of life, and the distal tibial physis closes between 14 and 15 years of age. Additional ossification centers are found occasionally in the medial malleolus and in the tibial tubercle.[51]

The tibia articulates with the condyles of the femur proximally, with the fibula at the knee and the ankle, and with the talus distally.[51] Twelve muscles have either their origin or insertion on the tibia (Table 25-1). The fibula articulates with the tibia and the talus. The fibular diaphysis ossifies at about 8 weeks of gestation. The distal epiphysis is visible at 2 years of age, and the proximal secondary ossification center at 4 years. The distal fibular physis closes at approximately 16 years; the proximal physis closes later, between the ages of 15 and 18 years.[51] Nine muscles have either their origin or insertion on the fibula (Table 25-2).[51]

VASCULAR ANATOMY

The popliteal artery descends vertically between the condyles of the femur and passes between the medial and lateral heads of the gastrocnemius muscle. It ends at the distal border of the popliteus muscle, where it divides into the anterior and posterior tibial arteries. The anterior tibial artery passes between the tibia and the fibula over the proximal aspect of the intraosseous membrane. The posterior tibial artery divides several centimeters distal to this point, giving rise to the peroneal artery (Fig. 25-1).[51]

TABLE 25-2 Muscle Origins and Insertions on the Fibula

Soleus, flexor hallucis longus	Arises from the posterior aspect of the diaphysis
Peroneus longus, peroneus brevis	Arises from the lateral aspect of the fibular diaphysis
Biceps femoris, soleus, peroneus longus	Attaches to the head of the fibula
Extensor digitorum longus, peroneus tertius, extensor hallucis longus	Attaches to the anterior surface of the fibular shaft
Tibialis posterior	Arises from the medial aspect of the fibular diaphysis

From Gray H. Anatomy: descriptive and surgical. In: Pick TP, Howden R, eds. Anatomy: Descriptive and Surgical. New York: Bounty Books, 1977:182, with permission.

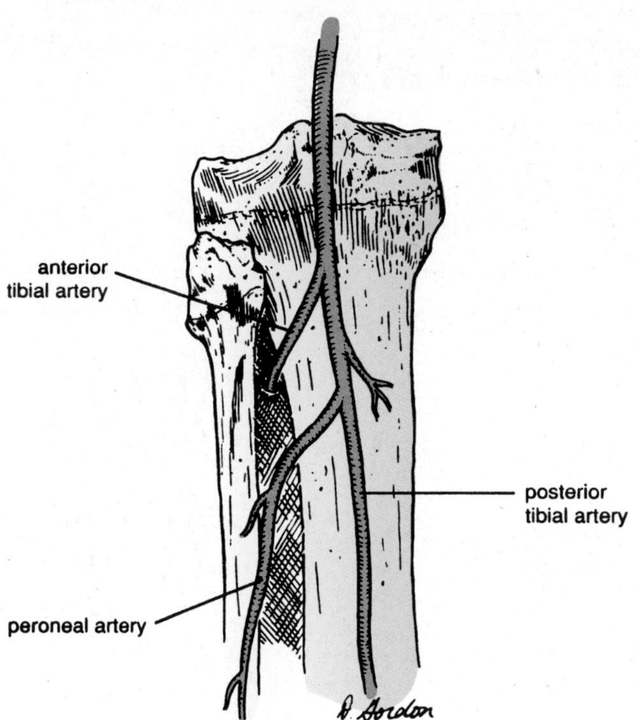

FIGURE 25-1 Vascular anatomy of the proximal tibia.

Nerves

The posterior tibial nerve runs adjacent and posterior to the popliteal artery in the popliteal fossa, and then enters the deep posterior compartment of the leg. This nerve provides innervation to the muscles of the deep posterior compartment and sensation to the plantar aspect of the foot. The common peroneal nerve passes around the proximal neck of the fibula. It divides into the deep and superficial branches, and then passes into the anterior and the lateral compartments of the lower leg,[51] respectively. Each branch innervates the muscles within its compartment. The deep peroneal nerve provides sensation to the first web space. The superficial branch is responsible for sensation across the dorsal surface of the foot.

Fascial Compartments

The lower leg has four fascial compartments (Fig. 25-2). The anterior compartment contains the extensor digitorum longus, the extensor hallucis longus, and the tibialis anterior muscles; the anterior tibial artery and deep peroneal nerve run in this compartment. The lateral compartment contains the peroneus longus and brevis muscles. The superficial peroneal nerve runs through this compartment. The superficial posterior compartment contains the soleus and gastrocnemius muscles. The deep posterior compartment contains the flexor digitorum longus, the flexor hallucis longus, and the tibialis posterior muscles.

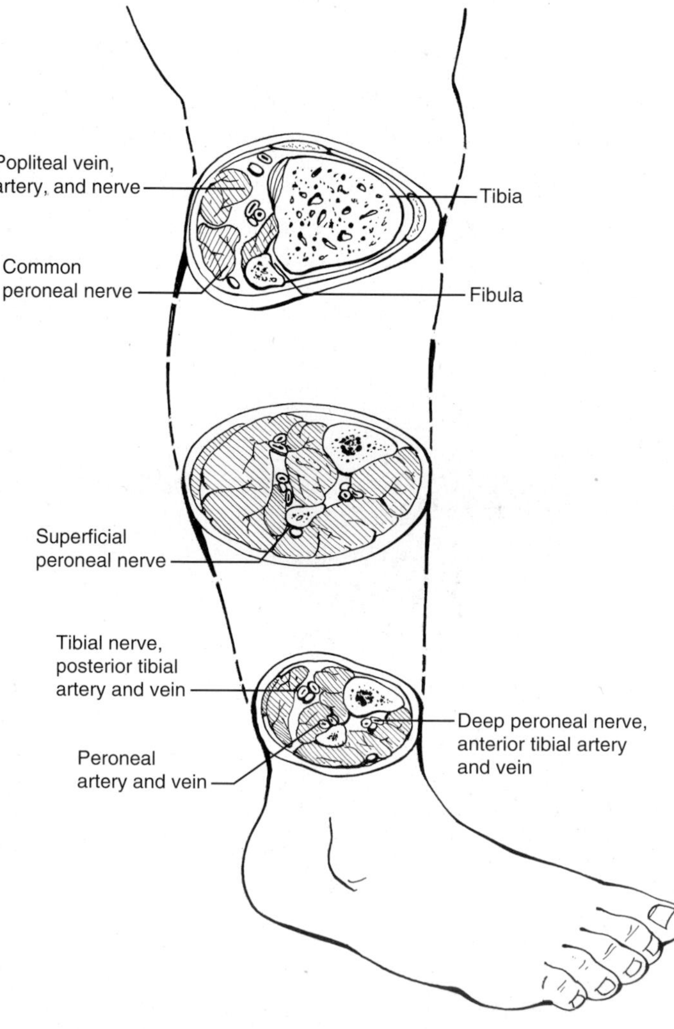

FIGURE 25-2 Fibroosseous compartments of the leg.

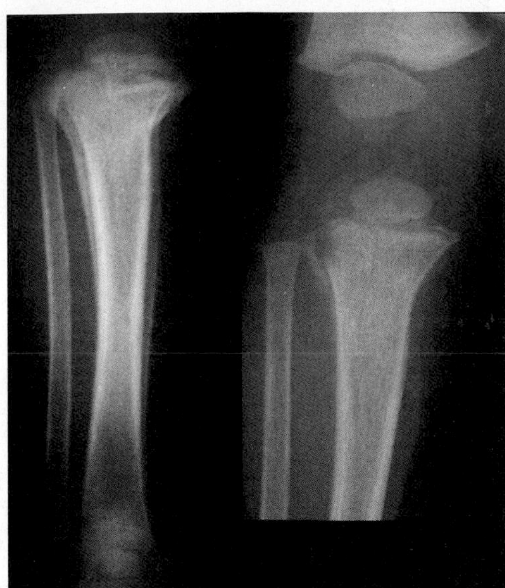

FIGURE 25-3 Anteroposterior radiographs of the knee in a 9-month-old child who was abused show a proximal tibial metaphyseal corner fracture with extension into the physis (right). The follow-up radiograph on the left demonstrates marked new bone formation, which suggests the degree of periosteal stripping that occurred at the time of the injury.

The posterior tibial artery, peroneal artery, and posterior tibial nerve run in this compartment.[51]

FRACTURES OF THE PROXIMAL TIBIAL METAPHYSIS

The peak incidence for proximal tibial metaphyseal fractures is between the ages of 3 and 6 years. The most common mechanism of injury is a force applied to the lateral aspect of the extended knee generating a valgus moment. The cortex of the medial tibial metaphysis fails in tension, often resulting in an incomplete fracture. The fibula generally escapes injury, although plastic deformation may occur.* Occasionally, a proximal tibial metaphyseal fracture may occur as the result of abuse (Fig. 25-3).

Children with proximal tibial metaphyseal fractures present with pain, swelling, and tenderness in the region of the fracture. Motion of the knee causes moderate pain, and in most cases the child will not walk. Crepitance is seldom identified on physical examination, especially if the fracture is incomplete.[2,4,21,22,52,71,76,81,110,135,141,146,150,154,155]

Radiographs usually show a complete or incomplete fracture of the proximal tibial metaphysis. The medial aspect of the fracture often is widened, producing a valgus deformity.[2,4,15,22,52,71,76,126,135,141,146,150,154,155]

An uncommon sequela of a proximal tibial metaphyseal fracture is development of a late valgus deformity (Fig. 25-4). In 1953, Cozen[22] reported 4 patients with valgus deformities after fractures of the proximal tibial metaphysis. Since that time, many other investigators[4,21,52,71,76,81,92,110,142,146,150] have reported development of tibia valga, even in fractures without any significant malalignment at the time of initial treatment.

*References 2,4,21,22,52,71,76,81,109,126,135,141,146,150,154,155.

Many theories have been proposed to explain the development of a valgus deformity after a proximal tibial metaphyseal fracture (Table 25-3). In some cases, proximal tibia valga can be the result of an inadequate reduction or the loss of satisfactory reduction in the weeks following the manipulation.[135,154] Lehner and Dubas[92] suggested that an expanding medial callus produced a valgus deformity, whereas Goff[46] and Keret et al.[81] believed that the lateral aspect of the proximal tibial physis was injured at the time of the initial fracture (Salter-Harris type V injury), resulting in asymmetric growth. Taylor[146] believed that the valgus deformity was secondary to postfracture stimulation of the tibial physis without a corresponding stimulation of the fibular physis. Pollen[115] suggested that premature weight bearing produced an angular deformity of the fracture before union. Rooker and Salter[123] believed that the periosteum was trapped in the medial aspect of the fracture, producing an increase in medial physeal growth and a developmental valgus deformity.

Another theory postulates that the progressive valgus deformity occurs secondary to an increase in vascular flow to the medial proximal tibial physis after fracture, producing an asymmetric physeal response that causes increased medial growth.[76] Support for this theory includes quantitative bone scans performed months after proximal tibial metaphyseal fractures that have shown increased tracer uptake in the medial aspect of the physis compared with the lateral aspect.[154] Ogden[109] identified an increase in the collateral geniculate vascularity to the medial proximal tibia in a cadaver angiography study of a 5-year-old child with a previous fracture. This further supports the theory that medial overgrowth occurs secondary to an increase in the blood flow supplying the medial aspect of the proximal tibia following injury.[101]

Recent studies suggest that the postfracture tibia valga is the result of an injury to the pes anserinus tendon plate. It is suggested that the pes anserinus tethers the medial aspect of the physis, just as the fibula appears to tether the lateral aspect of the proximal tibial physis. Multiple authors believe that the proximal tibial fracture disrupts the tendon plate, producing a loss of the tethering affect. This, then, may lead to medial physeal overgrowth and a functional hemichondrodiastasis.[4,25,26,150,155] Exploration of the fracture, followed by removal and repair of the infolded periosteum that forms the foundation of the pes anserinus tendon plate, has been suggested as an approach that may decrease the risk of a developmental valgus deformity.

Developmental tibia valga has been reported to occur after simple excision of a bone graft from the proximal tibial metaphysis,[146] proximal tibial osteotomy,[2,71] and osteomyelitis of the proximal tibial metaphysis.[2,146] Tibia valga deformity can occur after healing of a nondisplaced fracture, and can recur after corrective tibial osteotomy, further supporting the premise that asymmetric physeal growth is the cause of most posttraumatic tibia valga deformities.[154]

The natural history of postfracture proximal tibial valga is one of slow progression of the deformity, followed by gradual restoration of normal alignment over time. Zionts and MacEwen[155] followed 7 children with progressive valgus deformities of the tibia for an average of 39 months after metaphyseal fractures (Fig. 25-5). Most of the deformity developed during the first year after injury. The tibia continued to angulate at a slower rate for up to 17 months after injury. Six of their 7 patients

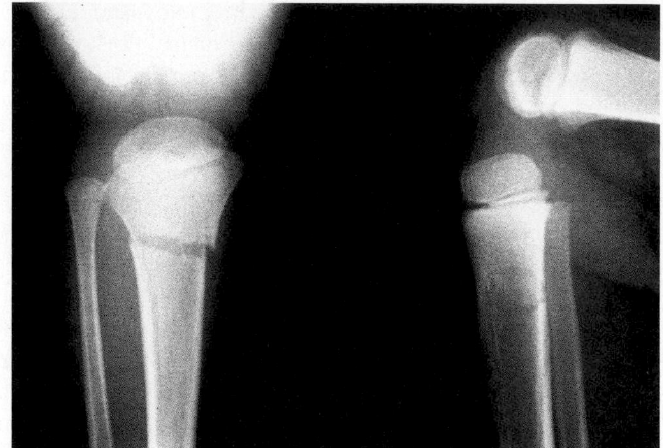

A

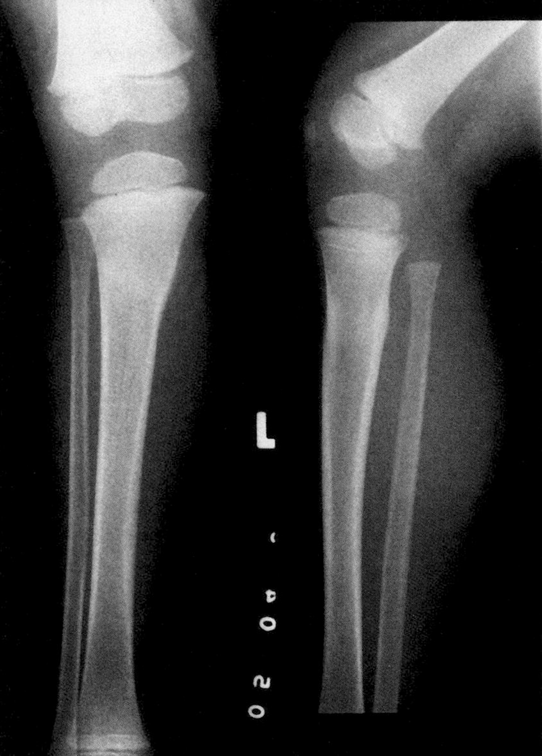

C

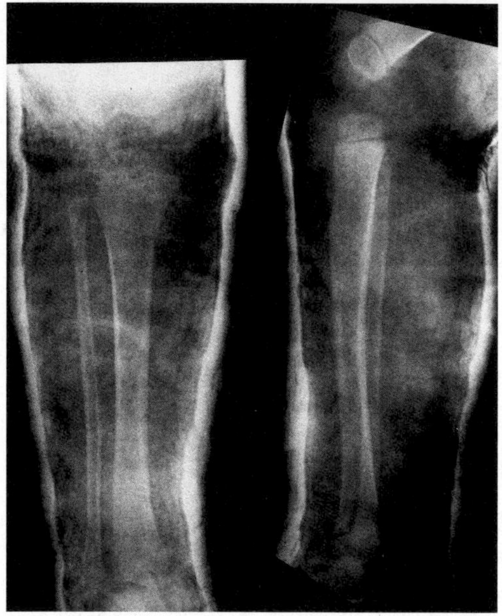

B

FIGURE 25-4 A. Anteroposterior and lateral radiographs of the proximal tibial metaphyseal fracture with an intact fibula in a 3-year-old child. **B.** Anteroposterior and lateral radiograph in the initial long-leg cast demonstrate an acceptable alignment. **C.** Posttraumatic tibia valga is present 1 year after fracture union. (From Sharps CH, Cardea JA. Fractures of the shaft of the tibia and fibula. In: MacEwen GD, Kasser JR, Heinrich SD, eds. Pediatric Fractures: A Practical Approach to Assessment and Treatment. Baltimore: Williams & Wilkins, 1993:321, with permission.)

had spontaneous clinical corrections. At follow-up, all children had less than a 10-degree deformity.

Robert et al.[119] analyzed 25 patients with proximal tibial fractures. Twelve children with a greenstick or a complete fracture developed valgus deformities, while no child with a torus fracture developed a deformity. Altered growth at the distal tibial physis appeared to compensate for the proximal tibia valga in three children. Corrective osteotomies were performed in four children. The valgus deformity recurred in two of these four children, and two had iatrogenic compartment syndromes. This study supports the premise that developmental tibia valga does not require correction in many patients. If correction is deemed necessary, it is important to remember that tibial osteotomy is not always a benign procedure without significant risk of complications. Gradual correction of the deformity with a proximal medial tibial hemiepiphysiodesis may be most appropriate treatment for recalcitrant postfracture tibia valga in a child with significant growth remaining.[10,110,119,141,146]

TABLE 25-3 Proposed Etiologies of Trauma-Induced Tibia Valgus

Asymmetric activity of medial portion of proximal tibial physis (overgrowth)
Tethering effect; fibula
Inadequate reduction
Interposed soft tissue (pes anserinus); medial collateral ligament
Loss of tethering effect of the pes anserinus
Early weight bearing producing developmental valgus
Physeal arrest of the lateral aspect of the proximal tibial physis

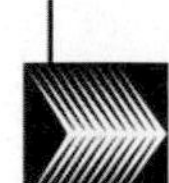

AUTHORS' PREFERRED TREATMENT

Nondisplaced proximal tibial metaphyseal fractures should be stabilized in a long-leg cast with the knee in 5 to 10 degrees of flexion and with a varus mold (Fig. 25-6). Displaced proximal tibial fractures require closed reduction with general anesthesia in the operating room or in an emergency room setting with adequate sedation. An anatomic reduction or slight varus positioning should be verified radiographically. If closed reduction to an anatomic or slight varus position

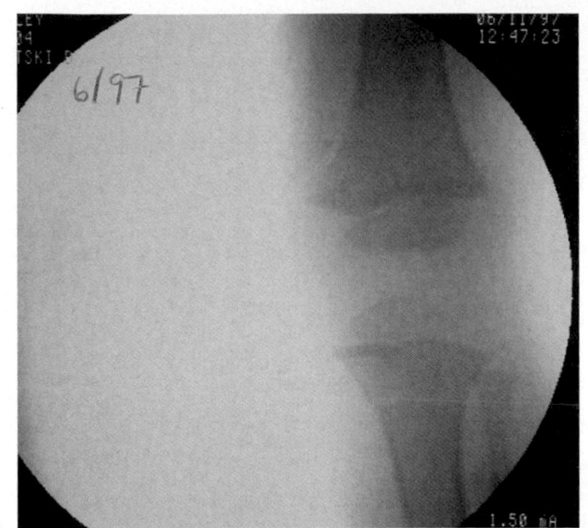

FIGURE 25-5 A–C. Anteroposterior radiographs demonstrating the development and subsequent spontaneous correction of postfracture tibia valga.

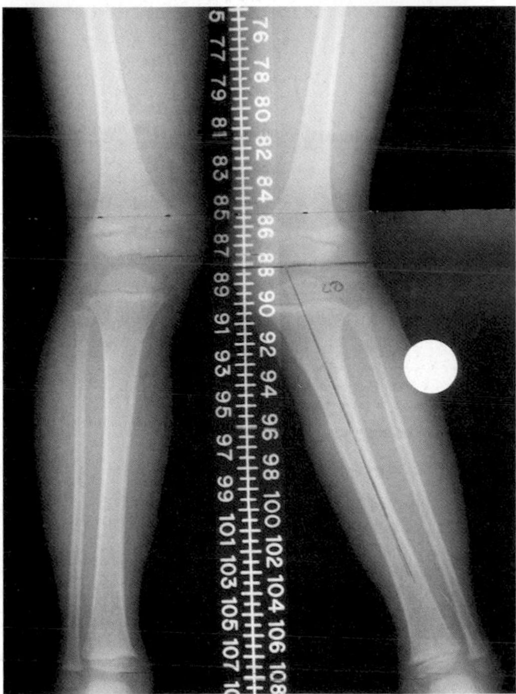

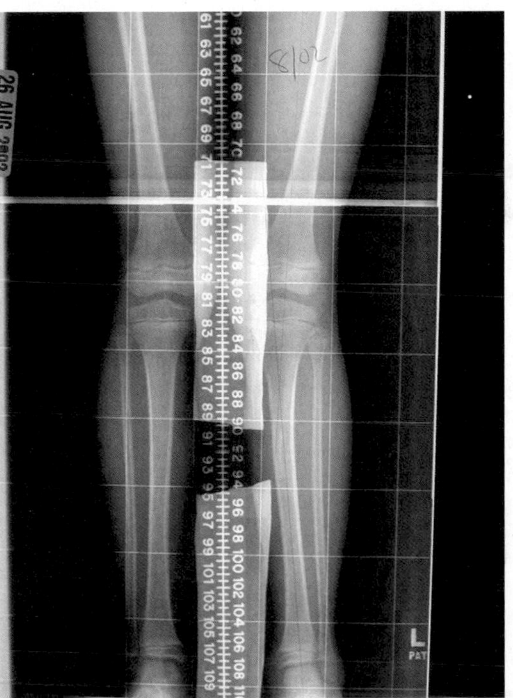

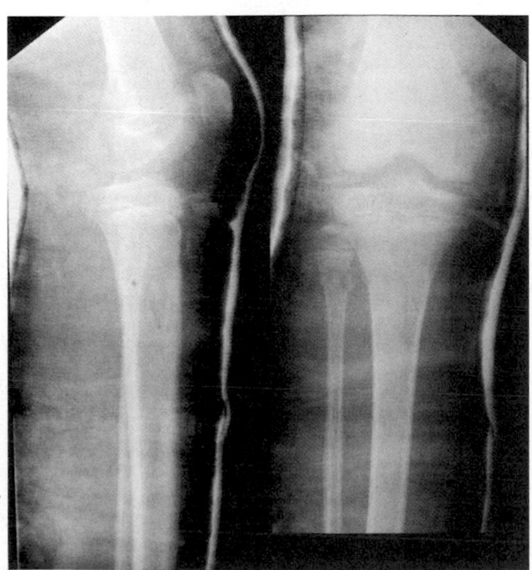

FIGURE 25-6 Anteroposterior and lateral radiographs of the proximal tibia and distal femur in a child who sustained a nondisplaced fracture of the proximal tibial and fibular metaphysis. The knee is casted in extension which facilitates accurate measurements of fracture alignment.

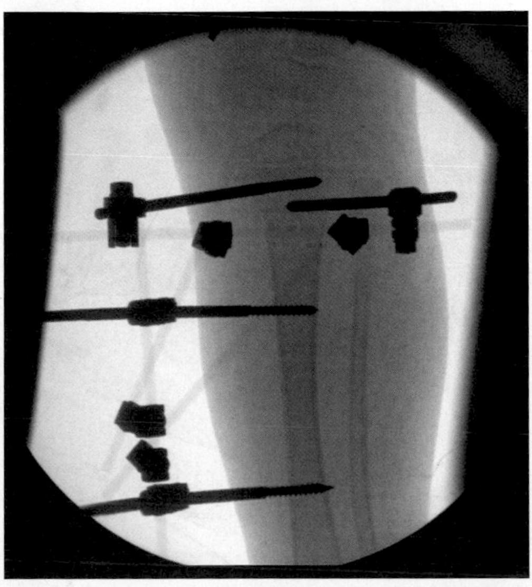

FIGURE 25-7 Anteroposterior radiograph of a 3-year-old female with a severe closed head injury, ipsilateral femur, and proximal tibial metaphyseal fractures. The tibia fracture was stabilized with a modified uniplanar external fixator.

cannot be obtained, open reduction is indicated. Open reduction includes removal of any soft tissue interposed within the fracture site and repair of the pes anserinus plate if ruptured. The child is placed into a long-leg, straight-knee cast after reduction, and the alignment is checked once again radiographically. In rare instances, percutaneous fixation with smooth pins, or an external fixator, may be required (Fig. 25-7). The goal is anatomic reduction or slight varus position at the fracture site. When the child initially presents for treatment of a tibia fracture at risk of developing genu valgum, it is imperative that the possibility of this unusual and unpredictable postfracture problem is discussed with the family. Frequent follow-up visits are required to verify maintenance of the reduction. The cast is removed approximately 6 weeks after injury. The child may return to normal activities after recovery of normal knee and ankle range of motion. Long-term follow-up with a warning to the family of possible growth abnormality is mandatory.

A child with a posttraumatic valgus deformity is followed until adequate spontaneous correction occurs. This may take 18 to 36 months. Surgical intervention may be indicated in patients more than 18 months postinjury with a mechanical axis deviation greater than 10 degrees as a result of tibial valgus. Tibial osteotomies are not indicated in patients with significant growth remaining (Fig. 25-8). A proximal tibial medial hemiepiphysiodesis can produce more anatomic alignment without many of the risks of osteotomy. Hemiepiphysiodesis may be accomplished through a variety of methods utilizing staples, screws, or newer plate and screw devices (Fig. 25-9A,B).[101,141] Orthotic devices do not alter the natural history of posttraumatic tibia valga and are not recommended. Since the valgus deformity usually is associated with some element of overgrowth, a contralateral shoe lift of appropriate size may make the deformity appear less apparent.

DIAPHYSEAL FRACTURES OF THE TIBIA AND FIBULA

Seventy percent of pediatric tibial fractures are isolated injuries.[133,151,153] The fractures can be incomplete (torus, greenstick) or complete. Most tibial fractures in children under 11 years of age are caused by a torsional force and occur in the distal third of the tibia. These oblique and spiral fractures occur when the body rotates with the foot in a fixed position on the ground. The fracture line generally starts in the distal anteromedial aspect of the bone and propagates proximally in a posterolateral direction. If there is not an associated fibula fracture, the intact fibula prevents significant shortening of the tibia; however, varus angulation develops in approximately 60% of isolated tibial fractures within the first 2 weeks after injury (Fig. 25-10).[153] In these cases, the forces of contraction of the long flexor muscles of the lower leg are converted into an angular moment by the intact fibula producing varus malalignment (Fig. 25-11A). Isolated transverse and comminuted fractures of the tibia most commonly are caused by direct trauma. Transverse fractures of the tibia with an intact fibula seldom displace significantly.[12,77] Comminuted tibial fractures with an intact fibula tend to drift into varus alignment similar to oblique and spiral fractures.[12,77,153]

Approximately 30% of pediatric tibial diaphyseal fractures have an associated fibular fracture.[133,151,153] The fibular fracture

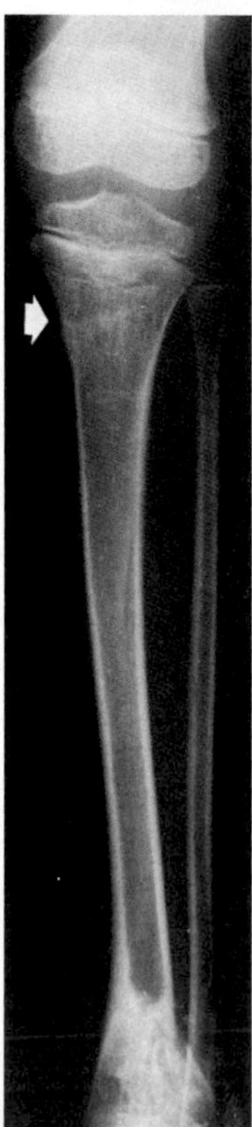

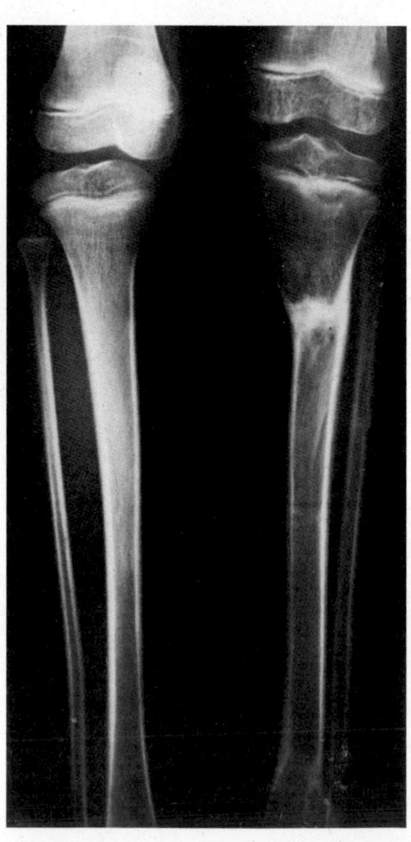

FIGURE 25-8 Developmental valgus after a proximal tibial metaphyseal fracture and subsequent corrective osteotomy. **A.** Radiograph taken 6 months after a fracture of the proximal tibia. The injury was nondisplaced. The scar from the initial proximal metaphyseal fracture is still seen (*arrow*). This child developed a moderate valgus deformity of the tibia within 6 months of fracture. **B.** A proximal tibial corrective osteotomy was performed. *(continues)*

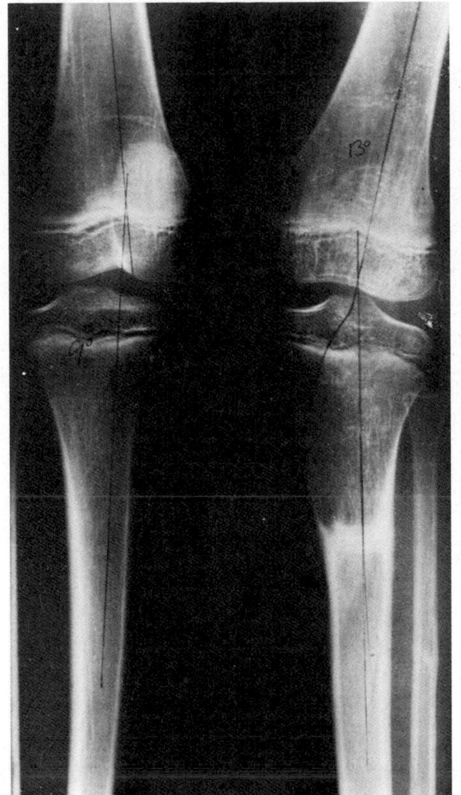

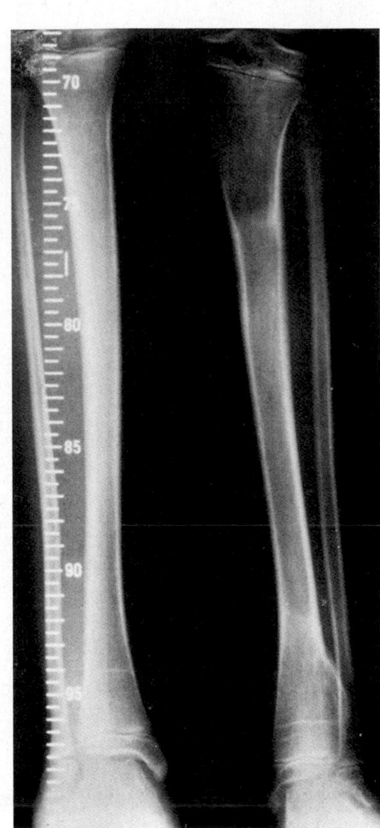

FIGURE 25-8 (*continued*) **C.** Two months postoperatively, the osteotomy was healed and the deformity corrected. **D.** Five months later, there was a recurrent valgus deformity of 13 degrees. (Courtesy of John J.J. Gugenheim, MD.)

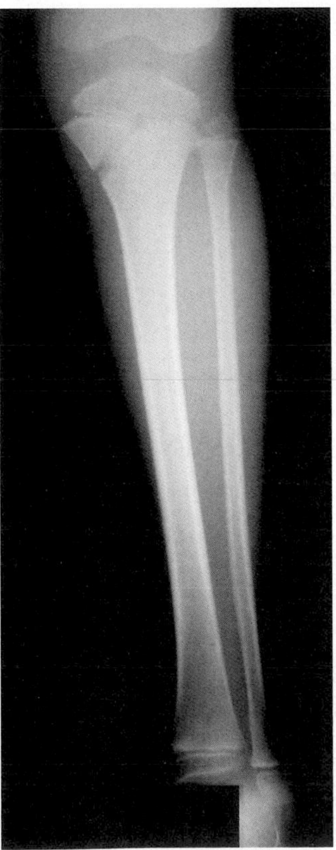

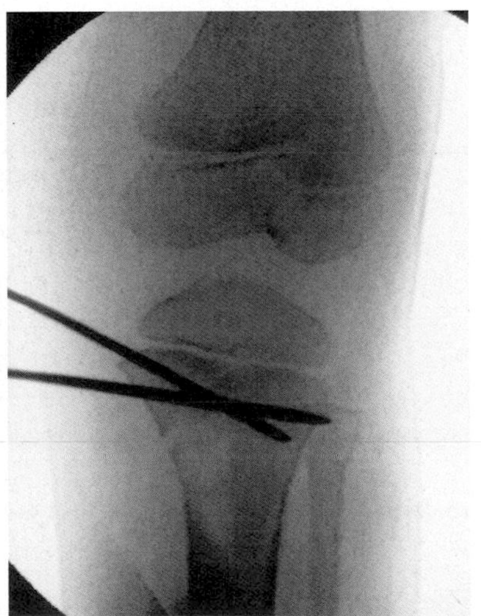

FIGURE 25-9 A. Anteroposterior image of a Salter-Harris type II fracture of the proximal tibia. Notice the valgus alignment. **B.** This fracture was treated with percutaneous pin fixation after reduction.

(*continues*)

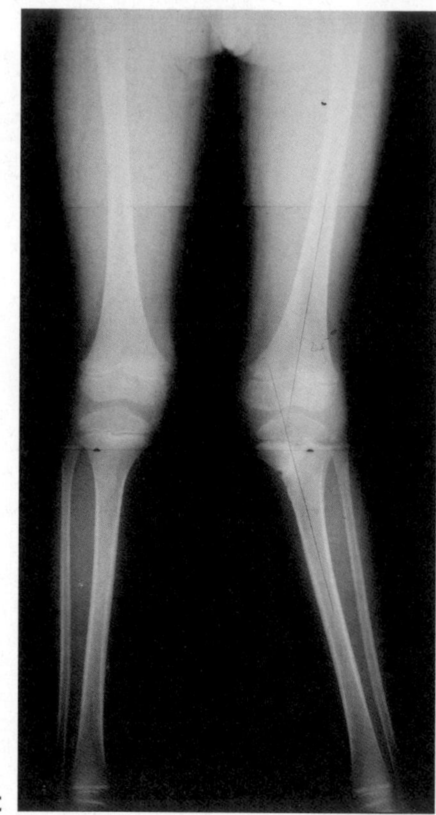

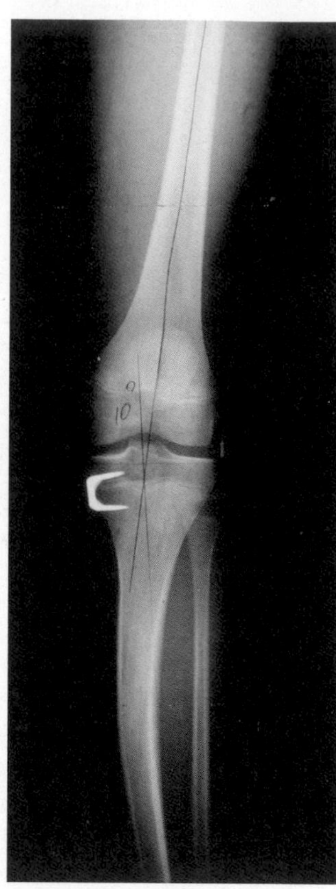

FIGURE 25-9 (*continued*) **C.** This patient developed tibia valga over a period of approximately 2 years following the injury. **D.** A medial proximal tibial hemiepiphysiodesis using a staple was performed.

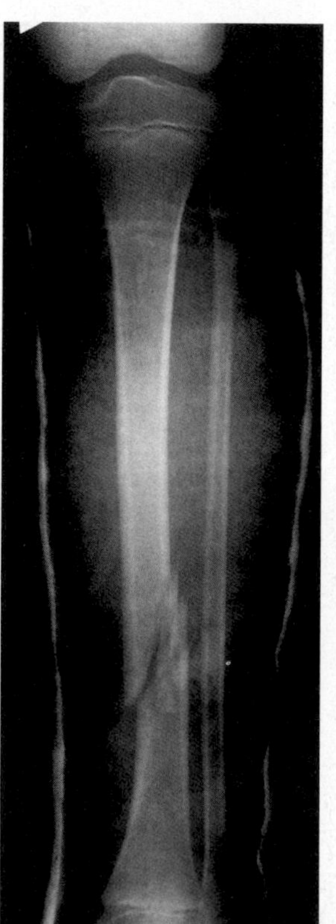

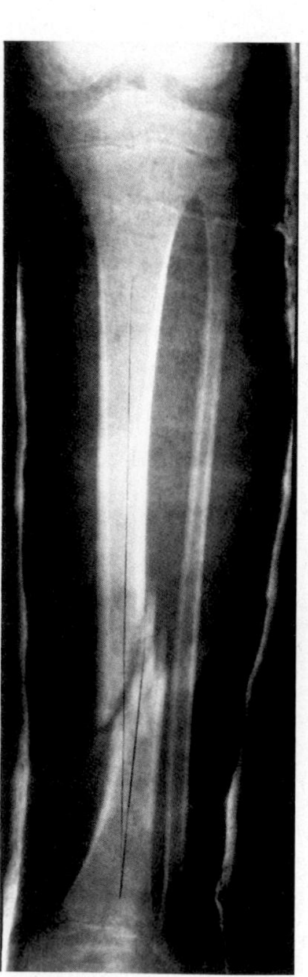

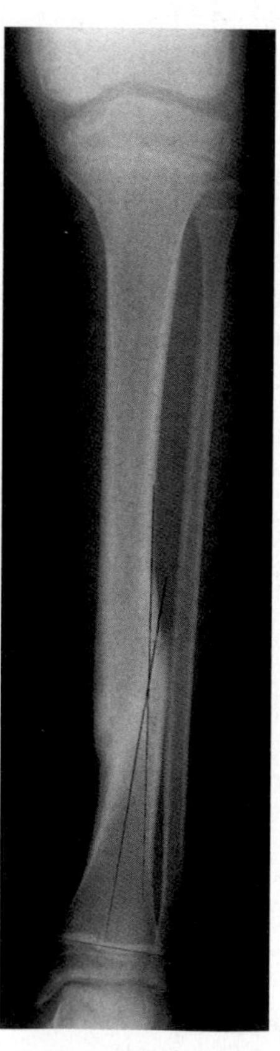

FIGURE 25-10 Anteroposterior radiograph of a distal one third tibial fracture without concomitant fibular fracture in a 10-year-old child. **A.** The alignment in the coronal plane is acceptable (note that the proximal and distal tibial growth physes are parallel). **B.** A varus angulation developed within the first 2 weeks after injury. **C.** A 10-degree varus angulation was present after union.

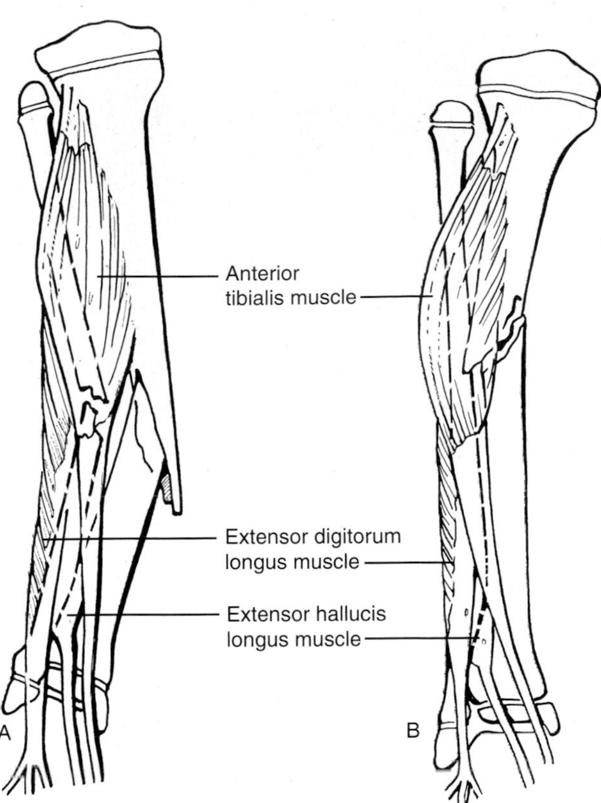

FIGURE 25-11 A. Fractures involving the middle third of the tibia and fibula may shift into a valgus alignment due to the activity of the muscles in the anterior and the lateral compartments of the lower leg. **B.** Fracture of the middle tibia without an associated fibular fracture tend to shift into varus due to the force created by the anterior compartment musculature of the lower leg and the tethering effect of the intact fibula.

may be either complete or incomplete with some element of plastic deformation. A tibial diaphyseal fracture with an associated complete fracture of the fibula usually results in valgus malalignment because of the action of the muscles in the anterolateral aspect of the leg (see Figs. 25-11B and 25-12). Any fibular injury must be identified and corrected to minimize the risk of recurrence of angulation after reduction (Fig. 25-13A–C).

An isolated fracture of the fibular shaft is rare in children and most commonly results from a direct blow to the lateral aspect of the leg (Fig. 25-14). Most isolated fractures of the fibular shaft are nondisplaced and heal quickly with symptomatic care and immobilization (Fig. 25-15). Rarely, compartment syndrome may accompany this injury.

Signs and Symptoms

The signs and symptoms associated with tibial and fibular diaphyseal fractures vary with the severity of the injury and the mechanism by which it was produced. Pain is the most common symptom. Children with fractures of the tibia or fibula have swelling at the fracture site, and the area is tender to palpation. Almost all children with a tibia fracture of any type will refuse to ambulate on that limb. If there is significant injury to the periosteum and fracture displacement, a bony defect or prominence may be palpable. Immediate neurologic impairment is rare except with fibular neck fractures caused by direct trauma.

Although arterial disruption is uncommon in pediatric tibial and fibular diaphyseal fractures, both the dorsalis pedis and the posterior tibial pulses should be assessed, and a Doppler examination should be performed if they are not palpable. Capillary refill, sensation, and pain response patterns, particularly pain with passive motion, should be monitored. Concomitant soft tissue injuries must be evaluated carefully. Open fractures must be treated aggressively to reduce the risk of late complications.

Radiographic Evaluation

Anteroposterior and lateral radiographs that include the knee and ankle joints (Fig. 25-16) should be obtained whenever a tibial and/or fibular shaft fracture is/are suspected. While uncommon, tibial shaft fractures may occur in combination with transitional fractures involving the distal tibial metaphysis, and as such, close evaluation of the ankle radiographs is essential (Fig 25-17A–D). Comparison views of the uninvolved leg normally are not indicated. Children with suspected fractures not

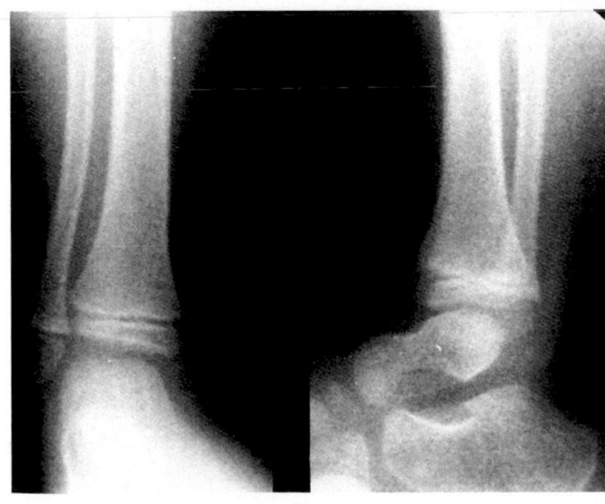
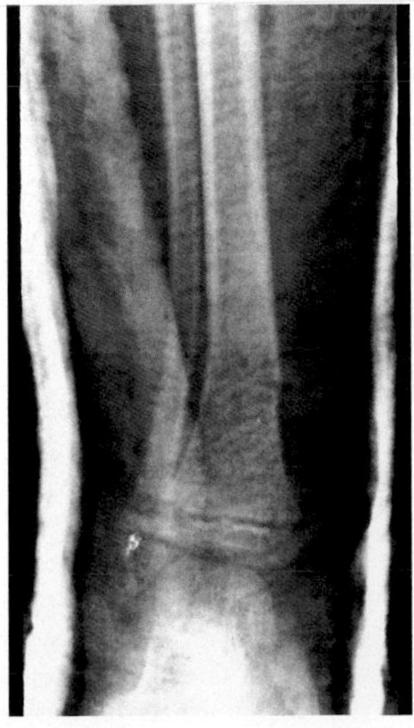

FIGURE 25-12 A. Nondisplaced distal tibia fracture with a plastic deformation of the fibula. **B.** The tibia fracture displaced in a cast 1 week later from the knee exerted by the plastically deformed fibula.

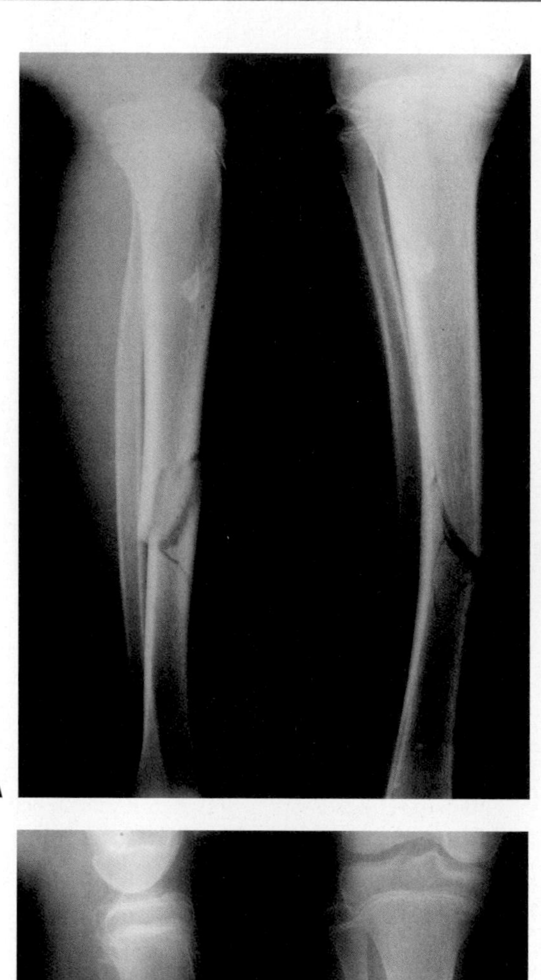

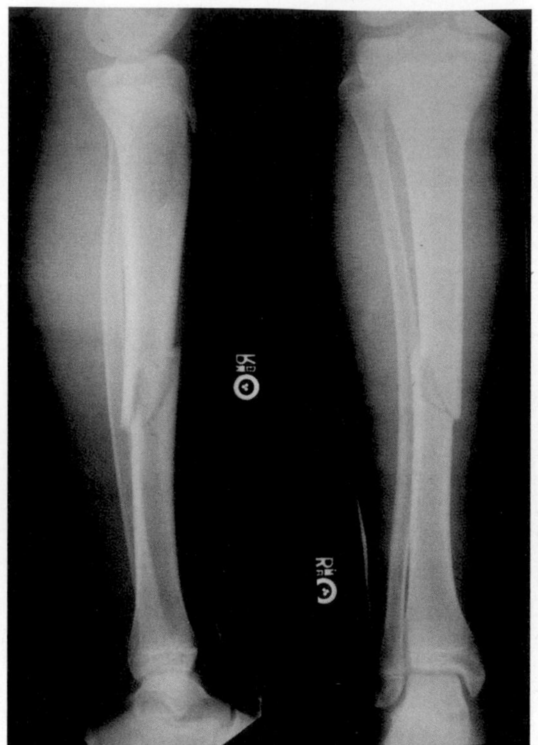

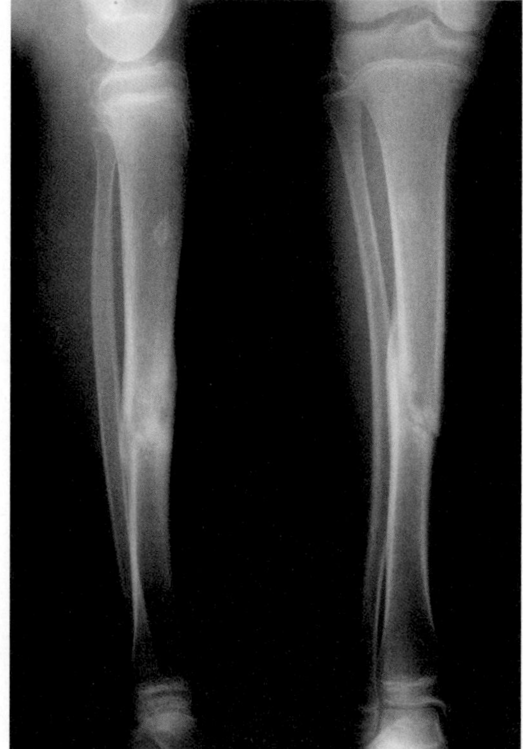

FIGURE 25-13 A. Anteroposterior and lateral radiograph of the lower leg in a 12-year-old child showing a comminuted tibial fracture with a concomitant plastic deformation of the fibula. Note the valgus alignment of the tibia. **B.** This patient had a closed manipulation and casting correcting the valgus alignment in the tibia and partially correcting the plastic deformation of the fibula. **C.** At union, there is an anatomic alignment of the tibia with a mild residual plastic deformation of the fibula.

apparent on the initial radiographs may need to be treated with supportive casting to control symptoms associated with the injuries. Technetium radionuclide scans obtained at least 3 days after injury are useful to identify fractures that are unapparent on radiographs; however, in most cases, patients with clinical findings consistent with a fracture are treated as though a fracture is present. Periosteal new bone formation on plain radiographs obtained 10 to 14 days after injury confirms the diagnosis.

Treatment

Cast Immobilization

The vast majority of uncomplicated pediatric tibial and fibular shaft fractures can be treated by manipulation and cast applica-

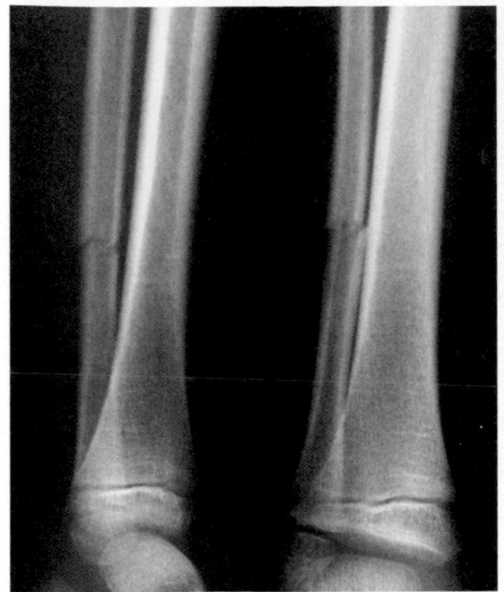

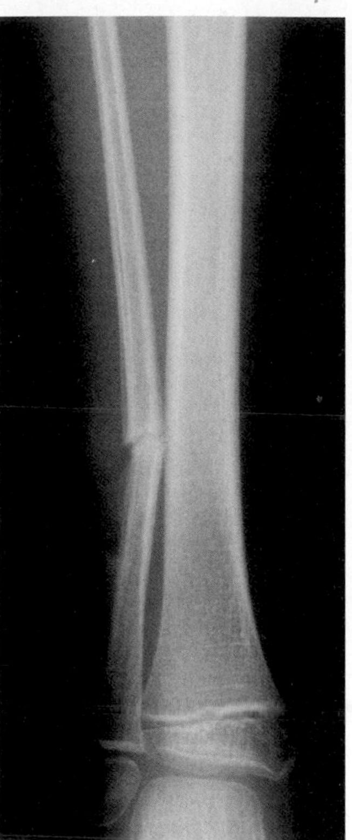

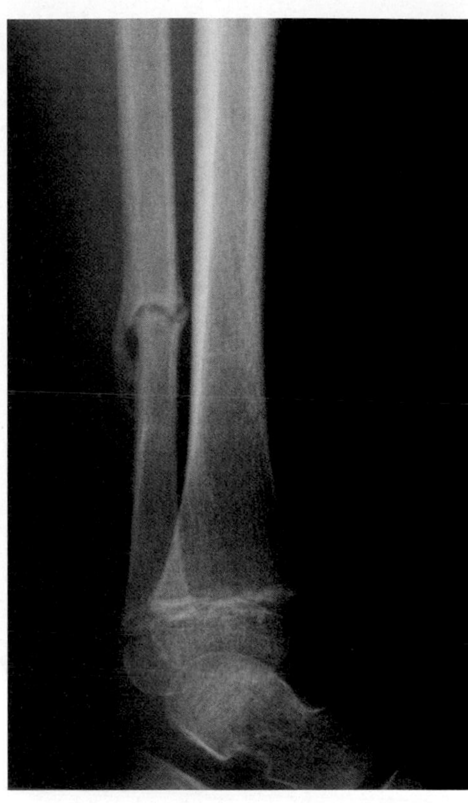

FIGURE 25-14 A. Anteroposterior and lateral radiograph of a 7-year-old child with an isolated open fibula fracture secondary to a bite by a pit bull. **B.** Anteroposterior radiograph 6 weeks after injury demonstrating consolidation at the fracture site. **C.** Lateral radiograph showing bridging callus 6 weeks after injury.

FIGURE 25-15 Distal one third fibular fracture in an 8-year-old who was struck on the lateral side of the leg (right). There is moderate new bone formation 6 weeks after injury (left).

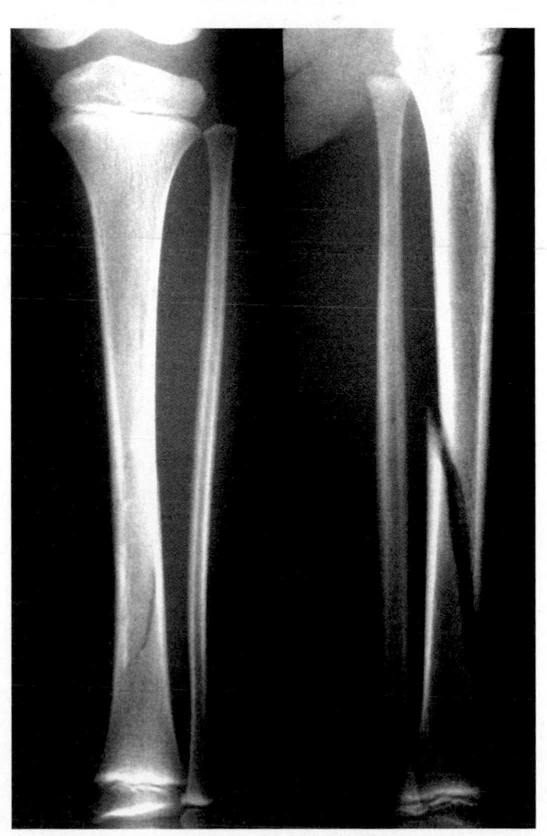

FIGURE 25-16 A. Spiral fracture of the distal tibia. The fracture is difficult to identify on the anteroposterior radiograph. **B.** The fracture is easily identified on the lateral radiograph.

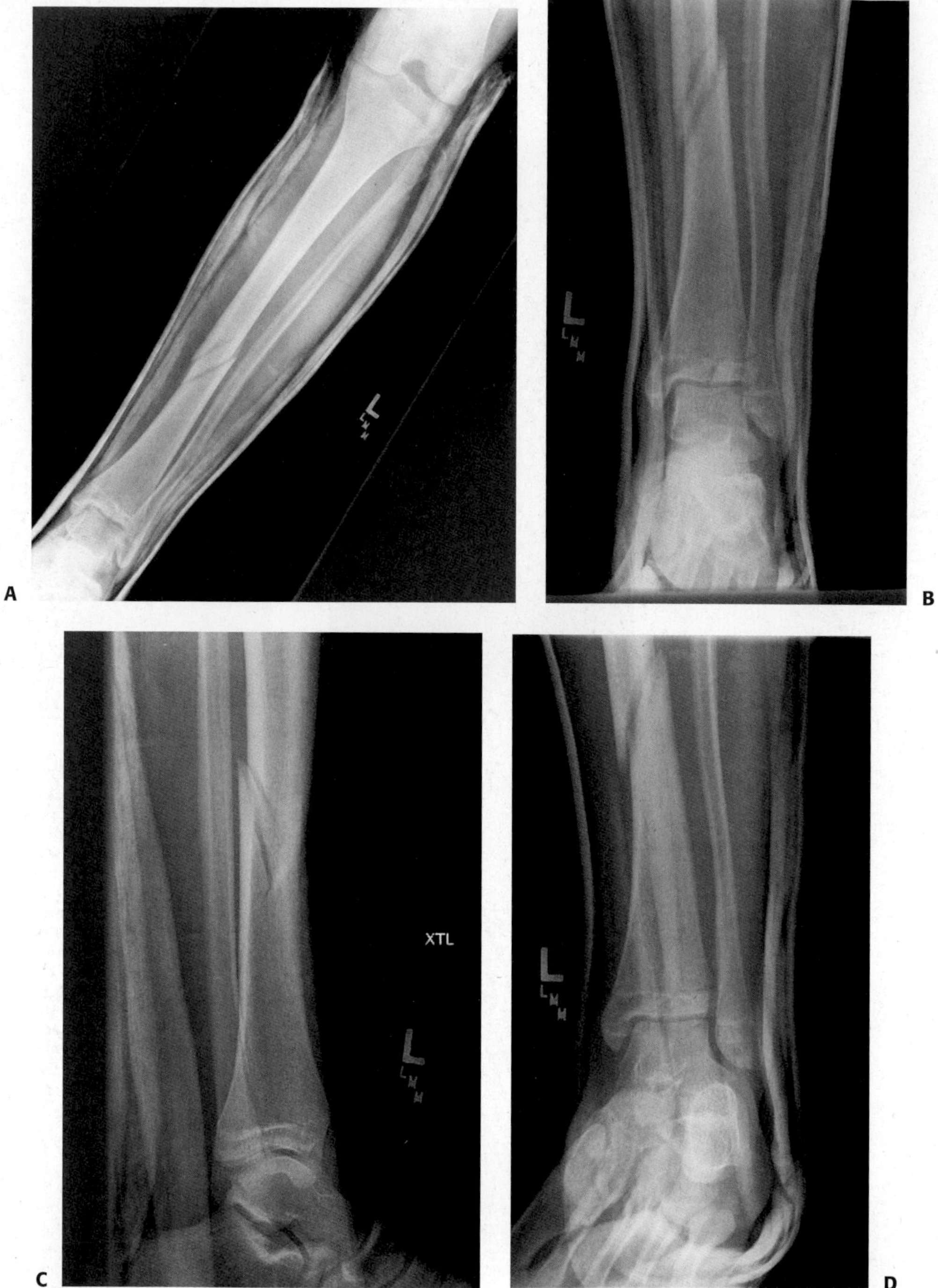

FIGURE 25-17 A. Anteroposterior radiograph of an adolescent patient with a tibial shaft fracture. **B–D.** Anteroposterior, lateral, and mortise views of the ankle demonstrate an associated triplane fracture.

tion.[64] Fractures of the tibial shaft without concomitant fibular fracture may develop varus malalignment. Valgus angulation and shortening can present a significant problem in children who have complete fractures of both the tibia and the fibula.

Displaced fractures should be managed with reduction under appropriate sedation, using fluoroscopic assistance when available. This can be done in the emergency room or in the operating room. A reduction plan should be made before manipulation based on review of the deforming forces apparent on the injury radiographs. A short-leg cast is applied with the foot in the appropriate position with either a varus or valgus mold, depending on the fracture pattern and alignment. The cast material is taken to the inferior aspect of the patella anteriorly and to a point 2 cm distal to the popliteal flexion crease posteriorly. It may be best to use plaster for the initial cast because of its ability to mold to the contour of the leg and the ease with which it can be manipulated while setting. The alignment of the fracture is reassessed after the short-leg cast has been applied. The cast is then extended to the proximal thigh with the knee flexed. Most children with complete, unstable diaphyseal tibial fractures are placed into a bent-knee (45-degree) long-leg cast to control rotation at the fracture site and to assist in maintaining non–weight bearing status during the initial healing phase. The child's ankle initially may be left in some plantar flexion (20 degrees for fractures of the middle and distal thirds, 10 degrees for fractures of the proximal third) to prevent apex posterior angulation (recurvatum) at the fracture site. In a child, there is little risk of developing a permanent equinus contracture, as any initial plantar-flexion can be corrected at a cast change once the fracture becomes more stable.

The alignment of the fracture should be checked weekly during the first 3 weeks after the cast has been applied. Muscle atrophy and a reduction in tissue edema may allow the fracture to drift into unacceptable alignment. Cast wedging may be indicated in an attempt to improve alignment, and in some cases a second cast application with remanipulation of the fracture under general anesthesia may be necessary to obtain acceptable alignment. Acceptable position is somewhat controversial and varies based on patient age as well as location and direction of the deformity.[35] Remodeling of angular deformity is limited in the tibia. No absolute numbers can be given, but the following general principles may be beneficial in decision making:

- Varus and valgus deformity in the upper and midshaft tibia remodel slowly, if at all. Up to 10 degrees of deformity can be accepted in patients less than 8 years old, and little more than 5 degrees of angulation in those older than 8 years of age.
- Moderate translation of the shaft of the tibia in a young child is satisfactory, whereas in an adolescent, at least 50% apposition is recommended.
- Up to 10 degrees of anterior angulation may be tolerated, although remodeling is slow.
- Little apex posterior angulation (recurvatum) can be accepted, as this forces the knee into extension at heel strike during gait.
- Up to 1 cm of shortening is acceptable.

Cast Wedging

Patients with a loss of fracture reduction and an unacceptable increase in angulation may benefit from remanipulation of the fracture. This can be attempted in the clinic setting through the use of cast "wedging." The fracture alignment in the cast can be changed by creating a closing wedge, an opening wedge, or a combination of wedges. Unfortunately, this technique is somewhat labor intensive and has become something of a lost art. The location for the wedge manipulation is determined by evaluating the child's leg under fluoroscopy and marking the midpoint of the tibial fracture on the outside of the cast. If fluoroscopy is not available, a series of paper clips are placed at 2-cm intervals on the cast and anteroposterior and lateral radiographs are then taken. The paper clips define the location of the fracture and the location most suitable for cast manipulation.

Closing Wedge Technique. A wedge of cast material is removed which encompasses 90% of the circumference of the leg with its base over the apex of the fracture. The exact width of the wedge is proportional to the amount of correction desired and therefore varies in each patient. The cast is left intact opposite the apex of the fracture in the plane of proposed correction. The edges of the cast are brought together to correct the angulation at the fracture. This wedging technique may produce mild fracture shortening, and care must be taken to avoid pinching the skin at the site of cast reapproximation. Theoretically, the closing wedge technique may increase exterior constrictive pressure, as the total volume of the cast is reduced. In light of these concerns, it may be preferable to use the opening wedge technique whenever possible.

Opening Wedge Technique. The side of the cast opposite the apex of the fracture is cut perpendicular to the long axis of the bone. A small segment of the cast is left intact directly over the apex of the malaligned fracture (~25%). A cast spreader is used to "jack" the cast open. Plastic blocks (Fig. 25-18) or a stack of tongue depressors of the appropriate size are placed into the open segment to maintain the distraction of the site, and the cast is wrapped with new casting material after the alignment has been assessed radiographically (Fig. 25-19). When using any wedging material, it is imperative that the edges do not protrude into the cast padding or cause pressure on the underlying skin. This wedging technique effectively lengthens the tibia while correcting the malalignment (Figs. 25-20A–D).

Combination Technique. Approximately 45% of the cast opposite the apex of the malaligned fracture is cut perpendicular to the shaft of the tibia. Two vertical cuts separated by approximately 0.5 cm are made 90 degrees from the first cut in both directions directly over the fracture. A wedge of casting material is removed from the apex side of the malaligned fracture and the cast opposite the apex of the fracture is opened. This closes the defect in the cast over the apex of the fracture, and produces a change in the angular alignment of the bone without a significant change in the length of the bone.

Operative Treatment

Historically, operative treatment has been recommended rarely for tibial shaft fractures in children. Weber et al.[151] reported that only 29 (4.5%) of 638 pediatric tibial fractures in their study required surgical intervention. However, in the last decade there has been an increasing interest in surgical stabilization, particularly for unstable closed tibial shaft fractures as well as open fractures or those with associated soft tissue injuries. The current indications for operative treatment include open fractures, some fractures with an associated compartment syndrome, some fractures in children with spasticity (head injury or cerebral palsy), fractures in which open treatment facilitates nursing care (floating knee, multiple long bone fractures, multiple system injuries), and unstable fractures in which adequate alignment can not be either attained or maintained.[3,9,24,36,40,43,53,68,80] Common methods of fixation for tibial fractures requiring operative treatment include percutaneous metallic pins, bioabsorbable pins,[6] external fixation,[28,106,130] and plates with screws; the use of flexible intramedullary titanium or stainless steel nails or, in some cases, intramedullary Steinmann pins, is becoming increasingly common.[44,48,49,88,106,108,117,125,148] Kubiak et al.[88] compared the use of titanium flexible nails with external fixation in a mixed group of patients with open and closed tibial fractures. While the groups were not matched and were reviewed retrospectively, the authors reported a clinically significant decrease in time to union with titanium nails compared to external fixation. Gordon et al.[49] retrospectively reviewed 60 pediatric patients with open or closed tibial shaft fractures managed with flexible nails. They found an 18% com-

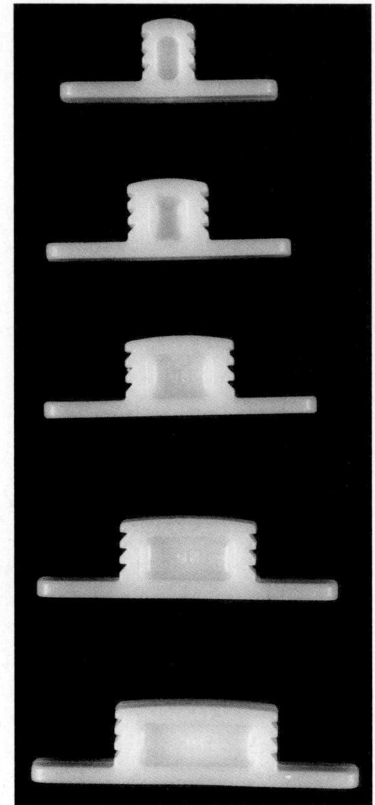

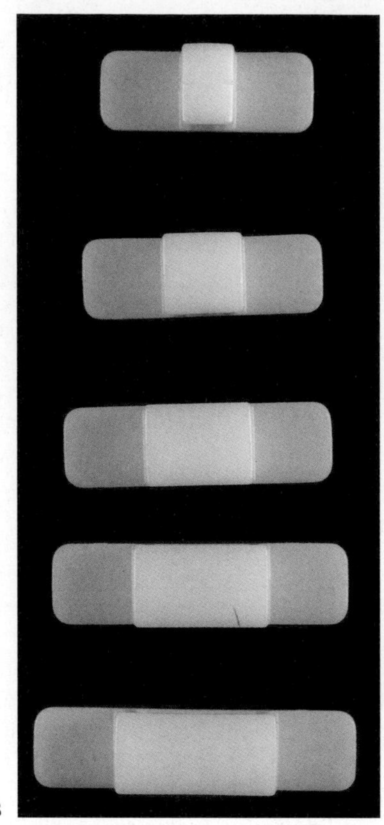

FIGURE 25-18 A,B. Blocks used to hold casts open after wedge corrections of malaligned fractures. The wings on the blocks prevent the blocks from migrating toward the skin.

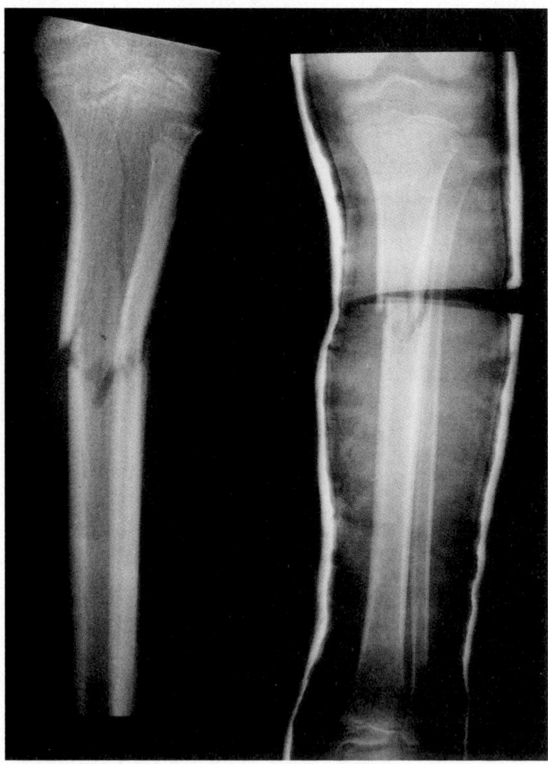

FIGURE 25-19 Comminuted fracture of the tibia and fibula in a 12-year-old boy struck by a car (left). Notice the extension of the fracture into the metaphysis from the diaphyseal injury. The fracture is in a valgus alignment. The fracture could not be maintained in an acceptable alignment (right). The cast was wedged with excellent result.

plication rate; the most common complication was delayed union. In this study, those patients with delayed time to union tended to be older (mean age 14.1 years) versus the mean age of the study population (11.7 years).

OPEN TIBIA FRACTURES

Open tibial fractures in children are treated similarly to comparable injuries in adults, and likewise, are classified by the Gustillo and Anderson System (Table 25-4 and Fig. 25-21).[56] Most open fractures of the tibia result from high-velocity/high-energy injuries.

Treatment Principles

Management principles for open tibial fractures include:

- Timely débridement, irrigation, and initiation of appropriate antibiotic therapy
- Fracture reduction followed by stabilization with either an internal or external device
- Intraoperative angiography (after rapid fracture stabilization) and management of possible elevation of compartment pressures when sufficiency of the vascular perfusion is unclear
- Open wound treatment with loose gauze packing or other methods[28,104]
- Staged débridement of necrotic soft tissue and bone in the operating room as needed until the wounds are ready for closure or coverage.
- Delayed closure or application of a split thickness skin graft when possible; use of delayed local or free vascularized flaps as needed
- Closed cancellous bone grafting for bone defects or delayed union after maturation of soft tissue coverage

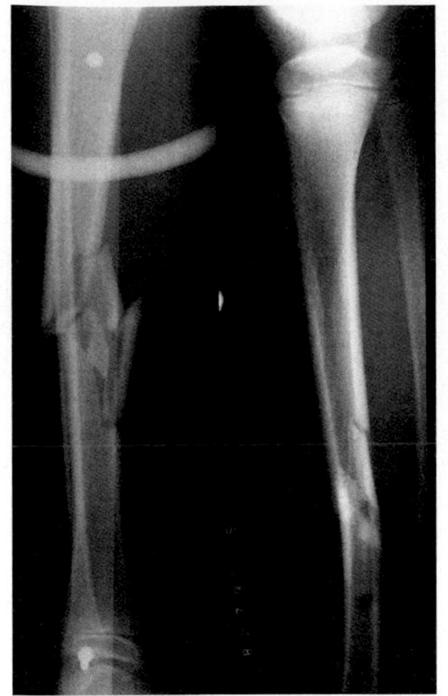

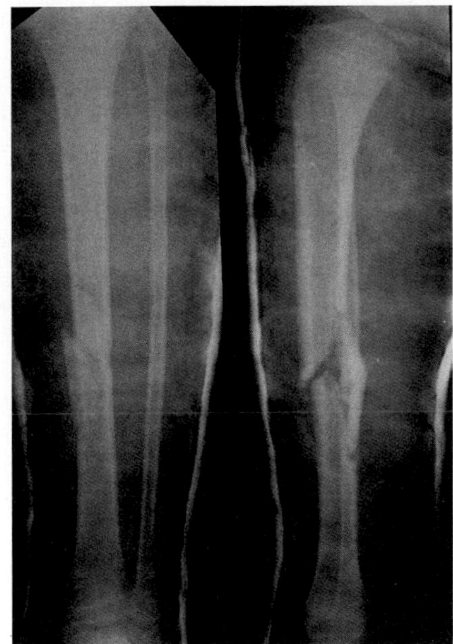

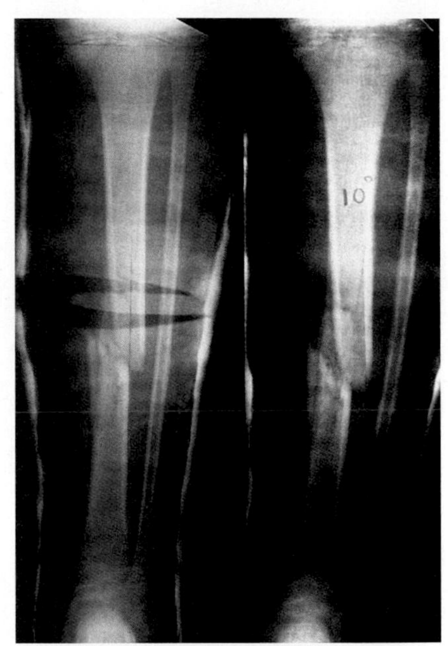

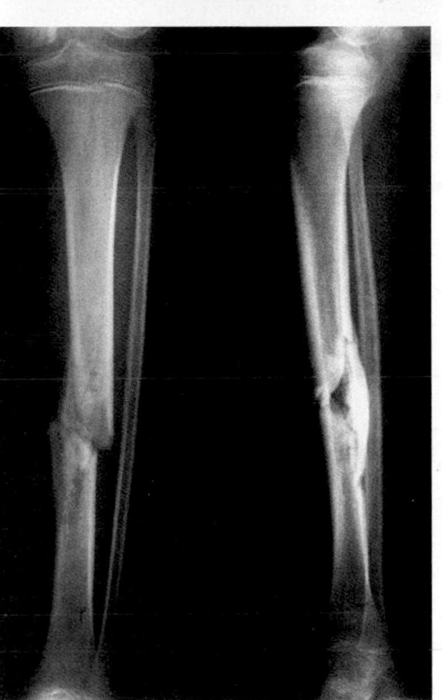

FIGURE 25-20 A. Anteroposterior and lateral tibial radiographs of an 11-year-old boy who was struck by an automobile, sustaining a markedly comminuted tibial fracture without concomitant fibular fracture. **B.** Despite the comminution, length and alignment were maintained in a cast. **C.** The patient's fracture shifted into a varus malalignment that measured 10 degrees (right). The cast was wedged, resulting in the re-establishment of an acceptable coronal alignment (left). **D.** The patient's fracture healed without malunion.

The principles of treatment for open tibial fractures in adults have been modified by the unique characteristics of the pediatric skeleton. These differences include the following[3,24,48,55,138]:

- Comparable soft tissue and bony injuries heal more reliably in children than in adults, particularly in patients less than 11 years of age.[75]
- Devitalized uncontaminated bone that can be covered with soft tissue can incorporate into the fracture callus, and in some cases may be left within the wound.
- External fixation can be maintained, when necessary, until fracture consolidation with fewer concerns about delayed or nonunions.
- Retained periosteum can reform bone even after segmental bone loss in younger children.
- After a thorough irrigation and débridement, many uncontaminated grade I open wounds may be closed primarily without an increased risk of infection.

Buckley et al.[14] reported 41 children with 42 open fractures of the tibia (18 grade II, 6 grade IIIA, 4 grade IIIB, and 2 grade IIIC). Twenty-two (52%) of the fractures were comminuted. All wounds were irrigated and débrided, and antibiotics were administered for at least 48 hours. Twenty-two fractures were treated with reduction and cast application, and 20 with external fixation. Three children had early infections, and one of these patients developed late osteomyelitis. All infections had resolved at final reported follow-up. The average time to union was 5 months (range, 2 to 21 months). The time to union was directly proportional to the severity of the soft tissue injury. Fracture pattern also had an effect on time to union. Segmental bone loss, infection, and the use of an external fixation device were associated with delayed union. Four angular malunions of more than 10 degrees occurred, three of which spontaneously corrected. Four children had more than 1 cm of overgrowth.

In a series of 40 open lower extremity diaphyseal fractures in 35 children, Cramer et al.[23] reported 22 tibial fractures

TABLE 25-4 Classification of Open Fractures

Grade I
Low-energy wound, <1 cm in length
Bone piercing skin from inside/out
Minimal muscle damage
Grade II
Wound >1 cm in length
Moderate soft tissue injury
Grade III
High-energy wound
Usually >10 cm in length
Extensive muscle devitalization
Bone widely displaced or comminuted
Special cases
Shotgun wound
High-velocity gunshot (>2000 ft/s)
Segmental fracture
Segmental diaphyseal loss
Farmyard environment
Associated vascular injury

From Gustillo RB, Anderson JT. Prevention of infection in the treatment of 1025 fractures of long bones. J Bone Joint Surg Am 1976;58:453, with permission.

(1 grade I, 10 grade II, and 11 grade III). External fixation was used for 15 fractures, casting for five, and internal fixation for two. Two children required early amputation, four required soft tissue flap coverage, and 13 children had skin grafts. Two additional children with initially closed injuries required fasciotomy for compartment syndrome and were included in the group of open tibial fractures. Ten of the 24 injuries healed within 24 weeks. Five children required bone grafting before healing.

Hope and Cole[66] reported the results of open tibial fractures in 92 children (22 grade I, 51 grade II, and 19 grade III). Irrigation and débridement were performed on admission, antibiotics were given for 48 hours, and tetanus prophylaxis was administered when necessary. Primary closure was performed in 51 children, and 41 fractures were left open. Eighteen soft tissue injuries healed secondarily, and 23 required either a split thickness skin graft or a tissue flap. Sixty-five (71%) of the 92 fractures were reduced and immobilized in an above-the-knee plaster cast. External fixation was used for unstable fractures, injuries with significant soft tissue loss, and fractures in patients with multiple system injuries. Early complications of open tibial fractures in these children were comparable with those in adults (Table 25-5).[9,14,17,20,29,57,63,65,90,107,114,127] Primary closure did not increase the risk of infection if the wound was small and uncontaminated.[3,24,65] At reevaluation 1.5 to 9.8 years after injury, the authors[23] found that 50% of the patients complained of pain at the fracture site; 23% reported decreased abilities to participate in sports, joint stiffness, and cosmetic defects; and 64% had leg length inequalities (Table 25-6). Levy et al.[93] found comparable late sequelae after open tibial fractures in children, including a 25% prevalence of nightmares surrounding the events of the accident. Blasier and Barnes[8] and Song et al.[138] found that most late complications associated with pediatric open tibial fractures occurred in children over the age 12 and 11 years, respectively.

Skaggs et al.[134] reviewed their experience with open tibial fractures and found no increased incidence of infection in patients initially débrided more than 6 hours after injury when compared to children treated similarly less than 6 hours after fracture. However, it appears that fractures with more severe soft tissue injuries were more likely to receive more expedient treatment, thereby complicating the analysis. This apparent selection bias in some ways limits the overall usefulness of the study.

Recent data demonstrates increasing concerns with the use of external fixators in tibia fractures in pediatric patients. Myers et al.[106] reviewed 31 consecutive high-energy tibia fractures in children treated with external fixation. Nineteen of the fractures were open, with mean follow-up of 15 months. The authors found a high rate of complications in this patient population, including delayed union (particularly in patients of at least 12 years of age), malunion, leg-length discrepancy, and pin track infections. To date, there are no published studies which directly and prospectively compare use of flexible intramedullary nails with external fixation for open pediatric tibial shaft fractures.

Open Tibia Fractures—Associated Issues

Soft Tissue Closure

Expedient coverage of an open tibial fracture that cannot be closed primarily reduces the morbidity associated with this injury.[83,105] Delayed primary closure can be performed if the wound is clean and does not involve significant muscle loss. In such cases, it is imperative that closure under tension is avoided. Other options include a wide variety of local rotational or pedicled myocutaneous flaps. Vascularized free flaps are viable options in cases for which no other method of closure is appropriate.

Most of the literature addressing the subject of soft tissue coverage for open tibia fractures involves adult patients, and as such, must be extrapolated to pediatric fracture management. In a series of 168 open tibial fractures with late secondary wound closure, Small and Mollan[136] found increased complications with early pedicled or rotational fasciocutaneous flaps and late free flaps, but no complications with fasciocutaneous flaps created more than 1 month after injury. Complications associated with free flaps were decreased if the procedure was performed within 7 days of injury. Hallock et al.[60] reviewed 11 free flaps for coverage in pediatric patients. They reported a 91% success rate, which was similar to their rate in adults. However, they reported a significant rate of complications at both the donor and the recipient sites.[60] Rinker et al.[118] reported their experience with free vascularized muscle transfers for traumatic lower extremity trauma in pediatric patients performed between 1992 and 2002. At their institution, 26 patients received 28 flaps during that period. The latissimus dorsi was used most commonly as the origin of the transfer. Twelve of the flaps were performed for coverage of open tibia fractures. There was a 62% overall complication rate, with infection and partial skin-graft loss being the most common problems. The authors concluded that patients receiving free flap coverage within 7 days of injury had a statistically significant lower complication rate than those covered later.[118]

Ostermann et al.[111] reported 115 grade II and 239 grade III tibial fractures in a series of 1085 open fractures. All patients

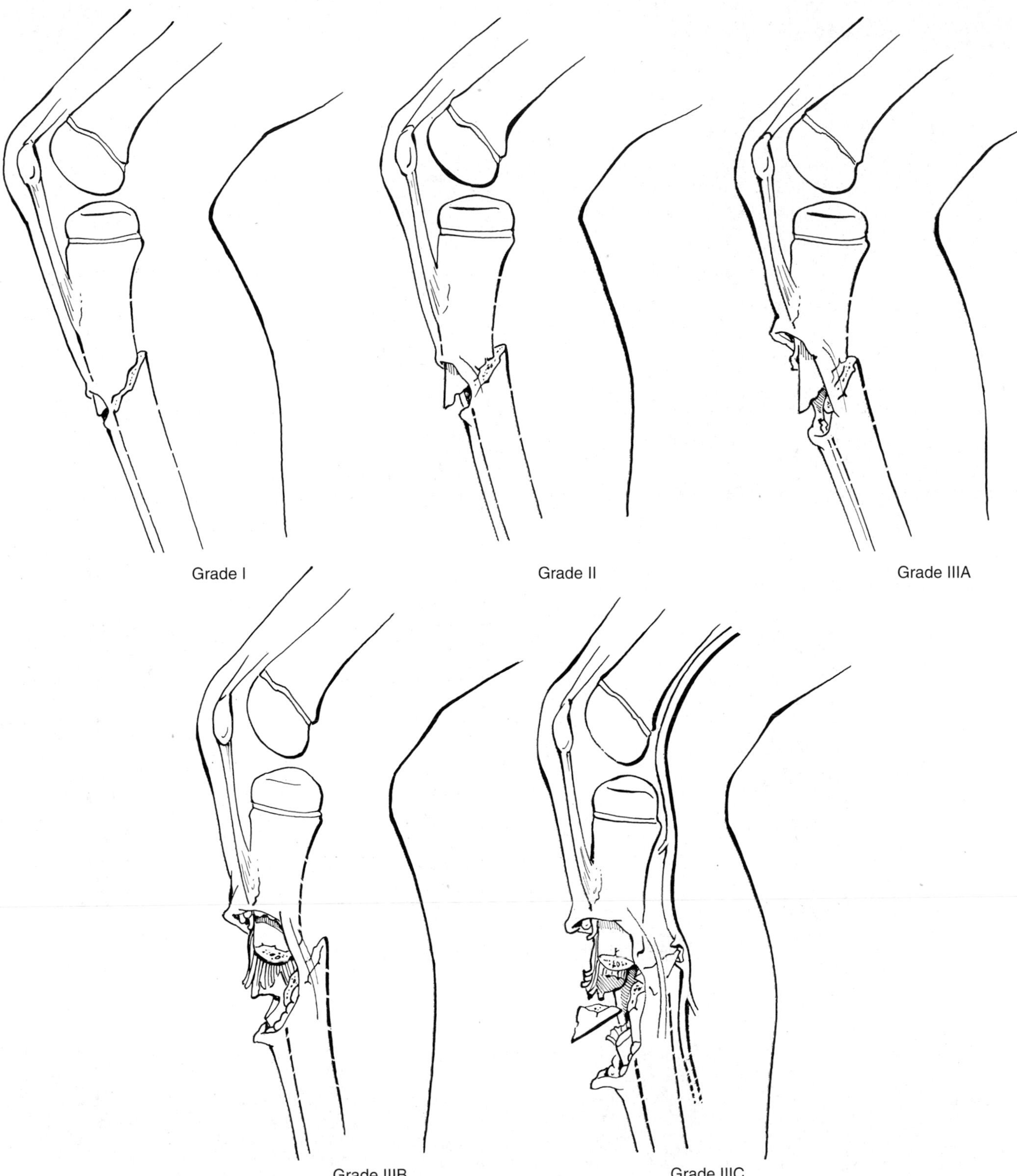

FIGURE 25-21 Gustilo and Anderson classification of open fractures. Grade I: The skin wound measures less than 1 cm long, usually from within, with little or no skin contusion. Grade II: The skin wound measures more than 1 cm long, with skin and soft tissue contusion but no loss of muscle or bone. Grade IIIA: There is a large severe skin wound with extensive soft tissue contusion, muscle crushing or loss, and severe periosteal stripping. Grade IIIB: Like grade IIIA but with bone loss and nerve or tendon injury. Grade IIIC: Like grade IIIA or B with associated vascular injury. (From Alonso JE. The initial management of the injured child: musculoskeletal injuries. In: MacEwen GD, Kasser J, Heinrich SD, eds. Pediatric Fractures: A Practical Approach to Assessment and Treatment. Baltimore: Williams & Wilkins, 1993:32, with permission.)

TABLE 25-5 Early Complications Associated with Open Pediatric Tibial Fractures

Complication	Grade I	II	III	Combined
Delayed union	18%	12%	26%	16%
Nonunion	5%	6%	16%	7.5%
Malunion	9%	4%	11%	6.5%
Infection	—	12%	21%	11%
Compartment syndrome	9%	2%	5%	4%
Physeal arrest	—	2%	5%	—
Weeks to union	13	12	17	13.5

From Hope PG, Cole WG. Open fractures of the tibia in children. J Bone Joint Surg Br 1992;74:546, with permission.

were treated with early broad-spectrum antibiotics, serial débridements, and the application of an external fixation device. Tobramycin-impregnated polymethylmethacrylate was placed into the wounds, and dressings were changed every 48 to 72 hours until the wounds spontaneously closed, underwent delayed primary closure, or received flap coverage. No infections occurred in grade I fractures; approximately 3% of grade II fractures and 8% of grade III fractures developed infections. No infections occurred in patients who had the wound closed within 8 days of injury. On the basis of these and other analyses, it now is recommended that wounds associated with open tibial fractures be covered within 7 days of injury whenever possible.[16,17,19,79,85,111,149]

Multiple authors have reported on the use of subatmospheric pressure dressings in the management of soft tissue injuries in pediatric patients. Dedmond et al.[28] reviewed the Wake Forest experience with negative pressure dressings in pediatric patients with type 3 open tibia fractures. They found that use of this device decreased the need for free tissue transfer to obtain coverage in this patient population.

TABLE 25-6 Late Complications Associated with Open Pediatric Tibial Fractures

Complication	Grade I	II	III	Combined
Pain	38%	48%	65%	—
Decreased athletic activity	19%	15%	47%	—
Decreased mobility (stiffness)	19%	20%	35%	—
Cosmetic complaints	6%	17%	53%	—
Leg length				
Short (0.5–2 cm)	22%	23%	40%	27%
Equal	14%	46%	33%	36%
Long (5.0–2 cm)	64%	31%	27%	37%

From Hope PG, Cole WG. Open fractures of the tibia in children. J Bone Joint Surg Br 1992;74:546, with permission.

Vascular Injuries

Vascular injuries have been reported in approximately 5% of children with open tibial fractures. Arterial injuries associated with open tibial fractures include those to the popliteal artery, the posterior tibial artery, the anterior tibial artery, and the peroneal artery. Complications are common in patients with open tibial fractures and associated vascular injuries. Amputation rates as high as 79% have been reported with grade IIIC fractures. Isolated anterior tibial and peroneal artery injuries generally have a good prognosis, whereas injuries of the posterior tibial and popliteal arteries have much less satisfactory prognoses, and more commonly require vascular repairs or reconstructions.[1,59,65] Patients with open tibial fractures and vascular disruption may benefit from arterial, and possibly venous, shunting before the bony reconstruction is performed. This allows meticulous débridement and repair of the fracture and maintains limb perfusion until the primary vascular repair is performed.[43] However, in most cases, rapid fracture stabilization, usually utilizing external fixation, can be performed prior to vascular reconstruction without the need for temporary shunts.

Compartment Syndrome

The prevalence of compartment syndromes in adults with open tibial fractures ranges from 6% to 9%.[9,29,90] The true incidence of compartment syndrome associated with open pediatric tibial fractures is unknown. Regardless, it is important to remember that compartment syndrome may occur in the face of significant soft tissue injury associated with extensively open fractures, as well as with closed injuries. Compartment pressures should be measured in all cases in which history and physical examination findings raise suspicion. In children, the cardinal initial finding is progressive pain in the limb, often signaled by increasing narcotic requirements. Signs such as motor and sensory deficits and loss of pulses are later findings. Unfortunately, despite physician experience and vigilance, compartment syndrome may be missed in pediatric patients. Fasciotomy is indicated for any patient with a significant elevation of compartment pressures or, more importantly, symptoms suggestive of a compartment syndrome. A more detailed review of the pathophysiology, diagnosis, and management of compartment syndrome is given in the later section regarding complications of closed, diaphyseal tibia fractures.

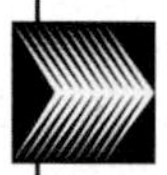

AUTHORS' PREFERRED TREATMENT

Closed Diaphyseal Fractures

Simple pediatric diaphyseal tibial fractures unite quickly in most cases, and cast immobilization can be used without affecting the long-term range of motion of the knee and the ankle. A bent-knee, long-leg cast provides maximal comfort to the patient and controls rotation of the fractured fragments. Children with nondisplaced or minimally dis-

TABLE 25-7 Acceptable Alignment of a Pediatric Diaphyseal Tibial Fracture

Patient Age	<8 Years	≥8 Years
Valgus	5 degrees	5 degrees
Varus	10 degrees	5 degrees
Angulation anterior	10 degrees	5 degrees
Posterior angulation	5 degrees	0 degrees
Shortening	10 mm	5 mm
Rotation	5 degrees	5 degrees

placed fractures that do not require manipulation generally do not need to be admitted to the hospital. Children with more extensive injuries should be admitted for neurovascular observation and instruction in wheelchair, crutch, or walker use.

Significantly displaced fractures disrupt the surrounding soft tissues and produce a large hematoma in the fascial compartments of the lower leg. Circulation, sensation, and both active and passive movement of the toes should be monitored carefully after injury. The child should be admitted to the hospital, and reduction should be performed with adequate sedation and fluoroscopy if available. Most fractures are casted after reduction, and the cast may be bivalved or split to allow room for swelling. The fracture must be evaluated clinically and radiographically within a week of manipulation to verify maintenance of the reduction. The cast can be wedged to correct minor alignment problems. Significant loss of reduction requires repeat reduction with adequate anesthesia (Table 25-7) and/or utilization of a more rigid fixation method. The long-leg cast may be changed to a short-leg, weight-bearing cast at 4 to 6 weeks after injury. Children over 11 years of age may be placed into a patellar tendon–bearing cast after removal of the long-leg cast.[127] Weight-bearing immobilization is maintained until sufficient callus is evident.

Fractures in patients with complicating factors including spasticity, a floating knee, multiple long-bone fractures, an associated transitional ankle fracture, extensive soft tissue damage, multiple system injuries, or an inability to obtain or maintain an acceptable reduction should be stabilized with a more rigid fixation method, such as external fixation, percutaneous Kirschner wires, or flexible intramedullary nails (Figs. 25-22 and 25-23).

Open Tibia Fractures

Open tibial fractures of any grade should have a thorough and expedient irrigation and débridement of the wound, although there is some evidence that infection rate is similar in injuries managed at less than 6 hours after injury and those treated later.[134] The patient's tetanus status is determined, and prophylaxis is administered as indicated. Appropriate intravenous antibiotic treatment is initiated as soon as possible and maintained as required based on the severity of the open fracture. The soft tissue wounds should be extended to be certain that the area is cleansed and débrided of all nonviable tissue and foreign material. Devitalized bone can be left in place if it is clean and can be covered by soft tissue. The operative wound extension may be closed along with the open segment in clean grade I injuries. The wound is allowed to heal by secondary intention if there is moderate contamination after irrigation and débridement. Patients with uncomplicated grade I fractures can be placed in a splint or a cast, or simple smooth pin fixation will prevent displace-

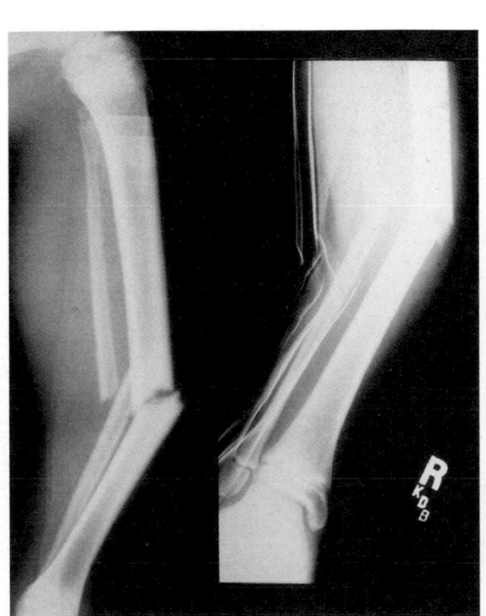

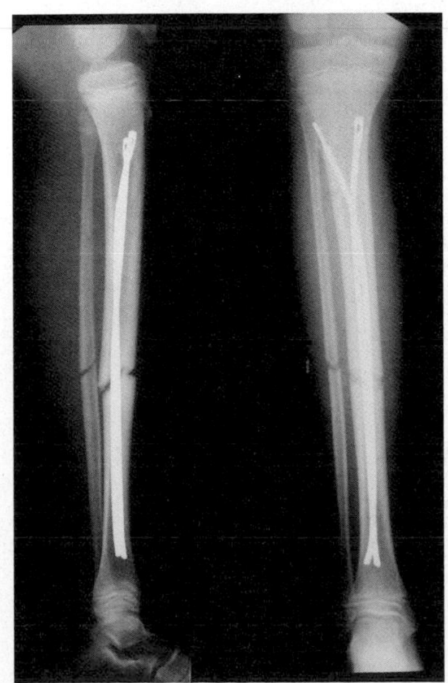

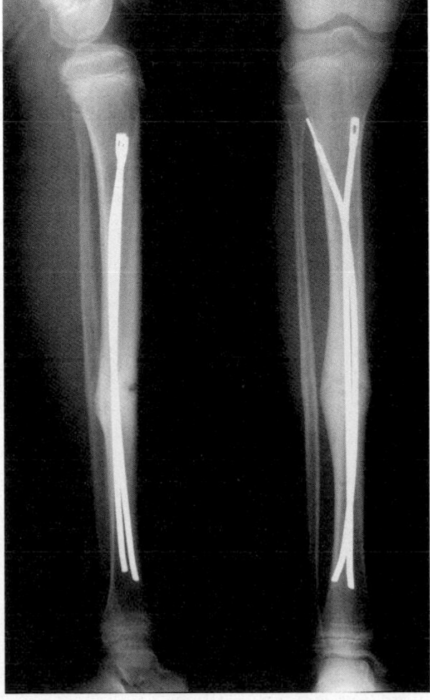

FIGURE 25-22 A. Anteroposterior and lateral radiographs of a 12-year-old who was involved in a motor vehicle accident sustaining a grade I open middle one third tibial and fibular fractures. **B.** This injury was treated with intramedullary nail fixation. **C.** At union, the patient has an anatomic alignment and no evidence of a growth disturbance.

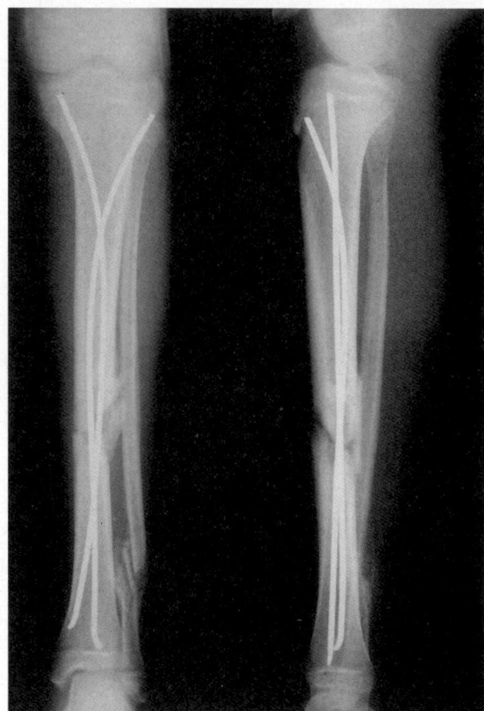

FIGURE 25-23 Anteroposterior radiograph of a 14-year-old who was involved in a motor vehicle accident sustaining a distal one third tibial fracture and comminuted distal fibular fracture. This was stabilized with titanium elastic nails.

ment of many unstable fractures (Fig. 25-24). Use of this limited fixation does not preclude supplemental splinting or casting. Wounds associated with grade II and III fractures are débrided of devitalized tissue and foreign material. Most children with grade II and all children with grade III wounds require more rigid fracture stabilization, usually with external fixation, although intramedullary nails may be used at the surgeon's discretion. More rigid fixation limits the need for significant external splinting, thereby allowing better access for wound care and sequential compartment evaluation as needed.

The most versatile external fixation device for open pediatric tibial fractures is a unilateral frame (Fig. 25-25). The unilateral frame is easy to apply and allows minor corrections in angular alignment and length. Secondary pins can be used for added support (Fig. 25-26); these are connected to the standard pins or the body of the external fixation device. This allows control of segmental fragments as needed. Fracture reduction tools can be applied to the pin clamps to assist in manipulating the fracture. A small-pin or thin-wire circular frame may be indicated for complicated fractures adjacent to the joint. Unilateral frames may be placed to span the joint in question so as to use ligamentotaxis as an indirect reduction method to establish and maintain alignment (Fig. 25-27).

If at all possible, external fixation pins are placed no closer than 1 cm to the physis. The external fixation device is applied, and a reduction maneuver is performed. All of the connections in the external fixation device are tightened after reduction has been obtained. Secondary pins to improve fracture stability are placed at this time. Limited internal fixation of the fracture can be used to aid in controlling fracture alignment. A posterior splint may be applied to prevent the foot from dropping into plantarflexion. This splint should be easy to remove for subsequent pin care and dressing changes of the open injury. Splinting of this type can be avoided by external fixation, be it unilateral or circular, to the forefoot.

Intramedullary fixation is performed most commonly in children using prebent stainless steel Enders nails or elastic titanium nails. In almost all cases, the implants are placed in

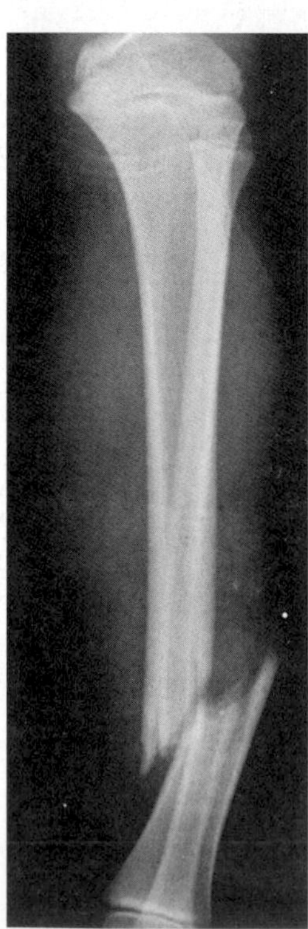

A

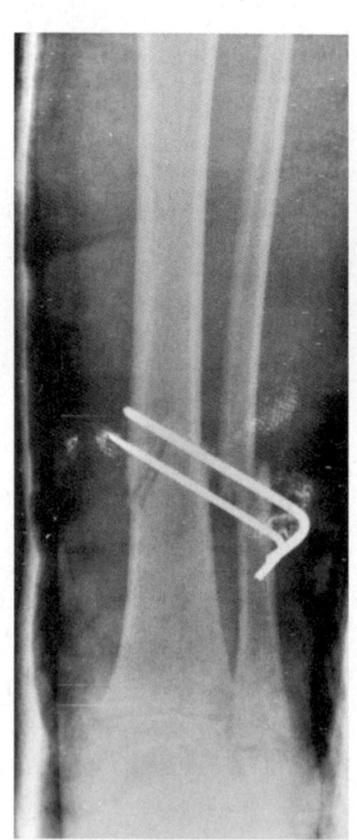

B

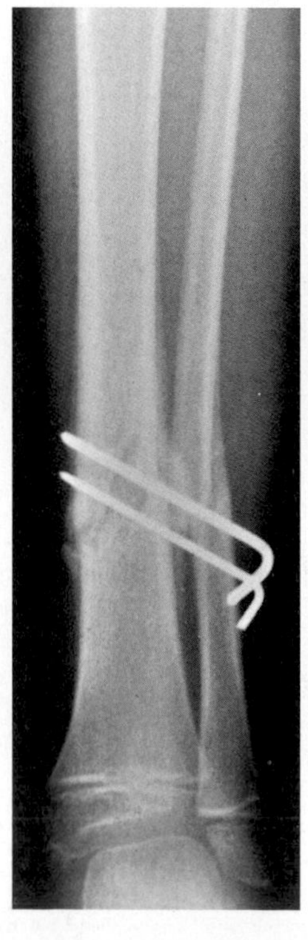

C

FIGURE 25-24 A. Anteroposterior radiograph of a grade I open distal one-third tibial fracture in a 7-year-old child. **B.** Two percutaneous pins were used to stabilize this fracture after irrigation and débridement. **C.** Good fracture callus was present and the pins were removed 4 weeks after injury.

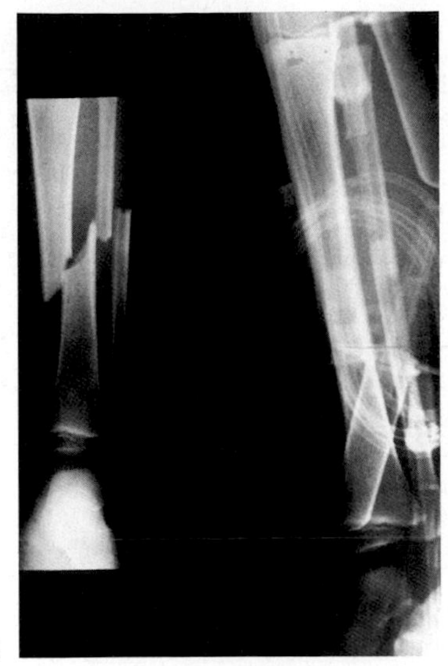
A

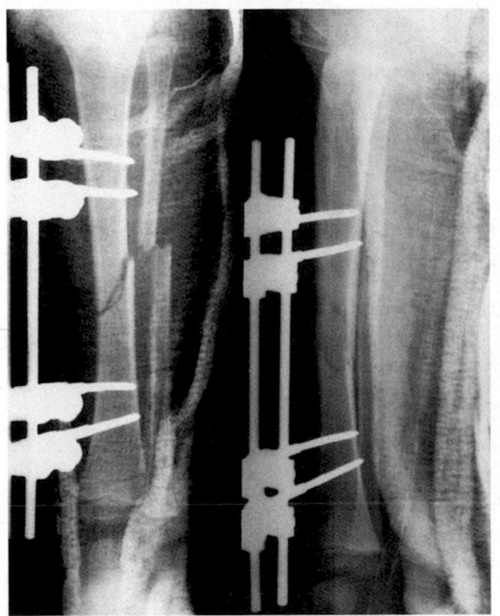
B

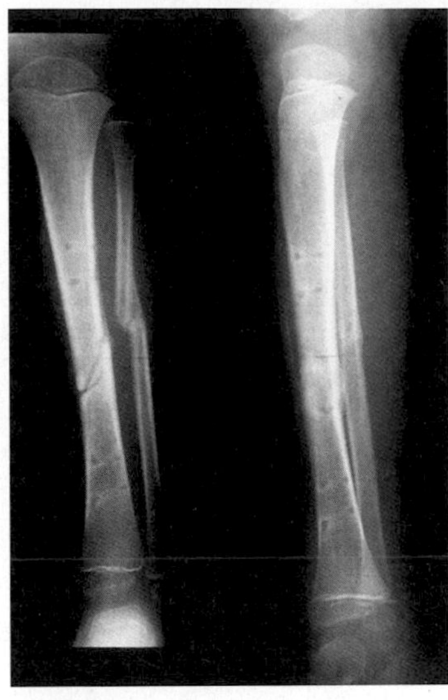
C

FIGURE 25-25 A,B. Type II open fracture of the tibia in a 5-year-old boy treated with débridement, unilateral external fixation, and split thickness skin graft. **C.** Four months after removal of the external fixation.

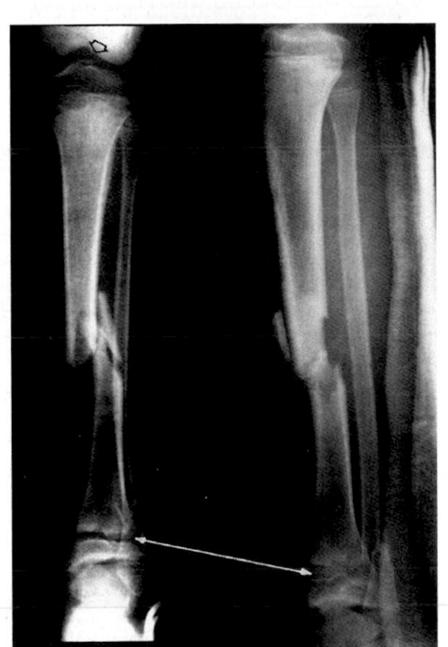
A

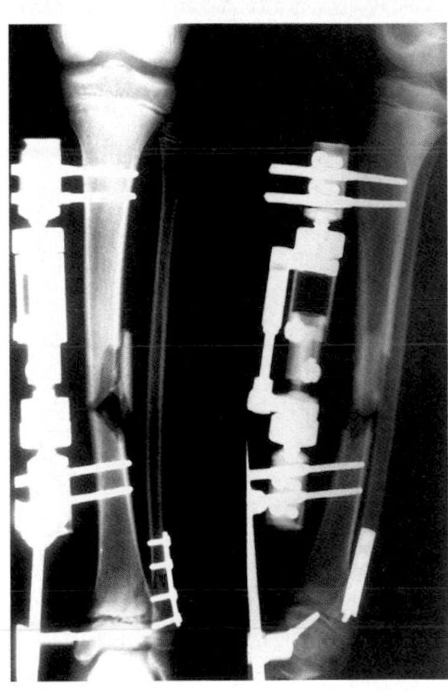
B

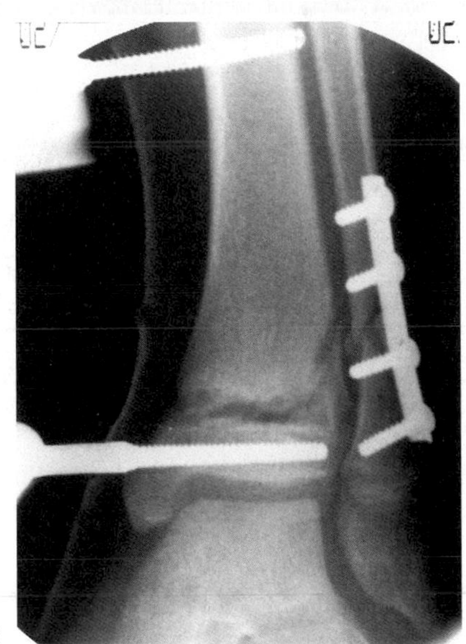
C

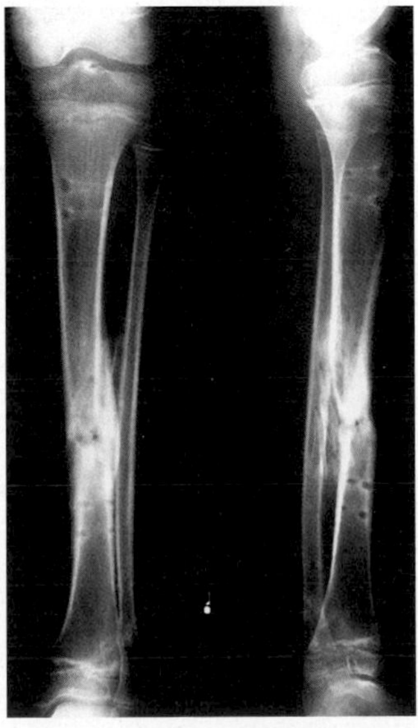
D

FIGURE 25-26 A. Anteroposterior and lateral radiographs of the tibia of a 12-year-old boy who was struck by a car. This child sustained a grade IIIB open middle one third tibial fracture, a Salter-Harris type II fracture of the distal tibial physis with associated distal fibular fracture (closed arrows), and a tibial eminence fracture (*open arrow*). **B.** Irrigation and débridement and application of an external fixation device were performed. **C.** The fracture of distal tibial physis was stabilized with a supplemental pin attached to the external fixation device. Open reduction and internal fixation of the fibula was performed to enhance the stability of the external fixator in the distal tibia. **D.** Anteroposterior and lateral radiogrphs of the tibia approximately 9 months after injury demonstrate healing of the tibial eminence fracture, the comminuted middle one third tibial fracture, and the distal tibial physeal fracture. The distal tibial physis remains open at this time.

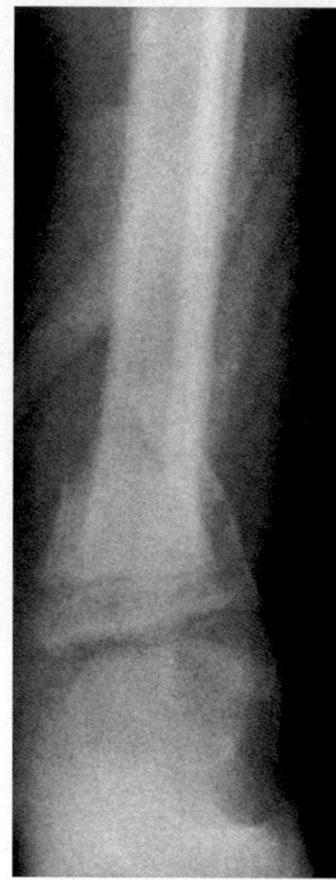

A

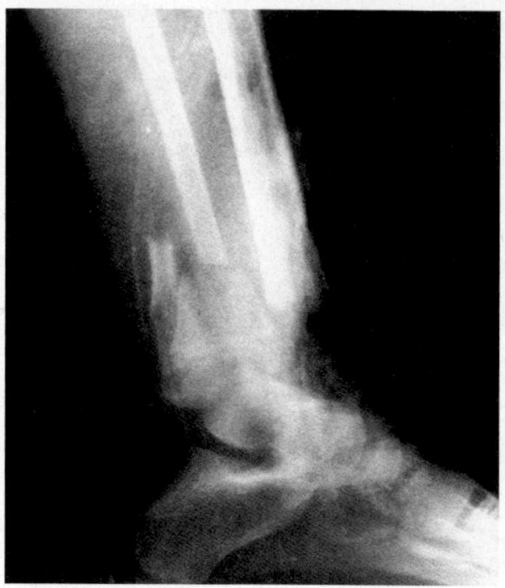

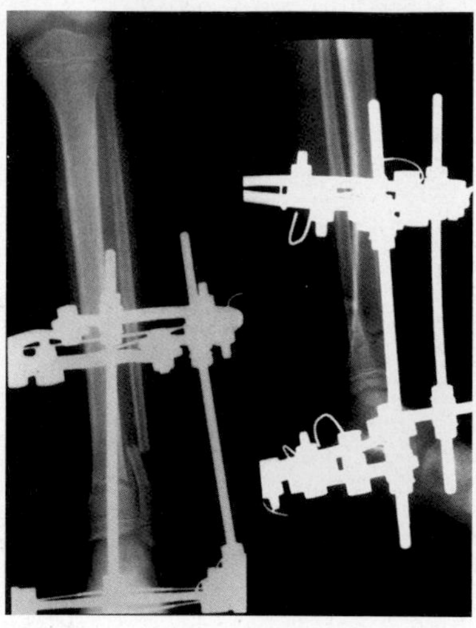

B

FIGURE 25-27 A. Anteroposterior and lateral radiographs of a grade IIIB open fracture of the distal tibia and fibula. **B.** Anteroposterior and lateral radiographs after fracture reduction and stabilization with an Ilizarov circular fixation frame. (From Sharps CH, Cardea JA. Fractures in the shaft of the tibia and fibula. In: MacEwen GD, Kasser J, Heinrich SD, eds. Pediatric Fractures: A Practical Approach to Assessment and Treatment. Baltimore: Williams & Wilkins, 1993:325, with permission.)

a proximal to distal fashion from medial and lateral proximal insertion points. Fluoroscopy is required for accurate placement. Care must be taken to avoid injury to the proximal tibial physes, including the tibial tubercle apophysis. Use of supplemental external splinting is at the discretion of the treating surgeon.

Immobilization

The length of immobilization varies with the child's age and the type of fracture. The duration of immobilization was 8 to 10 weeks in the Steinert and Bennek series.[142] Hansen et al.[61] found that healing time ranged from 5 to 8 weeks for "fissures and infractions" and from 5 to 13 weeks for oblique, transverse, and comminuted fractures. Hoaglund and States[63] reported that in 43 closed fractures in children, the average time in a cast was 2.5 months (range, 1.5 to 5.5 months), whereas the 5 children with open fractures were immobilized for 3 months.

Kreder and Armstrong[87] found an average time to union of 5.4 months (range, 1.5 to 24.8 months) in a series of 56 open tibial fractures in 55 children. The factor with the most effect on union time was the age of the patient. Grimard et al.[55] reported that the age of the patient and the grade of the fracture were significantly associated with union time. Blasier and Barnes[8] found that children under 12 years of age required less aggressive surgical treatment and healed faster than older children. They also found that younger children were more resistant to infection and had fewer complications than older children.

Rehabilitation

Most children with a tibial fracture do not require extensive rehabilitation. In the vast majority of cases, normal walking and running activities serve as therapy. Most children limp with an out-toeing rotation gait on the involved extremity for several weeks to a month after the cast is removed. This is secondary to muscle weakness, joint stiffness, and a tendency to circumduct the limb during swing phase, rather than a malalignment of the fracture. As the muscle atrophy and weakness resolve, the limp improves. In very rare situations, formal physical therapy may be required for some children after a tibial fracture. Knee range-of-motion exercises and quadriceps strengthening may be useful in an older child progressing from a bent-knee cast to weight bearing on a short-leg cast. Progressive weight bearing on a short-leg cast requires the patient to wean off crutches or a walker. In some children, this requires supervision. The child may return to sports when the fracture is healed and the patient has regained strength and function comparable to that of the uninjured leg.

FRACTURES OF THE DISTAL TIBIAL METAPHYSIS

Fractures of the distal tibial metaphysis are often greenstick injuries resulting from increased compressive forces along the anterior tibial cortex. The anterior cortex is impacted while the posterior cortex is displaced under tension, with a tear of the overlying periosteum. A recurvatum deformity may occur (Fig. 25-28). Reduction of these injuries should be performed with adequate sedation and maintained with a long-leg cast. The foot should be left in moderate plantarflexion to prevent recurrence of apex posterior angulation at the fracture site. The foot is brought up to neutral after 3 to 4 weeks, and a short-leg walking cast is applied. Unstable injuries can be treated with percutaneous pins (Fig. 25-29), antegrade flexible nails, or with open reduction and internal fixation as needed (Fig. 25-30). Open reduction and internal fixation of the distal fibula, if fractured, may prevent malalignment in an unstable distal tibia fracture.[37]

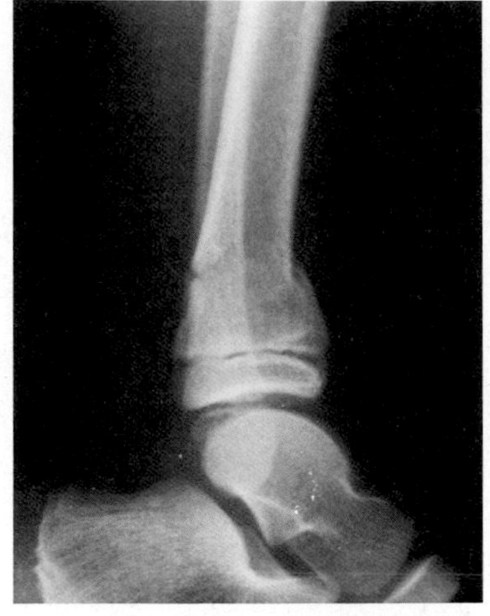

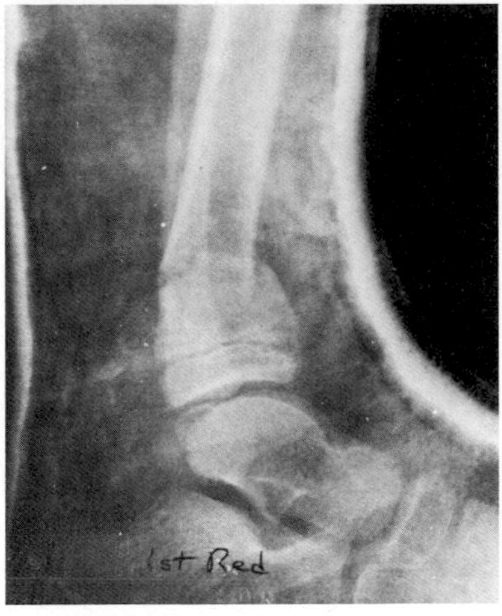

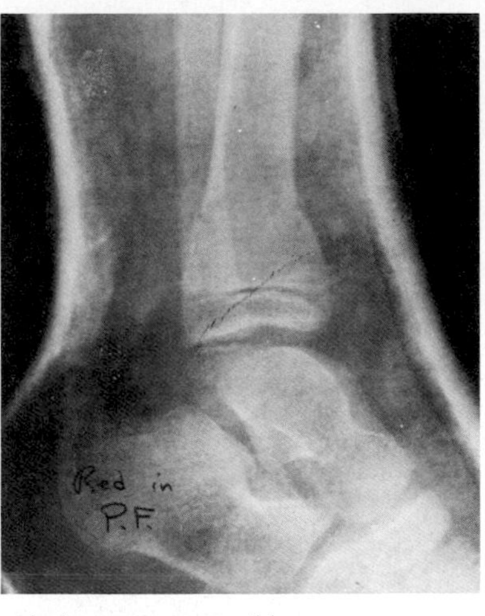

FIGURE 25-28 A. Fracture of the distal tibia in a 7-year-old child. The lateral radiograph demonstrates a mild recurvatum deformity. **B.** The ankle was initially immobilized in an ankle neutral position, producing an increased recurvatum deformity. The cast was removed and the ankle remanipulated into plantarflexion to reduce the deformity. **C.** The ankle was then immobilized in plantarflexion, which is the proper position for this type of fracture.

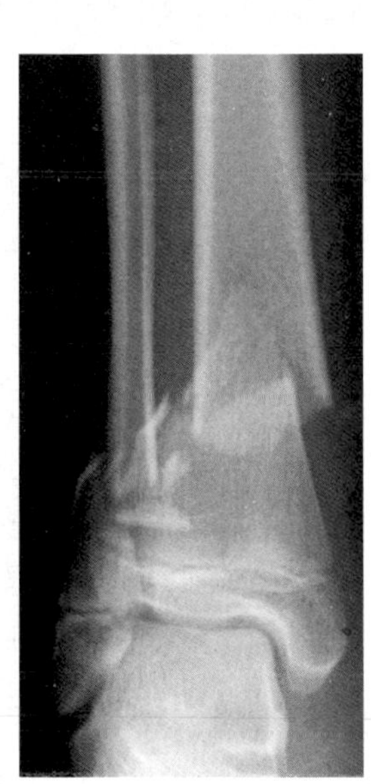

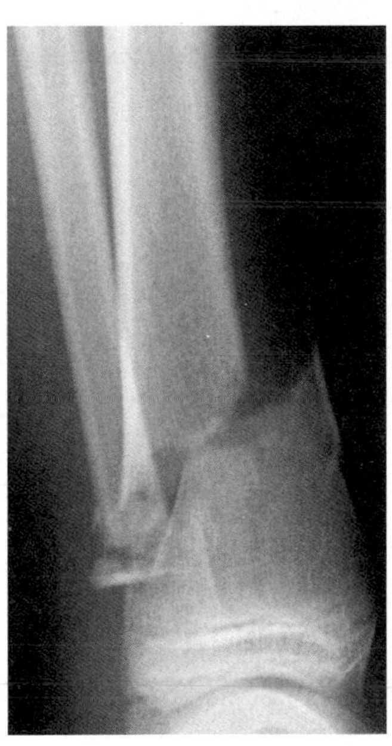

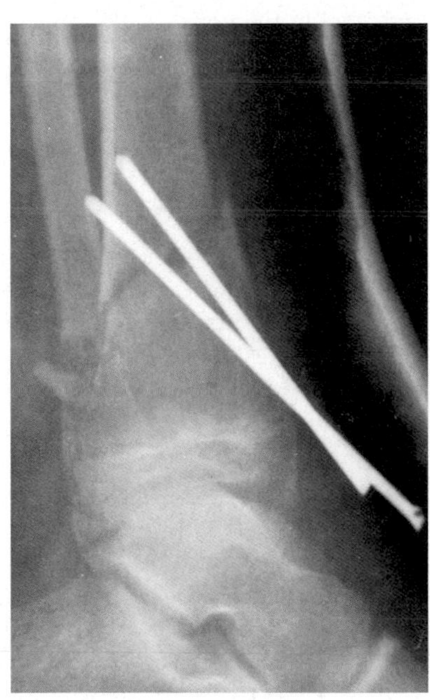

FIGURE 25-29 A,B. Unstable distal metadiaphyseal fractures of the tibia and fibula in a 15-year-old girl. **C.** This fracture was stabilized with percutaneous pins because of marked swelling and fracture instability.

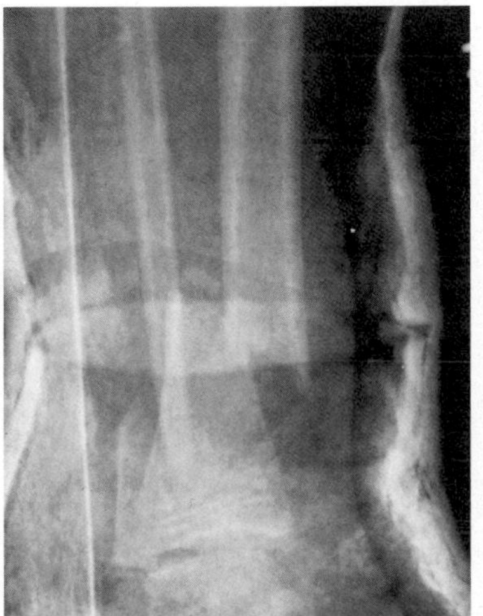

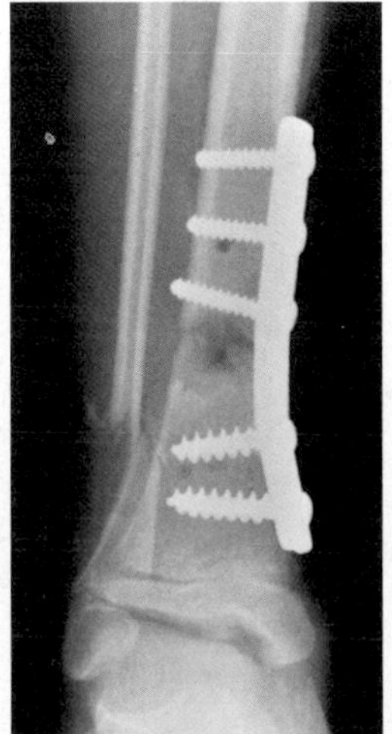

FIGURE 25-30 A. Anteroposterior radiograph of a distal one-third tibial and fibular fractures in a 9-year-old girl with a closed head injury and severe spasticity. The initial reduction in a cast could not be maintained. **B.** Open reduction and internal fixation with a medial buttress plate was used to achieve and maintain the alignment.

COMPLICATIONS ASSOCIATED WITH DIAPHYSEAL TIBIAL AND FIBULAR FRACTURES

Compartment Syndrome

A compartment syndrome may occur after any type of tibia fracture, ranging from a seemingly minor closed fracture to a severe, comminuted fracture.[91] Schrock[131] described compartment syndromes after derotational osteotomies of the tibia in children, and compartment syndrome is a well known complication of tibial osteotomy for angular correction.

Compartment syndromes may occur in any or all of the four compartments of the lower leg after trauma. Hemorrhage and soft tissue edema produce an elevation in the pressure within the myofascial compartment that impairs venous outflow. The small arterioles leading into the compartment become less efficient in delivering blood as venous outflow becomes occluded, and the vessels themselves become more permeable. The arterioles and capillaries close when the pressure in the compartment exceeds the pressure in the vessels with resultant ischemia of the surrounding soft tissue. Because tissue pressures can be elevated enough to produce an ischemic injury, but not high enough to occlude arterial inflow, the presence of peripheral pulses is unreliable evidence of adequate tissue perfusion.

Patients with a compartment syndrome often complain of pain out of proportion to the apparent severity of the injury. This increasing pain, often noted as increasing analgesic requirements, is the most important early sign of potential compartment syndrome in children. The compartment is firm to palpation. The patient may have a sensory deficit in the distribution of the nerves that traverse the compartment. Weakness of the muscles within the involved compartment and pain on passive motion of those muscles are common. Paralysis of the muscles in the involved compartment is a late finding. Pain with passive range of motion appears to be an early and strong clinical finding. As an example, patients with a compartment syndrome involving the deep posterior compartment have severe pain that increases with passive extension of the toes, plantar hyperesthesias, and weakness of toe flexion.[97] Late complications of untreated lower extremity compartment syndrome include clawed toes, a dorsal bunion, and limited subtalar motion secondary to necrosis and subsequent fibrous contracture of the muscles originating in the deep posterior compartment.[78]

Diagnosis

Direct intracompartmental pressure measurements at the level of the fracture provide the most accurate assessment of compartment conditions in those with clinically suspected compartment syndrome and allow early fasciotomy to reduce the pressure. Whitesides et al.[152] designed an inexpensive apparatus that permitted accurate measurement of compartment tissue pressure (Fig. 25-31). Small, portable devices or even an arterial monitoring set-up in the operating room are available to measure compartment pressures and are used most commonly at this time. When measuring compartment pressure in the leg after a tibial fracture, accurate placement of the needle is essential. Multiple measurements should be performed at different sites and depths within each compartment, due to apparent variations of pressure through the compartment.

Normal compartment tissue pressure in the adult lower leg is approximately 0 to 5 mm Hg. A small study of normal children demonstrated that baseline lower limb compartment pressures are higher (13 to 16 mm Hg).[140] The clinical application of this information is unclear at this time. Compartment blood inflow is decreased at 20 mm Hg, and prolonged pressures of 30 to 40 mm Hg, or within 30 mm Hg of diastolic blood pressure, may cause severe nonreversible injury to the muscles within a fascial compartment Vascular flow ceases in the microcirculation of an extremity muscular compartment by the time tissue pressures within the closed compartment reaches the diastolic blood pressure.

Treatment

Any cast should be bivalved and the padding divided in a patient with increased or increasing pain. If, after removal of all encircling wraps, there is no relief, compartment syndrome should be considered. Any child who has objective or subjective evidence of a compartment syndrome should undergo an emergent fasciotomy. While there is some controversy in the literature, symptomatic patients with compartment pressures greater than 30 mm Hg may benefit from fasciotomy.[73,152] In addition, release should be considered strongly if compartment pressures

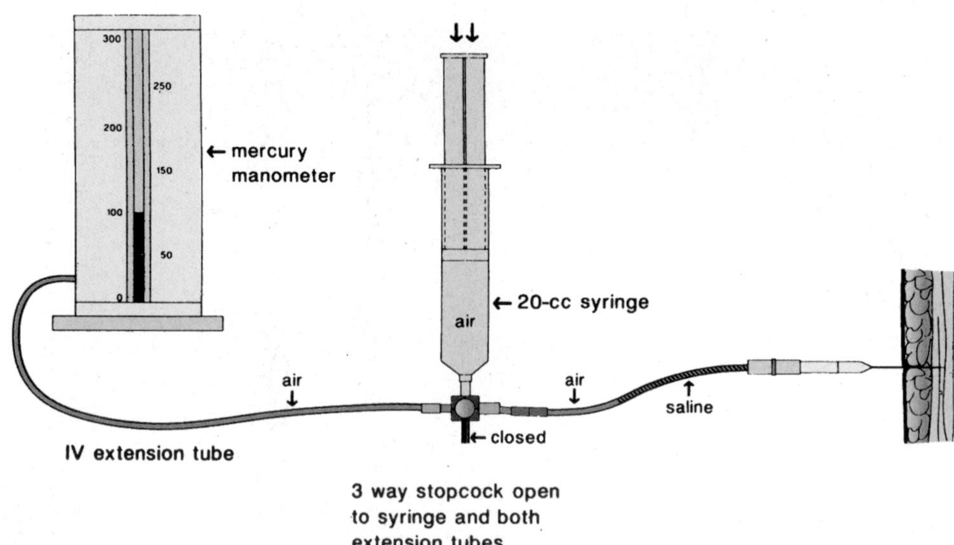

FIGURE 25-31 The Whitesides technique for measuring intracompartmental pressure. (From Whitesides TE, Hanley TC, Morinotok K, et al. Tissue pressure measurement as a determinant for the need for fasciotomy. Clin Orthop Relat Res 1975;113:43, with permission.)

are within 20 to 30 mm Hg of the diastolic pressure. This is especially critical in the hypotensive patient or those unable to communicate or undergo reliable serial examinations for any reason. In a dog model of ischemia, irreversible injury to muscles and nerves begins after approximately 5 hours.[132] How this animal data relates to children is unclear, but certainly the surgeon should assure rapid compartment release if muscle ischemia is suspected. Hyperesthesia, motor defects, and decreased pulses are late changes and denote significant tissue injury. These signs occur only after the ischemia has been well established and the injury is permanent.[78,152]

The two-incision technique is used most widely for fasciotomies, although a single incision, perifibular release is favored at some centers (Fig. 25-32A,B).[98] In the two-incision method, one incision is anterolateral and the second posteromedial. The fascia surrounding each of the four compartments should be opened widely. The wounds are left open and a delayed primary closure is performed when possible. Split thickness skin grafting of the wounds may be necessary in some cases. Fibulectomy has been recommended by some as a means by which all four compartments can be released through a single approach. Most literature does not support its use, and this procedure should not be performed in skeletally immature patients. Subsequent shortening of the fibula may occur, which can produce a valgus deformity at the ankle. Long-term significant ankle valgus may result in external tibial torsion, gait impairment, and potentially problematic foot and ankle deformity.[22,32]

Vascular Injuries

Vascular injuries associated with tibial fractures are uncommon in children; however, when they do occur, the sequelae can be devastating. In an evaluation of 14 patients with lower extremity fractures and concomitant vascular injuries, Allen et al.[1] noted that only three children returned to normal function. One factor leading to a poor outcome was a delay in diagnosis. Evaluation for vascular compromise is imperative (during the primary and secondary trauma surveys) in all children with tibial fractures.

The tibial fracture most frequently associated with vascular injury is that of the proximal metaphysis. The anterior tibial artery is in close proximity to the proximal tibia as it passes between the fibula and the tibia into the anterior compartment.[59,65] Distal tibial fractures also are associated with injuries to the anterior tibial artery. In these fractures, the vessels are injured when the distal fragment is translated posteriorly. Posterior tibial artery injuries are rare, except in fractures associated with crushing or shearing due to accidents involving heavy machinery, or those secondary to gunshot wounds involving the lower leg and ankle region.

Angular Deformity

Spontaneous correction of significant axial malalignment after a diaphyseal fracture of a child's forearm or femur is common. Remodeling of a angulated tibial shaft fracture, however, often is incomplete (Fig. 25-33).[11] As such, the goal of treatment should be to obtain as close to an anatomic alignment as possible. Swaan and Oppers[144] evaluated 86 children treated for fractures of the tibia. The original angulation of the fracture was measured on radiographs in the sagittal and frontal projections. Girls 1 to 8 years of age and boys 1 to 10 years of age demonstrated moderate spontaneous correction of residual angulation after union. In girls 9 to 12 years of age and boys 11 to 12 years of age, approximately 50% of the angulation was corrected. No more than 25% of the deformity was corrected in children over 13 years of age.

Bennek and Steinert[5] found that recurvatum malunion of more than 10 degrees did not correct completely. In this study,

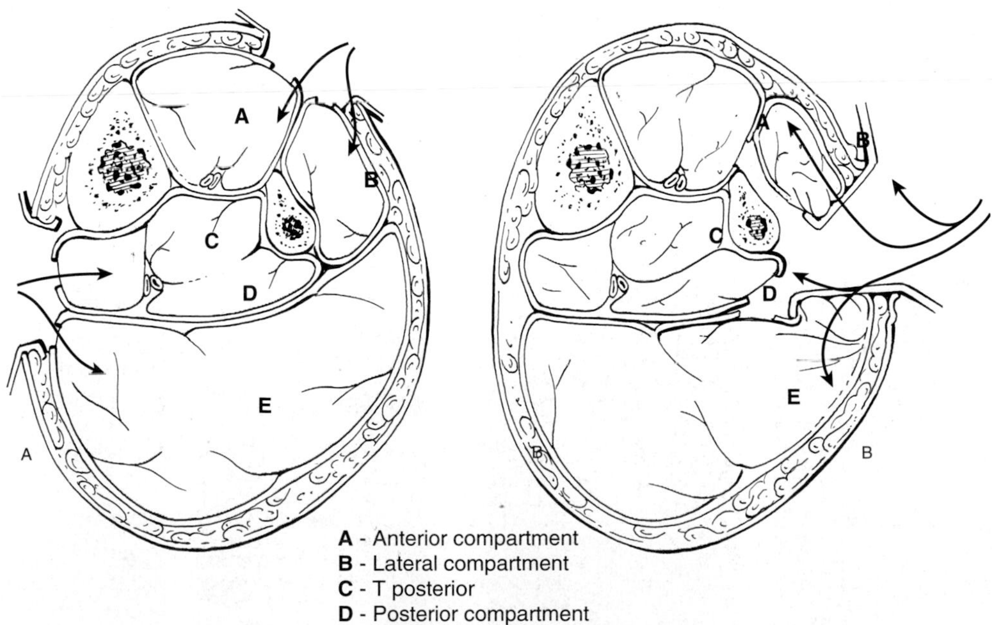

FIGURE 25-32 A. Decompressive fasciotomies through a two-incision approach. The anterior lateral incision allows decompression of the anterior and lateral compartments. The medial incision allows decompression of the superficial posterior and the deep posterior compartments. **B.** A one-incision decompression fasciotomy can be performed through a lateral approach that allows a dissection of all four compartments.

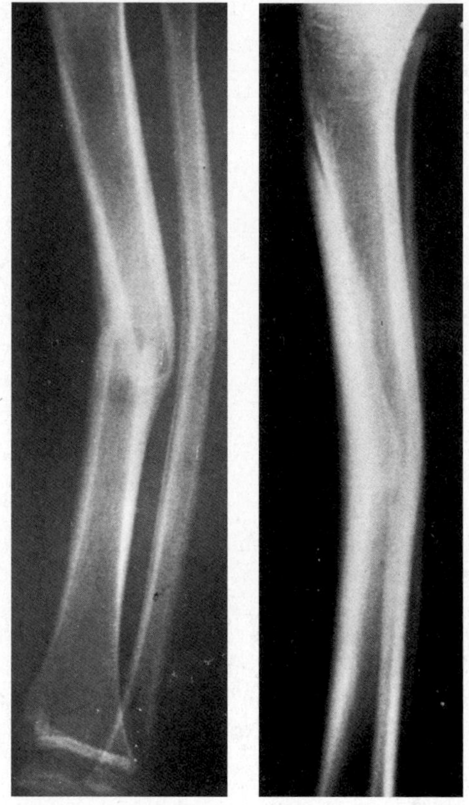

FIGURE 25-33 A 50-month-old child with a middle one-third transverse tibial fracture and a plastically deformed fibular fracture. **A.** Lateral view shows 20-degree posterior angulation. **B.** The deformity is still 15 degrees 4 years after the injury.

26 of 28 children with varus or valgus deformities at union had significant residual angular deformities at follow-up. Valgus deformities had a worse outcome because the tibiotalar joint was left in a relatively unstable position. Weber et al.[151] demonstrated that a fracture with varus malalignment of 5 to 13 degrees completely corrected at the level of the physis. Most children with valgus deformities of 5 to 7 degrees did not have a full correction.

Hansen et al.[61] reported 102 pediatric tibial fractures, 25 of which had malunions of 4 to 19 degrees. Residual angular malunions ranged from 3 to 19 degrees at final follow-up, without a single patient having a complete correction. The spontaneous correction was approximately 13.5% of the total deformity. Shannak[133] reviewed the results of treatment of 117 children with tibial shaft fractures treated in above-the-knee casts. Deformities in two planes did not remodel as completely as those in a single plane. The least correction occurred in apex posterior angulated fractures, followed by fractures with valgus malalignment (Fig. 25-34). Spontaneous remodeling of malunited tibial fractures in children appears to be limited to the first 18 months after fracture.[61]

Malrotation

Because rotational malalignment of the tibia does not correct spontaneously with remodeling,[61] any malrotation should be avoided. A computerized tomographic evaluation of tibial rotation can be performed if there is any question about the rotational alignment of the fracture that can not be determined on clinical examination.

Rotational malunion of more than 10 degrees may produce significant functional impairment and necessitate a late derotational osteotomy of the tibia. Most commonly, derotational osteotomy of the tibia is performed in the supramalleolar aspect of the distal tibia. The tibia is osteotomized, rotated, and internally fixed. The fibula may be left intact, particularly for planned derotation of less than 20 degrees. Maintaining continuity of the fibula adds stability and limits the possibility of introducing an iatrogenic angular deformity to the tibia.

Leg-Length Discrepancy

Hyperemia associated with fracture repair may stimulate the physes in the involved leg, producing growth acceleration. Tibial growth acceleration after fracture is less than that seen after

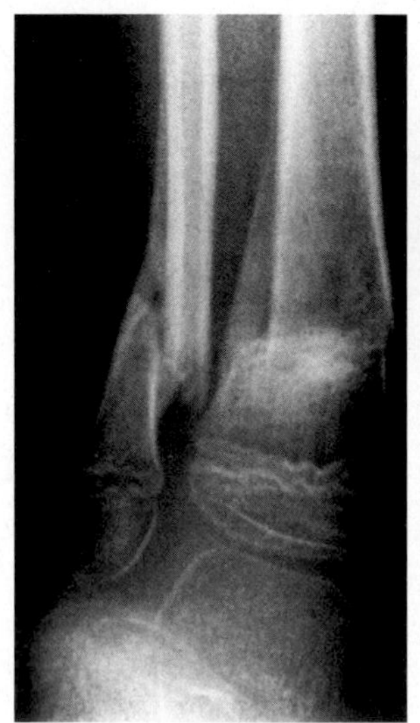

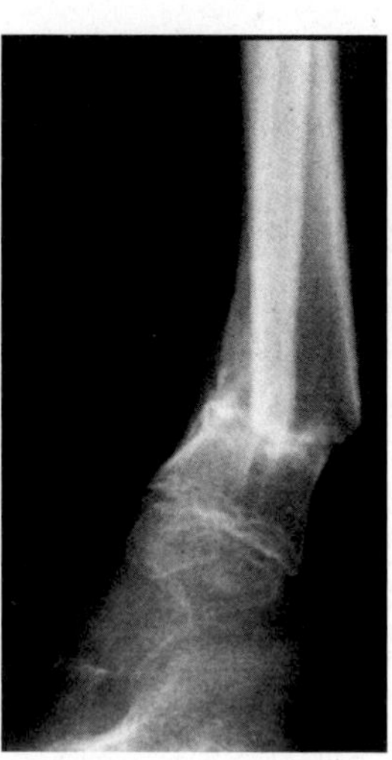

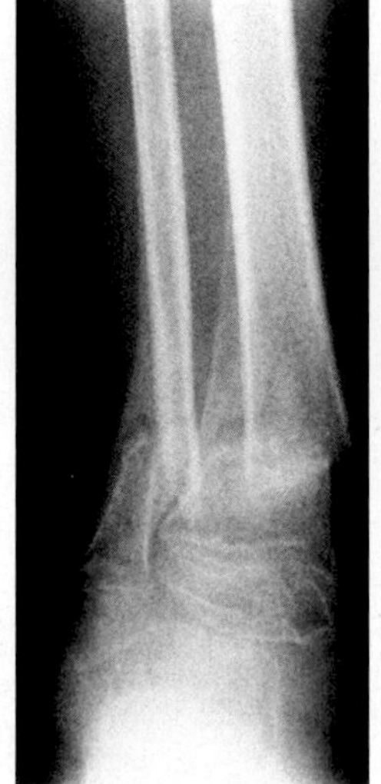

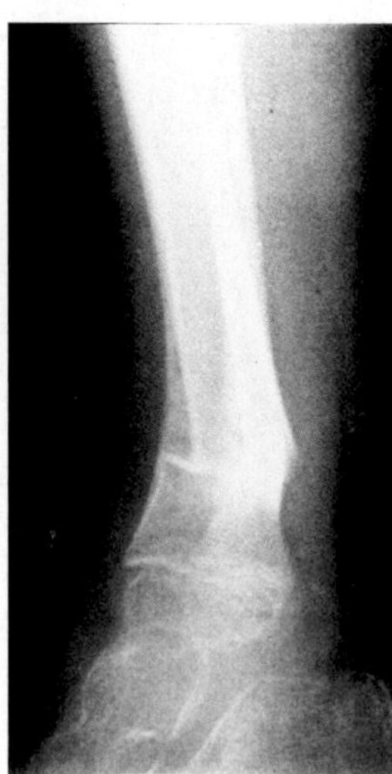

FIGURE 25-34 A. Anteroposterior and lateral radiographs 2 months after injury in a 6-year-old boy reveal a valgus and anterior malunion at the fracture. **B.** One year later, the child still has a moderate valgus and anterior malalignment of the distal fractured segment. This malalignment produced painful hyperextension of the knee at heel strike during ambulation.

femoral fractures in children of comparable ages. Shannak[133] showed that the average growth acceleration of a child's tibia after fracture is approximately 4.5 mm. Comminuted fractures have the greatest risk of accelerated growth and overgrowth.

Swaan and Oppers[144] reported that young children have a greater chance for overgrowth than older children. Accelerated growth after tibial fracture generally occurs in children under 10 years of age, whereas older children may have a mild growth inhibition associated with the fracture.[61] The amount of fracture shortening also has an effect on growth stimulation. Fractures with significant shortening have more physeal growth after fracture union than injuries without shortening at union.[100] The presence of angulation at union does not appear to affect the amount of overgrowth.[53]

Anterior Tibial Physeal Closure

Morton and Starr[105] reported closure of the anterior tibial physis after fracture in two children. Both patients sustained a comminuted fracture of the tibial diaphysis without a concomitant injury of the knee. The fractures were reduced and stabilized with Kirschner wires reportedly placed distal to the tibial tubercle. A genu recurvatum deformity developed after premature closure of the anterior physis. Smillie[137] reported one child who had an open tibial fracture complicated by a second fracture involving the supracondylar aspect of the femur. This patient also developed a recurvatum deformity secondary to closure of the anterior proximal tibial physis. At present, no universally acceptable explanation can be given for this phenomenon. Patients have demonstrated apparently iatrogenic closure after placement of a proximal tibial traction pin, the application of pins and plaster, and after application of an external fixation device. Some children may have an undiagnosed injury of the tibial physis at the time of the ipsilateral tibial diaphyseal fracture.[84] Regardless of etiology, premature closure of the physis produces a progressive recurvatum deformity and loss of the normal anterior to posterior slope of the proximal tibia as the child grows. Management requires surgical intervention including proximal tibial osteotomy with all the inherent risks and potential complications of that procedure.

Delayed Union and Nonunion

Delayed union and nonunion are uncommon after low-energy tibial fractures in children. The use of an external fixation device may lengthen the time to union in some patients, particularly those with open fractures resulting from high-energy injury.[50,94,106] Care must be taken to advance weight bearing appropriately and to dynamize the frame as soon as possible to maximize bone healing. Inadequate immobilization that allows patterned micro- or macromotion also can slow the rate of healing and lead to delayed or nonunion. In patients with a suspected delayed union or nonunion, a 1-cm fibulectomy will allow increased compression at the delayed union or nonunion site with weight bearing and often will induce healing (Fig. 25-35). A posterolateral bone graft also is an excellent technique to produce union in children (Fig. 25-36). Adolescents near skeletal maturity with a delayed or nonunion can be managed with a reamed intramedullary nail, concomitant fibular osteotomy, and correction of any angulation at the nonunion site as necessary (Fig. 25-37).

SPECIAL FRACTURES

Toddler's Fractures

External rotation of the foot with the knee fixed in an infant or toddler can produce a spiral fracture of the tibia without a concomitant fibular fracture, and is termed a "toddler's fracture" (Fig. 25-38). This fracture pattern was first reported by Dunbar et al.[34] in 1964. The traumatic episode often is unwitnessed by the adult caretaker. Of those injuries that are witnessed, most caregivers report a seemingly minor, twisting mechanism. Most

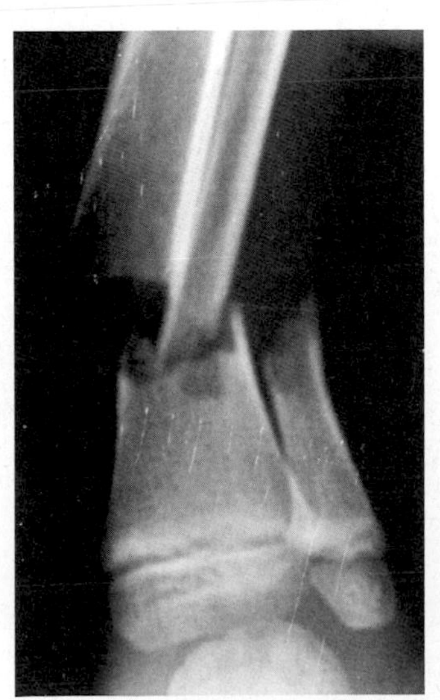
A

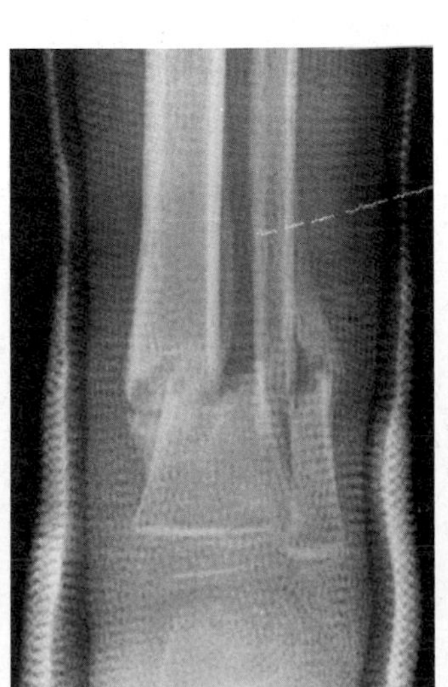
B

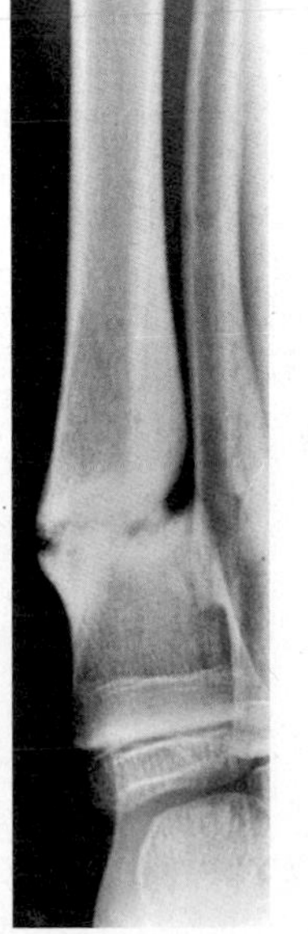
C

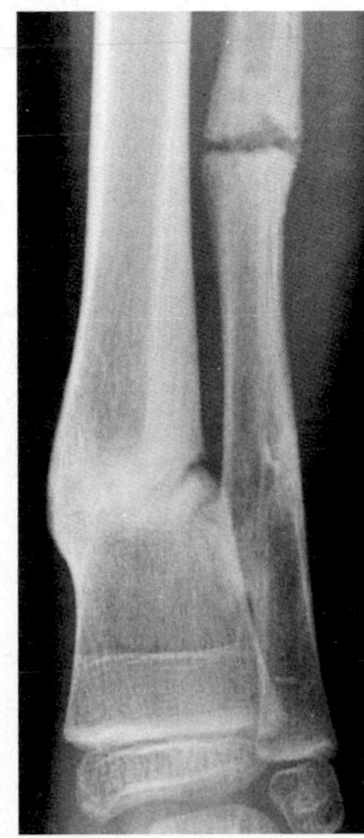
D

FIGURE 25-35 A. Anteroposterior radiograph of the distal tibia and fibula in a 5-year-old boy with an open fracture. **B.** Early callus formation is seen 1 month after injury. **C.** The tibia has failed to unite 10 months after injury. **D.** The patient underwent a fibulectomy 4 cm proximal to the tibial nonunion. The tibial fracture united 8 weeks after surgery.

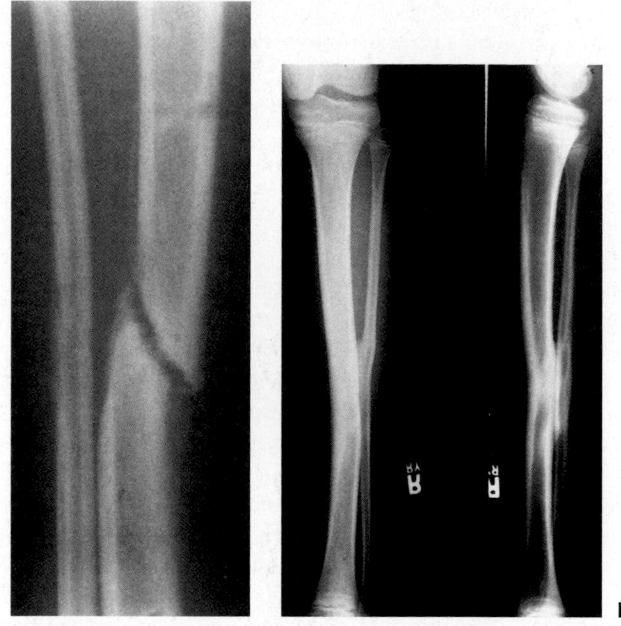

FIGURE 25-36 A. Nonunion of an open tibial fracture. **B.** After posterolateral tibial bone graft.

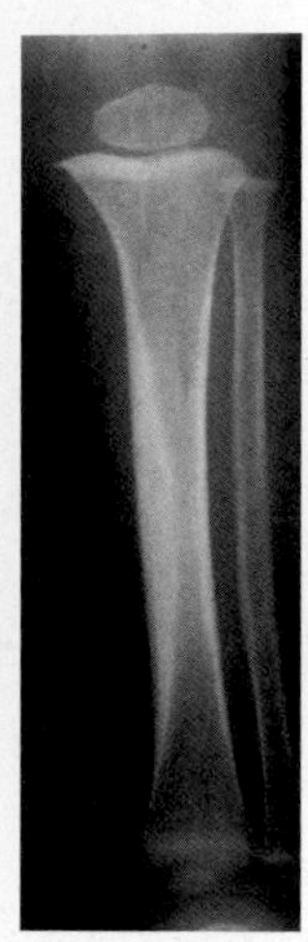

FIGURE 25-38 A. Anteroposterior and lateral radiographs of an 18-month-old child who presented with refusal to bear weight on her leg. Note the spiral middle one-third "toddler's" fracture (*arrows*). **B.** This fracture healed uneventfully after 4 weeks of immobilization in a cast.

children with this injury are under 6 years of age, and in one study the average age was 27 months. Sixty-three of 76 such fractures reported by Dunbar et al.[34] were in children under 2.5 years of age. Toddler's fractures occur in boys more often than in girls and in the right leg more often than in the left. Occasionally, a child may sustain a toddler's fracture in a fall from a height.[27,147]

Oujhane et al.[112] analyzed the radiographs of 500 acutely limping toddlers and identified 100 in whom a fracture was the etiology of the gait disturbance. The most common site of fracture was the distal metaphysis of the tibia. The fibula was fractured with the tibia in only 12 of the 56 tibial fractures. Only one physeal injury was noted.

The examination of a child with an acute limp begins with an evaluation of the uninvolved side. This serves as a control for the symptomatic extremity. The examination begins at the hip and proceeds to the thigh, knee, lower leg, ankle, and foot. It is important to note areas of point tenderness, any increase in local or systemic temperature, and any swelling or bruising of the leg.[147] Radiographs of the tibia and fibula should be obtained in both anteroposterior and lateral projections. An internally rotated oblique view can be helpful in identifying a nondisplaced toddler's fracture. Fluoroscopy also may assist in the identification of subtle fractures. Occasionally, a fracture line cannot be identified, and the first radiographic evidence of fracture becomes apparent when periosteal new bone forms 7

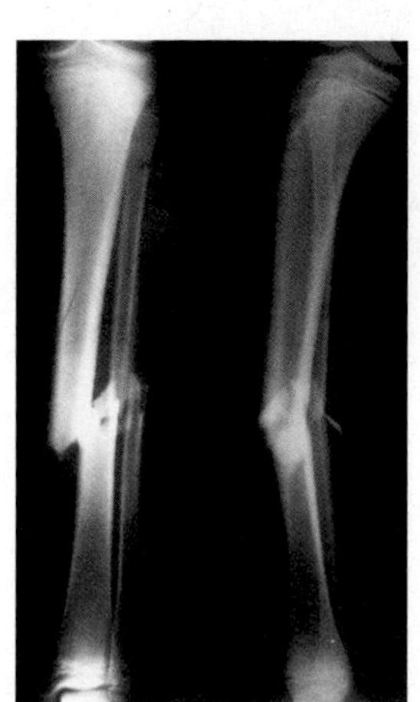

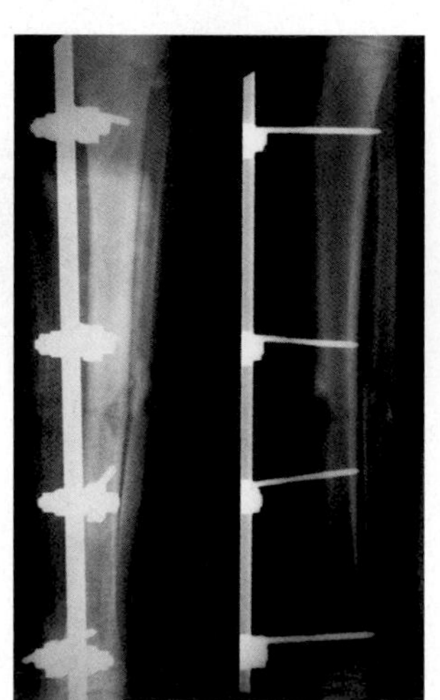

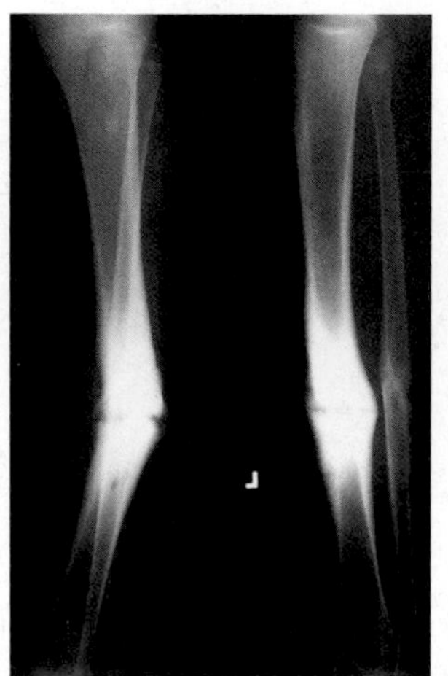

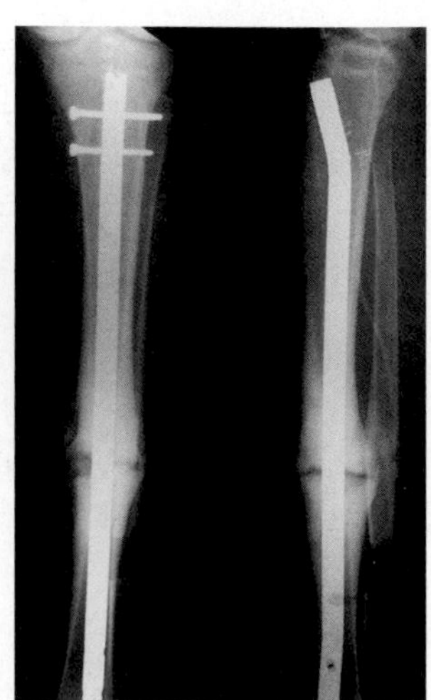

FIGURE 25-37 A. Anteroposterior and lateral radiographs of a 14-year-old adolescent who was struck by a car, sustaining a grade IIIB open fracture of the tibia. **B.** Anteroposterior and lateral radiographs of the tibia after irrigation and débridement, and application of an external fixation device. **C.** The patient developed a nonunion at the tibia, which progressively deformed into an unacceptable varus alignment. **D.** The nonunion was treated with a fibular osteotomy followed by a closed angular correction of the deformity and internal fixation with a reamed intramedullary nail.

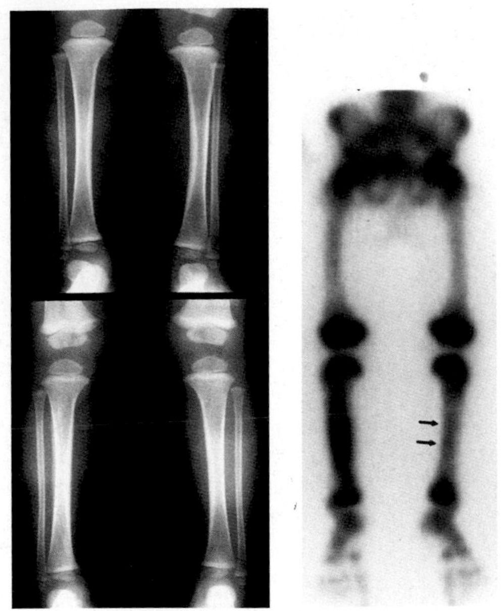

FIGURE 25-39 A. Anteroposterior radiograph of the tibia in a 3-year-old child who refused to bear weight on the right leg 3 weeks before presentation. The history of obvious trauma was absent. The radiographs revealed periosteal new bone formation in the midshaft of the right tibia. There was also tenderness to palpation in the left mid-tibia as well despite normal radiographs. **B.** A bone scan showed increased uptake in both the left and right tibia. There was significantly less uptake on the left side, the more recent injury.

to 14 days after the injury (Fig. 25-39). Technetium radionuclide bone scan can assist in the diagnosis of unapparent fractures, but is used rarely. A bone scan of a patient with such a spiral fracture of the tibia will demonstrate diffuse increased uptake of tracer throughout the affected bone ("black tibia"). This can be differentiated from infection as infection tends to produce a more localized area of increased tracer uptake.[34]

A child with a toddler's fracture should be immobilized in a bent-knee, long-leg cast for approximately 3 to 4 weeks. Some children may require an additional 2 weeks of immobilization in a below-the-knee walking cast once the above-the-knee cast is removed, but this is uncommon.

Bicycle Spoke Injuries

Bicycle spoke injuries normally occur when a child's foot is caught between the spokes of a turning bicycle wheel. This produces a severe compression or crushing injury to the soft tissues of the foot and ankle and occurs most commonly when two children are riding a bicycle designed for one, with the injured passenger riding on the handlebars or over the rear wheel.[41,99] An oblique or spiral fracture of the tibia also can occur secondary to the torsional forces on the limb. The injury to the foot, ankle, and lower leg can be exacerbated when the child's foot is extracted forcibly from the spokes of the bicycle.

The initial appearance of the extremity in a child with a bicycle spoke injury may be deceiving. The foot often appears normal or may show only minor skin abrasions. The patient often presents 24 to 48 hours after the accident complaining of a painful swollen foot and leg. This injury is similar to a "wringer" injury of the arm in that the initial examination may not reveal the true extent of the injury. Izant et al.[70] reviewed 60 bicycle spoke injuries in children under 14 years of age. The most common age range of injury was 2 to 8 years. Three components were identified to this trauma: (i) a laceration of the tissue from the knifelike action of the spoke, (ii) a crushing injury from the impingement between the wheel and the frame of the bicycle, and (iii) a shearing injury from the coefficient of these two forces. The laceration created by this injury often involves the malleoli, the Achilles tendon area of the heel, and the dorsum of the foot.

A child with an apparent bicycle spoke injury should be admitted to the hospital because the extent of the damage may not be identified initially. Initial therapy consists of a mild compression dressing with a multilayered cotton bandage. The extremity is elevated and the child is kept at bedrest during the first 24 hours. A long-leg splint is applied if a tibial fracture is present. After this period of bedrest and elevation, the child may ambulate nonweight bearing with crutches. Frequent inspection of the extremity must be made during the subsequent 48 hours. Débridement of devitalized tissue is performed as any necrosis becomes apparent. Large areas of hematoma formation may be treated with aspiration to prevent further elevation of the overlying skin. Multiple débridements may be required, and definitive treatment must await complete delineation of the necrotic area. Delayed wound closure, sometimes requiring skin grafting, may be necessary if full-thickness skin loss occurs. Occasionally, a free flap may be required however, this is rare.[41,70,99] A child with a concomitant tibial fracture is placed in an above-the-knee nonweight-bearing cast at the completion of care for the foot injury, particularly if the soft tissue injury is fairly minor.[41] The tibial fracture may require stabilization with an external fixator if the soft tissue loss on the foot and ankle is severe, and in these cases the external fixation device may be extended to include the foot and ankle.

Floating Knee

Significant trauma can cause ipsilateral fractures involving both the femur and the tibia. In the past, these injuries often were treated with traction and casting (Fig. 25-40). The extent of the injuries often left permanent functional deficits when not managed aggressively.[11,33]

Most children with ipsilateral femoral and tibial fractures are treated most appropriately with operative stabilization of the femur and either cast immobilization of the tibia after reduction or operative fixation. In pediatric patients, the femoral fracture can be stabilized with a unilateral external fixator, plate and screw constructs, or flexible nails. Patients near skeletal maturity may be candidates for lateral entry reamed femoral nails, although the other options remain viable as well. Plate fixation, either open or percutaneous, is useful for fractures in the subtrochanteric or supracondylar area of the femur in adolescents, while external fixation may be useful in these areas as well. The tibial fracture is reduced and stabilized after the femoral fracture has been stabilized. Closed tibia fractures in these situations may be treated with cast immobilization or operative intervention. Open tibial fractures associated with an ipsilateral femoral fracture should be stabilized with an external fixator or flexible intramedullary nails whenever possible (Fig. 25-41).

Tibial Fracture in Paraplegic Children

Motor paralysis from poliomyelitis was once the most common cause of lower extremity weakness in children. Because these patients had sensation, fractures were identified early. Disease

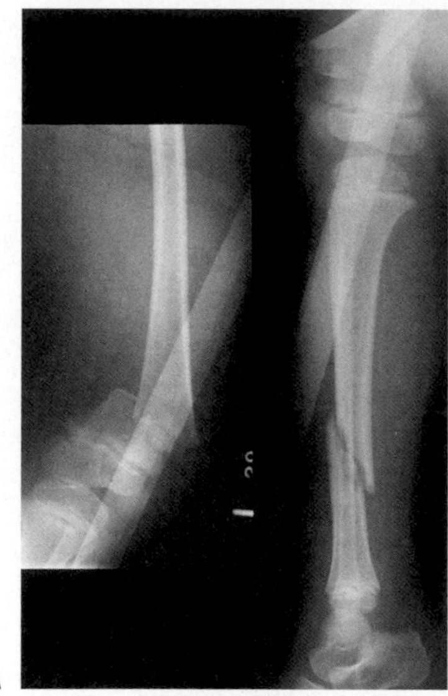

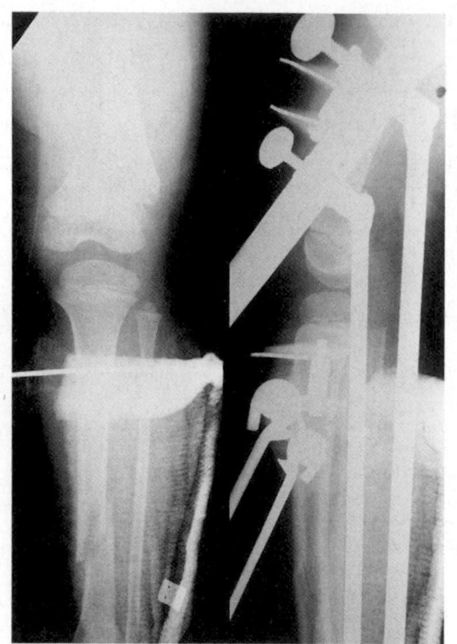

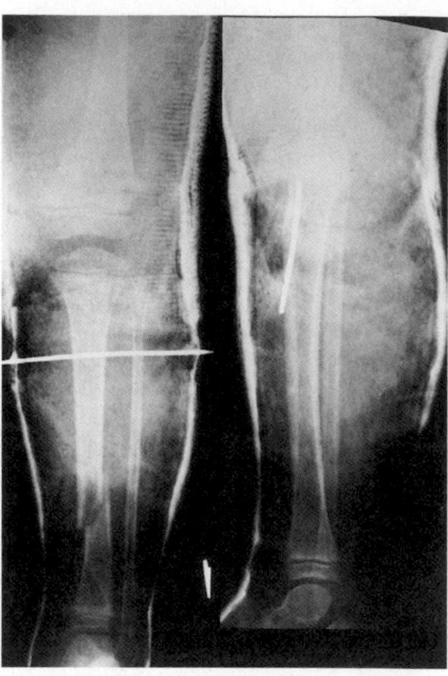

FIGURE 25-40 A. Ipsilateral fractures of the distal femur and tibia without an ipsilateral fibular fracture in a 5-year-old. **B.** The child was treated with tibial pin traction for the femoral injury (pin applied below the tibial tubercle) and a short-leg splint for the tibial fracture initially. **C.** The child was placed into a spica cast after 2 weeks of traction. The tibial traction pin was used to help stabilize both fractures.

trends have changed over time. As late as 1958, 90% to 95% of children with myelomeningocele died in the first year of life, usually from a neurologic complication. Advances in neurosurgery and urology have lengthened the lifespan of children with myelomeningocele significantly. The mortality rate in the first year of life for these children is now approximately 3% to 5%. Currently, pediatric orthopaedic surgeons manage a large number of paraplegic children who have sensory and/or motor deficits associated with myelomeningocele.[33,42,45]

Tibial fractures in paralyzed children without sensation require special attention. Gillies and Hartung[45] were the first to publish a report on children with myelomeningocele who sustained pathologic fractures of the proximal tibia. These two children had tense hyperemic skin and radiographic evidence of exuberant new bone formation, suggesting a malignant tumor (Fig. 25-42). Both children underwent a biopsy because of these radiographic findings.

Soutter[139] stressed that clinical findings such as swelling,

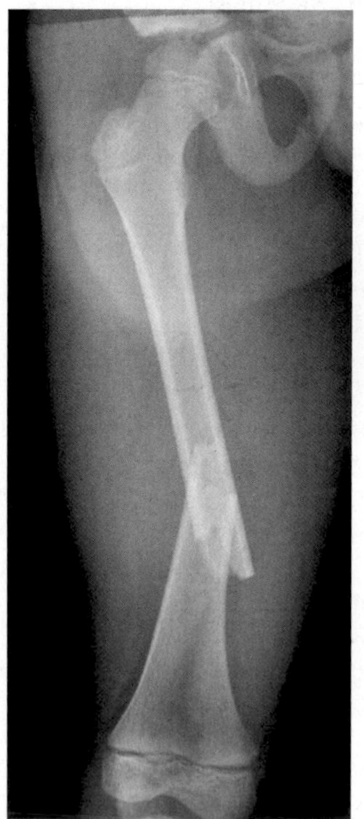

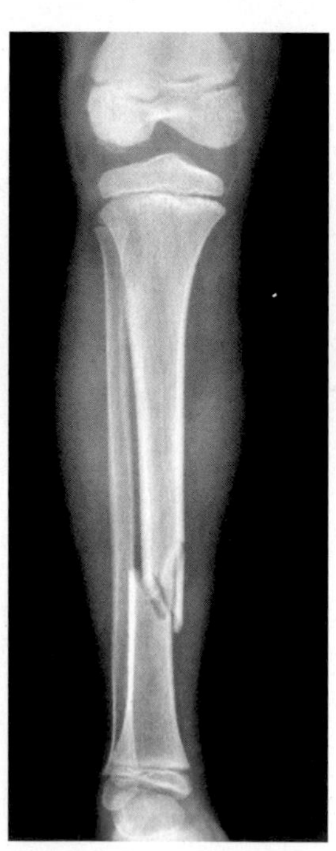

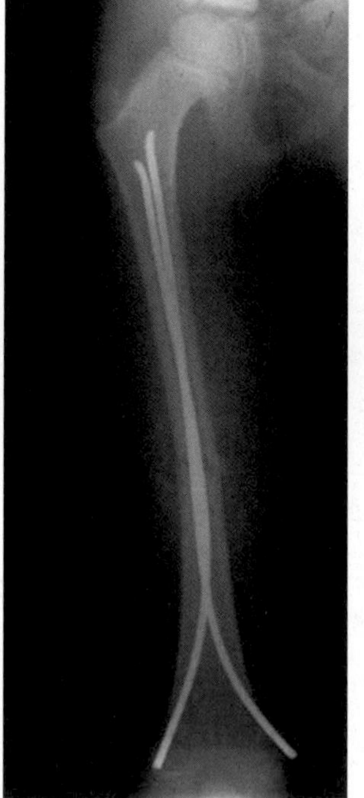

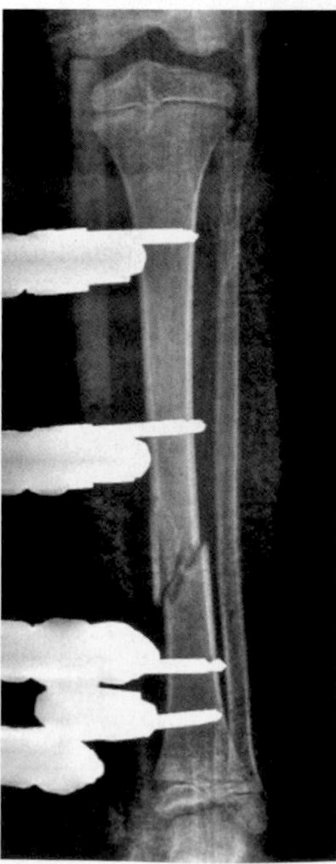

FIGURE 25-41 A,B. Floating knee injury in a 7-year-old boy. **C.** Femoral fracture was fixed with flexible intramedullary nails. **D.** Tibial fracture was stabilized with external fixation.

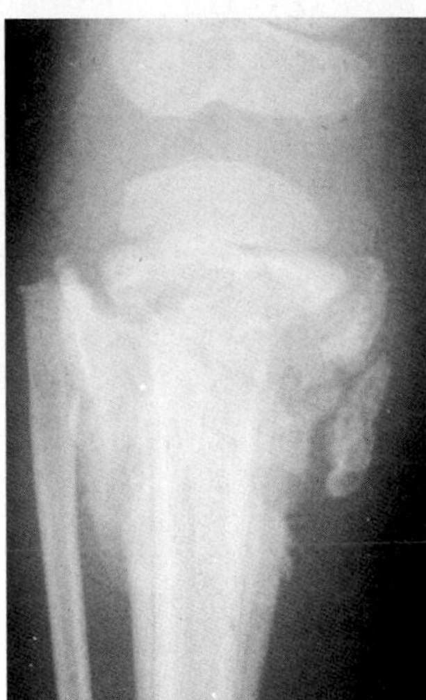

FIGURE 25-42 An undisplaced fracture of the proximal tibial metaphysis in a child with myelodysplasia. Note the exuberant new bone formation.

warmth, and erythema are common in paraplegic children with a fracture. He stated that "fractures to the growth plate in paraplegic children often resemble osteomyelitis."[139] Golding[47] reported one physeal injury to the distal tibia in a child with myelomeningocele. Gyepes et al.[47] reported seven metaphyseal and physeal injuries in patients with myelomeningocele. Stern et al.[143] reported bilateral distal tibial and fibular physeal injuries in a child with myelomeningocele. In most cases, these physeal fractures are chronic physeal injuries, which are characterized by an irregular, dense, widened physis and adjacent subperiosteal new bone formation.

Interestingly, these fractures are more common in children with flaccid paralysis than those with spastic paralysis.[72,122] James[72] reported 44 fractures in 22 children in a population of 122 children with myelomeningocele. The most common age range for fracture was 3 to 6 years. These fractures were more common in a flail limb. Only 6.6% of the patients with quadriceps activity had fractures, whereas 19% of those with no active muscle contraction (flail limb) had fractures. This incidence decreased to 12.5% in a group of children with spastic paralysis. The tibia and femur were the most common bones affected. The most common locations for tibial fractures were the distal diaphysis and distal metaphysis. Drennan and Freehafer[33] reported 58 fractures in 25 patients among 84 children with myelomeningocele. Ten fractures were of the tibia. Eleven of the 58 fractures occurred after the removal of a spica cast, suggesting that immobilization worsened osteopenia and increased the risk of subsequent fracture.

Incidental trauma appears to be the primary factor producing the complex findings associated with a tibial fracture in a paralytic child.[58] Repeated microtrauma can lead to a metaphyseal infarction, subperiosteal hemorrhage, and, perhaps, physeal hemorrhage. Subsequent healing produces endosteal and periosteal callus formation and further generalized osteopenia secondary to the immobilization. The widening of the physis most likely is secondary to a disturbance of the normal reabsorption mechanism during bone development at the metaphysis. This results from frequent subclinical metaphyseal infarctions and could be the result of hemorrhage into the physis itself.

Many fractures are nondisplaced, and nonoperative therapy is indicated. Displaced fractures are reduced closed and immobilized for 3 to 4 weeks in a bulky dressing or a posterior, molded, well-padded splint. As the underlying skin is insensate, care must be taken to avoid pressure areas which may lead to sores or skin breakdown. Healing is determined by the absence of local warmth and swelling and the reconstitution of the width of the physis on radiographs.[89] The child should be fitted with an orthosis or placed back into his or her prefracture orthosis soon after the immobilization is discontinued so as to return to prefracture activity level as soon as possible. Parsch and Rossak[113] reported 31 fractures in 120 patients with myelomeningocele. They emphasized treatment with a wrap and splint until early fracture consolidation. To prevent "fracture disease," they stressed early standing and walking to help minimize any further increases in existing osteopenia. Physeal injuries may require prolonged periods of immobilization and very rarely may be treated surgically to gain maximal stabilization. Complications in patients with paralysis and a tibial fracture are relatively uncommon, and usually are related to pressure sores produced by poorly padded casts. Early physeal arrest can occur, producing a leg-length discrepancy or angular deformity.[139]

Stress Fractures of the Tibia and Fibula

Roberts and Vogt[120] in 1939 reported an "unusual type of lesion" in the tibia of 12 children. All were determined to be stress fractures involving the proximal third of the tibial shaft. Since then, numerous reports of stress fractures involving the tibia and the fibula have been published.[7,31,36,39,62,69,86,96,102,103,116,124,128,145]

The pattern of stress fractures in children differs from that in adults.[30,31,129] In adults, the fibula is involved in stress fractures twice as often as the tibia; in children, the tibia is affected more often than the fibula (Fig. 25-43). The prevalence of stress fractures in boys and girls is equal.

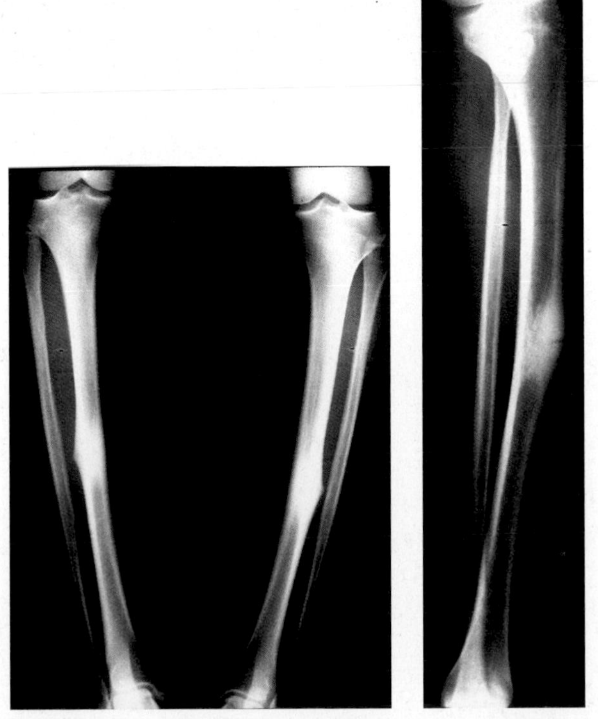

FIGURE 25-43 Bilateral midtibial stress fractures in an adolescent with genu varus.

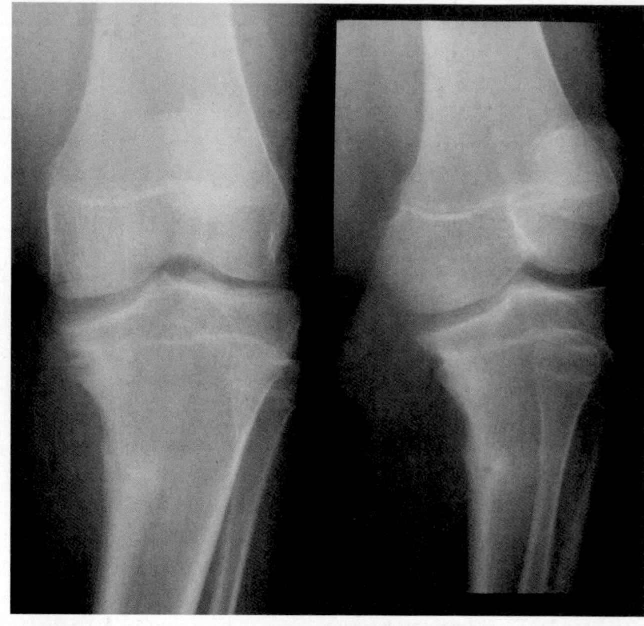

FIGURE 25-44 Anteroposterior and lateral radiographs of the knee of a 15-year-old with adolescent onset tibia vara. Note the posteromedial stress fracture.

A

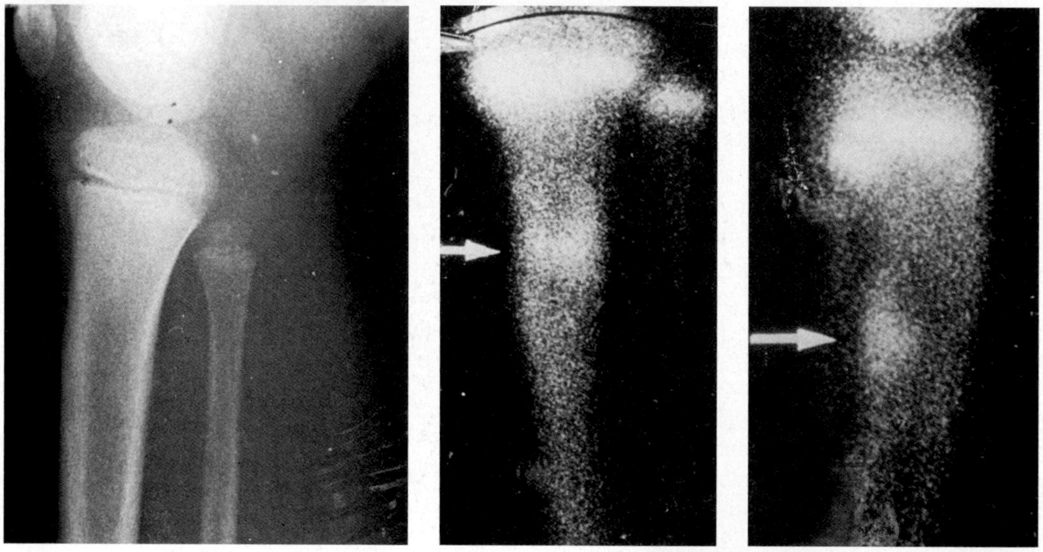

B

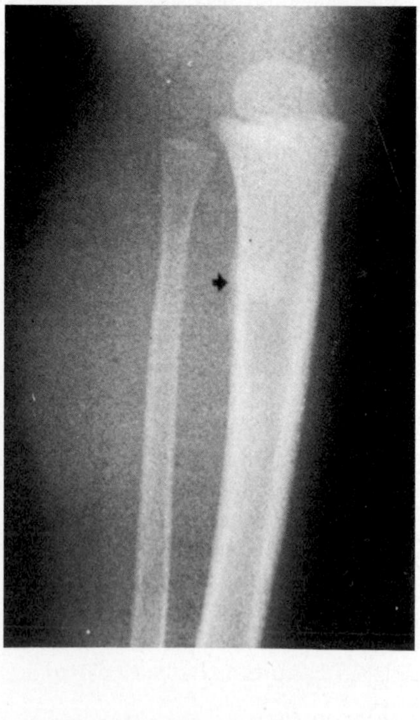

C

FIGURE 25-45 A. Lateral radiograph of the proximal tibia in a 9-year-old who complained of pain in the right leg. There was no history of trauma, and the radiographs were unremarkable. **B.** A bone scan 2 days after the onset of symptoms demonstrates increased tracer uptake in the proximal one third of the tibia in both the anteroposterior and lateral projections (*arrows*). **C.** Increased bone density and subtle periosteal new bone formation was identified in the proximal tibia 3 weeks later (*arrows*). (Courtesy of James Conway, MD.)

Stress fractures occur when the repetitive force applied to a bone is exceeded by the bone's capacity to withstand it. Initially, osteoclastic tunnel formation increases. These tunnels normally fill with mature bone. With continued force, cortical reabsorption accelerates. Woven bone is produced to splint the weakened cortex. This bone is disorganized, however, and does not have the strength of the bone it replaces. A fracture occurs when bone reabsorption outstrips bone production. When the offending force is reduced or eliminated, bone production exceeds bone reabsorption. This produces cortical and endosteal widening with dense repair bone that later remodels to mature bone.[38,74,112]

A child with a tibial stress fracture usually has an insidious onset of symptoms.[31,128] There is evidence of local tenderness that worsens with activity. The child may have a painful limp, while a toddler with a stress fracture will not bear weight on the involved extremity. The pain tends to be worse in the day and to improve at night and with rest. The knee and the ankle have full ranges of motion. Usually, there is minimal, if any, swelling at the fracture site.[15,30,39,67,85,120]

Radiographs reveal changes consistent with a stress fracture and generally become evident approximately 2 weeks after the onset of symptoms.[31] Radiographic findings consistent with fracture repair can manifest in one of three ways: localized periosteal new bone formation, endosteal thickening, or, rarely, a radiolucent cortical fracture line (Fig. 25-44).[30,31,33,85,128]

When utilized in this situation, technetium radionuclide bone scanning reveals a local area of increased tracer uptake at the site of the fracture (Fig. 25-45). Computerized tomography rarely demonstrates the fracture line, but often delineates increased marrow density, endosteal and periosteal new bone formation, and may show soft tissue edema within the area of concern. Magnetic resonance (MR) imaging[67,85] shows a localized band of very low signal intensity continuous with the cor-

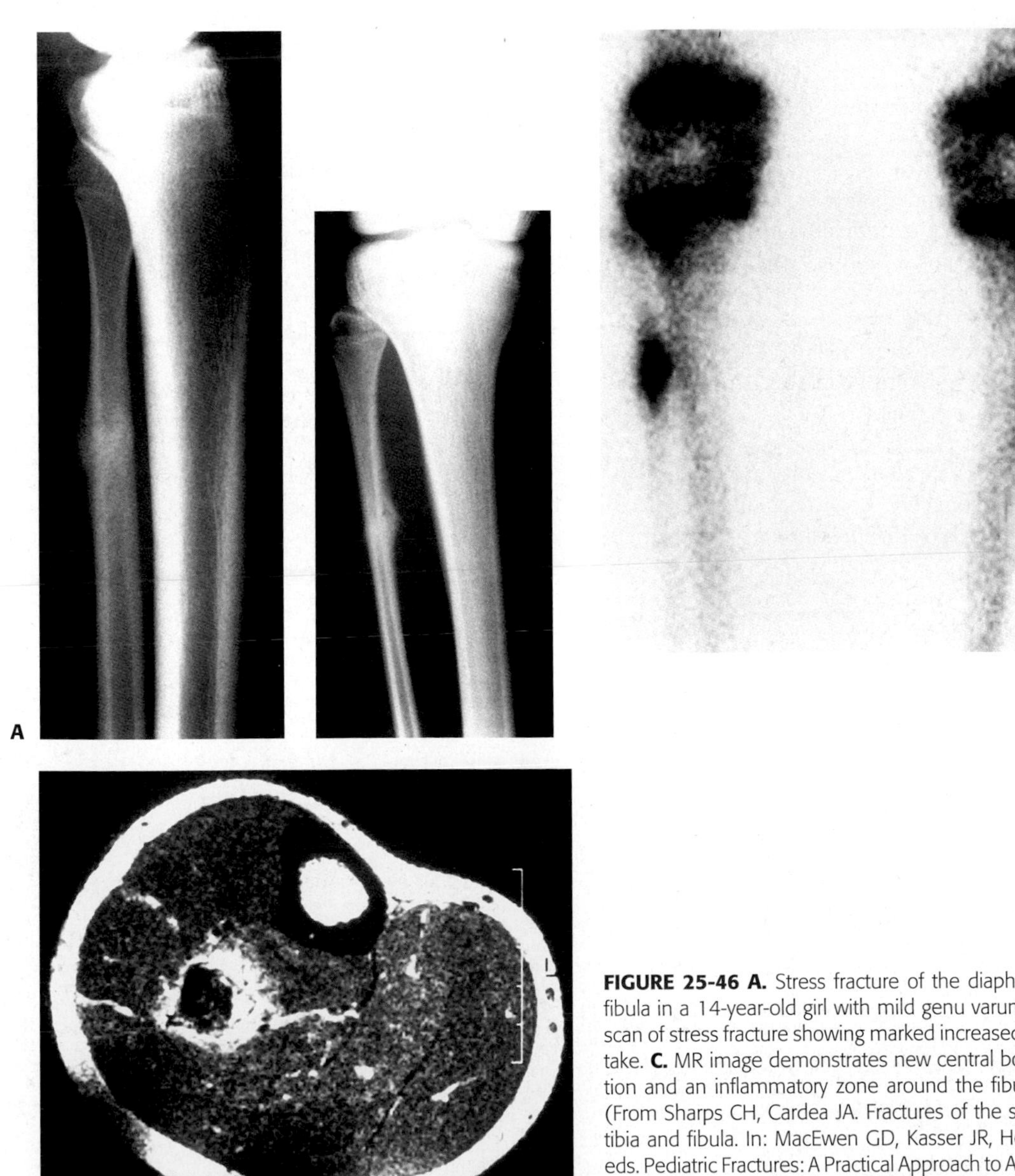

FIGURE 25-46 A. Stress fracture of the diaphysis of the fibula in a 14-year-old girl with mild genu varum. **B.** Bone scan of stress fracture showing marked increased tracer uptake. **C.** MR image demonstrates new central bone formation and an inflammatory zone around the fibular cortex. (From Sharps CH, Cardea JA. Fractures of the shaft of the tibia and fibula. In: MacEwen GD, Kasser JR, Heinrich SD, eds. Pediatric Fractures: A Practical Approach to Assessment and Treatment. Baltimore: Williams & Wilkins, 1993:324, with permission.)

tex. These MR findings can be diagnostic for a stress fracture, and will differentiate such lesions from malignancy, thereby obviating the need for biopsy.

Tibia

The most common location for a tibial stress fracture is in the upper third. The child normally has a painful limp of gradual onset with no history of a specific injury. The pain is described as dull, occurring in the calf near the upper end of the tibia on its medial aspect, and occasionally is bilateral. Physical findings include local tenderness on one or both sides of the tibial crest with a varying degree of swelling.

The treatment of a child with a stress fracture of the tibia begins with activity modification. An active child can rest in a long-leg walking cast for 4 to 6 weeks followed by gradual increase in activity. Nonunions of stress fractures of the tibia have been described. Green[52] reported six nonunions, three of which were in children. Two required excision of the nonunion site with iliac crest bone grafting. The third was treated by electromagnetic stimulation. In all three, the stress fractures occurred in the middle third of the tibia.

Fibula

Pediatric fibular stress fractures normally occur between the ages of 2 and 8 years.[54] The fractures are normally localized to the distal third of the fibula. The child presents with a limp and may complain of pain. Tenderness is localized to the distal half of the fibular shaft. Swelling normally is not present. The obvious bony mass commonly seen in a stress fracture of the fibula in an adult is normally not seen in a comparable fracture in a child.

No radiographic abnormalities are identified in the first 10 days to 2 weeks after the symptoms begin. The earliest sign of a stress fracture of the fibula is the presence of "eggshell" callus along the shaft of the fibula.[15] The fracture itself cannot always be seen because the periosteal callus may obscure the changes in the narrow canal. Radionuclide bone imaging can help to identify stress fractures before the presence of radiographic changes (Fig. 25-46).

The differential diagnosis includes sarcoma of bone, osteomyelitis, and a soft tissue injury without accompanying bony injury. Treatment consists of rest or, in the very active child, a short leg-walking cast for 4 to 6 weeks.

REFERENCES

1. Allen MJ, Nash JR, Ioannidies TT, et al. Major vascular surgeries associated with orthopaedic injuries to the lower limb. Ann R Coll Surg Engl 1984;66:101–104.
2. Balthazar DA, Pappas AM. Acquired valgus deformity of the tibia in children. J Pediatr Orthop 1984;4:538–541.
3. Bartlett GS III, Weiner LS, Yang EC. Treatment of type II and type III open tibia fractures in children. J Orthop Trauma 1997;11:357–362.
4. Bassey LO. Valgus deformity following proximal metaphyseal fractures in children: experiences in the African tropics. J Trauma 1990;30:102–107.
5. Bennek J, Steinert V. Knochenwachstam kindern. Zentralbl Chir 1966;91:633.
6. Benz G, Kallieris D, Seebock T, et al. Bioreabsorbable pins and screws in pediatric traumatology. Eur J Pediatr Surg 1994;4:103–107.
7. Berkebile RD. Stress fracture of the tibia in children. Am J Roentgenol Radium Ther Nucl Med 1964;91:588–596.
8. Blasier RD, Barnes CL. Age as a prognostic factor in open tibial fractures in children. Clin Orthop Relat Res 1996;331:261–264.
9. Blick SS, Brumback RJ, Poka A, et al. Compartment syndrome in open tibial fractures. J Bone Joint Surg Am 1986;68:1348–1353.
10. Blount WP. Fractures in Children. Baltimore: Williams & Wilkins, 1955.
11. Bohn WW, Durbin RA. Ipsilateral fractures of the femur and tibia in children and adolescents. J Bone Joint Surg Am 1991;73:429–439.
12. Briggs TWR, Orr MM, Lightowler CDR. Isolated tibial fractures in children. Injury 1992;23:308–310.
13. Buckley SL, Gotschall C, Robertson W, et al. The relationship of skeletal injuries with trauma score, injury severity score, length of hospital stay, hospital charges, and mortality in children admitted to a regional pediatric trauma center. J Pediatr Orthop 1994; 14:449–453.
14. Buckley SL, Smith G, Sponseller PD, et al. Open fractures of the tibia in children. J Bone Joint Surg Am 1990;72:1462–1469.
15. Burrows HJ. Fatigue fractures of the fibula. J Bone Joint Surg Br 1948;30:266–279.
16. Byrd HS, Spicer PJ, Cierney G. Management of open tibial fractures. Plast Reconstr Surg 1985;76:719–730.
17. Caudle RJ, Stern PJ. Severe open fractures of the tibia. J Bone Joint Surg Am 1987;69: 801–807.
18. Cheng JCY, Shen WY. Limb fracture pattern in different pediatric age groups: a study of 3350 children. J Orthop Trauma 1993;7:15–22.
19. Cierny G, Byrd HS, Jones RE. Primary versus delayed tissue coverage for severe open tibial fractures: a comparison of results. Clin Orthop Relat Res 1983;178:54–63.
20. Clancey GJ, Hansen ST Jr. Open fractures of the tibia: a review of 102 cases. J Bone Joint Surg Am 1978;60:118–122.
21. Coates R. Knock-knee deformity following upper tibial "greenstick" fractures. J Bone Joint Surg Br 1977;59:516.
22. Cozen L. Fracture of the proximal portion of the tibia in children followed by valgus deformity. Surg Gynecol Obstet 1953;97:183–188.
23. Cramer KE, Limbird TJ, Green NE. Open fractures of the diaphysis of the lower extremity in children. J Bone Joint Surg Am 1992;74:218–232.
24. Cullen MC, Roy DR, Crawford AH, et al. Open fractures of the tibia in children. J Bone Joint Surg Am 1996;78:1039–1047.
25. DeBastiani G, Aldegheiri R, Renzi-Brivio LR, et al. Chondrodiastasis-controlled symmetrical distraction of the epiphyseal plate. Limb lengthening in children. J Bone Joint Surg Br 1986;68:550–556.
26. DeBastiani G, Aldegheiri R, Renzi-Brivio L, et al. Limb lengthening by distraction of the epiphyseal plate. A comparison of two techniques in the rabbit. J Bone Joint Surg Br 1986;68:545–549.
27. DeBoeck K, van Eldere, DeVos P, et al. Radionuclide bone imaging in toddler's fracture. Eur J Pediatr 1991;150:166–169.
28. Dedmond BT, Kortesis B, Punger K, et al. Subatmospheric pressure dressing in temporary treatment of soft tissue injuries associated with type III open tibial shaft fractures in children. J Pediatr Ortho. 2006;26:728–732.
29. DeLee JC, Strehl JB. Open tibia fracture with compartment syndrome. Clin Orthop Relat Res 1981;160:175–184.
30. Devas MB. Stress fractures in children. J Bone Joint Surg Br 1963;45:528–541.
31. Devas MB, Sweetman R. Stress fracture of the fibula: a review of 50 cases in athletes. J Bone Joint Surg Br 1956;38:818–829.
32. Dias LS. Ankle valgus in children with myelomeningocele. Dev Med Child Neurol 1978;20:627–633.
33. Drennan JC, Freehafer AA. Fractures of the lower extremities in paraplegic children. Clin Orthop Relat Res 1971;77:211–217.
34. Dunbar JS, Owen HF, Nogrady MB, et al. Obscure tibial fracture of infants—the toddler's fracture. J Can Assoc Radiol 1964;25:136–144.
35. Dwyer AJ, John B, Mann M, Hora R. Remodeling of tibia fracture in children younger than 12 years. Orthopaedics 2007;30:393–396.
36. Edwards CC. Staged reconstruction of complex open tibial fractures using Hoffmann external fixation. Clin Orthop Relat Res 1983;178:130–161.
37. Egol KA, Weisz R, Hiebert R, et al. Does fibular plating improve alignment after intramedullary nailing of distal metaphyseal tibia fractures? J Orthop Trauma 2006;20: 94–103.
38. Elton RL. Stress reaction of bone in army trainees. JAMA 1968;204:314–316.
39. Engh CA, Robinson RA, Milgram J. Stress fractures in children. J Trauma 1970;10: 532–541.
40. Evanoff M, Strong ML, MacIntosh R. External fixation maintained until fracture consolidation in the skeletally immature. J Pediatr Orthop 1983;13:98–101.
41. Felman AH. Bicycle spoke fractures. J Pediatr 1973;82:302–303.
42. Freehafer AA, Mast WA. Lower extremity fractures in patients with spinal-cord injury. J Bone Joint Surg Am 1965;47:683–694.
43. Gates JD. The management of combined skeletal and arterial injuries of the lower extremity. Am J Orthop 1995;24:674–680.
44. Gicquel P, Giacomelli MC, Basic B, et al. Problems of operative and nonoperative treatment and healing in tibial fractures. Injury 2005;26(Suppl 1):A44–50.
45. Gillies CL, Hartung W. Fracture of the tibia in spina bifida vera. Radiology 1938;31: 621.
46. Goff CW. Surgical Treatment of Unequal Extremities. Springfield, IL: Charles C Thomas, 1960:135–136.
47. Golding C. Museum pages. III: spina bifida and epiphyseal displacement. J Bone Joint Surg Br 1960;42:387–389.
48. Goodwin RC, Gaynor T, Mahar A, et al. Intramedullary flexible nail fixation of unstable pediatric tibial diaphyseal fractures. J Pediatr Orthop 2005;25:570–576.
49. Gordon JE, Gregush RV, Schoenecker PL, et al. Complications after titanium elastic nailing of pediatric tibial fractures. J Pediatr Orthop 2007;27:442–446.
50. Gordon JE, Schoenecker PL, Oda JE, et al. A comparison of monolateral and circular external fixation of unstable diaphyseal tibial fractures in children. J Pediatr Orthop 2003;12:338–345.
51. Gray H. Anatomy: descriptive and surgical. In: Pick TP, Howden R, eds. Anatomy: Descriptive and Surgical. New York: Bounty Books, 1977:182.
52. Green NE. Tibia valga caused by asymmetrical overgrowth following a nondisplaced fracture of the proximal tibia metaphysis. J Pediatr Orthop 1983;3:235–237.
53. Greiff J, Bergmann F. Growth disturbance following fracture of the tibia in children. Acta Orthop Scand 1980;15:315–320.
54. Griffiths AL. Fatigue fracture of the fibula in childhood. Arch Dis Child 1952;27: 552–557.
55. Grimard G, Navdie D, Laberge LC, et al. Open fractures of the tibia in children. Clin Orthop Relat Res 1996;332:62–70.
56. Gustilo RB, Anderson JT. Prevention of infection in the treatment of 1025 fractures of

long bones: retrospective and prospective analyses. J Bone Joint Surg Am 1976;58: 453–458.

57. Gustilo RB, Mendoza RM, Williams PN. Problems in the management of type III (severe) open fractures: a new classification of type III open fractures. J Trauma 1984;24: 742–746.
58. Gyepes MT, Newbern DH, Neuhauser EBD. Metaphyseal and physeal injuries in children with spina bifida and meningomyeloceles. Am J Roentgenol Radium Ther Nucl Med 1965;95:168–177
59. Haas LM, Staple TW. Arterial injuries associated with fractures of the proximal tibia following blunt trauma. South Med J 1969;62:1439–1448.
60. Hallock GG. Efficacy of free flaps for pediatric trauma patients. J Reconstructive Microsurgery 1995;11:169–174.
61. Hansen BA, Greiff S, Bergmann F. Fractures of the tibia in children. Acta Orthop Scand 1976;47:448–453.
62. Hartley JB. Fatigue fracture of the tibia. Br J Surg 1942;30:9–14.
63. Hoaglund FT, States JD. Factors influencing the rate of healing in tibial shaft fractures. Surg Gynecol Obstet 1967;124:71–76.
64. Holderman WD. Results following conservative treatment of fractures of the tibial shaft. Am J Surg 1959;98:593–597.
65. Hoover NW. Injuries of the popliteal artery associated with fractures and dislocations. Surg Clin North Am 1961;41:1099–1112.
66. Hope PG, Cole WG. Open fractures of the tibia in children. J Bone Joint Surg Br 1992; 74:546–553.
67. Horev G, Korenreich L, Ziv N, et al. The enigma of stress fractures in the pediatric age: clarification or confusion through the new imaging modalities. Pediatr Radiol 1990;20:469–471.
68. Hull JB, Sanderson PL, Rickman M, et al. External fixation of children's fractures: use of the Orthofix Dynamic Axial Fixator. J Pediatr Orthop 1997;6:203–206.
69. Ingersoll CF. Ice skater's fracture. A form of fatigue fracture. Am J Roentgenol Radium Ther Nucl Med 1943;50:469–479.
70. Izant RJ, Rothman BF, Frankel V. Bicycle spoke injuries of the foot and ankle in children: an underestimated "minor" injury. J Pediatr Surg 1969;4:654–656.
71. Jackson DW, Cozen L. Genu valgum as a complication of proximal tibial metaphyseal fractures in children. J Bone Joint Surg Am 1971;53:1571–1578.
72. James CCM. Fractures of the lower limbs in spina bifida cystica: a survey of 44 fractures in 122 children. Dev Med Child Neurol Suppl 1970;22(Suppl 22):88.
73. Janzing HMJ, Boaos PLO. Routine monitoring of compartment pressures in patients with tibial fractures: beware of over treatment. Injury 2001;32:415–421.
74. Johnson LC. Morphologic analysis. In: Frost HM, ed. Pathology in Bone Biodynamics. Boston: Little & Brown, 1963.
75. Jones BG, Duncan RDD. Open Tibial Fractures in Children under 13 years of age—10-year experience. Injury 2003;34(10):776–780.
76. Jordan SE, Alonso JE, Cook FF. The etiology of valgus angulation after metaphyseal fractures of the tibia in children. J Pediatr Orthop 1987;7:450–457.
77. Karlsson MK, Nilsson BE, Obrant KJ. Fracture incidence after tibial shaft fractures: a 30-year follow-up study. Clin Orthop Relat Res 1993;287:87–89.
78. Karlström G, Lönnerholm T, Olerud S. Cavus deformity of the foot after fracture of the tibial shaft. J Bone Joint Surg Am 1975;57:893–900.
79. Karrholm J, Hansson LI, Svensson K. Incidence of tibiofibular shaft and ankle fractures in children. J Pediatr Orthop 1982;2:386–396.
80. Katzman SS, Dickson K. Determining the prognosis for limb salvage in major vascular injuries with associated open tibial fractures. Orthop Rev 1992;21:195–199.
81. Keret D, Harcke HT, Bowen JR. Tibia valga after fracture: documentation of mechanism. Arch Orthop Trauma Surg 1991;110:216–219.
82. King J, Defendorf D, Apthorp J, et al. Analysis of 429 fractures in 1889 battered children. J Pediatr Orthop 1988;8:585–592.
83. Klein DM, Caligiuri DA, Katzman BM. Local-advancement soft-tissue coverage in a child with ipsilateral grade IIIB open tibial and ankle fractures. J Orthop Trauma 1996; 10:577–580.
84. Knight JL. Genu recurvatum deformity secondary to partial proximal tibial epiphyseal arrest. Am J Knee Surg 1998;11:111–115.
85. Kozlowski K, Azouz M, Barrett IR, et al. Midshaft tibial stress fractures in children. Aust Radiol 1992;36:131–134.
86. Kozlowski K, Urbonaviciene A. Stress fracture of the fibula in the first few years of life (report of six cases). Aust Radiol 1996;40:261–263.
87. Kreder HJ, Armstrong P. A review of open tibia fractures in children. J Pediatr Orthop 1995;15:482–488.
88. Kubiak EM, Egal KA, Scher D, et al. Operative treatment of tibial fractures in children: are elastic stable intramedullary nails an improvement over external fixation? J Bone Joint Surg Am 2005;87:1761–1768.
89. Kumar SJ, Lowell HR, Townsend P. Physeal, metaphyseal, and diaphyseal injuries of the lower extremities in children with myelomeningocele. J Pediatr Orthop 1984;4: 25–27.
90. Larsson K, van der Linden W. Open tibial shaft fractures. Clin Orthop Relat Res 1983; 180:63–67.
91. Leach RE, Hammond G, Stryker WS. Anterior tibial compartment syndrome. Acute and chronic. J Bone Joint Surg Am 1967;49:451–462.
92. Lehner A, Dubas J. Sekundare Deformierungen nach Epiphysenlosungen und Epiphysenliniennahen Fraktunen. Helv Chir Acta 1954;21:388–410.
93. Levy AS, Wetzlan M, Lewars M, et.al. The orthopaedic and social outcome of open tibia fractures in children. Orthopaedics 1997;20:593–598.
94. Liow RU, Montgomery RJ. Treatment of established and anticipated nonunion of the tibia in childhood. J Pediatr Orthop 2002;22:754–760.
95. Loder RT, Bookout C. Fracture patterns in battered children. J Ortho Trauma 1991; 5:428–433.
96. Matin P. The appearance of bone scans following fractures, including immediate and long-term studies. J Nucl Med 1979;20:1227–1231.
97. Matsen FA III, Clawson DK. The deep posterior compartmental syndrome of the leg. J Bone Joint Surg Am 1975;57:34–39.
98. Matsen FA III, Winquist RA, Krugmire RTS. Diagnosis and management of compartment syndromes. J Bone Joint Surg Am 1980;62:286–291.
99. Mellick LB, Reesor K. Spiral tibial fractures of children: a commonly accidental spiral long bone fracture. Am J Emerg Med 1990;8:234–237.
100. Mellick LB, Reesor K, Demers D, et al. Tibial fractures of young children. Pediatr Emerg Care 1988;4:97–101.
101. Metaizeau JP, Wong-Chung J, Bertrand H, et al. Percutaneous epiphysiodesis using transphyseal screws (PETS). J Pediatric Ortho 1998;18:363–369.
102. Meurman KOA, Elfving S. Stress fracture in soldiers: a multifocal bone disorder. Radiology 1980;134:483–487.
103. Micheli LJ, Gerbino PG. Etiologic assessment of stress fractures of the lower extremity in young athletes. Orthop Trans 1980;4:1.
104. Mooney JF III, Argenta LC, Marks MW, et al. Treatment of soft tissue defects in pediatric patients using the VAC system. CORR 2000;376:26–31.
105. Morton KS, Starr DE. Closure of the anterior portion of the upper tibial epiphysis as a complication of tibial-shaft fracture. J Bone Joint Surg Am 1964;46:570–574.
106. Myers SH, Spiegel D, Flynn JM. External fixation of high-energy tibia fractures. J Pediatr Orthop 2007;27:537–539.
107. Nicoll EA. Fractures of the tibial shaft, a survey of 705 cases. J Bone Joint Surg Br 1964;46:373–387.
108. O'Brien T, Weisman DS, Ronchetti P, et al. Flexible titanium nailing for the treatment of the unstable pediatric tibial fracture. J Pediatr Orthop 2004;24:601–609.
109. Ogden JA. Tibia and fibula. In: Ogden JA. Skeletal Injury in the Child. Philadelphia: Lea & Febiger, 1982:587.
110. Ogden JA, Ogden DA, Pugh L, et al. Tibia valga after proximal metaphyseal fracture in childhood: a normal biologic response. J Pediatr Orthop 1995;15:489–494.
111. Ostermann PAW, Henry SL, et al. Timing of wound closure in severe compound fractures. Orthopedics 1994;17:397–399.
112. Oudjhane K, Newman B, Oh KS, et al. Occult fractures in preschool children. Trauma 1988;28:858–860.
113. Parsch K, Rossak K. Die pathologischen frakturen bei spina bifida. Arch DeVecchi Anat Pat 1970;68:165–178.
114. Patzakis MJ, Wilkins J, Moore TM. Used antibiotics in open tibial fractures. Clin Orthop Relat Res 1983;118:31–35.
115. Pollen AG. Fractures and Dislocations in Children. Baltimore: Williams & Wilkins, 1973:179.
116. Prather JL, Nusynowitz ML, Snowdy HA, et al. Scintigraphic findings in stress fractures. J Bone Joint Surg Am 1977;59:869–874.
117. Qidwai SA. Intramedullary Kirschner wiring for tibia fractures in children. J Pediatr Ortho 2001;21:294–297.
118. Rinker B, Valerio IL, Stewart DH, et al. Microvascular free flap reconstruction in pediatric lower extremity trauma: a 10-year review. Plast Reconstr Surg 2006;118:570–571.
119. Robert M, Khouri N, Carlioz H, et al. Fractures of the proximal tibial metaphysis in children: review of a series of 25 cases. J Pediatr Orthop 1987;7:444–449.
120. Roberts SM, Vogt EC. Pseudofracture of the tibia. J Bone Joint Surg 1939;21:891–901.
121. Robertson P, Karol LA, Rab GT. Open fractures of the tibia and femur in children. J Pediatr Orthop 1996;16:621–626.
122. Robin G. Fracture in childhood paraplegia. Paraplegia 1966;3:165–170.
123. Rooker G, Salter R. Presentation of valgus deformity following fracture of the proximal metaphysis of the tibia in children. J Bone Joint Surg Br 1980;62:527.
124. Roub LW, Gumerman LW, Hanley EN, et al. Bone stress: a radionuclide imaging perspective. Radiology 1979;132:431–438.
125. Salem KH, Lindemann I, Keppler P. Flexible intramedullary nailing in pediatric lower limb fractures. J Pediatr Orthop 2006;26:505–509.
126. Salter RB, Best T. The pathogenesis and prevention of valgus deformity following fractures of the proximal metaphyseal region in the tibia in children. J Bone Joint Surg Am 1973;55:1324.
127. Sarmiento A. A functional below-the-knee cast for tibial fractures. J Bone Joint Surg Am 1967;49:855–875.
128. Savoca CJ. Stress fractures. A classification of the earliest radiographic signs. Radiology 1971;100:519–524.
129. Sawmiller S, Michener WM, Hartman JT. Stress fracture in childhood. Cleveland Clin Q 1965;32:119–123.
130. Sayyad MJ. Taylor spatial frame in the treatment of pediatric and adolescent tibial shaft fractures. J Pediatr Orthop 2006;26:164–170.
131. Schrock RD Jr. Peroneal nerve palsy following derotation osteotomies for tibial torsion Clin Orthop Relat Res 1969;62:172–177.
132. Scully RE, Shannon JM, Dickerson JR. Factors involved in recovery from experimental skeletal muscle ischemia in dogs. Am J Pathol 1961;39:721–737.
133. Shannak AO. Tibial fractures in children: follow-up study. J Pediatr Orthop 1988;8: 306–310.
134. Skaggs DL, Kautz SM, Kay RM, et al. Effects of delay on surgical treatment on rate of infection in open fractures in children. J Pediatric Ortho 2000;20:19–22.
135. Skak SV. Valgus deformity following proximal tibial metaphyseal fracture in children. Acta Orthop Scand 1982;53:141–147.
136. Small JO, Mollan RAB. Management of the soft tissues in open tibial fractures. Br J Plast Surg 1992;45:571–577.
137. Smillie IS. Injuries of the Knee Joint. 2nd ed. Baltimore: Williams & Wilkins, 1951.
138. Song KM, Sangeorzan B, Benirschke S, et al. Open fractures of the tibia in children. J Pediatr Orthop 1996;16:635–638.
139. Soutter FE. Spina bifida and epiphyseal displacement. J Bone Joint Surg Br 1962;44: 106.
140. Staudt JM, Smeulders MJ, van der Horst CM. Normal compartment pressures of the lower leg in children. J Bone Joint Surg Br 2008;90(2):215–219.
141. Steel HH, Sandrow RE, Sullivan PD. Complications of tibial osteotomy in children for genu varum or valgum. Evidence that neurological changes are due to ischemia. J Bone Joint Surg Am 1971;53:1629–1635.
142. Steinert VV, Bennek J. Unterschenkelfrakturen im Kindesalter. Zentralbl Chir 1966; 91:1387–1392.
143. Stern MB, Grant SS, Isaacson AS. Bilateral distal tibial and fibular epiphyseal separation associated with spina bifida. Clin Orthop Relat Res 1967;50:191–196.
144. Swaan JW, Oppers VM. Crural fractures in children. A study of the incidence of changes of the axial position and of enhanced longitudinal growth of the tibia after the healing of crural fractures. Arch Chir Neerl 1971;23:259–272.
145. Taunton JE, Clement DB, Webber D. Lower extremity stress fractures in athletes. J Sports Med Phys Fitness 1981;9:77–86.

146. Taylor SL. Tibial overgrowth: a cause of genu valgum. J Bone Joint Surg Am 1963;45: 659.
147. Tenenbein M, Reed MH, Black GB. The toddler's fracture revisited. Am J Emerg Med 1990;8:208–211.
148. Vallamshetla VR, De Silva U, Bache CE, et al. Flexible intramedullary nails for unstable fractures of the tibia in children. An 8-year experience. J Bone Joint Surg 2006;88: 536–540.
149. Van der Werkon C, Meevwis JD, et al. The simple fix: external fixation of displaced isolated tibial fractures. Injury 1993;24:46–48.
150. Weber BG. Fibrous interposition causing valgus deformity after fracture of the upper tibial metaphysis in children. J Bone Joint Surg Br 1977;59:290–292.
151. Weber BG, Brunner C, Freuner F, eds. Treatment of Fractures in Children and Adolescents. Berlin: Springer-Verlag, 1980.
152. Whitesides TE Jr, Haney TC, Morimoto K, et al. Tissue pressure measurements as a determinant for the need of fasciotomy. Clin Orthop Relat Res 1975;113:43–51.
153. Yang J, Letts M. Isolated fractures of the tibia with intact fibula in children: a review of 95 patients. J Pediatr Orthop 1997;17:347–351.
154. Zionts LE, Harcke HT, Brooks KM, et al. Posttraumatic tibia valga: a case demonstrating asymmetric activity at the proximal growth plate on technetium bone scan. J Pediatr Orthop 1977;7:458–462.
155. Zionts LE, MacEwen GD. Spontaneous improvement of posttraumatic tibia valga. J Bone Joint Surg Am 1986;68:680–687.

SUGGESTED READINGS

Letts M, Vincent M. The "floating knee" in children. J Bone Joint Surg Br 1986;68:442–446.

Mars M, Hadley GP. Raised compartmental pressures in children: a basis for treatment. Injury 1998;24:183–185.

Siegmeth A, Wruhs O, Vecsei V. External fixation of lower limb fractures in children. Eur J Pediatr Surg 1998;8:35–41.

Wood D, Hoffer MH. Tibial fractures in head-injured children. J Trauma 1987;27:65–68.

26

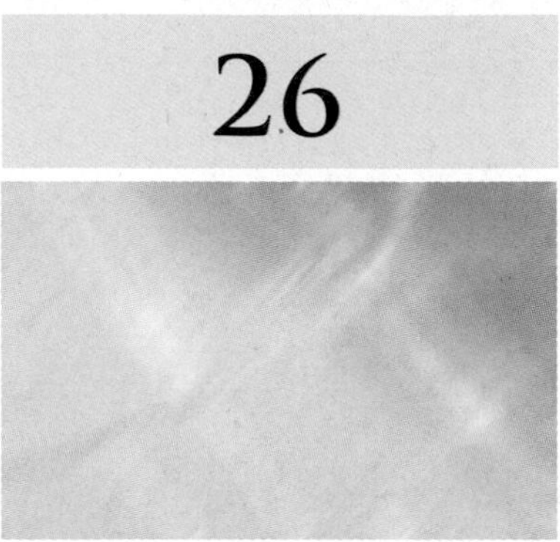

DISTAL TIBIAL AND FIBULAR FRACTURES

R. Jay Cummings and Kevin G. Shea

EPIDEMIOLOGY 967

HISTORICAL STUDIES 967

PRINCIPLES OF MANAGEMENT 968
Mechanism of Injury and Classification 968
Signs and Symptoms 974
Diagnostic Studies 975

ANATOMY 980

TREATMENT 981
Distal Tibial Fractures 982
Juvenile Tillaux Fractures 991
Triplane Fracture 991
Pilon Fractures 993
Fractures of the Incisura 994
Syndesmosis Injuries 994
Open Fractures and Lawnmower Injuries 995
Distal Fibula Fractures 996
Lateral Ankle Sprains 997
Ankle Dislocations 997

PROGNOSIS AND COMPLICATIONS 1009
Delayed Union and Nonunion 1009
Deformity Secondary to Malunion 1009
Physeal Arrest or Growth Disturbance 1010
Medial Malleolus Overgrowth 1011
Arthritis 1011
Chondrolysis 1013
Osteonecrosis of the Distal Tibial Epiphysis 1013
Compartment Syndrome 1013
Synostosis 1013
Reflex Sympathetic Dystrophy/Complex Regional Pain Syndrome 1013

CONTROVERSIES AND FUTURE DIRECTIONS 1013

EPIDEMIOLOGY

Injuries to the distal tibial and fibular physes are generally reported to account for 25% to 38% of all physeal fractures,[78,156] second in frequency only to distal radial physeal fractures[141]; however, Peterson and associates[143] reported that phalangeal physeal fractures were most common, followed by physeal injuries of the radius and ankle. Approximately 4% of all ankle fractures involve the physes.[31] In skeletally immature individuals, physeal ankle fractures are slightly more common than fractures of the tibial or fibular diaphysis.[116]

Participation in sports is associated with a significant number of ankle injuries, including sprains and fractures. Up to 58% of physeal ankle fractures occur during sports activities[64,193] and account for 10% to 40% of all injuries to skeletally immature athletes.[132,136,159,178] Physeal ankle fractures are more common in males than in females in some studies.[175] Other studies have demonstrated that ankle injuries may be more likely in young female soccer players compared with males.[103] Fractures of the ankle are associated with the following sport activities: trampolines,[169] scooters,[115] soccer,[103] basketball,[45] skating,[131] and downhill skiing.[13]

In addition to sports, higher-energy trauma is associated with a significant number of distal tibia and fibular fractures in children. These fractures occur in approximately 10% to 20% of trauma patients presenting to the emergency room.[13] Tibial physeal fractures are most common between the ages of 8 and 15 years, and fibular fractures are most common between 8 and 14 years of age.[175]

HISTORICAL STUDIES

Although Foucher[57] reported the first pathologic study of these injuries in 1863, Poland's 1898 monograph[147] is generally recognized as the most extensive early study of physeal fractures. He pointed out that in children, ligaments are stronger than physeal cartilage so that forces that result in ligament damage in adults cause fractures of the physes in children. In 1922, Ashhurst and Bromer[4] published a thorough review of the literature and the results of their own extensive investigations and described a classification of ankle injuries based on the mechanism of injury. This classification did not differentiate between ankle injuries in adults and those in children. Bishop,[10] in 1932, classified 300 ankle fractures according to Ashhurst and Bromer's system; 33 fractures were physeal injuries, and the grouping of these injuries according to mechanism of injury represents one of the first attempts to classify physeal ankle injuries.

Aitken's[2] study of 21 physeal ankle injuries in 1936 is one of the first to attempt to determine the results of treatment of these injuries; he also outlined an anatomic classification. Only one of his patients (5%) had a deformity after fracture, in contrast to McFarland,[120] who, in 1932, reported deformities in 40% of a larger series of patients. In 1955, Caruthers and Crenshaw[31] reported 54 physeal ankle fractures, which were classified according to their modification of Ashhurst and Bromer's system. They confirmed that growth-related deformities were frequent after adduction (Salter-Harris types III and IV injuries) fractures and infrequent after fractures caused by external rotation, abduction, and plantarflexion (Salter-Harris type II injuries). Spiegel and colleagues,[175] in a 1978 review of 237 physeal ankle fractures, reported a high incidence of growth abnormalities after Salter-Harris type III and IV injuries but also found complications in 11 (16.7%) of 66 patients with Salter-Harris type II fractures. Most of these patients had only mild shortening, but 6 had angular deformities that did not correct with growth.

PRINCIPLES OF MANAGEMENT

Mechanism of Injury and Classification

Fracture classifications are usually based on anatomic[2,134,142,175] or mechanism of injury descriptions[4,10,101] Anatomic classifications distinguish fractures based on the regions of the metaphysis, physis, and epiphysis. Mechanism-of-injury classifications incorporate the forces that produce the fracture and the anatomic position of the foot and ankle that existed at the time of the injury. Most mechanism-of-injury classifications include the anatomic type of injury produced by a particular mechanism.

Since its description, the Salter-Harris classification system has been widely used to describe the anatomic features of fractures associated with open physes. This straight forward anatomic classification (Fig. 26-1) is effective for rapid communication. It has five distinct categories, which can be applied to most periarticular regions.

Injury classifications based upon the mechanism of injury may have some advantages. The description of the injury includes the anatomic deformity and the forces that produced the injury. Reduction of the displaced fracture may be enhanced by an understanding of these forces and how they produced the distorted relationship between the displaced fragments. Advanced imaging techniques that allow for comprehensive three-dimensional visualization of the fracture anatomy also facilitate surgical planning and reduction techniques.

Both anatomic- and mechanism-of-injury classifications can provide useful information for determining appropriate treatment. The prognoses for growth and deformity have been predicted on the basis of both types of classification (Table 26-1).[88,89,175] A theoretical advantage of mechanism-of-injury classifications is that identification of the force producing the injury might give even more information about the possible development of growth arrest than anatomic classifications. For example, a Salter-Harris type III or IV fracture of the tibia produced by a shearing (Fig. 26-2) or crushing force might be more likely to result in growth arrest than a similar injury produced by an avulsion force. However, it is difficult to establish that one type of classification is superior to the other in this regard because of the relatively small numbers of patients reported, the varying ages of patients in most series, and questions about the reproducibility of various classifications.

Ideally, classifications systems should have high interobserver and intraobserver agreement. Thomsen and coworkers[183] studied the reproducibility of the Lauge-Hansen (mechanism-of-injury) and Weber (anatomic) classifications in a series of adult ankle fractures. After all investigators in the study had received a tutorial on both systems and their application, they were asked to classify 94 fractures. On the first attempt, only the Weber classification produced an acceptable level of interobserver agreement. On a second attempt, the Weber classification and most of the Lauge-Hansen classification achieved an acceptable level of interobserver agreement. These authors concluded that all fracture classification systems should have demonstrably acceptable interobserver agreement rates before they are adopted, an argument made even more forcefully in an editorial by Burstein.[27] Vahvanen and Aalto[185] compared their ability to

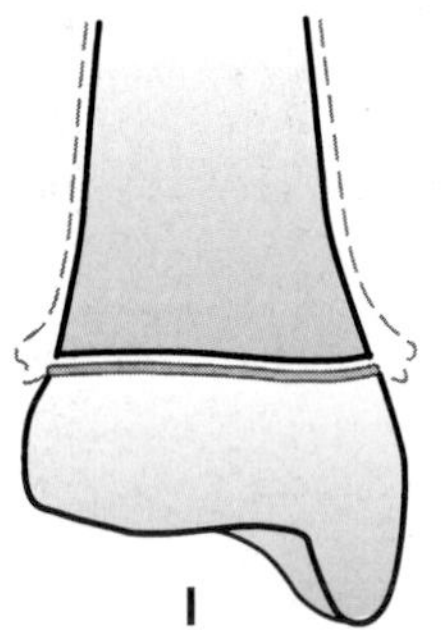

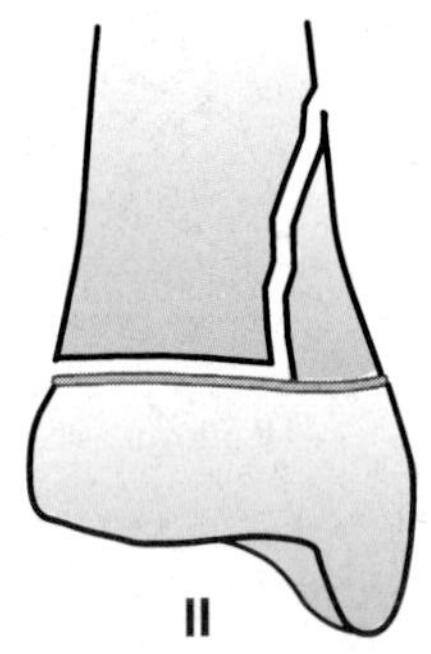

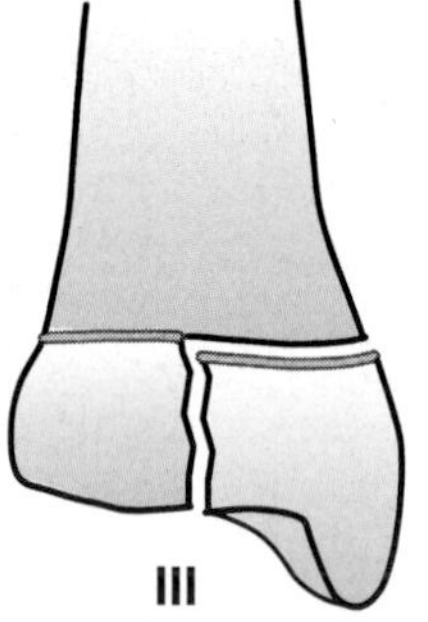

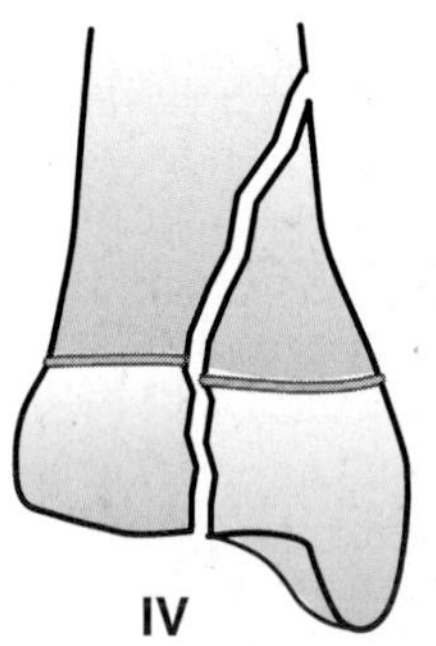

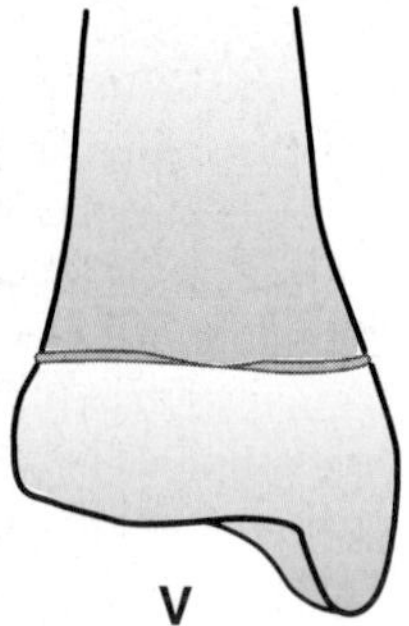

FIGURE 26-1 Salter-Harris anatomic classification as applied to injuries of the distal tibial epiphysis.

TABLE 26-1 Representative Mechanism of Injury Classifications: Applied Force

Ashhurst-Bromer (Adult)
External Rotation
Abduction
Adduction
Compression
Carothers-Crenshaw (Child)
External Rotation
Abduction
Adduction
Plantarflexion
Compression
Lauge-Hansen (Adult)
Supination
Pronation
Supination
Pronation
Eversion (External Rotation)
Abduction
Adduction
Compression
Eversion (External Rotation)
Dias-Tachdjian (Child)
Supination
External Rotation
Pronation Eversion (Abduction)
External Rotation
Supination
Inversion (Adduction)
Supination
Plantarflexion
Axial Compression
Juvenile Tillaux
Triplane

Lauge-Hansen Pronation: External rotation of foot, Abduction of hindfoot, Eversion of forefoot
Lauge Hansen Supination: External rotation of foot, Adduction of hindfoot, Inversion of forefoot

classify 310 ankle fractures in children with the Weber, Lauge-Hansen, and Salter-Harris classifications. They found that they were "largely unsuccessful" using the Weber and Lauge-Hansen classifications but could easily classify the fractures using the Salter-Harris system.

A commonly used mechanism-of-injury classification of ankle fractures in children is that described by Dias and Tachdjian,[49] who modified the Lauge-Hansen classification based on their review of 71 fractures (Fig 26-3). Their original classification (from 1978) consisted of four types in which the first word refers to the position of the foot at the time of injury and the second word refers to the force that produces the injury.

Other fracture types were subsequently added, including axial compression, juvenile Tillaux, triplane, and other physeal injuries, by Tachjidan.[179] Syndesmosis injuries have also been recently described.[43] Although these are designated differently, the first three have presumed mechanisms of injury. "Axial compression injury" describes the mechanism of injury but not the position of the foot. Juvenile Tillaux and triplane fractures are believed to be caused by external rotation. The final category, "other physeal injuries," includes diverse injuries, many of which have no specific mechanism of injury.

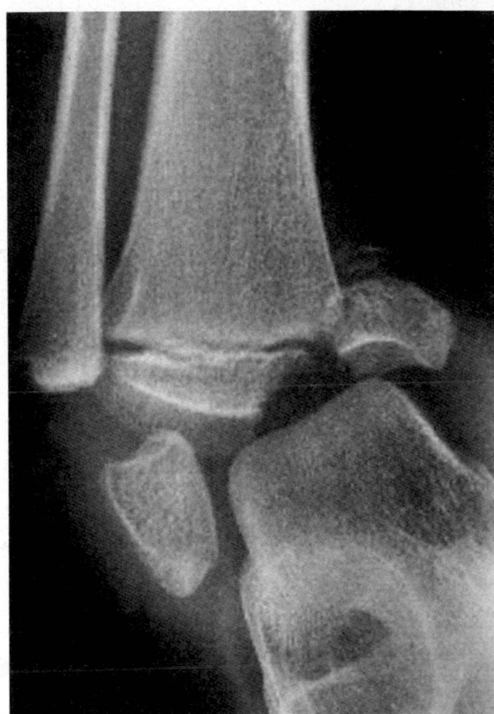

FIGURE 26-2 Comminuted Salter-Harris type IV fracture of the distal tibia and displaced Salter-Harris type I fracture of the distal fibula produced by an inversion (shearing) mechanism in a 10-year-old girl.

Classification of Ankle Fracture in Children (Dias-Tachdjian) (see Fig 26-3)

Supination–inversion

- Grade I: The adduction or inversion force avulses the distal fibular epiphysis (Salter-Harris type I or II fracture). Occasionally, the fracture is transepiphyseal; rarely, the lateral ligaments fail.
- Grade II (Fig. 26-4): Further inversion produces a tibial fracture, usually a Salter-Harris type III or IV and rarely a Salter-Harris type I or II injury, or the fracture passes through the medial malleolus below the physis (Fig. 26-5).

Supination–plantarflexion

The plantarflexion force displaces the epiphysis directly posteriorly, resulting in a Salter-Harris type I or II fracture. Fibular fractures were not reported with this mechanism. The tibial fracture may be difficult to see on anteroposterior radiographs (Fig 26-6).

Supination–external rotation

- Grade I: The external rotation force results in a Salter-Harris type II fracture of the distal tibia (Fig. 26-7). The distal fragment is displaced posteriorly, as in a supination–plantarflexion injury, but the Thurstan-Holland fragment is visible on the anteroposterior radiographs, with the fracture line ex-

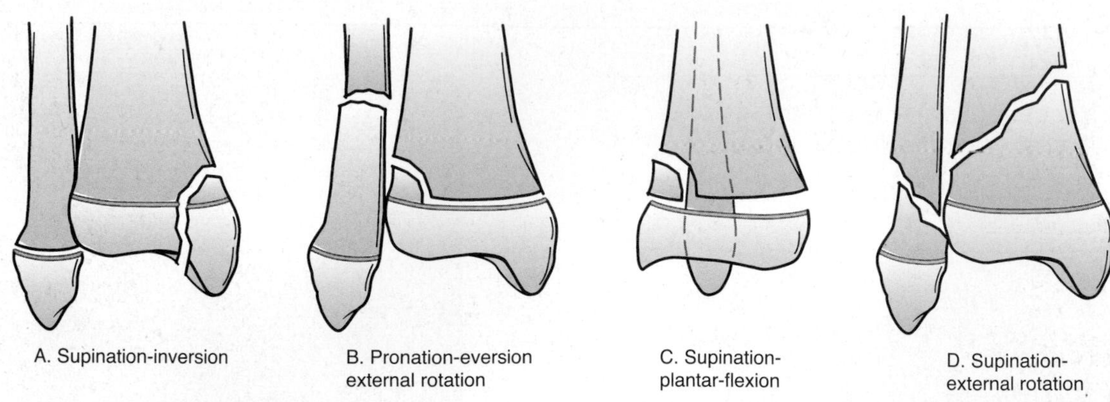

FIGURE 26-3 Dias-Tachdjian classification of physeal injuries of the distal tibia and fibula.

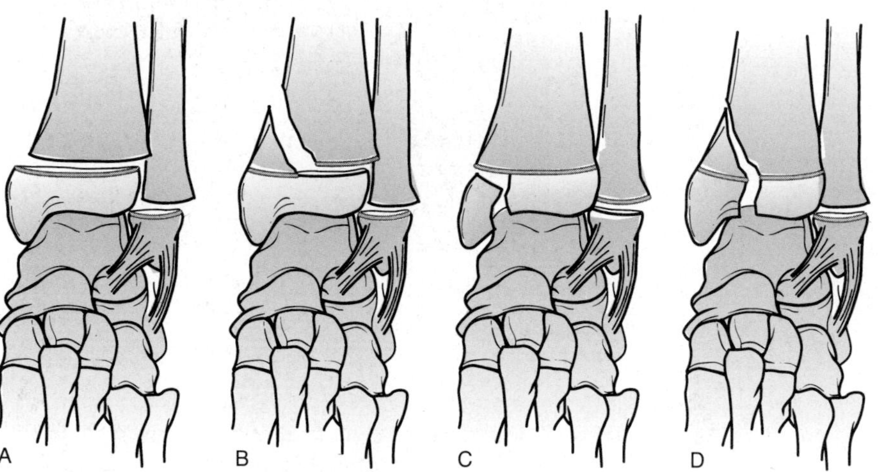

FIGURE 26-4 Variants of grade II supination–inversion injuries (Dias-Tachdjian classification). **A.** Salter-Harris type I fracture of the distal tibia and fibula. **B.** Salter-Harris type I fracture of the fibula, Salter-Harris type II tibial fracture. **C.** Salter-Harris type I fibular fracture, Salter-Harris type III tibial fracture. **D.** Salter-Harris type I fibular fracture, Salter-Harris type IV tibial fracture.

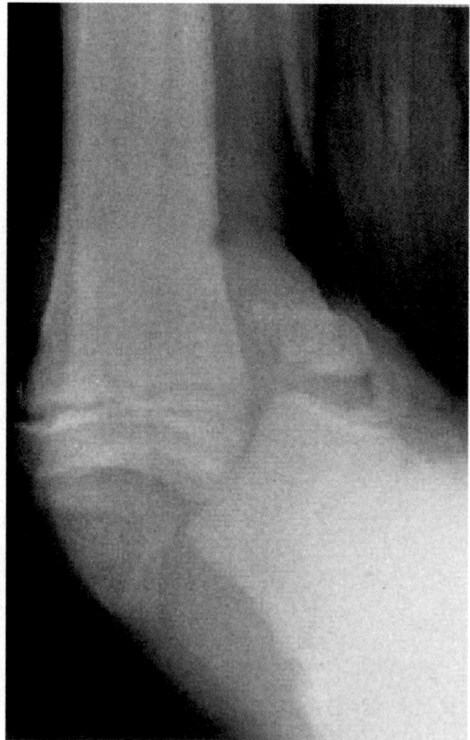

FIGURE 26-5 Severe supination–inversion injury with displaced fracture of the medial malleolus distal to the physis of the tibia.

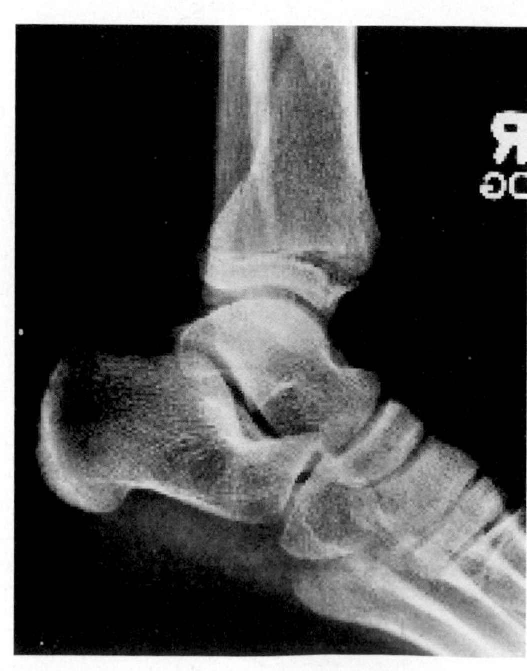

FIGURE 26-6 Lateral view of a supination plantarflexion injury.

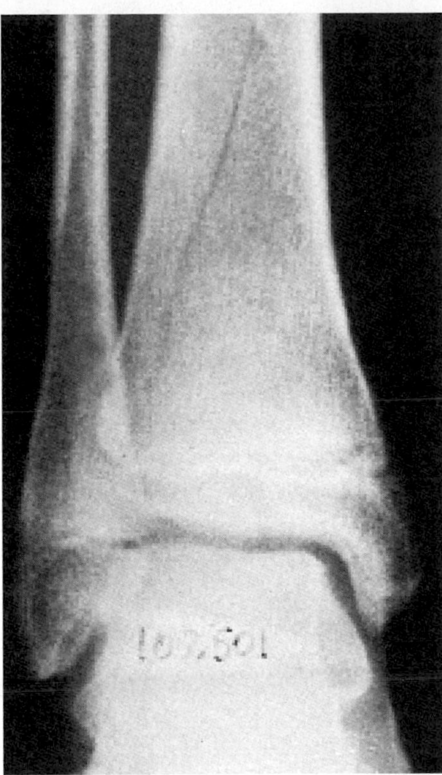

FIGURE 26-7 Stage I supination–external rotation injury in a 10-year-old child; the Salter-Harris type II fracture begins laterally.

tending proximally and medially. Occasionally, the distal tibial epiphysis is rotated but not displaced.

- Grade II: With further external rotation, a spiral fracture of the fibula is produced, running from anteroinferior to posterosuperior (Fig. 26-8).

Pronation–eversion–external rotation

A Salter-Harris type I or II fracture of the distal tibia occurs simultaneously with a transverse fibular fracture. The distal tibial fragment is displaced laterally and the Thurstan-Holland fragment, when present, is lateral or posterolateral (Fig. 26-9). Less frequently, a transepiphyseal fracture occurs through the medial malleolus (Salter-Harris type II). Such injuries may be associated with diastasis of the ankle joint, which is uncommon in children.

Transitional Fractures

Because the distal tibial physis closes in an asymmetric pattern over a period of about 18 months, injuries sustained during this period can produce fracture patterns that are not seen in younger children with completely open physes.[113] This group of fractures has been labeled "transitional" fractures because they occur during the transition from a skeletally immature ankle to a skeletally mature ankle. Such fractures, which include juvenile Tillaux and "triplane" fractures with two to four fracture fragments, have been described by Kleiger and Mankin,[97] Marmor,[117] Cooperman and coworkers,[39] Karrholm,[87] and Denton and Fischer.[46] The adolescent pilon fracture has been described by Letts et al.[105] The incisural and syndesmosis fractures have been described by Cummings and Hahn[44] and Cummings,[43] respectively, and these injuries are described below.

Classification of these fractures is even more confusing than

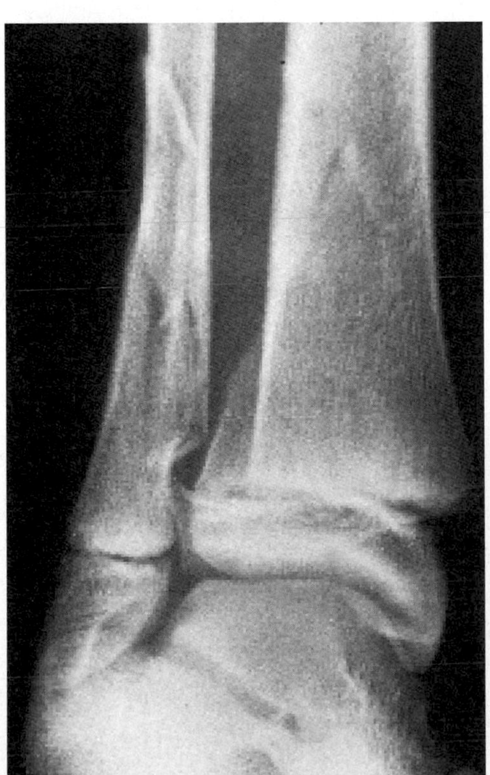

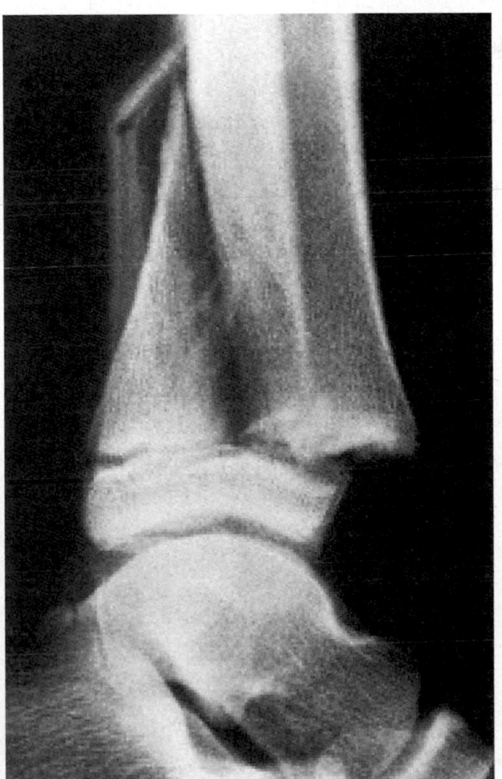

FIGURE 26-8 Stage II supination–external rotation injury. **A.** Oblique fibular fracture also is visible on anteroposterior view. **B.** Lateral view shows the posterior metaphyseal fragment and posterior displacement.

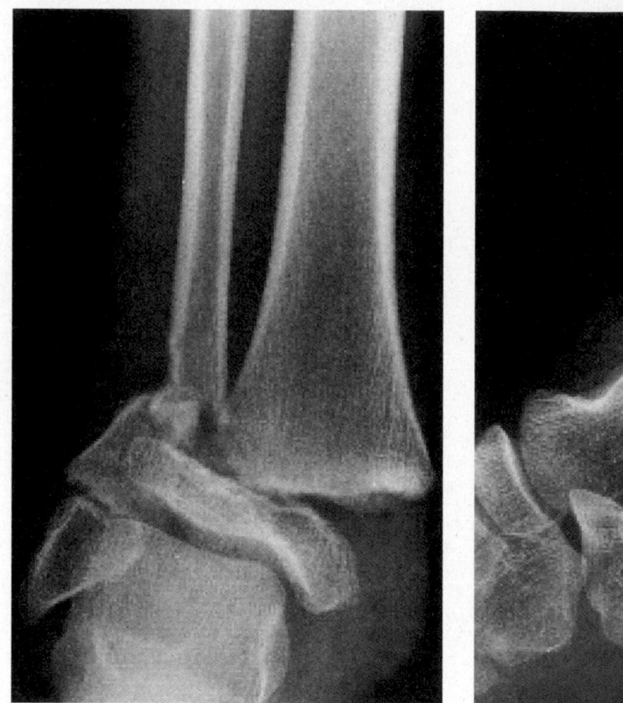

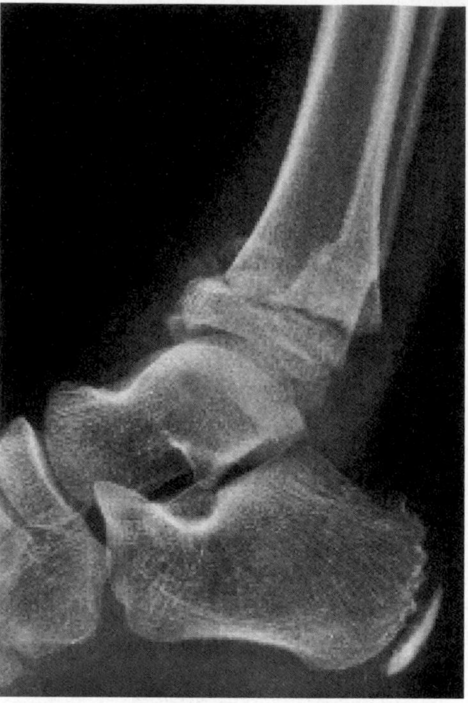

FIGURE 26-9 A. According to the Dias-Tachdjian classification, this injury in a 12-year-old boy would be considered a pronation–eversion–external rotation injury resulting in a Salter-Harris type II fracture of the distal tibia and a transverse fibular fracture. **B.** The anterior displacement of the epiphysis, visible on the lateral view, however, makes external rotation an unlikely component of the mechanism of injury; the mechanism is more likely pronation–dorsiflexion.

that of other distal tibial fractures. Advocates of mechanism-of-injury systems agree that most juvenile Tillaux and triplane fractures are caused by external rotation, but they disagree as to the position of the foot at the time of the injury.[47,48,148] Some authors[48] classify juvenile Tillaux fractures as stage I injuries, with further external rotation causing triplane fractures, and still further external rotation causing stage II injuries with fibular fracture. Others emphasize the extent of physeal closure as the only determinant of fracture pattern.[38]

Advocates of anatomic classifications are handicapped by the different anatomic configurations triplane fractures may exhibit on different radiographs projections, making tomography, computed tomography (CT) scanning, or examination at open reduction necessary to determine fracture anatomy and number of fragments. Because these fractures occur near the end of growth, growth disturbance is rare. Anatomic classification is, therefore, more useful for descriptive purposes than for prognosis.

Juvenile Tillaux Fractures

The juvenile Tillaux fracture is a Salter-Harris type III fracture involving the anterolateral distal tibia. The portion of the physis not involved in the fracture is closed (Fig. 26-10).

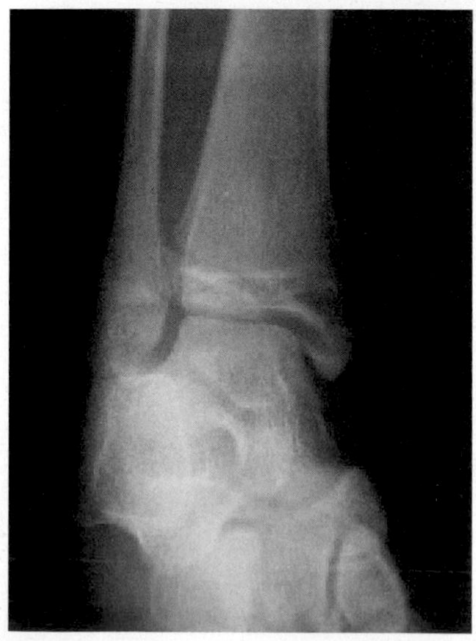

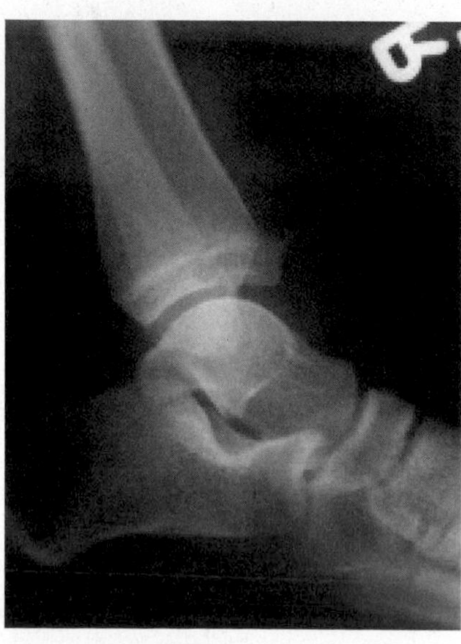

FIGURE 26-10 A. Anteroposterior radiograph of Salter Harris type III/juvenile Tillaux Fracture. **B.** Lateral radiograph of Salter Harris type III/juvenile Tillaux Fracture.

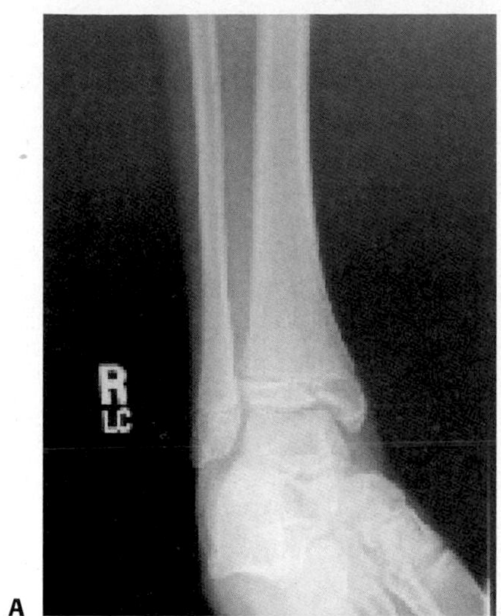

A

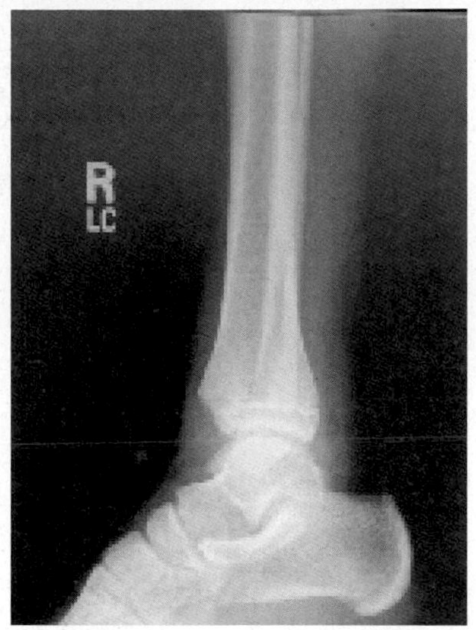

B

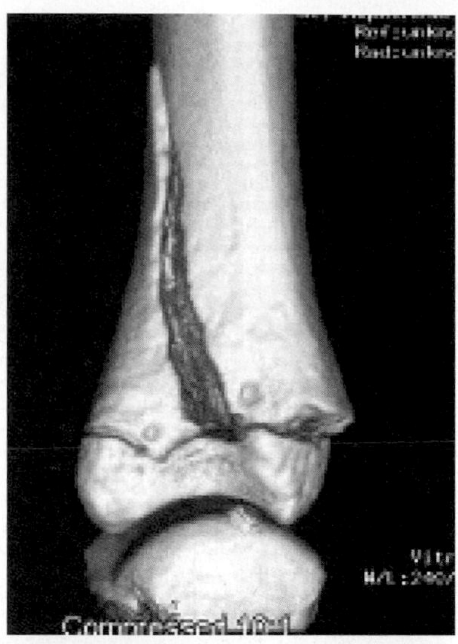

C

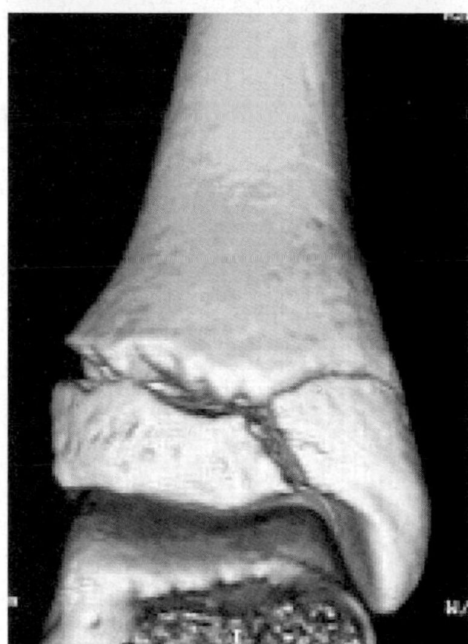

D

FIGURE 26-11 A. Anteroposterior view of triplane fracture. On this view, the fracture appears to be a Salter-Harris type III configuration. **B**. Lateral view of triplane fracture. On this view, the fracture appears to be a Salter-Harris type II configuration. **C**. Three-dimensional CT reconstruction can demonstrate significant metaphyseal displacement. **D**. Three-dimensional CT reconstruction can demonstrate intra-articular displacement.

Triplane Fractures

Triplane fractures are a group of fractures that have in common the appearance of a Salter-Harris type III fracture on the anteroposterior radiographs and of a Salter-Harris type II fracture on the lateral radiographs (Fig. 26-11). CT scans can be very helpful to understand the complex anatomy of these fractures (see Fig. 26-11). It has been proposed that the mechanism of injury for Tillaux and triplane fractures is external rotation.[47,148] Some classify juvenile Tillaux fractures as stage I injuries, with further external rotation leading to triplane fractures and stage three leading to fibula fractures.[47] Others suggest that the degree of physeal closure is the main determinant of fracture pattern.[38]

Adolescent Pilon Fractures

The pediatric/adolescent pilon fracture is defined as a fracture of the "tibial plafond with articular and physeal involvement, variable talar and fibular involvement, variable comminution, and greater than 5 mm of displacement" (Fig. 26-12).[105] Based upon a small number of cases, Letts et al.[105] developed a three part classification system. Type 1 fractures have minimal comminution and no physeal displacement. Type 2 fractures have marked comminution and less than 5 mm of physeal displacement. Type 3 fractures have marked comminution and more than 5 mm of physeal displacement.

Incisura Fractures

Incisural fractures are fractures that resemble Tillaux on standard radiographs, but the size of the fragment is smaller than that typically seen with the Tillaux fractures (Fig 26-13).[44] On the CT scan, this fracture does not extend to the anterior cortex of the distal tibia (Fig 26-14). The mechanism of injury may be an avulsion of the fragment by the interosseous ligament. This may be a variant of an adult tibia-fibular diastasis injury.

Syndesmosis Injuries

The authors have seen syndesmosis injuries in young patients. These have been associated with fractures of the distal fibula, Tillaux injuries, Salter-Harris type I fractures, and proximal fibula fractures (Figs. 26-15 to 26-17). These fractures are probably rare, and there is very limited literature on this injury.[140]

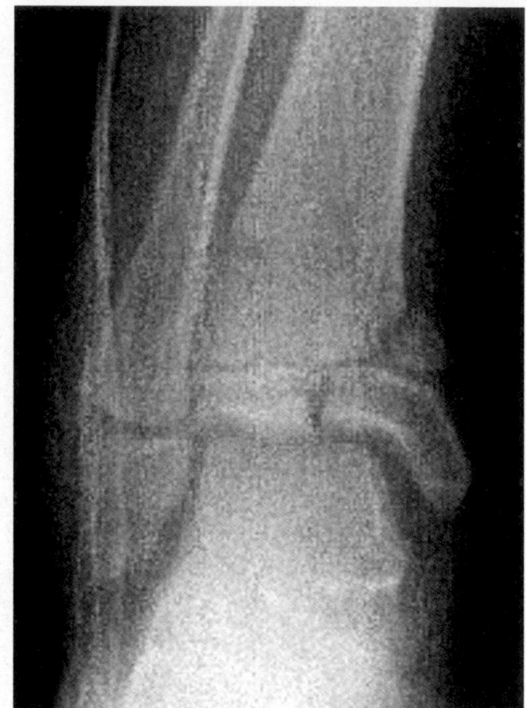

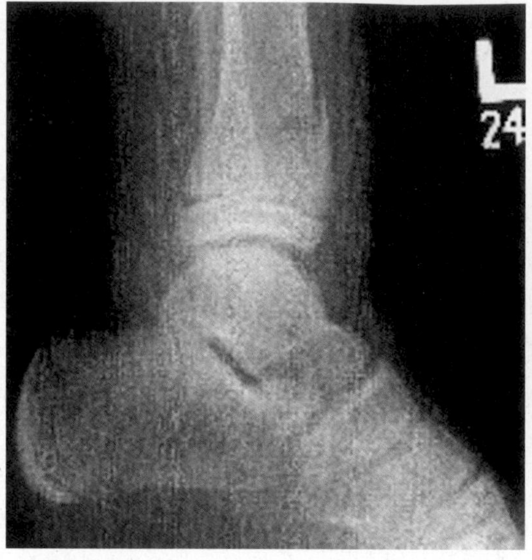

FIGURE 26-12 Anteroposterior and lateral radiographs of a pilon fracture in an adolescent.

Stress Fractures

Stress fractures can occur in the distal tibial metaphyseal area (Fig. 26-18) or through the distal fibular physis (Fig. 26-19). These patients may present with warmth, swelling, and pain around the metaphyseal or physeal regions. In our experience, these injuries are more common in running/endurance athletes. We have seen stress fractures through the distal fibular physeal scar in running athletes.

Ipsilateral triplane and diaphyseal fractures have been reported, and one of the fractures can be missed if adequate images are not obtained.[81]

Signs and Symptoms

Patients with significantly displaced fractures have severe pain and obvious deformity. The position of the foot relative to the leg may provide important information about the mechanism of injury (Fig. 26-20) and should be considered in planning

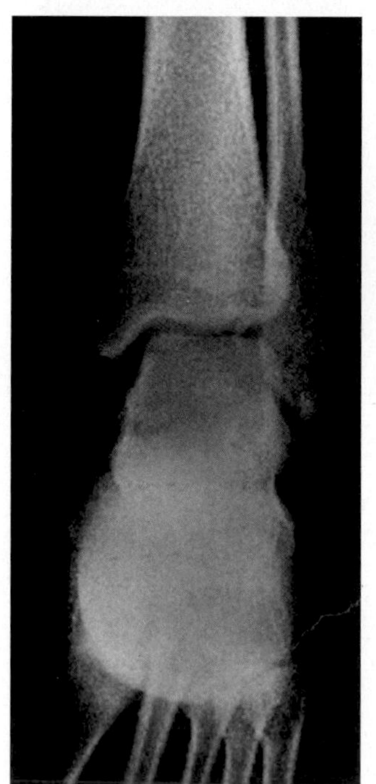

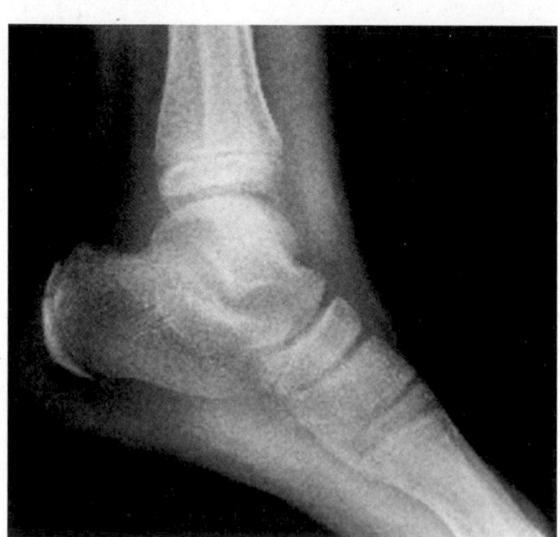

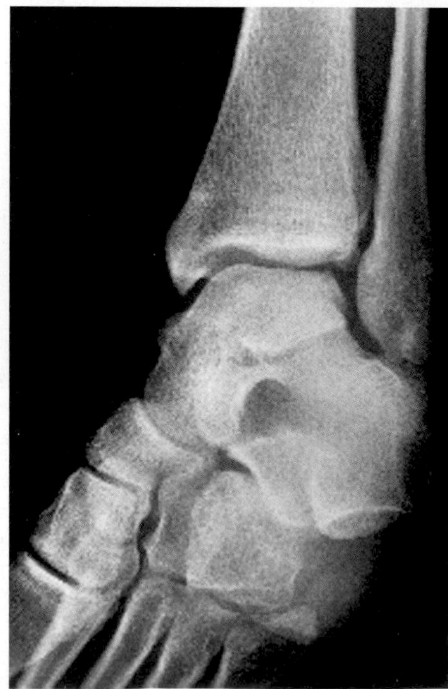

FIGURE 26-13 Anteroposterior **(A)**, lateral **(B)**, and oblique **(C)** views of the ankle demonstrating an apparent small juvenile Tillaux fracture in a 14-year-old girl.

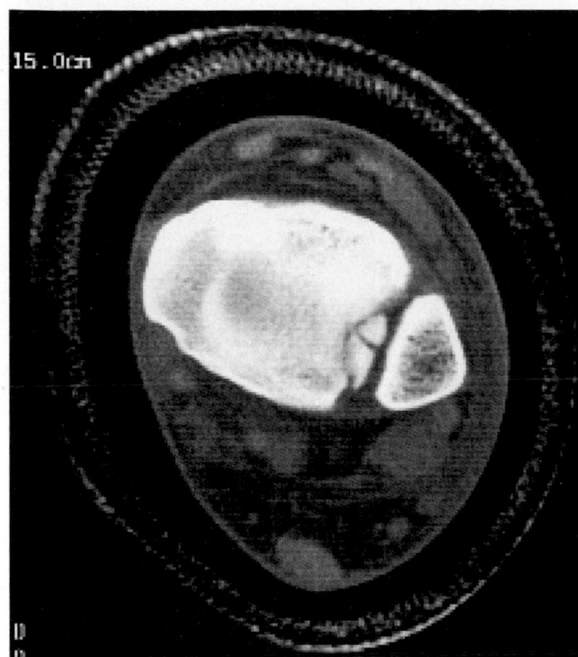

FIGURE 26-14 Incisural fracture: CT scan at the level of the tibiotalar joint demonstrates that the fracture fragment does not include the attachment of the anterior inferior tibiofibular ligament.

reduction. The status of the skin, pulses, and sensory and motor function should be determined and recorded. Tenderness, swelling, and deformity in the ipsilateral leg and foot should be noted. In patients with tibial shaft fractures, the ankle should be carefully evaluated clinically and radiographically.

Although compartment syndromes are rare, they do occur in these locations.[40,126] If patients are admitted to the hospital, discussion with the nursing staff about signs and symptoms of compartment syndrome are important. If patients are treated as outpatients, communication with the patient and family about the possibility of compartment syndrome is also important. These families should return to the hospital for evaluation if problems with pain control develop.

Diagnostic Studies

Patients with nondisplaced or minimally displaced ankle fractures often have no deformity, minimal swelling, and moderate pain. Because of their benign clinical appearance, such fractures may be easily missed if radiographs are not obtained. Petit et al.[145] reviewed 2470 radiographs from pediatric emergency rooms, demonstrating abnormal radiographic findings in 9%. Guidelines known as The Ottawa Ankle Rules have been established for adults to try to determine which injuries require radiographs.[177] The indications for radiographs according to the guidelines are complaints of pain near a malleolus with either inability to bear weight or tenderness to palpation at the malleolus. Chande[36] prospectively studied 71 children with acute ankle injuries to determine if these guidelines could be applied to pediatric patients with ankle injuries. It was determined that if radiographs were obtained only in children with tenderness over the malleoli and inability to bear weight, a 25% reduction in radiographic examinations could be achieved without missing any fractures. The physical examination should focus upon physeal areas of the tibia and fibula when evaluating ankle injuries to determine if radiographs are necessary. Interpretation of radiographs should focus upon signs of physeal injury, including soft tissues swelling in these regions.

For patients with obvious deformities or tenderness and swelling only about the ankle, anteroposterior, mortise, and lateral radiographs centered over the ankle may provide sufficient information to plan treatment. Although obtaining views of the joint above and below is recommended for most fractures, obtaining a film centered over the midtibia to include the knee and ankle joints on the radiographs significantly decreases the quality of ankle views and is not recommended.

For patients without obvious deformities, a high-quality mortise view of the ankle is essential in addition to anteroposterior and lateral views. On a standard anteroposterior view, the

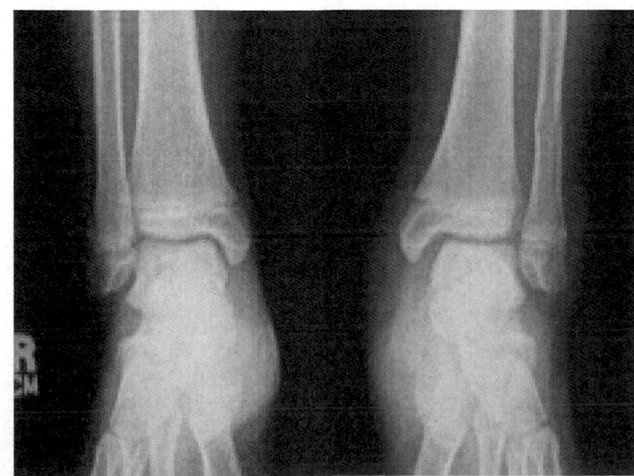

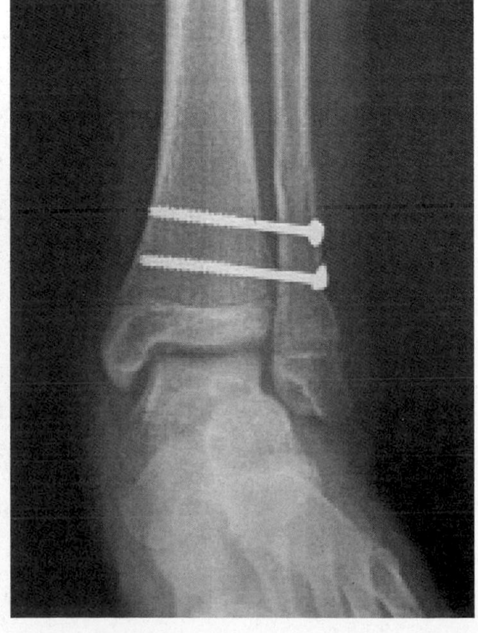

FIGURE 26-15 A. Syndesmosis injury with distal fibula fracture. Radiographs with comparison of right and left sides. Note the widening of the medial clear space and the syndesmosis. **B.** Use of two percutaneous placed cannulated screws to reduce the syndesmosis.

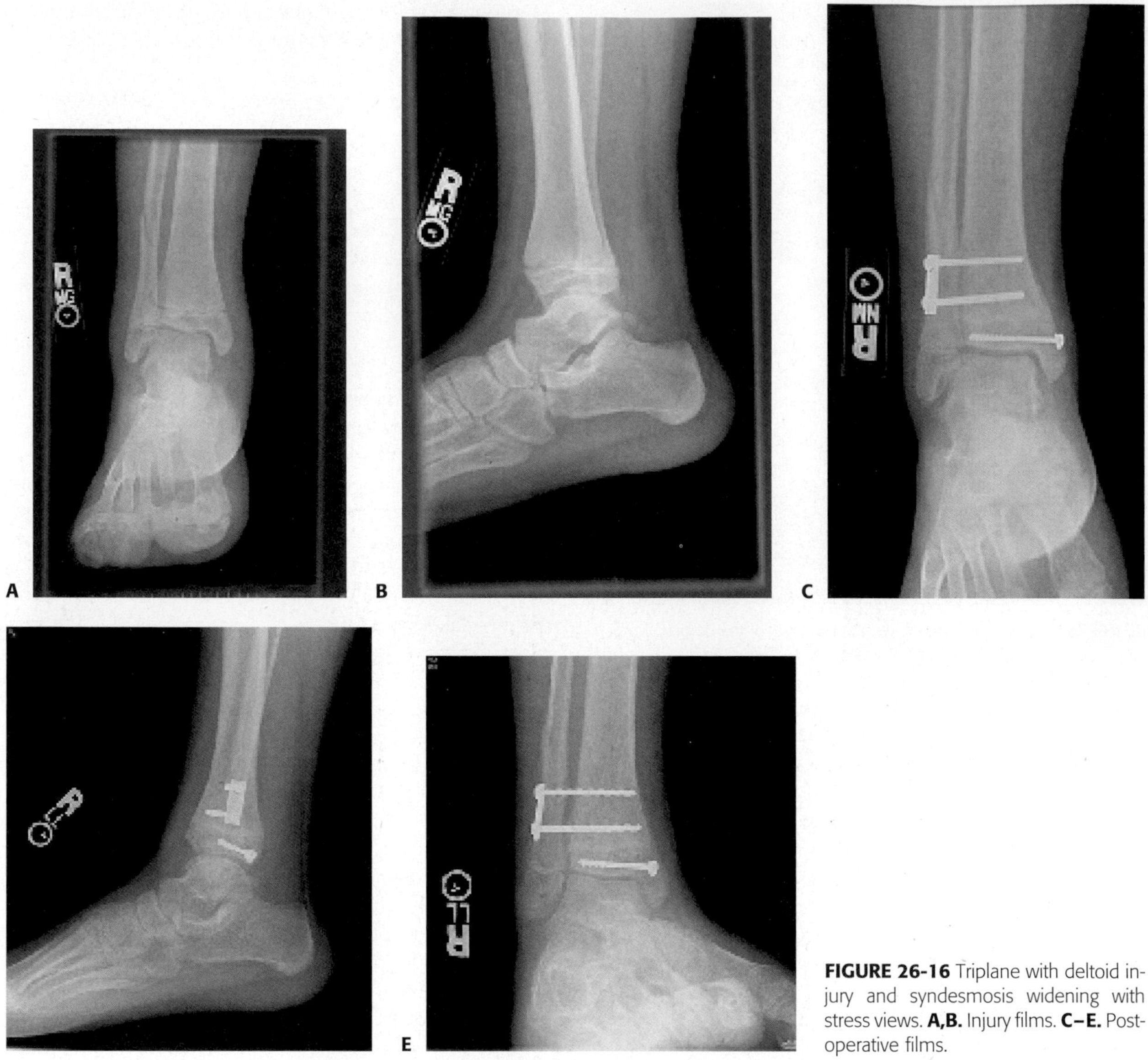

A B C D E

FIGURE 26-16 Triplane with deltoid injury and syndesmosis widening with stress views. **A,B.** Injury films. **C–E.** Postoperative films.

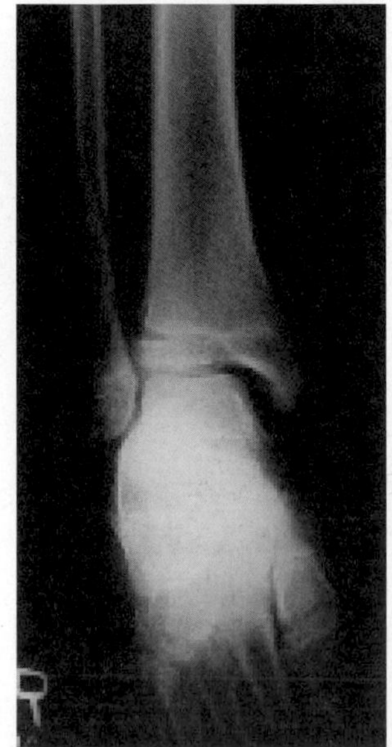

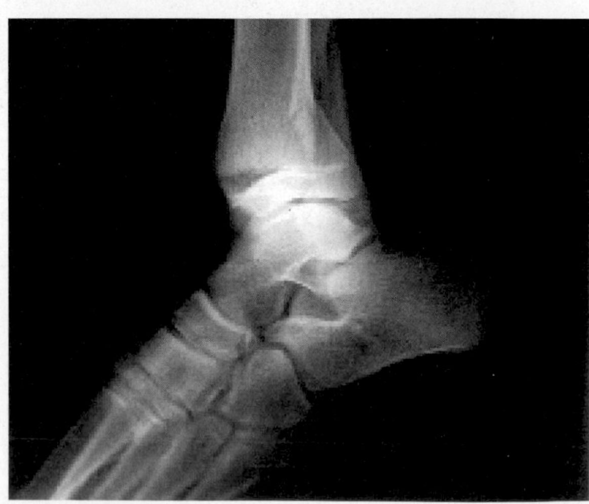

FIGURE 26-17 A,B. Deltoid and possible syndesmosis injury associated with triplane fracture pattern.

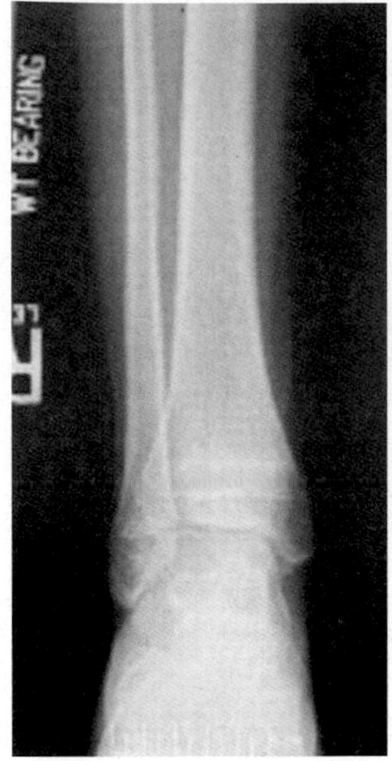

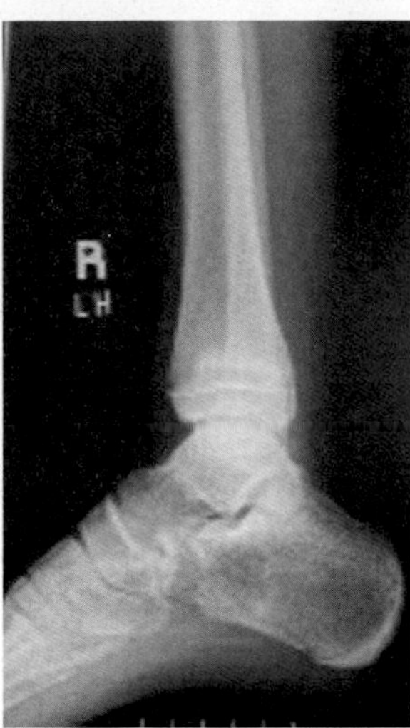

FIGURE 26-18 Distal tibia stress fracture. A 15-year-old male with 6 weeks of pain while running cross country. Anteroposterior radiograph shows callus formation in the distal tibia metaphysis.

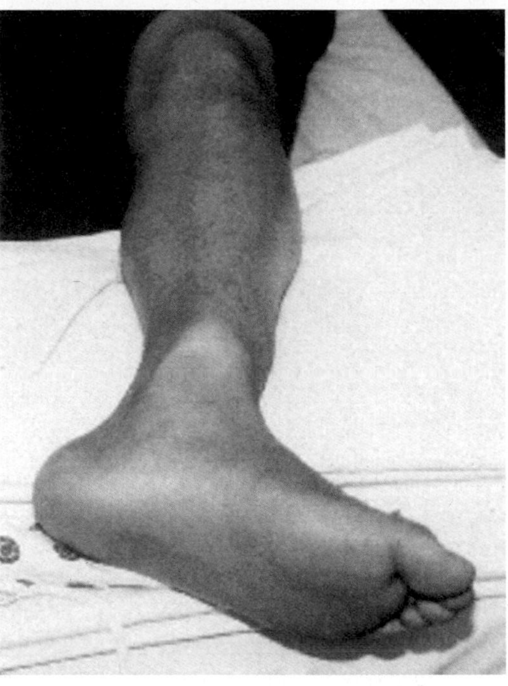

FIGURE 26-20 Severe clinical deformity in a 14-year-old boy with an ankle fracture. It is obvious without radiographs that internal rotation will be needed to reduce this fracture.

lateral portion of the distal tibial physis is usually partially obscured by the distal fibula. The vertical component of a triplane or Tillaux fracture can be hidden behind the overlying fibular cortical shadow.[107] A study by Vangsness and coworkers[186] found that diagnostic accuracy was essentially equal when using anteroposterior, lateral, and mortise views compared with using only mortise and lateral views. Therefore, if only two views are to be obtained, the anteroposterior view may be omitted and lateral and mortise views obtained.

Haraguchi et al.[69] described two special views designed to detect avulsion fractures from the lateral malleolus that are not visible on routine views and to distinguish whether they represent avulsions of the anterior tibiofibular ligament or the calcaneofibular ligament attachments. The anterior tibiofibular ligament view is made by positioning the foot in 45 degrees of plantarflexion and elevating the medial border of the foot 15 degrees. The calcaneofibular ligament view is obtained by rotating the leg 45 degrees inward.

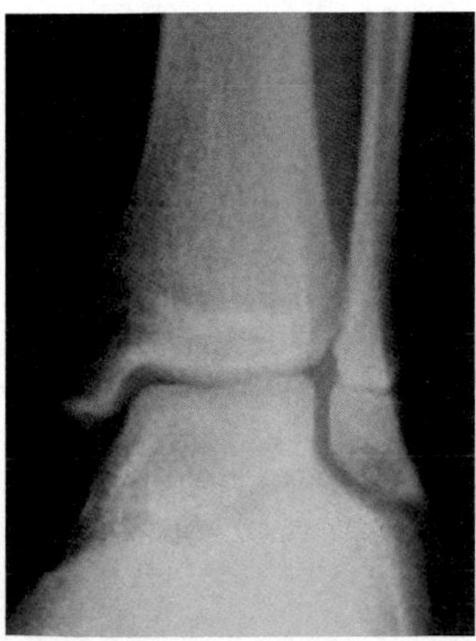

FIGURE 26-19 Stress fracture of distal fibula. A 16-year-old male with 6 weeks of pain while running track. Anteroposterior radiograph shows widened physis. The clinical exam shows point tenderness over the fibular physis.

Stress views may occasionally be needed to rule out ligamentous instability, although ligamentous injury at the ankle is infrequent in skeletally immature patients. Stress views may be considered to document a Salter-Harris type I fracture, but a patient with clinical signs of this fracture should be treated appropriately, regardless of stress-view findings.

Bozic et al.[21] studied the age at which the radiographic appearance of the incisura fibularis, tibiofibular clear space, and tibiofibular overlap develop in children. The purpose of their study was to facilitate the diagnosis of distal tibiofibular syndesmotic injury in children. They found that the incisura became detectable at a mean age of 8.2 for girls and 11.2 years for boys. The mean age at which tibiofibular overlap appeared on the anteroposterior view was 5 years for both sexes; on the mortise view, it was 10 years for girls and 16 years for boys. The range of clear space measurements in normal children was 2 to 8 mm with 23% of children having a clear space greater than 6 mm, a distance considered abnormal in adults.

CT is useful in the evaluation of intra-articular fractures, especially juvenile Tillaux and triplane fractures (Fig. 26-21).[6,25,56,85] In the past, some physicians have used plain tomograms,[192] although many imaging departments no longer provide this modality. CT evaluations involve less radiation to the patient. Cuts are generally made in the transverse plane. With thin cuts localized to the joint, it is possible to generate high-quality reconstructions that allow evaluation in the coronal and sagittal planes without repositioning the ankle. With plain tomography, the transverse anatomy can only be deduced from the anteroposterior and lateral tomograms. Three-dimensional CT reconstructions may add further useful information, and readily available software packages allow easy production of such images (Fig. 26-22). These images can assist with mini-

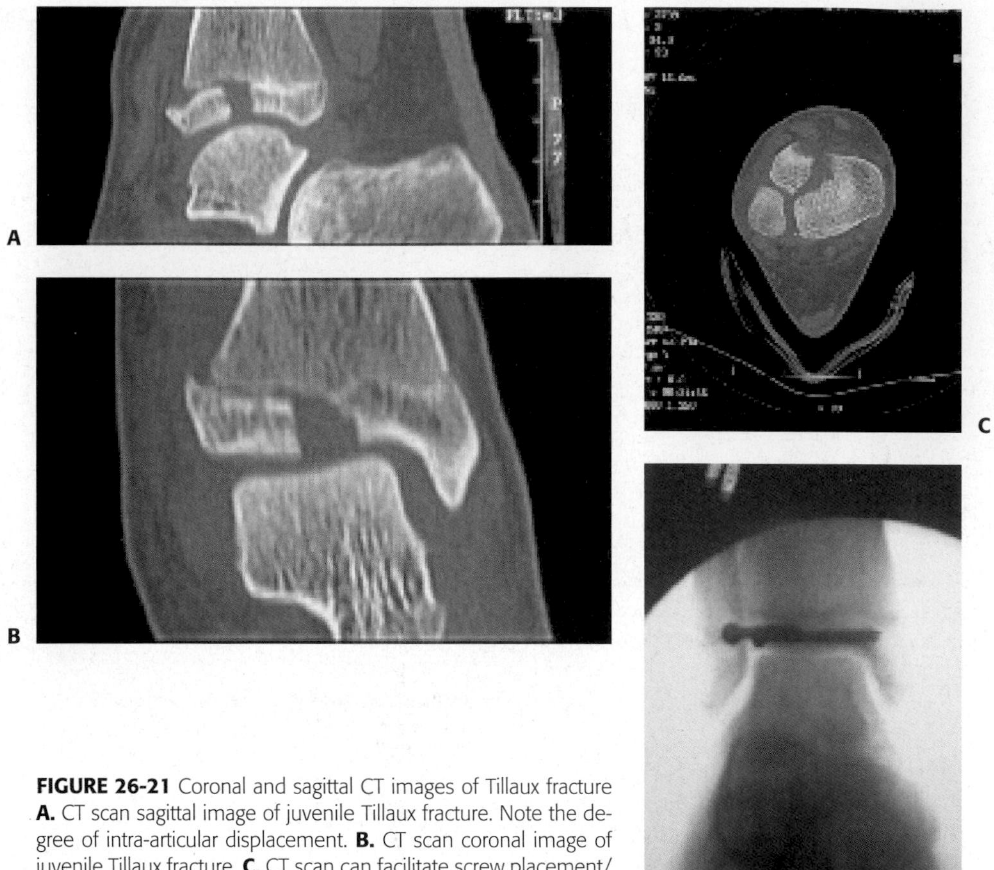

FIGURE 26-21 Coronal and sagittal CT images of Tillaux fracture **A.** CT scan sagittal image of juvenile Tillaux fracture. Note the degree of intra-articular displacement. **B.** CT scan coronal image of juvenile Tillaux fracture. **C.** CT scan can facilitate screw placement/orientation. **D.** Reduction with intraepiphyseal screws.

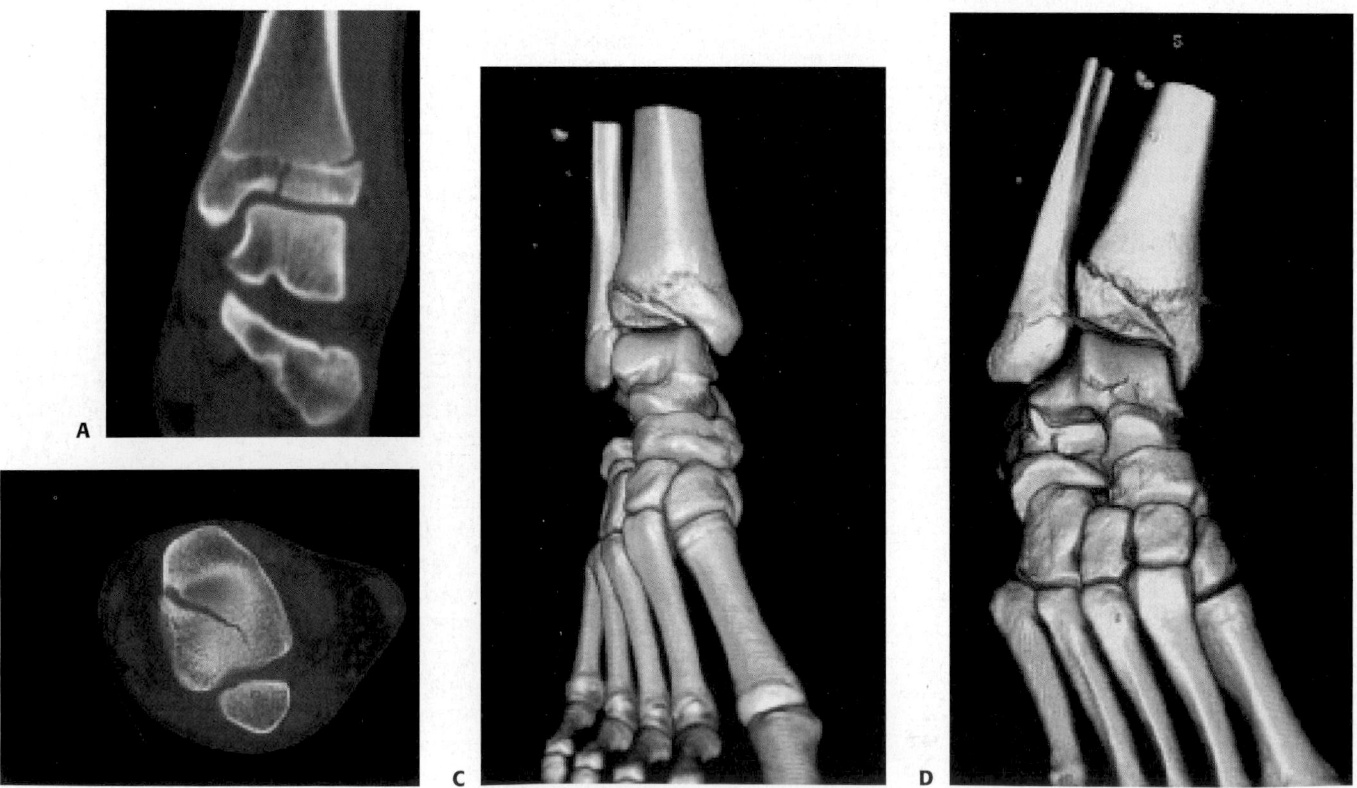

FIGURE 26-22 Three-dimensional CT reconstruction of juvenile Tillaux fracture. **A.** Coronal CT image of minimally displaced juvenile Tillaux fracture. **B.** Sagittal CT Image of minimally displaced juvenile Tillaux fracture. **C,D.** Three-dimensional reconstruction of juvenile Tillaux fracture.

mally invasive approaches and the use of percutaneous reduction clamps and screws.

Magnetic resonance imaging (MRI) may be useful for the evaluation of complex fractures of the distal tibia and ankle in patients with open physes. Smith and associates[174] found that of 4 patients with acute (3 to 10 days) physeal injuries, MRI showed that 3 had more severe fractures than indicated on plain films (Fig. 26-23). Early MRI studies (3 to 17 weeks after injury) not only added information about the pattern of physeal disruption but also supplied early information about the possibility of growth abnormality. MRI has been reported to be occasionally helpful in the identification of osteochondral injuries to the joint surfaces in children with ankle fractures.[95] Although these injuries may be more common in adolescent and adult fractures, we believe that these type of injuries are rare in younger patients.

Carey et al.[30] obtained MRI studies on 14 patients with known or suspected growth plate injury. The MRI detected five radiographically occult fractures in the 14 patients, changed the Salter-Harris classification in two cases, and resulted in a change in treatment plan in 5 of the 14 patients studied. These studies would seem to contradict an earlier study by Petit et al.[144] that showed only 1 patient in a series of 29 patients in whom MRI revealed a diagnosis different from that made on plain films. Iwinski-Zelder et al.[80] found that the MRI changed the management in 4 of 10 patients with ankle fractures seen on plain radiographs. Seifer et al.[168] found that MRI identified physeal injuries that were not identified by plain radiographs. At this time, the indications for MRI in the evaluation of ankle fractures in skeletally immature patients are still being defined, but this imaging modality may be a more sensitive tool for identification of minimally displaced or more complex injuries. If physeal arrest occurs, MRI scans have been reported useful for mapping physeal bars.[60,73]

Pitfalls in Diagnosis

A number of accessory ossification centers and normal anatomic variations may cause confusion in the interpretation of plain films of the ankle (Fig. 26-24). In a group of 100 children between the ages of 6 and 12 years, Powell[149] found accessory ossification centers on the medial side (os subtibiale) in 20% and on the lateral side (os subfibulare) in 1%. If they are asymptomatic on clinical examination, these ossification centers are of little concern, but tenderness localized to them may indicate an injury. Stress views to determine motion of the fragments or bone scanning may occasionally be considered if an injury to an accessory ossification center is suspected.

Clefts in the lateral side of the tibial epiphysis may simulate juvenile Tillaux fractures, and clefts in the medial side may simulate Salter-Harris type III fractures.[94] The presence of these

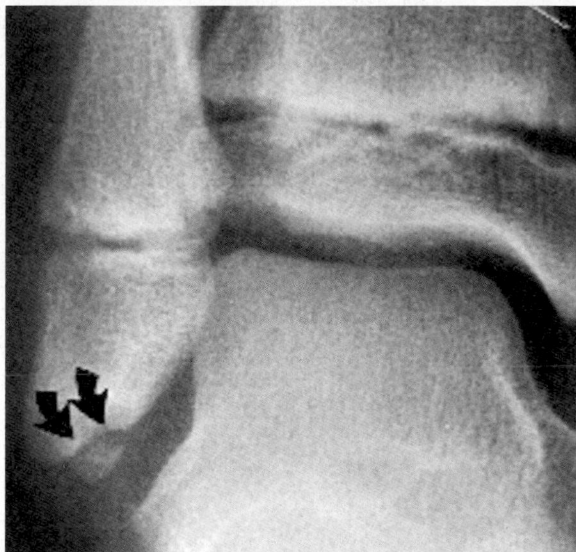

FIGURE 26-24 Secondary ossification center in the lateral malleolus (*arrows*) of a 10-year-old girl. Note the smooth border of the fibula and the ossification center. She also has a secondary ossification center in the medial malleolus.

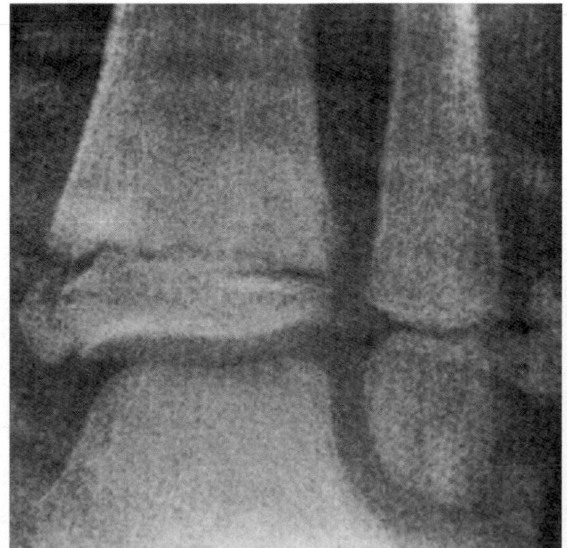

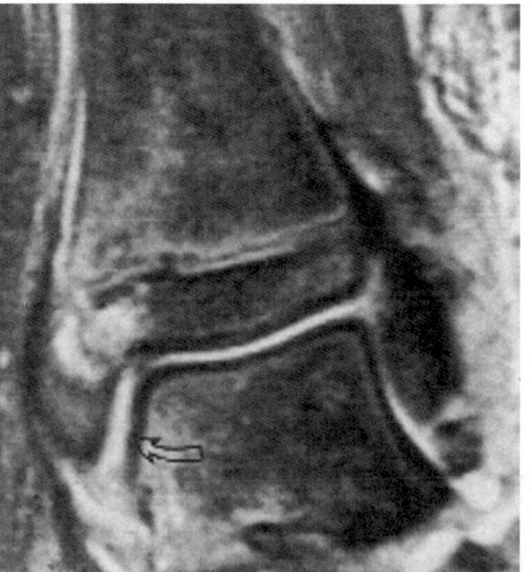

FIGURE 26-23 A. Follow-up radiograph of a 7-year-old boy 1 week after an initially nondisplaced Salter-Harris type III fracture from a supination–inversion injury of the distal tibia. **B.** Because of the incomplete ossification of this area and concern that the fracture might have displaced, MRI was performed. Note that the distance between the medial malleolus and the talus is greater than the distance between the talus and the distal tibia or lateral malleolus, confirming displacement of the fracture.

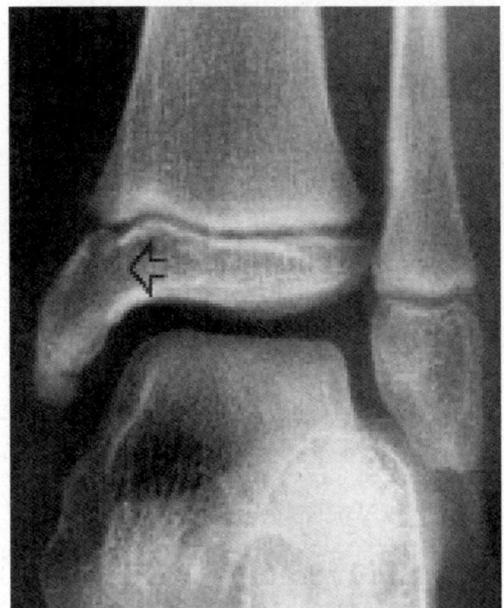
A

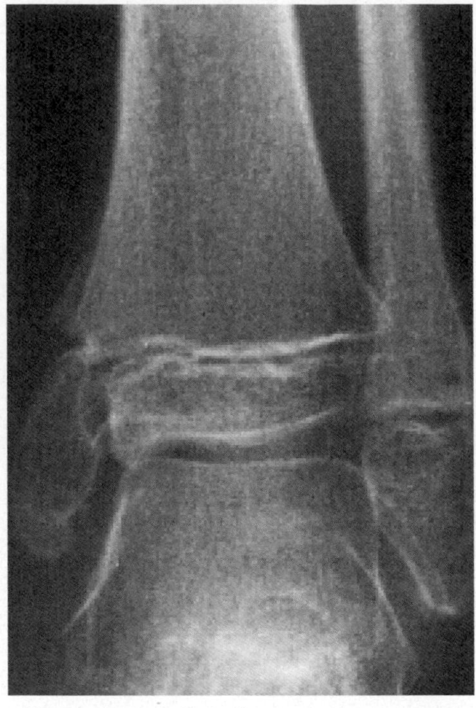
B

FIGURE 26-25 A. Mortise view of the ankle of a 10-year-old girl who had slight swelling and tenderness at the medial malleolus after an "ankle sprain." The ossicle at the tip of the medial malleolus was correctly identified as an os subtibiale. A subtle line extending from the medial physis to just distal to the medial tibial plafond (*arrow*) was believed to also be an anatomic variant. **B.** Four weeks after injury, soreness persisted and radiographs clearly demonstrated a displaced Salter-Harris type III fracture.

clefts on an radiographs of a child with an ankle injury may result in overtreatment if they are misdiagnosed as a fracture. Conversely, attributing a painful irregularity in these areas to anatomic variation may lead to undertreatment (Fig. 26-25). Other anatomic variations include a bump on the distal fibula that simulates a torus fracture and an apparent offset of the distal fibular epiphysis that simulates a fracture.

ANATOMY

The ankle is the joint that most closely approximates a hinge joint. It is the articulation between the talus and the ankle mortise, which is a syndesmosis consisting of the distal tibial articular surface, the medial malleolus, and the distal fibula or lateral malleolus.

Several ligamentous structures bind the distal tibia and fibula into the ankle mortise (Figs. 26-26 to 26-28). The anterior and posterior inferior tibiofibular ligaments course inferiorly from the anterior and posterior surfaces of the distal lateral tibia to the anterior and posterior surfaces of the lateral malleolus. The anterior ligament is important in the pathomechanics of "transitional" ankle fractures. Just anterior to the posteroinferior tibiofibular ligament is the broad, thick inferior transverse ligament, which extends down from the lateral malleolus along the posterior border of the articular surface of the tibia, almost to the medial malleolus. This ligament serves as a part of the articular surface for the talus. Between the anterior and posterior inferior tibiofibular ligaments, the tibia and fibula are bound by the interosseous ligament, which is continuous with the interosseous membrane above. This ligament may be important in the pathomechanics of what we have termed incisural fractures.

On the medial side of the ankle, the talus is bound to the ankle mortise by the deltoid ligament (see Fig. 26-27). This ligament arises from the medial malleolus and divides into superficial and deep layers. Three parts of the superficial layer are identified by their attachments: tibionavicular, calcaneotibial, and posterior talotibial ligaments. The deep layer is known as the anterior talotibial ligament, again reflecting its insertion and origin. On the lateral side, the anterior and posterior talofibular ligament, with the calcaneofibular ligaments, make up the lateral collateral ligament (see Fig. 26-28).

In children, all of the ligamentous structures that bind the medial and lateral malleolae to the talus, and the distal tibial epiphysis to the distal fibular epiphysis are attached to the malleolae distal to the physes. Because the ligaments are stronger than the

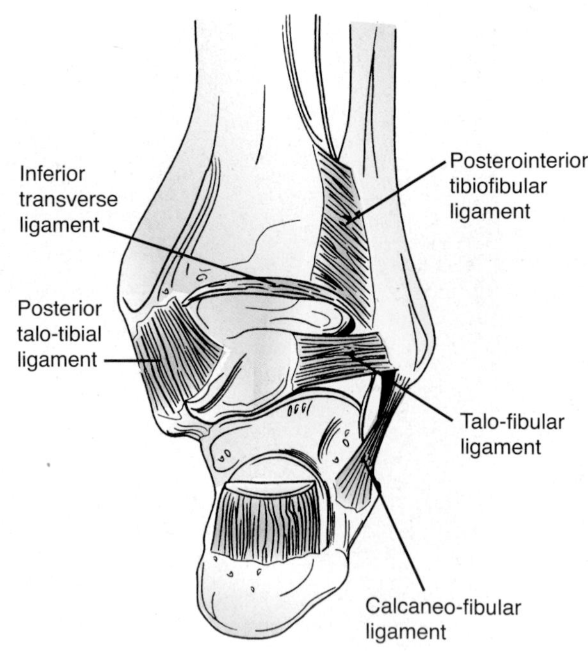

FIGURE 26-26 Posterior view of the distal tibia and fibula and the ligaments making up the ankle mortise.

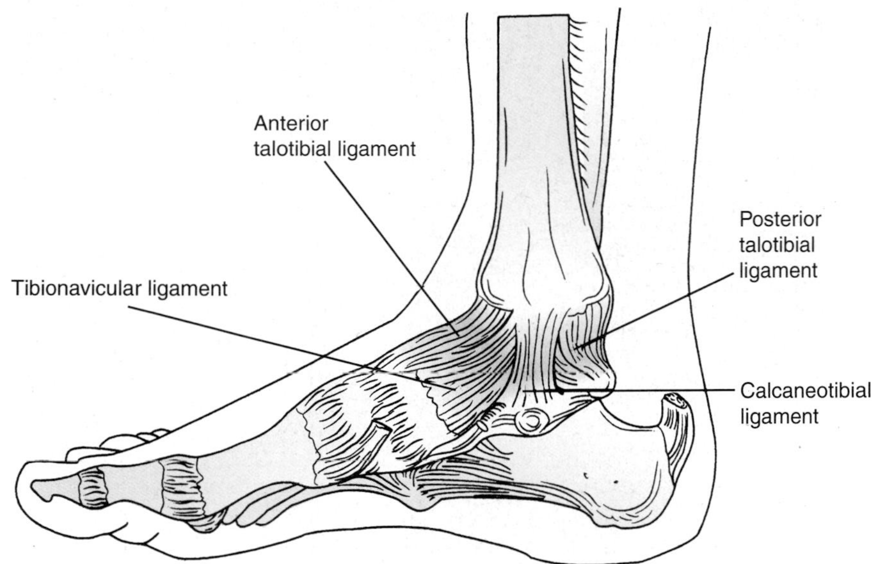

FIGURE 26-27 Medial view of the ankle demonstrating the components of the deltoid ligament.

physes, physeal fractures are more common than ligamentous injuries in children. When they accompany distal tibial physeal injuries, displaced diaphyseal fibular fractures are usually associated with injuries to and displacement of the entire distal tibial epiphysis rather than with injuries to the ligaments, making diastasis of the ankle uncommon in children (Fig. 26-29).

The distal tibial ossification center generally appears at 6 to 24 months of age. Its malleolar extension begins to form around the age of 7 or 8 years and is mature or complete at the age of 10 years. The medial malleolus develops as an elongation of the distal tibia ossific nucleus, although in 20% of cases, this may originate from a separate ossification center, the os tibial. This can be mistaken as a fracture.[92] The physis usually closes around the age of 15 years in girls and 17 years in boys. This process takes approximately 18 months and occurs first in the central part of the physis, extending next to the medial side, and finally ending laterally. This asymmetric closure sequence is an important anatomic feature of the growing ankle and is responsible for the Tillaux fracture in adolescents (Fig. 26-30).

The distal fibular ossification center appears around the age of 9 to 24 months. This physis is located at the level of the ankle joint. Closure of this physis generally follows closure of the distal tibial physis by 12 to 24 months.

The locations of the sensory nerves are important anatomic landmarks, as surgical exposures should aim to protect these structures. The superficial peroneal nerve branches may be most vulnerable around the ankle, especially during arthroscopic and arthrotomy approaches for triplane and Tillaux fractures.[11] This is important when arthroscopic and percutaneous reduction techniques are employed for fracture treatment (refer to section on arthroscopic and percutaneous reduction techniques.)

TREATMENT

Appropriate treatment of ankle fractures in children depends on the location of the fracture, the degree of displacement, and the age of the child (Table 26-2). Nondisplaced fractures may be

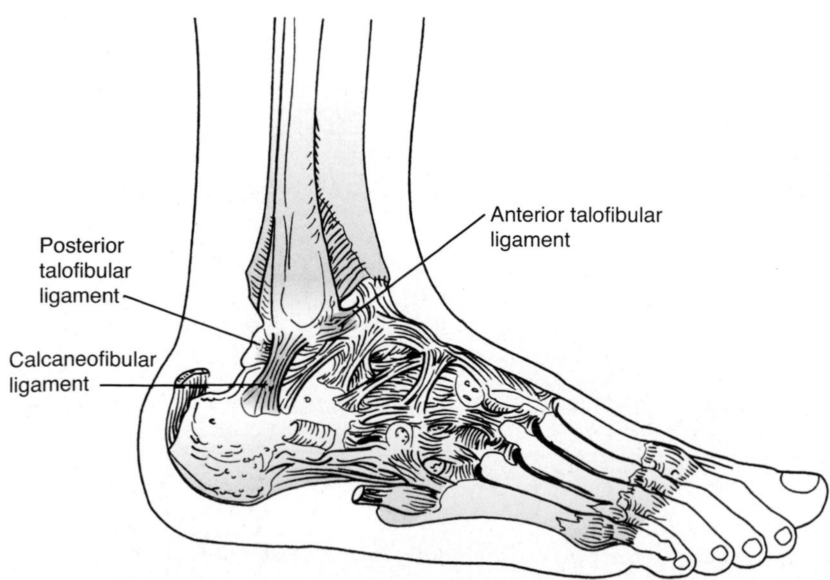

FIGURE 26-28 Lateral view of the ankle demonstrating the anterior and posterior talofibular ligaments and the calcaneofibular ligament.

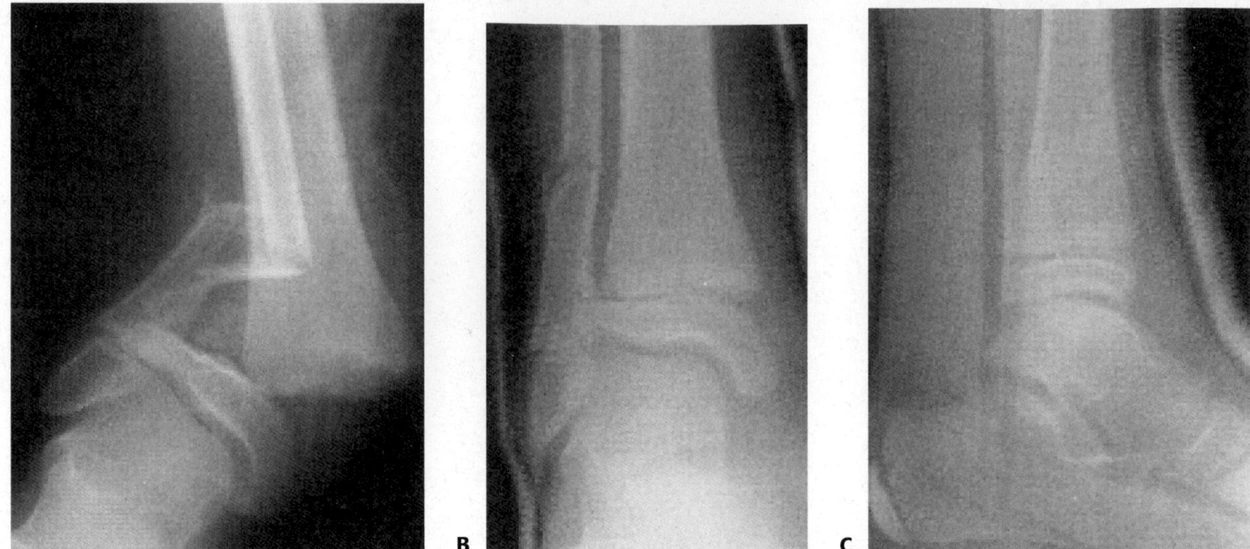

FIGURE 26-29 A. Pronation–external rotation injury resulting in a Salter-Harris type I fracture of the distal tibial physis. Note that despite this severe displacement, the relationship between the distal epiphysis of the tibia and distal fibula is preserved, and a diastasis is not present. **B,C.** Anteroposterior and lateral radiographs demonstrate satisfactory closed reduction.

simply immobilized. Closed reduction and cast immobilization may be appropriate for displaced fractures; if the closed reduction cannot be maintained with casting, skeletal fixation may be necessary. If closed reduction is not possible, open reduction may be indicated, followed by internal fixation or cast immobilization.

The anatomic type of the fracture (usually defined by the Salter-Harris classification), the mechanism of injury, and the amount of displacement of the fragments are important considerations. When the articular surface is disrupted, the amount of articular step-off or separation must be measured. The neurovascular status of the limb or the status of the skin may require emergency treatment of the fracture and associated problems. The general health of the patient and the time since injury must also be considered.

Distal Tibial Fractures

Salter-Harris Type I and II Fractures

According to Dias and Tachdjian,[49,179] Salter-Harris type I fractures of the distal tibia can be caused by any of four mechanisms: supination–inversion, supination–plantarflexion, supination–external rotation, or pronation–eversion–external rotation. Spiegel and associates[175] reported that these fractures accounted for 15.2% of 237 ankle injuries in their series and occurred in children significantly younger (average age, 10.5 years) than those with other Salter-Harris types of fractures.

The mechanism of injury is deduced primarily by the direction of displacement of the distal tibial epiphysis; for example, straight posterior displacement indicates a supination–plantarflexion mechanism. The type of associated fibular fracture is also indicative of the mechanism of injury; for example, a high, oblique, or transverse fibular fracture indicates a pronation–eversion–external injury, while a lower spiral fibular fracture indicates a supination–external rotation injury. Lovell,[112] Broock and Greer,[22] and Nevelos and Colton[130] reported unusual Salter-Harris type I fractures in which the distal tibial epiphysis was externally rotated 90 degrees without fracture of the fibula or displacement of the tibial epiphysis in any direction in the transverse plane.

Cast immobilization is generally sufficient treatment for non-

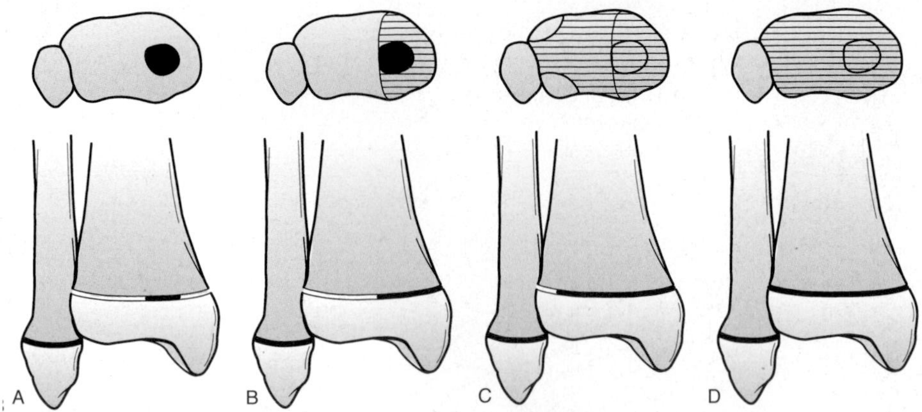

FIGURE 26-30 Closure of the distal tibial physis begins centrally **(A)**, extends medially **(B)** and then laterally **(C)** before final closure **(D)**.

TABLE 26-2 Current Treatment Options

Fracture	Options	Pros	Cons
Distal Tibia Physis	Above-knee versus below-knee cast	Below-knee casts may allow for less knee stiffness and muscle atrophy of the thigh	For fractures with potential for displacement, the below-knee cast may increase the risk of displacement
	Local anesthesia with sedation versus general anesthesia (closed reduction of fractures)	Local anesthesia techniques combined with sedation in the emergency room may be less expensive and allow for early reduction	Guidelines for sedation techniques must follow guidelines established by the American Society of Anesthesiologists, and adequate facilities and personnel may not be available in all emergency rooms
	Minimally invasive approaches (including arthroscopic assistance) versus traditional open surgical exposures	Arthroscopic-assisted procedures may allow for smaller incisions and better assessment of articular reductions than open exposures	Additional equipment and operating room staffing requirements for arthroscopy are necessary. Surgeon experience with arthroscopy may be more limited.
	Bioabsorbable versus metal implants	Bioabsorbable devices do not require removal, and subsequent imaging studies (CT, MRI) are not affected by these implants	First generation implants have a higher risk of local inflammation, and the quality of fixation may be less secure.

displaced Salter-Harris type I fractures of the distal tibia. A below-knee cast worn for 3 to 4 weeks may suffice, with the first 2 to 3 weeks limited to nonweight bearing. An above-knee cast may also be used, although this may not be necessary as these fractures are usually very stable. In very active patients that may not comply with activity/weight-bearing restrictions, this type of cast may be an advantage. After cast removal, use of a removable leg/ankle immobilizer may be used, followed by a therapy program in older patients or those trying to return to competitive sports at an earlier time. In our experience, formal supervised therapy is not usually necessary in younger patients. The normal activity of these children is usually sufficient therapy. For older children and adolescents, a formal supervised therapy program may be beneficial, especially in those trying to return to high-level sports.

Most displaced fractures can be treated with closed reduction and cast immobilization. An above-knee nonweight-bearing cast is preferable initially, as this should reduce the risk of displacement after reduction. These casts may be changed to a short-leg walking cast or removable walking boot at 3 to 4 weeks. These fractures can displace in the first 1 to 2 weeks postoperatively, and close follow-up for this is necessary. One of the authors (Kevin G. Shea) frequently places one or two Kirschner wires at the time of closed reduction, to prevent displacement after reduction, under anesthesia (Fig. 26-31). These pins are usually removed in the clinic 2 to 3 weeks after placement. As the pins are stabilizing the reduction, a below-knee cast can be used.

Salter-Harris Type II Fractures

Salter-Harris type II fractures can also be caused by any of the four mechanisms of injury described by Dias and Tachdjian.[48] In the series of Spiegel and associates,[175] Salter-Harris type II fractures were the most common injuries (44.8%). In addition to the direction of displacement of the distal tibial epiphysis and the nature of any associated fibular fracture, the location of the Thurstan-Holland fragment is helpful in determining the mechanism of injury; for example, a lateral fragment indicates a pronation–eversion–external rotation injury; a posteromedial

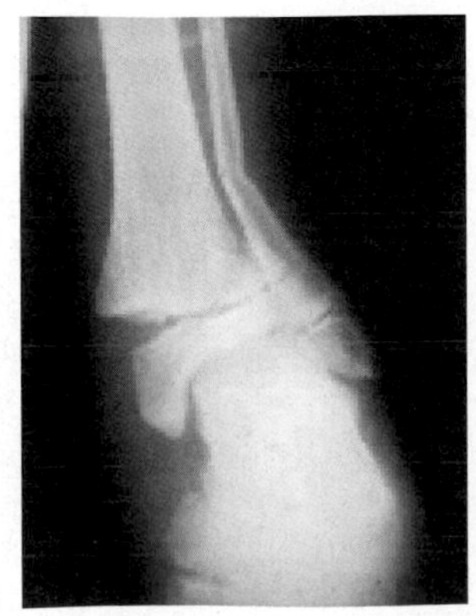
A

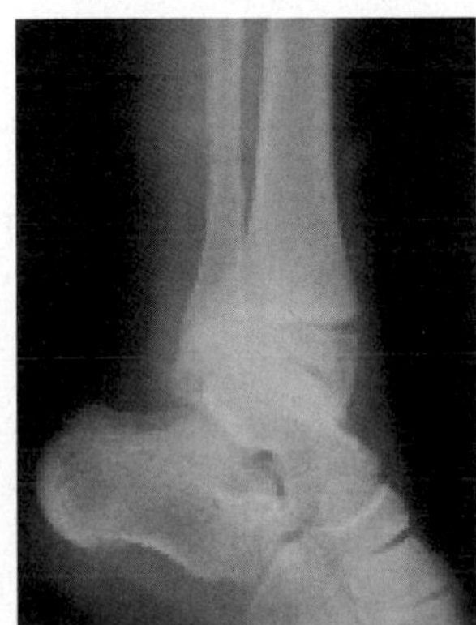
B

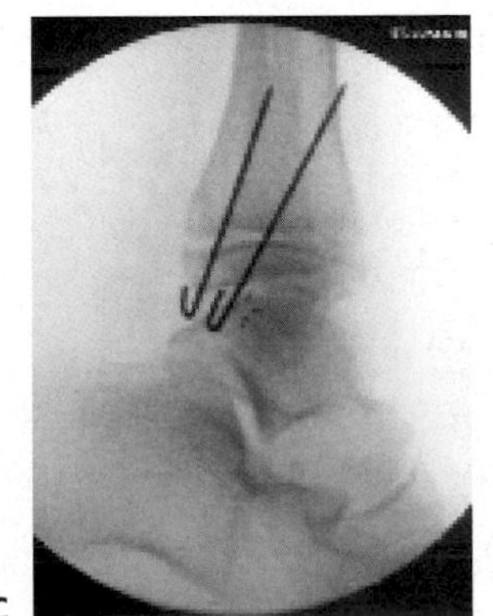
C

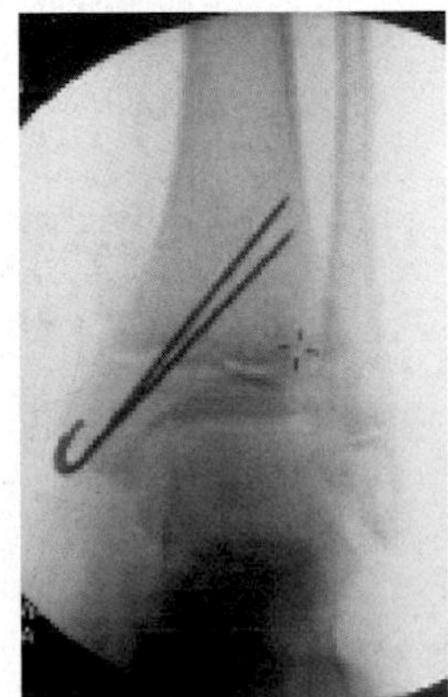
D

FIGURE 26-31 A,B. Displaced distal tibial Salter-Harris type II fracture, with distal diaphyseal fibula fracture. **C,D.** Fracture treated with closed reduction and internal fixation.

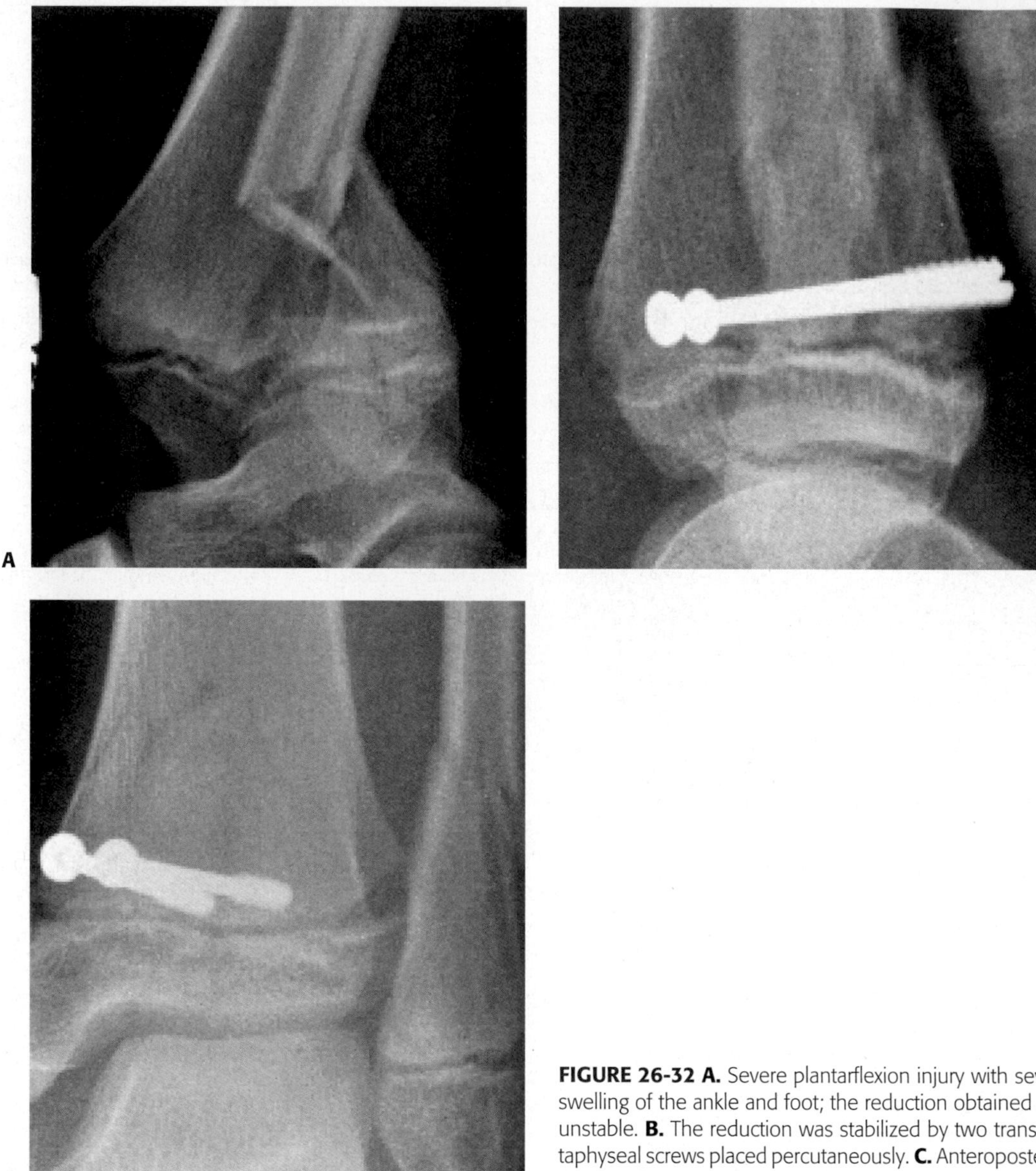

FIGURE 26-32 A. Severe plantarflexion injury with severe swelling of the ankle and foot; the reduction obtained was unstable. **B.** The reduction was stabilized by two transmetaphyseal screws placed percutaneously. **C.** Anteroposterior view confirms an anatomic reduction.

fragment, a supination-external rotation injury; and a posterior fragment, a supination–plantarflexion injury (Fig. 26-32).

Nondisplaced fractures can be treated with cast immobilization usually with an above-knee cast for approximately 3 weeks, followed by a below-knee walking cast or removable cast/walking boot for another 2 to 3 weeks.

Although most authors agree that closed reduction of a significantly displaced Salter-Harris type II ankle fracture should be attempted, opinions differ as to what degree of residual displacement or angulation is unacceptable and requires open reduction. Based on follow-up of 33 Salter-Harris type II ankle fractures, Caruthers and Crenshaw[31] concluded that "accurate reposition of the displaced epiphysis at the expense of forced or repeated manipulation or operative intervention is not indicated since spontaneous realignment of the ankle occurs even late in the growing period." They found no residual angulation at follow-up in patients who had up to 12 degrees of tilt after reduction, even in patients as old as 13 years of age at the time of injury. Spiegel and associates,[175] however, reported complications at follow-up in 11 of 16 patients with Salter-Harris type II ankle fractures. Because 6 of these 11 patients had angular deformities that were attributed to lack of adequate reduction of the fracture, Spiegel and associates recommend "precise anatomic reduction."

Barmada et al.[6] reviewed a series of Salter-Harris type I and II fractures. In patients with more than 3 mm of physeal widening, the risk of physeal arrest was 60%, compared with 17% in patients with less than 3 mm of physeal widening. Although they were unable demonstrate a significant decrease in partial physeal arrest in those treated with surgery, they recommended open reduction and removal of the entrapped periosteal flap.

Incomplete reduction is usually caused by interposition of soft tissue between the fracture fragments. Grace[65] reported 3 patients in whom the interposed soft tissue included the neurovascular bundle, resulting in circulatory embarrassment when closed reduction was attempted. In this situation, open reduction and extraction of the soft tissue obviously is required. A less definitive indication for open reduction is interposition of

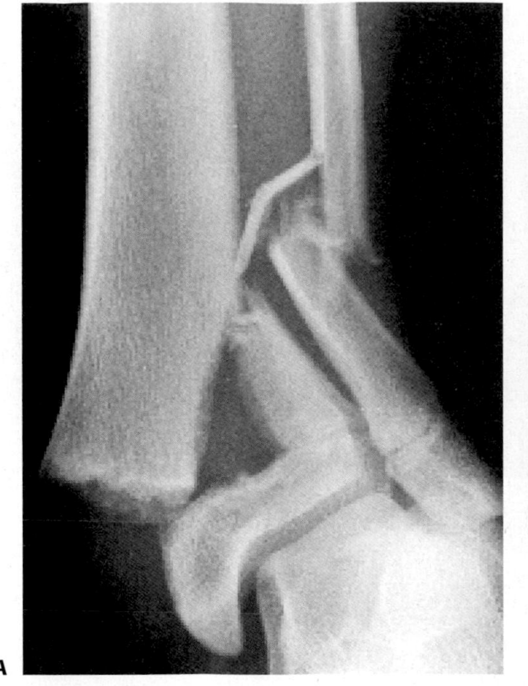

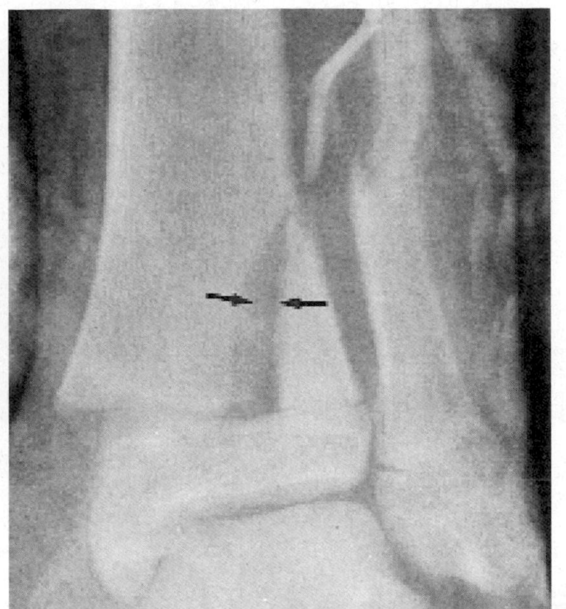

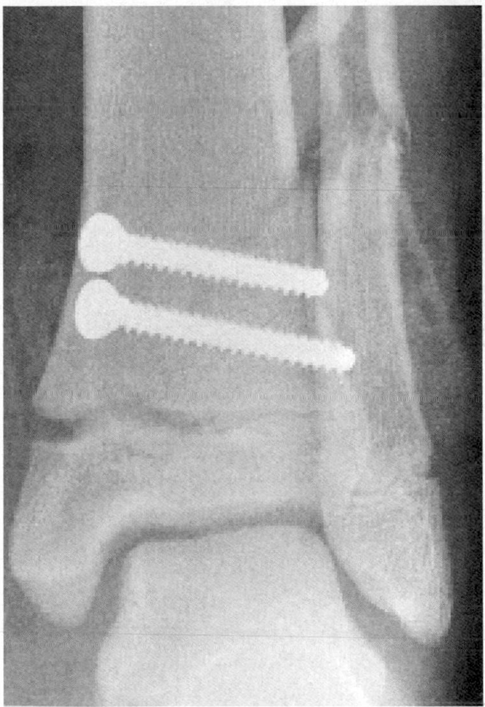

FIGURE 26-33 A. Severely displaced pronation–eversion–external rotation injury. **B.** Closed reduction was unsuccessful, and a valgus tilt of the ankle mortise was noted. At surgery, soft tissue was interposed laterally (*arrows*). **C.** Reduction completed and stabilized with two cancellous screws placed above the physis.

the periosteum, which causes physeal widening with no angulation or with minimal angulation. Good results have been reported after open reduction and extraction of the periosteal flap (Fig. 26-33).[99] It is not clear that failure to extract the periosteum in such cases results in problems sufficient to warrant operative treatment. Wattenbarger,[189] Pfieffer,[146] and others have attempted to determine the relationship between physeal bar formation and interposed periosteum, although at this time it is unclear if the periosteal flap increases the risk of physeal arrest.

Because of fears of iatrogenic damage to the distal tibial physis during closed reduction, many authors recommend the use of general anesthesia with adequate muscle relaxation for all patients with Salter-Harris type II distal tibial fractures. However, no study has compared the frequency of growth abnormalities in patients with these fractures reduced under sedation and local analgesia to those with fractures reduced with the use of general anesthesia. One of the authors (R. Jay Cummings) compared 9 patients who underwent closed reduction in the emergency department with the use of sedation and hematoma block to 9 patients who had closed reduction in the operating room with the use of general anesthesia. All fractures were reduced with a single manipulation, except for one in the emergency department group that required repeat manipulation. One patient in each group had a growth alteration. One of the authors uses general anesthesia, and an arthroscopic ankle

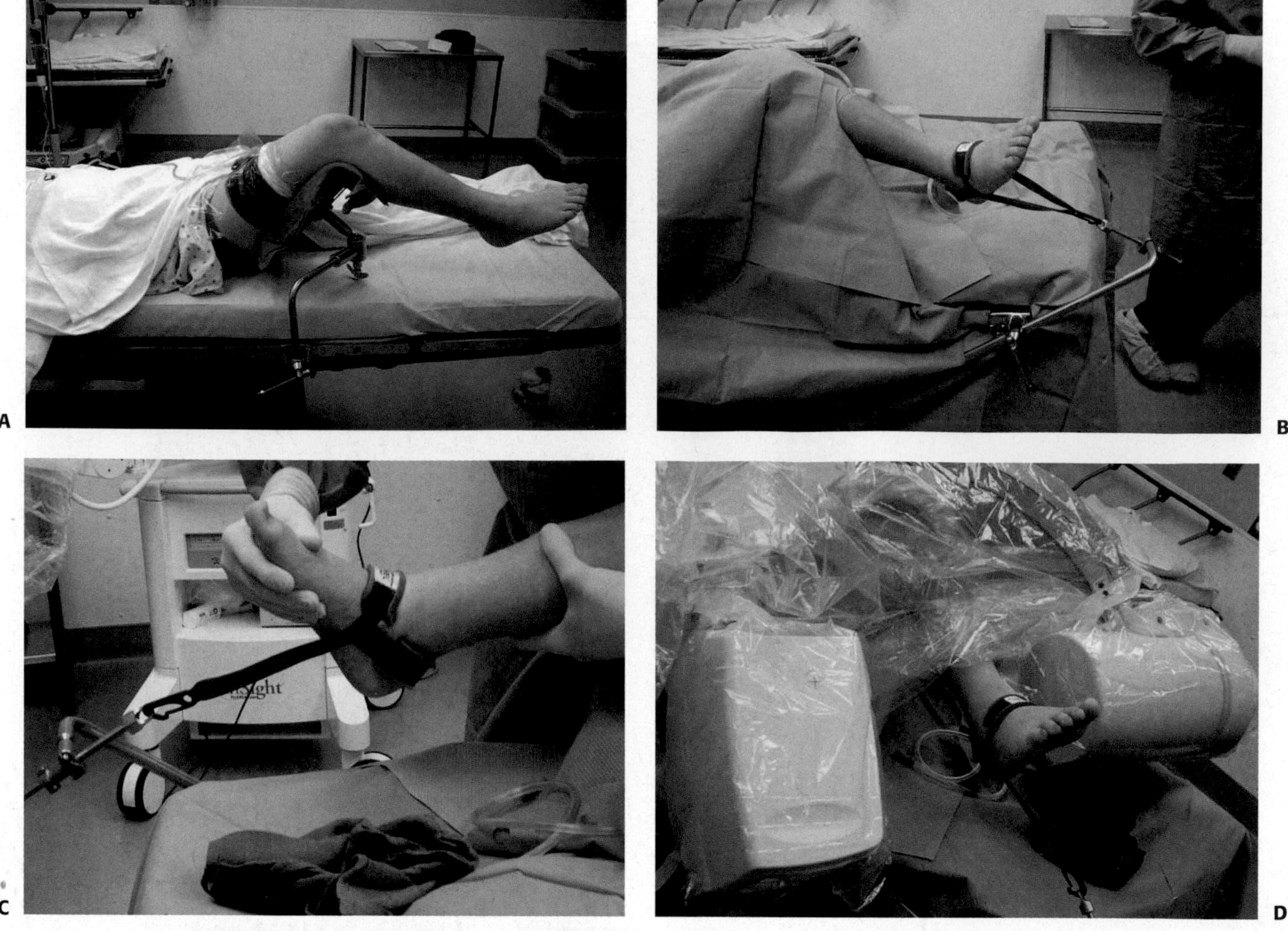

FIGURE 26-34 Use of ankle distractor **A.** Thigh positioner to allow for ankle distractor. **B.** Sterile ankle distractor in place. **C.** Distractor can remain in place during reduction maneuvers. **D.** C-arm can be brought into the field to evaluate the reduction.

distractor to distract the fracture before reduction, with the theoretical advantage of reducing the risk of physeal damage during the reduction maneuver (Fig. 26-34).

When closed reductions are not performed under general anesthesia, they are usually done under intravenous (IV) sedation. Furia et al.[41] demonstrated significantly improved pain relief with hematoma block for ankle fractures in a study comparing patients treated with IV sedation to patients receiving hematoma block. IV regional anesthesia or Bier block has also been reported to be effective for pain relief in lower extremity injuries.[102]

One advantage of reduction in the operating room with general anesthesia is the ease with which percutaneous pins can be placed to maintain reduction of the fractures. It is the experience of one of the authors that Salter-Harris type I and II fractures will occasionally displace after closed reduction and above-knee casting. If there is any concern about redisplacement or stability, pins can be placed at that time.

The use of regional block anesthesia within the first 2 to 3 days after the fracture should lead one to consider the potential for compartment syndrome. In fractures that have a higher risk of compartment syndrome, regional anesthesia, especially peripheral nerve blocks with longer acting agents, might delay the recognition of a compartment syndrome.

Salter-Harris Type III and IV Fractures

Salter-Harris type III and IV fracture are discussed together because their mechanism of injury is the same (supination–inversion) and their treatment and prognosis are similar. Juvenile Tillaux and triplane fractures are considered separately. In the series of Spiegel and associates,[175] 24.1% of the fractures were Salter-Harris type III injuries and 1.4% were type IV. These injuries are usually produced by the medial corner of the talus being driven into the junction of the distal tibial articular surface and the medial malleolus. As the talus shears off the medial malleolus, the physis may also be damaged (Fig. 26-35).

Nondisplaced Salter-Harris types III and IV fractures can be treated with above-knee cast immobilization, but care must be taken to be sure the significant intra-articular displacement is not present. Radiographs frequently underestimate the degree of intra-articular involvement and step-off of the articular surfaces. CT scans may be necessary to fully appreciate the degree of displacement (see Fig. 26-11). Follow-up radiographs and/or CT scans in the first 2 weeks may also be necessary to confirm that no displacement occurs after casting.

Salter-Harris type III fractures of the medial malleolus have a significant risk of physeal arrest. One study suggested that the rate of physeal arrest could be reduced by the use of open reduction and internal fixation.[92,100]

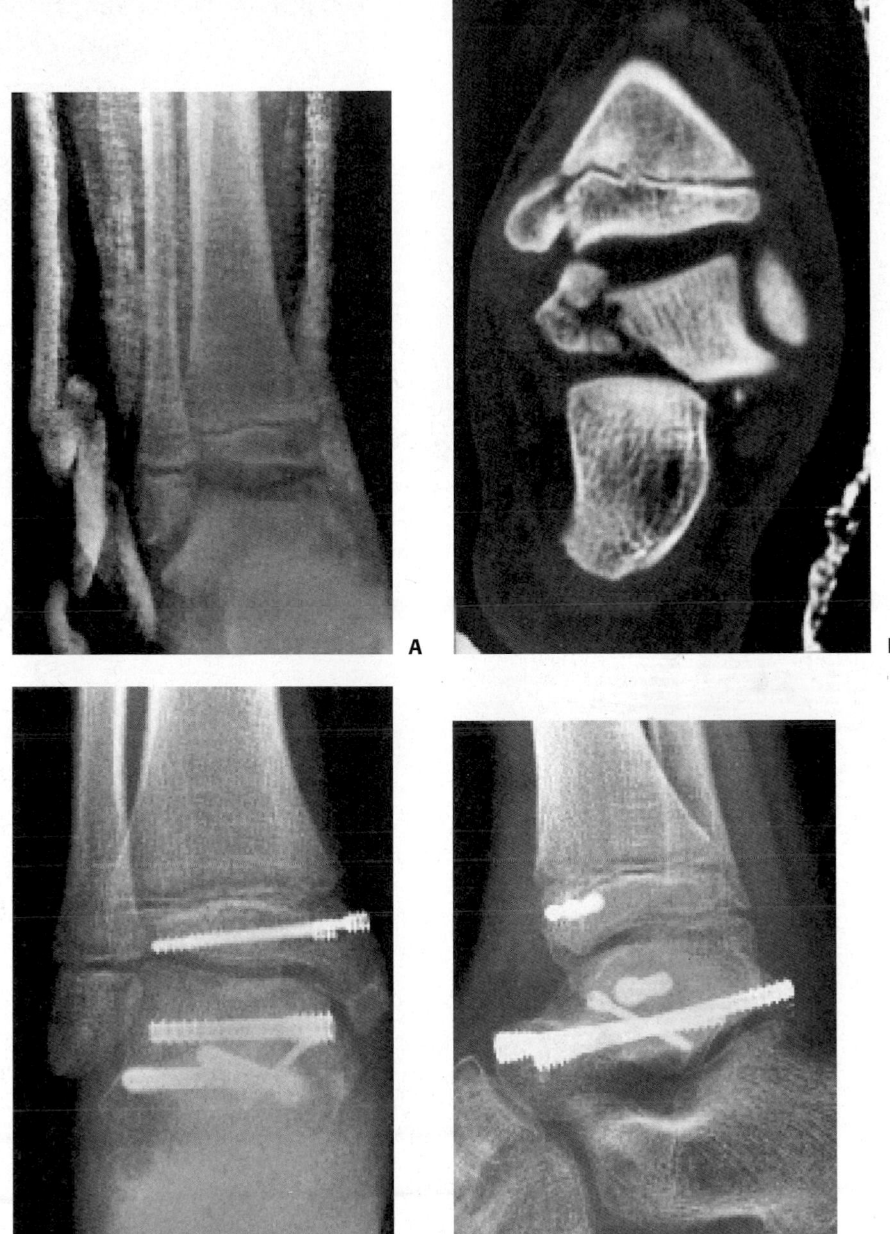

FIGURE 26-35 A. Severe ankle injury sustained by an 8-year-old involved in a car accident. The anteroposterior view in the splint does not clearly show the Salter-Harris type IV fracture of the tibia. The dome of the talus appears abnormal. **B.** CT scan shows the displaced Salter-Harris type IV fracture of the medial malleolus and a severe displaced intra-articular fracture of the body of the talus. **C,D.** Open reduction of both fractures was performed, and Herbert screws were used for internal fixation. (Courtesy of Armen Kelikian, MD.)

Based upon principles of fracture treatment in adults, displaced intra-articular fractures require as anatomic a reduction as possible. Studies in children confirming the importance of articular reduction to within 2 mm are lacking,[166] although most recommend articular reduction in displaced fractures involving the articular surface. Failure to obtain anatomic reduction may result in articular incongruity and posttraumatic arthritis, which often becomes symptomatic 5 to 8 years after skeletal maturity.[34] The risk of growth arrest has also been linked to the adequacy of reduction, although the literature is still unclear if anatomic reduction reduces the risk of physeal arrest (Fig. 26-36).[100] Closed reduction may be attempted but is likely to succeed only in minimally displaced fractures. If closed reduction is obtained, it can be maintained with a cast or with percutaneous pins or screws supplemented by a cast.

If anatomic reduction cannot be obtained by closed methods, open reduction and internal fixation or mini-open arthroscopic reduction should be carried out. Lintecum and Blasier[108] described a technique of open reduction achieved through a limited exposure of the fracture with the incision centered over the fracture site combined with percutaneous cannulated screw fixation. This technique was performed on 13 patients: eight Salter-Harris IV fractures, four Salter-Harris III fractures, and one triplane fracture. The authors reported one growth arrest at follow-up averaging 12 months. Beaty and Linton[8] reported a Salter-Harris type III fracture with an intra-articular fragment (Fig. 26-37); these fractures require open reduction for inspection of the joint to ensure that no osteochondral fragments are impeding reduction. Arthroscopic evaluation of the joint may also be an option. Internal fixation devices should be inserted

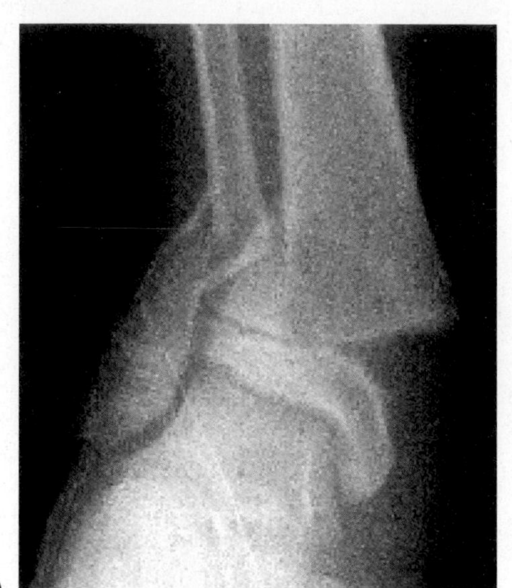

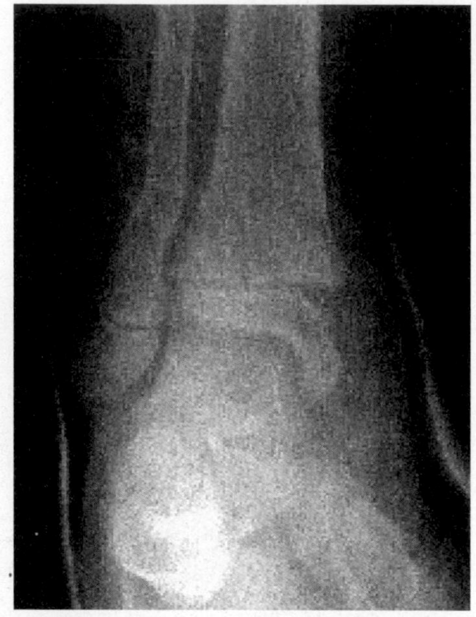

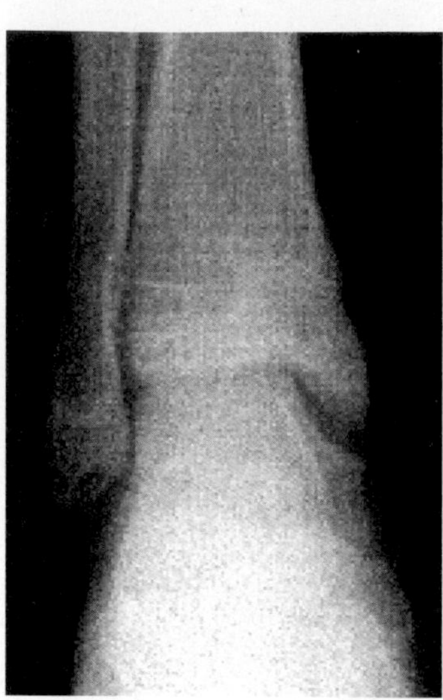

FIGURE 26-36 A. Anteroposterior view of a patient with a pronation–eversion external rotation fracture. **B.** Postreduction view shows residual gapping of physis suggesting periosteal interposition. **C.** Anteroposterior view obtained for a new injury (medial malleolar fracture) shows premature closure of the physis.

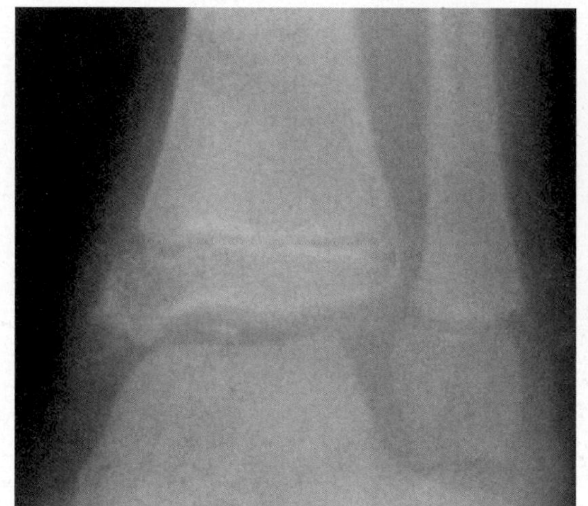

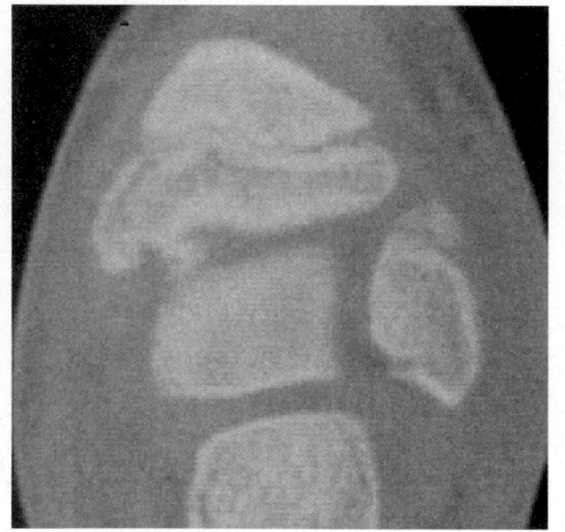

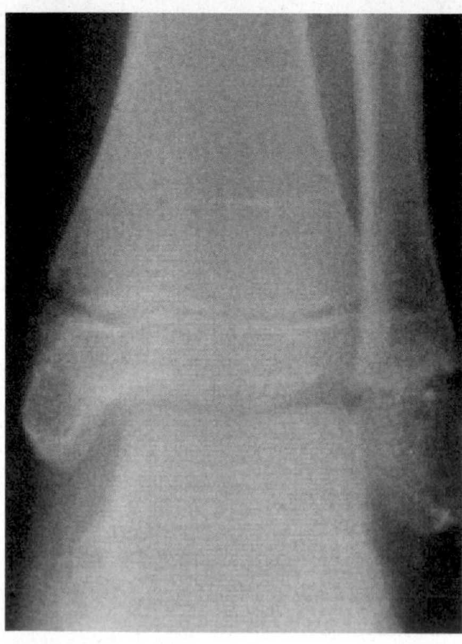

FIGURE 26-37 A. Salter-Harris type III fracture of the medial malleolus and Salter-Harris type I fracture of the fibula in a 9-year-old girl. An intra-articular fragment was visible only on a mortise view radiograph. **B.** CT scan outlined the Salter-Harris type III fracture of the medial malleolus and the fragment of bone. **C.** Two years after excision of the osteochondral fragment, open reduction of the malleolar fracture, and internal fixation. (A,B, reprinted from Beaty JH, Linton RC. Medial malleolar fracture in a child: a case report. J Bone Joint Surg Am 1988;70:1254–1255, with permission.)

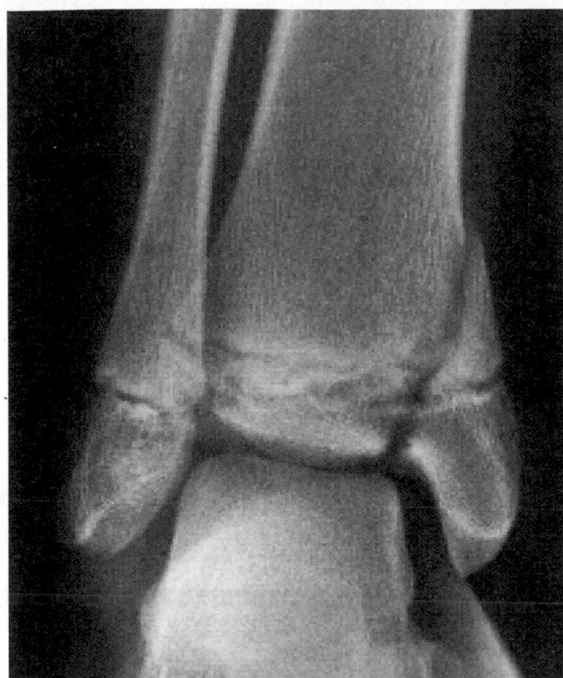

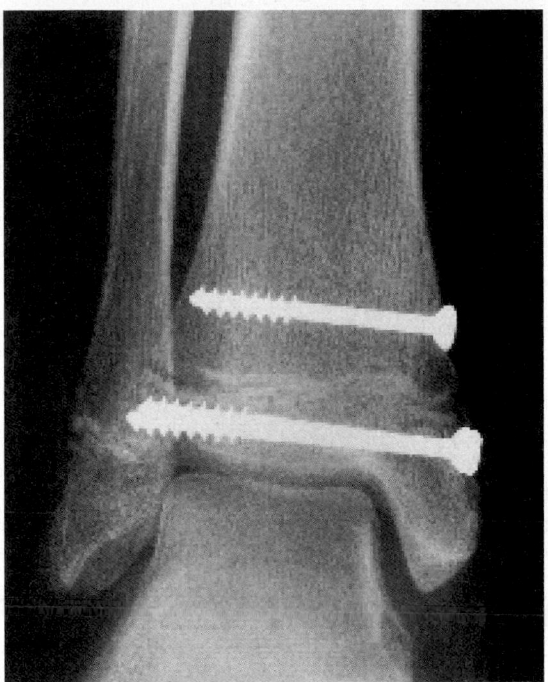

FIGURE 26-38 A. Grade II supination–inversion injury in a 12-year-old girl, resulting in a displaced Salter-Harris type IV fracture of the distal tibia and a nondisplaced Salter-Harris type I fracture of the distal fibula. **B.** After anatomic open reduction and stable internal fixation.

within the epiphysis, parallel to the physis, and should avoid the physis and ankle joint if possible (Fig. 26-38).

Arthroscopic assisted fixation of fractures with intra-articular involvement has been described by several centers. Jennings et al.[82] presented a series of five triplane and one Tillaux fractures treated with arthroscopic assistance. The outcome was excellent for fracture reduction and ankle function.[82] Kaya et al.[93] reviewed 10 patients with juvenile Tillaux fractures treated with arthroscopic assistance, demonstrating excellent reduction and clinical outcomes.[137] One of the primary advantages of arthroscopic fixation is that it allows for visualization of the articular surfaces, although the need for open reduction of the metaphyseal and epiphyseal regions may still require open incisions.

Options for internal fixation include smooth Kirschner-wires, small fragment cortical and cancellous screws, and 4-mm cannulated screws (Fig. 26-39). Several reports[9,18,26] have advocated the use of absorbable pins for internal fixation of ankle fractures. Benz and colleagues[9] reported no complications or growth abnormalities after the use of absorbable pins with metal screw supplementation for fixation of five ankle fractures in patients between the ages of 5 and 13 years. In reports of the use of absorbable pins without supplemental metal fixation in adults,[15,16,59,76] complications have included displacement (14.5%), sterile fluid accumulation requiring incision and drainage (8.1%), pseudarthrosis (8%), distal tibiofibular synostosis (3.8%), and infection (1.6%). Bucholz and coworkers[17] reported few complications in a series of fractures in adults fixed with absorbable screws made of polylactide and suggested that complications in earlier series might be related to the fact that those pins were made of polyglycolide. A report in 1993 by Bostman and associates,[18] however, included few complications in a series of fractures in children fixed with polyglycolide pins. A follow-up report by Rokkanen et al.[158] in 1996 reported 3.6% infection and 3.7% failure of fixation.

The main advantage of absorbable pins and screws is that hardware removal is avoided. Bostman[17] compared the cost effectiveness of absorbable implants in 994 patients treated with absorbable implants to 1173 patients treated with metallic implants. To be cost effective, the hardware removal rates required were calculated to range from 19% for metacarpal fractures to 54% for trimalleolar fractures.[17] At this time, the use of absorbable pins remains investigational.

Recent studies in the adult literature suggest second generation bioabsorbable screws have lower complication rates, and their use may be increasing.[150,173] Additional studies in adult patients using ultrasound and MRI have not detected deleterious effects on healing with newer screw designs.[68,118] Because children are typically smaller and lighter than adults, the implants used for fixation may not need to be as strong or large as those required by adult patients. This suggests that younger patients may be better candidates for these bioabsorbable implants. The presence of the physis and the low grade inflammation that may accompany the dissolution of these implants may increase the risk of physeal arrest, and additional studies in adult and pediatric patients will be necessary to confirm the effectiveness and safety of these devices.[91]

Salter-Harris Type V Fractures

Salter-Harris type V fractures of the ankle are believed to be caused by severe axial compression and crushing of the physis (Fig. 26-40). As originally described, these injuries are not associated with displacement of the epiphysis relative to the metaphysis, which make diagnosis of acute injury impossible from plain radiographs; the diagnosis can only be made on follow-up radiographs when premature physeal closure is evident. Spiegel and associates[175] have designated comminuted fractures that are otherwise unclassifiable as Salter-Harris type V injuries.

The incidence of Salter-Harris type V ankle fractures is diffi-

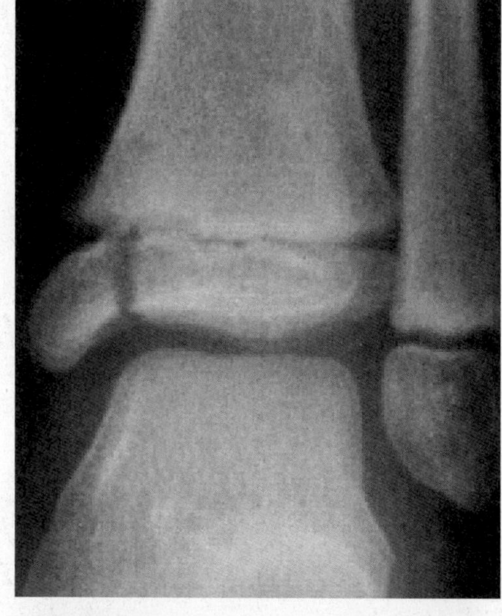

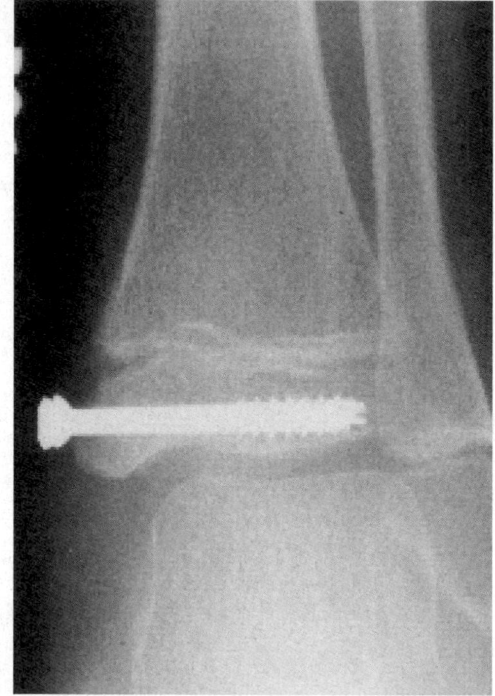

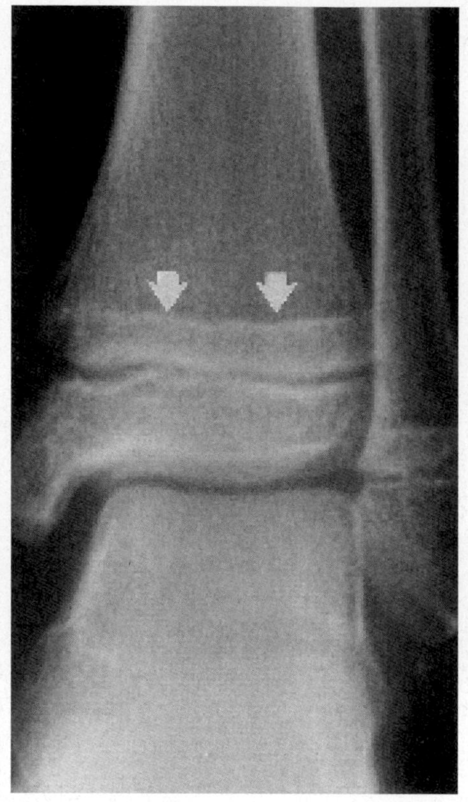

FIGURE 26-39 A. Supination–inversion injury with a Salter-Harris type III fracture of the medial malleolus. **B.** Six months after open reduction and internal fixation with two transepiphyseal cannulated screws. **C.** Eighteen months after injury, the fracture has healed with no evidence of growth arrest or angular deformity. (*Arrows* note normal, symmetric Park-Harris growth arrest line.)

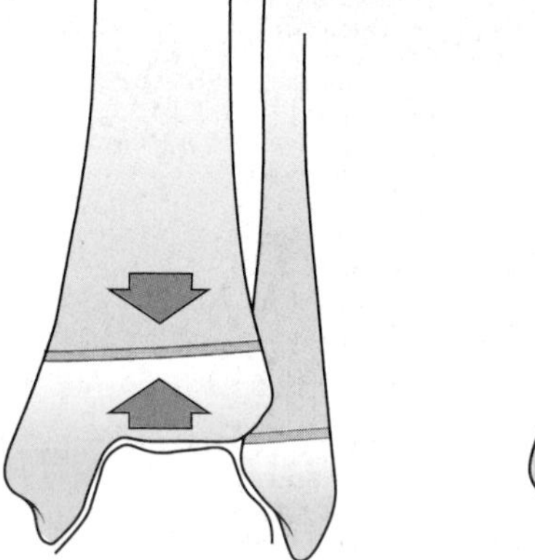

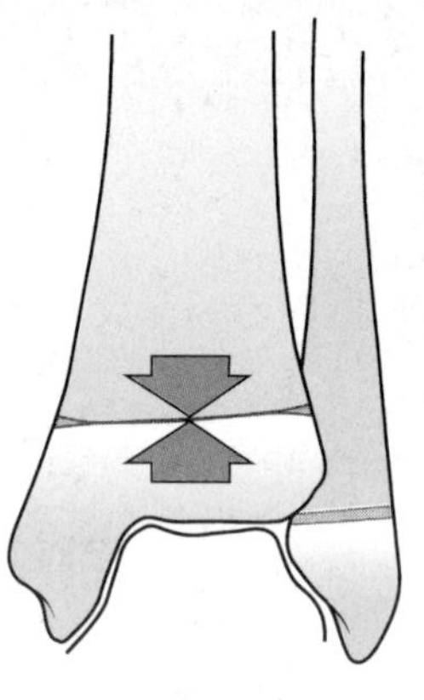

FIGURE 26-40 Compression-type injury of the tibial physis. Early physeal arrest can cause leg-length discrepancy.

cult to establish because of the difficulty of diagnosing acute injuries. Spiegel and associates[175] included two type V fractures in their series, but both were comminuted fractures rather than the classic crush injury.

Because of the uncertain nature of this injury, no specific treatment recommendations have been formulated. Treatment is usually directed primarily toward the sequelae of growth arrest that invariably follows Salter-Harris type V fractures. Perhaps more sophisticated scanning techniques will eventually allow identification and localization of areas of physeal injury so that irreparable damaged cells can be removed and replaced with interposition materials to prevent growth problems, but at present this diagnosis is made only several months after injury.

Other Fractures of the Distal Tibia

Accessory ossification centers of the distal tibia (os subtibiale) and distal fibula (os fibulare) are common and may be injured.

Treatment usually consists of cast immobilization for 3 to 4 weeks. Ogden and Lee[135] reported good results after cast immobilization in 26 of 27 patients with injuries involving the medial side of the tibia; only 1 patient required surgery. In contrast, 5 to 11 patients with injuries involving the lateral side had persistent symptoms that required excision. Bone scan may be used to help identify these injuries and to help to distinguish between normal accessory growth centers versus symptomatic accessory growth centers after injury. Ogden and Lee[135] recommend surgical excision in cases that do not respond to cast immobilization and remain chronically symptomatic.

Injuries to the perichondral ring of the distal tibial and fibular physes, with physeal disruption, have been described. Most of these injuries are caused by skiving of the bone by machinery such as lawn mowers. They may result in growth arrest or retardation and in angular deformities (see open fractures and lawn mower injuries.)

Juvenile Tillaux Fractures

This fracture is the adolescent counterpart of the fracture described in adults by the French surgeon Tillaux. It occurs when with external rotation of the foot, the anterior-inferior tibiofibular ligament through its attachments to the anterolateral tibia avulses a fragment of bone corresponding to the portion of the distal tibial physis that is still open (Fig. 26-41). In the series of Spiegel and associates,[175] these fractures occurred in 2.9% of patients.

Tillaux fractures may be isolated injuries or may be associated with ipsilateral tibial shaft fractures.[41] The fibula usually prevents marked displacement of the fracture and clinical deformity is generally absent. Swelling is usually slight, and local tenderness is at the anterior lateral joint line, in contrast to ankle sprains where the tenderness tends to be below the level of the ankle joint.

Mortise and anteroposterior views will usually identify these fractures (Fig. 26-42). Steinlauf et al.[176] reported a patient in whom the Tillaux fragment became entrapped between the distal tibia and fibula producing apparent diastasis of the ankle joint. To allow measurement of displacement from plain films, the radiograph beam would have to be directly in line with the fracture site, which makes CT confirmation of reduction mandatory after all closed reductions of these fractures.

Both below-knee and above-knee casts have been used for immobilization of nondisplaced juvenile Tillaux and triplane fractures. Fractures with more than 2 mm of displacement, associated with articular incongruity, may benefit from closed or open reduction.[93] Closed reduction is attempted by internally rotating the foot and applying direct pressure over the anterolateral tibia. A percutaneous pin or screw can be used for stabilization of the reduction. If closed reduction is not successful, open reduction or percutaneous reduction with arthroscopic assistance may be required. Occasionally, a percutaneously inserted pin can be used to manipulate the displaced fragment into anatomic position and then advanced to fix the fragment in place.[165] Screw fixation within the epiphysis is usually adequate (see Fig. 26-21 and section on arthroscopic treatment of intra-articular fractures).

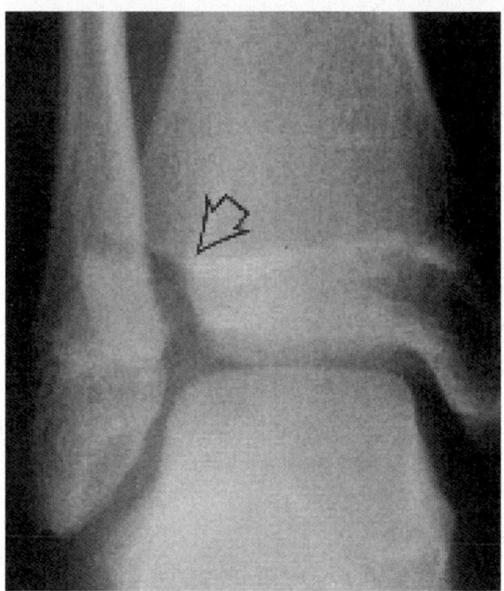

FIGURE 26-42 Anteroposterior mortise view of a 14-year-old who sustained a juvenile Tillaux fracture.

Triplane Fracture

Karrholm[86] attributed the original description of this injury to Bartl[7] in 1954 and noted that Gerner-Smidt,[62] in 1963, described triplane and Tillaux fractures as different stages of the same injury. In 1957, Johnson and Fahl[83] described a triplane fracture in their report of 27 physeal ankle injuries and reported that they had seen 10 such fractures. Despite these earlier reports, the nature of triplane fractures was not appreciated until Marmor's[117] report in 1970 of an irreducible ankle fracture that at surgery was found to consist of three parts (Fig. 26-43). Two years after Marmor's report, Lynn[113] reported two additional such fractures and coined the term triplane fracture. He described the fracture as consisting of three major fragments:

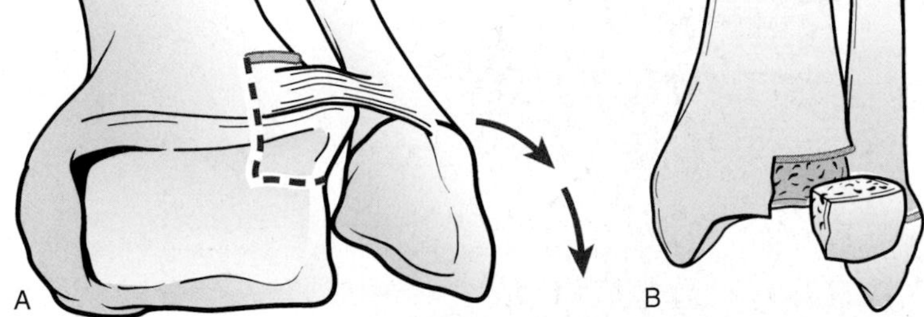

FIGURE 26-41 Juvenile Tillaux fracture. Mechanism of injury: the anteroinferior tibiofibular ligament avulses a fragment of the lateral epiphysis **(A)** corresponding to the portion of the physis that is still open **(B)**.

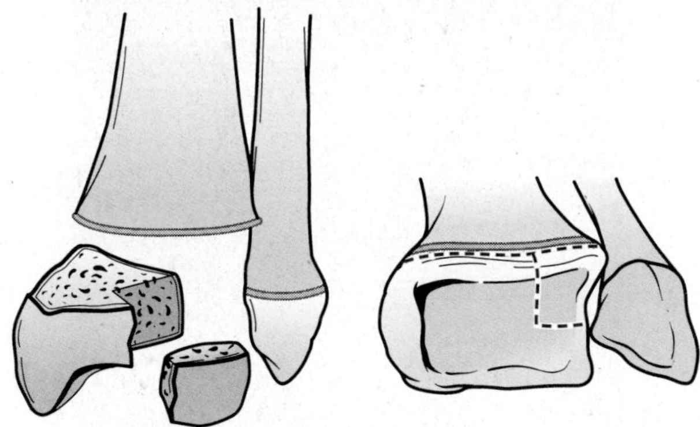

FIGURE 26-43 Anatomy of a three-part lateral triplane fracture (left ankle). Note the large epiphyseal fragment with its metaphyseal component and the smaller anterolateral epiphyseal fragment.

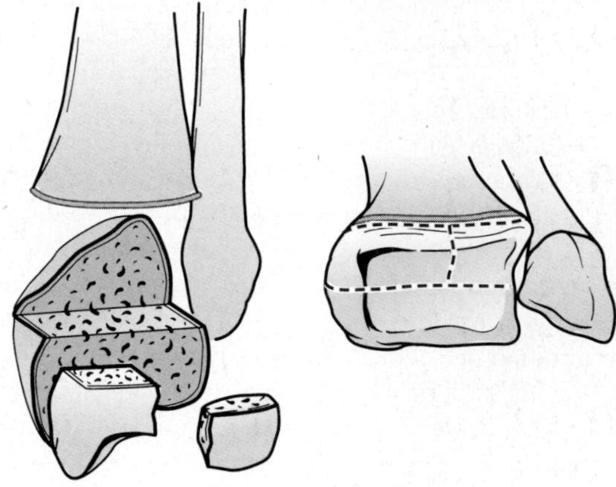

FIGURE 26-45 Anatomy of a four-part lateral triplane fracture (left ankle). The anterior epiphysis has split into two fragments, and the posterior epiphysis is the larger fragment with its metaphyseal component.

(i) the anterolateral quadrant of the distal tibial epiphysis, (ii) the medial and posterior portions of the epiphysis in addition to a posterior metaphyseal spike, and (iii) the tibial metaphysis. Cooperman and associates,[39] however, in their 1978 report of 15 such fractures concluded that, based on tomographic studies, most were two-part fractures produced by external rotation (Fig. 26-44). Variations in fracture patterns were attributed to the extent of physeal closure at the time of injury. Karrholm and colleagues[87] reported that CT evaluation of four adolescents with triplane fractures confirmed the existence of two-part and three-part fractures and also revealed four-part fractures (Fig.26-45). Denton and Fischer[46] described a two-part "medial triplane fracture" that they believed was caused by adduction and axial loading, and Peiro and associates[139] reported a three-part medial triplane fracture.

El-Karef et al.[52] studied 21 triplane fractures, identifying 19 as lateral triplane variants, and 2 as medial variants. Twelve were 2 part fractures, 6 were three-part fractures, and 3 were four-part fractures.

Von Laer[187] described a subgroup of two-part and three-part triplane fractures in which the fracture line on the anteroposterior radiographs did not extend into the ankle joint but into the medial malleolus instead (Fig. 26-46). Feldman and coworkers[54] also reported a case of an extra-articular triplane fracture in a skeletally immature patient. Shin et al.[170] reported 5 patients with intramalleolar triplane variants. They divided

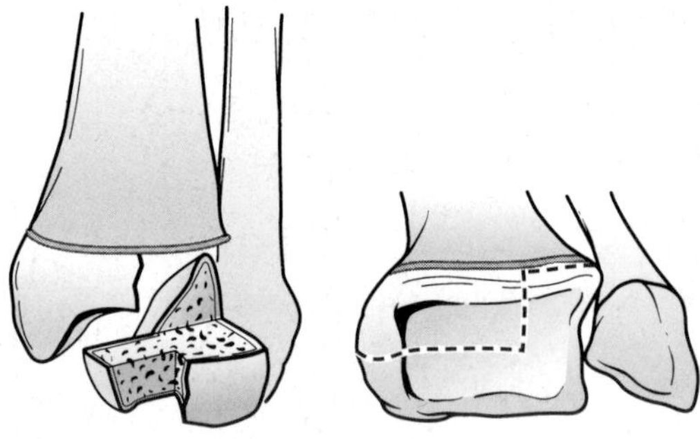

FIGURE 26-44 Anatomy of a two-part lateral triplane fracture (left ankle). Note the large posterolateral epiphyseal fragment with its posterior metaphyseal fragment. The anterior portion of the medial malleolus remains intact.

these into three types: type I, an intramalleolar intra-articular fracture, type II, an intramalleolar, intra-articular fracture outside the weight-bearing surface, and type III, an intramalleolar, extra-articular fracture (Fig. 26-47). These authors found that CT scans with three-dimensional reconstruction were helpful in determining displacement and deciding if surgery is indicated.

In the series of Spiegel and associates,[175] 7.3% were triplane fractures. Karrholm[86] reviewed 209 triplane fracture patients and found the mean age at the time of injury was 14.8 for boys and 12.8 for girls. This type injury did not occur in children younger than 10 or older than 16.7 years. The incidence is higher in males than females.[167] Patients with triplane fractures may have completely open physes. Swelling is usually more severe than with Tillaux fractures, and deformity may be more severe, especially if the fibula is also fractured. Radiographic views should include anteroposterior, lateral, and mortise views. Raparız et al.[152] found that 48% of triplane fractures were associated with fibular fracture and 8.5% were associated with ipsilateral tibial shaft fracture. Healy et al.[74] reported a triplane fracture associated with a proximal fibula fracture and syndesmotic injury (Maisonneuve equivalent). Failure to detect such injury may lead to chronic instability. Therefore, tenderness proximal to the ankle should be sought and if found is certainly an indication for radiographs of the proximal leg. CT scans have largely replaced plain tomograms for evaluation of the articular surface and the fracture anatomy (Fig. 26-48).

Nondisplaced triplane fractures, those with less than 2 mm of displacement, as well as extra-articular fractures can be treated with long-leg cast immobilization with the foot in internal rotation for lateral fractures and in eversion for medial fractures. Fractures with more than 2 mm of displacement, 65% of the injuries in the series by Karrholm et al.,[87] require reduction; this may be attempted in the emergency department or in the operating room with the use of general anesthesia. Closed reduction of lateral triplane fractures is attempted by internally rotating the foot. Based on the mechanism of injury, the most logical maneuver for reduction of medial triplane fractures is abduction. If closed reduction is shown to be adequate by image intensification as is the case in about half the time, a long-leg cast is applied or percutaneous screws are inserted for fixation if necessary. Well placed percutaneous screws will prevent sec-

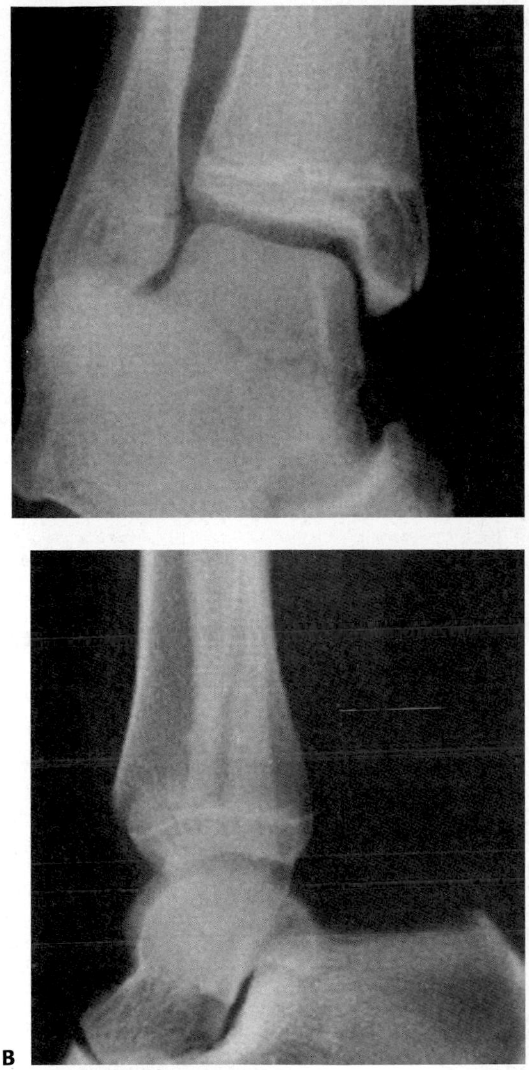

A

B

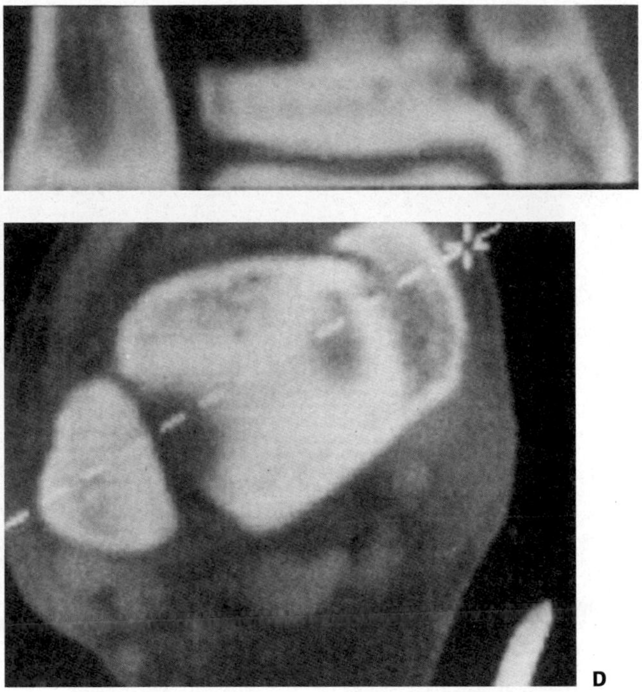

C

D

FIGURE 26-46 A,B. Anteroposterior and lateral radiographs of an "intramalleolar" variant triplane fracture in a 14-year-old boy. **C,D.** CT scans demonstrate extra-articular nature of the fracture.

ondary displacement in a cast, and may make follow-up radiographs and clinical visits less frequent. If closed reduction is unsuccessful, open reduction is required. This can be accomplished through an anterolateral approach for lateral triplane fractures or through an anteromedial approach for medial triplane fractures. Additional incisions may be necessary for adequate exposure.

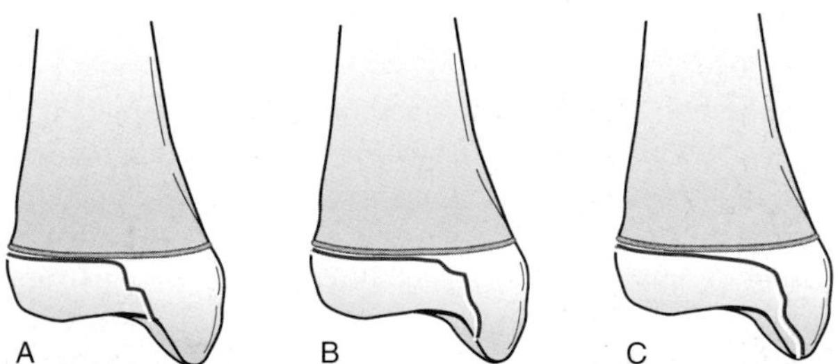

FIGURE 26-47 Schematic drawing of the immature distal tibial physis demonstrating types I, II, and III intramalleolar triplane fractures. **A.** Type I intramalleolar, intra-articular fracture at the junction of the tibial plafond and the medial malleolus. **B.** Type II intramalleolar, intra-articular fracture outside the weight-bearing zone of the tibial plafond. **C.** Type III intramalleolar, extraarticular fracture. (Adapted from Shin A, Moran ME, Wenger DR. Intramalleolar triplane fractures. J Pediatr Orthop 1997;17:352–355, with permission.)

Whipple and associates[190] described arthroscopic reduction of two-part triplane fractures in two patients. With the arthroscope in an anterolateral portal and an anteromedial portal used for inflow, two pins were inserted laterally into the epiphyseal fragment and used to maneuver it into proper position under direct arthroscopic vision. The pins were then advanced for fixation of the fragment.

The use of well-placed percutaneous clamps and arthroscopic assistance may help with the reduction and minimize the need for incisions. Careful review of the CT scans can help guide percutaneous clamp and screw placement that improves the biomechanics of clamp reduction and screw placement.[85] Care should be taken to avoid injury to neurovascular structures during clamp or percutaneous screw placement (see section on arthroscopy and surgical reduction tips).

Pilon Fractures

Although these fractures are relatively rare in young patients, these injuries can be associated with severe soft tissue swelling and edema. Similar to the treatment in adults with these injuries, management of the soft tissues is critical to prevent complications of skin loss, infection, wound healing problems, etc.[51,181]

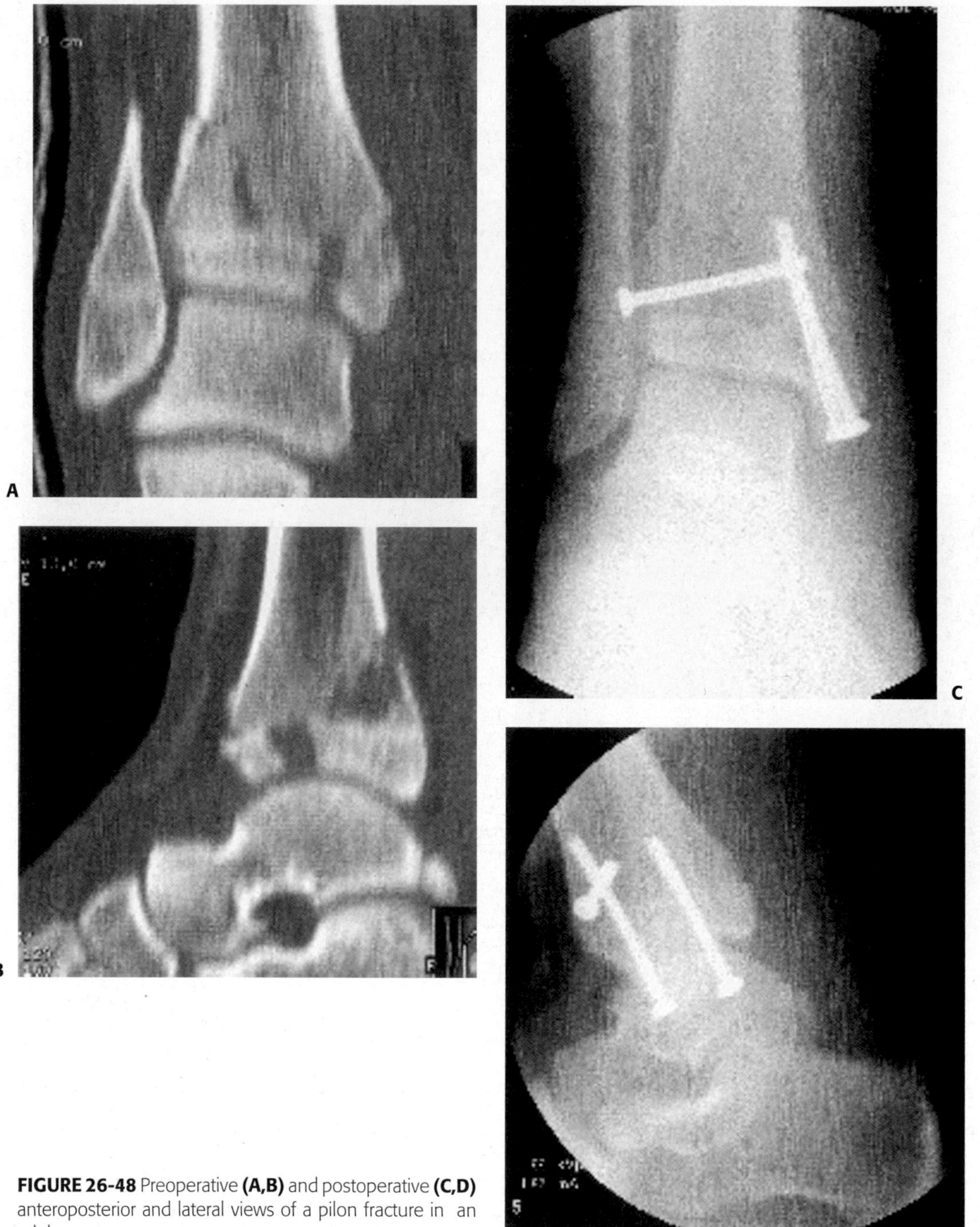

FIGURE 26-48 Preoperative **(A,B)** and postoperative **(C,D)** anteroposterior and lateral views of a pilon fracture in an adolescent.

Initial approaches may consist of application of external fixation or dressings to address swelling and edema, with delay of surgical intervention for 5 to 15 days (Fig. 26-49).[51]

Letts et al.[105] described a small series of pilon fractures in skeletally immature patients. The patients in this series did not have wound/skin complications, and only two of eight patients developed postoperative osteoarthritis at short-term follow-up. As these fractures may be higher risk for complications, we believe that treatment principles used in adult patients should be applied to this patient population as well.[5,12,104,105,138,155]

Fractures of the Incisura

One of the authors (R. Jay Cummings) has seen two patients with fractures of the incisura injuries.[44] Despite 12 weeks of immobilization, these fractures had not healed. Despite the appearance of nonunion on radiographs, these patients remained symptom free at 2-year follow-up. One patient developed mild symptoms of ankle pain several years later. If there is evidence of syndesmotic injury, syndesmosis reduction and internal fixation should probably be considered.

Syndesmosis Injuries

Healy[74] has reported a triplane fracture in association with a syndesmosis injury, and both authors have identified a small series of syndesmosis type injuries in their practice.[43] These have been associated with the following fracture patterns: distal fibula, Salter-Harris types I and II, triplane, and Tillaux. During surgical treatment of pediatric/adolescent ankle fractures, evalu-

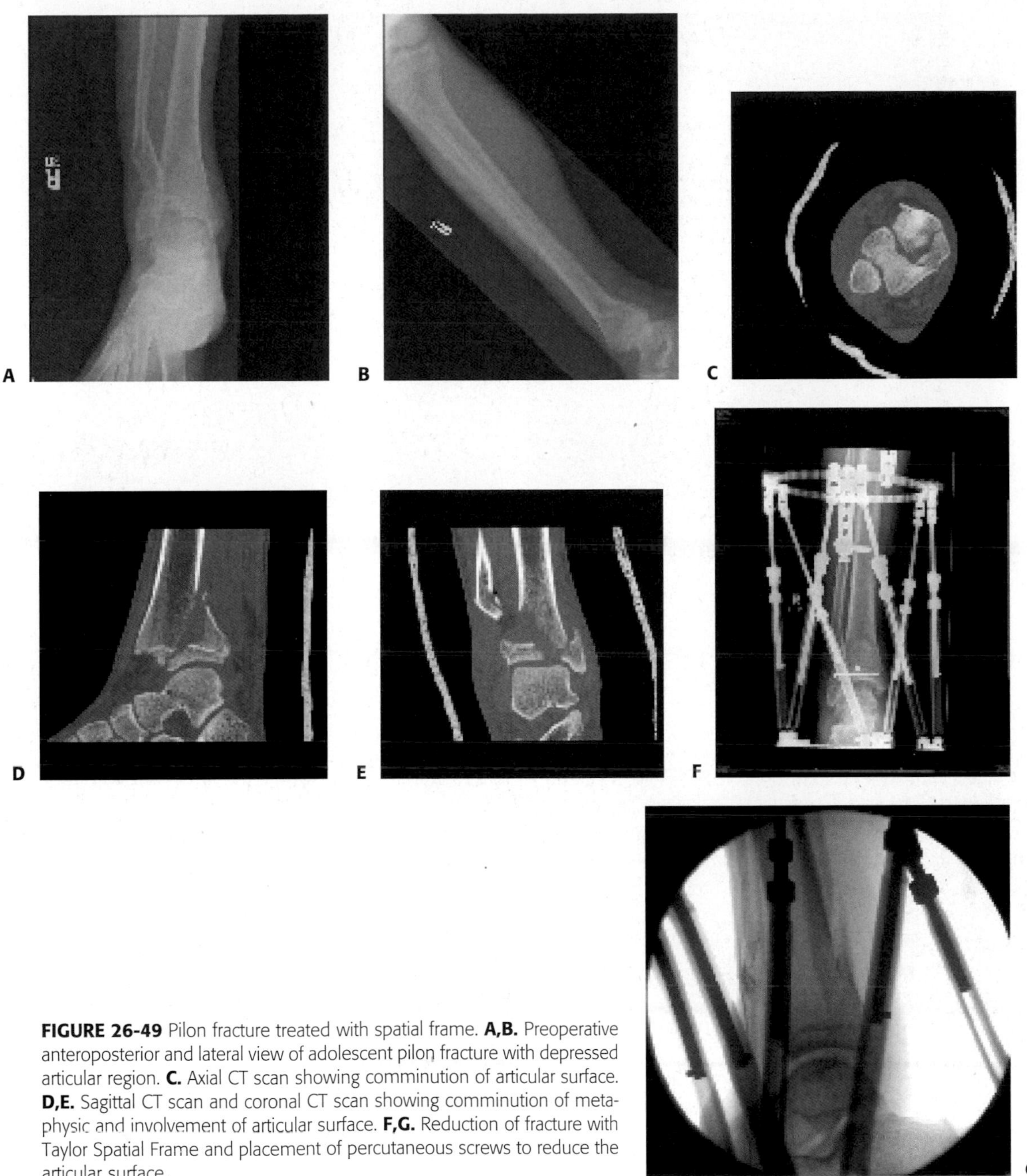

FIGURE 26-49 Pilon fracture treated with spatial frame. **A,B.** Preoperative anteroposterior and lateral view of adolescent pilon fracture with depressed articular region. **C.** Axial CT scan showing comminution of articular surface. **D,E.** Sagittal CT scan and coronal CT scan showing comminution of metaphysic and involvement of articular surface. **F,G.** Reduction of fracture with Taylor Spatial Frame and placement of percutaneous screws to reduce the articular surface.

ation for syndesmosis injuries should probably be performed in a manner similar to the treatment of adult fractures. Syndesmosis reduction and fixation may be necessary (see Fig. 26-15).

Open Fractures and Lawnmower Injuries

Severe open ankle fractures are often produced by high-velocity motor vehicular accidents or lawn mower injuries (Fig. 26-50).[66] Approximately 25,000 lawn mower injuries occur each year, 20% of which are in children. Ride-on mowers produce the most severe injuries, requiring more surgical procedures and resulting in more functional limitations.[1,3,50,57,161,188] Loder et al.[109] reviewed 144 children injured by lawn mowers. The average age at the time of injury was 7 years. The child was a bystander in 84 cases. Sixty-seven children required amputation. Soft tissue infection occurred in 8 of 118 and osteomyelitis in 6 of 117.

Principles of treatment are the same as in adults: copious irrigation and débridement, tetanus toxoid, and intravenous antibiotics. Gaglani et al.[61] reported the bacteriologic findings in three children with infections secondary to lawn mower injuries. They found that organisms infecting the wounds were frequently different than those found on initial débridement. Gram-negative organisms were common, and all three patients were infected with fungi as well. In children with lawn mower injuries, grass, dirt, and debris are blown into the wound under pressure, and removal of these embedded foreign objects requires meticulous mechanical débridement.

In most patients, the articular surface and physis should be aligned and fixed with smooth pins that do not cross the physis

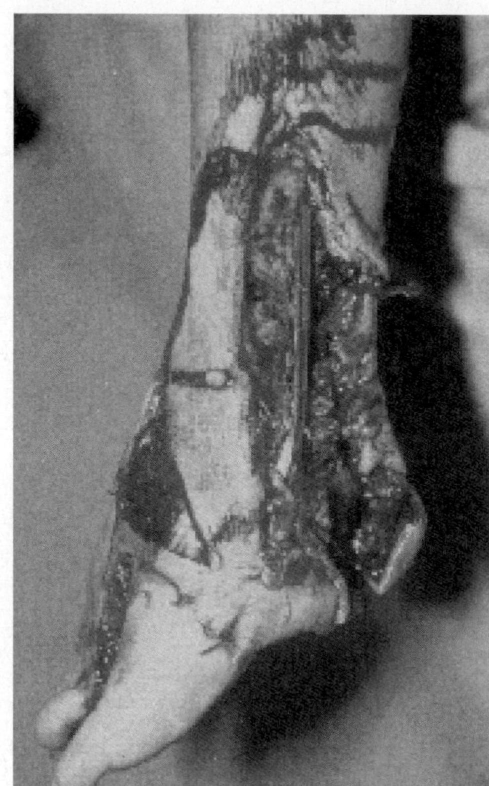

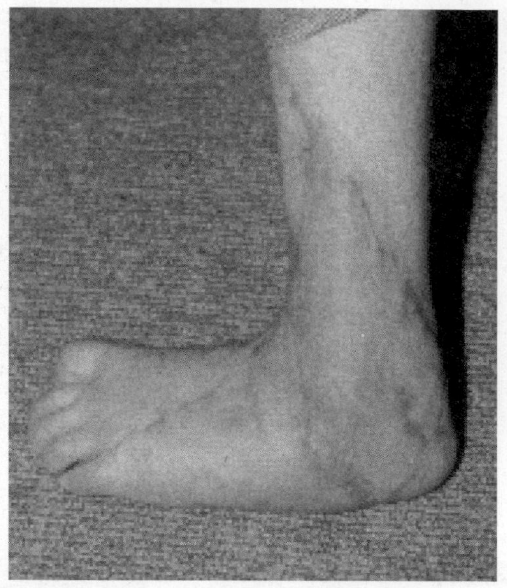

FIGURE 26-50 A. Severe lawn mower injury in a 5-year-old boy. **B.** One year after initial treatment with débridement, free flap, and skin graft coverage.

at the time of initial treatment. Exposed physeal surfaces should be covered with local fat to help prevent union of the metaphysis to the epiphysis. An external fixator may be used if neurovascular structures are injured, but small pins should be used through the metaphysis and epiphysis, avoiding the physis.[77,84,111,153,160] Wound closure may be a problem in cases with significant soft tissue injury and exposed bone. Skin coverage with local tissue is ideal; if local coverage is not possible, split-thickness skin grafting is generally the next choice. Free vascular flaps and rotational flaps may be required for adequate coverage. Klein et al.[98] reported two cases that had associated vascular injury precluding such flaps that were covered successfully with local advancement flaps made possible by multiple relaxing incisions. Mooney et al.[125] reported cross extremity flaps for such cases. They found external fixation for linkage of the lower extremities during the procedure to be valuable. After fixation removal, range of motion returned readily.

Vosburgh and associates[188] reported 33 patients with lawn mower injuries to the foot and ankle. They found that the most severe injuries were to the posterior-plantar aspect of the foot and ankle. Of their patients, five required split-thickness skin grafts and one required vascularized flap for soft tissue coverage. Two ultimately required Syme amputation. Four of the patients had complete disruption of the Achilles tendon. Three had no repair or reconstruction of the triceps surae tendon, and one had delayed reconstruction 3 months after injury. Vosburgh and associates[188] speculate that dense scarring in the posterior ankle results in a "physiologic tendon" and that extensive reconstructive surgery is not always necessary for satisfactory function. Boyer et al.[20] reported a patient with deltoid ligament loss due to a severe grinding injury that required free plantaris tendon graft to reconstruct the ligament. Soft tissue coverage was achieved using a free muscle transfer. Rinker et al.[154] also described the use of soft tissue transfer to assist pediatric patients with severe soft tissue loss.

The development of vacuum-assisted closure devices had been a dramatic improvement in the treatment of these injuries and may reduce the need for tissue transfers.[75] Referral to centers with experience with these treatment protocols may be necessary for these severe injuries. Our limited experience with the use of vacuum-assisted closure devices in high-energy trauma with severe soft tissue injury has shown very good results for limb salvage.

Distal Fibula Fractures

Fractures involving the fibular physis are most commonly Salter-Harris type I or II fractures that are caused by a supination–inversion injury. Isolated fibular fractures are usually minimally displaced and can be treated with immobilization in a below-knee cast for 3 to 4 weeks. Significantly displaced fibular fractures accompany Salter-Harris type III and IV tibial fractures and usually reduce when the tibial fracture is reduced. Internal fixation of the tibial fracture generally results in stability of the fibular fracture such that cast immobilization is sufficient. If the fibular fracture is unstable after reduction and fixation of the tibial fracture, fixation with a smooth intramedullary or obliquely inserted Kirschner wire is recommended (Fig. 26-51F). In older adolescents in whom growth is not a consideration, an intramedullary rod, screw, or plate-and-screw device may be used as in adults (Fig. 26-52).

Avulsion fractures from the lateral malleolus are seen in children with inversion "sprain" type injuries to the ankle. These may fail to unite with cast immobilization. Patients with such nonunions may have pain without associated instability. In such patients, simple excision of the ununited fragment usually relieves their pain.[46,71] When the nonunions are associated with

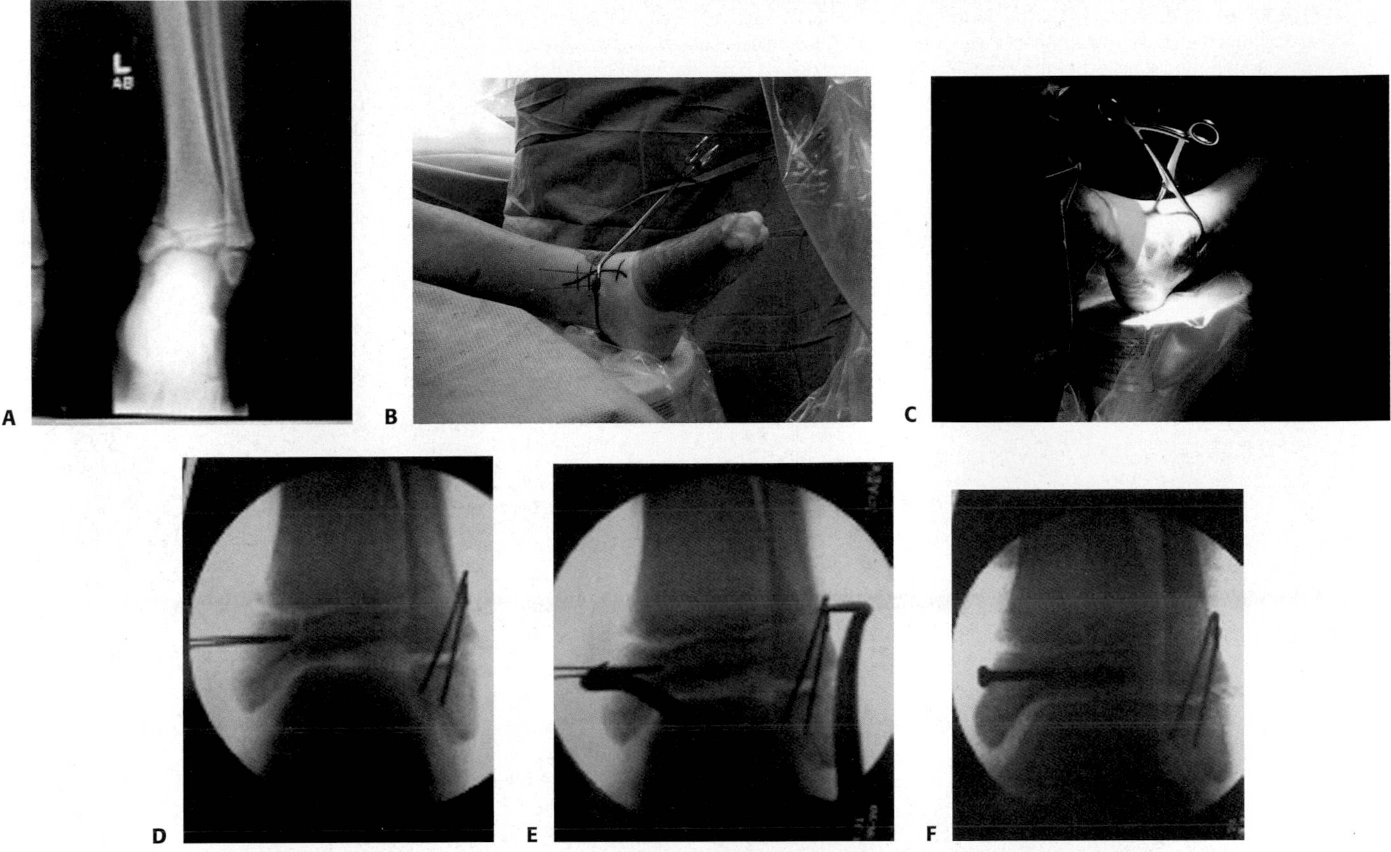

FIGURE 26-51 **A.** Anteroposterior view of displaced Salter-Harris type I fibula fracture and Salter-Harris type IV intra-articular medial malleolus fracture. **B.** Use of percutaneous clamps to facilitate reduction of medial malleolus fracture. **C.** Use of percutaneous clamps to facilitate reduction. **D.** Use of two pins as "joysticks" to guide reduction of the displaced medial malleolus fracture. **E.** Use of percutaneous clamps to facilitate reduction and compression across the epiphyseal fracture. **F.** Use of percutaneous epiphyseal screws to gain compression across the fracture and to facilitate reduction.

instability, reconstruction of one or more of the lateral ankle ligaments is required (see lateral ankle sprains).[23,24]

Avulsion fractures of the accessory ossification centers of the distal fibula (os subfibulare) are also common. In the series report by Ogden and Lee,[135] 5 of 11 patients with injures treated with casting had persistent symptoms and required excision.

Lateral Ankle Sprains

In 1984, Vahvanen[190] published a prospective study of 559 children who presented with severe supination injuries or sprains of the ankle. Forty patients, 28 boys and 12 girls, with an average age of 12 years (range 5 to 14) were surgically explored. The indications for surgery included swelling, pain over the anterior talofibular ligament, limp, clinical instability, and, when visible, a displaced avulsion fracture. Such fractures were visible radiographically in only 8 patients but were found at surgery in 19. Thirty-six ankles were found to have injury of the anterior talofibular ligament at surgery. Only 16 of these had either a positive lateral or anterior drawer stress test. At follow-up, all patients were pain free and none complained of instability. Based upon the incidence of residual disability after such injuries in adults reported in the literature (21% to 58%), these authors suggested primary surgical repair.

Busconi and Pappas[29] reported 60 skeletally immature children with chronic ankle pain and instability. Fifty of these children responded to rehabilitation, but 10 had persistent symptoms. While three of these patients' initial radiographs were within normal limits, all patients with persistent symptoms eventually were found to have ununited osteochondral fractures of the fibular epiphysis. All 10 patients with persistent symptoms were treated with excision of the ununited osteochondral fracture and a Broström reconstruction of the lateral collateral ligament. All were able to return to activities and none reported further pain or instability.

Ankle Dislocations

Nusem et al.[133] reported a 12-year-old girl who was seen with a posterior dislocation of the ankle without associated fracture. This was a closed injury and resulted from forced inversion of a maximally plantar flexed foot. The dislocation was reduced under IV sedation and the ankle immobilized in a short-leg cast for 5 weeks. The patient was asymptomatic at follow-up 4 years postinjury. The inversion stress views at that time revealed only a 3-degree increase laxity compared to the uninjured side. The anterior drawer sign was negative. There was no evidence of avascular necrosis of the talus on follow-up radiographs. Mazur et al.[119] also reported ankle dislocation without a fracture in a pediatric patient.

For Current Treatment Options, see Table 26-2.

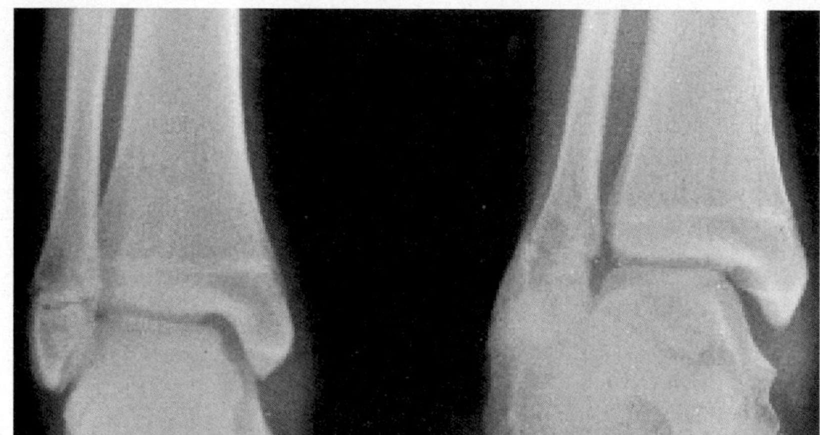

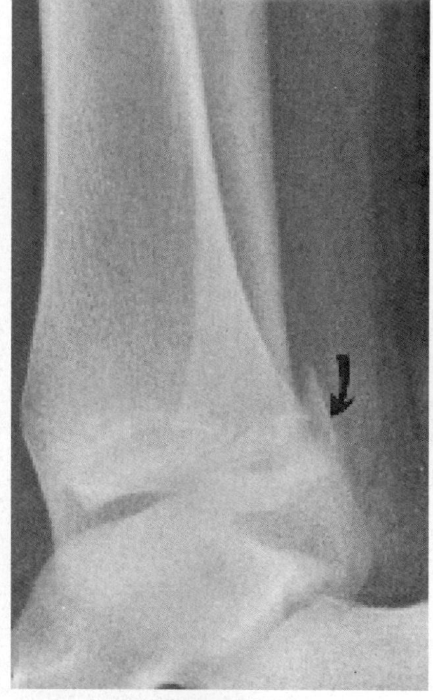

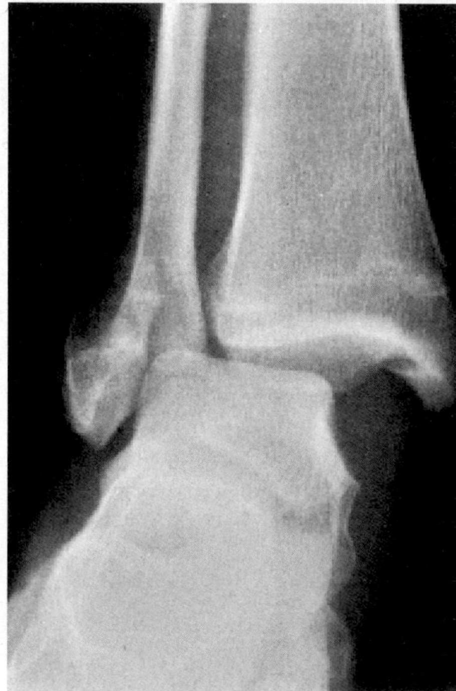

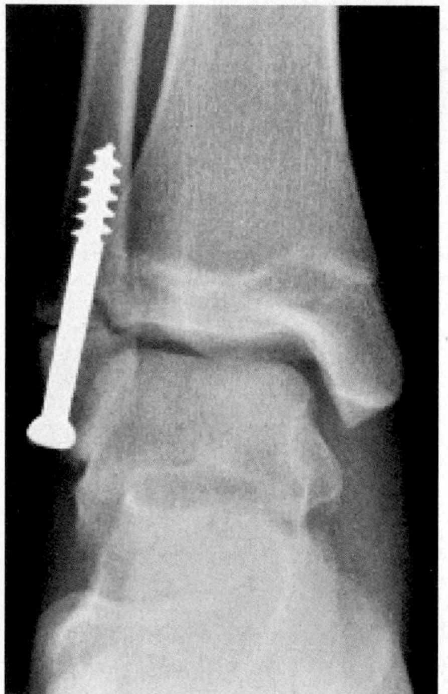

FIGURE 26-52 A. Salter-Harris type II fracture of the distal fibula in a 15-year-old. **B.** Lateral view shows the fibular metaphyseal fragment (*arrow*). Considerable soft tissue swelling was noted in the medial aspect of the ankle. **C.** Stress films showed complete disruption of the deltoid ligament. **D.** The fibular fracture was fixed with a cannulated screw; the deltoid ligament was not repaired.

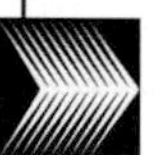

AUTHORS' PREFERRED METHOD OF TREATMENT

Salter-Harris Type I and II Fractures of the Distal Tibial

We prefer to treat nondisplaced Salter-Harris type I and II fractures initially with above-knee cast immobilization. Non-weight bearing is continued until 2 to 4 weeks postinjury, when the cast is changed to a below-knee walking cast or walking boot which is worn for an additional 2 to 3 weeks. Follow-up radiographs are obtained every 6 months for 2 years or until a Park-Harris growth arrest line parallel to the physis is visible and there is no evidence of physeal deformity.

For displaced fractures in children with at least 3 years of growth remaining, our objective is to obtain no more than 10–15 degrees of plantar tilt for posteriorly displaced fractures, 5–10 degrees of valgus for laterally displaced fractures, and 0 degrees of varus for medially displaced fractures (Fig. 26-53). Studies in the adult literature suggest that minor alteration in alignment of the ankle joint may have significant effect on tibiotalar contact pressures.[92,182,184] If a question exists as to whether the child has enough growth remaining to remodel the fracture, it is probably best to perform a reduction. For children with 2 years or less of growth remaining, the amount of acceptable angulation is

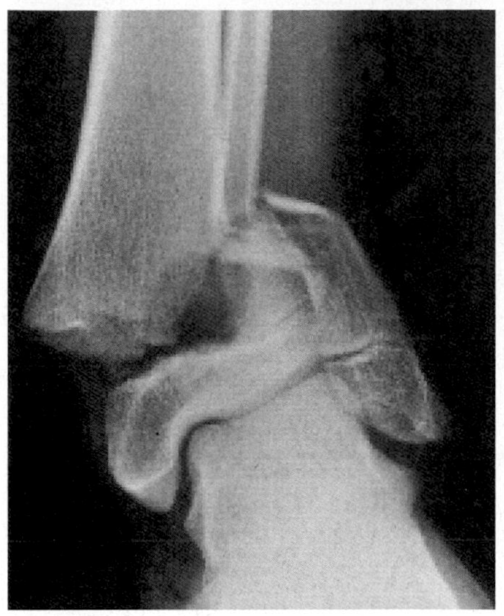
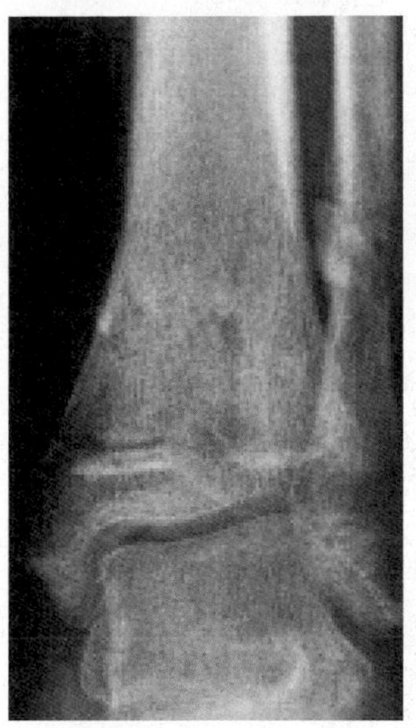
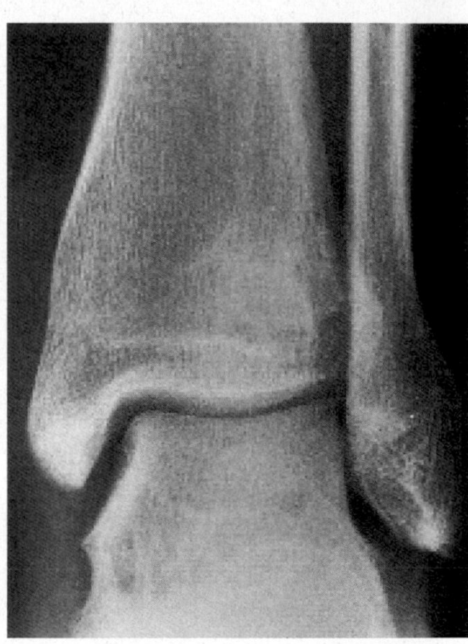

FIGURE 26-53 A. Displaced pronation–eversion–external rotation fracture of the distal tibia in a 12-year-old boy was treated with closed reduction and cast immobilization. **B.** After cast removal, a 10-degree valgus tilt was present. **C.** At maturity, the deformity has completely resolved.

reduced to less than 5 degrees. We prefer to attempt reduction of markedly displaced fractures with the use of general anesthesia with good muscle relaxation and image intensifier control. The use of an ankle distractor can facilitate distraction across the fracture, and may facilitate reduction (see Fig. 26-34). In children with mildly displaced fractures, especially if anesthesia is not going to be available for many hours, an attempt at gentle closed reduction under a hematoma block supplemented as needed by well-monitored IV sedation may be reasonable. Not all emergency rooms are equipped with appropriate sedation equipment for young patients. Once adequately reduced, the fractures are usually stable and a long-leg cast can be used for immobilization. Rarely, for markedly unstable fractures or severe soft tissue injuries that require multiple débridements, percutaneous screws are used when the Thurstan-Holland fragment is large enough to accept screw fixation. When the fragment is too small, smooth wire fixation across the physis is the only alternative. Repeated attempts at closed manipulation of these fractures may increase the risk of growth abnormality and should be avoided. In patients with fractures that are not seen until 7 to 10 days after injury, residual displacement is probably best accepted, unless very significant deformity or angulation is present, to avoid iatrogenic injury to the physis. If growth does not sufficiently correct malunion, corrective osteotomy can be performed later.

Open reduction of these fractures is occasionally indicated. The exception usually has been pronation–eversion–external rotation fractures with interposed soft tissue, which may include lateral and posterior displacement. For cases that have undergone an attempt at closed reduction, close inspection of the medial physis should be performed with image intensification. In some cases, the medial physeal space will appear abnormally widened, which may suggest incarceration of a large flap of periosteum in the physis. For these fractures, a small anteromedial incision is made and any interposed soft tissues, such as periosteum or tendons, are extracted. Even though reduction is usually stable, we generally use internal fixation. Fixation options include screw fixation through both the metaphyseal and epiphyseal fragments, avoiding fixation across the physis if possible (Fig. 26-54). Percutaneous smooth pins can also be placed from the medial malleolus, oriented proximally to engage the metaphysis (see Figs. 26-31and 26-55).

Salter-Harris Types III and IV Fractures of the Distal Tibia

Treatment of nondisplaced Salter-Harris type III and IV fractures is the same as for nondisplaced type I and II fractures with three modifications. Casting with a long-leg cast is confirmed with a CT scan and/or radiographs. These patients are examined more frequently (once a week) for the first 2–3 weeks after cast application to ensure that the fragments do not become displaced. Third, these patients are examined every 6 to 12 months after cast removal for 24 to 36 months to detect any growth abnormality.

Generally, only truly nondisplaced Salter-Harris types III and IV fractures, or those with 1 mm or less of displacement, can be treated closed. Fractures with 2 mm or more of displacement require open reduction and internal fixation with anatomical alignment of the physis and intra-articular fracture fragments. Arthroscopic assistance is also an option in these cases.

In cases where arthroscopic assistance is used, the visualization of the ankle joint can also assist with the evaluation of reduction. In some cases, the fractures may still have small gap present with the articular surface, but the presence of step-off or intra-articular incongruity can be clearly evaluated with arthroscopic visualization of the articular surface. It has been our experience that the C-arm views may show excellent reduction of the subchondral bone of the articular-

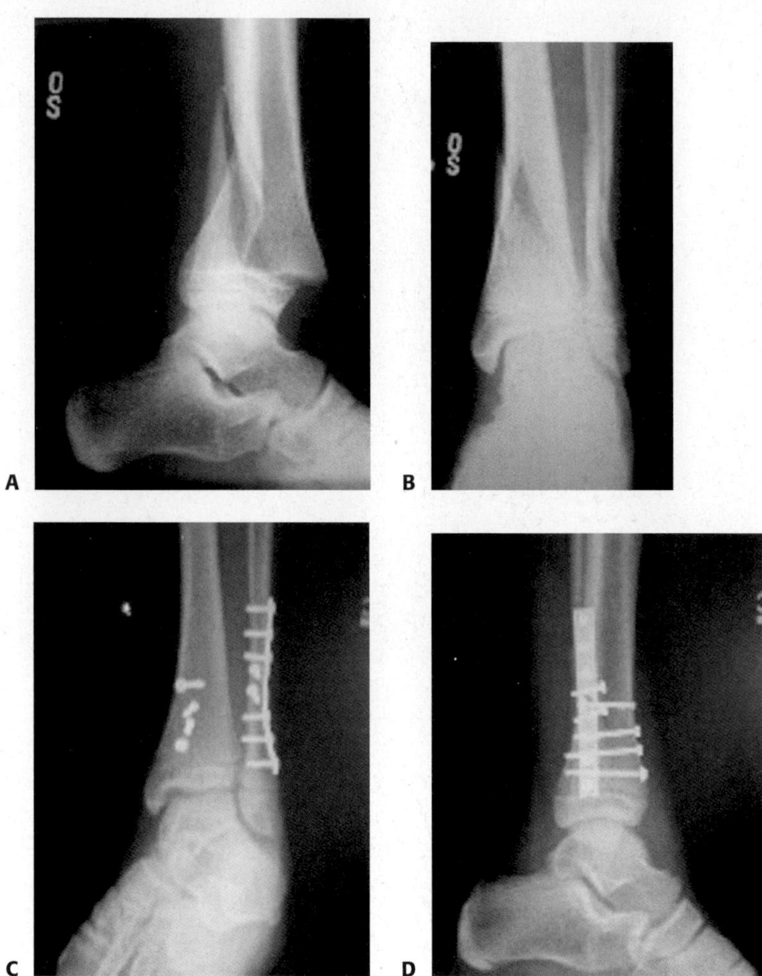

FIGURE 26-54 Salter-Harris type II distal tibial fracture with fibular fracture. **A.** Lateral view. **B.** Anteroposterior view. **C,D.** After percutaneous placement of tibial screws and plating of fibular fracture.

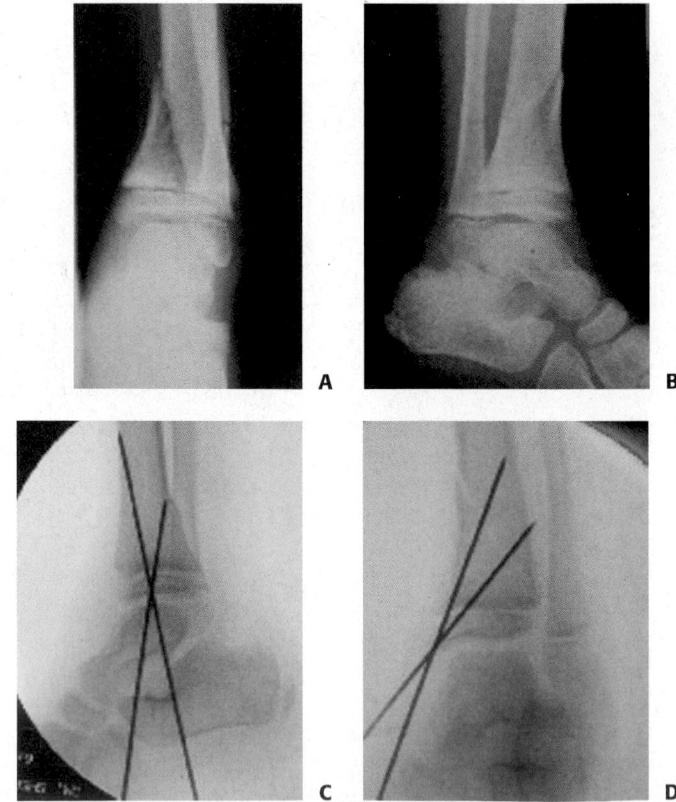

FIGURE 26-55 Salter-Harris type II distal tibial fracture with fibular fracture. **A.** Anteroposterior view. **B.** Lateral view. **C,D.** Percutaneous placement of Kirschner-wires.

surface, and the arthroscopic views may show that the cartilage surfaces are not as well reduced as one would expect based upon these radiographic images.

Fractures with more than 2 mm of displacement should be reduced, regardless of whether the fracture is acute or not. Closed reduction can be attempted, but these fractures usually require open reduction, arthroscopic assisted reduction, or mini-open reduction with arthroscopic assistance. Occasionally, primary débridement of callus and soft tissue back to normal-appearing physis and fat grafting have been successful for fractures that are more than 7 days old.

For fractures stabilized with internal fixation, below-knee casts may be used. If there is concern about fracture stability, above-knee casts can be used.

Open Reduction and Internal Fixation of Salter-Harris Type III or IV Fractures of the Distal Tibia

The patient is placed supine on an operating table that is radiolucent at the lower extremity. After exsanguination of the extremity and inflation of the tourniquet, longitudinal incisions are made to expose the fracture. Relatively small incisions may be acceptable, to allow for percutaneous or minimally invasive hardware placement. The use of the C-arm may assist with the use of smaller incision, allowing for visualization of the articular surface, with minimal exposure of the metaphyseal areas. The fracture site is identified, and an anteromedial capsulotomy of the ankle joint is performed. The fracture surfaces are exposed and gently cleaned with irrigation and forceps.

For Salter-Harris type IV fractures, the periosteum may be elevated several millimeters from the metaphyseal fracture edges. The epiphyseal edges and joint surfaces are examined through the arthrotomy. The perichondral ring should not be elevated from the physis. For Salter-Harris type III fractures, the reduction is evaluated by checking the joint surface and epiphyseal fracture edges through the arthrotomy. The epiphyseal fragment is grasped with a small towel clip or reduction forceps, and the fracture is reduced. Internal fixation is performed under direct vision and fluoroscopic control. It is important to view both the lateral and anteroposterior projections because of the curved shape of the distal tibial articular surface. If the fragment is large enough, 4.0-mm cannulated lag screws are inserted through the epiphyseal fragment; if the fragment is too small for screws, smaller screws or smooth Kirschner wires are used. The reduction and the position of the internal fixation are checked through the arthrotomy. In fractures with a significant Thurstan-Holland fragment, a metaphyseal screw may be used if a gap exists after the epiphyseal screws are inserted. After reduction of the tibial fracture, the associated Salter-Harris type I or II fibular fracture usually reduces and is stable. If it is not, closed reduction and fixation with percutaneous oblique smooth Kirschner-wires is performed.

The patient is kept nonweight bearing for 3 weeks, and then the cast is changed to a below-knee walking cast, which is worn for an additional 2 weeks. Frequent follow-up evaluations (every 3 months for the first year and yearly thereafter) are necessary to detect growth abnormalities until skeletal maturity.

Salter-Harris Type V Fractures

These injuries are quite rare. The risk of physeal arrest is thought to be quite high for this injury pattern, due to direct damage of the germinal layer of the physis.[92] We have seen these fractures associated with a varus load to the ankle joint, leading to a crush type injury to the medial malleolus (Figs. 26-56 and 26-57). These fractures can be treated with reduction of the joint and physeal surface, using minimally invasive techniques that avoid the physis and perichondral ring (see Fig. 26-57).

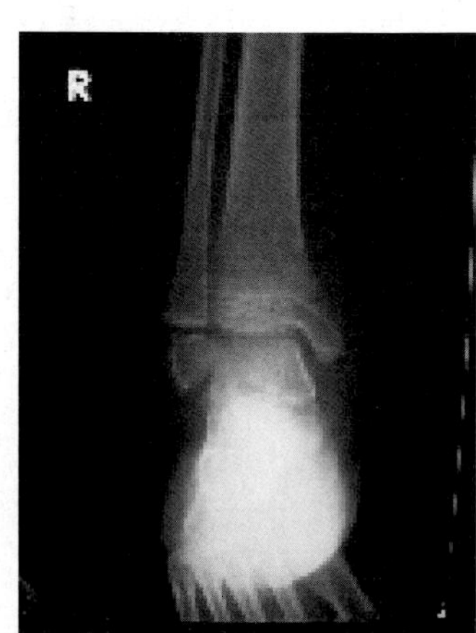

A

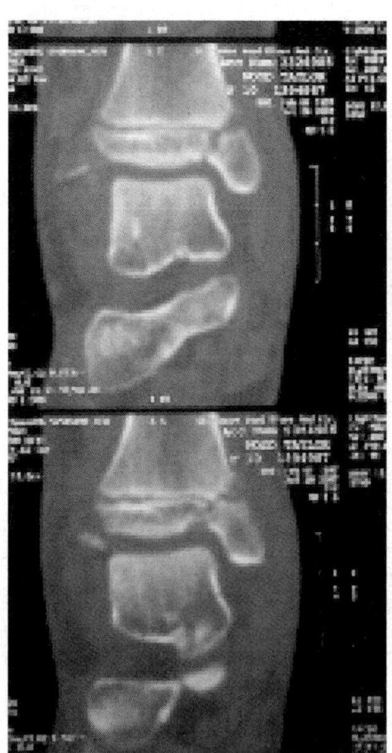

B

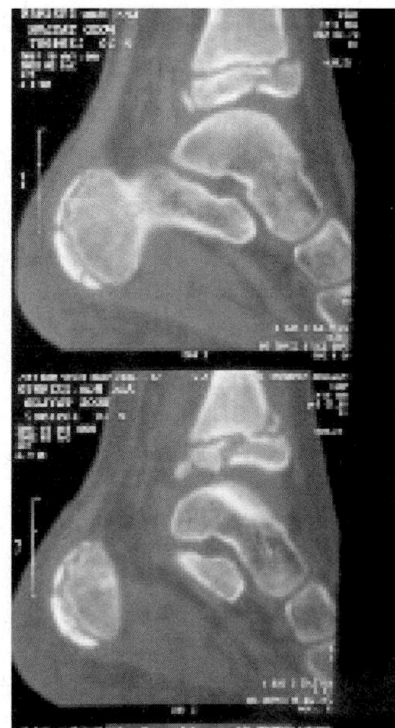

C

FIGURE 26-56 Salter-Harris type V distal fibula fracture. **A.** Anteroposterior ankle radiograph of crush injury to the medial malleolus. **B.** Coronal CT scan of medial malleolus crush injury. **C.** Sagittal CT scan of medial malleolus crush injury.

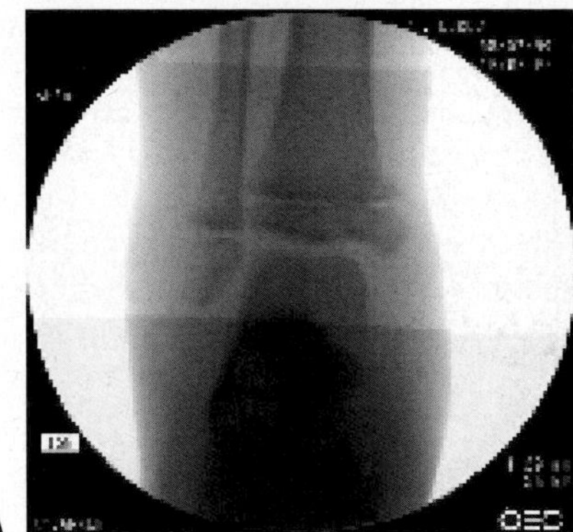

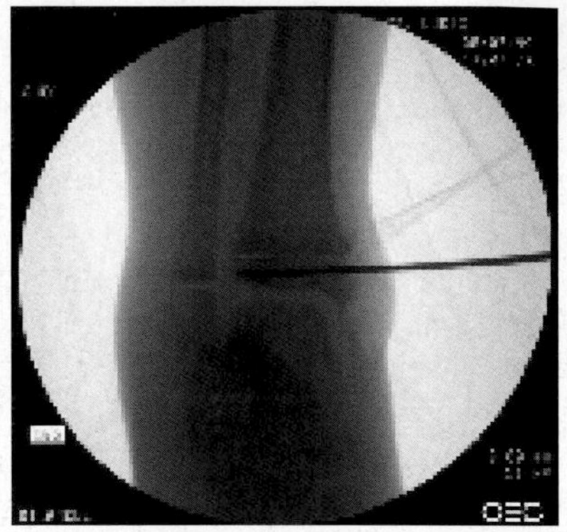

FIGURE 26-57 Salter-Harris type V patterns with crush injury to medial malleolus. **A.** Crush injury to medial malleolus and distal tibia metaphysis. **B.** The percutaneous pins can be used to manipulate the fracture.

In the rare case when the fracture is identified early, prophylactic surgery to excise the physeal bar and implantation of a fat graft might reduce the risk of physeal arrest. The prognosis for this injury is poor, and treatment is usually focused upon treating the complications of angular deformity and/or physeal arrest.[92]

Juvenile Tillaux Fractures

For nondisplaced fractures and fractures displaced less than 2 mm, we prefer immobilization in an above-knee cast with the knee flexed 30 degrees and the foot neutral or internally rotated. If the position appears acceptable on plain films, CT scanning in the transverse plane with coronal and sagittal reconstructions may be used to confirm acceptable reduction. For fractures with more than 2 mm of initial displacement, manipulation may be attempted by internal rotation of the foot and application of direct pressure over the anterolateral joint line. If reduction is not obtained with this maneuver, reduction can be attempted by dorsiflexing the pronated foot and then internally rotating the foot.[114] If successful reduction is obtained, percutaneous fixation (screws or pins) can be placed with C-arm guidance. In most cases, the medial portion of the physis is already closed or closing, so this is one of the rare times it is acceptable to cross the physis with screw fixation. Percutaneous clamps can be used to hold reduction during screw placement. If there are questions about the adequacy of reduction, this can be confirmed by use of an arthrotomy or ankle arthroscope.

In cases where the reduction is not ideal, several things can be attempted. Schlesinger and Wedge[165] have described a technique using percutaneous manipulation of a Tillaux fragment with a Steinman pin.[92] Small Kirschner wires or the threaded tip wires from a cannulated screw set can be inserted into the Tillaux fragment, to act as a "joystick" to reduce the fracture (Fig. 26-58). This is done under fluoroscopic control. Ideally, one or both of these pins can then be passed across the fracture site after reduction has been obtained, and the cannulated screw can then be placed over the pins (Figs. 26-59 and 26-60).

If reduction is not successful, open reduction is performed through an anterolateral approach or arthroscopic assistance can be used to obtain anatomic reduction. For open techniques, the following protocol is used. The patient is placed in a supine position, and an incision is placed in the region of the fracture. A small incision is made, perhaps 2 to 3 cm, to allow for visualization. The fracture plane is identified, and direct pressure or clamps can be applied to

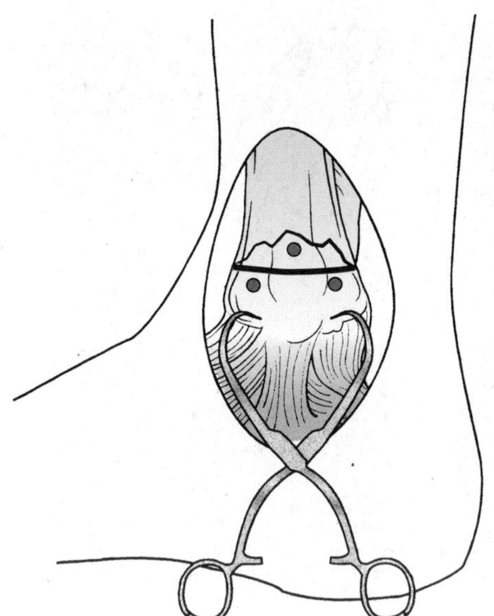

FIGURE 26-58 Technique for reduction of a Salter-Harris type IV fracture of the distal tibia.

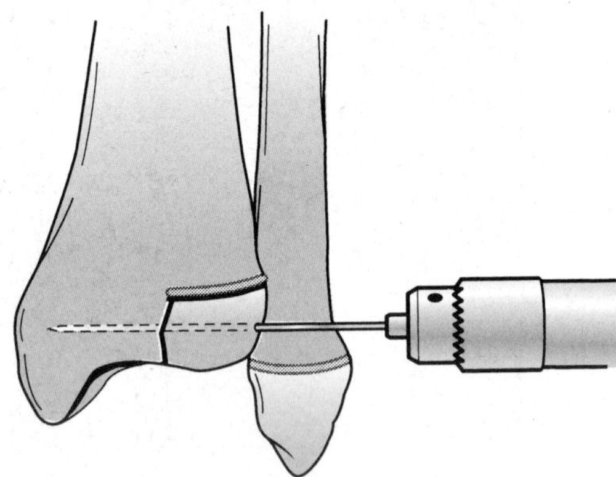

FIGURE 26-59 Advancement of pin after reduction of juvenile Tillaux fracture.

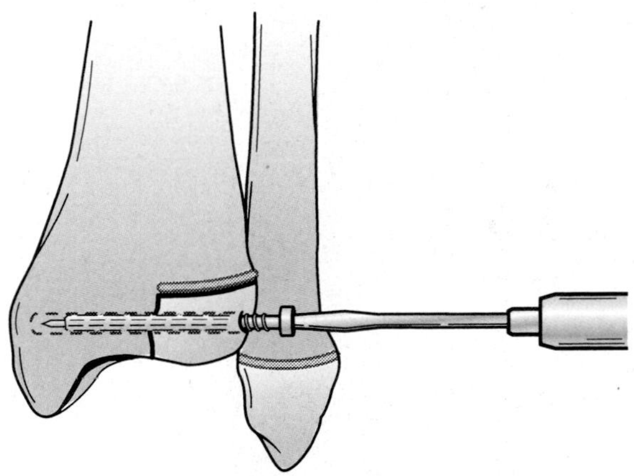

FIGURE 26-60 Percutaneous insertion of 4-mm cannulated screw over pin that has been advanced into the medial distal tibia after reduction of the juvenile Tillaux fracture fragment.

maintain the reduction. If necessary, a small arthrotomy or arthroscope can be used to evaluate the articular reduction. A guidewire from a cannulated screw system is used (a 4.0 mm cannulated system usually works well in this age group), followed by placement of the screw.

A short-leg, nonweight-bearing cast is worn for 3 weeks, followed by a weight-bearing cast or walking boot for another 2 to 3 weeks.

Triplane Fractures

For nondisplaced or minimally displaced (less than 2 mm) fractures, we prefer immobilization in a long-leg cast with the knee flexed 30 to 40 degrees. The position of the foot may be influenced by whether the fracture is lateral (internal rotation) or medial (eversion), though this is certainly inexact. A CT scan is usually obtained after casting to document adequate reduction. Plain films or CT scans are obtained approximately 7 days after cast application to verify that displacement has not recurred. At 3 to 4 weeks, the cast is changed to a below-knee walking cast or walking boot, which is worn another 2 to 3 weeks, though this may be delayed if there is concern over displacement of the weight-bearing surface.

The ability to reduce fractures in the emergency room with appropriate conscious sedation varies between institutions. For institutions that have such capabilities, fracture reduction can be attempted in the emergency room. For fractures with more than 2 mm of displacement, an attempt at closed reduction with sedation in the emergency department may be performed. An above-knee cast is applied. If plain radiographs show satisfactory reduction, a CT scan is obtained. If reduction is acceptable, treatment is the same as for nondisplaced fractures, though weight bearing could be delayed until 5 to 6 weeks.

If the reduction is unacceptable, closed reduction is attempted in the operating room with the use of general anesthesia. If fluoroscopy shows an acceptable reduction, percutaneous screws are inserted, avoiding the physis, and a short-leg cast is applied. If closed reduction is unacceptable, open reduction or mini-open reduction with the use of percutaneous clamps is performed. Preoperative CT scanning may be helpful for evaluating the position of the fracture fragments in the anteroposterior and lateral planes and for determining the appropriate skin incisions, percutaneous clamp placements, and screw location.

Open Reduction of Triplane Fracture

The patient is placed supine on a radiolucent operating table with padded elevation behind the hip on the affected side. The surgical approach depends on the fracture anatomy as determined by the preoperative CT scan can be quite variable, and may even require more than one incision. The goal is that the joint surface must be able to be assessed. A two-part medial triplane fracture can be approached through a hockey-stick anteromedial incision. The fracture fragments are irrigated to remove debris, and any interposed periosteum is removed. The fracture is reduced, and reduction is confirmed by direct observation through an anteromedial arthrotomy and by image intensification. Two 4-mm cancellous screws are inserted from medial to lateral or from anterior to posterior or both, depending on the fracture pattern (Fig. 26-61). Anterior to posterior screw placement may require an additional anterolateral incision or the screws may be inserted percutaneously making sure certain neurovascular structures are not damaged. Arthroscopic-assisted techniques with the use of percutaneous clamps and screws may also be used (Fig. 26-62).

For two-part lateral triplane fractures, these can be approached with a hockey-stick anterolateral approach. The fracture is reduced and stabilized with two screws placed from lateral to medial or from anterior to posterior or both, and reduction is confirmed through direct observation and by image intensification. In addition to open techniques, arthroscopic-assisted techniques with the use of percutaneous clamps and screws may also be used (see Fig. 26-62).

Fractures with three or more parts may occasionally require more exposure for reduction and internal fixation. Posteromedial approaches to the tibia can be used, with careful attention to the surrounding neurovascular bundle and tendons. If the fibula is fractured, posterior exposure of the tibial fracture can be readily obtained by detaching the anterior and posterior inferior tibiofibular ligaments and turning down the distal fibula on the lateral collateral ligament (Fig. 26-63). If the fibula is not fractured, a fibular osteotomy may be performed, though this is uncommonly necessary. Careful dissection is necessary to avoid iatrogenic fractures through the physis of the fibula. Medial exposure is obtained through an anteromedial or posteromedial incision. Reduction and internal fixation are carried out in a stepwise fashion. For typical three-part fractures, the Salter-Harris type II fracture may be reduced first by provisional fixation to the distal tibia through the metaphyseal fragment. Usually, the Salter-Harris type III fragment can then be reduced and provisionally fixed to the stabilized type II fragment (Fig. 26-64). Occasionally, the order of reduction and fixation should be reversed. Fractures with four or more fragments require additional steps, but fixation of the Salter-Harris type II or IV fragment through the metaphysis to the distal tibia is usually best performed first. This step can be followed by fixation of the Salter-Harris type III fragment or fragments (Fig. 26-65). After reduction, reliable patients may be treated with immobilization in a short-leg, nonweight-bearing cast

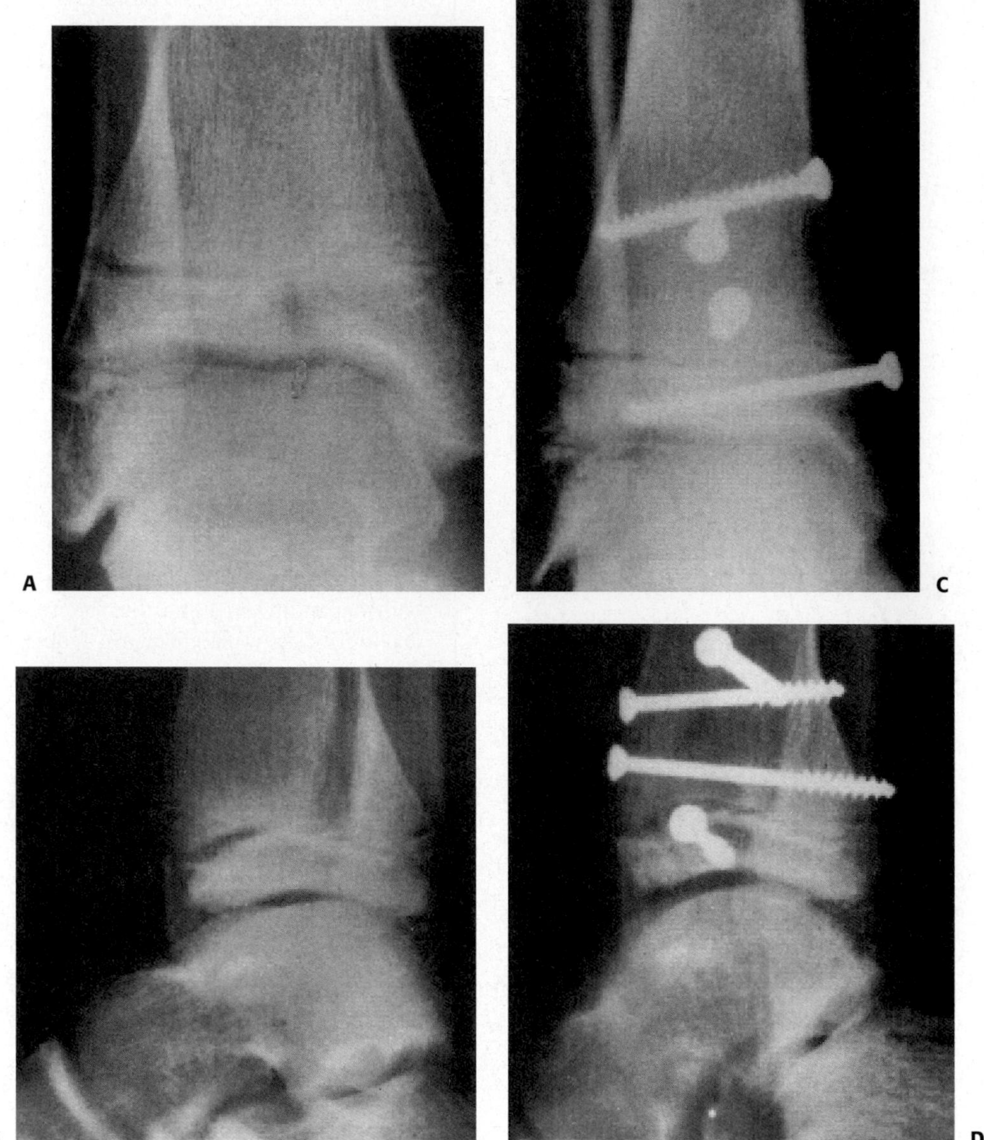

FIGURE 26-61 A,B. Irreducible three-part triplane fracture in a 13-year-old girl. **C,D.** After open reduction with internal fixation. Note anterior-to-posterior and medial-to-lateral screw placement that avoids the physis.

for 3 to 4 weeks. At 3–4 weeks, they may be converted to a weight-bearing cast or walking boot for an additional 2 to 4 weeks if there is stable fixation of the joint surface.

Pearls and Pitfalls: Open Reduction with Internal Fixation of Physeal Ankle Fractures

Soft Tissue Healing Problems

Under ideal circumstances, open reduction with internal fixation of ankle fractures is best done before excessive swelling occurs. Markedly swollen ankles often develop fracture blisters, which may become infected. The integrity of skin closure and, even more important, the vascularity of the wound edges also are threatened by excessive soft tissue swelling. When marked soft tissue swelling develops before surgery can be performed, elevation of the extremity in a soft compression bandage until swelling begins to subside is recommended, usually for no more than 5 days.

Partially Healed or Comminuted Physis

On occasion, inspection of the fractured fragments at the time of open reduction and internal fixation reveals comminution at the physeal line. In such cases, débridement of loose fragments back to normal-appearing physis and the insertion of a fat graft into the resulting void are recommended. This technique also can be useful for fractures that present for treatment a week or more after injury. Early callus that prevents the apposition of healthy physeal tissue at the fracture site is débrided and a fat graft is inserted (Fig. 26-66).

Fracture Reduction Tips, Arthroscopic Assistance, Use of Percutaneous Clamps, Implants

Ankle Distraction

Some advocate use of the ankle distractor (normally used for arthroscopy procedures) to assist with reduction of displaced

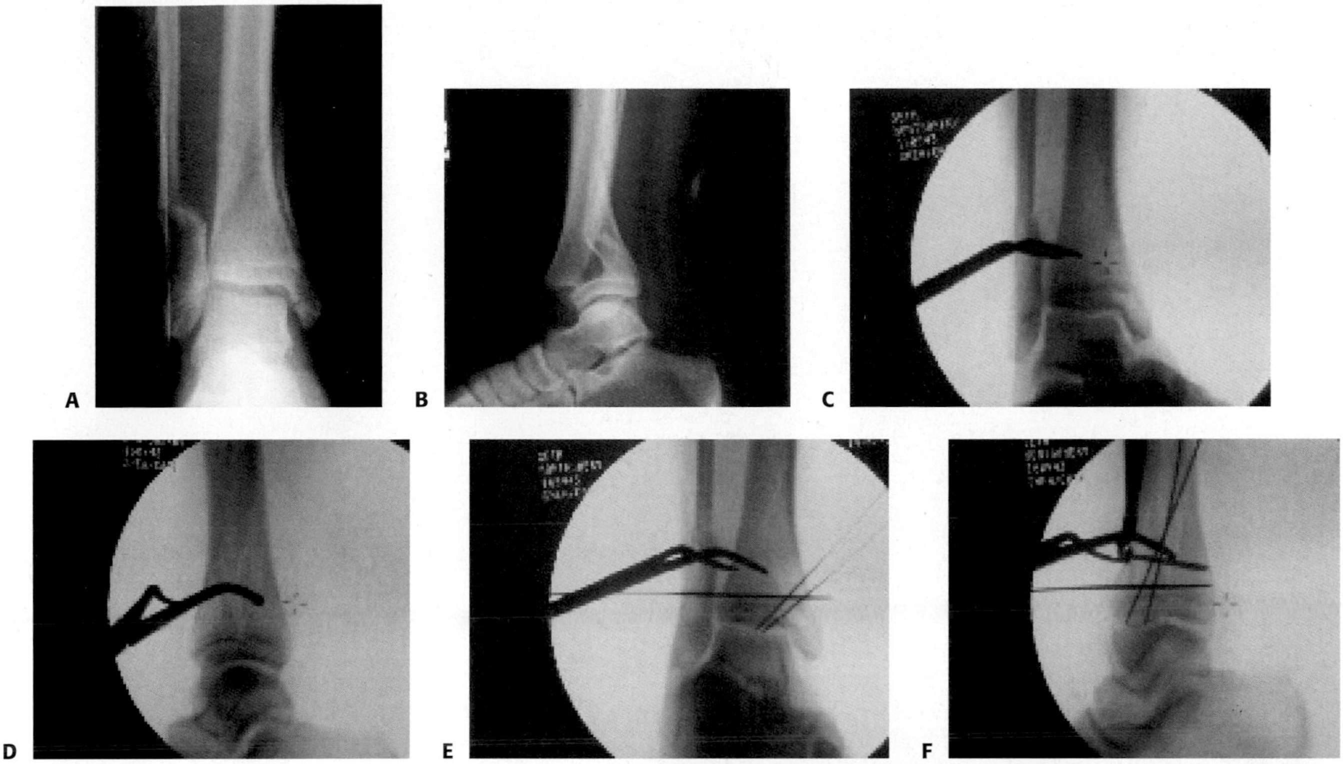

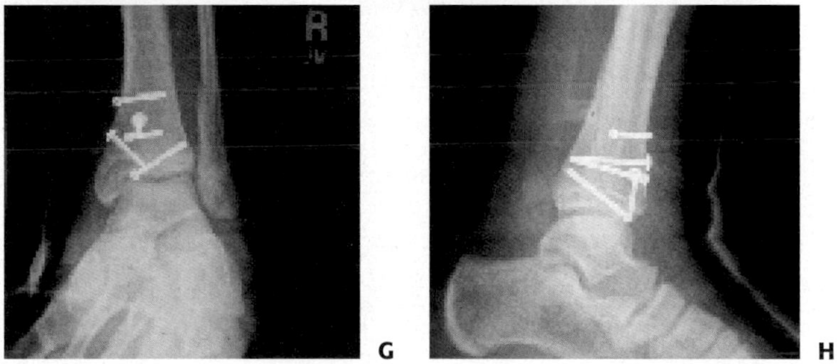

FIGURE 26-62 A,B. Anteroposterior and lateral radiograph of triplane fracture with involvement of medial malleolus. **C,D.** Use of percutaneous clamps for reduction, viewed in the anteroposterior plane **(C)** and in the lateral plane **(D)**. **E,F.** Use of percutaneous clamps for reduction, followed by placement of guidewires to hold reduction. **G,H.** Percutaneous and mini-open placement of cannulated screws, anteroposterior view **(G)** and lateral view **(H)**.

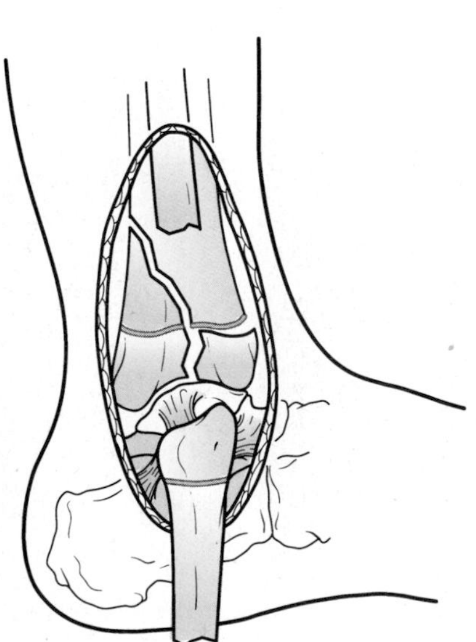

FIGURE 26-63 Transfibular approach to a complex triplane fracture.

extra-articular fractures, such as Salter-Harris type I or II patterns. When combined with the relaxation of general anesthesia, a few minutes of distraction across the physis may facilitate reduction. Some believe that distraction across the fracture may increase the likelihood that the first attempt at reduction will be successful; this may reduce the trauma to the physis during the reduction, perhaps reducing the risk of physeal arrest. Juvenile Tillaux and triplane fracture reduction can also be facilitated with ankle distraction, and this will also facilitate arthroscopic ankle visualization. Instead of having the surgeon pull manually for several minutes, the ankle distractor can provide this distraction force. The surgeon can then focus on the application of other forces, such as rotation or varus/valgus to facilitate fracture reduction. Although skeletal traction using a calcaneal pin is an option,[33] we prefer to use an ankle strap and special distractor routinely used for arthroscopy (Arthrex, Naples, FL). The ankle distractor can be position to allow for anteroposterior and lateral C-Arm images (see Fig. 26-34).

Imaging Studies

Use of CT scans can be very beneficial for evaluating intra-articular fractures or multiplanar fractures. High resolution scans with three-dimensional reconstructions provide excellent anatomic detail. For minimally invasive approaches using percutaneous screw fixation, these images can be used for precise screw

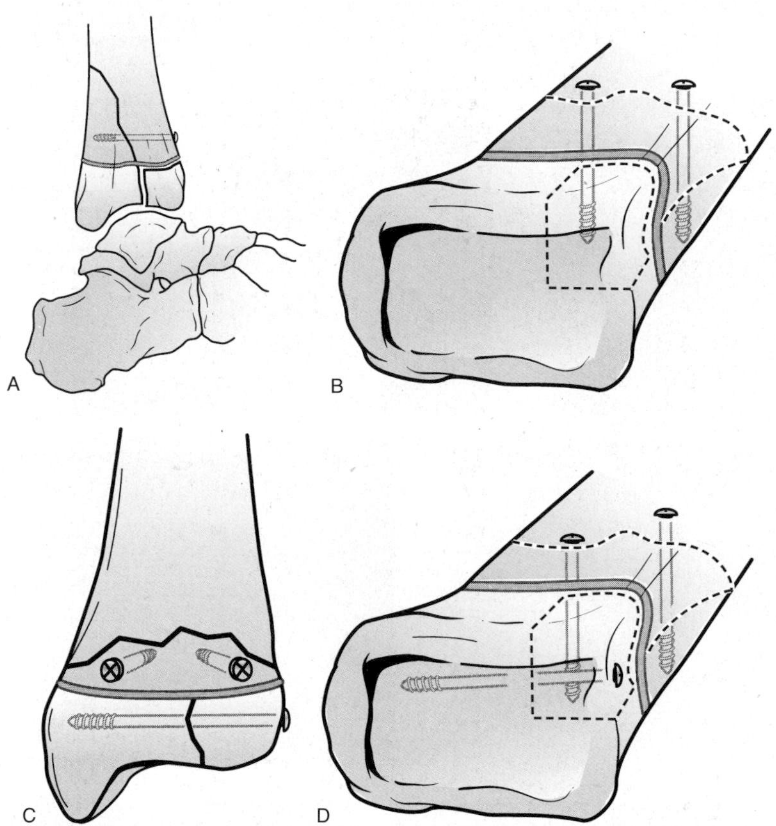

FIGURE 26-64 Open reduction with internal fixation of a three-part lateral triplane fracture. **A,B.** Reduction and fixation of the Salter-Harris type II fragment to the metaphysis. **C,D.** Reduction and internal fixation of the Salter-Harris type III fragment to the Salter-Harris type II fragment.

placement during surgery. The CT scan can also facilitate placement of clamp, to allow for compression in the plane perpendicular to the fracture. A clear preoperative evaluation should determine optimal screw position and orientation, and these images should also be available during the procedure to assist with screw placement.

Arthroscopy

The use of arthroscopy can facilitate minimally invasive procedures. Several clinical series document the effectiveness of arthroscopic assistance for Tillaux fractures[122,137] and triplane fractures.[79] The joint surfaces can be readily visualized through small incisions, avoiding the need for a larger arthrotomy. Even in cases where an arthrotomy is used, the scope can be utilized either with or without fluid to visualize the reduction of the fragments in the joint (Fig. 26-67). The fluid of the arthroscopy pump can also be used to wash out the fracture site, increasing visualization during reduction. Avoidance of high pump pressure will minimize the risks of soft tissue infiltration.

Different size scopes are available, including 2.8 and 5.0 mm. Both scopes work well, although in smaller children, the 2.8 mm scope may be a better choice. The smaller scope has a smaller field of view, but this does not seem to be much of a disadvantage

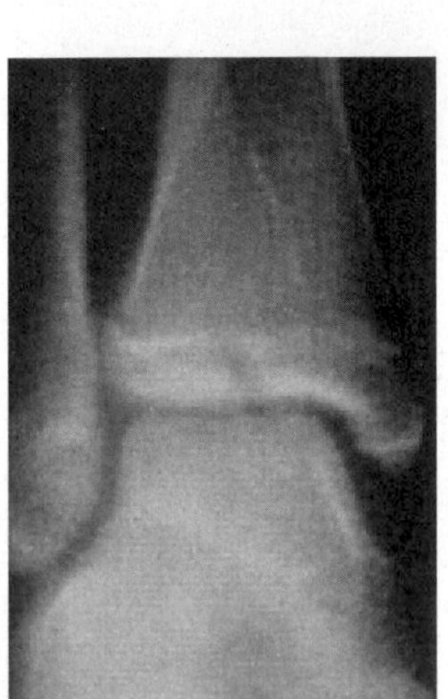

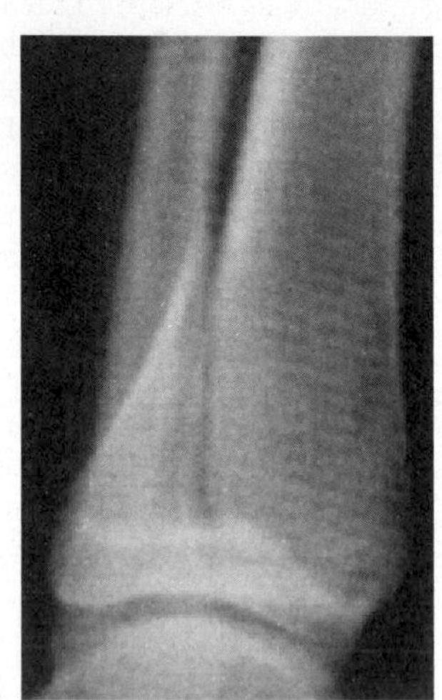

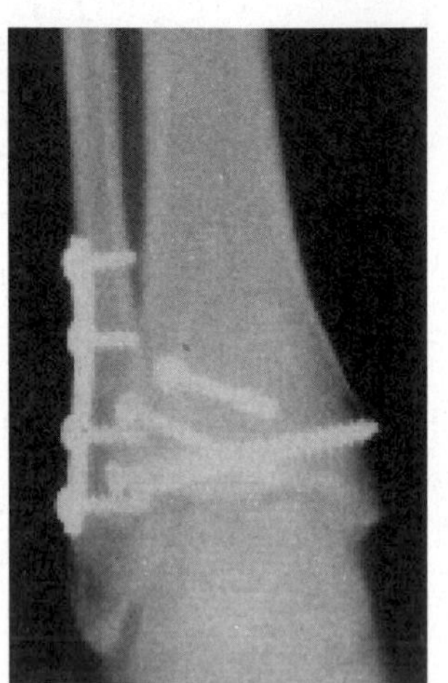

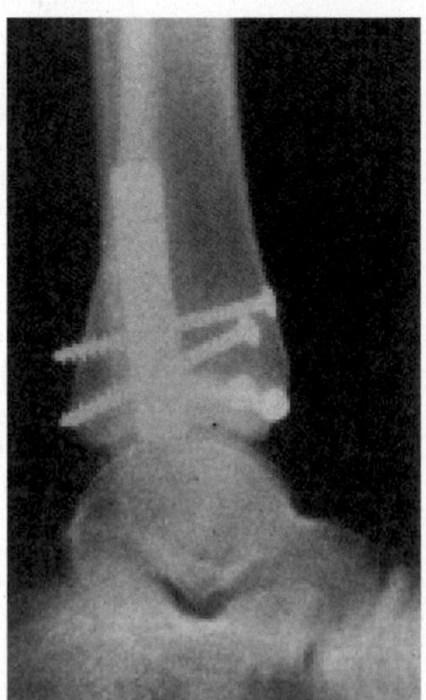

FIGURE 26-65 A,B. Irreducible three-part lateral triplane fracture in a 14-year-old boy. **C,D.** After open reduction through a transfibular approach and internal fixation with anterior-to-posterior and lateral-to-medial screws.

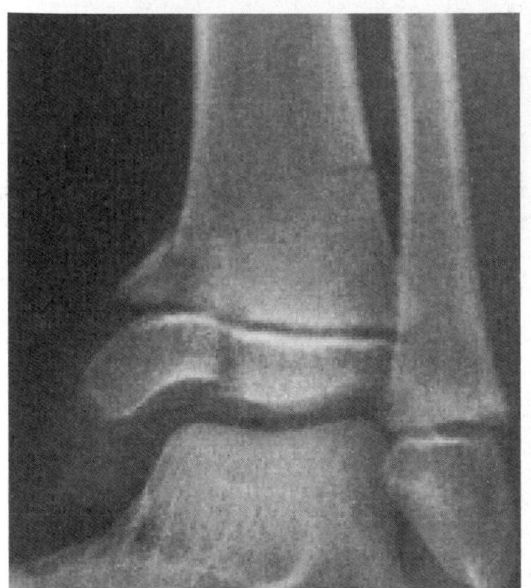
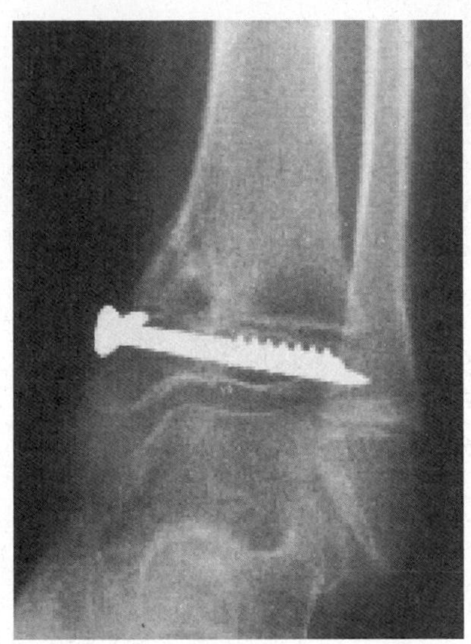
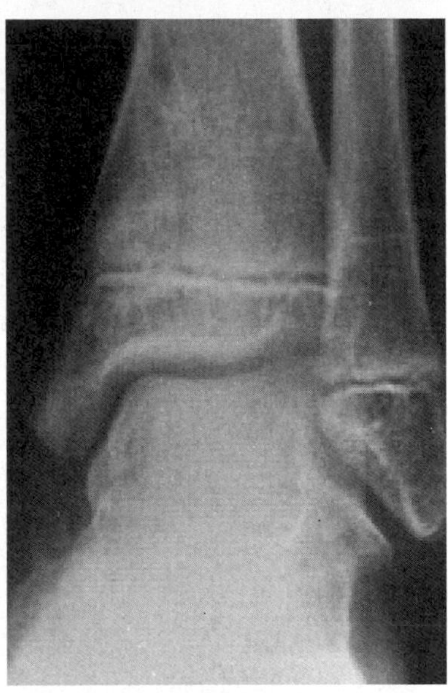

FIGURE 26-66 A. An 8-year-old girl who presented 10 days after a displaced Salter-Harris type IV fracture of the distal tibia. **B.** At open reduction, comminution of the physis was noted. The physis was débrided, and a fat graft was inserted before reduction and internal fixation of the fracture. **C.** Three years after injury, there is no evidence of physeal bar formation or growth abnormality.

for viewing the displaced cartilage surfaces. The smaller scope also delivers less fluid to the joint, which may require additional time to clean the hematoma from the joint and fracture, but has a lower risk of causing soft tissue infiltration around the joint.

Use of Small C-Arm Unit

The small C-arm unit will also assist with minimally invasive approaches. This can be easily rotated to allow for anteroposterior or lateral views. If the ankle distractor is used, position the foot and distractor to allow easy access by the C-arm (see Fig. 26-34).

Percutaneous Clamps

Precise placement of clamps can facilitate the reduction of fractures. Careful study of imaging studies, especially CT scans, can guide precise placement of clamps to provide maximal compression across fracture planes. Forces normal or near normal to the fracture planes are ideal. Care should be taken during placement to prevent injury to neurovascular structures, including sensory nerves. The skin can be divided, and then deeper dissection through the subcutaneous tissues can be performed with a hemostat. The hemostat is used to bluntly distract the tissues away from the skin portal and then advanced to the bone surface. The tips of the clamp can now be placed with minimal risk to neurovascular structures. The clamp can be compressed to facilitate reduction of triplane and Tillaux fractures (see Figs. 26-50, 26-51, and 26-62).

Implants

Different implants are available for fixation of ankle fractures. Smooth pins have the advantage that they do not place a threaded tip across the physis, therefore reducing the risk of iatrogenic physeal arrest. The main disadvantage of smooth pins is that they do not allow for compression. These pins can also migrate through bone and into soft tissues. Bending the ends at the surface of the bone to prevent migration is important. These pins should be removed early, as soon as the fracture stability is adequate.

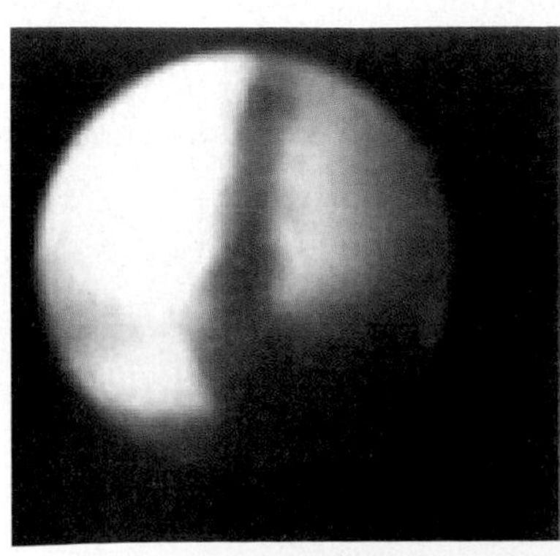
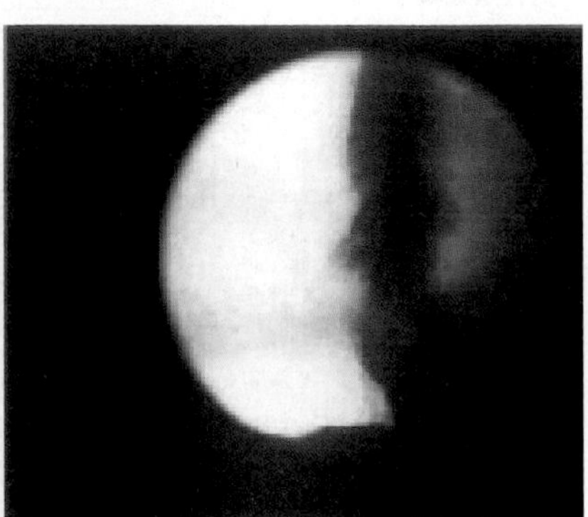
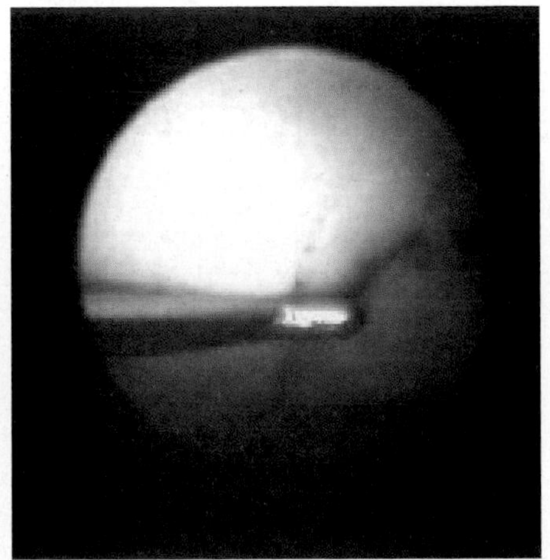

FIGURE 26-67 Ankle arthroscopy. **A.** Arthroscopic view of fracture gap in distal tibia articular surface. **B.** Arthroscopic view of fracture gap in distal tibial articular surface after reduction.

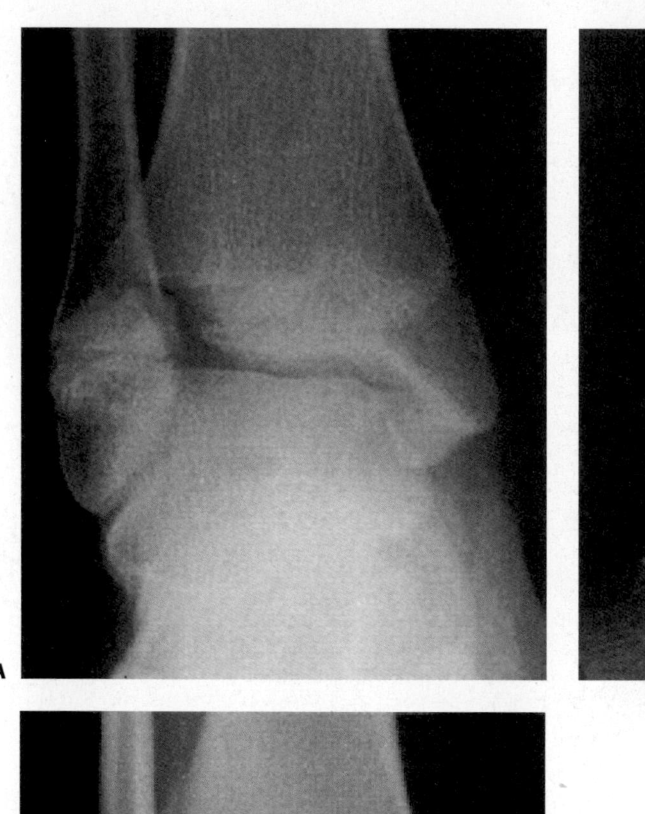

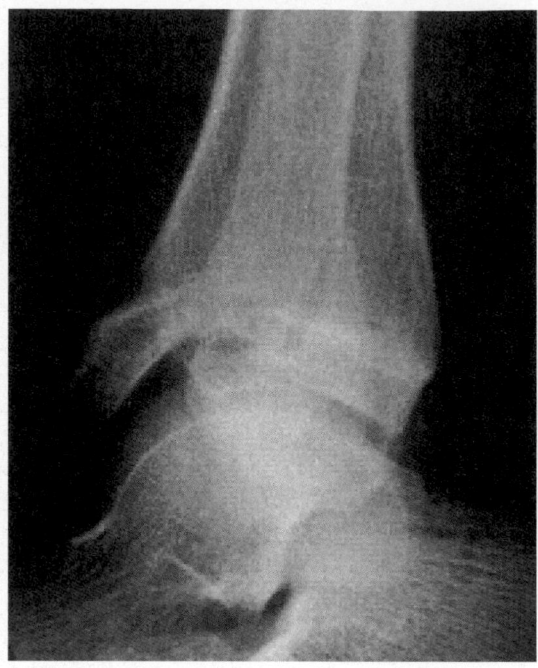

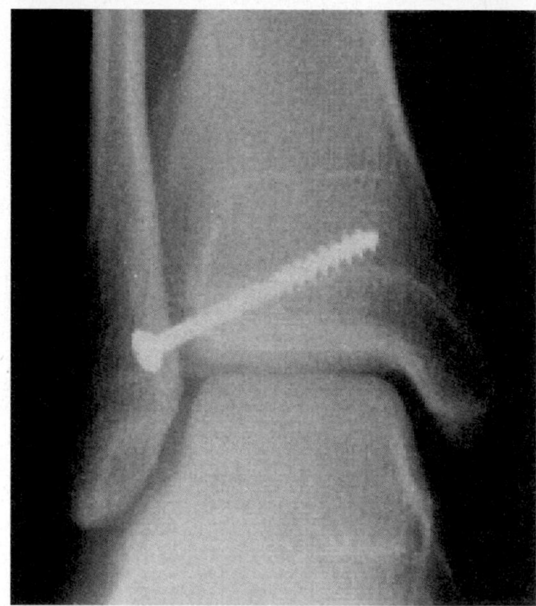

FIGURE 26-68 A,B. Displaced juvenile Tillaux fracture. Closed reduction was not successful. **C.** After open reduction with internal fixation with a small fragment screw.

In most physeal injuries, the use of screws or threaded devices across the physis should be avoided. In some cases, a screw implant may be necessary to cross a physis to maintain an articular reduction. The adequacy of reduction of the joint surface probably is probably more important than the physis. In patients approaching skeletally maturity, the use of screw implants across a physis that is approaching closure is probably a reasonable choice, especially in case where compression and/or stability are important, such as juvenile Tillaux fractures (Fig. 26-68).

Fractures Involving the Distal Fibula

We usually treat nondisplaced fibular physeal fractures with immobilization in a below-knee walking cast for 3 to 4 weeks. Closed reduction of displaced Salter-Harris types I and II fibular fractures is performed, but when reduction is unsuccessful, one of the authors (R. Jay Cummings) accepts up to 50% displacement without problems at long-term follow-up. Acceptance of this displacement may be more reasonable in young patients with significant remodeling potential, although in older patients, displaced fractures may have more affect on ankle function, and more anatomic reduction may be advantageous. Dias,[48] however, reported a patient with a symptomatic spike that required excision after inadequate reduction.

Lateral Ankle Sprains and Lateral Ligament Avulsion Injuries

The diagnosis of an ankle sprain is less common in younger patients, as these individuals are more likely to have nondisplaced distal fibular physeal injuries. If the pain can be localized to the ligaments and there is not pain over the distal fibular physis, then a true ankle sprain may be present. Chronic pain and instability can occur in young patients, especially adolescents. Brostom type reconstruction[24] may be appropriate in these patients, although Letts et al.[106] has described nonanatomic reconstruction in younger patients using nonanatomic reconstructions (Evans, Watson-Jones, Chrisman, and Snook techniques).

Avulsion fractures can be identified that originate from the distal fibula, and special radiographic views may facilitate diagnosis.[69] These avulsion type injuries can lead to symptoms, and a high index of suspicion is important in younger patients. Haraguchi et al.[70] evaluated a series of severe ankle sprains, and found that 26% had evidence of distal fibular avulsion injury. Children and adults over 40 years of age had the highest incidence of this injury. Patients were treated with weight-bearing casts for 3 to 4 weeks. Nonoperative treatment yielded satisfactory results in this series.

Rehabilitation

For patients treated with cast immobilization, quadriceps, hamstring, and abductor exercises are begun as soon as pain and swelling allow. Usually, a below-knee cast is worn during the last 2 to 3 weeks of immobilization, and weight bearing to tolerance is allowed during this time. After immobilization is discontinued, ankle range-of-motion exercises and strengthening exercises are begun. Protective splinting or bracing is usually not required after cast removal. Running is restricted until the patient demonstrates an essentially full, painless range of ankle and foot motion and can walk without a limp. Running progresses from jogging to more strenuous running and jumping as soreness and endurance dictate. For athletes, unrestricted running and jumping ability should be achieved before return to sports. Protective measures such as taping or bracing are recommended initially for return to most sports.

Younger patients with physeal ankle fractures recover quickly and require little or no formal physical therapy. For this reason, and because of compliance considerations, fractures treated with internal fixation are usually protected with below-knee casting instead of starting an early range-of-motion program in a removable splint. In older patients that may have a higher risk of arthrofibrosis, we may start early motion in a removable boot and start a formal supervised physical therapy program.

PROGNOSIS AND COMPLICATIONS

Delayed Union and Nonunion

Delayed union and nonunion are rare after distal tibial physeal fractures (Fig. 26-69). Dias[48] reported one patient with a delayed union and one patient with a previous physeal bar excision who had a nonunion that healed after open reduction, internal fixation, and bone grafting. Siffert[172] reported nonunion in a patient with avascular necrosis of the distal tibial epiphysis. We have seen two younger patients with Salter-Harris type III fractures that appeared to be progressing to nonunion. Because neither patient had any complaints of pain nor any evidence of progressive displacement of the fracture and stress views showed no instability, no treatment was undertaken. Both fractures eventually united. We have seen one patient with a nonunion after open reduction and internal fixation in whom pin

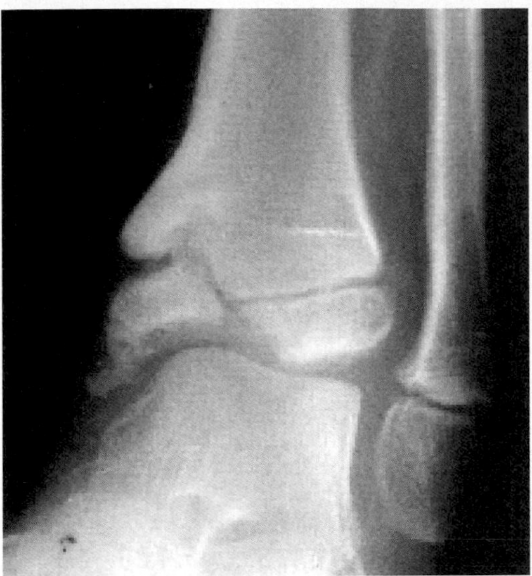

FIGURE 26-69 Complex nonunion of a Salter-Harris type III fracture of the medial malleolus in an 8-year-old boy. Note that the distal tibial epiphysis is in valgus, whereas the talus is in varus. (Courtesy of Brent Broztman, MD.)

fixation and cast immobilization were discontinued prematurely. The fracture healed after repeat open reduction and internal fixation.

Nonunion of a fracture of the fibular epiphysis has been reported by Mirimiran.[123] This was treated successfully with open reduction and internal fixation.

Deformity Secondary to Malunion

Rotational malunion usually occurs after triplane fractures that are either incompletely reduced or are initially immobilized in below-knee casts. It has also been reported after Salter-Harris type I and II injuries. Derotational osteotomy may be performed for extra-articular fractures if discomfort and stiffness occur. Guille et al.[67] reported a rotational malunion of lateral malleolar fracture that led to a stress fracture of the distal fibula that went on to delayed union. Their patient required correction of the malrotated distal fibula and bone grafting of the delayed union site.

Anterior angulation or plantarflexion deformity usually occurs after supination–plantarflexion Salter-Harris type II fractures. Theoretically, an equinus deformity might occur if the angulation exceeds the range of ankle dorsiflexion before fracture, but this is very rare, probably because the deformity is in the plane of joint motion and tends to remodel with growth.

Valgus deformity is most common after external rotation Salter-Harris type II fractures. The degree to which the deformity may spontaneously resolve or remodel with growth is controversial. Caruthers and Crenshaw[31] reported resolution of a 12 degrees valgus deformity in a 13.5-year-old boy, but Spiegel and associates[175] reported persistent residual deformity in a significant number of their patients (Fig. 26-70). Varus deformity most often results from growth abnormality and infrequently is the result of simple malunion.

If significant angular deformity persists at the completion of growth, supramalleolar osteotomy should be performed. Moon et al.[124] followed 9 children with posttraumatic varus deformi-

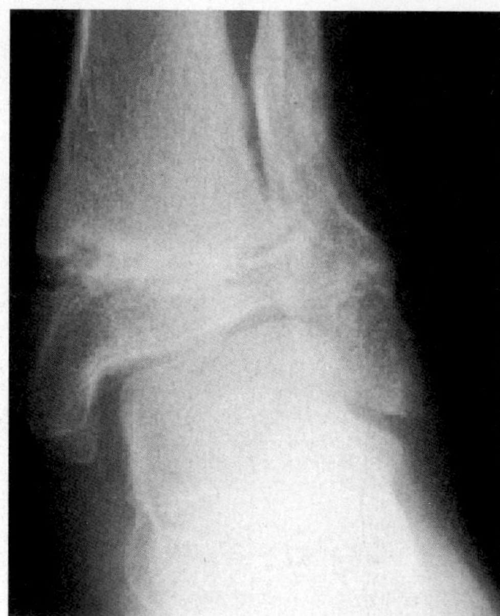

FIGURE 26-70 Radiograph of a 14-year-old boy, 4 months after pronation–eversion–external rotation injury, reveals 16 degrees of valgus angulation.

ties of the ankle secondary to supination inversion injuries. These patients went on to develop medial subluxation of their ankles with associated internal rotational deformity. Takakura et al.[180] described successful open wedge osteotomy for varus deformity in nine patients. Scheffer and Peterson[164] recommend opening wedge osteotomy when the angular deformity is 25 degrees or less and the limb length discrepancy is or will be 25 mm or less at maturity.[164] Preoperative planning should include templating the various types of osteotomies to determine which technique will maintain the proper mechanical alignment of the tibia and ankle joint and will not make the malleoli unduly prominent (Fig. 26-71).

The use of the Taylor Spatial Frame continues to evolve. Its use for correction of complex deformities can allow for multiplanar corrections, including rotation, length, and angular deformity. For more complex deformities, this device may be useful for correction.[55,171]

Physeal Arrest or Growth Disturbance

Deformity caused by growth arrest usually occurs after Salter-Harris types III and IV fractures in which a physeal bar develops at the fracture site, leading to varus deformity that progresses with continued growth. Spiegel and associates[175] reported growth problems in 9 of 66 patients with Salter-Harris type II fractures.

Earlier reports[31,42,63] attributed the development of physeal bars to crushing of the physis at the time of injury, but more recent reports[83,100] discount this explanation and claim that with anatomic reduction (open reduction and internal fixation if needed), the incidence of physeal bar formation can be decreased. The validity of this claim is difficult to determine from published reports. One problem is the small numbers of patients in all series and the even smaller numbers within each group in each series. Another problem is the age of the patients in operative and nonoperative groups in the various series; for example, many children reported to do well with a particular treatment method have so little growth remaining that treatment may have had little or no effect on growth.

A recent study by Rohmiller et al.[157] analyzed the outcome of 91 Salter-Harris type I and II fractures of the distal tibia. They identified premature physeal closure in 40%. This series identified a trend towards increased premature physeal closure in fractures that had worse displacement after reduction. They recommended operative reduction to restore anatomic alignment to reduce the risk of premature physeal closure.

Kling and coworkers[100] reported physeal bars in 2 of 5 patients treated nonoperatively and in none of 3 patients treated operatively in children 10 years of age and younger. In another series of 65 physeal ankle fractures, Kling and coworkers[99] concluded that the frequency of growth-related deformities could be reduced by open reduction and internal fixation of Salter-Harris type III and IV fractures.

However, in one of the author's experiences with 8 patients (R. Jay Cummings), 2 of 5 treated operatively developed physeal bars, while none of the 3 patients treated nonoperatively had physeal bars. This supports the conclusion of Cass and Peterson,[32] Ogden,[134] and others that growth problems after these injuries may not always be prevented by open reduction and internal fixation. Open reduction of displaced Salter-Harris type III and IV ankle fractures would seem advisable to restore joint congruity, regardless of whether growth potential can be preserved.

Harris growth lines have been reported to be reliable predictors of growth abnormality,[78] but one of the authors (R. Jay Cummings) has found that, although lines parallel to the physis are reliable, lines that appear to diverge from the physis may be misleading (Fig. 26-72). Harcke and colleagues[72] reported early detection of growth arrest with bone scanning techniques. The use of bone scan techniques may have very limited indications with the availability of MRI and CT Scans.

Spontaneous resolution of physeal bars has been reported[19,35] but is rare. Most patients require excision of small bony bars and may require correction of significant angular deformity with osteotomy (Fig. 26-73).

Karrholm and coworkers[90] reported progressive ankle deformity caused by complete growth arrest of the fibula with normal growth of the tibia (Fig. 26-74). They found that continued fibular growth with complete arrest of tibial growth was usually compensated by proximal migration of the fibula so that varus deformity did not occur.

Because the amount of growth remaining in the distal tibial physis is small (approximately 0.25 in per year) in most older patients with these injuries, the amount of leg-length discrepancy resulting from complete growth arrest tends to be relatively small. Treatment may be required if the anticipated discrepancy is projected to be clinically significant.

Imaging techniques to identify physeal arrest and bars include plane radiographs, tomography, CT, and MRI. In most imaging departments, standard tomography has been replaced by CT. CT scans can be useful for clear delineation of the anatomy, especially in cases in which surgical intervention is necessary. Recent studies have also used MRI scans.[60,110,163] Although the resolution capability is more limited, the avoidance of ionizing radiation is a major advantage of MRI scans over

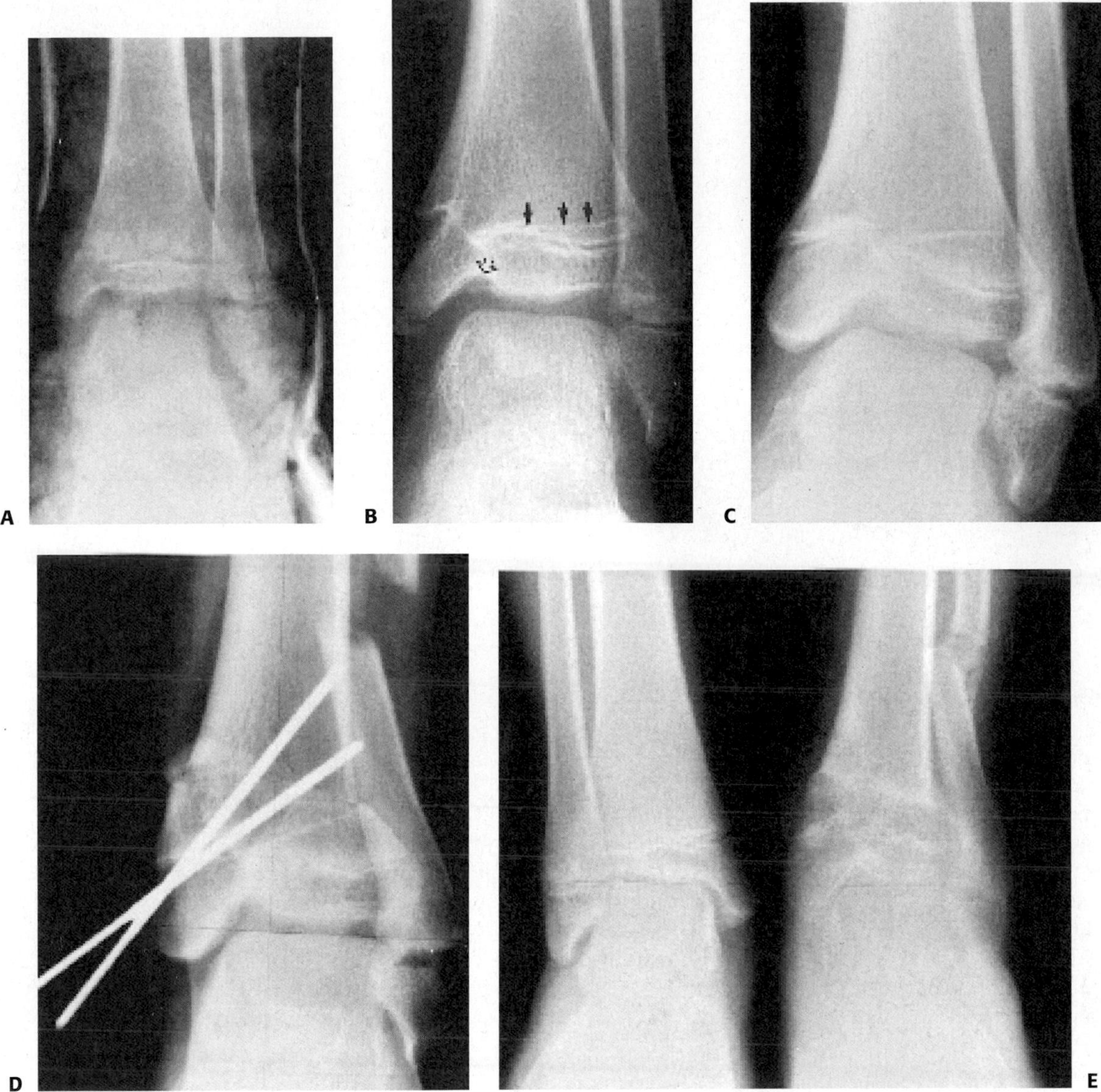

FIGURE 26-71 A. This apparently nondisplaced medial malleolar fracture in an 11-year-old boy was treated with immobilization in a long-leg cast. **B.** Fourteen months after injury, there is a clear medial osseous bridge and asymmetric growth of the Park-Harris growth arrest lines (*black arrows*). Note the early inhibition of growth on the subchondral surface of the fracture (*open arrow*). **C.** Five years after injury, the varus deformity has increased significantly and fibular overgrowth is apparent. **D.** The deformity was treated with a medial opening-wedge osteotomy of the tibia, an osteotomy of the fibula, and epiphysiodesis of the most lateral portion of the tibial physis and fibula. **E.** Three months after surgery, the osteotomies are healed and the varus deformity is corrected; the joint surface remains irregular. (Courtesy of Earl A. Stanley, Jr., MD.)

CT scans, though the ankle is much less sensitive to radiation than many central organs.

Physeal arrest of the distal tibia has been reported after fracture of the tibial diaphysis, in the absence of obvious physeal injury.[128]

Medial Malleolus Overgrowth

Overgrowth of the medial malleolus has been reported fractures of the distal tibia metaphysis and epiphysis. A recent series of 83 patients with fractures in this region demonstrated 2 patients with medial malleolus overgrowth. In both cases, there was no evidence of functional impairment.[129]

Arthritis

Epiphyseal ankle fractures that do not extend into the joint have a low risk of posttraumatic arthritis, but injuries that extend into the joint may produce this complication. Caterini and coworkers[34] found that 8 of 68 (12%) patients had pain and stiffness that began from 5 to 8 years after skeletal maturity. Ertl and associates[53] found that 18 to 36 months after injury 20 patients with triplane fractures were asymptomatic, but at 36 months to 13 years after injury only 8 of 15 patients evaluated were asymptomatic.[53]

Ramsey and Hamilton[151] demonstrated in a cadaver study that 1 mm of lateral talar displacement decreases tibiotalar contact area by 42%, which greatly increases the stress on

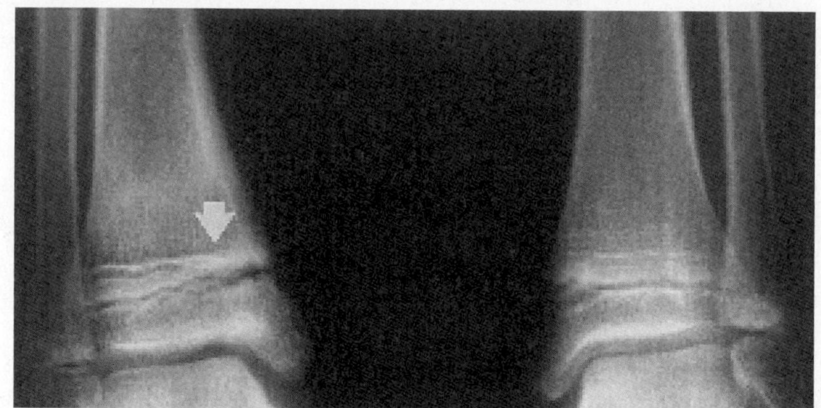

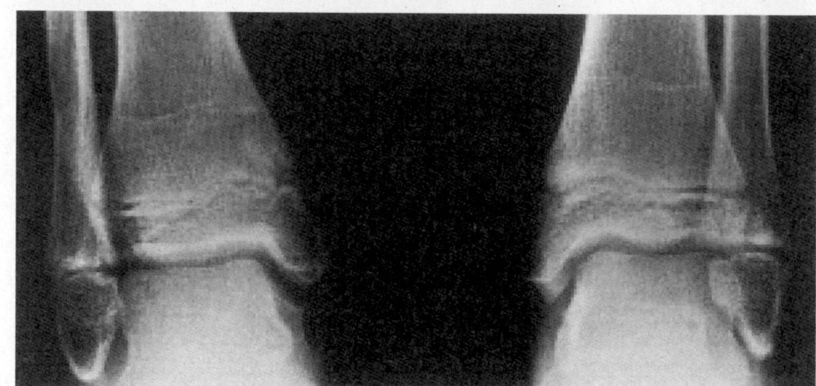

FIGURE 26-72 A. Six months after cast immobilization of a nondisplaced supination–inversion Salter-Harris type III fracture of the right distal tibia in an 8-year-old boy. The Park-Harris growth arrest line (*arrow*) appears to end in the physis medially and diverge from the physis laterally. **B.** Two years later, no physeal bar is present and growth is normal.

this weight-bearing joint. More recently, Michelson and colleagues[121] reported that a cadaver study using unconstrained specimens suggested that some lateral talar displacement occurs with normal weight bearing. Because of their findings, they questioned the current criterion of 2 mm of displacement for unstable ankle fractures. However, the results of Ramsey and Hamilton's[151] study correlate well with other studies that have shown increased symptoms in patients in whom more than 2 mm of displacement was accepted.[34,53]

Implant removal after fracture surgery remains controversial, and the indications for removal are not well-defined in the literature.[28] Charlton et al.[37] has demonstrated the periepiphyseal or subchondral screws may alter the joint contact pressures about the ankle. After removal of the screws from the subchon-

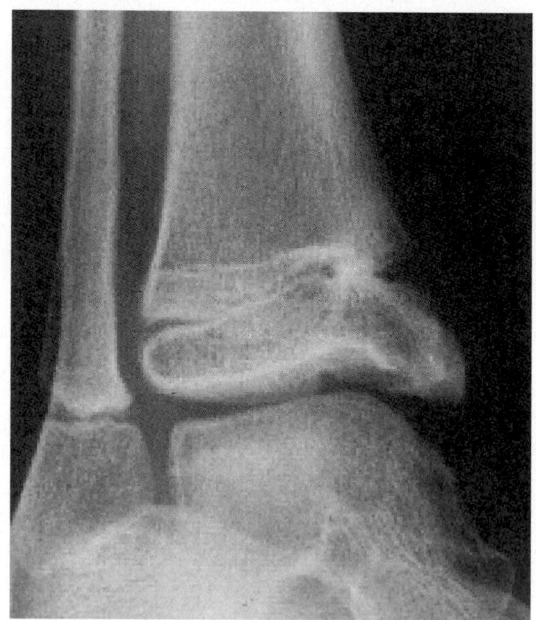

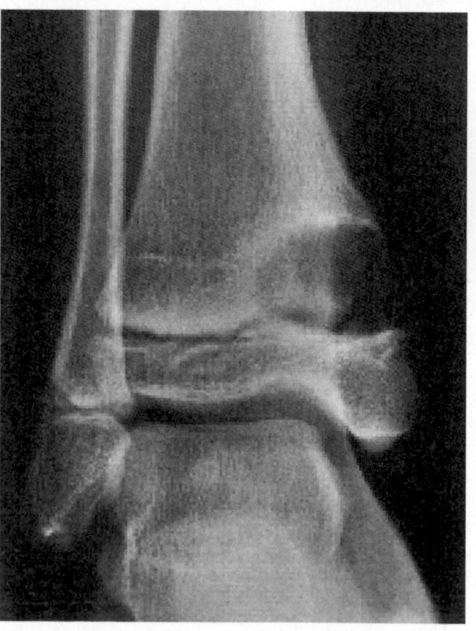

FIGURE 26-73 A. One year after open reduction and internal fixation of a Salter-Harris type III fracture of the distal tibia in a 7-year-old boy, varus deformity has been caused by a physeal bar. **B.** Two years after excision of the physeal bar and insertion of cranioplast, satisfactory growth has resumed and the deformity has resolved.

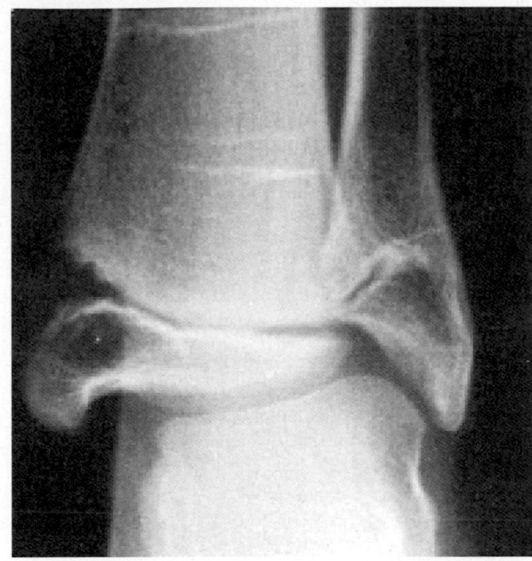

FIGURE 26-74 Valgus deformity of the ankle, lateral displacement of the talus with widening of the joint medially, and severe shortening of the fibula after early physeal arrest in a child who sustained an ankle injury at 6 years of age. (Courtesy of James Roach, MD.)

dral bone, the contact pressure normalized. For hardware in the subchondral bone, the study suggested that implant removal in transepiphyseal screws may be appropriate.[37]

Chondrolysis

Chondrolysis is a rare complication of adolescent ankle fractures.[14,162] Treatment options include therapy and nonsteroidal anti-inflammatory drugs, etc. Recent clinical studies have evaluated the affects of joint distraction for posttraumatic chondrolysis, although experience with this technique in young patients is very limited.[162]

Osteonecrosis of the Distal Tibial Epiphysis

Siffert and Arkin,[172] in 1950, were the first to call attention to this complication of distal tibial fractures. In their patient, the combination of nonunion of a medial malleolar fracture and avascular necrosis caused pain that required an arthrodesis 14 months after injury. Dias[47] reported a patient with this complication who did not require arthrodesis but who had a significant leg-length discrepancy that required epiphysiodesis of the contralateral tibia. We have seen one patient with this complication. The patient had significant joint stiffness and developed a valgus deformity secondary to collapse. After revascularization of the epiphysis, the ankle was realigned with a supramalleolar osteotomy, and 5 years later the patient had satisfactory function without pain.

Compartment Syndrome

Fractures of the distal tibia and ankle joint are associated with compartment syndromes,[40,126] similar to fractures in other regions of the leg. Mubarak[126] has described a unique compartment syndrome associated with distal tibial physeal fractures in 6 patients. These patients had clinical symptoms of severe pain and swelling, with associated sensory and motor deficits. The compartment pressure below the superior extensor retinaculum was above 40 mm in all cases, and the pressure was less than 20 mm in the anterior compartment. These patients were treated with limited fascial release of the superior extensor retinaculum and fracture stabilization.

Synostosis

Posttraumatic tibia-fibular synostosis is a rare complication of fractures in this region. This can lead to growth disturbance, including angular deformity and lower extremity length discrepancy.[58,127] Synostosis in this area alters the normal pattern of movement between the tibia and fibula and has been associated with pain in some patients. In a small clinical series, Frick et al.[58] demonstrated symptoms of pain, prominence of the fibula, and ankle deformity in 5 of 8 patients with this synostosis. In this series, the normal growth pattern of distal migration of the fibula was altered, resulting in decrease distances between the proximal physes of the tibia and fibula and proximal positioning of the distal fibula with respect to the distal tibia. Munjal et al.[127] demonstrated successful synostosis excision in a 7-year-old patient, which lead to normalization of the ankle joint at 16 months postsurgery.

Reflex Sympathetic Dystrophy/Complex Regional Pain Syndrome

Reflex sympathetic dystrophy or complex regional pain syndrome occasionally develops after these injuries and is treated initially with an intensive formal physical therapy regimen that encourages range of motion and weight bearing.[92,191] For patients who do not respond quickly to such a program, physical therapy in association with continuous epidural analgesia may be considered.[191]

CONTROVERSIES AND FUTURE DIRECTIONS

Many questions remain unanswered about the optimal treatment of ankle fractures in skeletally immature patients. The relationship between physeal displacement and the development of subsequent physeal arrest is still unclear. Interposition of periosteum in the fracture may place a role in physeal arrest, although this has not been clarified in animal models or clinical trials.

Recent studies in the adult literature have suggested that minimally angular deformities about the distal tibia can have pronounced effects on the tibiotalar contact pressures.[92,182,184] The limits of fracture remodeling and the magnitude of acceptable deformity in growing children are still not well-defined in the literature.

Advanced imaging techniques have improved our understanding of these fractures, and may play an increasing role in the use of computer-aided reduction techniques and other forms of minimally invasive surgery. CT scanning requires ionizing radiation, but provides high-resolution model reconstruction. Future MRI modalities may allow for higher quality images, including three-dimensional reconstructions; this would avoid the need for ionizing radiation.

The use of cultured chondrocytes and gene therapy may eventually play a role in the treatment of these fractures, either to prevent or treat a physeal arrest.[96]

ACKNOWLEDGMENTS

The authors and editors wish to acknowledge Dr. Luciano Dias' past contributions to this chapter.

REFERENCES

1. Adler P. Ride-on Mower Hazard Analysis (1987-1990). Washington, DC: Consumer Product Safety Commission, 1993:1–65.
2. Aitken AP. The end results of the fractured distal tibial epiphysis. J Bone Joint Surg 1936;18:685–691.
3. Alonso JE, Sanchez FL. Lawnmower injuries in children: a preventable impairment. J Pediatr Orthop 1995;15(1):83–89.
4. Ashhurst APC, Bromer, RS. Classification and mechanism of fractures of the leg bones involving the ankle. Arch Surg 1922;4:51–129.
5. Assal M, Ray A, Stern R. The extensile approach for the operative treatment of high-energy pilon fractures: surgical technique and soft-tissue healing. J Orthop Trauma 2007;21(3):198–206.
6. Barmada A, Gaynor T, Mubarak SJ. Premature physeal closure following distal tibia physeal fractures: a new radiographic predictor. J Pediatr Orthop 2003;23(6):733–739.
7. Bartl R. Die traumatische epiphysenlosung am distalen ende des schienbeines und des wadenbeines. Hefte Unfallheilkd 1957;54:228–257.
8. Beaty JH, Linton RC. Medial malleolar fracture in a child. A case report. J Bone Joint Surg Am 1988;70(8):1254–1255.
9. Benz G, Kallieris D, Seebock T, et al. Bioresorbable pins and screws in paediatric traumatology. Eur J Pediatr Surg 1994;4(2):103–107.
10. Bishop PA. Fractures and epiphyseal separation fractures of the ankle. Am J Roentgenol and Rad Therap 1932;28:49–67.
11. Blair JM, Botte MJ. Surgical anatomy of the superficial peroneal nerve in the ankle and foot. Clin Orthop Relat Res 1994;305:229–238.
12. Blauth M, Bastian L, Krettek C, et al. Surgical options for the treatment of severe tibial pilon fractures: a study of three techniques. J Orthop Trauma 2001;15(3):153–160.
13. Blitzer CM, Johnson RJ, Ettlinger CF, et al. Downhill skiing injuries in children. Am J Sports Med 1984;12(2):142–147.
14. Bojescul JA, Wilson G, Taylor DC. Idiopathic chondrolysis of the ankle. Arthroscopy 2005;21(2):224–227.
15. Böstman O, Hirvensalo E, Vainionpaa S, et al. Degradable polyglycolide rods for the internal fixation of displaced bimalleolar fractures. Int Orthop 1990;14(1):1–8.
16. Böstman OM. Distal tibiofibular synostosis after malleolar fractures treated using absorbable implants. Foot Ankle 1993;14(1):38–43.
17. Böstman OM. Metallic or absorbable fracture fixation devices. A cost minimization analysis. Clin Orthop Relat Res 1996;329:233–239.
18. Böstman O, Mäkelä EA, Söderg̊rd J, et ak. Absorbable polyglycolide pins in internal fixation of fractures in children. J Pediatr Orthop 1993;13:242–245.
19. Bostock SH, Peach BG. Spontaneous resolution of an osseous bridge affecting the distal tibial epiphysis. J Bone Joint Surg Br 1996;78(4):662–663.
20. Boyer MI, Bowen V, Weiler P. Reconstruction of a severe grinding injury to the medial malleolus and the deltoid ligament of the ankle using a free plantaris tendon graft and vascularized gracilis free muscle transfer: case report. J Trauma 1994;36(3):454–457.
21. Bozic KJ, Jaramillo D, DiCanzio J, et al. Radiographic appearance of the normal distal tibiofibular syndesmosis in children. J Pediatr Orthop 1999;19(1):14–21.
22. Broock GJ, Greer RB. Traumatic rotational displacements of the distal tibial growth plate. A case report. J Bone Joint Surg Am 1970;52(8):1666–1668.
23. Brostrom L. Sprained ankles. V. Treatment and prognosis in recent ligament ruptures. Acta Chir Scand 1966;132(5):537–550.
24. Brostrom L. Sprained ankles. VI. Surgical treatment of "chronic" ligament ruptures. Acta Chir Scand 1966;132(5):551–565.
25. Brown SD, Kasser JR, Zurakowski D, et al. Analysis of 51 tibial triplane fractures using CT with multiplanar reconstruction. AJR Am J Roentgenol 2004;183(5):1489–1495.
26. Bucholz RW, Henry S, Henley MB. Fixation with bioabsorbable screws for the treatment of fractures of the ankle. J Bone Joint Surg Am 1994;76(3):319–324.
27. Burstein AH. Fracture classification systems: do they work and are they useful? J Bone Joint Surg Am 1993;75(12):1743–1744.
28. Busam ML, Esther RJ, Obremskey WT. Hardware removal: indications and expectations. J Am Acad Orthop Surg 2006;14(2):113–120.
29. Busconi BD, Pappas AM. Chronic, painful ankle instability in skeletally immature athletes. Ununited osteochondral fractures of the distal fibula. Am J Sports Med 1996; 24(5):647–651.
30. Carey J, Spence L, Blickman H, et al. MRI of pediatric growth plate injury: correlation with plain film radiographs and clinical outcome. Skeletal Radiol 1998;27(5):250–255.
31. Caruthers CO, Crenshaw AH. Clinical significance of a classification of epiphyseal injuries at the ankle. Am J Surg 1955;89:879–889.
32. Cass JR, Peterson HA. Salter-Harris Type-IV injuries of the distal tibial epiphyseal growth plate, with emphasis on those involving the medial malleolus. J Bone Joint Surg Am 1983;65(8):1059–1070.
33. Casteleyn PP, Handelberg F. Distraction for ankle arthroscopy. Arthroscopy 1995; 11(5):633–634.
34. Caterini R, Farsetti P, Ippolito E. Long-term follow-up of physeal injury to the ankle. Foot Ankle 1991;11(6):372–383.
35. Chadwick CJ. Spontaneous resolution of varus deformity at the ankle following adduction injury of the distal tibial epiphysis. A case report. J Bone Joint Surg Am 1982; 64(5):774–776.
36. Chande VT. Decision rules for roentgenography of children with acute ankle injuries. Arch Pediatr Adolesc Med 1995;149(3):255–258.
37. Charlton M, Costello R, Mooney JF 3rd, et al. Ankle joint biomechanics following transepiphyseal screw fixation of the distal tibia. J Pediatr Orthop 2005;25(5):635–640.
38. Clement DA, Worlock PH. Triplane fracture of the distal tibia. A variant in cases with an open growth plate. J Bone Joint Surg Br 1987;69(3):412–415.
39. Cooperman DR, Spiegel PG, Laros GS. Tibial fractures involving the ankle in children. The so-called triplane epiphyseal fracture. J Bone Joint Surg Am 1978;60(8): 1040–1046.
40. Cox G, Thambapillay S, Templeton PA. Compartment syndrome with an isolated Salter Harris II fracture of the distal tibia. J Orthop Trauma 2008;22(2):148–150.
41. Cox PJ, Clarke NM. Juvenile Tillaux fracture of the ankle associated with a tibial shaft fracture: a unique combination. Injury 1996;27(3):221–222.
42. Crenshaw AH. Injuries of the distal tibial epiphysis. Clin Orthop Relat Res 1965;41: 98–107.
43. Cummings, RJ. Triplane ankle fracture with deltoid ligament tear and syndesmotic disruption. J Child Orthop 2008;2(1):11–14.
44. Cummings RJ, Hahn GA Jr. The incisural fracture. Foot Ankle Int 2004;25(3):132–135.
45. Damore DT, Metzl JD, Ramundo M, et al. Patterns in childhood sports injury. Pediatr Emer Care 2003;19(2):65–67.
46. Denton JR, Fischer SJ. The medial triplane fracture: report of an unusual injury. J Trauma 1981;21(11):991–995.
47. Dias L. Fractures of the tibia and fibula. In: Rockwood CA, Wilkins KE, King RE, eds. Fractures in Children. 3rd ed. Philadelphia: J.B. Lippincott, 1991.
48. Dias LS, Giegerich CR. Fractures of the distal tibial epiphysis in adolescence. J Bone Joint Surg Am983;65(4):438–444.
49. Dias LS, Tachdjian MO. Physeal injuries of the ankle in children: classification. Clin Orthop Relat Res 1978;136:230–233.
50. Donmans JP, Azzoni M, Davidson RS, et al. Major lower extremity lawn mower injuries in children. J Pediatr Orthop 1995;15 (1):78–82.
51. Dunbar RP, Barei DP, Kubiak EN, et al. Early limited internal fixation of diaphyseal extensions in select pilon fractures: upgrading AO/OTA type C fractures to AO/OTA type B. J Orthop Trauma 2008;22(6):426–429.
52. El-Karef E, Sadek HI, Nairn DS, et al. Triplane fracture of the distal tibia. Injury 2000; 31(9):729–736.
53. Ertl JP, Barrack RL, Alexander AH, et al. Triplane fracture of the distal tibial epiphysis. Long-term follow-up. J Bone Joint Surg Am 1988;70(7):967–976.
54. Feldman DS, Otsuka NY, Hedden DM. Extra-articular triplane fracture of the distal tibial epiphysis. J Pediatr Orthop 1995;15(4):479–481.
55. Feldman DS, Shin SS, Madan S, et al. Correction of tibial malunion and nonunion with six-axis analysis deformity correction using the Taylor Spatial Frame. J Orthop Trauma 2003;17(8):549–554.
56. Feldman F, Singson RD, Rosenberg ZS, et al. Distal tibial triplane fractures: diagnosis with CT. Radiology 1987;164(2):429–435.
57. Foucher J. De la divulsion des epiphyses. Clin Orthop Relat Res 1984;188:3–9.
58. Frick SL, Shoemaker S, Mubarak SJ. Altered fibular growth patterns after tibiofibular synostosis in children. J Bone Joint Surg Am 2001;83-A(2):247–254.
59. Frokjaer J, Moller BN. Biodegradable fixation of ankle fractures. Complications in a prospective study of 25 cases. Acta Orthop Scand 1992;63(4):434–436.
60. Gabel GT, Peterson HA, Berquist TH. Premature partial physeal arrest. Diagnosis by magnetic resonance imaging in two cases. Clin Orthop Relat Res 1991;272:242–247.
61. Gaglani MJ, Friedman J, Hawkins EP, et al. Infections complicating lawnmower injuries in children. Pediatr Infect Dis J 1996;15(5):452–455.
62. Gerner-Smidt M. Ankelbrud Hos Born. Copenhagen: Nytt Nordiskt Forlaz; 1963.
63. Gill GG, Abbott LC. Varus deformity of ankle following injury to distal epiphyseal cartilage of tibia in growing children. Surg Gynecol Obstet 1941;72:659–666.
64. Goldberg VM, Aadalen R. Distal tibial epiphyseal injuries: the role of athletics in 53 cases. Am J Sports Med 1978;6(5):263–268.
65. Grace DL. Irreducible fracture-separations of the distal tibial epiphysis. J Bone Joint Surg Br 1983;65(2):160–162.
66. Grosfeld JL, Morse TS, Eyring EJ. Lawnmower injuries in children. Arch Surg 1970; 100(5):582–583.
67. Guille JT, Lipton GE, Bowen JR, et al. Delayed union following stress fracture of the distal fibula secondary to rotational malunion of lateral malleolar fracture. Am J Orthop 1997;26(6):442–445.
68. Handolin L, Kiljunen V, Arnala I, et al. Effect of ultrasound therapy on bone healing of lateral malleolar fractures of the ankle joint fixed with bioabsorbable screws. J Orthop Sci 2005;10(4):391–395.
69. Haraguchi N, Kato F, Hayashi H. New radiographic projections for avulsion fractures of the lateral malleolus. J Bone Joint Surg Br 1998;80(4):684–688.
70. Haraguchi N, Toga H, Shiba N, et al. Avulsion fracture of the lateral ankle ligament complex in severe inversion injury: incidence and clinical outcome. Am J Sports Med 2007;35(7):1144–1152.
71. Haramati N, Roye DP, Adler PA, et al. Nonunion of pediatric fibula fractures: easy to overlook, painful to ignore. Pediatr Radiol 1994;24(4):248–250.
72. Harcke HT, Macy NJ, Mandell GA, et al. Quantitative assessment of growth plate activity (abstract). J Nucl Med 1984;25:P115.
73. Havranek P, Lizler J. Magnetic resonance imaging in the evaluation of partial growth arrest after physeal injuries in children. J Bone Joint Surg Am 1991;73(8):1234–1241.
74. Healy WA 3rd, Starkweather KD, Meyer J, et al. Triplane fracture associated with a proximal third fibula fracture. Am J Orthop 1996;25(6):449–451.
75. Herscovici D Jr, Sanders RW, Scaduto JM, et al. Vacuum-assisted wound closure (VAC therapy) for the management of patients with high-energy soft tissue injuries. J Orthop Trauma 2003;17(10):683–688.
76. Hirvensalo E. Fracture fixation with biodegradable rods. Forty-one cases of severe ankle fractures. Acta Orthop Scand 1989;60(5):601–606.
77. Horowitz JH, Nichter LS, Kenney JG, et al. Lawnmower injuries in children: lower extremity reconstruction. J Trauma 1985;25(12):1138–1146.
78. Hynes D, O'Brien T. Growth disturbance lines after injury of the distal tibial physis. Their significance in prognosis. J Bone Joint Surg Br 1988;70(2):231–233.
79. Imade S, Takao M, Nishi H, et al. Arthroscopy-assisted reduction and percutaneous fixation for triplane fracture of the distal tibia. Arthroscopy 2004;20(10):e123–128.
80. Iwinska-Zelder J, Schmidt S, Ishaque N, et al. [Epiphyseal injuries of the distal tibia. Does MRI provide useful additional information?]. Radiologe 1999;39(1):25–29.
81. Jarvis JG, Miyanji F. The complex triplane fracture: ipsilateral tibial shaft and distal triplane fracture. J Trauma 2001;51(4):714–716.
82. Jennings MM, Lagaay P, Schuberth JM. Arthroscopic assisted fixation of juvenile intra-articular epiphyseal ankle fractures. J Foot Ankle Surg 2007;46(5):376–386.

83. Johnson EW Jr, Fahl JC. Fractures involving the distal epiphysis of the tibia and fibula in children. Am J Surg 1957;93(5):778–781.
84. Johnstone BR, Bennett CS. Lawnmower injuries in children. Aust N Z J Surg 1989; 59(9):713–718.
85. Jones S, Phillips N, Ali F, et al. Triplane fractures of the distal tibia requiring open reduction and internal fixation. Preoperative planning using computed tomography. Injury 2003;34(4):293–298.
86. Karrholm J. The triplane fracture: four years of follow-up of 21 cases and review of the literature. J Pediatr Orthop B 1997;6(2):91–102.
87. Karrholm J, Hansson LI, Laurin S. Computed tomography of intraarticular supination–eversion fractures of the ankle in adolescents. J Pediatr Orthop 1981;1(2):181–187.
88. Karrholm J, Hansson LI, Laurin S. Pronation injuries of the ankle in children. Retrospective study of radiographical classification and treatment. Acta Orthop Scand. 1983; 54(1):1-17.
89. Karrholm J, Hansson LI, Laurin S. Supination–eversion injuries of the ankle in children: a retrospective study of radiographic classification and treatment. J Pediatr Orthop 1982;2(2):147–159.
90. Karrholm J, Hansson LI, Selvik G. Changes in tibiofibular relationships due to growth disturbances after ankle fractures in children. J Bone Joint Surg Am 1984;66(8): 1198–1210.
91. Kaukonen JP, Lamberg T, Korkala O, et al. Fixation of syndesmotic ruptures in 38 patients with a malleolar fracture: a randomized study comparing a metallic and a bioabsorbable screw. J Orthop Trauma 2005;19(6):392–395.
92. Kay RM, Matthys GA. Pediatric ankle fractures: evaluation and treatment. J Am Acad Orthop Surg 2001;9(4):268–278.
93. Kaya A, Altay T, Ozturk H, et al. Open reduction and internal fixation in displaced juvenile Tillaux fractures. Injury 2007;38(2):201–205.
94. Keats T. Atlas of Normal Roentgen Variants That may Simulate Disease. 5th ed. St. Louis, MO: MosbyYear Book, 1992.
95. Kerr R, Forrester DM, Kingston S. Magnetic resonance imaging of foot and ankle trauma. Orthop Clin North Am 1990;21(3):591–601.
96. Khoshhal KI, Kiefer GN. Physeal bridge resection. J Am Acad Orthop Surg 2005;13(1): 47–58.
97. Kleiger B, Mankin HJ. Fracture of the lateral portion of the distal tibial epiphysis. J Bone Joint Surg Am 1964;46:25–32.
98. Klein DM, Caligiuri DA, Katzman BM. Local-advancement soft-tissue coverage in a child with ipsilateral grade IIIB open tibial and ankle fractures. J Orthop Trauma 1996; 10(8):577–580.
99. Kling T. Fractures of the Ankle and Foot. In Drennan J, ed. The Child's Foot and Ankle. New York: Raven Press, 1992.
100. Kling TF Jr, Bright RW, Hensinger RN. Distal tibial physeal fractures in children that may require open reduction. J Bone Joint Surg Am 1984;66(5):647–657.
101. Lauge-Hansen N. Fractures of the ankle. II. Combined experimental-surgical and experimental-roentgenologic investigations. Arch Surg 1950;60(5):957–985.
102. Lehman WL, Jones WW. Intravenous lidocaine for anesthesia in the lower extremity. A prospective study. J Bone Joint Surg Am 1984;66(7):1056–1060.
103. Leininger RE, Knox CL, Comstock RD. Epidemiology of 1.6 million pediatric soccer-related injuries presenting to US emergency departments from 1990 to 2003. Am J Sports Med 2007;35(2):288–293.
104. Lerner A, Stein H. Hybrid thin wire external fixation: an effective, minimally invasive, modular surgical tool for the stabilization of periarticular fractures. Orthopaedics 2004; 27(1):59–62.
105. Letts M, Davidson D, McCaffrey M. The adolescent pilon fracture: management and outcome. J Pediatr Orthop 2001;21(1):20–26.
106. Letts M, Davidson D, Mukhtar I. Surgical management of chronic lateral ankle instability in adolescents. J Pediatr Orthop 2003;23(3):392–397.
107. Letts RM. The hidden adolescent ankle fracture. J Pediatr Orthop 1982;2(2):161–164.
108. Lintecum N, Blasier RD. Direct reduction with indirect fixation of distal tibial physeal fractures: a report of a technique. J Pediatr Orthop 1996;16(1):107–112.
109. Loder RT, Brown KL, Zaleske DJ, et al. Extremity lawnmower injuries in children: report by the Research Committee of the Pediatric Orthopaedic Society of North America. J Pediatr Orthop 1997;17(3):360–369.
110. Lohman M, Kivisaari A, Vehmas T, et al. MRI in the assessment of growth arrest. Pediatr Radiol 2002;32(1):41–45.
111. Love SM, Grogan DP, Ogden JA. Lawnmower injuries in children. J Orthop Trauma 1988;2(2):94–101.
112. Lovell E. An unusual rotatory injury of the ankle. J Bone Joint Surg 1968;50A:163–165.
113. Lynn MD. The triplane distal tibial epiphyseal fracture. Clin Orthop Relat Res 1972; 86:187–190.
114. Manderson EL, Ollivierre CO. Closed anatomic reduction of a juvenile tillaux fracture by dorsiflexion of the ankle. A case report. Clin Orthop Relat Res 1992,276:262–266.
115. Mankovsky AB, Mendoza-Sagaon M, Cardinaux C, et al. Evaluation of scooter-related injuries in children. J Pediatr Surg 2002;37(5):755–759.
116. Mann DC, Rajmaira S. Distribution of physeal and nonphyseal fractures in 2650 long-bone fractures in children aged 0 to 16 years. J Pediatr Orthop 1990;10(6):713–716.
117. Marmor L. An unusual fracture of the tibial epiphysis. Clin Orthop Relat Res 1970; 73:132–135.
118. Marumo K, Sato Y, Suzuki H, et al. MRI study of bioabsorbable poly-L-lactic acid devices used for fixation of fracture and osteotomies. J Orthop Sci 2006;11(2): 154–158.
119. Mazur JM, Loveless EA, Cummings RJ. Ankle dislocation without fracture in a child. Am J Orthop 2007;36(9):E138–140.
120. McFarland B. Traumatic arrest of epiphyseal growth at the lower end of the tibia. Br J Surg 1931;19:78.
121. Michelson JD, Clarke HJ, Jinnah RH. The effect of loading on tibiotalar alignment in cadaver ankles. Foot Ankle 1990;10(5):280–284.
122. Miller MD. Arthroscopically assisted reduction and fixation of an adult Tillaux fracture of the ankle. Arthroscopy 1997;13(1):117–119.
123. Mirmiran R, Schuberth JM. Nonunion of an epiphyseal fibular fracture in a pediatric patient. J Foot Ankle Surg 2006;45(6):410–412.
124. Moon MS, Kim I, Rhee SK, et al. Varus and internal rotational deformity of the ankle secondary to distal tibial physeal injury. Bull Hosp Jt Dis 1997;56(3):145–148.
125. Mooney JF 3rd, DeFranzo A, Marks MW. Use of cross-extremity flaps stabilized with external fixation in severe pediatric foot and ankle trauma: an alternative to free tissue transfer. J Pediatr Orthop 1998;18(1):26–30.
126. Mubarak SJ. Extensor retinaculum syndrome of the ankle after injury to the distal tibial physis. J Bone Joint Surg Br 2002;84(1):11–14.
127. Munjal K, Kishan S, Sabharwal S. Posttraumatic pediatric distal tibiofibular synostosis: a case report. Foot Ankle Int 2004;25(6):429–433.
128. Navascues JA, Gonzalez-Lopez JL, Lopez-Valverde S, et al. Premature physeal closure after tibial diaphyseal fractures in adolescents. J Pediatr Orthop 2000;20(2):193–196.
129. Nenopoulos SP, Papavasiliou VA, Papavasiliou AV. Outcome of physeal and epiphyseal injuries of the distal tibia with intra-articular involvement. J Pediatr Orthop 2005; 25(4):518–522.
130. Nevelos AB, Colton CL. Rotational displacement of the lower tibial epiphysis due to trauma. J Bone Joint Surg Br 1977;59(3):331–332.
131. Nguyen D, Letts M. In-line skating injuries in children: a 10-year review. J Pediatr Orthop 2001;21(5):613–618.
132. Nilsson S, Roaas A. Soccer injuries in adolescents. Am J Sports Med 1978;6(6): 358–361.
133. Nusem I, Ezra E, Wientroub S. Closed posterior dislocation of the ankle without associated fracture in a child. J Trauma 1999;46(2):350–351.
134. Ogden JA. Skeletal Injury in the Child. Philadelphia: Lea & Febiger, 1982.
135. Ogden JA, Lee J. Accessory ossification patterns and injuries of the malleoli. J Pediatr Orthop 1990;10(3):306–316.
136. Orava S, Saarela J. Exertion injuries to young athletes: a follow-up research of orthopaedic problems of young track and field athletes. Am J Sports Med 1978;6(2):68–74.
137. Panagopoulos A, van Niekerk L. Arthroscopic assisted reduction and fixation of a juvenile Tillaux fracture. Knee Surg Sports Traumatol Arthrosc 2007;15(4):415–417.
138. Papadokostakis G, Kontakis G, Giannoudis P, et al. External fixation devices in the treatment of fractures of the tibial plafond: a systematic review of the literature. J Bone Joint Surg Br 2008;90(1):1–6.
139. Peiro A, Aracil J, Martos F, et al. Triplane distal tibial epiphyseal fracture. Clin Orthop Relat Res 1981;160:196–200.
140. Pesl T, Havranek P. Rare injuries to the distal tibiofibular joint in children. Eur J Pediatr Surg 2006;16(4):255–259.
141. Peterson CA, Peterson HA. Analysis of the incidence of injuries to the epiphyseal growth plate. J Trauma 1972;12(4):275–281.
142. Peterson HA. Physeal fractures: part 3. Classification. J Pediatr Orthop 1994;14(4): 439–448.
143. Peterson HA, Madhok R, Benson JT, et al. Physeal fractures: part 1. Epidemiology in Olmsted County, Minnesota, 1979–1988. J Pediatr Orthop 1994;14(4):423–430.
144. Petit P, Panuel M, Faure F, et al. Acute fracture of the distal tibial physis: role of gradient-echo MR imaging versus plain film examination. AJR Am J Roentgenol 1996; 166(5):1203–1206.
145. Petit P, Sapin C, Henry G, et al. Rate of abnormal osteoarticular radiographic findings in pediatric patients. AJR Am J Roentgenol 2001;176(4):987–990.
146. Phieffer LS, Meyer RA Jr, Gruber HE, et al. Effect of interposed periosteum in an animal physeal fracture model. Clin Orthop Relat Res 2000;376:15–25.
147. Poland J. Traumatic Separation of the Epiphysis. London: Smith, Elder & Co, 1898.
148. Pollen AG. Fractures involving the epiphyseal plate. Reconstr Surg Traumatol 1979; 17:25–39.
149. Powell H. Extra centre of ossification for the medial malleolus in children: incidence and significance. J Bone Joint Surg 1961;43B:107–113.
150. Raikin SM, Ching AC. Bioabsorbable fixation in foot and ankle. Foot Ankle Clin 2005; 10(4):667–684, ix.
151. Ramsey PL, Hamilton W. Changes in tibiotalar area of contact caused by lateral talar shift. J Bone Joint Surg Am 1976;58(3):356–357.
152. Rapariz JM, Ocete G, Gonzalez-Herranz P, et al. Distal tibial triplane fractures: long-term follow-up. J Pediatr Orthop 1996;16(1):113–118.
153. Reff RB. The use of external fixation devices in the management of severe lower-extremity trauma and pelvic injuries in children. Clin Orthop Relat Res 1984;188:21–33.
154. Rinker B, Amspacher JC, Wilson PC, et al. Subatmospheric pressure dressing as a bridge to free tissue transfer in the treatment of open tibia fractures. Plast Reconstr Surg 2008;121(5):1664–1673.
155. Ristiniemi J. External fixation of tibial pilon fractures and fracture healing. Acta Orthop Suppl 2007,78(326):3, 5–34.
156. Rogers LF. The radiography of epiphyseal injuries. Radiology 1970;96(2):289–299.
157. Rohmiller MT, Gaynor TP, Pawelek J, et al. Salter-Harris I and II fractures of the distal tibia: does mechanism of injury relate to premature physeal closure? J Pediatr Orthop 2006;26(3):322–328.
158. Rokkanen P, Bostman O, Vainionpaa S, et al. Absorbable devices in the fixation of fractures. J Trauma 1996;40(Suppl 3):S123–127.
159. Roser LA, Clawson DK. Football injuries in the very young athlete. Clin Orthop Relat Res 1970;69:219–223.
160. Ross PM, Schwentker EP, Bryan H. Mutilating lawnmower injuries in children. JAMA 1976;236(5):480–481.
161. Rougraff BT, Kernek CB. Lawnmower injury resulting in Chopart amputation in a young child. Orthopaedics 1996;19(8):689–691.
162. Sabharwal S, Schwechter EM. Five-year follow-up of ankle joint distraction for post-traumatic chondrolysis in an adolescent: a case report. Foot Ankle Int 2007;28(8): 942–948.
163. Sailhan F, Chotel F, Guibal AL, et al. Three-dimensional MR imaging in the assessment of physeal growth arrest. Eur Radiol 2004;14(9):1600–1608.
164. Scheffer MM, Peterson HA. Opening-wedge osteotomy for angular deformities of long bones in children. J Bone Joint Surg Am 1994;76(3):325–334.
165. Schlesinger I, Wedge JH. Percutaneous reduction and fixation of displaced juvenile Tillaux fractures: a new surgical technique. J Pediatr Orthop 1993;13(3):389–391.
166. Schmittenbecher PP. What must we respect in articular fractures in childhood? Injury 2005;36(Suppl 1):A35–43.
167. Schnetzler KA, Hoernschemeyer D. The pediatric triplane ankle fracture. J Am Acad Orthop Surg 2007;15(12):738–747.
168. Seifert J, Laun R, Paris S, et al. [Value of magnetic resonance tomography (MRI) in diagnosis of triplane fractures of the distal tibia]. Unfallchirurg 2001;104(6):524–529.
169. Shankar A, Williams K, Ryan M. Trampoline-related injury in children. Pediatr Emerg Care 2006;22(9):644–646.

170. Shin AY, Moran ME, Wenger DR. Intramalleolar triplane fractures of the distal tibial epiphysis. J Pediatr Orthop 1997;17(3):352–355.
171. Siapkara A, Nordin L, Hill RA. Spatial frame correction of anterior growth arrest of the proximal tibia: report of three cases. J Pediatr Orthop B 2008;17(2):61–64.
172. Siffert RS, Arkin AM. Posttraumatic aseptic necrosis of the distal tibial epiphysis; report of a case. J Bone Joint Surg Am 1950;32-A(3):691–694.
173. Sinisaari IP, Luthje PM, Mikkonen RH. Ruptured tibiofibular syndesmosis: comparison study of metallic to bioabsorbable fixation. Foot Ankle Int 2002;23(8):744–748.
174. Smith BG, Rand F, Jaramillo D, et al. Early MR imaging of lower-extremity physeal fracture-separations: a preliminary report. J Pediatr Orthop 1994;14(4):526–533.
175. Spiegel PG, Cooperman DR, Laros GS. Epiphyseal fractures of the distal ends of the tibia and fibula. A retrospective study of 237 cases in children. J Bone Joint Surg Am 1978;60(8):1046–1050.
176. Steinlauf SD, Stricker SJ, Hulen CA. Juvenile Tillaux fracture simulating syndesmosis separation: a case report. Foot Ankle Int 1998;19(5):332–335.
177. Stiell IG, Greenberg GH, McKnight RD, et al. A study to develop clinical decision rules for the use of radiography in acute ankle injuries. Ann Emerg Med 1992;21(4): 384–390.
178. Sullivan JA, Gross RH, Grana WA, et al. Evaluation of injuries in youth soccer. Am J Sports Med 1980;8(5):325–327.
179. Tachdjian MO. The Child's Foot. Philadelphia: W.B. Saunders, 1985.
180. Takakura Y, Takaoka T, Tanaka Y, et al. Results of opening-wedge osteotomy for the treatment of a posttraumatic varus deformity of the ankle. J Bone Joint Surg Am 1998; 80(2):213–218.
181. Tarkin IS, Clare MP, Marcantonio A, et al. An update on the management of high-energy pilon fractures. Injury 2008;39(2):142–154.
182. Tarr RR, Resnick CT, Wagner KS, et al. Changes in tibiotalar joint contact areas following experimentally induced tibial angular deformities. Clin Orthop Relat Res 1985; 199:72–80.
183. Thomsen NO, Overgaard S, Olsen LH, et al. Observer variation in the radiographic classification of ankle fractures. J Bone Joint Surg Br 1991;73(4):676–678.
184. Ting AJ, Tarr RR, Sarmiento A, et al. The role of subtalar motion and ankle contact pressure changes from angular deformities of the tibia. Foot Ankle 1987;7(5):290–299.
185. Vahvanen V, Aalto K. Classification of ankle fractures in children. Arch Orthop Trauma Surg 1980;97(1):1–5.
186. Vangsness CT J, Carter V, Hunt T, et al. Radiographic diagnosis of ankle fractures: are three views necessary? Foot Ankle Int 1994;15(4):172–174.
187. von Laer L. Classification, diagnosis, and treatment of transitional fractures of the distal part of the tibia. J Bone Joint Surg Am 1985;67(5):687–698.
188. Vosburgh CL, Gruel CR, Herndon WA, et al. Lawnmower injuries of the pediatric foot and ankle: observations on prevention and management. J Pediatr Orthop 1995;15(4): 504–509.
189. Wattenbarger JM, Gruber HE, Phieffer LS. Physeal fractures, part I: histologic features of bone, cartilage, and bar formation in a small animal model. J Pediatr Orthop 2002; 22(6):703–709.
190. Whipple TL, Martin DR, McIntyre LF, et al. Arthroscopic treatment of triplane fractures of the ankle. Arthroscopy 1993;9(4):456–463.
191. Wilder RT, Berde CB, Wolohan M, et al. Reflex sympathetic dystrophy in children. Clinical characteristics and follow-up of 70 patients. J Bone Joint Surg Am 1992;74(6): 910–919.
192. Yao J, Huurman WW. Tomography in a juvenile Tillaux fracture. J Pediatr Orthop 1986;6(3):349–351.
193. Zaricznyj B, Shattuck LJ, Mast TA, et al. Sports-related injuries in school-aged children. Am J Sports Med 1980;8(5):318–324.

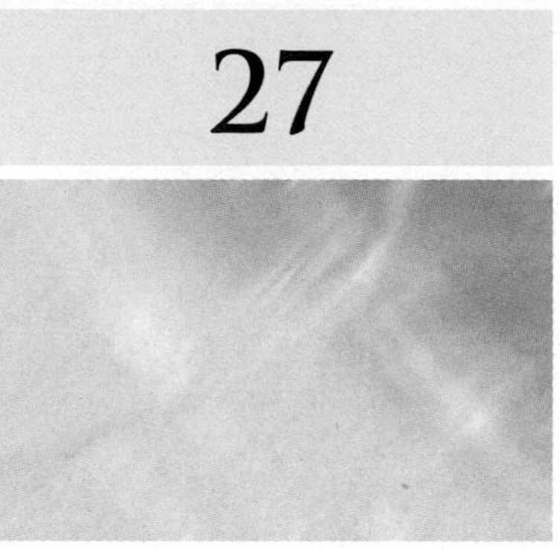

27

FRACTURES AND DISLOCATIONS OF THE FOOT

Haemish Crawford

INTRODUCTION 1018
Anatomy of the Growing Foot 1018

HISTORY AND EXAMINATION 1018

TALAR FRACTURES 1019
Management 1019
Signs and Symptoms 1019
Associated Injuries 1020
Imaging Evaluation 1020
Diagnosis and Classification 1020

FRACTURES OF THE TALAR NECK 1020
Treatment 1021
Surgical and Applied Anatomy 1022

FRACTURES OF THE TALAR BODY AND DOME 1024

FRACTURES OF THE LATERAL PROCESS OF THE TALAR BODY 1024

FRACTURES OF THE OSTEOCHONDRAL SURFACE OF THE TALUS 1025
Classification 1026
Treatment 1027
Complications 1028

CALCANEAL FRACTURES 1029
Epidemiology 1029
Management 1029
Signs and Symptoms 1029
Associated Injuries 1029
Diagnosis and Classification 1030
Classification 1031
Surgical and Applied Anatomy 1031
Current Treatment Options 1032
Complications 1034

SUBTALAR DISLOCATION 1037

MIDTARSAL INJURIES 1038
Cuboid Fractures 1039

TARSOMETATARSAL INJURIES (LISFRANC FRACTURE–DISLOCATION) 1039
Management 1039
Signs and Symptoms 1039
Classification 1040
Imaging Evaluation 1041
Surgical and Applied Anatomy 1041
Treatment Options 1042
Complications 1044

METATARSAL FRACTURES 1044
Management 1044
Signs and Symptoms 1044
Associated Injuries 1044
Imaging Evaluation 1045
Classification 1045
Current Treatment Options 1045
Fractures of the Base of the Fifth Metatarsal 1045

PHALANGEAL FRACTURES 1049
Great Toe Fractures 1049

LAWNMOWER AND OTHER MUTILATING INJURIES 1051
Treatment 1051

COMPARTMENT SYNDROME 1052

PUNCTURE WOUNDS 1053

STRESS FRACTURES 1054

INTRODUCTION

Trauma to the pediatric foot was traditionally treated nonoperatively by orthopaedic surgeons.[16,135] The dogma existed that the bones of the foot were predominantly cartilaginous and would remodel as the child matures. Few, if any, long-term studies exist to measure the outcomes of these treatments.

Children are now involved in sports and activities of greater physical intensity that lead to more complex fractures and dislocations.[4,38,41,130] It is not uncommon for young children to be competing in motocross, extreme skiing, and rock-climbing.[4,157] Professional sport has brought about more intense training and greater expectations from the child, the parent, and the coach. Injuries need to be treated "quicker" and rehabilitation time decreased to allow early return to the sport. These expectations should not get in the way of treating the child's foot injury in the best possible way.

As the child grows into a young adult, the largely cartilaginous foot becomes ossified and fracture and dislocation patterns change. Ogden[118] showed that the cartilaginous bones were elastic and absorbed the energy from the trauma and dissipated it differently from the adult foot. This resulted in different fracture patterns.[118] The management algorithms for the adolescent foot are therefore quite different from the infant's foot; however, the exact age at which this occurs needs to be individualized for each patient. The amount of fracture angulation and joint line displacement to accept is one of the real challenges in treating the skeletally immature foot. Some complex fractures of the talus and calcaneus in adolescents are in fact best internally fixed according to the priniciples used to treat adult trauma.

An in depth knowledge of the anatomy of the growing foot is helpful as the variable ossification centers, apophyses, and physes make fracture recognition difficult. Most of the papers quoted in this chapter are level IV (uncontrolled case series) or level V (expert consensus). One of the problems with pediatric foot and ankle research is that long follow-up intervals are necessary to validate treatments. There are no pediatric outcome scores for children's foot trauma, so prediction of outcome is dependent on orthopaedic first principles of anatomic reduction, union, and effective rehabilitation. Long-term retrospective studies also have the difficulty of locating children treated decades earlier and, therefore, the follow-up rate is low.

Anatomy of the Growing Foot

The child's foot is different from the adult foot in that the bones are largely cartilaginous until adolescence. Although the mechanisms of injury are similar, the resulting fracture is usually less severe in the child as the energy of the injury is dissipated by the elasticity of the cartilage. The cartilage also makes interpretation of imaging more difficult and fractures may not be appreciated on plain radiograph. Computed tomography (CT) and magnetic resonance imaging (MRI) scans assist in clarification of anatomy and identification of fractures. The remodeling potential of cartilage allows some displacement and angulation of fractures to be accepted in children, whereas in adults it may be unacceptable.

Secondary areas of ossification, accessory bones, and growth plates also make fracture recognition more difficult. The appearance of the ossification centers are summarized in Figure 27-1.[5] The calcaneus and talus are usually ossified at birth and the cuboid ossification center usually becomes evident shortly after. The navicular does not develop its primary ossification center until the child is around 3 years of age. Figure 27-2 shows the accessory ossicles and sesamoid bones in the foot which can also be confused with fractures especially if they are bipartite or if the accessory bones are closely adhered. It is useful clinically to radiograph the opposite foot if any doubt exists as to what may be normal or pathologic.

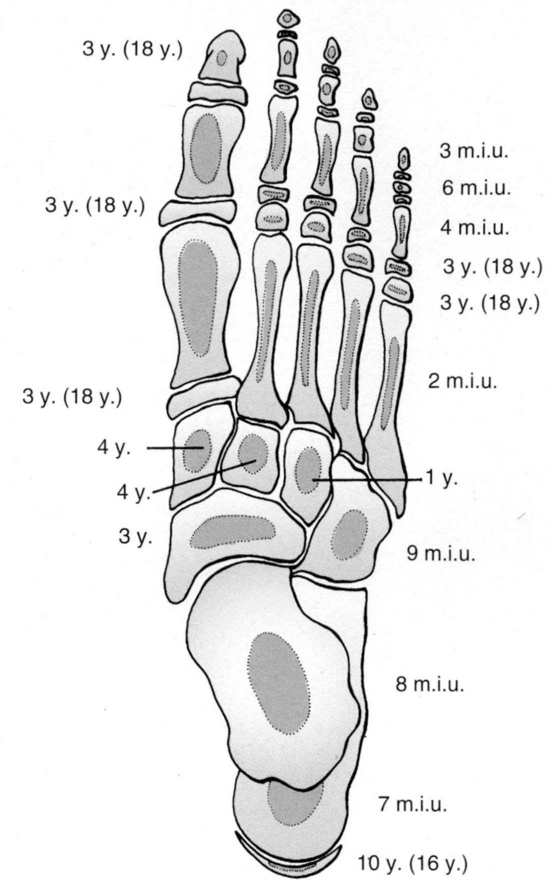

FIGURE 27-1 Appearance and fusion times of foot ossification centers, with figures in parentheses indicating the time of fusion of the primary and secondary ossification centers (y, years; m.i.u., months in utero). (From Aitken JT, Joseph J, Causey G, et al. A Manual of Human Anatomy. 2nd ed. London: E & S Livingstone, 1966:80, with permission).

HISTORY AND EXAMINATION

The history is not always accurate in childhood trauma; however, every attempt should be made to ascertain the mechanism of injury. Often, other children or adults who witnessed the accident can give a more accurate account than the patient. The degree of force, the speed and height of the fall, and the way the foot is twisted all help predict the degree of displacement or severity of the injury. In more subtle injuries, the ability to weight bear, degree of instability, and the location of the pain are vital parts of the history.

Careful examination of the foot will guide the surgeon to the site of injury. The child often complains of the whole foot "hurting"; however, systematic palpation helps localize the most painful site. Appropriate radiographs can then be taken. Bruis-

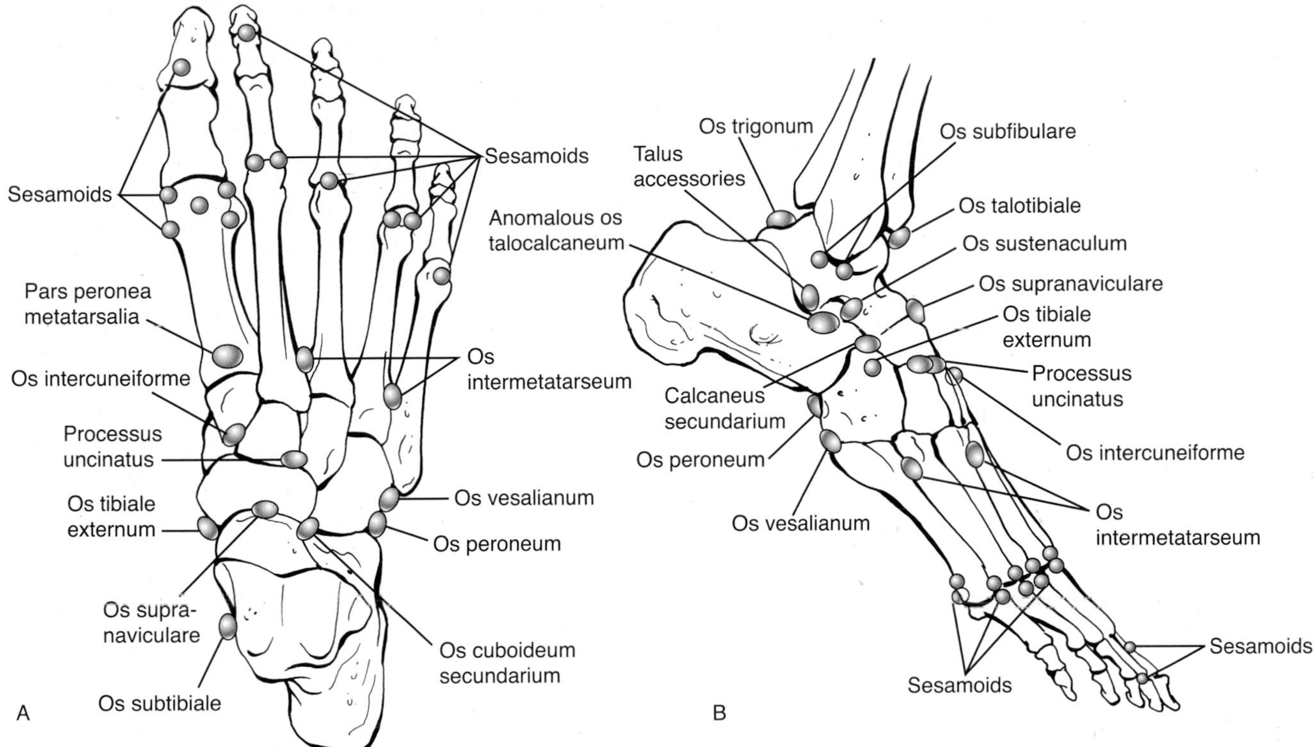

FIGURE 27-2 Diagrammatic representation of accessory ossicles and sesamoid bones about the foot and ankle. Note that the sesamoid bones can be bipartite and that accessory ossicles can be multicentric. (From Traughber PD. Imaging of the foot and ankle. In Coughlin MJ, Mann RA. Surgery of the Foot and Ankle. 7th ed. St. Louis: Mosby, 1999.)

ing and swelling will also help predict the injury pattern. Isolated bruising on the sole of the midfoot often overlies a subtle Lisfranc injury whereas excessive dorsal swelling may predict a more severe fracture dislocation.[139] In a soft tissue injury such as a crush injury, the possibility of increased compartment pressures should be considered.

Multiple trauma must also be ruled out. A complete secondary survey should be undertaken to exclude other injuries. For example, bilateral calcaneus fractures following a fall may be associated with a tibial fracture or spinal column injury.

TALAR FRACTURES

Management

Fractures of the talus are very rare in children and adolescents.[35,118] Talus fractures most commonly occur through the neck and occasionally the body. Although rare, talus fractures are important to recognize due to the possible complication of avascular necrosis (AVN). This can occur due to the precarious blood supply and fracture patterns. In children, AVN seems more prevalent in innocuous fractures when compared to adults with similar injuries.[134] The majority of talus fractures in children can be treated with cast immobilization whereas displaced fractures in adolescents need to be treated operatively similar to an adult fracture.

Mechanism of Injury

A fall from a height is the predominant mechanism of injury causing talar fractures.[74,92,105] The foot is forcibly dorsiflexed and the neck of the talus impinges against the anterior lip of the distal tibia. This shear force usually results in a vertical or slightly oblique fracture line at the junction of the body and neck of the talus. When the dorsiflexion is combined with supination of the foot, the impingement occurs more medially and the medial malleolus may be fractured as well. With displaced fractures, the subtalar joint may become subluxed. The force required to fracture a child's talus is almost twice that required to fracture the other ankle and tarsal bones.[125] One must be thorough in looking for other injuries that may coexist as a result of the severe trauma. The talus can also be fractured with crushing injuries, and open fractures are well described in lawnmower accidents.[118] Fractures of the lateral process of the talus have been described recently in snowboarding accidents where the mechanism appears to be forced dorsiflexion and inversion of the ankle.[89]

Signs and Symptoms

The history of forced dorsiflexion of the ankle especially associated with a fall from a height should lead to a suspicion of a talus fracture. The same mechanism of injury can cause other foot fractures and dislocations as well. The ankle and foot are extremely swollen and the foot is usually held plantarflexed. Due to this soft tissue swelling, the foot needs to be examined closely for increased compartment pressure. As with all fractures, the soft tissues need to be inspected for any puncture wounds, abrasions, or fracture blisters as these are important in determining the management of the patient.

In these patients, there may be less swelling so careful palpation around the talus is needed to detect the source of the pain.

Once the foot has been clinically assessed, the appropriate radiographic investigations can be performed.

Associated Injuries

Due to the level of force that is often required to fracture a talus, other injuries often coexist.[125] A number of studies have found fractures of the calcaneus, malleoli, tibia, and lumbar spine in the presence of a talus fracture.[20,26,61,121,122] Hawkins,[61] in his study, on adult talus fractures found 64% of the patients had an associated musculoskeletal injury.

Imaging Evaluation

The routine radiographs for a fractured talus include an anteroposterior (AP), lateral, and oblique views. Canale and Kelly[26] have described a pronated oblique view of the talus which may demonstrate the fracture more clearly. The fractures are not always easy to see in young children, as the talus is largely cartilaginous until the second decade.[105] The cartilage anlage often leads to an underestimation of fracture displacement. Some authors have even suggested the use of MRI to show the morphology better in children less than 10 years old.[118,166]

Once the fracture is identified, a CT scan is useful in assessing the fracture plane, communition, degree of displacement, and any other associated foot or ankle fractures. This is particularly useful preoperatively when pain prohibits the full range of radiographs mentioned above to be taken. If an open reduction is planned, the CT scan will also aid in the preoperative planning of the size and placement of the screws. Hawkins[61] described an x-ray classification to define the different types of fractures of the talar neck and used it to predict the risk of AVN (Fig. 27-3):

Type I fracture: undisplaced talar neck fracture
Type II fracture: displaced talar neck fracture with subtalar subluxation or dislocation
Type III fracture: displaced fracture of the talar neck with dislocation of both the subtalar and ankle joints

Hawkins[61] also described a subchondral lucent line, the "Hawkins sign," that indicates normal bloodflow to the talar body. The absence of this lucency may indicate the development of osteonecrosis (see complications of talar fractures).

Diagnosis and Classification

Fractures of the talus can be classified as occurring either in the body or the neck. Some authors suggest classifying talar fractures based on the age of the patient as children less than 6 years of age generally have a better prognosis.[105]

FRACTURES OF THE TALAR NECK

The majority of talar fractures in children are of the talar neck. Hawkins[61] has classified these into three different types depending on whether the fracture is displaced and the degree of subluxation of the subtalar and ankle joints (see Fig. 27-3). This classification was developed so it could be used to predict if the talus would become avascular due to the disruption of the tenuous blood supply. Canale and Kelly[26] later modified the classification (see Fig. 27-3) to include a type IV injury in which there is subluxation or dislocation of the ankle, subtalar, and talonavicular joints. In the adult literature, the majority of talar fractures are type II and III.[26,61] This classification of talus frac-

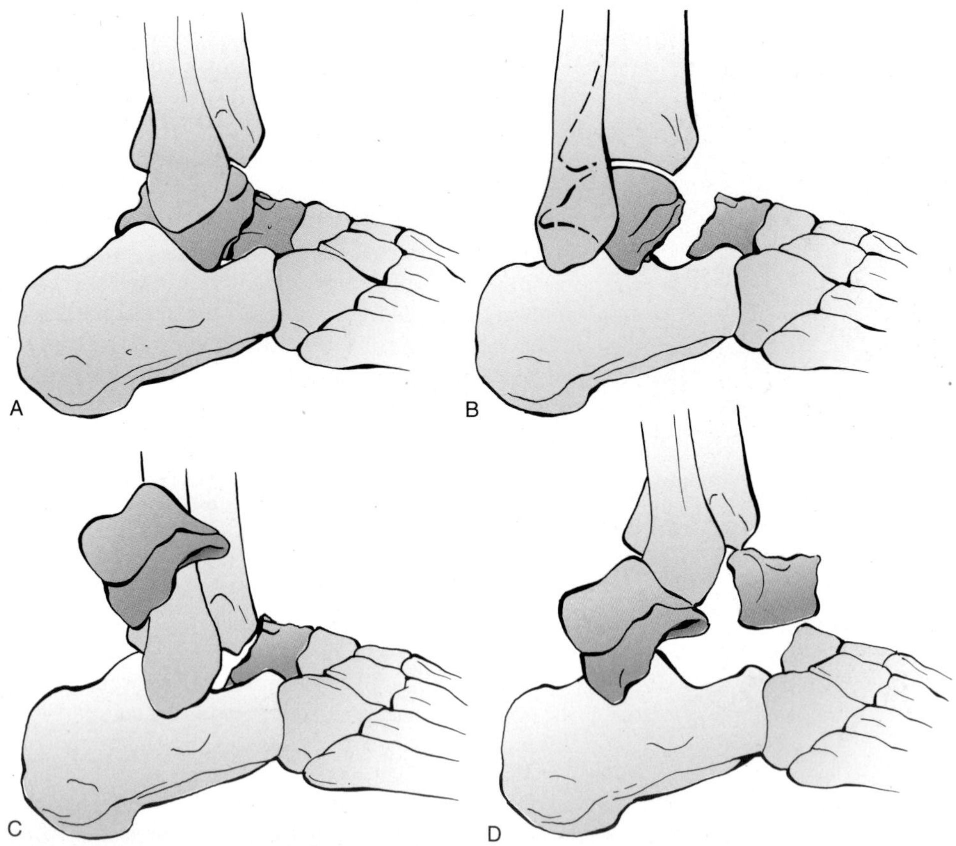

FIGURE 27-3 Hawkins classification of talar neck fractures (see text for details). **A.** Type I, nondisplaced fracture of the talar neck. **B.** Type II, displaced talar neck fracture with subluxation or dislocation of the subtalar joint. **C.** Type III, displaced talar neck fracture with associated dislocation of the talar body from both the subtalar and tibiotalar joints. **D.** Type IV, as suggested by Canale and Kelly, displaced talar neck fracture with an associated dislocation of the talar body from subtalar and tibiotalar joints and dislocation of the head and neck fragment from the talonavicular joint. (From Canale ST, Kelly FB Jr. Fractures of the neck of the talus: long-term evaluation of seventy-one cases. J Bone Joint Surg Am 1978; 60:143–156.)

TABLE 27-1 Hawkins Classification of Talar Neck Fractures

Type	Description	Treatment	Affect on Blood Supply*	Osteonecrosis Rate
Type I	Stable, undisplaced vertical fracture through talar neck.	8 weeks in cast, 4 weeks in CAM cast.	Theoretical damage to only one vessel entering talar neck.	0% to 10%
Type II	Displaced fracture with subtalar joint subluxation or dislocation; normal ankle joint.	Immediate closed reduction.† A near anatomic reduction delays surgical treatment.	Two of three blood supply vessels lost: neck vessel and one entering the tarsal canal.	20% to 50%
Type III	Same as type II but with subluxation or dislocation of both the ankle and subtalar joint.	Direct to operating room for combined anteromedial and anterolateral surgical approach (see text).	All three sources of blood affected.	80% to 100%
Type IV	Very rare; basically a type III with talonavicular joint displacement.	Same as type III.	Not related to blood supply.	100%

CAM, controlled active motion.
*See text for further details of blood supply to the talus.
†Reduction maneuver: maximal plantarflexion and foot traction to realign head and body in sagittal plane. Varus/valgus with or without supination/pronation stress realigns neck in coronal plane.

tures can help predict the type of treatment required and the outcome one can expect (Table 27-1).

Treatment

The treatment of talar fractures is based on the severity of the fracture and the age of the child. The Hawkins classification system is useful in directing the treatment. In a child less than 8 years of age, a less than perfect reduction of the fracture can be accepted due to the remodeling potential.[74,92,105] Adolescent fractures should be treated the same way as an adult injury.

Hawkins Type I Fractures

Undisplaced fractures of the talar neck can be treated for 6 to 8 weeks nonweight bearing in a below-knee cast. The child can then start taking full weight if the fracture has healed radiographically. Canale and Kelly[26] accepted 5 mm of displacement and 5 degrees of angulation of the talar neck in their series.

Hawkins Type II Fractures

A displaced or severely angulated talar neck fracture usually presents with significant soft tissue swelling and pain. This makes management more difficult than type I injuries. Achieving adequate radiographs to assess the degree of displacement is difficult without sedation. The distal fragment of the neck is usually displaced dorsally and medially.

The fracture and subluxation of the subtalar joint should be reduced under general anesthesia, most often by gentle plantarflexion and pronation of the foot. If a stable reduction is achieved, a well molded below-knee cast can be applied with the foot in plantarflexion. This initial cast is changed to a more neutral position at 4 weeks and then removed 8 weeks following fracture reduction. Postoperative serial radiographs or a CT scan should be performed as the fracture position may be lost when the soft tissue swelling subsides. If the fracture is unstable after reduction, percutaneous Kirschner wire (K-wire) fixation is useful to hold the fracture. Two K-wires can be passed through a small dorsomedial incision and across the fracture. The incision should be on the medial side of extensor hallucis longus to avoid damage to the tibial vessels. Although the amount of residual displacement or angulation acceptable is not clearly defined, it may be better to accept a few millimeters of offset and up to 10 degrees of angulation rather than perform an open reduction and risk devascularising the talus further.

Hawkins Type III fractures

These fractures are a result of a serious injury and require urgent surgery to openly reduce and internally fix the talus.

Surgical Approaches

There are three surgical approaches to the fractured talus:

1. Posterolateral
2. Anteromedial
3. Anterolateral

The decision on the approach depends on the condition of the soft tissues and the familiarity of the approach by the surgeon. Occasionally, more than one approach is required if adequate reduction cannot be achieved. It is preferable to use the posterolateral approach as this causes less potential disruption to the blood supply; however, direct visualization of the talar neck is not possible.The timing of the open reduction of these fractures is somewhat controversial. With such a tenuous blood supply, one would think that urgent reduction and internal fixation is indicated. Lindvall et al.[96] compared the results of surgery within 6 hours to delayed surgery in 26 fractures of the talus in adult patients and found no significant difference in outcome. Kellam et al.,[79] in another similar study, concluded that the severity of the injury, the quality of the reduction, and the surgical outcomes had a bigger influence on long-term outcome than if the surgery was fixed emergently or delayed (greater than 12 hours).

Posterolateral Approach. This approach is commonly used to internally fix fractures of the talar neck once it has been reduced. The patient is positioned supine so the other approaches can be utilized if necessary. The incision is made just lateral to the Achilles tendon. Blunt dissection is then carried out down to the joint capsule avoiding damage to the sural nerve. The posterior joint capsule can then be opened if not already torn by the injury and the posterior process of the talus can be identified. If possible, two partially threaded cannulated 4.5- or 6.5-mm screws can be used to provide compression across the fracture. It is preferable to use titanium screws which are MRI compatible to allow investigation of AVN during fracture healing if necessary. If only one screw is used, a separate K-wire should also be passed across the fracture for rotational stability. These posterior screws are more stable biomechanically than anterior screws (Fig. 27-4).[159]

Anteromedial Approach. This approach is useful to visualize the talar neck and directly reduce the fracture. Often, there is communition of the medial wall of the neck which makes restoring length difficult. With the patient supine, the incision is made from just anterior to the medial malleolus and directly distally down the midfoot. Deeper dissection is carried out medial to the tibialis anterior and the extensor hallucis longus tendons. The dissection down to the capsule is in the interval between the tibialis anterior and tibialis posterior tendons. This approach avoids damage to the deltoid branch of the posterior tibial artery and the medial branches of the anterior tibial artery. This approach is potentially less harmful to the blood supply of the talus when compared to the anterolateral approach.[3]

Anterolateral Approach. One advantage of this approach is that it permits excellent exposure of the lateral talar neck which is not usually comminuted allowing anatomic reduction. The approach also gives good access to the subtalar joint. The disadvantage to this approach is that it may disrupt the blood supply more than the other approaches. The incision starts at the tip of the lateral malleolus and extends to the base of the fourth metatarsal. Care must be taken to avoid damaging the sural nerve with deeper dissection. In the base of the incision is the artery of the sinus tarsi which should be visualized if possible.

Following open reduction and internal fixation of talar neck fractures, the foot is placed in a non–weight-bearing below-knee cast for 6 to 8 weeks. Radiographs are then taken to assess fracture healing and the presence or absence of the Hawkins sign. If the subchondral lucent line is present, one can assume there is adequate blood supply to the body of the talus and osteonecrosis is unlikely to occur. If the fracture has also healed, the child can start progressive weight bearing as tolerated. The absence of a subchondral lucency during healing should alert the surgeon to the possible development of osteonecrosis (Fig 27-5). The patient should continue to be nonweight bearing until the lucency is present. If it is still not present 3 months postinjury, an MRI scan should be performed which will assess the vascularity more accurately.[63] The use of titanium screws in the open reduction makes this possible. The decision on the amount of weight bearing in the presence of altered blood supply to the talus is not clear. AVN of the talus often takes 18 months to 2 years to revascularise so it would be impractical, if not impossible, to keep a child non–weight bearing for this period in the hope it will prevent premature collapse of the body.

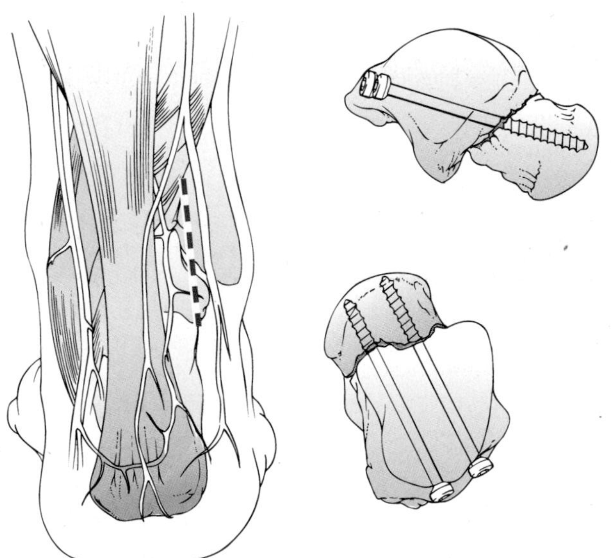

FIGURE 27-4 Posterolateral approach to the talus. Incision is based lateral to the Achilles tendon. The Achilles tendon and flexor hallucis longus are reflected medially. The posterolateral talar tubercle is the starting point for the guide pin. *Right*: Screws are directed in line with the long axis of the neck of the talus in a plantar-medial direction such that the distal threads of the screw are all in the distal fragment (talar head), beyond the fracture line to allow for compression. Combinations of two screws or one screw and one smooth pin are determined by size and anatomy. (From Adelarr RS. Complex fractures of the talus. Instr Course Lect 1997; 46:328, with permission.)

Surgical and Applied Anatomy

The talus is comprised of three parts: a body, neck, and head. Ossification starts from one center that appears in the sixth intrauterine month. The talus ossification process starts in the head and neck and proceeds in a retrograde direction towards the subchondral bone of the body. Approximately two thirds

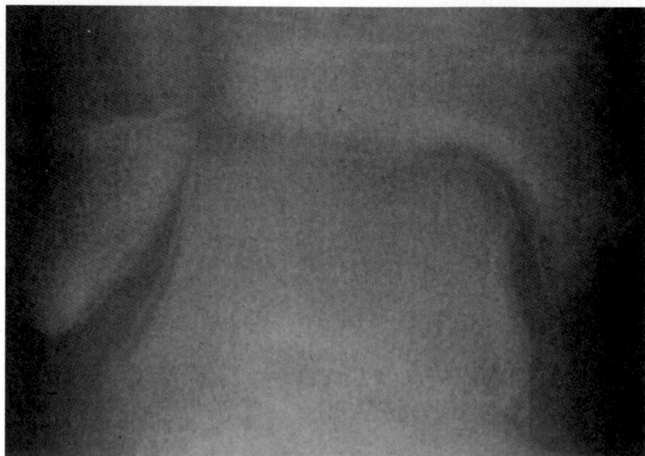

FIGURE 27-5 A 14-year-old girl with a talar neck fracture and a positive Hawkins sign. Disuse osteoporosis leads to halolike image of the talus on the AP view denoting adequate talar dome vascularization; if there had been no blood supply, there would be no bloodflow to loose calcium. If this happens, the dome of the talus would become denser and more radio-opaque than the surrounding bones that are undergoing diffuse osteoporosis.

of the talar body is articular cartilage with just a small area of bare bone on the neck where the bone receives its nutrient blood supply. There are no tendon insertions into the talus. The stability is provided by the capsular and ligamentous attachments to the surrounding bones.

The superior articular surface of the talus is wider anteriorly than it is posteriorly. Traditional teaching suggests the foot should generally be immobilized in neutral dorsiflexion so this widest part of the talus is engaged in the ankle mortise to help prevent an equinus contracture. This is of less importance in younger children who are less likely to develop equinus contractures.The lateral wall of the superior articular surface curves posteriorly whereas the medial wall is straight. The two walls converge posteriorly to form the posterior tubercle of the talus. Often, there is a separate ossification centre (os trigonum) that appears here on radiographs at 11 to 13 years of age in boys and 8 to 10 years of age in girls. It usually fuses to the talus 1 year after it appears (Fig. 27-6).[107]

The short neck of the talus is medially deviated approximately 10 to 44 degrees and plantarflexed between 5 and 50 degrees in relation to the axis of the body.[52] Beneath the talar neck is the tarsal canal, a funnel shaped area that contains the anastomotic ring formed between the artery of the tarsal canal and the artery of the tarsal sinus.[112] The broad interosseous ligament joining the calcaneus and talus is also within the canal.

The tarsal canal is conical in shape and runs from posteromedial (apex) to anterolateral where the base of the cone is known as the sinus tarsi (Fig. 27-7).

The lateral process of the talus is a large wedged-shaped process that is covered in articular cartilage. It articulates with the fibular superiorly and laterally and with the subtalar joint inferiorly. The lateral talocalcaneal ligament is attached to the most distal part of the process.[60,62]

The head of the talus is entirely cartilaginous, convex, and articulates with the concave surface of the navicular. The undersurface of the talus is comprised of three articulating surfaces for the calcaneus: the posterior, middle, and anterior facet. Between the posterior and middle facets is a transverse groove which forms the roof of the tarsal canal.

Blood Supply

The blood supply of the talus has been extensively studied.[9,58,112] The nutrient arteries are derived from the three major vessels that cross the ankle joint: posterior tibial artery, tibialis anterior artery, and peroneal artery (Fig. 27 -8). Branches of these three vessels perforate circumferentially the short talar neck which is the only part of the talus denude of articular cartilage. A fracture in this area can disrupt this intricate anastamosis of vessels and lead to AVN of the body of the talus.

The main blood supply to the talus is through the artery of the tarsal canal. This artery branches off the posterior tibial artery approximately 1 cm proximal to the origin of the medial and lateral plantar arteries. It passes between flexor digitorum

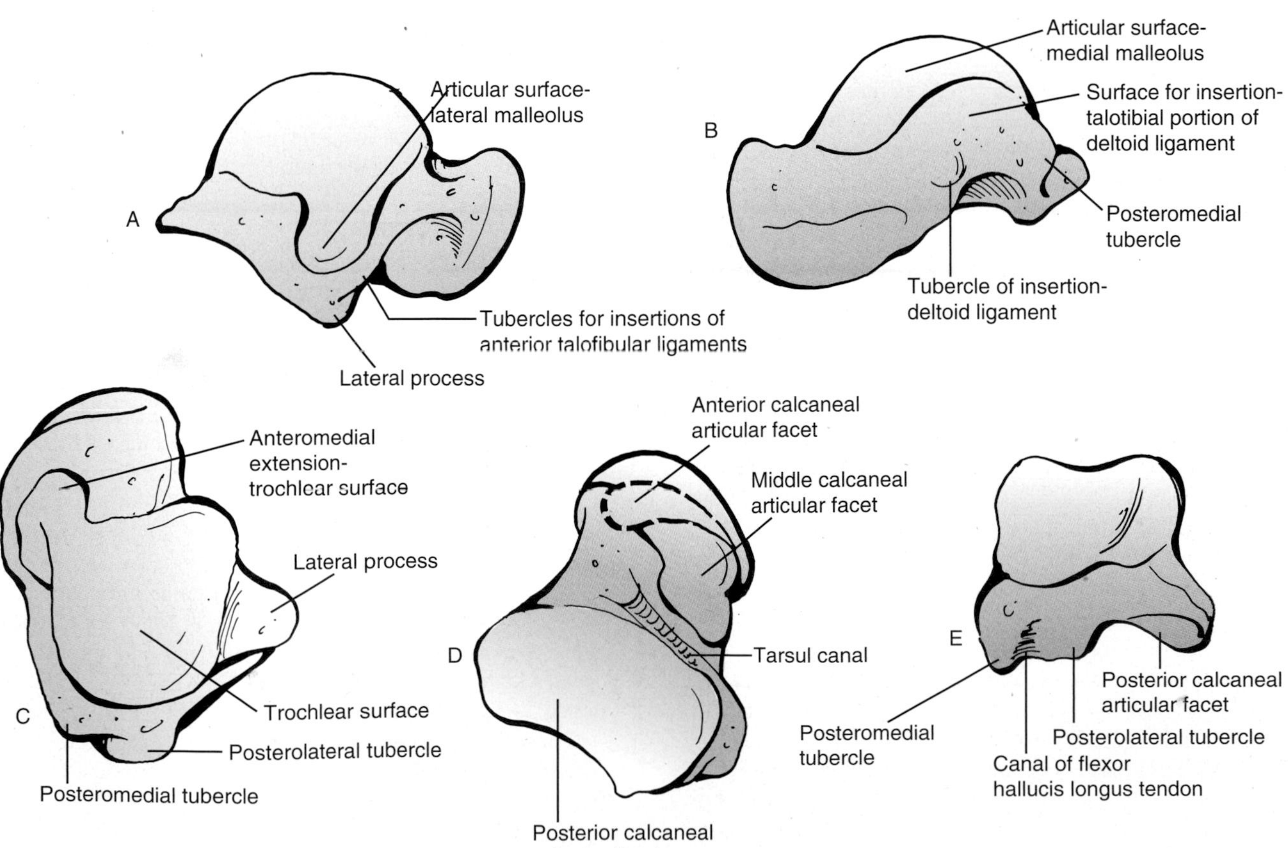

FIGURE 27-6 Anatomic details of the talus are important when correlating high-definition imaging, such as CT scans, with normal anatomy for the purposes of fracture management decision making.

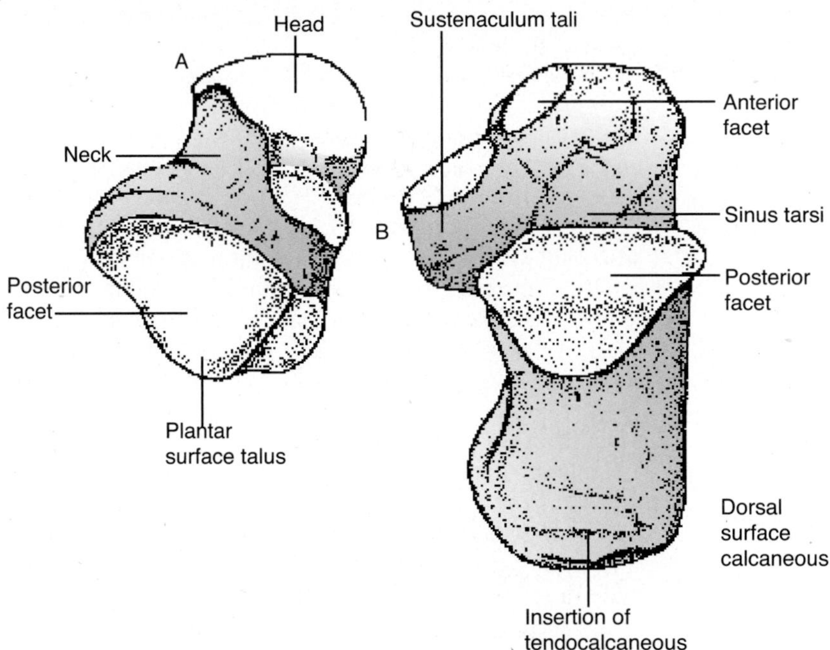

FIGURE 27-7 Subtalar joint opened such that the medial borders of the joint face each other. **A.** Plantar surface of the talus, which articulates with the dorsal surface of the calcaneus. Note the extensive area of the talus that is articular cartilage. **B.** Dorsal surface of the calcaneus with the articular facets occupying the anterior half of the calcaneus. (From Sammarco GJ. Anatomy. In: Helal B, Rowley D, Cracchiolo AC, et al, eds. Surgery of Disorders of the Foot and Ankle. Philadelphia: Lippincott-Raven, 1996.)

longus and flexor hallucis longus before entering the tarsal canal where it anastamoses with the artery of the tarsal sinus. Before entering the canal, the artery of the tarsal canal gives off a deltoid branch that penetrates the deltoid ligament and supplies the medial third of the talar body.[53] A dorsal vessel of the deltoid branch anastamoses with the medial branch of the dorsalis pedis artery to enter the talar neck.

The second source of blood supply is from the anterior tibial artery and its terminal extension, the dorsalis pedis artery. Multiple vessels from these arteries penetrate the dorsal neck of the talus. The third source of blood supply is from the peroneal artery. Small branches supply the posterior process of the talus and a larger branch forms the artery of the sinus tarsi to supply the lateral aspect of the talus.

Within the capsular and ligamentous attachments to the talus there are small vessels that also contribute to the blood supply.[124]

FRACTURES OF THE TALAR BODY AND DOME

Fractures of the talar body are less common than of the neck. In 1977, Sneppen et al.[156] described a classification system based on the anatomic position of the fracture in the talus. This was later modified by DeLee[39] and the result is a five-part classification.

Fractures of the talar body are rare in adults and children (Table 27-2). In a long-term follow-up of 14 talus fractures in children Jensen et al.[74] found only 4 (29%) were fractures through the body. Undisplaced fractures can be treated in a nonweight bearing below-knee cast for 6 to 8 weeks until the fracture is healed and the outcome is excellent. Undisplaced intra-articular fractures can be treated in the same way; however, serial radiographs must be taken to confirm displacement does not occur. Anatomic reduction of displaced fractures has been recommended because residual displacement of the articular surfaces leads to degenerative osteoarthritis.[91]

FRACTURES OF THE LATERAL PROCESS OF THE TALAR BODY

Fractures of the lateral process of the talus are rare in adults and children, and a high level of suspicion is required if the diagnosis is to be made. The lateral process is a wedged-shaped prominence that forms almost the whole lateral wall of the talus. It is covered entirely in articular cartilage and is the articulating surface of the talus with the fibular. The talocalcaneal ligament inserts into the tip of the lateral process. The mechanism of injury is a forced dorsiflexion injury with inversion of the foot.[60] The talocalcaneal ligament may avulse the lateral process.

Isolated fractures of the lateral process of the talus are often not recognized on the initial radiographs.[60,62,106] Leibner and colleagues[89] suggested that this may occur in 46% of the cases. The lateral process is best visualized on the mortise view so the fibula is not overlying it. On the lateral radiograph, the lateral process is seen just superior to the angle of Gissane.[62] This is the angle between a line drawn along the lateral border of posterior facet and a line drawn along the anterior process (Fig 27-9). If there is persistent pain laterally around the ankle following an inversion ankle injury, one should have a high suspicion for a lateral process fracture or an osteochondral injury. If not clearly seen on the plain films, a CT scan should be performed to assess the talus and rule out any other coexisting fractures.[81,117]

The incidence of this rare injury is increasing due to the increased popularity of snowboarding.[81,89,116] Kirkpatrick et al.[81] reviewed 3213 snowboarding injuries and found an unusually high incidence of lateral process fractures. They comprised 34% of all ankle fractures.[81]

The treatment of nondisplaced fractures of the lateral process is with a nonweight-bearing cast for 6 to 8 weeks. Displaced fractures are best treated with open reduction and internal fixation; however, the degree of displacement that is acceptable in a child is not clearly defined. What may be more important is the congruity of the joint surface of the talus. A step or gap in the articular surface of more than 2 to 3 mm may be useful criteria

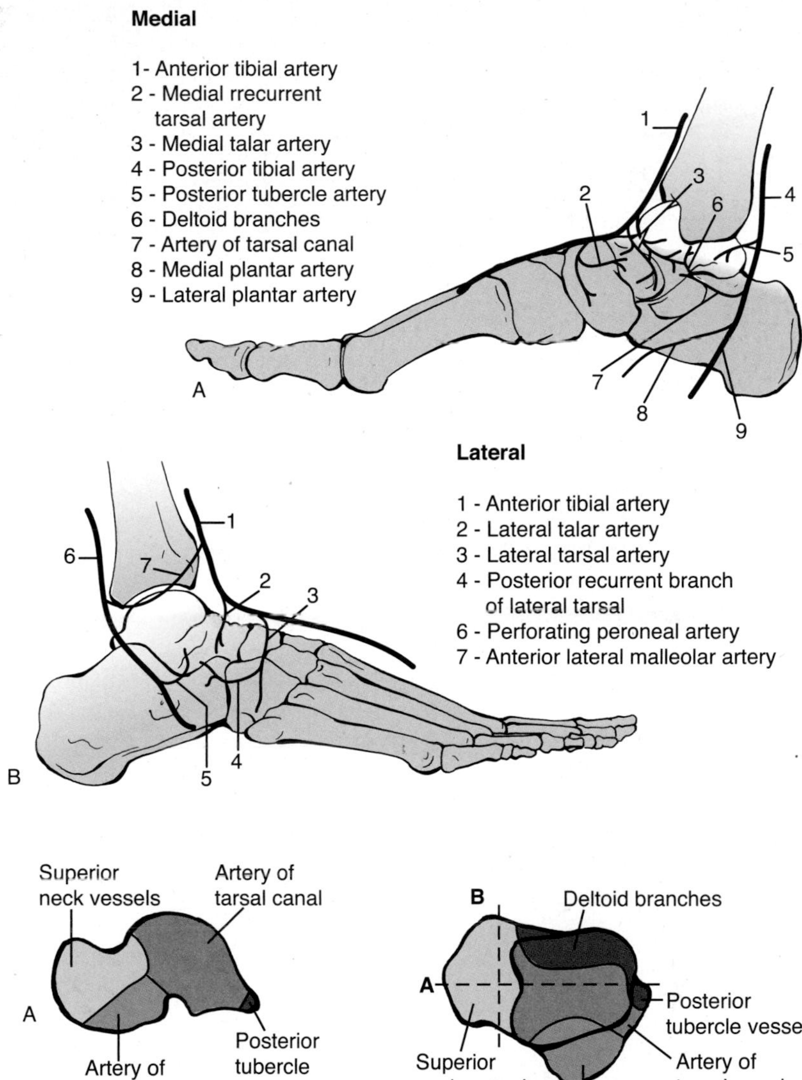

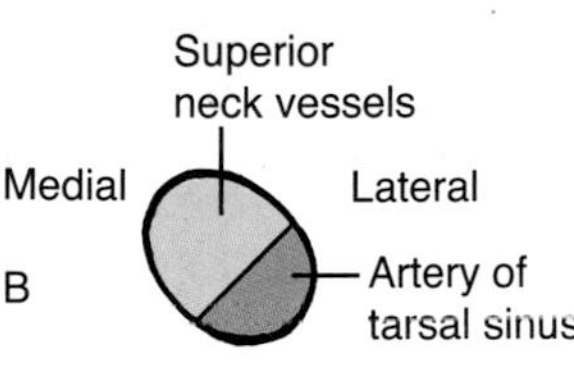

FIGURE 27-8 Arterial blood supply to the talus. Medial blood supply **(A)** and lateral blood supply **(B)**. Dorsal view with sagittal cut through length (*a*) of talus and transverse cut through neck of talus (*b*). (From Gelberman RH, Mortensen WW. The arterial anatomy of the talus. Foot Ankle 1983;4:64–72.)

as to when to open reduce the fracture. The fracture can be held with one 3.5-mm partially threaded cancellous screw inserted from lateral to medial perpendicular to the fracture line. A below-knee cast is then worn for 6 weeks.[60,62,89,165]

TABLE 27-2 Sneppen Classification System of Talar Body Fractures

Sneppen Grade	Fracture Type
1	Transchondral/osteochondral
2	Coronal, sagittal, or horizontal shear
3	Posterior tubercle
4	Lateral process
5	Crush fracture

FRACTURES OF THE OSTEOCHONDRAL SURFACE OF THE TALUS

Damage to the osteochondral surface of the talus can be caused by direct trauma or may be due to an underlying osteochondal lesion (osteochondritis dissecans [OCD]) that may have been present for some time and has been made symptomatic by the injury. The pathogenesis and etiology of OCD are controversial; however, most authors report preceding trauma as a cause of the defects (Canale and Bedding[25] 80%, Letts et al.[91] 79%, Higuera et al.[65] 63%, and Perumal et al.[123] 47%). The medial

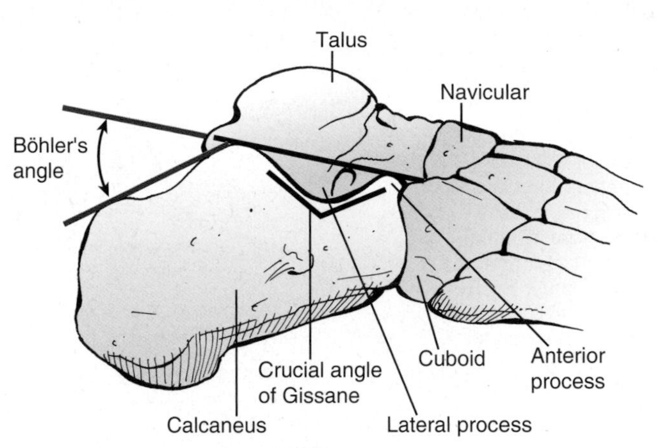

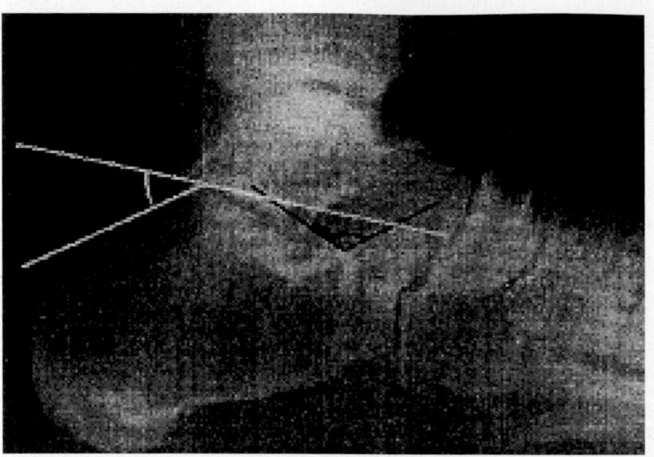

FIGURE 27-9 Diagrammatic depictions of the crucial angle of Gissane **(A)** and the Böhler angle **(B)**. The Böhler angle is more frequently used for decision making regarding fracture management. For measuring the Böhler angle, the landmarks on the lateral radiograph of the calcaneus are the anterior and posterior facets and the superior margin of the calcaneal tuberosity.

lesion is usually deeper and cup shaped compared to the thinner "wafer" type lateral lesion. The lateral lesion is more often associated with trauma and more symptomatic than the medial lesions. It is postulated that the medial lesions may be due to more repetitive microtrauma.[25,26] Berndt and Harty,[12] in 1959, used freshly amputated legs to biomechanically reproduce injuries to the ankle and observe the injuries inflicted. They showed that the anterolateral talus hits the medial aspect of the fibula with dorsiflexion and inversion and that plantarflexion and inversion caused posteromedial osteochondral lesions (Fig. 27-10).

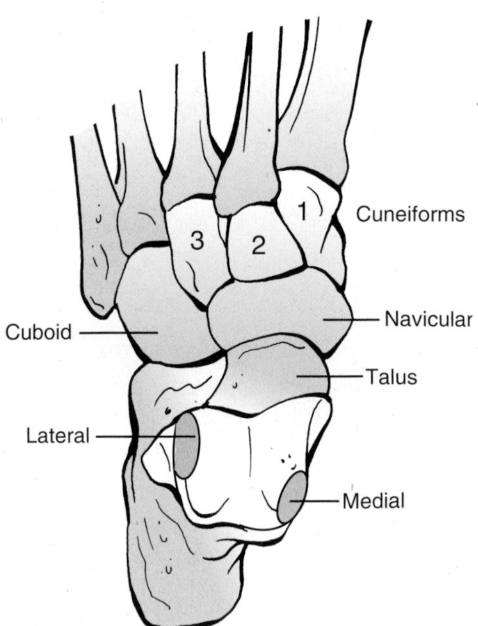

FIGURE 27-10 Typical positions of osteochondral lesions of the talus. Berndt et al.[48] found that of 201 osteochondral lesions in adults 56% were on the medial side and 44% on the lateral side. Letts et al. found medial lesions in 79% of 24 children, lateral lesions in 21%, and central lesions in 1%. (From Letts M, Davidson D, Ahmer A. Osteochondritis dissecans of the talus in children. J Pediatr Orthop 2003;23:617–625, with permission.)

The initial radiographs following an ankle injury in a child should be closely assessed for an osteochondral injury. If pain and swelling persist for over 2 months after an "ankle sprain," then further investigations should be carried out to look for an osteochondral lesion. This will initially be a further radiograph series; however, an MRI scan is often more useful at this stage to look for an osteochondral lesion as a small percentage are purely cartilaginous. Some consider an MRI arthrogram useful in further determining whether the fragment is detached or not as occasionally the arthrographic contrast can be seen deep to the osteochondral lesion. The bone scan has largely been superseded by the MRI scan in the diagnosis and assessment of these lesions. The bone scan is useful, however, when it is not clear if the pain in the child's ankle is coming from the osteochondral lesion or some other pathology. A normal bone scan in the presence of a stage I or II osteochondral lesion may indicate a soft tissue lesion as being a source of the pain.

Mechanical symptoms of locking and catching are not as common as one would think but can occur with these lesions if the loose fragment becomes trapped within the joint. The pain seems to be related to the synovitis and effusion that develops secondary to the uneven articular surface. On examination, the ankle is slightly swollen and can be painful on passive movement as the loose fragment passes under the tibia. With plant-erflexion of the foot, the anterolateral talus can be palpated directly and a lesion here can be painful on direct pressure.

Classification

Berndt and Harty[12] classified osteochondral fractures of the talar dome into four stages based on radiographic criteria (Fig. 27-11):

Stage I: subchondral trabecular compression fracture (not seen radiographically)
Stage II: incomplete separation of an osteochondral fragment
Stage III: the osteochondral fragment is unattached but undisplaced
Stage IV: a displaced osteochondral fragment

Anderson et al.[8] modified this classification after correlating clinical findings with radiographs and MRI scans. They described the stage I lesion as not visible on plain radiographs

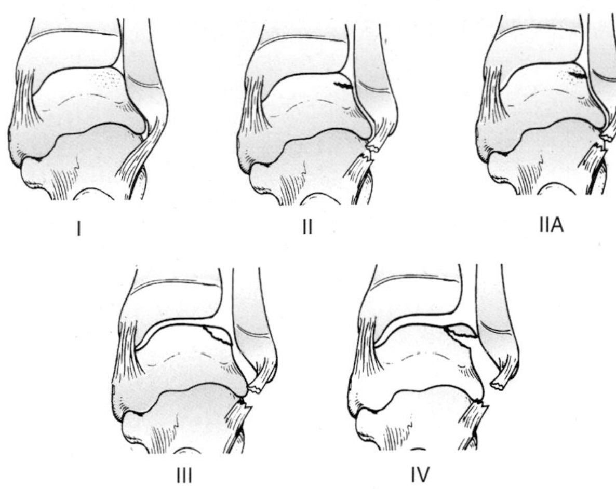

FIGURE 27-11 Adaptation of the Berndt and Hardy[12] (1951) classification of osteochondral injuries of the talus by Anderson et al.[8] Stage 1 is identified only by MRI scanning, which demonstrates trabecular compression of subchondral bone; stage 2 lesions have incomplete separation of the osteochondral fragment from the talus. If a subchondral cyst also is present, the lesion is designated stage 2a. Stage 3 lesions occur when the fragment is no longer attached to the talus but is undisplaced. Stage 4 indicates both complete detachment and displacement. (From Alexander IF, Chrichton KI, Grattan-Smith Y, et al. Osteochondral fractures of the dome of the talus. J Bone Joint Surg Am 1989;71:1143, with permission.)

but visible on an MRI scan. They also introduced a stage IIa lesion, which is an undisplaced osteochondral lesion with a subchondral cyst adjacent to the floor of the lesion. Anderson and his colleagues[8] felt a atage IIa lesion should be treated surgically whereas a atage II lesion can initially be treated nonoperatively (Fig. 27-12).

A further classification was proposed by Pritsch et al.[129] in 1986 based on the arthroscopic appearance of the articular cartilage at the time of surgery. The quality of the articular cartilage was placed into one of three grades:

Grade I: intact, firm, and shiny articular cartilage
Grade II: intact but soft articular cartilage
Grade III:frayed articular cartilage

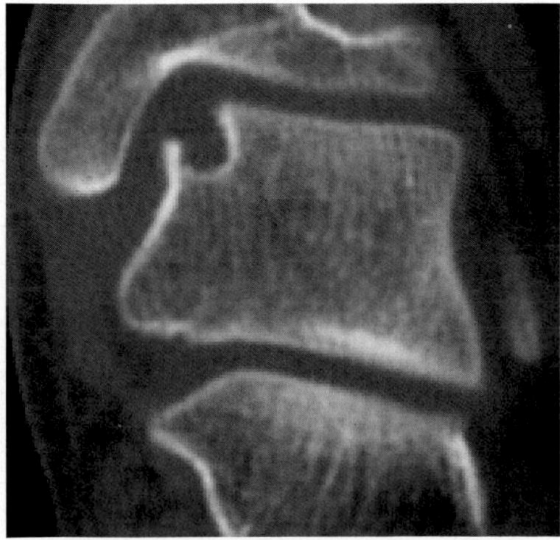

FIGURE 27-12 This CT scan clearly shows a well circumscribed cyst at the base of a stage II osteochondral lesion. This would be classified by Anderson et al.[8] as a stage IIa lesion.

They used this classification to determine which lesions should be treated with activity modification (grade I), who should have arthroscopic drilling (grade II), and finally which patients require arthroscopic curettage and microfracture (grade III).

Treatment

The treatment of osteochondral lesions of the talus in children is challenging. Only a few papers purely address this condition in children,[65,91,123] and the rest of the literature is a combination of adult and childhood lesions. It is important to distinguish between an acute osteochondral fracture and a chronic osteochondral lesion as the two may require different treatment strategies.

To enable thorough assessment, these patients need to be followed up for a minimum of 2 years as it takes this long for the lesion to become radiographically healed despite the child often being clinically normal.[123]

Nonoperative Management

Most authors agree that the primary treatment of stage I and stage II lesions is nonoperative.[12,65,91,123] The symptomatic patient can be immobilized for 6 weeks in a below-knee walking cast or a Cam walker (Fig. 27-13). This usually relieves the acute symptoms; over the next 6 weeks, the patient has activity modification maintaining a pain-free range of movement. This allows the fracture to heal before returning to active sport. Higuera et al.[65] treated their stage 3 lesions nonoperatively as well and all 7 patients had good outcomes.

Surgical Treatment

The outcomes of surgery for osteochondral fractures of the talus are controversial. It is hard to compare results between authors as they have often used different outcome measures. Some authors use pain as their primary outcome[91] whereas others also consider radiologic healing. The long term outcome of an asymptomatic subchondral lucency in the talar body is unknown. In some series, the patients have had arthrotomies[91] while others had arthroscopic débridement.[123] The staging of the lesions are also subject to interobserver variability.[91] Letts et al.[89] performed surgery in 24 patients with osteochondral lesions. They used arthroscopy in three patients only and two of those patients required arthrotomy as well.[89] With modern ankle arthroscopy equipment and newer surgical techniques, ankle arthroscopy has become the primary surgical treatment for both medial and lateral lesions of the talar dome. The anterolateral lesions are more accessible; however, with good ankle distraction and different portal placement posteromedial lesions are accessible.

Recently, Perumal et al.[123] reviewed 31 patients with juvenile OCD with a minimum of 6-months follow-up. They recommended nonoperative treatment with an ankle brace and activity modification in most cases for 6 months. Only 16% of the lesions healed radiographically in that timeframe. If pain continues after this time and the lesion is still present, further immobilization and activity modification is recommended. They recommend arthroscopic surgery for patients with type II lesions who are not prepared to modify their activities longer than 6 months and patients with type III lateral lesions and all stage IV lesions. Thirteen of the 31 patients were treated surgically.

Arthroscopic treatment options include:

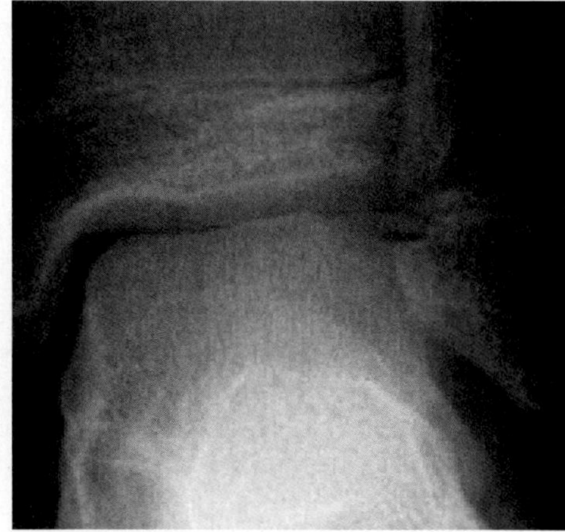

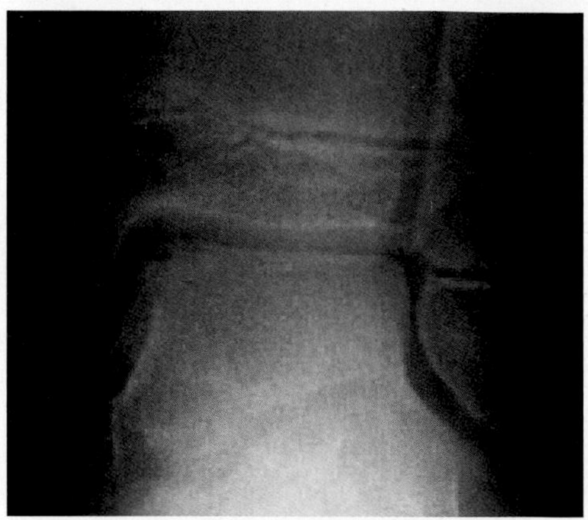

FIGURE 27-13 A. Anterolateral stage III osteochondral lesion that was treated by arthroscopic excision and microfracture. **B.** Posteromedial stage II osteochondral lesion that was treated successfully nonoperatively.

1. Drilling the lesion (antegrade or retrograde)
2. Curettage and microfracture
3. Internal fixation with bioabsorbable nails
4. Bone grafting and internal fixation

In stage II lesions with intact articular cartilage, Kumai et al.[82] showed excellent results drilling through the lesion into the subchondral bone. They also found that in skeletally immature patients, there may be an increased tendency for the lesion to heal when compared to the adult patients. Retrograde drilling can be performed using specific tip directed instrumentation.[161] This avoids damage to the articular cartilage and may prevent fragmentation of a small lesion. Access to a posteromedial lesion can be difficult. One approach is to use a transmalleolar portal after drilling a 3.5-mm drill through the medial malleolus or to use a posteromedial portal taking care to avoid damaging the neurovascular bundle.

Curettage and microfracture is a very effective, relatively straightforward procedure. It is particularly useful in small stage III and stage IV lesions where the fragment is too small to internally fix or there is no subchondral bone on the lesion for healing. The articular cartilage is débrided back to stable tissue and the subchondral bone is curettaged until bleeding occurs. Either a microfracture pick or 2-mm drill is then used in the subchondral bone. Anderson et al.[8] would suggest this treatment for all stage IIa lesions where a subchondral cyst is present.

Internal fixation with or without bone grafting is a difficult procedure for the inexperienced arthroscopist. It is preferable to use absorbable pegs or nails rather than metallic implants. In large stage III and IV acute osteochondral lesions, this is probably the treatment of choice rather than excising the fragment.

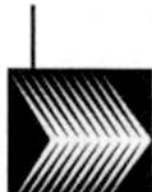

AUTHORS' PREFERRED TREATMENT

For simple undisplaced fractures, a below-knee nonwalking cast is applied for 6 weeks.

Displaced lateral process fractures need to be anatomically reduced especially if they are intra-articular and there is 2 to 3 mm of incongruity in the joint surface. A lateral approach is used and a single compression screw inserted across the fracture. The foot is immobilized in a below-knee cast for 6 weeks.

Displaced talar neck fractures should be operated on as soon as possible. If the fracture can be reduced closed, the author prefers a posterolateral approach to insert the compression screws as this helps preserve the tenuous blood supply (see Fig. 27-4). These screws are best inserted through this open approach so an accurate starting point can be found and neurovascular structures protected. The author has no hesitation to use an anteromedial approach as well to help with fracture reduction before inserting the screws. Through this approach, the neck fragment can be stabilized while the screws are being compressed and anatomic fracture reduction can be seen. Usually, two 4.5-mm partially threaded titanium screws are used depending on the size of the talus and degree of fragmentation. The titanium screws allows MRI postoperatively if osteonecrosis is suspected.

Acute osteochondral injuries need to be recognized and distinguished from OCD lesions. Acute lesions should be repaired after assessing the amount of bone present on the lesion. This can be initially assessed arthrocopically but is repaired through an arthrotomy depending on the position on the talus. The author prefers to repair the lesion with dissolvable nails.

The author treats types I to III OCD lesions nonoperatively for 6 months. Initially, the child or adolescent wears a Cam walker for 4 to 6 weeks to help the symptoms settle and then an elastic ankle support and activity modification. If symptoms persist, the author performs a repeat MRI scan and, if the staging has worsened, proceeds to an arthroscopic débridement and microfracture or stabilization. For patients with displaced fragments on presentation (stage IV), the author recommends arthroscopic removal and microfracture or repair if possible.

Complications

Osteonecrosis of the Talus

Osteonecrosis of the talus is the most serious complication of talus fractures. This has been reported in a number of large series of predominantly adult patients.[26,61] Osteonecrosis of the body of the talus occurs when the blood supply has been disrupted by a fracture of the talar neck. The result is necrosis of the talar dome and possible collapse of the articular surface. It appears that this process of necrosis can start as early as the first month following the fracture. Hawkins[61] described the presence of a subchondral lucent line, the "Hawkins sign," as prognostic of a good outcome as it indicates adequate blood flow to the talar body. The absence of the sign on a 6 to 8 week radiograph implies there is inadequate blood supply and osteonecrosis may evolve.

In adults, the incidence of osteonecrosis seems directly related to the degree of displacement of the femoral neck fracture. Hawkins[61] showed that type I fractures had a 0% to 10% AVN rate, type II fractures a 20% to 50% AVN rate, type III an 80% to 100% AVN rate, and all type IV fractures develop AVN. Canale and Kelly[26] had similar long-term results.

Osteonecrosis has also been seen in pediatric talus fractures; however, it does not seem to be as predictable as the adult literature suggests. The Hawkins sign was described in adults, and Ogden[118] suggests this sign may not be as reliable in the cartilaginous talar dome of a child. Mazel et al.[105] reported on seven complete fractures of the talar neck in children over 6 years of age and two developed AVN. Similarly, Letts and Gibeault[92] had 3 children with AVN after talus fractures. Interestingly, 2 of these patients had undisplaced fractures of the talus at the time of their injury that were not initially picked up. Subsequent radiographs revealed the AVN.[92] Rammelt and colleagues[134] also reported on a 5-year-old whose undisplaced talar neck fracture was missed who went on to develop AVN. In a literature search, they found a 16% incidence of AVN of the talus in undisplaced talar fractures in children. They suggest that the pediatric talus is more susceptible to AVN than the adult counterpart.[134] Jensen et al.,[74] on the other hand, had no cases of AVN in 14 children with talus fractures.

The dilemma for the treating surgeon is what to advise the patient regarding weight bearing when the Hawkins sign is not present by 8 weeks. Some of the above series report AVN occurring 6 months after the injury and not resolving for many years. There does not appear to be any series comparing outcomes in patients who bear weight over this period and those who do not. If the Hawkins sign is not present, it is advisable to perform an MRI scan at 3 months to establish if AVN is present or not.[63,163] If present, it may be advisable to encourage the child to avoid impact activities to prevent collapse rather than have a prolonged period of non–weight bearing.

CALCANEAL FRACTURES

Epidemiology

Fractures of the calcaneus are rare in children with an incidence of only 1 in 100,000 fractures.[174] The treatment of these fractures has historically been nonoperative, relying on the largely cartilaginous bone to remodel with time. The majority of fractures in children less than 14 years old are extra-articular whereas in older children the fracture pattern resembles those in adults. Children appear to have more coexisting lower limb fractures than adults but fewer fractures of the axial skeleton.[150]

Calcaneal fractures in young children are often missed or are diagnosed late on radiographs or bone scan when the child is still limping long after the injury. At the other end of the spectrum, the adolescent patient has often had a major fall and has a displaced intra-articular fracture. This older age group should be treated like the adult population with open reduction and internal fixation restoring the joint congruity and calcaneal height and width. The challenge for the surgeon is at what age and what degree of displacement is this more aggressive treatment indicated in a group of patients traditionally treated nonoperatively.

Management

Mechanism of Injury

The most common mechanism of injury is a fall from a height. This axial load drives the talus into the calcaneus resulting in the fracture. The degree of communition appears to be less in children even though they often fall from greater heights than adults.[20] Wiley and Profitt[174] found that in young children, the fall was usually less than 4 feet and in children older than 10 years the fall was greater than 14 feet. They noted that the minor falls in the younger children often resulted in undisplaced fractures that were diagnosed late.

Schmidt and Weiner[150] reviewed 56 children with calcaneal fractures of which 25 (45%) were due to a fall from a height. They also found that children less than 14 years of age predominantly had extra-articular fractures, hypothesizing that the calcaneus in this age bracket absorbs the compression force rather than dissipating it through the joint.

Vehicle-related injuries were the second biggest cause of calcaneal fractures in both Schmidt and Weiner[150] and Wiley and Profitt's reviews.[174]

Fractures of the calcaneus can also occur in major crush injuries when compartment syndrome may coexist and open fractures are common in lawnmower injuries.

Signs and Symptoms

Any child who has fallen from a height and landed on their feet should be examined carefully for a calcaneal fracture. Associated injuries should also be evaluated with a thorough secondary survey, especially of the lower limbs and spine.

The foot will often be extremely swollen with bruising around the heel and dorsum of the foot. Symptoms and signs of compartment syndrome, including excessive pain, pallor, parasthesia, and pulselessness should be assessed. In more subtle injuries, careful palpation is necessary to elucidate areas of pain which may disclose an underlying undisplaced fracture.

Many calcaneal fractures in children are initially missed and diagnosed late. Often, the fracture line is not evident on the initial radiographs. Inokuchi et al.[71] reported that 44% of fractures in their series were initially missed, as were 55% of those reported by Schantz and Rasmussen[148] and 44% of those reported by Wiley and Profitt.[174]

A differential diagnosis must be kept in mind for other causes of heel pain in a child. These include Sever disease, osteomyelitis, a unicameral bone cyst, or a stress fracture.

Associated Injuries

Schmidt and Weiner[150] reviewed 59 children with 62 calcaneal fractures and found a number of associated injuries. These included fractures of the lumbar spine, lower limb fractures, a pelvic fracture, and upper extremity fractures. These other skeletal injuries were more frequent in children over 13 years of age. Associated lower limb fractures occurred twice as frequently as in adults; however, injuries to the axial skeleton occurred half as often as in adults. Wiley and Profitt,[174] however, only had 2 patients with accompanying significant injuries in their series of 32 pediatric calcaneal fractures.

Diagnosis and Classification

Plain Radiographs

Calcaneal fractures in children are often missed as the radiographic findings are usually more subtle than in adults.[83,104,150,158,174] Subsequent radiographs at 10 to 14 days often show the fracture line. The majority of these missed fractures are extra-articular.[150]

The standard views for a suspected calcaneal fracture are posteroanterior, lateral, and axial views. The posteroanterior view shows the calcaneocuboid and talonavicular joints well. The lateral view is excellent at showing the congruity of the posterior articular facet and allows calculation of Böhler's angle (see Fig. 27-9). The axial view demonstrates the tuberosity, the body, the sustenaculum tali, and the posterior facet of the calcaneus.. Oblique views are also useful and will show a fracture of the anterior process more clearly (Fig. 27-14).[136] The oblique views also define the subtalar joint well so are very useful in intra-articular fractures. Broden views can also be taken that look at the posterior facet of the calcaneus. These are taken with the leg internally rotated 40 degrees and the x-ray beam angled between 15 to 40 degrees toward the head.[18] This is a difficult radiograph for the technicians to master and almost the same information can be achieved by ordering a mortise view of the ankle and looking at the posterior facet of the subtalar joint.

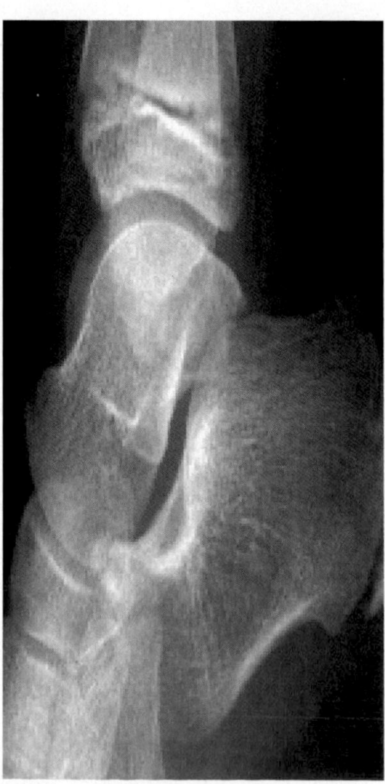

FIGURE 27-14 Fracture of the anterior process of the talus.

The lateral view is useful for measuring the Böhler angle. This is the angle between a line drawn from the highest point of the anterior process to the highest point of the posterior facet and a line drawn tangential to the highest point of the calcaneal tuberosity. The normal value in an adult is between 20 and 40 degrees. In a child, the angle is slightly less than in an adult and may be due to the incomplete ossification of the calcaneus. It is advisable to perform a lateral radiograph of the contralateral calcaneus to use as a comparison rather than accept the absolute value of Böhler's angle. The child's calcaneus does not resemble that of an adult until after 10 years of age.[67,69,118,166] Another angle which is not so easy to measure is "the crucial angle of Gissane". This is the angle formed by two strong cortical struts seen on the lateral radiograph. One runs along the lateral margin of the posterior facet and the other runs up to the anterior process of the calcaneus. The angle between them ranges from 95 to 105 degrees (see Fig. 27-9).[47]

When reviewing radiographs of children's feet, it is always important to be cognizant of the normally appearing ossification centers and accessory bones about the growing foot, which often are confused with fractures (see Figs. 27-1 and 27-2).[27] The os calcis is the earliest tarsal bone to ossify with the primary ossification center appearing in the third intrauterine month. The secondary ossification center appears around 6 to 8 years and is the crescentic epiphysis seen posteriorly that gives rise to Sever's disease. This epiphysis fuses to the body of the calcaneus when the adolescent is 14 to 16 years old.

The use of a technetium-labeled bone scan in diagnosing calcaneal fractures is uncommon with the ready availability of MRI scans. The bone scan is useful in evaluating a nonlocalized painful limp in a toddler and in this setting a calcaneal fracture may be diagnosed. Laliotis et al.[83] used bone scans and identified five calcaneal fractures in 7 toddlers less than 36 months of age who had no history of significant injury. Bone scanning is sensitive for bone pathology but not specific and will be positive when other conditions are present like infection, Sever disease, juvenile arthritis, and some neoplasms. A CT scan is a useful investigation to evaluate the positive bone scan.

Computed Tomography Scanning

CT scanning has evolved as the best method to evaluate the fractured calcaneus. Not only does it clearly show the fracture lines and altered anatomy, but also reveals injuries to adjacent bones. Sanders et al.[146] have used CT scans to develop a classification system that is particularly useful in the preoperative planning of open reduction of these fractures. The primary and secondary fracture lines are identified and the degree of communition and position of the fragments is more accurately seen than in the radiographs. The primary fracture line usually runs obliquely from plantar-medial to dorsolateral exiting the posterior facet. Secondary fracture lines that develop off this primary line are also seen and their pattern determines the classification of the fracture (Fig. 27-15). The CT scan also allows a three-dimensional reconstruction to be made which again is useful in visualizing the fracture lines for possible internal fixation.

Buckingham et al.[20] and Ogden[118] reviewed 9 patients with 10 calcaneal fractures and performed CT scans on all of them. They found the fracture patterns in these adolescents (average 13.4 years old) to be very similar to those found in adults. They did find less communition in children than in adults, even though the children reportedly had fallen from greater heights.

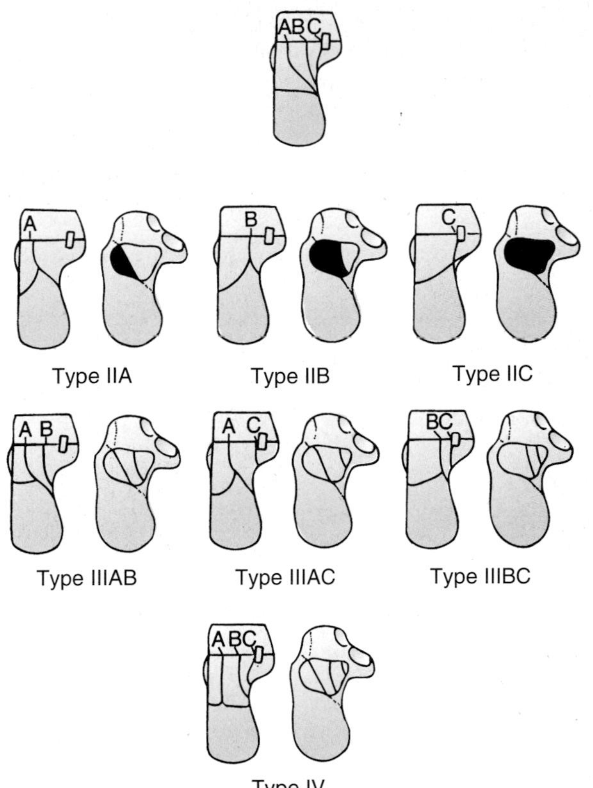

FIGURE 27-15 Sanders CT-based classification of intra-articular fractures of the calcaneus in adults. (From Sanders R. Intraarticular fractures of the calcaneus: present state of the art. J Orthop Trauma 1992;6:254, with permission.)

The use of MRI scans is largely unnecessary for the majority of calcaneal fractures. They can be useful in young children when the calcaneus is still largely cartilaginous and a fracture is not seen on plain films or CT.

Classification

Children's calcaneal fractures were traditionally classified according to their adult counterparts using the Essex-Lopresti[47] and Letournal[90] classifications. Schmidt and Weiner[150] reviewed 62 calcaneal fractures in children and compared them to the adult literature.[141] They used the classification systems of Essex-Lopresti[47] and Chapman and Galway[32] and added a new fracture type (type VI) to develop a classification for pediatric calcaneal fractures which is in routine use today (Fig. 27-16).

For adolescent fractures, it is probably more appropriate to use the Sanders classification.[146] This is an adult classification system that was developed after reviewing the CT scans on 120 cases preoperatively and at minimum 1-year follow-up. The follow up CT scans were correlated with the clinical outcome scores to help validate the classification system used.

Surgical and Applied Anatomy

The calcaneus is the largest tarsal bone and has quite an unusual shape. It has three articular facets (anterior, middle, and posterior) on the superior surface where it articulates with the talus to form the subtalar joint (see Fig. 27-7) and anteriorly there is a saddle-shaped articular surface for the cuboid. The posterior facet is the largest facet and is slightly convex. The middle facet is anterior and medial to the posterior facet lying on the sustenaculum tali. It is concave like the anterior facet with which it is often contiguous. Between the middle and posterior facets lies the calcaneal groove, which forms the inferior wall of the sinus

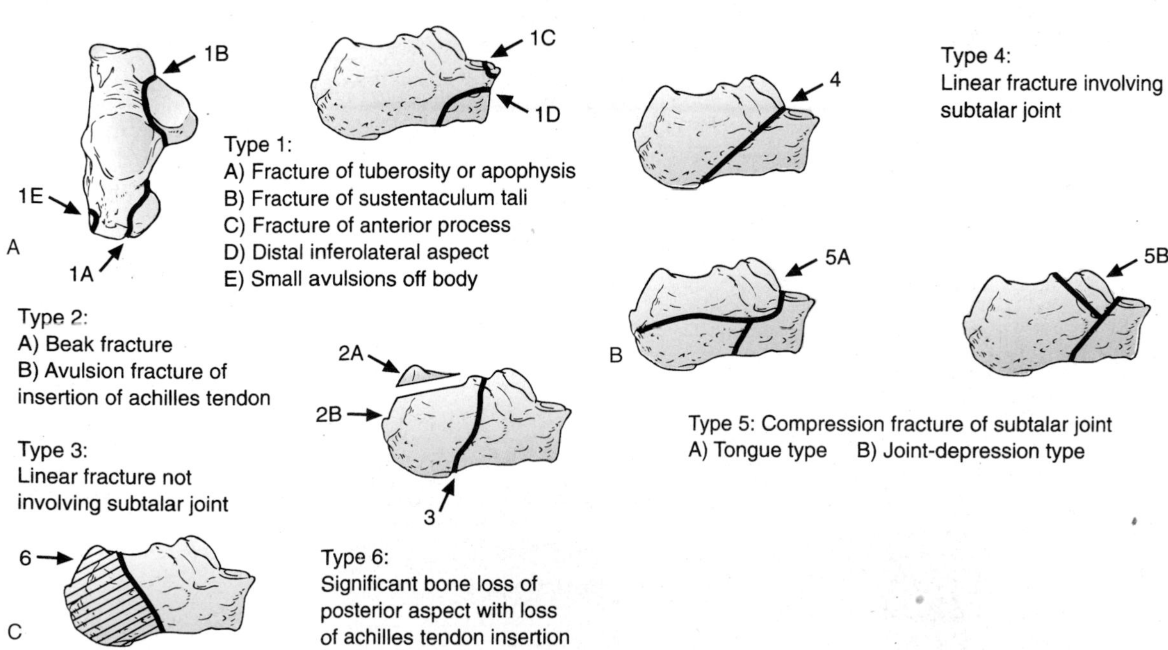

FIGURE 27-16 Schmidt and Weiner classification of calcaneal fracture patterns in children. **A.** Extra-articular fractures. **B.** Intra-articular fractures. **C.** Type 6 fracture pattern with significant bone loss, soft tissue injury, and loss of Achilles tendon insertion. (From Schmidt TL, Weiner DS. Calcaneus fractures in children: an evaluation of the nature of injury in 56 children. Clin Orthop Relat Res 1982;171:150, with permission.)

tarsi. Posteriorly, the tendoachilles inserts into the tuberosity of the calcaneus which is the whole area behind the posterior facet. On the lateral surface of the calcaneus are two shallow grooves with a small ridge in between (the peroneal trochlea). The peroneus longus and brevis run either side of this trochlea. The medial side is concave and is structurally stronger than the lateral side. The sustentaculum tali projects from the medial wall and supports the middle articular facet on its surface. The tendon of flexor hallucis longus runs on the undersurface of the sustenaculum. On the plantar surface are the medial and lateral processes for the origin of the abductor hallucis and abductor digiti minimi muscles, respectively (Fig. 24-17).

Secondary ossification occurs in the calcaneal apophysis between the ages of 6 and 10 years. Inflammation in the apophysis around this age causes heel pain and is referred to as Sever's disease.

The use of CT scans has defined the surgical anatomy of the calcaneus to help make treatment decisions. The coronal views show the important posterior facet and the sustenaculum tali and the height and width of the heel. The position of the peroneal tendons and flexor hallucis tendon can also be seen. The sagittal views provide additional information about the posterior facet and also show the anterior process well. The axial views visualize the calcaneocuboid joint well, the anteriorinferior aspect of the posterior facet, and the sustenaculum tali. This information can then be used in planning the reconstruction of the calcaneus.[144,145]

Current Treatment Options

Calcaneal fractures in growing children are usually less severe than in the adult population and often do well without operative intervention. The adolescent, on the other hand, often has fracture patterns similar to adults and requires open reduction and internal fixation. The challenge to the orthopaedic surgeon is to recognize the patient that requires this form of surgery. There is a degree of remodeling that will take place in the child and hence the amount of growth remaining, degree of ossification,

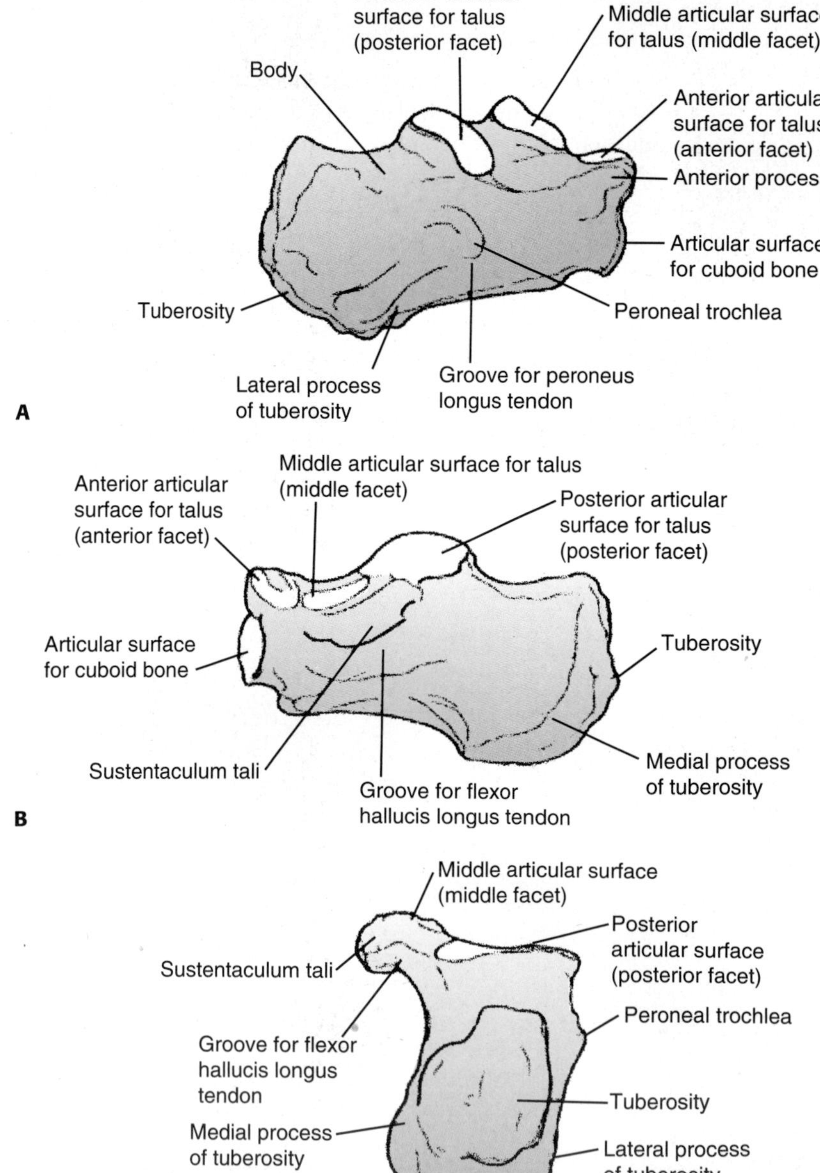

FIGURE 27-17 Anatomic details of various angles of the calcaneus including lateral **(A)**, medial **(B)**, and coronal **(C)** views through the level of the sustentaculum tali, which correlate with the CT scan view important in reconstruction of the posterior facet.

and difference in morphology from the contralateral side all need to be considered in making the treatment decisions.

Extra-articular fractures of the calcaneus are treated by cast immobilization for 6 weeks. The child can start weight bearing in this cast when comfortable and can be changed to a Cam walker for the final few weeks if necessary.[19,71]

Tongue-type fractures can be treated nonoperatively if the posterior gap is less than 1 cm and the Achilles tendon has not been significantly shortened by bringing the fragment up proximally. Occasionally, the technique described by Essex-Lopresti[47] for percutaneous reduction of tongue-type fractures (Fig. 27-18) is useful.

Open reduction and internal fixation is reserved for the severe intra-articular fractures with displacement of the fragments and depression of the joint surfaces. These fractures occur almost exclusively in the adolescent patient where the ossification process is complete. The adult literature abounds with indications for internal fixation, surgical approaches, rehabilitation, complications, and outcome measures (Fig. 27-19).[10,126,143–146] These series only have a few adolescent fractures among them, and therefore it is difficult to draw any conclusions specifically about children's calcaneal fractures. The literature on the management of displaced intra-articular fractures in children is somewhat conflicting in the indications for surgery. Schantz and Rasmussen[148] reported on the outcome of displaced intra-articular fractures in children less than 15 years old treated nonoperatively. The majority of the patients had a good outcome; however, 4 complained of pain an average of 12 years after injury.[148,162] Brunet[19] believes the outcome does not correlate to the severity of the fracture. This is most likely due to the remodeling potential of the calcaneus in this age group. This concept also was supported by Mora et al.,[111] who concluded that open reduction may be suitable only for severely displaced fractures in adolescents. The difficulty is defining the age or maturity of the patient that may predict a poor outcome if the fracture is left unreduced. Using validated quality-of-life scales 2 to 8 years after surgery, Buckley et al.[21] found that younger patients (adults under the age of 30 years) who had operative treatment had better gait satisfaction scores than those who did not have surgery. Allmacher et al.[6] questioned whether short-term or intermediate results of displaced intra-articular calcaneal fractures can predict long-term functional outcome. Using validated outcome instruments, they studied adult patients treated nonoperatively and found that nonoperative treatment often led to pain and loss of function, which increased in the second decade after injury.

Pickle et al.[126] reviewed the results of open reduction with internal fixation of displaced intra-articular calcaneal fractures in 6 adolescent patients (average age, 13 years) and found good short-term results at an average of 30 months after injury. None of the 6 patients (seven calcaneal fractures) developed any of the serious complications reported in adults. Four of the seven feet were completely pain-free, and three had some minor pain with sports or hard floors. Ceccarelli[28] found that adolescents with displaced intra-articular fractures had better clinical and radiologic outcomes if treated by open reduction rather than nonoperatively. Buckingham et al.[20] reviewed 10 adolescent patients and reported good or excellent outcomes in 8 patients. They had no wound complications and the range in motion was hardly affected in 7 patients. They recommended the routine removal of the screws and plates after fracture healing as this had improved the symptoms in 6 of 8 patients.[20]

The surgery for these fractures is technically demanding, and if the treating surgeon is not experienced with the approach, the child is best referred to a colleague who is.

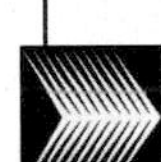

AUTHORS' PREFERRED TREATMENT

The key decision in treating children's calcaneal fractures is which ones require surgical intervention and which ones can be treated in a cast. Almost all closed fractures in children less than 10 years of age can be treated nonoperatively due to the remodeling potential. This includes intra-articular fractures that are displaced.

Extra-articular fractures of the calcaneus can be treated by nonoperative means with a below-knee cast for 6 weeks. Weight bearing in the cast can start after 2 to 3 weeks as the patient becomes more comfortable.

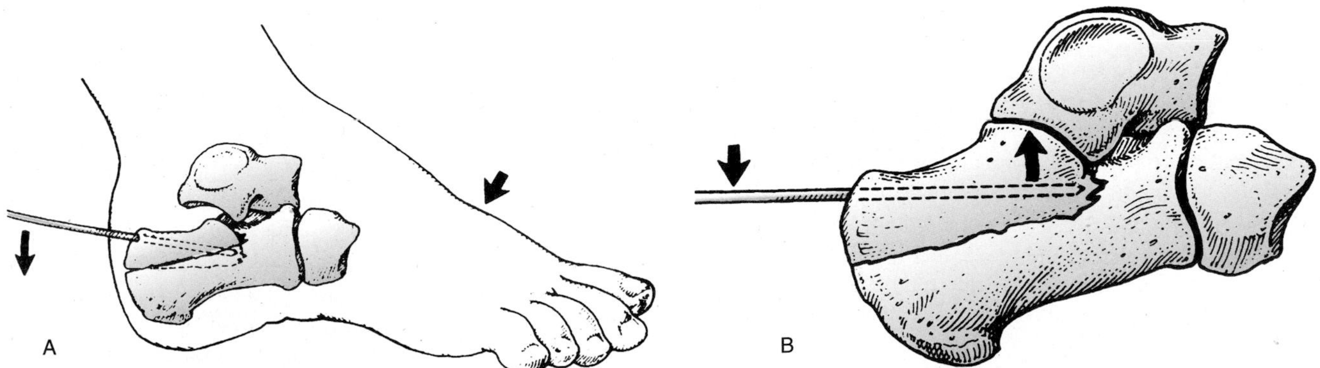

FIGURE 27-18 Percutaneous reduction technique for tongue-type fractures of the calcaneus, as described by Essex-Lopresti.[47] This technique remains an alternative to conservative treatment and open reduction with internal fixation of displaced, tongue-type fractures. **A.** A pin is inserted into the tongue fragment and used as a joystick to manipulate the fragment into better position, usually with a downward force on the pin and the forefoot (plantarflexion). **B.** After reduction, the pin is driven across the fracture to maintain reduction. (From Tornetta a III. The Essex-Lopresti reduction for calcaneal fractures revisited. J Orthop Trauma 1998;12: 471, with permission.)

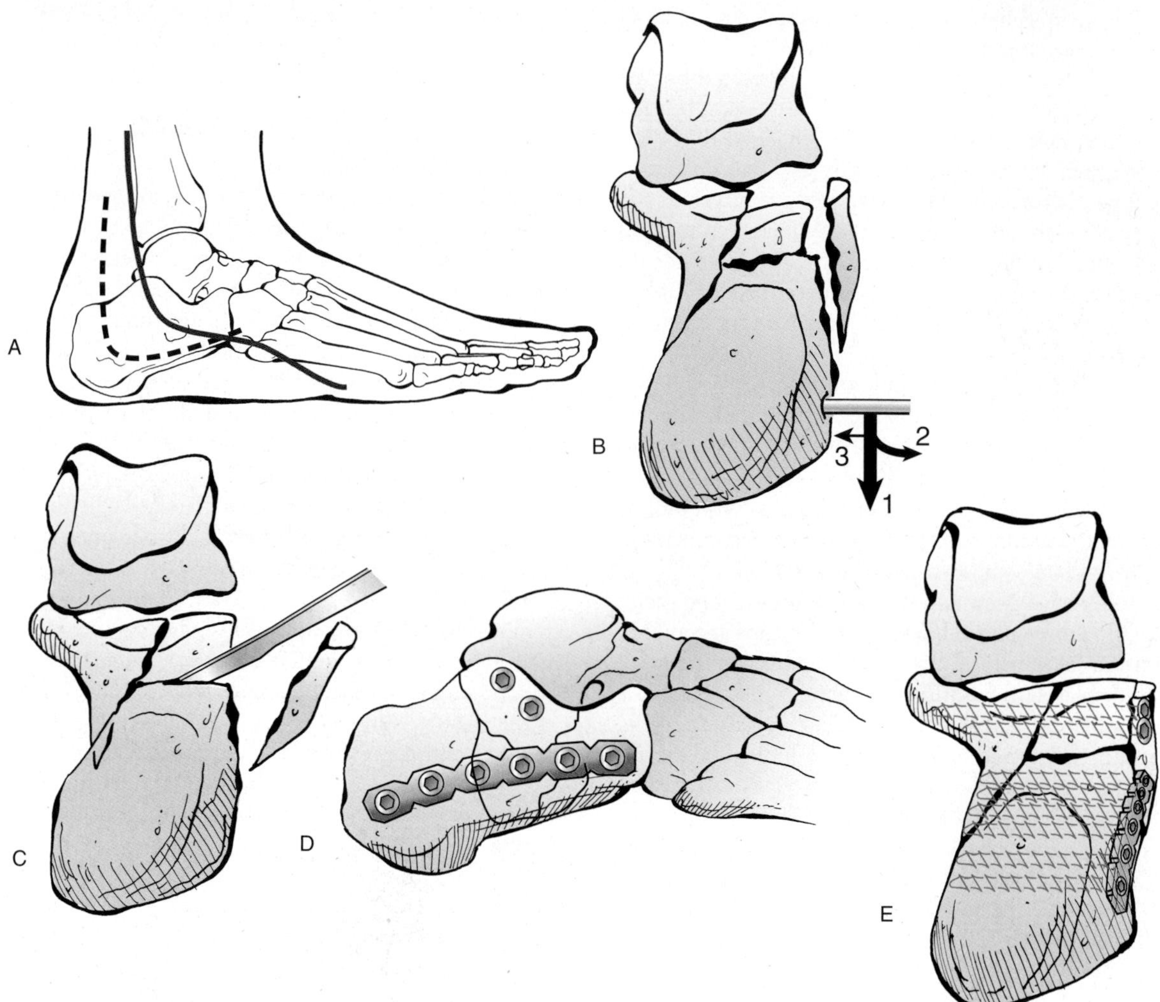

FIGURE 27-19 A. Lateral L-shaped approach to displaced intra-articular calcaneal fractures. The incision (*dashed line*) is laterally based, with the proximal arm approximately half the distance from the fibula to the posterior border of the foot and the distal arm halfway from the tip of the fibula to the sole of the foot. The sural nerve is illustrated. A full-thickness, subperiosteal flap exposes the entire lateral calcaneus. **B.** Reduction maneuvers 1, 2, and 3 (*densest arrow indicates greatest displacement*) with a Schantz screw are used to pull the tuberosity down and allow access to disimpact the posterior facet **(C)** after the lateral wall of the calcaneus is levered open. The posterior facet is then reduced anatomically, held provisionally with K-wires, and then fixed with two partially threaded cancellous screws (outside of plate) into the sustentaculum tali. Lateral view **(D)** of reduced calcaneus and axial view **(E)** of reduced fracture with hardware. (From Benirschke SK, Sangeorzan BJ. Extraarticular fractures of the foot: surgical management of calcaneal fractures [Review]. Clin Orthop Relat Res 1993;292:128–134; with permission.)

Undisplaced intra-articular fractures can also be treated in a below-knee cast. In this group of patients, it is advisable for them to be nonweight bearing for 6 weeks or until the fracture is healed to prevent further displacement.

Adolescent patients with displaced intra-articular fractures are best treated by open reduction and internal fixation (see Figs. 27-19 and 17-20). Before embarking on this surgery, a thorough assessment of the skin needs to be performed. Surgery should be delayed to allow swelling to subside and fracture blisters to resolve. This will decrease some of the wound complications commonly seen after open fixation of adult calcaneal fractures. The key point in performing this surgery is to maintain thick skin flaps, restore joint congruity, use specialized calcaneal plates, and be prepared to bone graft the defect. An outline of the surgical technique is in Table 27-3.

Complications

Wound Complications

Wound dehiscence is the most common complication following open reduction of adult calcaneal fractures.[10,68,93,146]

Although reported to occur in up to 25% of adult fractures, the incidence is lower in children. Pickle et al.[126] had no wound problems in the six adolescents (age range 11 to 16 years) they treated with open reduction and internal fixation. All the patients were treated with an extensile lateral approach an average of 10.5 days from the time of injury. The lower incidence in children reflects fewer risk factors in this group when compared to the adult population. Smoking, obesity, and diabetes all contribute to wound problems.

Wound dehiscence can be decreased by meticulous closure of the incision. In adults, it has been shown that a two layer closure is preferable to a single layer of sutures.[1,51] Wound

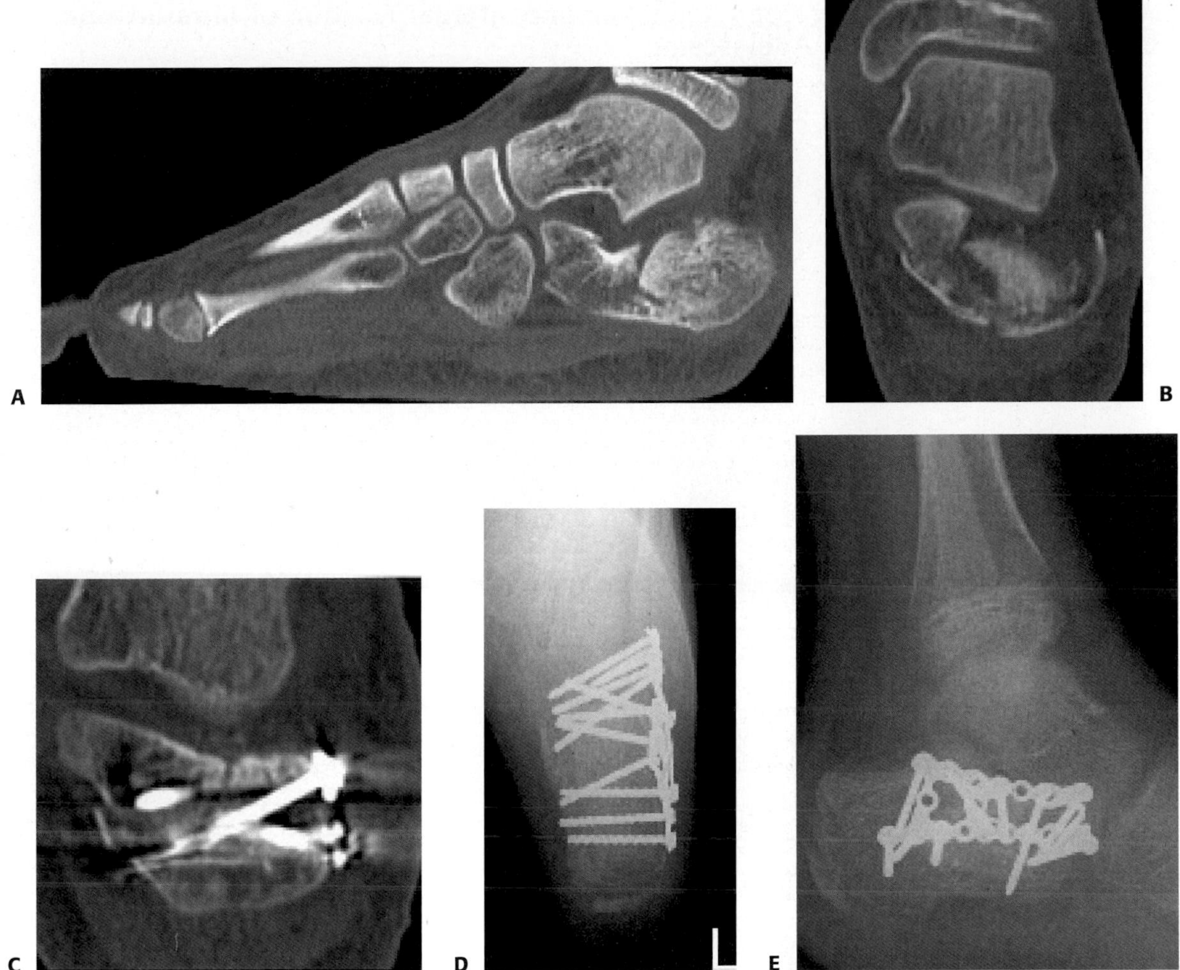

FIGURE 27-20 Intra-articular depressed fracture of the calcaneus in a 13-year-old boy. **A.** Preoperative sagittal CT shows the depression of the posterior facet into the body of the calcaneus. **B.** Coronal CT shows the displacement of the frature fragments. **C.** Postoperative CT scans are useful at checking the fracture reduction and length and position of the screws. **D,E.** Postoperative radiographs confirm restoration of the Böhler angle.

dehiscence can occur from days to weeks after the surgery. The best initial treatment is immobilization of the foot and ankle to decrease any tension on the wound edges. This is best accomplished in a below-knee cast with a large window cut around the entire incision. This allows space for wound dressing changes and débridements as necessary. Oral antibiotics may be required if superficial infection is also present. Once the wound is healed, gradual mobilization can be reinstated.

In serious deep wound infections, the patient will require rehospitalization, repeat surgical débridements, and intravenous antibiotics. Often, the use of a suction dressing (Vacuum-Assisted Closure [VAC], KCI, Inc., San Antonio, TX) is advisable in recalcitrant wounds. This VAC device has been shown to be safe and effective by Mooney et al.[110] for traumatic wounds in pediatric patients of all ages. Skin closure is usually not possible following such radical débridement. It is very helpful to consult with plastic surgeons early in the course of treatment as the patient often requires tissue transfer to cover the exposed metalware.

Complex Regional Pain Syndrome

This syndrome, previously known as reflex sympathetic dystrophy (RSD), is a devastating painful disorder that can occur following operative or nonoperative management of a calcaneal fractures or other trauma about the foot. The condition is usually diagnosed when there is severe pain present out of proportion to the severity of the injury following the acute phase of healing. The pain is difficult to control even with oral narcotics. The child will not bear weight or even allow the foot to be examined. Light touch even by water may stimulate an unusual pain response. The foot clinically demonstrates the signs of autonomic dysfunction. There is often a greyish discoloration, cold clammy skin, and decreased hair growth. Through disuse of the foot, the calf will atrophy. If radiographss are taken, the bones of the foot will show patchy disuse osteopenia.

There is a marked preponderance of lower extremity cases in children compared to adults.[170] Sarrail et al.[147] reviewed RSD in 24 children and adolescents and found that 73% had foot or ankle injuries. Wilder et al.[171] reviewed 70 children (average age, 12.5 years) with RSD and 87% had injuries to the lower limb. Eighty-four percent of their patients were girls, and on average the time from injury to a diagnosis of RSD was 12 months. Despite multidisciplinary treatments, 54% of patients still had persistent symptoms of RSD at 3 years after diagnosis. They emphasized that complex regional pain syndrome (CRPS) has a different disease course in children when compared with

TABLE 27-3 Operative Planning for Open Reduction and Internal Fixation of Intra-articular Calcaneal Fractures in Adolescents

Equipment	Radiolucent table Image Intensifier K-wires with driver Lambotte osteotomes Periosteal elevators AO modular foot set Synthes calcaneal plates, 2.7-mm reconstruction plates, H cervical plates
Positioning	Lateral decubitus on contralateral side Upper thigh pneumatic tourniquet Hip flexed 45 degrees, knee flexed 90 degrees Seattle cushions Radiolucent operating table
Incision	L-shaped incision (Letournel, Regazzoni, Bernirschke) Curved at apex Proximal extent 3 cm cephalid to tip of fibula anterior to lateral border of Achilles tendon Distal extent tip of base of fifth metatarsal
Exposure	Blunt dissection with scissors proximally to identify the short saphenous vein and sural nerve Sharp dissection with no. 15 blade direct to lateral wall of os calcaneus Subperiosteal reflection with scalpel Sharp dissection and reflection of peroneal tendons and attachment of calcaneofibular ligament dorsally Keep dorsal to the muscle belly of abductor digiti minimi Protect peroneal tendons with baby Hofmann's retractors when exposing the anterior process and calcaneocuboid joint Elevate flap dorsally to expose the posterior facet of the talus and sinus tarsi Maintain flap anteriorly with K-wires placed into the body and neck of the talus and the fibula Deflate tourniquet when exposure complete
Reduction	Place Schanz pin in inferior aspect of posterior tuber Reduce fracture by traction on the Schanz pin displacing posterior tuber inferiorly and thence medially Reflect lateral wall laterally if necessary Reduce anterior process first, then posterior facet, and finally restore alignment of the os calcis by confirming reduction and alignment of the crucial angle Thus reduce anterior to posterior, medial to lateral, and dorsal to plantar Provisional reduction maintained with multiple K-wires Reduction and alignment confirmed by screening with image intensifier
Fixation	Contour 2.7-mm reconstruction plate or an AO calcaneal plate to the lateral wall of the os calcis and fix to anterior process and the posterior tuber Maintain posterior facet reduction with two interfragmentary screws angled well inferiorly to avoid the inferiorly curved medial surface of the calcaneal posterior facet and to engage the sustenactulum
Closure	Irrigation Always drain Two-layered closure 2-0 Vicryl to the subcutaneous tissues (Interrupted vertical. Place all sutures on clips, tie individually commencing at the apex of the incision) Skin closure with interrupted 3-0 Nylon Donati Allgower sutures (all placed on clips and then tied individually commencing at the apex moving symmetrically to the proximal and distal extent of the wound holding multiple sutures to maintain even tension)
Dressings	Gelnet dressing Well padded below knee popliteal joint back slab supporting toes
Postoperative	Elevation on two pillows IV antibiotics CT scan to check reduction and exclude screw malposition Remove drain when drainage is less than 10 mLs over an 8-hour period Review wound for hematoma and skin viability within 48 hours Continue splintage, elevation, and restricted mobility nonweight bearing until sutures removed 14–18 days postsurgery

Courtesy of Dr. ACL Campbell, FRACS, Adult Foot and Ankle Surgeon, Auckland City Hospital, New Zealand.

adults and needs to be treated appropriately. CRPS occurs most commonly in girls with the incidence peaking at or just before puberty.[170]

Most tertiary children's hospitals now have multidisciplinary pain teams that treat CRPS. These comprise a physician (anesthetist or pediatrician), a psychiatrist or clinical psychologist, a physiotherapist, and sometimes an occupational therapist. The child initially undergoes a multidisciplinary assessment that involves both schooling and social circumstances. The physiotherapist carries out a thorough functional assessment.

The treatment focuses on improving function and therefore extensive physiotherapy is performed initially. Analgesics need to be used to facilitate this and include anti-inflammatory drugs, amitriptyline, and gabapentin. In severe cases, regional blocks occasionally need to be used to control the pain. Children appear to respond to physiotherapy better than adults and they require less medication and invasive procedures. On the other hand, the recurrence rate of CRPS is higher in children; however, they respond well to the reinitiation of treatment.[170]

Peroneal Tendonitis/Dislocation

Peroneal tendon pain can occur in both the operated and nonoperated foot. Pain in the peroneal tendons on movement or direct palpation may indicate prominent underlying metalware. Simply removing the offending screw or plate may help. Buckingham et al.[20] recommended the routine removal of metalware in their series of adolescent calcaneal fractures as this resulted in resolution of pain in their patients.

The extensile L-shaped lateral incision has largely prevented the peroneal tendon subluxation that used to occur with the Kocher incision. Care has to be taken at the proximal and distal ends of this incision as the sural nerve can be damaged and a painful neuroma develop.

In patients with calcaneal fractures treated nonoperatively, a displaced lateral wall can sublux or even dislocate the peroneal tendons. Lateral impingement pain can also result from the fragment coming in direct contact with the fibula.

Diagnostic local anesthetic injections have been useful in differentiating the cause of pain in the adult foot but its use in children is limited. It should, however, be considered in adolescents who are willing to cooperate.

SUBTALAR DISLOCATION

Subtalar dislocations (peritalar dislocation) occur infrequently and are particularly uncommon in children. They occur most often in young adult males. There are no series published on this condition in children; however, Dimentberg and Rosman[41] reported on five talonavicular dislocations.

A medial dislocation is the most common type (85%) and results from a forced inversion injury to the foot. The talonavicular and talocalcaneal ligaments rupture while the calcaneonavicular ligament stays intact. The result is that all the bones of the foot dislocate medially while the talus remains in the ankle mortise (Fig. 27-21). The foot looks markedly deformed and the talar head can be palpated laterally. A lateral dislocation is caused by a forced eversion injury and results in a laterally displaced "flatfoot."

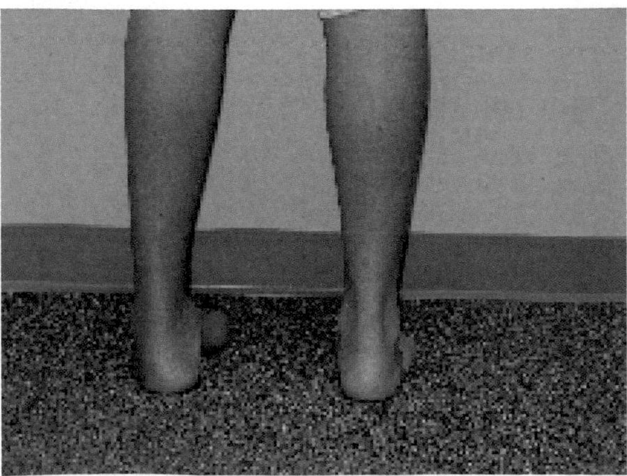

FIGURE 27-21 Posterior view demonstrating cavovarus deformity of the left foot. (Courtesy of Dr. Thomas Lee, MD.)

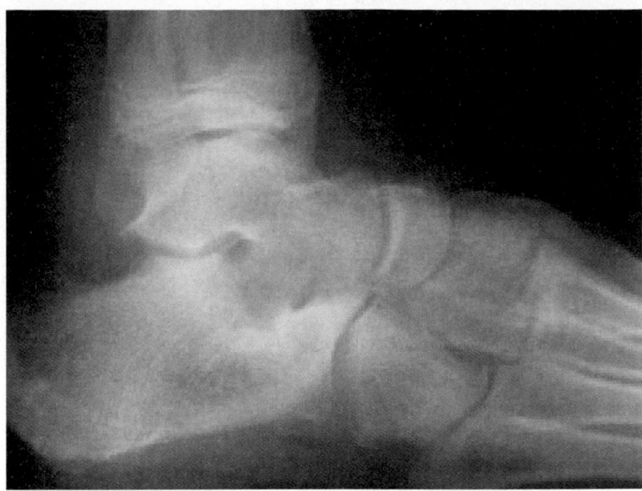

FIGURE 27-22 Lateral view showing subluxation of the subtalar joint. There is incongruity of the calcaneocuboid joint. (Courtesy of Dr. Thomas Lee, MD.)

Radiographs are difficult to interpret in this unusual injury (Figs. 27-22 and 27-23). The key is to look for the "empty navicular" where the talar head no longer articulates with it. A CT scan is useful to look for any associated fractures or osteochondral damage; however, it is probably more useful to perform this after a closed reduction to confirm anatomic alignment as well (Fig. 27-24).

The treatment for a closed subtalar dislocation is a reduction under general anesthetic. The knee should be flexed to relax the tendoachilles and then the deformity accentuated before a

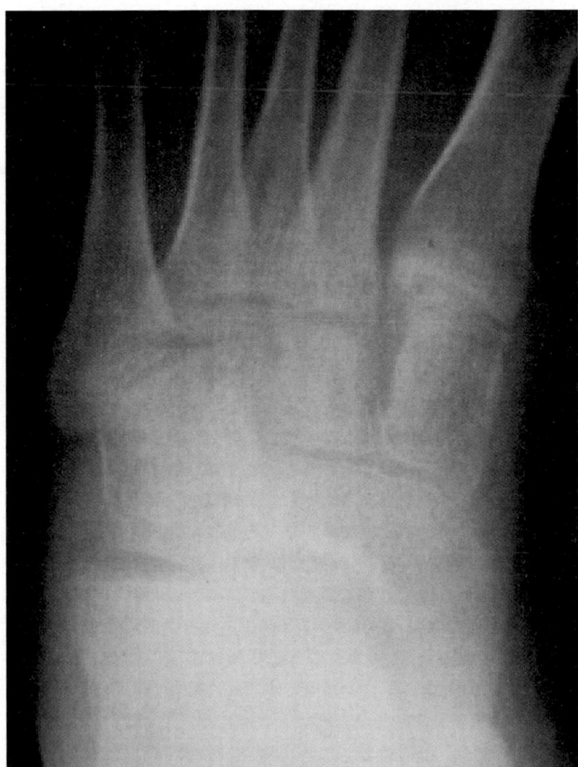

FIGURE 27-23 AP view demonstrating translation of the transverse tarsal joint. (Courtesy of Dr. Thomas Lee, MD.)

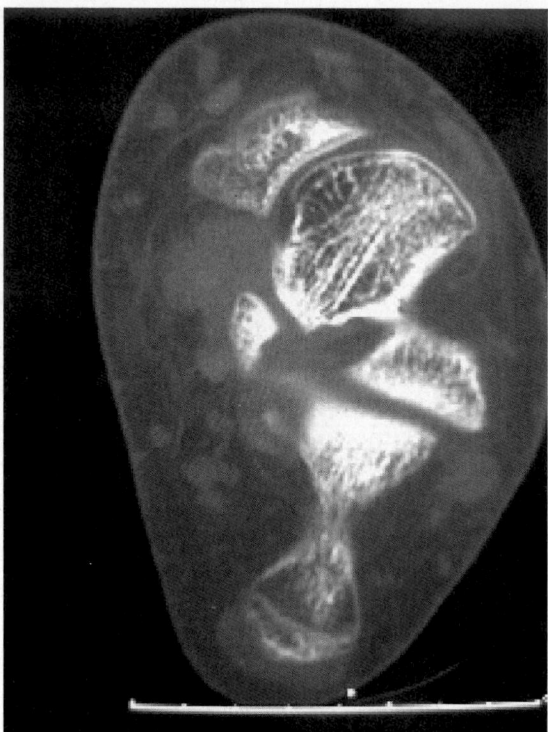

FIGURE 27-24 CT scan axial view shows marked talar head uncoverage ("ball is not in cup"). There is also significant incongruity of the subtalar joint. (Courtesy of Dr. Thomas Lee, MD.)

reduction is carried out by relocating the deformed foot. Usually, the reduction is stable and anatomic reduction can be confirmed by radiographs and CT scan. The foot is immobilized until the child is comfortable enough to start gentle mobilizations. K-wire stabilization and 6 weeks of immobilization are necessary for unstable dislocations.

Occasionally, the subtalar dislocation is irreducible by closed means and has to be opened through an anteromedial approach. The bone or soft tissue (often the tibialis posterior tendon) is removed from the joint and the foot reduced.

MIDTARSAL INJURIES

Fractures and dislocations of the navicular, cuboid, and cuneiforms are rare pediatric foot injuries. The midtarsal region extends from the calcaneocuboid and talonavicular joints (Chopart's joint) to the metatarsals. It includes the cuboid, navicular, and three cuneiform bones. These bones are interlinked by extremely strong ligaments especially on the plantar surface. The lateral side of the midfoot is more stable than the medial side. The shape of these small bones and strength of their ligaments help maintain the longitudinal and transverse arch of the foot. Disruption of this rigid anatomy therefore requires a large force especially in the cartilaginous bones of a child's foot. Isolated injuries to this area are rare and one needs to look for other associated fractures and dislocations.

Midtarsal injuries have been classified in adults by Main and Jowett.[100] This classification uses five broad categories based on the direction of the force causing the injury and the direction that the fragment is displaced. In parentheses are the percentages of this type of injury in Main and Jowett's[100] review of 71 midtarsal injuries.

Longitudinal stress (40%)
Medial stress (30%)
Lateral stress (17%)
Plantar stress (7%)
Crush injury (6%)

Hosking and Hoffman[66] reviewed four cases of midtarsal dislocations in children, and this is the only report in the literature of this injury in the pediatric age group. The children had an average age of 9.5 years, and the mechanism of injury was forced supination in 3 of the patients. They all had associated midtarsal injuries and presented with significant swelling. The key to making the diagnosis, which was delayed in 3 of the patients, was subluxation or dislocation of the calcaneocuboid joint on the lateral radiograph. The AP view only showed the dislocation in 2 patients and the oblique view showed it in only 1 patient.

The dislocation can usually be reduced closed and held with percutaneous K-wires. If an anatomic reduction is not possible closed, then one must proceed to an open reduction.

A CT scan should be performed to more clearly define the associated injuries to both the midtarsal bones and rest of the foot. One of the patients in Hosking and Hoffman's[66] series had an ipsilateral tibial fracture so associated injuries may be present due to the amount of force required to cause a midfoot disruption in a child.

Isolated fractures of the mid tarsal bones are rare. The navicular, cuboid, and cuneiforms are usually fractured in association with a Chopart joint (talonavicular and calcaneocuboid) dislocation or a serious Lisfranc injury. The navicular has a number of conditions that can mimic a fracture. Between the ages of 2 and 5 years, the navicular can become avascular (Kohler disease) and cause pain and limp while the changes seen on radiograph can look similar to a fracture (Fig. 27-25). Likewise, an

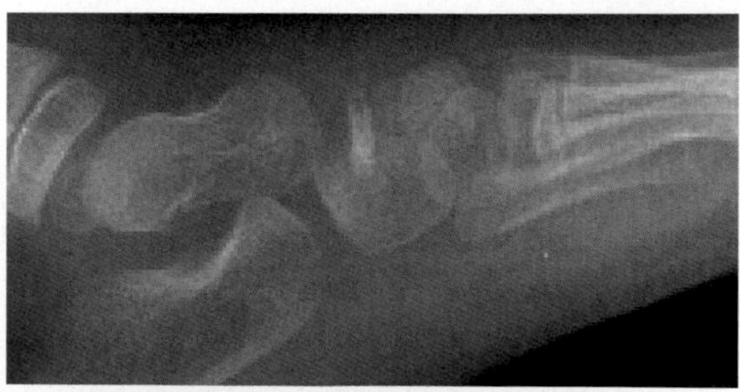

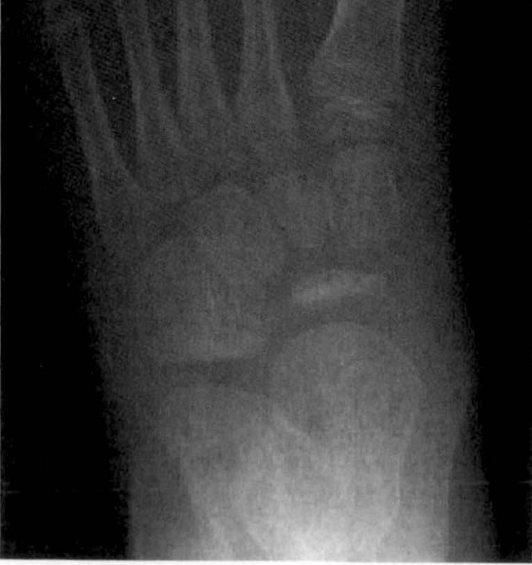

FIGURE 27-25 Kohler disease of the navicular that can occasionally be confused with a stress fracture.

accessory navicular may be present that may mimic an avulsion fracture of the navicular tuberosity. These can be differentiated from a fracture as they have smooth, rounded edges and are usually symmetrical when a radiograph is taken of the other foot. Stress fractures of the navicular are also becoming an increasingly common problem as children and adolescents train more aggressively for competitions (see stress fractures of the foot). These stress fractures usually run in the sagittal plane in the middle third of the bone. They are often difficult to see on plain radiographs but are more easily seen on bone scans, CT, and MRI.

Cuboid Fractures

Cuboid fractures were considered a rare foot injury in children and were usually associated with other foot fractures. Recent literature, however, reveals that this fracture may occur more often than we thought and commonly in isolation. Senaran et al.[152] reported on 28 consecutive cuboid fractures in preschool children from 1998 to 2004. They found most patients had an avoidance gait pattern and walked on the outside of their foot. They used the "nutcracker" maneuver to help diagnose the fracture. To perform this test, the heel is stabilized by the examiner and the forefoot is abducted. Pain in the lateral aspect of the foot usually confirms a fracture of the cuboid. The diagnosis was then confirmed on initial or subsequent radiographs. A below-knee cast or Cam walker was used for 2 to 3 weeks and all fractures healed without complications. Six patients had ipsilateral fractures in the tibia or foot. Interestingly, 8 patients had an associated genetic or systemic abnormality.[152] Cuboid fractures have been classified by Weber and Locher[169] into distal impaction shear-type fractures (type 1) and burst fractures (type 2).

Ceroni et al.[30] reported on 4 female teenagers who had equestrian injuries and cuboid fractures. The mechanism of the injury in all cases was a crush to the foot when the horse fell and abduction of the forefoot while it was still in the stirrup. All four cuboid fractures were associated with multiple midfoot fractures and the authors recommend CT scans in all patients in this age group with a cuboid fracture. Two patients required surgical reconstruction. This was performed through a lateral incision from the tip of the fibula to the base of the fifth metatarsal. The interval is then developed between the peroneal tendons and the extensor digitorum brevis. The lateral column length of is then restored using an allograft block.[30]

TARSOMETATARSAL INJURIES (LISFRANC FRACTURE–DISLOCATION)

Tarsometatarsal (TMT) injuries, more commonly referred to as a Lisfranc injury, are more common in adults than they are in children.[175] The degree of injury varies from a subtle disruption of the Lisfranc ligament to an extensive fracture–dislocation of the forefoot. Subtle injury can be difficult to diagnose especially if it is not thought about and if left untreated can develop into a painful chronic problem.

Although mostly described as isolated case reports,[17,29,133] a series of 18 TMT joint injuries in children was reported by Wiley[173] in 1981, and more recently Buoncristiani et al.[22] described an additional 8 such injuries in skeletally immature patients.

Management

Mechanism of Injury

TMT injuries are either due to a direct blow to the foot, usually secondary to a falling object, or indirect, where there is forced plantarflexion of the forefoot combined with a rotational force (Fig. 27-26).[172,173]

Traumatic Impact in the Tiptoe Position. This is an indirect injury where a load is applied to the foot while it is in the tiptoe position. A common example of this injury is jumping to the ground and landing awkwardly on the toes, producing acute plantarflexion at the TMT joint. The result is a TMT joint dislocation and usually a fracture at the base of the second metatarsal. Another example would be by putting the foot down suddenly to reduce speed while riding a bike.

Heel-to-Toe Compression. In this situation, the patient is in a kneeling position when the impact load strikes the heel. This is an example of a direct compression type injury and usually results in lateral dislocation of the lesser metatarsals and fracture of the base of the second metatarsal.

The Fixed Forefoot. In this third mechanism, the child falls backward while the forefoot is fixed to the ground by a heavy weight. An example would be a fall backwards while the foot was pinned under the wheel of a car. The patient's heel, which is resting on the ground, becomes the fulcrum for the forefoot injury.

In Wiley's[173] review of 18 patients with TMT joint injuries, 10 (56%) were a fall from a height in the "tiptoe" position, 3 (18%) suffered "heel to toe" compression, and 4 (22%) sustained a fall backwards while their forefoot was pinned to the ground. One patient could not recall their mechanism of injury following a motorbike collision.

Atypical Lisfranc injuries have recently been reported in mini-scooter injuries where the foot is planted to break speed. The resulting dorsiflexion, axial loading, and abduction cause the metatarsals to be impacted laterally. The result is a fracture of the base of the second metatarsal and a crush fracture of the cuboid.[13]

Signs and Symptoms

The diagnosis of these injuries may be difficult, and in adults as many as 20% of injuries are misdiagnosed or overlooked.[23,138] Some of the injuries are subtle and will present with minor pain and swelling at the base of the first and second metatarsals. This can be accompanied by ecchymosis on the plantar aspect of the midfoot where the TMT ligaments have been torn (Fig. 27-27).[139] This can be confirmed by gently abducting and pronating the forefoot while the hindfoot is held fixed with the other hand,[114] though this would be quite painful acutely. Alternatively, the child can be asked to try and perform a single limb heel lift. Pain in the midfoot often implies a TMT joint injury. With significant trauma, there is greater ligamentous injury and the resulting swelling makes it difficult to recog-

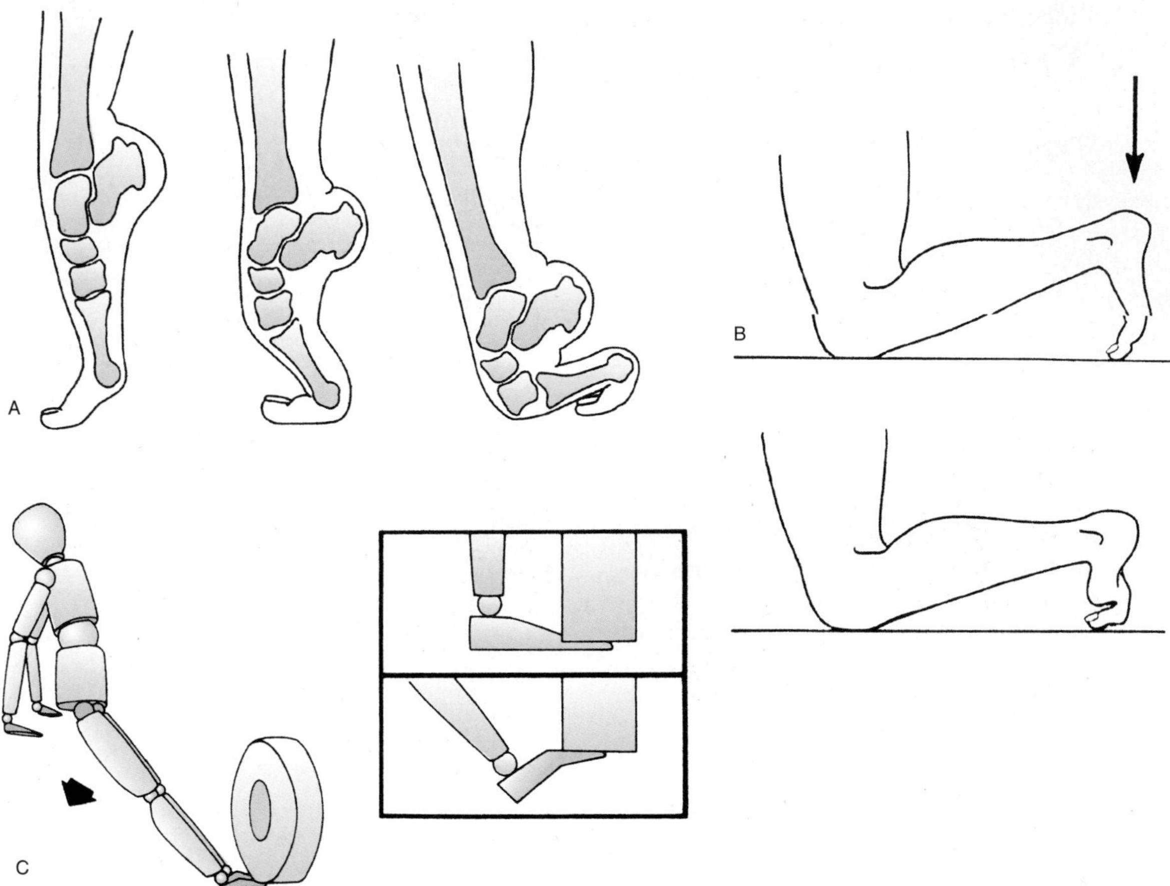

FIGURE 27-26 Mechanism of Lisfranc injuries. **A.** The most common mechanism of injury: progression from the "tiptoe" position to complete collapse of the TMT joint. **B.** Plantarflexion injury: direct heel-to-toe compression produces acute plantar flexion of the TMT joint. **C.** Backward fall with the forefoot pinned.

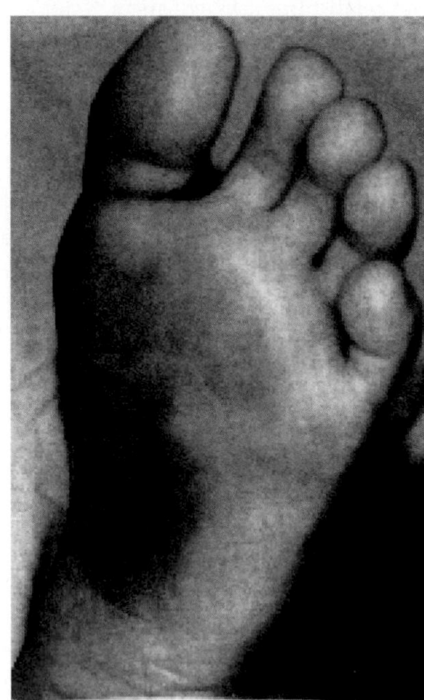

FIGURE 27-27 Plantar ecchymosis sign. Ecchymosis along the plantar aspect of the midfoot is an important clinical finding in subtle Lisfranc TMT injuries. (From Ross G, Cronin R, Hauzenblas J, et al. Plantar ecchymosis sign: a clinical aid to diagnosis of occult Lisfranc tarsometatarsal injuries. J Orthop Trauma 1996;10:120.)

nize any bony anatomy. It is important to assess the foot for a compartment syndrome in such circumstances, particularly when the foot has been crushed as part of the mechanism of injury.

The examiner of any child's foot following trauma needs to have a high level of suspicion for a Lisfranc injury as they are uncommon and difficult to diagnose but have a poor prognosis if left untreated.

Classification

Hardcastle et al.[59] developed a classification system based on the one developed by Queno and Kuss[131] in 1909 (Fig. 27-28). The classification comprises three types upon which treatment can be based.

Type A: Total incongruity. There is total incongruity of the entire metatarsal joint in a single plane. This can be either coronal or sagittal or combined.

Type B: Partial incongruity. Only partial incongruity of the joint is seen involving either medial displacement of the first metatarsal or lateral displacement to the four lateral metatarsals. The medial dislocation involves displacement of the first metatarsal from the first cuneiform because of disruption of the Lisfranc ligament or fracture at the base of the metatarsal, which remains attached to the ligament.

Type C: Divergent pattern. The first metatarsal is displaced medially; any combination of the lateral four metatarsals may

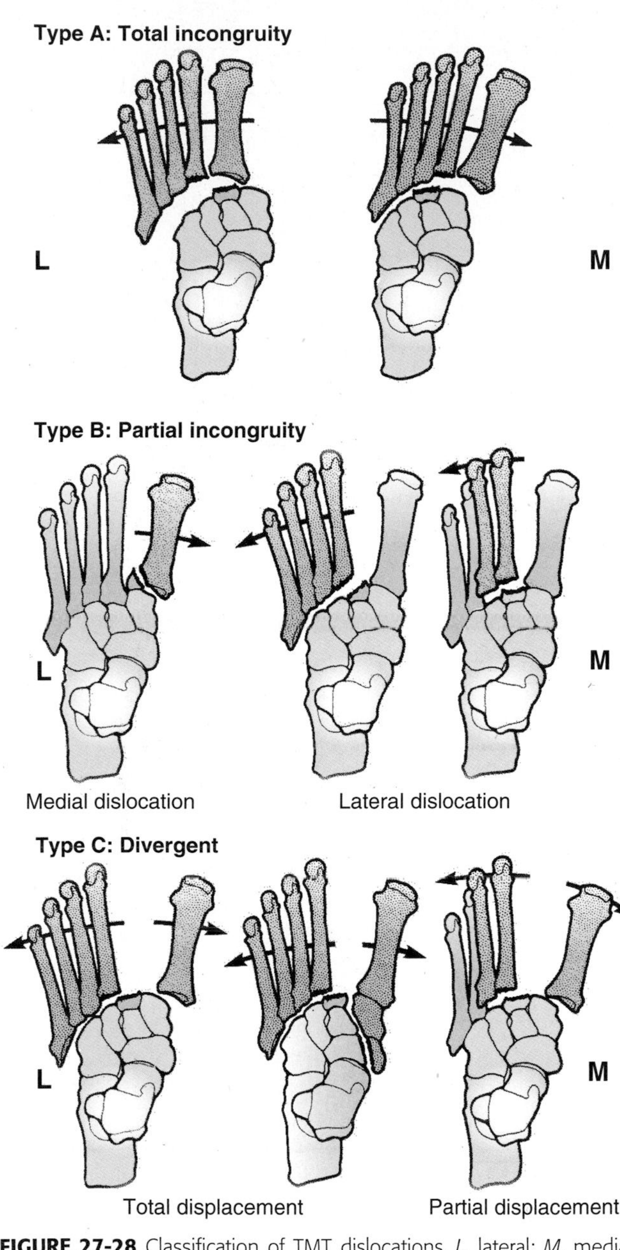

FIGURE 27-28 Classification of TMT dislocations. *L*, lateral; *M*, medial. (From DeLee JC. Fractures and dislocations of the foot. In: Mann RA, Coughlin MJ. Surgery of the Foot and Ankle. 6th ed. St. Louis: Mosby, 1993:1465–1703, with permission; From Hardcastle PH, Reschauer R, Kutscha-Lissberg E, et al. Injuries to the tarsometatarsal joint: incidence, classification, and treatment. J Bone Joint Surg Br 1982;64:349–356.)

be displaced laterally. This is associated with partial or total incongruity.

This classification does not address the nondisplaced TMT joint injury which can often be overlooked on initial assessment.

Most children's injuries are type B with minimal displacement, whereas types A and C are rare.[59,131,173]

Imaging Evaluation

The initial x-ray evaluation includes AP, lateral, and oblique views of the foot. These should be performed weight bearing if possible to stress the joint complex.

On the AP radiograph, the lateral border of the first metatarsal should be in line with the lateral border of the medial cuneiform and the medial border of the second metatarsal should line up with the medial border of the middle cuneiform. On the oblique radiograph, the medial border of the fourth metatarsal should be in line with the medial border of the cuboid. The examiner looks for a disruption in these lines or diastases of greater than 2 mm between the base of the first and second metatarsals. It is very useful to obtain a weight-bearing radiograph of the opposite foot for comparison (Fig. 27-29). When the radiographs appear normal or minimally displaced and a Lisfranc injury is still suspected, alternative imaging with CT or MRI scans is strongly recommended. The CT scan will often show a small avulsion fracture of the first TMT ligament and will show any other associated fractures in the foot.[55,87,99] The MRI scan can accurately visualize a partial tear or complete rupture of the first TMT ligament.[128]

A fracture of the base of the second metatarsal should alert the examiner to the possibility of a TMT dislocation because these injuries can spontaneously reduce. Likewise, a cuboid fracture in combination with a fracture of the base of the second metatarsal is highly suspicious for a Lisfranc injury (Fig. 27-30).

If weight-bearing radiographs are not possible, an abduction stress view can be obtained; however, in children these are difficult to obtain without general anesthesia. Bone scans may be helpful in the diagnosis of this injury when radiographs are normal, although they are not specific for the severity of the injury[57] and less useful than MRI or CT.

Surgical and Applied Anatomy

The TMT joint complex comprises the TMT joints, the intertarsal joints, and the intermetatarsal joints. The area represents

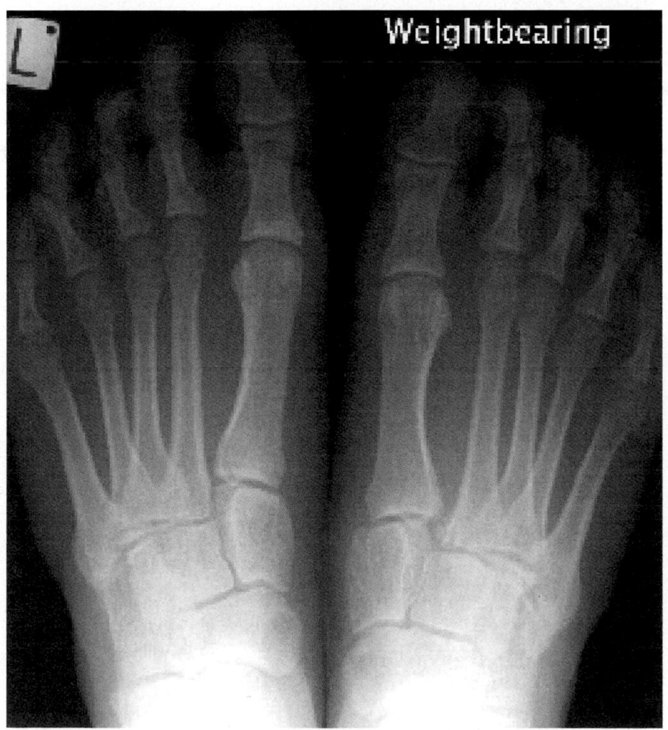

FIGURE 27-29 Weight-bearing radiographs show a subtle Lisfranc injury to the right foot. Weight-bearing radiographss are essential for diagnosis; using the opposite foot for comparison is also helpful.

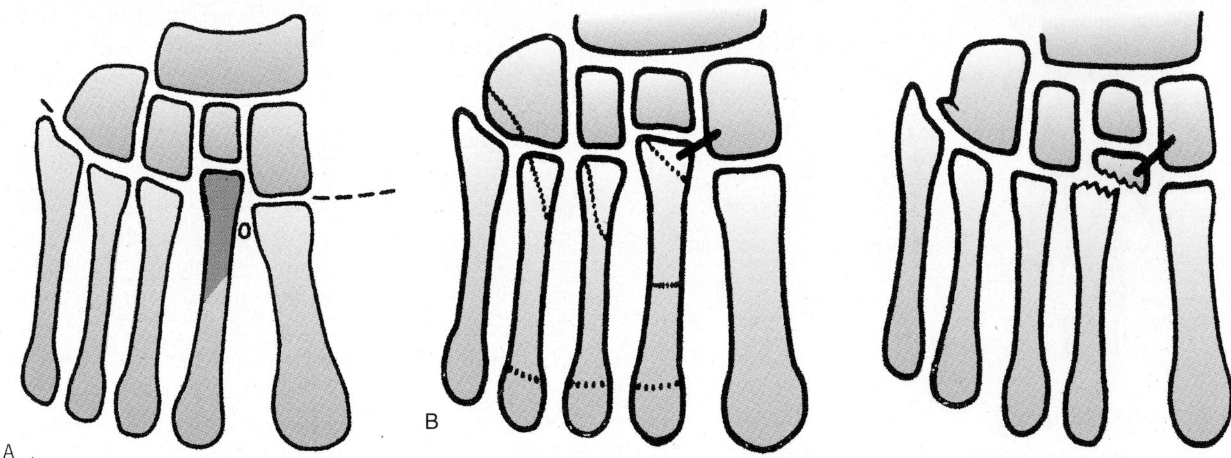

FIGURE 27-30 A. Second metatarsal is the "keystone" of the locking mechanism. **B.** Fractures of the cuboid and second metatarsal are pathognomonic signs of disruption of the TMT joints.

the apex of the longitudinal and transverse arches of the foot and therefore its structural integrity is crucial in maintaining normal foot function. At the same time, there needs to be enough motion between the joints to allow the transfer of weight evenly from the hindfoot to the forefoot during the walking cycle. This intricate relationship is achieved by the anatomy of the tarsal and metatarsal bones and the arrangement of the ligaments. These midfoot bones are trapezoidal in cross section with their base dorsal. This creates a "Roman arch" effect, which is structurally very strong and helps maintain the transverse arch in the midfoot. The TMT joint complex can be divided up into a medial column and a lateral column. The medial column is a continuation of the talus and navicular and includes the cuneiforms and the medial three metatarsals. The lateral column is a continuation of the calcaneus and comprises the cuboid and the fourth and fifth metatarsals which articulate with it. The medial column has far less mobility than the lateral column, reflecting the increased need for stability on the medial side of the foot to maintain the longitudinal arch. This stability is also provided by the second metatarsal which is "keyed" into the step formed by the cuneiforms. This explains why the second metatarsal is usually fractured when a dislocation occurs across the TMT joint. The ligaments also play a big role in maintaining stability medially and movement laterally. The plantar ligaments are extremely strong compared to the weaker dorsal ligaments. The intermetatarsal ligaments help bind the lateral four metatarsals together but are absent between the first and second metatarsals. Instead, the second metatarsal is connected to the medial cuneiform by Lisfranc's ligament (medial interosseous ligament) and an avulsion fracture of this strong ligament can sometimes be seen on radiograph (Fig. 27-31).[173]

The dorsalis pedis artery crosses the cuneiforms before it courses between the first and second metatarsals to form the plantar arterial branch. The deep peroneal nerve travels beside the artery but continues on to supply sensation to the first web space. This neurovascular bundle can be damaged by the injury and care must be taken protect these structures when internally fixing these fracture–dislocations. The tibialis anterior tendon inserts into the base of the first metatarsal and medial cuneiform. The peroneous longus tendon inserts into the plantar surface of the base of the first metatarsal and acts as a flexor of this bone. Together, these two muscles and their tendon insertions give added stability to the medial column of the foot.

Treatment Options

The key to treating these TMT injuries is to recognize the extent of the injury and the degree of instability. Once this is established, the appropriate treatment can be instigated. In all these injuries, a weight-bearing radiograph at the end of treatment should confirm anatomic congruency of the TMT joint complex.

When a clinical diagnosis of a "sprain" is made, the foot should be immobilized in a below-knee cast for 6 weeks. The MRI scan may confirm a partial tear of the first TMT ligament, but regardless this painful injury takes time to heal and immobilization is the best treatment. In young adult athletes, these injuries can take a long time to heal.[108] When there is complete intraligamentous rupture or an avulsion fracture of the first TMT ligament and no displacement of the joint surfaces, a below-

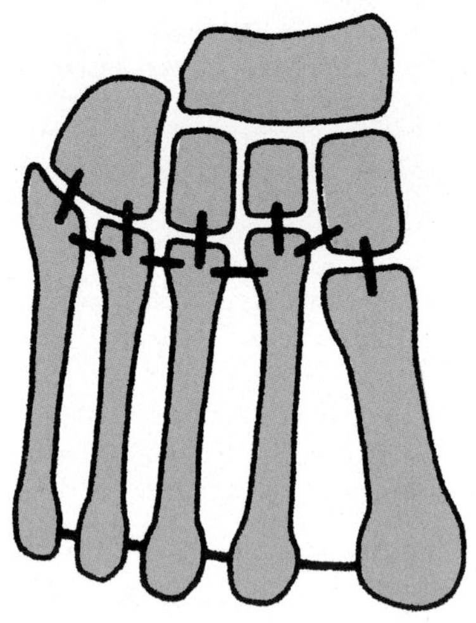

FIGURE 27-31 The ligamentous attachments at the TMT joints. There is only a flimsy connection between the bases of the first and second metatarsals (not illustrated). The second metatarsal is recessed and firmly anchored. (From Wiley JJ. The mechanism of tarsometatarsal joint injuries. J Bone Joint Surg Br 1971;53:474, with permission.)

knee cast for 6 weeks is advised. Whether the patient should be weight bearing or not for the entire 6 weeks is debatable. Wiley[173] treated the children with undisplaced TMT joint injuries in his series with 3 to 4 weeks of immobilization with good results.

Displaced fractures of the TMT joint need to be anatomically reduced and stabilized. Meyerson et al.[114] found that following a closed reduction greater than 2-mm displacement or a talometatarsal angle of greater than 15 degrees would lead to a poor outcome. A closed reduction is best carried out under a general anesthetic when the acute swelling has subsided. "Finger traps" can help with traction on the toes while the displaced metatarsals are manipulated into place. If a stable anatomic reduction is achieved clinically and this is confirmed radiologically, a well molded below-knee cast can be applied. Radiographs in the cast should also be taken while the patient is under anesthesia to confirm the reduction has been held. The nonweight-bearing cast is worn for 6 weeks with radiographs taken at 1 and 2 weeks to confirm the fracture–dislocation has remained reduced.

If the closed reduction results in an anatomic reduction but the fragments are unstable, then K-wire fixation is used to hold the alignment of the foot. Stout 0.062 in smooth K-wires should be used. Their placement is determined by the direction of displacement of the metatarsals and how many are involved. The most important wire is used to stabilize the second metatarsal to the medial cuneiform. Additional wires can be used between the first metatarsal and the medial cuneiform, and between the lesser metatarsals and their corresponding tarsal bones. A useful wire can also be passed from the first metatarsal to the second metatarsal. These K-wires are left bent over outside of the skin and are removed at 4 to 6 weeks when mobilization is initiated if the radiographs confirm healing. Again, full weight-bearing radiographs are necessary when comfort allows and after K-wire removal to confirm adequate stability. Wiley[173] used K-wire fixation in 4 patients. He removed these at 3 to 4 weeks and the alignment was maintained in all the children. There were some joint incongruities from intra-articular fractures that were not surgically addressed but they did not seem to alter the clinical outcome.

Open reduction and internal fixation is rarely required for these fractures. It is indicated if there is greater than 1 to 2 mm of joint displacement. The impediments to reduction are

1. Tibialis anterior tendon
2. Interposition of fracture fragments in the second metatarsal-middle cuneiform joint.
3. Incongruity of the first metatarsal-medial cuneiform articulation[15]

The entire TMT joint complex can be visualized using two longitudinal incisions.[149] One is made over the first–second metatarsal space and the second in line with the fourth metatarsal. The medial incision allows identification of the neurovascular bundle and access to the first and second metatarsal-cuneiform joints. The lateral incision allows the joints of the lesser TMT joints to be clearly seen. After anatomic reduction, the joints can held reduced with K-wires or internally fixed with 3.5 mm screws (Fig. 27-32). Small chondral defects can be excised and larger ones repaired. Care must be taken to avoid the proximal growth plate of the first metatarsal if screw fixation is used. The adult literature supports the use of K-wire stabilization of the lesser metatarsals rather than screws as it is important to maintain the mobility in these joints long-term.[43] Debate exists as to when to remove the screws across these weight-bearing joints. In a child, it would seem appropriate to remove the screws once pain free weight bearing is established as the ligaments and bone would have healed by this stage and further displacement is unlikely. Leaving the screws in longer than 3 months risks damage to the joint and possible screw breakage.

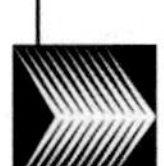

AUTHORS' PREFERRED TREATMENT

The majority of children have a type B TMT dislocation with minimal displacement. The most important step in treating

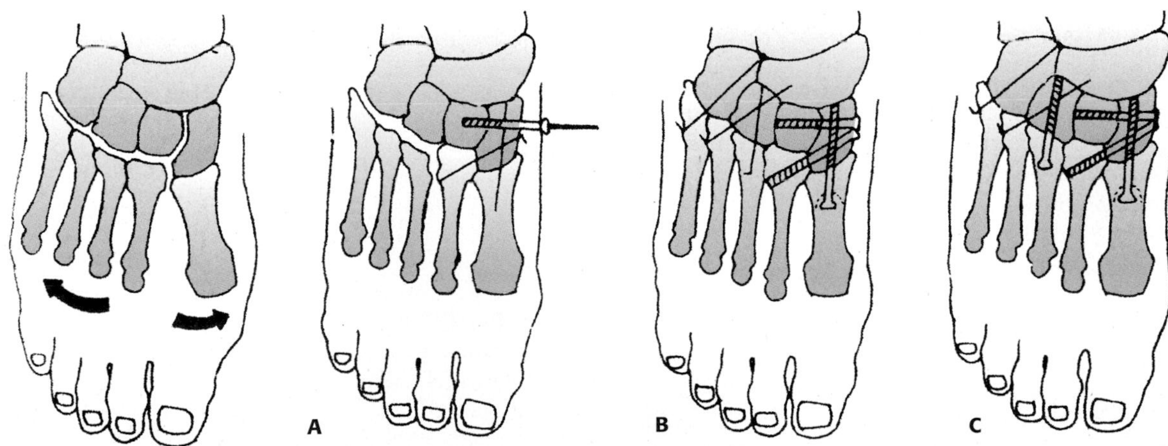

FIGURE 27-32 Sequence of repair for reduction and stabilization of TMT fracture dislocations. **A.** Stabilization of the first ray by alignment of the metatarsal, medial cuneiform, and navicular. **B.** Stabilization of the Lisfranc ligament by accurate alignment of the second metatarsal to the medial cuneiform, as well as the medial and middle cuneiforms. **C.** Alignment and stabilization of the third through fifth metatarsal rays. Cannulated screws can be used instead of pins as needed for stability and compression. (From Trevino SG, Kodros S. Controversies in tarsometatarsal injuries. Orthop Clin North Am 1995;26:229–238, with permission.)

these patients is confirming this diagnosis accurately and treating them until the joint is stable. If any doubt in the diagnosis exists, the author takes a comparable radiograph of the other foot. The author routinely orders a CT scan of the midfoot to assess the extent of the injury and to look for any associated injuries.

An injury with less than 1 to 2 mm of displacement is treated in a below-knee nonweight-bearing cast for 6 weeks. Weightbearing radiographs are taken on removal of the cast to assess stability. These radiographs are repeated 6 weeks later once pain free weight bearing is achieved to confirm no further displacement.

If the TMT joint is displaced greater than 1 to 2 mm, then the author performs a closed reduction and routinely uses percutaneous K-wire fixation with image intensifier control. Although these injuries can be held with cast immobilization, the author prefers the assurance of knowing the fracture–dislocation is being held internally. This is especially useful when the foot is very swollen and repeated assessments are necessary to rule out compartment syndrome. In the rare circumstance of an open reduction, the author prefers to use temporary screw fixation. These injuries are usually far more severe than a type B dislocation and the TMT joints are very unstable. After open reduction through two longitudinal incisions, 3.5-mm cortical screws are used to hold the reduction taking care to avoid the proximal growth plate of the first metatarsal. These screws are removed usually within a month of cast removal.

Regardless of the way the fracture–dislocation is treated, all these patients must be investigated at outpatient appointments with weight-bearing radiographs to confirm that the ligaments have healed and there is no residual subluxation.

Complications

The most common complication following TMT injuries is posttraumatic arthritis. This can often occur because the injury is "missed" and the subtle fracture–dislocation remains displaced. Another cause is a loss of reduction. Lastly, the trauma itself can damage the articular cartilage and, despite an anatomic reduction, arthritis can develop.

Hardcastle et al.[59] showed that the outcomes are poor if the diagnosis is made more than 6 weeks after the injury. Curtis et al.[36] found similar results in athletes who had a delayed diagnosis. This reinforces the importance of making the diagnosis early and treating appropriately.

Posttraumatic arthritis is known to occur after TMT injuries in a significant percentage of adults, and this is best prevented by achieving an anatomic reduction.[114] Wiss et al.[176] performed gait analysis on 11 adult patients with TMT joint fracture–dislocations and found that no patient walked normally after a displaced TMT fracture–dislocation. In Wiley's[173] series of 18 children, none of whom required open reduction, 14 patients were asymptomatic 3 to 8 months postinjury. Four patients had persisting pain of minor severity at the TMT joint 1 year following injury. Two of these patients had residual angulation at the injury site. One patient had an unrecognized dislocation and had not been treated; the other had not had an anatomic reduction due to extensive intra-articular fractures. One 16-year-old patient developed asymptomatic osteonecrosis of the second metatarsal head, and this was attributed to a possible compromise of the blood supply at the time of injury as the nutrient vessel to this area is a terminal branch of the dorsalis pedis. Buoncristiani et al.[22] followed 8 children (3 to 10 years old) with indirect TMT joint injuries treated in a below-knee cast and found 7 were asymptomatic at an average follow-up of 32 months. The one patient who had midfoot pain had developed early degenerative changes on the plain radiographs.

The treatment for painful TMT joint arthritis is arthrodesis if conservative care has failed. In children this would be extremely unusual. An arthrodesis often requires extensive soft tissue release to allow anatomic reduction of the joint and then rigid internal fixation with screws. It is important not to fuse the lesser TMT joints as mobility here is important for the long-term function of the foot.

METATARSAL FRACTURES

Fractures of the metatarsals are the most common fractures of the foot in children, accounting for up to 60% of all pediatric foot fractures.[35,36,119,155] Owen et al.[119] showed in an epidemiologic study that in children younger than 5 years of age, 73% of metatarsal fractures involve the first metatarsal, whereas in children older than 10 years these fractures accounted for only 12%. The most common metatarsal fracture for all 60 patients was a fracture of the fifth metatarsal (45%). Six and a half percent of all the fractures and 20% of first metatarsal fractures were not diagnosed at the initial consultation in their series.

Management

Mechanism of Injury

Metatarsal fractures result from either a direct or indirect injury. Direct injuries are usually caused by a heavy load falling on the forefoot or a crush injury (i.e., the foot being run over by a car). The metatarsals can be fractured anywhere along the shaft but typically they are fractured middiaphyseal. Indirect injuries are caused by axial loading or torsional forces and usually produce spiral fractures of the proximal shaft or neck of the metatarsal. Singer et al.[155] found in a recent study of 125 children that if the patient was less than 5 years of age, the primary mechanism was a fall from a height and this usually occurred within the home. In children older than 5 years of age, most injuries occurred while playing sport and occurred on a level playing surface.

Signs and Symptoms

Direct injuries can result in significant swelling and bruising of the foot due to the extensive soft tissue injury as well as the metatarsal fractures. Careful evaluation of a compartment syndrome should take place. An indirect injury usually has more subtle clinical findings and careful palpation will usually locate the site of the fracture. The infant with a metatarsal fracture due to an unwitnessed injury may present with minimal swelling but an inability to bear weight.

Associated Injuries

Proximal fractures of the metatarsals are often associated with tarsal fractures or fracture–dislocations, and this should be evaluated further with a CT scan. A fracture of the second metatarsal and a cuboid fracture are highly suggestive of a TMT joint dislocation rather than two isolated fractures. Singer et al.[155] found that the first and fifth metatarsals were usually isolated fractures, whereas if multiple metatarsals were fractured, they were always contiguous bones and involved the second, third, and fourth metatarsals.

Imaging Evaluation

Radiographic evaluation should consist of AP, lateral, and oblique views of the whole foot. The AP view often gives the impression that the fractures are minimally displaced; however, the lateral view often shows significant plantar or dorsal displacement. Other associated fractures may be apparent on the plain radiographs and if any doubt exists, especially if there has been significant trauma, a CT scan is advised. In a young child, if a fractured metatarsal is suspected but not visible on the initial radiograph, a repeat film can be taken 10 to 14 days later that often shows the fracture line or early callus.

Classification

No classification system exists for fractures of the first through fourth metatarsals. Fractures of the fifth metatarsal are classified according to their location along the bone (see section on treatment of the fifth metatarsal below).

Current Treatment Options

The majority of metatarsal fractures in children can be treated nonoperatively in a below-knee cast. The child with a displaced fracture often needs to be admitted overnight in the hospital for pain relief and observation for compartment syndrome.The initial treatment includes elevation for the severe swelling that coexists with the fractures. Immobilization may be performed by a well padded cast, splint, or a Cam walker.. Once the swelling subsides, a molded below-knee cast can be applied. Weight bearing can be initiated when pain allows, and the cast can usually be removed at 3 to 4 weeks at which time the patient can be transitioned to a Cam walker.

The amount of angulation or shortening to accept in a child has not been determined. A closed reduction of the central metatarsals is indicated in an adult if there is more than 10 degrees angulation in the dorsal plain or more than 4 mm of translation in any plane.[153] These criteria may be appropriate for an older adolescent whose growth plates had closed but are far too stringent for a skeletally immature patient. If there is severe dorsal angulation of greater than 20 degrees or "tenting" of the skin and shortening of greater than 5 mm, then a closed reduction is indicated. This is best performed under a general anesthetic when the swelling has subsided. Finger traps have been advocated by some surgeons to help with traction while the metatarsals are manipulated. A below-knee cast can be molded with pressure applied to both the dorsal and plantar aspects of the foot; however, the need to allow for swelling suggests implants should be used to hold fracture reduction rather than molding of a cast. To accomodate the swelling and to relax the plantar fascia, the cast can be applied with the ankle in slight equinus and when it is changed 2 weeks later, it can be bought up into a neutral position.

Fractures of the first metatarsal need careful attention especially in the adolescent patient. The first ray is important in maintaining the longitudinal arch of the foot and the position of the first metatarsal head in relation to the lesser metatarsal heads is also vitally important. A closed reduction should be considered if there is greater than 10 degrees of dorsal angulation or any shortening of the first metatarsal. It is unusual to have angulation in the coronal plane if the second metatarsal is intact and transverse displacement is acceptable if there is no shortening.

If a closed reduction is performed, K-wire fixation is at times required. Intramedullary placement is difficult to perform without opening the fracture and passing the wires under direct vision. Small, dorsal, longitudinal incisions are made over the fracture sites and dissection is carefully carried out down to the fracture. The wire is drilled down the distal fragment to exit the plantar skin. The wire is then withdrawn enough to allow the fracture to be reduced, then the wire is driven retrograde across the fracture site and sufficiently far enough into the proximal fragment. Another technique is to hold fracture reduction by placing K-wires across the fractured metatarsal to an adjacent nonfractured metatarsal both proximal and distal to the fracture. The K-wire is cut and bent outside the skin to facilitate removal in the outpatient clinic in 3 to 4 weeks when the patient can be placed in a walking cast for 2 further weeks to allow fracture consolidation. This is the same technique that can be used on the rare occurrence an open reduction is required for an irreducible fracture or when the fracture is open.

Fractures of the Base of the Fifth Metatarsal

Fractures of the fifth metatarsal are the most common metatarsal fracture in children, comprising almost 50% of all metatarsal fractures in some series.[64,119,155] Traditionally, treatment has been based on treatment algorithms from the adult literature. Fractures of the base of the fifth metatarsal are discussed separately from the other metatarsal fractures as the anatomy, fracture patterns, and treatment indications are quite different.

Surgical Anatomy

The fifth metatarsal has a number of tendinous insertions at its base. The peroneus brevis tendon inserts on the dorsal aspect of the tubercle and the peroneus tertius attaches on the dorsal aspect of the fifth metatarsal at the metaphyseal–diaphyseal junction. The strong plantar aponeurosis inserts into the plantar aspect of the tubercle at the base.

The nutrient artery enters the shaft of the fifth metatarsal medially at the junction of the proximal and middle thirds of the diaphysis and sends intraosseous branches proximally and distally (Fig. 27-33). Proximally within the bone are the me-

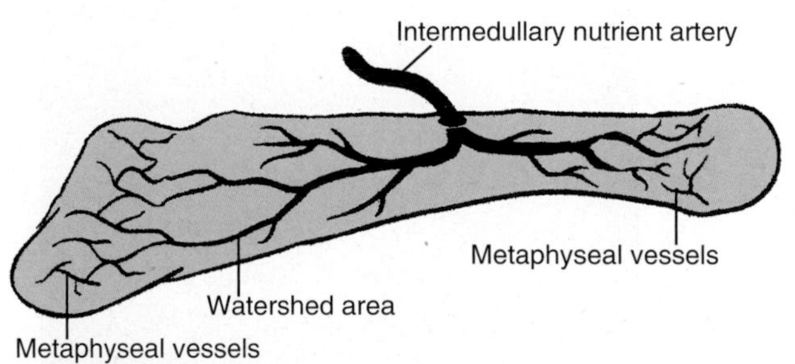

FIGURE 27-33 Blood supply of the proximal fifth metatarsal.

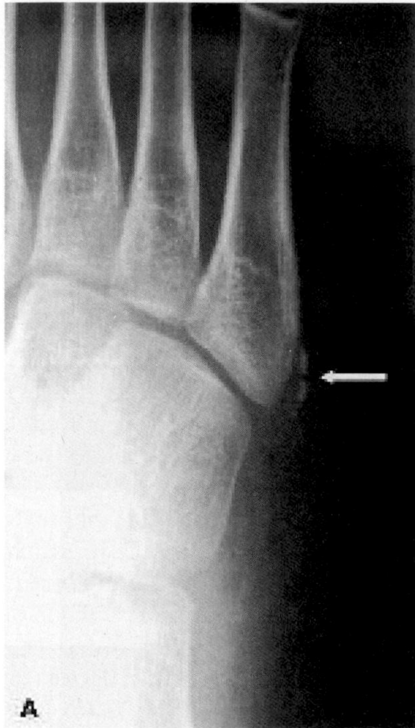

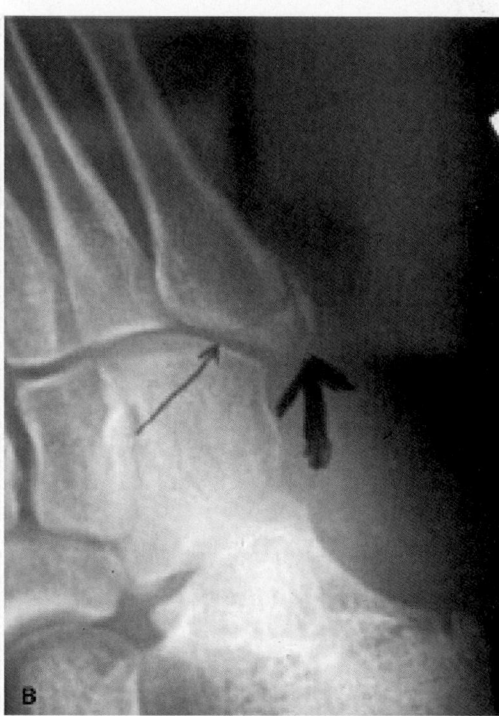

FIGURE 27-34 A. A normal apophysis of the base of the fifth metatarsal at the attachment of the peroneus brevis (*arrow*) in a 10-year-old girl. **B.** The *thicker arrow* points to the normal apophysis, which is roughly parallel to the metatarsal. The *thinner arrow* points towards a fracture, which is roughly perpendicular to metatarsal.

taphyseal vessels, and the small area where these overlap with the proximal vessels from the nutrient artery is known as the watershed area. This region corresponds with Zone 2 and fractures in this area have a higher rate delayed of union or nonunion in those close to maturity The proximal apophyseal growth center of the fifth metatarsal can often be confused for a fracture. The apophyseal growth center (os vesalianum) has a longitudinal orientation roughly parallel to the metarsal shaft and generally has smooth contours which distinguish it from a transverse orientated fracture (Fig. 27-34). The os vesalianum usually appears by the age of 9 years and unites with the metaphysis between the ages of 12 and 15 years (Fig. 27-35).

Classification

Fractures of the base of the fifth metatarsal are classified according to their location into one of three zones (Fig. 27-36). Zone 1 is the cancellous tuberosity, which includes the insertion of the peroneus brevis tendon, the abductor digiti minimi tendon, and the strong calcaneometatarsal ligament of the plantar fascia. Zone 2 is the distal aspect of the tuberosity where the dorsal and plantar ligamentous attachments to the fourth metatarsal attach to insert. Zone 3 is the region that extends from distal to these ligamentous attachments to approximately the middiaphyseal area. Herrera-Soto et al.[64] tried to define this classification further in their recent review of 103 children with fifth

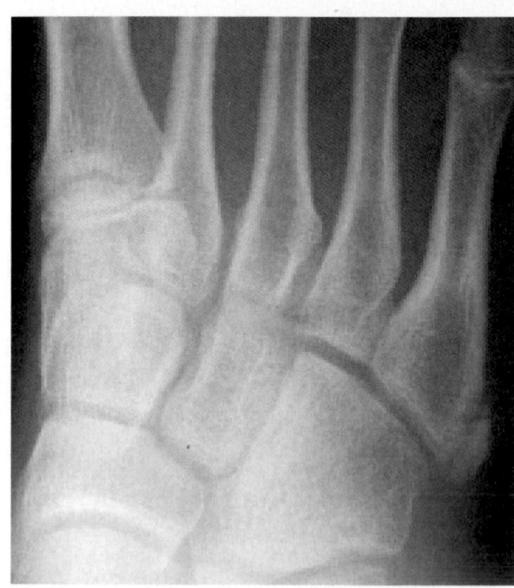

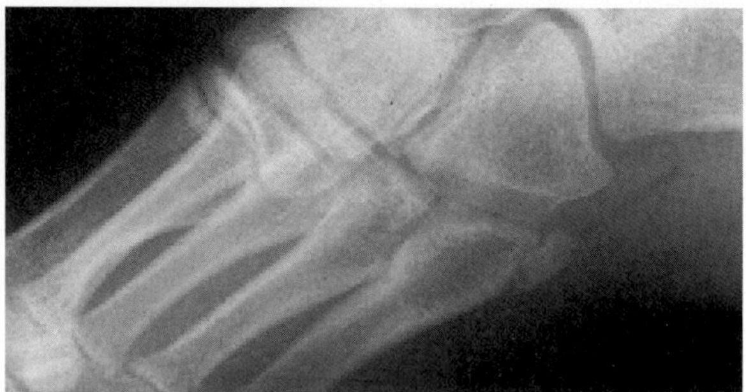

FIGURE 27-35 This 11-year-old girl had pain in her proximal fifth metatarsal after twisting her foot during physical education at school. No fracture was visible; however, her secondary ossification center is clearly seen running parallel to the shaft of the metatarsal.

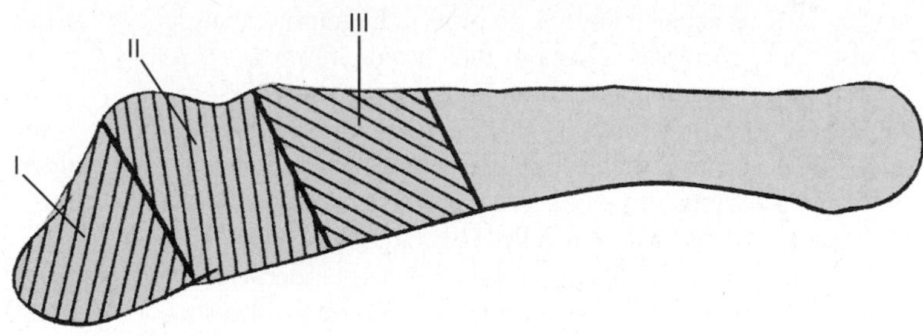

FIGURE 27-36 The three anatomic zones of the proximal fifth metatarsal.

metatarsal fractures. They define a type I fracture as a "fleck" injury. A type II fracture is a tubercle fracture with an intra-articular extension, and a type III fracture represents a fracture at the proximal diaphyseal region (Jones fracture).

Treatment

Traditionally, treatment has been based on treatment algorithms from the adult literature. Treatment of fractures of the base of the fifth metatarsal in children is determined primarily by the zone of the fracture, and somewhat by age.

Zone 1 Fractures. These injuries are usually traction-type injuries where the force from the peroneus brevis tendon and the pull from the plantar aponeurosis result in an avulsion fracture of the fifth metatarsal. Some authors suggest the fracture may be an avulsion at the origin of abductor digiti minimi.[78,137] Treatment involves a weight-bearing below-knee walking cast for 3 to 6 weeks. Herrera-Soto et al.[64] found all 30 of their children with an extra-articular type 1 fracture treated in this way healed with good outcomes even if they were displaced. Undisplaced intra-articular tuberosity fractures also healed well in the series[64]; however, displaced (>2 mm) intra-articular fractures took significantly longer to heal. Radiographic union usually lags behind resolution of symptoms, and most patients are asymptomatic after 3 weeks.[64] This delay in radiographic union should not prevent the child returning to full activities as symptoms allow. Treatment with a Cam walker rather than a cast may be considered. Nonunion can occur but usually is asymptomatic.[37] Although operative fixation of acute tuberosity avulsions rarely is indicated, it may be considered for significant displacement (more than 3-mm) in young active patients who want to return to competitive sports sooner (Fig. 27-37).

Zone 2 Fractures. Zone 2 fractures include the Jones fracture. This is an oblique fracture in the watershed area at the proximal metaphyseal-diaphyseal junction. It typically occurs in adolescents and is thought to be caused by a combination of vertical loading and coronal shear forces at the junction of the stable proximal metaphysis and the mobile fifth metatarsal diaphysis. Frequently, these fractures are stress injuries, usually involving athletic adolescents who present with a traumatic event superimposed on prior symptoms.[24,34,76,77,86,142] A good history is important to determine the duration of symptoms because chronic injuries are unlikely to respond to nonoperative treat-

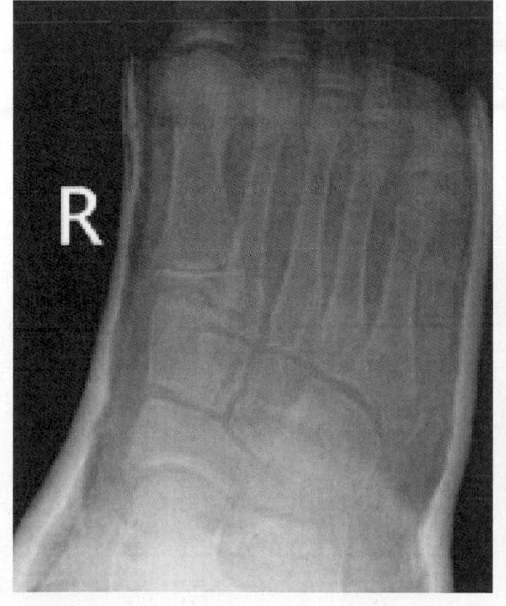

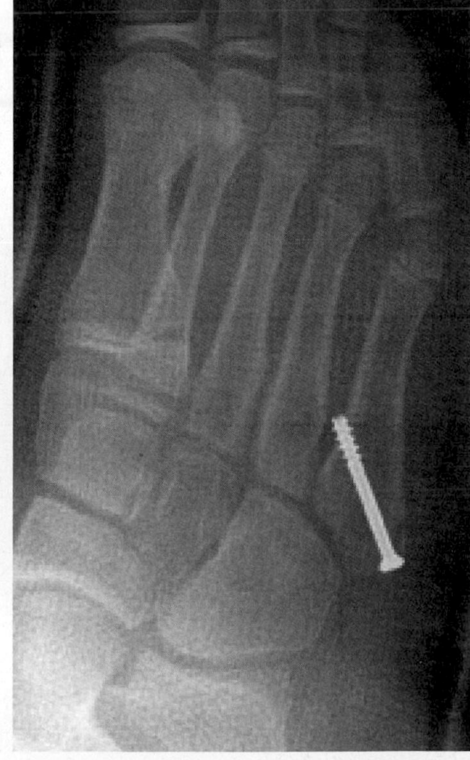

FIGURE 27-37 A. A 12-year-old boy who is a professional snowboarder with a displaced, intra-articular fifth metatarsal fracture. **B.** This was reduced open and internally fixed, which allowed him to compete 8 weeks after surgery.

ment as well as acute fractures. Critical radiographic analysis will also show cortical sclerosis in the chronic injuries.

Acute injuries should be immobilized in a short-leg non-weight-bearing cast for 6 weeks. Serial radiographs and examinations are necessary to determine adequate healing, and further non–weight-bearing immobilization may be necessary if the fracture has not healed clinically and radiographically at 6 weeks. With evidence of callus and diminished tenderness, the patient can begin protected weight bearing in a hard-soled shoe or Cam walker for an additional 4 weeks. This protected weight bearing may prevent refracture.[64] In a series of adults, Torg et al.[164] reported successful healing in 14 of 15 patients treated with non–weight-bearing casts, whereas only 4 of 10 who were allowed to bear weight went on to union. Herrera-Soto et al.[64] reported 15 fractures in this zone (type III) and found a higher rate of delayed union and refracture in patients over 13 years of age. They feel that primary internal fixation in this age group may be indicated.

For chronic fractures in zone 2 where the symptoms have been present for more than 3 months, nonoperative management is unlikely to be successful. Nonetheless, it is worthwhile initially trying 6 weeks immobilization in a non–weight-bearing below-knee cast or brace. If this fails, then internal fixation is required. A useful technique is to insert an intramedullary screw from proximal to distal which stabilizes the fracture site. A 4-mm cancellous screw is usually sufficient; however, in an older adolescent with a capacious intramedullary canal, a 6.5-mm cancellous screw may give better fixation and compression. It is beneficial to curette the intramedullary canal and use cancellous bone graft, which can be harvested from the distal tibia (Fig. 27-38).[88]

Zone 3 Fractures. Fractures in zone 3 are usually stress fractures in active athletes. Acute fractures in this zone with no prodromal symptoms can be treated with a below-knee non-weight-bearing cast for 6 weeks followed by protective weight bearing for 4 weeks. In the more common scenario, where the patient complains of pain with activity for several months, this period of casting is often unsuccessful but worth trying in the first instance. The stress fracture may heal clinically with 6 to 12 weeks of immobilization and radiographs will confirm the reconstitution of the medullary canal and less sclerosis at the fracture site. Electrical stimulation may be used. If the chronic stress fracture does not heal, then surgical intervention is re-

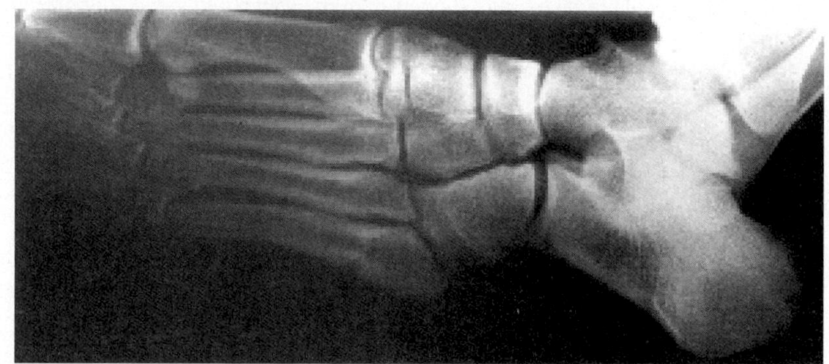
A

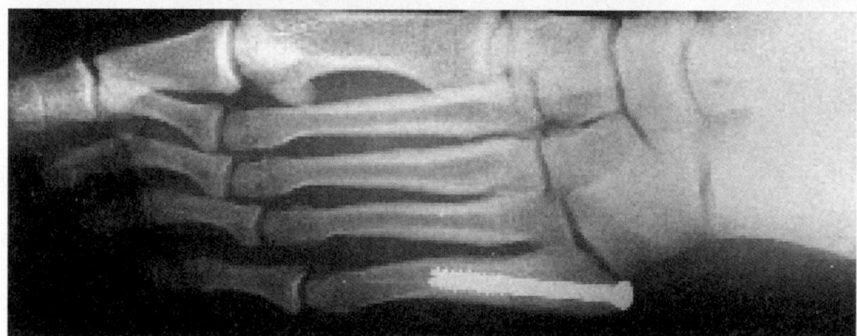
B

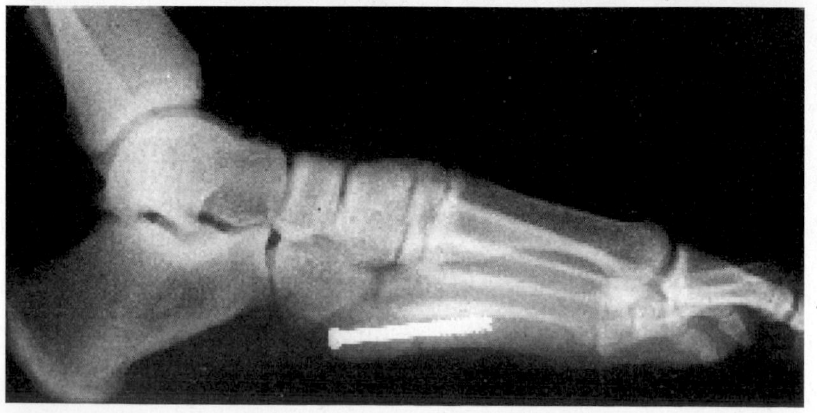
C

FIGURE 27-38 This 15-year-old high-level basketball player sustained a proximal fifth metatarsal fracture at the metaphyseal-diaphyseal junction. The patient chose intramedullary screw fixation because of his desire to return to sport as promptly as possible, lessen his time in immobilization, and lessen the risk of delayed union or nonunion. **A.** Radiograph at time of injury. **B,C.** After intramedullary screw fixation. (Courtesy of Keith S. Hechtman, MD.)

quired similar to that in a zone 2 fracture outlined above. Some authors advocate a more aggressive open débridement of the fracture site with bone grafting before introducing the intramedullary screw.[131,164]

Complications

The most common complication of treating fractures of the proximal fifth metatarsal is a painful nonunion. This is more common in zone 2 and zone 3 fractures and rarely occurs in zone 1. Herrera-Soto et al.[64] concluded that pediatric fifth metatarsal fractures behaved similarly to adult fractures and can be treated the same. If a symptomatic nonunion develops and surgery is indicated, a thorough débridement of the sclerotic medullary canal should be undertaken, the area bone grafted, and strong compression achieved across the fracture site with the appropriate size intramedullary screw.[54]

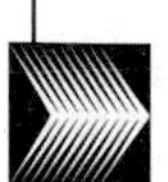

AUTHORS' PREFERRED TREATMENT

Lesser metatarsal fractures are usually treated nonoperatively in a below-knee walking cast for 3 to 4 weeks. Grossly displaced fractures in older children with greater than 20 degrees of dorsiflexion or more than 5 mm of shortening are treated with closed reduction under a general anesthetic and a well molded below-knee cast. If the reduction is difficult, percutaneous K-wires are used for supplementary support. Except for open injuries, rarely is an open reduction through longitudinal incisions required.

A shortened or rotated distal fracture of the first or fifth metatarsal is treated by closed reduction and crossed K-wire fixation.

Proximal fifth metatarsal fractures present a more challenging problem. Treatment is determined by the location of the fracture in the bone and the age and activity level of the child. If inadequately treated, they can go on to a delayed or nonunion. For zone 1 fractures that are intra-articular and displaced greater than 3 to 4 mm, the author recommends open reduction and internal fixation with a 3.5-mm partially threaded screw, especially if the child is involved in competitive sports, as this will allow an earlier return to sport. This fixation is perpendicular to the fracture line and gives maximum compression. The screw is inserted through a direct lateral approach. Care must be taken to identify and protect the sural nerve which is usually directly under the incision. The peroneous brevis and peroneous tertius tendons are identified, and the area between them at their insertion into the proximal fifth metatarsal is a good starting point for the screw. The author prefers to insert a bicortical cannulated compression screw, and this can either be a partially threaded cancellous screw or a fully threaded cortical screw. The fracture can usually be indirectly reduced and held with a K-wire. In difficult fracture patterns or in delayed presentations, the fracture line needs to be clearly seen and can be held reduced with a compression clamp.

In zone 2 fractures (Jones fracture), the author treats the patient in a nonweight-bearing cast for 6 weeks and then protected weight bearing in a moon-boot for 2 to 4 weeks as comfort allows. The recent study by Herrera-Soto et al.[64] showing poor results with this treatment in patients over 13 years old may make primary internal fixation a better option in this age group.

Chronic fractures or nonunions should be treated with internal fixation. The author prefers to perform this with an intramedullary screw which compresses the fracture site. If a 3.5-mm cancellous screw does not achieve adequate internal fixation in the medullary canal, the author increases the diameter of the screw until it does. Often, a 4.0-mm malleolar screw is used. A small curette is used down the medullary canal to help remove the sclerotic bone. If this is not possible, the fracture site should be débrided open with small osteotomes and rongeurs. Bone grafting is required for these chronic injuries and can be harvested from the distal tibia.

Grossly displaced shaft and distal metaphyseal fractures are treated with closed reduction and cast immobilization for 6 weeks. Occasionally, crossed K-wires are required.

PHALANGEAL FRACTURES

Phalangeal fractures are common in children and may account for up to 18% of pediatric foot fractures.[35] Most toe injuries are treated by primary care physicians, so orthopaedic surgeons only see the more severe fractures. Phalangeal fractures are the result of direct trauma by a falling object or indirect trauma when the unprotected toe is struck against a hard object (so-called "stubbing"). The proximal phalanx is more commonly injured than the distal phalanges.

The toes must be closely examined for any break in the skin especially at the base of the nail as this may indicate an open Salter-Harris fracture with an associated nailbed injury. These compound injuries require a thorough débridement, repair of the nailbed, and often a single longitudinal K-wire to stabilize the fracture (Fig. 27-39). IV antibiotics should be given for 24 hours followed by 7 days of oral antibiotics. Nailbed injuries should be repaired as meticulously as in the hand. A poorly repaired germinal matrix will cause abnormal nail growth and difficulty with shoewear long after the fracture has healed.

Closed fractures of the phalanges rarely require reduction and can be treated by simple "buddy strapping" to the adjacent toe and immediate mobilization. A hard sole shoe or Cam walker may help; however, crowding in the toe box may make this more uncomfortable than bare feet. An angulated toe in both the coronal and sagittal plane usually remodels well if the growth plate is still open. In adolescents, a percutaneous K-wire can be used if the fracture is grossly unstable and unable to be held reduced by strapping alone. This wire can be passed longitudinally through the tip of the affected toe or obliquely across the fracture. It is extremely unusual to get any growth disturbance from a smooth wire crossing the growth plate in the phalanges. These pins can be removed in clinic 4 to 6 weeks later. Laterally angulated fractures of the little toe sometimes need closed reduction before strapping them to the fourth toe.

Great Toe Fractures

The great toe is injured by the same mechanisms as the lesser toes. Standard AP and lateral radiographs are taken; however, it is useful to have the patient hold the lesser toes dorsiflexed with a small towel to maximize visualization on the lateral view. Intra-articular fractures of the proximal phalanx are more common in the great toe than the other toes. They are usually Salter-Harris type III or IV fractures (Fig. 27-40). Most of these frac-

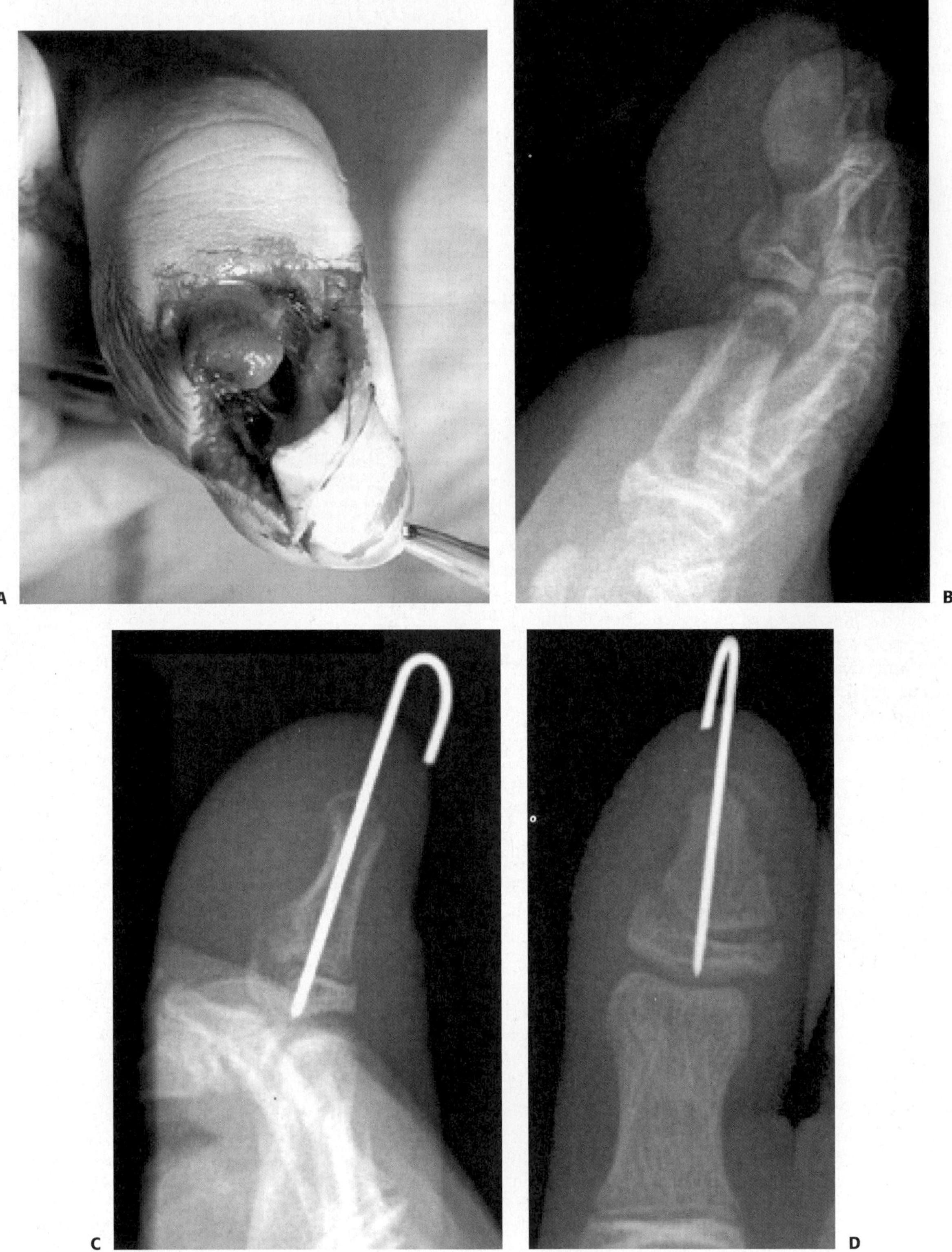

FIGURE 27-39 A. This 7-year-old boy "stubbed" his toe barefoot on his bike and sustained an open fracture of the tuft of the distal phalanx and associated laceration of the germinal matrix. **B.** Preoperative radiograph shows the small tuft fracture. **C,D.** The wound was thoroughly débrided, germinal matrix repaired, and a K-wire passed across the fracture to hold the fragment and soft tissues reduced.

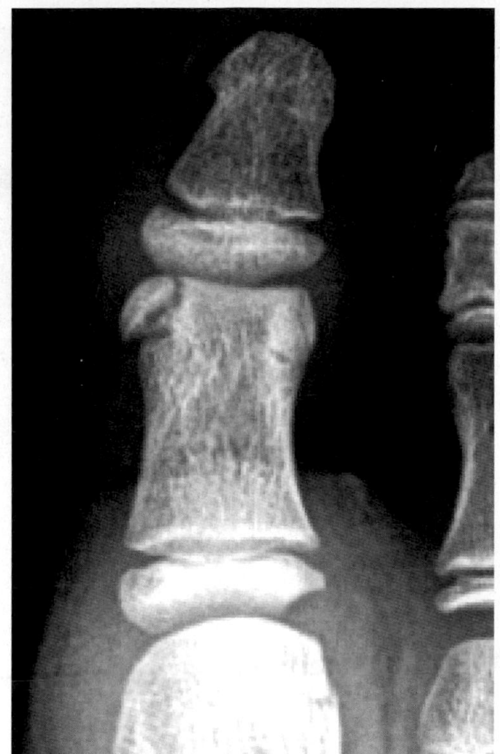

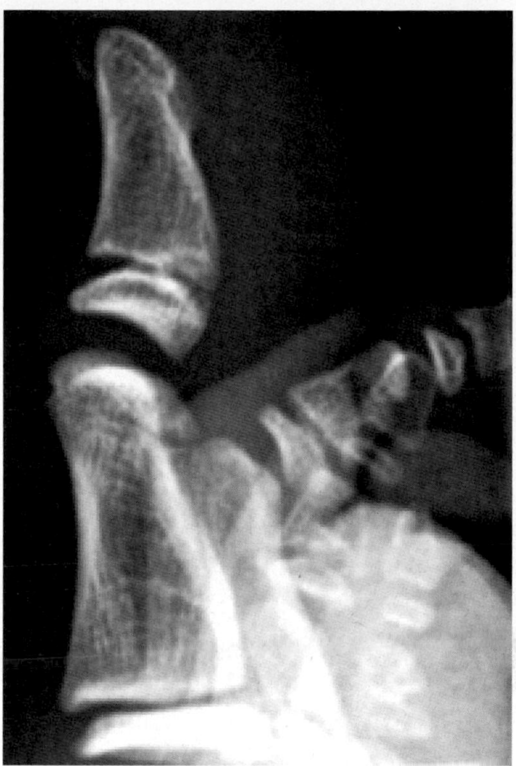

FIGURE 27-40 A. An 11-year old boy with an intra-articular fracture of the proximal phalanx of the great toe. Successful treatment was achieved with simple buddy strapping. **B.** A lateral radiograph of the great toe is best taken with the lesser toes held flexed with a bandage.

tures can be managed with "buddy-strapping" to the second toe; however, if greater than 25% of the joint surface is involved and there is displacement of more than 2 to 3 mm of the joint surface, reduction should be performed. Fracture reduction may be held by strapping to the second toe or a percutaneous K-wire. In the rare occasion that this is not successful, an open reduction can be performed either through a midlateral or dorsal incision. With diaphyseal fractures, axial alignment and rotation both need to be addressed with the closed reduction. Often, the clinical appearance of the toe following the reduction is more useful than the postreduction radiograph as the toe usually looks "fine" even though the radiograph shows malalignment.

LAWNMOWER AND OTHER MUTILATING INJURIES

There are approximately 9400 lawnmower injuries a year in the United States affecting children 20 years or younger with an average age of 10.7 years. This incidence has not changed in 15 years, indicating that new safety regulations have been ineffective.[167] These accidents occur with all types of lawnmowers; however, the most severe injuries are a result of a child being run over by a riding-mower.[97,168] Seventy-two percent of children who have severe lawnmower injuries are bystanders.[42,168] Ross et al.,[140] however, had a higher number of children in their series who fell off the riding-mowers and were run over. Seventy-eight percent of all lawnmower accidents occur in boys.[167] Loder and colleagues[97] reviewed 235 children who had a traumatic amputation and found that these injuries are more common in the spring and summer. Children under the age of 14 years are most susceptible to injury with those under the age of 6 years having the greatest risk of death.[115] The most common body region injured is the hand (34.6%), followed by the leg (18.9%) and the foot (17.7%) (Fig. 27-41).[167]

Treatment

The initial treatment for these children is a thorough assessment of the injuries suffered and appropriate resuscitation. Often, a large volume of blood has been lost from the time of the accident to arriving in the emergency department. Once the child is stabilized, a secondary survey can be conducted to assess the extent of the injury to each limb. With regard to the foot, these injuries are mutilating and heavily contaminated with soil and grass. After inspection, the wound should be dressed and a firm bandage applied to prevent further bleeding. Antibiotics need to be administered as soon as possible and include a cephalosporin, aminoglycoside, and penicillin. The patient's tetanus status should be ascertained and tetanus prophylaxis administered if unknown.

The child then needs to be taken urgently to the operating room for the initial débridement. Considerable time should be spent removing the foreign material as meticulously as possible. A water jet lavage system can be useful, but should be used with care as it can force debris further in to the soft tissue envelopes. Devitilized tissue should be débrided; however, questionable tissue should be left as there will be multiple return trips to the operating room when further débridements can take place. It is useful to involve a plastic surgeon even at this initial surgery so they can see the extent of the damage and start planning for definitive coverage. The child will generally need at least three trips to the operating room and some cases many more.[42] These return trips should be every 24 to 48 hours de-

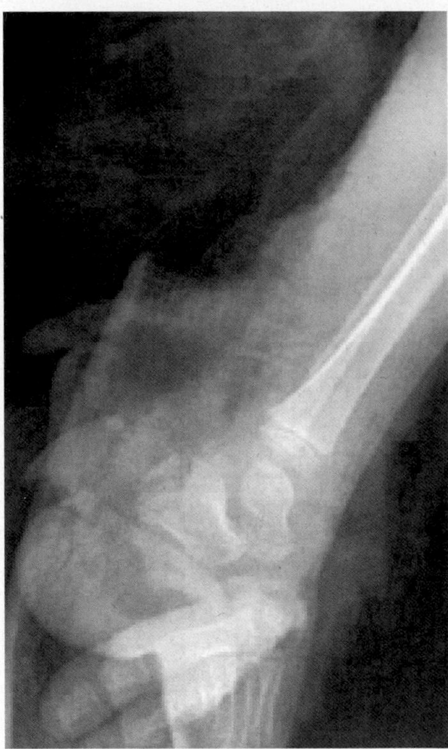

FIGURE 27-41 A 4-year-old boy with a severe lawnmower accident after being run over by the driver. There was extensive soft tissue loss and compound fractures to the foot. Despite multiple débridements, the leg was amputated below the knee.

pending on the state of the wound. Each débridement is important and should not be left to the most junior member of the surgical team to perform. Every piece of viable skin is vital and may be the difference between a primary closure over an amputation stump or a skin graft or tissue transfer. There is no hurry to close the wound until the soft tissue and bone is completely free of foreign material and the tissues are well perfused. Shilt and colleagues[154] have found the use of VAC safe and effective in managing these types of lawnmower injuries. Fractures need to be stabilized and initially external fixation is useful. This allows plenty of room for further débridements and does not compromise later internal fixation once the soft tissue coverage has been determined.

Skin grafting or flap coverage of lawnmower injuries is required in approximately 50% of cases.[42] Unlike adults, split-thickness skin grafting can function very well on the weight-bearing surfaces in children.[42,168] When the soft tissue defect is large or there is exposed bone that would be better to preserve than excise, a free tissue transfer is helpful.[46,94] Lin et al.[95] recently reviewed 93 microsurgical reconstructions of soft tissue defects of the pediatric foot. They reported excellent results with free musculocutaneous flaps or skin grafted muscle flaps. For plantar foot reconstructions, the musculocutaneous flaps had better results with fewer tropic ulcers and fewer resurfacing procedures. They also found that reconstruction of the tendons in the immediate setting led to fewer subsequent operations than staged tendon reconstructions.[95]

One of the most difficult decisions to make while treating these severe injuries is whether to salvage the affected part of the limb or amputate the questionable part. This decision is largely based on what the functional outcome will be with either treatment and what effect prolonged treatments and hospitalizations will have on the child. Amputation rates vary between 16% and 78% in the literature.[7,42,168] A mangled extremity severity score (MESS) has been developed in adults to help surgeons make these decisions.[75]. The MESS score was validated in children by Fagelman and coworkers[48]; however, they did not include fractures below the ankle. It is useful to ask for a colleague's advice when contemplating an amputation so the advantages and disadvantages can be freely debated. If an amputation is performed, as much length of the bone should be preserved as possible, and transdiaphyseal amputation should generally be avoided to prevent problems with stump overgrowth.[2,98]

The functional outcome for these patients is generally satisfactory. Vosburgh and colleagues[168] reviewed the functional outcome of 21 children with lawnmower accidents and found that patients who had their injury confined to the forefoot had 88% of normal function compared to 72% of normal function in patients who had sustained injuries to the posterior and plantar aspects of their foot.

COMPARTMENT SYNDROME

Compartment syndrome of the foot can occur in children with severe soft tissue injuries in the presence or absence of associated fractures. Most commonly, it occurs with severe crush injuries of the forefoot where there are multiple fractures and dislocations; however, it can occur without any fracture, such as the case of a car running over a foot causing crush and shear injury to soft tissue. The symptoms are not as obvious as they are in compartment syndrome of the forearm or leg, and increased pain with passive motion of the toes is not always present. There is significant pain from the injury itself, which often requires considerable amounts of pain relief. Pallor, pain on passive extension, parasthesia, and a dorsalis pedis pulse that is difficult to palpate likewise can all be clinical signs in a large number of foot injuries. The clinician needs to have a high index of suspicion for a compartment syndrome and if any doubt exists, the compartment pressures should be measured or the child taken urgently to the operating room for a decompression of the foot.

Compartment pressure measurements are difficult to perform with invasive catheterization in an awake child with trauma to the foot. Often, the compartments need to be measured under a general anesthetic, so the child and parents need to be warned that the surgeon may proceed to a decompression. There are nine compartments in the foot, and it is difficult to confirm exact compartment location. It is important, however, to measure the pressure in the calcaneal compartment because it appears to be the most sensitive.[103] When a pressure of greater than 30 mm Hg is measured in any compartment, a fasciotomy should be performed.[103,113] It may be more accurate to use a measurement that takes into account the patient's blood pressure. In adults, the threshold is a measured pressure that is less than 30 mm Hg below the patient's diastolic blood pressure.[102]

There are nine fascial compartments in the foot that contain the intrinsic muscles and short plantar flexors. When a decompression is carried out, all the compartments should be released regardless of the clinical findings or compartment measurements. The most thorough way to achieve this is by using

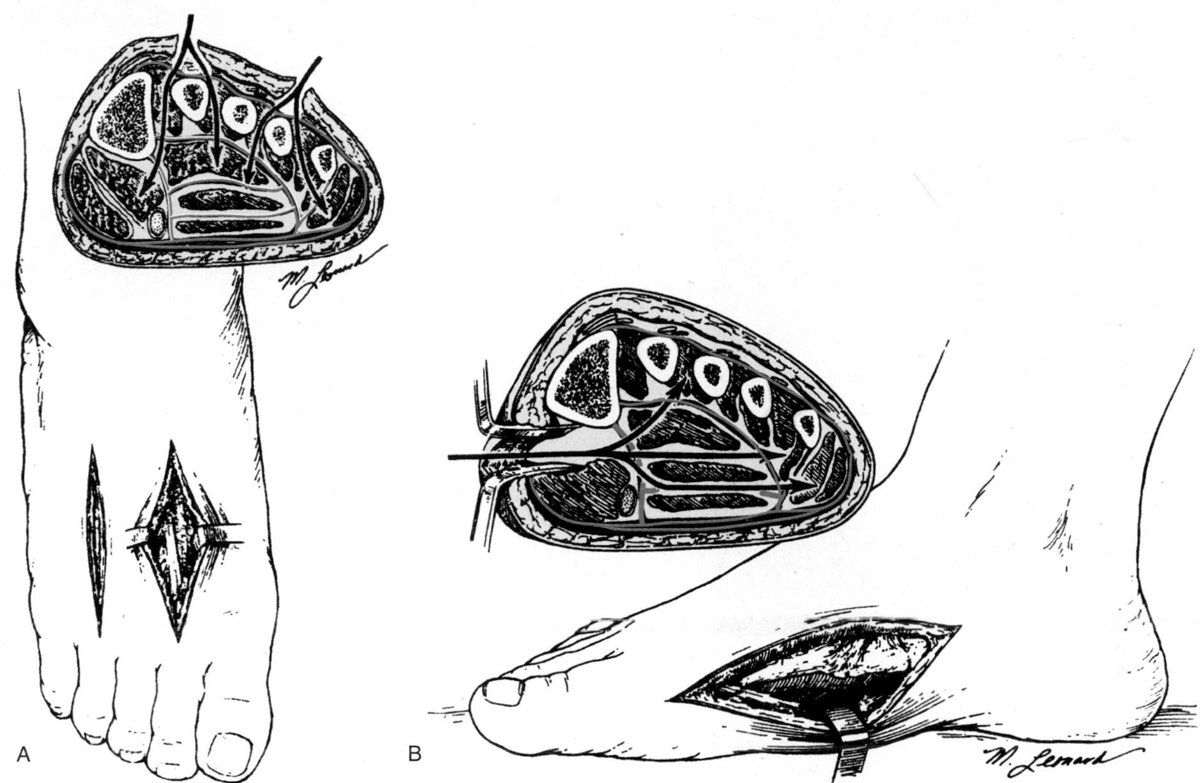

FIGURE 27-42 Surgical approaches for fasciotomy of the foot. **A.** The dorsal approach is made through an incision over the second and fourth metatarsal shafts and is more suitable for injuries of the forefoot or midfoot. **B.** The medial approach is more suitable for injuries of the hindfoot, with the incision extending from the base of the first metatarsal to the medial malleolus. A tarsal tunnel release can be done through this incision. (From Myerson MS. Experimental decompression of the fascial compartments of the foot: the basis for fasciotomy in acute compartment syndromes. Foot Ankle 1988;8:308–314, with permission.)

the three incision technique described by Myerson[113] (Fig. 27-42). Two dorsal longitudinal incisions are made in line with the second and fourth metatarsals. Dissection is then carried out through the interosseous compartments and fascia to enable decompression of the deep plantar compartments. Puncturing the fascia and spreading with a hemostat is an effective and safe technique. The lateral compartment is decompressed through the incision over the fourth metatarsal by dissecting deep to the fifth metatarsal. A medial incision is made along the arch of the foot as far posterior as the medial malleolus. This incision allows decompression of the medial compartment and a more thorough decompression of the deep compartments. It also allows decompression of the tarsal tunnel. Dissection is carried out on both the dorsal and plantar surfaces of the abductor hallucis muscle, freeing it from both the plantar fascia and bony attachments. Care must be taken to avoid damaging the lateral plantar nerve and vessels which lie on the quadrates plantae muscle. The deep compartments can now be easily released under direct vision. These three incisions are usually well placed to help with fracture reduction and K-wiring to stabilize the foot at the same time as the decompression. The wounds should be left open initially and closed 5 to 7 days later. Often, one of the wounds will require split-skin grafting.

Although uncommon in children, late sequelae of missed compartment syndrome can lead to disability including claw-toe deformity, paresthesia, cavus deformity, stiffness, and residual pain.[14,160]

PUNCTURE WOUNDS

Puncture wounds to the foot are extremely common in children and frequently treated by primary care physicians or in the emergency department. Most injuries can be treated by simply removing the offending foreign body, irrigating the entry site, giving tetanus prophylaxis if required, and a short course of oral antibiotics. It is important to carefully assess the foreign body that is removed to make sure a small part of it has not been retained in the foot. Often, the patient will bring the offending foreign body with them if it broke off or came out spontaneously. The depth of penetration should also be assessed by looking at the length of the foreign object as well as the point of entry. This may help predict if a joint or tendon sheath has been penetrated. The amount of contamination can also help determine if an open débridement is necessary and the length of administration of antibiotics.

Radiographs are useful in most cases of acute puncture wounds as occasionally a foreign body will be seen. If the foreign body has punctured a joint, air may be seen as well. When a retained foreign body is still suspected but not seen on radiograph, an ultrasound scan can be useful to identify its location. An MRI scan is even more useful at identifying foreign bodies and has the added advantage of showing secondary changes of septic arthritis or osteomyelitis if the puncture wound is more chronic (Fig. 27-43).

If a patient with a treated puncture wound does not rapidly

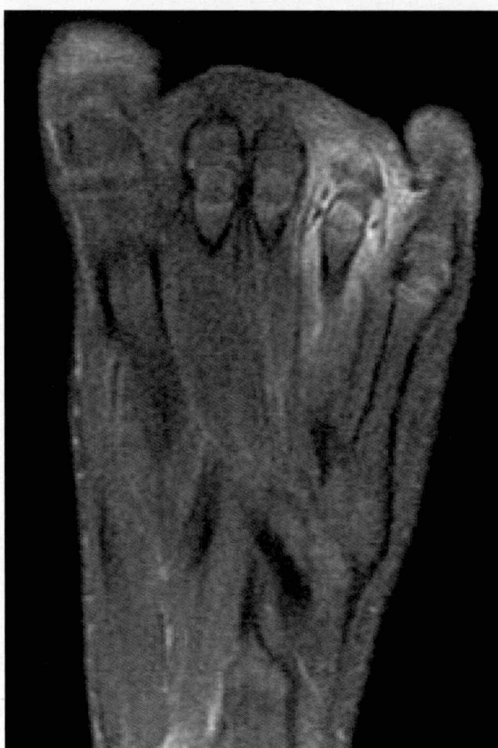

FIGURE 27-43 MRI scans are useful following penetrating foot injuries as the extent of the soft tissue or joint involment can be clearly seen. This 6-year-old boy had pain 4 days after standing on a nail in barefeet, and despite oral antibiotics he had developed a septic arthritis.

improve clinically, further investigation is required to rule out a retained foreign body, deep soft tissue infection, septic arthritis, or osteomyelitis. Eidelman et al.[44] recommend that patients who have an established infection 24 to 36 hours after a puncture wound should be admitted to hospital for IV antibiotics. In their series of 80 children with puncture wounds, a delay in diagnosis or presentation was associated with deep infection.[44] The most common organism causing deep infections in their study was *Staphylococcus aureus* and Group A *Streptococcus*. A complete blood count, erythrocyte sedimentation rate, and C-reactive protein should be performed, and an MRI scan is the most accurate radiologic investigation.[70,84] The patient can then be treated accordingly with IV antibiotics and open débridement of the entry site and deeper tissues.

Septic arthritis or osteomyelitis should be suspected if a child presents with foot pain and swelling following a puncture wound to the foot with a nail while wearing sneakers. Pseudomonas osteochondritis is thought to occur when the cartilage is damaged at the initial injury.[50] The source of the pseudomonas is debatable; however, some authors have postulated that it is from the sneakers.[49,85] The patient should be admitted to hospital and a thorough débridement of the affected soft tissues, cartilage, and bone should be carried out. IV antibiotics are administered often for 5 to 7 days or until the infection has clearly resolved.[72,73] The long-term sequelae of pain, growth arrests, chronic osteomyelitis, and recurrence make this an important infection to identify early and treat aggressively.

STRESS FRACTURES

Stress fractures in children are becoming more common due to overtraining in youth athletics and year-round participation in sports.[31] The tibia, fibula, femur, and pars interarticularis are the areas most commonly affected; however, stress fractures in the foot can also occur.[33,40,56,177]

The predominant symptom is "pain with weight bearing," and this usually coincides with the beginning of an intense period of training. The repetitive training results in bone fatigue and eventual partial or complete fracture. The normal cortical bone remodeling is accelerated and resorption occurs at a faster rate than the reparative process resulting in weakening of the bone and inevitable microfracture. Treatment, therefore, is aimed at breaking this cycle by activity modification and protected weight bearing to prevent further fracture and allow the reparative process to "catch up."

Patients with stress fractures in the foot present with pain on weight bearing and often no history of any particular injury that may have been the cause. A thorough history of their training regimen is essential, particularly any increases or changes in technique playing surface or footwear. On examination, there is point tenderness but minimal swelling. Radiographs taken early in the process are often normal but later show periosteal layering of new bone on the cortex and osteolysis at the fracture site. Bone scans are often more sensitive initially and a three-phase technetium bone scan is helpful when the radiographs are normal in the first 2 to 3 weeks after the onset of symptoms.[45] MRI has been shown to identify stress fractures before radiographic changes are evident, and in a prospective study of collegiate basketball players, MRI demonstrated marrow edema even before stress fractures were clinically evident.[101]

As well as concentrating on the fracture itself, the patient should be assessed for any conditions that could predispose them to stress fractures. These conditions include metabolic bone diseases, amenorrhea, eating disorders, and incorrect training techniques. There may have been as simple a cause as a change in footwear that has lead to increased stress in a particular bone in the foot.

The second metatarsal is the most common bone in the foot to get a stress fracture. This usually occurs at the neck of the metatarsal at the junction of the mobile shaft and rigid metaphysis. Treatment involves rest and partial weight bearing in a moonboot for 4–6 weeks. It is best to avoid a cast as during this time the athlete can maintain physical fitness with swimming, deep water running, and exercycling. A gradual return to activity can be restarted when radiographs confirm adequate healing and the symptoms have abated which often takes 8 to 12 weeks. Stress fractures of the navicular are disabling and difficult to treat. They occur most commonly in basketball players, hurdlers, and runners.[109] Bennell and Bruckner[11] reviewed 18 large studies of stress fractures and found that the incidence of navicular stress fractures can range between 0% and 28.6% of injuries among track and field athletes. These fractures are thought to arise due to overuse and the reduced vascularity that can exist in the central third of the navicular. They are difficult to diagnose and one needs to have a high level of suspicion as with any other stress fracture. The fracture is often diagnosed by technetium bone scan, and if this is positive in the region of the navicular, a CT scan is very helpful in delineating the stress response from an acute injury. The fracture line on CT, and if present on radiograph, is vertically orientated in the middle third of the bone. Most of these fractures heal with rest and protective weight bearing; however, some do go on to delayed or nonunion. The treatment for a painful nonunion is open reduction and internal fixation with autogenous bone grafting.[127] The average time for the return to activity following a navicular stress fracture in athletes is 5.6 months.[80] Stress fractures of the base of the fifth metatarsal usually occur in zone 2 or 3 and their treatment is discussed earlier in the chapter under the section sactures of the fifth metatarsal base.

Stress fractures can also occur in the cuboid, calcaneus, and sesamoid bones of the foot.

REFERENCES

1. Abidi NA, Dhawan S, Gruen GS, et al. Wound-healing risk factors after open reduction and internal fixation of calcaneal fractures. Foot Ankle Int 1998;19(12):856–861.
2. Abraham E, Pellicore RJ, Hamilton RC, et al. Stump overgrowth in juvenile amputees. J Pediatr Orthop 1986;6(1):66–71.
3. Adelaar RS. Complex fractures of the talus. Instr Course Lect 1997;46:323–338.
4. Adirim TA, Cheng TL. Overview of injuries in the young athlete. Sports Med 2003; 33(1):75–81.
5. Aitken AP. Fractures of the os calcis—treatment by closed reduction. Clin Orthop Relat Res 1963;30:67–75.
6. Allmacher DH, Galles KS, Marsh JL. Intra-articular calcaneal fractures treated nonoperatively and followed sequentially for 2 decades. J Orthop Trauma 2006;20(7):464–469.
7. Alonso JE, Sanchez FL. Lawn mower injuries in children: a preventable impairment. J Pediatr Orthop 1995;15(1):83–89.
8. Anderson IF, Crichton KJ, Grattan-Smith T, et al. Osteochondral fractures of the dome of the talus. J Bone Joint Surg Am 1989;71(8):1143–1152.
9. Aquino MD, Aquino L, Aquino JM. Talar neck fractures: a review of vascular supply and classification. J Foot Surg 1986;25(3):188–193.
10. Benirschke SK, Kramer PA. Wound healing complications in closed and open calcaneal fractures. J Orthop Trauma 2004;18(1):1–6.
11. Bennell KL, Brukner PD. Epidemiology and site specificity of stress fractures. Clin Sports Med 1997;16(2):179–196.
12. Berndt AL, Harty M. Transchondral fractures (osteochondritis dissecans) of the talus. J Bone Joint Surg Am 2004;86-A(6):1336.
13. Bibbo C, Davis WH, Anderson RB. Midfoot injury in children related to mini scooters. Pediatr Emerg Care 2003;19(1):6–9.
14. Bibbo C, Lin SS, Cunningham FJ. Acute traumatic compartment syndrome of the foot in children. Pediatr Emerg Care 2000;16(4):244–248.
15. Blair WF. Irreducible tarsometatarsal fracture-dislocation. J Trauma 1981;21(11): 988–990.
16. Blount W. Injuries of the foot. In: Beaty JH, Kasser JR, eds. Fractures in Children. Philadelphia: Williams and Wilkins, 1955:195-196.
17. Bonnel F, Barthelemy M. Injuries of Lisfranc's joint: severe sprains, dislocations, fractures. Study of 39 personal cases and biomechanical classification. J Chir (Paris) 1976; 111(5-6):573–592.
18. Broden B. Roentgen examination of the subtaloid joint in fractures of the calcaneus. Acta Radiol 1949;31(1):85–91.
19. Brunet JA. Calcaneal fractures in children. Long-term results of treatment. J Bone Joint Surg Br 2000;82(2):211–216.
20. Buckingham R, Jackson M, Atkins R. Calcaneal fractures in adolescents. CT classification and results of operative treatment. Injury 2003;34(6):454–459.
21. Buckley R, O'Brien J, McCormack R. Personal gait satisfaction of patients with displaced intraarticular calcaneal fractures: a 2- to 8-year follow-up. Poster Presentation 2770 in Orthopaedic Trauma Association Annual Meeting: Salt Lake City, Utah; October, 2003.
22. Buoncristiani AM, Manos RE, Mills WJ. Plantar-flexion tarsometatarsal joint injuries in children. J Pediatr Orthop 2001;21(3):324–327.
23. Burroughs KE, Reimer CD, Fields KB. Lisfranc injury of the foot: a commonly missed diagnosis. Am Fam Physician 1998;58(1):118–124.
24. Byrd T. Jones fracture: relearning an old injury. South Med J 1992;85(7):748–750.
25. Canale ST, Belding RH. Osteochondral lesions of the talus. J Bone Joint Surg Am 1980; 62(1):97–102.
26. Canale ST, Kelly FB Jr. Fractures of the neck of the talus. Long-term evaluation of 71 cases. J Bone Joint Surg Am 1978;60(2):143–156.
27. Carroll N. Fractures and dislocations of the tarsal bones. In: Letts RM, ed. Management of Pediatric Fractures. New York: Churchill Livingstone, 1994.
28. Ceccarelli F, Faldini C, Piras F, et al. Surgical versus nonsurgical treatment of calcaneal fractures in children: a long-term results comparative study. Foot Ankle Int 2000; 21(10):825–832.
29. Cehner J. Fractures of the tarsal bones, metatarsals, and toes. In: Weber B, Brunner C, Freuler F, eds. Treatment of Fractures in Children and Adolescents. New York: Springer-Verlag, 1980.
30. Ceroni D, De Rosa V, De Coulon G, et al. Cuboid nutcracker fracture due to horseback riding in children: case series and review of the literature. J Pediatr Orthop 2007;27(5): 557–561.
31. Chambers HG. Ankle and foot disorders in skeletally immature athletes. Orthop Clin North Am 2003;34(3):445–459.
32. Chapman H, Galway H. Os calcis fractures in childhood. J Bone Joint Surg 1977;59B: 510.
33. Childress H. March fracture in a 7-year-old boy. J Bone Joint Surg Am 1946;28:877.
34. Craigen MA, Clarke NM. Bilateral "Jones" fractures of the fifth metatarsal following relapse of talipes equinovarus. Injury 1996;27(8):599–601.
35. Crawford A. Fractures and dislocations of the foot and ankle. In: Green NE, ed. Skeletal Trauma in Children. Philadelphia: WB Saunders; 1994 :449–516.
36. Curtis MJ, Myerson M, Szura B. Tarsometatarsal joint injuries in the athlete. Am J Sports Med 1993;21(4):497–502.
37. Dameron TB Jr. Fractures of the proximal fifth metatarsal: selecting the best treatment option. J Am Acad Orthop Surg 1995;3(2):110–114.
38. Damore DT, Metzl JD, Ramundo M, et al. Patterns in childhood sports injury. Pediatr Emerg Care 2003;19(2):65–67.
39. DeLee J. Fracture and dislocations of the foot. In: Mann RA, ed. Surgery of the Foot and Ankle. St. Louis: Mosby, 1993.
40. Devas MB. Stress fractures in children. J Bone Joint Surg Br 1963;45:528–541.
41. Dimentberg R, Rosman M. Peritalar dislocations in children. J Pediatr Orthop 1993; 13(1): 89–93.
42. Dormans JP, Azzoni M, Davidsion RS, et al. Major lower extremity lawn mower injuries in children. J Pediatr Orthop 1995;15(1):78–82.
43. Early J. In: Rockwood CA, Green DP, Bucholz RW, et al, eds. Rockwood and Green's Fractures in Adults. Philadelphia: Lippincott Williams & Wilkins, 2006:2337–2400.
44. Eidelman M, Bialik V Miller Y, et al. Plantar puncture wounds in children: analysis of 80 hospitalized patients and late sequelae. Isr Med Assoc J 2003;5(4):268–271.
45. Englaro EE, Gelfand MJ, Paltiel HJ. Bone scintigraphy in preschool children with lower extremity pain of unknown origin. J Nucl Med 1992;33(3):351–354.
46. Erdmann D, Lee B, Roberts CD, et al. Management of lawnmower injuries to the lower extremity in children and adolescents. Ann Plast Surg 2000;45(6):595–600.
47. Essex-Lopresti P. The mechanism, reduction technique, and results in fractures of the os calcis. Br J Surg 1952;39:395.
48. Fagelman MF, Epps HR, Rang M. Mangled extremity severity score in children. J Pediatr Orthop 2002;22(2):182–184.
49. Fisher MC, Goldsmith JF, Gilligan PH. Sneakers as a source of *Pseudomonas aeruginosa* in children with osteomyelitis following puncture wounds. J Pediatr 1985;106(4): 607–609.
50. Fitzgerald RH Jr, Cowan JD. Puncture wounds of the foot. Orthop Clin North Am 1975;6(4):965–972.
51. Folk JW, Starr AJ, Early JS. Early wound complications of operative treatment of calcaneus fractures: analysis of 190 fractures. J Orthop Trauma 1999;13(5):369–372.
52. Fortin PT, Balazsy JE. Talus fractures: evaluation and treatment. J Am Acad Orthop Surg 2001;9(2):114–127.
53. Gelberman RH, Mortensen WW. The arterial anatomy of the talus. Foot Ankle 1983; 4(2):64–72.
54. Glasgow MT, Naranja RJ Jr, Glasgow SG, et al. Analysis of failed surgical management of fractures of the base of the fifth metatarsal distal to the tuberosity: the Jones fracture. Foot Ankle Int 1996;17(8):449–457.
55. Goiney RC, Connell DG, Nichols DM. CT evaluation of tarsometatarsal fracture-dislocation injuries. AJR Am J Roentgenol 1985;144(5):985–990.
56. Griffin LY. Common sports injuries of the foot and ankle seen in children and adolescents. Orthop Clin North Am 1994;25(1):83–93.
57. Groshar D, Alperson M, Mendes DG, et al. Bone scintigraphy findings in Lisfranc joint injury. Foot Ankle Int 1995;16(11):710–711.
58. Haliburton RA, Sullivan CR, Kelly PJ, et al. The extraosseous and intraosseous blood supply of the talus. J Bone Joint Surg Am 1958;40-A(5):1115–1120.
59. Hardcastle PH, Reschauer R, Kutshca-Lissberg E, et al. Injuries to the tarsometatarsal joint. Incidence, classification, and treatment. J Bone Joint Surg Br 1982;64(3): 349–356.
60. Hawkins LG. Fracture of the lateral process of the talus. J Bone Joint Surg Am 1965; 47:1170–1175.
61. Hawkins LG. Fractures of the neck of the talus. J Bone Joint Surg Am 1970;52(5): 991–1002.
62. Heckman JD, McLean MR. Fractures of the lateral process of the talus. Clin Orthop Relat Res 1985;199:108–113.
63. Henderson RC. Posttraumatic necrosis of the talus: the Hawkins sign versus magnetic resonance imaging. J Orthop Trauma 1991;5(1):96–99.
64. Herrera-Soto JA, Scherb M, Duffy MF, et al. Fractures of the fifth metatarsal in children and adolescents. J Pediatr Orthop 2007;27(4):427–431.
65. Higuera J, Laguna R, Peral M, et al. Osteochondritis dissecans of the talus during childhood and adolescence. J Pediatr Orthop 1998;18(3):328–332.
66. Hosking KV, Hoffman EB. Midtarsal dislocations in children. J Pediatr Orthop 1999; 19(5):592–595.
67. Howard CB, Benson MK. The ossific nuclei and the cartilage anlage of the talus and calcaneum. J Bone Joint Surg Br 1992;74(4):620–623.
68. Howard JL, Buckley R, McCormack R, et al. Complications following management of displaced intra-articular calcaneal fractures: a prospective randomized trial comparing open reduction internal fixation with nonoperative management. J Orthop Trauma 2003;17(4):241–249.
69. Hubbard AM, Meyer JS, Davidson RS, et al. Relationship between the ossification center and cartilaginous anlage in the normal hindfoot in children: study with MR imaging. AJR Am J Roentgenol 1993;161(4):849–853.
70. Imoisili MA, Bonwit AM, Bulas DI. Toothpick puncture injuries of the foot in children. Pediatr Infect Dis J 2004;23(1):80–82.
71. Inokuchi S, Usami N, Hiraishi E, et al. Calcaneal fractures in children. J Pediatr Orthop 1998;18(4):469–474.
72. Jacobs RF, McCarthy RE, Elser JM. Pseudomonas osteochondritis complicating puncture wounds of the foot in children: a 10-year evaluation. J Infect Dis 1989;160(4): 657–661.
73. Jarvis JG, Skipper J. Pseudomonas osteochondritis complicating puncture wounds in children. J Pediatr Orthop 1994;14(6):755–759.
74. Jensen I, Wester JU, Rasmussen F, et al. Prognosis of fracture of the talus in children. 21 (7- to 34-)-year follow-up of 14 cases. Acta Orthop Scand 1994;65(4):398–400.
75. Johansen K, Daines M, Howey T, et al. Objective criteria accurately predict amputation following lower extremity trauma. J Trauma 1990;30(5):568–572; discussion 572–573.

76. Josefsson PO, Karlsson M, Redlund-Johnell I, et al. Closed treatment of Jones fracture. Good results in 40 cases after 11-26 years. Acta Orthop Scand 1994;65(5):545–547.
77. Josefsson PO, Karlsson M, Redlund-Johnell I, et al. Jones fracture. Surgical versus nonsurgical treatment. Clin Orthop Relat Res 1994;299:252–255.
78. Kay RM, Tang CW. Pediatric foot fractures: evaluation and treatment. J Am Acad Orthop Surg 2001;9(5):308–319.
79. Kellam J, Bosse M, Obremskey W. Timing of surgical fixation of talar neck fractures. Paper 2745. Presented at: Orthopedic Trauma Association Annual General Meeting. Salt Lake City, Utah; October 9–11, 2003.
80. Khan KM, Fuller PJ, Brukner PD, et al. Outcome of conservative and surgical management of navicular stress fracture in athletes. Eighty-six cases proven with computerized tomography. Am J Sports Med 1992;20(6):657–666.
81. Kirkpatrick DP, Hunter RE, Janes PC, et al. The snowboarder's foot and ankle. Am J Sports Med 1998;26(2):271–277.
82. Kumai T, Takakura Y, Higashiyama I, et al. Arthroscopic drilling for the treatment of osteochondral lesions of the talus. J Bone Joint Surg Am 1999;81(9):1229–1235.
83. Laliotis N, Pennie BH, Carty H, et al. Toddler's fracture of the calcaneum. Injury 1993; 24(3):169–170.
84. Lau LS, Bin G, Jaovisidua S, et al. Cost effectiveness of magnetic resonance imaging in diagnosing *Pseudomonas aeruginosa* infection after puncture wound. J Foot Ankle Surg 1997;36(1):36–43.
85. Laughlin TJ, Armstrong DG, Caporusso J, et al. Soft tissue and bone infections from puncture wounds in children. West J Med 1997;166(2):126–128.
86. Lawrence SJ, Botte MJ. Jones' fractures and related fractures of the proximal fifth metatarsal. Foot Ankle 1993;14(6):358–365.
87. Leenen LP, van der Werken C. Fracture-dislocations of the tarsometatarsal joint, a combined anatomical and computed tomographic study. Injury 1992;23(1):51–55.
88. Lehman RC, Torg JS, Pavlov H, et al. Fractures of the base of the fifth metatarsal distal to the tuberosity: a review. Foot Ankle 1987;7(4):245–252.
89. Leibner ED, Simanovsky N, Abu-Sneinah K, et al. Fractures of the lateral process of the talus in children. J Pediatr Orthop B 2001;10(1):68–72.
90. Letournel E. Open treatment of acute calcaneal fractures. Clin Orthop Relat Res 1993; 290:60–67.
91. Letts M, Davidson D, Ahmer A. Osteochondritis dissecans of the talus in children. J Pediatr Orthop 2003;23(5):617–625.
92. Letts RM, Gibeault D. Fractures of the neck of the talus in children. Foot Ankle 1980; 1(2):74–77.
93. Levin LS, Nunley JA. The management of soft-tissue problems associated with calcaneal fractures. Clin Orthop Relat Res 1993;290:151–156.
94. Lickstein LH, Bentz ML. Reconstruction of pediatric foot and ankle trauma. J Craniofac Surg 2003;14(4):559–565.
95. Lin CH, Mardini S, Wei FC, et al. Free flap reconstruction of foot and ankle defects in pediatric patients: long-term outcome in 91 cases. Plast Reconstr Surg 2006;117(7): 2478–2487.
96. Lindvall E, Haidukewych G, DiPasquale T, et al. Open reduction and stable fixation of isolated, displaced talar neck and body fractures. J Bone Joint Surg Am 2004;86-A(10):2229–2234.
97. Loder RT. Demographics of traumatic amputations in children. Implications for prevention strategies. J Bone Joint Surg Am 2004;86-A(5):923–928.
98. Love SM, Grogan DP, Ogden JA. Lawnmower injuries in children. J Orthop Trauma 1988;2(2):94–101.
99. Lu J, Ebraheim NA, Skie M, et al. Radiographic and computed tomographic evaluation of Lisfranc dislocation: a cadaver study. Foot Ankle Int 1997;18(6):351–355.
100. Main BJ, Jowett RL. Injuries of the midtarsal joint. J Bone Joint Surg Br 1975;57(1): 89–97.
101. Major NM. Role of MRI in prevention of metatarsal stress fractures in collegiate basketball players. AJR Am J Roentgenol 2006;186(1):255–258.
102. Manoli A 2nd. Compartment syndromes of the foot: current concepts. Foot Ankle 1990;10(6):330–334.
103. Manoli A, Fakhouri A, Weber T. Compartmental catheterization and fasciotomy of the foot. Operative Tech Orthop 1992;2:203–210.
104. Matteri RE, Frymoyer JW. Fracture of the calcaneus in young children. Report of three cases. J Bone Joint Surg Am 1973;55(5):1091–1094.
105. Mazel C, Rigault P, Padovani JP, et al. [Fractures of the talus in children. Apropos of 23 cases]. Rev Chir Orthop Reparatrice Appar Mot 1986;72(3):183–195.
106. McCrory P, Bladin C. Fractures of the lateral process of the talus: a clinical review. "Snowboarder's ankle." Clin J Sport Med 1996;6(2):124–128.
107. McDougall A, The os trigonum. J Bone Joint Surg Br 1955;37-B(2):257–265.
108. Meyer SA, Callaghan JJ, Albright JP, et al. Midfoot sprains in collegiate football players. Am J Sports Med 1994;22(3):392–401.
109. Monteleone GP Jr. Stress fractures in the athlete. Orthop Clin North Am 1995;26(3): 423–432.
110. Mooney JF 3rd, Argenta LC, Marks MW, et al. Treatment of soft tissue defects in pediatric patients using the V.A.C. system. Clin Orthop Relat Res 2000;376:26–31.
111. Mora S, Thordorson DB, Zionts LE, et al. Pediatric calcaneal fractures. Foot Ankle Int 2001;22(6):471–477.
112. Mulfinger GL, Trueta J. The blood supply of the talus. J Bone Joint Surg Br 1970; 52(1):160–167.
113. Myerson MS. Experimental decompression of the fascial compartments of the foot—the basis for fasciotomy in acute compartment syndromes. Foot Ankle 1988;8(6):308–314.
114. Myerson MS, Fisher RT, Burgess AR, et al. Fracture dislocations of the tarsometatarsal joints: end results correlated with pathology and treatment. Foot Ankle 1986;6(5): 225–242.
115. Newman R, Miles R. Hazard Analysis: Injuries Associated with Riding Type Mowers. Washington, DC: U.S.C.P.S. Commission, 1981.
116. Nicholas R, Hadley J, Paul C, et al. "Snowboarder's fracture": fracture of the lateral process of the talus. J Am Board Fam Pract 1994;7(2):130–133.
117. Noble J, Royle SG. Fracture of the lateral process of the talus: computed tomographic scan diagnosis. Br J Sports Med 1992;26(4):245–246.
118. Ogden J. The foot. In: Ogden J. Skeletal Injury in the Child. New York: Springer Verlag, 2000:
119. Owen RJ, Hickey FG, Finlay DB. A study of metatarsal fractures in children. Injury 1995;26(8):537–538.
120. Paccola C, Kunioka C. Bifid calcaneus. The Foot 1991;1:49–50.
121. Pennal GF. Fractures of the talus. Clin Orthop Relat Res 1963;30:53–63.
122. Penny JN, Davis LA. Fractures and fracture-dislocations of the neck of the talus. J Trauma 1980;20(12):1029–1037.
123. Perumal V, Wall E, Babekir N. Juvenile osteochondritis dissecans of the talus. J Pediatr Orthop 2007;27(7):821–825.
124. Peterson L, Goldie IF. The arterial supply of the talus. A study on the relationship to experimental talar fractures. Acta Orthop Scand 1975;46(6):1026–1034.
125. Peterson L, Romanus B, Dahlberg E. Fracture of the collum tali—an experimental study. J Biomech 1976;9(4):277–279.
126. Pickle A, Benaroch TE, Guy P, et al. Clinical outcome of pediatric calcaneal fractures treated with open reduction and internal fixation. J Pediatr Orthop 2004;24(2): 178–180.
127. Pontell D, Hallivis R, Dollard MD. Sports injuries in the pediatric and adolescent foot and ankle: common overuse and acute presentations. Clin Podiatr Med Surg 2006; 23(1):209–231, x.
128. Potter HG, Deland JT, Gusmar PB, et al. Magnetic resonance imaging of the Lisfranc ligament of the foot. Foot Ankle Int 1998;19(7):438–446.
129. Pritsch M, Horoshovski H, Farine I. Arthroscopic treatment of osteochondral lesions of the talus. J Bone Joint Surg Am 1986;68(6):862–865.
130. Purvis JM, Burke RG. Recreational injuries in children: incidence and prevention. J Am Acad Orthop Surg 2001;9(6):365–374.
131. Quénu E, Küss G. Étude sur les luxations du metataese (luxations métatarsotariennes) du diastasis entre le 1er et la 2e metatarsien. Rev Chir Orthop Reparatrice Appar Mot 1909;39:281–336.
132. Quill GE Jr. Fractures of the proximal fifth metatarsal. Orthop Clin North Am 1995; 26(2):353–361.
133. Rainaut J, Cedard C, D'Hour J. Tarso-metatarsal luxations. Rev Chir Orthop Reparatrice Appar Mot 1966;52:449.
134. Rammelt S, Zwipp H, Gavlik JM. Avascular necrosis after minimally displaced talus fracture in a child. Foot Ankle Int 2000;21(12):1030–1036.
135. Rang M. The foot. In: Rang M. Children's Fractures. 2nd ed. Philadelphia: JB Lippincott, 1974.
136. Rasmussen F, Schantz K. Radiologic aspects of calcaneal fractures in childhood and adolescence. Acta Radiol Diagn (Stockh) 1986;27(5):575–580.
137. Richli WR, Rosenthal DI. Avulsion fracture of the fifth metatarsal: experimental study of pathomechanics. AJR Am J Roentgenol 1984;143(4):889–891.
138. Rosenberg GA, Patterson BM. Tarsometatarsal (Lisfranc's) fracture-dislocation. Am J Orthop 1995;Suppl:7–16.
139. Ross G, Cronin R, Hauzenblas J, et al. Plantar ecchymosis sign: a clinical aid to diagnosis of occult Lisfranc tarsometatarsal injuries. J Orthop Trauma 1996;10(2):119–122.
140. Ross PM, Schwentker EP, Bryan H. Mutilating lawnmower injuries in children. JAMA 1976;236(5):480–481.
141. Rowe C, Sakellarides H. Fractures of the os calcis, a long-term follow-up study of 146 patients. JAMA 1963;184:920.
142. Sammarco GJ. The Jones fracture. Instr Course Lect 1993;42:201–205.
143. Sanders R. Displaced intra-articular fractures of the calcaneus. J Bone Joint Surg Am 2000;82(2):225–250.
144. Sanders R. Fractures and fracture-dislocations of the calcaneus. In: Coughlin M, Mann R, eds. Surgery of the Foot and Ankle. 7th ed. St. Louis: Mosby, 1999.
145. Sanders R. Intra-articular fractures of the calcaneus: present state of the art. J Orthop Trauma 1992;6(2):252–265.
146. Sanders R, Fortin P, DiPasquale T, et al. Operative treatment in 120 displaced intra-articular calcaneal fractures. Results using a prognostic computed tomography scan. Clin Orthop Relat Res 1993;290:87–95.
147. Sarrail R, Launay F, Marez M. Reflex dystrophy in children and adolescents. J Bone Joint Surg Br 2004;86(Suppl):23.
148. Schantz K, Rasmussen F. Good prognosis after calcaneal fracture in childhood. Acta Orthop Scand 1988;59(5):560–563.
149. Schenck RC Jr, Heckman JD. Fractures and dislocations of the forefoot: operative and nonoperative treatment. J Am Acad Orthop Surg 1995;3(2):70–78.
150. Schmidt TL, Weiner DS. Calcaneal fractures in children. An evaluation of the nature of the injury in 56 children. Clin Orthop Relat Res 1982;171:150–155.
151. Schopfner C, Coin C. Effect of weight-bearing on the appearance and development of the secondary calcaneal epiphysis. Radiology 1968;86:201–206.
152. Senaran H, Mason D, De Pellegrin M. Cuboid fractures in preschool children. J Pediatr Orthop 2006;26(6):741–744.
153. Shereff MJ. Fractures of the forefoot. Instr Course Lect 1990;39:133–140.
154. Shilt JS, Yoder JS, Manuck TA, et al. Role of vacuum-assisted closure in the treatment of pediatric lawnmower injuries. J Pediatr Orthop 2004;24(5):482–487.
155. Singer G, Cichocki M, Schalamon J, et al. A study of metatarsal fractures in children. J Bone Joint Surg Am 2008;90(4):772–776.
156. Sneppen O, Christensen SB, Krogsoe O, et al. Fracture of the body of the talus. Acta Orthop Scand 1977;48(3):317–324.
157. Stanitski CL. Pediatric and adolescent sports injuries. Clin Sports Med 1997;16(4): 613–633.
158. Starshak RJ, Simons GW, Sty JR. Occult fracture of the calcaneus—another toddler's fracture. Pediatr Radiol 1984;14(1):37–40.
159. Swanson TV, Bray TJ, Holmes GB Jr. Fractures of the talar neck. A mechanical study of fixation. J Bone Joint Surg Am 1992;74(4):544–551.
160. Swoboda B, Scola E, Zwipp H. [Surgical treatment and late results of foot compartment syndrome]. Unfallchirurg 1991;94(5):262–266.
161. Taranow WS, Bisignani GA, Towers JD, et al. Retrograde drilling of osteochondral lesions of the medial talar dome. Foot Ankle Int 1999;20(8):474–480.
162. Thomas HM. Calcaneal fracture in childhood. Br J Surg 1969;56(9):664–666.
163. Thordarson DB, Triffon MJ, Terk MR. Magnetic resonance imaging to detect avascular necrosis after open reduction and internal fixation of talar neck fractures. Foot Ankle Int 1996;17(12):742–747.
164. Torg JS, Balduini FC, Zelko RR, et al. Fractures of the base of the fifth metatarsal distal to the tuberosity. Classification and guidelines for nonsurgical and surgical management. J Bone Joint Surg Am 1984;66(2):209–214.
165. Tucker DJ, Feder JM, Boylan JP. Fractures of the lateral process of the talus: two case reports and a comprehensive literature review. Foot Ankle Int 1998;19(9):641–646.

166. Vanderwilde R, Staheli LT, Chew DE, et al. Measurements on radiographs of the foot in normal infants and children. J Bone Joint Surg Am 1988;70(3):407–415.
167. Vollman D, Smith GA. Epidemiology of lawnmower-related injuries to children in the United States, 1990–2004. Pediatrics 2006;118(2):e273–278.
168. Vosburgh CL, Gruel CR, Herndon WA, et al. Lawnmower injuries of the pediatric foot and ankle: observations on prevention and management. J Pediatr Orthop 1995;15(4): 504–509.
169. Weber M, Locher S. Reconstruction of the cuboid in compression fractures: short to midterm results in 12 patients. Foot Ankle Int 2002;23(11):1008–1013.
170. Wilder RT. Management of pediatric patients with complex regional pain syndrome. Clin J Pain 2006;22(5):443–448.
171. Wilder RT, Berde CB, Wolohan M, et al. Reflex sympathetic dystrophy in children. Clinical characteristics and follow-up of 70 patients. J Bone Joint Surg Am 1992;74(6): 910–919.
172. Wiley JJ. The mechanism of tarsometatarsal joint injuries. J Bone Joint Surg Br 1971; 53(3):474–482.
173. Wiley JJ. Tarsometatarsal joint injuries in children. J Pediatr Orthop 1981;1(3): 255–260.
174. Wiley JJ, Profitt A. Fractures of the os calcis in children. Clin Orthop Relat Res 1984; 188:131–138.
175. Wilson DW. Injuries of the tarsometatarsal joints. Etiology, classification, and results of treatment. J Bone Joint Surg Br 1972;54(4):677–686.
176. Wiss DA, Kull DM, Perry J. Lisfranc fracture-dislocations of the foot: a clinical-kinesiological study. J Orthop Trauma 1987;1(4):267–274.
177. Yngve D. Stress fractures in the pediatric athlete. In: Sullivan J, Grana W, eds. The Pediatric Athlete. Park Ridge, IL: American Academy of Orthopaedic Surgeons, 1990: 235-240.

INDEX

Note: Page numbers followed by an f indicate figures; page numbers followed by a t indicate tables.

A

AAP. *See* American Academy of Pediatrics
Abbreviated Injury Scale (AIS), 75t
ABC. *See* Aneurysmal bone cysts
Abdominal injuries
  child abuse and, 202–203, 203f
  pelvic injuries and, 745
  polytrauma and, 79
Abuse. *See* Child abuse
Abusive head trauma (AHT), 195, 199–202, 200t, 201f, 202t
Accidents, motor vehicle. *See* Motor vehicle accidents
Acetabular fractures, 760f
  classification of, 760–761, 761f
  incidence of, 760
  postoperative management of, 767
  radiographic evaluation of, 761, 761f, 762f, 763f, 764f
  surgical treatment of, 765, 765f, 765t, 766f, 767
  treatment of, 761–762, 764
Acetaminophen, 53, 66t, 67, 67t
ACL. *See* Anterior cruciate ligament
Acromioclavicular joint. *See* Clavicle fractures
Acute respiratory distress syndrome, 79–80
ADI. *See* Atlanto-dens interval
Age
  cervical spine injuries and, 685–686
  distal femoral epiphyseal fractures classification and, 851, 851f
  femoral shaft fracture treatment and, 800, 800t, 802, 827, 928f
  fractures patterns and, 9
  hip fractures treatment and, 775
  skeleton staging by, 917, 917t
Aggrecan, 27t
AHT. *See* Abusive head trauma
Airway management equipment, 50, 50t
Airway status, 49–50, 50t
AIS. *See* Abbreviated Injury Scale
Aitken injury classification, 98
Alcohol abuse, 72, 193
Allis maneuver, 791
All-terrain vehicles (ATV), 13–14, 16
Aluminium toxicity, renal osteodystrophy and, 169
Amenorrhea, 783
American Academy Committee on Child Abuse and Neglect, 199
American Academy of Child and Adolescent Psychiatry, 212–213
American Academy of Orthopaedic Surgeons, 16
American Academy of Pediatrics (AAP), 16, 46, 206, 219, 711
American College of Radiology, 206
American Society for Internal Fixation, 575
Aminoglycoside, 82
Ampicillin, 156t
Amputation
  of fingertips, 237, 239, 240f
  NF and, 145
  of open fractures, 84
Analgesia, 46
  displaced fracture treatment and, 365–366
  postoperative, 65, 65t, 66t, 67–68, 67t
Anesthesia
  displaced fracture treatment and, 365–366
  for finger fractures, 230
  local
    axillary block, 62–63, 63f
    femoral nerve block, 64–65, 64f
    hematoma block, 62, 62f
    postoperative analgesia with, 65t, 66t, 67–68, 67t
    toxicity from, 59, 59t
    wrist/digital block, 63–64, 64f
  regional, 365
    agents for, 58–59
    intravenous, 59–61
    performing, 61
Aneurysmal bone cysts (ABC), 121t, 122t
  classification of, 126, 127f
  clinical features of, 125
  etiology of, 125
  natural history of, 126–128
  radiographs of, 125–126, 127f, 128f, 129f
  treatment of, 128
Angiogenic growth factors, 31
Angular deformity
  diaphyseal fibular shaft fractures and, 955–956, 956f
  diaphyseal tibial shaft fractures, 955–956, 956f
  femoral shaft fractures and, 829–830, 829f
Angulation limits
  femoral shaft fractures treatment, 804, 804t
  forearm fracture treatment and, 378
  radial shaft fractures, 378
  for radial/ulnar shaft fractures, 378
Ankle dislocations, 997
Ankle distractor, 985–986, 986f, 999, 1004–1005
Ankle fractures. *See* Distal fibular fractures; Distal tibial fractures
Ankle sprains, lateral, 997, 1008–1009
Annular ligament, 595, 597, 612–617. *See also* Pulled elbow syndrome
Anorexia nervosa, 783
Anterior cruciate ligament (ACL)
  injury to
    classification of, 914
    complications of, 925–926
    imaging of, 913
    incidence of, 911
    mechanism of, 911
    prognosis for, 925
    stress testing of, 913, 913f
    surgical/applied anatomy for, 915–916
    treatment of, 916, 917–919, 918f, 919f, 920f, 921–922, 921f, 922f, 923f, 924
  meniscal injuries and, 910
  tibial spine fractures and, 886, 887
Anterior elbow dislocation
  complications of, 611
  management of, 610
  mechanism of injury, 610
  postreduction care for, 611
  radiographic evaluation, 610, 610f
  signs/symptoms, 610
  treatment of, 610–611, 611f
Anticonvulsant therapy, 175
Apert syndrome, 710
Apophysis, 26, 26f, 27f
Arterial injuries, from posterior elbow dislocation, 605
Arthritis
  juvenile rheumatoid, 229
  posttraumatic, 1044
  psoriatic, 229
  septic, 213

Arthrodesis
atlanto-occipital, 702–703
occipitocervical, 701–702, 703, 703f, 704f
occiput to C2, 700–701, 701f, 702f
posterior subaxial cervical spine, 716, 717f, 718f
posterior subaxial cervical spine with lateral mass screw fixation, 716, 718, 718f, 719f
Arthrofibrosis, tibial spine injuries and, 895
Arthrography, elbow evaluation with, 485
Arthrogryposis, 181, 183–184, 183f
Arthropathies, 229
Aspirin, 66t, 67
Association for the Study of Internal Fixation, 657
Atlantoaxial joint, 690, 691t
congenital instability of, 710–711
odontoid fractures of
incidence of, 704–705
radiographic evaluation of, 705
treatment of, 705–706, 706f
operative treatment of
Brooks/Jenkins technique for, 707–708, 709f
Gallie technique for, 708–709, 709f
posterior C1–C2 polyaxial screw and rod fixation, 709–710, 711f
posterior C1–C2 transarticular screw fixation, 709, 710f
os odontoideum fractures
anatomy of, 706
diagnosis of, 706, 706f
treatment of, 706–707, 707f, 708f
traumatic ligamentous disruption, 707
Atlantoaxial rotatory subluxation
anatomy for, 711–712
classification of, 712, 712f
differential diagnosis of, 713
radiographic findings, 712–713, 714f
signs/symptoms of, 712, 712f, 713f
treatment of, 713
Atlanto-dens interval (ADI), 690, 691f
Atlanto-occipital instability
diagnosis of, 698, 698f
operative treatment of, 699
atlanto-occipital arthrodesis, 702–703
occipitocervical arthrodesis, 701–702, 703f
occipitocervical arthrodesis with contoured rod and segmental wire, 703, 704f
occiput to C2 arthrodesis, 700–701, 701f, 702f
radiographic evaluation of, 698–699, 699f, 700f
Atlanto-occipital junction, 690, 690t
Atlas fractures, 703–704, 705f
Atlas (C1) fractures, 703–704, 705f
ATV. *See* All-terrain vehicles
Avascular necrosis (AVN), 769, 771, 774
hip dislocation and, 794
hip fractures and, 780–782, 781f
AVN. *See* Avascular necrosis
Avulsion
lateral ligament, 1008–1009
medial epicondylar apophysis, 568–569, 569f
pelvic fractures
diagnosis of, 749
hip pain from, 785
incidence of, 748
mechanism of injury, 748, 749f
treatment/prognosis for, 749, 750f
tibial tuberosity
associated injuries, 871, 871f
compartment syndrome and, 876
complications of, 875–876, 875t
diagnosis/classification of, 871–872, 871f, 872f
incidence of, 870
mechanism of injury, 870
pearls/pitfalls of, 873, 875
postoperative management of, 873
signs/symptoms, 870, 870f
surgical applied anatomy, 872
treatment of, 873, 874f, 875f
Axillary block, 62–63, 63f
axis (C2)
crossing translaminar screw fixation of, 718, 719f, 720
occiput to C2 arthrodesis, 700–701, 701f, 702f
polyaxial screw and rod fixation to C1, 709–710, 711f
transarticular screw fixation to C1, 709, 710f

B
Backboards, 693
Bado, Jose Luis, 446–447
Barbiturates, 51
Baseball, Little League pathology from, 414, 415f, 580, 580t, 581f
Battered child syndrome, 7
Benzocaine, 58
Benzodiazepines, 47, 52–53, 53t, 55–56
Bicycle injuries, 12, 73
Bicycle spoke injuries, 959
Bier block, 59–60, 62
Biglycan, 27t, 28, 32
Birth injuries, humeral shaft fractures due to
mechanism of injury, 656
signs/symptoms of, 656
treatment of, 658–659, 659f
Bisphosphonate, 160
Blood pressure
ketamine and, 57
monitoring, 48, 48t
normal values for, 48, 48t
sedation and, 49
stabilizing, 74
Blount, Walter, 349
BMP. *See* Bone morphogenic proteins
Böhler, Lorenz, 348–349
Bone
anatomic regions of
apophysis, 26, 26f, 27f
diaphysis, 24, 24f, 25f
epiphysis, 19–20, 19f, 20f, 21f
metaphysis, 21–24, 22f, 23f
periosteum, 24–26, 25f
physis, 20–21, 20f, 21f
bruises of, 905
composition of, 27, 28t
defects in, 84
density of, 15
growth of
endochondral ossification, 31–32, 32f
membranous ossification, 34
physis regulatory mechanisms, 32–34
remodeling, 34, 35f, 37, 40
healing rate of, 74
molecular level of, cartilage/bone matrices, 26–31
molecular matrix of, 26–27
weakening conditions of
arthrogryposis, 181, 183–184, 183f
congenital primary hyperparathyroidism, 172, 172f
copper deficiency, 174–175
Cushing's syndrome, 173
osteogenesis imperfecta, 121t, 158–163, 159f, 161f, 162f, 213–216, 214f, 798, 835
osteopetrosis, 163–164, 163f, 164f, 165f
osteoporosis, 170–171, 171f, 730, 732f, 783
poliomyelitis, 181, 183–184
primary hyperparathyroidism, 171–173, 172f
pyknodysostosis, 164–165
rickets, 166–169, 166f, 167f, 168f, 169f
scurvy, 173–174, 174f
scurvy-like syndrome, 174–175
spinal cord injury in, 184
Bone cysts
aneurysmal, 121t, 122t
classification of, 126, 127f
clinical features of, 125
etiology of, 125
natural history of, 126–128
radiographs of, 125–126, 127f, 128f, 129f
treatment of, 128
classification of, 125f
unicameral, 121–122, 121t, 122t, 124f, 126f
classification of, 123
clinical features of, 122–123
femoral shaft fractures and, 798
natural history of, 123
staging of, 124t
treatment of, 123, 125, 125f
Bone density, child abuse screening and, 212
Bone infarct, 784
Bone marrow diseases, 121t
Gaucher's disease, 148, 150
hemophilia
clinical features of, 151–152
severity of, 152t
surgery in, 152–153
treatment of, 153
leukemia, 151, 152f
osteomyelitis, 121t, 122t
classification of, 153t, 154f, 154t
clinical features of, 153–154
radiographic evaluation of, 154–155, 155f
treatment of, 155–156, 156f, 156t
sickle cell disease, 150–151, 150f, 229
Bone mineral density, 399
Bone morphogenic proteins (BMP), 31, 32–33, 32f
Brooks/Jenkins technique, 707–708, 709f
Bruising, child abuse and, 197–198, 197f, 198t
Bupivacaine, 58–59, 60t, 61, 64
Burns
child abuse and, 198–199, 198f
hand injuries, 229
Butorphanol, 54

C
C1 (atlas) fractures, 703–704, 705f
C2 (axis)
crossing translaminar screw fixation of, 718, 719f, 720
occiput to C2 arthrodesis, 700–701, 701f, 702f
polyaxial screw and rod fixation to C1, 709–710, 711f
transarticular screw fixation to C1, 709, 710f
Caffey disease, 213. *See also* Infantile cortical hyperostosis
Calcaneal fractures
associated injuries, 1029–1030
complications of
complex regional pain syndrome, 1035–1037
peroneal tendonitis/dislocation, 1037
wound complications, 1034–1035
diagnosis/classification
classification, 1031, 1031f
CT, 1030–1031, 1031f
radiographs, 1030, 1030f
epidemiology of, 1029
mechanism of injury, 1029
signs/symptoms, 1029
surgical/applied anatomy, 1031–1032, 1032f

treatment of
cast immobilization, 1033, 1034
intervention selection, 1032–1033
open reduction/internal fixation, 1033, 1034, 1034f
operative planning for, 1036t
percutaneous reduction, 1033, 1033f
Campbell, Willis, 349
Cancer treatment, osteoporosis and, 170–171
Capitate fractures
diagnosis of, 277–278, 278f
epidemiology of, 276–277
mechanism of injury, 277
prognosis/complications of, 278
treatment of, 278
Capitellum fractures
associated injuries, 553
classification of, 552–553, 553f
complications of, 554
diagnosis of, 553
mechanism of injury, 553
scope of, 551–552, 552f
treatment of, 553–554, 554f
Carpal fractures
anatomy for, 268–269, 269f
capitate fractures
diagnosis of, 277–278, 278f
epidemiology of, 276–277
mechanism of injury, 277
prognosis/complications of, 278
treatment of, 278
epidemiology of, 267–268
hamate, pisiform, lunate, and trapezium fractures, 279
scaphoid fractures
bipartite scaphoid controversy, 270, 272
classification of, 272
complications of, 276, 276f, 277f
diagnosis of, 270f, 271f, 272f, 273f, 274f
epidemiology of, 269
mechanism of injury, 269–270
patterns of, 270
postoperative care/rehabilitation of, 275–276
prognosis for, 276
treatment of, 274–275, 275f
soft tissue injuries about carpus, ligamentous injuries, 279–280
triquetrum fractures
diagnosis of, 279
epidemiology of, 278
mechanism of injury, 278
treatment of, 279, 279f
Car seats, 72–73
Cartilage, matrix of, 26, 27t
Casts. *See specific fractures*
Cefazolin, 82, 156t
Cefotaxime, 156t
Celiac disease, 166–167
Central nervous system (CNS), injury to, 199
Cephalosporin, 82, 156t
Cerebral palsy (CP)
fractures in, 175–177, 176f, 177f, 178f
osteopenia and, 798
Cervical collars, 693
Cervical spine injuries
anatomy of
lower cervical spine, 687f, 688, 688f
upper cervical spine, 686–687, 686f, 687f
atlantoaxial joint, 690, 691t
congenital instability of, 710–711
odontoid fractures of, 704–706, 706f
operative treatment of, 707–710, 709f, 710f, 711f
os odontoideum fractures, 706–707, 706f, 707f, 708f
traumatic ligamentous disruption, 707
atlantoaxial rotatory subluxation
anatomy for, 711–712
classification of, 712, 712f
differential diagnosis of, 713
radiographic findings, 712–713, 714f
signs/symptoms of, 712, 712f, 713f
treatment of, 713
atlanto-occipital instability
diagnosis of, 698, 698f
operative treatment of, 699, 700--703, 701f, 702f, 703f, 704f
radiographic evaluation of, 698–699, 699f, 700f
atlas fractures, 703–704, 705f
child's age and, 685–686
evaluation of, 689
historical background, 688–689
immobilization for, 693–694, 693f, 694f
incidence of, 685
initial management of, 693–695, 693f, 694f, 695f
mechanism of injury, 686
multiple fracture evaluation and, 73, 75, 77
neurologic deficits and, 686
radiographic evaluation of
atlantoaxial joint, 690, 691t
atlanto-occipital junction, 690, 690t
lower cervical spine, 691–692, 692f
plain radiographs, 689–690, 690t
special imaging studies, 692–693, 693f
upper cervical spine, 690–691, 691f, 692f
subaxial
burst fractures, 716
compression fractures, 715
operative treatment of, 716, 717f, 718, 718f, 719f, 720
posterior ligamentous disruptions, 714–715
spondylolysis/spondylolisthesis, 716
unilateral/bilateral facet dislocations, 715, 715f
symptoms of, 689
Charnley, John, 349
Child abuse, 6–7
alcohol abuse and, 193
classic metaphyseal lesion of, 209, 209f, 210f
costs of, 193
deaths from, 193
differential diagnosis of, 212–214
distal femoral epiphyseal fractures from, 843, 843f
distal humeral physeal fractures and, 565
documenting, 197
drug abuse and, 193–194
fractures in, 204
dating of, 205–206
extremities, 208–209, 209t
femoral, 204–205, 204f
humeral, 205, 205f, 656, 798
long bone, 204–205, 204t
metatarsal, 205, 205f
multiple, 72, 205, 206f
pelvic, 744
rib, 209–211, 210f, 211f
skull, 208
spinal, 211–212, 212f
incidence of, 72
injury sites in, 72
legal reporting requirements for, 217–219
in medical settings, 194–195
orthopaedic investigative interview, 195–196, 196t
orthopaedists' role in recognition of, 193
parental predictors of, 194t
patient history and recognizing, 195
physical examination for
abdominal injuries, 202–203, 203f
abusive head trauma, 199–202, 200t, 201f, 202t
bruising, 197–198, 197f, 198t
burns, 198–199, 198f
genital injuries and, 203–204
soft tissue injuries, 197–198, 197f, 198t
postemergency room treatment, 217
prevention of, 219
risk factors for, 193–197
screening for
bone density tests, 212
laboratory studies in, 212
multidisciplinary approach for, 212
osteogenesis imperfecta in, 213, 214–216, 214f
skeletal survey in, 206–208
sudden unexpected death in infancy and, 216
temporary brittle bone disease and, 216
types of, 192
Childhood obesity, 399
Child maltreatment
defining, 192
epidemiology of, 192–193
types of, 192
Children's Fractures (Rang), 349
Chloral hydrate, 50–51, 51t
Chloramphenicol, 156t
Chloroprocaine, 58
Chlorpromazine, 50
Cholangitis, 167f
Choline magnesium, 67, 67t
Chondroblastoma, 122t
Chondrocytes, 31, 32f
Chondrolysis. *See also* Avascular necrosis
hip dislocation and, 794
hip fractures and, 782
Chondrosarcoma, 122t
Chronic sclerosing osteomyelitis, 784
Circulation, monitoring, 48–49, 48t
Classic metaphyseal lesions (CML), 205, 209, 209f, 210f
Clavicle fractures
anatomic factors for, 620, 621f
associated injuries, 621
classification of, 622–624, 623f, 624
complications from, 629
diagnosis of, 621–622, 622f, 623f
mechanism of injury, 620–621
signs/symptoms of, 621
surgical/applied anatomy, 624–625, 625f
treatment of
closed reduction for, 627
distal third fractures, 627
medial third fractures, 627
middle third fractures, 625–627, 626f
open reduction for, 628
options for, 625t, 626t
pearls/pitfalls for, 629
Clindamycin, 156t
Clonidine, 194
The Closed Treatment of Common Fractures (Charnley), 349
Clozapine, 194
CML. *See* Classic metaphyseal lesions
CNS. *See* Central nervous system
Cocaine, 58, 59, 194
Coccyx fractures, 759–760, 760f
Codeine, 54, 66t
Cold intolerance, 510
Collagen, 26, 27–28, 27t, 28f
Collateral ligaments
hand anatomy and, 227
lateral
injury to, 912–914, 915f, 922
knee dislocation and, 923–924, 924f
surgical/applied anatomy for, 915–916
tibial spine fractures and, 887
medial, 845
injury to, 912–914, 912f, 914f, 916–917
knee dislocation and, 924
surgical/applied anatomy for, 915–916
tibial spine fractures and, 887

Comminuted fractures
distal tibial fractures and, 1004
forearm, 368
medial column, 502, 508
Compartment syndrome, 364, 398, 426
distal tibial fractures and, 1013
femoral shaft fractures and, 832
fibular shaft fracture and
diagnosis of, 954, 954f
signs/symptoms of, 954
treatment of, 954–955, 955f
in foot fractures/dislocations, 1052–1053, 1053f
forearm fasciotomy for, 513–514, 514f
humeral shaft fractures and, 667
open tibial fractures and, 948
proximal tibial epiphyseal fractures and, 869
proximal ulnar fractures and, 440
supracondylar humeral fractures and, 491, 512–514, 514f
tibial shaft fracture and
diagnosis of, 954, 954f
signs/symptoms of, 954
treatment of, 954–955, 955f
tibial tuberosity avulsion and, 876
Complex regional pain syndromes, 398–399
calcaneal fractures and, 1035–1037
distal tibial fractures and, 1013
Compression plating, 85–86
femoral shaft fractures and, 824
Computed tomography (CT), 73, 74
of calcaneal fractures, 1030–1031, 1031f
of cervical spine injuries, 692
of distal femoral epiphyseal fractures, 862
elbow evaluation with, 485
of hip fractures, 770
multiple fracture evaluation with, 76–77, 77f
of osteochondral fractures, 896
of pelvic injuries, 745
of thoracolumbar spinal fractures, 724, 728
Condylar fractures
lateral physeal
anatomy/classification of, 534
closed reduction/percutaneous pinning of, 539–540, 541f
complications of, 546–549, 548f
cubitus valgus, 547–549, 548f
cubitus varus, 542, 543f, 546, 547, 548f, 549f
delayed union, 542–543, 543f
displacement stages, 534, 536f
fishtail deformity, 549, 549f
fracture/elbow joint displacement, 535, 537f, 538f
immobilization of, 538, 540–541
incidence/outcome, 534
ipsilateral injuries and, 551, 551f
late displacement of, 538
malunion from, 550
mechanism of injury, 535–537
neurologic complications, 549–550
nonunion, 543–546, 544f, 545f
open reduction/internal fixation, 540, 541–542, 542f
osteonecrosis in, 543, 544f, 550–551, 551f
osteotomy of, 543
physeal arrest and, 550
radiographic findings, 537, 538f, 539f
signs/symptoms, 537
soft tissue injuries, 534–535
spur formation in, 546, 547, 548f
treatment of, 537–542
medial physeal, 554
classification of, 557, 557f
complications of, 558–559, 559f, 560f, 561, 561f
cubitus valgus, 559
cubitus varus and, 559, 560f
diagnosis of, 557–558, 559f
incidence of, 555
mechanism of injury, 556–557, 556f
nonunion from, 559, 560f
surgical anatomy/pathology, 555–556, 555f
treatment of, 558, 558f, 560f
t-condylar
classification of, 584, 587f
complications of, 589
diagnosis of, 584–585
incidence of, 584
mechanism of injury, 584, 585f
patterns of, 584, 586f
treatment of, 585–589, 588f, 589f, 590f
Congenital elbow dislocation, 610
Congenital insensitivity to pain, 148, 149f, 213
Congenital primary hyperparathyroidism, 172, 172f
Congenital pseudarthrosis, 121t
Contractures, 78
Copper deficiency, 174–175
Coronoid process
fractures of
anatomy for, 440
associated injuries/complications, 444
classification of, 444, 444t
diagnosis of, 442, 443f, 444
incidence of, 440, 442
treatment of, 444
ossification of, 478
radiographic landmarks and, 483
Corticosteroids, muscular dystrophy and, 181, 182f
Covert in-hospital video surveillance (CVS), 195
Coxa magna, 794
Coxa vara, hip fractures and, 782
CP. *See* Cerebral palsy
Cross-union, of forearm fractures, 396–397
Cruciate ligament injuries
anterior
classification of, 914
complications of, 925–926
imaging of, 913
incidence of, 911
mechanism of, 911
meniscal injuries and, 910
prognosis for, 925
stress testing of, 913, 913f
surgical/applied anatomy for, 915–916
tibial spine fractures and, 886, 887
treatment of, 916, 917–919, 918f, 919f, 920f, 921–922, 921f, 922f, 923f, 924
posterior
classification of, 914
imaging of, 913
knee dislocation and, 924
mechanism of, 912
signs/symptoms of, 913, 914f
surgical/applied anatomy for, 915–916
treatment of, 923
Cryotherapy, of ABCs, 127–128
CT. *See* Computed tomography
Cubitus recurvatum, elbow dislocations and, 605
Cubitus valgus
lateral condylar physeal injury and, 547–549, 548f
medial condylar physeal injury and, 559
Cubitus varus
clinical presentation of, 520–521, 520f, 521f
distal humeral physeal fractures and, 566, 566f
lateral condylar physeal injury and, 546, 547, 548f, 549f
medial condylar physeal injury and, 559, 560f
treatment of
options for, 521–522
osteotomy for, 523–525, 523t, 524f, 525f, 526f
Cuboid fractures, 1039
Curettage
of ABCs, 128
of FD, 141
of UBCs, 4,6,6f, 127–128
Cushing's syndrome, 173
CVS. *See* Covert in-hospital video surveillance

D

Dactylitis, 229
Decorin, 27t, 28, 32
Deep venous thrombosis, 80
Delayed union
of distal tibial fractures, 1009
femoral shaft fractures and, 830, 830f
fibular/tibial fractures and, 957
of lateral condylar physeal injuries, 542–543, 543f
of radial shaft fractures, 396
of ulnar shaft fractures, 396
Diabetes insipidus, 136
Diaphysis, 24, 24f, 25f
Dias-Tachdjian classification, 969, 969t, 970f, 971, 972f
Diazepam, 52, 53t
Diet
deficiencies in, 121t
forearm fracture risk and, 399
Digital block, 63–64, 64f, 230
DIP joint. *See* Distal interphalangeal joint
Distal femoral epiphyseal fractures
associated injuries
ligamentous, 845, 847
peroneal nerve injury, 847
vascular impairment, 847
child abuse and, 843, 843f
classification/diagnosis of
by age, 851, 851f
by displacement, 851
by fracture pattern, 847–851, 847f, 848f, 849f, 850f
imaging for, 847, 851–852, 852t
complications of, 860t
leg-length discrepancy, 861
physeal arrest with progressive angulation, 861
physeal injury, 861
recurrent displacement/late reduction, 860–861
stiffness, 861–862
controversies in, 862
incidence of, 842–843
mechanism of injury
causes of, 843, 843t
compression, 844
ligament disruption and, 845
loading to failure, 843–844, 844f
varus/valgus stress, 843, 844f
signs/symptoms, 845, 845f, 846f
surgical/applied anatomy
bony anatomy, 853, 853f
neurovascular, 853–854
ossification, 852
physeal anatomy, 852–853
soft tissue, 853
treatment of
closed reduction and cast immobilization, 854–855, 855f
closed reduction and percutaneous fixation, 855–856, 856f
displaced fractures, 854–855, 859
external fixation, 857
follow-up imaging and clinical evaluation, 859
nondisplaced fractures, 854, 858–859, 858f
open reduction, 856–857, 857f

pearls/pitfalls for, 859–860, 860t
postreduction management of, 855, 859
principles for, 858
rationale for, 854, 854t
rigid plate fixation, 857
surgery for associated injuries, 857
Distal fibular fractures
classification of, 996
distal tibial fractures and, 1008
epidemiology of, 967
historical background for, 967–968
treatment of, 996–997, 997f, 998f, 1008
Distal humerus fractures, apophyseal
chronic tension stress injuries, 580, 580t, 581f
fractures through epicondylar apophysis
clinical findings, 572
complications of, 576–577, 576t, 577f
differential diagnosis, 573
fragmented apophysis in, 575–576
nonoperative management of, 573, 575f
operative intervention for, 573–575, 574t, 576f
radiographic findings, 572–573
lateral epicondylar apophysis
anatomy for, 577–578, 578f
complications of, 578
incidence of, 577
mechanism of injury, 578, 578f
radiographic findings, 578, 579f
treatment of, 578
medial epicondylar apophysis
avulsion mechanisms, 568–569, 569f
classification of, 570–572, 571f, 571t
elbow dislocation and, 567, 570, 572f
incidence of, 566–567, 567t
mechanism of injury, 568–570, 569f, 569t
ossification sequence and, 567–568, 567f
soft tissue attachments, 568, 568f
surgical anatomy for, 567
olecranon apophysis, 578–580
Distal humerus fractures, diaphyseal
diagnosis/classification of, 668, 668f
incidence of, 667
treatment of
nonoperative, 668, 668f, 669f, 670f
operative, 671–672, 671f, 672f, 673f
Distal humerus fractures, physeal
child abuse and, 565
classification of, 562
clinical signs/symptoms, 562
complications of, 565–566
cubitus varus and, 566, 566f
incidence of, 561
malunion of, 566
mechanism of injury, 562
nonunion of, 565
osteonecrosis in, 566, 566f
radiographic findings, 562–564, 563f, 564f
surgical anatomy for, 561–562, 562f
treatment of, 564–565, 564f, 565f
Distal interphalangeal joint (DIP joint), dislocation of, 281
Distal phalanx fractures
anatomy for, 233, 233f, 234f, 235f
classification of, 234t
complications of, 239–240
diagnosis of, 235–236, 235f, 236f
mechanism of injury, 233
patterns of, 233, 235
postoperative care/rehabilitation, 238
treatment of, 236–238, 236f, 237f, 238f, 239, 241f
Distal radioulnar joint (DRUJ), 293, 294
Distal radius fractures
classification of, 293t
diagnosis/classification of, 2t, 293–294
mechanism of injury, 292–293
physeal injuries, 294
signs/symptoms of, 293
surgical/applied anatomy for, 294
Distal tibial fractures
anatomy for, 980–981, 980f, 981f, 982f
classification/mechanism of injury, 968, 969t
adolescent pilon fractures, 973, 974f
Dias-Tachdjian, 969, 969t, 970f, 971, 972f
incisura fractures, 973, 975f
juvenile Tillaux fractures, 972, 972f, 974f
stress fractures, 974, 977f
syndesmosis fractures, 973, 975f, 976f
transitional fractures, 971–972
triplane fractures, 973, 973f, 976f
complications of
compartment syndrome, 1013
deformity/malunion, 1009–1010
delayed union/nonunion, 1009
osteonecrosis of epiphysis from, 1013
physeal arrest/growth disturbance, 1010–1011, 1012f, 1013f
reflex sympathetic dystrophy/complex regional pain syndrome, 1013
synostosis, 1013
controversies/future directions in, 1013
diagnostic studies of
clinical presentation, 975
CT for, 977, 978f
MRI for, 979, 979f
pitfalls in, 979–980
radiographic evaluation, 975, 977, 977f
epidemiology of, 967
historical background for, 967–968
pearls/pitfalls for
ankle distraction, 1004–1005
arthroscopy, 1006–1007, 1007f
imaging studies, 1005–1006
implants, 1007–1008
partially healed/comminuted physis, 1004
percutaneous clamps, 1007
small c-arm unit, 1007
soft tissue healing problems, 1004
signs/symptoms, 974–975, 977
treatment of
cast immobilization, 982–983, 984, 986, 992, 998
closed reduction, 983
distal fibula fractures and, 1008
incisura fractures, 994
internal fixation, 987, 989, 1001
juvenile Tillaux fractures, 991, 991f, 1002–1003, 1002f, 1003f, 1008f
lateral ankle sprains, 1008–1009
lateral ligament avulsion, 1008–1009
mechanism of injury and, 982, 983
open fractures, 995–996, 999
open reduction, 984–985, 987, 993, 1001, 1003–1004
options for, 981–982, 983t
pilon fractures, 993–994, 994f, 995f
rehabilitation, 1009
Salter-Harris type I/II, 982–986, 988f, 989f, 998–999, 999f, 1000f
Salter-Harris type III/IV, 986–987, 987f, 988f, 989, 990f, 999, 1001, 1002f
Salter-Harris type V, 989–990, 1001–1002, 1001f, 1002f
syndesmosis injuries, 994–995
triplane fractures, 991–993, 992f, 993f, 1003, 1005f, 1006
Disuse osteopenia, 121t
Divergent elbow dislocation
mechanism of injury, 612
radiographic evaluation of, 613f
treatment of, 613
Doris Duke Charitable Foundation, 219
Downs syndrome, 710–711
DPT. *See* Pediatric cocktail
Drug abuse, child abuse and, 193–194
DRUJ. *See* Distal radioulnar joint
Duchenne muscular dystrophy, 181, 182f

E

EG. *See* Eosinophilic granuloma
Ehlers-Danlos syndrome, 158, 216
Elastic stable intramedullary nailing (ESIN), 369–371, 371f, 372f, 373f, 374, 374f, 375f
Elbow dislocation, 413
anterior
complications of, 611
management of, 610
mechanism of injury, 610
postreduction care for, 611
radiographic evaluation, 610, 610f
signs/symptoms, 610
treatment of, 610–611, 611f
classification of, 595
congenital, 610
divergent
mechanism of injury, 612
radiographic evaluation of, 613f
treatment of, 613
incidence of, 594
medial epicondylar apophysis fractures and, 567, 570, 572f
medial/lateral
radiographic evaluation of, 612, 612f
signs/symptoms of, 611
treatment of, 612
posterior
arterial injuries in, 605
associated fractures, 596, 600
closed reduction of, 597–600
complications of, 602–605
cubitus recurvatum and, 605
loss of motion due to, 605
management principles for, 595
mechanism of injury, 595–596, 596f
myositis ossificans and, 605
neurologic injuries in, 603–605
neurovascular injuries in, 597
open dislocations, 600
pearls/pitfalls for, 602
postoperative care for, 600
postreduction care for, 600
puller technique for, 599f, 600–601, 600f
pusher technique for, 600, 602f
radiographic imaging of, 597, 598f, 603f
radioulnar synostosis in, 605
rationale for treatment of, 597
signs/symptoms, 596
soft tissue injury in, 596–597, 597f
surgical treatment, 600
treatment of, 597–601, 599f, 600f, 601f, 602f
proximal radioulnar
associated injuries, 613–614
closed v. open reduction for, 614
mechanism of injury, 613
signs/symptoms, 613
translocation in, 614, 614f
treatment of, 614
pulled elbow syndrome, 614
complications of, 617
imaging of, 616
mechanism of injury, 615, 615f
nonoperative treatment of, 616–617, 616f
signs/symptoms, 615–616
surgical treatment of, 617
recurrent posterior
complications of, 609, 609f
mechanism of injury, 605–606, 607f, 608
posttreatment care for, 609
treatment options for, 608–609, 608f
surgical and applied anatomy, 594–595, 595f

Elbow dislocation (*continued*)
unreduced posterior
diagnosis of, 609
treatment of, 609–610
Elbow injuries
anatomy of
blood supply, 479–480, 480f, 481f
fat pads, 481, 481f, 484, 484f
fusion process, 477–479, 479f
intra-articular structures, 480–481
ligaments, 481
neurovascular structures, 490, 490f
ossification process, 476–477, 476f, 476t, 477f, 478f, 479f
capitellum fractures
associated injuries, 553
classification of, 552–553, 553f
complications of, 554
diagnosis of, 553
mechanism of injury, 553
scope of, 551–552, 552f
treatment of, 553–554, 554f
distal humeral physeal fractures
child abuse and, 565
classification of, 562
clinical signs/symptoms, 562
complications of, 565–566
cubitus varus and, 566, 566f
incidence of, 561
malunion of, 566
mechanism of injury, 562
nonunion of, 565
osteonecrosis in, 566, 566f
radiographic findings, 562–564, 563f, 564f
surgical anatomy for, 561–562, 562f
treatment of, 564–565, 564f, 565f
epidemiology of, 475–476
hyperextension, 487
lateral condylar physeal injury
anatomy/classification of, 534
closed reduction/percutaneous pinning of, 539–540, 541f
complications of, 546–549, 548f
cubitus valgus, 547–549, 548f
cubitus varus, 542, 543f, 546, 547, 548f, 549f
delayed union, 542–543, 543f
displacement stages, 534, 536f
fishtail deformity, 549, 549f
fracture/elbow joint displacement, 535, 537f, 538f
immobilization of, 538, 540–541
incidence/outcome, 534
ipsilateral injuries and, 551, 551f
late displacement of, 538
malunion from, 550
mechanism of injury, 535–537
neurologic complications, 549–550
nonunion, 543–546, 544f, 545f
open reduction/internal fixation, 540, 541–542, 542f
osteonecrosis in, 543, 544f, 550–551, 551f
osteotomy of, 543
physeal arrest and, 550
radiographic findings, 537, 538f, 539f
signs/symptoms, 537
soft tissue injuries, 534–535
spur formation in, 546, 547, 548f
treatment of, 537–542
medial condylar physeal injuries, 554
classification of, 557, 557f
complications of, 558–559, 559f, 560f, 561, 561f
cubitus valgus, 559
cubitus varus and, 559, 560f
diagnosis of, 557–558, 559f
incidence of, 555
mechanism of injury, 556–557, 556f
nonunion from, 559, 560f
surgical anatomy/pathology, 555–556, 555f
treatment of, 558, 558f, 560f
physeal fractures, 533–534
pseudofracture, 483, 483f
radiographic findings
anteroposterior landmarks, 482–483, 482f
comparison radiographs, 485
Jones view, 481, 482f
lateral landmarks, 483–485, 483f, 484f
MRI, 485
other imaging modalities for, 485
standard views, 481
t-condylar fractures
classification of, 584, 587f
complications of, 589
diagnosis of, 584–585
incidence of, 584
mechanism of injury, 584, 585f
patterns of, 584, 586f
treatment of, 585–589, 588f, 589f, 590f
trochlear fractures, 561
osteonecrosis of, 580–581, 582f, 583f
Emergence phenomena, 56–57
Emotional abuse, 192
Enchondromatosis, 121t, 132, 134–135, 135f, 136f, 229
Endochondral ossification, 31–32, 32f
Eosinophilic granuloma (EG), 121t
clinical features of, 135–137
femoral shaft fractures and, 798
hip pain and, 785
radiographic findings in, 137–138
treatment of, 138
Epilepsy, 166
Epinephrine, 29, 64
Epiphysiodesis, completion of, 111
Epiphysis, 19–20, 19f, 20f, 21f
ESIN. *See* Elastic stable intramedullary nailing
Etidocaine, 58
Ewing's sarcoma, 121t, 122t, 138. *See also* Chondrosarcoma
Extension injuries, forearm fractures from
mechanism of, 433–435, 434f, 435f, 436f
treatment of, 438, 438f
External fixation, 86–87
femoral shaft fracture treatment with, 815
complications of, 818
external frame application, 817
fixator design for, 816–817
postoperative care, 817–818
Extra-articular knee injuries, 842
Extremity fractures, 208–209, 209t

F
Famotidine, 49
Fat embolism, 79–80
FCD. *See* Fibrous cortical defects
FD. *See* Fibrous dysplasia
Femoral epiphyseal fractures, distal
associated injuries
ligamentous, 845, 847
peroneal nerve injury, 847
vascular impairment, 847
child abuse and, 843, 843f
classification/diagnosis of
by age, 851, 851f
by displacement, 851
by fracture pattern, 847–851, 847f, 848f, 849f, 850f
imaging for, 847, 851–852, 852t
complications of, 860t
leg-length discrepancy, 861
physeal arrest with progressive angulation, 861
physeal injury, 861
recurrent displacement/late reduction, 860–861
stiffness, 861–862
controversies in, 862
incidence of, 842–843
mechanism of injury
causes of, 843, 843t
compression, 844
ligament disruption and, 845
loading to failure, 843–844, 844f
varus/valgus stress, 843, 844f
signs/symptoms, 845, 845f, 846f
surgical/applied anatomy
bony anatomy, 853, 853f
neurovascular, 853–854
ossification, 852
physeal anatomy, 852–853
soft tissue, 853
treatment of
closed reduction and cast immobilization, 854–855, 855f
closed reduction and percutaneous fixation, 855–856, 856f
displaced fractures, 854–855, 859
external fixation, 857
follow-up imaging and clinical evaluation, 859
nondisplaced fractures, 854, 858–859, 858f
open reduction, 856–857, 857f
pearls/pitfalls for, 859–860, 860t
postreduction management of, 855, 859
principles for, 858
rationale for, 854, 854t
rigid plate fixation, 857
surgery for associated injuries, 857
Femoral fractures. *See also* Distal femoral epiphyseal fractures
child abuse and, 204–205, 204f
compression plating for, 85, 86f
motor vehicle accidents and, 13
stress fractures of
classification of, 785, 786f
complications of, 786
differential diagnosis of, 784–785
incidence of, 783
mechanism of injury, 783
treatment of, 786
Femoral nerve block, 64–65, 64f
Femoral shaft fractures, 74
anatomy for, 798, 798f
classification of, 799, 800f
complications of
angular deformity, 829–830, 829f
compartment syndrome, 832
delayed union, 830, 830f
infection, 831–832
leg-length discrepancy, 827–829
muscle weakness, 831
neurovascular injury, 832
nonunion, 830–831, 831f
rotational deformity, 830
diagnosis of, 798–799
incidence of, 797
mechanism of injury, 798, 799f
metabolic/neuromuscular diseases and, 835, 838
multiple-system trauma and, 838
open, 834–835
osteopenia and, 798
radiographic evaluation, 799
stress fractures, 798
subtrochanteric, 832, 833f, 834f
supracondylar, 832, 834, 834f, 835f, 836f
treatment of
acceptable angulation, 804, 804t
age dependence of, 800, 800t
antegrade transtrochanteric intramedullary nailing, 819, 820f, 821, 821f, 822f, 823, 823f
casting technique for, 805–807, 806f, 807f
children 5–11 years of age, 802, 827, 928f

children 12 and up, 802–803
complications of casting, 809, 809f, 810f
complications of external fixation, 818
complications of flexible intramedullary nailing, 815
compression plating, 824
early spica casting, 804–805
external fixation, 815
external frame application, 817
fixator design for, 816–817
flexible intramedullary nail fixation, 809–811, 811f
infants, 800–801, 827
nail fixation technique for, 811–813, 812f, 813f, 814f, 815
outcomes, 808–809, 819t
Pharness for, 803–804
plate fixation, 823, 824
postoperative care, 808, 815, 817–818
preoperative planning for, 811
preschool children, 801–802, 801f, 802f, 827
rigid intramedullary rod fixation, 818–819
submuscular bridge plating, 824–827
tibial pin, 807–808, 808f
traction and casting, 807
Fentanyl citrate, 47, 54, 55t, 58
FGF. *See* Fibroblast growth factor
Fibroblast growth factor (FGF), 29, 30, 31, 34
Fibroma, nonossifying, 121t
Fibromodulin, 27t, 28, 32
Fibrous cortical defects (FCD)
clinical features of, 129
natural history of, 130
operative treatment of, 130–131
Fibrous dysplasia (FD), 121t, 122t. *See also* McCune-Albright syndrome
clinical presentation of, 141
radiographic appearance of, 141, 142f
treatment of, 141–143
Fibular fractures, distal
classification of, 996
distal tibial fractures and, 1008
epidemiology of, 967
historical background for, 967–968
treatment of, 996–997, 997f, 998f, 1008
Fibular shaft fractures
classification of, 931
diaphyseal
angular deformity from, 955–956, 956f
cast immobilization of, 941, 942–943
cast wedging of, 943, 944f
compartment syndrome in, 954–955
complications of, 943–944, 954–957
delayed union/nonunion in, 957
incidence of, 936
leg-length discrepancy due to, 956–957
malrotation in, 956
mechanism of injury, 939
operative treatment of, 943–944
radiographic evaluation of, 939–940, 939f, 940f, 941f
signs/symptoms of, 939
tibial shaft fractures and, 936, 939
treatment of, 941, 942–944
vascular injuries in, 955
epidemiology of, 930–931
stress fractures, 961, 962f, 963–964, 963f
surgical anatomy for
bony structure, 931
fascial compartments, 932–933, 932f
muscle origins/insertions on, 931, 931t
nerves, 932
vascular anatomy, 931, 932f
Finger fractures, anesthesia for, 230
Firearm injuries, 14–15
Flexible intramedullary nail fixation. *See also* Elastic stable intramedullary nailing
complications of, 815
femoral shaft treatment with, 809–813, 815
outcomes of, 810–811
postoperative management for, 815
preoperative planning for, 811
retrograde insertion of, 812–813, 815
rod bending for, 811–812
Flexion injuries
forearm fractures from, mechanism of, 433, 434f
supracondylar fractures
etiology/pathology of, 526, 526f
radiographic findings, 527, 527f
treatment of, 527–529, 528f, 529f
Floating knee injury, 86, 86f
femoral shaft fractures and, 838, 838f, 959
tibial fractures and, 959
Fluid replacement, 73–74
Flumazenil, 53, 55
Follicle-stimulating hormone, 29
Foot fractures/dislocations
anatomy for, 1018, 1018f, 1019f
compartment syndrome in, 1052–1053, 1053f
history/evaluation for, 1018–1019
lawn mower/mutilating injuries, 1051–1052, 1052f
puncture wounds, 1053–1054, 1054f
stress fractures, 1054–1055
trauma to, 1018
Forearm fasciotomy, 513–514, 514f
Forearm fractures
casting technique for, 365, 366f
classification of, 293t
comminuted, 368
complete, 367–368
displaced, 365
distal
associated injuries, 293
diagnosis/classification of, 293–294, 293t
mechanism of injury, 292–293
signs/symptoms of, 293
surgical/applied anatomy for, 294
in-line skating and, 399
intramedullary fixation of, 85
physeal injuries, 294
radial/ulnar shaft
angulation limits for, 378
associated injuries, 353–354
closed treatment of, 365–368
complications of, 381, 383–384, 387–388, 396–399
diagnosis and classification of, 354–355, 355f
epidemiology of, 350, 352f, 399
intramedullary fixation of, 369
intramedullary nailing, 369–371, 371f, 372f, 373f, 374, 374f, 375f
mechanism of injury, 350, 352, 352f, 353f
plate fixation of, 369, 370f
reduction of, 348, 364, 377–378
signs/symptoms, 352–353
surgical treatment of, 369–371, 374, 376–378, 380–381
treatment rationale for, 355–356, 356f, 357f, 358–360, 358f, 359t
range of motion losses from, 356, 356f, 359t
remodeling of, 359–360
risk factors for, 399
rotational malalignment from, 358
surgical/applied anatomy for
bony anatomy/static restraints, 360–361, 362f
muscle/nerve anatomy, 361, 363, 363f, 363t
surgical approaches, 364–365, 364f, 365f
Forearm malunion, 356, 356f, 357f
radial/ulnar fractures, 385, 387–388, 396
Fractures. *See also specific types and sites*
bicycle injuries and, 12
bone density and, 15
causes of, 11–15
comminuted, forearm, 368
complete, forearm, 368
dating of, 205–206
epidemiology of, 5–11
age patterns in, 9
classification bias in, 5
frequency of, 6–9, 6t, 7f, 8f, 9f, 10f, 10t, 11t
gender patterns in, 7
incidence, 6, 9–11, 14f
multiple, 10–11, 11t
physeal injuries, 9–10
socioclinical factors, 5
etiology of, 11–15, 14f, 14t
gunshot/firearm injuries, 15
healing mechanisms for, 36f
future methods for, 40
growth stimulation and, 40
inflammatory phase, 35–36
osseous, 35, 39f, 40f
phases of, 35, 36f
physeal patterns of, 38–40
remodeling phase, 37
reparative phase, 36–37
healing rates of, head injuries and, 79
home environment and, 11
incidence of, 72
in-line skating and, 399
intrinsic causes of, 15
management of, changes in philosophy of, 74–75
motor vehicle accidents and, 13–14
multiple
child abuse and, 72
epidemiology of, 10–11, 11t
external fixation for, 86–87
incidence of, 71–72
mechanisms of injury in, 72–73
operative fixation for, 84–86
outcomes of, 87
nutrition and, 15
open
epidemiology of, 10, 11t
management of, 81–84, 374, 376, 376f, 377f
operative intervention for, 74
play/recreational activities and, 12–13
premature infants and, 15
preventive programs for, 15–16, 399
risk factors for, 399
school environment and, 11–12
stabilizing
benefits of, 84
external fixation for, 86–87
open, 83
operative fixation for, 84–86
timing of, 84
Frostbite, 229

G
Gallie technique, 708–709, 709f
Gamekeeper's thumb. *See* Thumb metacarpophalangeal ulnar collateral ligament injury
Gaucher's disease, 148, 150
GCS. *See* Glasgow Coma Scale
Gene therapy, 41, 160
Genital injuries, child abuse and, 203–204
Genitourinary injuries, 79
Gentamicin, 82, 156t
GH. *See* Growth hormone
Giant cell tumor, 121t, 133t
Gla protein, 27t, 28
Glasgow Coma Scale (GCS), 74, 76t, 77

Glenohumeral subluxation/dislocation, 634
associated injuries, 637
atraumatic dislocations
mechanism of injury, 635, 636f
signs/symptoms, 636–637, 637f, 638f
classification of, 638–640, 641f
complications of, 644
diagnosis of, 638, 638f, 639f, 640f
signs/symptoms, 635–637, 637f, 638f
surgical/applied anatomy, 640, 641f, 642
traumatic dislocations
mechanism of injury, 635
recurrence rate of, 643
reduction of, 643
signs/symptoms, 635–636, 637f
treatment of
acute dislocation, 642, 642f
atraumatic instability, 643
determining traumatic v. atraumatic, 643
options for, 642t
recurrent dislocation, 642–643
rehabilitation after, 644
traumatic instability, 642
Glycopyrrolate, 57
Goldenhar syndrome, 710
Great toe fractures, 1049, 1051
Growth factors, 32f
cartilage/bone matrix and, 28–31
fracture therapy with, 40–41
Growth hormone (GH), 32f, 33
The Growth Plate and Its Disorders (Rang), 349
Growth plate cartilage regeneration, 41–42
Growth stimulation, 40
Gunshot injuries, 14
complications of, 15
etiology of, 15
prevention of, 15
Gunstock deformity. *See* Cubitus varus

H

Haemophilius influenza, 156t
Halo device, 694–696, 694f, 696f
Hamate fractures, 279
Hand anatomy
collateral ligaments, 227
epiphyses, 227, 227f
osseous, 226
periosteum, 227
physeal, 226–227
secondary ossification centers, 226, 226f
soft tissue, 227
tendons, 227
volar plate, 227
Hand and carpus dislocations
distal interphalangeal joint, 281
metacarpophalangeal
dorsal finger dislocation, 282–284, 284f, 285f
thumb ray, 284, 285f, 286f
proximal interphalangeal joint, 281–282, 281f
Hand injuries
carpal fractures
anatomy for, 268–269, 269f
epidemiology of, 267–268
congenital, 229
distal phalanx fractures
anatomy for, 233, 233f, 234f, 235f
classification of, 234t
complications of, 239–240
diagnosis of, 235–236, 235f, 236f
mechanism of injury, 233
patterns of, 233, 235
postoperative care/rehabilitation, 238
treatment of, 236–238, 236f, 237f, 238f, 239, 241f
epidemiology of
biphasic distribution, 225–226
incidence, 225–226, 226t
evaluation of
clinical examination, 228–229
differential diagnosis, 229
radiographic examination, 229, 230f
inflammatory/infectious, 229
management of
anesthesia for, 230
complications, 232–233
nonoperative, 229–232
rehabilitation, 232
surgical, 232
metacarpal fractures
anatomy for, 255
classification of, 256t
complications of, 262, 262t, 263f
diagnosis of, 256f, 257, 257f
mechanism of injury, 255
patterns of, 256–257
postoperative care/rehabilitation for, 261–262
treatment of, 257–261, 258f, 259f, 260f, 261f
osteochondrosis, 229
proximal/middle phalanx fractures, 287f, 288f
anatomy for, 240
classification of, 241t
complications of, 253–255, 254f, 255f
diagnosis of, 242, 242f, 243f, 244f, 245f, 246f, 251f
mechanism of injury, 240
patterns of, 240–242
postoperative care/rehabilitation for, 252–253
prognosis for, 253
treatment of, 242–243, 245, 246f, 247f, 248, 248f, 249f, 250–252, 250f, 252f, 253f
remodeling in, 227
thermal, 229
thumb metacarpal fractures
anatomy for, 262
classification of, 263f, 263t
complications of, 267–268
diagnosis of, 262, 264, 264f, 265f
mechanism of injury, 262
patterns of, 262
postoperative care/rehabilitation for, 267
prognosis for, 267, 268f
treatment of, 264–265, 265f, 266f, 267, 267f
tumors, 229
Hand-Schuller-Christian disease, 136
Hangman's fracture, 713–714, 714f
HCUP. *See* Healthcare Cost and Utilization Project
Head injuries, 49
delayed diagnosis of, 74–75
etiologies of, 199, 200t
fracture healing rates and, 79
incidence of, 744
intracranial pressure and, 78
pelvic fractures and, 744
prognosis for, 77–78
secondary orthopaedic effects of, 78–79
Healthcare Cost and Utilization Project (HCUP), 5, 6
Heart rate, normal values for, 48, 48t
Hemarthrosis, 771
Hematoma
formation of, 35–36
organization of, 36
Hematoma block, 52, 55, 62, 62f, 365
Hemifacial microsomy, 710
Hemodynamic status, sedation and, 49
Hemophilia
clinical features of, 151–152
severity of, 152t
surgery in, 152–153
treatment of, 153
Heterotopic bone formation, 78–79
Hip dislocations
associated injuries, 788, 788f
classification of, 789, 790f
complications of
avascular necrosis, 793, 793f
chondrolysis, 793–794
coxa magna, 794
habitual/recurrent dislocation, 794
heterotopic ossification, 794
late presentation, 794
soft tissue injury, 794
diagnosis of, 788–789, 789f
incidence of, 786
mechanism of injury, 786–787, 786f, 787f
signs/symptoms, 788
surgical/applied anatomy, 789
treatment of
closed reduction, 791
pearls/pitfalls for, 792–793, 792f
surgical procedures, 791–792
Hip fractures
associated injuries, 770
classification of, 771–773, 771f, 772f
complications of, 769
avascular necrosis, 780–782, 781f
chondrolysis, 782
coxa vara, 782
infection, 782
nonunion, 782
premature physeal closure, 782
slipped capital femoral epiphysis, 782–783
diagnosis of, 770–771
incidence of, 769
management rationale for, 770
mechanism of injury, 769–770
signs/symptoms of, 770
stress fractures, 773
classification of, 785, 786f
complications of, 786
incidence of, 783
mechanism of injury, 783–785
treatment of, 786
surgical/applied anatomy for
ossification, 773, 774f
preferred approaches, 775, 776f, 777f
soft tissue anatomy, 774–775
vascular anatomy, 774, 774f, 775f
treatment of
child's age and, 775
closed reduction, 779
displaced cervicotrochanteric fractures, 778
immobilization, 776, 779
internal fixation, 777–779
intertrochanteric fractures, 778
nondisplaced/minimally displaced, 778
pearls/pitfalls for, 779, 780t
physeal penetration in, 778
postoperative care for, 779
stabilization, 776
unusual patterns of, 773
Histamine-2-receptor blockers, 49
Histiocytosis, Langerhans cell, 122t
Home environment, fractures sustained in, 11
Hormones, 29, 32f
Humeral fractures. *See also* Supracondylar humeral fractures
apophyseal chronic tension stress injuries, 580, 580t, 581f
diaphyseal
diagnosis/classification of, 668, 668f
incidence of, 667
treatment of
nonoperative, 668, 668f, 669f, 670f
operative, 671–672, 671f, 672f, 673f
through epicondylar apophysis
clinical findings, 572
complications of, 576–577, 576t, 577f

differential diagnosis, 573
fragmented apophysis in, 575–576
nonoperative management of, 573, 575f
operative intervention for, 573–575, 574t, 576f
radiographic findings, 572–573
glenohumeral subluxation/dislocation, 634
associated injuries, 637
atraumatic dislocations, 635–637, 636f, 637f, 638f
classification of, 638–640, 641f
complications of, 644
diagnosis of, 638, 638f, 639f, 640f
signs/symptoms, 635–637, 637f, 638f
surgical/applied anatomy, 640, 641f, 642
traumatic dislocations, 635–636, 637f, 643
treatment of, 642–644, 642f, 642t
lateral epicondylar apophysis
anatomy for, 577–578, 578f
complications of, 578
incidence of, 577
mechanism of injury, 578, 578f
radiographic findings, 578, 579f
treatment of, 578
medial epicondylar apophysis
avulsion mechanisms, 568–569, 569f
classification of, 570–572, 571f, 571t
elbow dislocation and, 567, 570, 572f
incidence of, 566–567, 567t
mechanism of injury, 568–570, 569f, 569t
ossification sequence and, 567–568, 567f
soft tissue attachments, 568, 568f
surgical anatomy for, 567
nonaccidental trauma and, 205, 205f
olecranon apophysis, 578–580
physeal
child abuse and, 565
classification of, 562
clinical signs/symptoms, 562
complications of, 565–566
cubitus varus and, 566, 566f
incidence of, 561
malunion of, 566
mechanism of injury, 562
nonunion of, 565
osteonecrosis in, 566, 566f
radiographic findings, 562–564, 563f, 564f
surgical anatomy for, 561–562, 562f
treatment of, 564–565, 564f, 565f
proximal
associated injuries, 646
classification of, 647, 647f
complications of, 654–655
diagnosis of, 646–647, 646f
incidence of, 644
mechanism of injury, 644–645, 645f, 646f
signs/symptoms, 645–646
surgical/applied anatomy, 647–649, 648f, 649f
treatment of, 649–654, 650t, 651f, 652f, 653f, 654f, 656t
Humeral shaft fractures
birth injuries, 656
child abuse and, 656, 798
compartment syndrome and, 667
complications of, 667
diagnosis/classification of, 657
mechanism of injury, 656
radial nerve palsies with, 665–666, 665f, 667
signs/symptoms of, 656–657, 657f
surgical/applied anatomy for
embryology/development, 657
muscles, 658
nerves, 658
osseous, 657–658
treatment of
acceptable alignment in, 660–661, 660f, 661f
birth injuries, 658–659, 659f
nonoperative, 661, 662f, 663, 663f
operative, 663–664, 664f, 665f
operative v. conservative, 664–665
options for, 658t
pros/cons of, 658t
rehabilitation from, 666
stress fractures, 659–660
Hydrocodone, 66t
Hydromorphone, 66t
Hyperextension, supracondylar humeral fracture and, 520, 522f
Hyperparathyroidism
congenital primary, 172, 172f
primary, 171–173, 172f
treatment of, 173
Hyperthyroidism, 141
Hypophosphatasia, 158, 213, 213f
Hypovolemic shock, 74

I
Iatrogenic osteoporosis
cancer treatment and, 170–171
immobilization, 171
Ibuprofen, 53, 67t
Idiopathic osteoporosis
clinical features of, 170, 171f
treatment of, 170
Ifosfamide, 166
IGF. *See* Insulin-like growth factors
IHT. *See* Inflicted head trauma
Iliac wing fractures
displacement in, 750
incidence of, 749
treatment of, 750, 750f
Iliotibial friction band syndrome, 905
Immobilization osteoporosis, 171
Infantile Blount disease, 110, 110f, 110t, 115, 117
Infantile cortical hyperostosis, 213
Infection
femoral shaft fractures and, 831–832
forearm shaft fractures and, 397
hip fractures and, 771, 782
hip pain from, 785
humeral shaft fracture and, 667
of pin track, supracondylar humeral fractures and, 516
Inflammatory phase, 35–36
Inflicted head trauma (IHT), 199
Inflicted traumatic brain injury (ITBI), 199
Injury Severity Score (ISS), 74, 75t. *See also* Modified Injury Severity Score
In-line skates, 12–13, 399
Insufficiency fracture, 213
Insulin, 194
Insulin-like growth factors (IGF), 29, 30, 32–33, 32f
Intracranial pressure, 78
Intramedullary rod fixation, 74, 85
antegrade transtrochanteric intramedullary nailing
complications of, 821, 823, 823f
postoperative management, 821
technique for, 819, 820f, 821, 821f, 822f
femoral shaft fracture treatment with, 818–819
osteogenesis imperfecta and, 160
radial/ulnar shaft fractures, 369
Ipsilateral injuries, lateral condylar physeal injuries and, 551, 551f
Ischium fractures
clinical presentation of, 750–751
fractures near of subluxation of sacroiliac joint, 752–753, 753f
fractures near of subluxation of symphysis pubis, 752, 752f
incidence of, 750
ipsilateral rami, 751
ischium body, 751, 751f
stress fractures, 751–752, 752f
ISS. *See* Injury Severity Score
ITBI. *See* Inflicted traumatic brain injury
IV regional block, 61, 62. *See also* Bier block

J
Jersey finger, 239
Joint effusion, 229
Jones, Robert, 475
Juvenile rheumatoid arthritis, 229
Juvenile Tillaux fractures, 972, 972f, 974f

K
Ketamine hydrochloride, 47, 56–57, 56t, 58, 377
Ketofol, 58
Ketorolac, 60, 67, 67t
KID. *See* Kids' Inpatient Database
"Kids Can't Fly," 16
Kids' Inpatient Database (KID), 5, 6–7, 13
Kinky hair syndrome, 213
Kirner deformity, 229, 231f
Kirschner wires, 85
Klippel-Feil syndrome, 710
Knee, ligament injuries of
classification of, 913–915, 914f, 915f
complications of, 925–926
imaging of, 913
incidence of, 911
mechanism of injury, 911–912
prognosis for, 925
signs/symptoms, 912–913
surgical/applied anatomy for, 915–916
treatment of
ACL, 916–919, 918f, 919f, 920f, 921–922, 921t, 922f, 923f
controversies in, 916
knee dislocation, 923–924, 924f
LCL, 922
PCL, 923
pearls/pitfalls for, 924–925
Knee, meniscal injuries to
ACL injuries and, 910
adult v. children's patterns of, 904
classification of, 905–906, 906f
complications of, 911
defining, 904
differential diagnosis of, 905
imaging of, 905
incidence of, 904–905
mechanism of injury, 905
prognosis for, 910–911
signs/symptoms, 905
surgical/applied anatomy
blood supply, 906
composition of, 906–907
functional importance of menisci, 907
lateral meniscus, 906
medial meniscus, 906
treatment of
algorithm for, 909
discoid lateral meniscus, 907–908
nonoperative, 907
pearls/pitfalls for, 910
surgical, 907
technique for, 908–910, 909f, 910f, 911f
Knee, osteochondral fractures
classification of, 896, 897t
complications of, 899–900
imaging of, 896, 897f
incidence of, 895
locations of, 895, 895f
mechanism of injury, 895–896, 896f
meniscal injury v., 905
prognosis, 898–899
signs/symptoms, 896

Knee, osteochondral fractures (*continued*)
surgical/applied anatomy, 896–897
treatment of
algorithm for, 898f
options for, 897–898
pearls/pitfalls for, 898
technique for, 898, 899f, 900f, 901f
Knee, patellar dislocation
classification of, 902
imaging of, 901, 902f
incidence of, 900
mechanism of injury, 900
meniscal injury v., 905
signs/symptoms, 900–901
surgical/applied anatomy, 902, 902f
treatment of
chronic subluxation/dislocation, 903, 903f, 904f
pearls/pitfalls for, 903–904
prognosis/complications, 904
reduction, 902–903
surgical intervention, 903
Knee, patellar fractures
classification of
for management, 878
by mechanism of injury, 878–880
complications of, 883
diagnosis of, 877–878
incidence of, 876
mechanism of injury, 876, 877f
signs/symptoms
associated injuries, 877
clinical findings, 876–877
radiographic findings, 877, 878f, 879f
sleeve fracture, 876, 876f
surgical/applied anatomy, 880, 880f
treatment of
operative repair, 880–883, 881f, 882f
pearls/pitfalls for, 883
postoperative/postfracture care, 883
rationale for, 880
Knee injuries
degenerative changes, 869–870
dislocation, 923–924, 924f
floating, 86, 86f
femoral shaft fractures and, 838, 838f
tibial fractures and, 959
instability, 869–870
motor vehicle accidents and, 13
MRI evaluation of, 77
Kniest syndrome, 710
Kohler's disease, 1038, 1038f

L

Langerhans cell histiocytosis, 122t. *See also* Eosinophilic granuloma; Hand-Schuller-Christian disease; Letterer-Siwe disease
clinical features of, 135–137
radiographic findings in, 137–138
treatment of, 138
Lateral ankle sprains, 997
treatment of, 1008–1009
Lateral collateral ligament (LCL)
injury to
classification of, 914, 915f
imaging of, 913
mechanism of, 912
signs/symptoms of, 912–913
surgical/applied anatomy for, 915–916
treatment of, 922
knee dislocation and, 923–924, 924f
tibial spine fractures and, 887
Lateral/medial elbow dislocation
radiographic evaluation of, 612, 612f
signs/symptoms of, 611
treatment of, 612
Latex allergy, 180
Lawn mower injuries, 995–996, 996f
incidence of, 1051
treatment of, 1051–1052, 1052f
LCL. *See* Lateral collateral ligament
Legal reporting requirements, child abuse and, 217–219
Legg-Calvé-Perthes disease, 785
Leg-length discrepancy
diaphyseal fibular shaft fractures and, 956–957
diaphyseal tibial shaft fractures and, 956–957
distal femoral epiphyseal fractures and, 861
femoral shaft fractures and, 827–829
proximal tibial epiphyseal fractures and, 869
Letterer-Siwe disease, 136
Leukemia, 121t, 122t, 151, 152f, 213–214, 214f
Lidocaine, 58, 60, 60t, 61, 62–63, 64
Ligament injuries
classification of, 913–915, 914f, 915f
complications of, 925–926
imaging of, 913
incidence of, 911
mechanism of injury, 911–912
prognosis for, 925
signs/symptoms, 912–913
surgical/applied anatomy for, 915–916
treatment of
ACL, 916–919, 918f, 919f, 920f, 921–922, 921f, 922f, 923f
controversies in, 916
knee dislocation, 923–924, 924f
LCL, 922
PCL, 923
pearls/pitfalls for, 924–925
Ligamentous injuries
carpal fractures and, 279–280
distal femoral epiphyseal fractures and, 845, 847
distal tibial fractures and, 1008–1009
proximal tibial epiphyseal fractures and, 862
subaxial disruptions, 714–715
thumb metacarpophalangeal ulnar collateral (Gamekeeper's thumb), 284–287, 286f
Limb-length discrepancy
diaphyseal fibular shaft fractures and, 956–957
diaphyseal tibial shaft fractures and, 956–957
distal femoral epiphyseal fractures and, 861
femoral shaft fractures and, 827–829
proximal tibial epiphyseal fractures and, 869
Limb lengthening
methods of, 156
pathologic fractures after, 156–157, 157f, 158f
Linfranc injury. *See* Tarsometatarsal injuries
Little League pathology, 414, 415f, 580, 580t, 581f
Load-sharing devices, 160
Local anesthesia
agents for, 58–59
postoperative analgesia with, 65t, 66t, 67–68, 67t
recommended doses for, 59, 60t
toxicity from, 59, 59t
Locking plating, 85
Lunate fractures, 279
Lymphoma, 121t

M

Magnetic resonance angiography (MRA), 692
Magnetic resonance imaging (MRI), 74
of cervical spine injuries, 692, 693f
of distal femoral epiphyseal fractures, 862
elbow evaluation with, 485
of femoral shaft fractures, 799
of foot stress fractures, 1054
of hip fractures, 770
of ligamentous injuries, 913
of meniscal injuries, 905
multiple fracture evaluation with, 77
of osteochondral fractures, 896
of pelvic injuries, 745
of penetrating food injuries, 1053, 1054f
of thoracolumbar spinal fractures, 725, 728–729
of tibial spine fracture, 887
Malignant bone tumors, 138–141, 139f, 140f. *See also* Ewing's sarcoma; Osteogenic sarcoma
Malunion
of distal tibial fractures, 1009–1010
humeral shaft fracture and, 667
lateral condylar physeal injury and, 550
radial head injuries and, 427
of tibial spine fractures, 894, 895
Mangled Extremity Severity Score (MESS), 84, 1052
Marfan's syndrome, 158
Marrow diseases, 121t
Gaucher's disease, 148, 150
hemophilia
clinical features of, 151–152
severity of, 152t
surgery in, 152–153
treatment of, 153
leukemia, 151, 152f
osteomyelitis, 121t, 122t
classification of, 153t, 154f, 154t
clinical features of, 153–154
radiographic evaluation of, 154–155, 155f
treatment of, 155–156, 156f, 156t
sickle cell disease, 150–151, 150f, 229
McCune-Albright syndrome, 141
MCL. *See* Medial collateral ligament
MCP joint. *See* Metacarpophalangeal joint
MDCT. *See* Multidetector computed tomography
Medial collateral ligament (MCL), 845
injury to
classification of, 914, 914f
imaging of, 913
mechanism of, 912
signs/symptoms of, 912, 912f
surgical/applied anatomy for, 915–916
treatment of, 916–917
knee dislocation and, 924
tibial spine fractures and, 887
Medial column, comminution of, 502, 508
Medial/lateral elbow dislocation
radiographic evaluation of, 612, 612f
signs/symptoms of, 611
treatment of, 612
Membranous ossification, 34, 39f, 40f
Meniscal injuries
ACL injuries and, 910
adult v. children's patterns of, 904
classification of, 905–906, 906f
complications of, 911
defining, 904
differential diagnosis of, 905
imaging of, 905
incidence of, 904–905
mechanism of injury, 905
prognosis for, 910–911
signs/symptoms, 905
surgical/applied anatomy
blood supply, 906
composition of, 906–907
functional importance of menisci, 907
lateral meniscus, 906
medial meniscus, 906
treatment of
algorithm for, 909
discoid lateral meniscus, 907–908
nonoperative, 907
pearls/pitfalls for, 910

surgical, 907
technique for, 908–910, 909f, 910f, 911f
Meperidine, 50, 54, 55, 55t, 65, 65t, 66t
Mepivacaine, 58, 60t
MESS. *See* Mangled Extremity Severity Score
Metacarpal fractures
anatomy for, 255
classification of, 256t
complications of, 262, 262t, 263f
diagnosis of, 256f, 257, 257f
mechanism of injury, 255
patterns of, 256–257
postoperative care/rehabilitation for, 261–262
thumb
anatomy for, 262
classification of, 263f, 263t
complications of, 267–268
diagnosis of, 262, 264, 264f, 265f
mechanism of injury, 262
patterns of, 262
postoperative care/rehabilitation for, 267
prognosis for, 267, 268f
treatment of, 264–265, 265f, 266f, 267, 267f
treatment of, 257–261, 258f, 259f, 260f, 261f
Metacarpophalangeal dislocations, dorsal finger, 282–284, 284f, 285f
Metacarpophalangeal joint (MCP joint), 231
Metacarpophalangeal joint dislocation
dorsal finger dislocation, 282–284, 284f, 285f
neglected, 284
thumb ray, 284, 285f, 286f
Metaphysis, 21–24, 22f, 23f
Metastatic bone tumors, 138–141, 139f, 140f
Metastatic neuroblastoma, 213
Metatarsal fractures
associated injuries, 1044–1045
classification of, 1045
fifth metatarsal
classification of, 1046–1047, 1047f
complications of, 1049
incidence of, 1045
surgical anatomy for, 1045–1046, 1045f, 1046f
treatment of, 1047–1049, 1047f, 1048f
imaging evaluation of, 1045
incidence of, 1044
mechanisms of injury, 1044
nonaccidental trauma and, 205, 205f
signs/symptoms, 1044
treatment of, 1045
Metoclopramide, 49
Midazolam, 47, 52–53, 53t, 55, 58, 377
Middle phalanx fractures, 287f, 288f
anatomy for, 240
classification of, 241t
complications of, 253–255, 254f, 255f
diagnosis of, 242, 242f, 243f, 244f, 245f, 246f, 251f
mechanism of injury, 240
patterns of, 240–242
postoperative care/rehabilitation for, 252–253
prognosis for, 253
treatment of, 242–243, 245, 246f, 247f, 248, 248f, 249f, 250–252, 250f, 252f, 253f
Midtarsal injuries
associated injuries, 1038–1039
classification of, 1038
incidence of, 1038
MISS. *See* Modified Injury Severity Score
Modified Injury Severity Score (MISS), 80
Monteggia, Giovanni Batista, 446
Monteggia fracture-dislocations, 446
anatomy/biomechanics for
bones/joints, 449, 451f
ligaments, 448–449, 450f, 451f
muscles, 449–450
nerves, 450, 452f
associated fractures and unusual lesions, 472–473
chronic fracture-dislocations
late presentation of, 467, 467f
osteotomy for, 469–470, 469f
postoperative care, 472
surgical approach for, 470, 471f, 472
surgical reconstruction of, 468–470, 468f, 469f, 471f, 472
treatment indications for, 468
classification of
author's classification of, 448, 450t
Bado classification, 447, 447f
Letts classification, 448, 450f
Monteggia equivalent lesions, 447–448, 448f, 449f
Monteggia equivalent lesions
clinical findings, 466
mechanism of injury, 467
radiographic evaluation, 467
treatment of, 467
nerve injuries in, 472
periarticular ossification and, 472–473
type I
clinical findings, 450–451
closed reduction/cast immobilization of, 456, 456f, 457f, 458f
mechanism of injury, 452–454, 455f
operative treatment of, 456, 458–459, 459f, 460f
radiographic evaluation, 451–452, 452f, 453f
type II
clinical findings, 459
incidence of, 459
mechanism of injury, 460–461, 461f
radiographic evaluation, 459–460, 460f
treatment of, 461–462, 461f
type III
clinical findings, 462
incidence, 462
mechanism of injury, 462, 462f
radiographic evaluation, 462
treatment of, 462–464, 463f, 464f, 465f
type IV
clinical findings, 464
mechanism of injury, 464
postoperative care for, 466
radiographic evaluation, 464, 465f, 466f
treatment of, 464, 466, 466f
Morphine, 54, 55, 55t, 65, 65t, 66t, 67
Motor vehicle accidents (MVA), 13–14, 72–73, 744
MRA. *See* Magnetic resonance angiography
MRI. *See* Magnetic resonance imaging
Multidetector computed tomography (MDCT), 485
Multiple fractures
child abuse and, 72, 205, 206f
epidemiology of, 10–11, 11t
evaluation of
imaging studies for, 75–77, 77f
physical assessment for, 74–75
trauma rating systems for, 74, 75t, 76t
femoral shaft fractures and, 838
head injury evaluation and, 74–75
incidence of, 71–72
initial resuscitation and evaluation for, 73–74
mechanisms of injury in, 72–73
nonorthopaedic conditions and, 77–80
nutrition requirements and, 80
outcomes for, 87
pediatric trauma center's role in, 73
stabilization of
external fixation for, 86–87
operative fixation for, 84–86
Münchhausen syndrome by proxy, 194
Muscle/tendon entrapment, 397–398
Muscular dystrophy. *See also* Duchenne muscular dystrophy
fractures in, 181, 182f
Mutilating injuries, 1051–1052, 1052f. *See also* Lawn mower injuries
MVA. *See* Motor vehicle accidents
Myelodysplasia, 961f
Myelomeningocele, 960
fractures in
diagnosis of, 179
predisposing factors for, 177–178
preventive measures for, 178–179
treatment of, 180–181
osteopenia and, 798
Myositis ossificans, 426
posterior elbow dislocation and, 605
supracondylar humeral fracture and, 516, 516f

N

NAI. *See* Nonaccidental injury
Nail bed, repair of, 236
Nalbuphine, 54, 55t
Naloxone, 54–55
Naproxen, 67t
NAT. *See* Nonaccidental trauma
National Child Abuse and Neglect Data System (NCANDS), 192–193
National Electronic Injury Surveillance system (NEISS), 12
National Pediatric Trauma Registry (NPTR), 5
Nationwide Inpatient Sample (NIS), 5
NCANDS. *See* National Child Abuse and Neglect Data System
Neglect, 192, 193
NEISS. *See* National Electronic Injury Surveillance system
Neurapraxia, 397
Neuroblastoma, 121t, 122t, 213
Neurofibromatosis (NF), 121t
clinical presentation of, 143–144
radiographic findings in, 144–145
treatment of, 145–147, 146f, 147f
Neuroleptics, 47
Neurologic deficits, cervical spine injuries and, 686
Neurologic injury
elbow dislocation and, 603–605
lateral condylar physeal injury and, 549–550
supracondylar humeral fracture and, 514–515
NF. *See* Neurofibromatosis
NIS. *See* Nationwide Inpatient Sample
Nitrous oxide, 46, 51–52
NOF. *See* Nonossifying fibroma
Nonaccidental injury (NAI), 192, 217–219
Nonaccidental trauma (NAT), 6–7, 11, 192, 204f
humerus shaft fractures and, 205, 205t
legal responsibilities in, 217–219
metatarsal fractures and, 205, 205f
Nonossifying fibroma (NOF), 121t
clinical features of, 129
femoral shaft fractures and, 798
natural history of, 130
operative treatment of, 130–131
Nonsteroidal anti-inflammatory drug (NSAID), 60
postoperative analgesia with, 67, 67t
Nonunion, 396
distal humeral physeal fractures and, 565
femoral shaft fractures and, 830–831, 831f
fibular/tibial fractures and, 957
of hip fractures, 782
of humeral shaft fracture, 667
of lateral condylar physeal injuries, 543–546, 544f, 545f
medial condylar physeal injury and, 559, 560f
of proximal ulnar fractures, 440

Nonunion (*continued*)
of radial neck, 425
supracondylar humeral fracture and, 517
of tibial spine fractures, 895
NPTR. *See* National Pediatric Trauma Registry
NSAID. *See* Nonsteroidal anti-inflammatory drug
Nursemaid's elbow, 595. *See also* Pulled elbow syndrome
Nutritional requirements
deficiencies in, 121t
copper, 174–175
scurvy, 173–174, 174f
polytrauma and, 80
Nutritional rickets, 166

O
Obesity, 399
Occipital condylar fracture, 697, 698t
OD. *See* Osteofibrous dysplasia
Odontoideum, 710
OI. *See* Osteogenesis imperfecta
Ollier's disease, 121t
Open fractures
amputation of, 84
ankle fractures, 995–996, 996f
classification of, 81, 81t
epidemiology of, 10, 11t
femoral, 834–835
infections and, 397
management of, 81–84, 374, 376, 376f, 377f
stabilizing, 83
tibial
classification of, 945–946, 946t, 947f
comminution of, 945
compartment syndrome and, 948
complications of, 948, 948t
external fixation of, 946
immobilization for, 952
outcomes of, 946
rehabilitation of, 952
soft tissue closure in, 946, 948
treatment principles for, 944–945
treatment technique for, 949–950, 950f, 951f, 952, 952f
vascular injuries in, 948
wound management for, 83–84
Operative fixation, 84
compression plating, 85–86
intramedullary rod, 85
Kirschner wires, 85
locking plating, 85
myelomeningocele and, 180
Steinmann pins, 85
Operative intervention, improvement of results with, 74
Operative Orthopaedics (Campbell), 349
Opioids, 47, 52, 54–56, 55t
postoperative analgesia with, 65, 65t, 66t, 67
Orthopaedic Trauma Association (OTA), 354
Osteoblasts, 34, 35f
Osteochondral fractures
classification of, 896, 897t
complications of, 899–900
imaging of, 896, 897f
incidence of, 895
locations of, 895, 895f
mechanism of injury, 895–896, 896f
meniscal injury v., 905
prognosis, 898–899
signs/symptoms, 896
surgical/applied anatomy, 896–897
treatment of
algorithm for, 898f
options for, 897–898
pearls/pitfalls for, 898
technique for, 898, 899f, 900f, 901f
Osteochondritis dissecans, 905
Osteochondroma, 121t, 135, 137f
Osteochondrosis, 229
Osteoclasts, 34, 35f
Osteodystrophy, renal, rickets and, 140f, 167–168, 168f
Osteofibrous dysplasia (OD), 122t, 143, 144f
Osteogenesis imperfecta (OI), 121t
child abuse screening and, 213, 214–216, 214f
clinical presentation of, 158
femoral shaft fractures and, 798, 835
radiographic findings in, 158, 159f
treatment of, 158–163, 161f, 162f
Osteogenic sarcoma, 121t, 138
Osteoid osteoma, 122t, 213, 784
Osteomyelitis, 121t, 122t, 213
chronic sclerosing, 784
classification of, 153t, 154f, 154t
clinical features of, 153–154
radial neck fractures and, 427
radiographic evaluation of, 154–155, 155f
treatment of, 155–156, 156f, 156t
Osteonecrosis
distal humeral physeal fracture and, 566, 566f
of distal tibial epiphysis, 1013
intramedullary nailing and, 821, 823f
lateral condylar physeal injury and, 543, 544f, 550–551, 551f
of radial head, 425
supracondylar humeral fracture and, 517–518, 517f
of talus, 1028–1029
trochlear
patterns of, 581, 583f
theories of, 580
treatment of, 581
vascular anatomy of, 580–581, 582f
Osteopenia, 213
disuse, 121t
femoral shaft fractures and, 798
Osteopetrosis, 121t, 158, 213
clinical features of, 163
radiographic appearance of, 163, 163f, 164f, 165f
treatment of, 163–164
Osteopontin, 28
Osteoporosis
femoral neck stress fractures and, 783
iatrogenic, 170–171
cancer treatment and, 170–171
immobilization, 171
idiopathic, 170
clinical features of, 170, 171f
treatment of, 170
thoracolumbar fractures and, 730, 732f
Osteosarcoma, 122t, 784, 798
Osteotomies, 111
chronic Monteggia fracture-dislocations and, 469–470, 469f
cubitus varus treatment with, 523–525, 523t, 524f, 525f, 526f
for lateral condylar physeal injury, 543
OTA. *See* Orthopaedic Trauma Association
Oxacillin, 156t
Oxycodone, 66t
Oxygenation monitoring, 47

P
Pain management. *See also* Analgesia; Procedural sedation and analgesia; Sedation
principles of, 46
undertreatment in, 46
Pain relief, 45–46
analgesia, 46
displaced fracture treatment and, 365–366
postoperative, 65, 65t, 66t, 67–68, 67t
anesthesia
displaced fracture treatment and, 365–366
for finger fractures, 230
local
axillary block, 62–63, 63f
femoral nerve block, 64–65, 64f
hematoma block, 62, 62f
postoperative analgesia with, 67–68
toxicity from, 59, 59t
wrist/digital block, 63–64, 64f
regional, 365
agents for, 58–59
intravenous, 59–61
performing, 61
sedation, 365
classification of, 46, 46f
comparative studies of, 58
forearm fracture treatment and, 377–378
guidelines for
airway status, 49–50, 50t
coexisting nonmusculoskeletal injuries, 49
definitions for, 46–47, 46f
discharge criteria for, 47, 47t, 49
hemodynamic status, 49
monitoring, 47–49
oral intake precautions, 49
patient assessment, 49
inhalational, 46
medications for, 50–58
parenteral, 46–47
principles of, 46
respiratory depression due to, 55
Pamidronate, 160
Paraplegic children, 959–961, 961f
Patellar dislocation
classification of, 902
imaging of, 901, 902f
incidence of, 900
mechanism of injury, 900
meniscal injury v., 905
signs/symptoms, 900–901
surgical/applied anatomy, 902, 902f
treatment of
chronic subluxation/dislocation, 903, 903f, 904f
pearls/pitfalls for, 903–904
prognosis/complications, 904
reduction, 902–903
surgical intervention, 903
Patellar fractures
classification of
for management, 878
by mechanism of injury, 878–880
complications of, 883
diagnosis of, 877–878
incidence of, 876
mechanism of injury, 876, 877f
signs/symptoms
associated injuries, 877
clinical findings, 876–877
radiographic findings, 877, 878f, 879f
sleeve fracture, 876, 876f
surgical/applied anatomy, 880, 880f
treatment of
operative repair, 880–883, 881f, 882f
pearls/pitfalls for, 883
postoperative/postfracture care, 883
rationale for, 880
Patellofemoral dislocation, 905
Pathologic fractures. *See also specific types*
bone marrow diseases
Gaucher's disease, 148, 150
hemophilia, 151–153, 152t
leukemia, 151, 152f
osteomyelitis, 153–156, 153t, 154t, 155f, 156f, 156t
sickle cell disease, 150–151, 150f, 229
bone-weakening conditions
arthrogryposis, 181, 183–184, 183f

congenital primary hyperparathyroidism, 172, 172f
copper deficiency, 174–175
Cushing's syndrome, 173
iatrogenic osteoporosis, 170–171
idiopathic osteoporosis, 170, 171f
osteogenesis imperfecta, 121t, 158–163, 159f, 161f, 162f, 213–216, 214f, 798, 835
osteopetrosis, 163–164, 163f, 164f, 165f
poliomyelitis, 181, 183–184
primary hyperparathyroidism, 171–173, 172f
pyknodysostosis, 164–165
rickets, 166–169, 166f, 167f, 168f, 169f
scurvy, 173–174, 174f
scurvy-like syndrome, 174–175
spinal cord injury in, 184
after limb lengthening, 156–157, 157f, 158f
neuromuscular disease
cerebral palsy, 175–177, 176f, 177f, 178f
muscular dystrophy, 181, 182f
myelomeningocele, 177–181, 180f
pain characterization in, 121
predisposing factors for, 121t
radiographic evaluation of, 121–122
schematic distribution of, 122t
tumors/tumor-like
aneurysmal bone cysts, 121t, 122t, 125–128, 127f, 128f, 129f
congenital insensitivity to pain, 148, 149f
enchondromatosis, 132, 134–135, 135f, 136f
eosinophilic granuloma, 121t, 135–138
fibrous cortical defects, 129–131
fibrous dysplasia, 141–143, 142f
giant cell tumor, 131–132, 133f, 133t
hand injuries from, 229
Langerhans cell histiocytosis, 122t, 135–138
malignant bone tumors/metastasis, 138–141, 139f, 140f
neurofibromatosis, 144–147, 146f, 147f
nonossifying fibroma, 129–131, 130f, 131f, 132f
osteochondroma, 135, 137f
osteofibrous dysplasia, 143, 144f
unicameral bone cyst, 122–123, 124f, 124t, 125, 125f, 126f
Patient assessment
child abuse recognition and, 195
sedation and, 49
Patient-controlled analgesia (PCA), 65, 66t
PCA. *See* Patient-controlled analgesia
PCL. *See* Posterior cruciate ligament
PDGF. *See* Platelet-derived growth factor
Pediatric cocktail (DPT), 50
Pediatric intensive care unit (PICU), 73
Pediatric trauma centers, 73
Pediatric Trauma Score (PTS), 74, 76t
Pelvic fractures
acetabular fractures, 760f
classification of, 760–761, 761f
incidence of, 760
postoperative management of, 767
radiographic evaluation of, 761, 761f, 762f, 763f, 764f
surgical treatment of, 765, 765f, 765t, 766f, 767
treatment of, 761–762, 764
applied anatomy for, 747–748, 748f
associated injuries, 744–745
avulsion fractures
diagnosis of, 749
hip pain from, 785
incidence of, 748
mechanism of injury, 748, 749f
treatment/prognosis for, 749, 750f
child abuse and, 744
classification of, 746–747, 746f, 746t, 747t
of coccyx, 759–760, 760f
complications of, 767
genitourinary injuries and, 79
iliac wing fractures
displacement in, 750
incidence of, 749
treatment of, 750, 750f
imaging studies of, 745–746
incidence of, 743
management of, 80
mechanism of injury, 744
motor vehicle accidents and, 13
pubis/ischium fractures
clinical presentation of, 750–751
fractures near of subluxation of sacroiliac joint, 752–753, 753f
fractures near of subluxation of symphysis pubis, 752, 752f
incidence of, 750
ipsilateral rami, 751
ischium body, 751, 751f
stress fractures, 751–752, 752f
of sacrum, 759, 759f
severe multiple/open, 758–759
signs/symptoms of, 745
unstable (ring disruption)
bilateral fractures of inferior and superior pubic rami, 753–754, 754f
complex fracture patterns, 754–757, 754f, 755f, 756f, 757f
types of, 753
urologic injury and, 77, 79
Penicillin, 156t
Periarticular ossification, Monteggia fracture-dislocations and, 472–473
Periosteum, 24–26, 25f
Peripheral nerve injuries, 79
Perthes disease, 771
Peterson injury classification, 103–104, 104f, 105f, 105t
Phalangeal fractures
evaluation of, 1049, 1050f
incidence of, 1049
treatment of, 1049, 1051
Phalanx fractures
distal
anatomy for, 233, 233f, 234f, 235f
classification of, 234t
complications of, 239–240
diagnosis of, 235–236, 235f, 236f
mechanism of injury, 233
patterns of, 233, 235
postoperative care/rehabilitation, 238
treatment of, 236–238, 236f, 237f, 238f, 239, 241f
proximal/middle, 287f, 288f
anatomy for, 240
classification of, 241t
complications of, 253–255, 254f, 255f
diagnosis of, 242, 242f, 243f, 244f, 245f, 246f, 251f
mechanism of injury, 240
patterns of, 240–242
postoperative care/rehabilitation for, 252–253
prognosis for, 253
treatment of, 242–243, 245, 246f, 247f, 248, 248f, 249f, 250–252, 250f, 252f, 253f
Phencyclidine, 56
Phenothiazines, 50
Physeal anatomy, 20–21, 20f, 21f. *See also* Classic metaphyseal lesions
distal femoral epiphyseal fractures and, 852–853
growth of, 94, 95f, 95t
healing patterns in, 38–40
mechanical features of, 92, 94
normal
gross, 91–92, 92f, 93f, 94f
microscopic, 92, 93f
regulatory mechanisms in, 32–34
Physeal growth disturbance
without arrest, 115, 117
distal tibial fractures and, 1010–1011, 1012f, 1013f
etiology of, 108, 110t
evaluation of, 108–110, 109f
physeal arrests
classification of, 110, 111f
distraction of, 111
lateral condylar physeal injury and, 550
management of, 110–111
osteotomies for, 111
preoperative planning/surgical principles for, 112–115, 113f, 114f, 115f, 116f
prevention of, 111
resection of, 111–112
Physeal injuries, 9–10, 91. *See also specific fractures*
classification of, 534
Aitken, 98
Peterson, 103–104, 104f, 105f, 105t
Poland, 97–98, 98f
Salter-Harris, 98f, 99–101, 100f, 101f, 102f, 103, 103f, 104, 104f, 105t
complications of, 107–108
distal phalanx fractures and, 239
epidemiology of, 105, 105t, 106f
etiology of
fracture, 94
infection, 94, 96f
miscellaneous, 97, 97f
repetitive stress, 95, 97, 97f
tumors, 94–95, 96f
vascular insult, 95, 96f
evaluation of, 105–106
historical review of, 97
lateral condylar fractures
anatomy/classification, 534, 535f
displacement stages, 534, 536f
incidence/outcome, 534
patterns of, 92, 94
radial
diagnosis of, 294, 296
treatment of, 296–297, 299–301, 303, 305–312
treatment of, 106–108
Physical abuse, 192
PICU. *See* Pediatric intensive care unit
PIP joint. *See* Proximal interphalangeal joint
Pisiform fractures, 279
Plastic deformation, 378
Plate fixation, 369, 370f
distal femoral epiphyseal fractures, 857
femoral shaft fracture treatment with, 823, 824, 827
Platelet-derived growth factor (PDGF), 31, 32–33, 32f
Play and recreational activities, fractures from, 12–13, 16
Playground equipment, 12
Plica syndrome, 905
Poland injury classification, 97–98, 98f
Poliomyelitis, 181, 183–184, 959
Posterior cruciate ligament (PCL)
injury to
classification of, 914
imaging of, 913
mechanism of, 912
signs/symptoms of, 913, 914f
surgical/applied anatomy for, 915–916
treatment of, 923
knee dislocation and, 924

Posterior elbow dislocation
arterial injuries in, 605
associated fractures, 596, 600
closed reduction of, 597–600
complications of, 602–605
cubitus recurvatum and, 605
loss of motion due to, 605
management principles for, 595
mechanism of injury, 595–596, 596f
myositis ossificans and, 605
neurologic injuries in, 603–605
neurovascular injuries in, 597
open dislocations, 600
pearls/pitfalls for, 602
postoperative care for, 600
postreduction care for, 600
puller technique for, 599f, 600–601, 600f
pusher technique for, 600, 602f
radiographic imaging of, 597, 598f, 603f
radioulnar synostosis in, 605
rationale for treatment of, 597
recurrent
complications of, 609, 609f
mechanism of injury, 605–606, 607f, 608
posttreatment care for, 609
treatment options for, 608–609, 608f
signs/symptoms, 596
soft tissue injury in, 596–597, 597f
surgical treatment, 600
treatment of, 597–601, 599f, 600f, 601f, 602f
Postoperative analgesia
with local anesthetics, 67–68
NSAID for, 67, 67t
opioids for, 65, 65t, 66t, 67
Posttraumatic arthritis, 1044
Powers ratio, 690, 690t, 698
Practicing Safety, 219
Premature infants, 15
Preventive programs, 15–16
Prilocaine, 58, 60t
Procaine, 58
Procedural sedation and analgesia (PSA), 47
Promethazine, 50
Propofol, 47, 57–58
Prostaglandin, 29, 213
Proteoglycans, 26, 27t, 28, 29f
Proximal humerus fractures
associated injuries, 646
classification of, 647, 647f
complications of
early, 654–655
late, 655
diagnosis of, 646–647, 646f
incidence of, 644
mechanism of injury, 644–645, 645f, 646f
signs/symptoms, 645–646
surgical/applied anatomy, 647–649, 648f, 649f
treatment of
algorithm for, 654f
nonoperative, 649–650
options for, 650t
pearls/pitfalls for, 653–654
pros/cons for, 656t
surgical, 650–653, 651f, 652f, 653f
Proximal interphalangeal joint (PIP joint), dislocation of, 281–282, 281f
Proximal phalanx fractures, 287f, 288f
anatomy for, 240
classification of, 241t
complications of, 253–255, 254f, 255f
diagnosis of, 242, 242f, 243f, 244f, 245f, 246f, 251f
mechanism of injury, 240
patterns of, 240–242
postoperative care/rehabilitation for, 252–253
prognosis for, 253
treatment of, 242–243, 245, 246f, 247f, 248, 248f, 249f, 250–252, 250f, 252f, 253f
Proximal radioulnar elbow dislocation
associated injuries, 613–614
closed v. open reduction for, 614
mechanism of injury, 613
signs/symptoms, 613
translocation in, 614, 614f
treatment of, 614
Proximal radius
fractures of
anatomy for, 406
associated injuries/complications, 425–427, 425t
cam effect in, 406, 407f
classification of, 407–408, 410t
diagnosis of, 406
incidence of, 405–406
mechanism of injury, 410, 411f, 412f, 412t
radial head displacement, 410–413
radial neck displacement, 413–414, 414f
radiographic evaluation of, 407, 407f, 408f, 409f, 410f
stress injuries, 414
treatment of, 414–418, 416f, 417f, 418f, 419f, 420–423, 420f, 421f, 422f, 422t, 423f, 424f, 425
malunion of, 427
normal angulation of, 406
ossification patterns in, 406, 406f
soft tissue attachments, 406
Proximal tibial epiphyseal fractures
associated injuries
ligamentous, 862
nerve, 863
vascular, 863, 863f, 864f
complications of, 869t
compartment syndrome, 869
growth disturbance/leg-length discrepancy, 869
knee instability/degenerative changes, 869–870
loss of reduction, 869
diagnosis/classification of, 863, 865–866, 865f, 865t
incidence of, 862
mechanism of injury, 862
signs/symptoms, 862
surgical/applied anatomy, 866
treatment of
closed reduction and fixation, 866
closed reduction and immobilization, 866, 867
open reduction, 867
options for, 867t
pearls/pitfalls for, 869
surgical treatment, 867, 868f, 869
Proximal ulna (olecranon)
elbow dislocation and, 597f
epiphyseal fractures of
anatomy for, 427–428, 429f
associated injuries/complications, 431
classification of, 430, 430t, 431f
incidence of, 427
mechanism of injury, 428, 430
signs/symptoms of, 428, 430f
treatment of, 430–431
extension injuries
mechanism of, 433–435, 434f, 435f, 436f
treatment of, 438, 438f
flexion injuries
mechanism of, 433, 434f
treatment of, 435, 438, 438f
metaphyseal fractures
anatomy for, 433
associated injuries/complications, 439–440, 442, 444
classification of, 433t
incidence of, 431, 433, 433t
mechanism of injury, 433–435, 434f, 435f, 436f, 437f
signs/symptoms, 433
treatment of, 435, 438–439, 438f, 439f
ossification of, 478
shear injuries
mechanism of, 435
treatment of, 438–439, 439f
PSA. *See* Procedural sedation and analgesia
Pseudarthrosis, 349
Psoriatic arthritis, 229
PTS. *See* Pediatric Trauma Score
Pubis fractures
clinical presentation of, 750–751
fractures near of subluxation of sacroiliac joint, 752–753, 753f
fractures near of subluxation of symphysis pubis, 752, 752f
incidence of, 750
ipsilateral rami, 751
ischium body, 751, 751f
stress fractures, 751–752, 752f
Pulled elbow syndrome, 614
complications of, 617
imaging of, 616
mechanism of injury, 615, 615f
nonoperative treatment of, 616–617, 616f
signs/symptoms, 615–616
surgical treatment of, 617
Pulmonary embolism, 79–80
Pulmonary thromboembolism, 80
Pyelography, multiple fracture evaluation with, 77
Pyknodysostosis, 164–165

R

Radial head displacement/fractures. *See also* Monteggia fracture-dislocations
associated injuries/complications, 425–427, 425t
during dislocation, 413
elbow dislocation and, 597f
malunion from, 427
neck migration in, 412–413, 414f
nonunion after, 425
osteonecrosis from, 425
patterns of, 412, 413f
during reduction, 413
treatment of
fixation methods, 420–421, 420f
nonoperative methods, 416–417, 416f, 417f, 422
operative methods, 417–420, 418f, 419f, 422–423, 425
options for, 414–415
prognostic factors for, 415–416
radial head fractures, 421–422, 421f, 422t
type B injuries, 421
valgus injuries
angular force on neck, 410
associated injuries, 410–411
fracture patterns in, 411–412, 412f, 413f
Radial head overgrowth, 425
Radial head subluxation, 595
Radial neck displacement/fractures
angular forces in, 413–414, 414f
notching, 425
rotational forces, 414
Radial nerve palsies, humeral shaft fractures and, 665–666, 665f, 667
Radial shaft fractures, 74, 347–348
associated injuries, 353–354
complications of
compartment syndrome, 398
complex regional pain syndromes, 398–399
cross-union/synostosis, 396–397

delayed union/nonunion, 396
forearm stiffness, 383
infection, 397
malunion, 384, 387–388, 396
muscle/tendon entrapment/tendon rupture, 397–398
neurapraxia, 397
redisplacement/malalignment, 381, 383
refracture, 383–384
diagnosis and classification of, 354–355, 355f
epidemiology of, 350, 352f
historical overview of, 348–350, 348f, 349f, 350f, 351f
mechanism of injury, 350, 352, 352f, 353f
remodeling of, 359–360
signs/symptoms, 352–353
surgical/applied anatomy for
bony anatomy/static restraints, 360–361, 362f
muscle/nerve anatomy, 361, 363, 363f, 363t
surgical approaches, 364–365, 364f, 365f
treatment of
angulation limits for, 378
closed, 365–368
comminuted fractures, 368
complete fractures, 367–368
greenstick fractures, 366–367
intramedullary fixation, 369
intramedullary nailing, 369–371, 371f, 372f, 373f, 374, 374f, 375f
plate fixation, 369, 370f
rationale for, 355–356, 356f, 357f, 358–360, 358f, 359t
reduction, 377–378
surgical, 369–371, 374, 376–378, 380–381
traumatic bowing/plastic deformation, 366, 366f, 367f
Radiographs. *See also specific injuries and sites*
multiple fracture evaluation with, 75–76
of pathologic fractures, 121–122
Radionuclide scans, multiple fracture evaluation with, 77
Radioulnar synostosis, 426, 427f
Radius
distal fractures of
classification of, 293t
diagnosis/classification of, 2t, 293–294
mechanism of injury, 292–293
physeal injuries, 294
signs/symptoms of, 293
surgical/applied anatomy for, 294
proximal fractures of
anatomy for, 406
associated injuries/complications, 425–427, 425t
cam effect in, 406, 407f
classification of, 407–408, 410t
diagnosis of, 406
incidence of, 405–406
malunion of, 427
mechanism of injury, 410, 411f, 412f, 412t
normal angulation of, 406
ossification patterns in, 406, 406f
radial head displacement, 410–413
radial neck displacement, 413–414, 414f
radiographic evaluation of, 407, 407f, 408f, 409f, 410f
soft tissue attachments, 406
stress injuries, 414
treatment of, 414–418, 416f, 417f, 418f, 419f, 420–423, 420f, 421f, 422f, 422t, 423f, 424f, 425
Rang, Mercer, 349–350
Range-of-motion losses, 356, 356f, 359t
Recurrent posterior elbow dislocation
complications of, 609, 609f
mechanism of injury, 605–606, 607f, 608
posttreatment care for, 609
treatment options for, 608–609, 608f
Reduction
closed
clavicle fractures, 627
distal femoral epiphyseal fractures, 854–856, 855f, 856f
distal tibial fractures, 983
hip dislocations, 791
hip fractures, 779
lateral condylar physeal injury, 539–540, 541f
lateral physeal condylar fractures, 539–540, 541f
posterior elbow dislocation, 597–600
proximal radioulnar elbow dislocation, 614
proximal tibial epiphyseal fractures, 866, 867
supracondylar humeral fractures, 496, 502–507, 504f, 505f, 506f, 510
type I Monteggia fracture-dislocations, 456, 456f, 457f, 458f
of forearm shaft fractures, 348, 364, 377–378
of glenohumeral subluxation/dislocation, 643
loss of
proximal tibial epiphyseal fractures, 869
supracondylar humeral fractures, 518, 518f, 519f, 520
open
calcaneal fractures, 1033, 1034, 1034f
clavicle fractures, 628
distal femoral epiphyseal fractures, 856–857, 857f
distal tibial fractures, 984–985, 987, 993, 1001, 1003–1004
lateral condylar physeal injury, 540, 541–542, 542f
lateral physeal condylar fractures, 540, 541–542, 542f
proximal radioulnar elbow dislocation, 614
proximal tibial epiphyseal fractures, 867
supracondylar humeral fractures, 498–499, 499f, 502, 508–510
of patellar dislocation, 902–903
percutaneous, 1033, 1033f
plate fixation and, 369
posterior elbow dislocation
puller technique for, 599f, 600–601, 600f
pusher technique for, 600, 602f
radial head displacement/fractures, 413
of radial shaft fractures, 377–378
radial/ulnar shaft fractures, 348, 364, 377–378
tarsometatarsal injuries, 1043–1044
ulnar shaft fractures, 377–378
Reflex sympathetic dystrophy, 1013. *See also* Complex regional pain syndromes
Refracture, of forearm fractures, 384–385
Rehabilitation, hand injuries, 232
Relative head injury severity scale (RHISS), 74
Remodeling, 6, 34, 35f, 74
bone healing and, 37
in children, 40
of forearm fractures, 359–360
hand injuries and, 227
Renal osteodystrophy
aluminium toxicity complicating, 169
rickets and, 140f, 167–168, 168f
Respiratory depression, sedation and, 55
Resuscitation, multiple fractures and, 73–74
Rhabdomyosarcoma, 122t
RHISS. *See* Relative head injury severity scale
Rib fractures, 72, 209–211, 210f, 211f
Rickets, 121t, 214
child abuse screening and, 212
clinical features of, 165–166
drug-induced, 213, 216f
malabsorption and, 166–167, 167f
nutritional, 166
radiographic appearance of, 166f, 167f, 168f, 169f
renal osteodystrophy and, 167–168, 168f, 169f
types of, 166t
very-low-birth-weight infants and, 167–168
Rodenticide-induced coagulopathy, 194
Roller skates, 12–13
Ropivacaine, 58–59

S

Sacrum fractures, 759, 759f
Salmonella, 156t
Salsalate, 67, 67t
Salter-Harris fracture classification, 92, 94, 847–851, 847f, 848f, 849f, 850f
physeal injury classification, 98f, 99–101, 100f, 101f, 102f, 103, 103f, 104, 104f, 105f
tibial fracture classification
type I/II, 982–986, 988f, 989f, 998–999, 999f, 1000f
type III/IV, 986–987, 987f, 988f, 989, 990f, 999, 1001, 1002f
type V, 989–990, 1001–1002, 1001f, 1002f
SBS. *See* Shaken baby syndrome
Scaphoid fractures
bipartite scaphoid controversy, 270, 272
classification of, 272
complications of, 276, 276f, 277f
diagnosis of, 270f, 271f, 272f, 273f, 274f
epidemiology of, 269
mechanism of injury, 269–270
patterns of, 270
postoperative care/rehabilitation of, 275–276
prognosis for, 276
treatment of, 274–275, 275f
Scapula fractures
associated injuries, 630
classification of, 630, 631f, 632
complications of, 634
diagnosis of, 630
mechanism of injury, 629–630
signs/symptoms, 630
surgical/applied anatomy, 632–633, 633f
treatment of, 631t, 633–634
SCD. *See* Sickle cell disease
SCFE. *See* Slipped capital femoral epiphysis
School environment, fractures sustained in, 11–12
SCI. *See* Spinal cord injury
SCIWORA. *See* Spinal cord injury without radiographic abnormality
Scleroderma, 229
Scurvy, 173–174, 174f, 213, 215f
Scurvy-like syndrome, 174–175
Sedation, 365. *See also specific sedatives*
classification of, 46, 46f
comparative studies of, 58
forearm fracture treatment and, 377–378
guidelines for
airway status, 49–50, 50t
coexisting nonmusculoskeletal injuries, 49
definitions for, 46–47, 46f
discharge criteria for, 47, 47t, 49
hemodynamic status, 49
monitoring, 47–49
oral intake precautions, 49
patient assessment, 49
inhalational, 46
medications for, 50–58
parenteral, 46–47
principles of, 46
respiratory depression due to, 55

Septic arthritis, 213
Sexual abuse, 192, 195
Shaken baby syndrome (SBS), 199. *See also* Abusive head trauma
Shear injuries, forearm fractures from
  mechanism of, 435, 436f, 437f
  treatment of, 438–439, 439f
Short Musculoskeletal Function Assessment (SMFA), 754
Sickle cell disease (SCD), 150–151, 150f, 229
SICU. *See* Surgical intensive care unit
SID. *See* State Inpatient Databases
SIDS. *See* Sudden infant death syndrome
Skateboarding, 12, 16
Skate parks, 13
Skeletal survey
  child abuse screening and, 206–208
  radiographic protocol for, 201, 201t
Skeleton
  age staging of, 917, 917t
  immature, 18–19
Skiing injuries, 13
Skull fractures, child abuse and, 208
Slipped capital femoral epiphysis (SCFE), 773, 782–783, 785
SMFA. *See* Short Musculoskeletal Function Assessment
Sniffing position, 48, 48f
Snowboarding injuries, 13, 399
Society for Pediatric Radiology, 216
Somatropin, 29
Sonography, elbow evaluation with, 485
Spasticity, 78
Special Olympics, 711
Spinal cord injury (SCI). *See also* Cervical spine injuries; Thoracolumbar spinal fractures
  in children, 696–697
  neonatal, 697
  pathologic fractures and, 184
Spinal cord injury without radiographic abnormality (SCIWORA), 77, 200, 201, 212, 692, 696, 724, 727
Spinal injury
  child abuse and, 211–212, 212f
  motor vehicle accidents and, 13
  multiple fracture evaluation and, 74–75, 77
Splinting, 74, 84
Spondylolisthesis, 716
Spondylolysis, 716
Stabilization
  external fixation for, multiple injuries and, 86–87
  of open fractures, 83
  operative fixation for, multiple injuries and, 84–86
Staphylococcus aureus, 156t
State Inpatient Databases (SID), 5
Steinmann pins, 85
Stem cell therapy, 41
Streptococcus, Group B, 156t
Stress fractures, 121t
  distal tibial, 974, 977f
  distal tibial fractures, 974, 977f
  femoral fractures
    classification of, 785, 786f
    complications of, 786
    differential diagnosis of, 784–785
    incidence of, 783
    mechanism of injury, 783
    treatment of, 786
  femoral shaft fractures, 798
  fibular, 961, 962f, 963–964, 963f
  fibular shaft fractures, 961, 962f, 963–964, 963f
  foot, 1054–1055
  foot fractures/dislocations, 1054–1055
  hip fractures, 773
    classification of, 785, 786f
    complications of, 786
    incidence of, 783
    mechanism of injury, 783–785
    treatment of, 786
  humeral shaft fractures, 659–660
  ischium fractures, 751–752, 752f
  osteoporosis, 783
  proximal radius, 414
  pubis fractures, 751–752, 752f
  pubis/ischium fractures, 751–752, 752f
  tibial, 961, 962f, 963–964, 963f
Stress x-rays, 862
Subaxial injuries
  burst fractures, 716
  compression fractures, 715
  operative treatment of
    crossing translaminar screw fixation of C2, 718, 719f, 720
    posterior arthrodesis, 716, 717f, 718f
    posterior arthrodesis with lateral mass screw fixation, 716, 718, 718f, 719f
  posterior ligamentous disruptions, 714–715
  spondylolysis/spondylolisthesis, 716
  unilateral/bilateral facet dislocations, 715, 715f
Subdural hemorrhage, 202t
Submuscular bridge plating, femoral shaft fractures and, 824–827
Subtalar dislocation
  incidence of, 1037
  radiographic evaluation of, 1037, 1037f
  treatment of, 1037–1038
Sudden infant death syndrome (SIDS), 193, 216
Sudden unexpected death in infancy (SUDI), 216. *See also* Sudden infant death syndrome
SUDI. *See* Sudden unexpected death in infancy
Supracondylar humeral fractures, 74
  anatomy for, 487–489, 489f, 490f
  classification of, 490, 491f, 491t
  complications
    compartment syndrome, 513–514, 514f
    cubitus varus, 520–522, 520f, 521f
    elbow stiffness, 515
    hyperextension, 520, 522f
    loss of reduction, 518, 518f, 519f, 520
    myositis ossificans, 516–517, 516f
    neurologic deficit, 514–515
    nonunion, 517
    osteonecrosis, 517–518, 517f
    pin track infection, 516
    vascular injury, 510–513, 510f, 511f
  controversies related to, 525–526
  extension-type, posteromedial v. posterolateral displacement, 489–490, 490f
  flexion-type
    etiology/pathology of, 526, 526f
    radiographic findings, 527, 527f
    treatment of, 527–529, 528f, 529f
  mechanism of injury, 487–489, 488f
  operative intervention for, 74
  overview of, 487, 488t
  postoperative care for, 502, 507
  radiographic evaluation, 493–494, 493f, 495f
  signs/symptoms of
    associated forearm fractures, 491, 492f
    compartment syndrome, 491
    elbow displacement, 490, 492f
    examination for, 490–491
    pucker sign, 490, 492f
  treatment
    casting technique, 507–508, 507f
    closed reduction and pinning, 496, 502–507, 504f, 505f, 506f, 510
    imaging during, 503f, 506f
    initial management, 496
    medial column comminution and, 502, 508
    open reduction of, 498–499, 499f, 508–510
    options for, 496t
    pin configuration for, 496–498, 497f
    traction, 499, 500f
    type I fracture, 499–500, 502
    type II fracture, 500–501, 501f, 502, 503f
    type III fracture, 501–507, 501f
    type IV fracture, 502
Supracondyloid process fractures
  anatomy of, 672–673
  diagnosis/classification of, 674, 674f
  treatment of, 674
Surgical intensive care unit (SICU), 73
Synostosis, 396–397
  distal tibial fractures and, 1013
  radioulnar, 426, 427f, 605
Synovial cell sarcoma, 122t
Synovitis, 229, 771
Systemic lupus, 229

T

Talar fractures
  associated injuries, 1020
  classification of, 1020–1021, 1021t
  complications of, osteonecrosis, 1028–1029
  diagnosis/classification, 1020
  imaging evaluation of, 1020, 1020f
  incidence of, 1019, 1024
  mechanism of injury, 1019
  osteochondral surface
    anatomy for, 1026, 1026f
    classification of, 1026–1027, 1027f
    mechanism of injury, 1025–1026
    radiographic evaluation, 1026, 1027, 1027f
    treatment of, 1027–1028, 1028f
  signs/symptoms, 1019–1020
  surgical/applied anatomy for
    blood supply, 1023–1024, 1025f
    bony anatomy, 1023, 1023f, 1024f
    cartilage, 1023
    ossification, 1022
  talar body
    classification of, 1025t, 1026f
    lateral process, 1024–1025
  treatment of
    surgical approaches for, 1021–1022, 1022f
    by type, 1021
Tarsometatarsal injuries (TMT)
  classification of, 1040–1041, 1041f
  complications of, 1044
  imaging evaluation of, 1041, 1041f, 1042f
  incidence of, 1039
  mechanism of injury, 1039, 1040f
  signs/symptoms, 1039–1040, 1040f
  surgical/applied anatomy for, 1041–1042, 1042f
  treatment of
    immobilization, 1042–1043
    reduction and stabilization, 1043–1044
TBI. *See* Traumatic brain injury
T-condylar fractures
  classification of, 584, 587f
  complications of, 589
  diagnosis of, 584–585
  incidence of, 584
  mechanism of injury, 584, 585f
  patterns of, 584, 586f
  treatment of
    principles of, 585–586
    type I, 586–587, 588f
    type II, 587–589, 589f, 590f
    type III, 589
Temporary brittle bone disease, 216
Tendonitis, peroneal, 1037
Tendon rupture, 397–398
Tenosynovitis, 229

Testosterone, 29
Tetracaine, 58
TFCC. *See* Triangular fibrocartilage complex
TGF-β. *See* Transforming growth factor-β
Thermal injury, 229
Thiemann disease. *See* Osteochondrosis
Thoracolumbar spinal fractures
associated injuries, 724–725
classification of, 725, 726f, 728
burst fractures, 726–727
compression fractures, 725–726
flexion-distraction injuries, 727
fracture-dislocations, 727
controversies/future directions for, 736–738
incidence of, 723
mechanism of injury, 723–724, 724f
osteoporosis and, 730, 732f
radiographic evaluation of, 728–729
signs/symptoms, 724
surgical/applied anatomy for, 729–730, 729f
treatment of
burst fractures, 730–733, 733f, 734, 734f, 736
compression fractures, 730, 731f, 732f, 734
flexion-distraction injuries, 733–734, 735f, 736
fracture-dislocations, 734, 736, 736f, 737f, 738f
pearls/pitfalls for, 736
treatment rationale for, 725, 725f
Thoracolumbosacral orthosis (TLSO), 730
Thromboembolism, pulmonary, 80
Thumb metacarpal fractures
anatomy for, 262
classification of, 263f, 263t
complications of, 267–268
diagnosis of, 262, 264, 264f, 265f
mechanism of injury, 262
patterns of, 262
postoperative care/rehabilitation for, 267
prognosis for, 267, 268f
treatment of, 264–265, 265f, 266f, 267, 267f
Thumb metacarpophalangeal ulnar collateral ligament injury (Gamekeeper's thumb), 284–287, 286f
Tibial fractures. *See also* Distal tibial fractures; Proximal tibial epiphyseal fractures
associated injuries, 887–888, 887f
bicycle spoke injuries, 959
classification of, 888, 888f, 889f
complications of
malunion, 894, 895
nonunion, 895
recurvatum deformity/shortening, 893–894
residual knee laxity, 892–893
stiffness/arthrofibrosis, 895
floating knee injury, 959
imaging of, 887
immobilization for, 952
metaphyseal, 952, 953f
motor vehicle accidents and, 13
open
classification of, 945–946, 946t, 947f
comminution of, 945
compartment syndrome and, 948
complications of, 948, 948t
external fixation of, 946
outcomes of, 946
soft tissue closure in, 946, 948
treatment principles for, 944–945
treatment technique for, 949–950, 950f, 951f, 952, 952f
vascular injuries in, 948
paraplegic children and, 959–961, 961f
prognosis for, 892
rehabilitation of, 952
stress fractures, 961, 962f, 963–964, 963f
surgical/applied anatomy, 888, 889f, 890f
toddler's fractures, 957–959, 959f
treatment of
algorithm for, 890f
arthroscopic, 890
arthroscopic with internal fixation, 891, 892f, 893f
closed, 888, 890–891, 890f
open, 890
pearls/pitfalls for, 891–892
Tibial shaft fractures
classification of, 931
diaphyseal
angular deformity from, 955–956, 956f
anterior physeal closure in, 957
cast immobilization of, 941, 942–943
cast wedging of, 943, 944f
compartment syndrome in, 954–955
complications of, 943–944, 954–957
delayed union/nonunion in, 957
fibular shaft fractures and, 936, 939
incidence of, 936
leg-length discrepancy due to, 956–957
malrotation in, 956
mechanism of injury, 939
operative treatment of, 943–944
radiographic evaluation of, 939–940, 939f, 940f, 941f, 942f
signs/symptoms of, 939
treatment of, 941, 942–944, 948–949, 949t
vascular injuries in, 955
epidemiology of, 930–931
metaphyseal
clinical presentation of, 933
etiology of, 933–934, 934t
incidence of, 933
treatment of, 934, 935f, 936
valgus deformity and, 933, 934f
surgical anatomy for
bony structure, 931
fascial compartments, 932–933, 932f
muscle origins/insertions on, 931, 931t
nerves, 932
vascular anatomy, 931, 932f
Tibial spine fractures
historical background for, 886
incidence of, 886
mechanism of injury, 887
prognosis for, 887
signs/symptoms, 887
Tibial tuberosity avulsion
associated injuries, 871, 871f
complications of, 875t
compartment syndrome, 875–876
growth disturbance, 875
loss of fixation, 876
loss of motion, 876
prominent screw heads, 876
refracture, 876
diagnosis/classification of, 871–872, 871f, 872f
incidence of, 870
mechanism of injury, 870
pearls/pitfalls of, 873, 875
postoperative management of, 873
signs/symptoms, 870, 870f
surgical applied anatomy, 872
treatment of, 873, 874f, 875f
Tissue engineering, 41
TLSO. *See* Thoracolumbosacral orthosis
TMT. *See* Tarsometatarsal injuries
Toddler's fractures, 957–959, 959f
Traction, 348
Trampoline-related injuries, 13, 399
Transforming growth factor-β (TGF-β), 29, 30–31, 32–34, 32f
Trapezium fractures, 279
Trauma. *See also* Abusive head trauma
accidental, 11–15
cellular response to, 35
epidemiology of, 5
to foot, 1018
glenohumeral dislocation due to, 635
incidence of, 47, 71–72
inflammatory/infectious processes resembling, 229
nonaccidental, 6–7, 11, 192
patellar dislocation due to, 900
pelvic injuries and, 744
Traumatic brain injury (TBI), 75. *See also* Abusive head trauma
diagnosing, 202t
peripheral nerve injury and, 79
The Treatment of Fractures (Böhler), 348
Triangular fibrocartilage complex (TFCC), 294
anatomy of, 280
tears of
classification of, 280
diagnosis of, 281
epidemiology of, 280
mechanism of injury, 280
treatment of, 281
Trigger thumb, 229
Triquetrum fractures
diagnosis of, 279
epidemiology of, 278
mechanism of injury, 278
treatment of, 279, 279f
Trisalicylate, 67, 67t
Trochlea
fractures of, 561
osteonecrosis of
patterns of, 581, 583f
theories of, 580
treatment of, 581
vascular anatomy of, 580–581, 582f
Tumors/tumor-like conditions
aneurysmal bone cysts, 121t, 122t, 125–128, 127f, 128f, 129f
chondrosarcoma, 122t
congenital insensitivity to pain, 148, 149f
enchondromatosis, 132, 134–135, 135f, 136f
eosinophilic granuloma, 121t, 135–138
Ewing's sarcoma, 121t, 122t, 138
fibrous cortical defects, 129–131
fibrous dysplasia, 141–143, 142f
giant cell, 121t, 131–132, 133f, 133t
hand injuries from, 229
Langerhans cell histiocytosis, 122t, 135–138
malignant bone tumors/metastasis, 138–141, 139f, 140f
neurofibromatosis, 144–147, 146f, 147f
nonossifying fibroma, 129–131, 130f, 131f, 132f
osteochondroma, 135, 137f
osteofibrous dysplasia, 143, 144f
osteogenic sarcoma, 121t, 138
osteosarcoma, 122t, 784, 798
rhabdomyosarcoma, 122t
synovial cell sarcoma, 122t
unicameral bone cyst, 122–123, 124f, 124t, 125, 125f, 126f
Wilm's tumor, 121t, 122t
Turco casting technique, 368, 368t

U

UBC. *See* Unicameral bone cysts
Ulna. *See also* Proximal ulna (olecranon)
distal fractures of
classification of, 293t
diagnosis/classification of, 2t, 293–294

Ulna (*continued*)
- mechanism of injury, 292–293
- physeal injuries, 294
- signs/symptoms of, 293
- surgical/applied anatomy for, 294
- proximal (olecranon)
  - epiphyseal fractures of, 427–428, 429f, 430–431, 430f, 430t, 431f
  - extension injuries, 433–435, 434f, 435f, 436f, 438, 438f
  - flexion injuries, 433, 434f, 435, 438, 438f
  - metaphyseal fractures, 433–435, 433t, 434f, 435f, 436f, 437f, 438–440, 438f, 439f, 442, 444
  - shear injuries, 435, 438–439, 439f

Ulnar shaft fractures, 74, 347–348
- associated injuries, 353–354
- complications of
  - compartment syndrome, 398
  - complex regional pain syndromes, 398–399
  - cross-union/synostosis, 396–397
  - delayed union/nonunion, 396
  - forearm stiffness, 383
  - infection, 397
  - malunion, 384, 387–388, 396
  - muscle/tendon entrapment/tendon rupture, 397–398
  - neurapraxia, 397
  - redisplacement/malalignment, 381, 383
  - refracture, 383–384
- diagnosis and classification of, 354–355, 355f
- epidemiology of, 350, 352f
- historical overview of, 348–350, 348f, 349f, 350f, 351f
- mechanism of injury, 350, 352, 352f, 353f
- remodeling of, 359–360
- signs/symptoms, 352–353
- surgical/applied anatomy for
  - bony anatomy/static restraints, 360–361, 362f
  - muscle/nerve anatomy, 361, 363, 363f, 363t
  - surgical approaches, 364–365, 364f, 365f
- treatment of
  - angulation limits for, 378
  - closed, 365–368
  - comminuted fractures, 368
  - complete fractures, 367–368
  - intramedullary fixation, 369
  - intramedullary nailing, 369–371, 371f, 372f, 373f, 374, 374f, 375f
  - plate fixation, 369, 370f
  - rationale for, 355–356, 356f, 357f, 358–360, 358f, 359t
  - reduction, 377–378
  - surgical, 369–371, 374, 376–378, 380–381
  - traumatic bowing/plastic deformation, 366, 366f, 367f

Ultrasonography
- of hip fractures, 770, 773
- multiple fracture evaluation with, 77
- of physeal injuries, 107f
- of pulled elbow syndrome, 616

Unicameral bone cysts (UBC), 121–122, 121t, 122t, 124f, 126f
- classification of, 123
- clinical features of, 122–123
- femoral shaft fractures and, 798
- natural history of, 123
- staging of, 124t
- treatment of, 123, 125, 125f

Urologic injury, 77, 79

V

Valgus injuries
- angular force on neck, 410
- associated injuries, 410–411
- extension fractures and, 434–435, 435f
- fracture patterns in, 411–412, 412f, 413f

Vancomycin, 156t

van Neck disease, 751

Vascular endothelial growth factor (VEGF), 31, 32–34, 32f

Vascular injury
- cold intolerance and, 511
- supracondylar humeral fractures and, 510–513, 510f, 511f

VEGF. *See* Vascular endothelial growth factor

Vehicle-bicycle accidents, 13

Vehicle-pedestrian accidents, 13

Ventilation
- ketamine and, 57
- monitoring, 47–48, 48f

Verbrugge, Jean, 349

Vertebra plana, 137, 138f

Very low birth weight infants, rickets and, 167–168

Vitamin C, 173–174

Vitamin D, 165–166, 212, 213

Volar plate, 227

von Münchhausen (Baron), 194

von Recklinghausen's disease. *See* Neurofibromatosis

W

Wackenheim line, 698

Wilm's tumor, 121t, 122t

Wound management, for open fractures, 83–84

Wrist block, 63–64, 64f

Wrist fractures, intramedullary fixation and, 85

Wrist guards, 399